P9-EGL-157

THE MERCK MANUAL
HOME HEALTH HANDBOOK

THE
MERCK MANUAL
HOME
HEALTH
HANDBOOK

Robert S. Porter, MD, *Editor-in-Chief*
Justin L. Kaplan, MD, *Senior Assistant Editor*
Barbara P. Homeier, MD,

Editorial Board

Richard K. Albert, MD

Marjorie A. Bowman, MD, MPA

Glenn D. Braunstein, MD

Sidney Cohen, MD

Linda Emanuel, PhD

Jan Fawcett, MD

Eugene P. Frenkel, MD

Susan L. Hendrix, DO

Michael Jacewicz, MD

Brian F. Mandell, MD, PhD

Gerald L. Mandell, MD

Judith S. Palfrey, MD

Albert A. Rundio, Jr., PhD

David A. Spain, MD

Paul H. Tanser, MD

WILEY

John Wiley & Sons, Inc.

This book is printed on acid-free paper. ♾

Copyright © 2009, Merck Sharp & Dohme Corp., a subsidiary of Merck & Co., Inc., Whitehouse Station, NJ, U.S.A. All rights reserved

Published by John Wiley & Sons, Inc., Hoboken, New Jersey
Published simultaneously in Canada

No part of this publication may be reproduced, stored in a retrieval system, or transmitted in any form or by any means, electronic, mechanical, photocopying, recording, scanning, or otherwise, except as permitted under Section 107 or 108 of the 1976 United States Copyright Act, without either the prior written permission of the Publisher, or authorization through payment of the appropriate per-copy fee to the Copyright Clearance Center, 222 Rosewood Drive, Danvers, MA 01923, (978) 750-8400, fax (978) 646-8600, or on the web at www.copyright.com. Requests to the Publisher for permission should be addressed to the Permissions Department, John Wiley & Sons, Inc., 111 River Street, Hoboken, NJ 07030, (201) 748-6011, fax (201) 748-6008, or online at http://www.wiley.com/go/permissions.

Limit of Liability/Disclaimer of Warranty: While the publisher and the author have used their best efforts in preparing this book, they make no representations or warranties with respect to the accuracy or completeness of the contents of this book and specifically disclaim any implied warranties of merchantability or fitness for a particular purpose. No warranty may be created or extended by sales representatives or written sales materials. The advice and strategies contained herein may not be suitable for your situation. You should consult with a professional where appropriate. Neither the publisher nor the author shall be liable for any loss of profit or any other commercial damages, including but not limited to special, incidental, consequential, or other damages.

For general information about our other products and services, please contact our Customer Care Department within the United States at (800) 762-2974, outside the United States at (317) 572-3993 or fax (317) 572-4002.

Wiley also publishes its books in a variety of electronic formats and by print-on-demand. Some content that appears in standard print versions of this book may not be available in other formats. For more information about Wiley products, visit us at www.wiley.com.

ISBN 978-1-11811-542-8 (paper: alk. paper); ISBN 978-1-11817-123-3 (ebk); 978-1-11817-124-0 (ebk); 978-1-11817-125-7 (ebk)

Printed in the United States of America

10 9 8 7 6 5 4 3 2 1

PREFACE

People are now taking increasing responsibility for their own health care. Many come to their doctor's office with printouts from the Internet of the latest scientific studies. People now evaluate options—such as whether to have surgery, radiation therapy, or drug therapy for cancer—to a depth and extent that was unheard of in their parents' generation. Then, people did what their doctor recommended, asked few questions, and sought little outside information about their medical problems.

Although that earlier era may have been a more trusting time, one of the main reasons people gathered little information on their own was that there was little understandable material readily available. Back then, some people turned to *The Merck Manual* for help. Even though it was a book for health care professionals, its straightforward style and minimal use of dense medical jargon helped make it understandable and useful to some of the general public.

To make *The Merck Manual*'s content even more helpful to the public, in 1997 we "translated" it into everyday language, creating *The Merck Manual of Medical Information, Home Edition*. The current book, *The Merck Manual Home Health Handbook*, represents the 3rd edition of that first home version.

However, we were not the only ones to respond to the public's need. By the end of the 1990s, bookstores had entire sections devoted to health care with hundreds of titles. And then came the Internet, with thousands of web sites by doctors, patients, caregivers, hospitals, professional societies, patient advocacy groups, and seemingly almost everyone with an opinion, idea, or product related to health care.

Now, everyone everywhere has access to a depth and breadth of medical information that most doctors would have been hard pressed to find a generation ago. The current problem seems to be too much information rather than too little. Where do we go? Where do we start? The answer, of course, varies from person to person. Different people need different types and amounts of information. If people have had a disorder for a long time, they usually want very specialized information about it—they already know the basics. On the other hand, people who have just learned that they have a disorder usually first want general information.

In this wide range of information needs, *The Merck Manual Home Health Handbook* is designed to be the starting point on the road to understanding. For many people, it will be all the information they need. For others, it will be the foundation that helps them understand more complex information from other books and web sites. For all, it will improve communication with health care practitioners by providing full explanations of medical problems in clear, plain language, thus taking the mystery out of medical terms and jargon and also by raising awareness of questions and issues in medicine that people can then discuss in depth with their doctor. Our hope is that this book enlightens and empowers people and contributes to a healthier future.

Robert S. Porter, MD
Editor-in-Chief

Special Note to Readers

The authors, reviewers, editors, and publisher have made extensive efforts to ensure that the information is accurate and conforms to the standards accepted at the time of publication. However, constant changes in information resulting from continuing research and clinical experience, reasonable differences in opinions among authorities, unique aspects of individual situations, and the possibility of human error in preparing such an extensive text require that the reader exercise judgment when making decisions and consult and compare information from other sources. In particular, the reader is advised to discuss information obtained in this book with a doctor, pharmacist, nurse, or other health care practitioner.

CONTENTS

EDITOR-IN-CHIEF
Robert S. Porter, MD

Merck & Co., Inc, and Clinical Assistant Professor, Department of Emergency Medicine, Jefferson Medical College

SENIOR ASSISTANT EDITOR
Justin L. Kaplan, MD

Merck & Co., Inc, and Clinical Associate Professor, Department of Emergency Medicine, Jefferson Medical College

ASSISTANT EDITOR
Barbara P. Homeier, MD

Merck & Co., Inc, and Clinical Instructor, Department of Pediatrics, Jefferson Medical College

Executive Editor	**Keryn A.G. Lane**
Senior Staff Writers	**Susan T. Schindler**
	Susan C. Short
Staff Editor	**Michelle A. Steigerwald**
Senior Operations Manager	**Diane C. Zenker**
Senior Project Manager	**Diane Cosner-Bobrin**
Manager, Electronic Publications	**Michael A. DeFerrari**
Executive Assistant	**Jean Perry**
Designer	**Jerilyn Bockorick**
Illustrators	**Michael Reingold**
	Christopher C. Butts
Indexers	**Keryn A.G. Lane**
	Susan Thomas, PhD
Publisher	**Gary Zelko**
Advertising and Promotions Supervisor	**Pamela J. Barnes-Paul**
Subsidiary Rights Coordinator	**Jeanne Nilsen**
Systems Administrator	**Leta S. Bracy**

ACKNOWLEDGMENTS

We thank Beth Datskovsky Ben-Avraham, Enid Jacobus, Elizabeth LoMastro, Alisa Gayle Mayor, Beth Mescolotto, and Regina Stamatis for their assistance with proofreading and Alisa Gayle Mayor for her assistance with editing. We also thank Paul Fennessy, Brielle Matson, and the team at Nesbitt Graphics for their assistance in producing this book.

EDITORIAL BOARD

Richard K. Albert, MD
Professor, Department of Medicine, University of Colorado Health Sciences Center; Chief of Medicine, Denver Health Medical Center

Marjorie A. Bowman, MD, MPA
Professor and Founding Chair of Family Medicine and Community Health, University of Pennsylvania School of Medicine

Glenn D. Braunstein, MD
Professor of Medicine, David Geffen School of Medicine at University of California, Los Angeles; Chairman, Department of Medicine, Cedars-Sinai Medical Center

Sidney Cohen, MD
Professor of Medicine and Director, Research Programs, Thomas Jefferson University

Linda Emanuel, PhD
Professor of Medicine, Northwestern University, Feinberg School of Medicine, Buehler Center on Aging

Jan Fawcett, MD
Professor of Psychiatry, University of New Mexico School of Medicine

Eugene P. Frenkel, MD
Professor of Internal Medicine and Radiology, Patsy R. and Raymond D. Nasher Distinguished Chair in Cancer Research, Elaine Dewey Sammons Distinguished Chair in Cancer Research in honor of Eugene P. Frenkel, MD; A. Kenneth Pye Professorship in Cancer Research, Harold C. Simmons Comprehensive Cancer Center, The University of Texas Southwestern Medical Center at Dallas

Susan L. Hendrix, DO
Clinical Professor, Department of Obstetrics and Gynecology, Michigan State University School of Osteopathic Medicine and Detroit Medical Center/Hutzel Women's Hospital

Michael Jacewicz, MD
Professor of Neurology, University of Tennessee Health Science Center and Veterans Administration Medical Center, Memphis

Brian F. Mandell, MD, PhD
Professor and Vice Chairman of Medicine, Department of Rheumatic and Immunologic Diseases, Cleveland Clinic Lerner College of Medicine at Case Western Reserve University

Gerald L. Mandell, MD
Professor of Medicine (Emeritus), Owen R. Cheatham Professor of the Sciences (Emeritus), and Chief of Infectious Diseases (Emeritus), University of Virginia Health Center

Judith S. Palfrey, MD
T. Berry Brazelton Professor of Pediatrics, Harvard Medical School; General Pediatrics Division, Children's Hospital, Boston

Albert A. Rundio, Jr., PhD
Associate Professor of Nursing, The Richard Stockton College of New Jersey; Nurse Practitioner, Lighthouse at Mays Landing

David A. Spain, MD
Professor of Surgery and Chief of Trauma/Surgical Critical Care, Stanford University

Paul H. Tanser, MD
Professor of Medicine (Emeritus), McMaster University, Hamilton, Ontario; Cardiology Consultant, North Shore and Waitakere Hospitals, Auckland

CONSULTANTS

Noel A. Armenakas, MD
Clinical Associate Professor, Department of Urology, Weill Cornell Medical School; Lenox Hill Hospital and New York Presbyterian Hospital

Robert B. Cohen, DMD
Clinical Assistant Professor and Practice Coordinator, Tufts University School of Dental Medicine

Ralph E. Cutler, MD *(Deceased)*
Professor of Medicine (Emeritus), Loma Linda University School of Medicine; Consultant in Nephrology, Loma Linda VA Medical Center

Sidney N. Klaus, MD
Professor of Medicine, Department of Dermatology, Dartmouth Medical School

Melvin I. Roat, MD
Clinical Associate Professor, Department of Ophthalmology, Thomas Jefferson University; Cornea Service, Wills Eye Institute

James R. Roberts, MD
Professor and Vice Chairman, Department of Emergency Medicine, Drexel University College of Medicine; Chair, Department of Emergency Medicine and Director, Division of Toxicology, Mercy Catholic Medical Center

Robert J. Ruben, MD
Distinguished University Professor, Department of Otolaryngology–Head and Neck Surgery, Albert Einstein College of Medicine and Montefiore Medical Center

Stewart Shankel, MD
Clinical Professor of Medicine and Director of Clinical Medicine, University of California at Riverside

Eva M. Vivian, PharmD
Clinical Associate Professor, University of Wisconsin School of Pharmacy

Reviewers for Selected Chapters

William E. Brant, MD
Deborah M. Consolini, MD
Arthur Coverdale, MD
Albert T. Derivan, MD
Ara DerMarderosian, PhD
Denis J. Dollard, MD
Margery Gass, MD
George M. Grames, MD
Norton J. Greenberger, MD
Donald Hanson, DMD

Randall Hughes, MD
Karen Birckelbaw Kopacek, RPh
Diane Kraft, MS, RD, LDN
Anil K. Lalwani, MD
Douglas Lanska, MD, MS, MSPH
Edwin M. Leidholdt, Jr., PhD
James I. McMillan, MD
David S. Rootman, MD
James Wayne Warnica, MD

CONTRIBUTORS

Bola Adamolekun, MD
Director of Epilepsy, Department of
Neurology, University of Tennessee Health
Science Center
Seizure Disorders

Neil B. Alexander, MD
Professor, Department of Internal Medicine,
Division of Geriatric Medicine, University of
Michigan; Associate Professor for Research;
Director, VA Ann Arbor Health Care System,
Geriatrics Research Education and Clinical
Center
Falls

Roy D. Altman, MD
Professor of Medicine, Division of
Rheumatology and Immunology, University of
California, Los Angeles
Paget's Disease of Bone; Joint Disorders

Mary Ann Anderson, PhD, RN
Associate Professor, University of Chicago,
College of Nursing, Quad Cities Regional
Program
Provision of Care

Gerald L. Andriole, MD
Professor and Chief of Urologic Surgery,
Barnes-Jewish Hospital, Washington University
School of Medicine
Prostate Disorders

Parswa Ansari, MD
Assistant Program Director, Department of
Surgery, Lenox Hill Hospital, New York
*Anal and Rectal Disorders; Gastrointestinal
Emergencies*

Brian R. Apatoff, MD, PhD
Director of Multiple Sclerosis Clinical Care
and Research Center, Department of
Neurology and Neuroscience, Weill Medical
College of Cornell University, New York
Presbyterian Hospital
Multiple Sclerosis and Related Disorders

Noel A. Armenakas, MD
Clinical Associate Professor, Department of
Urology, Weill Cornell Medical College;
Attending Physician, Lenox Hill Hospital and
New York Presbyterian Hospital
Injury to the Urinary Tract

J. Malcolm O. Arnold, MD
Professor of Medicine, Physiology and
Pharmacology, University of Western Ontario;
Cardiologist, London Health Sciences Center,
Ontario
Heart Failure; Cardiomyopathy

George L. Bakris, MD
Professor of Medicine and Director,
Hypertension Unit, Section of Endocrinology,
Diabetes and Metabolism, University of
Chicago-Pritzker School of Medicine
High Blood Pressure; Low Blood Pressure

Robert Barish, MD, MBA
Professor of Emergency Medicine and Medicine
and Vice Dean for Clinical Affairs, University
of Maryland School of Medicine
Bites and Stings

John G. Bartlett, MD
Professor of Medicine, Johns Hopkins
University School of Medicine
*Abscess in the Lungs; Acute Bronchitis;
Pneumonia*

Rosemary Basson, MD
Clinical Professor, Department of Psychiatry,
University of British Columbia and Vancouver
Hospital
Sexual Dysfunction in Women

Mark H. Beers, MD (Deceased)
Clinical Professor of Medicine, Drexel
University
The Human Body

Joshua O. Benditt, MD
Professor of Medicine, Division of Pulmonary
and Critical Care, University of Washington
School of Medicine; Director of Respiratory
Care Medicine, University of Washington
Medical Center
Atelectasis; Bronchiectasis

James R. Berenson, MD
Medical and Scientific Director, Institute for
Myeloma and Bone Cancer Research, West
Hollywood
Plasma Cell Disorders

Richard W. Besdine, MD
Professor of Medicine, Greer Professor of Geriatric Medicine, and Director, Division of Geriatrics (Medicine) and of Center for Gerontology and Health Care Research, The Warren Alpert Medical School of Brown University
The Aging Body

Adil E. Bharucha, MD, MBBS
Professor of Medicine, Division of Gastroenterology and Hepatology, Mayo Clinic College of Medicine
Irritable Bowel Syndrome

Albert W. Biglan, MD
Adjunct Associate Professor of Ophthalmology, University of Pittsburgh School of Medicine; Staff Physician, Children's Hospital of Pittsburgh
Eye Disorders

Joseph J. Biundo, MD
Clinical Professor of Medicine, Tulane Medical Center
Muscle, Bursa, and Tendon Disorders

Sean C. Blackwell, MD
Assistant Professor, Department of Obstetrics, Gynecology, and Reproductive Sciences, University of Texas Health Sciences Center at Houston
Pregnancy Complicated by Disease

Russell Blair, MD
Fellow, Department of Pulmonary and Critical Care, Wake Forest University Baptist Medical Center
Asthma

Ann S. Botash, MD
Professor of Pediatrics, State University of New York, Upstate Medical University
Child Neglect and Abuse

Alfred A. Bove, MD, PhD
Chief of Cardiology, Cardiology Section, Temple University School of Medicine
Diving and Compressed Air Injuries

Marjorie A. Bowman, MD, MPA
Professor and Founding Chair of Family Practice and Community Medicine, University of Pennsylvania School of Medicine
Making the Most of Health Care

Thomas G. Boyce, MD, MPH
Associate Professor of Pediatrics and Consultant in Pediatric Infectious Diseases and Immunology, Mayo Clinic College of Medicine
Gastroenteritis

Joseph D. Brain, ScD
Drinker Professor of Environmental Physiology and Chair of Environmental Health, Harvard School of Public Health
Biology of the Lungs and Airways

Peter C. Brazy, MD
Professor of Medicine, University of Wisconsin at Madison
Tubular and Cystic Kidney Disorders

Jeremy S. Breit, MD
Fellow, Department of Pulmonary and Critical Care, Wake Forest University Baptist Medical Center
Asthma

Christian M. Briery, MD
Assistant Professor of Obstetrics and Gynecology, Division of Maternal-Fetal Medicine, University of Tennessee–Chattanooga Unit
High-Risk Pregnancy

George R. Brown, MD
Professor and Associate Chairman, Department of Psychiatry, East Tennessee State University; Chief of Psychiatry, James H. Quillen VA Medical Center
Sexuality

Haywood L. Brown, MD
Roy T. Parker Professor and Chair, Department of Obstetrics and Gynecology, Duke University Medical Center
Normal Pregnancy; Normal Labor and Delivery

Rebecca H. Buckley, MD
J. Buren Sidbury Professor of Pediatrics and Professor of Immunology, Duke University School of Medicine
Immunodeficiency Disorders

Jerrold T. Bushberg, PhD, DABMP
Clinical Professor of Radiology, Clinical Professor of Radiation Oncology, University of California, Davis School of Medicine
Radiation Injury

Juan R. Bustillo, MD
Associate Professor of Psychiatry and
Neurosciences, University of New Mexico
Schizophrenia and Delusional Disorder

David B. Carr, MD
Associate Professor of Internal Medicine and
Neurology, Washington University School of
Medicine–Older Adult Health Center
Driving

Mary T. Caserta, MD
Associate Professor of Pediatrics, University of
Rochester School of Medicine and Dentistry;
Attending Physician, Golisano Children's
Hospital at Strong
Viral Infections

Bartolome R. Celli, MD
Professor of Medicine, Tufts University; Chief,
Pulmonary, Critical Care and Sleep Study,
St. Elizabeth's Medical Center, Boston
Rehabilitation for Lung and Airway Disorders

Bruce A. Chabner, MD
Professor of Medicine, Harvard Medical
School; Clinical Director, Massachusetts
General Hospital Cancer Center
*Overview of Cancer; Prevention and Treatment
of Cancer*

Ian M. Chapman, MBBS, PhD
Associate Professor in Endocrinology,
University of Adelaide, Department of
Medicine, Royal Adelaide Hospital, Australia
Pituitary Gland Disorders

William J. Cochran, MD
Vice Chairman, Department of Pediatrics,
Geisinger Clinic, Danville
Digestive Disorders

Alan S. Cohen, MD
Distinguished Professor of Medicine
(Emeritus), Conrad Wessolhoeft Professor of
Medicine, Boston University School of
Medicine; Editor-in-Chief of Amyloid, The
Journal of Protein Folding Disorders
Amyloidosis

Philip L. Cohen, MD
Professor of Medicine, University of
Pennsylvania; Chief of Rheumatology Section,
Philadelphia VA Medical Center
Autoimmune Disorders

Robert B. Cohen, DMD
Clinical Associate Professor and Practice
Coordinator, Tufts University School of Dental
Medicine
*Lip and Tongue Disorders; Salivary Gland
Disorders; Mouth Sores; Mouth Growths*

Sidney Cohen, MD
Professor of Medicine, Division of
Gastroenterology and Hepatology, Thomas
Jefferson University Hospital
*Peptic Disorders; Hiatus Hernia, Bezoars, and
Foreign Bodies; Biology of the Liver and
Gallbladder; Manifestations of Liver Disease;
Hepatitis*

Kathryn Colby, MD, PhD
Director, Clinical Research Center,
Massachusetts Eye and Ear Infirmary;
Assistant Professor of Ophthalmology,
Harvard Medical School
*Symptoms and Diagnosis of Eye Disorders;
Injuries to the Eye; Cataract*

Daniel W. Collison, MD
Associate Professor of Medicine and Surgery,
Section of Dermatology, Dartmouth Medical
School
*Sweating Disorders; Pressure Sores;
Noncancerous Skin Growths*

Eve R. Colson, MD
Associate Professor of Pediatrics, Yale
University School of Medicine; Director of Well
Newborn Nursery, Yale-New Haven Children's
Hospital
Preschool and School-Aged Children

Mary Ann Cooper, MD
Professor, Department of Emergency Medicine,
University of Illinois at Chicago
Electrical and Lightning Injuries

Bryan D. Cowan, MD
Professor and Chairman, Department of
Obstetrics and Gynecology, University of
Mississippi Medical Center
Fibroids

Jill P. Crandall, MD
Associate Professor of Clinical Medicine,
Albert Einstein College of Medicine
Hypoglycemia

Emmett T. Cunningham, Jr., MD, PhD, MPH
Professor of Ophthalmology, Stanford
University; Director, The Uveitis Service,
California Pacific Medical Center and Clinic
Uveitis

Ralph E. Cutler, MD (Deceased)
Professor of Medicine (Emeritus), Loma Linda
University School of Medicine; Consultant in
Nephrology, Loma Linda VA Medical Center
Biology of the Kidneys and Urinary Tract;
Symptoms and Diagnosis of Kidney and
Urinary Tract Disorders

Patricia A. Daly, MD
Visiting Assistant Professor of Medicine,
University of Virginia; Clinical
Endocrinologist, Front Royal Internal
Medicine, VA
Multiple Endocrine Neoplasia Syndromes

Daniel F. Danzl, MD
Professor and Chair of Emergency Medicine,
University of Louisville School of Medicine
Cold Injuries

Norman L. Dean, MD
Fellow (Emeritus), American College of Chest
Physicians; Lifetime Fellow, American College
of Physicians
Drowning

Peter J. Delves, PhD
Reader in Immunology, Department of
Immunology and Molecular Pathology,
Division of Infection and Immunity, University
College, London
Biology of the Immune System; Allergic
Reactions

Ara DerMarderosian, PhD
Professor of Pharmacognosy and Medicinal
Chemistry, Roth Chair of Natural Products,
and Scientific Director of Complementary and
Alternative Medicine Institute, University of
the Sciences in Philadelphia
Medicinal Herbs and Nutraceuticals

Deepinder K. Dhaliwal, MD
Associate Professor, Department of
Ophthalmology, University of Pittsburgh
School of Medicine; Director of Cornea/
External Disease and Director of Refractive
Surgery, University of Pittsburgh Medical
Center, Eye Center; Medical Director,
University of Pittsburgh Medical Center, Laser
Center; Director and Founder, Center for
Integrative Eye Care, University of Pittsburgh
Refractive Disorders

A. Damian Dhar, MD, JD
Private Practice, Atlanta Dermatology, Vein
and Research Center
Bacterial Skin Infections; Fungal Skin
Infections

Michael C. DiMarino, MD
Clinical Assistant Professor of Medicine,
Division of Gastroenterology and Hepatology,
Department of Medicine, Thomas Jefferson
University
Esophageal Disorders; Diverticular Disease

James G. H. Dinulos, MD
Assistant Professor of Medicine and Pediatrics
(Dermatology), Dartmouth-Hitchcock Clinic
Parasitic Skin Infections; Viral Skin Infections

Caroline Carney Doebbeling, MD, MSc
Associate Professor of Internal Medicine and
Psychiatry, Indiana University School of
Medicine; Research Scientist, Regenstrief
Institute
Overview of Mental Health Care

Karl Doghramji, MD
Professor of Psychiatry and Human Behavior
and Medical Director, Jefferson Sleep
Disorders Center, Thomas Jefferson University
Sleep Disorders

Jeffrey S. Dungan, MD
Associate Professor, Department of Obstetrics
and Gynecology, Northwestern University
Feinberg School of Medicine
Detection of Genetic Disorders

David Eidelberg, MD
Susan and Leonard Feinstein Professor of
Neurology and Neurosurgery, New York
University School of Medicine; Director, Center
for Neurosciences, The Feinstein Institute for
Medical Research, North Shore–Long Island
Jewish Health System
Movement Disorders

Sherman Elias, MD
John J. Sciarra Professor and Chair,
Department of Obstetrics and Gynecology,
Northwestern University Feinberg School of
Medicine; Chairman, Obstetrics and
Gynecology, Prentice Women's Hospital of
Northwestern Memorial Hospital
Detection of Genetic Disorders

Jan Fawcett, MD
Professor of Psychiatry, University of New
Mexico School of Medicine
Mood Disorders

Norah C. Feeny, PhD
Associate Professor, Department of Psychiatry
and Psychology, Case Western Reserve
University
Violence Against Women

James H. Fisher, MD
Professor of Internal Medicine, University of
Colorado School of Medicine; Pulmonary and
Critical Care, Denver Health Medical Center
Symptoms and Diagnosis of Lung Disorders

Michael R. Foley, MD
Clinical Professor, University of Arizona School
of Medicine; Medical Director for Academic
Affairs, Scottsdale Healthcare
Pregnancy and Drug Use

Steven D. Freedman, MD, PhD
Associate Professor of Medicine, Harvard
Medical School; Director, The Pancreas Center,
Beth Israel Deaconess Medical Center
Pancreatitis

Emil J. Freireich, MD
Professor, Department of Leukemia, and
Director, Adult Leukemia Research Programs,
University of Texas, MD Anderson Cancer
Center
Leukemias

Eugene P. Frenkel, MD
Professor of Internal Medicine and Radiology,
Patsy R. and Raymond D. Nasher
Distinguished Chair in Cancer Research; Elaine
Dewey Sammons Distinguished Chair in
Cancer Research in honor of Eugene P. Frenkel,
MD; and A. Kenneth Pye Professorship in
Cancer Research, Harold C. Simmons
Comprehensive Cancer Center, The University
of Texas Southwestern Medical Center at
Dallas
Biology of Blood

Marvin P. Fried, MD
Professor and Chairman, Department of
Otorhinolaryngology–Head and Neck Surgery,
Albert Einstein College of Medicine and
Montefiore Medical Center
Nose, Sinus, and Taste Disorders

Mitchell H. Friedlaender, MD
Adjunct Professor, The Scripps Research
Institute; Head of Ophthalmology, Scripps
Clinic, La Jolla
Conjunctival and Scleral Disorders

Edmund F. Funai, MD
Associate Chair for Clinical Affairs,
Department of Obstetrics, Gynecology, and
Reproductive Sciences, Yale University School
of Medicine; Chief of Obstetrics, Yale-New
Haven Hospital
Complications of Pregnancy

Matthew G. Fury, MD
Assistant Attending Physician, Memorial
Sloan-Kettering Cancer Center; Instructor,
Department of Medicine, Weill Medical
College of Cornell University
Symptoms and Diagnosis of Cancer

Pierluigi Gambetti, MD
Professor and Director, National Prion Disease
Pathology Surveillance Center, Institute of
Pathology, Division of Neuropathology, Case
Western Reserve University
Prion Diseases

Sunir J. Garg, MD
Assistant Professor of Ophthalmology, Thomas
Jefferson University; Assistant Surgeon, The
Retina Service of Wills Eye Institute
Retinal Disorders

James Garrity, MD
Whitney and Betty MacMillan Professor of
Ophthalmology, Mayo Clinic, Rochester
*Biology of the Eyes; Optic Nerve Disorders;
Eye Socket Disorders; Eyelid and Tearing
Disorders*

Brian K. Gehlbach, MD
Assistant Professor of Medicine, Section of
Pulmonary and Critical Care Medicine,
University of Chicago
*Respiratory Failure and Acute Respiratory
Distress Syndrome*

David M. Gershenson, MD
Professor and Chairman, Department of
Gynecologic Oncology and J. Taylor Wharton,
MD, Distinguished Chair in Gynecologic
Oncology, The University of Texas M.D.
Anderson Cancer Center
Cancers of the Female Reproductive System

Kenneth A. Getz, MBA
Senior Research Fellow, Tufts Center for the
Study of Drug Development; Founder and
Chairman, The Center for Information and
Study on Clinical Research Participation
The Science of Medicine and Clinical Trials

Elias A. Giraldo, MD
Assistant Professor of Neurology and
Neurosurgery; Director, Stroke and
Neurological Critical Care Programs,
University of Tennessee Health Science
Center at Memphis
Stroke

Anne Carol Goldberg, MD
Associate Professor of Medicine, Washington
University School of Medicine, St. Louis
Cholesterol Disorders

Stephen E. Goldfinger, MD
Professor of Medicine, Harvard Medical
School; Physician, Massachusetts General
Hospital
Hereditary Periodic Fever Syndromes

Steven A. Goldman, MD, PhD
Dean Zutes Chair and Professor of Neurology
and Neurosurgery, University of Rochester
Medical Center; Adjunct Professor of
Neurology and Neuroscience, Weill Medical
College of Cornell University
Biology of the Nervous System

M. Jay Goodkind, MD
Associate Professor (Emeritus) of Clinical
Medicine, University of Pennsylvania School of
Medicine; Chairman (Emeritus) of Clinical
Cardiology, Capital Health System, Mercer
Hospital Campus, Trenton
Heart Tumors

Carmen E. Gota, MD
Staff Physician, Department of Rheumatology,
Cleveland Clinic Foundation
Vasculitic Disorders

John H. Greist, MD
Clinical Professor of Psychiatry, University of
Wisconsin Medical School; Distinguished
Senior Scientist, Madison Institute of Medicine
Anxiety Disorders

Ashley B. Grossman, MD
Professor of Neuroendocrinology and
Honorary Consultant Physician,
St. Bartholomew's Hospital, London
Adrenal Gland Disorders

John Gunderson, MD
Professor of Psychiatry, Harvard Medical
School; Director of Center for Treatment and
Research on Borderline Personality Disorder,
McLean Hospital
Personality Disorders

Rula A. Hajj-ali, MD
Staff Physician, Center of Vasculitis Care and
Research, Department of Rheumatic and
Immunologic Disease, Cleveland Clinic
Foundation
Autoimmune Disorders of Connective Tissue

Jesse B. Hall, MD
Professor of Medicine, Department of
Anesthesia and Critical Care; Chief, Section of
Pulmonary and Critical Care Medicine,
University of Chicago
*Respiratory Failure and Acute Respiratory
Distress Syndrome*

Judith G. Hall, OC, MD
Professor of Pediatrics and Medical Genetics
(Emeritus), University of British Columbia,
British Columbia Children's Hospital
Genetics

John W. Hallett, Jr., MD
Clinical Professor of Surgery, Medical
University of South Carolina; Medical Director
and Vascular Surgeon, Roper St. Francis Heart
and Vascular Center
*Aneurysms and Aortic Dissection; Peripheral
Arterial Disease*

Susan L. Hendrix, DO
Clinical Professor, Department of Obstetrics
and Gynecology, Michigan State University
School of Osteopathic Medicine and Detroit
Medical Center/Hutzel Women's Hospital
Menopause

Steven K. Herrine, MD
Professor of Medicine, Division of
Gastroenterology and Hepatology, Thomas
Jefferson University; Assistant Dean for
Academic Affairs, Jefferson Medical College
Tumors of the Liver

Jerome M. Hershman, MD
Distinguished Professor of Medicine, David
Geffen School of Medicine, University of
California at Los Angeles; Associate Chief,
Endocrinology and Diabetes Division,
West Los Angeles VA Medical Center
Thyroid Gland Disorders

Martin Hertl, MD, PhD
Assistant Professor of Surgery, Harvard
Medical School; Surgical Director, Liver
Transplantation Program, Massachusetts
General Hospital
Transplantation

Paula J. Adams Hillard, MD
Professor of Obstetrics and Gynecology and of
Pediatrics, University of Cincinnati; Director of
Obstetrics and Gynecology, Cincinnati
Children's Hospital Medical Center
*Symptoms and Diagnosis of Gynecologic
Disorders*

Robert M. A. Hirschfeld, MD
Harry K. Davis Professor, Titus H. Harris
Chair, Department of Psychiatry and
Behavioral Sciences, University of Texas
Medical Branch at Galveston
Suicidal Behavior

Brian D. Hoit, MD
Professor of Medicine, Case Western Reserve
University; Director of Echocardiography,
University Hospitals of Cleveland
Pericardial Disease

Waun Ki Hong, MD
American Cancer Society Professor and
Samsung Distinguished University Chair in
Cancer Medicine; Professor of Medicine,
Department of Thoracic/Head and Neck
Medical Oncology, and Head, Division of
Cancer Medicine, University of Texas M.D.
Anderson Cancer Center
Cancer of the Lungs

Juebin Huang, MD, PhD
Research Associate, Department of Neurology,
University of Tennessee Health Science Center
Brain Dysfunction; Delirium and Dementia

Daniel A. Hussar, PhD
Remington Professor of Pharmacy,
Philadelphia College of Pharmacy, University of
the Sciences in Philadelphia
*Factors Affecting Response to Drugs;
Adherence to Drug Treatment; Over-the-
Counter Drugs*

Masayoshi Itoh, MD, MPH
Clinical Professor of Rehabilitation Medicine,
New York University School of Medicine;
Consultant, Coler/Goldwater Specialty
Hospital and Nursing Facility
Rehabilitation

Michael Jacewicz, MD
Professor of Neurology, University of
Tennessee Health Science Center and Veterans
Administration Medical Center, Memphis
*Symptoms and Diagnosis of Musculoskeletal
Disorders; Diagnosis of Brain, Spinal Cord,
and Nerve Disorders; Dizziness and Vertigo;
Infections of the Brain and Spinal Cord; Nose,
Sinus, and Taste Disorders* (Smell and Taste
Disorders portion)

Harry S. Jacob, MD
Professor of Medicine, University of Minnesota
Medical School; Editor-in-Chief, Hematology/
Oncology Today
Spleen Disorders

Jon A. Jacobson, MD
Associate Professor of Radiology, University of
Michigan
Common Imaging Tests

James W. Jefferson, MD
Clinical Professor of Psychiatry, University of
Wisconsin Medical School; Distinguished
Senior Scientist, Madison Institute of Medicine
Anxiety Disorders

Larry E. Johnson, MD, PhD
Associate Professor of Geriatrics and Family
and Preventive Medicine, University of
Arkansas for Medical Sciences; Attending
Physician, Central Arkansas Veterans
Healthcare System
Vitamins; Minerals and Electrolytes

Robert G. Johnson, MD
C. Rollins Hanlon Professor and Chair,
Department of Surgery, Saint Louis University
Surgery

Brian D. Johnston
Fitness Clinician and President and Director of
Education, International Association of
Resistance Trainers Certification Institute,
Ontario
Exercise and Fitness

Hugh F. Johnston, MD
Clinical Associate Professor, Department of
Psychiatry and Office of Continuing Medical
Education, University of Wisconsin Medical
School; Medical Director, Bureau of Mental
Health and Substance Abuse
Mental Health Disorders

Thomas V. Jones, MD, MPH
Director, Musculoskeletal and Inflammatory
Diseases, Global Medical Affairs, Wyeth
Medical Decision Making

Nicholas Jospe, MD
Professor of Pediatrics, University of Rochester
School of Medicine and Dentistry
Diabetes Mellitus

Michael J. Joyce, MD
Orthopaedic Surgeon, Cleveland Clinic;
Associate Clinical Professor, Orthopaedic
Surgery, Case Western Reserve University
Bone and Joint Tumors

Fran E. Kaiser, MD
Clinical Professor of Medicine, University of
Texas Southwestern Medical Center; Adjunct
Professor of Medicine, Saint Louis University;
Executive Medical Director, Merck & Co., Inc.
Sexual Dysfunction in Men

Anand D. Kantak, MD
Clinical Associate Professor of Pediatrics,
Northeastern Ohio Universities Colleges of
Medicine and Pharmacology; Director,
Division of Neonatology, Akron Children's
Hospital
Respiratory Disorders

Harold S. Kaplan, MD
Professor of Clinical Pathology, Columbia
University; Director of Transfusion Medicine,
Columbia University Medical Center
Blood Transfusion

Justin L. Kaplan, MD
Clinical Associate Professor of Emergency
Medicine, Jefferson Medical College; Senior
Assistant Editor, The Merck Manuals,
Merck & Co., Inc.
First Aid

Paul R. Katz, MD
Professor of Medicine, University of Rochester
School of Medicine; Medical Director, Monroe
Community Hospital; Director, Finger Lakes
Geriatric Education Center of Upstate New
York; Associate Chief of Staff/Research,
Canandaigua VA Medical Center
Long-Term Care

Talmadge E. King, Jr., MD
Chief, Department of Medicine, Julius R.
Krevans Distinguished Professorship in Internal
Medicine, University of California at
San Francisco
Interstitial Lung Diseases

Preeti Kishore, MD
Assistant Professor of Medicine, Division
of Endocrinology, Albert Einstein College
of Medicine
Diabetes Mellitus

James P. Knochel, MD
Clinical Professor of Internal Medicine,
University of Texas Southwestern Medical
Center; Past Chairman, Department of Internal
Medicine, Presbyterian Hospital of Dallas
Heat Disorders

Karen Birckelbaw Kopacek, RPh
Clinical Assistant Professor and Clinical
Pharmacist, Division of Pharmacy Practice,
University of Wisconsin School of Pharmacy
Administration and Kinetics of Drugs

Arthur E. Kopelman, MD
Professor of Pediatrics and Neonatology
(Emeritus), The Brody School of Medicine at
East Carolina University
Problems in Newborns

David N. Korones, MD
Associate Professor of Pediatrics, Oncology,
and Neurology, University of Rochester
Medical Center
Childhood Cancers

Steven H. Kroft, MD
Associate Professor of Pathology, Medical
College of Wisconsin; Director of
Hematopathology, Dynacare Laboratories/
Froedtert Hospital
Symptoms and Diagnosis of Blood Disorders

Mark S. Lachs, MD, MPH
Irene F. and I. Roy Psaty Distinguished
Professor of Medicine and Director of
Geriatrics, New York Presbyterian Health
System
Elder Mistreatment

Jules Y. T. Lam, MD
Associate Professor of Medicine, University of
Montreal; Cardiologist, Montreal Heart
Institute, Montreal, Quebec, Canada
Atherosclerosis

Lewis Landsberg, MD
Irving S. Cutter Professor of Medicine and
Dean (Emeritus), Northwestern University
Multiple Endocrine Neoplasia Syndromes

Ruth A. Lawrence, MD
Professor of Pediatrics, Obstetrics and
Gynecology, University of Rochester School of
Medicine and Dentistry; Director of Normal
Newborn Nursery, Strong Memorial Hospital
Newborns and Infants

Mathew H. M. Lee, MD
Howard A. Rusk Professor of Rehabilitation
Medicine and Chairman, Department of
Rehabilitation Medicine, New York University
School of Medicine
Rehabilitation

Wendy S. Levinbook, MD
Assistant Professor of Dermatology, University
of Connecticut Health Center
Hair Disorders

Matthew E. Levison, MD
Adjunct Professor of Medicine, Drexel
University College of Medicine; Professor of
Public Health, Drexel University School of
Public Health
Antibiotics; Bacterial Infections

Sharon Levy, MD, MPH
Assistant Professor of Pediatrics, Harvard
Medical School; Associate Researcher, Center
for Adolescent Substance Abuse Research;
Medical Director, Adolescent Substance Abuse
Program, Children's Hospital
Adolescents; Problems in Adolescents

James L. Lewis III, MD
Nephrology Associates, PC, Birmingham
Water Balance; Acid-Base Balance

Alan E. Lichtin, MD
Associate Professor, Department of Medicine,
Cleveland Clinic Lerner College of Medicine of
Case Western Reserve; Staff Physician,
Hematologic Oncology and Blood Disorders,
Cleveland Clinic
Anemia

Paul L. Liebert, MD
Private Practice, Tomah Memorial Hospital,
Tomah, WI
Sports Injuries

Richard W. Light, MD
Professor of Medicine, Division of Allergy,
Pulmonary, and Critical Care Medicine,
Vanderbilt University Medical Center
Pleural Disorders

Gregory S. Liptak, MD, MPH
Professor of Pediatrics, Upstate Medical
University; Chief, Center for
Neurodevelopmental Pediatrics
*Birth Defects; Chromosomal and Genetic
Abnormalities*

Elliot M. Livstone, MD
Attending Physician, Sarasota Memorial
Hospital
Tumors of the Digestive System

Phillip Low, MD
Professor of Neurology, Mayo Clinic College of Medicine
Autonomic Nervous System Disorders

Paul D. Lui, MD
Associate Professor of Urology, Loma Linda University School of Medicine
Male Reproductive System; Penile and Testicular Disorders

Joanne Lynn, MD
Bureau Chief, Chronic Disease and Cancer, Community Health Administration, Department of Health, Washington, DC
Death and Dying

Robert J. MacNeal, MD
Assistant Professor, Department of General Internal Medicine; Resident Physician, Section of Dermatology, Dartmouth–Hitchcock Medical Center
Biology of the Skin; Diagnosis and Treatment of Skin Disorders; Sunlight and Skin Damage

Kenneth Maiese, MD
Professor and Director, Neurology, Anatomy, and Cell Biology, Center for Molecular Medicine and Institute for Environmental Health Sciences, Wayne State University School of Medicine
Head Injuries; Stupor and Coma

Scott Manaker, MD, PhD
Associate Professor of Medicine; Vice Chair for Regulatory Affairs, Department of Medicine, University of Pennsylvania Health System
Shock

James F. Markmann, MD, PhD
Professor of Surgery, Harvard Medical School; Clinical Director, Division of Transplantation, Massachusetts General Hospital
Transplantation

John T. McBride, MD
Professor of Pediatrics, Northeastern Ohio Universities Colleges of Medicine and Pharmacology; Vice Chair, Department of Pediatrics, Akron Children's Hospital
Respiratory Disorders

Margaret C. McBride, MD
Professor of Pediatrics (Neurology), Northeastern Ohio Universities Colleges of Medicine and Pharmacology; Director, Neurodevelopmental Center, Akron Children's Hospital
Neurologic Disorders

Daniel J. McCarty, MD
Will and Cava Ross Professor of Medicine (Emeritus), Medical College of Wisconsin
Gout and Pseudogout

J. Allen McCutchan, MD, MSc
Professor of Medicine, Division of Infectious Diseases, School of Medicine, University of California at San Diego
Human Immunodeficiency Virus Infection; Sexually Transmitted Diseases

Daniel E. McGinley-Smith, MD
Private Practice, New England Dermatology, Lebanon, NH; Staff Dermatologist, New London Hospital
Pigment Disorders

Karen McKoy, MD, MPH
Assistant Clinical Professor in Dermatology, Harvard Medical School; Senior Staff, Group Practice, Lahey Clinic Department of Dermatology, Burlington, MA
Acne

James I. McMillan, MD
Associate Professor of Medicine, Loma Linda University; Chief, VA Loma Linda Healthcare System
Kidney Failure; Dialysis

S. Gene McNeeley, MD
Chief of Gynecology, Hutzel Women's Hospital; Clinical Professor, Michigan State University, College of Osteopathic Medicine, Hutzel Women's Health Specialists
Pelvic Floor Disorders; Noncancerous Gynecologic Abnormalities

Noshir R. Mehta, DMD, MDS, MS
Professor and Chairman of General Dentistry; Assistant Dean, International Relations; Director, Craniofacial Pain Center, Tufts University School of Dental Medicine
Temporomandibular Disorders

Daniel R. Mishell Jr., MD
Lyle G. McNeile Professor, Department of
Obstetrics and Gynecology, Keck School of
Medicine, University of Southern California;
Chief Physician, Womens and Childrens
Hospital, Los Angeles County and University of
Southern California Medical Center
Family Planning

L. Brent Mitchell, MD
Professor and Head, Department of Cardiac
Sciences, University of Calgary; Director, Libin
Cardiovascular Institute of Alberta, Calgary
Health Region and University of Calgary
Abnormal Heart Rhythms

Richard T. Miyamoto, MD
Arilla Spence DeVault Professor and
Chairman, Department of Otolaryngology–
Head and Neck Surgery, Indiana University
School of Medicine
Middle and Inner Ear Disorders

Joel L. Moake, MD
Professor of Medicine, Baylor College of
Medicine; Associate Director, Biomedical
Engineering Laboratory, Rice University
Bleeding and Clotting Disorders

Julie S. Moldenhauer, MD
Assistant Professor of Obstetrics and
Gynecology, University of North Carolina
*Complications of Labor and Delivery;
Postdelivery Period*

Pekka Mooar, MD
Associate Professor, Department of
Orthopaedics and Sports Medicine, Temple
University School of Medicine
Biology of the Musculoskeletal System

John E. Morley, MB, BCh
Dammert Professor of Gerontology, St. Louis
University Health Sciences Center; Director of
Geriatric Research, Education and Clinical
Center, St. Louis VA Medical Center
Biology of the Endocrine System

Angela Cafiero Moroney, PharmD
Assistant Professor of Clinical Pharmacy,
Philadelphia College of Pharmacy, University of
the Sciences in Philadelphia; Clinical Pharmacy
Specialist-Geriatrics, Philadelphia VA Medical
Center
Drug Dynamics

John Morrison, MD
Professor of Obstetrics and Gynecology and
Pediatrics, University of Mississippi Medical
Center
High-Risk Pregnancy

David F. Murchison, DDS, MMS
Colonel, USAF, DC; Director, Air Force Dental
Operations, USAF Dental Service, Lackland-
Kelly Air Force Base
Urgent Dental Problems

Edward A. Nardell, MD
Associate Professor, Harvard Medical School
and Harvard School of Public Health;
Department of Social Medicine and Health
Inequalities, Brigham and Women's Hospital
Tuberculosis; Leprosy

Linda P. Nelson, DMD, MScD
Assistant Professor of Pediatric Dentistry,
Harvard School of Dental Medicine; Associate
Pediatric Dentist, Children's Hospital
Biology of the Mouth

John H. Newman, MD
Elsa S. Hanigan Professor of Pulmonary
Medicine, Vanderbilt University School of
Medicine
*Pulmonary Embolism; Pulmonary
Hypertension*

Lee S. Newman, MD, MA
Professor, Department of Preventive Medicine
and Biometrics and Department of Medicine,
University of Colorado at Denver and Health
Sciences Center
*Allergic and Autoimmune Diseases of the
Lungs; Environmental Lung Diseases*

Patrick G. O'Connor, MD, MPH
Professor of Medicine; Chief, Section of
General Internal Medicine, Yale University
School of Medicine
Drug Use and Abuse

Gerald F. O'Malley, DO
Clinical Associate Professor, Department of
Emergency Medicine, Thomas Jefferson
University Hospital; Director of Research,
Department of Emergency Medicine, Albert
Einstein Medical Center
Poisoning

Joseph G. Ouslander, MD
Professor of Medicine and Director, Division of Geriatric Medicine and Gerontology, Emory University School of Medicine
Urinary Incontinence

James T. Pacala, MD
Associate Professor and Distinguished University Teaching Professor, Family Practice and Community Health, University of Minnesota Medical School
Prevention

Robert M. Palmer, MD, MPH
Visiting Professor of Medicine and Clinical Director, Division of Geriatric Medicine, Department of Medicine, University of Pittsburgh
Hospital Care

Elizabeth J. Palumbo, MD
Private Practice, The Pediatric Group, Fairfax, VA
Problems in Infants and Very Young Children

Richard D. Pearson, MD
Professor of Medicine and Pathology; Senior Associate Dean for Education, University of Virginia School of Medicine
Parasitic Infections

Lawrence L. Pelletier, Jr., MD
Professor of Internal Medicine, University of Kansas School of Medicine; Staff Physician, Robert J. Dole VA Medical and Regional Office Center, Wichita
Infective Endocarditis

Frank Pessler, MD, PhD
Pediatric Rheumatologist, Klinik und Polyklinik für Kinder und Jagendmedizin, Medizinische Fakultät Carl-Gustav-Carus, Technische Universität, Dresden
Juvenile Idiopathic Arthritis; Bone Disorders; Hereditary Connective Tissue Disorders

Stephen P. Peters, MD, PhD
Professor of Medicine and Pediatrics and Associate Director, Center for Human Genomics, Wake Forest University Health Sciences
Asthma

Hart Peterson, MD
Clinical Professor of Neurology in Pediatrics (Retired), Cornell University; Attending Neurologist and Pediatrician (Retired), New York Hospital
Cerebral Palsy

William A. Petri, Jr., MD, PhD
Wade Hampton Frost Professor of Epidemiology and Chief, Division of Infectious Diseases and International Health, University of Virginia School of Medicine
Rickettsial and Related Infections

David G. Pfister, MD
Professor, Weill Medical College of Cornell University; Member and Attending Physician and Chief, Head and Neck Medical Oncology, Memorial Sloan-Kettering Cancer Center
Symptoms and Diagnosis of Cancer

Katharine A. Phillips, MD
Professor of Psychiatry and Human Behavior, Butler Hospital and The Warren Alpert Medical School of Brown University
Somatoform Disorders

Harold C. Pillsbury III, MD
Thomas J. Dark Distinguished Professor and Chairman, Department of Otolaryngology–Head and Neck Surgery, University of North Carolina, Chapel Hill
Biology of the Ears, Nose, and Throat

JoAnn V. Pinkerton, MD
Professor of Obstetrics and Gynecology and Director, Midlife Health, University of Virginia Health System
Menstrual Disorders and Abnormal Vaginal Bleeding

Russell K. Portenoy, MD
Professor of Neurology and Anesthesiology, Albert Einstein College of Medicine; Chairman, Department of Pain Medicine and Palliative Care, Beth Israel Medical Center
Pain

Carol S. Portlock, MD
Professor of Clinical Medicine, New York Weill Cornell University Medical College; Attending Physician, Lymphoma Service, Memorial Sloan-Kettering Cancer Center
Lymphomas

Michael Pourfar, MD
Assistant Professor, Department of Medicine,
New York University School of Medicine
Movement Disorders

Josef T. Prchal, MD
Professor of Medicine, Division of Hematology,
University of Utah; George E. Wahlen Veterans
Administration Medical Center
Myeloproliferative Disorders

Glenn M. Preminger, MD
Professor of Urologic Surgery and Director,
Comprehensive Kidney Stone Center, Duke
University Medical Center
Obstruction of the Urinary Tract

Sally Pullman-Mooar, MD
Clinical Associate Professor, Department of
Medicine, Division of Rheumatology,
University of Pennsylvania; Chief, Department
of Rheumatology, Philadelphia Veterans
Administration Medical Center
Low Back and Neck Pain

Lawrence G. Raisz, MD
Board of Trustees Distinguished Professor of
Medicine and Director, UConn Center for
Osteoporosis, University of Connecticut Health
Center
Osteoporosis

Pedro T. Ramirez, MD
Assistant Professor, Gynecologic Oncology
Department, The University of Texas M.D.
Anderson Cancer Center
Cancers of the Female Reproductive System

Robert W. Rebar, MD
Executive Director, American Society for
Reproductive Medicine; Volunteer Clinical
Professor, Department of Obstetrics and
Gynecology, University of Alabama,
Birmingham
Endometriosis; Infertility

Wingfield E. Rehmus, MD, MPH
Clinical Assistant Professor of Dermatology,
Stanford University; Ministry of Health, Koror,
Palau
Nail Disorders

Douglas J. Rhee, MD
Assistant Professor, Massachusetts Eye and Ear
Infirmary, Harvard Medical School
Glaucoma

Melvin I. Roat, MD
Clinical Associate Professor, Department of
Ophthalmology, Thomas Jefferson University;
Cornea Service, Wills Eye Institute
Corneal Disorders

James R. Roberts, MD
Professor and Vice Chairman, Department of
Emergency Medicine, Drexel University
College of Medicine; Chair, Department of
Emergency Medicine and Director, Division of
Toxicology, Mercy Catholic Medical Center
Fractures

Austin S. Rose, MD
Assistant Professor, Department of
Otolaryngology–Head and Neck Surgery,
University of North Carolina, Chapel Hill
Biology of the Ears, Nose, and Throat

Peter L. Rosenblatt, MD
Assistant Professor, Obstetrics, Gynecology and
Reproductive Biology, Harvard Medical
School; Director of Urogynecology, Mount
Auburn Hospital, Beth Israel Deaconess
Medical Center
Female Reproductive System

Beryl J. Rosenstein, MD
Professor of Pediatrics, Johns Hopkins
University School of Medicine
Cystic Fibrosis

Steven Rosenzweig, MD
Clinical Associate Professor, Drexel University
College of Medicine
Complementary and Alternative Medicine

Robert J. Ruben, MD
Distinguished University Professor,
Department of Otolaryngology–Head and
Neck Surgery, Albert Einstein College of
Medicine and Montefiore Medical Center
*Hearing Loss and Deafness; Ear, Nose, and
Throat Disorders*

Fred H. Rubin, MD
Professor of Medicine, University of Pittsburgh
School of Medicine; Chair, Department of
Medicine, University of Pittsburgh Medical
Center, Presbyterian Shadyside Hospital,
Shadyside Campus
Immunization

Michael Rubin, MD
Professor of Clinical Neurology, Weill Cornell
Medical College; Director, Neuromuscular
Service and EMG Laboratory, New York
Presbyterian Hospital–Cornell Medical Center
Muscular Dystrophies and Related Disorders;
Spinal Cord Disorders; Peripheral Nerve
Disorders; Cranial Nerve Disorders

Atenodoro R. Ruiz, Jr., MD
Attending Physician, Department of Medicine-
Gastroenterology, Kaiser Permanente,
Santa Clara
Malabsorption

J. Mark Ruscin, PharmD
Professor, Department of Pharmacy Practice,
Southern Illinois University Edwardsville
School of Pharmacy
Aging and Drugs

Julie E. Russack, MD
Melanoma Fellow, Rigel Dermatology (private
practice associated with New York University
Medical Center)
Blistering Diseases

Paul S. Russell, MD
John Homans Distinguished Professor of
Surgery, Harvard Medical School; Senior
Surgeon, Massachusetts General Hospital
Transplantation

Charles Sabatino, JD
Adjunct Professor, Georgetown University Law
Center; Director, Commission on Law and
Aging, American Bar Association
Legal and Ethical Issues

David B. Sachar, MD
Clinical Professor of Medicine, Mount Sinai
School of Medicine; Director (Emeritus) of the
Dr. Henry D. Janavitz Division of
Gastroenterology, The Mount Sinai Hospital
Inflammatory Bowel Diseases; Clostridium
difficile-*Induced Colitis*

Seyed-Ali Sadjadi, MD
Associate Professor of Medicine, Loma Linda
University School of Medicine
Blood Vessel Disorders of the Kidneys; Kidney
Filtering Disorders

Lee M. Sanders, MD, MPH
Associate Professor of Pediatrics, University of
Miami, Miller School of Medicine; Associate
Professor of Pediatrics, Holtz Children's
Hospital
Hereditary Metabolic Disorders

Christopher Sanford, MD, MPH, DTM & H
Clinical Assistant Professor, Department of
Family Medicine, University of Washington;
Co-Director, Travel Clinic, Hall Health Center,
University of Washington
Travel and Health

Clarence T. Sasaki, MD
The Charles W. Ohse Professor, Chief of
Otolaryngology, and Director, Head and Neck
Unit of the Yale Comprehensive Cancer Center
Throat Disorders

Peter C. Schalock, MD
Instructor in Dermatology, Harvard Medical
School; Assistant in Dermatology,
Massachusetts General Hospital
Itching and Noninfectious Rashes

Steven Schmitt, MD
Head, Section of Bone and Joint Infections,
Department of Infectious Disease, Cleveland
Clinic
Bone and Joint Infections

Eldon A. Shaffer, MD
Professor of Medicine, Faculty of Medicine,
University of Calgary
Diagnostic Tests for Liver, Gallbladder, and
Biliary Disorders; Fatty Liver, Cirrhosis, and
Related Disorders; Blood Vessel Disorders of
the Liver; Gallbladder Disorders

Nicholas J. Shaheen, MD, MPH
Associate Professor of Medicine and
Epidemiology, University of North Carolina
School of Medicine; Director, Center for
Esophageal Diseases and Swallowing,
University of North Carolina Hospitals
Biology of the Digestive System; Symptoms and
Diagnosis of Digestive Disorders

Stewart Shankel, MD
Clinical Professor of Medicine and Director of
Clinical Medicine, University of California at
Riverside
Urinary Tract Infections

William R. Shapiro, MD
Professor of Clinical Neurology, University of Arizona College of Medicine, Tucson; Chief, Neuro-Oncology, Barrow Neurological Institute
Tumors of the Nervous System

David D. Sherry, MD
Professor of Pediatrics, The Children's Hospital of Philadelphia, University of Pennsylvania
Juvenile Idiopathic Arthritis; Bone Disorders; Hereditary Connective Tissue Disorders

Stephen D. Silberstein, MD
Professor of Neurology, Headache Center, Thomas Jefferson University
Headaches

Harold M. Silverman, PharmD
Editor-in-Chief, The Pill Book
Trade-Name and Generic Drugs

Daphne Simeon, MD
Associate Professor, Department of Psychiatry, Mount Sinai School of Medicine
Dissociative Disorders

Ashish C. Sinha, MD, PhD
Assistant Professor, Anesthesiology and Critical Care, University of Pennsylvania School of Medicine
Obesity and the Metabolic Syndrome (Bariatric Surgery portion)

Donna L. Skerrett, MD
Associate Professor of Clinical Pathology and Laboratory Medicine and Director of Transfusion Medicine and Cellular Therapy, Weill Cornell Medical College
Blood Transfusion

Richard V. Smith, MD
Vice Chair, Department of Otorhinolaryngology, Head and Neck Surgery, Albert Einstein College of Medicine; Director, Head and Neck Service, Montefiore Medical Center
Nose and Throat Cancers

Norman Sohn, MD
Clinical Assistant Professor of Surgery, New York University School of Medicine; Attending Surgeon, Lenox Hill Hospital
Anal and Rectal Disorders

David E. Soper, MD
Professor and Vice Chairman for Clinical Affairs, Department of Obstetrics and Gynecology, Medical University of South Carolina
Pelvic Inflammatory Disease; Vaginal Infections

David R. Steinberg, MD
Associate Professor, Department of Orthopaedic Surgery, and Director, Hand and Upper Extremity Fellowship Program, Department of Orthopaedic Surgery, University of Pennsylvania School of Medicine
Hand Disorders

Marvin E. Steinberg, MD
Professor (Emeritus) of Orthopaedic Surgery, University of Pennsylvania School of Medicine
Osteonecrosis

Kingman P. Strohl, MD
Professor of Medicine and Director, Center for Sleep Disorders Research, Case Western Reserve University
Sleep Apnea

Albert J. Stunkard, MD
Professor of Psychiatry, University of Pennsylvania School of Medicine
Eating Disorders

Alan M. Sugar, MD
Professor of Medicine (Emeritus), Boston University School of Medicine; Medical Director, Infectious Disease Clinical Services and HIV/AIDS Program, Cape Cod Healthcare
Fungal Infections

Stephen Brian Sulkes, MD
Professor of Pediatrics, Division of Neurodevelopmental and Behavioral Pediatrics, Golisano Children's Hospital at Strong, University of Rochester School of Medicine and Dentistry
Mental Retardation/Intellectual Disability; Behavioral and Developmental Problems in Young Children; Learning and Developmental Disorders

David A. Swanson, MD
Clinical Professor, Department of Urology, The University of Texas, M.D. Anderson Cancer Center
Cancers of the Kidney and Urinary Tract

Moira Szilagyi, MD, PhD
Associate Professor of Pediatrics, University of
Rochester; Medical Director, Starlight
Pediatrics, Monroe County Health Department
*Social Issues Affecting Children and Their
Families*

Paul H. Tanser, MD
Professor of Medicine (Emeritus), McMaster
University, Hamilton, Ontario; Cardiology
Consultant, North Shore and Waitakere
Hospitals, Auckland
*Biology of the Heart and Blood Vessels;
Symptoms and Diagnosis of Heart and Blood
Vessel Disorders; Heart Valve Disorders*

Joan B. Tarloff, PhD
Professor, Department of Pharmaceutical
Sciences, University of the Sciences in
Philadelphia
Adverse Drug Reactions

Mary Territo, MD
Professor of Medicine, Director of
Hematopoietic Stem Cell Transplantation,
University of California, Los Angeles
White Blood Cell Disorders

David R. Thomas, MD
Professor of Internal Medicine, Division of
Geriatrics, Saint Louis University Health
Sciences Center
Undernutrition

Elizabeth Chabner Thompson, MD, MPH
Private Practice, NY Group for Plastic Surgery
*Overview of Cancer; Prevention and Treatment
of Cancer*

Stig Thunell, MD, PhD
Professor, Karolinska Institute; Senior
Consultant, Porphyria Center Sweden,
Karolinska University Hospital Huddinge,
Stockholm
Porphyrias

Courtney M. Townsend, Jr., MD
Professor and John Woods Harris
Distinguished Chairman, Department of
Surgery, The University of Texas Medical
Branch at Galveston
Carcinoid Tumors

Oren Traub, MD, PhD
Attending Physician, Department of Internal
Medicine, Pacific Medical Centers and
University of Washington
The Science of Medicine and Clinical Trials

Amal Trivedi, MD, MPH
Assistant Professor of Community Health,
The Warren Alpert Medical School of Brown
University; Investigator, REAP on Outcomes
and Quality in Chronic Disease and
Rehabilitation, Providence VA Medical Center
Health Care Coverage for Older People

Anne S. Tsao, MD
Assistant Professor, Department of Thoracic/
Head and Neck Oncology, Division of Cancer
Medicine, University of Texas M.D. Anderson
Cancer Center
Cancer of the Lungs

Allan R. Tunkel, MD, PhD
Chair, Department of Medicine, Monmouth
Medical Center; Professor of Medicine, Drexel
University College of Medicine
Biology of Infectious Disease

Alexander G. G. Turpie, MD
Professor of Medicine, McMaster University
and Hamilton Health Sciences General
Hospital
Venous Disorders; Lymphatic Disorders

James T. Ubertalli, DMD
Assistant Clinical Professor, Tufts University
School of Dental Medicine; Private Practice,
Hingham, MA
Periodontal Diseases; Tooth Disorders

Marguerite A. Urban, MD
Associate Professor of Medicine, University of
Rochester School of Medicine
Viral Infections

Eva M. Vivian, PharmD
Clinical Associate Professor, University of
Wisconsin School of Pharmacy
Overview of Drugs

Victor G. Vogel, MD, MHS
National Vice President for Research,
American Cancer Society
Breast Disorders

Aaron E. Walfish, MD
Division of Digestive Diseases, Department of
Medicine, Beth Israel Medical Center,
Manhattan Campus of Albert Einstein College
of Medicine
Inflammatory Bowel Diseases; Clostridium
difficile-*Induced Colitis*

James Wayne Warnica, MD
Professor of Medicine, Department of Cardiac
Science, University of Calgary; Director,
Cardiac Intensive Care Unit, Foothills Medical
Centre
Coronary Artery Disease

Geoffrey A. Weinberg, MD
Professor of Pediatrics, University of Rochester
School of Medicine and Dentistry; Director,
Pediatric HIV Program, Golisano Children's
Hospital at Strong
Bacterial Infections

Gregory L. Wells, MD
Resident in Dermatology, Dartmouth Medical
School and Dartmouth-Hitchcock Medical
Center
Skin Cancers

John B. West, MD, PhD, DSc
Professor of Medicine and Physiology,
University of California, San Diego
Altitude Sickness

Terrie Fox Wetle, PhD, MS
Associate Dean of Medicine for Public Health,
The Warren Alpert Medical School; Professor,
Department of Community Health, Division of
Biology and Medicine, Brown University
Coping with Changes Related to Aging

Kendrick Alan Whitney, DPM
Assistant Professor, Department of Medicine
and Orthopedics, Temple University School of
Podiatric Medicine
Foot Problems

Margaret-Mary G. Wilson, MD
Medical Director, Health Services,
UnitedHealthcare, Maryland Heights
*Overview of Nutrition; Disorders of Unknown
Cause*

Robert A. Wise, MD
Professor of Medicine, Pulmonary and Critical
Care, Johns Hopkins University School of
Medicine
Chronic Obstructive Pulmonary Disease

Steven E. Wolf, MD
Betty and Bob Kelso Distinguished Chair in
Burns and Trauma, Vice-Chair for Research
and Professor, Department of Surgery,
University of Texas Health Science Center–San
Antonio; Chief, Clinical Research, United
States Army Institute of Surgical Research
Burns

Eiji Yanagisawa, MD
Clinical Professor of Otolaryngology, Yale
University School of Medicine
Outer Ear Disorders

Heidi Yeh, MD
Instructor in Surgery, Harvard Medical
School; Assistant in Surgery, Massachusetts
General Hospital
Transplantation

Adrienne Youdim, MD
Director, Medical Weight Loss, Cedars-Sinai
Center for Weight Loss
Obesity and the Metabolic Syndrome

Lowell S. Young, MD
Clinical Professor of Medicine, University of
California at San Francisco; Director, Kuzell
Institute, California Pacific Medical Center
Bacteremia, Sepsis, and Septic Shock

A GUIDE FOR READERS

The Merck Manual Home Health Handbook is organized into sections and chapters. Understanding this organization will help the reader navigate through the book and find the most information. Topics of interest may be quickly located by consulting the Contents or Index.

Sections

The first section—Fundamentals—covers many general topics important to health care, such as making the most of health care, prevention of disease and disability, exercise and fitness, rehabilitation, and death and dying.

Most sections cover the disorders of one organ or organ system, such as those of the eye, skin, or heart and blood vessels. A few sections cover one type of disorder, such as hormonal disorders or infectious diseases. Four separate sections cover health issues specific to men, women, children, and older people.

The Injuries and Poisoning section includes first aid, burns, fractures, sports injuries, poisoning, and bites and stings, among other topics. The last section—Special Subjects—provides an overview of clinical trials, medical decision making, imaging tests, hospital care, surgery, complementary and alternative medicine, medicinal herbs, and travel and health, as well as other topics.

Chapters

Most chapters begin with a brief introduction, which contains background information relating to all the topics in that chapter. Some chapters describe a single disorder. Other chapters cover a group of related disorders. In either case, the discussion of a disorder usually starts with a definition. If the topic is lengthy, then the definition is followed by summary bullets. The information that follows is typically organized under headings, such as causes, symptoms, diagnosis, prevention, treatment, and prognosis. Bold-faced type within the text indicates topics of major importance. For ease of reading, text bullets are frequently used.

In sections about disorders of an organ or organ system, the first chapter describes the organ's normal structure and function. Reading about how the heart works or looking at illustrations of the heart, for example, may make reading about a specific heart disorder more understandable. Many sections also include a chapter describing symptoms and relevant medical tests.

Information on Aging

Many topics contain a "Spotlight on Aging" to address specific aging-related information. In addition, a section called Older People's Health Issues covers such topics as health care coverage for older people, long-term care, coping with changes related to aging, driving, and falls, among others.

Cross-references

Throughout the book are cross-references that identify other important or related discussions of a topic. Some cross-references point the reader to a figure, sidebar, or table.

Medical Terms

Medical terms are often provided, usually in parentheses after the common term. On the next page is a list of prefixes, roots, and suffixes used in medical terminology. This list can help take the mystery out of medicine's multisyllabic vocabulary.

Figures, Sidebars, and Tables

The many figures, sidebars, and tables help explain material in the text or give additional, related information.

Drug Information

The Drugs section provides comprehensive information about drugs. Also, scattered throughout the book are many drug tables, marked by an Rx symbol. These drug tables provide additional information about a class or group of drugs.

Individual drugs are almost always referred to by their generic name rather than by their brand or trade names. Appendix III contains a table of the generic drugs mentioned in the book along with some of their corresponding trade names. Appendix III also provides a separate table of drug trade names with their corresponding generic name.

Drug doses are not provided because doses can vary greatly, depending on individual circumstances. For example, doses are affected by age, sex, weight, height, the presence of more than one disorder, and the use of other drugs. Therefore, health care practitioners tailor the dose of a drug to the individual.

Diagnostic Tests

Diagnostic tests are mentioned throughout the book. Usually, an explanation is provided the first time a test is mentioned in a chapter. On page 2034, the chapter on Common Imaging Tests gives detailed information about computed tomography, magnetic resonance imaging, radionuclide scanning, as well as other imaging tests. In addition, Appendix II lists many common diagnostic tests and procedures and explains what they are used for.

Did You Know

A feature called "Did You Know?" provides interesting tidbits of information related to a specific topic. Hundreds of such boxes are scattered throughout the book.

Resources for Help and information

Appendix IV lists the contact information for many organizations that help people who have specific disorders. These organizations can provide additional information about a disorder or help locate support services.

UNDERSTANDING MEDICAL TERMS

At first glance, medical terminology can seem like a foreign language. But often the key to understanding medical terms is focusing on their components (prefixes, roots, and suffixes). For example, spondylolysis is a combination of "spondylo," which means vertebra, and "lysis," which means dissolve, and so means dissolution of a vertebra.

The same components are used in many medical terms. "Spondylo" plus "itis," which means inflammation, forms spondylitis, an inflammation of the vertebrae. The same prefix plus "malacia," which means soft, forms spondylomalacia, a softening of the vertebrae.

Knowing the meaning of a small number of components can help with interpretation of a large number of medical terms. The following list defines many commonly used medical prefixes, roots, and suffixes.

a(n)	absence of	cut	skin
acou, acu	hear	cyan(o)	blue
aden(o)	gland	cyst(o)	bladder
aer(o)	air	cyt(o)	cell
alg	pain	dactyl(o)	finger or toe
andr(o)	man	dent	tooth
angi(o)	vessel	derm(ato)	skin
ankyl(o)	crooked, curved	dipl(o)	double
ante	before	dors	back
anter(i)	front, forward	dys	bad, faulty, abnormal
anti	against	ectomy	excision (removal by cutting)
arteri(o)	artery		
arthr(o)	joint	emia	blood
articul	joint	encephal(o)	brain
ather(o)	fatty	end(o)	inside
audi(o)	hearing	enter(o)	intestine
aur(i)	ear	epi	outer, superficial, upon
aut(o)	self	erythr(o)	red
bi, bis	double, twice, two	eu	normal
brachy	short	extra	outside
brady	slow	gastr(o)	stomach
bucc(o)	cheek	gen	become, originate
carcin(o)	cancer	gloss(o)	tongue
cardi(o)	heart	glyc(o)	sweet, or referring to glucose
cephal(o)	head		
cerebr(o)	brain	gram, graph	write, record
cervic	neck	gyn	woman
chol(e)	bile, or referring to gallbladder	hem(ato)	blood
		hemi	half
chondr(o)	cartilage	hepat(o)	liver
circum	around, about	hist(o)	tissue
contra	against, counter	hydr(o)	water
corpor	body	hyper	excessive, high
cost(o)	rib	hypo	deficient, low
crani(o)	skull	hyster(o)	uterus
cry(o)	cold	iatr(o)	doctor

infra	beneath	phleb(o)	vein
inter	among, between	phob(ia)	fear
intra	inside	plasty	repair
itis	inflammation	pleg(ia)	paralysis
lact(o)	milk	pnea	breathing
lapar(o)	flank, abdomen	pneum(ato)	breath, air
latero	side	pneumon(o)	lung
leuk(o)	white	pod(o)	foot
lingu(o)	tongue	poie	make, produce
lip(o)	fat	poly	much, many
lys(is)	dissolve	post	after
mal	bad, abnormal	poster(i)	back, behind
malac	soft	presby	elder
mamm(o)	breast	proct(o)	anus
mast(o)	breast	pseud(o)	false
megal(o)	large	psych(o)	mind
melan(o)	black	pulmon(o)	lung
mening(o)	membranes	pyel(o)	pelvis of kidney
my(o)	muscle	pyr(o)	fever, fire
myc(o)	fungus	rachi(o)	spine
myel(o)	marrow	ren(o)	kidneys
nas(o)	nose	rhag	break, burst
necr(o)	death	rhe	flow
nephr(o)	kidney	rhin(o)	nose
neur(o)	nerve	scler(o)	hard
nutri	nourish	scope	instrument
ocul(o)	eye	scopy	examination
odyn(o)	pain	somat(o)	body
oma	tumor	spondyl(o)	vertebra
onc(o)	tumor	steat(o)	fat
oophor(o)	ovaries	sten(o)	narrow, compressed
ophthalm(o)	eye	steth(o)	chest
opia	vision	stom	mouth, opening
opsy	examination	supra	above
orchi(o)	testes	tachy	fast, quick
osis	condition	therap	treatment
osse(o)	bone	therm(o)	heat
oste(o)	bone	thorac(o)	chest
ot(o)	ear	thromb(o)	clot, lump
path(o)	disease	tomy	incision (operation by cutting)
ped(o)	child		
penia	deficient, deficiency	tox(i)	poison
peps, pept	digest	uria	urine
peri	around	vas(o)	vessel
phag(o)	eat, destroy	ven(o)	vein
pharmaco	drug	vesic(o)	bladder
pharyng(o)	throat	xer(o)	dry

Fundamentals

1   The Human Body

The human body is a complex, highly organized structure made up of unique cells that work together to accomplish the specific functions necessary for sustaining life. The biology of the human body includes structure (anatomy) and function (physiology). Physiology is discussed in greater detail in the first chapter of each section of this book.

Anatomy is organized by levels, from the smallest components of cells to the largest organs and their relationships to other organs. Gross anatomy is the study of the body's organs as seen with the naked eye during visual inspection and when the body is cut open for examination (dissection). Cellular anatomy is the study of cells and their components, which can be observed only with the use of special techniques and special instruments such as microscopes. Molecular anatomy (often called molecular biology) is the study of the smallest components of cells at the biochemical level.

Anatomy and physiology change remarkably between fertilization and birth. After birth, the rate of anatomic and physiologic changes slows, but childhood is still a time of remarkable growth and development. Some anatomic changes occur past adulthood, but the physiologic changes in the body's cells and organs are what contribute most to what we experience as aging (see page 1884).

Cells

Often thought of as the smallest unit of a living organism, a cell is made up of many even smaller parts, each with its own function. Human cells vary in size, but all are quite small. Even the largest, a fertilized egg, is too small to be seen with the naked eye.

Human cells have a membrane that holds the contents together. However, this membrane is not just a sac. It has receptors that identify the cell to other cells. The receptors also react to substances produced in the body and to drugs taken into the body, selectively allowing these substances or drugs to enter and leave the cell. Reactions that take place at the receptors often alter or control a cell's functions. An example of this is when insulin binds to receptors on the cell membrane to maintain appropriate blood sugar levels and to allow glucose to enter cells.

Within the cell membrane are two major compartments, the cytoplasm and the nucleus. The cytoplasm contains structures that consume and transform energy and perform the cell's functions. The nucleus contains the cell's genetic material and the structures that control cell division and reproduction. Inside every cell are mitochondria. Mitochondria are tiny structures that provide the cell with energy.

The body is composed of many different types of cells, each with its own structure and function. Some, such as white blood cells, move freely, unattached to other cells. Others, such as muscle cells, are firmly attached one to another. Some cells, such as skin cells, divide and reproduce quickly. Others, such as nerve cells, do not divide or reproduce except under usual circumstances. Some cells, especially glandular cells, have as their primary function the production of complex substances, such as a hormone or an enzyme. For example, some cells in the breast produce milk, some in the pancreas produce insulin, some in the lining of the lungs produce mucus, and some in the mouth produce saliva. Other cells have primary functions that are not related to the production of substances—for example, muscle cells contract, allowing movement. Nerve cells generate and conduct electrical impulses, allowing communication between the central nervous system (brain and spinal cord) and the rest of the body.

Tissues and Organs

Related cells joined together are collectively referred to as a tissue. The cells in a tissue are not identical, but they work together to accomplish specific functions. A sample of tissue removed for examination under a microscope (biopsy) contains many types of cells, even though a doctor may be interested in only one specific type.

Connective tissue is the tough, often fibrous tissue that binds the body's structures together and provides support. It is present in almost every organ, forming a large part of skin, tendons, and muscles. The characteristics of connective tissue and the types of cells it contains vary, depending on where it is found in the body.

The body's functions are conducted by organs. Each organ is a recognizable structure—for example, the heart, lungs, liver, eyes, and stomach—that performs specific functions. An organ is made of several types of tissue and therefore several types of

Inside a Cell

Although there are different types of cells, most cells have the same components. A cell consists of a nucleus and cytoplasm and is contained within the cell membrane, which regulates what passes in and out. The nucleus contains chromosomes, which are the cell's genetic material, and a nucleolus, which produces ribosomes. Ribosomes produce proteins, which are packaged by the Golgi apparatus so that they can leave the cell. The cytoplasm consists of a fluid material and organelles, which could be considered the cell's organs. The endoplasmic reticulum transports materials within the cell. Mitochondria generate energy for the cell's activities. Lysosomes contain enzymes that can break down particles entering the cell. Centrioles participate in cell division.

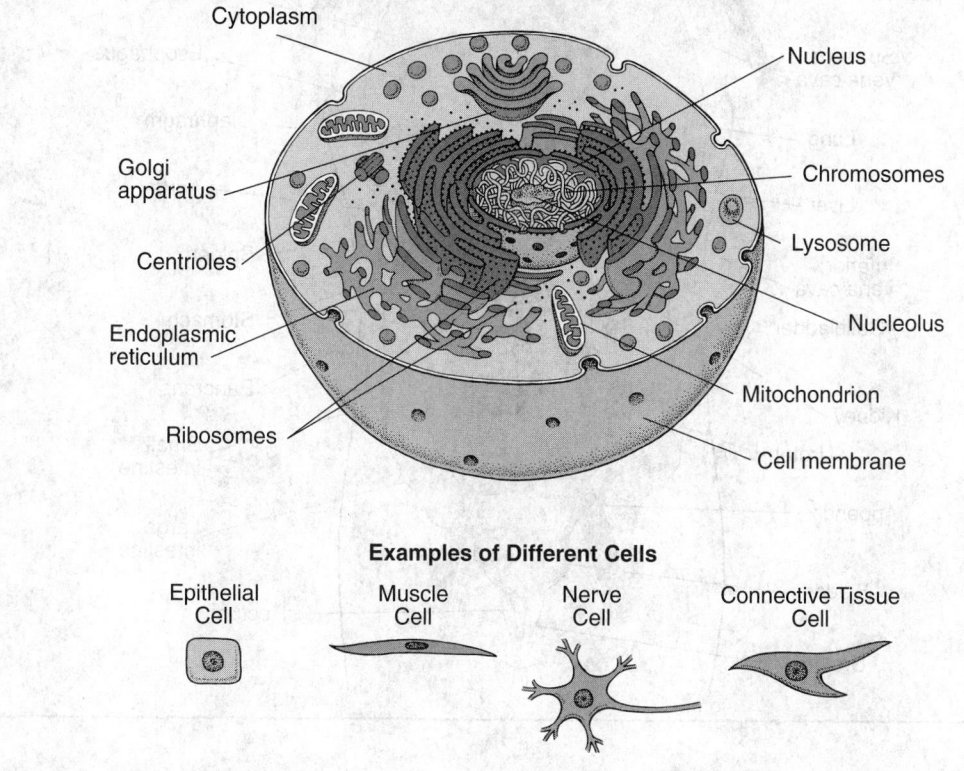

Examples of Different Cells

Epithelial Cell   Muscle Cell   Nerve Cell   Connective Tissue Cell

cells. For example, the heart contains muscle tissue that contracts to pump blood, fibrous tissue that makes up the heart valves, and special cells that maintain the rate and rhythm of heartbeats. The eye contains muscle cells that open and close the pupil, clear cells that make up the lens and cornea, cells that produce the fluid within the eye, cells that sense light, and nerve cells that conduct impulses to the brain. Even an organ as apparently simple as the gallbladder contains different types of cells, such as those that form a lining resistant to the irritative effects of bile, muscle cells that contract to expel bile, and cells that form the fibrous outer wall holding the sac together.

Organ Systems

Although an organ has a specific function, organs also function as part of a group, called an organ system. The organ system is the organizational unit by which medicine is studied, diseases are generally categorized, and treatments are planned. This book is, in large part, organized around the concept of organ systems.

Inside the Torso

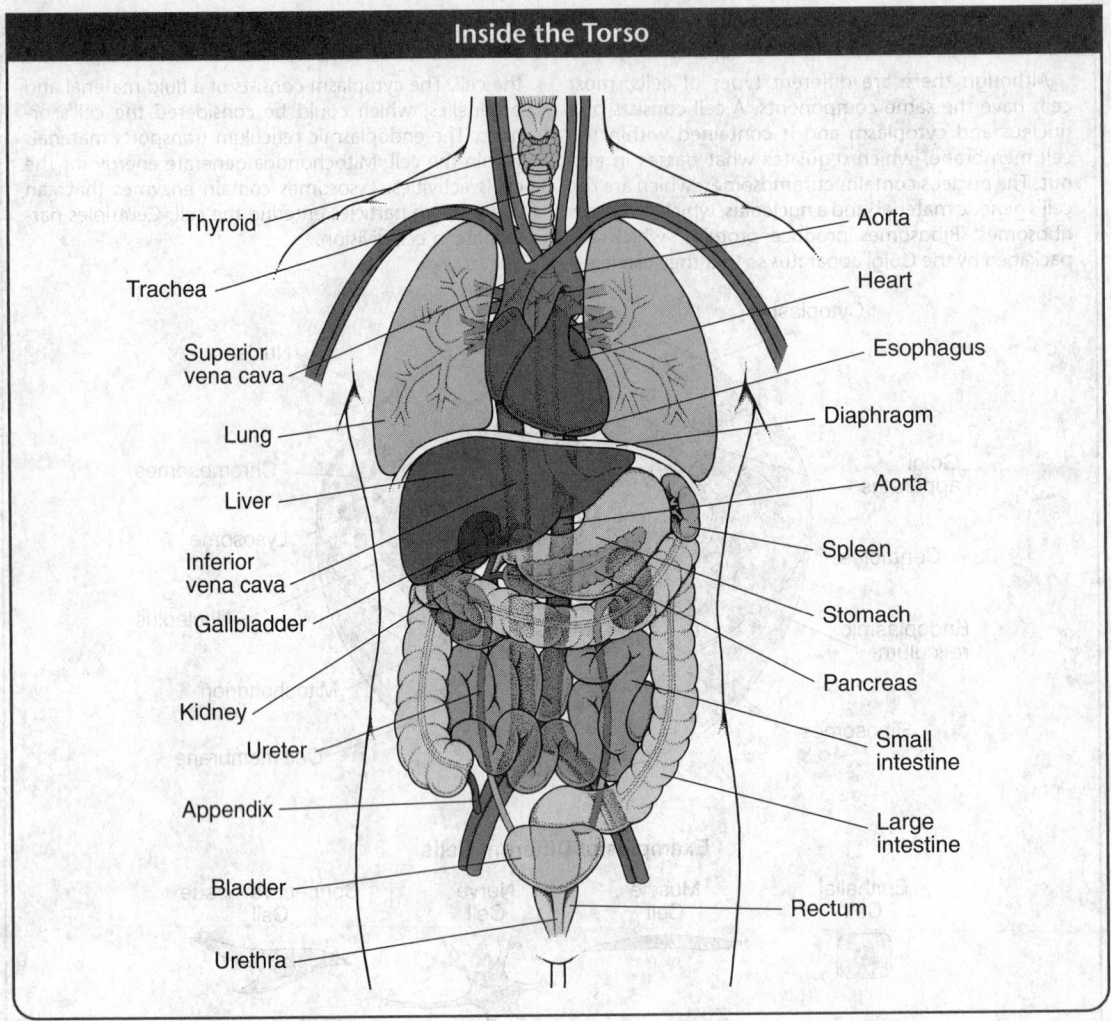

Thyroid

Trachea

Superior
vena cava

Lung

Liver

Inferior
vena cava

Gallbladder

Kidney

Ureter

Appendix

Bladder

Urethra

Aorta

Heart

Esophagus

Diaphragm

Aorta

Spleen

Stomach

Pancreas

Small
intestine

Large
intestine

Rectum

An example of an organ system is the cardiovascular system, which includes the heart (cardio) and blood vessels (vascular). The cardiovascular system is responsible for pumping and circulating the blood. The digestive (or gastrointestinal) system, extending from the mouth to the anus, is responsible for receiving and digesting food and excreting waste. This system includes not only the stomach, small intestine, and large intestine, which move and absorb food, but associated organs such as the pancreas, liver, and gallbladder, which produce digestive enzymes, remove toxins, and store substances necessary for digestion. The musculoskeletal system includes the bones, muscles, ligaments, tendons, and joints, which support and move the body.

Of course, organ systems do not function alone. For example, after a large meal is eaten, the digestive system needs more blood to perform its functions. Therefore, it enlists the aid of the cardiovascular system and the nervous system. Blood vessels of the digestive system widen to transport more blood. Nerve impulses are sent to the brain, notifying it of the increased work. The digestive system even directly stimulates the heart through nerve impulses and chemicals released into the bloodstream. The heart responds by pumping more blood. The brain responds by perceiving less hunger, more fullness, and less interest in vigorous activity.

Communication between organs and organ systems is vital. Communication allows the body to adjust the function of each organ according to the needs of the whole body. The heart must know when the body is resting so that it can slow down and when organs need more blood so that it can speed up. The kidneys must know when the body has too much fluid, so that they can produce more dilute urine, and when the body is dehydrated, so that they can conserve water.

Through communication, the body keeps itself in balance—a concept called homeostasis. Through homeostasis, organs neither underwork nor overwork, and each organ facilitates the functions of every other organ.

Communication to maintain homeostasis can occur through the nervous system or through chemical stimulation. One part of the nervous system, the autonomic nervous system, largely controls the complex communication network that regulates bodily functions. This part of the nervous system functions without a person's thinking about it and without much noticeable indication that it is working. Chemicals used to communicate are called transmitters. Transmitters that are produced by one organ and travel to other organs through the bloodstream are called hormones. Transmitters that conduct messages between parts of the nervous system are called neurotransmitters.

One of the best known transmitters is the hormone epinephrine (adrenaline). When a person is suddenly stressed or frightened, the brain instantly sends a message to the adrenal glands, which quickly release epinephrine. Within moments, this chemical has the entire body on alert, a response sometimes called the fight-or-flight response. The heart beats more rapidly and powerfully, the eyes dilate to allow more light in, breathing quickens, and the activity of the digestive system decreases to allow more blood to go to the muscles. The effect is rapid and intense.

Other chemical communications are less dramatic but equally effective. For example, when the body becomes dehydrated and needs more water, the volume of blood circulating through the cardiovascular system decreases. This decreased blood volume is perceived by receptors in the arteries in the neck. They respond by sending impulses through nerves to the pituitary gland, at the base of the brain, which then produces antidiuretic hormone. This hormone signals the kidneys to concentrate urine and retain more water. Simultaneously, the brain senses thirst, stimulating a person to drink.

The body also has a group of organs—the endocrine system—whose primary function is to produce hormones that regulate the function of other organs. For example, the thyroid gland produces thyroid hormone, which controls the metabolic rate (the speed at which the body's chemical functions proceed); the pancreas produces insulin, which controls the use of sugar; and the adrenal glands produce epinephrine, which stimulates many organs to prepare the body for stress.

Barriers on the Outside and the Inside

As strange as it may seem, defining what is outside and what is inside the body is not always easy, because the body has many surfaces. The skin, which is actually an organ system, is obviously outside the body. It forms a barrier that prevents many harmful substances from entering the body. The digestive system is a long tube that begins at the mouth, winds through the body, and exits at the anus. Is food as it passes through this tube inside or outside of the body? Nutrients and fluid are not really inside the body until they are absorbed into the bloodstream.

Air passes through the nose and throat into the windpipe (trachea), then into the extensive, branching airways of the lungs (bronchi). At what point is this passageway inside the body? Oxygen in the lungs is not useful to the body until it enters the bloodstream. To enter the bloodstream, oxygen must cross through a thin layer of cells lining the lungs. This layer acts as a barrier to viruses and bacteria, such as those that cause tuberculosis, which may be carried into the lungs with air. Unless these organisms penetrate the cells or enter the bloodstream, they generally do not cause disease. Because the lungs have many protective mechanisms, such as antibodies to fight infection and cilia to sweep debris out of the airways, most airborne infectious organisms never cause disease.

Body surfaces not only separate the outside from the inside but also keep structures and substances in their proper place so that they can function properly. For example, internal organs do not float in a pool of blood; blood is normally confined to blood vessels. If blood leaks out of the vessels into other parts of the body (hemorrhage), it not only fails to bring oxygen and nutrients to tissues but also can cause severe harm. For example, a very small amount of blood leaking into the brain destroys brain tissue because there is no room for expansion in the skull. On the other hand, a similar amount of blood leaking into the abdomen does not destroy tissue because the abdomen has room for expansion.

Saliva, so important in the mouth, can cause severe damage if inhaled into the lungs, because saliva carries bacteria that can cause an abscess to form in the lung. The hydrochloric acid produced by the stomach rarely causes harm there. However,

MAJOR ORGAN SYSTEMS

SYSTEM	ORGANS IN THE SYSTEM	SYSTEM	ORGANS IN THE SYSTEM
Cardiovascular	Heart Blood vessels (arteries, capillaries, veins)	Digestive	Mouth Esophagus Stomach Small intestine Large intestine Rectum Anus Liver Gallbladder Pancreas (the part that produces enzymes) Appendix
Respiratory	Nose Mouth Pharynx Larynx Trachea Bronchi Lungs		
Nervous	Brain Spinal cord Nerves (both those that carry impulses to the brain and those that carry impulses from the brain to muscles and organs)	Endocrine	Thyroid gland Parathyroid gland Adrenal glands Pituitary gland Pancreas (the part that produces insulin) Stomach (the cells that produce gastrin) Pineal gland Ovaries Testes
Skin	Skin (both the surface that is generally thought of as skin and the underlying structures of connective tissue, including fat, glands, and blood vessels)	Urinary	Kidneys Ureters Bladder Urethra
Musculoskeletal	Muscles Tendons and ligaments Bones Joints	Male reproductive	Penis Prostate gland Seminal vesicles Vasa deferentia Testes
Blood	Blood cells and platelets Plasma (the liquid part of blood) Bone marrow (where blood cells are produced) Spleen Thymus	Female reproductive	Vagina Cervix Uterus Fallopian tubes Ovaries

the acid can burn and damage the esophagus if it flows backward and can damage other organs if it leaks through the stomach wall. Stool, the undigested part of food expelled through the anus, can cause life-threatening infections if it leaks through a hole in the intestinal wall into the abdominal cavity.

Mind-Body Interactions

The mind and body interact in powerful ways that affect a person's health. The digestive system is profoundly controlled by the mind (brain); anxiety, depression, and fear dramatically affect the function of this system (see page 110). Social and psychologic stress can trigger or aggravate a wide variety of diseases and disorders, such as diabetes mellitus, high blood pressure, and migraine headache. However, the relative importance of psychologic factors varies widely among different people with the same disorder.

Most people, on the basis of either intuition or personal experience, believe that emotional stress can cause or alter the course of even major physical diseases. How these stressors do this is not clear. Emotions obviously can affect certain body functions, such as heart rate, blood pressure, sweating, sleep patterns, stomach acid secretion, and bowel movements, but other relationships are less obvious. For example, the pathways and mechanisms by which the brain and immune system interact are only beginning to be identified. It is remarkable that the brain can alter the activity of white blood cells and thus an immune response, because white blood cells travel through the body in blood or lymph vessels and are not attached to nerves. Nevertheless, research has shown that the brain does communicate with the white blood cells. For example, depression may suppress the immune system, making a person more susceptible to infections, such as those by the viruses that cause the common cold.

Stress can cause physical symptoms even though no physical disease may be present, because the body responds physiologically to emotional stress. For example, stress can cause anxiety, which then triggers the autonomic nervous system and hormones such as epinephrine to speed up the heart rate and to increase the blood pressure and the amount of sweating. Stress can also cause muscle tension, leading to pain in the neck, back, head, or elsewhere.

The mind-body interaction is a two-way street. Not only can psychologic factors contribute to the onset or aggravation of a wide variety of physical disorders, but also physical diseases can affect a person's thinking or mood. People with life-threatening, recurring, or chronic physical disorders commonly become depressed. The depression may worsen the effects of the physical disease and add to a person's misery.

Anatomy and Disease

The human body is remarkably well designed. Most of its organs have a great deal of extra capacity or reserve: They can still function adequately even when damaged. For example, more than two thirds of the liver must be destroyed before serious consequences occur, and a person can usually live with only one lung or kidney. Other organs can tolerate little damage before they malfunction and symptoms occur. For example, if a an artery in the brain becomes blocked or ruptures (stroke) and even a small amount of tissue in a vital part of the brain is destroyed, a person may be unable to speak, move a limb, or maintain balance. If a heart attack destroys a small amount of tissue in the part of the heart that creates or carries the signals to beat, the heart rate may become dangerously slow and the person may even die.

Disease often affects anatomy, and changes in anatomy can cause disease. If the blood supply to a tissue is blocked or cut off, the tissue dies (infarction), as in a heart attack (myocardial infarction) or stroke (cerebral infarction). An abnormal heart valve can cause heart malfunction. Trauma to the skin may damage its ability to act as a barrier, which may lead to infection. Abnormal growths, such as cancer, can directly destroy normal tissue or produce pressure that ultimately destroys it.

Because of the relationship between disease and anatomy, methods of seeing into the body have become a mainstay in the diagnosis and treatment of disease. The first breakthrough came with x-rays, which enabled doctors to see into the body and examine internal structures without surgery. Another major advance was computed tomography (CT), in which x-rays are linked with computers. A CT scan produces detailed cross-sectional (two-dimensional) images of the body's interior.

Other methods of producing images of internal structures include ultrasound scanning, which uses sound waves; magnetic resonance imaging (MRI), which uses the movement of atoms in a magnetic field; and radionuclide imaging, which uses radioactive chemicals injected into the body (see page 2043). These are noninvasive ways to see into the body, in contrast to surgery, which is an invasive procedure.

2   Genetics

A person's genetic makeup is a complete set of instructions on how the body is "supposed" to be built. The body's genetic material consists of genes, made up of coils of deoxyribonucleic acid (DNA). Genes are contained in chromosomes, which are mainly in the cell nucleus.

Chromosomes and Genes

- A gene is a segment of DNA containing the code used to synthesize a protein.
- A chromosome contains hundreds to thousands of genes.
- Every human cell contains 23 pairs of chromosomes, for a total of 46 chromosomes.
- A trait is any gene-determined characteristic and is usually determined by more than one gene.
- Some traits are caused by abnormal genes that are inherited or that are the result of a mutation.

Proteins are probably the most important class of material in the body. Proteins are not just building blocks for muscles, connective tissues, skin, and other structures. They also are needed to make enzymes. Enzymes are complex proteins that control and carry out nearly all chemical processes and reactions within the body. The body produces thousands of different enzymes. Thus, the entire structure and function of the body is governed by the types and amounts of proteins the body synthesizes. Protein synthesis is controlled by genes, which are contained on chromosomes.

The **genotype** is a person's unique combination of genes or genetic makeup. Thus, the genotype is a complete set of instructions on how that person's body synthesizes proteins and thus how that body is *supposed* to function and be built.

The **phenotype** is the *actual* structure and function of a person's body. The phenotype typically differs somewhat from the genotype because not all the instructions in the genotype may be carried out (or expressed). Whether and how a gene is expressed is determined not only by the genotype, but also by the environment (including illnesses and diet) and other factors.

Genes

DNA: Genes consist of deoxyribonucleic acid (DNA). DNA contains the code, or blueprint, used to synthesize a protein. Genes vary in size, depending on the sizes of the proteins for which they code. Each DNA molecule is a long double helix that resembles a spiral staircase containing millions of steps. The steps of the staircase consist of pairs of four types of molecules called bases (nucleotides). In each step, the base adenine (A) is paired with the base thymine (T), or the base guanine (G) is paired with the base cytosine (C).

Synthesizing Proteins: Proteins are composed of a long chain of amino acids linked together one after another. There are 20 different amino acids that can be used—some come from the diet, and some are made by enzymes in the body. As a chain of amino acids is put together, it folds upon itself to create a complex three-dimensional structure. It is the shape of the folded structure that determines its function in the body. Because the folding is determined by the precise sequence of amino acids, each different sequence results in a different protein. Some proteins (such as hemoglobin) contain several different folded chains. Instructions for synthesizing proteins are coded within the DNA.

Coding: Information is coded within DNA by the sequence in which the bases (A, T, G, and C) are arranged. The code is written in triplets. That is, the bases are arranged in groups of three. Particular sequences of three bases in DNA code for specific instructions, such as the addition of one amino acid to a chain. For example, GCT (guanine, cytosine, thymine) codes for the addition of the amino acid alanine, and GTT (guanine, thymine, thymine) codes for the addition of the amino acid valine. Thus, the sequence of amino acids in a protein is determined by the order of triplet base pairs in the gene for that protein on the DNA molecule. The process of turning coded genetic information into a protein involves transcription and translation.

Transcription and Translation: Transcription is the process in which information coded in DNA is transferred (transcribed) to ribonucleic acid (RNA). RNA is a long chain of nucleotides just like a strand of DNA, except that the base uracil (U) replaces the base thymine (T). Thus, RNA contains triplet-coded information just like DNA.

When transcription is initiated, part of the DNA double helix splits open and unwinds. One of the unwound strands of DNA acts as a template against which a complementary strand of RNA forms. The complementary strand of RNA is called messenger RNA (mRNA). The mRNA separates from the DNA, leaves the nucleus, and travels into the cell cytoplasm (the part of the cell outside the nucleus). There, the

Structure of DNA

DNA (deoxyribonucleic acid) is the cell's genetic material, contained in chromosomes within the cell nucleus and mitochondria.

Except for certain cells (for example, sperm and egg cells and red blood cells), the cell nucleus contains 23 pairs of chromosomes. A chromosome contains many genes. A gene is a segment of DNA that provides the code to construct proteins.

The DNA molecule is a long, coiled double helix that resembles a spiral staircase. In it, two strands, composed of sugar (deoxyribose) and phosphate molecules, are connected by pairs of four molecules called bases, which form the steps of the staircase. In the steps, adenine is paired with thymine, and guanine with cytosine. Each pair of bases is held together by a hydrogen bond. A gene consists of a sequence of bases. Sequences of three bases code for an amino acid (amino acids are the building blocks of proteins) or other information.

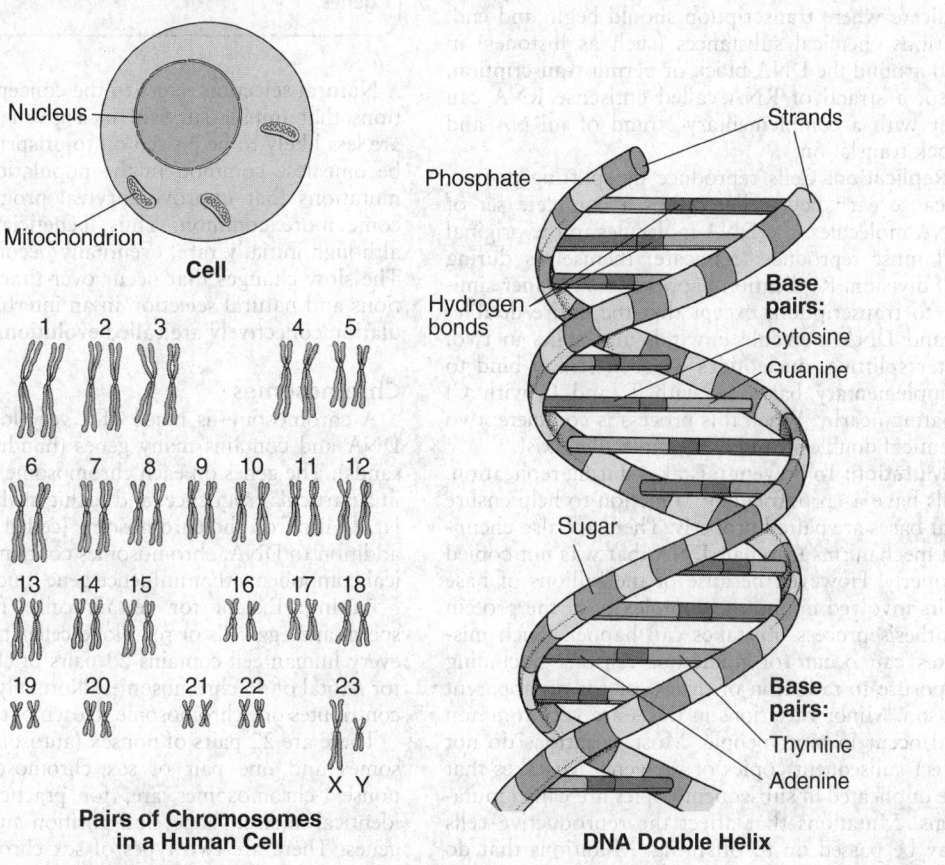

Cell

Nucleus

Mitochondrion

Pairs of Chromosomes in a Human Cell

1 2 3 4 5

6 7 8 9 10 11 12

13 14 15 16 17 18

19 20 21 22 23

X Y

Strands

Phosphate

Hydrogen bonds

Sugar

Base pairs:
Cytosine
Guanine

Base pairs:
Thymine
Adenine

DNA Double Helix

mRNA attaches to a ribosome, which is a tiny structure in the cell where protein synthesis occurs.

With translation, the mRNA code (from the DNA) tells the ribosome the order and type of amino acids to link together. The amino acids are brought to the ribosome by a much smaller type of RNA called transfer RNA (tRNA). Each molecule of tRNA brings one amino acid to be incorporated into the growing chain of protein, which is folded into a precise shape under the influence of nearby molecules ("chaperone" molecules).

Control of Gene Expression: There are many types of cells in a person's body, such as heart cells, liver cells, and muscle cells. These cells look different, act differently, and produce very different chemical substances. However, every cell is the descendant of a single fertilized egg cell, and as such contains the exact same DNA. Cells acquire their very different appearances and functions because different genes are expressed in different cells (and at different times in the same cell). The information about when a gene should be expressed is also coded in the DNA. Gene expression depends on the type of tissue, the age of the person, the presence of specific chemical signals, and numerous other factors, many of which are still poorly understood.

The mechanisms by which genes control each other are very complicated. Genes have markers to indicate where transcription should begin and end. Various chemical substances (such as histones) in and around the DNA block or permit transcription. Also, a strand of RNA called antisense RNA can pair with a complementary strand of mRNA and block translation.

Replication: Cells reproduce by splitting in two. Because each new cell requires a complete set of DNA molecules, the DNA molecules in the original cell must reproduce (replicate) themselves during cell division. Replication happens in a manner similar to transcription, except that the entire double-strand DNA molecule unwinds and splits in two. After splitting, nucleotides on each strand bind to complementary bases (A with T, and G with C) floating nearby. When this process is complete, two identical double-strand DNA molecules exist.

Mutation: To prevent mistakes during replication, cells have a "proofreading" function to help ensure that bases are paired properly. There are also chemical mechanisms to repair DNA that was not copied properly. However, because of the billions of base pairs involved in and the complexity of the protein synthesis process, mistakes can happen. Such mistakes can occur for numerous reasons (including exposure to radiation or drugs) or for no apparent reason. Minor variations in DNA are very common and occur in most people. Most variations do not affect subsequent copies of the gene. Mistakes that are duplicated in subsequent copies are called mutations. Mutations that affect the reproductive cells may be passed on to offspring. Mutations that do not affect reproductive cells die out with the affected person.

Mutations may involve small or large segments of DNA. Depending on its size and location, the mutation may have no apparent effect, or it may alter the amino acid sequence in a protein or decrease the amount of protein produced. If the protein has a different amino acid sequence, it may function differently or not at all. An absent or nonfunctioning protein is often harmful or fatal. For example, in phenylketonuria, a mutation results in the deficiency or absence of the enzyme phenylalanine hydroxylase. This deficiency allows the amino acid phenylalanine (absorbed from the diet) to accumulate in the body, ultimately causing severe mental retardation. In rare cases, a mutation introduces a change that is advantageous to the cell.

?   **Did You Know...**

Not all gene abnormalities are purely harmful—the gene that causes sickle cell disease also provides protection against malaria.

People carry an average of six to eight abnormal genes.

Natural selection refers to the concept that mutations that impair survival in a given environment are less likely to be passed on to offspring (and thus become less common in the population), whereas mutations that improve survival progressively become more common. Thus, beneficial mutations, although initially rare, eventually become common. The slow changes that occur over time from mutations and natural selection in an interbreeding population collectively are called **evolution**.

Chromosomes

A chromosome is made of a very long strand of DNA and contains many genes (hundreds to thousands). The genes on each chromosome are arranged in a particular sequence, and each gene has a particular location on the chromosome (called its locus). In addition to DNA, chromosomes contain other chemical components that influence gene function.

Pairing: Except for certain cells (for example, sperm and egg cells or red blood cells), the nucleus of every human cell contains 23 pairs of chromosomes, for a total of 46 chromosomes. Normally, each parent contributes one chromosome to each of the 23 pairs.

There are 22 pairs of nonsex (autosomal) chromosomes and one pair of sex chromosomes. Paired nonsex chromosomes are, for practical purposes, identical in size, shape, and position and number of genes. There are two types of sex chromosomes, X and Y, each very different from the other. Because each member of a pair of nonsex chromosomes contains one of each corresponding gene, there is in a sense a backup for the genes on those chromosomes.

Sex Chromosomes: The pair of sex chromosomes determines whether a fetus becomes male or female. Males have one X and one Y chromosome. A male's X comes from his mother and the Y from his father. Females have two X chromosomes, one from the mother and one from the father. In certain ways, sex chromosomes function differently than nonsex chromosomes.

The Y chromosome carries relatively few genes other than the ones that determine male sex. The X chromosome contains many more genes than the Y chromosome, many of which have functions besides determining sex and have no counterpart on the Y chromosome. In males, because there is no second X chromosome, these extra genes on the X chromosome are not paired and virtually all of them are expressed. Genes on the X chromosome are referred to as sex-linked, or X-linked, genes.

Normally, in the nonsex chromosomes, the genes on both of the pairs of chromosomes are capable of being fully expressed. However, in females, most of the genes on one of the two X chromosomes are turned off through a process called X inactivation (except in the eggs in the ovaries). X inactivation occurs early in the life of the fetus. In some cells, the X from the father becomes inactive, and in other cells, the X from the mother becomes inactive. Thus, one cell may have a gene from the person's mother and another cell has the gene from the person's father. Because of X inactivation, the absence of one X chromosome usually results in relatively minor abnormalities (such as Turner's syndrome—see page 1728). Thus, missing an X chromosome is far less harmful than missing a nonsex chromosome.

If a female has a disorder in which she has more than two X chromosomes, the extra chromosomes tend to be inactive. Thus, having one or more extra X chromosomes causes far fewer developmental abnormalities than having one or more extra nonsex chromosomes. For example, women with three X chromosomes (triple X syndrome) are often physically and mentally normal (see page 1729).

Mitochondrial Chromosomes: Mitochondria are tiny structures inside cells that synthesize molecules used for energy. Unlike other structures inside cells, each mitochondrion contains its own circular chromosome. This chromosome contains DNA (mitochondrial DNA) that codes for some, but not all, of the proteins that make up that mitochondrion. Mitochondrial DNA usually comes only from the person's mother because, in general, when an egg is fertilized, only mitochondria from the egg become part of the developing embryo. Mitochondria from the sperm usually do not become part of the developing embryo.

Chromosomal Abnormalities: There are several types of chromosomal abnormalities (see page 1726). A person may have an abnormal number of chromosomes or have abnormal areas on one or more chromosomes. Many such abnormalities can be diagnosed before birth.

Abnormal numbers of nonsex chromosomes usually result in severe abnormalities. For example, receiving an extra nonsex chromosome can be fatal to a fetus or can lead to abnormalities such as Down syndrome, which commonly results from a person having three copies of chromosome 21. Absence of a nonsex chromosome is always fatal to the fetus.

Large areas on a chromosome may be abnormal, usually because a whole section was left out (deletion) or mistakenly placed in another chromosome (translocation). For example, chronic myelogenous leukemia is sometimes caused by translocation of part of chromosome 9 onto chromosome 22. This abnormality can be inherited or be the result of a new mutation.

Traits

A trait is any gene-determined characteristic. Many traits are determined by the function of more than one gene. For example, a person's height is likely to be determined by genes affecting growth, appetite, muscle mass, and activity level. However, some traits are determined by the function of a single gene.

Variation in some traits, such as eye color or blood type, is considered normal. Other variations, such as albinism, Marfan syndrome, and Huntington's disease, harm body structure or function and are considered disorders. However, not all such gene abnormalities are uniformly harmful. For example, the sickle cell gene causes disease (sickle cell anemia) but also provides protection against malaria.

Genetic Disorders

A genetic disorder is a detrimental trait caused by an abnormal gene. The abnormal gene may be inherited or may arise spontaneously as a result of a mutation. Abnormalities of one or more genes are fairly common. Humans carry an average of six to eight abnormal genes. However, most of the time the corresponding gene on the other chromosome in the pair is normal and prevents any harmful effects. In the general population, the chance of a person having two copies of the same abnormal gene (and hence a disorder) is very small, but in children of close relatives, the chances are higher. Chances are also high among children of parents who have married within an isolated population, such as the Amish or Mennonites.

Inheritance of Single-Gene Disorders

The traits produced by a gene can be characterized as dominant or recessive. Dominant traits can be expressed when only one copy of the gene for that trait is present. Recessive traits carried on autosomal chromosomes can be expressed only when two copies of the gene are present (because the gene on the paired chromosome is usually expressed instead). People with one copy of an abnormal gene for a recessive trait (and who thus do not have the disorder) are called carriers.

How Genes Affect People: Penetrance and Expressivity

People who have the same gene may be affected differently. Two terms explain these differences: penetrance and expressivity.

Penetrance refers to whether the gene is expressed or not. That is, it refers to how many people with the gene have the trait associated with the gene. Penetrance is complete (100%) if everyone with the gene has the trait. Penetrance is incomplete if only some people with the gene have the trait. For example, 50% penetrance means that only half the people with the gene have the trait.

Expressivity determines how much the trait affects (or, is expressed in) a person. A trait may be very pronounced, barely noticeable, or in between. Various factors, including genetic makeup, exposure to harmful substances, other environmental influences, and age, can affect expressivity.

Both penetrance and expressivity can vary. People with the gene may or may not have the trait, and in people with the trait, how the trait appears varies.

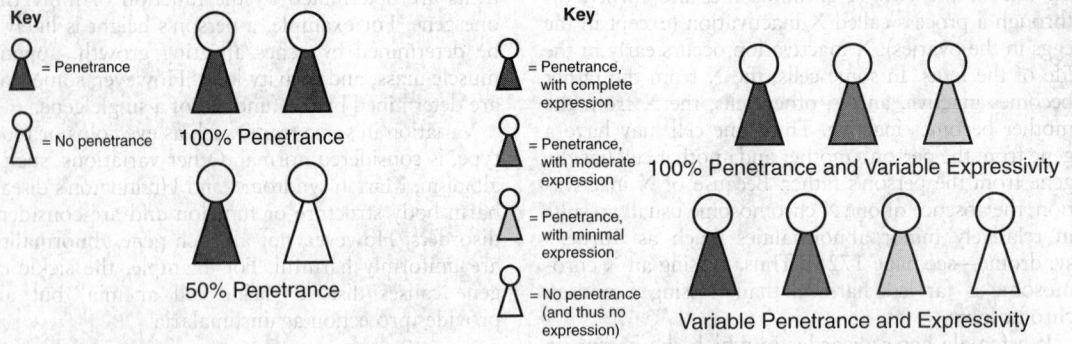

Key
- = Penetrance
- = No penetrance

100% Penetrance

50% Penetrance

Key
- = Penetrance, with complete expression
- = Penetrance, with moderate expression
- = Penetrance, with minimal expression
- = No penetrance (and thus no expression)

100% Penetrance and Variable Expressivity

Variable Penetrance and Expressivity

With codominant traits, both copies of a gene are expressed to some extent. An example of a codominant trait is blood type. If a person has one gene coding for blood type A and one gene coding for blood type B, the person has both blood types (blood type AB).

Whether a gene is X-linked (sex-linked) also determines expression. Among males, almost all genes on the X chromosome, whether the trait is dominant or recessive, are expressed because there is no paired gene to offset their expression.

Penetrance and Expressivity: Penetrance refers to how often a trait is expressed in people with the gene for that trait. Penetrance may be complete or incomplete. A gene with incomplete penetrance is not always expressed even when the trait it produces is dominant or when the trait is recessive and present on both chromosomes. If half the people with a gene show its trait, its penetrance is said to be 50%. Expressivity refers to how much a trait affects a person—whether the person is greatly, moderately, or mildly affected.

INHERITANCE PATTERNS

Many genetic disorders, particularly those involving traits controlled by multiple genes or those that are highly susceptible to environmental influences, do not have an obvious pattern of inheritance. However, some single-gene disorders display characteristic patterns, particularly when penetrance is high and expressivity is full. In such cases, patterns can be identified based on whether the trait is dominant or recessive, and whether the gene is X-linked or carried on a mitochondrial chromosome.

Non–X-Linked Inheritance

Dominant Disorders: The following principles generally apply to dominant disorders determined by a dominant non–X-linked gene:

- When one parent has the disorder and the other does not, each child has a 50% chance of inheriting the disorder.
- People who do not have the disorder usually do not carry the gene and thus do not pass the trait on to their offspring.
- Males and females are equally likely to be affected.
- Many people with the disorder have at least one parent with the disorder. However, sometimes the disorder arises as a new genetic mutation.

Recessive Disorders: The following principles generally apply to recessive disorders determined by a recessive non–X-linked gene:

- Virtually everyone with the disorder has parents who both carry the abnormal gene, even though

Non–X-Linked Recessive Disorders

Some disorders represent a non–X-linked recessive trait. To have the disorder, a person usually must receive two abnormal genes, one from each parent. If both parents carry one abnormal gene and one normal gene, neither has the disorder but each has a 50% chance of passing the abnormal gene to their children. Therefore, each child has a 25% chance of inheriting two abnormal genes (and thus of developing the disorder), a 25% chance of inheriting two normal genes, and a 50% chance of inheriting one normal and one abnormal gene (thus becoming a carrier of the disorder like the parents). Therefore, among the children, the chance of not developing the disorder (that is, being normal or a carrier) is 75%.

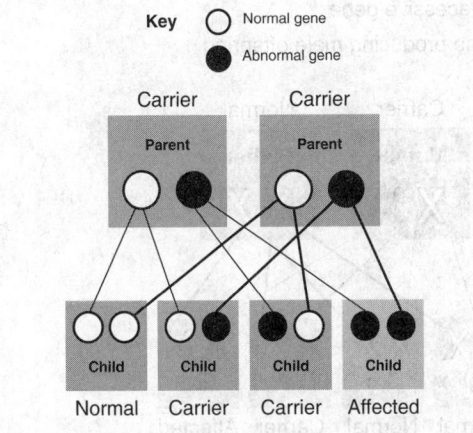

| Key | ○ Normal gene |
| | ● Abnormal gene |

Carrier — Parent
Carrier — Parent

Child — Normal
Child — Carrier
Child — Carrier
Child — Affected

usually neither parent has the disorder (because two copies of the abnormal gene are necessary for the gene to be expressed).

- Single mutations are less likely to result in the disorder than in dominantly inherited disorders (because expression in recessive disorders requires that both genes be abnormal).
- When one parent has the disorder and the other parent carries one abnormal gene but does not have the disorder, half of their children are likely to have the disorder. Their other children will be carriers with one abnormal gene. If the parent without the disorder does not carry the abnormal gene, none of the children will have the disorder, but all of the children will inherit and carry an abnormal gene that they may pass on to their offspring.
- A person who does not have the disorder and whose parents do not have it but whose siblings do have it has a 66% chance of being a carrier of the abnormal gene.
- Males and females are equally likely to be affected.

X-Linked Inheritance

Dominant Disorders: The following principles generally apply to dominant disorders determined by a dominant X-linked gene:

- Affected males transmit the disorder to all of their daughters but to none of their sons. (The sons of the affected male receive his Y chromosome, which does not carry the abnormal gene.)
- Affected females with only one abnormal gene transmit the disorder to, on average, half their children, regardless of sex.
- Many X-linked dominant disorders are lethal among affected males. Among females, even though the gene is dominant, having a second normal gene on the other X chromosome offsets the effect of the dominant gene to some extent, decreasing the severity of the resulting disorder.
- More females have the disorder than males. The difference between the sexes is even larger if the disorder is lethal in males.

Dominant X-linked severe diseases are rare. Examples are familial rickets (familial hypophosphatemic rickets—see page 287) and hereditary nephritis (Alport's syndrome—see page 273). Females with hereditary rickets have fewer bone symptoms than do affected males. Females with hereditary nephritis usually have no symptoms and little abnormality of kidney function, whereas affected males develop kidney failure in early adult life.

Recessive Disorders: The following principles generally apply to recessive disorders determined by a recessive X-linked gene:

- Nearly everyone affected is male.
- All daughters of an affected male will carry the abnormal gene.
- Normally, an affected
- male does not transmit the disorder to his sons.
- Females who carry the gene do not have the disorder (unless they have the abnormal gene on

EXAMPLES OF GENETIC DISORDERS

GENE	DOMINANT	RECESSIVE
Non–X-linked	Marfan syndrome Huntington's disease	Cystic fibrosis
X-linked	Familial rickets Hereditary nephritis	Red–green color blindness Hemophilia

X-Linked Recessive Disorders

If a gene is X-linked, it is present on the X chromosome. Recessive X-linked disorders usually develop only in males. This male-only development occurs because males have only one X chromosome, so there is no paired gene to offset the effect of the abnormal gene. Females have two X chromosomes, so they usually receive a normal or offsetting gene on the second X chromosome. The normal or offsetting gene normally prevents females from developing the disorder (unless the offsetting gene is inactivated or lost).

If the father has the abnormal X-linked gene (and thus the disorder) and the mother has two normal genes,

all of their daughters receive one abnormal gene and one normal gene, making them carriers. None of their sons receive the abnormal gene because they receive the father's Y chromosome.

If the mother is a carrier and the father has the normal gene, any son has a 50% chance of receiving the abnormal gene from the mother (and developing the disorder). Any daughter has a 50% chance of receiving one abnormal gene and one normal gene (becoming a carrier) or a 50% chance of receiving two normal genes.

Key X̶ Normal gene

X Abnormal recessive gene

Y̶ Normal gene producing male offspring

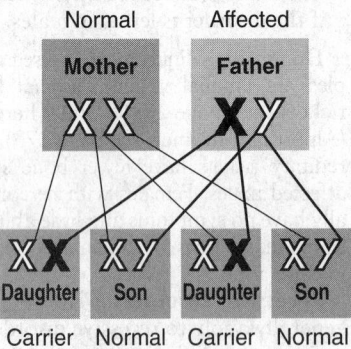

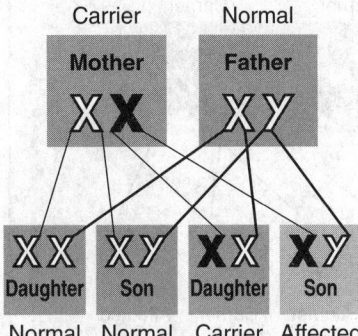

both X chromosomes or there is inactivation of the other normal chromosome). However, they transmit the gene to half their sons, who usually have the disorder. Their daughters, like their mothers, usually do not have the disorder, but half are carriers.

An example of a common X-linked recessive trait is red–green color blindness, which affects about 10% of males but is unusual among females. In males, the gene for color blindness comes from a mother who usually has normal vision but is a carrier of the color-blind gene. It never comes from the father, who instead supplies the Y chromosome. Daughters of color-blind fathers are rarely color-blind but are always carriers of the color-blind gene. An example of a serious disease caused by an X-linked recessive gene is hemophilia.

Abnormal Mitochondrial Genes

Several rare diseases are caused by abnormal genes carried by the chromosome inside a mitochondrion.

An example is Leber's hereditary optic neuropathy, which causes a variable but often devastating loss of vision in both eyes that typically occurs during the teenage years. Another example is a disorder characterized by type 2 diabetes and deafness.

Because the father generally cannot pass mitochondrial deoxyribonucleic acid (DNA) to the child, diseases caused by abnormal mitochondrial genes are almost always transmitted by the mother. However, not all mitochondrial disorders are caused by abnormal mitochondrial genes (some are caused by genes in the cell nucleus that affect the mitochondria). Thus, the father's DNA may contribute to some mitochondrial disorders.

Unlike the DNA in the nucleus of cells, the number of abnormal mitochondrial DNA occasionally varies from cell to cell throughout the body. Thus, an abnormal mitochondrial gene in one body cell does not necessarily mean it will cause disease in another cell. Even when two people seem to have the same mitochondrial gene abnormality, the expression of disease may be very different in the two people. This variation makes genetic testing and genetic counseling of limited value in making predictions for people with known or suspected mitochondrial gene abnormalities.

Gene Technology

Gene technology is rapidly improving. The polymerase chain reaction (PCR) is a laboratory technique that can produce large numbers of copies of a gene, which makes studying the gene much easier. A specific segment of deoxyribonucleic acid (DNA), such as a specific gene, can be copied (amplified) in a laboratory. Starting with one DNA molecule, at the end of 30 doublings (only a few hours later) about a billion copies are produced.

> **?** **Did You Know...**
> Obtaining detailed information about one's own genotype may be commercially feasible in the foreseeable future.

A gene probe can be used to locate a specific part of a gene (a segment of the gene's DNA) or a whole gene in a particular chromosome. Probes can be used to find normal or mutated segments of DNA. A DNA segment that has been cloned or copied becomes a labeled probe when a radioactive atom or fluorescent dye is added to it. The probe will seek out its mirror-image segment of DNA and bind to it. The labeled probe can then be detected by sophisticated microscopic and photographic techniques. With gene probes, a number of disorders can be diagnosed before and after birth. In the future, gene probes will probably be used to test people for many major genetic disorders simultaneously.

Microchips are powerful new tools that can be used to identify DNA mutations, pieces of ribonucleic acid (RNA), or proteins. A single chip can test for 30,000 different DNA changes by using only one sample.

Uses of Genetics

The potential for understanding human genetics increased greatly when the Human Genome Project successfully identified and mapped all the genes on human chromosomes in 2003. Genetic techniques can be used to study individual genes to learn more about specific disorders. For example, some kinds of disorders that have been classified based on what symptoms they caused have been reclassified based on what the genetic abnormality is.

Genetic tests are used to diagnose certain disorders (for example, hemochromatosis and chromosomal disorders such as Down syndrome and Turner's syndrome). Genetics is also increasing the ability to predict what disorders a person is likely to develop. For example, women with certain abnormalities in the *BRCA* genes are prone to develop breast and ovarian cancers. These predictions may allow disease prevention and screening to be tailored much more to each person. Advances in techniques that assess people's genetic characteristics and increased understanding of human genetics have improved diagnosis of genetic disorders before birth. Genetic screening can be used to counsel parents about the risks of passing on a genetic disorder to their offspring (see page 1607). Screening can also be used to detect fetal abnormalities (see page 1608).

Increased understanding of human genetics has the potential to predict how people, depending on their precise genetic makeup, will respond to certain treatments. For example, specific genes can predict how much warfarin, a blood thinner, a person is likely to require. This prediction is important because taking too much warfarin can cause serious bleeding and taking too little makes the drug ineffective, which is also risky. Gene analysis can also predict whether a person will have intolerable or only minor side effects when taking irinotecan, an anticancer drug. People likely to have intolerable side effects can be treated with a different drug.

> **?** **Did You Know...**
> Genetics may be able to help predict what disorders a person is likely to develop or how the person will respond to certain treatments.

Gene Therapy

Although gene therapy is defined as any treatment that changes gene function, it is often thought of as the insertion of normal genes into the cells of a person who lacks such normal genes because of a specific genetic disorder (gene insertion therapy). The normal genes can be manufactured, using polymerase chain reaction (PCR), from normal deoxyribonucleic acid (DNA) donated by another person. Currently, such gene insertion therapy is most likely to be effective in the prevention or cure of single-gene defects, such as cystic fibrosis.

The transfer of the normal DNA into a person's cells can be done by several methods. One method is to use a virus, because certain viruses have the

Cloning

A clone is a group of genetically identical cells or organisms derived from a single cell or individual. Cloning (the producing of clones) has been commonplace for many years in agriculture. A plant can be propagated (cloned) by simply taking a small piece of the original plant and growing a new one from it. The new plant is thus an exact genetic copy of the original one. Such propagation is also possible with simple animals such as flatworms: cut a flatworm in two, and the tail grows a new head and the head grows a new tail. However, such simple techniques do not work with higher animals, such as sheep or humans.

In the now-famous "Dolly" experiments, cells from a sheep (donor cells) were fused with unfertilized sheep eggs from another sheep (recipient cells) from which the natural genetic material was removed by microsurgery. Then the genetic material from the donor cells was transferred into the unfertilized eggs. Unlike unfertilized eggs, these laboratory-made eggs had a complete set of chromosomes and genes. Unlike eggs fertilized naturally (with sperm), the laboratory-made eggs received genetic material from only one source. The eggs then started to develop into embryos. The developing embryos were transplanted into a female sheep (the surrogate mother), where they developed naturally. One of the embryos survived, and the resulting lamb was named Dolly. As expected, Dolly was an exact genetic copy of the original sheep from which the donor cells were taken, not of the sheep that provided the eggs.

Research on cloning continues, but cloning of humans is technically difficult and ethically controversial. Studies suggest that cloned higher animals (and thus humans) are more likely to have serious genetic defects than normally conceived offspring. Governments have attempted to make cloning humans illegal. However, cloning need not only be used to create a whole organism. It can, theoretically, also be used to create a single organ. Thus, one day a person may be able to receive "spare parts" manufactured in the laboratory, using the person's own genes.

Whether a cell used for a clone produces a specific type of tissue, a specific organ, or an entire organism depends on the potential of the cell—that is, how highly the cell has developed into a particular type of tissue. For example, certain cells (stem cells) have the potential to produce a wide variety of tissue types or even possibly an entire organism. They have not yet differentiated into specific types of tissues. Other cells have differentiated and can develop into only those specific tissue types. Stem cells have stimulated interest because of their potential to generate tissue that can replace diseased or damaged tissues. Because stem cells tend to be less differentiated, they can thus potentially replace a wide or unlimited variety of types of tissue.

---

ability to insert their genetic material into human DNA. The normal DNA is inserted by a chemical reaction into the virus, which then infects (transfects) the person's cells, thereby transmitting the DNA into the nucleus of those cells. One of the concerns about insertion using a virus is potential reactions to the virus, similar to an infection. Another concern is that the new, normal DNA may become "lost" or may fail to be incorporated into new cells after some period of time, leading to the reappearance of the genetic disorder. Also, antibodies may develop against the virus, causing a reaction similar to the rejection of a transplanted organ.

Another method for inserting genes uses liposomes, which are microscopic sacs containing the DNA that are absorbed by the person's cells, thereby delivering their DNA to the cell nucleus. Sometimes this method does not work because the liposomes are not absorbed into the person's cells, the new gene does not work as intended, or the new gene is eventually lost. A third method is called naked plasmid DNA injection, in which plasmid DNA (a special circular form of DNA) is injected into a person's muscle.

A different method of gene therapy uses antisense technology, in which, rather than inserting normal genes, the abnormal genes are simply switched off. Using antisense technology, drugs can combine with specific parts of the DNA, preventing the affected genes from functioning. Antisense technology is currently being tried for cancer therapy but is still very experimental. However, it seems to have the potential to be more effective or safer than gene insertion therapy.

Another approach to gene therapy is to increase or decrease the activities of certain genes by modifying chemical reactions in the cell that control gene expression. For example, modifying a chemical reaction called methylation can change the function of a gene, causing it to increase or decrease production of certain proteins or to produce different kinds of proteins. Such methods are being tried experimentally to treat certain cancers.

Gene therapy is also being studied experimentally in transplantation surgery. By altering the genes of the transplanted organs to make them more compatible with the recipient's genes, the organ recipient is less likely to reject the transplanted organ. Thus, the recipient may not need to receive drugs that suppress the immune system, which can have serious side effects. However, this type of treatment is usually unsuccessful.

Ethical Controversies

With the new genetic diagnostic and therapeutic capabilities come many controversies about how they should be used. Concerns have been raised that knowledge of a person's genetic information might be used improperly. For instance, people whose genetic characteristics make them prone to particular disorders might be denied employment or health insurance coverage.

Prenatal screening for genetic abnormalities that cause serious disorders is widely supported. However, concern exists that screening could also be used to select for traits that are desirable (for example, physical appearance and intelligence).

Cloning of humans is highly controversial. Creating a human being by cloning is still technically impossible. Animal studies suggest it is much more likely than natural methods to result in severe defects that are lethal or cause serious health problems. Creating a human by cloning is widely seen as unethical and is usually illegal.

CHAPTER

3   Making the Most of Health Care

Gone are the days when people can rely solely on their family doctor with the help of a nurse to take charge of their health care. To obtain the best health care today, people must participate actively in the process. Active participation means many things:

- Learning about health care issues (including how care can be paid for)
- Visiting a health care practitioner regularly
- Communicating effectively with health care practitioners
- Obtaining appropriate preventive care (see page 28)
- Remaining watchful for signs of ill health or bodily changes (such as a change in the color of a mole or detection of a lump in a breast or testis)
- Keeping a record of personal medical information

For people with a specific disorder, active participation also means monitoring their health. For example, people with hypertension regularly measure their blood pressure, and people with diabetes regularly measure their blood sugar level.

Good communication—open, honest sharing of information—with health care practitioners is crucial because it can mean better health. With good communication, practitioners better understand the problems a person is having and the person better understands how problems should be treated. It also fosters trust and confidence between the practitioner and the person, making the person more likely to follow the treatment regimen.

Where to Start

Typically, the entry point into the health care system is a primary care practitioner, usually a doctor but sometimes a nurse practitioner or physician's assistant. Having a primary care doctor has many advantages that can lead to better care. People who have a primary care doctor are less likely to go to an emergency department unnecessarily and less likely to be seen by a doctor they do not know. When people see a doctor they do not know, the doctor may not have all the background information necessary to diagnose and treat the problem. Consequently, the doctor may repeat tests or do unnecessary tests.

Communication is often better and medical decisions are more easily made when people have an established relationship with a primary care doctor. People are more likely to trust a doctor they know and to experience less anxiety when a medical problem develops. Primary care doctors often have long-standing relationships with their patients. They are familiar with what their patients want and value, how they best receive information, how they cope with adversity, whether they are able to purchase prescribed drugs, and which family members they rely on.

Primary care doctors explain what type of care is needed, why it is needed, and how often visits should be scheduled. They can refer people to specialists when needed and coordinate care with other health care practitioners. Some health care

Is This Doctor the Right One?

Helpful questions to ask a doctor include the following:

- Does the doctor participate in my health insurance plan?
- What are the doctor's normal office hours?
- What is the usual wait to obtain a routine visit? An urgent visit?
- Does the doctor respond to phone calls or e-mail (during office hours and after office hours)? If so, how quickly does the doctor respond?
- Will the doctor take care of me if I need to be hospitalized, or will I be referred to another doctor? At what hospitals is the doctor on staff?
- Is the doctor board-certified?
- Is the doctor's office easy to get in and out of?
- Does the doctor keep office appointments on time?
- Who takes care of the doctor's patients when the office is closed (at night or on weekends) or when the doctor is away? When care is provided by another practitioner, does that practitioner know the patients or have access to the patients' medical records?
- Who else is routinely involved in taking care of the doctor's patients? For example, are nurses or physician's assistants involved?
- How are test results (normal and abnormal) communicated, and who (doctor or patient) initiates the communication?

Helpful questions to ask the doctor's patients include the following:

- Does the doctor take time to listen to concerns?
- Does the doctor adequately explain a diagnosis?
- Do you trust the doctor's opinion?
- Before a prescribing a drug, does the doctor discuss its benefits and risks?
- Before a prescribing a drug, does the doctor discuss alternatives?

plans require people to see their primary care doctor to get a referral before they see a specialist.

To find a primary care doctor, people can begin by asking friends and relatives for recommendations. Or they can call a medical school and ask for a department, such as pediatrics, internal medicine, or family practice. Older people may want a doctor who specializes in treatment of their age group (a geriatrician) as their primary care doctor. Many health insurance plans limit the choice of doctors and other practitioners. In such cases, people should consult the plan to obtain a list of participating practitioners. Sometimes people cannot see the doctor they have chosen because the practice no longer accepts new patients.

For information about a doctor's credentials, people can call the American Board of Medical Specialties (866-275-2267 toll-free) or check that organization's web site (www.abms.org) or book, which is available in many public and medical libraries.

When choosing a primary care doctor, people should consider what is most important to them in a doctor (for example, friendliness, thoroughness, patience, or promptness). Some people prefer a doctor who spends extra time with them, even if doing so tends to make the doctor run late keeping office appointments. Other people prefer a doctor who keeps appointments on time, even though doing so may limit the time the doctor spends with them.

People should look for a doctor they feel comfortable with and have confidence in.

When to See a Doctor

Routine Visits: Generally, everyone should routinely see their doctor, dentist, and eye doctor for preventive care. Women should routinely see their primary care doctor or gynecologist for gynecologic examinations. People can obtain a schedule of what type of care is required and how often visits are needed from their primary care doctor. Usually, infants and older people need more frequent preventive visits, but frequency also depends on a person's health conditions. For example, a person with diabetes or a heart disorder (or risk factors for them) may need to have checkups relatively frequently.

Visits for a Problem: When symptoms or other medical problems develop between preventive visits, people may be unsure whether they need to see a doctor. Many symptoms and problems can be handled at home. For example, most routine colds do not require a doctor's attention. Many small cuts and abrasions can be handled by first cleaning them with mild soap and water, then applying an antibiotic ointment and a protective covering (see page 1946).

People with certain disorders should see a doctor sooner rather than later when new symptoms develop.

For example, if people with a chronic lung disorder (such as asthma or chronic obstructive pulmonary disease) begin to have difficulty breathing or if people with a weakened immune system get a fever, they should see a doctor promptly. The immune system may be weakened by diabetes, human immunodeficiency virus (HIV) infection, use of chemotherapy drugs, or other conditions.

When unsure about the need to see a doctor or other practitioner, people can sometimes call their primary care doctor for guidance. Some doctors can be contacted by e-mail for nonemergency questions. Others prefer to be contacted by telephone. Doctors cannot give set guidelines for when to see a doctor and when it is unnecessary because symptoms with the same cause vary too much and symptoms with different causes overlap too much. However, some problems clearly require a call to a health care practitioner.

Visits to the Emergency Department: In general, true emergencies should be handled by calling 911 or the local emergency service to provide ambulance service to the nearest hospital. However, deciding what qualifies as an emergency is sometimes difficult because symptoms vary greatly. Learning as much as possible about symptoms of life-threatening disorders (such as heart attack and stroke) in advance is useful, and good judgment is often required. If the problem seems possibly life threatening, the emergency department is the place to go. The following examples clearly require a visit to the emergency department:

- Signs of a heart attack (see page 411)
- Signs of a stroke (see page 720)
- Difficulty breathing
- Heavy bleeding
- Burns that are open, char, or blister the skin; that result from inhalation; that cover a large area; or that are on the hands, face, feet, or genitals
- Severe injury (as in a motor vehicle accident)
- Poisoning that causes symptoms (if symptoms are minor or do not develop, the poison control center can be called first at 800-222-1222 for advice)
- A severe allergic reaction (see page 1123)
- Shock (see page 350)
- Sudden, severe pain anywhere
- Vomiting blood or coughing up a relatively large amount of blood (more than a few streaks in sputum)
- Sudden, severe worsening of a serious chronic disorder, such as asthma or diabetes

Going to the emergency department for less serious problems may be appropriate when the primary care doctor is unavailable, as on weekends or during the night. In some health insurance plans, calling the primary care doctor first is required in order to be reimbursed for a visit to the emergency department, unless symptoms suggest a life-threatening disorder. People should know the requirements of their insurance plan before an emergency develops.

Making the Most of a Health Care Visit

Preparing for a health care visit helps people get the most out of time spent with a doctor or another health care practitioner. Preparing ahead also helps people communicate with a practitioner more effectively. Information and questions for the practitioner should be written down before the visit.

First Visit: The first time people visit their primary care doctor, they should ask any of the questions that are relevant to choosing a doctor and that they have not asked or need to ask again (see box on page 18). In addition, several other questions may be helpful:

- How are sudden urgent health problems that occur at night or during weekends handled?
- How are test results obtained? (For example, where to call or e-mail if the person is responsible for asking for these results.)
- Why should I have an advance directive (such as a living will or a durable power of attorney agreement—see page 69)? How do I go about preparing one?

If people already have an advance directive, they should bring a copy or the original to be copied for the doctor's records. They should also collect all drugs they are currently taking, including over-the-counter drugs, medicinal herbs, and vitamins, and bring them to the doctor's office.

At the first visit, the doctor asks about topics such as past and present health, the health of close relatives, treatments, tests, and lifestyle. Even if the doctor does not ask, people should make sure the doctor has certain information about them:

- Any personal, spiritual, or ethnic considerations that might affect health care decisions
- Information about past hospitalizations, use of home health services, or care received from any specialists or other health care practitioners (including alternative medicine practitioners), with the names, addresses, and phone numbers of these sources of health care
- Information about any diagnostic tests and treatments already planned
- Exercise habits, sleep habits, diet (including consumption of caffeine), sexual practices, and use of

SOME REASONS TO CALL A DOCTOR*

PROBLEM	REASONS TO CALL
Cold or influenza	Vomiting or inability to keep fluids down Painful swallowing Coughing that lasts more than 2 or 3 weeks Earache Symptoms that last more than 7 days
Diarrhea	Black or bloody stools More than 6 to 8 watery stools in children Symptoms of dehydration (such as very dry mouth and armpits, confusion, and decreased urination), particularly in children and older people
Digestive problems	A feeling that food is stuck in the throat Development of or change in heartburn, particularly during exercise Frequent heartburn, belching, or regurgitation Persistent or severe abdominal pain Persistent nausea
General problems	Symptoms that prevent participation in usual activities Unexplained weight loss Dizziness or an about-to-faint feeling Persistent fatigue Sweating, especially heavy or cold sweats
Headaches	Severe headache that peaks in intensity within seconds Memory loss or confusion Blurred or double vision Slurred speech Loss of balance or dizziness Seizures Numbness in the arms, legs, or face Nausea
Heart problems	Rapid or galloping heartbeats (palpitations) Chest pain
Leg problems	Pain in the calves that worsens when walking Swelling in the ankles or legs
Menstrual problems	No periods by age 16 Sudden stopping of periods A period that lasts much longer than usual or is excessively heavy A sudden feeling of illness while using tampons Severe or disabling cramps
Rash	Fever of 100.4° F (38° C) or above A rash that is painful, involves swelling, or oozes
Sinusitis	Swelling or redness in or around an eye Problems with vision
Vomiting	Moderate or severe abdominal pain Symptoms of dehydration, particularly in children and older people Green, black, or bloody vomit

*The list of problems and the reasons to call a doctor are only a small sample.

tobacco and drugs not prescribed by a health care practitioner (including alcohol, over-the-counter drugs, and medicinal herbs)

Providing this information helps improve the quality of care and ensure that any change in practitioners is smooth. For example, people should give their primary care doctor contact information for other health care practitioners and facilities they have visited. Then, the involved practitioners can communicate with each other more easily. Contact information also helps the primary care doctor obtain copies of pertinent information for the medical record.

Subsequent Visits: Each time people see their doctor, they should prepare a list to make sure the doctor knows everything relevant to their health care. The list should include the following:

- Any health-related questions
- Any symptoms or medical problems, including mental health problems
- Any side effects experienced while taking drugs
- Any diagnostic testing or new treatments recommended by another health care practitioner
- Any time they are not taking drugs as prescribed and the reason for it (for example, "I seem to get stomach cramps from the drug" or "I cannot afford the drug")
- Any changes in personal information, including major life events (such as retirement, change in marital status, a death in the family, or a move to a different home)

Lists should be written down. During a busy office visit, people can easily forget what they want to say. The list should also be prioritized, with the most important items listed first. Symptoms should be described as accurately and precisely as possible, being careful not to minimize or exaggerate them. Reading about or talking with someone who has had a disorder or a recommended diagnostic test or treatment before a visit may enable people to ask more specific, useful questions.

Any forms (such as insurance, school, or preemployment forms) that need to be completed by the doctor or office staff should be brought. People should also bring current insurance cards, any required referrals, and a means of payment for any required fees.

Arriving at the doctor's office 10 to 15 minutes before the scheduled appointment (particularly for the first visit) gives the office staff time to make sure that insurance information is current and that any required forms are completed.

During the visit, listening carefully to the doctor and responding as honestly and completely as possi-

ble, even about sensitive issues (such as bladder control or sexual practices), is essential. If a treatment or an invasive diagnostic test is being considered, people should ask about the following:

- How effective is the treatment or how accurate is the diagnostic test?
- How will the test results change treatment?
- What are the possible side effects?
- What other choices are available?
- What are the specific goals for the treatment?
- How will the response to treatment be followed or monitored?
- Any other questions they have about the treatment or test

People should request an explanation of anything that is not understood and ask for a patient education sheet or handout on the subject if available. Asking the doctor to write out instructions and reading them back to the doctor at the end of the visit help make sure the instructions are understood. Reading them back gives the doctor the opportunity to correct any miscommunication. Taking notes during a visit may also help. For people who cannot use written materials or who have problems with vision, speech, or hearing, other approaches may be needed to keep track of the information. For example, the instructions may be recorded on tape, or a family member or friend may agree to read the instructions when needed. When people go to the pharmacy for drugs, they can use the same approaches.

Before leaving, people should check their list of questions and symptoms and talk to the doctor about anything that was not covered. If many questions remain, the doctor may have to schedule another appointment or write a referral to another health care practitioner, such as a nurse, pharmacist, or dietitian, for further information and education.

After the visit, any recommended follow-up appointments should be scheduled. Any prescriptions should be filled, and any written materials provided by the doctor or pharmacist should be read. Also, people may want to consider keeping a diary of important aspects of their care. For example, a person with constant headaches may want to record when headaches occur, what triggers them, and how they respond to drugs.

Getting a Second Opinion

Despite many similarities in training, doctors may vary in their opinions about how to diagnose or treat certain disorders. Such differences can occur among the best of doctors. Differences often occur because the evidence for benefits and risks is not clear. For example, opinions can differ about whether or when to measure prostate-specific antigen (PSA) to check for prostate cancer in men who have no symptoms (see page 1083). Differences in recommendations may also be based on how familiar a doctor is with a test or treatment or on how willing a doctor is to use the latest tests and treatments.

For these reasons, getting a second opinion from a different doctor can give a person additional insight and more information about what to do. If the second opinion is the same, it can reassure the person and reduce anxiety. If it differs, options can be weighed, and the result is a more informed choice about what to do. Also, a person can get a third opinion, particularly if the second opinion is different from the first.

Handling Medical Records

People may not have total access to their medical record kept in the doctor's office. But usually the person owns the medical information, and the doctor or institution owns the document itself. The courts can require submission of copies or summaries of the records, but only in certain specific legal situations that most people do not experience. When people request their medical record, a staff member at the doctor's office usually copies and releases the record to them or creates a summary of all or part of the record to send to other health care practitioners. People who want a copy of their whole medical record for personal use may or may not be entitled to it, depending on state law. Generally, people need only the most useful medical

information. They do not need a complete record, which may contain a lot of information that is not useful to them.

To make sure they have what they need, people should maintain a personal medical record of the most significant information. They should not rely on memory. Immunization records, which are traditionally kept for children, should be kept current throughout life. People should write or ask someone to write their drug regimen on one sheet of paper to keep with their medical record. They should also keep a copy of their drug regimen with them at all times in case they need emergency medical care. This information can be updated as the regimen changes. Copies of laboratory results should be included with the medical record for future reference. People may also want to keep a diary of their symptoms with their medical record. Computer software and Internet programs are available to record most medical information, or a file box or binder may be used.

Keeping a copy of their medical record helps people participate in their health care. For example, it helps them better explain a problem to a health care practitioner.

Confidentiality laws and ethical principles protect the privacy of communication between people and their doctor. These laws also protect the contents of the medical record that is maintained by a doctor or hospital. One such law is the Health Insurance Portability and Accountability Act (HIPAA) of 1996. HIPAA states that disclosing a person's medical information normally requires the person's written consent. In the doctor's waiting room, people are asked to sign a form confirming that they are

How to Get a Second Opinion

- People should check with their health insurance provider to make sure the cost of a second opinion is covered. Usually it is. They should also ask about and follow any special procedures for getting a second opinion.
- People can ask their doctor to recommend another doctor or specialist. Most doctors welcome another opinion. However, the second doctor should not be a close associate of the first because they may share the same perspective. If people do not feel comfortable asking their doctor, they may be able to ask another doctor they trust. If not, university teaching hospitals, specialty medical societies (such as the American College of Surgeons), or insurance providers can often provide names of doctors.
- People should have their medical records sent to the

second doctor before the visit. That doctor then has time to look at the records, preventing unnecessary repetition of diagnostic tests. Because of the Health Insurance Portability and Accountability Act (HIPAA), people are required to give written permission to their original doctor to forward any records or test results.
- People should write down questions and concerns about their disorder and bring the list to discuss with the second doctor.
- People should go to the doctor to get the second opinion. They should not rely on the telephone or Internet. For a second opinion to be meaningful, the doctor should thoroughly review the medical records and do all relevant parts of a physical examination.

What Should Be in a Personal Medical Record?

- Significant or chronic medical problems
- Current drug regimen
- Other treatments
- Allergic reactions to drugs
- Hospitalizations, including operations (dates, location, attending doctor's name, and diagnoses)
- Laboratory and other test results
- Family medical history
- Immunizations, including dates
- Visits to any doctor's office (dates, reason, test results, diagnosis, and recommendations)
- Payments made

aware of HIPAA and their privacy rights. The form also states how their medical information can be used and shared. HIPAA allows medical information to be shared in certain specified cases. For example, it can be shared

- To coordinate and facilitate a person's treatment (especially important when different practitioners and health care facilities are involved)
- To enable doctors, other practitioners, and hospitals to be paid for health care

Thus, information needed to authorize payment may be shared with managed care organizations and health insurance providers, who may require medical information as a condition of payment for a claim. Sharing this information also requires the person's consent, which is usually obtained before health care is provided. A person's medical information cannot be shared with the person's employer or marketeers unless the person gives written consent.

Increasingly, health care practitioners are recording and storing medical records electronically. This practice has the potential to enable different practitioners who care for the same person to share information about the person more easily and with fewer errors.

Researching a Disorder

When a disorder is first diagnosed, the doctor often gives a handout that summarizes key points of information. People may also have some general knowledge of the disorder from newspaper or magazine articles or television or radio shows.

If people want to learn more about their disorder, many other sources of information are avail-able. People can ask doctors, nurses, or other practitioners to tell them about the disorder or to recommend reliable sources of information. Many books provide helpful, general information about disorders. Some local, university, or hospital libraries have useful resources, including a research librarian. The Internet provides a lot of information. However, judging the credibility of these sources is not always easy.

Generally, governmental medical sources are authoritative and reliable. On the Internet, the National Institutes of Health (NIH), the Agency for Healthcare Research and Quality (AHRQ), and the Centers for Disease Control and Prevention (CDC) provide a large amount of useful and accurate information to the public. These sites also provide links to other helpful and reliable sites. Many disease-specific, patient-oriented sites (such as the National Multiple Sclerosis Society) provide information for people with a particular disorder (see page 2151). In contrast, sites designed to sell specific products or a specific service may be less reliable. Their information may be biased or inaccurate.

Support groups may provide helpful information, as well as psychologic support. Such groups can be found through local newspapers, phone directories, hospitals, offices of doctors or other health care practitioners, and the Internet. Most cities have support groups, sometimes for specific disorders. For example, Gilda's Club, which is located in several cities, offers support for people living with cancer. Other people who have the same disorder or who care for someone with the same disorder may have many practical and useful suggestions for day-to-day living, such as where to find pieces of specialized equipment, what equipment works best, and how to interact with or care for someone with a disorder. Another resource is chat rooms on the Internet. They enable people to communicate with one another about specific disorders and to share possible resources.

How Health Care Is Paid For

Health care, particularly hospitalization, advanced technologies, and complicated treatments, is so expensive that most people cannot afford to pay for it by themselves. Total health care costs annually in the United States were about $1.9 trillion in 2004, and the cost of providing high-quality (not even the best quality) health care to everyone in the United States would be very much higher. Consequently, the cost of health care is usually shared by some combination of the person who is receiving care, employers, health insurance providers (including managed care organizations and private insurance companies), and the government.

Many people who are employed full-time (and often their family members) receive health insurance through their employer as an employee benefit. Many employers require employees to contribute some of the cost of the coverage through salary deductions. Such contributions may enable employers to offer plans with a range of benefits depending on how much the employee chooses to pay. Plans with more comprehensive coverage have higher employee costs, sometimes amounting to several thousand dollars per year. Other people purchase insurance privately. However, private insurance may be very expensive or unavailable, particularly for people who have preexisting disorders or risk factors for certain disorders. Also, it may not cover certain disorders. If people are eligible for government aid because they have limited financial means, are disabled, or are older than 65, health care costs may be covered by plans such as Medicare and Medicaid.

Whatever the source of health care coverage, most people have to pay some part of the costs themselves (called out-of-pocket costs). Typically, there are three sources of out-of-pocket costs:

- **Deductibles:** A certain amount of the initial cost is paid by the person before an insurance plan pays any benefits. A deductible may have to be paid only once during a given time (usually yearly) or each time certain services are provided.

- **Copayments:** Part of the cost of each service provided is usually paid by the person. A copayment may be a fixed amount or a percentage of the cost.

- **Costs that exceed those covered by a plan:** Plans may limit what they will pay for a given service (called the allowable amount). If a practitioner charges more than this limit, the person must pay it. Sometimes the limit is based on what the plan defines as usual, customary, and reasonable for a given service. Sometimes plans set a relatively low limit (which means people are likely to have to pay extra charges). However, people often pay extra charges only if the service is provided by a practitioner outside the plan's network because practitioners in the network have agreed not to charge more than the plan allows them to. Thus, people can usually avoid the extra charges by using practitioners in the network.

Care sometimes includes all three sources of out-of-pocket costs. For example, a person has an x-ray that costs $275. The person's plan has a $50 deductible, a 20% copayment, and a limit of $200 for this type of x-ray. Thus, the person pays the following charges:

- $50 for the deductible (the initial $50 of the cost) plus

- $30 as the copayment, which is 20% of the plan's allowable amount for the service minus the deductible ($200 minus $50, or $150) plus

- $75, the difference between the charge ($275) and the plan's allowable amount ($200)

The total charges are thus $155, which the person must pay out-of-pocket.

Traditionally, most people have had access to some type of plan. However, health care costs have been increasing much faster than the rate of inflation and are expected to continue to increase rapidly, partly because the population is aging and partly because advanced tests and treatments are increasingly available. As a result, many employers have eliminated or reduced health care insurance for their employees or retirees, and private insurance has become more expensive and difficult to qualify for. Thus, increasing numbers of people do not have insurance from their employer, cannot obtain or afford private insurance, and are not eligible for government coverage. In 2004, about 16% of the U.S. population was without health care insurance. Ironically, people without health care plans may be charged much more for services than people with plans because plans have bargaining power to negotiate low rates for their members.

CONTROLLING HEALTH CARE COSTS

Because health care is very expensive, all who are involved in health care—health insurance providers, health care practitioners, institutions, employers, and people who use health care—are looking for ways to reduce or at least control costs. One method for controlling cost is competition. For example, employers encourage competition between health insurance providers by comparing the costs of plans and choosing the cheapest that provides the desired services. People who have a choice between plans can similarly choose one that minimizes their costs. People also can help reduce costs by actively participating in their own care. They can learn to maintain good health, prevent disorders, and, if they have a disorder, manage it.

Health insurance providers, including managed care organizations and private insurance companies, can have a big effect on health care costs. Their strategies include reducing their costs and reducing the use of health care.

Reducing Their Costs: Health insurance providers try to reduce what they pay out in several ways:

- They can limit what they pay for specific services. Also, providers can require that practitioners agree to accept the lower payment to be able to receive any payment from the provider's plan.

- They can limit the services they pay for. For example, providers may pay for only a few days of hospitalization.
- They can pay a fixed amount for all people with certain diagnoses, such as pneumonia, regardless of what tests and treatments are used. This arrangement, called diagnosis-related groups, is usually made with hospitals.
- They can negotiate lower rates of reimbursement with groups of practitioners and hospitals.

These strategies give practitioners and hospitals a financial incentive to lower their costs and to treat people efficiently and rapidly.

Reducing Use of Health Care Services: Health insurance providers use several strategies:

- They can decrease the need for health care by encouraging good health. For example, they may set up wellness programs that encourage people to eat healthfully and exercise. They may provide educational materials to teach people to take preventive measures, such as visiting a primary care doctor regularly or getting an influenza (flu) vaccination. Providers may set up disease management programs, which can help people with a chronic disorder, such as diabetes, asthma, or hypertension, manage their disorder and thus prevent complications (and high costs).
- They can deny or limit coverage. For example, they can make eligibility requirements for the plan more restrictive. People with preexisting disorders can be denied coverage or given limited coverage. Coverage may be stopped if health care costs exceed a fixed amount during a year or a lifetime.
- They can limit access. For example, to be reimbursed, people may be required to get a referral before they see a specialist or get an approval before they have certain tests or procedures.

- They can increase how much the people who use health care pay. Health insurance providers or employers who provide health care plans for employees can increase deductibles and copayments. Payment for certain services (such as psychotherapy) may be limited or eliminated. This strategy may reduce the use of health care services because people have to pay for more costs out-of-pocket and thus may use services more selectively.

However, encouraging people to use health care services less and choose services more selectively has disadvantages:

- People may not get the services they need to maintain health or to prevent disorders. Then, health may eventually worsen, resulting in even higher costs to the health care system.
- Making good health care choices is difficult because people cannot easily compare the quality of health care. Also, people cannot easily access the costs of comparable services and thus cannot compare costs.
- Usually, people do not determine which health care services they need. Doctors do.

HOW HEALTH CARE PRACTITIONERS ARE PAID

Generally, health care practitioners and institutions can be paid in two very different ways: as fee for service or by capitation. Many payment plans use aspects of both fee for service and capitation. Each system has advantages and disadvantages, and whether one is better than another is unclear.

Fee for Service: Each hospital stay, each visit to a health care practitioner, each test, and each treatment is paid for individually. Fee for service is the way people purchase most services, such as car repairs and consultations with lawyers or accountants. This

What Is a Flexible Spending Account?

An employer may set up a flexible spending account to help their employees reduce what they pay for health care. These accounts enable people to set aside some of their salary before taxes to pay for health care costs that are not covered by their health insurance plan, such as copayments, deductibles, and over-the-counter drugs. The amount is deducted from their paychecks before federal income and Social Security taxes are withheld, so people pay less in taxes. Employers may limit the amount of money employees can contribute to the account.

People must estimate how much they think they will need for health care in the coming year and designate this amount to be put in their flexible spending account. They must use the full amount put in the account by the end of each year, or the money is lost. The money cannot be carried over to cover costs in the next year.

To be reimbursed for costs, people submit itemized receipts for services and drugs to the account's administrator.

system gives practitioners and institutions an incentive to work harder and to provide the type and quality of service that people want. However, there is no incentive to limit the type or amount of treatment provided. Thus, when there is a question of whether to do more tests or procedures in a borderline case, practitioners in this system tend to provide the additional care even when it is unclear that it will provide a real benefit. Because people with many types of health care insurance pay little or nothing for the additional care, they also tend to want the additional care. As a result, expenditures tend to be high and difficult to limit.

Many fee-for-service plans limit the amount that they pay for certain services. Sometimes the limit is based on what the plan deems to be a usual, customary, and reasonable charge for that service. The plan may require practitioners and institutions not to charge people any amounts above this limit. In such cases, the limit is called the contracted rate. If the plan allows practitioners to charge more, people must pay the difference.

Capitation: In capitated plans, practitioners and institutions are paid a fixed amount to provide health care for a specific group of people regardless of the number or cost of health care services provided. Unlike fee-for-service plans, plans that use capitation (capitated plans) give a financial incentive to minimize costs and tend not to provide services when the benefit is likely to be low or absent. Also, capitated plans often include a financial incentive to provide preventive care. Thus, these plans can minimize costs to those who receive care and potentially to society. However, the tendency to limit care can go too far. For example, if getting referrals to specialists or advanced medical centers is too hard, some people are discouraged and do not get the care that would benefit them. If practitioners are not rewarded for seeing or attracting more patients, the type and quality of service may suffer. For example, practitioners are not motivated to expand their office hours or provide on-call availability, and hospitals are not motivated to provide convenient times for diagnostic tests, good-tasting food, or liberal visitation policies.

Many people think managed care and capitated plans are the same. Managed care often uses capitation, but it is not the same thing.

An arrangement for reimbursing hospitals called diagnosis-related groups is related to capitation. The hospital is paid a fixed amount for all patients with a particular diagnosis (such as pneumonia) regardless of services provided or the length of the hospital stay.

Incentives: In some plans, whether fee-for-service or capitated, the amount practitioners and institutions are paid depends partly on how well they provide care—a practice called pay for performance. Payment is increased or decreased based on the practitioner's or institution's performance. Health insurance providers use several measures to judge performance, such as the following:

- Measures of patient health, such as changes in blood sugar levels to evaluate control of diabetes, changes in blood pressure to evaluate control of hypertension, or the percentage of people who need influenza vaccination and receive it
- The efficiency of the care provided, such as how quickly people with pneumonia are discharged from the hospital

UNDERSTANDING MANAGED CARE

Managed care has many variations. It is often thought of as capitation (paying a fixed amount to provide health care for a specific group of people regardless of the number or cost of health care services provided), but this definition is incorrect. Any plan that systematically directs the provision of care can be called managed care. Managed care is used to provide better, more consistent care and to control costs.

Managed care organizations improve care by providing practitioners and institutions with guidelines for care, which reflect what the current best practices are. Practitioners and institutions are monitored to determine how well they are complying with the guidelines.

Managed care organizations control costs in several ways:

- By encouraging and paying for recommended preventive measures
- By evaluating how well practitioners provide care and paying accordingly (pay for performance)
- By developing cost-saving arrangements (for example, by negotiating a lower rate of payment) with groups of practitioners
- By paying a fixed amount for all people with certain diagnoses, thus giving doctors and hospitals a financial incentive to lower their costs and to treat people efficiently and rapidly
- By using capitation

When people are choosing a managed care organization, they should choose one that best suits their needs and preferences.

Managed care organizations include health maintenance organizations (HMOs), preferred provider organizations (PPOs), and point-of-service (POS) plans. There are many more HMOs than PPOs or POS plans. Plans may combine various features. For example, an HMO may have POS and pay-for-performance features.

HMOs: HMOs can be less expensive than other managed care organizations but are restrictive. They have a list of practitioners, hospitals, and pharmacies (called a network) that have accepted their terms for payments. Typically, people must choose a primary care doctor or other practitioner and pharmacy and use a hospital from the list. People must see their primary care doctor before they see specialists or other practitioners. The primary care doctor must write a referral for care from other practitioners and sometimes writes orders for diagnostic or screening tests done at other facilities. Without a referral, the specialist or testing facility usually refuses to see the person unless the person pays the full cost of the service. Each person is responsible for having the correct referral form. The exception is emergencies. If people think their symptoms could represent a true emergency and go to the nearest emergency department and if the HMO agrees that the visit is appropriate (sometimes after the fact), the HMO usually partly or fully covers the costs. Sometimes whether symptoms represent a true emergency is unclear. In such cases, some plans do not reimburse people for an emergency department visit unless they first obtain authorization over the telephone from the primary care doctor. Thus, people should make sure they know in advance what their plan requires for reimbursement for an emergency department visit.

HMOs may have lower premiums. Copayments are typically very low or free. However, some HMOs (and some other plans, particularly Medicaid) keep costs low by paying practitioners a low rate for visits. Thus, practitioners may have an incentive to see more patients per hour.

PPOs: In PPOs, people are not restricted as in HMOs. They can choose their own practitioners. They do not have to choose a primary care doctor, and they do not need referrals. However, PPOs have a group of practitioners who have agreed to provide health care for members of the PPO at a discounted fee. People can see practitioners outside of the group, but care from these practitioners is more expensive than that from practitioners in the PPO group because people typically must pay the difference between the outside practitioner's fee and what the PPO allows.

POS: In POS plans, people can choose their own primary care doctor, as long as that doctor agrees to participate in the POS. When care from other practitioners is needed, the copayment is lowest if people go through their primary care doctor, who may direct them to practitioners in or outside the POS network. If people go directly to another network practitioner (without going through their primary care doctor), the copayment is higher. If people go directly to a practitioner who is not in the network, the copayment is the highest. Nonetheless, the plan still partly reimburses that practitioner.

Variations in Plans: Most managed care plans do not cover all types of health care, and what is covered varies from plan to plan. For example, coverage of certain kinds of care, such as mental health or physical therapy, may be limited. The total number of physical therapy treatments or mental health sessions may be limited during a year or over a lifetime, and copayments or deductibles may be higher than those for other types of care. Managed care does not usually cover assisted living or long-term nursing home care. Managed care organizations provide a list of tests, treatments, and other resources that are covered, and people can talk to their doctor about what types of care are covered. Most established diagnostic tests and treatments are covered. If people want a test or treatment that is not covered, they must pay for it.

Reimbursement procedures can vary greatly. For example, in some plans, people pay for their care when they receive it and are reimbursed for it later after the practitioner's office submits the required forms to the plan. In other plans, the practitioner's office is reimbursed directly by the managed care organization.

The variations in plans can be confusing and can lead to many problems (often in communication) for people and health care practitioners. Whether certain tests and treatments are covered is a common topic of discussion between people and their primary care doctor because no doctor can remember all the policies of the various plans. Thus, people who have a managed care plan should keep a summary of it handy for easy reference and should make sure they know what to do if a health emergency occurs.

Advantages: Managed care may have several advantages, in addition to lower costs:

- **Prevention:** Some managed care organizations emphasize prevention. For example, members may be notified when they need a particular screening test, such as mammography to check for breast cancer. Practitioners and members may be sent information about the benefit of annual influenza (flu) vaccination. The information often includes specific steps to follow so that members know how to get vaccinated. Practitioners may be sent current guidelines about tests and treatments.

- **Individualized health care guidelines:** Some managed care organizations try to identify members who have specific needs, who need complex health care, or who are likely to develop a disorder. To identify such people, these organizations may periodically send members health appraisals to fill out. Information is also collected from health care visits, insurance claims, and pharmacies. The information is used to develop and then distribute guidelines for managing the specific health care needs of certain members. For example, members who take many drugs may be sent a letter describing the risks of taking many drugs simultaneously. They may be advised to bring all their drugs (prescription and nonprescription) to their primary care doctor. The doctor can then check to make sure the drugs the person is taking are necessary and not likely to interact harmfully with one another. Sometimes the doctor can eliminate unnecessary or similar drugs, simplify the drug regimen, or recommend strategies for remembering to take drugs as prescribed.

- **Coordinated health care:** Records of a person's health care visits, insurance claims, and pharmacy visits may be kept in a central database that can be accessed from different places of care. If so, many health care practitioners can access complete medical information about the person, potentially avoiding duplicate, unnecessary, or harmful treatments, tests, and drugs.

- **Care for older people:** Some managed care plans are designed specifically for older people. Some of these plans coordinate the services of all involved health care practitioners at the appropriate sites of care (such as a hospital, rehabilitation facility, or long-term care facility). Also, managed care organizations tend to encourage access to health care services in the home. As a result, older people may be able to avoid a stay in a hospital or long-term care facility. Many plans include drug benefits under a special plan coordinated by the government

called Medicare Part D. The reminders and guidelines for preventive care and coordination of care provided by some managed care organizations are particularly useful for older people. Organizations may also send practitioners guidelines about which tests and treatments are helpful for older people and which are unnecessary or may do more harm than good.

PAYING FOR DRUGS

The cost of prescribed drugs may be covered by health plans (government, employer-sponsored, or private) or by separate prescription plans. However, many plans do not cover drug costs. Plans that cover drug costs vary, but most have certain things in common:

- Over-the-counter drugs are usually not covered.
- Some plans cover only certain drugs. This list of drugs is called a formulary. Plans may exclude a drug that is more expensive than other similar drugs and that has no or only minor advantages. The drugs included in a formulary vary from plan to plan.
- Usually, people must pay a copayment each time they get a prescription filled.
- The copayment is often higher for a brand-name than a generic drug if an equivalent generic drug is available.
- Drugs prescribed for reasons other than a medical need (such as drugs used to treat baldness or minor cosmetic problems) are often not covered.

People eligible for Medicare are also eligible to participate in Medicare Part D. Part D is a government plan that supplements drug coverage provided by private prescription plans. Thus, to receive benefits from Medicare Part D, people must have a prescription plan supplied by a private insurer, such as their managed care organization.

CHAPTER 4   Prevention

Traditional medical care focuses on improving health by identifying and treating health problems that have already produced symptoms or complications. In contrast, preventive medical care focuses on preventing health problems from occurring. Preventive care also focuses on diagnosing problems before symptoms or complications arise, when the

chances of recovery are greatest. When done well, prevention improves overall health and reduces health care costs.

The general goal of prevention is to reduce a person's likelihood of becoming ill or disabled or of dying prematurely. Preventive medical care is not a case of "one size fits all"; specific goals are devel-

EXAMPLES OF RISK FACTORS FOR HEALTH PROBLEMS

CATEGORY	RISK FACTORS
Diet	Eating an imbalanced, improper diet
Genetic	Family predisposition to specific disease, such as heart disease, colon cancer, breast cancer, cervical cancer, diabetes, mental health disorders, and substance abuse
Mental health	Stressful situations such as ■ A new job ■ Difficulty at work ■ Death of a loved one ■ Not getting sufficient sleep ■ Getting married or divorced
Physical activity	Sedentary lifestyle (not getting enough exercise)
Physical environment	Failure to maintain a safe environment, which would include the following: ■ For all people: Failing to keep firearms locked; not using bicycle helmets and seat belts; not having working smoke detectors and fire extinguishers in the home; not having heating systems and fireplaces inspected and cleaned periodically ■ For children: Not using child safety seats, bicycle helmets, flame-retardant sleepwear, window and chair guards; not assessing the home for leaded paint and removing if applicable; not safely storing drugs and toxic substances ■ For older adults: Not protecting against falls
Race and sex	White men: Higher risk of heart attack Black men: Higher risk of high blood pressure
Social environment	Neighborhood violence Family violence High-risk sexual behavior (such as multiple partners or not using condoms) Difficulty getting along with others
Substance use	Smoking cigarettes, cigars, or pipes Chewing tobacco Using illicit drugs Misusing alcohol or prescription drugs
Vaccinations	Not having received all recommended vaccinations
Weight	Weight that is above what is recommended for height and gender, particularly by 20% or more
Work environment	Working with potential toxins (for example, asbestos or ionizing radiation), machinery, power tools, farm equipment, and other possibly dangerous objects

oped by and for each person. Specific goals depend heavily on a person's risk profile, that is, the person's risk of developing a disease based on such factors as age, sex, genetic background, lifestyle, and physical and social environment. Factors that increase risk are called risk factors.

Some risk factors are beyond a person's control, such as age, sex, and family history. Other risk factors, such as a person's lifestyle and physical and social environment, can be altered, potentially decreasing risk of developing disorders.

In addition, risk can be reduced through good medical care.

Most of the medical care that infants (see page 1682), older children (see page 1744), and adolescents (see page 1754) receive (specifically well-child care) is aimed at recognizing and preventing problems. For example, examination focuses on detecting early signs of developing problems. Most vaccinations are given during childhood. Health care practitioners counsel parents about preventing accidents and injuries for children and adolescents.

Tools of Prevention

Prevention includes four major tools. One tool is establishing a healthful lifestyle, which includes habits such as wearing a seat belt, eating a healthy diet, getting enough physical exercise, wearing sunscreen, and not smoking. Another tool is getting vaccinated to prevent infectious diseases such as influenza, pneumococcal pneumonia, and childhood infections. A third tool is participating in screening efforts so that diseases such as high blood pressure and cancer are detected early. The fourth tool is taking drug therapy recommended to prevent disorders from developing or worsening (preventive drug therapy, also known as chemoprevention) for people at high risk. Examples of chemoprevention include cholesterol-lowering drugs to prevent atherosclerosis, aspirin to prevent heart attacks or strokes, tamoxifen to prevent breast cancer, and antihypertensive drugs to reduce blood pressure and prevent strokes.

> ### ❓ Did You Know...
> Improving diet and exercise habits and stopping smoking help prevent all three leading causes of death in the United States (heart disease, cancer, and stroke).

Healthful Lifestyle

Lifestyle and disease are clearly linked. Particular lifestyle changes can help prevent particular disorders. Also, some lifestyle changes improve fitness and quality of life and decrease risks of many different disorders. For example, the three leading causes of death in the United States—heart disease, cancer, and stroke—are more likely to occur in people who make poor lifestyle choices, especially eating a diet high in calories, saturated fats, trans fatty acids, and cholesterol (such a diet increases the risk of having high cholesterol levels in the blood); not exercising regularly; and smoking. By having informative discussions with doctors and other health care practitioners, people can make good decisions and establish healthful habits. Establishing and maintaining a healthful lifestyle can be done only by the person. Consistently eating a healthy diet and getting enough exercise are difficult for many people. However, doing so can prove to be exciting, rewarding, and affordable. Some important parts of maintaining a healthful lifestyle follow.

Healthful eating habits can help people prevent or control diseases such as high blood pressure, heart disease, diabetes, osteoporosis, and certain cancers. A diet that includes plenty of vegetables, fruits, and whole-grain cereals and breads is recommended, in part because such a diet is high in fiber (see page 907). Cutting down on harmful types of fat (saturated fats and trans fatty acids—see page 905) and instead eating fish, skinless poultry, and very lean meat and choosing low-fat dairy foods are recommended as well. Calories are best limited to maintain a recommended body weight. Limiting salt and getting adequate amounts of calcium and vitamin D are also recommended.

Physical activity and exercise can help prevent obesity, high blood pressure, heart disease, stroke, diabetes, some types of cancer, constipation, falls, and other health problems. The best routine includes moderate physical activity for 60 minutes or more on all or most days of the week. However, getting even a little bit of exercise is much better than none at all. For example, people who can devote only 10 minutes at a time to physical activity may still reap important benefits, particularly if the exercise is vigorous or if they repeat the activity throughout the day (see page 38). Walking is one simple, effective exercise that many people enjoy. Certain types of exercise can also target specific problems. For example, stretching improves flexibility, which can help prevent falls. Aerobic exercise may decrease the risk of heart attacks and angina.

Quitting smoking is important to a healthful lifestyle. A doctor can offer encouragement and advice on ways to successfully quit smoking, including information and recommendations on the use of nicotine replacement products, bupropion and varenicline (drugs that help reduce cravings), and other tools (see page 2096).

Safe sex practices remain important. Key safe sex practices are avoiding risky sex partners and remaining mutually monogamous. People who have more than one sex partner can greatly reduce their risk of contracting a sexually transmitted disease by using a latex condom properly every time they have sex (see box on page 1265). People who are allergic to latex can use other kinds of condoms.

Limiting alcohol use is important. Although small amounts of alcohol, particularly red wine, may have some health benefits, drinking more than moderate amounts (for example, 1 to 2 drinks per day, possibly less for women) is often harmful (see page 2083). Each drink is about 12 ounces of beer, 5 ounces of wine, or 1.5 ounces of more concentrated liquor, such as whiskey.

Injury prevention plays a major role in maintaining a healthful lifestyle. For example, people can lower their risk of injury by taking certain precautions.

Adequate sleep is also an important part of a healthful lifestyle, particularly affecting mood and mental state. Insufficient sleep is a risk factor for injuries.

Vaccination

Vaccines have been enormously successful. Dangerous and sometimes fatal infectious diseases such as diphtheria, pertussis, tetanus, mumps, measles, rubella, and polio have decreased by more than 99% from their peak number of cases, thanks to the availability of effective and safe vaccines and their widespread use. Furthermore, vaccinations save about $14 in health care costs for every $1 spent.

Many side effects have been attributed to vaccines. Actual side effects that occur depend on the vaccine, but common side effects are usually minor, such as swelling, soreness, allergic reactions at the injection site, and sometimes fever or chills. More serious side effects can occur, such as autoimmune reactions (for example, Guillain-Barré syndrome, which causes temporary weakness or paralysis). However, serious side effects are very rare if vaccines are given properly. Through systematic and extensive research, vaccines have not been linked to other serious side effects such as autism. Reports that vaccines cause side effects such as AIDS and sterility are "urban legends" that have no factual basis in developed countries. (If contaminated needles are improperly reused, however, infectious diseases can be spread, but this infection is not caused by a vaccine.) People who refuse vaccination to avoid complications place their health at much greater risk from the infection that the vaccine is designed to prevent.

Did You Know...
Vaccinations can benefit people other than those receiving the vaccine.

Children and adolescents, older adults, and people whose immune system is impaired are often the most vulnerable to developing vaccine-preventable infections. They are also often the most vulnerable to developing serious symptoms from those infections. For example, whooping cough (pertussis) can develop in people of any age but may be mistaken for a cold in otherwise healthy people because the symptoms are so mild. Although it is most important to vaccinate the most vulnerable people, vaccinating other people is also important. Doing so prevents illness in the vaccinated person and also decreases the number of people in the community who could develop and thus transmit infection to more vulnerable people. Thus, deaths and serious complications in the community are reduced by vaccinating as many people as possible. This effect is called herd immunity. See page 1144 for an in-depth discussion on vaccination.

Screening

Screening is testing of people who are at risk of a disorder but do not have any symptoms. Screening can allow for early treatment, sometimes keeping disorders from turning deadly. For example, abnormalities of the cervix or colon can be diagnosed and cured before they turn cancerous. Screening programs have greatly reduced the number of deaths associated with some disorders. For example, deaths due to cervical cancer, once the most common cause of cancer death among American women, have decreased 75% since 1955. Screening can also diagnose disorders that are not curable but that can be treated before they cause too much damage (for example, high blood pressure).

Did You Know...
It is often helpful to avoid tests designed to diagnose disorders before symptoms occur (screening tests).

People might think that any test capable of diagnosing a serious disorder should be performed. However, this is not true. Although screening can offer great benefits, it can also create problems. Some screening tests have a small risk of causing harm (for example, a colonoscopy can perforate or tear the colon). If such a test is performed on a large number of people who do not have any disease, then the small number of people who have the complication can outweigh the even smaller number who benefit by having the disease diagnosed. Similarly, because test results are sometimes positive in people who do not have disease, a certain number of people undergo unnecessary (and expensive and possibly painful or dangerous) tests or treatment in follow-up. Also, sometimes screening reveals abnormalities that cannot or need not be treated. For example, prostate cancer often grows so slowly that in older men the cancer is unlikely to affect their health before they die from another cause. In such cases, the treatment can be worse than the disease. Whole-body computed tomography scans are not recommended because they do not have benefits (such as saving lives) that exceed the risks (such as disorders caused by the radiation exposure, including cancer). In addition, when people are told they could have a serious disorder, they can become anxious, which can affect health. Because of these issues, screening is recommended only when

- The person has some real risk of the disorder.
- The screening test is accurate.
- The disorder can be more effectively treated when diagnosed before symptoms develop.

Safety 101

Practicing common-sense safety measures can help prevent injuries. Following simple preventive measures can greatly decrease the risk of injury in various situations. Here are some specific examples.

GENERAL SAFETY

- Learn first aid
- Prepare or purchase a first aid kit
- Learn cardiopulmonary resuscitation (CPR) and other methods to relieve airway obstruction, such as the Heimlich maneuver
- Wear a helmet when riding a bike or motorcycle and additional protective equipment as indicated for the sport, such as wrist guards for roller blading or skate boarding
- Store firearms safely
- Never swim alone
- If repetitive wrist motion (such as typing) is necessary, use a position unlikely to increase risk of carpal tunnel syndrome
- Exercise regularly and safely
- Eliminate or moderate alcohol intake

HOME SAFETY

Childhood Falls

- Install safety locks on basement doors
- Close and lock windows when children are present
- Replace or cover sharp-edged furniture
- Do not use baby walkers
- Install window guards, especially above the first floor
- Use stair gates at the top and bottom of stairs

Poisoning

- Never mix cleaning products
- Keep oven and toilet bowl cleaners, pesticides, alcohol, and antifreeze tightly sealed and out of the reach of children
- Keep all drugs in their original containers, and use child protective pill containers if small children are in or visiting the household
- Carefully dispose of expired drugs and drugs that are no longer necessary in the trash (never flush them down the toilet)—alternatively, some pharmacies accept them for disposal

Fires

- Install operational smoke detectors on every floor in the home, including the basement, and in every bedroom
- Test batteries every month and install new batteries every 6 months

- Plan an escape route and practice it
- Keep a fire extinguisher in or near the kitchen
- Have the electrical system inspected by a professional
- Do not leave lit candles unattended
- Do not smoke in bed

Carbon Monoxide Poisoning

- Ensure adequate ventilation for indoor sources of combustion (such as furnaces, hot-water heaters, wood- or charcoal-burning stoves, and kerosene heaters)
- Clean flues and chimneys regularly and inspect them for leaks
- Use a carbon monoxide detector in the home

Radon

- Have the radon level in the home checked
- Ensure adequate ventilation, especially in the basement

Lead Poisoning

- Consult the local health department and ask how to detect toxic levels of lead in the home's drinking water
- Find out whether the paint in the house is lead-based (present in older houses); if there is any question, test paint chips
- Have children tested for lead levels if recommended by the children's doctor

Other

- Set the maximum hot water heater temperature at 130° F (54.44° C) or less

FOOD SAFETY

- Pay attention to "sell by" dates on packaging
- Refrigerate perishable food immediately
- Do not buy dented canned goods or anything with a loose or bulging lid
- Keep the refrigerator at 40° F (4.44° C) and the freezer at 0° F (–17.78° C)
- Freeze fresh meats (including fish and poultry) that will not be used in 2 days
- Do not let the juices from raw meats drip on other foods
- Wash hands before and after preparing food
- Cook foods thoroughly
- Do not use the same utensils or platters for raw and cooked meats
- Wash all countertops, cutting boards, and utensils in hot soapy water after use

(continued on the following page)

Safety 101 (*Continued*)

CAR SAFETY

- Obey speed limits and drive defensively
- Make sure all passengers wear seat belts
- Put children in car seats or other restraints appropriate for their height and weight

- Do not allow a baby or child to sit on someone's lap in a moving vehicle
- Do not drink or use drugs before driving

- The health care benefits of appropriate screening make it relatively cost-effective.

Some screening tests (such as tests for cervical and colon cancers) are recommended for all people of a certain age or sex. For people at increased risk because of other factors, tests may be recommended at an earlier age or at more frequent intervals or additional tests may be recommended. For example, a person with a family history of colorectal cancer or with a disease that increases the chances of developing colorectal cancer, such as ulcerative colitis, would be advised to undergo a screening colonoscopy more often than is normally recommended for people at average risk. A woman with a strong family history of breast cancer would likely be advised to undergo screening mammography at an earlier age. Some screening measures are recommended for people with certain disorders. For example, people with diabetes should check their feet at least once daily for redness and ulcers, which, if ignored, may potentially result in severe infection and ultimately amputation.

Three Levels of Prevention

The three levels of prevention are primary, secondary, and tertiary.

In **primary prevention**, a disorder is actually prevented from developing. Vaccinations, counseling to change high-risk behaviors, and sometimes chemoprevention are types of primary prevention.

In **secondary prevention**, disease is detected and treated early, often before symptoms are present, thereby minimizing serious consequences. Secondary prevention can involve screening programs, such as mammography to detect breast cancer; dual x-ray absorptiometry (DEXA) scanning to detect osteoporosis; and tracking down the sex partners of a person diagnosed with a sexually transmitted disease (contact tracing) to treat these people, if necessary, and to minimize spread of the disease.

In **tertiary prevention**, an existing, usually chronic disease is managed to prevent complications or further damage. For example, tertiary prevention for people with diabetes focuses on tight control of blood sugar, excellent skin care, frequent examination of the feet, and frequent exercise to prevent heart and blood vessel disease. Tertiary prevention for a person who has had a stroke may involve taking aspirin to prevent a second stroke from occurring. Tertiary prevention can involve providing supportive and rehabilitative services to prevent deterioration and maximize quality of life, such as rehabilitation from injuries, heart attack, or stroke. It also includes preventing complications among people with disabilities, such as preventing bed sores in those confined to bed.

Preventive Drug Therapy

Preventive drug therapy (also known as chemoprevention) is the use of drugs to prevent disease. For such therapy to be recommended, the person must be at risk of the disorder being prevented and be at low risk of side effects caused by the drug being considered. Preventive drug therapy is clearly helpful in, for example, prevention of infection in people with certain disorders (such as AIDS), prevention of headache in people with migraines, and many other specific situations. Although preventive drug therapy is effective only in specific situations, some of those situations are common, so the therapy is useful for many people. For example, for adults at risk of coronary artery disease or stroke, aspirin is usually recommended. Newborns routinely receive eye drops to prevent gonococcal infection of the eyes. Women who are at high risk of breast cancer may benefit from preventive drug therapy (for example, with the drug tamoxifen).

Prevention in Pregnant Women

Prenatal care is focused on recognizing and preventing problems that can complicate pregnancy (see page 1622). For example, pregnant women are screened for high blood pressure, diabetes, sexually transmitted diseases, $Rh_o(D)$ blood incompatibility (which can cause hemolytic disease of the newborn), urinary bacteria, genetic variations that could result in birth defects or chromosomal abnormalities in the fetus, toxemia of pregnancy, and usually placental

SELECTED SCREENING SCHEDULE FOR ADULTS*†

CONDITION	TEST	FOR	HOW OFTEN
Abdominal aortic aneurysm	Abdominal ultrasonography	Men age 65 to 75 who smoke or have previously smoked	Once
Alcohol misuse	Questioning	Adults	Once and periodically, such as if circumstances change (for example, when under new stresses or if lifestyle changes)
Amblyopia and strabismus	Vision testing and eye examination	Children age 5 or younger	Once
Breast and ovarian cancers	Genetic counseling and possible genetic testing for *BRCA* mutation, which indicates increased risk of breast and ovarian cancers	Women with a strong family history of breast cancer (see box on page 1551) or ovarian cancer (see page 1573)	Once
Breast cancer	Mammography and clinical breast examination	Women 40 and older	Every 1 to 2 years
Cervical cancer	Papanicolaou (Pap) smear or liquid cervical cytology test	All women who have ever been sexually active and have not had their cervix removed	Every 1 to 3 years Most women can stop having Pap smears after age 65
Chlamydial infection	Culture or DNA test	Sexually active women age 25 or younger or who have risk factors (such as multiple sex partners or a sexually transmitted disease)	Once and periodically, such as when circumstances change (for example, new sex partners or after becoming pregnant)
Colorectal cancer	Colonoscopy or other testing (such as virtual colonoscopy or computed tomography scan)	Adults age 50 or older	Every 5 to 10 years
Dental problems	Check-up with dentist	All	Every 3 to 12 months for those under age 18 Every 3 to 24 months for age 18 and older
Depression	Questioning	Adults	Once and periodically, such as during stressful circumstances (for example, divorce, job or lifestyle change, or death in the family)
Diabetes	Blood tests to measure blood sugar level	Adults who are overweight or have high blood pressure or high levels of lipids in their blood	At least once
Glaucoma	Eye examination and eye pressure test	Adults age 40 and older	Every 2 to 4 years for adults age 40 to 64 Every 1 to 2 years for those age 65 and older
Gonorrhea	Culture or tests such as DNA testing	Pregnant women and young women who are sexually active	Once and periodically, such as when circumstances change (such as with new sex partners or after becoming pregnant)

(continued on the following page)

SELECTED SCREENING SCHEDULE FOR ADULTS*† *(Continued)*

CONDITION	TEST	FOR	HOW OFTEN
Hearing loss	Hearing tests	Adults age 65 or older	Yearly
Hemolytic disease of the newborn	$Rh_o(D)$ incompatibility screening	Pregnant women	First prenatal visit; for most $Rh_o(D)$-negative women, test again at 24 to 28 weeks of pregnancy
Hepatitis B	Blood test for infection with the virus	Pregnant women	At first prenatal visit
High blood pressure (hypertension)	Blood pressure measurement	Adults	Every office visit or annually
High levels of lipids (fats) and cholesterol in the blood	Blood tests to measure lipid (including cholesterol) levels	Men age 35 and older and women age 45 and older	Every 5 years; more often if levels are abnormal
Human immunodeficiency virus (HIV) infection, including AIDS	Blood test for infection with the virus	Adolescents and adults at risk of HIV infection and all pregnant women	Once and if new high-risk activity occurs (for example, those with multiple sex partners or injection drug use and in men having sex with men)
Osteoporosis	Dual-energy x-ray absorptiometry (DEXA) scan to measure bone density	Women age 60 and older who are at risk for osteoporotic fractures and all women age 65 and older (see page 546)	At least once
Overweight in adults and children; growth disturbance in children	Measurement of height and weight	All	Weight: every scheduled office visit or annually Height: every scheduled office visit in children and adolescents
Refractive errors (poor vision)	Vision testing (screening examinations do not require an optometrist or ophthalmologist)	All	Once for age 0 to 6 months Once at age 3 Every 2 years for age 6 to 17 Every 2 to 3 years for age 18 to 40 Every 2 years for age 41 to 60 Every year for age 61 and older
Syphilis	Blood test	Adults with risk factors (such as multiple sex partners or a previous sexually transmitted disease), all pregnant women, and those who have other diagnosed sexually transmitted diseases	Once and periodically, such as when circumstances change (such as with new sex partners or after becoming pregnant)
Tobacco use	Questioning	Adolescents and adults	Every office visit

*Based on recommendations by most major authorities in the United States. However, differences do exist among their recommendations.
†Screening measures that can be done at home include regularly measuring weight and, once yearly, checking skin for signs of change and for bleeding skin lesions, perhaps having another person (such as a spouse) look at locations that are difficult to see, such as the back or behind the ears.

SELECTED STRATEGIES FOR PREVENTING SOME MAJOR HEALTH PROBLEMS*

HEALTH PROBLEM	PREVENTIVE MEASURES
Heart disease	Maintain normal lipid and cholesterol levels through diet and drugs (if necessary) Maintain normal blood pressure through diet, exercise, stress reduction, and drugs (if necessary) Consume a balanced diet high in fiber and limited in fat, cholesterol, and calories Avoid smoking Undergo sufficient regular exercise Take aspirin if recommended (most adults at high risk of coronary artery disease)
Cancer	Avoid smoking (lung cancer) Eat a balanced diet high in fiber and limited in fat, cholesterol, and calories (breast cancer, colorectal cancer) Avoid too much sun exposure and use sunscreens with a high sun-protection factor (skin cancer) Take recommended chemoprevention such as tamoxifen (women at high risk of breast cancer and who choose to do this) Get recommended screening tests
Stroke	Avoid smoking Maintain normal blood pressure through diet, exercise, stress reduction, and drugs (if necessary) Maintain normal cholesterol through diet, exercise, and drugs (if necessary) Avoid cocaine
Chronic obstructive pulmonary disease	Avoid smoking Avoid exposure to toxic substances (especially in industrial settings)
Diabetes	Exercise regularly Eat a balanced diet Maintain recommended body weight
Osteoporosis	Consume adequate amounts of calcium and vitamin D Do weight-bearing exercises (for example, walking, jogging, tennis, dancing) every day for at least 30 minutes Take bone-strengthening drugs if prescribed by a doctor
Pneumonia	Receive pneumonia (pneumococcal) vaccine once, repeated once after 5 years for those at high risk, including those over age 65
Influenza	Receive influenza vaccine every year (particularly infants, older adults, and people who have heart, lung, or immune system disorders)
Tooth loss	Brush teeth and use dental floss regularly Avoid frequent sweets Visit a dentist regularly Take supplemental fluoride (preschool children older than 6 months whose water source is fluoride-deficient)
Sexually transmitted diseases	Practice abstinence or limit the number of sex partners Use condoms and follow safe sex practices
Liver disease	Drink alcohol in moderation if at all Receive vaccination against hepatitis A and B (all children and high-risk adults)

*In addition to these preventive measures, people should undergo recommended screening tests (see table on page 34).

and fetal abnormalities (using ultrasonography). Before (if possible) and during pregnancy, women are given folate (folic acid) to prevent birth defects. Often during pregnancy, women also are given iron to prevent anemia. They are counseled to stop using tobacco, alcohol, and recreational drugs before becoming pregnant and during pregnancy.

Prevention in Older Adults

The goals of prevention in an older adult usually depend on the person's health, level of function, and risk profile. For example, a healthy, independent person with no serious disorders may focus mainly on preventing disorders from developing. A person with several mild chronic disorders who remains independent may focus more on preventing or slowing decline in function and avoiding frailty than on preventing new disorders. A frail person with several advanced chronic diseases who has become mostly dependent on others may focus mainly on preventing accidents and complications that could cause further loss of independence or death.

Lifestyle: Exercise, including aerobic exercise, is still important. Weight lifting helps protect against muscle weakness, age-related loss of muscle tissue, and osteoporosis by strengthening muscles and increasing bone density. Aerobic exercise increases endurance and may slightly lower the risk of some heart and blood vessel disorders. In older adults, dancing and tai chi may be enjoyable forms of exercise and may have additional benefits, such as enhancing balance and preventing falls.

> ### ? Did You Know...
> Preventing falls, restricting driving (when necessary), and understanding the side effects of drug therapy can greatly increase good health for certain older adults.

Stopping smoking is helpful even in older adults. It can help improve endurance at any age, decrease symptoms of certain disorders (such as angina and claudication), and may decrease risks of certain disorders developing (such as heart attacks).

Alcohol is metabolized differently in older adults. Older adults who drink alcohol need to be aware that more than one drink per day may increase their risk of injuries and other health problems.

Drugs and Vaccines: Understanding drug therapy is particularly important for older adults because

they are more susceptible to adverse drug effects (see page 1896). Factors that can increase susceptibility include age-related differences in drug metabolism and use of many drugs (which can lead to drug interactions). A primary care doctor and pharmacist can provide information on all prescription and nonprescription drugs. Knowing the brand and generic name of all drugs taken; each drug's purpose; the length of time each drug is to be taken; and what activities, foods, drinks, and other drugs are to be avoided while taking a drug can help older adults avoid problems. Older adults should bring all of their drugs, both prescription and nonprescription, to their doctor appointments so that they can be reviewed with their doctor.

Vaccines for influenza, pneumococcal pneumonia (a bacterial lung infection), and the combination of pertussis and tetanus are important for older adults because of their increased susceptibility to pneumonia and tetanus.

> ## SPOTLIGHT ON AGING
>
> Measures that prevent injuries in younger adults are also important in older adults. So are some additional measures. For example, driving should be avoided in people whose vision, reflexes, or overall function is poor. Driving should also be avoided when taking drugs that cause sedation and at night if night vision is poor.
>
> Falls are a leading cause of serious health problems in older adults. Health risks can be reduced by preventing falls in the following ways:
>
> - Clean up cluttered areas in the home
> - Remove or secure throw rugs, edges of carpet, and uncovered phone and electrical cords to the floor
> - Maintain adequate lighting
> - Add handrails, grab bars, and traction/non-skid surfaces (such as strips or nonslip bathmats) to stairways and bathtubs as needed
> - Install handrails near the toilet and in the tub and shower
> - Avoid use of slippery bath oils
> - Review drugs to eliminate unnecessary ones and reduce others to lowest effective dose
> - Preserve or improve balance (for example, by exercise, dance, or tai chi) to decrease the risk of falls

5   Exercise and Fitness

Exercise is physical activity done regularly to improve, maintain, or slow the loss of fitness. Physical fitness is the capacity to perform physical activities with vigor and alertness and without undue fatigue. Fit people have more energy to pursue leisure activities. Fitness is also the degree to which people can withstand stress and persevere under difficult or emergency circumstances. Regular exercise is one of the best things that people can do to help prevent illness, preserve health and longevity, and enhance quality of life. Exercise comes in many forms and can vary in intensity of effort. With so many ways to exercise, almost everyone can participate in some way.

Benefits of Exercise

Regular exercise makes the heart stronger and the lungs fitter, enabling the cardiovascular system to deliver more oxygen to the body with every heartbeat and the pulmonary system to increase the maximum amount of oxygen that the lungs can take in. Exercise lowers blood pressure, somewhat decreases the levels of total and low-density lipoprotein (LDL) cholesterol (the bad cholesterol), and increases the level of high-density lipoprotein (HDL) cholesterol (the good cholesterol). These beneficial effects in turn decrease the risk of heart attack, stroke, and coronary artery disease. In addition, colon cancer and some forms of diabetes are less likely to occur in people who exercise regularly.

> **? Did You Know...**
>
> Most frail, older people benefit from exercise at least as much as younger people.

Exercise makes muscles stronger, allowing people to do tasks that they otherwise might not be able to do or to do them more easily. Every physical task requires muscle strength and some degree of range of motion in joints. Regular exercise can improve both.

Exercising stretches muscles and joints, which in turn can increase flexibility and help prevent injuries. Weight-bearing exercise, such as brisk walking and weight training, strengthens bones and helps prevent osteoporosis. Exercise can improve function and reduce pain in people with osteoarthritis, although exercises that put undue strain on joints, such as jumping and running, may need to be avoided.

Exercise increases the body's level of endorphins, chemicals in the brain that reduce pain and induce a sense of well-being. Thus, exercise appears to help improve mood and energy levels and may even help relieve depression. Exercise may also help boost self-esteem by improving a person's overall health and appearance.

In addition to all its other benefits, regular exercise helps older people remain independent by improving functional ability and by preventing falls and fractures. It can strengthen the muscles of even the frailest older person living in a nursing or retirement home. It tends to increase appetite, reduce constipation, and promote sleep.

The benefits of exercise diminish within months after a person stops exercising. Heart strength, muscle strength, and the level of HDL cholesterol (the good cholesterol) decrease, whereas blood pressure and body fat increase. Even former athletes who stop exercising do not retain measurable long-term benefits. However, people who were physically active in the past regain fitness faster.

Starting an Exercise Program

People should consult their doctors before beginning competitive sports or an exercise program. Doctors ask about known medical disorders in the person and family members and symptoms the person has. They do a physical examination, including listening to the heart with a stethoscope. This evaluation identifies some of the rare young people who could have a previously unsuspected heart disorder that can lead to serious heart rhythm abnormalities or sudden, unexpected death with strenuous exercise. It also detects conditions that could restrict activities. For example, overweight people are more likely to develop musculoskeletal injuries after activities involving sudden starts and stops (such as tennis and basketball) as well as those that involve impact (such as jogging).

People older than age 40 who are starting an exercise program should report any diagnoses of heart disorders or arthritis and describe any symptoms of chest pain, shortness of breath, leg pains with walking, palpitations (awareness of heartbeat) or irregular heartbeats, joint pain or swelling, and inability to exercise for long periods (for example, because of weakness, shortness of breath, sweating, or leg pains). Certain drugs may limit the ability to

Athletic Heart Syndrome

Athletic heart syndrome refers to the normal changes that the heart undergoes in people who regularly do strenuous aerobic exercise (for example, very well conditioned athletes) and, to a variable extent, in those who do extensive weight training.

In a person with athletic heart syndrome, the heart is larger and its walls thicker than in a nonathlete. The chambers inside the heart get somewhat larger. This increase in size and thickening of walls allow the heart to pump substantially more blood per heartbeat without much increase in heart rate. The large volume of blood flowing through the heart results in a slower, stronger pulse (which can be felt at the wrist and elsewhere on the body) and sometimes in a heart murmur. These murmurs, which are specific sounds created as blood flows through the valves of the heart, are perfectly normal in an athlete and are not dangerous. The heartbeat of a person with athletic heart syndrome may be irregular at rest but becomes regular when exercise begins. Blood pressure is virtually the same as in any other healthy person.

The enlarged heart can be seen on an echocardiogram and sometimes on a chest x-ray. A variety of changes are detectable on an electrocardiogram. These changes would be considered abnormal in a nonathlete but are perfectly normal in an athlete.

When an athlete stops training, the athletic heart syndrome slowly disappears—that is, heart size and heart rate tend to return gradually to those of the nonathlete.

Athletic heart syndrome is not thought to affect health in any way. The rare sudden deaths of athletes are usually due to underlying heart disease that was not previously detected rather than to any danger resulting from athletic heart syndrome.

---

exercise, such as beta-blockers, which slow heart rate, and sedatives, which can cause drowsiness and increase the risk of falling.

Conditions that make exercise too risky to recommend in children include heart inflammation (myocarditis), which is uncommon. It increases the risk of sudden death due to heart dysfunction. Fever is another, because it impairs ability to exercise, may be a sign of serious illness, and may lead to heat-related illness such as heatstroke. Conditions that lead to dehydration (for example, vomiting and diarrhea) are also risky, because sweating during exercise can worsen dehydration.

Conditions that make exercise too risky to recommend and that occur mainly in adults include angina pectoris and a heart attack in the previous 6 weeks.

People should take precautions when they have certain other conditions. For example:

- People with cystic fibrosis or diabetes, which can lead to dehydration, should drink large amounts of fluids around the time of exercise.
- People who have had several concussions or a recent concussion should avoid contact sports.
- People with seizures should avoid swimming and weight lifting alone to prevent injuring themselves and should avoid riflery and archery to prevent injuring others.
- People with an enlarged spleen (for example, after infectious mononucleosis) should avoid contact sports because being hit or falling may rupture the enlarged spleen.

Doctors can provide specific instructions on the type of activity as well as the level of intensity (how hard the exercise should be), the duration of activity (how long the exercise should last), and the frequency (how often the exercise should be done). In some cases, exercise should be supervised by a physical therapist or other health care practitioner or by an experienced, licensed fitness professional.

The safest way to start an exercise program is to do the chosen exercise or sport at a low intensity of effort. Beginning at a low intensity allows time to learn proper body mechanics, which helps to prevent future injuries when training at a higher intensity. Beginning at a low intensity also prevents excessive muscle strain. The exercise should be done until the legs or arms ache or feel heavy. If muscles ache after just a few minutes, the first workout should last only that long. As fitness increases, a person should be able to exercise longer without feeling muscle pain. However, some discomfort is necessary for developing stronger, larger muscles. Over time, a person can increase exercise demands as needed or required to achieve fitness goals.

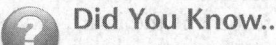 **Did You Know...**

Stretching exercises are more beneficial when done after rather than before other exercises.

Sustained, high-intensity weight training can be at least as beneficial for the heart as aerobic exercise.

Estimating Target Heart Rate

To estimate target heart rate, calculate the maximum heart rate (the heart rate estimated to correspond to the rate of maximum oxygen use), which is 220 minus age. Then, multiply the maximum heart rate by 60 to 85% (or by 0.6 and 0.85, respectively). For example, for a 40-year-old, the maximum heart rate is 180, so the target heart rate is 108 to 153 (60 to 85% of 180).

Screening for Sports Participation: Most schools and organized sports organizations require that people have a doctor evaluate whether they can safely participate before they join the program. Doctors ask questions about general health and do an examination as previously described. Adolescents and young adults are often asked about use of illicit and performance-enhancing drugs. In girls and women, doctors look for delays in the onset of menarche and presence of the female athlete triad (eating disorders, amenorrhea or other menstrual dysfunction, and diminished bone mineral density), which is becoming more common as more adolescent and young women engage in overly intensive physical activity and overly zealous loss of body fat.

Type of Exercise

A major distinction among different types of exercise is whether they are aerobic (low intensity, steady state) or strength training (also sometimes called anaerobic exercise). Most forms of exercise have components of both.

Aerobic Exercise: This term refers to exercise that requires more than the usual amount of oxygen to get to the muscles, thus the heart and lungs are forced to work harder. Running, biking, swimming, skating, and using aerobic exercise machines (such as treadmill, stair-climbing, and elliptical training machines) are activities that people do to experience aerobic exercise. Aerobic exercise tends to expend a great deal of calories, improves cardiac function, and decreases slightly the risk of death from cardiac causes. However, it is less effective than strength training at building strength and muscle mass. Too much weight-bearing aerobic exercise causes excessive wear on the joints and surrounding tissues, so trying to improve muscle strength through frequent, repetitive bouts of aerobic activity must be done cautiously if at all.

For aerobic exercise to benefit the heart, oxygen use should be increased to a rate that is within about 15 to 40% of the maximum rate the body can sustain. This maximum rate can be estimated in several ways:

- The heart rate increases by 20 beats per minute more than the resting heart rate.

- Exercise is accompanied by reasonably heavy breathing and sweating, presuming that the environmental temperature is not inordinately hot.
- A "target" heart rate is reached.

The target heart rate is only an estimate. Overweight or deconditioned people reach their target heart rate more quickly and with less effort. Athletic people reach their target heart rate more slowly. It is also probably safer for athletes to exceed the target heart rate, because such targets take into consideration the conditioning of average people. People taking drugs that slow heart rate (such as beta-blockers or calcium channel blockers) may not reach their target heart rate despite intense exercise. They should discuss with their doctors what target heart rate is desirable.

Did You Know...

The maximum possible benefit from aerobic exercise can be obtained by doing just 10 to 15 minutes of interval cycling a few times a week.

Tension time (how long a set lasts) may be the best way to gauge how much weight to use when strength training.

A typical recommendation is to do 30 minutes of aerobic exercise at sufficient intensity about 2 to 3 times per week, with 5-minute warm-up (gradual increase to peak intensity) and 5-minute cool-down (gradual decrease in intensity) periods. However, the 30-minute length of time is arbitrary. Maximum aerobic conditioning can be achieved by doing as little as 10 to 15 minutes of activity per session 2 to 3 times per week if interval cycling is used. In interval cycling, moderate aerobic exercise is alternated with intense exertion. For example, about 90 seconds of moderate activity (60 to 80% of maximum heart rate) is alternated with 20 to 30 seconds of all-out sprinting (85 to 95% of maximum heart rate or as hard as the person can exercise while maintaining correct exercise form). Sprinting, however, can strain joints and thus should be done for only limited times or, perhaps, avoided completely if joint pain occurs or if the person has certain joint disorders. Proper body mechanics should be maintained to avoid injury. Sometimes aerobic exercise can be done while strength training (for example, if little time is taken to rest between doing strength training exercises).

Different aerobic exercises work different muscle groups. For example, running works primarily the lower leg muscles. Landing on the heels and rising on the toes exerts the greatest force on the ankle. Riding a bicycle works primarily the upper leg muscles because pedaling works the front thigh muscles (quadriceps) and hips. Rowing and swimming work the upper body and the back predominantly. These exercises can be alternated daily to avoid injury.

Strength Training: Strength training (also called resistance training or anaerobic exercise) involves forceful muscular contraction against resistance, usually using free or machine weights. Depending on how it is done, strength training may be somewhat less beneficial for cardiovascular fitness than aerobic exercise. However, it develops muscle strength, size, endurance, and flexibility and still benefits the heart and lungs. In the long run, increased muscle mass helps a person become leaner and lose weight, because muscle uses more calories, even at rest, than do other types of tissues, particularly fat. More muscle mass also means more functional ability into later years, which helps people remain independent as they age.

Individual exercises are designed to strengthen particular muscles or muscle groups. Usually, larger muscle groups are exercised first, then smaller ones. Maximum benefit is obtained by exercising at a high workload, but not necessarily to failure (that is, the point at which another repetition in good form is impossible). Traditionally, particular exercises are done in sets. Each set includes 8 to 12 repetitions of the exercise, done continuously (that is, no rest, including joint "locking," between repetitions). The amount of weight used is the maximum that the person can use and still do 8 to 12 repetitions in a relatively slow and controlled manner, without heaving, throwing, or dropping the weight. Doing one set with steady tension results in about 75 to 85% of the benefit of doing 3 sets, the maximum recommended.

Tension time is another way to determine recommended muscle workload (the amount of weight lifted and the amount of work the muscle does). Tension time refers to the total duration of lifting and lowering the weight in one set. Tension time should be briefer if the goal is moderate exercise and building strength than if the goal is more muscular endurance than strength (for example, during rehabilitation from injury). Tension time is a better way to gauge recommended muscle workload for increasing strength than are sets and repetitions. To continue to increase strength, after the recommended tension time is achieved with good technique, weight should be increased to the maximum at which the person can maintain or be challenged again with the same tension time. Recommended tension time is ideally 40 to 60 seconds for the upper body and, because the lower body has greater endurance, about 60 to 90 seconds for the lower body. If the goal is muscular endurance, tension time is usually about 90 to 120 seconds. Strength athletes, such as power lifters, respond better and

USUAL MAXIMUM AND TARGET HEART RATES		
AGE	MAXIMUM HEART RATE	TARGET HEART RATE
20	200	120 to 170
30	190	114 to 162
40	180	108 to 153
50	170	102 to 145
60	160	96 to 136
70	150	90 to 128

favor briefer tension times of 10 to 30 seconds, because the concurrently heavier loads stimulate superior strength increases, although with less muscle growth and endurance responses.

Frequency of exercise is a critical factor. Muscles start to break down when exercised at sufficient workloads more often than every other day. The day after an adequate workout, bleeding and microscopic tearing occur in muscle fibers, which is probably why muscles feel sore. This soreness (also called an alarm reaction) stimulates muscles to repair themselves and grow to adapt to a higher state of function. Exercisers should allow about 48 hours for muscles to recover after exercise. After very vigorous exercise, a muscle group may take several days to heal completely, thus allowing the muscles to heal and to become stronger. Hence, in strength training, it is usually best to alternate the muscle groups being exercised. An ideal schedule, for example, alternates exercise for the upper body on one day with exercise for the lower body on the next, with each muscle trained no more than twice per week. The more intense and the more exercise done for a muscle, the less often it should be worked. People who train with a very high level of intensity of effort likely should not train each muscle any more than once a week.

Injury rehabilitation may not aim for development of large muscles. Exercising with less weight but increased numbers of repetitions can increase strength and endurance, provide some aerobic exercise, and increase blood flow to the area, which accelerates healing. This approach may be tolerated better than exercising muscles more intensely, which requires a high degree of motivation. Once confidence and function increase in the injured person, intensity of effort and work loads should increase in order to optimize results.

In **circuit training**, the large muscles of the legs, hips, back, and chest are exercised followed by the smaller muscles of the shoulders, arms, abdomen, and neck. Some people prefer to train legs last because they require so much energy and are so fatiguing to work. Circuit training of only 15 to 20 minutes can benefit the cardiovascular system more than jogging or using aerobic exercise machines for the same time. The workout is often more intense, and heart rate can increase even more as a result.

Safe technique is important. Jerking or dropping weights can cause minor injury due to sudden starts and stops. Controlled breathing prevents dizziness (and, in extreme cases, fainting), which can occur when forcefully exhaling or bearing down. Specifically, people should exhale while lifting a weight and inhale when lowering a weight. If a movement is slow, such as lowering a weight for 5 seconds or longer, people may need to breathe in and out more than once, but breathing should still be coordinated so that a final breath is taken in just before the lifting phase and released during lifting. Blood pressure increases during resistance training, particularly when working the large muscles of the lower body and while gripping very hard with the hands, as can be experienced when doing the leg press exercise. However, blood pressure returns to normal quickly after exercise. And the increase in blood pressure is smaller when breathing technique is correct, no matter how hard a person exerts. Most people who intend to lift weights benefit from initial supervision that includes instruction on how to set the weights and seat levels, how to maintain proper body mechanics, and how to breathe during exercises. Having a professional trainer observe the person as the exercise is being done is usually most helpful, so that improper mechanics can be identified and corrected.

Stretching and Flexibility: Stretching reduces stiffness of muscles and tendons and thereby improves flexibility. Flexibility is important for comfortable performance of physical activities. Although stretching itself does not strengthen muscles, it can increase the area over which the muscle contracts, which allows muscle force to be exerted more effectively and with less risk of injury. Stretching may help people jump higher, lift heavier weights, run faster, and throw farther.

Specific flexibility exercises involve slowly and steadily stretching groups of muscles without jerking, bouncing, or causing excess pain (minor discomfort is normal when stretching current limits of a joint, but pain should never be intolerable). These exercises can be done before or after other forms of training or as a program itself, as occurs in yoga and Pilates sessions. Although stretching before exercise enhances mental preparedness, there is no evidence that stretching decreases risk of injury. General warming-up (for example, with low-intensity simulation of the exercise to be performed, jogging on the spot, calisthenics, or other light activities that increase core temperature) appears to be more effective than stretching for facilitating safe exercise. Stretching after exercise is preferred because tissues stretch more effectively when warmed.

Workload and Variation

In general, if the intensity of an exercise increases, duration, frequency, or both may need to decrease and vice versa. For most people who participate in weight training, the amount of weight lifted should continue to increase as they get stronger, whereas duration and frequency typically remain constant once a certain level is reached. Exercise that involves too low a workload provides fewer rewards. Exercise that involves too high a workload increases risk of improper mechanics and thus injury. Additionally, people should vary the way they train their muscles over time. The body adapts to routine, so that doing the same exercises in the same way over time becomes less effective in building strength, muscle, and cardiovascular fitness. Therefore, people who engage in resistance exercises should alter their routines every few weeks, and aerobic exercisers should alternate among the different forms of aerobic exercise available.

Exercising Safely

Exercising without proper safety precautions often leads to injury. Scheduling workouts 48 hours apart, to allow muscles to recover, and keeping workouts varied in regard to exercise method and equipment choices may help prevent muscle overuse and repetitive strain injuries. In addition, people should stop exercising immediately if they feel pain other than the usual burning sensation in muscles caused by lactate buildup, which is the "burn" that occurs because exercise is intense.

Two types of muscle discomfort may be felt after exercise. The desirable or at least expected type, delayed-onset muscle soreness, does not start until several hours after exercising intensely. Usually it peaks within 48 hours, goes away 72 hours later, and feels better after the warm-up for the next workout. The undesirable type, in which pain indicates injury, is usually felt soon after injury occurs, may not disappear 72 hours later, and may become much more severe if a person tries to exercise.

Warming Up: Warming up is meant literally. Warm muscles are more pliable and less likely to tear than cold muscles, which contract sluggishly. Starting exercise at lower intensity (for example, walking rather than running or using lighter weights) raises the temperature of muscles by increasing blood flow. Therefore, warming up helps prevent injuries. Activities that do not raise muscle temperature do not provide such benefit. Warm-up activities also help prepare the mind for more intense activity, thus increasing confidence, motivation, and improving the mind-muscle link for higher quality activity.

> **? Did You Know...**
>
> During exercise, people should drink about ½ to 1 cup (120 to 240 milliliters) every 15 to 20 minutes, even if they are not thirsty.

Cooling Down: Slowing down gradually (cooling down) at the end of exercise helps prevent dizziness. When the leg muscles relax, blood collects (pools) in the veins near them. To return the blood toward the heart, the leg muscles must contract. When exercise is suddenly stopped, blood pools in the legs and not enough blood goes to the brain, causing dizziness. By preventing blood from pooling, cooling down also helps the bloodstream speed up its removal of lactic acid, a natural chemical product that builds up in the muscles during exercise and that can unduly strain the body if it accumulates.

Hydration: Proper hydration is important, particularly when exertion is prolonged or occurs in a hot environment. People should be well-hydrated before activity, drink fluids regularly during extended exertion, and continue to drink fluids after activity. During exercise, people should drink about ½ to 1 cup (120 to 240 milliliters) every 15 to 20 minutes, depending on heat and exertion level. They should drink these amounts regardless of thirst, which may be absent or minimal sometimes even when a person is dehydrated. Another way to estimate the amount of fluids needed is to subtract body weight after exercise from body weight before exercise. Then, about 2 cups of fluid is drunk per pound lost (about 1 liter for each kilogram lost).

However, people need to be careful to avoid drinking too much water because overhydration can cause the level of salt in the blood to fall too low (a condition called hyponatremia—see page 948) and lead to nausea or even seizures. Overhydration and hyponatremia are usually only a problem for people who engage in prolonged outdoor exertion (for example, long-distance runners or sport teams playing long games).

To replace lost fluids, plain water is usually fine, unless very large amounts are necessary (several quarts, for example). Such a large fluid requirement is unusual unless a person exercises outdoors in high heat and humidity. In this case, electrolyte-containing sports drinks may be preferred. However, if the sports drink has a lot of sugar (more than 8% glucose), it should be mixed with plain water at a 50:50 ratio so that the fluids are not absorbed too slowly.

Choosing the Right Exercise

There are many forms of exercise, and each type has its advantages and disadvantages. Some people prefer to exercise in a gym or at home, whereas others prefer to exercise outdoors. Some people have a very structured exercise routine, whereas others simply incorporate exercise into their lifestyle, for example, by walking rather than driving, parking farther away from their destination, or walking up stairs rather than using an elevator. Choosing the right exercise is a matter of finding an activity that helps people achieve their fitness goals and is safe, sustainable, and enjoyable (or at least tolerable). Exercise should also offer some degree of challenge; if not, then the benefits will be few.

Walking: Walking is a well-balanced form of exercise for most people, regardless of age. Many older people are able to keep fit through a regular walking program. Walking is relatively easy on the joints. During walking, at least one foot is on the ground at all times, so the force with which the foot strikes the ground is never much more than the person's weight. However, walking expends fewer calories than does running and places fewer demands on the heart. Walking slowly will not make a person very fit. To walk faster, a person can take longer steps in addition to moving the legs faster. Steps can be lengthened by swiveling the hips from side to side so that the feet can reach further forward. Swiveling the hips tends to make the toes point outward when the feet touch the ground, so the toes do not reach as far forward as they would if they were pointed straight ahead. Therefore, a person walking should always try to point the toes straight ahead. Moving the arms faster helps the feet move faster. To move the arms faster, a person bends the elbows to shorten the swing and reduce the time the arms take to swing back and forth from the shoulder. People with instability or severe joint injury may find walking difficult. Also, even vigorous walking does not strengthen the upper body and has little strengthening effect on the lower body unless the person is initially very deconditioned.

Swimming: Swimming exercises the whole body— the legs, arms, and back—without straining the joints and muscles. Often, swimming is recommended for people who have muscle and joint problems. Swimmers, moving at their own pace and using any stroke, can gradually increase endurance until they can swim for 30 minutes continuously. If weight loss is one of the main goals of exercise, however, swimming is not the best choice. Exercise out of water is more effective because air insulates the body, increasing body temperature and metabolism for up to 18 hours. This process expends extra calories after exercise as well as during exercise. In contrast, water conducts heat away from the body, so that body temperature does not rise and metabolism does not remain increased after swimming. Also, swimming tends not to build muscle, because the muscles are supported by the water, which restricts the type of movements the muscles make. And because swimming is not a weight-bearing exercise, it does not help prevent osteoporosis.

> **? Did You Know...**
> Swimming is a less effective way to lose weight and build muscle than exercise out of water.

Bicycling: Riding a bicycle is good exercise for cardiovascular fitness. Pedaling a bicycle strengthens the upper leg muscles. Bicycles are pedaled in a smooth circular motion that does not jolt the muscles. A rider can enjoy the variety and challenges of different scenes and terrains. However, bicycling can be harmful in some people with knee disorders because there is greater shearing force on the knee joint than with some other activities, such as walking. Bicycling requires balance. Some people cannot maintain balance, even on a stationary bicycle, and others find the pressure of the narrow seat against the pelvis uncomfortable. Also, outdoor bicycling may involve risks of cars and traffic.

With a stationary bicycle, the tension on the bicycle wheel should be set so that the rider can pedal at a cadence of 60 rotations per minute. As they progress, riders can gradually increase the tension and the cadence up to 90 rotations per minute. A recumbent stationary bicycle is both secure and comfortable. It has a contoured chair that even a person who has had a stroke can sit in. Also, if one leg is paralyzed, toe clips can hold both feet in place, so that the person can pedal with one leg. A recumbent stationary bicycle is a particularly good choice for older people, many of whom have weak upper leg muscles. Having weak upper leg muscles makes rising from a squatting position, getting up from a chair without using the hands, or walking up stairs without holding on to the railing difficult.

CALORIES EXPENDED DURING EXERCISE*

Activity	125-lb (57-kilogram) person	175-lb (80-kilogram) person
Aerobics	283	396
Biking	453	635
Cross-country skiing	453	635
Downhill skiing	340	476
Golf		
Riding cart	198	277
Carrying clubs	311	436
Hiking	340	476
Ice skating	396	555
In-line skating	283	396
Running		
8-minute mile	708	992
12-minute mile	453	635
Softball	283	396
Swimming	453	635
Swing dancing	226	317
Tae kwon do	283	396
Tennis (singles)	453	635
Walking	198	277
Weight lifting	170	238
Yoga	226	317

* Average calories expended in 1 hour. Calories expended are calculated based on moderate intensity.

Aerobic Dancing: This popular type of exercise, offered in many communities, exercises the whole body. Dancing with light to moderate weights can offer extra benefit because it increases the challenge and overall demands on the muscles. People can exercise at their own pace with guidance from experienced instructors. Lively music and familiar routines make the workout fun. Committing to a schedule and exercising with friends can improve motivation. Aerobic dancing also can be done at home with videotapes. Low-impact aerobic dancing eliminates the jumping and pounding of regular aerobic dancing, thus decreasing strain on the knee and hip joints. However, the benefits of aerobic dancing, especially in terms of weight loss, are proportional to the intensity. Consequently, muscle strengthening does not increase much with this type of activity.

Step Aerobics: Step aerobics works primarily the muscles in the front and back of the upper legs (the quadriceps and hamstrings) as a person steps up and down on a raised platform (a step) in a routine set to music at a designated pace. As soon as these muscles start to feel sore, exercisers should stop, do something else, and return to step aerobics a couple of days later. High-intensity step aerobics can strain the joints, particularly the knees and hips.

Water Aerobics: Water aerobics is an excellent choice for older people and for those with weak muscles, because it prevents falls on a hard surface and provides support for the body. It is often used for people with arthritis and sometimes for injury rehabilitation. Water aerobics involves doing various types of muscle movements or simply walking in waist- to shoulder-deep water. Aerobic exercises done out of the water, however, are more effective for weight loss.

Cross-Country Skiing: Cross-country skiing exercises the upper body and the legs. Many people enjoy using machines that simulate cross-country skiing, but others find the motions difficult to master and stressful around the hip joints and inner thighs (although working with shorter leg strokes often helps). Because using these machines requires more coordination than most types of exercise, a person should try out a machine before buying one. Cross-country skiing outdoors is more enjoyable to some people but adds the challenges of exercising in the cold while maintaining balance.

Rowing: Rowing strengthens the large muscles of the legs and upper arms and back. More people use rowing machines than row on water, although rowing outdoors adds the challenge of coordinating the oars and the joys of spending time in a boat. However, if the boat does not have a sliding seat, the leg muscles will not be strengthened. People who have back problems should not row without a doctor's approval.

Strength Training: Strength training is meant to build strength and muscle mass. It is described elsewhere (see page 41).

Yoga: Yoga is not exercise. It is mental and physical relaxation used to stretch muscles. Many people enjoy yoga. However, yoga does not benefit the heart, increase endurance, or help build muscle or improve muscle function.

6   Rehabilitation

Rehabilitation services are needed by people who have lost the ability to function normally, often because of trauma, a stroke, an infection, a tumor, surgery, or a progressive disorder (such as arthritis). A pulmonary rehabilitation program (see page 459) is often appropriate for people who have chronic obstructive lung disease. People who become weak after prolonged bed rest (for example, because of a severe injury or after surgery) also need rehabilitation. Physical therapy, occupational therapy, treatment of any pain and inflammation, and retraining to compensate for specific lost functions are the typical focus of rehabilitation. Treatment usually involves continued sessions of one-on-one training for many weeks.

The need for rehabilitation crosses all age groups, although the type, level, and goals of rehabilitation often differ by age. People with chronic impairments, often older people, have different goals and require less intensive rehabilitation or a longer period of rehabilitation than do younger people with a temporary impairment (such as that due to a fracture or burn). For example, the goal of an older person who has severe heart failure and has had a stroke may simply be to regain the ability to do as many self-care activities—such as eating, dressing, bathing, transferring between a bed and a chair, using the toilet, and

> **? Did You Know...**
> After a major disorder, injury, or surgical procedure, people must follow the recommended rehabilitation program if they want to recover as fully as possible.
>
> Rehabilitation can be done in a doctor's office or at home as well as in rehabilitation centers.

controlling bladder and bowel function—as possible. The goal of a younger person who has had a fracture is often to regain all functions as quickly as possible. Nonetheless, age alone is not a reason to alter goals or the intensity of rehabilitation, but the presence of other disorders or limitations may be.

To initiate a formal rehabilitation program, a doctor writes a referral (similar to a prescription) to a physiatrist (a doctor who is board-certified in rehabilitation medicine), an occupational or physical therapist, or a rehabilitation center. The referral establishes the goals of therapy, a description of the type of illness or injury, and its date of onset. The referral also specifies the type of therapy needed, such as ambulation training (help with walking) or training in activities of daily living.

Setting: Where rehabilitation takes place depends on the person's needs. Many people recovering from injuries can be treated as outpatients in a therapist's office. People with severe disabilities may need care in a hospital or inpatient rehabilitation center. In such settings, a rehabilitation team provides care. With the doctor or therapist, this team may include nurses, psychologists, social workers, speech pathologists (who evaluate speech, language, and voice), audiologists (who evaluate hearing), other health care practitioners, and family members. A team approach is best because significant loss of function can lead to other problems, such as depression, apathy, and financial problems.

Care at home can be appropriate for people who cannot travel easily but who require less care, such as those who can transfer from bed to a chair or from a chair to a toilet. However, family members or friends must be willing to participate in the rehabilitation process. Providing rehabilitation at home with the help of family members is highly desirable, but it can be physically and emotionally taxing for all involved. Sometimes a visiting physical therapist or occupational therapist can help with home care.

Many nursing homes have less intensive rehabilitation programs, which are better suited to people less able to tolerate therapy, such as frail or older people.

Goals: The rehabilitation team or therapist sets both short-term and long-term goals for each problem. For example, a person with a hand injury may have restricted range of motion and weakness. The short-term goals may be to increase the range of motion by a certain amount and grip strength by so many pounds. The long-term goal may be to play the piano again. Short-term goals are set to provide an immediate, achievable target. Long-term goals are set to help people understand what they can expect from rehabilitation and where they can expect to be in several months. People are encouraged to achieve each short-term goal, and the team closely monitors the progress. The goals may be changed if people become unwilling or unable (financially or otherwise) to continue or if they progress more slowly or quickly than expected.

Regardless of the severity of the disability or the skill of the rehabilitation team, the final outcome of rehabilitation depends on the person's motivation. Some people delay recovery to gain attention from family members or friends.

Treatment of Pain and Inflammation

Therapists treat pain and inflammation. Such treatment makes movement easier and enables people to participate more fully in rehabilitation. Techniques used include heat therapy, cold therapy, electrical stimulation, traction, massage, and acupuncture. For therapists, whether to use heat or cold therapy is often a personal choice, although cold therapy seems to be more effective for acute pain.

Heat Therapy: Heat increases blood flow and makes connective tissue more flexible. It temporarily decreases joint stiffness, pain, and muscle spasms. Heat also helps reduce inflammation and the buildup of fluid in tissues (edema). Heat therapy is used to treat inflammation (including various forms of arthritis), muscle spasm, and injuries such as sprains and strains.

Heat may be applied to the body's surface or to deep tissues. Hot packs, infrared heat, paraffin (heated wax) baths, and hydrotherapy (agitated warm water) provide surface heat. Heat may be generated in deep tissues by electric currents (diathermy) or high-frequency sound waves (ultrasound).

Cold Therapy (Cryotherapy): Applying cold may help numb tissues and relieve muscle spasms, acute low back pain, and acute inflammation. Cold may be applied using an ice bag, a cold pack, or fluids (such as ethyl chloride) that cool by evaporation. The therapist limits the time and amount of cold exposure to avoid damaging tissues and reducing body temperature (causing hypothermia). Cold is not applied to tissues with a reduced blood supply (for example, when the arteries are narrowed by peripheral arterial disease).

Electrical Stimulation: If muscles lack proper nerve input (because of a peripheral nerve injury, spinal cord disorder, or stroke), the muscles quickly waste away (atrophy), and become stiff and contracted (spastic). Electrical stimulation by electrodes placed on the skin causes the muscles to contract, providing a form of exercise that helps prevent atrophy and spasticity.

One form of electrical stimulation—called transcutaneous electrical nerve stimulation (TENS)—uses

TYPES OF HEAT THERAPY

TYPE	DESCRIPTION	COMMENT	USES
Heat applied to the body's surface			
Infrared heat	Heat applied with a lamp	Care needed to avoid burns Not used in people with a severe heart, liver, or kidney disorder, peripheral vascular disease, or reduced skin sensation	Arthralgia Arthritis (various forms) Back pain Fibromyalgia Muscle spasm Myositis Neuralgia Sprains Strains
Hot packs	Cotton cloth containers filled with silicate gel, usually warmed in a microwave oven	Same as for infrared heat	Tenosynovitis Whiplash injuries
Paraffin bath	Dipping in, immersion in, or painting with melted wax	Usually applied to small joints, such as those of the hand, knee, or elbow Not used for open wounds	
Hydrotherapy	Immersion in agitated warm water in a large industrial whirlpool	Enhances wound healing by stimulating blood flow and helping clean out burns and wounds Relaxes muscles and relieves pain Helps with range-of-motion exercises	
Heat applied to deep tissues			
Diathermy, shortwave	Heat produced by an oscillating, high-frequency electromagnetic field	Not used in people with cancer, bleeding disorders, peripheral vascular disease, reduced skin sensation, nonremovable prostheses, or implanted metal devices (such as pacemakers)	Pain due to kidney stones, pelvic infections, or sinusitis (short-term or chronic)
Diathermy, microwave	Heat produced by microwaves	Simpler to apply and more comfortable than shortwave diathermy Evenly warms deep tissues (such as muscles) without undue heating of the skin Same limits to use as for shortwave diathermy	
Ultrasound	High-frequency sound waves to penetrate deep into tissues, vibrating them and producing heat, which draws blood (with oxygen and nutrients) to the area	Not applied to tissues whose blood supply has been reduced (ischemia), numbed or actively infected areas, bones that are healing, or certain parts of the body (such as the eyes, brain, spinal cord, ears, heart, or reproductive organs) Not used in people with a tendency to bleed or cancer	Bone injuries Bursitis Complex regional pain syndrome Contractures Osteoarthritis Tendinitis

low current that does not cause muscles to contract. TENS may be useful for chronic back pain, rheumatoid arthritis, a sprained ankle, shingles, or a localized area of pain. For TENS, a handheld, battery-powered device produces the current, which is applied through electrodes placed on the skin. The device produces a tingling sensation but is not painful.

TENS may be applied several times a day for 20 minutes to several hours, depending on the severity of the pain. Often, people can be taught to use the TENS device at home as needed. Most people tolerate the therapy well, but not all people experience pain relief. TENS may cause abnormal heart rhythms (arrhythmias). Thus, people who have a severe heart disorder or a pacemaker should not use it. TENS should not be applied to or near the eyes.

Traction: Neck (cervical) traction may be used in a hospital, rehabilitation center, or at home to treat chronic neck pain due to cervical spondylosis, disk prolapse, whiplash injuries, or torticollis. Traction is more effective when people are sitting than when they are lying in bed. A system that uses a motor is usually most effective. Typically, traction is combined with other physical therapy, including exercises and manual stretching. Although cervical traction devices are available through consumer catalogues, therapists should select the type of device and determine the amount of weight to be used. People should not use such devices alone. A family member should be available to release the weight gently, which reduces the risk of injury.

Massage: Massage may relieve pain, reduce swelling, and help loosen tight (contracted) tissue. Only a licensed massage therapist should perform massage for treatment of an injury. Massage should not be used to treat infections or thrombophlebitis.

Acupuncture: Thin needles are inserted through the skin at specific body sites, often far from the site of pain. The needles may be twirled rapidly and intermittently for a few minutes, or a low electric current is applied through the needles. Acupuncture may stimulate the brain to produce endorphins. Endorphins, produced naturally in the brain, block pain sensations and reduce inflammation (see page 2061). Acupuncture is sometimes used with other treatments to manage chronic pain and to help with rehabilitation after stroke. Acupuncture should be done by a certified acupuncturist and with sterile needles.

Physical Therapy

Physical therapy involves exercising and manipulating the body. It can improve joint and muscle function, helping people stand, balance, walk, and climb stairs better. Techniques include range-of-motion exercises, muscle-strengthening exercises, coordination and balance exercises, ambulation (walking) exercises, general conditioning exercises, transfer training, and use of a tilt table.

Range-of-Motion Exercises: Range of motion commonly becomes restricted after a stroke or prolonged bed rest. Restricted range of motion can cause pain, interfere with a person's ability to function, and increase the risk of skin being worn away (skin breakdown) and pressure sores. Range of motion typically decreases as people age, although this decrease does not usually prevent healthy older people from being able to care for themselves.

Before beginning therapy, the physical therapist evaluates range of motion with an instrument called a goniometer, which measures the largest angle a joint can move through. The therapist also determines whether restricted motion results from tight muscles or from tight ligaments and tendons. If tight muscles are the cause, a joint may be stretched more vigorously. If tight ligaments or tendons are the cause, gentle stretching is attempted, but surgery is sometimes needed before progress can be made with range-of-motion exercises. Stretching is usually most effective and least painful when tissues are warmed up. Thus, therapists may apply heat first.

There are three types of range-of-motion exercises:

- **Active exercise:** This type is for people who can exercise a muscle or joint without help. They must move their limbs themselves.

Some Uses for Massage

- Amputation
- Arthritis
- Bruises
- Bursitis
- Cerebral palsy
- Fibromyalgia
- Fractures
- Hemiplegia
- Joint injuries
- Low back pain
- Multiple sclerosis
- Neuritis
- Paraplegia
- Periarthritis
- Peripheral nerve injuries
- Quadriplegia
- Sprains
- Strains
- Tight (contracted) tissues

Increasing the Shoulder's Range of Motion

A therapist stabilizes the person's shoulder with one hand while slowly raising the person's elbow as high as possible with the other. Over several sessions, the elbow is gradually moved higher, increasing the joint's range of motion.

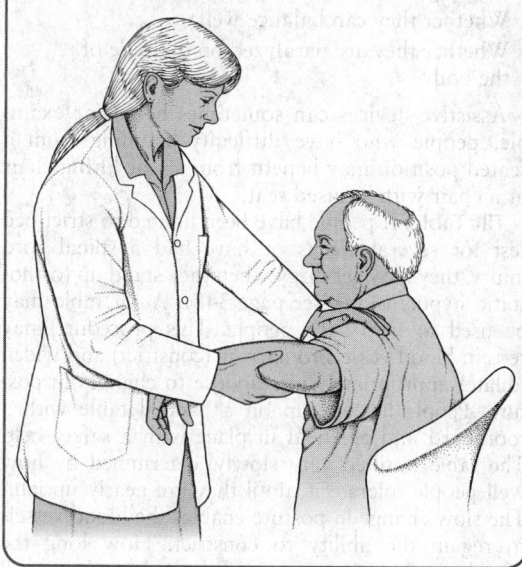

- **Active-assistive exercise:** This type is for people who can move their muscles with a little help or who can move their joints but feel pain when they do. People move their limbs themselves, but a therapist helps them do so, by hand or with bands or other equipment.
- **Passive exercise:** This type is for people who cannot actively participate in exercise. No effort is required from them. The therapist moves their limbs.

Active-assistive and passive range-of-motion exercises are done very gently to avoid injury, although some discomfort may be unavoidable.

To increase range of motion, the therapist must move an affected joint beyond the point of pain, but the movement should not cause residual pain (pain that continues once the movement is stopped). Sustained moderate stretching is more effective than momentary forceful stretching. For sustained stretching, appropriately heavy weights with pulleys are applied for about 20 minutes per day.

Muscle-Strengthening Exercises: Many forms of exercise increase muscle strength. All involve pro-

gressively increased resistance. When a muscle is very weak, movement against gravity alone is sufficient. As muscle strength increases, resistance is gradually increased by using stretchy bands or weights. In this way, muscle size (mass) and strength are increased, and endurance improves.

Coordination and Balance Exercises: These exercises can help people who have problems with coordination and balance, usually because of a stroke or brain damage. Coordination exercises aim to help people do specific tasks. The exercises involve repeating a meaningful movement that works more than one joint and muscle, such as picking up an object or touching a body part. Balance exercises are initially done using parallel bars, with a therapist standing right behind the person. The person shifts weight between the right and left legs in a swaying motion. Once this exercise can be done safely, weight can be shifted forward and backward. When these exercises are mastered, the person can do them without parallel bars.

Ambulation Exercises: Walking (ambulation)—independently or with assistance—may be the main goal of rehabilitation. Before starting ambulation exercises, people must be able to balance while standing. To improve balance, people usually hold onto parallel bars and shift weight from side to side and from front to back. To keep them safe, the therapist stands in front of or behind them. Some people need to improve a joint's range of motion or muscle strength. Some people need an orthotic device such as a brace.

> ### ❓ Did You Know...
> For people who have difficulty walking, learning to safely move from bed to chair or from chair to toilet can help them live independently.

When people are ready for ambulation exercises, they may begin on parallel bars, then progress to walking with mechanical aids, such as a walker, crutches, or a cane. Some people need to wear an assistive belt, which the therapist uses to prevent them from falling.

As soon as people can walk safely on a level surface, they may be taught how to step over curbs or to climb stairs. When climbing up stairs, they are instructed to step up with the unaffected leg first. To climb down stairs, they are instructed to step down with the affected leg first. The phrase "good is up, bad is down" can help people remember. Family members and caregivers who help people walk should learn how to support them correctly.

Helping a Person Walk

If a person needs support while walking, family members or caregivers can place their arm under the person's arm and gently grasp the forearm. Then they should lock their arm, pressing their upper arm firmly against the person's upper arm. Thus, if the person starts to fall, support is provided at the person's shoulder. The person may wear a special belt that caregivers can grasp from the back, if needed, to steady the person.

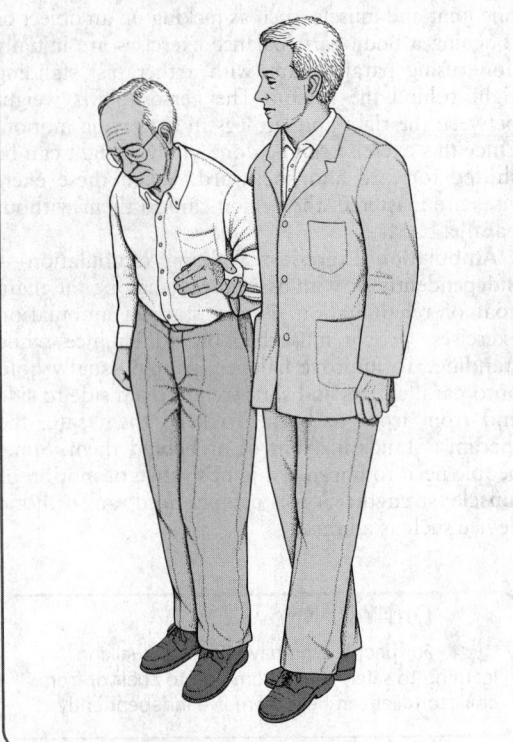

General Conditioning Exercises: A combination of range-of-motion, muscle-strengthening, and ambulation exercises is used to counter the effects of prolonged bed rest or immobilization. General conditioning exercises help improve cardiovascular fitness (the ability of the heart, lungs, and blood vessels to deliver oxygen to working muscles), as well as maintain flexibility and muscle strength.

Transfer Training: For many people (particularly those who have had a hip fracture, an amputation, or a stroke), transfer training is a critical goal of rehabilitation. Being able to transfer safely and independently from bed to chair, chair to toilet, or chair to a standing position is essential to remaining at home. People who cannot transfer without help usually require 24-hour assistance. Caregivers may help them transfer using special devices, such as a gait belt or harness.

The techniques used in transfer training depend on the following:

- Whether people can bear weight on one or both legs
- Whether they can balance well
- Whether they are paralyzed on one side of the body

Assistive devices can sometimes help. For example, people who have difficulty standing from a seated position may benefit from a seat-lifting chair or a chair with a raised seat.

Tilt Table: If people have been limited to strict bed rest for several weeks or have had a spinal cord injury, they may get dizzy when they stand up (orthostatic hypotension—see page 348). A tilt table may be used to help such people. This procedure may retrain blood vessels to narrow (constrict) and widen (dilate) appropriately in response to changes in posture. People lie face up on a padded table with a footboard and are held in place with a safety belt. The table is tilted very slowly, determined by how well people tolerate it, until they are nearly upright. The slow change in posture enables the blood vessels to regain the ability to constrict. How long the upright position is maintained depends on how well people tolerate it, but it should not exceed 45 minutes. The tilt-table procedure is done once or twice a day. Its effectiveness varies depending on the type and degree of disability.

Occupational Therapy

Occupational therapy is intended to enhance a person's ability to do basic self-care activities, useful work, and leisure activities. This therapy focuses on the coordination of many abilities required for even simple activities:

- The ability to feel and move
- The ability to create and execute a plan
- The ability to want to do the task and to persevere until it is completed

These abilities can be impaired in many ways.

Occupational therapists may detect impairments by observing the person, by doing specific tests (such as balance tests), and by talking with other health care practitioners, family members, or caregivers. Therapists assess needs by observing the person doing a task in a natural environment. They try to identify potential problems with the social and phys-

WHAT CAN INTERFERE WITH DOING A SIMPLE TASK?

ABILITY NEEDED	TYPE OF ABILITY	POSSIBLE IMPAIRMENTS
To feel and move	Sensorimotor	Impaired sensation and perception Restricted range of motion Weak muscles Short endurance Poor balance Loss of dexterity and coordination
To create and execute a plan	Cognitive	Difficulty paying attention Distractibility Loss of concentration Impaired judgment Indecision Memory problems Poor problem-solving skills
To want to do the task and to persevere until it is completed	Psychologic	Apathy Depression Anxiety Perceived incompetence Frustration Lack of persistence Decreased coping skills

ical environment. For example, family members' attitudes or inadequate lighting may interfere with the person's ability to do a task, or electrical cords across walkways may make walking hazardous.

Did You Know...

Occupational therapists focus on helping people do specific daily tasks that have become difficult to do because of a disorder or injury.

Many specialized devices, such as grabbers and large-handled utensils and tools, are available to help people function.

People with impairments work with the occupational therapist to determine and prioritize goals and to select appropriate techniques and activities. For example, if people have difficulty eating with utensils, therapy may include activities that develop fine motor skills, such as inserting pegs on a peg board. A memory game may improve recognition and recall.

Adaptive techniques can help people use their strengths to compensate for impairments. For example, a person with a paralyzed arm can learn new ways to dress, tie shoes, and fasten buttons. Activities are made more challenging as people improve.

Assistive Devices: Occupational therapists recommend devices that can help people function more independently (assistive devices). For example, a person with arthritis can be fitted with a splint to prevent joints from freezing in an abnormal position (deformity) or with a device to support damaged joints, ligaments, tendons, muscles, and bones (orthoses). Therapists may construct as well as fit such devices. Or for a person who has had an arm amputated, therapists may recommend an artificial arm (prosthesis) that includes a pincer needed to hold a utensil. Most occupational therapists can recommend appropriate wheelchairs and train people who have had an arm amputated to use their artificial limb or other devices to help them with daily tasks.

Specific Problems

For many problems—for example, heart disorders, stroke, other brain injuries, spinal injuries, hip fractures,

DEVICES THAT HELP PEOPLE FUNCTION

PROBLEM	DEVICE
Poor balance, weak legs, or dizziness	Canes, walkers, or wheelchairs Shower chairs Grab bars on the side and back of the bathtub or toilet
Weak grip	Built-up handles on eating utensils or shoehorns
Limited reach or movement	Grabbers that can pick items off the floor or from a shelf
Hand problems	Tools with built-up handles or with spring-loaded or electronic controls
Difficulty standing up because of back problems or weak legs	Raised toilet seats Seat-lifting chairs Chair leg extenders (to make the seat higher)
Paralysis (including quadriplegia) and other disorders that severely limit function	Sophisticated computer-assisted devices
Impaired vision	Larger dials on telephones
Impaired hearing	Telephones with a flashing light to replace the ring
Impaired memory	Automatic dialing telephones Drug organizers and reminders Pocket devices that record and play back messages (reminders, instructions, and lists) at the appropriate time

amputation, and loss of hearing, speech, or vision—specific rehabilitation programs are available. Rehabilitation is sometimes needed for other types of fractures (see page 1958).

Heart Disorders

Cardiac rehabilitation is useful for some people who have had a recent heart attack (see page 418), sudden onset or worsening of heart failure, or heart surgery. The goal is to maintain or regain independence or, at the least, to do basic activities of daily living, within the constraints of abnormal heart function.

Remaining in bed for longer than 2 or 3 days can lead to weakening of muscles and the heart (deconditioning) and even depression. Therefore, cardiac rehabilitation is started as soon as possible after the person has been stabilized, if needed (as after a heart attack), and usually while the person is still in the hospital.

Rehabilitation programs typically begin with light activity, such as transferring to and sitting in a chair. When these activities can be done comfortably, usually by the second or third day, more moderate activities, such as dressing, grooming, and walking short distances, are begun. If fatigue or discomfort occurs as activity is increased (as when walking the length of the hall), the person is instructed to stop immediately and rest until symptoms disappear. A doctor then reassesses the person's readiness to continue rehabilitation.

After discharge, the amount and intensity of activity are slowly increased, and a full range of normal activities can be resumed after about 6 weeks. Most people benefit from an outpatient cardiac rehabilitation program, which is usually about 12 weeks long, because they receive instruction and are monitored. For example, they may receive help with handling the psychologic effects of having had a heart attack or heart surgery. People learn why changes in lifestyle are necessary and how to make them, so that risk factors are modified. Quitting smoking, losing weight, controlling blood pressure, reducing blood cholesterol levels through diet or drugs, and doing daily aerobic exercises all help prevent or slow the progression of coronary artery disease and reduce the risk of another heart attack. Similarly, modifying risk factors may help slow the progression of heart failure.

Brain Injuries

If a stroke or head injury damages but does not destroy brain tissue, the tissue can gradually recover its function. Recovery can take 6 months to several years, but rehabilitation can speed recovery and make it more complete. Brain tissue that is destroyed cannot recover its function, but other parts of the brain sometimes learn to take over some of the duties of the destroyed area. Rehabilitation can help this learning process. The amount and rate of recovery of function cannot be predicted with certainty. Thus, rehabilitation is begun as soon as people are medically stable. Early rehabilitation also helps prevent complications such as shortened muscles (contractures), weakened muscles, and depression.

? Did You Know...

Rehabilitation for many serious disorders, such as a heart attack or hip fracture, is begun soon after the initial treatment.

People who have lost a limb may choose artificial limbs with microprocessors or bionic parts that provide more precise control of movements.

A detailed evaluation of the person, including psychologic testing, helps the rehabilitation team identify the type and severity of damage. Members of the team then assess which lost functions may benefit from rehabilitation therapy and create a program focusing on the person's specific needs. The success of rehabilitation depends on the person's general condition, range of motion, muscle strength, bowel and bladder function, functional ability before the brain injury, social situation, learning ability, motivation, coping skills, and readiness to participate in a rehabilitation program.

If brain injury results in weakened or paralyzed limbs, therapists move the affected limbs or encourage the person to move them. Moving the affected limbs helps prevent or relieve contractures and maintain the joints' range of motion. Usually, the unaffected limbs should also be exercised regularly to maintain muscle tone and strength. The person is expected to practice other activities, such as moving in bed, turning, changing position, and sitting up. Being able to get out of bed and transfer to a chair or wheelchair safely and independently is important to a person's physical and mental health. Coordination exercises may also be needed. Sometimes therapists restrain the unaffected limb (called constraint-induced movement therapy). For example, people with a partially paralyzed arm may wear a mitt or sling on their unaffected arm as they repeatedly practice daily activities, such as eating, washing, grooming, writing, and opening doors. This strategy helps rewire the brain to use the weakened or paralyzed limb.

Some problems due to brain injury require specific therapies—for example, to help with walking (gait or ambulation training), to improve coordination and balance, to reduce spasticity (continuous contraction of muscles), or to compensate for vision or speech problems. For example, people who are having trouble walking may be taught how to prevent falls. Occupational therapy may improve coordination. Heat or cold therapy may temporarily decrease spasticity in muscles and allow muscles to be stretched. People with one-sided blindness may be taught how to avoid bumping into door frames or other obstacles—for example, by turning the head toward the affected side.

A stroke or another brain injury, especially concussion (see page 737), can impair the ability to think (cognition). People may have problems with orientation, attention and concentration, perception, comprehension, learning, organization of thought, problem solving, memory, and speech (see page 56). Which problems people have depends on the injury. Cognitive rehabilitation is a very slow process, has to be tailored to each person's situation, and requires one-on-one treatment. The goals are to retrain the brain and to teach ways to compensate for problems. For example, tasks, such as tying a shoe, are broken down into simple parts and practiced. Verbal, visual, and tactile (touch) cues, such as verbal hints, gestures, and color-coding items, also help people learn and remember how to do the task.

Spinal Injuries

Recovery from spinal cord injury depends on the location (level) and degree of damage (see page 793). The higher the level of injury, the greater the physical impairment. Injury at the level of the chest or below usually causes weakness or paralysis of the legs (paraplegia). Injury at the level of the neck usually causes weakness or paralysis of all four limbs (quadriplegia). If the level of injury is very high in the neck, the muscles that control breathing may be paralyzed, and a ventilator may be needed to assist breathing. Sensation also is impaired below the level of injury, and bladder and bowel control is usually lost.

The two most important aspects of caring for people with quadriplegia or paraplegia are the following:

- **Preventing pressure sores:** To prevent pressure sores, people move or are turned frequently, and a special bed or bedding material is used (see page 1300). When people are seated in a wheelchair, a special cushion that contains water, air, or gel is used to reduce pressure on areas where sores tend to form.

- **Maintaining joint mobility (range of motion):** To maintain joint mobility and prevent spasticity, the person or a caregiver must frequently move joints through their range of motion. Heat, massage, and some drugs may also be used.

People with paraplegia can live independently. Range-of-motion and strengthening exercises of the arms and hands enable them to use a wheelchair and to transfer from bed to a wheelchair and from a wheelchair to a toilet or a car seat. They can do many activities of daily living on their own, and many return to work. Some paraplegics can drive a car with the help of assistive devices.

People with quadriplegia can use a motorized wheelchair to move independently, but they must be lifted into the wheelchair manually or mechanically. Some quadriplegics can move their hands or fingers slightly and thus can operate the motorized wheel-chair with a hand switch. If the hands and arms are completely paralyzed, quadriplegics can use a special device that enables them to control the motorized wheelchair with chin movements or even their breath. However, this method requires very intensive training. Most quadriplegics need support 24 hours a day.

Hip Fracture

Rehabilitation is begun as soon as possible after hip fracture surgery, often within a day. The initial goals are to help people retain the level of strength they had before the fracture (by keeping them mobile and by preventing loss of muscle tone) and to prevent problems that result from bed rest. The ultimate goal is to restore their ability to walk as well as they were able to before the fracture.

As soon as possible, sometimes within hours of surgery, people are encouraged to sit in a chair. Sitting reduces the risk of pressure sores and blood clots and eases the transition to standing. They are taught to do daily exercises to strengthen the trunk and arm muscles and are sometimes taught exercises

Just the Right Height

For people who are recovering from a leg injury or surgery, using a cane that is the correct height is important. A cane that is too long or too short can cause low back pain, poor posture, and instability. The cane should be held on the side opposite the injured leg.

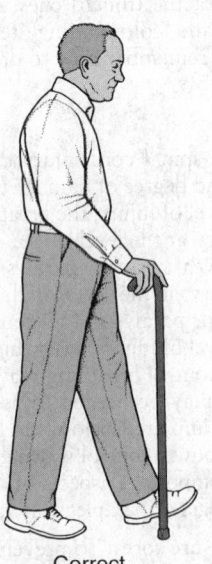

Correct

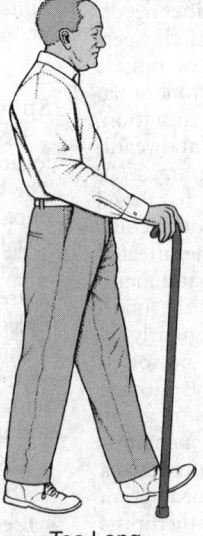

Too Long

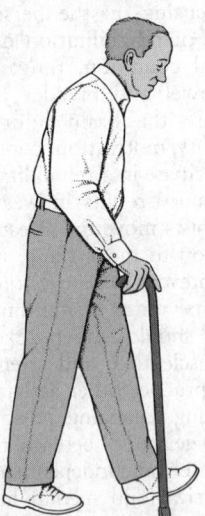

Too Short

to strengthen the large muscles of both legs. Usually within the first day after surgery, they are encouraged to stand on the uninjured leg, often with the assistance of another person or while holding onto a chair or a bed rail. While doing these exercises, people are directed to touch only the tips of the toes of the injured leg to the floor. Putting their full weight on the injured leg is often encouraged on the second day after surgery but depends on the kind of fracture and repair.

Ambulation (walking) exercises are started after 4 to 8 days as long as people can bear full weight on the injured leg without discomfort and can balance well enough. Stair-climbing exercises are started soon after walking is resumed. In addition, people may be taught how to use a cane or another assistive device and how to reduce the risk of falls.

Limb Amputation

Before surgery, a surgeon, prosthetist, and physical therapist discuss plans and goals with the person who requires amputation. A prosthetist is an expert who fits, builds, and adjusts artificial limbs (prostheses) and provides advice about how to use them. The exercises used in rehabilitation may be started before the amputation.

A prosthesis for a limb (arm or leg) consists of a socket in a rigid frame (interface), components, and a cover. The interface enables the prosthesis to be attached to the body. Components include terminal devices (such as artificial hands, feet, fingers, or toes) and artificial joints.

Arm (Upper-Limb) Amputation: Most arm amputations result from occupational injuries. Rarely, all or part of an arm is removed surgically to treat a disorder (such as cancer). The arm can be amputated below the elbow, above the elbow, or at the shoulder. Or a hand or one or more figures can be amputated.

After arm amputation, most people are fitted for an artificial arm (an upper-limb prosthesis). Components may include fingers, a hook or hand, a wrist unit, and, for an above-the-elbow amputation, an elbow unit. Movement of the hook or hand is controlled by movement of the shoulder muscles. A hook may be more functional, but most people prefer the way a hand looks. Control of an above-the-elbow prosthesis is more complicated than that of a below-the-elbow prosthesis. Newer prostheses that are controlled by microprocessors and powered myoelectrically (using energy produced by the person's muscles) have been developed, enabling the person to control movements with more precision. Bionic components, which are just now becoming available, may enable people to function even better. Rehabilitation includes general conditioning exercises and exercises to stretch the shoulder and elbow and to strengthen arm muscles. Endurance exercises may also be necessary. The specific exercise program prescribed depends on whether one or both arms were amputated and how much of the arm was amputated. People learn how to do activities of daily living using the prosthesis, adaptive devices, or other parts of the body (such as the mouth and feet).

Leg (Lower-Limb) Amputation: These amputations result almost equally from an injury (as in a motor vehicle crash or during combat) or from a surgical procedure to treat a complication of a disorder (such as decreased circulation due to atherosclerosis or diabetes). The leg can be amputated below the knee, above the knee, or at the hip. Or a foot or one or more toes may be amputated.

After leg amputation, most people are fitted for an artificial leg (a lower-limb prosthesis). Components may include toes, a foot, and, for an above-the-knee amputation, a knee unit. Newer prostheses that are controlled by microprocessors and powered myoelectrically or prostheses with bionic components enable people to control movements with more precision.

Rehabilitation includes exercises for general conditioning and exercises to stretch the hip and knee and to strengthen all arm and leg muscles. The person is encouraged to begin standing and balancing exercises with parallel bars as soon as possible. Endurance exercises may be needed. The specific program prescribed depends on whether one or both legs were amputated and how much of the leg was amputated.

The muscles near the amputated limb or at the hip or knee joint tend to shorten. This shortening (called contractures) usually results from sitting in a chair or wheelchair for a long time or from lying in bed with the body out of alignment. Contractures limit the range of motion. If a contracture is severe, a prosthesis may not fit correctly, or the person may become unable to use the prosthesis. Therapists or nurses teach the person ways to prevent contractures.

Therapists help people learn how to condition the stump, which promotes the natural process of stump shrinking. The stump must shrink before a prosthesis is fitted. An elastic stump shrinker or bandages worn 24 hours a day can help shape the stump and prevent fluid buildup in tissues. Soon after the amputation, people may be given a temporary prosthesis so that they may begin walking sooner and thus help the stump shrink. With a temporary prosthesis, people can start ambulation exercises on parallel bars and progress to walking with crutches or a cane until a permanent prosthesis is made. Sometimes people use a prosthesis with permanent components but with a temporary socket and frame. Because some parts remain the same, people may adjust to the new parts more quickly.

If a permanent prosthesis is made before the stump stops shrinking, adjustments may be needed to make it comfortable and to enable people to walk well. A permanent prosthesis is usually made several weeks after amputation to give the stump time to shrink completely.

When people receive the prosthesis, they are taught the basics of using it:

- How to put the prosthesis on
- How to take it off
- How to walk with it
- How to care for the prosthesis and the skin of the stump

Training is usually continued, preferably by a team of specialists. A physical therapist develops a program of exercises to improve strength, balance, flexibility, and cardiovascular fitness. The therapist teaches people more about how to walk with a prosthesis. Walking begins with direct assistance and progresses to walking with a walker, then with a cane. Within a few weeks, many people walk without a cane. The therapist teaches them to use stairs, walk up and down hills, and cross other uneven surfaces. Younger people may be taught to run and participate in athletic activities. Progress is slower and more limited for people who have above-the-knee amputation, for older people, and for people who are weak or poorly motivated.

The prosthesis needed for an above-the-knee amputation weighs much more than that for a below-the-knee amputation, and controlling a prosthetic knee joint requires skill. Walking requires 10 to 40% more energy after a below-the-knee amputation and 60 to 100% more energy after an above-the-knee amputation.

Pain: After an arm or a leg amputation, people may feel pain that seems to be in amputated limb (phantom pain). The pain is real, but the location is wrong. Phantom pain is more likely if pain before amputation was severe or lasted a long time. Phantom pain is often more severe soon after the amputation, then decreases over time. For many people, phantom pain is more common when the prosthesis is not being worn (for example, during the night). If a spinal anesthetic and a general anesthetic are used during surgery, the risk of having this pain is reduced.

Some people experience phantom limb sensation, which is not painful but feels as if the amputated limb is still there. When people with an amputated leg have this sensation, they may stand up (and thus fall back

down). This experience usually occurs at night when people wake to use the bathroom. Phantom limb sensation is more common than phantom pain.

The stump itself may be painful. Massaging the stump sometimes helps relieve this pain. The pain may be due to infection or wearing away of the skin (skin breakdown). In such cases, people may need to see a doctor.

Speech Disorders

Aphasia: Aphasia is partial or complete loss of the ability to express or understand spoken or written words. It often results from a stroke or another brain injury that affects the language center in the brain (see art on page 678).

The goal of rehabilitation is to establish the most effective means of communication. For people with mild impairment, a speech therapist uses an approach that emphasizes ideas and thoughts rather than words. Pointing to an object or picture, gesturing, nodding, and relying on facial expressions are often sufficient for basic communication. For people with more severe impairment, a stimulation approach (frequently repeating words to the person) and a programmed stimulation approach (speaking words and presenting objects that can be touched and seen) help people regain some ability to use language. People with aphasia may use a letter or picture board to communicate.

Caregivers of a person with aphasia need to be very patient and to understand the person's frustration. Caregivers must also realize that the person is not mentally impaired and should not be spoken to in baby language, which is insulting. Instead, caregivers should speak normally and, if necessary, use gestures or point to objects.

Dysarthria: People cannot articulate words normally because part of the nervous system that controls muscles used in speech is damaged.

Rehabilitation goals depend on the cause of the dysarthria. If the cause is a stroke, a head injury, or brain surgery, the goal is to restore and preserve speech. If dysarthria is mild, repetition of words or sentences may enable people to relearn to use facial muscles and the tongue for correct pronunciation. If dysarthria is severe, people may be taught to use a letter or picture board or electronic communication device.

If dysarthria is caused by a progressive disorder of the nervous system, such as amyotrophic lateral sclerosis (Lou Gehrig's disease) or multiple sclerosis, the goal of therapy is to maintain speech function for as long as possible. People are taught exercises that increase control of the mouth, tongue, and lips and to speak more slowly and use shorter phrases. Poor control of breathing muscles may force people to take a breath in the middle of a sentence. Planning punctuation in a sentence can help. Doing breathing exercises can also help, sometimes by breathing through handheld assistive devices, which help dislodge mucus in the airways.

Verbal Apraxia: Verbal apraxia is the inability to produce the basic sound units of speech because of an abnormality in initiating, coordinating, or sequencing the muscle movements needed to talk. Verbal apraxia is often caused by brain injury, as results from a stroke or head injury. A therapist may have people practice making sound patterns over and over or teach them to use the natural melody and rhythm of common phrases. Every phrase has its own melody and rhythm depending on the mood of the speaker. For example, "Good morning! How are you?" has a particular melody and rhythm when the speaker is feeling cheerful than it does when the speaker is feeling unsociable. The therapist encourages people with verbal apraxia to exaggerate the natural melody and rhythm of phrases. As people progress, the exaggeration of melody and rhythm is gradually toned down.

Blindness

Rehabilitation for people who are blind depends on whether blindness was present at birth (congenital) or at a very young age or whether it developed later in life. Children who are born blind or who become blind at a very young age usually receive special education about how to function without sight from the beginning. Thus, most of them become well adjusted. However, people who become blind later in life must learn new ways of dealing with daily living, such as how to feed themselves. Usually, people are taught the clock method. The dinner plate is pictured as a clock, and the meat is always placed at 8 o'clock, with the vegetable at 4 o'clock and the beverage at 1 o'clock.

Blind people also have to learn how to use a cane, and family members and other caregivers must learn how to walk with them. Family members are instructed not to change the location of furniture or other objects without telling the blind person. Learning how to use a seeing eye dog and Braille comes much later. In the interim, audio books help the blind participate in reading.

CHAPTER

7 Death and Dying

A century ago, most people who suffered major injuries or contracted serious infections died soon afterward. Most people expected little more than comfort measures from doctors. Today, because medical procedures commonly extend the lives of people who have serious illnesses, death is often seen as an event that can be deferred indefinitely. However, death is an intrinsic part of life, and talking about the likely outcomes of illness, including death and dying, is an important part of health care.

Doctors and patients vary in the language they use and in their comfort level regarding such discussions. People also vary in their comfort level regarding the amount of information and involvement in decision making that they want. Dying people and their loved ones should generally try to understand their situation and likely future course and to make any preferences about treatment and family support known (see page 69). People who do not wish to talk about death and dying with their doctor should understand that major decisions will often then be made without their input.

Time Course of Dying

A prognosis is a prediction of the probable course and outcome of a disease or the likelihood of recovery from a disease. People often think that the doctor knows and can predict how long an ill person will live but is withholding this information from them. The truth is that, generally, no one knows when an ill person will die. Families should not press for exact predictions or rely on those that are offered. Such exact predictions are often wrong because there is so much variation in how long people can live with a disease. Sometimes very sick people live a few months or years, well past what seems possible. Other people die quickly. If a dying person wants a particular person there at the time of death, arrangements may have to accommodate that

Communicating With a Dying Person

Many people find it difficult to discuss death openly with a dying person, mistakenly believing that the dying person does not want to discuss the condition or will be hurt by such a discussion. However, dying people usually do better when family members continue to speak with them and include them in decision making. The following suggestions can help people to feel more comfortable when communicating with a dying person:

- Listen to what the person is saying. Ask, for example, "What are you thinking?" rather than shutting down communication with such comments as "Don't talk that way."
- Talk about what the person would envision for surviving family members at a time long after death has occurred and work back toward events nearer to death. This allows for a gentle introduction to a discussion of more immediate concerns, such as the person's preferences regarding funeral arrangements and support for loved ones.
- Reminisce with the dying person; this is a way of honoring the person's life.
- Continue to speak with the dying person, even if the person is unable to speak. Other ways of communicating, such as holding the person's hand, giving the person a massage, or just being near the person, can be very comforting.

wish for an indefinite amount of time. Yet, predicting when a person will die of a disease is sometimes necessary. For example, hospice care usually requires a doctor's prognosis of less than 6 months to live.

Rather than asking their doctor "How much time do I have?" or "Am I likely to die within 6 months?," people might ask for the typical range of survival—the shortest and longest amount of time a person has lived with a similar illness. Another prediction doctors can often make is whether the ill person is now sick enough that they would not be surprised if death were to occur within a year. At that point, life is tenuous, and the possibility of worsening health and likely death lets the person plan to live as fully and comfortably as possible.

Sometimes, doctors offer hope by describing remarkable recoveries without also mentioning the high likelihood that most people who have such serious conditions will die much more quickly. Gravely ill people and their families eventually find this "hope" to have been misleading and belittling. Instead, ill people and their family members are entitled to the

most complete information available and the most realistic prognosis possible. However, they may have to clearly express their preference for such information over an excessively optimistic account.

Symptoms progress differently with different diseases. For a person dying of cancer, energy, function, and comfort usually decrease substantially only in the last month or two before death. The person then is visibly failing, and the fact that death is near becomes obvious to all. Other diseases, such as Alzheimer's disease, liver failure, and kidney failure, follow a steady decline from the beginning. Severe heart disease and chronic obstructive pulmonary disease cause a steady decline, but with episodes of serious worsening. These episodes are often followed by improvement, but usually death comes within a few days of being stable.

Choices to Make Before Death

Sick people and their families may feel swept along by the fatal illness and the various treatments, as if they have no control over the events. Some people seem to prefer this sense of having no control because it relieves them of the responsibility of deciding what should be done. Others prefer to determine all aspects of their care, sometimes even including the specifics of their funeral and burial.

Honest, open communication between patients and doctors about preferences for care at the end of life helps to ensure the best possible quality of life during a fatal illness. The doctors provide a candid assessment of the likely benefits of end-of-life treatments and their disadvantages, including effects on quality of life. People express what they do and do not want to experience. People have the chance to state their preferences for treatment, place limits on that treatment, express wishes concerning where they want to die and what they want done when death is expected, and decide whether they want to donate organs after death.

Most people who become seriously or terminally ill receive care from their regular doctor, with whom they may have a long-standing, trusting relationship. However, there are some exceptions. For example, some doctors may object to using terminal

Did You Know...

Doctors usually cannot accurately predict precisely how long an ill person will live.

Doctors are often more helpful by giving the boundaries of reasonably anticipated outcomes—the best and the worst that would not be surprising.

sedation or high doses of opioids to control pain. Both of these treatments can make dying more comfortable but have the potential to hasten death slightly. If a person prefers such treatments and their doctor cannot provide them, the person may choose to obtain medical care from another doctor. Sometimes a hospice (see page 60) can provide such care if the dying person's regular doctor can cooperate in coordinating care with the hospice team.

Choosing a Set of Health Care Practitioners to Provide Care: A system of care includes a care delivery program made up of doctors, a hospital, a nursing home, and home health care agencies. Systems of care may vary in their costs, insurance reimbursements, and patient deductibles and copayments. Asking questions of doctors, nurses, other patients and families, social workers, and case managers can help a person find the best available clinical team and their network, which makes up a system of care:

- What treatments are more readily available in different networks?
- What is the usual practice in providing information about the merits of possible treatments?
- How can a person talk to other patients and families who have been treated there?
- What experimental treatments are available?
- Does the team regularly attend to patients and families through the end of life?
- Are they proud of ensuring reliable comfort and dignity and care that matches patient and family preferences?

Choosing to Donate Organs After Death: The dying person may wish to donate organs after death. This decision is best made before death occurs and with the family in accord.

In general, people dying of a chronic illness can donate only corneas, skin, and bone. People who die more suddenly can donate more organs, such as kidneys, liver, heart, and lungs. To become an organ donor, the person usually needs only to sign a standard organ donor card and to let the doctor and family know.

Common concerns that may prevent some people from becoming organ donors can be allayed: Organ donation usually does not affect the appearance of the body at the funeral and does not cost the family any money. Also, organs are never taken until after death. The doctor should know how to arrange for organ donation, even for people who die at home or in a nursing home.

Treatment Options

Quantity Versus Quality: Often, the available choices involve a decision whether to accept the

Choosing a Doctor

When choosing a doctor (or a whole care team), a person with a potentially fatal condition or just advanced old age should ask several questions about care at the end of life:

- Does the doctor offer to treat symptoms fully (palliative care) at the end of life and provide strong opioids to fully manage pain?
- Does the doctor have substantial experience caring for dying people?
- Does the doctor care for the person until death in all settings—hospital, nursing home, or home?
- Is the doctor flexible enough to accommodate the person's prioritized treatment options for end-of-life care?
- Is the doctor familiar with home health, physical therapy, and occupational therapy services in the community—who qualifies for them, how they are paid for, and how to help people and families get more intensive services when needed?

In some cases, what a doctor may lack in experience is offset by a trusting, long-standing relationship that exists between the doctor and a patient and family and by the doctor's willingness to consult other experts.

likelihood of dying sooner but to be more comfortable or attempt to live slightly longer by receiving aggressive therapy that may increase discomfort and dependence. For example, a person dying of severe lung disease may live longer if placed on a mechanical ventilator (a machine that helps people breathe). However, most people find being on a ventilator very unpleasant and often require heavy sedation.

Some dying people and their families feel that they must try any treatment that might prolong survival, even when hope for gaining more than a little time is unrealistic. Such treatment often sacrifices the person's last few days to side effects without gaining quality time. In many cases, as a person nears death, the focus of care should shift entirely to providing comfort measures to ensure that the dying person does not suffer and has every opportunity to experience the closure that honors the life lived. Personal philosophy, values, and religious beliefs become more important when such decisions are made by and for a dying person.

People usually do best when they discuss their wishes for end-of-life care well in advance of a crisis

Services to Know About

- **Home care** is medically supervised care in a person's home by professional caregivers, who may help give drugs, assess the person's condition, and provide baths and other personal services.
- **Hospice care** is care at the end of life that emphasizes relief of symptoms and provides emotional, spiritual, and social support for a dying person and family members. The setting may be the person's home, a hospice facility, or another institution, such as a nursing home. Hospice-type care is provided in some hospitals. To obtain hospice care, a person usually has to be expected to live less than 6 months.
- **Nursing home** care is residential care in a licensed facility with nurses and support workers.
- **Respite care** is temporary care at home, in a nursing home, or in a hospice facility that enables family members or other caregivers to travel, rest, or attend to other matters. It may last days or weeks, depending on the care delivery system and funding.
- **Voluntary organizations** provide a variety of financial and support services to people who are ill and their families. Such organizations usually focus on people who have a certain disease.

electrical shocks applied to someone whose heart has stopped beating. It is the only treatment provided automatically in the hospital unless specifically decided otherwise in advance (called a do-not-resuscitate [DNR] order—see page 72). Resuscitation efforts can be prohibited by advance care planning, whether a formal advance directive (see page 69) or an agreement between the patient (or proxy if the patient is unable to make decisions) and the doctor. Once decided, the doctor writes the needed order in the patient's medical record.

Because resuscitation at best returns people to the state they were in before their heart stopped, it is not beneficial for people who are coming close to death, for whom the stopping of their heart is simply the final event. Such people are overwhelmingly unlikely to respond to resuscitation. The very few who do respond survive only briefly and often without return of full consciousness.

The decision to forgo resuscitation makes sense for most people expected to die soon, and such a decision need not weigh heavily on the family.

Location: Sometimes dying people and their family members may prefer to have the final days at home—a familiar, supportive setting—and not in a hospital. For people who are at home, this usually requires a reminder to all caregivers not to call an ambulance when symptoms indicate the approach of death (see page 65). For people who are in the hospital, staff can help families arrange for the person to go home with all necessary treatments for comfort, such as medications and a hospital bed. If hospitalization is preferred, or is unavoidable, it is especially important to have the person's decisions regarding undesired interventions documented.

that makes their decisions urgent. Such early discussions are very important because, later on, illness often prevents people from explaining their wishes. Family members are often reluctant to decline life-prolonging treatment without clear prior direction from the ill person. This process is called advance care planning, and it can result in legally enforceable advance directives (see page 69). Advance directives should be in writing and comply with legal requirements whenever possible. However, even a conversation among the patient, family, and health care practitioners about the best course of care creates an advance care plan that is usually sufficient to guide care decisions later, when the patient is unable to make such decisions.

Feeding Tubes: Food and water given through tubes (artificial nutrition and hydration) do not usually make a dying person feel better (see page 62) or live significantly longer, though some people do benefit. If undesired, these measures can be prohibited by advance directives or by decisions at the time when tube feeding might otherwise be used.

Resuscitation: The act of trying to revive a person who has died (resuscitation) includes measures such as chest compressions, rescue breathing, drugs, and

Hospice Care

- Hospice programs focus on symptom relief, comfort care, and emotional support for the patient and family.
- Hospice programs do not emphasize diagnostic testing and prolonging life.

Hospice is a concept and a program of care that is specifically designed to minimize suffering for dying people and their family members. In the United States, hospice is the only widely available comprehensive program to support very sick people at home. Hospice programs forgo most diagnostic testing and life-prolonging treatments in favor of symptom relief. They also educate dying people and family members about appropriate care and comfort care.

Hospice always involves different types of professionals, such as doctors, nurses, social workers, and attendants (for example, home health aides). Pharmacists, nutritionists, and therapists may also be involved. Hospice program personnel care for people at home, in nursing homes, or in other care facilities. Although hospice program personnel do not usually care for people in hospitals and rehabilitation centers, many hospitals are establishing care programs that treat symptoms fully (palliative care services) to address the same care issues.

Hospice programs differ from each other in the services they readily provide and in treatments and devices they support and use. Whether hospice care serves a particular person and family best depends on their needs and wishes, on financial considerations, and on the skills and capacity of the local programs.

Hospice care can provide most necessary medical treatments, and doctors stay involved. Nurses ordinarily oversee the general plan of care, including drug use, oxygen therapy, and intravenous lines or other special equipment. Social workers, chaplains, and volunteers help address interpersonal, spiritual, and financial issues. Bereavement counselors provide support and insight during the grieving process. Hospice plans of care help family members prepare for the challenges of facing the death of a loved one and dealing with the situation at the time of death, including their roles and how to obtain needed help.

Most people ill enough to require hospice also require some assistance with daily activities (for example, dressing, bathing, and preparing food), and some may be completely dependent. Family members and friends often provide this care, and the hospice or the family can provide additional paid help from home health aides.

Medicare or insurance pays for most hospice services, but usually only after a doctor certifies that the person has a fatal disorder and is expected to live less than 6 months.

Doctors may be reluctant to use hospice because a treatable condition outside of the hospice program's capabilities could develop. However, many treatable conditions are within the scope of hospice care, and people can leave hospice at any time to try a promising treatment and re-enroll later. Therefore, this reluctance is not justified.

Symptoms During a Fatal Illness

Many fatal illnesses cause similar symptoms, including pain, shortness of breath, digestive problems, incontinence, skin breakdown, and fatigue. Depression, anxiety, confusion, unconsciousness, and disability may also occur.

Pain

Most people fear pain as they confront dying. However, nearly all people can be comfortable, and most can also remain awake and involved in the world. However, aggressive pain therapy may sometimes cause sedation or confusion.

The doctor's choice of pain reliever (analgesic) depends largely on the intensity of the pain and its cause, which the doctor determines by talking with and observing the person. Aspirin, acetaminophen, or nonsteroidal anti-inflammatory drugs (NSAIDs) are effective in relieving mild pain. However, many people need more powerful pain relievers such as opioids to treat moderate to severe pain. Opioids given by mouth, such as oxycodone, hydromorphone, morphine, and methadone, can relieve pain conveniently and effectively for many hours. More severe pain usually requires more potent opioids given by skin patch, injection, or continuous infusion into a vein. Injections into the muscle are painful and are not reliably absorbed.

Adequate drug therapy should be given early, rather than held off until the pain is intolerable. There is no usual dose. Some people need only small doses, whereas others need much larger doses for the same effect. If a lower opioid dose is no longer effective, doctors usually should increase the dose. Drug dependence may result from regular opioid use but causes no problems in dying people except the need to avoid sudden withdrawal and its uncomfortable symptoms. Drug addiction simply is not a concern when a person is close to death.

Opioids may cause side effects such as nausea, sedation, confusion, constipation, or slow or shallow breathing (respiratory depression). Most side effects other than constipation usually resolve over time or when another opioid is substituted. People who have severe or persistent side effects or inadequate pain relief often benefit from treatment by a pain specialist.

Using other drugs in addition to opioids often increases comfort and reduces the opioid dosage and side effects. Corticosteroids (such as prednisone or methylprednisolone) can reduce the pain of inflammation and swelling. Antidepressants (such as nortriptyline and doxepin) or gabapentin helps manage pain caused by abnormalities in the nerves, spinal cord, or brain. Some antidepressants such as doxepin can be given at night to help people sleep as well. Benzodiazepines (such as lorazepam) are useful for people whose pain is worsened by anxiety.

For severe pain located in one spot, a local anesthetic injected into or around a nerve (a "nerve block") given by an anesthesiologist (a doctor with special training in managing pain and supporting people during surgery) may provide relief with few side effects.

Pain-modification techniques (such as guided imagery, hypnosis, acupuncture, relaxation, and biofeedback—see page 2063) help some people.

Counseling for stress and anxiety may be very helpful as well.

> **? Did You Know...**
> Most of the distressing symptoms that occur near death can be relieved, at least to a large extent.

Shortness of Breath

Although particularly frightening to dying people, the sensation of shortness of breath and struggling to breathe (dyspnea) can usually be relieved. Various methods can usually ease dyspnea—for example, relieving fluid buildup, changing the person's position, and providing supplemental oxygen. Opioids (such as morphine) may help to ensure comfort for people who have mild, persistent dyspnea, even if they do not have pain. Taking opioids at bedtime can promote comfortable sleep by preventing the person from waking up frequently, fighting to breathe. Benzodiazepines (such as lorazepam) often help relieve the anxiety caused by dyspnea. Other useful measures include providing a cool draft from an open window or fan and maintaining a calming presence.

When these treatments are not effective, most doctors who work in hospice programs agree that a person suffering by struggling to breathe should be given an opioid dose that is high enough to relieve the perception of dyspnea, even if the person might become unconscious. A person who wants to avoid dyspnea at the end of life should make sure the doctor will treat this symptom fully, even if such a treatment leads to unconsciousness or hastens death somewhat.

Digestive Tract Problems

Digestive tract problems, including a dry mouth, nausea, constipation, and loss of appetite, are common among people who are very sick. Some of these problems are caused by the disease. Others, such as constipation, can be side effects of drugs.

Dry Mouth: A dry mouth can be relieved with wet swabs, ice chips, or hard candy. Various commercially available products can soothe chapped lips. To prevent dental problems, a caregiver should brush the person's teeth or use mouth sponges frequently to clean the teeth, gums, inside of the cheeks, and tongue.

Nausea and Vomiting: These may be caused by drugs, an intestinal obstruction, stomach disorders, a chemical imbalance, increased pressure in the skull (which occurs with certain brain tumors), or many advanced diseases. Identifiable causes of nausea or vomiting should usually be treated. A doctor

may have to change drugs or prescribe an antinausea (antiemetic) drug.

An **intestinal obstruction** may cause nausea and vomiting. The most common cause of intestinal obstruction at the end of life is cancer. Nausea and vomiting caused by an intestinal obstruction may be less troubling when treated with antiemetic drugs and sometimes corticosteroids. However, symptom relief may be only temporary. Surgical repair may be needed to open an obstruction. However, depending on the person's overall condition, likely life expectancy, and reason for the obstruction, the use of drugs to paralyze the intestine and decrease stomach secretions, sometimes with continuous suctioning of stomach secretions with a tube inserted through the nose into the stomach (nasogastric tube), may be preferable. Opioids are useful for pain relief.

Constipation: Constipation is very uncomfortable and common among dying people. A limited intake of food, fluids, and dietary fiber; a lack of physical activity; and certain drugs cause the intestine to be sluggish. Abdominal cramping may occur. A regimen of stool softeners, laxatives, and enemas may be needed to relieve constipation, especially when caused by opioids. Relief of constipation is usually beneficial, even at late stages of a disease.

Difficulty Swallowing: Difficulty swallowing (dysphagia) occurs in some people, especially after a stroke, in those with advanced dementia, or from an obstruction of the tube that connects the throat with the stomach (esophagus) with cancer. Sometimes the person can swallow safely by maintaining a certain body position while eating or by having only foods that are easy to swallow. If the problem persists, some families may want the ill relative to try a feeding tube (a tube placed directly into the stomach or small intestine).

Loss of Appetite: Loss of appetite (anorexia) eventually occurs in most people who are dying. Many conditions that cause poor food and liquid intake can be relieved, including inflammation of the stomach lining, constipation, toothache, a yeast infection in the mouth, pain, and nausea. Some people benefit from appetite stimulants such as corticosteroids taken by mouth (dexamethasone or prednisone), megestrol, or dronabinol. People who are close to dying should not have to force themselves to eat, but they may especially enjoy eating small amounts of favorite home-cooked dishes.

If death is not expected to occur within hours or days, artificial nutrition or hydration—given by vein (intravenously) or via a nasogastric tube—may also be tried for a limited time to see whether the person's comfort, mental clarity, or energy improves. Improvement often does not happen; thus many people opt not to continue. The dying person and family members should have an explicit agreement with the doctor about what they are trying to accomplish with these measures and when the artificial nutrition and hydration should be stopped if they are not helping.

During the last few days of life, anorexia is quite common and does not cause additional physical problems or suffering, even though the ill person's lack of eating or drinking may distress family members. Anorexia probably even helps people die more comfortably. As the heart and kidneys fail, an otherwise normal intake of liquids often causes dyspnea, because fluid accumulates in the lungs. A reduced food and liquid intake may lessen the need for suctioning because of less fluid in the throat and may reduce pain in people with cancer because of reduced swelling around tumors. Dehydration may even help the body release larger amounts of the body's natural pain-relieving chemicals (endorphins). Therefore, people who are dying should not usually be forced to eat or drink, especially if doing so requires restraints, intravenous or nasogastric tubes, or hospitalization.

Incontinence

Many dying people lose the ability to control bowel and bladder function (incontinence), either because of the disease or general weakness. Disposable adult diapers and attentive hygiene measures usually address the problem. Incontinent people should be kept as dry as possible, usually with frequent bedding and diaper changes. A catheter (a small tube placed into the bladder) should be used only when bedding changes cause pain or when dying people or their family members strongly prefer it.

Bedsores

Dying people are susceptible to bedsores (also called pressure ulcers), which cause discomfort and can lead to infections. Those who are very ill, move very little, are confined to bed, incontinent, poorly nourished, or sit much of the time are at greatest risk. Ordinary pressure on the skin from sitting or moving across sheets may tear or damage the skin. Every effort should be made to protect the skin, and reddened or broken skin should be reported to the doctor or nurse promptly (see page 1299). Position changes every 2 hours decrease the likelihood of bedsores. A specialized mattress or continuously inflated air-suspension bed may also help.

Fatigue

Most fatal illnesses cause fatigue. A person who is dying can try to save energy for activities that really matter. Often, making a trip to the doctor's office or continuing an exercise that is no longer helping is not essential, especially if doing so saps the energy needed for more satisfying activities. Sometimes, stimulant drugs help.

Depression and Anxiety

Feeling sad when contemplating the end of life is a natural response, but this sadness is not depression. People who are depressed usually lack interest in what is going on and may see only the bleak side of life or feel no emotions (see page 863). Providing psychologic support and allowing people to express concerns and feelings are usually the best approach. A skilled social worker, doctor, nurse, or chaplain can help with these concerns. Dying people and their family should talk to the doctor about such feelings so that depression can be diagnosed and treated. Treatment (usually a combination of antidepressant drugs and counseling) is often effective, even in the last weeks of life, because it improves the quality of the time remaining.

Anxiety is more than normal worry: Anxiety is feeling so worried and fearful that it interferes with daily activities (see page 853). Feeling uninformed or overwhelmed can cause anxiety, which may be relieved by asking caregivers for more information or help. People who typically feel anxiety during periods of stress may be more likely to feel anxiety when dying. Strategies that have helped people in the past—including reassurance, drugs, and channeling worries into productive endeavors—will probably help them when dying. Dying people troubled by anxiety should get help from counselors and may need antianxiety drugs.

Confusion and Unconsciousness

People who are very sick become confused easily. Confusion may be triggered by a drug, a minor infection, a chemical imbalance, or even a change in living arrangements. Reassurance and reorientation may relieve the confusion, but the doctor should evaluate the possibility of treatable causes. People who are very confused may need to be mildly sedated or constantly attended by a caregiver.

A dying person who is confused does not understand dying and is often unaware of any confusion. Near death, a confused person sometimes has surprising periods of clear thinking. These episodes may be very meaningful to family members but can be misunderstood as improvement. The family should be prepared for the possibility of such episodes but should not count on them happening.

Almost half of dying people are unconscious most of the time during their last few days. If family members believe that a dying person who is unconscious is still able to hear, they can say their goodbyes as if the person hears them. Drifting off while unconscious is a peaceful way to die, especially if the person and family are at peace and all plans have been made.

Disability

Progressive disability often accompanies fatal illnesses. People may gradually become unable to tend to a house or an apartment, prepare food, handle financial matters, walk, or care for themselves. Most people who are dying need help, at least during their last weeks. Such disability should be anticipated, perhaps by choosing housing that is accessible to wheelchairs and close to family caregivers. Services such as occupational or physical therapy and home health nursing may help a person remain at home, even when the disability progresses.

Stress

A few people approach death peacefully, but most dying people and their family members experience stressful periods. Death is particularly stressful when interpersonal conflicts keep dying people and family members from sharing their last moments together in peace. Such conflicts can lead to excessive guilt or inability to grieve in survivors and can cause anguish in dying people. A family member who is caring for a dying relative at home may experience physical and emotional stress. Usually, stress in dying people and family members can be relieved somewhat with counseling or brief psychotherapy. Community services may be available to help relieve caregiver burden. If sedatives are prescribed, they usually should be taken sparingly and briefly.

When a partner dies, the survivor may be overwhelmed by having to make decisions about legal or financial matters or household management. For an older couple, the death of one may reveal the survivor's thought impairment, for which the deceased partner had compensated. If such a situation is suspected, friends and family should tell the care team before death occurs, so that resources needed to prevent undue suffering and dysfunction can be obtained.

Financial Concerns

Medicare does not pay for some services dying people need, such as long-term care in nursing homes or home health aides at home. Services provided by a hospice program are the exception in that they are usually quite comprehensive. However, hospice programs mostly provide services in the home, not all people qualify for a hospice program,

and doctors are often reluctant to certify the 6-month prognosis required for hospice coverage.

The family should investigate the cost of care for a family member's serious illness. Information about coverage and regulations can take substantial and diligent work to obtain. Consulting the doctor and care team and often involving the local Area Agency on Aging (visit the National Association for Area Agencies on Aging at www.n4a.org) or a social worker from a hospital or health plan are good places to start.

> **? Did You Know...**
> In one large study, about one third of families caring for a dying relative spent nearly all their savings.

Family members often provide most of the care at the end of life for free, but they should explore how professional caregivers can help them so that the burdens are tolerable. There may be costs of giving up employment as well as expenses of drugs, home care, and travel. The family should talk openly about costs with the doctor, insisting on reasonable attention to costs and planning ahead to limit or prepare for them.

Planning for the dying person's estate is advisable. Although discussing property and financial issues is hard to do when death is impending, it is usually a good idea. Doing so often reveals things that could be signed or arranged by the dying person, easing the burden on the family. Some attorneys specialize in elder care and can help people deal with financial and legal concerns.

Legal and Ethical Concerns

- Advance directives instruct family members and health care practitioners about a person's decisions for medical care, if the person is unable to make such decisions when they are needed.
- The Death with Dignity Act in Oregon allows terminally ill citizens of that state to end their lives through the voluntary self-administration of lethal drugs prescribed by a doctor for that purpose.

Advance Directives: People can give written directions called advance directives (see page 69) about the type of care they do and do not want to receive when dying. Advance directives are legal written agreements that will be honored in the future when people can no longer communicate their wishes. For example, advance directives can prohibit resuscitation (the act of trying to revive a person whose heart has stopped) or tube feeding, if this is the person's wish. Advance directives may be in the form of a living will, which expresses the person's preferences for medical care; a durable power of attorney, in which the ill person designates another person to make health care decisions; or both. In most states, less formal decisions made during advance care planning among a person, family, and doctor are also powerfully helpful in shaping care to suit the person's preferences.

Suicide: Although very few people actually take any steps toward causing their own deaths, many dying people at least consider suicide—even more so as the public debate about assisted suicide grows. Discussing suicide with a doctor may help sort out the issues and often correct certain problems that prompted consideration of suicide. The doctor can increase efforts to control pain, depression, and other troubling symptoms. Other members of the care team, such as clergy members, can assure the person and family that they are cherished and help them find meaning. Nevertheless, some people opt for suicide to relieve an intolerable situation or to retain control of when and how they wish to die. Most people find that they have enough control by refusing treatments that might prolong life, including feeding tubes and ventilators. Making decisions to forgo life-sustaining treatment is not considered suicide.

The Death With Dignity Act was passed in Oregon in 1997, and similar measures are being considered in other states. This law has made it legal for doctors in Oregon to prescribe lethal combinations of drugs for competent terminally ill people (a phrase that has a specific legal definition) to take when they decide to die. This law includes several measures to prevent potential abuses:

- A mandatory waiting period
- Counseling
- A second medical opinion

Acceptance

- Dying people and their family members can often achieve a deep sense of peace by mending relationships.
- Grieving often progresses through five emotional stages: denial, anger, bargaining, depression, and acceptance.

Preparing for death often means finishing a life's work, setting things right with family and friends, and making peace with the inevitable. Spiritual and religious issues are important to many dying people and their families. Members of the clergy are part of the care team in some hospice and hospital facilities, and professional caregivers can help people and their families find appropriate spiritual assistance if they do not have a relationship with a minister or other spiritual leader.

The prospect of dying raises questions about the nature and meaning of life and the reasons for suffering and dying. No easy answers to these fundamental questions exist. In their pursuit of answers, seriously ill people and their families can use or turn to their own resources, religion, counselors, friends, and research. They can talk, participate in religious or family rituals, or engage in meaningful activities. The most effective antidote to despair is often feeling cherished by another person. The torrents of medical diagnoses and treatments should not be allowed to obliterate larger questions, meaningful experiences, and the importance of human relationships.

Grieving is a normal process that usually begins before an anticipated death. According to Elisabeth Kübler-Ross, a pioneer in death and dying studies, dying people often experience five emotional stages. These stages generally occur in the following order: denial, anger, bargaining, depression, and acceptance. People in denial may act, talk, or think as though they are not dying. Denial is usually a temporary response to overwhelming fears about loss of control, separation from loved ones, an uncertain future, and suffering. Talking to a doctor or other health care practitioner can help dying people understand that they can remain in control and can count on being comfortable and comforted. Anger may be expressed as a sense of injustice: "Why me?" Bargaining can be a sign of reasoning with death—that is, seeking more time. When dying people realize that bargaining and other strategies are not working, depression may develop. Acceptance, sometimes described as facing the inevitable, may come after discussions with family, friends, and care providers. Within this general pattern, the course varies a great deal among people, and the stages may occur in different sequences than usual.

Preparing for death is hard work, with many emotional ups and downs. However, for most people, it is a time of new understanding and growth. By dealing with past hurts and mending relationships, dying people and their family members often achieve a profound sense of peace.

When Death Is Near

At some point, deciding not to undergo cardiopulmonary resuscitation (CPR—an emergency procedure that restores heart and lung function) is appropriate for virtually all people who are dying and who can accept death. Dying people, families, and the care team should also make and record other important decisions about medical care (such as whether the dying person should be hospitalized or use a ventilator). Often, implementing these decisions requires specific actions (for instance, having the drugs at home, ready to manage symptoms).

If a person is expected to die at home, family members should rehearse whom to call (such as a doctor or hospice nurse) and know whom not to call (such as an ambulance service). They should also have help in obtaining legal advice and arranging burial or cremation services. The person or family and the care team should discuss organ and tissue donation, if appropriate, before death or immediately after death. These discussions are ordinarily mandated by law. Religious practices may affect after-death care of the body. Unusual practices should be discussed before death with the care team, as well as the dying person or family members.

Dying people and their family members should also be prepared for the characteristic physical signs that death is near. Consciousness may decrease. The limbs may become cool and perhaps bluish or mottled. Breathing may become irregular. Confusion and sleepiness may occur in the last hours.

Secretions in the throat or the relaxing of the throat muscles can lead to noisy breathing, sometimes called the death rattle. Repositioning the person or using drugs to dry secretions can minimize the noise. Such treatment is aimed at the comfort of the family or caregivers, because noisy breathing occurs at a time when the dying person is unaware of it. This breathing can continue for hours.

At the time of death, a few muscle contractions may occur, and the chest may heave as if to breathe. The heart may beat a few minutes after breathing stops, and a brief seizure may occur. Unless the dying person has a contagious infectious disease that poses a risk to others, family members should be assured that touching, caressing, and holding the body of a dying person, even for a while after the death, are acceptable. Generally, seeing the body after death is helpful to those close to the person. Doing so seems to counter the common but irrational idea later on that the person really did not die.

The last moments of a person's life can have a lasting effect on family members, friends, and caregivers. When possible, the person should be in an area that is peaceful, quiet, and physically comfortable. If desired by the person, family members, friends and clergy should be present.

When Death Occurs

Death must be pronounced in an official and timely way by an authorized person (such as a doctor or nurse), and the cause and circumstances of death must be certified. Fulfilling these requirements varies substantially in different parts of the United States. If a person plans to die at home, the family should know ahead of time what to expect and what to do. When a person has hospice care, the hospice nurse generally explains the protocol. If police or other public officials must be called, the family should know this and the officials should be notified in advance that the person is dying at home. Hospice and home care programs often have routines for notifying officials that spare the family uncomfortable encounters. If no hospice or home care agency is involved, the family should contact the medical examiner or funeral home director, preferably before death occurs, to learn what to expect. A death certificate is necessary for making insurance claims, getting access to financial accounts, conveying real property titled to the deceased, and settling the estate, so the family often needs a few dozen copies.

The family may be reluctant to ask for or approve an autopsy. Although it does not help the deceased, an autopsy may help advance knowledge about the diseases contributing to death and can help family members clear up any uncertainties about what caused death. After the autopsy, the body can be prepared by the funeral home or family for burial or cremation. Incisions made during the autopsy are hidden by clothing.

Prearranging and even prepaying for funeral services can be very helpful to the family, as can knowing the dying person's preferences for the handling of the body after death. The options can range from burial to cremation to donating the body to research. Many families have a funeral or some gathering to honor the memory of the loved one. Some choose to have a funeral service soon after the person has died, whereas others choose to have a planned memorial service a few weeks or even months later.

Getting on with life after a loved one has died depends on the nature of the relationship with the deceased, the age of the deceased, experiences near the time of the loved one's death, and the emotional and financial resources available. Also, the family often needs to examine whether they did what was expected of them and to seek reassurance. Having a talk with the doctor a few weeks after the death can help answer lingering questions. Most people who have lost a close family member experience at least 6 months of grief, which can involve disbelief, anger, depression, loneliness, disorientation, and yearning. Grief abates with time, but a sense of loss persists. People do not "get over" a death as much as they make sense of it and go on with life.

CHAPTER 8 Legal and Ethical Issues

The law has a lot to say about personal decision-making. For example, people have the legal right to make their own health care decisions. However, poor health can jeopardize people's ability to defend their legal rights. Safeguarding these rights requires advance thinking and planning. Sudden or chronic illness can cause profound weakness and confusion, which makes people vulnerable and can lead to the unwilling loss of control. Conducting personal affairs, making wishes known, and making sure those wishes are respected may be impossible for people who are physically or mentally impaired. Nevertheless, adults of any age can take steps to protect themselves against losing control over their life, and such steps are especially important for older people.

For health-related personal matters, the key planning tool is a health care advance directive, which includes both a living will and a durable power of attorney for health care. For financial and other property matters, the key legal planning tools are a durable power of attorney, a revocable trust (or living trust), and a will. Together, these legal tools help direct family, friends, health care practitioners, and the legal system so that decisions affecting health care, personal affairs, and property management and distribution are made in accordance with a person's wishes.

The legal system in the United States operates on federal, state, and local levels. State law and especially federal law dictate how property is taxed when it is given away, either while the owner is alive or after death. Federal law controls Medicare, a program that provides health care coverage for most people aged 65 and older. State laws determine how people can direct their own care if they become incapacitated. Under broad federal guidelines, state laws also determine who is qualified for benefits under Medicaid, a program that provides health care coverage for some of the poor and disabled. In addition, state laws control property distribution if a person dies with no will or trust. Because state laws differ significantly, it is important to seek an attorney's advice concerning property matters. Regarding health care matters, people can take many steps on their own and can enlist the help of their doctor, nurse, or social worker. A living will or a durable power of attorney for health care can be prepared without an attorney. However, an attorney may be helpful, especially if a person's wishes are complex or family members are not likely to be in agreement. Complex financial documents should be written by an attorney.

Capacity to Make Health Care Decisions

The law recognizes that adults—in most states, people over age 18—have the right to manage their own affairs and conduct business, including the right to make health care decisions. Emancipated minors are people below the age of adulthood (usually 18) who are also considered legally capable. The definition of this group varies by state but generally includes minors who are married or who are in the armed forces or who have obtained a court decree of emancipation.

Legal Incapacity: Legal capacity and all the rights that go with it remain in effect until death, unless a court of law determines that a person can no longer manage personal affairs in his own best interest and court intervention is necessary to protect the person (a status called legal incapacity or incompetency). Health care practitioners, even if they think the person is incapable of making a decision, cannot override the person's expressed wishes unless a court declares the person legally incapacitated. Today, state laws favor the term "incapacity" rather than

---

Legal Terms Related to Health Care

Legal capacity (competency): The right to manage one's own affairs (bestowed at age 18 in most states).

Legal incapacity (incompetency): The inability to manage one's own affairs because of injury or disability; declared by a court of law.

Clinical incapacity: The inability to make appropriate decisions regarding health care or to carry them out, as determined by a doctor or other health care practitioner.

Advance directives: Documents in the form of either a living will or a durable power of attorney for health care.

Living will: A document, sometimes called a directive to doctors, that expresses a person's wishes regarding future medical interventions when the person can no longer communicate those decisions.

Durable power of attorney for health care: A document that allows people to designate someone else to make medical treatment decisions on their behalf. Also called a proxy.

"incompetency" and define the term as task-specific—that is, every task requires different capabilities to accomplish. For example, a person may be declared legally incapacitated regarding financial affairs, yet still retain legal capacity to make medical decisions or decisions about where to live. A finding of legal incapacity by a court of law takes away all or part of a person's right to make decisions. Legal incapacity normally results in the appointment of a guardian or conservator to make necessary decisions for the person.

Clinical Incapacity: Clinical incapacity to make health care decisions is the medical judgment of a qualified doctor or other health care practitioner who determines a person is unable to do the following:

- Understand his or her medical condition or the significant benefits and risks of proposed treatment and its alternatives
- Make or communicate appropriate medical decisions

A person in a coma cannot make *any* decisions, whereas a person with a severe language problem may be able to make decisions but may be unable to communicate them. People with mild dementia may think clearly enough to understand discussions with their doctors and make some medical decisions. Also, clinical incapacity is not necessarily permanent. People who are intoxicated, delirious, comatose, severely depressed, agitated, or otherwise impaired are likely to lack the capacity to make health care decisions but may later regain that capacity. A person's ability to carry out a decision is also important for doctors to assess. For example, a person with a broken leg may be able to make decisions but be unable to carry them out. Providing the necessary support to carry out a decision becomes an important goal of care.

People with dementia may require an evaluation of their level of cognition, memory, and judgment before their doctors can proceed with medical care. Likewise, a clinical evaluation of the person's ability to conduct major legal and business transactions may be needed before a lawyer or accountant can proceed with transactions. For medical decisions, if doctors find that a person lacks capacity, they turn to someone appointed by the person or to a close relative or friend to act as substitute decision maker. This process of making health care decisions for people who cannot make decisions for themselves is rarely litigated in court. However, if the person or other appropriate party objects to a particular medical decision or to the determination of clinical incapacity, the courts may become involved. A doctor cannot go against the person's wishes unless a court declares the person legally incapacitated.

Informed Consent

Before performing any invasive tests or providing medical treatment, doctors must obtain permission from the patient in a manner that is informed, voluntary, and competent. The process is known as informed consent. People have the right to information about risks, benefits, and alternative treatments when making decisions about medical care and the freedom to choose. If the patient is not capable of understanding these elements or making a decision, the doctor turns to the person named in a durable power of attorney for health care. If none exists, the doctor may turn to another authorized surrogate decision maker.

Self-determination means that adults of sound mind have the right to decide what shall be done to their body. It is the foundation of the legal and ethical doctrine of informed consent. The process of informed consent should grow out of discussion between patients and doctors. Patients ask questions about their condition and treatment options, and doctors share facts and insights along with support and advice. Doctors should present the information in a way that is understandable to the patient and truly communicate the risks and benefits. The law requires that doctors take reasonable steps to communicate adequately with patients who do not speak English or who have other communication barriers. Informed consent is substantially achieved when patients understand:

- Their current medical status, including its likely course if no treatment is pursued
- Potentially helpful treatments, including a description and explanation of potential risks and benefits
- Usually, the practitioner's professional opinion as to the best alternative
- Uncertainties associated with each of these elements

Normally a document summarizing the discussion is signed by the patient for any major treatment decisions.

Refusing Care: Along with the right of informed consent comes the right of informed refusal. People who have legal and clinical capacity may refuse any medical care. They may refuse care even if it is something almost everyone else would accept or something that is clearly life-saving. For example, a person having a severe heart attack can decide to leave the hospital even if that is likely to lead to death. Even if other people think the decision is wrong or irrational, the decision to refuse treatment cannot be used by itself as proof that the person is incapacitated. In many cases, people refuse treatment based on fear, misunderstanding, or lack of trust. But refusal may also be a product of depression, delirium, or other medical condition. A refusal of care should prompt the doctor to initiate further discussion. A person's competent refusal of treatment is not considered to be attempted suicide, nor is the doctor's compliance with the person's wishes legally considered doctor-assisted suicide. Rather, the subsequent death is legally considered to be a natural consequence of the disease process itself.

Sometimes, a person's refusal of treatment may harm others. For example, people who refuse treatment of certain infectious diseases, such as tuberculosis, place other people at risk of infection. Also, people who refuse to allow treatment of others, such as a minor child or a dependent adult, may place that other person's health at risk. In such cases, doctors often consult lawyers, judges, and experts in ethics.

Confidentiality and HIPAA

Health care practitioners have a duty to keep personal medical information confidential. Communication between the patient and doctor is strictly confidential. Even well-meaning family members are not necessarily allowed to have information about a person's medical condition. All people are entitled to confidentiality unless they give permission for disclosure or they clearly can no longer express a preference (for example, if they are severely confused or comatose). A federal law called the Health Insurance Portability and Accountability Act (HIPAA) applies to most health care practitioners and sets detailed rules regarding privacy, access, and disclosure of information. For example, HIPAA specifies the following:

- People should normally be able to see and obtain copies of their medical records and request corrections if they find mistakes.
- Health care practitioners should routinely disclose their practices regarding privacy of personal medical information.
- Health care practitioners may share the person's medical information, but only among themselves and only as much as is necessary to provide medical care.
- Personal medical information may not be disclosed for marketing purposes.
- Health care practitioners should take reasonable precautions to ensure that their communications with the person are confidential.
- People may file complaints about privacy practices of health care practitioners.

At the same time, HIPAA rules should not be read to create barriers to normal communications with a patient's family or friends. The rules permit doctors or other health care practitioners to share information that is directly relevant to the involvement of a spouse, family members, friends, or other people identified by a patient. If the patient has the capacity to make health care decisions, the doctor may discuss this information with the family or others present if the patient agrees or, when given the opportunity, does not object. Even when the patient is not present or it is not practical to ask the patient's permission because of emergency or incapacity, a doctor may share this information with family members or friends when, in exercising professional judgment, the doctor determines that doing so would be in the best interest of the patient.

Health care practitioners are sometimes required by law to disclose certain information, usually because the condition may present a danger to others. For example, certain infectious diseases, such as human immunodeficiency virus (HIV) infection, syphilis, and tuberculosis, must be reported to state or local public health agencies. Conditions that might seriously impair a person's ability to drive, such as dementia or recent seizures, must be reported to the Department of Motor Vehicles in some states.

Advance Directives

Health care advance directives are documents that communicate a person's wishes about health care decisions in the event the person becomes incapable of making health care decisions. There are two basic kinds of advance directives: living wills and durable powers of attorney for health care.

- A living will expresses, in advance, a person's instructions or preferences about health care.
- A durable power of attorney for health care appoints a person (called an agent or proxy) to make decisions for the patient (the principal) in the event of incapacity.

Normally, people communicate their wishes directly to their doctors. But when a person can no longer communicate sufficiently, another process for decision making is needed. That is the role advance directives play. If no advance directive has been prepared, someone else may be called on to make health care decisions that the person may not want. Many states authorize default surrogate decision makers (see page 71), usually next of kin. When state law is silent, doctors and hospitals still usually turn to next of kin, although the extent of their legal authority becomes less clear. In the rare event that the issue is referred to a court, courts generally prefer to name a family member as guardian or conservator, but they may also turn to a friend or a stranger to oversee care. A durable power of attorney for health care (and, in some cases, a living will) eliminates almost any need for the courts to get involved and helps ensure that the person's health care decisions will be respected.

Management of Property: People who are incapacitated by illness may also have difficulty with nonmedical affairs. Someone may need to pay bills, manage finances, take care of property, and handle business affairs. Having plans to turn over legal authority to a trusted decision maker can minimize disruption and expenses. Three principal mechanisms allow a person to arrange in advance for property and business to be overseen by someone else: a power of attorney, a revocable trust, and joint tenancy. These arrangements are best made with the help of an attorney.

Living Will

A living will expresses a person's preferences for medical care (it is called a "living" will because it is in effect while the person is still alive). In some states, the document is called a directive to doctors or a declaration. Living wills become effective only when the person has lost capacity to make health care decisions and the person has a particular condition defined by state law—usually a terminal condition or permanent unconsciousness. Some states recognize additional conditions such as an end-stage condition (for example, advanced Alzheimer's disease) or any condition specified in the living will.

Many people believe that death is preferable to being perpetually dependent on medical equipment or having no hope of returning to a certain quality of life. Others feel just as strongly that extreme heroic measures and technology should be used to extend life as long as possible, regardless of the degree of medical intervention required or the quality of life that results. A living will allows a person to express either of these preferences (or any intermediate measure that the person finds acceptable).

To be valid, a living will must comply with state law. Many states have specific forms available for people to complete. Some states require that living wills be written in a standardized way. Most are more flexible, permitting any language as long as the document is appropriately signed and witnessed.

Examples of Language: Typically, language addresses specific issues such as cardiopulmonary resuscitation (CPR), mechanical ventilation, and artificial nutrition and hydration. Language may also address general preferences, particular combinations of circumstances, or both. For example, to indicate preferences for aggressive medical treatment, the document

might state: "I want my life to be prolonged to the greatest extent possible without regard to my condition, the chances I have for recovery, the burdens of the treatment, or the cost of the procedures." It should be noted, however, that the person's choice has certain limits. For example, health care practitioners are not required to provide treatments that are medically inappropriate or clearly futile.

To prevent heroic attempts to extend life, the document might state: "I do not want my life to be prolonged, and I do not want life-sustaining treatment (including artificial feeding and hydration) to be provided or continued if I can no longer recognize friends and loved ones and am not expected to resume an independent lifestyle." A person can also state that interventions should be limited if a disorder severely limits quality of life or a certain stage of a terminal illness has been reached. However, most living wills stipulate that comfort measures should always be given.

To express a preference for an intermediate position, the document might state: "I want my life to be prolonged, and I want life-sustaining treatment to be provided unless I am in a coma or in a persistent vegetative state that my doctors reasonably believe to be irreversible. After my doctors have reasonably concluded that I am in an irreversible condition, I do not want life-sustaining treatment (including artificial feeding and hydration) to be provided or continued."

Limitations: Living wills have substantial limitations. For example, they generally address only a narrow range of end-of-life decisions; they cannot realistically anticipate all the serious medical circumstances the person may face in the future; and the written document may not be available at the time and place needed. Nevertheless, a living will can provide general guidance to health care practitioners and the person's substitute decision makers in the face of serious illness.

Durable Power of Attorney for Health Care

A durable power of attorney for health care is a document in which one person (the principal) names another person (the agent, or the attorney-in-fact, or proxy) to make decisions about health care. A power is *durable* if it remains legally effective or becomes effective, when the principal becomes incapable of making health care decisions. Like the living will, this document may be called by different names in different states.

A durable power of attorney for health care differs from a living will in that it focuses on the decision-making process and not on a specific decision. No living will can anticipate all possible circumstances. Thus, the power of attorney can cover a far broader

? Did You Know...
Although having both is desirable, a durable power of attorney for health care usually is preferable to a living will because it is far more flexible and responsive to changing medical circumstances.

range of health care decisions. Once in effect, the agent can act in the here-and-now, review the medical record, serve as an advocate, discuss care and questions with the medical staff, and decide what the patient would want or what is in the best interest of the patient. The durable power of attorney for health care can include a living will provision—a description of health care preferences—or any other instructions but should, preferably, do so only as guidance for the agent, rather than as a binding selection.

The agent should be selected with great care. A person who strongly wishes to avoid aggressive medical treatment should not name an agent who might not carry out such wishes. For example, selecting as agent a person who believes that every possible medical intervention should be used to prolong life, or a spouse whose emotional state might make it difficult to limit or terminate care, may not be wise. A better choice for a person who has strong preferences but who does not want the limitations of a living will might be a trusted associate, advisor, or a longtime friend. An ideal agent has the ability to talk effectively with health care practitioners and act as a strong advocate, even when faced with resistance from the person's family members, friends, or health care practitioners. A person should discuss the details of possible future medical choices with the agent, because the agent should be guided by the person's preferences. In addition, a person should make sure that the agent is willing to act in this role.

If feasible, the durable power of attorney for health care should name an alternate or successor agent in case the first-named person is unable or unwilling to serve. Two or more people may be named to serve together (jointly) or alone (severally). However, such joint appointments can create conflicts and complications and should probably be avoided or discussed with an attorney.

The law of each state prescribes the essential formalities for a valid durable power of attorney for health care and should be carefully followed. Most states require two witnesses, and a few permit notarization as an alternative. A person who has capacity can cancel the durable power of attorney at any time. The choice of agent does not have to be

permanent. If circumstances change, the person can and should create a new durable power of attorney for health care.

The durable power of attorney for health care is important for younger as well as older adults. It is especially important for anyone who wants someone other than next of kin to control decision making (for example, a partner, friend, or anyone else legally unrelated). It is the only way, outside of a court proceeding (which is a complicated process), to give that person the legal authority to make health care decisions and to ensure rights of visitation and access to medical information.

Ideally, copies of the living will or durable power of attorney for health care should be given to every doctor providing care for the person and to the hospital upon admission. Copies should also be placed in the person's permanent medical record, given to the person's lawyer and the appointed agent, and placed with important papers.

Having multiple advance directives or ones that are overly complicated can create confusion. If there is both a living will and a durable power of attorney for health care, the person should stipulate which should be followed if the documents seem to conflict. In general, a durable power of attorney for health care is preferable if the patient has a trusted person to appoint as agent.

? Did You Know...
A durable power of attorney for health care is particularly important for all adults, even younger adults, who want someone other than next of kin to control decision making (for example, a partner, friend, or anyone else legally unrelated).

Surrogate Decision Making

If a person is unable to make decisions about personal health care, some other person or persons must provide direction in decision making. Such a person is called the surrogate decision maker. If there is a durable power of attorney for health care, the agent appointed by that document is authorized to make health care decisions within the scope of authority granted by the document. If the person has a court-appointed guardian with authority to make health care decisions, the guardian is the authorized surrogate.

If there is no appointed surrogate, the normal custom and practice, as well as the law in most states, permits health care practitioners to turn to next of kin as default surrogate decision makers. States that provide this option by statute typically

Medical Terms Related to Life-Sustaining Treatment

Cardiopulmonary resuscitation (CPR): An action taken to revive a person whose heart stops (cardiac arrest), whose breathing stops (respiratory arrest), or whose heart and breathing stop (cardiopulmonary arrest).

Code: The summoning of professionals trained in CPR to revive a person in cardiac, respiratory, or cardiopulmonary arrest.

No code: An order signed by a person's doctor stating that CPR should not be performed. (Also called a do-not-resuscitate [DNR] order.)

Irreversible coma: A coma or persistent vegetative state from which the person will not recover.

Terminally ill: The medical state of being near death where there is no hope of cure.

Life-sustaining treatment: Any treatment given to postpone the death of a terminally ill person.

Palliative care: Measures taken to keep a terminally ill person as comfortable as possible.

provide an order of priority of surrogates, starting with the person's spouse (or domestic partner in jurisdictions that recognize this status), then an adult child, a parent, a sibling, and then possibly other relatives. A growing number of states also authorize a close friend to act as default surrogate. If more than one person has the same priority (such as several adult children), consensus is preferred, but some states allow health care practitioners to rely on a majority decision or to request that one person be selected to decide for the group. Doctors are more likely to accept the judgment of a person who understands the person's medical situation and seems to have the best interest of the person in mind. People with no family or close friends who are alone in the hospital are far more likely to receive a court-appointed guardian. If it is not clear who should make decisions, doctors may need to consult with hospital ethics boards or lawyers.

Children also require a decision maker in medical situations. For most nonemergency medical decisions affecting children and minors, medical care cannot be given without a parent's or guardian's consent. The parent's or guardian's decision can be overridden only if a court determines that the decision constitutes neglect or abuse of the child. In some states, children can consent to certain medical treatments (such as treatment of sexually transmitted diseases, prescriptions for birth control, and abortion) without parental permission.

All surrogates, whether appointed by the person, by default, or by the court, have an obligation to follow the expressed wishes of the adult person and to act in the person's best interests, taking into account the person's values if known. Health care practitioners are responsible for honoring these wishes as well. However, health care practitioners are not required to provide treatments that are medically inappropriate, such as those that are against generally accepted health care standards. If a particular treatment is against a practitioner's conscience but is still within generally accepted health care standards, the practitioner should try to transfer a person to another doctor or institution of the surrogate's choice.

Do-Not-Resuscitate Orders

A do-not-resuscitate (DNR) order placed in a person's medical record by a doctor informs the medical staff that cardiopulmonary resuscitation (CPR— see page 1942) should not be performed. This order has been useful in preventing unnecessary and unwanted invasive treatment at the end of life.

Doctors discuss with patients the possibility of cardiopulmonary arrest (when the heart stops and breathing ceases), describe CPR procedures, and ask patients about treatment preferences. If a person is incapable of making a decision about CPR, a surrogate may make the decision based on the person's previously expressed preferences or, if such preferences are unknown, in accordance with the person's best interests.

A DNR order does not mean "do not treat." Rather, it means only that CPR will not be performed. Other treatments (for example, antibiotic therapy, transfusions, dialysis, or use of a ventilator) that may prolong life can still be provided. Treatment that keeps the person free of pain and comfortable (called palliative care) should always be given.

Most states also provide for special DNR orders that are effective outside of hospitals, wherever the person may be in the community. These are called out-of-hospital DNR orders, Comfort Care orders, No CPR orders, or other terms. Generally, they require the signature of the doctor and patient (or patient's surrogate), and they provide the patient with a visually distinct quick identification form or bracelet or necklace that emergency medical services personnel can identify and comply with. These orders are especially important for terminally ill people living in the community who want only comfort care and no resuscitation if their heart or breathing stops. Living wills and durable powers of attorney for health care are not generally effective in emergency situations.

Medical Malpractice

People can sue health care practitioners if they feel they have been injured. A wide variety of causes of action and legal proceedings may be involved. However, successful medical malpractice lawsuits generally require proof of all of the following:

- The care provided was below the ordinary standard of care that would be provided by similar health care practitioners under similar circumstances.
- A professional relationship existed between the health care practitioner and the injured person.

- The person was harmed because of the deviation from the standard of care.

Concern about lawsuits sometimes puts pressure on doctors to act in ways that are not necessarily in the best interest of their patients. For example, doctors may order tests or treatments that are not clearly medically necessary to avoid even a remote possibility of missing something and thus leaving themselves open to a lawsuit. However, most doctors understand that the best defense against malpractice lawsuits is providing excellent medical care and building close, trusting, collaborative relationships with their patients.

Drugs

9   Overview of Drugs

A drug is defined by U.S. law as any substance (other than a food or device) intended for use in the diagnosis, cure, relief, treatment, or prevention of disease or intended to affect the structure or function of the body. (Oral contraceptives are an example of drugs that affect the function of the body rather than a disease.) This comprehensive definition of a drug, although important for legal purposes, is rather complex for everyday use. A simpler but workable definition of a drug is any chemical substance that affects the body and its processes.

Some people incorrectly use the word *drug* to mean only a substance that produces a pleasurable sensation. Drug abuse—the excessive and persistent use of mind-altering substances without medical need—has accompanied the appropriate medical use of drugs throughout recorded history. Some drugs with potential for abuse have legitimate medical purposes, and others do not (see page 2078).

Prescription or Nonprescription: By law, drugs are divided into two categories: prescription drugs and nonprescription drugs. Prescription drugs—those considered safe for use only under medical supervision— may be dispensed only with a prescription from a licensed professional with governmental privileges to prescribe (for example, a physician, dentist, podiatrist, nurse practitioner, physician's assistant, or veterinarian). Nonprescription drugs—those considered safe for use without medical supervision (such as aspirin)—are sold over the counter (see page 104). In the United States, the Food and Drug Administration (FDA) is the government agency that decides which drugs require a prescription and which may be sold over the counter.

Dietary supplements (medicinal herbs and nutraceuticals—see page 2067) are products intended to supplement the diet. These products may contain vitamins, amino acids, minerals, and herbs or other plant-derived material (botanicals). Because dietary supplements do not require FDA approval before marketing, they do not have to meet the same standards as drugs for safety and effectiveness (efficacy). Although these products are not classified as drugs, they can act in the same way as a drug does in the body and may cause health problems if not used correctly or if taken in large amounts. Because these products do not meet the FDA standards for safety and efficacy, they may not claim to treat specific medical conditions.

Drug Names: Some knowledge of drug names can help in understanding drug product labels. Every drug has at least three names—a chemical name, a generic (nonproprietary or official) name, and a trade (proprietary or brand) name (see box on page 100).

The chemical name describes the atomic or molecular structure of the drug. This name is usually too complex and cumbersome for general use. So an official body assigns a generic name to a drug. The generic names for drugs of a particular type (class) usually have the same ending. For example, the names of all beta-blockers, which are used to treat such disorders as high blood pressure, end in "lol."

The trade name is chosen by the pharmaceutical company that manufactures or distributes the drug. Patented drugs are usually sold under a trade name. Generic versions of trade-name drugs—manufactured after expiration of the pharmaceutical company's patent—may be sold under the generic name (for example, ibuprofen) or under the manufacturer's own trade name (for example, Advil).

Drug Groups: Understanding what group a drug belongs to is also useful. Broadly, drugs are classified by therapeutic group—that is, by what disorder or symptom they are used to treat. For example, drugs used to treat high blood pressure are called antihypertensives, and drugs used to treat nausea are called antiemetics (emesis is the medical term for vomiting). Within each therapeutic group, drugs are categorized by classes. Some classes are based on how the drugs work in the body to produce their effect. For example, diuretics, calcium channel blockers, beta-blockers, and angiotensin-converting enzyme (ACE) inhibitors are all classes of antihypertensives that work differently.

Design and Development

Many of the drugs in current use were discovered by experiments conducted in animals and humans. However, many drugs are now being designed with the specific disorder in view. Abnormal biochemical and cellular changes caused by disease are identified, and then compounds that may specifically prevent or correct these abnormalities (by interacting with specific sites in the body) can be designed. When a new compound shows promise, its structure is usually modified many times to optimize its ability to target the intended site (selectivity), remain attached to the site (affinity), and optimize its strength (potency), effectiveness (efficacy), and safety (side effects). Other factors, such as whether the compound is absorbed through the intestinal wall and whether it is stable in body tissues and fluids, are also considered. These factors involve what the body does to the drug (drug kinetics—see page 80) and what the drug does to the body (drug dynamics—see page 85).

Ideally, a drug is highly selective for its target site, so that it has little or no effect on other body systems—that is, it has minimal or no side effects (see page 93). The drug should also be very potent and effective, so that low doses can be used, even for disorders that are difficult to treat. The drug should be effective when taken by mouth (for convenient use), absorbed well from the digestive tract, and reasonably stable in body tissues and fluids so that, ideally, one dose a day is adequate.

During drug development, standard or average doses are determined. However, people respond to drugs differently. Many factors, including age (see page 1896), weight, genetic make-up, and the presence of other disorders, affect drug response (see page 88). These factors must be considered when doctors determine the dose for a particular person.

Placebos

Placebos are substances that are made to resemble drugs but do not contain an active drug.

A placebo is made to look exactly like a real drug but is made of an inactive substance, such as a starch or sugar. Placebos are now used only in research studies (see page 2024).

Despite there being no active ingredients, some people who take a placebo feel better. Some others develop "side effects." This phenomenon, called the placebo effect, appears to occur for two reasons. The first reason is coincidental change. Many medical conditions and symptoms come and go without treatment, so a person taking a placebo may just coincidentally feel better or worse. When this change occurs, the placebo may incorrectly be credited with or blamed for the result. The second reason is anticipation (sometimes called suggestibility). Anticipating that a drug will work often actually makes people feel better. The placebo effect is mainly on symptoms rather than the actual disease. For example, a placebo will never make a broken bone heal faster, but it may make the pain seem less. Some people seem more susceptible to the placebo effect than others. People who have a positive opinion of drugs, doctors, nurses, and hospitals are more likely to respond favorably to placebos than are people who have a negative opinion.

When a new drug is being developed, investigators conduct studies to compare the effect of the drug with that of a placebo because any drug can have a placebo effect, unrelated to its action. The true drug effect must be distinguished from a placebo effect. Typically, half the study's participants are given the drug, and half are given an identical-looking placebo. Ideally, neither the participants nor the investigators know who received the drug and who received the placebo (this type of study is called a double-blind study).

When the study is completed, all changes observed in participants taking the active drug are compared with those in participants taking the placebo. The drug must perform significantly better than the placebo to justify its use. In some studies, as many as 50% of participants taking the placebo improve (an example of the placebo effect), making it difficult to show the effectiveness of the drug being tested.

Effectiveness and Safety

The main goals of drug development are effectiveness (efficacy) and safety. Because all drugs can harm as well as help, safety is relative. The difference between the usual effective dose and the dose that produces severe or life-threatening side effects is called the margin of safety. A wide margin of safety is desirable, but when treating a dangerous condition or when there are no other options, a narrow margin of safety often must be accepted. If a drug's usual effective dose is also toxic, doctors do not use the drug unless the situation is serious and there is no safer alternative.

The most useful drugs are effective and, for the most part, safe. Penicillin is such a drug. Except for people who are allergic to it, penicillin is virtually nontoxic, even in large doses. On the other hand, barbiturates, which were once commonly used as sleep aids, can interfere with breathing, dangerously lower blood pressure, and even cause death if taken in excess. Newer sleep aids such as temazepam and zolpidem have a wider margin of safety than barbiturates do.

Designing effective drugs with a wide margin of safety and few side effects cannot always be achieved. Consequently, some drugs must be used even though they have a very narrow margin of safety. For example, warfarin, which is taken to prevent blood clotting, can cause bleeding, but it is used when the need is so

---

Placebo: I Shall Please

In Latin, *placebo* means "I shall please." In 1785, the word placebo first appeared in a medical dictionary as "a commonplace method or medicine." Two editions later, the placebo had become "a make-believe medicine," allegedly inactive and harmless. Now, the profound effects of placebos, both good and bad, are well known.

FROM LABORATORY TO MEDICINE CABINET

Early Development: After a drug that may be useful in treating a disorder is identified or designed, it is studied in laboratory animals (a phase called early development). Early development gathers information about how the drug works, how effectively it works, and what toxic effects it produces, including possible effects on reproductive capacity and the health of offspring. Many drugs are rejected at this stage because they are shown to be too toxic or not effective.

If a drug seems promising after early development, an investigational new drug application is filed with the Food and Drug Administration (FDA), which, if approved, allows the drug to be tested in people (a phase called clinical studies).

Clinical Studies: These occur in several phases and only in volunteers who have given their full consent.

- Phase I evaluates the drug's safety and toxicity in people. Different amounts of the drug are given to a small number of healthy, young people to determine the dose at which toxicity first appears.
- Phase II evaluates what effect the drug has on the target disorder and what the right dose might be. Different amounts of the drug are given to a small number of selected people who have the target disorder to see whether there is any benefit. Just because a drug is effective in animals in early development does not mean it is effective in people.
- Phase III tests the drug in a much larger group of people who have the target disorder. These people are selected to be as similar as possible to the people who might use the drug in the real world. The drug's effectiveness is studied further, and any new side effects are noted. Phase III tests usually compare the new drug against an established drug, a placebo, or both.

In addition to determining a drug's effectiveness, studies in people focus on the type and frequency of side effects and on factors that make people susceptible to these effects (such as age, sex, other disorders, and the use of other drugs).

Approval: If studies indicate that the drug is effective and safe, a new drug application (including data from the animal and human tests, intended drug manufacturing procedures, prescribing information, and product labeling) is filed with the FDA, which reviews all the information and decides whether the drug is sufficiently effective and safe to be marketed. If the FDA approves, the drug becomes available for use. The whole process usually takes about 10 years. On average, only about 5 out of 4,000 drugs studied in the laboratory are studied in people, and only about 1 out of 5 drugs studied in people is approved and prescribed.

Postmarketing: After a new drug is approved, the manufacturer must monitor the use of the drug and promptly report any additional, previously undetected side effects to the FDA. Doctors and pharmacists are encouraged to participate in the ongoing monitoring of the drug. Such monitoring is important because before the drug is marketed, even comprehensive studies can detect only relatively common side effects (that occur about once in every 1,000 doses). Important side effects that occur once in every 10,000 (or more) doses can be detected only when a large number of people use the drug, that is, after it is on the market. The FDA may withdraw approval if new evidence indicates that a drug may cause severe side effects. For example, the diet aid fenfluramine was withdrawn from the market because some people who took it developed serious heart disorders.

PHASE	TEST GROUP	PURPOSE	LENGTH
Early development			
	Laboratory settings (such as cell cultures and animals)	To determine the chemical and physical characteristics of the drug and to assess the safety and effects of the drug in living organisms	2–6.5 years
Clinical studies			
Phase I	20–80 healthy volunteers	To establish basic safety and blood levels achieved with different doses of the drug	1.5 years
Phase II	Up to 100 people who have or who might develop the disorder being studied	To establish the drug's effectiveness and dosage range and to identify side effects	2 years
Phase III	300–30,000 people who have the disorder being studied	To confirm the most effective dosage regimen; to obtain more information about the drug's effectiveness and side effects not seen during phases I and II; and to compare the drug with existing drugs, a placebo, or both	3.5 years

(continued on the following page)

FROM LABORATORY TO MEDICINE CABINET (*Continued*)

PHASE	TEST GROUP	PURPOSE	LENGTH
FDA review			
	Government review of all information from early development and clinical studies	To determine whether the drug has been proven to be effective and safe	0.5–1 years
Postmarketing surveillance (sometimes called phase IV)			
	All people taking the drug, particularly subgroups such as pregnant women, children, and older people	To identify any problems that did not occur in phases I, II, or III, such as those that take a long time to appear and those that occur rarely	Ongoing

great that the risk must be tolerated. People who take warfarin need frequent checkups to see whether the drug is causing the blood to clot too much, too little, or appropriately.

Clozapine is another example. This drug often helps people with schizophrenia when all other drugs have proved ineffective. But clozapine has a serious side effect: It can decrease the production of white blood cells, which are needed to protect against infection. Because of this risk, people who take clozapine must have their blood tested frequently as long as they take the drug.

To help ensure that their treatment plan is as safe and effective as possible, people should keep their health care practitioners well informed about their medical history, drugs (including over-the-counter drugs) and dietary supplements (including medicinal herbs—see page 2067) that they are currently taking, and any other relevant health information. In addition, they should not hesitate to ask a doctor, nurse, or pharmacist to explain the goals of treatment, the types of side effects and other problems that may develop, and the extent to which they can participate in the treatment plan.

Making the Most of Drug Treatment

People can help make their treatment plan as safe and effective as possible by doing the following:

- Telling the doctor, nurse, or pharmacist:
  - What medical problems they have
  - What drugs (prescription and nonprescription) and dietary supplements (including medicinal herbs) they have taken in the previous few weeks
  - Whether they have or have had any allergies or unusual reactions to drugs, foods, or other substances
  - Whether they follow special diets or have food restrictions
  - Whether they are pregnant, plan to become pregnant, or are breastfeeding
- Knowing the brand names and generic names of a drug
- Reading the label on drug containers carefully before taking a drug whether prescription or nonprescription
- Understanding what a drug is being taken for, how to know whether the drug is working, and what side effects are possible

- Knowing how long the drug should be taken
- Not drinking alcohol if so advised
- Not chewing, cutting, or crushing a capsule or tablet unless so instructed
- Not using household spoons to measure liquid drugs
- Knowing what to do if a dose is missed
- Using simple tools like charts or drug boxes to remember to take doses at the correct times
- Storing drugs in the correct place (cool, dry place; out of sunlight; and away from children and pets)
- Disposing of expired drugs properly
- Never taking someone else's prescription drugs
- Taking recommended preventive steps and participating in recommended health programs
- Keeping a wallet-size drug list handy
- Keeping appointments
- Seeking medical care promptly when a problem develops

10 Administration and Kinetics of Drugs

Drug administration is the giving of a drug by one of several means (routes). *Drug kinetics (pharmacokinetics)* involves what the body does to a drug, including the processes of absorption, distribution, metabolism, and elimination, and how long these processes take.

Drug treatment requires getting a drug to its target site or sites—specific sites in tissues where the drug performs its action. Typically, the drug is introduced (the process of administration) into the body far from this site. The drug must move into the bloodstream (the process of absorption) and be transported to the target sites where the drug is needed (the process of distribution). Some drugs are chemically altered (the process of metabolism) by the body before they perform their action; others are metabolized afterward; and still others are not metabolized at all. The final step is the removal of the drug and its metabolites from the body (the process of elimination).

Many factors, including a person's genetic makeup, can influence these processes (see page 88). Changes due to aging also affect how the body processes drugs (see page 1896).

Administration

Drugs are introduced into the body by several routes. They may be taken by mouth (orally); given by injection into a vein (intravenously), into a muscle (intramuscularly), into the space around the spinal cord (intrathecally), or beneath the skin (subcutaneously); placed under the tongue (sublingually); inserted in the rectum (rectally) or vagina (vaginally); instilled in the eye (by the ocular route); sprayed into the nose and absorbed through the nasal membranes (nasally); breathed into the lungs, usually through the mouth (by inhalation); applied to the skin (cutaneously) for a local (topical) or bodywide (systemic) effect; or delivered through the skin by a patch (transdermally) for a systemic effect. Each route has specific purposes, advantages, and disadvantages.

Oral Route: Because the oral route is the most convenient and usually the safest and least expensive, it is the one most often used. However, it has limitations because of the way a drug typically moves through the digestive tract. For drugs administered orally, absorption may begin in the mouth and stomach. Usually, however, most of the drug is absorbed from the small intestine. The drug passes through the intestinal wall and travels to the liver before it is transported via the bloodstream to its target site. The intestinal wall and liver chemically alter (metabolize) many drugs, decreasing the amount of drug reaching the bloodstream. Consequently, these drugs are often given in smaller doses when injected intravenously to produce the same effect.

When a drug is taken orally, food and other drugs in the digestive tract may affect how much of and how fast the drug is absorbed. Thus, some drugs should be taken on an empty stomach, others should be taken with food, others should not be taken with certain other drugs, and still others cannot be taken orally at all.

Some orally administered drugs irritate the digestive tract. For example, aspirin and most other nonsteroidal anti-inflammatory drugs (NSAIDs— see page 644) can harm the lining of the stomach and small intestine and can cause or aggravate preexisting ulcers (see page 139). Other drugs are absorbed poorly or erratically in the digestive tract or are destroyed by the acid and digestive enzymes in the stomach.

Other routes of administration may be required when the oral route cannot be used: for example, when a person cannot take anything by mouth, when a drug must be administered rapidly or in a precise or very high dose, or when a drug is poorly or erratically absorbed from the digestive tract.

Injection Routes: Administration by injection (parenteral administration) includes the subcutaneous, intramuscular, intravenous, and intrathecal routes. A drug product can be prepared or manufactured in ways that prolong drug absorption from the injection site for hours, days, or longer. Such products do not need to be administered as often as drug products with more rapid absorption.

For the subcutaneous route, a needle is inserted into fatty tissue just beneath the skin. The drug is injected, then moves into small blood vessels (capillaries) and is carried away by the bloodstream or reaches the bloodstream through the lymphatic vessels. Protein drugs that are large in size, such as insulin, usually reach the bloodstream through the lymphatic vessels because these drugs move slowly from the tissues into capillaries. The subcutaneous route is used for many protein drugs because such drugs would be digested in the digestive tract if they were taken orally.

Certain drugs (such as progestin, used for birth control—see page 1598) may be given by inserting plastic capsules under the skin (subcutaneously). This route of administration is rarely used.

Through the Skin

Sometimes a drug is given through the skin—by needle (subcutaneous, intramuscular, or intravenous route), by patch (transdermal route), or by implantation.

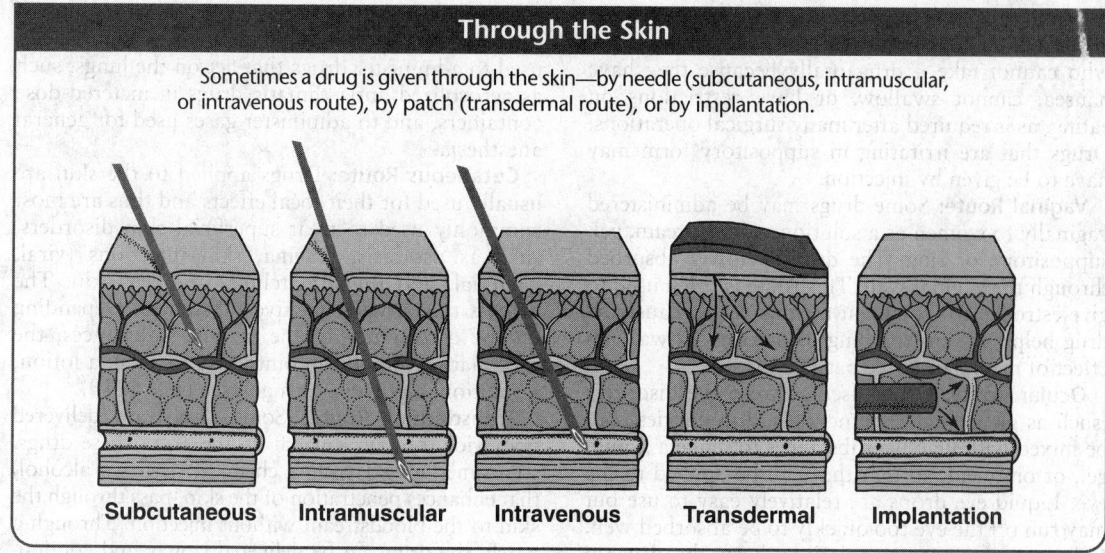

Subcutaneous **Intramuscular** **Intravenous** **Transdermal** **Implantation**

The intramuscular route is preferred to the subcutaneous route when larger volumes of a drug product are needed. Because the muscles lie below the skin and fatty tissues, a longer needle is used. Drugs are usually injected into the muscle of the upper arm, thigh, or buttock. How quickly the drug is absorbed into the bloodstream depends, in part, on the blood supply to the muscle: The sparser the blood supply, the longer it takes for the drug to be absorbed.

For the intravenous route, a needle is inserted directly into a vein. A solution containing the drug may be given in a single dose or by continuous infusion. For infusion, the solution is moved by gravity (from a collapsible plastic bag) or by an infusion pump through thin flexible tubing to a tube (catheter) inserted in a vein, usually in the forearm. Intravenous administration is the best way to deliver a precise dose quickly and in a well-controlled manner throughout the body. It is also used for irritating solutions, which would cause pain and damage tissues if given by subcutaneous or intramuscular injection. An intravenous injection can be more difficult to administer than a subcutaneous or intramuscular injection, because inserting a needle or catheter into a vein may be difficult, especially if the person is obese.

When given intravenously, a drug is immediately delivered to the bloodstream and tends to take effect more quickly than when given by any other route. Consequently, health care practitioners closely monitor people who receive an intravenous injection for signs that the drug is working or is causing undesired side effects. Also, the effect of a drug given by this route tends to last for a shorter time. Therefore, some drugs must be given by continuous infusion to keep their effect constant.

For the intrathecal route, a needle is inserted between two vertebrae in the lower spine and into the space around the spinal cord. The drug is then injected into the spinal canal. A small amount of local anesthetic is often used to numb the injection site. This route is used when a drug is needed to produce rapid or local effects on the brain, spinal cord, or the layers of tissue covering them (meninges)—for example, to treat infections of these structures. Anesthetics and analgesics (such as morphine) are sometimes given this way.

Sublingual Route: A few drugs are placed under the tongue (taken sublingually) so that they can be absorbed directly into the small blood vessels that lie beneath the tongue. The sublingual route is especially good for nitroglycerin—which is used to relieve angina (chest pain caused by an inadequate blood supply to the heart muscle)—because absorption is rapid and the drug immediately enters the bloodstream without first passing through the intestinal wall and liver. However, most drugs cannot be taken this way because they may be absorbed incompletely or erratically.

Rectal Route: Many drugs that are administered orally can also be administered rectally as a suppository. In this form, a drug is mixed with a waxy substance that dissolves or liquefies after it is inserted into the rectum. Because the rectum's wall is thin and its blood supply rich, the drug is readily absorbed. A suppository is prescribed for people who cannot take a drug orally because they have nausea, cannot swallow, or have restrictions on eating, as is required after many surgical operations. Drugs that are irritating in suppository form may have to be given by injection.

Vaginal Route: Some drugs may be administered vaginally to women as a solution, tablet, cream, gel, suppository, or ring. The drug is slowly absorbed through the vaginal wall. This route is often used to give estrogen to women at menopause, because the drug helps prevent thinning of the vaginal wall, an effect of menopause (see page 1514).

Ocular Route: Drugs used to treat eye disorders (such as glaucoma, conjunctivitis, and injuries) can be mixed with inactive substances to make a liquid, gel, or ointment, so that they can be applied to the eye. Liquid eye drops are relatively easy to use but may run off the eye too quickly to be absorbed well. Gel and ointment formulations keep the drug in contact with the eye surface longer. Solid inserts, which release the drug continuously and in slow amounts, are also available, but they may be hard to put in and keep in place. Ocular drugs are almost always used for their local effects. For example, artificial tears are used to relieve dry eyes. Other drugs (for example, those used to treat glaucoma [see table on page 1450], such as acetazolamide and betaxolol, and those used to dilate pupils, such as phenylephrine and tropicamide), produce a local effect after they are absorbed through the cornea and conjunctiva. Some of these drugs then enter the bloodstream and may have unwanted effects on other parts of the body.

Nasal Route: If a drug is to be breathed in and absorbed through the thin mucous membrane that lines the nasal passages, it must be transformed into tiny droplets in air (atomized). Once absorbed, the drug enters the bloodstream. Drugs administered by this route generally work quickly. Some of them irritate the nasal passages. Drugs that can be administered by the nasal route include nicotine (for smoking cessation), calcitonin (for osteoporosis), sumatriptan (for migraine headaches), and corticosteroids (for allergies).

Inhalation: Drugs administered by inhalation through the mouth must be atomized into smaller particles than those administered by the nasal route, so that the drug can pass through the windpipe (trachea) and into the lungs. How deeply into the lungs they go depends on the size of the droplets. Smaller droplets go deeper, which increases the amount of drug absorbed. Inside the lungs, they are absorbed into the bloodstream.

Relatively few drugs are administered this way because inhalation must be carefully monitored to ensure that a person receives the right amount of drug within a specified time. Usually, this method is used to administer drugs that act on the lungs, such as aerosolized antiasthmatic drugs in metered-dose containers, and to administer gases used for general anesthesia.

Cutaneous Route: Drugs applied to the skin are usually used for their local effects and thus are most commonly used to treat superficial skin disorders, such as psoriasis, eczema, skin infections (viral, bacterial, and fungal), itching, and dry skin. The drug is mixed with inactive substances. Depending on the consistency of the inactive substances, the formulation may be an ointment, a cream, a lotion, a solution, a powder, or a gel (see page 1279).

Transdermal Route: Some drugs are delivered bodywide through a patch on the skin. These drugs, sometimes mixed with a chemical (such as alcohol) that enhances penetration of the skin, pass through the skin to the bloodstream without injection. Through a patch, the drug can be delivered slowly and continuously for many hours or days or even longer. As a result, levels of a drug in the blood can be kept relatively constant. Patches are particularly useful for drugs that are quickly eliminated from the body because such drugs, if taken in other forms, would have to be taken frequently. However, patches may irritate the skin of some people. In addition, patches are limited by how quickly the drug can penetrate the skin. Only drugs to be given in relatively small daily doses can be given through patches. Examples of such drugs include nitroglycerin (for chest pain), scopolamine (for motion sickness), nicotine (for smoking cessation), clonidine (for high blood pressure), and fentanyl (for pain relief).

Absorption

Drug absorption is the movement of a drug into the bloodstream.

Absorption affects bioavailability—how quickly and how much of a drug reaches its intended target (site) of action. Factors that affect absorption (and therefore bioavailability) include the way a drug product is designed and manufactured, its physical and chemical properties, and the physiologic characteristics of the person taking the drug. Physiologic characteristics that may affect the absorption of drugs taken by mouth include how long the stomach takes to empty, what the acidity (pH) of the stomach is, and how quickly the drug is moved through the digestive tract.

A drug product is the actual dosage form of a drug—a tablet, capsule, suppository, transdermal patch, or solution. It consists of the drug (active ingredient) and additives (inactive ingredients). For example, tablets are a mixture of drug and diluents, stabilizers, disintegrants, and lubricants. The mixture is granulated and compressed into a tablet. The type and amount of additives and the degree of compression affect how quickly the tablet disintegrates and how quickly the drug is absorbed. Drug manufacturers adjust these variables to optimize absorption.

If a tablet releases the drug too quickly, the blood level of the drug may become too high, causing an excessive response. If the tablet does not release the drug quickly enough, much of the drug may be eliminated in the feces without being absorbed, and blood levels may be too low. Drug manufacturers formulate the tablet to release the drug at the desired speed.

Capsules consist of drugs and additives within a gelatin shell. The shell swells and releases its contents when it becomes wet, usually eroding quickly. The size of the drug particles and the properties of the additives affect how quickly the drug dissolves and is absorbed. Drugs tend to be absorbed more quickly from capsules filled with liquid than from those filled with solid particles.

Because drug products that contain the same drug (active ingredient) may have different inactive ingredients, absorption of the drug from different products may vary. Thus, a drug's effects, even at the same dose, may vary from one drug product to another. Drug products that not only contain the same active ingredient but also produce virtually the same blood levels at the same points in time are considered bioequivalent. Bioequivalence ensures therapeutic equivalence (that is, production of the same medicinal effect), and bioequivalent products are interchangeable.

If an orally administered drug can harm the stomach lining or decomposes in the acidic environment of the stomach, a tablet or capsule of the drug can be coated with a substance intended to prevent it from dissolving until it reaches the small intestine. These protective coatings are described as enteric, which refers to the small intestine. For the coatings to dissolve, they must come in contact with the less acidic environment of the small intestine or with the digestive enzymes there. However, the coatings do not always dissolve as intended. The tablet or capsule may be passed intact in the feces, especially in older people.

Some drug products are specially formulated to release their active ingredients slowly or in repeated small amounts over time—usually for a period of 12 hours or more. This dosage form is called modified-release, controlled-release, sustained-release, or extended-release.

Food, other drugs, and digestive disorders can affect drug absorption and bioavailability. For example, high-fiber foods may bind with a drug and prevent it from being absorbed. Laxatives and diarrhea, which speed up the passage of substances through the digestive tract, may reduce drug absorption. Surgical removal of parts of the digestive tract (such as the stomach or colon) may also affect drug absorption.

Where and how long a drug product is stored can affect drug bioavailability. The drug in some products deteriorates and becomes ineffective or harmful if stored improperly or kept too long. Some products must be stored in the refrigerator or in a cool, dry, or dark place. Storage directions should be followed, and expiration dates should be observed.

Distribution

Drug distribution refers to the movement of a drug to and from the blood and various tissues of the body (for example, fat, muscle, and brain tissue) and the relative proportions of drug in the tissues.

After a drug is absorbed into the bloodstream, it rapidly circulates through the body. The average circulation time of blood is 1 minute. As the blood recirculates, the drug moves from the bloodstream into the body's tissues.

Once absorbed, most drugs do not spread evenly throughout the body. Drugs that dissolve in water (water-soluble drugs), such as the antihypertensive drug atenolol, tend to stay within the blood and the fluid that surrounds cells (interstitial space). Drugs that dissolve in fat (fat-soluble drugs), such as the anesthetic drug halothane, tend to concentrate in fatty tissues. Other drugs concentrate mainly in only one small part of the body (for example, iodine concentrates mainly in the thyroid gland), because the tissues there have a special attraction for (affinity) and ability to retain the drug.

Drugs penetrate different tissues at different speeds, depending on the drug's ability to cross membranes. For example, the anesthetic thiopental, a highly fat-soluble drug, rapidly enters the brain, but the antibiotic penicillin, a water-soluble drug, does not. In general, fat-soluble drugs can cross cell membranes more quickly than water-soluble drugs can. For some drugs, transport mechanisms aid movement into or out of the tissues.

Some drugs leave the bloodstream very slowly, because they bind tightly to proteins circulating in the blood. Others quickly leave the bloodstream and enter other tissues, because they are less tightly bound to blood proteins. Some or virtually all molecules of a drug in the blood may be bound to blood proteins. The protein-bound part is generally inactive. As unbound drug is distributed to tissues and its level in the bloodstream decreases, blood proteins gradually release the drug bound to them. Thus, the bound drug in the bloodstream may act as a reservoir for the drug.

Some drugs accumulate in certain tissues, which can also act as reservoirs of extra drug. These tissues slowly release the drug into the bloodstream, keeping blood levels of the drug from decreasing rapidly and thereby prolonging the effect of the drug. Some drugs, such as those that accumulate in fatty tissues, leave the tissues so slowly that they circulate in the bloodstream for days after a person has stopped taking the drug.

Distribution of a given drug may also vary from person to person. For instance, obese people may store large amounts of fat-soluble drugs, whereas very thin people may store relatively little. Older people, even when thin, may store large amounts of fat-soluble drugs because the proportion of body fat increases with aging.

Metabolism

Drug metabolism is the chemical alteration of a drug by the body.

Some drugs are chemically altered by the body (metabolized). The substances that result from metabolism (metabolites) may be inactive, or they may be similar to or different from the original drug in therapeutic activity or toxicity. Some drugs, called prodrugs, are administered in an inactive form, which is metabolized into an active form. The resulting metabolites produce the desired therapeutic effects. Metabolites may be metabolized further instead of being excreted from the body. The subsequent metabolites are then excreted.

A vast majority of drugs must pass through the liver, which is the site of most drug metabolism. Once in the liver, enzymes convert prodrugs to active metabolites or convert active drugs to inactive forms. The liver's primary mechanism for metabolizing drugs is via a specific group of cytochrome P-450 enzymes. The level of these cytochrome P-450 enzymes controls the rate at which many drugs are metabolized. The capacity of the enzymes to metabolize is limited, so they can become overloaded when blood levels of a drug are high (see page 89).

Because metabolic enzyme systems are only partially developed at birth, newborns have difficulty metabolizing certain drugs. As people age, enzymatic activity decreases, so that older people, like newborns, cannot metabolize drugs as well as younger adults and children do (see page 1896). Consequently, newborns and older people often need smaller doses per pound of body weight than do young or middle-aged adults.

Elimination

Drug elimination is the removal of drugs from the body.

All drugs are eventually eliminated from the body. They may be eliminated after being chemically altered (metabolized), or they may be eliminated intact. Most drugs, particularly water-soluble drugs and their metabolites, are eliminated largely by the kidneys in urine. Some drugs are eliminated by excretion in the bile (a greenish yellow fluid secreted by the liver and stored in the gallbladder).

Elimination in the Urine: Several factors, including certain characteristics of the drug, affect the kidneys' ability to excrete drugs. To be extensively excreted in urine, a drug or metabolite must be water soluble and must not be bound too tightly to proteins in the bloodstream. The acidity of urine, which is affected by diet, drugs, and kidney disorders, can affect the rate at which the kidneys excrete some drugs. In the treatment of poisoning with some drugs, the acidity of the urine is changed by giving antacids (such as sodium bicarbonate) or acidic substances (such as ammonium chloride) orally to speed up the excretion of the drug.

The kidneys' ability to excrete drugs also depends on urine flow, blood flow through the kidneys, and the condition of the kidneys. Kidney function can be impaired by many disorders (especially high blood pressure, diabetes, and recurring kidney infections), by exposure to high levels of toxic chemicals, and by age-related changes. As people age, kidney function slowly declines. For example, the kidneys of an 85-year-old person excrete drugs only about half as efficiently as those of a 35-year-old person.

In people whose kidney function has declined, the "normal" dosage of a drug that is eliminated primarily through the kidneys may be too much and may cause side effects. Therefore, health care practitioners sometimes must adjust the drug dosage based on the amount of decline in the person's kidney function. Health care practitioners have several ways to estimate the decline in kidney function. Sometimes they base an estimate solely on the person's age. However, they can get a more accurate estimate of kidney function by using the results of tests that measure the level of creatinine (a waste product) in the blood and sometimes also the urine. They use these results to calculate how effectively creatinine is removed from the body (called creatinine clearance), which reflects how well the kidneys are functioning.

Elimination in the Bile: Some drugs pass through the liver unchanged and are excreted in the bile. The bile then enters the digestive tract. From there, drugs are either eliminated in feces or reabsorbed into the bloodstream and thus recycled. Other drugs are converted to metabolites in the liver and excreted in the bile. These metabolites may be excreted in the feces or can be converted back to the drug, which is then reabsorbed into the bloodstream and recycled.

If the liver is not functioning normally, the dosage of a drug that is eliminated primarily by metabolism in the liver may need to be adjusted. However, there are no simple ways to estimate liver function quantitatively for drug metabolism comparable to those for kidney function.

Other Forms of Elimination: Some drugs are excreted in saliva, sweat, breast milk, and even exhaled air. Most are excreted in small amounts. The excretion of drugs in breast milk is significant only because the drug may affect the breastfeeding infant. Excretion in exhaled air is the main way that inhaled anesthetics are eliminated.

11 Drug Dynamics

Drug dynamics (pharmacodynamics) involves what a drug does to the body.

Drug dynamics describes the therapeutic effects of drugs (such as relief of pain and reduction of blood pressure) and their side effects. But drug dynamics also describes where (the site) and how (the mechanism) a drug acts on the body. A drug's effects on the body may be influenced by many factors, such as a person's age (see pages 89 and 1896), genetic makeup, and other medical conditions the person has other than the one being treated.

Site Selectivity

After being swallowed, injected, inhaled, or absorbed through the skin, most drugs enter the bloodstream and circulate throughout the body. Some drugs are administered directly to the area where they are wanted—for example, to the eyes in eyedrops. The drugs then interact with cells or tissues where they produce their intended effects (target sites). Some drugs are relatively nonselective. They affect many different tissues or organs. For example, atropine, a drug given to relax muscles in the digestive tract, may also relax muscles in the eyes and in the respiratory tract. Other drugs are relatively selective. For example, nonsteroidal antiinflammatory drugs (NSAIDs), such as aspirin and ibuprofen (see page 644), target any area where inflammation is present. Still other drugs are highly selective. They affect mainly a single organ or system. For example, digoxin, a drug given to manage heart failure, affects mainly the heart, increasing its pumping efficiency. Sleep aids target certain nerve cells of the brain.

How do drugs know where to exert their effects? The answer involves how they interact with cells or substances such as enzymes.

Receptors on Cells

On their surface, most cells have many different types of receptors. A receptor is a molecule with a specific three-dimensional structure, which allows only substances that fit precisely to attach to it—as a key fits in its lock. Receptors enable natural (originating in the body) substances outside the cell, such as neurotransmitters and hormones, to influence the activity of the cell. That influence may be to stimulate or inhibit a process inside the cell. Drugs tend to mimic these natural substances and thus use receptors in the same way. For example, morphine and related pain-relieving drugs act on or affect the same receptors in the brain used by endorphins, which are substances produced by the body to help control pain. Some drugs attach to only one type of receptor. Other drugs, like a master key, can attach to several types of receptors throughout the body. A drug's selectivity can often be explained by how selectively it attaches to receptors.

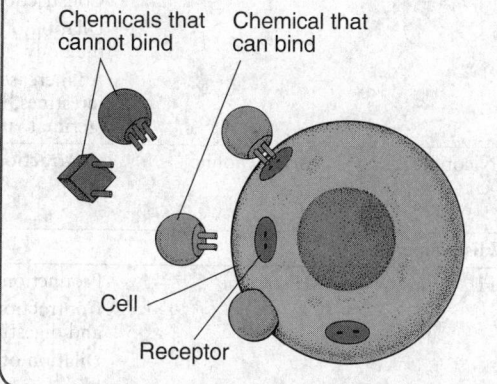

A Perfect Fit

A receptor on the cell's surface has a three-dimensional structure that allows a specific substance, such as a drug, hormone, or neurotransmitter, to bind to it because the substance has a three-dimensional structure that perfectly fits the receptor, as a key fits a lock.

Chemicals that cannot bind

Chemical that can bind

Cell

Receptor

TARGETS IN THE BODY: CELL RECEPTORS

Certain natural substances in the body, such as neurotransmitters and hormones, target specific receptors on the surface of cells. When these substances bind with the receptor on a cell, they stimulate that receptor to perform its function, which is to produce or to inhibit a specific action in the cell. Drugs can also target and bind with these receptors.

Some drugs act as agonists, stimulating the receptor in the same way that the body's natural substances do. Others act as antagonists, blocking the action of the natural substance on the receptor. Each type of receptor has many subtypes, and drugs may act on one or several subtypes of receptors.

TYPE OF RECEPTOR	BODY'S NATURAL AGONIST	RESULTING ACTION	DRUGS THAT TARGET THE RECEPTOR
Adrenergic			
Alpha$_1$	Epinephrine and norepinephrine	"Fight-or-flight" reactions: Constriction of the blood vessels in the skin, digestive tract, and urinary tract Breakdown of glucose in the liver (releasing energy) A decrease in activity of the stomach and intestines Contraction of smooth muscle in the genital and urinary organs	Agonist: Methoxamine and phenylephrine Antagonist: Doxazosin, prazosin, tamsulosin, and terazosin
Alpha$_2$	Epinephrine and norepinephrine	A decrease in insulin secretion, in the clumping of platelets, in the constriction of blood vessels in the skin and intestines, and in the release of norepinephrine from nerves	Agonist: Clonidine Antagonist: Yohimbine
Beta$_1$	Epinephrine and norepinephrine	An increase in heart rate, in the force of heart contraction, and in secretion of renin (a hormone involved in controlling blood pressure)	Agonist: Dobutamine and isoproterenol Antagonist: Beta-blockers (used to treat hypertension and heart disease), such as atenolol and metoprolol
Beta$_2$	Epinephrine and norepinephrine	Dilation of smooth muscle in the blood vessels, airways, digestive tract, and urinary tract Breakdown of glycogen in skeletal muscles (releasing glucose for energy)	Agonist: Albuterol, isoetharine, and terbutaline Antagonist: Propranolol
Cholinergic			
Muscarinic	Acetylcholine	A decrease in heart rate and the force of the heart's contraction Constriction of airways Dilation of blood vessels throughout the body An increase in activity of the stomach, intestines, bladder, and salivary, lacrimal, and sweat glands	Agonist: Bethanechol and carbachol Antagonist: Atropine, ipratropium, and scopolamine
Nicotinic	Acetylcholine	Contraction of skeletal muscles	Agonist: None commonly used Antagonist: Atracurium, pancuronium, and tubocurarine
Histaminergic			
H$_1$	Histamine	Production of an allergic response Contraction of muscles in the airways and digestive tract Dilation of small blood vessels Drowsiness (sedation)	Agonist: None commonly used Antagonist: Cetirizine, chlorpheniramine, clemastine, diphenhydramine, fexofenadine, and loratadine

(continued on the following page)

TARGETS IN THE BODY: CELL RECEPTORS (Continued)

TYPE OF RECEPTOR	BODY'S NATURAL AGONIST	RESULTING ACTION	DRUGS THAT TARGET THE RECEPTOR
H$_2$	Histamine	Stimulation of stomach secretions	Agonist: None commonly used Antagonist: Cimetidine, famotidine, nizatidine, and ranitidine
Serotoninergic			
	Serotonin	Constriction of blood vessels within the brain Stimulation of activity (motility) in the digestive tract Contraction of blood vessels Effects on sleep, memory, sensory perception, temperature regulation, mood, appetite, and hormone secretion	Partial agonist: Buspirone Agonist*: Sumitriptan and zomitriptan Antagonist: Methysergide and ondansetron
Dopaminergic			
	Dopamine	Involved in movement, mood, thinking, learning, and reward-seeking. Also increases blood flow to the kidneys, which allows for increased urine excretion	Agonist: Pramipexole and ropinirole Antagonist: Olanzapine and risperidone

*Antidepressants called serotonin reuptake inhibitors (SSRIs) act by enhancing the effects of serotonin but are not agonists (they do not act on the serotonin receptor).

Agonists and Antagonists: Drugs that target receptors are classified as agonists or antagonists. Agonist drugs activate, or stimulate, their receptors, triggering a response that increases or decreases the cell's activity. Antagonist drugs block the access or attachment of the body's natural agonists, usually neurotransmitters, to their receptors and thereby prevent or reduce cell responses to natural agonists.

Agonist and antagonist drugs can be used together in patients with asthma. For example, albuterol can be used with ipratropium. Albuterol, an agonist, attaches to specific (adrenergic) receptors on cells in the respiratory tract, causing relaxation of smooth muscle cells and thus widening of the airways (bronchodilation). Ipratropium, an antagonist, attaches to other (cholinergic) receptors, blocking the attachment of acetylcholine, a neurotransmitter that causes contraction of smooth muscle cells and thus narrowing of the airways (bronchoconstriction). Both drugs widen the airways (and make breathing easier) but in different ways.

Beta-blockers, such as propranolol, are a widely used group of antagonists. These drugs are used to treat high blood pressure, angina (chest pain caused by an inadequate blood supply to the heart muscle), and certain abnormal heart rhythms and to prevent migraines. They block or reduce stimulation of the heart by the agonist hormones epinephrine (adrenaline) and norepinephrine (noradrenaline), which are released during stress. Antagonists such as betablockers are most effective when the concentration of the agonist is high in a specific part of the body. Similar to the way a roadblock stops more vehicles during the 5:00 PM rush hour than at 3:00 AM, betablockers, given in doses that have little effect on normal heart function, may have a greater effect during sudden surges of hormones released during stress and thereby protect the heart from excess stimulation.

Enzymes

Instead of receptors, some drugs target enzymes, which regulate the rate of chemical reactions. Drugs that target enzymes are classified as inhibitors or activators (inducers). For example, the cholesterol-lowering drug lovastatin inhibits an enzyme called HMG-CoA reductase, which is critical in the body's production of cholesterol. A side effect of the antibiotic rifampin is the activation of the enzymes involved in metabolizing oral contraceptives. When women who are taking an oral contraceptive also take rifampin, the contraceptive is metabolized (that is, broken down into inactive components) and removed from the body more quickly than usual and may therefore be ineffective.

Drug Action

Drugs affect only the rate at which existing biologic functions proceed. Drugs do not change the basic nature of these functions or create new functions. For example, drugs can speed up or slow down the biochemical reactions that cause muscles to contract, kidney cells to regulate the volume of water and salts retained or eliminated by the body, glands to secrete substances (such as mucus, stomach acid, or insulin), and nerves to transmit messages.

Drugs cannot restore structures or functions already damaged beyond repair by the body. This fundamental limitation of drug action underlies much of the current frustration in trying to treat tissue-destroying or degenerative diseases such as heart failure, arthritis, muscular dystrophy, multiple sclerosis, and Alzheimer's disease. Nonetheless, some drugs can help the body repair itself. For example, by stopping an infection, antibiotics can allow the body to repair damage caused by the infection.

Some drugs are hormones, such as insulin, thyroid hormones, estrogens, or cortisol. They can be used to replace hormones that are missing from the body.

Reversibility

Most interactions between a drug and a receptor or between a drug and an enzyme are reversible: After a while, the drug disengages, and the receptor or enzyme resumes normal function. Sometimes an interaction is largely irreversible, and the drug's effect persists until the body manufactures more enzyme. For example, omeprazole, a drug used in the management of gastroesophageal reflux and ulcers, irreversibly inhibits an enzyme involved in the secretion of stomach acid.

Affinity and Intrinsic Activity

A drug's action is affected by the quantity of drug that reaches the receptor and the degree of attraction (affinity) between it and its receptor on the cell's surface. Once bound to their receptor, drugs vary in their ability to produce an effect (intrinsic activity). Drugs vary in their affinity and intrinsic activity.

Drugs that activate receptors (agonists) must have both great affinity and intrinsic activity: They must bind effectively to their receptors, and the drug bound to its receptor (drug-receptor complex) must be capable of producing an effect in the targeted area. In contrast, drugs that block receptors (antagonists) must bind effectively but have little or no intrinsic activity, because their function is to prevent an agonist from interacting with its receptors.

Potency and Efficacy

A drug's effects can be evaluated in terms of strength (potency) or effectiveness (efficacy).

Potency refers to the amount of drug (usually expressed in milligrams) needed to produce an effect, such as relief of pain or reduction of blood pressure. For instance, if 5 milligrams of drug A relieves pain as effectively as 10 milligrams of drug B, drug A is twice as potent as drug B.

Efficacy refers to the potential maximum therapeutic response that a drug can produce. For example, the diuretic furosemide eliminates much more salt and water through urine than does the diuretic chlorothiazide. Thus, furosemide has greater efficacy than chlorothiazide. However, greater potency or efficacy does not necessarily mean that one drug is preferable to another. When judging the relative merits of drugs for a person, doctors consider many factors, such as side effects, potential toxicity, duration of effect (which determines the number of doses needed each day), and cost.

CHAPTER

12   Factors Affecting Response to Drugs

Everyone responds to drugs differently. The way a person responds to a drug is affected by many factors, including genetic makeup, age, body size, the use of other drugs and dietary supplements (such as medicinal herbs—see page 2067), the consumption of food (including beverages), the presence of diseases (such as kidney or liver disease), storage of the drug (whether the drug was stored too long or in the wrong environment), and the development of tolerance and resistance. For example, a large person generally needs more of a drug than a smaller person needs for the same effect. Whether people take a drug as instructed (see page 97) also affects their response to it. These factors may affect how the body absorbs the drug (see page 82), how the body breaks down (metabolizes—see page 84) and eliminates the drug (see page 84), or what effects the drug has on the body.

Because so many factors affect drug response, doctors must choose a drug appropriate for each person and must adjust the dose carefully. This process is more complex if the person takes other drugs and has other diseases, because drug-drug and drug-disease interactions are possible.

A standard or average dose is determined for every new drug. But the concept of an average dose can be like "one size fits all" in clothing: It may fit a range of people well enough, but it may fit almost no one perfectly. For some drugs, however, the dose does not have to be adjusted, because the same dose works well in virtually everyone.

Effects of Age: Infants and older people particularly have problems with drug response. Their liver and kidneys function less effectively, so drugs that are broken down by the liver or excreted by the kidney tend to accumulate, thus potentially causing problems.

Older people typically have more disorders than children and younger adults and thus usually take more drugs (see page 1896). The more drugs people take, the more likely they are to have problems caused by one drug interfering with another drug or disease. With aging, people also may have more difficulty following complicated instructions for taking drugs, such as to take the drug at very specific times or to avoid certain foods.

Genetic Makeup

Differences in genetic (inherited) makeup among individuals affect what the body does to a drug and what the drug does to the body. The study of genetic differences in the response to drugs is called pharmacogenetics.

Because of their genetic makeup, some people process (metabolize) drugs slowly. As a result, a drug may accumulate in the body, causing toxicity. Other people metabolize drugs so quickly that after they take a usual dose, drug levels in the blood never become high enough for the drug to be effective.

In about half of the people in the United States, N-acetyltransferase, a liver enzyme that metabolizes certain drugs, works slowly. Such people are called slow acetylators. Drugs, such as isoniazid (which is used to treat tuberculosis), that are metabolized by this enzyme tend to reach higher blood levels and remain in the body longer in slow acetylators than they do in people in whom this enzyme metabolizes drugs rapidly (fast acetylators).

About 1 of 1,500 people have low levels of pseudocholinesterase, a blood enzyme that inactivates drugs such as succinylcholine, which is given to temporarily relax muscles during many surgical procedures. If succinylcholine is not rapidly inactivated, muscle relaxation may be prolonged, and people may not be able to breathe on their own as soon after surgery as is usual. They may need a ventilator for an extended time.

About 10% of black men and fewer black women have a deficiency of glucose-6-phosphate dehydrogenase (G6PD), an enzyme that protects red blood cells from certain toxic chemicals. For example, in people with G6PD deficiency, some drugs (such as chloroquine and primaquine, which are used to treat malaria) destroy red blood cells and cause hemolytic anemia (see page 1031).

About 1 of 20,000 people have a genetic defect that makes muscles overly sensitive to anesthetics such as halothane, isoflurane, and sevoflurane. When such people are given one of these anesthetics with a muscle relaxant (usually succinylcholine), a life-threatening disorder called malignant hyperthermia may develop. It produces a very high fever. Muscles stiffen, the heart races, and blood pressure falls.

Drug Interactions

The effect a drug has on a person may be different than expected because that drug interacts with

- Another drug the person is taking (drug-drug interaction)
- Food, beverages, or supplements the person is consuming (drug-nutrient interaction)
- Another disease the person has (drug-disease interaction)

The effects of drug interactions are usually unwanted and sometimes harmful. Interactions may increase or decrease the actions of one or more drugs, resulting in side effects or failed treatment.

DRUG-DRUG INTERACTIONS

Drug-drug interactions can involve prescription or nonprescription (over-the-counter) drugs. Types of drug-drug interactions include duplication, opposition (antagonism), and alteration of what the body does to one or both drugs.

Duplication: When two drugs with the same effect are taken, their side effects may be intensified. Duplication may occur when people inadvertently take two drugs (often at least one is an over-the-counter drug) that have the same active ingredient. For example, people may take a cold remedy and a sleep aid, both of which contain diphenhydramine, or a cold remedy and a pain reliever, both of which contain acetaminophen. This type of duplication is particularly likely with the use of drugs that contain multiple ingredients or that are sold under brand names (thus appearing to be different but actually containing the same ingredients). Awareness of drug ingredients is important, as is checking each new drug to avoid duplication. For

Many Factors Affect Drug Response

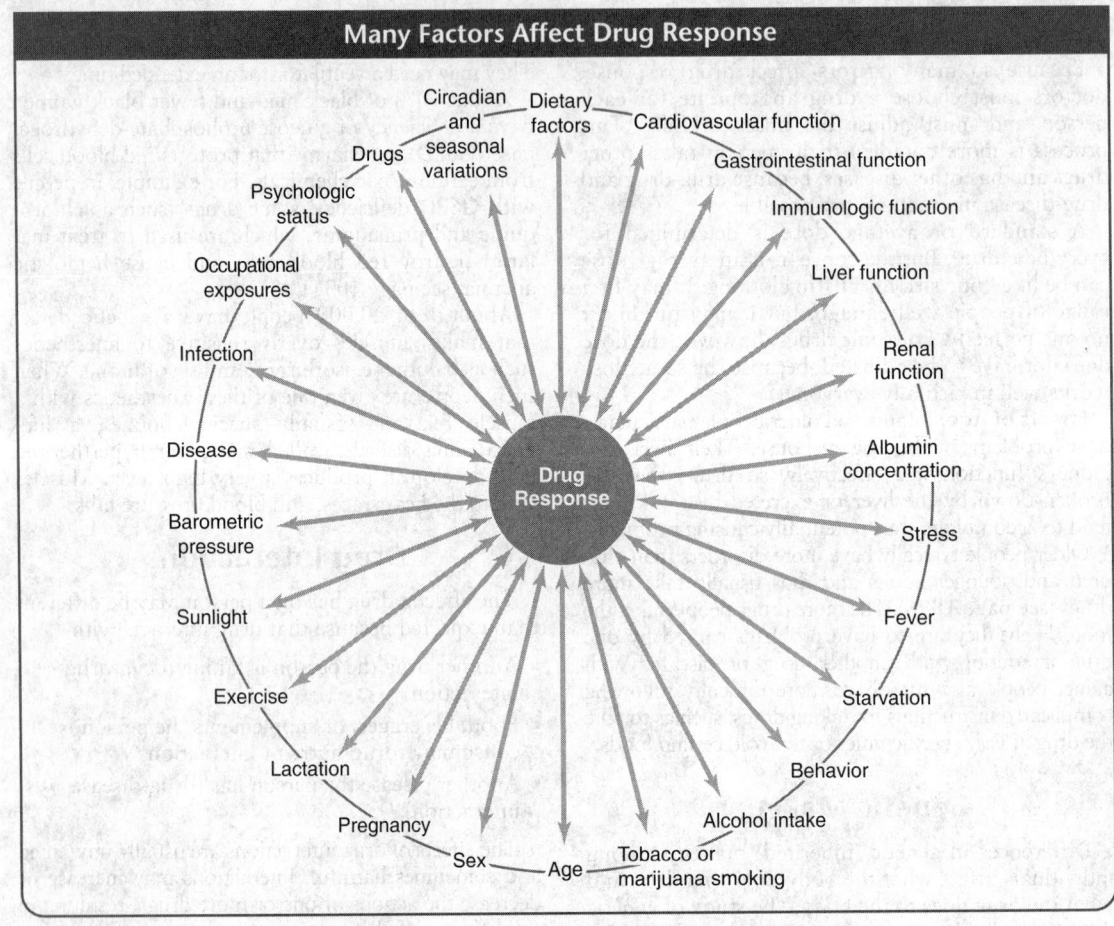

example, many prescription-strength pain relievers contain an opioid plus acetaminophen. People taking such a product who do not know its ingredients might take over-the-counter acetaminophen for extra relief, risking toxicity.

Similar problems with duplication can arise when two different drugs with the same effect are taken. This is most likely to occur when people see several doctors, obtain prescriptions at more than one pharmacy, or both. Doctors who are not aware of what others have prescribed may inadvertently prescribe similar drugs. For example, excessive sedation and dizziness can occur when two doctors both prescribe a sleep aid or when one prescribes a sleep aid and the other prescribes another drug (such as an antianxiety drug) that has similar sedative effects. People can reduce this risk by keeping each doctor informed about all drugs being taken and by using one pharmacy to obtain all prescriptions. It is helpful to keep

an up-to-date written list of all drugs being taken and to bring the list along on each doctor visit. Also, people should not take previously prescribed drugs (such as a sleeping pill or pain reliever) without checking with the doctor or pharmacist because that drug may duplicate or otherwise interact with one of their current drugs.

Opposition (Antagonism): Two drugs with opposing actions can interact, thereby reducing the effectiveness of one or both. For example, nonsteroidal anti-inflammatory drugs (NSAIDs—see page 644), such as ibuprofen, which are taken to relieve pain, may cause the body to retain salt and fluid. Diuretics, such as hydrochlorothiazide and furosemide, help rid the body of excess salt and fluid. If a person takes both types of drug, the NSAID may reduce the diuretic's effectiveness. Certain beta-blockers (such as propranolol), taken to control high blood pressure and heart disease, counteract beta-adrenergic stimulants, such as albuterol, taken to manage asthma. Both types of drugs target the same cell receptors—beta-2 receptors (see table on page 86)—but one type blocks them, and the other stimulates them.

Alteration: One drug may alter how the body absorbs, distributes, metabolizes, or excretes another drug.

Acid-blocking drugs, such as histamine-2 (H_2) blockers and proton pump inhibitors, raise the pH of the stomach and decrease absorption of some drugs, such as ketoconazole, a drug for fungal infections.

Many drugs are broken down and inactivated (metabolized) by certain enzymes in the liver. Some drugs affect these liver enzymes, either increasing or decreasing their activity, and may cause another drug to be inactivated more quickly or more slowly than usual. For example, by increasing the activity of liver enzymes, barbiturates such as phenobarbital cause the anticoagulant warfarin to be inactivated more quickly and thus to be less effective when taken during the same time period. Conversely, by decreasing the activity of the enzyme system, drugs such as erythromycin and ciprofloxacin can increase the activity of warfarin, risking bleeding. When drugs that affect liver enzymes are used in people taking warfarin, doctors monitor the people more closely and adjust the dose of warfarin to compensate for this effect. The warfarin dose is adjusted again when other drugs are stopped. Many other drugs affect liver enzymes.

Chemicals in cigarette smoke can increase the activity of some liver enzymes. As a result, smoking decreases the effectiveness of some drugs, including propoxyphene (an analgesic) and theophylline (a drug that widens the airways called a bronchodilator).

Some drugs affect the rate at which the kidneys excrete another drug. For example, large doses of vitamin C increase the urine's acidity and thus may change the rate of excretion and activity of certain drugs. For example, the rate of excretion may be decreased for acidic drugs such as aspirin but may be increased for basic drugs such as pseudoephedrine.

Because there are so many drug interactions, many doctors and pharmacists reduce the risk of problems by checking reference books and computer software programs when prescribing or dispensing prescriptions for additional drugs. In most pharmacies, drug orders and prescriptions are reviewed using a computer system that automatically checks for drug interactions.

DRUG-NUTRIENT INTERACTIONS

Nutrients include food, beverages (including alcohol), and dietary supplements. Consumption of these substances may alter the effects of drugs the person takes.

How to Reduce the Risk of Drug-Drug Interactions

- Consult the doctor or pharmacist before taking any new drugs, including over-the-counter drugs and dietary supplements, such as medicinal herbs.
- Keep a list of all drugs being taken. Periodically discuss this list with the doctor or pharmacist.
- Keep a list of all disorders. Periodically discuss this list with the doctor.
- Select a pharmacy that provides comprehensive services (including checking for possible interactions) and that maintains a complete drug profile for each person. Have all prescriptions dispensed in this pharmacy.
- Learn about the purpose and actions of all drugs prescribed.
- Learn about the possible side effects of the drugs.
- Learn how to take the drugs, what time of day they should be taken, and whether they can be taken during the same time period as other drugs.
- Review the use of over-the-counter drugs with the pharmacist. Discuss any disorders present and any prescription drugs being taken.
- Take drugs as instructed.
- Report to the doctor or pharmacist any symptoms that might be related to the use of a drug.
- If seeing more than one doctor, make sure each doctor knows all the drugs being taken.

Food: Like food, drugs taken by mouth must be absorbed through the lining of the stomach or the small intestine. Consequently, the presence of food in the digestive tract may reduce absorption of a drug. Often, such interactions can be avoided by taking the drug 1 hour before or 2 hours after eating.

Dietary Supplements: Dietary supplements, including medicinal herbs, are products (besides tobacco) that contain a vitamin, mineral, herb, or amino acid and that are intended as a supplement to the normal diet (see page 2067). Supplements are regulated as foods, not as drugs, so they are not tested as comprehensively. However, they may interact with prescription or over-the-counter drugs. People who take dietary supplements should tell their doctors and pharmacists, so that interactions can be avoided.

Alcohol: Although many people do not consider alcohol a nutrient, it affects body processes and interacts with many drugs. For example, taking alcohol with the antibiotic metronidazole can cause flushing, headache, palpitations, and nausea and vomiting. Doctors or pharmacists can answer questions about possible alcohol and drug interactions.

SOME DRUG-FOOD INTERACTIONS

AFFECTED DRUG	INTERACTING FOOD	INTERACTION
Bisphosphonates (such as alendronate, ibandronate, and risedronate)	Any food	Food, even orange juice, coffee, or mineral water, may markedly reduce the absorption and effectiveness of these drugs. Alendronate and risedronate must be taken with plain water at least ½ hour before the first food, beverage, or drug of the day is taken, and ibandronate must be taken at least 1 hour before.
Anticoagulants	Foods high in vitamin K (such as broccoli, brussels sprouts, spinach, and kale)	Such foods may reduce the effectiveness of anticoagulants (such as warfarin), increasing the risk of clotting. Intake of such foods should be limited, and the amount consumed daily should remain constant.
Certain benzodiazepines (such as triazolam)　Calcium channel blockers (such as felodipine, nifedipine, and nisoldipine)　Cyclosporine　Estrogen and oral contraceptives　Certain statins (such as atorvastatin, lovastatin, and simvastatin)	Grapefruit juice	Grapefruit juice inhibits enzymes involved in drug metabolism and thereby intensifies the effect of certain drugs, many of which are not listed here.
Digoxin	Oatmeal	The fiber in oatmeal and other cereals, when consumed in large amounts, can interfere with the absorption of digoxin.
MAO inhibitors (such as phenelzine and tranylcypromine)	Foods high in tyramine, including many cheeses (such as American processed, cheddar, blue, brie, mozzarella, and Parmesan), yogurt, sour cream, cured meats (such as sausage and salami), liver, dried fish, caviar, avocados, bananas, yeast extracts, raisins, sauerkraut, soy sauce, fava beans, red wine, certain beers, and products containing caffeine	Severe headache and a potentially fatal increase in blood pressure (hypertensive crisis) can occur if people taking an MAO inhibitor (used most often to treat depression) consume these foods. These foods must be avoided.
Tetracycline	Calcium or foods containing calcium, such as milk and other dairy products	These foods can reduce the absorption of tetracycline, which should be taken 1 hour before or 2 hours after eating.

MAO = monoamine oxidase.

DRUG-DISEASE INTERACTIONS

Sometimes, drugs that are helpful in one disease are harmful in another disorder. For example, some beta-blockers taken for heart disease or high blood pressure can worsen asthma and make it hard for people with diabetes to tell when their blood sugar is too low. Some drugs taken to treat a cold may worsen glaucoma. People should tell their doctor all of the diseases they have before the doctor prescribes a new drug. Diabetes, high or low blood pressure, an ulcer, glaucoma, an enlarged prostate, poor bladder control, and insomnia are particularly important, because people with such diseases are more likely to have a drug-disease interaction.

Drug-disease interactions can occur in any age group but are common among older people, who tend to have more diseases (see page 1896).

Tolerance and Resistance

Tolerance is a person's diminished response to a drug, which occurs when the drug is used repeatedly and the body adapts to the continued presence of the drug. Resistance refers to the ability of microorganisms or cancer cells to withstand the effects of a drug usually effective against them.

Tolerance: A person may develop tolerance to a drug when the drug is used repeatedly. For instance, when morphine or alcohol is used for a long time, larger and larger doses must be taken to produce the same effect. Usually, tolerance develops because metabolism of the drug speeds up (often because the liver enzymes involved in metabolizing drugs become more active) and because the number of sites (cell receptors) that the drug attaches to or the strength of the bond (affinity) between the receptor and drug decreases (see page 85).

Tolerance is not the same as dependence or addiction. Dependence, which may be physical or psychologic, refers to a strong desire to experience the effects of the drug (see page 2079). In physical dependence, the person may experience symptoms of withdrawal when the drug is stopped. Addiction is compulsive use and overwhelming involvement with a drug (see page 2080).

Resistance: Strains of microorganisms (bacteria or viruses) are said to develop resistance when they are no longer killed or inhibited by the antibiotics and antiviral drugs that are usually effective against them (or, in practice, when significantly higher than normal doses are required to have an effect). Similarly, cancer cells may develop resistance to chemotherapy drugs.

Resistance appears because of the mutations that take place spontaneously in any group of growing cells, whether exposed to drugs or not. Most such mutations change the cell's structure or biochemical pathways in a harmful way. But some mutations change the parts of the cell that are affected by drugs, decreasing the drug's ability to work (that is, causing resistance). Because such mutations are very rare, there are normally only a few such resistant cells in any group. However, if all or many of the "normal" cells are killed by a drug, a much higher proportion of the survivors are likely to be resistant. If the resistant survivors are not killed by the body's natural defenses, which is more likely when drugs are stopped too soon or not taken in the proper manner, they may reproduce and pass on the resistant trait to their descendants.

Prevention and Treatment

To prevent the development of resistance, doctors try to use antibiotics only when necessary (not for viral infections such as a cold) and have people take them for a full course of treatment. In the treatment of certain serious infections, such as HIV, doctors usually give two or more different drugs at the same time because it is very unlikely that a cell would spontaneously be resistant to two drugs at the same time. However, giving one drug for a short time followed by another can produce resistance to multiple drugs—this has become a problem with tuberculosis in particular.

Once tolerance or resistance has developed to a drug, doctors may increase the dose or use a different drug.

13 Adverse Drug Reactions

In the early 1900s, German scientist Paul Ehrlich described an ideal drug as a "magic bullet"; such a drug would be aimed precisely at a disease site and would not harm healthy tissues. Although many new drugs are aimed more accurately than their predecessors, none of them, as of yet, hit the target precisely.

Most drugs produce several effects, but usually only one effect—the therapeutic effect—is wanted for the treatment of a disorder. The other effects may be regarded as unwanted, whether they are intrinsically harmful or not. For example, certain antihistamines cause drowsiness as well as control the symptoms of allergies. When an over-the-counter sleep aid containing an antihistamine is taken, drowsiness is considered a therapeutic effect. But when an antihistamine is taken to control allergy symptoms during the daytime, drowsiness is considered an annoying, unwanted effect.

Most people, including health care practitioners, refer to unwanted effects as side effects; another term used is adverse drug event. However, the term *adverse drug reaction* is technically more appropriate for drug effects that are unwanted, unpleasant, noxious, or potentially harmful.

Not surprisingly, adverse drug reactions are common. Most adverse drug reactions are relatively mild, and many disappear when the drug is stopped or the dose is changed. Some gradually subside as the body adjusts to the drug. Other adverse drug reactions are more serious

SOME SERIOUS ADVERSE DRUG REACTIONS

ADVERSE DRUG REACTION	TYPES OF DRUGS	EXAMPLES
Peptic ulcers or bleeding from the stomach	Corticosteroids taken by mouth or by injection (not those applied to the skin in creams or lotions)	Hydrocortisone Prednisone
	Nonsteroidal anti-inflammatory drugs	Aspirin Ibuprofen Ketoprofen Naproxen
	Anticoagulants	Heparin Warfarin
Anemia (resulting from decreased production or increased destruction of red blood cells)	Certain antibiotics	Chloramphenicol
	Some nonsteroidal anti-inflammatory drugs	Phenylbutazone (not available in the United States)
	Drugs used to treat malaria and tuberculosis in people with G6PD enzyme deficiency	Chloroquine Isoniazid Primaquine
Decreased production of white blood cells, with increased risk of infection	Certain antipsychotic drugs	Clozapine
	Chemotherapy drugs	Cyclophosphamide Mercaptopurine Methotrexate Vinblastine
	Some drugs used to treat thyroid disorders	Propylthiouracil
Liver damage	Some analgesics	Acetaminophen (use of excessive doses)
	Some drugs used to treat tuberculosis Iron supplements (in excessive amounts)	Isoniazid
Kidney damage	Nonsteroidal anti-inflammatory drugs (repeated use of excessive doses)	Ibuprofen Ketoprofen Naproxen
	Aminoglycoside antibiotics	Gentamicin Kanamycin
	Some chemotherapy drugs	Cisplatin
Confusion and drowsiness	Sedatives, including many antihistamines	Diphenhydramine
	Antidepressants (especially in older people)	Amitriptyline Imipramine

and last longer. About 3 to 7% of all hospital admissions in the United States are for treatment of adverse drug reactions. Adverse drug reactions occur during 10 to 20% of hospital admissions, and about 10 to 20% of these reactions are severe.

Digestive disturbances—loss of appetite, nausea, a bloating sensation, constipation, and diarrhea—are particularly common adverse drug reactions, because most drugs are taken by mouth and pass through the digestive tract. However, almost any organ system can be affected. In older people, the brain is commonly affected, often resulting in drowsiness and confusion.

Types of Adverse Drug Reactions

Many adverse drug reactions represent an exaggeration of the drug's therapeutic effects (called type 1 or overdose reactions). For example, a person taking a drug to reduce high blood pressure may feel dizzy or light-headed if the drug reduces blood pressure too much. A person with diabetes may develop weakness, sweating, nausea, and palpitations if insulin or an oral antidiabetic drug reduces the blood sugar level too much. This type of adverse drug reaction is usually predictable but sometimes unavoidable. It may occur if a drug dose is too high, if the person is unusually sensitive to the drug, or if another drug slows the metabolism of the first drug and thus increases its level in the blood (see page 89). Type 1 reactions are usually not serious but are relatively common.

Some adverse drug reactions result from mechanisms that are not currently understood (called type 2 or idiosyncratic reactions). This type of adverse drug reaction is largely unpredictable. Examples of such adverse drug reactions include skin rashes, jaundice, anemia, a decrease in the white blood cell count, kidney damage, and nerve injury that may impair vision or hearing. These reactions tend to be more serious but typically occur in a very small number of people. Affected people may be allergic or hypersensitive to the drug because of genetic differences in the way their body metabolizes or responds to drugs.

Some adverse drug reactions are not related to the drug's therapeutic effect but are usually predictable, because the mechanisms involved are largely understood. For example, stomach irritation and bleeding often occur in people who regularly use aspirin or other nonsteroidal anti-inflammatory drugs (NSAIDs— see page 644). The reason is that these drugs reduce the production of prostaglandins, which help protect the digestive tract from stomach acid.

Severity of Adverse Drug Reactions

There is no universal scale for describing or measuring the severity of an adverse drug reaction. Assessment is largely subjective. Reactions can be described as mild, moderate, severe, or lethal.

Reactions usually described as mild and of minor significance include digestive disturbances, headaches, fatigue, vague muscle aches, malaise (a general feeling of illness or discomfort), and changes in sleep patterns. However, such reactions can be very distressing to people who experience them. As a result, people may be less willing to take their drug as instructed, and the goals of treatment may not be achieved.

Reactions that are usually described as mild are considered moderate if the person experiencing them considers them distinctly annoying, distressing, or intolerable. Other moderate reactions include skin rashes (especially if they are extensive and persistent), visual disturbances (especially in people who wear corrective lenses), muscle tremor, difficulty with urination (a common effect of many drugs in older men), any perceptible change in mood or mental function, and certain changes in blood components, such as a temporary, reversible decrease in the white blood cell count or in blood levels of some substances, such as glucose.

Mild or moderate adverse drug reactions do not necessarily mean that a drug must be discontinued, especially if no suitable alternative is available. However, doctors are likely to reevaluate the dose, frequency of use (number of doses a day), and timing of doses (for example, before or after meals; in the morning or at bedtime). Other drugs may be used to control the adverse drug reaction (for example, a stool softener to relieve constipation).

Severe reactions include those that may be life threatening (such as liver failure, abnormal heart rhythms, certain types of allergic reactions), that result in persistent or significant disability or hospitalization, and that cause a birth defect. Severe reactions are relatively rare. People who develop a severe reaction usually must stop using the drug and must be treated. However, doctors must sometimes continue giving high-risk drugs (for example, chemotherapy to people with cancer or immunosuppressants to people undergoing organ transplantation). Doctors use every possible means to control a severe adverse drug reaction.

Benefits Versus Risks

Every drug has the potential to do harm as well as good. When doctors consider prescribing a drug, they must weigh the possible risks against the expected benefits. Use of a drug is not justified unless the expected benefits outweigh the possible risks. Doctors must also consider the likely outcome of withholding the drug. Potential benefits and risks can never be determined with mathematical precision.

When assessing the benefits and risks of prescribing a drug, doctors consider the severity of the disorder being treated and the effect it is having on the person's quality of life. For example, for relatively minor disorders—such as coughs and colds, muscle strains, or infrequent headaches—only a very low risk of adverse drug reactions is acceptable. For such symptoms, over-the-counter drugs are usually effective and well tolerated. When used according to directions, over-the-counter drugs for treating minor disorders have a wide safety margin (the difference between the usual effective dose and the dose that produces severe adverse drug reactions). In contrast, for serious or life-threatening disorders (such as a heart attack, stroke, cancer, or organ transplant rejection), a higher risk of a severe adverse drug reaction is usually acceptable.

Risk Factors

Many factors can increase the likelihood of an adverse drug reaction. They include the simultaneous use of several drugs, very young or old age, pregnancy, and breastfeeding. Hereditary factors make some people more susceptible to the toxic effects of certain drugs. Certain diseases can alter drug absorption, metabolism, and elimination and the body's response to drugs (see page 92), increasing the risk of adverse drug reactions. How mind-body interactions, such as mental attitude, outlook, belief in self, and confidence in health care practitioners, influence adverse drug reactions remains largely unexplored.

Use of Several Drugs

Taking several drugs, whether prescription or over-the-counter, contributes to the risk of having an adverse drug reaction. The number and severity of adverse drug reactions increase disproportionately as the number of drugs taken increases. The use of alcohol, which is technically a drug, also increases the risk. Asking a doctor or pharmacist to periodically review all the drugs a person is taking and to make appropriate adjustments can reduce the risk of an adverse drug reaction.

> **? Did You Know...**
> In the United States, 3 to 7% of all hospitalizations are for treatment of adverse drug reactions.

Age

Infants and very young children are at high risk of adverse drug reactions because their capacity to metabolize drugs is not fully developed. For example, newborns cannot metabolize and eliminate the antibiotic chloramphenicol. Newborns who are given the drug may develop gray baby syndrome, a serious and often fatal reaction. If tetracycline, another antibiotic, is given to infants and young children during the period when their teeth are being formed (up to about age 8), it may permanently discolor tooth enamel. Children under age 18 are at risk of Reye's syndrome if they are given aspirin while they have influenza or chickenpox.

Older people are at high risk of having an adverse drug reaction for several reasons (see page 1896). They are likely to have many health problems and thus to be taking several prescription and over-the-counter drugs. Also, as people age, the liver is less able to metabolize many drugs, and the kidneys are less able to eliminate drugs from the body, increasing the risk of kidney damage by a drug and other adverse drug reactions. These age-related problems are often made worse by malnourishment and dehydration, which tend to become more common as people age.

Older people are also more sensitive to the effects of many drugs. For example, older people are more likely to experience light-headedness, loss of appetite, depression, confusion, and impaired coordination, putting them at risk of falling and fracturing a bone. Drugs that can cause these reactions include many antihistamines, sleep aids, antianxiety drugs, antihypertensives, and antidepressants (see table on page 1899).

Pregnancy and Breastfeeding

Many drugs—for example, antihypertensive drugs such as angiotensin-converting enzyme (ACE) inhibitors and angiotensin II receptor blockers—pose a risk to the health and normal development of a fetus. To the extent possible, pregnant women should not take any drugs, especially during the first trimester (see table on page 1638). However, for some drugs, including ACE inhibitors and angiotensin II receptor blockers, risk is greatest during the last trimester of pregnancy. Use of any prescription drugs, over-the-counter drugs, and dietary supplements (including medicinal herbs) during pregnancy requires a doctor's supervision. Social drugs (alcohol and nicotine) and illicit drugs (cocaine and opioids such as heroin) also pose risks to the pregnancy and the fetus.

Drugs and medicinal herbs may be transmitted through breast milk to a baby (see box on page 1641). Some drugs should not be taken by women who are breastfeeding, whereas others can be taken but require a doctor's supervision. Some drugs do not usually harm the breastfed baby. However, women who are breastfeeding should consult with a health care practitioner before they take any drugs. Social and illicit drugs may harm a breastfeeding baby.

Allergies to Drugs

People sometimes mistake many adverse drug reactions for allergies. For example, people who experience stomach discomfort after taking aspirin (a common adverse reaction) often say they are "allergic" to aspirin. However, this is not a true allergic reaction. True allergic reactions involve activation of the immune system by the drug. Aspirin use can cause stomach discomfort because aspirin interferes with the stomach's natural barrier defenses against stomach acid.

Allergic (hypersensitivity) reactions to a drug are relatively uncommon. In contrast to other types of adverse drug reactions, the number and severity of allergic reactions do not usually correlate with the amount of drug taken. For people who are allergic to a drug, even a small amount of the drug can trigger an allergic reaction (see page 1112). These reactions range from minor and simply annoying to severe and life threatening. Examples are skin rashes and itching; fever; constriction of the airways and wheezing; swelling of tissues (such as the voice box [larynx] and the opening between the vocal cords that closes to stop the flow of air to the lungs [glottis]), which impairs breathing; and a fall in blood pressure, sometimes to dangerously low levels.

Drug allergies cannot be anticipated, because reactions occur after a person has been previously exposed to the drug (whether it was applied to the skin, taken by mouth, or injected) one or more times without any allergic reaction. However, appropriate skin tests can sometimes help predict allergic adverse drug reactions. A mild reaction may be treated with an antihistamine. A severe or life-threatening reaction may require an injection of epinephrine (also called adrenaline) or a corticosteroid, such as hydrocortisone.

Before prescribing a new drug, doctors usually ask whether a person has any known drug allergies. People who have had severe allergic reactions should wear a Medic Alert necklace or bracelet inscribed with their drug allergies. This information (for example, penicillin allergy) can alert medical and paramedical personnel in case of an emergency.

Overdose Toxicity

Overdose toxicity refers to serious, often harmful, and sometimes fatal toxic reactions to an accidental overdose of a drug (because of a doctor's, pharmacist's, or patient's error) or to an intentional overdose (homicide or suicide).

A lower risk of overdose toxicity is often the reason doctors prefer one drug to another when both drugs are equally effective. For example, if a sedative, antianxiety drug, or sleep aid is needed, doctors usually prescribe benzodiazepines, such as diazepam and temazepam, rather than barbiturates, such as pentobarbital. Benzodiazepines are not more effective than barbiturates, but they have a wider margin of safety and are much less likely to cause severe toxicity in case of an accidental or intentional overdose. Safety is also the reason that newer antidepressants, such as fluoxetine and paroxetine, have largely replaced older but equally effective antidepressants, such as imipramine and amitriptyline (see table on page 868).

Young children are at high risk of overdose toxicity. Brightly colored tablets and capsules, most of which are adult-dose formulations, can attract the attention of toddlers and young children. In the United States, federal regulations require that all prescription drugs taken by mouth be dispensed in childproof containers unless a person signs a waiver to the effect that such a container presents a handicap.

Most metropolitan areas in the United States have poison control centers that provide information about chemical and drug poisoning, and most telephone directories list the number of the local center. This number should be copied and placed near a telephone or programmed into an automatic-dialing telephone or cellular phone.

CHAPTER

14 Adherence to Drug Treatment

Adherence is the degree to which a person takes prescribed drugs as directed.

Adherence to (compliance with) drug treatment is important. However, only about half the people who leave a doctor's office with a prescription take the drug as directed. Among the many reasons people give for not adhering to drug treatment, forgetfulness is the most common. The key question then is: Why do people forget? Sometimes, the psychologic mechanism of denial is at work. Having a disorder causes concern, and having to take a drug is a constant reminder of the disorder. Or, something about the treatment, such as possible side effects, may greatly concern the person, resulting in a reluctance to follow the plan.

Results of Not Adhering

Most obviously, if a person does not adhere to treatment, symptoms may not be relieved or the disorder may not be cured. However, not adhering may have other serious or costly consequences. It is estimated to result in 125,000 deaths due to cardiovascular disease (such as heart attack and stroke)

Reasons for Not Adhering to Drug Treatment

- Forgetting to take the drug
- Not understanding or misinterpreting the instructions
- Experiencing side effects (the treatment may be perceived as worse than the disorder)
- Finding the drug to taste or smell bad
- Finding restrictions on treatment to be inconvenient (for example, having to avoid sunlight, alcohol, or milk products)
- Having to take the drug very frequently or follow complicated instructions
- Denying the disorder (repressing the diagnosis or its significance)
- Believing that the drug cannot help or is not needed
- Mistakenly believing that the disorder has been sufficiently treated (for example, thinking an infection is over just because the fever disappears)
- Fearing dependence on the drug
- Worrying about the expense
- Not caring (being apathetic) about getting better
- Encountering obstacles (for example, having difficulty swallowing tablets or capsules, having problems opening bottles, or being unable to obtain the drug)
- Distrusting the health care practitioner

---

each year. In addition, it is thought that up to 23% of nursing home admissions, 10% of hospital admissions, and many doctor visits, diagnostic tests, and unnecessary treatments could be avoided if people took their drugs as directed.

Not only does not adhering add to the cost of medical care, but it can also worsen the quality of life. For example, missed doses can lead to optic nerve damage and blindness in people with glaucoma, to an erratic heart rhythm and cardiac arrest in people with heart disease, and to stroke in people with high blood pressure. Not taking all prescribed doses of an antibiotic can cause an infection to flare up again and may be contributing to the problem of drug-resistant bacteria.

Children and Adherence

Children are less likely than adults to take or be given drugs as directed. In a study of children who had streptococcal infections and for whom a 10-day course of penicillin was prescribed, 56% were not taking the drug by the third day, 71% were not taking the drug by the sixth day, and 82% were not taking the drug by the ninth day. For children with chronic diseases such

as type 1 diabetes or asthma, adherence is difficult to achieve because their treatment plan is complex and must be continued for a long time. Getting children to take drugs that do not taste good, seem frightening (such as eye drops or those that require a mask over the face), or require injections can also be difficult.

Sometimes parents do not understand a doctor's instructions. Also, parents (and patients) forget, on average, about half the information 15 minutes after meeting with a doctor. They remember the first third of the discussion best and remember more about diagnosis than about the details of treatment. That is why doctors try to keep the treatment plan simple and often provide written instructions.

Older People and Adherence

Although adherence is probably not affected by old age itself, it is affected by several factors that are common among older people, such as physical or mental impairments, the use of more drugs, and an increased risk of drug-drug interactions and side effects. Taking several drugs makes remembering when to take each drug harder and increases the risk of adverse drug-drug interactions (see page 89), particularly when over-the-counter drugs are also being taken. Doctors may be able to simplify the drug regimen—by using one drug that serves two purposes or by reducing the number of times a drug must be taken—to improve adherence and to reduce the risk of interactions.

Because older people are generally more sensitive to drugs than younger people, they are more likely to have adverse drug reactions and may require a lower dose of certain drugs (see page 1896).

Improving Adherence

People are more likely to adhere to treatment if they have a good relationship with their doctor and pharmacist. Such relationships involve two-way communication.

Communication can start with an information exchange. By asking questions, people can come to terms with the severity of their disorder, intelligently weigh the advantages and disadvantages of a treatment plan, and ensure that they understand their situation correctly. By discussing concerns, people can learn that denial of their disorder and misconceptions about their treatment can lead to forgetting to take drugs as directed, resulting in unwanted effects. Doctors and pharmacists can encourage adherence by providing clear explanations about how to take the drugs, why the drugs are necessary, and what to expect during treatment. When people know what to expect from a drug, good and bad, they and the health care practitioners involved in their care can better judge how well the drug is working and whether potentially serious problems are developing. Written instructions help people avoid mistakes caused by poor recall of their discussions with the doctor and pharmacist.

Good communication is important, particularly when people have more than one health care practitioner, because it ensures that all practitioners know all the drugs prescribed by the others, and an integrated treatment plan can be developed. Such a plan can help reduce the number of side effects and drug-drug interactions and possibly result in a simpler drug regimen.

When people participate in decisions about their treatment plan, they are more likely to adhere. By participating, people take responsibility for the plan and are therefore more likely to follow it. Taking responsibility includes helping monitor the good and bad effects of treatment and discussing concerns with at least one of their health care practitioners—doctor, physician assistant, pharmacist, or nurse. People should report unwanted or unexpected effects to a health care practitioner rather than adjust a drug dose or discontinue a drug on their own. When a person has good reasons for not following a plan and explains them, the doctor or other health care practitioner can usually make an appropriate adjustment. It is wise for people to keep an up-to-date list of all of their drugs and to take it with them to any health care appointments.

People are also more likely to adhere if they believe that their health care practitioner cares whether they follow the plan. People who receive explanations from a concerned practitioner are more likely to be satisfied with the care they receive and to like the practitioner more. The more people like the practitioner, the more likely they are to adhere.

Obtaining all drugs from one pharmacist can also help, because pharmacists keep computerized records of the drugs a person is taking and can monitor them for possible duplication and for drug-drug interactions. People taking prescription drugs should inform their pharmacist about what over-the-counter drugs and dietary supplements (such as medicinal herbs)

they are taking. Also, people can ask the pharmacist about what to expect from a drug, how to take it correctly, and which drugs interact with each other.

Support groups for people with particular disorders are often available. These groups can often reinforce the importance of following a treatment plan and provide suggestions for coping with problems. Names and telephone numbers of support groups can be obtained through local hospitals and community councils.

Memory aids can help people remember to take their drugs. For example, reminder cards can be placed in different areas of the home, or taking a drug can be associated with a specific daily task, such as brushing teeth. A wristwatch that beeps can be used as a reminder of when to take a drug. A health care practitioner or the person can mark the drug dose and the time of day to take it on a calendar. When the drug is taken, the person checks the appropriate space.

A pharmacist can provide containers that help people take drugs as instructed. Daily doses for a month may be packaged in a blister pack marked with calendar days, so that people can keep track of doses taken by noting the empty spaces. Caps or stickers the same color as the tablet or capsule can be placed on each container to help people match the drug to the instructions on the container. Multicompartment boxes or trays that contain compartments for each day of the week and/or for different times of each day can be used. The person or caregiver fills the compartments on a regular basis, such as at the beginning of each week. By looking at the box, the person can determine whether the pills have been taken.

Containers with a computerized cap are available. These caps beep or flash at dosing time and can record how many times a container is opened each day and how many hours have passed since the last time the container has been opened. Another alternative is a paging service with a beeper (available from subscriber-based telecommunications companies).

CHAPTER

15 Trade-Name and Generic Drugs

Drugs often have several names. When a drug is first discovered, it is given a chemical name, which describes the atomic or molecular structure of the drug. The chemical name is thus usually too complex and cumbersome for general use. Next, a shorthand version of

the chemical name or a code name (such as RU 486) is developed for easy reference among researchers.

When a drug is approved by the Food and Drug Administration (FDA—the government agency responsible for ensuring that drugs marketed in the United

WHAT'S IN A NAME?

CHEMICAL NAME	GENERIC NAME	TRADE NAME
N-(4-hydroxyphenyl) acetamide	Acetaminophen	Tylenol
7-chloro-1,3-dihydro-1-methyl-5-phenyl-2H-1, 4-benzodiazepin-2-one	Diazepam	Valium
4-[4-(p-chlorophenyl)-4-hydroxypiperidino] -4'-fluorobutyrophenone	Haloperidol	Haldol
5-thia-1-azabicyclo [4.2.0]-oct-2-ene-2 carboxylic acid, 7-[(aminophenylacetyl)amino]-3-methyl-8-oxo-, monohydrate	Cephalexin	Keflex, Keforal, or Keftabs
dl-threo-2-(methylamino)-1-phenylpropan-1-ol	Pseudoephedrine	Sudafed
N"-cyano-N-methyl-N'-[2-[[(5-methyl-1H-imidazol-4-yl) methyl]thio]ethyl]guanidine	Cimetidine	Tagamet

States are safe and effective), it is given a generic (official) name and a trade (proprietary or brand) name. The trade name is developed by the company requesting approval for the drug and identifies it as the exclusive property of that company. For example, phenytoin is the generic name and Dilantin is a trade name for the same drug. When a drug is under patent protection, the company markets it under its trade name. When the drug is off-patent (no longer protected by patent), the company may market its product under either the generic name or trade name. Other companies that file for approval to market the off-patent drug must use the same generic name but can create their own trade names. As a result, the same generic drug may be sold under either the generic name or one of many trade names.

In the United States, an official body—the United States Adopted Names (USAN) Council—assigns the generic name. The company that manufactures the drug develops the trade name. Generic and trade names must be unique to prevent one drug from being mistaken for another when drugs are prescribed and prescriptions are dispensed. To prevent this possible confusion, the FDA must agree to every proposed trade name.

Government officials, doctors, researchers, and others who write about the new compound use the drug's generic name because it refers to the drug itself, not to a particular company's brand of the drug or a specific product. However, doctors often use the trade name on prescriptions, because it is easier to remember and doctors usually learn about new drugs by the trade name.

Generic names are usually more complicated and harder to remember than trade names. Many generic names are a shorthand version of the drug's chemical name, structure, or formula. In contrast, trade names are usually catchy, often related to the drug's intended use, and relatively easy to remember, so that doctors will prescribe the drug and consumers will look for it by name. Trade names often suggest a characteristic of the drug. For example, Lopressor lowers blood pressure, Vivactil is an antidepressant that might make a person more vivacious, Glucotrol controls high blood sugar (glucose) levels, and Skelaxin relaxes skeletal muscles. Sometimes, the trade name is simply a shortened version of the drug's generic name—for example, Minocin for minocycline.

The term *generic*, when applied to such items as foods and household products, is used to describe a less expensive, sometimes less effective or lower-quality copycat version of a trade-name product. However, most generic drugs, although less expensive than the comparable trade-name drug, are as effective and of the same quality as the trade-name drug. In fact, generic drug makers manufacture many trade-name products for companies that control the trade names. Sometimes, more than one generic version of a drug is available. For example, many manufacturers sell versions of acetaminophen.

Patent Protection

In the United States, a company that develops a new drug can be granted a patent for the drug itself, for the way the drug is made, for the way the drug is to be used, and even for the method of delivering and releasing the drug into the bloodstream. Thus, a company often owns more than one patent for a drug. Patents grant the company exclusive rights to a drug for 20 years. Additional patents can sometimes be filed to extend the patent life. Usually, about 10 years elapse between the time a drug is discovered (when the patent is obtained) and the time the drug is approved for human use, leaving the company only about half of the patent time to exclusively market a new drug. The FDA may choose to accelerate the approval process for drugs to treat AIDS, cancer, and other life-threatening disorders when no current effective treatment exists.

After a patent has expired, other companies may produce and sell a generic version of the drug as long as the FDA has approved it. They typically sell their product at a lower price than the original trade-name drug because the generic manufacturer does not have to recover the original costs of drug development and usually spends much less on marketing. A generic drug may be sold under its generic name or under a trade name (a branded generic drug) but not under the trade name used by the original patent-holder.

Not all off-patent drugs have generic versions. Sometimes a drug is too hard to duplicate, or adequate tests are not available to prove that the generic drug acts the same as the trade-name drug. Sometimes the market for the drug is so small that producing another version does not make good business sense.

Nonprescription Generic Drugs

Generic versions of some nonprescription (over-the-counter) drugs are often sold as house brands by drug chains or cooperatives, usually at a lower cost. These drugs are evaluated in the same way that generic prescription drugs are evaluated and must meet the same requirements.

Pharmacists can advise which generic over-the-counter drug products should be as effective as the original. However, a consumer may prefer one product to another because of appearance, taste, consistency, or other characteristics.

Bioequivalence and Interchangeability of Generic Drugs

When a company develops a generic version of a trade-name drug, the company's experts in drug formulation must figure out how to make it. It is not enough for them to simply reproduce the trade-name drug's chemical structure or to buy the active ingredient from a chemical manufacturer. Although 250 milligrams (mg) of a trade-name chemical is identical to 250 mg of the same generic chemical, a 250-mg generic pill containing that chemical may or may not have the same effect in the body as a 250-mg trade-name pill. That is because everything that is used in a particular product formulation affects how it is absorbed into the bloodstream. Inactive ingredients such as coatings, stabilizers, fillers,

binders, flavorings, diluents, and others are necessary to turn a chemical into a usable drug product. These ingredients may be used to provide bulk so that a tablet is large enough to handle, to keep a tablet from crumbling between the time it is manufactured and the time it is used, to help a tablet dissolve in the stomach or intestine, or to provide a pleasant taste and color. Inactive ingredients are usually harmless substances that do not affect the body. However, because inactive ingredients can cause unusual and sometimes severe allergic reactions in a few people, one version, or brand, of a drug may be preferable to another. For example, chemicals called bisulfites (such as sodium metabisulfite), which are used as preservatives in many products, cause asthmatic allergic reactions in many people. Consequently, drug products containing bisulfites are prominently labeled as such.

Bioequivalence: Manufacturers must conduct studies to determine whether their version is bioequivalent to the original drug—that is, that the generic version releases its active ingredient (the drug) into the bloodstream at virtually the same speed and in virtually the same amounts as the original drug. Because the active ingredient in the generic drug has already been shown in testing of the trade-name drug to be safe and effective, bioequivalence studies only have to show that the generic version produces virtually the same levels of drug in the blood over time and thus require only a relatively small number (24 to 36) of healthy volunteers.

Although people generally think of oral dosage forms, such as tablets, capsules, and liquids, when they think about generic prescription drugs, generic versions of other drug dosage forms, such as injections, patches, inhalers, and others, must also meet a bioequivalence standard. The FDA sets bioequivalence standards for different drug dosage forms.

The manufacturer of the trade-name drug also must prove bioequivalence before a new form of an approved drug can be sold. New forms include new dosage forms or strengths of an existing trade-name drug product and any other modified form that is developed, as well as new generic drugs. Sometimes the form that was originally tested is modified for commercial reasons. For example, tablets may need to be made sturdier, flavoring or coloring may be added or changed, or inactive ingredients may be changed to increase consumer acceptance.

Evaluation and Approval Procedures: The FDA evaluates every generic version of a drug. The FDA approves a generic drug if studies indicate that the original trade-name drug and the generic version are essentially bioequivalent. The FDA also makes sure that a new generic drug contains the appropriate amount of the active (drug) ingredient, that it is manufactured according to federal standards (Good

WHEN GENERIC SUBSTITUTION MAY NOT BE APPROPRIATE

DRUG CATEGORY	EXAMPLES	COMMENTS
Drugs on the market before the 1938 Federal Food, Drug, and Cosmetic Act	Despite efforts by the FDA, some brands of thyroid hormone replacement products, which are still not bioequivalent	Pre-1938 drugs are exempt from generic drug requirements, but only a few of these are still prescribed. Switching among different versions is unwise because no standards are available by which to compare them. Caution is needed when switching brands.
Drugs with little difference between a toxic dose and an effective dose (a narrow margin of safety)	Anticonvulsants such as phenytoin, carbamazepine, and valproate; digoxin (for heart failure and a very rapid heart rate); and the anticoagulant warfarin	The margin of safety is relatively small. Too little drug may not work, and too much drug may have side effects.
Antihypertensive drugs	Reserpine and reserpine plus polythiazide	Generic versions are not bioequivalent to trade-name drugs.
Antiasthmatic drugs taken by mouth	Theophylline, dyphylline, and some brands of aminophylline	Different versions are generally not bioequivalent. If one version is working, it should not be interchanged for another unless absolutely necessary.
Corticosteroid creams, lotions, and ointments	Alclometasone, amcinonide, betamethasone, clocortolone, desonide, desoximetasone, dexamethasone, diflorasone, fluocinolone, fluocinonide, flurandrenolide, fluticasone, halcinonide, halobetasol, hydrocortisone, mometasone, and triamcinolone	These products are standardized by tests of skin response, and many have been rated as bioequivalent by the FDA. But response varies, and different drug vehicles (creams, ointments, gels) can affect product potency. Response may be unpredictable. So, if one version is effective, it should not be interchanged for another.
Corticosteroid tablets	Dexamethasone, triamcinolone, and others	Many generic versions are not bioequivalent to trade-name drugs and should not be freely interchanged for them.
Hormones	Esterified estrogen (estrogen therapy in postmenopausal women), some brands of medroxyprogesterone, and most generic brands of methyltestosterone	The two brands of esterified estrogen are not bioequivalent. Hormones are usually taken in small doses, so differences in brands could produce major swings in response.
Antihyperglycemic drugs	Glyburide (for type 2 diabetes)	One version of glyburide, Diabeta, may not be interchanged for any other. All other versions are considered interchangeable.
Drugs to control gout	Colchicine	Generic versions of individual drugs are not bioequivalent to one another.
Antipsychotic drugs	Chlorpromazine tablets	Generic versions are not bioequivalent to the trade-name version.
Antidepressants	A few brands of amitriptyline and one brand of amitriptyline plus perphenazine	Not all versions are interchangeable. A pharmacist can advise whether the FDA considers a particular generic drug bioequivalent to the trade-name drug.
Potassium	Most long-acting potassium replacement products in tablet form	Long-acting potassium products in capsule (not tablet) form are considered bioequivalent and may be interchanged.
Other drugs	Fluoxymesterone, some brands of promethazine tablets and suppositories, chloramphenicol capsules, and clozapine	Generic versions may not bioequivalent. Although any version can be effective, versions should not be interchanged.

FDA = Food and Drug Administration.

Manufacturing Practices), and that the generic version differs from its trade-name counterpart in size, color, and shape—a legal requirement.

Interchangeability and Substitution: Theoretically, any generic drug that is bioequivalent to its trade-name counterpart may be interchanged with it. For drugs that are off-patent, the generic drug may be the only form available. To limit costs, many doctors write prescriptions for generic drugs whenever possible. Even if the doctor has prescribed a trade-name drug, the pharmacist may dispense a generic drug unless the doctor wrote on the prescription that no substitution can be made. Also, insurance plans and managed care organizations may require that generic drugs be prescribed and dispensed whenever possible to save money. Some plans may allow a consumer to select a more expensive trade-name product prescribed by the doctor as long as the consumer pays the difference in cost. However, in some state-run programs, the consumer has no say. If the doctor prescribes a generic drug, the pharmacist must dispense a generic drug. In most states, the consumer may insist on a trade-name drug even if the doctor and pharmacist recommend a generic drug.

Sometimes generic substitution may not be appropriate. For example, some available generic versions may not be bioequivalent to the trade-name drug. Such generic drugs may still be used, but they may not be substituted for the trade-name product. In cases in which small differences in the amount of drug in the bloodstream can make a very large difference in the drug's effectiveness, generic drugs are often not substituted for trade-name drugs, although bioequivalent generic products are available. Warfarin, an anticoagulant, and phenytoin, an anticonvulsant, are examples of such drugs. Finally, a generic product may not be appropriate if it contains an inactive ingredient that the person is allergic to. Thus, if a doctor specifies a trade-name drug on the prescription and the consumer wants an equivalent generic version, the consumer or pharmacist should discuss the matter with the doctor.

Drugs that must be given in very precise amounts are less likely to be interchangeable, because the difference between an effective dose and a harmful or an ineffective dose (the margin of safety) is small. Digoxin, used to treat people with heart failure, is an example. Switching from the trade-name version of digoxin to a generic product may cause problems, because the two versions may not be sufficiently bioequivalent. However, some generic versions of digoxin have been certified as bioequivalent by the FDA. Pharmacists and doctors can answer questions about which generic drugs are interchangeable for their trade-name counterparts and which are not.

A book published by the FDA each year and updated periodically also provides guidance about which drugs are interchangeable. This book, *Approved Drug Products With Therapeutic Equivalence Evaluations* (also known as "the orange book" because it has a bright orange cover), is available both in print and online to anyone but is intended for use by doctors and pharmacists.

The substitution of a generic drug can sometimes cause other problems for the consumer. A doctor may write a prescription for a trade-name product and discuss the trade-name product with the consumer. If a pharmacist dispenses an equivalent generic product and the label does not also list the reference (trade-name product), the consumer may not know how the generic product relates to the drug the doctor prescribed. To prevent this confusion, pharmacists should include the reference trade name on the label when a generic product is substituted.

Generic Biologic Drugs

Traditional drugs are called small-molecule agents because the active ingredient is usually a single, discrete chemical entity. Biologic drugs are complex products that can be derived from viruses, blood and body tissues, antibodies, toxins and antitoxins, vaccines, and related products used for treating disease. Until now, it has not been possible to develop generic versions of these products because of their complex manufacturing requirements and the difficulty in defining their exact composition. Companies have made several attempts to get approval for generic equivalent biological products, such as human growth hormone. However, the Food and Drug Administration has required manufacturers of the proposed products to submit for approval under new drug regulations rather than as a generic equivalent. Ongoing scientific developments may allow the creation of generic biologic products in the next several years. The advantage of generic biologic drugs for manufacturers, pharmacies, and consumers is that they could be freely interchanged and compete against one another for inclusion on a hospital or health plan drug list. Having different brands of very similar biologic products, as with epoetin, a hormone to increase red blood cell count, does not offer all the benefits of generically equivalent products.

16 Over-the-Counter Drugs

Over-the-counter (OTC) drugs are those available without a prescription.

OTC drugs enable people to relieve many annoying symptoms and to cure some diseases simply and without the cost of seeing a doctor. However, safe use of these drugs requires knowledge, common sense, and responsibility.

In addition to the substances such as aspirin and acetaminophen that people typically think of as OTC drugs, many other commonly available products are considered OTC drugs by the federal Food and Drug Administration (FDA). Some toothpastes, some mouthwashes, some types of eye drops, wart removers, first aid creams and ointments that contain antibiotics, and even dandruff shampoos are considered OTC drugs. Some OTC drugs were originally available only by prescription. After many years of use under prescription regulation, drugs with excellent safety records may be approved by the FDA for over-the-counter sale. The analgesic ibuprofen and the indigestion remedy famotidine are examples of such drugs. Often, the OTC version has a substantially lower amount of active ingredient in each tablet, capsule, or caplet than does the prescription drug. When establishing appropriate doses of OTC drugs, manufacturers and the FDA try to balance safety and effectiveness.

OTC drugs are not always better tolerated than similar prescription drugs. For example, the OTC sleep aid diphenhydramine is neither as effective nor as safe, especially for older people, as many prescription sleep aids.

Historical Background

At one time, most drugs were available without a prescription. Before the FDA existed, just about anything could be put in a bottle and sold as a sure-fire cure. Alcohol, cocaine, marijuana, and opium were included in some OTC products without notification to users. The Food, Drug, and Cosmetic (FD&C) Act, enacted in 1938, gave the FDA some authority to issue regulations, but the act did not provide clear guidelines as to which drugs could be sold by prescription only and which could be sold over the counter.

An amendment to the FD&C Act in 1951 attempted to clarify the difference between OTC and prescription drugs and to deal with issues of drug safety. Prescription drugs were defined as compounds that could be habit forming, toxic, or unsafe for use except under a doctor's supervision. Anything else could be sold over the counter.

As noted by an amendment to the FD&C Act of 1962, OTC drugs were required to be both effective and safe (see page 77). However, determining effectiveness and safety can be difficult. What is effective for one person may not be for another, and any drug may cause unwanted side effects (also called adverse effects, adverse events, or adverse drug reactions—see page 93). There is no organized system for reporting the side effects of OTC drugs. Consequently, the FDA and drug manufacturers have virtually no way of knowing how common or serious the side effects are.

Safety Considerations

Safety is a major concern when the FDA considers reclassifying a prescription drug as OTC. Most OTC drugs—unlike health foods, dietary supplements

---

Guidelines for Choosing and Using Over-the-Counter Drugs

- Make sure that the self-diagnosis is as accurate as possible. Do not assume the problem is "something that is going around."
- Choose a product because the ingredients are appropriate for the condition, not because the product has a familiar brand name.
- Choose a product with the fewest appropriate ingredients. Products that attempt to relieve every possible symptom are likely to expose people to unnecessary drugs, pose additional risks, and cost more.
- Read the label carefully to determine the correct dose and precautions, including what conditions would make the drug a poor choice.
- When in doubt, ask a pharmacist or doctor what the most appropriate ingredient or product is.
- Ask a pharmacist to check for potential interactions with other drugs being used.
- Ask a pharmacist to identify possible side effects.
- Do not take more than the recommended dose.
- Do not take an over-the-counter drug longer than the maximum time suggested on the label. Stop taking the drug if symptoms worsen.
- Keep all drugs, including over-the-counter drugs, out of the reach of children.

(including medicinal herbs—see page 2067) and complementary therapies (see page 2059)—have been studied scientifically and extensively. However, all drugs have benefits and risks, and some degree of risk has to be tolerated if people are to receive a drug's benefits. Defining an acceptable degree of risk is a judgment call.

Safety depends on using a drug properly. For OTC drugs, proper use often relies on consumer self-diagnosis, which leaves room for error. For example, most headaches are not dangerous, but in rare cases, a headache is an early warning of a brain tumor or hemorrhage. Similarly, what seems like severe heartburn may signal an impending heart attack. Ultimately, people must use common sense in determining when a symptom or ailment is minor and when it requires medical attention and consult a doctor if they are unsure.

People who purchase OTC drugs should read and follow the instructions carefully. Because different formulations—such as immediate-release and controlled-release (slow-release) formulations—may have the same brand name, the label should be checked each time a product is purchased, and the dosage should be noted. Assuming that the dosage is the same is not safe. Also, different formulations with the same brand name may have different ingredients, so checking the ingredients on the label is important. For example, there are several dozen different Tylenol formulations with a vast array of ingredients. Some Maalox products contain aluminum and magnesium hydroxides, while others contain calcium carbonate. When selecting a product, people should read the label carefully to determine which product is most appropriate for their particular problem. Labels on OTC drugs, which are required by the FDA, can help people understand a drug's benefits and risks as well as how to use the drug correctly. People should ask a pharmacist if they have any questions about an OTC product.

Often, the labels of OTC drugs do not list the full range of possible side effects. As a result, many people assume that these drugs have few, if any, side effects. For example, the package insert for one analgesic cautions people not to take the drug for more than 10 days for pain. However, the possible serious side effects that can occur with long-term use (such as life-threatening bleeding from the digestive tract) are not mentioned—not on the box, bottle, or package insert. Consequently, people with chronic pain or inflammation may take the drug for a long time without realizing that such use could lead to serious problems.

Precautions With Over-the-Counter Drugs

Certain groups of people, such as the very young, the very old, the very sick, and pregnant and breast-

---

Considerations in Reclassifying a Drug as Over-the-Counter

SAFETY

- Has the drug been used for a long enough time so that any harmful effects are fully understood?
- What harmful effects (including effects from misuse or abuse) may the drug produce?
- Is the drug habit forming?
- Do the benefits of over-the-counter status outweigh the risks?

EASE OF DIAGNOSIS AND TREATMENT

- Can the average person self-diagnose the condition that calls for the drug?
- Can the average person treat the condition without the help of a doctor or other health care practitioner?

LABELING

- Can adequate directions for use be written?
- Can warnings against unsafe use be written?
- Can the average person understand the information on the label?

---

feeding women, are more vulnerable to harm from drugs, including OTC drugs. When such people use drugs, special precautions, which may include a doctor's supervision, should be taken.

To avoid dangerous drug-drug interactions, people should consult a pharmacist or doctor before they take prescription drugs and OTC drugs at the same time. People who have chronic disorders should also consult a pharmacist or doctor. OTC drugs are not designed to treat serious disorders and can make some disorders worse. An unanticipated reaction, such as a rash or insomnia, is a signal to stop taking the drug immediately and obtain medical advice.

CHILDREN

Children's bodies metabolize and react to drugs differently from the way adults' bodies do. A drug may be used by many people for many years before its hazards to children are discovered. For example, many years passed before researchers confirmed that the risk of Reye's syndrome was linked to the use of aspirin in children who had chickenpox or influenza. Doctors and parents alike are often surprised to learn that most OTC drugs, even those drugs with recommended dosages for children, have not been thoroughly tested in children. The effectiveness of some cough and cold remedies is unproved, especially in children, so that giving these drugs to children may unnecessarily expose them to harmful effects of a drug and may be a waste of money.

Giving a child a correct drug dose can be tricky. Although children's doses are often expressed in terms of age ranges (for example, children aged 2 to 6 or 6 to 12), age is not the best criterion. Children can vary greatly in size within any age range, so experts advise using the child's weight to determine doses of OTC drugs.

If the label does not give instructions on how much drug to give the child, a parent should not guess. When in doubt, a parent should consult a pharmacist or doctor. Such consultation may prevent a child from receiving a dangerous drug or a dangerously high dose of a potentially helpful drug.

Many drugs for treating children come in liquid form. Even though the label should give clear guidelines about the dose, a child may be given the wrong dose because the adult in charge uses an ordinary teaspoon. The only kitchen spoons accurate enough to measure liquid drugs are measuring spoons. However, a cylindrical measuring spoon is far better for measuring a child's dose, and an oral syringe is preferred for measuring and squirting a precise amount of drug into an infant's mouth. The cap should always

be removed from the tip of an oral syringe before use. A child can choke if the cap is accidentally propelled into the windpipe. Sometimes, drugs intended for treating children come with a measuring device packaged with the product. If so, the device that is in the package should be used to measure the appropriate dose.

Several children's drugs are available in more than one form. Adults must read labels carefully every time a new children's drug is used.

OLDER PEOPLE

Normal aging changes the speed and ways in which the body metabolizes drugs (see page 1896), and older people tend to have more diseases and to take more than one drug at a time. For these reasons, older people may be more likely than younger ones to experience side effects or drug interactions. More and more prescription drug labels specify whether different doses are needed for older people, but such information is rarely included on OTC drug labels.

Many OTC drugs are potentially hazardous for older people. The risk increases when drugs are taken regularly at the maximum dose. For example, an older person who has arthritis may frequently use an analgesic or anti-inflammatory drug, with potentially

---

Reading a Drug Label

Nonprescription drugs are required to have labels that explain what a drug's benefits and risks are and how to use the drug correctly. The label is entitled "Drug Facts." Active ingredients are listed at the top, followed by uses, warnings, directions, other information, and inactive ingredients.

Active ingredient: The drug itself is the active ingredient. Combination products have more than one active ingredient. The drug's generic name is listed with the amount of drug in each tablet, capsule, or dose unit. The same generic drug may be sold under several different trade (brand) names.

Uses: Symptoms or disorders for which the drug product is recommended are listed.

Warnings: When the drug should not be used, when a doctor or pharmacist should be consulted (and after how long), and which factors can alter the expected response to the drug are listed, usually in four sections.

- "Ask a doctor before use if you have" lists conditions that can make taking the drug more problematic or unsafe. This section refers to drug-disease interactions.
- "Ask a doctor or a pharmacist before use if you are taking" lists other drugs that can interfere with the drug's effectiveness or safety. This section refers to drug-drug interactions.

- "When using this product" includes common side effects, foods that may interfere with the drug's effectiveness or safety (drug-food interactions), and special precautions to take (for example, not driving while taking the drug).
- The last section lists special warnings for women who are pregnant or breastfeeding and for children, with instructions about what to do in case of an overdose.

Directions: How much of the drug and how often to take the drug are given for different age groups, because size and age, among other factors, affect how a person responds to a drug.

Other information: Special instructions, such as how to store the drug so that it does not deteriorate, are listed.

Inactive ingredients: In addition to the drug, drug products—the tablets, capsules, or other formulations that consumers buy—contain substances added to facilitate the administration of the drug, such as ingredients that provide bulk or a pleasant taste and color. Products with the same active ingredient may contain different inactive ingredients. Inactive ingredients are usually harmless, but some of them cause an allergic reaction in a few people, who should look for products made without those ingredients.

serious consequences, such as a bleeding peptic ulcer. Such an ulcer is life threatening for an older person and can occur without warning.

Antihistamines, such as diphenhydramine, also pose special risks for older people. Many nighttime pain relief formulas, cough and cold remedies, allergy drugs, and sleep aids contain antihistamines. Antihistamines may worsen some disorders common among older people, such as closed-angle glaucoma and an enlarged prostate gland. They can also make a person dizzy or unsteady, leading to falls and broken bones. Antihistamines, particularly at a high dose or in combination with other drugs, can sometimes cause blurred vision, light-headedness, dry mouth, difficulty with urination, constipation, and confusion in older people.

Older people may be more susceptible to the possible side effects of antacids. Antacids that contain aluminum are more likely to cause constipation, and antacids that contain magnesium are more likely to cause diarrhea and dehydration.

During visits to the doctor, older people should mention all OTC products they are taking, including vitamins, minerals, and medicinal herbs. This information helps the doctor evaluate the entire drug regimen and determine whether or not an OTC drug may be responsible for certain symptoms.

PREGNANT AND BREASTFEEDING WOMEN

Drugs can move from a pregnant woman to her fetus (primarily through the placenta—see art on page 1637), and drugs can be transmitted through breast milk to the baby. Some such drugs can affect or harm the fetus or baby, so pregnant women and breastfeeding women should consult their doctor or pharmacist before taking any OTC drug or medicinal herb. OTC drug labels should be checked because they contain warnings against use during pregnancy and breastfeeding, if applicable.

Certain types of drugs are particularly problematic. They include antihistamines (commonly contained in cough and cold remedies, allergy drugs, motion sickness drugs, and sleep aids) and nonsteroidal anti-inflammatory drugs (NSAIDs). NSAIDs should not be used during the last 3 months of pregnancy unless specified by a doctor, because they may cause problems in the fetus or complications during delivery.

PEOPLE WITH CHRONIC DISORDERS

A number of chronic disorders can become worse if an OTC drug is taken inappropriately. Because OTC drugs are intended primarily for occasional use by people who are essentially healthy, people who have a chronic or serious disorder or who plan to take an OTC drug every day should consult a

---

Recognizing Antihistamines

Many different types of OTC products (such as cold and allergy remedies, motion sickness drugs, and sleep aids) contain antihistamines. Most antihistamines decrease alertness and have many other side effects, and they may be dangerous for people with certain disorders. Consequently, being able to identify which products contain these antihistamines is useful. OTC antihistamines are listed under active ingredients on the package. Antihistamines that have such side effects include the following:

- Brompheniramine
- Chlorpheniramine
- Dexbrompheniramine
- Diphenhydramine
- Doxylamine
- Phenindamine
- Pheniramine
- Pyrilamine
- Triprolidine

---

health care practitioner before they purchase OTC products. In such cases, drug use is beyond the normal boundaries of self-care and requires the advice of an expert.

DRUG-DRUG INTERACTIONS

Many people neglect to mention their use of OTC drugs to their doctor or pharmacist. Drugs taken intermittently, such as drugs for colds, constipation, or an occasional headache, are mentioned even less often. Health care practitioners may not think of asking about use of OTC drugs or medicinal herbs when they are prescribing or dispensing a prescription. Yet many OTC drugs and medicinal herbs can interact adversely with a wide range of drugs (see page 89).

Some of these interactions can be serious, interfering with the effectiveness of a drug or causing side effects. For example, taking aspirin with the anticoagulant warfarin can increase the risk of abnormal bleeding. An antacid containing aluminum or magnesium can reduce the absorption of digoxin, taken for heart disease. Taking a multiple vitamin and mineral supplement can interfere with the action of some prescription drugs. For example, the antibiotic tetracycline may be ineffective if swallowed with a product that contains calcium, magnesium, or iron.

OTC drug-drug interactions have not been studied systematically. Many serious problems have

CHRONIC DISORDERS AND OVER-THE-COUNTER DRUGS

DISORDER	OTC DRUGS	PRECAUTIONS
Alcoholism	Cold remedies	Recovering alcoholics need to be vigilant about avoiding cold remedies that contain alcohol. Some products contain as much as 25% alcohol.
Diabetes	Decongestants	People with diabetes should consult a doctor before they take decongestants because these drugs can worsen diabetes and have dangerous side effects.
	Cough syrups	People with diabetes may need help locating a cough syrup that does not contain sugar.
Enlarged prostate	Antihistamines Decongestants	People with an enlarged prostate should consult a doctor or pharmacist before they take antihistamines and decongestants because side effects can be dangerous.
Glaucoma	Antihistamines	Taking an antihistamine can complicate certain types of glaucoma.
Heart disease	Antacids Cold remedies	People with heart disease should consult a doctor or pharmacist to help them select an antacid or cold remedy that does not interact with their prescription drugs.
	Decongestants	People with heart disease should consult a doctor or pharmacist before they take decongestants because side effects can be dangerous.
High blood pressure (hypertension)	Antacids	People with high blood pressure should consult a doctor or pharmacist before they select an antacid.
	Decongestants	People with high blood pressure should consult a doctor or pharmacist before they take decongestants because side effects can be dangerous.
Hyperthyroidism	Decongestants	People with hyperthyroidism should consult a doctor or pharmacist before they take decongestants because side effects can be dangerous.
Kidney disorders	Antacids	People with kidney disorders should consult a doctor or pharmacist before they select an antacid.

OTC = over-the-counter.

been discovered accidentally, after side effects or deaths were reported. Even when interaction warnings are printed on the label for OTC drugs, the language may be meaningless to most people. For example, the labels of some cold remedies that contain pseudoephedrine caution against using the product with a monoamine oxidase inhibitor (MAOI—given for depression) or during the 2 weeks after discontinuing the MAOI. For the many people who do not know that the antidepressant they are taking is an MAOI (such as phenelzine and tranylcypromine), this important warning is not helpful.

The best way to reduce the risk of drug-drug interactions is to ask the pharmacist to check for them. Additionally, the doctor should be told about all drugs being taken, both prescription and OTC (see box on page 91).

DRUG OVERLAP

Another potential problem is drug overlap. OTC products used to treat different problems may contain the same active ingredient. Unless people read the labels on everything they take, they can accidentally overdose themselves. For example, a person who takes a sleep aid and a cold remedy, both of which contain diphenhydramine, may take double the dose considered safe. Many products contain acetaminophen. A person who simultaneously takes two different products that contain acetaminophen— one for a headache and another for allergies or sinus problems—may exceed the recommended dose.

Digestive Disorders

CHAPTER
17 Biology of the Digestive System

The digestive system, which extends from the mouth to the anus, is responsible for receiving food, breaking it down into nutrients (a process called digestion), absorbing the nutrients into the bloodstream, and eliminating the indigestible parts of food from the body. The digestive tract consists of the mouth (see page 1343), throat, esophagus, stomach, small intestine, large intestine, rectum, and anus. The digestive system also includes organs that lie outside the digestive tract: the pancreas, the liver, and the gallbladder.

The digestive system is sometimes called the gastrointestinal system, but neither name fully describes the system's functions or components. The organs of the digestive system also produce clotting factors and hormones unrelated to digestion, help remove toxic substances from the blood, and chemically alter (metabolize) drugs.

The abdominal cavity is the space that holds the digestive organs. It is bordered by the abdominal wall (composed of layers of skin, fat, muscle, and connective tissue) in front, the spinal column in back, the diaphragm above, and the pelvic organs below. It is lined, as is the outer surface of the digestive organs, by a membrane called the peritoneum.

Experts have recognized a powerful connection between the digestive system and the brain. For example, psychologic factors greatly influence contractions of the intestine, secretion of digestive enzymes, and other functions of the digestive system. Even susceptibility to infection, which leads to various digestive system disorders, is strongly influenced by the brain. In turn, the digestive system influences the brain. For example, long-standing or recurring diseases such as irritable bowel syndrome, ulcerative colitis, and other painful diseases affect emotions, behaviors, and daily functioning. This two-way association has been called the brain-gut axis.

Throat and Esophagus

The throat (pharynx) lies behind and below the mouth. When food and fluids leave the mouth, they pass through the throat. Swallowing of food and fluids begins voluntarily and continues automatically. A small muscular flap (epiglottis) closes to prevent food and fluids from going down the windpipe (trachea) toward the lungs. The back portion of the roof of the mouth (soft palate) lifts to prevent food and fluids from going up the nose.

The esophagus—a thin-walled, muscular channel lined with mucous membranes—connects the throat with the stomach. Food and fluids are propelled through the esophagus not only by gravity but also by waves of rhythmic muscular contractions, called peristalsis. At either end of the esophagus are ring-shaped muscles (the upper and lower esophageal sphincters),

Digestive System

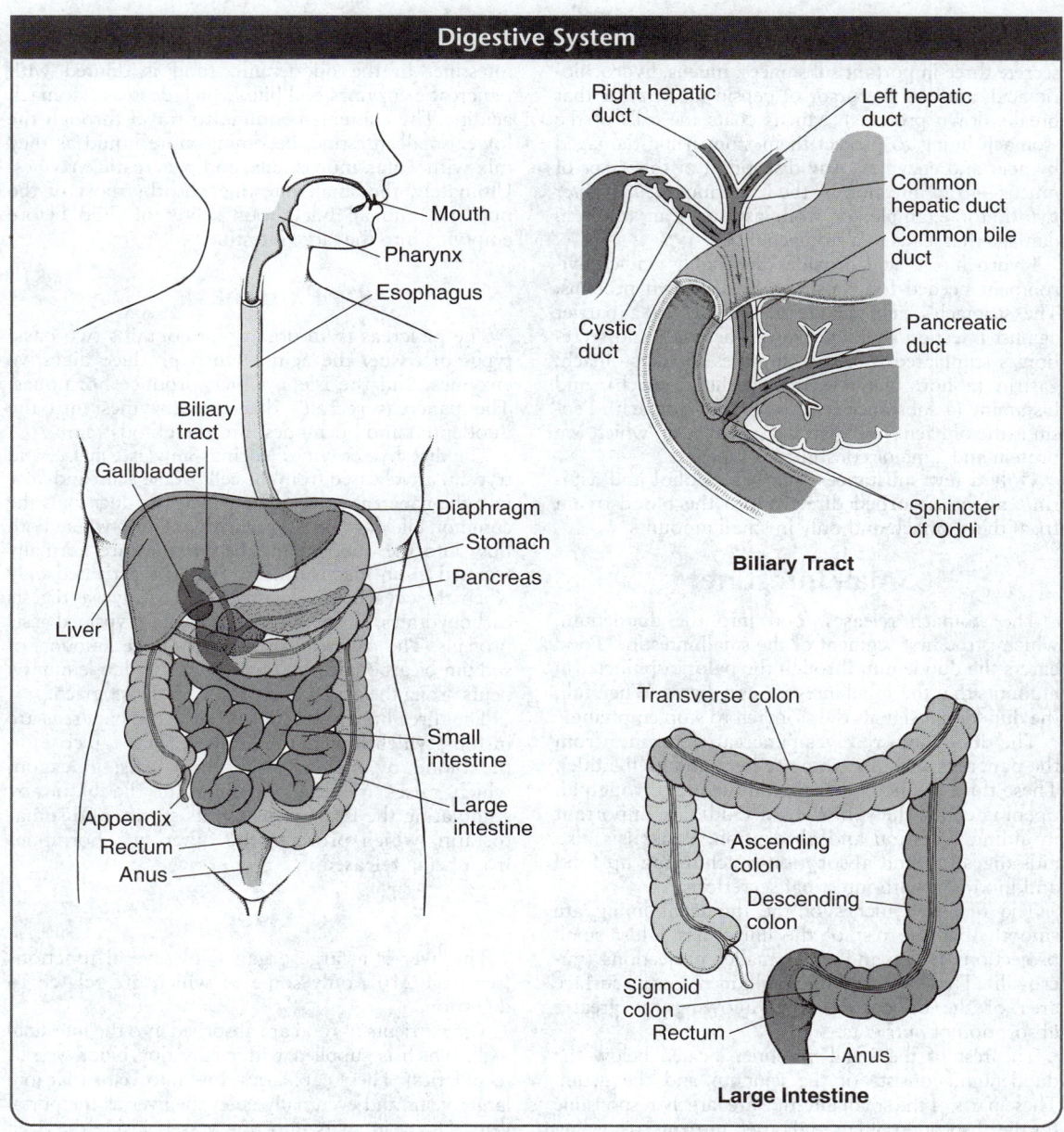

Biliary Tract

Large Intestine

which open and close. The esophageal sphincters normally prevent the contents of the stomach from flowing back into the esophagus or throat.

Stomach

The stomach is a large, bean-shaped, hollow muscular organ consisting of three regions: the cardia,

the body (fundus), and the antrum. Food and fluids enter the stomach from the esophagus by passing through the lower esophageal sphincter.

The upper stomach serves as a storage area for food. Here, the cardia and body of the stomach relax to accommodate food that enters the stomach. Then the antrum (lower stomach) contracts rhythmically, mixing the food with acid and enzymes (stomach juices) and grinding the food down into small pieces so that it is more easily digested. The cells lining the stomach secrete three important substances: mucus, hydrochloric acid, and the precursor of pepsin (an enzyme that breaks down proteins). Mucus coats the cells of the stomach lining to protect them from being damaged by acid and enzymes. Any disruption of this layer of mucus—from infection by the bacterium *Helicobacter pylori*, for example, or from aspirin—can result in damage that leads to a stomach ulcer.

Hydrochloric acid provides the highly acidic environment needed for pepsin to break down proteins. The stomach's high acidity also serves as a barrier against infection by killing most bacteria. Acid secretion is stimulated by nerve impulses to the stomach, gastrin (a hormone released by the stomach), and histamine (a substance released by the stomach). Pepsin is the only enzyme that digests collagen, which is a protein and a major constituent of meat.

Only a few substances, such as alcohol and aspirin, can be absorbed directly into the bloodstream from the stomach and only in small amounts.

Small Intestine

The stomach releases food into the duodenum, which is the first segment of the small intestine. Food enters the duodenum through the pyloric sphincter in amounts that the small intestine can digest. When full, the duodenum signals the stomach to stop emptying.

The duodenum receives pancreatic enzymes from the pancreas and bile from the liver and gallbladder. These fluids, which enter the duodenum through an opening called the sphincter of Oddi, are important in aiding digestion and absorption. Peristalsis also aids digestion and absorption by churning up food and mixing it with intestinal secretions.

The first few inches of the duodenal lining are smooth, but the rest of the lining has folds, small projections (villi), and even smaller projections (microvilli). These villi and microvilli increase the surface area of the duodenal lining, allowing for greater absorption of nutrients.

The rest of the small intestine, located below the duodenum, consists of the jejunum and the ileum. These parts of the small intestine are largely responsible for the absorption of fats and other nutrients. Churning movements facilitate absorption. Absorption is also enhanced by the vast surface area made up of folds, villi, and microvilli. The intestinal wall is richly supplied with blood vessels that carry the absorbed nutrients to the liver through the portal vein. The intestinal wall releases mucus, which lubricates the intestinal contents, and water, which helps dissolve the digested fragments. Small amounts of enzymes that digest proteins, sugars, and fats are also released.

The consistency of the intestinal contents changes gradually as the contents travel through the small intestine. In the duodenum, food is diluted with pancreatic enzymes and bile, which decrease stomach acidity. The contents continue to travel through the lower small intestine, becoming more liquid as they mix with water, mucus, bile, and pancreatic enzymes. Ultimately, the small intestine absorbs most of the nutrients and all but about 1 liter of fluid before emptying into the large intestine.

Pancreas

The pancreas is an organ that contains two basic types of tissue: the acini, which produce digestive enzymes, and the islets, which produce hormones. The pancreas secretes digestive enzymes into the duodenum and hormones into the bloodstream.

The digestive enzymes (such as amylase, lipase, and trypsin) are released from the cells of the acini and flow into the pancreatic duct. The pancreatic duct joins the common bile duct at the sphincter of Oddi, where both flow into the duodenum. The enzymes are normally secreted in an inactive form. They are activated only when they reach the digestive tract. Amylase digests carbohydrates; lipase digests fats; and trypsin digests proteins. The pancreas also secretes large amounts of sodium bicarbonate, which protects the duodenum by neutralizing the acid that comes from the stomach.

The three hormones produced by the pancreas are insulin, which lowers the level of sugar (glucose) in the blood by moving sugar into cells; glucagon, which raises the level of sugar in the blood by stimulating the liver to release its stores; and somatostatin, which prevents the other two hormones from being released.

Liver

The liver is a large organ with several functions (see page 210), only some of which are related to digestion.

The nutrients of food are absorbed into the intestinal wall, which is supplied with many tiny blood vessels (capillaries). These capillaries flow into veins that join larger veins and eventually enter the liver as the portal vein. This vein splits into tiny vessels inside the liver, where the incoming blood can be processed.

Blood in the liver is processed in two ways: Bacteria and other foreign particles absorbed from the intestine are removed, and many nutrients absorbed from the intestine are further broken down so they can be used by the body. The liver performs the necessary processing at high speed and passes the blood, laden with nutrients, into the general circulation.

The liver manufactures about half of the body's cholesterol; the rest comes from food. About 80% of the cholesterol made by the liver is used to make bile. The liver secretes bile, which is stored in the gallbladder until it is needed.

Gallbladder and Biliary Tract

Bile flows out of the liver through the right and left hepatic ducts (see page 210), which come together to form the common hepatic duct. This duct then joins with a duct coming from the gallbladder, called the cystic duct, to form the common bile duct. The pancreatic duct joins the common bile duct just where it empties into the duodenum through the sphincter of Oddi.

Between meals, bile salts are stored in the gallbladder, and only a small amount of bile flows into the intestine. Food that enters the duodenum triggers a series of hormonal and nerve signals that cause the gallbladder to contract. As a result, bile flows into the duodenum and mixes with food contents.

Bile has two important functions: It assists in the digestion and absorption of fats, and it is responsible for the elimination of certain waste products from the body—particularly hemoglobin from destroyed red blood cells and excess cholesterol. Specifically, bile is responsible for these actions:

- Bile salts increase the solubility of cholesterol, fats, and fat-soluble vitamins to aid in their absorption.
- Bile salts stimulate the secretion of water by the large intestine to help move the contents along.
- Bilirubin (the main pigment in bile) is excreted in bile as a waste product of destroyed red blood cells, giving stool a green-brown color.
- Drugs and other waste products are excreted in bile and later eliminated from the body.
- Various proteins that play important roles in bile's absorptive function are secreted in bile.

Bile salts are reabsorbed by the last portion of the small intestine, extracted by the liver, and resecreted into bile. This recirculation of bile salts is known as the enterohepatic circulation. All the bile salts in the body circulate about 10 to 12 times a day. During each pass, small amounts of bile salts reach the large intestine, where bacteria break them down into various constituents. Some constituents are reabsorbed; the rest are excreted with the stool.

Large Intestine

The large intestine consists of the cecum and ascending (right) colon, the transverse colon, the descending (left) colon, and the sigmoid colon, which is connected to the rectum. The cecum, which is at the beginning of the ascending colon, is the point at which the small intestine joins the large intestine. Projecting from the cecum is the appendix, which is a small finger-shaped tube that serves no known function. The large intestine secretes mucus and is largely responsible for the absorption of water from the stool.

Intestinal contents are liquid when they reach the large intestine but are normally solid by the time they reach the rectum as stool. The many bacteria that inhabit the large intestine can further digest some material, creating gas. Bacteria in the large intestine also make some important substances, such as vitamin K, which plays an important role in blood clotting. These bacteria are necessary for healthy intestinal function, and some diseases and antibiotics can upset the balance among the different types of bacteria in the large intestine. The result is irritation that leads to the secretion of mucus and water, causing diarrhea.

Rectum and Anus

The rectum is a chamber that begins at the end of the large intestine, immediately following the sigmoid colon, and ends at the anus. Ordinarily, the rectum is empty because stool is stored higher in the descending colon. Eventually, the descending colon becomes full, and stool passes into the rectum, causing an urge to move the bowels (defecate). Adults and older children can withstand this urge until they reach a bathroom. Infants and young children lack the muscle control necessary to delay bowel movement.

The anus is the opening at the far end of the digestive tract through which stool leaves the body. The anus is formed partly from the surface layers of the body, including the skin, and partly from the intestine. The anus is lined with a continuation of the external skin. A muscular ring (anal sphincter) keeps the anus closed until the person has a bowel movement.

Effects of Aging

Because the digestive system has a lot of reserve built into it, aging has relatively little effect on its function compared to its effects on other organ systems. Nonetheless, aging is a factor in several digestive system disorders. In particular, older adults are more likely to develop diverticulosis and to experience digestive tract disorders (for example, constipation) as a side effect of taking certain drugs.

Esophagus: With age, the strength of esophageal contractions and the tension in the upper esophageal sphincter decrease, but the movement of food is not impaired by these changes. However, many older adults are likely to be affected by diseases that interfere with esophageal contractions.

Stomach: With age, the stomach lining's capacity to resist damage decreases, which in turn may increase the risk of peptic ulcer disease, especially in people who use aspirin and other nonsteroidal anti-inflammatory drugs (NSAIDs). Also with age, the stomach cannot accommodate as much food (because of decreased elasticity), and the rate at which the stomach empties food into the small intestine decreases, but these changes generally do not produce any noticeable symptoms. Aging has little effect on the secretion of stomach juices such as acid and pepsin, but conditions that decrease acid secretion, such as atrophic gastritis, become more common.

Small Intestine: Aging has only minor effects on the structure of the small intestine, so movement of contents through the small intestine and absorption of most nutrients do not change much. However, lactase levels decrease, leading to intolerance of dairy products by many older adults (lactose intolerance). Excessive growth of certain bacteria (bacterial overgrowth) becomes more common with age and can lead to pain, bloating, and weight loss. Bacterial overgrowth may also lead to decreased absorption of certain nutrients, such as folic acid, iron, and calcium.

Pancreas, Liver, and Gallbladder: With age, the pancreas decreases in overall weight, and some tissue is replaced by scarring (fibrosis). However, these changes do not decrease the ability of the pancreas to produce digestive enzymes and sodium bicarbonate. As the liver and gallbladder age, a number of structural and microscopic changes occur (see page 212).

Large Intestine and Rectum: The large intestine does not undergo much change with age. The rectum does enlarge somewhat. Constipation becomes more common. This may be due partly to a slight slowing in the movement of contents through the large intestine and a modest decrease in the contractions of the rectum when filled with stool.

CHAPTER 18

Symptoms and Diagnosis of Digestive Disorders

Disorders that affect the digestive (gastrointestinal) system are called digestive disorders. Some disorders simultaneously affect several parts of the digestive system, whereas others affect only one part or organ.

Symptoms

Some symptoms, such as diarrhea, constipation, bleeding from the digestive tract, regurgitation, and difficulty swallowing, usually suggest a digestive disorder. More general symptoms, such as abdominal pain, flatulence, loss of appetite, and nausea, may suggest a digestive disorder or another type of disorder.

Indigestion is an imprecise term that is used by different people to mean different things. The term covers a wide range of symptoms, including dyspepsia, nausea and vomiting, regurgitation, and the sensation of having a lump in the throat (globus sensation).

Bowel (intestinal) function varies greatly not only from one person to another but also for any one person at different times. Most people find it easiest to move their bowels in the morning. The urge tends to be strongest about 30 to 60 minutes after first eating in the morning. Bowel function can be affected by diet, stress, drugs, disease, and even social and cultural patterns. In most Western societies, the normal number of bowel movements ranges from 2 or 3 a week to as many as 2 or 3 a day. Changes in the frequency, consistency, or volume of bowel movements or the presence of blood, mucus, pus, or excess fatty material (oil or grease) in the stool may indicate a disorder.

ABDOMINAL PAIN

Abdominal pain is common and often minor. Severe abdominal pain of rapid onset, however, almost always indicates a significant problem. The pain may be the only sign of the need for surgery and must be attended to swiftly. Abdominal pain is of particular concern in people who are very young or very old and those who have human immunodeficiency virus (HIV) infection or are taking drugs that suppress the immune system. Older adults may have less abdominal pain than younger adults, and, even if the condition is serious, the pain may develop more gradually. Abdominal pain also affects children, including newborns and infants—who cannot communicate the cause of their distress.

Causes

Pain can arise from any of several causes, including infection, inflammation, formation of sores (ulcers), perforation or rupture of organs, muscle contractions that are uncoordinated or blocked by an obstruction, and blockage of blood flow to organs.

Examples of disorders that are immediately life threatening, requiring rapid diagnosis and surgery, include a ruptured abdominal aortic aneurysm, perforated stomach or intestine, blockage of blood flow to the intestine (mesenteric ischemia), and ruptured ectopic pregnancy (see page 1644). Disorders that are also serious and nearly as urgent include intestinal obstruction, appendicitis, and acute inflammation of the pancreas (pancreatitis).

Peritonitis is pain caused by inflammation of the lining of the abdominal cavity (peritoneum), which occurs with many disorders that result in inflammation or infection of abdominal organs (such as appendicitis and diverticulitis) or leakage of intestinal contents into the abdomen (such as a perforated ulcer).

Sometimes, disorders outside the abdomen also produce abdominal pain. Examples include heart attack, pneumonia, and twisting of the testes (testicular torsion). Other problems that cause abdominal pain include diabetic ketoacidosis, porphyria, sickle cell disease, and certain bites and poisons (such as a black widow spider bite, heavy metal or methanol poisoning, and some scorpion stings).

ABDOMINAL PAIN IN NEWBORNS, INFANTS, AND YOUNG CHILDREN

CAUSE OF PAIN	DESCRIPTION	COMMENTS
Meconium peritonitis	Inflammation and sometimes infection of the abdominal cavity and its lining (peritonitis) caused by a perforation in the intestine and leakage of meconium, the dark green fecal material that is produced in the intestines before birth	Occurs while infants are still in the womb or shortly after birth
Pyloric stenosis	A blockage at the stomach outlet (duodenum)	Forceful (projectile) vomiting occurs after feedings Usually begins between birth and 4 months of age
Esophageal webs	Thin membranes that grow across the inside of the upper one third of the esophagus from its surface lining (mucosa)	Solids are difficult to swallow
Volvulus	Twisting of a loop of the intestines	Causes intestinal obstruction and cuts off blood supply to intestines Vomiting, diarrhea, abdominal swelling, and episodic and excessive crying (colic) are common
Imperforate anus (anal atresia)	Narrowing or blockage of the anal opening	Normally detected by doctors when infants are examined after birth and usually requiring immediate surgery
Intussusception	The condensing and overlapping (telescoping) of one portion of the intestine into another	Causes obstruction of the bowel and blockage of its blood flow, sudden pain, vomiting, bloody stools, and fever Typically affects children between the ages of 6 months and 2 years
Intestinal obstruction	A blockage that completely stops or seriously impairs the passage of intestinal contents	Commonly caused by a birth defect, meconium, or volvulus in newborns and infants Symptoms vary by type of obstruction but may include cramping pain in the abdomen, bloating, disinterest in eating, vomiting, severe constipation, diarrhea, and fever

Causes of Abdominal Pain by Location

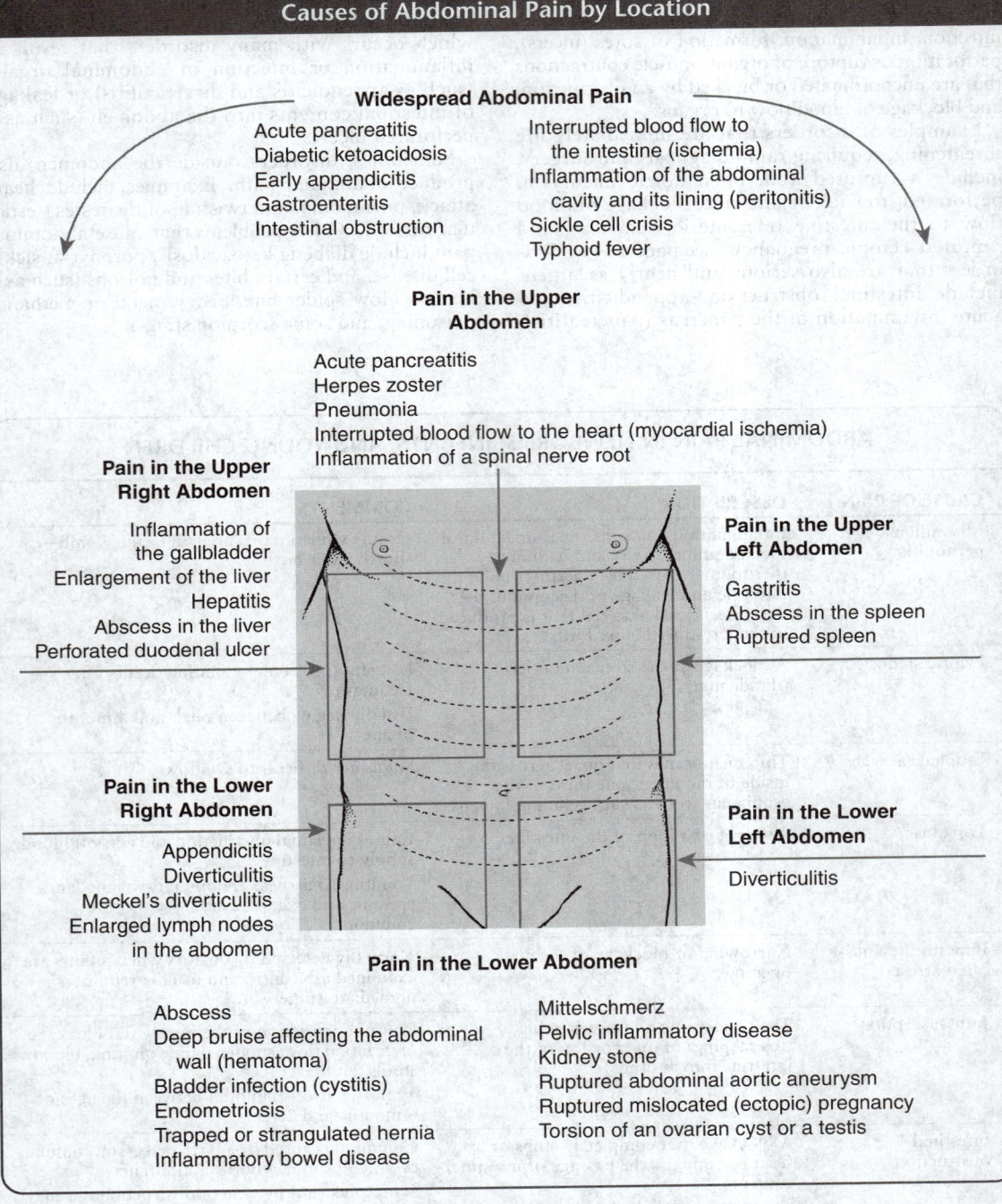

Widespread Abdominal Pain

Acute pancreatitis
Diabetic ketoacidosis
Early appendicitis
Gastroenteritis
Intestinal obstruction

Interrupted blood flow to
the intestine (ischemia)
Inflammation of the abdominal
cavity and its lining (peritonitis)
Sickle cell crisis
Typhoid fever

Pain in the Upper Abdomen

Acute pancreatitis
Herpes zoster
Pneumonia
Interrupted blood flow to the heart (myocardial ischemia)
Inflammation of a spinal nerve root

Pain in the Upper Right Abdomen

Inflammation of
the gallbladder
Enlargement of the liver
Hepatitis
Abscess in the liver
Perforated duodenal ulcer

Pain in the Upper Left Abdomen

Gastritis
Abscess in the spleen
Ruptured spleen

Pain in the Lower Right Abdomen

Appendicitis
Diverticulitis
Meckel's diverticulitis
Enlarged lymph nodes
in the abdomen

Pain in the Lower Left Abdomen

Diverticulitis

Pain in the Lower Abdomen

Abscess
Deep bruise affecting the abdominal
wall (hematoma)
Bladder infection (cystitis)
Endometriosis
Trapped or strangulated hernia
Inflammatory bowel disease

Mittelschmerz
Pelvic inflammatory disease
Kidney stone
Ruptured abdominal aortic aneurysm
Ruptured mislocated (ectopic) pregnancy
Torsion of an ovarian cyst or a testis

Evaluation

Sometimes, the nature and location of the pain help doctors identify the cause. Pain that comes and goes in waves suggests an organ is blocked, which might occur with gallstones, kidney stones, or intestinal obstruction. Pain produced by a peptic ulcer is often characterized as burning. Pain that accompanies diverticulitis is often limited to the lower left abdomen, whereas the pain of peritonitis is frequently felt throughout the abdomen. Pancreatitis often produces pain that is worsened by rolling over in bed and is relieved somewhat by sitting upright and leaning forward.

Often, the doctor must perform tests to help choose among several different causes suggested by the person's symptoms and physical examination results. An abdominal computed tomography (CT) scan helps identify many, but not all, causes of abdominal pain. Blood and urine tests are frequently obtained. An ultrasound is helpful if gynecologic disorders are suspected.

Treatment

The specific cause of the pain is treated. Until recently, doctors thought that it was not wise to give pain medicine to people with severe abdominal pain until a diagnosis was made because the medicine might mask important symptoms. Pain relievers are often now be given while tests are in progress.

BLEEDING FROM THE DIGESTIVE TRACT

Bleeding may occur anywhere along the digestive tract, from the mouth to the anus. Blood may be visible in vomit (hematemesis). When blood is vomited, it may be bright red if bleeding is brisk and ongoing. Alternatively, vomited blood may have the appearance of coffee grounds if bleeding has slowed or stopped, due to the partial digestion of the blood by acid in the stomach.

Blood may also be passed from the rectum, either as black, tarry stools (melena), as bright red blood (hematochezia), or in apparently normal stool if bleeding is less than a few teaspoons per day. Melena is more likely when bleeding comes from the esophagus, stomach, or small intestine. The black color of melena is caused by blood that has been exposed for several hours to stomach acid and enzymes and to bacteria that normally reside in the large intestine. Hematochezia is more likely when bleeding comes from the large intestine, although it can be caused by very rapid bleeding from the upper portions of the digestive tract as well.

Serious and sudden blood loss may be accompanied by a rapid pulse, low blood pressure, and reduced urine flow. A person may also have cold, clammy hands and feet. Severe bleeding may lead to reduced flow of blood to the brain, causing confusion, disori-

COMMON CAUSES OF GASTROINTESTINAL BLEEDING	
REGION	**CAUSE**
Upper digestive tract	Doudenal ulcer
	Erosions of esophagus, stomach, or duodenum
	Esophageal varices
	Stomach ulcer
Lower digestive tract	Abnormal blood vessels
	Anal fissures
	Colon cancer
	Colon polyps
	Diverticulosis
	Inflammatory bowel disease
	Internal hemorrhoids
	Large-bowel inflammation from radiation or poor blood supply

entation, sleepiness, and even extremely low blood pressure (shock). Slow, chronic blood loss may cause symptoms and signs of anemia (such as weakness, easy fatigue, pallor, chest pain, and dizziness).

Causes

Bleeding can have many causes, including peptic ulcers; abnormal connections between the arteries and veins of the intestines (arteriovenous malformations); dilated veins in the esophagus (esophageal varices); irritation from use of certain drugs, such as aspirin and other nonsteroidal anti-inflammatory drugs (NSAIDs); inflammatory bowel disease; small balloon-like sacs in the wall of the colon (diverticulosis); and cancer.

Bleeding from any cause is more likely, and potentially more severe, in people who have chronic liver disease or hereditary disorders of blood clotting and in those who are taking certain drugs. Drugs that can cause bleeding include anticoagulants (such as heparin and warfarin) and those that affect platelet function (such as aspirin and certain other NSAIDs and clopidogrel).

Evaluation

The doctor tries to find out exactly where the bleeding is coming from, how rapid it is, and what is causing it. The person's symptoms and physical examination (including a digital rectal examination to feel for masses and test the stool for blood) sometimes suggest a cause and location and may suggest which tests are needed.

If the person has vomited blood or dark material (which may represent partially digested blood), the doctor passes a small, hollow plastic tube through the person's nose down into the stomach (nasogastric tube—see page 131) and suctions out the stomach contents. Bloody contents indicate active bleeding, and dark material may indicate that bleeding is slow or has stopped. Sometimes, there is no sign of blood even though the person was bleeding very recently. A nasogastric tube is also inserted in anyone who has not vomited but has passed a large amount of blood from the rectum (if not from an obvious hemorrhoid) because this blood may have originated in the upper digestive tract. The nasogastric tube is usually left in place until it is clear that all bleeding has stopped.

If the nasogastric tube reveals signs of active bleeding, or the person's symptoms strongly suggest the bleeding is originating in the upper digestive tract, the doctor usually performs upper endoscopy. Upper endoscopy is a visual examination of the esophagus, stomach, and the first segment of the small intestine (duodenum) using a flexible tube called an endoscope (see page 129). An upper endoscopy allows the doctor to see the bleeding source and often treat it. Similarly, colonoscopy (see page 129) is performed if symptoms suggest the bleeding is originating in the lower digestive tract, or if upper endoscopy does not reveal a bleeding site.

Rarely, endoscopy (both upper and lower) does not show the cause of bleeding. For such people, if bleeding is severe, doctors sometimes perform angiography or inject the person with red blood cells labeled with a radioactive marker. With the use of a special scanning camera, the radioactive marker can sometimes show the approximate location of the bleeding. If bleeding is slow, doctors may instead take x-rays after the person drinks liquid barium (see page 130). Another option is capsule endoscopy (see page 130). Capsule endoscopy is especially useful in the small intestine, but it is not very useful in either the colon or stomach, because these organs are too big to get good pictures of their inner lining.

Doctors also obtain blood tests. The person's blood count helps indicate how much blood has been lost. A low platelet count is a risk factor for bleeding. Other blood tests include prothrombin time (PT), partial thromboplastin time (PTT), and tests of liver function, which help detect problems with blood clotting.

Treatment

People with sudden, severe blood loss require intravenous fluids and sometimes an emergency blood transfusion to stabilize their condition. Those with blood clotting abnormalities may require transfusion of platelets or fresh frozen plasma or injections of vitamin K.

Most gastrointestinal bleeding stops on its own. If it does not, the doctor can often stop it during endoscopy by using an electrocautery device, laser, or injections of certain drugs. Bleeding polyps can be removed with a wire snare or other device. If these methods do not stop the bleeding, the person may require surgery.

CHEST OR BACK PAIN

Pain in the middle of the chest or upper back can result from disorders of the esophagus or from disorders of the heart or aorta. Symptoms may be similar. Gastroesophageal reflux disease (GERD), caused by stomach acid splashing up into the esophagus, can produce a burning sensation or a tightness under the breastbone (sternum), which may resemble the pain of heart disease. Spasms of the esophagus and other esophageal muscle disorders can cause a severe squeezing sensation also resembling the pain of heart disease.

Some symptoms are more suggestive of esophageal disorders. Heartburn is a burning pain caused by GERD that rises into the chest and sometimes the neck and throat, usually after meals or when lying down. Heartburn is among the most common digestive symptoms in the United States. Discomfort that occurs only with swallowing also suggests an esophageal disorder. Chest discomfort that occurs routinely with exertion and goes away after a brief rest suggests a heart problem. However, because symptoms frequently overlap, and because heart disease is particularly dangerous, doctors often obtain a chest x-ray, electrocardiogram (ECG), and sometimes a cardiac stress test before doing tests to look for esophageal disease.

Treatment is usually given only when the cause is known, although people with very typical symptoms of GERD may be given a trial of acid-blocking drugs.

CONSTIPATION

Constipation is a condition in which a person has uncomfortable or infrequent bowel movements.

Constipation may be acute or chronic. Acute constipation begins suddenly and conspicuously. Chronic constipation may begin gradually and persists for months or years.

A person with constipation often or always produces hard stools that may be difficult to pass. The rectum may not feel completely empty. Bowel movements are likely to be infrequent. Many people believe they are constipated if they do not have a bowel movement (defecate) every day. However, daily bowel movements are not normal for everyone, and having less frequent bowel movements does not necessarily indicate a problem unless there has been a substantial change from previous patterns. The same is true of the color and consistency of stool; unless there is a substantial change, the person probably does not have constipation. Constipation is blamed for many symptoms (such as abdominal discomfort, nausea, fatigue, and poor appetite—although constipation can cause nausea and poor appetite) that are actually the result of other disorders (such as irritable bowel syndrome and depression). People should not expect all symptoms to be relieved by a daily bowel movement.

Complications: Straining during a bowel movement increases pressure on the veins around the anus and can lead to hemorrhoids. Straining also increases blood pressure, which, although temporary, may be extreme.

Constipation is one of the major risk factors for the development of diverticular disease. The walls of the large intestine are damaged by the increased pressure required to move small, hard stools. Damage to the walls of the large intestine leads to the formation of balloon-like sacs or outpocketings (diverticula), which can become clogged and inflamed.

Fecal impaction, in which stool in the last part of the large intestine and rectum hardens and blocks the passage of other stool, sometimes develops in people with constipation. This condition is particularly common among older people, pregnant women, and people with an inactive colon (colonic inertia). Fecal impaction leads to cramps, rectal pain, and strong but futile efforts to defecate. Often, watery mucus or liquid stool oozes around the blockage, sometimes giving the false impression of diarrhea. Fecal impaction can aggravate or further worsen constipation.

Overconcern with regular bowel movements causes many people to abuse their bowels with laxatives, suppositories, and enemas. Overusing these treatments can actually inhibit the bowel's normal contractions and worsen constipation.

Causes

Constipation can result when the passage (transit) of stool through the large intestine is slowed by disease or certain drugs. Sometimes constipation is caused by dehydration or a low-fiber diet. Pain and mental disorders, such as depression, may also contribute to constipation. In many cases, however, the cause of constipation is unknown.

Slowed Transit of Stool: Constipation tends to occur when the passage of stool along the large intestine slows. Under normal circumstances, water is pulled from the stool as it passes through the large intestine. Slowed transit of stool allows the large intestine to pull more water from the stool, resulting in the hard, dry stools and difficult passage of stools that characterize constipation.

Drugs that can slow transit of stool include aluminum hydroxide (common in over-the-counter antacids), bismuth subsalicylate, iron salts, drugs with anticholinergic effects (such as many antihistamines and some antidepressants), certain antihypertensives, opioids, and many sedatives. Because physical activity helps the intestines move stool along, lack of activity tends to slow transit and lead to constipation. For this reason, people who are confined to bed because of illness often are constipated.

Disorders and diseases that can slow transit of stool include an underactive thyroid gland (hypothyroidism), high blood calcium levels (hypercalcemia), and Parkinson's disease. People with diabetes often develop a condition in which parts of the digestive system slow down. Other conditions, including poor blood supply to the large intestine and nerve or spinal cord injury, can also cause constipation by slowing transit.

In an extreme case of slowed transit, called colonic inertia, the large intestine stops responding to the stimuli that usually cause bowel movements: eating, a full stomach, a full large intestine, and stool in the rectum. A decrease in contractions in the large intestine or an insensitivity of the rectum to the presence of stool results in severe, chronic constipation. Colonic inertia often occurs in people who are older, debilitated, or bedridden, but it occasionally occurs in otherwise healthy younger women (and, much less commonly, in healthy younger men). Colonic inertia sometimes occurs in people who habitually delay moving their bowels or who have used laxatives or enemas for a long time.

Dehydration and Low-Fiber Diet: Dehydration causes constipation because the body tries to conserve water in the blood by removing additional water from the stool. Lack of fiber (the indigestible part of food) in the diet can lead to constipation because fiber helps hold water in the stool and increases its bulk, making it easier to pass.

Obstruction: Constipation is sometimes caused by obstruction of the large intestine. Obstruction can be caused by cancer, especially in the last portion of the large intestine, if a tumor blocks the movement of stool. People who previously had abdominal surgery may develop obstruction, usually of the small intestine, because of formation of bands of fibrous tissues (adhesions), which impede the flow of the stool.

Dyschezia: Dyschezia is difficulty in defecating caused by an inability to control the pelvic and anal muscles. Having a normal bowel movement requires relaxing the pelvic floor muscles (the muscles that support the bladder, uterus, and rectum) and the circular muscles (sphincters) that keep the anus closed. Otherwise, efforts to defecate are futile, even with severe straining. People with dyschezia sense the need

CAUSES OF CONSTIPATION

CAUSE	EXAMPLES OR COMMENTS
Acute constipation	
Acute bowel obstruction	Twisting of a loop of intestine (volvulus), hernia, adhesions, fecal impaction
Ileus (temporary absence of the contractile movements of the intestinal wall)	Inflammation of the lining of the abdominal cavity (peritonitis), head or spinal trauma, bed rest
Drugs	Drugs with anticholinergic effects (antihistamines, some antidepressants, antipsychotics, antiparkinsonians, antispasmodics), metallic ions (iron, aluminum, calcium, barium, bismuth), opioids, general anesthesia
Chronic constipation	
Colon cancer	Often, constipation gradually worsens as tumor grows
Metabolic disorders	Diabetes mellitus, underactive thyroid gland (hypothyroidism), high levels of calcium in the blood (hypercalcemia), build up of toxic substances in the blood (uremia), porphyria (a group of disorders caused by deficiencies of enzymes)
Central nervous system disorders	Parkinson's disease, multiple sclerosis, stroke, spinal cord injury or disease
Peripheral nervous system disorders	Hirschsprung's disease, neurofibromatosis, autonomic neuropathy
Systemic disorders	Systemic sclerosis, amyloidosis, skin inflammation plus muscle inflammation and muscle degeneration (dermatomyositis), weakness and stiff muscles (myotonic dystrophy)
Functional disorders	Inactive colon (colonic inertia), irritable bowel syndrome
Diet	Low fiber, chronic laxative abuse

to have a bowel movement but cannot. Even stool that is not hard may be difficult to pass.

Conditions that can cause dyschezia include pelvic floor dyssynergia (a disturbance of muscle coordination), anismus (a failure of the sphincter muscles to relax during defecation), rectocele (hernia of the rectum into the vagina), enterocele (bulging of the small intestine and the lining of the abdominal cavity between the uterus and the rectum or between the bladder and the rectum), rectal ulcer, and rectal prolapse (protrusion of the rectal lining through the anus).

Aging: Constipation is particularly common among older people. Age-related changes in the large intestine (see page 114) along with increased use of drugs, a low-fiber diet, and reduced physical activity tend to slow the transit of stool through the large intestine. Slowed transit is particularly common during periods of illness. The rectum enlarges with age, and increased storage of stool in the rectum allows hard stool to become impacted.

Pain and Psychologic Factors: Chronic pain and psychologic conditions, especially depression, are common causes of acute and chronic constipation. Changes in the levels of certain substances in the brain, such as serotonin, can affect the intestinal tract.

Evaluation

When constipation develops in someone who has not had it before, the doctor first looks for an easy explanation, such as a change in diet or physical activity or new use of a drug known to cause constipation. Then, the doctor may perform blood tests to check for an underactive thyroid gland (hypothyroidism) or high calcium levels in the blood (hypercalcemia), both of which can cause constipation. If there is any question about cancer as a cause, a colonoscopy is performed.

Prevention

Constipation is best prevented and treated with a combination of exercise, a high-fiber diet, an adequate intake of fluids, and the occasional use of laxatives.

When a potentially constipating drug has been prescribed, a laxative along with increased intake of dietary fiber and fluids help to prevent constipation.

Vegetables, fruits, and bran are excellent sources of fiber. Many people find it convenient to sprinkle 2 or 3 teaspoons of unrefined miller's bran on high-fiber cereal or fruit 2 or 3 times a day. To work well, fiber must be consumed with plenty of fluids.

Treatment

When an underlying disorder is causing constipation, the disorder must be treated.

Dyschezia is not easily treated with laxatives. Relaxation exercises and biofeedback are effective for some people with pelvic floor dyssynergia. Surgery may be needed to repair an enterocele or a large rectocele.

Fecal impaction cannot be treated by modifying the diet or simply by taking laxatives. The hard stool usually has to be removed by a doctor or nurse using a gloved finger. Often an enema is given after the hard stool is removed.

Overzealous treatment, especially the long-term use of stimulant laxatives, irritant suppositories, and enemas, can lead to diarrhea, dehydration, cramps, or dependence on laxatives.

Laxatives: Many people use laxatives to relieve constipation. Some laxatives are safe for long-term use; others should be used only occasionally. Some are good for preventing constipation, others for treating it.

Bulking agents, such as bran and psyllium (also available in the fiber of many vegetables), add bulk to the stool. The increased bulk stimulates the natural contractions of the intestine, and bulkier stools are softer and easier to pass. Bulking agents act slowly and gently and are among the safest ways to promote regular bowel movements. These agents generally are taken in small amounts at first. The dose is increased gradually until regularity is achieved. People who use bulking agents should always drink plenty of fluids. These agents may cause problems with increased gas (flatulence).

Stool softeners, such as docusate, increase the amount of water that the stool can hold. Actually, these laxatives are detergents that decrease the surface tension of the stool, allowing water to penetrate the stool more easily and soften it. In addition, the slightly increased bulk that results from these drugs stimulates the natural contractions of the large intestine and thus promotes easier elimination. Some people, however, find the softened nature of the stool unpleasant. Stool softeners are best reserved for people who must avoid straining, such as people who have hemorrhoids or have recently had surgery.

Osmotic agents pull large amounts of water into the large intestine, making the stool soft and loose.

The excess fluid also stretches the walls of the large intestine, stimulating contractions. These laxatives consist of salts or sugars that are poorly absorbed. They may cause fluid retention in people who have kidney disease or heart failure, especially when given in large or frequent doses. Osmotic agents that contain magnesium and phosphate are partially absorbed into the bloodstream and can be harmful to people who have kidney failure. Although a rare occurrence, phosphate laxatives taken by mouth have caused kidney failure. These laxatives usually work within 3 hours. They are also used to clear stool from the intestine before x-rays of the digestive tract are taken or before a colonoscopy is performed.

Stimulant laxatives contain irritating substances, such as senna and cascara. These substances stimulate the walls of the large intestine, causing them to contract and move the stool. Taken by mouth, stimulant laxatives usually cause a semisolid bowel movement in 6 to 8 hours, but they often cause cramping as well. As suppositories, stimulant laxatives often work in 15 to 60 minutes. Prolonged use of stimulant laxatives can create abnormal changes in the lining of the large intestine caused by deposits of a pigment (a condition called melanosis coli). Also, stimulant laxatives can become addictive, leading to the development of lazy bowel syndrome, which in turn causes the large intestine to become dependent on the laxatives. Therefore, stimulant laxatives should be used only for brief periods of time to treat constipation. They are useful for preventing constipation in people who are taking drugs that will almost certainly cause constipation, such as opioids. Stimulant laxatives are often used to empty the large intestine before diagnostic procedures are performed. A newer stimulant laxative, lubiprostone, works by making the large intestine secrete extra fluid, which makes stool easier to pass. Unlike other stimulant laxatives, lubiprostone is safe for prolonged use.

Enemas: Enemas mechanically flush stool from the rectum and lower part of the large intestine. Small-volume enemas can be purchased in squeeze bottles at a pharmacy. They can also be given with a reusable squeeze-ball device. However, small-volume enemas are often inadequate, especially for older people, whose rectal capacity increases with age, thus making the rectum more easily stretched. Larger-volume enemas are given with an enema bag.

Plain water is often the best fluid to be used as an enema. The water should be room temperature to slightly warm, not hot or cold. About 5 to 10 fluid ounces (150 to 300 milliliters) is gently directed into the rectum. (CAUTION: Additional force is dangerous.) The water is then expelled, washing stool out with it.

Prepackaged enemas often contain small amounts of salts, often phosphates. Appropriate salts can also

℞ DRUGS USED TO PREVENT OR TREAT CONSTIPATION

DRUG	SOME SIDE EFFECTS	COMMENTS
Bulking agents		
Bran Polycarbophil Methylcellulose Psyllium	Flatulence, bloating	Bulking agents generally are used to prevent or control chronic constipation.
Stool softeners		
Docusate	Nausea (especially with syrup/liquid formulation)	Stool softeners may be used to treat constipation and are often used to help prevent it.
Osmotic agents		
Lactulose Magnesium salts (magnesium hydroxide, magnesium citrate) Polyethylene glycol Sodium phosphate Sorbitol	Cramps, flatulence (lactose, sorbitol)	Osmotic agents are better for treating constipation than for preventing it.
Stimulant laxatives		
Bisacodyl Cascara Castor oil Lubiprostone Senna	Abdominal pain (cramps); prolonged use can damage large intestine	Stimulant laxatives are not used if there is a possibility of an intestinal obstruction. Lubiprostone can be used for chronic constipation.

be added to homemade enemas. They offer little advantage, however, to plain water.

The addition of small amounts of soap to the water (soap-suds enema) adds the stimulant laxative effects of soap. Soap-suds enemas are sometimes useful when plain water enemas fail, but they can cause cramping.

Many other substances, including mineral oil, are sometimes added to water-based enemas. However, they offer little advantage.

Very large-volume enemas, called colonic enemas, are rarely used in medical practice. Doctors use colonic enemas in people with very severe constipation (obstipation). Some practitioners of alternative medicine use colonic enemas in the belief that cleansing the large intestine is beneficial. Tea, coffee, and other substances are often added to colonic enemas but have no proven health value and may be dangerous.

DIARRHEA

Diarrhea is an increase in the volume, wateriness, or frequency of bowel movements.

The frequency of bowel movements alone is not the defining feature of diarrhea. Some people normally move their bowels 3 to 5 times a day. People who eat large amounts of vegetable fiber may produce more than a pound of stool a day, but the stool in such cases is well formed and not watery. Diarrhea occurs when not enough water is removed from the stool, making the stool loose and poorly formed. Diarrhea is often associated with gas, cramping, an urgency to defecate, and, if the diarrhea is caused by an infectious organism or a toxic substance, nausea and vomiting.

Diarrhea can lead to dehydration and a loss of electrolytes, such as sodium, potassium, magnesium, chloride, and bicarbonate, from the blood. If large amounts of fluid and electrolytes are lost, the person feels weak, and blood pressure can drop enough to cause fainting (syncope), heart rhythm abnormalities (arrhythmias), and other serious disorders. At particular risk are the very young, the very old, the debilitated, and people with very severe diarrhea. Diarrhea is a major cause of infant mortality in developing countries and results in many hospitalizations in the United States.

Causes

Normally, stool is 60 to 90% water. Diarrhea mainly occurs when the percentage is over 90%. Stool may contain too much water if it travels too quickly through the digestive tract, if certain components of the stool prevent the large intestine from absorbing water, or if water is being secreted by the large intestine into the stool. There are many different causes, including drugs and chemicals; infection with viruses, bacteria, or parasites (gastroenteritis—see page 145); some foods; stress; tumors; and chronic disorders such as irritable bowel syndrome, inflammatory bowel disease, and malabsorption syndromes.

Rapid passage (transit) of stool is one of the most common causes of diarrhea. For stool to have normal consistency, it must remain in the large intestine for a certain amount of time. Stool that leaves the large intestine too quickly is watery. Many medical conditions and treatments can decrease the amount of time that stool stays in the large intestine, including an overactive thyroid (hyperthyroidism); Zollinger-Ellison syndrome (a condition of over-production of acid secondary to a tumor); surgical removal of part of the stomach, small intestine, or large intestine; surgical bypass of part of the intestine; and drugs such as antacids containing magnesium, laxatives, prostaglandins, serotonin, and even caffeine. Many foods, especially those that are acidic, can increase the rate of transit. Some people are intolerant of specific foods and always develop diarrhea after eating them. Stress and anxiety are also common causes.

Osmotic diarrhea occurs when certain substances that cannot be absorbed through the colon wall remain in the intestine. These substances cause excessive amounts of water to remain in the stool, leading to diarrhea. Certain foods (such as some fruits and beans) and hexitols, sorbitol, and mannitol (used as sugar substitutes in dietetic foods, candy, and chewing gum) can cause osmotic diarrhea. Also, lactase deficiency can lead to osmotic diarrhea. Lactase is an enzyme normally found in the small intestine that converts lactose (milk sugar) to glucose and galactose, so that it can be absorbed into the bloodstream. When people with lactase deficiency drink milk or eat dairy products, lactose is not digested. As lactose accumulates in the intestine, it causes osmotic diarrhea—a condition known as lactose intolerance. The severity of osmotic diarrhea depends on how much of the osmotic substance is consumed. Diarrhea stops soon after the person stops eating or drinking the substance. Blood in the digestive tract also acts as an osmotic agent and results in black, tarry stools (melena). Another cause of osmotic diarrhea is an overgrowth of normal intestinal bacteria or the growth of bacteria normally not found in the intestines. Antibiotics can cause osmotic diarrhea by destroying the normal intestinal bacteria.

FOODS AND DRUGS THAT CAN CAUSE DIARRHEA	
FOOD OR DRUG	**INGREDIENT CAUSING DIARRHEA**
Apple juice, pear juice, sugar-free gum, mints	Hexitols, sorbitol, mannitol
Apple juice, pear juice, grapes, honey, dates, nuts, figs, soft drinks (especially fruit flavors)	Fructose
Table sugar	Sucrose
Milk, ice cream, yogurt, frozen yogurt, soft cheese, chocolate	Lactose
Antacids containing magnesium	Magnesium
Coffee, tea, cola drinks, some over-the-counter headache remedies	Caffeine
Fat-free potato chips, fat-free ice cream	Olestra

Secretory diarrhea occurs when the small and large intestines secrete salts (especially sodium chloride) and water into the stool. Certain toxins—such as the toxin produced by a cholera infection or during some viral infections—can cause these secretions. Infections by certain bacteria (for example, *Campylobacter*) and parasites (for example, *Cryptosporidium*) can also stimulate secretions. The diarrhea can be massive—more than a quart of stool an hour in cholera. Other substances that cause salt and water secretion include certain laxatives, such as castor oil, and bile acids (which may build up after surgery to remove part of the small intestine). Certain rare tumors—such as carcinoid, gastrinoma, and vipoma—also can cause secretory diarrhea, as can some polyps.

Inflammatory diarrhea occurs when the lining of the large intestine becomes inflamed, ulcerated, or engorged and releases proteins, blood, mucus, and other fluids, which increase the bulk and fluid content of the stool. This type of diarrhea can be caused by many diseases, including ulcerative colitis, Crohn's disease (regional enteritis), tuberculosis, and cancers such as lymphoma and adenocarcinoma. When the lining of the rectum is affected, people often feel an urgent need to move their bowels and have frequent bowel movements because the inflamed rectum is more sensitive to expansion (distention) by stool.

℞ DRUGS USED TO TREAT DIARRHEA

DRUG	SOME SIDE EFFECTS	COMMENTS
Adsorbents		
Bismuth subsalicylate Kaolin Pectin	Well tolerated	Adsorbents are less potent than intestinal muscle relaxants.
Intestinal muscle relaxants		
Codeine Diphenoxylate Loperamide* Paregoric (tincture of opium)	Obstruction of the large intestine	Doctors use these drugs carefully if they suspect infectious cause of diarrhea.

*Some formulations of loperamide are available over-the-counter.

Evaluation

The evaluation depends on whether the diarrhea is acute (sudden and present for a short time) or chronic (persistent).

For acute diarrhea that lasts for more than 72 hours (or sooner if blood is present, or the person is weak or has a fever, rash, or severe pain), a doctor should be consulted. If, on the doctor's examination, the person does not appear to be dehydrated or seriously ill, and the diarrhea is not severe and has lasted for less than a week, testing is usually not needed. Other people may need blood tests for electrolyte abnormalities or stool tests for blood, white blood cells, and the presence of infectious organisms (for example, bacteria such as *Campylobacter* and *Yersinia* and parasites such as amebas, *Giardia*, and *Cryptosporidium*). Some causes of infection are detected by looking under the microscope, whereas others require a culture (growing the organism in the laboratory) or special enzyme tests (for example, *Shigella* or *Giardia*). If the person has taken antibiotics recently, the doctor may test the stool for *Clostridium difficile* toxin. A colonoscopy is usually not necessary.

For chronic diarrhea, similar tests are performed. In addition, the doctor may test the stool for fat (indicating malabsorption) and perform a sigmoidoscopy or colonoscopy to examine the lining of the rectum and colon. Sometimes a biopsy (removal of a tissue specimen for examination under a microscope) of the rectal lining is performed. Sometimes the volume of stool over a 24-hour period is determined. Secret (surreptitious) use of a laxative also can be identified in the stool sample.

Treatment

Diarrhea is a symptom, and its treatment depends on its cause. For most people, treating diarrhea involves only removing the cause to suppress the diarrhea until the body heals itself. A viral cause usually resolves by itself in 24 to 48 hours. Extra fluids containing a balance of water, sugars, and salts are needed for people who are dehydrated. As long as the person is not vomiting excessively, these fluids can be given by mouth (see box on page 1733). Seriously ill people and those with significant electrolyte abnormalities require intravenous fluid and sometimes hospitalization.

Many prescription and over-the-counter drugs are available for the treatment of diarrhea. Over-the-counter drugs include adsorbents (for example, kaolin-pectin), which adhere to chemicals, toxins, and infectious organisms. Some adsorbents also help firm up the stool. Bismuth helps many people with diarrhea. It has a normal side effect of turning the stool black. Other drugs used are loperamide, codeine, and diphenoxylate.

Prescription drugs used to treat diarrhea include opioids and other drugs that relax the muscles of the intestines. Bulking agents used for chronic constipation, such as psyllium or methylcellulose, can sometimes help relieve chronic diarrhea as well.

DIFFICULTY SWALLOWING

Difficulty swallowing (dysphagia) is the sensation that food is not moving normally through the esophagus (the tube that connects the throat to the stomach) or that the food has become stuck on the way down.

Causes

A swallowing difficulty can result from a physical blockage or a problem with the nerves or muscles of the esophagus (esophageal motility [movement] disorder). Sometimes, a swallowing difficulty may be imagined (psychogenic).

Mechanical blockage can result from cancer of the esophagus, rings or webs of tissue across the inside of the esophagus, and scarring of the esophagus from chronic acid reflux or from swallowing caustic solutions. Sometimes the esophagus is compressed by an enlarged thyroid, a bulge in the large artery in the chest (aortic aneurysm), or a tumor in the chest, such as one caused by lung cancer.

Esophageal motility disorders include achalasia (in which the rhythmic contractions of the esophagus are greatly decreased and the lower esophageal muscle does not relax normally) and esophageal spasm. Systemic sclerosis may also cause a motility disorder.

Evaluation and Treatment

Equal difficulty swallowing liquids and solids suggests a motility disorder. Gradually increasing difficulty swallowing first solids and then liquids suggests a worsening physical obstruction, such as a tumor. Doctors usually take x-rays while the person swallows a marshmallow or tablet along with barium liquid (which shows up on x-rays). Or they look in the esophagus and stomach with a flexible tube (upper endoscopy).

The specific cause is treated. To relieve symptoms, doctors usually advise the person to take small bites and chew food thoroughly.

DYSPEPSIA

Dyspepsia is pain or discomfort in the middle of the upper abdomen.

The sensation may be described as indigestion, gassiness, a sense of fullness, or a gnawing or burning pain. Other symptoms may include a poor appetite, nausea, constipation, diarrhea, flatulence, belching, and loud intestinal sounds (borborygmi). For some people, eating makes symptoms worse; for others, eating relieves symptoms.

Causes

Dyspepsia has many causes, including stomach ulcers, duodenal ulcers, and stomach cancer. Stomach inflammation (gastritis) may also cause dyspepsia. *Helicobacter pylori* bacteria may contribute to dyspepsia by causing inflammation and ulcers of the stomach and duodenum (the first segment of the small intestine). Gallstones, when present in the tubes (ducts) that drain bile from the gallbladder, sometimes produce dyspepsia. Some drugs, especially aspirin and other NSAIDs, cause symptoms. In many people, however, no abnormality can be found (a condition called functional dyspepsia), and symptoms are linked to increased sensitivity in the stomach or increased contractions (spasms).

Anxiety can cause or worsen dyspepsia—possibly because anxiety can increase a person's perception of unpleasant sensations, so that minor discomfort becomes very distressing. Sometimes, anxiety may worsen the abnormal stomach sensitivity and contractions or cause a person to sigh or gasp and swallow air (aerophagia).

Evaluation and Treatment

Symptoms that suggest a more serious cause of dyspepsia include prolonged loss of appetite, nausea and vomiting, weight loss, anemia, blood in the stools, and difficulty or pain with swallowing. For people with these symptoms and those over age 45, doctors typically look in the esophagus and stomach with a flexible tube (upper endoscopy). Those who are younger and have no symptoms other than dyspepsia are often given a course of treatment with acid-blocking drugs. If this treatment is unsuccessful, doctors usually perform endoscopy.

FECAL INCONTINENCE

Fecal incontinence is the loss of control over bowel movements.

Causes

Fecal incontinence can occur briefly during bouts of diarrhea or when hard stool becomes lodged in the rectum (fecal impaction). Persistent fecal incontinence can develop in people who have injuries to the anus or spinal cord, rectal prolapse (protrusion of the rectal lining through the anus), dementia, neurologic injury from diabetes, tumors of the anus, or injuries to the pelvis during childbirth.

Evaluation

A doctor examines the person for any structural or neurologic abnormality. This involves examining the anus and rectum, checking the extent of sensation around the anus, and usually performing a sigmoidoscopy. Other tests, including an ultrasound of the anal sphincter, magnetic resonance imaging (MRI), and an examination of the function of nerves and muscles lining the pelvis, may be needed.

Treatment

The first step in correcting fecal incontinence is to try to establish a regular pattern of bowel movements that produces well-formed stool. Dietary changes, including the addition of a small amount of fiber, often help. If such changes do not help, a drug that slows bowel movements, such as loperamide, may be successful.

Exercising the anal muscles (sphincters) by squeezing and releasing them increases their tone and strength. Using a technique called biofeedback, a person can retrain the sphincters and increase the sensitivity of the rectum to the presence of stool. About 70% of well-motivated people benefit from biofeedback.

If fecal incontinence persists, surgery may help—for instance, when the cause is an injury to the anus or an anatomic defect in the anus. As a last resort, a colostomy (the surgical creation of an opening between the large intestine and the abdominal wall—see art on page 194) may be performed. The anus is sewn shut, and stool is diverted into a removable plastic bag attached to the opening in the abdominal wall.

GAS-RELATED COMPLAINTS

Gas is normally present in the digestive system and may be expelled through the mouth (belching) or through the anus (flatus).

There are three main gas-related complaints: excessive belching, the sensation of abdominal distention or bloating, and excessive flatus (known colloquially as farting).

Belching is more likely to occur shortly after eating or during periods of stress. Some people feel a tightness in their chest or stomach just before belching that is relieved as the gas is expelled.

People normally pass gas through the anus more than 10 times a day, but some people pass gas more often. Gas passed through the anus may or may not have an odor. On occasion, fecal incontinence occurs as a person tries to pass gas, only to be surprised by the expulsion of stool as well.

Causes

Increased amounts of gas can gather in the stomach or farther along the digestive tract.

Belching results from swallowed air or from gas generated by carbonated beverages. Swallowing small amounts of air is normal, but some people unconsciously swallow large amounts (aerophagia) while eating or smoking and also at other times, especially when they feel anxious. Excessive salivation, which may occur with gastroesophageal reflux, ill-fitting dentures, and gum chewing, increases air swallowing. Most swallowed air is later belched up, and very little passes from the stomach into the rest of the digestive system. Most of the swallowed air that makes it into the intestines is absorbed through the walls of the intestines into the bloodstream, and very little is passed through the anus.

Flatus results from hydrogen, methane, and carbon dioxide gases that are produced by bacterial breakdown of food in the intestine, especially after a person eats certain foods such as beans and cabbage. Almost anyone who eats large amounts of proteins or fruits will develop some degree of flatulence. People who have deficiencies of the enzymes that break down certain sugars (such as those with lactase deficiency) also tend to produce large amounts of gas when they eat foods containing these sugars. Other malabsorption syndromes, such as tropical sprue and pancreatic insufficiency, also may lead to the production of large amounts of gas.

A **bloating** sensation can be present in people who have digestive disorders such as poor stomach emptying (gastroparesis) or irritable bowel syndrome. Sometimes, the only symptom in heart disease is a feeling of bloating. However, aside from those who drink carbonated beverages or swallow excessive air, most people who have a sensation of bloating do not seem to have excessive gas in their digestive system. Some people, such as those who have irritable bowel syndrome, are particularly sensitive to normal amounts of gas.

Evaluation and Treatment

Doctors do not usually perform any testing on people who belch. Those who have flatus may require tests if their symptoms suggest a malabsorption syndrome.

Bloating and belching are difficult to relieve. If belching is the main problem, reducing the amount of air being swallowed can help, which is difficult because people usually are not aware of swallowing air. Avoiding chewing gum and eating more slowly in a relaxed atmosphere may help. Avoiding carbonated beverages helps some people.

People who pass flatus excessively may need to change their diet by avoiding foods that are difficult to digest. Discovering which foods cause a problem may require eliminating one food or group of foods at a time. A person can start by eliminating foods containing hard-to-digest carbohydrates (such as beans and cabbage), milk and dairy products, then fresh fruits, and then certain vegetables and other foods.

Simethicone, which is present in some antacids and is also available by itself, may provide some minor relief. Sometimes other drugs—including other types of antacids (including those that contain baking soda), metoclopramide, and bethanechol—may help. Aromatic oils, such as peppermint oil, help some people, especially those who experience cramps with flatulence. Eating more fiber helps some people but worsens the symptoms in others. Chlorophyll, an ingredient in many over-the-counter products, and charcoal tablets do not decrease flatulence but help reduce its offensive odor.

GLOBUS SENSATION

Globus sensation (previously called globus hystericus) is the feeling of having a lump in the throat when there is no lump.

The feeling produced by globus sensation is similar to that experienced when feeling emotionally choked up, such as during events that trigger grief, anxiety, anger, pride, or happiness. Food does not stick in the throat, and the person is able to swallow liquids without difficulty. Eating and drinking may actually provide relief.

Globus sensation may result from abnormal muscle activity or sensitivity of the esophagus. It sometimes occurs when stomach acid and enzymes flow backward from the stomach into the esophagus (gastroesophageal reflux). Globus sensation also may occur with frequent swallowing and drying of the throat caused by anxiety or another strong emotion or by rapid breathing.

Doctors do not usually perform tests as long as the person is able to swallow normally and has no other symptoms such as pain, weight loss, or blood in the stool.

LOSS OF APPETITE

Loss of appetite (anorexia) implies that hunger is absent—a person with anorexia has no desire to eat. In contrast, a person with an eating disorder such as anorexia nervosa or bulimia nervosa (see page 876) is hungry but restricts food intake or vomits after eating because of overconcern about weight gain.

A brief period of anorexia usually accompanies almost all sudden (acute) illnesses. Long-lasting (chronic) anorexia usually occurs only in people with a serious underlying disorder such as cancer; AIDS; chronic lung disease; and severe heart, kidney, or liver failure. Disorders that affect the part of the brain where appetite is regulated can cause anorexia as well. Anorexia is common in people who are dying. Some drugs, such as digoxin, fluoxetine, quinidine, and hydralazine, cause anorexia.

Most often, anorexia occurs in a person with a known underlying disorder. Unexplained chronic anorexia is a signal to the doctor that something is wrong. A thorough evaluation of the person's symptoms and a complete physical examination often suggest a cause and help the doctor decide which tests are needed.

Underlying causes are treated to the extent possible. Steps that can help increase a person's desire to eat include providing favorite foods, a flexible meal schedule, and, if the person desires, a small amount of an alcoholic beverage served 30 minutes before meals. In certain situations, doctors may use drugs, such as cyproheptadine, low-dose corticosteroids, megestrol, and dronabinol, to help stimulate the appetite.

NAUSEA AND VOMITING

Nausea is an unpleasant feeling that may include dizziness, vague discomfort in the abdomen, an unwillingness to eat, and a sensation of needing to vomit. Vomiting is the forceful contraction of the stomach that propels its contents up the esophagus and out through the mouth. Vomiting serves to empty the stomach of its contents and often makes a person with nausea feel considerably better, at least temporarily. Vomiting is not the same as regurgitation, which is the spitting up of stomach contents without forceful abdominal contractions and nausea.

Vomitus—the material that is vomited up—usually reflects what was recently eaten. Sometimes it contains chunks of food. When blood is vomited, the vomitus is usually bright red (hematemesis). When bile is present, the vomitus is green.

Even normal vomiting can be violent. A person who is vomiting typically doubles over and makes considerable noise. Severe vomiting can project food many feet (projectile vomiting). Vomiting greatly increases pressure within the esophagus, and severe vomiting can tear or even rupture the lining of the esophagus. People who are unconscious can inhale their vomitus. The acidic nature of the vomitus can severely irritate the lungs. Frequent vomiting can cause dehydration and electrolyte abnormalities; newborns and infants are particularly susceptible to these complications.

Causes

Nausea and vomiting result when the vomiting center in the brain is activated. These symptoms commonly occur with any dysfunction of the digestive tract but are particularly common with gastroenteritis and bowel obstruction. Obstruction of the intestine causes vomiting because food and fluids back up into the stomach from the blockage. The vomiting center also can be activated by certain brain disorders, including infections (such as meningitis and encephalitis), brain tumors, and migraines.

The balance organs of the inner ear (vestibular apparatus) are connected to the vomiting center. This connection is why some people become nauseated by the movement of a boat, car, or airplane and by certain disorders of the inner ear (such as labyrinthitis and positional vertigo). Nausea and vomiting may also occur during pregnancy, particularly during the early weeks and especially in the morning. Many drugs, including opioid analgesics, such as morphine, and chemotherapy drugs, can cause nausea.

Psychologic problems also can cause nausea and vomiting (known as functional, or psychogenic, vomiting). Such vomiting may be intentional—for instance, a person who has bulimia vomits to lose weight. Or it may be unintentional—a conditioned response to address psychologic distress, such as to avoid going to school.

Evaluation

Otherwise healthy adults and older children who have only a few episodes of vomiting (with or without diarrhea) and no other symptoms may not require evaluation. Young children and older people, and those in whom vomiting lasts more than 1 day or who have any other symptoms, particularly abdominal pain, headache, weakness, or confusion, are evaluated by the doctor. If the person's symptoms and physical examination show no signs of dehydration or serious underlying illness, doctors may not perform any testing. Women of childbearing age may receive a pregnancy test. In others, blood tests may be obtained to look for signs of dehydration or abnormal electrolyte levels. If bowel obstruction is suspected, x-rays are obtained.

Treatment

Specific conditions are treated. If there is no serious underlying disorder and the person is not dehydrated, small amounts of clear liquids may be given an hour or so after the last bout of vomiting. If these liquids are tolerated, the amounts are increased gradually. When these increases are tolerated, the person may resume eating normal foods. If the person is dehydrated and can tolerate some liquids by mouth, doctors usually recommend oral rehydration solutions. Those with significant dehydration or electrolyte abnormalities and those who cannot tolerate liquids by mouth usually require intravenous fluids.

For some adults and adolescents, doctors use antinausea drugs such as metoclopramide or prochlorperazine. For people whose vomiting is caused by chemotherapy, doctors usually use stronger drugs such as odansetron or granisetron.

REGURGITATION

Regurgitation is the spitting up of food from the esophagus or stomach without nausea or forceful contractions of the abdominal muscles.

A ring-shaped muscle (sphincter) between the stomach and esophagus normally helps prevent regurgitation. Regurgitation of sour or bitter-tasting material can result from acid coming up from the stomach. Regurgitation of tasteless fluid containing mucus or undigested food can result from a narrowing (stricture) or a blockage of the esophagus. The blockage may result from acid damage to the esophagus, ingestion of caustic substances, cancer of the esophagus, or abnormal nerve control that interferes with coordination between the esophagus and its sphincter at the opening to the stomach.

Regurgitation sometimes occurs with no apparent physical cause. Such regurgitation is called rumination. In rumination, small amounts of food are regurgitated from the stomach, usually 15 to 30 minutes after eating. The material often passes all the way to the mouth where a person may chew it again and reswallow it. Rumination occurs without pain or difficulty in swallowing. Rumination is common in infants. In adults, rumination most often occurs among people who have emotional disorders, especially during periods of stress.

Diagnosis

Usually, a doctor can determine whether a person has a digestive disorder based on a medical history and a physical examination. The doctor can then select appropriate procedures that help to confirm the diagnosis, determine the extent and severity of the disorder, and aid in planning treatment.

MEDICAL HISTORY AND PHYSICAL EXAMINATION

A doctor identifies symptoms by interviewing a person to obtain the medical history. Doctors ask specific questions to gain additional information. For example, in speaking with a person who has abdominal pain, the doctor might first ask, "What is the pain like?" This question might be followed by questions such as, "Does the pain get better after you eat?" or "Does the pain get worse when you bend over?"

During the physical examination, the doctor notes the person's weight and overall appearance, which may be indicators of digestive disorders. Although the doctor may examine the entire body, emphasis is placed on examining the abdomen, anus, and rectum.

First, the doctor observes the abdomen from different angles, looking for expansion (distention) of the abdominal wall that might accompany abnormal growth or enlargement of an organ. A stethoscope is placed on the abdomen, through which the doctor listens for sounds that normally accompany the movement of material through the intestines and for any abnormal sounds. The doctor feels for tenderness and any abnormal masses or enlarged organs. Pain that is caused by gentle pressure on the abdomen and that is relieved when the pressure is released (rebound tenderness) usually indicates inflammation and sometimes infection of the lining of the abdominal cavity (peritonitis).

The anus and rectum are examined with a gloved finger, and a small sample of stool is sometimes tested for hidden (occult) blood. In women, a pelvic examination often helps distinguish digestive problems from gynecologic ones.

PSYCHOLOGIC EVALUATION

Because the digestive system and the brain are highly interactive, a psychologic evaluation is sometimes needed in the evaluation of digestive problems. In such cases, doctors are not implying that the digestive problems are made up or imagined. Rather, the digestive problems may be the result of anxiety, depression, or other treatable mental disorders, which seems to be true for as many as 50% of people with symptoms of a digestive disorder.

DIAGNOSTIC PROCEDURES

Based on the findings of the medical history, physical examination, and, if applicable, psychologic evaluation, doctors choose appropriate tests. Tests performed on the digestive system make use of endoscopes (flexible tubes that doctors use to view internal structures and to obtain tissue samples from inside the body), x-rays, ultrasound scans, tiny amounts of radioactive materials, capsule endoscopy, and chemical measurements. These tests can help a doctor locate, diagnose, and sometimes treat a problem. Some tests require the digestive system to be cleared of stool, some require 8 to 12 hours of fasting, and others require no preparation.

Although diagnostic tests can be very accurate, they can also be quite expensive and, in rare cases, can cause bleeding or injury.

Endoscopy

Endoscopy is an examination of internal structures using a flexible viewing tube (endoscope). When passed through the mouth, an endoscope can be used to examine the esophagus (esophagoscopy), the stomach (gastroscopy), and part of the small intestine (upper gastrointestinal endoscopy). When passed through the anus, an endoscope can be used to examine the rectum (anoscopy); the lower portion of the large intestine, the rectum, and the anus (sigmoidoscopy); and the entire large intestine, the rectum, and the anus (colonoscopy). For procedures other than anoscopy and sigmoidoscopy, the person is given drugs intravenously to prevent discomfort.

Endoscopes range in diameter from about 1/4 inch (a bit more than 1/2 centimeter) to about 1/2 inch (1 1/4 centimeters) and range in length from about 1 foot (about 30 1/2 centimeters) to about 6 feet (almost 2 meters). The choice of endoscope depends on which part of the digestive tract is to be examined. The endoscope is flexible and provides both a lighting source and a small camera, which allows doctors to get a good view of the tract lining. The doctor can see areas of irritation, ulcers, inflammation, and abnormal tissue growth.

Viewing the Digestive Tract With an Endoscope

A flexible tube called an endoscope is used to view different parts of the digestive tract. The tube contains several channels along its length. The different channels are used to transmit light to the area being examined, to view the area through a camera lens (with a camera at the tip of the tube), to pump fluids or air in or out, and to pass biopsy or surgical instruments through.

When passed through the mouth, an endoscope can be used to examine the esophagus, the stomach, and some of the small intestine. When passed through the anus, an endoscope can be used to examine the rectum and the entire large intestine. The instrument used in the different procedures varies in length and size of the tube.

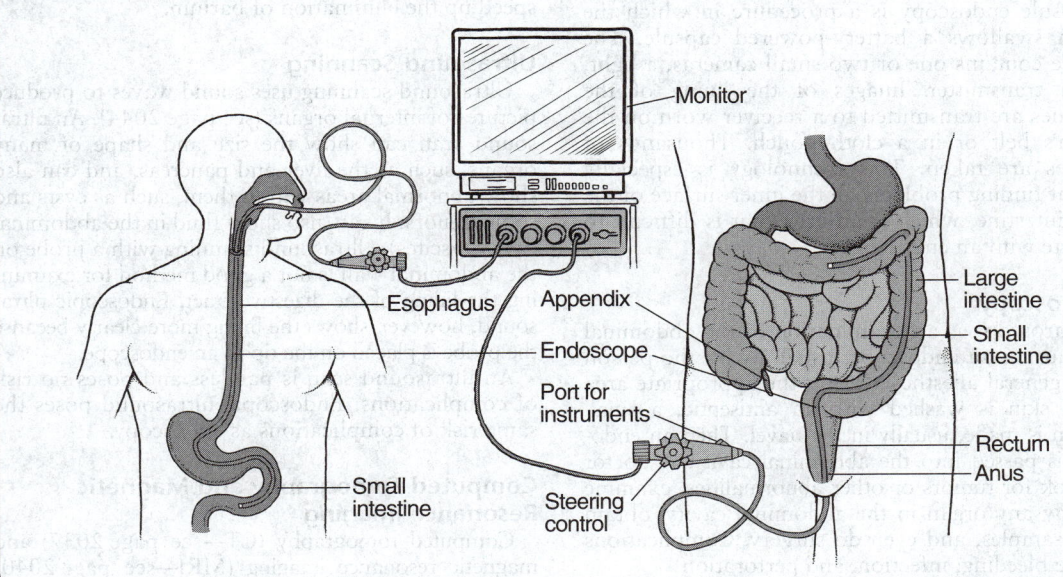

Monitor

Esophagus

Appendix

Endoscope

Port for instruments

Small intestine

Steering control

Large intestine

Small intestine

Rectum

Anus

Many endoscopes are equipped with a small clipper with which tissue samples can be taken (endoscopic biopsy). These samples can then be evaluated for inflammation, infection, or cancer. Because the lining and the inner layers of the walls of the digestive tract do not have nerves that sense pain (with the exception of the lower part of the anus), this procedure is painless.

Endoscopes can also be used for treatment. A doctor can pass different types of instruments through a small channel in the endoscope. An electric probe at the tip of the endoscope can be used to destroy abnormal tissue, to remove small growths, or to close off a blood vessel. A needle at the tip can be used to inject drugs into dilated veins in the esophagus and stop their bleeding. A laser mounted at the end can be used to destroy abnormal tissue.

Before having an endoscope passed through the mouth, a person usually must avoid food for several hours. Food in the stomach can obstruct the doctor's view and might be vomited up during the procedure. Before having an endoscope passed into the rectum and colon, a person usually takes laxatives and is sometimes given enemas to clear out any stool. In addition, the person must avoid food for several hours because it might be vomited up and because it would reduce the effectiveness of the laxatives and enemas.

Complications from endoscopy are relatively rare. Although endoscopes can injure or even perforate the digestive tract, they more commonly cause irritation of the tract lining and a little bleeding.

Capsule Endoscopy

Capsule endoscopy is a procedure in which the person swallows a battery-powered capsule. The capsule contains one or two small cameras, a light, and a transmitter. Images of the lining of the intestines are transmitted to a receiver worn on the person's belt or in a cloth pouch. Thousands of pictures are taken. This technology is especially good at finding problems on the inner surface of the small intestine, which is an area that is difficult to evaluate with an endoscope.

Laparoscopy

Laparoscopy is an examination of the abdominal cavity using an endoscope, usually with the person under general anesthesia. After the appropriate area of the skin is washed with an antiseptic, a small incision is made, usually in the navel. Then an endoscope is passed into the abdominal cavity. A doctor can look for tumors or other abnormalities, examine virtually any organ in the abdominal cavity, obtain tissue samples, and even do surgery. Complications include bleeding, infection, and perforation.

X-ray Studies

X-rays often are used to evaluate digestive problems. Standard x-rays do not require any special preparation (see page 2042). These x-rays usually can show an obstruction or paralysis of the digestive tract or abnormal air patterns in the abdominal cavity. Standard x-rays can also show enlargement of the liver, kidneys, and spleen.

Barium studies often provide more information. X-rays are taken after a person swallows barium in a flavored liquid mixture or as barium-coated food. The barium looks white on x-rays and outlines the digestive tract, showing the contours and lining of the esophagus, stomach, and small intestine. Barium collects in abnormal areas, showing ulcers, tumors, obstructions, erosions, and enlarged, dilated esophageal veins.

X-rays may be taken at intervals to determine where the barium is. In a continuous x-ray technique called fluoroscopy, the barium is observed as it moves through the digestive tract. With this technique, doctors can see how the esophagus and stomach function, determine whether their contractions are normal, and tell whether food is getting blocked. The doctor may film this process for later review.

Barium also can be given in an enema to outline the lower part of the large intestine. Then, x-rays can show polyps, tumors, or other structural abnormalities. This procedure may cause crampy pain, producing slight to moderate discomfort.

Barium taken by mouth or as an enema is eventually excreted in the stool, making the stool chalky white. Because barium can cause significant constipation, the doctor may give a gentle laxative to speed up the elimination of barium.

Ultrasound Scanning

Ultrasound scanning uses sound waves to produce pictures of internal organs (see page 2044). An ultrasound scan can show the size and shape of many organs, such as the liver and pancreas, and can also show abnormal areas within them, such as cysts and some tumors. It can also show fluid in the abdominal cavity (ascites). Ultrasound scanning with a probe on the abdominal wall is not a good method for examining the lining of the digestive tract. Endoscopic ultrasound, however, shows the lining more clearly because the probe is placed on the tip of an endoscope.

An ultrasound scan is painless and poses no risk of complications. Endoscopic ultrasound poses the same risk of complications as endoscopy.

Computed Tomography and Magnetic Resonance Imaging

Computed tomography (CT—see page 2037) and magnetic resonance imaging (MRI—see page 2040) scans are good tools for assessing the size and location of abdominal organs. Additionally, growths such as cancerous (malignant) or noncancerous (benign) tumors are often detected by these tests. Changes in blood vessels can be detected as well. Inflammation, such as that of the appendix (appendicitis) or diverticula (diverticulitis), is usually evident. Sometimes, these tests are used to help guide radiologic or surgical procedures.

Paracentesis

Paracentesis is the insertion of a needle into the abdominal cavity for the removal of fluid. Normally, the abdominal cavity contains only a small amount of fluid. However, fluid can accumulate in certain circumstances, such as when a person has liver disease, heart failure, a ruptured stomach or intestine, cancer, or a ruptured spleen. A doctor may use paracentesis to aid in diagnosis (for example, to obtain a fluid sample for analysis) or as part of treatment (for example, to remove excess fluid).

Before paracentesis, a physical examination, sometimes accompanied by an ultrasound scan, is performed to confirm that the abdominal cavity contains excess fluid. Next, an area of the skin, usually just below the navel, is washed with an antiseptic solution and numbed with a small amount of anesthetic. A doctor then pushes a needle attached to a syringe through the skin and muscles of the abdominal wall and into the area of fluid accumulation. A small amount of fluid may be removed for laboratory testing, or up to several quarts may be removed to relieve distention. Complications include perforation of the digestive tract and bleeding.

Occult Blood Tests

Bleeding in the digestive system can be caused by something as insignificant as a little irritation or as serious as cancer. Amounts of blood too small to be seen or to change the appearance of stool can be detected chemically. The detection of such small amounts may provide early clues to the presence of ulcers, cancers, and other abnormalities.

During a rectal examination, the doctor may obtain a small amount of stool on a gloved finger. This sample is placed on a piece of filter paper impregnated with a chemical (guaiac). After another chemical is added, the sample will change color if blood is present. More preferably, the person can take home a kit containing the filter papers. The person places samples of stool from about three different bowel movements on the filter papers, which are then mailed in special containers back to the doctor for testing. If blood is detected, further examinations are needed to determine the source.

Intubation of the Digestive Tract

Intubation of the digestive tract is the process of passing a small, flexible plastic tube (nasogastric tube) through the nose or mouth into the stomach or small intestine. This procedure may be used for diagnostic or treatment purposes. Intubation typically causes gagging and nausea, so a numbing spray is usually applied into the nose and back of the throat. The tube size varies according to the purpose.

Nasogastric intubation can be used to obtain a sample of stomach fluid. The tube is passed through the nose rather than through the mouth, primarily because the tube can be more easily guided to the esophagus. Also, passage of a tube through the nose is less irritating and less likely to trigger coughing. Doctors can determine whether the stomach contains blood, or they can analyze the stomach's secretions for acidity, enzymes, and other characteristics. In people with poisoning, samples of the stomach fluid can be analyzed to identify the poison. In some cases, the tube is left in place so that samples can be obtained over several hours.

Nasogastric intubation may also be used to treat certain conditions. For example, poisons can be pumped out or neutralized with activated charcoal, or liquid food can be given to people who cannot swallow.

Sometimes nasogastric intubation is used to continuously remove the contents of the stomach. The end of the tube is usually attached to a suction device, which removes gas and fluid from the stomach. This helps relieve pressure when the digestive system is blocked or otherwise not functioning properly. This type of tube is often used after abdominal surgery until the digestive system can resume its normal function.

In a procedure called 24-hour pH testing, a tube is placed through the nose into the esophagus, where it sits for 24 hours. The tube frequently samples the fluid of the esophagus, allowing detection of stomach acid that comes up into the chest (esophageal reflux). This test allows the doctors to measure the severity and frequency of reflux.

In nasoenteric intubation, a longer tube is passed through the nose, through the stomach, and into the small intestine. This procedure can be used to remove a sample of intestinal contents, continuously remove fluids, or provide food.

Manometry

Manometry is a test in which a tube with pressure gauges along its surface is placed in the esophagus. Using this device (manometer), a doctor can determine whether contractions of the esophagus can propel food normally. Sometimes a doctor uses a similar device to measure pressure in the anal sphincter to determine whether the muscle opens normally.

19 Esophageal Disorders

The esophagus is the hollow tube that leads from the throat (pharynx) to the stomach. The walls of the esophagus propel food to the stomach not by gravity, but by rhythmic waves of muscular contractions called peristalsis.

Just below the junction of the throat and the esophagus is a band of muscle called the upper esophageal sphincter. Slightly above the junction of the esophagus and the stomach is another band of muscle called the lower esophageal sphincter. When the esophagus is not in use, these sphincters contract so that food and stomach acid do not flow up from the stomach to the mouth. During swallowing, the sphincters relax so food can pass to the stomach.

With aging, the strength of esophageal contractions and the tension in the sphincters decrease. This condition, called presbyesophagus, makes older people more prone to backflow of acid from the stomach (gastroesophageal reflux or GERD—see page 144), especially when lying down after eating.

Two of the most common symptoms of esophageal disorders are dysphagia (an awareness of swallowing difficulty) and chest or back pain. Dysphagia and chest or back pain may occur in any esophageal disorder, the most serious of which is esophageal cancer.

The esophageal disorders discussed in this chapter are propulsion-related, infection-related, injury-related, or obstruction-related. In another esophageal disorder, called esophageal varices, the veins at the lower end of the esophagus become dilated and bleed easily (see page 217).

Abnormal Propulsion of Food

The movement of food from mouth to stomach requires normal and coordinated action of the mouth and throat, propulsive waves of the esophagus, and relaxation of the sphincters. A problem with any of these functions can cause difficulty swallowing (dysphagia), regurgitation (the spitting up of food from the esophagus or stomach without nausea or forceful contractions of abdominal muscles), vomiting, or aspiration of food (sucking food into the airways when inhaling).

ACHALASIA

Achalasia (also called cardiospasm, esophageal aperistalsis, or megaesophagus) is a disorder in which the rhythmic contractions of the esophagus are greatly decreased, the lower esophageal sphincter does not relax normally, and the resting pressure of the lower esophageal sphincter is increased.

Achalasia results from a malfunction of the nerves controlling the rhythmic contractions of the esophagus. The cause of the nerve malfunction is not known, but a viral cause is suspected. Certain tumors may cause achalasia either by directly constricting (narrowing) the lower esophageal sphincter or by infiltrating the nerves of the esophagus. Chagas' disease, which causes the destruction of clusters of nerve cells (autonomic ganglia), may also result in achalasia.

Symptoms

Achalasia may occur at any age but usually begins, almost unnoticed, between the ages of 20 and 60 and then progresses gradually over many months or years. The tight lower esophageal sphincter causes the part of the esophagus above it to enlarge greatly. This enlargement contributes to many of the symptoms. Difficulty swallowing both solids and liquids is the main symptom. Other symptoms may include chest pain; regurgitation of the bland, nonacidic contents of the enlarged esophagus; and coughing at night. Although uncommon, chest pain may occur during swallowing or for no apparent reason. About one third of people who have achalasia regurgitate undigested food while sleeping. They may inhale food into their lungs, which can cause coughing, a lung abscess, infection of the airways, bronchiectasis, or aspiration pneumonia. Undigested food typically remains in the esophagus. Mild to moderate weight loss also occurs. When people have significant weight loss, especially older people whose symptoms of dysphagia developed rapidly, doctors consider and look for a tumor at the gastroesophageal junction (the place where the esophagus connects to the stomach).

Diagnosis

X-rays of the esophagus taken while the person is swallowing barium (a barium swallow—see page 130) show an absence of the normal rhythmic waves of muscular contractions (peristalsis). The esophagus is widened, usually only moderately but occasionally to enormous proportions, but is narrow at the lower esophageal sphincter.

Doctors usually also insert a small tube into the esophagus to take pressure measurements of the contractions (esophageal manometry—see page 131). Often, doctors examine the esophagus through a flexible viewing tube (esophagoscopy—see page 129). During an esophagoscopy, the doctor performs a biopsy (removal of tissue samples for examination under a microscope) to make sure the symptoms are not caused by cancer at the lower end of the esophagus.

Achalasia that is caused by cancer at the gastroesophageal junction can be diagnosed by computed tomography (CT) of the chest and abdomen or by an endoscopic ultrasound (a tiny ultrasound probe on the tip of an endoscope that is passed through the mouth into the stomach).

Treatment

No treatment restores peristalsis. The aim of treatment is to relieve symptoms by decreasing pressure in the lower esophageal sphincter. Nitrates (for example, nitroglycerin placed under the tongue before meals) or calcium channel blockers (for example, nifedipine) are of limited effectiveness but may delay the need for dilation by helping to relax the sphincter.

Dilation widens the sphincter mechanically—for example, by inflating a large balloon inside it. This procedure helps about 85% of the time, but repeated dilations may be needed. In fewer than 2% of people with achalasia, the esophagus ruptures during the dilation procedure. Esophageal rupture leads to severe inflammation in the chest outside the esophagus (mediastinitis) and, in rare cases, is fatal if not treated appropriately. Immediate surgery is needed to close the rupture in the wall of the esophagus.

As an alternative to mechanical dilation, a doctor may inject botulinum toxin into the lower esophageal sphincter. This therapy is as effective as mechanical dilation with balloons. Botulinum toxin seems to be successful in providing sustained symptom relief for 70 to 80% of people, but the relief may last only 6 months to 1 year.

If dilation or botulinum toxin therapy does not work, a surgical procedure to cut the muscular fibers in the lower esophageal sphincter (myotomy) is usually performed. The procedure can be done with a laparoscope (see page 130) or a thoracoscope (see page 457). This procedure is successful about 85% of the time. A procedure (called a fundoplication) to prevent backflow of acid from the stomach (gastroesophageal reflux or GERD) is usually performed during the same surgery. About 15% of people experience episodic backflow of acid (reflux) after surgery.

ESOPHAGEAL POUCHES

Esophageal pouches (diverticula) are abnormal protrusions from the esophagus that in rare cases cause swallowing difficulties and regurgitation (the spitting up of food from the esophagus or stomach without nausea or forceful contractions of abdominal muscles).

There are several types of esophageal diverticula. Each has a different cause, but probably all are related

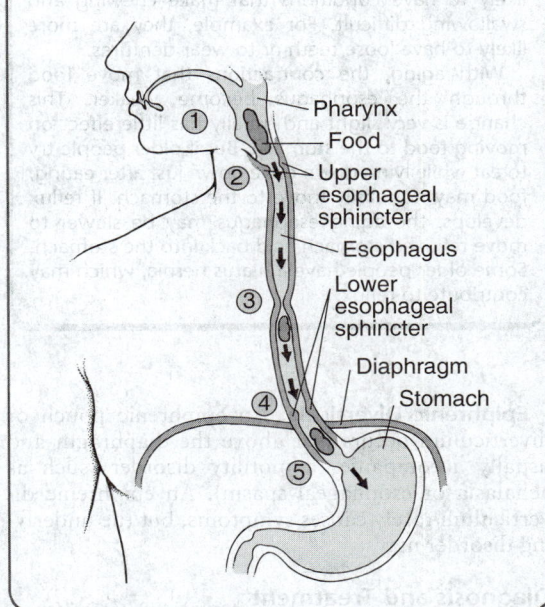

How the Esophagus Works

As a person swallows, food moves from the mouth to the throat, also called the pharynx (1). The upper esophageal sphincter opens (2) so that food can enter the esophagus, where waves of muscular contractions, called peristalsis, propel the food downward (3). The food then passes through the lower esophageal sphincter (4) and moves into the stomach (5).

Pharynx
Food
Upper esophageal sphincter
Esophagus
Lower esophageal sphincter
Diaphragm
Stomach

to uncoordinated swallowing and muscle relaxation. Most of these diverticula are associated with motility disorders of the esophagus, such as esophageal spasm and achalasia.

Zenker's Diverticula: A pharyngeal pouch or Zenker's diverticulum is probably caused by an incoordination between movement of food out of the mouth and relaxation of the cricopharyngeal muscle. This diverticulum can fill with food, which may be regurgitated when the person bends over or lies down. This may also cause food to be inhaled into the lungs during sleep, resulting in aspiration pneumonia. Rarely, the pouch enlarges and causes swallowing difficulty and sometimes a swelling in the neck.

Midesophageal Diverticula: A midesophageal pouch or traction diverticulum is caused by traction from inflamed lesions located in the chest outside the esophagus (mediastinum) or, secondarily, by esophageal movement (motility) disorders. A traction diverticulum rarely causes symptoms, but the underlying disorder may.

SPOTLIGHT ON AGING

As people age, several changes may affect the ability to swallow. Slightly less saliva is produced. As a result, food is softened (macerated) less well and is drier before it is swallowed. The muscles in the jaws and throat may weaken slightly, making chewing and swallowing less efficient. Also, older people are more likely to have conditions that make chewing and swallowing difficult. For example, they are more likely to have loose teeth or to wear dentures.

With aging, the contractions that move food through the esophagus become weaker. This change is very slight and usually has little effect on moving food to the stomach. But if older people try to eat while lying down or lie down just after eating, food may not easily move to the stomach. If reflux develops, the aging esophagus may be slower to move refluxed stomach acid back into the stomach. Some older people have a hiatus hernia, which may contribute to reflux.

Epiphrenic Diverticula: An epiphrenic pouch or diverticulum occurs just above the diaphragm and usually accompanies a motility disorder (such as achalasia or esophageal spasm). An epiphrenic diverticulum rarely causes symptoms, but the underlying disorder may.

Diagnosis and Treatment

All diverticula can be diagnosed with a videotaped barium swallow.

Treatment is not usually needed. If symptoms are severe, however, the pouch can be removed surgically. Diverticula associated with motility disorders require treatment of the underlying disorder. For example, if a Zenker's diverticulum is caused by an abnormally functioning cricopharyngeal muscle, a doctor can cut the muscle (myotomy) when removing the Zenker's diverticulum. When esophageal spasm or achalasia is present, treatment of sphincter tightness may be needed.

ESOPHAGEAL SPASM

Esophageal spasm (also called spastic pseudodiverticulosis, rosary bead or corkscrew esophagus, or symptomatic diffuse esophageal spasm) is a disorder of the propulsive movements (peristalsis) of the esophagus.

In this disorder, the normal propulsive contractions that move food through the esophagus are replaced periodically by nonpropulsive contractions or excessive muscular contractions (hyperdynamia). In 30% of people with this disorder, the lower esophageal sphincter opens and closes abnormally. The exact cause is not known but is suspected to be a nerve defect.

Symptoms

Muscle spasms throughout the esophagus typically are felt as chest pain under the breastbone coinciding with difficulty in swallowing liquids (especially those that are very hot or cold) and solids. Pain also occurs at night and may be severe enough to awaken a person. Esophageal spasm also may cause severe pain without swallowing difficulty. This pain, often described as a squeezing pain under the breastbone, may accompany exercise or exertion, making it difficult for a doctor to distinguish it from angina (chest pain stemming from heart disease). Over many years, this disorder may evolve into achalasia (see page 132), a disorder in which the rhythmic contractions of the esophagus are greatly decreased. Some people have symptoms that combine those of achalasia and diffuse esophageal spasm. One such combination of symptoms has been called vigorous achalasia. It features both food retention, which can lead to aspiration, as well as severe chest pain from diffuse esophageal spasm.

Diagnosis

X-rays taken while the person swallows a barium drink (a barium swallow—see page 130) may show that liquid barium does not move normally down the esophagus and that contractions of the esophageal wall are uncoordinated and do not propel the barium. Pressure measurements by manometry (a test in which a tube placed in the esophagus measures the pressure of contractions—see page 131) provide the most sensitive and detailed analysis of the spasms.

Treatment

Esophageal spasm is often difficult to treat. Calcium channel blockers such as nifedipine may relieve the symptoms by relaxing the muscles of the esophagus. Sometimes, injecting botulinum toxin into the muscles of the esophagus is helpful. Other drugs such as nitroglycerin, long-acting nitrates, and drugs with anticholinergic effects (such as dicyclomine) are less successful. Sometimes people need strong analgesics. In many cases, a narrowing is treated by inflating a balloon inside the esophagus or by inserting bougies (progressively larger dilators) to dilate the esophagus. In rare cases, if other less radical forms of treatment are not effective, a surgeon may cut the muscle layer along the full length of the esophagus (surgical myotomy).

PROPULSION DISORDERS OF THE THROAT

Propulsion disorders of the throat can cause trouble moving food from the upper part of the throat into the esophagus. Such problems occur most often in people who have disorders of the throat muscles or the nerves that serve them. The most common cause is stroke. Dermatomyositis, scleroderma, myasthenia gravis, muscular dystrophy, polio, pseudobulbar palsy, Parkinson's disease, and amyotrophic lateral sclerosis (Lou Gehrig's disease) all can affect the throat muscles or nerves. Difficulty swallowing may also result from the use of a phenothiazine (a class of antipsychotic drug), because these drugs can impair the normal function of the throat muscles. People with a propulsion disorder of the throat often regurgitate food through the back of the nose or inhale it into the windpipe (trachea), which causes them to cough.

In cricopharyngeal incoordination, the upper esophageal sphincter (cricopharyngeal muscle) remains closed, or it opens in an uncoordinated way. An abnormally functioning sphincter may allow food to repeatedly enter the windpipe and lungs, which may lead to recurring lung infections and eventually to chronic lung disease. A surgeon can cut the sphincter so that it is permanently relaxed. If left untreated, the condition may lead to the formation of a diverticulum (see page 133), a pouch formed when the lining of the esophagus pushes outward and backward through the cricopharyngeal muscle.

Infection

Infection of the esophagus occurs mainly in people who have impaired host defenses. The main causes are Candida albicans, herpes simplex virus infections, and cytomegalovirus infection.

There are several defense mechanisms that protect the esophagus against infection. These defenses include saliva, the normal movement (motility) of the esophagus, and the cells of the immune system. Thus, people at risk include those who have AIDS, an organ transplant, alcoholism, diabetes, malnutrition, cancer, or motility disorders. *Candida* infection may occur in any of these people. Herpes simplex virus infections (see page 1245) and cytomegalovirus infection (see page 1250) occur mainly in people who have AIDS or who have had an organ transplant and are on immunosuppressant medications.

Pain with swallowing (odynophagia) is the typical symptom. Some people also notice difficulty swallowing (dysphagia).

 Did You Know...
Saliva helps protect the esophagus from infection.

Sometimes, the doctor can see signs of *Candida* infection in the mouth (thrush) in people who have *Candida* infection of the esophagus. Usually there

are no abnormalities in the mouths of people with herpes simplex virus infections or cytomegalovirus infection. To diagnose an infection of the esophagus, usually the doctor looks down the esophagus using a flexible viewing tube with a camera on the end (esophagoscopy—see page 129).

People with *Candida* are given an antifungal drug such as fluconazole. The drug is given by mouth or, if people are having trouble swallowing, by injection into a vein.

People with herpes simplex virus infections or cytomegalovirus infection are given antiviral drugs such as acyclovir or ganciclovir by injection into a vein.

Injury

The esophagus is relatively impervious to injury but can be harmed gradually by backflow of acid from the stomach (gastroesophageal reflux or GERD—see page 144). The esophagus may also be harmed suddenly, by caustic or acidic chemicals, irritating drugs, a sharp object, or extreme pressure. Extreme pressure can occur during violent vomiting.

The more sudden types of injuries can cause pain, often experienced as sharp pain under the breastbone. It may also cause bleeding, which would be evident in vomited material or stool. Fainting may occur due to this pain, especially if the esophagus ruptures. This rupture allows food contents to spill into the mediastinum (the area of the chest bordered by the sternum in front, the spinal column in back, the entrance to the chest cavity above, and the diaphragm below) and causes mediastinitis.

 Did You Know...
Forceful vomiting can tear the esophagus.

EROSIVE ESOPHAGITIS

Erosive esophagitis is a condition in which areas of the esophageal lining are inflamed and ulcerated.

The most common cause of erosive esophagitis is chronic acid reflux. Corrosive substances, such as cleaning solutions, can erode the esophagus if they are swallowed accidentally or deliberately. Some pills (for example, aspirin or other nonsteroidal anti-inflammatory drugs [NSAIDs], alendronate, doxycycline, tetracycline, and certain large iron and potassium tablets) can cause painful erosions if they lodge temporarily in the esophagus.

The diagnosis of erosive esophagitis is made by esophagoscopy (see page 129). If a pill becomes stuck in the esophagus, it usually can be washed down with large quantities of water, and the pain often resolves within hours. Rarely, erosions caused by corrosive substances or pills persist, leading to narrowing of the esophagus.

ESOPHAGEAL LACERATION

An esophageal laceration (Mallory-Weiss syndrome) is a tear that does not penetrate the wall of the esophagus.

A laceration of the lower esophagus and the upper part of the stomach during forceful vomiting, retching, or hiccups is called Mallory-Weiss syndrome. The tear may rupture blood vessels, which then bleed. This syndrome was initially described in alcoholics but can occur in anyone who vomits forcefully.

The first symptom is usually the appearance of blood in vomited material. Mallory-Weiss syndrome is the cause of about 5% of bleeding episodes in the upper digestive tract.

The diagnosis is made by esophagoscopy or angiography (a catheter is used to inject an artery with a dye that can be seen on x-rays). The laceration cannot be detected on routine x-rays.

Most bleeding episodes stop by themselves, but sometimes the doctor must perform esophagoscopy and stop the bleeding by cauterizing the bleeding vessel or injecting a drug into it. Alternatively, the doctor may inject vasopressin or epinephrine during angiography to reduce blood flow into the bleeding vessel. People who lose a lot of blood require a transfusion. Surgical repair is rarely required.

ESOPHAGEAL RUPTURES

Esophageal ruptures are tears that penetrate the wall of the esophagus.

Ruptures of the esophagus are usually caused during endoscopy (examination of the esophagus with a flexible viewing tube—see page 129) or other procedures in which instruments are inserted through the mouth and throat. Ruptures also may occur during vomiting, retching, or swallowing a large mass of food. Such rupture is called Boerhaave's syndrome.

An esophageal rupture leads to severe inflammation in the chest outside the esophagus (mediastinitis). This inflammation allows fluid to enter the space between the membrane layers (pleura) covering the lungs, a condition called pleural effusion (see page 518). People also have chest pain, abdominal pain, and shock.

Because swallowing barium (a contrast agent that makes the lining of the esophagus visible on x-ray) is too irritating, doctors confirm the diagnosis by performing an x-ray or video of the esophagus after the person swallows a different type of contrast agent (gastrographin). Surgical repair of the esophagus and drainage of the area surrounding it are performed immediately. Before surgical repair, broad-spectrum antibiotics and fluids as needed are given to treat shock. Even with treatment, the risk of death from a large rupture is very high.

Obstruction

The esophagus can be narrowed or completely blocked. In rare cases, the cause is hereditary (for example, congenital rings). In most cases, the cause is progression of an injury to the esophagus or tumor growth. Food and foreign bodies may obstruct the esophagus as well. Injuries that can progress to obstruction can result from damage caused by the repeated backflow of acid from the stomach (gastroesophageal reflux or GERD), usually over years. Injury can also result from damage caused by drugs taken in pill form or ingestion of corrosive substances (see page 135). Narrowing may also be caused by compression against the outside of the esophagus. Compression can result from a number of causes, such as enlargement of the left atrium of the heart, an aortic aneurysm, an abnormally formed blood vessel (dysphagia lusoria), an abnormal thyroid gland, a bony outgrowth from the spine, or cancer—most commonly lung cancer. Another serious cause of narrowing is noncancerous (benign) and cancerous (malignant) tumors of the esophagus.

Because all these conditions decrease the diameter of the esophagus, people with one of them usually have difficulty swallowing solid foods—particularly meat and bread. Difficulty in swallowing liquids develops much later, if at all.

A type of barium x-ray called a barium swallow (see page 130) is usually taken to find the cause and location of the narrowing or obstruction. Treatment and outcome depend on the cause.

DYSPHAGIA LUSORIA

Dysphagia lusoria is difficulty swallowing caused by compression of the esophagus by an abnormally formed blood vessel, which is present at birth.

Dysphagia lusoria is a birth defect. However, the swallowing difficulty may not appear until childhood or later in life because that is when degenerative changes occur in the abnormally formed blood vessel. A barium swallow x-ray shows the compression, but angiography (injecting a blood vessel with a dye that can be seen on x-rays) is necessary for an accurate diagnosis. Most people require no treatment, but surgical repair is sometimes performed.

ESOPHAGEAL WEBS

Esophageal webs (also called Plummer-Vinson syndrome, Paterson-Kelly syndrome, or sideropenic dysphagia) are thin membranes that grow across the inside of the upper one third of the esophagus from its surface lining (mucosa).

Although rare, esophageal webs occur most often in people who have untreated severe iron deficiency anemia. Why anemia leads to the development of webs is unknown. Webs in the upper esophagus usually make swallowing solids difficult. A barium swallow x-ray is usually the best procedure with which to diagnose the problem.

Once the iron deficiency has been treated, the web usually disappears. If not, a doctor can rupture it using a dilator or an endoscope.

LOWER ESOPHAGEAL RING

A lower esophageal ring (also called Schatzki's ring or B ring) narrows the lower esophagus and is most likely present at birth.

Normally, the lower esophagus has a diameter of 1½ to 2 inches (about 3½ to 5 centimeters).

However, it may be narrowed to ½ inch in diameter (about 1¼ centimeters) or less by a ring of tight tissue, which may cause difficulty in swallowing solids. This symptom can begin at any age but usually does not begin until after age 25. The swallowing difficulty comes and goes and is especially aggravated by meat and dry bread. Often, barium swallow x-rays are done to show the ring.

Chewing food thoroughly followed by sips of water usually prevents symptoms. A doctor may fix the narrowing by passing an endoscope (a flexible viewing tube—see page 129) through the mouth and throat and into the esophagus or may use a dilator (called a bougie) to widen the passageway. In rare cases, the constricting ring is opened via a surgical procedure.

CHAPTER 20 Peptic Disorders

Peptic disorders include gastritis, peptic ulcer, and gastroesophageal reflux. They involve damage to the lining of the esophagus, stomach, or duodenum (the first segment of the small intestine). These disorders are usually caused by stomach acids (especially hydrochloric acid), digestive enzymes (especially pepsin), infection with the bacterium *Helicobacter pylori*, and use of certain drugs, such as nonsteroidal anti-inflammatory drugs (NSAIDs).

Gastritis

Gastritis is inflammation of the stomach lining.

- The inflammation can be caused by many factors, including infection, injury, certain drugs, and disorders of the immune system.
- When symptoms do occur, they include abdominal pain or discomfort and sometimes nausea or vomiting.
- Doctors often base the diagnosis on the person's symptoms, but sometime they need to examine the stomach by using a flexible viewing tube (endoscopy).
- Treatment is with drugs that reduce stomach acid.

The stomach lining resists irritation and can usually withstand very strong acid. Nevertheless, in gastritis, the stomach lining becomes irritated and inflamed.

Causes

Gastritis can be caused by many factors, including infection, injury, certain drugs, and disorders of the immune system.

Infections with bacteria, viruses, or fungi can cause gastritis. Worldwide, the most common cause of gastritis is infection with *Helicobacter pylori* bacteria. Viral or fungal gastritis may develop in people who have had a prolonged illness or an impaired immune system, such as those who have AIDS or cancer or those who take immunosuppressant drugs.

Erosive gastritis involves both inflammation and wearing away of the stomach lining. Erosive gastritis results from irritants such as drugs, especially aspirin and other nonsteroidal anti-inflammatory drugs (NSAIDs—see page 644); Crohn's disease; bacterial and viral infections; and the ingestion of corrosive substances. In some people, even a baby aspirin taken daily can injure the stomach lining. Erosive gastritis can develop suddenly but more commonly develops slowly, usually in people who are otherwise healthy.

Acute stress gastritis, actually a form of erosive gastritis, is caused by a sudden illness or injury. The injury may not even be to the stomach. For example, extensive skin burns and injuries involving major bleeding are typical causes. Exactly why serious illness can lead to gastritis is not known but may be related to decreased blood flow to the stomach or to impairment of the stomach lining's ability to protect and renew itself.

Radiation gastritis can occur if radiation is delivered to the lower left side of the chest or upper abdomen, where it can irritate the stomach lining.

Postgastrectomy gastritis occurs in people who have had part of their stomach surgically removed (a procedure called partial gastrectomy). The inflammation usually occurs where tissue has been sewn back together. Postgastrectomy gastritis is thought to result when surgery impairs blood flow to the stomach lining or exposes the stomach lining to an excessive amount of bile (the greenish yellow digestive fluid produced by the liver).

Atrophic gastritis causes the stomach lining to become very thin and to lose many or all of the cells that produce acid and enzymes. This condition can occur when antibodies (see page 1124) attack the stomach lining (termed autoimmune metaplastic atrophic gastritis). Atrophic gastritis can also occur in people who are chronically infected with *Helicobacter pylori* bacteria. It also tends to occur in those who have had part of their stomach removed.

Eosinophilic gastritis may result from an allergic reaction to an infestation with roundworms. In other cases, the cause is unknown. In this type of gastritis, eosinophils (a type of white blood cell) accumulate in the stomach wall.

Ménétrier's disease, whose cause is unknown, is a type of gastritis in which the stomach wall develops thick, large folds; enlarged glands; and fluid-filled cysts. The disease may be due to an abnormal immune reaction and has also been associated with *Helicobacter pylori* infection.

In lymphocytic gastritis, lymphocytes (another type of white blood cell) accumulate in the stomach wall and other organs. This lymphocyte accumulation also occurs in celiac sprue (a malabsorptive disorder), but the cause is frequently unknown.

Symptoms and Complications

Gastritis usually causes no symptoms. When symptoms do occur, they vary depending on the cause and may include pain or discomfort (dyspepsia) or nausea or vomiting, problems that are often simply referred to as indigestion. Gastritis can lead to ulcers, which may cause the symptoms to get worse.

Nausea and intermittent vomiting can result from erosive gastritis, radiation gastritis, Ménétrier's disease, and lymphocytic gastritis. Dyspepsia can occur, especially with erosive gastritis, radiation gastritis, postgastrectomy gastritis, and atrophic gastritis. Very mild dyspepsia also occurs with acute stress gastritis.

Ulcers can develop with several types of gastritis, especially acute stress gastritis, erosive gastritis, and radiation gastritis. Ulcers may bleed, causing a person to vomit blood (hematemesis) or pass tarry black stools (melena). Acute stress gastritis may lead to bleeding from ulcers within a few days after an illness or injury, whereas bleeding tends to develop more slowly in the case of erosive gastritis or radiation gastritis. Persistent

bleeding can lead to symptoms of anemia, including fatigue, weakness, and light-headedness. If an ulcer goes through (perforates) the stomach wall, stomach contents may spill into the abdominal cavity, resulting in inflammation and usually infection of the lining of the abdominal cavity (peritonitis) and sudden worsening of pain.

Some complications of gastritis are slow to develop. The scarring and narrowing of the stomach outlet that can result from gastritis, especially from radiation gastritis and eosinophilic gastritis, can cause severe nausea and frequent vomiting. In Ménétrier's disease, fluid retention and swelling of the tissues (edema) may occur because of loss of protein from the inflamed stomach lining. About 10% of people with Ménétrier's disease develop stomach cancer some years later. Postgastrectomy gastritis and atrophic gastritis may cause symptoms of anemia, such as fatigue and weakness, because of decreased production of intrinsic factor (a protein that binds vitamin B_{12}, allowing the B_{12} to be absorbed and used in the production of red blood cells). A small percentage of people with atrophic gastritis develop a condition called metaplasia, in which cells lining the stomach change and become precancerous. In an even smaller percentage of people, metaplasia leads to stomach cancer.

Diagnosis

A doctor suspects gastritis when a person has upper abdominal discomfort or pain or nausea. Tests usually are not needed. However, if the doctor is uncertain of the diagnosis, or if symptoms do not resolve with treatment, an examination of the stomach using an endoscope (a flexible viewing tube—see page 129) may be needed. If necessary, the doctor can perform a biopsy (removal of a tissue sample for examination under a microscope) of the stomach lining.

Treatment

Regardless of the cause of gastritis, symptoms can be relieved by taking drugs that neutralize or reduce the production of stomach acid and by discontinuing drugs that cause symptoms (see page 145). For mild symptoms, taking antacids, which neutralize acid that has already been produced and released in the stomach, is often sufficient. However, antacids have to be taken several times a day and often produce diarrhea or constipation. Drugs that reduce acid production include histamine-2 (H_2) blockers and proton pump inhibitors. H_2 blockers are usually more effective than antacids in relieving symptoms, and many people find them far more convenient. Proton pump inhibitors are prescribed when the strongest treatment is needed. When infection is a part of gastritis, antibiotics are also prescribed. Doctors may prescribe sucralfate, which

When the Stomach Is Infected

Infection with *Helicobacter pylori,* a type of bacteria, is the most common cause of gastritis and peptic ulcer worldwide. Infection is very common and increases with age; by age 60, about 50% of people are infected. Long-term infection increases the risk of stomach cancer.

H. pylori bacteria grow in the protective mucus layer of the stomach lining, where they are less exposed to the highly acidic juices produced by the stomach. Virtually all people who have *H. pylori* infection have gastritis, which may affect the entire stomach or only the lower part (antrum). Infection can sometimes lead to erosive gastritis. *H. pylori* contributes to ulcer formation by increasing acid production, interfering with the normal defenses against stomach acid, and producing toxins.

Most people with gastritis from *H. pylori* infection do not develop symptoms, but people who do develop symptoms experience those typical of gastritis, such as indigestion and pain or discomfort in the upper abdomen. Ulcers caused by *H. pylori* infection produce symptoms similar to ulcers caused by other disorders, including pain in the upper abdomen.

H. pylori can be detected with tests that use blood, breath, or stool samples. However, because blood tests can remain positive for years after the *H. pylori* infection has been eliminated, the breath test is often used to confirm treatment success.

H. pylori infection must be treated with antibiotics. The most popular treatment for *H. pylori* infection includes a proton pump inhibitor to reduce acid production combined with two antibiotics, such as amoxicillin and clarithromycin given twice daily for 7 to 14 days. The combination of bismuth subsalicylate (a drug similar to sucralfate), tetracycline (an antibiotic), metronidazole (an antibiotic), and a proton pump inhibitor is another popular option. However, this treatment requires people to take a total of four drugs up to 4 times a day for 7 to 14 days.

The likelihood that a peptic ulcer will recur during the course of 1 year is about 60 to 80% in people who have not been treated with antibiotics. This percentage decreases to less than 20% in people who have been treated with antibiotics. In addition, treatment of *H. pylori* infection may heal ulcers that have resisted previous treatment.

---

helps to prevent irritation. When gastritis leads to ulceration that perforates the stomach wall, immediate surgery is usually needed.

People with erosive gastritis must avoid taking drugs that irritate the stomach lining (such as NSAIDs). Some doctors prescribe proton pump inhibitors or misoprostol to help protect the stomach lining. The coxibs (COX-2 inhibitors such as celecoxib) are less likely to irritate the stomach lining than the older NSAIDs, but studies have shown that coxibs appear to increase the risk of heart attack and stroke with long-term use. Therefore, caution should be taken with use of coxibs.

Most people with acute stress gastritis recover fully when the underlying illness, injury, or bleeding is controlled. However, 2% of people in intensive care units have heavy bleeding from acute stress gastritis, which is often fatal. Therefore, doctors try to prevent acute stress gastritis after a major illness, major injury, or severe burn. Drugs that reduce acid production are commonly given after surgery and to people in most intensive care units to prevent acute stress gastritis. These drugs are also used to treat any ulcers that form. For people with heavy bleeding from acute stress gastritis, a wide variety of treatments have been used. Few of these treatments, however, improve the outcome. Blood transfusions may actually make bleeding worse. Bleeding points can be temporarily heat-sealed (cauterized) during an endoscopy, but bleeding often starts again if the underlying illness persists. If bleeding continues, the entire stomach may have to be removed as a lifesaving measure.

There is no cure for postgastrectomy gastritis or atrophic gastritis. People with anemia resulting from decreased absorption of vitamin B_{12} that occurs with atrophic gastritis must take supplemental injections of the vitamin for the rest of their lives.

Corticosteroids or surgery may be needed to relieve a blocked stomach outlet caused by eosinophilic gastritis. Removing part or all of the stomach may cure Ménétrier's disease. There is no effective drug treatment.

Peptic Ulcer

A peptic ulcer is a round or oval sore where the lining of the stomach or duodenum has been eaten away by stomach acid and digestive juices.

- Peptic ulcers can result from an infection with *Helicobacter pylori* or from drugs that weaken the lining of the stomach or duodenum.
- Discomfort caused by ulcers tends to come and go.
- The diagnosis is based on symptoms of stomach pain and on the results of an examination of the stomach by using a flexible viewing tube (endoscopy).
- Antacids and other drugs are given to reduce acid in the stomach, and antibiotics are given to eliminate *Helicobacter pylori*.

Ulcers penetrate into the lining of the stomach or duodenum (the first part of the small intestine). Gastritis may develop into ulcers.

The names given to specific ulcers identify their anatomic locations or the circumstances under which they developed. Duodenal ulcers, the most common type of peptic ulcer, occur in the first few inches of the duodenum. Gastric ulcers, which are less common, usually occur along the upper curve of the stomach. Marginal ulcers can develop when part of the stomach has been removed surgically, at the point where the remaining stomach has been reconnected to the intestine. Stress ulcers, like acute stress gastritis, can occur as a result of the stress of severe illness, skin burns, or trauma. Stress ulcers occur in the stomach and the duodenum.

Causes

Ulcers develop when the normal defense and repair mechanisms of the lining of the stomach or duodenum are weakened, making the lining more likely to be damaged by stomach acid.

By far, the two most common causes of peptic ulcer are infection of the stomach with *Helicobacter pylori* bacteria and use of certain drugs.

Before current treatments for *Helicobacter pylori* infection were used, these bacteria were present in nearly 90% of people with duodenal ulcers and in 75% of people with stomach ulcers. Currently, the percentage is lower, about 50 to 75%.

Many drugs, especially aspirin, other nonsteroidal anti-inflammatory drugs (NSAIDs), and corticosteroids, irritate the stomach lining and can cause ulcers. However, most people who take NSAIDs or corticosteroids do not develop peptic ulcers. Regardless, some experts suggest that people at high risk of developing peptic ulcers should use a type of NSAID called a coxib (COX-2 inhibitor), rather than one of the older types of NSAIDs, because coxibs are less likely to irritate the stomach (see page 646). However, studies have shown that coxibs appear to increase the risk of heart attack and stroke with long-term use and, therefore, caution should be taken with their use. Because of these complications, most doctors now use a standard NSAID plus a strong acid inhibitor (such as a proton pump inhibitor) for people at high risk of developing peptic ulcers.

People who smoke are more likely to develop a peptic ulcer than people who do not smoke, and their ulcers heal more slowly. Although psychologic stress can increase acid production, no link has been found between psychologic stress and peptic ulcers.

A rare cause of peptic ulcers is a type of cancer that causes excess acid production (Zollinger-Ellison syndrome—see box on page 142). The symptoms of cancerous ulcers are very similar to those of noncancerous ulcers. However, cancerous ulcers usually do not respond to the treatments used for noncancerous ulcers.

Symptoms

The typical ulcer tends to heal and recur. Thus, pain may occur for days or weeks and then wane or disappear. Symptoms can vary with the location of the ulcer and the person's age. For example, children and older people may not have the usual symptoms or may have no symptoms at all. In these instances, ulcers are discovered only when complications develop.

Only about half of the people with duodenal ulcers have the typical symptoms of gnawing, burning, aching, soreness, an empty feeling, and hunger. The pain is steady and mild or moderately severe and usually located just below the breastbone. For many people with a duodenal ulcer, pain is usually absent on awakening but appears by midmorning. Drinking milk or eating (which buffers stomach acid) or taking antacids generally relieves the pain, but it usually returns 2 or 3 hours later. Pain that awakens the person during the night is common. Frequently, the pain erupts once or more a day over a period of one to several weeks and then may disappear without treatment. However, pain usually recurs, often within the first 2 years and occasionally after several years. People generally develop patterns and often learn by experience when a recurrence is likely (commonly in spring and fall and during periods of stress).

The symptoms of gastric, marginal, and stress ulcers, unlike those of duodenal ulcers, do not follow any pattern. Eating may relieve pain temporarily or may cause pain rather than relieve it. Gastric ulcers sometimes cause swelling of the tissues (edema) that lead into the small intestine, which may prevent food from easily passing out of the stomach. This blockage may cause bloating, nausea, or vomiting after eating.

Complications of peptic ulcers, such as bleeding or rupture, are accompanied by symptoms of low blood pressure, such as dizziness and fainting.

Diagnosis

A doctor suspects an ulcer when a person has characteristic stomach pain. Sometimes the doctor simply treats the person for an ulcer to see whether the symptoms resolve, which suggests that the person had an ulcer that has healed.

Tests may be needed to confirm the diagnosis, especially when symptoms do not resolve after a few weeks of treatment, or when they first appear in a person who is over age 45 or who has other symptoms such as weight loss, because stomach cancer can cause similar symptoms. Also, when severe ulcers

What Are the Complications of Peptic Ulcers?

Most ulcers can be cured without complications. However, in some cases, peptic ulcers can develop potentially life-threatening complications, such as penetration, perforation, bleeding (hemorrhage), obstruction, and cancer.

Penetration

An ulcer can go through (penetrate) the muscular wall of the stomach or duodenum (the first segment of the small intestine) and continue into an adjacent organ, such as the liver or pancreas. This penetration causes intense, piercing, persistent pain, which may be felt outside of the area involved—for example, the back may hurt when a duodenal ulcer penetrates the pancreas. The pain may intensify when the person changes position. If drugs do not heal the ulcer, surgery may be needed.

Perforation

Ulcers on the front surface of the duodenum, or less commonly the stomach, can go through the wall, creating an opening (perforation) to the free space in the abdominal cavity. The resulting pain is sudden, intense, and steady. The pain rapidly spreads throughout the abdomen. The person may feel pain in one or both shoulders, which may intensify with deep breathing. Changing position worsens the pain, so the person often tries to lie very still. The abdomen is tender when touched, and the tenderness worsens if a doctor presses deeply and then suddenly releases the pressure. (Doctors call this rebound tenderness.) Symptoms may be less intense in older people, in people taking corticosteroids, or in very ill people. A fever indicates an infection in the abdominal cavity. If the condition is not treated, shock may develop. This emergency situation requires immediate surgery and intravenous antibiotics.

Bleeding

Bleeding (hemorrhage) is a common complication of ulcers even when they are not painful. Vomiting bright red blood or reddish brown clumps of partially digested blood that look like coffee grounds and passing black or obviously bloody stools can be symptoms of a bleeding ulcer. However, small amounts of blood in the stool may not be noticeable but, if persistent, can still lead to anemia. Bleeding may result from other digestive conditions as well, but doctors begin their investigation by looking for the source of bleeding in the stomach and duodenum. Unless bleeding is massive, a doctor performs an endoscopy (an examination using a flexible viewing tube). If a bleeding ulcer is seen, the endoscope can be used to cauterize it (that is, destroy it with heat). A doctor may also use the endoscope to inject a material that causes a bleeding ulcer to clot. If the source cannot be found and the bleeding is not severe, treatments include taking ulcer drugs, such as histamine-2 (H_2) blockers or proton pump inhibitors. The person also receives intravenous fluids and takes nothing by mouth, so the digestive tract can rest. If these measures fail, surgery is needed.

Obstruction

Swelling of inflamed tissues around an ulcer or scarring from previous ulcer flare-ups can narrow the outlet from the stomach or narrow the duodenum. A person with this type of obstruction may vomit repeatedly—often regurgitating large volumes of food eaten hours earlier. A feeling of being unusually full after eating, bloating, and a lack of appetite are symptoms of obstruction. Over time, vomiting can cause weight loss, dehydration, and an imbalance in body chemicals (electrolytes). Treating the ulcers relieves the obstruction in most cases, but severe obstructions may require endoscopy or surgery.

Cancer

People with ulcers caused by *Helicobacter pylori* have 3 to 6 times the chance of developing stomach cancer later in life. There is no increased risk of developing cancer from ulcers that have other causes.

---

resist treatment, particularly if a person has several ulcers or the ulcers are in unusual places, a doctor may suspect an underlying condition that causes the stomach to overproduce acid.

To help diagnose ulcers and determine their cause, the doctor may use endoscopy (a procedure performed using a flexible viewing tube) or barium contrast x-rays (x-rays taken after a substance that outlines the digestive tract has been swallowed).

Endoscopy is usually the first diagnostic procedure ordered by a doctor. Endoscopy is more reliable than barium contrast x-rays for detecting ulcers in the duodenum and on the back wall of the stomach; endoscopy is also more reliable if the person has had stomach surgery. However, even a highly skilled endoscopist may miss a small number of gastric and duodenal ulcers. With an endoscope, a doctor can perform a biopsy (removal of a tissue sample for examination under a microscope) to determine if a gastric ulcer is cancerous and to help identify the presence of *Helicobacter pylori* bacteria. An endoscope also can be used to stop active bleeding and decrease the likelihood of recurring bleeding from an ulcer.

Barium contrast x-rays of the stomach and duodenum (also called a barium swallow or an upper gastrointestinal series) can help determine the severity and size of an ulcer, which sometimes cannot be

Zollinger-Ellison Syndrome: An Acid-Stimulating Cancer

Zollinger-Ellison syndrome causes the stomach to produce too much acid. In this syndrome, a tumor, usually in the duodenum, pancreas, or adjacent structures, produces gastrin. Gastrin is a hormone that stimulates the stomach to produce large amounts of acid. About half of the tumors are cancerous (malignant). People with Zollinger-Ellison syndrome frequently develop many ulcers that recur despite treatment to control ulcer disease. They may also develop diarrhea that is difficult to control.

People with this disease typically have an elevated level of gastrin in their blood, which can be measured to make the diagnosis. Sometimes, testing involves giving the person a hormone called secretin. In people with Zollinger-Ellison syndrome, gastrin levels in the bloodstream greatly increase when secretin is injected into a vein. In addition, testing can reveal increased production of stomach acid. A number of tests can be performed in an attempt to find the tumor's location, including computed tomography (CT) scanning, endoscopic ultrasound, and radionuclide scanning.

Proton pump inhibitors help control the excess production of stomach acid. Surgery to remove the tumor can be curative. Even when not curative, surgery can reduce the tumor size, which in turn reduces the amount of acid produced by the stomach and prevents local complications, such as blockage of the intestine. Radiation and chemotherapy are not helpful. Although chemotherapy may reduce tumor size, it is not curative.

completely seen during an endoscopy because it is further down the duodenum or hidden by a fold.

Treatment

Because infection with *Helicobacter pylori* bacteria is a major cause of ulcers, antibiotics are often used. Sometimes bismuth subsalicylate is used in combination with antibiotics. Neutralizing or reducing stomach acid by taking drugs that directly inhibit the stomach's production of acid promotes healing of peptic ulcers regardless of the cause. In most people, treatment is continued for 4 to 8 weeks. Although bland diets may help reduce acid, no evidence supports the belief that such diets speed healing or keep ulcers from recurring. Nevertheless, it makes sense for people to avoid foods that seem to make pain and bloating worse. Eliminating possible stomach irritants, such as NSAIDs, alcohol, and nicotine, is also important.

Antacids: Antacids do not effectively heal ulcers but they do relieve symptoms of ulcers by neutralizing stomach acid and thereby raising the pH level in the stomach. Their effectiveness varies with the amount of antacid taken and the amount of acid a person produces. Almost all antacids can be purchased without a doctor's prescription and are available in tablet or liquid form. However, antacids can interact with many different prescription drugs, so a pharmacist should be consulted about possible drug-drug interactions before antacids are taken.

Sodium bicarbonate (baking soda) and calcium carbonate, the strongest antacids, may be taken occasionally for fast, short-term relief. However, because they are absorbed by the bloodstream, continual use of these drugs may make the blood too alkaline (alkalosis—see page 974), resulting in nausea, headache, and weakness. Therefore, these antacids generally should not be used in large amounts for more than a few days. These products also contain a lot of salt and should not be used by people who need to follow a low-sodium diet or who have heart failure or high blood pressure.

Aluminum hydroxide is a relatively safe, commonly used antacid. However, aluminum may bind with phosphate in the digestive tract, thereby depleting the body of calcium, reducing phosphate levels in the blood, and causing weakness and a loss of appetite. The risk of these side effects is greater in people with alcoholism and in people with kidney disease, including those receiving dialysis. Aluminum hydroxide may also cause constipation.

Magnesium hydroxide is a more effective antacid than aluminum hydroxide. This antacid acts fast and neutralizes acids effectively. Bowel movements usually remain regular if only a few tablespoons a day are taken; more than four doses a day may cause diarrhea. Because small amounts of magnesium are absorbed into the bloodstream, people with kidney damage should take magnesium hydroxide only in small doses. Many antacids contain both magnesium hydroxide and aluminum hydroxide.

Anyone who has heart disease, high blood pressure, or a kidney disorder should consult a doctor before selecting an antacid.

Acid-reducing Drugs: Proton pump inhibitors are the most potent of the drugs that reduce acid production. Proton pump inhibitors promote healing of ulcers in a greater percentage of people in a shorter period of time than do histamine-2 (H_2) blockers. They are also very useful in treating conditions that cause excessive stomach acid secretion, such as Zollinger-Ellison syndrome.

Histamine-2 (H_2) blockers, such as cimetidine, famotidine, nizatidine, and ranitidine, relieve symptoms and promote ulcer healing by reducing the production of stomach acid. These highly effective drugs are taken once or twice a day. H_2 blockers usually do not cause serious side effects. However, cimetidine is more likely to cause side effects, particularly in older people, in whom the drug may cause confusion. In addition, cimetidine may interfere with the body's elimination of certain drugs—such as theophylline for asthma, warfarin for excessive blood clotting, and phenytoin for seizures.

Miscellaneous Drugs: Sucralfate may work by forming a protective coating in the base of an ulcer to promote healing. It works well on peptic ulcers and is a reasonable alternative to antacids. Sucralfate is taken 2 to 4 times a day and is not absorbed into the bloodstream, so it causes few side effects. It may, however, cause constipation, and in some cases it reduces the effectiveness of other drugs.

Misoprostol may be used to reduce the likelihood of developing stomach and duodenal ulcers caused by NSAIDs. Misoprostol may work by reducing production of stomach acid and by making the stomach lining more resistant to acid. Older people, people taking corticosteroids, and people who have a history of ulcers are at higher risk of developing an ulcer when they take NSAIDs and may also be potential candidates for misoprostol. However, misoprostol causes diarrhea and other digestive problems in more than 30% of people who take it. In addition, this drug can cause spontaneous abortions in pregnant women. Alternatives to misoprostol are available for people taking aspirin, NSAIDs, or corticosteroids. These alternatives, such as proton pump inhibitors, are just as effective for reducing the likelihood of developing an ulcer and cause fewer side effects.

℞ DRUGS USED TO TREAT PEPTIC DISORDERS

DRUG	SOME SIDE EFFECTS	COMMENTS
Antacids		
Aluminum hydroxide Calcium carbonate Magnesium hydroxide Sodium bicarbonate	Nausea, headache, weakness, loss of appetite, and constipation (aluminum hydroxide) or diarrhea (magnesium hydroxide)	These drugs are used mainly to relieve symptoms, not as a cure.
Histamine-2 blockers		
Cimetidine Famotidine Nizatidine Ranitidine	Rash, fever, muscle pains, and confusion (cimetidine or ranitidine) May cause breast enlargement and erectile dysfunction in men May interfere with elimination of certain drugs (cimetidine)	The once-daily dose is taken in the evening or at bedtime. Doses taken in the morning are less effective.
Proton pump inhibitors		
Lansoprazole Omeprazole Pantoprazole Rabeprazole Esomeprazole	Diarrhea, constipation, and headache	These drugs are usually well tolerated and are most effective means of reducing stomach acid.
Antibiotics		
Amoxicillin Clarithromycin Metronidazole Tetracycline	Diarrhea (amoxicillin, clarithromycin, or tetracycline), altered taste, and nausea	These drugs are effective for treating peptic ulcers caused by *Helicobacter pylori* infection.
Miscellaneous		
Bismuth subsalicylate Misoprostol Sucralfate	Diarrhea (bismuth subsalicylate, misoprostol), darkening of the tongue and stool (bismuth subsalicylate), spontaneous abortion (misoprostol), and constipation (bismuth subsalicylate) May reduce effectiveness of other drugs (sucralfate)	Bismuth subsalicylate is used in combination with antibiotics to cure *Helicobacter pylori* infection.

Surgery: Surgery for ulcers is now seldom needed because drugs so effectively heal peptic ulcers and endoscopy so effectively stops active bleeding. Surgery is used primarily to deal with complications of a peptic ulcer, such as a perforation, an obstruction that fails to respond to drug therapy or that recurs, two or more major episodes of bleeding ulcers, a gastric ulcer suspected of being cancerous, or severe and frequent recurrences of peptic ulcers. A number of different surgical procedures may be performed to treat these complications. However, ulcers may recur after surgery, and each procedure may cause problems of its own, such as weight loss, poor digestion, and anemia.

Gastroesophageal Reflux

In gastroesophageal reflux (gastroesophageal reflux disease [GERD]), stomach acid and enzymes flow backward from the stomach into the esophagus, causing inflammation and pain in the esophagus.

- Reflux occurs when the ring-shaped muscle that normally prevents the contents of the stomach from flowing back into the esophagus (lower esophageal sphincter) does not function properly.
- The most typical symptom is heartburn (a burning pain behind the breastbone).
- The diagnosis is based on symptoms.
- Treatment is avoiding trigger substances (such as alcohol and fatty foods) and taking drugs that reduce stomach acid.

The stomach lining protects the stomach from the effects of its own acid. Because the esophagus lacks a similar protective lining, stomach acid and enzymes that flow backward (reflux) into the esophagus routinely cause symptoms and in some cases damage.

Acid and enzymes reflux when the lower esophageal sphincter, the ring-shaped muscle that normally prevents the contents of the stomach from flowing back into the esophagus, is not functioning properly. When a person is standing or sitting, gravity helps to prevent the reflux of stomach contents into the esophagus, which explains why reflux can worsen when a person is lying down. Reflux is also more likely to occur soon after meals, when the volume and acidity of contents in the stomach are higher and the sphincter is less likely to work properly. Factors contributing to reflux include weight gain, fatty foods, chocolate, caffeinated and carbonated beverages, alcohol, tobacco smoking, and certain drugs. Types of drugs that interfere with lower esophageal sphincter function include those that have anticholinergic effects (such as many antihistamines and some antidepressants), calcium channel blockers, progesterone, and nitrates. Alcohol and coffee also contribute by stimulating acid production. Delayed emptying of the stomach (for example, due to diabetes or use of opioids) can also worsen reflux.

Symptoms and Complications

Heartburn (a burning pain behind the breastbone) is the most obvious symptom of gastroesophageal reflux. Sometimes the pain even extends to the neck, throat, and face. Heartburn may be accompanied by regurgitation, in which the stomach contents reach the mouth.

Inflammation of the esophagus (esophagitis) may cause bleeding that is usually slight but can be massive. The blood may be vomited up or may pass through the digestive tract, resulting in the passage of dark, tarry stools (melena) or bright red blood, if the bleeding is heavy enough.

Esophageal ulcers, which are open sores on the lining of the esophagus, can result from repeated reflux. They can cause pain that is usually located behind the breastbone or just below it, similar to the location of heartburn.

Narrowing (stricture) of the esophagus caused by reflux makes swallowing solid foods increasingly more difficult. Narrowing of the airways can cause shortness of breath and wheezing. Other symptoms of gastroesophageal reflux include chest pain, sore throat, hoarseness, excessive salivation (water brash), a sensation of a lump in the throat (globus sensation), and inflammation of the sinuses (sinusitis).

With prolonged irritation of the lower part of the esophagus caused by repeated reflux, the cells lining the esophagus may change (resulting in a condition called Barrett's esophagus). Changes may occur even without symptoms. These abnormal cells are precancerous and progress to cancer in some people.

Diagnosis

The symptoms point to the diagnosis, and treatment can be started without detailed diagnostic testing. Specific testing is usually reserved for situations in which the diagnosis is not clear or treatment has not controlled symptoms. Examination of the esophagus using an endoscope (a flexible viewing tube), x-ray studies, pressure measurements (manometry) of the lower esophageal sphincter, and esophageal pH (acidity) tests are sometimes needed to help confirm the diagnosis and check for complications.

Endoscopy may confirm the diagnosis if the doctor finds that the person has esophagitis or Barrett's esophagus. Endoscopy also helps to exclude the presence of esophageal cancer. X-rays taken after a person drinks a barium solution (a substance that outlines the digestive tract) and then lies on an incline with the head lower than the feet may show reflux of the barium from the stomach into the esophagus. A doctor may press on the abdomen to increase the likelihood of reflux. The x-rays taken after the barium is swallowed also can reveal esophageal ulcers or a narrowed esophagus.

Pressure measurements at the lower esophageal sphincter indicate the strength of the sphincter and can distinguish a normal sphincter from a poorly functioning one. The information gained from this test helps the doctor decide whether surgery is an appropriate treatment.

Some doctors believe that the best test for gastroesophageal reflux is esophageal pH testing. In this test, a thin, flexible tube with a sensor probe on the tip is placed through the nose and into the lower esophagus. The other end of this tube is attached to a monitor that the person wears on a belt. The monitor records the acid levels in the esophagus, usually for 24 hours. Besides determining how much reflux is occurring, this test identifies the relationship between symptoms and reflux and is particularly helpful for people who have symptoms that are not typical of reflux. The esophageal pH test is needed for all people being considered for surgery to correct gastroesophageal reflux. A new device (using a small implanted pH electrode that transmits a signal) is available for people who cannot tolerate a tube in their nose.

Prevention and Treatment

Several measures may be taken to relieve gastroesophageal reflux. Raising the head of the bed about 6 inches (about 15 centimeters) can prevent acid from flowing into the esophagus as a person sleeps. Causative foods and drugs should be avoided, as should smoking. A doctor may prescribe a drug (for example, bethanechol or metoclopramide) to make the lower sphincter close more tightly. Coffee, alcohol, acid-containing beverages such as orange juice, cola drinks, and vinegar-based salad dressings, and other substances that strongly stimulate the stomach to produce acid or that delay stomach emptying should be avoided as well.

Many of the drugs used to treat gastritis and peptic ulcers also help prevent and treat gastroesophageal reflux (see table on page 142). Antacids taken at bedtime, for example, are often helpful. Antacids can usually relieve the pain of esophageal ulcers by reducing the amount of acid that reaches the esophagus. However, proton pump inhibitors, the most powerful drugs for reducing acid production, are usually the most effective treatment for gastroesophageal reflux, because even a small amount of acid can cause significant symptoms. Healing requires drugs that reduce stomach acid over a 4- to 12-week period. The ulcers heal slowly, tend to recur, and, when chronic and severe, can leave a narrowed esophagus after healing.

Esophageal narrowing is treated with drugs and repeated dilation, which may be performed using balloons or progressively larger dilators (bougies). If dilation is successful, narrowing does not seriously limit what a person can eat.

Barrett's esophagus does not disappear when treatment relieves symptoms. Therefore, people with Barrett's esophagus are asked to undergo an endoscopic examination every 2 to 3 years to ensure that the condition is not progressing to cancer.

Surgery is an option for people whose symptoms are unresponsive to drugs or for people who have esophagitis that persists even after symptoms are relieved. In addition, surgery may be the preferred treatment for people who do not like the prospect of having to take drugs for many years. A minimally invasive procedure performed through a laparoscope is available. However, 20 to 30% of people who undergo this procedure experience side effects, most commonly difficulty swallowing and a feeling of bloating or abdominal discomfort after eating.

CHAPTER

21 Gastroenteritis

Gastroenteritis is inflammation of the lining of the stomach and small and large intestines. It is usually caused by infection with a microorganism but can also be caused by ingestion of chemical toxins or drugs.

- The infection is usually caused by an infection but can be caused by ingesting toxins or drugs.
- Typically, people have diarrhea, nausea, vomiting, and abdominal pain.
- The diagnosis is based on some laboratory tests and a person's history of recent contact with contaminated people, food, or water or antibiotic use.

- Thoroughly washing the hands after a bowel movement or contact with fecal matter is the best way to prevent infection.
- Antibiotics are used to eliminate only certain kinds of bacteria.

Gastroenteritis usually consists of mild to severe diarrhea that may be accompanied by loss of appetite, nausea, vomiting, cramps, and discomfort in the abdomen. Although gastroenteritis usually is not serious in a healthy adult, causing only discomfort and inconvenience, it can cause life-threatening

MICROORGANISMS THAT CAUSE GASTROENTERITIS

MICROORGANISM	COMMON SOURCES	SYMPTOMS	ANTIMICROBIAL USE
Campylobacter	Eating contaminated meat (especially undercooked poultry) Drinking contaminated water or unpasteurized milk	Often bloody, sometimes watery diarrhea lasting 1 day to a week or more	Antibiotics given in the early stages of illness may shorten the duration of symptoms (for example, azithromycin or ciprofloxacin).
Salmonella	Eating contaminated food Contact with reptiles (for instance iguanas, snakes, and turtles)	High fever, exhaustion, abdominal cramps, nausea, vomiting, diarrhea that may or may not be bloody Symptoms usually last 3 to 7 days	Antibiotics usually are not given.
Shigella	Person-to-person contact, especially in day care centers	May be mild or severe In mild cases, watery, loose stools In severe cases, high fever, exhaustion, severe abdominal cramps, painful passage of stool containing blood and mucus Symptoms usually last about a week without treatment	Antibiotics shorten the duration of the illness and decrease chance of spread to another person (for example, ciprofloxacin or trimethoprim-sulfamethoxazole).
Enterohemorrhagic *Escherichia coli* O157:H7	Eating undercooked ground beef or drinking unpasteurized milk or juice Swimming in contaminated pools Person-to-person contact Touching infected animals and then putting fingers in the mouth	Sudden abdominal cramps, watery diarrhea that usually becomes bloody within 24 hours, and hemolytic-uremic syndrome	Antibiotics are not given.
Clostridium difficile	Usually due to bacterial overgrowth in people who have been taking antibiotics	Diarrhea	Antibiotic use is stopped. In some cases, metronidazole is given by mouth.
Entamoeba histolytica	Eating or drinking contaminated food or water	Bloody diarrhea, abdominal pain, weight loss lasting 1 to 3 weeks Can cause infection in liver and other organs	Antiparasitic drugs are given (for example, metronidazole, iodoquinol, or paromomycin).
Enterotoxigenic *Escherichia coli* (causes traveler's diarrhea)	Eating or drinking contaminated food or water	Frequent watery diarrhea Usually lasts 3 to 5 days	Antibiotics (for example, ciprofloxacin or levofloxacin) may help shorten duration of illness. Azithromycin is given to children.
Vibrio cholerae	Eating or drinking contaminated food or water	Painless, watery diarrhea and vomiting Can lead to massive fluid loss and shock	Antibiotics are given (for example, ciprofloxacin or doxycycline).
Other types of *Vibrio*	Shellfish	Watery diarrhea, often with little nausea or vomiting	Antibiotics are given (for example, ciprofloxacin, doxycycline, or trimethoprim-sulfamethoxazole).

(continued on the following page)

MICROORGANISMS THAT CAUSE GASTROENTERITIS (*Continued*)

MICROORGANISM	COMMON SOURCES	SYMPTOMS	ANTIMICROBIAL USE
Staphylococcus aureus *Bacillus cereus* *Clostridium perfringens*	Eating food contaminated by toxins produced by bacteria	Severe nausea, vomiting, and diarrhea Symptoms begin within 12 hours after eating contaminated food and lessen within 36 hours	Antibiotics are not given.
Rotavirus	Epidemic and often seasonal	Frequent watery diarrhea Vomiting and fever higher than 102° F (about 39° C) Symptoms begin 1 to 3 days after infection May last 5 to 7 days	Antibiotics and antiviral drugs are not given. A vaccine is available for infants.
Norovirus	Epidemic and often seasonal	Frequent watery diarrhea Vomiting occurs in 90% of people Stomach cramps, headache, and aches and pains Fever higher than 102° F (about 39° C) occurs in about 30% of people Diarrhea usually affects adults Symptoms begin 1 to 2 days after infection Usually lasts 2 to 7 days	Antibiotics and antiviral drugs are not given.
Astrovirus	Epidemic and often seasonal	Milder watery diarrhea Vomiting and fever Symptoms begin 3 to 4 days after infection Usually lasts 2 to 7 days Similar to rotavirus	Antibiotics and antiviral drugs are not given.
Intestinal adenovirus	Epidemic and often seasonal	Frequent watery diarrhea lasts 1 to 2 weeks Mild vomiting begins 1 to 2 days after diarrhea Fever affects 50% of people Symptoms begin 3 to 10 days after infection Usually lasts 10 days or more	Antibiotics and antiviral drugs are not given.
Giardia	Drinking contaminated stream water Person-to-person contact, particularly in day care centers	Diarrhea, nausea, and loss of appetite More long-term illness (lasting several days to several weeks) may occur, with greasy stools, abdominal bloating, gas, fatigue, and weight loss	Antiparasitic drugs are given (for example, metronidazole or nitazoxanide).
Cryptosporidium	Drinking contaminated water Person-to-person contact People with AIDS particularly susceptible	Watery diarrhea, crampy abdominal pain, nausea, fatigue, and vomiting Usually lasts about 2 weeks	Antiparasitic drugs are sometimes given (for example, nitazoxanide).

dehydration (see page 970) and electrolyte imbalance (see page 933) in the very ill or weak, the very young, and the very old. About 3 to 6 million children around the world die each year from infectious gastroenteritis.

Causes

Infections that cause gastroenteritis can be transmitted from person to person, especially if people with diarrhea do not thoroughly wash their hands after a bowel movement. Infection also can occur if people touch their mouth after touching an object (such as a diaper or toy) contaminated by infected stool. All such transmission involving infected stool is termed fecal-oral transmission. A person, and sometimes large numbers of people (in which case an outbreak of illness is called an epidemic), can also become infected by eating food or drinking water that has been contaminated by infected stool. Most foods can be contaminated with bacteria and cause gastroenteritis if not cooked thoroughly or pasteurized. Contaminated water is sometimes ingested in unexpected ways, such as when swimming in a pond contaminated by stool from an animal or in a swimming pool contaminated by stool from another person. In some cases, gastroenteritis is acquired through contact with animals that carry the infectious microorganism.

> **? Did You Know...**
> Worldwide, about 3 to 6 million children die each year from gastroenteritis caused by an infection.

Infectious gastroenteritis may be caused by viruses, bacteria, or parasites. Chemical toxins and drugs can also cause gastroenteritis.

Viruses: Viruses are the most common cause of gastroenteritis in the United States. Certain viruses infect cells in the lining of the small intestine where they multiply and cause watery diarrhea, vomiting, and fever. Four categories of viruses cause most gastroenteritis: rotavirus, calicivirus (predominantly the norovirus), and less commonly, astrovirus, and enteric (intestinal) adenovirus.

Rotavirus (see page 1782) is the most common cause of severe, dehydrating diarrhea among young children. It usually affects those between the ages of 3 months and 15 months. Rotavirus is highly contagious. Most infections are spread by fecal-oral transmission. Adults may be infected after close contact with an infected infant, but the illness is generally mild. During the winter in temperate climates, rotavirus causes most cases of diarrhea that are serious enough to send infants and toddlers to the hospital. Each year in the United States, a wave of rotavirus illness begins in the Southwest in November and ends in the Northeast in March.

Norovirus most commonly infects older children and adults. Infections occur year-round. Most people are infected after swallowing contaminated food or water. Because norovirus is highly contagious, infection can easily be spread from person to person.

Astrovirus can infect people of all ages but usually infects infants and young children. Infection is most common in the winter and is spread by fecal-oral transmission.

Adenovirus most commonly affects children under the age of 2. Infections occur year-round and increase slightly in the summer. The infection is spread by fecal-oral transmission.

Other viruses (such as cytomegalovirus and enterovirus) can cause gastroenteritis in people who have an impaired immune system.

Bacteria: Bacterial gastroenteritis is less common than viral gastroenteritis.

Some bacteria (such as certain strains of *Escherichia coli* [*E. coli*], *Campylobacter*, *Shigella*, and *Salmonella*) invade the lining of the small intestine or colon. There, they damage cells, causing tiny sores (ulcerations) that bleed, and allow a considerable leakage of fluid containing proteins, electrolytes, and water. The diarrhea contains white and red blood cells and sometimes visible blood.

Salmonella and *Campylobacter* are the most common bacterial causes of diarrhea in the United States. Both infections are most frequently acquired from undercooked poultry. Unpasteurized milk is also a possible source. *Campylobacter* is occasionally transmitted by dogs or cats with diarrhea. *Salmonella* can be transmitted by undercooked eggs and by having contact with reptiles (such as turtles or lizards).

Species of *Shigella* are the third most common bacterial cause of diarrhea in the United States and are usually transmitted person to person, although food-borne epidemics occur.

Several different subtypes of *E. coli* cause diarrhea. Enterohemorrhagic *E. coli* is the most significant subtype of *E. coli* in the United States and causes hemorrhagic colitis (see page 150) and sometimes hemolytic-uremic syndrome (see page 1042). The strain *E. coli* O157:H7 is the most common strain of this subtype in the United States. Undercooked ground beef, unpasteurized milk and juice, and contaminated water are possible sources. Person-to-person transmission is common in day care centers. Another subtype of *E. coli* (called enterotoxigenic *E. coli*) produces two toxins that cause watery diarrhea. This subtype is the most common cause of traveler's diarrhea (see page 152). A third subtype of *E. coli* also causes watery diarrhea. It was once a common cause of diarrhea outbreaks in nurseries but is now rare. A fourth subtype of *E. coli* causes bloody or nonbloody diarrhea, primarily in developing countries. It is rare in the United States.

Other bacteria (such as *Staphylococcus aureus*, *Bacillus cereus*, and *Clostridium perfringens*) produce a toxin that can be present in contaminated food. The toxin can cause gastroenteritis without causing a bacterial infection. These toxins generally cause severe nausea, vomiting, and diarrhea. Symptoms begin within 12 hours of ingestion of contaminated food and lessen within 36 hours.

Several other bacteria cause gastroenteritis, but most are rare in the United States. *Yersinia enterocolitica* can cause gastroenteritis or a syndrome that mimics appendicitis. A person is infected after ingesting undercooked pork, unpasteurized milk, or contaminated water. Several *Vibrio* species (such as *Vibrio parahaemolyticus*) cause diarrhea after ingestion of undercooked seafood. *Vibrio cholerae*, which is responsible for the watery diarrhea that is the main symptom of cholera, sometimes causes severe dehydrating diarrhea in developing countries. *Listeria* causes food-borne gastroenteritis. *Aeromonas* is acquired from swimming in or drinking contaminated fresh water or briny, salty water. *Plesiomonas shigelloides* can cause diarrhea in people who have eaten raw shellfish or traveled to tropical regions in developing countries.

Parasites: Certain intestinal parasites, particularly *Giardia lamblia*, stick to or invade the lining of the intestine and cause nausea, vomiting, diarrhea, and a general sick feeling. The resulting infection, called giardiasis, is more common in cold climates but occurs in every region of the United States and throughout the world. If the disease becomes persistent (chronic), it can keep the body from absorbing nutrients, a condition known as a malabsorption syndrome. Infection is usually spread through person-to-person contact (often in day care centers) or from contaminated water.

Another intestinal parasite, called *Cryptosporidium parvum*, causes watery diarrhea that is sometimes accompanied by abdominal cramps, nausea, and vomiting. The resulting infection, called cryptosporidiosis, is usually mild in otherwise healthy people, but it may be severe or even fatal in people with a weakened immune system. It is most commonly acquired by drinking contaminated water.

Other parasites that can cause symptoms similar to those of cryptosporidiosis include *Cyclospora cayetanensis* and, in people with an impaired immune system, *Isospora belli* and a collection of organisms referred to as microsporidia. *Entamoeba histolytica* causes amebiasis, an infection of the large intestine and sometimes the liver and other organs. Amebiasis is a common cause of bloody diarrhea in developing countries and occasionally occurs in the United States.

Chemical Gastroenteritis: Gastroenteritis may result from ingesting chemical toxins. These toxins are usually produced by a plant, such as poisonous mushrooms, or by certain kinds of exotic seafood and thus are not the product of an infection. Gastro-

Gastroenteritis as a Side Effect of Drugs

Nausea, vomiting, and diarrhea are common side effects of many drugs. Common culprits include antacids containing magnesium as a major ingredient, antibiotics, chemotherapy drugs, radiation therapy, colchicine (for gout), digoxin (usually used for heart failure or certain irregular heart rhythms), drugs used to remove or destroy internal parasitic worms, and laxatives. Laxative abuse can lead to weakness, vomiting, diarrhea, electrolyte loss, and other disturbances. Antibiotic use may cause *Clostridium difficile*–induced diarrhea.

Recognizing that a drug is causing gastroenteritis can be difficult. In mild cases, a doctor can have a person stop taking the drug and later start taking it again. If the symptoms subside when the person stops taking the drug and resume when the person starts taking the drug again, then the drug may be the cause of the gastrointestinal symptoms. In severe cases of gastroenteritis, a doctor may instruct the person to stop taking the drug permanently.

enteritis due to chemical toxicity can also occur after ingesting water or food contaminated by chemicals such as arsenic, lead, mercury, or cadmium. Heavy-metal poisoning frequently causes nausea, vomiting, abdominal pain, and diarrhea. Eating large amounts of acidic foods, such as citrus fruits and tomatoes, gives some people gastroenteritis.

Symptoms

The type and severity of the symptoms depend on the type and quantity of microorganism or toxin ingested. Symptoms also vary according to the person's resistance. Symptoms often begin suddenly—sometimes dramatically—with a loss of appetite, nausea, or vomiting. Audible rumbling of the intestine and abdominal cramping may occur. Diarrhea is the most common symptom and may be accompanied by visible blood and mucus. Loops of intestine may be painfully swollen (distended) with gas. The person may have a fever, feel generally sick, and experience aching muscles and extreme exhaustion.

Severe vomiting and diarrhea can lead to marked dehydration (see page 970). Symptoms of dehydration include weakness, decreased frequency of urination, dry mouth, and, in infants, lack of tears when crying. Excessive vomiting or diarrhea can result in low levels of potassium in the blood (hypokalemia). Low blood pressure and a rapid heart rate can also develop. Low levels of sodium in the blood (hyponatremia) also may develop, particularly if the person replaces lost fluids by drinking fluids that contain little or no salt, such as water and tea. Water and electrolyte imbalances are potentially serious, especially in the young, the old, and people with chronic diseases. Shock and kidney failure can occur in severe cases.

Diagnosis

The diagnosis of gastroenteritis is usually obvious from the symptoms alone, but the cause often is not. Sometimes other family members or coworkers have recently been ill with similar symptoms. Other times, gastroenteritis can be traced to contaminated water or inadequately cooked, spoiled, or contaminated food, such as raw seafood or mayonnaise left out of the refrigerator too long. Recent travel, especially to certain foreign countries, and recent antibiotic use may give clues as well.

If the symptoms are severe or last for more than 48 hours, stool samples may be cultured and examined in a laboratory for white blood cells and bacteria, viruses, or parasites.

If the symptoms persist beyond a few days, a doctor may need to examine the large intestine with a colonoscope (a flexible viewing tube used to view the lower part of the digestive tract) to determine whether the person has a disease such as ulcerative colitis.

Prevention

A rotavirus vaccine given by mouth is now available that is safe and effective against most strains of rotavirus. This vaccine is now part of the recommended infant vaccination schedule and is given at 2, 4, and 6 months of age (see art on page 1685).

For infants, a simple and effective way to prevent gastroenteritis is breastfeeding. Caregivers should wash their hands thoroughly with soap and water after changing diapers, and diaper-changing areas should be disinfected with a freshly prepared solution of household bleach (1/4 cup bleach diluted in 1 gallon of water). Children with diarrhea should be excluded from day care centers for the duration of their symptoms. Children infected with *E. coli* that causes bloody diarrhea or *Shigella* should also have two negative stool cultures before they are allowed to return to the center.

Because most infections that cause gastroenteritis are transmitted by person-to-person contact, particularly through direct or indirect contact with infected stool, good hand washing with soap and water after a bowel movement is the most effective means of prevention. To prevent food-borne infections, hands should be washed before touching food, knives and cutting boards used to cut raw meat should be washed before use with any other food, meat and eggs should be cooked thoroughly, and leftovers should be refrigerated promptly after cooking. Only pasteurized dairy products and pasteurized apple juice should be used. Travelers should try to avoid possibly contaminated food and drink.

Treatment

Usually the only treatment needed for gastroenteritis is getting bed rest and drinking an adequate amount of fluids. Even a person who is vomiting should drink as much as can be tolerated, taking small frequent sips. If vomiting or diarrhea is prolonged or the person becomes severely dehydrated, fluids and electrolytes given by vein (intravenously) may be needed. Because children can become dehydrated more quickly, they should be given fluids with the appropriate mix of salts and sugars. Any of the commercially available solutions designed to replace lost fluids and electrolytes (rehydration solutions) are satisfactory. Carbonated beverages, teas, sports drinks, beverages containing caffeine, and fruit juices are not appropriate. If the child is breastfed, breastfeeding should continue. Drugs that control severe vomiting are not generally given to young children. For adults, a doctor may give a drug, either as an injection or as a suppository, to control severe vomiting.

As the symptoms subside, the person may gradually add foods to the diet. Traditionally, bland foods such as cereal, gelatin, bananas, rice, applesauce, and toast are given, but there is no evidence that these are superior to other foods. If the diarrhea continues for 24 to 48 hours and there is no blood in the stool to indicate a more serious bacterial infection, the doctor may prescribe a drug to control the diarrhea, such as diphenoxylate, or instruct the person to use an over-the-counter drug, such as loperamide. Again, these drugs usually are not given to children under the age of 5.

Because antibiotics can cause diarrhea and may encourage the growth of organisms resistant to antibiotics, they are rarely appropriate, even when a known bacterium is causing gastroenteritis. Antibiotics may be used, however, when certain bacteria, such as *Campylobacter*, *Shigella*, and *Vibrio*, are the cause, and for people who have traveler's diarrhea.

Parasitic infections are treated with antiparasitic drugs such as metronidazole and nitazoxanide.

Some bacteria are naturally found in the body and promote the growth of good bacteria (probiotics). The use of probiotics, such as lactobacillus (normally found in the mouth, digestive tract, and vagina), is generally safe and may relieve symptoms. They can be given in the form of yogurt with active cultures.

Hemorrhagic Colitis

Hemorrhagic colitis is a type of gastroenteritis in which certain strains of the bacterium Escherichia coli (E. coli) *infect the large intestine and produce a toxin (Shiga toxin) that causes bloody diarrhea and other serious complications.*

Hemorrhagic colitis can occur in people of all ages but is most common among children and older people. In North America, the most common strain of *E. coli* that causes hemorrhagic colitis is *E. coli* O157:H7. These bacteria naturally occur in the intestines of healthy cattle. Outbreaks can be caused by eating undercooked ground beef or by drinking unpasteurized milk or juice and contaminated water. The disease can be transmitted from person to person, particularly among children in diapers.

E. coli toxins damage the lining of the large intestine. If they are absorbed into the bloodstream, they can also affect other organs, such as the kidney.

Symptoms

Severe abdominal cramps begin suddenly along with watery diarrhea, which typically becomes bloody within 24 hours. The diarrhea usually lasts 1 to 8 days. Fever is usually absent or mild but occasionally can exceed 102° F (38.9° C).

About 2 to 7% of people with hemorrhagic colitis develop a severe complication called hemolytic-uremic syndrome (see page 1042). Symptoms include anemia (characterized by fatigue, weakness, and light-headedness) caused by the destruction of red blood cells (hemolytic anemia), a low platelet count (thrombocytopenia), and sudden kidney failure. Some people with hemolytic-uremic syndrome also develop complications of nerve or brain damage, such as seizures or strokes. These complications typically develop in the second week of illness and may be preceded by increasing fever. Hemolytic-uremic syndrome is more likely to occur in children younger than 5 years and in older people. Even without hemolytic-uremic syndrome and its complications, hemorrhagic colitis may cause death in older people.

Diagnosis

A doctor usually suspects hemorrhagic colitis when a person reports bloody diarrhea. To make the diagnosis, a doctor has stool specimens tested for strains of *E. coli*. Sometimes, the doctor performs a stool test to detect the toxin produced by the *E. coli*. Other tests, such as colonoscopy, may be performed if a doctor suspects that other diseases may be causing the bloody diarrhea.

Treatment

The most important aspect of treatment is drinking enough fluids. Sometimes so much fluid is lost, however, that a doctor has to replace them intravenously. Antibiotics are not given because they increase the risk of developing hemolytic-uremic syndrome. People who develop complications are likely to require intensive care in the hospital and may need kidney dialysis (see page 265).

Staphylococcal Food Poisoning

Staphylococcal food poisoning results from eating food contaminated with toxins produced by certain types of staphylococci, resulting in diarrhea and vomiting.

The staphylococci bacteria grow in food, in which they produce toxins. Thus, staphylococcal food poisoning does not result from ingesting the bacteria but rather from ingesting the toxins that are already present in the contaminated food. Typical contaminated foods include custard, cream-filled pastry, milk, processed meats, and fish. The risk of an outbreak is high when food handlers with skin infections contaminate foods that are undercooked or left at room temperature.

Symptoms and Diagnosis

Symptoms usually begin abruptly with severe nausea and vomiting starting about 2 to 8 hours after the contaminated food is eaten. Other symptoms may include abdominal cramping, diarrhea, and sometimes headache and fever. Severe fluid and electrolyte loss may cause weakness and very low blood pressure (shock). Symptoms usually last less than 12 hours, and recovery is usually complete. Occasionally, staphylococcal food poisoning is fatal, especially in the very young, the very old, and people weakened by long-term illness.

The symptoms are usually all a doctor needs to diagnose gastroenteritis. A more specific diagnosis of staphylococcal food poisoning may be suspected when other people who ate the same food are similarly affected and when the disorder can be traced to a single source of contamination. To confirm the diagnosis, a laboratory analysis must identify staphylococci in the suspected food, but this analysis is not usually performed.

Prevention and Treatment

Careful food preparation can prevent staphylococcal food poisoning. Anyone who has a skin infection should not prepare food for others until the infection heals. Food should be consumed immediately or refrigerated and not kept at room temperature.

Treatment usually consists of only drinking an adequate amount of fluids. A doctor may give an antinausea drug, either as an injection or as a suppository, to help control severe nausea and vomiting. Sometimes so much fluid is lost that fluids have to be given intravenously.

Clostridium perfringens Food Poisoning

Clostridium perfringens food poisoning results from eating food contaminated by the bacterium Clostridium perfringens. *Once in the small intestine, the bacterium releases a toxin that often causes diarrhea.*

Some strains cause mild to moderate disease that gets better without treatment, whereas other strains cause severe gastroenteritis that can damage the small intestine and sometimes lead to death. Contaminated meat is usually responsible for outbreaks of *Clostridium perfringens* food poisoning. Some strains cannot be destroyed by cooking the food thoroughly, whereas others can.

Symptoms

The gastroenteritis starts about 6 to 24 hours after contaminated food is eaten. The most common symptoms are watery diarrhea and abdominal cramps. Although usually mild, the infection also can cause abdominal pain, abdominal expansion (distention) from gas, severe diarrhea, dehydration, and a severe decrease in blood pressure (shock). Symptoms usually last about 24 hours.

Diagnosis and Treatment

A doctor usually suspects the diagnosis when a local outbreak of the disease has occurred. The diagnosis is confirmed by testing contaminated food or the stool of affected people for *Clostridium perfringens*.

To prevent infection, leftover cooked meat should be refrigerated promptly and reheated thoroughly before serving. The person is given fluids and is encouraged to rest. Antibiotics are not given.

Traveler's Diarrhea

Traveler's diarrhea (turista) is characterized by diarrhea, nausea, and vomiting that commonly occur in travelers to areas of the world with poor water purification.

- Traveler's diarrhea can be caused by bacteria, parasites, or viruses.
- Organisms that cause the disorder are usually acquired from food or water, especially in developing countries where the water supply may be inadequately treated.
- Nausea, vomiting, abdominal cramping, and diarrhea can occur with any degree of severity.
- Preventive measures include drinking only bottled carbonated beverages, avoiding uncooked vegetables or fruits, not using ice cubes, and using bottled water to brush teeth.
- Treatment involves drinking plenty of fluids and sometimes taking antidiarrheal drugs or antibiotics.

Traveler's diarrhea occurs when people are exposed to bacteria or, less commonly, parasites to which they have had little exposure and thus no immunity. The bacteria (or parasites) are usually acquired from food or water (including water used to wash foods). Traveler's diarrhea occurs mostly in developing countries where the water supply is inadequately treated. The organisms most likely to cause traveler's diarrhea are the types of *Escherichia coli* (*E. coli*) that produce certain toxins and some viruses such as norovirus, which has been a particular problem on some cruise ships.

Travelers who avoid drinking local water may still become infected by brushing their teeth with an improperly rinsed toothbrush, drinking bottled drinks with ice made from local water, or eating food that is improperly handled or washed with local water.

Symptoms and Diagnosis

Nausea, vomiting, intestinal rumbling, abdominal cramping, and diarrhea can occur in any combination and with any degree of severity. These symptoms begin 12 to 72 hours after ingesting contaminated food or water. Vomiting, headache, and muscle pain are particularly common in infections caused by norovirus. Most cases are mild and disappear without treatment within 3 to 5 days. Diagnostic tests are rarely needed.

Prevention

Travelers should patronize only those restaurants with a reputation for safety and should not consume any food or beverages from street vendors. Cooked foods that are still hot when served are generally safe. Salads containing uncooked vegetables or fruit and salsa left on the table in open containers should be avoided. Any fruit should be peeled by the traveler. Travelers should drink only bottled carbonated beverages or beverages made with water that has been boiled. Even ice cubes should be made with water that has been boiled. Buffets and fast food restaurants pose an increased risk of infection.

Preventive antibiotics are recommended only for people who are particularly susceptible to the consequences of traveler's diarrhea, such as those whose immune system is impaired. The antibiotic most commonly recommended is ciprofloxacin.

Treatment

When symptoms occur, treatment includes drinking plenty of fluids and taking drugs to reduce stomach muscle spasms (such as loperamide). These drugs cannot be given to people who have a fever or bloody stools or to children under 2 years of age. In addition, antibiotics (for adults, ciprofloxacin, levofloxacin, azithromycin, or rifaximin; for children, azithromycin) and antidiarrheal drugs (such as loperamide) are usually recommended. Travelers are encouraged to seek medical care if they develop fever or blood in the stool.

Chemical Food Poisoning

Chemical food poisoning results from eating a plant or animal that contains a toxin.

- The poisoning occurs after ingesting poisonous species of mushrooms or plants or contaminated fish or shellfish.
- The most common symptoms are diarrhea, nausea, and vomiting and sometimes seizures and paralysis.
- The diagnosis is based on symptoms and examination of the ingested substance.

- Avoiding wild or unfamiliar mushrooms and plants and contaminated fish reduces the risk of poisoning.
- Replacing fluids and ridding the stomach of the toxic substance are the best forms of treatment; however, some substances are deadly.

Mushroom (Toadstool) Poisoning

Many species of mushroom are poisonous. The potential for poisoning may vary within the same species, at different times of the growing season, and with cooking. It is difficult to differentiate poisonous from nonpoisonous mushrooms in the wild, even for highly knowledgeable people. Folklore rules are unreliable.

All poisonous mushrooms cause vomiting and abdominal pain. Other symptoms vary greatly depending on mushroom type. Generally, mushrooms that cause symptoms early (within 2 hours) of ingestion are less dangerous than those that cause symptoms later (usually after 6 hours).

Mushrooms that cause early gastrointestinal symptoms (such as *Chlorophyllum molybdates*, the little brown mushrooms that often grow on lawns) cause vomiting and diarrhea. The diarrhea is occasionally bloody. Some people have headaches or body aches. Symptoms usually go away within 24 hours.

Mushrooms that cause early symptoms that affect the brain and spine include hallucinogenic mushrooms, which contain the hallucinogen psilocybin. The most common are members of the *Psilocybe* genus, but some other mushrooms also contain psilocybin. Symptoms begin within 15 to 30 minutes of ingestion and include euphoria, enhanced imagination, and hallucinations. A rapid heart beat and high blood pressure often develop, and some children develop a fever. However, these symptoms go away without treatment, and serious consequences are rare, so specific treatment is usually not needed. However, if the person is very agitated, the doctor may prescribe a sedative (such as lorazepam).

In poisoning caused by many species of *Inocybe* and some species of *Clitocybe*, the dangerous substance is muscarine. Symptoms, which begin a few minutes to 2 hours after eating, may include increased tearing and salivation, narrowing (constriction) of the pupils, sweating, vomiting, stomach cramps, diarrhea, dizziness, confusion, coma, and, occasionally, seizures. Symptoms are usually mild and go away within 12 hours. Doctors give atropine intravenously to people who have severe symptoms, and nearly all people recover in 24 hours. Without treatment, death can occur in a few hours with severe poisoning.

Mushrooms that cause delayed gastrointestinal symptoms include *Amanita phalloides* and related types of mushroom (members of the *Amanita*, *Gyromitra*, and *Cortinarius* genera). *Amanita phalloides* causes 95% of mushroom poisoning deaths. Vomiting and

---

Chinese Restaurant Syndrome

What is popularly called the Chinese restaurant syndrome refers to symptoms such as facial pressure, chest pain, burning sensations throughout the body, and anxiety after eating Chinese food. These symptoms are thought to be a hypersensitivity reaction to monosodium glutamate (MSG), a flavor enhancer often used in Chinese cooking. This reaction is uncommon.

---

diarrhea start in 6 to 24 hours. Sometimes the blood sugar level drops dangerously low. Symptoms subside for a few days, but then people develop liver failure and sometimes kidney failure. Liver failure causes the skin to turn yellow (jaundice). People with kidney failure may reduce or stop urination. Sometimes the symptoms disappear on their own, but about half of the people who have this type of poisoning die in 5 to 8 days. Those with liver failure may survive if given a liver transplant.

Gyromitra mushrooms also cause delayed vomiting and diarrhea and a low blood sugar level. Other problems include brain toxicity (such as seizures) and, after a few days, liver and kidney failure.

Most *Cortinarius* mushrooms originate in Europe. Symptoms of gastroenteritis may last for 3 days. Kidney failure, with symptoms of flank pain and decreased urine output, may occur 3 to 20 days after ingestion. Kidney failure often resolves spontaneously.

Plant and Shrub Poisoning

A few commonly grown plants are poisonous. Highly toxic and potentially fatal plants include castor beans, jequirity beans, poison hemlock, and water hemlock, as well as oleander and foxglove, which contain digitalis glycosides. Few plant poisonings can be cured by specific antidotes.

Castor beans contain ricin, an extremely concentrated poison. Ricin has been used in assassination attempts. Castor bean seeds have a very tough shell so the bean must be chewed to release the poison. Jequirity beans can cause death after swallowing. Children can die after chewing only one bean. Poisoning from castor beans or jequirity beans may cause severe vomiting and diarrhea (often bloody) after a delayed period. People later become delirious and have seizures. They may become comatose and die. Doctors sometimes try to flush the beans out of the stomach and intestines before they are absorbed.

Hemlock poisoning can cause symptoms within 15 minutes. People develop a dry mouth and later a rapid heart beat, tremors, sweating, seizures, and

MODERATELY POISONOUS PLANTS

PLANT	SYMPTOMS	TREATMENT
Aloe and related plants	Gastroenteritis (see page 145), kidney inflammation, and skin irritation	Supportive care* if the plant is swallowed and flushing (irrigation) with soap and water if the skin is irritated
Azalea	Cholinergic† symptoms	Supportive care* and atropine
Cactus and related plants	Infection and formation of abnormal lumps in the skin (granulomas)	Removal of plant spines
Caladium and related plants	Irritation of the mouth due to calcium oxalate crystals in the leaves	Supportive care* and use of milk or ice cream to help dissolve the irritant
Capsicum and related plants (peppers)	Irritation of the skin and mucous membranes	Supportive care,* irrigation, and possibly use of an agent to help dissolve the irritant
Colchicine (autumn crocus, meadow saffron, or glory lily)	Delayed gastroenteritis and malfunction (failure) of many organ systems	Supportive care*
Deadly nightshade	Anticholinergic‡ symptoms, a high body temperature, seizures, and hallucinations	Supportive care* For a very high body temperature or seizures, possibly physostigmine
Dumbcane (dieffenbachia)	Damage to the mouth due to calcium oxalate crystals in the leaves	Supportive care* and use of milk or ice cream to help dissolve the irritant
Fava beans	In people with a deficiency of the enzyme G6PD (which protects red blood cells), gastroenteritis, fever, headache, and hemolytic anemia	Supportive care* For severe anemia and poisoning, gradual removal and replacement of blood with equal volumes of fresh donor blood (exchange transfusion) considered
Green potatoes and potato sprouts	Gastroenteritis, hallucinations, and delirium	Supportive care*
Holly berries	Gastroenteritis	Supportive care*
Jimsonweed	Anticholinergic‡ symptoms, a high body temperature, seizures, and hallucinations	Supportive care* For a very high body temperature or seizures, possibly physostigmine
Lily of the valley	Too much potassium in blood and abnormal heart rhythms (arrhythmias)	Supportive care* and antibodies against digitalis
Mistletoe	Gastroenteritis	Supportive care*
Nettle	Stinging and burning of the skin	Supportive care*
Nightshade, common or woody	Gastroenteritis, hallucinations, and delirium	Supportive care*
Nightshade, deadly	Anticholinergic‡ symptoms, a high body temperature, seizures, and hallucinations	Supportive care* For a very high body temperature or seizures, possibly physostigmine
Philodendron and related plants	Damage to the mouth due to calcium oxalate crystals in the leaves	Supportive care* and use of milk or ice cream to help dissolve the irritant
Poinsettia	Mild irritation of the mucous membranes of the mouth, nasal passages, vagina, and urethra	Unnecessary

(continued on the following page)

MODERATELY POISONOUS PLANTS (*Continued*)

PLANT	SYMPTOMS	TREATMENT
Poison ivy	Inflammation of the skin	See box on page 1286
Pokeweed	Irritation of the mucous membranes of the mouth, nasal passages, vagina, and urethra and gastroenteritis	Supportive care*
Pothos	Damage to the mouth due to calcium oxalate crystals in the leaves	Supportive care* and use of milk or ice cream to help dissolve the irritant
Yew	Gastroenteritis Rarely, seizures, abnormal heart rhythms, and coma	Supportive care*

*Supportive care may include intravenous administration of fluids, treatments to maintain body functions (such as drugs to lower fever), drugs if blood pressure drops, and a ventilator.

†Cholinergic symptoms include a slow heart rate, weakened contraction of the heart, difficulty breathing (because airways are constricted), flushing, abdominal cramps, diarrhea, increased urination and salivation, watery eyes, increased sweating, and muscle cramping.

‡Anticholinergic symptoms include confusion, blurred vision, constipation, dry mouth, light-headedness, difficulty starting and continuing to urinate, and loss of bladder control.

G6PD = glucose-6-phosphate dehydrogenase.

muscle weakness. Water hemlock may cause vomiting and diarrhea, delirium, seizures, and coma.

Oleander, foxglove, and the similar but less toxic lily of the valley can cause vomiting and diarrhea, confusion, irregular heartbeat, and high levels of potassium in the bloodstream. These plants contain a substance very similar to the heart drug digoxin. Doctors sometimes treat people who are poisoned by these plants with a drug used to treat digoxin overdose.

Many other plants cause less serious toxic effects.

Seafood Poisoning

Gastroenteritis may be caused by eating bony fish or shellfish. There are 3 common types of poisoning caused by eating bony fish—ciguatera, tetrodotoxin, and scombroid.

Ciguatera Poisoning: This type of poisoning can occur after eating any of the more than 400 species of fish from the tropical reefs of Florida, the West Indies, or the Pacific. The toxin is produced by certain dinoflagellates, microscopic sea organisms that the fish eat and that accumulate in their flesh. Larger, older fish are more toxic than smaller, younger ones. The flavor of the fish is not affected. Current processing procedures, including cooking, cannot destroy the toxin. The initial symptoms—abdominal cramps, nausea, vomiting, and diarrhea—may begin 2 to 8 hours after the person eats the fish and last 6 to 17 hours. Later symptoms may include itchiness, a pins-and-needles sensation, headache, muscle aches, a reversal

of sensations of hot and cold, and facial pain. For months afterward, the sensations may be disabling. Doctors sometimes try to treat affected people with intravenous mannitol (a drug that reduces swelling and pressure), but it is unclear whether this provides any benefit.

Tetrodotoxin Poisoning: Symptoms caused by the toxin in the puffer fish (fugu, a sushi delicacy), which is found most commonly in the seas surrounding Japan, are similar to those caused by fish in ciguatera poisoning. Death may result from paralysis of the muscles that regulate breathing. The toxin cannot be destroyed by cooking or freezing.

Scombroid Poisoning: After fish such as mackerel, tuna, bonito, skipjack, and blue dolphin (mahi mahi) have been caught, the tissues of the fish break down, producing high levels of histamine. When ingested, histamine causes immediate facial flushing. It can also cause nausea, vomiting, stomach pain, and hives (urticaria) a few minutes after the fish is eaten. Symptoms, which are often mistaken for a seafood allergy, usually last less than 24 hours. The fish may taste peppery or bitter.

Unlike other fish poisonings, this poisoning can be prevented by properly storing the fish after it is caught. Antihistamine drugs such as diphenhydramine and ranitidine may help.

Shellfish Poisoning: Shellfish poisoning can occur from June to October, especially on the Pacific and New England coasts. Shellfish such as mussels, clams, oysters, and scallops may ingest certain poisonous dinoflagellates at certain times when the water has a red cast, called the red tide. The dinoflagellates produce a toxin that attacks nerves (such toxins are called neurotoxins. The toxin, saxitoxin, which causes paralytic shellfish poisoning, persists even after the food has been cooked. The first symptom, a pins-and-needles sensation around the mouth, begins 5 to 30 minutes after eating. Nausea, vomiting, and abdominal cramps develop next, followed by muscle weakness. Occasionally, the weakness progresses to paralysis of the arms and legs. Weakness of the muscles needed for breathing may even be severe enough to cause death. Those who survive usually recover completely.

Contaminant Poisoning

Gastroenteritis may affect people who have ingested unwashed fruits and vegetables sprayed with arsenic, lead, or organic insecticides; acidic fluids served in lead-glazed pottery; or food stored in cadmium-lined containers.

Treatment

Most people with chemical food poisoning recover fully and rapidly with nothing more than replacement of fluids and electrolytes. As soon as symptoms begin, a person should try to consume large amounts of fluids. If fluids cannot be tolerated, the person needs to go to an emergency department for intravenous fluids.

If possible, it is often a good idea to rid the stomach of the toxic substance as quickly as possible. For most people, vomiting accomplishes this task. Saving a small amount of the first vomitus may be useful if tests are needed later. If a person cannot vomit adequately and symptoms are severe, a doctor may empty the stomach by placing a small tube through the nose or mouth into the stomach. A laxative helps to pass the toxins from the intestines more quickly.

Specific treatments are sometimes given when the toxin is known.

---

22 Hiatus Hernia, Bezoars, and Foreign Bodies

The stomach is a large, bean-shaped organ that receives food and fluids after they are eaten. Normally, the stomach is located below the diaphragm in the abdomen, and food is partly digested in the stomach, then passes into the small intestine. However, the stomach may move upward through the diaphragm or become clogged with undigested material.

Hiatus Hernia

Hiatus hernia is a protrusion of a portion of the stomach across the opening in the diaphragm that the esophagus normally passes through.

- This cause of this disorder usually is not known, but age, obesity, and smoking are common factors.
- Some people have no symptoms or minor ones such as reflux and indigestion, whereas others have more serious symptoms such as chest pain, bloating, belching, and difficulty swallowing.
- The diagnosis is based on results of a barium x-ray.
- Treatment is aimed at relieving symptoms, sometimes by using drugs and rarely by performing surgery.

Protrusion of any structure in the abdomen through the diaphragm (the sheet of muscle that separates the chest cavity from the abdomen) is called a diaphragmatic hernia. The diaphragm has an opening that the esophagus normally passes through (the hiatus). A diaphragmatic hernia that occurs through this opening is called a hiatus hernia. The cause of hiatus hernia is usually unknown, but the condition is more common among people who are older than 50, who are overweight (particularly women), or who smoke. Other types of diaphragmatic hernia may result from a birth defect (see page 1721) or from an injury.

There are two main types of hiatus hernia. In a sliding hiatus hernia, the junction between the esophagus and the stomach as well as a portion of the stomach itself, all of which are normally below the diaphragm, protrude above it. More than 40% of people in the United States have a sliding hiatus hernia. The frequency increases with aging, so that the rate climbs to 60% of people older than 60.

In a paraesophageal hiatus hernia, the junction between the esophagus and stomach is in its normal

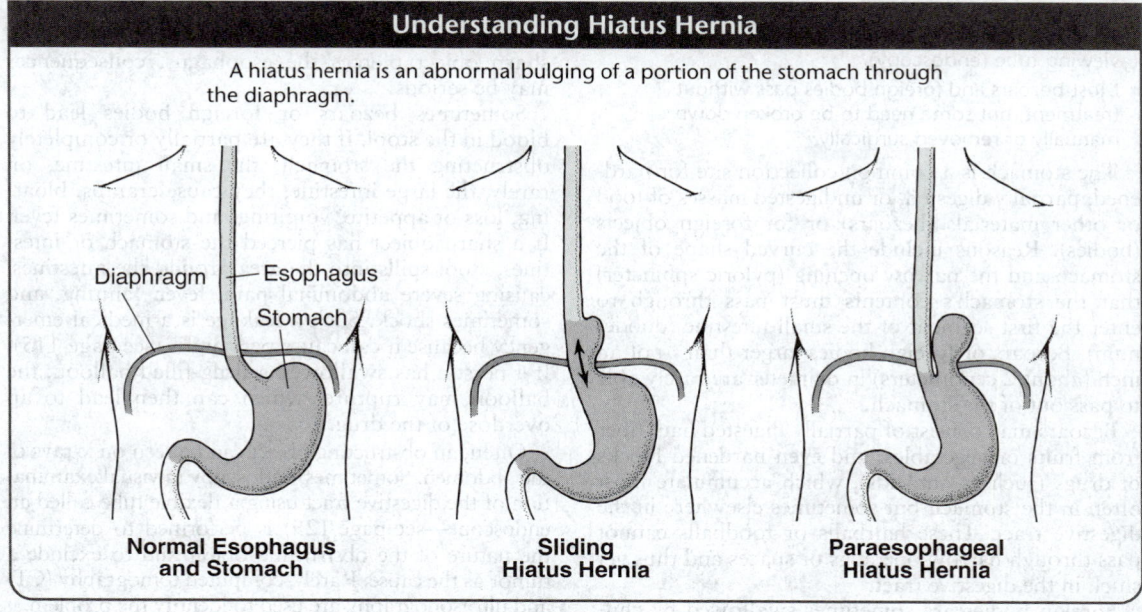

Understanding Hiatus Hernia

A hiatus hernia is an abnormal bulging of a portion of the stomach through the diaphragm.

Diaphragm — Esophagus
Stomach

Normal Esophagus and Stomach

Sliding Hiatus Hernia

Paraesophageal Hiatus Hernia

place below the diaphragm, but a portion of the stomach is pushed above the diaphragm and lies beside the esophagus.

Symptoms

Most sliding hiatus hernias are very small, and most people with a sliding hiatus hernia have no symptoms. Symptoms that do occur are usually minor. They are usually related to gastroesophageal reflux (see page 144) and include indigestion, typically when a person lies down after eating. Leaning forward, straining, and lifting heavy objects make symptoms worse, as does pregnancy.

A paraesophageal hiatus hernia may get trapped or pinched by the diaphragm and lose its blood supply. This serious and painful condition, called strangulation, requires immediate surgery. Symptoms may include chest pain, bloating, belching, and difficulty swallowing.

Rarely, microscopic or massive bleeding from the lining of the hernia occurs with either type of hiatus hernia.

Diagnosis and Treatment

Usually, x-rays clearly reveal a hiatus hernia, although a doctor may have to press on the abdomen during the procedure to make the hernia visible. Often, people are given barium in a liquid before the x-ray. Barium outlines the digestive tract, making abnormalities easier to see.

Most sliding hiatus hernias do not require treatment, but if symptoms of reflux occur, elevating the head of the bed while sleeping often helps. Other helpful measures for reflux include eating small meals, losing excess weight, stopping smoking, not lying down or exercising after meals, and not wearing tight-fitting clothes. Eliminating or limiting intake of beverages that contain acid (such as orange juice and colas), alcohol, coffee, and certain foods (such as onions, chocolate, and spicy, acidic, and fatty foods) is recommended. Antacids and drugs that prevent acid production also relieve symptoms (see table on page 143).

A paraesophageal hiatus hernia that causes symptoms should be corrected surgically to prevent strangulation. Surgery may be done through a tiny incision in the chest or abdomen and using a small viewing tube (laparoscopic surgery) or may require a full open operation.

Bezoars and Foreign Bodies

Bezoars are tightly packed collections of partially digested or undigested material stuck in the stomach or other parts of the digestive tract. *Foreign bodies* are small ingested objects that can also get stuck in the digestive tract and sometimes perforate (pierce) it.

- Masses of undigestible materials can get stuck in various parts of the digestive tract.
- Most bezoars and foreign bodies cause no symptoms.

- The diagnosis is based on x-rays and sometimes on a visual examination of the digestive tract using a flexible viewing tube (endoscopy).
- Most bezoars and foreign bodies pass without treatment, but some need to be broken down manually or removed surgically.

The stomach is a common collection site for hardened, partially digested, or undigested masses of food or other materials (bezoars) or for foreign objects (bodies). Reasons include the curved shape of the stomach and the narrow opening (pyloric sphincter) that the stomach's contents must pass through to enter the first segment of the small intestine (duodenum). Bezoars or foreign bodies larger than 3/4 of an inch (about 2 centimeters) in diameter are rarely able to pass out of the stomach.

Bezoars may consist of partially digested hair, fiber from fruits or vegetables, and even hardened blocks of drugs (such as antacids), which accumulate most often in the stomach but sometimes elsewhere in the digestive tract. These hairballs or foodballs cannot pass through narrow openings or spaces and thus get stuck in the digestive tract.

Foreign bodies are sometimes swallowed by children and even adults, especially intoxicated adults. If these undigestible objects are small, they pass through the digestive system until they are excreted with stool. However, larger objects or sharp ones, such as fish bones, may get stuck in the esophagus or stomach or, less often, in other parts of the digestive tract (see page 185). Sometimes foreign bodies are swallowed purposely, as when smugglers swallow balloons filled with illegal drugs to get through customs.

Food or other materials can collect in anyone but do so more often under certain circumstances. People who have undergone surgery to their digestive tract, particularly if they have had part of their stomach or intestines removed, are particularly prone to bezoars and foreign bodies becoming stuck. People with diabetes sometimes develop a condition in which the stomach does not empty properly, resulting in problematic collections of food.

Symptoms and Diagnosis

Most bezoars and foreign bodies cause no symptoms. A small blunt object that is swallowed may produce the sensation of something being stuck in the esophagus. This feeling may persist for a short time even after the object has passed into the stomach. A small sharp object that is swallowed may become lodged in the esophagus and cause pain, even though the person is able to swallow normally. When the esophagus is completely blocked, the person is unable to swallow anything, even saliva, and drools and spits constantly. The person may try to vomit, but nothing comes up. If a sharp object pierces the esophagus, consequences may be serious.

Sometimes bezoars or foreign bodies lead to blood in the stool. If they are partially or completely obstructing the stomach, the small intestine, or, rarely, the large intestine, they cause cramps, bloating, loss of appetite, vomiting, and sometimes fever. If a sharp object has pierced the stomach or intestines, stool spills into the area around the intestines, causing severe abdominal pain, fever, fainting, and sometimes shock. Such a leakage is a medical emergency because it can cause peritonitis (see page 115). If a person has swallowed a drug-filled balloon, the balloon may rupture, which can then lead to an overdose of the drug.

Often, an obstructing object can be seen on x-rays of the abdomen. Sometimes, endoscopy (a visual examination of the digestive tract using a flexible tube called an endoscope—see page 129) is performed to determine the nature of the obstructing object and to exclude a tumor as the cause. Rarely, computed tomography (CT) and ultrasonography are used to identify the problem.

Treatment

Most bezoars and foreign bodies require no treatment. Even a small coin is likely to pass without a problem. A doctor advises the person to check the stool to see when the object is excreted. Sometimes a doctor recommends that the person consume a liquid diet to help excrete the object.

To help break down a bezoar, a doctor may prescribe a regimen of cellulase or meat tenderizer, which is dissolved in a liquid and taken by mouth for several days. Sometimes doctors use forceps, a laser, or other instruments to break up bezoars so that they can pass through or be removed more easily.

When a doctor suspects that a blunt foreign body is stuck in the esophagus, the drug glucagon may be given intravenously to relax the esophagus and allow the object to pass through the digestive tract. Other drugs such as metoclopramide taken by mouth can help bezoars or blunt foreign objects pass through the digestive tract by causing muscles to contract.

Doctors can remove some objects that are stuck in the esophagus with forceps or a basket passed through an endoscope.

Because sharp objects may pierce the wall of the esophagus, they must be removed, either by endoscopy or surgery. Batteries are also removed from the esophagus because they can cause internal burns. When an object suspected of being a drug-filled balloon is detected, it is removed to prevent the drug overdose that can occur if such a balloon ruptures.

23 Pancreatitis

Pancreatitis is inflammation of the pancreas.

The pancreas is a leaf-shaped organ about 5 inches (about 13 centimeters) long. It is surrounded by the lower edge of the stomach and the wall of the duodenum (the first portion of the small intestine leading out of the stomach). The pancreas has three major functions:

- To secrete fluid containing digestive enzymes into the duodenum
- To secrete the hormones insulin and glucagon, which help regulate sugar levels in the bloodstream
- To secrete into the duodenum the large quantities of sodium bicarbonate (the chemical in baking soda) needed to neutralize the acid coming from the stomach

Inflammation of the pancreas can be caused by gallstones, alcohol, various drugs, some viral infections, and digestive enzymes. Pancreatitis usually develops quickly and subsides within a few days but can last for a few months (acute pancreatitis). In some cases, however, inflammation persists and gradually destroys pancreatic function (chronic pancreatitis).

Acute Pancreatitis

Acute pancreatitis is sudden inflammation of the pancreas that may be mild or life threatening but usually subsides.

- Gallstones and alcohol abuse are the main causes of acute pancreatitis.
- Severe abdominal pain is the predominant symptom.
- Blood tests and imaging tests, such as x-rays and computed tomography, help the doctor make the diagnosis.
- Whether mild or severe, acute pancreatitis usually requires hospitalization.

Gallstones (biliary tract disease—see page 243) and alcohol abuse account for almost 80% of hospital admissions for acute pancreatitis. About 1½ times as many women as men have acute pancreatitis caused by gallstones. Normally, the pancreas secretes pancreatic fluid through the pancreatic duct to the duodenum. This pancreatic fluid contains digestive enzymes in an inactive form and inhibitors that inactivate any enzymes that become activated on the way to the duodenum. Blockage of the pancreatic duct by a gallstone stuck in the sphincter of Oddi stops the flow of pancreatic fluid. Usually, the blockage is temporary and causes limited damage, which is

soon repaired. But if the blockage remains, activated enzymes accumulate in the pancreas, overwhelm the inhibitors, and begin to digest the cells of the pancreas, causing severe inflammation.

Drinking as little as 2 ounces of alcohol a day (half a bottle of wine, 4 bottles of beer, or 5 ounces of liquor) for several years may cause the small ductules in the pancreas that drain into the pancreatic duct to clog, eventually causing acute pancreatitis. An attack of pancreatitis may be precipitated by an alcoholic binge or by an excessively large meal. Many other conditions can also cause acute pancreatitis.

Many drugs can irritate the pancreas. Usually, the inflammation resolves when the drugs are stopped. Viruses can cause pancreatitis, which is usually short-lived.

Symptoms

Almost everyone with acute pancreatitis suffers severe abdominal pain in the upper abdomen, below the breastbone (sternum). The pain often penetrates to the back in about 50% of people. Rarely, the pain is first felt in the lower abdomen. When acute pancreatitis is caused by gallstones, the pain usually starts suddenly and reaches its maximum intensity in minutes. When pancreatitis is caused by alcoholism, pain develops over a few days. The pain then

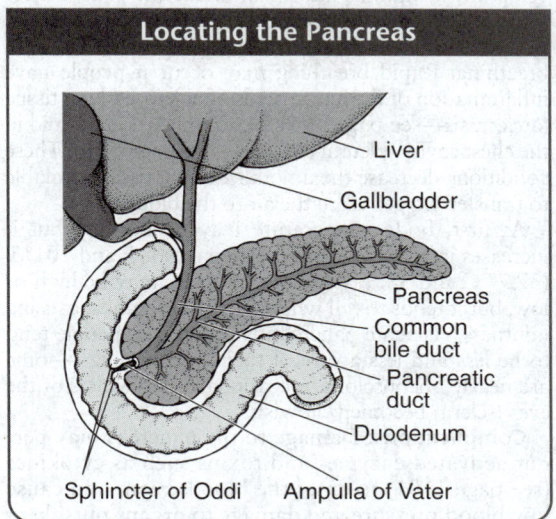

Locating the Pancreas

Liver
Gallbladder
Pancreas
Common bile duct
Pancreatic duct
Duodenum
Sphincter of Oddi
Ampulla of Vater

Some Causes of Acute Pancreatitis

- Gallstones
- Alcohol abuse
- Drugs such as furosemide and azathioprine
- Estrogen use in women with high levels of lipids in the blood
- Hyperparathyroidism and high levels of calcium in the blood
- Mumps
- High levels of lipids (especially triglycerides) in the blood
- Damage to the pancreas from surgery or endoscopy
- Damage to the pancreas from blunt or penetrating injuries
- Cancer of the pancreas
- Reduced blood supply to the pancreas, for example, from severely low blood pressure
- Hereditary pancreatitis
- Kidney transplantation

remains steady and severe, has a penetrating quality, and persists for days.

Coughing, vigorous movement, and deep breathing may worsen the pain. Sitting upright and leaning forward may provide some relief. Most people feel nauseated and have to vomit, sometimes to the point of dry heaves (retching without producing any vomit). Often, even large doses of an injected opioid analgesic (see page 642) do not relieve pain completely.

Some people, especially those who develop acute pancreatitis because of alcohol abuse, may never develop any symptoms other than moderate pain. Others feel terrible. They look sick and sweaty and have a fast pulse (100 to 140 beats a minute) and shallow, rapid breathing. Rapid breathing may occur if people have inflammation of the lungs, areas of collapsed lung tissue (atelectasis—see page 495), or accumulation of fluid in the chest cavity (pleural effusion—see page 518). These conditions decrease the amount of lung tissue available to transfer oxygen from the air to the blood.

At first, body temperature may be normal, but it increases in a few hours to between 100° F and 101° F (37.7° C and 38.3° C). Blood pressure may be high or low, but it tends to fall when the person stands, causing faintness. As acute pancreatitis progresses, people tend to be less and less aware of their surroundings—some are nearly unconscious. Occasionally, the whites of the eyes (sclera) become yellowish.

Complications: Damage to the pancreas may permit activated enzymes and toxins such as cytokines (see page 1101) to enter the bloodstream and cause low blood pressure and damage to organs outside of the abdominal cavity, such as the lungs and kidneys. The part of the pancreas that produces hormones, especially insulin, tends not to be damaged or affected. One of five people with acute pancreatitis develops some swelling in the upper abdomen. This swelling may occur because the movement of stomach and intestinal contents stops (a condition called ileus—see page 204).

In severe acute pancreatitis, parts of the pancreas die (necrotizing pancreatitis), and blood and pancreatic fluid may escape into the abdominal cavity, which decreases blood volume and results in a large drop in blood pressure, possibly causing shock (see page 350). Severe acute pancreatitis can be life threatening.

Infection of an inflamed pancreas is a risk, particularly after the first week of illness. Sometimes, a doctor suspects an infection because the person's condition worsens and because a fever and high white blood cell count develop after other symptoms had initially started to subside. The diagnosis is made by culturing blood samples (growing large numbers of bacteria) to identify bacteria that are causing the infection and performing a computed tomography (CT) scan. A doctor may be able to withdraw a sample of infected material from the pancreas by inserting a needle through the skin and into the pancreas. An infection is treated with antibiotics, and surgical removal of infected and dead tissue usually is necessary.

Sometimes, a collection of pancreatic enzymes, fluid, and tissue debris resembling a cyst (a pseudocyst) forms in the pancreas and expands like a balloon. If a pseudocyst grows larger and causes pain or other symptoms, a doctor drains it quickly because death can result if the pseudocyst expands further, becomes infected, bleeds, or ruptures. Depending on its location, the pseudocyst is drained either by performing a surgical procedure or by inserting a catheter through the skin or through an endoscope (a flexible viewing tube) that is passed through the mouth and into the stomach or intestine and allowing the pseudocyst to drain for several weeks.

Diagnosis

Characteristic abdominal pain leads a doctor to suspect acute pancreatitis, especially in a person who has gallbladder disease or who is an alcoholic. On examination, a doctor often notes that the abdominal wall muscles are rigid. When listening to the abdomen with a stethoscope, a doctor may hear few or no bowel (intestinal) sounds.

No single blood test proves the diagnosis of acute pancreatitis, but certain tests corroborate it. Blood levels of two enzymes produced by the pancreas, amylase and lipase, usually increase on the first day of the illness but return to normal in 3 to 7 days. If the person has had other flare-ups (bouts or attacks) of pancreatitis, however, the levels of these enzymes may not increase, because so much of the pancreas may have been destroyed that few cells are left to release the enzymes. The white blood cell count is usually increased.

X-rays of the abdomen may show dilated loops of intestine or, rarely, one or more gallstones. Chest x-rays may reveal areas of collapsed lung tissue or an accumulation of fluid in the chest cavity. An ultrasound may show gallstones in the gallbladder or sometimes in the common bile duct and also may detect swelling of the pancreas.

A CT scan is particularly useful in detecting inflammation of the pancreas and is used in people with severe acute pancreatitis and in people with complications, such as extremely low blood pressure. Because the images are so clear, a CT scan helps a doctor make a precise diagnosis.

Prognosis

In severe acute pancreatitis, a CT scan helps determine the outlook, or prognosis. If the scan indicates that the pancreas is only mildly swollen, the prognosis is excellent. If the scan shows large areas of destroyed pancreas, the prognosis is poor.

When acute pancreatitis is mild, the death rate is about 5% or less. However, in pancreatitis with severe damage and bleeding, or when the inflammation is not confined to the pancreas, the death rate can be as high as 10 to 50%. Death during the first several days of acute pancreatitis is usually caused by failure of the heart, lungs, or kidneys. Death after the first week is usually caused by pancreatic infection or by a pseudocyst that bleeds or ruptures.

Treatment

Treatment of mild pancreatitis usually involves short-term hospitalization where analgesics are given for pain relief and the person fasts to try to rest the pancreas. Usually, normal eating can resume after 2 to 3 days without further treatment.

People with moderate to severe pancreatitis need to be hospitalized. They must initially avoid food and liquids, because eating and drinking stimulate the pancreas. Symptoms such as pain and nausea are controlled with intravenous drugs. Intravenous fluids are given as well. People with severe acute pancreatitis are admitted to an intensive care unit, where vital signs (pulse, blood pressure, and rate of breathing) and urine production can be monitored continuously. Blood samples are repeatedly drawn to monitor various components of the blood, including hematocrit, sugar (glucose) levels, electrolyte levels, white blood cell count, and amylase and lipase levels. A tube may be inserted through the

nose and into the stomach (nasogastric tube) to remove fluid and air, particularly if nausea and vomiting persist and gastrointestinal ileus is present. Nutrition is given intravenously, via a nasogastric tube, or by both means.

For people with a drop in blood pressure or who are in shock, blood volume is carefully maintained with intravenous fluids, and heart function is closely monitored. Some people need supplemental oxygen, and the most seriously ill require a ventilator.

When acute pancreatitis results from gallstones, treatment depends on the severity. If the pancreatitis is mild, removal of the gallbladder can usually be delayed until symptoms subside. Severe pancreatitis caused by gallstones can be treated with endoscopic retrograde cholangiopancreatography (ERCP—see art on page 213). Although more than 80% of people with gallstone pancreatitis pass the stone spontaneously, ERCP with stone removal is usually needed for people who do not improve over the initial 24 hours of hospitalization and who have an infection of the bile duct system (cholangitis).

Chronic Pancreatitis

Chronic pancreatitis is long-standing inflammation of the pancreas that results in irreversible deterioration of pancreatic structure and function.

- Abdominal pain may be persistent or intermittent.
- The diagnosis is usually based on the symptoms, but blood tests may be helpful.
- Treatment involves allowing the pancreas to rest and taking drugs to relieve the pain.

In the United States, most chronic pancreatitis has no clear cause (idiopathic) or is due to alcohol abuse. Other less common causes include a hereditary predisposition; hyperparathyroidism (see box on page 937); and an obstruction of the pancreatic duct caused by a narrowing of the duct, gallstones, or cancer. Rarely, an attack of severe acute pancreatitis makes the pancreatic duct so narrow that chronic pancreatitis results. In tropical countries (for example, India, Indonesia, and Nigeria), chronic pancreatitis of unknown cause occurs among children and young adults.

Symptoms

Symptoms of chronic pancreatitis may be identical to those of acute pancreatitis and generally fall into two patterns. In one pattern, a person has persistent midabdominal pain that varies in intensity. In this pattern, a complication of chronic pancreatitis, such as an inflammatory mass, a cyst, or even pancreatic cancer, is more likely. In the second pattern, a person has intermittent flare-ups (bouts or attacks) of pancreatitis with symptoms similar to those of mild to moderate acute pancreatitis. The pain sometimes is severe and lasts for many hours or several days. With either pattern, as chronic pancreatitis progresses, cells that secrete the digestive enzymes are slowly destroyed, so eventually the pain may stop.

As the number of digestive enzymes decreases (a condition called pancreatic insufficiency), food is inadequately broken down. Food that is inadequately broken down is not absorbed properly (malabsorption), and the person may produce bulky, unusually foul-smelling, greasy stools (steatorrhea). The stool is light-colored and may even contain oil droplets. Undigested muscle fibers may also be found in the feces. The inadequate absorption of food also leads to weight loss. Eventually, the insulin-secreting cells of the pancreas may be destroyed, gradually leading to diabetes.

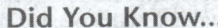

Did You Know...

Anyone who has chronic pancreatitis should avoid alcohol.

Diagnosis

A doctor suspects chronic pancreatitis because of a person's symptoms or history of acute pancreatitis flare-ups or alcohol abuse. Blood tests are less useful in diagnosing chronic pancreatitis than in diagnosing acute pancreatitis, but they may indicate elevated levels of amylase and lipase. Also, blood tests can be used to check the level of sugar (glucose) in the blood, which may be elevated.

Computed tomography (CT) may be done to show changes of chronic pancreatitis. When available, many doctors now perform a special magnetic resonance imaging (MRI) test called magnetic resonance cholangiopancreatography (MRCP) instead of CT. MRCP shows the bile and pancreatic ducts more clearly than does CT.

People with chronic pancreatitis are at increased risk of pancreatic cancer. Worsening of symptoms, especially narrowing of the pancreatic duct, makes doctors suspect cancer. In such cases, a doctor is likely to do an MRI scan, CT scan, or endoscopic study.

Treatment

Treatment of repeated flare-ups of chronic pancreatitis is similar to that of acute pancreatitis. Even if alcohol is not the cause, all people with chronic pancreatitis should avoid drinking alcohol. Avoiding all food and receiving only intravenous fluids can rest the pancreas and intestine and may relieve a painful flare-up. In addition, opioid analgesics (see page 642) are sometimes needed to relieve the pain. Too often,

these measures do not relieve the pain, requiring increased amounts of opioids, which may put the person at risk of addiction. Medical treatment of chronic pancreatic pain is often unsatisfactory.

Later, eating four or five meals a day consisting of food low in fat may help reduce the frequency and intensity of the flare-ups. If pain continues, a doctor searches for complications, such as an inflammatory mass in the head of the pancreas or a pseudocyst (a collection of pancreatic enzymes, fluid, and tissue debris resembling a cyst). An inflammatory mass may require surgical treatment. A pancreatic pseudocyst that causes pain as it expands may have to be drained (decompressed).

If the person has continuing pain and no complications, the doctor may recommend injecting a combination of the anesthetic lidocaine and corticosteroids into the nerves from the pancreas to block pain impulses from reaching the brain. If this procedure does not work, which is frequently the case, surgical treatment may be an option if the pancreatic ducts are dilated or if there is an inflammatory mass in one region of the pancreas. For instance, when the pancreatic duct is dilated, creating a bypass from the pancreas to the small intestine relieves the pain in about 70 to 80% of people. When the duct is not dilated, part of the pancreas may have to be removed. Removing part of the pancreas means that cells that produce insulin are removed as well, and diabetes may develop. Doctors reserve surgical treatment for people who have stopped using alcohol and who can manage any diabetes that develops. For people who no longer produce adequate digestive enzymes, taking tablets or capsules of pancreatic enzyme extracts with meals can make the stool less greasy and improve food absorption, but these problems are rarely eliminated. If necessary, a histamine-2 (H_2) blocker or a proton pump inhibitor (drugs that reduce or prevent the production of stomach acid) may be taken with the pancreatic enzymes. With such treatment, the person usually gains some weight, has fewer daily bowel movements, has no more oil droplets in the stool, and generally feels better. If these measures are ineffective, the person can try decreasing fat intake. Supplements of the fat-soluble vitamins (A, D, E, and K) also may be needed.

Oral hypoglycemic drugs rarely can be used in the treatment of diabetes caused by chronic pancreatitis. Insulin is generally needed but can cause a problem, because affected people also have decreased levels of glucagon, which is a hormone that acts to balance the effects of insulin. An excess of insulin in the bloodstream causes low sugar levels in the blood, which can result in a hypoglycemic coma (see page 1015).

24 Malabsorption

Malabsorption syndrome refers to a number of disorders in which nutrients from food are not absorbed properly in the small intestine.

- Certain disorders, infections, and surgical procedures can cause malabsorption.
- Malabsorption causes diarrhea, weight loss, and bulky, extremely foul-smelling stools.
- The diagnosis is based on typical symptoms along with testing of stool samples for fat and sometimes examination of a tissue specimen removed from the lining of the small intestine.
- The treatment depends on the cause.

Normally, foods are digested and nutrients are absorbed into the bloodstream mainly in the small intestine. Malabsorption may occur if a disorder interferes with the digestion of food or interferes directly with the absorption of nutrients.

Digestion can be affected by disorders that prevent adequate mixing of food with digestive enzymes and acid from the stomach. Inadequate mixing may occur in a person who has had part of the stomach surgically removed. In some disorders, the body produces inadequate amounts or types of digestive enzymes, which are necessary for the breakdown of food. For example, a common cause of malabsorption is insufficient production of digestive enzymes by the pancreas, as occurs with some pancreatic diseases, or by the small intestine, as occurs in lactase deficiency. Decreased production of bile, too much acid in the stomach, or too many of the wrong kinds of bacteria growing in the small intestine may also interfere with digestion.

Absorption of nutrients into the bloodstream can be affected by disorders that injure the lining of the small intestine. The normal lining consists of small projections called villi and even smaller projections called microvilli, which create an enormous surface area for absorption. Surgical removal of a large section of the small intestine substantially reduces the surface area for absorption (short bowel syndrome). Infections (bacterial, viral, or parasitic), drugs such as neomycin and alcohol, celiac sprue, and Crohn's disease all may injure the intestinal lining. Disorders that affect the remaining layers of the intestinal wall, such as blockage of the lymph vessels by lymphoma (cancer of the lymphatic system) or poor blood supply to the small intestine, also reduce absorption.

Symptoms

Symptoms of malabsorption are caused by the increased passage of unabsorbed nutrients through the digestive tract or by the nutritional deficiencies that result from inadequate absorption.

The inadequate absorption of fats in the digestive tract results in stool that is light-colored, soft, bulky, and unusually foul smelling (such stool is called steatorrhea). The stool may float or stick to the side of the toilet bowl and may be difficult to flush away. The inadequate absorption of certain sugars can cause explosive diarrhea, abdominal bloating, and flatulence.

SYMPTOMS OF NUTRIENT DEFICIENCIES	
NUTRIENT	**SYMPTOMS**
Calcium	Bone pain and deformities, greater likelihood of fractures (due to bone thinning or osteoporosis), muscle spasms, and tooth discoloration and greater susceptibility to painful tooth decay
Folate (folic acid)	Fatigue and weakness (due to anemia)
Iron	Fatigue and weakness (due to anemia)
Magnesium	Muscle spasms
Niacin	Diarrhea, skin disorders, confusion (pellagra), and sore tongue
Protein	Tissue swelling (edema), usually in legs; dry skin; and hair loss
Vitamin A	Night blindness
Vitamin B_1	Pins-and-needles sensation, especially in the feet, and heart failure
Vitamin B_2	Sore tongue and cracks at edge of mouth
Vitamin B_{12}	Fatigue and weakness (due to anemia), pins-and-needles sensation, and confusion
Vitamin C	Weakness and bleeding gums
Vitamin D	Bone thinning and bone pain
Vitamin K	Tendency to bruise and bleed

Malabsorption can cause deficiencies of all nutrients or selective deficiencies of proteins, fats, sugars, vitamins, or minerals. People with malabsorption usually lose weight. The symptoms vary depending on the specific deficiencies. For example, a protein deficiency can cause swelling (edema) anywhere throughout the body, dry skin, and hair loss.

Diagnosis

A doctor suspects malabsorption when a person has chronic diarrhea, nutritional deficiencies, and substantial weight loss despite a healthy diet. Malabsorption is less obvious and often more difficult to recognize in older people than in younger people.

Laboratory tests can help confirm the diagnosis. Tests that directly measure fat in stool samples collected over 2 or 3 days are the most reliable ones for diagnosing malabsorption of fat, which is present in almost all malabsorption disorders. A finding of more than 7 grams of fat in the stool daily is the hallmark of malabsorption. Several other tests for measuring fat in stool are available that do not require the messy 3-day collection of stool. Other laboratory tests can detect malabsorption of other specific substances, such as lactose or vitamin B_{12}.

Stool samples are examined with the unaided eye as well as under the microscope. Undigested food fragments may mean that food passes through the intestine too rapidly. In a person with jaundice, stool with excess fat indicates decreased production or secretion of bile. Sometimes parasites or their eggs are seen under the microscope, suggesting that malabsorption is caused by a parasitic infection.

A biopsy may be needed to detect abnormalities in the lining of the small intestine. The tissue is removed through an endoscope (a flexible viewing tube equipped with a light source and a small clipper) passed through the mouth and into the small intestine.

Pancreatic function tests are performed if the doctor thinks that the cause of malabsorption may be the insufficient production of digestive enzymes by the pancreas. However, some of these tests are complex, time-consuming, and invasive. In one test, a tube is passed through the mouth and guided to the small intestine, so that intestinal fluids containing pancreatic secretions can be collected and measured. In another test, the person swallows a substance that requires pancreatic enzymes for its digestion. The products of digestion are then measured in the urine.

Lactose Intolerance

Lactose intolerance is the inability to digest the sugar lactose (which is present in all dairy products) because of a deficiency of the digestive enzyme lactase, leading to diarrhea and abdominal cramping.

- Lactose intolerance is caused by a lack of the enzyme lactase.
- Children have diarrhea and may not gain weight, whereas adults have abdominal bloating, cramps, diarrhea, flatulence, nausea, audible bowel sounds (borborygmi), and an urgent need to have a bowel movement.
- The diagnosis is based on recognizing that symptoms occur after a person has consumed dairy products.
- Treatment involves taking supplemental lactase enzymes and avoiding lactose, particularly in dairy products.

Lactose, the predominant sugar found in milk and other dairy products, is broken down by the enzyme lactase, which is produced by the cells in the inner lining of the small intestine. Lactase breaks down lactose, a complex sugar, into its two components, glucose and galactose. These simple sugars are then absorbed into the bloodstream through the intestinal wall. If lactase is lacking, lactose cannot be digested and absorbed. The resulting high concentration of lactose draws fluid into the small intestine, causing diarrhea. The unabsorbed lactose then passes into the large intestine, where it is fermented by bacteria, resulting in flatulence and acidic stool.

Lactase levels are high in infants, permitting them to digest milk. However, in most ethnic groups (80% of blacks and Hispanics, almost 100% of Asians), lactase levels decrease after weaning. These decreased levels mean that older children and adults in these ethnic groups are unable to digest much lactose. However, 80 to 85% of whites of Northwest European descent produce lactase throughout life and are thus able to digest milk and milk products as adults. Therefore, because of the ethnic composition of the United States population, it is likely that between 30 million and 50 million people in the United States are lactose intolerant. It is interesting to note that this "intolerance" is really the normal state for more than 75% of the world's population.

Intolerances to other sugars can also occur but are relatively rare. For example, a lack of the enzyme sucrase prevents the sugar sucrose from being absorbed into the bloodstream, and a lack of the enzymes maltase and isomaltase prevents the sugar maltose from being absorbed into the bloodstream.

Symptoms

People with lactose intolerance usually cannot tolerate milk and other dairy products, all of which contain lactose. Some people recognize this early in life and consciously or unconsciously avoid dairy products.

A child who is lactose intolerant has diarrhea and may not gain weight when milk is part of the diet. An adult may have abdominal bloating, cramps, diarrhea, flatulence, nausea, audible bowel sounds (borborygmi), and an urgent need to have a bowel movement between 30 minutes and 2 hours after eating a meal containing lactose. For some people, severe diarrhea may prevent proper absorption of nutrients because they are expelled from the body too quickly. However, the symptoms that result from lactose intolerance are usually mild. In contrast, symptoms that result from malabsorption in such conditions as celiac disease, tropical sprue, and infections of the intestine are more severe.

Diagnosis and Treatment

A doctor suspects lactose intolerance when a person has symptoms after consuming dairy products. If a 3- to 4-week trial period of a diet free of dairy products eliminates the symptoms, the diagnosis is confirmed. Specific tests are rarely necessary.

Lactose intolerance can be controlled through diet by avoiding foods containing lactose, primarily dairy products. Lactase enzymes are available in liquid and tablet forms without a prescription and can be added to milk. Lactose-reduced milk and other products are available at many supermarkets. People who must avoid dairy products should take calcium supplements to prevent calcium deficiency.

Celiac Sprue

Celiac sprue (nontropical sprue, gluten enteropathy, celiac disease) is a hereditary intolerance to gluten (a protein found in wheat, barley, and oats) that causes characteristic changes in the lining of the small intestine, resulting in malabsorption.

- The intestinal lining becomes inflamed after a person ingests the protein gluten.
- Symptoms in adults include diarrhea, undernutrition, and weight loss, and symptoms in children include abdominal bloating and bulky, very foul-smelling stools.
- The diagnosis is based on typical symptoms and examination of a tissue specimen removed from the lining of the small intestine.
- Most people do well if they maintain a gluten-free diet.

Celiac sprue affects as many as 1 out of 150 people in southwestern Ireland, 1 out of 300 people in Europe, and perhaps 1 out of 250 people in the United States, yet it is extremely rare in Africa, Japan, and China. There is a genetic component. About 10% of people with celiac sprue have a close relative with the disease. In this disease, gluten—a protein found in wheat and, to a lesser extent, barley, rye, and oats—stimulates the immune system to produce certain antibodies. These antibodies damage the inner lining of the small intestine, resulting in flattening of the villi. The resulting smooth surface leads to malabsorption of nutrients.

However, the small intestine's normal brushlike surface and function are restored when the person stops eating foods containing gluten.

Symptoms

Some people develop symptoms as children. Others do not develop symptoms until adulthood. The severity of symptoms depends on how much of the small intestine is affected.

Adults with the more classic or typical form of the disease experience diarrhea, undernutrition, and weight loss. However, some people have no digestive symptoms at all. About 10% of people with celiac sprue develop a painful, itchy skin rash with small blisters—a disease called dermatitis herpetiformis (see page 1310).

In children, symptoms do not appear until foods containing gluten are introduced. Some children experience only mild upset stomach, whereas others develop painful abdominal bloating and have light-colored, unusually foul-smelling, bulky stools (steatorrhea).

The nutritional deficiencies resulting from malabsorption in celiac sprue can cause additional symptoms, which tend to be more prominent in children. Some children develop growth abnormalities, such as short stature. Anemia, causing fatigue and weakness, develops as a result of iron deficiency. Low protein levels in the blood can lead to fluid retention and tissue swelling (edema). Malabsorption of vitamin B_{12} can lead to nerve damage, causing a pins-and-needles sensation in the arms and legs. Poor calcium absorption results in abnormal bone growth, a higher risk of broken bones, and painful bones and joints. Lack of calcium can also cause tooth discoloration and greater susceptibility to painful tooth decay. Girls with celiac sprue may not have menstrual periods because of a low production of hormones, such as estrogen.

Diagnosis

Doctors suspect the diagnosis when a person has the previously mentioned symptoms. Measurement of the level of specific antibodies produced when a person with celiac sprue consumes gluten is a helpful test. The diagnosis is confirmed by an initial microscopic examination of a biopsy specimen revealing flattened villi of the small intestine and by a subsequent improvement in the lining after the person stops eating foods containing gluten.

Prognosis and Treatment

Although most people do well if they avoid gluten, long-standing celiac sprue can be fatal in a small percentage of people who develop intestinal lymphoma. Whether strictly adhering to a gluten-free diet decreases the risk of long-term complications such as intestinal cancers or lymphoma is not known.

People with celiac sprue must exclude all gluten from their diet, because eating even small amounts may cause symptoms. The response to a gluten-free diet is usually rapid. Once gluten is avoided, the brushlike surface of the small intestine and its absorptive function return to normal. Gluten is so widely used in food products that people with celiac sprue need detailed lists of foods to be avoided and expert advice from a dietitian. Gluten is found, for example, in commercial soups, sauces, ice cream, and hot dogs.

Some people continue to have symptoms even when gluten is avoided. In such cases, either the diagnosis is incorrect or the disease has progressed to a condition called refractory celiac sprue. In refractory celiac sprue, treatment with corticosteroids, such as prednisone, may help. In rare cases, if there is no response to either gluten withdrawal or drug treatment, intravenous feeding is needed. Sometimes children are seriously ill when first diagnosed and need a period of intravenous feeding before starting a gluten-free diet.

Tropical Sprue

Tropical sprue is a disorder of unknown cause affecting people living in tropical and subtropical areas who develop abnormalities of the lining of the small intestine, leading to malabsorption and deficiencies of many nutrients.

- This disorder might be caused by an infection, but the real cause is not known.
- Typical symptoms include anemia, light-colored stools, chronic diarrhea, and weight loss.
- A doctor bases the diagnosis on symptoms in a person who lives in or has recently visited one of the areas in which the disorder commonly occurs.
- The antibiotic tetracycline treats the disorder.

Tropical sprue occurs chiefly in the Caribbean, southern India, and Southeast Asia. Both natives and visitors may be affected, but children are rarely affected. The cause is unknown, but available evidence suggests an infectious cause.

Symptoms and Diagnosis

Light-colored stools, chronic diarrhea, and weight loss are typical symptoms of tropical sprue. Other symptoms of malabsorption of specific nutrients may also develop. A sore tongue develops from vitamin B_2 deficiency. Anemia usually develops as a result of iron, vitamin B_{12}, or folate (folic acid) deficiency, causing fatigue and weakness.

A doctor considers the diagnosis of tropical sprue in a person with anemia and symptoms of malabsorption who lives in or has recently visited one of the areas in which the disorder commonly occurs. X-rays of the small intestine may or may not be abnormal. An endoscopic biopsy (in which a tissue sample is obtained through a flexible tube and examined microscopically) of the small intestine can show some characteristic but not specific abnormalities. A stool sample may be analyzed to exclude parasites or bacteria as a cause.

Treatment

A person suspected of having tropical sprue is treated with an antibiotic. Tetracycline is given over several months. Nutritional supplements, especially folate and vitamin B_{12}, are given as needed. Treatment usually results in a full recovery.

Whipple's Disease

Whipple's disease (intestinal lipodystrophy) is the result of a rare bacterial infection that damages the lining of the small intestine and may involve other organs of the body.

- This disease is caused by a bacterial infection.
- Typical symptoms include diarrhea, inflamed and painful joints, fever, and skin darkening.
- The diagnosis is based on the results of different biopsies.
- If left untreated, the disease is progressive and fatal.
- Antibiotics can eliminate the infection, but the disease can recur.

Whipple's disease affects mainly white men aged 30 to 60. It is caused by an infection with the organism *Tropheryma whippelii*. The infection usually involves the small intestine but can affect other organs, such as the heart, lungs, brain, joints, and eyes.

Symptoms

Symptoms of Whipple's disease include diarrhea, inflamed and painful joints, fever, and skin darkening. Severe malabsorption results in weight loss along with fatigue and weakness caused by anemia. Other common symptoms are abdominal pain, cough, and pain when breathing caused by inflammation of the membrane layers covering the lungs (pleura). Fluid may collect in the space between the pleural layers (a condition called pleural effusion—see page 518). The lymph nodes may become enlarged. People with Whipple's disease may develop heart murmurs. Confusion, memory loss, or uncontrolled eye movements indicate that the infection has spread to the brain. If left untreated, the disease is progressive and fatal.

Diagnosis and Treatment

A doctor can make the diagnosis of Whipple's disease when an endoscopic biopsy (in which a tissue sample is obtained through a flexible tube and examined microscopically) of the small intestine or a biopsy of an enlarged lymph node shows the bacteria.

Whipple's disease can be cured with antibiotics. Usually people are given ceftriaxone initially by vein, followed by trimethoprim/sulfamethoxazole taken orally for at least 12 months. Symptoms subside rapidly. Despite an initial response to antibiotics, however, the disease can recur.

Intestinal Lymphangiectasia

Intestinal lymphangiectasia (idiopathic hypoproteinemia) is a disorder in which the lymph vessels supplying the lining of the small intestine become enlarged and obstructed.

- This disorder is the result of improperly formed lymph vessels.
- Diarrhea is the main symptom.
- The diagnosis is based on the results of a biopsy.
- Once the specific cause of the disorder is treated, following a low-fat, high-protein diet and taking supplements can help manage symptoms.

The lymph vessels from the digestive tract carry digested fats that were absorbed by the small intestine. Sometimes, these lymph vessels are improperly formed at birth, causing them to be enlarged. Less commonly, these lymph vessels may enlarge later in life as a result of such conditions as inflammation of the pancreas (pancreatitis) or stiffening of the sac that envelops the heart (constrictive pericarditis). The enlarged lymph vessels carry lymphatic fluid poorly, and the fluid leaks back into the intestine, preventing fat and proteins from being absorbed into the bloodstream.

Symptoms and Diagnosis

A person with intestinal lymphangiectasia has diarrhea. Nausea, vomiting, fatty stools, and abdominal pain may also develop. The person may also have swelling (edema) if lymph vessels elsewhere in the body are blocked.

Levels of protein in the blood are low. The low protein levels result in tissue swelling. The number of lymphocytes in the blood is decreased, and cholesterol levels in the blood may be normal or low.

The diagnosis is established by a biopsy of the small intestine showing enlargement of the lymph vessels. Measurement of a certain protein, called alpha$_1$-antitrypsin, in the stool can indicate the severity of protein loss into the intestines.

Treatment

When intestinal lymphangiectasia is caused by a specific condition, the underlying condition is treated. Symptoms can be helped by eating a low-fat, high-protein diet and taking supplements of calcium, vitamins, and certain triglycerides (medium-chain triglycerides), which are absorbed directly into the blood and not through the lymph vessels.

Short Bowel Syndrome

Short bowel syndrome is a disorder causing diarrhea and poor absorption of nutrients (malabsorption), which often occurs after surgical removal of a large portion of the small intestine.

- This disorder often occurs after a large part of the small intestine is removed.
- Diarrhea is the main symptom.
- After surgery, people are given food and fluids by vein (intravenously).
- Some people must continue the intravenous feedings for life.
- Drugs such as loperamide and cholestyramine can help reduce diarrhea.

Common reasons for removing a large portion of small intestine are Crohn's disease, a blockage of an artery that supplies blood to a large part of the intestine (mesenteric infarction), inflammation of the intestine caused by radiation (radiation enteritis), cancer, a twisted loop of intestine (volvulus), and birth defects.

Most digestion and absorption of food takes place in the small intestine. The consequences of removing a portion of the small intestine depend on how much is removed and its location. If the middle part (jejunum) is removed, sometimes the last part (ileum) can adapt and absorb more nutrients. If more than about 3 feet (about 1 meter) of ileum is removed, the remaining small intestine usually cannot adapt. Before adaptation occurs, or if it does not, the intestines have difficulty absorbing many nutrients, including fats, proteins, and vitamins. The intestines also cannot absorb bile acids secreted by the liver, which aid digestion.

Malabsorption causes diarrhea, typically beginning immediately after the surgery. Later, people develop undernutrition and vitamin deficiencies.

Treatment

Immediately after surgery, when diarrhea is typically severe, doctors give intravenous fluids to replace losses and usually also give intravenous feedings. These feedings, called total parenteral nutrition (TPN), contain all necessary nutrients, including proteins, fats, carbohydrates, vitamins, and minerals. As people recover and their stool output lessens, they are slowly given fluids by mouth.

The small intestine is about 12 to 21 feet (about 4 to 7 meters) in length. People who have had a large amount of small intestine removed (such as those with less than 3.3 feet [about 1 meter] of remaining jejunum) and those who continue to have excessive fluid losses require TPN for life. Others eventually tolerate food by mouth. The recommended diet usually has more fat and protein than carbohydrate. Small, frequent meals are better than fewer, large ones.

People who have diarrhea after meals should take antidiarrheal drugs such as loperamide 1 hour before eating. Cholestyramine can be taken with meals to reduce diarrhea caused by malabsorption of bile acid. Most people should take supplemental vitamins, calcium, and magnesium. Some people require monthly injections of vitamin B_{12}.

Small-intestine transplantation is an alternative for people who do not adapt to their short bowel and who cannot tolerate long-term TPN.

Bacterial Overgrowth Syndrome

Bacterial overgrowth syndrome is a disorder in which poor movement of intestinal contents allows certain normal intestinal bacteria to grow excessively, causing diarrhea and poor absorption of nutrients (malabsorption).

- Some conditions and disorders slow or stop the movement of contents through the intestines.
- Some people have no symptoms, whereas others have weight loss, nutritional deficiencies, and diarrhea.
- The diagnosis is based on symptoms that occur after people have had certain types of surgery.
- Antibiotics can eliminate the excess bacteria.

The normal steady movement of intestinal contents (peristalsis) is important to help maintain a proper balance of bacteria in the small intestine. Conditions in which intestinal contents slow or pool in one place allow excess bacteria to grow. Such conditions include certain types of surgery on the stomach, intestines, or both. Disorders such as diabetes, systemic sclerosis, and amyloidosis also can slow peristalsis, causing bacterial overgrowth.

The excess bacteria consume nutrients, including vitamin B_{12} and carbohydrates, leading to lower calorie intake and vitamin B_{12} deficiency. The bacteria also split bile salts, which are secreted by the liver to aid digestion. The loss of bile salts causes difficulty absorbing fats, leading to diarrhea and poor nutrition.

Some people have few symptoms or only weight loss. Others have severe nutritional deficiencies, diarrhea, or both.

Diagnosis and Treatment

Doctors base the diagnosis on typical symptoms that occur in people who have had certain types of surgery. Sometimes they take a fluid sample from the small intestine by means of a thin plastic tube passed through the nose. Some doctors instead perform breath tests, such as the ^{14}C-xylose breath test. In this test, the person drinks a liquid containing a special, faintly radioactive marker (carbon-14) attached to a sugar (xylose). If the xylose is broken down by the excess bacteria, the carbon-14 can be detected in the person's breath.

Most people get better with antibiotics given by mouth for 10 to 14 days. Doctors prescribe supplements to correct any nutritional deficiencies.

CHAPTER 25 Inflammatory Bowel Diseases

In inflammatory bowel diseases, the intestine (bowel) becomes inflamed, often causing recurring abdominal cramps and diarrhea.

The two primary types of inflammatory bowel disease are Crohn's disease and ulcerative colitis. These two diseases have many similarities and sometimes are difficult to distinguish from each other. However, there are several differences. For example, Crohn's disease can affect almost any part of the digestive tract, whereas ulcerative colitis almost always affects only the large intestine. The cause of these diseases is not known but may involve an overactive immune reaction to intestinal bacteria or other agents in people with a genetic predisposition. More recently recognized inflammatory bowel diseases include collagenous colitis, lymphocytic colitis, and diversion colitis.

To make a diagnosis of inflammatory bowel disease, a doctor must first exclude other possible causes of inflammation. For example, infection with parasites or bacteria may cause inflammation. Therefore, the doctor performs several tests. Stool samples are analyzed for evidence of a bacterial or parasitic infection (acquired during travel, for example), including a type of bacterial infection (*Clostridium difficile* infection) that can result from antibiotic use (see page 176). A doctor also checks for sexually transmitted diseases of the rectum, such as gonorrhea, herpesvirus infection, and chlamydial infection. Tissue samples (biopsies) may be taken from the lining of the rectum during a sigmoidoscopy (an examination of the sigmoid colon using a viewing tube) and examined microscopically for evidence of other causes of colon inflammation (colitis). Other possible causes of similar abdominal symptoms that a doctor tries to exclude are ischemic colitis, which occurs more often in people older than 50; certain gynecologic disorders in women; celiac disease; and irritable bowel syndrome.

Crohn's Disease

Crohn's disease (regional enteritis, granulomatous ileitis, ileocolitis) is a chronic inflammation of the intestinal wall that may affect any part of the digestive tract.

- Although the exact cause is unknown, an improperly functioning immune system may result in Crohn's disease.
- Typical symptoms include chronic diarrhea (which sometimes is bloody), crampy abdominal pain, fever, loss of appetite, and weight loss.
- The diagnosis is based on an examination of the large intestine with a flexible viewing tube (colonoscopy) and barium x-rays.
- There is no cure for Crohn's disease.
- Treatment is aimed at relieving symptoms and reducing inflammation, but some people require surgery.

The cause of Crohn's disease is not known for certain, but many researchers believe that a dysfunction of the immune system causes the intestine to overreact to an environmental, dietary, or infectious agent. Certain people may have a hereditary predisposition to this immune system dysfunction. Cigarette smoking seems to contribute to both the development and the periodic flare-ups (bouts or attacks) of Crohn's disease.

In the past few decades, Crohn's disease has become more common worldwide. However, it is most common among populations living in northern climates in developed areas of the world. It occurs about equally in both sexes, often runs in families, and seems to be more common among Ashkenazi Jews. Most people develop Crohn's disease before age 35, usually between the ages of 15 and 25.

Most commonly, Crohn's disease occurs in the last portion of the small intestine (ileum) and in the large intestine, but it can occur in any part of the digestive tract, from the mouth to the anus and even in the skin around the anus. Crohn's disease affects the small intestine alone (35% of people), the large intestine alone (20% of people), or both the last portion of the small intestine and the large intestine (45% of people). The disease may affect some segments of the intestinal tract while leaving normal segments (skip areas) between the affected areas. Where Crohn's disease is active, the full thickness of the bowel is usually involved.

Symptoms

The most common early symptoms of Crohn's disease are chronic diarrhea (which sometimes is bloody), crampy abdominal pain, fever, loss of appetite, and weight loss. Symptoms may continue for days or weeks and may resolve without treatment. Complete and permanent recovery after a single attack is extremely rare. Crohn's disease almost always flares up at irregular intervals throughout a person's life. Flare-ups can be mild or severe, brief or prolonged. Severe flare-ups can lead to intense pain, dehydration, and blood loss. Why the symptoms come and go and what triggers new flare-ups or determines their severity is not known. Recurrent inflammation tends to appear in the same area of the intestine, but it may spread to adjacent areas after a diseased segment has been removed surgically.

In children, gastrointestinal symptoms such as abdominal pain and diarrhea often are not the main symptoms and may not appear at all. Instead, the main symptoms may be slow growth, joint inflammation, fever, or weakness and fatigue resulting from anemia.

Complications: Common complications of inflammation include scarring, which can cause intestinal blockage (obstruction), and deep ulcers penetrating through the bowel wall that can create pus-filled pockets of infection (abscesses) or abnormal connecting channels between the intestine and other organs (fistulas). Fistulas may connect two different parts of the intestine. Fistulas also may connect the intestine and bladder or the intestine and the skin surface, especially around the anus. Although fistulas from the small intestine are common, wide-open holes (perforations) are rare.

When the large intestine is affected extensively by Crohn's disease, rectal bleeding commonly occurs. After many years, the risk of colon cancer (cancer of the large intestine) is greatly increased. About one third of people who develop Crohn's disease have problems around the anus, especially fistulas and cracks (fissures) in the lining of the mucus membrane of the anus. Crohn's disease may lead to complications in other parts of the body. These complications include gallstones, inadequate absorption of nutrients, urinary tract infections, kidney stones, and deposits of the protein amyloid in several organs (amyloidosis).

When Crohn's disease causes a flare-up of gastrointestinal symptoms, the person may also experience inflammation of the joints (arthritis), inflammation of the whites of the eyes (episcleritis), mouth sores (aphthous stomatitis), inflamed skin nodules on the arms and legs (erythema nodosum), and blue-red skin sores containing pus (pyoderma gangrenosum). Even when Crohn's disease is not causing a flare-up of gastrointestinal symptoms, the person still may experience inflammation of the spine (ankylosing spondylitis), inflammation of the pelvic joints (sacroiliitis), inflammation inside the eye (uveitis), or inflammation of the bile ducts (primary sclerosing cholangitis) entirely without relation to the bowel disease.

Diagnosis

A doctor may suspect Crohn's disease in a person with recurring crampy abdominal pain and diarrhea, particularly if the person has a family history of Crohn's disease or a history of problems around the anus. Other clues to the diagnosis may include inflammation in the joints, eyes, or skin. The doctor may feel a lump or fullness in the lower part of the abdomen, most often on the right side.

No laboratory test specifically identifies Crohn's disease, but blood tests may show anemia, abnormally high numbers of white blood cells, low levels of the protein albumin, and other indications of inflammation such as an elevated level of C-reactive protein (CRP).

A colonoscopy (an examination of the large intestine with a flexible viewing tube) and a biopsy (removal of a tissue specimen for microscopic examination) are usually the first tests performed after a physical examination and blood tests have been completed.

If Crohn's disease is limited to the small intestine, a colonoscopy will not detect the disease unless the colonoscope is advanced all the way through the colon into the last part of the small intestine where the inflammation most often resides. However, Crohn's disease can almost always be detected on x-rays after barium is swallowed. X-rays taken after barium is given by enema can reveal the characteristic appearance of Crohn's disease in the large intestine. Computed tomography (CT) can show changes that are helpful in distinguishing between Crohn's disease and ulcerative colitis and is the best way to identify complications that occur outside the walls of the intestinal tract, such as abscesses or fistulas. Another way in which the small intestine can be evaluated is with wireless capsule endoscopy (see page 129).

Prognosis and Treatment

Crohn's disease usually does not shorten a person's life. However, some people die of cancer of the digestive tract, which may develop in long-standing Crohn's disease.

Although Crohn's disease has no known cure, many treatments help reduce inflammation and relieve symptoms.

Antidiarrheal Drugs: These drugs, which may relieve cramps and diarrhea (see box on page 124), include drugs that have anticholinergic effects (drugs that block certain pathways of the nervous system—see page 1897) such as diphenoxylate, loperamide, deodorized opium tincture, and codeine. They are taken by mouth—preferably before meals. Taking methylcellulose or psyllium preparations sometimes helps prevent anal irritation by making the stool firmer.

Anti-Inflammatory Drugs: Sulfasalazine and related drugs such as mesalamine, olsalazine, and balsalazide reduce inflammation. These drugs can suppress symptoms when they occur and reduce inflammation, especially in the large intestine. Mesalamine may be effective in preventing recurrences. These drugs do not work as well for relieving severe flare-ups.

Corticosteroids such as prednisone, which is given by mouth, may dramatically reduce fever and diarrhea, relieve abdominal pain and tenderness, and improve appetite and sense of well-being. However, long-term corticosteroid therapy invariably results in side effects (see box on page 568). Usually, high doses are taken initially to relieve major inflammation and symptoms. The dose is then reduced and the drug is discontinued as soon as possible. A corticosteroid called budesonide has fewer side effects than prednisone, but it may not be quite as rapidly effective and usually does not prevent relapses beyond 6 to 9 months.

If the disease becomes severe, the person is hospitalized and corticosteroids are given intravenously. Initially, the person is given nothing by mouth, and intravenous fluids are given to restore and maintain body fluids (hydration). People with heavy rectal bleeding may require blood transfusions. People who have more chronic anemia may require iron supplements by mouth or intravenously.

Immunomodulating Drugs: Drugs such as azathioprine and mercaptopurine, which modify the actions of the immune system, are effective for people with Crohn's disease who do not respond to other drugs and are especially effective for maintaining long periods of remission. They significantly improve the person's overall condition, decrease the need for corticosteroids, and often heal fistulas. However, these drugs may not produce clinical benefits for 1 to 3 months and may have potentially serious side effects. Therefore, a doctor closely monitors the person for allergy, inflammation of the pancreas (pancreatitis), and a low white blood cell count. Genetic testing that detects variations in one of the enzymes that metabolize azathioprine and mercaptopurine and blood tests that directly measure metabolite levels may sometimes help the doctor ensure safe and effective drug dosages.

Methotrexate, given by injection or by mouth once a week, often benefits people who do not respond to or who cannot tolerate corticosteroids, azathioprine, or mercaptopurine.

Cyclosporine in high doses may help heal fistulas, but it cannot safely be used long-term.

Infliximab, which is derived from monoclonal antibodies, is another modifier of the immune system's actions. Infliximab infused intravenously can be given to treat moderate to severe Crohn's disease that has not responded to other drugs, to treat people with fistulas, and to maintain response when

℞ DRUGS THAT REDUCE BOWEL INFLAMMATION

DRUG	SOME SIDE EFFECTS	COMMENTS
Aminosalicylates		
Sulfasalazine	Common: Nausea, headache, dizziness, fatigue, fever, rash, and reversible male infertility Uncommon: Inflammation of the liver (hepatitis), pancreas (pancreatitis), or lung (pneumonitis); and hemolytic anemia	Abdominal pain, dizziness, and fatigue are related to dose. Hepatitis and pancreatitis are unrelated to dose.
Balsalazide Mesalamine Olsalazine	Common: Fever and rash Uncommon: Pancreatitis, inflammation of the pericardium (pericarditis), and pneumonitis For olsalazine: Watery diarrhea	Most side effects seen with sulfasalazine may occur with any of the other aminosalicylates but much less frequently.
Corticosteroids		
Prednisone	Diabetes mellitus, high blood pressure, cataracts, osteoporosis (decreased bone density), thinning of skin, mental problems, acute psychosis, mood swings, infections, acne, excessive body hair (hirsutism), menstrual irregularities, gastritis, and peptic ulcer disease	Diabetes and high blood pressure are more likely to occur in people who have other risk factors.
Budesonide	Diabetes mellitus, high blood pressure, cataracts, and osteoporosis	Budesonide causes the same side effects as prednisone but to a lesser degree.
Immunomodulators		
Azathioprine Mercaptopurine	Anorexia, nausea, vomiting, infection, cancer, allergic reactions, pancreatitis, low white blood cell count, bone marrow suppression, and liver dysfunction	Side effects that are usually dose dependent include bone marrow suppression and liver dysfunction. Interval blood monitoring is required.
Cyclosporine	High blood pressure, nausea, vomiting, diarrhea, kidney failure, tremors, infections, seizures, neuropathy, and development of lymphomas (cancers of the lymphatic system)	Side effects become more likely with long-term use.
Methotrexate	Nausea, vomiting, abdominal distress, headache, rash, soreness of the mouth, fatigue, scarring of the liver (cirrhosis), low white blood cell count, and infections	Liver toxicity is likely dose dependent. Not prescribed for pregnant women because it causes abortions and birth defects during pregnancy.
Infliximab	Infusion reactions, infections, cancer, abdominal pain, liver dysfunction, and low white blood cell count	Infusion reactions are potentially immediate side effects that occur during the infusion (such as fever, chills, hives, decreased blood pressure, or difficulty breathing). People should be screened for tuberculosis before initiating treatment.
Adalimumab	Pain or itching at the injection site, headache, infections, cancer, and hypersensitivity reactions	Side effects are similar to infliximab except adalimumab does not cause infusion reactions. Hypersensitivity reactions include rash, urticaria, pruritus, and hives.

the disease is difficult to control. However, because the benefits of each infusion of infliximab are short-lived, other treatments are needed between infusions. Such treatments may include other immunomodulating drugs such as azathioprine, mercaptopurine, or methotrexate. Because infliximab is a relatively new drug, its long-term benefit and all of its side effects are not yet known, but it may worsen an existing uncontrolled bacterial infection, may reactivate tuberculosis, and may increase the risk of some types of cancer. Some people have reactions such as fever or rash during the infusion.

Adalimumab is a drug related to infliximab, which focuses on regulating the immune system. Adalimumab is particularly helpful for people who cannot tolerate or who no longer respond to infliximab.

Broad-Spectrum Antibiotics: Antibiotics that are effective against many types of bacteria are often prescribed. The antibiotic metronidazole is the most common choice for the treatment of abscesses and fistulas around the anus. Metronidazole may also help relieve the noninfectious symptoms of Crohn's disease, such as diarrhea and abdominal cramps. However, when used for a long time, metronidazole can damage nerves, resulting in a pins-and-needles feeling in the arms and legs. This side effect usually disappears when the drug is stopped, but relapses of Crohn's disease after discontinuing metronidazole are common. Some other antibiotics, such as ciprofloxacin or levofloxacin, may be used in place of or in combination with metronidazole. Rifaximin, a nonabsorbable antibiotic, is also sometimes used in treating active Crohn's disease.

Dietary Regimens: Defined-formula liquid diets, in which each nutritional component is precisely measured, may improve the condition of an intestinal obstruction or fistula at least for a short time. Nutritional therapy also may help children grow more than they might otherwise, especially when given at nighttime by tube feeding. These diets may be tried before or in addition to surgery. Occasionally, concentrated nutrients are given intravenously to compensate for the poor absorption of nutrients that is typical of Crohn's disease.

Surgery: Most people with Crohn's disease require surgery at some point during their illness. Surgery is needed when the intestine is obstructed or when abscesses or fistulas do not heal. An operation to remove diseased sections of the intestine may relieve symptoms indefinitely, but it does not cure the disease. Crohn's disease tends to recur where the remaining intestine is rejoined, although several drug therapies initiated after surgery reduce this tendency. A second operation is ultimately needed in nearly half of the people. Consequently, surgery is performed only if specific complications or the failure of

drug therapy makes it necessary. Still, most people who have undergone surgery consider their quality of life to be better than it was before the operation.

Ulcerative Colitis

Ulcerative colitis is a chronic disease in which the large intestine becomes inflamed and ulcerated (pitted or eroded), leading to flare-ups (bouts or attacks) of bloody diarrhea, abdominal cramps, and fever. The long-term risk of colon cancer is increased.

- The exact cause of this disease is not known.
- Typical symptoms during flare-ups include abdominal cramps, an urge to move the bowels, and diarrhea (typically bloody).
- The diagnosis is based on an examination of the sigmoid colon using a flexible viewing tube (sigmoidoscopy) or an examination of the large intestine using a flexible viewing tube (colonoscopy).
- People who have had ulcerative colitis for a long time may develop colon cancer.
- Treatment is aimed at controlling the inflammation, reducing symptoms, and replacing any lost fluids and nutrients.

Ulcerative colitis may start at any age but usually begins between the ages of 15 and 30. A small group of people have their first attack between the ages of 50 and 70.

Ulcerative colitis usually does not affect the full thickness of the wall of the large intestine and hardly ever affects the small intestine. The disease usually begins in the rectum or the rectum and the sigmoid colon (the lower end of the large intestine) but may eventually spread along part or all of the large intestine.

Ulcerative proctitis, which is confined to the rectum, is a very common and relatively benign form of ulcerative colitis. In some people, most of the large intestine is affected early on.

The cause of ulcerative colitis is not known for certain, but heredity and an overactive immune response in the intestine seem to be contributing factors. Cigarette smoking, which is detrimental in Crohn's disease, seems to decrease the risk of ulcerative colitis. However, smoking to reduce the risk of ulcerative colitis is ill-advised in light of the many health problems that smoking can cause.

Symptoms

The symptoms of ulcerative colitis occur in flare-ups. A flare-up may be sudden and severe, causing violent diarrhea (typically bloody), high fever, abdominal pain, and peritonitis (inflammation of the lining of the abdominal cavity). During such flare-ups, the person is profoundly ill. More often, a flare-up begins gradually, and the person has an urgency to have a bowel movement (defecate), mild cramps in the lower abdomen, and visible blood and mucus in the stool. A flare-up can last days or weeks and can recur at any time.

When the disease is limited to the rectum and the sigmoid colon, the stool may be normal or hard and dry; however, mucus containing large numbers of red and white blood cells is discharged from the rectum during or between bowel movements. General symptoms of illness, such as fever, are mild or absent.

If the disease extends farther up the large intestine, the stool is looser, and the person may have as many as 10 to 20 bowel movements a day. Often, the person has severe abdominal cramps and distressing, painful spasms that accompany the urge to defecate. There is no relief at night. The stool may be watery and contain pus, blood, and mucus. Frequently, the stool consists almost entirely of blood and pus. The person also may have a fever and a poor appetite and may lose weight.

Complications: Bleeding, the most common complication, often causes iron deficiency anemia. In nearly 10% of people with ulcerative colitis, a rapidly progressive first attack becomes very severe, with massive bleeding, perforation, or widespread infection.

Toxic colitis, a particularly severe complication, involves damage to the entire thickness of the intestinal wall. The damage causes ileus—a condition in which the normal contractile movements of the intestinal wall temporarily stop—so that the intestinal contents are not propelled along their way. Abdominal expansion (distention) develops. As toxic colitis worsens, the large intestine loses muscle tone, and within days—or even hours—it starts to dilate. X-rays of the abdomen show gas inside the paralyzed sections of intestine.

Toxic megacolon occurs when the large intestine greatly expands (distends). The person is severely ill and may have a high fever. The person also has pain and tenderness in the abdomen and a high white blood cell count. If the intestine ruptures, the risk of death is great. However, of the people who receive prompt treatment before rupture occurs, fewer than 2% die.

Colon cancer occurs in as many as 1 of 100 to 200 people with ulcerative colitis each year in the later stages of their illness. The risk of colon cancer is highest when the entire large intestine is affected and the person has had ulcerative colitis for more than 8 years, even if the disease has not always been clinically active. Colonoscopy (examination of the large intestine using a flexible viewing tube) every 1 to 2 years is advised for people who have had ulcerative colitis for at least 8 years. During

colonoscopy, tissue samples (biopsies) are obtained from areas throughout the large intestine for microscopic examination to detect the early warning signs of cancer (dysplasia). Most people survive if the diagnosis of dysplasia or even cancer is made during the early stages and the colon is removed in time.

Other complications can occur, as in Crohn's disease. When ulcerative colitis causes a flare-up of gastrointestinal symptoms, the person also may experience inflammation of the joints (arthritis), inflammation of the whites of the eyes (episcleritis), inflamed skin nodules (erythema nodosum), and blue-red skin sores containing pus (pyoderma gangrenosum). When ulcerative colitis is not causing a flare-up of gastrointestinal symptoms, the person still may experience pyoderma gangrenosum, and inflammation of the spine (ankylosing spondylitis), inflammation of the pelvic joints (sacroiliitis), and inflammation of the inside of the eye (uveitis) are liable to occur entirely without relation to the bowel disease. Rarely, blood clots develop in the veins.

Although people with ulcerative colitis commonly have minor liver dysfunction, only about 1 to 3% have symptoms of mild to severe liver disease. Severe liver disease can include inflammation of the liver (chronic active hepatitis); inflammation of the bile ducts (primary sclerosing cholangitis), which narrow and eventually close; and replacement of functional liver tissue with scar tissue (cirrhosis). Inflammation of the bile ducts may appear many years before any intestinal symptoms of ulcerative colitis. The inflammation greatly increases the risk of cancer of the bile ducts and also seems to be associated with a sharp increase in the risk of colon cancer.

Diagnosis

The person's symptoms and a stool examination help the doctor suspect the diagnosis. A sigmoidoscopy (an examination of the sigmoid colon using a flexible viewing tube) confirms the diagnosis and permits a doctor to directly observe the severity of the inflammation. Even during symptom-free intervals, the intestine rarely appears entirely normal, and tissue samples removed for microscopic examination usually show chronic inflammation. Blood tests do not confirm the diagnosis but may reveal that the person has anemia, increased numbers of white blood cells, a low level of the protein albumin, and an elevated erythrocyte sedimentation rate (ESR), which indicates active inflammation.

X-rays of the abdomen may indicate the severity and extent of the disease. Barium enema x-ray studies and colonoscopy are not usually done during the active stages of the disease. At some point, however, the entire large intestine is usually evaluated by colonoscopy to determine the extent of the disease.

Prognosis and Treatment

Ulcerative colitis is usually chronic, with repeated flare-ups and remissions. A rapidly progressive initial attack results in serious complications in about 10% of people. Complete recovery after a single attack may occur in another 10%. However, some people who have only a single attack may actually have had an acute undetected infection rather than true ulcerative colitis. Biopsies of the colon can be helpful in making this distinction.

People who have ulcerative proctitis have the best prognosis. Severe complications are unlikely; however, in about 10 to 30% of people, the disease eventually spreads to the large intestine (thus evolving into ulcerative colitis).

Treatment aims to control the inflammation, reduce symptoms, and replace any lost fluids and nutrients.

Dietary Restrictions: Iron supplements may offset anemia caused by ongoing blood loss in the stool. Raw fruits and vegetables should be avoided to reduce injury to the inflamed lining of the large intestine. A diet free of dairy products may decrease symptoms and is worth trying but need not be continued if no benefit is noted.

Antidiarrheal Drugs: Drugs with anticholinergic effects (such as many antihistamines and some antidepressants) or small doses of loperamide or diphenoxylate are taken for relatively mild diarrhea. For more intense diarrhea, higher doses of diphenoxylate or deodorized opium tincture, loperamide, or codeine may be needed. In severe cases, however, a doctor must closely monitor the person taking these antidiarrheal drugs to avoid precipitating toxic megacolon.

Anti-Inflammatory Drugs: Drugs such as sulfasalazine, olsalazine, mesalamine, and balsalazide are used to reduce the inflammation of ulcerative colitis and to prevent flare-ups of symptoms. These drugs usually are taken by mouth (orally), but mesalamine can also be given as an enema or a suppository (rectally). Whether given orally or rectally, these drugs are at best moderately effective for treating mild or moderately active disease, but they are more effective for maintaining remission and possibly even reducing the long-term risk of colorectal cancer.

People with moderately severe disease who are not confined to bed usually take oral corticosteroids such as prednisone. Prednisone in fairly high doses frequently induces a dramatic remission. After prednisone controls the inflammation of ulcerative colitis, sulfasalazine, olsalazine, or mesalamine often is given to maintain the improvement. Gradually, the prednisone dosage is decreased, and ultimately, the prednisone is discontinued. Prolonged corticosteroid treatment almost always causes side effects. When mild or moderate ulcerative colitis is limited to the left side of the large intestine (descending colon) and the rectum, enemas or suppositories with a corticosteroid or mesalamine may be helpful.

If the disease becomes severe, the person is hospitalized, and corticosteroids and fluids are given intravenously. People with heavy rectal bleeding may require blood transfusions.

Immunomodulating Drugs: Drugs such as azathioprine and mercaptopurine have been used to maintain remissions in people with ulcerative colitis who would otherwise need long-term corticosteroid therapy. These drugs inhibit the function of T cells, which are an important component of the immune system. However, these drugs are slow to act, and a benefit may not be seen for 1 to 4 months. They also have potentially serious side effects that require close monitoring by the doctor.

Cyclosporine has been given to some people who have severe flare-ups and have not responded to corticosteroid therapy. Most of these people respond initially to the cyclosporine, but some may still ultimately require surgery.

Infliximab, which is derived from monoclonal antibodies and given intravenously, is beneficial for some people with ulcerative colitis. This drug may be given to people who do not respond to corticosteroids or who develop symptoms whenever corticosteroid doses are lowered, despite the optimal use of other immunomodulating drugs.

Surgery: About 30% of people with extensive ulcerative colitis require surgery. Emergency surgery may be necessary for acute life-threatening attacks with massive bleeding, perforations, toxic megacolon, or blood clotting. Nonemergency reasons for surgery include unremitting chronic disease that is disabling or that constantly requires high doses of corticosteroids.

Surgery is also performed on a nonemergency basis when cancer is diagnosed or dysplasia is identified in the large intestine, and sometimes when there is narrowing of the large intestine or growth retardation in children.

Complete removal of the large intestine and rectum permanently cures ulcerative colitis. Living with a permanent ileostomy (a surgically created connection between the lowest portion of the small intestine and an opening in the abdominal wall) and an ileostomy bag used to be the traditional price of this cure. However, various alternative procedures are now available, the most common one being a procedure called ileo-anal anastomosis. In this procedure, the large intestine and most of the rectum are removed, and a small reservoir is created out of the small intestine and attached to the remaining rectum just above the anus. This procedure maintains continence, although some complications, such as inflammation of the reservoir (pouchitis), may occur.

For people with ulcerative proctitis, surgery is rarely needed, and life expectancy is normal. In some people, though, the symptoms may prove exceptionally resistant to treatment.

Toxic megacolon is an emergency that may require surgery. As soon as a doctor detects it or suspects impending toxic megacolon, all antidiarrheal drugs are discontinued; the person is given nothing to eat; a tube is inserted through the nose and into the stomach or small intestine and attached to intermittent suction; and all fluids, nutrition, and drugs are given intravenously. The person is monitored closely for signs of peritonitis or a perforation. If time and the person's condition permit, drug therapy with cyclosporine or infliximab is sometimes given. If these measures are inappropriate or ineffective, however, emergency surgery is needed: All or most of the large intestine is removed.

Collagenous Colitis and Lymphocytic Colitis

Collagenous colitis and lymphocytic colitis are chronic diseases, characterized by watery diarrhea, in which certain kinds of white blood cells infiltrate the lining of the large intestine.

These chronic diseases can affect the entire length of the large intestine, including the sigmoid colon and the rectum, but often in a patchy distribution. The lining of the intestine develops a thicker layer of a type of connective tissue (collagen) or an accumulation of lymphocytes (a certain type of white blood cell).

The cause is unknown, although an overactive immune response to some unidentified triggering factor seems possible. Many people who develop collagenous colitis or lymphocytic colitis have been regular users of nonsteroidal anti-inflammatory drugs (NSAIDs), but these drugs have not been proven to be a cause of the diseases. Unlike Crohn's disease and ulcerative colitis, collagenous colitis and lymphocytic colitis do not increase the risk of colon cancer.

Collagenous colitis develops primarily in middle-aged or older women, whereas lymphocytic colitis may develop in younger people and occurs in both sexes equally.

Symptoms and Diagnosis

In addition to nonbloody, watery diarrhea, people with collagenous colitis or lymphocytic colitis often experience crampy abdominal pain, nausea, abdominal expansion (distention), and weight loss. Fasting for a few days often leads to a decrease in the frequency and amount of diarrhea. Diarrhea and other symptoms often fluctuate, with periods of worsening symptoms and periods of improvement or complete resolution.

A doctor considers the diagnosis of collagenous colitis or lymphocytic colitis when a person has persistent watery diarrhea and when tests do not reveal another cause. The diseases are diagnosed by microscopic examination of several samples of tissue taken from the lining of the large intestine obtained during colonoscopy (examination of the large intestine with a flexible viewing tube).

Treatment

Antidiarrheal drugs, such as drugs with anticholinergic effects (for example, many antihistamines and some antidepressants) or small doses of loperamide or diphenoxylate, are effective for many people with these diseases. Anti-inflammatory drugs such as bismuth subsalicylate, sulfasalazine, and mesalamine are sometimes effective as well. Budesonide, a newer corticosteroid with fewer side effects, may be very helpful. Otherwise, cholestyramine, a drug that binds bile acids, or antibiotics may be useful. Corticosteroids (such as prednisone) also work well but, because of their serious possible side effects, are usually reserved for people who do not respond to other drug treatment.

Diversion Colitis

Diversion colitis is inflammation that develops in a lower part of the large intestine after the passage of stool above this part has been surgically diverted.

Some people undergo an ileostomy (a surgically created connection between the lowest portion of the small intestine and an opening in the abdominal wall) or a colostomy (the surgical creation of an opening between the large intestine and the abdominal wall). Ileostomies and colostomies may be performed to treat diseases such as cancer, ulcerative colitis, and diverticulitis or to treat damage to the intestine due to an injury. In many people, especially when the doctor expects the need for the bypass of the large intestine to be temporary, either the entire large intestine or a portion of the large intestine is left in place below the point where the flow of stool is diverted.

In about one third of people who have all or a portion of their large intestine left in place after an ileostomy or colostomy, symptoms of diversion colitis, ranging from passage of mucus from the rectum to rectal bleeding and pain, may develop within 1 year after surgery. Most people do not require treatment because the symptoms remain mild. Surgery to reattach the two separated portions of the intestine and restore the normal flow of stool usually leads to resolution of the inflammation and symptoms.

Clostridium difficile–Induced Colitis

Clostridium difficile–*induced colitis (also called antibiotic-associated colitis and pseudomembranous colitis) is inflammation of the large intestine that results in diarrhea. The inflammation is caused by the growth of unusual bacteria, which usually results from antibiotic use.*

- The colitis usually is caused by taking antibiotics.
- Typical symptoms range from slightly loose stools to bloody diarrhea, abdominal pain, and fever.
- Doctors test the stool and examine the large intestine of people who have symptoms of Clostridium difficile–induced colitis.
- Most people who have mild Clostridium difficile–induced colitis get better after the causative antibiotic has been discontinued, but those with a severe infection require other antibiotics.

Many antibiotics alter the balance among the types and quantity of bacteria in the intestine, thus allowing certain disease-causing bacteria to multiply and replace other bacteria. The type of bacteria that most commonly overgrows and causes infection is *Clostridium difficile. Clostridium difficile* infection releases two toxins that can cause inflammation of the protective lining of the large intestine (colitis).

Almost any antibiotic can cause this disorder, but clindamycin, penicillins (such as ampicillin and amoxicillin), and cephalosporins (such as cephalexin) are implicated most often. Other commonly involved antibiotics include erythromycin, sulfonamides (such as sulfamethoxazole), chloramphenicol, tetracycline, and quinolones (such as norfloxacin). *Clostridium difficile* colitis also may follow the use of certain cancer chemotherapy drugs.

Clostridium difficile infection is most common when an antibiotic is taken by mouth, but it also occurs when antibiotics are injected or given intravenously. The risk of developing *Clostridium difficile*–induced colitis increases with age. Other risk factors include having a severe underlying disease, staying for an extended time in the hospital, living in a nursing home, and undergoing gastrointestinal surgery. Drugs and conditions that decrease gastric acidity may also increase susceptibility, particularly proton pump inhibitor drugs.

Sometimes the source of the bacteria is the person's own intestinal tract. *Clostridium difficile* is normally present in the intestines of about 15 to 70% of newborns and a considerable proportion of healthy adults. These populations of people, known as carriers, have the bacteria but do not show any signs of illness. Other times, carriers spread the infection to at-risk people. Additionally, the bacteria are commonly found in soil, water, and household pets. Spread among people can be prevented by meticulous hand washing.

> **Did You Know...**
>
> Many healthy people have *Clostridium difficile* bacteria living in their intestines.

Colitis caused by *Clostridium difficile* infection rarely occurs when there has not been any recent use of antibiotics. Physically stressful events, such as surgery (typically involving the stomach or bowels), can likely lead to the same kind of imbalance among the type and quantity of bacteria in the intestine or can interfere with the intestine's intrinsic defense mechanisms, which in turn allows *Clostridium difficile* infection and colitis to develop.

Symptoms

Symptoms typically begin 5 to 10 days after starting antibiotics but may occur on the first day. However, in one third of people who have this disorder, symptoms do not appear until 1 to 10 days after treatment has stopped, and in some people, symptoms do not appear for as long as 2 months afterward.

Symptoms vary according to the degree of inflammation caused by the bacteria, ranging from slightly loose stools to bloody diarrhea, abdominal pain, and fever. Nausea and vomiting are rare. The most severe cases may involve life-threatening dehydration, low blood pressure, toxic megacolon (see page 173), and perforation of the large intestine.

Diagnosis

Clostridium difficile–induced colitis should be suspected in anyone who develops diarrhea within 2 months of using an antibiotic or within 72 hours of being admitted to a hospital. The diagnosis is confirmed when one of the toxins produced by *Clostridium difficile* is identified in a stool sample. A toxin is found in about 20% of people with mild antibiotic-associated colitis and in more than 90% of those with severe antibiotic-associated colitis. Sometimes two or three stool samples must be obtained before the toxin is detected.

A doctor can also diagnose *Clostridium difficile*–induced colitis by inspecting the lower part of the inflamed large intestine (the sigmoid colon), usually through a sigmoidoscope (a rigid or flexible viewing tube) and observing a specific type of inflammation called pseudomembranous colitis. A colonoscope (a longer flexible viewing tube) is used to examine the entire large intestine if the diseased section of intestine is higher than the reach of the sigmoidoscope. These procedures, however, usually are not required.

Treatment

If a person with *Clostridium difficile*–induced colitis has diarrhea while taking antibiotics, the drugs are discontinued immediately unless they are essential. Drugs that slow the movement of the intestine, such as diphenoxylate, usually are avoided because they may prolong the disorder by keeping the disease-causing toxin in contact with the large intestine. *Clostridium difficile*–induced colitis without complications usually subsides on its own within 10 to 12 days after the antibiotic has been stopped. When it does, no other therapy is required. However, if mild symptoms persist, cholestyramine resin may be effective, probably because it binds itself to the toxin.

For most cases of more severe *Clostridium difficile*–induced colitis, the antibiotic metronidazole is usually effective against *Clostridium difficile*. The antibiotic vancomycin is reserved for the most severe or resistant cases. Some people require bacitracin or *Saccharomyces boulardii*, a yeast probiotic. Symptoms return in up to 20% of people with this disorder, and treatment with antibiotics is repeated. If diarrhea returns repeatedly, prolonged antibiotic therapy may be needed. In very rare instances, people are treated with preparations of lactobacillus given by mouth; an enema of fecal material, which recolonizes the intestine with normal bacteria; or intravenous gamma globulin. Doctors are studying whether the antibiotic rifaximin will prove effective in treating *Clostridium difficile*–induced colitis and whether vaccination against *Clostridium difficile* may help in the treatment of refractory (treatment-resistant) disease and even prevent the disease in people at risk.

Rarely, *Clostridium difficile*–induced colitis is so severe that the person must be hospitalized to receive intravenous fluids, electrolytes (such as sodium, magnesium, calcium, and potassium), and blood transfusions. A temporary ileostomy (a surgically created connection between the small intestine and an opening in the abdominal wall that diverts stool from the large intestine and rectum) or surgical removal of the large intestine (colectomy) occasionally is needed in these severe cases as a lifesaving measure.

CHAPTER

27 / Diverticular Disease

Diverticular disease is characterized by small, balloon-like sacs (diverticula) protruding through the muscular layer of the gastrointestinal (digestive) tract.

By far, the most common site for diverticula to develop is in the large intestine. Rarely, diverticula develop in the stomach and small intestine. Meckel's diverticulum is the most common diverticular disease of the small intestine. It is present at birth in about 2 to 3% of people (see page 1798). The presence of diverticula is called diverticulosis—a condition that tends to develop during middle age. If diverticula become inflamed, the condition is called diverticulitis.

Diverticulosis

Diverticulosis is the presence of multiple balloon-like sacs (diverticula), usually in the large intestine.

- Spasms of the muscular layer of the intestine are thought to cause diverticula.

- Diverticula usually cause no symptoms, but sometimes they bleed, causing blood in the stool or bleeding from the rectum.
- Typically, the diagnosis is confirmed by colonoscopy or a barium enema x-ray.
- A high-fiber diet and stool-bulking agents are given, but sometimes bleeding requires colonoscopy or even surgery.

Diverticula may develop anywhere in the large intestine, but they are more common in the sigmoid colon, which is the last part of the large intestine just before the rectum. Diverticula vary in diameter from 1/10 inch to 1 inch (about 1/4 to 2 1/2 centimeters). They are uncommon before age 40 but become more common rapidly thereafter. Just about everyone who reaches age 90 has many diverticula. Giant diverticula, which are rare, range from 1 to 6 inches (about 2 1/2 to 15 centimeters) in diameter. A person may have only a single giant diverticulum.

Causes

Diverticula are thought to be caused by spasms of the muscular layer of the intestine. The cause of these intestinal spasms is unknown but may be related to a low-fiber diet. The resulting pressure that these spasms exert on the intestinal wall causes a part of the wall to bulge at a point of weakness, usually near to where an artery penetrates the muscular layer of the large intestine. An increase in the thickness of the muscular layer is a common finding in the sigmoid colon of people with diverticulosis. The cause of a giant diverticulum is unclear.

Symptoms

Diverticula themselves are not dangerous. In fact, most people with diverticulosis do not have symptoms. However, diverticulosis can sometimes cause unexplained painful cramps, bowel movement disturbances, and blood in the stool. The narrow opening of a diverticulum can bleed, sometimes heavily, into the intestine and out through the rectum. Bleeding may also result when stool gets wedged in the diverticulum and damages a blood vessel (usually the artery beside the diverticulum). Stool that is trapped in a diverticulum may cause not only bleeding but also inflammation and infection, resulting in diverticulitis.

What Is Diverticulosis?

In diverticulosis, many balloon-like sacs (diverticula) develop in the large intestine, most commonly in the last part of it (sigmoid colon). Most diverticula vary in diameter from 1/10 inch to more than 1 inch (about 1/4 centimeter to more than 2 1/2 centimeters). For unclear reasons, some diverticula become very large—up to 6 inches (about 15 centimeters) in diameter.

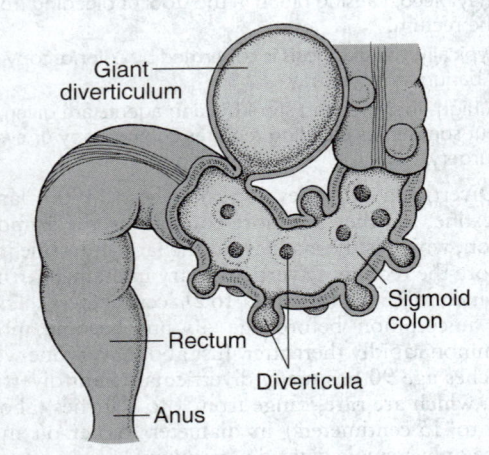

Giant diverticulum

Sigmoid colon

Rectum

Diverticula

Anus

Diagnosis

Diverticulosis is suspected when symptoms such as unexplained painful cramps, bowel movement disturbances, or rectal bleeding are present. The diagnosis is usually confirmed by colonoscopy or sometimes a barium enema x-ray study (see page 130). However, if the person has severe abdominal pain, computed tomography (CT) is performed instead, so as not to rupture the inflamed intestine.

If blood is present in the stool, a colonoscopy is usually the best method with which to identify the source. However, angiography or radionuclide scans taken after an intravenous injection of radioactive red blood cells may be required to determine the source of bleeding.

Treatment

The goal of treatment is usually to reduce intestinal spasms, which is best achieved by maintaining a high-fiber diet (which consists of vegetables, fruits, and whole grains) and drinking plenty of fluids. An increased bulk in the large intestine reduces spasms, which in turn decreases the pressure on the walls of the large intestine. If a high-fiber diet alone is not effective, a diet supplemented daily with bran or a bulking agent, such as psyllium or methylcellulose, may help.

Uncomplicated diverticulosis, in which a person has no evidence of inflammation, infection, or complications, does not require surgery. Most bleeding stops without treatment, but if it does not, doctors often perform a colonoscopy to clot (coagulate) the bleeding area by injecting the area with a drug. If bleeding recurs often or if the source of the bleeding cannot be determined, surgery to remove most of the large intestine may be needed, but such surgery is not commonly done.

A giant diverticulum usually requires surgery, because it is likely to become infected and to rupture.

Diverticulitis

Diverticulitis is inflammation or infection of one or more balloon-like sacs (diverticula).

- Diverticulitis usually affects the colon.
- Pain and tenderness (usually in the left lower part of the abdomen) and fever are the typical symptoms.
- The diagnosis is usually confirmed by CT scan, often followed later by colonoscopy.
- People with mild symptoms are treated with rest, a liquid diet, and oral antibiotics, whereas those with severe symptoms are hospitalized for treatment with intravenous antibiotics and sometimes surgery.

Diverticulitis occurs in people with diverticulosis. It most commonly affects the sigmoid colon, which is the last part of the large intestine just before the rectum. Diverticulitis is more common among people

Complications of Diverticular Disease

In diverticular disease, a diverticulum may bleed into the intestine. If a diverticulum ruptures, the contents of the intestine, including bacteria and blood, spill into the abdominal cavity, often causing infection. An abnormal channel (fistula) may form between the large intestine and another organ, usually when a diverticulum that touches another organ ruptures.

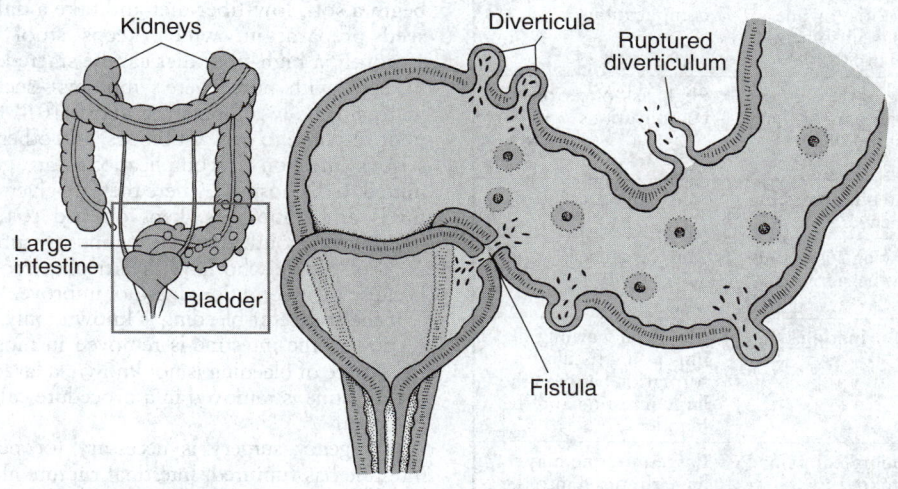

Once inflammation has subsided or infection has been treated, a doctor may perform a colonoscopy older than 40. It can be severe in people of any age, although it is most serious in the elderly, especially those taking corticosteroids or other drugs that suppress the immune system and thus increase the risk of infection. Among people younger than 50 who must undergo surgery for diverticulitis, men outnumber women 3 to 1. Among those older than 70, women outnumber men 3 to 1.

Symptoms and Diagnosis

Diverticulitis typically causes pain, tenderness (usually in the left lower part of the abdomen), and fever. Unlike diverticulosis, diverticulitis generally does not cause gastrointestinal bleeding.

If a doctor knows that the person already has diverticulosis, a diagnosis of diverticulitis may be based almost entirely on the symptoms. However, many other conditions involving the large intestine and other organs in the abdomen and pelvis can cause symptoms similar to diverticulitis, including appendicitis, colon or ovarian cancer, a pus-filled pocket of infection (abscess), and noncancerous (benign) growths on the wall of the uterus (uterine fibroids).

A computed tomography (CT) or ultrasound scan may be helpful in determining that the problem is diverticulitis and not appendicitis or an abscess.

Once inflammation has subsided or infection has been treated, a doctor may perform a colonoscopy (an examination of the large intestine using a flexible viewing tube) or a barium enema x-ray study (see page 130). These tests are performed to either confirm the presence or assess the severity of diverticula and to rule out colon cancer. Colonoscopy or barium enema x-rays usually need to be delayed for several weeks after treatment, because they could damage or rupture an inflamed intestine. Exploratory surgery is rarely needed to confirm the diagnosis.

Complications: The inflammation of the intestinal wall can lead to the development of fistulas (abnormal channels) that connect the large intestine with other organs. Fistulas usually form when a diverticulum in the large intestine is touching another organ (such as the bladder) and the diverticulum ruptures. The resulting inflammation along with the bacterial contents of the large intestine slowly penetrate the adjacent organ, resulting in a fistula. Most fistulas form between the sigmoid colon and the bladder. These fistulas are more common among men than women, although women who have had a hysterectomy (removal of the uterus) are at increased risk, because the large intestine and bladder are no longer separated by the uterus. When fistulas form between the large intestine and bladder, intestinal contents, including normal bacteria, enter the bladder and cause urinary tract infections. Less commonly, a fistula can develop

DIVERTICULITIS: REASONS FOR ELECTIVE SURGERY

CONDITION	REASON
Two or more severe attacks of diverticulitis (or one severe attack in someone younger than 50)	High risk of serious complications
Narrowing of the sigmoid colon (lower part of the large intestine) due to scarring	High risk of serious complications
Persistent tender mass in the abdomen	May be cancer
X-ray showing suspicious changes in the sigmoid colon	May be cancer
Pain when urinating	May be a warning of impending fistula formation between the large intestine and the bladder
Sudden abdominal pain in people taking corticosteroids	Large intestine may have ruptured into the abdominal cavity

between the large intestine and the small intestine, uterus, vagina, abdominal wall, or even the thigh or chest.

Other possible complications of diverticulitis include inflammation of nearby organs (such as the uterus, bladder, or other areas of the digestive tract), rupture of the wall of a diverticulum, abscess (a pus-filled pocket of infection), infection of the lining of the abdominal cavity (peritonitis), and bleeding. Repeated bouts of diverticulitis can lead to intestinal obstruction, because the resulting scarring and muscle thickening can narrow

the inside of the large intestine and prevent solid stool from passing through.

Treatment

Mild diverticulitis can be treated with rest, a liquid diet, and oral antibiotics. Symptoms usually disappear rapidly. After a few days, the person can begin a soft, low-fiber diet and take a daily psyllium seed preparation, which keeps stool soft. After 1 month, a high-fiber diet can be started.

People with more severe symptoms—such as abdominal pain, body temperature above 101° F (38.3° C), poor response to oral antibiotics, and other evidence of serious infection or complications—are generally admitted to the hospital. There they are given intravenous fluids and antibiotics, kept on bed rest, and given nothing by mouth until the symptoms subside. About 20% of people who have diverticulitis require surgery because their condition does not improve.

If the source of bleeding is known, only the affected section of the intestine is removed in most people. If the source of bleeding is not known, a larger section of the intestine is removed in a procedure called subtotal colectomy.

Emergency surgery is necessary for people whose intestine has ruptured. Intestinal rupture always results in infection of the abdominal cavity. The surgeon generally removes the ruptured section and creates an opening between the large intestine and the skin surface. This opening is called a colostomy (see art on page 194). About 10 to 12 weeks later (or sometimes longer), the cut ends of the intestine are rejoined during a follow-up operation, and the colostomy is closed.

Surgery may be optional for some people with diverticulitis. If an abscess is discovered, draining it with a needle inserted through the skin and guided by a CT scan might be attempted before surgery is considered.

Treatment of a fistula involves removing the section of large intestine where the fistula begins, rejoining the cut ends of the large intestine, and repairing the other affected area (for example, the bladder or small intestine).

28 Irritable Bowel Syndrome

Irritable bowel syndrome (IBS) is a disorder of the entire digestive tract that causes abdominal pain and constipation or diarrhea.

- Symptoms vary but often include lower abdominal pain, bloating, gas, and constipation or diarrhea.
- A variety of substances and emotional factors can trigger symptoms of IBS.
- A doctor usually diagnoses IBS based on the symptoms but performs tests to rule out other problems.
- A regular diet is often best, and drugs can usually relieve specific symptoms.

IBS affects about 10 to 15% of the general population. Some but not all studies suggest women with IBS are more likely to consult a doctor. IBS is the most common disorder diagnosed by gastroenterologists (doctors who specialize in disorders of the digestive tract).

IBS is generally classified as a functional disorder because it impairs the functioning of the body's normal activities, such as the movement of the intestines, the sensitivity of the nerves of the intestines, or the way in which the brain controls some of these functions. Although the normal functioning is impaired, there are no structural abnormalities that can be seen with an endoscope (a flexible viewing tube), x-rays, or blood tests. Thus, IBS is identified by the characteristics of the symptoms and, when needed, the results of limited tests.

Causes

The cause of IBS is not clear. In many people with IBS, the digestive tract is especially sensitive to many stimuli. People may experience discomfort caused by intestinal gas or contractions that other people do not find distressing. Although the changes in bowel movements that occur with IBS might seem to be related to abnormal intestinal contractions, not all people with IBS have abnormal contractions, and in many of those that do, the abnormal contractions do not always coincide with symptoms.

Emotional factors (for example, stress, anxiety, depression, and fear), diet, drugs, hormones, or minor irritants may trigger or worsen a flare-up (a bout or attack) of IBS. For some people, high-calorie meals or a high-fat diet may be a trigger (precipitating factor). For other people, wheat, dairy products, coffee, tea, or citrus fruits seem to aggravate the symptoms. Because many food products contain several ingredients, it may be difficult to identify the specific trigger. Others find that eating too quickly or eating after too long a period

without food stimulates a flare-up. However, the relationship is inconsistent. A person does not always get symptoms after a usual trigger, and symptoms often appear without any obvious trigger. It is not clear how all the triggers relate to the cause of IBS.

Symptoms

IBS tends to begin in the teens and 20s, causing bouts of symptoms that recur at irregular periods. Onset in late adult life is less common but not rare. Flare-ups almost always occur when a person is awake, and they rarely wake a person from sleep.

Symptoms include abdominal pain related to or relieved by having a bowel movement (defecation), change in stool frequency (such as constipation or diarrhea) or consistency, abdominal expansion (distention), mucus in the stool, and the sensation of incomplete emptying after defecation. The pain may come in bouts of continuous dull aching or cramps, usually over the lower abdomen. Bloating, gas, nausea, headaches, fatigue, depression, anxiety, and difficulty concentrating are other possible symptoms. In general, the character and location of pain, triggers, and the pattern of bowel movements are relatively consistent over time. However, symptoms may increase or decrease in severity and also change over time.

Diagnosis

Most people with IBS appear healthy. A physical examination generally does not reveal anything unusual except sometimes tenderness over the large intestine. Doctors usually perform some tests—for example, blood tests, a stool examination, and a sigmoidoscopy (see page 129)—to differentiate IBS from Crohn's disease, ulcerative colitis, cancer (mainly in people over age 40), collagenous colitis, lymphocytic colitis, and the many other diseases that can cause abdominal pain and changes in bowel habits. These test results are usually normal in people with IBS, although the stool may be watery, and the sigmoidoscopy procedure may cause an unusual amount of spasms and pain. Doctors usually perform more tests—such as abdominal ultrasound, x-rays of the intestines, or a colonoscopy (see page 129)—in older people and in those who have symptoms that are unusual for IBS, such as fever, bloody stools, weight loss, and vomiting.

Other digestive tract disorders (such as appendicitis, gallbladder disease, ulcers, and cancer) may develop in a person with IBS, particularly after age 40. Thus, if a person's symptoms change significantly or are unusual for IBS, further testing may be needed.

Treatment

Treatment differs from person to person. If particular foods or types of stress appear to bring on the problem, they should be avoided if possible. For most people, especially those who tend to be constipated, regular physical activity helps keep the digestive tract functioning normally.

In general, a normal diet is best. Many people do better eating frequent, smaller meals rather than less frequent, larger meals (for example, five or six small meals rather than three large meals a day). People with bloating and increased gas (flatulence) should avoid beans, cabbage, and other foods that are difficult to digest. Sorbitol, an artificial sweetener used in dietetic foods and in some drugs and chewing gums, should not be consumed in large amounts. Fructose, a sugar found in fruits, berries, and some plants, should be eaten only in small amounts. A low-fat diet helps some people, particularly those whose stomach empties too slowly or too quickly. People who have both IBS and lactase deficiency should consume dairy products in moderation. Even patients with lactase deficiency can probably tolerate a glass of milk consumed in small amounts during the day.

Constipation can often be relieved by eating more fiber. People with constipation can take a tablespoon of raw bran with plenty of water and other fluids at each meal, or they can take psyllium mucilloid supplements with two glasses of water. Increasing the dietary fiber may aggravate flatulence and bloating. Occasionally, such flatulence may be reduced by switching to a synthetic fiber preparation (such as methylcellulose). Certain laxatives are often effective and reasonably safe. Such laxatives include those containing sorbitol, lactulose, or polyethylene glycol, and stimulant laxatives such as those containing bisacodyl or glycerin. Lubiprostone, a newer laxative, may also relieve constipation.

Smooth-muscle relaxants, such as dicyclomine, can relieve abdominal pain but often cause anticholinergic side effects (see box on page 1897), such as dry mouth, blurred vision, or difficulty urinating.

Antidiarrheal drugs, such as diphenoxylate or loperamide, help people with diarrhea, as may drugs such as alosetron, which decrease the effects of serotonin, a chemical messenger in the body. Aromatic oils, such as oil of peppermint, often help symptoms of flatulence and cramping. Antidepressants, behavior modification techniques (such as cognitive-behavioral therapy), psychotherapy, and hypnosis are often extremely effective for managing symptoms of IBS. Long-term use of antidepressants in low or higher doses is reasonably safe. Antidepressants may not only relieve pain and other symptoms but also may help relieve sleep problems and depression or anxiety.

CHAPTER 29

Anal and Rectal Disorders

The anus is the opening at the end of the digestive tract where stool leaves the body. The rectum is the section of the digestive tract above the anus where stool is held before it passes out of the body through the anus.

The anus is formed partly from the surface layers of the body, including the skin, and partly from the intestine. The rectal lining consists of glistening red tissue containing mucus glands—much like the rest of the intestinal lining. The lining of the rectum is relatively insensitive to pain, but the nerves from the anus and nearby external skin are very sensitive to pain.

The veins from the rectum and anus drain into the portal vein, which leads to the liver, and then into the general circulation. The lymph vessels of the rectum drain into lymph nodes in the lower abdomen. Those of the anus drain into the lymph nodes in the groin.

A muscular ring (anal sphincter) keeps the anus closed. This sphincter is controlled subconsciously by the autonomic nervous system (see page 831); however, the lower part of the sphincter can be relaxed or tightened at will.

To diagnose disorders of the anus and rectum, a doctor inspects the skin around the anus for any abnormality. With a gloved finger, the doctor probes the rectum. For women, this is often done along with a manual examination of the vagina.

Next, a doctor looks into the anus and rectum with a 3- to 10-inch (about 7.6- to 25-centimeter) rigid viewing tube (anoscope or proctoscope). A longer, flexible tube (sigmoidoscope—see page 129) may then be inserted so that the doctor can observe as much as 2 or more feet of the large intestine. An anoscopy or sigmoidoscopy is generally uncomfortable but not painful. However, if the area in or around the anus is painful because of an abnormal condition, the doctor may give a local, regional, or even general anesthetic before proceeding with the examination. Sometimes a cleansing enema to rid the lower part of the large intestine of stool is given before sigmoidoscopy. Tissue and stool samples for microscopic examination and cultures may be obtained during sigmoidoscopy. A barium enema x-ray may also be performed.

Anal Fissure

An anal fissure is a tear or ulcer in the lining of the anus.

Anal fissures may be caused by an injury from a hard or large bowel movement. Uncommonly, they may also be caused by penetration of the anus during anal sex. Fissures cause the anal sphincter to go into spasm, which worsens pain and prevents healing.

Fissures cause pain and bleeding, usually during or shortly after a bowel movement. The pain lasts for several minutes to several hours and then subsides until the next bowel movement. A doctor diagnoses a fissure by gently inspecting the anus.

Treatment

A stool softener or psyllium or increased dietary fiber may reduce the possibility of reinjury by hard bowel movements. Healing is aided by use of protective zinc oxide ointments or bland suppositories (such as glycerin) that lubricate the lower rectum and soften stool. A warm sitz bath for 10 to 15 minutes after each bowel movement eases discomfort and helps increase blood flow, which promotes healing.

Treatments to reduce sphincter spasm and promote healing of fissures include injecting the sphincter with botulinum toxin and applying nitroglycerin ointment or calcium channel blockers to the area of the fissure.

If these measures do not work, surgery may be needed. Sphincter spasm can be relieved either by stretching (dilating) the anus or by cutting the internal sphincter (internal anal sphincterotomy).

Anal Itching

Itchy skin around the anus (pruritus ani) can have many causes.

After bowel movements, the anal area should be cleaned with absorbent cotton or soft, plain toilet or facial tissue, which may be moistened with warm water. Frequent dusting with cornstarch or talcum

CAUSES OF ANAL ITCHING	
CATEGORY	**EXAMPLES**
Disorders	
Anal disorders	Bowen's disease
	Fistulas that drain
	Inflammation of a follicle in the rectum (cryptitis)
	Paget's disease of the anal sweat glands
Bacterial infections*	
Fungal infections	Yeast infection (candidiasis)
Parasitic infections	Pinworms
	Scabies
Skin disorders	Atopic dermatitis
	Psoriasis
	Skin tags
Other disorders	Diabetes
	Liver disorders
Other factors	
Anxiety	Anxiety about itching (anxiety-itch-anxiety cycle)
Drugs	Antibiotics
Foods and dietary supplements	Beer
	Caffeinated beverages (such as coffee and cola)
	Citrus fruits
	Spices
	Vitamin C tablets
Hygiene-related problems	Excessive sweating
	Overly meticulous cleansing
	Poor cleansing
	Tight undergarments
Skin irritants	Anesthetic preparations
	Ointments
	Soaps

*Bacterial infections around the anus often start when scratching breaks the skin so that bacteria can enter the body.

powder helps combat moisture. Corticosteroid creams, antifungal creams such as miconazole, or soothing suppositories may be used. Foods that can cause anal itching are avoided for a while to see whether the condition improves. Clothing should be loose, and bed clothing should be lightweight. If the condition does not improve and a doctor suspects cancer, a skin specimen may be obtained for examination.

Anorectal Abscess

An anorectal abscess is a pus-filled cavity caused by bacteria invading a mucus-secreting gland in the anus and rectum.

- Bacteria infect a gland in the anus or rectum and create an abscess.
- The infection produces pus and causes pain and swelling.
- The diagnosis is based on an examination and the results of imaging tests if needed.
- Cutting and draining the abscess is the best form of treatment.

An abscess may be deep in the rectum or close to the opening of the anus. An abscess develops when bacteria invade a mucus-secreting gland in the anus or rectum, where they multiply. Although the anus is an area that is rich in bacteria, infection generally does not occur because the internal sphincter acts as a barrier and blood flow to the area is rich. When infection does occur, it usually is caused by a combination of different types of bacteria. An abscess can cause substantial damage to nearby tissues and may lead to fecal incontinence. People who have Crohn's disease are at particular risk of abscesses. Sometimes, abscesses are a complication of diverticulitis or pelvic inflammatory disease.

Symptoms and Diagnosis

Abscesses just under the skin can be swollen, red, tender, and very painful. Abscesses deep in the rectum often cause fewer symptoms but may cause fever and pain in the lower abdomen. A doctor can usually see an abscess if it is in the skin around the anus. When no external swelling or redness is seen, however, a doctor can make the diagnosis by examining the rectum with a gloved finger. A tender swelling in the rectum indicates an abscess. If the doctor suspects a deep abscess, magnetic resonance imaging (MRI), computed tomography (CT), or ultrasonography can determine the extent and location.

Treatment

Antibiotics have limited value except for people who have a fever, diabetes, or an infection elsewhere in the body. For an abscess just under the skin, treatment consists of cutting into the abscess and draining the pus after a local anesthetic has been given. For a deeper abscess, the person is usually hospitalized, and the abscess is drained in the operating room after general anesthesia has been given. Even with proper treatment, in about two thirds of people, an abscess leads to the formation of an abnormal channel from the anus or rectum to the skin (anorectal fistula).

Anorectal Fistula

An anorectal fistula is an abnormal channel that leads from the anus or rectum usually to the skin near the anus but occasionally to another organ, such as the vagina.

- Anorectal fistulas are common among people who have an anorectal abscess, Crohn's disease, or tuberculosis.
- Anorectal fistulas can cause pain and produce pus.
- The diagnosis is based on an examination and other viewing techniques.
- Treatment may involve surgery, but some nonsurgical alternatives now exist.

Most fistulas begin in a deep gland in the wall of the anus or rectum. Sometimes fistulas occur after drainage of an anorectal abscess, but often the cause cannot be identified. Fistulas are more common among people with Crohn's disease or tuberculosis. They also occur in people with tumors, diverticulitis, cancer, or an anal or rectal injury. A fistula in an infant is usually a birth defect and is more common among boys than girls. Fistulas that connect the rectum and vagina may result from radiation therapy, cancer, Crohn's disease, or an injury to a mother during childbirth.

Symptoms and Diagnosis

An infected fistula may be painful and may discharge pus. A doctor can usually see one or more openings of a fistula or can feel the fistula beneath the surface. A probe may be inserted to determine its depth and direction. Looking through an anoscope inserted into the rectum and exploring with the probe, a doctor may locate the internal opening. Inspection with a sigmoidoscope, which is a much longer viewing scope, helps a doctor determine whether the problem is being caused by cancer, Crohn's disease, or another disorder.

Treatment

Previously, the only effective treatment was surgery to open the fistula (fistulotomy). During surgery, sometimes the sphincter is partially cut. If too much of the sphincter is cut, the person may have difficulty controlling bowel movements. Newer surgical procedures use advancement flaps (flaps are stretched over the opening of the fistula). Biologic plugs and fibrin glue instillations are alternatives to surgery.

If the person has diarrhea or Crohn's disease, which may delay wound healing, surgery usually is not performed. Drug treatment for Crohn's disease (see page 170) can help a fistula close.

Foreign Objects

Swallowed objects, such as toothpicks, chicken bones, or fish bones, may become lodged at the junction between the anus and rectum (anorectal junction). Also, enema tips, surgical sponges or instruments, thermometers, and objects used for sexual stimulation may become lodged unintentionally in the rectum after being passed through the anus.

Sudden, excruciating pain during bowel movements suggests that a foreign object, usually at the anorectal junction, is penetrating the lining of the anus or rectum. Other symptoms depend on the size and shape of the object, how long it has been there, and whether it has perforated (pierced) the anus or rectum or caused an infection.

A doctor can feel the object by probing with a gloved finger during an examination. An abdominal examination, sigmoidoscopy, and x-rays may be needed to make sure the wall of the large intestine has not been perforated.

Treatment

If a doctor can feel the object, a local anesthetic is usually injected under the skin and lining of the anus to numb the area. The anus can then be spread wider with an instrument called a rectal retractor, and the object can be grasped and removed. Natural movements of the wall of the large intestine (peristalsis) generally bring higher foreign objects down, making removal possible.

Occasionally, if a doctor cannot feel the object or if the object cannot be removed through the anus, exploratory surgery is needed. The person is given a regional or general anesthetic so that the object can be gently moved toward the anus or so that the rectum can be cut open to remove the object. After the object is removed, the doctor performs a sigmoidoscopy (a flexible tube is inserted into the anus to view the lower portion of the large intestine, the rectum, and the anus) to determine whether the rectum has been perforated or otherwise injured.

Hemorrhoids

Hemorrhoids are dilated, twisted (varicose) veins located in the wall of the rectum and anus.

- The swollen veins are caused by an increase in pressure.
- Lumps form inside or outside of the anus, which can cause pain or bleeding.

- The diagnosis is based on an examination of the anus and rectum with an anoscope, sigmoidoscope, or colonoscope.
- Most hemorrhoids go away without treatment, but stool softeners and sitz baths can help relieve symptoms.
- Some hemorrhoids are treated with a rubber band procedure or surgery.

Hemorrhoids occur when the veins in the rectum or anus become enlarged. Hemorrhoids that form above the boundary between the rectum and anus (anorectal junction) are called internal hemorrhoids. Hemorrhoids that form below the anorectal junction are called external hemorrhoids. Both internal and external hemorrhoids may remain in the anus or protrude outside the anus. External hemorrhoids may become inflamed or develop a blood clot (thrombus). Internal hemorrhoids may bleed.

Causes

Increased pressure in the veins of the anorectal area leads to hemorrhoids. This pressure may result from pregnancy, frequent heavy lifting, or repeated straining during bowel movements (defecation). Constipation may contribute to straining. In a few people, hemorrhoids develop from increased blood pressure in the portal vein.

Symptoms and Diagnosis

External hemorrhoids form a lump on the anus. If a thrombus forms (thrombosed external hemorrhoid), the lump becomes quite painful and more swollen. Internal hemorrhoids often do not cause a visible lump or pain, but they can bleed. Bleeding from internal hemorrhoids typically occurs with bowel movements, causing blood-streaked stool or toilet paper. The blood may turn water in the toilet bowl red. However, the amount of blood is usually small, and hemorrhoids rarely lead to severe blood loss or anemia.

Hemorrhoids may discharge mucus and create a feeling that the rectum is not completely emptied after a bowel movement. Itching in the anal region (pruritus ani) is usually not a symptom of hemorrhoids, but itching may develop if hemorrhoids make proper cleaning of the anal region difficult.

A doctor can readily diagnose swollen, painful hemorrhoids by inspecting the anus and rectum. An examination with an anoscope (a short, rigid tube used to view the rectum) or sigmoidoscope (a flexible tube used to view the lower portion of the large intestine, the rectum, and the anus) helps a doctor determine whether the person has a more serious condition, such as a tumor. People who have bleeding from the rectum often require a sigmoidoscopy or colonoscopy.

Banding a Hemorrhoid

Some internal hemorrhoids are removed by tying them off with rubber bands in an outpatient procedure called rubber band ligation. The instrument used (ligator) consists of forceps surrounded by a cylinder with 1/2-inch (1/2-centimeter) rubber bands placed on one end. The ligator is inserted into the anus through an anoscope (a short, rigid viewing tube), and the hemorrhoid is grasped with the forceps. The cylinder is slid upward over the forceps and the hemorrhoid, pushing the rubber bands off the cylinder and around the base of the hemorrhoid. The rubber bands cut off the hemorrhoid's blood supply, causing it to wither and drop off painlessly in a few days. One hemorrhoid is ligated about every 2 weeks. Several treatments may be required. Sometimes, multiple hemorrhoids can be ligated at a single visit.

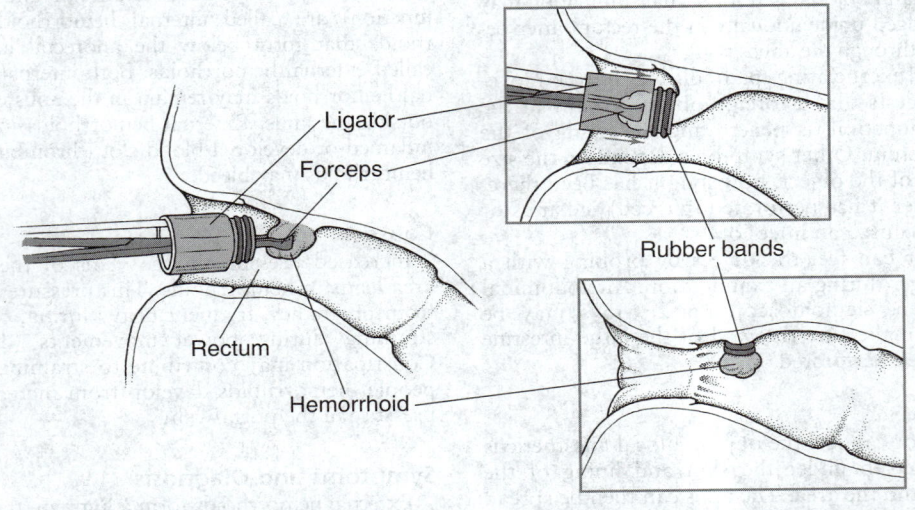

Ligator

Forceps

Rubber bands

Rectum

Hemorrhoid

Treatment

Usually, hemorrhoids do not require treatment unless they cause symptoms. Taking stool softeners or a bulking type of laxative (such as psyllium) may relieve straining with bowel movements. Symptoms can sometimes be relieved by soaking the anus in warm water in what is known as a sitz bath. The soaking is accomplished by squatting or sitting in a partially filled tub or using a container filled with warm water placed on the toilet bowl or commode.

Bleeding hemorrhoids can be treated with an injection of a substance that causes the hemorrhoids to become obliterated with scar tissue. This procedure is called injection sclerotherapy.

Large internal hemorrhoids and those that do not respond to injection sclerotherapy can be tied off with rubber bands (a procedure called rubber band ligation). The band causes the hemorrhoid to wither and drop off painlessly. The treatment is usually applied to one hemorrhoid at a time at intervals of 2 weeks or longer. Internal hemorrhoids may also be destroyed with a laser (laser destruction), an infrared light (infrared photocoagulation), or an electrical current (electrocoagulation).

Surgery to remove the hemorrhoids may be used if other treatments do not work. However, hemorrhoid surgery may result in severe pain, as well as urine retention and constipation. Less painful techniques are being investigated, such as Doppler-guided hemorrhoid artery ligation, in which hemorrhoid arteries are identified and tied off, thus reducing the blood supply to the hemorrhoids. Another technique is called circumferential stapled hemorrhoidopexy, in which a circular surgical stapler is used to remove or resuspend protruding hemorrhoids, but its advantages and indications have yet to be defined.

When a hemorrhoid with a blood clot causes pain, it is treated with nonsteroidal anti-inflammatory drugs, warm sitz baths, local anesthetic ointments, or witch hazel compresses. Pain and swelling usually diminish after a short while, and clots disappear over 4 to 6 weeks. Alternatively, especially when the pain is severe, a doctor may inject a local anesthetic and cut out the hemorrhoid, which sometimes relieves the pain rapidly.

Levator Syndrome

Levator syndrome is sporadic pain in the rectum caused by spasm of a muscle near the anus (the levator ani muscle).

Proctalgia fugax (fleeting pain in the rectum) and **coccydynia** (pain near the tailbone [coccyx]) are variations of levator syndrome. The muscle spasm causes pain that typically is not related to defecation. The pain usually lasts less than 20 minutes. Pain may be brief and intense or a vague ache high in the rectum. It may occur spontaneously or with sitting and can waken a person from sleep. The pain may feel as if it would be relieved by the passage of gas or a bowel movement. In severe cases, the pain can persist for many hours and can recur frequently. A person may have undergone various unsuccessful rectal operations to relieve these symptoms.

Diagnosis

A doctor performs a physical examination to exclude other painful rectal conditions (such as thrombosed hemorrhoids, fissures, or abscesses). The physical examination is often normal, although the muscle may be tender or tight. Occasionally, the pain is caused by low back or prostate disorders.

Treatment

The doctor explains the benign nature of the condition. An episode may be relieved by the passage of gas or a bowel movement, by a sitz bath, or by a mild pain reliever (such as aspirin). When the symptoms are more intense, people can undergo therapy with electrogalvanic stimulation, in which a high-voltage current is delivered to the muscle via a probe inserted into the anus. Such stimulation helps stop muscle spasms.

Pilonidal Disease

Pilonidal disease is an infection caused by a hair that injures the skin at the top of the cleft between the buttocks.

A pilonidal abscess is a collection of pus at the infection site. A pilonidal sinus is a chronic draining wound at the site.

Pilonidal disease usually occurs in young, hairy, white men but can also occur in women. A pilonidal sinus can cause pain and swelling. To distinguish pilonidal disease from other infections, a doctor looks for pits—tiny holes in or next to the infected area.

Generally, a pilonidal abscess must be cut and drained by a doctor. Usually, a pilonidal sinus must be removed surgically.

Proctitis

Proctitis is inflammation of the lining of the rectum (rectal mucosa).

- The inflammation has many causes ranging from infection to radiation therapy.
- Depending on its cause, proctitis can be painless or very painful.
- A doctor makes the diagnosis after examining the inside of the rectum.
- Antibiotics can treat proctitis caused by an infection.

Proctitis, which is becoming increasingly common, has several causes. It may result from Crohn's disease or ulcerative colitis. It can also result from a sexually transmitted disease (such as gonorrhea, syphilis, *Chlamydia trachomatis* infection, herpes simplex virus infection, or cytomegalovirus infection), especially among homosexual men.

A person whose immune system is impaired is also at increased risk of developing proctitis, particularly from infections by herpes simplex virus or cytomegalovirus. Proctitis may also be caused by some bacteria not transmitted sexually, such as *Salmonella*, or by the use of an antibiotic that destroys normal intestinal bacteria, thus allowing other bacteria to grow in their place (see page 176). Another cause of proctitis is radiation therapy directed at or near the rectum, which is commonly used to treat prostate and rectal cancer.

Symptoms and Diagnosis

Proctitis typically causes painless bleeding or the passage of mucus from the rectum. When the cause is gonorrhea, herpes simplex virus, or cytomegalovirus, the anus and rectum may be intensely painful.

To make the diagnosis, a doctor looks inside the rectum with an anoscope or sigmoidoscope (a tube used to view the rectum or anus) and takes swabs and a tissue sample of the rectal lining for examination. The laboratory then can identify the bacterium, fungus, or virus that may be causing the proctitis. A doctor may also examine other areas of the intestine using colonoscopy.

Treatment

Antibiotics are the best treatment for proctitis caused by a specific bacterial infection. When proctitis is caused by use of an antibiotic that destroys normal intestinal bacteria, a doctor may prescribe metronidazole or vancomycin, which should destroy the harmful bacteria that have displaced the normal ones.

When the cause is radiation therapy or is unknown, anti-inflammatory drugs such as hydrocortisone (a corticosteroid) or mesalamine may provide relief. Both hydrocortisone and mesalamine can be given as either an enema or a suppository. Some corticosteroids are available in a foam preparation that can be inserted with a cartridge and plunger. Mesalamine and other anti-inflammatory drugs, such as sulfasalazine and olsalazine, may be taken by mouth at the same time that drugs are given rectally, for added benefit. If these forms of treatment do not relieve the inflammation, formalin can be applied directly to the area or corticosteroids taken by mouth may be used. Laser or Argon plasma coagulation has also been used.

Rectal Prolapse

Rectal prolapse is a painless protrusion of the rectum through the anus.

- A rectal prolapse is often caused while straining, such as during a bowel movement.
- The diagnosis is based on an examination and various viewing and imaging tests.
- Rectal prolapse in infants and children usually heals without surgery.
- Rectal prolapse in adults is treated surgically.

Rectal prolapse causes the rectum to turn inside out, so that the rectal lining is visible outside the body as a dark red, moist, fingerlike projection from the anus. Bleeding from the rectum can occur, and an uncontrolled loss of urine (urinary incontinence) is a frequent symptom. Less commonly, the rectum protrudes into the vagina (rectocele—see page 1544).

A temporary prolapse of only the rectal lining (mucosa) often occurs in otherwise healthy infants, probably when the infant strains during a bowel movement, and is rarely serious. In adults, prolapse of the rectal lining tends to persist and may worsen, so that more of the rectum protrudes. A complete prolapse of the rectum is called procidentia. This condition occurs most often in women older than age 60.

To determine the extent of a prolapse, a doctor examines the area while the person is standing or squatting and straining. By feeling the anal sphincter with a gloved finger, a doctor often detects diminished muscle tone. A sigmoidoscopy, colonoscopy, or barium enema x-rays of the large intestine may reveal an underlying disease.

Treatment

In infants and children, a stool softener eliminates the urge to strain. Strapping the buttocks together between bowel movements usually helps the prolapse heal on its own.

In adults, surgery is usually needed to correct the problem. Surgery often cures procidentia. During one kind of abdominal operation, the entire rectum is lifted, pulled back, and attached to the sacral bone in the pelvis. In another, a segment of the rectum is removed, and the remainder of the rectum is stitched to the sacral bone.

For people who are too weak to undergo surgery because of extreme old age or poor health, surgery to the rectum is preferred to surgery to the abdomen. One type of surgery to the rectum is performed by inserting a wire or plastic loop to encircle the sphincter in a technique called the Thiersch procedure. Alternatively, a segment of the rectum or the excess lining of the rectum may be cut out (excised).

CHAPTER 30   Tumors of the Digestive System

A variety of abnormal growths (tumors) can develop throughout the digestive system, from the esophagus to the anus, as well as in the liver (see page 238), gallbladder (see page 247), and pancreas. Some of these tumors are noncancerous (benign), whereas others are cancerous (malignant).

Esophageal Tumors That Are Noncancerous

Noncancerous (benign) tumors of the esophagus are rare and are usually more bothersome than harmful.

The most common type of noncancerous tumor is a leiomyoma, a tumor of the smooth muscle. It occurs most frequently in people between the ages of 30 and 60. Most leiomyomas are small and do not require treatment. A small number of leiomyomas grow large enough to cause partial obstruction of the esophagus, which may lead to difficulty swallowing (dysphagia) and pain or discomfort. Analgesics (pain relievers) may provide temporary relief, but surgical removal is needed for permanent relief.

Other types of noncancerous tumors, including those consisting of connective tissue (fibrovascular polyps) and tissues related to nerves (schwannomas), are rare.

Esophageal Cancer

- Esophageal cancers usually develop in the cells that line the wall of the esophagus (the tube that connects the throat to the stomach).
- Tobacco and alcohol use, certain infections, disorders, and other cancers are major risk factors for certain types of esophageal cancer.

- Typical symptoms include difficulty swallowing, weight loss, and, later, pain.
- The diagnosis is based on an endoscopy.
- Unless discovered early, almost all cases of esophageal cancer are fatal.
- Surgery, chemotherapy, and various other therapies can help relieve the symptoms.

The most common types of esophageal cancer are squamous cell carcinoma and adenocarcinoma, which develop in the cells that line the wall of the esophagus. These cancers may develop anywhere in the esophagus and may appear as a narrowing (stricture) of the esophagus, a lump, an abnormal flat area (plaque), or an abnormal connection (fistula) between the esophagus and the airways that supply the lungs. Less common types of esophageal cancer include leiomyosarcomas (cancers of the smooth muscle of the esophagus) and metastatic cancer (cancer that has spread from elsewhere in the body).

Cancer of the esophagus affects about 15,500 people each year in the United States. Both squamous cell carcinoma and adenocarcinoma are more common among men than women. Squamous cell carcinoma is more common among blacks, whereas adenocarcinoma is more common among whites. The frequency of adenocarcinoma has been increasing rapidly in the United States since the 1970s, especially among white men and is now more common than squamous cell carcinoma in the lower part of the esophagus.

Risk Factors

Tobacco use (any kind) and alcohol are the most important risk factors for developing esophageal cancer, although more so for squamous cell carcinoma than for adenocarcinoma. People who have had certain human papillomavirus infections, who have had head and neck cancer, or who have undergone radiation therapy to the esophagus for treatment of other nearby cancers are at greater risk of developing esophageal cancer.

People with an existing disorder of the esophagus, such as achalasia, esophageal webs (Plummer-Vinson syndrome), or narrowing due to having once swallowed a corrosive substance (such as lye), are also at greater risk of developing esophageal cancer. Prolonged irritation of the esophagus caused by the repeated backflow of stomach acid (gastroesophageal reflux) can cause a precancerous condition called Barrett's esophagus. Although esophageal cancer caused by Barrett's esophagus remains relatively rare in most industrialized countries, its frequency is increasing faster than all other esophageal cancers.

Symptoms

Early-stage esophageal cancer may go unnoticed. The first symptom is usually difficulty in swallowing solid foods, which develops as the growing cancer narrows the esophagus. Several weeks later, swallowing soft foods and then liquids and saliva becomes difficult. Weight loss is common, even when the person continues to eat well. People may have chest pain, which feels like it travels to the back.

As the cancer progresses, it commonly invades various nerves and other tissues and organs. The tumor may compress the nerve that controls the vocal cords, which can lead to hoarseness. Compression of surrounding nerves may cause Horner's syndrome (see page 834), spinal pain, and hiccups. The cancer usually spreads to the lungs, where it may cause shortness of breath, and to the liver, where it may cause fever and abdominal swelling. Spread to bones may cause pain. Spread to the brain may cause headache, confusion, and seizures. Spread to the intestines may cause vomiting, blood in the stool, and iron deficiency anemia. Spread to the kidneys often causes no symptoms.

In late stages, the cancer may completely block the esophagus. Swallowing becomes impossible so that secretions build up in the mouth, which can be very distressing.

Diagnosis

Endoscopy, in which a flexible viewing tube (endoscope) is passed through the mouth to view the esophagus, is the best diagnostic procedure if esophageal cancer is suspected. Endoscopy also allows the doctor to remove a tissue sample (biopsy) and loose cells (brush cytology) for examination under a microscope. An x-ray procedure called a barium swallow (in which the person swallows a solution of barium, which shows up on x-rays) can also show the obstruction. Computed tomography (CT) and ultrasonography scans performed through an endoscope inserted in the esophagus may be used to further assess the extent of the cancer.

Prognosis and Treatment

Because esophageal cancer usually is not diagnosed until the disease has spread, the death rate is high. Fewer than 5% of people survive more than 5 years. Many die within a year of noticing the first symptoms. Because nearly all cases of esophageal cancer are fatal, the doctor's main objective is to control symptoms, especially pain (see page 61) and the inability to swallow (see page 62), which can be very frightening to the person and loved ones.

Surgery to remove a tumor offers the most prolonged relief but seldom cures, because the cancer usually has spread by the time of surgery. Chemotherapy, alone or with radiation therapy, may relieve symptoms and lengthen survival time by a few months. Sometimes preoperative radiation therapy combined with chemotherapy can increase the surgical cure rate. Other measures that aim only to relieve symptoms include widening (dilating) the narrowed area of the esophagus and then inserting a tube (a stent) to keep the esophagus open; bypassing the tumor using a loop of intestine; and performing laser phototherapy, in which a high-energy beam of light is directed at the growth to destroy the cancer tissue obstructing the esophagus.

Another technique for symptom relief is photodynamic therapy, in which a light-sensitive dye (contrast agent) is given by vein (intravenously) 48 hours before treatment. The dye is absorbed by cancer cells to a much greater degree than by the cells of normal surrounding esophageal tissue. When activated by light from a laser passed into the esophagus through an endoscope, the dye destroys cancer tissue, thus opening the esophagus. Photodynamic therapy destroys obstructing lesions more rapidly than radiation or chemotherapy in people who cannot tolerate surgery because of poor health.

Adequate nutrition makes any type of treatment more feasible and tolerable. People who can swallow may receive concentrated liquid nutritional supplements. People who cannot swallow may need temporary tube feeding or intravenous feeding.

Because death is likely, a person with esophageal cancer should make all necessary plans. The person should have frank discussions with the doctor about wishes for medical care (advance directives—see page 69) and the need for end-of-life care.

Stomach Tumors That Are Noncancerous

Noncancerous (benign) tumors of the stomach are unlikely to cause symptoms or medical problems, so they often remain undiagnosed and untreated. Occasionally, however, some bleed and are then removed during endoscopy (in which a flexible viewing tube [endoscope] is passed through the mouth to view the esophagus) or surgery.

Stomach polyps, uncommon noncancerous round growths that project into the stomach cavity, may become cancerous (that is, they are precancerous). Therefore, polyps are usually removed using endoscopy. Through the endoscope, an electrical current (electrocautery) or heat (thermal obliteration) is applied directly to the growth, or a high-energy beam of light is directed at the growth (laser phototherapy).

Stomach Cancer

- A *Helicobacter pylori* infection seems to be the cause of most stomach cancer.

- Vague abdominal discomfort, weight loss, and weakness are some typical symptoms.
- The best diagnostic procedure is an endoscopy.
- The survival rate is low because the cancer tends to spread early to other sites.
- Surgery is performed to eliminate the cancer or relieve symptoms.

About 95% of stomach cancers are adenocarcinomas. Adenocarcinomas of the stomach originate from the glandular cells of the stomach lining.

In the United States, adenocarcinoma of the stomach occurs in about 21,000 people each year and is the seventh most common cause of cancer death. It is more common among certain populations: people aged 50 and older, poor people, blacks, Hispanics, American Indians, and people who live in northern climates. For unknown reasons, adenocarcinoma of the stomach is becoming less common in the United States. It is far more common in Japan, China, Chile, and Iceland. In these nations, screening programs are an important means of early detection.

Causes and Risk Factors

Adenocarcinoma of the stomach often begins at a site where the stomach lining is inflamed. Many experts now believe that an infection with the bacterium *Helicobacter pylori* is the cause of most stomach cancer.

Stomach polyps may become cancerous (malignant) and are thus removed. Adenocarcinoma of the stomach is particularly likely to develop if the polyps consist of glandular cells, if the polyps are larger than 3/4 inch (2 centimeters), or if several polyps exist.

Certain dietary factors were once thought to play a role in the development of adenocarcinoma of the stomach. These factors included a high intake of salt, a high intake of carbohydrates, a high intake of preservatives called nitrates (often present in smoked foods), and a low intake of fruit and green leafy vegetables. However, none of these factors has proven to be a cause.

Symptoms

In the early stages, symptoms are vague and easily ignored. Early symptoms may mimic peptic ulcer disease, with burning abdominal pain. Therefore, peptic ulcer symptoms that do not resolve with treatment may indicate stomach cancer. The person may notice a feeling of fullness after a small meal (early satiety).

Weight loss or weakness usually results from difficulty in eating or from an inability to absorb some vitamins and minerals. Anemia, characterized by fatigue, weakness, and light-headedness, may result from very gradual bleeding that causes no

Rare Types of Stomach Cancer

Lymphoma is cancer of the lymphatic system. Lymphoma can develop within the stomach. The bacterium *Helicobacter pylori* is believed to play a role in the development of some lymphomas of the stomach. Surgery is often the initial treatment. Chemotherapy and radiation therapy are more successful in treating lymphoma than adenocarcinoma. Longer survival and even cure are possible.

Leiomyosarcoma (also called stromal cell tumor or spindle cell tumor) is cancer of the smooth muscle of the stomach. It is best treated with surgery. If cancer has already spread (metastasized) to other parts of the body at the time a leiomyosarcoma is found, then chemotherapy may lead to slightly longer survival. A newer drug, imatinib, has been found to be effective in treating leiomyosarcoma that cannot be treated with surgery.

other symptoms, from malabsorption of vitamin B_{12} (a vitamin needed for red blood cell formation), or from malabsorption of iron (a mineral needed for red blood cell formation) due to a lack of stomach acid. Uncommonly, a person may vomit large amounts of blood (hematemesis) or pass black tarry stools (melena). When adenocarcinoma is advanced, a doctor may be able to feel a mass when pressing on the abdomen.

Even in the early stages, a small adenocarcinoma may spread (metastasize) to distant sites. The spread of the tumor may cause liver enlargement, a yellowish discoloration of the skin and the whites of the eyes (jaundice), fluid accumulation and swelling in the abdominal cavity (ascites), and cancerous skin nodules. The spreading cancer also may weaken bones, leading to bone fractures.

Diagnosis

Endoscopy (an examination in which a flexible tube is used to visualize the inside of the digestive tract) is the best diagnostic procedure. It allows a doctor to view the stomach directly, to check for *Helicobacter pylori*, and to remove tissue samples for examination under a microscope (biopsy). Barium x-rays are used less often because they rarely reveal small early-stage cancers and do not allow for biopsy. If cancer is found, people usually have a computed tomography (CT) scan of the chest and abdomen to determine the extent to which the tumor has spread to other organs. If the CT scan does not show the tumor has spread, doctors usually perform an endoscopic ultrasound (which shows the lining of the digestive tract more clearly because the probe is placed on the tip of the endoscope) to determine the depth of the tumor and the involvement of nearby lymph nodes.

Prognosis and Treatment

Fewer than 15% of people with adenocarcinoma of the stomach survive longer than 5 years. The cancer tends to spread early to other sites. If the cancer is confined to the stomach, surgery is usually performed to try to cure it. Removal of the entire tumor before it has spread offers the only hope of cure. Most or all of the stomach and nearby lymph nodes are removed. The prognosis is good if the cancer has not penetrated the stomach wall too deeply. In the United States, the results of surgery are often poor, because most people have extensive cancer by the time a diagnosis is made. In Japan, where stomach cancer is very common, mass public health screening programs help to detect it early so that a cure is more likely. Chemotherapy and radiation therapy may help in certain circumstances.

If the cancer has spread beyond the stomach, surgery cannot cure the condition, but it is sometimes used to relieve symptoms. For example, if the passage of food is obstructed at the far end of the stomach, a bypass operation, in which an alternate connection is made between the stomach and the small intestine, allows food to pass. This connection relieves the symptoms of obstruction—pain and vomiting—at least for a while. Chemotherapy and radiation therapy may relieve symptoms as well, but their effectiveness is limited.

Small-Intestine Tumors That Are Noncancerous

Most tumors of the small intestine are noncancerous (benign). These include tumors of fat cells (lipomas), nerve cells (neurofibromas), connective tissue cells (fibromas), and muscle cells (leiomyomas).

Most noncancerous tumors of the small intestine do not cause symptoms. However, larger ones may cause blood in the stool, a partial or complete intestinal obstruction, or intestinal strangulation if one part of the intestine telescopes into an adjacent part (a condition called intussusception).

Small noncancerous growths may be destroyed by treatments applied through a flexible viewing tube (endoscope) inserted into the intestine. These treatments include applying an electrical current (electrocautery) or heat (thermal obliteration) directly to the growth and directing a high-energy beam of light at the growth (laser phototherapy). For large growths, surgery may be needed.

Small-Intestine Cancer

■ Blood in the stool is a common symptom, but sometimes the cancer blocks the intestine, causing crampy abdominal pain and vomiting.

- The diagnosis is based on various intestinal viewing techniques, including endoscopy and barium x-rays.
- Surgical removal is the best form of treatment.

Cancerous (malignant) tumors in the small intestine are very uncommon, occurring in fewer than 6,000 people in the United States each year. Adenocarcinoma is the most common type of cancer of the small intestine. Adenocarcinomas develop in the glandular cells of the lining of the small intestine. People with Crohn's disease of the small intestine are more likely than others to develop adenocarcinoma.

Symptoms and Diagnosis

Adenocarcinoma may cause bleeding into the intestine, which shows up as blood in the stool, and obstruction, which in turn may lead to crampy abdominal pain, expansion (distention) of the abdomen, and vomiting.

A doctor may use an endoscope (a flexible viewing tube) passed through the mouth and down to the duodenum and part of the jejunum (the upper and middle sections of the small intestine) to locate the tumor and perform a biopsy (remove a tissue sample for examination under a microscope). A doctor can sometimes see tumors of the ileum (the lower section of the small intestine) by passing a colonoscope (an endoscope used to view the lower part of the digestive tract) through the anus, through the entire large intestine, and up into the ileum. A barium x-ray can show the entire small intestine and may be used to outline the tumor. A wireless video capsule camera (see page 130) can also be used to show tumors of the small intestine. Arteriography (an x-ray taken after a radiopaque dye is injected into an artery) of the intestinal arteries may be performed, especially if the tumor is bleeding. Similarly, radioactive technetium can be injected into the artery and observed on x-rays as it leaks into the intestine. This procedure helps locate sites where the tumor is bleeding. The bleeding can then be corrected surgically. Sometimes exploratory surgery is needed to identify a tumor in the small intestine.

Treatment

The best treatment for all types of cancerous growths is surgical removal of the tumor. Chemotherapy and radiation therapy after surgery do not lengthen survival time.

Colorectal Polyps

- Some polyps are caused by hereditary conditions.
- Bleeding from the rectum is the most common symptom.
- A colonoscopy is performed to make the diagnosis.
- Surgical removal is the best form of treatment.

A polyp is a growth of tissue from the intestinal or rectal wall that protrudes into the intestine or rectum and may be noncancerous (benign) or cancerous (malignant). Polyps vary considerably in size, and the bigger the polyp, the greater the risk that it is cancerous or precancerous. Polyps may grow with or without a stalk. Those without a stalk are more likely to be cancerous than those with a stalk. Adenomatous polyps, which consist primarily of glandular cells that line the inside of the large intestine, are likely to become cancerous (that is, they are precancerous). Serrated adenomas are a particularly aggressive form of adenoma.

Hereditary Conditions: Some polyps are the result of hereditary conditions, such as familial adenomatous polyposis and Peutz-Jeghers syndrome.

In **familial adenomatous polyposis**, 100 or more precancerous polyps develop throughout the large intestine and rectum during childhood or adolescence. In nearly all untreated people, the polyps develop into cancer of the large intestine or rectum (colorectal cancer) before age 40. People with familial adenomatous polyposis can develop other complications (previously termed Gardner's syndrome), particularly various types of noncancerous tumors. These noncancerous tumors develop elsewhere in the body (for example, on the skin, skull, or jaw).

In **Peutz-Jeghers syndrome**, people have many small polyps in the stomach, small intestine, large intestine, and rectum. They also have numerous bluish black spots on their face, inside their mouth, and on their hands and feet. The spots tend to fade by puberty except for those inside the mouth. People

---

Rare Types of Small-Intestine Cancer

Carcinoid tumors can develop in the glandular cells that line the small intestine. Carcinoid tumors often secrete hormones that cause diarrhea and flushing of the skin. Chemotherapy and other types of drugs sometimes help control the symptoms caused by carcinoid tumors.

Lymphoma (cancer of the lymphatic system) may develop in the middle section (jejunum) or the lower section (ileum) of the small intestine. Lymphoma may cause a segment of intestine to become rigid or elongated. This cancer is more common among people with celiac sprue. Chemotherapy and radiation therapy can help control symptoms and sometimes lengthen survival time.

Leiomyosarcomas develop in the muscle cells in the wall of the small intestine. Chemotherapy may slightly lengthen survival time after surgery to remove leiomyosarcomas.

with Peutz-Jeghers syndrome have an increased risk of developing cancer in many organs, particularly the pancreas, small intestine, colon, breast, lung, ovary, and uterus.

> ### ? Did You Know...
> There is an inherited disorder that causes people to develop hundreds of polyps in their colon. Without treatment, nearly all of these people develop cancer by age 40.

Symptoms and Diagnosis

Most polyps do not cause symptoms. When they do, the most common symptom is bleeding from the rectum. A large polyp may cause cramps, abdominal pain, or obstruction. Large polyps with tiny, fingerlike projections (villous adenomas) may excrete water and salts, causing profuse watery diarrhea that may result in low levels of potassium in the blood (hypokalemia). Rarely, a rectal polyp on a long stalk drops down and dangles through the anus.

A doctor may be able to feel polyps by inserting a gloved finger into the rectum, but usually polyps are discovered during flexible sigmoidoscopy (examination of the lower portion of the large intestine with a viewing tube). If flexible sigmoidoscopy reveals a polyp, colonoscopy is performed to examine the entire large intestine. This more complete and reliable examination is performed because more than one polyp is usually present and any may be cancerous. Colonoscopy also allows a doctor to perform a biopsy (removal of a tissue sample for examination under a microscope) of any area that appears cancerous.

Treatment

Doctors generally recommend removing all polyps from the large intestine and rectum because of their potential to become cancerous. Polyps are removed during a colonoscopy procedure using a cutting instrument or an electrified wire loop. If a polyp has no stalk or cannot be removed during colonoscopy, abdominal surgery may be needed.

If a polyp is found to be cancerous, treatment depends on whether the cancer is likely to have spread. The risk of spread is determined by microscopic examination of the polyp. If the risk is low, no further treatment is necessary. If the risk is high, particularly if the cancer has invaded the polyp's stalk, the affected segment of the large intestine is removed surgically, and the cut ends of the intestine are rejoined.

When a person has a polyp removed, the entire large intestine and rectum are examined by colonoscopy a year later and then at intervals determined by the doctor. If such an examination is impossible because of a narrowing of the large intestine, a barium enema may be used to view the large intestine on x-ray.

For people with familial adenomatous polyposis, complete removal of the large intestine and rectum eliminates the risk of cancer. Alternatively, the large intestine is removed and the rectum is joined to the small intestine. This procedure sometimes eliminates the rectal polyps and thus is preferred by many experts. The remaining part of the rectum is inspected by sigmoidoscopy every 3 to 6 months, so that new polyps can be removed. If new polyps appear too rapidly, however, the rectum must also be removed. If the rectum is removed, a surgical opening is created through the abdominal wall from the small intestine (ileostomy). Bodily wastes are eliminated through the ileostomy into a disposable bag.

Some nonsteroidal anti-inflammatory drugs (NSAIDs) are being studied for their ability to reverse the growth of polyps in people with familial adenomatous polyposis. Their effects are temporary, however, and once these drugs are discontinued, the polyps begin to grow again.

Colorectal Cancer

- Family history and some dietary factors increase a person's risk of colorectal cancer.
- Typical symptoms include bleeding during a bowel movement, fatigue, and weakness.
- Screening tests are important for people over 50.
- Colonoscopy is often used to make the diagnosis.
- Cancer that is caught early is most curable.
- Surgery is usually performed to remove the cancer.

Almost all cancers of the large intestine and rectum (colorectal) are adenocarcinomas, which develop from the lining of the large intestine (colon) and rectum. Colorectal cancer usually begins as a buttonlike swelling on the surface of the intestinal or rectal lining or on a polyp. As the cancer grows, it begins to invade the wall of the intestine or rectum. Nearby lymph nodes also may be invaded. Because blood from the wall of the intestine and much of the rectum is carried to the liver, colorectal cancer usually spreads (metastasizes) to the liver soon after spreading to nearby lymph nodes.

In Western countries, cancer of the large intestine and rectum is one of the most common types of cancer and the second leading cause of cancer death. The incidence of colorectal cancer begins to rise at age 40 and peaks between the ages of 60 and 75.

Understanding Colostomy

In a colostomy, the large intestine (colon) is cut. The part that remains connected to the colon is brought to the skin surface through an opening that has been formed.

The part is then stitched to the skin. Stool passes through the opening and into a disposable bag.

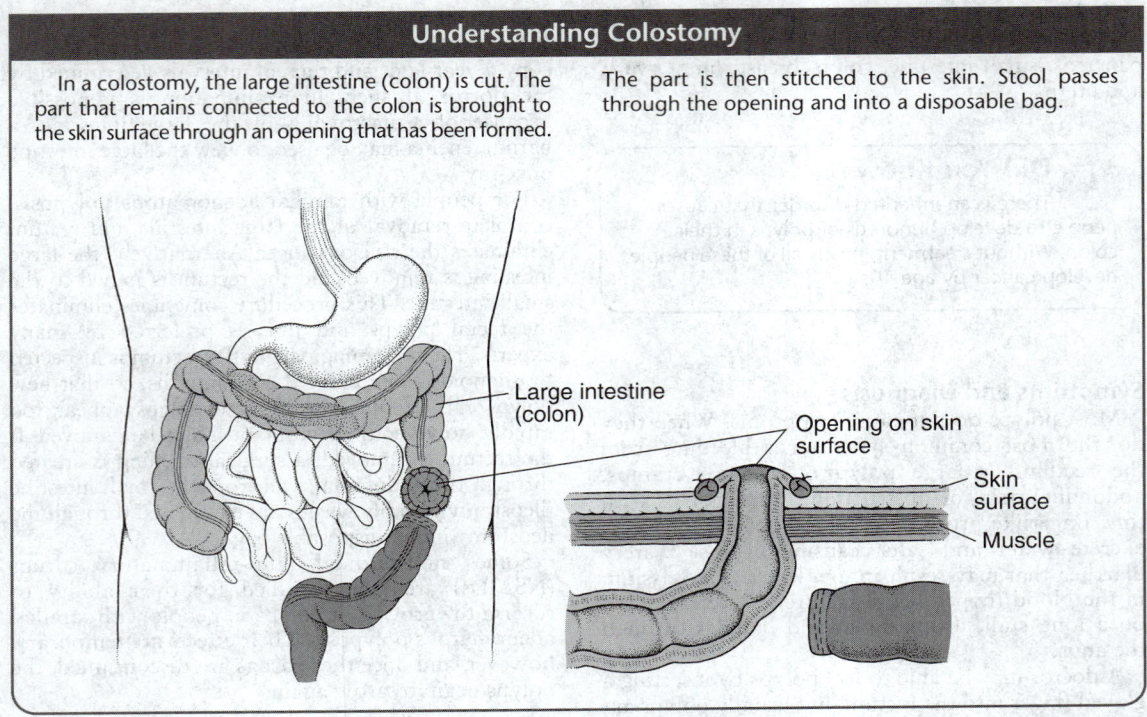

Large intestine (colon)

Opening on skin surface

Skin surface

Muscle

Each year, about 153,000 people in the United States develop colorectal cancer and about 52,000 die. Colon cancer is more common among women, and rectal cancer is more common among men. About 5% of people with colon cancer or rectal cancer have cancer in two or more sites in the colon and rectum that do not seem to simply have spread from one site to another.

Risk Factors

People with a family history of colorectal cancer have a higher risk of developing the cancer themselves. A family history of polyps (see page 192) also increases the risk of colorectal cancer.

People with ulcerative colitis or Crohn's disease are at greater risk as well. This risk is related to the person's age when the disease developed and the length of time the person has had the disease.

People at highest risk tend to consume a high-fat, low-fiber diet. Greater exposure to air and water pollution, particularly to industrial cancer-causing substances (carcinogens), may play a role.

Hereditary Nonpolyposis Colorectal Carcinoma (HNPCC): HNPCC comes from an inherited gene mutation that causes cancer in 70 to 80% of the people with that mutation. People with HNPCC often develop colorectal cancer before age 50. They are also at increased risk of other types of cancer, particularly endometrial cancer, stomach cancer, cancer of the small intestine, and ovarian cancer.

Symptoms

Colorectal cancer grows slowly and does not cause symptoms for a long time. Symptoms depend on the type, location, and extent of the cancer.

Fatigue and weakness resulting from occult bleeding (bleeding not visible to the naked eye) may be the person's only symptoms. A tumor in the left (descending) colon is likely to cause obstruction at an earlier stage, because the left colon has a smaller diameter and the stool is semisolid. Cancer tends to encircle this part of the colon, causing alternating constipation and frequent bowel movements before obstruction. The person may seek medical treatment because of crampy abdominal pain or severe abdominal pain and constipation. A tumor in the right (ascending) colon does not cause obstruction until late in the course of the cancer, because the ascending colon has a large diameter and the contents flowing through it are liquid. By the time the tumor is discovered, therefore, it may be so large that a doctor can feel it through the abdominal wall.

Staging Colon Cancer

STAGE 0: Cancer is limited to the inner layer (lining) of the large intestine (colon) covering the polyp. More than 95% of people with cancer at this stage survive at least 5 years.

STAGE 1: Cancer spreads to the space between the inner layer and muscle layer of the large intestine. (This space contains blood vessels, nerves, and lymph vessels.) More than 90% of people with cancer at this stage survive at least 5 years.

STAGE 2: Cancer invades the muscle layer and outer layer of the colon. About 55 to 85% of people with cancer at this stage survive at least 5 years.

STAGE 3: Cancer extends through the outer layer of the colon into nearby lymph nodes. About 20 to 55% of people with cancer at this stage survive at least 5 years.

STAGE 4 (not shown): Cancer spreads to other organs, such as the liver, lungs, or ovaries, or to the lining of the abdominal cavity (peritoneum). Fewer than 1% of people with cancer at this stage survive at least 5 years.

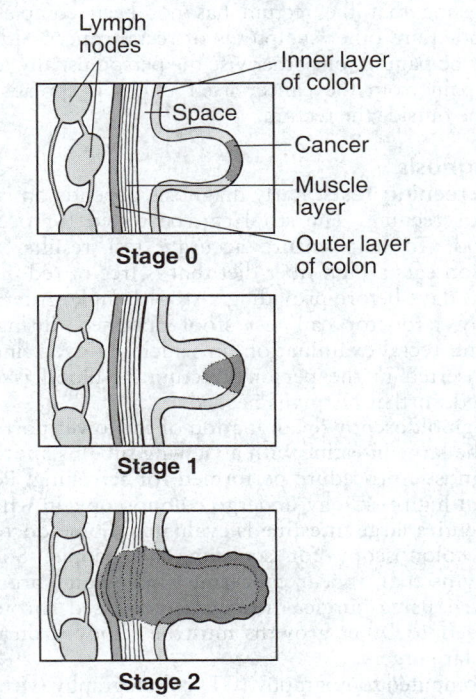

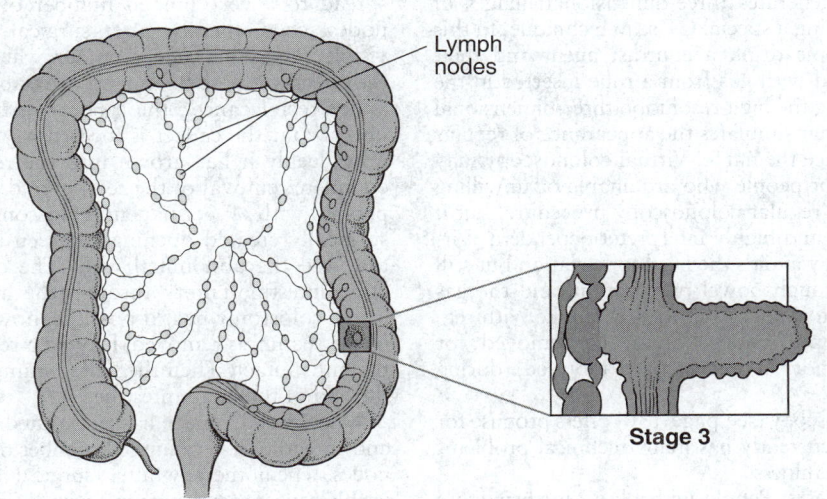

Most colon cancers bleed, usually slowly. The stool may be streaked or mixed with blood, but often the blood cannot be seen. Testing the stool for occult blood is needed (see page 131). The most common first symptom of rectal cancer is bleeding during a bowel movement. Whenever the rectum bleeds, even if the person is known to have hemorrhoids or diverticular disease, doctors must consider cancer as part of their diagnosis. Painful bowel movements and a feeling that the rectum has not been completely emptied are other symptoms of rectal cancer. Sitting may be painful, but otherwise the person usually feels no pain from the cancer itself unless it spreads to tissue outside the rectum.

Diagnosis

Screening Tests: Early diagnosis depends on routine screening. The stool can be tested for occult blood. To help ensure accurate test results, the person eats a high-fiber diet that is free of red meat for 3 days before providing a stool sample. Alternatively, a doctor can test stool obtained during a digital rectal examination, in which a gloved finger is inserted in the person's rectum. If blood is detected, further testing is needed.

Sigmoidoscopy (examination of the lower portion of the large intestine with a viewing tube) is another diagnostic procedure performed for screening. People at high risk may undergo colonoscopy, in which the entire large intestine is evaluated. Some doctors use colonoscopy for screening all people. Some growths that appear cancerous (malignant) are removed using surgical instruments passed through the scope. Other growths must be removed during regular surgery.

Computed tomography (CT) colonography (virtual colonoscopy) generates three-dimensional images of the colon by using a special CT scan technique. In this technique, people drink a contrast agent and their colon is inflated with gas from a tube inserted in the rectum. Viewing the high-resolution three-dimensional images somewhat simulates the appearance of regular endoscopy, hence the name. Virtual colonoscopy may be an option for people who are unable or unwilling to undergo the regular colonoscopy procedure, but it is less sensitive and highly interpreter-dependent. Virtual colonoscopy avoids the need for sedation but still requires a thorough bowel preparation, and the gas may be uncomfortable. Additionally, unlike with regular colonoscopy, lesions cannot be removed for examination under a microscope (biopsied) during the procedure.

Capsule endoscopy (see page 130) offers promise for the future but currently has many technical problems that limit its usefulness.

Diagnostic Tests: People with blood in their stool require colonoscopy, as do those with abnormalities seen during a sigmoidoscopy. Any lesions seen should be completely removed during the colonoscopy.

Once cancer is diagnosed, doctors usually perform an abdominal CT, chest x-ray, and routine laboratory tests to look for cancer that has spread, to detect a low blood count (anemia), and to evaluate the person's overall condition.

Blood tests are not used to diagnose colorectal cancer, but they can help the doctor monitor the effectiveness of treatment after a tumor has been removed. For example, if levels of carcinoembryonic antigen (CEA) are high before surgery to remove a known cancer and low after surgery, monitoring for another increase in the CEA level may help detect an early recurrence of the cancer. Two other cancer markers, CA 19-9 and CA 125, are similar to CEA and are sometimes elevated in colorectal cancer.

Prognosis and Treatment

Colon cancer is most likely to be cured if it is removed early, before it has spread. Cancers that have grown deeply or through the wall of the colon have often spread, even if metastases (spread) cannot be detected. Surgery, the main treatment for colorectal cancer, cures about 90% of cases when the cancer is only in the lining of the bowel wall, about 70% of cases when the cancer extends through the bowel wall, and only about 30 to 50% of cases when the cancer has spread to the lymph nodes in the abdomen.

In most cases of colon cancer, the cancerous segment of the intestine and any nearby lymph nodes are removed surgically, and the remaining ends of the intestine are joined. When people have colon cancer that has penetrated the wall of the large intestine and spread to a very limited number of nearby lymph nodes, chemotherapy after surgical removal of all visible cancer may lengthen survival time, although the effects of these treatments are often modest.

For rectal cancer, the type of operation depends on how far the cancer is located from the anus and how deeply it has grown into the rectal wall. The complete removal of the rectum and anus leaves the person with a permanent colostomy, which is a surgically created opening between the large intestine and the abdominal wall. The contents of the large intestine empty through the abdominal wall into a colostomy bag. If possible, however, only part of the rectum is removed, leaving a rectal stump and the anus intact. Then the rectal stump is rejoined to the end of the large intestine.

When rectal cancer has penetrated the rectal wall and spread to a very limited number of nearby lymph nodes, chemotherapy after surgical removal of all visible cancer may lengthen survival time. Also, radiation therapy after surgical removal of visible rectal cancer may help control the growth of any residual tumors, delay a recurrence, and lengthen survival time.

When cancer has spread to lymph nodes far from the colon or rectum, to the lining of the abdominal cavity, or to other organs, the cancer cannot be cured by surgery alone. Survival time is typically only about 7 months. Chemotherapy with fluorouracil (sometimes also with another drug) may be given after surgery as part of the treatment for colorectal cancer that has spread widely, but the chemotherapy usually has little effect on how long the person survives. The doctor usually discusses end-of-life care with the person, the family, and other health care practitioners (see page 57). Even when the cancer has spread widely, surgery is sometimes performed to relieve the intestinal obstruction and ease symptoms.

When the cancer has spread only to the liver, chemotherapy drugs can be injected directly into the artery supplying the liver. A small pump inserted surgically beneath the skin or an external pump worn on a belt allows the person to be mobile during the treatment. This treatment may provide more benefit than ordinary chemotherapy, but more research is needed. When cancer has spread beyond the liver, this approach has no advantage.

For people who cannot tolerate surgery because of poor health, treatment may involve drying out and shrinking the tumor in a procedure called desiccation. Desiccation is performed either with a probe that applies an electrical charge to the surface of the tumor (cautery device) or with a device that dries the tumor with electrified Argon gas (Argon plasma coagulator). Both devices can be passed through a colonoscope. Desiccation may relieve symptoms and lengthen survival time modestly by reducing tumor mass but rarely cures the cancer.

Anal Cancer

- Risk factors for anal cancer include certain sexually transmitted diseases.
- Bleeding with bowel movements, pain, and sometimes itching around the anus are typical symptoms.
- A manual examination and a biopsy are performed to verify the diagnosis.
- Treatment may involve either surgery alone or a combination of radiation therapy and chemotherapy or radiation therapy and surgery.

Anal cancer develops in the skin cells of the immediate area around the anus or in the lining of the transitional zone between the anus and the rectum (the anal canal). Unlike in the rectum and the large intestine, in which cancers are almost always adenocarcinomas, cancers of the anus are primarily squamous cell carcinomas.

Anal cancer occurs in somewhat over 4,000 people in the United States each year. Anal cancer is almost twice as common among women. The cause of anal cancer is unclear, but people who practice receptive anal intercourse are at increased risk, as

are those who have certain types of sexually transmitted infections, particularly human papillomavirus (HPV type 16) and lymphogranuloma venereum (see page 1271).

Symptoms and Diagnosis

People with anal cancer often experience bleeding with bowel movements, pain, and sometimes itching around the anus. About 25% of people with anal cancer have no symptoms. In this instance, the cancer is found only during a routine examination.

To diagnose anal cancer, a doctor first inspects the skin around the anus for any abnormalities. With a gloved hand, the doctor probes the anus and lower rectum, checking for any portions of the lining that feel different from surrounding areas. The doctor then removes a sample of tissue from an abnormal area and examines it under a microscope (performs a biopsy).

Treatment

Radiation therapy combined with chemotherapy may be used instead of or in addition to surgery. Surgery alone is often satisfactory treatment, although the doctor must be careful not to interfere with the functioning of the muscular ring that keeps the anus closed until the person has a bowel movement (the anal sphincter), which could lead to loss of control over bowel movements (fecal incontinence). A combination of radiation with chemotherapy, or radiation with surgery, cures many anal cancers, with 70% or more of people surviving longer than 5 years. More extensive surgery is sometimes needed if the results of follow-up biopsies performed after initial treatment show recurrence of the cancer.

Pancreatic Cancer

- Smoking, chronic pancreatitis, and possibly long-standing diabetes are risk factors for pancreatic cancer.
- Pain, weight loss, jaundice, and vomiting are some typical symptoms.
- Computed tomography is the most accurate diagnostic technique.
- Pancreatic cancer is usually fatal.
- Surgery may cure those whose cancer has not spread.

About 95% of cancerous (malignant) tumors of the pancreas are adenocarcinomas. Adenocarcinomas usually originate in the glandular cells lining the pancreatic duct. Most adenocarcinomas occur in the head of the pancreas, the part nearest the first segment of the small intestine (duodenum).

Adenocarcinoma of the pancreas has become increasingly common in the United States, occurring in an estimated 37,000 people each year. Adenocarcinoma usually does not develop before age 50. The average

Rare Types of Pancreatic Cancer

Cystadenocarcinoma of the pancreas is a rare type of pancreatic cancer that develops from a fluid-filled noncancerous (benign) tumor called a cystadenoma. It often causes upper abdominal pain and may grow large enough for a doctor to feel it through the abdominal wall. The diagnosis is usually made by an ultrasound or computed tomography (CT) scan of the pancreas. Only 20% of these cancers have spread by the time surgery is performed. Therefore, cystadenocarcinoma has a much better prognosis than adenocarcinoma. If the cancer has not spread and the whole pancreas is removed surgically, the person has a 65% chance of surviving for at least 5 years.

Intraductal papillary-mucinous tumor is a rare type of pancreatic tumor characterized by enlargement (dilation) of the main pancreatic duct, mucus overproduction, and occasional pain. More than 30% of these tumors are cancerous (malignant), but because diagnostic tests cannot distinguish between noncancerous and cancerous forms of this tumor, surgery is the best diagnostic and treatment option for all people suspected of having an intraductal papillary-mucinous tumor.

age at diagnosis is 55. These tumors are nearly twice as common among men. Adenocarcinoma of the pancreas is 2 to 3 times more common among smokers than in nonsmokers. Alcohol and caffeine consumption do not seem to be risk factors. People with chronic pancreatitis and possibly those with long-standing diabetes (primarily women) are at greater risk as well.

Symptoms

Tumors in the head of the pancreas can interfere with the drainage of bile (the digestive fluid produced by the liver) into the small intestine (see pages 159 and 210). Therefore, jaundice (a yellowish discoloration of the skin and the whites of the eyes) caused by obstruction of bile flow is typically an early symptom. The jaundice is accompanied by itchiness all over the body resulting from the deposit of bile salt crystals under the skin. Vomiting may result from instances when cancer in the head of the pancreas obstructs the flow of stomach contents into the small intestine (gastric outlet obstruction) or obstructs the small intestine itself.

Complications: Adenocarcinoma of the body or tail of the pancreas (the middle part of the pancreas and the part farthest from the duodenum) typically causes no symptoms until the tumor has grown large. Thus, at the time of diagnosis, the tumor has already spread (metastasized) beyond the pancreas in 90% of cases. It usually spreads to the neighboring lymph nodes, the liver, or the lung. Typically, the first symptoms are pain and weight loss. At the time of diagnosis, 90% of people have abdominal pain—usually severe pain in the upper abdomen that penetrates to the back—and significant weight loss.

Adenocarcinoma of the body or tail of the pancreas may obstruct the vein draining the spleen (the organ that produces, monitors, stores, and destroys blood cells), resulting in enlargement of the spleen (splenomegaly). Obstruction can also cause the veins to become swollen and twisted (varicose) around the esophagus (esophageal varices) and stomach. Severe bleeding may result, particularly from the esophagus, if these varicose veins rupture.

Diagnosis

Early diagnosis of tumors in the body or tail of the pancreas is difficult because symptoms occur late and physical examination and blood test results are often normal. When adenocarcinoma of the pancreas is suspected, the most accurate diagnostic test is computed tomography (CT). Other commonly used tests are ultrasound scans, endoscopic retrograde cholangiopancreatography (see art on page 213), and magnetic resonance imaging (MRI).

To confirm the diagnosis, a doctor may obtain a sample of the pancreas for examination under a microscope (biopsy) by inserting a needle through the skin using a CT or ultrasound scan as a guide. However, this approach often misses the tumor and may spread cancer cells out of the local area along the track of the needle. The same approach may be used to obtain a biopsy sample from the liver to look for cancer that has spread to the pancreas. If the results of these tests are normal but the doctor still strongly suspects adenocarcinoma, the pancreas may be evaluated surgically.

Prognosis and Treatment

Because adenocarcinoma of the pancreas has usually spread to other parts of the body before it is discovered, the prognosis is very poor. Fewer than 2% of people with adenocarcinoma of the pancreas survive for 5 years after the diagnosis. The only hope of a cure is surgery, which is performed on the 10 to 20% of people in whom it is believed that the cancer has not spread. Either the pancreas alone or the pancreas and the duodenum are removed. After such surgery, only 15 to 20% of people live for 5 years. Additional chemotherapy and radiation therapy are usually given but are not likely to improve survival time or rates substantially.

Mild pain may be relieved by aspirin or acetaminophen. Most often, stronger painkillers, such as codeine or morphine taken by mouth, are needed. For 70 to 80% of people with severe pain, injections into nerves to block pain sensations may provide relief. The lack of pancreatic digestive enzymes can be treated with oral enzyme preparations. If diabetes develops, insulin treatment may be needed.

Obstruction of bile flow may be temporarily relieved by placement of a tube (stent) in the lower portion of the duct that drains bile from the liver and gallbladder. In most cases, however, the tumor eventually obstructs the duct above and below the stent. An alternative treatment method is the surgical creation of a channel that bypasses the obstruction. For example, an obstruction of the small intestine can be bypassed by a channel that connects the stomach with a portion of the small intestine that is beyond the obstruction.

Because adenocarcinoma of the pancreas is fatal in most cases, a doctor usually discusses end-of-life care with the person, family members, and other health care practitioners (see page 57).

Pancreatic Endocrine Tumors

Pancreatic endocrine tumors are those that arise from the types of pancreatic cells that produce hormones. These tumors may or may not secrete hormones themselves and may or may not be cancerous (malignant). Even if they do not secrete hormones (nonfunctioning tumors) and are not cancerous, these tumors may cause symptoms by blocking the biliary tract or small intestine or by bleeding into the gastrointestinal tract. Functioning tumors secrete large amounts of a particular hormone, causing various syndromes.

INSULINOMA

An insulinoma is a rare type of pancreatic tumor that secretes insulin, a hormone that lowers the levels of sugar (glucose) in the blood.

Only 10% of insulinomas are cancerous.

Symptoms

Symptoms result from low levels of sugar (glucose) in the blood, which occur when the person does not eat for several hours (most often in the morning after an all-night fast). The symptoms include faintness, weakness, trembling, awareness of the heartbeat (palpitations), sweating, nervousness, and profound hunger. Other symptoms include headache, confusion, vision abnormalities, unsteadiness, and marked changes in personality. The low levels of sugar in the blood may even lead to a loss of consciousness, seizures, and coma.

Diagnosis and Treatment

Diagnosing an insulinoma can be difficult. Doctors try to perform blood tests while the person has symptoms. Blood tests include measurements of blood glucose levels and insulin levels. Very low levels of glucose and high levels of insulin in the blood indicate the presence of an insulinoma. Because many people have symptoms only occasionally, doctors may admit them to the hospital. In the hospital, the person fasts for at least 24 hours, sometimes up to 72 hours, and is closely monitored. During that time, the symptoms usually appear, and blood tests are performed to measure the levels of glucose and insulin.

If the blood tests suggest the person has an insulinoma, the location must then be pinpointed. Imaging tests, such as endoscopic ultrasonography (which shows the lining of the digestive tract more clearly because the ultrasound probe is placed on the tip of the endoscope) or positron emission tomography (PET) scans, can be used to locate the tumor, but sometimes exploratory surgery is needed.

The primary treatment for an insulinoma is surgical removal, which has a cure rate of about 90%. When the insulinoma cannot be completely removed and symptoms continue, drugs such as diazoxide and octreotide can help keep blood glucose from falling too low. Chemotherapy drugs such as streptozotocin and 5-fluorouracil may help control the tumor.

GASTRINOMA

A gastrinoma is a tumor usually in the pancreas or duodenum (the first segment of the small intestine) that produces excessive levels of the hormone gastrin, which stimulates the stomach to secrete acid and enzymes, causing peptic ulcers.

Most people with gastrinomas have several tumors clustered in or near the pancreas. About half of the tumors are cancerous. Sometimes a gastrinoma occurs as part of multiple endocrine neoplasia, a hereditary disorder in which tumors arise from the cells of various endocrine glands, such as the insulin-producing cells of the pancreas.

Symptoms and Diagnosis

The excess gastrin secreted by the gastrinoma causes Zollinger-Ellison syndrome (see box on page 142), in which a person suffers the symptoms of aggressive peptic ulcers in the stomach, duodenum, and elsewhere in the intestine. However, as many as 25% of people with Zollinger-Ellison syndrome may not have an ulcer when the diagnosis is made. Rupture, bleeding, and obstruction of the intestine can occur and are life threatening. For more than half of the people with a gastrinoma, symptoms are no worse than those experienced by people with ordinary peptic ulcer disease. In 25 to 40% of people, diarrhea is the first symptom.

A doctor suspects a gastrinoma when a person has frequent peptic ulcers or several peptic ulcers that do not respond to the usual ulcer treatments. Blood tests to detect abnormally high levels of gastrin are the most reliable diagnostic tests.

Once blood tests diagnose gastrinoma, doctors use several imaging techniques, such as computed tomography (CT), endoscopic ultrasonography, PET scans, and arteriography (an x-ray taken after a radiopaque dye is injected into an artery), to locate tumors. These tumors may be difficult to find, however, because usually they are small.

Treatment

High doses of proton pump inhibitors (see page 142 and table on page 143) may be effective for reducing acid levels and relieving symptoms temporarily. About 20% of people who do not have multiple endocrine neoplasia can be cured with surgical removal of the gastrinoma. If these treatments do not work, an operation to remove the stomach completely (total gastrectomy) may be necessary. This operation does not remove the tumor, but the gastrin can no longer create ulcers after the acid-producing stomach is removed. If the stomach is removed, daily iron and calcium supplements taken by mouth and monthly injections of vitamin B_{12} are needed, because absorption of these nutrients is impaired when stomach juices that prepare these nutrients for absorption are no longer available.

If cancerous tumors have spread to other parts of the body, chemotherapy may help reduce the number of tumor cells and the levels of gastrin in the blood. However, such therapy does not cure the cancer, which is ultimately fatal.

VIPOMA

A vipoma is a rare type of pancreatic tumor that produces vasoactive intestinal peptide (VIP), a substance that causes severe watery diarrhea.

About 50 to 75% of these tumors are cancerous. In about 6% of people, vipoma occurs as part of multiple endocrine neoplasia (see page 1016).

Symptoms

The major symptoms are prolonged massive watery diarrhea. People produce 1 to 3 quarts (1,000 to 3,000 milliliters) of stool per day, causing dehydration. In 50% of people, diarrhea is constant, and in the rest, the severity of the diarrhea varies over time.

Because the diarrhea removes many of the body's normal salts, people often develop low blood levels of potassium (hypokalemia) and excessively acidic blood (acidosis). These changes can cause lethargy, muscular weakness, nausea, vomiting, and crampy abdominal pain. Some people have flushing.

Diagnosis and Treatment

A doctor bases the diagnosis on the person's symptoms and finding elevated levels of VIP in the blood. People with elevated levels of VIP should also have an endoscopic ultrasound or PET scan to detect the location of the vipoma.

Initially fluids and electrolytes must be replaced. Bicarbonate must be given to replace that lost in the stool and avoid acidosis. Because water and electrolytes continue to be lost in the stool as rehydration is achieved, doctors may find it difficult to continually replace water and electrolytes.

The drug octreotide usually controls diarrhea, but large doses may be needed. Surgical removal of the vipoma cures about 50% of people whose tumor has not spread. Surgery may temporarily relieve symptoms in people whose tumor has spread. Chemotherapy does not cure the disease.

GLUCAGONOMA

A glucagonoma is a tumor of the pancreas that produces the hormone glucagon, which raises the level of sugar (glucose) in the blood and causes a distinctive rash.

About 80% of glucagonomas are cancerous. However, they grow slowly, and many people survive for 15 years or more after the diagnosis. The average age at which symptoms begin is 50. About 80% of people with glucagonomas are women.

Symptoms and Diagnosis

High levels of glucagon in the blood cause the symptoms of diabetes mellitus. Often, the person loses weight. In 90% of people, the most distinctive features are a chronic brownish red skin rash (necrolytic migratory erythema) and a smooth, shiny, bright red-orange tongue. The mouth also may have cracks at the corners. The rash, which causes scaling, starts in the groin and moves to the buttocks, forearms, and legs.

The diagnosis is made by identifying high levels of glucagon in the blood and then locating the tumor by performing an abdominal CT followed by an endoscopic ultrasound. An MRI or PET scan may be used if the CT scan does not show a tumor.

Treatment

Ideally, the tumor is surgically removed, which eliminates all symptoms. However, if removal is not possible or if the tumor has spread, chemotherapy may reduce the levels of glucagon and lessen the symptoms. However, chemotherapy does not improve survival.

The drug octreotide can be used to reduce glucagon levels, may clear up the rash, and may restore appetite, facilitating weight gain. But octreotide may elevate the levels of glucose in the blood even more. Zinc ointment may be used to treat the skin rash. Sometimes the rash is treated with intravenous amino acids or fatty acids.

31 Gastrointestinal Emergencies

Certain gastrointestinal disorders can be life threatening and require emergency treatment—surgery, in many cases.

Abdominal pain (see page 114), often severe, usually accompanies gastrointestinal emergencies. If a person is experiencing abdominal pain, a doctor must decide whether immediate surgery is needed to both identify and treat the problem or whether surgery can wait until diagnostic test results are available. Emergency surgery of the abdomen is often performed when the abdominal pain seems to result from an intestinal obstruction; a ruptured organ, such as the gallbladder, appendix, or intestine; or an abscess (a pus-filled pocket of infection).

Gastrointestinal bleeding (see page 117), which is typically painless, also can be life threatening. Doctors usually perform an endoscopy (an examination of internal structures using a flexible viewing tube) to find and treat the source of bleeding.

Abdominal Abscesses

An abscess is a pocket of pus, usually caused by a bacterial infection.

- Most people have constant abdominal pain and a fever.
- Computed tomography or another imaging test can distinguish an abscess from other problems.
- Treatment involves draining pus from the abscess and taking antibiotics.

Abdominal abscesses may form below the diaphragm, in the middle of the abdomen, in the pelvis, or behind the abdominal cavity. Abscesses also may form in or around any abdominal organ, such as the kidneys, spleen, pancreas, or liver, or in the prostate gland.

Causes and Symptoms

Often, abdominal abscesses are caused by injury, infection, or rupture of the intestine or by spread of infection from another abdominal organ. Sometimes abscesses form after injury to the abdomen or after surgery on the abdomen. Specific symptoms depend on the location of the abscess, but most people have constant discomfort or pain, feel generally sick (malaise), and often have a fever. Other symptoms include loss of appetite and weight loss.

An abscess below the diaphragm may form when infected fluid, for example, from a ruptured appendix, is moved upward by the pressure of abdominal organs and by the suction created when the diaphragm moves during breathing. Symptoms may include a cough, painful breathing, and pain in one shoulder—an example of referred pain that occurs because the shoulder and the diaphragm share the same nerves, and the brain incorrectly interprets the source of the pain (see art on page 639).

Abscesses in the mid-abdomen may result from a ruptured appendix, a ruptured intestine, inflammatory bowel disease, diverticular disease, or an abdominal wound. The abdomen is usually painful in the area of the abscess.

Pelvic abscesses can result from the same disorders that cause abscesses in the mid-abdomen or from gynecologic infections. Symptoms may include abdominal pain, diarrhea caused by intestinal irritation, and an urgent or frequent need to urinate caused by bladder irritation.

Abscesses behind the abdominal cavity (called retroperitoneal abscesses) lie behind the peritoneum, the membrane that lines the abdominal cavity and organs. The causes, which are similar to those of abscesses in the abdomen, include inflammation and infection of the appendix (appendicitis) and of the pancreas (pancreatitis). Pain, usually in the lower back, worsens when the person moves the leg at the hip.

Abscesses inside the pancreas typically form after an attack of acute pancreatitis. Symptoms such as fever, abdominal pain, nausea, and vomiting often begin a week or more after a person recovers from pancreatitis.

Liver abscesses may be caused by bacteria or by amebas (single-celled parasites). Bacteria can reach the liver from an infected gallbladder; a penetrating or blunt wound; an infection in the abdomen, such as a nearby abscess; or an infection carried by the bloodstream from elsewhere in the body. Amebas from an intestinal infection reach the liver through the lymph vessels. Symptoms of liver abscesses include loss of appetite, nausea, and a fever. A person may or may not have abdominal pain.

Abscesses in the spleen are caused by an infection traveling through the bloodstream to the spleen, by an injury to the spleen, or by the spread of an infection from a nearby abscess, such as one below the diaphragm. Pain may occur in the left side of the abdomen, the back, or the left shoulder.

Diagnosis

Doctors can easily misdiagnose an abscess, because the first symptoms it causes are usually vague and mild and may be mistaken for less serious problems that are more common. If doctors suspect a person has an abscess, they usually perform computed tomography

(CT) or sometimes ultrasound scanning or magnetic resonance imaging (MRI). These tests can help distinguish an abscess from other problems (for example, tumors or cysts), as well as determine the size and position of an abscess. Because abscesses and tumors often cause the same symptoms and show similar results on imaging tests, a definitive diagnosis sometimes requires that a doctor obtain a sample of the pus or surgically remove the abscess for examination under a microscope.

Treatment

To treat an abdominal abscess, the pus must be drained, either by surgery or by a needle inserted through the skin. To guide the placement of the needle, a doctor uses CT or ultrasound scanning. Antibiotics are usually used in conjunction with drainage to prevent the infection from spreading and to help completely eliminate the infection. Laboratory analysis of the pus identifies the infecting organism so that the most effective antibiotic can be selected. It is uncommon for antibiotics to cure an abscess without drainage. If the abscess cannot be reached safely by a needle, surgery may be necessary.

Maintaining proper nutrition is important. People may receive nutrition through a tube (enteral) or a vein (parenteral).

Abdominal Wall Hernias

An abdominal wall hernia is a protrusion of the intestine through an opening or area of weakness in the abdominal wall.

- An abdominal wall hernia causes a noticeable bulging but little discomfort.
- The diagnosis is made by physical examination and sometimes ultrasonography.
- Treatment involves surgery to repair the hernia.

Abdominal hernias are very common, particularly among men. There are about 700,000 hernia operations each year in the United States. Hernias are usually named for the area in which they occur.

The abdominal wall is thick and tough in most places, so hernias usually occur in an area of weakness where a previous opening has closed. Heavy lifting or straining may make a hernia more obvious but does not cause a hernia to form.

Inguinal Hernia: Inguinal hernias appear in the crease of the groin or in the scrotum. They are more common among men. There are two types, direct and indirect, depending on exactly where the hernia occurs.

Umbilical Hernia: Umbilical hernias occur around the bellybutton (umbilicus). Many babies have a small umbilical hernia because the opening for the umbilical cord blood vessels did not close completely. Some adults have an umbilical hernia because of obesity, pregnancy, or excess fluid in the abdomen (ascites).

Femoral Hernia: A hernia may develop just below the crease of the groin in the middle of the thigh where the femoral artery and vein leave the abdomen to go into the leg. This type of hernia is more common among women.

Incisional Hernia: Sometimes hernias form through a surgical incision in the abdominal wall. This type of hernia may develop many years after surgery.

Incarceration and Strangulation: Sometimes, a loop of intestine becomes stuck in the hernia, a condition called incarceration. Rarely, the hernia traps the intestine so tightly that it cuts off the blood supply, a condition called strangulation. With strangulation, the trapped piece of intestine can develop gangrene in as few as 6 hours. With gangrene, the intestinal wall dies, usually causing rupture, which leads to peritonitis (inflammation and usually infection of the abdominal cavity), shock, and, if untreated, death.

Symptoms

Most people usually notice only a bulge at the site of the hernia. Sometimes the hernia appears only with lifting, coughing, or straining. There is usually little or no discomfort, and the bulge can be pushed back in (reduced) by the person or a doctor. An incarcerated hernia has no additional symptoms, but the bulge cannot be reduced. A strangulated hernia causes steady, gradually increasing pain, typically with nausea and vomiting, cannot be reduced, and is tender when touched.

Diagnosis

Doctors base the diagnosis on an examination. Lumps in the groin that resemble hernias may be swollen lymph nodes or undescended testes. A swelling in the scrotum may be a varicocele (a condition in which the blood supply of the testis develops varicose veins) or a spermatocele (a collection of sperm in a sac that develops next to the epididymis). Sometimes the doctor performs an ultrasound to help make the diagnosis.

Treatment

Umbilical hernias in infants rarely strangulate and are not treated. Most go away without treatment within several years. Very large umbilical hernias may be repaired after the infant is 2 years old.

Because other types of hernias are more likely to strangulate, doctors usually repair them surgically when they are diagnosed. If the hernia is incarcerated or strangulated, surgery is performed immediately. Otherwise, repair is done at a time convenient for the person (elective surgery).

Holding the hernia in by tape, bandages, or other means sometimes makes the person more comfortable but does not lower the risk of strangulation or allow the opening to close; therefore, these are not recommended treatments. Only umbilical hernias go away without treatment.

Acute Mesenteric Ischemia

Acute mesenteric ischemia is sudden blockage of blood flow to part of the intestines, which may lead to gangrene and perforation (puncture).

- Severe abdominal pain develops suddenly.
- Angiography may be performed.
- Immediate surgery is needed.

Acute mesenteric ischemia has several causes. It can be caused by an arterial embolism, which is a blood clot or piece of atherosclerotic plaque material (the buildup of cholesterol and other fatty materials in an artery) that travels from its origin in the heart or aorta to lodge in the smaller arteries (in this case those of the intestines). A blood clot may form spontaneously in the arteries or veins of the intestines, blocking flow. Sometimes flow is not blocked completely but is simply too low because of low heart output (as in heart failure or shock—see page 350) or because certain drugs (such as cocaine) narrow the blood vessels. In general, people older than 50 years are at greatest risk.

Blockage of blood flow for more than 10 to 12 hours causes the affected area of intestine to die, allowing intestinal bacteria to invade the person's system. Shock, organ failure, and death are likely if intestinal death occurs.

Symptoms

At first, the person has severe abdominal pain, usually developing suddenly, but the abdomen is only slightly tender when the doctor presses it. This pain out of proportion to tenderness is an important clue for the doctor. Later, as the intestine starts to die, the person's abdomen becomes tender to the touch.

Diagnosis and Treatment

If the doctor can make the diagnosis early, people usually recover well. If the diagnosis is not made until some of the affected intestine has died, 70 to 90% of people die. If the person has typical symptoms and the abdomen is very tender, doctors usually take the person right to surgery. At surgery, the blood vessel blockage can sometimes be removed or bypassed but sometimes the affected intestine must be removed. If the symptoms suggest acute ischemia but the abdomen is not tender, doctors may perform angiography, in which they thread a small catheter through the artery in the groin and into the arteries of the intestines and inject a contrast agent that outlines the blood vessels. If a blockage is seen, sometimes it can be opened by injecting certain drugs—if not, the person needs surgery. After recovery, many people need to take a drug to help prevent blood clotting. A person cannot survive if almost all the small intestine dies or is removed.

Appendicitis

Appendicitis is inflammation and infection of the appendix.

- Often a blockage inside the appendix causes the appendix to become inflamed and infected.
- Abdominal pain, nausea, and fever are common.
- Exploratory surgery or an imaging test, such as computed tomography or ultrasonography, is done.
- Treatment involves surgery to remove the appendix and antibiotics to treat the infection.

The appendix is a small finger-shaped tube projecting from the large intestine near the point where it joins the small intestine. The appendix may have some immune function, but it is not an essential organ.

Except for trapped hernias, appendicitis is the most common cause of sudden, severe abdominal pain and abdominal surgery in the United States. Over 5% of the population develops appendicitis at some point. Appendicitis most commonly occurs in the teens and 20s but may occur at any age.

The cause of appendicitis is not fully understood. However, in most cases, a blockage inside the appendix probably starts a process. The blockage may be from a small, hard piece of stool, a foreign body, or, rarely, even worms. As a result of the blockage, the appendix becomes inflamed and infected. If inflammation continues without treatment, the appendix can rupture. A ruptured appendix spills bacteria-laden intestinal contents into the abdominal cavity, causing peritonitis (inflammation and usually infection of the abdominal cavity), which may result in a life-threatening infection. A rupture also may cause a pus-filled pocket of infection (abscess) to form. In a woman, the ovaries and fallopian tubes may become infected, and the resulting blockage of the fallopian tubes may cause infertility. A ruptured appendix also may allow bacteria to infect the bloodstream—a life-threatening condition called sepsis (see page 1186).

Symptoms

Fewer than 50% of people with appendicitis have the traditionally described symptoms in which pain begins in the upper abdomen or around the navel; then nausea and vomiting develop; and then, after a few hours, the nausea passes, and the pain shifts to the right lower portion of the abdomen. When a doctor presses on this area, it is tender, and when the pressure is released, the pain may increase sharply (rebound tenderness). A fever of 100° to 101° F (37.7° to 38.3° C) is common. Moving and coughing increase the pain.

In many people, particularly infants and children, the pain may be widespread rather than confined to the right lower portion of the abdomen. In older people and in pregnant women, the pain may be less severe, and the area is less tender.

If the appendix is ruptured, pain and fever may become severe. Worsening infection can lead to shock (see page 350).

Diagnosis

A doctor may suspect appendicitis after reviewing the person's symptoms and examining the abdomen. Typically, exploratory surgery is performed immediately if the doctor strongly suspects appendicitis. If the diagnosis is not clear, doctors usually perform an imaging test such as computed tomography (CT) or ultrasonography. Doctors can also perform a laparoscopy (see page 130) to help determine the diagnosis. A blood test often shows a moderate increase in the white blood cell count in response to the infection.

> **? Did You Know...**
> In the United States, over 5% of the population eventually develops appendicitis.

Treatment

Surgery is the main treatment. In nearly 15% of operations for appendicitis, the appendix is found to be normal. However, delaying surgery until the cause of the abdominal pain is certain can be fatal: An infected appendix can rupture less than 24 hours after symptoms begin. If appendicitis is found, antibiotics are given by vein and the appendix is removed (appendectomy). If the doctor performs an operation and appendicitis is not found, the appendix is usually removed anyway.

With an early operation, the chance of death from appendicitis is very low. The person can usually leave the hospital in 1 to 3 days, and convalescence is normally quick and complete. However, without surgery or antibiotic drugs, more than 50% of people with appendicitis die.

For a ruptured appendix, the prognosis is more serious. Decades ago, a rupture often was fatal. Surgery and antibiotics have lowered the death rate to nearly zero, but repeated operations and a long convalescence may be necessary.

Ileus

Ileus (paralytic ileus, adynamic ileus) is temporary absence of the normal contractile movements of the intestinal wall.

- Abdominal surgery and drugs that interfere with the intestine's movements are a common cause.
- Bloating, vomiting, constipation, cramps, and loss of appetite occur.
- The diagnosis is made by x-ray.
- People are given nothing to eat or drink, and a thin suction tube is passed through the nose into the stomach.

Like an obstruction of the intestines, ileus prevents the passage of intestinal contents. Unlike a mechanical obstruction, though, ileus rarely leads to rupture.

Ileus commonly occurs for 24 to 72 hours after abdominal surgery, particularly when the intestines have been manipulated. Drugs, especially opioid analgesics and anticholinergic drugs (see box on page 1897), are a common cause. Ileus may also be caused by an infection or a blood clot inside the abdomen, atherosclerosis that reduces the blood supply to the intestine, or an injury to an intestinal artery or vein. Disorders outside the intestine may cause ileus, such as kidney failure, an underactive thyroid gland, or abnormal levels of blood electrolytes (low potassium levels or high calcium levels, for example).

Symptoms and Diagnosis

The symptoms of ileus are abdominal bloating, vomiting, severe constipation, loss of appetite, and cramps.

A doctor hears few bowel sounds or none at all through a stethoscope. An x-ray of the abdomen shows bulging loops of intestine. Occasionally, doctors evaluate the situation using colonoscopy (examination of the large intestine with a flexible viewing tube).

Treatment

The buildup of gas and liquid caused by ileus must be relieved. Usually, a tube is passed through the nose into the stomach or small intestine, and suction is applied to relieve pressure and expansion (distention). The person is not allowed to eat or drink anything until intestinal function normalizes (or returns). Fluids and electrolytes (such as sodium, chloride, and potassium) are given intravenously. Sometimes, if the problem involves mainly the large intestine, a tube is passed through the anus into the large intestine to relieve the pressure.

Intestinal Obstruction

An obstruction of the intestine is a blockage that completely stops or seriously impairs the passage of intestinal contents.

- The most common causes in adults are scar tissue from previous abdominal surgery, hernias, and tumors.
- Pain, fever, bloating, and a lack of interest in eating are common.

- The diagnosis is based on the results of a physical examination and x-rays.
- Surgery to remove the obstruction is often needed.

An obstruction may occur anywhere along the small or large intestine and can be partial or complete. The part of the intestine above the obstruction continues to function. This part of the intestine enlarges as it fills with food, fluid, digestive secretions, and gas. The intestinal lining becomes swollen and inflamed. If the condition is not treated, the intestine can rupture, leaking its contents and causing inflammation and infection of the abdominal cavity (peritonitis).

Causes

In newborns and infants, intestinal obstruction is commonly caused by a birth defect, a hard mass of intestinal contents (meconium), a twisting of a loop of intestine (volvulus), or a telescoping of one segment of intestine into another (intussusception).

In adults, the most common causes overall are bands of internal scar tissue from previous abdominal surgery (adhesions), parts of the intestine bulging through an abnormal opening (hernias), and tumors. The likelihood of a particular cause varies depending on the part of the intestine affected.

An obstruction of the first segment of the small intestine (duodenum) may be caused by cancer of the pancreas; scarring from an ulcer, a previous operation, or Crohn's disease; or adhesions. Rarely, a gallstone, a mass of undigested food, or a collection of parasitic worms may block the intestine.

An obstruction of the large intestine is commonly caused by cancer, diverticulitis, or a hard lump of stool (fecal impaction). Adhesions and volvulus are less common causes of large-intestinal obstruction.

Strangulation: If an obstruction cuts off the blood supply to the intestine, the condition is called strangulation. Strangulation occurs in nearly 25% of people with small-intestinal obstruction. Usually, strangulation results when part of the intestine becomes trapped in an abnormal opening (strangulated hernia); volvulus; or intussusception. Gangrene can develop in as few as 6 hours. With gangrene, the intestinal wall dies, usually causing rupture, which leads to peritonitis, shock, and, if untreated, death.

Symptoms and Diagnosis

Intestinal obstruction usually causes cramping pain in the abdomen, accompanied by bloating and disinterest in eating (anorexia). Vomiting is common with small-intestinal obstruction but is less common and begins later with large-intestinal obstruction. Complete obstruction causes severe constipation, whereas partial obstruction may cause diarrhea. With strangulation, pain may become severe and steady. A fever is common and is particularly likely if the intestinal wall ruptures.

A doctor examines the abdomen for tenderness, swelling, or masses. When an obstruction occurs, the abdomen is almost always swollen. The sounds normally made by a functioning intestine (bowel sounds), which can be heard through a stethoscope, may be much louder and higher pitched, or they may be absent. The abdomen is usually not very tender when the doctor presses on it unless rupture has caused peritonitis.

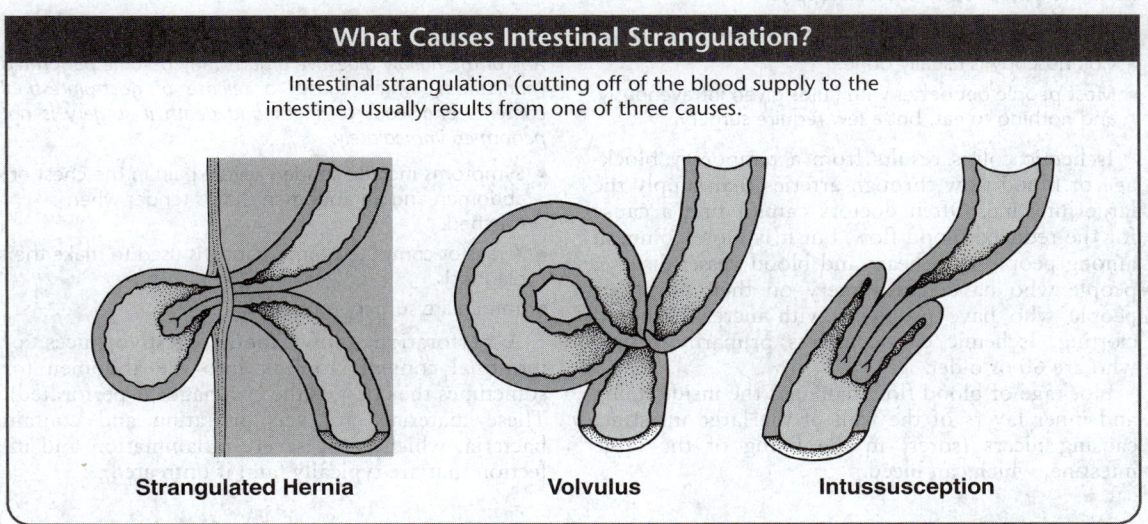

What Causes Intestinal Strangulation?

Intestinal strangulation (cutting off of the blood supply to the intestine) usually results from one of three causes.

Strangulated Hernia　　　**Volvulus**　　　**Intussusception**

X-rays may show dilated loops of intestine that indicate the location of the obstruction. The x-rays also may reveal air around the intestine or under the layer of muscle that separates the abdomen and the chest (diaphragm). Air normally is not found in those places and thus is a sign of rupture.

Treatment

Anyone suspected of having an intestinal obstruction is hospitalized. Usually, a long, thin tube is passed through the nose and placed in the stomach or intestine. Suction is applied to the tube to remove the material that has accumulated above the blockage. Fluid and electrolytes (sodium, chloride, and potassium) are given intravenously to replace water and salts lost from vomiting or diarrhea.

Sometimes an obstruction resolves without further treatment, especially if caused by scarring or adhesions. Occasionally, an endoscope (a flexible viewing tube), which is advanced through the anus, or a barium enema, which inflates the large intestine, may be used to treat some disorders, such as a twisted intestinal segment in the lower part of the large intestine. Most often, however, surgery is performed as soon as possible. The cause of the obstruction determines whether the surgeon can relieve the blockage without removing a segment of the intestines. Sometimes adhesions can be cut to release the trapped segment of intestine, although they tend to recur. In some cases, a colostomy (see art on page 194) is required.

Ischemic Colitis

Ischemic colitis is injury of the large intestine that results from an interruption of its blood supply.

- Abdominal pain and bloody stools are common.
- Colonoscopy is usually done.
- Most people get better with fluids given intravenously and nothing to eat, but a few require surgery.

Ischemic colitis results from a temporary blockage of blood flow through arteries that supply the large intestine. Often doctors cannot find a cause for the reduced blood flow, but it is more common among people with heart and blood vessel disease, people who have had surgery on their aorta, or people who have problems with increased blood clotting. Ischemic colitis affects primarily people who are 60 or older.

Blockage of blood flow damages the inside lining and inner layers of the wall of the large intestine, causing ulcers (sores) in the lining of the large intestine, which can bleed.

Symptoms and Diagnosis

Usually, the person experiences abdominal pain. The pain is felt more often on the left side, but it can occur anywhere in the abdomen. The person frequently passes loose stools that are often accompanied by dark red clots. Sometimes bright red blood is passed without stool. Low-grade fevers (usually below 100° F [37.7° C]) are common.

A doctor may suspect ischemic colitis on the basis of the symptoms of pain and bleeding, especially in a person older than 60. It is important for doctors to distinguish ischemic colitis from acute mesenteric ischemia, a more dangerous condition in which blood flow to part of the intestine is completely and irreversibly blocked (see page 203). They use colonoscopy (examination of the large intestine with a flexible viewing tube) to distinguish ischemic colitis from other forms of inflammation, such as infection or inflammatory bowel disease.

Prognosis and Treatment

People with ischemic colitis are hospitalized. Initially, the person is given neither fluids nor food by mouth so that the intestine can rest. Instead, fluids, electrolytes, and nutrients are given intravenously. Antibiotics are often given to prevent infection that might follow the inflammation. Within a few days, antibiotics are usually stopped and eating is resumed. Nearly all people with ischemic colitis improve and recover over a period of 1 to 2 weeks. However, when the interruption to the blood supply is more severe or more prolonged, the affected portion of the large intestine may have to be surgically removed. Rarely, people get better but later on develop a scar in the affected area, causing a partial obstruction requiring surgical repair.

Perforation

Any of the hollow digestive organs may become perforated (punctured), which causes a release of gastrointestinal contents and leads to shock and death if surgery is not performed immediately.

- Symptoms include sudden severe pain in the chest or abdomen and an abdomen that is tender when touched.
- X-rays or computed tomography is used to make the diagnosis.
- Immediate surgery is needed.

A perforation allows food, digestive juices, or intestinal contents to leak into the abdomen (or sometimes the chest, if the esophagus is perforated). These materials are very irritating and contain bacteria, which cause severe inflammation and infection that are typically fatal if untreated.

SOME CAUSES OF PERFORATION

AREA OF PERFORATION	CAUSES	COMMENTS
Anywhere along the digestive tract	Trauma Foreign bodies	
Esophagus	Forceful vomiting	Called Boerhaave's syndrome
	Injury caused by a medical procedure	Typically caused by an esophagoscope, balloon dilator, or bougie (a thin cylinder-shaped instrument)
	Swallowing strong corrosive material	Typical substances are battery acid or lye
Stomach or small intestine (duodenum)	Peptic ulcer disease	About one third of people have had no previous ulcer symptoms
	Swallowing strong corrosive material	Typically affects the stomach rather than the small intestine
Intestine	Strangulating obstruction	
	Possibly acute appendicitis and Meckel's diverticulitis	
	Obstruction	High risk: People receiving prednisone or other immunosuppressants (these people may have few symptoms)

Causes

Causes vary depending on the location of the perforation, but trauma can affect any part of the digestive system. Swallowed foreign bodies usually pass through a person without difficulty but occasionally become stuck and lead to perforation.

Symptoms

Perforation of the esophagus, stomach, or duodenum causes sudden severe pain, which may travel (radiate) to the shoulder. The person appears very ill, with rapid heart rate, sweating, and an abdomen that is tender and firm to the touch. Because perforation of the small or large intestine often occurs during the course of another painful condition, and is sometimes walled off, symptoms may be less dramatic and can be mistaken for a worsening of the original problem.

In all types of perforation, the person usually has nausea, vomiting, and loss of appetite.

Diagnosis and Treatment

The doctor usually takes x-rays of the chest and abdomen, which may show air that has leaked from the digestive system, a sure sign of perforation. Sometimes, the doctor needs to perform a computed tomography (CT) scan to confirm the diagnosis.

If doctors diagnose a perforation, immediate surgery is needed. Before surgery, the person receives intravenous fluids and antibiotics. Also, a small tube is placed through the nose into the stomach to suction out stomach juices so they do not flow out the perforation.

Liver and Gallbladder Disorders

CHAPTER 32

Biology of the Liver and Gallbladder

Located in the upper right portion of the abdomen, the liver and gallbladder are interconnected by ducts known as the biliary tract, which drains into the first segment of the small intestine (the duodenum). Although the liver and gallbladder participate in some of the same functions, they are very different.

Liver

The wedge-shaped liver is the largest—and, in some ways, the most complex—organ in the body. It serves as the body's chemical factory, performing many vital functions, from regulating the levels of chemicals in the body to producing substances that make blood clot (clotting factors) during bleeding.

Functions of the Liver

The liver manufactures about half of the body's cholesterol. The rest comes from food. Most of the cholesterol made by the liver is used to make bile, a greenish yellow, thick, sticky fluid that aids in digestion. Cholesterol is also needed to make certain hormones, including estrogen, testosterone, and the adrenal hormones, and is a vital component of every cell membrane. The liver manufactures other substances, including proteins needed by the body for its functions. For example, clotting factors are proteins needed to stop bleeding. Albumin is a protein needed to maintain fluid pressure in the bloodstream.

Sugars are stored in the liver as glycogen and then broken down and released into the bloodstream as glucose when needed—for example, during sleep when a person spends many hours without eating and sugar levels in the blood become too low.

The liver also breaks down harmful or toxic substances (toxins) absorbed from the intestine or manufactured elsewhere in the body and then excretes them as harmless by-products into the bile or blood. By-products excreted into bile enter the intestine, then leave the body in stool. By-products excreted into blood are filtered out by the kidneys, then leave the body in urine. The liver also chemically alters (metabolizes) drugs (see page 84), often making them inactive or easier to excrete from the body.

Blood Supply of the Liver

The liver receives blood directly from the intestines, as well as from the heart, as do all other organs. Blood from the intestines contains nearly everything absorbed by the intestines, including nutrients, drugs, and sometimes toxins. This blood flows through tiny capillaries in the intestinal wall into the portal vein, which enters the liver. The blood then flows through a latticework of tiny channels inside the liver, where digested nutrients and toxins are processed.

The hepatic artery brings blood to the liver from the heart. This blood carries oxygen to the liver tissues as well as cholesterol and other substances for processing. Blood from the intestines and heart then mix together in the liver tissues and flow back to the heart through the hepatic vein.

Gallbladder and Biliary Tract

The gallbladder is a small, pear-shaped, muscular storage sac that holds bile. Bile is a greenish yellow, thick, sticky fluid. It consists of bile salts, electrolytes (dissolved charged particles, such as sodium and bicarbonate), bile pigments, cholesterol, and other fats (lipids). Bile has two main functions: aiding in digestion and eliminating certain waste products (mainly hemoglobin and excess cholesterol) from the body. Bile salts aid in digestion by making cholesterol, fats, and fat-soluble vitamins easier to absorb from the intestine. The main pigment in bile, bilirubin, is a waste product that is formed from hemoglobin (the protein that carries oxygen in the blood) and is excreted in bile. Hemoglobin is released when old or damaged red blood cells are destroyed.

Bile flows out of the liver through the left and right hepatic ducts, which come together to form the common hepatic duct. This duct then joins with a duct connected to the gallbladder, called the cystic duct, to form the common bile duct. The common bile duct enters the small intestine at the sphincter of Oddi (a ring-shaped muscle), located a few inches below the stomach.

About half the bile secreted between meals flows directly through the common bile duct into the small intestine. The rest of the bile is diverted through the cystic duct into the gallbladder to be stored. In the gallbladder, up to 90% of the water in bile is absorbed into the bloodstream, making the remaining bile very concentrated. When food enters the small intestine, a series of hormonal and nerve signals triggers the gallbladder to contract and the sphincter of Oddi to relax and open. Bile then flows from the gallbladder into the small intestine to mix with food contents and perform its digestive functions.

After bile enters and passes down the small intestine, about 90% of bile salts are reabsorbed into the blood-

View of the Liver and Gallbladder

Liver cells produce bile, which flows into small channels called bile canaliculi. These small channels drain into bile ducts. The ducts join to form larger and larger channels and eventually form the left and right hepatic ducts, which join to form the common hepatic duct. The common hepatic duct joins with a duct connected to the gallbladder, called the cystic duct, to form the common bile duct. The common bile duct is joined by the pancreatic duct just before it enters the small intestine at the sphincter of Oddi.

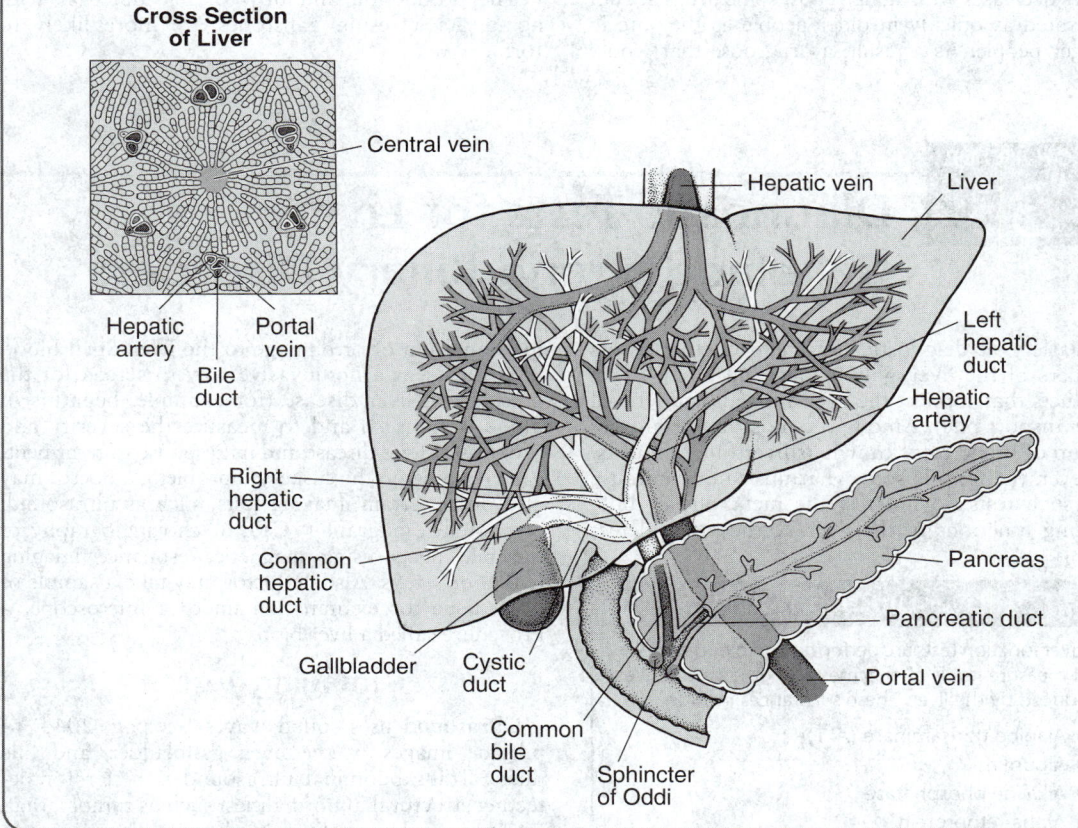

Cross Section of Liver

Central vein

Hepatic artery

Portal vein

Bile duct

Hepatic vein

Liver

Left hepatic duct

Hepatic artery

Right hepatic duct

Common hepatic duct

Gallbladder

Cystic duct

Common bile duct

Sphincter of Oddi

Pancreas

Pancreatic duct

Portal vein

stream through the wall of the lower small intestine. The liver extracts these bile salts from the blood and resecretes them back into the bile. Bile salts go through this cycle about 10 to 12 times a day. Each time, small amounts of bile salts escape absorption and reach the large intestine, where they are broken down by bacteria. Some bile salts are reabsorbed in the large intestine. The rest are excreted in the stool.

The gallbladder, although useful, is not necessary. If the gallbladder is removed (for example, in a person with cholecystitis), bile can move directly from the liver to the small intestine.

Hard masses consisting mainly of cholesterol (gallstones) may form in the gallbladder or bile ducts. Gallstones usually cause no symptoms. However, gallstones may block the flow of bile from the gallbladder, causing pain (biliary colic) or inflammation. They may also migrate from the gallbladder to the bile duct, where they can block the normal flow of bile to the intestine, causing jaundice (a yellowish discoloration of the skin and whites of the eyes) in addition to pain and inflammation. The flow of bile can also be blocked by tumors. Other causes of blocked flow are less common.

Effects of Aging

A number of structural and microscopic changes occur as the liver ages. For example, the color of the liver changes from lighter to darker brown. Its size and blood flow decrease. However, liver function test results generally remain normal.

The ability of the liver to metabolize many substances decreases with aging. Thus, some drugs are not inactivated as quickly in older people as they are in younger people. As a result, a drug dose that would not have side effects in younger people may cause dose-related side effects in older people (see page 1896). Thus, drug dosages often need to be decreased in older people. Also, the liver's ability to withstand stress decreases. Thus, substances that are toxic to the liver can cause more damage in older people than in younger people. Repair of damaged liver cells is also slower in older people.

The production and flow of bile decrease with aging. As a result, gallstones are more likely to form.

CHAPTER

33 Diagnostic Tests for Liver, Gallbladder, and Biliary Disorders

A variety of diagnostic tests help doctors assess disorders of the liver, gallbladder, and biliary tract (the ducts that connect the liver and gallbladder and that transport bile). Among the most important are a group of blood tests known as liver function tests. However, the term is somewhat misleading because most such tests do not test the metabolic or bile-secreting functions of the liver. Rather, they detect inflammation of or damage to the liver. Such blood tests represent a noninvasive way to screen for the presence of liver disease (for example, hepatitis in blood donations) and to measure the severity and progress of liver disease and its response to treatment.

Depending on the suspected problem, a doctor may also order certain imaging tests, such as ultrasound, computed tomography (CT), or cholangiography of the bile ducts using magnetic resonance imaging (MRI) or x-rays. Also, a doctor may take a sample of liver tissue for examination under a microscope, a procedure called a liver biopsy.

Imaging Tests

Ultrasound uses sound waves (see page 2044) to provide images of the liver, gallbladder, and bile ducts. Transabdominal ultrasound is better for detecting structural abnormalities, such as tumors, than for diffuse abnormalities, such as cirrhosis (severe scarring of the liver) or fatty liver (excess fat in the liver). It is the least expensive and safest technique for creating images of the gallbladder and bile ducts.

Using ultrasound, a doctor can readily detect gallstones in the gallbladder. Ultrasound of the abdomen can distinguish whether jaundice (a yellowish discoloration of the skin and the whites of the eyes) is caused by bile duct obstruction or by liver cell malfunction. If ultrasound shows ducts that are dilated (widened), the cause is obstruction. Ultrasound also provides guidance when inserting a needle to obtain a tissue sample for biopsy. A type of ultrasound, called Doppler ultrasound, can show blood flow in the blood vessels of the liver. Doppler ultrasound can detect blockages in the liver's arteries and veins, particularly

---

Liver Function Tests

Liver function tests are performed on blood samples and measure levels of enzymes and other substances produced by the liver. These substances include

- Alanine transaminase (ALT)
- Albumin
- Alkaline phosphatase
- Alpha-fetoprotein
- Aspartate transaminase (AST)
- Bilirubin
- Gamma-glutamyl transpeptidase
- Lactic dehydrogenase
- Mitochondrial antibodies
- 5'-Nucleotidase

Levels of some of these substances measure how well the liver performs its normal functions of making proteins and secreting bile. Levels of other substances detect the presence and degree of liver inflammation.

One test of liver function is the prothrombin time (PT), which is used to calculate the international normalized ratio (INR). Both the PT and the INR are measures of the time needed for blood to clot.

the portal vein, which brings blood from the intestine to the liver. Doppler ultrasound can also detect the effects of high blood pressure in the portal vein (portal hypertension). Endoscopic ultrasound uses a tiny probe on the top of an endoscope that is passed through the mouth into the stomach and the first segment of the small intestine (duodenum), bringing the probe closer to the liver and its surrounding organs.

Radionuclide (radioisotope) imaging (see page 2043) uses a substance containing a radioactive tracer that, when injected intravenously into the body, collects in a particular organ. The radioactivity is detected by a gamma-ray camera, which is positioned over the upper abdomen and is attached to a computer that generates an image. A liver scan uses a radioactive substance that collects in liver cells. Cholescintigraphy (hepatobiliary scintigraphy or scan), another type of radionuclide imaging, follows the movement of a radioactive substance as it is secreted from the liver and passes into the gallbladder and through the bile ducts into the duodenum. This technique can detect a blocked cystic duct (which joins the gallbladder to the major bile duct). Such a blockage indicates acute inflammation of the gallbladder (cholecystitis—see page 245).

Computed tomography (CT—see page 2037) provides excellent images of the liver. It is particularly useful for detecting tumors. It can also detect collections of pus (abscesses) and some diffuse disorders, such as a fatty liver (excess fat in the liver).

Magnetic resonance imaging (MRI—see page 2040) can detect diffuse liver disorders, such as hepatitis, hemochromatosis, and Wilson's disease, which affect all areas of the liver about equally. MRI shows blood flow, providing information about blood vessel disorders. MRI technology can also provide images of the bile ducts and nearby structures, using a technique called **magnetic resonance cholangiopancreatography (MRCP)**. The images produced are as good as those produced by more invasive tests, in which dye is directly injected into the biliary and pancreatic ducts. Unlike CT, MRI tests do not involve exposure to x-rays, though they are more expensive than CT and take longer to perform.

Endoscopic retrograde cholangiopancreatography (ERCP) involves passing an endoscope (a flexible viewing tube) through the mouth, esophagus, and stomach into the duodenum. A thin tube is then inserted through the endoscope into the biliary tract. A radiopaque dye is injected through the tube into the biliary tract, and x-rays are taken of the biliary tract and pancreatic duct. ERCP is occasionally used simply to see the biliary tract structures, although MRCP is usually preferred when available because it is just as good and is safer. However, unlike other diagnostic tests, ERCP allows doctors to do biopsies and certain treatments. For example, a stone in a bile duct can be removed, or a tube

Understanding Endoscopic Retrograde Cholangiopancreatography

In endoscopic retrograde cholangiopancreatography (ERCP), a radiopaque dye is introduced through an endoscope (a flexible viewing tube), which is inserted into the mouth and through the stomach into the duodenum (the first segment of the small intestine). The radiopaque dye is injected into the biliary tract just past the sphincter of Oddi. The dye then flows back up the biliary tract and often shows the pancreatic ducts. Surgical instruments can also be used with the endoscope, allowing a doctor to remove a stone in a bile duct or insert a tube (stent) to bypass a bile duct blocked by scarring or cancer.

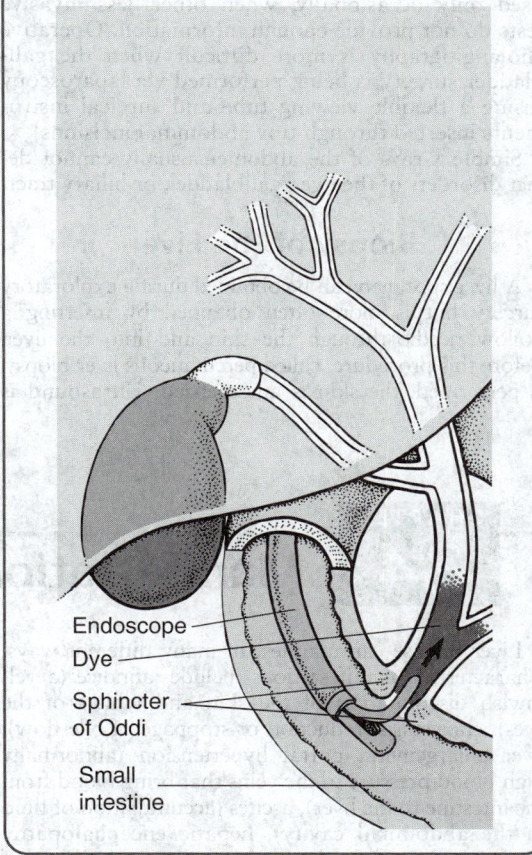

Endoscope
Dye
Sphincter of Oddi
Small intestine

(stent) can be inserted to bypass a bile duct blockage caused by cancer. With ERCP, complications (such as inflammation of the pancreas [pancreatitis] or bleeding) occur about 1% of the time. If a treatment is performed during ERCP, such complications can occur more often.

Percutaneous transhepatic cholangiography involves inserting a long needle through the skin into the liver and then injecting a radiopaque dye into a bile duct in the liver, using ultrasound for guidance. The x-rays clearly reveal the biliary tract, particularly any blockage within the bile ducts. Like ERCP, percutaneous transhepatic cholangiography is used more often for treatment or biopsy than to obtain images of the biliary tract. Complications of percutaneous transhepatic cholangiography, such as bleeding and internal damage, make it a less desirable method than ERCP, except in special circumstances.

Operative cholangiography involves the injection of a radiopaque dye directly into the ducts of the biliary tract during gallbladder surgery. X-rays then reveal clear images of the biliary tract. This test is used only occasionally, when other, less invasive tests do not provide enough information. Operative cholangiography is more difficult when the gallbladder surgery is being performed via laparoscopy (using a flexible viewing tube and surgical instruments inserted through tiny abdominal incisions).

Simple x-rays of the abdomen usually cannot detect disorders of the liver, gallbladder, or biliary tract.

Biopsy of the Liver

A liver specimen can be obtained during exploratory surgery but is more often obtained by inserting a hollow needle through the skin and into the liver. Before this procedure, called percutaneous liver biopsy, is performed, the skin is anesthetized. Ultrasound is usually used to locate the liver and guide the needle to biopsy any abnormal area. Liver biopsy can be performed as an outpatient procedure. After the specimen is obtained, the person remains in the outpatient department for 3 to 4 hours because of a small risk of complications, such as tearing (laceration) of the liver. If the liver is torn, bleeding into the abdomen may occur. If severe, bleeding can lead to shock. Because bleeding can start up to 15 days after the biopsy, the person is instructed to stay within an hour's drive of the hospital during that period. These complications, though infrequent, can cause serious problems; 1 of 10,000 people die as a result of the procedure. Mild pain in the upper right abdomen, sometimes extending to the right shoulder, is common after a liver biopsy and is usually relieved by analgesics.

In transvenous liver biopsy, a catheter is inserted into a neck vein, threaded through the heart, and placed into one of the hepatic veins that drain the liver. A needle on the tip of the catheter is then inserted through the wall of the vein into the liver. This procedure is less likely to injure the liver than is percutaneous liver biopsy. It is especially useful in people who bleed easily, a complication of severe liver disease.

Liver biopsy can detect information about the liver that may not be evident from other tests. It is commonly used to detect excess fat in the liver (fatty liver), chronic liver inflammation (chronic hepatitis), metabolic liver diseases such as Wilson's disease (an excess of copper) and hemochromatosis (iron overload), complications following liver transplantation, and cancer that has spread to the liver.

CHAPTER

34 Manifestations of Liver Disease

Liver disease can manifest in many different ways. Characteristic manifestations include jaundice (a yellowish discoloration of the skin and whites of the eyes), cholestasis (reduction or stoppage of bile flow), liver enlargement, portal hypertension (abnormally high blood pressure in the veins that bring blood from the intestine to the liver), ascites (accumulation of fluid in the abdominal cavity), hepatic encephalopathy (deterioration of brain function due to buildup of toxic substances normally removed by the brain), and liver failure.

Sometimes the manifestations of liver disease are not obvious. For example, symptoms may include fatigue, a feeling of unwellness, loss of appetite, and mild weight loss. However, these symptoms are also typical of many other diseases. Thus, liver disease can easily be overlooked, particularly in its early stages.

Jaundice

Jaundice is a yellowish discoloration of the skin and of the whites of the eyes caused by abnormally high levels of the pigment bilirubin in the bloodstream.

- Liver damage or a blockage in a bile duct can cause jaundice.
- The skin and whites of the eyes look yellow, the skin may itch, and urine is often dark.
- Laboratory and often imaging tests help identify the cause.
- Often, jaundice disappears as its cause resolves, but surgery or endoscopy is sometimes needed.

SOME MAJOR FEATURES OF LIVER DISEASE

FEATURE	DESCRIPTION
Jaundice	A yellowish discoloration of the skin and whites of the eyes
Hepatomegaly	Liver enlargement
Ascites	Fluid in the abdominal cavity
Hepatic encephalopathy	Confusion caused by deterioration of brain function due to buildup of toxic substances in the blood
Gastrointestinal bleeding	Bleeding from large, tortuous veins (varices) in the esophagus and stomach
Portal hypertension	Abnormally high blood pressure in the veins that bring blood from the intestine to the liver (branches of the portal vein)
Skin symptoms	Spiderlike blood vessels on the face and chest Red palms Bright red complexion Itching
Blood abnormalities	Decreased number of red blood cells (anemia) Decreased number of white blood cells (leukopenia) Decreased number of platelets (thrombocytopenia) A tendency to bleed (coagulopathy)
Hormonal abnormalities	High levels of insulin but a poor response to it, leading to high blood sugar levels Cessation of menstrual periods and decreased fertility in women Erectile dysfunction and feminization in men
Heart and blood vessel abnormalities	Increased heart rate and amount of blood pumped Low blood pressure (hypotension)
General symptoms	Fatigue Weakness Weight loss Poor appetite Nausea Fever Abdominal pain

Old or damaged red blood cells are constantly being removed from the circulation, mainly by the spleen. During this process, hemoglobin, the part of red blood cells that carries oxygen, is broken down into a dark greenish yellow pigment called bilirubin. Bilirubin is then carried in the bloodstream to the liver and is excreted into the intestine as a component of bile (the digestive fluid produced by the liver). If bilirubin cannot be excreted into bile quickly enough, it builds up in the blood. The excess bilirubin is deposited in the skin, resulting in the yellowish discoloration called jaundice.

Causes

High levels of bilirubin in the blood may result from problems originating either within the liver or outside the liver. Damage to the liver, such as that due to inflammation or scarring, can impair its ability to excrete bilirubin into bile. Alternatively, the bile ducts, which carry bile from the liver to the small intestine, may be blocked, for example, by a gallstone or a tumor. Less commonly, overproduction of bilirubin, due to excessive breakdown of red blood cells, can overwhelm the liver with more bilirubin than the liver is capable of processing. Overproduction is most common in newborns with jaundice (see page 1700).

In Gilbert's syndrome, bilirubin levels are slightly increased but usually not enough to cause jaundice. This disorder, which is sometimes hereditary, is most often detected in young adults during routine screening tests. It causes no other symptoms and no problems.

The skin of people who eat large amounts of food rich in beta-carotene (such as carrots, squash, and some melons) may develop a mild yellow tint, but their eyes do not turn yellow. This condition is not jaundice and is unrelated to liver disease.

> **? Did You Know...**
> Eating too many carrots can make the skin look yellow but does not cause jaundice.

Symptoms

In jaundice, the skin and whites of the eyes appear yellow. Urine is often dark because excess bilirubin is excreted through the kidneys. People may have itching, light-colored stools, or other symptoms, depending on the cause of jaundice. For example, acute inflammation of the liver (acute hepatitis) may cause loss of appetite, nausea, vomiting, and fever. Blockage of bile may result in abdominal pain and fever.

Diagnosis and Treatment

A doctor uses laboratory tests and imaging studies to determine the cause of the jaundice. If the problem is a disease of the liver, such as acute viral hepatitis, the jaundice usually disappears gradually as the condition of the liver improves. If the problem is blockage of a bile duct, surgery or surgical endoscopy (using a flexible viewing tube with surgical instruments attached—see page 129) is usually performed as soon as possible to reopen the affected bile duct. Itching caused by jaundice can be treated with cholestyramine taken by mouth. Usually, the itching gradually disappears as the liver's condition improves.

Cholestasis

Cholestasis is reduction or stoppage of bile flow.

- Disorders of the liver, bile duct, or pancreas can cause cholestasis.
- The skin and whites of the eyes look yellow, the skin itches, urine is dark, and stools may become light-colored and smell foul.
- Laboratory and often imaging tests are needed to identify the cause.
- Treatment depends on the cause, but drugs can help relieve itching.

With cholestasis, the flow of bile (the digestive fluid produced by the liver) is impaired at some point between the liver cells and the duodenum (the first segment of the small intestine). When bile flow is stopped, the pigment bilirubin (a waste product formed when old or damaged red blood cells are broken down) escapes into the bloodstream and accumulates.

Causes

The causes of cholestasis are divided into two groups: those originating within the liver and those originating outside the liver.

Within the Liver: Causes include acute hepatitis, alcoholic liver disease, primary biliary cirrhosis with inflammation and scarring of the bile ducts, cirrhosis due to viral hepatitis B or C (also with inflammation and scarring of the bile ducts), drugs, hormonal effects on bile flow during pregnancy (a condition called cholestasis of pregnancy—see page 1634), and cancer that has spread to the liver.

Outside the Liver: Causes include a stone in a bile duct, narrowing (stricture) of a bile duct, cancer of a bile duct, cancer of the pancreas, and inflammation of the pancreas (pancreatitis).

Symptoms

Jaundice, dark urine, light-colored stools, and generalized itchiness are characteristic symptoms of cholestasis. Jaundice results from excess bilirubin deposited in the skin, and dark urine results from excess bilirubin excreted by the kidneys. Retention of bile products in the skin may cause itching, with subsequent scratching and skin damage. Stools may become light-colored because the passage of bilirubin into the intestine is blocked. Stools may contain too much fat (a condition called steatorrhea) because bile cannot enter the intestine to help digest fat in foods. Fatty stools may be foul-smelling. The lack of bile in the intestine also means that calcium and vitamin D are poorly absorbed. If cholestasis persists, a deficiency of these nutrients can cause loss of bone tissue. Vitamin K, which is needed for blood clotting, is also poorly absorbed from the intestine, causing a tendency to bleed easily.

Prolonged jaundice due to cholestasis produces a muddy skin color and fatty yellow deposits in the skin. Whether the person has other symptoms, such as abdominal pain, loss of appetite, vomiting, or fever, depends on the cause of cholestasis.

Diagnosis

A doctor tries to determine whether the cause is within or outside the liver on the basis of symptoms and the results of a physical examination.

Recent use of drugs that can cause cholestasis suggests a cause within the liver. Small, spiderlike blood vessels visible in the skin, an enlarged spleen, and fluid in the abdominal cavity (ascites), which are signs of chronic liver disease, also suggest a cause within the liver.

Findings that suggest a cause outside the liver include certain kinds of abdominal pain (such as intermittent pain in the upper right side of the abdomen and sometimes also in the right shoulder) and an enlarged gallbladder (felt during the physical examination or detected by imaging studies).

Some findings do not indicate whether the cause is within or outside the liver. They include heavy alcohol intake, loss of appetite, nausea, and vomiting.

Typically, the blood levels of two enzymes, alkaline phosphatase and gamma-glutamyl transpeptidase, are very high in people with cholestasis. A blood test that measures the level of bilirubin indicates the severity of the cholestasis but not its cause. An imaging study, usually ultrasonography, is almost always done if blood test results are abnormal. Computed tomography (CT) or sometimes magnetic resonance imaging (MRI) may be done in addition to or instead of ultrasonography. If the cause appears to be within the liver, a liver biopsy (see page 214) may be done and usually establishes the diagnosis. If the cause appears to be blockage of the bile ducts, more precise images of these ducts are usually needed. Typically, either endoscopic retrograde cholangiopancreatography (ERCP) or magnetic resonance cholangiopancreatography (MRCP) is done. MRCP uses magnetic resonance imaging (see page 213). In ERCP, a contrast agent is injected and x-rays are taken (see art on page 213).

Treatment

A blockage of the bile ducts can usually be treated with surgery or endoscopy (using a flexible viewing tube with surgical instruments attached). A blockage within the liver may be treated in various ways depending on the cause. If a drug is the suspected cause, the doctor stops its use. If acute hepatitis is the cause, cholestasis and jaundice usually disappear when hepatitis has run its course. A person with cholestasis is advised to avoid or stop using any substance that is toxic to the liver, such as alcohol and certain drugs.

Cholestyramine, taken by mouth, can be used to treat itchiness. This drug binds with certain bile products in the intestine, so they cannot be reabsorbed to irritate the skin. Unless the liver is severely damaged, taking vitamin K can improve blood clotting. Supplements of calcium and vitamin D are often taken if the cholestasis persists, but they are not very effective in preventing loss of bone tissue.

Portal Hypertension

Portal hypertension is abnormally high blood pressure in branches of the portal vein, the large vein that brings blood from the intestine to the liver.

- Cirrhosis is the most common cause in Western countries.
- Portal hypertension can lead to an enlarged abdomen, abdominal discomfort, confusion, and internal bleeding.

- Doctors base the diagnosis on symptoms and results of a physical examination, sometimes with ultrasonography.
- Drugs can reduce blood pressure in the portal vein, but if internal bleeding occurs, emergency treatment is required.

The portal vein receives blood from the entire intestine and from the spleen, pancreas, and gallbladder. After entering the liver, the vein divides into right and left branches and then into tiny channels that run through the liver. When blood leaves the liver, it flows back into the general (systemic, or bodywide) circulation through the hepatic vein (see art on page 233).

Two factors can increase blood pressure in the portal blood vessels:

- Increased volume of blood flowing through the vessels
- Increased resistance to the blood flow through the liver

In Western countries, the most common cause of portal hypertension is increased resistance to blood flow caused by extensive scarring of the liver in cirrhosis, which is most often due to chronic excessive alcohol intake.

Portal hypertension leads to the development of new veins (called collateral vessels) that directly connect the portal blood vessels to the general circulation, bypassing the liver. Because of this bypass, substances (such as toxins) that are normally removed from the blood by the liver can pass into the general circulation. Collateral vessels develop at specific places. The most important are located at the lower end of the esophagus and at the upper part of the stomach. Here, the vessels become engorged and full of twists and turns—that is, they become varicose veins of the esophagus (esophageal varices) or stomach (gastric varices). These engorged vessels are fragile and prone to bleeding, sometimes seriously and occasionally with fatal results. Other collateral vessels may develop on the abdominal wall and at the rectum.

Portal hypertension often causes the spleen to enlarge because the pressure interferes with blood flow from the spleen into the portal blood vessels. Pressure in the portal blood vessels may cause protein-containing (ascitic) fluid from the surface of the liver and intestine to leak into the abdominal cavity. This condition is called ascites (see page 218).

Symptoms and Diagnosis

Portal hypertension itself does not cause symptoms, but some of its consequences do. If a large amount of ascitic fluid accumulates, the person's abdomen swells (distends), sometimes noticeably and sometimes enough to make the abdomen greatly enlarged and taut. This distention is painless.

An enlarged spleen may cause a vague sense of discomfort in the upper left part of the abdomen. Esophageal and gastric varices bleed easily and sometimes massively. Much less commonly, varicose veins in the rectum bleed.

When substances that are normally removed from the liver pass into the general circulation and reach the brain, they may cause confusion or drowsiness (hepatic encephalopathy). Collateral vessels may be visible on the skin over the abdominal wall or around the rectum. Because most people with portal hypertension also have severe liver dysfunction, they may have symptoms of liver failure, such as a tendency to bleed.

Doctors can usually recognize hepatic encephalopathy based on symptoms and findings during the physical examination. Doctors can usually feel an enlarged spleen through the abdominal wall. They can detect fluid in the abdomen by noting abdominal swelling and by listening for a dull sound when tapping (percussing) the abdomen. An ultrasound scan may be used to examine blood flow in the portal vein and nearby blood vessels and to detect fluid in the abdomen. An ultrasound or computed tomography (CT) scan can be used to look for and examine collateral vessels. Rarely, a catheter is inserted through an incision in the neck and threaded through blood vessels into the liver or spleen to directly measure pressure in the portal blood vessels (manometry).

Treatment

To reduce the risk of bleeding from esophageal varices, a doctor may try to reduce pressure in the portal vein. One way is to give drugs such as propranolol or nadolol.

Bleeding from esophageal varices is a medical emergency. Drugs such as vasopressin or octreotide may be given intravenously to constrict the bleeding veins, and blood transfusions are given to replace lost blood. An endoscopic examination is usually done to confirm that the bleeding is from varices. The veins can then be blocked off with rubber bands or with injections of a chemical given through the endoscope.

If the bleeding continues or recurs repeatedly, a surgical procedure may be done to create a bypass (called a shunt) between the portal venous system and the general (systemic, or bodywide) venous system. This bypass lowers pressure in the portal vein because pressure is much lower in the general venous system.

There are various types of portal-systemic shunt procedures. In one type, called transjugular intrahepatic portal-systemic shunting (TIPS), an x-ray-guided needle is passed through the liver to create a shunt connecting the portal vein directly with one of the hepatic veins. Shunt procedures are usually successful in stopping the bleeding but pose certain risks, such as hepatic encephalopathy (see page 219). The TIPS procedure, although less dangerous than other portal-systemic shunt procedures, may need to be repeated periodically because the shunt narrows in some people.

Ascites

Ascites is the accumulation of protein-containing (ascitic) fluid in the abdominal cavity.

- Many disorders can cause ascites, but cirrhosis is the most common.
- If large amounts of fluid accumulate, the abdomen becomes very large, sometimes making people lose their appetite and feel short of breath.
- Analysis of the fluid can help determine the cause.
- Usually, bed rest, a low-salt diet, and diuretics help eliminate excess fluid.

Ascites tends to occur in long-standing (chronic) rather than in short-lived (acute) disorders. It occurs most commonly in cirrhosis (severe scarring of the liver), especially in cirrhosis caused by alcoholism or viral hepatitis. It may occur in other liver disorders, such as severe alcoholic hepatitis without cirrhosis, chronic hepatitis, and obstruction of the hepatic vein (Budd-Chiari syndrome). Ascites can also occur in disorders unrelated to the liver, such as cancer, heart failure, kidney failure, inflammation of the pancreas (pancreatitis), and tuberculosis affecting the lining of the abdominal cavity.

In people with a liver disorder, ascitic fluid leaks from the surface of the liver and intestine. A combination of factors is responsible. They include portal hypertension, decreased ability of the blood vessels to retain fluid, fluid retention by the kidneys, and alterations in various hormones and chemicals that regulate bodily fluids.

Symptoms and Diagnosis

Small amounts of fluid in the abdominal cavity usually produce no symptoms, but massive amounts may cause abdominal swelling (distention) and discomfort. Pressure on the stomach from the swollen abdomen may lead to loss of appetite, and pressure on the lungs may lead to shortness of breath. When a doctor taps (percusses) the abdomen, the fluid makes a dull sound. When the abdominal cavity contains large amounts of fluid, the abdomen is taut, and the navel is flat or even pushed out. In some people with ascites, the ankles swell with excess fluid (edema). However, a doctor may not be able to detect ascitic fluid unless the volume is about a quart or more.

If the presence of ascites or its cause is not clear, the doctor may use ultrasonography. In addition, a small sample of ascitic fluid can be withdrawn by inserting a needle through the abdominal wall—a procedure called diagnostic paracentesis (see page 131). Laboratory analysis of the fluid can help determine the cause.

Treatment

The basic treatment for ascites is bed rest and a salt-restricted diet, usually combined with drugs called diuretics, which make the kidneys excrete more water into the urine. If ascites makes breathing or eating difficult, the fluid may be removed through a needle inserted into the abdomen—a procedure called therapeutic paracentesis. The fluid tends to reaccumulate unless the person also restricts salt consumption and takes a diuretic. Because a large amount of albumin (the major protein in plasma) is usually lost from the blood into the abdominal fluid, albumin may be administered intravenously.

An infection called spontaneous bacterial peritonitis occasionally develops in ascitic fluid for no apparent reason, especially in people with alcoholic cirrhosis. Untreated, this infection can be fatal. Survival depends on early vigorous treatment with antibiotics.

Hepatic Encephalopathy

Hepatic encephalopathy (portal-systemic encephalopathy, liver encephalopathy, hepatic coma) is deterioration of brain function that occurs because toxic substances normally removed by the liver build up in the blood and reach the brain.

- Hepatic encephalopathy may be triggered by an alcohol binge, a drug, or another stress in people who have a long-standing liver disorder.
- People become confused, disoriented, and drowsy, with changes in personality, behavior, and mood.
- Doctors base the diagnosis on results of a physical examination, electroencephalography, and blood tests.
- Eliminating the trigger and reducing protein in the diet may help symptoms resolve.

Substances absorbed into the bloodstream from the intestine pass through the liver, where toxins are normally removed. Many of these toxins are normal breakdown products of the digestion of protein. In hepatic encephalopathy, toxins are not removed because liver function is impaired. Also, some toxins may bypass the liver altogether through connections formed between the portal venous system (which supplies blood to the liver) and the general (systemic, or bodywide) venous system as a result of liver disease and portal hypertension. A surgical bypass (portal-systemic shunt) to correct portal hypertension may have the same effect. Whatever the cause, the outcome is the same: Toxins can reach the brain and affect its function. Exactly which substances are toxic

to the brain is not known. However, high levels of protein breakdown products in the blood, such as ammonia, appear to play a role.

In a person with a long-standing (chronic) liver disorder, encephalopathy is usually triggered by an event such as an acute infection or an alcoholic binge, which increases liver damage. Or encephalopathy may be triggered by eating too much protein, which increases the levels of protein breakdown products in the blood. Bleeding in the digestive tract, such as bleeding from dilated, twisted veins in the esophagus (esophageal varices), can also lead to a buildup of protein breakdown products, which may directly affect the brain. Dehydration, an electrolyte imbalance, and certain drugs—especially some sedatives, analgesics, and diuretics—may also trigger encephalopathy. When such a trigger is eliminated, the encephalopathy may disappear.

Symptoms and Diagnosis

Symptoms are those of decreased brain function, especially reduced alertness and confusion. In the earliest stages, subtle changes appear in logical thinking, personality, and behavior. The person's mood may change, and judgment may be impaired. Normal sleep patterns may be disturbed. At any stage of encephalopathy, the person's breath may have a musty sweet odor. As the disorder progresses, the hands cannot be held steady when the person stretches out the arms, resulting in a crude flapping motion of the hands (asterixis). Also, the person usually becomes drowsy and confused, and movements and speech become sluggish. Disorientation is common. Uncommonly, a person with encephalopathy becomes agitated and excited. Seizures are also uncommon. Eventually, the person may lose consciousness and lapse into a coma.

An electroencephalogram (EEG—see page 636) may help in diagnosing early encephalopathy. Even in mild cases, an EEG shows abnormal slowing of brain waves. Blood tests usually show abnormally high levels of ammonia, but measuring the level is not always a reliable way to diagnose encephalopathy.

In an older person, hepatic encephalopathy may be more difficult to recognize in its early stages because its initial symptoms (such as disturbed sleep patterns and mild confusion) may be attributed to dementia or erroneously labeled as delirium (see page 682).

Treatment

A doctor looks for and tries to eliminate any triggers for the encephalopathy, such as an infection or a drug. A doctor also tries to eliminate toxic substances from the intestines, usually by restricting the person's diet. Protein is reduced or eliminated from the diet, and oral or intravenous carbohydrates serve as the main source of calories. Later, a doctor may increase the amount of vegetable protein (such as soy protein) rather than animal protein, to provide adequate protein without worsening the encephalopathy. The higher fiber content of a vegetable diet tends to speed up the passage of food through the intestine and alter the acidity in the intestine, thereby helping reduce absorption of ammonia. A synthetic sugar (lactulose), taken by mouth, has similar beneficial effects: It alters the acidity of the intestine and acts as a laxative, speeding up the passage of food. Cleansing enemas also may be given. Occasionally, a person who has difficulty tolerating lactulose is given an antibiotic by mouth.

With treatment, hepatic encephalopathy is frequently reversible. In fact, complete recovery is possible, especially if the encephalopathy was triggered by a reversible cause. However, people with a chronic liver disorder are susceptible to future episodes of encephalopathy. In up to 80% of people in a coma due to acute liver inflammation, the disorder is fatal despite intensive treatment.

Liver Failure

Liver failure is severe deterioration in liver function.

- Liver failure is caused by a disorder or substance that damages the liver.
- Common symptoms include jaundice, fatigue, weakness, and loss of appetite.
- Severe symptoms include fluid build-up in the abdomen (ascites) and easy bruising and bleeding.
- The diagnosis is usually based on symptoms, the results of a physical examination, and blood tests.
- Treatment usually involves controlling protein consumption, restricting salt in the diet, and completely avoiding alcohol, in addition to treating the cause.

Liver failure can result from any type of liver disorder, including viral hepatitis, cirrhosis, and liver damage from alcohol or drugs such as acetaminophen. A large portion of the liver must be damaged before liver failure occurs. Liver failure may develop rapidly over days or weeks (acute) or gradually over months or years (chronic).

Many effects occur because the liver malfunctions:

- The liver can no longer adequately process bilirubin (a waste product formed when old red blood cells are broken down) to be excreted. The result is jaundice.

- The liver can no longer synthesize enough of the proteins that help blood clot. The result is a tendency to bruise and bleed (coagulopathy).
- Portal hypertension often occurs. It can result in fluid in the abdominal cavity (ascites), hepatic (liver) encephalopathy, or both.

Symptoms and Diagnosis

A person with liver failure usually has jaundice, ascites, hepatic encephalopathy, and generally failing health. Other common symptoms include fatigue, weakness, nausea, and loss of appetite. In acute liver failure, a person may go from being healthy to near death within a few days. In chronic liver failure, the deterioration in health may be very gradual until a dramatic event, such as bleeding varices (large, tortuous veins), occurs. The person may tend to bruise and bleed easily. Bleeding that would be slight in other people (for example, bleeding from a small cut or a nosebleed) may not stop on its own and may even be difficult for doctors to control.

Doctors can usually diagnose liver failure based on symptoms and the results of a physical examination. Blood tests are done to evaluate liver function, which is usually severely impaired.

Prognosis and Treatment

Treatment depends on the cause and on the specific symptoms. The urgency of treatment depends on whether liver failure is acute or chronic, but the principles of treatment are the same. The person is usually placed on a restricted diet. Protein consumption is carefully controlled: Too much protein can cause brain dysfunction, and too little can cause weight loss. Salt (sodium) consumption is kept low to help prevent ascitic fluid from accumulating in the abdomen. Alcohol is completely avoided because it can worsen liver damage.

Ultimately, liver failure is fatal if it is not treated or if the liver disorder is progressive. Even after treatment, liver failure may be irreversible. Some people die of kidney failure (hepatorenal syndrome) because liver failure can eventually lead to kidney failure. Liver transplantation (see page 1132) if performed soon enough, can restore liver function, sometimes enabling people to live as long as they would have if they did not have a liver disorder. However, liver transplantation is suitable for only a small number of people with liver failure.

Fatty Liver, Cirrhosis, and Related Disorders

Most liver diseases, including fatty liver, cirrhosis, primary biliary cirrhosis and primary sclerosing cholangitis, result from injury to the liver. If damage is acute (sudden) and limited, the liver commonly repairs itself by regenerating new liver cells onto the scaffolding (internal structure) left when liver cells die. Repair and full recovery occur if the person can survive long enough to allow this renewal. However, repeated damage, particularly with disruption of the liver scaffolding, leads to scarring (fibrosis) and erratic attempts at regenerating, resulting in cirrhosis.

Injury to the liver can follow exposure to any of the following:

- Alcohol (a common cause)
- Toxins in the environment and as contaminants in foods
- Certain drugs, such as aspirin (given to infants), corticosteroids, tamoxifen, and tetracycline
- Some medicinal herbs (for example, bush tea, which contains pyrrolizidine alkaloids)
- Metabolic problems
- Certain viral infections
- Inflammation due to malfunction of the immune system, causing the body to attack its own tissues (an autoimmune reaction—see page 1124)

Sometimes the exact cause of liver injury is not known.

Fatty Liver

Fatty liver (steatosis) is an abnormal accumulation of certain fats (triglycerides) inside liver cells.

- People with fatty liver may feel tired or have mild abdominal discomfort but otherwise have no symptoms.
- A liver biopsy may be needed to confirm the diagnosis and provide valuable information.
- Treatment involves eliminating the cause of fatty liver, such as alcohol.

In the United States and other Western countries, the most common causes of fatty liver are alcoholism, toxins, certain drugs, hereditary metabolic disorders, and metabolic abnormalities, such as excess body weight, insulin resistance, and high triglyceride levels in the blood. This combination of metabolic abnormalities is called the metabolic syndrome (see page 960). These conditions cause fat to accumulate in liver cells either by causing the body to synthesize more fat or by processing (metabolizing) and excreting fat more slowly. As a result, fat accumulates and is then stored inside liver cells. Just consuming a high-fat diet does not result in fatty

---

Medicinal Herbs and the Liver

Some medicinal herbs (plant parts taken for medicinal purposes) contain substances that can damage the liver. These substances may also be consumed in contaminated foods. The liver is a prime target for damage because it processes everything that enters the mouth and is swallowed.

Herbs that contain pyrrolizidine alkaloids may damage the liver. Hundreds of herbs contain pyrrolizidine alkaloids. These herbs include borage, comfrey, and certain Chinese herbs, such as zi cao (groomwell), kuan dong hua (coltsfoot), qian li guang (liferoot), and pei lan (*Eupatorium*). Some of the herbs that contain pyrrolizidine alkaloids are used to make teas. Sometimes milk, honey, and cereals are contaminated with pyrrolizidine alkaloids, which are then consumed unknowingly.

Pyrrolizidine alkaloids can damage the liver gradually if small amounts are consumed for a long time or more quickly if a large amount is consumed. They may cause the hepatic vein to become clogged, blocking the blood supply to the liver.

Affected people have abdominal pain and may vomit. Fluid accumulates in the abdomen and legs. Eventually, scar tissue in the liver (cirrhosis), liver failure, and even death may result.

Other herbs that can damage the liver include *Atractylis gummifera*, *Camellia sinensis* (used to make black tea), celandine (greater), chaparral, germander, jin bu huan, kava, ma huang (*Ephedra*), mistletoe, pennyroyal oil (used to make teas), and syo-saiko-to (a mixture of herbs).

Common Causes of Fatty Liver

Alcoholism

Metabolic abnormalities

- Excess body weight
- Insulin resistance (as occurs in diabetes)
- High levels of triglycerides (a fat) in the blood

Drugs

- Aspirin
- Corticosteroids
- Tamoxifen
- Tetracycline

Pregnancy

Toxins

Viruses

liver. Microvesicular steatosis, a rare form of fatty liver, can develop in certain genetically susceptible women during pregnancy.

The fatty liver may or may not be inflamed. Inflammation may then develop into scarring (fibrosis). Fibrosis often progresses into cirrhosis. Fatty liver (with or without fibrosis) due to any condition except alcoholism is called nonalcoholic steatohepatitis. This disorder develops most often in people with the metabolic syndrome.

Symptoms and Diagnosis

Fatty liver usually causes no symptoms. Some people may feel tired or have vague abdominal discomfort. The liver tends to enlarge and can be detected by the doctor during a physical examination. If doctors suspect fatty liver, they ask about alcohol use. This information is crucial. Continued and excessive alcohol use causes severe liver damage.

Blood tests to detect liver abnormalities, such as inflammation, are important because this type of hepatitis may lead to cirrhosis. Additional blood tests help exclude other causes of liver abnormalities, such as viral hepatitis. Ultrasonography, computed tomography (CT), or magnetic resonance imaging (MRI) of the abdomen can detect excess fat in the liver but cannot determine whether inflammation or fibrosis is present.

Liver biopsy may be necessary to confirm the diagnosis. For the biopsy, a doctor inserts a long hollow needle through the skin (after giving a local anesthetic to lessen any pain) and into the liver to

obtain a small piece of liver tissue for examination under a microscope (see page 214). The biopsy can help determine whether fatty liver is present, whether it resulted from alcohol or certain other specific causes, and how severe the liver damage is.

Prognosis and Treatment

Excess fat in the liver alone is not necessarily a serious problem. For example, if alcoholism is the cause, the fat can disappear, usually within 6 weeks, when people stop drinking. If the cause is not identified and remedied, fatty liver can have serious consequences. For example, if excessive alcohol use continues or a drug causing fatty liver is not stopped, repeated liver injury may eventually lead to cirrhosis. Microvesicular steatosis has a worse prognosis.

Treatment focuses on minimizing or eliminating the cause of fatty liver. People should stop taking a drug, lose weight, or take measures to control diabetes, lower triglyceride levels, or stop drinking.

Cirrhosis

Cirrhosis is the irreversible replacement of a large amount of normal liver tissue with nonfunctioning scar tissue. It develops because the liver is damaged. Attempts at regenerating new liver cells are not effective.

- Alcoholism and hepatitis are the most common causes of cirrhosis.
- Symptoms, when they occur, include poor appetite, weight loss, and feeling weak, sick, and tired.
- Many serious complications can occur, causing additional problems.
- The diagnosis is based on symptoms, a physical examination, blood tests, and sometimes imaging tests or a biopsy.
- Stopping all alcohol intake is critical.

Liver damage, when repeated or sustained, can result in cirrhosis. In the United States, the most common cause of cirrhosis is alcoholism—continued excessive intake of alcohol for a long time. Viral hepatitis is also a common cause: chronic hepatitis C in developed countries and chronic hepatitis B in many parts of Asia and Africa. Fatty liver (nonalcoholic steatohepatitis) and other metabolic problems such as iron overload (hemochromatosis) can also cause cirrhosis.

Cirrhosis is the third most common cause of death after heart disorders and cancer among people aged 45 to 65. The scar tissue forms bands throughout the liver, destroying the liver's internal structure and impairing the liver's ability to regenerate itself or function. The liver is less able to do the following:

- Break down waste products made in the body
- Produce enough bile salts, which help the body absorb fats (in disorders of bile excretion)

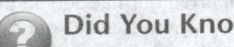 **Did You Know...**

Metabolic syndrome causes fat to accumulate in the liver.

- Remove toxins
- Process (metabolize) drugs
- Produce proteins that help blood clot (clotting factors) and albumin for holding fluid in blood vessels

The scar tissue also blocks blood flow through the portal vein (which carries blood from the intestines to the liver). The result is high blood pressure in that vein (portal hypertension—see page 217). In addition, the scar tissue can block the flow of bile (a greenish yellow digestive fluid produced by the liver) out of the liver.

Symptoms

Many people with mild cirrhosis have no symptoms and appear to be well for years. About one third never develop symptoms. Others are weak, feel sick and fatigued, have a poor appetite, and lose weight. The tips of the fingers may enlarge (called clubbing). If the flow of bile is chronically blocked, people develop jaundice (see page 214), overall itchiness, and small yellow skin bumps (nodules), especially around the eyelids. Because the damaged liver cannot produce enough bile salts, absorption of fats and fat-soluble vitamins (A, D, E, and K) is impaired. As a result, people may feel weak, have stools that are greasy and foul-smelling (steatorrhea), and lose their appetite. Undernutrition and weight loss commonly result from the impaired absorption of fats and vitamins and from loss of appetite.

People with cirrhosis may have other symptoms due to severe liver failure or alcoholism:

- Muscles waste away (atrophy).
- The palms become red (called palmar erythema).
- The tendons of the hand shrink, causing the fingers to curl up (called Dupuytren's contracture).
- Small spiderlike blood vessels appear in the skin.
- Salivary glands in the cheeks enlarge.
- The nerves outside the brain and spinal cord (peripheral nerves) malfunction (causing neuropathy).
- Men have enlarged breasts (gynecomastia) and shrunken testes (testicular atrophy) because the damaged liver cannot break down estrogens. Hair in the armpits decreases.
- The spleen enlarges.
- Fluid inside the abdomen accumulates (ascites).
- The liver usually shrinks but sometimes enlarges.

Complications: Advanced cirrhosis causes additional problems. The high blood pressure in the portal veins can cause dilated, twisted veins to form at the lower end of the esophagus (esophageal varices—see page 217), in the stomach (gastric varices), or in the rectum (rectal varices). People may vomit large amounts of blood if esophageal or gastric varices bleed. High blood pressure in the portal vein plus impaired liver function may lead to fluid accumulation in the abdomen (ascites—see page 218). Kidney failure may develop, and brain function may deteriorate (causing hepatic encephalopathy—see page 219).

Because vitamin D is poorly absorbed with impaired bile excretion, osteoporosis can develop. Because vitamin K is poorly absorbed, people have a tendency to bleed easily. The spleen, if enlarged, may trap blood cells and platelets, preventing them from entering the bloodstream. Platelets (important for blood clotting) in the blood decrease, making the tendency to bleed worse. Bleeding into the gastrointestinal tract can result in anemia.

Liver cancer (hepatocellular carcinoma or hepatoma) can develop, particularly when cirrhosis is due to chronic hepatitis B or hepatitis C or alcoholism.

> **? Did You Know...**
> Cirrhosis can turn the skin and eyes yellow and cause the tips of the fingers to enlarge.

Diagnosis

Cirrhosis is usually diagnosed based on symptoms, results of the physical examination, and a history of risk factors such as alcoholism. During the physical examination, a doctor may feel a small, firm liver. Occasionally, the doctor feels small lumps (nodules) on the surface of the liver or an enlarged spleen.

Blood tests to evaluate liver function are done. Results are often normal because these tests are relatively insensitive and the liver has a tremendous reserve. The liver can carry out essential functions even when its total activity is 85% below normal. A complete blood cell count (CBC) is done to check for anemia and other blood abnormalities. Blood tests may be done to check for hepatitis and other possible causes. Ultrasonography or computed tomography (CT) can determine whether the liver is shrunken or abnormally patterned, suggesting cirrhosis. Radionuclide scanning (using a radioactive isotope) can show which areas of the liver are functioning and which are scarred. If the diagnosis is still uncertain, a liver biopsy (removal of a tissue sample for examination under a microscope) is done to confirm it. Biopsy and sometimes blood tests can also help doctors determine the cause of cirrhosis.

If cirrhosis is confirmed, screening tests for liver cancer should be done every 6 to 12 months. Tests include blood tests to measure alpha-fetoprotein levels and ultrasonography. Levels of alpha-fetoprotein (a protein normally produced by immature liver cells in fetuses) increase when liver cancer develops.

Alcohol's Toll on the Liver

In alcoholic liver disease, damage to the liver results from excessive and prolonged alcohol use. In general, the amount of alcohol consumed (how much and how often) determines the risk and degree of liver damage. Women are more vulnerable to liver damage than men. Over a period of years, drinking as little as 2/3 ounce of pure alcohol (6 1/2 ounces of wine, 13 ounces of beer, or 2 ounces of whiskey) a day for women or 2 ounces (20 ounces of wine, 40 ounces of beer, or 6 ounces of whiskey) a day for men can damage the liver. The amount of alcohol that causes liver damage varies from person to person. Heavy drinkers usually first develop symptoms during their 30s and tend to develop severe problems by their 40s.

Alcohol may cause three types of liver damage:

- **Fat accumulation (fatty liver or steatosis):** People usually have no symptoms. In some people, the liver is enlarged, tender, or both.

- **Inflammation (alcoholic hepatitis):** People may have a fever, jaundice, fatigue, undernutrition, and a tender, painful, enlarged liver. Spiderlike veins may appear.

- **Cirrhosis:** People may have few symptoms or the same symptoms as those of people with alcoholic hepatitis. Complications of cirrhosis develop in some but not all.

If people with alcoholic liver disease continue to drink alcohol, liver damage progresses and is usually fatal. If drinking stops, some damage may be reversed, and such people are likely to live longer.

The only effective treatment is to stop drinking alcohol. Doing so can be extremely difficult. Participating in a formal recovery program, such as Alcoholics Anonymous (AA), can help.

Prognosis and Treatment

Cirrhosis is usually progressive. Stopping all alcohol intake halts further liver scarring but cannot reverse damage already done. Continued alcohol use, even small amounts, leads to progressive disease and serious complications. Once a major complication occurs—such as vomiting of blood, accumulation of fluid in the abdominal cavity, or deterioration in brain function—the outlook is grim.

No cure exists for cirrhosis. The liver will never again be normal. Cirrhosis is best arrested at its earliest stages to stop any further injury. Treatment includes eliminating the cause (such as alcohol) and treating complications as they develop. People need to inform their doctor of all the drugs they are taking, including over-the-counter drugs and dietary supplements because the damaged liver may not be able to metabolize them. If people need to take drugs that are metabolized by the liver, much smaller doses are used to avoid further damage to the liver. People with advanced cirrhosis should limit the protein and sodium in their diet and should take supplemental vitamins.

Liver transplantation can be lifesaving for people with advanced cirrhosis. If they continue to drink too much alcohol or if another cause cannot be altered, a transplanted liver also eventually develops cirrhosis. Thus, liver transplantation is not done unless the person has abstained from alcohol for at least 6 months.

Primary Biliary Cirrhosis

Primary biliary cirrhosis is inflammation with progressive scarring of the bile ducts in the liver. Eventually, the ducts are blocked, the liver becomes scarred, and liver failure develops.

- An autoimmune reaction is the likely cause of primary biliary cirrhosis.
- Itchiness, fatigue, a dry mouth and eyes, and jaundice are common.
- A blood test to measure certain antibodies is highly accurate for the diagnosis.
- Treatment focuses on relieving symptoms, slowing liver damage, and treating complications.

Primary biliary cirrhosis is most common among women aged 35 to 70, although it can occur in men and women of any age. It tends to occur in families. The cause is not clear but is probably an autoimmune reaction (in which the immune system attacks the body's own tissues—see page 1124). About 95% of people with primary biliary cirrhosis have antibodies against mitochondria (tiny structures that produce energy in cells) in their blood. This disorder often occurs in people with autoimmune disorders, such as rheumatoid arthritis, scleroderma, Sjögren's syndrome, or autoimmune thyroiditis. Primary biliary cirrhosis affects only the small bile ducts inside the liver and the nearby liver cells. Another inflammatory bile duct disorder, primary sclerosing cholangitis, affects bile ducts inside and outside the liver.

Primary biliary cirrhosis begins with inflammation of the bile ducts. The inflammation blocks the flow of bile (a greenish yellow digestive fluid) out of the liver. Thus, toxic bile products are retained in the liver cells and spill over into the bloodstream. As inflammation spreads from the bile ducts to the rest of the liver, a latticework of scar tissue develops throughout the liver.

Symptoms

Usually, primary biliary cirrhosis starts very gradually. Some people have no symptoms at first.

The first symptoms often include itchiness, fatigue, and a dry mouth and eyes. Others have jaundice (a yellowish discoloration of the skin and whites of the eyes).

Other problems may not occur until months or years later. Some people have enlarged fingertips (clubbing), osteoporosis, nerve damage (neuropathy), and kidney abnormalities. People may feel discomfort in the upper abdomen. Retained fats accumulate as small yellow deposits of fat in the skin (xanthoma) or eyelids (xanthelasma).

Eventually, any of the symptoms and complications of cirrhosis can develop (see page 223). If bile is not able to reach the small intestine, fat absorption is impaired, including the absorption of fat-soluble vitamins (A, D, E, and K). Fat malabsorption results in osteoporosis, easy bruising and bleeding, and stools that are greasy and foul-smelling (steatorrhea). The liver and spleen may enlarge. But as scarring progresses, the liver shrinks.

Diagnosis

A doctor may suspect this disorder in middle-aged women who have typical symptoms such as fatigue and itchiness (pruritus). However, in many people, the disorder is discovered well before symptoms appear because abnormalities in liver function are detected during routine blood testing.

During the physical examination, the doctor may feel an enlarged, firm liver (in about 50% of people) or an enlarged spleen (in about 25%).

Ultrasonography or magnetic resonance imaging (MRI) of the bile duct system (called magnetic resonance cholangiography) is done to check for abnormalities or obstruction of bile ducts outside the liver. Finding no obstruction outside the liver supports the diagnosis of primary biliary cirrhosis because it identifies the liver as the site of the problem. A blood test is done to measure antibodies against mitochondria. This test is highly accurate for the diagnosis. A liver biopsy (removal of a tissue sample for examination under a microscope—see page 214) may be done to confirm the diagnosis. Biopsy also helps doctors determine how advanced the disorder is (the stage).

Prognosis

The progression of primary biliary cirrhosis varies greatly but usually is slow. Symptoms may not appear for 2 years or up to 10 to 15 years. Some people become very ill in 3 to 5 years. Once symptoms develop, life expectancy is about 10 years. When itching disappears, xanthomas shrink, and jaundice develops, the disorder is advanced.

Treatment

No cure is known. Treatment focuses on relieving symptoms, slowing liver damage, and treating complications. Cholestyramine or another treatment (such as ursodeoxycholic acid plus ultraviolet light, rifampin, or naltrexone) may control itchiness. Ursodeoxycholic acid appears to reduce liver damage, prolong life, and delay the need for liver transplantation.

No alcohol should be consumed. Drugs that may damage the liver are stopped.

Supplements of calcium and vitamin D are needed to help prevent osteoporosis or slow its progression. Weight-bearing exercises, bisphosphonates, or raloxifene may also help prevent or slow osteoporosis. Vitamin A, D, E, and K supplements may be needed to correct vitamin deficiencies. Vitamins A, D, and E can be taken by mouth in a water-soluble form. Vitamin K is given by injection.

Liver transplantation (see page 1132) is the best treatment when the disorder is advanced.

Primary Sclerosing Cholangitis

Primary sclerosing cholangitis is inflammation with progressive scarring and narrowing of the bile ducts in and outside the liver. Eventually, the ducts become blocked and then obliterated. Cirrhosis, liver failure, and sometimes bile duct cancer develop.

- Symptoms begin gradually and include worsening fatigue, itchiness, and, later, jaundice.
- An imaging test can confirm the diagnosis.
- Treatment focuses on relieving symptoms, but liver transplantation can prolong life.

In primary sclerosing cholangitis, scarring worsens, eventually becoming severe (cirrhosis). The scar tissue narrows and blocks the bile ducts. As a result, bile salts, which help the body absorb fats, are not secreted normally. The disorder resembles primary biliary cirrhosis except that it affects the bile ducts outside the liver as well as those in the liver. The cause is not known but is likely to be autoimmune (when the immune system attacks the body's own tissues—see page 1124).

Primary sclerosing cholangitis most often affects young men, usually aged 30 to 60. It commonly occurs in people with inflammatory bowel disease, especially ulcerative colitis. It tends to occur in families. An infection or injury of the bile ducts may trigger the disorder in certain people. The bile ducts may also be injured during an endoscopic procedure, such as placement of tubes (stents) intended to keep the bile ducts open.

Symptoms

Symptoms usually begin gradually with worsening fatigue and itchiness. Jaundice (yellowish discoloration of the skin and whites of the eyes) tends to develop later.

Inflammation and recurring infection of the bile ducts (bacterial cholangitis) sometimes occur when the bile ducts are injured during a procedure. Bacterial cholangitis causes attacks of pain in the upper abdomen, jaundice, and fever.

Because bile salts are not secreted normally, people may be unable to absorb enough fats and fat-soluble vitamins (A, D, E, and K). Such impaired bile secretion results in osteoporosis, easy bruising and bleeding, and stools that are greasy and foul-smelling (steatorrhea). Gallstones and bile duct stones may develop. The liver and spleen may enlarge.

As the disorder progresses, symptoms of cirrhosis (see page 223) develop. Advanced cirrhosis causes the following:

- Increased blood pressure in the vein that carries blood from the intestines to the liver (portal hypertension)
- Accumulation of fluid in the abdominal cavity (ascites)
- Liver failure, which can be fatal

Some people have no symptoms until the disorder is advanced and cirrhosis is present. Symptoms may not appear for up to 10 years.

Cancer of the bile ducts (cholangiocarcinoma) develops in 10 to 15% of people with primary sclerosing cholangitis.

Diagnosis

The disorder may be suspected when results of liver function tests, done as part of an annual physical examination or for some unrelated reason, are abnormal. Then, ultrasonography is typically done first to check for blockage of bile ducts outside the liver. Tests that can confirm the diagnosis include the following:

- **Magnetic resonance cholangiopancreatography (MRCP):** Magnetic resonance imaging (MRI) is used to obtain images of the bile ducts and the pancreatic duct. This test helps confirm primary

sclerosing cholangitis and rule out other causes of bile duct obstruction.

- **Endoscopic ultrasonography:** A flexible viewing tube (endoscope) is passed through the mouth into the stomach and upper small intestine. A tiny ultrasound probe at the tube's tip is used to obtain images.
- **Endoscopic retrograde cholangiopancreatography (ERCP):** X-rays are taken after a radiopaque dye, which is visible on x-rays, is injected into the bile ducts through an endoscope (see art on page 213). ERCP is less desirable than MRCP because ERCP is more invasive and requires injection of a dye. However, ERCP can also be used in treatment.

Once primary sclerosing cholangitis is confirmed, the person must have yearly evaluations to monitor the progression of the disorder. MRCP may also be done regularly to check for cancer of the bile ducts.

Prognosis and Treatment

Usually, primary sclerosing cholangitis worsens gradually. Liver failure occurs about 12 years after the disorder is diagnosed.

The drug ursodeoxycholic acid may help relieve itching. Recurring bacterial cholangitis is treated with antibiotics Blocked ducts can be widened (dilated) during ERCP. Sometimes tubes to keep the ducts open (stents) are inserted temporarily.

Liver transplantation (see page 1132) is the only treatment that prolongs life. It can cure some types of this otherwise fatal disorder. People with cirrhosis that causes serious complications or those with recurrent bacterial cholangitis may require liver transplantation.

If cancer of the bile ducts develops and surgery to remove the cancer is not possible, stents may be passed through an endoscope and placed in bile ducts that are blocked by the cancer. These stents open the ducts.

CHAPTER 36

Hepatitis

Hepatitis is inflammation of the liver.

Hepatitis commonly results from a virus, particularly one of the five hepatitis viruses—A, B, C, D, or E. Other common causes of hepatitis are excessive alcohol intake and use of certain drugs, such as isoniazid (used to treat tuberculosis). Less commonly, hepatitis results from other viral infections, such as infectious mononucleosis, herpes simplex, or cytomegalovirus infection. Various other infections and disorders can result in small areas of inflammation in the liver but rarely cause symptoms or problems.

Hepatitis can be acute (short-lived) or chronic (lasting at least 6 months). It is common throughout the world.

Acute Viral Hepatitis

Acute viral hepatitis is inflammation of the liver caused by infection with one of the five hepatitis viruses. In most people, the inflammation begins suddenly and lasts only a few weeks.

- Symptoms range from none to very severe.
- Affected people may have a poor appetite, nausea, vomiting, fever, pain in the upper right abdomen, and jaundice.
- Doctors do a physical examination and take blood samples to analyze.
- Vaccines can prevent hepatitis A, B, and E.
- Usually, specific treatment is not needed.

Acute viral hepatitis can be caused by many different viruses (see table on page 228). Hepatitis A is the most common cause, followed by hepatitis B.

Symptoms

Acute viral hepatitis can cause anything from a minor flu-like illness to fatal liver failure. Sometimes there are no symptoms. The severity of symptoms and speed of recovery vary considerably, depending on the particular virus and on the person's response to the infection. Hepatitis A and C often cause very mild symptoms or none at all and may be unnoticed. Hepatitis B and E are more likely to produce severe symptoms. Co-infection with hepatitis B and D may make the symptoms even more severe.

Symptoms usually begin suddenly. They include a poor appetite, nausea, vomiting, and often a fever and pain in the upper right of the abdomen (where the liver is located). In people who smoke, a distaste for cigarettes is a typical symptom. Occasionally, especially with hepatitis B, infected people develop joint pains and itchy red hives on the skin (wheals or urticaria).

Typically, after a few days, the urine becomes dark, and jaundice (a yellowish discoloration of the skin and whites of the eyes) develops. Both of these symptoms occur because bilirubin builds up in the blood. Bilirubin is the main pigment in bile, the greenish yellow digestive fluid produced by the liver. Most symptoms usually disappear at this point, and people feel better even though the jaundice may worsen. The jaundice usually peaks in 1 to 2 weeks, then fades over 2 to 4 weeks. Symptoms of cholestasis (a reduction or stoppage of bile flow)—such as pale stools and overall itchiness—may develop, particularly in people with hepatitis A.

Rarely, particularly with hepatitis B, symptoms become extremely severe (fulminant). Liver failure may occur and may be fatal, especially in adults.

Did You Know...

Vaccines can prevent most types of hepatitis or decrease its severity.

A few simple, common-sense precautions can also help prevent hepatitis.

Diagnosis

Doctors suspect acute viral hepatitis on the basis of symptoms. During the physical examination, a doctor presses on the abdomen above the liver, which is tender and somewhat enlarged in about half of the people with acute viral hepatitis. Blood tests to evaluate liver function are done. They can indicate whether the liver is inflamed and often help doctors distinguish hepatitis due to alcohol abuse from that due to a virus. Blood tests help doctors identify which hepatitis virus is causing the infection. These tests can detect parts of the viruses or specific antibodies produced by the body to fight the viruses. Occasionally, if the diagnosis is unclear, a biopsy is done: A sample of liver tissue is removed with a needle and examined.

Prevention

Vaccines, given by injection into muscle, are available to prevent hepatitis A, B, and E infections. The hepatitis A vaccine is recommended for all children and for adults likely to be exposed to the virus. Hepatitis B vaccine is recommended for everyone. Hepatitis E vaccine, a new vaccine, is most likely to

THE HEPATITIS VIRUSES

TRANSMISSION	SYMPTOMS AND PROGNOSIS	PREVENTION
Hepatitis A		
Hepatitis A is spread primarily from the stool of one person to the mouth of another, usually because of poor hygiene—for example, when an infected person prepares food with unwashed hands. Hepatitis A is sometimes spread in day care centers, where caregivers and children can come in contact with infected stool in diapers. Shellfish taken from waters where raw sewage drains are sometimes contaminated and can cause infection when they are eaten raw. Epidemics, usually linked to contamination of water supplies by stool, are common, especially in developing countries.	Most hepatitis A infections cause no symptoms and are unrecognized. However, typical symptoms of acute hepatitis can occur. Recovery from the acute infection is usually complete except when the infection is very severe (fulminant). Such cases are rare (rarer than with hepatitis B). Also, people with hepatitis A do not become carriers, and the virus does not cause chronic hepatitis.	Good hygiene in handling food and avoiding contamination of water supplies are important. Vaccination against hepatitis A is recommended for all children. It is also recommended for adults at high risk of exposure to the infection: ■ Travelers to parts of the world where hepatitis A is widespread ■ Military personnel ■ Day care center employees ■ Sanitation workers ■ People who work in diagnostic or research laboratories that handle hepatitis A virus ■ People with chronic liver disorders or bleeding disorders ■ Men who have sex with men ■ People who use illicit drugs (who are often infected for reasons other than drug use) Standard immune globulin* is given to people exposed to hepatitis A. This treatment prevents or decreases the severity of infection and can be given in addition to the vaccine.
Hepatitis B		
Hepatitis B is less easily transmitted than hepatitis A. Transmission commonly occurs when needles are reused without being first sterilized—as when people share needles to inject drugs or when needles are reused to apply tattoos or to inject a vaccine. Transmission through blood transfusions is possible but is now rare in the United States because blood is screened. Hepatitis B is also spread through contact with saliva, tears, breast milk, urine, vaginal fluid, and semen. Transmission commonly occurs between sex partners, both heterosexual and homosexual. Also at increased risk are people in closed environments (such as prisons and institutions for the mentally retarded) because contact with another person's body fluid is more likely. A pregnant woman infected with hepatitis B can transmit the virus to her baby during birth.	In general, hepatitis B is more serious than hepatitis A and is occasionally fatal, especially in older people. The infection can be mild or very severe. When people with hepatitis B also have hepatitis D, symptoms are more severe. Joint pains and itchy red hives on the skin (wheals) are more likely in people with hepatitis B than with other hepatitis viruses. About 5 to 7% of infected adults develop chronic hepatitis B. The rate is higher among children, and the younger the child, the greater the chance of developing chronic hepatitis B.	High-risk behavior, such as sharing needles to inject drugs and having several sex partners, should be avoided, as should unnecessary blood transfusions. Vaccination against hepatitis B protects most people but may provide less protection for people undergoing dialysis, people with cirrhosis, and people with a weakened immune system. These people may need booster doses. In the United States, vaccination is recommended for all people younger than 18 (starting at birth), but it is especially important for people at risk of exposure to hepatitis B. Worldwide vaccination of all people against hepatitis B is desirable but expensive.

(continued on the following page)

THE HEPATITIS VIRUSES (*Continued*)

TRANSMISSION	SYMPTOMS AND PROGNOSIS	PREVENTION
Hepatitis B (*continued*)		
Hepatitis B can be transmitted by healthy people who have the virus (carriers). Whether insect bites can transmit this virus is not clear. Many cases of hepatitis B have no known source.	In the Far East and parts of Africa, hepatitis B virus accounts for many cases of chronic hepatitis, cirrhosis, and liver cancer.	People who have been exposed to hepatitis B, including infants born to mothers with hepatitis B, are given hepatitis B immune globulin and the vaccine. This combination prevents chronic hepatitis B in more than 80%.
Hepatitis C		
Hepatitis C is most commonly transmitted among people who share needles to inject drugs. The infection can also be transmitted through needles used for tattoos and body piercings. Transmission through blood transfusions is possible but is now rare. Transmission through sexual contact is uncommon, as is transmission from an infected pregnant woman to her baby. For unknown reasons, about one of five people with alcoholic liver disease has hepatitis C. A small proportion of healthy people appear to be carriers.	Hepatitis C is somewhat unpredictable. At first, the infection is usually mild and often without symptoms. However, liver function may fluctuate repeatedly for several months or years. Hepatitis C becomes chronic in about 75% of people. Chronic infection is usually mild. However, about 20 to 30% of affected people develop cirrhosis, and liver cancer may occur once cirrhosis has developed.	High-risk behavior, such as sharing needles to inject drugs and getting tattoos and body piercings, should be avoided, as should unnecessary blood transfusions. No vaccine is currently available. Standard immune globulin* is not useful.
Hepatitis D		
Hepatitis D occurs most often among people who share needles to inject illicit drugs.	Hepatitis D occurs only as a co-infection with hepatitis B and usually makes the hepatitis B infection more severe.	Measures that protect against hepatitis B (such as avoiding high-risk behavior and receiving hepatitis B vaccine and hepatitis B immune globulin) also protect against hepatitis D.
Hepatitis E		
Hepatitis E is spread primarily from the stool of one person to the mouth of another. It occasionally causes epidemics, which are often linked to water contaminated by stool. Epidemics have occurred only in Mexico, Peru, and parts of Asia and Africa, not in the United States or western Europe.	Hepatitis E may cause severe symptoms, especially in pregnant women. Hepatitis E does not become chronic, and people do not become carriers.	A new vaccine is available. Standard immune globulin* is ineffective.

*Standard immune globulin is a preparation containing antibodies obtained from the blood (plasma) of people with a normal immune system. It is used to treat a variety of diseases.

be used in endemic areas. As with most vaccines, protection requires allowing a number of weeks for the vaccine to reach its full effect as the immune system gradually creates antibodies against the particular virus.

People who have not been vaccinated and who are exposed to hepatitis A virus can obtain protec-tion with an injection of an antibody preparation called standard immune globulin. It prevents infection or decreases its severity. However, the amount of protection varies, and the protection is only temporary.

If people who have not been vaccinated are ex-posed to hepatitis B virus, they are given hepatitis B immune globulin and are vaccinated. Hepatitis B immune globulin contains antibodies to hepatitis B, which help the body fight the infection. This preparation prevents symptoms or decreases their severity, although it is unlikely to prevent infection. Some people need a booster dose of the vaccine.

No vaccines against hepatitis C or D virus are available. However, vaccination against hepatitis B virus also reduces the risk of infection with hepatitis D virus.

Other preventive measures against infection with the hepatitis viruses can be taken:

- Washing hands thoroughly before handling food
- Not sharing needles to inject drugs
- Not sharing toothbrushes, razors, or other items that could get blood on them
- Practicing safe sex—for example, using barrier protection such as a condom
- Limiting the number of sex partners

Donated blood is unlikely to be contaminated because it is screened. Nonetheless, doctors help reduce the risk of hepatitis by ordering blood transfusions only when essential. Before surgery, people can also sometimes prevent the need for transfusion of blood from an unknown donor by donating their own blood weeks before the operation.

Treatment and Prognosis

In most people, special treatment is not necessary, although people with unusually severe acute hepatitis may require hospitalization. After the first several days, appetite usually returns and people do not need to stay in bed. Severe restrictions of diet or activity are unnecessary, and vitamin supplements are not required. Most people can safely return to work after the jaundice clears, even if their liver function test results are not quite normal.

People with hepatitis should not drink alcohol until they have fully recovered (see box on page 224). A doctor may need to stop a drug or reduce the dosage of a drug that could accumulate to harmful levels in the body (such as warfarin or theophylline) because the infected liver cannot process (metabolize) them. Thus, people should tell their doctor all the drugs they are taking (both prescription and nonprescription, including any medicinal herbs), so that the dosage can be adjusted if necessary.

People with acute viral hepatitis usually recover in 4 to 8 weeks, even without treatment. However, people infected with hepatitis C and, to a lesser extent, those infected with hepatitis B may become carriers of the virus. Carriers have no symptoms but are still infected and can transmit the virus to others. Carriers may develop chronic hepatitis even though the disease is not apparent. Carriers may eventually develop cirrhosis (severe scarring of the liver—see page 222) or

liver cancer (see page 238). Carriers of hepatitis B are also more likely than other people to develop liver cancer.

Chronic Hepatitis

Chronic hepatitis is inflammation of the liver that lasts at least 6 months.

- Common causes are hepatitis B and C viruses and drugs.
- Many people have no symptoms until the liver has become severely scarred.
- Chronic hepatitis can result in cirrhosis, with an enlarged spleen, fluid accumulation in the abdominal cavity, and deterioration of brain function.
- A biopsy is done to confirm the diagnosis.
- Drugs, such as antiviral drugs or corticosteroids, may be used, and for advanced disease, liver transplantation may be needed.

Chronic hepatitis, although much less common than acute hepatitis, can persist for years, even decades. In most people, it is quite mild and does not cause significant liver damage. However, in some people, continued inflammation slowly damages the liver, eventually resulting in cirrhosis (severe scarring of the liver), liver failure, and sometimes liver cancer.

Causes

Chronic hepatitis is usually caused by one of the hepatitis viruses (see table on page 228). Hepatitis C virus causes about 60 to 70% of cases, and at least 75% of acute hepatitis C cases become chronic. About 5 to 7% of hepatitis B cases, sometimes with hepatitis D co-infection, become chronic. Hepatitis A and E viruses do not cause chronic hepatitis.

Certain drugs can cause chronic hepatitis, particularly when they are taken for a long time. They include isoniazid, methyldopa, nitrofurantoin, and, rarely, acetaminophen. Wilson's disease, a rare hereditary disorder involving abnormal retention of copper in the liver (see page 938), may cause chronic hepatitis in children and young adults. Other causes include alcoholic hepatitis, fatty liver not due to alcohol use (nonalcoholic steatohepatitis), and alpha$_1$-antitrypsin deficiency (a hereditary disorder).

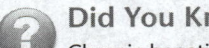

Did You Know...

Chronic hepatitis may not be diagnosed until after cirrhosis develops.

No one knows exactly why a particular virus or drug causes chronic hepatitis in some people but not in others or why the degree of severity varies. In many people with chronic hepatitis, no obvious cause can be found. In some of these people, the chronic inflammation resembles inflammation caused by the body attacking its own tissues (an autoimmune reaction (see page 1124), but this connection has not been proven. This type of inflammation called autoimmune hepatitis, is more common among women than men.

Symptoms

In about two thirds of people, chronic hepatitis develops gradually without causing any obvious symptoms until cirrhosis occurs. In the remaining one third, it develops after a bout of acute viral hepatitis that persists or returns (often several weeks later).

Symptoms often include a vague feeling of illness (malaise), poor appetite, and fatigue. Sometimes affected people also have a low-grade fever and some upper abdominal discomfort. Jaundice is rare. Complications of chronic liver disease and cirrhosis may eventually develop. They can include an enlarged spleen, spiderlike blood vessels in the skin, redness of the palms, and accumulation of fluid in the abdominal cavity (ascites—see page 218). Liver malfunction may lead to deterioration of brain function (hepatic encephalopathy—see page 219), particularly in people with cirrhosis due to hepatitis C.

Autoimmune hepatitis may cause other symptoms that can involve virtually any body system, especially in young women. Such symptoms include acne, cessation of menstrual periods, joint pain, lung scarring, inflammation of the thyroid gland and kidneys, and anemia.

In many people, chronic hepatitis does not progress for years. In others, it gradually worsens. The outlook depends partly on which virus is the cause:

- Chronic hepatitis C leads to cirrhosis, which develops over a period of years, in about 15 to 25% of people. The risk of liver cancer is increased but only if cirrhosis is present.
- Chronic hepatitis B tends to worsen, sometimes rapidly, and increases the risk of liver cancer.
- Chronic co-infection with hepatitis B and D causes cirrhosis in up to 70%.
- Autoimmune hepatitis can be effectively treated in most people, but some develop cirrhosis, with or without liver failure.
- Chronic hepatitis caused by a drug may completely resolve once the drug is stopped.

Diagnosis

Doctors may suspect hepatitis C when people have typical symptoms, when blood tests to evaluate liver function are abnormal, or when people have had hepatitis C before. Blood tests are done and may help establish the diagnosis, identify the cause, and determine the severity of liver damage. However, a liver biopsy (see page 214) is essential for a definite diagnosis. The liver biopsy also enables a doctor to determine how severe the inflammation is and whether any scarring or cirrhosis has developed. The biopsy may help identify the cause of hepatitis. Occasionally, a biopsy needs to be done more than once.

If people have chronic hepatitis B, ultrasonography and blood tests to measure alpha-fetoprotein levels are done annually to screen for liver cancer. Levels of alpha-fetoprotein—a protein normally produced by immature liver cells in fetuses—usually increase when liver cancer is present. People with chronic hepatitis C are screened similarly, but only if they have cirrhosis.

Treatment

If a drug is the cause, the drug is stopped. If another disorder is the cause, it is treated.

Hepatitis B and C: People with progressive chronic hepatitis B or C are usually given antiviral drugs. For hepatitis B, entecavir, adefovir, or lamivudine is usually used. These drugs are taken by mouth, as is telbivudine, a new drug for which little information is available. Interferon-alpha or pegylated interferon-alpha, given by injection under the skin, may be used instead. Hepatitis B tends to recur once drug treatment is stopped and may be even more severe. Thus, an antiviral drug may need to be taken indefinitely.

For hepatitis C, pegylated interferon-alpha plus ribavirin is most effective. This combination may stop the inflammation. After taking these drugs for 6 months to 1 year, 45 to 75% of people improve and have no further problems.

Antiviral drugs used to treat chronic hepatitis commonly cause side effects. Lamivudine may have fewer side effects than the others. These drugs should not be taken by people who have certain conditions:

- Advanced cirrhosis due to hepatitis B
- A transplanted organ
- A reduced number of blood cells (cytopenia), such as red blood cells (anemia)
- Substance abuse

If family members and close contacts of people with chronic hepatitis B have not been vaccinated, they should be. They are also given hepatitis B immune globulin. Such measures are not necessary for chronic hepatitis C.

Autoimmune Hepatitis: Usually, corticosteroids (such as prednisone) are used, sometimes with azathioprine, a drug used to suppress the immune system. These drugs suppress the inflammation, relieve symptoms, and improve long-term survival. Nevertheless, scarring in the liver may gradually worsen. Stopping these drugs usually leads to recurrence of the inflammation, so most people have to take the drugs indefinitely.

Treatment of Complications: Regardless of the cause or type of chronic hepatitis, complications require treatment. For example, treating ascites involves restriction of salt consumption, bed rest, and sometimes drugs. If brain function deteriorates, eliminating protein from the diet can help.

Liver Transplantation: Transplantation (see page 1132) may be considered for people with severe liver failure. However, in people who have hepatitis B or hepatitis C, the virus tends to infect the transplanted liver. In people with hepatitis B, the virus tends to severely damage the transplanted liver over months or a few years, but taking lamivudine may improve the outcome. In people with hepatitis C, the virus virtually always recurs in the transplanted liver, but the infection is usually so mild that people are likely to survive for many years.

(see page 1132)

CHAPTER 37

Blood Vessel Disorders of the Liver

The liver receives the oxygen and nutrients it needs in blood that comes from two large blood vessels. The portal vein, provides about two thirds of the blood. This blood contains oxygen and many nutrients brought to the liver from the intestine for processing. The other, the hepatic artery, provides the remaining one third of blood. This oxygen-rich blood comes from the heart and provides the liver with about one half of its oxygen supply. Receiving blood from two blood vessels helps protect the liver: If one of these blood vessels is damaged, the liver can often continue to function because it receives oxygen and nutrients from the other blood supply.

> **? Did You Know...**
> Unlike the rest of the body, the liver is the only organ in the body that gets most of its oxygen supply from a vein.

Blood leaves the liver through the hepatic veins. This blood is a mixture of blood from the hepatic artery and from the portal vein. The hepatic veins carry blood to the inferior vena cava—the largest vein in the body—which then carries blood from the abdomen and lower extremities to the right side of the heart.

Blood vessel (vascular) disorders of the liver usually result from inadequate blood flow.

- If blood flow (and thus oxygen supply) to the liver is inadequate, ischemia results.
- If blood flow out of the liver is inadequate, blood backs up in the liver, causing congestion.

For example, in heart failure, blood flow to (pump failure) and from the liver (congestion) is inadequate. Both can result in ischemia. In people with blood clotting disorders, blood flow to the liver through the obstructed portal vein or from the liver through the hepatic veins may be slowed or blocked.

Ischemic Hepatitis

Ischemic hepatitis is damage throughout the liver caused by an inadequate blood or oxygen supply.

- Heart or respiratory failure may reduce the blood flow or oxygen supply to the liver.
- People feel nauseated and vomit, and the liver may be tender and enlarged.

In ischemic hepatitis, liver cells are damaged or die because the liver does not receive enough blood or oxygen.

Ischemic hepatitis differs from other types of hepatitis. Usually, "hepatitis" implies inflammation of the liver, which can have many causes, most commonly a virus (as in hepatitis A or B). In ischemic hepatitis, however, the liver is not inflamed. Rather, liver cell death (necrosis) occurs. It is termed hepatitis because, as in viral and other types of hepatitis, liver enzymes called aminotransferases leak from damaged liver cells into the blood.

Causes

For ischemic hepatitis to develop, the liver's requirements for blood, oxygen, or both are not being met. The most common cause for such unmet needs is decreased blood flow throughout the body. Causes include the following:

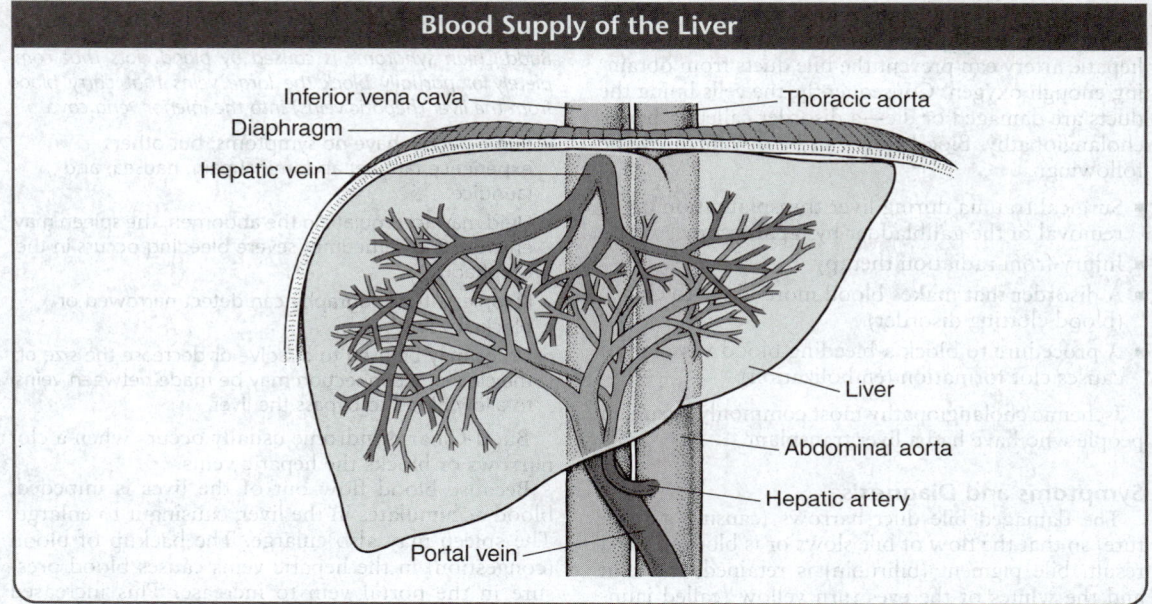

Blood Supply of the Liver

- Inferior vena cava
- Diaphragm
- Hepatic vein
- Thoracic aorta
- Liver
- Abdominal aorta
- Hepatic artery
- Portal vein

- Heart failure
- Respiratory failure
- Shock
- Massive bleeding
- Severe dehydration

A severe infection that affects all or most of the body, such as sepsis, can increase the liver's need for oxygen and thus contribute to ischemic hepatitis.

Because the liver receives blood from the hepatic artery and portal vein, narrowing or blockage of one of these vessels does not usually cause ischemic hepatitis. This disorder results when blood flow in both vessels is reduced or blocked. The most common cause of blocked blood vessels is a blood clot. (Blockage by a blood clot is termed thrombosis.) Blood clots in the hepatic artery can have many causes, such as the following:

- Injury of blood vessels (as occurs during liver transplantation surgery)
- Aneurysms of the hepatic artery
- Inflammation of the artery (vasculitis)
- Use of cocaine (causing spasm of the artery)
- Tumors, certain medical procedures, or heart infections (endocarditis) that cause emboli—clumps of material, such as a piece of fatty material or blood clot on the wall of an artery—to break off and travel through the bloodstream and become lodged in a blood vessel

Disorders that make blood more likely to clot (blood clotting disorders) can cause blockages in arteries or veins. These disorders may be inherited or acquired.

Symptoms and Diagnosis

Symptoms include nausea and vomiting. The liver may be tender and enlarged.

Doctors suspect ischemic hepatitis when results of liver biochemical and blood clotting tests are abnormal, especially in people who have a condition that can cause the disorder. Blockage of the hepatic artery can be detected using ultrasonography, magnetic resonance angiography, or x-rays taken after a radiopaque dye (which is visible on x-rays) is injected into an artery (arteriography).

Treatment

Doctors focus on treating the condition that is reducing blood flow to the liver. If blood flow can be restored, ischemic hepatitis commonly resolves. Liver failure can occur if people already have severe scarring of the liver (cirrhosis).

Ischemic Cholangiopathy

Ischemic cholangiopathy is damage to one or more bile ducts caused by inadequate blood flow.

Bile ducts (such as the hepatic ducts and the common bile duct), unlike the liver, are supplied with blood from only one major blood vessel, the hepatic artery. Thus, disruption of blood flow through the hepatic artery can prevent the bile ducts from obtaining enough oxygen. Consequently, the cells lining the ducts are damaged or die—a disorder called ischemic cholangiopathy. Blood flow can be disrupted by the following:

- Surgical trauma during liver transplantation or removal of the gallbladder by laparoscopy
- Injury from radiation therapy
- A disorder that makes blood more likely to clot (blood clotting disorder)
- A procedure to block a bleeding blood vessel that causes clot formation (embolization)

Ischemic cholangiopathy most commonly occurs in people who have had a liver transplant.

Symptoms and Diagnosis

The damaged bile duct narrows (causing a stricture) so that the flow of bile slows or is blocked. As a result, bile pigment (bilirubin) is retained, the skin and the whites of the eyes turn yellow (called jaundice), and the urine becomes dark. Because bile (containing pigment such as bilirubin) does not enter the small intestine, the stools become pale. Itching (pruritus) is common, often beginning in the hands and feet but usually affecting the whole body. Itching is especially worse at night. Bile duct infection (cholangitis—see page 225) may also occur, producing abdominal pain, chills, and fever.

The diagnosis is based on the symptoms and abnormal blood test results, especially in people who have conditions that make ischemic cholangiopathy more likely (such as liver transplant recipients).

Ultrasonography helps doctors visualize the ducts, but the results may be inconclusive. Better definition often requires magnetic resonance imaging of the bile ducts (a procedure called magnetic resonance cholangiopancreatography or MRCP) or endoscopic retrograde cholangiopancreatography (ERCP—see art on page 213). ERCP involves inserting a flexible viewing tube (endoscope) through the mouth and into the small intestine and injecting dye into the bile duct system.

Treatment

In addition to detecting narrowing of the bile ducts, ERCP can be used in treatment. A wire with a deflated balloon at its end is introduced through the endoscope. Doctors inflate the balloon to widen (dilate) the narrowing. A mesh tube (stent) is then inserted to keep the duct open.

Some people who have had a liver transplant require another transplant.

Budd-Chiari Syndrome

Budd-Chiari syndrome is caused by blood clots that completely or partially block the large veins that carry blood from the liver (hepatic veins) into the inferior vena cava.

- Some people have no symptoms, but others experience fatigue, abdominal pain, nausea, and jaundice.
- Fluid may accumulate in the abdomen, the spleen may enlarge, and sometimes severe bleeding occurs in the esophagus.
- Doppler ultrasonography can detect narrowed or blocked veins.
- Drugs may be used to dissolve or decrease the size of the clot, or a connection may be made between veins to allow blood to bypass the liver.

Budd-Chiari syndrome usually occurs when a clot narrows or blocks the hepatic veins.

Because blood flow out of the liver is impeded, blood accumulates in the liver, causing it to enlarge. The spleen may also enlarge. The backup of blood (congestion) in the hepatic veins causes blood pressure in the portal vein to increase. This increased pressure, called portal hypertension, can result in dilated, twisted (varicose) veins in the esophagus (esophageal varices). Portal hypertension, plus the engorged and damaged liver, leads to fluid accumulating in the abdomen, a condition termed ascites. The kidneys contribute to the problem by causing salt and water to be retained.

The clot may extend to also block the inferior vena cava (the large vein that carries blood from the lower parts of the body, including the liver, to the heart). Varicose veins in the abdomen near the skin's surface may develop and become visible.

Eventually, severe scarring of the liver (cirrhosis) occurs.

Causes

Usually, the cause is a disorder that makes blood more likely to clot, such as the following:

- Excess red cells (polycythemia)
- Sickle cell disease
- Inflammatory bowel disease
- Connective tissue disorders
- Injury

Sometimes Budd-Chiari syndrome begins suddenly and rather severely, typically during pregnancy. During pregnancy, the blood normally coagulates more readily. In some women, a blood clotting disorder may first become apparent during pregnancy. Other causes include disorders that develop near the hepatic veins, such as parasitic infections and liver or kidney tumors that press on or invade the veins. In Asia and

South Africa, the cause is commonly a membrane (web) that blocks the inferior vena cava. Often, the cause is unknown.

Symptoms

Symptoms vary somewhat depending on whether they appear suddenly or develop more slowly.

Usually, symptoms develop gradually over weeks or months. Fatigue is common. The enlarged liver becomes tender, and people have abdominal pain.

Fluid may accumulate in the legs, causing swelling (edema), or in the abdomen, causing ascites. Varicose veins in the esophagus can rupture and bleed, sometimes profusely. People may vomit blood. Such bleeding is a medical emergency.

If cirrhosis develops, it can lead to liver failure with deterioration of brain function (hepatic encephalopathy), resulting in confusion and even coma (see page 219).

Sometimes symptoms begin suddenly, as in hepatic vein thrombosis during pregnancy. In this case, people feel tired, and the liver is enlarged and tender. Abdominal pain occurs in the upper abdomen. Additional symptoms include vomiting and a yellow discoloration of the skin and whites of the eyes—a condition called jaundice. Liver failure infrequently develops.

Diagnosis

Doctors suspect the Budd-Chiari syndrome in people with either of the following:

- An enlarged liver, ascites, liver failure, or cirrhosis when there is no obvious cause, even after testing
- Abnormal results of blood tests done to evaluate liver function plus conditions that increase the risk of blood clots

If results of liver function tests are abnormal, an imaging test, typically Doppler ultrasonography, is done. If results are unclear, magnetic resonance imaging of blood vessels (magnetic resonance angiography) or computed tomography (CT) is done.

If surgery is planned, venography is necessary. For this procedure, x-rays of the veins are taken after a radiopaque dye (which is visible on x-rays) is injected into a vein in the groin.

A liver biopsy may be done to confirm the diagnosis and determine whether cirrhosis has developed.

Prognosis

When the vein remains completely blocked, most people, if untreated, die of liver failure within 3 years. When the blockage is incomplete, life expectancy is longer but varies.

Treatment

Treatment depends on how rapidly the disorder developed and how severe it is.

When symptoms begin suddenly and the cause is a clot, fibrinolytic (thrombolytic) drugs, which dissolve clots, help. For long-term treatment, anticoagulant drugs prevent clots from enlarging or recurring.

If a vein is narrowed or blocked by a web, angioplasty may be done to widen it. For this procedure (called percutaneous transluminal angioplasty), a catheter with a deflated balloon at its tip is inserted through the skin into a blood vessel (such as a vein in the groin) and threaded to the blocked vein. The balloon is inflated, widening the vein. A wire mesh tube (stent) is then inserted and left in place to keep the vein open.

Another solution is to create an alternate route for blood flow, bypassing the liver. This procedure, called transjugular intrahepatic portal-systemic shunting (TIPS), reduces pressure in the portal vein. For the procedure, a local anesthetic is used to numb the neck, and a catheter with a cutting needle is inserted into a vein in the neck (jugular vein). The catheter is threaded through the inferior vena cava to the hepatic vein. The needle is used to create a connection (called a shunt) between two veins, usually a branch of the hepatic vein and the portal vein, so that blood can bypass the liver. Then, a stent is threaded to and placed in the shunt to keep it open. The shunt enables blood to bypass the liver, flowing from the portal vein (which normally brings blood to the liver) directly to the hepatic veins (which drain blood away from the liver). The blood returns to the heart through the inferior vena cava. However, such shunts increase the risk of hepatic encephalopathy (deterioration of brain function due to liver dysfunction). Also, shunts occasionally become blocked, especially in people who have a tendency to form blood clots.

Liver transplantation (see page 1132) can be lifesaving, particularly for people with severe liver failure.

Problems resulting from the disorder are also treated:

- Bleeding from varicose veins in the esophagus: Several techniques can be used to stop the bleeding (see page 218). Usually, rubber bands are inserted through a flexible viewing tube (endoscope), placed through the mouth into the esophagus. The bands are used to tie off the varicose veins (termed ligation).
- Fluid accumulation in the abdomen: A low-salt (sodium) diet and diuretics can help prevent too much fluid from accumulating in the abdomen.

Most people need to take anticoagulants indefinitely to prevent new blockages from developing.

Veno-Occlusive Disease of the Liver

Veno-occlusive disease of the liver is blockage of the very small (microscopic) veins in the liver.

- Fluid tends to accumulate in the abdomen, the spleen may enlarge, and severe bleeding may occur in the esophagus.
- The skin and whites of the eyes may turn yellow, and the abdomen may enlarge.
- Doctors base the diagnosis on symptoms and results of Doppler ultrasonography.
- If possible, the cause is corrected or eliminated, and symptoms are treated.

Veno-occlusive disease is similar to Budd-Chiari syndrome except that blood flow is blocked within (rather than outside of) the liver. That is, blockages do not affect the large hepatic veins and the inferior vena cava (the large vein that carries blood from the lower parts of the body, including the liver, to the heart).

Veno-occlusive disease may occur at any age. It is more common among people who are malnourished.

Because flow out of the liver is blocked, blood backs up in the liver. This backup (congestion) then reduces the amount of blood entering the liver. Liver cells are damaged because they do not get enough blood (ischemia). The congestion causes the liver to become engorged and enlarged. The congestion also causes increased pressure in the portal vein (portal hypertension). Portal hypertension can result in dilated, twisted (varicose) veins in the esophagus (esophageal varices). The elevated pressure in the portal vein and the liver congestion lead to fluid accumulating in the abdomen—a disorder called ascites. The spleen also tends to enlarge.

Such congestion reduces blood flow into the liver. The resulting liver damage leads eventually to severe scarring (cirrhosis).

> **? Did You Know...**
> Some herbal teas can cause veno-occlusive disease of the liver.

Causes

Common causes include the following:

- Ingestion of pyrrolizidine alkaloids, which are found in crotalaria and senecio plants (used in Jamaica to make herbal tea) and in other herbs, such as comfrey (see box on page 221)
- Use of certain drugs that occasionally have toxic effects on the liver, including cyclophosphamide

and azathioprine (used to suppress the immune system)

- Radiation therapy (used to suppress the immune system before bone marrow or stem cell transplantation)
- A reaction after bone marrow or stem cell transplantation (graft-versus-host disease)

In graft-versus-host disease, white blood cells in the transplanted tissue attack the recipient's tissues. This reaction tends to occur about 3 weeks after transplantation.

Symptoms

Symptoms may begin suddenly. The liver enlarges and becomes tender. The abdomen may swell because of fluid accumulating there. The skin and the whites of the eyes may become yellow—a condition called jaundice.

Varicose veins in the esophagus may rupture and bleed, sometimes profusely, causing people to vomit blood and often go into shock. The blood may pass through the digestive tract, making stools black, tarry, and foul-smelling (called melena). When bleeding is severe, shock ensues. A few people develop liver failure with deterioration of brain function (hepatic encephalopathy), resulting in confusion and coma (see page 219).

Other people develop cirrhosis with time, usually over months, depending on the cause and repeated exposure to toxic agents.

Diagnosis

Doctors suspect veno-occlusive disease based on symptoms or blood test results that suggest liver dysfunction, particularly if people have ingested substances or have conditions (particularly following bone marrow transplantation) that may cause the disease. Blood tests evaluate the liver and blood clotting.

Doppler ultrasonography often confirms the diagnosis. Occasionally, invasive tests may be necessary. Liver biopsy or blood pressure measurements of the hepatic veins and portal veins rarely are necessary. These measurements are done by inserting a catheter into a vein in the neck (jugular vein) and threading it to the hepatic veins. A biopsy of the liver can be taken at the same time.

Prognosis

The prognosis depends on how extensive the damage is and whether the condition causing it recurs or continues—for example, when people continue to drink senecio tea.

Overall, about one fourth of people with veno-occlusive disease die of liver or other organ failure within 3 months. When the cause is graft-versus-host disease after bone marrow transplantation, veno-occlusive disease often resolves on its own within a few weeks. Increasing the dose of drugs used to suppress the immune system can also cause graft-versus-host disease to resolve. If the cause is an ingested substance, stopping its use helps prevent further liver damage.

Treatment

There is no specific treatment for the blockage. If possible, the cause should be eliminated.

Ursodeoxycholic acid helps prevent veno-occlusive disease from developing after bone marrow or stem cell transplantation.

Problems resulting from the blocked vessels are treated. For example, a low-salt (low-sodium) diet and diuretics help keep fluid from accumulating in the abdomen.

An alternate route for blood flow, bypassing the liver, may be created by directly connecting the portal vein to the inferior vena cava. A catheter is inserted in a neck vein (jugular vein), threaded to the portal vein, and used to make this connection (shunt). Then a wire mesh tube (called a transjugular intrahepatic stent) is inserted to keep the shunt open. The effectiveness of such shunts is unclear.

Liver transplantation may be necessary in extreme cases.

Portal Vein Thrombosis

Portal vein obstruction results from thrombosis (blood clot) or narrowing of the portal vein, which brings blood to the liver from the intestines.

- Most people have no symptoms. Fluid may accumulate in the abdomen, the spleen may enlarge, and severe bleeding may occur in the esophagus.
- Doppler ultrasonography can usually confirm the diagnosis.
- If possible, the cause is treated, and drugs may be used to prevent the clot from enlarging or to dissolve the clot.

Because the portal vein is narrowed or blocked, pressure in the portal vein increases. This increased pressure (called portal hypertension) causes the spleen to enlarge (splenomegaly). It also results in dilated, twisted (varicose) veins in the esophagus (esophageal varices) and often in the stomach (portal hypertensive gastropathy). These veins can bleed profusely. Fluid accumulation in the abdomen (called ascites) is not common but may develop when the blockage of the portal vein is accompanied by liver congestion or damage or when large amounts of fluids are given intravenously to treat major bleeding from ruptured varices in the esophagus or stomach. Portal vein thrombosis that develops in people with cirrhosis causes their condition to deteriorate.

Causes

About 25% of adults with cirrhosis have portal vein thrombosis, usually due to sluggish blood flow. Portal vein thrombosis also can be caused by any condition that makes blood more likely to clot. Common causes differ by age group:

- Newborns: Infection of the umbilical cord stump (at the navel)
- Older children: Appendicitis
- Adults: Excess red blood cells (polycythemia), certain cancers (liver, pancreas, kidney, or adrenal gland), surgery, and pregnancy

Often, several conditions work together to cause the blockage. The cause is unknown in about one third of people.

Symptoms

Most people do not have any symptoms. In some people, problems gradually develop, resulting from portal hypertension. If varicose veins develop in the esophagus or stomach, they may rupture and bleed, sometimes profusely. People then vomit blood. The blood may also pass through the digestive tract, making stools black, tarry, and foul-smelling (called melena). Another vascular complication of portal hypertension is the development of abnormal small veins and capillaries in the stomach (portal hypertensive gastropathy), which may result in gastrointestinal bleeding.

Diagnosis

Doctors suspect portal vein thrombosis in people who have some combination of the following:

- Bleeding from esophageal or gastric varices
- An enlarged spleen
- High-risk conditions (for example, children with umbilical cord infection or acute appendicitis)

Blood tests to evaluate the liver often are normal.

Doppler ultrasonography usually confirms the diagnosis. It shows that blood flow through the portal vein is reduced or absent. In some people, magnetic resonance imaging (MRI) or computed tomography (CT) is necessary.

Angiography is done if a procedure to create an alternate route for blood flow is planned. For angiography, x-rays of the veins are taken after a radiopaque dye (which is visible on x-rays) is injected into the portal vein.

Treatment

If a blood clot suddenly blocks the vein, a drug that dissolves clots (such as tissue plasminogen activator) is sometimes used. The effectiveness of this treatment (called thrombolysis) is unclear.

If the disorder develops gradually, an anticoagulant, such as heparin, is sometimes used long term to help prevent clots from recurring or enlarging. Anticoagulants do not dissolve existing clots.

In newborns and children, the cause (usually an infected umbilical cord or acute appendicitis) is treated.

Problems caused by portal hypertension are also treated. Bleeding from varicose veins in the esophagus can be stopped using several techniques (see page 218):

- Usually, rubber bands are inserted through a flexible viewing tube (endoscope), placed through the mouth into the esophagus. The bands are used to tie off the varicose veins.
- Antihypertensive drugs, such as beta-blockers and nitrates, reduce pressure in the portal vein and thus prevent bleeding in the esophagus. (Beta-blockers also are used in portal hypertensive gastropathy.)
- Octreotide, a drug that also reduces blood flow to the liver and thus decreases blood pressure in the abdomen, may be given intravenously to help stop bleeding.

Occasionally, when these treatments are ineffective, a procedure to create an alternate route for blood flow, bypassing the liver, may be done. Here, the intent is to reduce pressure in the portal vein by creating a connection (shunt) to the inferior vena cava. Creating a shunt when the portal vein is blocked is difficult. Also, shunts tend to become blocked.

For some people, liver transplantation is necessary.

Congestive Hepatomegaly

Congestive hepatomegaly is a backup of blood in the liver, resulting from heart failure.

Severe heart failure causes blood to back up from the heart into the inferior vena cava (the large vein that carries blood from the lower parts of the body to the heart). Such congestion increases pressure in this vein and other veins that carry blood to it, including the hepatic veins (which drain blood from the liver). If this pressure is high enough, the liver becomes engorged (congested) with blood and malfunctions.

In most people, the congested liver causes only mild abdominal discomfort. The liver (in the upper right part of the abdomen) is tender and enlarged. In severe cases, the skin and whites of the eyes may turn yellow—a disorder called jaundice. Fluid may accumulate in the abdomen—a disorder called ascites. The spleen also tends to enlarge. If congestion is severe and chronic, liver damage or even severe scarring (cirrhosis) develops.

Doctors suspect the disorder in people with heart failure who have typical symptoms and abnormal results on blood tests done to evaluate the liver.

Management focuses on treating the heart failure (see page 357). Such treatment may restore normal liver function.

38 Tumors of the Liver

Liver tumors may be noncancerous (benign) or cancerous (malignant). Cancerous liver tumors are classified as primary (originating in the liver) or metastatic (spreading from elsewhere in the body). Most liver cancers are metastatic. Cancers often spread to the liver because when cancer cells break away from cancer elsewhere in the body, they often enter and travel through the bloodstream, and the liver filters most of the blood from the rest of the body.

Noncancerous liver tumors are relatively common and usually cause no symptoms. Most are detected only when an imaging test—such as ultrasonography, computed tomography (CT), or magnetic resonance imaging (MRI)—is done for an unrelated reason.

However, rarely, noncancerous tumors cause the liver to enlarge or to bleed into the abdominal cavity. The liver usually functions normally even when a noncancerous tumor is present. Thus, results of liver function tests are usually normal.

 Did You Know...

Most liver cancers start in other parts of the body.

Most noncancerous liver tumors are detected by accident, when an imaging test, such as ultrasonography, is done for another reason.

Fluid-filled sacs (cysts) sometimes form in the liver. Most cause no symptoms or health problems. They are detected incidentally by imaging tests. Rarely, people are born with many cysts in the liver (a disorder called polycystic liver). Usually, cysts also form in other organs, such as the kidneys (a disorder called polycystic kidney disease). The liver enlarges but usually continues to function well.

Hemangioma

A hemangioma is a noncancerous liver tumor composed of a mass of abnormal blood vessels.

In the United States, about 1 to 5% of adults have small hemangiomas that cause no symptoms. These tumors are usually detected only when ultrasonography or computed tomography (CT) is done for unrelated reasons. Such tumors do not require treatment.

Hemangiomas that cause symptoms are very rare. In infants, hemangiomas usually disappear on their own. However, occasionally hemangiomas are large and cause symptoms, such as widespread blood clotting and heart failure. These tumors require treatment, which may include drugs, a procedure to block the hemangioma's blood supply, and sometimes surgery.

Hepatocellular Adenoma

A hepatocellular adenoma is a relatively uncommon noncancerous liver tumor that may be mistaken for cancer. Rarely, it ruptures and bleeds or becomes cancerous.

Hepatocellular adenomas occur mainly in women of childbearing age, particularly those who use oral contraceptives.

Usually, these tumors cause no symptoms, so most remain undetected. Large adenomas may cause pain in the upper right part of the abdomen. Rarely, a hepatocellular adenoma suddenly ruptures and bleeds into the abdominal cavity, requiring emergency surgery. Very rarely, these tumors become cancerous.

An adenoma is usually suspected when an imaging test, such as ultrasonography or computed tomography (CT), is done and shows an abnormality. Sometimes a biopsy is needed to confirm the diagnosis.

Hepatocellular adenomas caused by oral contraceptive use may disappear when the woman stops taking the drug. If adenomas are large or located near the surface of the liver, surgery is recommended because bleeding and cancer are risks.

Hepatic Granulomas

Hepatic granulomas are abnormal small clumps of cells that form when certain disorders are present.

Granulomas themselves usually cause no problems, but the disorders that cause them may. Granulomas have many causes. The most common are drugs, infections, and certain disorders that affect the whole body, such as tuberculosis and schistosomiasis (which are infections) and sarcoidosis (see page 511). Granulomas can occur in primary biliary cirrhosis (see page 224).

Granulomas may form when cells of the immune system gather to respond to irritants or to defend the body against foreign substances in the liver. Inflammation can result. If it is widespread, the liver may malfunction. Rarely, fibrous tissue and portal hypertension develop.

Symptoms

Granulomas themselves typically cause no symptoms. The liver may enlarge slightly, and mild jaundice (a yellowish discoloration of the skin and the whites of the eyes) may develop. Other symptoms, if they develop, result from the disorder causing the granulomas. Granulomas caused by sarcoidosis may disappear spontaneously or persist for years without causing any noticeable symptoms.

Idiopathic granulomatous hepatitis is a rare disorder of unknown cause. It causes granulomas, fever, muscle aches, and fatigue. These symptoms often occur intermittently for years.

Diagnosis

Doctors ask questions about drug use and other disorders that could cause granulomas. Doctors also do blood tests to evaluate liver function and imaging tests, such as ultrasonography, computed tomography (CT), or magnetic resonance imaging (MRI). However, the results are inconclusive. Biopsy (removal of a small sample of liver tissue with a needle for examination under a microscope) is needed to confirm the diagnosis. Other tests, such as cultures, may be needed to identify the cause.

Treatment

The underlying disorder is treated. Stopping a drug or treating an infection usually causes the granulomas to disappear. Sometimes corticosteroids are used to treat sarcoidosis, but whether they prevent the disorder from progressing is uncertain.

Primary Liver Cancers

Primary liver cancers are cancers that originate in the liver. The most common is a hepatoma (hepatocellular carcinoma). At first, liver cancer usually causes only vague symptoms (such as weight loss, loss of appetite, and fatigue). As a result, the diagnosis is often made late, and the prognosis is usually poor.

HEPATOMA

A hepatoma (hepatocellular carcinoma) is a cancer that begins in the liver cells.

- Having hepatitis B or hepatitis C or drinking excess alcohol increases the risk of developing a hepatoma.
- People may have abdominal pain, lose weight, and feel a large mass in the upper right abdomen.
- Doctors base the diagnosis on results of a blood test and imaging tests.
- Hepatomas are usually fatal unless they are diagnosed early.

Hepatomas are the most common type of cancer originating in the liver. They usually occur in people who have severe scarring of the liver (cirrhosis—see page 222).

In certain areas of Africa and East Asia, hepatomas are more common than metastatic liver cancer and are a common cause of death. In these areas, many people have chronic infection with the hepatitis B virus. The presence of this virus in the body increases the risk of hepatomas more than 100-fold. Hepatitis B can cause cirrhosis but can lead to hepatomas whether cirrhosis develops or not and whether the infection is chronic or not. Cirrhosis due to chronic hepatitis C also increases the risk of hepatomas.

Hepatomas sometimes result from exposure to certain cancer-causing substances (carcinogens). In subtropical regions where hepatomas are common, food is often contaminated by carcinogens called aflatoxins, substances that are produced by certain types of fungi.

In North America, Europe, and other geographic areas where hepatomas are less common, most people with hepatomas are alcoholics with long-standing cirrhosis. Other types of cirrhosis may also lead to hepatomas, but the risk is lower with primary biliary cirrhosis than with other types.

Symptoms

Usually, the first symptoms are abdominal pain, weight loss, and a large mass that can be felt in the upper right abdomen. Or people who have had cirrhosis for a long time may unexpectedly become much more ill. A fever may occur. Occasionally, the first symptoms are sudden abdominal pain and shock (dangerously low blood pressure) caused by rupture or bleeding of the hepatoma.

Occasionally, hepatomas interfere with how the body processes certain substances (metabolism). For example, hepatomas can lead to low sugar levels (hypoglycemia), high calcium levels (hypercalcemia), and high fat levels (hyperlipoproteinemia) in the blood.

Diagnosis

Detecting a hepatoma early is difficult because at first, the symptoms do not provide many clues. If a doctor feels an enlarged liver or an imaging test detects a mass in the upper right abdomen during an examination for other purposes, the doctor may suspect a hepatoma, especially in people with long-standing cirrhosis.

If a hepatoma is suspected, the following are done:

- **Blood tests to measure levels of alpha-fetoprotein:** This protein is normally produced by the fetus, and levels decrease markedly by age 1 year. Levels are high in about half the people with a hepatoma.
- **Physical examination:** Doctors feel the upper right abdomen to check for an enlarged liver or mass. They may place a stethoscope over the liver to check for sounds caused by hepatomas. For example, they occasionally hear rushing sounds (hepatic bruits, which are due to blood rushing through blood vessels inside the cancer) or scratchy sounds (friction rubs, which are due to the cancer rubbing against the liver surface and surrounding structures).
- **Imaging tests:** Ultrasonography, computed tomography (CT), or magnetic resonance imaging (MRI) of the abdomen can sometimes detect hepatomas that have not yet caused symptoms. If the diagnosis is unclear, x-rays may be taken after a radiopaque dye (a dye visible on x-rays) is injected into the main artery in the liver (hepatic artery) to check for a hepatoma. This procedure (called hepatic arteriography) is particularly useful before surgical removal of the hepatoma because the x-rays show the precise location of the liver's blood vessels.

If the diagnosis is still unclear, a liver biopsy (removal of a small sample of liver tissue with a needle for examination under a microscope) can confirm the diagnosis (see page 214). The risk of bleeding or other injury during a liver biopsy is usually low.

Staging: If cancer is diagnosed, doctors determine how large the hepatoma is and whether it has spread to nearby structures or other parts of the body. The imaging tests used for diagnosis can provide some of this information. Doctors may also use a small viewing tube (laparoscope), inserted through a small incision in the abdomen, to look directly at the liver and nearby organs.

The cancer is classified ranging from stage I (a single tumor that has not spread) to stage IV (spread to distant parts of the body). Staging helps doctors decide on treatment and estimate survival.

Screening: In some areas where the hepatitis B virus is common, ultrasonography is used to screen people with hepatitis B for liver cancer. Screening usually involves measurement of the alpha-fetoprotein level and ultrasonography every 6 or 12 months.

Prognosis

In the United States, most people with a hepatoma do not live for more than a few years because the hepatoma is detected at a late stage. Screening and early detection result in a better prognosis. In some areas of East Asia, routine screening is more common. If the hepatoma is small and has not spread and liver transplantation can be done, the person can often live a number of years.

Prevention

Use of the vaccine against hepatitis B virus eventually reduces the incidence of hepatomas, especially in areas where they are common. Preventing the development of cirrhosis regardless of cause can also help. For example, treating chronic hepatitis C and alcoholism can help prevent hepatomas from developing.

Treatment

Only liver transplantation or surgical removal of the hepatoma offers any hope of cure. However, when the hepatoma is surgically removed, it often recurs. Also, removing the hepatoma in people who have cirrhosis may not be possible because too much of their liver is damaged.

If transplantation or surgery is not possible or if people are waiting for liver transplantation, treatments may be used to slow the hepatoma's growth and relieve symptoms. For example, the hepatoma's blood supply may be blocked by inserting particles into blood vessels to the hepatoma (a procedure called selective hepatic artery embolization). As a result, the hepatoma shrinks. Cold (cryoablation) or electrical energy (radiofrequency ablation) may be directly applied to the hepatoma to destroy cancer cells. These methods do not destroy all the cancer cells.

Chemotherapy drugs can be injected into a vein or into the hepatic artery, providing a high concentration of the drugs directly to cancer cells in the liver. Chemotherapy drugs can temporarily slow the growth of the hepatoma.

Radiation therapy is usually ineffective.

OTHER PRIMARY LIVER CANCERS

Other primary liver cancers are uncommon or rare. For diagnosis, a biopsy is usually needed. Most people with these cancers have a poor prognosis. If the cancer has not spread, it can sometimes be removed. When it can be, people may live several years or longer.

A **cholangiocarcinoma** is a relatively slow-growing cancer that originates in the lining of the bile ducts in or outside the liver. In China, infestation with liver flukes (a parasite) contributes to the development of this cancer. People with primary sclerosing cholangitis are at risk of developing cholangiocarcinoma. Symptoms of the cancer are often vague but may include sudden deterioration of the person's general health, a mass in the upper right abdomen, jaundice (a yellowish discoloration of the skin and the whites of the eyes), weight loss, and abdominal discomfort.

A **fibrolamellar carcinoma** is a rare type of hepatoma that usually affects relatively young adults. It is not caused by preexisting cirrhosis, hepatitis B or C, or other known risk factors. People with fibrolamellar carcinoma usually fare better than those with other types of hepatoma. Many live several years after this hepatoma is removed.

A **hepatoblastoma** is a relatively common cancer in infants. Boys are affected twice as often as girls. Occasionally, it occurs in older children and may produce hormones (called gonadotropins) that result in early (precocious) puberty (see box on page 1755). No cause has been identified. Doctors may be able to diagnosis this cancer based on elevated alpha-fetoprotein levels and results of imaging tests.

An **angiosarcoma** is a rare cancer originating in the blood vessels of the liver. An angiosarcoma may be caused by exposure to vinyl chloride in the workplace, as occurs in the manufacture of polyvinyl chloride (PVC), or by exposure to arsenic. However, in most people, no cause is identified.

Diagnosis and Treatment

A hepatoblastoma is usually suspected when a doctor feels a large mass in an infant's upper right abdomen and the infant's general health is deteriorating.

Cholangiocarcinoma in the liver, hepatoblastoma, and angiosarcoma are diagnosed by liver biopsy (removal of a sample of liver tissue with a needle for examination under a microscope—see page 214).

Cholangiocarcinoma of the bile ducts outside the liver is usually diagnosed with special x-ray techniques (such as endoscopic retrograde cholangiopancreatography [ERCP] or percutaneous transhepatic cholangiography) or during surgery. In two thirds of people with this type of cancer, the cancer has already spread to nearby lymph nodes by the time it is detected.

Usually, treatment of these cancers has little effect, and most people die within a few months of when the cancer was detected. However, if the cancer is detected relatively early, it may be surgically removed, offering the hope of long-term survival.

Metastatic Liver Cancer

Metastatic liver cancer is a cancer that has spread to the liver from elsewhere in the body.

- Weight loss and a poor appetite may be the first symptoms.
- Doctors base the diagnosis on results of blood tests and usually biopsy.
- Chemotherapy drugs and radiation therapy may help relieve symptoms but do not cure the cancer.

Metastatic liver cancer most commonly originates in the lungs, breasts, large intestine, pancreas, or stomach. Leukemia (a cancer of white blood cells) and lymphoma (a cancer of the lymph system), especially Hodgkin lymphoma (Hodgkin's disease), may involve the liver. Cancers spread to the liver because the liver filters most of the blood from the rest of the body, and when cancer cells break away from a primary cancer, they often enter and travel through the bloodstream. Sometimes the discovery of metastatic liver cancer is the first indication that a person has cancer.

Symptoms

Often, the first symptoms are vague. They include weight loss, poor appetite, and sometimes fever. Typically, the liver is enlarged and hard. It may feel tender and often lumpy. Occasionally, the spleen is enlarged, especially if the cancer originated in the pancreas. At first, unless the cancer is blocking the bile ducts, the person has mild or no jaundice (a yellowish discoloration of the skin and the whites of the eyes). Later, the abdominal cavity may become swollen (distended) with fluid (a condition called ascites—see page 218).

In the weeks before death, jaundice progressively worsens. People may become confused and drowsy as toxins accumulate in the brain because the liver is too damaged to remove them from the blood. This condition is called hepatic encephalopathy (see page 219).

> **(?) Did You Know...**
> Sometimes the discovery of metastatic liver cancer is the first indication of cancer elsewhere in the body.

Diagnosis

Doctors often have difficulty diagnosing the cancer until it is advanced. Liver function tests, which are simple blood tests, are done. Results may be abnormal, as they are in many disorders. Thus, this finding cannot confirm the diagnosis. Ultrasonography, computed tomography (CT), and magnetic resonance imaging (MRI) of the liver may detect the cancer, but these tests cannot always detect small tumors or distinguish cancer from cirrhosis or other abnormalities.

A liver biopsy (removal of a sample of liver tissue with a needle for examination under a microscope—see page 214) is done if the diagnosis is unclear after imaging tests or if more information is needed to help with treatment decisions. To improve the chances of obtaining cancerous tissue, a doctor uses ultrasonography or CT to guide the placement of the biopsy needle. Alternatively, doctors may insert a flexible viewing tube (laparoscope) through a tiny incision in the abdomen to better identify and obtain cancerous tissue.

Treatment

Treatment depends on how far the cancer has spread and what the primary cancer is. Options include the following:

- **Chemotherapy drugs:** These drugs may be used to temporarily shrink the tumor and prolong life, but they do not cure the cancer. Chemotherapy drugs may be injected into the liver's main artery (the hepatic artery), providing a high concentration of the drugs directly to the cancer cells in the liver.
- **Radiation therapy to the liver:** Sometimes this treatment reduces severe pain, but it has little other benefit.
- **Surgery:** If only a single tumor or a few tumors are found in the liver, they may be surgically removed, especially if they originated in the intestines. However, not all experts consider this surgery worthwhile.

If cancer has spread extensively, usually all a doctor can do is relieve the symptoms (see page 61). People may prepare an advance directive (see page 69) to specify the type of care they desire if they become unable to make decisions about care.

Gallbladder and Bile Duct Disorders

The liver produces bile, a greenish yellow, thick, sticky fluid. Bile aids digestion by making cholesterol, fats, and fat-soluble vitamins easier to absorb from the intestine. Bile also helps eliminate certain waste products (mainly bilirubin and excess cholesterol) and by-products of drugs from the body.

The biliary tract consists of small tubes (ducts) that carry bile from the liver to the gallbladder and then to the small intestine. The gallbladder is a small, pear-shaped sac located beneath the liver. It stores bile (see page 210). When bile is needed, as when people eat, the gallbladder contracts, pushing bile through the bile ducts into the small intestine.

The flow of bile can be blocked by the following:

- Gallstones that pass out of the gallbladder into the ducts
- Injury to the bile ducts during gallbladder surgery
- Disorders of the pancreas, which can narrow the bile ducts that pass through the pancreas
- Tumors in the pancreas or bile ducts
- Infestation by parasites (in Asia)

If the bile ducts are blocked, the gallbladder may become inflamed.

Gallstones

Gallstones are collections of solid material (predominantly crystals of cholesterol) in the gallbladder.

- The liver can secrete too much cholesterol, which precipitates from bile in the gallbladder.
- Gallstones sometimes cause upper abdominal pain that can last for hours.
- Ultrasonography is quite accurate in detecting gallstones.
- If gallstones cause recurrent pain or other problems, the gallbladder is removed.

Most disorders of the gallbladder and bile ducts result from gallstones. Gallstones are more common among women and among certain groups of people, such as American Indians. The risk factors for gallstones include the following:

- Female sex
- Older age
- Obesity
- A typical western diet
- A family history of gallstones

In the United States, about 20% of people older than age 65 have gallstones.

Stones in the gallbladder (called cholelithiasis) sometimes pass into the bile ducts. Stones in the bile ducts are called choledocholithiasis. These stones sometimes block a bile duct.

Most gallstones do not cause symptoms. But if symptoms or other problems occur, treatment is necessary. Each year, more than half a million people in the United States have their gallbladder surgically removed.

In the Western world, the major component of most gallstones is cholesterol, a fat (lipid) that normally is dissolved in bile (but not in water). When the liver secretes excess cholesterol, bile becomes oversaturated with cholesterol. The excess forms

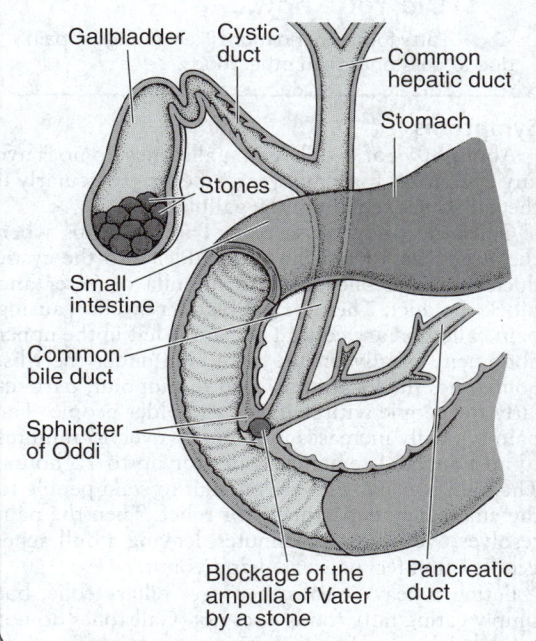

What Are Gallstones?

Gallstones are usually composed of cholesterol that has crystallized from bile. They form in the gallbladder. They may leave the gallbladder and lodge in the cystic duct, the common bile duct, or the ampulla of Vater.

solid particles (cholesterol crystals). These microscopic crystals accumulate in the gallbladder, where they clump and grow into gallstones. Other types of gallstones begin with precipitates of calcium compounds and bilirubin (the main pigment in bile). Stones composed of bilirubin, called pigment stones, are either black (forming in the gallbladder) or brown (forming in the bile ducts).

The stones may stay in the gallbladder or pass into bile ducts. Stones can block the cystic duct, common bile duct, or ampulla of Vater (where the common bile duct and pancreatic duct join). Most cholesterol stones in the bile ducts came from the gallbladder. Any narrowing (stricture) of the bile ducts can lead to a blockage or slow bile flow. Bacterial infections can develop when bile flow is slowed or blocked. Bile duct strictures, in turn, can lead to infection, inflammation, and thus brown pigment stones in the bile ducts.

Sometimes microscopic particles of cholesterol, calcium compounds, bilirubin, and other materials accumulate but do not form stones. This material is called biliary sludge. Sludge develops when bile remains in the gallbladder too long, for example, as it does during pregnancy. Gallbladder sludge usually disappears when its cause resolves, for example, when pregnancy ends. Sludge, however, can evolve into gallstones or pass into the biliary tract and block the ducts.

> **Did You Know...**
>
> Fatty foods are no more likely to trigger pain due to gallstones than other foods.

Symptoms

About 80% of people with gallstones do not have any symptoms for many years, if ever, particularly if the gallstones remain in the gallbladder.

Gallstones may cause pain. Pain develops when the stones pass from the gallbladder into the cystic duct, common bile duct, or ampulla of Vater and block the duct. Then the gallbladder swells, causing pain called biliary colic. The pain is felt in the upper abdomen, usually on the right side under the ribs. Sometimes the location is hard to pinpoint, particularly for people with diabetes and older people. The pain typically increases in intensity over 15 minutes to an hour and remains steady for up to 12 hours. The pain is usually severe enough to send people to the emergency department for relief. Then the pain resolves over 30 to 90 minutes, leaving a dull ache. People often feel nauseated and vomit.

Eating a heavy meal can trigger biliary colic, but simply eating fatty foods does not. Gallstones do not cause belching or bloating. Nausea occurs only when biliary colic occurs.

Although most episodes of biliary colic resolve spontaneously, pain returns in 20 to 40% of people each year, and complications may develop. Between episodes, people feel well.

If the blockage persists, the gallbladder becomes inflamed (a condition called acute cholecystitis, see page 245). When the gallbladder is inflamed, bacteria flourish, and infection may develop. The inflammation usually causes fever.

Blockage of the common bile duct or the ampulla of Vater is more serious than blockage of the cystic duct. Blockage of a bile duct can cause the ducts to widen (dilate). It can also cause fever, chills, and jaundice (a yellowish discoloration of the skin and the whites of the eyes). This combination of symptoms indicates that a serious infection called acute cholangitis has developed. Bacteria can spread to the bloodstream and cause serious infections elsewhere in the body. Also, pockets of pus (abscesses) can develop in the liver.

Stones that block the ampulla of Vater also can block the pancreatic duct, causing inflammation of the pancreas (pancreatitis), as well as pain.

Inflammation of the gallbladder caused by gallstones can erode the gallbladder wall, sometimes resulting in a hole (perforation). Perforation results in leakage of the gallbladder contents throughout the abdominal cavity, causing severe inflammation (peritonitis). A large gallstone that enters the small intestine can cause intestinal blockage, called a gallstone ileus. Though rare, this complication is more likely to occur in older people.

Diagnosis

Doctors suspect gallstones in people with the characteristic pain in the upper abdomen (caused by a swollen gallbladder). Sometimes gallstones are detected when an imaging test such as ultrasonography is done for other reasons.

Ultrasonography is essential. It is 95% accurate in detecting gallstones in the gallbladder. It is less accurate in detecting stones in the bile ducts, but it may show that the blockage has caused the ducts to dilate. Other diagnostic tests may be necessary. They include magnetic resonance imaging (MRI) of the bile and pancreatic ducts, computed tomography (CT), and endoscopic retrograde cholangiopancreatography (ERCP—see art on page 213).

Blood test results are usually normal unless stones block the bile ducts. Then, the liver tests are abnormal, suggesting a backup of bile in the liver (cholestasis). Results often include an increase in bilirubin and certain liver enzymes.

> **Did You Know...**
>
> Gallstones do not cause belching and bloating.
>
> About 80% of gallstones cause no symptoms or other problems.

Treatment

Gallstones that do not cause symptoms (silent gallstones) do not require treatment. If gallstones cause pain, changing the diet (for example, to a low-fat diet) does not help.

Gallstones in the Gallbladder: If gallstones cause disruptive, recurring episodes of pain, a doctor may recommend surgical removal of the gallbladder (cholecystectomy). Removal of the gallbladder prevents episodes of biliary colic yet does not affect digestion. No special dietary restrictions are required after surgery. During cholecystectomy, the doctor may also check for stones in the bile ducts.

About 90% of cholecystectomies are done using a flexible viewing tube called a laparoscope. After small incisions are made in the abdomen, the laparoscope is inserted. Surgical tools are passed through the incisions and used to remove the gallbladder. Laparoscopic cholecystectomy has lessened the discomfort after surgery, shortened the length of hospital stays, provided better cosmetic results, and reduced the time needed to recover.

The rest of cholecystectomies are done by open abdominal surgery, which requires a larger incision in the abdomen.

Alternatively, gallstones can be dissolved with drugs, such as bile acids (ursodeoxycholic acid). Such a drug, taken daily, can dissolve tiny stones in 6 months. Larger stones may take up to 1 to 2 years. Many never dissolve. Dissolving gallstones with drugs works only when stones are made of cholesterol and the opening of the gallbladder is not blocked. Even if the stones are successfully dissolved, half of these people develop gallstones again within 5 years. This treatment has limited use, and doctors reserve it for the few in whom surgery is too risky (for example, for those with major medical problems).

Gallstones in the Bile Ducts: Stones in the bile ducts are removed during ERCP. With ERCP, a flexible viewing tube (endoscope) with surgical attachments is passed through the mouth, down the esophagus, through the stomach, and into the small intestine (see art on page 213). A thin catheter is passed through the endoscope, into the sphincter of Oddi, and up into the common bile duct. A dye that is visible on x-rays (radiopaque dye) is then injected through the catheter into the bile ducts, and x-rays are taken to detect any abnormalities.

Most stones can be removed during ERCP. An instrument passed through the endoscope is used to cut the sphincter of Oddi, where the ampulla of Vater (lower bile duct) joins the small intestine—a procedure called endoscopic sphincterotomy. If the stones do not spill out into the small intestine on their own after the cut is made, a catheter with a small basket at its tip can be used to trap and then pull the stone out of the duct. Cutting the end of the bile duct leaves the opening wide enough to let any future stones pass more easily into the small intestine. Gallstones located in the gallbladder cannot be removed by this technique.

ERCP with endoscopic sphincterotomy is successful in 90% of people. It is far safer than open abdominal surgery. Fewer than 1% of people die from this procedure, and 1 to 2% experience complications. Immediate complications include bleeding, inflammation of the pancreas (pancreatitis), and perforation or infection of the bile ducts. Later on, some (2 to 6%) of the people who have this procedure develop narrowing of the inflamed ducts (strictures). Narrowing leads to stones forming in the ducts, causing further duct blockages.

Most people who have had ERCP and endoscopic sphincterotomy later have their gallbladder removed, typically using a laparoscope. If the gallbladder remains, they are at risk of later developing acute gallbladder problems or passing stones into the ducts, causing repeated blockages.

Cholecystitis

Cholecystitis is inflammation of the gallbladder, usually resulting from a gallstone blocking the cystic duct.

- Gallbladder inflammation usually results from a gallstone blocking the flow of bile.
- Typically, people have abdominal pain that lasts more than 6 hours, fever, and nausea.
- Ultrasonography can usually detect signs of gallbladder inflammation.
- The gallbladder is removed, often using a laparoscope.

Cholecystitis is the most common problem resulting from gallbladder stones. It occurs when a stone blocks the cystic duct, which carries bile from the gallbladder. Cholecystitis is classified as acute or chronic.

Acute Cholecystitis: Acute cholecystitis begins suddenly, resulting in severe, steady pain in the upper abdomen. At least 95% of people with acute cholecystitis have gallstones. The inflammation almost always begins without infection, although infection may follow later. Inflammation may cause the gallbladder to fill with fluid and its walls to thicken.

Rarely, a form of acute cholecystitis without gallstones (acalculous cholecystitis) occurs. Acalculous cholecystitis is more serious than other types of cholecystitis. It tends to occur after the following:

- Major surgery
- Critical illnesses such as serious injuries, major burns, and bodywide infections (sepsis)
- Intravenous feedings for a long time
- Fasting for a prolonged time
- A deficiency in the immune system

It can occur in young children, perhaps developing from a viral or another infection.

Chronic Cholecystitis: Chronic cholecystitis is gallbladder inflammation that has lasted a long time. It almost always results from gallstones. It is characterized by repeated attacks of pain (biliary colic). In chronic cholecystitis, the gallbladder is damaged by repeated attacks of acute inflammation, usually due to gallstones, and may become thick-walled, scarred, and small. The gallbladder usually contains sludge (microscopic particles of materials similar to those in gallstones) or gallstones that block its opening into the cystic duct or reside in the cystic duct itself.

Symptoms

A gallbladder attack, whether in acute or chronic cholecystitis, begins as pain. The pain of cholecystitis is similar to that caused by gallstones but is more severe and lasts longer—more than 6 hours and often more than 12 hours. The pain peaks after 15 to 60 minutes and remains constant. It usually occurs in the upper right part of the abdomen. The pain may become excruciating. Most people feel a sharp pain when a doctor presses on the upper right part of the abdomen. Breathing deeply may worsen the pain. The pain often extends to the lower part of the right shoulder blade or to the back. Nausea and vomiting are common.

Within a few hours, the abdominal muscles on the right side may become rigid. Fever occurs in about one third of people with acute cholecystitis. The fever tends to rise gradually to above 100.4° F (38° C) and may be accompanied by chills. Fever rarely occurs in people with chronic cholecystitis.

In older people, the first or only symptoms of cholecystitis may be rather general. For example, older people may lose their appetite, feel tired or weak, or vomit. They may not develop a fever.

Typically, an attack subsides in 2 to 3 days and completely resolves in a week. If the acute episode persists, it may signal a serious complication. A high fever, chills, a marked increase in the white blood cell count, and cessation of the normal rhythmic contractions of the intestine (ileus—see page 204) suggest pockets of pus (abscesses) in the abdomen near the gallbladder or a perforated gallbladder. Abscesses result from gangrene, which develops when tissue dies.

If people develop jaundice (see page 214) or pass dark urine and light-colored stools, the common bile duct is probably blocked by a stone, causing a backup of bile in the liver (cholestasis). Inflammation of the pancreas (pancreatitis) can develop. It is caused by a stone blocking the ampulla of Vater, near the exit of the pancreatic duct.

Acalculous cholecystitis typically causes sudden, excruciating pain in the upper abdomen in people with no previous symptoms or other evidence of a gallbladder disorder. The inflammation is often very severe and can lead to gangrene or rupture of the gallbladder. In people with other severe problems (including people in the intensive care unit for another reason), acalculous cholecystitis may be overlooked at first. The only symptoms may be a swollen (distended), tender abdomen or a fever with no known cause. If untreated, acalculous cholecystitis results in death for 65% of people.

Diagnosis

Doctors diagnose cholecystitis based mainly on symptoms and results of imaging tests. Ultrasonography is the best way to detect gallstones in the gallbladder. Ultrasonography can also detect fluid around the gallbladder or thickening of its wall, which are typical of acute cholecystitis. Often, when the ultrasound probe is moved across the upper abdomen above the gallbladder, people report tenderness.

Cholescintigraphy, another imaging test, is useful when acute cholecystitis is difficult to diagnose. For this test, a radioactive substance (radionuclide) is injected intravenously. A gamma camera detects the radioactivity given off, and a computer is used to produce an image. Thus, movement of the radionuclide from the liver through the biliary tract can be followed. Images of the liver, bile ducts, gallbladder, and upper part of the small intestine are taken. If the radionuclide does not fill the gallbladder, the cystic duct is probably blocked by a gallstone.

Liver blood tests are often normal unless the person has an obstructed bile duct. Other blood tests can detect some complications such as a high level of a pancreatic enzyme (lipase or amylase) in pancreatitis. A high white blood cell count suggests inflammation, an abscess, gangrene, or a perforated gallbladder.

Treatment

People with acute or chronic cholecystitis need to be hospitalized. They are not allowed to eat or drink and are given fluids and electrolytes intravenously. A doctor may pass a tube through the nose and into the stomach, so that suctioning can be used to keep the stomach empty and reduce fluid accumulating in the intestine if the intestine is not contracting normally. Usually, antibiotics are given intravenously, and pain relievers are given.

If acute cholecystitis is confirmed and the risk of surgery is small, the gallbladder is usually removed within 24 to 48 hours after symptoms start. If necessary, surgery can be delayed for 6 weeks or more while the attack subsides. Delay is often necessary for people with a disorder that makes surgery too risky (such as a heart, lung, or kidney disorder). If a complication such as an abscess, gangrene, or perforated gallbladder is suspected, immediate surgery is necessary.

In chronic cholecystitis, the gallbladder is usually removed after the acute episode subsides.

In acalculous cholecystitis, immediate surgery is necessary to remove the diseased gallbladder.

Surgical removal of the gallbladder (cholecystectomy) is usually done using a flexible viewing tube called a laparoscope. After small incisions are made in the abdomen, the laparoscope and other tubes are inserted, and surgical tools are passed through the incisions and used to remove the gallbladder.

Pain After Surgery: A few people have new or recurring episodes of pain that feel like gallbladder attacks even though the gallbladder (and the stones) have been removed. The cause is not known, but it may be malfunction of the sphincter of Oddi, the muscles that control the release of bile and pancreatic secretions through the opening of the bile and pancreatic ducts into the small intestine. Pain may occur because pressure in the ducts is increased by sphincter spasms, which hinder the flow of bile and pancreatic secretions. Pain may also result from small gallstones that remain in the ducts after the gallbladder is removed. More commonly, the cause is another problem, such as irritable bowel syndrome or even peptic ulcer disease.

Endoscopic retrograde cholangiopancreatography (ERCP) may be necessary to determine whether the cause of pain is increased pressure. For this procedure, a flexible viewing tube (endoscope) is inserted through the mouth and into the intestine, and a device to measure pressure is inserted through the tube. If pressure is increased, surgical instruments are inserted into the tube and used to cut and thus widen the sphincter of Oddi. This procedure (called endoscopic sphincterotomy) can relieve symptoms in people who have an abnormality of the sphincter.

Tumors of the Bile Ducts and Gallbladder

- Cancer of the bile ducts or gallbladder is rare.
- Ultrasonography can usually detect a tumor in the bile ducts or gallbladder.
- These cancers are usually fatal, but symptoms can be treated.

Cancer of the bile ducts (cholangiocarcinoma) can originate anywhere along the biliary tract, particularly outside of the liver to where it enters the small intestine. It can complicate primary sclerosing cholangitis (see page 225)

Cancer of the gallbladder is rare. Nearly everyone with gallbladder cancer has gallstones. Many people live only a few months after this cancer develops.

Polyps, which are noncancerous (benign) outgrowths of tissue, may develop in the gallbladder. They rarely cause symptoms or require treatment. They are found in about 5% of people during ultrasonography.

Sometimes cancers can block the flow of bile, but most blockages are caused by gallstones. Even less often, cancer can spread (metastasize) from elsewhere in the body to adjacent structures or nearby lymph nodes, causing blockage. Noncancerous tumors in bile ducts also cause blockages.

Symptoms

Early symptoms include the following:

- Worsening jaundice (yellowish discoloration of the skin and the whites of the eyes)
- Abdominal discomfort
- Loss of appetite
- Weight loss
- Itchiness

Symptoms gradually worsen. Abdominal pain may become severe and constant. It is usually caused by blockage of the bile ducts. People feel tired and uncomfortable. They may feel a mass in their abdomen.

Diagnosis

Doctors suspect bile duct cancer when no other cause of a bile duct blockage is identified, especially in people with primary sclerosing cholangitis. Ultrasonography is the first test to check for a tumor in the bile ducts. Magnetic resonance cholangiopancreatography (MRCP) or computed tomography (CT) may be done instead (see page 212).

If a tumor is found, doctors take a tissue sample by inserting a thin needle through the skin. Ultrasonography or CT is used to guide the needle. Endoscopic retrograde cholangiopancreatography (ERCP), using a flexible viewing tube inserted through the mouth and into the small intestine, may also be used to obtain images and a tissue sample (see page 213).

If gallbladder cancer is suspected, CT is usually done. It provides more information than ultrasonography.

Treatment

Most bile duct and gallbladder cancers are fatal, but treatment can help control symptoms.

Tubes (stents) inserted into a duct allows bile to flow past the blockage. This procedure helps control pain and relieves itchiness. Blockages can be opened during ERCP.

Surgery to remove a cancerous tumor may be done, but usually the tumor cannot be completely removed. Chemotherapy and radiation therapy for cholangiocarcinoma are being studied. If tumors have spread from other parts of the body (metastasized), chemotherapy may provide some symptom relief but does not dramatically improve survival.

Very early gallbladder cancer that is found during surgery for gallstones can often be cured by removing the gallbladder.

Kidney and Urinary Tract Disorders

CHAPTER
40   Biology of the Kidneys and Urinary Tract

Normally, a person has two kidneys. The rest of the urinary tract consists of two ureters (the tubes connecting each kidney to the bladder), the bladder, and the urethra (a tube attached to the bladder that leads to the outside of the body). Each kidney continuously produces urine, which then drains through the ureter into the bladder at a low pressure. From the bladder, urine drains through the urethra and exits the body through the penis in males and at the vulva in females. Usually, urine is free of bacteria and other infectious organisms.

Kidneys

The kidneys are bean-shaped organs, each about 4 to 5 inches (12 centimeters) long. One lies on each side of the spinal column, just behind the abdominal cavity, which contains the digestive organs. Each kidney receives blood through a branch of the aorta, called the renal artery. Blood flows from the renal artery into progressively smaller arteries, the smallest being the arterioles. From the arterioles, blood flows into glomeruli, which are tufts of microscopic blood vessels called capillaries. Blood exits each glomerulus through an arteriole that connects to a small vein. The small veins join to form a single large renal vein, which carries blood away from each kidney.

Nephrons are microscopic units that filter the blood and produce urine. Each kidney contains about one million nephrons. Each nephron contains a glomerulus surrounded by a thin-walled, bowl-shaped structure (Bowman's capsule). Also in the nephron is a tiny tube (tubule) that drains fluid (now considered urine) from the space in Bowman's capsule (Bowman's space). A third part of the nephron is a collecting duct that drains urine from the tubule.

Each tubule has three interconnected parts: the proximal convoluted tubule, the loop of Henle, and the distal convoluted tubule.

The kidneys consist of an outer part (cortex) and an inner part (medulla). All glomeruli are located in the cortex, while tubules are located in both the cortex and the medulla. The urine drains from the collecting ducts of many thousands of nephrons into a cuplike structure (calix). Each kidney has several calices, all of which drain into a single central chamber (renal pelvis). Urine drains from the renal pelvis of each kidney into a ureter.

FUNCTIONS OF THE KIDNEYS

All of the functions normally performed by two kidneys can be carried out adequately by one healthy kidney. Some people are born with only one kidney and others choose to donate one kidney. In other cases, one kidney may be severely damaged by disease or injury.

The primary function of the kidneys is to maintain the proper balance of water and minerals (including electrolytes) in the body. Additional functions include filtration and excretion of waste products from the processing of food, drugs, and harmful substances (toxins); regulation of blood pressure; and secretion of certain hormones.

Water and Electrolyte Balance: People consume water regularly in order to maintain life. More water is produced by the processing (metabolism) of food. If the amount of water added to the body is not matched by an equal amount going out, water accumulates rapidly and the person becomes ill and may even die. Excess water dilutes the body's electrolytes, whereas water restriction concentrates them. The

Viewing the Urinary Tract

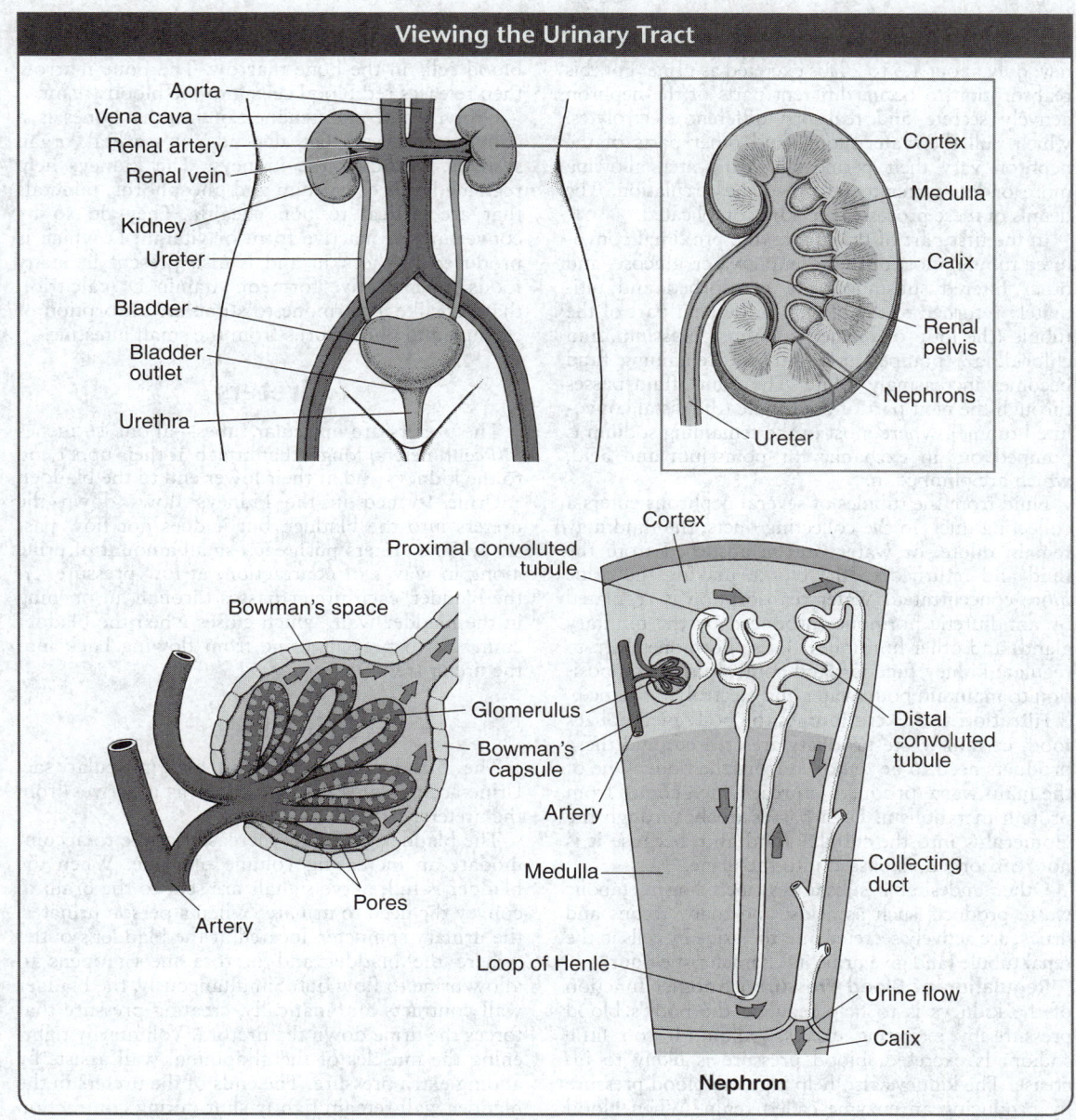

Nephron

body's electrolytes must be maintained at very precise concentrations. The kidneys regulate and help maintain the proper balance of water and electrolytes.

Blood enters a glomerulus at high pressure. Much of the fluid part of blood is filtered through small pores in the glomerulus, leaving behind blood cells and most large molecules, such as proteins. The clear, filtered fluid enters Bowman's space and passes into the tubule leading from Bowman's capsule. In healthy adults, about 47 gallons (180 liters) of fluid is filtered into the kidney tubules each day. Nearly all this fluid (and the electrolytes contained in it) is reabsorbed by the kidney; only about 1.5 to 2% is excreted as urine. For this reabsorption to occur, different parts of the nephron actively secrete and reabsorb different electrolytes, which pull the water along, and other parts of the nephron vary their permeability to water, allowing more or less water to return to the circulation. The details of these processes are a bit complicated.

In the first part of the tubule (the proximal convoluted tubule) most of the sodium, water, glucose, and other filtered substances are reabsorbed and ultimately returned to the blood. In the next part of the tubule (the loop of Henle), sodium, potassium, and chloride are pumped out; thus the remaining fluid becomes increasingly dilute. The dilute fluid passes through the next part of the tubule (the distal convoluted tubule), where most of the remaining sodium is pumped out in exchange for potassium and acid, which are pumped in.

Fluid from the tubules of several nephrons enters a collecting duct. In the collecting ducts, the fluid may remain dilute, or water can be absorbed from the fluid and returned to the blood, making the urine more concentrated. Water reabsorption is regulated by antidiuretic hormone (produced by the pituitary gland) and other hormones. These hormones help to regulate kidney function and control urine composition to maintain body water and electrolyte balance.

Filtration and Excretion: As the body metabolizes food, certain waste products are created, and these products need to be removed from the body. One of the main waste products is urea, which comes from protein metabolism. Urea passes freely through the glomerulus into the tubular fluid and, because it is not reabsorbed, is passed into the urine.

Other undesirable substances, including metabolic waste products such as acids, and many toxins and drugs, are actively secreted into the urine by cells in the renal tubule (and give urine its characteristic odor).

Regulation of Blood Pressure: Another function of the kidneys is to help regulate the body's blood pressure by excreting excess sodium. If too little sodium is excreted, blood pressure is likely to increase. The kidneys also help regulate blood pressure by producing an enzyme called renin. When blood pressure falls below normal levels, the kidneys secrete renin into the bloodstream, thereby activating the renin-angiotensin-aldosterone system, which in turn raises blood pressure (see art on page 334). A person with kidney failure is less able to regulate blood pressure and tends to have high blood pressure.

Secretion of Hormones: Through the secretion of hormones, the kidneys help regulate other important functions, such as the production of red blood cells and the growth and maintenance of bones.

The kidneys produce a hormone called erythropoietin, which stimulates the production of red blood cells in the bone marrow. The bone marrow then releases red blood cells into the bloodstream.

Growth and maintenance of healthy bones is a complex process that depends on several organ systems, including the kidneys. The kidneys help regulate levels of calcium and phosphorus, minerals that are critical to bone health. They do so by converting an inactive form of vitamin D which is produced in the skin and is also present in many foods, to an active form of vitamin D (calcitriol) that acts like a hormone to stimulate absorption of calcium and phosphorus from the small intestine.

Ureters

The ureters are muscular tubes—about 16 inches (40 centimeters) long—that attach at their upper end to the kidneys and at their lower end to the bladder.

Urine formed in the kidneys flows down the ureters into the bladder, but it does not flow passively. The ureters push each small amount of urine along in waves of contraction, at low pressure. At the bladder, each ureter passes through an opening in the bladder wall, which closes when the bladder contracts to prevent urine from flowing back into the ureter (reflux).

Bladder

The bladder is an expandable, muscular sac. Urine accumulates in the bladder as it arrives from the ureters.

The bladder gradually increases in size to accommodate an increasing volume of urine. When the bladder is full, nerve signals are sent to the brain to convey the need to urinate. When a person urinates, the urinary sphincter, located at the bladder's outlet (where the bladder and urethra meet), opens to allow urine to flow out. Simultaneously, the bladder wall contracts automatically, creating pressure that forces the urine down the urethra. Voluntarily tightening the muscles of the abdominal wall assists by adding extra pressure. The ends of the ureters in the bladder wall remain tightly shut during contraction of the bladder to prevent urine from flowing back into the ureters toward the kidneys.

Urethra

The urethra is a tube that drains urine from the bladder out of the body. In men, the urethra is about 8 inches (20 centimeters) long, ending at the tip of the penis. In women, the urethra is about 1 1/2 inches (4 centimeters) long, ending at the vulva.

Effects of Aging

As people age, there is a slow, steady decline in the weight of the kidneys. After about age 30 to 40, about two thirds of people (even those who do not have kidney disease) undergo a gradual decline in the rate at which their kidneys filter blood. However, the rate does not change in the remaining one third of older people, which suggests that factors other than age may affect kidney function.

As people age, the arteries supplying the kidneys narrow, decreasing the size of the kidneys. Also, the walls of the small arteries that flow into the glomeruli thicken, which decreases the function of the remaining glomeruli. Accompanying these losses is a decline in the ability of the nephrons to concentrate or dilute urine and to excrete acid. Despite age-related changes, however, sufficient kidney function is preserved to meet the needs of the body. Changes that occur with age do not in and of themselves cause disease, but the changes do reduce the amount of reserve kidney function that is available. In other words, performing all of the normal kidney functions may require that both kidneys work at nearly their full capacity. Thus,

even minor damage to one or both of the kidneys may result in a loss of kidney function.

The ureters do not change much with age, but the bladder and the urethra do undergo some changes. The maximum volume of urine that the bladder can hold decreases. A person's ability to delay urination after first sensing a need to urinate also declines. The rate of urine flow out of the bladder and into the urethra slows. Throughout life, sporadic contractions of bladder wall muscles occur separately from any need or appropriate opportunity to urinate. In younger people, most of these contractions are blocked by spinal cord and brain controls, but the number of sporadic contractions that are not blocked rises with age. The amount of urine that remains in the bladder after urination is completed (residual urine) increases. In women, the urethra shortens and its lining becomes thinner. These changes in the urethra decrease the ability of the urinary sphincter to close tightly. The trigger for these changes in a woman's urethra seems to be a declining level of estrogen during menopause.

In men, the prostate gland tends to enlarge with aging, gradually blocking the flow of urine (see page 1474).

Symptoms and Diagnosis of Kidney and Urinary Tract Disorders

Kidney and urinary tract disorders can affect one or both kidneys, one or both ureters, the bladder, or the urethra.

Symptoms

Some urinary tract disorders rarely cause symptoms until the problem is very advanced. These include kidney failure, tumors and stones that do not block urine flow, and some low-grade infections. Sometimes, symptoms occur but are very general and difficult for the doctor to connect to the kidney. For example, a general feeling of illness (malaise), loss of appetite, nausea, or generalized itching may be the only symptoms of chronic kidney failure. In older people, mental confusion may be the first recognized symptom of infection or kidney failure. Symptoms that are more suggestive of a kidney or urinary problem include pain in the side (flank), swelling of the lower extremities, and problems with urination.

BURNING OR PAIN WITH URINATION

Burning or pain with urination (dysuria) may be felt at the opening to the urethra or, less often, over the bladder (in the pelvis, the lower part of the abdomen just above the pubic bone). Occasionally, if a woman has vaginal irritation (for example, due to inflammation or infection of the vagina or of the area surrounding the vaginal opening, called vulvovaginitis), she may feel a burning sensation when urinating.

Causes

Dysuria is very common, particularly among adult women, in whom it is often caused by urinary tract infections, such as cystitis and urethritis. However, dysuria can occur in men and women of any age and can have many noninfectious causes.

Evaluation

Doctors can sometimes get clues to the cause based on where symptoms are most severe. For example, if

COMMON CAUSES OF DYSURIA

TYPE	EXAMPLES
Infectious*	Cervicitis
	Cystitis (more common among women)
	Epididymo-orchitis
	Prostatitis
	Urethritis
	Vulvovaginitis
Inflammatory	Inflammatory connective tissue disorders (reactive arthritis or Behçet's syndrome)
	Interstitial cystitis (noninfectious bladder inflammation)
	Vulvar vestibulitis (increased vulvar sensitivity to pain)
Physical	Catheterization of the bladder
	Obstruction of the bladder neck (for example, due to benign prostatic hyperplasia) or urethra (due to strictures)
Other	Atrophic vaginitis or urethritis
	Tumors

*Common infectious organisms include nonsexually transmitted bacteria (mostly *Escherichia coli*) and sexually transmitted organisms (such as those that cause gonorrhea, chlamydial infection, and trichomoniasis).

symptoms are most severe just above the pubic bone, a bladder infection (cystitis) may be the cause. Women with frequent episodes of cystitis may recognize characteristic symptoms that suggest another episode. If symptoms are most severe at the opening of the urethra, urethritis may be the cause. In men with a penile discharge, urethritis is often the cause. If burning affects mainly the vagina and the woman has a discharge, vaginitis may be the cause.

Examination may confirm a condition that could be causing dysuria. For example, vaginal or penile discharge can be confirmed. Inflammation or atrophy of the vagina or vulva may confirm vulvovaginitis. An enlarged prostate may confirm benign prostatic hyperplasia. Tenderness of the epididymis or testes may suggest epididymo-orchitis, and tenderness of the prostate may suggest prostatitis.

Doctors do not always agree on the need for tests. Some doctors just treat adult women who have symptoms that suggest cystitis. Other doctors usually do testing for all people or for people in whom the diagnosis is not clear. The first test is usually a urinalysis. Urine culture is often done to identify the organism causing infection and to determine which antibiotics will be effective. For women, a sample of vaginal discharge is examined on a slide using a microscope. Men and women with a urethral discharge are tested for gonorrhea and chlamydia.

Treatment

The cause is treated. Often, the cause is an infection, and treatment produces relief in 1 or 2 days. If dysuria is severe, phenazopyridine can be taken for the first 2 days to relieve discomfort. Phenazopyridine turns the urine a red-orange color.

FLANK PAIN

Pain caused by kidney disorders usually is felt in the side (flank) or small of the back. Occasionally, the pain radiates to the center of the abdomen. Usually pain occurs because the kidney's outer covering (renal capsule) is stretched by a disorder that causes rapid swelling of the kidney. Severe kidney pain is often accompanied by nausea and vomiting.

Causes

A kidney stone causes excruciating pain when it enters a ureter. The ureter contracts in response to the stone, causing severe, crampy pain (renal or ureteral colic) in the flank or lower back that often radiates to the groin or, in men, to the testis. The pain typically comes in waves. A wave may last 20 to 60 minutes and then stop. The pain stops without resuming again when the ureter relaxes or the stone passes into the bladder.

A kidney infection (pyelonephritis) causes swelling of the kidney tissue, which stretches the renal capsule, causing steady, aching pain. Kidney tumors do not usually cause pain until they have become very large.

Other disorders that cause pain in the flank include acute blockage of blood flow to the kidney or intestine, ruptured and occasionally unruptured abdominal aortic aneurysms, problems with the spine or spinal nerves, musculoskeletal injuries, and tumors that involve the back of the abdomen (retroperitoneum).

Evaluation and Treatment

After noting symptoms, the doctor examines the person and usually obtains a urinalysis to check for red blood cells or excess white blood cells, which suggest an infection, and a urine culture when appropriate. A person with very severe, colicky pain and blood in the urine is very likely to have a kidney stone. A person with milder, steady pain, tenderness when the doctor taps over one kidney, fever, and excess white blood cells in the urine is likely to have a kidney infection. If a kidney stone is suspected, the doctor usually obtains a computed tomography (CT) scan to determine the size and location of the stone and whether it significantly obstructs urine flow. An intravenous contrast agent is not used for this CT scan. If the doctor is not sure of the cause of pain, often a CT scan that uses an intravenous contrast agent or another imaging test is done.

The underlying disorder is treated. Mild pain can be relieved by taking acetaminophen or nonsteroidal anti-inflammatory drugs (NSAIDs). Pain from kidney stones may be severe and may require use of intravenous opioids.

SWELLING

Swelling results from accumulation of fluid in the tissues (edema). The swelling may cause weight gain. Swelling is usually most noticeable in the ankles and feet, but it may also involve the abdomen, lower back, hands, and face. If swelling is particularly severe, fluid may accumulate in the lungs, causing difficulty breathing.

Causes

Swelling may occur if the kidneys are unable to excrete excess water and sodium from the body, as in kidney failure. Swelling may also develop from a kidney disorder that causes the loss of large amounts of blood protein (especially albumin) in the urine (nephrotic syndrome). When the albumin level in the blood drops sufficiently, swelling occurs as fluid leaks from the circulation into the tissues.

Other disorders may also cause swelling. Heart failure, caused by inadequate pumping by the heart, signals the kidneys to retain salt and fluid, which may accumulate in tissues. Advanced liver disease also signals the kidneys to retain salt and fluid; swelling is worsened by the reduction in blood protein that occurs. This protein decrease causes fluid to leak into the tissues. If swelling occurs in only one limb, the cause is probably something related to the limb (such as a blood clot in a vein or an injury) rather than a kidney, heart, or liver problem.

Evaluation and Treatment

Doctors usually assess the presence and degree of swelling by pressing on the person's shins. If the skin retains the impression of the doctor's finger, extra fluid is present. The person's symptoms and the doctor's physical examination suggest whether the kidneys, liver, or heart is the cause, but doctors also obtain a urinalysis and blood tests of liver and kidney function. If heart failure is suspected, a chest x-ray and sometimes an echocardiogram are obtained. To diagnose nephrotic syndrome, doctors may assess urinary loss of protein by calculating the ratio of total protein to creatinine in a urine specimen.

The underlying disorder is treated when possible. Swelling can often be relieved by a diuretic if the kidneys are working properly. If the kidneys are not working properly and fluid has collected in the lungs, the person may need dialysis.

INCREASED URINATION

Most people urinate about 4 to 6 times a day, mostly in the daytime. Normally, adults pass between 3 cups (700 milliliters) and 2 quarts (2 liters) of urine a day. Infants may pass as little as 1 cup (230 milliliters) per day. Urination can be increased if a person produces an excess volume of urine or produces a normal volume of urine but feels the need to go more often (urinary frequency).

Causes

Increased Volume: Excess urine can be caused by drinking too much fluid (polydipsia), by taking diuretic drugs or substances that have a diuretic effect, such as alcohol or caffeine, or by having a high level of sugar in the blood (as in diabetes mellitus). A rare condition called diabetes insipidus causes excess urine because of problems with a brain hormone called antidiuretic hormone (also called vasopressin). Antidiuretic hormone helps the kidney reabsorb fluid. If too little antidiuretic hormone is produced (a condition called central diabetes insipidus—see page 986) or if the kidney is unable to properly respond to it (nephrogenic diabetes insipidus—see page 285), the person urinates excessively.

Increased Frequency: A frequent need to urinate without an increase in the total daily output of urine can occur when something irritates or presses on the bladder. A urinary tract infection (UTI) is the most common cause of bladder irritation. Rarer causes include a stone or tumor in the bladder. A tumor or other mass (or even the uterus if a woman is pregnant) pressing on the outside of the bladder can also cause a frequent urge to urinate because the mass reduces the capacity of the bladder. An inability to fully empty the bladder because of partial obstruction, often from an enlarged prostate (in men), can cause frequency.

Evaluation and Treatment

The doctor asks about the use of diuretics. Symptoms such as pain or burning may indicate infection. For men, the doctor examines the prostate by putting a gloved, lubricated finger in the man's rectum. If the prostate is enlarged, a blood test (prostate specific antigen, or PSA, test) and sometimes a prostate ultrasound are done. The doctor usually checks the urine for glucose (suggesting diabetes mellitus) and bacteria or excess white blood cells (indicating infection). If the cause is not clear, the doctor may measure levels of electrolytes in the blood and urine and sometimes perform imaging tests of the kidney, ureters, or bladder (such as CT, ultrasound, or magnetic resonance imaging [MRI]).

Treatment is directed at the underlying disorder.

URINATING AT NIGHT

Needing to urinate during the night (nocturia) is more common among older people. It can contribute to sleep problems and to falls, especially if a person is rushing to the bathroom or if the area is not well lit.

Causes

Nocturia may occur in the early stages of many kidney disorders. Nocturia is also common among people with heart failure, liver failure, poorly controlled diabetes mellitus, or diabetes insipidus. A person may have nocturia if the kidneys cannot concentrate urine normally. Frequent urination of very small amounts at night may result when the flow of urine into and through the urethra is obstructed and urine backs up in the bladder. An enlarged prostate is the most common cause of obstruction in older men (see page 1474). Sometimes, however, the cause of nocturia may simply be drinking a large amount of fluids, especially alcohol or caffeinated beverages (such as coffee or tea), in the late evening.

Bed-wetting (enuresis) is normal in young children. After about age 5 or 6, it may indicate a delay in the maturation of the muscles and nerves of the lower urinary tract, which most often resolves without treatment. If bed-wetting persists, other causes are considered, such as UTI, diabetes, inadequate control of the nerves of the bladder, or psychologic causes.

Evaluation and Treatment

The cause of nocturia is often evident from the person's symptoms and the results of the examination. In men, doctors examine the prostate. Testing may be needed, depending on what possible causes are suspected.

Treatment is directed at the underlying disorder. In all people, minimizing intake of fluids, alcohol, and caffeinated beverages during the late evening and voiding immediately before going to bed may help limit nocturia.

HESITATING, STRAINING, AND DRIBBLING

A hesitating start when urinating, a need to strain, a weak and trickling stream of urine, and dribbling at the end of urination are common symptoms of a partially obstructed urethra. In men, these symptoms are caused most commonly by an enlarged prostate that compresses the urethra and less often by a narrowing (stricture) of the urethra. Similar symptoms in a boy may mean that he was born with an abnormally narrow urethra or has a urethra with an abnormally narrow external opening. The opening may also be abnormally narrow in women.

A doctor examines the prostate by inserting a gloved, lubricated finger into the man's rectum. If the prostate is enlarged, a blood test to measure the PSA level and sometimes a prostate ultrasound are obtained. If a urethral stricture is suspected, the doctor may insert a flexible viewing tube into the bladder (cystoscopy).

To treat an enlarged prostate, drugs or surgery can be used. To treat a urethral stricture in a man, doctors may insert a catheter into the bladder through the penis and perform dilation (stretching the urethra). It may be necessary to insert a hollow tube to hold the urethra open (a stent). Surgeons may rebuild the urethra or perform other surgical treatments.

URGENCY

A compelling need to urinate (urgency), which may feel like almost constant painful straining (tenesmus), can be caused by bladder irritation. Incontinence may occur if a person does not urinate immediately. Urgency may be caused by a bladder infection. Caffeine and alcohol use may contribute to urgency but rarely cause severe urgency by themselves. Rarely, a poorly understood inflammation of the bladder (interstitial cystitis) is the cause.

Doctors can usually determine the cause of urgency by the person's symptoms, the results of the physical examination, and urinalysis. If infection is suspected, urine culture may be needed. Sometimes, particularly if interstitial cystitis is suspected, cystoscopy and bladder biopsy are necessary.

Treatment is directed at the underlying disorder.

INCONTINENCE

An uncontrollable loss of urine (incontinence) can have a variety of causes (see page 290).

BLOOD IN THE URINE

Blood in the urine (hematuria) can make the urine appear red or brown, depending on the amount of blood, how long it has been in the urine, and how acidic the urine is. An amount of blood too small to turn the urine red may be detected by chemical tests or microscopic examination.

Causes

Blood in the urine may be caused by infection, stones, tumors, injuries, or other problems in the bladder, urethra, ureters, or kidneys. About half of the people who have blood in the urine without pain have a disorder affecting primarily certain specialized blood vessels of the kidney (glomeruli). Sometimes, sickle cell anemia or a related disorder is the cause. Blood in the urine with pain is often the result of a kidney, bladder, or prostate infection or a stone or a blood clot moving through one of the ureters or the urethra.

Evaluation and Treatment

Sometimes, a diagnosis can be made on the basis of the person's symptoms and the results of the doctor's physical examination, urinalysis, and, if infection is suspected, urine culture. Often, however, cystoscopy, imaging studies (such as CT, ultrasound, or MRI), or other tests are needed. If a tumor is suspected, urine is examined for tumor cells. A blood test for sickle cell anemia may be needed for people of African descent who are not known to have the disease.

Treatment is directed at the underlying disorder.

GAS IN THE URINE

Passing gas (air) in the urine, a rare symptom, usually indicates an abnormal connection (fistula) between the urinary tract and the intestine, which normally contains gas. A fistula may be a complication of diverticulitis, other types of intestinal inflammation, an abscess, or cancer. A fistula between the bladder and the vagina may also cause gas to escape into the urine. Rarely, certain bacteria in the urine may produce gas.

Doctors perform a pelvic examination in affected women. To diagnose fistulas, doctors may perform cystoscopy, sigmoidoscopy, or both and obtain imaging studies, such as CT, MRI, or ultrasound.

Fistulas are usually repaired surgically.

CHANGES IN THE URINE'S COLOR

Normally, dilute urine is nearly colorless. Concentrated urine is deep yellow. Colors other than yellow are abnormal.

Food pigments can make the urine red, and drugs can produce a variety of colors: brown, black, blue, green, orange, or red. Brown urine may contain broken-down hemoglobin (the protein that carries oxygen in red blood cells). Broken-down hemoglobin can leak into the urine when bleeding occurs in the kidney, ureter, or bladder, or it can be excreted into the urine as the result of certain disorders that damage or destroy red blood cells (hemolytic anemia). Brown urine may contain muscle protein (myoglobin), which is excreted into the urine after severe muscle injury. Urine may be red because of pigments produced by porphyria, or black because of pigments produced by melanoma. Cloudy urine suggests the presence of excess white blood cells from a UTI, the presence of crystals of salts from uric acid or from phosphoric acid, or the presence of a vaginal discharge.

Doctors usually can identify the cause of an abnormal color by examining the urine under a microscope or by performing chemical tests. Treatment is unnecessary except if needed to treat the underlying disorder.

CHANGES IN THE URINE'S ODOR

The odor of urine can vary and does not usually indicate a disorder except in people who have certain rare metabolic disorders.

Diagnosis

During a physical examination of a person whose symptoms may indicate a kidney disorder, a doctor may attempt to feel the kidneys. Normal kidneys cannot usually be felt in children or adults (though they may be felt in newborn infants). Enlarged kidneys or a kidney tumor may be detectable. Often, a distended bladder can be detected. The doctor may perform a rectal examination in a man to determine whether the prostate is abnormal or enlarged, although the size of the prostate does not always correlate with the degree of urethral obstruction. The doctor may perform a pelvic examination in a woman to determine whether vaginitis or the genital organs are contributing to urinary tract symptoms.

Additional procedures may need to be performed to diagnose a kidney or urinary tract disorder.

URINALYSIS

Urinalysis is testing of the urine. A urine sample is usually collected using the clean-catch method or another sterile method. For example, a method to obtain an uncontaminated urine sample involves passing a catheter through the urethra into the bladder.

Urinalysis can be used to detect and measure the level of various substances in the urine, including protein, glucose (sugar), ketones, blood, and other substances. These tests use a thin strip of plastic (dipstick) impregnated with chemicals that react with substances in the urine and quickly change color. Sometimes, the test results are confirmed with more sophisticated and accurate laboratory analysis of the urine. The urine may be examined under a microscope to check for the presence of red and white blood cells, crystals, and casts (impressions of the

Obtaining a Clean-Catch Urine Sample

1. The head of a man's penis or opening of a woman's urethra is cleansed, usually with a small pad that contains an antiseptic substance.
2. The first few drops of urine are allowed to flow into the toilet, washing out the urethra.
3. Urination is resumed, and a sample is collected from the stream into a sterile cup. Usually the sample is obtained before the stream ends (midstream).

kidney tubules created when urinary cells, protein, or both precipitate out in the tubules and are passed in the urine).

Protein in the urine (proteinuria) can usually be detected by dipstick. Protein may appear constantly or only intermittently in the urine, depending on the cause. Proteinuria is usually a sign of kidney disorders, but it may occur normally after strenuous exercise, such as marathon running.

Glucose in the urine (glucosuria) can be accurately detected by dipstick. The most common cause of glucose in the urine is diabetes mellitus, but absence of glucose does not mean a person does not have diabetes or that the diabetes is well controlled.

Ketones in the urine (ketonuria) can often be detected by dipstick. Ketones are formed when the body breaks down fat. Ketones can appear in the urine from starvation, uncontrolled diabetes mellitus, and occasionally after drinking significant amounts of alcohol.

Blood in the urine (hematuria) is detectable by dipstick and confirmed by viewing the urine with a microscope and other tests. Sometimes the urine contains enough blood to be visible, making the urine appear red or brown.

Nitrites in the urine (nitrituria) are also detectable by dipstick. High nitrite levels indicate a urinary tract infection.

Leukocyte esterase (an enzyme found in certain white blood cells) in the urine can be detected by dipstick. Leukocyte esterase is a sign of inflammation, which is most commonly caused by a urinary tract infection.

The **acidity** of urine is measured by dipstick. Certain foods, chemical imbalances, and metabolic disorders may change the acidity of urine.

The **concentration** of urine (also called the osmolality or specific gravity) can vary widely depending on whether a person is dehydrated, how much fluid a person has drunk, and other factors. Urine concentration is also sometimes important in diagnosing abnormal kidney function. The kidneys lose their capacity to concentrate urine at an early stage

of a disorder that leads to kidney failure. In one special test, a person drinks no water or other fluids for 12 to 14 hours. In another test, a person receives an injection of antidiuretic hormone (also called vasopressin). Afterward, urine concentration is measured. Normally, either test should make the urine highly concentrated. However, in certain kidney disorders (such as nephrogenic diabetes insipidus), the urine cannot be concentrated even though other kidney functions are normal.

Sediment in urine can be examined under a microscope to provide information about a possible kidney or urinary tract disorder. Normally, urine contains a small number of cells and other debris shed from the inside of the urinary tract. A person who has a kidney or urinary tract disorder usually sheds more cells, which form a sediment if urine is centrifuged or allowed to settle.

URINE CULTURE

Urine cultures, in which bacteria from a urine sample are grown in a laboratory, are performed to diagnose a urinary tract infection. Cultures are not part of routine urinalysis. The sample of urine must be obtained by the clean-catch method or by briefly inserting a sterile catheter through the urethra into the bladder.

KIDNEY FUNCTION TESTS

Doctors can assess kidney function by performing tests on blood and urine samples. Creatinine, a waste product, is increased in the blood when the kidney filtration rate is decreased by a large amount. Creatinine clearance—a more accurate test—can be approximated from a blood sample using a formula that relates the creatinine level in the blood to a person's age, weight, and sex. Determining creatinine clearance more precisely requires an accurately timed urine collection in conjunction with the blood creatinine determination. The level of blood urea nitrogen (BUN) can also indicate how well the kidneys are functioning, although many other factors can alter the BUN level.

IMAGING TESTS

Plain X-rays: X-rays are usually not helpful in evaluating urinary tract disorders.

Ultrasonography: Ultrasonography is often the initial imaging technique because it can be performed safely even when kidney function is impaired. It is noninvasive and painless and requires no radiopaque contrast agent (see page 2044). Ultrasound scans provide some indirect information about kidney function, are an excellent way to estimate kidney size and position, readily detect obstruction, and help diagnose structural abnormalities. Ultrasonography is not as accurate as computed tomography (CT) in the diagnosis of kidney tumors. Doctors also use ultrasonography to locate the best place for a kidney biopsy.

Urinary tract stones may be detected by ultrasonography, although stones smaller than about 1/4 inch (5 millimeters) may be missed. When doctors suspect that the flow of urine from the bladder is obstructed, they sometimes use ultrasonography to measure the amount of urine that remains in the bladder after a person makes every effort possible to urinate. Ultrasonography is not as accurate as CT in the diagnosis of bladder tumors.

Computed Tomography (see page 2037): CT is used to evaluate kidney masses. Helical CT (sometimes called spiral CT), performed by continuously moving the person through the CT scanner, permits special images of certain structures and more rapid completion of the scanning process. Helical CT without the use of a radiopaque contrast agent is useful for people who may have kidney stones or for people who have suffered trauma in whom bleeding into the kidney or surrounding tissues must be identified rapidly. A radiopaque contrast agent is often used in CT examinations. The intravenous contrast agent provides extra detail about the kidney arteries and veins, about certain kidney tumors (such as renal cell cancer), and about polycystic kidney disease. Use of contrast agents may result in allergic-type reactions or, rarely, kidney damage.

Magnetic Resonance Imaging (see page 2040): MRI can provide three-dimensional images of the kidneys, blood vessels, and structures surrounding the kidneys. MRI helps distinguish tumors from cysts. When used with a paramagnetic contrast agent to enhance images, MRI can identify disorders of kidney blood vessels. People who require evaluation of the kidney blood vessels and who are at risk of reactions to radiopaque contrast agents can undergo MRI rather than CT.

Intravenous Urography: Intravenous urography (IVU, also called intravenous pyelography or IVP) uses a radiopaque contrast agent given through a vein to provide an x-ray image of the kidneys, ureters, and bladder. Usually, an ultrasound, CT scan, or MRI scan is done instead. However, IVU can better detect small abnormalities of the ureters and some abnormalities of the kidneys. IVU is often done for people with blood in the urine, even if the blood is not visible to the naked eye. It is also often done for people who doctors suspect may have cancer involving the ureters or other urinary passages. Use of contrast agents may result in allergic-type reactions or, rarely, kidney damage.

Cystourethrography: In cystourethrography, a radiopaque contrast agent similar to that used in IVU is injected directly through a scope or catheter passed through the urethra and into the bladder. When x-ray films of the bladder and urethra are taken during and immediately after urination, the study is called a voiding cystourethrogram, which is especially useful in evaluating recurring urinary tract infections. Cystourethrography may result in infection. Use of contrast agents may result in allergic-type reactions or, rarely, kidney damage.

Radionuclide Scanning (see page 2043): A radionuclide scan of the kidneys is an imaging technique that relies on the detection of small amounts of radiation by a special gamma camera after the injection of a radioactive chemical. One type of radionuclide study assesses kidney blood flow (renogram). Radionuclide scans are useful in evaluating other kidney problems.

Angiography (see page 2036): Angiography involves injecting a radiopaque contrast agent into an artery. Because it involves inserting a catheter into an artery and injecting the contrast agent under high pressure, angiography has higher risks than all other kidney imaging procedures. Thus, angiography is reserved for special situations (such as prior to balloon angioplasty and following angioplasty for the placement of a stent) to hold one of the kidney arteries open or to provide detailed information about the kidney arteries before kidney surgery. Complications of angiography may include injury to the injected arteries and neighboring organs, bleeding, and reactions to radiopaque contrast agents.

CYSTOSCOPY

A doctor can diagnose some disorders of the bladder and urethra by looking through a flexible viewing tube (cystoscope, a type of endoscope). A cystoscope, which has a diameter about the size of a pencil, may be between 1 and 5 feet (30 to 150 centimeters) in length, but only 6 to 12 inches (about 15 to 30 centimeters) of the scope are inserted into the urethra and bladder. Most contain a light source and a small camera, which allows the doctor to view the inside of the bladder and urethra. Many cystoscopes also contain a small clipping device on the tip, allowing the doctor to obtain a sample (biopsy) of the bladder lining. Cystoscopy can be done while a person is awake and causes only minor discomfort. The doctor usually inserts an anesthetic gel into the urethra before the procedure. Possible complications include bleeding in the urine and, rarely, perforation of the bladder.

TISSUE AND CELL SAMPLING

Kidney Biopsy: A kidney biopsy (in which a sample of kidney tissue is removed and examined under a microscope) is primarily used to help the doctor diagnose disorders that affect the specialized blood vessels of the kidney (glomeruli) and tubules and unusual causes of acute kidney failure. A biopsy is often performed on a transplanted kidney to look for signs of rejection.

When undergoing a kidney biopsy, the person lies face down, and a local anesthetic is injected into the skin and muscles of the back over the kidney. Ultrasonography or CT is used to locate the part of the kidney where the glomeruli are located and to avoid large blood vessels. The biopsy needle is inserted through the skin and into the kidney.

This procedure is not recommended for anyone with uncontrolled high blood pressure, bleeding disorders, active urinary tract infection, or only one kidney (except for a transplanted kidney). Compli-cations include bleeding into the urine around the kidney and formation of small arteriovenous fistu-las (abnormal connections between very small arter-ies and veins) within the kidney.

Urine Cytology: Urine cytology (microscopic ex-amination of the urine to look for cancer cells) is sometimes useful in diagnosing cancers of the kidneys and urinary tract. For people at high risk—for exam-ple, smokers, petrochemical workers, and people with painless bleeding—urine cytology may be used to screen for cancer. For people who have had a bladder or kidney tumor removed, the technique may be used for follow-up evaluation. However, the results can sometimes indicate cancer when none is present, or they can fail to indicate cancer when it is present, especially if the cancer is very new or slow growing.

CHAPTER 42 Kidney Failure

Kidney (renal) failure is the inability of the kidneys to adequately filter metabolic waste products from the blood.

Kidney failure has many possible causes. Some lead to a rapid decline in kidney function (acute kidney failure). Others lead to a gradual decline in kidney function (chronic kidney failure, also called chronic kidney disease). In addition to the kidneys being unable to filter metabolic waste products (such as creatinine and urea nitrogen) from the blood, the kidneys are less able to control the amount and distribution of water in the body (fluid balance) and the levels of electrolytes (sodium, potassium, calcium, phosphate) in the blood.

When kidney failure becomes chronic, blood pressure often rises. The kidneys lose their ability to produce sufficient amounts of a hormone (erythro-poietin) that stimulates the formation of new red blood cells, resulting in a low red blood cell count (anemia). In children, kidney failure affects the growth of bones. In both children and adults, kidney failure can lead to weaker, abnormal bones.

Although kidney failure can affect people of all ages, both acute and chronic kidney failure are more common in older than in younger people. Many causes of kidney failure can be treated, and kidney function may recover. The availability of dialysis has transformed kidney failure from a fatal disease to a chronic one.

Acute Kidney Failure

Acute kidney failure is a rapid (days to weeks) decline in the kidneys' ability to filter metabolic waste products from the blood.

- Causes include disorders that decrease blood flow to the kidneys, that damage the kidneys themselves, or that block drainage of urine from the kidneys.
- Symptoms may include swelling, nausea, fatigue, itching, difficulty breathing, and symptoms of the disorder that caused the kidney failure.
- Serious complications include heart failure and high levels of potassium in the blood.
- Diagnosis is with blood and urine tests and usually imaging studies.
- Treatment involves correcting the cause of the kidney failure and sometimes doing dialysis.

Acute kidney failure can result from any condi-tion that decreases the blood supply to the kidneys, any disease affecting the kidneys themselves, or any condition that obstructs urine flow anywhere along the urinary tract. In many people, no cause of acute kidney failure can be identified. Kidney failure develops only if both kidneys are affected.

Symptoms

Symptoms depend on the severity of kidney fail-ure, its rate of progression, and its cause.

MAJOR CAUSES OF ACUTE KIDNEY FAILURE

CAUSE	UNDERLYING PROBLEM
Insufficient blood supply to the kidneys	Blood loss Loss of large amounts of sodium and fluid Physical injury that blocks blood vessels Inadequate pumping of the heart (heart failure) Extremely low blood pressure (shock) Liver failure (hepatorenal syndrome)
Injury to the kidneys	Blood supply to the kidneys decreased long enough to damage the kidneys Toxic substances (for example, drugs, radiopaque dyes used in imaging tests, and poisons) Allergic reactions (for example, to certain antibiotics) Disorders affecting the filtering units (nephrons) of the kidneys (for example, acute glomerulonephritis, tumors damaging the kidneys, or vascular injury as occurs with hemolytic-uremic syndrome, systemic lupus erythematosus [lupus], atheroembolic kidney disease, Goodpasture's syndrome, Wegener's granulomatosis, or polyarteritis nodosa)
Obstructed urine flow	Enlarged prostate Tumor pressing on the urinary tract Stones Obstruction within the kidneys (for example, by stones such as oxalate or uric acid)

In some people, the first symptom of acute kidney failure is water retention, with swelling of the feet and ankles or puffiness of the face and hands. People may pass cola-colored urine, which may indicate a number of kidney diseases. The amount of urine (which for most healthy adults is between 3 cups [about 750 milliliters] and 2 quarts [about 2 liters] per day) often decreases to less than 2 cups (about 500 milliliters) per day or stops completely. Very little urine production is called oliguria, and no urine production is called anuria. However, some people with acute kidney failure continue to produce normal amounts of urine.

As acute kidney failure persists and metabolic waste products accumulate in the body, people may experience fatigue, a decreased ability to concentrate on mental tasks, loss of appetite, nausea, and overall itchiness (pruritus). People with acute kidney failure may experience a rapid heart rate (tachycardia) and light-headedness.

If the cause is an obstruction, the backup of urine within the kidneys causes the drainage system to stretch (a condition called hydronephrosis). Urinary obstruction often causes a constant dull ache under the lower ribs but may cause crampy pain—ranging from mild to excruciating—usually along the sides (flanks) of the body. Some people with hydronephrosis have blood in their urine. If the obstruction is located below the bladder, the bladder will enlarge. If the bladder enlarges rapidly, people are likely to feel severe pain in the pelvis, just above the pubic bone. If the bladder enlarges slowly, pain may be minimal, but the lower part of the abdomen may swell because of the markedly distended bladder.

If acute kidney failure develops during hospitalization, the condition often relates to some recent injury, surgery, drug, or illness such as infection. The symptoms of the cause of the acute kidney failure may predominate. For example, high fever, life-threatening low blood pressure (shock), and symptoms of heart failure or liver failure may occur before symptoms of kidney failure and be more obvious and urgent.

Some of the conditions that cause acute kidney failure also affect other parts of the body. For example, Goodpasture's syndrome or Wegener's granulomatosis, which damages blood vessels in the kidneys, may also damage blood vessels in the lungs, causing a person to cough up blood. Rashes are typical of some causes of acute kidney failure, including polyarteritis nodosa, systemic lupus erythematosus, and some toxic drugs.

Diagnosis

Blood tests that measure levels of creatinine and urea nitrogen in the blood are needed to confirm the diagnosis. A progressive daily rise in creatinine indicates acute kidney failure. The level of creatinine is also the best indicator of the degree or severity of kidney failure. The higher the level, the more severe the failure is likely to be. Other blood tests detect metabolic imbalances that occur as kidney failure persists, such as an increase in blood acidity (acidosis, which causes a low bicarbonate level), a high potassium level (hyperkalemia), a low sodium level (hyponatremia), and a high phosphorus level (hyperphosphatemia).

The physical examination findings may help doctors identify the cause of the acute kidney failure. For example, enlarged or tender kidneys may indicate obstruction with hydronephrosis. Urine tests, such as a urinalysis and measurement of certain electrolytes, may enable doctors to determine whether the cause of kidney failure is insufficient blood flow to the kidneys, damage to the kidneys, or urinary obstruction.

Imaging of the kidneys using ultrasonography or computed tomography (CT) is helpful, sometimes by identifying hydronephrosis or an enlarged bladder. Imaging can also reveal the size of the kidneys. X-rays of the arteries or veins that lead to and from the kidneys (angiography) may be done if obstruction of blood vessels is the suspected cause. However, angiography is done only when other tests do not provide enough information, because angiography uses radiopaque dye (contrast agent) that contains iodine, which carries a risk of additional kidney damage. Magnetic resonance imaging (MRI) can provide the same type of information. However, MRI has traditionally used gadolinium, a substance that rarely causes a disorder that triggers production of scar tissue in the body (nephrogenic fibrosing dermopathy). Thus, MRI is now less likely to be used. If other tests do not reveal the cause of kidney failure, a biopsy may be necessary to determine the diagnosis and the prognosis.

Prognosis

Acute kidney failure and its immediate complications, such as water retention, high acid and potassium levels in the blood, and increased urea nitrogen in the blood, can often be treated successfully. The overall survival rate is about 60%. Survival is less than 50% for people who have several organs failing at the same time. Yet, survival is about 90% for people whose kidney failure is due to decreased blood flow because body fluids have been lost through bleeding, vomiting, or diarrhea—conditions that are reversible with treatment.

Treatment

Any treatable cause of kidney failure is treated as soon as possible. For example, if obstruction is the cause, a catheter (a tube placed into the bladder), endoscopy, or surgery may be needed to relieve the obstruction.

Often, the kidneys can heal themselves, especially if the kidney failure has existed for less than 5 days and there are no complicating problems such as infection. During this time, measures are taken to prevent kidney failure from causing serious problems. Such measures may include the following:

- Restricting use of certain drugs
- Restricting fluids, sodium, and potassium in the diet
- Maintaining good nutrition
- Giving drugs if blood levels of potassium or phosphate are too high
- Giving dialysis

Doctors strictly limit the intake of all substances that are eliminated through the kidneys, including a large number of drugs. Salt (sodium) and potassium intake is usually restricted. Fluid intake is restricted to replacing the amount lost from the body, unless fluid is needed because there is too little blood flowing to the kidneys. Weight is measured every day because a change in weight is a good indicator of whether there is too much or too little water in the body.

A healthy diet is provided to people whose condition allows them to eat. Moderate amounts of protein are acceptable, typically 0.8 to 1 grams per kilogram of body weight (0.4 to 0.5 grams per pound).

Sodium polystyrene sulfonate is sometimes given by mouth or rectally to treat a high level of potassium in the blood. Calcium salts (calcium carbonate or calcium acetate) or sevelamer may be given by mouth to prevent or treat a high level of phosphorus in the blood.

> **Did You Know...**
>
> To cause kidney failure, a disorder must affect both kidneys.

Fluids are not restricted in people who are recovering from acute kidney failure caused by obstruction. During the recovery period, the kidneys are unable to reabsorb sodium and water normally, and a large amount of urine is produced for a period of time after the obstruction is relieved. During recovery, people may also need replacement of fluids and electrolytes, such as sodium, potassium, and magnesium.

Acute kidney failure may be prolonged, necessitating removal of waste products and excess water.

Waste removal can be done through dialysis, usually hemodialysis (see page 266). If kidney failure is predicted to be prolonged, dialysis is started as soon as possible after diagnosis. Dialysis may be needed only temporarily, until the kidneys recover their function, usually in several days to several weeks. If the kidneys are too badly damaged to recover, then the acute kidney failure becomes chronic.

Chronic Kidney Failure

Chronic kidney failure (also called chronic kidney disease) is a slowly progressive (months to years) decline in the kidneys' ability to filter metabolic waste from the blood.

- Major causes are diabetes and high blood pressure.
- Blood becomes more acidic, anemia develops, nerves are damaged, bone tissue deteriorates, and risk of atherosclerosis increases.
- Symptoms can include urinating at night, fatigue, nausea, itching, muscle twitching and cramps, loss of sensation, confusion, difficulty breathing, and yellow skin.
- Diagnosis is by blood and urine tests.
- Treatment aims to restrict fluids, sodium, and potassium in the diet, use drugs to correct other conditions (such as diabetes, high blood pressure, anemia, and electrolyte imbalances), and, when necessary, use dialysis.

Many diseases can irreversibly damage or injure the kidneys. Acute kidney failure can become chronic if kidney function does not recover after treatment. Therefore, anything that can cause acute kidney failure can cause chronic kidney failure. However, the most common cause of chronic kidney failure is diabetes mellitus, followed by high blood pressure (hypertension). Both of these conditions directly damage the kidneys' small blood vessels. Other causes of chronic kidney failure include urinary tract obstruction, kidney abnormalities (such as polycystic kidney disease and glomerulonephritis), and autoimmune disorders (such as systemic lupus erythematosus) in which antibodies damage the tiny blood vessels (glomeruli) and the tiny tubes (tubules) of the kidneys.

When kidney failure is mild or moderately severe, the kidneys cannot absorb water from the urine to reduce the volume of urine and concentrate it. Later, the kidneys have less ability to excrete the acids normally produced by the body and the blood becomes more acidic, a condition called acidosis. Production of red blood cells decreases, leading to anemia. High levels of metabolic wastes in the blood can damage nerve cells in the brain, trunk, and limbs. Diseased kidneys produce hormones that increase blood pressure. In addition, diseased kidneys cannot excrete excess salt and water. Salt and water retention can lead to heart failure. The sac that surrounds the heart (pericardium) may become inflamed (pericarditis). The level of triglycerides in the blood is often elevated, which, along with high blood pressure, increases the risk of atherosclerosis.

The formation and maintenance of bone tissue may be impaired (renal osteodystrophy) if certain conditions that accompany chronic kidney failure are present for a long time. These conditions include a high level of parathyroid hormone, a low concentration of calcitriol (the active form of vitamin D) in the blood, impaired absorption of calcium, and a high concentration of phosphate in the blood. Renal osteodystrophy may lead to bone pain and an increased risk of fractures.

Symptoms

Symptoms usually develop very slowly. People with mild to moderately severe kidney failure may have only mild symptoms, such as the need to urinate several times during the night (nocturia). Nocturia occurs because the kidneys cannot absorb water from the urine to reduce the volume and concentrate it as normally occurs during the night.

As kidney failure progresses and metabolic wastes build up in the blood, people may feel fatigued and generally weak and may become less mentally alert. Some have a loss of appetite and shortness of breath. Anemia also contributes to fatigue and generalized weakness. The buildup of metabolic waste also causes nausea, vomiting, and an unpleasant taste in the mouth, which may lead to undernutrition and weight loss. People with chronic kidney failure tend to bruise easily or bleed for an unusually long time after cuts or other injuries. Chronic kidney failure also diminishes the body's ability to fight infections.

As metabolic wastes build up to higher levels in the blood, damage to muscles and nerves can cause muscle twitches, muscle weakness, cramps, and pain. People may also feel a pins-and-needles sensation in the arms and legs and may lose sensation in certain areas of the body. Encephalopathy, a condition in which the brain malfunctions, may ensue and lead to confusion, lethargy, and seizures.

Heart failure may cause shortness of breath. Pericarditis may cause chest pain and low blood pressure. People who have advanced chronic kidney failure commonly develop gastrointestinal ulcers and bleeding. The skin may turn yellow-brown, and occasionally, the concentration of urea is so high that it crystallizes from sweat, forming a white powder on the skin. Some people with chronic kidney failure itch all over their body. Their breath may also be foul.

Diagnosis

Blood and urine tests are essential. They confirm the presence of kidney failure and can help determine whether it is acute or chronic.

In chronic kidney failure, blood levels of urea and creatinine, metabolic waste products that are normally filtered out by the kidneys, are increased. Typically, the blood becomes moderately acidic. The level of potassium in the blood is often normal or only slightly increased but can become dangerously high when kidney failure reaches an advanced stage or if people ingest large amounts of potassium or take a drug that prevents the kidneys from excreting the potassium. Usually, people have some degree of anemia. The levels of calcium and calcitriol in the blood decrease, and the phosphate and parathyroid hormone levels increase. Analysis of the urine may detect many abnormalities, including protein and abnormal cells.

Ultrasonography is often done to rule out obstruction and check the size of the kidneys. Small, scarred kidneys often indicate that kidney failure is chronic. Determining a precise cause becomes increasingly difficult as kidney failure reaches an advanced stage. Removing a sample of tissue from a kidney for examination (kidney biopsy) may be the most accurate test, but it is not recommended if results of an ultrasound examination show that the kidneys are small and scarred.

Prognosis

Ultimately, chronic kidney failure progresses in most people regardless of treatment. The rate of decline in kidney function depends somewhat on the underlying disorder causing the kidney failure and on how well it is controlled. For example, diabetes and high blood pressure, particularly if poorly controlled, cause kidney failure to progress more rapidly. Kidney failure is fatal if not treated. Survival when kidney failure is severe (sometimes called end-stage kidney failure) is usually limited to several months in people who are not treated, but those who are treated with dialysis can live much longer. However, even with dialysis, most people with end-stage kidney failure die within 5 to 10 years. Most die from heart or blood vessel disorders or infections.

Treatment

Conditions that can cause or worsen kidney failure and consequences of the kidney failure that might adversely affect overall health should be treated promptly. For example, bacterial infections are treated with antibiotics, and any obstructions in the urinary tract are removed or relieved.

Measures are also taken to prevent worsening of kidney function or complications of kidney failure. These measures often include

- Controlling diabetes, blood pressure, and cholesterol and triglyceride levels
- Restricting dietary protein, salt, potassium, phosphorus, and fluids
- Using drugs to control potassium, phosphorus, triglyceride, cholesterol, and parathyroid hormone levels and to treat heart failure or anemia
- Eventually, giving dialysis

Controlling the level of sugar in the blood as well as high blood pressure in people with diabetes substantially slows deterioration in kidney function. Drugs called angiotensin-converting enzyme (ACE) inhibitors and angiotensin II receptor blockers may decrease the rate of decline in kidney function in some people with chronic kidney failure. However, people with severe kidney failure should not take these drugs.

Meticulous attention to diet helps control several potential problems. Sometimes, mild acidosis can be controlled by increasing the intake of carbohydrates and reducing the intake of protein. However, moderate or severe acidosis may require treatment with sodium bicarbonate. The decline in kidney function can be slowed slightly by restricting the amount of protein consumed daily. People need to consume sufficient carbohydrates to offset the reduction in protein. The triglyceride and cholesterol levels may be controlled somewhat by limiting fat in the diet. Drugs such as statins, ezetimibe, and, occasionally clofibrate or gemfibrozil may be required to correct the levels of triglycerides, cholesterol, or both.

The restriction of salt (sodium) is usually beneficial, especially if heart failure occurs. Diuretics may also relieve symptoms of heart failure, even when kidney function is poor, but dialysis may be needed to remove the excess body water in severe kidney failure.

During chronic kidney failure, fluid intake may need to be restricted to prevent the sodium concentration in the blood from becoming too low. Foods that are extremely high in potassium, such as salt substitutes, must be avoided, and foods that are somewhat high in potassium, such as dates, figs, and many other fruits, should not be consumed in excess. A high potassium level in the blood increases the risk of abnormal heart rhythms and cardiac arrest. If the potassium level becomes too high, drugs such as sodium polystyrene sulfonate may help, but emergency dialysis may be required.

The elevated phosphorus level in the blood can cause deposits of calcium and phosphorus to form in tissues, including the blood vessels. Restricting the intake of foods that are high in phosphorus, such as dairy products, liver, legumes, nuts, and most soft drinks, lowers the phosphate concentration in the blood. Drugs that bind phosphate, such as calcium carbonate, calcium acetate, and sevelamer, taken by mouth, may also lower the phosphorus level in the blood. Calcium citrate should be avoided. Calcium citrate is found in many calcium supplements and is in many products as a food additive (sometimes called E333). Vitamin D and similar drugs are often taken by mouth to reduce high levels of parathyroid hormone.

The anemia caused by kidney failure responds to the drugs erythropoietin and darbepoietin. Blood transfusions are given only if the anemia is severe, is causing symptoms, and does not respond to erythropoietin or darbepoietin. Doctors also look for and treat other causes of anemia, particularly dietary deficiencies of iron, folate (folic acid), and vitamin B_{12}. Most people who take erythropoietin or darbepoietin regularly need to be given iron intravenously to prevent iron deficiency, which impairs the body's response to these drugs. Anemia often requires more aggressive treatment in older people, because they are more likely to have heart disease, which can be aggravated by the anemia. The tendency to bleed

can be temporarily suppressed by transfusions of fresh frozen plasma or by such drugs as desmopressin or estrogens. Such treatment may be needed after an injury or before a surgical procedure or a tooth extraction.

Doctors avoid prescribing drugs that are excreted by the kidneys, or they prescribe lower doses of such drugs. Many other drugs may need to be avoided. For example, ACE inhibitors, angiotensin II receptor blockers, and the diuretics spironolactone and triamterene may need to be discontinued in people with severe kidney failure and high potassium levels because these drugs can increase potassium levels. High blood pressure is treated with antihypertensive drugs to prevent further impairment of heart and kidney function.

When the treatments for chronic kidney failure are no longer effective, the only options are long-term dialysis (see below) and kidney transplantation (see page 1131). End-of-life care is important (see page 57).

CHAPTER

43 Dialysis

Dialysis is an artificial process for removing waste products and excess fluids from the body, a process that is needed when the kidneys are not functioning properly.

There are a number of reasons why people may need dialysis, but kidney failure is the most common. For kidney failure, many doctors recommend dialysis when urine output is low and certain conditions develop. For acute kidney failure, doctors continue dialysis until the person's blood test results indicate that adequate kidney function has been restored. For people with chronic kidney failure, dialysis may be used as long-term therapy or as a temporary measure until a kidney can be transplanted. Short-term or urgent dialysis can also be used to remove certain drugs or poisons from the body.

Making the decision to begin long-term dialysis is not easy because it entails a major change in lifestyle, including a dependency on machines to maintain life. However, for most people, a successful dialysis program results in an acceptable quality of life. Most people undergoing dialysis are able to eat a tolerable diet, have normal blood pressure, and avoid progression of nerve damage, severe anemia, and other severe complications.

Reasons for Dialysis in Kidney Failure

Doctors decide to place a person on dialysis when kidney failure is causing certain conditions:

- Abnormal brain function (uremic encephalopathy)
- Certain other severe symptoms, such as loss of appetite or vomiting with weight loss
- Inflammation of the sac around the heart (pericarditis)
- A high level of acid in the blood (acidosis) that does not respond to other treatments
- Heart failure
- Total body fluid overload
- Fluid overload in the lungs (pulmonary edema) that does not respond to other treatments
- A very high level of potassium in the blood (hyperkalemia)
- A high level of calcium in the blood (hypercalcemia)
- Greatly reduced kidney function

Dialysis usually requires the effort of a team of people. A doctor completes a dialysis prescription, manages complications, and monitors the medical care. A nurse monitors the person's general well-being and mental health and educates the person about dialysis and what needs to be done to maintain the best possible health. A social worker arranges transportation and home assistance. A dietitian recommends an appropriate diet and monitors the person's response to dietary changes.

Types of Dialysis

There are two types of dialysis: hemodialysis and peritoneal dialysis.

Hemodialysis: In hemodialysis, blood is removed from the body and pumped by a machine outside the body into a dialyzer (artificial kidney). The dialyzer filters metabolic waste products from the blood and then returns the purified blood to the person. The total amount of fluid returned can be adjusted. Hemodialysis requires repeated access to the bloodstream. Doctors can achieve temporary access by inserting a large intravenous catheter in a big vein, usually one near the neck. An artificial connection between an artery and a vein (an arteriovenous fistula) is surgically created to make long-term access easier. In this procedure, typically the radial artery in the forearm is joined with the cephalic vein. As a result, the cephalic vein subsequently enlarges and blood flow through the vein increases, making the vein suitable for repeated puncture with a needle. When a fistula cannot be created, an artery and a vein may be surgically connected to each other using a synthetic connector (graft). In this situation, the synthetic graft is punctured by the needle for hemodialysis.

Heparin, a drug that prevents clotting, is given during hemodialysis to prevent blood from clotting in the dialyzer. Inside the dialyzer, a porous artificial membrane separates the blood from a fluid (the dialysate). Fluid, waste products, and electrolytes in the blood filter through the membrane into the dialysate. Blood cells and large proteins are unable to filter through the small pores of the membrane and so remain in the blood. The dialyzed (purified) blood is then returned to the person's body.

Dialyzers have different sizes and degrees of efficiency. Dialysis treatment time is usually about 3 to 4 hours. Most people who have chronic kidney failure need hemodialysis 3 times a week.

Peritoneal Dialysis: In peritoneal dialysis, the peritoneum—a membrane that lines the abdomen and covers the abdominal organs—acts as a filter. This membrane has a large surface area and a rich network of blood vessels. Substances from the blood can easily pass through the peritoneum into the abdominal cavity. A fluid (dialysate) is infused through a catheter inserted through the abdominal wall into the peritoneal space within the abdomen. The dialysate must be left in the abdomen for a sufficient time to allow waste products from the bloodstream to pass slowly into it. Then the dialysate is drained out, discarded, and replaced with fresh dialysate.

A soft silicone rubber or porous polyurethane catheter allows the dialysate to flow smoothly and is unlikely to cause damage. A catheter can be put in place temporarily at the person's bedside, or it may be surgically put in place permanently. One type of permanent catheter eventually forms a seal with the skin and can be capped when not in use.

Various techniques are used for peritoneal dialysis.

Manual intermittent peritoneal dialysis is the simplest technique. In manual intermittent peritoneal dialysis, bags containing dialysate are warmed to body temperature and infused into the peritoneal (abdominal) cavity, which takes about 10 minutes. The dialysate is allowed to remain there (dwell time) for 60 to 90 minutes and then is drained out in about

POSSIBLE COMPLICATIONS OF HEMODIALYSIS

COMPLICATION	USUAL CAUSE
Fever	Bacteria or fever-causing substances (pyrogens) in the bloodstream Overheated dialysate
Life-threatening allergic reaction (anaphylaxis)	Allergy to a substance in the dialyzer or blood tubing
Low blood pressure	Removal of too much fluid or excessive fluid gain between dialysis
Abnormal heart rhythms	Abnormal levels of potassium and other substances in the blood Low blood pressure
Air embolus	Air entering blood in the machine
Bleeding in the intestine, brain, eyes, or abdomen	Use of heparin to prevent clotting in the machine
Infection	Bacteria entering the bloodstream through a dialysis catheter or through a needle inserted into veins for hemodialysis access

10 to 20 minutes. This process is then repeated. The entire treatment can take 12 to 24 hours.

Automated cycler intermittent peritoneal dialysis is another technique. This technique uses a machine (cycler) to do automated exchanges of dialysate. Use of an automated cycler can reduce the need for nursing attention.

In **continuous ambulatory peritoneal dialysis**, the dialysate is kept in the abdomen for much longer intervals. Typically, the dialysate is drained and replenished 4 or 5 times a day. Generally three of these dialysate exchanges are performed during the day, with dwell times of 4 hours or longer. An exchange is performed at night with a long dwell time of 8 to 12 hours during sleep.

Continuous cycler-assisted peritoneal dialysis uses an automated cycler to perform short exchanges at night during sleep, whereas longer exchanges are performed manually—without the cycler—during the day. This technique minimizes the number of exchanges during the day but prevents mobility at night because of cumbersome equipment.

Choice of Method: Many factors, including lifestyle, must be considered in determining which type of dialysis is best for a person. People typically undergo hemodialysis at a dialysis center, usually outside of a hospital. Peritoneal dialysis can be performed at home, eliminating the need for travel to a hemodialysis center.

Doctors recommend hemodialysis for people with recent abdominal wounds or abdominal surgery or defects in the abdominal wall that make peritoneal dialysis difficult. Peritoneal dialysis is better tolerated in people whose blood pressure fluctuates frequently between periods of high or normal pressure and periods of low blood pressure.

Special Considerations

Diet: People undergoing dialysis need a special diet. In people undergoing peritoneal dialysis, appetite is generally poor, and protein is lost during dialysis. The diet should be relatively high in protein, roughly 1/2 gram of protein per pound of ideal body weight a day. (The American Association of Kidney Patients has a food guide.) Salt, both the usual salt containing sodium and the salt containing potassium, is restricted.

For those undergoing hemodialysis, daily consumption of sodium and potassium is even more restricted. Foods high in phosphorus also may have to be limited. Daily fluid intake is limited for people who have very little urine output or a persistently low or decreasing sodium concentration in the blood. Daily weighing is important to monitor weight gain. Excessive weight gain between hemodialysis treatments indicates that the person is consuming excessive fluid.

POSSIBLE COMPLICATIONS OF PERITONEAL DIALYSIS

COMPLICATION	CAUSE
Bleeding	Unintentional perforation of an internal organ during placement of the catheter Removal of the catheter from the body Irritation and inflammation of the internal lining of the abdomen (peritoneum) or the area around the insertion site (when the catheter does not seal to the abdominal wall)
Infection	Unsterile techniques during dialysis
Low level of albumin (a protein) in the blood	Loss of protein in fluid removed during dialysis along with inadequate protein in diet
Scarring of the peritoneum	Inflammation and infection Electrolytes in the dialysis fluid Use of certain drugs
A high sugar (glucose) level in the blood	Use of a peritoneal dialysate that has a high concentration of glucose (used to remove water and sodium during dialysis)
Hernias in the abdomen or groin	Increased pressure within the abdomen caused by continued exposure to high fluid levels, which weaken the barriers that normally prevent excessive movement of organs and other structures
Constipation	Intake of inadequate fiber or use of calcium salts to treat high phosphate levels in the blood, causing the intestine to widen, which possibly interferes with dialysate flow in and out of the abdomen

Usually, excessive fluid intake is the result of excessive sodium intake, which makes a person thirsty.

Multivitamin supplements are needed to replace the nutrients lost through hemodialysis or peritoneal dialysis.

Comparing Hemodialysis With Peritoneal Dialysis

When the kidneys fail, waste products and excess water can be removed from the blood by hemodialysis or peritoneal dialysis.

In hemodialysis, blood is removed from the body into a dialyzer (called an artificial kidney), which filters the blood. An artificial connection between an artery and a vein (arteriovenous fistula) is made to facilitate the removal of blood.

In peritoneal dialysis, the peritoneum is used as a filter. The peritoneum is a membrane that lines the abdomen and covers the abdominal organs, creating a space within the abdomen called the peritoneal space or abdominal cavity.

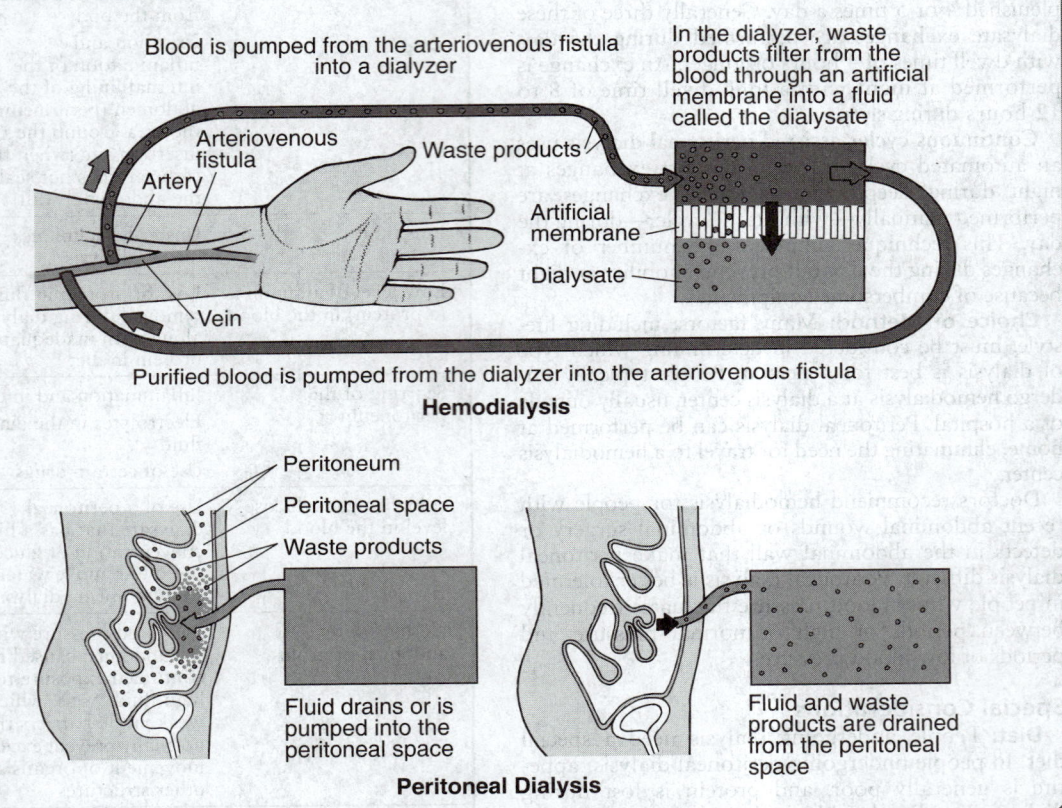

Blood is pumped from the arteriovenous fistula into a dialyzer

In the dialyzer, waste products filter from the blood through an artificial membrane into a fluid called the dialysate

Arteriovenous fistula

Artery

Waste products

Artificial membrane

Dialysate

Vein

Purified blood is pumped from the dialyzer into the arteriovenous fistula

Hemodialysis

Peritoneum

Peritoneal space

Waste products

Fluid drains or is pumped into the peritoneal space

Fluid and waste products are drained from the peritoneal space

Peritoneal Dialysis

Medical Considerations: Erythropoietin or darbepoietin may be given to stimulate the production of red blood cells. Iron may also be needed to help the body produce new red blood cells. Phosphate binders, most often those such as calcium carbonate or calcium acetate, are used to remove excess dietary phosphate.

Normally, the body's bone tissue is continually replaced, helping bones remain strong and dense. The kidneys secrete hormones that help regulate the production of bone tissue. In people with kidney failure, the kidneys are not able to regulate hormone production, so parathyroid hormone levels may increase. The active form of vitamin D (calcitriol) or a similar substance is given to control high parathyroid hormone levels because high parathyroid hormone levels can weaken bones by decreasing their density, a bone condition called renal osteodystrophy.

Psychosocial Considerations: People undergoing dialysis may experience losses in every aspect of their life. The potential loss of independence can be especially distressing. Coping with disruptions in lifestyle can be difficult. Many people undergoing dialysis become depressed and anxious. Psychologic and social counseling is often helpful to families as well as to those undergoing dialysis. Many dialysis centers provide psychologic and social support. Dealing with a loss of independence is helped when people are encouraged to pursue their previous interests. People undergoing hemodialysis need to arrange for transportation to and from dialysis centers on a regular basis. Dialysis sessions may interfere with work, school, or leisure activities.

More than half of the people on long-term dialysis are 60 years of age or older. Older people often are better able to adapt to long-term dialysis and the loss of independence than are younger people. However, older people undergoing dialysis may become more dependent on their grown children or may not be able to continue living alone. Older people are more likely to experience fatigue from treatments. Often, family roles and responsibilities must be modified to fit the dialysis routine, creating stress and feelings of guilt and inadequacy.

Considerations in Children: Children whose growth has been stunted may feel isolated and different from their peers. Young adults and adolescents coping with identity, independence, and body image issues may find these issues further complicated by dialysis. Diet is an important issue for children undergoing dialysis because children must receive enough nutrients to support their growth.

Each kidney contains about 1 million filtering units (glomeruli). The glomeruli are made up of many microscopic clusters of tiny blood vessels (capillaries) with small pores. These blood vessels are designed to leak fluid from the bloodstream into a system of miniature tubules that process the fluid to become urine. Normally this filtering system permits fluid and small molecules (but almost no protein or blood cells) to leak into the tubules. Diseases that affect the kidneys can be divided into three categories based on the way they affect different parts of the kidneys:

- Glomerulonephritis (or nephritic syndrome) is inflammation of the glomeruli, which causes blood cells and protein to escape from the glomerular capillaries into the urine.

- In nephrotic syndrome, damage to the capillaries of the glomeruli causes proteins to leak into the urine.

- Tubulointerstitial nephritis is inflammation of the tubules and the tissues surrounding the tubules (interstitium).

With **glomerulonephritis**, the inflammation is often the result of an abnormal immune reaction. Such a reaction can occur in two ways: (1) Antibodies (proteins made by the body to attack specific molecules called antigens) may attach directly to cells of the kidney or molecules trapped in them, causing inflammation. (2) Antibodies attach to antigens outside the kidney, and these antigen-antibody (or immune) complexes are carried to the kidney by the bloodstream and get trapped in the glomeruli, causing inflammation.

If enough glomeruli are damaged, kidney function is decreased. As a result, urine production falls and waste products build up in the blood. Also, when damage is severe, inflammatory cells and injured glomerular cells accumulate, compressing the capillaries within the glomerulus and interfering with filtration. Scarring may develop, which also impairs kidney function and reduces urine production. In some cases, tiny blood clots (microthrombi) may form in the small blood vessels, further decreasing kidney function. Rarely, glomerulonephritis can result from a hereditary condition. In other cases, glomerulonephritis is caused by inflammation of the blood vessels (vasculitis).

Nephrotic syndrome causes large amounts of protein to leak from blood into the urine. This leakage can be caused by damage to the glomeruli by inflammatory or noninflammatory processes. In inflammatory processes, red blood cells appear in the urine. Nephrotic syndrome caused by inflammation therefore has characteristics similar to those of glomerulonephritis. With noninflammatory processes, no red blood cells appear in the urine. Some forms of nephrotic syndrome can be severe. The glomeruli become scarred, and kidney failure develops. In less severe forms of nephrotic syndrome, kidney function decreases very little.

Tubulointerstitial nephritis often is caused by a toxic or allergic reaction to a drug. White blood cells or scar tissue appears in the kidney's tissues. Infection of the kidneys (pyelonephritis—see page 306) can also cause tubulointerstitial nephritis. When inflammation damages the tubules and surrounding tissues, the kidneys may become unable to perform their normal functions, such as concentrating urine, eliminating (excreting) waste products from the body, or balancing the excretion of sodium and other electrolytes, such as potassium. If the damage is severe and affects both kidneys, the result is kidney failure.

Glomerulonephritis

Glomerulonephritis (nephritic syndrome) is a disorder of glomeruli (clusters of microscopic blood vessels in the kidneys with small pores through which blood is filtered). It is characterized by body tissue swelling (edema), high blood pressure, and the presence of red blood cells in the urine.

- Glomerulonephritis can be caused by various disorders, such as infections, an inherited genetic disorder, or autoimmune disorders.
- People may have tissue swelling, headaches, visual disturbances, and seizures.
- Diagnosis is based on tests of blood and urine and sometimes imaging tests, a biopsy of the kidneys, or both.
- People need to restrict salt and protein intake and take diuretics or antibiotics until kidney function improves.

Glomerulonephritis can develop over a short time period (acute glomerulonephritis) or develop and progress slowly (chronic glomerulonephritis). In 1% of children and 10% of adults who have acute glomerulonephritis, it evolves into rapidly progressive glomerulonephritis, in which most of the glomeruli are destroyed, resulting in kidney failure.

Causes

Glomerulonephritis can be primary, affecting only the kidneys, or secondary, caused by a vast array of disorders that affect other parts of the body.

Acute Glomerulonephritis: Acute glomerulonephritis most often occurs as a complication of throat or skin infection by streptococcus, a type of bacteria. Acute glomerulonephritis that occurs after a streptococcal infection (poststreptococcal glomerulonephritis) typically develops in children between the ages of 2 and 10 following recovery from the infection. Infections with other types of bacteria, such as staphylococcus and pneumococcus, viral infections, such as chickenpox, and parasitic infections, such as malaria, can also result in acute glomerulonephritis. Acute glomerulonephritis that results from any of these infections is called postinfectious glomerulonephritis. Noninfectious causes of acute glomerulonephritis include membranoproliferative glomerulonephritis, immunoglobulin A (IgA) nephropathy, thin basement membrane disease, Henoch-Schönlein purpura, systemic lupus erythematosus (lupus), cryoglobulinemia, Goodpasture's syndrome, and Wegener's granulomatosis.

Acute glomerulonephritis that develops into rapidly progressive glomerulonephritis most often results from conditions that involve an abnormal immune reaction.

Chronic Glomerulonephritis: Often, chronic glomerulonephritis seems to result from one of the same conditions that cause acute glomerulonephritis, such as IgA nephropathy or membranoproliferative glomerulonephritis. Sometimes, acute glomerulonephritis does not resolve and instead becomes chronic. Occasionally, chronic glomerulonephritis is caused by hereditary nephritis, an inherited genetic disorder. In many people, the cause of chronic glomerulonephritis cannot be identified.

Symptoms

About half of the people with **acute glomerulonephritis** have no symptoms. If symptoms do occur, the first to appear are tissue swelling (edema) due to fluid retention, low urine volume, and production of urine that is dark because it contains blood.

Secondary Causes of Glomerulonephritis

INFECTIONS

- Bacterial infections (streptococcus, staphylococcus, or pneumococcus)
- Fungal infections
- Parasitic infections (malaria)
- Viral infections (hepatitis B and C or HIV)

VASCULITIS

- Churg-Strauss syndrome
- Cryoglobulinemia
- Microscopic polyangiitis
- Wegener's granulomatosis

IMMUNE DISORDERS

- Goodpasture's syndrome
- Serum sickness
- Systemic lupus erythematosus (lupus)

HEREDITARY DISORDERS

- Hereditary nephritis
- Nail-patella syndrome

DRUGS

- Gold
- Pamidronate
- Penicillamine
- Propylthioracil

Edema may first appear as puffiness of the face and eyelids but later is prominent in the legs. Blood pressure increases as kidney function becomes impaired. In turn, high blood pressure and swelling of the brain may cause headaches, visual disturbances, and more serious disturbances of brain function (for example, seizures or coma). In older people, nonspecific symptoms, such as nausea and a general feeling of illness (malaise), are more common.

When **rapidly progressive glomerulonephritis** develops, weakness, fatigue, and fever are the most frequent early symptoms. Loss of appetite, nausea, vomiting, abdominal pain, and joint pain are also common. About 50% of people have a flu-like illness in the month before kidney failure develops. These people have edema and usually produce very little urine. High blood pressure is uncommon and rarely severe when it does occur.

Because **chronic glomerulonephritis** usually causes only very mild or subtle symptoms, it goes undetected for a long time in most people. Edema may occur. High blood pressure is common. The disease may progress to kidney failure, which can cause itchiness, fatigue, decreased appetite, nausea, vomiting, and difficulty breathing.

Diagnosis

Doctors investigate the possibility of acute glomerulonephritis in people whose laboratory test results indicate kidney dysfunction or blood in the urine and in people who develop symptoms of the disorder, particularly those who have had strep throat or other infections. Laboratory tests show variable amounts of protein and blood cells in the urine and often kidney dysfunction, as shown by a high concentration of urea and creatinine (waste products) in the blood.

In people with rapidly progressive glomerulonephritis, casts (clumps of red blood cells or white blood cells) are almost always visible in a urine sample that is examined under a microscope. Blood tests detect anemia and often an abnormally high number of white blood cells. When doctors suspect glomerulonephritis, a biopsy of the kidney is usually done to confirm the diagnosis, help determine the cause, and determine the amount of scarring and potential for reversibility. Kidney biopsy is done by inserting a needle in one of the kidneys under ultrasound or computed tomography (CT) guidance to obtain a small amount of kidney tissue. Although kidney biopsy is an invasive procedure and occasionally can become complicated, it is usually safe.

Additional tests are sometimes helpful for identifying the cause. For example, a throat culture may provide evidence of streptococcal infection. Blood levels of antibodies against streptococci may be higher than normal or progressively increase over several weeks. Acute glomerulonephritis that follows an infection other than strep throat is usually easier to diagnose, because its symptoms often begin while the infection is still obvious. Cultures and blood tests that help identify the organisms that cause these other types of infections are sometimes needed to confirm the diagnosis.

Chronic glomerulonephritis develops gradually, and therefore, a doctor may not be able to tell exactly when it began. It may be discovered when a urine test, done as part of a medical examination, reveals the presence of protein and blood cells in a person who is feeling well, has normal kidney function, and has no symptoms. Doctors usually do an imaging test of the kidneys, such as an ultrasound, CT scan, or magnetic resonance imaging (MRI) scan. A kidney biopsy is the most reliable way to distinguish chronic glomerulonephritis from other kidney diseases. A biopsy, however, is rarely done in advanced stages. In these cases, the kidneys are shrunken and scarred, and the chance of obtaining specific information about the cause is small. Doctors suspect that the kidneys are shrunken and scarred if kidney function has been poor for a long time and the kidneys appear abnormally small on an imaging test.

Prognosis

Acute poststreptococcal glomerulonephritis resolves completely in most cases, especially in children. About 0.1% of children and 25% of adults develop chronic kidney failure.

The prognosis for people with rapidly progressive glomerulonephritis depends on the severity of glomerular scarring and whether the underlying disease, such as infection, can be cured. In about 75% of the people who are treated early (within weeks to a few months), kidney function is preserved and dialysis is not needed. However, because the early symptoms can be subtle and vague, many people who have rapidly progressive glomerulonephritis are not aware of the underlying disease and do not seek medical care until kidney failure develops. If treatment occurs late, the person is more likely to develop chronic kidney failure. The prognosis also depends on the cause, the person's age, and any other diseases the person might have. When the cause is unknown or the person is older, the prognosis is worse.

In some children and adults who do not recover completely from acute glomerulonephritis, other types of kidney disorders develop, such as asymptomatic proteinuria and hematuria syndrome or nephrotic syndrome. Other people with acute glomerulonephritis, especially older adults, often develop chronic glomerulonephritis.

PRIMARY GLOMERULAR DISORDERS THAT CAN CAUSE GLOMERULONEPHRITIS

DISORDER	DESCRIPTION	PROGNOSIS
Fibrillary glomerulonephritis	In this rare disease, abnormal proteins are deposited around the glomerulus. It may also cause nephrotic syndrome.	The prognosis is poor. End-stage kidney failure occurs in half of people within 4 years. It is not clear how much treatment (with corticosteroids and immunosuppressants) helps.
Primary rapidly progressive glomerulonephritis	This group of disorders causes microscopic damage to the glomeruli and progress rapidly. Sometimes they are caused by an infection or other treatable disorder.	The prognosis is poor. At least 80% of people develop end-stage kidney failure within 6 months without treatment. The prognosis is better for people younger than 60 years or if an underlying disorder causing the glomerulonephritis responds to treatment.
Immunoglobulin A (IgA) nephropathy	The most common form of glomerulonephritis in the world is caused by immune complexes (combinations of antigens and antibodies) deposited in the kidney.	Usually the disorder progresses slowly. End-stage kidney failure develops in about 20% to 40% of people after 5 to 25 years. The disorder progresses more slowly in children.
Thin basement membrane disease (benign familial hematuria)	This hereditary disorder is caused by thinning of a part of the glomerulus called the basement membrane.	The prognosis is excellent. Most people do not develop end-stage kidney failure.
Membranoproliferative glomerulonephritis	This uncommon type of glomerulonephritis occurs primarily between the ages of 8 and 30. Sometimes the cause is unknown, or the disorder may be caused by immune complexes (combinations of antigens and antibodies) attaching to the kidney.	If caused by immune complex disease, a partial remission may occur. The outcome is not as good in people in whom the cause remains unknown. About half of untreated people progress to end-stage kidney failure within 10 to 15 years, while in most others, the kidney function stabilizes or improves.

Treatment

No specific treatment is available in most cases of acute glomerulonephritis. Following a diet that is low in protein and sodium may be necessary until kidney function recovers. Diuretics may be prescribed to help the kidneys excrete excess sodium and water. High blood pressure needs to be treated.

When a bacterial infection is suspected as the cause of acute glomerulonephritis, antibiotics are usually ineffective because the nephritis begins 1 to 6 weeks (average, 2 weeks) after the infection, which has, by then, usually resolved. However, if a bacterial infection is still present when acute glomerulonephritis is discovered, antibiotic therapy is started. Antimalarial drugs may be beneficial if the cause of the syndrome is malaria.

For rapidly progressive glomerulonephritis, drugs to suppress the immune system are started promptly. High doses of corticosteroids are usually given intravenously for about a week, followed by a variable period of time when they are taken by mouth. Cyclophosphamide, an immunosuppressant, may also be given. In addition, plasmapheresis is sometimes used to remove antibodies from the blood. The sooner treatment occurs, the less likely are kidney failure and the need for dialysis. Kidney transplantation is sometimes considered for people who develop chronic kidney failure, but rapidly progressive glomerulonephritis may recur in the transplanted kidney.

Angiotensin-converting enzyme (ACE) inhibitors and angiotensin II receptor blockers (ARBs) either alone or in combination often slow progression of chronic glomerulonephritis. Taking drugs to reduce high blood pressure and reducing sodium intake are considered beneficial. Restricting the amount of protein in the diet is modestly helpful in reducing the rate of kidney deterioration. End-stage kidney failure can be treated with dialysis or a kidney transplant.

ASYMPTOMATIC PROTEINURIA AND HEMATURIA SYNDROME

Asymptomatic proteinuria and hematuria syndrome is the result of diseases of glomeruli (clusters of microscopic blood vessels in the kidneys that have small pores through which blood is filtered). It is characterized by steady or intermittent loss of small amounts of protein and blood in the urine.

Small amounts of protein excreted in the urine (proteinuria) or blood excreted in the urine (hematuria) are sometimes discovered in people without symptoms, when urine tests are done for some routine purpose. The presence of casts (clumps of red blood cells) or abnormally shaped red blood cells is a clue for doctors that the blood in the urine came from glomeruli. Casts and proteinuria may be present because the person is recovering from a recent undiagnosed episode of nephritis. If this situation seems likely, a doctor needs only to recheck the person over the next weeks or months to make sure that the abnormalities resolve.

If casts and proteinuria persist, the cause is usually one of three disorders. One is immunoglobulin A (IgA) nephropathy, a type of nephritis caused by deposition of immune complexes (combinations of antibodies and antigens) in the kidney that can be very mild and nonprogressive or become a severe disease leading to kidney failure. Another is hereditary nephritis (Alport's syndrome), a progressive disorder that can be severe and lead to kidney failure. The third disorder is thin basement membrane disease (benign familial hematuria). Thin basement membrane disease is a hereditary disorder caused by thinning of a part of the glomerulus called the basement membrane. It follows a mild and nonprogressive course. The diagnosis can usually be made with a kidney biopsy. However, a kidney biopsy is rarely done because the likelihood of finding a treatable disease is very low.

Doctors usually recommend that people with asymptomatic proteinuria and hematuria have a physical examination and undergo urine testing once or twice a year. Additional tests are done if the amount of protein or blood increases much, or if symptoms occur that suggest the development of a specific disease. Most people with asymptomatic proteinuria and hematuria syndrome do not worsen, and the condition may persist indefinitely.

HEREDITARY NEPHRITIS (ALPORT'S SYNDROME)

Hereditary nephritis (Alport's syndrome) is a genetic disorder in which kidney function is poor, blood is present in the urine, and deafness and eye abnormalities sometimes occur.

Hereditary nephritis is usually caused by a defective gene on the X chromosome, but it sometimes results from an abnormal gene on a nonsex (autosomal) chromosome. Other factors influence how severe the disorder is in a person who has the gene. Females with the defective gene on one of their two X chromosomes usually do not have symptoms, although their kidneys may function somewhat less efficiently than normal. Most of these females have some blood in the urine. Males with the defective gene develop more severe problems because males do not have a second X chromosome to compensate for the defect. Males usually develop kidney failure between the ages of 20 and 30. Many people with the defective gene on only one autosomal chromosome have no symptoms other than blood in the urine, but the urine may also contain varying amounts of protein, white blood cells, and casts (small clumps of cells) that are visible under a microscope. Kidney function in people who have the defective gene on two autosomal chromosomes slowly worsens, and kidney failure usually occurs.

Hereditary nephritis can affect other organs. Hearing problems, usually an inability to hear sounds in the higher frequencies, are common. Cataracts can also occur, although less often than hearing loss. Abnormalities of the cornea, lens, or retina sometimes cause blindness. Other problems include a low number of platelets in the blood (thrombocytopenia) and abnormalities that affect several nerves (polyneuropathy).

People who develop kidney failure need to undergo dialysis or receive a kidney transplant. Genetic testing is usually offered to people who want to have children.

NAIL-PATELLA SYNDROME

Nail-patella syndrome (also called osteo-onychodysplasia, arthro-onychodysplasia, and onycho-osteodysplasia) is a rare hereditary disorder that results in abnormalities of the kidneys, bones, joints, and fingernails.

The gene that causes nail-patella syndrome is dominant. Commonly, people who have this syndrome have one or both kneecaps (patellas) missing, one of the arm bones (the radius) dislocated at the elbow, and the pelvic bone abnormally shaped. They have either no fingernails or poorly developed ones, with pitting and ridges. About 30% to 40% of people with this syndrome have blood or protein in their urine, which may prompt the doctor to order kidney function tests. Kidney failure eventually develops in about 30% of the people with affected kidneys by the time they are 50 or 60. The diagnosis is confirmed by bone x-rays and a biopsy of kidney tissue.

There is no effective treatment for this syndrome. Controlling blood pressure may slow the rate that kidney function deteriorates. Those who develop kidney failure need dialysis or a kidney transplant. Genetic testing is usually offered to people who want to have children.

Nephrotic Syndrome

Nephrotic syndrome is a disorder of the glomeruli (clusters of microscopic blood vessels in the kidneys that have small pores through which blood is filtered) in which excessive amounts of protein are excreted in the urine. This typically leads to accumulation of fluid in the body (edema) and low levels of the protein albumin and high levels of fats in the blood.

- Drugs and disorders that damage the kidneys may cause nephrotic syndrome.
- People feel tired and have tissue swelling and sometimes muscle wasting.
- Diagnosis is based on blood and urine tests and sometimes imaging of the kidneys, a biopsy of the kidneys, or both.
- People who have disorders that may cause nephrotic syndrome are given angiotensin-converting enzyme (ACE) inhibitors or angiotensin II receptor blockers (ARBs) to prevent kidney damage.
- ACE inhibitors and ARBs are used to treat this disorder.

Secondary Causes of Nephrotic Syndrome

DISEASES

- Amyloidosis
- Cancer (lymphoma, leukemia, or various solid tumors)
- Diabetes mellitus*
- Pre-eclampsia (also called toxemia of pregnancy)
- Some glomerulonephritis (including rapidly progressive glomerulonephritis)
- Systemic lupus erythematosus (lupus)*
- Vasculitic disorders (Henoch-Schönlein purpura, Wegener's granulomatosis, or microscopic polyangiitis)
- Viral infections (hepatitis B,* hepatitis C,* or HIV*)

DRUGS

- Gold
- Nonsteroidal anti-inflammatory drugs (NSAIDs)*
- Penicillamine
- Heroin taken intravenously

ALLERGIES

- Insect bites
- Pollens
- Poison ivy and poison oak

*Asterisks indicate the most common causes.

Nephrotic syndrome can develop gradually or suddenly. Nephrotic syndrome can occur at any age. In children, it is most common between the ages of 18 months and 4 years, and more boys than girls are affected. In older people, both sexes are equally affected.

Protein excretion into the urine (proteinuria) is accompanied by low levels of important proteins, such as albumin, in the blood, increased levels of fats (lipids) in the blood, a tendency for increased blood clotting, and a greater susceptibility to infection. The decreased level of albumin in the blood leads to edema and to the retention of excess sodium.

Causes

Nephrotic syndrome can be primary, affecting only the kidneys, or secondary, caused by a vast array of disorders that affect other parts of the body, most commonly diabetes mellitus, systemic lupus erythematosus, and certain viral infections. Nephrotic syndrome can also result from glomerulonephritis. A number of drugs that are toxic to the kidneys can also cause nephrotic syndrome, especially nonsteroidal anti-inflammatory drugs (NSAIDs). The syndrome may be caused by certain allergies, including allergies to insect bites and to poison ivy or poison oak. Some types of nephrotic syndrome are hereditary.

Symptoms

Early symptoms include loss of appetite, a general feeling of illness (malaise), puffy eyelids and tissue swelling from excess sodium and water retention, abdominal pain, wasting of muscles (atrophy), and frothy urine. The abdomen may be swollen because of a large accumulation of fluid in the abdominal cavity (ascites). Shortness of breath may develop because fluid accumulates in the space surrounding the lungs (pleural effusion). Other symptoms may include swelling of the knees and, in men, the scrotum. Most often, the fluid that causes tissue swelling is affected by gravity and therefore moves around. During the night, fluid accumulates in the upper parts of the body, such as the eyelids. During the day, when the person is sitting or standing, fluid accumulates in the lower parts of the body, such as the ankles. Swelling may hide the muscle wasting that is progressing at the same time.

In children, blood pressure is generally low, and blood pressure may fall when the child stands up (orthostatic hypotension). Shock occasionally develops. Adults may have low, normal, or high blood pressure. Urine production may decrease, and kidney failure may develop if the leakage of fluid from blood vessels into tissues depletes the liquid component of blood and the blood supply to the kidney is diminished. Occasionally, kidney failure with low urine output occurs suddenly.

Nutritional deficiencies may result because nutrients are excreted in the urine. In children, growth may be stunted. Calcium may be lost from bones. The hair and nails may become brittle, and some hair may fall out. Horizontal white lines may develop in fingernail beds for unknown reasons.

The membrane that lines the abdominal cavity and abdominal organs (peritoneum) may become inflamed and infected. Opportunistic infections—infections caused by normally harmless bacteria—are common. The higher likelihood of infection is thought to occur because the antibodies that normally combat infections are excreted in the urine or not produced in normal amounts. The tendency for blood clotting (thrombosis) increases, particularly inside the main vein from the kidney. Less commonly, the blood may not clot when clotting is needed, generally leading to excessive bleeding. High blood pressure accompanied by complications affecting the heart and brain is most likely to occur in people who have diabetes or systemic lupus erythematosus.

Diagnosis

A doctor bases the diagnosis of nephrotic syndrome on the symptoms, physical examination findings, and laboratory findings. Sometimes nephrotic syndrome is at first mistaken for heart failure in older adults because swelling occurs in both disorders and heart failure is common among older people. A laboratory test of urine collected over a 24-hour period is useful for measuring the degree of protein loss, but collection of urine over such a long period is difficult for many people to accomplish. Alternatively, to estimate protein loss, a randomly collected urine specimen can be tested to measure the ratio of the level of protein to that of creatinine (a waste product). Blood tests and other urine tests detect additional characteristics of the syndrome. The level of albumin in the blood is low because this vital protein is excreted in the urine and its production is impaired. The urine often contains clumps of cells that may be combined with protein and fat (casts). The urine contains low levels of sodium and high levels of potassium.

Concentrations of lipid in the blood are high, sometimes exceeding 10 times that of a normal concentration. Levels of lipid in the urine are also high. Anemia may be present. Levels of blood clotting proteins may be increased or decreased.

The doctor investigates possible causes of nephrotic syndrome, including drugs. Analysis of the urine and blood may reveal an underlying disorder. An imaging test of the kidney, such as ultrasound, computed tomography (CT), or magnetic resonance imaging (MRI), is usually done. If the person has lost weight or is older, a search for cancer is undertaken. A kidney biopsy is especially useful in determining the cause and extent of kidney damage.

Prognosis

The prognosis varies depending on the cause of the nephrotic syndrome, the person's age, and the type and degree of kidney damage. Symptoms may disappear completely if the nephrotic syndrome is caused by a treatable disorder, such as an infection, cancer, or drugs. This situation occurs in about half the cases in children but less often in adults. If the underlying disorder responds to corticosteroids, sometimes progression of the disease is halted, and less often the condition partially or, rarely, completely reverses. When the syndrome is caused by HIV infection, it usually progresses relentlessly, often resulting in complete kidney failure in 3 or 4 months. Children born with the nephrotic syndrome rarely live beyond their first birthday, although a few have survived by means of dialysis treatments or a kidney transplant.

When the cause is systemic lupus erythematosus or diabetes mellitus, drug treatment often stabilizes or decreases the amount of protein in the urine. However, some people do not respond to drug treatment and develop progressive kidney failure within a few years.

In cases of nephrotic syndrome resulting from conditions such as an infection, allergy, or intravenous heroin use, the prognosis varies, depending on how early and effectively the underlying condition is treated.

Prevention and Treatment

Use of an angiotensin-converting enzyme (ACE) inhibitor, such as enalapril, quinapril, or lisinopril, or an angiotensin II receptor blocker (ARB), such as candesartan, losartan, or valsartan, alone or in combination is the mainstay of both prevention and treatment. When a person with a disease such as systemic lupus erythematosus or diabetes mellitus has mild or moderate proteinuria, an ACE inhibitor or ARB is used as soon as possible because it may prevent proteinuria from increasing and kidney function from worsening.

When a person who already has nephrotic syndrome is treated with an ACE inhibitor or ARB, symptoms may improve, the amount of protein excreted in the urine usually decreases, and lipid concentrations in the blood are likely to decline. However, these drugs can increase the potassium levels in the blood in people who have moderate to severe kidney failure, which can cause potentially dangerous heart rhythm abnormalities.

General therapy for nephrotic syndrome includes a diet that contains normal amounts of protein and potassium but that is low in saturated fat and cholesterol and sodium. Some doctors recommend limiting the amount of protein in the diet.

PRIMARY GLOMERULAR DISORDERS THAT CAN CAUSE NEPHROTIC SYNDROME

GLOMERULAR DISORDER	DESCRIPTION	PROGNOSIS
Minimal change disease	This mild disease of the glomerulus is more common in children but also affects adults.	The prognosis is good; 90% of children and nearly as many adults respond to treatment. In 30 to 50% of adults, disease relapses. After treatment for 1 or 2 years, more than 80% of people have permanent remission.
Focal segmental glomerulosclerosis	This disease damages glomeruli. It affects mainly adolescents but also young and middle-aged adults. It is more common in blacks.	The prognosis is poor because treatment is not very effective. In most adults and children, the disease progresses to end-stage kidney failure 5 to 20 years after diagnosis.
Membranous glomerulopathy	This serious type of glomerular disease affects mainly adults. It is more common in whites.	Spontaneous remission of proteinuria occurs in 30 to 40% of people. The likelihood of end-stage kidney failure rises steadily over time to about 40% at 15 years.
Congenital and infantile nephrotic syndrome	This rare disease is inherited. Congenital nephrotic syndrome (Finnish type) and diffuse mesangial sclerosis are the two main causes. They closely resemble focal segmental glomerulosclerosis. Symptoms are present at birth in the Finnish type and develop during childhood in the infantile variety.	The disorder does not respond to corticosteroids. Because the level of albumin in the blood is extremely low, removal of both kidneys is often considered. Supportive therapy, including dialysis, is given until the child is eligible for a kidney transplant.
Membranoproliferative glomerulonephritis	This uncommon type of glomerulonephritis occurs primarily between the ages of 8 and 30. Sometimes the cause is unknown, or it may be caused by immune complex disease, which is caused by immune complexes (combinations of antigens and antibodies) attaching to the kidney.	If caused by immune complex disease, a partial remission may occur. The outcome is not as good in people in whom the cause remains unknown. About half of untreated people progress to end-stage kidney failure within 10 to 15 years, while in most others, kidney function stabilizes or improves.
Mesangial proliferative glomerulonephritis	This disorder accounts for about 3 to 5% of people with nephrotic syndrome of unknown cause. It affects all ages. It is sometimes considered a subtype of membranoproliferative glomerulonephritis but may be a severe form of minimal change disease.	About 50% of people initially respond to corticosteroids; 10 to 30% develop progressive kidney failure. Relapses may respond to cyclophosphamide.

If fluid accumulates in the abdomen, the person may need to eat frequent, small meals because of the reduced capacity of the stomach. High blood pressure is usually treated with diuretics. Diuretics can also reduce fluid retention and tissue swelling but may increase the risk of blood clots. Anticoagulants may help control clot formation if it occurs. Infections can be life threatening and must be treated promptly.

Whenever possible, specific treatment is aimed at the cause. Treating an infection that causes nephrotic syndrome may cure the syndrome. If a treatable dis-

ease, such as certain cancers, causes the syndrome, treating that disease can eliminate the syndrome. If a heroin user with nephrotic syndrome stops using heroin in the early stages of the disease, the syndrome may resolve. If other drugs are responsible for the syndrome, discontinuing the drugs may be curative. People who are sensitive or allergic to poison oak, poison ivy, or insect bites should avoid these irritants. If no reversible cause can be found, the person may be given corticosteroids and other drugs that suppress the immune system, such as cyclophosphamide. However, corticosteroids cause problems, particularly for children, in whom these drugs can stunt growth and suppress sexual development (see box on page 568).

Tubulointerstitial Nephritis

Tubulointerstitial nephritis is inflammation that affects the tubules of the kidneys and the tissues that surround them (interstitial tissue).

- This disorder may be caused by diseases, drugs, and toxins that damage the kidneys.
- People may have painful urination, pain in the lower back or side, fever, and a rash.
- Laboratory tests of blood and urine are used to detect kidney damage.
- Stopping exposure to harmful drugs and toxins and treating underlying disorders improve kidney function.

Tubulointerstitial nephritis may be acute or chronic, and it often results in kidney failure. It may be caused by various diseases, drugs, toxins, or radiation that damages the kidneys. Damage to the tubules results in changes in the concentrations of electrolytes in the blood or in problems with the kidney's ability to concentrate urine. There are two parts of the kidney tubules, the proximal and the distal. When the proximal tubule is damaged, the normal reabsorption into the blood of sodium, potassium, bicarbonate, uric acid, and phosphate may be altered, resulting in low levels in the blood of these substances. Injuries to the distal tubule are usually associated with a loss of urine-concentrating ability and an increase in daily urine volume (polyuria).

Causes

The most common cause of acute tubulointerstitial nephritis is an allergic reaction to a drug. Antibiotics such as penicillin and the sulfonamides, diuretics, and nonsteroidal anti-inflammatory drugs (NSAIDs)—including aspirin—may trigger an allergic reaction. The interval between the exposure to the allergen that caused the reaction and the development of acute tubulointerstitial nephritis varies from 5 days to 5 weeks.

Drugs can also cause tubulointerstitial nephritis through nonallergic mechanisms. For example, NSAIDs can damage the tissues gradually, taking up to 18 months to cause chronic tubulointerstitial nephritis.

Infection of the kidneys (pyelonephritis) can also cause acute or chronic tubulointerstitial nephritis. Kidney failure is unlikely unless inflammation causes a blockage in the urinary tract or pyelonephritis occurs in both kidneys.

Secondary Causes of Tubulointerstitial Nephritis

DISEASES

- Pyelonephritis
- Sarcoidosis
- Sickle cell disease
- Sjögren's syndrome
- Systemic lupus erythematosus (lupus)

DRUGS

- Lithium
- Nonsteroidal anti-inflammatory drugs (NSAIDs)
- Chemotherapy drugs
- Anti-rejection drugs for transplant recipients (such as cyclosporine and tacrolimus)

TOXINS

- Aristolochic acid
- Cadmium
- Lead

Symptoms and Diagnosis

Some people have few or no symptoms. When symptoms develop, they are highly variable and may develop suddenly or gradually.

When tubulointerstitial nephritis develops suddenly, the amount of urine produced may be normal or less than normal. Some people develop the symptoms of pyelonephritis: fever, painful urination, pus in the urine, and pain in the lower back or side (flank). If the cause is an allergic reaction, symptoms may include fever and a rash.

When tubulointerstitial nephritis develops gradually, the first symptoms to appear are those of kidney failure, such as itchiness, fatigue, decreased appetite, nausea, vomiting, and difficulty breathing. Blood pressure is normal or only slightly above normal in the early stages of the disease. The amount of urine produced may be greater than normal.

Laboratory tests usually detect signs of kidney failure, such as an increase in the level of waste products in the blood, or other characteristic abnormalities, such as metabolic acidosis, hypokalemia, hypouricemia, or hypophosphatemia. A kidney biopsy is the only conclusive means of diagnosing tubulointerstitial nephritis, although a biopsy is rarely done except when the cause cannot be found or treatment with corticosteroids is being considered.

When tubulointerstitial nephritis develops suddenly, the urine may be almost normal, with only a trace of protein or pus, but often the abnormalities are striking. The urine may show large numbers of white blood cells, including eosinophils. Eosinophils rarely appear in the urine, but when they do, a person usually has acute tubulointerstitial nephritis caused by an allergic reaction. Also, the number of eosinophils in the blood may be increased.

When an allergic reaction is the cause, the kidneys usually are large because of inflammation caused by the allergic reaction. This enlargement can be seen with x-rays or ultrasound scanning.

Prognosis and Treatment

Kidney function usually improves when an offending drug is discontinued or treatment of the underlying disease is effective, although some kid-

ney scarring is common. Treatment with a corticosteroid may speed the recovery of kidney function when the disorder is caused by an allergic reaction. If kidney function worsens and kidney failure develops, dialysis is usually needed. In some cases, the damage is irreversible, and kidney failure becomes chronic.

When the inflammation occurs gradually, kidney damage may develop at different rates in different portions of the kidney. The person may develop abnormalities characteristic of damage to different portions of the kidney at different times. However, kidney damage usually progresses to involve most or all of the kidney and becomes irreversible. Irreversible kidney damage, whatever the cause, results in the need for dialysis or kidney transplantation.

CHAPTER
45   Blood Vessel Disorders of the Kidneys

The blood flow to the kidneys needs to be intact for the kidneys to function properly. Any interruption of or reduction in the blood flow can cause kidney damage or dysfunction and, if long-standing, increased blood pressure. When blood flow in the arteries supplying the kidneys is completely blocked, the entire kidney or a portion of the kidney supplied by that artery dies (kidney infarction). Kidney infarction can lead to kidney failure.

Blood vessel disorders of the kidneys have a number of causes, including blockages in the renal arteries or veins, inflammation of blood vessels (vasculitis), injury to the kidneys or blood vessels, and other disorders. For example, systemic sclerosis (scleroderma) and sickle cell anemia can affect the kidneys, sometimes leading to chronic kidney failure. Systemic sclerosis that affects the kidneys can also cause malignant hypertension.

Blockage of the Renal Arteries

- Gradual narrowing or sudden, complete blockage may affect arteries that supply the right or the left kidney, their branches, or a combination.
- Kidney failure or high blood pressure may result.
- An imaging test can show the narrowing or blockage.
- Eliminating a blockage or widening a narrowed artery may be possible and helpful.

There are two renal arteries—one supplies blood to the right kidney, the other to the left kidney. These arteries branch into many smaller arteries.

A gradual narrowing of one or both of the renal arteries may cause high blood pressure or a worsening of previously controlled high blood pressure. Blood pressure may remain high despite treatment with multiple antihypertensive drugs. In people who are given an angiotensin-converting enzyme (ACE) inhibitor, an angiotensin II receptor blocker, or a renin inhibitor to treat high blood pressure, kidney function may decline rapidly. The effect is reversible if the drug is stopped promptly.

Causes

Blockage of the renal artery or one of its large or medium-sized branches is unusual. Most often such blockages occur when a clot moves through the bloodstream from elsewhere in the body (becoming an embolus) and lodges in the renal artery. Typically, such clots originate as fragments from a larger clot in the heart or from the breakup of a fatty deposit (atheroma) in the aorta.

Alternatively, a blockage may result when a blood clot forms in the renal artery itself, usually where the artery has been injured. A sudden injury may be caused by a medical procedure, such as surgery, angiography, or angioplasty. A clot may also develop where the renal artery has been gradually injured or damaged by atherosclerosis, arteritis (inflammation of arteries), or an aneurysm (a slow-forming bulge in the wall of the artery).

A tear in the lining of the aorta or the renal artery can cause a sudden obstruction of blood flow. A tear may also cause the artery to rupture. Diseases that cause the walls of arteries to become thicker and less elastic because of deposits of fatty material (atherosclerosis) or the development of fibrous material (fibromuscular dysplasia) may predispose vessels to tears. These disorders can lead to significant narrowing and partial blockage of the renal arteries even when there is no blood clot. When narrowing or blockage occurs but no blood clot exists, the condition is called renal artery stenosis.

Symptoms

A partial blockage of the renal arteries usually does not cause any symptoms. If blockage is sudden and complete, the person may have a steady aching pain in the lower back or occasionally in the lower abdomen. A complete blockage may cause fever, nausea, vomiting, and back pain. Rarely, a blockage causes bleeding that turns the urine red or dark brown. Complete blockage of both renal arteries—or of one renal artery in people who have only one kidney—completely stops urine production and shuts down the kidneys (a condition called acute kidney failure).

If a blockage is the result of a clot that has moved to and lodged in one of the renal artery branches, the person may have clots elsewhere in the body, such as in the intestine, brain, and the skin of the fingers and toes. These clots may cause pain in these areas as well as small ulcers or gangrene or a small stroke.

Diagnosis

Doctors may suspect a blockage because of the symptoms. Laboratory tests, such as a complete blood count and urinalysis (microscopic examination of the urine), may add further clues.

Because none of the symptoms or laboratory tests can specifically identify a blockage, doctors need to perform imaging tests of the kidneys to show that they are not functioning properly. Computed tomography (CT) angiography, magnetic resonance (MR) angiography, Doppler ultrasonography, and an isotope perfusion scan can show absent or diminished blood flow to the affected kidney. All of these tests have advantages and disadvantages. For example, CT angiography and MR angiography are very accurate. However, CT angiography involves using an intravenous radiopaque dye (contrast agent), which increases the risk of kidney damage in people with decreased kidney function. MR angiography involves use of an intravenous contrast agent (gadolinium), which increases the risk of nephrogenic systemic fibrosis in people with de-

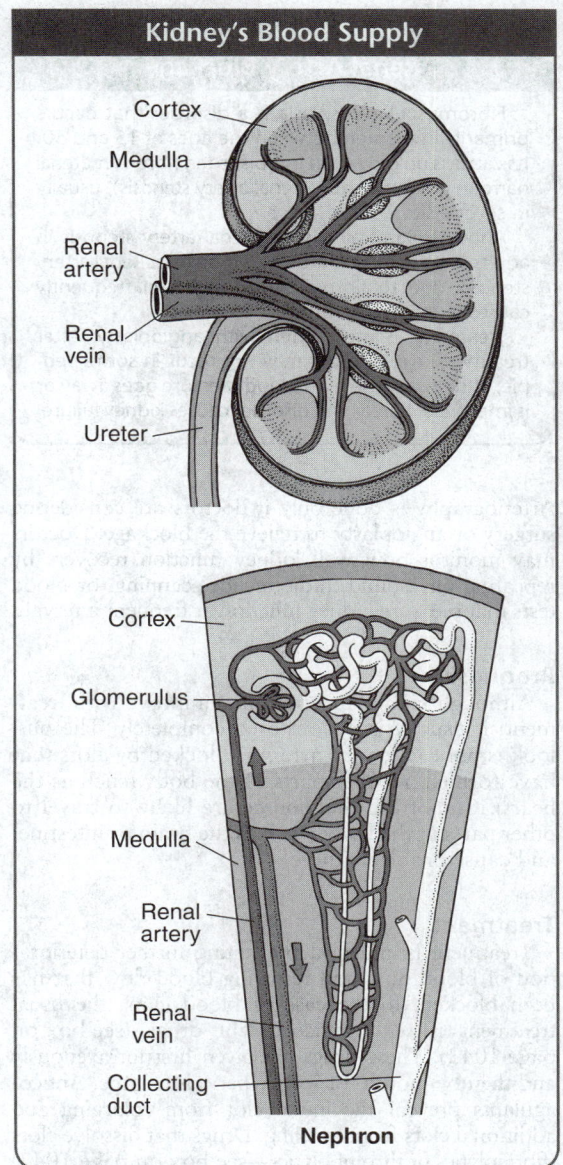

Kidney's Blood Supply

Cortex
Medulla
Renal artery
Renal vein
Ureter

Cortex
Glomerulus
Medulla
Renal artery
Renal vein
Collecting duct

Nephron

creased kidney function. Nephrogenic systemic fibrosis causes scar tissue to form throughout the body and is not easily reversed or cured.

Arteriography is the most accurate test doctors can use to confirm the diagnosis. With arteriography, a catheter is inserted into an artery, which occasionally causes injury to the artery. In addition, as with CT angiography, arteriography involves use of a radiopaque dye that increases risk of kidney damage.

Fibromuscular Dysplasia: A Cause of Renal Artery Blockage

Fibromuscular dysplasia is a disorder that occurs primarily in women between the ages of 15 and 50. Its cause is unknown. In this disorder, fibrous material narrows the renal artery (renal artery stenosis), usually in several sites.

About 10% of all cases of renal artery stenosis in adults are due to fibromuscular dysplasia. Renal artery stenosis due to fibromuscular dysplasia frequently causes high blood pressure.

Treatment is most often with angioplasty. After treatment, the disorder may not recur in some people, and usually the high blood pressure goes away or is improved. Rarely, this disorder causes kidney failure.

Arteriography is done only if doctors are considering surgery or angioplasty to relieve the blockage. Doctors may monitor how well kidney function recovers by repeating ultrasound, radionuclide scanning, or blood tests that measure kidney function at frequent intervals.

Prognosis

Although kidney function may improve with treatment, it usually is not restored completely. The outlook is poor when the artery is blocked by clots that have formed in other parts of the body (such as the heart). Clots from that source are likely to travel to other parts of the body (such as the brain or intestine) and cause problems there.

Treatment

Treatment is aimed at preventing further deterioration of blood flow and restoring blood flow that has been blocked. In the case of blood clots, the usual treatment is with anticoagulant drugs (see box on page 1043). These drugs are given first intravenously and then by mouth for longer periods of time. Anticoagulants prevent the initial clot from enlarging and additional clots from forming. Drugs that dissolve clots (fibrinolytics or thrombolytics—see box on page 1043) may be more effective than anticoagulants. However, fibrinolytic drugs improve kidney function only when the artery is not completely blocked or when clots can be dissolved quickly. After 30 to 60 minutes of complete blockage, permanent damage is likely. However, fibrinolytic drugs can be helpful only if given within 3 hours.

Surgery is sometimes done to open an artery blocked by a clot, but this treatment has a greater risk of complications and death and does not improve kidney function more than anticoagulant or fibrinolytic drugs

alone. Drug treatment is almost always preferred to surgery. However, when the cause is injury, the artery must be surgically repaired.

To relieve a blockage caused by atherosclerosis or fibromuscular dysplasia of a renal artery, doctors may thread a balloon catheter from the femoral artery in the groin to the renal artery. The balloon is then inflated to force open the obstructed area. This procedure is called percutaneous transluminal angioplasty. When doctors perform this procedure, they may place a short hollow tube (stent) in the artery to prevent the blockage from occurring again. When angioplasty is unsuccessful, surgery may be considered to remove or bypass a blockage caused by atherosclerosis or fibromuscular dysplasia.

Atheroembolic Kidney Disease

In atheroembolic kidney disease, numerous small pieces of fatty material (atheroemboli) travel from arteries above the kidneys to clog the smallest branches of the renal arteries, causing the kidneys to fail.

- Usually atheroemboli occur as a complication of surgery or a procedure on an atherosclerotic aorta.
- Symptoms of kidney failure, blue toes, or a lacy purplish discoloration of the skin of the feet and legs may develop.
- Removing and analyzing a piece of kidney tissue (biopsy) may be done to confirm the diagnosis.

Tiny pieces of hard fatty material adhering to a hardened (atherosclerotic) blood vessel wall, usually the aorta, break off and travel through the bloodstream, becoming emboli (atheroemboli). Some emboli travel to the smallest renal arteries, blocking parts of the kidney's blood supply. Usually, this process affects both kidneys about equally and at the same time.

The fatty material may break off spontaneously when there is severe atherosclerosis of the aorta. It more commonly occurs as a complication of surgery or angioplasty or of imaging procedures that involve the aorta, such as arteriography, when pieces of fatty material adhering to the walls of the aorta are unintentionally broken off. Atheroembolic kidney disease is much more common in older people.

Symptoms

Atheroembolic kidney disease usually causes acute or slowly progressive failure of the kidneys. If the blockage of arteries results from a surgical or imaging procedure involving the aorta, the kidneys often fail suddenly. Urine production is often decreased.

As the duration and severity of kidney failure increase, various symptoms may appear, beginning with fatigue, nausea, loss of appetite, itching, and difficulty concentrating. The symptoms reflect disturbances in the muscles, brain and nerves, heart, digestive tract, and skin that result from kidney failure.

Atheroemboli may cause symptoms in other organs. If atheroemboli travel to the arms or legs, such symptoms as blue toes or a lacy purplish discoloration of the skin and even gangrene may result. Pieces of atheroemboli that travel to an eye may cause sudden blindness.

Diagnosis

An imaging test may be done to exclude the possibility of renal artery blockage, which can sometimes cause similar symptoms. A kidney biopsy is the best way for doctors to make the diagnosis of atheroembolic kidney disease. A tissue sample examined with a microscope shows characteristic evidence of fatty material in the smallest arteries. Examination of skin or muscle specimens may also help to establish the diagnosis.

Prognosis and Treatment

In the past, people with atheroembolic kidney disease tended to die within weeks or months. However, more recently, treatment has improved. Most people live at least a year. About half live 4 years or more.

The treatment is to support the person as well as possible. For example, high blood pressure is treated. Dialysis may be needed during kidney failure, but sometimes the kidneys eventually resume functioning.

Renal Cortical Necrosis

Renal (kidney) cortical necrosis is death of the tissue in the outer part of kidney (cortex) that results from blockage of the small arteries that supply blood to the cortex and that causes acute kidney failure.

- Usually the cause is a major, catastrophic disorder that decreases blood pressure.
- Symptoms may include dark urine, decreased urine volume, fever, and pain in the side of the body.
- Sometimes an imaging test or tissue analysis (biopsy) is done to confirm the diagnosis.

Renal cortical necrosis can occur at any age. About 10% of the cases occur in infants and children. More than half of the newborns with this condition had deliveries complicated by premature detachment of the placenta. The next most common cause is a bacterial infection of the bloodstream (sepsis). In children, renal cortical necrosis may occur after severe infection, severe dehydration, shock, or the hemolytic-uremic syndrome (see page 1042).

In adults, sepsis causes one third of all cases of renal cortical necrosis. Other causes in adults include rejection of a transplanted kidney, burns, inflammation of the pancreas, injury, snakebite, use of certain drugs, and poisoning caused by certain chemicals.

About half of the cases in women occur after complications of pregnancy, such as premature detachment of or abnormal position of the placenta, bleeding from the uterus, infections immediately after childbirth, blockage of arteries by amniotic fluid, death of the fetus within the uterus, and preeclampsia.

Symptoms

The urine often becomes red or dark brown because of the presence of blood. Pain along both sides of the lower back may occur. A fever is often present. Changes in blood pressure, including mildly high pressure or even low pressure, are common. Urine flow may slow or stop.

Diagnosis

Doctors may have difficulty making a diagnosis of renal cortical necrosis because it may resemble other types of acute kidney failure. Doctors may suspect renal cortical necrosis based on symptoms in people who have predisposing conditions. The diagnosis is often confirmed with an imaging test such as computed tomography (CT) angiography. Kidney biopsy can give doctors the most accurate diagnostic information, but a biopsy involves removing kidney tissue and may be unnecessary if the diagnosis is evident. Thus, a biopsy is not done in most people.

Blood tests may reveal abnormally shaped red blood cells circulating in the blood. The small amount of urine that is produced contains protein and many white and red blood cells, along with kidney cells and other debris.

Prognosis and Treatment

In recent years, with improved treatment, prognosis has improved. About 80% of people live a year or longer, although most people need permanent dialysis or kidney transplantation.

Treatment is supportive care, which may involve giving intravenous fluids, blood transfusion, antibiotics, dialysis, or a combination.

Malignant Hypertensive Nephrosclerosis

In malignant hypertensive nephrosclerosis, severe high blood pressure (malignant hypertension) damages the smallest arteries in the kidneys, and kidney failure progresses rapidly.

- Severe high blood pressure can rapidly damage organs, including the kidneys.
- Headache, restlessness, blurred vision, confusion, nausea, and sleepiness may develop.

- Diagnosis is usually based on symptoms and the results of routine blood and urine tests.
- Blood pressure is lowered rapidly, and dialysis may be necessary.

Malignant hypertensive nephrosclerosis occurs in about 1 out of 200 people with high blood pressure and is more common among blacks than whites. It is most common in men during their 40s and 50s and women during their 30s.

High blood pressure (hypertension) causes damage to body organs. However, usually the damage takes months or years to develop. In malignant hypertension, organ damage develops over hours or days. Because hypertension causes damage so rapidly, it is described as malignant, but in this case, malignant does not mean cancerous. Malignant hypertension most commonly results from poorly controlled high blood pressure. It may also result from other conditions, such as glomerulonephritis, chronic kidney failure, narrowing of the renal artery causing renovascular hypertension, inflammation of renal blood vessels (vasculitis), or, rarely, hormonal disorders such as pheochromocytoma, primary aldosteronism, or Cushing's syndrome.

Symptoms

Symptoms initially are caused by the effects of the severe high blood pressure on the brain, eye, and heart. Some symptoms, which may include restlessness, blurred vision, headache, nausea, vomiting, sleepiness, and confusion, result from swelling of brain and eye tissue. Seizures and coma may also occur if swelling is severe or if there is bleeding within the brain. Heart failure may cause difficulty breathing. Damage to the kidneys eventually causes the symptoms of kidney failure, such as fatigue, weakness, and itching.

Diagnosis

Malignant hypertensive nephrosclerosis is likely in people who have malignant hypertension and symptoms of kidney failure or laboratory evidence of kidney failure. By viewing the back of the eye with an ophthalmoscope, doctors can see areas of bleeding, collections of fluid, and swelling of the optic nerve. Doctors may also detect heart enlargement and heart strain or failure. These findings in the eye and heart indicate malignant hypertension.

Blood tests show elevated levels of creatinine and urea nitrogen, indicating kidney failure. Protein leaking from the kidneys can be detected in the urine, along with blood cells. Anemia often results from the breakdown and impaired production of red blood cells. Widespread clotting within the blood vessels is also common (disseminated intravascular coagulation—

see page 1046). Blood levels of substances produced by the kidneys that help regulate blood pressure (renin and aldosterone) are extremely high.

Prognosis

If malignant nephrosclerosis is not treated, 40 to 80% of people die within one year. However, with the best medical care, including rigorous control of high blood pressure with diet and drugs and treatment of the kidney failure, average survival can be up to 12 years. People who have less severe kidney failure improve the most with treatment.

Treatment

Treatment includes aggressive lowering of blood pressure with drugs. Lifestyle changes (for example, diet and exercise) also help lower blood pressure but rarely enough without drugs. Treating the kidney failure is also essential. Occasionally, people improve enough that dialysis can be stopped.

Renal Vein Thrombosis

Renal vein thrombosis is blockage of the renal vein, which carries blood away from the kidney, by a blood clot.

- The clot can damage the kidney or can break off, causing a piece of it to travel through the bloodstream (becoming an embolus).
- Symptoms may be minimal unless the clot develops suddenly.
- Diagnosis is with computed tomography angiography or magnetic resonance angiography.
- Treatment includes anticoagulant drugs and sometimes clot-dissolving (fibrinolytic) drugs.

In adults, renal vein thrombosis usually occurs with other kidney disorders that cause nephrotic syndrome, in which large amounts of protein are lost in the urine. Renal vein thrombosis may also be caused by kidney cancer or conditions that put pressure on the renal vein (for example, a tumor) or on the inferior vena cava, which the renal vein drains into. Other possible causes are blood clotting disorders (hypercoagulability disorders), vasculitis, sickle cell disease or diabetes that affects the kidney, oral contraceptive use, injury, cocaine abuse, or, rarely, thrombophlebitis migrans—a condition in which clotting occurs sequentially in different veins all over the body.

Symptoms

Renal vein thrombosis occurs most often in adults. In adults, onset and progression are usually gradual and without symptoms. An occasional clue to doctors is when a piece of clot breaks off and travels from the renal vein to the lungs (pulmonary embolism—see page 488). This event causes sudden pain in the chest that is made worse by breathing, along with shortness of breath. In other people, urine production diminishes.

In most children and a limited number of adults, onset and progression are usually sudden. Pain, often the first symptom, typically occurs in the back behind the lower ribs and in the hips. The person may have fever, less than a normal amount of urine, and blood in the urine.

Diagnosis

Blood tests may indicate evidence of kidney failure.

Computed tomography (CT) angiography and magnetic resonance (MR) angiography are the tests doctors use to diagnose renal vein thrombosis. They are highly accurate and do not require insertion of a catheter into an artery or a vein deep in the body, so they are usually the preferred tests. Ultrasonography is not as accurate, but it is very safe. An ultrasound scan shows enlarged kidneys if the blockage developed suddenly. Doppler ultrasonography may show that there is no blood flowing in the kidney vein. X-rays of the inferior vena cava or the renal vein that are taken after a radiopaque dye is injected into an artery or deep vein (venography) is the most accurate test but may cause clots to break off and travel through the bloodstream, becoming emboli, which can cause complications.

Prognosis

The outcome depends on the cause of the thrombosis, complications, and the degree of kidney damage. Death from renal vein thrombosis is rare and usually results from a fatal underlying disorder or from complications, such as a pulmonary embolism. The effects on kidney function depend on whether one or both kidneys are affected, whether blood flow is restored, and what the state of kidney function was before the blockage occurred.

Treatment

The primary treatment is with anticoagulant drugs, which usually improve kidney function by preventing the formation of additional clots and reducing the risk of pulmonary embolism. Use of drugs that dissolve clots (fibrinolytics) is a newer treatment that is becoming more widespread but is still not routine. Rarely, surgery is done to remove clots in the renal vein. A kidney is rarely removed and then only if other complications, such as high blood pressure, develop.

CHAPTER

46 Tubular and Cystic Kidney Disorders

The kidneys filter and cleanse the blood. They also maintain the body's balance of water, dissolved salts (electrolytes, such as sodium, potassium, and calcium), and nutrients in the blood. The kidneys begin these tasks by filtering the blood as it flows through microscopic tufts of blood vessels with small pores (glomeruli). This process moves a large amount of water and electrolytes and other substances into small tubules. The cells lining these tubules reabsorb and return needed water, electrolytes, and nutrients (such as glucose and amino acids) to the blood. The cells also move waste products and drugs from the blood into the fluid (which becomes urine) as it flows through the tubules as well as add hormones that maintain blood supply (erythropoietin), blood pressure, and electrolyte balance.

Disorders that interfere with the function of the cells lining the tubules are called tubular disorders. Some conditions, called cystic disorders, interfere with these tubular cell functions by causing fluid-filled sacs (cysts) to form and replace or compress normal tubules.

Many of these tubular and cystic disorders are hereditary. Of the hereditary disorders, some are detected at birth, and others are not obvious until years later.

Renal Tubular Acidosis

In renal tubular acidosis, the kidney tubules cannot adequately remove acids from the blood to excrete them in the urine.

- The tubules of the kidneys that remove acid from the blood are damaged when a person takes certain drugs or has another disorder that affects the kidneys.
- Typically muscle weakness and diminished reflexes occur when the disorder has been present for a long time.
- Blood tests are done to detect high acid levels.
- Some people drink a solution of baking soda every day to neutralize the acid.

Normally, the breakdown of food produces acids that circulate in the blood. The kidneys remove acids from the blood and excrete them in the urine.

SOME TYPES OF RENAL TUBULAR ACIDOSIS

TYPE	CAUSE	UNDERLYING ABNORMALITY	RESULTING SYMPTOMS AND METABOLIC ABNORMALITIES
1	May be hereditary or may be triggered by an autoimmune disease or certain drugs Cause usually not known, especially in women	Inability to excrete acid into the urine	High blood acidity Mild dehydration Low potassium levels in the blood, leading to muscle weakness and paralysis Fragile bones Bone pain Calcium deposits, leading to kidney stones Kidney failure
2	Usually caused by a hereditary disease such as Fanconi syndrome, hereditary fructose intolerance, Wilson's disease, or oculocerebrorenal syndrome (Lowe syndrome) May also be caused by heavy metal poisoning or certain drugs	Inability to reabsorb bicarbonate from the urine, so too much bicarbonate is excreted	High blood acidity Mild dehydration Low potassium levels in the blood
4	Not hereditary Caused by diabetes, an autoimmune disease, sickle cell disease, or an obstruction in the urinary tract Worsened by certain drugs, including potassium-sparing diuretics, angiotensin-converting enzyme inhibitors, and angiotensin II receptor blockers	Deficiency of or inability to respond to aldosterone, a hormone that helps regulate potassium and sodium excretion by the kidneys	High blood acidity and high potassium levels in the blood that rarely cause symptoms, unless the potassium level is unusually high (in that case, irregular heartbeats and muscle paralysis develop)

Note: Type 3 is a mixture of Types 1 and 2 and is extremely rare.

This function is predominantly performed by the kidney tubules. In renal tubular acidosis, the ability of the kidneys to excrete acids is partially impaired, and acid levels build up in the blood (metabolic acidosis). The balance of electrolytes is also affected. Renal tubular acidosis may lead to the following problems:

- Low or high potassium levels in the blood
- Calcium deposits in the kidneys, which may lead to kidney stones
- Dehydration
- Painful softening and bending of the bones (osteomalacia or rickets)

Renal tubular acidosis may be a permanent, inherited disorder. However, it may be an intermittent problem in people who have other disorders, such as diabetes mellitus, sickle cell disease, or an autoimmune disorder (such as systemic lupus erythematosus). Renal tubular acidosis may also be a temporary condition brought on by an obstruction of the urinary tract or by drugs, such as acetazolamide, amphotericin B, angiotensin-converting enzyme (ACE) inhibitors, angiotensin receptor blockers (ARBs), and diuretics that conserve the body's potassium (so-called potassium-sparing diuretics).

There are four types of renal tubular acidosis, types 1 through 4. The types are distinguished by the particular abnormality in kidney function that causes acidosis. All four types are uncommon, but type 3 is extremely rare.

Symptoms and Diagnosis

Many people have no symptoms. Most others develop symptoms only after the disorder has been present for a long time. Which symptoms eventually develop depend on the type of renal tubular acidosis. When potassium levels in the blood are low, as occurs in types 1 and 2, neurologic problems may develop, including muscle weakness, diminished reflexes, and even paralysis. In type 4, potassium levels typically increase, although it is uncommon for the level to rise high enough to cause symptoms. If the level becomes too high, irregular heartbeats and muscle paralysis may develop. In type 1, kidney stones may develop, causing damage to kidney cells and, in some cases, chronic kidney failure.

A doctor considers the diagnosis of type 1 or type 2 renal tubular acidosis when a person has certain characteristic symptoms (such as muscle weakness and diminished reflexes) and when tests reveal high levels of acid and low levels of bicarbonate and potassium in the blood. Type 4 renal tubular acidosis is usually suspected when high potassium levels accompany high acid levels and low bicarbonate levels in the blood. Special tests help to determine the type of renal tubular acidosis.

Treatment

Treatment depends on the type. Types 1 and 2 are treated by drinking a solution of sodium bicarbonate (baking soda) every day to neutralize the acid that is produced from food. This treatment relieves the symptoms and prevents kidney failure and bone disease or keeps these problems from becoming worse. Other specially prepared solutions are available, and potassium supplements may also be required. In type 4, the acidosis is so mild that bicarbonate may not be needed. High potassium levels in the blood can usually be kept in check by restricting potassium intake, avoiding dehydration, and substituting different drugs or adjusting drug dosages.

Renal Glucosuria

In renal glucosuria (glycosuria), glucose (sugar) is excreted in the urine, despite normal or low glucose levels in the blood.

Normally, the body excretes glucose in the urine only when glucose levels in the blood are very high. In most healthy people, glucose that is filtered from the blood by the kidneys is completely reabsorbed back into the blood. In people with renal glucosuria, glucose may be excreted in the urine despite normal or low levels of glucose in the blood. This happens because of a defect in the tubular cells that decreases the reabsorption of glucose. Renal glucosuria may be a hereditary condition.

Renal glucosuria has no symptoms or serious consequences. A doctor makes the diagnosis when a routine urine test detects glucose in the urine even though glucose levels in the blood are normal. In a small number of people, renal glucosuria may be an early sign of diabetes mellitus. No treatment is needed.

Nephrogenic Diabetes Insipidus

In nephrogenic diabetes insipidus, the kidneys produce a large volume of dilute urine because they fail to respond to antidiuretic hormone and are unable to concentrate urine.

- Often this disorder is hereditary, but it can be caused by drugs or disorders that affect the kidneys.
- Symptoms include excessive thirst and excretion of large amounts of urine.

- Diagnosis is based on tests of blood and urine.
- Drinking large amounts of water, restricting salt in the diet, and sometimes taking drugs reduce urine volume.

Both diabetes insipidus and the better-known type of diabetes, diabetes mellitus, result in the excretion of large volumes of urine. Otherwise, the two types of diabetes are very different.

Two types of diabetes insipidus exist. In nephrogenic diabetes insipidus, the kidneys do not respond to antidiuretic hormone (vasopressin), so they continue to excrete a large amount of dilute urine. In the other, more common, type (central diabetes insipidus), the pituitary gland fails to secrete antidiuretic hormone (see page 986).

> **? Did You Know...**
>
> Nephrogenic diabetes insipidus and diabetes mellitus are very different, except that both cause people to excrete large amounts of urine.

Causes

Normally, the kidneys adjust the concentration of urine according to the body's needs. The kidneys make this adjustment in response to the level of antidiuretic hormone in the blood. Antidiuretic hormone, which is secreted by the pituitary gland, signals the kidneys to conserve water and concentrate the urine. In nephrogenic diabetes insipidus, the kidneys fail to respond to the signal.

Nephrogenic diabetes insipidus may be hereditary. The gene that causes the disorder is recessive and carried on the X chromosome, one of the two sex chromosomes, so usually only males develop symptoms. However, females who carry the gene can transmit the disease to their sons. In other people, nephrogenic diabetes insipidus may be caused by certain drugs that block the action of antidiuretic hormone, such as lithium. Also, high levels of calcium or low levels of potassium in the blood partially block the action of antidiuretic hormone. Nephrogenic diabetes insipidus can also occur if the kidney is affected by disorders such as polycystic kidney disease, sickle cell anemia, medullary sponge kidney, infections (pyelonephritis) that are severe, amyloidosis, Sjögren's syndrome, or myeloma.

Symptoms and Diagnosis

The symptoms of nephrogenic diabetes insipidus are excessive thirst (polydipsia) and the excretion of large volumes of dilute urine (polyuria). When nephrogenic diabetes insipidus is hereditary, symptoms usually start soon after birth. Because infants cannot communicate thirst, they may become very dehydrated. They may develop a fever accompanied by vomiting and seizures.

If hereditary nephrogenic diabetes insipidus is not quickly diagnosed and treated, the brain may be damaged, leaving the infant with permanent mental retardation. Frequent episodes of dehydration can also retard physical development. With treatment, however, an infant who has this disorder is likely to develop normally.

Laboratory tests reveal high sodium levels in the blood and very dilute urine. A doctor may use a water deprivation test to help make the diagnosis (see page 987).

Prognosis and Treatment

The prognosis is good if nephrogenic diabetes insipidus is diagnosed before the person suffers severe episodes of dehydration. In cases in which the disorder is not inherited, correction of the underlying abnormality usually helps kidney function return to normal.

To prevent dehydration, people with nephrogenic diabetes insipidus must drink adequate amounts of water as soon as they feel thirsty. Infants, young children, and very sick older people must be given water often. People who drink enough water are not likely to become dehydrated, but several hours without water can lead to serious dehydration. A diet low in salt may help. Nonsteroidal anti-inflammatory drugs (NSAIDs) and thiazide diuretics are sometimes used to treat this disorder. NSAIDs and thiazide diuretics act by different mechanisms to increase the amounts of sodium and water that are reabsorbed by the kidney. These changes decrease the volume of urine.

Cystinuria

Cystinuria is a rare disorder that results in excretion of the amino acid cystine into the urine, often causing cystine stones to form in the urinary tract.

Cystinuria is caused by an inherited defect of the kidney tubules. The gene that causes cystinuria is recessive, so people with the disorder must have inherited two abnormal genes, one from each parent (see art on page 13). People who carry the gene but do not have the disorder have one normal and one abnormal gene. These people may excrete larger than normal amounts of cystine into the urine, but seldom enough to form cystine stones.

Cystine stones form in the bladder, renal pelvis (the area where urine collects and flows out of the kidney), or ureters (the long, narrow tubes that carry urine from the kidneys to the bladder). Occasionally, kidney failure develops.

Symptoms and Diagnosis

Symptoms usually start between the ages of 10 and 30. Often, the first symptom is intense pain caused by a spasm of the ureter where a stone becomes lodged. The stone may also become a site where bacteria collect and cause a serious infection.

A doctor tests for cystinuria when a person has recurring kidney stones. Cystine crystals may be seen during a microscopic examination of the urine (urinalysis), and high cystine levels are found in the urine.

Treatment

Treatment consists of preventing cystine stones from forming by keeping the concentration of cystine in the urine low. To keep the cystine concentration low, a person must drink enough fluids to produce at least 8 pints (4 liters) of urine each day. During the night, however, when the person is not drinking, less urine is produced and stone formation is more likely. This risk is reduced by drinking fluids before going to bed. Another treatment approach involves taking potassium citrate or sodium bicarbonate to make the urine more alkaline, because cystine dissolves more easily in alkaline urine than in acidic urine. Efforts to increase intake of water and make the urine more alkaline can lead to abdominal bloating, making the treatment difficult for some people to tolerate.

If stones continue to form despite these measures, drugs such as penicillamine, tiopronin, or captopril may be tried. These drugs react with cystine to keep it dissolved. Captopril is slightly less effective than the other drugs, but it has fewer serious side effects. Although the treatments are usually effective, there is a fairly high risk that stones will continue to form.

Fanconi Syndrome

Fanconi syndrome is a rare disorder of tubule function that results in excess amounts of glucose, bicarbonate, phosphates (phosphorus salts), uric acid, potassium, sodium, and certain amino acids being excreted in the urine.

Fanconi syndrome may be hereditary or may be caused by exposure to heavy metals or other chemical agents, vitamin D deficiency, kidney transplantation, multiple myeloma, or amyloidosis. Fanconi syndrome usually occurs with another hereditary disorder, such as cystinuria.

Symptoms and Diagnosis

In hereditary Fanconi syndrome, symptoms usually begin during infancy. A child with Fanconi syndrome may excrete a large amount of urine. Other symptoms include weakness and bone pain.

The symptoms and a test that shows a high level of acid in the blood may lead a doctor to suspect Fanconi syndrome. The diagnosis is confirmed when high levels of glucose, bicarbonate, phosphates, uric acid, potassium, and sodium are detected in the urine. Most often, some damage to bones or kidney tissue has occurred before the diagnosis is made.

Treatment

Fanconi syndrome cannot be cured, but it can be controlled with proper treatment. Effective treatment can keep the damage to bones and kidney tissue from getting worse and in some cases correct it. The high acid level of the blood (acidosis) may be neutralized by drinking sodium bicarbonate. People with low potassium levels in the blood may need to take potassium supplements by mouth. Bone disease requires treatment with phosphates and vitamin D supplements given by mouth. Kidney transplantation may be lifesaving if a child with the disorder develops kidney failure.

Hypophosphatemic Rickets

Hypophosphatemic rickets (previously called vitamin D–resistant rickets) is a disorder in which the bones become painfully soft and bend easily because the blood contains low levels of phosphate.

This very rare disorder is nearly always hereditary, passed as a dominant gene that is carried on the X chromosome, one of the two sex chromosomes. The genetic defect causes a kidney abnormality that allows an inappropriately high amount of phosphate to be excreted into the urine, resulting in low levels of phosphate in the blood. Because bones need phosphate for growth and strength, this deficiency causes defective bones. Females with hypophosphatemic rickets have less severe bone disease than do males. In rare cases, the disorder develops as a result of certain cancers, such as giant cell tumors of bone, sarcomas, prostate cancer, and breast cancer. Hypophosphatemic rickets is not the same as rickets caused by vitamin D deficiency (see page 929).

Symptoms and Diagnosis

Hypophosphatemic rickets usually begins to cause abnormalities in the first year of life. Abnormalities may be so mild that they cause no noticeable symptoms or so severe that they cause bowing of the legs and other bone deformities, bone pain, and a short stature. Bony outgrowth where muscles attach to bones may limit movement at those joints. The space between a baby's skull bones may close too soon, leading to seizures. Laboratory tests show that calcium levels in the blood are normal but phosphate levels are low.

Treatment

The aim of treatment is to raise phosphate levels in the blood, which promotes normal bone formation. Phosphate can be taken by mouth and should be combined with calcitriol, the activated form of vitamin D. Taking vitamin D alone is not sufficient. The amounts of phosphate and calcitriol must be adjusted carefully because this treatment often leads to high levels of calcium in the blood, the accumulation of calcium in kidney tissue, or kidney stones. These effects can harm the kidneys and other tissues. In some adults, hypophosphatemic rickets resulting from cancer improves dramatically after the cancer is removed.

Hartnup Disease

Hartnup disease is a rare hereditary disorder that results in a skin rash and brain abnormalities because tryptophan and certain other amino acids are not well absorbed from the intestine and not well reabsorbed by the kidneys.

Hartnup disease occurs when a person inherits two copies of the abnormal gene for the disorder, one from each parent. The defective gene controls the absorption of certain amino acids from the intestine and the reabsorption of those amino acids in the kidneys. Consequently, a person with Hartnup disease cannot absorb amino acids properly from the intestine and cannot reabsorb them properly from tubules in the kidneys. Excessive amounts of amino acids, such as tryptophan, are excreted in the urine. The body is thus left with inadequate amounts of amino acids, which are the building blocks of protein. With too little tryptophan in the blood, the body is unable to make a sufficient amount of the B-complex vitamin niacinamide, particularly under stress when more vitamins are needed.

Symptoms

Hartnup disease is a disorder of amino acid transport in the intestine and kidneys; otherwise, the intestine and kidneys function normally, and the effects of the disease occur mainly in the brain and skin. Symptoms may begin in infancy or early childhood, but sometimes they begin as late as early adulthood. Symptoms may be triggered by sunlight, fever, drugs, or emotional or physical stress. A period of poor nutrition nearly always precedes an attack. The attacks usually become progressively less frequent with age. Most symptoms occur sporadically and are caused by a deficiency of niacinamide. A rash develops on parts of the body exposed to the sun. Mental retardation, short stature, headaches, an unsteady gait, and collapsing or fainting are common. Psychologic problems (such as anxiety, rapid mood changes, delusions, and hallucinations) may also result.

Diagnosis and Treatment

Laboratory tests performed on urine samples reveal abnormally high excretion of amino acids and their breakdown products.

People with Hartnup disease can prevent attacks by maintaining good nutrition and supplementing their diet with niacinamide or niacin, a B-complex vitamin very similar to niacinamide. A diet that is adequate in protein can overcome the deficiency caused by poor intestinal absorption and excess excretion of amino acids into the urine.

Bartter Syndrome

In Bartter syndrome, the kidneys excrete excessive amounts of electrolytes (potassium, sodium, and chloride), resulting in electrolyte abnormalities in the blood.

Bartter syndrome is usually hereditary and is caused by a recessive gene. Thus, a person with the disorder has inherited two recessive genes for the disorder, one from each parent. In affected people, the kidneys excrete excessive amounts of sodium, chloride, and potassium. The loss of sodium and chloride leads to excessive urine production and thus mild dehydration, which causes the body to produce more renin and aldosterone. The increase in aldosterone increases potassium and acid secretion in the kidneys, leading to low blood potassium (hypokalemia) and loss of acids in the blood that causes blood pH to be alkaline (metabolic alkalosis—see page 974).

Symptoms and Diagnosis

Children with Bartter syndrome grow slowly and appear malnourished. They may have muscle weakness and excessive thirst, may produce large amounts of urine, and may be mentally retarded. The loss of sodium and chloride leads to chronic mild dehydration. Abnormally low blood pressure (hypotension) may occur.

The diagnosis of Bartter syndrome in young children is based on a physical examination and on the characteristic abnormalities of electrolytes in blood and urine. Abnormal results are confirmed by finding high levels of certain hormones (renin, aldosterone) on blood tests. However, similar findings may occur when children with certain eating disorders, such as bulimia nervosa, self-induce vomiting and misuse diuretics.

Treatment

Many of the consequences of Bartter syndrome can be prevented by taking potassium supplements and a drug that reduces excretion of potassium into the urine, such as spironolactone (which also blocks the action of aldosterone), triamterene, amiloride, angiotensin-converting enzyme (ACE) inhibitors, or nonsteroidal anti-inflammatory drugs (NSAIDs), such as indomethacin. Drinking adequate amounts of fluids is necessary to compensate for the excessive fluid losses.

Liddle Syndrome

Liddle syndrome is a rare hereditary disorder in which the kidneys excrete potassium but retain too much sodium and water, leading to high blood pressure.

The gene that causes Liddle syndrome is dominant, meaning that children of a person with the disorder have a 50% chance of inheriting the defective gene. The disorder does not always cause symptoms. When it does, symptoms such as high blood pressure often begin during childhood. Some people have low levels of potassium in the blood.

The condition is effectively treated by drugs that increase sodium excretion and lessen potassium excretion, such as triamterene or amiloride. These drugs effectively lower the blood pressure. The prognosis is very good.

Polycystic Kidney Disease

Polycystic kidney disease is a hereditary disorder in which many fluid-filled sacs (cysts) form in both kidneys. The kidneys grow larger but have less functioning tissue.

- Polycystic kidney disease is caused by an inherited gene defect.
- Some people have such mild symptoms that they do not realize they have a disorder, but others have pain in the side, blood in the urine, and crampy pain caused by kidney stones.
- Diagnosis is based on laboratory tests of kidney function and ultrasonography or computed tomography scans of the kidneys.
- The kidney stones and infections are treated, but more than half of affected people eventually need dialysis or kidney transplantation.

There are several genetic defects that causes polycystic kidney disease. Several types are caused by dominant genes, and one rare type is caused by a recessive gene. That is, a person with the disease has inherited either one copy of a dominant gene from one parent or two copies of a recessive gene, one from each parent. People with dominant gene inheritance usually have no symptoms until adulthood. Those with recessive gene inheritance develop severe illness in childhood.

The genetic defect leads to the widespread formation of cysts in the kidneys. Gradual enlargement of the cysts with increasing age is accompanied by a reduction of blood flow and scarring within the kidneys. Kidney stones may develop. Kidney failure can occur eventually. The genetic defect may also cause cysts to develop in other parts of the body, such as the liver and pancreas.

Polycystic Kidney Disease

In polycystic kidney disease, many cysts form in both kidneys. The cysts gradually enlarge, destroying some or most of the normal tissue in the kidneys.

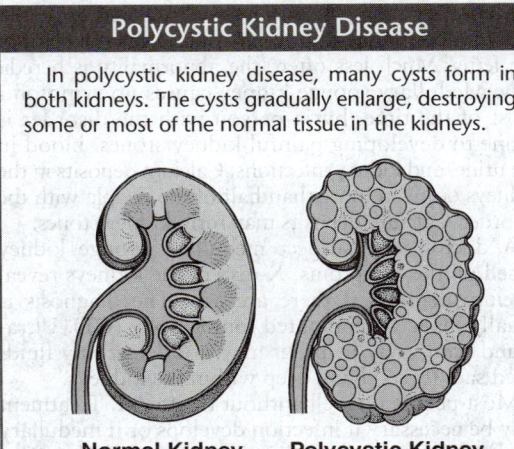

Normal Kidney   Polycystic Kidney

Symptoms

In the rare, recessive form of this disease that begins during childhood, the cysts become very large and cause the abdomen to protrude. A severely affected newborn may die shortly after birth, because kidney failure can develop in the fetus, leading to poor development of the lungs. The liver is also affected, and at 5 to 10 years of age, a child with this disorder tends to develop high pressure in the blood vessels that connect the intestine and the liver (portal system). Eventually, liver failure and kidney failure occur.

In the more common, dominant form of polycystic kidney disease, the cysts develop slowly in number and size. Typically, symptoms begin in early or middle adulthood. Sometimes symptoms are so mild that people with the disease will live their whole life without ever having known that they had the disorder. Symptoms usually include discomfort or pain in the abdomen or side (flank), blood in the urine, frequent urination, and intense crampy (colicky) pain from kidney stones. In other cases, fatigue, nausea, and other consequences of slowly developing kidney failure may result because the person has less functioning kidney tissue. Repeated urinary tract infections can worsen the kidney failure. At least half of the people with polycystic kidney disease have high blood pressure by the time the disorder is recognized.

Complications: About one third of people who have the dominant form of polycystic kidney disease also have cysts in their liver, but these cysts do not affect liver function. As many as 10% of people have dilated blood vessels (aneurysms) in their brain. Usually, the dilated blood vessels cause headaches when they expand. Many of these brain aneurysms bleed and cause strokes.

Diagnosis, Prognosis, and Treatment

A doctor suspects this disease on the basis of family history and laboratory tests of kidney function. Ultrasonography and computed tomography (CT) reveal the characteristic appearance of cysts in the kidneys and liver.

Effective treatment of urinary tract infections and high blood pressure slows the rate of kidney destruction. However, more than half of the people who have this disease develop kidney failure at some time in their life. Without dialysis or kidney transplantation, kidney failure is fatal.

Genetic testing is available to help people with polycystic kidney disease understand the probability that their children will inherit the condition.

Nephronophthisis–Medullary Cystic Disease Complex

Nephronophthisis–medullary cystic disease complex is a group of disorders in which fluid-filled sacs (cysts) develop deep within the kidneys, leading to kidney failure.

Nephronophthisis–medullary cystic disease complex is a group of hereditary disorders that affect the development of microscopic tubules deep within the kidneys that concentrate the urine and reabsorb sodium. The damaged tubules become inflamed and scarred, eventually causing kidney failure.

Nephronophthisis is inherited as an autosomal recessive disease, so one defective gene must be received from each parent. It causes symptoms that usually begin during childhood or early adolescence and usually leads to kidney failure in early adolescence.

Medullary cystic disease is inherited as an autosomal dominant disorder, so a defective gene from only one parent is necessary, and it usually causes symptoms that begin in adulthood. Occasionally, the disorder occurs in a person with no family history of kidney disease. These people may have developed the gene defect as a new mutation (the gene becomes abnormal for no apparent reason) or the defect was present but not recognized in one or both parents.

Symptoms and Diagnosis

A person starts to produce excessive amounts of urine and becomes excessively thirsty because the kidneys become unable to concentrate urine and conserve sodium.

With nephronophthisis, the symptoms begin in children age one year or older and are associated with retarded growth. People with nephronophthisis may have eye disorders, liver disorders, and mental retardation. Later in childhood, kidney failure may cause anemia, nausea, and weakness.

With medullary cystic disease, the symptoms develop in adolescence or early adulthood. Excessive thirst and abnormal urine production are not as severe as with nephronophthisis. Other organs are not affected. Kidney failure occurs usually between the ages of 34 and 65. Some people develop gout.

Family history of this type of kidney disease is an important clue to the diagnosis. Laboratory tests indicate poor kidney function and a low level of sodium in the blood. Computed tomography (CT) is the imaging test that is most likely to detect cysts. In the future, genetic testing may become the most precise method of making the diagnosis.

Treatment

When kidney failure occurs, dialysis or kidney transplantation is needed. Particularly in nephronophthisis, large daily intake of fluids and salt (sodium) is needed to compensate for the excessive excretion of sodium and the production of large volumes of dilute urine.

Medullary Sponge Kidney

Medullary sponge kidney is an uncommon disorder in which the urine-containing tubules of the kidneys are dilated.

Medullary sponge kidney is usually caused by a nongenetic abnormality that occurs during development of the fetus. Much less often, the abnormality is hereditary. Medullary sponge kidney causes no symptoms most of the time, but a person with the disorder is prone to developing painful kidney stones, blood in the urine, and kidney infections. Calcium deposits in the kidneys occur in more than half of the people with the disorder. Calcium deposits may form kidney stones.

A doctor may suspect medullary sponge kidney based on the symptoms. X-rays of the kidneys reveal calcium deposits if there are any. The diagnosis is usually made by computed tomography (CT). Ultrasound scans may help but may not detect tiny fluid-filled sacs (cysts) lying deep within the kidneys.

Most people do well without treatment. Treatment may be necessary if infection develops or if medullary sponge kidney causes calcium to deposit and repeatedly form stones. Treatment for calcium stones is high fluid intake (more than 2 quarts [2 liters] per day) and a diet that is low in sodium, normal in calcium, and low to normal in protein. Sometimes a thiazide diuretic or amiloride is recommended. Surgery may be needed if the urinary tract becomes obstructed. Infections are treated with antibiotics.

CHAPTER

47 Urinary Incontinence

Urinary incontinence is the uncontrollable loss of urine.

- Urinary incontinence can be caused by a bladder infection, certain drugs, brain and spinal cord disorders, diseases that affect the nerves leading to and from the bladder, conditions in the lower urinary tract such as an enlarged prostate, and conditions that impair mental function or mobility.

- Symptoms depend on the type of incontinence but may include a sudden uncontrollable urge to urinate or constant leak of urine.

- Doctors ask about the pattern of urine leakage, may ask the person to keep a record of episodes of incontinence, and do some basic examinations to help determine the cause and treatment.

- Some general measures, including urinating at regular intervals, regulating fluid intake, and practicing pelvic muscle exercises, help many people.

- Other treatments are available including various drugs and surgical procedures.

Urinary incontinence affects as many as 1 in 3 older people, and fewer, but many, younger people. In most age groups, urinary incontinence is more common among women than men.

Urinary incontinence differs somewhat among age groups. Incontinence experienced by younger adults tends to begin suddenly, and it often resolves quickly with little or no treatment. Also, when younger adults experience incontinence, they usually maintain control without leakage for most of their episodes of urination. Older adults are often more frequently and severely affected. In addition, incontinence is less likely to resolve quickly or without treatment in older adults.

Although urinary incontinence is common, highly treatable, and very often curable, it is often not diagnosed or treated. People often live with incontinence without seeking professional help because they are afraid, embarrassed, or mistakenly believe it is a normal part of aging. A person with incontinence often feels isolated or depressed. In addition, urinary incontinence is often a reason for institutionalization because of the substantial burden it places on caregivers. More than 50% of nursing home residents are incontinent.

Urinary incontinence can lead to many complications. For example, incontinence that is not properly managed can contribute to the development of bladder and kidney infections. Particularly among older adults, incontinence can also increase the risk of skin rashes and pressure sores (because urine can irritate the skin) and falls (because an incontinent person may fall when rushing to use the toilet).

Control of Urination

The kidneys constantly produce urine, which flows through two tubes (the ureters) to the bladder, where urine is stored. The lowest part of the bladder (the neck) is encircled by a muscle (the urinary sphincter) that remains contracted to close off the channel that carries urine out of the body (the urethra), so that urine is retained in the bladder until it is full.

When the bladder is full, messages travel along nerves from the bladder to the spinal cord. The messages are then relayed to the brain, and the person becomes aware of the urge to urinate. A person who has control of urination can consciously and voluntarily decide whether to release the urine from the bladder or to hold it for a while. When the decision is made to urinate, the sphincter muscle relaxes, allowing urine to flow out through the urethra, and the bladder wall muscles contract to push the urine out. Muscles in the abdominal wall and floor of the pelvis can be contracted to increase the pressure on the bladder.

Types and Causes

Incontinence can be categorized according to whether it is temporary (transient incontinence) or caused by a long-standing problem (established incontinence).

A bladder infection is the most common cause of transient incontinence. Other reversible factors that can contribute to incontinence include conditions that result in confusion (for example, a severe infection such as pneumonia) or impaired mobility (for example, because of a leg or hip fracture). Additional causes of transient incontinence include excess intake of alcohol or beverages that contain caffeine and conditions that can result in irritation of the bladder or urethra, such as atrophic vaginitis or severe constipation.

Established incontinence may be caused by brain and spinal cord disorders such as stroke, Alzheimer's disease, and multiple sclerosis; diseases that affect the nerves leading to and from the bladder such as diabetes; conditions in the lower urinary tract such as an enlarged prostate; and conditions that permanently impair mental function or mobility.

Urinary incontinence can also be categorized into five basic types based on the pattern of symptoms:

- Urge
- Stress
- Overflow
- Functional
- Mixed

Urge Incontinence: Urge incontinence is an abrupt and intense urge to urinate that is usually followed by an uncontrollable loss of urine. People with urge incontinence usually have little time to get to the bathroom before they have an "accident." An illness or injury that interferes with mobility makes it even harder for a person to get to the bathroom quickly. Use of a diuretic can aggravate the problem.

Urge incontinence is the most common type of established incontinence in older people and often has no clear cause. In most older people with urge incontinence, the bladder muscles are overactive (the muscles contract involuntarily before the bladder is full). Part of the cause of persistent urge incontinence may be changes in the part of the brain in the frontal lobe that inhibits urination. These changes, which disrupt the nervous system's ability to inhibit the bladder, may accompany brain disorders, especially stroke and dementia. Chronic overactivity of the bladder—overactive bladder—is common among older people and causes the abrupt and intense urge to urinate as well as frequent urination during the day and night. In postmenopausal women, a lack of estrogen contributes to atrophic vaginitis (thinning of the vaginal tissue), which causes irritation and can worsen urinary urgency and contribute to incontinence.

SPOTLIGHT ON AGING

Several changes occur with aging that may affect a person's ability to control urination. With aging, the maximum amount of urine that the bladder can hold (bladder capacity) tends to decline. Also, the ability to postpone urination after feeling the need to urinate may decrease. In addition, the amount of urine remaining in the bladder after urination is finished (residual urine) increases with aging.

In women, the urethra shortens and its lining becomes thinner as the level of estrogen declines during menopause. These changes decrease the ability of the urinary sphincter to close tightly.

In men, the rate of urine flow out of the bladder and through the urethra slows, especially when the prostate gland enlarges. This change becomes common as men age.

All of these age-related changes increase the odds that people will develop incontinence as they get older.

DRUGS THAT MAY CAUSE OR WORSEN URINARY INCONTINENCE

TYPE OF DRUG	EXAMPLES	EFFECTS
Alcohol	Beer, liquor, and wine	Increases urine production
Alpha-adrenergic agonists	Nasal decongestants that contain pseudoephedrine	Tighten the urinary sphincter Can cause urinary retention and overflow incontinence
Alpha-adrenergic blockers	Doxazosin, prazosin, and terazosin	Relax the bladder outlet and urethra Can cause stress incontinence in women
Angiotensin-converting enzyme (ACE) inhibitors	Benazepril and captopril	Can cause cough and worsen stress incontinence
Caffeine	Coffee, tea, colas, and chocolate	Increases urine production
Cholinesterase inhibitors	Donepezil	Can increase bladder contractility and contribute to urge incontinence
Diuretics	Bumetanide, furosemide, theophylline, and thiazides	Increase urine production
Drugs with anticholinergic effects*	Antihistamines, benztropine, some antidepressants (such as amitriptyline, desipramine, and nortriptyline), and some antipsychotics (such as haloperidol, risperidone, thioridazine, and thiothixene)	Interfere with bladder contraction, sometimes causing urinary retention and overflow incontinence Can worsen constipation, worsening urge or overflow incontinence
Hormonal therapy in women (given orally)	Estrogen-progestin combination therapy, which is used to treat hot flashes and other menopausal symptoms	When estrogen-progestin therapy is taken by mouth, new or worsening incontinence in some women When topical estrogen is applied locally by cream or other methods, less severe symptoms of incontinence in some women
Opioids	Codeine, morphine, and oxycodone	Interfere with bladder contraction, sometimes causing urinary retention and overflow incontinence Can worsen constipation and thus worsen urge or overflow incontinence
Sedatives and sleep aids (hypnotics)	Diazepam, eszopiclone, flurazepam, lorazepam, and zoldipem	Can cause slow mobility and make people less aware of the need to urinate

*Drugs with anticholinergic effects can have side effects such as confusion, memory problems, blurred vision, constipation, dry mouth, and retention of urine.

Stress Incontinence: Stress incontinence is the uncontrollable loss of small amounts of urine, such as with coughing, straining, sneezing, lifting heavy objects, or performing any maneuver that suddenly increases pressure within the abdomen. Stress incontinence is the most common type of incontinence among young and middle-aged women. It can be caused by weakness of the urinary sphincter, which sometimes results from childbirth, pelvic surgery, or an abnormal position of the urethra or uterus. In postmenopausal women, a lack of estrogen reduces the urethra's resistance to urine flow. In men, stress incontinence may follow prostate surgery if the upper part of the urethra or the bladder neck is injured. In both men and women, obesity can cause or worsen stress incontinence because extra weight stresses the bladder.

Some people with severe stress incontinence have nearly constant urine loss (sometimes referred to as total incontinence). In adults, this usually occurs because the urinary sphincter does not close adequately.

Overflow Incontinence: Overflow incontinence is the uncontrollable leakage of small amounts of urine from a bladder that does not empty well. Overflow incontinence is usually caused by some type of blockage or by weak bladder contraction caused by nerve damage or bladder muscle weakness. When urine flow is blocked or the bladder muscles can no longer contract, the bladder becomes overfilled and enlarged. Pressure increases in the bladder until small amounts of urine dribble out.

> **? Did You Know...**
> People often live with incontinence because they mistakenly believe it is a normal part of aging.

In men, an enlarged prostate can block the opening into the urethra from the bladder. Less commonly, blockage is caused by narrowing of the bladder neck or the urethra (urethral stricture), which may occur after prostate surgery or radiation therapy for prostate cancer. In men and women, constipation can cause overflow incontinence if stool fills the rectum to the point of putting pressure on the bladder neck and urethra. A number of drugs that affect the brain or spinal cord or that interfere with nerve messages—such as drugs with anticholinergic effects (for example, benztropine, most antihistamines, some antidepressants, and some antipsychotics) and opioids—may impair bladder contractions and cause overflow incontinence. Nerve damage that paralyzes the bladder (neurogenic bladder) can also cause overflow incontinence. Diabetes mellitus can also cause a form of neurogenic bladder and overflow incontinence.

Functional Incontinence: Functional incontinence refers to urine loss resulting from the inability (or sometimes unwillingness) to get to a toilet. The most common causes are conditions that cause immobility, such as stroke or severe arthritis, and conditions that interfere with mental function, such as dementia due to Alzheimer's disease. In rare situations, people may become so depressed or otherwise emotionally disturbed that they do not go to the toilet. This is sometimes referred to as psychogenic incontinence.

Mixed Incontinence: Mixed incontinence involves more than one type of incontinence. The most common type of mixed incontinence occurs in older women, who often have a mixture of urge and stress incontinence. Also, many older people have both urge and functional incontinence.

Diagnosis

Ideally, a doctor asks about incontinence. If not, however, the person should bring up the subject. The doctor asks specific questions about the history of the problem. The doctor also asks how much the incontinence is affecting the person's quality of life and ability to function and how long incontinence has been occurring. People with urinary incontinence may be asked to record the pattern of urination for at least 3 days (a "bladder diary"). This diary can help doctors evaluate the cause of the incontinence. Useful information might include the following:

- What symptoms are associated with the incontinence? For example, before urination or episodes of incontinence, is there an abrupt and intense urge to urinate? If so, how much time typically passes after the urge to urinate before urination begins?
- Do episodes of incontinence occur with laughing, coughing, sneezing, or bending?
- When episodes of incontinence occur, are undergarments typically damp or are they soaked? This can help estimate how much urine leaked.
- Does there seem to be a relationship between urination and taking drugs or drinking alcohol or caffeinated beverages? The time the person eats, drinks, takes drugs, and sleeps helps determine whether urination is related to any of these activities.
- What is the frequency of urination or episodes of incontinence during a typical day? A typical night? If people urinate frequently at night but in much smaller amounts than when awake, the cause may be that sleep is disturbed. That is, people urinate because they are awake rather than being awakened to urinate.

A physical examination can provide valuable information. A rectal examination can confirm whether the person is severely constipated, determine whether the nerves to the bladder are damaged, and, in men, determine whether the prostate is enlarged. A pelvic examination in women can help identify problems that may contribute to or cause incontinence, such as atrophy of the lining of urethra, prolapse of the bladder (cystocele), and damage affecting the nerves to the bladder. Examination may also help determine if a problem with mental function or immobility is contributing to incontinence.

Stress incontinence is sometimes diagnosed simply by observing the loss of urine while the person is coughing or straining. The amount of urine left in the bladder after urination (residual urine) can be measured using ultrasonography or urinary catheterization (placing a small tube called a catheter into the bladder). A large amount of residual urine indicates an obstruction or a problem with nerves or the bladder muscle, which may indicate overflow incontinence. Urinalysis is performed to determine whether an infection is present.

Doctors often test urine for evidence of a urinary tract infection and test blood for evidence of impaired kidney function. They may also test for the bladder's ability to empty completely by using an ultrasound or inserting a catheter in the bladder (a test called post-void residual determination). For some people, special tests during urination (urodynamic evaluation) and cystoscopy may be helpful. Urodynamic tests measure the pressure in the bladder at rest and when filling. A catheter is inserted through the urethra into the bladder and water is passed through the catheter while the pressure within the bladder is recorded. Normally, the pressure increases only when the bladder is relatively full. In some people, pressure builds in sudden spasms or rises too sharply before the bladder is completely filled. The pattern of pressure change helps the doctor determine the type of incontinence and the best treatment. The rate of urine flow can also be measured. This measurement can help determine whether urine flow is obstructed and whether the bladder muscles can contract strongly enough to expel the urine. Additionally, the function of the urethral sphincter muscle, which helps retain urine in the bladder, can be assessed. A weak urethral sphincter muscle may cause or contribute to incontinence. Cystoscopy involves looking directly into the bladder with a flexible viewing tube (similar to colonoscopy) to identify abnormalities that may be contributing to the incontinence and related symptoms.

Treatment

Treatment varies according to the type and cause of incontinence. Most people can be either cured or helped considerably.

People should receive education about bladder functioning, the effects of drugs and fluid intake, and bladder and bowel habits. Prevention of constipation is especially important because a full bowel can irritate the bladder more. Treatment often requires only taking some simple steps to change behavior, such as deliberately urinating at regular intervals—every 2 to 3 hours (sometimes called scheduled voiding)—to keep the bladder relatively empty. Avoiding fluids that may irritate the bladder, such as beverages that contain caffeine, may help. People should drink adequate amounts of fluids (for many people, six to eight 8-ounce [or about 250-milliliter] glasses a day) to prevent the urine from becoming too concentrated—which can irritate the bladder. Drugs that adversely affect bladder function can often be stopped. For people taking diuretics, the timing of the dose can be adjusted so that the person can be close to a bathroom when the drug takes effect.

Specially designed incontinence pads and undergarments can protect the skin and enable people to remain dry, comfortable, and socially active. These items are unobtrusive and readily available.

Bladder training techniques, which include pelvic muscle (Kegel) exercises (see page 1545), can be very helpful, particularly for urge or stress incontinence. The exercises involve repeatedly contracting the muscles many times a day to build up strength and learning to use the muscles properly in situations that cause incontinence, such as coughing. Nurses or physical therapists can help teach these exercises. People who have trouble learning how to contract these muscles may find biofeedback helpful. With biofeedback, electrodes are temporarily placed near the sphincter muscles at the outside of the anus. The electrodes transmit signals that display muscle activity and allow the person to better identify and contract the appropriate muscles.

Drugs may also be useful for certain types of incontinence. It may seem confusing that some drugs that can cause incontinence, such as alpha-adrenergic agonists, alpha-adrenergic blockers, and drugs with anticholinergic effects, can also be used to treat incontinence. Doctors choose drugs based on the type of incontinence and the symptoms that are most troublesome. For example:

- Alpha-adrenergic agonists tighten the urinary sphincter, which can help prevent stress incontinence caused by a weak urinary sphincter.
- Alpha-adrenergic blockers relax the urinary sphincter. Relaxing the urinary sphincter can be helpful in men who have urinary symptoms associated with an enlarged prostate.
- Drugs with anticholinergic effects decrease bladder contractions, which can help people with urge incontinence by decreasing the strong urge to urinate.

Urge Incontinence: Episodes of urge incontinence often can be prevented by urinating at regular intervals before the urge occurs (scheduled voiding). Pelvic muscle (Kegel) exercises, which can strengthen bladder muscles and help inhibit involuntary urination, may also help. Drugs that relax the bladder, such as the anticholinergic drugs used to treat incontinence, are the ones most commonly prescribed. The two most commonly used drugs of this class are oxybutynin and tolterodine. Both can be taken once a day. Oxybutynin can be used as a skin patch that is applied twice a week, or the drug can be administered directly into the bladder. Newer drugs in this category include solifenacin, darifenacin, and trospium. Alternatively, botulinum toxin, which paralyzes muscles, can be injected into the bladder to help relax the overactive bladder muscles. Although this treatment is too new to be recommended routinely, results with it so far suggest that it may be effective for 6 to 9 months. Although all of these drugs can help reduce bladder irritability and the strong urge to urinate, they have potential side effects, such as dryness of the mouth, constipation, gastroesophageal reflux, and even retention of urine.

Stress Incontinence: For people with stress incontinence, urinating frequently to avoid a full bladder

SOME DRUGS USED TO TREAT URINARY INCONTINENCE

EXAMPLES	SOME SIDE EFFECTS	COMMENTS
Drugs with anticholinergic effects		
Darifenacin Hyoscyamine Oxybutynin Solifenacin Tolterodine Trospium	Dry mouth, constipation, worsening of glaucoma, confusion, memory problems, worsening of heartburn, and urinary retention	Can decrease the strong urge to urinate in people with urge incontinence Equally effective overall, although some people may respond better to one drug than to another Effective in older and younger people Oxybutynin more likely to have side effects, especially dry mouth
Serotonin-norepinephrine reuptake inhibitor (an antidepressant) for women		
Duloxetine	Nausea	Used to treat stress incontinence due to weak bladder outlet Not yet widely used in the United States
Alpha-adrenergic agonist for women		
Pseudoephedrine	Insomnia, anxiety, awareness of heart beats, high blood pressure, and, in men, urinary retention	Used to treat stress incontinence due to a weak bladder outlet Not recommended for people with heart disorders, high blood pressure, glaucoma, or diabetes
Alpha-adrenergic blockers for men		
Alfuzosin Doxazosin Prazosin Tamsulosin Terazosin	Low blood pressure (especially after standing up), fatigue, weakness, and dizziness	Used to relieve blockage of the bladder in men with urge or overflow incontinence May take days to a few weeks to become effective May increase the rate of urine flow If taken with drugs that lower blood pressure, can cause blood pressure to become too low With alfuzosin and tamsulosin, less of an effect on blood pressure than the other drugs listed
5-Alpha-reductase inhibitors for men		
Dutasteride Finasteride	Decreased libido and erectile dysfunction	Used to treat an enlarged prostate that is blocking urine flow out of the bladder in men with urge or overflow incontinence May enable men to postpone or avoid prostate surgery May take months to become effective

and pelvic muscle (Kegel) exercises are often helpful. In women with stress incontinence and thinning of the vagina or urethra due to a lack of estrogen, applying estrogen cream or inserting a rubber ring with estrogen or estrogen tablets into the vagina may be helpful. Risks and benefits should be discussed thoroughly (see page 1517). However, using estrogen cream or an estrogen ring or tablet does not have as many side effects or as much risk as does taking estrogens by mouth. Other drugs that help tighten the sphincter, such as pseudoephedrine and duloxetine, may also help. Incontinence pads may be used to absorb the small amount of urine that usually leaks during stress.

More severe cases of stress incontinence that do not respond to other treatments can be corrected with surgery. By using any of several procedures, doctors can strengthen or tighten the tissues around the urethra. Injections of bulk-forming agents, such as collagen, around the urethra are effective in some people. A urinary sphincter that does not close adequately may be replaced with an artificial one.

Overflow Incontinence: For overflow incontinence caused by an enlarged prostate or other blockage, surgery is usually necessary. Several procedures are available to remove part or all of the prostate. Dutasteride or finasteride, when taken over a period of months, can reduce the size of the prostate or stop its growth, so that surgery can be avoided or deferred. Drugs that relax the prostate, such as alfuzosin, doxazosin, prazosin, terazosin, and tamsulosin, may help the bladder empty more efficiently.

When the cause of overflow incontinence is weak contraction of the bladder muscles, drugs are usually not helpful. Gentle pressure applied by squeezing the lower abdomen with the hands just over the bladder may help, especially for people who can empty the bladder but have difficulty emptying it completely. In some cases, a catheter may need to be inserted into the bladder to drain the bladder and prevent complications, such as recurring infections and kidney damage. The catheter may be placed permanently, or it may be inserted and removed several times a day (intermittent catheterization).

Functional Incontinence: Treatment for functional incontinence involves regular toileting assistance. For example, another person can remind the incontinent person to urinate on a schedule, usually every 3 to 4 hours, so that the bladder is emptied before episodes of incontinence can occur (prompted scheduled voiding). Sometimes, a bedside commode or a hand-held urinal is useful for people who have difficulty getting to the toilet. If depression is a contributing factor, it should be treated. The use of garments and pads is also helpful; however, a person should not become unnecessarily dependent on them.

Incontinence in Children

- The pattern of incontinence helps the doctor determine the *likely* cause.
- The child's history and results of a physical examination, laboratory tests, and imaging tests help the doctor determine the *specific* cause.
- Treatment includes behavioral changes, dietary changes, and sometimes drugs.

Incontinence in children has different causes and treatment than that in adults. Incontinence can occur at night (bed-wetting, also called nocturnal enuresis—see page 1746). Nocturnal enuresis is more common among boys, and children usually outgrow this type of incontinence by age 9. Incontinence during the daytime is sometimes called diurnal enuresis. Diurnal enuresis tends to be more common among girls and has a number of different causes.

Causes

The pattern of incontinence helps the doctor determine the likely cause. If the child has never had a consistent dry period during the day, the doctor considers the possibility of a birth defect, an anatomic abnormality, or certain behaviors that can lead to incontinence. A spinal cord defect such as spina bifida can cause nerve damage to the bladder and lead to incontinence, but such a defect is usually obvious. Some infants have a birth defect that prevents the bladder or urethra from developing completely, leading to nearly constant urine loss (total incontinence). Another type of birth defect causes the ureter to end outside the bladder, causing incontinence. Some children have an overactive bladder that easily spasms, or they have difficulty emptying their bladder.

Certain behaviors can lead to daytime incontinence, especially in girls. Such behaviors include urinating infrequently and urinating using an incorrect position, which can cause urine to leak into the vagina, then dribble out after standing. Some girls experience bladder spasm when laughing, resulting in "giggle incontinence."

If the child has been dry for a long time and the incontinence is new, the doctor considers conditions that intermittently cause difficulties. These include constipation, diet, emotional stress, infections, and sexual abuse. Bacterial urinary tract infections and viral infections that lead to bladder irritation (viral cystitis) are common infectious causes. To prevent urine from leaking, many children with incontinence cross their legs or use other postures, which may increase the chance of developing a urinary tract infection. Sexually active adolescents can have urinary difficulties from certain sexually transmitted diseases. Caffeine and acidic juices, such as orange and tomato juice, can irritate the bladder and lead to leakage of urine. Children with diabetes mellitus or diabetes insipidus (a disorder resulting in excessive amounts of dilute urine) can develop incontinence because these disorders result in production of excessive amounts of urine.

Diagnosis

Sometimes doctors can diagnose the cause by the child's symptoms and the results of an examination. To check for an infection, a urinalysis and sometimes a urine culture is done. To check for diabetes mellitus and diabetes insipidus, doctors use blood and urine tests to check sugar and electrolyte levels. If a birth defect is suspected, an ultrasound examination of the kidneys and bladder and x-rays of the spine may be necessary. A special x-ray of the bladder and kidneys, called a voiding cystourethrogram, may also be necessary. With this test, a dye is injected into the bladder using a catheter, which shows the anatomy of the urinary tract, as well as the direction of urine flow.

Treatment

Treatment depends on the cause of the incontinence. An infection is usually treated with antibiotics. Relieving and preventing constipation, urinating at 2- to 3-hour intervals, using a technique called biofeedback for an overactive bladder, and changing other behaviors may be effective depending on the cause. Dietary changes can help decrease bladder irritants. If behavioral interventions are not effective, certain drugs (such as oxybutynin) may help if the cause is bladder spasm. Children with birth defects or anatomic abnormalities may need surgery, drugs, or intermittent catheterization.

CHAPTER 48 Obstruction of the Urinary Tract

An obstruction anywhere along the urinary tract—from the kidneys, where urine is produced, to the urethra, through which urine leaves the body—can increase pressure inside the urinary tract and slow the flow of urine. An obstruction may occur suddenly or develop slowly over days, weeks, or even months. An obstruction may completely or only partially block part of the urinary tract.

Urinary tract obstruction can make the kidneys distend (dilate). Distention damages the kidneys. Although the kidneys can usually recover if the obstruction is relieved quickly, permanent damage may occur. Severe damage can result in loss of kidney function (kidney failure). Obstruction can also lead to stone formation and urinary tract infections. An infection may develop because bacteria that enter the urinary tract are not flushed out when the flow of urine is obstructed.

Hydronephrosis

Hydronephrosis is distention (dilation) of the kidney with urine, caused by backward pressure on the kidney when the flow of urine is obstructed.

- Kidney stones are common causes of urinary tract obstruction.
- When hydronephrosis occurs quickly, people may have excruciating pain, most often in the flank (the area between the ribs and the hips).
- When hydronephrosis occurs more gradually, people may have no symptoms or experience attacks of dull, aching discomfort in the flank.
- Doctors initially use bladder catheterization (or ultrasonography) to detect hydronephrosis, and they may use ultrasonography or another imaging test to determine the site of the blockage.
- Treatment depends on the cause of the obstruction.

Normally, urine flows out of the kidneys at extremely low pressure. If the flow of urine is obstructed, urine backs up behind the point of blockage, eventually reaching the small tubes of the kidney and its collecting area (renal pelvis), distending the kidney and increasing the pressure on its internal structures. The elevated pressure from obstruction may ultimately damage the kidney and can result in loss of its function. When the flow of urine is obstructed, urinary tract infections are fairly common and stones are more likely to form. If both kidneys are obstructed, kidney failure may result.

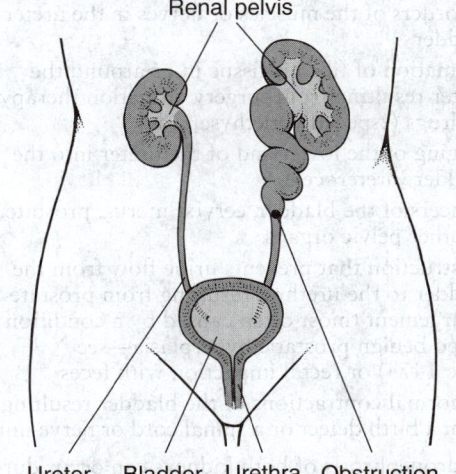

Hydronephrosis: A Distended Kidney

In hydronephrosis, the kidney is distended because the flow of urine is obstructed and urine backs up in the kidney's small tubes and central collecting area (renal pelvis).

Normal Kidney   Distended Kidney

Renal pelvis

Ureter   Bladder   Urethra   Obstruction

Long-standing distention of the renal pelvis and ureter can also inhibit the rhythmic muscular contractions that normally move urine down the ureter from the kidney to the bladder (peristalsis). Scar tissue may then replace the normal muscular tissue in the walls of the ureter, resulting in permanent damage.

Causes

Hydronephrosis commonly results from an obstruction located at the junction of the ureter and renal pelvis (ureteropelvic junction). Causes of this type of obstruction include the following:

- Structural abnormalities—for example, a birth defect in which the insertion of the ureter into the renal pelvis is too high or there is inadequate development of the ureteral muscles (congenital ureteropelvic junction obstruction)
- Kinking at the ureteropelvic junction resulting from a kidney shifting downward (ptosis of the kidney)
- Stones (calculi) or a blood clot in the renal pelvis
- Compression of the ureter by bands of fibrous tissue, an abnormally located artery or vein, or a tumor

Hydronephrosis can also result from an obstruction below the ureteropelvic junction or from backflow (reflux) of urine from the bladder. Causes of this type of obstruction include the following:

- Stones in the ureter
- Blood clot in the ureter
- Tumors in or near the ureter
- Narrowing of the ureter resulting from a birth defect, an injury, an infection, radiation therapy, or surgery
- Disorders of the muscles or nerves in the ureter or bladder
- Formation of fibrous tissue in or around the ureter resulting from surgery, radiation therapy, or drugs (especially methysergide)
- Bulging of the lower end of the ureter into the bladder (ureterocele)
- Cancers of the bladder, cervix, uterus, prostate, or other pelvic organs
- Obstruction that prevents urine flow from the bladder to the urethra, resulting from prostate enlargement (most often caused by a condition called benign prostatic hyperplasia—see page 1474) or rectal impaction with feces
- Abnormal contractions of the bladder resulting from a birth defect or a spinal cord or nerve injury

Hydronephrosis of both kidneys can occur during pregnancy as the enlarging uterus compresses the ureters. Hormonal changes during pregnancy may aggravate the problem by reducing the muscular contractions that normally move urine down the ureters. This condition, commonly called hydronephrosis of pregnancy, usually ends when the pregnancy ends, although the renal pelvis and ureters may remain somewhat distended afterward.

Symptoms

Symptoms depend on the cause, location, and duration of the obstruction. When the obstruction begins quickly (acute hydronephrosis), it usually causes renal colic—an excruciating, intermittent pain in the flank (the area between the ribs and hip) on the affected side. Obstruction on one side does not reduce urine flow. Obstruction can stop or reduce urine flow if blockage affects the ureters from both kidneys or if it affects the urethra. Obstruction of the urethra or bladder outlet may cause pain, pressure, and distention of the bladder.

People who have slowly progressive (chronic) hydronephrosis may have no symptoms, or they may have attacks of dull, aching discomfort in the flank on the affected side. Sometimes a kidney stone temporarily blocks the ureter and causes painful hydronephrosis that occurs intermittently.

Hydronephrosis may cause vague intestinal symptoms, such as nausea, vomiting, and abdominal pain. These symptoms sometimes occur in children when hydronephrosis results from a birth defect in which the junction of the ureter and renal pelvis is too narrow (ureteropelvic junction obstruction).

People who have urinary tract infections may have pus in the urine, fever, and discomfort in the area of the bladder or kidneys.

Diagnosis

Early diagnosis is important, because most cases of obstruction can be corrected and because a delay in treatment can lead to irreversible kidney damage. Doctors may suspect hydronephrosis because of a person's symptoms and sometimes because of findings discovered during a physical examination. A distended kidney can occasionally be felt in the flank, particularly if the kidney is greatly enlarged in an infant or a child or a thin adult. A distended bladder can sometimes be felt in the lower part of the abdomen just above the pubic bone.

Doctors depend on testing to make the diagnosis. Bladder catheterization (insertion of a hollow, flexible tube through the urethra) is often the first diagnostic test done in people with renal colic, pelvic pressure, or distention. If the catheter drains a large amount of urine from the bladder, then either the bladder outlet or the urethra is obstructed. Many doctors do ultrasonography to determine whether the bladder is filled with a large amount of urine before doing bladder catheterization.

If the presence or site of obstruction is in doubt, various imaging tests can be done to identify evidence of obstruction such as hydronephrosis or a site of blockage. For example, ultrasonography is a very useful test in most people (particularly children and pregnant women) because it is fairly accurate and does not expose the person to any radiation. Computed tomography (CT) scanning is an alternative. It is rapid and highly accurate, particularly at identifying stones. Other imaging tests, such as intravenous urography, may be performed to identify the site of obstruction, if it is not visible with ultrasonography or CT.

An endoscope (a rigid or flexible telescope) is sometimes used to look at possible sites of obstruction as closely as possible. An endoscope can be used to examine the urinary tract.

Blood and urine tests are done. Blood test results are usually normal, but tests may reveal high levels of urea nitrogen (sometimes called BUN), creatinine, or both if obstruction affects both kidneys. Results from an analysis of urine (urinalysis) are usually normal, but white blood cells and red blood cells may be present when a stone or a cancer is the cause of obstruction or when the obstruction is complicated by an infection.

Prognosis

Permanent kidney damage is unlikely to result unless both kidneys are obstructed for at least a few weeks. The prognosis is less certain for chronic hydronephrosis.

Treatment

Treatment usually aims to relieve the cause of obstruction. For example, if the urethra is obstructed because of an enlarged or cancerous prostate, treatment can include drugs, such as hormone therapy for prostate cancer (see page 1480), surgery, or enlargement of the urethra with dilators. Other treatments, such as lithotripsy or endoscopic surgery, may be needed for stones that block the flow of urine. If the cause of obstruction cannot be rapidly corrected, particularly if there is infection, kidney failure, or severe pain, the urinary tract is drained. In acute hydronephrosis, urine that has accumulated above the obstruction can be drained with a soft tube inserted through the skin into the kidney (nephrostomy tube) or by insertion of a soft plastic tube that connects the bladder with the kidney (ureteral stent). Complications of nephrostomy tubes or ureteral stents can include displacement of the tube, infection, and discomfort.

Urgent relief of chronic hydronephrosis is usually not required. Complications of hydronephrosis, such as urinary tract infections and kidney failure, if present, are treated promptly.

Stones in the Urinary Tract

Stones (calculi) are hard masses that form anywhere in the urinary tract and may cause pain, bleeding, obstruction of the flow of urine, or an infection.

- Tiny stones may cause no symptoms, but larger stones can cause excruciating pain in the area between the ribs and hips.
- Usually, an imaging test and an analysis of urine are done to diagnose stones.
- Sometimes, stone formation can be prevented by changing the diet.
- Stones that do not pass on their own are removed with lithotripsy or an endoscopic technique.

Depending on where a stone forms, it may be called a kidney stone, ureteral stone, or bladder stone. The process of stone formation is called urolithiasis, renal lithiasis, or nephrolithiasis.

Every year, about 1 of 1,000 adults in the United States is hospitalized because of stones in the urinary tract. Stones are more common among middle-aged and older adults and men. Stones vary in size from too small to be seen with the naked eye to 1 inch (2.5 centimeters) or more in diameter. A large so-called staghorn stone may fill almost the entire renal pelvis (small tubes of the kidney and its collecting area) and the tubes that drain into it (calices).

A urinary tract infection may result when bacteria become trapped in urine that pools above a blockage. When stones block the urinary tract for a long time, urine backs up in the tubes inside the kidney, producing excessive pressure that can distend the kidney (hydronephrosis) and eventually damage it.

Causes

Stones may form because the urine becomes too saturated with salts that can form stones or because the urine lacks the normal inhibitors of stone formation. Citrate is such an inhibitor, because it normally binds with the calcium that is often involved in forming stones. About 80% of the stones are composed of calcium, and the remainder are composed of various substances, including uric acid, cystine, and struvite. Stones are more common among people with certain disorders (for example, hyperparathyroidism and short bowel syndrome) and among people whose diet is very high in protein or vitamin C or who do not consume enough water or calcium. People who have a family history of stone formation are more likely to have calcium stones and to have them more often.

Struvite stones—a mixture of magnesium, ammonium, and phosphate—are also called infection stones, because they form only in infected urine.

Symptoms

Stones, especially tiny ones, may not cause any symptoms. Stones in the bladder may cause pain in the lower abdomen. Stones that obstruct the ureter or renal pelvis or any of the kidney's drainage tubes may cause back pain or renal colic. Renal colic is characterized by an excruciating intermittent pain, usually in the flank (the area between the ribs and hip), that spreads across the abdomen, often to the genital area and inner thigh. The pain tends to come in waves, gradually increasing to a peak intensity, then fading, over about 20 to 60 minutes. The pain may radiate down the abdomen toward the groin or testis or vulva.

Other symptoms include nausea and vomiting, restlessness, sweating, and blood in the urine. A person may have an urge to urinate frequently, particularly as a stone passes down the ureter. Chills, fever, and abdominal distention sometimes occur.

> **? Did You Know...**
> People who have recurrent kidney stones should consider limiting the number of CT scans they get to prevent excessive radiation exposure.

Diagnosis

Doctors usually suspect stones in people with renal colic. Sometimes doctors suspect stones in people with tenderness over the back and groin or pain in the genital area without an obvious cause. Occasionally, the symptoms and physical examination findings are so distinctive that no additional tests are needed, particularly in people who have had urinary tract stones before. However, most people are in so much pain and have symptoms and findings that make other causes for the pain seem likely enough that testing is necessary to exclude these other causes. Helical (also called spiral) computed tomography (CT) that is done without the use of radiopaque contrast material is usually the best diagnostic procedure. CT can locate a stone and also indicate the degree to which the stone is blocking the urinary tract. CT can also detect many other disorders that can cause pain similar to the pain caused by stones. The disadvantage of CT is that it exposes people to radiation. Still, this risk seems prudent when possible causes include another serious disorder that would be diagnosed by CT, such as an aortic aneurysm or appendicitis. Ultrasonography is an alternative to CT and does not expose people to radiation. However, ultrasonography, compared with CT, more often misses small stones (especially when located in the ureter), the location of urinary tract blockage, and other, serious disorders that could be causing the symptoms.

Urinalysis is usually done. It may show blood or pus in the urine whether or not symptoms are present.

For people with diagnosed stones, doctors often do tests to determine the type of stones. People should attempt to retrieve stones that are passed. They can retrieve stones by straining all urine. Stones found can be analyzed. Depending on the type of stone, urine tests and tests of blood chemistries and hormone levels may be necessary.

Prevention

Measures to prevent the formation of new stones vary, depending on the composition of the existing stones.

Drinking large amounts of fluids—8 to 10 ten-ounce (300-milliliter) glasses a day—is recommended for prevention of all stones, although it is not clear whether and how much this helps. Many people with calcium stones have a condition called hypercalciuria, in which excess calcium is excreted in the urine. For them, a diet that is low in sodium and high in potassium may also help. Calcium intake should be about normal—1,000 to 1,500 milligrams daily (see page 933). Restricting dietary protein from red meat may help reduce the risk of stone formation. Thiazide diuretics, such as chlorthalidone or indapamide, reduce the concentration of calcium in the urine and help prevent the formation of new stones in such people. Potassium citrate may be given to increase a low urine level of citrate, a substance that inhibits calcium stone formation.

A high level of oxalate in the urine, which contributes to calcium stone formation, may result from excess consumption of foods high in oxalate, such as rhubarb, spinach, cocoa, nuts, pepper, and tea, or from certain intestinal disorders. Calcium citrate, cholestyramine, and a low-oxalate, low-fat diet may help to reduce urinary oxalate levels in some people. Sometimes pyridoxine decreases the amount of oxalate the body makes.

In rare cases, when calcium stones result from hyperparathyroidism, sarcoidosis, vitamin D toxicity, renal tubular acidosis, or cancer, the underlying disorder must be treated.

For stones that contain uric acid, a diet low in red meat is recommended, because red meat increases the level of uric acid in the urine. If this is not effective, allopurinol may be given to reduce the production of uric acid. Potassium citrate should be given to all people who have uric acid stones to make the urine alkaline, because uric acid stones form when urine acidity increases. Maintaining a large fluid intake is also very important.

For stones made of cystine, urinary cystine levels must be kept low by maintaining a large fluid intake and sometimes taking α-mecaptopropionylglycine (tiopronin) or penicillamine.

People with recurrent struvite stones may need to take antibiotics continually to prevent urinary tract infections. Acetohydroxamic acid may also be helpful.

Treatment

Small stones that are not causing symptoms, obstruction, or an infection usually do not need to be treated. Drinking plenty of fluids or receiving large amounts of fluids intravenously has been recommended to help stones pass, but it is not clear that this approach is helpful. Drugs that may help the stone pass include alpha-adrenergic blockers (such as tamsulosin) and calcium channel blockers (such as diltiazem, nifedipine, and verapamil). Once a stone has passed, no other immediate treatment is needed. The pain of renal colic may be relieved with nonsteroidal anti-inflammatory drugs (NSAIDs) or opioids.

Often, a stone in the renal pelvis or uppermost part of the ureter that is ½ inch (1 centimeter) or less in diameter can be broken up by shock waves directed at the body by a sound wave generator (a procedure called extracorporeal shock wave lithotripsy). The pieces of stone are then passed in the urine. Sometimes, a stone is removed with grasping forceps using an endoscope (viewing tube) through a small incision in the skin, or the stone can be shattered into fragments using a probe from a lithotripsy machine and then the pieces are passed in the urine.

Small stones in the lower part of the ureter that require removal may be removed with a small, flexible scope (called a ureteroscope, a kind of endoscope) that is inserted into the urethra and through the bladder. In some instances, the ureteroscope can also be used with a device to break up stones into smaller pieces that can be removed with the ureteroscope or passed in the urine (a procedure called intracorporeal lithotripsy). Most commonly, the device is a laser. When a laser is used, the procedure is called holmium laser lithotripsy.

Uric acid stones may sometimes be dissolved gradually by making the urine more alkaline (for example, with potassium citrate taken for 4 to 6 months by mouth), but other types of stones cannot be dissolved this way. Sometimes, larger stones that are causing an obstruction may need to be removed surgically.

Removing a Stone With Sound Waves

Kidney stones can sometimes be broken up by sound waves produced by a lithotriptor in a procedure called extracorporeal shock wave lithotripsy. After an ultrasound device or fluoroscope is used to locate the stone, the lithotriptor is placed against the back, and the sound waves are focused on the stone, shattering it. Then the person drinks fluids to flush the stone fragments out of the kidney, to be eliminated in the urine. Sometimes blood appears in the urine or the abdomen is bruised after the procedure, but serious problems are rare.

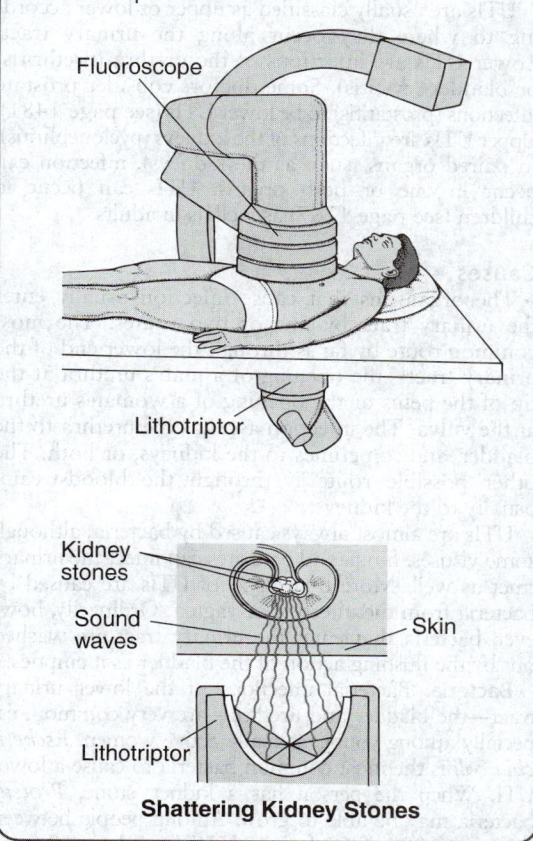

Shattering Kidney Stones

Struvite stones usually need to be removed by endoscopic surgery. Antibiotics are not helpful for urinary tract infections until the stones are removed.

CHAPTER

49   Urinary Tract Infections

In healthy people, urine in the bladder is sterile—no bacteria or other infectious organisms are present. The tube that carries urine from the bladder out of the body (urethra) contains no bacteria or too few to cause an infection. However, any part of the urinary tract can become infected. An infection anywhere along the urinary tract is called a urinary tract infection (UTI).

UTIs are usually classified as upper or lower according to where they occur along the urinary tract. Lower UTIs are infections of the urethra (urethritis) or bladder (cystitis). Some doctors consider prostate infections (prostatitis) to be lower UTIs (see page 1481). Upper UTIs are infections of the kidneys (pyelonephritis). In paired organs (such as the kidneys), infection can occur in one or both organs. UTIs can occur in children (see page 1767) as well as in adults.

Causes

The organisms that cause infection usually enter the urinary tract by one of two routes. The most common route by far is through the lower end of the urinary tract—the opening of a man's urethra at the tip of the penis or the opening of a woman's urethra at the vulva. The infection ascends the urethra to the bladder, and sometimes to the kidneys, or both. The other possible route is through the bloodstream, usually to the kidneys.

UTIs are almost always caused by bacteria, although some viruses, fungi, and parasites can infect the urinary tract as well. More than 85% of UTIs are caused by bacteria from the intestine or vagina. Ordinarily, however, bacteria that enter the urinary tract are washed out by the flushing action of the bladder as it empties.

Bacteria: Bacterial infections of the lower urinary tract—the bladder and urethra—are very common, especially among young, sexually active women. *Escherichia coli* is the most common bacteria to cause a lower UTI. When the person has a kidney stone, *Proteus* bacteria may be able to grow. Among people between the ages of 20 and 50, bacterial UTIs are about 50 times more common among women than men. In men, the urethra is longer, so it is more difficult for bacteria to ascend far enough to cause an infection. In people older than 50, UTIs become more common among both men and women, with less difference between the sexes.

Viruses: The herpes simplex virus type 2 (HSV-2) may infect the urethra, making urination painful and emptying of the bladder difficult.

Fungi: Certain fungi, or yeasts, can infect the urinary tract. This type of infection is often called a yeast infection (yeasts can also cause vaginitis). The fungus *Candida* is the organism most likely to cause urinary tract yeast infections. *Candida* frequently infects people who have an impaired immune system or a bladder catheter in place. Rarely, other types of fungi, including those that cause blastomycosis (*Blastomyces*) or coccidiomycosis (*Coccidioides*), infect the urinary tract. Fungi and bacteria may infect the kidneys at the same time.

Parasites: A number of parasites, including certain types of worms, can infect the urinary tract.

Trichomoniasis, caused by a type of microscopic parasite, is a sexually transmitted disease that can cause a copious greenish yellow, frothy discharge from the vagina in women. Occasionally, the bladder or urethra becomes infected. Trichomoniasis can infect the urethra in men. It usually causes no symptoms, although it can cause inflammation of the prostate (prostatitis).

Factors Contributing to Bacterial Urinary Tract Infections

ASCENDING INFECTIONS

- Blockage (for example, by stones) anywhere in the urinary tract
- Abnormal bladder function that prevents proper emptying, such as occurs in neurologic diseases
- Leaking of the valve-like mechanism between the ureter and the bladder, allowing urine and bacteria to flow backward from the bladder up the ureters, possibly reaching the kidneys (more common among children who have a UTI)
- Insertion of a urinary catheter or any instrument by a doctor
- Sexual intercourse
- Use of a diaphragm with spermicide
- Presence of an abnormal connection (fistula) between the vagina and the bladder or the intestine and the bladder
- Among men, prostatitis

BLOOD-BORNE INFECTIONS

- Infection in the bloodstream (septicemia)
- Infection of the heart valves (infective endocarditis)

Schistosomiasis, an infection caused by a type of worm called a fluke, can affect the kidneys, ureters, and bladder. This infection is a common cause of severe kidney failure among people who live in Africa, South America, and Asia. Persistent bladder schistosomiasis often causes blood in the urine or blockage of the ureters and may eventually result in bladder cancer.

Filariasis, a threadworm infection, obstructs lymphatic vessels, causing lymph fluid to enter the urine (chyluria). Filariasis can cause enormous swelling of tissues (elephantiasis), which, in men, may involve the scrotum.

Urethritis

Urethritis is infection of the urethra, the tube that carries urine from the bladder out of the body.

- Bacteria, including those that are sexually transmitted, are the most common cause of urethritis.
- Symptoms include pain while urinating, a frequent need to urinate, and sometimes a discharge.
- Antibiotics are usually given to treat the infection.

Causes

Urethritis may be caused by bacteria, fungi, or viruses (for example, herpes simplex virus). In most women, the bacteria involved are those that normally live in the lower intestine. These bacteria reach the urethra from the anus. Men are much less likely to develop urethritis because the opening of the male urethra is far removed from the anus, and thus bacteria from the anus less often reach the urethra. Bladder infection (cystitis) develops in most women who have urethritis but not in most men who have urethritis.

Sexually transmitted organisms—such as *Neisseria gonorrhoeae*, which causes gonorrhea—can spread to the urethra during sexual intercourse with an infected partner (see page 1269). *Chlamydia* and the herpes simplex virus are also commonly transmitted sexually and can cause urethritis (see page 1266). When men develop urethritis, the gonorrheal organism is a very common cause. Although this organism may infect the urethra in women, the vagina, cervix, uterus, ovaries, and fallopian tubes are more likely to be infected. *Trichomonas*, a type of microscopic parasite, also causes urethritis in men. Urethritis may also be caused by the bacteria that commonly cause other urinary tract infections, such as *Escherichia coli*.

Symptoms

In both men and women, there is usually pain with urination and a frequent, urgent need to urinate. Sometimes people have no symptoms. In men, when gonorrhea or chlamydia is the cause, there is usually a discharge from the urethra. The discharge is often yellowish green when the gonococcal organism is involved and may be clear when other organisms are involved. In women, discharge is less common.

Other disorders that cause pain with urination include bladder infection and vaginitis. In vaginitis, urination may cause pain because urine, which is acidic, irritates the inflamed vulva and lining of the vagina.

Complications: Infections of the urethra that are not treated or are inadequately treated eventually can cause a narrowing (stricture) of the urethra. A stricture increases the risk that infections will develop in the bladder or the kidneys. Untreated gonorrhea occasionally leads to an accumulation of pus (abscess) around the urethra. An abscess can cause outpouchings from the urethral wall (urethral diverticula), which can also become infected. If the abscess perforates the skin, the vagina, or the rectum, urine may flow through a newly created abnormal connection (urethral fistula).

Diagnosis

Doctors can usually make a diagnosis of urethritis based on the symptoms and examination. A sample of the discharge, if present, is collected by inserting a soft-tipped swab into the end of the urethra. The urethral swab is then sent to a laboratory for analysis so that the infecting organism can be identified.

Prevention and Treatment

Sexually transmitted diseases that cause urethritis may be prevented by using a condom.

Treatment depends on the cause of the infection. However, identification of the organism causing urethritis can take days. Thus, doctors usually begin treatment with antibiotics that cure the most common causes. For sexually active men, treatment is usually with a ceftriaxone injection for gonorrhea plus oral azithromycin or oral doxycycline for chlamydia. If tests exclude the possibility of gonorrhea and chlamydia, trimethoprim/sulfamethoxazole or a fluoroquinolone antibiotic (such as ciprofloxacin) may be used. Women are treated as if they had cystitis. An antiviral drug, such as acyclovir, may be needed for a herpes simplex infection.

Cystitis

Cystitis is infection of the bladder.

- Usually, bacteria are the cause of cystitis.
- A frequent need to urinate and pain or burning while urinating are the most common symptoms.
- Doctors can base the diagnosis on the symptoms, but they usually examine a urine specimen.
- Drugs are needed to treat the infection and often the symptoms.

Interstitial Cystitis: Bladder Inflammation, Not Infection

Interstitial cystitis is painful inflammation of the bladder without evidence of infection. It is usually chronic. The cause is unknown. No infectious organisms are found in the urine. Typically, middle-aged women are affected. It is very unusual for men to be affected.

Symptoms include very frequent, painful urination. The urine may contain pus and blood, which are detected by microscopic examination. Over time, the inflammation may cause the bladder to shrink. An examination of the bladder by cystoscopy may detect small, shallow areas of bleeding and ulceration.

A number of treatments have been tried, but none is routinely satisfactory. Drugs to relieve pain, anticholinergic drugs, or antidepressants sometimes help. Pentosan is a drug taken by mouth that may provide pain relief for some people. Dimethyl sulfoxide, a drug instilled directly into the bladder, can also be of benefit. In extreme cases, when the person has intolerable symptoms that do not respond to treatment, the bladder may need to be surgically removed. In such instances, a new bladder is created from a segment of the intestine.

Causes

Women: Cystitis is common among women, particularly during the reproductive years. Some women have recurring episodes of cystitis. There are a number of reasons why women are susceptible, including the short length of the urethra and the closeness of the urethra to the vagina and anus, where bacteria are commonly found. Sexual intercourse can contribute, too, because the motion can cause a tendency for bacteria to reach the urethra, from which they ascend to the bladder. Pregnant women are especially likely to develop cystitis because the pregnancy itself can interfere with emptying of the bladder.

Use of a diaphragm increases the risk of developing cystitis, possibly because spermicide used with the diaphragm suppresses the normal vaginal bacteria and allows bacteria that cause cystitis to flourish in the vagina.

The decrease in estrogen production that occurs after menopause can thin the vaginal and vulvar tissues around the urethra (atrophic vaginitis and atrophic urethritis), which can predispose a woman to repeated episodes of cystitis. In addition, a drooping (prolapsed) uterus or bladder may cause poor emptying of the bladder and predispose to cystitis. A prolapsed uterus or bladder is more common among women who have had many children.

Rarely, cystitis recurs because of an abnormal connection between the bladder and the vagina (vesicovaginal fistula).

Men: Cystitis is less common among men. In men, cystitis generally starts with an infection in the urethra that moves into the prostate, then into the bladder. The most common cause of recurring cystitis in men is a persistent bacterial infection of the prostate. Although antibiotics quickly clear bacteria from the urine in the bladder, most of these drugs cannot penetrate well enough into the prostate to quickly cure an infection there. Usually antibiotics must be taken for weeks at a time. Consequently, if drug therapy is stopped prematurely, bacteria that remain in the prostate tend to reinfect the bladder.

Both Sexes: If the flow of urine becomes partly obstructed because of a stone in the bladder or urethra, an enlarged prostate (in men), or a stricture in the urethra, bacteria that enter the urinary tract are less likely to be flushed out with urine. Bacteria that are left in the bladder after voiding can multiply rapidly. The more bacteria in the bladder, the more likely is infection. People with longstanding or repeated obstruction of urine flow may develop a bladder outpouching (diverticulum). This pocket retains urine after voiding, further increasing the risk of infection.

Cystitis can also be caused by a catheter or any instrument inserted into the urinary tract that introduces bacteria into the bladder. In men and women, an abnormal connection between the bladder and the intestine (vesicoenteric fistula) can develop, allowing fecal material to pass from the intestine into the bladder, causing bladder infection.

Sometimes the bladder can become inflamed without an infection being present (interstitial cystitis).

Symptoms

Cystitis usually causes a frequent, urgent need to urinate and a burning or painful sensation while urinating. These symptoms usually develop over several hours or a day. The urgent need to urinate may cause an uncontrollable loss of urine (urge incontinence), especially in older people. Fever is rarely present. Pain is usually felt above the pubic bone and often in the lower back as well. Frequent urination during the night (nocturia) may be another symptom. The urine is often cloudy and contains visible blood in about 30% of people. Air can be passed in the urine (pneumaturia) when infection results from an abnormal connection between the bladder and the intestine or the vagina (fistula).

Symptoms of cystitis may disappear without treatment. Sometimes cystitis causes no symptoms, particularly in older people, and is discovered when urine tests are performed for other reasons. A person whose bladder is malfunctioning because of nerve damage (neurogenic bladder—see page 293) or a person who has a permanently placed catheter may have cystitis with no symptoms until a kidney infection or an unexplained fever develops.

Diagnosis

Doctors can usually diagnose cystitis based on its typical symptoms. A midstream (clean-catch) urine specimen (see box on page 258) is collected so that the urine is not contaminated with bacteria from the vagina or the tip of the penis. A strip of test paper is sometimes dipped into the urine to perform two quick and simple tests for substances that are normally not found in the urine. The testing strip can detect nitrites that are released by bacteria. The testing strip can also detect leukocyte esterase (an enzyme found in certain white blood cells), which may indicate that the body is trying to clear the urine of bacteria. In adult women, these may be the only tests necessary.

In addition, the urine specimen can be examined under a microscope to see whether it contains red or white blood cells or other substances. Bacteria are counted, and the sample can be cultured to identify the numbers and type of bacteria. If the person has an infection, one type of bacteria is usually present in large numbers.

> ### ❓ Did You Know...
>
> It is not clear whether wiping from front to back or avoiding the use of tight, nonporous underwear helps women prevent bladder infections.
>
> In contrast, cranberry juice does seem to help prevent infections.

In men, a midstream urine specimen is usually sufficient for a urine culture. In women, a specimen is more likely to be contaminated with bacteria from the vagina or vulva. When the urine contains only small numbers of bacteria, or several different types of bacteria simultaneously, the urine has likely been contaminated during the collection process. To ensure that the urine is not contaminated, doctors sometimes must obtain a specimen directly from the bladder with a catheter.

It is important for doctors to find the cause of cystitis in several different groups. The cause should be found in children, in men of any age, and in some women with frequently recurring infections (3 or more per year), especially when accompanied by symptoms of obstruction, an upper urinary tract infection, or infection with the *Proteus* bacteria. In these types of people, there is a greater likelihood of finding a cause that requires treatment other than simply giving drugs to treat the infection (for example, a large kidney

stone). Doctors may perform an x-ray study in which a radiopaque dye, visible on x-rays, is injected into a vein, then excreted into the urine by the kidneys (intravenous urogram, or IVU). The x-rays then provide images of the kidneys, ureters, and bladder. Ultrasonography or computed tomography (CT) may be done instead of IVU. Performing voiding cystourethrography, which involves injecting a radiopaque dye into the bladder and filming its exit, is a good way to investigate the backflow (reflux) of urine from the bladder, up the ureters, particularly in children, and may also identify any narrowing (stricture) of the urethra. Retrograde urethrography, in which the radiopaque dye is injected directly into the urethra, is useful for detecting stricture, outpouching, or an abnormal connection (fistula) of the urethra in both men and women. Looking directly into the bladder with a flexible viewing tube (cystoscopy) may help diagnose the problem when cystitis does not resolve with treatment.

Prevention

People who have frequent bladder infections may continuously take low doses of antibiotics. The antibiotic can be taken daily, 3 times a week, or immediately after sexual intercourse. Postmenopausal women

---

Preventing Bladder Infections in Women

In women who experience three or more bladder infections in a year, these measures may help:

- Drinking cranberry juice (about 10 ounces [about 300 milliliters] of juice or 2 ounces [about 50 milliliters] of concentrate per day) or taking cranberry pills, because cranberry fruit contains a substance that directly inhibits bacterial attachment to the bladder and because it acidifies the urine (making it a less hospitable environment for bacterial growth)
- Increasing the intake of fluids
- Urinating often
- Urinating within a short time after sexual intercourse
- Avoiding the use of spermicides (used with a diaphragm for birth control)
- Taking antibiotics continually in low doses. Typically, the antibiotic is taken daily, 3 times a week, or immediately after sexual intercourse
- For postmenopausal women who have atrophic vaginitis or atrophic urethritis, applying estrogen cream to the vulva or inserting estrogen suppositories into the vagina

with frequent bladder infections and atrophic vaginitis or atrophic urethritis may benefit from estrogen creams applied to the vulva or estrogen suppositories inserted into the vagina.

Drinking plenty of fluids may help to prevent cystitis. The flushing action of the urine washes many bacteria out of the bladder. The body's natural defenses eliminate the remainder of the bacteria. It is commonly believed that wiping from front to back, urinating soon after sexual intercourse, and avoiding the use of tight, nonporous underwear helps women prevent bladder infections. However, it is not clear whether any of these strategies is effective.

Treatment

Cystitis is usually treated with antibiotics. Before prescribing antibiotics, the doctor determines whether the person has a condition that would make cystitis more severe, such as diabetes or a weakened immune system (which reduces the person's ability to fight infection), or more difficult to eliminate, such as a structural abnormality. Such conditions may require more potent antibiotics taken for a longer period of time, particularly because the infection is likely to return as soon as the person stops taking antibiotics.

For women, taking an antibiotic by mouth for 3 days is usually effective if the infection has not led to any complications, although some doctors prefer to give a single dose. For more stubborn infections, an antibiotic is usually taken for 7 to 10 days. For men, cystitis usually is caused by prostatitis, and antibiotic treatment is usually required for weeks.

A variety of drugs can relieve symptoms, especially the frequent, insistent urge to urinate and painful urination. Drugs that have anticholinergic effects (such as oxybutynin and tolterodine) may relieve bladder spasms that cause the sense of urgency. These drugs should be used with caution in men with a large prostate gland because the drugs may cause urinary retention. Other drugs, such as phenazopyridine, reduce the pain by soothing the inflamed tissues.

Surgery may be necessary to relieve any physical obstruction to the flow of urine or to correct a structural abnormality that makes infection more likely, such as a drooping uterus or bladder. Until surgery can occur, draining urine from an obstructed area through a catheter helps control the infection. Usually, an antibiotic is given before surgery to reduce the risk of the infection spreading throughout the body.

Pyelonephritis

Pyelonephritis is a bacterial infection of one or both kidneys.

- Infection can spread up the urinary tract to the kidneys, or the kidneys may become infected through bacteria in the bloodstream.

- Chills, fever, back pain, nausea, and vomiting can occur.
- Urine and sometimes blood tests are done to diagnose pyelonephritis.
- Antibiotics are given to treat the infection.

Causes

Pyelonephritis is more common among women than men. *Escherichia coli*, a type of bacteria normally in the large intestine, causes about 90% of cases of pyelonephritis among people who are not hospitalized or living in a nursing home. Infections usually ascend from the genital area through the urethra to the bladder, up the ureters, into the kidneys. In a person with a healthy urinary tract, an infection is usually prevented from moving up the ureters into the kidneys by the flow of urine washing organisms out and by closure of the ureters at their entrance to the bladder. However, any physical obstruction to the flow of urine, such as a structural abnormality, kidney stone, or an enlarged prostate, or the backflow (reflux) of urine from the bladder into the ureters increases the likelihood of pyelonephritis. The risk of pyelonephritis is increased during pregnancy. During pregnancy, the enlarging uterus puts pressure on the ureters, which partially obstructs the normal downward flow of urine. Pregnancy also increases the risk of reflux of urine up the ureters by causing the ureters to dilate and reducing the muscle contractions that propel urine down the ureters into the bladder.

Infections can also be carried to the kidneys from another part of the body through the bloodstream. For instance, a staphylococcal skin infection can spread to the kidneys through the bloodstream.

The risk and severity of pyelonephritis are increased in people with diabetes or a weakened immune system (which reduces the body's ability to fight infection). Pyelonephritis is usually caused by bacteria, but rarely it is caused by tuberculosis, fungal infections, and viruses.

Some people develop long-standing infection (chronic pyelonephritis). Almost all of them have major underlying abnormalities, such as a urinary tract obstruction, large kidney stones that persist, or, more commonly, reflux of urine from the bladder into the ureters (which occurs mostly in young children). Chronic pyelonephritis can cause bacteria to be released into the bloodstream, sometimes resulting in infections in the opposite kidney or elsewhere in the body. Rarely, chronic pyelonephritis can eventually severely damage the kidneys.

Some people develop xanthogranulomatous pyelonephritis, an unusual type of chronic pyelonephritis that is usually caused by kidney stones. Severe kidney scarring (causing permanent kidney damage) and kidney abscesses (causing fever and severe pain) often develop.

Symptoms

Symptoms of pyelonephritis often begin suddenly with chills, fever, pain in the lower part of the back on either side, nausea, and vomiting.

About one third of people with pyelonephritis also have symptoms of cystitis, including frequent, painful urination. One or both kidneys may be enlarged and painful, and doctors may find tenderness in the small of the back on the affected side. Sometimes the muscles of the abdomen are tightly contracted. Irritation from the infection or the passing of a kidney stone (if one is present) can cause spasms of the ureters. If the ureters go into spasms, people may experience episodes of intense pain (renal colic). In children, symptoms of a kidney infection often are slight and more difficult to recognize (see page 1767). In older people, pyelonephritis may not cause any symptoms that seem to indicate a problem in the urinary tract. Instead, older people may have delirium or an infection of the bloodstream (sepsis).

In chronic pyelonephritis, the pain may be vague, and fever may come and go or not occur at all.

Diagnosis

The typical symptoms of pyelonephritis lead doctors to perform two common laboratory tests to determine whether the kidneys are infected: examining a urine specimen under a microscope and culturing bacteria in a urine specimen to determine which bacteria are present. Blood tests may be performed to check for elevated white blood cells or bacteria in the blood.

Additional tests are performed in people who have intense back pain typical of renal colic, in those who do not respond to antibiotic treatment within 48 hours, in those whose symptoms return shortly after antibiotic treatment is finished, in those with long-standing or recurrent pyelonephritis, and in men (because they so rarely develop pyelonephritis). Ultrasonography or helical (spiral) computed tomography (CT) studies performed in these situations may reveal kidney stones, structural abnormalities, or other causes of urinary obstruction.

Prognosis

Most people recover fully. Delayed recovery and the chance of complications are more likely if the person needs hospitalization, the infecting organism is resistant to commonly used antibiotics, or the person has a disorder that weakens the immune system (such as certain cancers, diabetes mellitus, or AIDS) or a kidney stone.

Prevention and Treatment

Antibiotics are started as soon as the doctor suspects pyelonephritis and samples have been taken for laboratory tests. The choice of drug or its dosage may be modified based on the laboratory test results (including culture results), how sick the person is, and whether the infection started in the hospital, where bacteria tend to be more resistant to antibiotics.

Outpatient treatment with antibiotics given by mouth is usually successful if the person has:

- No nausea or vomiting
- No signs of dehydration
- No other disorders that weaken the immune system, such as certain cancers, diabetes mellitus, or AIDS
- No signs of very severe infection, such as low blood pressure or confusion
- Pain that is controlled with drugs taken by mouth

Otherwise, the person is usually treated initially in the hospital. If hospitalization is needed and the person needs antibiotics, the antibiotics are given intravenously for 1 or 2 days, then they can usually be given by mouth.

Antibiotic treatment of pyelonephritis is given for 14 days so that infection will not recur. However, antibiotic therapy may continue for up to 6 weeks for men in whom the infection is due to prostatitis, which is more difficult to eradicate. A final urine sample is usually taken shortly after the antibiotic treatment is finished to make sure the infection has been eradicated.

Surgery may be needed if tests reveal a predisposing condition, such as an obstruction, a structural abnormality, or a stone. Surgical removal of the infected kidney is usually necessary for people with xanthogranulomatous pyelonephritis because repeated infections are likely. Removal of the infected kidney may also be necessary for people with chronic pyelonephritis who are about to undergo a kidney transplant. Spread of infection to the transplanted kidney is particularly risky because the person takes immunosuppressant drugs, which prevent rejection of the transplanted kidney but also weaken the body's ability to fight infection.

People who have frequent episodes of pyelonephritis or whose infection returns after antibiotic treatment is finished may be advised to take a small dose of antibiotic every day as preventive therapy. The ideal duration of such therapy is unknown, but it is often stopped after a year. If the infection returns, preventive therapy may be continued indefinitely. If a woman of child-bearing age is taking an antibiotic, she should avoid pregnancy or talk to her doctor about whether to use an antibiotic that is safe during pregnancy in case she becomes pregnant.

Asymptomatic Bacteriuria

Asymptomatic bacteriuria is a condition in which larger than normal numbers of bacteria are present in the urine but symptoms do not result.

Asymptomatic bacteriuria is not normally treated because eradicating the bacteria can be difficult and complications are usually rare. Also, giving antibiotics can alter the balance of bacteria in the body, sometimes allowing bacteria to flourish that are more difficult to eliminate.

> **? Did You Know...**
> Most people who have excess bacteria in the urine and have no symptoms should not be treated.

An exception is if the person has a condition that makes a urinary tract infection particularly risky. Such conditions may include pregnancy, a kidney transplant, taking drugs that suppress the immune system, or having a condition that suppresses the immune system (for example, AIDS, certain cancers, or having a low white blood cell count). For example, cystitis can seriously complicate pregnancy by ascending to the kidneys and causing pyelonephritis, leading to early labor. Also, a urinary tract infection can permanently damage one or both kidneys after a kidney transplant. A urinary tract infection can cause potentially fatal bloodstream infection in people whose immune system is suppressed by a drug or disorder. Sometimes, the immune system becomes suppressed after cancer chemotherapy. Asymptomatic bacteriuria is also sometimes treated in people who have certain kinds of kidney stones that cannot be eliminated and cause repeated urinary tract infections.

CHAPTER 50 Injury to the Urinary Tract

The kidneys and the rest of the urinary tract may become injured in a number of ways. Examples include injuries from a blunt force (most commonly motor vehicle collisions, falls, or sports injuries) or a pentrating force (most commonly gunshot or stab wounds), or surgery. Injuries to the urinary tract often occur with injuries to other organs, especially abdominal organs. In men, the penis and testes may also be injured (see page 1470).

Because the function of the kidneys is to continuously filter out metabolic wastes from the blood and remove them from the body through the urinary tract, injuries to the kidneys or urinary tract can lead to the inability to perform these functions (kidney failure). Other complications of injury include bleeding, leakage of urine from the urinary tract into surrounding tissues, and infection. Preventing permanent damage to the urinary tract and even death may depend on prompt diagnosis and treatment.

Bladder Injuries

A bladder injury often occurs when the pelvis is injured, as in a high-speed motor vehicle collision or a fall. Penetrating wounds, usually from gunshots, also can injure the bladder. In addition, a bladder injury may occur unintentionally during surgery involving the pelvis or lower abdomen (such as hysterectomy, cesarean section, or colectomy).

If bladder injuries are not promptly treated, complications, such as frequent and urgent urination, uncontrollable loss of urine (urinary incontinence), and infection, may develop.

Symptoms and Diagnosis

The most common symptoms of a bladder injury are blood in the urine, difficulty in urinating, and pain in the pelvis and lower abdomen. If the lowermost portion of the bladder (where the muscle that helps to control urination is located) has been injured, the person may experience frequent urination or urinary incontinence.

The diagnosis of a bladder injury is best established by cystography, a procedure in which a radiopaque dye (contrast agent), which is visible on x-rays, is injected into the bladder and a computed tomography (CT) scan or x-rays are taken to look for leakage. Bladder injuries that occur during a surgical procedure are usually recognized promptly and imaging tests are not needed.

Treatment

Minor bladder injuries, either bruises or tears (lacerations), may be treated by inserting a catheter into the urethra for 5 to 10 days while the bladder heals. For more extensive bladder injuries or any injury resulting in leakage of urine into the abdominal cavity, surgery should be performed to determine the extent of the injury and to repair all tears. The urine can then be more effectively drained from the bladder using two catheters, one inserted through the urethra (a transurethral catheter) and one inserted directly into the bladder through the skin over the lower abdomen (a suprapubic catheter). These catheters are removed in 7 to 10 days or once the bladder has healed satisfactorily. If complications develop, they must be treated.

When a bladder injury is recognized during a surgical procedure, it is treated at that time.

Kidney Injuries

The kidney is injured more often than any of the organs along the urinary tract. Blunt force due to motor vehicle collisions, falls, or sports injuries is the usual cause of injury. Penetrating kidney injuries can result from gunshot or stab wounds. Less commonly, injuries can occur during diagnostic tests, such as a kidney biopsy, or during various treatments, such as those for kidney stones, including extracorporeal shock wave lithotripsy. Most blunt kidney injuries are minor. However, some are serious. If serious blunt or penetrating kidney injuries are not treated, complications, such as kidney failure, high blood pressure, delayed bleeding, and infection, may result.

Symptoms and Diagnosis

Symptoms of a blunt kidney injury may include pain in the upper abdomen or flank (the area between the ribs and hip), bruising of the flank, blood in the urine, marks near a kidney made by a seat belt, or pain resulting from fractures of the lower ribs. With severe kidney injuries, low blood pressure (shock) and anemia may occur if the person loses a significant amount of blood.

The history of events that led to the injury, the person's symptoms, and a physical examination help doctors recognize kidney injuries. A sample of urine is taken and examined to see whether blood is present. Blood in the urine in a person with an injury to the trunk suggests that the injury involves the kidney. The blood may be visible with the naked eye (gross hematuria) or visible only using a microscope (microscopic hematuria). With penetrating injuries, the location of the wound (whether in the upper or mid part of the abdomen, back, or flank) may help doctors determine whether the kidney is involved.

Adults who have mild symptoms and blood in the urine that is visible only with a microscope probably have a minor bruise that will heal on its own. Further tests are usually not needed. For children, and for adults in whom doctors suspect a more serious injury, computed tomography (CT) with radiopaque dye (contrast agent) is done. Occasionally, additional imaging tests may be needed to confirm the diagnosis.

Treatment

For minor kidney injuries, careful control of fluid intake and bed rest are often the only treatment needed, because these measures allow the kidney to heal itself. For more serious injuries, treatment begins with steps to control blood loss and to prevent shock.

Kidney Injuries: Minor to Severe

The severity of kidney injuries varies widely. When an injury is minor, the kidney may only be bruised. When an injury is more severe, the kidney may be cut or torn (lacerated), and urine and blood may leak into the surrounding tissue. If the kidney is torn from its attachment to blood vessels, bleeding may be profuse, resulting in shock or death. Most kidney injuries result in blood in the urine.

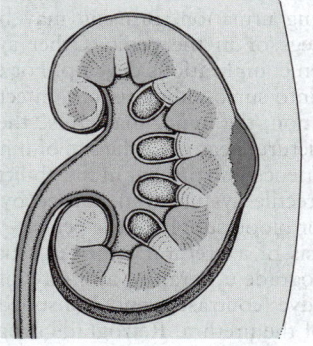

Bruise

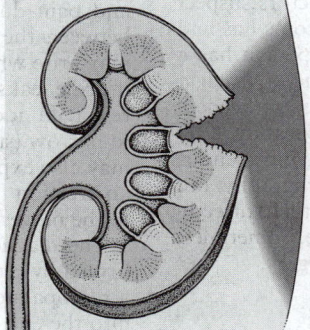

Laceration

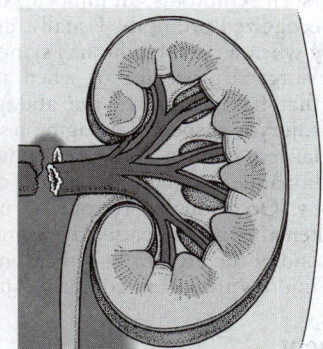

Torn Attachment

Fluids and sometimes blood are given intravenously to help keep blood pressure within a normal range and stimulate urine production. Only the most serious injuries, such as when the kidney is torn from its attachments to blood vessels, require surgical repair. Rarely, the injured kidney needs to be removed.

Most people recover from even serious kidney injuries, provided the injuries are diagnosed and treated promptly. Kidney failure, when it develops, may require lifelong treatment. Other complications of kidney injuries that require treatment include high blood pressure, delayed bleeding, and infection.

Ureteral Injuries

Most injuries to the ureter occur during pelvic or abdominal operations, such as removal of the uterus (hysterectomy) or the colon (colectomy) or repair of an abdominal aortic aneurysm, or during ureteroscopy (an examination of the ureter with a rigid or flexible viewing tube). Another cause of ureteral injury is penetration by either a gunshot or stab wound. A ureteral injury from a direct blow to the body is uncommon. Rarely, blunt injuries, particularly those that cause the trunk to bend backward, can separate the upper part of the ureter from the kidney.

If ureteral injuries are untreated, complications, such as formation of a fistula (abnormal connection to another abdominal structure), stricture (narrowing of the ureter), or persistent urinary leakage and infection, may result.

Symptoms and Diagnosis

People may complain simply of pain in the abdomen or flank (the area between the ribs and hip), or they may notice urine leaking from their wound. Fever may accompany an infection caused by persistent urinary leakage. Blood may appear in the urine.

Because ureteral injury is rarely the most likely cause of such symptoms, an injury to the ureter may not be recognized promptly. Usually, doctors suspect an injury when a person who has symptoms has had a recent surgical procedure or when a person has a wound that has penetrated the abdomen. When a ureteral injury is suspected, imaging tests are needed. The initial test is often computed tomography (CT) with radiopaque dye (contrast agent) or intravenous urography. Occasionally, retrograde urography (an x-ray taken after a radiopaque dye is instilled directly into the end of the urethra) may be done. Sometimes, ureteral injuries are identified during surgery.

Treatment

Some minor ureteral injuries can be treated by placing a flexible tube (stent) in the ureter either through the bladder or through the kidney via a small incision in the side (percutaneous nephrostomy). These treatments divert urine from flowing through the ureter, usually for 2 to 6 weeks, allowing the ureter to heal. If the ureteral injury does not heal despite the use of a stent, additional surgery may be needed. In people with more severe injuries, surgery may be required to reconstruct the ureter.

Treatment helps to prevent complications of ureteral injuries. If complications occur despite efforts to prevent them, they must be treated.

Urethral Injuries

Most urethral injuries occur in men. Common causes include pelvic fractures and straddle injuries (injuries to the area between the legs). The urethra can also be injured unintentionally during surgical procedures performed directly on the urethra or during procedures in which instruments are passed into the urethra, such as bladder catheterization or cystoscopy (passing a flexible viewing tube through the urethra into the bladder). Occasionally, injuries result from gunshot wounds. Rarely, urethral injuries can be self-inflicted when a person inserts a foreign object directly into the urethra.

Some injuries to the urethra are limited to bruising. Injury to the urethra can also tear the lining, resulting in leakage of urine into the tissues of the penis, scrotum, abdominal wall, or perineum (the area between the anus and vulva or scrotum).

Complications that can result from urethral injuries include infection, bleeding, permanent narrowing (stricture), erectile dysfunction, and uncontrollable loss of urine (urinary incontinence).

Symptoms and Diagnosis

The most common symptoms include blood at the tip of the penis in men or the urethral opening in women, blood in the urine, an inability to urinate, and pain during urination. Bruising may be visible between the legs or in the penis. Other symptoms may arise when complications develop. For example, if urine leaks into surrounding tissues, infection may result. In addition, the injury may cause the urethra to narrow (stricture) near or at the site of injury. Men may also experience impairment in the ability to have an erection (erectile dysfunction), caused by damage to the nerves or blood supply to the penis.

The diagnosis of a urethral injury is usually confirmed by retrograde urography, an x-ray taken after a radiopaque dye (contrast agent) is instilled directly into the end of the urethra. Retrograde urography is done before a catheter is passed through the urethra into the bladder.

Treatment

For urethral bruises that do not result in any leakage of urine, a doctor can place a catheter through the urethra into the bladder for several days to drain the urine while the urethra heals. For urethral tears, the urine should be diverted from the urethra using a catheter placed directly into the bladder through the skin over the lower abdomen. The urethra is repaired surgically after all other injuries have healed or after 8 to 12 weeks (when inflammation has resolved). Rarely, urethral tears heal without surgery.

Treatment helps to prevent some complications of urethral injuries. Complications that cannot be prevented are treated.

CHAPTER

51 Cancers of the Kidney and Urinary Tract

Most tumors of the kidney and urinary tract affect men and women alike and may occur in people of any age. Most of these tumors are cancerous (malignant).

Kidney Cancer

- Kidney cancer may cause blood in the urine, pain in the side, or fever.
- Cancer may be detected by accident when an imaging test is done for another reason.
- Diagnosis is by computed tomography or magnetic resonance imaging.
- If cancer has not spread, removing the kidney may be curative.

Kidney cancer accounts for about 2 to 3% of cancers in adults, affecting about 50% more men than women. Smokers are about twice as likely to develop kidney cancer as nonsmokers. Other risk factors include exposure to toxic chemicals and obesity. People affected are usually between 50 and 70 years of age.

Most solid kidney tumors are cancerous, but fluid-filled tumors (cysts) generally are not. Almost all kidney cancer is renal cell carcinoma. Another kind of kidney cancer, Wilms' tumor, occurs in children (see page 1848).

Symptoms

Blood in the urine is the most common first symptom, but the amount of blood may be so small that it can be detected only under a microscope. On the other hand, the urine may be visibly red. The next most common symptoms are pain in the flank (the area between the ribs and hip), fever, and weight loss. Infrequently, a kidney cancer is first detected when a doctor feels an enlargement or lump in the abdomen.

The red blood cell count may become abnormally high (polycythemia) because high levels of the hormone erythropoietin (which is produced by the diseased kidney or by the tumor itself) stimulate the bone marrow to increase the production of red blood cells. Symptoms of a high red blood cell count may be absent or may include headache, fatigue, dizziness, and visual disturbances. Conversely, kidney cancer may lead to a drop in the red blood cell count (anemia) because of slow bleeding into the urine. Anemia may cause easy fatigability or dizziness. Some people develop high levels of calcium in the blood (hypercalcemia), which may cause weakness, fatigue, slowed reaction times, and constipation.

Diagnosis

Today, most kidney cancers are discovered by chance when an imaging test such as computed tomography (CT) or ultrasonography is done to evaluate another problem, such as high blood pressure. If doctors suspect kidney cancer based on a person's symptoms, they use CT or magnetic resonance imaging (MRI) to confirm the diagnosis. Ultrasonography or intravenous urography may also be used initially, but doctors must use CT to verify the diagnosis. If cancer is diagnosed, other imaging tests (for example, chest x-ray, bone scan, or CT of the head, chest, or both) may be done to determine whether and where the cancer has spread. However, sometimes cancer that has recently spread cannot be detected.

Prognosis

Many factors affect prognosis, but the 5-year survival rate for people with cancer confined to the kidney is 85% or better. If the cancer has spread into the renal vein or the vena cava but has not spread to distant sites, the 5-year survival rate is 35 to 60%. When cancer has spread to distant sites, the 5-year survival rate is no higher than 10%. In some instances, the goal is to focus on pain relief and other means to improve the person's comfort (see page 61). As with all terminal illnesses, planning for end-of-life issues, including creating advance directives, is essential (see page 69).

Treatment

When the cancer has not spread (metastasized) beyond the kidney, surgically removing the affected kidney provides a reasonable chance of cure. Alternatively, surgeons may remove only the tumor with a rim of adjacent normal tissue, which spares the remainder of the kidney.

If the cancer has spread into adjacent sites such as the renal vein or even the large vein that carries blood to the heart (vena cava) but has not spread to distant sites, surgery may still provide a chance for cure. However, kidney cancer has a tendency to spread early, especially to the lungs, sometimes before symptoms develop. Because kidney cancer that has spread to distant sites may escape early diagnosis, metastasis sometimes becomes apparent only after doctors have surgically removed all of the kidney cancer that could be found.

Treating the cancer by enhancing the immune system's ability to destroy it causes some cancers to shrink and may prolong survival (see page 1092). One such treatment, interleukin-2, is used for kidney cancer. Various combinations of interleukin-2, interferon, and other biologic agents and even vaccines developed from cells removed from the kidney cancer are being investigated. These treatments may be helpful for metastatic cancer, although the benefit is usually small. For people with metastatic cancer, recently developed treatments include the drugs sunitinib, sorafenib, and temsirolimus. These drugs alter molecular pathways that affect the tumor and are thus called targeted therapies. Rarely (in less than 1% of people), removing the affected kidney causes tumors elsewhere in the body to shrink. However, the slim possibility that tumor shrinkage will occur is not considered sufficient reason to remove a cancerous kidney when the cancer has already spread, unless removal is part of an overall plan that includes other systemic therapies.

Renal Pelvis and Ureter Cancer

- Cancers may cause blood in the urine or crampy pain in the side.
- Diagnosis is by computed tomography.
- Treatment is removal of the kidney and ureter.

Cancer can occur in the cells lining the central collecting area of the kidney (the renal pelvis—usually a type called transitional cell carcinoma of the renal pelvis) and in the slender tubes that carry urine from the kidney to the bladder (ureters). Cancers of the renal pelvis and ureter are much less common than cancers of the rest of the kidney or bladder. They probably occur in fewer than 6,000 people in the United States each year.

Symptoms

Blood in the urine is usually the first symptom. Crampy pain in the flank (the space between the ribs and hip) or lower abdomen may occur if the flow of urine is obstructed (for example, because a blood clot blocks the ureter).

Diagnosis

The cancer is usually detected by using computed tomography (CT) scanning. CT can help doctors distinguish other noncancerous (benign) kidney and ureteral problems such as stones or blood clots. Microscopic examination of a urine sample may reveal cancer cells. A flexible viewing tube—a ureteroscope—threaded up through the bladder may be used to view, and occasionally even treat, small cancers.

Prognosis

If the cancer has not spread and if it can be completely removed surgically, cure is likely. However, if the cancer has spread into the wall of the renal pelvis or ureter or to distant sites, cure is unlikely.

Treatment

If the cancer has not spread beyond the area of the renal pelvis and ureter, the usual treatment is surgical removal of the entire kidney and ureter (nephroureterectomy) along with a small part of the bladder. However, in some situations—for example, when the kidneys are not functioning well or a person has only one kidney—the kidney is usually not removed, because the person would then become dependent on dialysis. Some cancers in the renal pelvis and ureter may be treated with a laser to destroy the cancer cells or with surgery that removes only the cancer itself while leaving the kidney, the noncancerous portion of the ureter, and the bladder in place. If the cancer has spread, chemotherapy is also used.

A cystoscopy (insertion of a flexible viewing tube to examine the inside of the bladder) is done periodically after surgery, indefinitely, because people who have had this type of cancer are at risk of developing bladder cancer.

Bladder Cancer

- Bladder cancer most often causes blood in the urine.
- To make the diagnosis, a thin, flexible viewing tube (cystoscope) is inserted through the urethra into the bladder.
- Many cancers are treated with removal, using a cystoscope (for surface cancers) or by removing the bladder (for deeper cancers).

An estimated 67,000 new cases of bladder cancer are diagnosed every year in the United States. About 3 times as many men as women develop bladder cancer. Smoking is the greatest single risk factor and seems to be one of the causes in at least half of all new cases. Certain chemicals that are used in industry can become concentrated in the urine and cause cancer, although exposure to these chemicals is decreasing. The chronic irritation that occurs with a parasitic infection called schistosomiasis or with a bladder stone also predisposes people to bladder cancer, although irritation accounts for only a small proportion of all cases.

Most bladder cancers are of a type called transitional cell, affecting the same kinds of cells (transitional cells) that are usually the cancerous cells responsible for renal pelvis and ureter cancers.

Symptoms

Bladder cancer most often causes blood in the urine. Later symptoms may include pain and burning during urination and an urgent, frequent need to urinate. The symptoms of bladder cancer may be identical to those of a bladder infection (cystitis—see page 303), and the two problems may occur together. A low blood count (anemia) may cause fatigue, paleness, or both.

Diagnosis

The diagnosis is often first suspected when blood is found in the urine. Blood may be detected when a routine microscopic examination of a urine specimen detects red blood cells, or sometimes the urine may be visibly red. Bladder cancer may be suspected if the symptoms of cystitis do not disappear with treatment. Special microscopic evaluation of urine (such as cytology—see page 260) may detect cancer cells. Sometimes bladder cancer is detected when an imaging study such as computed tomography (CT) or ultrasonography is done for another reason.

Most bladder cancers are diagnosed by cystoscopy. This examination involves passing a thin, flexible viewing tube through the urethra into the bladder. The person is awake. The urethra is anesthetized somewhat so the procedure is not very uncomfortable.

Prognosis

For cancers that remain on the bladder's inner surface (superficial tumors) and grow and divide slowly, the risk of death from bladder cancer is less than 5% in the 5 years after diagnosis. The 5-year death rate for tumors that invade the bladder muscle is significantly higher (40 to 55%). Bladder cancers that have spread beyond the bladder wall (such as to the lymph nodes or other abdominal or pelvic organs) have a much poorer prognosis.

Treatment

Cancers that are on only the bladder's inner surface may be removed completely during cystoscopy. However, people commonly develop new cancers later within the bladder. Doctors may be able to prevent the recurrence of these cancers by repeatedly putting anticancer drugs or bacille Calmette-Guérin (BCG—a substance that stimulates the body's immune system) into the bladder after all of the cancer has been removed.

Cancers that have grown into the bladder wall cannot be completely removed through a cystoscope. They are usually treated by total or partial removal of the bladder (cystectomy). Radiation therapy alone or in combination with chemotherapy may also be used in an attempt to cure the cancer.

If the entire bladder needs to be removed, doctors must devise a method for the person to be able to drain urine. The usual way has been to route the urine to an opening (stoma) made in the abdominal wall through a passageway made of intestine, called an ileal loop. The urine is then collected in a bag worn on the outside of the body.

Several alternative methods of diverting urine are becoming increasingly common and are appropriate for most people. These methods can be grouped into two categories: an orthotopic neobladder and a continent urinary diversion. In both, an internal reservoir for urine is constructed from the intestine.

For an orthotopic neobladder, the reservoir is connected to the urethra. The person learns to empty this reservoir by relaxing the pelvic floor muscles and increasing pressure within the abdomen, so that urine passes through the urethra very much as it would naturally. Most people are dry during the day, but some urine leakage may occur at night.

For a continent urinary diversion, the reservoir is connected to a stoma in the abdominal wall. A collecting bag is not needed, because the urine remains in the reservoir until the person empties it by inserting a catheter through the stoma into the reservoir, which is done at regular intervals throughout the day.

Cancer that has spread beyond the bladder to the lymph nodes or other organs is treated with chemotherapy. Several different combinations of drugs are active against this type of cancer, particularly when the spread is confined to the lymph nodes. Cystectomy or radiation may be offered to people who respond well to chemotherapy. However, a relatively small number of people are cured. For people who are not cured, efforts are directed at pain relief and end-of-life issues (see page 57).

Urethral Cancer

Cancer of the urethra (the channel that carries urine from the bladder out of the body) is rare, occurring most commonly after age 50. It can occur in men and women. Certain types of human papillomavirus are implicated as the cause of cancer of the urethra in some people. Otherwise, the cause is unknown.

The first symptom is usually blood in the urine. The amount of blood may be so small that it can be detected only under a microscope. On the other hand, the urine may be visibly red. The flow of urine may become obstructed, making urination difficult or the stream of urine slow and thin. Fragile, bleeding growths at the external opening of a woman's urethra may be cancerous. A biopsy must be performed to positively identify a cancer.

Radiation therapy, surgical removal, or a combination of both has been used to treat cancer of the urethra with variable results. The prognosis of cancer of the urethra depends on the precise location and extent of the cancer.

Heart and Blood Vessel Disorders

CHAPTER

52   Biology of the Heart and Blood Vessels

The heart and blood vessels constitute the cardiovascular (circulatory) system. The blood circulating in this system delivers oxygen and nutrients to the tissues of the body and removes waste products from the tissues.

Heart

The heart, a hollow muscular organ, is located in the center of the chest. The right and left sides of the heart each have an upper chamber (atrium), which collects blood and pumps it into a lower chamber (ventricle), which pumps blood out.

To ensure that blood flows in only one direction, each ventricle has an "in" (inlet) valve and an "out" (outlet) valve. In the left ventricle, the inlet valve is the mitral valve, and the outlet valve is the aortic valve. In the right ventricle, the inlet valve is the tricuspid valve, and the outlet valve is the pulmonary (pulmonic) valve. Each valve consists of flaps (cusps or leaflets), which open and close like one-way swinging doors. The mitral valve has two cusps; the others (tricuspid, aortic, and pulmonary) have three. The large inlet valves (mitral and tricuspid) have tethers—consisting of the papillary muscles and cords of tissue—which prevent the valves from swinging backward into the atria. If a papillary muscle is damaged (for example, by a heart attack), the valve may then swing backwards and start leaking. If a valve opening is narrowed, blood flow through the valve is reduced. A valve may have both problems.

The heartbeats are evidence that the heart is pumping. The first sound (the lub of lub-dub) is the

A Look Into the Heart

This cross-sectional view of the heart shows the direction of normal blood flow.

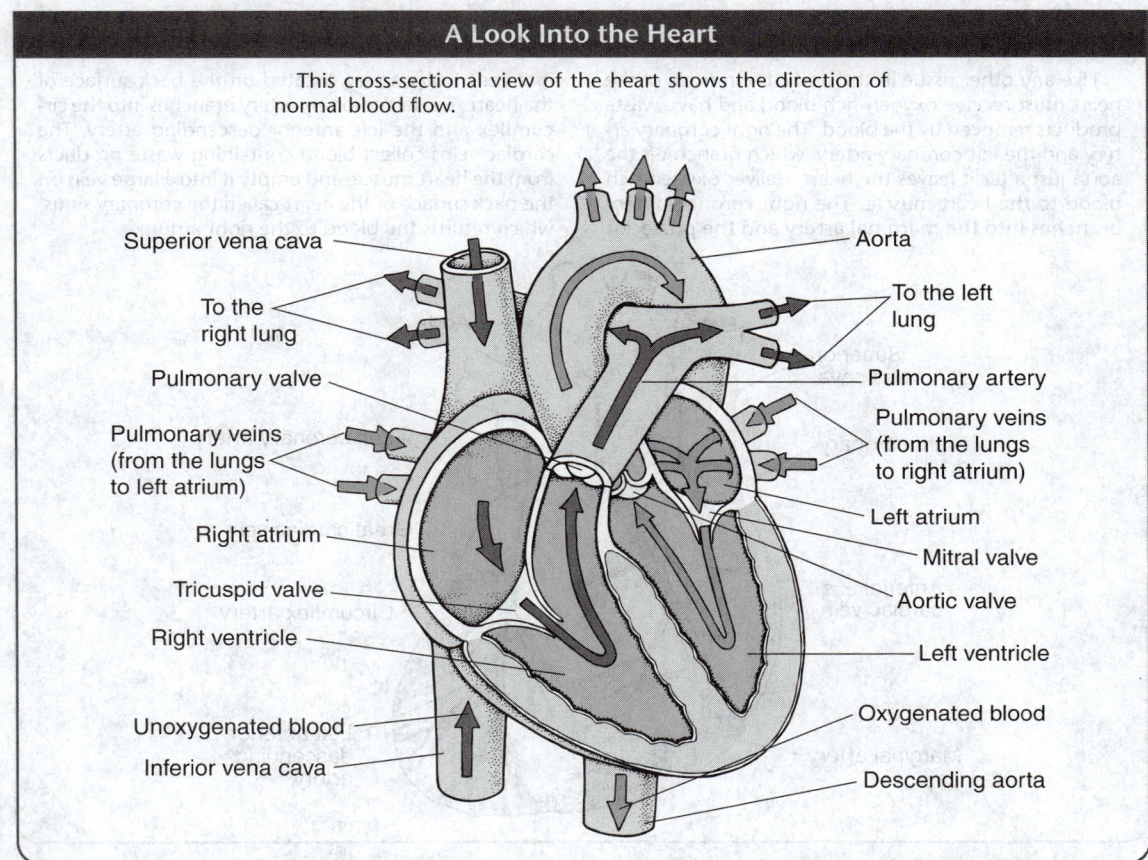

- Superior vena cava
- To the right lung
- Pulmonary valve
- Pulmonary veins (from the lungs to left atrium)
- Right atrium
- Tricuspid valve
- Right ventricle
- Unoxygenated blood
- Inferior vena cava
- Aorta
- To the left lung
- Pulmonary artery
- Pulmonary veins (from the lungs to right atrium)
- Left atrium
- Mitral valve
- Aortic valve
- Left ventricle
- Oxygenated blood
- Descending aorta

sound of the mitral and tricuspid valves closing. The second sound (the dub) is the sound of the aortic and pulmonary valves closing. Each heartbeat has two parts: diastole and systole. During diastole, the ventricles relax and fill with blood; then the atria contract, forcing more blood into the ventricles. During systole, the ventricles contract and pump blood, and the atria relax and begin filling with blood again.

FUNCTION OF THE HEART

The heart's only function is to pump blood. The right side of the heart pumps blood to the lungs, where oxygen is added to the blood and carbon dioxide is removed from it. The left side pumps blood to the rest of the body, where oxygen and nutrients are delivered to tissues and waste products (such as carbon dioxide) are transferred to the blood for removal by other organs (such as the lungs and kidneys).

Blood travels the following circuit: Blood from the body, which is depleted of oxygen and laden with carbon dioxide, flows through the two largest veins (the venae cavae) into the right atrium. When the right ventricle relaxes, blood in the right atrium pours through the tricuspid valve into the right ventricle. When the right ventricle is nearly full, the right atrium contracts, propelling additional blood into the right ventricle, which then contracts. This contraction propels blood through the pulmonary valve into the pulmonary arteries, which supply the lungs. In the lungs, blood flows through the tiny capillaries that surround the air sacs. Here, the blood absorbs oxygen and gives up carbon dioxide, which is then exhaled.

Blood from the lungs, which is now oxygen-rich, flows through the pulmonary veins into the left atrium. When the left ventricle relaxes, the blood in the left atrium pours through the mitral valve into the left ventricle. When the left ventricle is nearly full, the left atrium contracts, propelling additional blood into the left ventricle, which then contracts. (In older people, the left ventricle does not fill as

Supplying the Heart With Blood

Like any other tissue in the body, the muscle of the heart must receive oxygen-rich blood and have waste products removed by the blood. The right coronary artery and the left coronary artery, which branch off the aorta just after it leaves the heart, deliver oxygen-rich blood to the heart muscle. The right coronary artery branches into the marginal artery and the posterior interventricular artery, located on the back surface of the heart. The left coronary artery branches into the circumflex and the left anterior descending artery. The cardiac veins collect blood containing waste products from the heart muscle and empty it into a large vein on the back surface of the heart called the coronary sinus, which returns the blood to the right atrium.

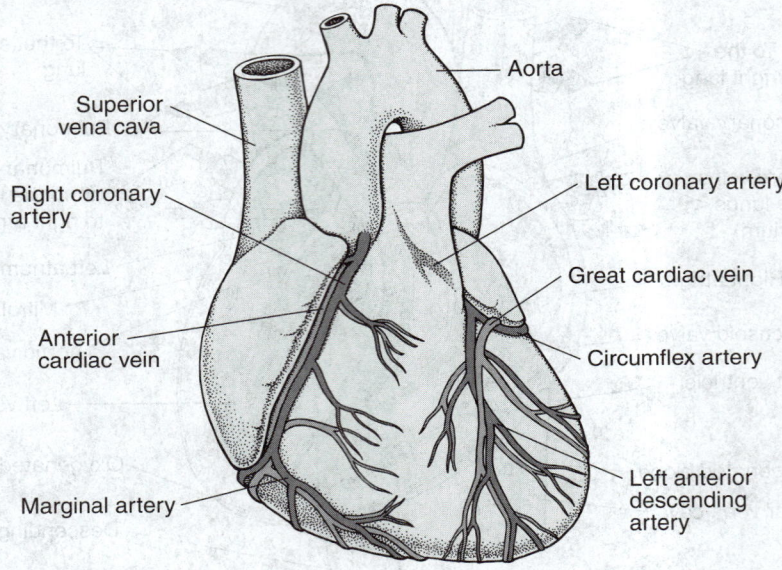

Superior vena cava

Right coronary artery

Anterior cardiac vein

Marginal artery

Aorta

Left coronary artery

Great cardiac vein

Circumflex artery

Left anterior descending artery

well before the left atrium contracts, making this contraction of the left atrium especially important.) The contraction of the left ventricle propels blood through the aortic valve into the aorta, the largest artery in the body. This blood carries oxygen to all of the body except to the lungs.

The circuit through the right side of the heart, the lungs, and the left atrium is called the pulmonary circulation. The circuit through the left side of the heart, most of the body, and the right atrium is called the systemic circulation.

BLOOD SUPPLY OF THE HEART

Like all organs, the heart needs a constant supply of oxygen-rich blood. A system of arteries and veins, called the coronary circulation, supplies the heart muscle (myocardium) with oxygen-rich blood and then returns oxygen-depleted blood to the right atrium. The right coronary artery and the left coro-

nary artery branch off the aorta (just after it leaves the heart) to deliver oxygen-rich blood to the heart muscle. These two arteries branch into other arteries, including the circumflex artery, that also supply blood to the heart. The cardiac veins collect blood from the heart muscle and empty it into a large vein on the back surface of the heart called the coronary sinus, which returns the blood to the right atrium. Because of the great pressure exerted in the heart as it contracts, most blood flows through the coronary circulation only while the heart is relaxing between beats (during diastole).

REGULATION OF THE HEART

The contraction of the muscle fibers in the heart is very organized and highly controlled. Rhythmic electrical impulses (discharges) flow through the heart in a precise manner along distinct pathways and at a controlled speed. The impulses originate in the heart's pacemaker (the sinus or sinoatrial node—a small mass of tissue in the wall of the right atrium), which generates a tiny electrical current (see page 366).

The rate at which the pacemaker sends out its impulses (and thus governs the heart rate) is determined by two opposing systems—one to speed the heart rate up (the sympathetic division of the nervous system) and one to slow it down (the parasympathetic division—see page 628). The sympathetic division works through a network of nerves called the sympathetic plexus and through the hormones epinephrine (adrenaline) and norepinephrine (noradrenaline), which are released by the adrenal glands and the nerve endings. The parasympathetic division works through a single nerve—the vagus nerve—which releases the neurotransmitter acetylcholine.

Blood Vessels

The blood vessels consist of arteries, arterioles, capillaries, venules, and veins. All blood is carried in these vessels. The arteries, which are strong, flexible, and resilient, carry blood away from the heart and bear the highest blood pressures. Because arteries are elastic, they narrow (recoil) passively when the heart is relaxing between beats and thus help maintain blood pressure. The arteries branch into smaller and smaller vessels, eventually becoming very small vessels called arterioles. Arteries and arterioles have muscular walls that can adjust their diameter to increase or decrease blood flow to a particular part of the body.

Capillaries are tiny, extremely thin-walled vessels that act as a bridge between arteries (which carry

Blood Vessels: Circulating the Blood

Blood travels from the heart in arteries, which branch into smaller and smaller vessels, eventually becoming arterioles. Arterioles connect with even smaller blood vessels called capillaries. Through the thin walls of the capillaries, oxygen and nutrients pass from blood into tissues, and waste products pass from tissues into blood. From the capillaries, blood passes into venules, then into veins to return to the heart.

Arteries and arterioles have relatively thick muscular walls because blood pressure in them is high and because they must adjust their diameter to maintain blood pressure and to control blood flow. Veins and venules have much thinner, less muscular walls than arteries and arterioles, largely because the pressure in veins and venules is much lower. Veins may dilate to accommodate increased blood volume.

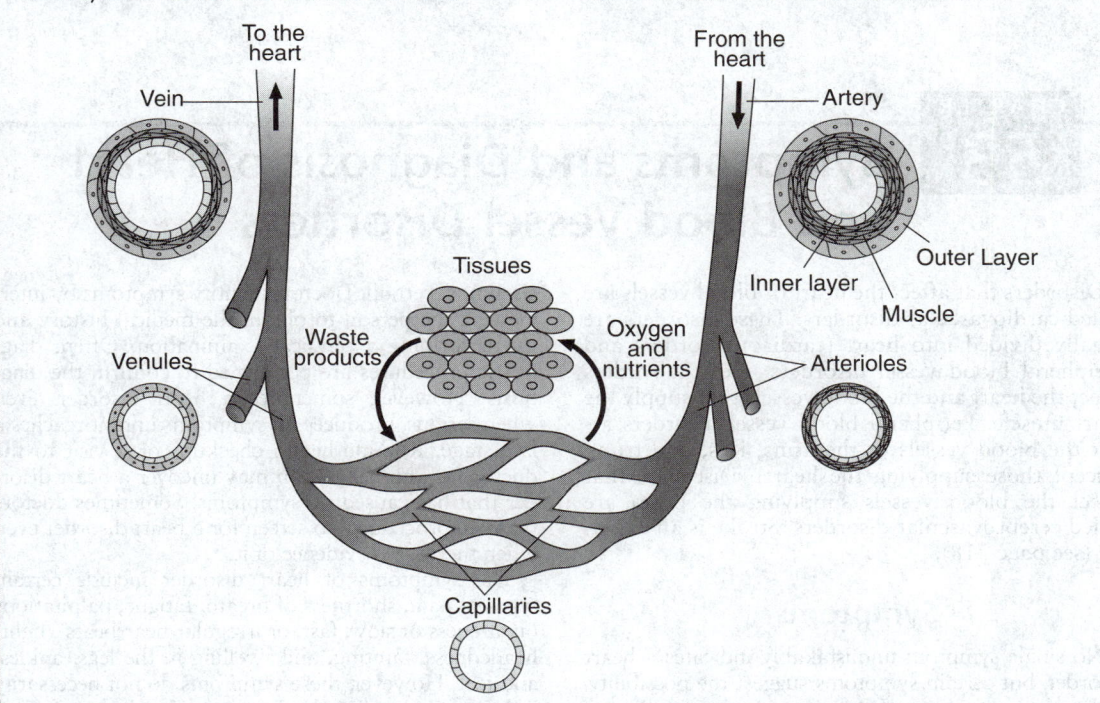

blood away from the heart) and veins (which carry blood back to the heart). The thin walls of the capillaries allow oxygen and nutrients to pass from the blood into tissues and allow waste products to pass from tissues into the blood.

Blood flows from the capillaries into very small veins called venules, then into the veins that lead back to the heart. Veins have much thinner walls than do arteries, largely because the pressure in veins is so much lower. Veins can widen (dilate) as the amount of fluid in them increases. Some veins, particularly veins in the legs, have valves in them, to prevent blood from flowing backward. When these valves leak, the backflow of blood can cause the veins to stretch and become elongated and convoluted (tortuous). Stretched, tortuous veins near the body's surface are called varicose veins (see page 437).

If a blood vessel breaks, tears, or is cut, blood leaks out, causing bleeding. Blood may flow out of the body, as external bleeding, or it may flow into the spaces around organs or directly into organs, as internal bleeding.

Effects of Aging

As people age, the heart tends to enlarge slightly, developing thicker walls and slightly larger chambers.

The increase in size is mainly due to an increase in the size of individual heart muscle cells.

During rest, the older heart functions in almost the same way as a younger heart, except the heart rate is slightly lower. However, during exercise, the older heart cannot increase the amount of blood pumped out as much as a younger heart can.

The walls of the arteries and arterioles become thicker, and the space within the arteries expands slightly. Elastic tissue within the walls of the arteries and arterioles is lost. Together, these changes make the vessels stiffer and less resilient.

Because arteries and arterioles become less elastic as people age, they cannot relax as quickly during the rhythmic pumping of the heart. As a result, blood pressure increases more when the heart contracts (during systole)—sometimes above normal—than it does in younger people. Abnormally high blood pressure during systole with normal blood pressure during diastole is very common among older people; this disorder is called isolated systolic hypertension (see page 333).

Many of the effects of aging on the heart and blood vessels can be reduced by regular exercise. Exercise helps people maintain cardiovascular fitness as well as muscular fitness as they age. Exercise is beneficial regardless of the age at which it is started.

CHAPTER

53 Symptoms and Diagnosis of Heart and Blood Vessel Disorders

Disorders that affect the heart or blood vessels are called cardiovascular disorders. These disorders are usually divided into heart (cardiac) disorders and peripheral blood vessel disorders. Heart disorders affect the heart and the blood vessels that supply the heart muscle. Peripheral blood vessel disorders affect the blood vessels of the arms, legs, and trunk (except those supplying the heart). Disorders that affect the blood vessels supplying the brain are called cerebrovascular disorders. Stroke is an example (see page 718).

Symptoms

No single symptom unmistakably indicates a heart disorder, but certain symptoms suggest the possibility, and several symptoms together may make the diagno-

sis almost certain. Doctors identify symptoms by interviewing the person to obtain the medical history and by performing a physical examination. Often, diagnostic procedures are performed to confirm the diagnosis. However, sometimes a heart disorder, even when serious, produces no symptoms until it reaches a late stage. Routine health checkups or a visit to the doctor for another reason may uncover a heart disorder that has caused no symptoms. Sometimes doctors perform procedures to screen for a heart disorder even when there is no evidence of it.

The symptoms of heart disorder include certain types of pain, shortness of breath, fatigue, palpitations (awareness of slow, fast, or irregular heartbeats), lightheadedness, fainting, and swelling in the legs, ankles, and feet. However, these symptoms do not necessarily indicate a heart disorder. For example, chest pain may be due to a respiratory or digestive disorder rather than to a heart disorder.

Symptoms of peripheral blood vessel disorders vary depending on where the affected blood vessels are located. Symptoms may include pain, shortness of breath, muscle cramps, muscle fatigue, light-headedness, swelling, numbness, and a change in skin color of the affected part of the body.

CHEST PAIN

Pain due to a disorder of the heart, lungs, esophagus, or large blood vessels of the trunk is usually felt in the chest, although it can seem to be located anywhere between the upper abdomen and the jaw, including the arms or shoulders. The discomfort may be described as pressure, gas, burning, aching, or sometimes sharp pain.

Causes

Chest pain has many causes. Immediately life-threatening causes include a heart attack, separation of the layers of the aorta's wall (aortic dissection), rupture of the esophagus, a blood clot in the lungs (pulmonary embolism), and a type of collapsed lung in which pressure builds up enough to obstruct blood flow returning to the heart (tension pneumothorax). Less immediately dangerous causes include an inadequate blood supply to the heart (ischemia), inflammation of the sac that envelops the heart (pericarditis), pneumonia, inflammation of the pancreas (pancreatitis), and certain cancers. Uncomfortable but rarely dangerous causes include acid reflux in the esophagus, peptic ulcer, inflammation of rib cartilage (costochondritis) or of the membranes covering the lungs (pleuritis), strained chest muscles, and a gallbladder disorder. In some people, the valve between the left atrium and left ventricle (mitral valve) bulges back into the left atrium when the left ventricle contracts. This disorder, called mitral valve prolapse, sometimes causes brief episodes of stabbing or needle-like pain.

Evaluation

Sometimes the symptoms suggest a cause to the doctor. For example, tightness or a squeezing sensation in the chest that occurs during physical activity and that is relieved by a few minutes of rest suggests angina, which results from an inadequate blood supply to the heart. A sharp pain that worsens when the person lies down or breathes deeply, decreases when the person sits up and leans forward, and is not related to physical activity suggests pericarditis. Pain increased by inhaling deeply can also be caused by pleuritis. A sudden sharp, excruciating pain in the back of the neck, between the shoulder blades, down the back, or in the abdomen that begins fairly quickly may be due to an aortic dissection.

Symptoms due to dangerous and not dangerous chest disorders overlap and vary greatly. Consequently, tests are usually done if people have chest pain. Evaluation and testing are usually done in the hospital or emergency department if a dangerous cause is suspected. The tests are chosen based on the person's physical examination, age, overall health, other symptoms, and risk factors. But most often, an electrocardiogram (ECG), chest x-ray, and measurement of oxygen levels with a small sensor placed over a finger (pulse oximetry) are done. If the doctor suspects a heart attack, blood tests to measure levels of heart muscle enzymes and proteins may be done several times. High levels of these enzymes indicate damage to heart muscle. If angina is suspected, exercise stress testing may be done (see page 326).

PAIN IN THE LIMBS

Pain may occur when tissues do not get enough blood (a condition called ischemia). Pain occurs because the tissues do not get enough oxygen, which is carried to tissues by the blood, and because waste products, which are carried away from tissues by the blood, accumulate.

If blood flow is completely blocked, as from a blood clot in a large artery, severe constant pain occurs suddenly, and the affected arm or leg becomes pale and cool. If blood flow is only partly blocked, as may occur with atherosclerosis (usually a problem in the legs), the person usually feels a tightening, fatiguing pain in the calf muscle during physical activity. This pain, called claudication, is rapidly relieved by rest and comes back during similar activity.

Pain in the limbs may also result from strained muscles, injury to certain nerves near the spinal cord, formation of blood clots in veins (venous thrombosis), or skin or muscle infections. If doctors suspect that the pain is caused by a blood vessel disorder, ultrasonography to evaluate blood flow in the affected area may be done.

SHORTNESS OF BREATH

Shortness of breath (dyspnea) is the sensation of difficult or labored breathing (see page 450).

Causes

Any disorder that upsets the normal, delicate balance between the body's oxygen supply and oxygen requirement can cause shortness of breath. It is a common symptom of lung disorders, including infections, asthma, and allergies. Shortness of breath can also occur in people who have a disorder of the respiratory muscles, a disorder of the nervous system that interferes with breathing, or too few red blood cells to carry oxygen to tissues (anemia).

Shortness of breath is also a common symptom of heart disorders, mainly heart failure (see page 352) and coronary artery disease (see page 401).

In heart failure, shortness of breath results from fluid seeping into the air spaces of the lungs—a condition called pulmonary congestion or pulmonary edema. Ultimately, this process is similar to drowning. In the early stages of heart failure, shortness of breath may occur only during physical activity. As heart failure worsens, shortness of breath occurs with less and less activity and eventually occurs at rest. Shortness of breath at rest occurs mostly when people lie down because fluid seeps throughout the lung tissue. This symptom often occurs at night and is then called nocturnal dyspnea. When people sit up and dangle their legs, gravity causes fluid to collect at the base of the lungs, reducing symptoms. Consequently, people with nocturnal dyspnea usually sleep propped up by pillows to avoid lying flat.

In coronary artery disease, shortness of breath usually occurs during physical activity, but in people with severe disease, it may occur during minimal activity or during rest.

Evaluation

Sometimes the symptoms suggest a cause to the doctor. Nocturnal dyspnea that is relieved by sitting up and dangling the legs suggests heart failure. Shortness of breath that occurs during physical activity and is accompanied by chest pain suggests coronary artery disease. Shortness of breath with cough and fever suggests a lung infection. Shortness of breath that seems to be triggered by exposure to something in the environment, such as smoke or animal hair, suggests asthma or an allergic disorder.

If the cause is not obvious, tests are usually done. The tests are chosen based on the person's particular symptoms, physical examination, and other factors suggesting a specific disorder. But most often, a chest x-ray and measurement of oxygen levels with a small sensor placed over a finger (pulse oximetry) are done. Electrocardiography (ECG) is commonly performed in adults, particularly if they have risk factors for heart disorders.

FATIGUE

When the heart pumps inefficiently as it does in heart failure, blood flow to the muscles may be inadequate during physical activity, causing feelings of weakness and fatigue. Symptoms are often subtle. People usually compensate by gradually reducing their activity level, or they may blame the symptoms on increasing age.

LIMITATION OF PHYSICAL ACTIVITY

Heart disorders can limit a person's ability to perform physical activities. One way to evaluate the severity of a heart disorder is to determine how limited this ability is. Doctors may use the New York Heart Association (NYHA) functional class system to make this evaluation. In mild disease (class I), ordinary physical activity may not be limited. In moderate disease (class II), ordinary activity causes symptoms, and in moderately severe disease (class III), less-than-ordinary activity causes symptoms. In severe disease (class IV), symptoms occur during rest, and any physical activity makes them worse. However, this system is not foolproof, because even serious heart disorders may produce no symptoms if people reduce their activity level to compensate for the disorder.

PALPITATIONS

Palpitations are the awareness of heart activity. The sensation may feel like pounding, fluttering, racing, or skipping beats.

Causes

Ordinarily, people do not notice the beating of their heart, but sometimes awareness of normal heart activity is heightened. Many people can feel heartbeats when they lie on their left side. Also, under certain circumstances—for example, when exercising strenuously or having a dramatic emotional experience—healthy people may become aware of their heartbeats. They may feel the heart beating very forcefully or rapidly or sense an irregular heartbeat.

Palpitations may result from a disturbance of heart rhythm (arrhythmia). Arrhythmias range from harmless to life threatening. The most common are premature atrial contractions (PACs) and premature ventricular contractions (PVCs), which are usually harmless. These arrhythmias usually occur in people without a heart disorder, as does paroxysmal supraventricular tachycardia.

Other arrhythmias, such as atrial fibrillation, atrial flutter, and ventricular tachycardia, usually occur in people with a heart disorder such as coronary artery disease, a heart valve disorder, or a disorder that affects the heart's electrical conduction system.

Caffeine, alcohol, and some drugs (such as amphetamines, cocaine, epinephrine, ephedrine, and theophylline) can cause palpitations. Palpitations may also result from an overactive thyroid gland (hyperthyroidism), anemia, a low oxygen level in the blood (hypoxia), and a low potassium level in the blood (hypokalemia).

Evaluation

Determining whether palpitations are abnormal depends on answers to a number of questions, such as whether they started suddenly or gradually, whether something seems to trigger them, how fast the heart beats, and whether and to what extent the beat seems to be irregular. An occasional skipped heartbeat suggests PACs or PVCs. A constant sensation of irregular heartbeats suggests atrial fibrillation. Regular heartbeats that suddenly become rapid, then suddenly slow to the normal rate, suggest supraventricular or ventricular tachycardia. Palpitations that occur with other symptoms, such as shortness of breath, pain, weakness, fatigue, or fainting, are more likely to result from an abnormal heart rhythm or a serious disorder.

Doctors also listen to the heart with a stethoscope. Electrocardiography (ECG) is usually done, but unless symptoms occur during the test, ECG does not usually help with a diagnosis. If symptoms are significant but intermittent, continuous ambulatory ECG may be done (see art on page 327). Other possible tests include ultrasonography of the heart (echocardiography) and certain blood tests.

LIGHT-HEADEDNESS AND FAINTING

Light-headedness (near-syncope) is the feeling that one is about to faint. Fainting (syncope) is a sudden, brief loss of consciousness followed by spontaneous return of consciousness.

Causes

The causes of light-headedness and fainting tend to be the same. A person cannot lose consciousness unless brain function is generally disturbed. This disturbance usually occurs because blood flow to the brain is reduced. Brain blood flow can be reduced by a heart disorder or, more commonly, by something that interferes with the normal return of blood to the heart and thus reduces blood flow to the brain. Older people are particularly susceptible because blood flow to the brain decreases as people age. Brain disorders by themselves rarely cause fainting, unless they also affect the blood vessels. Seizures, a brain disorder, can cause loss of consciousness but are not considered fainting.

In heart disorders, blood flow to the brain may be reduced when the heart rate or rhythm is abnormal (too slow or too fast) or when the heart cannot pump blood adequately because blood flow is blocked. Blood flow can be blocked by a defective heart valve (most commonly, the aortic valve), by blood clots in

the lungs or sometimes the heart, and, rarely, by certain heart tumors such as an atrial myxoma.

Many factors can interfere with the return of blood to the heart. Coughing or straining during bowel movements can increase chest pressure, reducing the return of blood to the heart. Healthy soldiers may feel faint or may faint when standing still for a long time (a phenomenon called parade ground syncope), because the leg muscles have to be active to help return blood to the heart. Strong emotion (particularly that triggered by viewing a bloody or gruesome scene) or pain can activate the vagus nerve. As a result, blood vessels widen (dilate), reducing the return of blood to the heart and sometimes causing fainting (called vasovagal syncope). Certain brain and spinal cord disorders and drugs (particularly those used to treat blood pressure) can also dilate blood vessels and cause fainting.

Sitting or standing up too quickly can cause a feeling of faintness or fainting, because the change in position causes blood to pool in the legs, resulting in a fall in blood pressure. Normally, the body quickly adjusts to maintain blood pressure. Inability to adjust quickly is called orthostatic hypotension. This disorder is particularly common among older people.

People are more likely to feel faint or to faint when they are standing up. When they lie or fall down, blood flow to the brain is increased, usually restoring consciousness.

Evaluation

Doctors must distinguish dangerous causes of fainting from relatively harmless ones. If fainting is preceded by brief warning symptoms such as light-headedness, nausea, yawning, blurred vision, or sweating and occurs during a painful or unpleasant situation, it is probably vasovagal, which is not dangerous. In such cases, doctors perform a physical examination. If results are normal, usually no further testing is needed. Fainting is worrisome in adolescents because it more often indicates a serious heart disorder.

Further testing is needed if fainting occurs without any warning symptoms (particularly during physical activity), is acc5ompanied by shortness of breath or chest pain, or results in injury to the person or if the results of a heart or neurologic examination are abnormal. Electrocardiography (ECG) is often done. Other tests, such as ultrasonography of the heart (echocardiography), tilt table testing (see page 328), and electrophysiologic testing (see page 327) are sometimes useful.

SWELLING, NUMBNESS, AND CHANGES IN SKIN COLOR

Swelling is due to the accumulation of fluid (edema) in tissues. It occurs when blood pools in the leg veins, increasing pressure in the leg veins and forcing fluids out of the veins into tissues. Blood may pool because the heart cannot pump out all of the blood it receives from the rest of the body (in heart failure) or because a deep vein in the leg is blocked (in deep vein thrombosis).

Swelling in the legs, ankles, and feet or in the abdomen may indicate heart failure or a venous disorder, such as deep vein thrombosis. However, such swelling is most commonly caused by standing or sitting in one position too long or by age-related changes in leg veins. Swelling of the legs is also common during pregnancy. Swelling may also be due to liver or kidney disorders.

If the blood supply is inadequate, the affected part of the body may feel numb.

If the blood supply is inadequate, if anemia is present, or if the veins do not drain adequately, the skin may appear pale or bluish (or purplish).

Diagnosis

Usually, doctors can tell whether a person has a heart or blood vessel disorder on the basis of the medical history and the physical examination. Diagnostic procedures are used to confirm the diagnosis, determine the extent and severity of the disease, and help in planning treatment.

MEDICAL HISTORY AND PHYSICAL EXAMINATION

A doctor first asks about symptoms. Chest pain, shortness of breath, palpitations, and swelling in the legs, ankles, and feet or abdomen suggest a heart disorder. Other, more general symptoms, such as fever, weakness, fatigue, lack of appetite, and a general feeling of illness or discomfort (malaise), may suggest a heart disorder. Pain, numbness, or muscle cramps in a leg may suggest peripheral arterial disease, which affects the arteries of the arms, legs, and trunk (except those supplying the heart).

Next, the doctor asks about past infections; previous exposure to chemicals; use of drugs, alcohol, and tobacco; home and work environments; and recreational activity. The doctor also asks whether family members have had a heart disorder or any other disorders that may affect the heart or blood vessels.

During the physical examination, the doctor notes the person's weight and overall appearance and looks for paleness (pallor), sweating, or drowsiness, which may be subtle indicators of heart disorders. The person's general mood and feeling of well-being, which also may be affected by heart disorders, are noted.

Assessing skin color is important because pallor or a bluish or purplish coloration (cyanosis) may indicate anemia or inadequate blood flow. These findings may indicate that the skin is not receiving enough oxygen from the blood because of a lung disorder, heart failure, or various circulatory problems.

The doctor feels the pulse in arteries in the neck, beneath the arms, at the elbows and wrists, in the abdomen, in the groin, at the knees, and in the ankles and feet to assess whether blood flow is adequate and equal on both sides of the body. The blood pressure and body temperature are also checked. An abnormality may suggest a heart or blood vessel disorder.

The doctor inspects the veins in the neck while the person is lying down with the upper part of the body elevated at a 45° angle. These veins are inspected because they are directly connected to the right atrium (the upper chamber of the heart that receives oxygen-depleted blood from the body) and thus give an indication of the volume and pressure of blood entering the right side of the heart.

The doctor presses the skin over the ankles and legs and sometimes over the lower back to check for fluid accumulation (edema) in the tissues beneath the skin.

An ophthalmoscope (see art on page 1422) is used to view the blood vessels of the retina (the light-sensitive membrane on the inner surface of the back of the eye). The retina is the only place a doctor can directly view veins and arteries. Visible abnormalities in the retina are common among people with high blood pressure, diabetes, arteriosclerosis, and bacterial infections of the heart valves.

The doctor observes the chest to determine whether the breathing rate and movements are normal. By tapping (percussing) the chest with the fingers, the doctor can determine if the lungs are filled with air, which is normal, or if they contain fluid, which is abnormal. Percussion also helps determine whether the sac that envelops the heart (pericardium) or the layers of membranes covering the lungs (pleura) contain fluid. Using a stethoscope, the doctor also listens to the breathing sounds to determine whether airflow is normal or obstructed and whether the lungs contain fluid as a result of heart failure.

By placing a hand on the person's chest, the doctor can feel (palpate) where the heartbeat is strongest and thus determine heart size. The quality and force of contractions during each heartbeat can also be determined. Sometimes abnormal, turbulent blood flow within vessels or between heart chambers causes a vibration (called a thrill) that can be felt with the fingertips or palm.

By listening to (auscultating) the heart with a stethoscope, the doctor can hear the distinctive sounds caused by the opening and closing of the heart valves. Abnormalities of the valves and heart structures create turbulent blood flow that causes characteristic sounds called murmurs. Turbulent blood flow typically occurs as blood moves through narrowed or leaking valves. However, not all heart disorders cause murmurs, and not all murmurs indicate a heart disorder. For example, pregnant women usually have heart murmurs because of a normal increase in blood flow. Harmless heart murmurs also are common among infants and children because of the rapid flow of blood through their heart's smaller structure. As blood vessel walls, valves, and other tissues gradually stiffen in older people, blood may flow turbulently, even when no serious heart disorder is present. Also, the doctor may hear clicks and opening snaps when an abnormal valve opens. A gallop rhythm (a sound resembling that of a galloping horse), due to one or two extra heart sounds, is often heard in people who have heart failure.

ECG: Reading the Waves

An electrocardiogram (ECG) represents the electrical current moving through the heart during a heartbeat. The current's movement is divided into parts, and each part is given an alphabetic designation in the ECG.

Each heartbeat begins with an impulse from the heart's pacemaker (sinus or sinoatrial node). This impulse activates the upper chambers of the heart (atria). The P wave represents activation of the atria.

Next, the electrical current flows down to the lower chambers of the heart (ventricles). The QRS complex represents activation of the ventricles.

The electrical current then spreads back over the ventricles in the opposite direction. This activity is called the recovery wave, which is represented by the T wave.

Many kinds of abnormalities can often be seen on an ECG. They include a previous heart attack (myocardial infarction), an abnormal heart rhythm (arrhythmia), an inadequate supply of blood and oxygen to the heart (ischemia), and excessive thickening (hypertrophy) of the heart's muscular walls.

Certain abnormalities seen on an ECG can suggest bulges (aneurysms) that develop in weak areas of the heart's walls. Aneurysms may result from a heart attack. If the rhythm is abnormal (too fast, too slow, or irregular), the ECG may also indicate where in the heart the abnormal rhythm starts. Such information helps doctors begin to determine the cause.

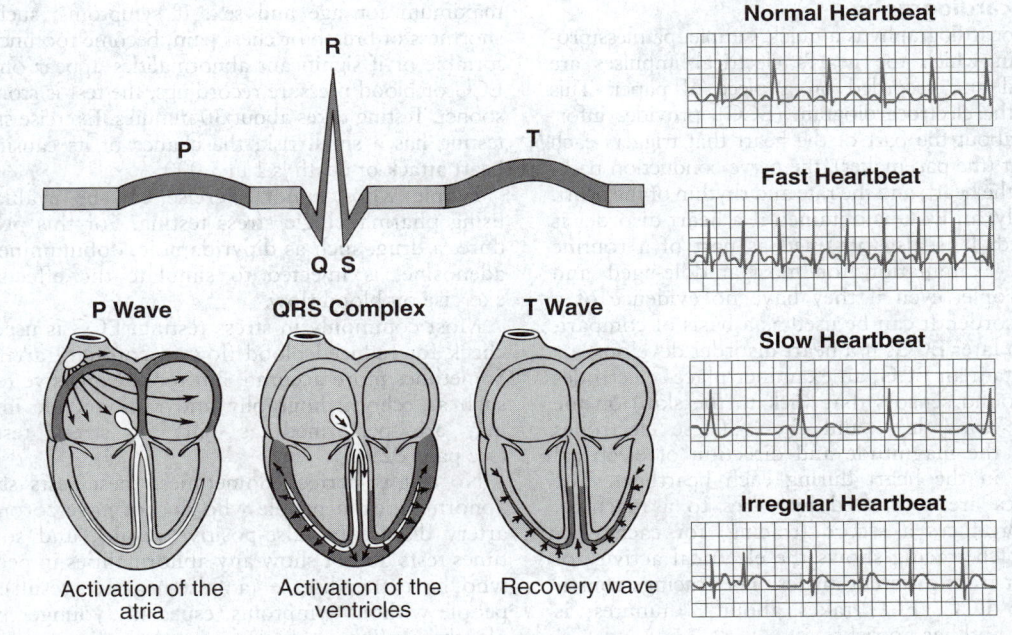

P Wave — Activation of the atria

QRS Complex — Activation of the ventricles

T Wave — Recovery wave

Normal Heartbeat

Fast Heartbeat

Slow Heartbeat

Irregular Heartbeat

By placing the stethoscope over arteries and veins elsewhere in the body, the doctor can listen for sounds of turbulent blood flow (bruits). Bruits may be caused by narrowing of blood vessels, increased blood flow, or an abnormal connection between an artery and a vein (arteriovenous fistula).

The doctor feels the abdomen to determine if the liver is enlarged. Enlargement may indicate that blood is pooled in the major veins leading to the heart. Swelling of the abdomen due to fluid accumulation may indicate heart failure. By pressing gently on the abdomen, the doctor checks the pulse and determines the width of the abdominal aorta.

DIAGNOSTIC PROCEDURES

There are many diagnostic procedures that can help doctors make a rapid, precise diagnosis. They include electrocardiography (ECG), stress testing, electrophysiologic testing, tilt table testing, radiologic procedures (x-rays), ultrasonography (including echocardiography), magnetic resonance imaging (MRI), radionuclide imaging, positron emission tomography (PET), cardiac catheterization, central venous catheterization, angiography, and computed tomography (CT). Fluoroscopy is used infrequently. Blood tests to measure levels of sugar (to test for diabetes), cholesterol, and other substances are often performed.

Most of these procedures carry very small risk, but the risk increases with the complexity of the procedure and the severity of the heart disorder.

Electrocardiography

Electrocardiography is a quick, simple, painless procedure in which the heart's electrical impulses are amplified and recorded on a piece of paper. This record, the electrocardiogram (ECG), provides information about the part of the heart that triggers each heartbeat (the pacemaker), the nerve conduction pathways of the heart, and the rate and rhythm of the heart.

Usually, an ECG is obtained if a heart disorder is suspected. It is also obtained as part of a routine physical examination for most middle-aged and older people, even if they have no evidence of a heart disorder. It can be used as a basis of comparison with later ECGs if a heart disorder develops.

To obtain an ECG, an examiner places electrodes (small round sensors that stick to the skin) on the person's arms, legs, and chest. These electrodes measure the magnitude and direction of electrical currents in the heart during each heartbeat. The electrodes are connected by wires to a machine, which produces a record (tracing) for each electrode. Each tracing shows the electrical activity of the heart from different angles. The tracings constitute the ECG. ECG takes about 3 minutes, is painless, and has no risks.

Exercise Stress Testing

Testing the heart during exercise can help identify coronary artery disease. In coronary artery disease, blood flow through the coronary arteries (which supply blood to the heart muscle) is partly or completely blocked. If the coronary arteries are only partly blocked, the heart may have an adequate blood supply when the person is resting but not when the person exercises. Thus, testing the heart during exercise can help identify coronary artery disease. Because exercise stress testing specifically monitors how the heart is functioning, the testing helps doctors distinguish between problems due to a heart disorder and those due to other problems that limit exercise, such as lung disorders, anemia, and poor general fitness.

Exercise testing has two components. Exercise or a drug is used to stress the heart, making it beat faster, and the person is tested for signs of inadequate blood flow to the heart. The person is also monitored for symptoms that suggest coronary artery disease, such as low blood pressure, shortness of breath, and chest pain.

To stress the heart, most people walk on a treadmill or pedal an exercise bicycle. People who cannot use their legs can use an arm crank. Gradually, the pace of the exercise and the force required to do it (workload) are increased. The ECG is monitored continuously, and blood pressure is measured at intervals. Usually, the person being tested is asked to keep going until the heart rate reaches between 80% and 90% of the maximum for age and sex. If symptoms, such as shortness of breath or chest pain, become too uncomfortable or if significant abnormalities appear on the ECG or blood pressure recordings, the test is stopped sooner. Testing takes about 30 minutes. Exercise stress testing has a small risk; the chance of its causing a heart attack or death is 1 in 5,000.

People who cannot exercise can be evaluated using pharmacologic stress testing. For this procedure, a drug, such as dipyridamole, dobutamine, or adenosine, is injected to simulate the effects of exercise on blood flow.

Most commonly in stress testing, ECG is used to check for reduced blood flow in coronary arteries. Sometimes more accurate but more expensive tests, such as echocardiography and radionuclide imaging, are performed as part of stress testing (see page 329).

No test is perfect. Sometimes, these tests show abnormalities in people who do not have coronary artery disease (a false-positive result), and sometimes tests do not show any abnormalities in people who have the disease (a false-negative result). In people without symptoms, especially younger people, the likelihood of coronary artery disease is low, despite an abnormal test result. In such cases, a positive result is usually more likely to be false than true. These false-positive results may cause considerable worry and medical expense. For these reasons, most experts discourage routine exercise stress testing (such as for screening purposes before an exercise program is begun or during an evaluation for life insurance) in people who do not have symptoms.

Continuous Ambulatory Electrocardiography

Abnormal heart rhythms and inadequate blood flow to the heart muscle may occur only briefly or unpredictably. To detect such problems, doctors may use continuous ambulatory ECG, in which the ECG is recorded continuously for 24 hours while the person engages in normal daily activities.

For this procedure, the person wears a small battery-powered device (Holter monitor) held on with a shoulder strap. The monitor detects the heart's electrical activity through electrodes attached to the chest and records the ECG. While wearing the monitor, the person notes in a diary the time and type of any symptoms. Subsequently, the ECG is run through a computer, which analyzes the rate and rhythm of the heart, looks for changes in electrical activity that could indicate inadequate blood flow to the heart muscle, and produces a record of every heartbeat during the 24 hours. Symptoms recorded in the diary can then be correlated with changes in the ECG.

If necessary, the ECG can be transmitted by telephone to a computer at the hospital or doctor's office for an immediate reading as soon as symptoms occur.

An event monitor is used when a person must be monitored longer than 24 hours. It is similar to a Holter monitor, but it records only when the user activates it—that is, when symptoms occur. If symptoms occur so rarely that they cannot be captured during 24-hour monitoring, an event monitor may be placed under the skin for up to a year. A small magnet is used to activate this monitor.

Continuous Ambulatory Blood Pressure Monitoring

If the diagnosis of high blood pressure is in doubt (for example, if the measurements taken in the office vary too much), a 24-hour blood pressure monitor may be used. The monitor is a portable battery-operated device, worn on the hip, connected to a blood pressure cuff, worn on the arm. This monitor repeatedly records blood pressure throughout the day and night over a 24- or 48-hour period. The readings determine not only whether high blood pressure is present but also how severe it is.

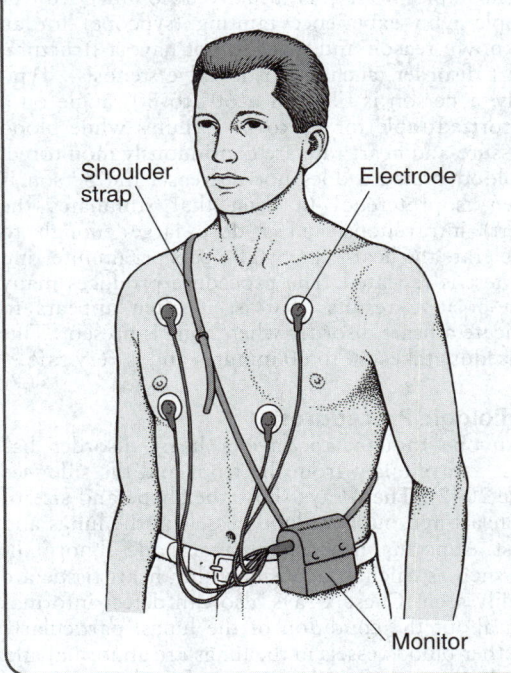

Holter Monitor: Continuous ECG Readings

The small monitor is attached to a strap worn over one shoulder. Through electrodes attached to the chest, the monitor continuously records the electrical activity of the heart.

Shoulder strap

Electrode

Monitor

Electrophysiologic Testing

Electrophysiologic testing is used to evaluate serious abnormalities in heart rhythm or electrical conduction. Testing is performed in the hospital. After injecting a local anesthetic, a doctor inserts a catheter with tiny electrodes at its tip through an incision, usually in the groin, into a vein or sometimes an artery. The catheter is threaded through the major blood vessels into the heart chambers, using fluoroscopy (a continuous x-ray procedure) for guidance. The catheter is used to record the ECG from within the heart and to identify the precise location of the electrical conduction pathways.

Usually, a doctor intentionally provokes an abnormal heart rhythm during testing to find out whether a particular drug can stop the disturbance or whether an operation will help by eliminating abnormal electrical connections within the heart. If necessary, a doctor can quickly restore a normal rhythm with a brief electrical shock to the heart (cardioversion). Although electrophysiologic testing is an invasive procedure and an anesthetic is required, the procedure is very safe: The risk of death is 1 in 5,000. This procedure usually takes 1 to 2 hours.

Tilt Table Testing

Tilt table testing is usually recommended for people who experience fainting (syncope) for an unknown reason and who do not have a structural heart disorder (such as aortic valve stenosis). Typically, a person is tilted at a 60° to 80° angle on a motorized table for 15 to 20 minutes while blood pressure and heart rate are continuously monitored. If blood pressure does not decrease, the person is given isoproterenol (a drug that stimulates the heart) intravenously in a dose large enough to accelerate the heart rate by 20 beats per minute, and the test is repeated. The procedure produces many false-positive results; that is, it often appears to indicate a heart disorder when none is present. This procedure takes 30 to 60 minutes and is very safe.

Radiologic Procedures

Anyone thought to have a heart disorder has chest x-rays taken from the front and the side (see page 2042). The x-rays show the shape and size of the heart and outline blood vessels in the lungs and chest. Abnormal heart shape or size and abnormalities such as calcium deposits within heart tissue are readily seen. Chest x-rays also can detect information about the condition of the lungs, particularly whether blood vessels in the lungs are abnormal and whether there is fluid in or around the lungs.

X-rays can detect enlargement of the heart, which is often due to heart failure or a heart valve disorder. The heart does not enlarge when heart failure results from constrictive pericarditis, in which scar tissue forms throughout the sac that envelops the heart (pericardium).

The appearance of blood vessels in the lungs is often more useful in making a diagnosis than the appearance of the heart itself. For instance, enlargement of the pulmonary arteries (the arteries that carry blood from the heart to the lungs) and narrowing of the arteries within the lung tissue suggest high blood pressure in the pulmonary arteries, which may lead to thickening of the muscle of the right ventricle (the lower heart chamber that pumps blood through the pulmonary arteries to the lungs). X-rays of other parts of the body may be taken to detect blockages in other blood vessels.

Computed Tomography

Spiral (helical) computed tomography (CT—see page 2037) may be used to detect structural abnormalities of the heart, the sac that envelops the heart (pericardium), major blood vessels, lungs, and supporting structures in the chest. Typically, a dye that can be seen on x-rays (radiopaque dye or contrast agent) is injected into the person's vein. The person is asked not to breathe during a scan so that the image will not be blurred.

Newer electron beam CT, previously called ultrafast or cine-computed tomography, is used mainly to detect calcium deposits in arteries that supply blood to the heart (coronary arteries), an early sign of coronary artery disease. This type of scanning is not widely available.

Computed tomography angiography (CTA) is a type of CT that is used to produce three-dimensional images of the major arteries of the body, except the coronary arteries. The images are similar in quality to those produced by conventional angiography (see page 332). CTA can be used to detect narrowing of the arteries supplying organs and aneurysms and tears in major arteries. CTA can also detect clots that have broken off within an artery, traveled through the bloodstream, and lodged in the small arteries of the lungs (pulmonary emboli).

Unlike conventional angiography, CTA is not an invasive procedure. The radiopaque dye is injected into a vein rather than into an artery as in angiography. CTA usually takes less than 1 to 2 minutes.

Fluoroscopy

Fluoroscopy is a continuous x-ray procedure that shows the heart beating and the lungs inflating and deflating on a screen. However, fluoroscopy, which involves a relatively high dose of radiation, has been largely replaced by echocardiography and other procedures. Fluoroscopy is still used as a component of cardiac catheterization and electrophysiologic testing.

Echocardiography and Other Ultrasound Procedures

Ultrasonography (see page 2044) uses high-frequency (ultrasound) waves bounced off internal structures to produce a moving image. It uses no x-rays. Ultrasonography of the heart (echocardiography) is one of the most widely used procedures for diagnosing heart disorders because it is noninvasive, harmless, relatively inexpensive, and widely available and because it provides excellent images. Ultrasonography is also used in the diagnosis of disorders affecting blood vessels in other parts of the body.

Echocardiography can be used to detect abnormalities in heart wall motion and to measure the volume of blood being pumped from the heart with each beat. This procedure can also detect abnormalities in the heart's structure, such as defective heart valves, birth defects, and enlargement of the heart's walls or chambers, as occurs in people with high blood pressure, heart failure, or impairment of the heart's muscular walls (cardiomyopathy). Echocardiography can also be used to detect pericardial effusion, in which fluid accumulates between the two layers of the sac that envelops the heart (pericardium), and constrictive pericarditis, in which scar tissue forms throughout the pericardium.

The main types of ultrasonography are M-mode, two-dimensional, Doppler, and color Doppler. In M-mode ultrasonography, the simplest technique, a single beam of ultrasound is aimed at the part of the heart being studied. Two-dimensional ultrasonography, the most widely used technique, produces realistic two-dimensional images in computer-generated "slices." Stacking the slices together can re-create a three-dimensional structure.

Doppler ultrasonography shows the direction and velocity of blood flow and thus can detect turbulent flow due to narrowing or blockage of blood vessels. Color Doppler ultrasonography shows the different rates of blood flow in different colors. Doppler ultrasonography and color Doppler ultrasonography are commonly used to help diagnose disorders affecting the heart and the arteries and veins in the trunk, legs, and arms. Because these procedures can show the direction and rate of blood flow in the chambers and blood vessels of the heart, they enable doctors to evaluate the structure and function of these parts. For example, doctors can determine if the heart valves open and close properly, if and how much they leak when closed, and if blood flows normally. Abnormal connections between an artery and a vein or between heart chambers can also be detected.

The ultrasound waves are emitted by a handheld recording probe (transducer). For echocardiography, the examiner places gel on the chest over the heart and moves the probe over that area. The probe is connected to a monitor that displays an image. The image is recorded on a videocassette, a computer disk, or paper. By varying the placement and angle of the probe, doctors can view the heart and nearby major blood vessels from various angles and thus get an accurate picture of heart structure and function. Echocardiography is painless and takes 20 to 30 minutes.

If doctors need to obtain greater clarity or to analyze the aorta or structures at the back of the heart (particularly the left atrium or left ventricle), transesophageal echocardiography can be used. For this procedure, a probe is passed down the person's throat into the esophagus and stomach. The probe records signals from just behind the heart. Transesophageal echocardiography is also used when regular echocardiography is difficult to perform because of obesity, lung disorders, or other technical problems.

Magnetic Resonance Imaging

With magnetic resonance imaging (MRI—see page 2040), a powerful magnetic field and radio waves are used to produce detailed images of the heart and chest. This expensive and sophisticated procedure is used predominantly for the diagnosis of complex heart disorders that are present at birth (congenital) and to differentiate between normal and abnormal tissue.

MRI has some disadvantages. It takes longer to produce MRI images than computed tomography (CT) images. Because of the movement of the heart, the images obtained with MRI are fuzzier than those obtained with CT. However, newer MRI scans that are timed to match specific parts of the ECG (called gated MRI) are much clearer than conventional MRI scans.

Magnetic resonance angiography (MRA) is a type of MRI that focuses on blood vessels rather than organs. MRA produces images of blood vessels and blood flow similar in quality to those produced by conventional angiography but is not an invasive procedure (see page 332). MRA can be used to detect bulges (aneurysms) in the aorta, narrowing of the arteries supplying the kidneys (renal stenosis), and a narrowing or blockage in the arteries that supply blood to the heart (coronary arteries) or the arms and legs (peripheral arteries).

Radionuclide Imaging

In radionuclide imaging (see page 2043), a tiny amount of a radioactive substance (radionuclide), called a tracer, is injected into any vein. The amount of radiation the person receives is tiny—less than that produced by most x-rays. The tracer emits gamma rays, which are detected by a gamma camera. A computer analyzes this information and constructs an image to show the different amounts of tracer taken up by tissues.

Radionuclide imaging of the heart is particularly useful in the diagnosis of chest pain when the cause is unknown. If the coronary arteries are narrowed, radionuclide imaging is used to learn how the narrowing is affecting the heart's blood supply and function. Radionuclide imaging is also used to assess improvement in blood supply to the heart muscle after bypass surgery or similar procedures and may be used to help determine a person's prognosis after a heart attack.

Different tracers are used depending on which disorder is suspected. For evaluating blood flow through heart muscle, the tracers typically used are technetium-99 sestamibi or thallium-201, and images are obtained after the person has an exercise stress test (see page 326). The amount of tracer absorbed by the heart muscle cells depends on the blood flow. At peak exercise, an area of heart muscle that has an inadequate blood supply (ischemia) absorbs less tracer—and produces a fainter image—than neighboring muscle with a normal supply. In people unable to exercise, an intravenous injection of a drug, such as dipyridamole, dobutamine, or adenosine, may be used to simulate the effects of exercise on blood flow. These drugs divert the blood supply from abnormal to normal blood vessels, depriving the area with inadequate blood flow even further.

After the person rests for a few hours, a second scan is performed, and the resulting image is compared with that obtained during exercise. Doctors can then distinguish areas of the heart where inadequate blood flow is reversible (usually caused by narrowing of the coronary arteries) from areas where it is irreversible (usually caused by scarring due to a previous heart attack).

If a heart attack may have occurred very recently, technetium-99m is used instead of thallium-201. With technetium, damage due to a heart attack can be detected after 12 to 24 hours and up to about 1 week. Unlike thallium, which accumulates primarily in normal tissue, technetium accumulates primarily in abnormal tissue. However, because technetium also accumulates in bone, the ribs somewhat obscure the image of the heart.

A specialized type of radionuclide imaging called single-photon emission computed tomography (SPECT) can produce a series of computer-enhanced cross-sectional images. A three-dimensional image can also be produced. SPECT provides more information about function, blood flow, and abnormalities than does conventional radionuclide imaging.

Positron Emission Tomography

In positron emission tomography (PET—see page 2044), a substance necessary for heart cell function (such as oxygen or sugar) is labeled with a radioactive substance (radionuclide) that gives off positrons (electrons with a positive charge). The labeled nutrient is injected into a vein and reaches the heart in a few minutes. PET is used to determine how much blood is reaching different parts of the heart muscle and how different parts of the heart muscle process (metabolize) various substances. For example, when labeled sugar is injected, doctors can determine which parts of the heart muscle have an inadequate blood supply because those parts use more sugar than normal.

PET scans produce clearer images than do other radionuclide procedures. However, the procedure is very expensive and not widely available. It is used in research and in cases in which simpler, less expensive procedures are inconclusive.

Cardiac Catheterization and Coronary Angiography

Cardiac catheterization used with coronary angiography is the most accurate method of diagnosing coronary artery disease. Used together, the two procedures are the only way to directly measure the pressure of blood in each chamber of the heart and to obtain an image of the interior of coronary arteries. These procedures are performed to determine whether angioplasty or coronary artery bypass surgery is technically feasible. They may be performed to confirm the diagnosis of other heart disorders, to determine the severity of a heart disorder, or to detect the cause of worsening symptoms.

More than a million cardiac catheterizations and angiographic procedures are performed every year. They are relatively safe, and complications are rare. With cardiac catheterization and angiography, the chance of a serious complication—such as stroke, heart attack, or death—is 1 in 1,000. Fewer than 0.01% of people undergoing these procedures die; most of those who die already have a severe heart disorder or other disorder. The risk of complications and death is increased for older people.

Cardiac Catheterization: Cardiac catheterization is used extensively for the diagnosis and treatment of heart disorders that are not due to disease of the coronary arteries. Cardiac catheterization can be used to measure how much blood the heart pumps out per minute (cardiac output) and to detect birth defects of the heart and tumors, such as a myxoma.

In cardiac catheterization, a thin catheter (a tubular, flexible surgical instrument) is inserted into an artery or vein through a puncture made with a needle or a tiny incision. A local anesthetic is given to numb the insertion site. The catheter is then threaded through the major blood vessels and into the heart chambers. The procedure is performed in the hospital and takes 40 to 60 minutes.

Various instruments may be placed at the tip of the catheter. They include instruments to measure the pressure of blood in each heart chamber and in blood vessels connected to the heart, to view or take ultrasound images of the interior of blood vessels, to take blood samples from different parts of the heart, or to remove a tissue sample from inside the heart for examination under a microscope (biopsy).

When a catheter is used to inject a dye that can be seen on x-rays, the procedure is called **angiography.** When a catheter is used to widen a narrowed heart valve opening, the procedure is called **valvuloplasty.** When a catheter is used to clear a narrowed or blocked artery, the procedure is called **angioplasty** (see page 404).

If an artery is used for catheter insertion, the puncture or incision site must be steadily compressed for 10 to 20 minutes after all the instruments are removed. Compression prevents bleeding and bruise formation. However, bleeding occasionally occurs at the incision site, leaving a large bruise that can persist for weeks but that almost always goes away on its own.

Because inserting a catheter into the heart may cause abnormal heart rhythms, the heart is monitored with electrocardiography (ECG). Usually, doctors can correct an abnormal rhythm by moving the catheter to another position. If this maneuver does not help, the catheter is removed. Very rarely, the heart wall is damaged or punctured when a catheter is inserted; immediate surgical repair may be required.

Cardiac catheterization may be performed on the right or left side of the heart.

Catheterization of the right side of the heart is performed to obtain information about the heart chambers on the right side (right atrium and right ventricle) and the tricuspid valve (located between these two chambers). The right atrium receives oxygen-depleted blood from the body, and the right ventricle pumps the blood into the lungs, where blood takes up oxygen and drops off carbon dioxide. In this procedure, the catheter is inserted into a vein, usually in an arm or the groin. Pulmonary artery catheterization (see below), in which the balloon at the catheter's tip is passed through the right atrium and ventricle and lodged in the pulmonary artery, is sometimes performed during certain major operations and in intensive care units.

Catheterization of the left side is performed to obtain information about the heart chambers on the left side (left atrium and left ventricle), the mitral valve (located between the left atrium and left ventricle), and the aortic valve (located between the left ventricle and the aorta). The left atrium receives oxygen-rich blood from the lungs, and the left ventricle pumps the blood into the rest of the body. The left side is catheterized more often than the right. For example, catheterization of the left side is performed when coronary artery disease has been detected (to determine the extent of the disease) or is suspected (to confirm the diagnosis). This procedure is usually combined with coronary angiography to obtain information about the coronary arteries.

For catheterization of the left side of the heart, the catheter is inserted into an artery, usually in an arm or the groin. Less commonly, the catheter is inserted into a vein in the groin and threaded into the right side of the heart (as in catheterization of the right side). The catheter is then threaded into the left side by puncturing the wall (septum) separating the right atrium from the left.

Coronary Angiography (see page 2036): This procedure provides information about the coronary arteries, which supply the heart with oxygen-rich blood. Coronary angiography is similar to catheterization of the left side of the heart, and the two procedures are almost always performed at the same time. After injecting a local anesthetic, a doctor inserts a thin catheter into an artery through an incision in an arm or the groin. The catheter is threaded toward the heart, then into the coronary arteries. During insertion, the doctor uses fluoroscopy (a continuous x-ray procedure) to observe the progress of the catheter as it is threaded into place. After the catheter tip is in place, a radiopaque dye, which can be seen on x-rays, is injected through the catheter into the coronary arteries, and the outline of the arteries appears on a video screen and is recorded on a tape or disk. Usually, motion picture techniques that produce continuous images are used; this procedure is then called **cineangiography.** It provides clear pictures of the heart chambers and coronary arteries as they move.

Coronary angiography is seldom uncomfortable and usually takes 30 to 50 minutes. It is performed as an outpatient procedure unless the person is very ill.

When the radiopaque dye is injected into the aorta or heart chambers, the person has a temporary feeling of warmth throughout the body as the dye spreads through the bloodstream. The heart rate may increase, and blood pressure may fall slightly. Rarely, the dye causes the heart to slow briefly or even stop. The person may be asked to cough vigorously during the procedure to help correct such problems, which are rarely serious. Rarely, mild complications, such as nausea, vomiting, and coughing, occur. Serious complications, such as shock (see page 350), seizures, kidney problems, and sudden cessation of the heart's pumping (cardiac arrest), are very rare. Allergic reactions to the dye range from skin rashes to a rare life-threatening reaction called anaphylaxis (see page 1123). The team performing the procedure is prepared to treat the complications of coronary angiography immediately.

Risk of complications is higher in older people, although it is still low. Coronary angiography is essential when angioplasty or coronary artery bypass surgery is being considered (see page 404).

Ventriculography is a type of angiography in which x-rays are taken as a radiopaque dye is injected into the left or right ventricle of the heart through a catheter. It is performed during cardiac catheterization. With this procedure, doctors can see the motion of the left or right ventricle and can thus evaluate the pumping ability of the heart. Based on the heart's pumping ability, doctors can calculate the ejection fraction (the percentage of blood pumped out by the left ventricle with each heartbeat). Evaluation of the heart's pumping helps determine how much of the heart has been damaged.

Pulmonary Artery Catheterization

Pulmonary artery catheterization is a useful measure of overall heart function in people who are critically ill, particularly when fluids are being given intravenously. Such people include those who have severe heart or pulmonary disorders (such as heart failure, heart attack, abnormal heart rhythms, or pulmonary embolism when these disorders are accompanied by complications), those who have just undergone heart surgery, those who are in shock (see page 350), and those who have severe burns.

Pulmonary artery catheterization is also performed to measure pressure in the right heart chambers and to estimate pressure in the left heart chambers, the amount of blood the heart pumps per minute (cardiac output), resistance to blood flow in the arteries that carry blood from the heart (peripheral resistance), and the volume of blood. This procedure can provide useful information about cardiac tamponade (see box on page 391) and pulmonary embolism (see page 488).

As in right heart catheterization, a catheter with a balloon at its tip is inserted into a vein, usually in the neck (under the collarbone) or an arm, and is threaded toward the heart. The tip of the catheter may be passed through the superior vena cava or inferior vena cava (the large veins that return blood to the heart from the upper and lower parts of the body) and through the right atrium and right ventricle to the pulmonary artery. The balloon at the catheter's tip is lodged in the pulmonary artery. A chest x-ray is taken or fluoroscopy may be used to make sure the tip is placed correctly.

The balloon is inflated to temporarily block the pulmonary artery, so that pressure in the capillaries of the lungs (pulmonary capillary wedge pressure) can be measured. This measurement is an indirect way to determine pressure in the left atrium. Blood samples can be taken through the catheter, so that the oxygen and carbon dioxide levels in the blood can be measured.

The procedure may cause many complications, but they are usually rare. They include an air pocket between the layers of membranes covering the lungs (pneumothorax), abnormal heart rhythms (arrhythmias), infection, damage or clotting in the pulmonary artery, and injury to an artery or vein.

Central Venous Catheterization

In central venous catheterization, a catheter is inserted into one of the large veins of the neck, upper chest, or groin. This procedure is most often used to give intravenous fluids or drugs when a catheter cannot be inserted into an arm or a leg vein (peripheral intravenous catheter). Central venous catheterization is occasionally used to monitor central venous pressure (pressure in the superior vena cava, the large vein that returns blood to the heart from the upper part of the body). Central venous pressure reflects the pressure in the right atrium when it is filled with blood. This measurement helps doctors estimate whether the person is dehydrated and how well the heart is functioning. But it has largely been replaced by pulmonary artery catheterization.

Angiography of Peripheral Blood Vessels

Angiography of the peripheral arteries (those of the arms, legs, and trunk—except those supplying the heart) is similar to coronary angiography, except the catheter is threaded to the artery being investigated (see page 2036). Angiography may be performed to detect narrowing or blockage of an artery, a bulge (aneurysm) in an artery, or an abnormal channel between an artery and a vein (arteriovenous fistula). Angiography is often performed to determine whether angioplasty (see page 404) or coronary artery bypass grafting (see art on page 406) is needed.

Angiography of the aorta (**aortography**) can be used to detect abnormalities (such as an aneurysm or a dissection) in the aorta. It can also be used to detect leakage of the valve between the left ventricle and the aorta (aortic regurgitation).

Digital subtraction angiography may be performed before selective angiography to detect and visualize problems such as narrowing or blockage of an artery. However, this type of angiography is seldom adequate to determine whether surgery (with or without angioplasty) is needed. Digital subtraction angiography is not used for coronary arteries because it is unnecessary; clear images of these arteries can be obtained when a radiopaque dye is injected directly into a coronary artery.

In digital subtraction angiography, images of arteries are obtained before and after a radiopaque dye is injected, and a computer subtracts one image from the other. Images of tissues other than the arteries (such as bones) are thus eliminated. As a result, the arteries can be seen more clearly, much less dye is required, and the procedure may be safer than standard angiography.

CHAPTER 54 | High Blood Pressure

High blood pressure (hypertension) is abnormally high pressure in the arteries.

- Often no cause for high blood pressure can be identified, but sometimes it occurs as a result of an underlying disorder of the kidneys or a hormonal disorder.
- Obesity, a sedentary lifestyle, stress, smoking, and excessive amounts of alcohol or salt in the diet all can play a role in the development of high blood pressure in people who have an inherited tendency to develop it.
- In most people, high blood pressure causes no symptoms.
- Doctors make the diagnosis after measuring blood pressure on two or more occasions.
- People are advised to lose weight, stop smoking, and decrease the amounts of salt and fats in their diets.
- Antihypertensive drugs are given.

To many people, the word hypertension suggests excessive tension, nervousness, or stress. In medical terms, hypertension refers to high blood pressure, regardless of the cause. Because it usually does not cause symptoms for many years—until a vital organ is damaged—it has been called "the silent killer." Uncontrolled high blood pressure increases the risk of problems such as stroke, aneurysm, heart failure, heart attack, and kidney damage.

More than 65 million Americans are estimated to have high blood pressure. High blood pressure occurs more often in blacks—in 32% of black adults compared with 23% of whites and 23% of Mexican Americans. It also occurs with high frequency in people whose ancestors are from China or Japan. The consequences of high blood pressure are worse for blacks. High blood pressure occurs more often in older people—in about three fourths of women and almost two thirds of men aged 75 or older, compared with only about one fourth of people aged 20 to 74. People who have normal blood pressure at age 55 have a 90% risk of developing high blood pressure. High blood pressure is twice as common among people who are obese as among those who are not.

In the United States, only an estimated 70% of people with high blood pressure have been diagnosed. Of people with a diagnosis of high blood pressure, about 84% receive treatment, and of the people receiving treatment, about 58% have adequately controlled blood pressure.

When blood pressure is checked, two values are recorded. The higher value reflects the highest pressure in the arteries, which is reached when the heart contracts (during systole). The lower value reflects the lowest pressure in the arteries, which is reached just before the heart begins to contract again (during diastole). Blood pressure is written as systolic pressure/diastolic pressure—for example, 120/80 mm Hg (millimeters of mercury). This reading is referred to as "120 over 80."

High blood pressure is defined as a systolic pressure at rest that averages 140 mm Hg or more, a diastolic pressure at rest that averages 90 mm Hg or more, or both. However, the higher the blood pressure, the greater the risk of complications—even within the normal blood pressure range—so these limits are somewhat arbitrary. In most young people with high blood pressure, both systolic and diastolic pressures are high. In contrast, many older people with high blood pressure have high systolic pressure (140 mm Hg or more) with normal or low diastolic pressure (less than 90 mm Hg). This disorder is called **isolated systolic hypertension.**

A **hypertensive urgency** is blood pressure that is more than 180/120 mm Hg but has not yet produced any organ damage that is apparent to people or their doctors. A hypertensive urgency usually does not produce symptoms.

A **hypertensive emergency** is a particularly severe form of high blood pressure. Blood pressure is at least 180/120 mm Hg, and there is evidence of progressive damage in one or more vital organs, often accompanied by a variety of symptoms. Malignant hypertension is one type of hypertensive emergency. It occurs in only about 1 of 200 people who have high blood pressure. However, it is several times more common among blacks than among whites, among men than among women, and among people in lower socioeconomic groups than among those in higher socioeconomic groups. Malignant hypertension typically involves

SPOTLIGHT ON AGING

Changes due to aging may contribute to primary hypertension. As people age, large arteries gradually stiffen and small arteries may become partially blocked. Some experts think that this stiffening combined with the narrowing of small arteries may partly explain why blood pressure increases as people age.

damage to the eyes, and in some cases, damage to the kidneys. If untreated, malignant hypertension usually leads to death in 3 to 6 months.

The Body's Control of Blood Pressure

The body has many mechanisms to control blood pressure: The body can change the amount of blood the heart pumps, the diameter of arteries, and the volume of blood in the bloodstream. To increase blood pressure, the heart can pump more blood by pumping more forcefully or more rapidly. Small arteries (arterioles) can narrow (constrict), forcing the blood from each heartbeat through a narrower space than normal. Because the space in the arteries is narrower, the same amount of blood passing through them increases the blood pressure. Veins can constrict to reduce their capacity to hold blood, forcing more blood into the arteries. As a result, blood pressure increases. Fluid can be added to the bloodstream to increase blood volume and thus increase blood pressure. Conversely, to decrease blood pressure, the heart can pump less forcefully

---

Regulating Blood Pressure: The Renin-Angiotensin-Aldosterone System

The renin-angiotensin-aldosterone system is a series of reactions designed to help regulate blood pressure.

1. When blood pressure falls (for systolic, to 100 mm Hg or lower), the kidneys release the enzyme renin into the bloodstream.
2. Renin splits angiotensinogen, a large protein that circulates in the bloodstream, into pieces. One piece is angiotensin I.
3. Angiotensin I, which is relatively inactive, is split into pieces by angiotensin-converting enzyme (ACE). One piece is angiotensin II, a hormone, which is very active.

4. Angiotensin II causes the muscular walls of small arteries (arterioles) to constrict, increasing blood pressure. Angiotensin II also triggers the release of the hormone aldosterone from the adrenal glands and antidiuretic hormone from the pituitary gland.
5. Aldosterone causes the kidneys to retain salt (sodium) and excrete potassium. The sodium causes water to be retained, thus increasing blood volume and blood pressure.

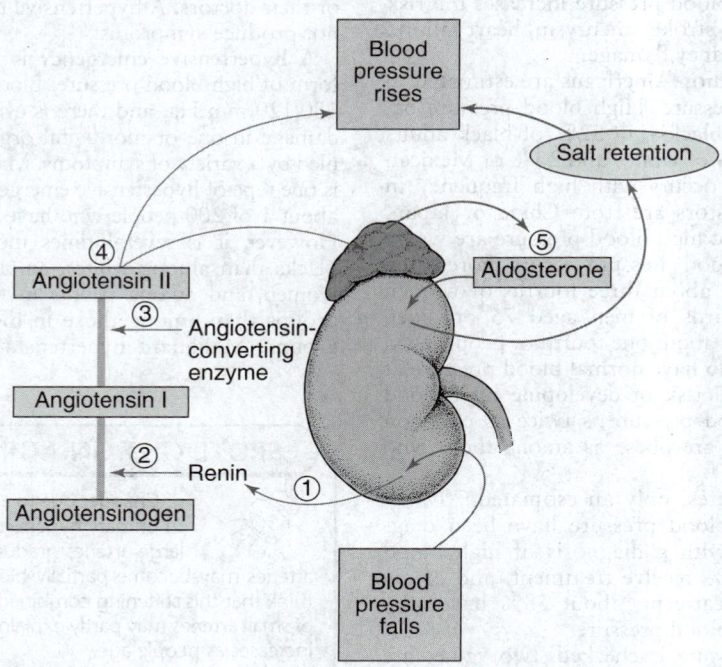

or rapidly, arterioles and veins can widen (dilate), and fluid can be removed from the bloodstream.

These mechanisms are controlled by the sympathetic division of the autonomic nervous system (the part of the nervous system that regulates internal body processes requiring no conscious effort) and by the kidneys. The sympathetic division uses several means to temporarily increase blood pressure during the fight-or-flight response (the body's physical reaction to a threat). The sympathetic division stimulates the adrenal glands to release the hormones epinephrine (adrenaline) and norepinephrine (noradrenaline). These hormones stimulate the heart to beat faster and more forcefully, most arterioles to constrict, and some arterioles to dilate. The arterioles that dilate are those in areas where an increased blood supply is needed (such as in skeletal muscle—the muscles controlled by conscious effort). The sympathetic division also stimulates the kidneys to decrease their excretion of salt (sodium) and water, thereby increasing blood volume. The body controls the movement of salt in and out of cells, to prevent an excess of salt inside cells. Excessive amounts of salt inside cells can cause the body to become overly sensitive to stimulation by the sympathetic division.

The kidneys also respond directly to changes in blood pressure. If blood pressure increases, the kidneys increase their excretion of salt and water, so that blood volume decreases and blood pressure returns to normal. Conversely, if blood pressure decreases, the kidneys decrease their excretion of salt and water, so that blood volume increases and blood pressure returns to normal. The kidneys can increase blood pressure by secreting the enzyme renin, which eventually results in the production of the hormone angiotensin II. Angiotensin II helps increase blood pressure by causing the arterioles to constrict, by triggering the sympathetic division of the autonomic nervous system, and by triggering the release of two other hormones, aldosterone and antidiuretic hormone (also called vasopressin), which cause the kidneys to increase the retention of salt and water. The kidneys normally produce substances that cause arterioles within the kidney to dilate. This helps balance the effects of hormones that cause constriction of arterioles.

Normally, whenever a change (for example, increased activity or a strong emotion) causes a transient increase in blood pressure, one of the body's compensatory mechanisms is triggered to counteract the change and keep blood pressure at normal levels. For example, an increase in the amount of blood pumped out by the heart—which tends to increase blood pressure—causes dilation of blood vessels and an increase in the kidneys' excretion of salt and water—which tend to reduce blood pressure.

Ups and Downs of Blood Pressure

Blood pressure varies naturally over a person's life. Infants and children normally have much lower blood pressure than adults. For almost everyone living in industrialized countries such as the United States, blood pressure increases with aging. Systolic pressure increases until at least age 80, and diastolic pressure increases until age 55 to 60, then levels off or even decreases. However, for people living in some developing countries, neither systolic nor diastolic pressure increases with aging, and high blood pressure is practically nonexistent, possibly because salt (sodium) intake is low and the physical activity level is higher.

Activity temporarily affects blood pressure, which is higher when a person is active and lower when a person rests. Blood pressure also varies with the time of day: It is highest in the morning and lowest at night during sleep. These variations are normal.

Causes

Primary Hypertension: High blood pressure with no known cause is called primary (formerly called essential) hypertension. Between 85% and 95% of people with high blood pressure have primary hypertension. Several changes in the heart and blood vessels probably combine to increase blood pressure. For instance, the amount of blood pumped per minute (cardiac output) may be increased, and the resistance to blood flow may be increased because blood vessels are constricted. Blood volume may be increased also. The reasons for such changes are not fully understood but appear to involve an inherited abnormality affecting the constriction of arterioles, which help control blood pressure. Other changes may contribute to increases in blood pressure, including accumulation of excessive amounts of salt inside cells and decreased production of substances that dilate arterioles.

Secondary Hypertension: High blood pressure with a known cause is called secondary hypertension. Between 5% and 15% of people with high blood pressure have secondary hypertension. In many of these people, high blood pressure results from a kidney disorder. Many kidney disorders can cause high blood pressure, because the kidneys are important in controlling blood pressure. For example, damage to the kidneys from inflammation or other disorders may impair their ability to remove enough salt and water from the body, increasing blood volume and blood pressure. Other kidney disorders that cause high blood pressure include renal artery stenosis (narrowing of the artery supplying one

Some Causes of Secondary Hypertension

Kidney disorders
Renal artery stenosis
Pyelonephritis
Glomerulonephritis
Kidney tumors
Polycystic kidney disease (usually inherited)
Injury to a kidney
Radiation therapy affecting the kidneys

Hormonal disorders
Hyperthyroidism
Hyperaldosteronism
Cushing's syndrome
Pheochromocytoma
Acromegaly

Other disorders
Coarctation of the aorta
Arteriosclerosis
Preeclampsia (a complication of pregnancy)
Acute intermittent porphyria
Acute lead poisoning

Drugs
Nonsteroidal anti-inflammatory drugs
Oral contraceptives
Corticosteroids
Cyclosporine
Erythropoietin
Cocaine
Alcohol abuse
Licorice (excessive amounts)

of the kidneys), which may be due to atherosclerosis, injury, or other disorders.

In a few patients, secondary hypertension is caused by another disorder, such as a hormonal disorder, or by the use of certain drugs, such as birth control pills (oral contraceptives). Hormonal disorders that cause high blood pressure include Cushing's syndrome (a disorder characterized by high levels of cortisol), hyperthyroidism (an overactive thyroid gland), hyperaldosteronism (overproduction of aldosterone, often by a tumor in one of the adrenal glands), and, rarely, a pheochromocytoma (a tumor that is located in an adrenal gland and that produces the hormones epinephrine and norepinephrine). Severe hyperthyroidism can also cause systolic hypertension.

Arteriosclerosis interferes with the body's control of blood pressure, increasing the risk of high blood pressure. Arteriosclerosis makes arteries stiff, preventing the dilation that would otherwise return blood pressure to normal (see box on page 398).

Aggravating Factors: Obesity, a sedentary lifestyle, stress, smoking, and excessive amounts of alcohol or salt in the diet all can play a role in the development of high blood pressure in people who have an inherited tendency to develop it. Stress tends to cause blood pressure to increase temporarily, but blood pressure usually returns to normal once the stress is over. An example is "white coat hypertension," in which the stress of visiting a doctor's office causes blood pressure to increase enough to be diagnosed as high blood pressure in someone who has normal blood pressure at other times. In susceptible people, these brief increases in blood pressure are thought to cause damage that eventually results in permanent high blood pressure, even when no stress is present. This theory has not been proved.

Symptoms

In most people, high blood pressure causes no symptoms, despite the coincidental occurrence of certain symptoms that are widely, but erroneously, attributed to high blood pressure: headaches, nosebleeds, dizziness, a flushed face, and fatigue. People with high blood pressure may have these symptoms, but the symptoms occur just as frequently in people with normal blood pressure.

Severe or long-standing high blood pressure that is untreated can produce symptoms because it can damage the brain, eyes, heart, and kidneys. Symptoms include headache, fatigue, nausea, vomiting, shortness of breath, and restlessness. In people who have malignant hypertension, severe high blood pressure causes bleeding and swelling of the retina (the light-sensitive membrane on the inner surface of the back of the eye), resulting in blurred vision. Occasionally, severe high blood pressure causes the brain to swell, resulting in nausea, vomiting, worsening headache, drowsiness, confusion, seizures, sleepiness, and even coma. This condition is called hypertensive encephalopathy. Malignant hypertension and hypertensive encephalopathy are types of hypertensive emergencies and, as such, require emergency treatment.

Did You Know...

Certain symptoms, such as headaches, nosebleeds, dizziness, a flushed face, and fatigue, are commonly attributed to high blood pressure but actually occur equally often in people who do not have high blood pressure.

If high blood pressure is due to a pheochromocytoma, symptoms may include severe headache, anxiety, an awareness of a rapid or irregular heart rate (palpitations), excessive perspiration, tremor, and paleness. These symptoms result from high levels of the hormones epinephrine and norepinephrine, which are secreted by the pheochromocytoma.

Complications: Long-standing high blood pressure can damage the heart and blood vessels.

When pressure in the arteries is increased above 140/90 mm Hg, the heart enlarges and the heart's walls thicken because the heart has to work harder to pump blood. The thickened walls are stiffer than normal. Consequently, the heart's chambers do not expand normally and are harder to fill with blood, further increasing the heart's workload. These changes in the heart may result in abnormal heart rhythms (see page 366) and heart failure (see page 352).

High blood pressure causes thickening of the walls of blood vessels and also makes them more likely to develop hardening of the arteries (atherosclerosis). When these things have occurred, people are at risk of stroke, heart attack, and kidney failure.

Diagnosis

Blood pressure is measured after a person sits or lies down for 5 minutes. It should be measured again after the person stands for a few minutes, especially if the person is older or has diabetes. A reading of 140/90 mm Hg or more is considered high, but a diagnosis cannot be based on a single high reading. Sometimes, even several high readings are not enough to make the diagnosis—because, for example, the readings may vary too much. If a person has an initial high reading, blood pressure is measured again during the same visit and then measured twice on at least two other days to make sure that the high blood pressure persists.

If there is still doubt, a 24-hour blood pressure monitor may be used. It is a portable battery-operated device, worn on the hip, connected to a blood pressure cuff, worn on the arm. This monitor repeatedly records blood pressure throughout the day and night over a 24-hour or 48-hour period. The readings determine not only whether high blood pressure is present but also how severe it is.

In people with very stiff arteries (most commonly, in older people), blood pressure may be measured as high when it is not. This phenomenon is called **pseudohypertension.** It occurs when the artery in the arm is too stiff to be compressed by the blood pressure cuff, and as a result, blood pressure cannot be measured accurately.

After high blood pressure has been diagnosed, its effects on key organs, especially the blood vessels, heart, brain, eyes, and kidneys, are usually evaluated. Doctors also look for the cause of high blood pressure. The number and type of tests that are performed to look for organ damage and to determine the cause of high blood pressure vary from person to person. In general, routine evaluation for all people with high blood pressure involves a medical history, a physical examination, electrocardiography (ECG), blood tests (including the hematocrit level, potassium and sodium levels, and tests of kidney function), and urine tests.

The physical examination includes checking the area of the abdomen over the kidneys for tenderness and placing a stethoscope over the abdomen to listen for a bruit (the sound caused by blood rushing through a narrowed artery) in the artery supplying each kidney.

The retina in each eye is examined with an ophthalmoscope (see art on page 1422). The retina is the only place doctors can directly view the effects of high blood pressure on arterioles. The assumption is that the changes in the arterioles of the retina are similar to changes in arterioles and other blood vessels elsewhere in the body, such as in the kidneys. By determining the degree of damage to the retina (retinopathy—see page 1456), doctors can classify the severity of high blood pressure.

A stethoscope is used to detect heart sounds. An abnormal heart sound, called the fourth heart sound, is one of the earliest changes in the heart caused by high blood pressure. This sound develops because the left atrium of the heart has to contract harder to fill the enlarged, stiff left ventricle, which pumps blood to all of the body except the lungs.

Electrocardiography (ECG—see page 326) is usually performed to detect changes in the heart—particularly thickening (hypertrophy) of the heart muscle or heart enlargement. If enlargement is suspected, the person may undergo echocardiography (see page 328).

Kidney damage can be detected by urine and blood tests. Urine tests can detect early evidence of kidney damage. The presence of blood cells and albumin (the most abundant protein in blood) in the urine may indicate such damage. Symptoms of kidney damage (such as lethargy, poor appetite, and fatigue) do not usually develop until 70 to 80% of kidney function is lost.

Diagnosis of Cause: The higher the blood pressure and the younger the person, the more extensive the search for a cause is likely to be, even though a cause is identified in less than 10% of people. A more extensive evaluation may include x-ray, ultrasonography, and radionuclide imaging of the kidneys and their blood supply as well as a chest x-ray. Blood and urine tests are done to measure the levels of certain hormones, such as epinephrine, aldosterone, and cortisol.

The cause may be suggested by abnormal results of a physical examination or by the symptoms. For

Measuring Blood Pressure

Several instruments can measure blood pressure quickly and with little discomfort. A sphygmomanometer is commonly used. It consists of a soft rubber cuff connected to a rubber bulb that is used to inflate the cuff and a meter that registers the pressure of the cuff. The meter may be a dial or a glass column filled with mercury. Blood pressure is measured in millimeters of mercury (mm Hg) because the first instrument used to measure it was a mercury column.

When a sphygmomanometer is used, a person sits with legs uncrossed and back supported. An arm is bared (if a sleeve is rolled up, caution is needed to ensure that it is not tight around the arm), bent, and resting on a table, so that the arm is about the same level as the heart. The cuff is wrapped around the arm. Using a cuff that is proportional to the size of the arm is important. If the cuff is too small, the blood pressure reading is too high. If the cuff is too large, the reading is too low.

Listening with a stethoscope placed over the artery below the cuff, a health care practitioner inflates the cuff by squeezing the bulb until the cuff compresses the artery tightly enough to temporarily stop blood flow, usually to a pressure that is about 30 mm Hg higher than the person's usual systolic pressure (the pressure exerted when the heart beats). Then the cuff is gradually deflated. The pressure at which the practitioner first hears a pulse in the artery is the systolic pressure. The cuff continues to be deflated, and at some point, the sound of blood flowing stops. The pressure at this point is the diastolic pressure (the pressure exerted when the heart relaxes, between beats).

Some instruments can measure blood pressure automatically, without use of a stethoscope or rubber bulb. These devices may fit around the upper arm, finger, or wrist. For people older than 50, blood pressure measured at the upper arm is the most accurate. Sometimes a precise measurement of blood pressure is needed—for example, for a person in an intensive care unit. In such cases, a catheter can be inserted inside an artery to measure blood pressure directly.

Instruments to measure blood pressure are available for home use by people who have high blood pressure.

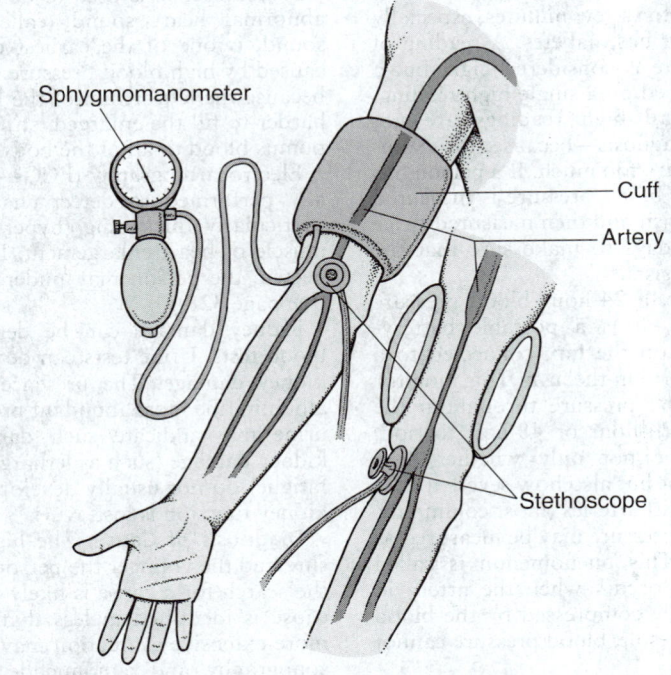

Sphygmomanometer

Cuff

Artery

Stethoscope

example, a bruit in the artery to a kidney may suggest renal artery stenosis (narrowing of the artery supplying a kidney). Various combinations of symptoms may suggest high levels of the hormones epinephrine and norepinephrine, produced by a pheochromocytoma. The presence of a pheochromocytoma is confirmed when the breakdown products of these hormones are detected in the urine.

Other rare causes of high blood pressure may be detected by certain routine tests. For example, measuring the potassium level in the blood can help detect hyperaldosteronism (see page 1003).

Treatment

Primary hypertension cannot be cured, but it can be controlled to prevent complications. Because high blood pressure itself has no symptoms, doctors try to avoid treatments that cause side effects or interfere with a person's lifestyle. Alternative measures are usually tried before any drugs are prescribed. However, drug therapy is usually started at the same time as alternative measures in all people with blood pressure at or above 160/100 mm Hg and in people with blood pressure at or above 120/80 mm Hg who also have diabetes, a kidney disorder, evidence of damage to a vital organ, or other risk factors for coronary artery disease.

Overweight people with high blood pressure are advised to lose weight. Losing as few as 10 pounds (4.5 kilograms) can lower blood pressure. For people who are obese or who have diabetes or high cholesterol levels, changes in diet (to a diet rich in fruits, vegetables, and low-fat dairy products, with reduced saturated and total fat content) are important for reducing the risk of heart and blood vessel disease. Smokers should stop smoking.

Reducing the intake of alcohol and sodium (while maintaining an adequate intake of calcium, magnesium, and potassium) may make drug therapy for high blood pressure unnecessary. Daily alcohol intake should be reduced to no more than 2 drinks (a daily total of 24 ounces [about 1 liter] of beer, 8 ounces [about 240 milliliters] of wine, or 2 ounces [about 60 milliliters] of 100-proof whiskey or other liquor) in men and 1 drink in women. Daily sodium intake should be reduced to less than 2½ grams, or sodium chloride intake, to 6 grams.

Moderate aerobic exercise is helpful. People with primary hypertension do not have to restrict their physical activity as long as their blood pressure is controlled. Regular exercise helps reduce blood pressure and weight and improves the functioning of the heart and overall health (see page 38).

Doctors often recommend that people with high blood pressure monitor their own blood pressure at home. Self-monitoring probably helps motivate people to follow a doctor's recommendations regarding treatment.

CLASSIFYING BLOOD PRESSURE IN ADULTS

Blood pressure is classified by its severity because treatment is based, in part, on severity. When a person's systolic and diastolic pressures fall into different categories, the higher category is used to classify blood pressure. For instance, 150/88 mm Hg is classified as stage 1 hypertension, and 150/105 mm Hg is classified as stage 2 hypertension.

The optimal blood pressure for minimizing the risk of cardiovascular problems (such as heart attack and heart failure) and stroke is below 115/75 mm Hg.

CATEGORY	SYSTOLIC BLOOD PRESSURE (mm Hg)	DIASTOLIC BLOOD PRESSURE (mm Hg)	RECOMMENDED FOLLOW-UP
Normal blood pressure	Below 120	Below 80	Blood pressure is rechecked in 2 years.
Prehypertension	120–139	80–89	Blood pressure is rechecked in 1 year, and advice about lifestyle changes is provided.
Stage 1 hypertension	140–159	90–99	The high blood pressure is confirmed within 2 months, and advice about lifestyle changes is provided.
Stage 2 hypertension	Above 160	Above 100	The person is evaluated or referred to a source of care within 1 month. For people with higher pressures (eg, 180/110 mm Hg or higher), evaluation or treatment is immediate or within 1 week, depending on the person's condition.

℞ ANTIHYPERTENSIVE DRUGS

TYPE	EXAMPLES	SOME SIDE EFFECTS
Diuretics		
Loop diuretics	Bumetanide Ethacrynic acid Furosemide Torsemide	Decreased levels of potassium and magnesium, temporarily increased levels of blood sugar and cholesterol, an increased level of uric acid, sexual dysfunction in men, and digestive upset
Potassium-sparing diuretics	Amiloride Eplerenone Spironolactone Triamterene	With all, a high potassium level and digestive upset With spironolactone, breast enlargement in men (gynecomastia) and menstrual irregularities in women
Thiazide and thiazide-like diuretics	Chlorothiazide Chlorthalidone Hydrochlorothiazide Indapamide Metolazone	Decreased levels of potassium and magnesium, increased levels of calcium and uric acid, sexual dysfunction in men, and digestive upset
Adrenergic blockers		
Alpha-blockers	Doxazosin Prazosin Terazosin	Fainting (syncope) with the first dose, awareness of rapid heartbeats (palpitations), dizziness, low blood pressure when the person stands (orthostatic hypotension), and fluid retention (edema)
Beta-blockers	Acebutolol Atenolol Betaxolol Bisoprolol Carteolol Metoprolol Nadolol Penbutolol Pindolol Propranolol Timolol	Spasm of the airways (bronchospasm), an abnormally slow heart rate (bradycardia), heart failure, possible masking of low blood sugar levels after insulin injections, impaired peripheral circulation, insomnia, fatigue, shortness of breath, depression, Raynaud's syndrome, vivid dreams, hallucinations, and sexual dysfunction With some beta-blockers, an increased triglyceride level
Alpha-beta blockers	Carvedilol Labetalol	Low blood pressure when the person stands and spasm of the airways
Peripherally acting adrenergic blockers	Guanadrel Guanethidine Reserpine	With guanadrel and guanethidine, diarrhea, sexual dysfunction, low blood pressure when the person stands, and fluid retention With reserpine, depression, nasal congestion, lethargy, and bleeding of a peptic ulcer
Centrally acting alpha-agonists		
	Clonidine Guanabenz Guanfacine Methyldopa	Drowsiness, dry mouth, fatigue, an abnormally slow heart rate, rebound high blood pressure when the drug is withdrawn (except with methyldopa), and sexual dysfunction With methyldopa, depression, low blood pressure when the person stands, and liver and autoimmune disorders
Angiotensin-converting enzyme (ACE) inhibitors		
	Benazepril Captopril Enalapril Fosinopril Lisinopril Moexipril	Cough (in up to 20% of people), low blood pressure, an increased potassium level, rash, angioedema (allergic swelling that affects the face, lips, and windpipe and may interfere with breathing), and, in pregnant women, serious injury to the fetus

(continued on the following page)

℞ ANTIHYPERTENSIVE DRUGS (*Continued*)

TYPE	EXAMPLES	SOME SIDE EFFECTS
Angiotensin-converting enzyme (ACE) inhibitors (*continued*)		
	Perindopril Quinapril Ramipril Trandolapril	
Angiotensin II receptor blockers (ARBs)		
	Candesartan Eprosartan Irbesartan Losartan Olmesartan Telmisartan Valsartan	Dizziness, an increased potassium level, angioedema (rare), and, in pregnant women, serious injury to the fetus
Calcium channel blockers		
Dihydropyridines	Amlodipine Felodipine Isradipine Nicardipine Nifedipine (sustained-release only) Nisoldipine	Dizziness, fluid retention in the ankles, flushing, headache, heartburn, enlarged gums, and an abnormally fast heart rate (tachycardia)
Nondihydropyridines	Diltiazem (sustained-release only) Verapamil	Headache, dizziness, flushing, fluid retention, problems in the heart's electrical conduction system (including heart block), an abnormally slow heart rate (bradycardia), heart failure, and enlarged gums With verapamil, constipation
Direct vasodilators		
	Hydralazine Minoxidil	Headache, an abnormally fast heart rate (tachycardia), and fluid retention

Drug Therapy: Drugs that are used in the treatment of high blood pressure are called antihypertensives. With the wide variety of antihypertensives available, high blood pressure can be controlled in almost anyone, but treatment has to be tailored to the individual. Treatment is most effective when patient and doctor communicate well and collaborate on the treatment program.

The blood pressure goal for antihypertensive therapy is to decrease blood pressure to below 140/90 mm Hg. For people with diabetes or a kidney disorder, the goal is below 130/80 mm Hg. Some experts believe that the goal should also be below 130/80 mm Hg for people with coronary artery disease or angina. Doctors try to avoid decreasing diastolic blood pressure below 65, especially in older people and in people with coronary artery disease or angina.

Different types of antihypertensives reduce blood pressure by different mechanisms, so many different treatment strategies are possible. For some people, doctors use a stepped approach to drug therapy: They start with one type of antihypertensive and add others as necessary. For other people, doctors find a sequential approach is preferable: They prescribe one antihypertensive, and if it is ineffective, they discontinue it and prescribe another type. For people with blood pressure at or above 160/100 mm Hg, usually two drugs are started at the same time. In choosing an antihypertensive, doctors consider such factors as

- The person's age, sex, and race
- The severity of high blood pressure
- The presence of other conditions, such as diabetes or high blood cholesterol levels

- Potential side effects, which vary from drug to drug
- The costs of the drugs and of tests needed to check for certain side effects

A majority of people (more than 74%) ultimately require two or more drugs to reach their blood pressure goal.

Most people tolerate their prescribed antihypertensive drugs without problems. But any antihypertensive drug can cause side effects. So if side effects develop, a person should tell the doctor, who can adjust the dose or substitute another drug. Usually, an antihypertensive drug must be taken indefinitely to control blood pressure.

A **thiazide diuretic** is often the first drug given to treat high blood pressure. Diuretics cause blood vessels to dilate. Diuretics also help the kidneys eliminate salt and water, decreasing fluid volume throughout the body and thus lowering blood pressure. Because thiazide diuretics cause potassium to be excreted in the urine, potassium supplements or a diuretic that does not cause potassium loss or that causes potassium levels to increase (a potassium-sparing diuretic) sometimes must be taken with a thiazide diuretic. Usually, potassium-sparing diuretics are not used alone because they do not control blood pressure as well as thiazide diuretics do; however, the potassium-sparing diuretic spironolactone is sometimes used alone. Diuretics are particularly useful for blacks, older people, obese people, and people with heart failure or chronic kidney failure.

Adrenergic blockers include alpha-blockers, beta-blockers, alpha-beta blockers, and peripherally acting adrenergic blockers. These drugs block the effects of the sympathetic division, the part of the nervous system that can rapidly respond to stress by increasing blood pressure. The most commonly used adrenergic blockers, the beta-blockers, are particularly useful for whites, young people, and people who have had a heart attack. They are also useful for people who have a rapid heart rate, angina pectoris (chest pain due to inadequate blood supply to the heart muscle), or migraine headaches. The risk of side effects is higher for older people. Alpha-blockers are no longer used as the main therapy because they do not decrease the risk of death. Peripherally acting adrenergic blockers are usually only used if a third or fourth type of drug is needed to control blood pressure.

Centrally acting alpha-agonists lower blood pressure through a mechanism that somewhat resembles that of adrenergic blockers. By stimulating certain receptors in the brain stem, these agonists inhibit the effects of the sympathetic division of the nervous system. These drugs are rarely used now.

Angiotensin-converting enzyme (ACE) inhibitors lower blood pressure in part by dilating arterioles.

They dilate arterioles by preventing the formation of angiotensin II, which causes arterioles to constrict. Specifically, these inhibitors block the action of angiotensin-converting enzyme, which converts angiotensin I to angiotensin II (see art on page 334). These drugs are particularly useful for people with coronary artery disease or heart failure, whites, young people, people with protein in their urine because of chronic kidney disease or diabetic kidney disease, and men who develop sexual dysfunction as a side effect of another antihypertensive drug.

Angiotensin II receptor blockers (ARBs) lower blood pressure by a mechanism similar to the one used by angiotensin-converting enzyme inhibitors: They directly block the action of angiotensin II, which causes arterioles to constrict. Because the mechanism is more direct, angiotensin II receptor blockers may cause fewer side effects.

Calcium channel blockers cause arterioles to dilate by a completely different mechanism. They are particularly useful for blacks and older people. Calcium channel blockers are also useful for people who have angina pectoris, certain types of rapid heart rate, or migraine headaches. Calcium channel blockers may be short-acting or long-acting. Short-acting calcium channel blockers are not used to treat high blood pressure. Reports suggest that people using short-acting calcium channel blockers may have an increased risk of death due to heart attack, but no reports suggest such effects for long-acting calcium channel blockers.

Direct vasodilators dilate blood vessels by another mechanism. A drug of this type is almost never used alone; rather, it is added as a second drug when another drug alone does not lower blood pressure sufficiently.

Aspirin is not an antihypertensive, but some doctors recommend that people who have high blood pressure take a low-dose aspirin tablet once a day.

Treatment of Secondary Hypertension

The cause of the high blood pressure is treated if possible. Treating kidney disease can sometimes return blood pressure to normal or at least lower it, so that antihypertensive therapy is more effective. A narrowed artery to the kidney may be dilated by inserting a balloon-tipped catheter and inflating the balloon (angioplasty—see art on page 405). Or the narrowed part of the artery supplying the kidney can be bypassed. Often such surgery cures high blood pressure. Tumors that cause high blood pressure, such as a pheochromocytoma, usually can be removed surgically (see page 1003).

Treatment of Hypertensive Urgencies and Emergencies

Hypertensive urgencies are treated with clonidine, an adrenergic blocker, given by mouth. The calcium channel blocker nifedipine, given under the tongue (sublingually), has been used but is less safe.

In hypertensive emergencies, such as malignant hypertension and hypertensive encephalopathy, blood pressure must be lowered rapidly. Hypertensive emergencies are treated in hospital intensive care units. Most drugs used to rapidly lower blood pressure, such as fenoldopam, nitroprusside, nicardipine, or labetalol, are given intravenously.

Prognosis

Untreated high blood pressure increases a person's risk of developing heart disease (such as heart failure, heart attack, or sudden cardiac death), kidney failure, or stroke at an early age. High blood pressure is the most important risk factor for stroke. It is also one of the three most important risk factors for heart attack that a person can modify (the other two are smoking and high cholesterol levels in the blood).

Treatment that lowers high blood pressure greatly decreases the risk of stroke and heart failure. Such treatment may also decrease the risk of a heart attack, although not as dramatically. Without treatment, fewer than 5% of people with malignant hypertension survive for a year.

CHAPTER

55 Low Blood Pressure

Low blood pressure (hypotension) is blood pressure low enough to cause symptoms such as dizziness and fainting.

- Various drugs and disorders can cause the body's system for maintaining blood pressure to malfunction.
- When blood pressure is too low, the brain malfunctions and fainting may occur.

Normally, the body maintains the pressure of blood in the arteries within a narrow range. If blood pressure is too high, it can damage a blood vessel and even rupture it, causing bleeding or other complications. If blood pressure is too low, not enough blood reaches all parts of the body. As a result, cells do not receive enough oxygen and nutrients, and waste products are not adequately removed. Very low blood pressure can be life threatening because it can lead to shock (see page 350). Healthy people who have blood pressure that is low but still in the normal range (when measured at rest) tend to live longer than people who have higher normal blood pressure.

The body has several compensatory mechanisms that control blood pressure (see page 334). They involve changing the diameter of veins and small arteries (arterioles), the amount of blood pumped from the heart (cardiac output), and the volume of blood in the blood vessels. These mechanisms return blood pressure to normal after it increases or decreases during normal activities, such as exercise or sleep.

Veins can widen (dilate) and narrow (constrict) to change how much blood they can hold (capacity). When veins constrict, their capacity to hold blood is reduced, allowing more blood to return to the heart from which it is pumped into the arteries. As a result, blood pressure increases. Conversely, when veins dilate, their capacity to hold blood is increased, allowing less blood to return to the heart. As a result, blood pressure decreases.

Arterioles can also dilate and constrict. The more constricted arterioles are, the greater their resistance to blood flow and the higher the blood pressure. Constriction of arterioles increases blood pressure because more pressure is needed to force blood through the narrower space. Conversely, dilation of arterioles reduces resistance to blood flow, thus reducing blood pressure.

The more blood pumped from the heart per minute (that is, the larger the cardiac output), the higher the blood pressure—as long as resistance to blood flow in the arteries remains constant. The body can change the amount of blood pumped during each heartbeat by making each contraction weaker or stronger.

The higher the volume of blood in the blood vessels, the higher the blood pressure—as long as resistance to blood flow in the arteries remains constant. To increase or decrease blood volume, the kidneys can vary the amount of fluid excreted in urine.

The compensatory mechanisms are activated by specialized cells that act as sensors, called baroreceptors. Located within arteries, these sensors constantly monitor blood pressure. Those in the large arteries of the neck and chest are particularly important. When sensors detect a change in blood pressure, they trigger a change in one of the compensatory mechanisms and so maintain a steady blood pressure. Nerves carry signals from these sensors and the brain to several key organs, which control the compensatory mechanisms:

- The heart is signaled to change the rate and force of heartbeats (thus changing the amount of blood pumped). This change is one of the first, and it corrects low blood pressure quickly.
- The arterioles are signaled to constrict or dilate (thus changing the resistance of blood vessels).
- The veins are signaled to constrict or dilate (thus changing their capacity to hold blood).
- The kidneys are signaled to change the amount of fluid excreted (thus changing the volume of blood in blood vessels). This change takes a long time to produce results and thus is the slowest mechanism for blood pressure control.

For example, when a person is bleeding, blood volume and thus blood pressure decrease. In such cases, sensors activate the compensatory mechanisms to prevent blood pressure from decreasing too much: The heart rate increases, increasing the amount of blood pumped; the veins constrict, reducing their capacity to hold blood; and the arterioles constrict, increasing their resistance to blood flow. If the bleeding is stopped, fluids from the rest of the body move into the blood vessels to begin restoring blood volume and thus blood pressure. The kidneys decrease their production of urine. Thus, they help the body retain as much fluid as possible to return to the blood vessels. Eventually, the bone marrow and spleen produce new blood cells, and blood volume is fully restored.

Nonetheless, these compensatory mechanisms have limitations. For example, if a person loses a lot of blood quickly, these mechanisms cannot compensate quickly enough, blood pressure falls, and organs may begin to malfunction (shock).

Causes

Various disorders and drugs can cause the compensatory mechanisms to malfunction, and low blood pressure may result. For example, cardiac output may be reduced as a result of heart disease, such as a heart attack (myocardial infarction), a heart valve disorder, an extremely rapid heartbeat (tachycardia), a very slow heartbeat (bradycardia), or another abnormal heart rhythm (arrhythmia). These disorders impair the heart's pumping ability. Arterioles may be dilated by toxins produced by bacteria during a bacterial infection. Blood volume can be reduced as a result of dehydration, bleeding, or kidney disorders. Some kidney disorders impair the kidneys' ability to return fluid to the blood vessels, resulting in the loss of large amounts of fluid in the urine. (Conversely, kidney failure, in which the kidneys cannot remove fluid from the blood, may result in overhydration that leads to

high blood pressure.) The ability of the nerves to conduct signals between sensors and the organs that control the compensatory mechanisms may be impaired by neurologic disorders (a condition called autonomic nervous system failure). In addition, as people age, compensatory mechanisms respond to changes in blood pressure more slowly.

Symptoms

When blood pressure is too low, the first organ to malfunction is usually the brain. The brain malfunctions first because it is located at the top of the body and blood flow must fight gravity to reach the brain. Consequently, most people with low blood pressure feel dizzy or light-headed, particularly when they stand, and some may even faint. People who faint fall to the floor, usually bringing the brain to the level of the heart. As a result, blood can flow to the brain without having to fight gravity, and blood flow to the brain increases, helping protect it from injury. However, if blood pressure is low enough, brain damage can still occur.

Low blood pressure occasionally causes shortness of breath or chest pain due to an inadequate blood supply to the heart muscle (angina).

All organs begin to malfunction if blood pressure becomes sufficiently low and remains low. This condition is called shock (see page 350).

The disorder causing low blood pressure may produce many other symptoms, which are not due to low blood pressure itself. For example, an infection may produce a fever.

Some symptoms occur when the body's compensatory mechanisms try to increase blood pressure that is low. For example, when arterioles constrict, blood flow to the skin, feet, and hands decreases. These areas may become cold and turn blue. When the heart beats more quickly and more forcefully, a person may feel palpitations (awareness of heartbeats).

Fainting

Fainting (syncope) is a sudden, brief loss of consciousness.

- Fainting occurs if brain function is disturbed.
- Dizziness and light-headedness are common, but other symptoms can occur depending on the cause of fainting.
- Doctors may use tilt-table testing and tests of heart function to try to determine the cause of fainting.
- Usually, lying flat causes the person to regain consciousness, but underlying disorders may need to be treated.

Fainting is a symptom of an inadequate supply of oxygen and other nutrients to the brain, usually caused by a temporary decrease in blood flow.

SOME CAUSES OF LOW BLOOD PRESSURE

CHANGE IN COMPENSATORY MECHANISM	CAUSES
Decrease in cardiac output	Abnormal heart rhythms Heart muscle damage or malfunction (such as that due to a heart attack or viral infection) Heart valve disorders Pulmonary embolism
Dilation of blood vessels	Alcohol Some allergic reactions Some antidepressants, such as amitriptyline Antihypertensive drugs that dilate blood vessels (such as calcium channel blockers, angiotensin-converting enzyme inhibitors, and angiotensin II receptor blockers) Nitrates Bacterial infections Exposure to heat Nerve damage (such as that due to diabetes, amyloidosis, or spinal cord injuries)
Decrease in blood volume	Diarrhea Diuretics (such as furosemide and hydrochlorothiazide) Excessive bleeding Excessive sweating Excessive urination (a common symptom of untreated diabetes or Addison's disease)
Blockage of blood flow back to the heart	During pregnancy, pressure on the inferior vena cava (the main vein that carries blood from the legs) from the uterus when women lie in certain positions Increased abdominal pressure when straining to move bowels or pass urine or when lifting heavy weights
Inhibition of the brain centers that control blood pressure	Alcohol Antidepressants Antihypertensive drugs such as methyldopa and clonidine Barbiturates
Impairment of the autonomic nervous system	Amyloidosis Diabetes Multiple system atrophy (Shy-Drager syndrome) Parkinson's disease

Blood flow to the brain can decrease whenever the body cannot quickly compensate for a fall in blood pressure.

Causes

A person cannot lose consciousness unless there is a general disturbance of brain function. This disturbance usually involves a reduction in blood flow to the brain. Blood flow to the brain can be reduced by a heart disorder or, more commonly, by something that interferes with the normal return of blood to the heart, which necessarily reduces blood flow to the brain (and the rest of the body). Rarely, blood flow to the brain is reduced by a disorder of the blood vessels at the base of the brain. Although seizures—a brain disorder—can cause loss of consciousness, they are not considered fainting. People and their doctors may not be able to differentiate between fainting and seizures without careful testing.

Problems With the Heart's Pumping: Fainting may occur if the heart cannot pump enough blood to maintain a normal blood pressure. For example, an abnormal heart rhythm or a heart valve disorder may impair the heart's pumping ability. People with such disorders may feel fine when resting. However, they feel faint or actually faint when exercising because the heart cannot pump enough blood to meet the body's increased demand for oxygen. This type of fainting is called exertional or effort syncope. People with these disorders may also faint *after* exercising. During exercise, the increase in heart rate may enable the heart to pump enough blood to maintain adequate blood pressure, although just barely. When exercise stops, the heart rate (and the amount of blood pumped) begins to decrease. However, the blood vessels in muscles, which dilate (widen) during exercise to move more blood to and from the muscles, remain dilated. (The arterioles in muscles remain dilated to help supply oxygen and nutrients to muscle tissue, and the veins remain dilated to remove metabolic waste products produced during exercise.) The decrease in the amount of blood pumped out combined with dilation of the arterioles and veins causes blood pressure to fall, and fainting results.

An abnormality of the heart called hypertrophic cardiomyopathy (see page 363) can also cause fainting that usually occurs during exercise. Severe narrowing (stenosis) of the aortic valve can have the same effect. These disorders may occur in younger people as well as older people, particularly those who have high blood pressure. If untreated, they can lead to death.

Low Volume of Blood: Fainting may occur if the blood volume is too low. An obvious cause of low blood volume is bleeding. Another cause is dehydration, which may be due to diarrhea, excessive sweating, inadequate intake of fluids, or excessive urination (which is a common symptom of untreated diabetes—see page 1005—or Addison's disease—see page 999). In older people, the use of diuretics is a common cause of dehydration, particularly during warm weather or during an illness when obtaining or drinking enough fluids may be difficult. (Diuretics help the kidneys eliminate salt and water by increasing urine formation and thus decrease fluid volume in the body.)

Vagus Nerve Stimulation: Fainting may occur if the vagus nerve, which supplies the neck, chest, and intestine, is stimulated. When stimulated, the vagus nerve slows the heart. Such stimulation also causes nausea and cool, clammy skin. This type of fainting is called vasovagal (vasomotor) syncope. The vagus nerve is stimulated by pain, fear, other distress (such as that due to the sight of blood), vomiting, a large bowel movement, and urination. Fainting during or immediately after urination is called micturition syncope. Rarely, vigorous swallowing causes fainting due to stimulation of the vagus nerve.

Reduced Blood Flow: Fainting may also occur if straining reduces the amount of blood flowing back to the heart. Fainting due to coughing (cough syncope) usually results from such straining. Fainting after urination (micturition syncope) or after a bowel movement is partly due to straining (in addition to stimulation of the vagus nerve). Older men who must strain to empty their bladder because of a large prostate gland are particularly susceptible. Fainting when lifting weights (weight lifter's syncope) results from the strain of trying to lift or push heavy weights without breathing adequately during the exercise.

Problems With Blood Pressure: Fainting that occurs when a person sits or stands up too quickly is called orthostatic (postural) syncope. It is particularly common among older people. It is caused by orthostatic hypotension (see page 348). In orthostatic hypotension, the compensatory mechanisms, particularly the constriction of blood vessels and the increase in heart rate, do not adequately restore blood pressure when a person stands and gravity causes blood to pool in the leg veins. A related form of fainting, called parade ground syncope, occurs when people stand still for a long time on a hot day. If the leg muscles are not used, blood is not pumped back to the heart. As a result, blood pools in the leg veins, and blood pressure falls.

In older people, an excessive decrease in blood pressure after eating a meal (postprandial hypotension—see page 349) may cause fainting.

Other Problems: Fainting may result from very rapid breathing (hyperventilation, or overbreathing), which may be due to anxiety. This type of fainting is called hyperventilation syncope. Hyperventilation removes large amounts of carbon dioxide from the body. The decreased level of carbon dioxide causes blood vessels in the brain to constrict, and the person may feel faint or actually faint.

Rarely, fainting results from a mild stroke in which blood flow to a certain part of the brain (at the base) suddenly decreases. Fainting due to a stroke is more common among older people. Many other disorders, such as a deficiency of red blood cells (anemia), lung disorders, a decreased blood sugar level (hypoglycemia), and diabetes can cause fainting, especially if the compensatory mechanisms are also impaired.

Certain drugs may cause fainting. They include many of those used to treat high blood pressure, angina, and heart failure. Doses of these drugs must be carefully adjusted to prevent blood pressure from decreasing too much.

Symptoms

Dizziness or light-headedness may precede fainting, especially if the person is standing. After the person falls, blood pressure increases, partly because the person is lying down (and blood can flow to the brain without having to fight gravity) and often because the cause of fainting has passed. However, getting up too quickly may make the person faint again.

When the cause is an abnormal heart rhythm (arrhythmia), fainting usually begins and ends suddenly. Sometimes the person feels palpitations (awareness of heartbeats) just before fainting.

Vasovagal syncope may occur when a person is sitting or standing. It is often preceded by nausea, weakness, yawning, blurring of vision, and sweating. The skin may become cool and clammy. The person becomes ghostly pale, the pulse becomes very slow, and the person faints.

Fainting that begins gradually with warning symptoms and also disappears gradually suggests changes in the blood, such as a decreased level of sugar (hypoglycemia) or carbon dioxide (hypocapnia). Hypocapnia is often preceded by a pins-and-needles sensation in the fingertips and around the lips.

Diagnosis

Doctors try to determine the cause of fainting because some causes are more serious than others. Heart disease, such as an abnormal heart rhythm or narrowing (stenosis) of the aortic valve, can be fatal. Other causes are much less worrisome.

Sometimes the nature of the symptoms suggests a cause to the doctor. Descriptions from witnesses of the fainting episode may be helpful. Of concern is fainting that occurs without any warning symptoms (particularly during exertion), is accompanied by shortness of breath or chest pain, results in injury, or occurs in a person with an abnormal finding during an examination of the heart or nervous system. Doctors also need to know whether the person has any disorders and whether the person is taking any prescription or over-the-counter drugs.

If the fainting occurs during emotionally stressful situations or is preceded by symptoms of vasovagal syncope (such as nausea, sweating, cool and clammy skin, and paleness), fainting usually is not serious, and extensive diagnostic procedures and treatment are rarely necessary.

Doctors will often obtain an electrocardiogram (ECG), which records the electrical activity of the heart and can detect an underlying heart disorder. Continuous ECG may be required to determine the cause of fainting. For this procedure, the person wears a small battery-powered device (Holter monitor). It records the heart's electrical activity for 24 hours or more as the person engages in normal daily activities (see page 327). If an irregular heart rhythm coincides with a fainting episode, it is probably—but not necessarily—the cause.

Other procedures, such as echocardiography, which uses ultrasound waves to produce an image

SPOTLIGHT ON AGING

Low blood pressure may be caused by many disorders that affect the heart. Because many heart disorders are common among older people, older people are also more likely to have low blood pressure.

A heart muscle that is weakened because of a heart attack can pump less blood, leading to low blood pressure. Infections, heart valve disorders, and drugs that damage the heart may also decrease the pumping ability. Pericarditis causes fluid to build up within the sac surrounding the heart (the pericardium), compressing the heart and restricting its ability to pump blood.

An abnormally slow or an abnormally fast heart rate can cause low blood pressure. If the heart rate is slow (bradycardia), the heart does not pump sufficient blood to the body. If the heart rate is fast, as happens in atrial fibrillation, the ventricles do not have time to fill completely with blood before each heartbeat and cannot pump enough blood to the body.

Some drugs, such as calcium channel blockers and angiotensin-converting enzyme inhibitors that are used to treat heart disorders, diuretics, and drugs for Parkinson's disease, may also lower blood pressure.

Orthostatic hypotension is particularly common among older people who take drugs to treat high blood pressure. Older people are also more likely to experience low blood pressure and loss of consciousness during urination (micturition syncope) and after eating (postprandial hypotension).

The body has many mechanisms to help prevent low blood pressure, but these mechanisms work less well in older people.

of the heart (see page 328), can detect whether the heart has a structural or functional abnormality. Blood tests may show that the person has hypoglycemia or anemia.

Loss of consciousness due to a seizure (see page 709) is distinguished from fainting because the causes and treatment are different. To distinguish between the two, doctors may use electroencephalography (EEG), which records the brain's electrical activity (see page 636). Also, after a seizure, recovery from unconsciousness is much slower, causing drowsiness that usually lasts for at least 10 minutes.

To confirm a suspected cause, doctors may attempt to re-create a fainting episode under safe conditions. For example, the person may be asked to breathe quickly and deeply. Or, while monitoring the heartbeat with ECG, a doctor may press gently over the carotid sinus (a part of the internal carotid artery containing sensors that monitor blood pressure). This pressure temporarily increases blood pressure inside the carotid sinus, tricking the body into thinking that blood pressure has increased throughout the body. The sinus then sends signals to the brain to reduce blood pressure, and faintness or fainting may result.

Tilt table testing (see page 328) is commonly done to determine the cause of fainting. The person is strapped to a motorized table. Then the table tilts until the person is almost standing. This position is held for up to 45 minutes. Blood pressure and heart rate are continuously monitored during the test. If blood pressure does not decrease, the person is given isoproterenol (a drug that stimulates the heart), and the test is repeated. Use of this drug makes the test more sensitive.

Treatment

Usually, lying flat restores consciousness. Raising the legs can speed recovery by increasing blood flow to the heart and brain. If the person sits up too rapidly or is propped up or carried in an upright position, another fainting episode may occur. Therefore, the person should remain lying down until fully recovered.

A heart rate that is too slow can be corrected by surgically implanting a pacemaker, an electronic device that stimulates heartbeats (see art on page 369). A heart rate that is too rapid can be slowed by using drugs, particularly a beta-blocker (such as atenolol or metoprolol). A defibrillator can be implanted to restore normal rhythm if the heart beats irregularly (see page 368). Other causes of fainting—such as hypoglycemia and anemia—can be treated. If blood volume is very low, fluids may be given intravenously. Surgery may be considered for heart valve disorders.

Orthostatic Hypotension

Orthostatic hypotension is an excessive decrease in blood pressure that occurs when a person stands up, resulting in reduced blood flow to the brain and dizziness or fainting.

- Dizziness or light-headedness that occurs when a person sits up or stands abruptly is the most common symptom.
- Measuring blood pressure while the person is sitting and standing may reveal orthostatic hypotension.
- When the cause cannot be cured, people are taught to stand up gradually and to drink plenty of fluids.

Orthostatic hypotension is particularly common among older people.

Orthostatic hypotension is not a specific disease but an inability to compensate quickly for changes in blood pressure. When a person stands up suddenly, gravity causes about a pint of blood to pool in the veins of the legs and lower body. As a result, the amount of blood returned to the heart and pumped out by the heart is reduced, and blood pressure falls. Normally, the body quickly responds to a decrease in blood pressure: The heart beats faster and more forcefully to increase its output of blood and the arterioles (small arteries) constrict to increase resistance to blood flow (see page 343). If these compensatory mechanisms malfunction or function too slowly—both of which commonly occur in older people—orthostatic hypotension may occur.

Causes

Orthostatic hypotension is caused by conditions that interfere with the compensatory mechanisms that control blood pressure. These conditions include many disorders and drugs as well as normal age-related changes.

Some conditions cause orthostatic hypotension by affecting the heart's ability to increase its output enough when a person stands. This problem can be caused by heart disease, such as abnormal heart rhythms and heart valve disorders. Also, with aging, the body becomes less able to increase the heart rate (and thus the heart's output) when a person stands.

Some conditions cause orthostatic hypotension by reducing blood volume. Diuretics, which are used to treat high blood pressure, can reduce blood volume by removing fluid from the body. Diuretics, especially potent ones given in high doses, are a common cause of orthostatic hypotension. Other causes of reduced blood volume include bleeding and an excessive loss of fluid due to severe vomiting, diarrhea, excessive sweating, or excessive urination (which is a common symptom of untreated diabetes or Addison's disease). Among older people, dehydration during an illness is a common cause of low blood volume leading to orthostatic hypotension. People who are ill may not be able to obtain fluids without assistance. Also, during an illness, the leg muscles are not used regularly. As a result, blood pools in the leg veins and is not pumped back to the heart (see page 433). Because this pooling reduces the amount of blood returning to the heart, it, in effect, reduces blood volume and thus reduces blood pressure.

Some conditions cause orthostatic hypotension by dilating arterioles and veins. Drugs that dilate arterioles (vasodilators) can cause orthostatic hypotension. They include nitrates, calcium channel blockers, angiotensin-converting enzyme (ACE) inhibitors, angiotensin II receptor blockers, alpha blockers, alcohol, and antidepressants. Disorders such as diabetes, amyloidosis, and spinal cord injuries may damage the nerves that regulate blood vessel diameter. In addition, veins dilate when body temperature increases, for example, because of a warm day, a warm room, or too much clothing. Fever also has this effect.

Fatigue, exercise (which causes blood vessels to dilate), or consumption of a heavy meal (which requires increased blood flow to the intestine) can contribute to orthostatic hypotension.

Symptoms and Diagnosis

Most people with orthostatic hypotension experience some faintness, light-headedness, dizziness, confusion, or blurred vision when they get out of bed abruptly or stand up after sitting for a long time. Symptoms are worse if people are tired, have been exercising, have consumed alcohol, or have eaten a heavy meal. A severe decrease in blood flow to the brain can cause the person to faint and even to have seizures.

These symptoms suggest orthostatic hypotension. The diagnosis can be confirmed if the blood pressure falls significantly when the person stands and returns to normal when the person lies down. Doctors then look for the cause of orthostatic hypotension, because treatment and prognosis depend on the cause.

Treatment

Even when the cause of orthostatic hypotension cannot be treated, certain measures can often reduce or eliminate symptoms. For example, susceptible people should not sit or stand up rapidly or remain standing still for long periods. They should sit or stand up slowly. Wearing fitted elastic stockings up to the waist may help reduce pooling of blood in the leg veins. If orthostatic hypotension results from prolonged bed rest, gradually increasing the time spent sitting up each day may help.

Several measures help maintain blood volume. People with orthostatic hypotension should drink plenty of fluids and little or no alcohol. People who do not have heart failure or high blood pressure are often told to salt their food liberally or to take salt tablets. However, a doctor's supervision is necessary, because a high-salt diet can lead to heart failure in certain people, particularly older people. For people who have severe symptoms, taking hormones that cause salt to be retained, such as fludrocortisone, can increase blood volume. However, use of such hormones increases the risk of heart failure, particularly for older people and people who have heart disease. Use of fludrocortisone can also cause a loss of potassium, so taking a potassium supplement may be necessary. Midodrine may be taken with fludrocortisone to help prevent blood pressure from falling. Midodrine constricts arterioles, thereby reducing their capacity to hold blood and increasing resistance to blood flow.

If these measures are ineffective, other drugs (such as pindolol and clonidine), which work in various ways, may help relieve orthostatic hypotension in certain people. However, the risk of side effects from these drugs may make their use undesirable, particularly by older people.

Postprandial Hypotension

Postprandial hypotension is an excessive decrease in blood pressure that occurs after a meal.

- Dizziness, light-headedness, and falls may occur.
- Doctors measure blood pressure before and after a meal to diagnose postprandial hypertension.
- Eating small, low-carbohydrate meals frequently may help.

Postprandial hypotension occurs in up to one third of older people but virtually never occurs in younger people. It is more likely to occur in people who have high blood pressure or disorders that impair the brain centers controlling the autonomic nervous system (which regulates internal body processes). Examples of such disorders are Parkinson's disease, multiple system atrophy (Shy-Drager syndrome), and diabetes.

The intestine requires a large amount of blood for digestion. When blood flows to the intestine after a meal, the heart rate increases and blood vessels in other parts of the body constrict to help maintain blood pressure. However, in some older people, such mechanisms may be inadequate. Blood flows normally to the intestine, but the heart rate does not increase adequately and blood vessels do not constrict enough to maintain blood pressure. As a result, blood pressure falls.

Postprandial hypotension can cause dizziness, light-headedness, faintness, and falls. If an older person experiences these symptoms after eating, doctors measure blood pressure before and after meals to determine if postprandial hypotension is the cause.

People who have symptoms of postprandial hypotension should not take antihypertensive drugs before meals and should lie down after meals. Taking a smaller dose of the antihypertensive drugs and eating small, low-carbohydrate meals more frequently may help reduce the effects of this disorder. For some people, walking after a meal helps improve blood flow, but blood pressure may fall when they stop walking.

Taking certain drugs before a meal may help. For example, nonsteroidal anti-inflammatory drugs (NSAIDs) cause salt to be retained and thus increase blood volume. Caffeine causes blood vessels to constrict. Caffeine should be taken only before breakfast so that sleep is not affected and the person does not become tolerant of caffeine's effects. For people who have severe symptoms that do not respond to other measures and who are in the hospital, injections of the drug octreotide may help by reducing the amount of blood flowing to the intestine.

CHAPTER 56

Shock

Shock is a life-threatening condition in which blood pressure is too low to sustain life.

- Shock has several causes: a low blood volume, which causes hypovolemic shock; inadequate pumping action of the heart, which causes cardiogenic shock; or excessive widening of blood vessels, which causes distributive shock.
- When shock is caused by low blood volume or inadequate pumping of the heart, people may feel lethargic, sleepy, or confused, and their skin becomes cold and sweaty and often bluish and pale.
- When shock results from excessive dilation of blood vessels, the skin may be warm and flushed, and the pulse may be strong and forceful (bounding) rather than weak.
- People who are in shock should be kept warm and positioned so their legs are elevated, and then they are given intravenous fluids, oxygen, and sometimes drugs to help restore the blood pressure.

In the United States, hospital emergency departments report more than 1 million cases of shock each year. People go into shock when their blood pressure becomes so low that the body's cells do not receive enough blood and therefore do not receive enough oxygen. As a result, cells in numerous organs, including the brain, kidneys, liver, and heart, stop functioning normally. If blood flow (perfusion) to these cells is not quickly restored, they become irreversibly damaged and die. If enough cells are damaged or dead, the organ they are in may fail and the person may die. People in shock require immediate emergency treatment. The medical disorder of shock has nothing to do with the "shock" that people feel from a sudden emotional stress.

Causes

Shock has several causes: a low blood volume, which causes hypovolemic shock; inadequate pumping action of the heart, which causes cardiogenic shock; or excessive widening of blood vessels, which causes distributive shock.

Hypovolemic Shock: Low blood volume results in less-than-normal amounts of blood entering the heart with every heartbeat and therefore less-than-normal amounts of blood being pumped out to the body and its cells.

Blood volume may be low because of severe bleeding, an excessive loss of body fluids, or, less commonly, inadequate fluid intake. Blood may be rapidly lost because of external bleeding, such as that caused by an accident, or internal bleeding, such as that caused by an ulcer in the stomach or intestine, a ruptured blood vessel, or a ruptured ectopic pregnancy (a pregnancy outside the uterus). An excessive loss of body fluids other than blood can result from major burns, inflammation of the pancreas (pancreatitis), perforation of the intestinal wall, severe diarrhea, kidney disease, or excessive use of loop diuretics, which increase the output of urine. Fluid intake may be inadequate because a physical disability (such as severe joint disease) or a mental disability (such as Alzheimer's disease) may prevent people from obtaining enough fluids even though they feel thirsty.

Cardiogenic Shock: Inadequate pumping action of the heart can also result in less-than-normal amounts of blood being pumped out with every heartbeat. The inadequate pumping action usually results from complications of a heart attack (see box on page 415) or a blood clot in the lungs (pulmonary embolism). Other causes include malfunction of a heart valve (particularly an artificial valve), rupture of the wall between the two sides of the heart (septum), an abnormal heart rhythm (arrhythmia), and inability of the heart to fill (cardiac tamponade).

Distributive Shock: Excessive dilation of blood vessels (vasodilation) increases the capacity of blood vessels, so that blood meets with less resistance as it flows through them. Blood pressure in the dilated vessels is lower, so the cells fed by those vessels get less blood.

Blood vessels may be excessively dilated because of a serious allergic reaction (anaphylaxis—see page 1123), a severe bacterial infection (shock caused by such an infection is called septic shock—see page 1186), overdose of drugs or poisons that dilate blood vessels, and injuries to the spinal cord and rarely the brain. The mechanisms by which these conditions cause vasodilation vary. For example, a spinal cord

---

? Did You Know...

Shock is very low blood pressure that often cannot be measured with a blood pressure cuff.

Shock has nothing to do with sudden emotional stress.

injury interrupts the nerves that maintain the tone of arteries; poisons or toxins released by bacteria can cause the blood vessels to dilate.

Symptoms and Diagnosis

Symptoms of shock are similar when the cause is low blood volume or inadequate pumping action of the heart. The condition may begin with lethargy, sleepiness, and confusion. The skin becomes cold and sweaty and often bluish and pale. If the skin is pressed, color returns much more slowly than normal. Blood vessels may become more visible as a bluish network of lines under the skin. The pulse is weak and rapid, unless a slow heartbeat is causing the shock. Usually, the person cannot sit up without feeling light-headed or passing out. Breathing is rapid, but breathing and the pulse may both slow down if death is imminent. Blood pressure drops so low that it often cannot be measured with a blood pressure cuff. Eventually, the person may die.

When shock results from excessive dilation of blood vessels, the symptoms are somewhat different. The skin may be warm and flushed, and the pulse may be strong and forceful (bounding) rather than weak, particularly at first. However, later on, shock due to excessive dilation of blood vessels also produces cold, clammy skin and lethargy.

In the earliest stages of shock, especially septic shock, many symptoms may be absent or may be undetected unless they are specifically looked for. In older people, the only symptom may be confusion. The blood pressure is very low. Urine flow is significantly reduced (because blood supply to the kidneys is reduced), and waste products build up in the blood.

Prognosis and Treatment

If untreated, shock is usually fatal. If shock is treated, the outlook depends on the cause, the other disorders the person has, the presence and severity of any organ failure, the amount of time that passes before treatment begins, and the type of treatment given. Regardless of treatment, the likelihood of death due to shock after a massive heart attack or due to septic shock, especially in older people, is great.

The first person to arrive on the scene can take several measures that help, including calling for additional help. A person who is in shock should be laid down and kept warm, with the legs elevated about 12 to 24 inches (about 30 to 60 centimeters) to facilitate the return of blood to the heart. Any bleeding should be stopped, and breathing should be checked. The head should be turned to the side to prevent inhalation of vomit. Nothing should be given by mouth.

When emergency medical personnel arrive, they may provide oxygen through a face mask or provide a mechanical device to assist breathing. Fluids are given intravenously at a fast rate and in large volumes to raise blood pressure. For shock caused by bleeding, a blood transfusion may be given. Usually, blood is cross-matched before transfusion, but in an emergency when there is no time for crossmatching, type O negative blood can be given to anyone. Drugs, if needed, are given intravenously. Opioids and sedatives are usually not used because they tend to decrease blood pressure.

Shock caused by excessive dilation of the blood vessels also may require drugs that constrict the vessels, such as epinephrine for people with anaphylaxis or low-dose dopamine for people with other forms of shock. The cause of the excessive dilation is also treated. For example, a bacterial infection is treated with antibiotics.

The intravenous fluid and blood transfusion may not be enough to counteract the shock if bleeding or fluid loss continues or if the shock is caused by a heart attack or another problem unrelated to blood volume. Drugs that constrict the blood vessels may be given to boost blood flow to the brain or heart. However, such drugs should be used as briefly as possible because they can reduce blood flow to other tissues in the body.

When shock is caused by an inadequate pumping action of the heart, efforts are made to improve the heart's performance. The rate and rhythm abnormalities of the heartbeat are corrected, and blood volume is increased if necessary. Atropine may be used to increase a slow heart rate, and other drugs may be given to improve the ability of the heart muscle to contract.

If the cause is a heart attack and shock persists after emergency treatment, a balloon pump may be inserted into the aorta to reverse shock temporarily. After this procedure, emergency percutaneous transluminal coronary angioplasty (PTCA—see art on page 405) or coronary artery bypass surgery (see art on page 406) may be needed. By opening a blocked coronary artery (one of the arteries supplying the heart muscle), emergency PTCA can improve the heart's pumping action and can reverse the shock. If emergency PTCA or bypass surgery is not performed, a drug that helps break up clots (thrombolytic drug) is given as soon as possible, unless it could worsen problems in people who have another disorder, such as a bleeding ulcer, or who have had a stroke recently.

If the cause is a malfunctioning heart valve or rupture of the septum, surgery may also be needed. If the heart is unable to fill because of blood or fluid in the pericardium (the sac surrounding the heart), the fluid can be removed through a needle inserted into the pericardium.

Heart failure is a disorder in which the heart pumps blood inadequately, leading to reduced blood flow, back-up (congestion) of blood in the veins and lungs, and other changes that may further weaken the heart.

- Many disorders that affect the heart can cause heart failure.

- Most people have no symptoms at first, and shortness of breath and fatigue develop gradually over days to months.

- Doctors usually suspect heart failure on the basis of symptoms, but procedures, such as echocardiography, are usually done to evaluate heart function.

- Treatment focuses on treating the disorder causing heart failure, making lifestyle changes, and treating heart failure with drugs or with surgery or other interventions.

Heart failure can occur in people of any age, even in young children (especially those born with a heart defect). However, it is much more common among older people, because older people are more likely to have disorders that damage the heart muscle and the heart valves. Also, age-related changes in the heart tend to make the heart pump less efficiently. Heart failure develops in about 1 of 100 people. The disorder is likely to become more common because people are living longer and because, in some countries, certain risk factors for heart disease (such as smoking, high blood pressure, and a high-fat diet) are affecting more people.

Heart failure does not mean that the heart has stopped. It means that the heart cannot keep up with the work required to pump adequate blood to all parts of the body (its workload). However, this definition is somewhat simplistic. Heart failure is extremely complex, and no simple definition can encompass its many causes, aspects, forms, and consequences.

The function of the heart is to pump blood (see page 317). A pump moves fluid out of one place and into another. For example, the right side of the heart pumps blood from the veins into the lungs. The left side of the heart pumps blood from the lungs out through the arteries to the rest of the body. Blood goes out when the heart muscle contracts (called systole) and comes in when the heart muscle relaxes (called diastole). Heart failure develops when the pumping action of the heart is inadequate, typically because the heart muscle is weaker,

stiffer, or both. As a result, blood may not flow out in adequate amounts. Blood may also build up in the tissues from which it is coming, causing congestion in those tissues. That is why heart failure is sometimes known as congestive heart failure.

Accumulation of blood coming into the left side of the heart causes congestion in the lungs, making breathing difficult. Accumulation of blood coming into the right side of the heart causes congestion and fluid accumulation in other parts of the body, such as the legs and the liver. Heart failure usually affects both the right and left sides of the heart to some degree. However, one side may be affected by disease more than the other. In such cases, heart failure may be described as right-sided heart failure or left-sided heart failure.

In heart failure, the heart may not pump enough blood to meet the body's need for oxygen and nutrients, which are supplied by the blood. As a result, arm and leg muscles may tire more quickly, and the kidneys may not function normally. The kidneys filter fluid and waste products from the blood into the urine, but when the heart cannot pump adequately, the kidneys malfunction and cannot remove excess fluid from the blood. As a result, the amount of fluid in the bloodstream increases, and the workload of the failing heart increases, creating a vicious circle. Thus, heart failure becomes even worse.

Types of Heart Failure: Heart failure has two main forms: systolic dysfunction and diastolic dysfunction. Some people with heart failure have both types of dysfunction.

In **systolic dysfunction,** the heart contracts less forcefully and cannot pump out as much of the blood that is returned to it as it normally does. As a result, more blood remains in the lower chambers of the heart (ventricles). Blood then accumulates in the lungs, veins, or both.

In **diastolic dysfunction,** the heart is stiff and does not relax normally after contracting, which impairs its ability to fill with blood. The heart contracts normally, so it is able to pump a normal proportion of blood out of the ventricles. Sometimes the stiff heart compensates for its poor filling by pumping out an even higher proportion of the blood than it normally does. However, eventually, as in systolic dysfunction, the blood returning to the heart accumulates in the lungs or veins. Often, both forms of heart failure occur together.

Heart Failure: Pumping and Filling Problems

Normally, the heart stretches as it fills with blood (during diastole), then contracts to pump out the blood (during systole). The main pumping chambers in the heart are the ventricles.

Heart failure due to systolic dysfunction usually develops because the heart cannot contract normally. It may fill with blood, but the heart cannot pump out as much of the blood it contains because the muscle is weaker or because a heart valve malfunctions. As a result, the amount of blood pumped to the body and to the lungs is reduced, and the ventricle usually enlarges.

Heart failure due to diastolic dysfunction develops because the heart muscle stiffens (particularly the left ventricle) and may thicken so that the heart cannot fill normally with blood. Consequently, blood backs up in the left atrium and lung (pulmonary) blood vessels and causes congestion. Nonetheless, the heart may be able to pump out a normal percentage of the blood it receives (but the total amount pumped out may be less).

The heart chambers always contain some blood, but different amounts of blood may enter or leave the chambers with each heartbeat as indicated by the thickness of the arrows.

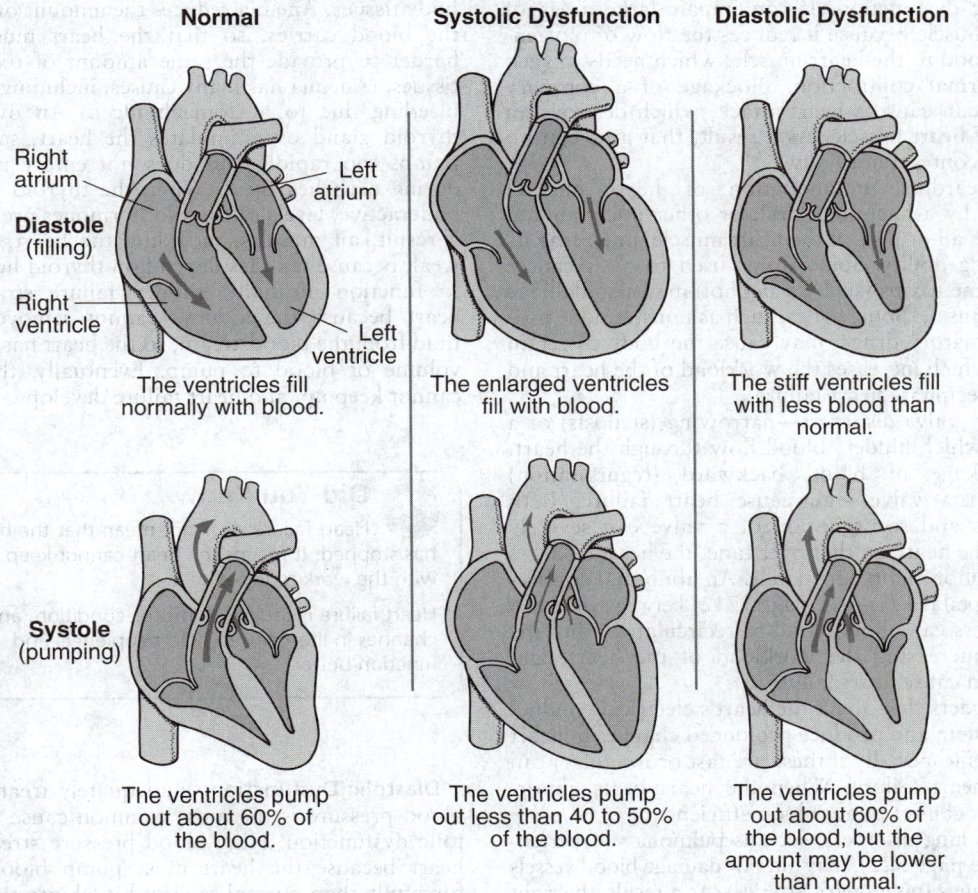

Normal

Systolic Dysfunction

Diastolic Dysfunction

Right atrium

Left atrium

Diastole (filling)

Right ventricle

Left ventricle

The ventricles fill normally with blood.

The enlarged ventricles fill with blood.

The stiff ventricles fill with less blood than normal.

Systole (pumping)

The ventricles pump out about 60% of the blood.

The ventricles pump out less than 40 to 50% of the blood.

The ventricles pump out about 60% of the blood, but the amount may be lower than normal.

Causes

Any disorder that directly affects the heart can lead to heart failure, as can some disorders that indirectly affect the heart. Some disorders cause heart failure quickly; others do so only after many years. Some disorders cause systolic dysfunction, others cause diastolic dysfunction, and some disorders, such as high blood pressure and some heart valve disorders, can cause both types of dysfunction.

Systolic Dysfunction: Disorders that cause systolic dysfunction may impair the entire heart or one area of the heart. As a result, the heart does not contract normally. In many cases, a combination of factors results in heart failure.

Coronary artery disease is a common cause of systolic dysfunction. It can impair large areas of heart muscle because it reduces the flow of oxygen-rich blood to the heart muscle, which needs oxygen for normal contraction. Blockage of a coronary artery can cause a heart attack, which destroys an area of heart muscle. As a result, that area can no longer contract normally.

Myocarditis (inflammation of heart muscle) caused by a bacterial, viral, or other infection can damage all or part of the heart muscle, impairing its pumping ability. Some drugs used to treat cancer and some toxins (such as alcohol) may also damage heart muscle. Some drugs, such as nonsteroidal anti-inflammatory drugs, may cause the body to retain fluid, which increases the workload of the heart and may precipitate heart failure.

Heart valve disorders—narrowing (stenosis) of a valve, which hinders blood flow through the heart, or leakage of blood backward (regurgitation) through a valve—can cause heart failure. Both stenosis and regurgitation of a valve can severely stress the heart, so that over time, the heart enlarges and cannot pump adequately. An abnormal connection (septal defects—see page 1712) between the heart chambers can allow blood to recirculate within the heart, increasing the workload of the heart, and thus can cause heart failure.

Disorders that affect the heart's electrical conduction system and produce prolonged changes in heart rhythms (especially if these are fast or irregular) can cause heart failure. When the heart beats abnormally, it cannot pump blood efficiently.

Some lung disorders, such as pulmonary hypertension (see page 522), may alter or damage blood vessels in the lungs (pulmonary arteries). As a result, the right side of the heart has to work harder to pump blood into the lungs. The person may then develop cor pulmonale (see box on page 523), in which the right ventricle is enlarged and there is right-sided heart failure.

Sudden, usually complete blockage of a pulmonary artery by several small blood clots or one very large clot (pulmonary embolism) also makes pumping blood into the pulmonary arteries difficult. A very large clot can be immediately life threatening. The increased effort required to pump blood into the blocked pulmonary arteries can cause the right side of the heart to enlarge and may cause the walls of the right ventricle to thicken, resulting in right-sided heart failure.

Disorders that indirectly affect the heart's pumping ability include a severe deficiency of red blood cells or hemoglobin (anemia), an overactive thyroid gland (hyperthyroidism), an underactive thyroid gland (hypothyroidism), and kidney failure. Red blood cells contain hemoglobin, which enables them to carry oxygen from the lungs and deliver it to body tissues. Anemia reduces the amount of oxygen the blood carries, so that the heart must work harder to provide the same amount of oxygen to tissues. (Anemia has many causes, including chronic bleeding due to a stomach ulcer.) An overactive thyroid gland overstimulates the heart, so that it pumps too rapidly and does not empty normally during each heartbeat. When the thyroid gland is underactive, levels of thyroid hormones are low. As a result, all muscles, including the heart, become weak because muscles depend on thyroid hormones to function normally. Kidney failure strains the heart because the kidneys cannot remove excess fluid from the bloodstream, so the heart has a larger volume of blood to pump. Eventually, the heart cannot keep up, and heart failure develops.

> **? Did You Know...**
>
> Heart failure does not mean that the heart has stopped. It means the heart cannot keep up with the work required of it.
>
> Heart failure is usually a chronic condition, and changes in lifestyle can help people feel and function better.

Diastolic Dysfunction: Inadequately treated high blood pressure is the most common cause of diastolic dysfunction. High blood pressure stresses the heart because the heart must pump blood more forcefully than normal to eject blood into the arteries against the higher pressure. Eventually, the heart's walls thicken (hypertrophy), then stiffen. The stiff heart does not fill quickly or adequately, so that with each contraction, the heart pumps less blood than it normally does. Diabetes causes other changes that stiffen the walls of the ventricle.

SPOTLIGHT ON AGING

Aging alone does not cause heart failure. But older people are more likely to have the most common causes of heart failure, which are long-standing high blood pressure and heart attacks (due to coronary artery disease).

Disorders can cause heart failure in two ways. They can cause problems with the heart's ability to fill with blood or to pump blood out. Among older people, filling problems (called diastolic dysfunction) and pumping problems (called systolic dysfunction) are equally common.

Filling problems usually occur because the walls of the ventricles have become stiff. As a result, the ventricles cannot fill with blood normally, and too little blood is pumped out. As people age, heart muscle tends to become stiffer, making heart failure due to filling problems more likely. High blood pressure can cause filling problems because it makes the heart muscle thicker and stiffer.

Filling problems are not always caused by a stiff heart. In atrial fibrillation (an abnormal heart rhythm more common with aging), the atria beat rapidly and irregularly. As a result, the atria do not move enough blood into the ventricles. If atrial fibrillation occurs suddenly in older people, heart failure may result.

Pumping problems usually occur when the heart muscle has been damaged. A damaged heart pumps less blood, causing pressure inside the heart to increase and the heart's chambers to enlarge. The most common cause of heart damage in older people is a heart attack (due to a blockage in an artery that supplies the heart with blood). Heart valve disorders can also cause pumping problems.

In aortic stenosis (a heart valve disorder), the opening between the left ventricle and the aorta (aortic valve) narrows. As a result, pumping blood out of the heart is harder. Aortic stenosis is a common cause of heart failure in older people.

If a lung disorder such as emphysema or scarring (pulmonary fibrosis) has been present for a long time, blood pressure in the lungs increases. As a result, pumping blood to the lungs is harder for the right ventricle.

As people age, the heart's walls also tend to stiffen. The combination of high blood pressure and diabetes, which are common among older people, and age-related stiffening makes heart failure particularly common among older people.

Heart failure may result from other disorders that cause the heart's walls to stiffen, such as infiltrations and infections. For example, in amyloidosis, amyloid, an unusual protein not normally present in the body, infiltrates many tissues in the body. If amyloid infiltrates the heart's walls, they stiffen, and heart failure results. In tropical countries, infiltration by certain parasites into heart muscle can cause heart failure, even in young people. Some heart valve disorders, such as aortic valve stenosis, hinder blood flow out of the heart. As a result, the heart muscle thickens and has to work harder, and diastolic dysfunction develops. Eventually, systolic dysfunction also develops.

In constrictive pericarditis, the sac that envelops the heart (pericardium) stiffens, preventing even a healthy heart from pumping and filling normally.

Compensatory Mechanisms

The body has several mechanisms to compensate for heart failure. The body's first response to stress, including that due to heart failure, is to release the fight-or-flight hormones, epinephrine (adrenaline) and norepinephrine (noradrenaline). For example, these hormones may be released immediately after a heart attack damages the heart. Epinephrine and norepinephrine cause the heart to pump faster and more forcefully. They help the heart increase the amount of blood pumped out (cardiac output), sometimes to a normal amount, and thus initially help compensate for the heart's impaired pumping ability.

People who do not have heart disease usually benefit from release of these hormones when more work is temporarily required of the heart. However, for people who have chronic heart failure, this sustained response increases demands on an already damaged heart. Over time, the increased demands lead to further deterioration of heart function.

Another of the body's main compensatory mechanisms for the reduced blood flow in heart failure is to increase the amount of salt and water retained by the kidneys. Retaining salt and water instead of excreting it into urine increases the volume of blood in the bloodstream and helps maintain blood pressure. However, the larger volume of blood also stretches the heart muscle, enlarging the heart chambers, particularly the ventricles. At first, the more the heart muscle is stretched, the more forcefully it contracts, which improves heart function. However, after a certain amount of stretching, stretching no longer helps but instead weakens the heart's contractions (as when a rubber band is overstretched). Consequently, heart failure worsens.

Another important compensatory mechanism is enlargement of the muscular walls of the ventricles (ventricular hypertrophy). When the heart must work harder, the heart's walls enlarge and thicken, as biceps muscles enlarge after months of weight training. At first, the thickened heart walls can contract more forcefully. However, the thickened heart walls eventually become stiff, causing or worsening diastolic dysfunction.

Symptoms

Symptoms of heart failure may begin suddenly, especially if the cause is a heart attack. However, most people have no symptoms when the heart first begins to develop problems. Symptoms then develop gradually over days to months or years. The most common symptoms are shortness of breath and fatigue, but in older people, heart failure sometimes causes vague symptoms such as sleepiness, confusion, and disorientation. Heart failure may stabilize for periods of time but often progresses slowly and insidiously.

Right-sided heart failure and left-sided heart failure produce different symptoms. Although both types of heart failure may be present, the symptoms of failure of one side often predominate. Eventually, left-sided heart failure causes right-sided failure.

The main symptoms of right-sided heart failure are fluid accumulation and swelling (edema) in the feet, ankles, legs, liver, and abdomen. Where the fluid accumulates depends on the amount of excess fluid and the effects of gravity. If a person is standing, fluid accumulates in the legs and feet. If a person is lying down, fluid usually accumulates in the lower back. If the amount of fluid is large, fluid also accumulates in the abdomen. Fluid accumulation in the liver or stomach can cause nausea and loss of appetite. Eventually, food is not absorbed well, resulting in loss of weight and muscle. This condition is called cardiac cachexia.

Left-sided heart failure leads to fluid accumulation in the lungs, which causes shortness of breath. At first, shortness of breath occurs only during exertion, but as heart failure progresses, it occurs with less and less exertion and eventually occurs even at rest. People with severe left-sided heart failure may be short of breath when lying down (a condition called orthopnea—see page 450), because gravity causes more fluid to move into the lungs. Such people often wake up, gasping for breath or wheezing (a condition called paroxysmal nocturnal dyspnea). Sitting up causes some of the fluid to drain to the bottom of the lungs and makes breathing easier. People with left-sided heart failure also feel tired and weak when performing physical activities, because their muscles are not receiving enough blood.

A sudden accumulation of a large amount of fluid in the lungs (acute pulmonary edema) causes extreme difficulty breathing, rapid breathing, bluish skin, and feelings of restlessness, anxiety, and suffocation. Some people have severe spasms of the airways (bronchospasms) and wheezing. Acute pulmonary edema is a life-threatening emergency.

When heart failure is advanced, Cheyne-Stokes respiration (periodic breathing) may develop. In this unusual pattern of breathing, a person breathes rapidly and deeply, then more slowly, then not at all for several seconds. Cheyne-Stokes respiration develops because blood flow to the brain is reduced and the areas of the brain that control breathing therefore do not receive enough oxygen.

When the heart is severely damaged, blood clots can form because blood flow within the chambers is sluggish. Clots may break loose (becoming emboli), travel through the bloodstream, and partially or completely block an artery elsewhere in the body. If a clot blocks an artery to the brain, a stroke may result.

Depression and decline in mental function are common in people with severe heart failure, particularly the elderly, and require careful evaluation and treatment.

Diagnosis

Doctors usually suspect heart failure on the basis of symptoms alone. The diagnosis is supported by the results of a physical examination, including a weak, often rapid pulse, reduced blood pressure, abnormal heart sounds and fluid accumulation in the lungs (both heard through a stethoscope), an enlarged heart, swollen neck veins, an enlarged liver, and swelling in the abdomen or legs. A chest x-ray can show an enlarged heart and fluid accumulation in the lungs.

Procedures to evaluate heart function are usually done. Electrocardiography (ECG—see page 326) is almost always performed to determine whether the heart rhythm is normal, whether the walls of the ventricles are thickened, and whether the person has had a heart attack.

Echocardiography (see page 328), which uses sound waves to produce an image of the heart, is one of the best procedures for evaluating heart function, including the pumping ability of the heart and the functioning of heart valves. Echocardiography can show the following:

- Whether the heart walls are thickened and relax normally
- Whether the valves are functioning normally
- Whether contractions are normal
- Whether any area of the heart is contracting abnormally

Echocardiography may help determine whether heart failure is due to systolic or diastolic dysfunction by enabling doctors to estimate the thickness and stiffness of the heart walls and the ejection fraction. The ejection fraction, an important measure of heart function, is the percentage of blood pumped out by the heart with each beat. A normal left ventricle ejects about 60% of the blood in it. If the ejection fraction is low, systolic dysfunction is confirmed. If the ejection fraction is normal or high in a person who has symptoms of heart failure, diastolic dysfunction is likely.

Other procedures, such as radionuclide, magnetic resonance, or computed tomography imaging and cardiac catheterization with angiography (see page 330), may be done to identify the cause of heart failure. Rarely, a biopsy of heart muscle is needed, usually when doctors suspect infiltration of the heart (as occurs in amyloidosis) or myocarditis due to a bacterial, viral, or other infection.

Prevention

Preventing heart failure involves treating disorders that can cause heart failure before they lead to heart failure. Disorders that can be treated include heart valve disorders, an abnormal connection between heart chambers, blockage of a coronary artery, high blood pressure, infections, thyroid disorders, anemia, and alcoholism.

Treatment

Treatment of heart failure requires several general measures, along with treatment of the disorder causing heart failure, lifestyle changes, and drugs for heart failure.

General Measures: Although heart failure is a chronic disorder for most people, much can be done to make physical activity more comfortable, improve the quality of life, and prolong life. Affected people and their family members should learn all they can about heart failure because much care occurs at home. In particular, they should know how to recognize the early warning symptoms of worsening heart failure and should be aware of the actions they need to take (for example, take an extra dose of a diuretic or contact their doctor).

Regular communication with health care practitioners and examinations by doctors are critical because heart failure can worsen suddenly. For example, nurses may regularly call people who have heart failure to ask about changes in weight and in symptoms. Thus, they can gauge whether people need to see a doctor.

People may also go to specialized heart failure clinics. These clinics have doctors with expertise in heart failure who work closely with specially trained nurses and other health care practitioners, such as pharmacists, dietitians, and social workers, to care for people with heart failure. These clinics can help decrease symptoms, reduce hospitalizations, and improve life expectancy by making sure that people receive the most effective treatments.

This care complements rather than replaces care provided by primary care doctors.

People with heart failure should always check with their doctor before taking a new drug, even a nonprescription drug. Some drugs (including many used to treat arthritis) can cause salt and fluid retention, and other drugs may make the heart function more slowly. Forgetting to take necessary drugs is a common cause of worsening symptoms, and people should be given ways to remind themselves to take their drugs.

Treatment of the Cause: If the cause of heart failure is a narrowed or leaking heart valve or an abnormal connection between heart chambers, surgery can often correct the problem. Blockage of a coronary artery may require treatment with drugs, surgery, or angioplasty (see page 409). Antihypertensive drugs can reduce and control high blood pressure. Antibiotics can eliminate some infections. Treatment of a stomach ulcer or use of an iron supplement may correct anemia. Drugs, surgery, or radiation therapy can be used to manage an overactive thyroid gland, and thyroid hormones can be given to manage an underactive thyroid gland.

Lifestyle Changes: Changes in lifestyle can help people with heart failure feel and function better.

People who have heart failure should stay as physically fit as possible, even if they cannot exercise vigorously. People who have mild heart failure should follow an exercise program as described by a doctor. Those with more severe heart failure may need to exercise in a cardiovascular rehabilitation facility under the supervision of a trained attendant.

If people with heart failure are overweight, the heart must work harder during activity, worsening heart failure. Such people should follow a weight loss diet (see page 909) to attain and maintain ideal weight.

Smoking damages blood vessels. Large amounts of alcohol can act as a direct toxin to the heart. Thus, smoking and drinking alcohol can worsen heart failure and should be stopped.

Excess salt (sodium) in the diet can cause fluid retention, which counteracts drugs given to increase the excretion of water (such as diuretics) and relieve fluid accumulation. Thus, consuming excess salt worsens symptoms. Almost all people with heart failure should limit their intake of table salt and salty foods and their use of salt in cooking. The sodium content of packaged foods can be determined by reading the label. People with severe heart failure are usually given detailed information about how to limit salt intake. People who limit their salt intake can usually consume a normal amount of water unless fluid retention is severe. Drinking extra amounts of water is not recommended.

SOME DRUGS USED TO TREAT HEART FAILURE

DRUG*	COMMENTS†
Angiotensin-converting enzyme (ACE) inhibitors	
Captopril Enalapril Lisinopril Perindopril Ramipril Trandolapril	ACE inhibitors cause blood vessels to widen (dilate), thus decreasing the amount of work the heart has to do. They may also have direct beneficial effects on the heart. These drugs are the mainstay of heart failure treatment. They reduce symptoms and the need for hospitalization, and they prolong life.
Angiotensin II receptor blockers	
Candesartan Losartan Valsartan	Angiotensin II receptor blockers have effects similar to those of ACE inhibitors and may be tolerated better. They may be used with an ACE inhibitor or used alone in people who cannot take an ACE inhibitor.
Beta-blockers	
Bisoprolol Carvedilol Metoprolol	Beta-blockers slow the heart rate and block excessive stimulation of the heart. They may be appropriate for most people with heart failure. These drugs are usually used with ACE inhibitors and provide an added benefit. They may temporarily worsen symptoms but result in long-term improvement in heart function.
Other vasodilators	
Hydralazine Isosorbide dinitrate Nitroglycerin	Vasodilators cause blood vessels to dilate. These vasodilators are usually given to people who cannot take an ACE inhibitor or angiotensin II receptor blocker. Nitroglycerin is particularly useful for people who have heart failure and angina and for those who have acute heart failure. The combination of hydralazine and nitrates has been shown to be effective, particularly in blacks.
Cardiac glycosides	
Digoxin	Cardiac glycosides increase the force of each heartbeat and slow the heart rate in people with atrial fibrillation.
Aldosterone receptor blockers	
Eplerenone Spironolactone	These drugs block the action of the hormone aldosterone, which promotes salt and fluid retention and may have direct adverse effects on the heart. Both are potassium-sparing diuretics and improve survival. Eplerenone is less likely than spironolactone to cause breast tenderness or enlargement in men.
Loop diuretics	
Bumetanide Ethacrynic acid Furosemide Torsemide	These diuretics help the kidneys eliminate salt and water, thus decreasing the volume of fluid in the bloodstream.
Potassium-sparing diuretics	
Amiloride Triamterene	Because these diuretics prevent potassium loss, they may be given in addition to thiazide or loop diuretics, which cause potassium to be lost. Spironolactone is a potassium-sparing diuretic that is also an aldosterone receptor blocker. It is particularly useful in the treatment of severe heart failure.

(continued on the following page)

SOME DRUGS USED TO TREAT HEART FAILURE (Continued)

DRUG*	COMMENTS†
Thiazide and thiazide-like diuretics	
Chlorthalidone Hydrochlorothiazide Indapamide Metolazone	The effects of these diuretics are similar to but milder than those of loop diuretics. The two types of diuretics are particularly effective when used together.
Anticoagulants	
Heparin Warfarin	Anticoagulants may be given to prevent clots from forming in the heart chambers. Heparin is only given for a short time because it is given by injection.
Opioids	
Morphine	Morphine is given to relieve anxiety in a medical emergency, such as acute pulmonary edema.
Positive inotropic drugs (drugs that make muscle contract more forcefully)	
Dobutamine Dopamine Milrinone	For people who have severe symptoms, these drugs may be given intravenously to stimulate heart contractions and help keep blood circulating. They are only used temporarily because long-term use shortens life. Digoxin (a cardiac glycoside) has some positive inotropic effect and is sometimes given orally in low doses.

*These specific drugs have been better studied to prevent or treat heart failure.

†Selected side effects for ACE inhibitors, angiotensin II receptor blockers, diuretics, and beta-blockers are listed in the table on page 340.

A simple, reliable way to check whether the body is retaining fluid is to check body weight daily. Doctors often ask people with heart failure to weigh themselves as accurately as possible every day, typically once in the morning, after they arise and urinate and before they eat breakfast. Trends are easier to spot when people weigh themselves at the same time every day, use the same scale, wear a similar amount of clothing, and keep a written record of their daily weight. Increases of more than 2 pounds (about 1 kilogram) per day are early warning signs of fluid retention. A consistent, rapid weight gain (such as 2 pounds per day) is a clue that heart failure is worsening.

Many people who limit their salt intake still have swelling. Swollen legs should be kept elevated on a stool when sitting. This position helps the body reabsorb and eliminate the excess fluid. Some people also need to wear full-length supportive stockings that help prevent accumulation of fluid. If fluid accumulates in the lungs, sleeping with several pillows or elevating the head of the bed makes sleeping easier.

Drugs for Heart Failure: Heart failure can be treated with several different types of drugs, including diuretics, angiotensin-converting enzyme (ACE) inhibitors, angiotensin II receptor blockers, beta-blockers, digoxin, and others.

When salt restriction alone does not reduce fluid retention, doctors often prescribe diuretics (see page 342). These drugs help the kidneys eliminate salt and water by increasing urine formation and thus decreasing fluid volume throughout the body. The diuretics most commonly used for heart failure are loop diuretics. These diuretics are usually taken by mouth on a long-term basis, but in an emergency, they are very effective when given intravenously. Loop diuretics are preferred for moderate to severe heart failure. Thiazide diuretics, which have milder effects and can lower blood pressure, may be prescribed particularly for people who also have high blood pressure. Loop and thiazide diuretics can cause potassium to be lost in the urine. Consequently, a potassium supplement or a diuretic that does not cause potassium loss or that causes potassium levels to increase (a potassium-sparing diuretic) may be given as well. For people with severe heart failure due to systolic dysfunction, spironolactone is the preferred potassium-sparing diuretic. It can prolong life in people with severe heart failure. Taking diuretics can worsen urinary incontinence. However, a dose of a diuretic can usually be timed so that the risk of incontinence does not occur when a bathroom is unavailable or when access to one is inconvenient.

The mainstay of heart failure treatment is a group of drugs called ACE inhibitors (see page 342). These drugs not only reduce symptoms and the need for hospitalization but also prolong life. ACE inhibitors reduce blood levels of the hormones angiotensin II and aldosterone (which normally help increase blood pressure (see art on page 334). By doing so, ACE inhibitors cause arteries and veins to widen (dilate) and help the kidneys excrete excess water, thus decreasing the amount of work the heart has to do. These drugs also may have direct beneficial effects on the heart and blood vessel walls.

Angiotensin II receptor blockers (see page 342) have effects similar to those of ACE inhibitors. Angiotensin II receptor blockers are used with ACE inhibitors in some people with persistent symptoms of heart failure or are used alone in people who cannot tolerate ACE inhibitors because of cough, a side effect of ACE inhibitors.

Drugs that dilate blood vessels (vasodilators) are not used as often as ACE inhibitors or angiotensin II receptor blockers, which are more effective. Nonetheless, people who do not respond to or cannot take ACE inhibitors or angiotensin II receptor blockers can benefit from vasodilators, such as hydralazine, isosorbide dinitrate, and nitroglycerin patches or spray.

Beta-blockers are often used with ACE inhibitors to treat heart failure. By blocking the action of the hormone norepinephrine (which causes the heart to pump faster and more forcefully), these drugs produce long-term improvement in heart function and survival. Beta-blockers may reduce the force of the heart's contractions initially, so they are usually introduced after heart failure has first been stabilized with other drugs. In people with heart failure due to diastolic dysfunction, beta-blockers are used to slow the heart rate and relax the stiff or thickened muscle. Thus, the heart can fill with blood more completely.

Digoxin, one of the oldest treatments for heart failure, increases the force of each heartbeat and slows a heart rate that is too rapid. Digoxin helps relieve symptoms for some people with systolic dysfunction, especially if atrial fibrillation is present, but it does not prolong life.

Anticoagulants, such as warfarin, may be given to prevent clots from forming in the heart chambers. If the heart rhythm is abnormal, antiarrhythmic drugs (see table on page 370) may be given, or an implantable cardioverter-defibrillator (see page 368) may be recommended. Doctors may consider an implantable cardioverter-defibrillator in people with poor heart function despite the best medical treatment, as their risk of sudden death is increased. In some people with severe symptoms, a pacemaker that stimulates both ventricles may be recommended because it coordinates heart contraction and function better.

Other Measures: People with pulmonary edema require oxygen, which is sometimes given by special nasal masks. Occasionally, a tube may be inserted into the airway so that a mechanical ventilator can help with the increased work of breathing.

Heart transplantation may be an option for a few otherwise healthy people who have very severe, worsening heart failure and who have not responded to drug therapy. Mechanical assist devices that help pump blood are used in specialized centers for certain patients with very severe heart failure that is not responding to drug therapy. Other mechanical and novel treatments are being studied.

Treatment of Acute Heart Failure: Heart failure that develops or worsens quickly requires emergency treatment in a hospital.

If acute pulmonary edema develops (see page 356), oxygen is given through a face mask. Diuretics given intravenously and other drugs such as nitroglycerin given intravenously or under the tongue can produce rapid, dramatic improvement. Morphine relieves the anxiety that usually accompanies acute pulmonary edema. It also decreases the rate of breathing, slows the heart rate, dilates blood vessels, and thereby reduces the amount of work the heart has to do. If these measures do not adequately improve breathing, a specialized mask to deliver oxygen at controlled pressures may be used or a tube may be inserted into the person's airway so that a mechanical ventilator can assist breathing.

For people who have severe symptoms and have not responded well to treatments, drugs that are similar to epinephrine and norepinephrine (such as dopamine or dobutamine) or other drugs that make cardiac muscle contract more forcefully (such as milrinone) are sometimes used for a short time to stimulate heart contractions. These drugs are not useful for long-term treatment.

End-of-Life Issues: Although many people with heart failure live for many years, up to 70% of people die of the disorder within 10 years. Life expectancy depends on how severe the heart failure is, whether its cause can be corrected, and which treatment is used. About half of people who have mild heart failure live at least 10 years, and about half of those who have severe heart failure live at least 2 years. Life expectancy does improve with treatment. Eventually, for a person with chronic heart failure, quality of life may deteriorate and the possibilities for further treatment may become limited, especially for an older person for whom heart transplantation may not be feasible. Keeping the person comfortable may eventually become more important than trying to prolong life. The person and the family members should be involved in these decisions. Much can be done to provide com-

passionate care, relieve symptoms, and maintain the person's dignity (see page 57).

Heart failure can cause death suddenly and unexpectedly, without symptoms worsening. Consequently, when possible, people who have heart failure should prepare advance directives about the type of care desired in case they are no longer able to make decisions about their care (see page 69). Also, making or updating a will is important.

CHAPTER

58 Cardiomyopathy

Cardiomyopathy refers to progressive impairment of the structure and function of the muscular walls of the heart chambers.

Cardiomyopathy can be caused by many disorders, or it may have no identifiable cause. The main types of cardiomyopathy—which may overlap—are dilated, hypertrophic, and restrictive. Cardiomyopathies often cause symptoms of heart failure (see page 356). Some cardiomyopathies may also cause chest pain, fainting, or sudden death.

Dilated Cardiomyopathy

Dilated (congestive) cardiomyopathy is a group of heart muscle disorders in which the ventricles enlarge but are not able to pump enough blood for the body's needs, resulting in heart failure.

- Coronary artery disease, viral infections, and some hormonal disorders are common causes of dilated cardiomyopathy.
- Shortness of breath and fatigue are often the first symptoms.
- Electrocardiography and echocardiography are used to diagnose dilated cardiomyopathy.
- Doctors try to treat the cause of this cardiomyopathy, usually by giving drugs.

Dilated cardiomyopathy can develop at any age but is more common among people aged 20 to 60 years. About 10% of people who develop dilated cardiomyopathy are older than 65. The disorder occurs in about 3 times as many men as women and 3 times as many blacks as whites. About 5 to 8 of every 100,000 people develop the disorder each year.

Causes

In North America, the most common identifiable cause of dilated cardiomyopathy is extensive coro-

nary artery disease. Such coronary artery disease results in an inadequate blood supply to the heart muscle, which leads to permanent injury and death of heart muscle. As a result, the heart cannot pump as forcefully. The dead heart muscle is replaced by fibrous (scar) tissue. The remaining uninjured heart muscle then stretches and thickens (hypertrophies) to compensate for the lost pumping action. The more the heart muscle is stretched, the more forcefully it contracts or pumps but only up to a point. After that point, the stretching and thickening do not adequately compensate, and dilated cardiomyopathy with heart failure develops.

Dilated cardiomyopathy also may be caused by an acute inflammation of the heart muscle (myocarditis) due to a viral infection. This disorder is called viral cardiomyopathy. In North America, infection with coxsackie B virus is the most common cause of viral cardiomyopathy. In other parts of the world, other viral infections are more common causes. The virus infects and weakens the heart muscle. As in coronary artery disease, the weakened heart stretches in an attempt to compensate, resulting in dilated cardiomyopathy and often heart failure. Occasionally, dilated cardiomyopathy results from a bacterial infection.

Other causes of dilated cardiomyopathy include certain chronic hormonal disorders such as long-standing, poorly controlled diabetes, morbid obesity, a persistently rapid heart rate, or thyroid disease. Dilated cardiomyopathy also can be caused by use of certain substances, especially alcohol (when intake is heavy and malnutrition is also present), cocaine, antidepressants, and a few chemotherapy drugs. Rare causes of dilated cardiomyopathy include pregnancy and connective tissue disorders such as rheumatoid arthritis. When no specific cause can be identified, the disorder is called an idiopathic dilated cardiomyopathy.

Types of Cardiomyopathy

There are three main types of cardiomyopathy—dilated, hypertrophic, and restrictive.

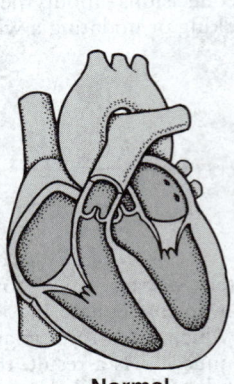

Normal

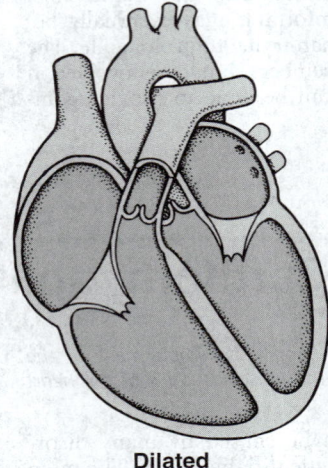

Dilated Cardiomyopathy

The ventricles enlarge.

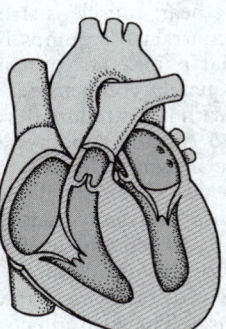

Hypertrophic Cardiomyopathy

The walls of the ventricles thicken and become stiff.

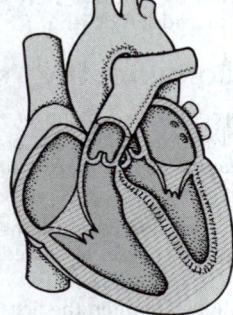

Restrictive Cardiomyopathy

The walls of the ventricles become stiff, but not necessarily thickened.

Symptoms

Usually, the first symptoms of dilated cardiomyopathy are becoming short of breath during exertion and tiring easily. They result from a weakening of the heart's pumping action, which is called heart failure (see page 352). When cardiomyopathy results from an infection, the first symptoms may be a sudden fever and flu-like symptoms. Whatever the cause of dilated cardiomyopathy, if the heart damage is severe enough, the heart rate eventually speeds up, blood pressure is normal or low, fluid is retained in the legs and abdomen, and the lungs fill with fluid.

Because the heart is enlarged, the heart valves may be unable to close normally and often leak. The valves most often affected are the mitral valve, which is positioned between the left atrium (upper heart chamber) and the left ventricle (lower heart chamber), and the tricuspid valve, which is positioned between the right atrium and the right ventricle. Leakage causes murmurs, which doctors can hear with a stethoscope. Damage to and stretching of the heart muscle may result in abnormal heart rhythms (arrhythmias), which may cause awareness of heartbeats (palpitations) or death. The leakage of the valves and the abnormal heart rhythms may interfere further with the heart's pumping action.

Blood pools in the enlarged heart, increasing the risk of blood clots forming on heart chamber walls. The clots can break into pieces (becoming emboli), travel from the heart to blood vessels elsewhere in the body, and block them, causing damage to the organ they supply. If the blood supply to the brain is blocked, a stroke can result.

Diagnosis

The diagnosis is based on the symptoms and the results of a physical examination. Electrocardiography (ECG) may detect abnormalities in the electrical activity of the heart. However, these abnormalities are usually not sufficient evidence for a diagnosis. Echocardiography which uses ultrasound waves to produce an image of the heart, is the most useful procedure because it can show the size and pumping action of the heart. Magnetic resonance imaging (MRI), which produces very detailed images of the heart, may be used to confirm the diagnosis (and sometimes identify the cause).

If the diagnosis remains in doubt, cardiac catheterization, an invasive procedure in which a catheter is threaded into the heart, can provide additional information about the pumping ability of the heart. During cardiac catheterization, doctors can also measure pressures in the heart chambers and determine the extent of coronary artery disease. During catheterization, doctors sometimes remove a tissue sample for examination under a microscope (biopsy). A biopsy can sometimes identify the characteristic microscopic changes of some disorders that cause dilated cardiomyopathy (such as a viral infection that has just developed) and thus confirm the diagnosis. However, usually, the results of a biopsy are not specific enough to help with the diagnosis.

Prognosis

About 70% of people die within 5 years of when their symptoms begin, and the prognosis worsens as the heart becomes more dilated and functions less well. Abnormal heart rhythms also indicate a worse prognosis. Overall, men survive only half as long as women, and blacks survive half as long as whites.

About 50% of deaths are sudden, probably resulting from an abnormal heart rhythm.

Treatment

If possible, doctors treat the underlying cause.

General treatment measures include avoiding stress, limiting salt in the diet, and having periods of rest, which help reduce strain on the heart, particularly when the cardiomyopathy is acute or severe.

Drugs, such as angiotensin-converting enzyme (ACE) inhibitors, angiotensin II receptor blockers, beta-blockers, spironolactone or eplerenone, and low-dose digoxin, improve the heart's pumping function, prolong life, and decrease persistent symptoms. Diuretics are used to reduce excess fluid in the lungs and decrease symptoms of swelling due to fluid retention, but they do not prolong life.

Antiarrhythmic drugs may be given to prevent abnormal heart rhythms. Most of these drugs are prescribed in small doses. Doses are increased in small increments, because if the dose is too large, an antiarrhythmic drug may worsen heart rhythm abnormalities or depress pumping function. Some people have an abnormality of the electrical conduction in the heart, which can be helped by a pacemaker. Doctors may consider an implantable cardioverter-defibrillator pacemaker in patients with persistent poor heart function and an increased risk of sudden death.

Regardless of the cause of dilated cardiomyopathy, doctors may give anticoagulants, such as warfarin, to prevent blood clots, which may form on the heart chamber walls of very dilated and poorly contracting ventricles.

Unless a specific cause of dilated cardiomyopathy can be treated, heart failure in dilated cardiomyopathy is often fatal. Because of this poor prognosis, dilated cardiomyopathy is the most common reason for heart transplantation (see page 1132). Successful heart transplantation cures the disorder, but it has its own complications and limitations.

Hypertrophic Cardiomyopathy

Hypertrophic cardiomyopathy includes a group of heart disorders in which the walls of the ventricles thicken (hypertrophy) and become stiff, even though the workload of the heart is not increased.

- Most cases of hypertrophic cardiomyopathy are caused by an inherited genetic defect.

- People experience fainting, chest pain, shortness of breath, and awareness of irregular heartbeats.

- Doctors can usually make a diagnosis based on physical examination findings, but they use echocardiography to confirm the diagnosis.

- Drugs that reduce the force of the heart's contractions are given.

Generally, hypertrophic cardiomyopathy affects men and women equally. But among older people, it is more common among women than among men, mainly because women live longer than men. It occurs in about 4% of older people.

Causes

Hypertrophic cardiomyopathy may be present at birth (congenital) or acquired later in life. Hypertrophic cardiomyopathy that is congenital and most cases that develop later are caused by an inherited genetic defect. Acquired hypertrophic cardiomyopathy may be caused by such disorders as acromegaly (excessive growth due to overproduction of growth hormone, usually by a benign pituitary tumor) and a pheochromocytoma (a tumor that overproduces the hormone epinephrine). Neurofibromatosis, a hereditary disorder, may also cause hypertrophic cardiomyopathy.

Symptoms

Symptoms include fainting (syncope), chest pain, shortness of breath, and awareness of irregular heartbeats (palpitations) produced by an abnormal heart rhythm (arrhythmia). Fainting usually occurs during exertion.

Shortness of breath develops because fluid accumulates in the lungs. Fluid accumulates because the thickened, stiff heart resists filling with blood from the lungs and blood consequently pools in the lungs.

Because the ventricle walls thicken, the mitral valve (the valve that opens between the left atrium and the left ventricle) may be unable to close normally, resulting in leakage of a small amount of blood back into the left atrium. In some people, the thickened muscle obstructs the flow of blood out of the heart below the aortic valve. This variation is called hypertrophic obstructive cardiomyopathy.

Diagnosis

Doctors can usually make a preliminary diagnosis of hypertrophic cardiomyopathy based on the results of a physical examination. For example, the heart sounds heard through a stethoscope are usually characteristic. Echocardiography is the best way to confirm the diagnosis. Electrocardiography (ECG) and a chest x-ray are also helpful. Cardiac catheterization, an invasive procedure, is performed to measure pressures in the heart chambers only if surgery is being considered.

Prognosis

About 4% of people with hypertrophic cardiomyopathy die each year. Death is usually sudden, presumably due to an abnormal heart rhythm. Death due to chronic heart failure is less common. People who learn that they have inherited this disorder may wish to obtain genetic counseling when they plan a family. Family members of people who have this inherited disorder may wish to consider genetic testing. Hypertrophic cardiomyopathy increases the risk of sudden death in young athletes.

Treatment

If possible, doctors treat the underlying cause.

Treatment of hypertrophic cardiomyopathy is aimed primarily at reducing the heart's resistance to filling with blood between heartbeats. Beta-blockers and the calcium channel blocker verapamil—taken separately or together—are the main treatment. Both reduce the extent to which heart muscle contracts, so that the heart contracts less forcefully. As a result, the heart can fill better and, if the thickened muscle was blocking blood flow, blood can flow out of the heart more easily. Also, beta-blockers and verapamil slow the heart rate, so that the heart has more time to fill. Sometimes, disopyramide, a drug that decreases the strength of heart contractions, is also used.

In people who are thought to have an increased risk of sudden death, doctors may recommend an implantable cardioverter-defibrillator.

Surgery to remove some of the thickened heart muscle (myectomy) can improve the flow of blood from the heart, but it is done only when symptoms are incapacitating despite drug therapy. Surgery can relieve symptoms, but it does not reduce the risk of death. Alcohol ablation (controlled destruction of a small area of heart muscle) is increasingly being used in certain people to improve blood flow from the heart because it can be done by using cardiac catheterization. Although cardiac catheterization is an invasive procedure in which a catheter is threaded into the heart, it has fewer risks than surgery.

Restrictive Cardiomyopathy

Restrictive (infiltrative) cardiomyopathy includes a group of heart disorders in which the walls of the ventricles become stiff, but not necessarily thickened, and resist normal filling with blood between heartbeats.

- Restrictive cardiomyopathy may occur when heart muscle is gradually infiltrated or replaced by scar tissue or when abnormal substances accumulate in the heart muscle.
- Shortness of breath, fluid accumulation in the tissues, abnormal heart rhythms, and awareness of heartbeats are common symptoms.
- The diagnosis is based on results of a physical examination, electrocardiography, echocardiography and cardiac catheterization.
- Treatment is not often helpful, although sometimes doctors are able to treat the cause.

The least common form of cardiomyopathy, restrictive cardiomyopathy, shares many features with hypertrophic cardiomyopathy. Its cause is usually unknown.

There are two basic types of restrictive cardiomyopathy. In one type, the heart muscle is gradually replaced by scar tissue. Scarring may result from injury due to radiation therapy for cancer. In the other type, abnormal substances accumulate in or infiltrate the heart muscle. For example, if the body contains too much iron, iron may accumulate in the heart muscle, as it does in people who have iron overload (hemochromatosis—see page 942). Eosinophils, a type of blood cell, may infiltrate the heart muscle in people who have the hypereosinophilic syndrome (see page 1050), which most often occurs in tropical regions. Amyloid, an unusual protein not normally present in the body, may accumulate in heart muscle and other tissues, causing amyloidosis (see page 2107). Amyloidosis is more common among older people. Other examples are tumors and granuloma tissue (abnormal collections of certain white blood cells that form in response to chronic inflammation), which, for example, develops in people who have sarcoidosis (see page 511). A congenital form of restrictive cardiomyopathy occurs in infants who have endocardial fibroelastosis. In this rare disorder, a thickened layer of fibrous tissue lines the left ventricle.

Symptoms

Restrictive cardiomyopathy causes heart failure (see page 352), with shortness of breath and fluid accumulation in tissues (edema). Chest pain and fainting (syncope) are less likely than in hypertrophic cardiomyopathy, but abnormal heart rhythms (arrhythmias) and awareness of heartbeats (palpitations) are common. Usually, symptoms do not occur during rest because in restrictive cardiomyopathy, the heart can supply the body with enough blood and oxygen during rest, even though the stiff heart resists filling with blood. Symptoms occur during exercise, when the stiff heart cannot pump enough blood to meet the body's increased need for blood and oxygen.

Diagnosis

Restrictive cardiomyopathy is one of the possible causes investigated when a person has heart failure. The diagnosis is based largely on the results of a physical examination, electrocardiography (ECG), and echocardiography. ECG can typically detect abnormalities in the heart's electrical activity, but they are not specific enough for a diagnosis. Echocardiography shows that the atria are enlarged and that the heart is functioning normally only when the heart contracts (during systole). Magnetic resonance imaging (MRI) can detect abnormal texture in heart muscle due to accumulation of or infiltration with abnormal substances, such as iron and amyloid. Although the procedure is not often necessary, doctors sometimes do cardiac catheterization to measure pressures in the heart chambers and remove a sample of heart muscle for examination under a microscope (biopsy), which may enable doctors to identify the infiltrating substance.

Prognosis and Treatment

About 70% of people with restrictive cardiomyopathy die within 5 years after symptoms begin.

For most people, treatment is not very helpful. For example, diuretics, which are usually taken to treat heart failure, may help people who have troublesome leg swelling or lung congestion but also reduce the amount of blood entering the heart, which can worsen restrictive cardiomyopathy instead of improving it. Drugs commonly used in heart failure to reduce the heart's workload, such as angiotensin-converting enzyme (ACE) inhibitors, are usually not helpful because they reduce blood pressure too much. As a result, not enough blood reaches the rest of the body. Similarly, digoxin is usually not helpful and is sometimes harmful.

Sometimes, the disorder causing restrictive cardiomyopathy can be treated to prevent heart damage from worsening or even to partially reverse it. For example, removing blood at regular intervals reduces the amount of stored iron in people with iron overload. People who have sarcoidosis may take corticosteroids, which cause the granuloma tissue to disappear. However, many cases of restrictive cardiomyopathy have no specific treatment.

Abnormal Heart Rhythms

Abnormal heart rhythms (arrhythmias) are sequences of heartbeats that are irregular, too fast, too slow, or conducted via an abnormal electrical pathway through the heart.

- Heart disorders are the most common cause of an abnormal heart rhythm.
- Sometimes people are aware of abnormal heart rhythms, but many times they feel only their consequences, such as weakness or fainting.
- The diagnosis is based on electrocardiography.
- Treatment involves restoring the heart to a normal rhythm and preventing further episodes.

The heart is a muscular organ with four chambers designed to work efficiently, reliably, and continuously over a lifetime. The muscular walls of each chamber contract in a regulated sequence, pumping blood as required by the body while expending as little energy as possible during each heartbeat.

Contraction of the muscle fibers in the heart is controlled by electricity that flows through the heart in a precise manner along distinct pathways and at a controlled speed. The electrical current that begins each heartbeat originates in the heart's pacemaker (sinus or sinoatrial node), located in the top of the upper right heart chamber (right atrium). The rate at which the pacemaker discharges the electrical current determines the heart rate. This rate is influenced by nerve impulses and by levels of certain hormones in the bloodstream.

The heart rate is regulated automatically by the autonomic nervous system (see page 627), which consists of the sympathetic and parasympathetic divisions. The sympathetic division increases the heart rate through a network of nerves called the sympathetic plexus. The parasympathetic division decreases the heart rate through a single nerve, the vagus nerve.

Heart rate is also influenced by hormones released into the bloodstream by the sympathetic division: epinephrine (adrenaline) and norepinephrine (noradrenaline), which increase the heart rate. Thyroid hormone, which is released into the bloodstream by the thyroid gland, also increases the heart rate.

In an adult at rest, the normal heart rate is usually between 60 and 100 beats per minute. However, lower rates may be normal in young adults, particularly those who are physically fit. A person's heart rate varies normally in response to exercise and such stimuli as pain and anger. Heart rhythm is considered abnormal only when the heart rate is inappropriately fast (called tachycardia), slow (called bradycardia), or irregular or when electrical impulses travel along abnormal pathways.

Normal Electrical Pathway

The electrical current from the pacemaker flows first through the right atrium and then through the left atrium, causing the muscles of these chambers to contract and blood to be pumped from the atria into the lower heart chambers (ventricles). The electrical current then reaches the atrioventricular

Tracing the Heart's Electrical Pathway

The sinoatrial node (1) initiates an electrical impulse that flows through the right and left atria (2), making them contract. When the electrical impulse reaches the atrioventricular node (3), it is delayed slightly. The impulse then travels down the bundle of His (4), which divides into the right bundle branch for the right ventricle (5) and the left bundle branch for the left ventricle (5). The impulse then spreads through the ventricles, making them contract.

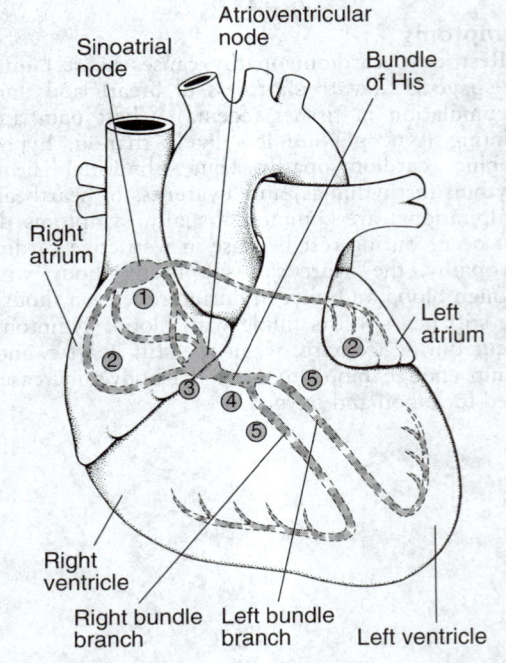

node, located in the lower part of the wall between the atria near the ventricles. The atrioventricular node provides the only electrical connection between the atria and ventricles; otherwise, the atria are insulated from the ventricles by tissue that does not conduct electricity. The atrioventricular node delays transmission of the electrical current so that the atria can contract completely and the ventricles can fill with as much blood as possible before the ventricles are electrically signaled to contract.

After passing through the atrioventricular node, the electrical current travels down the bundle of His, a group of fibers that divide into a left bundle branch for the left ventricle and a right bundle branch for the right ventricle. The electrical current then spreads in a regulated manner over the surface of the ventricles, from the bottom up, initiating contraction of the ventricles, which ejects blood from the heart.

Causes

The most common cause of arrhythmias is a heart disorder, particularly coronary artery disease, heart valve disorders, and heart failure. Many drugs, prescription or nonprescription, including those used to treat heart disorders, can lead to arrhythmias. Some arrhythmias are caused by anatomic abnormalities present at birth (congenital birth defects). Age-related changes in the heart's electrical system make some arrhythmias more likely. An overactive thyroid gland (hyperthyroidism), producing high levels of thyroid hormone, may cause fast arrhythmias. An underactive thyroid gland (hypothyroidism), producing low levels of thyroid hormone, may cause slow arrhythmias. Sometimes no cause for an arrhythmia can be identified.

Fast arrhythmias (tachyarrhythmias) may be triggered by exercise, emotional stress, excessive alcohol consumption, smoking, or use of drugs that contain stimulants, such as cold and hay fever remedies. Slow arrhythmias (bradyarrhythmias) may be triggered by pain, hunger, fatigue, digestive disorders (such as diarrhea and vomiting), or swallowing, which can stimulate the vagus nerve excessively. (With enough stimulation, which is rare, the vagus nerve can cause the heart to stop.) In most of these circumstances, the arrhythmia tends to resolve on its own.

Symptoms

Some people who have abnormal heartbeats may be aware of them. However, awareness of heartbeats (called palpitations) varies widely among people. Some people can feel normal heartbeats, and most people can feel heartbeats when they lie on their left side.

Arrhythmias have consequences that range from harmless to life threatening. The seriousness of an arrhythmia may not be closely linked with the severity of the symptoms it causes. Some life-threatening arrhythmias cause no symptoms, and some otherwise inconsequential arrhythmias may cause severe symptoms. Often, the nature and severity of the underlying heart disorder are more important than the arrhythmia itself

When arrhythmias impair the heart's ability to pump blood, they can produce weakness, a reduced capacity for exercise, shortness of breath, light-headedness, dizziness, and fainting (syncope—see page 344). Fainting occurs when the heart is pumping so inefficiently that it can no longer maintain adequate blood pressure. If such an arrhythmia persists, death may result. Arrhythmias may also aggravate the symptoms of an underlying heart disorder, including chest pain and shortness of breath. Arrhythmias that produce symptoms require prompt attention.

> **? Did You Know...**
> Some life-threatening arrhythmias cause no symptoms, and some otherwise inconsequential ones may cause severe symptoms.

Diagnosis

Often, a person's description of symptoms can help doctors make a preliminary diagnosis and determine the severity of the arrhythmia. The most important considerations are whether the palpitations are fast or slow, regular or irregular, or brief or prolonged and whether the arrhythmia produces symptoms. Doctors also need to know whether the palpitations occur at rest or only during strenuous or unusual activity and whether they start and stop suddenly or gradually. However, certain diagnostic procedures are often needed to determine the exact nature of the arrhythmia and its cause.

Electrocardiography (ECG—see page 326) is the main diagnostic procedure for detecting arrhythmias and determining their cause. This procedure provides a graphic representation of the electrical current producing each heartbeat. Usually, ECG records the heart rhythm for only a very short time. Because arrhythmias are often intermittent, a portable ECG monitor (Holter monitor—see page 327) may be used to record heart rhythm continuously or when the wearer senses an abnormal heart rhythm and activates the monitor. This monitor, usually worn for 24 hours, can record sporadic arrhythmias as the person engages in normal daily activities. During the 24-hour period, the person also keeps a diary of symptoms and activities, which are correlated with the arrhythmias. To detect dangerous arrhythmias that occur very infrequently, doctors sometimes implant a recording device under the skin below the left collarbone (clavicle). The device can be left in place for long periods. It electronically transmits stored recordings of abnormal heart rhythms painlessly through the skin.

People with suspected life-threatening arrhythmias are usually hospitalized. Their heart rhythm is continuously recorded and displayed on a television-type monitor by the bedside or at the nursing station. Thus, any problems can be identified promptly.

Other diagnostic procedures include exercise stress testing (ECG and blood pressure measurement during exercise—see page 326) and electrophysiologic testing (see page 327). During electrophysiologic testing, catheters with tiny electrodes at their tip are inserted through a vein and threaded into the heart. The electrodes are used to stimulate the heart, and the heart's response is monitored, so that the type of arrhythmia and the preferred treatment options can be determined.

Prognosis

Most arrhythmias neither cause symptoms nor interfere with the heart's ability to pump blood. Thus, they usually pose little or no risk, although they can cause considerable anxiety if a person becomes aware of them. However, some arrhythmias, harmless in themselves, can lead to more serious arrhythmias. Any arrhythmia that impairs the heart's ability to pump blood adequately is serious. How serious depends in part on whether the arrhythmia originates in the heart's normal pacemaker, in the atria, or in the ventricles. Generally, arrhythmias that originate in the ventricles are more serious than those that originate in the atria, which are more serious than those that originate in the pacemaker. However, there are many exceptions.

Treatment

For people who have a harmless yet worrisome arrhythmia, reassurance that the arrhythmia is harmless may be treatment enough. Sometimes arrhythmias occur less often or even stop when doctors change a person's drugs or adjust the dosages. Avoiding alcohol, caffeine (in beverages and foods), or smoking may also help. Avoiding strenuous exercise may help if palpitations occur only with exercise.

Drugs: Antiarrhythmic drugs are useful for suppressing fast arrhythmias that cause intolerable symptoms or pose a risk. No single drug cures all arrhythmias in all people. Sometimes several drugs must be tried until the response is satisfactory. Sometimes antiarrhythmic drugs can worsen or even cause arrhythmias. This effect is called proar-

rhythmia. Antiarrhythmic drugs also produce other side effects.

Pacemakers: Artificial pacemakers are electronic devices that act in place of the heart's own pacemaker. These devices are implanted surgically under the skin, usually below the left or right collarbone. They are connected to the heart by wires running inside a vein. Because of new low-energy circuitry and battery designs, these units now last about 10 to 15 years. New circuitry has almost completely eliminated the risk of interference from cell phones, automobile ignition systems, radar, microwaves, and airport security detectors. However, some equipment may interfere with pacemakers. Examples are machines used in magnetic resonance imaging (MRI) and in diathermy (physical therapy in which heat is applied to muscles).

The most common use of pacemakers is to treat slow arrhythmias. When the heart slows below a set threshold, the artificial pacemaker begins to produce electrical impulses. Less commonly, pacemakers are used to treat fast arrhythmias by delivering a series of impulses to decrease the heart rate.

Restoring Normal Rhythm: Sometimes an electrical shock to the heart can stop a fast arrhythmia and restore normal rhythm. Using an electrical shock for this purpose is called cardioversion, defibrillation, or electroversion. Cardioversion may be used for arrhythmias starting in the atria or the ventricles. The machine that delivers the shock (a defibrillator) is used by a team of doctors and nurses, by paramedics, or by firefighters.

An **implantable cardioverter-defibrillator** (ICD), which is about one half the size of a deck of cards, can be placed. Most devices are implanted through the blood vessels just as a pacemaker is, thus eliminating the need for open chest surgery. ICDs continually monitor the rate and rhythm of the heart, automatically detect fast arrhythmias, and deliver a shock to convert the arrhythmia back to a normal rhythm. Most commonly, these devices are used in people who might otherwise die of the arrhythmia. An ICD can also act like a pacemaker, sending electrical impulses to overcome a slow arrhythmia. When an ICD delivers a shock, it can feel like a mild thump in the chest. When a stronger shock is given, people may feel as if they have been kicked. People who have ICDs can safely be around most home electronic devices, including microwaves, and airport security detectors. However, some equipment with strong magnetic fields or strong electric fields may interfere with ICDs. Examples are machines used in magnetic resonance imaging (MRI) and in diathermy (physical therapy in which heat is applied to muscles). Because implantable defibrillators do not prevent arrhythmias, drugs often must be taken as well. These devices last for about 5 years.

Keeping the Beat: Artificial Pacemakers

Artificial pacemakers are electronic devices that act in place of the heart's natural pacemaker (the sinus or sinoatrial node). They generate electrical impulses that initiate each heartbeat. Pacemakers consist of a battery, an impulse generator, and wires that connect the pacemaker to the heart.

An artificial pacemaker is implanted surgically. After a local anesthetic is used to numb the insertion site, the wires that connect the pacemaker are usually inserted into a vein near the collarbone and threaded toward the heart. Through a small incision, the impulse generator, which is about the size of a silver dollar, is inserted just under the skin near the collarbone and connected to the wires. The incision is stitched closed. Usually, the procedure takes

about 30 to 60 minutes. The person may be able to go home shortly afterward or may briefly stay in the hospital. The battery for a pacemaker usually lasts 10 to 15 years. Nevertheless, the battery should be checked regularly. Battery replacement is a quick procedure.

There are different types of pacemakers. Some take over the control of the heart rate, overriding the electrical impulses generated by the heart. Others, called demand pacemakers, allow the heart to beat naturally unless it skips a beat or begins to beat at an abnormal rate. Still others, called programmable pacemakers, can do either. Some pacemakers can adjust their rate depending on the wearer's activity, increasing the heart rate during exercise and decreasing it during rest.

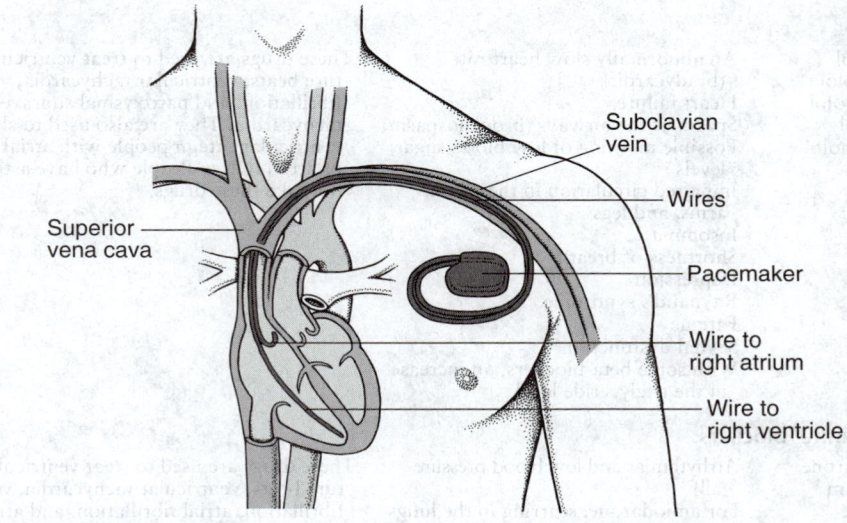

Subclavian vein

Wires

Superior vena cava

Pacemaker

Wire to right atrium

Wire to right ventricle

A newer type of defibrillator, called an automated external defibrillator (AED), requires only minimal training for its use. For example, AEDs can be used by people who receive first-aid instruction in its use (see art on page 1940). AEDs can detect the presence of an arrhythmia, determine if a shock is advisable, and deliver the shock automatically. They are being placed in many public places, such as airports, sports arenas, hotels, and shopping malls.

Destroying Abnormal Tissue: Certain types of arrhythmias can be controlled by performing surgical and other invasive procedures. An arrhythmia due to a localized abnormal area in the heart's electrical system can be controlled by destroying or

removing that area (ablation). Most often, the abnormal area is destroyed by radiofrequency ablation (delivery of energy of a specific frequency through an electrode catheter inserted in the heart). This procedure is successful in 90 to 95% of people, takes 2 to 4 hours, and requires only 1 to 2 days in the hospital. Less commonly, the area is destroyed or removed during open-heart surgery.

Atrial Premature Beats

An atrial premature beat (atrial ectopic beat, premature atrial contraction) is an extra heartbeat caused by electrical activation of the atria from an abnormal site before a normal heartbeat would occur.

SOME DRUGS USED TO TREAT ARRHYTHMIAS

EXAMPLES	SOME SIDE EFFECTS	COMMENTS
Sodium channel blockers		
Disopyramide Flecainide Lidocaine Mexiletine Moricizine Phenytoin Procainamide Propafenone Quinidine Tocainide	Arrhythmias (which can be fatal, particularly in people who have a heart disorder) Digestive upset Dizziness Light-headedness Tremor Retention of urine Increased intraocular pressure in people who have glaucoma Dry mouth	These drugs slow the conduction of electrical impulses through the heart. These drugs are used to treat ventricular premature beats, ventricular tachycardia, and ventricular fibrillation and to convert atrial fibrillation or atrial flutter to normal rhythm (cardioversion).
Beta-blockers		
Atenolol Bisoprolol Metoprolol Nadolol Propranolol	An abnormally slow heart rate (bradycardia) Heart failure Spasm of the airways (bronchospasm) Possible masking of low blood sugar levels Impaired circulation in the trunk, arms, and legs Insomnia Shortness of breath Depression Raynaud's syndrome Fatigue Sexual dysfunction With some beta-blockers, an increase in the triglyceride level	These drugs are used to treat ventricular premature beats, ventricular tachycardia, ventricular fibrillation, and paroxysmal supraventricular tachycardia. They are also used to slow the ventricular rate in people with atrial fibrillation or atrial flutter. People who have asthma should not take these drugs.
Potassium channel blockers		
Amiodarone Bretylium Ibutilide Sotalol	Arrhythmias and low blood pressure (all) For amiodarone, scarring in the lungs (pulmonary fibrosis) For sotalol (also a beta-blocker), also the same side effects as beta-blockers	These drugs are used to treat ventricular premature beats, ventricular tachycardia, ventricular fibrillation, atrial fibrillation, and atrial flutter. Because amiodarone can be toxic, it is used for long-term treatment only in some people who have serious or very bothersome arrhythmias. Bretylium is used only for short-term treatment of life-threatening ventricular tachycardias.
Calcium channel blockers		
Diltiazem Verapamil	Constipation Diarrhea Low blood pressure Swollen feet	Only certain calcium channel blockers, such as diltiazem and verapamil, are useful. They are used to slow the ventricular rate in people who have atrial fibrillation or atrial flutter and to treat paroxysmal supraventricular tachycardia. Diltiazem and verapamil slow the conduction of electrical impulses through the atrioventricular node. Certain people with Wolff-Parkinson-White syndrome should not take verapamil or diltiazem.

(continued on the following page)

R℞ SOME DRUGS USED TO TREAT ARRHYTHMIAS (*Continued*)

EXAMPLES	SOME SIDE EFFECTS	COMMENTS
Digoxin		
	Nausea Vomiting Serious arrhythmias If the dose is too high, xanthopsia (a condition in which objects appear greenish yellow)	Digoxin slows conduction of electrical impulses through the atrioventricular node. Digoxin is used to decrease the ventricular rate in people who have atrial fibrillation or atrial flutter and to treat paroxysmal supraventricular tachycardia. The drug is given to infants and children younger than 10 years who have Wolff-Parkinson-White syndrome, but older people with the syndrome should not take digoxin.
Purine nucleoside		
Adenosine	Spasm of the airways (bronchospasm) Flushing (for a short time)	Adenosine slows conduction of electrical impulses through the atrioventricular node. Adenosine is used to end episodes of paroxysmal supraventricular tachycardia. People who have asthma are not given this drug.

Atrial premature beats occur in many healthy people and rarely cause symptoms. Atrial premature beats are common among people who have lung disorders and are more common among older people than among younger people. These beats may be caused or worsened by consuming coffee, tea, or alcohol and by using some cold, hay fever, and asthma remedies.

Atrial premature beats may be detected during a physical examination and are confirmed by electrocardiography (ECG). Rarely, when these beats occur frequently and cause intolerable palpitations, treatment is necessary. Antiarrhythmic drugs are usually effective.

Atrial Fibrillation and Atrial Flutter

Atrial fibrillation and atrial flutter are very fast electrical discharge patterns that make the atria contract very rapidly, with some of the electrical impulses reaching the ventricles and causing them to contract faster and less efficiently than normal.

- These disorders often result from conditions that cause the atria to enlarge.
- Symptoms depend on how fast the ventricles contract and may include palpitations, weakness, and chest pain.
- Electrocardiography confirms the diagnosis.
- Treatment includes drugs to slow the ventricles' contractions and sometimes electrical shocks (cardioversion) to restore normal heart rhythm.

Atrial fibrillation and atrial flutter are more common among older people.

Atrial fibrillation and atrial flutter may be intermittent or sustained. During atrial fibrillation or flutter, the contractions of the atria are so fast that the atrial walls quiver. As a result, blood is not pumped effectively to the ventricles. During atrial fibrillation, the atrial rhythm is irregular, so the ventricular rhythm is also irregular. During atrial flutter, the atrial rhythm is regular, and the ventricular rhythm may be regular or irregular. In both cases, the ventricles beat more slowly than the atria because the atrioventricular node cannot conduct electrical impulses at such a fast rate. As a result, only some impulses get through. Even though the ventricles beat more slowly than the atria, the ventricles often still beat too fast to fill completely. Therefore, the heart pumps inefficiently, blood pressure may fall, and heart failure may occur.

Causes: Atrial fibrillation or flutter may occur even when there is no other sign of a heart disorder. However, more often, these arrhythmias are caused by such conditions as rheumatic heart disease, high blood pressure, coronary artery disease, alcohol abuse, an overactive thyroid gland (hyperthyroidism), or a birth defect of the heart. Rheumatic heart disease (heart valve disorders resulting from previous acute rheumatic fever) and high blood pressure cause the atria to enlarge, making atrial fibrillation or flutter more likely.

Complications: In atrial fibrillation or flutter, the atria do not empty completely into the ventricles with each beat. Over time, some blood inside the atria may stagnate, and clots may form. Pieces of the clot may break off, often shortly after atrial fibrillation converts back to normal rhythm—whether spontaneously or because of treatment. These pieces may pass into the left ventricle, travel through the bloodstream (becoming emboli), and block a smaller artery. If pieces of a clot block an artery in the brain, a stroke results. Rarely, a stroke is the first sign of atrial fibrillation or flutter.

> ### ? Did You Know...
> Because blood can pool inside the heart's atria and form clots, atrial fibrillation is a strong risk factor for stroke.

Symptoms and Diagnosis

Symptoms of atrial fibrillation or flutter depend largely on how fast the ventricles beat. A modest increase in the ventricular rate—to less than about 120 beats per minute—may produce no symptoms. Higher rates cause unpleasant palpitations or chest discomfort.

In people with atrial fibrillation, the pulse is irregular and usually fast. In people with atrial flutter, the pulse is more likely to be regular and fast.

The reduced pumping ability of the heart may cause weakness, faintness, and shortness of breath. Some people, especially older people, develop heart failure or chest pain. Very rarely, shock (very low blood pressure—see page 350) occurs in people who have atrial fibrillation or flutter and a very severe heart disorder.

Symptoms suggest the diagnosis of atrial fibrillation or flutter, and electrocardiography (ECG) confirms it.

Treatment

Treatment of atrial fibrillation or flutter is designed to control the rate at which the ventricles contract, to restore the normal rhythm of the heart, and to treat the disorder causing the arrhythmia. Drugs to prevent the formation of clots and emboli (anticoagulants or aspirin) usually are given.

Treatment of the underlying disorder is important but does not always alleviate atrial arrhythmias. However, treatment of an overactive thyroid gland or surgery to correct a heart valve disorder or a birth defect of the heart may help.

Slowing the Heart Rate: Usually, the first step in treating atrial fibrillation or flutter is to slow the beating of the ventricles so that the heart pumps blood more efficiently. Often, the first drug tried is a calcium channel blocker, such as diltiazem or verapamil, which may slow the conduction of impulses to the ventricles. A beta-blocker, such as propranolol or atenolol, may be used. For people who have heart failure, digoxin may be used.

Restoring the Rhythm: Atrial fibrillation or flutter may spontaneously convert to a normal rhythm. However, these arrhythmias must often be actively converted to normal. Certain antiarrhythmic drugs (most commonly, amiodarone, flecainide, propafenone, or sotalol) may be effective, but cardioversion, or defibrillation (delivery of an electrical shock to the heart), is the most effective approach. Conversion to a normal rhythm by any means becomes less likely the longer the arrhythmia has been present (especially after 6 months or more), the larger the atria become, and the more severe the underlying heart disorder becomes. When conversion is successful, the risk of recurrence is high, even if people are taking a drug to prevent recurrence (typically one of the same drugs used to convert the arrhythmia to a normal rhythm).

Destroying the Atrioventricular Node: Rarely, when all other treatments of atrial fibrillation are ineffective, the atrioventricular node can be destroyed by radiofrequency ablation (delivery of energy of a specific frequency through an electrode catheter inserted in the heart). This procedure completely stops conduction from the atria to the ventricles and slows the ventricular rate. However, a permanent artificial pacemaker is required to activate the ventricles afterward. Another type of ablation procedure destroys atrial tissue near the pulmonary veins (pulmonary vein isolation). Pulmonary vein isolation spares the atrioventricular node but is less often successful (60 to 80%) and carries a significant risk of serious complications (1 to 5%). Accordingly, this ablation procedure is often reserved for the best candidates—young patients with drug-resistant atrial fibrillation who do not have other serious heart disorders.

For people who have atrial flutter, radiofrequency ablation may be used to interrupt the flutter circuit in the atrium and permanently re-establish normal rhythm. This procedure is successful in about 90% of people

Preventing Blood Clots: When atrial fibrillation or flutter is converted back to normal rhythm, the risk that a clot will be dislodged and cause a stroke is particularly high. Most people with atrial fibrillation or flutter and one or more risk factors for developing clots are given an anticoagulant to prevent clots, because they are at risk of a stroke. (Risk factors for developing blood clots include advancing age, high blood pressure, diabetes, an enlarged left atrium, and a structural heart disorder, especially mitral valve disorders—see page 378). Unless conversion to a normal rhythm is needed immediately, doctors recommend that most people take an anticoagulant for about 3 weeks before cardioversion of established atrial fibrillation or flutter is attempted. However, sometimes there is a specific reason not to use an anticoagulant. For example, people who have uncontrolled high blood pressure or a bleeding disorder should not be given anticoagulants. Anticoagulant therapy can cause bleeding, which can lead to hemorrhagic stroke and other bleeding complications, such as excessive bleeding after surgery. Therefore, doctors balance the potential benefits and risks for each person.

Even after atrial fibrillation or flutter converts to normal rhythm, doctors usually continue anticoagulant treatment, often for the remainder of the person's life. This anticoagulant treatment is needed because the arrhythmia may come back without the person being aware of it. Dangerous clots can form during these episodes.

Paroxysmal Supraventricular Tachycardia

Paroxysmal supraventricular (atrial) tachycardia is a regular, fast (160 to 220 beats per minute) heart rate that begins and ends suddenly and originates in heart tissue other than that in the ventricles.

- Most people have uncomfortable palpitations, shortness of breath, and chest pain.
- Episodes can often be stopped by maneuvers that stimulate the vagus nerve, which slows the heart rate.
- Sometimes, people are given drugs to stop the episode.

Paroxysmal supraventricular tachycardia is most common among young people and is more unpleasant than dangerous. It may occur during vigorous exercise.

Paroxysmal supraventricular tachycardia may be triggered by a premature heartbeat that repeatedly activates the heart at a fast rate. This repeated, rapid activation may be caused by several abnormalities. There may be two electrical pathways in the atrioventricular node (an arrhythmia called atrioventricular nodal reentrant supraventricular tachycardia). There may be an abnormal electrical pathway between the atria and the ventricles (an arrhythmia called atrioventricular reciprocating supraventricular tachycardia). Much less commonly, the atria may generate abnormal rapid or circling impulses (an arrhythmia called true paroxysmal atrial tachycardia).

The fast heart rate tends to begin and end suddenly and may last from a few minutes to many hours. It is almost always experienced as an uncomfortable palpitation. It is often associated with other symptoms, such as weakness, light-headedness, shortness of breath, and chest pain. Usually, the heart is otherwise normal. The doctor confirms the diagnosis by doing an electrocardiogram (ECG).

Treatment

Episodes of paroxysmal supraventricular tachycardia often can be stopped by one of several maneuvers that stimulate the vagus nerve and thus decrease the heart rate. These maneuvers are usually conducted or supervised by a doctor, but people who repeatedly experience the arrhythmia often learn to do the maneuvers themselves. Maneuvers include straining as if having a difficult bowel movement, rubbing the neck just below the angle of the jaw (which stimulates a sensitive area on the carotid artery called the carotid sinus), and plunging the face into a bowl of ice-cold water. These maneuvers are most effective when they are used shortly after the arrhythmia starts.

If these maneuvers are not effective, if the arrhythmia produces severe symptoms, or if the episode lasts more than 20 minutes, people are advised to seek medical intervention to stop the episode. Doctors can usually stop an episode promptly by giving an intravenous injection of a drug, usually adenosine or verapamil. Rarely, drugs are ineffective, and cardioversion (delivery of an electrical shock to the heart) may be necessary.

Prevention is more difficult than treatment, but almost any antiarrhythmic drug may be effective. Drugs commonly used include beta-blockers, digoxin, diltiazem, verapamil, propafenone, and flecainide. Increasingly, radiofrequency ablation (delivery of energy of a specific frequency through an electrode catheter inserted in the heart) is being used to destroy the tissue in which paroxysmal supraventricular tachycardia originates.

Wolff-Parkinson-White Syndrome

Wolff-Parkinson-White syndrome is a disorder in which an extra electrical connection between the atria and the ventricles is present at birth. People may have episodes of a very rapid heartbeat.

- Most people have palpitations, and some feel weak or short of breath.
- Electrocardiography is used to make the diagnosis.
- Usually, episodes can be stopped by maneuvers that stimulate the vagus nerve, which slows the heart rate.

Wolff-Parkinson-White syndrome is the most common of several disorders that involve an extra (accessory) pathway between the atria and the ventricles. (Such disorders are called atrioventricular reciprocating supraventricular tachycardias.) This extra pathway makes fast arrhythmias more likely to occur. Wolff-Parkinson-White syndrome is present at birth, but the arrhythmias it causes usually become apparent during the teens or early twenties. However, arrhythmias may occur during the first year of life or not until after age 60.

Symptoms

Wolff-Parkinson-White syndrome is a common cause of paroxysmal supraventricular tachycardia (see page 373). Very rarely, this syndrome results in a very fast, life-threatening heart rate during atrial fibrillation.

When infants develop arrhythmias due to this syndrome, they may become short of breath or lethargic, stop eating well, or have rapid, visible pulsations of the chest. Heart failure may develop.

Typically, when teenagers or people in their early 20s first experience an arrhythmia due to this syndrome, it is an episode of palpitations that begins suddenly, often during exercise. The episode may last for only a few seconds or may persist for several hours. For most people, the very fast heart rate is uncomfortable and distressing. A few people faint.

In older people, episodes of paroxysmal supraventricular tachycardia due to Wolff-Parkinson-White syndrome tend to produce more symptoms, such as fainting, shortness of breath, and chest pain.

Atrial Fibrillation and Wolff-Parkinson-White Syndrome: Atrial fibrillation may be particularly dangerous for people with Wolff-Parkinson-White syndrome. The extra pathway can conduct the rapid impulses to the ventricles at a much faster rate than the normal pathway (through the atrioventricular node) can. The result is an extremely fast ventricular rate that may be life threatening. Not only is the heart very inefficient when it beats so rapidly, but this extremely fast heart rate may also progress to ventricular fibrillation, which is fatal unless treated immediately.

Diagnosis

Because Wolff-Parkinson-White syndrome changes the pattern of electrical activation in the heart, it can be diagnosed using electrocardiography (ECG—see page 326), which records the electrical activity of the heart.

Treatment

Episodes of paroxysmal supraventricular tachycardia due to Wolff-Parkinson-White syndrome can often be stopped by one of several maneuvers that stimulate the vagus nerve and thus slow the heart rate (see page 373). The maneuvers are most effective when they are used shortly after the arrhythmia starts. When these maneuvers are ineffective, drugs such as verapamil or adenosine are usually given intravenously to stop the arrhythmia. Antiarrhythmic drugs may then be continued indefinitely to prevent episodes of a fast heart rate.

In infants and children younger than 10 years, digoxin may be given to suppress episodes of paroxysmal supraventricular tachycardia due to Wolff-Parkinson-White syndrome. However, adults with the syndrome should not take digoxin because it can facilitate conduction by the extra pathway and increase the risk that atrial fibrillation will degenerate into ventricular fibrillation. For this reason, digoxin is usually stopped before people with this syndrome reach puberty.

Destruction of the extra conduction pathway by radiofrequency ablation (delivery of energy of a specific frequency through an electrode catheter inserted in the heart) is successful in more than 95% of people. The risk of death during the procedure is less than 1 in 1,000. Radiofrequency ablation is particularly useful for young people who might otherwise have to take antiarrhythmic drugs for a lifetime.

Ventricular Premature Beats

A ventricular premature beat (ventricular ectopic beat, premature ventricular contraction) is an extra heartbeat resulting from abnormal electrical activation originating in the ventricles before a normal heartbeat would occur.

- The main symptom is a perception of a skipped heartbeat.
- Electrocardiography is used to make the diagnosis.
- Avoiding things that trigger these beats, such as stress, caffeine, and alcohol, is usually sufficient treatment.

Ventricular premature beats are common, particularly among older people. This arrhythmia may be caused by physical or emotional stress, intake of caffeine (in beverages and foods) or alcohol, or use of cold or hay fever remedies containing drugs that stimulate the heart, such as pseudoephedrine. Other causes include coronary artery disease (especially during or shortly after a heart attack) and disorders that cause ventricles to enlarge, such as heart failure and heart valve disorders.

Symptoms and Diagnosis

Isolated ventricular premature beats have little effect on the pumping action of the heart and usually do not cause symptoms, unless they are extremely frequent. The main symptom is the perception of a strong or skipped beat. Ventricular premature beats are not dangerous for people who do not have a heart disorder. However, when they occur frequently in people who have a structural heart disorder, they may be followed by more dangerous arrhythmias such as ventricular tachycardia or ventricular fibrillation, which can cause sudden death.

Electrocardiography (ECG—see page 326) is used to diagnose ventricular premature beats.

Treatment

In an otherwise healthy person, no treatment is needed other than decreasing stress and avoiding caffeine, alcohol, and over-the-counter cold or hay fever remedies containing drugs that stimulate the heart. Drug therapy is usually prescribed only if symptoms are intolerable or if the pattern of ventricular premature beats suggests a risk of progression to ventricular tachycardia or ventricular fibrillation. For example, the presence of a structural heart disorder or episodes of consecutive ventricular beats suggest this risk. Beta-blockers are usually tried first because they are relatively safe drugs. However, some people do not want to take them because they can cause sluggishness.

After a heart attack, people who have frequent ventricular premature beats can reduce the risk of sudden death due to ventricular tachycardia or ventricular fibrillation by taking beta-blockers or undergoing angioplasty or coronary artery bypass surgery to treat coronary artery disease (see page 409). Anti-arrhythmic drugs can suppress ventricular premature beats, but they also may increase the risk of a fatal arrhythmia. Therefore, doctors prescribe them only for carefully selected people who have been evaluated for risk of developing serious arrhythmias.

Ventricular Tachycardia

Ventricular tachycardia is a heart rhythm that originates in the ventricles and produces a heart rate of at least 120 beats per minute.

- People almost always have palpitations.
- Electrocardiography is used to make the diagnosis.
- Drugs and procedures to destroy abnormal areas of the ventricles are usually needed, but usually an automatic defibrillator is used.

Ventricular tachycardia may be thought of as a sequence of consecutive ventricular premature beats. Sometimes only a few such beats occur together, and then the heart returns to a normal rhythm. Ventricular tachycardia that lasts more than 30 seconds is called sustained ventricular tachycardia. Sustained ventricular tachycardia usually occurs in people with a structural heart disorder that has damaged the ventricles. Most commonly, it occurs weeks or months after a heart attack. It is more common among older people. However, rarely, ventricular tachycardia develops in young people who do not have a structural heart disorder.

Symptoms and Diagnosis

People with ventricular tachycardia almost always have palpitations. Sustained ventricular tachycardia can be dangerous because the ventricles cannot fill adequately or pump blood normally. Blood pressure tends to fall, and heart failure follows. Sustained ventricular tachycardia is also dangerous because it can worsen until it becomes ventricular fibrillation—a form of cardiac arrest. Sometimes ventricular tachycardia causes few symptoms, even at rates of up to 200 beats per minute, but it may still be extremely dangerous.

Electrocardiography (ECG—see page 326) is used to diagnose ventricular tachycardia and to help determine whether treatment is required. A portable ECG (Holter) monitor may be used to record heart rhythm over a 24-hour period.

Treatment

Ventricular tachycardia is treated when it causes symptoms or when episodes last more than 30 seconds even without causing symptoms. Sustained ventricular tachycardia often requires emergency treatment. If episodes cause blood pressure to fall to a low level, cardioversion is needed immediately. Drugs may be given intravenously to end or suppress ventricular tachycardia. The most commonly used drugs are amiodarone, lidocaine, and procainamide.

Certain procedures may be used to destroy the small abnormal area in the ventricles, identified by ECG, that is usually responsible for sustained ventricular tachycardia. They include radiofrequency ablation (delivery of energy of a specific frequency through an electrode catheter inserted in the heart) and open-heart surgery.

In people with ventricular tachycardia who have an underlying heart disorder, particularly if their heart does not pump well, an automatic defibrillator (a small device that can detect an arrhythmia and deliver a shock to correct it) is often implanted. This procedure is similar to implantation of an artificial pacemaker.

Ventricular Fibrillation

Ventricular fibrillation is a potentially fatal, uncoordinated series of very rapid, ineffective contractions of the ventricles caused by many chaotic electrical impulses.

- Ventricular fibrillation causes unconsciousness in seconds, and if the disorder is not rapidly treated, death follows.
- Electrocardiography helps determine the cause of cardiac arrest.
- Cardiopulmonary resuscitation must be started within a few minutes, and it must be followed by defibrillation (an electrical shock delivered to the chest) to restore normal heart rhythm.

In ventricular fibrillation, the ventricles merely quiver and do not contract in a coordinated way. No blood is pumped from the heart, so ventricular fibrillation is a form of cardiac arrest. It is fatal unless treated immediately.

The most common cause of ventricular fibrillation is inadequate blood flow to the heart muscle due to coronary artery disease, as occurs during a heart attack. Other causes include the following:

- Shock (very low blood pressure—see page 350), which can result from coronary artery disease and other disorders
- Electrical shock
- Drowning
- Very low levels of potassium in the blood (hypokalemia)
- Drugs that affect electrical currents in the heart (such as sodium or potassium channel blockers—see table on page 370)

Symptoms and Diagnosis

Ventricular fibrillation causes unconsciousness in seconds. If untreated, the person usually has seizures and develops irreversible brain damage after about 5 minutes because oxygen no longer reaches the brain. Death soon follows.

Cardiac arrest is diagnosed when a person suddenly collapses, turns deathly pale, has very dilated pupils, and has no detectable pulse, heartbeat, or blood pressure. Ventricular fibrillation is diagnosed as the cause of the cardiac arrest by electrocardiography (ECG).

Treatment

Ventricular fibrillation must be treated as an extreme emergency. Cardiopulmonary resuscitation (CPR) must be started as soon as possible—within a few minutes. It must be followed by defibrillation (an electrical shock delivered to the chest), as soon as the defibrillator is available. Antiarrhythmic drugs may then be given to help maintain the normal heart rhythm.

When ventricular fibrillation occurs within a few hours of a heart attack in people who are not in shock and who do not have heart failure, prompt cardioversion restores normal rhythm in 95% of people, and the prognosis is good. Shock and heart failure suggest major damage to the ventricles. If they are present, even prompt cardioversion has only a 30% success rate, and 70% of resuscitated survivors die without regaining normal function.

People who are successfully resuscitated from ventricular fibrillation and survive are at high risk of another episode. If ventricular fibrillation is caused by a reversible disorder, that disorder is treated.

Otherwise, most people have an automatic defibrillator surgically implanted to correct the problem, if it recurs, by delivering a shock. Such people are often also given drugs to prevent recurrences.

Pacemaker Dysfunction

- People may have no symptoms, or they may feel weak or tired or have palpitations.
- Electrocardiography is used to make the diagnosis.
- A permanent artificial pacemaker is usually needed.

Dysfunction of the heart's pacemaker (sinus or sinoatrial node) may result in a persistently slow heartbeat (sinus bradycardia) or complete cessation of normal pacemaker activity (sinus arrest). When activity ceases, another area of the heart usually takes over the function of the pacemaker. This area, called an escape pacemaker, may be located lower in the atrium, in the atrioventricular node, in the conduction system, or even in the ventricle.

All types of pacemaker dysfunction are more common among older people. Some drugs and an underactive thyroid gland (hypothyroidism) can cause pacemaker dysfunction. However, the cause is usually unknown. When the cause is unknown, the disorder is called **sick sinus syndrome.**

An important subtype of the sick sinus syndrome is the bradycardia-tachycardia syndrome, in which periods of slow heart rhythms (bradycardia) alternate with periods of fast atrial arrhythmias (tachycardia), such as atrial fibrillation and atrial flutter.

Symptoms and Diagnosis

Many types of pacemaker dysfunction cause no symptoms. A persistent slow heart rate commonly causes weakness and tiredness. Fainting may occur if the rate becomes very slow. A fast heart rate is often perceived by the person as palpitations. When the fast heart rate stops, fainting may occur if the pacemaker is slow in restarting normal heart rhythm.

A slow pulse (especially an irregular one), a pulse that varies greatly without any change in the person's activity, or a pulse that does not increase during exercise suggests pacemaker dysfunction. Doctors can usually diagnose pacemaker dysfunction based on symptoms and the results of electrocardiography (ECG—see page 326), particularly when heart rhythm is recorded over a 24-hour period with a Holter monitor.

Treatment

People with symptoms are usually given a permanent artificial pacemaker to accelerate the heart rate. If they also sometimes have a fast rate, they may also need drugs to slow the heart rate (such as a beta-blocker or a calcium channel blocker—see table on page 370).

Heart Block

Heart block is a delay in the conduction of electrical current as it passes through the atrioventricular node, bundle of His, or both bundle branches, all of which are located between the atria and the ventricles.

- Some types of heart block cause no symptoms, but others cause fatigue, dizziness, and fainting.
- Electrocardiography is used to detect heart block.
- Some people require an artificial pacemaker.

Heart block is classified as first-degree when electrical conduction to the ventricles is slightly delayed, second-degree when conduction is intermittently blocked, or third-degree (complete) when conduction is completely blocked. Most types of heart block are more common among older people.

In **first-degree heart block**, every electrical impulse from the atria reaches the ventricles, but each is slowed for a fraction of a second as it moves through the atrioventricular node. First-degree heart block is common among well-trained athletes, teenagers, young adults, and people with a highly active vagus nerve. However, the disorder also occurs in people with rheumatic heart disease, sarcoidosis that affects the heart (see page 511), or other structural heart disorders. It may be caused by drugs, particularly those that slow conduction of electrical impulses through the atrioventricular node (such as beta-blockers, diltiazem, verapamil, digoxin, and amiodarone). This disorder rarely causes symptoms and can be detected only by electrocardiography (ECG), which shows the conduction delay.

In **second-degree heart block**, only some electrical impulses reach the ventricles. The heart may beat slowly, irregularly, or both. Some forms of second-degree heart block progress to third-degree heart block.

In **third-degree heart block**, no impulses from the atria reach the ventricles, and the ventricular rate and rhythm are controlled by the atrioventricular node, bundle of His, or the ventricles themselves. These substitute pacemakers are slower than the heart's normal pacemaker (sinus or sinoatrial node) and are often irregular and unreliable. Thus, the ventricles beat very slowly—less than 50 beats per minute and sometimes as slowly as 30 beats per minute. Third-degree heart block is a serious arrhythmia that can affect the heart's pumping ability. Fatigue, dizziness, and fainting are common. When the ventricles beat faster than 40 beats per minute, symptoms are less severe.

Treatment

First-degree heart block requires no treatment even when it is caused by a heart disorder. Some people with second-degree heart block require an artificial pacemaker. Almost all people with third-degree heart block require an artificial pacemaker.

A temporary pacemaker may be used in an emergency until a permanent one can be implanted. Most people need an artificial pacemaker for the rest of their lives, although heart rhythm may return to normal if the cause of the heart block resolves—for example, after recovery from a heart attack.

Bundle Branch Block

Bundle branch block is a type of conduction block involving partial or complete interruption of the flow of electrical impulses through the right or left bundle branches.

The bundle of His is a group of fibers that conducts electrical impulses from the atrioventricular node. The bundle of His divides into two bundle branches. The left bundle branch conducts impulses to the left ventricle, and the right bundle branch conducts impulses to the right ventricle. Conduction may be blocked in the left or right bundle branch.

Bundle branch block usually causes no symptoms. Right bundle branch block is not serious in itself and may occur in apparently healthy people. However, it may also indicate significant heart damage due to, for example, a previous heart attack. Left bundle branch block tends to be more serious. In older people, it often indicates coronary artery disease due to high blood pressure or atherosclerosis.

Bundle branch block can be detected by electrocardiography (ECG—see page 326). Each type of block produces a characteristic pattern. Usually, no treatment is needed for either type. However, an artificial pacemaker (see art on page 369) may be implanted in people who are at high risk of complete heart block (such as people with certain types of second-degree heart block) to maintain the heart rate if complete heart block occurs.

60 Heart Valve Disorders

Heart valves regulate the flow of blood through the heart's four chambers—two small, round upper chambers (atria) and two larger, cone-shaped lower chambers (ventricles—see art on page 317). Each ventricle has a one-way "in" (inlet) valve and a one-way "out" (outlet) valve. In the right ventricle, the inlet valve is the tricuspid valve, which opens from the right atrium, and the outlet valve is the pulmonary (pulmonic) valve, which opens into the pulmonary artery. In the left ventricle, the inlet valve is the mitral valve, which opens from the left atrium, and the outlet valve is the aortic valve, which opens into the aorta. Each valve consists of flaps (cusps or leaflets) that open and close like one-way swinging doors.

The heart valves can malfunction either by leaking (termed regurgitation) or by not opening adequately and thus partially blocking the flow of blood through the valve (termed stenosis). Either problem can greatly interfere with the heart's ability to pump blood. Sometimes a valve has both problems. Faulty valves generally create murmurs and other abnormal heart sounds that a doctor can hear with a stethoscope; faulty valves can be identified by using echocardiography. Often, minor degrees of regurgitation are not detected with a stethoscope but are detected during an echocardiogram. Doctors often regard this as a normal finding.

A faulty valve may be repaired or replaced. Repair may require surgery but may sometimes be accomplished during heart catheterization, particularly when the problem is a valve with stenosis. A stenotic valve can sometimes be stretched open using a procedure called balloon valvuloplasty. In this procedure, a balloon-tipped catheter is threaded through a vein and eventually into the heart. Once inside the faulty valve, the balloon is inflated, separating the valve cusps. This procedure does not require a general anesthetic and allows a quick recovery.

Two types of valves are available for replacement, a mechanical type and one made from the heart valve of a pig (bioprosthetic). Mechanical valves last for many years, but people with mechanical valves must take anticoagulants for the rest of their lives to prevent blood clots from forming in the valve. Bioprosthetic valves generally deteriorate and require replacement after 10 to 12 years but do not require use of anticoagulants for more than a few months after surgery. Abnormal valves and all replacement valves can become infected, and people need to take prophylactic antibiotics, which are antibiotics taken at certain times (for example, before some dental or medical procedures) in order to prevent bacterial infection of the valves (infective endocarditis).

Changes With Aging: As people age, the mitral and aortic valves thicken. The aorta becomes stiffer, which increases blood pressure and stress on the mitral valve, and the heart requires additional oxygen to pump blood effectively. These age-related changes may lead to symptoms and complications in older people with heart disease.

Mitral Regurgitation

Mitral regurgitation (mitral valve regurgitation, mitral incompetence, mitral insufficiency) is leakage of blood backward through the mitral valve each time the left ventricle contracts.

- Heart attack is the most common cause of mitral regurgitation except in places where antibiotics are not readily available to treat strep infections.
- When regurgitation is severe, people may have shortness of breath.
- Mild regurgitation may not need treatment, but people with more severe regurgitation may need to take angiotensin-converting enzyme inhibitors or have surgery to replace the damaged heart valve.

As the left ventricle pumps blood into the aorta, some blood leaks backward into the left atrium, increasing blood volume and pressure there. The increased blood pressure in the left atrium increases blood pressure in the veins leading from the lungs to the heart (pulmonary veins) and causes the left atrium to enlarge to accommodate the extra blood leaking back from the ventricle. An extremely enlarged atrium often beats rapidly in an irregular pattern (a disorder called atrial fibrillation), which reduces the heart's pumping efficiency because the fibrillating atrium is quivering rather than pumping. Consequently, blood does not flow through the atrium normally, and blood clots may form inside the chamber. If a clot breaks loose (becoming an embolus), it is pumped out of the heart and may block an artery, possibly causing a stroke or other damage.

Severe regurgitation can result in heart failure, in which increased pressure in the atrium causes fluid accumulation (congestion) in the lungs, or in which reduced forward flow of blood from the ventricle to the body deprives organs of the proper amount of blood. The left ventricle may gradually dilate and weaken, further worsening heart failure.

Understanding Stenosis and Regurgitation

The heart valves can malfunction either by leaking (causing regurgitation) or by not opening adequately and thus partially blocking the flow of blood through the valve (causing stenosis). Stenosis and regurgitation can affect any of the heart valves. These two disorders are shown below affecting the mitral valve.

Normal Valve Mechanisms

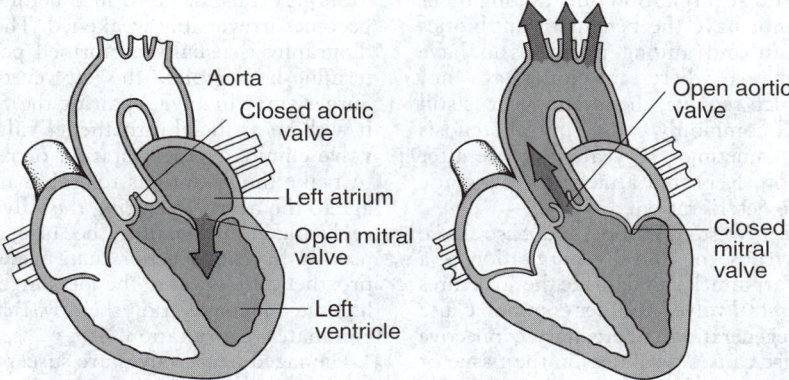

Normally, just after the left ventricle finishes contracting and starts to relax and fill with blood again (during diastole), the aortic valve closes, the mitral valve opens, and some blood flows from the left atrium into the left ventricle. Then the left atrium contracts, ejecting more blood into the left ventricle.

As the left ventricle begins to contract (during systole), the mitral valve closes, the aortic valve opens, and blood is ejected into the aorta.

Mitral Stenosis

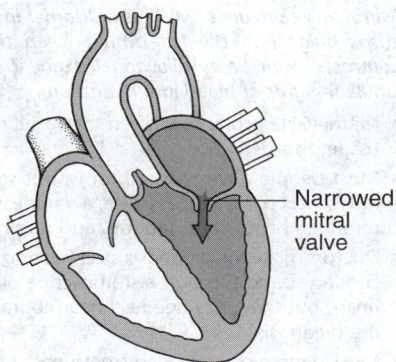

In mitral stenosis, the mitral valve opening is narrowed, and blood flow from the left atrium into the left ventricle during diastole is reduced.

Mitral Regurgitation

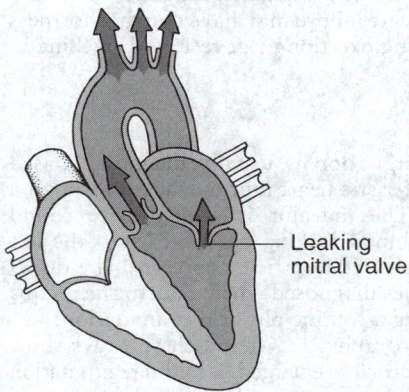

In mitral regurgitation, the mitral valve leaks when the left ventricle contracts (during systole), and some blood flows backward into the left atrium.

Cause

Rheumatic fever (see page 1765)—a childhood illness that sometimes occurs after untreated strep throat or scarlet fever—used to be the most common cause of mitral regurgitation. But today, rheumatic fever is rare in North America, Australasia, Western Europe, and other regions where antibiotics are widely used to treat infections such as strep throat. In these regions, rheumatic fever is a common cause of mitral regurgitation only among older people who did not have the benefit of antibiotics during their youth and among people who have moved from regions where antibiotics are not widely used. In such regions, rheumatic fever is still common and still commonly causes mitral stenosis or regurgitation, sometimes 10 years or more after the initial infection. Repeated attacks of rheumatic fever hasten valve deterioration.

In North America, Western Europe, and Australasia, a more common cause of mitral regurgitation is a heart attack. A heart attack can damage the structures that support the mitral valve. Another common cause is myxomatous degeneration, a hereditary connective tissue disorder that causes weakness in the tissue of the valve. As a result, the heart valve gradually becomes floppy and does not close properly.

Symptoms

Mild mitral regurgitation may not produce any symptoms. When regurgitation is more severe or when there is atrial fibrillation, people may have palpitations (an awareness that their heart beat has changed rhythm) or unexplained shortness of breath. People with heart failure may have cough, shortness of breath during exertion or at rest, and swelling in the legs.

Diagnosis

Mitral regurgitation is usually diagnosed based on the characteristic heart murmur heard through a stethoscope. The murmur is a distinctive sound produced by blood leaking backward into the left atrium when the left ventricle contracts. The disorder is sometimes diagnosed when a doctor hears this murmur during a routine physical examination.

Electrocardiography (ECG) and chest x-rays show that the left ventricle is enlarged. If mitral regurgitation is severe, the chest x-ray may also show fluid accumulation in the lungs. Echocardiography (see page 328), which uses ultrasound waves to produce an image of the heart structures and blood flow, provides the most information. This procedure can show the size of the atrium and ventricle and the amount of blood leaking, so that the severity of the regurgitation can be determined.

Treatment

If regurgitation is mild, no specific treatment may be required; however, the person may need to be evaluated periodically and may need to take antibiotics before dental and medical procedures. More serious regurgitation may be treated with an angiotensin-converting enzyme (ACE) inhibitor, such as enalapril or lisinopril, with or without digoxin. Sometimes surgery is necessary for those with severe regurgitation.

Surgery must be performed before the left ventricle becomes irreversibly weakened. Therefore, echocardiography is usually performed periodically to determine how rapidly the left ventricle is enlarging. Surgery may involve repairing the valve or replacing it with an artificial (prosthetic) valve. Repairing the valve eliminates regurgitation or reduces it enough to make the symptoms tolerable and prevent damage to the heart. Repairing the valve is preferable to replacing it, if possible, because a repaired valve usually functions better than a mechanical or bioprosthetic valve and the person does not require lifetime anticoagulation therapy. Replacing the valve eliminates regurgitation.

Damaged heart valves are susceptible to a serious infection by bacteria (infective endocarditis). People with a damaged or an artificial valve should take antibiotics before surgical, dental, or medical procedures (see box on page 388) to reduce the risk of an infection on a valve, even though this risk is small. Atrial fibrillation, if present, may require treatment (see page 371), including use of anticoagulants to prevent clots.

Mitral Valve Prolapse

Mitral valve prolapse (MVP) is a disorder in which the valve cusps bulge into the left atrium when the left ventricle contracts, sometimes allowing leakage (regurgitation) of small amounts of blood into the atrium.

- Mitral valve prolapse is often the result of a connective tissue disorder.
- Most people have no symptoms, but some people have chest pain, a rapid pulse, awareness of heartbeats, migraine headaches, fatigue, and dizziness.
- Doctors make the diagnosis after hearing a characteristic clicking sound through a stethoscope placed over the heart, but they may need echocardiography to confirm the diagnosis.
- Most people do not need treatment.

About 2 to 5% of people have mitral valve prolapse. The cause is redundancy of the valve tissue often from myxomatous degeneration, a hereditary connective tissue disorder that causes weakness in the tissue of the valve. It causes serious heart problems only if the regurgitation becomes severe, infection of the valve occurs, or myxomatous tissue ruptures.

Replacing a Heart Valve

A damaged heart valve may be replaced with a mechanical valve made of plastic and metal or with a bioprosthetic valve made of heart valve tissue, usually from pigs, placed in a synthetic ring. There are many types of mechanical valves. A St. Jude valve is commonly used.

Choice of a valve depends on many factors, including characteristics of the valve. A mechanical valve lasts longer than a bioprosthetic valve but requires that anticoagulants be taken indefinitely to prevent the formation of blood clots on the valve. A bioprosthetic valve rarely requires the use of anticoagulants. So whether a person can take anticoagulants is an important factor. For example, anticoagulants may not be appropriate for women of childbearing age because anticoagulants cross the placenta and may affect the fetus. Also considered are how old the person is, what the person's activity level is, how well the heart is working, and which heart valve is damaged.

For heart valve replacement, a general anesthetic is given. The heart must be still to be operated on, so a heart-lung machine is used to pump blood through the bloodstream. The damaged valve is removed, and the replacement valve is sewn in place. The incisions are closed, the heart-lung machine is disconnected, and the heart is restarted. The operation takes from 2 to 5 hours. For some people, a heart valve can be replaced using a less invasive procedure (without cutting through the sternum), available at some medical centers. The length of the hospital stay varies from person to person. Full recovery may take 6 to 8 weeks.

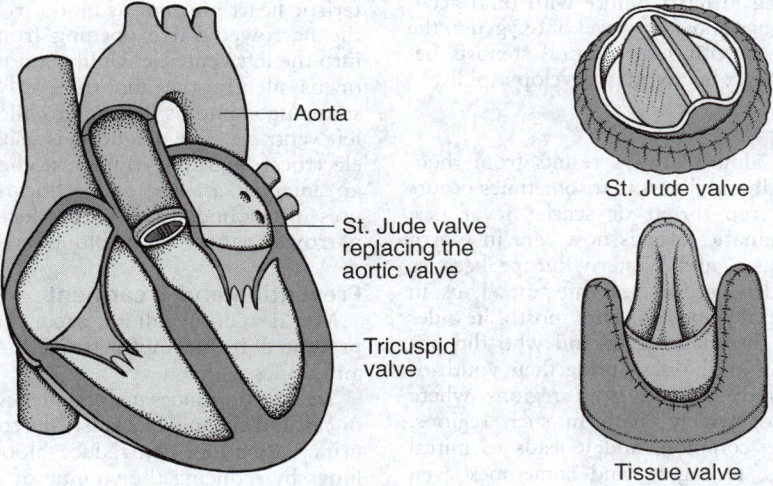

Aorta

St. Jude valve replacing the aortic valve

Tricuspid valve

St. Jude valve

Tissue valve

Symptoms and Diagnosis

Most people with mitral valve prolapse have no symptoms. Others have symptoms that are difficult to explain on the basis of the mechanical problem alone; these symptoms include chest pain, a rapid pulse, palpitations (awareness of heartbeats), migraine headaches, fatigue, and dizziness. In some people, blood pressure may fall below normal when they stand up (a disorder called orthostatic hypotension).

Doctors diagnose mitral valve prolapse after hearing the characteristic clicking sound through a stethoscope. Regurgitation is diagnosed if a murmur is heard when the left ventricle contracts. Echocardiography (see page 328) enables doctors to view the prolapse and determine the severity of regurgitation if present.

Treatment

Most people with mitral valve prolapse do not need treatment. If the heart is beating too fast, a beta-blocker may be taken to slow the heart rate and to reduce palpitations and other symptoms.

If regurgitation is also present, antibiotics should be taken before surgical, dental, or medical procedures (see box on page 388) because bacterial infection of the heart valve (infective endocarditis) is a risk, although a small one.

Mitral Stenosis

Mitral stenosis (mitral valve stenosis) is a narrowing of the mitral valve opening that increases resistance to blood flow from the left atrium to the left ventricle.

- Mitral stenosis usually results from rheumatic fever, but infants can be born with the condition.
- Mitral stenosis does not usually cause symptoms unless it is severe.
- Doctors make the diagnosis after hearing a characteristic heart murmur through a stethoscope placed over the heart.
- Treatment includes use of diuretics and beta-blockers or calcium channel blockers.

In mitral stenosis, blood flow through the narrowed valve opening is reduced. As a result, the volume and pressure of blood in the left atrium increases, and the left atrium enlarges. The enlarged left atrium often beats rapidly in an irregular pattern (a disorder called atrial fibrillation). As a result, the heart's pumping efficiency is reduced. If mitral stenosis is severe, pressure increases in the blood vessels of the lungs, resulting in heart failure with fluid accumulation in the lungs and a low level of oxygen in the blood. If a woman with severe mitral stenosis becomes pregnant, heart failure may develop rapidly.

Cause

Mitral stenosis almost always results from rheumatic fever, a childhood illness that sometimes occurs after untreated strep throat or scarlet fever (see page 1765). Rheumatic fever is now rare in North America, Australasia, and Western Europe because antibiotics are widely used to treat infection. Thus, in these regions, mitral stenosis occurs mostly in older people who had rheumatic fever and who did not have the benefit of antibiotics during their youth or in people who have moved from regions where antibiotics are not widely used. In such regions, rheumatic fever is common, and it leads to mitral stenosis in adults, teenagers, and sometimes even children. Typically, when rheumatic fever is the cause of mitral stenosis, the mitral valve cusps are partially fused together.

Mitral stenosis can rarely be present at birth (congenital). Infants born with the disorder rarely live beyond age 2, unless they have surgery.

Three rare conditions unrelated to mitral stenosis can produce the same effects as the stenosis. They include a myxoma (a noncancerous tumor in the left atrium), cor triatriatum (a rare developmental abnormality in which a membrane goes across the left atrium), and pulmonary veno-occlusive disease (a narrowing of the veins that lead from the lungs into the left atrium).

Symptoms and Diagnosis

Mild mitral stenosis does not usually cause symptoms. Some people with more severe mitral stenosis have atrial fibrillation or heart failure. People with atrial fibrillation may feel palpitations (awareness of heartbeats). People with heart failure become easily fatigued and short of breath. Shortness of breath may occur only during physical activity at first, but later, it may occur even during rest. Some people can breathe comfortably only when they are propped up with pillows or sitting upright. Those people with a low level of oxygen in the blood and high blood pressure in the lungs may have a plum-colored flush in the cheeks (called mitral facies). People may cough up blood (hemoptysis) if the high pressure causes a vein or capillaries in the lungs to burst. The resulting bleeding into the lungs is usually slight, but if hemoptysis occurs, the person should be evaluated by a doctor promptly because hemoptysis indicates severe mitral stenosis or another serious problem.

With a stethoscope, doctors may hear the characteristic heart murmur as blood tries to pass through the narrowed valve opening from the left atrium into the left ventricle. Unlike a normal valve, which opens silently, the abnormal valve often makes a snapping sound as it opens to allow blood into the left ventricle. The diagnosis is usually confirmed by electrocardiography (ECG), a chest x-ray showing an enlarged atrium, and echocardiography, which uses ultrasound waves to produce an image of the narrowed valve and the blood passing through it.

Prevention and Treatment

Mitral stenosis will not occur if rheumatic fever is prevented by promptly treating strep throat with antibiotics.

Treatment includes use of diuretics and beta-blockers or calcium channel blockers. Diuretics, which increase urine formation, can reduce blood pressure in the lungs by reducing the volume of circulating blood. Beta-blockers, digoxin, and calcium channel blockers help control heart rhythms. Anticoagulants may be needed to prevent clot formation in people with atrial fibrillation.

If drug therapy does not reduce the symptoms satisfactorily, the valve may be repaired or replaced. Sometimes the valve can be stretched open using a procedure called balloon valvuloplasty. In this procedure, a balloon-tipped catheter is threaded through a vein and eventually into the heart (see page 330). Once inside the valve, the balloon is inflated, separating the valve cusps. Alternatively, heart surgery may be performed to separate the fused cusps. If the valve is too badly damaged, it may be surgically replaced with an artificial valve.

People with mitral stenosis are given antibiotics before a surgical, dental, or medical procedure (see box on page 388) to reduce the small risk of developing a heart valve infection (infective endocarditis).

Aortic Regurgitation

Aortic regurgitation (aortic incompetence, aortic insufficiency) is leakage of blood back through the aortic valve each time the left ventricle relaxes.

- Rheumatic fever and syphilis are the most common causes.
- Aortic regurgitation causes no symptoms unless heart failure develops.
- Doctors suspect the diagnosis because of physical examination findings, and they use echocardiography to confirm the diagnosis.
- The damaged heart valve must be replaced surgically.

As the left ventricle relaxes to fill with blood from the left atrium, blood leaks backward from the aorta into the left ventricle, increasing the volume and pressure of blood in the left ventricle. As a result, the amount of work the heart has to do increases. To compensate, the muscular walls of the ventricles thicken (hypertrophy), and the chambers of the ventricles enlarge (dilate). Eventually, despite this compensation, the heart may be unable to meet the body's need for blood, leading to heart failure, with fluid accumulation in the lungs.

Cause

Rheumatic fever and syphilis used to be the most common causes of aortic regurgitation in North America, Australasia, and Western Europe, where both disorders are now rare because of the widespread use of antibiotics. In regions where antibiotics are not widely used, aortic regurgitation due to rheumatic fever or syphilis is still common. Aside from these infections, the most common causes of severe aortic regurgitation are weakening of the valve's usually tough, fibrous tissue due to myxomatous degeneration (a hereditary connective tissue disorder in which the valve gradually becomes floppy); degeneration of the valve due to unknown factors; aortic aneurysms; and aortic dissection. Common causes of mild aortic regurgitation are severe high blood pressure and a birth defect in which the aortic valve consists of two cusps (bicuspid valve) instead of the usual three (tricuspid valve). About 2% of boys and 1% of girls are born with this defect. Other causes of aortic regurgitation include bacterial infection of the valve (infective endocarditis) and injury.

Symptoms and Diagnosis

Mild aortic regurgitation produces no symptoms other than a characteristic heart murmur that can be heard with a stethoscope each time the left ventricle relaxes. People with severe regurgitation may develop symptoms when heart failure results. Heart failure causes shortness of breath during exertion. Lying flat, especially at night, makes breathing difficult. Sitting up allows backed-up fluid to drain out of the upper part of the lungs, restoring normal breathing. About 5% of people with aortic regurgitation have chest pain due to an inadequate blood supply to the heart muscle (angina), especially at night.

The pulse, sometimes called a collapsing pulse, is momentarily strong, then disappears quickly because the blood leaks backward through the aortic valve, causing blood pressure to decrease sharply.

Doctors usually suspect the diagnosis based on the results of a physical examination (such as the collapsing pulse and characteristic heart murmur) and an enlarged heart seen on an x-ray. Electrocardiography (ECG) may show signs of an enlarged left ventricle. Echocardiography can show the faulty valve and help doctors determine how severe regurgitation is and whether heart valve replacement surgery is needed. Coronary angiography is performed in older people before surgery because about 20% of people with aortic regurgitation also have coronary artery disease.

Treatment

Unless aortic regurgitation is mild, surgery is ultimately almost always required. Drug treatment is not especially effective in slowing the progression of heart failure and does not eliminate the need for timely valve replacement, but various drugs may be used to control symptoms prior to surgery. The damaged valve should be surgically replaced with an artificial valve before the left ventricle becomes irreversibly damaged and heart failure becomes too severe. Usually, echocardiography is performed periodically to determine how rapidly the left ventricle is enlarging, so that surgery can be scheduled at an appropriate time.

People with aortic regurgitation, even when mild, are given antibiotics before surgical, dental, or medical procedures (see box on page 388) to reduce the risk of infection of the damaged heart valve.

Aortic Stenosis

Aortic stenosis is a narrowing of the aortic valve opening that increases resistance to blood flow from the left ventricle to the aorta.

- The most common cause in people younger than 70 is a congenital abnormality of the valve. In people over 70, the most common cause is aortic sclerosis.
- People may have chest pain or feel short of breath or faint.
- Doctors usually base the diagnosis on a characteristic heart murmur heard through a stethoscope, on pulse abnormalities, and on results of echocardiography.
- People see their doctors regularly so their condition can be monitored, and people with symptoms may undergo surgical replacement of the valve.

In aortic stenosis, the wall of the left ventricle usually thickens because the ventricle must work harder to pump blood through the narrowed valve opening into the aorta. The thickened heart muscle requires an increasing supply of blood from the coronary arteries, and sometimes, especially during exercise, the blood supply does not meet the needs of the heart muscle, and chest pain, fainting, and sometimes sudden death may occur. The heart muscle may also begin to weaken, leading to heart failure. The abnormal aortic valve can rarely become infected by bacteria (infective endocarditis).

Cause

In North America, Australasia, and Western Europe, aortic stenosis is mainly a disease of older people—the result of scarring and calcium accumulation (calcification) in the valve cusps. In such cases, aortic stenosis begins after age 60 but does not usually produce symptoms until age 70 or 80. Aortic stenosis may also result from rheumatic fever contracted in childhood. When rheumatic fever is the cause, aortic stenosis is usually accompanied by mitral stenosis, leakage (regurgitation), or both.

In younger people, the most common cause is a birth defect, such as a valve with only two cusps instead of the usual three or a valve with an abnormal funnel shape (see page 1715). The narrowed aortic valve opening may not be a problem in infancy, but problems occur as a person grows. The valve opening remains the same size, but the heart grows and enlarges further as it tries to pump increasing amounts of blood through the small valve opening. Over the years, the opening of a defective valve often becomes stiff and narrow because calcium accumulates.

Symptoms and Diagnosis

Chest pain (angina) may occur during exertion. This pain goes away with several minutes of rest. People with heart failure develop fatigue and shortness of breath during exertion.

People who have severe aortic stenosis may faint during exertion because blood pressure may fall suddenly. Fainting usually occurs without any warning symptoms (such as dizziness or light-headedness) or with any symptoms after awakening.

Doctors usually base the diagnosis on a characteristic heart murmur heard through a stethoscope, on pulse abnormalities, and on results of electrocardiography (ECG) indicating thickening of the heart wall. For people who experience angina, shortness of breath, or faintness, echocardiography (see page 328) is the best procedure for assessing the severity of aortic stenosis (by measuring how small the valve opening is) and the function of the left ventricle.

SPOTLIGHT ON AGING

Sometimes calcium accumulates on the aortic valve, and the valve thickens. But the thickening does not interfere with blood flow through the valve. This disorder is called aortic sclerosis. About 1 out of 4 people over 65 have this disorder.

Aortic sclerosis does not cause symptoms. It may cause a soft heart murmur, heard by a doctor through a stethoscope. Aortic sclerosis may not make a person feel any different, but it increases the risk of a heart attack and death. Consequently, identifying and eliminating or controlling risk factors for coronary artery disease are important for people with aortic sclerosis. These risk factors include smoking, high blood pressure, abnormal cholesterol and triglyceride levels, and diabetes.

Cardiac catheterization (see page 330) is usually necessary as the doctor is not sure whether the person also has coronary artery disease.

Treatment

Adults who have aortic stenosis but no symptoms should see their doctor regularly and should avoid overly stressful exercise. Echocardiography is performed periodically to monitor heart and valve function.

In adults who have aortic stenosis that causes shortness of breath on exertion, angina, or fainting, the aortic valve is surgically replaced, preferably before the left ventricle is irreversibly damaged. Echocardiography, usually performed periodically, can help doctors determine when to schedule surgery. Surgical replacement of the abnormal valve is the best treatment for adults of all ages, and the prognosis after valve replacement is excellent.

Before surgery, heart failure is treated with diuretics (see page 359). Treating angina is often difficult, because nitroglycerin, which is used to treat angina in people who have coronary artery disease, can rarely cause dangerously low blood pressure and worsen the angina in people with aortic stenosis.

People with an artificial valve must take antibiotics before a surgical, dental, or medical procedure (see box on page 388) to reduce the risk of an infection on the valve (infective endocarditis).

For children who have severe stenosis, surgery may be performed even before symptoms develop, because sudden death may occur before symptoms develop. Safe, effective alternatives to valve replacement are surgical repair of the valve and balloon valvuloplasty.

In balloon valvuloplasty, a balloon-tipped catheter is threaded through a vein and eventually into the heart (see page 330). Once inside the valve, the balloon is inflated to expand the valve opening. However, later, when children are fully grown, the valve usually must be replaced. In adults, stenosis always recurs after balloon valvuloplasty; so among adults, this procedure is used only for frail older people who cannot tolerate surgery.

Tricuspid Regurgitation

Tricuspid regurgitation (tricuspid incompetence, tricuspid insufficiency) is leakage of blood backward through the tricuspid valve each time the right ventricle contracts.

- Tricuspid regurgitation is caused by disorders that enlarge the right ventricle.
- Symptoms are vague, such as weakness and fatigue.
- Doctors suspect the diagnosis because of physical examination findings, and they use echocardiography to confirm the diagnosis.
- The underlying disorder needs to be treated.

As the right ventricle contracts to pump blood forward to the lungs, some blood leaks backward into the right atrium, increasing the volume of blood there and resulting in less blood being pumped through the heart and to the body. As a result, the right atrium enlarges, and blood pressure increases in the right atrium and the large veins that enter it from the body. The liver may swell because of this increased pressure. Enlargement of the right atrium also can result in atrial fibrillation, a rapid, irregular heartbeat. Eventually, heart failure develops.

Cause

Tricuspid regurgitation usually results when the right ventricle enlarges and resistance to blood flow from the right ventricle to the lungs is increased. Resistance may be increased by a severe, long-standing lung disorder, such as emphysema or pulmonary hypertension, by disorders involving the left side of the heart, or rarely by narrowing of the pulmonary valve (pulmonic stenosis). To compensate, the right ventricle enlarges, stretching the tricuspid valve and causing regurgitation.

Other, less common causes are infection of the heart valves (infective endocarditis most often due to intravenous injection of illicit drugs), use of fenfluramine (no longer available), birth defects of the tricuspid valve, injury, and myxomatous degeneration (a hereditary disorder in which the valve gradually becomes floppy).

Symptoms and Diagnosis

Tricuspid regurgitation can cause vague symptoms, such as weakness and fatigue. They develop because the heart is pumping a smaller amount of blood. Usually, the only other symptoms are pulsations in the neck from the elevated right atrial pressure and discomfort in the right upper part of the abdomen due to an enlarged liver. Heart failure results in accumulation of fluid in the body, mainly in the legs.

The diagnosis is based on the person's medical history and results of a physical examination, electrocardiography (ECG), and chest x-ray. Through a stethoscope, doctors may hear a characteristic murmur produced by the blood leaking backward through the tricuspid valve, but the murmur tends to disappear as the regurgitation worsens. Echocardiography (see page 328) can produce an image of the leaky valve and the amount of blood leaking, so that the severity of the regurgitation can be determined.

Treatment

Usually, mild tricuspid regurgitation requires little or no treatment. However, the underlying disorder, such as emphysema, pulmonary hypertension, pulmonic stenosis, or abnormalities of the left side of the heart, is likely to require treatment. Treatment of atrial fibrillation and heart failure is also necessary, but surgery to repair the tricuspid valve is rarely done unless surgery on another heart valve (for example, mitral valve replacement) is also needed.

Tricuspid Stenosis

Tricuspid stenosis is a narrowing of the tricuspid valve opening that increases resistance to blood flow from the right atrium to the right ventricle.

Over many years, the right atrium enlarges because blood flow through the narrowed valve opening is partially blocked, increasing the volume of blood in the atrium. In turn, this increased volume causes an increase in pressure in the veins bringing blood back to the heart from the body (except the lungs). However, the right ventricle shrinks, because the amount of blood entering it from the right atrium is reduced. Tricuspid regurgitation rarely occurs.

Nearly all cases are caused by rheumatic fever, which has become rare in North America, Australasia, and Western Europe. Rarely, the cause is a tumor in the right atrium, a connective tissue disorder, or, even more rarely, a birth defect of the heart.

Symptoms are usually mild. They include palpitations (awareness of heartbeats), a fluttering discomfort in the neck, cold skin, and fatigue. Abdominal discomfort may result if the increased pressure in the veins causes the liver to enlarge.

Through a stethoscope, doctors may hear the characteristic murmur of tricuspid stenosis. A chest x-ray shows that the right atrium is enlarged.

Echocardiography (see page 328) can produce an image of the narrowed valve opening and show the amount of blood passing through the valve, so that the severity of the stenosis can be determined. Electrocardiography (ECG—see page 326) shows changes indicating that the right atrium is strained.

Tricuspid stenosis is rarely severe enough to require surgical repair.

Pulmonic Stenosis

Pulmonic (pulmonary) stenosis is a narrowing of the pulmonary valve opening that increases resistance to blood flow from the right ventricle to the pulmonary artery. It is often present at birth (congenital) and thus affects children.

Pulmonic stenosis, which is rare among adults, is usually due to a birth defect (see page 1716). When the stenosis is severe, it is usually diagnosed during childhood, because it produces a loud heart murmur. Severe pulmonic stenosis occasionally causes heart failure in children but often does not produce symptoms until adulthood. Symptoms include chest pain (angina), shortness of breath, and fainting.

Young children with this disorder often require heart surgery. In adults and older children, balloon valvuloplasty may be done. In this procedure, the valve is stretched open using a balloon-tipped catheter threaded through a vein and eventually into the heart. Once inside the valve, the balloon is inflated, separating the valve cusps.

CHAPTER

61 Infective Endocarditis

Infective endocarditis is an infection of the lining of the heart (endocardium) and usually also of the heart valves.

- Infective endocarditis occurs when bacteria enter the bloodstream and travel to previously injured heart valves.
- Acute bacterial endocarditis usually begins suddenly with a high fever, fast heart rate, fatigue, and rapid and extensive heart valve damage.
- Subacute bacterial endocarditis causes such symptoms as fatigue, mild fever, a moderately fast heart rate, weight loss, sweating, and a low red blood cell count.
- Echocardiography is used to detect the damaged heart valves.
- People with heart valve problems or artificial valves need to take antibiotics before they undergo dental or surgical procedures to prevent endocarditis.
- High doses of antibiotics are given intravenously, but sometimes surgery is needed to repair damaged heart valves.

Infective endocarditis affects twice as many men as women of all ages but 8 times as many older men as older women. It has become more common among older people: More than one fourth of all cases occur in people older than 60.

Infective endocarditis refers specifically to infection of the lining of the heart, but the infection usually also affects the heart valves, muscles of the heart, and any birth defects that involve abnormal connections between the chambers of the heart or its blood vessels. There are two forms of infective endocarditis. One form, called acute infective endocarditis, develops suddenly and may become life threatening within days. The other form, called subacute infective endocarditis or subacute bacterial endocarditis, develops gradually and subtly over a period of weeks to several months.

Bacteria (or, less often, fungi) may be introduced into the bloodstream. These organisms can then lodge on heart valves and infect the endocardium. Abnormal, damaged, or artificial valves are more susceptible to infection than normal valves. The bacteria that cause subacute bacterial endocarditis nearly always infect abnormal, damaged, or artificial valves. However, normal valves can be infected by some aggressive bacteria, especially if many bacteria are present.

Risk factors for children and young adults include birth defects, particularly a defect that allows blood to leak from one part of the heart to another. One risk factor for older people is degeneration of the valves or calcium deposits in the mitral valve (which opens from the left atrium into the left ventricle) or in the aortic valve (which opens from the left ventricle into the aorta). Damage to the heart by rheumatic fever during childhood (rheumatic heart disease—see page 1765) is also a risk factor. Rheumatic fever has become a less common risk factor in countries where antibiotics have become widely available. In such countries, rheumatic fever is a risk factor for people who did not have the benefit of antibiotics during their childhood (such as immigrants).

An Inside View of Infective Endocarditis

This cross-sectional view shows vegetations (accumulations of bacteria and blood clots) on the four valves of the heart.

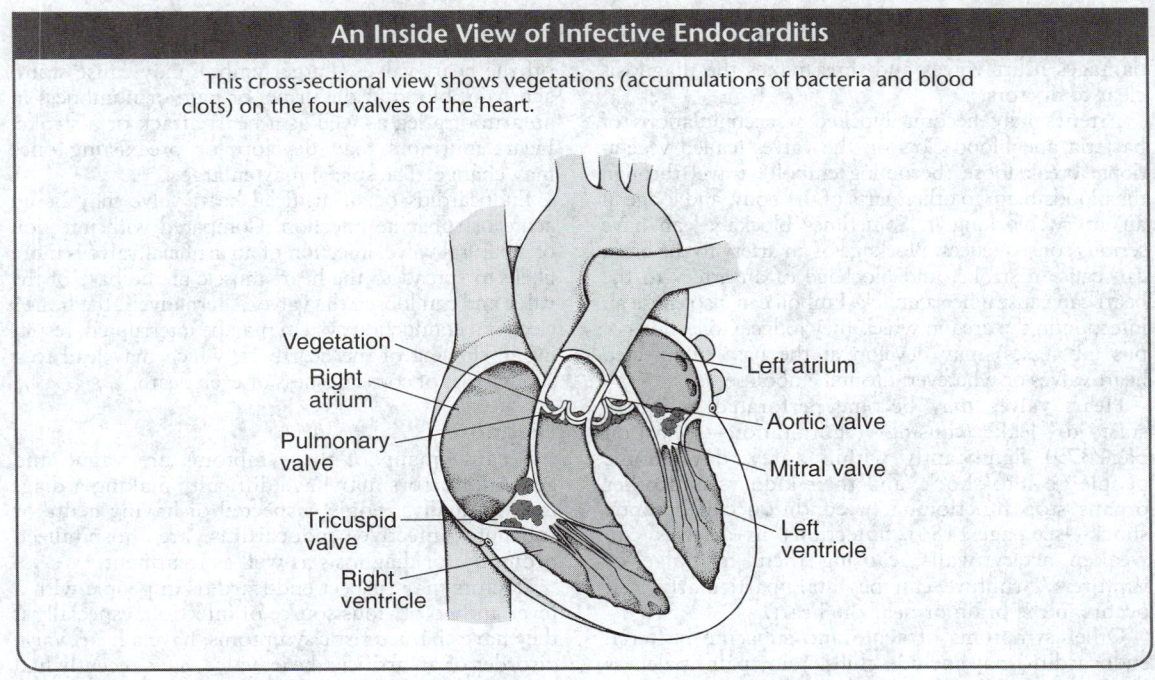

Vegetation

Right atrium

Pulmonary valve

Tricuspid valve

Right ventricle

Left atrium

Aortic valve

Mitral valve

Left ventricle

People who inject illicit drugs are at high risk of endocarditis because they are likely to inject bacteria directly into their bloodstream through dirty needles, syringes, or drug solutions. People who have an artificial (prosthetic) heart valve are also at high risk. For them, the risk of infective endocarditis is greatest during the first year after heart valve surgery; after that, the risk decreases but remains slightly higher than normal. For unknown reasons, the risk is always greater with an artificial aortic valve than with an artificial mitral valve and with a mechanical valve rather than with a valve made from an animal.

Causes

Although bacteria are not normally found in the blood, an injury to the skin, lining of the mouth, or gums (even an injury from a normal activity such as chewing or brushing the teeth) can allow a small number of bacteria to enter the bloodstream. Gingivitis (inflammation of the gums) with infection, minor skin infections, and infections elsewhere in the body may introduce bacteria into the bloodstream.

Certain surgical, dental, and medical procedures may also introduce bacteria into the bloodstream. Rarely, bacteria are introduced into the heart during open-heart surgery or heart valve replacement sur-gery. In people with normal heart valves, usually no harm is done, and the body's white blood cells and immune responses rapidly destroy these bacteria. However, damaged heart valves may trap the bacteria, which can then lodge on the endocardium and start to multiply. Sepsis (see page 1186), a severe blood infection, introduces a large number of bacteria into the bloodstream. When the number of bacteria in the bloodstream is large enough, endocarditis can develop, even in people who have normal heart valves.

If the cause of infective endocarditis is injection of illicit drugs or prolonged use of intravenous lines, the tricuspid valve (which opens from the right atrium into the right ventricle) is most often infected. In most other cases of endocarditis, the mitral valve or the aortic valve is infected.

Symptoms

Acute bacterial endocarditis usually begins suddenly with a high fever (102° to 104°F [38.9° to 40°C]), fast heart rate, fatigue, and rapid and extensive heart valve damage.

Subacute bacterial endocarditis may produce such symptoms as fatigue, mild fever (99° to 101° F [37.2° to 38.3°C]), a moderately fast heart rate, weight loss, sweating, and a low red blood cell count (anemia).

These symptoms may occur for months before the endocarditis results in blockage of an artery or damages heart valves and thus makes the diagnosis clear to doctors.

Arteries may become blocked if accumulations of bacteria and blood clots on the valves (called vegetations) break loose (becoming emboli), travel through the bloodstream to other parts of the body, and lodge in an artery, blocking it. Sometimes blockage can have serious consequences. Blockage of an artery to the brain can cause a stroke, and blockage of an artery to the heart can cause a heart attack. Emboli can also cause an infection in the area in which they lodge. Collections of pus (abscesses) may develop at the base of infected heart valves or wherever infected emboli settle.

Heart valves may become perforated and may start to leak (causing regurgitation—see art on page 379) significantly within a few days. Some people go into shock, and their kidneys and other organs stop functioning (a condition called septic shock—see page 1186). Infections in arteries can weaken artery walls, causing them to bulge or rupture. A rupture can be fatal, particularly if it occurs in the brain or near the heart.

Other symptoms of acute and subacute bacterial endocarditis may include chills, joint pain, paleness (pallor), painful nodules under the skin, and confusion. Tiny reddish spots that resemble freckles may appear on the skin and in the whites of the eyes. Small streaks of red (called splinter hemorrhages) may appear under the fingernails. These spots and streaks are caused by tiny emboli that have broken off the heart valves. Larger emboli may cause stomach pain, blood in the urine, or pain or numbness in an arm or a leg as well as a heart attack or a stroke. Heart murmurs may develop, or preexisting ones may change. The spleen may enlarge.

Endocarditis of an artificial heart valve may be an acute or subacute infection. Compared with infection of a natural valve, infection of an artificial valve is more likely to spread to the heart muscle at the base of the valve and can loosen the valve. Alternatively, the heart's electrical conduction system may be interrupted, resulting in slowing of the heartbeat, which may lead to a sudden loss of consciousness or even death.

Diagnosis

Because many of the symptoms are vague and general, doctors may have difficulty making a diagnosis. Usually, people suspected of having acute or subacute infective endocarditis are hospitalized promptly for diagnosis as well as treatment.

Doctors may suspect endocarditis in people with a fever and no obvious source of infection, especially if they have characteristic symptoms; have a heart valve disorder or an artificial heart valve; have recently had certain surgical, dental, or medical procedures; or inject illicit drugs. Development of a heart murmur or a change in a preexisting heart murmur further supports the diagnosis.

WHICH PROCEDURES REQUIRE PREVENTIVE ANTIBIOTICS?*

SURGICAL PROCEDURES	DENTAL PROCEDURES	MEDICAL PROCEDURES
Heart valve replacement	Tooth extraction	Use of catheters or intravenous lines to provide fluids, nutrition, or drugs
Open-heart surgery	Periodontal procedures such as gum surgery, scaling, root planing, and probing	Bronchoscopy
Removal of tonsils or adenoids		
Lung surgery	Placement of dental implants	Cystoscopy
Surgery on the intestines or bile ducts	Replacement of a tooth that was knocked out	Dilation of the esophagus
Prostate surgery	Root canal surgery beyond the end of the root	Dilation of the urethra
	Placement of orthodontic bands beneath the gums	Endoscopic retrograde cholangiopancreatography (endoscopy, with injection of a dye that can be seen on x-rays, to remove gallstones in the bile duct)
	Injection of an anesthetic into a ligament	Sclerotherapy for varicose veins in the esophagus
	Cleanings if bleeding is expected to result	

*As a preventive measure before certain procedures, antibiotics are given to people at risk of developing infective endocarditis.

To help make the diagnosis, doctors usually perform echocardiography and obtain blood samples to test for the presence of bacteria. Usually, three or more blood samples are taken at different times on the same day. These blood tests (blood cultures) may identify the specific disease-causing bacteria and the best antibiotics to use against them. In people with heart abnormalities, doctors test their blood for bacteria before giving them antibiotics.

Echocardiography, which uses ultrasound waves (see page 328), can produce images showing heart valve vegetations and damage to the heart. Typically, transthoracic echocardiography (a procedure in which the ultrasound probe is placed on the chest) is done. If this procedure doesn't provide enough information, the person may undergo transesophageal echocardiography (a procedure in which the ultrasound probe is passed down the throat into the esophagus just behind the heart). Transesophageal echocardiography is more accurate and detects smaller bacterial deposits, but it is invasive and more costly.

Sometimes bacteria cannot be cultured from blood samples. Special techniques may be needed to grow the particular bacteria, or the person may have taken antibiotics that did not cure the infection but did reduce the number of bacteria enough to be undetectable. Another possible explanation is that the person does not have endocarditis but has a disorder, such as a heart tumor (see page 393), that produces symptoms very similar to those of endocarditis.

Prognosis

If untreated, infective endocarditis is always fatal. When treatment is given, the risk of death depends on factors such as the person's age, duration of the infection, the presence of an artificial heart valve, and the type of infecting organism. Nonetheless, with aggressive antibiotic treatment, most people survive.

Prevention

As a preventive measure, people with heart valve abnormalities, artificial valves, or congenital heart defects are given antibiotics before certain surgical, dental, and medical procedures. Consequently, surgeons, dentists, and other health care practitioners need to know if a person has had a heart valve disorder. Although the risk of endocarditis is not very high for these procedures and preventive antibiotics are not always effective, the consequences of endocarditis are so severe that most doctors believe that giving antibiotics before these procedures is a reasonable precaution.

Treatment

Treatment usually consists of at least 2 weeks and often up to 8 weeks of antibiotics given intrave-

---

Endocarditis Without Infection

Another form of endocarditis is noninfective endocarditis. It develops when blood clots form on damaged heart valves. Damage may be due to a birth defect, rheumatic fever, or an autoimmune disorder (in which antibodies attack the heart valves). Rarely, damage results from insertion of a catheter into the heart. People most at risk include those with the following:

- Systemic lupus erythematosus (an autoimmune disorder)
- Antiphospholipid syndrome (a disorder of excessive blood clots)
- Lung, stomach, or pancreatic cancer
- Tuberculosis
- Pneumonia
- Sepsis (a severe blood infection)
- Uremia (the buildup of wastes in the blood)
- Burns

Noninfective endocarditis, like infective endocarditis, may cause heart valves to leak or not open normally. The risk of a blood clot breaking off (becoming an embolus) and causing a stroke or heart attack is high.

Distinguishing between noninfective and infective endocarditis is difficult but important because treatment differs. Noninfective endocarditis may be diagnosed when echocardiography detects vegetations on heart valves, but no bacteria are detected in blood samples. Anticoagulants may be used to prevent clotting, but their benefits have not been confirmed. Prognosis is generally poor, more because of the seriousness of the underlying disorder than because of the heart problem.

---

nously in high doses. Antibiotic therapy is almost always started in the hospital but may be finished at home with the help of a home nurse.

Antibiotics alone do not always cure an infection, particularly if the valve is artificial. One reason is that the bacteria that cause endocarditis in a person with an artificial valve are often resistant to antibiotics. Because antibiotics are given before heart valve replacement surgery to prevent infection, any bacteria that survive this treatment to cause infection are probably resistant. Another reason is that it is generally harder to cure infection on artificial, implanted material than in human tissue.

Heart surgery may be needed to repair or replace damaged valves, remove vegetations, or drain abscesses if antibiotics do not work, a valve leaks significantly, or a birth defect connects one chamber to another. Heart failure from significant valvular leaks can be fatal.

CHAPTER

62 Pericardial Disease

Pericardial disease affects the pericardium, which is the flexible two-layered sac that envelops the heart.

The pericardium helps keep the heart in position, prevent the heart from overfilling with blood, and protect the heart from being damaged by chest infections. However, the pericardium is not essential to life; if the pericardium is removed, there is little measurable effect on the heart's performance.

Normally, the pericardium contains just enough lubricating fluid between its two layers for them to slide easily over one another. There is very little space between the two layers. However, in some disorders, extra fluid accumulates in this space (called the pericardial space), causing it to expand.

Rarely, the pericardium is missing at birth or has defects, such as weak spots or holes. These defects can be dangerous because the heart or a major blood vessel may bulge (herniate) through a hole in the pericardium and become trapped. In such cases, death can occur in minutes. Therefore, these defects are usually surgically repaired; if repair is not feasible, the whole pericardium may be removed. Other diseases of the pericardium may result from infections, injuries, or spread of cancer.

Acute Pericarditis

Acute pericarditis is inflammation of the pericardium that begins suddenly, is often painful, and causes fluid and blood components such as fibrin, red blood cells, and white blood cells to pour into the pericardial space.

- Infection and other conditions that can irritate the pericardium cause pericarditis.
- Fever and chest pain, which may feel like a heart attack, are common symptoms.
- Diagnosis is based on symptoms and by hearing a telltale sound when listening to the heartbeat with a stethoscope.
- People are hospitalized and given drugs to reduce pain and inflammation.

Acute pericarditis usually results from infection or other conditions that irritate the pericardium. Infection is usually due to a virus but may be caused by bacteria, parasites (including protozoa), or fungi.

In some inner city hospitals, AIDS is the most common cause of pericarditis with extra fluid in the pericardial space (pericardial effusion). In people who have AIDS, a number of infections, including tuberculosis, may result in pericarditis. Pericarditis due to tuberculosis (tuberculous pericarditis) accounts

for less than 5% of cases of acute pericarditis in the United States but accounts for the majority of cases in some areas of India and Africa.

Other conditions can irritate the pericardium and thus can cause acute pericarditis. These conditions include a heart attack, heart surgery, systemic lupus erythematosus, rheumatoid arthritis, kidney failure, injury, cancer (such as leukemia and, in people with AIDS, Kaposi's sarcoma), rheumatic fever, an underactive thyroid gland (hypothyroidism), radiation therapy, and leakage of blood from an aortic aneurysm (a bulge in the wall of the aorta). After a heart attack, acute pericarditis develops during the first day or two in 10 to 15% of people and after about 10 days to 2 months in 1 to 3%. Acute pericarditis may occur as a side effect of certain drugs, including anticoagulants (such as warfarin and heparin), penicillin, procainamide (an antiarrhythmic drug), phenytoin (an anticonvulsant), and phenylbutazone (a nonsteroidal anti-inflammatory drug).

Symptoms

Usually, acute pericarditis causes fever and chest pain, which typically extends to the left shoulder and sometimes down the left arm. The pain may be similar to that of a heart attack, except that it tends to be made worse by lying down, swallowing food, coughing, or even deep breathing. The accumulating fluid or blood in the pericardial space puts pressure on the heart, interfering with its ability to pump blood. If the pressure is too high, cardiac tamponade—a potentially fatal condition—may occur.

Acute pericarditis due to tuberculosis begins insidiously, sometimes without obvious symptoms of lung infection. It may produce fever and symptoms of heart failure, such as weakness, fatigue, and difficulty breathing. Cardiac tamponade may occur.

Acute pericarditis due to a viral infection is usually painful but short-lived and has no lasting effects.

When acute pericarditis develops in the first day or two after a heart attack, symptoms of pericarditis are seldom noticed, because symptoms of the heart attack are the main concern (see page 411). Pericarditis that develops about 10 days to 2 months after a heart attack is usually accompanied by Dressler's syndrome (post-myocardial infarction syndrome), which includes fever, pericardial effusion (extra fluid in the pericardial space), pleurisy (inflammation of the pleura, which are the membranes covering the lungs), pleural effusion (fluid between the two layers of the pleura), and joint pain.

Cardiac Tamponade: The Most Serious Complication of Pericarditis

Cardiac tamponade is caused by accumulation of fluid or blood between the two layers of the pericardium. The accumulating fluid or blood puts pressure on the heart, interfering with its ability to pump blood. As a result, when a person breathes in, blood pressure may fall rapidly to abnormally low levels and the pulse may correspondingly weaken. When a person breathes out, blood pressure increases and the pulse becomes stronger. This exaggeration in the variation in blood pressure and pulse that occurs with breathing is called a paradoxical pulse. Later, as the heart is compressed more, the blood pressure remains low, and the person may pass out or die.

The most common causes of such significant fluid accumulation are cancer, heart injury, or heart surgery. Viral and bacterial pericardial infections and kidney failure are other common causes.

Echocardiography (which uses ultrasound waves to produce an image of the heart) may be used to confirm the diagnosis. This procedure can detect characteristic changes, such as compression of the heart and the variations in blood flow in the heart that occur with breathing.

Cardiac tamponade is usually a medical emergency. Doctors treat it immediately by removing fluid from the pericardium using a needle or catheter inserted through the chest wall to relieve the pressure in a procedure called pericardiocentesis. When time permits, fluid removal is closely monitored using echocardiography. Fluid may be surgically drained using a balloon-tipped catheter inserted through the skin (a procedure called percutaneous balloon pericardiotomy) or using a tube inserted through a small incision in the chest (a procedure called subxiphoid limited pericardiotomy). If the cause of pericarditis is unknown, doctors may send a sample of the fluid or a piece of tissue removed from the pericardium for examination under a microscope. This examination may provide information that helps identify the cause.

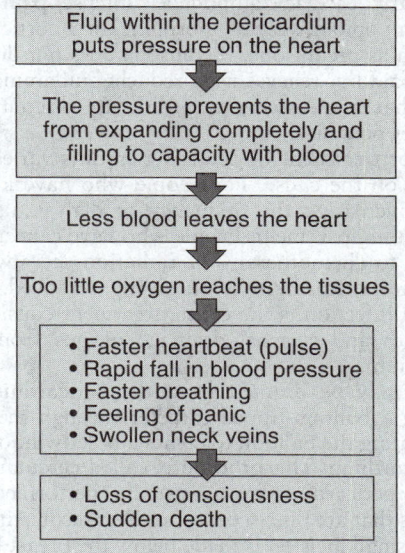

Fluid within the pericardium puts pressure on the heart

↓

The pressure prevents the heart from expanding completely and filling to capacity with blood

↓

Less blood leaves the heart

↓

Too little oxygen reaches the tissues

↓

- Faster heartbeat (pulse)
- Rapid fall in blood pressure
- Faster breathing
- Feeling of panic
- Swollen neck veins

↓

- Loss of consciousness
- Sudden death

After the pressure is relieved, the person is usually kept in the hospital in case cardiac tamponade recurs. The person is usually monitored for 24 hours. The length of the hospital stay depends on the cause of tamponade. If a drain is in place, the person stays in the hospital until no more drainage occurs and the drain is removed.

If cardiac tamponade recurs, the same procedures may be performed again, or a different procedure may be tried. Other procedures include injection of a solution that obliterates the pericardium by causing scar tissue to form (sclerotherapy) and removal of the pericardium (pericardiectomy).

Diagnosis

Doctors can diagnose acute pericarditis based on the person's description of the pain and the sounds heard by listening through a stethoscope placed on the person's chest. Pericarditis can produce a crunching sound similar to the creaking of a leather shoe or a scratchy sound similar to the rustling of dry leaves (pericardial rub). Doctors can often diagnose pericarditis a few hours to a few days after a heart attack based on hearing these sounds.

A chest x-ray and echocardiography (a procedure that uses ultrasound waves to produce an image of the heart—see page 328) may be useful because they can usually detect too much fluid in the pericardial space. Echocardiography may suggest the cause—for example, cancer. Electrocardiography (ECG) may be performed. ECG results may suggest pericarditis, but distinguishing pericarditis from a heart attack based on ECG results may be difficult. Blood tests can detect some of the conditions that cause pericarditis—for example, leukemia, AIDS, other infections, rheumatic fever, and increased levels of urea in the blood resulting from kidney failure.

Treatment and Prognosis

Regardless of the cause, doctors usually hospitalize people with pericarditis, give them drugs that reduce inflammation and pain (such as aspirin, ibuprofen, or another nonsteroidal anti-inflammatory drug—see page 644), and watch for complications, particularly cardiac tamponade. Intense pain may require an opioid, such as morphine, or a corticosteroid, such as prednisone. Prednisone does not directly reduce pain but relieves it by reducing inflammation. Drugs that may cause pericarditis are discontinued whenever possible.

Further treatment of acute pericarditis varies, depending on the cause. For people who have kidney failure, increasing the frequency of dialysis usually results in improvement. People who have cancer may respond to chemotherapy or radiation therapy, but often the pericardium is surgically removed. If a bacterial infection is the cause, treatment consists of antibiotics and surgical drainage of pus from the pericardium.

Fluid may be drained from the pericardium by inserting a balloon-tipped catheter through the skin and inflating the balloon to create a hole (window) in the pericardium. This procedure, called percutaneous balloon pericardiotomy, is usually performed for effusions that are due to cancer or that recur. Alternatively, a small incision is made below the breast bone, and a piece of the pericardium is removed. Then a tube is inserted into the pericardial space. This procedure, called a subxiphoid pericardiotomy, is often performed for effusions due to bacterial infections. Both procedures require a local anesthetic, can be performed at the bedside, allow fluid to drain continuously, and are effective.

If pericarditis resulting from a virus, an injury, or an unidentified disorder recurs, aspirin, ibuprofen, or corticosteroids may provide relief. For some people, colchicine is effective. If drug treatment is ineffective, the pericardium is usually removed surgically.

When acute pericarditis occurs within the first few hours or days after a heart attack, treatment for the heart attack, including aspirin and stronger analgesics such as morphine, can usually reduce any discomfort due to pericarditis.

The prognosis for people who have pericarditis depends on the cause. When pericarditis is caused by a virus or when the cause is not apparent, recovery usually takes 1 to 3 weeks. Complications or recurrences can slow recovery. People with cancer that has invaded the pericardium rarely survive beyond 12 to 18 months.

Chronic Pericarditis

Chronic pericarditis is inflammation that begins gradually, is long-lasting, and results in fluid accumulation in the pericardial space or thickening of the pericardium.

- Symptoms include shortness of breath, coughing, and fatigue.

- Echocardiography is used to make the diagnosis.
- The cause, if known, is treated, or rest, salt restriction, and diuretics may be used to relieve symptoms.
- Sometimes surgery to remove the pericardium is needed.

There are two main types of chronic pericarditis. In **chronic effusive pericarditis**, fluid slowly accumulates in the pericardial space, between the two layers of the pericardium.

Chronic constrictive pericarditis is a rare disease that usually results when scarlike (fibrous) tissue forms throughout the pericardium. The fibrous tissue tends to contract over the years, compressing the heart. Thus, the heart does not enlarge as it does in most types of heart disease. Because higher pressure is needed to fill the compressed heart, pressure in the veins that return blood to the heart increases. Fluid accumulates in the veins, then leaks out, and accumulates in other areas of the body, such as under the skin.

Causes

Usually, the cause of chronic effusive pericarditis is unknown, but it may be cancer, tuberculosis, or an underactive thyroid gland (hypothyroidism).

Usually, the cause of chronic constrictive pericarditis is also unknown. The most common known causes are viral infections and radiation therapy for breast cancer or lymphoma. Chronic constrictive pericarditis may also result from any condition that causes acute pericarditis, such as rheumatoid arthritis, systemic lupus erythematosus, a previous injury, heart surgery, or a bacterial infection. Previously, tuberculosis was the most common cause of chronic pericarditis in the United States, but today tuberculosis accounts for only 2% of cases. In Africa and India, tuberculosis is still the most common cause of all forms of pericarditis.

> **? Did You Know...**
> People can actually live without a pericardium, but surgery to remove it is risky.

Symptoms

Symptoms include shortness of breath, coughing, and fatigue. Coughing occurs because the high pressure in the veins of the lungs forces fluid into the air sacs. Fatigue occurs because the abnormal pericardium interferes with the heart's pumping action, so that the heart cannot pump enough blood to meet the body's needs. Other common symptoms are accumulation of fluid in the abdomen (ascites) and in the legs (edema). Sometimes fluid accumulates in the space between the two layers of the pleura, the membranes covering the lungs (a condition called pleural effusion—see page 518). However, chronic pericarditis does not cause pain.

Chronic effusive pericarditis may produce few symptoms if fluid accumulates slowly. The reason is that the pericardium can stretch gradually, so that cardiac tamponade may not occur. However, if fluid accumulates rapidly, the heart can become compressed and cardiac tamponade may occur.

Diagnosis

Symptoms provide important clues that a person has chronic pericarditis, particularly if there is no other reason for reduced heart performance—such as high blood pressure, coronary artery disease, or a heart valve disorder.

Echocardiography (see page 328) is often performed to confirm the diagnosis. It can detect the amount of fluid in the pericardial space and the formation of fibrous tissue around the heart. It can confirm the presence of cardiac tamponade. Chest x-rays may detect calcium deposits in the pericardium. These deposits develop in nearly half of the people who have chronic constrictive pericarditis.

The diagnosis can be confirmed in one of two ways. Cardiac catheterization can be used to measure blood pressure in the heart chambers and major blood vessels. These measurements help doctors distinguish pericarditis from similar disorders. Alternatively, magnetic resonance imaging (MRI) or computed tomography (CT) can be used to determine the thickness of the pericardium. Normally, the pericardium is less than 1/8 inch (3 millimeters) thick, but in chronic constrictive pericarditis, it is usually 1/4 inch (6 millimeters) thick or more.

A biopsy may be performed to help determine the cause of chronic pericarditis—for example, tuberculosis. A small sample of the pericardium is removed during exploratory surgery and examined under a microscope. Alternatively, a sample can be removed using a pericardioscope (a fiber-optic tube used to view the pericardium and to obtain tissue samples) inserted through an incision in the chest.

Treatment

Known causes of chronic effusive pericarditis are treated when possible. If heart function is normal, doctors take a wait-and-see approach. If the disorder causes symptoms or if an infection is suspected, surgical drainage may be performed (see page 392).

For people with chronic constrictive pericarditis, bed rest, restriction of salt in the diet, and diuretics (drugs that increase the excretion of fluid) may relieve symptoms. However, the only possible cure is surgical removal of the pericardium. Surgery cures about 85% of people. However, because the risk of death from surgery is 5 to 15%, most people do not have surgery unless the disease substantially interferes with daily activities. Surgery is not performed in the early stages of the disorder (before significant symptoms appear) or in the late stages (when symptoms occur at rest).

CHAPTER

63 Heart Tumors

A tumor is any type of abnormal growth, whether cancerous (malignant) or noncancerous (benign). Tumors that originate in the heart are called primary tumors. They may develop in any of the heart tissues and may be cancerous or noncancerous. Primary heart tumors are rare, occurring in fewer than 1 of 2,000 people. In adults, about half of noncancerous primary heart tumors are myxomas. Myxomas usually develop in the heart's left upper chamber (atrium). They may develop from embryonic cells located in the inner layer (lining) of the heart's wall.

In infants and children, the most common type of noncancerous primary heart tumor is a rhabdomyoma. Rhabdomyomas, which typically occur in groups, usually grow within the heart wall and develop directly from the heart's muscle cells. Rhabdomyomas commonly develop during infancy or childhood, often as part of a rare disease called tuberous sclerosis. The second most common noncancerous primary tumors in infants and children are fibromas. Fibromas, which typically occur as a single tumor, usually grow on heart valves and develop from the heart's fibrous tissue cells.

Several other types of primary heart tumors can develop, but all are rare. Some are cancerous and some benign.

Tumors that originate in some other part of the body—usually the lung, breast, blood, or skin—and then spread (metastasize) to the heart are called secondary tumors. They are always cancerous. Secondary heart tumors are 30 to 40 times more common than primary heart tumors but are still uncommon. About 10% of people who have lung or breast cancer—two of the most common cancers—and about 75% of people with malignant melanoma have metastases to the heart.

Both primary and secondary tumors may develop in the sac that surrounds the heart (pericardium). Tumors in the pericardium may squeeze (constrict) the heart, preventing it from filling properly. Chest pain and heart failure may develop.

Symptoms

Heart tumors may cause no symptoms, minor symptoms, or symptoms of life-threatening heart malfunction, which resemble those of other heart diseases but which develop suddenly. For example, tumors may cause heart failure, abnormal heart rhythms (arrhythmias), or a decrease in blood pressure caused by bleeding into the pericardium. Heart murmurs develop in about half of the people who have tumors that develop near or on a heart valve (such as myxomas and fibromas), because blood does not flow through the valve normally. Noncancerous tumors can be as deadly as cancerous ones if they interfere with the function of the heart.

Heart tumors, especially myxomas, may degenerate so that pieces of them break off and travel through the bloodstream (becoming emboli). Emboli may lodge in small arteries and block blood flow. Also, blood clots that form on the surface of tumors, such as myxomas, may break off as emboli and block arteries. Symptoms due to emboli depend on where the clot goes and therefore which tissues or organs are affected by the blocked artery.

> **? Did You Know...**
>
> Noncancerous tumors can be as deadly as cancerous ones if they interfere with the heart's function.

Diagnosis

Primary heart tumors are difficult to diagnose because they are relatively uncommon and because their symptoms resemble those of many other disorders. Doctors may suspect a primary heart tumor in people who have heart murmurs, abnormal heart rhythms, unexplained symptoms of heart failure, or unexplained fever (which may be due to a myxoma). Secondary heart tumors are suspected when people who have cancer elsewhere in the body come to a doctor with symptoms of heart malfunction.

If a tumor is suspected, echocardiography (see page 328) is usually performed to confirm the diagnosis. For this procedure, a probe that emits ultrasound waves is passed over the chest, producing an image of heart structures. If another view of the heart is needed, the probe can be passed down the throat into the esophagus to record signals from just behind the heart. This procedure is called transesophageal echocardiography. Computed tomography (CT) (see page 328) or magnetic resonance imaging (MRI) (see page 329) can provide additional information. Coronary angiography (see page 331) can produce an outline of a heart tumor that can be seen on x-rays, but this procedure is rarely needed.

If a tumor is detected in the right side of the heart, a small sample may be removed for examination under a microscope (biopsy). The sample is removed with a catheter that is inserted into a vein, usually in the leg, and threaded toward the heart in a procedure called cardiac catheterization (see page 330). This procedure helps doctors identify the type of tumor and select the appropriate treatment. Biopsy of tumors on the left side is rarely performed, because the risks of the procedure outweigh the benefits.

Treatment

A single small noncancerous primary heart tumor can be surgically removed, usually resulting in a cure. If a large noncancerous primary tumor is significantly reducing blood flow through the heart, removal of the part of the tumor that does not grow into the heart wall may improve heart function. However, if a large part of the heart wall is involved, surgery may be impossible.

In about half of newborns who have noncancerous rhabdomyomas, tumors regress without treatment; in the other half, the tumors do not grow any larger and do not require treatment. In infants and children, a fibroma may be successfully removed if it does not affect the wall between the ventricles (septum). Tumors that affect this wall usually also affect the electrical conduction system of the heart and cannot be surgically removed. Children with this type of tumor usually die of an abnormal heart rhythm at an early age. If a fibroma is large, blocks blood flow, and has grown into the surrounding tissue, heart transplantation may be required.

Primary cancerous tumors cannot be surgically removed and are usually fatal; chemotherapy or radiation therapy is sometimes used. Noncancerous tumors in the pericardium can be removed surgically, but cancerous tumors are not removed, as they have usually spread elsewhere in the body. If the tumor secretes fluid that interferes with heart motion, this fluid can be drained with a small plastic tube inserted by needle into the space between the pericardium and the heart (the pericardial space). Sometimes drugs are injected into the pericardial space to slow the tumor's growth.

Myxomas

A myxoma is a noncancerous primary tumor, usually irregular in shape and jellylike in consistency.

- People may feel short of breath or faint, or they may have fever or weight loss.
- Doctors confirm the diagnosis with echocardiography.
- Surgery is needed to remove a myxoma.

Half of all primary heart tumors are myxomas. Three fourths of myxomas occur in the left atrium, the chamber of the heart that receives oxygen-rich blood from the lungs. Some types of myxomas tend to run in families. These hereditary myxomas usually develop in young men in their mid-20s. Myxomas that are not hereditary usually develop in women, typically between the ages of 40 and 60. These myxomas are more likely to occur in the left atrium than are hereditary myxomas. All myxomas are more common in women.

Myxomas in the left atrium often grow from a stalk and swing freely with the flow of blood, as a tetherball does. As they swing, they may move in and out of the nearby mitral valve, the valve that opens from the left atrium into the left ventricle. This swinging motion may plug and unplug the valve over and over again, so that blood flow stops and starts intermittently.

Symptoms

When they stand, people with a myxoma in the left atrium may feel short of breath or may faint. With standing, the force of gravity pulls the myxoma into the opening of the mitral valve, blocking blood flow through the heart. This blockage causes transient heart failure. Lying down typically causes the myxoma to move away from the valve and relieves the symptoms.

Pieces of a myxoma or blood clots that form on the surface of the myxoma may break off (becoming emboli), travel through the bloodstream to other organs, and block arteries there. The resulting symptoms depend on which artery is blocked. For example, a blocked artery in the brain may cause a stroke; a blocked artery in the lung may cause pain and coughing up of blood.

Other symptoms of myxomas include fever, weight loss, Raynaud's syndrome (the fingers and toes become cold and painful when exposed to cold), a low red blood cell count (anemia), a high white blood cell count, and a low platelet count.

How a Myxoma Can Block Blood Flow in the Heart

A myxoma in the left atrium often grows from a stalk and swings freely with the flow of blood. As it swings, the myxoma may move in and out of the nearby mitral valve, which opens from the left atrium into the left ventricle. This swinging motion may plug and unplug the valve over and over again, so that blood flow stops and starts intermittently.

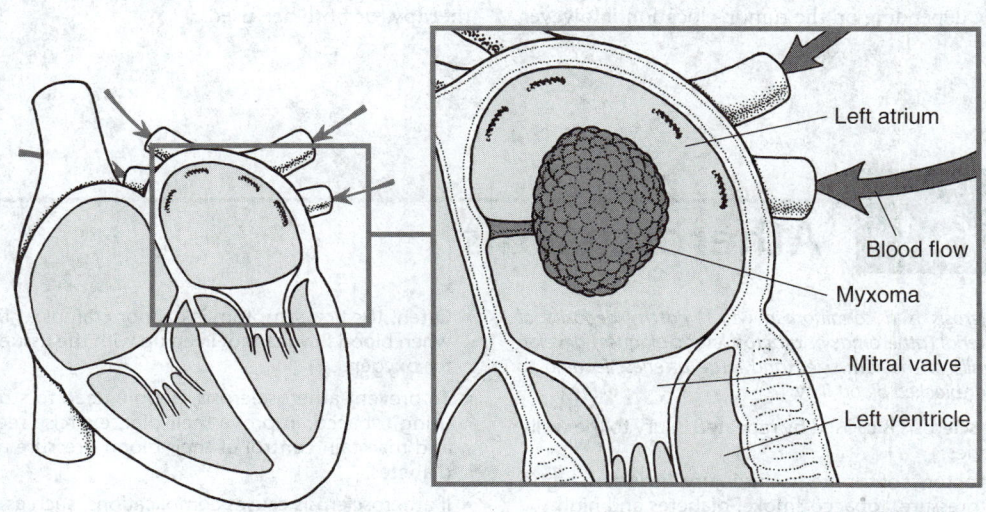

Left atrium

Blood flow

Myxoma

Mitral valve

Left ventricle

Diagnosis and Treatment

Myxomas are suspected based on the symptoms. With a stethoscope, doctors may hear a sound (heart murmur) produced by abnormal blood flow. The myxoma may block blood flow to or from the heart.

Blood tests may show inflammation, anemia, and a low number of platelets in the blood. But none of these tests is conclusive. The diagnosis is confirmed by echocardiography. Other procedures, including angiography, computed tomography (CT), magnetic resonance imaging (MRI), and biopsy, are sometimes necessary.

Surgical removal of the myxoma usually cures the person. After surgery, echocardiography is performed periodically for about 5 years to be sure that the myxoma does not recur.

Cancerous Tumors

- People may feel short of breath or faint, or they may have fever or weight loss or develop heart failure or abnormal heart rhythms.
- Doctors use echocardiography to confirm a heart tumor.
- Surgery, and sometimes chemotherapy or radiation therapy, is used to treat cancerous tumors.

Cancerous primary heart tumors are extremely rare, accounting for about one fourth of primary heart tumors. The most common are sarcomas that develop from blood vessel tissue. Secondary heart tumors are far more common, but how common is difficult to determine.

Symptoms

The symptoms of cancerous heart tumors are essentially the same as those of noncancerous heart tumors and vary depending on the tumor's location. However, the symptoms of cancerous tumors tend to worsen more quickly than those of noncancerous tumors, because cancerous tumors grow much faster. Other symptoms include sudden development of heart failure, abnormal heart rhythms, and bleeding into the sac that surrounds the heart (pericardium), which may interfere with the heart's functioning and cause cardiac tamponade (see box on page 391). Cancerous primary heart tumors may spread (metastasize) to the spine, nearby tissues, or organs such as the lungs and brain.

Symptoms of a secondary heart tumor often include those caused by the original tumor and may include those caused by metastases elsewhere in the body. Cancers, such as lung or breast cancer, may spread to the heart by direct invasion, often into the pericardium; the heart may be compressed because cancers cause blood and fluid to accumulate. Cancers may also spread to heart muscle and chambers through the bloodstream or through the lymph system; these cancers may produce symptoms of heart failure.

Diagnosis and Treatment

The procedures used to diagnose cancerous heart tumors are the same as those used for noncancerous heart tumors. For secondary tumors, procedures are performed to find the original tumor, unless its location is already known. If tumors in the pericardium cause fluid to accumulate around the heart, that fluid may have to be drained. Other treatment is usually needed and depends on the type of tumor. Often, however, treatment requires surgery.

Because cancerous heart tumors—both primary and secondary—are almost always incurable, treatment is designed to reduce symptoms. Depending on the type of tumor, radiation therapy, chemotherapy, or both are used.

CHAPTER

64 Atherosclerosis

Atherosclerosis is a condition in which patchy deposits of fatty material (atheromas or atherosclerotic plaques) develop in the walls of medium-sized and large arteries, leading to reduced or blocked blood flow.

- Atherosclerosis is caused by repeated injury to the walls of arteries.
- Many factors contribute to this injury, including high blood pressure, tobacco smoke, diabetes and high levels of cholesterol in the blood.

- Often, the first symptom is pain or cramps at times when blood flow cannot keep up with the tissues' need for oxygen.
- To prevent atherosclerosis, people need to stop using tobacco, improve their diet, exercise regularly, and maintain control of their blood pressure and diabetes.
- If atherosclerosis causes complications, such as a heart attack or stroke, these are treated.

How Atherosclerosis Develops

The wall of an artery is composed of several layers. The lining or inner layer (endothelium) is usually smooth and unbroken. Atherosclerosis begins when the lining is injured or diseased. Then certain white blood cells called monocytes and T cells are activated and move out of the bloodstream and through the lining of an artery into the artery's wall. Inside the lining, they are transformed into foam cells, which are cells that collect fatty materials, mainly cholesterol.

In time, smooth muscle cells move from the middle layer into the lining of the artery's wall and multiply there. Connective and elastic tissue materials also accumulate there, as may cell debris, cholesterol crystals, and calcium. This accumulation of fat-laden cells, smooth muscle cells, and other materials forms a patchy deposit called an atheroma or atherosclerotic plaque. As they grow, some plaques thicken the artery's wall and bulge into the channel of the artery. These plaques may narrow or block an artery, reducing or stopping blood flow. Other plaques do not block the artery very much but may split open, triggering a blood clot that suddenly blocks the artery.

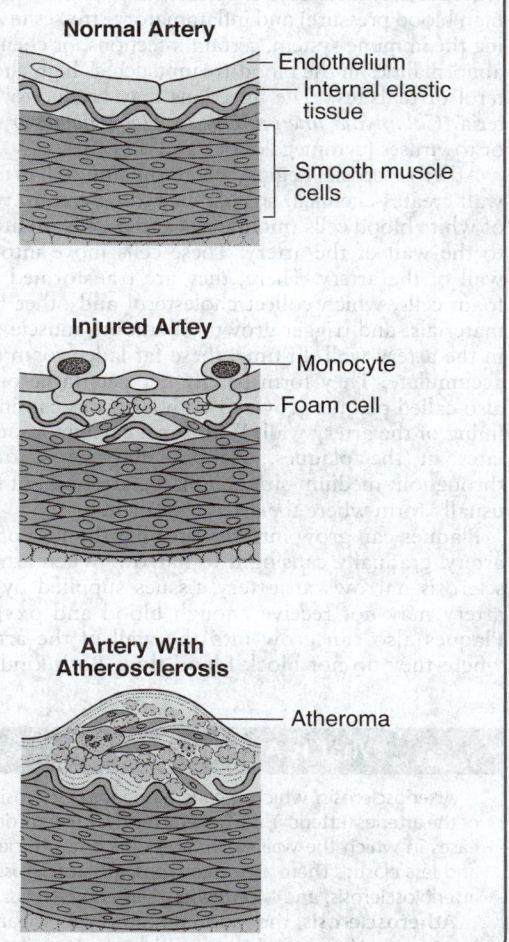

Normal Artery
— Endothelium
— Internal elastic tissue
— Smooth muscle cells

Injured Artey
— Monocyte
— Foam cell

Artery With Atherosclerosis
— Atheroma

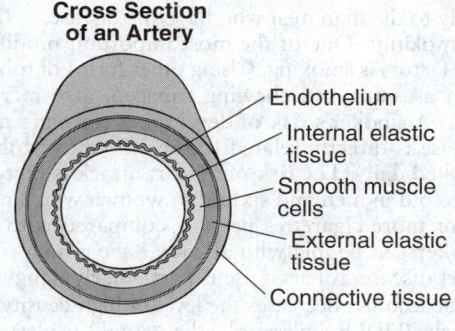

Cross Section of an Artery
— Endothelium
— Internal elastic tissue
— Smooth muscle cells
— External elastic tissue
— Connective tissue

In the United States and most other developed countries, atherosclerosis is the leading cause of illness and death. Estimates for 2005 in the United States alone are that about 16 million people have atherosclerotic heart disease and 5.8 million have stroke. Cardiovascular disease, primarily coronary and cerebrovascular atherosclerosis, caused almost 870,000 deaths in 2005—almost twice as many as cancer caused and 9 times as many as injuries caused. This year an estimated 1.2 million Americans will have a new or recurrent heart attack. Despite significant medical advances, heart attacks due to coronary artery disease (atherosclerosis that affects the arteries supplying blood to the heart—see page 401) and stroke (due to atherosclerosis that affects the arteries to the brain—see page 718) are responsible for more deaths than all other causes combined.

Atherosclerosis can affect the medium-sized and large arteries of the brain, heart, kidneys, other vital organs, and legs. It is the most important and most common type of **arteriosclerosis,** a general term for several diseases in which the wall of an artery becomes thicker and less elastic.

Causes

The development of atherosclerosis is complicated, but the primary event seems to be repeated, subtle injury to the artery's wall through various mechanisms. These mechanisms include physical stresses from turbulent blood flow (such as occurs where arteries branch, particularly in people who have high blood pressure) and inflammatory stresses involving the immune system, certain infections, or chemical abnormalities in the bloodstream (such as high cholesterol or diabetes). The infections may be due to bacteria (*Chlamydia pneumoniae* or *Helicobacter pylori*) or to viruses (cytomegalovirus and others).

Atherosclerosis begins when the injured arterial wall creates chemical signals that cause certain types of white blood cells (monocytes and T cells) to attach to the wall of the artery. These cells move into the wall of the artery. There, they are transformed into foam cells, which collect cholesterol and other fatty materials, and trigger growth of smooth muscle cells in the artery wall. In time, these fat-laden foam cells accumulate. They form patchy deposits (atheromas, also called plaques) covered with a fibrous cap in the lining of the artery wall. With time, calcium accumulates in the plaques. Plaques may be scattered throughout medium-sized and large arteries, but they usually form where the arteries branch.

Plaques can grow into the opening (lumen) of the artery, gradually causing it to narrow. When atherosclerosis narrows an artery, tissues supplied by the artery may not receive enough blood and oxygen. Plaques also can grow into the wall of the artery, where they do not block blood flow. Both kinds of plaques can split open (rupture), exposing the material within to the bloodstream. This material triggers blood clot formation. These blood clots can suddenly block all blood flow through the artery, which is the main cause of a heart attack or stroke. Sometimes these blood clots break off, travel through the bloodstream, and block an artery elsewhere in the body. Similarly, pieces of the plaque can break off and travel through the bloodstream and block an artery elsewhere.

Risk Factors

Risk factors for atherosclerosis include tobacco use, high levels of cholesterol in the blood, high blood pressure, diabetes, obesity, physical inactivity, and diet. Dietary factors include low daily consumption of fruits and vegetables and other than moderate alcohol consumption (that is, none or too much). These risk factors can usually be modified (see page 402). Risk factors that cannot be modified include having a family history of early atherosclerosis (that is, having a close relative who developed the disease at a young age), advancing age, and male sex. Men have a higher risk than women, although women who have coronary artery disease are more likely to die than men who have the disease.

Smoking: One of the most important modifiable risk factors is smoking. (Using other forms of tobacco, such as snuff and chewing tobacco, also increases risk.) A smoker's risk of developing coronary artery disease is directly related to the amount of tobacco smoked daily. The risk of a heart attack is increased threefold in men and sixfold in women who smoked 20 or more cigarettes per day compared with nonsmokers. In people who already have a high risk of heart disease, tobacco use is particularly dangerous.

Tobacco use decreases the level of high-density lipoprotein (HDL) cholesterol—the "good" cholesterol—and increases the level of low-density lipoprotein (LDL) cholesterol—the "bad" cholesterol. Smoking increases the level of carbon monoxide in the blood, which may increase the risk of injury to the lining of the artery's wall. Tobacco use causes arteries already narrowed by atherosclerosis to constrict, further decreasing the amount of blood reaching the tissues. In addition, tobacco use increases the blood's tendency to clot (by making platelets stickier), so that it increases the risk of peripheral arterial disease (atherosclerosis affecting arteries other than those that supply the heart and brain—see page 418), coronary artery disease (see page 401), stroke (see page 718), and blockage of an arterial graft placed during bypass surgery (see art on page 406 and on page 423).

People who quit using tobacco have only half the risk of those who continue to use tobacco—regardless of how long they smoked before quitting. Quitting

---

What Is Arteriosclerosis?

Arteriosclerosis, which means hardening (sclerosis) of the arteries (arterio-), is a general term for several diseases in which the wall of an artery becomes thicker and less elastic. There are three types: atherosclerosis, arteriolosclerosis, and Mönckeberg's arteriosclerosis.

Atherosclerosis, the most common type, means hardening related to plaques, which are deposits of fatty materials. It affects medium-sized and large arteries.

Arteriolosclerosis means hardening of the arterioles, which are small arteries. It affects primarily the inner and middle layers of the walls of arterioles. The walls thicken, narrowing the arterioles. As a result, organs supplied by the affected arterioles do not receive enough blood. The kidneys are often affected. This disorder occurs mainly in people who have high blood pressure or diabetes. Either of these disorders may stress the walls of arterioles, resulting in thickening.

Mönckeberg's arteriosclerosis affects small to medium-sized arteries. Calcium accumulates within the walls of arteries, making them stiff but not narrow. This essentially harmless disorder usually affects men and women older than 50.

also decreases the risk of death after coronary artery bypass surgery or a heart attack and the risk of illness and death in people who have peripheral arterial disease. The benefits of quitting tobacco use begin immediately and increase with time.

Secondhand smoke (smoke breathed in from someone else's smoking) appears to increase risk also. It should be avoided.

> **? Did You Know...**
> Smoking is an important risk factor for atherosclerosis.

Cholesterol Levels (see page 961): A high level of LDL cholesterol level is another important modifiable risk factor. A diet that is high in saturated fats causes LDL cholesterol levels to increase in susceptible people. Cholesterol levels also increase as people age and are normally higher in men than in women, although levels increase in women after menopause. Several hereditary disorders result in high levels of cholesterol or other fats. People with these hereditary disorders can have extremely high levels of cholesterol and (if untreated) die of coronary artery disease at an early age.

Lowering high LDL cholesterol levels through the use of drugs called statins (see table on page 967) can significantly reduce the risk of heart attacks, strokes, and death.

Not all types of cholesterol increase the risk of atherosclerosis. A high level of HDL (good) cholesterol decreases the risk of atherosclerosis, and a low level increases the risk.

The desired level of total cholesterol, which includes LDL and HDL cholesterol and triglycerides, is 140 to 200 mg/dL (3.6 to 5.2 mmol/L). Risk of a heart attack more than doubles when the total cholesterol level approaches 300 mg/dL (7.8 mmol/L). The risk is decreased when the LDL cholesterol level is below 130 mg/dL (3.4 mmol/L), and the HDL cholesterol level is above 40 mg/dL (1 mmol/L). In high-risk people, such as those who have diabetes or who already have atherosclerotic heart disease, heart attacks, stroke, or bypass surgery, LDL cholesterol should be below 70 mg/dL (1.8 mmol/L). However, the percentage of HDL cholesterol in relation to total cholesterol is a more reliable measure of risk than is the total or LDL cholesterol level. HDL cholesterol should account for more than 25% of total cholesterol. High triglyceride levels are often associated with low HDL cholesterol levels. However, evidence suggests that high triglyceride levels alone may also increase the risk of atherosclerosis.

High Blood Pressure: Uncontrolled high diastolic or systolic blood pressure is a risk factor for heart attack and stroke, which are caused by atherosclerosis. The risk of cardiovascular disease starts increasing when blood pressure levels are above 110/75 mm Hg. Reducing high blood pressure clearly lowers risk. Doctors usually try to achieve a blood pressure of less than 140/90 mm Hg, and often less than 130/80 mm Hg in those with diabetes or kidney disease.

Diabetes Mellitus: People who have type 1 diabetes (see page 1005) tend to develop disease that affects small arteries, such as those in the eyes, nerves, and kidneys, leading to vision loss, nerve damage, and kidney failure. Some people with type 1 diabetes and most people with type 2 diabetes tend to develop atherosclerosis in large arteries. These people also tend to develop atherosclerosis at an earlier age and more extensively than do people who do not have diabetes. The risk of developing atherosclerosis is 2 to 6 times higher for people with diabetes, particularly women. Women who have diabetes, unlike those who do not, are not protected from atherosclerosis before menopause. People who have diabetes have the same risk of death as someone who has had a prior heart attack, and doctors usually try to help these people keep other risk factors (such as high cholesterol levels and high blood pressure) under careful control.

Obesity: Obesity, particularly abdominal (truncal) obesity, increases the risk of coronary artery disease (atherosclerosis of the arteries that supply blood to the heart). Abdominal obesity increases the risk of other risk factors for atherosclerosis: high blood pressure, type 2 diabetes, and high cholesterol levels. Losing weight reduces the risk of all these disorders.

Physical Inactivity: Physical inactivity appears to increase the risk of developing coronary artery disease, and much evidence suggests that regular exercise even to a moderate degree reduces this risk and decreases mortality. Exercise can also help modify other risk factors for atherosclerosis—by lowering blood pressure and cholesterol levels and by helping with weight loss and decreasing insulin resistance.

Diet: There is substantial evidence that regular vegetable and fruit consumption can decrease coronary artery disease risk. It is unclear whether fruits and vegetables appear beneficial due to the substances (phytochemicals) they contain, or whether people who eat a lot of fruits and vegetables also eat less saturated fat and are more likely to take fiber and vitamins. However, phytochemicals called flavonoids (in red and purple grapes, red wine, black teas, and dark beers) appear especially protective. High concentrations in red wine may help explain why the French have a relatively low incidence of coronary artery disease, even though they use more tobacco and consume more fat than Americans do. But no studies prove that eating flavonoid-rich foods or using supplements instead of foods prevents atherosclerosis. Increased fiber content in certain vegetables may decrease total cholesterol and may decrease blood glucose and insulin levels. However, excessive fiber interferes with the absorption of certain minerals and vitamins. In general, foods rich in phytochemicals and vitamins are also rich in fiber.

Fat is an essential part of the diet. The notion that eating less fat is important to a healthy diet is only partly true because the type of fat also matters. The main types of fats are

- Saturated and trans fats
- Unsaturated fats (polyunsaturated and monounsaturated—see box on page 403)

Fats may be soft (or liquid) or firm at room temperature. Soft fats, such as oils and some margarines, tend to be higher in polyunsaturated and monounsaturated fats. Hard fats, such as butter and shortening, tend to be higher in saturated and trans fats. Saturated and trans fats are more likely to cause atherosclerosis. Thus, whenever possible, people should limit the amount of saturated and trans fats in their diet and choose foods with monounsaturated or polyunsaturated fats instead. Saturated and trans fats are found in red meat, many fast food and junk food items, full-fat dairy products (such as cheese, butter, and cream), and hard (stick) margarines. Monounsaturated fats are found in canola and olive oil, soft margarines with no trans fat, nuts, and olives. Polyunsaturated fats are found in nuts, seeds, oils, and mayonnaise. Two types of polyunsaturated fats—omega-3 and omega-6 fats—are essential to a healthy diet. Omega-3 fats are found in fatty fish such as salmon, omega-3 eggs, canola oil, and walnuts. Omega-6 fats are found in some nuts and seeds and in safflower, sunflower, and corn oils.

Alcohol Intake: People who drink a moderate amount of alcohol seem to have a lower risk of coronary artery disease than do people who drink too much or do not drink at all. Alcohol increases the level of good cholesterol (HDL), and it also decreases the risk of blood clots and inflammation and helps protect the body from the by-products of cell activity. However, more than moderate alcohol consumption (more than 14 drinks per week for men and more than 9 drinks per week for women) can cause significant health problems and increase the risk of death.

High Blood Levels of Homocysteine (Hyperhomocysteinemia): People who have very high levels of homocysteine (an amino acid) in their blood, usually because of a hereditary disorder, have an increased risk of coronary artery disease, usually at a young age. High levels of homocysteine may directly injure the lining of arteries, making the formation of plaques more likely. High homocysteine levels may also promote the formation of blood clots. However, giving people drugs that lower homocysteine levels does not seem to reduce risk of death.

Symptoms

Symptoms depend on where the affected artery is located and whether it is gradually narrowed or suddenly blocked.

With narrowing, atherosclerosis usually does not produce symptoms until the interior of an artery is narrowed by more than 70%. The first symptom of a narrowed artery may be pain or cramps at times when blood flow cannot keep up with the tissues' need for oxygen. For instance, during exercise, a person may feel chest pain because the oxygen supply to the heart is inadequate. While walking, a person may feel leg cramps (intermittent claudication—see page 419) because the oxygen supply to the leg muscles is inadequate. If the arteries supplying one or both kidneys become narrowed, kidney failure or dangerously high blood pressure can result.

If the arteries supplying the heart (coronary arteries) are blocked, a heart attack can result. Blockage in the arteries supplying the brain can cause a stroke. Blockage of the arteries in the legs can cause gangrene of a toe, foot, or leg.

Diagnosis

People who have symptoms that suggest a blocked artery have tests to look for the location and extent of the blockage. Different tests are used depending on what organ seems to be involved. People with atherosclerotic arteries in one organ often have atherosclerosis in other arteries. Therefore, when doctors find atherosclerotic blockage in one artery, for example in the leg, they usually do tests to look for blockage in other arteries, such as those in the heart. Doctors also test for certain risk factors in people who have an atherosclerotic blockage. For example, they measure the fasting levels of blood glucose, cholesterol, and triglycerides. Doctors usually also do these tests as part of the routine yearly examination in adults.

Some doctors recommend tests to look for atherosclerotic blockage in people who have no symptoms as part of a prevention strategy. Such tests include an electron beam computed tomography (CT) scan or magnetic resonance imaging (MRI) of the heart and ultrasound of the arteries in the neck (carotid arteries). Electron beam CT and MRI can detect hardened (calcified) plaque in the coronary arteries.

Ultrasonography of the carotid arteries can detect thickening of the artery wall, which suggests atherosclerosis. However, many doctors think that these tests rarely change the advice they would give based on the person's other, more easily recognized, risk factors.

Prevention and Treatment

To help prevent atherosclerosis, people need to stop tobacco use (see page 402), lower LDL cholesterol levels (see page 964), lower blood pressure (see page 339), lose weight (see page 954), and exercise (see page 38). People who have diabetes must maintain strict control of their blood sugar (glucose). People who are at high risk for atherosclerosis also may benefit from taking certain drugs. Helpful drugs include the statins (even if cholesterol levels are normal or only slightly high) and aspirin or other antiplatelet drugs (see table on page 967).

When atherosclerosis becomes severe enough to cause complications, the complications themselves must be treated. Complications include angina, heart attack, abnormal heart rhythms, heart failure, kidney failure, stroke, and leg cramps (intermittent claudication) or gangrene.

CHAPTER
65 Coronary Artery Disease

Coronary artery disease is a condition in which the blood supply to the heart muscle is partially or completely blocked.

The heart muscle needs a constant supply of oxygen-rich blood. The coronary arteries (see page 318), which branch off the aorta just after it leaves the heart, deliver this blood. Coronary artery disease can block blood flow, causing chest pain (angina) or a heart attack (also called myocardial infarction, or MI).

Coronary artery disease was once widely thought to be a man's disease. On average, men develop it about 10 years earlier than women because, until menopause, women are protected by high levels of estrogen. However, after menopause, coronary artery disease becomes more common among women. Among people aged 75 and older, a higher proportion of women have the disease, because women live longer.

In developed countries, coronary artery disease is the leading cause of death in both men and women. Coronary artery disease, specifically coronary atherosclerosis (literally "hardening of the arteries," which involves fatty deposits in the artery walls and may progress to narrowing and even blockage of blood flow in the artery), occurs in about 5 to 9% (depending on sex and race) of people aged 20 and older. The death rate increases with age and overall is higher for men than for women, particularly between the ages of 35 and 55. After age 55, the death rate for men declines, and the rate for women continues to climb. After age 70 to 75, the death rate for women exceeds that for men who are the same age.

Coronary artery disease affects people of all races, but the incidence is extremely high among blacks and Southeast Asians. The death rate is higher for black men than for white men until age 60 and is higher for black women than for white women until age 75.

Causes

Coronary artery disease is almost always due to the gradual buildup of cholesterol and other fatty materials (called atheromas or atherosclerotic plaques) in the wall of a coronary artery. This process is called atherosclerosis (see page 396) and can affect many arteries, not just those of the heart.

Occasionally, however, coronary artery disease is caused by spasm of a coronary artery, which can occur spontaneously, or from use of certain drugs such as cocaine and nicotine. Rarely, the cause is a birth defect, a viral infection (such as Kawasaki disease), systemic lupus erythematosus (lupus), inflammation of the arteries (arteritis), a blood clot that traveled from a heart chamber into one of the coronary arteries, or physical damage (from an injury or radiation therapy).

As an atheroma grows, it may bulge into the artery, narrowing the interior (lumen) of the artery and partially blocking blood flow. With time, calcium accumulates in the atheroma. As an atheroma blocks more and more of a coronary artery, the supply of oxygen-rich blood to the heart muscle (myocardium) can become inadequate. The blood supply is more likely to be inadequate during exertion, when the heart muscle requires more blood. An inadequate blood supply to the heart muscle (from any cause) is called myocardial ischemia. If the heart does not receive enough blood, it can no longer contract and pump blood normally.

An atheroma, even one that is not blocking very much blood flow, may rupture suddenly. The rupture of an atheroma often triggers the formation of a blood clot (thrombus). The clot further narrows or completely blocks the artery, causing acute myocardial ischemia. The consequences of this acute ischemia are referred to as **acute coronary syndromes** (see page 410). These syndromes include unstable angina and several types of heart attack, depending on the location and degree of the blockage. In a heart attack, the area of the heart muscle supplied by the blocked artery dies.

Sometimes an acute coronary syndrome is caused by coronary artery spasm or another type of coronary artery disease.

Risk Factors

Some factors that affect whether a person develops coronary artery disease cannot be modified. They include

- Advancing age
- Male sex
- Family history of early coronary artery disease (that is, having a close relative who developed the disease before age 50 to 55)

Other risk factors for coronary artery disease can be modified or treated. These factors include

- High blood levels of low-density lipoprotein (LDL) cholesterol
- High blood levels of lipoprotein a
- Low blood levels of high-density lipoprotein (HDL) cholesterol
- Diabetes mellitus
- Smoking
- High blood pressure
- Obesity
- Physical inactivity
- Dietary factors

Smoking more than doubles the risk of developing coronary artery disease and having a heart attack. Secondhand smoke appears also to increase risk.

Dietary risk factors include a diet that is low in fiber, vitamins C and E, and phytochemicals (which are present in fruits and vegetables and are thought to promote health). For some people, a diet low in fish oils (omega-3 polyunsaturated fatty acids) increases risk.

Having one or two drinks of alcohol a day appears to slightly reduce the risk of coronary artery disease (while slightly increasing that of stroke). However, having more than two drinks a day increases the risk, and the larger the amount, the greater the risk.

Certain metabolic disorders, such as hypothyroidism, hyperhomocysteinemia, and a high level of apoprotein B (apo B), also are risk factors.

Whether infection with certain organisms contributes to the development of coronary artery disease is uncertain. The organisms suspected include *Chlamydia pneumoniae* (which can cause pneumo-

nia), *Helicobacter pylori* (which can contribute to stomach ulcers), and a virus (as yet unidentified). One example of the relationship between infection and premature coronary artery disease is the finding that people who have poor dental health, particularly periodontal disease (infection of the gums), appear somewhat more likely to have a heart attack. Nonetheless, inflammation, whether caused by infection or not, appears to contribute to the development of acute coronary syndromes. If an atheroma becomes inflamed, it softens and is more likely to rupture, and blood clots are more likely to form.

Prevention

Modifying risk factors can help prevent coronary artery disease. Some of these factors are interrelated, so that modifying one also modifies another.

Smoking: Quitting smoking is most important. People who quit smoking decrease their risk of developing coronary artery disease by half compared with those who continue to smoke. How long people smoked before quitting does not matter. Quitting also decreases the risk of death after coronary artery bypass surgery or after a heart attack. Avoiding secondhand smoke is also important.

Diet: Limiting the amount of fat to no more than 25 to 35% of daily calories is recommended to promote good health. However, some experts believe that fat must be limited to 10% of daily calories to reduce the risk of coronary artery disease. A low-fat diet also helps lower high total and LDL (the bad) cholesterol levels, another risk factor for coronary artery disease. The type of fat consumed is as important as the amount of fat. Thus, eating oily fish, such as salmon, which are high in omega-3 fats (good fats), regularly and strictly avoiding the more harmful trans fats are recommended. Trans fats are being removed from ingredients in many fast food sites and restaurants.

Eating at least five servings of fruits and vegetables daily can decrease the risk of coronary artery disease. Such foods contain many phytochemicals. Whether the phytochemicals are responsible for the risk reduction is unclear because people who consume such diets also tend to eat less fat, more fiber, and more foods containing vitamins C and E. One group of phytochemicals called flavonoids (found in red and purple grapes, red wine, and black teas) appears to be particularly protective.

A high-fiber diet is also recommended. There are two kinds of fiber. Soluble fiber (which dissolves in liquid) is found in oat bran, oatmeal, beans, peas, rice bran, barley, citrus fruits, strawberries, and apple pulp. It helps lower high cholesterol levels. It may decrease or stabilize high blood sugar (glucose) levels and increase low insulin levels. Thus, soluble

Types of Fat

There are three types of fat: saturated, monounsaturated, and polyunsaturated.

"Saturated" refers to the number of hydrogen atoms in a molecule of fat. Saturated fats contain as many hydrogen atoms as they can. They are usually solid at room temperature. Saturated fats are present in meats, dairy products, and artificially hydrogenated vegetable oils. The more solid the product, the higher is the proportion of saturated fats. A diet high in saturated fats promotes coronary artery disease.

Unsaturated fats (monounsaturated and polyunsaturated) do not contain as many hydrogen atoms as they could. Monounsaturated fats could contain one more hydrogen atom. They are usually liquid at room temperature but start to solidify in the refrigerator. Olive oil and canola oil are examples. Polyunsaturated fats could contain more than one additional hydrogen atom. These fats are usually liquid at room and refrigerator temperatures. They tend to become rancid at room temperature. Corn oil is an example. Other polyunsaturated fats include omega-3 fats, contained in deep-sea fatty fish (such as mackerel, salmon, and tuna), and omega-6 fats, contained in vegetable oils.

In a process called hydrogenation, hydrogen atoms are artificially added to polyunsaturated oils so that these oils may be used to make food products that do not become rancid and to make solid fat products, such as margarine. Trans fats result from this process. ("Trans" refers to where the hydrogen atoms are added to the fat molecule.) Trans fats are particularly common in commercial baked and fried foods, such as cookies, crackers, doughnuts, french fries, and other similar foods.

Trans fats increase low-density lipoprotein (LDL—the bad) cholesterol levels and decrease high-density lipoprotein (HDL—the good) cholesterol levels, and these effects appear to increase the risk of coronary artery disease. Avoiding products that contain trans fats is wise. Trans fats are now listed on food labels. Also, if hydrogenated fat or partially hydrogenated fat is the first fat on the list of ingredients, the product contains trans fats. Some restaurants also provide information on which menu items contain trans fats. Several cities in the United States have barred restaurants from using trans fats in their food, and more cities are likely to follow this trend. Many manufacturers are changing their products to eliminate trans fats. The appearance of a margarine or oil can also help identify foods containing these fats—the softer or more liquid, the smaller the trans fat content. For example, the trans fat content of tub margarines is lower than that of stick margarines.

Some margarine products contain a plant sterol or stanol, which can lower total and LDL cholesterol levels. Plant sterols and stanols may have this effect because they are not absorbed well in the digestive tract and they interfere with the absorption of cholesterol. These margarine products have been approved as heart healthy foods when they are used as part of a healthy diet. These products are made from unsaturated fat, contain less saturated fat than butter, and do not contain trans fats. However, they are expensive.

The ideal combination of types of fats is unknown. However, a diet high in monounsaturated or omega-3 fats and low in trans fats is probably desirable.

---

fiber may help people with diabetes reduce their risk of coronary artery disease. Insoluble fiber (which does not dissolve in liquid) is found in most grains and grain products and in fruits and vegetables such as apple skin, cabbage, beets, carrots, brussels sprouts, turnips, and cauliflower. It helps with digestive function. However, eating too much fiber can interfere with the absorption of certain vitamins and minerals.

The diet should contain the recommended daily requirements of vitamins and minerals. Vitamin supplements are not considered an acceptable substitute for a healthy diet. The role of supplements in reducing the risk of coronary artery disease is somewhat controversial. Taking supplements of vitamin E or vitamin C does not seem to prevent coronary artery disease. Taking folate or vitamins B_6 and B_{12} may lower homocysteine levels, but studies have not shown that taking these supplements decreases the risk of coronary artery disease.

Limiting the amount of simple sugar carbohydrates (such as refined white flour, white rice, processed foods) and increasing the amount of whole grains may help reduce the risk of coronary artery disease because it reduces the risk of obesity and possibly of diabetes, which are also risk factors for coronary artery disease.

Overall, people should maintain a healthy weight and eat a variety of foods. The Mediterranean diet, which consists of large portions of fruits, vegetables, nuts, and olive oil, appears to reduce the risk of coronary artery disease.

Physical Inactivity: People who are physically active are less likely to develop coronary artery disease and high blood pressure. Exercise that promotes endurance (aerobic exercise such as brisk walking, bicycling, and jogging) or muscle strength (resistance training with free weights or weight machines) helps prevent coronary artery disease (see page 40). Walking just 30 minutes each day can be beneficial. People who are out of shape or who have not exercised in a long time should consult their doctor before they start an exercise program.

Obesity: Modifying the diet and engaging in physical activity can help control obesity. Decreasing alcohol consumption can also help because alcohol is high in calories. A loss of even 10 to 20 pounds (4½ to 9 kilograms) can reduce the risk of coronary artery disease.

High Cholesterol Levels: High total and LDL (the bad) cholesterol levels can be lowered by exercising and by quitting smoking as well as by reducing the amount of fat in the diet. Drugs that lower levels of total and LDL cholesterol in the blood (lipid-lowering drugs) may be used (see table on page 967). The benefits of lowering cholesterol levels are greatest in people with other risk factors, such as smoking, high blood pressure, obesity, and physical inactivity.

Increasing the level of HDL (the good) cholesterol also helps reduce the risk of coronary artery disease. The same lifestyle changes that lower total and LDL cholesterol levels can help increase HDL cholesterol levels, as can certain drugs. For people who are overweight, losing weight can also help.

High Blood Pressure: Lowering high blood pressure reduces the risk of coronary artery disease. Treatment of high blood pressure begins with lifestyle changes: eating a healthy diet that is low in salt and, if needed, losing weight and increasing physical activity. Drug therapy (see table on page 340) may also be necessary.

Diabetes Mellitus: Good control of diabetes reduces the risk of some complications of diabetes, but the effects of such control on the development of coronary artery disease are less clear. Good control of diabetes may also reduce the risk of complications of coronary artery disease.

Treatment

Doctors try to do three things for people with coronary artery disease. They try to reduce the heart's workload, improve coronary artery blood flow, and slow down or reverse the buildup of atherosclerosis. The heart's workload can be reduced by controlling the person's blood pressure and using certain drugs such as beta-blockers or calcium channel blockers that keep the heart from pumping as hard. Coronary blood flow can be improved by percutaneous coronary intervention (PCI) or coronary artery bypass grafting (CABG). A coronary artery blood clot may sometimes be dissolved by drugs (see page 417). Modifying the diet, exercising, and taking certain drugs can help reverse atherosclerosis.

Percutaneous Coronary Intervention

In PCI (also called percutaneous transluminal coronary angioplasty—PTCA), doctors insert a large needle into the main artery of the thigh (femoral artery). Then a long guide wire is threaded through the needle, into the artery, and up through the aorta into the narrowed coronary artery. A catheter with a balloon attached to the tip is threaded over the guide wire and into the narrowed coronary artery. The catheter is positioned so that the balloon is at the level of the narrowing. The balloon is then inflated for several seconds. The inflated balloon compresses the atheroma that is narrowing the artery and widens the artery. Inflation and deflation may be repeated several times. In 80 to 90% of people, the narrowed arteries that are reached are opened.

To help keep the coronary artery open, doctors usually insert a tube made of wire mesh (a stent) into the artery. About 75% of the time, doctors use stents that are coated with a drug. The drug is released slowly to help prevent the coronary artery from becoming blocked again, a common problem with bare-metal stents. However, although these drug-releasing stents are very helpful in keeping the artery open, people who have a drug-releasing stent have a slightly higher risk of developing a blood clot in the stent than do people who have a bare metal stent. To decrease the risk of such clots, people who have a drug-releasing stent are given an antiplatelet drug for at least a year after the stent is inserted. If the artery becomes blocked again, whether from a clot or other causes, doctors may do a second PCI.

Generally, PCI is preferred to bypass grafting because it is a less invasive procedure. However, the affected area of the coronary artery may not be suited to PCI because of its location, its length, the amount of calcium that accumulates, or other conditions. Thus, doctors carefully determine whether a person is a good candidate for the procedure.

Other Techniques: Doctors have tried other techniques to remove atheromas. These include the use of tiny blades, burrs, or lasers to remove thick, fibrous, and calcified atheromas by cutting, shaving, crushing, or dissolving them. Some of these techniques are still being evaluated, but so far, the results, especially over the long term, have been disappointing.

Coronary Artery Bypass Grafting

Coronary artery bypass grafting (CABG) is also called bypass surgery or coronary artery bypass surgery. In the procedure, doctors take an artery or vein from another part of the body to connect the aorta (the major artery that takes blood from the heart to the rest of the body) to a coronary artery

Understanding Percutaneous Coronary Intervention (PCI)

Doctors insert a balloon-tipped catheter into a large artery (usually the femoral artery) and thread the catheter through the connecting arteries and the aorta to the narrowed or blocked coronary artery. Then doctors inflate the balloon to force the atheroma against the arterial wall and thus open the artery. Usually, a collapsed tube made of wire mesh (a stent) is placed over the deflated balloon at the catheter's tip and inserted with the catheter. When the catheter reaches the atheroma, the balloon is inflated, opening up the stent. Then the balloon-tipped catheter is removed, and the stent is left in place to help keep the artery open.

People are usually awake during the procedure, but doctors may give a drug to help them relax. People are closely monitored during PCI because balloon inflation momentarily blocks blood flow in the affected coronary artery. This blockage can produce chest pain and changes in the heart's electrical activity (detected by ECG) in some people. Fewer than 1 to 2% of people die during PCI, and 3 to 5% have nonfatal heart attacks. Coronary artery bypass surgery becomes necessary immediately after PCI for fewer than 3% of people.

Site of a blocked artery

Femoral artery

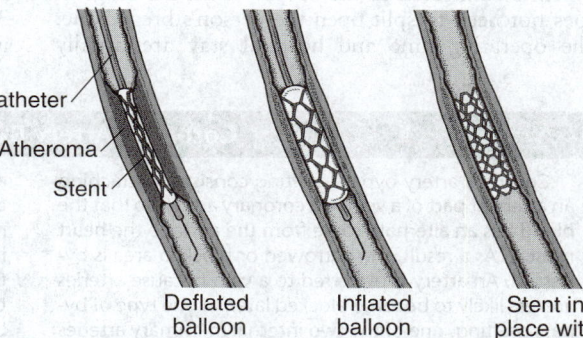

Catheter

Atheroma

Stent

Deflated balloon surrounded by stent

Inflated balloon surrounded by stent

Stent in place with balloon removed

---

past the point of its blockage. Blood flow is thus rerouted, skipping over (bypassing) the narrowed or blocked area. Veins are usually taken from the leg. Arteries are usually taken from beneath the breastbone (sternum) or from the forearm. Artery grafts rarely develop coronary artery disease, and more than 90% of them still work properly 10 years after the bypass surgery. However, vein grafts may gradually become narrowed by atheromas, and after 5 years, one third or more may be completely blocked.

The operation takes 2 to 4 hours, depending on the number of blood vessels to be grafted. A numeric modifier (for example, triple or quadruple) before bypass refers to the number of arteries (for example, 3 or 4) that are bypassed. The person is given a general anesthetic. Then, an incision is made down the center of the chest from the neck to the top of the stomach, and the breastbone is parted. This type of surgery is called open-heart surgery. Usually, the heart is stopped so that it is not moving and thus easier to operate on. A heart-lung machine is then used to put oxygen into the blood and pump the blood through the bloodstream. When only one or two blood vessels require grafting, the heart may be left pumping. The hospital stay is typically 5 to 7 days, usually less if a heart-lung machine was not used during surgery.

The risks from surgery include stroke and heart attack. For people who have a normal-sized and normally functioning heart, have never had a heart attack, and have no additional risk factors, risk is less than 5% for a heart attack during surgery, 2 to

3% for stroke, and less than 1% for death. Risk is somewhat higher for people with reduced pumping ability of the heart (poor left ventricular function), damaged heart muscle from a previous heart attack, or other cardiovascular problems. However, if these people survive the surgery, their prospects for long-term survival are improved.

Other Techniques: With new techniques, chest incisions can be much smaller, resulting in minimally invasive bypass surgery. One technique involves robotics. While sitting at a computer console, a surgeon uses pencil-sized robotic arms to do the operation. The arms hold specially designed surgical instruments that can do intricate movements, mimicking those of the surgeon's hands. Through a viewing scope, the surgeon watches a magnified three-dimensional image of the operation. The operation requires three 1-inch (about 2½-centimeter) incisions—one for each of the two robotic arms and one for a camera, which is connected to the scope. Thus, the surgeon does not need to split open the person's breastbone. The operating time and hospital stay are usually shorter with the newer procedures than with open-heart surgery.

Angina

Angina, also called angina pectoris, is temporary chest pain or a sensation of pressure that occurs while the heart muscle is not receiving enough oxygen.

- A person with angina has discomfort or pressure beneath the breastbone (sternum).
- Angina typically occurs in response to exertion and is relieved by rest.
- Doctors diagnose angina based on symptoms, electrocardiography, and imaging tests.
- Treatment may include nitrates, beta-blockers, calcium channel blockers, and percutaneous coronary intervention or coronary artery bypass graft surgery.

In the United States, almost 6.5 million people have angina, and it is newly diagnosed in about 350,000 people each year. Angina tends to develop in women at a later age than in men.

Coronary Artery Bypass Grafting

Coronary artery bypass grafting consists of attaching an artery or part of a vein to a coronary artery, so that the blood has an alternate route from the aorta to the heart muscle. As a result, the narrowed or blocked area is bypassed. An artery is preferred to a vein because arteries are less likely to become blocked later. In one type of bypass grafting, one of the two internal mammary arteries is cut, and one of the cut ends is attached to a coronary artery beyond the blocked area. The other end of this artery is tied off. If an artery cannot be used or if there is more than one blockage, a section of a vein—usually, from the saphenous vein, which runs from the groin to the ankle—is used. One end of the section (graft) is attached to the aorta, and the other to a coronary artery beyond the blocked area. Sometimes a vein graft is used in addition to the mammary artery graft.

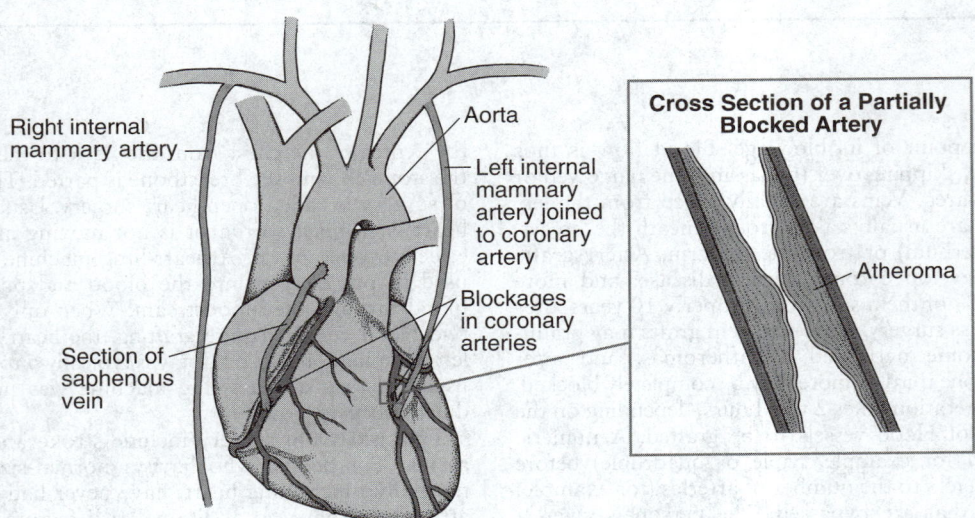

Right internal mammary artery

Aorta

Left internal mammary artery joined to coronary artery

Blockages in coronary arteries

Section of saphenous vein

Cross Section of a Partially Blocked Artery

Atheroma

Causes

Usually, angina occurs when the heart's workload (and need for oxygen) exceeds the ability of the coronary arteries to supply an adequate amount of blood to the heart. Coronary blood flow can be limited when the arteries are narrowed. Narrowing usually results from fatty deposits in the arteries (atherosclerosis—see page 396) but may result from coronary artery spasm. Inadequate blood flow to any tissue is termed ischemia.

When angina is due to atherosclerosis, it usually first occurs during physical exertion or emotional distress, which make the heart work harder and increase its need for oxygen. If the artery is narrowed enough (usually by more than 70%), angina can occur even at rest, when the demands on the heart are at their minimum.

Severe anemia increases the likelihood of angina. In anemia, the number of red blood cells (which contain hemoglobin—the molecule that carries oxygen) or the amount of hemoglobin in the cells is below normal. As a result, the oxygen supply to the heart muscle is reduced.

Unusual Causes: Syndrome X is a form of angina caused neither by spasm nor by any apparent blockage in the large coronary arteries. Temporary narrowing of much smaller coronary arteries may be responsible, at least in some people. The reasons for the temporary narrowing are unknown but may involve a chemical imbalance in the heart or abnormalities in the functioning of small arteries (arterioles). This syndrome is sometimes called cardiac syndrome X to distinguish it from another disorder also called syndrome X (metabolic syndrome or the syndrome of insulin resistance—see page 960).

Other unusual causes of angina include the following:

- Severe high blood pressure
- Narrowing of the aortic valve (aortic valve stenosis)
- Leakage of the aortic valve (aortic valve regurgitation)
- Thickening of the walls of the ventricles (hypertrophic cardiomyopathy), especially thickening of the wall separating the ventricles (hypertrophic obstructive cardiomyopathy).

These conditions increase the heart's workload and thus the amount of oxygen needed by the heart muscle. When the need for oxygen exceeds the supply, angina results. Abnormalities of the aortic valve may reduce blood flow through the coronary arteries, because the openings of the coronary arteries are located just beyond this valve.

Classification

Nocturnal angina is angina that occurs at night, during sleep.

Stable angina is chest pain or discomfort that typically occurs with activity or stress. Episodes of pain or discomfort are provoked by similar or consistent amounts of activity or stress.

Angina decubitus is angina that occurs when a person is lying down (not necessarily only at night) without any apparent cause. Angina decubitus occurs because gravity redistributes fluids in the body. This redistribution makes the heart work harder.

Variant angina results from a spasm of one of the large coronary arteries on the surface of the heart. It is called variant because it is characterized by pain during rest, not during exertion, and by specific changes detected with electrocardiography (ECG) during an episode of angina.

Unstable angina refers to angina in which the pattern of symptoms changes. Because the characteristics of angina in a particular person usually remain constant, any change—such as more severe pain, more frequent attacks, or attacks occurring with less exertion or during rest—is serious. Such change usually reflects a sudden narrowing of a coronary artery because an atheroma has ruptured or a clot has formed. The risk of a heart attack is high. Unstable angina is considered an acute coronary syndrome (see page 410).

> **? Did You Know...**
>
> Women experieznce the discomfort of angina differently than men and are more likely to have a burning sensation or tenderness in the back, shoulders, arms, or jaw.

Symptoms

Most commonly, a person feels angina as pressure or an ache beneath the breastbone (sternum). People often interpret the sensation as discomfort or heaviness rather than pain. Discomfort also may occur in either shoulder or down the inside of either arm; through the back; and in the throat, jaw, or teeth.

Symptoms are very often different in women. Women are more likely to have a burning sensation or tenderness in the back, shoulders, arms, or jaw.

Typically, angina is triggered by exertion, lasts no more than a few minutes, and subsides with rest. Some people experience angina predictably with a specific degree of exertion. In other people, episodes occur unpredictably. Often, angina is worse when exertion follows a meal. It is usually worse in cold weather. Walking into the wind or moving from a warm room into the cold air may trigger angina. Emotional stress may also cause or worsen angina. Sometimes, experiencing a strong emotion while

SPOTLIGHT ON AGING

In older people, symptoms of angina may be different and therefore easily misdiagnosed. For instance, the pain is less likely to occur beneath the breastbone. Pain may occur in the back and shoulders and may be incorrectly blamed on arthritis. Discomfort, bloating, and gas may occur in the stomach area, particularly after meals (because extra blood is needed to help in digestion). People may mistake such discomfort for indigestion or blame it on a stomach ulcer. Belching may even seem to relieve these symptoms. Also, older people who have confusion or dementia may have difficulty in communicating that they have pain.

resting or having a bad dream during sleep can cause angina.

Silent Ischemia: Not everyone with ischemia experiences angina. Ischemia without angina is called silent ischemia. Doctors do not understand why ischemia is sometimes silent, and some debate its significance. However, most experts consider silent ischemia as serious as ischemia with angina.

Diagnosis

Doctors diagnose angina largely based on a person's description of the symptoms. A physical examination and ECG (see page 326) may detect little, if anything, abnormal between and sometimes even during attacks of angina, even in people with extensive coronary artery disease. During an attack, the heart rate may increase slightly, blood pressure may go up, and with a stethoscope, doctors may hear a change in the heartbeat. ECG may detect changes in the heart's electrical activity.

When symptoms are typical, the diagnosis is usually easy for doctors. The kind of pain, its location, and its association with exertion, meals, weather, and other factors help doctors make the diagnosis. The presence of risk factors for coronary artery disease also helps establish the diagnosis. If a person experiences chest pain during the examination, a doctor may place a dose of nitroglycerin (a drug that dilates blood vessels) under the person's tongue as a test, because if the pain is due to angina, relief should occur in less than 3 minutes.

The following procedures may help evaluate the inadequate blood supply (ischemia) to the heart muscle and determine whether coronary artery disease is present and how extensive it is.

For **exercise stress testing** (see page 326), the person walks on a treadmill or rides a stationary bicycle while being monitored by ECG. This procedure can help doctors determine whether coronary angiography or coronary artery bypass grafting (CABG) is needed. If people cannot exercise, testing is done after a drug that makes the heart work harder is injected (a procedure called pharmacologic stress testing).

For **radionuclide imaging** (see page 329), a tiny amount of a radioactive substance is injected into a vein. Radionuclide imaging can identify the location and extent of ischemia and show the amount of blood reaching the heart muscle. This procedure is usually combined with stress testing.

Echocardiography (see page 328) uses ultrasound waves to produce images of the heart (echocardiograms). This procedure shows heart size, movement of the heart muscle, blood flow through the heart valves, and valve function. Echocardiography is done during rest and exercise. When ischemia is present, the pumping motion of the left ventricle is abnormal.

For **coronary angiography** (see page 331), x-rays of arteries are taken after a radiopaque dye is injected. Coronary angiography, the most accurate procedure for diagnosing coronary artery disease, may be done when a diagnosis is uncertain. Coronary angiography is commonly used to help evaluate whether CABG or percutaneous coronary intervention (PCI) is appropriate. Angiography can also detect spasm of an artery. A drug that can produce a spasm may be used during angiography if a spasm does not occur.

In a few people who have typical symptoms of angina and abnormal results on an exercise stress test, coronary angiography does not confirm the presence of coronary artery disease. Some of these people have syndrome X, but for most, the source of the symptoms does not involve the heart.

Continuous ECG monitoring with a Holter monitor (see page 327) may detect abnormalities indicating symptomatic or silent ischemia or variant angina (which typically occurs during rest).

Electron beam computed tomography (CT) scans can detect the amount of calcium deposits in the coronary arteries. The amount of calcium present (the calcium score) is roughly proportional to the likelihood of the person having angina or a heart attack. However, because calcium deposits may be present even in people whose arteries are not very narrowed, the score does not reliably predict the need for PCI or CABG. Electron beam CT scans are not recommended for screening all people, in part because it exposes people to a significant amount of radiation. However, the test is often valuable for evaluating people who have a relatively high risk of death or heart attack. People at risk include those who have diabetes, high blood pressure, or both; high cholesterol levels; and abnormal or unclear stress test results.

Multidetector row CT is a new technique that uses a high-speed CT scanner with many small detectors that can accurately identify coronary artery narrowing. The technique is noninvasive and highly accurate in excluding coronary artery narrowing as a source of a person's symptoms (particularly in those who were not able to have a stress test or had a stress test that was inconclusive). It can also be used to determine whether a stent or bypass graft is unobstructed, to display cardiac and coronary venous anatomy, and to assess whether atheromas contain calcium. However, the technique cannot be used in women who are pregnant or in people who are unable to hold their breath for 15 to 20 seconds three or four times during the procedure. Also, because the test does not work well if the heart is beating fast, people whose heart rate is above 65 beats per minute are given drugs to slow the heart rate. People who cannot tolerate such drugs or a low heart rate cannot have the test. People are also exposed to significant amounts of radiation.

Cardiac magnetic resonance imaging (MRI) is valuable in evaluating the heart and the large vessels coming from the heart (the aorta and the pulmonary arteries). This technique avoids any radiation exposure. In people with coronary artery disease, MRI may be used to evaluate narrowing of the arteries, measure the blood flow in the coronary arteries, and test how well the heart is being supplied with oxygen. MRI can also be used to assess abnormalities of heart wall motion during stress (which may indicate poor blood supply to that area) and whether areas of heart muscle damaged by a heart attack may recover (testing viability).

Prognosis

Key factors that can worsen the outcome (prognosis) for people who have angina include advancing age, extensive coronary artery disease, diabetes, other risk factors (particularly smoking), severe pain, and, most importantly, reduced pumping ability of the heart (ventricular function). For example, the more coronary arteries affected or the larger the blockage of the arteries, the worse is the prognosis. The prognosis is surprisingly good for people with stable angina and normal pumping ability. Reduced pumping ability dramatically worsens the prognosis. The prognosis for people with syndrome X does not differ from that for people without coronary artery disease.

The death rate each year for people with angina and no other risk factors is about 1.4%. The rate is higher for people with risk factors such as high blood pressure, abnormal ECG results, or a previous heart attack, particularly in those who have diabetes.

Treatment

Treatment begins with attempts to slow or reverse the progression of coronary artery disease by dealing with risk factors. Risk factors, such as high blood pressure and high cholesterol levels, are treated promptly. Quitting smoking is crucial. A low-fat, varied diet that is low in simple sugar carbohydrates and exercise (for most people) are recommended. Weight loss, if needed, is also recommended.

Treatment of angina depends partly on the stability and severity of the symptoms. When symptoms are stable and mild to moderate, the most effective treatment may be modification of risk factors and the use of certain drugs. If modification of risk factors and drug therapy do not cause symptoms to subside markedly, a procedure to restore blood flow to affected areas of the heart (a revascularization procedure) may be needed. When symptoms worsen rapidly, immediate hospitalization is usually required and the person is evaluated for an acute coronary syndrome (see page 410).

Drug Therapy

Drug treatment of stable angina is designed to prevent or reduce ischemia and to minimize symptoms. Five types of drugs are available: beta-blockers, nitrates (including nitroglycerin and long-acting nitrates), calcium channel blockers, angiotensin-converting enzyme (ACE) inhibitors, and antiplatelet drugs.

Beta-blockers interfere with the effects of the hormones epinephrine (adrenaline) and norepinephrine (noradrenaline) on the heart and other organs. These hormones stimulate the heart to beat faster and more forcefully and most arterioles to constrict (causing blood pressure to increase—see table on page 340). Thus, beta-blockers reduce the resting heart rate and blood pressure. During exercise, they limit the increase in heart rate and in blood pressure and so reduce the demand for oxygen. Beta-blockers reduce the risk of heart attacks and sudden death, improving the long-term outcome for people with coronary artery disease.

Nitroglycerin is a very short-acting nitrate drug that dilates blood vessels. Taking nitroglycerin usually relieves an episode of angina in 1 to 3 minutes, and the effects last 30 minutes. Nitroglycerin is usually taken as a tablet placed under the tongue (sublingual administration) or as a spray inhaled through the mouth. Alternatively, the tablet may be placed next to the gum. People with chronic stable angina should keep nitroglycerin tablets or spray with them at all times. Taking nitroglycerin just before reaching a level of exertion known to induce angina may be useful.

Long-acting nitrates (such as isosorbide) are taken by mouth 1 to 4 times a day. Nitrate skin patches and paste, in which the drug is absorbed through the skin over many hours, are also effective. Long-acting nitrates taken regularly can soon lose their ability to provide relief. Most experts recommend that people not take the drug for an 8- to 12-hour period each day, usually at night unless that is when angina occurs. This approach helps maintain the long-term effectiveness of the drug. Unlike beta-blockers, nitrates do not reduce the risk of heart attacks and sudden death, but they greatly reduce symptoms in people with coronary artery disease.

Calcium channel blockers prevent blood vessels from narrowing (constricting) and can counter coronary artery spasm. These drugs are also effective in treating variant angina. All calcium channel blockers reduce blood pressure. Some of these drugs, such as verapamil and diltiazem, may also reduce the heart rate. This effect can be useful to many people, especially those who cannot take beta-blockers or who do not get enough relief from nitrates.

ACE inhibitors, such as ramipril, are often given to people who have evidence of coronary artery disease, including angina. These drugs do not treat angina itself, but they can reduce the risk of heart attack and of death due to coronary artery disease.

Antiplatelet drugs, such as aspirin, ticlopidine, and clopidogrel, modify platelets so that they do not clump and stick on blood vessel walls. Platelets, which circulate in the blood, promote clot formation (thrombosis) when a blood vessel is injured. However, when platelets collect on atheromas in an artery's walls, the resulting clot can narrow or block the artery and result in a heart attack. Aspirin modifies platelets irreversibly and thus reduces the risk of death from coronary artery disease. Doctors recommend that most people who have coronary artery disease take both aspirin and clopidogrel daily to reduce the risk of a heart attack. Ticlopidine, which has similar effects but more potential side effects than clopidogrel, may be used if the person is allergic or cannot tolerate clopidogrel. Antiplatelet drugs are given to people with angina unless there is a reason not to. For example, they are not given to people who have a bleeding disorder.

Revascularization Procedures

These procedures include percutaneous coronary intervention (PCI) procedures (also called angioplasty) and coronary artery bypass grafting (CABG). These invasive techniques are effective, but they are only mechanical measures for correcting the immediate problem. They do not stop the progression of the underlying disease. People still need to modify risk factors.

PCI (see page 404) is often preferred to CABG because it is less invasive, although it is not appropriate for every situation. PCI is usually preferred when only one or two arteries are affected, and the blocked area is not very long. However, new technology and increasing experience are allowing doctors to use PCI for more and more people.

CABG (see page 404) is highly effective for people who have angina and coronary artery disease. It can improve exercise tolerance, relieve symptoms, and decrease the number or dose of drugs needed. CABG is most likely to benefit people who have severe angina that is not relieved by drug therapy, a normally functioning heart, no previous heart attacks, and no other conditions that would make surgery hazardous (such as chronic obstructive pulmonary disease). For such people, CABG that is not done on an emergency basis carries a risk of death of 1% or less and a risk of heart damage (such as a heart attack) during surgery of less than 5%. About 85% of people have complete or dramatic relief of symptoms after surgery.

Acute Coronary Syndromes

Acute coronary syndromes result from a sudden blockage in a coronary artery. This blockage causes unstable angina or heart attack (myocardial infarction) depending on the location and amount of blockage.

- People who experience an acute coronary syndrome usually have chest pressure or ache, shortness of breath, and fatigue.
- People who think they are experiencing an acute coronary syndrome should call for emergency help and then chew an aspirin tablet.
- Doctors use electrocardiography and measure substances in the blood to determine whether a person is experiencing an acute coronary syndrome.
- Treatment varies depending on the type of syndrome but usually includes attempts to increase blood flow to affected areas of the heart.

In the United States, more than 1.5 million people have a heart attack each year. About 400,000 to 500,000 of them die, half before they reach the hospital. Almost all of them have underlying coronary artery disease and about two thirds of them are men.

Causes

An acute coronary syndrome occurs when a sudden blockage in a coronary artery greatly reduces or cuts off the blood supply to an area of the heart muscle (myocardium). The lack of blood supply to any tissue is termed ischemia. If the supply is greatly reduced or cut off for more than a few minutes, heart tissue dies. A heart attack, also termed myocardial infarction (MI), is death of heart tissue from ischemia.

A blood clot is the most common cause of a blocked coronary artery. Usually, the artery is already partially narrowed by atheromas. An atheroma may rupture or tear, which releases substances that make platelets stickier, encouraging clots to form. In about 2/3 of people, the blood clot dissolves on its own, typically within a day or so. However, by this time, some heart damage has usually occurred.

Uncommonly, a heart attack results when a clot forms in the heart itself, breaks away, and lodges in a coronary artery. Another uncommon cause is a spasm of a coronary artery that stops blood flow. Spasms may be caused by drugs such as cocaine. Sometimes the cause is unknown.

Classification: Doctors classify acute coronary syndromes based on an electrocardiogram (ECG) and on the presence of substances in the blood (serum markers) released by the damaged heart. The classification is important because treatments differ depending on the specific acute coronary syndrome. The classification consists of unstable angina and two types of heart attack.

- **Unstable angina** is a change in the pattern of angina symptoms (see page 407), including prolonged or worsening angina and new onset of severe angina symptoms. People who have unstable angina do not have signs of heart attack on their ECG or blood tests.
- **Non-ST-segment elevation MI** is a heart attack that doctors can identify by blood tests but that does not produce typical changes (ST-segment elevation) on an ECG.
- **ST-segment elevation MI** is a heart attack that doctors can identify by blood tests and also produces typical changes on an ECG.

Symptoms

Symptoms of the acute coronary syndromes are similar, and it is usually impossible to distinguish the syndromes based on symptoms alone. Symptoms of unstable angina are the same as those of angina pectoris, intermittent pressure, or an ache beneath the breastbone (sternum). However, in people with unstable angina, the pattern changes. People experience more frequent or more severe episodes of angina, or episodes occur at rest or after less physical exertion. About two of three people who have heart attacks experience unstable angina, shortness of breath, or fatigue a few days or weeks beforehand. Such a change in the pattern of chest pain discomfort may culminate in a heart attack.

Usually, the most recognizable symptom of a heart attack is pain in the middle of the chest that may spread to the back, jaw, or left arm. Less often, the pain spreads to the right arm. The pain may occur in one or more of these places and not in the chest at all. The pain of a heart attack is similar to the pain of angina but is generally more severe, lasts

longer, and is not relieved by rest or nitroglycerin. Less often, pain is felt in the abdomen, where it may be mistaken for indigestion, especially because belching may bring partial or temporary relief. For unknown reasons, women often have different, less identifiable symptoms.

About one third of people who have a heart attack do not have chest pain. Such people are more likely to be women, people who are not white, those who are older than 75, those who have heart failure or diabetes, and those who have had a stroke.

Other symptoms include a feeling of faintness or actually fainting, sudden heavy sweating, nausea, shortness of breath, and a heavy pounding of the heart (palpitations).

During a heart attack, a person may become restless, sweaty, and anxious and may experience a sense of impending doom. The lips, hands, or feet may turn slightly blue.

 Did You Know...
About one third of people who have a heart attack do not have chest pain.

Older people may have unusual symptoms. In many, the most obvious symptom is breathlessness. Symptoms may resemble those of a stomach upset or a stroke. Older people may become disoriented. Nonetheless, about two thirds of older people have chest pain, as do younger people. Older people, especially women, often take longer than younger people to admit they are ill or to seek medical help.

Despite all the possible symptoms, as many as one of five people who have a heart attack have only mild symptoms or none at all. Such a silent heart attack may be recognized only when ECG is routinely done some time afterward.

During the early hours of a heart attack, heart murmurs and other abnormal heart sounds may be heard through a stethoscope.

Complications

The complications of acute coronary syndromes depend on how much, how long, and where a coronary artery is blocked. If the blockage affects a large amount of heart muscle, the heart will not pump effectively. If the blockage shuts off blood flow to the electrical system of the heart, the heart rhythm may be affected.

Pumping Problems: In a heart attack, part of the heart muscle dies. Dead tissue, and the scar tissue

DRUGS USED TO TREAT CORONARY ARTERY DISEASE

EXAMPLES	SOME SIDE EFFECTS	COMMENTS
Anticoagulants		
Argatroban Bivalirudin Enoxaparin Fondaparinux Heparin Warfarin	Bleeding, especially when used with other drugs that have a similar effect (such as aspirin and other nonsteroidal anti-inflammatory drugs)	These drugs prevent blood from clotting. They are used to treat people who have unstable angina or who have had a heart attack.
Antiplatelet drugs		
Aspirin Clopidogrel Ticlopidine	Bleeding, especially when used with other drugs that have a similar effect (such as anticoagulants) With aspirin, stomach irritation With ticlopidine and less so with clopidogrel, a small risk of reducing the white blood cell count	These drugs prevent platelets from clumping and blood clots from forming. They also reduce the risk of a heart attack. They are used to treat people who have stable or unstable angina or who have had a heart attack. Aspirin is taken as soon as a heart attack is suspected. People with an allergy to aspirin may take clopidogrel or ticlopidine as an alternative.
Glycoprotein IIb/IIIa inhibitors (a type of antiplatelet drug)		
Abciximab Eptifibatide Tirofiban	Bleeding, especially when used with other drugs that have a similar effect (such as anticoagulants or thrombolytic drugs) Reduction of the platelet count	These drugs prevent platelets from clumping and blood clots from forming. They are used to treat people who have unstable angina or who are undergoing percutaneous coronary intervention after a heart attack.
Beta-blockers		
Acebutolol Atenolol Betaxolol Bisoprolol Carteolol Carvedilol Celiprolol Metoprolol Nadolol Penbutolol Propranolol Timolol	Spasm of airways (bronchospasm) Abnormally slow heart rate (bradycardia) Heart failure Cold hands and feet Insomnia Fatigue Shortness of breath Depression Raynaud's syndrome Vivid dreams Hallucinations Sexual dysfunction With many beta-blockers, an increase in the triglyceride level and a decrease in the HDL level	These drugs reduce the workload of the heart and the risk of a heart attack and sudden death. They are used to treat people who have stable or unstable angina or syndrome X or who have had a heart attack.
Calcium channel blockers		
Amlodipine Diltiazem Felodipine Nifedipine (sustained-release only) Verapamil	Dizziness Fluid accumulation (edema) in the ankles Flushing Headache Heartburn Enlarged gums Abnormal heart rhythms (arrhythmias) With verapamil, constipation	These drugs prevent blood vessels from narrowing and can reverse artery spasm. Diltiazem and verapamil reduce the heart rate. Calcium channel blockers are used to treat people who have stable angina.

(continued on the following page)

Rx DRUGS USED TO TREAT CORONARY ARTERY DISEASE (*Continued*)

EXAMPLES	SOME SIDE EFFECTS	COMMENTS
Calcium channel blockers (*continued*)		
	With short-acting, but not long-acting, calcium channel blockers, possible increased risk of death due to heart attack, especially in people who have unstable angina or who have had a heart attack recently	
Nitrates		
Isosorbide dinitrate Isosorbide mononitrate Nitroglycerin	Flushing Headache Temporarily fast heart rate (tachycardia)	These drugs relieve angina, prevent episodes of angina, and reduce the risk of a heart attack and sudden death. (However, risk reduction is much less than that with beta-blockers.) They are used to treat people who have stable or unstable angina or syndrome X. For these drugs to remain effective over the long term, people need to go 8 to 12 hours without taking the drug each day.
Opioids		
Morphine	Low blood pressure when a person stands Constipation Nausea Vomiting Confusion (especially in older people)	In people who have had a heart attack, these drugs are used to relieve anxiety and pain if the pain persists despite use of other drugs.
Thrombolytic drugs		
Anistreplase Recombinant tissue plasminogen activator (alteplase) Reteplase Streptokinase Tenecteplase	Bleeding after injuries Rarely, bleeding within the brain (intracerebral hemorrhage)	These drugs dissolve blood clots. They are used to treat people who have had a heart attack.
Angiotensin-converting enzyme (ACE) inhibitors		
Benazepril Captopril Enalapril Fosinopril Lisinopril Moexipril Perindopril Quinapril Ramipril Trandolapril	Cough, usually dry and metallic Rash Rarely, a severe allergic reaction (angioedema) Possibly worsening of kidney function when people already have kidney disease or when the artery to one of the kidneys is greatly narrowed	These drugs lower blood pressure and treat heart failure and prevent kidney damage in people with high blood pressure or diabetes. They also benefit people who have had heart attacks. People who have high blood pressure, heart failure, or prior heart attacks and who are treated with an ACE inhibitor live longer than people who do not take an ACE inhibitor.
Angiotensin II receptor blockers		
Candesartan Irbesartan Losartan Telmisartan Valsartan	Similar to ACE inhibitors, but cough is much less common	These drugs have equivalent effects and benefits to those of ACE inhibitors. In people with severe high blood pressure or heart failure, these drugs may be used in combination with an ACE inhibitor.

(continued on the following page)

℞ DRUGS USED TO TREAT CORONARY ARTERY DISEASE (*Continued*)

EXAMPLES	SOME SIDE EFFECTS	COMMENTS
Statins*		
Atorvastatin Fluvastatin Lovastatin Pravastatin Simvastatin Rosuvastatin	Occasionally, muscle aches and pains, but rarely severe muscle pain (myositis) Rarely, liver damage, but not more commonly than in people who are not taking the drug	These drugs lower cholesterol levels and help heal damaged arteries, decreasing the chance of having a first or repeated heart attack or stroke.

*Also known as hydroxymethylglutaryl-CoA (HMG-CoA) reductase inhibitors.
HDL = high-density lipoprotein.

that eventually replaces it, does not contract. The scar tissue sometimes even expands or bulges when the rest of the heart contracts. Consequently, there is less muscle to pump blood. If enough muscle dies, the heart's pumping ability may be so reduced that the heart cannot meet the body's need for blood and oxygen. Heart failure, low blood pressure, or both develop. If more than half of the heart tissue is damaged or dies, the heart generally cannot function, and severe disability or death is likely.

Drugs such as beta-blockers and especially angiotensin-converting enzyme (ACE) inhibitors can reduce the extent of the abnormal areas by reducing the workload of and the stress on the heart. Thus, these drugs help the heart maintain its shape and function more normally.

The damaged heart may enlarge, partly to compensate for the decrease in pumping ability (a larger heart beats more forcefully). Enlargement of the heart makes abnormal heart rhythms more likely.

Rhythm Problems: Abnormal heart rhythms (arrhythmias) occur in more than 90% of people who have had a heart attack. These abnormal rhythms may occur because the heart attack damaged part of the heart's electrical system. Sometimes there is a problem with the part of the heart that triggers the heartbeat, so heart rate may be too slow. Other problems can cause the heart to beat rapidly or irregularly. Sometimes the signal to beat is not conducted from one part of the heart to the other, and the heartbeat may slow or stop.

In addition, areas of heart muscle that have poor blood flow but that have not died can be very irritable. This irritability can cause heart rhythm problems, such as ventricular tachycardia or ventricular fibrillation. These rhythm problems greatly interfere with the heart's pumping ability and may cause the heart to stop beating (cardiac arrest). A loss of consciousness or death can result. These rhythm disturbances are a particular problem in people who have an imbalance in blood chemicals, such as a low potassium level.

Other Problems: Pericarditis (inflammation of the membranes enveloping the heart) may develop in the first day or two after a heart attack or about 10 days to 2 months later. People seldom notice symptoms of early developing pericarditis, because their heart attack symptoms are more prominent. However, pericarditis produces a scratchy rhythmic sound that can sometimes be heard through a stethoscope 2 to 3 days after a heart attack. Later developing pericarditis is usually called Dressler's (post-myocardial infarction) syndrome. This syndrome causes fever, pericardial effusion (extra fluid in the space between the two layers of the pericardium), pleurisy (inflammation of the pleura, which are the membranes covering the lungs), pleural effusion (extra fluid in the space between the two layers of the pleura), and joint pain.

Other complications after a heart attack include rupture of the heart muscle, a bulge in the wall of the ventricle (ventricular aneurysm), blood clots (emboli), and low blood pressure (hypotension). Nervousness and depression are common after a heart attack. Depression after a heart attack may be significant and may persist.

Diagnosis

Whenever a man over age 35 or a woman over age 40 reports chest pain, doctors usually consider the possibility of an acute coronary syndrome. But several other conditions can produce similar pain: pneumonia, a blood clot in the lung (pulmonary embolism), pericarditis, a rib fracture, spasm of the

Complications of a Heart Attack

A person who has a heart attack may experience any of the following complications:

- Rupture of the heart muscle (myocardial rupture)
- A bulge in the wall of the ventricle (ventricular aneurysm)
- Blood clots
- Heart failure (see page 352)
- Low blood pressure (hypotension—see page 343)
- Abnormal heart rhythms (see page 366), particularly originating in the ventricles (ventricular arrhythmias)
- Shock (see page 350)
- Inflammation of the two-layered sac that envelops the heart (pericarditis—see page 390)

Myocardial Rupture

Rarely, the heart muscle ruptures under the pressure of the heart's pumping action because the damaged heart muscle is weak. Rupture usually occurs 1 to 10 days after a heart attack and is more common among women. The wall separating the two ventricles (septum), the external heart wall, and the muscles that open and close the mitral valve are particularly susceptible to rupture during or after a heart attack.

Rupture of the septum results in too much blood being diverted to the lungs, causing accumulation of fluid (pulmonary edema). A rupture of the septum can sometimes be repaired surgically.

Rupture of the external wall almost always causes rapid death. Doctors rarely have time to attempt surgery, and even then, surgery is rarely successful.

If the mitral valve muscles rupture, the valve cannot function—the result is sudden and severe heart failure. Doctors can sometimes repair the damage surgically.

Ventricular Aneurysm

The damaged muscle may form a thin bulge (aneurysm) on the wall of the ventricle. Doctors may suspect an aneurysm based on abnormal results of electrocardiography (ECG), but echocardiography is done to be sure. These aneurysms may cause episodes of abnormal heart rhythms and may reduce the heart's pumping ability. Because blood flows more slowly through aneurysms, blood clots can form in the heart's chambers. If heart failure or abnormal heart rhythms develop, the aneurysm may be removed surgically.

Blood Clots

In about 20% of people who have had a heart attack, clots form inside the heart, over the area of dead heart muscle. In about 10% of these people, parts of the clots break off, travel through the bloodstream, and lodge in smaller blood vessels throughout the body. They may block the blood supply to part of the brain (causing a stroke) or to other organs. Echocardiography may be done to detect clots forming in the heart or to determine whether a person has factors that make clots more likely to form. For example, an area of the left ventricle may not be beating as well as it should. For people who have clots and those at risk of clots, doctors often prescribe anticoagulants such as heparin and warfarin. Heparin is given intravenously in the hospital for at least 2 days. Then, warfarin is given by mouth for 3 to 6 months. If the heart attack was massive or if areas of the heart are not beating well, warfarin is continued indefinitely. Aspirin also is taken indefinitely.

---

esophagus, indigestion, or chest muscle tenderness after injury or exertion.

ECG (see page 326) and certain blood tests can usually confirm the diagnosis within a few hours.

ECG is the most important initial diagnostic procedure when doctors suspect an acute coronary syndrome. This procedure provides a graphic representation of the electrical current producing each heartbeat. In many instances, it immediately shows that a person is having a heart attack. Abnormalities detected by ECG help doctors determine the type of treatment needed. The abnormalities on ECG also help show where the heart muscle was damaged. If a person has had previous heart problems, which can alter the ECG, the most recent damage may be harder for doctors to detect. Such people should carry a small copy of their ECG in their wallets, so that if they have symptoms of an acute coronary syndrome, doctors can compare the previous ECG with the current ECG. If a few ECGs recorded over several hours are completely normal, doctors consider a heart attack unlikely.

Measuring levels of certain substances (called cardiac markers) in the blood also helps doctors diagnose acute coronary syndromes. These substances are normally found in heart muscle but are released into the bloodstream only when heart muscle is damaged or dead. Most commonly measured are a heart muscle proteins called troponin I and troponin T and an enzyme called CK-MB (creatinine kinase, muscle and brain subunits). Levels in the blood are elevated within 6 hours of a heart attack and remain elevated for 36 to 48 hours. Levels of cardiac markers are usually measured when the person is admitted to the hospital and at 6- to 8-hour intervals for the next 24 hours.

When ECG and serum marker measurements do not provide enough information, echocardiography or radionuclide imaging may be done. Echocardiography may show reduced motion in part of the wall of the left ventricle (the heart chamber that pumps blood to the body). This finding suggests damage due to a heart attack.

Dressler's syndrome (pericarditis that develops 10 days to 2 months after a heart attack) is diagnosed based on the symptoms it produces and on the time it occurs.

Other Testing: Other tests may be done during or shortly after hospitalization. These tests are used to determine whether a person needs additional treatment or is likely to have more heart problems. For instance, a person may have to wear a Holter monitor, which records the heart's electrical activity for 24 hours (see box on page 327). This procedure enables doctors to detect whether the person has abnormal heart rhythms (arrhythmias) or episodes of inadequate blood supply without symptoms (silent ischemia). An exercise stress test (electrocardiography done during exercise—see page 326) before or shortly after discharge can help determine how well the person is doing after the heart attack and whether ischemia is continuing. If these procedures detect abnormal heart rhythms or ischemia, drug therapy may be recommended. If ischemia persists, doctors may recommend coronary angiography to evaluate the possibility of doing percutaneous coronary intervention or bypass grafting to restore blood flow to the heart.

Prognosis

Many people who have unstable angina go on to have a heart attack within about 3 months.

Most people who survive for a few days after a heart attack can expect a full recovery, but about 10% die within a year. Most deaths occur in the first 3 or 4 months, typically in people who continue to have angina, abnormal heart rhythms originating in the ventricles (ventricular arrhythmias), and heart failure. The prognosis is worse if the heart has enlarged after a heart attack than if heart size remains normal. Older people are more likely to die after a heart attack and to have complications, such as heart failure. The prognosis for smaller people is worse than that for larger people. This finding may help explain why the prognosis for women who have had a heart attack is, on average, worse than that for men. Women also tend to be older and to have more serious disorders when they have a heart attack. Also, they tend to wait longer after a heart attack to go to the hospital than do men.

Prevention

Taking one baby aspirin, one half of an adult aspirin, or one full adult aspirin daily after a heart attack is recommended. Because aspirin prevents platelets from forming clots, it reduces the risk of death and the risk of a second heart attack by 15 to 30%. People who have not yet had a heart attack or stroke who are over 50 years of age and have 2 or more risk factors (see page 402) should take low-dose aspirin every day to prevent heart attacks and stroke. People with an allergy to aspirin may take clopidogrel or ticlopidine instead.

Usually, doctors also prescribe a beta-blocker (such as metoprolol, propranolol, or timolol) because these drugs reduce the risk of death by about 25%. The more serious the heart attack, the more benefit beta-blockers provide. However, some people cannot tolerate the side effects (such as wheezing, tiredness, and cold limbs), and not everyone benefits.

Taking lipid-lowering drugs and modifying diet will reduce the risk of death after a heart attack. People at high risk (especially obese people with diabetes) who have not yet had a heart attack or stroke may benefit from lipid-lowering drugs.

Angiotensin-converting enzyme (ACE) inhibitors, such as captopril, enalapril, lisinopril, and ramipril, are often prescribed after a heart attack. They help prevent death and the development of heart failure, particularly in people who have had a massive heart attack or who have heart failure.

People should also make changes in their lifestyle. They should eat a low-fat diet and increase the amount of exercise they get. People who have high blood pressure of diabetes should try to keep those disorders under control. People who smoke should quit.

Treatment

Acute coronary syndromes are medical emergencies. Half of deaths due to a heart attack occur in the first 3 or 4 hours after symptoms begin. The sooner treatment begins, the better the chances of survival. Anyone having symptoms that might indicate an acute coronary syndrome should obtain prompt medical attention. Prompt transportation to a hospital's emergency department by an ambulance with trained personnel may save the person's life. Trying to contact the person's doctor, relatives, friends, or neighbors is a dangerous waste of time.

People who may be having a heart attack are usually admitted to a hospital that has a cardiac care unit. Heart rhythm, blood pressure, and the amount of oxygen in the blood are closely monitored so that heart damage can be assessed. Nurses in these units are specially trained to care for people with heart problems and to handle heart emergencies.

If no complications occur during the first few days, most people can safely leave the hospital within a few more days. If complications such as abnormal heart rhythms develop or the heart can no longer pump adequately, hospitalization can be prolonged.

Drug Treatment: People who think they may be having a heart attack should chew an aspirin tablet immediately after calling an ambulance. If aspirin is not taken at home or given by emergency personnel, it is immediately given at the hospital. This therapy improves the chances of survival by reducing the size of the clot (if present) in the coronary artery. People with an allergy to aspirin may be given clopidogrel or ticlopidine instead. Some people are given both aspirin and clopidogrel.

Because decreasing the heart's workload also helps limit tissue damage, a beta-blocker is usually given to slow the heart rate. Slowing the rate enables the heart to work less hard and reduces the area of damaged tissue.

Most people are also given an anticoagulant drug, such as heparin, to help prevent the formation of additional blood clots.

Often, oxygen is given through nasal prongs or a face mask. Providing more oxygen to the heart helps keep heart tissue damage to a minimum.

Because most people who have had a heart attack are experiencing severe discomfort and anxiety, morphine is often used. This drug has a calming effect and reduces the workload of the heart. Most people are given nitroglycerin, which relieves pain by reducing the workload of the heart and possibly by dilating arteries. Usually, it is first given under the tongue, then intravenously.

ACE inhibitors (see page 342) can reduce heart enlargement and increase the chance of survival for many people. Therefore, these drugs are usually given in the first few days after a heart attack and prescribed indefinitely.

Opening the Arteries: The decision on the timing and method of opening a blocked coronary artery depends on the type of acute coronary syndrome and on how quickly the person got to the hospital.

In people who have an ST-segment elevation MI, immediately clearing the coronary artery blockage saves heart tissue and improves survival. Doctors try to clear the blockage within 90 minutes after the person arrives at the hospital. Because the sooner the artery is cleared the better the outcome, the method of clearing is probably not as important as the timing. If available within 90 minutes, percutaneous cardiac interventions (PCI) such as angioplasty and stent placement (see page 404) appear to be the best way to open blocked arteries during an ST-segment elevation MI. If these procedures are not available within that time frame, doctors give clot-dissolving (thrombolytic, or fibrinolytic) drugs intravenously to open the arteries. Thrombolytic drugs include streptokinase, tenecteplase (TNK-tPA), recombinant tissue plasminogen activator (alteplase), and reteplase. Although better if given immediately, these drugs can work well within 3 hours and may be of some benefit for up to 12 hours after arriving at the hospital. In some areas, thrombolytic drugs are given before hospital arrival by specially trained paramedics. Most people who are given a thrombolytic drug still need to have PCI before they leave the hospital.

Because thrombolytic drugs can cause bleeding, they are not usually given to people who have bleeding in the digestive tract, who have severe high blood pressure, who have recently had a stroke, or who have had surgery during the month before the heart attack. Older people who do not have any of these conditions can be safely given a thrombolytic drug.

People who have a non-ST-segment elevation MI or unstable angina do not usually benefit from immediate PCI or thrombolytic drugs. However, doctors usually do PCI within the first day or two of hospitalization. If the person's symptoms worsen or certain complications develop, doctors may do PCI earlier.

In some people, coronary artery bypass grafting (CABG—see page 404) is done during an acute coronary syndrome instead of using PCI or a thrombolytic drug. For example, CABG may be used for people who cannot be given a thrombolytic drug (for example, because they have a bleeding disorder or have had a recent stroke or recent major surgery). CABG may also be used for those who cannot undergo PCI because of the severity of their arterial disease (for example, because two or three arteries are blocked, the blockage is severe, or heart function is poor, especially if the person also has diabetes).

General Measures: Because physical exertion, emotional distress, and excitement stress the heart and make it work harder, a person who has just had a heart attack should stay in bed in a quiet room for a few days. Visitors are usually limited to family members and close friends. Watching television may be permitted if the programs do not cause stress.

Smoking, a major risk factor for coronary artery disease, is prohibited in hospitals. Moreover, an acute coronary syndrome is a compelling reason to stop smoking.

Stool softeners and gentle laxatives may be used to prevent constipation, so that the person does not have to strain. If the person cannot pass urine or if the doctors and nurses need to keep track of the precise amount of urine produced, a urinary catheter is used.

For severe nervousness (which can stress the heart), a mild antianxiety drug (for example, a benzodiazepine such as lorazepam) may be prescribed. To deal with mild depression and denial of illness, which are common after acute coronary syndromes, people are encouraged to talk about their feelings with doctors, nurses, social workers, and their family members and friends. Some people require an antidepressant.

Discharge: After about 3 to 4 days in the hospital, people who have had an uncomplicated heart attack and successful PCI are usually discharged. Other people may require a longer stay.

Nitroglycerin, aspirin and sometimes clopidogrel, a beta-blocker, an ACE inhibitor, and a lipid-lowering drug (most often, a statin—see table on page 967) are usually prescribed.

People who develop Dressler's syndrome are usually given aspirin. Even with treatment, the syndrome can recur. If Dressler's syndrome is severe, a corticosteroid or a nonsteroidal anti-inflammatory drug other than

aspirin (such as ibuprofen) may be needed for a short time.

Rehabilitation: Cardiac rehabilitation, an important part of recovery, begins in the hospital. Remaining in bed for longer than 2 or 3 days leads to physical deconditioning and sometimes to depression and a sense of helplessness. Barring complications, people who have had a heart attack can usually progress to sitting in a chair, passive exercise, use of a commode chair, and reading on the first day. By the second or third day, people are encouraged to walk to the bathroom and engage in nonstressful activities, and they can do more activities each day (see page 52). If everything goes well, people are usually back to their normal activities within about 6 weeks. Participation in a regular exercise program consistent with the person's age and heart health is beneficial.

CHAPTER

66   Peripheral Arterial Disease

Peripheral arterial disease results in reduced blood flow in the arteries of the trunk, arms, and legs.

Most often, doctors use the term peripheral arterial disease to describe poor circulation in the arteries of the legs that results from atherosclerosis. However, peripheral arterial disease can affect other arteries and can have other causes. Disorders affecting arteries that supply the brain are considered separately as cerebrovascular disease.

Peripheral arterial disease may be described as occlusive or functional. Occlusive peripheral arterial disease is due to structural changes that narrow or block arteries. Functional peripheral arterial disease is usually due to a sudden temporary narrowing (spasm) or, rarely, to a widening (vasodilation) of arteries.

Occlusive Peripheral Arterial Disease

- Occlusive peripheral arterial disease often results from atherosclerosis.
- Symptoms depend on which artery is blocked and how severe the blockage is.
- To make a diagnosis, doctors measure blood flow to affected areas.
- Drugs, angioplasty, or surgery is used to relieve the blockage and reduce symptoms.

Occlusive peripheral arterial disease is common among older people because it often results from

atherosclerosis, which becomes more common with aging. Occlusive peripheral arterial disease may affect 15 to 20% of people older than 70. The disease is particularly common among people who have ever smoked regularly and among those who have diabetes, whether type 1 or type 2 (see page 1005).

Occlusive peripheral arterial disease is also common among men and among

- People who have a family history of atherosclerosis, high blood pressure, high cholesterol levels, or high homocysteine levels
- People who are obese
- People who are physically inactive

Each of these factors contributes not only to the development of occlusive peripheral arterial disease but also to the worsening of the disease.

Occlusive peripheral arterial disease may result from gradual narrowing or sudden blockage of an artery. When an artery narrows, the parts of the body it supplies may not receive enough blood. An inadequate blood supply is called ischemia. Ischemia may develop suddenly or gradually. When an artery is suddenly or completely blocked, the tissue it supplies may die.

Gradual narrowing of arteries is usually due to atherosclerosis, in which deposits of cholesterol and other fatty materials (atheromas or atherosclerotic plaques) develop in the walls of arteries. Atheromas may gradually narrow the interior (lumen) of the artery and reduce blood flow (see art on page 397). Calcium may accumulate in the atheromas, making the arteries stiff.

Less commonly, arteries are gradually narrowed by an abnormal growth of muscle in the artery's wall (fibromuscular dysplasia), inflammation (vasculitis), or pressure from an expanding mass, such as a tumor or fluid-filled sac (cyst), outside the artery.

Sudden, complete blockage may result when a blood clot (thrombus) forms in an artery that is already narrowed. A sudden blockage may also result when a clot breaks off (becoming an embolus) from a site such as the heart or aorta, travels through the bloodstream, and lodges in an artery downstream. Some disorders increase the risk of blood clot formation. They include atrial fibrillation, other heart disorders, clotting disorders, and inflammation of blood vessels (vasculitis), which may be due to an autoimmune disorder.

Sometimes a piece of fatty material breaks off from an atheroma and suddenly blocks an artery. Sudden blockage may also result from an aortic dissection (see page 431), in which the inner layer of the aorta tears, allowing blood to surge through the tear into the middle layer. As the dissection enlarges, it can block one or more arteries connected to the aorta.

Obstructive peripheral arterial disease may also be caused by the thoracic outlet syndrome (see page 823). In this syndrome, blood vessels (as well as nerves) in the passageway between the neck and the arm become compressed.

Obstructive peripheral arterial disease can affect arteries in different parts of the body. It commonly develops in the arteries of the legs, including the main arteries of the thighs (femoral arteries), of the knees (popliteal arteries), and of the calves (tibial and peroneal arteries). Much less commonly, the disease develops in the arteries of the shoulders or arms. It may develop in the part of the aorta that passes through the abdomen (abdominal aorta) or in its branches, including the lower aorta where it divides into two branches that supply blood to the legs (common iliac arteries). The branches that supply the kidneys (renal arteries) are a relatively common site of gradual narrowing due to atherosclerosis. But sudden, complete blockage of one of the renal arteries is relatively rare. The branch that supplies the intestines (superior mesenteric artery) is also blocked less commonly. Blockage of the branches that supply the liver (hepatic artery) and spleen (splenic artery) is very rare.

Symptoms

Symptoms vary depending on which artery is affected, how completely the artery is blocked, and whether the artery is gradually narrowed or suddenly blocked. Usually, about 70% of the artery's interior has to be blocked before symptoms occur. Gradual narrowing of an artery may result in less severe symptoms than sudden blockage—even if the artery eventually becomes completely blocked. Symptoms may be less severe because gradual narrowing allows time for nearby blood vessels to expand or new blood vessels (called collateral vessels) to grow. Thus, the affected tissue can still be supplied with blood. If an artery is suddenly blocked, there is no time for collateral vessels to develop, so symptoms are usually severe.

Arteries of the Legs and Arms: Sudden, complete blockage of an artery in a leg or an arm may cause severe pain, coldness, and numbness in the affected limb. The person's leg or arm is either pale or bluish (cyanotic). No pulse can be felt below the blockage. The sudden, drastic decrease in blood flow to the limb is a medical emergency. The absence of blood flow can quickly result in loss of sensation in or paralysis of a limb.

Intermittent claudication, the most common symptom of peripheral arterial disease, results from gradual narrowing of a leg artery. It is a painful, aching, cramping, or tired feeling in the muscles of the leg—not in the joints. Intermittent claudication occurs regularly and predictably during physical activity but is always relieved promptly by rest. The muscles ache when a person walks, and the pain begins more quickly and is more severe when the person walks quickly or uphill. Usually, after 1 to 5 minutes of rest (sitting is not necessary), the person can walk the same distance already covered, although continued walking will again provoke the pain at a comparable distance. Most commonly, the pain occurs in the calf, but it can also occur in the thigh, hip, or buttock, depending on the location of the blockage. Very rarely, pain occurs in the foot.

As a leg artery is narrowed further, the distance a person can walk without pain decreases. Eventually, as the disease becomes very severe, leg muscles may ache even at rest, especially when the person is lying down. Such pain usually begins in the lower leg or front of the foot, is severe and unrelenting, and worsens when the leg is elevated. The pain often interferes with sleep. For relief, the person may hang the feet over the side of the bed or rest sitting up with the legs hanging down.

Large blockages of the arm arteries, which are rare, may cause fatigue, cramping, or pain felt in the arm muscles when the arm is used repeatedly.

When the blood supply is only mildly or moderately reduced, the leg or arm may look almost normal. When the blood supply to a foot is severely reduced, the foot may be cold. The skin of the foot or leg may be dry, scaly, shiny, or cracked. Nails may not grow normally, and the hair on the limb may not grow. As the artery is narrowed further, a person may develop sores that do not easily heal, typically on the toes or heel and occasionally on the lower leg, especially after an injury. Infections occur easily and become serious quickly. In people with severe occlusive peripheral arterial disease, wounds in the skin may take weeks or months to heal or may not heal. Foot ulcers may develop. Leg muscles usually shrink (atrophy). A large blockage may cause gangrene.

In some people who have had predictable, stable claudication, claudication can suddenly worsen. For example, calf pain that occurs after walking 10 blocks may suddenly occur after walking one block. This change may indicate that a new clot has formed in a leg artery. Such people should be evaluated by a specialist as soon as possible.

Lower Aorta and Common Iliac Arteries: Sudden blockage of the lower aorta where it divides into the common iliac arteries causes both legs to suddenly become painful, pale, and cold. No pulse can be felt in the legs, which may become numb.

Gradual narrowing of the lower aorta or of both common iliac arteries can cause intermittent claudication that affects the buttocks and thighs of both legs. The legs may also feel cold or appear pale, although they usually appear normal. This combination of symptoms is sometimes called Leriche syndrome. Leriche syndrome usually occurs in men and commonly also causes erectile dysfunction.

Renal Arteries: Sudden, complete blockage of one of the renal arteries, which supply the kidneys, may cause a sudden pain in the side, and the urine may become bloody. These symptoms indicate a medical emergency.

Gradual, moderate narrowing of one or both renal arteries may not cause symptoms or affect kidney function. Rarely, more complete narrowing of one or both renal arteries contributes to the development of kidney failure or high blood pressure (a disorder called renovascular hypertension). Less than 5% of people with high blood pressure have renovascular hypertension.

Superior Mesenteric Artery: Sudden, complete blockage of the superior mesenteric artery is a medical emergency. Initially, most people with such a blockage vomit and feel an urgent need to have a bowel movement. They may become seriously ill and have severe abdominal pain because the superior mesenteric artery supplies a large part of the intestine. The abdomen may feel tender when a doctor presses on it, but the severe abdominal pain is usually more prominent than the tenderness, which is widespread and vague. The abdomen may

be slightly swollen (distended). Through a stethoscope, a doctor initially hears fewer bowel sounds in the abdomen than normal. Later, no bowel sounds can be heard. The stool initially contains small amounts of blood but soon looks bloody. Blood pressure falls, and shock may result as gangrene develops in the intestine.

Gradual narrowing of the superior mesenteric artery typically causes pain about 30 to 60 minutes after each meal, because the intestine requires more blood during digestion. The pain is steady, severe, and usually centered at the navel. This pain makes people afraid to eat, so they may lose considerable weight. Because the blood supply to the intestine is reduced, nutrients may be poorly absorbed into the bloodstream, contributing to the weight loss.

Hepatic and Splenic Arteries: Blockage of the hepatic artery, which supplies the liver, or the splenic artery, which supplies the spleen, is usually not as dangerous as blockage of the major arteries that supply the intestine. However, parts of the liver or spleen may be damaged.

Diagnosis

The diagnosis of occlusive peripheral arterial disease is based on the symptoms and the results of a physical examination. Procedures that directly measure blood pressure or blood flow are also done.

A doctor or nurse assesses each pulse, including those at the armpits, elbows, wrists, groin, and ankles and those behind the knees. The pulse in arteries beyond the blockage may be weak or absent. For example, if doctors suspect a blockage in a leg artery, they check the pulse below a certain point in the leg. (For arteries in which the pulse is inaccessible, such as the renal arteries, procedures that provide images of blood flow are done.) A stethoscope is used to listen for abnormal sounds caused by turbulent blood flow through a narrowed artery (bruits). Doctors examine the skin of the limbs, noting the color and temperature and pressing gently to see how quickly color returns after pressure is removed. These observations can help doctors determine whether circulation is adequate.

Most of the procedures used in the diagnosis of peripheral arterial disease are noninvasive and can be done in a doctor's office or in a hospital on an outpatient basis. Most commonly, a standard blood pressure cuff and a special electronic stethoscope are used to measure the systolic blood pressure in both arms and both legs. If blood pressure in the ankle is lower than that in the arms by a certain amount, blood flow to the legs is inadequate, and occlusive peripheral arterial disease is diagnosed. If doctors suspect a blockage in an arm artery, they measure systolic blood pressure in both arms. Pressure

When the Blood Supply to the Intestine Is Blocked

The superior mesenteric artery supplies a large part of the intestine with blood.
When this artery is blocked, intestinal tissue begins to die.

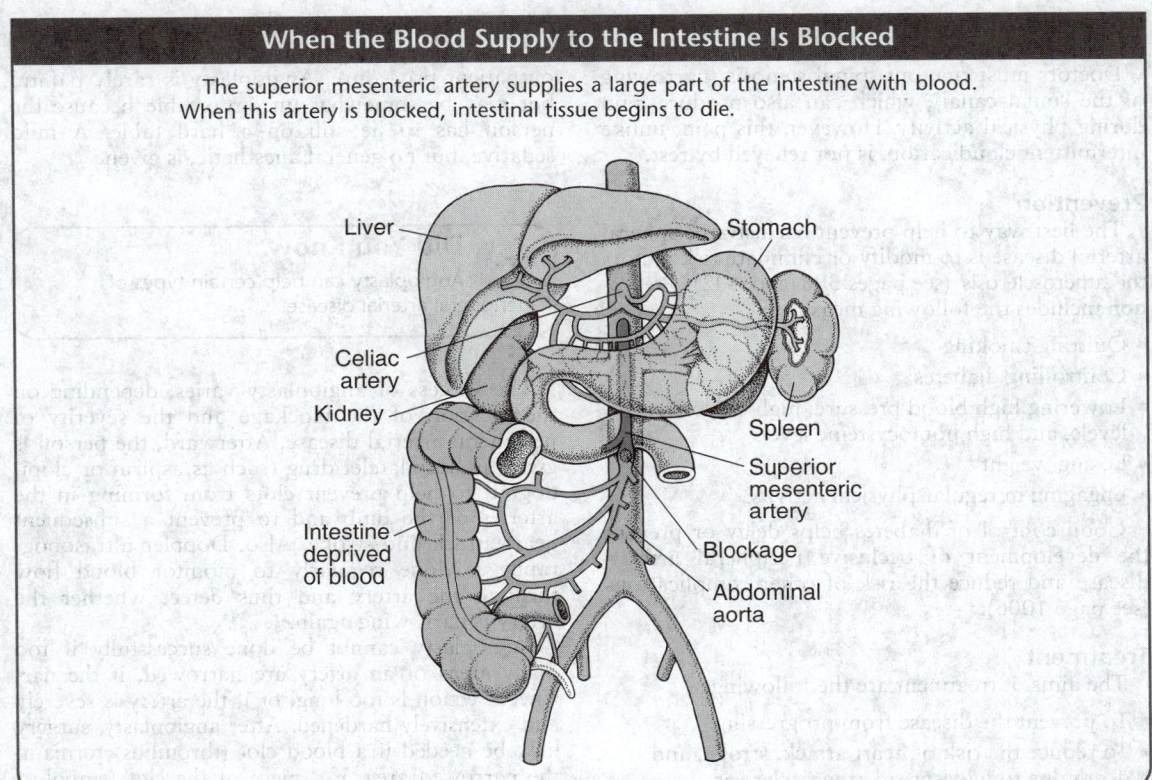

Liver

Stomach

Celiac
artery

Kidney

Spleen

Superior
mesenteric
artery

Intestine
deprived
of blood

Blockage

Abdominal
aorta

that is consistently higher in one arm suggests a blockage in the arm with lower blood pressure, and occlusive peripheral arterial disease is diagnosed.

Doppler ultrasonography (see page 329) can be used to directly measure blood flow and can confirm the diagnosis of occlusive peripheral arterial disease. This procedure can accurately detect narrowing or blockage of blood vessels. Color Doppler is useful because it shows different rates of blood flow in different colors. Doppler ultrasonography to measure blood flow also may be done during exercise stress testing (see page 326), because some problems appear only during exercise. X-rays and other noninvasive procedures (for example, procedures to evaluate blood flow or to measure the amount of oxygen in the blood) may be done.

Usually, angiography (see page 332), an invasive procedure, is done only after the need for surgery or angioplasty has been established. In such cases, its purpose is to provide doctors with clear images of the affected arteries before surgery or angioplasty is done. Rarely, angiography is needed to determine whether surgery or angioplasty is possible. In an-

giography, a radiopaque dye, which can be seen on x-rays, is injected into an artery. The dye outlines the artery. Thus angiography can show the precise diameter of the artery and is more accurate than Doppler ultrasonography in detecting some blockages. At some medical centers, a less invasive type of angiography can be done with helical (spiral) computed tomography (called CT angiography) or with a type of magnetic resonance imaging (called magnetic resonance angiography, or MRA—see page 329).

For people with atherosclerosis, doctors try to identify risk factors, often by doing blood tests to measure levels of cholesterol, sugar (glucose), and, occasionally, homocysteine. Blood pressure is measured on more than one occasion to determine if it is consistently high.

Blood tests also may be done to identify other causes of narrowed or blocked arteries, such as inflammation of blood vessels due to an autoimmune disorder. Such procedures include the erythrocyte sedimentation rate (ESR) and tests for C-reactive protein, which is produced only when inflammation is present. For blockage of an arm artery, doctors try to determine if the cause is atherosclerosis, thoracic outlet syndrome, or arteritis.

Doctors must rule out spinal stenosis (narrowing of the spinal canal), which can also produce pain during physical activity. However, this pain, unlike intermittent claudication, is not relieved by rest.

Prevention

The best way to help prevent occlusive peripheral arterial disease is to modify or eliminate risk factors for atherosclerosis (see pages 398 and 402). Prevention includes the following measures:

- Quitting smoking
- Controlling diabetes
- Lowering high blood pressure, high cholesterol levels, and high homocysteine levels
- Losing weight
- Engaging in regular physical activity

Good control of diabetes helps delay or prevent the development of occlusive peripheral arterial disease and reduce the risk of other complications (see page 1006).

Treatment

The aims of treatment are the following:

- To prevent the disease from progressing
- To reduce the risk of heart attack, stroke, and death due to widespread atherosclerosis
- To prevent amputation
- To improve the quality of life by relieving symptoms (such as intermittent claudication)

Treatments include drugs such as those that relieve claudication and those that cause clots to dissolve (thrombolytic or fibrinolytic drugs—see page 417), angioplasty, surgery, and other measures, such as exercise and foot care. Which treatments are used depends on the severity of the symptoms, the severity and location of the blockage, the risks related to the treatment (particularly for surgery), and the overall health of the person. Regardless of the specific treatments used, people still need to modify risk factors for atherosclerosis to improve their overall prognosis. Angioplasty and surgery are only mechanical measures for correcting the immediate problem. They do not cure the underlying disease.

Angioplasty is often done immediately after angiography. Angioplasty may be done to relieve symptoms and thus postpone or avoid surgery. Sometimes it is used in combination with surgery. Angioplasty consists of inserting a catheter with a balloon at its tip into the narrowed part of the artery and then inflating the balloon to clear the blockage (see page 404). To keep the artery open, doctors may insert a permanent wire mesh (a stent) into the artery. Angioplasty is usually done as an outpatient procedure. Angioplasty is rarely painful but may be somewhat uncomfortable because the person has to lie still on a hard table. A mild sedative, but no general anesthetic, is given.

> ### ? Did You Know...
> Angioplasty can help certain types of peripheral arterial disease.

The success of angioplasty varies, depending on the location of the blockage and the severity of peripheral arterial disease. Afterward, the person is given an antiplatelet drug (such as aspirin or clopidogrel) to help prevent clots from forming in the arteries of the limb and to prevent a subsequent heart attack and stroke. Also, Doppler ultrasonography is done regularly to monitor blood flow through the artery and thus detect whether the artery is narrowing again.

Angioplasty cannot be done successfully if too many areas of an artery are narrowed, if the narrowed section is too long, or if the artery is severely and extensively hardened. After angioplasty, surgery may be needed if a blood clot (thrombus) forms in the narrowed area, if a piece of the clot (embolus) breaks off and blocks an artery downstream, if blood seeps into the lining of the artery causing a bulge inward that blocks blood flow (a disorder called dissection), or if severe bleeding occurs.

Other devices—including lasers, mechanical cutters, ultrasonic catheters, and rotational sanders—can be used instead of a balloon catheter during angioplasty, but none appear to be more effective.

Surgery to remove blood clots (thromboendarterectomy) can be done when thrombolytic drugs are ineffective or too dangerous. Surgery to remove atheromas (endarterectomy) or other blockages may also be done. Alternatively, bypass surgery may be done. In bypass surgery, a graft consisting of a tube made of a synthetic material or a part of a vein from another part of the body is joined to the blocked artery above and below the blockage. Thus, blood is rerouted around the blocked artery. Another approach is to remove the narrowed or blocked section and insert a graft in its place. Usually before surgery, doctors assess heart function and blood flow through the heart to determine the relative safety of surgery, because many people with occlusive peripheral arterial disease also have coronary artery disease.

Arteries of the Legs and Arms: For sudden, complete blockage of these arteries, surgery is done as soon as possible to prevent irreversible loss of limb function or amputation.

For most people with intermittent claudication, exercise or drugs can relieve the pain. Exercise is the most effective treatment and may be appropriate for motivated people who can follow a prescribed daily exercise program. Exactly how exercise relieves claudication is not well understood, but exercise probably improves muscle function. There is no evidence that exercise improves blood flow or causes new (collateral) blood vessels to grow. People with claudication should walk at least 30 minutes a day at least 3 times a week, if possible. For most people, following this routine increases the distance they can walk comfortably. Discomfort felt during walking is not dangerous. When discomfort is felt, a person should stop walking until the discomfort subsides and then walk again. The total walking time (excluding rest periods) must be at least 30 minutes to improve walking distance.

Exercise is usually most effective when it is supervised by a trained therapist in a rehabilitation program. Doctors recommend that people with claudication undergo an exercise stress test (see page 326) before they begin a rehabilitation program to make sure that the blood supply to heart muscle is adequate.

People should minimize exposure to cold, which causes blood vessels to narrow (constrict), and avoid the use of drugs that cause blood vessels to constrict. These drugs include ephedrine or pseudoephedrine, which are components of some sinus congestion and cold remedies.

Pentoxifylline or cilostazol may be used to treat claudication. These drugs may increase blood flow and thus the oxygen supply to muscles. Both drugs must be taken for 2 to 3 months to determine whether they are effective. However, the usefulness of pentoxifylline is now in doubt, and many experts no longer recommend its use. In contrast, cilostazol may result in a 50 to 100% increase in the distance that can be walked without pain. Cilostazol should not be used by people with heart failure.

Aspirin or clopidogrel is usually given because these drugs help prevent clot formation and reduce the risk of heart attack or stroke. They modify platelets so that they do not adhere to blood vessel walls. Normally, platelets, which circulate in the blood, gather and form a clot to stop bleeding when a blood vessel is injured.

Surgery to remove the blockage or bypass surgery may be done if other treatments do not relieve claudication. Surgery is usually done to avoid amputation of a leg when blood flow is greatly reduced—that is, when claudication is incapacitating or occurs during rest, when wounds do not heal, or when gangrene develops.

Bypass Surgery in the Leg

Bypass surgery may be done to treat arteries that are narrowed or blocked. In this procedure, blood is rerouted around the affected artery—for example, around part of the femoral artery in the thigh or part of the popliteal artery in the knee. A graft consisting of a tube made of a synthetic material or part of a vein from another part of the body is joined to the blocked artery above and below the blockage.

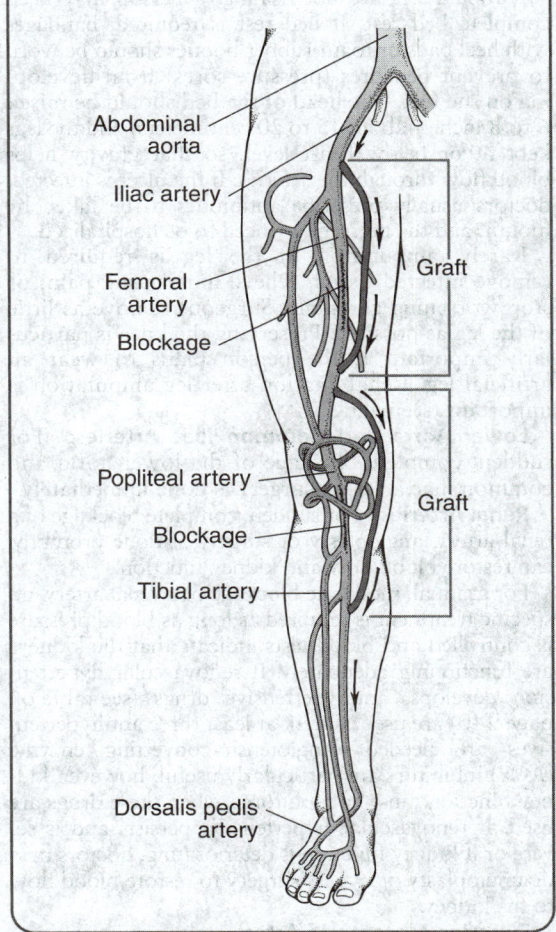

Good foot care is important. It helps prevent wounds or foot ulcers from becoming infected and painful or resulting in gangrene. Good foot care also helps prevent amputation. Foot ulcers require meticulous care. Such care is needed to treat infection, to protect the skin from further damage, and to enable the person to continue to walk.

A foot ulcer must be kept clean: It should be washed daily with a mild soap or antibacterial solution and covered daily with clean, dry dressings. The legs should be kept below the level of the heart to help improve blood flow. People with diabetes must control blood sugar levels as well as possible. As a rule, anyone with poor circulation to the feet or with diabetes should have a doctor check a foot ulcer that is not healing after about 7 days. Often, doctors prescribe an antibiotic ointment.

If foot ulcers are not healing, a person may need complete bed rest. If bed rest is required, bandages with heel pads or foam-rubber booties should be worn to prevent bedsores (pressure sores) from developing on the feet. The head of the bed should be raised 6 to 8 inches (about 15 to 20 centimeters) and the legs kept at or below heart level, so that gravity helps blood flow through the arteries. If the ulcer is infected, doctors usually prescribe antibiotics to be taken by mouth, and the person may need to be hospitalized.

Rarely, amputation of the leg is required to remove infected tissue, relieve unrelenting pain, or stop worsening gangrene. Surgeons remove as little of the leg as possible. Preserving the knee is particularly important if the person plans to wear an artificial leg. Rehabilitation after leg amputation is important (see page 55).

Lower Aorta and Common Iliac Arteries: For sudden, complete blockage of the lower aorta and common iliac arteries, surgery is done immediately.

Renal Arteries: For sudden, complete blockage of a renal artery, angioplasty or surgery, if done promptly, can restore blood flow and kidney function.

For gradual, moderate blockage of a renal artery, no specific treatment is required as long as blood pressure is controlled and blood tests indicate that the kidneys are functioning adequately. If renovascular hypertension develops, antihypertensive drugs (see table on page 340) are used. Often, at least three antihypertensives are needed. Angiotensin-converting enzyme (ACE) inhibitors are particularly useful; however, kidney function must be monitored when these drugs are used. If renovascular hypertension persists and is severe or if kidney function is deteriorating, doctors may do angioplasty or bypass surgery to restore blood flow to the kidney.

Superior Mesenteric Artery: If the superior mesenteric artery is suddenly and completely blocked, only immediate treatment can restore the blood supply fast enough to save the person's life. Often, to save time, doctors send people straight to surgery rather than do diagnostic tests first. During surgery, doctors may remove or bypass the blockage, or they sometimes remove the affected piece of intestine. If the diagnosis of blockage is made by angiography, sometimes doctors can open the blockage during the

---

Caring for the Feet

Foot care is essential for people with peripheral arterial disease of the leg arteries. The following self-care measures and precautions can help:

- Inspect the feet daily for cracks, sores, corns, and calluses.
- Wash the feet daily in lukewarm water with mild soap, and dry them gently and thoroughly.
- Use a lubricant, such as lanolin, for dry skin.
- Use unmedicated powder to keep the feet dry.
- Cut toenails straight across and not too short. (A podiatrist may have to cut the nails. Tell the podiatrist that peripheral arterial disease is present.)
- Have a podiatrist treat corns or calluses.
- Do not use adhesive or harsh chemicals to remove corns or calluses.
- Change socks or stockings daily and shoes often.
- Wear loose wool socks to keep the feet warm.
- Do not wear tight garters or stockings with tight elastic tops.
- Wear shoes that fit well and have wide toe spaces.
- Do not wear open shoes or walk barefoot.
- Ask the podiatrist about a prescription for special shoes if the feet are deformed.
- Do not use hot water bottles or heating pads.
- Do not soak feet in hot water or chemical solutions.

---

angiography procedure by giving clot-dissolving drugs or artery-dilating drugs directly into the artery. This may avoid the need for surgery. Whether a person survives and whether the intestine can be saved depend on how fast the blood supply is restored.

If the superior mesenteric artery has gradually narrowed, nitroglycerin may relieve the abdominal pain, but angioplasty or surgery is needed to widen the artery. Doppler ultrasonography and angiography can determine how narrow the artery is and help doctors decide whether to operate.

Hepatic and Splenic Arteries: Surgery is needed to clear a blockage of the hepatic or splenic artery.

THROMBOANGIITIS OBLITERANS

Thromboangiitis obliterans (Buerger's disease) is inflammation and subsequent blockage of small and medium-sized arteries of the legs or arms.

- Thromboangiitis obliterans commonly develops in smokers.

- Symptoms are those of reduced blood flow to an extremity: coldness, numbness, tingling or a burning sensation.
- Ultrasonography is often used to detect decreased blood flow in the affected extremity.
- Stopping smoking is the most important part of treatment.
- People may also need to take drugs.

Thromboangiitis obliterans is a rare disease that usually develops in smokers, most commonly in men aged 20 to 40. Thromboangiitis obliterans was once considered a man's disease, but it is becoming increasingly common among women who smoke. Now, about 5% of people with the disease are women, perhaps because more women are smoking.

How cigarette smoking relates to thromboangiitis obliterans is poorly understood, and what causes the disease is unknown. One theory is that smoking triggers inflammation and constriction of arteries. However, only a small number of smokers develop thromboangiitis obliterans. Some people may be more susceptible than others for as yet unknown reasons. Nonetheless, thromboangiitis obliterans invariably worsens in people who continue to smoke, and amputation is commonly required. In contrast, if people with thromboangiitis obliterans quit smoking, amputation is rarely required.

Symptoms

Usually, symptoms of a reduced blood supply to the arms or legs—coldness, numbness, tingling, a burning sensation, or pain—develop gradually. These abnormal sensations start at the fingertips or toes and progress up the legs or arms. The legs are affected more often than the arms. People may feel abnormal sensations before their doctor sees any skin changes indicating an inadequate blood supply (ischemia) or gangrene. Raynaud's syndrome (see page 426) and muscle discomfort during exertion (intermittent claudication—see page 419) may develop. Cramps occur in the calf muscles or feet if the legs are affected and in the hands or forearms if the arms are affected.

As the disease progresses, cramps become more painful and last longer. Late in the disease, skin ulcers, gangrene, or both may appear, usually on one or more toes or fingers. The foot or hand feels cold and may turn bluish, probably because blood flow is greatly reduced.

Some patients with this disease also have episodes of inflammation in the veins (migratory phlebitis), usually in the superficial veins.

Diagnosis

Usually, doctors suspect thromboangiitis obliterans on the basis of symptoms and results of the physical examination. In most people, the pulse is weak or absent in one or more arteries of the feet or wrists. Often, the affected hands, feet, fingers, or toes become pale when raised above the heart and red when lowered.

Ultrasonography detects a substantial decrease in blood pressure and blood flow in the affected feet, toes, hands, and fingers. Angiography (see page 332) can detect specific patterns of narrowing and thus can help confirm the diagnosis. Sometimes a biopsy (removal of a tissue sample for examination under a microscope) of the affected artery or referral to a specialist is needed to confirm the diagnosis.

Treatment

A person with thromboangiitis obliterans must stop smoking immediately, or symptoms will relentlessly worsen. Amputation is then likely to become necessary. Exposure to cold, which causes blood vessels to narrow (constrict), and use of certain drugs should be avoided. These drugs include those that cause blood vessels to constrict (such as ephedrine or pseudoephedrine, which are components of some sinus congestion and cold remedies) and those that increase the tendency of blood to clot (such as estrogen). Care should be taken to prevent any injury to the affected limb, including burns and injuries from cold or minor surgery (such as trimming calluses). Corns and calluses should be treated by a podiatrist. Wearing shoes that fit well and have wide toe spaces can help prevent injury to the feet.

For people who quit smoking but still have blocked arteries, doctors sometimes give drugs such as iloprost, which may help prevent amputation. Other drugs, such as pentoxifylline and calcium channel blockers, may be tried to help open blood vessels but are probably not very effective. Surgeons may cut certain nearby nerves (a procedure called sympathectomy) to prevent blood vessels from constricting. These procedures are seldom done, because they usually improve blood flow only temporarily.

Functional Peripheral Arterial Disease

Functional peripheral arterial disease is much less common than occlusive peripheral arterial disease. Normally, the arteries of the arms and legs widen (dilate) and narrow (constrict) in response to changes in the environment, such as a change in temperature. Functional peripheral arterial disease usually occurs when the normal mechanisms that dilate and constrict these arteries are exaggerated. The affected arteries constrict more tightly and more often. These changes in constriction can be caused by an inherited defect in the blood vessels, by disturbances of the nerves that control the dilation and constriction of arteries (sympathetic nervous system), by injuries, or by drugs.

RAYNAUD'S SYNDROME

Raynaud's syndrome is a condition in which small arteries (arterioles), usually in the fingers or toes, constrict more tightly in response to exposure to cold.

- Constriction of small arteries causes fingers (or toes) to become pale or bluish, numb, and tingle.
- Doctors can often make a diagnosis on the basis of the person's symptoms.
- Keeping warm, avoiding smoking, and sometimes taking drugs may help.

Doctors use the term primary Raynaud's syndrome when no cause is apparent. They use the term secondary Raynaud's syndrome when a cause is known. Primary Raynaud's syndrome is much more common then secondary Raynaud's syndrome. Between 60% and 90% of cases of primary Raynaud's syndrome occur in women aged 15 to 40.

Anything that stimulates the sympathetic nervous system, particularly exposure to cold but also strong emotion, can cause arteries to constrict and thus trigger primary Raynaud's syndrome.

Secondary Raynaud's syndrome may be caused by scleroderma, rheumatoid arthritis, atherosclerosis, cryoglobulinemia, an underactive thyroid gland (hypothyroidism), injury, or reactions to certain drugs, such as beta-blockers, clonidine, and the antimigraine drugs ergotamine and methysergide. Use of such drugs, which constrict blood vessels, can also make Raynaud's syndrome worse. Some people with Raynaud's syndrome also have other disorders that occur when arteries are prone to constrict. These disorders include migraine headaches, variant angina, and high blood pressure in the lungs (pulmonary hypertension). The association of Raynaud's syndrome with these disorders suggests that the cause of arterial constriction may be the same in all of them.

Symptoms and Diagnosis

Constriction of small arteries in the fingers and toes begins quickly, most often triggered by exposure to cold. It may last minutes or hours. The fingers and toes become pale or bluish, usually in patches. Only one finger or toe or parts of one or more may be affected. The fingers or toes usually do not hurt, but numbness, tingling, a pins-and-needles sensation, and a burning sensation are common. As the episode ends, the affected areas may be redder than usual or bluish. Rewarming the hands or feet restores normal color and sensation. However, if episodes of Raynaud's syndrome recur and are prolonged (especially in people with scleroderma), the skin of the fingers or toes may become smooth, shiny, and tight. Small painful sores may appear on the tips of the fingers or toes.

Often, no procedures are needed to make the diagnosis. If doctors suspect an artery is blocked, color Doppler ultrasonography (see page 329) may be done before and after the person is exposed to cold. Doctors may also order blood tests to check for conditions that can cause Raynaud's syndrome.

Treatment

People can control mild Raynaud's syndrome by protecting their head, trunk, arms, and legs from cold. For those who experience symptoms when they get excited, mild sedatives or biofeedback may help. People who have the disorder must stop smoking because nicotine constricts blood vessels.

Primary Raynaud's syndrome is commonly treated with a calcium channel blocker (see table on page 341), such as nifedipine, amlodipine, diltiazem, or verapamil. Prazosin may also be effective.

If the disorder becomes progressively disabling and other treatments do not work, certain sympathetic nerves may be temporarily blocked or even cut to relieve the symptoms in a procedure called sympathectomy. However, even when this procedure is effective, relief may last only 1 to 2 years. This procedure is usually more effective for people with primary Raynaud's syndrome than for those with secondary Raynaud's syndrome. For people with secondary Raynaud's syndrome, the disorder causing it is treated.

ACROCYANOSIS

Acrocyanosis is a persistent, painless bluish discoloration of both hands and, less commonly, of both feet, caused by spasm of the small blood vessels within the skin, usually in response to cold.

The disorder usually occurs in women. The fingers and hands or toes and feet tend to feel cold and to be bluish. They sometimes sweat profusely and may swell. Exposure to cold usually intensifies the bluish discoloration, and warming reduces it. The disorder is not painful and does not damage the skin.

Doctors diagnose the disorder based on symptoms that are limited to the person's hands or feet and that persist even though pulses are normal. Treatment is usually unnecessary. Doctors may prescribe drugs that dilate the arteries (such as calcium channel blockers—see table on page 341), but these drugs usually do not help. Usually, reassurance that the bluish skin discoloration does not indicate a serious disorder is all that is necessary.

ERYTHROMELALGIA

Erythromelalgia is a rare syndrome in which arterioles of the skin dilate periodically, causing a burning pain, making the skin feel hot, and making the feet and, less often, the hands turn red.

Usually, the cause of erythromelalgia is unknown. In such cases, the disorder tends to start when people are in their 20s or older. A rare hereditary form of erythromelalgia starts at birth or during childhood. Less commonly, the disorder is related to the use of some drugs, such as nifedipine (an antihypertensive) or bromocriptine (a drug used to treat Parkinson's disease). It also occurs in people who have certain blood disorders (myeloproliferative disorders), high blood pressure, venous insufficiency, diabetes mellitus, systemic lupus erythematosus (lupus), rheumatoid arthritis, lichen sclerosus, gout, spinal cord disorders, or multiple sclerosis. Erythromelalgia usually develops 2 to 3 years before the underlying disorder is diagnosed.

Symptoms include burning pain in the feet or hands, which feel hot and appear red. Attacks are usually triggered by environmental temperatures of over 84° F (over about 29° C). Symptoms may remain mild for years or may progress and become completely incapacitating.

Diagnosis of erythromelalgia is based on the symptoms and the increase in skin temperature. Tests, such as blood cell counts, are usually done to help identify a cause.

Treatment includes resting, elevating the legs or arms, and applying cold packs to the legs or arms or immersing them in cold water. These measures sometimes relieve symptoms or prevent attacks. If no underlying disorder is identified, aspirin or gabapentin may relieve symptoms. However, aspirin does not relieve symptoms for the form that starts at birth or during childhood. If an underlying disorder is identified, treating that disorder may relieve symptoms.

Aneurysms and Aortic Dissection

The aorta, which is about 1 inch (2.5 centimeters) in diameter, is the largest artery of the body. It receives oxygen-rich blood from the left ventricle and distributes it to all of the body except the lungs (which receive blood from the right ventricle). Just after the aorta leaves the heart, smaller arteries that carry blood to the head and arms branch off. The aorta then arches down, with additional smaller arteries branching off along its route from the left ventricle to the lower abdomen at the top of the hipbone (pelvis). At this point, the aorta divides into the two iliac arteries, which supply blood to the legs.

Disorders of the aorta include bulges (aneurysms) in weak areas of its walls and separation of the layers of its wall (dissection). These disorders can be immediately fatal, but they usually take years to develop. Aneurysms may also develop in other arteries.

Aneurysms

An aneurysm is a bulge (dilation) in the wall of an artery, usually the aorta.

The bulge usually occurs in a weak area of the artery's wall. The pressure of blood inside the artery forces the weak area to balloon outward. If untreated, an aneurysm may rupture, resulting in internal bleeding. Consequences depend on the size of the rupture. A large rupture may be rapidly fatal, and a small one (sometimes termed a "leak") may produce warning symptoms that allow people to seek medical care.

Aneurysms can develop anywhere along the aorta. Three fourths of aortic aneurysms develop in the part that passes through the abdomen (the abdominal aorta), and the rest develop in the part that passes through the chest (thoracic aorta). Aneurysms can also develop in the arteries at the back of the knee (popliteal arteries), the main arteries of the thighs (femoral arteries), the arteries supplying the head (carotid arteries), the arteries supplying the brain (cerebral arteries), and the arteries supplying the heart muscle (coronary arteries). In older people, aneurysms are most likely to occur in areas where arteries branch (for example, where the abdominal aorta branches into the iliac arteries) or in areas of stress (for example, in the popliteal artery). Aneurysms may be round (saccular) or tubelike (fusiform). Most are fusiform.

The most common cause of aortic aneurysms is atherosclerosis, which weakens the wall of the aorta. Less common causes include injuries, inflammatory diseases of the aorta (aortitis), hereditary

Where Do Aortic Aneurysms Occur?

Aneurysms can develop anywhere along the aorta. Most develop in the abdominal aorta. The rest develop in the thoracic aorta, most commonly in the ascending aorta.

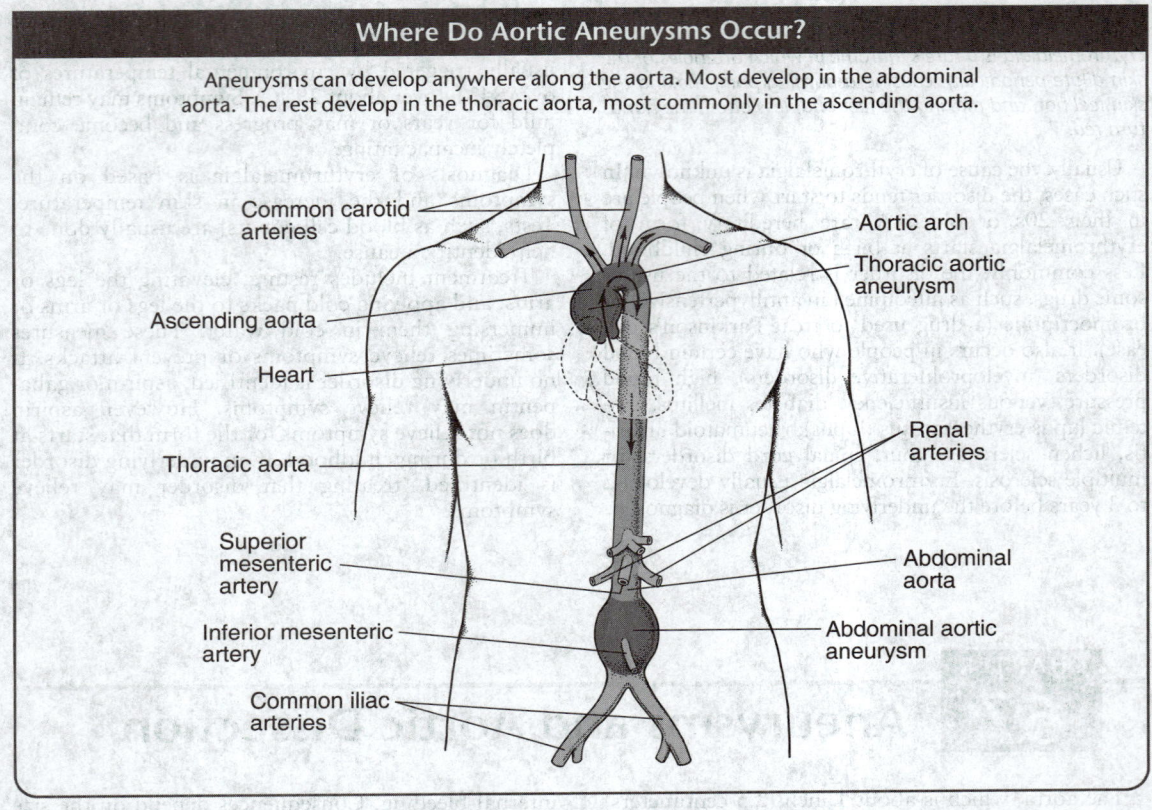

connective tissue disorders such as Marfan syndrome, and some infectious diseases such as syphilis. In people with Marfan syndrome, an aneurysm is most likely to develop in the first part of the aorta, where it emerges from the heart (the ascending aorta). In older people, almost all aneurysms are associated with atherosclerosis. High blood pressure, which is common among older people, and cigarette smoking increase the risk of an aneurysm.

A blood clot (thrombus) often develops in the aneurysm because blood flow inside the aneurysm is sluggish. The clot may extend along the entire wall of the aneurysm. A blood clot may break loose (becoming an embolus), travel through the bloodstream, and block arteries. Aneurysms in the popliteal arteries are more likely to produce emboli than aneurysms in other arteries. Occasionally, calcium is gradually deposited in the wall of an aneurysm.

ABDOMINAL AORTIC ANEURYSMS

Abdominal aortic aneurysms are aneurysms that occur in the part of the aorta that passes through the abdomen (abdominal aorta).

- Aneurysms may cause a pulsing sensation in the abdomen and, when they rupture, cause deep, excruciating pain.
- Doctors often detect an aneurysm during an examination or imaging procedure that is done for another purpose.
- Drugs to lower blood pressure are given, and aneurysms that are large or growing are repaired by either open or endovascular stent-graft surgery.

Abdominal aortic aneurysms may occur at any age but are most common among men aged 50 to 80 years. Abdominal aortic aneurysms may run in families and occur in people who have high blood pressure, especially those who also smoke. About 20% of abdominal aneurysms eventually rupture.

Symptoms

People who have an abdominal aortic aneurysm often have no symptoms, but some people become aware of a pulsing sensation in their abdomen. The aneurysm may cause pain, typically a deep, penetrating pain mainly in the back. The pain can be severe and is usually unrelenting if the aneurysm is leaking.

When an aneurysm ruptures, the first symptom is usually excruciating pain in the lower abdomen and back and tenderness in the area over the aneurysm. If the resulting internal bleeding is severe, a person may rapidly go into shock (see page 350). A ruptured abdominal aortic aneurysm is often fatal.

Did You Know...

Small aneurysms rarely rupture.

A person can live with a small abdominal aortic aneurysm, but doctors recommend treatment once the aneurysm reaches a certain size.

Diagnosis

Pain is a useful but late clue. However, many people with aneurysms have no symptoms and are diagnosed by chance when a routine physical examination or an imaging procedure (such as x-rays or ultrasonography) is done for another reason. Doctors may feel a pulsating mass in the midline of the abdomen. With a stethoscope placed on the middle of the abdomen, doctors can usually hear a whooshing sound (bruit) caused by turbulence as blood rushes past the aneurysm. However, in obese people, even large aneurysms may not be detected. Rapidly enlarging aneurysms that are about to rupture commonly hurt or feel tender when pressed during an abdominal examination.

Occasionally, an abdominal x-ray detects an aneurysm that has calcium deposits in its wall, but this procedure provides little other information. Other procedures are more useful for detecting aneurysms and determining their size. Usually, ultrasonography can clearly show the size of an aneurysm. If an aneurysm is detected, ultrasonography may be repeated every few months to determine if and how quickly the aneurysm is enlarging. Computed tomography (CT) of the abdomen, particularly if done after a radiopaque dye is injected intravenously, can determine the size and shape of an aneurysm more accurately than ultrasonography but exposes the person to radiation. Magnetic resonance imaging (MRI) is also accurate but may not be available as quickly as ultrasonography or CT.

Treatment

Aneurysms that are less than 2 inches (5 centimeters) wide rarely rupture. The only treatments required may be antihypertensive drugs (see table on page 340) to lower blood pressure and smoking cessation. Imaging procedures are done to estimate the rate of enlargement and determine when repair will be necessary. At first, procedures are done every 3 to 6 months, then at various intervals, depending on how quickly the aneurysm is enlarging.

Aneurysms that are wider than about 2 to 2½ inches (5 to 5.5 centimeters) may rupture, so doctors usually recommend surgery, unless surgery is too risky for a particular patient. Surgery consists of inserting a synthetic graft to repair the aneurysm. There are two approaches. With the traditional approach, a general anesthetic is given, and an incision is made from below the breastbone to just below the navel. The graft is stitched into place in the aorta, the walls of the aneurysm are wrapped around the graft, and the incision is closed. This procedure takes 3 to 6 hours, and the hospital stay is usually 5 to 8 days. A newer, less invasive approach is called endovascular stent grafting. A regional (epidural) anesthetic, which causes loss of sensation only from the waist down, is used. Through a small incision made in the groin, a long, thin guide wire is threaded through the femoral artery into the aorta to the aneurysm. A tube (catheter) containing the stent-graft (which resembles a meshed, collapsible straw) is guided over the wire and positioned inside the aneurysm. Then the stent-graft is opened, forming a stable channel for blood flow. This procedure takes 2 to 5 hours, and the hospital stay is usually 2 to 5 days. The risk of death during surgery to insert a graft is about 2 to 5%.

Rupture or threatened rupture of an abdominal aortic aneurysm requires emergency open surgery or placement of an endovascular stent-graft. The risk of death during an emergency repair of a ruptured aneurysm is about 50%. The risk of death may be lower with endovascular stent-graft placement (20 to 30%). When an aneurysm ruptures, the kidneys may be affected because their blood supply is disrupted or because blood loss results in shock. If kidney failure develops after the operation, the chances of survival are very poor. Untreated ruptured abdominal aortic aneurysms are always fatal.

THORACIC AORTIC ANEURYSMS

Thoracic aortic aneurysms are aneurysms in the part of the aorta that passes through the chest (thorax).

- Thoracic artery aneurysms may not cause symptoms, or they may cause pain, coughing, and wheezing.

- If an aneurysm ruptures, people may have excruciating pain that begins high in the back and spreads down the back and into the abdomen.

- Aneurysms are often discovered by chance, but doctors do x-rays, computed tomography, or another imaging procedure to determine the size and precise location.

- Doctors try to repair aneurysms surgically before the aneurysm ruptures.

Thoracic aortic aneurysms are being identified more often than in the past because computed tomography (CT) of the chest to screen for other disorders is used more widely. In a common form of thoracic aortic aneurysm, the walls of the aorta degenerate (a condition called cystic medial necrosis), and the part of the aorta nearest the heart enlarges. This enlargement may cause a malfunction of the valve between the heart and the aorta (aortic valve), allowing blood to leak backward into the heart when the valve is closed. This disorder is called aortic valve regurgitation. About half of the people with this form of aneurysm also have Marfan syndrome. In the other half, no cause is apparent, although many of these people have high blood pressure. Rarely, syphilis causes an aneurysm to form in the part of the aorta nearest the heart. Thoracic aneurysms that develop further away from the heart may result from a blunt injury to the chest.

Symptoms

Thoracic aortic aneurysms may become huge without causing symptoms. When they do occur, symptoms result from the pressure of the enlarging aorta against nearby structures and thus depend on where the aneurysm develops. Typical symptoms are pain (usually high in the back), coughing, and wheezing. Rarely, a person coughs up blood because of pressure on or erosion of the windpipe (trachea) or nearby airways. Swallowing may be difficult if an aneurysm puts pressure on the esophagus, which carries food to the stomach. Hoarseness may result from pressure on the nerve to the voice box (larynx). A group of symptoms called Horner's syndrome (see page 834) may result from pressure on certain nerves in the chest. Symptoms include a constricted pupil, drooping eyelid, and sweating on one side of the face. Abnormal pulsations felt in the chest may indicate a thoracic aortic aneurysm. A displaced windpipe may be seen on chest x-rays.

When a thoracic aortic aneurysm ruptures, excruciating pain usually begins high in the back. It may radiate down the back and into the abdomen as the rupture progresses. The pain may also be felt in the chest and arms, as it is during a heart attack. A person can quickly go into shock (see page 350) and die because of internal bleeding.

Diagnosis

Doctors may diagnose a thoracic aortic aneurysm based on symptoms, or they may discover the aneurysm by chance during a routine physical examination. A chest x-ray taken for another reason may detect an aneurysm. Computed tomography (CT), magnetic resonance imaging (MRI), or transesophageal ultrasonography (in which the ultrasound probe is passed down the throat into the esophagus) is used to determine the precise size of the aneurysm. Aortography or CT angiography (an x-ray procedure or CT scan done after injection of a radiopaque dye that outlines the aneurysm) is usually done to help doctors determine what type of surgery, if any, is needed. Alternatively, magnetic resonance angiography may be done.

Treatment

It is much better to treat a thoracic aortic aneurysm before it ruptures, so once it becomes 2½ inches (5.5 centimeters) wide or larger, open surgical or endovascular stent-graft repair using a synthetic graft is usually done, as for an abdominal aortic aneurysm. Before surgery, a beta-blocker, calcium channel blocker, or another antihypertensive drug (see table on page 340) may be given to reduce the heart rate and blood pressure and thus reduce the risk of a rupture. The hospital stay is 5 to 8 days for traditional surgery (in which the chest in opened) and 2 to 5 days for stent-graft placement (in which a collapsible graft is threaded to the aorta through a small incision, usually in the groin). In people who have Marfan syndrome, a rupture is more likely, so doctors may recommend surgical repair even for smaller aneurysms.

The risk of death is about 5 to 15% during repair of thoracic aortic aneurysms but is about 50% during an operation for a ruptured thoracic aneurysm. Untreated ruptured thoracic aortic aneurysms are always fatal.

ANEURYSMS IN OTHER ARTERIES

Aneurysms may occur in arteries other than the aorta, such as the popliteal arteries (at the back of the knees), the femoral arteries (in the thighs), the coronary arteries (around the heart), and, rarely, the carotid arteries (in the neck). Older people are more likely to have aneurysms in these arteries than are younger people.

Many of these aneurysms result from a weakness present at birth (congenital) or arteriosclerosis. Others result from injuries caused by stab or gunshot wounds or from bacterial or fungal infections in the wall of the artery. Such infections usually start elsewhere in the body, typically in a heart valve (see page 386).

Most popliteal and femoral aneurysms do not produce symptoms. However, blood clots can form within the aneurysm, break loose (becoming emboli), and block an artery in the lower leg or foot. Emboli from carotid aneurysms can block an artery in the brain and cause a stroke. Popliteal, femoral, coronary, and carotid aneurysms rarely rupture.

Doctors may feel a pulsating mass in the affected artery. Ultrasonography or computed tomography (CT) can confirm the diagnosis. For popliteal aneurysms larger than 1 inch (2.5 centimeters) in diameter, open surgery or endovascular stent grafting to repair the aneurysm is usually done. Usually, femoral and carotid aneurysms are surgically repaired.

Aneurysms may also occur in the arteries of the brain (cerebral arteries). Rupture of a cerebral aneurysm may cause bleeding into the brain tissue (intracerebral hemorrhage), resulting in a stroke. Because cerebral aneurysms are near the brain and are usually small, their diagnosis and treatment differ from those of other aneurysms (see page 731). Infected aneurysms of the cerebral arteries are particularly dangerous, making early treatment important. Treatment often involves surgical repair.

Aortic Dissection

An aortic dissection (dissecting aneurysm, dissecting hematoma) is an often fatal disorder in which the inner layer (lining) of the aortic wall tears.

- Most aortic dissections occur because high blood pressure causes the artery's wall to deteriorate.
- People have sudden, excruciating pain, most commonly across the chest but also in the back between the shoulder blades.
- Doctors usually do x-rays or computed tomography scans to confirm the diagnosis.
- People usually take drugs to decrease blood pressure, and doctors do surgery or place stent grafts to repair the tear.

When the lining of the aorta tears, blood can surge through, separating (dissecting) the middle layer of the wall from the still intact outer layer. As a result, a new, false channel forms in the wall of the aorta. Aortic dissections are 3 times more common among men and are more common among blacks (specifically African-Americans) and less common among Asians. About three fourths of aortic dissections occur in people aged 40 to 70.

Most aortic dissections occur because the artery's wall deteriorates. Most commonly, such deterioration is associated with high blood pressure, which is present in more than two thirds of people who have an aortic dissection. Aortic dissection may be caused by hereditary connective-tissue disorders, especially Marfan syndrome (see page 1827) and Ehlers-Danlos syndrome (see page 1826). It may also be caused by birth defects of the heart and blood vessels (see page 1709), such as coarctation of the aorta, patent ductus arteriosus (a connection between the aorta and the pulmonary artery), and defects of the aortic valve. Other causes include arteriosclerosis and injury (such as a car crash or fall causing a strong

Understanding Aortic Dissection

In an aortic dissection, the inner layer (lining) of the aortic wall tears, and blood surges through the tear, separating (dissecting) the middle layer from the outer layer of the wall. As a result, a new, false channel forms in the wall.

blow to the chest). Rarely, a dissection occurs accidentally when doctors are inserting a catheter into an artery (for example, during aortography or angiography) or performing surgery on the heart or blood vessels.

Symptoms

Virtually everyone who has an aortic dissection experiences pain—typically sudden, excruciating pain, often described as tearing or ripping. Most commonly, the pain is felt across the chest but is often also felt in the back between the shoulder blades. The pain frequently travels along the path of the dissection as it advances along the aorta.

As the dissection advances, it can close off the points at which one or more arteries branch off from the aorta, blocking blood flow. The consequences vary depending on which arteries are blocked. Consequences include stroke (if the cerebral arteries, which supply the brain, are blocked), heart attack (if the coronary arteries, which supply the heart muscle, are blocked), sudden abdominal pain (if the mesentery arteries, which supply the intestines, are blocked), lower back pain (if the renal arteries, which supply the kidneys, are blocked) and nerve damage that causes tingling or an inability to move a limb (if the spinal arteries are blocked).

Blood may leak from the dissection and accumulate in the chest. Blood leaking from a dissection near the heart may enter the pericardial space (between the two layers of membranes that surround

SPOTLIGHT ON AGING

About half of aortic dissections occur in people who are over 60. Aortic dissection becomes more likely as people age.

In older people, aortic dissection often results from high blood pressure. The high pressure can cause part of the aorta's wall to deteriorate. Aging itself can cause similar deterioration. Although birth defects and connective tissue disorders can also cause aortic dissection, these disorders usually cause dissection before people reach old age.

the heart), preventing the heart from filling properly and causing cardiac tamponade—a life-threatening disorder (see box on page 391).

Diagnosis

The distinctive symptoms of an aortic dissection usually make the diagnosis obvious to doctors, although the disorder produces a variety of symptoms that sometimes resemble those of other disorders. In about two thirds of people with aortic dissection, pulses in the arms and legs are diminished or absent. A dissection that is moving backward toward the heart may cause a murmur that can be heard through a stethoscope.

Chest x-rays are the first step in detecting aortic dissection. X-rays show a widened aorta in 90% of people with symptoms. However, this finding may be due to other disorders. Computed tomography (CT) done after injecting a radiopaque dye can quickly and reliably detect aortic dissection and thus is useful in an emergency. Standard or transesophageal echocardiography (see page 328) can also reliably detect aortic dissections, even very small ones.

Treatment and Prognosis

People with an aortic dissection are admitted to an intensive care unit, where their vital signs (pulse, blood pressure, and rate of breathing) are closely monitored. Death can occur a few hours after an aortic dissection begins. Therefore, as soon as possible, drugs, usually nitroprusside plus a beta-blocker, are given intravenously to reduce the heart rate and blood pressure to the lowest level that can maintain a sufficient blood supply to the brain, heart, and kidneys. The lower heart rate and blood pressure help limit the spread of the dissection. Soon after drug therapy begins, doctors must decide whether

to recommend surgery or to continue drug therapy without surgery.

Doctors almost always recommend surgery for dissections that involve the first few inches of the aorta closest to the heart, unless complications of the dissection make the risk of surgery too high. For dissections farther from the heart, doctors usually continue drug therapy without surgery. However, surgery is necessary if the dissection causes the artery to leak blood, blocks the blood supply to the legs or to vital organs in the abdomen, causes symptoms, is enlarging, or occurs in a person with Marfan syndrome. In specialized major medical centers, the risk of death during surgery is about 15% for aortic dissections close to the heart and is somewhat higher for those farther away (because the risk of complications is higher).

During surgery, surgeons remove the largest possible area of dissected aorta, close the false channel between the middle and outer layers of the aorta's wall, and rebuild the aorta with a synthetic graft. If the aortic valve is leaking, surgeons repair or replace it. Removal and repair of a dissected aorta usually takes 3 to 6 hours, and the hospital stay is usually 7 to 10 days. Newer endovascular stent-grafts can be inserted through tubes (catheters) inserted into the blood vessels in the groin in some people. This procedure takes 2 to 4 hours, and the hospital stay is usually 1 to 3 days.

All people who have an aortic dissection, including those treated surgically, have to take drug therapy to keep their blood pressure down, usually for the rest of their lives. Such therapy helps reduce stress on the aorta. Drug therapy usually consists of a beta-blocker or calcium channel blocker plus another antihypertensive drug such as an angiotensin-converting enzyme (ACE) inhibitor (see table on page 340). Cholesterol-lowering drugs and diet modification (see page 399) are used if the person has atherosclerosis.

Doctors watch closely for late complications. The most important are another dissection, development of aneurysms in the weakened aorta, and increasing leakage backward through the aortic valve. Any of these complications may require surgical repair.

Without treatment, about 75% of people who have an aortic dissection die within the first 2 weeks. With treatment, about 70% who have dissection of the first part of the aorta and about 90% of those who have dissection of the aorta farther from the heart survive to leave the hospital. About 60% of people who survive the first 2 weeks are still alive 5 years after treatment, and 40% live at least 10 years. Of people who die after the first 2 weeks, about one third die of complications of the dissection, and the other two thirds die of other disorders.

CHAPTER
68 Venous Disorders

Veins return blood to the heart from all the organs of the body. The large veins parallel the large arteries and often share the same name, but the pathways of the venous system are more difficult to trace than those of the arteries. Many unnamed small veins form irregular networks and connect with the large veins.

Many veins, particularly those in the arms and legs, have one-way valves. Each valve consists of two flaps (cusps or leaflets) with edges that meet. Blood, as it moves toward the heart, pushes the cusps open like a pair of one-way swinging doors. If gravity or muscle contractions try to pull the blood backward or if blood begins to back up in a vein, the cusps are pushed closed, preventing backward flow. Thus, valves help the return of blood to the heart—by opening when the blood flows toward the heart and closing when it might flow backward because of gravity.

The main problems that affect the veins include the following:

- Abnormal connections of the arterial blood flow into veins called arteriovenous malformations or shunts, which are present at birth
- Inflammation
- Clotting
- Defects that lead to swelling (distention) and varicose veins

The veins in the legs are particularly affected because when a person is standing, blood must flow upward from the leg veins, against gravity, to reach the heart.

The body has superficial veins, located in the fatty layer under the skin, and deep veins, located in the muscles and along the bones. Short veins, called connecting veins, link the superficial and deep veins.

The deep veins play a major role in propelling blood toward the heart. The one-way valves in deep veins prevent blood from flowing backward, and the muscles surrounding the deep veins compress them, helping force the blood toward the heart, just as squeezing a toothpaste tube ejects toothpaste. The powerful calf muscles are particularly important, forcefully compressing the deep veins in the legs with every step. The deep veins carry 90% or more of the blood from the legs toward the heart.

Superficial veins have the same type of valves as deep veins, but they are not surrounded by muscle. Thus, blood in the superficial veins is not forced toward the heart by the squeezing action of muscles,

One-Way Valves in the Veins

One-way valves consist of two flaps (cusps or leaflets) with edges that meet. These valves help veins return blood to the heart. Blood, as it moves toward the heart, pushes the cusps open like a pair of one-way swinging doors (shown on the left). If gravity momentarily pulls the blood backward or if blood begins to back up in a vein, the cusps are immediately pushed closed, preventing backward flow (shown on the right).

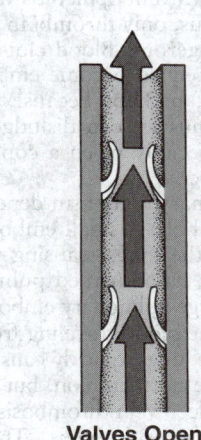
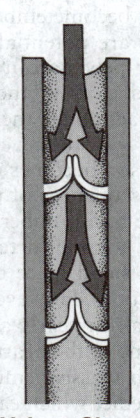

Valves Open   **Valves Closed**

and it flows more slowly than blood in the deep veins. Much of the blood that flows through the superficial veins is diverted into the deep veins through the many connecting veins between the deep and superficial veins. Valves in the connecting veins allow blood to flow from the superficial veins into the deep veins but not vice versa.

Deep Vein Thrombosis

Deep vein thrombosis is the formation of blood clots (thrombi) in the deep veins.

- Blood clots may form in veins if the vein is injured, a disorder causes the blood to clot, or something slows the return of blood to the heart.
- Blood clots may cause the leg or arm to swell.
- A blood clot can break loose and travel to the lungs, which is called a pulmonary embolism.

- Doppler ultrasonography and blood tests are used to detect deep vein thrombosis.
- Anticoagulants are given to prevent pulmonary embolism.

Blood clots (thrombi) can occur in the deep veins, termed deep vein thrombosis, or in the superficial veins, termed superficial thrombophlebitis (see page 437). Deep vein thrombosis occurs most often in the legs or pelvis but may also occasionally develop in the arms.

Pulmonary Embolism: A blood clot in a deep vein sometimes will break loose, becoming an embolus. The embolus can travel through the bloodstream, through the heart, and into the lungs, where it lodges in a blood vessel in the lung, blocking blood flow. This blockage is called pulmonary embolism (see page 488) and can be fatal. The small blood clots that occur in superficial thrombophlebitis usually do not become emboli. Thus, only thrombi in the deep veins are potentially dangerous. Blood clots in the legs or pelvis are more likely to become emboli than blood clots in the arms, perhaps because the squeezing action of the calf muscles can dislodge a blood clot in a deep vein, especially when a convalescing person becomes more active.

The consequences of pulmonary embolism depend on the size and number of emboli. A small embolus may block a small artery in the lungs, causing the death of a small piece of lung tissue (called pulmonary infarction). However, a large pulmonary embolus can block all or nearly all of the blood traveling from the right side of the heart to the lungs, quickly causing death. Such massive emboli are not common, but no one can predict which case of deep vein thrombosis, if untreated, will lead to a massive embolus. Thus, doctors are greatly concerned about every person who has deep vein thrombosis.

Sometimes, people have an abnormal opening, called a patent foramen ovale, between the right and left sides of the heart. If this opening is present, an embolus can pass into the arterial circulation and block a blood vessel in another part of the body, such as the brain where it will cause a stroke.

Causes

Three main factors (known as Virchow's triad) can contribute to deep vein thrombosis:

- Injury to the vein's lining
- An increased tendency for blood to clot
- Slowing of blood flow

Veins may be injured during surgery, by the injection of irritating substances, or by certain disorders, such as thromboangiitis obliterans (Buerger's disease). They may also be injured by a clot, making formation of a second clot more likely.

Some disorders, such as cancer and certain inherited disorders, cause blood to clot when it should not. Some drugs, including oral contraceptives, estrogen therapy, or drugs that act like estrogen (such as tamoxifen and raloxifene), can cause blood to clot more readily. Smoking is also a risk factor. Sometimes blood clots more readily after childbirth or surgery. Among older people, dehydration commonly causes the blood to clot more readily and can therefore contribute to deep vein thrombosis.

During prolonged bed rest and other occasions when the legs are not moving normally (such as after a leg injury), blood flow slows, because the calf muscles are not contracting and squeezing the blood toward the heart. For example, deep vein thrombosis may develop in people who have had a heart attack and lie in a hospital bed for several days without sufficiently moving their legs or in people whose legs and lower body are paralyzed (paraplegics). Deep vein thrombosis can develop after pelvic, hip, or knee surgery. Thrombosis can even occur in healthy people who sit for long periods, for example, during long drives or airplane flights, but thrombosis is extremely uncommon in this circumstance and usually occurs in people with other risk factors.

> **? Did You Know...**
>
> Although uncommon, thrombosis can occur in healthy people who sit for long periods, such as during long drives or flights.

Symptoms

About half of the people with deep vein thrombosis have no symptoms at all. In these people, chest pain or shortness of breath caused by pulmonary embolism may be the first indication that something is wrong. In other people, if a deep leg vein is involved, the calf swells and may be painful, tender to the touch, and warm. The ankle, foot, or thigh may also swell, depending on which veins are involved. Similarly, if an arm vein is involved, the arm may swell.

Chronic Deep Vein Insufficiency: Some blood clots heal by being converted to scar tissue, which may damage the valves in the veins. Because the damaged valves prevent the veins from functioning normally, fluid accumulates (a condition called edema) and the ankle swells. The edema can extend up the leg and even affect the thigh if the blockage is high enough in the vein. Edema is worse toward the end of the day, because blood must flow upward, against gravity, to reach the heart when a person is standing or sitting. Overnight, edema subsides because the veins empty well when the legs are horizontal.

Sometimes, the affected veins are obliterated (destroyed). In people whose veins are obliterated, leg edema is always present, generally worsening at the end of the day. The skin on the inside of the ankle becomes scaly and itchy and may turn a reddish brown. The discoloration is caused by red blood cells that escape from swollen (distended) veins into the skin. The discolored skin is vulnerable, and even a minor injury, such as that from scratching or a bump, can break it open, resulting in an ulcer. Varicose veins may be present. In addition to ulcer pain, there may be throbbing pain when standing or walking.

If edema is severe and persistent, scar tissue develops and traps fluid in the tissues. As a result, the calf permanently enlarges and feels hard. In such cases, ulcers are more likely to develop, and they heal less easily.

Diagnosis

Deep vein thrombosis may be difficult for doctors to detect, especially when pain and swelling are absent or very slight. When this disorder is suspected, Doppler ultrasonography (see page 329) can confirm the diagnosis. Sometimes doctors do a blood test to measure a substance called D-dimer that is released from blood clots. If the level of D-dimer in the blood is not increased, the person probably does not have a deep vein thrombosis.

If the person has symptoms of pulmonary embolism, a computed tomography (CT) scan or chest scanning using a radioactive marker (see page 455) is done to detect pulmonary embolism, and Doppler ultrasonography is done to check the legs for clots. These procedures are done except when a person collapses. Collapse suggests massive pulmonary embolism and requires immediate treatment.

Prevention

Although the risk of deep vein thrombosis cannot be entirely eliminated, it can be reduced in several ways. People at risk of deep vein thrombosis should flex and extend their ankles about 10 times every 30 minutes. Such people include those who have just had major surgery and those taking long trips. During long flights, everyone should walk and stretch every 2 hours while awake.

Continuously wearing elastic stockings (support hose) makes the veins narrow slightly and the blood flow more rapidly. As a result, clotting is less likely. However, elastic stockings are not sufficient protection against developing deep vein thrombosis. Also, they may give a false sense of security and discourage more effective methods of prevention. If not worn correctly, they may bunch up and aggravate the problem by blocking blood flow in the legs.

Pneumatic compression stockings are an effective way to prevent clots. Usually made of plastic, these stockings are automatically pumped up and emptied by an electric pump. They repeatedly squeeze the calves and empty the veins. The stockings are put on before surgery and kept on during and after surgery, until the person can walk again.

An anticoagulant drug (see page 490), such as heparin, fondaparinux, or warfarin, is given to people at high risk of developing deep vein thrombosis before, during, and sometimes after surgery. Such people include those who have clotting disorders (see page 1040) and those who have recently had one or more episodes of deep vein thrombosis. For certain types of surgery (such as hip replacement surgery), the risk is particularly high. People who are at particularly high risk may be given an anticoagulant when they are hospitalized even though they are not undergoing surgery. Anticoagulants reduce blood clotting much more effectively than wearing elastic stockings.

Treatment

For deep vein thrombosis, a doctor's main goal is to prevent pulmonary embolism. Hospitalization may be necessary at first, but because of the advances in treatment, most people with deep vein thrombosis can be treated at home. Bed rest is unnecessary except to help relieve symptoms.

Treatment usually consists of anticoagulant therapy with low-molecular-weight heparin or fondaparinux given by injection under the skin (subcutaneously), accompanied by warfarin taken by mouth. The injectable drug works immediately, but warfarin takes several days to be fully effective. Once the warfarin has taken effect, people stop taking the injectable drug. For some people, doctors simply use the injectable drug and do not start warfarin. How long people continue drug treatment (with warfarin or an injectable drug) varies according to the degree of risk. Patients whose deep vein thrombosis resulted from a specific cause (such as surgery or a drug they have stopped taking) should continue for 3 to 6 months. Patients in whom a specific cause is not found should take warfarin for at least 6 months. People who have had two or more episodes of deep vein thrombosis should continue warfarin indefinitely.

Use of warfarin increases the risk of bleeding, both internally and externally. To minimize the risk, people taking warfarin must have periodic blood tests to see how much their blood is anticoagulated. Doctors then use the blood test result to adjust the dose of warfarin.

Doctors are studying the use of intravenous drugs, such as tissue plasminogen activator, to dissolve blood clots. These drugs (thrombolytic, or fibrinolytic, drugs), may be given if the blood clot has been present for less than 48 hours. After 48 hours, scar tissue begins to develop in the blood clot, making it less likely to dissolve.

Very rarely, a filter (umbrella) is placed inside a large vein between the heart and the area affected by deep vein thrombosis, usually the inferior vena cava, which returns blood to the heart from the lower part of the body. A filter can trap emboli, preventing them from reaching the lungs.

Complications: If pulmonary embolism occurs, treatment usually includes oxygen (usually given by a face mask or nasal prongs), analgesics to relieve pain, and the anticoagulant drug heparin followed by warfarin. If pulmonary embolism is life threatening, thrombolytic drugs are given or surgery is done to remove the embolus.

The veins never completely recover after deep vein thrombosis develops, and surgery to repair the valves of the veins is experimental. Elastic compression stockings worn below the knee may be helpful.

If painful skin ulcers develop, properly applied compression bandages can help. When these bandages are applied once or twice a week, the ulcer almost always heals because blood flow in the veins improves. The ulcers are almost always infected, and pus and a foul-smelling discharge appear on the bandage each time it is changed. The pus and discharge can be washed off the skin with soap and water. Skin creams, balms, and skin medications of any kind have little effect.

Umbrellas: One Way to Prevent Pulmonary Embolism

In people who have deep vein thrombosis, a blood clot may break loose from an affected vein in the leg and travel through the bloodstream. A clot that breaks loose is called an embolus.

The embolus travels toward the heart and passes through the right atrium and ventricle and into one of the pulmonary arteries, which carry blood to the lungs. The clot may lodge in an artery in a lung and block blood flow, resulting in pulmonary embolism. Pulmonary embolism may be life threatening, depending on the size of the blocked artery.

To prevent pulmonary embolism, doctors usually use drugs that limit blood clotting. However, for some people, doctors may recommend that a filter, called an umbrella, be permanently placed in the inferior vena cava. The filter traps emboli before they reach the heart but allows blood to flow through freely. Emboli that are trapped sometimes dissolve on their own.

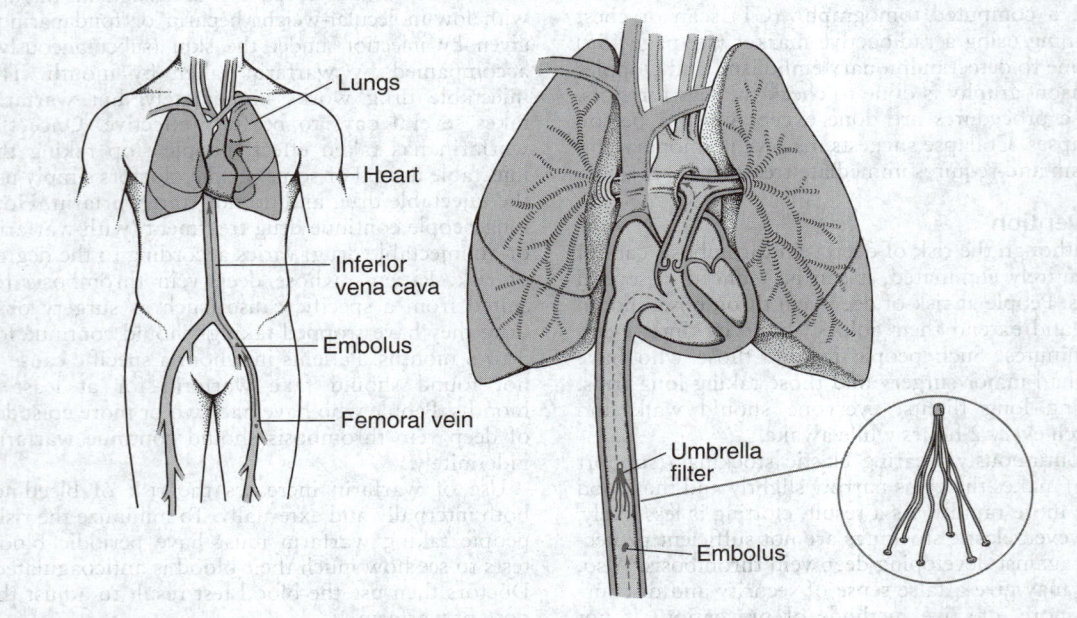

Lungs

Heart

Inferior vena cava

Embolus

Femoral vein

Umbrella filter

Embolus

Once blood flow in the veins has improved, the ulcer heals by itself. After it has healed, wearing an elastic stocking daily can prevent a recurrence. The stocking must be replaced as soon as it becomes too loose. If possible, the person should purchase seven stockings or pairs of stockings (if both legs are involved)—one for each day of the week so that stockings remain effective considerably longer.

Rarely, ulcers that do not heal require skin grafting. After grafting, an elastic stocking must be worn to prevent ulcers from returning.

Superficial Thrombophlebitis

Superficial thrombophlebitis (superficial phlebitis) is inflammation and clotting in a superficial vein.

- The skin over the vein becomes red, swollen, and painful.
- Doctors examine the area, but tests are not usually needed.
- People may need to take analgesics to relieve pain until the disorder resolves.

Superficial thrombophlebitis most often affects the superficial veins in the legs but may also affect superficial veins in the groin or in the arms. Superficial thrombophlebitis in the arms usually results from having an intravenous catheter. Often, thrombophlebitis occurs in people with varicose veins. However, most people with varicose veins do not develop thrombophlebitis.

Even a slight injury can cause a varicose vein to become inflamed. Unlike deep vein thrombosis, which causes very little inflammation, superficial thrombophlebitis involves a sudden (acute) inflammatory reaction that causes the thrombus (blood clot) to adhere firmly to the vein wall and lessens the likelihood that it will break loose. Unlike deep veins, superficial veins have no surrounding muscles to squeeze and dislodge a thrombus. For these reasons, superficial thrombophlebitis rarely causes embolism.

Thrombophlebitis that repeatedly occurs in normal veins is called migratory phlebitis or migratory thrombophlebitis. It may indicate a serious underlying disorder, such as cancer of an internal organ. When migratory phlebitis and cancer of an internal organ occur together, the disorder is called Trousseau's syndrome.

Symptoms and Diagnosis

Localized pain and swelling develop rapidly, the skin over the vein becomes red, and the area feels warm and is very tender. Because blood in the vein is clotted, the vein feels like a hard cord under the skin, not soft like a normal or varicose vein. The vein may feel hard along its entire length. The diagnosis is usually obvious to doctors just from examining the painful area. However, doctors must distinguish superficial thrombophlebitis from cellulitis, which is treated differently.

Treatment

Most often, superficial thrombophlebitis subsides by itself. Taking an analgesic, such as aspirin or another nonsteroidal anti-inflammatory drug (NSAID—see page 644), usually helps relieve the pain. Although the inflammation generally subsides in a matter of days, several weeks may pass before the lumps and tenderness subside completely. To provide early relief, doctors may inject a local anesthetic, remove the thrombus, and then apply a compression bandage, which the person wears for several days.

Varicose Veins

Varicose veins are abnormally enlarged superficial veins in the legs.

- Varicose veins may ache or cause itching or a sensation of tiredness.
- Doctors can detect varicose veins by examining the skin.
- Surgery or injection therapy can remove varicose veins, but new ones often form.

The precise cause of varicose veins is unknown, but the main problem is probably a weakness in the walls of superficial veins. This weakness may be inherited. Over time, the weakness causes the veins to lose their elasticity. They stretch and become longer and wider. To fit in the same space that they occupied when they were normal, the elongated veins become convoluted. They may appear as a snakelike bulge beneath the skin. Varicose veins often develop during pregnancy and resolve shortly after childbirth.

More important than the elongation is the widening of the veins, which causes the valve cusps to separate. When the person stands, the blood is pulled backward by gravity and is not stopped because the valve cusps are separated. Thus, blood flows backward, rapidly filling the veins and causing the thin-walled, convoluted veins to enlarge even more. Some of the connecting veins, which normally allow blood to flow only from the superficial veins into the deep veins, also enlarge. If they enlarge, their valve cusps also separate. Consequently, blood squirts backward into the superficial veins when the muscles squeeze the deep veins, causing the superficial veins to stretch further.

Many people with or without varicose veins may have spider veins, which are enlarged capillaries. Spider veins may be caused by the pressure from

Valves in Varicose Veins

In a normal vein, the cusps of the valves close to prevent backward flow of blood. In a varicose vein, the cusps cannot close because the vein is abnormally widened. Consequently, blood can flow in the wrong direction.

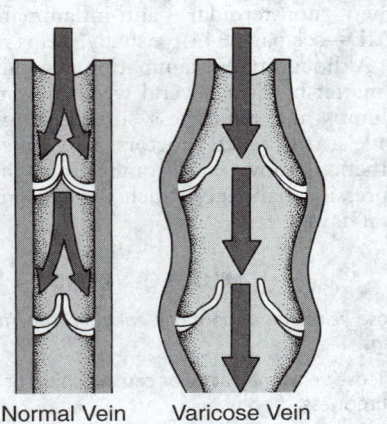

Normal Vein   Varicose Vein

blood in varicose veins, but the cause is generally thought to be hormonal factors that are not yet understood. A hormonal cause would explain why spider veins most commonly occur in women, particularly during pregnancy.

Symptoms and Complications

Besides being unsightly, varicose veins commonly ache and cause a sensation of tiredness in the legs. However, many people, even some with very large veins, have no pain. The lower part of the leg and ankle may itch, especially if the leg is warm after a person has been wearing socks or stockings. Itching can lead to scratching and can cause redness or a rash, which is often incorrectly attributed to dry skin. The pain is sometimes worse when varicose veins are developing than when they are fully stretched.

Only a small percentage of people with varicose veins have complications, such as dermatitis, inflammation of the veins (phlebitis), or bleeding. Dermatitis produces a red, scaling, itchy rash or a brown area, usually on the inside of the leg above the ankle. Scratching or a minor injury, particularly from shaving, can cause bleeding or development of a painful ulcer that does not heal. Ulcers may also bleed. Phlebitis may occur spontaneously or result from an injury. Although usually painful, phlebitis that occurs with varicose veins is rarely harmful.

Diagnosis

Varicose veins can usually be seen bulging under the skin, but symptoms may develop before the veins become visible. When varicose veins are not visible, doctors experienced in checking for them can feel the leg to determine the extent of the problem.

X-rays or ultrasonography may be done to assess the functioning of the deep veins prior to surgery. Usually, such procedures are necessary only if malfunction of the deep veins is suggested by changes in the skin or by swollen ankles. The ankles swell because fluid accumulates in the tissue under the skin—a condition called edema. Varicose veins alone do not cause edema.

Treatment

Although individual varicose veins can be removed or eliminated by surgery or injection therapy, the disorder cannot be cured. Thus, treatment mainly relieves symptoms, improves appearance, and prevents complications. Elevating the legs—by lying down or using a footstool when sitting—relieves the symptoms of varicose veins but does not prevent new varicose veins from forming. Usually, varicose veins that appear during pregnancy largely subside during the 2 or 3 weeks after delivery. During this time, they should not be treated.

Elastic stockings (support hose) compress the veins and prevent them from stretching and hurting. People who do not want surgery or injection therapy or who have a medical condition that prevents them from having these treatments may choose to wear elastic stockings.

Surgery: Surgery aims to remove as many of the varicose veins as possible. However, surgeons try to preserve the saphenous vein because it can be used as a bypass graft in case coronary artery or peripheral artery disease ever develops. This vein is the longest superficial vein in the body, extending from the ankle to the groin, where it joins the femoral vein (the main deep vein in the leg). If the saphenous vein must be removed, a procedure called stripping is done. The surgeon makes two incisions, one at the groin and one at the ankle, and opens the vein at each end. A flexible wire is threaded through the entire vein and then pulled out to remove the vein.

To remove other varicose veins, the surgeon makes incisions in other areas. Because the superficial veins play a less significant role than the deep veins in returning blood to the heart, their removal does not impair circulation if the deep veins are functioning normally.

Removal of varicose veins is a lengthy procedure, so the person is usually given a general anesthetic. This procedure relieves the symptoms and prevents complications, but it leaves scars. The more extensive the procedure, the longer the time before new varicose veins develop. However, removal of varicose veins does not eliminate the tendency to develop new varicose veins.

Injection Therapy (Sclerotherapy): An alternative to surgery is injection therapy, which seals the veins, so that blood can no longer flow through them. A solution is injected into the vein to irritate it and produce a thrombus (blood clot). In essence, this procedure produces a harmless kind of superficial thrombophlebitis. Healing of the thrombus leads to formation of scar tissue, which blocks the vein. However, the thrombus may dissolve instead of becoming scar tissue, and the varicose vein then reopens.

Injection therapy was common in the United States between the 1930s and 1950s but fell out of favor because of poor results and complications. Current techniques are more likely to be successful and are safe for varicose veins of all sizes.

Current techniques include special bandaging that reduces the size of the thrombus by compressing the diameter of the injected vein. A smaller thrombus is more likely to form scar tissue, as desired. A further advantage of this technique is that adequate compression virtually eliminates the pain usually associated with superficial phlebitis.

Although injection therapy is more time-consuming than surgery, it has several advantages: Anesthesia is not necessary, new varicose veins can be treated as they develop, and people can go about their normal daily activities between treatments. However, even with current techniques, some doctors consider injection therapy only when varicose veins return after surgery or when a person desires cosmetic improvement.

If spider veins cause pain or a burning sensation or are unsightly, they also may be treated with injection therapy.

Laser Therapies: Laser therapy is being used experimentally by some surgeons for the treatment of varicose veins. This therapy uses a highly focused, continuous stream of high-intensity light to cut or destroy tissue. However, the usefulness of this therapy has not yet been determined. Intense pulsed light therapy can be used to treat small spider veins. This therapy is similar to laser therapy except that the light is applied in short bursts.

Arteriovenous Fistula

An arteriovenous fistula is an abnormal channel between an artery and a vein.

- Although doctors may be able to hear the distinctive sound of blood flow though a fistula by using a stethoscope, imaging tests are often needed.

- Fistulas can be cut out or eliminated with laser therapy, or sometimes substances are injected into the fistula to block the blood flow.

Normally, blood flows from arteries into capillaries and then into veins. When an arteriovenous fistula is present, blood flows directly from an artery into a vein, bypassing the capillaries. A person may be born with an arteriovenous fistula (congenital fistula), or a fistula may develop after birth (acquired fistula).

Congenital arteriovenous fistulas are uncommon. Acquired arteriovenous fistulas can be caused by any injury that damages an artery and a vein that lie side by side. Typically, the injury is a piercing wound, as from a knife or bullet. The fistula may appear immediately or may develop after a few hours. The area can swell quickly if blood escapes into the surrounding tissues.

Some medical treatments, such as kidney dialysis, require that a vein be pierced for each treatment. With repeated piercing, the vein becomes inflamed and clotting can develop. Eventually, scar tissue may develop and destroy the vein. To avoid this problem, doctors may deliberately create an arteriovenous fistula, usually between an adjoining vein and artery in the arm. This procedure widens the vein, making needle insertion easier and enabling the blood to flow faster. Faster flowing blood is less likely to clot. Unlike some large arteriovenous fistulas, these small, intentionally created fistulas do not lead to heart problems, and they can be closed when no longer needed.

Symptoms and Diagnosis

When congenital arteriovenous fistulas are near the surface of the skin, they may appear swollen and reddish blue. In conspicuous places, such as the face, they appear purplish and may be unsightly.

If a large acquired arteriovenous fistula is not treated, a large volume of blood flows under high pressure from the artery into the vein network. Vein walls are not strong enough to withstand such high pressure, so the walls stretch and the veins enlarge and bulge (sometimes resembling varicose veins). In addition, blood flows more freely into the enlarged veins than it would if it continued its normal course through the arteries. As a result, blood pressure falls. To compensate for this fall in blood pressure, the heart pumps more forcefully and more rapidly, thus greatly increasing its output of blood. Eventually, the increased effort may strain the heart, causing heart failure. The larger the fistula, the more quickly heart failure can develop.

With a stethoscope placed over a large acquired arteriovenous fistula, doctors can hear a distinctive "to-and-fro" sound, like that of moving machinery. This sound is called a machinery murmur. Doppler ultrasonography is used to confirm the diagnosis and to determine the extent of the problem. For fistulas between deeper blood vessels (such as the aorta and vena cava), magnetic resonance imaging (MRI) is more useful.

Treatment

Small congenital arteriovenous fistulas can be cut out or eliminated with laser coagulation therapy. This procedure must be done by a skilled vascular surgeon, because the fistulas are sometimes more extensive than they appear to be on the surface. Arteriovenous fistulas near the eye, brain, or other major structures can be especially difficult to treat.

Acquired arteriovenous fistulas are corrected by a surgeon as soon as possible after diagnosis. Before the surgery, a radiopaque dye, which can be seen on x-rays, may be injected to outline the fistula more clearly in a procedure called angiography (see page 332). If the surgeon cannot reach the fistula easily (for example, if it is in the brain), complex injection techniques that cause clots to form may be used to block blood flow through the fistula. For example, coils or plugs may be inserted into the fistula at the various points where the vein and the artery meet. This procedure is done using x-rays for guidance and does not require open surgery.

CHAPTER

69 Lymphatic Disorders

Like the venous system, the lymphatic system transports fluids throughout the body. The lymphatic system consists of thin-walled lymphatic vessels, lymph nodes, and two collecting ducts (see art on page 1098). Lymphatic vessels, located throughout the body, are larger than capillaries, and most are smaller than the smallest veins. Most of the lymphatic vessels have valves like those in veins to keep the lymph, which can clot, flowing in the one direction (toward the heart). Lymphatic vessels drain fluids from tissues throughout the body that have diffused through the very thin walls of capillaries. The fluids contain proteins, minerals, nutrients, and other substances, which provide nourishment to tissues. However, most of the fluid is reabsorbed into the capillaries. The rest of the fluid (lymph) is drained from the spaces surrounding the cells into the lymphatic vessels, which eventually return it to the veins. Lymphatic vessels also collect and transport damaged cells, cancer cells, and foreign particles (such as bacteria and viruses) that may have entered the tissue fluids.

All lymph passes through strategically placed lymph nodes, which filter damaged cells, cancer cells, and foreign particles out of the lymph. Lymph nodes also produce specialized blood cells designed to engulf and destroy damaged cells, cancer cells, infectious organisms, and foreign particles. Thus, important functions of the lymphatic system are to remove damaged cells from the body and to provide protection against the spread of infection and cancer.

The lymph vessels drain into collecting ducts, which empty their contents into the two subclavian veins, located under the collarbones. These veins join to form the superior vena cava, the large vein that drains blood from the upper body into the heart.

The lymphatic system may not perform its function adequately when the quantity of fluid is excessive or when the lymph vessels or nodes are damaged or removed during surgery, become blocked by a tumor, or become inflamed.

Lymphedema

Lymphedema is the accumulation of lymph resulting in swelling.

- Lymph fluid does not drain from tissues, causing swelling.
- Compression bandages or pneumatic stockings can reduce the swelling.

Lymphedema results when the lymphatic system cannot adequately drain lymph from the tissues, causing swelling. Lymphedema may be due to conditions present at birth (congenital) or to conditions that develop later (acquired).

Congenital Lymphedema: This disorder results from having so few lymphatic vessels that they cannot handle all the lymph. The problem almost always affects the legs; rarely, it affects the arms. Women are much more likely than men to have congenital lymphedema.

Rarely, the swelling is obvious at birth, but usually, the lymphatic vessels can handle the small amount of lymph produced in an infant. More often, the swelling appears later in life, as the volume of lymph increases and overwhelms the small number of lymph vessels. The swelling starts gradually in one or both legs. The first sign of lymphedema may be puffiness of the foot, making the shoe feel tight at the end of the day. The shoe may leave indentations in the skin of the foot. (Many people who do not have lymphedema experience swelling after they stand for prolonged periods. They may have indentations around their ankles after they wear ankle socks, but the indentations are much less deep than those of lymphedema, and the surrounding area is not puffy.)

In the early stages of congenital lymphedema, the swelling goes away when the leg is elevated. This disorder worsens with time: The swelling becomes more obvious and does not disappear completely, even after a night's rest.

Acquired Lymphedema: Acquired lymphedema is more common than congenital lymphedema. It typically appears after major surgical treatment, especially after cancer treatment in which lymph nodes and lymphatic vessels are removed or treated with radiation. For example, the arm tends to swell after removal of a cancerous breast and lymph nodes in the armpit. Scarring of lymphatic vessels from repeated infection also may cause lymphedema, but this type of scarring is very uncommon except among people who have an infection due to the tropical parasite *Filaria* (filariasis).

In acquired lymphedema, the skin looks healthy but is puffy or swollen. Pressing the area with a finger does not leave a significant indentation, as it does when edema results from inadequate blood flow in the veins. Rarely, especially in filariasis, the swollen limb becomes extremely large and the skin is so thick and ridged that it looks almost like elephant skin. This disorder is called **elephantiasis**.

Treatment

Lymphedema has no cure. For people with mild lymphedema, compression bandages can reduce the swelling. People who are more severely affected may wear pneumatic stockings (see page 435) every day for an hour or two to reduce the swelling. Once the swelling has been reduced, the person must wear elastic stockings up to the knee every day from the moment of rising until bedtime. This measure controls the swelling to some degree. For lymphedema in the arm, pneumatic sleeves—like pneumatic stockings—can be used every day to reduce the swelling; elastic sleeves are also available. For elephantiasis, an extensive operation may be performed to remove most of the swollen tissues under the skin.

Lung and Airway Disorders

CHAPTER

70   Biology of the Lungs and Airways

To sustain life, the body must produce sufficient energy. Energy is produced by burning molecules in food, which is done by the process of oxidation (whereby food molecules are combined with oxygen). Oxidation involves carbon and hydrogen being combined with oxygen to form carbon dioxide and water. The consumption of oxygen and the production of carbon dioxide are thus indispensable to life. It follows that the human body must have an organ system designed to exchange carbon dioxide and oxygen between the circulating blood and the atmosphere at a rate rapid enough for the body's needs, even during peak exercise. The respiratory system enables oxygen to enter the body and carbon dioxide to leave the body.

Respiratory System

The respiratory system starts at the nose and mouth and continues through the airways and the lungs. Air enters the respiratory system through the nose and mouth and passes down the throat (pharynx) and through the voice box, or larynx. The entrance to the larynx is covered by a small flap of tissue (epiglottis) that automatically closes during swallowing, thus preventing food or drink from entering the airways.

The largest airway is the windpipe (trachea), which branches into two smaller airways: the left and right bronchi, which lead to the two lungs. Each lung is divided into sections (lobes): three in the right lung and two in the left lung. The left lung is a little smaller than the right lung because it shares space in the left side of the chest with the heart.

The bronchi themselves branch many times into smaller airways, ending in the narrowest airways (bronchioles), which are as small as one half of a millimeter across. The airways resemble an upside-down tree, which is why this part of the respiratory system is often called the bronchial tree. Large

Inside the Lungs and Airways

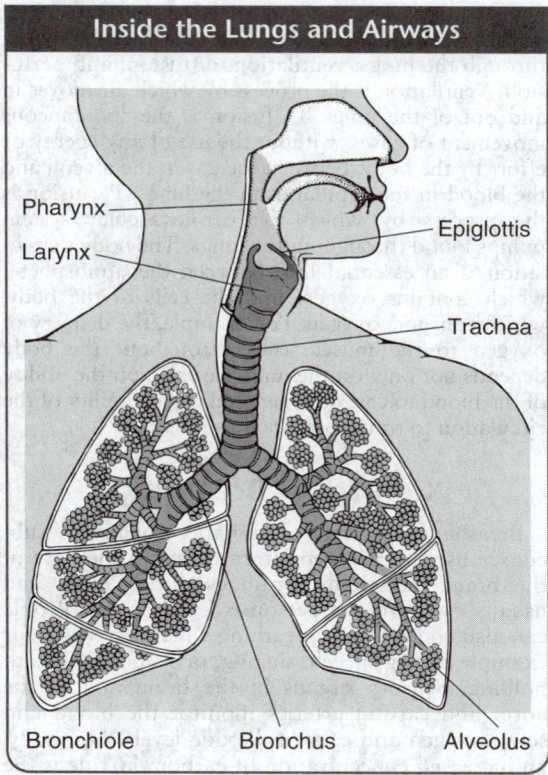

Pharynx

Epiglottis

Larynx

Trachea

Bronchiole   Bronchus   Alveolus

airways are held open by semiflexible, fibrous connective tissue called cartilage. Smaller airways are supported by the lung tissue that surrounds and is attached to them. Circular airway smooth muscle can dilate or constrict, thus changing airway size.

At the end of each bronchiole are thousands of small air sacs (alveoli). Together, the millions of alveoli of the lungs form a surface of more than 100 square meters. Within the alveolar walls is a dense network of tiny blood vessels called capillaries. The extremely thin barrier between air and capillaries allows oxygen to move from the alveoli into the blood and allows carbon dioxide to move from the blood in the capillaries into the air in the alveoli.

The pleura is a slippery membrane that covers the lungs as well as the inside of the chest wall. It allows the lungs to move smoothly during breathing and as the person moves. Normally, the two layers of the pleura have only a small amount of lubricating fluid between them. The two layers glide smoothly over each other as the lungs change size and shape.

Chest Cavity

The lungs are housed in the chest cavity, a space that also includes the mediastinum. The mediastinum is in the center of the chest and contains the heart, thymus, and lymph nodes, along with portions of the aorta, vena cava, trachea, esophagus, and various nerves. It encompasses the area bordered by the breastbone (sternum) in front, the spinal column in back, the entrance to the chest cavity above, and the diaphragm below. Functionally, the mediastinum isolates the left and right lung from each other. For example, if the chest wall is punctured on one side, causing the lung on that side to collapse, the other lung remains inflated and functioning, because the two lungs are separated by the mediastinum.

The lungs and other organs in the chest are protected by a bony cage, which is formed by the sternum, ribs, and spine. The 12 pairs of ribs curve around the chest from the back. Each pair is joined to the bones (vertebrae) of the spine. In the front of the body, the upper seven pairs of ribs are attached to the sternum by cartilage. The eighth, ninth, and tenth pairs of ribs join the cartilage of the pair above; the last two pairs (floating ribs) are shorter and do not join in the front (see page 447).

Exchanging Oxygen and Carbon Dioxide

The primary function of the respiratory system is to exchange oxygen and carbon dioxide. Inhaled oxygen enters the lungs and reaches the alveoli. The layers of cells lining the alveoli and the surrounding capillaries are each only one cell thick and are in very close contact with each other. This barrier between air and blood averages about 1 micron (1/10,000 of a centimeter) in thickness. Oxygen passes quickly through this air-blood barrier into the blood in the capillaries. Similarly, carbon dioxide passes from the blood into the alveoli and is then exhaled.

Oxygenated blood travels from the lungs through the pulmonary veins and into the left side of the heart, which pumps the blood to the rest of the body (see page 317). Oxygen-deficient, carbon dioxide-rich blood returns to the right side of the heart through two large veins, the superior vena cava and the inferior vena cava. Then the blood is pumped through the pulmonary artery to the lungs, where it picks up oxygen and releases carbon dioxide.

To support the exchange of oxygen and carbon dioxide, about 6 to 10 liters of air per minute are brought in and out of the lungs, and about three tenths of a liter of oxygen is transferred from the alveoli to

Gas Exchange Between Alveolar Spaces and Capillaries

The function of the respiratory system is to exchange two gases: oxygen and carbon dioxide. The exchange takes place in the millions of alveoli in the lungs and the capillaries that envelop them. As shown below, inhaled oxygen moves from the alveoli to the blood in the capillaries, and carbon dioxide moves from the blood in the capillaries to the air in the alveoli.

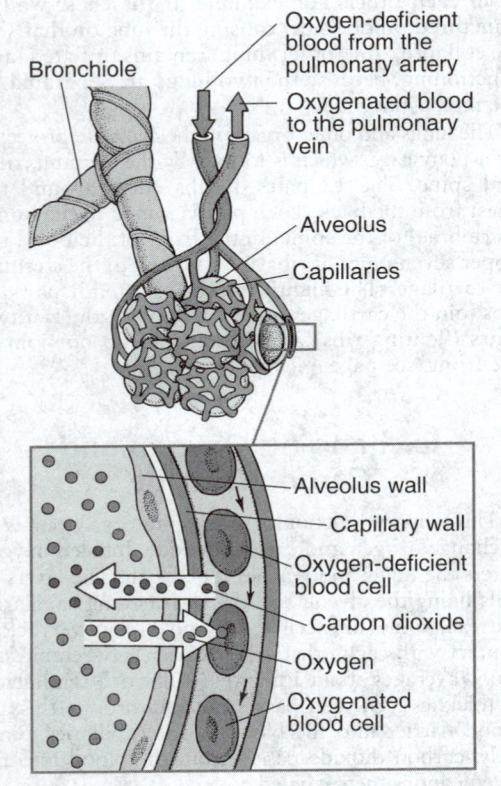

Bronchiole

Oxygen-deficient blood from the pulmonary artery

Oxygenated blood to the pulmonary vein

Alveolus

Capillaries

Alveolus wall

Capillary wall

Oxygen-deficient blood cell

Carbon dioxide

Oxygen

Oxygenated blood cell

Three processes are essential for the transfer of oxygen from the outside air to the blood flowing through the lungs: ventilation, diffusion, and perfusion. Ventilation is the process by which air moves in and out of the lungs. Diffusion is the spontaneous movement of gases, without the use of any energy or effort by the body, between the gas in the alveoli and the blood in the capillaries in the lungs. Perfusion is the process by which the cardiovascular system pumps blood throughout the lungs. The body's circulation is an essential link between the atmosphere, which contains oxygen, and the cells of the body, which consume oxygen. For example, the delivery of oxygen to the muscle cells throughout the body depends not only on the lungs but also on the ability of the blood to carry oxygen and on the ability of the circulation to transport blood to muscle.

Control of Breathing

Breathing is usually automatic, controlled subconsciously by the respiratory center at the base of the brain. Breathing continues during sleep and usually even when a person is unconscious. People can also control their breathing when they wish, for example during speech, singing, or voluntary breath holding. Sensory organs in the brain and in the aorta and carotid arteries monitor the blood and sense oxygen and carbon dioxide levels. Normally, an increased concentration of carbon dioxide is the strongest stimulus to breathe more deeply and more frequently. Conversely, when the carbon dioxide concentration in the blood is low, the brain decreases the frequency and depth of breaths. During breathing at rest, the average adult inhales and exhales about 15 times a minute.

The lungs have no skeletal muscles of their own. The work of breathing is done by the diaphragm, the muscles between the ribs (intercostal muscles), the muscles in the neck, and the abdominal muscles. The diaphragm, a dome-shaped sheet of muscle that separates the chest cavity from the abdomen, is the most important muscle used for breathing in (called inhalation or inspiration). The diaphragm is attached to the base of the sternum, the lower parts of the rib cage, and the spine. As the diaphragm contracts, it increases the length and diameter of the chest cavity and thus expands the lungs. The intercostal muscles help move the rib cage and thus assist in breathing. The muscles used in breathing can contract only if the nerves connecting them to the brain are intact. In some neck and back injuries, the spinal cord can be severed, which breaks the nervous system connection between the brain and the muscles, and the person will die unless artificially ventilated.

the blood each minute, even when the person is at rest. At the same time, a similar volume of carbon dioxide moves from the blood to the alveoli and is exhaled. During exercise, it is possible to breathe in and out more than 100 liters of air per minute and extract 3 liters of oxygen from this air per minute. The rate at which oxygen is used by the body is one measure of the rate of energy expended by the body. Breathing in and out is accomplished by respiratory muscles.

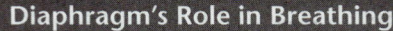

Diaphragm's Role in Breathing

When the diaphragm contracts and moves lower, the chest cavity enlarges, reducing the pressure outside the lungs. To equalize the pressure, air enters the lungs.

When the diaphragm relaxes and moves back up, the elasticity of the lungs and chest wall pushes air out of the lungs.

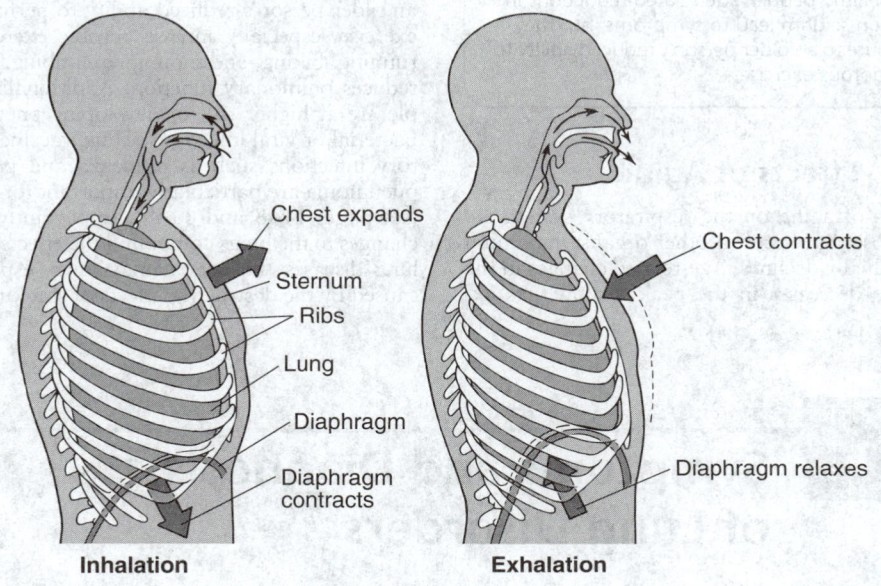

Chest expands
Sternum
Ribs
Lung
Diaphragm
Diaphragm contracts

Inhalation

Chest contracts

Diaphragm relaxes

Exhalation

The process of breathing out (called exhalation or expiration) is usually passive when a person is not exercising. The elasticity of the lungs and chest wall, which are actively stretched during inhalation, causes them to expel air out of the lungs when inspiratory muscles are relaxed. Therefore, when a person is at rest, no effort is needed to breathe out. During vigorous exercise, however, a number of muscles participate in exhalation. The abdominal muscles are the most important of these. Abdominal muscles contract, raise abdominal pressure, and push a relaxed diaphragm against the lungs, causing air to be pushed out.

Defense Mechanisms

The average person who is moderately active during the daytime breathes about 20,000 liters of air every 24 hours. Inevitably, this air (which would weigh more than 20 kilograms) contains potentially harmful particles and gases. Particles, such as dust and soot, mold, fungi, bacteria, and viruses, deposit on airway and alveolar surfaces. Only small particles less than 3 to 5 microns in diameter penetrate

to the deep lung. Fortunately, the respiratory system has defense mechanisms to clean and protect itself.

One such defense mechanism involves tiny muscular projections (cilia) on the cells that line the airways. The airways are covered by a liquid layer of mucus that is propelled by the cilia. These tiny muscles beat more than 1,000 times a minute, moving the mucus that lines the trachea about 0.5 to 1 centimeter per minute. Particles and pathogens that are trapped on this mucus layer are cleared to the mouth and swallowed.

Because of the requirements of gas exchange, alveoli are not protected by mucus and cilia—mucus is too thick and would slow movement of oxygen and carbon dioxide. Instead, the body has another defense system. Mobile cells on the alveolar surface called phagocytes seek out deposited particles, bind to them, ingest them, kill any that are living, and digest them. Phagocytes in alveoli of the lungs are called alveolar macrophages. When the lungs are exposed to serious threats, additional white blood cells in the circulation, especially neutrophils, can be recruited to help ingest and kill pathogens (foreign particles). For example, when the person inhales a great deal of dust or is fighting a respiratory infection, more macrophages are produced and neutrophils are recruited.

? Did You Know...

In healthy people, age-related reductions in lung function seldom lead to symptoms, but they can contribute to an older person's reduced ability to perform vigorous exercise.

Effects of Aging

The effects of aging on the respiratory system are similar to those that occur in other organs: maximum function gradually declines. Age-related changes in the lungs include decreases in the peak airflow, gas exchange, and vital capacity (the maximum amount of air that can be breathed out following a maximum inhalation); weakening of the respiratory muscles; and a decline in the effectiveness of lung defense mechanisms. In healthy people, these age-related changes seldom lead to symptoms, but they can contribute to an older person's reduced ability to perform vigorous exercise, especially intense aerobic exercise, such as running, biking, and mountain climbing. Obesity also reduces pulmonary function. Additionally, older people are at higher risk of developing pneumonia after bacterial or viral infections. Thus, vaccines for respiratory infections such as influenza and pneumococcal pneumonia are particularly important for older people (see pages 1148 and 1149). Importantly, age-related changes in the lungs compound the effects of heart and lung diseases the person may have, especially those caused by the destructive effects of smoking.

CHAPTER

71   Symptoms and Diagnosis of Lung Disorders

Disorders that affect the lungs and airways are called lung, respiratory, or pulmonary disorders. Depending on the person's symptoms, a doctor usually recommends various tests to help determine the exact disorder.

Symptoms

Among the most common symptoms of lung disorders are cough, shortness of breath (dyspnea), and wheezing. Less commonly, a blockage in the airways between the mouth and lungs results in a gasping sound when breathing (stridor). Problems in the lungs can also lead to coughing up of blood (hemoptysis), a bluish discoloration of the skin due to a lack of oxygen in the blood (cyanosis), or chest pain. Prolonged lung disease can even produce changes in other parts of the body, including finger clubbing. Some of these symptoms do not always indicate a respiratory problem. Chest pain, for example, may also result from a heart or gastrointestinal disorder, and shortness of breath can be caused by a heart or blood problem.

COUGH

A cough is a sudden, explosive exhalation of air; the function of a cough is to clear material from the airways.

Coughing, a familiar but complicated reflex, is one way in which the lungs and airways are protected. Along with other mechanisms, coughing helps to protect the lungs from particles that have been inhaled. Coughing sometimes brings up sputum (also called phlegm)—a mixture of mucus, debris, and cells expelled by the lungs.

Causes

Coughing occurs when the airways are irritated. Respiratory infections—usually bacterial or viral—irritate the airways and are a common cause of coughing. Allergies can irritate the airways as well. People who smoke often cough. Smoke not only irritates the airways but also damages the cells that line the airways, including the hairlike projections that normally cleanse the airways of debris (cilia). Coughing may also result from postnasal drip, in which nasal secretions drain down the back of the nose into the throat and sometimes into the trachea and other airways, where they produce irritation. Coughing may result from gastroesophageal reflux, in which stomach or esophageal contents flow backward from the esophagus into the trachea and airways, producing irritation. Another cause of cough can be drugs, for example, angiotensin-converting enzyme (ACE) inhibitors (see table on page 340). Narrowing of the airways below the windpipe (bronchoconstriction), foreign bodies, or tumors in the airway can cause cough, wheezing, or both. Bronchoconstriction occurs in asthma, in chronic obstructive pulmonary disease, and heart failure (when fluid accumulates in the lungs).

Coughs vary considerably. A cough may be distressing, especially if coughing episodes are accompanied by chest pain, shortness of breath, blood, or unusually large amounts of or very sticky sputum. However, if coughing increases slowly over decades, as it may in a smoker, the person may hardly be aware of it.

Evaluation

Information about a cough helps a doctor determine its cause. Therefore, a doctor may ask:

- How long has the cough been present?
- At what time of day does the cough occur?
- What factors—such as cold air, body position, talking, eating, or drinking—influence the cough?
- Is the cough accompanied by chest pain, shortness of breath, hoarseness, dizziness, or wheezing?
- Does the cough bring up sputum or blood?
- Are there symptoms of another disorder that could cause a cough (for example, gastroesophageal reflux or postnasal drip)?
- Could a drug be causing the cough?
- What color is the sputum?

The appearance of the sputum, especially a change in color or consistency, occasionally helps the doctor identify the cause. A yellowish, greenish, or brownish appearance may indicate a bacterial infection. Clear but very sticky (mucoid) sputum is characteristic of asthma. Occasionally, a doctor may use a microscope to examine a sputum sample. Bacteria and white blood cells are additional indications of infection. The presence of a specific type of white blood cell (eosinophil) suggests asthma. A cough may also produce blood, which commonly suggests bronchitis but may also suggest more serious disorders. Usually, a chest x-ray or other tests are done when a person develops a cough that is severe or persistent or has no obvious cause.

Treatment

Because coughing plays an important role in bringing up sputum and clearing the airways, a cough should not be suppressed unless it interferes with sleep. Treating an underlying disorder—such as an infection, fluid in the lungs, or asthma—is more important. For example, antibiotics can be given for an infection, or inhalers can be used for asthma. Depending on the severity of the cough and its cause,

a variety of drugs may be used for treatment. When cough results from narrowing of the airways, bronchodilators may provide relief. It is not clear how well other drugs relieve cough.

Antitussive Therapy: Antitussive drugs are given to suppress cough. All **opioids** are antitussives because they suppress the cough center in the brain. Codeine is the opioid used most often for cough. Codeine may cause nausea, vomiting, and constipation; it may also be addictive. If codeine is taken for a prolonged period, the dose needed to suppress a cough may need to be increased. Opioid cough suppressants can cause drowsiness, particularly when the person also is taking other drugs that reduce concentration (such as alcohol, sedatives, sleep aids, antidepressants, and certain antihistamines). Opioids are not always safe, and doctors usually reserve them for special situations.

Several **non-opioid cough suppressants,** such as dextromethorphan and benzonatate, are antitussives that also suppress the cough center in the brain. These drugs, and others, are the active ingredients in many over-the-counter and prescription cough medications. They are not addictive and, when used correctly, produce little drowsiness. In certain people, especially those who are coughing up an abundant amount of sputum, frequent use of these cough suppressants is not recommended.

Steam inhalation, for example from a vaporizer, can help stop a cough by reducing irritation in the throat (pharynx) and airways. The moisture from the steam also loosens secretions, making them easier to cough up. A cool-mist humidifier can achieve the same result. Some doctors believe that drinking sufficient water can produce good hydration and is as effective as steam inhalation for loosening secretions.

Expectorants: Some doctors recommend expectorants (sometimes called mucolytics) to help loosen mucus by making bronchial secretions thinner and easier to cough up, although these drugs do not suppress a cough. It is not clear how effective these drugs are. A saturated solution of potassium iodide may be prescribed. The most commonly used over-the-counter preparations contain guaifenesin or terpin hydrate. A small dose of syrup of ipecac may help in children, especially in those who have croup.

In cystic fibrosis, dornase alfa (inhaled recombinant human deoxyribonuclease I) is used to help thin the pus-filled mucus that results from chronic respiratory infections. Also, inhalation of a saline (salt) solution or use of acetylcysteine (for up to a few days) sometimes helps thin excessively thick and troublesome mucus.

Bronchodilators, Corticosteroids, Antihistamines, and Decongestants: Bronchodilators, such as inhaled albuterol and similar drugs, and inhaled corticosteroids are effective if a cough occurs as a result of airway narrowing (bronchoconstriction), as happens in asthma and chronic obstructive pulmonary disease. Theophylline, which is taken by mouth, is sometimes helpful. Some people who develop wheezing or prolonged cough after viral respiratory infections appear to benefit from short-term use of bronchodilators.

Antihistamines, which dry the respiratory tract, have little or no value in treating a cough, except when it is caused by an upper airway allergy. With coughs from other causes, such as bronchitis, the drying action of antihistamines can be harmful, thickening respiratory secretions and making them difficult to cough up.

Decongestants such as phenylephrine that relieve a stuffy nose are only useful in relieving a cough that is caused by postnasal drip.

DYSPNEA

Dyspnea (shortness of breath) is the unpleasant sensation of difficulty in breathing.

An increase in the rate and depth of breathing occurs normally during exercise and at high altitudes, but the increase seldom causes discomfort. Breathing is also increased at rest in people with many illnesses, whether of the lungs or of other parts of the body. For example, people with a fever generally breathe faster.

With dyspnea, faster breathing is accompanied by the sensation of running out of air. The person feels a sensation of not being able to breathe fast enough or deeply enough. Other sensations include an awareness of increased muscular effort to expand the chest when breathing in or to expel air when breathing out, the uncomfortable sensation that inhaling (inspiration) is urgently needed before exhaling (expiration) is completed, and various sensations often described as tightness in the chest.

Causes

Lung Disorders: People who have lung disorders often experience dyspnea when they physically exert themselves. During exercise, the body makes more carbon dioxide and uses more oxygen. The respiratory center in the brain accelerates breathing when blood levels of oxygen are low or blood levels of carbon dioxide are high. If the heart or lungs are not functioning properly, even a little exertion can lead to dramatic increases in breathing rates and dyspnea. Dyspnea is so unpleasant that the person avoids exertion. As the lung disorder becomes more severe, dyspnea may even occur at rest.

Dyspnea may result from restrictive or obstructive lung disorders. In restrictive lung disorders (such as idiopathic pulmonary fibrosis), lungs become stiff and require increased effort to expand during inhalation. Severe curvature of the spine (scoliosis) also restricts breathing by reducing the movement of the rib cage. In obstructive disorders (such as chronic obstructive pulmonary disease or asthma), resistance to airflow is increased because the airways are narrowed. Because airways widen on inhalation, air can usually be pulled in. However, because airways narrow on exhalation, air cannot be exhaled from the lungs as fast as normal, and breathing becomes labored.

Heart Failure: The heart pumps blood through the lungs. The heart must function properly for the lungs to function normally. If the heart is pumping inadequately (heart failure), fluid may accumulate in the lungs, a condition called pulmonary edema. This condition causes dyspnea that is often accompanied by a feeling of smothering or heaviness in the chest. The fluid accumulation in the lungs may also lead to airway narrowing and wheezing—a condition called cardiac asthma.

Some people with heart failure experience orthopnea, paroxysmal nocturnal dyspnea, or both. Orthopnea is shortness of breath when a person lies down that is relieved by sitting up. Paroxysmal nocturnal dyspnea is a sudden, often terrifying, attack of shortness of breath during sleep. The person awakens gasping and must sit or stand to take a breath. This condition is an extreme form of orthopnea and a sign of severe heart failure (see page 356).

Anemia: Dyspnea can also occur in people who have anemia or blood loss because of a decreased number of red blood cells, which carry oxygen to the tissues. The person breathes rapidly and deeply, in a reflex effort to try to increase the amount of oxygen in the blood.

Other Causes: Someone with severe kidney failure or sudden worsening of diabetes mellitus or someone who has taken certain drugs or poisons feels out of breath and may begin to pant quickly because of an accumulation of a large amount of acids in the blood (a condition called **metabolic acidosis**). Anemia and heart failure may also contribute to dyspnea in people with kidney failure.

Hyperventilation syndrome causes people to feel that they cannot get enough air, and they breathe heavily and rapidly. This condition is commonly caused by anxiety rather than a physical problem. Many people who experience this syndrome are frightened, may have chest pain, and may believe they are having a heart attack. People may experience a change in consciousness usually described as a feeling that events occurring around them are far away, and they may experience tingling in the hands and feet and around the mouth.

Evaluation and Treatment

Doctors can usually get an idea of what is causing dyspnea from the person's symptoms and the results of a physical examination. A chest x-ray and measurement of levels of oxygen in the blood with arterial blood gas testing or pulse oximetry help determine the cause. The chest x-ray can show evidence of pneumonia and many other lung abnormalities and can often show evidence of heart failure. A low blood oxygen level usually indicates a heart or lung problem. Pulmonary function testing (see page 454) can measure the degree of restriction or obstruction and the ability of the lungs to transport oxygen from the air to the blood. A lung problem may include both restrictive and obstructive defects as well as abnormal oxygen transport. Other tests may be necessary to diagnose and further evaluate anemia, heart problems, certain specific lung problems, and kidney failure.

Treatment of dyspnea is directed at the cause. People with a low blood oxygen level are given supplemental oxygen using plastic nasal prongs or a plastic mask worn over the face. In severe cases, particularly if a person cannot breathe deeply or rapidly enough, doctors may assist breathing by mechanical ventilation administered through a breathing tube inserted into the trachea or through a tight-fitting face mask.

CHEST PAIN

Chest pain may be described as sharp (possibly knifelike), dull, burning, or squeezing; it may be located in a specific spot on the chest (such as the chest wall) or may be difficult to locate, often feeling like a deep ache. The pain may be constant or intermittent, lasting seconds, minutes, or longer. It may be worsened by breathing, changes in body position, exertion, eating, or other factors.

Pleuritic pain is a sharp pain that is made worse by deep breathing and coughing. Keeping the chest wall still—for example, by holding the side that hurts and avoiding deep breathing or coughing—can reduce the pain. Usually, the site of the pain can be pinpointed, although it may move over time. Pain may occur in the part of the chest supplied by a nerve between the ribs (intercostal nerve). This pain runs from the spine across the back to the chest in a path roughly parallel to a rib, usually affecting an area no wider than two or three ribs.

Causes

Chest pain may arise from structures in the respiratory system, including the pleura (the two-layered membrane covering the lungs). Chest pain can also arise from structures not related to the respiratory system, such as the chest wall, heart, major blood vessels, or esophagus. Some disorders of the heart and major blood vessels are serious; a person may need immediate testing and treatment.

Pleuritic pain often results from inflammation of the pleura (pleurisy). There are many causes of pleuritic pain, including viral and bacterial infections, cancer, and inflammation from disorders that can affect many organs, such as rheumatoid arthritis and systemic lupus erythematosus. Blood clots can travel through the bloodstream to the lungs (pulmonary embolism (see page 488)), lodge in the pulmonary arteries, and cause pleuritic chest pain. Air in the chest cavity (pneumothorax) and inflammation of the membrane surrounding the heart (pericarditis) can also cause chest pain that worsens during deep breathing. Pleural effusion, a fluid buildup in the space between the two layers of pleura (see page 518), may produce pleuritic pain at first, but the pain may subside as accumulating fluid separates the two layers.

Pain arising from other lung disorders (such as a lung abscess or tumor) is usually more difficult to describe than pleuritic pain. The pain is often described as a vague, deep-seated ache in the chest. Almost any disorder that damages the lungs or airways can cause such pain.

Pain originating in the chest wall may worsen with deep breathing or coughing and often is confined to one area in the chest wall, which also feels sore when pressed. The most common causes are chest wall injuries, such as broken ribs and torn or injured muscles located between the ribs (intercostal muscles). Even hard coughing can injure these muscles, causing pain for days or weeks. Pain along the area supplied by an intercostal nerve occurs if the nerve is irritated by a tumor or affected by shingles, which is caused by the varicella-zoster virus. In shingles, pain may occur before the tell-tale rash appears.

Evaluation and Treatment

Characteristics of the pain that a person describes provide clues to help doctors determine the cause. A chest x-ray is usually done. It often reveals the cause of chest pain, particularly pain caused by respiratory system problems. If serious disorders of the heart or major blood vessels are suspected, tests that help diagnose them are done, such as an electrocardiogram (ECG) or blood tests. Treatment is directed at the underlying disorder. Until the underlying disorder is controlled, drugs can relieve pain.

WHEEZING

Wheezing is a whistling, musical sound during breathing resulting from partially obstructed airways.

Wheezing results from an obstruction somewhere in the airways. It may be caused by widespread narrowing of the airways (as in asthma, chronic obstructive pulmonary disease, and some severe allergic reactions), by a local narrowing (as with a tumor), or by a foreign object lodged in an airway. The most common cause of recurrent wheezing is asthma, although many people who have never had asthma wheeze at some time in their lives. Infections such as pneumonia or bronchitis and, in infants, bronchiolitis can sometimes cause wheezing.

A doctor usually is able to detect wheezing by listening with a stethoscope as the person breathes. Loud wheezing can be heard easily, sometimes even without a stethoscope. To hear mild wheezing, the doctor may need to listen with a stethoscope while the person exhales forcefully. A persistent wheeze that occurs in one location in a smoker may be due to lung cancer. If a person develops wheezing suddenly for the first time, a chest x-ray may help in diagnosis. In people with persistent or repeated episodes of wheezing, pulmonary function testing (see page 456) may be needed to help measure the extent of airway narrowing and to assess the benefits of treatment. If doctors suspect a foreign object is lodged in an airway, they can insert a flexible viewing tube (bronchoscope) into the airway to diagnose the problem and remove the object.

Wheezing is relieved with bronchodilators, such as inhaled albuterol. Corticosteroids, taken by mouth for a week or two, can often help relieve an acute episode of wheezing if it is due to asthma or chronic obstructive pulmonary disease.

STRIDOR

Stridor is a gasping sound during inhalation resulting from a partial blockage of the throat (pharynx), voice box (larynx), or windpipe (trachea).

Stridor is usually loud enough to be heard at some distance. The sound is caused by turbulent airflow through a narrowed upper airway. In children, the cause may be croup, an inhaled foreign object, or, rarely, an infection of the epiglottis. In adults, the cause may be a tumor, an abscess, swelling (edema) in the upper airway, or a malfunction of the vocal cords.

Stridor causing dyspnea when the person is at rest is a medical emergency. In such cases, a tube may be inserted through the person's mouth or nose (tracheal intubation) or by a small surgical incision directly into the trachea (tracheostomy) to allow air to get past the blockage and prevent suffocation. The cause usually becomes clear during tracheal intubation, during which a doctor can see the upper airway directly. If tracheal intubation is not done, the diagnosis is usually determined by inserting a flexible viewing tube through

the nose and upper airway (a procedure called nasopharyngeal laryngoscopy).

HEMOPTYSIS

Hemoptysis is the coughing up of blood from the respiratory system.

Although hemoptysis can often be frightening, most causes turn out not to be serious.

Causes

Infection is the most common cause. Sometimes the cause is blood from the nose that has traveled down to the airways and then is coughed up. Unexplained or large amounts of blood in the sputum require evaluation by a doctor.

Tumors, especially those due to lung cancer, account for up to 20% of cases of hemoptysis. Death of lung tissue from blockage of an artery by a blood clot (pulmonary embolism—see page 488) may also cause hemoptysis.

Other causes include high blood pressure in the pulmonary veins, as may occur in heart failure and mitral valve stenosis. Other lung circulation problems, including arteriovenous malformations or inflammatory conditions of the pulmonary blood vessels, may also cause hemoptysis.

Evaluation

If hemoptysis is severe, persistent, or unexplained, a diagnostic evaluation is necessary. Doctors check for lung cancer in smokers older than 40 (and even in younger smokers if the person started smoking in adolescence) who develop hemoptysis, even if the sputum is only blood streaked. A chest x-ray is usually the first test done. A flexible viewing tube (bronchoscope) may be needed to identify the bleeding site. A scan using a radioactive marker (lung perfusion scan (see page 490) or other imaging test may reveal a pulmonary embolism. Despite testing, the cause of hemoptysis is not found in 30 to 40% of cases. When hemoptysis is severe, however, the cause is usually found.

Treatment

Bleeding may produce clots that block the airways and lead to further breathing problems. Therefore, coughing is important to keep the airways clear and should not be suppressed with antitussive drugs.

Hemoptysis is usually mild and usually stops by itself or when the disorder causing the bleeding (for example, heart failure or infection) is successfully treated.

If a large clot blocks a major airway, doctors may have to remove the clot using bronchoscopy. Rarely, hemoptysis is severe or does not stop by itself. If so, a tube may need to be inserted through the mouth or nose into the windpipe or lower into the airways to help keep the airways open. If the source of bleeding is a major blood vessel, a doctor may try to close off the bleeding vessel using a procedure called bronchial artery embolization. Using x-rays for guidance, the doctor passes a catheter into the vessel and then injects a chemical, fragments of a gelatin sponge, or a wire coil to block the blood vessel and thereby stop the bleeding. Sometimes bronchoscopy or surgery may be needed to stop severe or continuing bleeding, or surgery may be needed to remove a diseased portion of the lung. These high-risk procedures are used only as last resorts. If clotting abnormalities are contributing to the bleeding, a transfusion of plasma, clotting factors, or platelets may be needed.

CYANOSIS

Cyanosis is a bluish discoloration of the skin resulting from an inadequate amount of oxygen in the blood.

Cyanosis occurs when oxygen-depleted (also called deoxygenated) blood, which is bluish rather than red, circulates through the skin. Cyanosis can be caused by many types of severe lung or heart disease that produce low levels of oxygen in the blood. It can also result from certain blood vessel and heart malformations that allow blood to flow directly to the heart without ever flowing past the air sacs of the lung (alveoli) where oxygen is extracted from the air. This abnormal blood flow is called a shunt. In a shunt, blood from veins in the body, which is oxygen-depleted, may flow directly into blood vessels returning blood from the lungs to the left side of the heart or directly into the left side of the heart itself. The oxygen-depleted blood then is pumped out to the body, to circulate through the skin and other tissues.

The amount of oxygen in the blood can be estimated by pulse oximetry, in which a sensor is attached to a finger or an earlobe, or it can be measured directly by arterial blood gas analysis (see page 455). Chest x-rays, echocardiography, cardiac catheterization, pulmonary function tests, and sometimes other tests may be needed to determine the cause of decreased oxygen in the blood and the resulting cyanosis.

Oxygen therapy is often the first treatment given, in a similar fashion as for other conditions in which the blood oxygen level is low. Many malformations that cause shunts can be treated with surgery or other procedures.

CLUBBING

Clubbing is an enlargement of the tips of the fingers or toes and a change in the angle where the nails emerge.

Recognizing Finger Clubbing

Finger clubbing is characterized by enlarged fingertips and a loss of the normal angle at the nail bed.

160   180+

Normal Finger   **Clubbed Finger**

Clubbing occurs when the amount of soft tissue beneath the nail beds increases. Why this increase occurs is not clear but may relate to the levels of proteins that stimulate blood vessel growth. Clubbing seems to occur with some lung disorders (lung cancer, lung abscess, bronchiectasis), but not with others (pneumonia, asthma, chronic obstructive pulmonary disease). Clubbing also occurs with some congenital heart disorders and liver disorders, or in some cases, it may be inherited and not indicate any disorder. Clubbing itself does not need treatment.

Diagnosis

A doctor usually can tell whether a person has a lung or airway disorder based on the medical history and physical examination. Diagnostic procedures are used to confirm the diagnosis, determine the extent and severity of the disorder, and help in planning treatment.

MEDICAL HISTORY AND PHYSICAL EXAMINATION

A doctor first asks the person about symptoms. Chest pain, shortness of breath (dyspnea) either at rest or during exertion, cough, coughing up of sputum or blood (hemoptysis), and wheezing may indicate a lung or airway disorder. Other, more general symptoms, such as fever, weakness, fatigue, or a general feeling of illness or discomfort (malaise), sometimes also reflect a lung or airway disorder.

Next, the doctor asks the person about past infections; previous exposure to chemicals; use of drugs, alcohol, and tobacco; home and work environments; travels; and recreational activities. A doctor asks whether family members have had lung or airway disorders or any other disorders that may affect the lungs or airways (such as clotting and generalized inflammatory disorders). The doctor also asks about other common symptoms, even those that do not seem related to the respiratory system.

During the physical examination, a doctor notes the person's weight and overall appearance. The person's general mood and feeling of well-being, which also may be affected by a lung or airway disorder, are also noted. A doctor may ask a person to walk around or climb a flight of stairs to see if either activity causes shortness of breath.

Assessing skin color is important because paleness (pallor) may indicate anemia or poor blood flow, and a bluish discoloration (cyanosis) may indicate an inadequate amount of oxygen in the blood. Fingers are examined for clubbing.

A doctor observes the chest to determine if the breathing rate and movements are normal. Using a stethoscope, a doctor listens to the breath sounds to determine whether airflow is normal or obstructed and whether the lungs contain fluid. By tapping (percussing) the chest, a doctor can often determine if the lungs are filled with air or collapsed and if the space around the lungs contains fluid. In addition to examination of the chest, a complete physical examination may be needed, because disorders of the lungs may affect other parts of the body. Additionally, for some disorders not related to the lungs, the first symptoms may suggest a lung problem. For example, shortness of breath might reflect an abnormality of the kidneys or heart, and pneumonia might reflect an abnormality of the immune system.

PULMONARY FUNCTION TESTING

Pulmonary function tests measure the lungs' capacity to hold air, to move air in and out, and to exchange oxygen and carbon dioxide. These tests are better at detecting the general type and severity of lung disorder than at defining the specific cause of problems; however, these tests can be used to diagnose some specific disorders, such as asthma.

Lung Volume and Flow Rate Measurements: The assessment of a lung disorder often involves testing how much air the lungs can hold as well as how much and how quickly air can be exhaled. These measurements are made with a spirometer, which consists of a mouthpiece and tubing connected to a recording device. The person's lips should be held tightly around the mouthpiece, and nose clips should be worn to ensure that all the air inhaled or exhaled goes through the mouth. A person inhales deeply, then exhales forcefully as quickly as possible through the tubing while measurements are taken. The volume of air inhaled and exhaled and the length of time each breath takes are recorded and analyzed. Often, the tests are repeated after a person takes a drug that opens the airways of the lungs (bronchodilator).

A simpler device for measuring how quickly air can be exhaled is the small, hand-held peak flow

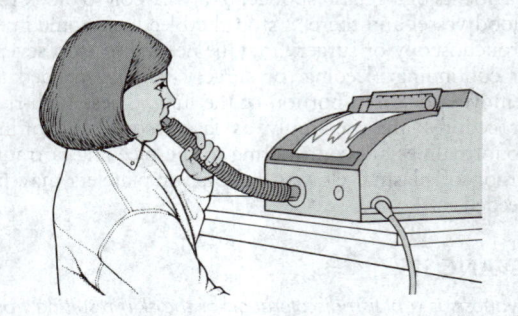

Using a Spirometer

A spirometer consists of a mouthpiece, tubing, and a recording device. To use a spirometer, a person inhales deeply, then exhales vigorously and as quickly as possible through the tubing. The recording device measures the volume of air inhaled or exhaled and the length of time each breath takes.

meter. After inhaling deeply, a person blows into this device as hard as possible.

Lung volume measurements reflect the stiffness or elasticity of the lungs and rib cage as well as the strength of respiratory muscles. The lungs are abnormally stiff in disorders such as pulmonary fibrosis, and the chest wall is abnormally stiff in disorders such as curvature of the spine (scoliosis). Various neuromuscular disorders can cause weakness of the diaphragm and other respiratory muscles, such as myasthenia gravis (see page 818) and Guillain-Barré syndrome (see page 828).

Flow rate measurements reflect the degree of narrowing or obstruction of the airways. The measurements are abnormal in obstructive disorders, such as chronic obstructive pulmonary disease and asthma.

Flow Volume Testing: Most spirometers can continuously display lung volumes and flow rates during a forced breathing maneuver. These flow rates can be particularly helpful in detecting abnormalities that partially block the voice box (larynx) and windpipe (trachea).

Muscle Strength Assessment: The strength of the respiratory muscles can be measured by having the person forcibly inhale and exhale against a pressure gauge. Disorders that weaken the muscles, such as muscular dystrophy and amyotrophic lateral sclerosis (ALS, or Lou Gehrig's disease), make breathing more difficult and result in low pressures during inhalation and exhalation.

Diffusing Capacity Measurement: A diffusing capacity test can estimate how efficiently oxygen is transferred from the air sacs of the lungs (alveoli) to the bloodstream. Because the diffusing capacity of oxygen is difficult to measure directly, a person inhales a small amount of carbon monoxide, holds the breath for 10 seconds, and then exhales into a carbon monoxide detector.

If the test shows that carbon monoxide is not well absorbed, oxygen will not be exchanged normally between the lungs and the bloodstream either. The diffusing capacity is characteristically abnormal in people with pulmonary fibrosis, in those with disorders affecting the blood vessels of the lungs, and in some people with chronic obstructive pulmonary disease.

Maximal Voluntary Ventilation (MVV): MVV measures a person's maximum ability to breathe. This test is done in the sitting position. A person is instructed to breathe as rapidly and deeply as possible through a spirometer for a predetermined period of time, usually 15 to 30 seconds. The volume of air moved over that period of time is measured. This test is dependent upon the ability of a person to cooperate but is useful in certain situations.

SLEEP STUDIES

Breathing is usually automatic and controlled by centers in the brain that respond to the levels of oxygen and carbon dioxide in the blood. However, in some people, breathing may stop for prolonged periods, especially during sleep—a condition called sleep apnea (see page 485). The best test for sleep apnea consists of monitoring brain wave activity (with an electroencephalogram, also called an EEG), the oxygen concentration in the blood (with pulse oximetry, which uses a sensor clipped on a finger or an earlobe), the movement of air during breathing (using a device placed in one nostril), chest wall motion, and sometimes other measurements. Combining all these measurements as part of a single test is called a polysomnogram. Because polysomnography is not always available, other tests are sometimes used during sleep to see whether a person has sleep apnea.

ARTERIAL BLOOD GAS ANALYSIS

Arterial blood gas tests measure the levels of oxygen and carbon dioxide in the arterial blood and determine the acidity (pH) of the blood. Taking a sample from an artery requires skill and may cause a few minutes of discomfort. Usually the sample is taken from an artery in the wrist (radial artery). Oxygen, carbon dioxide, and acidity levels are important indicators of lung function because they reflect how well the lungs are getting oxygen into the blood and getting carbon dioxide out of it.

Oxygenation of the blood can be monitored using a sensor placed on a finger or an earlobe—a procedure called pulse oximetry. When a doctor also needs a carbon dioxide or blood acidity measurement (for example, in certain people who are seriously ill), an arterial blood gas measurement is needed.

CHEST IMAGING

Chest x-rays are routinely taken from the back to front. Usually a view from the side is taken also. Chest x-rays provide a good outline of the heart and major blood vessels and usually can reveal a serious disorder in the lungs, the adjacent spaces, or the chest wall, including the ribs. For example, chest x-rays can clearly show most pneumonias, lung tumors, chronic obstructive pulmonary disease, a collapsed lung (atelectasis), and air (pneumothorax) or fluid (pleural effusion) in the pleural space. Although chest x-rays seldom give enough information to determine the exact cause of the abnormality, they can help a doctor determine whether and which other tests are needed to make a diagnosis.

Computed tomography (CT—see page 2037) of the chest provides more detail than a plain x-ray. With CT, a series of x-rays is analyzed by a computer, which then provides several views in different planes, such as longitudinal and cross-sectional views. During CT, a radiopaque dye may be injected into the bloodstream or given by mouth to help clarify certain abnormalities in the chest.

Magnetic resonance imaging (MRI—see page 2040) also produces highly detailed pictures that are especially useful when a doctor suspects blood vessel abnormalities in the chest, such as an aortic aneurysm. Unlike CT, MRI does not use radiation.

Ultrasonography (see page 2044) creates a picture from the reflection of sound waves in the body. Ultrasonography is often used to detect fluid in the pleural space (the space between the two layers of pleura covering the lung and inner chest wall). Ultrasonography can also be used for guidance when using a needle to remove the fluid.

Nuclear lung scanning (see page 2043) is particularly useful in detecting blood clots in the lungs (pulmonary emboli); it also may be used during the preoperative evaluation of people who have lung cancer. This type of imaging uses minute amounts of short-lived radioactive materials to depict the flow of air and blood through the lungs. Usually, the test is done in two stages. In the first stage (lung perfusion scan), a radioactive substance is injected into a vein, and a scanner creates a picture of how it is distributed throughout the blood vessels of the lung. If the perfusion scan is abnormal, a second stage is necessary (lung ventilation scan); the person inhales a radioactive gas, and a scanner creates a picture of how the gas is distributed throughout the lungs.

Pulmonary artery angiography (also called pulmonary artery arteriography) is done by injecting a radiopaque dye into the pulmonary artery and using conventional x-rays to view the dye in the lungs (see page 2036). Angiography is used most often when pulmonary embolism is suspected, usually on the basis of abnormal lung scan results, and is considered the best test for diagnosing or excluding pulmonary embolism. Increasingly, angiography of the pulmonary arteries is being done instead with pictures obtained from a CT scan (CT angiography). CT angiography is less invasive, because in this procedure, radiopaque dye is injected into a small peripheral vein rather than a central pulmonary artery.

Positron emission tomography (PET—see page 2044) scanning may be used when cancer is suspected. This radiographic imaging technique relies on different metabolic rates of malignant (cancerous) compared with benign (noncancerous) tissues. Glucose molecules are combined with a compound that is visible using PET. These molecules are injected intravenously, where they accumulate in rapidly metabolizing tissue (such as in cancerous lymph nodes), making these tissues visible on PET scans. Benign growths usually do not accumulate enough molecules to be visible.

THORACENTESIS

In thoracentesis, fluid that has collected abnormally in the pleural space (pleural effusion—see page 518) is removed. The two principal reasons to perform thoracentesis are to obtain a fluid sample for diagnostic testing or to relieve shortness of breath caused by fluid compressing lung tissue.

During the procedure, the person sits comfortably and leans forward, resting the arms on supports. A small area of skin on the back is cleaned and numbed with a local anesthetic. Then a doctor inserts a needle between two ribs into the chest cavity, but not into the lung, and withdraws some fluid into a syringe. Sometimes the doctor uses ultrasound for guidance (to determine where to insert the needle). The collected fluid is analyzed to assess its chemical makeup and to determine whether bacteria or cancerous cells are present.

If a large volume of fluid has accumulated, it may need to be removed through a plastic catheter and it may be necessary to use a fluid container that is larger than a syringe. The fluid may need to be drained over several days, in which case a larger tube (chest tube or drainage catheter) is left in the chest and suctioned continuously.

The risk of complications during and after thoracentesis is low. A person may feel some pain as the lung fills with air and expands against the chest wall or may feel the need to cough. Also, a person may

briefly feel light-headed and short of breath. Other possible complications include puncture of the lung with leakage of air into the pleural space (pneumothorax), bleeding into the pleural space or chest wall, fainting, infection, puncture of the spleen or liver, and, if a large amount of fluid that has been present for weeks to months is withdrawn rapidly, accumulation of fluid within the lung itself (pulmonary edema). A chest x-ray may be performed after the procedure to determine whether any of these complications has occurred.

NEEDLE BIOPSY OF THE PLEURA OR LUNG

If thoracentesis does not uncover the cause of a pleural effusion (a fluid buildup in the space between the two layers of the pleura), a doctor may do a pleural biopsy. First, the skin is cleaned and anesthetized as for thoracentesis. Then using a larger cutting needle, a doctor takes a small sample of tissue from the pleura and sends it to a laboratory to be examined for signs of disorders, such as cancer or tuberculosis. About 80 to 90% of the time, a pleural biopsy is accurate in diagnosing tuberculosis, but it is less accurate for diagnosing cancer and other disorders.

If a tissue specimen needs to be obtained from a lung tumor, a doctor may do a needle biopsy. After anesthetizing the skin, a doctor, often using chest computed tomography (CT) for guidance, directs a biopsy needle into a tumor and obtains cells or a small piece of tissue to be sent to the laboratory for analysis. If a lung infection is suspected, tissue can also be sent for culture (a procedure in which a tissue sample is placed in a container containing nutrients and the container is observed to detect bacterial growth). Complications of pleural and lung biopsies are similar to those for thoracentesis.

BRONCHOSCOPY

Bronchoscopy is a direct visual examination of the voice box (larynx) and airways through a flexible viewing tube (a bronchoscope). A bronchoscope has a light at the end that allows a doctor to look down through the larger airways (bronchi) into the lungs.

A bronchoscope can be used to investigate the source of bleeding in the lungs. If a doctor suspects lung cancer, the airways can be examined and specimens can be taken from any areas that look cancerous. Bronchoscopy can be used for collecting the organisms causing pneumonia that are difficult to collect and identify in other ways. Bronchoscopy is especially helpful for obtaining specimens from the lungs in people who have AIDS and other immune deficiencies. When people have been burned or have inhaled smoke, bronchoscopy helps doctors

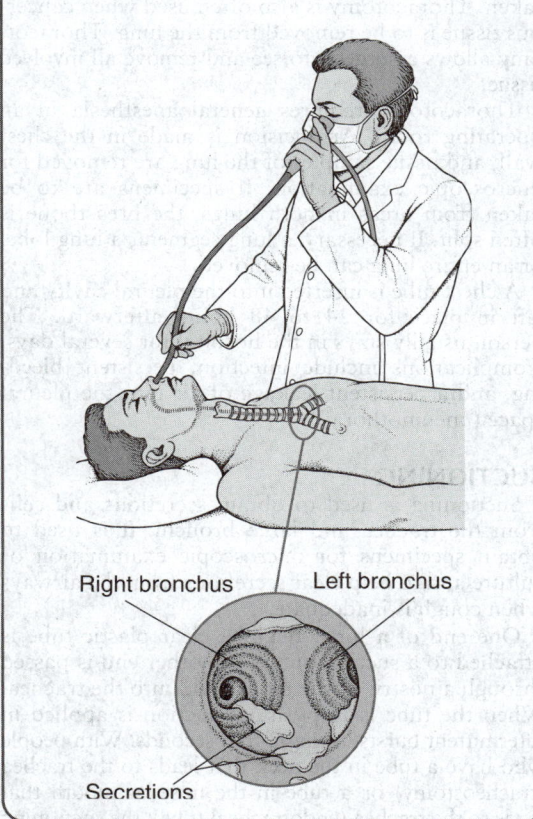

Understanding Bronchoscopy

To view the airways directly, a doctor passes a flexible bronchoscope through a person's nostril and down into the airways. The circular inset shows the doctor's view.

Right bronchus   Left bronchus

Secretions

assess for burns and smoke injury of the larynx and airways. Bronchoscopy can help a doctor treat certain conditions. For example, the bronchoscope can also be used to remove secretions, blood, pus, and foreign bodies; to place drugs in specific areas of the lung; and as a guide over which a tube can be inserted to assist breathing (tracheal intubation).

For at least 4 hours before bronchoscopy, the person should not eat or drink. A sedative is often given to ease anxiety, and atropine may be given to reduce the risks of spasm of the voice box and slowing of the heart rate, which sometimes occur during the procedure. The throat and nasal passage are sprayed with an anesthetic, and the bronchoscope is passed through a nostril and into the airways of the lungs.

Bronchoalveolar lavage is a procedure doctors can use to collect specimens from the smaller airways and alveoli that cannot be seen through the bronchoscope. After wedging the bronchoscope into a small airway, a doctor instills salt water (saline) through the instrument. The fluid is then suctioned back into the bronchoscope, bringing cells and any bacteria with it. Examination of the material under the microscope helps in diagnosing infections and cancers. The fluid can also be placed into containers containing special nutrients and left alone for a period of time to see if bacteria grow (culturing), which is a better way to diagnose infections.

Transbronchial lung biopsy involves obtaining a specimen (pieces) of lung tissue by using forceps passed through a bronchoscope. The forceps is threaded through a channel in the bronchoscope into progressively smaller airways until reaching the area of concern. A doctor may use a fluoroscope (an imaging device that uses x-rays to show internal body structures on a screen) for guidance in identifying the area of concern. Such guidance can also decrease the risk of accidentally perforating the lung and causing leakage of air into the pleural space (pneumothorax—see page 520). Although transbronchial lung biopsy increases the risk of complications during bronchoscopy, it provides additional diagnostic information and may make major surgery unnecessary.

Transbronchial needle aspiration is sometimes done. In this procedure, a needle is passed through the bronchoscope into the bronchial wall. The needle may be passed through the wall of a large airway under direct visualization or through the wall of a small airway using an x-ray machine for visualization. A doctor may be able to extract cells from suspicious lymph nodes to examine under a microscope.

After bronchoscopy, the person is observed for several hours. If a tissue specimen was removed, a chest x-ray may be taken to check for complications, such as bleeding or leakage of air into the pleural space (pneumothorax).

THORACOSCOPY

Thoracoscopy is the visual examination of the lung surfaces and pleural space through a viewing tube (a thoracoscope). The most common means for obtaining a sample of lung tissue for a biopsy is with a thoracoscope. A thoracoscope also may be used in treating accumulations of fluid in the pleural space (pleural effusions).

The person usually is given general anesthesia for this procedure. Then a surgeon makes up to three small incisions in the chest wall and passes a thoracoscope into the pleural space; this allows air to enter, collapsing the lung. Besides being able to view the lung surface and pleura, a doctor may take samples of tissue for microscopic examination and culture. In certain cases, the doctor may give drugs through the thoracoscope to prevent a reaccumulation of fluid in the pleural space. After the thoracoscope is removed, a chest tube is inserted to remove air that entered the pleural space during the procedure, enabling the collapsed lung to reinflate.

Complications are similar to those for thoracentesis and needle biopsy of the pleura. However, this procedure is more invasive, leaves a small wound, and requires hospitalization.

MEDIASTINOSCOPY

Mediastinoscopy is the direct visual examination of the area of the chest between the two lungs (the mediastinum) through a viewing tube (mediastinoscope). The mediastinum contains the heart, trachea, esophagus, thymus, and lymph nodes. Nearly all mediastinoscopies are used to diagnose the cause of enlarged lymph nodes deep in the chest or to evaluate how far lung cancer has spread before chest surgery (thoracotomy) is done.

Mediastinoscopy is done in an operating room with the person under general anesthesia. A small incision is made in the notch just above the breastbone (sternum). The instrument then is passed down into the chest in front of the windpipe, allowing the doctor to observe the contents of the mediastinum next to the windpipe and to obtain specimens for diagnostic tests if necessary. Complications are similar to those for thoracentesis and needle biopsy of the pleura.

THORACOTOMY

Thoracotomy is an operation in which the chest wall is opened to view the internal chest organs, to obtain samples of tissue for laboratory examination, and to treat disorders of the lungs, heart, or major arteries.

Thoracotomy is a major operation and therefore is used less often than other diagnostic techniques.

Thoracotomy is used when procedures such as thoracentesis, bronchoscopy, or mediastinoscopy fail to provide adequate information. The lung problem is identified in more than 90% of people who undergo this operation because the sample site can be seen and selected and because large tissue samples can be taken. Thoracotomy is also often used when cancerous tissue is to be removed from the lung. Thoracotomy allows a surgeon to see and remove all involved tissue.

Thoracotomy requires general anesthesia in an operating room. An incision is made in the chest wall, and tissue samples of the lung are removed for microscopic examination. If specimens are to be taken from areas in both lungs, the breastbone is often split. If necessary, a lung segment, a lung lobe, or an entire lung can be removed.

A chest tube is inserted into the pleural cavity and left in place for 24 to 48 hours afterward. The person usually stays in the hospital for several days. Complications include infection, persistent bleeding, and a persistent leakage of air into the pleural space (pneumothorax).

SUCTIONING

Suctioning is used to obtain secretions and cells from the trachea and large bronchi. It is used to obtain specimens for microscopic examination or culture and to help clear secretions from the airways when cough is inadequate.

One end of a long, flexible, clear plastic tube is attached to a suction pump; the other end is passed through a nostril or the mouth and into the trachea. When the tube is in position, suction is applied in intermittent bursts lasting 2 to 5 seconds. With people who have a tube in the neck that leads to the trachea (tracheostomy) or a tube in the nose or mouth that leads to the trachea (endotracheal tube), the suctioning tube can be inserted directly into the tube that leads to the trachea. Sometimes inserting some salt water into the tube that leads to the trachea eases removal of secretions and cells via suctioning.

72 Rehabilitation for Lung and Airway Disorders

Pulmonary rehabilitation is a program designed for people who have chronic lung disease. Its primary goal is to enable people to achieve and maintain their maximum level of independence and functioning. Although most pulmonary rehabilitation programs focus on people who have chronic obstructive pulmonary disease, people with other types of lung disease may benefit as well. People in all age groups can benefit, including those older than 70.

Pulmonary rehabilitation programs may improve quality of life by reducing shortness of breath, increasing exercise tolerance, promoting a sense of well-being, and, to a lesser extent, decreasing the number of hospitalizations. However, these programs do not significantly improve survival.

Pulmonary rehabilitation programs are usually conducted in an outpatient setting or in the person's home. Inpatient services often take place in special rehabilitation centers. Inpatient services are used mainly for people who are recovering from a hospitalization, often because of a severe lung problem. These people are often not stable enough to go home but no longer require care in an intensive care unit. The most successful rehabilitation programs are those in which services are provided by a respiratory or physical therapist, a nurse, a doctor, a psychologist or social worker, and a dietitian working as the pulmonary rehabilitation team to coordinate complex medical services. Most people are enrolled in these programs for 8 to 12 weeks. However, the techniques learned during the program have to be continued at home after the rehabilitation program ends or the gains made will be lost.

Supportive respiratory therapy, which includes oxygen therapy and chest physical therapy, can be used in conjunction with pulmonary rehabilitation. Supportive therapy can also be used for people not enrolled in these programs but who have chronic lung disorders (such as cystic fibrosis or bronchiectasis) or acute lung conditions (such as pneumonia).

Enrollment and Goal Setting

The first step for the team members is to determine the person's short-term and long-term goals. For example, an older person may desire to travel by air to visit a grandchild. If the person can walk only 300 feet (about 90 meters) because of shortness of breath but must be able to walk 1,000 feet

(300 meters) to board the airplane, the initial short-term goal may be to increase the walking distance by small increments. Team members must be encouraging while also setting realistic goals. Periodic reevaluation (weekly) is important to ensure that these goals are being met.

It is also important for team members to identify factors that may limit the program's effectiveness for a particular person. These factors may include problems with financial resources, transportation to the rehabilitation center, cognition, and family dynamics. An example of a problem with cognition would be when a person who has lung problems also has dementia. Such a person may need a specific approach to enhance comprehension. An example of a problem with family dynamics would be when a person who is enrolled in a program is dependent on a caregiver who is not able to help the person with rehabilitation at home. It is important for team members to recognize such problems and plan ways to help the person.

Long-term goals are also established, and team members teach people to recognize changes in their lung condition, so that they will contact their doctor promptly. Treatment may need to be modified in response to changes in symptoms.

Exercise Training

Exercise training is probably the most important component of pulmonary rehabilitation. It reduces the effects of inactivity and deconditioning, resulting in less shortness of breath and an increased ability to exercise. However, physical limitations may restrict the types of exercise training that can be used. Exercise training may help some people who are dependent on ventilators to function without ventilator assistance.

Exercise of the legs is the cornerstone of training. Because walking is necessary for most activities of daily living, many rehabilitation programs use walking (sometimes on a treadmill) as the preferred mode of training. Some people may prefer exercising on a stationary bicycle. Choosing an exercise that is comfortable and satisfying for the person enhances willingness to participate long-term.

Exercise training of the arms is also beneficial for people with chronic lung diseases who have shortness of breath or other symptoms during their normal activities of daily living, such as washing their hair or shaving. Such training is needed because some of the shoulder muscles are used in breathing as well as in moving the arms, and arm work can quickly overexert these muscles.

Psychosocial Counseling

Because strong emotions tend to worsen shortness of breath, some people suppress their emotions, but depression and anxiety are common reactions to the life changes a person with lung disease experiences. In addition, shortness of breath itself may cause anxiety and depression, interfere with sexual activity, and cause difficulty managing stress and relaxing. Through counseling, group therapy, and, when needed, drug treatment, people may be able to better cope with these psychosocial problems. Sometimes family members participate in counseling to help them cope with the stress involved in caring for a person with lung disease.

Nutritional Evaluation and Counseling

People who have lung disease often need nutritional evaluation and counseling. For example, those with the most severe chronic obstructive pulmonary disease often experience weight loss. Pulmonary rehabilitation programs help people avoid weight loss and maintain muscle mass. People must be taught to eat in such a way that they maintain adequate caloric intake while avoiding becoming too full, which can interfere with breathing. Alternatively, some people gain weight because of a reduced activity level. In this case, breathing places a greater demand on an already taxed respiratory system. Weight reduction benefits such people.

Drug Use and Education

People with severe lung disease usually take several drugs. Often these drugs must be taken according to precise instructions and a complex schedule. Through a rehabilitation program, people can learn about the appropriate timing and doses of all drugs they need to take. Education often includes information about the nature of the lung disease and the role of drug therapy, including expected benefits, potential side effects, and the proper technique for use of inhaled drugs. Programs closely monitor how well people follow instructions and teach them and their families about the importance of appropriate drug use.

Oxygen Therapy

Some people with chronic lung disease need only a brief period of oxygen therapy during an acute exacerbation of their lung disease. Others, in whom oxygen levels in the blood are consistently low, may require oxygen therapy on a daily basis. In these people, oxygen use improves survival. The more hours a day the oxygen is used, the better the result. Survival is better when 12 hours of oxygen are used than when no oxygen is used. Survival is even better when oxygen is used continuously (24 hours per day). Long-term oxygen use decreases shortness of breath and reduces the strain on the heart that lung disease causes. Both sleep and the ability to exercise tend to improve.

Some people with chronic lung disease have low levels of oxygen only when they physically exert themselves. These people can limit their oxygen use to periods of exertion. Other people have low oxygen levels only when they are sleeping. These people can limit their oxygen use to overnight hours.

Once the critical level of oxygen is determined, oximetry may be used to adjust oxygen flow settings over time. Oximetry is painless and uses a simple device that is attached to a finger or ear to measure the concentration of oxygen in the blood.

Oxygen for long-term home use is available from three different delivery systems: electrically driven oxygen concentrators, liquid systems, and compressed gas. Inside the home, liquid and compressed gas systems use large tanks to store oxygen. Small, portable tanks of compressed oxygen also may be needed for brief periods—a few hours—outside the home. Each system has advantages and disadvantages.

Oxygen is typically administered with continuous flow through a two-pronged nasal tube (cannula), even though this system is highly wasteful of oxygen. To improve efficiency and increase the person's mobility, several devices, including reservoir cannulas, demand-type systems, and transtracheal catheters, can be used. Usually, a respiratory therapist or physician instructs the person about proper oxygen use.

While using oxygen therapy at home, it is important to stabilize the tank (possibly using a stand) and store it in an area that is out of the way so it will not fall. Tanks should be closed tightly when not in use. Because oxygen can cause an explosion, it is also important to keep tanks away from any flammable source, such as matches, heaters, or hair dryers. No one in the house should smoke when oxygen is in use.

Chest Physical Therapy

Respiratory therapists use several different techniques to help treat lung disease, including postural drainage, suctioning, and breathing exercises. The choice of therapy is based on the underlying disease and the person's overall condition.

Postural Drainage: In postural drainage, the person is tilted or propped at an angle selected to help drain secretions from the lungs. The chest or back may also be clapped with a cupped hand to help loosen secretions—a technique called chest percussion. Alternatively, the therapist may use a mechanical chest vibrator or teach a family member to use one.

These techniques are used at intervals on people who have conditions, such as cystic fibrosis, bronchiectasis, or lung abscess, that cause a great deal of sputum to be produced. The techniques may also be used when a person cannot cough up sputum effectively, as may happen with older people or with people who have muscle weakness or who are recovering from surgery, injury, or severe illness.

Postural drainage cannot be used for people who are unable to tolerate the position required, those taking anticoagulation drugs, those who have recently vomited up blood, those who have had a recent rib or vertebral fracture, or those who have severe osteoporosis. Postural drainage also should not be used for people who are unable to produce any secretions.

Suctioning: Respiratory therapists, nurses, and family members who have been taught the procedure may use suctioning to help remove secretions from the airways. A small plastic tube is introduced through the nose and extended a few inches into the windpipe (trachea). A gentle vacuum sucks out the secretions that cannot be coughed up. Suctioning is also used to remove secretions in someone who has a tracheostomy (a surgical opening in the trachea to allow breathing) or who has a breathing tube inserted through the nose or mouth and into the trachea (endotracheal tube) while on a ventilator.

Breathing Exercises: Breathing exercises may help strengthen the muscles that inflate and deflate the lungs, but they do not directly improve lung function. Still, breathing exercises decrease the likelihood of lung complications after surgery in heavy smokers and other people with lung disease. Such exercises are particularly helpful for sedentary people who have chronic obstructive pulmonary disease or those who have just been taken off of a ventilator.

Often, these exercises involve using an instrument called an incentive spirometer (see art on page 454). A person breathes in as deeply as possible through a tube that is attached to a hand-held plastic chamber. The chamber houses a ball, and each breath lifts the ball. Ideally, this maneuver is done 5 to 10 consecutive times each hour while the person is awake. This device is used routinely in hospitals before and after surgery. However, deep breathing exercises encouraged by nurses and respiratory therapists may be more effective than self-directed breathing exercises using an incentive spirometer.

Pursed-lip breathing is a type of breathing pattern that may be helpful when people who have chronic obstructive pulmonary disease overinflate their lungs during attacks of airway narrowing, panic, or exercise. It also can function as an additional breathing exercise for people undergoing pulmonary rehabilitation. People are taught—or often discover by themselves—to exhale against partially closed (pursed) lips, as if preparing to whistle. This measure increases pressure in the airways and helps prevent them from collapsing. The exercise causes no ill effects, and some people adopt the habit without instruction. People may also benefit from bending forward while performing pursed-lip breathing. In this position, the person stands with the arms and hands outstretched and supports the body on a table or similar structure. This position improves functioning of the diaphragm (the most important breathing muscle) and reduces shortness of breath.

CHAPTER

73 Acute Bronchitis

Bronchitis is inflammation of the large airways that branch off the trachea (bronchi), usually caused by infection but sometimes caused by irritation from inhaling gases, smoke, dust particles, or some types of pollution.

- Acute bronchitis is usually caused by viral infections.
- Symptoms of the common cold that are followed by a cough usually indicate acute bronchitis.
- The diagnosis is made based primarily on symptoms.

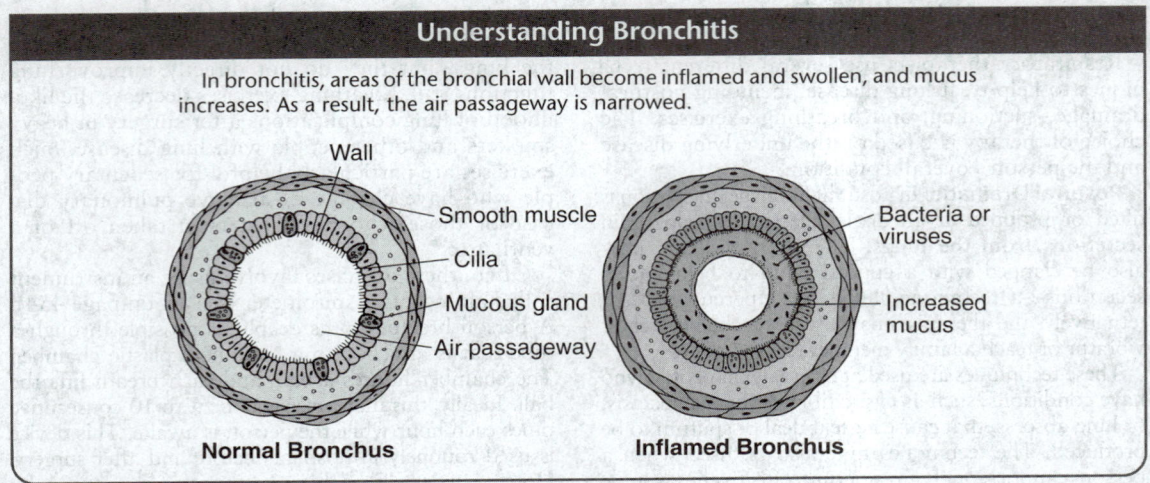

Understanding Bronchitis

In bronchitis, areas of the bronchial wall become inflamed and swollen, and mucus increases. As a result, the air passageway is narrowed.

Wall
Smooth muscle
Cilia
Mucous gland
Air passageway

Normal Bronchus

Bacteria or viruses

Increased mucus

Inflamed Bronchus

- Most treatments, such as cough suppressants and drugs to reduce fever, are used to make the person more comfortable until the episode ends.
- Antibiotics are almost never needed.

Symptoms lasting up to 90 days are usually classified as acute bronchitis; symptoms lasting longer, sometimes for months or years, are usually classified as chronic bronchitis. When chronic bronchitis occurs with decreased expiratory airflow, it is considered a defining characteristic of chronic obstructive pulmonary disease (see page 480). This chapter discusses acute bronchitis only.

Causes

Acute bronchitis can be caused by infection or by exposure to irritants.

Infectious Bronchitis: Infectious bronchitis occurs most often during the winter and is most often caused by viruses. Viral bronchitis may be caused by a number of common viruses, including the influenza virus. Even after a viral infection has resolved, the irritation it causes can continue to cause symptoms for weeks.

Infectious bronchitis may also be caused by bacteria. Often bacterial bronchitis follows a viral upper respiratory infection. Acute bronchitis is more likely to be caused by bacteria in people who smoke. *Mycoplasma pneumoniae* and *Chlamydia pneumoniae* are the bacteria that often cause acute bronchitis in young adults. In rare cases, *Bordetella pertussis* infection (whooping cough) may cause acute bronchitis.

Smokers and people who have chronic lung diseases may have repeated attacks of acute bronchitis. These episodes may be caused by bacteria, viruses, irritation

from inhaling smoke, or a combination of factors. Undernutrition increases the risk of upper respiratory tract infections and subsequent acute bronchitis, especially in children and older people. Chronic sinus infections, bronchiectasis (see page 491), and allergies also increase the risk of repeated episodes of acute bronchitis. Children with enlarged tonsils and adenoids may have repeated episodes of bronchitis.

Irritative Bronchitis: Irritative bronchitis (also called industrial or environmental bronchitis) may be caused by exposure to various mineral and vegetable dusts as well as cigarette smoke and smog. Exposure to fumes from strong acids, ammonia, some organic solvents, chlorine, hydrogen sulfide, sulfur dioxide, and bromine can also cause irritative bronchitis.

Symptoms

Infectious bronchitis generally begins with the symptoms of a common cold: runny nose, sore throat, fatigue, and chilliness. Back and muscle aches together with a slight fever (100° to 101° F, or 37.5° to 38° Celsius [C]) may be present, particularly if the infection is due to influenza. The onset of cough (usually dry at first) signals the beginning of acute bronchitis. With viral bronchitis, small amounts of white mucus are often coughed up. This mucus often changes from white to green or yellow. The color change does not mean there is a bacterial infection. Color change means only that cells associated with inflammation have moved into the airway and are coloring the sputum.

With severe bronchitis, fever may be slightly higher at 101° to 102° F (38° to 39° C) and may last for 3 to 5 days, but higher fevers are unusual unless bronchitis is caused by influenza. Cough is the last symptom to subside and often takes several weeks or even longer to do so. Viruses can damage the epithelial cells lining the bronchi, and the body needs time to repair the damage. Airway hyperreactivity, which is a short-term narrowing of the airways with impairment or limitation of the amount of air flowing into and out of the lungs, is common with acute bronchitis. The impairment of airflow may be triggered by common exposures, such as inhaling mild irritants (for example, perfume, strong odors, or exhaust fumes) or cold air. If the impairment of airflow is severe, the person may be short of breath. Wheezing, especially after coughing, is common.

Complications: Serious complications, such as acute respiratory failure (see page 524) or pneumonia (see page 463), usually occur only in people who have advanced underlying chronic lung disease (such as chronic obstructive pulmonary disease), who are older, or who have problems with immune defenses.

Diagnosis

Doctors usually make a diagnosis of bronchitis based on the symptoms. Fevers that are high or prolonged or both could indicate the presence of pneumonia. Doctors may hear wheezing during the physical examination. A chest x-ray is sometimes done to exclude pneumonia, mainly when doctors hear wheezing or congestion in the lungs or when the person is short of breath.

A sample taken from the throat can be used to detect influenza. Sputum is generally only examined if doctors find evidence of pneumonia on a chest x-ray or during the examination. If a cough persists for more than 2 months, a chest x-ray is done to exclude an underlying lung disease, such as lung cancer.

Treatment

Cough medicines can be used to suppress a dry, disturbing cough, particularly when it interferes with sleep (see page 449). However, a cough that produces a lot of sputum usually should not be suppressed. Expectorants may help to thin secretions and make them easier to cough up, but whether this is helpful is not clear. Adults may take aspirin, acetaminophen, or ibuprofen to reduce fever and general feelings of illness, but children should take only acetaminophen or ibuprofen, not aspirin. People with acute bronchitis, especially those who have a fever, should drink plenty of fluid.

Antibiotics are not used to treat bronchitis except for people whose infection is caused by *Bordetella pertussis* or for some people with chronic obstructive pulmonary disease. Antibiotics do not help people with viral bronchitis. However, if influenza is the suspected cause, treatment with an antiviral drug may be helpful if given within 48 hours of onset of symptoms.

In children, very mild symptoms of limited airflow can be helped with cool-mist humidifiers or steam vaporizers. In more severely affected children and adults who are wheezing, inhaled bronchodilators, which widen the bronchi, can be used to open the airways and reduce wheezing. Corticosteroids, usually given by means of a metered-dose inhaler (see art on page 476), are also sometimes used to diminish cough and inflammation and hyperreactivity of the airways, especially when the cough persists after the infection has resolved.

74   Pneumonia

Pneumonia is an infection of the small air sacs of the lungs (alveoli) and the tissues around them.

- Pneumonia is one of the most common causes of death worldwide.
- Often, pneumonia is the final illness in people who have other serious, chronic diseases.
- Some types of pneumonia can be prevented by immunization.

In the United States, about 2 to 3 million people develop pneumonia each year, and 45,000 of them die. Pneumonia is the sixth most common cause of death overall, and the most common fatal infection acquired in hospitals. In developing countries, pneumonia is either the leading cause of death or second only to dehydration from severe diarrhea.

The setting in which pneumonia develops is one of the most important features to doctors. Pneumonia

Preventing Certain Pneumonias With Vaccines

Certain pneumonias can be prevented with immunizations.

Pneumococcal pneumonia vaccine: Pneumococcal pneumonia, which is caused by *Streptococcus pneumoniae*, can sometimes be prevented with the pneumococcal pneumonia vaccine. The organism that causes pneumococcal pneumonia can also cause many other infections (such as infections of the blood and meningitis). The pneumococcal pneumonia vaccine also protects people from many of these serious pneumococcal infections. Vaccination is recommended for people at high risk of pneumococcal pneumonia—such as all those older than 65 and younger adults who have lung or heart disease, a weakened immune system, or diabetes or who have had their spleen removed. The protection from vaccination may last a lifetime, although it is recommended that people at highest risk be revaccinated after 5 years. Although temporary soreness at the site of injection is common, only 1% of people develop a fever and muscle pain after vaccination. Even fewer people have a severe allergic reaction. Pregnant women should not receive this vaccine.

Pneumococcal conjugate vaccine: Pneumococcal conjugate vaccine also protects against pneumococcal infections, including pneumonia. This vaccine is given to children younger than 2 years old.

Haemophilus influenzae type b vaccine: Pneumonia caused by *Haemophilus influenzae* type b strain can be prevented with the *Haemophilus influenzae* type b vaccine. This vaccine is recommended for all children to prevent pneumonia as well as other infections caused by this organism. The vaccine is given in two or three doses—at ages 2 months, 4 months, and sometimes 6 months.

Influenza vaccine: Pneumonia caused by the influenza virus can usually be prevented with the influenza vaccine. Annual influenza vaccinations are recommended for health care workers, older people, and people with chronic conditions such as emphysema, diabetes, heart disease, and kidney disease. Some experts recommend vaccination for all people if enough vaccine is available. Vaccination should take place every year during the fall (September through November), so that levels of antibodies will be highest during the peak influenza months—November through March. A different vaccine is introduced every year based on predictions of which strains are most likely to cause influenza.

Chickenpox vaccine: Pneumonia caused by the chickenpox virus may be prevented with the chickenpox vaccine. Pneumonia caused by this virus is very rare. One dose of the vaccine is given between ages 12 and 15 months and another between ages 4 and 6 years. Children between 6 and 12 years who have not already received the vaccine should be vaccinated, unless testing indicates a natural immunity from a previous infection. Vaccination without testing is acceptable because vaccination appears to be safe even if a person has had chickenpox. In people 13 years and older, the vaccine should be given only if testing does not indicate natural immunity. For these people, two doses are given 4 to 8 weeks apart.

---

may develop in people living in the community (community-acquired pneumonia), in the hospital (hospital-acquired pneumonia), or in some other institutional setting, such as a nursing home (nursing home–acquired pneumonia). The setting often helps determine what infecting organism is responsible for the pneumonia. For example, community-acquired pneumonia is more likely to stem from infection with the bacterium *Streptococcus pneumoniae*. Hospital-acquired pneumonia is more likely to be caused by *Staphylococcus aureus* or a gram-negative bacterium, such as *Klebsiella pneumoniae* or *Pseudomonas aeruginosa*. Depending on the infecting organism, there is usually a difference in the severity of pneumonia and the way it is treated (for example, whether with oral drugs at home or with intravenous drugs in the hospital).

Another critical feature is whether the pneumonia occurs in a healthy person or in someone who has an impaired immune system. Certain drugs (such as oral or intravenous corticosteroids) can impair the immune system, as can the presence of diseases, such as AIDS or various types of cancer. Sometimes the immune system can be worn down by a severe acute or chronic illness, as is often the case with older people. A person who has an impaired immune system is far more likely to contract pneumonia, including pneumonia caused by unusual organisms. Also, a person whose immune system is impaired may not respond as well to treatment as someone whose immune system is healthy.

Other conditions that predispose people to pneumonia include alcoholism, cigarette smoking, diabetes, heart failure, and chronic obstructive pulmonary disease. The very young and very old are at higher-than-average risk.

Causes

Pneumonia is not a single illness but rather many different ones, each caused by a different microscopic organism—whether it is a bacterium, virus, fungus, or parasite. Usually pneumonia starts after organisms are inhaled into the lungs, but sometimes the infection is carried to the lungs by the bloodstream or organisms migrate to the lungs directly from a nearby infection. Pneumonia may follow surgery, particularly abdominal surgery, or an injury (trauma), particularly a chest injury, because of the resulting shallow breathing, impaired ability to cough, and retention of mucus. Also at risk are people who are debilitated, bedridden, paralyzed, or unconscious, because the cough reflex may be impaired or breathing may be shallow. Sometimes pneumonia occurs when particles from the mouth are inhaled and are not cleared or when an obstruction (such as a tumor blocking one of the tubes in the lungs) causes bacteria to accumulate behind the obstruction. The former type is called aspiration pneumonia, and the latter type is called obstructive pneumonia.

Symptoms

The most common symptom of pneumonia is a cough that produces sputum. Other common symptoms include chest pain, chills, fever, and shortness of breath. These symptoms may vary, however, depending on how extensive the disease is and which organism is causing it.

Symptoms vary even more in infants and older people. Fever may not occur. Chest pain may not occur, or people may not be able to communicate that they have chest pain. Sometimes the only symptom is rapid breathing or a sudden refusal to eat. An older person may suddenly become confused.

Complications: A severe pneumonia can prevent oxygen from getting to the bloodstream, causing people to feel short of breath. Low levels of oxygen can be life threatening.

Some pneumonias can lead to lung abscesses (see page 472), or pus can collect around the lung, a condition called empyema (see page 518).

Diagnosis

A doctor or nurse checks for pneumonia by listening to the chest with a stethoscope. Pneumonia usually produces distinctive sounds. These abnormal sounds are caused by narrowing of airways or filling of the normally air-filled parts of the lungs with inflammatory cells and fluid, a process called consolidation. In most cases, the diagnosis of pneumonia is confirmed with a chest x-ray.

In people who are sick enough to require hospitalization, doctors often culture specimens of sputum, blood, and urine in an attempt to identify the organism causing pneumonia. They often will obtain sputum samples by giving a vapor treatment that causes the person to cough deeply (inducing sputum production) or insert a bronchoscope into the airways (see page 456). Sputum samples obtained by inducing a cough, particularly those obtained with a bronchoscope, are less likely to contain saliva and are more likely than expectorated sputum samples to allow doctors to identify the organism causing pneumonia. It is particularly important to identify the causative organism when people are severely ill, do not have a normal immune system, or are not responding well to treatment. However, despite these tests, the precise organism cannot be identified conclusively in most people who have pneumonia.

What Is Legionnaires' Disease?

Legionnaires' disease is caused by the bacterium *Legionella*. It accounts for about 1 to 8% of all pneumonias and about 4% of fatal pneumonias acquired in hospitals. *Legionella* bacteria live in water, and outbreaks have occurred primarily in hotels and hospitals when the organism has spread through the air conditioning systems or water supplies, such as showers. No cases have been identified in which one person directly infected another.

Although Legionnaires' disease may occur at any age, people who are middle-aged and older have been affected most often. People who smoke tobacco, take corticosteroids, have chronic kidney failure, or have undergone organ transplantation seem to be at greater risk. Legionnaires' disease can be life threatening.

The first symptoms, appearing 2 to 10 days after the infection is transmitted, include fatigue, fever, headache, and muscle aches. A dry cough later becomes productive of sputum. People with serious infections can become extremely short of breath and may have diarrhea or mental disturbances.

Laboratory tests are done on sputum and urine samples to confirm the diagnosis. Because people infected with *Legionella* produce antibodies to fight the disease, blood tests show an increasing concentration of these antibodies. However, the results of antibody tests usually are not available until after the pneumonia has run its course.

Antibiotics, such as the fluoroquinolones, erythromycin, or azithromycin, are used for treatment. About 20% of the people who develop the disease die. The death rate is much higher among people who contract the disease in the hospital or who have an impaired immune system.

Prevention

The most effective way to prevent pneumonia is to stop smoking. Vaccines are available that offer partial protection against pneumococcal pneumonia (caused by the bacterium *Streptococcus pneumoniae*) and almost 100% protection against pneumonia caused by the bacterium *Haemophilus influenzae*. The ability of vaccines to prevent pneumonia caused by the influenza virus depends on how well the strains used in the vaccine match the epidemic strain that occurs in a particular year. Protection has been very good in 9 of the past 10 years. Vaccination can also help prevent pneumonia caused by chickenpox.

Deep-breathing exercises and therapy to clear secretions help prevent pneumonia in people at high risk, such as those who have had chest or abdominal surgery and those who are debilitated.

Treatment

People with pneumonia also need to clear secretions and benefit from deep-breathing exercises and therapy. People with pneumonia who are short of breath or have low levels of oxygen in their blood are given supplemental oxygen. Although rest is an important part of treatment, moving often and getting out of bed and into a chair are encouraged.

Usually antibiotics are started whenever bacterial pneumonia is suspected, even before the organism is identified. The prompt use of antibiotics likely reduces the severity of pneumonia and the chance of developing complications, some of which can lead to death.

When choosing an antibiotic, doctors consider which organism is likely to be the cause. Doctors can give a different antibiotic later, after the organism has been identified and its susceptibility to various antibiotics is known. Often, people who have pneumonia but are not very sick can take oral antibiotics and remain at home. Older people, infants, and those who are short of breath, are very sick, or have preexisting heart or lung disease are usually hospitalized and given intravenous antibiotics to start. Those antibiotics are usually switched to oral ones after a few days. These people may also need supplemental oxygen, intravenous fluids, and, if they are very sick, mechanical respiratory support (see page 527).

Antibiotics are not helpful for viral pneumonias. However, antibiotics are given for viral pneumonias that are likely to be followed by bacterial infections, such as those caused by respiratory syncytial virus infection in infants and sometimes those caused by the influenza virus, at least in some people who are very susceptible to pneumonia.

Community-Acquired Pneumonia

Community-acquired pneumonia develops in people with limited or no contact with medical institutions or settings.

- Many bacteria, viruses, and fungi can cause pneumonia.
- The most common symptom of pneumonia is a cough that produces sputum, but chest pain, chills, fever, and shortness of breath are also common.
- Doctors diagnose community-acquired pneumonia by listening to the lungs with a stethoscope and by reading x-rays of the chest.
- Antibiotics, antiviral drugs, or antifungal drugs are used depending on which organism doctors believe has caused the pneumonia.

Causes

Many organisms cause community-acquired pneumonia, including bacteria, viruses, fungi, and parasites. Causative organisms vary depending on the person's age and other factors, such as whether the person also has other disorders. The term community-acquired pneumonia is usually reserved for people who have pneumonia caused by one of the more common bacteria or viruses.

Bacteria: *Streptococcus pneumoniae, Haemophilus influenzae, Chlamydia pneumoniae,* and *Mycobacterium pneumoniae* are the most common bacterial causes.

C. pneumoniae accounts for a small percentage of community-acquired pneumonia and is the second most common cause of lung infections in healthy people aged 5 to 35 years. *C. pneumoniae* is commonly responsible for outbreaks of respiratory infection within families, in college dormitories, and in military training camps. It causes a pneumonia that is rarely severe and infrequently requires hospitalization. *Chlamydia psittaci* pneumonia (psittacosis) is rare and occurs in people who own or are often exposed to birds.

Viruses: Common viral causes include respiratory syncytial virus (RSV), adenoviruses, influenza viruses, metapneumovirus, and parainfluenza viruses. The virus that causes chickenpox can also cause a lung infection. Hantavirus and severe acute respiratory syndrome (SARS) are also types of lung infections. A bacterium can infect people with pneumonia originally caused by a virus.

Fungi: Common fungal causes include *Histoplasma capsulatum* (histoplasmosis) and *Coccidioides immitis* (coccidioidomycosis). Less common fungi include *Blastomyces dermatitidis* (blastomycosis) and *Paracoccidioides braziliensis* (paracoccidioidomycosis). *Pneumocystis jiroveci* commonly causes pneumonia in people who have HIV infection or are immunosuppressed.

Parasites: Parasites that cause lung infection in people who live in developed countries include *Toxocara canis* and *T. catis* (visceral larva migrans), *Dirofilaria immitis*

Psittacosis: An Unusual Type of Pneumonia

Psittacosis (parrot fever) is a rare pneumonia caused by *Chlamydia psittaci*, a bacterium present mainly in birds such as parrots, parakeets, and lovebirds. It is also present in other birds, such as pigeons, finches, chickens, and turkeys. Usually, people are infected by inhaling dust from the feathers or the waste of infected birds. The organism also may be transmitted by a bite from an infected bird and, rarely, from person to person in cough droplets. Psittacosis mainly occurs in bird fanciers or in people who work in pet shops or on poultry farms.

About 1 to 3 weeks after being infected, a person develops a fever, chills, fatigue, and loss of appetite. A cough develops, which is initially dry but later brings up greenish sputum. The fever persists for 2 to 3 weeks and then slowly subsides. The disease may be mild or severe, depending on the person's age and the extent of lung tissue involved. Blood antibody tests are the most reliable method for confirming the diagnosis, but doctors usually suspect the infection in people who have a history of exposure to birds.

Bird breeders and owners can protect themselves by avoiding the dust from the feathers and the cages of sick birds. Importers are required to treat susceptible birds with a 45-day course of tetracycline, which generally gets rid of the organism. People with psittacosis are treated with tetracycline taken by mouth for at least 10 days. Recovery may take a long time, especially in severe cases. The death rate may reach 30% in severe untreated cases.

(dirofilariasis), and *Paragonimus westermani* (paragonimiasis).

Symptoms

Symptoms include a general feeling of weakness (malaise), cough, shortness of breath, and chest pain. Cough typically produces sputum in older children and adults, but it is dry in infants, young children, and older people. Shortness of breath usually is mild and occurs mainly during exertion. Chest pain is typically worse when breathing in or coughing. Sometimes people have upper abdominal pain.

Symptoms vary at the extremes of age. Infants may be irritable and restless, and older people may be confused or have a decreased level of consciousness. These people may be unable to communicate chest pain and shortness of breath. Fever is common but may not occur in older people.

Diagnosis

No matter what type of pneumonia is suspected, doctors listen to a person's chest with a stethoscope to make a diagnosis. Chest x-rays are usually also done to confirm the diagnosis. Doctors usually do not need to do additional tests to determine what organism is causing the pneumonia. However, if doctors do need to identify the organism, they usually try to grow the organism from a specimen of sputum, blood, or urine. Even when such testing is done, the organism is identified less than half the time.

Sometimes the likely cause is evident from the person's symptoms. For example, a bird fancier may have psittacosis. Certain combinations of risk factors and symptoms may suggest Legionnaire's disease. In people who have symptoms typical of influenza (see page 1242), influenza is a likely cause of pneumonia. In people with a rash characteristic of chickenpox and pneumonia, chickenpox is probably the cause of the pneumonia. However, a bacterium may have also infected the lung after a virus such as influenza or chickenpox first caused pneumonia.

Prevention

Stopping smoking is the best way to prevent pneumonia. Some pneumonias can be prevented by vaccination. Oseltamivir or zanamivir can be given to prevent influenza in household contacts of people who have influenza and in people with heart or lung disorders who have not been vaccinated because these people would be at risk of severe pneumonia if they developed influenza.

Treatment

Doctors evaluate many factors to determine whether people can be safely treated at home or whether they should be hospitalized because of high risk of complications. Some of the factors include the following:

- Age
- Whether another disorder, such as cancer or a liver, heart, or lung disease, is also present
- Whether there are worrisome findings on physical examination or testing
- Whether people are able to care for themselves or have someone to help them

Antibiotics are started as soon as possible. People are also given fluids, drugs to relieve fever and pain, and supplemental oxygen if needed.

HOW IS COMMUNITY-ACQUIRED PNEUMONIA TREATED?

SEVERITY	POSSIBLE DRUGS	COMMENTS
Mild pneumonia in otherwise healthy people with no risk factors*	Azithromycin Clarithromycin Doxycycline	Drugs are taken by mouth. People are treated at home.
Mild pneumonia in people with risk factors*	Amoxicillin Amoxicillin plus clavulanate Azithromycin Cefpodoxime Cefuroxime Clarithromycin Doxycycline Levofloxacin Moxifloxacin	Drugs are usually taken by mouth. Often, more than one drug is taken. People are treated at home.
Moderate pneumonia or Pneumonia in people who cannot care for themselves	Azithromycin Cefotaxime Ceftriaxone Levofloxacin Moxifloxacin	Drugs are usually given intravenously in a hospital. Often, more than one drug is given.
Severe pneumonia in people with many risk factors*	Some of the same drugs used for moderate pneumonia Aztreonam Cefepime Ciprofloxacin Gentamicin Imipenem Meropenem Piperacillin plus tazobactam	Drugs are usually given intravenously in an intensive care unit. Usually, more than one drug is given.

*Risk factors include heart or lung disorders, cancer, alcoholism, age older than 65, recent use of antibiotics, and a weakened immune system (for example, because of AIDS, organ transplantation, or use of drugs that suppress the immune system).

Because the causative organism is difficult to identify, doctors choose antibiotics based on the organisms that are most likely to be causing pneumonia and the severity of illness.

With antibiotic treatment, most people with bacterial pneumonia improve. In people who do not improve, doctors look for unusual organisms, resistance to the antibiotic used for treatment, infection with a second organism, or some other disorder (such as a problem with the immune system or a lung abnormality) that is delaying recovery.

To treat influenza pneumonia, oseltamivir or zanamivir can be given. To treat chickenpox pneumonia, acyclovir is given. If a person with a viral pneumonia is very sick or does not improve within a few days after beginning treatment, doctors may prescribe antibiotics in case a bacterium has also infected the lung.

Doctors usually do follow-up chest x-rays about 6 weeks after treatment in people older than 35 to ensure that the infection has been cured.

Prognosis

Most people with community-acquired pneumonia recover. However, pneumonia can be fatal, most often in infants and in older people. Mortality is higher in Legionnaires' disease, possibly because people who develop the disease are less healthy even before they become sick.

Hospital-Acquired and Institution-Acquired Pneumonia

Hospital-acquired pneumonia develops in people who have been hospitalized, typically after about 2 days or more of *hospitalization. **Institution-acquired pneumonia** develops in people who reside in nursing homes or who have contact with medical settings, such as dialysis centers.*

- Many bacteria, viruses, and even fungi can cause pneumonia in people who are hospitalized or have visited medical institutions.

- The most common symptom of pneumonia is a cough that produces sputum, but chest pain, chills, fever, and shortness of breath are also common.

- Diagnosis is made by listening to the lungs with a stethoscope and by examining x-rays of the chest.

- Antibiotics, antiviral drugs, or antifungal drugs are used, depending on which organism has most likely caused the pneumonia.

One reason that pneumonia acquired in the hospital is more severe is that the infecting organisms tend to be more aggressive and harder to treat. Additionally, people in hospitals and nursing homes tend to be sicker even without pneumonia than those living in the community and therefore are not as able to fight the infection.

Cause

People who are hospitalized and seriously ill, especially if they require assistance in breathing from a mechanical ventilator, are at greatest risk of acquiring pneumonia. Other risk factors include previous antibiotic treatment and coexisting illness such as heart, lung, liver, or kidney dysfunction. People who are older than 70, have had abdominal or chest surgery, take proton pump inhibitors, or have a combination of these factors are at particularly high risk.

People who are debilitated, such as those living in nursing homes, are also at risk.

Organisms that do not normally cause pneumonia in healthy people can cause pneumonia in people who are hospitalized or debilitated. Many such people have an immune system that is not able to resist even mild infectious challenges. The most likely organisms depend on what organisms are prevalent in the hospital and sometimes depend on what other illnesses the person has.

Hospital-acquired pneumonia is more likely than community-acquired pneumonia to be caused by *Staphylococcus aureus* or a gram-negative bacterium, such as *Klebsiella pneumoniae* or *Pseudomonas aeruginosa*. Sometimes pneumonia is caused by *Legionella* or methicillin-resistant *Staphylococcus aureus* (MRSA, the super-bug).

Symptoms

Symptoms are generally the same as those for community-acquired pneumonia: a general feeling of weakness (malaise), cough, shortness of breath, and chest pain. Pneumonia in critically ill people, especially those who are on a mechanical ventilator, causes fever and increases the respiratory rate and the heart rate.

Pneumonia acquired in an institutional setting may be more difficult for doctors to recognize than pneumonia acquired in other settings. For example, many people in institutional settings who develop pneumonia, such as the elderly, those with breathing tubes who are receiving mechanical ventilation, and those with dementia, may be unable to describe symptoms such as chest pain, shortness of breath, and weakness.

> **? Did You Know...**
>
> Pneumonia that is acquired in the hospital or another type of institution tends to be far more severe than pneumonia acquired in the community.

Diagnosis

Hospital-acquired and institution-acquired pneumonia is suspected on the basis of a person's symptoms. The diagnosis is confirmed with a chest x-ray. Blood tests are done. However, these methods are not always accurate. Also, because people may be very sick, doctors may need to identify the organism that is causing pneumonia so that they can determine the best treatment. For these reasons, sometimes doctors use bronchoscopy to confirm pneumonia and obtain a sputum specimen to try to identify the organism. During bronchoscopy, a flexible viewing tube is inserted into the trachea and lungs. Samples of pus, secretions, or even lung tissue can be collected for examination. If no secretions are visible, an area of the lung can be washed with a solution, which can then be retrieved for analysis (bronchoalveolar lavage).

Treatment

Treatment is with antibiotics that are chosen based on which organisms are most likely to be the cause and the specific risk factors the person has. Because of the seriousness of the infection, people in nursing homes are often treated in the hospital. People who are seriously ill may be placed in an intensive care unit and sometimes put on a ventilator. Treatments include intravenous antibiotics, supplemental oxygen, and intravenous fluids. There are several drugs that can be used, including the following:

- Imipenem plus cilastatin
- Meropenem
- Aztreonam

- Piperacillin plus tazobactam
- Ceftazidime
- Cefepime

These drugs are given alone or combined with vancomycin. If MRSA is suspected, an antibiotic called linezolid may be used.

End-of-life Issues: Because some people who live in nursing homes are very ill, pneumonia can be extremely serious. In order to treat pneumonia with the most powerful treatments available, doctors usually have nursing home residents transferred to a hospital. However, pneumonia is often fatal despite such treatment, and the treatment itself may be difficult to tolerate, especially if a mechanical ventilator is needed. People who are expected to die soon may not wish to receive such aggressive treatment. People with severe or terminal disorders should discuss with their doctors and family members their wishes for treatment of pneumonia when they enter a nursing home.

Prognosis

Despite receiving excellent treatment, about 25 to 50% of people who develop hospital-acquired pneumonia die. Whether the cause of death is due to underlying illness or to the pneumonia itself can be difficult to tell.

Pneumonia in Immunocompromised People

Pneumonia in people whose immune system is weakened (for example, by AIDS, organ transplantation, or the use of certain drugs) is usually caused by different organisms than those that cause pneumonia in healthy people.

- *Pneumocystis jiroveci* pneumonia often occurs in people who have a weakened immune system.
- People have shortness of breath, a dry cough, and often fever.
- X-rays of the chest are not as helpful as microscopic examinations of sputum samples for making the diagnosis.
- Trimethoprim-sulfamethoxazole is often used to treat this pneumonia.

Pneumocystis jiroveci is a common fungus that may reside harmlessly in the lungs of healthy people. It usually causes pneumonia only when the body's defenses are weakened because of cancer, drugs that alter the immune system, or AIDS. Drugs that alter the immune system include corticosteroids, chemotherapy drugs, and drugs used to treat autoimmune disorders. Often, *P. jiroveci* pneumonia is the first indication that a person with human immunodeficiency virus (HIV) infection has developed AIDS.

SPOTLIGHT ON AGING

Pneumonia occurs more commonly in older than in younger people, and it also tends to be more serious. In many older people, the infection spreads beyond the lungs.

Older people have weakened defenses against infection. The mechanisms that clear microorganisms from the airways are not as effective in older people as they are in younger people. Weakness may make coughing less vigorous. Aging also weakens the immune system. Older people at greater risk of developing pneumonia include those

- Whose lungs have been damaged by smoking or chronic obstructive pulmonary disease (smoking irritates the lining of the lungs and paralyzes the cells that normally sweep and cleanse the airways)
- Whose lungs have recently been irritated by a mild infection, such as a cold or, especially, influenza
- Who have a poor cough reflex or who are too weak (or who are in pain from recent surgery or an accident) to cough vigorously
- Who are less able to fight off infections, including people who are undernourished
- Who are taking certain drugs, such as corticosteroids
- Who have certain diseases, such as heart failure or diabetes
- Who have cancer in or near the airways of the lungs (the cancer may block the airways and trap any microorganisms that have reached the air sacs)
- Who are paralyzed (for example, because of a spinal injury or stroke)
- Who are unconscious (in part because they are unable to cough)

Infection with some of the microorganisms that cause pneumonia can be prevented with vaccinations. So doctors recommend that people who are 65 or older receive the pneumococcal vaccine. Doctors also recommend that older people in particular receive an annual influenza vaccine because the influenza virus can also cause or contribute to pneumonia.

Most older people who get pneumonia are treated in the hospital with intravenous antibiotics. Pneumonia can cause older people to get very sick very quickly, and older people tend to respond less well to oral antibiotics.

Most people develop a fever, shortness of breath, and a dry cough. These symptoms usually arise over several weeks. The lungs may not be able to deliver sufficient oxygen to the blood, leading to shortness of breath that is sometimes severe.

X-rays show either no abnormality or patchy infection, similar to that which occurs in some viral infections. The diagnosis is made by microscopic examination of expectorated sputum or from sputum obtained by induction (in which a vapor is used to stimulate coughing) or bronchoscopy (in which an instrument is inserted into the airways to collect a specimen—see page 456).

The combination antibiotic trimethoprim-sulfamethoxazole can be used to help prevent *Pneumocystis* pneumonia in people at risk. This drug's side effects, which are particularly common in people who have AIDS, include rashes, a reduced number of infection-fighting white blood cells, and fever. Alternative preventive drug treatments are dapsone, atovaquone, and pentamidine (which can be taken as an aerosol, inhaled directly into the lungs).

Drugs used to treat *Pneumocystis* pneumonia are trimethoprim-sulfamethoxazole, dapsone combined with trimethoprim, clindamycin and primaquine, atovaquone, or intravenous pentamidine. When the level of oxygen in the blood falls below a certain level, corticosteroids may also be given.

Even when the pneumonia is treated, the overall death rate is 15 to 20%.

Aspiration Pneumonia

Aspiration pneumonia is lung infection caused by inhaling mouth secretions, stomach contents, or both. Chemical pneumonitis is lung irritation caused by inhalation of substances toxic to the lungs.

- Symptoms include cough and shortness of breath.
- Doctors make the diagnosis on the basis of the person's symptoms and a chest x-ray.
- Treatment and prognosis differ depending on the substance that was aspirated.

Aspiration Pneumonia: Tiny particles from the mouth frequently dribble or are inhaled (aspirated) into the airways. Usually they are cleared out by normal defense mechanisms (such as coughing) before they can get into the lungs and cause inflammation or infection. When such particles are not cleared (because of impaired defense mechanisms or because the volume of aspirated material is so large), they can cause aspiration pneumonia. Older people and people who are debilitated, have trouble swallowing (as may happen from a stroke), are intoxicated by alcohol or drugs, or are unconscious from anesthesia or a medical condition are especially at risk for this type of pneumonia.

Symptoms of pneumonia do not begin for at least a day or two. The sputum may smell foul. Treatment requires antibiotics. Many antibiotics, including clindamycin, amoxicillin plus clavulanate, ampicillin, and imipenem, can be used. If a solid particle was inhaled, bronchoscopy may be needed to remove it (see page 456).

Chemical Pneumonitis: Chemical pneumonitis occurs when a person inhales (aspirates) material that is toxic to the lungs. The problem is more the result of irritation than infection. A commonly inhaled toxic material is stomach acid, so that chemical pneumonitis may result whenever a person inhales what has been vomited up. Inhalation of vomit can occur when a person who vomits is not completely awake, as can happen after a seizure, stroke, or drug or alcohol overdose. Chemical pneumonitis may also be caused by inhalation of laxative oils (such as mineral, castor, and paraffin oils) and hydrocarbons (such as gasoline, kerosene, and petroleum products). Sudden shortness of breath and a cough develop within minutes or hours. Other symptoms may include fever and pink frothy sputum. In less severe cases, the symptoms of aspiration pneumonia may occur a day or two after inhalation of the toxin.

The diagnosis of chemical pneumonitis is usually obvious from the sequence of events if this information is available. Chest x-rays and measurements of oxygen concentrations in arterial blood may help. When the diagnosis remains unclear, bronchoscopy is sometimes done.

Treatment consists of oxygen therapy (see page 460) and mechanical ventilation (see page 527) if necessary. The windpipe (trachea) may be suctioned to clear secretions and aspirated food particles out of the airways. Bronchoscopy may also be used for this purpose.

Antibiotics are usually given because doctors cannot easily distinguish this form of aspiration pneumonia from a bacterial infection. Up to 30 to 50% of people with serious chemical pneumonitis due to inhaled stomach acid die.

Abscess in the Lungs

A lung abscess is a pus-filled cavity in the lung surrounded by inflamed tissue and caused by an infection.

- A lung abscess is usually caused by bacteria that normally live in the mouth and are inhaled into the lungs.
- Symptoms include fatigue, loss of appetite, sweating, fever, and a cough that brings up sputum.
- Diagnosis is usually determined with a chest x-ray.
- People usually need to take antibiotics for several weeks before a lung abscess disappears.

Causes

A lung abscess is usually caused by bacteria that normally live in the mouth or throat and that are aspirated into the lungs, resulting in an infection. Often, gum (periodontal) disease is the source of the bacteria that cause a lung abscess. The body has many defenses (such as a cough) to help prevent bacteria from getting into the lungs. Infection occurs primarily when a person is unconscious or very drowsy because of sedation, anesthesia, alcohol or drug abuse, or a disease of the nervous system. In people whose immune system functions poorly, a lung abscess may be caused by organisms that are not typically found in the mouth or throat, such as fungi or *Mycobacterium tuberculosis* (the organism that causes tuberculosis). Another cause of lung abscess is *Staphylococcus aureus* as well as methicillin-resistant *Staphylococcus aureus* (MRSA), which is a serious infection. This usually occurs in young, previously healthy adults or children, especially if they have influenza.

Obstruction of the airways also can lead to abscess formation. If the branches of the windpipe (bronchi) are blocked by a tumor or a foreign object, an abscess can form because secretions (mucus) can accumulate behind the tumor. Bacteria sometimes enter these secretions. The obstruction prevents the bacteria-laden secretions from being coughed back up through the airway.

Less commonly, abscesses result when bacteria or infected blood clots travel through the bloodstream to the lung from another infected site in the body (septic pulmonary emboli).

Usually, people develop only one lung abscess as a result of aspiration or airway obstruction. If several abscesses develop, they are usually in the same lung. When an infection reaches the lung through the bloodstream, however, many scattered abscesses may develop in both lungs. This problem is most common among people who inject drugs using dirty needles or unsterile methods.

Eventually, most abscesses rupture into an airway, producing a lot of sputum that gets coughed up. A ruptured abscess leaves a cavity in the lung that is filled with fluid and air. The cavity may become an inactive part of the lung, or it may require surgical removal. Sometimes an abscess ruptures into the space between the lungs and the chest wall (pleural space), filling the space with pus, a condition called empyema. Very rarely, if an abscess destroys a blood vessel wall, it may lead to serious bleeding.

Symptoms

Symptoms most commonly start slowly. However, depending on the cause of the abscess, symptoms can occur suddenly. Early symptoms resemble those of pneumonia: fatigue, loss of appetite, sweating, fever, and a cough that brings up sputum. The sputum may be foul smelling (because bacteria from the mouth or throat tend to produce foul odors) or streaked with blood. People also may feel chest pain with breathing, especially if the lining on the outside of the lungs and inside of the chest wall (pleura) is inflamed (a condition called pleurisy—see page 518).

Many people have these symptoms for weeks or months before seeking medical attention. These people have chronic abscesses and, in addition to the other symptoms, lose a substantial amount of weight and have daily fever and night sweats. In contrast, lung abscesses caused by *Staphylococcus aureus* or MRSA can be fatal within days, sometimes even hours.

Diagnosis

Chest x-rays nearly always reveal a lung abscess. However, how a lung abscess appears on an x-ray is sometimes similar to how other conditions, such as cancer, sarcoidosis, or Wegener's granulomatosis, appear on x-ray. Sometimes, an abscess is only found when computed tomography (CT) of the chest is done. Cultures of sputum may help identify the organism causing the abscess, but this test is usually not useful except for excluding MRSA, tuberculosis, and fungal infections.

Treatment

Treatment requires antibiotics. Antibiotics are initially given intravenously in most cases and later by mouth when the person has improved and the fever has resolved. Antibiotic treatment continues until the symptoms disappear and a chest x-ray shows that the abscess has disappeared. Such improvement may require several weeks or even months of antibiotic therapy.

Bronchoscopy (see page 456) is often done when the abscess is thought to be the result of a tumor or a foreign object blocking the airway. Rarely, a lung abscess may have to be drained through a tube inserted through the chest wall and into the abscess, or infected lung tissue may have to be removed surgically. Sometimes an entire lobe of a lung or even an entire lung has to be removed.

Most people are cured. Treatment is less likely to be successful when the person is debilitated or has an impaired immune system, lung cancer, or a very large abscess.

76 Asthma

Asthma is a condition in which the airways narrow—usually reversibly—in response to certain stimuli.

- Coughing, wheezing, and shortness of breath that occur in response to specific triggers are the most common symptoms.
- Doctors confirm the diagnosis of asthma by doing pulmonary function tests.
- To prevent attacks, people should avoid substances that trigger asthma and should take drugs that help keep airways open.
- During an asthma attack, people need to take a drug that quickly opens the airways.

Asthma affects more than 20 million people in the United States, and it is becoming more common. Although it is one of the most common chronic diseases of childhood, adults can also develop asthma, even at an old age. Asthma affects more than 6 million children and occurs more frequently in boys before puberty and in girls after puberty. It also occurs more frequently in blacks and Puerto Ricans. Although the number of people affected by asthma has increased, the number of deaths has decreased.

The reason for the increase in asthma in children is not known, but it may relate to more widespread use of vaccines and antibiotics, to the fact that children are spending more time indoors, or to both. Increased use of vaccines and antibiotics may have shifted the activity of a special subgroup of white blood cells (called lymphocytes) in the body from fighting infection to releasing chemical substances that promote the development of allergies. Alternatively, because children are spending more time indoors and living in better-insulated homes than they were in the past, the exposure to potentially allergic substances is increased. There are few data to support either theory.

The most important characteristic of asthma is narrowing of the airways that can be reversed. The airways of the lungs (the bronchi) are basically tubes with muscular walls (see page 444). Cells lining the bronchi have microscopic structures, called receptors. There are two main types of receptors: beta-adrenergic and cholinergic. These receptors sense the presence of specific substances and stimulate the underlying muscles to contract and relax, thus altering the flow of air. Beta-adrenergic receptors respond to chemicals such as epinephrine and make the muscles relax, thereby widening (dilating) the airways and increasing airflow. Cholinergic receptors respond to a chemical called acetylcholine, making the muscles contract, thereby decreasing airflow.

Did You Know...

Coughing may be the only symptom of asthma.

Causes

Narrowing of the airways is often caused by abnormal sensitivity of cholinergic receptors, which cause the muscles of the airways to contract when they should not. Certain cells in the airways, particularly mast cells, are thought to be responsible for initiating the response. Mast cells throughout the bronchi release substances such as histamine and leukotrienes, which cause smooth muscle to contract, mucus secretion to increase, and certain white blood cells to migrate to the area. Eosinophils, a type of white blood cell found in the airways of people with asthma, release additional substances, contributing to airway narrowing.

In an asthma attack, the smooth muscles of the bronchi contract, causing the bronchi to narrow (called bronchoconstriction), and the tissues lining the airways swell from inflammation and mucus secretion into the airways. The top layer of the airway lining can become damaged and shed cells, further narrowing the diameter

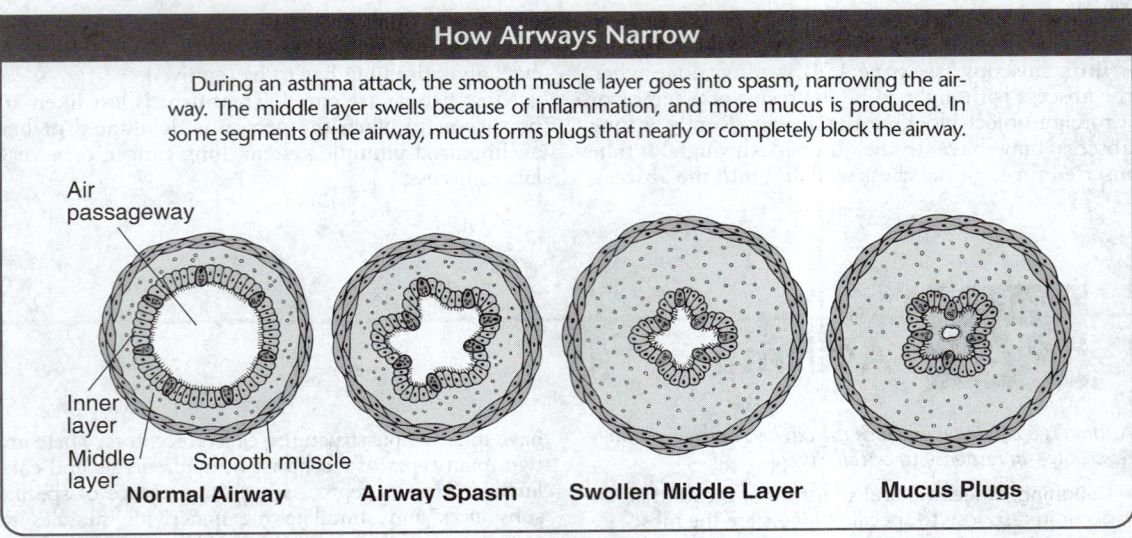

How Airways Narrow

During an asthma attack, the smooth muscle layer goes into spasm, narrowing the airway. The middle layer swells because of inflammation, and more mucus is produced. In some segments of the airway, mucus forms plugs that nearly or completely block the airway.

Air passageway

Inner layer

Middle layer

Smooth muscle

Normal Airway   **Airway Spasm**   **Swollen Middle Layer**   **Mucus Plugs**

of the airway. A narrower airway requires the person to exert more effort to move air in and out of the lungs. In asthma, the narrowing is reversible, meaning that with appropriate treatment or on their own, the muscular contractions of the airways stop, the airways widen again, and the airflow into and out of the lungs returns to normal.

In people who have asthma, the airways narrow in response to stimuli that usually do not affect the airways in normal lungs. The narrowing can be triggered by many inhaled allergens, such as pollens, particles from dust mites, body secretions from cockroaches, particles from feathers, and animal dander. These allergens combine with immunoglobulin E (a type of antibody) on the surface of mast cells to trigger the release of asthma-causing chemicals from these cells. (This type of asthma is called allergic asthma.) Although food allergies induce asthma only rarely, certain foods (such as shellfish and peanuts) can induce severe attacks in people who are sensitive to these foods.

Cigarette smoke, cold air, and viral infections can also provoke asthma attacks. Additionally, people who have asthma can develop bronchoconstriction when exercising. Stress and anxiety can trigger mast cells to release histamine and leukotrienes and stimulate the vagus nerve (which connects to the airway smooth muscle), which then contracts and narrows the bronchi. Gastroesophageal reflux disease (GERD) is a common trigger of asthma.

Symptoms

Asthma attacks vary in frequency and severity. Some people who have asthma are symptom-free most of the time, with only an occasional, brief, mild episode of shortness of breath. Other people cough and wheeze most of the time and have severe attacks after viral infections, exercise, or exposure to allergens or irritants, including cigarette smoke. Coughing may be the only symptom in some people (cough-variant asthma). Crying or hearty laughing may bring on symptoms in some people. Some people with asthma produce a clear, sometimes sticky (mucoid) phlegm (sputum). Asthma attacks occur most often in the early morning hours when the effects of protective drugs wear off and the body is least able to prevent bronchoconstriction.

An asthma attack may begin suddenly with wheezing, coughing, and shortness of breath. Wheezing is particularly noticeable when the person breathes out. At other times, an asthma attack may come on slowly with gradually worsening symptoms. In either case, people with asthma usually first notice shortness of breath, coughing, or chest tightness. The attack may be over in minutes, or it may last for hours or days. Itching on the chest or neck may be an early symptom, especially in children. A dry cough at night or while exercising may be the only symptom. Symptoms of asthma can also be caused by other disorders. Symptoms are reversible with timely treatment and typically occur after exposure to one or more triggers.

During an asthma attack, shortness of breath may become severe, creating a feeling of severe anxiety. The person instinctively sits upright and leans forward, using the neck and chest muscles to help in breathing, but still struggles for air. Sweating is a common reaction to the effort and anxiety. The pulse usually quickens, and the person may feel a pounding in the chest.

In a very severe asthma attack, a person is able to say only a few words without stopping to take a breath. Wheezing may diminish, however, because hardly any air is moving in and out of the lungs. Confusion, lethargy, and a blue skin color (cyanosis) are signs that the person's oxygen supply is severely limited, and emergency treatment is needed. Usually, a person recovers completely with appropriate treatment, even from a severe asthma attack. Rarely, some people develop attacks so quickly that they may lose consciousness before they can give themselves effective therapy. Such people should wear a medical alert bracelet and carry a cellular phone to call for emergency medical assistance.

Diagnosis

Doctors suspect asthma based largely on a person's report of characteristic symptoms. Doctors confirm the diagnosis by doing pulmonary function tests (see page 454). These tests are done before and after giving the person an inhaled drug, called a beta-adrenergic agonist, that reverses bronchoconstriction. If test results are significantly better after the person receives the drug, asthma is thought to be present. If the airways are not narrowed at the time of the test, a diagnosis can be confirmed by doing a challenge test. In a challenge test, pulmonary function is measured before and after the person inhales a chemical (usually methacholine but histamine may be used) that can narrow the airways. The chemical is given in doses that are too low to affect a person with healthy lungs but that cause the airways to narrow in a person with asthma. If the challenge test shows airway narrowing, asthma is thought to be present.

An abbreviated form of pulmonary function testing, spirometry, is used in people known to have asthma. Spirometry can help assess the severity of the airway obstruction and monitor effectiveness of treatment.

Peak expiratory flow (the fastest rate at which air can be exhaled) can be measured using a small handheld peak flow meter. Often, this test is used at home to monitor the severity of asthma. Usually, peak flow rates are lowest between 4 AM and 6 AM and highest at 4 PM. However, more than a 30% difference in rates at these times is considered evidence of moderate to severe asthma.

Determining what triggers a person's asthma is often difficult. Allergy testing is appropriate when there is a suspicion that some avoidable substance is stimulating attacks (for example, exposure to cat dander). Skin testing can help identify allergens that may trigger asthma symptoms. However, an allergic response to a skin test does not necessarily mean that the allergen being tested is causing the asthma. The person still has to note whether attacks occur after exposure to this allergen. If doctors suspect a particular allergen, a blood test that measures the level of antibody produced in response to the allergen (the radioallergosorbent test [RAST]) can be done to determine the degree of sensitivity.

To test for exercise-induced asthma, an examiner uses spirometry before and after exercise on a treadmill or stationary bicycle to measure how much air the person can exhale in 1 second (forced expiratory volume in 1 second). If the forced expiratory volume in 1 second decreases more than 15%, the person's asthma can be induced by exercise.

A chest x-ray is not generally helpful in diagnosing asthma. Doctors use chest x-rays when considering another diagnosis. However, a chest x-ray is often obtained when a person with asthma needs to be hospitalized for severe asthma.

Prevention and Treatment

An array of drugs can be used to prevent and treat asthma. Most of the drugs used to prevent asthma are also used to treat an asthma attack but in higher doses or in different forms. Some people need to use more than one drug to prevent and treat their symptoms.

Therapy is based on two classes of drugs: anti-inflammatory drugs and bronchodilators. Anti-inflammatory drugs suppress the inflammation that narrows the airways. Bronchodilators help to relax

---

Status Asthmaticus

The most severe form of asthma is called status asthmaticus. In this condition, the lungs are no longer able to provide the body with adequate oxygen or adequately remove carbon dioxide. Without oxygen, many organs begin to malfunction. The buildup of carbon dioxide leads to acidosis, an acidic state of the blood that affects the function of almost every organ. Blood pressure may fall to low levels. The airways are so narrowed that it is difficult to move air in and out of the lungs.

Status asthmaticus requires that an artificial airway be passed through the person's mouth and throat (intubation) and that a mechanical ventilator be used to assist breathing. Maximum doses of several drugs are also needed. Support is also given to correct acidosis.

How to Use a Metered-Dose Inhaler

- Shake the inhaler after removing the cap.
- Breathe out for 1 or 2 seconds.
- Put the inhaler in your mouth or 1 to 2 inches from it and start to breathe in slowly, like sipping hot soup.
- While starting to breathe in, press the top of the inhaler.

- Breathe in slowly until your lungs are full. (This should take about 5 or 6 seconds.)
- Hold your breath for 4 to 6 seconds.
- Breathe out and repeat the procedure.
- If this method is difficult, a spacer can be used.

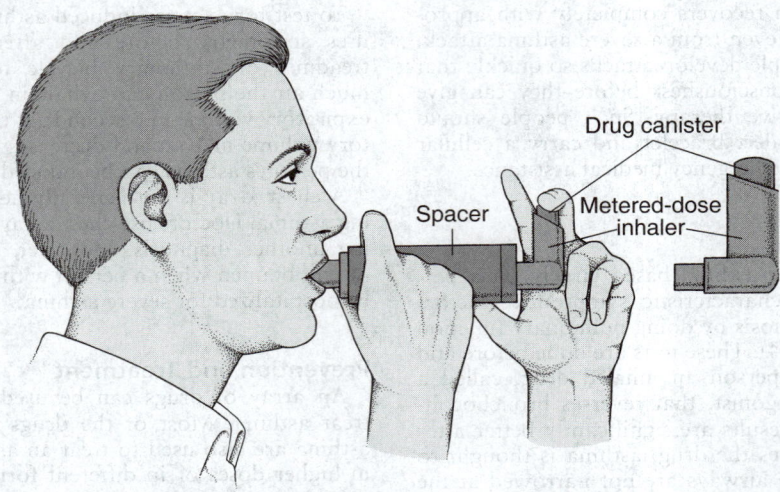

Drug canister

Spacer

Metered-dose inhaler

and widen (dilate) the airways. Anti-inflammatory drugs include corticosteroids (which can be inhaled, taken by mouth, or given intravenously), leukotriene modifiers, and mast cell stabilizers. Bronchodilators include beta-adrenergic agonists (both those for quick relief of symptoms and those for long-term control), drugs with anticholinergic effects, and methylxanthines.

Education about how to prevent and treat asthma attacks is beneficial for all people who have asthma and often for their family members. Proper use of inhalers is essential for effective treatment. People should know what can stimulate an attack, what helps to prevent an attack, how to use drugs properly, and when to seek medical care. Many people use a handheld peak flow meter to evaluate their breathing and determine when they need intervention, before their symptoms get extreme. People who experience frequent, severe asthma attacks should know how to reach help quickly.

Many people have a written treatment plan that was devised in collaboration with their doctor. Such a plan allows them to take control of their own treatment and has been shown to decrease the number of times people need to seek care for asthma in the emergency department.

Preventing Attacks

Asthma is a chronic condition that cannot be cured, but individual attacks can often be prevented. Asthma attacks may commonly be prevented if the factors that trigger them are identified and eliminated or avoided. People who have asthma should avoid cigarette smoke. Often, attacks triggered by exercise can be blocked by taking medication beforehand. When dust and allergens are the problem, air filters, air conditioners, and other types of barriers (such as mattress covers, which reduce the amount of particles from dust mites that are in the air) can help considerably. For people whose asthma is stimulated by allergies, desensitization through the use of allergy shots may prevent attacks.

Some people who have asthma may have a sensitivity to aspirin or other nonsteroidal anti-inflammatory drugs (NSAIDs) and must avoid using these drugs. Drugs that block the beneficial effects of beta-adrenergic agonists (called beta-blockers) may worsen asthma.

Most people with asthma take drugs, such as inhaled or oral corticosteroids, leukotriene modifiers, long-acting beta-adrenergic agonists, methylxanthines, antihistamines, or mast cell stabilizers to prevent attacks. Prevention efforts are individualized according to the frequency of attacks and the stimuli that trigger the attacks.

Treating Attacks

An asthma attack can be frightening, both to the person experiencing it and to others around. Even when relatively mild, the symptoms provoke anxiety and alarm. A severe asthma attack is a life-threatening emergency that requires immediate, skilled, professional care. If not treated adequately and quickly, a severe asthma attack can cause death.

People who have asthma are generally able to treat most attacks without assistance from a health care practitioner. Typically, they use an inhaler to deliver a dose of a short-acting beta-adrenergic agonist, move into fresh air (away from cigarette smoke or other irritants), and sit down and rest. An attack usually subsides in 5 to 10 minutes. An attack that does not subside in 15 minutes or that gets worse is likely to require additional treatment supervised by a doctor.

Because people with severe asthma commonly have low blood oxygen levels, doctors may check the level of oxygen by using a sensing monitor on a finger or ear. Supplemental oxygen may be given during attacks. However, in severe attacks, doctors also need to monitor levels of carbon dioxide in the blood, and this test requires a sample of blood from an artery (see page 455). Doctors may also check lung function, usually with a spirometer or a peak flow meter. Usually, a chest x-ray is needed only in severe asthma attacks. People experiencing very severe asthma attacks may need to have an artificial airway passed through their mouth and throat (intubation) and be placed on a mechanical ventilator (see page 527). Generally, people who have severe asthma are admitted to the hospital if their lung function does not improve after they have received an inhaled beta-adrenergic agonist and corticosteroids by mouth or vein. People also are hospitalized if they have a seriously low blood oxygen level or a high blood carbon dioxide level.

Intravenous fluids may be needed if the person is dehydrated. Antibiotics also may be needed if a doctor suspects a lung infection; however, most such infections are due to viruses for which (with a few exceptions) no treatment exists.

Drugs for Preventing or Treating Attacks

Drugs allow most people with asthma to lead relatively normal lives. Most of the drugs used to treat an asthma attack can be used (often in lower doses) to prevent attacks.

Beta-Adrenergic Agonists: Short-acting beta-adrenergic agonists are usually the best drugs for relieving asthma attacks. They also are used to prevent exercise-induced asthma. These drugs are referred to as bronchodilators because they stimulate beta-adrenergic receptors to widen (dilate) the airways. Bronchodilators that act on all beta-adrenergic receptors throughout the body, such as epinephrine, cause side effects such as rapid heartbeat, restlessness, headache, and muscle tremors. Bronchodilators (such as albuterol) that act mainly on beta$_2$-adrenergic receptors, which are found primarily on cells in the lungs, have little effect on other organs and thus cause fewer side effects. Most beta-adrenergic agonists, especially the inhaled ones, act within minutes, but the effects last only 2 to 6 hours.

Long-acting bronchodilators are available, but because they do not begin to act as quickly, they are used for prevention rather than for attacks of asthma. The long-acting beta-adrenergic agonists are not used alone because people using only long-acting bronchodilators have a slightly higher risk of death. Thus, doctors usually give them together with inhaled corticosteroids.

Most often, beta-adrenergic agonists are inhaled using metered-dose inhalers (handheld cartridges containing gas under pressure). The pressure turns the

---

Avoiding Common Causes of Asthma Attacks

The most common indoor allergens are house dust mites, feathers, cockroaches, and animal dander. Anything that can be done to reduce exposure to these allergens may reduce the number or severity of asthma attacks. Exposure to house dust mites can be reduced by removing wall-to-wall carpets and using air conditioning to keep the relative humidity low (preferably below 50%) in the summer. Also, special pillow and mattress covers can help reduce exposure to these dust mites. Animals with fur or hair, most commonly cats and dogs, often must be given away to decrease the overall exposure to animal dander.

Irritating fumes such as cigarette smoke should also be avoided. In some people with asthma, aspirin and other nonsteroidal anti-inflammatory drugs trigger attacks. Tartrazine, a yellow coloring used in some drug tablets and food, may also bring on an attack. Sulfites—commonly added to foods as a preservative—may trigger attacks after a susceptible person eats a certain food or drinks beer or red wine.

For outdoor activity in cold weather, people with asthma can wear a ski mask or scarf that covers the nose and mouth to help keep the air being breathed in warm and moist.

drug into a fine spray containing a measured dose of drug. Inhalation deposits the drug directly in the airways, so that it acts quickly, but the drug may not reach airways that are severely narrowed. For people who have difficulty using a metered-dose inhaler, spacers or holding chambers can be used. These devices increase the amount of drug delivered to the lungs. With any type of inhaler, proper technique is vital. If the device is not used properly, the drug will not reach the airways. A dry powder drug formulation is also available. The powder formulation is easier for some people to use, in part because it requires less coordination with breathing.

Beta-adrenergic agonists can also be delivered directly to the lungs using a nebulizer. A nebulizer uses pressurized air to create a continuous mist of drug that is inhaled without having to coordinate dosing with breathing. Nebulizers are more portable than they were in the past, and some units can even be plugged into a cigarette lighter in a car. Nebulizers and metered-dose inhalers deliver equivalent amounts of drug to the lungs.

Beta-adrenergic agonists can also be taken in liquid or tablet form or injected. However, the oral drugs tend to work slower than the inhaled or injected ones and are more likely to cause side effects. Side effects include abnormal heart rhythms, which may suggest excessive use.

Other bronchodilators may be combined with beta-adrenergic agonists for acute attacks, including nebulized ipratropium. A combination of ipratropium with albuterol in a metered-dose inhaler is also available.

Quick medical attention should be sought when a person who has asthma feels the need to use more of a beta-adrenergic agonist than is recommended. Overusing these drugs can be very dangerous. The need for continuous use indicates severe bronchoconstriction, which can lead to respiratory failure and death.

Methylxanthines: Theophylline, a methylxanthine, is another drug that produces bronchodilation. It is now used less frequently than in the past. Theophylline is usually taken by mouth but can be given intravenously in the hospital. Oral theophylline comes in many forms, from short-acting tablets and syrups to longer-acting sustained release capsules and tablets. Theophylline is used for both prevention and treatment of asthma.

The amount of theophylline in the blood can be measured in a laboratory and must be closely monitored by a doctor. Too little drug in the blood may provide little benefit, and too much drug may cause life-threatening abnormal heart rhythms or seizures. When first taking theophylline, a person who has asthma may feel slightly jittery and may develop headaches. These side effects usually disappear as the body adjusts to the drug. Larger doses may cause a rapid heartbeat, nausea, or palpitations. A person may also experience insomnia, agitation, vomiting, and seizures.

Drugs With Anticholinergic Effects: Drugs with anticholinergic effects, such as ipratropium, block acetylcholine from causing smooth muscle contraction and from producing excess mucus in the bronchi. These drugs are usually inhaled but can be given intravenously in the hospital. These drugs further widen (dilate) the airways in people who have already been given beta-adrenergic agonists. However, doctors use drugs with anticholinergic effects mainly in the emergency department in combination with a beta-adrenergic agonist.

Leukotriene Modifiers: Leukotriene modifiers, such as montelukast, zafirlukast, and zileuton also help control asthma. They are anti-inflammatory drugs, preventing the action or synthesis of leukotrienes, chemicals made by the body that cause bronchoconstriction. These drugs, which are taken by mouth, are used more to prevent asthma attacks than to treat them, although because leukotrienes are increased in acute asthma, these drugs potentially can be used during an attack as well.

Mast Cell Stabilizers: These drugs, which are inhaled, include cromolyn and nedocromil. Mast cell stabilizers are thought to inhibit the release of inflammatory chemicals from mast cells and make the airways less likely to narrow. Thus, they are also anti-inflammatory drugs. They are useful for preventing but not treating an attack. These drugs may be helpful for children who have asthma and for people who develop asthma from exercise. Mast cell stabilizers are very safe and must be taken regularly even when a person is free of symptoms.

Corticosteroids: These drugs block the body's inflammatory response and are exceptionally effective at reducing asthma symptoms. They are the most potent form of anti-inflammatory drugs and have been an important part of asthma treatment for decades. They are given in the inhaled form to prevent attacks and improve lung function. They are given by mouth in higher doses for people experiencing severe attacks. Corticosteroids given by mouth are generally continued for at least several days after a severe attack. Corticosteroids can be taken in several different forms. Often, inhaled versions are best because they deliver the drug directly to the airways and minimize the amount sent throughout the body. They come in several strengths and are generally used twice a day. People should rinse their mouth after use to decrease the likelihood that a fungal infection of the mouth (thrush) develops. Oral or injected corticosteroids may be used in high doses to

℞ DRUGS USED TO TREAT ASTHMA

DRUG	SOME SIDE EFFECTS	COMMENTS
Short-acting beta-adrenergic agonists		
Albuterol Levalbuterol Pirbuterol	Increased heart rate Shakiness	For immediate relief of acute attack
Long-acting beta-adrenergic agonists		
Formoterol Salmeterol	Increased heart rate Shakiness	For ongoing treatment, not for acute relief Not recommended for use alone (without other asthma drugs)
Methylxanthines		
Theophylline	Increased heart rate Shakiness Stomach upset Seizures (if the blood level is high) Serious heartbeat irregularities (if the blood level is high)	Can be used for prevention and treatment Taken by mouth but can be given intravenously in a hospital
Drugs with anticholinergic effects		
Ipratropium	Dry mouth Rapid heart rate	Used mainly in the emergency department in combination with a beta-adrenergic agonist
Mast cell stabilizers		
Cromolyn Nedocromil	Coughing or wheezing	Useful for preventing attacks, often related to exercise, but not for treatment of an acute attack
Corticosteroids (inhaled)		
Beclomethasone Budesonide Flunisolide Fluticasone Mometasone Triamcinolone	Fungal infection of the mouth (thrush) A change in the voice	Inhaled for prevention (long-term control) of asthma
Corticosteroids (oral)		
Methylprednisolone Prednisolone Prednisone	Weight gain Elevated blood sugar levels Rarely, psychosis	Used for acute attacks and for asthma that cannot be controlled with inhaled therapy
Leukotriene modifiers		
Montelukast Zafirlukast Zileuton	Churg-Strauss syndrome With zileuton, elevated liver enzymes	Used more for prevention (long-term control) than for treatment
Immunomodulator		
Omalizumab	Discomfort at the injection site Rarely, anaphylactic reactions	Used in people with severe asthma to decrease use of oral corticosteroids

relieve a severe asthma attack and are generally continued for 1 to 2 weeks. Oral corticosteroids are prescribed on a long-term basis only when no other treatments can control the symptoms.

If taken for long periods, corticosteroids gradually reduce the likelihood of an asthma attack by making the airways less sensitive to a number of provocative stimuli. Long-term use of corticosteroids, especially larger doses taken by mouth, can produce side effects including obesity, osteoporosis, elevated blood sugar levels, and, very rarely, psychosis.

Immunomodulators: Omalizumab is a drug that is an antibody. This antibody is directed against a group of other antibodies called immunoglobulin E (IgE). Omalizumab is used in people with asthma who also have severe allergies and high levels of IgE in their blood. Omalizumab prevents IgE from binding to mast cells and thus prevents the release of inflammatory chemicals that can narrow the airways. It can decrease requirements for oral corticosteroids and help relieve symptoms. The drug is injected subcutaneously every 2 weeks.

CHAPTER 77

Chronic Obstructive Pulmonary Disease

Chronic obstructive pulmonary disease is persistent obstruction of the airways occurring with emphysema, chronic bronchitis, or both disorders.

- Cigarette smoking is the most important cause of chronic obstructive pulmonary disease.
- People develop a cough and eventually become short of breath.
- Diagnosis is made with chest x-rays and tests of lung function.
- Stopping smoking and taking drugs that help keep airways open are important.
- People who have severe disease may need to take other drugs, use oxygen, or have pulmonary rehabilitation.

In the United States, about 12 million people suffer from chronic obstructive pulmonary disease (COPD). It is second only to heart disease as a cause of disability that forces people to stop working. It is the fourth most common cause of death, accounting for more than 120,000 deaths per year in the United States. The number of deaths from COPD has increased more than 60% over the last 20 years, and more than 95% of all COPD-related deaths occur in people older than age 55. COPD affects men more often than women, but men and women die as a result of COPD at about equal rates. COPD is more often fatal in whites than in nonwhites and in blue-collar workers than in white-collar workers.

COPD leads to chronic airflow obstruction, which is defined as a persistent decrease in the rate of airflow from the lungs when the person breathes out (exhales). This airflow obstruction is partially reversible in most people, either spontaneously or with treatment. COPD includes the diagnoses of chronic obstructive bronchitis and emphysema. Many people have both disorders. **Chronic bronchitis** is defined as cough that produces sputum repeatedly during two successive years. When chronic bronchitis involves airflow obstruction, it qualifies as chronic obstructive bronchitis. **Emphysema** is defined as widespread and irreversible destruction of the alveolar walls (the cells that support the air sacs, or alveoli, that make up the lungs) and enlargement of many of the alveoli.

The small airways (bronchioles) of the lungs contain smooth muscles and are normally held open by their attachments to alveolar walls. In emphysema, the destruction of alveolar wall attachments results in collapse of the bronchioles, causing permanent airflow obstruction. In chronic bronchitis, the glands lining the larger airways (bronchi) of the lungs enlarge and increase their secretion of mucus. Inflammation of the bronchioles develops and causes smooth muscle to contract (spasm), further obstructing airflow. Inflammation also causes airflow to be blocked by secretions. Asthma is also characterized by airflow obstruction (see page 473). However, in contrast with the airflow obstruction of COPD, the airflow obstruction of asthma is completely reversible in most people, either spontaneously or with treatment.

The airflow obstruction of COPD causes air to become trapped in the lungs after a full exhalation, increasing the effort required to breathe. Also in COPD, the number of capillaries in the walls of the alveoli decreases. These abnormalities impair the exchange of oxygen and carbon dioxide between the alveoli and the blood. In the earlier stages of COPD, oxygen levels in the blood may be decreased, but carbon dioxide levels remain normal. In the later stages, carbon dioxide levels increase and oxygen levels fall.

The decrease in oxygen levels in the blood stimulates the bone marrow to send more red blood cells into the bloodstream, a condition known as secondary polycythemia (see box on page 1069). The decrease in oxygen levels in the blood also increases the pressure in the artery through which blood flows from the heart to the lungs (pulmonary artery). As a result of the increased pressure, pulmonary hypertension and cor pulmonale can occur (see box on page 523). People with COPD also have an increased risk of developing heart rhythm abnormalities (arrhythmias). For smokers, the risk of developing lung cancer is higher than it would be on the basis of cigarette smoking alone.

Causes

Cigarette smoking is the most important cause of COPD, although only about 15% of smokers develop the disease. Pipe and cigar smokers develop COPD more often than nonsmokers but not as often as cigarette smokers. With aging, susceptible cigarette smokers lose lung function more rapidly than nonsmokers. Lung function improves only a little if people stop smoking. However, the rate of decline of lung function returns to that of nonsmokers when people stop smoking, thus delaying development and progression of symptoms.

COPD tends to occur more often in some families, so there may be an inherited tendency. Working in an environment polluted by chemical fumes or dust may increase the risk of COPD (see page 496). Exposure to air pollution and to smoke from nearby cigarette smokers (secondhand or passive smoke exposure) may cause COPD (and also worsens the disease).

A rare cause of COPD is a hereditary condition in which the body produces a markedly decreased amount of the protein alpha$_1$-antitrypsin. The main role of this protein is to prevent neutrophil elastase (an enzyme in certain white blood cells) from damaging the alveoli. Consequently, emphysema develops by early middle age in people with severe alpha$_1$-antitrypsin deficiency (also called alpha$_1$-antiprotease inhibitor deficiency), especially in those who also smoke.

Symptoms

In people with COPD, a mild cough that produces clear sputum develops by around age 45. The cough usually occurs when the person first gets out of bed in the morning. Cough and sputum production persist. Shortness of breath may occur with exertion. Sometimes, shortness of breath first occurs only with a lung infection, during which time the person coughs more and has an increased amount of sputum. The color of the sputum changes from clear or white to yellow or green.

By the time people with COPD reach their middle to late 60s, especially if they continue smoking, shortness of breath with exertion becomes more troublesome. Pneumonia and other lung infections occur more often. They may result in severe shortness of breath even when the person is at rest and may require hospitalization. Shortness of breath during activities of daily living, such as toileting, washing, dressing, and sexual activity, may persist after the person has recovered from the lung infection.

About one third of people with severe COPD experience severe weight loss, in part because shortness of breath makes eating difficult and in part because of increased levels in the blood of a substance called tumor necrosis factor. Swelling of the legs often develops, which may be due to cor pulmonale. People with COPD may intermittently cough up blood, which is usually due to inflammation of the bronchi, but which always raises the concern of lung cancer. Morning headaches may occur because breathing decreases during sleep, which causes increased retention of carbon dioxide.

As COPD progresses, some people, especially those who have emphysema, develop unusual breathing patterns. Some people breathe out through pursed lips. Others find it more comfortable to stand over a table with their arms outstretched and weight on their palms, a maneuver that improves the function of the respiratory muscles. Over time, many people develop a barrel chest as the size of the lungs increases because of trapped air. Low oxygen levels in the blood can give a blue tint to the skin (cyanosis). Clubbing of the fingers is rare (see page 453) and raises the suspicion of lung cancer.

Fragile areas in the lungs may rupture, permitting air to leak from the lung into the pleural space, a condition called pneumothorax (see page 520). This condition often causes sudden pain and shortness of breath and requires immediate intervention by a doctor to remove the air from the pleural space.

A flare-up of COPD is a worsening of symptoms, usually cough, increased sputum, and shortness of breath. Sputum color often changes to yellow or green, and fever and body aches sometimes occur. Shortness of breath may be present when the person is at rest and may be severe enough to require hospitalization. Severe air pollution, common allergens, and viral or bacterial infections may cause flare-ups. During severe flare-ups, people may develop a life-threatening condition called acute respiratory failure. Among the possible symptoms are severe shortness of breath (a feeling likened to being drowned), severe anxiety, sweating, cyanosis, and confusion.

Diagnosis

Chronic bronchitis is diagnosed by the history of a prolonged productive cough. People with chronic obstructive bronchitis have chronic bronchitis and evidence of airflow obstruction on pulmonary function tests. Emphysema is diagnosed on the basis of findings observed during a physical examination and on pulmonary function test results. However, by the time the doctor notices these abnormalities, emphysema is moderately severe. It is not important for doctors to differentiate between chronic obstructive bronchitis and emphysema. The most important determinant of how the person feels and functions is the severity of the airflow obstruction.

In mild COPD, a doctor may find nothing unusual during the physical examination. As the disease progresses, wheezes may be heard through the stethoscope, and prolonged expiration and decreased breath sounds become apparent. Chest movement diminishes during breathing, and use of the neck and shoulder muscles in breathing may occur.

In mild COPD, the chest x-ray is usually normal. As COPD worsens, the chest x-ray shows over-inflation of the lungs. Thinning of blood vessels suggests the presence of emphysema.

Doctors can evaluate airflow obstruction with forced expiratory spirometry (see page 454). Decrease in the forced expiratory volume in 1 second (FEV_1) and the ratio of the FEV_1 to the forced vital capacity (FVC) are required to demonstrate airflow obstruction and to make the diagnosis.

A blood test may show an abnormally high level of red blood cells (polycythemia). Pulse oximetry or a sample of blood taken from an artery often shows low levels of oxygen. High levels of carbon dioxide in the arteries occur late in the course of the disease.

In people who develop COPD at a young age, especially when there is a family history of COPD, the alpha$_1$-antitrypsin blood level is measured to determine whether alpha$_1$-antitrypsin deficiency is present. This genetic disorder is also suspected when COPD develops in people who have never smoked.

Treatment

The most important treatment for COPD is to stop smoking. Stopping smoking when the airflow obstruction is mild or moderate often lessens cough, reduces the amount of sputum, and slows the development of shortness of breath. Stopping smoking at any point in the disease process provides some benefit. Trying several strategies at once is most likely to be effective. Among these strategies are committing to a specific date for quitting, using behavioral modification techniques (for example, making cigarettes difficult to obtain or rewarding oneself for abstaining for increasingly long periods of time), group counseling and support sessions, and nicotine replacement (for example, by chewing nicotine gum, wearing a nicotine skin patch, or using a nicotine inhaler, nicotine lozenge, or nicotine nasal spray). The drugs varenicline and bupropion may also help decrease tobacco craving. However, even with the most effective methods, less than half of people have quit smoking after one year.

People should also try to avoid exposure to other airborne irritants, including secondhand smoke and air pollution.

Contracting influenza or developing pneumonia may worsen COPD markedly. Therefore, all people with COPD should receive an influenza vaccination every year and a pneumococcal vaccination every 5 or 6 years.

Treatment of Symptoms: Wheezing and shortness of breath are relieved when airflow obstruction improves. Although airflow obstruction due to emphysema is not reversible, bronchial smooth muscle spasm, inflammation, and increased secretions are all potentially reversible.

Inhaled bronchodilators are given with a device that allows the user to spray a specific and consistent dose of a drug into the airways via the mouth and throat (metered-dose inhaler). Inhaled bronchodilators include anticholinergic and beta-adrenergic agonist drugs. Both relax muscles around the bronchioles. Anticholinergic drugs include ipratropium and tiotropium. Ipratropium is given about 4 times daily, and tiotropium is given once daily. Inhaled short-acting beta-adrenergic agonists, such as albuterol, more rapidly relieve shortness of breath than anticholinergic drugs and so can be most useful during flare-ups. Salmeterol, a long-acting beta-adrenergic agonist with a delayed onset of action, can be given by inhalation every 12 hours. This drug is useful for prolonged relief of symptoms in some people, especially at night.

Many people can use metered dose inhalers more effectively when they inhale the drug through a delivery device called a spacer (see art on page 476). Inhaled bronchodilators may also be given using nebulizers. This mode of therapy should be reserved for people who have severe disease or for those who cannot use a metered-dose inhaler properly. A nebulizer creates a mist of drug, and the timing of its inhalation does not have to be coordinated with breathing. Nebulizers are more portable than they were in the past; some units can even be plugged into the cigarette lighter in a car.

Corticosteroids are helpful for many people with moderate and severe COPD whose symptoms cannot be controlled by the other drugs or for those who get frequent flare-ups despite the use of other drugs. Inhaled corticosteroids do not prevent decline of lung function over time. However, their use improves symptoms and results in decreased frequency of COPD flare-ups. Because the drug is delivered to the lungs, inhaled corticosteroids produce fewer side effects than treatment given by mouth. However, high doses of inhaled corticosteroids can have effects throughout the body, such as worsening of osteoporosis. Corticosteroids given by mouth are largely restricted to treatment of COPD flare-ups or are given to people who continue to have symptoms from airflow obstruction and who are not responding to a simpler regimen.

Theophylline is given only to people who do not respond to other drugs. The dose must be carefully controlled by the doctor, and, in some patients, levels of the drug in the blood must be measured periodically. A long-acting form of the drug permits once-daily or twice-daily dosing in many people and helps to control shortness of breath at night.

There is no reliable therapy for thinning secretions so they can be coughed up more easily. However, avoiding dehydration may prevent thickening of secretions. A rule of thumb is to drink enough fluids to keep the urine pale except for that passed first in the morning. In severe COPD, respiratory therapy may help loosen secretions in the chest.

Spirometry and pulse oximetry are often used to monitor symptoms. Arterial blood gas measurements add information that is useful in severe disease.

Treatment of Flare-ups: Flare-ups should be treated as soon as possible. When bacterial infection is suspected, a 7- to 10-day course of antibiotic treatment is usually prescribed. Many doctors give people who have COPD a supply of an antibiotic to be kept on hand and taken early in a flare-up. A number of antibiotics can be taken by mouth, including trimethoprim-sulfamethoxazole, doxycycline, amoxicillin-clavulanate, and ampicillin. Many doctors reserve more expensive antibiotics, such as azithromycin, clarithromycin, and levofloxacin, for more severe lung infections, for people in whom treatment with the older and less expensive drugs has not worked, for those who have severe symptoms, and for those at risk of infection with organisms that are not likely to be eliminated by the older drugs (resistant bacteria). People whose immune system is suppressed or those who live in nursing homes are most likely to be infected with resistant bacteria.

People with severe flare-ups require hospitalization and treatment with short-acting beta-adrenergic agonist drugs and ipratropium, oral or intravenous corticosteroids, and oxygen. They may require machine-assistance with breathing (mechanical ventilation) and sometimes placement of an endotracheal (breathing) tube. Although many people with COPD think they should take antibiotics to prevent flare-ups, there is no indication that this practice is effective.

Oxygen Therapy: Long-term oxygen therapy (see page 460) prolongs the life of people who have advanced COPD and severely reduced oxygen levels in their blood. Although round-the-clock therapy is best, using oxygen 12 hours a day also has some benefits. This therapy reduces the excess of red blood cells caused by low blood oxygen levels and helps to relieve cor pulmonale caused by COPD. Oxygen therapy may also improve shortness of breath during exercise.

Different devices are available for oxygen therapy. Electrically driven oxygen concentrators are used when electrical outlets are available. Compressed oxygen is available in small tanks that permit people to travel outside of their homes for 2 to 6 hours. Liquid oxygen systems are more expensive but are preferable for active people as they permit several hours away from the source reservoir. People must never use oxygen therapy near open flames or while smoking.

Pulmonary Rehabilitation: Pulmonary rehabilitation can help people who have COPD (see page 459), but it does not improve lung function. Programs encompass education about the disease, exercise, and nutritional and psychosocial counseling. These programs can improve independence and quality of life, decrease the frequency and length of hospital stays, and improve the ability to exercise. Exercise programs can be carried out in an outpatient setting or at home. Walking (sometimes on a treadmill) is usually used to exercise the legs. Sometimes stationary bicycling and stair climbing are also used. Weight lifting is used for the arms. Often, oxygen is recommended during exercise. As with any exercise program, gains in conditioning are quickly lost if the person stops exercising. Special techniques are taught for decreasing shortness of breath during activities, such as cooking, engaging in hobbies, and sexual activity.

Other Treatments: Over-the-counter cough suppressants usually help little and are not recommended. For people with a severe alpha$_1$-antitrypsin deficiency, the missing protein can be replaced. The treatment, which requires weekly intravenous infusions of the protein, is expensive.

Single lung transplantation may be used in certain people who are usually younger than 60 and have severe airflow obstruction. The goal of lung transplantation is to improve quality of life, because survival time is rarely increased. Lifelong immunosuppression is required, placing people at risk of infections.

Lung volume reduction surgery can be carried out in people with severe emphysema in the upper portions of their lungs. In this operation, the most severely diseased portions of the lungs are removed, thus permitting the remaining portions of the lungs and the diaphragm to function better. It is not known how long the improvement lasts. People are required to stop smoking for at least 6 months before surgery. They should undergo an intense rehabilitation program to determine whether overall function can be improved significantly without surgery before undertaking this operation, which carries a risk of death of about 5%.

Prognosis and End-of-Life Issues

COPD itself usually does not cause death or severe symptoms if the person stops smoking at a time when airflow is only mildly obstructed. Continued smoking, however, virtually assures that symptoms will worsen. With moderate and severe airflow obstruction, the prognosis becomes progressively worse. People in advanced stages of COPD are likely to need considerable help with medical care and with activities of daily living. They may, for example, arrange to live on a single floor of their house, eat several small meals rather than one large meal, and avoid wearing shoes that must be tied. Death may result from respiratory failure, lung cancer, heart disorders (for example, heart failure or heart rhythm abnormalities), pneumonia, pneumothorax, or blockage of the arteries leading to the lungs (pulmonary embolism).

People with end-stage disease who develop flare-ups may need a breathing tube and mechanical ventilation. The duration of mechanical ventilation may be prolonged, and some people remain ventilator-dependent until death. It is important for people to consider with their doctors and loved ones whether or not they wish this kind of supportive therapy and to do so before a flare-up occurs. The best way to ensure that the person's wishes regarding prolonged mechanical ventilation are carried out is to prepare an advance directive (see page 69) and appoint a health care proxy (see page 70).

Alpha₁-Antitrypsin Deficiency

Alpha₁-antitrypsin deficiency is a hereditary disorder in which a lack or low level of the enzyme alpha₁-antitrypsin damages the lungs and liver.

- Alpha₁-antitrypsin deficiency is caused by an inherited gene mutation.
- Infants may develop jaundice and cirrhosis.
- Adults commonly develop emphysema, with shortness of breath, wheezing, and coughing; some adults develop cirrhosis.
- Tests that measure the amount of the enzyme in the blood and that detect the gene mutations are used for diagnosis.

- People with emphysema take drugs to improve breathing and sometimes receive infusions of alpha₁-antitrypsin by vein.
- Some people need lung or liver transplants.

Alpha₁-antitrypsin is an enzyme produced by the liver that inhibits the action of other enzymes called proteases. Proteases break down proteins as part of normal tissue repair. Alpha₁-antitrypsin protects the lungs from the damaging effects of proteases.

Alpha₁-antitrypsin deficiency results from an inherited mutation in the gene that controls production and release of the enzyme. There are many subtypes of alpha₁-antitrypsin deficiency, but in all, levels of active enzyme in the blood are insufficient, the enzyme is structurally abnormal (and thus functions poorly), or both. Whites are affected more often than blacks or Asians.

The most common problems caused by the deficiency are

- Liver damage
- Emphysema

If the enzyme is structurally abnormal, it may clump in the liver, causing the liver to malfunction. In some people, liver malfunction leads to cirrhosis (see page 222) and to an increased risk of liver cancer.

The low levels of alpha₁-antitrypsin allow proteases to damage the lungs, resulting in emphysema (see page 480). Emphysema is more common (and worse) in people who smoke. Emphysema in nonsmokers is often caused by alpha₁-antitrypsin deficiency.

Disorders of other organs sometimes occur. These disorders include inflammation of fat under the skin (panniculitis), life-threatening hemorrhage, aneurysms, ulcerative colitis, vasculitis, and kidney disease.

Symptoms

Symptoms may first appear during infancy, childhood, or adulthood. About 20% of affected people have symptoms during infancy. Affected infants develop yellowing of the skin and the whites of the eyes (jaundice) and an enlarged liver during the first week of life. Jaundice disappears at about age 2 to 4 months. However, about 20% of these infants later develop cirrhosis, and some die before reaching adulthood.

Adults commonly develop emphysema, with progressively increasing shortness of breath, difficulty breathing, coughing, and wheezing. Emphysema rarely develops before age 25. It develops earlier and is more severe in smokers than in nonsmokers. The severity of symptoms also varies depending on the form of the deficiency, other disorders people have, environmental exposure to lung irritants, and other factors. If people have never smoked, their symptoms tend to be moderate, and most have a normal life expectancy.

Even if they did not have liver problems during infancy, about 10% of adults develop cirrhosis, which may eventually lead to liver cancer.

People with panniculitis have painful, tender bumps or discolored patches on the lower abdomen, buttocks, and thighs. The bumps may feel hard to the touch.

Diagnosis

Alpha$_1$-antitrypsin deficiency is suspected in the following:

- Infants who have typical symptoms
- Smokers who develop emphysema before age 45
- Nonsmokers who develop emphysema at any age
- People with an unexplained liver disorder

Because the deficiency is inherited, doctors usually ask whether any family members have had emphysema or cirrhosis with no known cause.

The deficiency is often confirmed by genetic testing, which also can determine the specific form of the deficiency. Doctors also usually do blood tests to measure the level of alpha$_1$-antitrypsin.

Treatment

Emphysema: People who smoke are advised to stop. Bronchodilators such as albuterol may help ease breathing and relieve cough. Lung infections that develop are treated promptly.

Alpha$_1$-antitrypsin may be given by vein to replace the deficient enzyme. It is collected from a group of donors and screened for bloodborne disorders. Thus, it is expensive and is most beneficial to people who have only moderate symptoms due to emphysema and do not smoke. This treatment is thought to prevent further damage but does not reverse damage already done.

If people are younger than 60 and have severe symptoms, lung transplantation may be done. A few medical centers sometimes do transplantations in highly selected people as old as 70.

Liver Damage: Taking alpha$_1$-antitrypsin does not treat or prevent liver damage because liver damage is caused by production of an abnormal enzyme, not by enzyme deficiency. If the liver is severely damaged, liver transplantation may be done (see page 1132). The transplanted liver does not become damaged because the alpha$_1$-antitrypsin it produces is normal and thus does not accumulate in the liver.

Panniculitis: Doctors may give corticosteroids, antimalarial drugs, or certain antibiotics (tetracyclines) to relieve inflammation. But whether these drugs are effective is unclear.

CHAPTER

78 Sleep Apnea

Sleep apnea is a serious disorder in which breathing repeatedly stops long enough to disrupt sleep and temporarily decrease the amount of oxygen and increase the amount of carbon dioxide in the blood.

- People with sleep apnea often are very sleepy during the day, snore loudly, and have episodes of gasping or choking, pauses in breathing, and sudden awakenings with a snort.
- Although the diagnosis of sleep apnea can often be based on symptoms, doctors usually use polysomnography to confirm the diagnosis and determine the severity.
- Continuous positive airway pressure, oral appliances fitted by dentists, and sometimes surgery are used to treat sleep apnea.

Sleep apnea occurs when breathing is interrupted during sleep for periods of more than 10 seconds. There are three types: obstructive sleep apnea, central sleep apnea, and a mixed type.

Obstructive sleep apnea, the most common type, is caused by repeated closure of the throat or upper airway during sleep. This type of apnea affects about 4 to 9% of middle-aged people in the United States. Obstructive sleep apnea is more common in obese people. Obesity, perhaps in combination with aging and other factors, leads to narrowing of the upper airway. Excessive use of alcohol worsens obstructive sleep apnea. Having a narrow throat, thick neck, and round head—features that tend to run in families—increases the risk of sleep apnea. Hypothyroidism or excessive and abnormal growth due to excessive production of growth hormone (acromegaly) can contribute to obstructive sleep apnea. In children, enlarged tonsils or adenoids, some dental conditions (such as a large overbite), and some birth defects (such as an abnormally small lower jaw) can cause obstructive sleep apnea.

Central sleep apnea, a much rarer type, is caused by a problem with the control of breathing in the brain (which is accomplished in the brain stem). Normally, the brain stem is very sensitive to changes in the blood level of carbon dioxide (a by-product of metabolism). When levels are high, the brain stem signals the respiratory muscles to breathe harder and faster to remove carbon dioxide through exhalation, and vice versa. In central sleep apnea, the brain stem is less sensitive to changes in the carbon dioxide level. Because the brain stem responds slowly to the buildup of carbon dioxide in the blood, the body's response is exaggerated, resulting in overventilation. Similarly, because the brain stem responds slowly to the removal of carbon dioxide from the blood, the body's response—a pause in breathing—is prolonged. People who have heart failure or severe brain disease, such as a stroke that affects the brain stem, may have central sleep apnea. In one form of central sleep apnea, called Ondine's curse, which usually occurs in newborns, people may breathe inadequately or not at all except when they are fully awake. Using an opioid, a strong prescription pain reliever, can cause central sleep apnea. Being at high altitude can also cause central sleep apnea. A brain tumor is very rare cause. Unlike obstructive sleep apnea, central sleep apnea is not associated with obesity.

Mixed sleep apnea, the third type, is a combination of central and obstructive factors occurring in the same episode of sleep apnea. Episodes of mixed sleep apnea are most often begin as obstructive apneas and are treated like obstructive apneas.

> **? Did You Know...**
>
> People who have excessive daytime sleepiness and who snore should discuss these symptoms with their doctor.
>
> People with obstructive sleep apnea should avoid alcohol and sedating drugs, particularly before bedtime.

Symptoms

Symptoms during sleep are usually first noticed by a sleep partner, roommate, or housemate. In all types of sleep apnea, breathing may become abnormally slow and shallow, or breathing may suddenly stop (sometimes for up to 1 minute), then resume.

In obstructive sleep apnea, the most common symptom is disruptive snoring, with episodes of gasping or choking, pauses in breathing, and sudden awakenings with a snort. The person may awaken choking and frightened. When obstructive sleep apnea is severe, repeated bouts of sleep-related snorts and loud snores occur at night, and sleepiness or involuntary naps occur during the day. In people who live alone, daytime sleepiness may be the most noticeable symptom. Eventually, sleepiness interferes with daytime work and reduces the quality of life. For example, the person may fall asleep while watching television, while attending a meeting, or in more extreme sleepiness even while stopped at a red light when driving. Memory may be impaired, sex drive may be reduced, and interpersonal relationships suffer because the person is unable to participate actively in relationships due to sleepiness and irritability. In obstructive sleep apnea, the risk of stroke, heart attack, and high blood pressure is increased. If episodes of obstructive sleep apnea are more frequent than about 15 per hour, the risk of premature death is increased, often in the next 5 to 10 years.

People who are extremely obese can have obesity-hypoventilation syndrome (termed the Pickwickian syndrome) alone, or in combination with obstructive sleep apnea. Excess body fat interferes with the movement of the chest and excess body fat below the diaphragm compresses the lungs, which combine to cause shallow, less effective breathing. Excess body fat around the throat compresses the upper airway, reducing air flow.

Almost all affected children snore. Other sleep symptoms may include restless sleep and sweating at night. Daytime symptoms may include mouth breathing, morning headache, and problems concentrating. Excessive daytime sleepiness is less common than among adults with obstructive sleep apnea.

In central sleep apnea, snoring is not as prominent. However, the tempo of breathing is irregular and interrupted by pauses. Cheyne-Stokes respiration (periodic breathing) is one type of central apnea. In Cheyne-Stokes respiration, breathing gradually becomes more rapid, gradually slows down, stops for a short period, then starts again. Then the cycle repeats. Each cycle lasts 30 seconds to 2 minutes.

In all types of sleep apnea, the disturbances in sleep can result in daytime sleepiness, fatigue, irritability, headaches in the mornings, slowness of thought, and difficulty concentrating. Because oxygen levels in the blood may decrease significantly, abnormal heart rhythms may develop, and blood pressure may increase.

Prolonged, severe sleep apnea of any type increases the risk of heart failure and constriction of lung blood vessels. Then the heart cannot pump enough blood to the body, and the lungs cannot provide enough oxygen to or remove enough carbon dioxide from the body.

Diagnosis

In its early stages, sleep apnea is often diagnosed on the basis of symptoms. The diagnosis is confirmed and severity is best determined in a sleep laboratory by using a test called polysomnography. In this test, electroencephalography (EEG—see page 636) is used to monitor changes in levels of sleep and eye movements, The oxygen level in the blood is measured with an electrode placed on a finger or an earlobe (a procedure called oximetry). Airflow is measured with a device placed in front of the nostrils, and the motion and pattern of breathing are measured with a monitor placed on the chest. This evaluation can help doctors distinguish between obstructive and central sleep apnea.

Because there are too few sleep laboratories to test all people, portable monitors are often used at home to help diagnose sleep apnea. These monitors measure heart rate, level of oxygen in the blood, effort of breathing, position, and nasal airflow.

Treatment

With treatment, the prognosis is excellent. Life span is not affected, and most serious complications can be prevented.

People should be warned of the risks of driving, operating heavy machinery, or engaging in other activities during which falling asleep would be hazardous. People who are undergoing surgery should inform their anesthesiologist that they have sleep apnea, because anesthesia can sometimes cause additional airway narrowing.

Support groups can provide information and help people with sleep apnea and their family members cope with the condition.

Obstructive Sleep Apnea: Losing weight, quitting smoking, and not using alcohol excessively can help. Nasal infections and allergies should be treated. Hypothyroidism and acromegaly should be treated. Weight loss (bariatric) surgery reduces sleep apnea and reverses symptoms in about 85% of people who are very overweight (morbidly obese).

Heavy snorers and people who often choke in their sleep should not consume alcohol or take sleep aids, sedating antihistamines, or other drugs that cause drowsiness. Sleeping on the side or elevating the head of the bed can help reduce snoring. Special devices strapped on the back help prevent people from sleeping on their back. The various other devices and sprays marketed to reduce snoring may help simple snoring, but they have not been shown to relieve obstructive sleep apnea. There are several surgical procedures marketed for snoring as well, but there is little proof of how well they work and how long they are effective.

People with obstructive sleep apnea, particularly those who have excessive daytime sleepiness, benefit most predictably from continuous positive airway pressure (CPAP). With CPAP, people breathe through a face or nose mask that provides a slightly higher pressure in the airway. This increased pressure props the throat open as the person breathes in. CPAP can be given with or without humidifying the delivered air. Close follow-up by a health care practitioner is needed during the first 2 weeks of use to ensure proper mask fit and provide appropriate encouragement as the person learns to sleep with the mask.

Removable oral appliances, fitted by dentists, can help relieve obstructive sleep apnea (and snoring) in people with mild to moderate sleep apnea. These appliances, which are worn only while sleeping, help keep the airway open. Most appliances separate the jaws and push the lower jaw forward so the tongue cannot move backward to block the throat. Others hold the tongue forward.

Surgery of the head or neck as a treatment for sleep apnea is useful if there are enlarged tonsils or an obvious blockage of the upper airway by another structure. Surgery is sometimes used in people without obvious blockage if no other treatments have worked. The most common procedure is a uvulopalatopharyngoplasty, in which tissue from around the upper airways (for example, the tonsils and adenoids) is removed. It is most often helpful in people who have mild sleep apnea. Other surgical procedures are sometimes used, but they have not been studied as thoroughly. In children, removal of the adenoids and tonsils usually relieves sleep apnea.

Central Sleep Apnea: The underlying disorder is treated if possible. For example, drugs may be given to reduce the severity of heart failure (see table on page 358). Otherwise, there are few, well-conducted clinical trials. Oxygen delivered by nasal prongs (not under pressure) may reduce events. Acetazolamide has some benefit for central sleep apnea, at sea level as well as high altitude. Some people with central sleep apnea may benefit from CPAP. Patients with central apnea of the Cheyne-Stokes type have fewer events and show improvements in heart failure with this treatment but do not survive longer.

CHAPTER 79 Pulmonary Embolism

Pulmonary embolism is the sudden blocking of an artery of the lung (pulmonary artery) by a collection of solid material brought through the bloodstream (embolus)—usually a blood clot (thrombus) or rarely other foreign material.

- Pulmonary embolism is usually caused by a blood clot, although other substances can also form emboli and block an artery.
- Symptoms vary but usually include shortness of breath.
- Doctors often diagnose pulmonary embolism by looking for blockage of the pulmonary artery using a lung scan or CT angiogram.
- Blood thinners (anticoagulants) can be given to people at high risk to prevent pulmonary embolism.
- Anticoagulant drugs are used to keep emboli from enlarging while the body dissolves the clots; other measures (such as drugs to break up blood clots or surgery) may be needed for people who appear to be at risk of dying.

The pulmonary arteries carry blood from the heart to the lungs. The blood picks up oxygen from the lungs and travels back to the heart. From the heart, the blood is pumped to the rest of the body to provide oxygen to the tissues (see page 445). When a pulmonary artery is blocked by an embolus, people may not be able to get sufficient oxygen into the blood. Large emboli may cause so much blockage that the heart has to strain to pump blood through the pulmonary arteries that remain open. If too little blood is pumped or the heart is strained excessively, the person can go into shock and die. Sometimes, the blockage of blood flow causes lung tissue to die (a condition called **pulmonary infarction**).

The body usually breaks up small clots quickly, keeping damage to a minimum. Large clots take much longer to disintegrate, so more damage is done.

About 1% of people admitted to the hospital have a pulmonary embolism. In about 5% of people in whom autopsy is done to find the cause of death, pulmonary embolism is unexpectedly found to be the cause.

Causes

The most common type of pulmonary embolism is a blood clot, usually one that forms in a leg or pelvic vein (see page 433) when blood flow slows down or stops, as may occur in the leg veins when a person stays in one position for a long time. People who have been on prolonged bed rest and those recovering from major surgery are at risk. Those sitting for long time periods without moving around (as may happen during air travel) are at slightly increased risk. Far less often, blood clots form in the veins of the arms or in the right side of the heart. Once a clot breaks free into the bloodstream, it usually travels to the lungs.

Unusual Types of Emboli: The sudden blocking of an artery of the lung is not only caused by blood clots. Other material can also form emboli.

- **Fat** can escape into the blood from the bone marrow when a long bone is fractured or during bone surgery and form an embolus.
- **Amniotic fluid** that is forced into the pelvic veins during a tumultuous childbirth can form an embolus.
- **Cancer cells** in clumps may break free into the circulation to form tumor emboli.
- **Air bubbles** may form emboli if a catheter in one of the large veins (central veins) is inadvertently opened to air. Air emboli may also form when a vein is operated on (such as when a blood clot is being removed) or when a person is being resuscitated (because of the force of chest compressions). An additional risk is underwater diving (see page 1996).
- **Infected material** may also form emboli and travel to the lung. Causes include intravenous drug use, certain heart valve infections, and inflammation of a vein with blood clot formation and infection (septic thrombophlebitis).
- **A foreign substance** can be introduced into the bloodstream, usually by intravenous injection of inorganic substances such as talc by injection drug users, where it can form emboli and travel to the lung.

Symptoms

Symptoms depend on the extent that the pulmonary artery is blocked and on the person's overall health. For example, people who have another disease such as chronic obstructive pulmonary disease or coronary artery disease may have more disabling symptoms.

Small emboli may not cause any symptoms, but when symptoms do occur, they usually develop abruptly. Shortness of breath may be the only symptom, especially if pulmonary infarction does not develop. Often, the breathing is very rapid, and the person may feel anxious or restless and appear to have an anxiety attack. Some people have pain in the chest. In some people, the first symptoms are light-headedness, fainting, or seizures. In older people, the first symptom may

What Predisposes Someone to Blood Clots?

The cause of blood clots in the veins may not be discernible, but many times predisposing conditions (risk factors) are obvious. These conditions include

- Advanced age, particularly older than 60 years
- Atrial fibrillation (a type of irregular heartbeat)
- Blood clotting disorder (increased risk of clotting, called a hypercoagulable state)
- Cancer
- Cigarette smoking (including passive smoke inhalation)
- Heart failure
- Immobility
- Injury to the pelvis, hip, or leg
- Indwelling venous catheters
- A kidney disorder called nephrotic syndrome
- Major surgery within the past 3 months
- Myeloproliferative disease, which can make the blood too thick (hyperviscosity)
- Obesity
- Pregnancy or the period after delivery
- Prior blood clot
- Sickle cell anemia
- Use of estrogens, for example, as treatment for menopausal symptoms or as contraception (in which case the risk is particularly high among women who are older than 35 or who smoke)
- Use of estrogen receptor modulators (such as raloxifene or tamoxifen)

be confusion or deterioration of mental function. These symptoms usually result from a sudden decrease in the heart's ability to deliver enough oxygen-rich blood to the brain and other organs.

The heartbeat may become rapid, irregular, or both. With very large emboli, blood pressure may be dangerously low (shock), the skin may have a blue color (cyanosis), or the person may suddenly die.

The symptoms of pulmonary infarction develop over hours. If pulmonary infarction occurs, the person experiences coughing that may produce blood-stained sputum, sharp chest pain when breathing in, and in some cases fever. Symptoms of infarction often last several days but usually become milder every day.

In people who have recurring episodes of small pulmonary emboli, symptoms such as chronic shortness of breath, swelling of the ankles or legs, and weakness tend to develop progressively over weeks, months, or years.

Diagnosis

Doctors suspect pulmonary embolism based on the person's symptoms and risk factors, such as recent surgery, a prolonged period of bed rest, or an inherited tendency to form blood clots. A large pulmonary embolism may be relatively easy for doctors to diagnose, especially when there are obvious preconditions, such as signs of a blood clot in a leg. However, in many cases, symptoms are absent or not very characteristic, which is an important reason why pulmonary embolism is often difficult to diagnose. Indeed, pulmonary embolism is one of the most difficult serious disorders for doctors to recognize and diagnose.

A chest x-ray may reveal subtle changes in the blood vessel patterns after embolism and signs of pulmonary infarction. However, the x-ray results are often normal, and even when they are abnormal, they rarely enable doctors to establish the diagnosis with certainty.

An electrocardiogram may show abnormalities, but often these abnormalities are transient and can only support the possibility of pulmonary embolism.

The person's symptoms and risk factors and the results of tests help doctors estimate the likelihood of a pulmonary embolism. This estimate determines what other tests are done. Doctors try to use tests that do not involve making an incision or entering the person's body (noninvasive tests) before they use an invasive test. Noninvasive tests are usually easier to perform and carry less risk of side effects. For example, if pulmonary embolism appears unlikely, testing may be limited to a blood test that measures a substance called D-dimer. If pulmonary embolism seems more likely or if the result of the D-dimer test is abnormal, further testing is done, which may include a CT angiogram, an ultrasound examination of the legs, or a lung perfusion scan. These are noninvasive tests. If the diagnosis is still unclear after noninvasive tests are done, an invasive test (for example, pulmonary angiography) may be done.

A CT angiogram is a type of computed tomography (CT) scan. It is fast, noninvasive, and fairly accurate, particularly for large clots. In this test, contrast material is injected into a vein. The contrast material travels to the lungs, and a CT scanner generates images of blood in the arteries to determine if a pulmonary embolism is blocking blood flow. A CT angiogram is the imaging test most often used to diagnose pulmonary embolism.

An ultrasound examination of the legs is noninvasive and can identify clots in the legs, which are the usual sources of pulmonary embolism. The absence of clots on this test does not rule out pulmonary embolism. However, if the ultrasound examination reveals blood clots, people are usually treated as they would be for pulmonary embolism without any further testing.

A lung perfusion scan is noninvasive and fairly accurate but is not very rapid. A tiny amount of radioactive substance is injected into a vein and travels to the lungs, where it outlines the blood supply (perfusion) of the lung. Completely normal scan results indicate that the person does not have a significant blood vessel obstruction. Abnormal scan results support the possibility of pulmonary embolism but may also reflect disorders other than pulmonary embolism, such as emphysema, which can result in decreased blood flow to areas where lung tissue has been damaged.

Usually, the perfusion scan is done with a lung ventilation scan. The person inhales a harmless gas containing a trace amount of radioactive material, which is distributed throughout the small air sacs of the lungs (alveoli). The areas where carbon dioxide is being released and oxygen is taken up can then be seen on a scanner. By comparing this scan to the pattern of blood supply shown on the perfusion scan, doctors can usually determine whether a person has had a pulmonary embolism.

Pulmonary angiography (see page 456) is the most accurate means of diagnosing pulmonary embolism, but it is invasive and poses some risk and is more uncomfortable than the other tests. It is usually performed only if the results of other tests are not conclusive.

Prognosis

The likelihood of dying from pulmonary embolism is very low, but massive pulmonary embolism can cause sudden death. Most deaths occur before the diagnosis is made, often within 1 to 2 hours of the embolism occurring. If a person is alive when diagnosed, the chance of survival is about 95%. Important factors include the size of the embolus, the size and number of pulmonary arteries blocked, and the person's overall health status. Anyone with a serious heart or lung problem is at greater risk of dying from pulmonary embolism. A person with normal heart and lung function usually survives unless the embolus blocks half or more of the pulmonary arteries.

Prevention

Given the danger of pulmonary embolism and the limitations of treatment, doctors try to prevent blood clots from forming in the veins of people at risk. In general, people, particularly those who are prone to clotting, should try to be active and move around as much as possible. For example, when traveling on an airplane for a long period, people should try to get up and move around every 2 hours.

Anticoagulation: For certain people, an anticoagulant drug is given, most often heparin. Heparin comes in two forms: traditional and low molecular weight. They appear equally effective. Heparin is the most widely used drug for reducing the likelihood of clots forming in calf veins after any type of major surgery, especially surgery on the legs. Small doses are injected just under the skin shortly before surgery, and ideally additional doses are given until the person is up and walking again. Hospitalized people at high risk of developing pulmonary embolism (such as those with heart failure, immobility, obesity, or who have had clots in the past) benefit from small doses of heparin even if they are not undergoing surgery. Low-dose heparin does not increase the frequency of major bleeding complications, but heparin can increase minor oozing of blood from wounds.

Warfarin, an anticoagulant given by mouth, may be given to people with one or more risk factors. It is also given to those who have undergone certain kinds of surgery that are particularly likely to result in clots, such as surgery for a hip fracture or a joint replacement. Warfarin therapy may need to be continued for several weeks or months. Low-molecular-weight heparin is also effective for people in this situation.

Newer anticoagulants include those such as hirudin, which inhibits the production of thrombin (a substance that promotes the formation of blood clots), and danaparoid and fondaparinux, which inhibit the formation of other substances that enhance the body's production of clots. These drugs are effective in prevention but are still being studied to determine whether they have advantages compared with heparin.

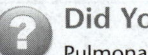

Did You Know...

Pulmonary embolism is one of the most common causes of unexplained deaths.

Physical Measures: For people who have undergone surgery—especially older people—the risk of clot formation can be reduced by wearing compression elastic stockings, doing leg exercises, and getting out of bed and becoming active as soon as possible. For people who cannot move their legs, intermittent air compression devices can provide rhythmic external pressure to keep blood moving in the legs. However, these devices alone are inadequate to prevent clot formation in people who have undergone hip or knee surgery.

Treatment

Treatment of pulmonary embolism begins with treating the symptoms. Oxygen is given if blood oxygen levels are low. Analgesics are given to relieve pain. If blood pressure is low, intravenous fluids are given, and sometimes drugs that increase blood pressure are given. Mechanical ventilation (a breathing tube) may be needed if respiratory failure develops.

Anticoagulation: Anticoagulant drugs such as heparin are given to prevent existing blood clots from enlarging and additional clots from forming. Heparin is given intravenously to achieve a rapid effect, and doctors carefully regulate the dose. Doctors strive to achieve a full anticoagulant effect within the first 24 hours of treatment. Low-molecular-weight heparin is probably as effective as traditional heparin and does not require the blood test monitoring that is commonly recommended for conventional heparin. Warfarin, which also inhibits clotting but takes longer to start working, is given next. Because warfarin is taken by mouth, it can be used long-term. Heparin and warfarin are given together for 5 to 7 days, until blood tests show that the warfarin is effectively preventing clotting. Then, the heparin is discontinued.

How long anticoagulants are given depends on the person's situation. If pulmonary embolism is caused by a temporary risk factor, such as surgery, treatment is given for 2 to 3 months. If the cause is some longer-term problem, such as prolonged bed rest, treatment usually is given for 3 to 6 months, but sometimes it must continue indefinitely. For example, people who have recurrent pulmonary embolism, often because of a hereditary clotting disorder, usually take anticoagulants indefinitely. While taking warfarin, people periodically have to have a blood test to determine if the dose needs to be adjusted.

Changes in diet and use of other drugs may affect warfarin's anticoagulant effects. If excessive anticoagulation occurs, severe bleeding in a number of body organs can develop. Because many drugs can interact with warfarin, people who take anticoagulants should be sure to check with their doctor before taking any other drugs, including drugs that can be obtained without a prescription (over-the-counter drugs) such as acetaminophen or aspirin, herbal preparations, and dietary supplements. Foods that are high in vitamin K (which affects blood clotting), such as broccoli, spinach, kale, and other leafy green vegetables, liver, grapefruit and grapefruit juice, and green tea, may also need to be avoided.

Thrombolytic Therapy: Thrombolytic drugs such as streptokinase or tissue plasminogen activator (TPA) break up and dissolve blood clots. They can be used for people who appear to be in danger of dying of pulmonary embolism. However, except in the most dire situations, these drugs cannot be given to people who have had surgery in the preceding 2 weeks, are pregnant, have had a recent stroke, or tend to bleed excessively.

Physical Measures: In some centers, if a person appears to be in danger of dying from a massive pulmonary embolism, doctors may try to shatter the embolus using a catheter inserted into the pulmonary artery. Surgery may be needed to save someone with severe embolism. Removal of the embolus from the pulmonary artery may be lifesaving. Surgery is also used to remove long-standing pulmonary artery clots that cause persistent shortness of breath and high pressures in the pulmonary artery (pulmonary hypertension).

A filter can be surgically placed in the main vein in the abdomen that drains blood from the legs and pelvis to the right side of the heart (see art on page 436). Such a filter can be used if emboli recur despite anticoagulant treatment or if anticoagulants cannot be used or cause significant bleeding. Because clots generally originate in the legs or pelvis, this filter usually prevents them from being carried into the pulmonary artery. Newer filters are removable. Removal helps prevent some complications that can occur when filters are left in place permanently.

80 Bronchiectasis

Bronchiectasis is an irreversible widening (dilation) of portions of the breathing tubes or airways (bronchi) resulting from damage to the airway wall.

- The most common cause is severe or repeated respiratory infections.
- Most people develop a chronic cough, and some also cough up blood and have chest pain and recurrent episodes of pneumonia.

- Chest x-rays are usually done to determine the extent and severity of the disorder.
- People usually take antibiotics and drugs to suppress the build-up of mucus.

Bronchiectasis can result when conditions directly injure the bronchial wall or indirectly lead to injury by interfering with normal airway defenses. Airway defenses include tiny projections (cilia) on the cells that line the airways. These cilia beat back and forth, moving the thin liquid layer of mucus that normally coats the airways. Harmful particles and bacteria trapped in this mucus layer are moved up to the throat and coughed out or swallowed.

Whether airway injury is direct or indirect, areas of the bronchial wall are damaged and become chronically inflamed. The inflamed bronchial wall becomes less elastic, resulting in the affected airways becoming wider and flabby and developing small outpouchings or sacs that resemble tiny balloons. Inflammation also increases secretions (mucus). Because cells with cilia are damaged or destroyed, these secretions accumulate in the widened airways and serve as a breeding ground for bacteria. The bacteria further damage the bronchial wall, leading to a vicious circle of infection and airway damage.

Bronchiectasis may affect many areas of the lung (diffuse bronchiectasis), or it may appear in only one or two areas (focal bronchiectasis). Typically, bronchiectasis causes widening of medium-sized airways, but often smaller airways become scarred and destroyed.

Complications: The inflammation and infection can extend to the small air sacs of the lungs (alveoli) and cause pneumonia, scarring, and a loss of functioning lung tissue. Severe scarring and loss of lung tissue can ultimately strain the right side of the heart as the heart tries to pump blood through the altered tissue. The right-sided heart strain can lead to a form of heart failure called cor pulmonale (see box on page 523).

Very severe cases of bronchiectasis, which occur more commonly in underdeveloped countries and in people who have advanced cystic fibrosis, may impair breathing enough to cause abnormally low levels of oxygen and high levels of carbon dioxide in the blood, a condition called respiratory failure (see page 524).

> **? Did You Know...**
>
> Bronchiectasis was first identified in 1819 by the same man who invented the stethoscope.

Causes

The most common cause is severe or repeated respiratory infections. Other causes include

- Immune deficiency disorders
- Hereditary disorders, such as primary ciliary dyskinesia or cystic fibrosis, in which the ability to clear the airway of organisms that cause infection is impaired

- Mechanical factors, such as airway obstruction caused by an inhaled object or a lung tumor
- Inhaling toxic substances that injure the airways, such as noxious fumes, gases, smoke (including tobacco smoke), and injurious dust (for example, silica and coal dust)

Occasionally, a condition that affects larger airways, called allergic bronchopulmonary aspergillosis, occurs in people with asthma. Allergic bronchopulmonary aspergillosis (see page 516) is an allergic reaction to *Aspergillus* species, which is a fungal organism. It can cause mucus plugs that obstruct the airways and lead to bronchiectasis.

Symptoms

Bronchiectasis can develop at any age, but the process often begins in early childhood. However, symptoms may not appear until much later. In most people, symptoms begin gradually, usually after a respiratory infection, and tend to worsen over the years. Most people develop a chronic cough that produces sputum. The amount and type of sputum depend on the extent of the disease and whether there is a complicating infection. Often, people have coughing spells only early in the morning and late in the day. Coughing up of blood (hemoptysis) is common because the damaged airway walls are fragile and have increased numbers of blood vessels. Hemoptysis may be the first or only symptom.

Recurrent fever or chest pain, with or without frequent bouts of pneumonia, may also occur. People with widespread bronchiectasis may develop wheezing or shortness of breath. People whose bronchiectasis progresses to cor pulmonale or respiratory failure also have fatigue, lethargy, and worsening shortness of breath, particularly with exertion.

Diagnosis

Doctors may suspect bronchiectasis because of a person's symptoms or the presence (currently or in the past) of a condition thought to cause bronchiectasis. Tests are done to confirm the diagnosis and assess the extent and location of the disease. Chest x-rays can often detect the lung changes caused by bronchiectasis. However, occasionally, x-ray results are normal. Computed tomography (CT) is the most sensitive test to identify and confirm the diagnosis and to determine the extent and severity of the disease.

After bronchiectasis is diagnosed, tests are often done to check for disorders that may be causing or contributing to it. Such tests may include the following:

- Measuring certain proteins in blood
- Testing for HIV infection and other immune system disorders

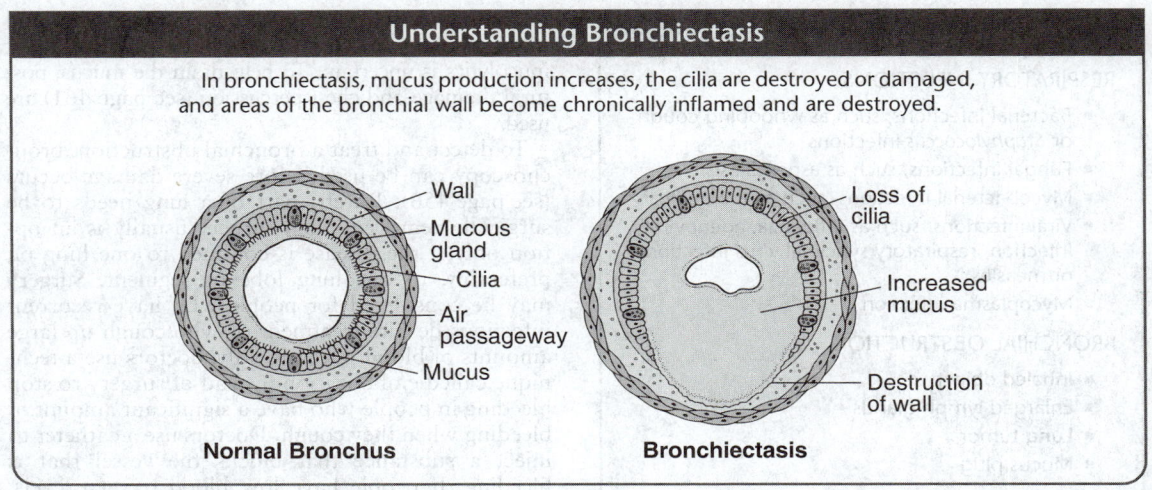

Understanding Bronchiectasis

In bronchiectasis, mucus production increases, the cilia are destroyed or damaged, and areas of the bronchial wall become chronically inflamed and are destroyed.

Normal Bronchus — Wall, Mucous gland, Cilia, Air passageway, Mucus

Bronchiectasis — Loss of cilia, Increased mucus, Destruction of wall

- Measuring the salt level in sweat (which is abnormal in people with cystic fibrosis)
- Examining nasal, bronchial, or sperm specimens with a special microscope
- Other tests to determine if the cilia are structurally or functionally defective

When bronchiectasis is limited to one area—for example, a lung lobe or segment—doctors may do a bronchoscopy (see page 456) to determine whether an inhaled foreign object or lung tumor is the cause. Other tests may be done to identify underlying disorders, such as allergic bronchopulmonary aspergillosis or tuberculosis.

Genetic testing for cystic fibrosis may be needed when there is a family history, repeated respiratory infections, or other unusual findings in a child or young adult, even when other typical features of cystic fibrosis are absent.

Prevention

Early identification and treatment of conditions that tend to cause bronchiectasis may prevent its development or reduce its severity. More than half the cases of bronchiectasis in children can be accurately diagnosed and promptly treated.

Childhood immunizations against measles and whooping cough, improved living conditions, and good nutrition have markedly reduced the number of people who develop bronchiectasis. Annual influenza vaccines, pneumococcal vaccine, and use of appropriate antibiotics early in the course of lung infections help to prevent bronchiectasis or reduce its severity. Receiving immunoglobulin for an immunoglobulin deficiency syndrome may prevent re-

curring infections. In people who have allergic bronchopulmonary aspergillosis, the appropriate use of corticosteroids and perhaps the antifungal drug itraconazole may reduce the bronchial damage that results in bronchiectasis.

Avoiding toxic fumes, gases, smoke, and injurious dusts also helps prevent bronchiectasis or reduce its severity. Inhalation of foreign objects into the airways by children may be prevented by watching what they put in their mouth. Avoiding over-sedation from drugs or alcohol and seeking medical care for neurologic symptoms (such as impaired consciousness) or gastrointestinal symptoms (such as difficulty in swallowing and regurgitation or coughing after eating) may help to prevent aspiration. Also, drops of mineral oil or petroleum jelly should never be placed in the nose because they can be inhaled into the lungs.

Treatment and Prognosis

Treatment of bronchiectasis is directed toward eradicating infections, decreasing the build-up of mucus and inflammation, and relieving airway obstruction. Drugs that suppress coughing may worsen the condition and generally should not be used. Early, effective treatment can reduce complications such as hemoptysis, low oxygen levels in the blood, respiratory failure, and cor pulmonale.

Infections are treated with antibiotics, bronchodilators, and physical therapy to promote drainage of secretions. Sometimes antibiotics are prescribed for a long period to prevent recurring infections, especially in people who have cystic fibrosis.

For inflammation and the build-up of mucus, anti-inflammatory drugs such as inhaled corticosteroids and

Some Causes of Bronchiectasis

RESPIRATORY INFECTIONS

- Bacterial infections, such as whooping cough or *Staphylococcus* infections
- Fungal infections, such as aspergillosis
- Mycobacterial infections, such as tuberculosis
- Viral infections, such as influenza, adenoviral infection, respiratory syncytial virus infection, or measles
- Mycoplasma infection

BRONCHIAL OBSTRUCTION

- Inhaled object
- Enlarged lymph glands
- Lung tumor
- Mucus plug

INHALATION INJURIES

- Injury from noxious fumes, gases, or particles
- Inhalation of stomach acid and food particles

HEREDITARY CONDITIONS

- Cystic fibrosis
- Primary ciliary dyskinesia, including Kartagener's syndrome
- Marfan syndrome

IMMUNOLOGIC ABNORMALITIES

- Immunoglobulin deficiency syndromes
- White blood cell dysfunction
- Complement deficiencies
- Certain autoimmune or hyperimmune disorders, such as rheumatoid arthritis and ulcerative colitis

OTHER CONDITIONS

- Drug abuse, such as heroin abuse
- Human immunodeficiency virus (HIV) infection
- Young's syndrome (obstructive azoospermia)
- Yellow nail syndrome (with lymphedema)

drugs that thin the pus and mucus (mucolytics and saline) may also be given, although the effectiveness of mucolytics is uncertain. To help drain the mucus, postural drainage and chest percussion (see page 461) are used.

To detect and treat a bronchial obstruction, bronchoscopy can be used before severe damage occurs (see page 456). Rarely, part of a lung needs to be surgically removed. Such surgery usually is an option only if the disease is confined to one lung or, preferably, to one lung lobe or segment. Surgery may be considered for people who have recurrent infections despite treatment or who cough up large amounts of blood. Occasionally, doctors use a technique called embolization instead of surgery to stop bleeding in people who have a significant amount of bleeding when they cough. Doctors use a catheter to inject a substance that blocks the vessel that is bleeding. If people have low blood oxygen levels, doctors give oxygen therapy (see page 460). Appropriate use of oxygen may help prevent complications such as cor pulmonale. If people have wheezing or shortness of breath, oral and inhaled corticosteroids taken with or without bronchodilators often help. Respiratory failure, if present, should be treated (see page 524).

Lung transplantation can be done in some people who have advanced bronchiectasis, mostly those who also have advanced cystic fibrosis. Five-year survival rates as high as 65 to 75% have been reported when a heart-lung or a double lung transplantation is used. Pulmonary function (as measured by the amount of air in the lungs and the rate and amount of air moving in and out of the lungs with each breath) usually improves within 6 months, and the improvement may be sustained for at least 5 years.

Prognosis for people with bronchiectasis depends on how well infections and other complications are prevented or controlled. People with co-existing conditions, such as chronic bronchitis or emphysema, and people who have complications, such as pulmonary hypertension or cor pulmonale, tend to have a worse prognosis.

81 Atelectasis

Atelectasis is a condition in which all or part of a lung becomes airless and collapses.

- Blockage of the bronchial tubes is a common cause of atelectasis.
- Shortness of breath is the only symptom that atelectasis itself causes.
- Chest x-ray is used to confirm the diagnosis.
- Treatment may involve making sure deep breathing occurs, relieving airway blockages, or both.

The main function of the lungs is to absorb oxygen into the bloodstream from the atmosphere and to expel carbon dioxide from the blood into the exhaled breath (gas exchange—see art on page 446). For gas exchange to occur, the small air sacs within the lungs (alveoli) must remain open and filled with air. Alveoli are kept open by the elastic structure of the lung and by a liquid lining called surfactant. Surfactant counters the natural tendency of the alveoli to close (collapse). Periodic deep breaths, which people take unconsciously, and cough also help keep alveoli open. Cough expels any mucus or other secretions that could block the airways leading to the alveoli. If the alveoli are closed for any reason, they cannot participate in gas exchange. The more alveoli that are closed, the less gas exchange occurs. Accordingly, atelectasis can decrease the level of oxygen in the blood. The body compensates for a small amount of atelectasis by constricting the blood vessels in the affected area. This constriction redirects blood flow to alveoli that are open so that gas exchange can occur.

Causes

A common cause of atelectasis is a blockage of one of the tubes (bronchi) that branch off from the trachea (windpipe) and lead to the lung tissue. The blockage may be caused by something inside the bronchus, such as a plug of mucus, a tumor, or an inhaled foreign object (such as a coin, piece of food, or a toy). Alternatively, the bronchus may be blocked by something pressing from the outside, such as a tumor or enlarged lymph nodes. Blockage from the outside can also occur if the pleural space (the space outside of the lung but inside of the chest) contains a large amount of fluid (pleural effusion) or air (pneumothorax— see page 520). When a bronchus or bronchiole becomes blocked, the air in the alveoli beyond the blockage is absorbed into the bloodstream, causing the alveoli to shrink and collapse. The area of collapsed lung may become infected because bacteria and white blood cells can build up behind (to the inside of) the blockage. Infection is particularly likely if atelectasis persists for several days or more. If atelectasis persists for months, the lung may not easily re-expand.

Any condition that decreases deep breathing or suppresses a person's ability to cough can cause or contribute to atelectasis. Large doses of opioids or sedatives can decrease deep breathing. Atelectasis is common after general anesthesia, which temporarily suppresses a person's cough and drive to breathe. Atelectasis is particularly common after chest or abdominal surgery because the effects of receiving general anesthesia may be added to the pain of deep breathing, so people take only small breaths. Chest or abdominal pain from other causes (for example, from injury or pneumonia) also makes taking a deep breath painful. Certain neurologic conditions and chest deformities can limit chest movement and thus decrease deep breathing, as can abdominal swelling, immobility of the body, and some tight bandages. People who smoke or who have lung disorders (eg, chronic obstructive pulmonary disease, cystic fibrosis) have a greater risk of developing atelectasis.

> **? Did You Know...**
>
> Taking deep breaths after surgery can help prevent atelectasis.
>
> People who smoke can decrease their risk of atelectasis after surgery by stopping smoking, ideally 6 to 8 weeks before the surgery.

Symptoms

The only symptom a person with atelectasis may feel is shortness of breath. The presence and severity of shortness of breath depend on how rapidly atelectasis develops and how much of the lung is affected. If atelectasis involves a small number of alveoli or develops slowly, symptoms may be mild or not even noticed. If a large number of alveoli are affected, particularly if atelectasis occurs rapidly, shortness of breath may be severe. The heart rate and breathing rate may increase, and sometimes the person may look bluish (a condition called cyanosis) because oxygen levels in the blood are low.

Symptoms may also reflect the disorder that caused atelectasis (for example, chest pain due to an injury) or a disorder that results from atelectasis (for example, chest pain with deep breathing, due to pneumonia).

Diagnosis

Doctors suspect atelectasis based on a person's symptoms, the physical examination findings, and the setting in which the symptoms occurred. A chest x-ray that shows the airless area confirms the diagnosis. When bronchial blockage is suspected, computed tomography (CT), bronchoscopy (inserting a viewing tube into the bronchus), or both may be performed to find the cause, especially when the collapse persists despite treatment.

Prevention

People who smoke can decrease their risk of atelectasis after surgery by stopping smoking, ideally 6 to 8 weeks before surgery. After surgery, people are encouraged to breathe deeply, cough regularly, and move about as soon as possible. The use of devices to encourage voluntary deep breathing (incentive spirometry) and certain exercises, including changing position to increase the drainage of lung mucus and other secretions, may help to prevent atelectasis.

Atelectasis may be prevented by making sure deep breathing occurs. Whenever possible, conditions that cause shallow breathing for long periods should be treated. Some people affected by these disorders may

benefit from mechanical assistance with breathing. One method is continuous positive airway pressure, which delivers air or a mixture of air and oxygen through the nose or a face mask under continuous pressure, even during exhalation, to help ensure that the airways do not collapse and the lung stays expanded.

Treatment

Treatment of atelectasis may involve making sure deep breathing occurs, relieving airway blockages, or both.

Sometimes blockages can be relieved when a patient's airway is suctioned by a health care practitioner. A blockage that cannot be removed by suctioning may require removal by bronchoscopy (see page 456). Sometimes other methods are necessary. For example, if a tumor is blocking an airway, the obstruction can sometimes be relieved by surgery, radiation therapy, chemotherapy, or laser therapy.

Symptoms and complications of atelectasis may require treatment. Patients may require supplemental oxygen, continuous positive airway pressure, or, rarely, insertion of a breathing tube (endotracheal intubation) and mechanical ventilation. If a bacterial infection is suspected, antibiotics are almost always given.

CHAPTER

82 Environmental Lung Diseases

Environmental lung diseases are caused by harmful particles, mists, vapors, or gases that are inhaled, usually while people work. If the lung disease is due to inhaled particles, the term pneumoconiosis is often used. Where within the airways or lungs an inhaled substance ends up and what type of lung disease develops depend on the size and kind of particles inhaled. Large particles may get trapped in the nose or large airways, but very small ones may reach the lungs. There, some particles dissolve and may be absorbed into the bloodstream. Most solid particles that do not dissolve are removed by the body's defenses.

The body has several means of getting rid of inhaled particles. In the airways, an accumulation of secretions (mucus) coats particles so that they can be coughed up more easily. Additionally, tiny cells lining the airways (cilia) are able to brush inhaled particles upward, out of the lungs. In the small air sacs of the lungs (alveoli), special scavenger cells (macrophages) engulf most particles and render them harmless.

Many different kinds of particles can harm the lungs. Some are organic, meaning that they are made of materials that contain carbon and are part of living organisms (such as grain dusts, cotton dust, or animal dander). Some are inorganic, meaning that they usually come from nonliving sources, such as metals or minerals (for example, asbestos).

Different types of particles produce different reactions in the body. Some particles—animal dander, for example—can cause allergic reactions, such as hay fever–like symptoms or a type of asthma. Other particles cause harm not by triggering allergic reactions but by being toxic to the cells of the airways and air sacs in the lung. Some particles, such as quartz dust and asbestos, may cause chronic irritation that can lead to scarring of lung tissue (pulmonary fibrosis—see page 507). Certain toxic particles, such as asbestos, can cause lung cancer, especially in people who smoke, or cancer of the lining of the chest and lung (mesothelioma), regardless of the person's smoking history.

Who Is at Risk of Environmental Lung Diseases?

ASBESTOSIS

- Construction workers who install or remove materials (including insulation) that contain asbestos
- Shipyard workers
- Workers who mine, mill, or manufacture asbestos

BENIGN PNEUMOCONIOSIS

- Barium workers
- Iron miners
- Tin workers
- Welders

BERYLLIUM DISEASE

- Aerospace workers
- Metallurgical (castings) workers

BRONCHIOLITIS OBLITERANS

- Flavorings workers (popcorn workers' lung)

BYSSINOSIS

- Cotton, hemp, jute, and flax workers

COAL WORKERS' PNEUMOCONIOSIS

- Coal workers

HYPERSENSITIVITY PNEUMONITIS

- Office workers (because of air-conditioning systems contaminated by certain fungi and bacteria)

- Swimming pool and spa workers (because of contaminated sprays)
- Farmers, mushroom workers, bird keepers, people exposed to isocyanates (urethanes)

OCCUPATIONAL ASTHMA

- People who work with grains, western red cedar wood, castor beans, isocyanates (urethanes), dyes, antibiotics, epoxy resins, tea, and enzymes used in manufacturing detergent, malt, leather goods, latex, jewelry, abrasives and paints used in automobile body repairs, animals, shellfish, irritating gases, vapors, and mists

SILICOSIS

- Certain coal miners (for example, those who drill or blast rock)
- Foundry workers
- Lead, copper, silver, and gold miners
- Potters
- Sandblasters
- Sandstone or granite cutters
- Tombstone makers
- Tunnel workers
- Workers who make abrasive soaps

SILO FILLER'S DISEASE

- Farmers

Air Pollution-Related Illness

The major components of air pollution in developed countries are nitrogen dioxide (from combustion of fossil fuels), ozone (from the effect of sunlight on nitrogen dioxide and hydrocarbons), and suspended solid or liquid particles. Burning of biomass fuel is an important source of particulate matter indoors in developing countries. Secondhand smoke is also an important source of indoor air pollution.

High levels of air pollution can trigger exacerbations in people with asthma or chronic obstructive pulmonary disease. People living in areas with high traffic are at particular risk. Most air pollutants cause airways to narrow (airway hyperreactivity). Long-term exposure may increase respiratory infections and symptoms in the general population, especially children.

Ozone, which is the major component of smog, is a strong lung irritant. Levels tend to be highest in

the summer compared to other seasons and relatively higher in the late morning and early afternoon compared to other times of the day. Short-term exposures can cause breathing difficulties, chest pain, and airway hyperreactivity. Children who participate in outdoor sports on days on which ozone pollution is high are more likely to develop asthma. Long-term exposure to ozone produces a small, permanent decrease in lung function.

Combustion of fossil fuels that are high in sulfur can create acid particles that are easily deposited in the upper airway. These particles, called sulfur oxides, can cause the airways to become inflamed and constricted and increase the risk for chronic bronchitis.

Particulate air pollution derived from fossil fuel combustion (especially diesel fuel) is a complex mixture. The particles can cause inflammation of the airways or can affect other parts of their body, such

Nanoparticles: A New Cause of Environmental Lung Disease?

Particles affect the lung differently depending on what substances they are made from. Particles of the same material also may have different effects depending on their size and shape. For example, the risk from inhaling asbestos varies with the size and length of the asbestos fibers.

The nanotechnology industry creates extremely small particles of different substances, such as carbon, for various uses. These particles are called nanoparticles when they are less than 100 nanometers in size. For comparison, a human hair is about 100,000 nanometers in diameter, so it would take 1000 nanoparticles to equal the thickness of one hair. Animal and laboratory tests show that high concentrations of nanoparticles can be dangerous. But doctors do not know for certain the effects on workers in the nanotechnology industry of the amounts and types of nanoparticles that they are exposed to. Studies are being designed to evaluate the risks and to ensure that workers are protected.

as the heart. Data from some studies suggest that particulate air pollution increases death rates from all causes, especially heart and lung disorders.

Asbestosis

Asbestosis is widespread scarring of lung tissue caused by breathing asbestos dust.

- Asbestosis causes shortness of breath and a decreased ability to exercise.
- Diagnosis is usually made with chest x-rays and computed tomography.
- Asbestosis can be prevented by minimizing exposure to asbestos.
- Treatments include giving oxygen and draining fluid from around the lungs to ease breathing.
- Asbestosis exposure can also cause mesothelioma and lung cancer.

Asbestos is composed of fibrous mineral silicates of different chemical compositions. When inhaled, asbestos fibers settle deep in the lungs, causing scars. Asbestos inhalation also can cause the two layers of membranes covering the lungs (the pleura) to thicken. These thickenings are called pleural plaques. These plaques do not become cancerous.

Inhaling asbestos fibers can occasionally cause fluid to accumulate in the space between the two pleural layers of the lungs (pleural space). This fluid accumulation is called a noncancerous (benign) asbestos effusion.

Asbestos also causes cancer in the pleura, called mesothelioma, or in the membranes of the abdomen, called peritoneal mesothelioma. In the United States, asbestos is the only known cause of mesothelioma. Smoking is not a cause of mesothelioma. Mesotheliomas most commonly occur after exposure to crocidolite, one of four types of asbestos. Amosite, another type, also causes mesotheliomas. Chrysotile probably causes fewer cases of mesotheliomas than other types, but chrysotile is often contaminated with tremolite,

which does. Mesotheliomas usually develop 30 to 40 years after exposure and can occur after low levels of exposure.

Asbestos can also cause lung cancer. Lung cancer from asbestos is related in part to the level of exposure to asbestos fibers. Among people with asbestosis, lung cancer occurs most commonly in those who also smoke cigarettes, particularly those who smoke more than a pack a day (see page 528).

Although the public has become alarmed about the risks of asbestos, people who have no occupational exposure have a very low risk of developing asbestos-related lung disease. The asbestos must be broken into tiny pieces to be inhaled into the lungs. Workers who demolish buildings that have insulation containing asbestos are at increased risk. People who regularly work with asbestos are at greatest risk of developing lung disease. The more a person is exposed to asbestos fibers, the greater the risk of developing an asbestos-related disease.

 Did You Know...

Smoking is not a cause of mesothelioma.

Most people have a very low risk of developing asbestosis-related lung disorders.

Symptoms

Symptoms of asbestosis appear gradually only after large areas of the lung become scarred. The scarring causes the lungs to lose their elasticity. The first symptoms are a mild shortness of breath and a decreased ability to exercise. Smokers who have chronic bronchitis along with asbestosis may cough and wheeze. Gradually, breathing becomes more and more difficult. In about 15% of people with asbestosis, severe shortness of breath and respiratory failure develop.

People with a noncancerous asbestos effusion may have difficulty breathing because of fluid accumulation. Pleural plaques cause only mild breathing difficulty resulting from stiffness of the chest wall. Persistent pain in the chest and shortness of breath are the most common symptoms of mesothelioma.

Diagnosis

People with asbestosis usually have abnormal lung function, and a doctor listening with a stethoscope placed over the lungs can usually hear abnormal sounds called crackles. In people who have a history of exposure to asbestos, doctors sometimes can diagnose asbestosis with a chest x-ray or a chest computed tomography (CT) scan that shows characteristic changes. Pleural plaques that develop in many people with exposure to asbestos often contain calcium, which makes them easy to see on chest x-rays and CT scans. A lung biopsy is rarely needed to make the diagnosis.

If a tumor of the pleura is found on the x-ray, doctors must do a biopsy (remove a small piece of pleura and examine it under a microscope) to determine if it is cancerous. Fluid around the lungs may be removed with a needle and analyzed for cancer cells (a procedure called thoracentesis). However, thoracentesis is not usually as accurate as a pleural biopsy. If a chest x-ray reveals something that looks like a tumor, there is a good possibility that the area is a lung cancer, and it should be evaluated fully.

Prevention and Treatment

Diseases caused by asbestos inhalation can be prevented by minimizing asbestos dust and fibers in the workplace. Because industries that use asbestos have improved dust control, fewer people develop asbestosis today, but mesotheliomas are still occurring in people who were exposed as many as 30 to 50 years ago. Asbestos-containing materials in a home are typically only a concern if the materials are going to be removed or the home renovated, in which case they should be removed by workers trained in safe removal techniques. Smokers who have been in contact with asbestos can reduce their risk of lung cancer by giving up smoking and should probably have a chest x-ray annually. Pneumococcal and influenza vaccination are recommended for people who have been in contact with asbestos to help protect against infections to which workers may be more vulnerable.

Most treatments for asbestosis ease symptoms. Oxygen therapy relieves shortness of breath. Draining fluid from around the lungs may make breath-

ing easier. Occasionally, lung transplantation has been successful in treating asbestosis.

Mesotheliomas are invariably fatal within 1 to 4 years of diagnosis. Chemotherapy and radiation therapy do not work well, and surgical removal of the tumor does not cure the cancer. Other treatment is focused on controlling pain and shortness of breath in an effort to preserve as much quality of life as possible (see pages 61 and 62).

Beryllium Disease

Beryllium disease (sometimes called berylliosis) is a lung inflammation caused by inhaling dust or fumes that contain beryllium.

- Most people with beryllium disease have gradual development of coughing, difficulty breathing, fatigue, and night sweats.
- Diagnosis is based on a person's history of exposure, chest x-rays, computed tomography, and tests of the immune system's reaction to beryllium.
- Oxygen and corticosteroids may be needed for treatment.
- Some people need to take corticosteroids for the rest of their lives, and others may need lung transplantation.

In the past, beryllium was commonly mined and extracted for use in the electronics and chemical industries and in the manufacture of fluorescent light bulbs. Today, it is used mainly in the aerospace industry and in beryllium–aluminum castings. Besides workers in these industries, a few people living near beryllium refineries also have developed beryllium disease.

Beryllium disease differs from other environmental lung diseases in that at low levels of exposure, lung problems seem to occur only in people who are sensitive to beryllium—about 2 to 6% of those who come in contact with it. The disease can occur in such people even with a relatively brief exposure to beryllium dust.

Symptoms and Diagnosis

In some people, beryllium disease develops suddenly (acute beryllium disease), mainly as an inflammation of the lungs (pneumonitis). In these people, the lungs are stiff and function poorly. People with acute disease have an abrupt onset of coughing, difficulty in breathing, and weight loss. Acute beryllium disease also can affect the skin and eyes. This form of beryllium disease is now rare.

More commonly, people develop chronic beryllium disease, in which abnormal tissue forms in the lungs and the lymph nodes enlarge. In these people, coughing, difficulty breathing, weight loss, night sweats, and fatigue develop gradually, often 10 to 20 years after exposure. When detected early, people may initially have no symptoms.

The diagnosis is based on the person's history of exposure to beryllium and on results of a blood test, called the beryllium lymphocyte proliferation test (BeLPT), which tests for allergy to beryllium. If the disease is at a more advanced stage, characteristic changes on a chest x-ray or computed tomography (CT) helps doctors make the diagnosis. However, x-rays and CT scans of people with beryllium disease resemble those of people with sarcoidosis (another lung disease—see page 511). Definitive diagnosis is made by doing a test in which a tube, called a bronchoscope, is inserted into the lungs to obtain pieces of lung tissue and cells to test for an allergic reaction to beryllium.

Prognosis, Prevention, and Treatment

Acute beryllium disease may be severe. Most people recover in 7 to 10 days, with appropriate treatment, such as ventilator support and corticosteroid drugs. However, some people with severe acute disease die or develop chronic beryllium disease.

The course of people who develop symptoms years after exposure is completely different. People with chronic beryllium disease continue to have symptoms, which tend to progress. If the lungs are severely damaged, the heart may become strained, causing a type of heart failure (cor pulmonale—see box on page 523) and death. Sometimes corticosteroids, such as oral prednisone, are prescribed for chronic beryllium disease. Some people need to take corticosteroids for the rest of their lives. In some people with very severe chronic beryllium disease, lung transplantation can be life saving. Other supportive measures, such as supplemental oxygen therapy, pulmonary rehabilitation, and drugs for treatment of right-sided heart failure, are used as needed.

Beryllium disease can be prevented by strictly limiting exposure to beryllium.

Building-Related Illnesses

Building-related illnesses are disorders that affect the lungs as well as other parts of the body and are caused by exposure to substances within modern airtight buildings.

- Building-related illnesses are caused by exposure to substances within airtight buildings that have poor ventilation.
- Symptoms vary depending on the cause but may include fever, difficulty breathing, runny nose or congestion, headaches, skin problems, and difficulty concentrating.
- Diagnosis usually includes evaluating the air quality of the building and determining how many people experience building-related symptoms.

- Treatment is usually removal from the building or improvement of air quality within the building.

Building-related illnesses are a group of disorders whose cause is linked to the environment of modern airtight, energy-efficient buildings. Such buildings are characterized by sealed windows and dependence on heating, ventilation, and air conditioning systems for circulation of air. Most cases occur in nonindustrial office buildings, but illnesses can occur in apartment buildings, single-family homes, schools, museums, and libraries.

Building-related illnesses can be specific or nonspecific.

Specific Building-Related Illnesses

Specific building-related illnesses are those illnesses for which a link between building-related exposure and illness is proved. Examples include Legionnaires' disease (see box on page 465), occupational asthma (see page 503), hypersensitivity pneumonitis (see page 514), and inhalational fever.

Inhalational fever is a fever caused by exposure to organic (made of materials that contain carbon and are part of living organisms) aerosols or dusts. Metal fumes and polymer fumes can also produce fever.

In nonindustrial buildings, **humidifier fever** occurs as a consequence of humidifiers or other types of ventilation units serving as a reservoir for the growth of bacteria or fungi and as a method of aerosolizing these contaminants. People with humidifier fever have a low-grade fever, malaise, cough, and shortness of breath. Improvement that occurs when exposure stops (for example, after a weekend away from the building) is often an indication of the cause. The condition starts abruptly and usually lasts a few days. Symptoms may be absent or subtle. Clusters of cases are common. Disease can occur after initial exposure. Acute episodes do not generally require treatment apart from removal from the contaminated environment and drugs to reduce the fever. If symptoms persist, testing may be required to determine if infection or another condition is causing symptoms. Sampling to detect airborne organisms can be costly and time consuming but is necessary in some cases to document the source of contaminated air. Inhalational fevers are usually prevented by good maintenance of ventilation systems.

Nonspecific Building-Related Illnesses

Nonspecific building-related illnesses are those for which a link between building-related exposure and illness is difficult to prove. The term **sick building syndrome** has been used to refer to illnesses that occur in clusters within a building. The symptoms are often very general and may include the following:

- Itchy, irritated, dry, or watery eyes
- Runny nose or nasal congestion

- Throat soreness or tightness
- Dry itchy skin or unexplained rashes
- Headache, lethargy, or difficulty concentrating

Some building-related factors, including higher building temperature, higher humidity, and poor ventilation, typically with a failure to incorporate sufficient fresh air from outdoors, appear to account for symptoms in some instances. Women, people with allergies, people who have increased sensitivity to body sensations or worry about the meaning of symptoms, and some people with anxiety or depression are more likely to experience building-related symptoms.

No specific clinical tests can be used to diagnose a building-related illness. Testing the air quality of the building and finding high rates of symptoms among the building occupants can allow doctors to surmise that building-related factors may be causing the problems. Treatment involves reducing exposure to the building or improving building ventilation and conditions. Depending on the illness, recovery may require a prolonged period of time.

Byssinosis

Byssinosis is a narrowing of the airways caused by inhaling cotton, flax, or hemp particles.

- Byssinosis may cause wheezing and tightness in the chest, usually on the first day of work after a break.
- The diagnosis is made by using a test that shows decreasing lung capacity over the course of a workday.
- Exposure should be stopped, then wheezing and chest tightness can be treated with drugs used for asthma.

In the United States and Great Britain, byssinosis occurs almost exclusively in people who work with unprocessed cotton. People who work with flax and hemp may also develop the condition. People who open bales of raw cotton or who work in the first stages of cotton processing seem to be most affected. Apparently, something in the raw cotton causes the airways of susceptible people to narrow. Variations of this condition may occur in people exposed to grain dusts in agricultural environments (grain worker's lung).

Symptoms and Diagnosis

Byssinosis may cause wheezing and tightness in the chest, usually on the first day of work after a break. Unlike with asthma, the symptoms tend to diminish after repeated exposure, and the chest tightness may disappear by the end of the workweek. However, after a person has worked with cotton for many years, the chest tightness may last for 2 or 3 workdays or even the whole week. Prolonged

exposure to cotton dust increases the frequency of symptoms (wheezing, chest tightness) and leads to permanent lung disease, which can sometimes be disabling.

The diagnosis is made by using pulmonary function tests that show decreasing lung capacity over the course of a workday. Usually, the decrease in lung capacity is greatest on the first day of the workweek.

Prevention and Treatment

Controlling dust is the best way to prevent byssinosis. Workers with symptoms who also experience sudden drops in lung function on the first day of the workweek should be removed from exposure. Wheezing and chest tightness can be treated with the drugs used for asthma. Drugs that open the airways (bronchodilators) may be given.

Coal Workers' Pneumoconiosis

Coal workers' pneumoconiosis (black lung) is a lung disease caused by deposits of coal dust in the lungs.

- People generally have no symptoms, but people who have severe disease cough and become short of breath.
- Chest x-rays and computed tomography are used to make the diagnosis.
- Prevention by minimizing exposure is important.
- People may need to take drugs to keep the airways open and free of mucus.

Coal workers' pneumoconiosis results from inhaling coal dust or graphite over a long time. Although coal dust is relatively inert and does not provoke much reaction, it spreads throughout the lungs and shows up as tiny spots on an x-ray. Coal dust may block the airways. In simple coal workers' pneumoconiosis, coal dust collects around the small airways (bronchioles) of the lungs. Every year, 1 to 2% of people with simple coal workers' pneumoconiosis develop a more serious form of the disease called progressive massive fibrosis, in which large scars (at least 1/2 inch [about 1.3 centimeters] in diameter) develop in the lungs as a reaction to the dust. Progressive massive fibrosis may worsen even after exposure to coal dust stops. Lung tissue and the blood vessels in the lungs can be destroyed by the scarring.

In Caplan's syndrome, a rare disorder that can affect coal miners who also have rheumatoid arthritis, large round nodules of scarring develop quickly in the lung. Such nodules may form in people who have had significant exposure to coal dust, even if they do not have coal workers' pneumoconiosis.

Symptoms and Diagnosis

Simple coal workers' pneumoconiosis usually does not cause symptoms. However, many people with this disease cough and easily become short of breath because they also have an airway disease, such as bronchitis or emphysema. These disorders are more likely to occur in smokers, so smokers with coal workers' pneumoconiosis are more likely to have symptoms. The severe stages of progressive massive fibrosis, on the other hand, cause coughing and often disabling shortness of breath.

Doctors make the diagnosis after noting characteristic spots on a chest x-ray or computed tomography (CT) scan of a person who has been exposed to coal dust for a long time—usually someone who has worked in a coal mine for at least 10 years.

Prevention and Treatment

Prevention is crucial because there is no cure for coal workers' pneumoconiosis. The disorder can be prevented by adequately suppressing coal dust at a work site. Ventilation systems may help. Face pieces (masks) that filter and purify the air may provide some additional benefit, but the protection is limited.

Doctors usually recommend that coal workers have chest x-rays every year, so that the disease can be detected at a relatively early stage. If the disease is detected, the worker should be transferred to an area where coal dust levels are low to help prevent progressive massive fibrosis. Coal workers who smoke are encouraged to stop. Workers may be given the pneumococcal vaccine and an annual influenza vaccination to help protect against infections to which workers may be more vulnerable.

A person who is short of breath may benefit from drugs to keep the airways open and free of mucus (bronchodilators—see page 482).

Gas and Chemical Exposure

- Symptoms depend on which gas or chemical is inhaled and how deeply and for how long it was inhaled.
- Symptoms may include irritation of the eyes or nose, cough, blood in the sputum, and shortness of breath.
- Chest x-rays, computed tomography, and breathing tests are used to determine how much lung damage has occurred.
- Oxygen and drugs to open the airways and decrease inflammation are given.

Many types of gases—such as chlorine, phosgene, sulfur dioxide, hydrogen sulfide, nitrogen dioxide, and ammonia—may suddenly be released during industrial accidents and may severely irritate the lungs. Gases such as chlorine and ammonia easily dissolve and immediately irritate the mouth, nose, and throat. The more peripheral parts of the lungs are affected only when the gas is inhaled deeply. Radioactive gases, which may be released in a nuclear reactor accident, may cause lung and other cancers many years after the exposure.

Some gases—for instance, nitrogen dioxide—do not dissolve easily. Therefore, they do not produce early warning signs of exposure, such as irritation of the nose and eyes, and they are more likely to be inhaled deeply into the lungs. Such gases can cause inflammation of the small airways (bronchiolitis) or lead to fluid accumulation in the lungs (pulmonary edema).

Silo filler's disease (which mostly affects farmers) results from inhaling fumes that contain nitrogen dioxide given off by moist silage. Fluid may develop in the lungs as late as 12 hours after exposure. The condition may temporarily improve and then recur 10 to 14 days later, even without further contact with the gas. A recurrence tends to affect the small airways (bronchioles).

Inhalation of some gases and chemicals may also trigger an allergic response that leads to inflammation and, in some cases, scarring in and around the tiny air sacs (alveoli) and bronchioles of the lung. This condition is called hypersensitivity pneumonitis (see page 514).

In some people, inhalation of small amounts of gas or other chemicals over a long period may result in chronic bronchitis. Also, inhalation of some chemicals, such as arsenic compounds and hydrocarbons, can cause cancer. Cancer may develop in the lungs or elsewhere in the body, depending on the substance inhaled.

Symptoms and Diagnosis

Soluble gases such as chlorine, ammonia, and hydrofluoric acid cause severe burning in the eyes, nose, throat, windpipe, and large airways within minutes of exposure to them. In addition, they often produce a cough and blood in the sputum (hemoptysis). Retching and shortness of breath also are common. Less soluble gases such as nitrogen dioxide and ozone produce shortness of breath, which may be severe, after a delay of 3 to 4 hours and sometimes up to 12 hours after exposure. Chronic wheezing and shortness of breath can occur with long-term lung damage.

A chest x-ray can show whether pulmonary edema or bronchiolitis has developed. Computed tomography is especially helpful when people have symptoms but their chest x-ray looks normal.

Prognosis, Prevention, and Treatment

Most people recover completely from accidental exposure to gases. The most serious complications are lung infection or severe damage with scarring of the small airways (bronchiolitis obliterans). Some studies have shown long-term impairment of the lung function years after episodes of exposure to gases.

The best way to prevent exposure is to use extreme care when handling gases and chemicals. Gas masks with their own air supply should be available in case of accidental spillage. Farmers need to know that accidental exposure to toxic gases in silos is dangerous, even fatal.

Oxygen is the mainstay of treatment for people who are exposed to gases. If lung damage is severe, a person may need mechanical ventilation (see page 525). Drugs that open the airways (bronchodilators), intravenous fluids, and antibiotics may be helpful. Corticosteroids such as prednisone are often prescribed to reduce inflammation in the lungs.

Occupational Asthma

Occupational asthma is a reversible narrowing of the airways caused by inhaling work-related particles or vapors that act as irritants or cause an allergic reaction.

- Occupational asthma may cause shortness of breath, tightness in the chest, wheezing, and coughing.
- People are tested for allergies to substances known to cause asthma.
- Treatment involves drugs to open the airways and reduce inflammation.

Many substances in the workplace can cause narrowing of the airways, which makes breathing difficult. Some people are particularly sensitive to airborne allergens, some develop disease from very high exposures to airborne irritants even if they do not have an allergy, and some develop building-related illness (see page 500). Examples of workers at risk for occupational asthma from exposure to allergens include animal handlers and bakers.

Occupational asthma is different from occupationally aggravated asthma in which people who have a history of asthma have an increase in their symptoms while they are at work because they are exposed to a substance that triggers an asthma attack.

Symptoms

Occupational asthma may cause shortness of breath, tightness in the chest, wheezing, and coughing. Sometimes people show signs of allergy to dust at work, with symptoms of sneezing, runny nose, and watery eyes. For some people, wheezing at night is the only symptom. Symptoms may develop during work hours but often do not start until a few hours after work. In some people, symptoms begin as much as 24 hours after exposure. Also, symptoms may come and go for a week or more after exposure. Commonly, people who have daytime exposures start having symptoms at nighttime. Thus, the link between the workplace and the symptoms is often obscured. Symptoms often become milder or disappear on weekends or over holidays. They worsen with repeated exposure.

Diagnosis

To make a diagnosis, doctors ask about the symptoms and about exposure to any substances known to cause asthma. Occasionally, the allergic reaction can be detected with a skin test (patch test), in which a small amount of a substance that is suspected of causing a reaction is placed on the skin. When making the diagnosis is more difficult, doctors in specialized centers use an inhalation challenge test, in which the person inhales small amounts of the substance being tested and is observed for wheezing and shortness of breath and tested for decreased lung function.

Because the airways may begin to narrow before symptoms appear, a person with delayed symptoms may use a device to monitor the airways while at work. This device, a portable peak flow meter, measures the speed at which a person can blow air out of the lungs. When the airways narrow, the rate slows significantly, suggesting occupational asthma.

Prevention and Treatment

Industries using substances that can cause asthma must have dust and vapor control measures, but sometimes eliminating the dusts and vapors may be impossible. Workers with occupational asthma should change jobs, if possible. Continued exposure often leads to more severe and persistent asthma.

Treatments are the same as for other types of asthma (see page 475). Drugs that open the airways (bronchodilators) may be given, preferably in an inhaler (for example, albuterol). Drugs that reduce inflammation may be given, either in an inhaler (for example, the corticosteroid triamcinolone) or as a tablet (for example, montelukast). For severe attacks, corticosteroids such as prednisone may be taken by mouth for a short time. For long-term management, inhaled corticosteroids are preferred.

Silicosis

Silicosis is permanent scarring of the lungs caused by inhaling silica (quartz) dust.

- People develop difficulty breathing during exercise that sometimes progresses to shortness of breath even at rest, and some people also have a cough that may or may not produce sputum.
- Diagnosis is made with a chest x-ray or computed tomography.
- Doctors can sometimes give drugs to help keep airways clear.

Silicosis is the oldest known environmental lung disease. It is caused by inhalation of tiny particles of silica (usually quartz) or, less commonly, by inhalation of silicates, such as talc. Workers at greatest risk are those who move or blast rock and sand (miners, quarry workers, stonecutters) or who use silica-containing rock or sand abrasives (sand blasters; glass makers; foundry, gemstone, and ceramic workers; potters). Coal miners are at risk of mixed silicosis and coal workers' pneumoconiosis (see page 501).

Chronic silicosis is the most common form and generally develops only after exposure over decades. Accelerated silicosis, which is rare, and acute silicosis may develop after more intense exposures over several years or months. Silica is also a cause of lung cancer.

When inhaled, silica dust passes into the lungs, and scavenger cells such as macrophages engulf it (see table on page 1097). Enzymes released by the scavenger cells cause the lung tissue to scar. At first, the scarred areas are tiny round lumps (simple chronic silicosis), but eventually they may combine into larger masses (complicated chronic silicosis). These scarred areas cannot transfer oxygen into the blood normally. The lungs become less flexible, and breathing takes more effort.

Symptoms

People who have chronic silicosis often do not have symptoms for years, but many people eventually develop difficulty breathing during exercise that sometimes progresses to shortness of breath even at rest. Some people have a cough that may produce sputum. Breathing may worsen for years after the person stops working with silica. The lung damage can lead to lower levels of oxygen in the blood and can also strain the right side of the heart. This strain can lead to a type of heart failure called cor pulmonale (see box on page 523), which can be fatal. People with accelerated silicosis experience the same symptoms as people with chronic silicosis, but symptoms develop and worsen over a shorter period.

In acute silicosis, shortness of breath worsens rapidly. People also lose weight and have fatigue. Respiratory failure often develops within 2 years.

People with silicosis are many times more likely to develop tuberculosis when exposed to the organism that causes it than are people without silicosis.

Diagnosis

Diagnosis is made when someone who has worked with silica has a chest x-ray that shows distinctive patterns consistent with the disease. When x-ray findings are unclear, samples of lung tissue can help confirm the diagnosis. Additional tests, including computed tomography (CT), are done to distinguish silicosis from other disorders.

Prevention

Controlling silica dust in the workplace is key to preventing silicosis. When dust cannot be controlled, as may be true in the sandblasting industry, workers should wear protective gear, such as hoods that supply clean external air or special masks that efficiently filter out tiny particles. Such protection may not be available to all people working in a dusty area (for example, painters and welders), so whenever possible abrasives other than sand should be used.

Workers exposed to silica dust should have regular chest x-rays so that problems can be detected early. Workers who smoke should be encouraged to stop. Other preventive measures include pneumococcal vaccine and an annual influenza vaccination to help protect against infections to which workers may be more vulnerable.

Treatment

Silicosis cannot be cured, but its progression can be slowed if exposure to silica is avoided, especially at an early stage of the disease. A whole lung lavage (washing) can be used to treat the acute form of silicosis. During this procedure, doctors fill the lung with a salt (saline) solution and then drain it to clear material from the air spaces. Some people with acute or accelerated silicosis benefit from taking corticosteroids. People who have difficulty breathing may benefit from drugs to keep the airways open and free of mucus (bronchodilators—see page 482). Lung transplantation is a last resort. Because people with silicosis have a high risk of developing tuberculosis, they should have regular checkups that include a tuberculosis skin test.

People should be monitored and treated for low oxygen levels in the blood. Pulmonary rehabilitation may help people carry out activities of daily living.

83 Interstitial Lung Diseases

Interstitial lung disease (also called diffuse parenchymal or infiltrative lung disease) is a term used to describe a number of different disorders that affect the interstitial space. The interstitial space consists of the air sacs of the lungs (alveoli), the walls of alveoli, and the spaces around blood vessels and small airways. Interstitial lung diseases result in abnormal accumulation of inflammatory cells in lung tissue, cause shortness of breath and cough, and have similarities in their appearances on imaging studies but are otherwise unrelated. Some of these diseases are very unusual.

Early in the course of these diseases, white blood cells, macrophages, and protein-rich fluid accumulate in the interstitial space, causing inflammation.

If the inflammation persists, scarring (fibrosis) may replace the normal lung tissue. As alveoli are progressively destroyed, thick-walled cysts (called honeycombing because they resemble the cells of a beehive) are left in their place. The condition resulting from these changes is called pulmonary fibrosis.

Although the various interstitial lung diseases are separate and have different causes, they have some similar features. All lead to a decreased ability to transfer oxygen to the blood, and all cause stiffening and shrinkage of the lungs, which makes breathing difficult and causes cough. However, the elimination of carbon dioxide from the blood is usually not a problem.

UNUSUAL INTERSTITIAL LUNG DISEASES

DISORDER	SYMPTOMS	TREATMENT	COMMENTS
Drug-induced interstitial lung disease	Slow-developing (over weeks to months) or sudden, severe symptoms Shortness of breath Cough	Stopping the drug that is causing symptoms Corticosteroids (sometimes effective)	Many classes of drugs may cause this disease. The disease is often more severe in older people. The effects of some drugs on the lung are similar to those of systemic lupus erythematosus (lupus). The extent and severity of the disease are sometimes related to how large the drug dose was and how long the drug was taken.
Alveolar hemorrhage syndromes (iron in the lungs)	Most commonly, coughing up blood (hemoptysis) Anemia due to chronic blood loss Kidney failure (sometimes)	Corticosteroids and cytotoxic drugs (such as azathioprine) during flare-ups Blood transfusions if needed because of blood loss Oxygen therapy for a low level of oxygen in the blood	In this rare disorder, blood leaks from the capillaries into the lungs for unknown reasons. People may also have Goodpasture's syndrome, Wegener's granulomatosis, systemic lupus erythematosus, idiopathic pulmonary hemosiderosis, or drug reactions. Massive bleeding can cause death.
Lymphangiomyomatosis	Difficulty breathing Cough Chest pain Sometimes coughing up blood	Lung transplantation	This rare disorder occurs in young women. It may worsen during pregnancy.

CAUSES OF INTERSTITIAL LUNG DISEASES

TYPE	EXAMPLES
Autoimmune disorders	Ankylosing spondylitis, Behçet's syndrome, Goodpasture's syndrome, mixed connective tissue disease, polymyositis and dermatomyositis, relapsing polychondritis, rheumatoid arthritis, scleroderma, Sjögren's syndrome, and systemic lupus erythematosus (lupus)
Infections	Fungal, mycoplasmal (a type of bacterial), parasitic, rickettsial, or viral infections and tuberculosis
Organic dust	Bird droppings and molds
Drugs	Amiodarone, bleomycin, busulfan, carbamazepine, chlorambucil, cocaine, cyclophosphamide, gold, methotrexate, nitrofurantoin, sulfasalazine, and sulfonamides
Gases, fumes, and vapors	Chlorine and sulfur dioxide
Therapeutic or industrial radiation	Radiation therapy for cancer
Idiopathic* interstitial pneumonias	Acute interstitial pneumonia, cryptogenic organizing pneumonia, desquamative interstitial pneumonia, idiopathic pulmonary fibrosis, lymphoid interstitial pneumonia, nonspecific interstitial pneumonia, and respiratory bronchiolitis-associated interstitial lung disease
Other disorders	Alveolar proteinosis, amyloidosis, chronic gastric microaspiration, lymphangiomyomatosis, neurofibromatosis, pulmonary Langerhans' cell granulomatosis (histiocytosis), sarcoidosis, and vasculitic disorders (which cause inflammation of blood vessels) such as Churg-Strauss syndrome and Wegener's granulomatosis

* Idiopathic means with no known cause.

Diagnosis

Because interstitial lung diseases cause symptoms that are similar to those of much more common disorders (for example, pneumonia, chronic obstructive pulmonary disease), they may not be suspected at first. When interstitial lung disease is suspected, diagnostic testing is done. Testing can vary by the disease suspected but tends to be similar. Most people have a chest x-ray, computed tomography (CT), pulmonary function tests (see page 454), and often arterial blood gas analysis. CT is more sensitive than chest x-ray and helps doctors make a more specific diagnosis. CT is done using techniques that maximize resolution (high-resolution CT). Pulmonary function tests often show that the volume of air that the lungs can hold is abnormally small. In addition, the person's response to exercise is commonly tested.

To confirm the diagnosis, doctors may remove a small sample of lung tissue for microscopic examination (lung biopsy) using a procedure called fiberoptic bronchoscopy. A lung biopsy done this way is called transbronchial lung biopsy (see page 457). Many times, a larger tissue sample is needed and must be removed surgically, sometimes with use of a thoracoscope (a procedure called video-assisted thoracoscopic lung biopsy.

Blood tests are usually done. They usually cannot confirm the diagnosis but are done as part of the search for other, similar disorders. Doctors may also order electrocardiography (ECG) or echocardiography to determine whether the heart has been affected by the lung disease.

Idiopathic Interstitial Pneumonias

Idiopathic interstitial pneumonias are interstitial lung diseases that have no known cause and that affect the lungs similarly.

- Some types of these pneumonias are much more serious than others.
- Diagnosis requires chest x-rays, computed tomography, and usually analysis of a sample of lung tissue (biopsy).

The word *idiopathic* means of unknown cause, so when the cause of interstitial lung disease is not

COMPARING TYPES OF IDIOPATHIC INTERSTITIAL PNEUMONIAS

DISORDER	PEOPLE MOST OFTEN AFFECTED	PERCENTAGE OF AFFECTED PEOPLE WHO SMOKE CIGARETTES	TREATMENT	OUTLOOK
Idiopathic pulmonary fibrosis	Men over 60	More than 60%	Possibly lung transplantation (most other treatments appear ineffective)	50–70% die in 5 years
Nonspecific interstitial pneumonia	Women aged 40–60	Fewer than 40%	Corticosteroids	Fewer than 10% die in 5 years
Cryptogenic organizing pneumonia	People aged 40–50	Fewer than 50%	Corticosteroids	Two thirds completely recover, but the disorder recurs in many Death is rare
Desquamative interstitial pneumonia	Men aged 40–50	More than 90%	Smoking cessation Corticosteroids	5% die in 5 years
Respiratory bronchiolitis–associated interstitial lung disease	People aged 40–50 (slightly more men)	More than 90%	Smoking cessation Corticosteroids	Death is rare
Acute interstitial pneumonia	People of any age	Unknown	Best treatment unknown	60% die in less than 6 months

identified, idiopathic interstitial pneumonia is diagnosed. Pneumonias are often thought of as infections, but these diseases do not appear to result from infection.

There are six types of idiopathic interstitial pneumonias. In decreasing order of frequency, they are

- Idiopathic pulmonary fibrosis
- Nonspecific interstitial pneumonia
- Cryptogenic organizing pneumonia
- Respiratory bronchiolitis-associated interstitial lung disease
- Desquamative interstitial pneumonia
- Acute interstitial pneumonia

Some experts also consider lymphoid interstitial pneumonia to be a type of idiopathic interstitial pneumonia.

All types cause shortness of breath and affect the lungs similarly. However, they differ in how quickly they develop, how they are treated, and how serious they are. For example, most diseases take weeks to months to develop, but idiopathic pulmonary fibrosis takes more than 12 months to fully develop. Acute interstitial pneumonia takes only 1 to 2 weeks.

Diagnosis

Chest x-rays, pulmonary function tests (see page 454), and computed tomography (CT) are done. CT may be diagnostic. If not, doctors remove a small sample of lung tissue for examination under a microscope (lung biopsy). Usually, biopsy is done surgically with use of a thoracoscope (see page 457).

Blood tests are usually done. They usually cannot confirm the diagnosis but are done as part of the search for other, similar disorders. Doctors may also order an electrocardiogram (ECG) or echocardiogram to determine whether the heart has been affected by the lung disease.

IDIOPATHIC PULMONARY FIBROSIS

Idiopathic pulmonary fibrosis is the most common form of idiopathic interstitial pneumonia.

- Idiopathic pulmonary fibrosis affects mostly people in their 50s and 60s, usually men and usually smokers.
- People may cough, lose weight, have difficulty breathing, and feel tired.
- Lung transplantation may be the only effective treatment.

The lungs suffer progressive injury for a long period of time. The injury causes chronic inflammation that eventually leads to lung scarring (fibrosis).

Symptoms

Symptoms depend on the extent of the lung damage, the rate at which the disease progresses, and whether complications, such as lung infections and right-sided heart failure (cor pulmonale—see box on page 523) develop. The main symptoms start insidiously as shortness of breath on exertion, cough, and diminished stamina. Other common complaints include weight loss and fatigue. In most people, symptoms worsen over a period ranging from about 6 months to several years.

As the disease progresses, the level of oxygen in the blood decreases, and the skin may take on a bluish tinge (called cyanosis) and the ends of the fingers may become thick or club-shaped (see art on page 453). Strain on the heart may cause the right ventricle to enlarge, eventually resulting in right-sided heart failure. Through a stethoscope, doctors often hear crackling sounds. These sounds are called Velcro crackles, described as such because the sound is similar to that of Velcro when it is pulled apart.

Diagnosis

A chest x-ray may show widespread tiny white lines, often in a netlike pattern, most profuse in the lower parts of both lungs. Computed tomography (CT) typically shows a pattern of patchy, white lines in the lower lungs. In areas of more severe involvement, the thick scarring often creates a honeycombing appearance. Pulmonary function tests (see page 454) show that the amount of air the lungs can hold is below normal. Analysis of a blood sample or use of an oximeter (see page 455) shows a low level of oxygen with minimal exercise (walking at a normal pace) and, as the disease progresses, even when the person is resting.

To confirm the diagnosis, doctors may do a lung biopsy by using a procedure called bronchoscopy (see page 456). Many times, a larger tissue sample is needed and must be removed surgically, sometimes with use of a thoracoscope (see page 457).

Blood tests cannot confirm the diagnosis but are done as part of the search for other disorders that may cause a similar pattern of inflammation and scarring. For example, doctors do blood tests to screen for certain autoimmune disorders.

Prognosis and Treatment

Most people continue to get worse. On average, people live less than 3 years after diagnosis. A few people survive for more than 5 years after diagnosis. A few die within several months.

If a chest x-ray or lung biopsy shows that scarring is not extensive, the usual treatment is a corticosteroid (such as prednisone), with or without azathioprine, N-acetylcysteine, or both. Doctors evaluate the person's response using chest x-rays, CT, and pulmonary function tests. High doses of prednisone are usually given for about 3 months, and then the dose is gradually reduced over another 3 months. Much lower doses are then continued for 6 more months. However, this combination treatment fails to help most people. Promising treatments that appear to decrease lung fibrosis and prolong survival include pirfenidone and bosentan.

Other treatments are aimed at relieving symptoms: pulmonary rehabilitation for improving ability to carry out activities of daily life (see page 459), oxygen therapy for low blood oxygen levels, antibiotics for infection, and drugs for the heart failure that is produced by cor pulmonale. Lung transplantation (often with a single lung) has been successful in some people with severe idiopathic pulmonary fibrosis.

RESPIRATORY BRONCHIOLITIS–ASSOCIATED INTERSTITIAL LUNG DISEASE AND DESQUAMATIVE INTERSTITIAL PNEUMONIA

Respiratory bronchiolitis-associated interstitial lung disease and desquamative interstitial pneumonia are rare conditions that cause chronic lung inflammation and occur mostly in current or former cigarette smokers.

These conditions have many similarities, so that some experts think they may be part of the same disorder. However, desquamative interstitial pneumonia is often more severe. Both disorders affect cigarette smokers in their 30s and 40s, with most people developing shortness of breath with even minimal exertion. Men are affected more often than women (ratio of almost 2:1).

A chest x-ray shows less severe changes than in idiopathic pulmonary fibrosis and may show no changes in up to 20% of people. Pulmonary function tests show a decline in the amount of air contained in the lungs. The amount of oxygen in a blood sample is low.

A lung biopsy is often needed to confirm the diagnosis.

About 70% of people who have respiratory bronchiolitis-associated interstitial lung disease or desquamative interstitial pneumonia survive for 10 years or longer. The response is even better when people stop smoking.

Some doctors give corticosteroids because they may be effective in other interstitial lung diseases, but the effectiveness is unknown.

CRYPTOGENIC ORGANIZING PNEUMONIA

Cryptogenic organizing pneumonia (also called bronchiolitis obliterans organizing pneumonia) is a rapidly developing idiopathic interstitial pneumonia characterized by lung inflammation and scarring that obstructs the small airways and air sacs of the lungs (alveoli).

The disease usually begins between the ages of 40 and 60 and affects men and women equally. Cigarette smoking does not appear to increase the risk of developing the disease.

Almost 75% of people have symptoms for less than 2 months before seeking medical attention. A flu-like illness, with a cough, fever, a feeling of illness (malaise), fatigue, and weight loss, heralds the onset in about 50% of people.

Diagnosis and Treatment

Doctors do not find any specific abnormalities on routine laboratory tests or on a physical examination, except for the frequent presence of crackling sounds (called Velcro crackles) when the doctor listens with a stethoscope. Pulmonary function tests usually show that the amount of air the lungs can hold is below normal. The amount of oxygen in the blood is often low at rest and is even lower with exercise.

The chest x-ray is distinctive with features that appear similar to an extensive pneumonia, with both lungs showing widespread white patches. The white patches may seem to migrate from one area of the lung to another as the disease persists or progresses. Computed tomography (CT) may be used and sometimes confirms the diagnosis. Often, the findings are typical enough to allow doctors to make a diagnosis without ordering additional tests.

In other cases, to confirm the diagnosis, doctors do a lung biopsy using a bronchoscope (see page 456). Many times, a larger sample is needed and must be removed surgically.

When treated with corticosteroids, about two thirds of people recover. However, symptoms may later return. If so, repeat treatment with corticosteroids is usually effective.

NONSPECIFIC INTERSTITIAL PNEUMONIA

Nonspecific interstitial pneumonia is an idiopathic interstitial pneumonia that occurs mainly in women, people who do not smoke, and people younger than 50 years.

Nonspecific interstitial pneumonia seems to be the second most common kind of idiopathic interstitial pneumonia. Most people are between the ages of 40 and 50. Most people have no known cause or

risk factor. However, a similar process can develop in people with connective tissue disorders (in particular, systemic sclerosis and polymyositis or dermatomyositis), in some forms of drug-induced lung injury, and in people with hypersensitivity pneumonitis (see page 514).

A dry cough and shortness of breath develop over 6 to 18 months. Low-grade fever and a feeling of illness (malaise) may occur, but high fever, weight loss, and other general symptoms of illness are unusual.

Diagnosis and Treatment

As with other idiopathic interstitial pneumonias, chest x-rays are done, and CT is usually also done. Pulmonary function tests usually show that the amount of air the lungs can hold is below normal. The amount of oxygen in the blood is often low at rest and is even lower with exercise. Doctors often do bronchoscopy (see page 456) and wash segments of the lung with a salt-water solution and then collect the washings (bronchoalveolar lavage) for testing. More than half of people have more lymphocytes (a type of white blood cell) than normal in the washings. Lung biopsy is often necessary.

Corticosteroids are usually effective. More than 80% of people survive for more than 10 years after being diagnosed.

ACUTE INTERSTITIAL PNEUMONIA

Acute interstitial pneumonia (also called accelerated interstitial pneumonia or Hamman-Rich syndrome) is an idiopathic interstitial pneumonia that develops suddenly and is severe.

Acute interstitial pneumonia causes the same type of symptoms as the acute respiratory distress syndrome (see page 525). It tends to affect healthy men and women who are usually older than 40. Fever, cough, and difficulty breathing develop over 1 to 2 weeks, typically progressing to acute respiratory failure.

When possible, the diagnosis is confirmed with CT, lung biopsy, and pulmonary function tests.

Treatment aims to keep the person alive until the disorder resolves. Mechanical ventilation is needed if there is respiratory failure. Corticosteroids are generally used, but it is not clear whether they are effective.

More than 60% of affected people die within 6 months, usually from respiratory failure. In people who survive, lung function usually improves with time. However, the disease may recur.

Pulmonary Langerhans' Cell Granulomatosis

Pulmonary Langerhans' cell granulomatosis (histiocytosis or eosinophilic granuloma) is a disorder in which cells called histiocytes and eosinophils proliferate in the lung, often causing scarring.

- People may have no symptoms or may cough and have difficulty breathing.
- Diagnosis requires computed tomography and sometimes analysis of a sample of lung tissue (biopsy).
- Whether and which treatments help are unknown.

Pulmonary Langerhans' cell granulomatosis (histiocytosis) is one form of Langerhans' cell granulomatosis, which can affect other organs (such as the pituitary gland and the white blood cells) as well as the lungs. The cause is unknown, and the disorder is rare. It occurs almost exclusively in whites aged 20 to 40 who smoke cigarettes. It starts with infiltration of the lung by histiocytes, which are cells that scavenge for foreign materials, and to a lesser extent by eosinophils, which are cells that are normally involved in allergic reactions.

Symptoms

About 15% of people have no symptoms and the disorder is first recognized when an imaging study of the chest is done for another reason. The remainder develop coughing, shortness of breath, fever, chest pain, fatigue, and weight loss. Pneumothorax is a common complication due to rupture of a lung cyst. It occurs in 15 to 25% of people with the disorder and may be the cause of the first symptoms that develop. Scarring makes the lungs stiff and impairs their ability to transfer oxygen into and out of the blood. A few people cough up blood (hemoptysis).

Some people have localized bone pain or a pathologic bone fracture (a fracture that occurs with only a minor injury because the bone has been thinned by a disorder). Diabetes insipidus occurs in about 15% of people. This condition results when histiocytes also affect the hypothalamus in the brain. The person makes excessive amounts of urine that is dilute. People with diabetes insipidus probably have a worse prognosis than those who do not.

Diagnosis

Chest x-rays show nodules, small lung cysts (honeycombing), and other changes that are typical of this disorder. Computed tomography (CT) may show these changes in enough detail to establish the diagnosis. X-rays may also show that the bones are affected. Pulmonary function tests show that the amount of air the lungs can hold is below normal. If CT is not diagnostic, biopsy is required. Biopsy can usually be done during bronchoscopy (see page 456).

Prognosis and Treatment

Half of people are alive more than 12 years after diagnosis. Death usually results from respiratory failure or cor pulmonale (see box on page 523). When people stop smoking, improvement occurs in about one third of cases.

The disorder may be treated with corticosteroids and immunosuppressants such as cyclophosphamide, although no therapy is clearly beneficial.

Lymphoid Interstitial Pneumonia

Lymphoid interstitial pneumonia is an uncommon lung disease in which mature lymphocytes (a type of white blood cell) accumulate in the alveoli.

- People usually have cough and difficulty breathing.
- Diagnosis requires chest x-ray, computed tomography, pulmonary function tests, and often bronchoscopy.
- Treatment involves corticosteroids, immunosuppressants, or both.

Lymphoid interstitial pneumonia can occur in children, usually those infected with the human immunodeficiency virus (HIV). Lymphoid interstitial pneumonia can also occur in adults, often those with autoimmune disorders such as plasma cell disorders, Sjögren's syndrome (see page 577), Hashimoto's thyroiditis, rheumatoid arthritis, and systemic lupus erythematosus (lupus). Average age of affected adults is 54.

Symptoms

Children develop wheezing, cough, and difficulty breathing, and they may not grow and gain weight. Adults develop difficulty breathing and cough over months or, in some cases, years. Less common symptoms include weight loss, fever, joint pain, and night sweats.

Diagnosis

Doctors can sometimes hear crackles in the lungs using a stethoscope.

Diagnosis requires chest x-ray, computed tomography (CT), and pulmonary function tests. Pulmonary function tests usually show a decrease in the amount of air the lungs can hold. Doctors often do bronchoscopy (see page 456) and wash segments of the lung with a salt-water solution and then collect the washings (bronchoalveolar lavage) for testing. Children may have abnormalities in their blood proteins that can help establish the diagnosis. If not, and for all adults, lung biopsy is usually necessary.

Prognosis and Treatment

The prognosis is difficult to predict. The disorder may resolve on its own or after treatment, or it may progress to lung fibrosis or lymphoma (a cancer). One half to two thirds of people are alive 5 years after diagnosis.

Treatment is with corticosteroids, other immuno-suppressants, or both, but the effectiveness of these drugs is unknown.

Sarcoidosis

Sarcoidosis is a disease in which abnormal collections of inflammatory cells (granulomas) form in many organs of the body.

- Sarcoidosis usually develops in people aged 20 to 40, most often people of Scandinavian ancestry and American blacks.
- It can affect many organs, most commonly the lungs.
- People cough and have difficulty breathing but can have various symptoms depending on which organs are affected.
- Diagnosis usually requires chest x-ray, computed tomography, and analysis of a sample of tissue (biopsy), usually from the lungs.
- Symptoms eventually subside without treatment in most people.
- Treatment, when necessary, begins with corticosteroids.

The cause of sarcoidosis is unknown. It may result from an infection or from an abnormal response of the immune system. Inherited factors may be important. Sarcoidosis typically develops between the ages of 20 and 40. It is most common among people of Scandinavian ancestry and American blacks, although it can occur in anyone.

Sarcoidosis is characterized by the presence of collections of inflammatory cells (granulomas). The disease is primarily one of the lungs, but granulomas can also form in the lymph nodes, lungs, liver, eyes, and skin, and less often in the spleen, bones, joints, sinuses, skeletal muscles, kidneys, heart, reproductive organs, salivary glands, and nervous system. The granulomas may eventually disappear completely or become scar tissue.

Symptoms

Many people with sarcoidosis have no symptoms, and the disorder is discovered on a chest x-ray that is taken for other reasons. Most people develop minor symptoms that do not progress. Serious symptoms are rare.

The symptoms of sarcoidosis vary greatly according to the site and extent of the disease.

General: Fever, fatigue, vague chest pain, a feeling of illness (malaise), weight loss, and aching joints may be the first indications of a problem in about one third of people. Enlarged lymph nodes are common but do not often cause symptoms. Fever and night sweats may recur throughout the illness.

Lungs: The organ most affected by sarcoidosis is the lung. Enlarged lymph nodes at the place where the lungs meet the heart or to the right of the windpipe (trachea) may be seen on a chest x-ray. Sarcoidosis produces inflammation in the lungs that may eventually lead to scarring and the formation of cysts, which can cause coughing and shortness of breath. Fortunately, such progressive scarring occurs infrequently. Occasionally, the fungus *Aspergillus* can settle in (colonize) the lung cysts, grow, and cause bleeding. Breathing can become difficult, and sometimes the person may cough blood. Severe involvement of the lung by sarcoidosis can eventually strain the right side of the heart, causing right-sided heart failure (cor pulmonale—see box on page 523).

Skin: The skin is frequently affected by sarcoidosis. In people of Scandinavian ancestry, sarcoidosis often starts as raised, tender, red lumps, usually on the shins (erythema nodosum—see page 1292), accompanied by a fever and joint pain. This set of symptoms is less common in American blacks. Prolonged sarcoidosis may lead to the formation of flat patches (plaques), raised patches, or lumps just under the skin with discoloration of the nose, cheeks, lips, and ears (lupus pernio). Lupus pernio is most common in black women.

Liver and Spleen: About 70% of people with sarcoidosis have granulomas in their liver. These granulomas often produce no symptoms, and the liver seems to function normally. Fewer than 10% of people with sarcoidosis have an enlarged liver. Jaundice caused by liver malfunction is rare. The spleen also is enlarged in some people.

Eyes: The eyes are affected in 15% of people with sarcoidosis. Inflammation of certain internal eye structures (uveitis) makes the eyes red and painful and interferes with vision. Inflammation that persists for a long time may block fluid from draining from the eye, causing glaucoma (see page 1448), which can lead to blindness. Granulomas may form in the conjunctiva (the membrane over the eyeball and inside the eyelids). Such granulomas often do not cause symptoms, but the conjunctiva is an accessible site from which doctors can take tissue samples for examination. Some people with sarcoidosis complain of dry, sore, and red eyes, probably because sluggish tear glands that have been affected by the disorder no longer produce enough tears to keep the eyes lubricated.

Heart: Granulomas that form in the heart may cause chest pain (angina) or heart failure. Granulomas that form near the heart's electrical conducting system can trigger potentially fatal irregularities in the heartbeat.

Joints and Bones: Inflammation can cause widespread pain in the joints. The joints in the hands and feet are most commonly affected. Cysts form in the bones and can make nearby joints swollen and tender.

Nervous System: Sarcoidosis can affect the cranial nerves (nerves of the head), causing double vision and making one side of the face droop. If the pituitary gland or the bones surrounding it are affected, diabetes insipidus (see page 986) may result. The pituitary gland stops producing vasopressin, a hormone needed by the kidney to concentrate urine, causing frequent urination and excessive amounts of urine.

High Calcium Levels: Sarcoidosis can cause high levels of calcium to accumulate in the blood and urine. These high levels occur because sarcoid granulomas produce activated vitamin D, which enhances calcium absorption from the intestine. High blood calcium levels lead to a loss of appetite, nausea, vomiting, thirst, and excessive urine production. If present for a long time, high blood calcium levels may lead to the formation of kidney stones or calcium deposits in the kidney and, eventually, to kidney failure.

Diagnosis

Doctors most often diagnose sarcoidosis by observing its distinctive changes, including enlarged lymph nodes and abnormal findings on a chest x-ray or on computed tomography (CT). When further testing is necessary, microscopic examination of a tissue sample showing inflammation and granulomas confirms the diagnosis. Bronchoscopy with transbronchial lung biopsy (see page 457) is 90% accurate and is the best procedure for people whose lungs are involved. Other possible sources of tissue specimens are skin abnormalities, enlarged lymph nodes close to the skin, and granulomas on the conjunctiva. A liver biopsy is rarely needed even if there is evidence that the liver is affected.

Tuberculosis can cause many changes similar to those caused by sarcoidosis. Therefore, doctors also do a tuberculin skin test (and sometimes a lung biopsy) to make sure the problem is not tuberculosis.

Other methods that can help doctors diagnose sarcoidosis or assess its severity include measuring the level of angiotensin-converting enzyme (ACE) in the blood, irrigating the lungs and examining the fluid, and using a whole-body gallium scan. In many people with sarcoidosis, the level of ACE in the blood is usually high, but this test is not always accurate. The washings from a lung with active sarcoidosis contain a large number of lymphocytes, but this finding is not unique to sarcoidosis. Because gallium scanning shows abnormal patterns in the lungs or lymph nodes of people with sarcoidosis in those places, this test is sometimes used when the diagnosis is uncertain.

In people with lung scarring, pulmonary function tests may show that the amount of air the lung can hold is below normal. Blood tests may reveal a low number of white blood cells, red blood cells, or platelets. Immunoglobulin levels are often high, especially in blacks.

Levels of calcium in the blood may be high. The levels of liver enzymes, particularly alkaline phosphatase, may be high if the liver is affected.

Prognosis

Sarcoidosis improves or clears up spontaneously in nearly two thirds of people with lung sarcoidosis. Even enlarged lymph nodes in the chest and extensive lung inflammation may disappear in a few months or years. The course can be chronic or progressive in 10 to 30% of people. Serious involvement outside of the chest (for example, of the heart, nervous system, eyes, or liver) occurs in 4 to 7% of people at the beginning of their illness. The chance of involvement outside of the chest increases if lung disease persists.

People who have sarcoidosis that has not spread beyond the chest do better than those who also have sarcoidosis elsewhere in the body. People with enlarged lymph nodes in the chest but no sign of lung disease have a very good prognosis. People whose disease began with erythema nodosum and tender, swollen joints often have the best prognosis. About 50% of people who once had sarcoidosis have relapses.

About 10% of people with sarcoidosis develop a serious disability from damage to the eyes, respiratory system, or elsewhere. Lung scarring leading to respiratory failure and cor pulmonale is the most common cause of death, followed by bleeding from lung infection caused by *Aspergillus*.

Treatment

Most people with sarcoidosis do not need treatment. Corticosteroids are given to suppress severe symptoms such as shortness of breath, joint pain, and fever. These drugs also are given if

- Tests show high levels of calcium in the blood, even if symptoms are mild.
- Function of the heart, liver, or nervous system is affected.
- Sarcoidosis causes disfiguring skin lesions or eye disease that corticosteroid eye drops do not cure.
- Lung disease worsens.

People who have no symptoms should not take corticosteroids. Although corticosteroids control symptoms well, they do not prevent lung scarring over the years. About 10% of people who need treatment do not respond to corticosteroids alone, and they are also given methotrexate, which may be very effective. Hydroxychloroquine is sometimes helpful in eliminating disfiguring skin lesions.

The success of treatment can be monitored with chest x-rays, CT, pulmonary function tests, and measurements of calcium or ACE levels in the blood. These tests are repeated regularly to detect relapses after treatment stops.

Pulmonary Alveolar Proteinosis

Pulmonary alveolar proteinosis is a rare disorder in which the air sacs of the lungs (alveoli) become plugged with a protein-rich fluid.

- Pulmonary alveolar proteinosis typically affects people who are aged 20 to 60 and who have not had lung disease.
- People have difficulty breathing and cough.
- Diagnosis is by computed tomography and testing a sample of lung fluid obtained using a bronchoscope.
- If symptoms are severe, the lungs are washed out, one at a time.

The cause of pulmonary alveolar proteinosis is almost always unknown, but recent studies have linked it to production of an antibody directed against a protein that seems to be involved with the production or the breakdown of surfactant (a substance normally produced in the lungs). Occasionally, development of pulmonary alveolar proteinosis is related to exposure to toxic substances, such as inorganic dusts, infection with *Pneumocystis jiroveci* (see page 470), certain cancers, and immunosuppressants. Rarely, it occurs in newborns.

The protein in the lungs plugs up the alveoli and small airways. In rare instances, lung tissue becomes scarred. The disease may progress, remain stable, or disappear spontaneously.

Symptoms

When the alveoli are plugged, the transfer of oxygen to the blood from the lungs is severely impaired. Consequently, most people with pulmonary alveolar proteinosis experience shortness of breath when they exert themselves. Some people have severe difficulty breathing, even at rest. Other symptoms may include fatigue, weight loss, and low-grade fever. Most people also have a cough that often does not produce sputum, but occasionally people expectorate chunky gelatinous material. People often have severe disability from inadequate lung function. Lung infections may quickly worsen symptoms of shortness of breath and produce fever.

Diagnosis

A chest x-ray shows extensive dense white patches in both lungs, usually located centrally near the heart. Computed tomography (CT) shows this and other changes that suggest the disease. Pulmonary function tests (see page 454) reveal that the volume of air that the lungs can hold is abnormally small. Tests show low levels of oxygen in the blood, at first only during exercise but later also when the person is at rest. The elimination of carbon dioxide from the lungs may be impaired. Blood test results are not specific for the diagnosis, although levels of some substances (for example, lactic dehydrogenase, red blood cells, serum surfactant proteins, and gamma globulin) are often elevated.

To make a definitive diagnosis, doctors examine a sample of the fluid from the alveoli. To obtain a sample, doctors use a bronchoscope (see page 456) to wash segments of the lung with a salt-water solution and then collect the washings (bronchoalveolar lavage). The washings are often opaque or milky because the fluid is rich in protein and fats. Sometimes doctors obtain a lung tissue sample for microscopic examination (lung biopsy) during bronchoscopy. Occasionally, a larger sample is needed, which must be removed surgically.

Treatment

People who have few or no symptoms do not require treatment. For people with disabling symptoms, the protein- and fat-rich fluid in the alveoli can be washed out with a salt solution during bronchoscopy or through a special tube inserted through the mouth or through the windpipe (trachea) and into one lung. Sometimes only a small section of the lung must be washed, but if symptoms are severe and the levels of oxygen in the blood are very low, the person is given general anesthesia, so that one entire lung can be washed. About 3 to 5 days later, the other lung is washed, again after the person has been given general anesthesia. One washing is enough for some people, but others need washings every 6 to 12 months for many years.

Corticosteroids, such as prednisone, are not effective and may actually increase the chance of infection. Bacterial infections are treated with antibiotics, usually taken by mouth.

Some people with pulmonary alveolar proteinosis are short of breath indefinitely, but the disease is rarely fatal as long as they have regular lung washings.

84 Allergic and Autoimmune Diseases of the Lungs

The lungs are particularly prone to allergic reactions because they are exposed to large quantities of airborne substances that commonly cause allergic reactions (called antigens), including dusts, pollens, fungi, and chemicals. Exposure to irritating dusts or airborne substances, often when a person is at work, may increase the likelihood of an allergic respiratory reaction. Allergic reactions involving the lungs may also occur from eating a certain food or taking a certain drug.

The body reacts to an antigen by forming proteins that react with antigens (antibodies). In a normal immune response, antibodies typically bind to an antigen, thereby rendering it harmless (see page 1096). Sometimes, however, when the antibody and antigen interact, inflammation and tissue damage occur; this is called an allergic reaction. Allergic reactions are classified by the various mechanisms that are involved in causing the tissue damage. Many allergic reactions involve a combination of more than one type of tissue damage. Some allergic reactions depend on antigen-specific lymphocytes (a type of white blood cell) rather than on antibodies. It is believed that some types of allergic reactions decrease as people age.

Hypersensitivity Pneumonitis

Hypersensitivity pneumonitis (extrinsic allergic alveolitis) is a type of inflammation in and around the tiny air sacs (alveoli) and smallest airways (bronchioles) of the lung caused by an allergic reaction to inhaled organic dusts or, less commonly, chemicals.

- Dusts that contain microorganisms or proteins may cause an allergic reaction in the lungs.
- People may develop fever, cough, chills, and shortness of breath within 4 to 8 hours of re-exposure to substances to which they are sensitized.
- Doctors use chest x-rays and tests of lung function to determine whether there is a problem with the lungs.
- The substance that is causing the reaction can often be identified by using a blood test.
- People who work with substances that are likely to cause allergic reactions should use protective equipment, such as face masks, during work.
- People who can avoid re-exposure usually recover, but they sometimes need to take corticosteroids to reduce lung inflammation.

Causes

Many types of dust can cause allergic reactions in the lungs. Organic dusts that contain microorganisms or proteins and chemicals, such as isocyanates, may cause hypersensitivity pneumonitis. Farmer's lung, which results from repeated inhalation of heat-loving (thermophilic) bacteria in moldy hay, is a well-known example of hypersensitivity pneumonitis. Air conditioner lung is another example. It occurs when contaminated humidifiers or air conditioners (especially large systems in office buildings) circulate antigens that are capable of causing a hypersensitivity reaction.

Only a small number of people who inhale these common dusts develop allergic reactions. Only a small percentage of those people who develop allergic reactions suffer irreversible damage to the lungs. Generally, a person must be exposed repeatedly over time before sensitivity and resultant disease develop.

Lung damage appears to result from damage done by lymphocytes, a type of white blood cell. Initial exposures to the dusts sensitize lymphocytes. Some lymphocytes then help to produce antibodies that play a role in tissue damage. Other lymphocytes participate directly in inflammation after subsequent antigen exposure. Recurrent exposure to the antigen results in a chronic inflammatory response, which is manifested by a buildup of white blood cells in the walls of the alveoli and small airways. This buildup leads progressively to symptoms and disease.

Symptoms and Diagnosis

If a person has developed hypersensitivity to an organic dust, then fever, cough, chills, and shortness of breath typically appear 4 to 8 hours after re-exposure to it. Wheezing is unusual. If the person has no further contact with the antigen, symptoms usually diminish over a day or two, but complete recovery may take weeks.

In a slower form of hypersensitivity pneumonitis (subacute form), cough and shortness of breath may develop over days or weeks and sometimes may be so severe that the person needs to be hospitalized.

With chronic hypersensitivity pneumonitis, a person repeatedly comes in contact with an antigen over months to years, and lung scarring (fibrosis) may result. Shortness of breath during exercise, cough, fatigue, and weight loss may gradually progress over months or years. Eventually, the disease may lead to

WHAT CAUSES HYPERSENSITIVITY PNEUMONITIS?

DISEASE	SOURCE OF DUST PARTICLES OR ANTIGENS
Air conditioner lung	Humidifiers and air conditioners
Bagassosis	Sugarcane
Bird fancier's lung, pigeon breeder's lung, hen worker's lung	Droppings from parakeets, pigeons, and chickens
Cheese washer's lung	Cheese mold
Chemical worker's lung	Chemicals used in manufacturing polyurethane foam, molding, insulation, synthetic rubber, and packaging materials
Coffee worker's lung	Unroasted coffee beans
Cork worker's lung (suberosis)	Moldy cork
Farmer's lung	Moldy hay
Hot tub lung	Bacteria-contaminated hot tubs and therapy pools
Malt worker's lung	Moldy barley or malt
Maple bark stripper's lung	Infected maple bark
Miller's lung	Weevil-infested wheat flour
Mushroom worker's lung	Mushroom compost
Sequoiosis	Moldy sawdust from redwoods
Woodworker's lung	Wood dust

pulmonary function tests (see page 454)—which measure the lungs' capacity to hold air and their ability to move air in and out and to exchange oxygen and carbon dioxide—are used to assess how well the lungs work and may help support a diagnosis of hypersensitivity pneumonitis. When the antigen cannot be identified and the diagnosis is in doubt, re-exposing the recovered person to the antigen that is thought to be responsible and observing the person for symptoms or changes in lung function may occasionally be useful to confirm the diagnosis.

In cases that are not clear, especially when an infection is suspected, doctors may remove small pieces of lung tissue for examination under a microscope (lung biopsies). They may remove the tissue while examining the airways using a viewing tube (bronchoscopy—see page 456). Sometimes, rather than (or in addition to) removing tissue by using a sharp instrument, the person performing bronchoscopy may wash out the lung with fluid (bronchoalveolar lavage) to extract cells for examination. Rarely, a different type of viewing tube (thoracoscope) may be used to examine the lung surface and pleural space, or an operation in which the chest wall is opened (thoracotomy) may be needed to obtain larger pieces of lung tissue (see page 458).

Prevention and Treatment

The best prevention is to avoid exposure to the antigen, but this may be impractical if the person cannot change jobs. Eliminating or reducing dust, wearing protective masks, and using good ventilation systems may help prevent both sensitization and recurrence. However, even the best prevention methods may not be effective.

People who have an acute episode of hypersensitivity pneumonitis usually recover if further contact with the substance is avoided. If the episode is severe, corticosteroids, such as prednisone, reduce symptoms and may help reduce severe inflammation. Prolonged or recurring episodes may lead to irreversible disease and progressive disability.

Eosinophilic Pneumonia

Eosinophilic pneumonia (also called pulmonary infiltrates with eosinophilia syndrome) comprises a group of lung diseases in which eosinophils (a type of white blood cell) appear in increased numbers in the lungs and usually in the bloodstream.

- Certain drugs, chemicals, fungi, and parasites may cause eosinophils to accumulate in the lungs.
- People may cough, wheeze, or feel short of breath, and some people develop respiratory failure.
- Doctors use x-rays and laboratory tests to detect the disorder and determine the cause, especially if parasites are suspected as the cause.
- Corticosteroids are usually given.

respiratory failure (see page 524). Older people may be more prone to chronic, progressively worsening disease because they have been exposed to an antigen for a long period of time.

The diagnosis of hypersensitivity pneumonitis depends on the clinical features, identification (if possible) of the dust or other substance causing the problem, and evidence of the person's exposure to the suspected agent, as determined by the presence of antibodies on a blood test.

Doctors may suspect the diagnosis based on finding something abnormal on a chest x-ray. Results of

Eosinophils participate in the immune response of the lung. The number of eosinophils increases during many inflammatory and allergic reactions, including asthma, which frequently accompanies certain types of eosinophilic pneumonia. Eosinophilic pneumonia differs from typical pneumonias in that there is no suggestion that the tiny air sacs of the lungs (alveoli) are infected by bacteria, viruses, or fungi. However, the alveoli and often the airways do fill with eosinophils. Even the blood vessel walls may be invaded by eosinophils, and the narrowed airways may become plugged with an accumulation of secretions (mucus) if asthma develops.

The exact reason that eosinophils accumulate in the lungs is not well understood, and often it is not possible to identify the substance that is causing the allergic reaction. However, there are some known causes of eosinophilic pneumonia, including certain drugs (penicillin, aminosalicylic acid, carbamazepine, naproxen, isoniazid, nitrofurantoin, chlorpropamide, and sulfonamides [such as trimethoprim-sulfamethoxazole]); chemical fumes (nickel inhaled as a vapor); fungi (*Aspergillus fumigatus*); and parasites (roundworms, including nematodes).

Symptoms and Diagnosis

Symptoms may be mild or life threatening. Simple eosinophilic pneumonia (Löffler's syndrome) and similar pneumonias (such as tropical eosinophilia, which is due to infestation by any of several species of nematode worms called filaria) may produce a slight fever and mild respiratory symptoms, if any. A person may cough, wheeze, and feel short of breath but usually recovers quickly. Another disease, known as acute eosinophilic pneumonia, may cause the level of oxygen in the blood to decrease severely and can progress to acute respiratory failure in a few hours or days if not treated.

Chronic eosinophilic pneumonia, which slowly progresses over weeks to months, is a distinct disorder that may also become severe. Life-threatening shortness of breath can develop if the condition is not treated.

With acute eosinophilic pneumonia, tests show large numbers of eosinophils in the blood, sometimes as many as 10 to 15 times the normal number. However, with chronic eosinophilic pneumonia, the numbers of eosinophils in the blood may be normal.

The most conclusive evidence for the diagnosis is that the person's symptoms occur within a relatively short time after taking a drug or after travel to an area in which exposure to worms was possible. A chest x-ray is abnormal in eosinophilic pneumonia, but similar abnormalities can occur in other conditions. In acute eosinophilic pneumonia, a chest x-ray usually shows small white lines and hazy patches in the lungs, sometimes with large white patches that are characteristic of fluid in the lungs (called edema). Fluid in the chest cavity (pleural effusion) may also develop and be visible on chest x-ray. In chronic eosinophilic pneumonia, the chest x-ray shows white patches located mainly in the outer zones of the lungs that may appear to migrate to new areas of the lung when x-rays are taken later.

Microscopic examination of cells from coughed-up sputum or washings of the alveoli obtained during bronchoscopy typically shows clumps of eosinophils. Other laboratory tests may be performed to search for an infection with fungi or parasites; these tests may include microscopic examination of stool specimens to look for worms and other parasites.

Prognosis and Treatment

Eosinophilic pneumonia may be mild, and people with the disease may get better without treatment. For acute cases, a corticosteroid such as prednisone is usually needed. In chronic eosinophilic pneumonia, prednisone may be needed for many months or even years. If a person develops wheezing, the same treatments used for asthma are given as well (see page 475). If worms or other parasites are the cause, the person is treated with appropriate drugs. Ordinarily, drugs that may be causing the illness are discontinued.

Allergic Bronchopulmonary Aspergillosis

Allergic bronchopulmonary aspergillosis is an allergic lung reaction to a type of fungus (most commonly Aspergillus fumigatus) that occurs in some people with asthma or cystic fibrosis.

- People may cough and wheeze, and they sometimes have fever or cough up flecks of blood.
- Doctors use chest x-rays, blood tests, and skin tests to make a diagnosis.
- Antiasthma drugs are usually given.
- If untreated, chronic lung damage may develop.

The fungus *Aspergillus fumigatus* flourishes in soil, decaying vegetation, foods, dusts, and water. Certain people who inhale the fungus may become sensitized and develop a chronic allergic reaction. Other fungi, including *Penicillium*, *Candida*, *Curvularia*, and *Helminthosporium*, can cause an identical illness. In some people, the effects of the allergic reaction combine with the effects of the fungus to damage the airways and lungs.

The disorder differs from typical pneumonias caused by bacteria, viruses, and most fungi, in that the fungus does not actually invade the lung tissue and directly destroy it. The fungus colonizes the mucus in the airways of people with asthma or cystic fibrosis (both of whom tend to have increased amounts of mucus) and causes recurrent allergic inflammation in the lung. The tiny air sacs of the lungs (alveoli) become packed primarily with eosinophils. Increased numbers of mucus-producing cells may also appear. If the disease has caused extensive damage, inflammation may cause the central airways to widen permanently, a condition called bronchiectasis (see page 491). Eventually, the lungs are likely to become scarred.

Other forms of aspergillosis can occur. *Aspergillus* can invade the lungs and cause serious pneumonia in people with an impaired immune system. This condition is an infection, not an allergic reaction (see page 1229). *Aspergillus* can also form fungus balls (aspergillomas) in cavities and cysts of lungs damaged by another disease, such as tuberculosis; severe bleeding may result.

Symptoms and Diagnosis

The first indications of allergic bronchopulmonary aspergillosis are usually progressive symptoms of asthma, such as wheezing and shortness of breath, and a mild fever. The person usually does not feel well. Brownish flecks or plugs may appear in coughed-up sputum.

Repeated chest x-rays show areas that look like pneumonia, but they appear to migrate to new areas of the lung, most often in the upper parts. With long-standing disease, chest x-rays or computed tomography (CT) may show widened airways, which are often plugged with mucus; this appearance is similar to one that would be found in a person who has a lung tumor. The fungus itself, along with excess eosinophils, may be seen when the sputum is examined under the microscope. Blood tests reveal high levels of eosinophils and antibodies to *Aspergillus*. Skin testing can determine if the person is allergic to *Aspergillus*, but the test does not distinguish between allergic bronchopulmonary aspergillosis and a simple allergy to *Aspergillus*, which may occur in people who have allergic asthma without aspergillosis.

Treatment

Because *Aspergillus* appears in many places in the environment, the fungus is difficult to avoid. Antiasthma drugs, especially corticosteroids, are used to treat allergic bronchopulmonary aspergillosis (see table on page 479). Antiasthma drugs also open up the airways, making it easier to cough up mucus plugs and clear out the fungus. The corticosteroid prednisone, taken initially in high doses, and then over a long period of time in lower doses, may prevent progressive lung damage. Most specialists recommend oral corticosteroids; the inhaled kind has not been shown to work well for this condition. The antifungal drug itraconazole is sometimes used in addition to corticosteroids to help eliminate the fungus from the lung. Allergy shots (desensitization) may cause complications and are not recommended.

Because the lung damage may worsen gradually without causing any noticeable changes in symptoms, chest x-rays, pulmonary function tests (see page 454), levels of eosinophils in the blood, and amounts of immunoglobulin E (IgE) antibody are regularly monitored. As the disease is controlled, the eosinophil and antibody levels usually fall, but they may rise again as an early sign of flare-ups.

Goodpasture's Syndrome

Goodpasture's syndrome is an uncommon autoimmune disorder in which bleeding into the lungs and progressive kidney failure occur.

- People usually are short of breath and cough up blood.
- Laboratory tests on samples of blood and urine and chest x-rays are needed to make the diagnosis.
- Corticosteroids, cyclophosphamide (a chemotherapy drug), and plasmapheresis are used to try to prevent permanent lung and kidney damage.

This disease usually affects young men. Some people appear to be genetically susceptible to Goodpasture's syndrome. In these people, substances in the environment, such as tobacco smoke and some solvents, or a viral upper respiratory infection can cause them to produce antibodies against certain parts of their own bodies. Thus, Goodpasture's syndrome is actually an autoimmune rather than an allergic disease. These antibodies usually damage certain structures in the walls of the tiny air sacs (alveoli) and capillaries of the lungs and in the filtering apparatus of the kidneys. The antibodies trigger inflammation that interferes with lung and kidney function. Presumably, they are the direct cause of the disease.

Symptoms and Diagnosis

A person with this disease typically develops shortness of breath and coughs up blood. Symptoms can quickly become severe: Breathing can fail, and large amounts of blood can be lost. At the same time, the kidneys can rapidly fail. There may be small amounts of blood in the urine.

Laboratory tests reveal the characteristic antibodies in the blood. Urine examination reveals blood and protein in the urine. Anemia is often present. A chest x-ray shows abnormal white patches (due to lung bleeding) in both lungs. A needle biopsy specimen of kidney tissue shows microscopic deposits of antibodies in a specific pattern.

Treatment

The disease may very rapidly lead to severe loss of lung function, a complete loss of kidney function, and death. High doses of corticosteroids (such as prednisone) and cyclophosphamide are given intravenously to suppress the activity of the immune system, and the person undergoes plasmapheresis—a procedure in which blood is removed from the circulation, the unwanted antibodies are removed, and the blood cells are returned to the circulation (see box on page 1030). The early use of this combination of treatments may help preserve lung and kidney function. Once damage occurs to the kidneys, it is usually permanent.

Many people may need supportive care until the disease runs its course. People may require supplemental oxygen or may need to be on a ventilator for a period of time. Blood transfusions may also be needed. If the kidneys fail, kidney dialysis or a kidney transplant may be required.

CHAPTER

85   Pleural Disorders

The pleura is a thin, transparent, two-layered membrane that covers the lungs and also lines the inside of the chest wall. The layer that covers the lungs lies in close contact with the layer that lines the chest wall. Between the two thin flexible layers is a small amount of fluid that lubricates them as they slide smoothly over one another with each breath.

In abnormal circumstances, air or excess fluid can get between the pleural surfaces, creating a space. If excess fluid accumulates (called pleural effusion) or if air accumulates (called pneumothorax), one or both lungs may not be able to expand normally with breathing, resulting in the collapse of lung tissue.

Pleural Effusion

Pleural effusion is the abnormal accumulation of fluid in the pleural space.

- Fluid can accumulate in the pleural space as a result of a large number of disorders, including infections, injuries, heart or liver failure, blood clots in the lung blood vessels (pulmonary emboli), and drugs.
- Symptoms may include difficulty breathing and chest pain, particularly when breathing and coughing.
- Diagnosis is by chest x-rays, laboratory testing of the fluid, and often computed tomography.
- Large amounts of fluid are drained with a tube inserted into the chest.

Normally, only a thin layer of fluid separates the two layers of the pleura. An excessive amount of fluid may accumulate for many reasons, including heart failure, cirrhosis, pneumonia, and cancer.

Types of Fluid: Depending on the cause, the fluid may be either rich in protein (exudate) or watery (transudate). Doctors use this distinction to help determine the cause.

Blood in the pleural space (hemothorax) usually results from a chest injury. Rarely, a blood vessel ruptures into the pleural space when no injury has occurred, or a bulging area in the aorta (aortic aneurysm) leaks blood into the pleural space.

Pus in the pleural space (empyema) can accumulate when pneumonia or a lung abscess spreads into the space. Empyema may also complicate an infection from chest wounds, chest surgery, rupture of the esophagus, or an abscess in the abdomen.

Lymphatic (milky) fluid in the pleural space (chylothorax) is caused by an injury to the main lymphatic duct in the chest (thoracic duct) or by a blockage of the duct by a tumor.

Fluid in the pleural space that contains excessive amounts of cholesterol results from a long-standing pleural effusion caused by a condition such as tuberculosis or rheumatoid arthritis.

Symptoms

Many people with pleural effusion have no symptoms at all. The most common symptoms, regardless of the type of fluid in the pleural space or its cause, are shortness of breath and chest pain. Chest pain is usually of a type called pleuritic pain. It may be felt only when the person breathes deeply or coughs, or it may be felt continuously but may be worsened by deep breathing and coughing. The pain is usually felt in the chest wall right over the site of the inflammation. However, the pain may be felt also or only in the upper abdominal region or neck and shoulder as referred pain (see box on page 639). Pleuritic pain is also called **pleurisy**. Pleurisy can be caused by disorders other than pleural effusion.

Pleuritic chest pain due to a pleural effusion may disappear as fluid accumulates. Large amounts of

Two Views of the Pleura

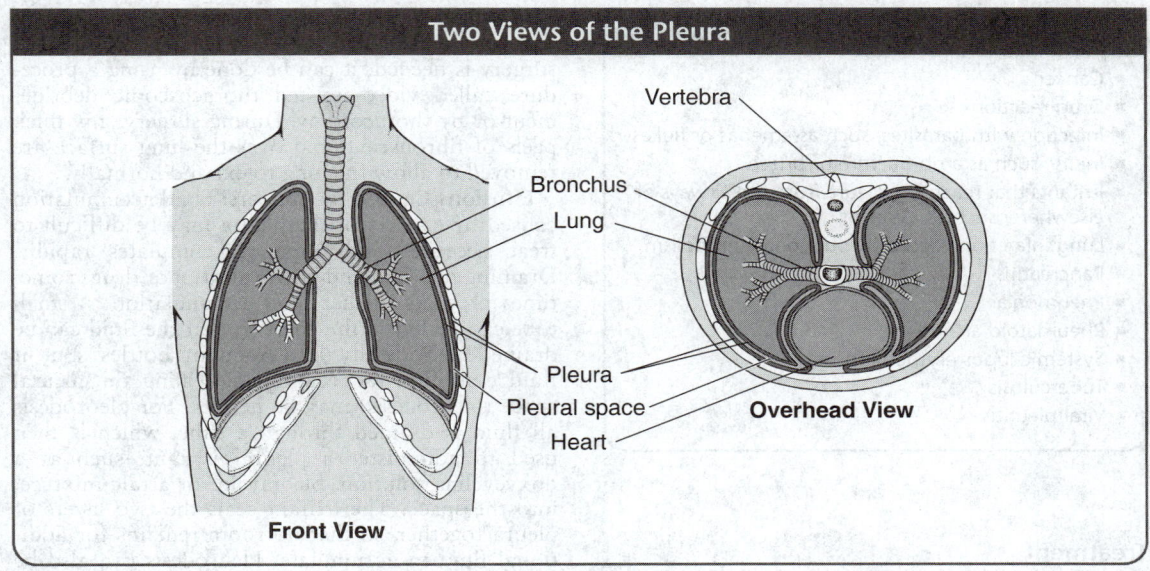

Front View

Overhead View

Vertebra

Bronchus

Lung

Pleura

Pleural space

Heart

fluid can cause difficulty in expanding one or both lungs when breathing, causing shortness of breath.

Diagnosis

A chest x-ray, which shows fluid in the pleural space, is usually the first step in making the diagnosis. However, small amounts of fluid may not be visible on a chest x-ray. Computed tomography (CT) more clearly shows the lung and the fluid and may show evidence of pneumonia, a pulmonary embolus, a lung abscess, or a tumor. An ultrasound examination may help doctors determine the position of a small accumulation of fluid.

A specimen of the fluid is almost always removed for examination using a needle, a procedure called thoracentesis (see page 456). The appearance of the fluid may help doctors determine its cause. Certain laboratory tests evaluate the chemical composition of the fluid and determine the presence of bacteria, including the bacteria that cause tuberculosis. The fluid specimen is also examined for the number and types of cells and for the presence of cancerous cells.

If these tests cannot identify the cause of the pleural effusion, other tests may be done. Sometimes a sample is obtained using a thoracoscope (a viewing tube that allows doctors to examine the pleural space and obtain tissue samples of the covering of the chest wall or the lung—see page 457). This procedure is called thoracoscopy and can detect cancer and tuberculosis. If thoracoscopy is unavailable, a needle biopsy of the pleura may be done (see page 456). Occasionally, bronchoscopy (a direct visual examination of the airways through a viewing tube) helps doctors find the cause of the fluid. In about 20% of people with pleural effusion, the cause is not obvious after initial testing, and in some people a cause is never found, even after extensive testing.

Common Causes of Pleural Effusion*

- Heart failure
- Tumors
- Pneumonia
- Pulmonary embolus
- Surgery, such as recent coronary artery bypass surgery
- Injury to the chest
- Cirrhosis
- Kidney failure
- Systemic lupus erythematosus (lupus)
- Pancreatitis
- Rheumatoid arthritis
- Tuberculosis
- Nephrotic syndrome (protein in the urine and high blood pressure)
- Peritoneal dialysis
- Drugs such as hydralazine, procainamide, isoniazid, phenytoin, chlorpromazine, methysergide, interleukin-2, nitrofurantoin, bromocriptine, dantrolene, and procarbazine

*Listed as most common to least common.

Major Causes of Pleurisy

- Cancer
- Drug reactions
- Infection with parasites, such as amebas or flukes
- Injury, such as a rib fracture or bruise
- Irritants that reach the pleura from the airways or elsewhere, such as asbestos
- Lung infarction caused by pulmonary embolism
- Pancreatitis
- Pneumonia
- Rheumatoid arthritis
- Systemic lupus erythematosus
- Tuberculosis
- Viral pleuritis

Treatment

Small pleural effusions may not require treatment, although the underlying disorder must be treated. Larger pleural effusions, especially those that cause shortness of breath, may require drainage of the fluid. Usually, drainage dramatically relieves shortness of breath. Often, fluid can be drained using thoracentesis. An area of skin between two lower ribs is anesthetized, then a small needle is inserted and gently pushed deeper until it reaches the fluid. A thin plastic catheter is often guided over the needle into the fluid to lessen the chance of puncturing the lung and causing a pneumothorax. Although thoracentesis is usually done for diagnostic purposes, doctors can safely remove as much as about 1½ quarts (1.5 liters) of fluid at a time using this procedure.

When larger amounts of fluid must be removed, a tube (chest tube) may be inserted through the chest wall. After numbing the area by injecting a local anesthetic, doctors insert a plastic tube into the chest between two ribs. Then doctors connect the tube to a water-sealed drainage system that prevents air from leaking into the pleural space. A chest x-ray is taken to check the tube's position. Drainage can be blocked if the chest tube is incorrectly positioned or becomes kinked. If the fluid is very thick or full of clots, it may not flow out.

Effusions Caused by Pneumonia: An accumulation of fluid from pneumonia requires intravenous antibiotics and sampling of the fluid. If the fluid is pus or if the fluid has certain characteristics, the fluid needs to be drained, usually with a chest tube. If the fluid has formed within scars (fibrous compartments) in the pleural space, drainage is more difficult. Sometimes drugs called thrombolytics (fi-brinolytics) are instilled into the pleural space to help drainage, which may avoid the need for surgery. If surgery is needed, it can be done by using a procedure called video-assisted thoracoscopic debridement or by thoracotomy. During surgery, any thick peels of fibrous material over the lung surface are removed to allow the lung to expand normally.

Effusions Caused by Cancers: Fluid accumulation caused by cancers of the pleura may be difficult to treat because fluid often reaccumulates rapidly. Draining the fluid and giving antitumor drugs sometimes prevents further fluid accumulation. A small tube can be left in the chest so that the fluid can be drained periodically into vacuum bottles. But if fluid continues to accumulate, sealing the pleural space (pleurodesis) may be helpful. For pleurodesis all fluid is drained through a tube, which is then used to administer a pleural irritant, such as a doxycycline solution, bleomycin, or a talc mixture, into the space. The irritant seals the two layers of pleura together, so that no room remains for additional fluid to accumulate. Pleurodesis can also be done using thoracoscopy.

Chylothorax: Treatment of chylothorax focuses on eliminating the leakage from the lymphatic duct. Such treatment may consist of surgery, chemotherapy, or radiation treatment for a cancer that is blocking lymph flow.

Pneumothorax

A pneumothorax is the presence of air between the two layers of pleura, resulting in partial or complete collapse of the lung.

- Symptoms include difficulty breathing and chest pain.
- Diagnosis is by chest x-ray.
- Treatment is usually draining the air with a tube or sometimes a plastic catheter inserted into the chest.

Normally, the pressure in the pleural space is lower than that inside the lungs or outside the chest. If a perforation develops that causes a connection between the pleural space and the inside of the lungs or outside the chest, air enters the pleural space until the pressures become equal or the connection closes. When there is air in the pleural space, the lung partially collapses. Sometimes most or all of the lung collapses, leading to severe shortness of breath.

A pneumothorax that occurs without any apparent cause in people without a known lung disorder is called a primary spontaneous pneumothorax. Primary spontaneous pneumothorax usually occurs when a small weakened area of lung (bulla) ruptures. The condition is most common in tall men younger than age 40 who smoke. Most people recover fully; however, primary spontaneous pneumothorax recurs in up to 50% of people.

Spontaneous pneumothorax also occurs in people with an underlying lung disorder (secondary spontaneous pneumothorax). This type of pneumothorax most often results from the rupture of a bulla in older people who have emphysema, but it also occurs in people with other lung conditions, such as cystic fibrosis, asthma, Langerhans' cell granulomatosis, sarcoidosis, lung abscess, tuberculosis, and *Pneumocystis* pneumonia. Because of the underlying lung disorder, the symptoms and outcome are generally worse in secondary spontaneous pneumothorax. The recurrence rate is similar to that of primary spontaneous pneumothorax.

A pneumothorax may also occur after an injury or a medical procedure that introduces air into the pleural space, such as thoracentesis, bronchoscopy, or thoracoscopy. Ventilators can cause pressure damage to the lungs (barotrauma) that leads to a pneumothorax—most often in people with emphysema or severe acute respiratory distress syndrome (see page 525). Changes in lung pressure (as occur in divers and airline pilots), can increase the risk of pneumothorax.

Symptoms

Symptoms vary greatly depending on how much air enters the pleural space, how much of the lung collapses, and the person's lung function before the pneumothorax occurred. They range from a little shortness of breath or chest pain to severe shortness of breath, shock, and life-threatening cardiac arrest. Most often, sharp chest pain and shortness of breath and occasionally a dry hacking cough begin suddenly. Pain may also be felt in the shoulder, neck, or abdomen. Symptoms tend to be less severe in a slowly developing pneumothorax than in a rapidly developing one. Except with a very large pneumothorax or a tension pneumothorax, symptoms usually subside as the body adapts to the lung collapse, and the lung slowly begins to reinflate as the air is reabsorbed from the pleural space.

Diagnosis

A physical examination can usually confirm the diagnosis if the pneumothorax is large. Using a stethoscope, a doctor may note that one part of the chest does not transmit the normal sounds of breathing, while tapping (percussing) the chest produces a hollow, drumlike sound. A chest x-ray shows the air pocket and the collapsed lung outlined by the thin inner pleural layer. A chest x-ray can also show if the trachea (the large airway that passes through the front of the neck) is being pushed to one side.

Treatment

A small primary spontaneous pneumothorax usually requires no treatment. It usually does not cause serious breathing problems, and the air is absorbed in several days. The full absorption of air in a larger

---

What Is Tension Pneumothorax?

Tension pneumothorax is a serious and potentially life-threatening form of pneumothorax. In this condition, the tissues surrounding the area where air is entering the pleural space act as a one-way valve, allowing air to enter but not to exit. This situation causes such high pressure in the pleural cavity that the lung completely collapses, and the heart and other structures in the chest cavity are pushed over to the opposite side of the chest.

If not relieved, tension pneumothorax can cause death in minutes. A doctor immediately inserts a needle into the chest to relieve the pressure. Then, a chest tube is inserted separately to drain the air continuously.

---

pneumothorax may take 2 to 4 weeks. However, the air can be removed more quickly by inserting a catheter or chest tube into the pneumothorax.

If a primary spontaneous pneumothorax is large enough to impair breathing, the air can be removed (aspirated) with a large syringe attached to a plastic catheter inserted into the chest. The catheter can be sealed and then left in place for a time so that any air that reaccumulates can be removed. If catheter aspiration is unsuccessful and for any other type of pneumothorax (such as a secondary spontaneous pneumothorax or a traumatic pneumothorax), a chest tube is used to drain the air. The chest tube is inserted through an incision in the chest wall and is connected to a water-sealed drainage system or a one-way valve that allows the air to exit without allowing any air to get back in. A suction pump may be attached to the chest tube if air keeps leaking in from an abnormal connection (fistula) between an airway and the pleural space. Occasionally, surgery is necessary. Often the surgery is done by using a thoracoscope inserted through the chest wall and into the pleural space.

A recurring pneumothorax can cause considerable disability. Surgery can be done to prevent pneumothorax from recurring. Usually surgery involves repairing leaking areas of the lung and firmly attaching the inner layer of pleura to the outer layer. This surgery is usually done by using a thoracoscope (a tube that allows doctors to view the pleural space—see page 457. People who may need the surgery include

- People at high risk—for example, divers and airplane pilots—after the first episode of pneumothorax
- People who have secondary spontaneous pneumothorax—after the first episode of pneumothorax, if the person is healthy enough to undergo surgery
- People who have a pneumothorax that will not heal or a pneumothorax that has occurred twice on the same side

If a person with recurring pneumothorax cannot tolerate surgery because of poor health, the pleural space can be sealed by administering a talc mixture or the drug doxycycline through a chest tube that is draining air from the space. However, sealing the space this way is less effective than surgery. When sealed this way, pneumothorax eventually develops again in 25% of people. In contrast, when surgery is done, pneumothorax develops again in only 5% of people.

Viral Pleuritis

Viral pleuritis is a viral infection of the pleurae, which typically causes chest pain when breathing or coughing.

Viral pleuritis is most commonly caused by infection with coxsackie B virus. Occasionally, echovirus causes a rare condition known as epidemic or Bornholm's pleurodynia. It occurs in the late summer and affects adolescents and young adults.

The primary symptom of viral pleuritis is chest pain. The pain is usually worse when breathing in or coughing and is often sharp. Epidemic or Bornholm's pleurodynia also causes fever and chest muscle spasms. Chest x-ray is usually done. Viral pleuritis resolves on its own after a few days or more. Analgesics can help relieve the pain.

---

86 Pulmonary Hypertension

Pulmonary hypertension is a condition in which blood pressure in the arteries of the lungs (the pulmonary arteries) is abnormally high.

- Many disorders can cause pulmonary hypertension.
- People usually have shortness of breath upon exertion and loss of energy, and some people feel light-headed or fatigued on exertion.
- Chest x-rays, electrocardiography, and echocardiography give clues to the diagnosis, but measurement of blood pressure in the right ventricle and the pulmonary artery is needed for confirmation.
- Treatment of the cause and use of drugs that improve blood flow through the lungs are helpful.

Blood travels from the right side of the heart through the pulmonary arteries into the lungs. There, carbon dioxide is removed from the blood and oxygen is added. Normally, the pressure in the pulmonary arteries is low, allowing the right side of the heart to be less muscular than the left side (because relatively little muscle and effort are needed to push the blood through the lungs via the pulmonary arteries). In contrast, the left side of the heart is more muscular because it has to push blood through the entire body against a much higher pressure.

If the pressure of the blood in the pulmonary arteries increases to a sufficiently high level, the condition is called pulmonary hypertension. With pulmonary hypertension, the right side of the heart must work harder to push the blood through the pulmonary arteries into the lungs. Over time, the right ventricle becomes thickened and enlarged and heart failure develops (see page 352).

Causes

There are many causes of pulmonary hypertension, including HIV infection, drugs and toxins, lung disorders, and low blood oxygen levels (hypoxia). One of the most common causes of pulmonary hypertension is left-sided heart failure, which can occur if

- One of the heart valves does not work properly
- The left ventricle is stressed by high blood pressure
- A heart attack or some other disorder involving the heart diminishes the ability of heart muscle to pump

Lung disorders can also lead to pulmonary hypertension. One of the most common conditions is chronic obstructive pulmonary disease (COPD—see page 480). When the lungs are impaired by a disorder, more effort is needed to pump blood through them. Over time, COPD destroys the small air sacs (alveoli) together with their small vessels (capillaries) in the lungs. The single most important cause of pulmonary hypertension in COPD is the narrowing (constriction) of the pulmonary arteries that occurs as a result of low blood oxygen levels. Having sleep apnea and living in or prolonged visiting in places that are at high altitudes can also cause pulmonary hypertension by lowering levels of oxygen in the blood. Other lung disorders that may cause pulmonary hypertension include pulmonary fibrosis, cystic fibrosis, sarcoidosis, and Langerhans' cell granulomatosis (histiocytosis).

Less often, pulmonary hypertension is caused by extensive loss of lung tissue from surgery or trauma. Other causes include heart failure, scleroderma, obesity with reduced ability to breathe (pickwickian syndrome), neurologic diseases involving the respiratory muscles,

Cor Pulmonale: A Disorder Stemming From Pulmonary Hypertension

Cor pulmonale is pulmonary hypertension related to the underlying lung disorder. The right ventricle of the heart becomes enlarged and thickened, eventually resulting in heart failure.

Cor pulmonale develops because the pulmonary arteries constrict and become thickened in response to low oxygen levels. This thickening narrows the passageway through which blood flows through the lung, and this narrowing, in turn, increases the pressure in the pulmonary arteries. Once pulmonary hypertension develops, the right side of the heart has to work harder to compensate, but the increased effort causes it to become enlarged and thickened. These changes can lead to right-sided heart failure.

The failing right ventricle places a person at risk of pulmonary embolism because blood flow is abnormally low, so blood tends to pool in the legs. If clots form in the pooled blood, they may eventually travel to and lodge in the lungs, with dangerous consequences.

There may be few symptoms of cor pulmonale until the disorder is quite advanced. When symptoms do occur, people describe shortness of breath during exertion, light-headedness, fatigue, and chest pain. Symptoms of heart failure, such as swelling (edema) in the legs and progressively worse shortness of breath, also develop.

A number of tests are available to help doctors diagnose cor pulmonale, but the diagnosis is often suspected on the basis of the physical examination. By listening through a stethoscope, doctors can hear certain characteristic heart sounds that occur when the right ventricle becomes strained. Chest x-rays can show the enlarged right ventricle and pulmonary arteries. Doctors evaluate the function of the left and right ventricles with echocardiography, radionuclide studies, and cardiac catheterization.

Treatment is usually directed at the underlying lung disorder. Measures to relieve right-sided heart failure are also taken. Because people with cor pulmonale are at increased risk of pulmonary embolism, doctors may prescribe an anticoagulant to be taken long-term.

chronic liver disease, and HIV infection. Pulmonary hypertension also occurred in some people who took the diet drugs dexfenfluramine and phentermine (fen-phen) during the 1990s. A cause of sudden pulmonary hypertension is pulmonary embolism, a condition in which blood clots become lodged in the arteries of the lung (see page 488). In the tropics, schistosomiasis, a parasite disorder, is a common cause.

A small group of people have pulmonary hypertension without any identifiable cause (called idiopathic pulmonary hypertension). Women are affected by idiopathic pulmonary hypertension twice as often as men, and the average age at which the diagnosis is made is about 35 years.

Symptoms

Shortness of breath upon exertion is the most common symptom of pulmonary hypertension, and virtually everyone who has the condition develops it. Some people feel light-headed or fatigued on exertion. The person is likely to feel weak because body tissues are not receiving enough oxygen. Other symptoms, such as coughing and wheezing, are usually caused by the underlying lung disorder. Swelling (edema), particularly of the legs, may occur because fluid may leak out of the blood vessels and into the tissues. Swelling is usually a sign that right-sided heart failure has developed.

Some people with pulmonary hypertension have connective tissue disorders, especially systemic sclerosis (scleroderma—see page 575).

Diagnosis

Based on the symptoms, doctors may suspect pulmonary hypertension in people who have an underlying lung disorder. A chest x-ray may show that the pulmonary arteries are enlarged. Electrocardiography (ECG) and echocardiography enable doctors to look for certain problems with the right side of the heart before cor pulmonale develops. For example, thickening of the right ventricle or a partial reversal (back flow) of blood through the tricuspid valve between the right atrium and right ventricle may be detected on an echocardiogram. Pulmonary function tests help doctors assess the extent of lung damage. A sample of blood may be taken from an artery in an arm to measure the level of oxygen in the blood.

A definite diagnosis of pulmonary hypertension usually requires passing a tube through a vein in an arm or a leg into the right side of the heart to measure the blood pressure in the right ventricle and the pulmonary artery.

Treatment

Treatment of pulmonary hypertension is best directed at the cause when the cause has been identified. Vasodilators (drugs to dilate blood vessels), such as calcium channel blockers and prostacyclin analogs, are often helpful for pulmonary hypertension that occurs in people with scleroderma, chronic liver disease, and HIV infection. In contrast, these drugs have not proved effective for people with pulmonary hypertension due to an underlying lung disorder. For most people with idiopathic pulmonary hypertension, vasodilators, such as prostacyclin, drastically reduce blood pressure in the pulmonary arteries. Prostacyclin given intravenously through a catheter that is surgically implanted in the skin improves the quality of life, increases survival, and prolongs the time until lung transplantation needs to be considered. Before administering vasodilators, however, doctors usually first test the effectiveness of these drugs while the person is in a cardiac catheterization laboratory, because their use may be dangerous in some people. Subcutaneous (under the skin) and inhaled forms of prostacyclin are now available and are effective in some people.

Endothelin (a substance in the blood that causes constriction of the vessels) receptor blockers, bosentan and ambrisentan, given by mouth, have been effective in some people with mild disease. A drug similar to prostacyclin, called iloprost, can be administered by inhalation and, as a result, has a much lower risk of complications than prostacyclin. Oral sildenafil is very effective in some people with pulmonary arterial hypertension.

In people with pulmonary hypertension who have a low level of oxygen in the blood, the continuous use of oxygen through nasal prongs or an oxygen mask may reduce blood pressure in the pulmonary arteries and may relieve shortness of breath. A diuretic drug is usually given to assist the right ventricle in maintaining a normal volume for effective beating and to reduce leg swelling. An anticoagulant may also be given to reduce the risk of blood clots and subsequent pulmonary embolism (see page 488).

Lung transplantation is an established procedure for treating people with pulmonary hypertension. Lung transplantation can be used only in people with severe disease who are healthy enough to withstand the potential consequences and difficulties with the procedure.

CHAPTER

87 Respiratory Failure and Acute Respiratory Distress Syndrome

Lung (or respiratory) failure is a condition in which the level of oxygen in the blood becomes too low or the level of carbon dioxide in the blood becomes too high. Acute respiratory distress syndrome (ARDS) is a cause of sudden and severe lung failure.

Respiratory Failure

Respiratory failure (lung failure) is a condition in which the level of oxygen in the blood becomes dangerously low or the level of carbon dioxide becomes dangerously high.

- Conditions that block the airways, damage lung tissue, weaken the muscles that control breathing, or decrease the drive to breathe may cause lung failure.
- People may be very short of breath, have a bluish coloration to the skin, and be confused or sleepy.
- Doctors use blood tests to detect low levels of oxygen or high levels of carbon dioxide in the blood.
- Oxygen is given.
- Sometimes people need the help of a machine to breathe until the underlying problem can be treated.

Respiratory failure is a medical emergency that can result from long-standing, progressively worsening lung disease or from severe lung disease that develops suddenly, such as the acute respiratory distress syndrome (see page 525), in otherwise healthy people.

Causes

Almost any condition that affects breathing or the lungs can lead to respiratory failure. Certain disorders, such as hypothyroidism or sleep apnea, can decrease the unconscious reflex that drives people to breathe. An overdose of opioids or alcohol also can decrease the drive to breathe by causing profound sedation. Obstruction of the airways, injury to the lung tissues, damage to the bones and tissues around the lungs, and weakness of the muscles that normally inflate the lungs are also common causes. Respiratory failure can occur if blood flow through the lungs becomes abnormal, as happens in pulmonary embolism

> ### ? Did You Know...
> Age-related reductions in lung function place older people at higher risk of severe symptoms after developing pneumonia.

WHAT CAUSES RESPIRATORY FAILURE?

UNDERLYING PROBLEM	CAUSE
Airway obstruction	Chronic obstructive pulmonary disease, asthma, bronchiectasis, cystic fibrosis, bronchiolitis, or inhaled foreign bodies
Poor breathing (decrease in the drive to breathe)	Obesity, sleep apnea, hypothyroidism, or drug or alcohol intoxication
Muscle weakness	Myasthenia gravis, muscular dystrophy, polio, Guillain-Barré syndrome, polymyositis, certain strokes, amyotrophic lateral sclerosis (ALS), or spinal cord injury
Abnormality of lung tissue	Acute respiratory distress syndrome (ARDS), pneumonia, pulmonary edema (excess fluid in the lungs) due to heart or kidney failure, a drug reaction, pulmonary fibrosis, widespread tumors, radiation, sarcoidosis, or burns
Abnormality of the chest wall	Scoliosis, a chest wound, extreme obesity, or deformities resulting from chest surgery

(see page 488). This disorder does not stop air from moving in and out of the lungs, but without blood flow to a portion of the lungs, oxygen is not properly extracted from the air.

Symptoms

Low oxygen levels in the blood can cause shortness of breath and result in a bluish coloration to the skin (cyanosis). Low oxygen levels, high carbon dioxide levels, and increasing acidity of the blood cause confusion and sleepiness. If the drive to breathe is normal, the body tries to rid itself of carbon dioxide by deep, rapid breathing. If the lungs cannot function normally, however, this breathing pattern may not help. Eventually, the brain and heart malfunction, resulting in drowsiness (sometimes to the point of becoming unconscious) and abnormal heart rhythms (arrhythmias), both of which can lead to death.

Some symptoms of respiratory failure vary with the cause. A child with an obstructed airway due to the inhalation (aspiration) of a foreign object (such as a coin or a toy) may suddenly gasp and struggle for breath. People with acute respiratory distress syndrome may become severely short of breath over a period of hours. Someone who is intoxicated or weak may quietly slip into a coma.

Diagnosis

A doctor may suspect respiratory failure because of the symptoms and physical examination findings. A blood test done on a sample taken from an artery confirms the diagnosis when it shows a dangerously low level of oxygen or a dangerously high level of carbon dioxide. Chest x-rays and other tests are done to determine the cause of respiratory failure.

Treatment

People with respiratory failure are treated in an intensive care unit. Oxygen is given initially, usually in a greater amount than is needed, but the amount of oxygen can be adjusted at a later time. Occasionally, in people in whom carbon dioxide levels have remained high for some time, excess oxygen can result in slowing of the movement of air (ventilation) in and out of the lungs and a dangerous further increase in the carbon dioxide level. In such people, the dosage of oxygen needs to be more carefully regulated.

The underlying disorder causing the respiratory failure must also be treated. For example, antibiotics are used to fight bacterial infection, and bronchodilators are used in people with asthma to open the airways. Other drugs may be given, for example, to decrease inflammation or treat blood clots. Mechanical ventilation is necessary unless respiratory failure resolves rapidly.

Acute Respiratory Distress Syndrome

Acute respiratory distress syndrome is a type of respiratory (lung) failure resulting from many different disorders that cause fluid to accumulate in the lungs and oxygen levels in the blood to be too low.

- The person experiences shortness of breath, usually with rapid, shallow breathing, the skin may become mottled or blue (cyanosis), and other organs such as the heart and brain may malfunction.
- A blood sample is taken from an artery and analyzed to determine the levels of oxygen in the blood, and a chest x-ray is also taken.

Causes of Acute Respiratory Distress Syndrome

- Aspiration (inhalation) of food into the lung
- Burns
- Coronary bypass surgery
- Chest injury (pulmonary contusion)
- Inflammation of the pancreas (pancreatitis)
- Inhalation of large amounts of smoke
- Inhalation of other toxic gas
- Injury to the lungs from inhaling high concentrations of oxygen
- Major trauma
- Near drowning
- Overdose of certain drugs, such as heroin, methadone, propoxyphene, or aspirin
- Pneumonia
- Prolonged or severe low blood pressure (shock)
- Pulmonary embolism
- Severe, widespread infection (sepsis)
- Stroke or seizure
- Transfusions of more than about 15 units of blood in a short period of time

- People are treated in an intensive care unit because they may need mechanical ventilation.
- Oxygen is given and the cause of the lung failure is treated.

The acute respiratory distress syndrome (ARDS) is a medical emergency. It may occur in people who already have lung disease or in those with previously normal lungs. This syndrome used to be called the adult respiratory distress syndrome, although it can occur in children. The less severe form of this syndrome is called acute lung injury (ALI).

Causes

Any disease or condition that injures the lungs can cause ARDS. More than half of the people with ARDS develop it as a consequence of a severe, widespread infection (sepsis) or pneumonia.

When the small air sacs (alveoli) and tiny blood vessels (capillaries) of the lungs are injured, blood and fluid leak into the spaces between the air sacs and eventually into the sacs themselves. Collapse of many alveoli (a condition called atelectasis—see page 495) may also result because of a reduction in surfactant, a liquid that coats the inside surface of the alveoli and helps to keep them open. Fluid in the alveoli and the collapse of many alveoli interfere with the movement of oxygen from inhaled air into the blood, causing oxygen levels in the blood to decrease sharply. Movement of

carbon dioxide from the blood to air that is exhaled is affected less, and levels of carbon dioxide in the blood change very little.

The decreased blood oxygen levels caused by ARDS and the leakage into the bloodstream of certain proteins (cytokines) produced by injured lung cells and white blood cells can lead to inflammation and complications in other organs. Failure of several organs (a condition called multiple organ system failure) may also result. Organ failure can begin soon after the onset of ARDS or days or weeks later. Additionally, people with ARDS are less able to fight lung infections, and they tend to develop bacterial pneumonia.

Symptoms

ARDS usually develops within 24 to 48 hours of the original injury or disease but may take as long as 4 or 5 days to occur. The person first experiences shortness of breath, usually with rapid, shallow breathing. Using a stethoscope, a doctor may hear crackling or wheezing sounds in the lungs. The skin may become mottled or blue (cyanosis) because of low oxygen levels in the blood, and other organs such as the heart and brain may malfunction, resulting in a rapid heart rate, abnormal heart rhythms (arrhythmias), confusion, and lethargy.

Diagnosis

Analysis of a blood sample taken from an artery indicates low levels of oxygen in the blood, and chest x-rays show fluid in spaces that should be filled with air. Further tests may be needed to ensure that heart failure is not the cause of the problem (see page 352).

Prognosis

Without prompt treatment, the severe oxygen deprivation causes death in 90% of people with ARDS. However, with appropriate treatment, about three fourths of people with ARDS survive.

People who respond promptly to treatment usually recover completely with few or no long-term lung abnormalities. Those whose treatment involves long periods on a ventilator are more likely to develop lung scarring. Such scarring may decrease over a few months after the person is taken off the ventilator. Lung scarring, if extensive, can impair lung function in ways that are noticeable during certain day-to-day activities. Less extensive scarring may impair lung function only when the lungs are stressed, such as during exercise or an illness.

Many people lose large amounts of weight and muscle during the illness. Rehabilitation in the hospital can help them regain their strength and independence.

Treatment

People with ARDS are treated in an intensive care unit. Successful treatment usually depends on treating the underlying disorder (for example, pneumonia). Oxygen therapy, which is vital to correcting low oxygen levels, also is given.

If oxygen delivered by a face mask or nasal prongs does not correct the low blood oxygen levels, or if very high doses of inhaled oxygen are required, mechanical ventilation must be used. Usually a ventilator delivers oxygen-rich air under pressure using a tube inserted through the mouth into the windpipe (trachea). For people who have ARDS, the ventilator pressure is delivered during the inhaled breath and at a lower pressure during exhalation (called positive end-expiratory pressure), which helps keep the alveoli open at the end of exhalation.

Mechanical Ventilation

Mechanical ventilation is use of a machine to aid the movement of air into and out of the lungs.

Some people with respiratory failure (see page 524) need a mechanical ventilator (a machine that helps air get in and out of the lungs) to aid breathing. Mechanical ventilation can be lifesaving.

Mechanical ventilation can be delivered many ways. Usually a plastic tube is inserted through the nose or mouth into the windpipe (trachea). If people need mechanical ventilation for more than a few days, doctors may insert the tube directly into the trachea through a small incision in the front of the neck (tracheostomy). A tracheostomy is safer and more comfortable for long-term ventilation. The tube is then attached to the ventilator. Exhalation occurs passively because of the elastic recoil of the lungs. Many types of ventilators and modes of operation may be used, depending on the underlying disorder. Depending on the person's needs, the ventilator delivers pure oxygen or a mixture of oxygen and air.

Alternatives: Some people do not require complete support of their breathing. These people may be treated with a tight-fitting mask placed over the nose or nose and mouth. A mixture of oxygen and air is delivered under pressure through the mask. The pressure assists the person's own breathing efforts and prevents fatigue of the respiratory muscles. In about half of the people with respiratory failure, this technique (called bilevel positive airway pressure or continuous positive airway pressure) can avoid the need to intubate the trachea. Use of bilevel positive airway pressure at night can help people whose respiratory failure is caused by muscle weakness, because after resting at night, the respiratory muscles are able to function more effectively during the day.

Complications: Pushing air into the lungs under too much pressure or with too high a volume can overstretch the lungs and cause lung damage. Sometimes the fragile alveoli (small air sacs in the lungs) rupture, allowing air to accumulate around the lung and collapse it, a condition called pneumothorax (see page 520). To avoid these problems, doctors try to limit the volume and pressure of air delivered by the ventilator. On the other hand, too little pressure and volume may not move enough air in and out, causing the blood to become too acidic and letting the small airways and alveoli close. Doctors constantly monitor and adjust the frequency and size of breaths delivered by the ventilator and the ventilator pressure to strike a careful balance.

Although most people undergoing mechanical ventilation need extra oxygen, too much oxygen actually can damage the lungs. Doctors monitor the person's oxygen level to ensure that just the right amount is given.

People undergoing mechanical ventilation, particularly with intubation of the trachea, may experience agitation, which can be controlled with sedating drugs, such as propofol, lorazepam, and midazolam, or opioids, such as morphine or fentanyl. These drugs can also help relieve breathlessness.

When the trachea is intubated, bacteria from the nose and mouth can easily enter the lungs and cause serious infection. These infections must be diagnosed and treated as quickly as possible.

Because people on mechanical ventilation cannot eat, nutritional support is usually provided by giving liquid supplements through a tube positioned in the stomach.

88 Cancer of the Lungs

- Cigarette smoking is the most common cause of lung cancer.
- One common presenting symptom is a persistent cough.
- Chest x-rays can detect most lung cancers, but other additional imaging tests and biopsies are needed.
- Surgery, chemotherapy, targeted agents, and radiation therapy may all be used to treat lung cancer.

Lung cancer is the leading cause of cancer death in both men and women. It occurs most commonly between the ages of 45 and 70 and has become more prevalent in women in the last few decades because more women are smoking cigarettes.

Cancer that originates from lung cells is called a primary lung cancer. Primary lung cancer can start in the airways that branch off the trachea to supply the lungs (the bronchi) or in the small air sacs of the lung (the alveoli). Cancer may also spread (metastasize) to the lung from other parts of the body (most commonly from the breasts, colon, prostate, kidneys, thyroid gland, stomach, cervix, rectum, testes, bone, or skin).

There are two main categories of lung cancer.

- **Non–small cell lung carcinoma:** About 85 to 87% of lung cancers are in this category. This cancer grows more slowly than small cell lung carcinoma. Nevertheless, by the time about 40% of people are diagnosed, the cancer has spread to other parts of the body outside of the chest. The most common types of non–small cell lung carcinoma are squamous cell carcinoma, adenocarcinoma, and large cell carcinoma.
- **Small cell lung carcinoma:** Also called oat cell carcinoma, this cancer accounts for about 13 to 15% of all lung cancers. It is very aggressive and spreads quickly. By the time that most people are diagnosed, the cancer has metastasized to other parts of the body.

Causes

Cigarette smoking is the leading cause of cancer, accounting for about 85% of all lung cancer cases. About 10% of all smokers (former or current) eventually develop lung cancer, and both the number of cigarettes smoked and number of years of smoking seem to correlate with the increased risk. In people who quit smoking, the risk of developing lung cancer decreases, but former smokers will still always have a higher risk of developing lung cancer than people who never smoked.

About 15% of people who develop lung cancer have never smoked. In these people, the reason why they develop lung cancer is unknown. Recent studies have found that some people with lung cancer who have never smoked have genetic mutations in the epidermal growth factor receptor (*EGFR*) gene. Although an environmental association has not clearly been established, it is believed that exposure to radon gas in the home may be a risk factor. Other possible risk factors include exposure to secondhand smoke and exposure to carcinogens such as asbestos, radiation, arsenic, chromates, nickel, chloromethyl ethers, mustard gas, or coke-oven emissions, encountered or breathed in at work. It is believed that the risk of contracting lung cancer is greater in people who are exposed to these substances and who also smoke cigarettes. Air pollution and cigar smoke also contain carcinogens, and exposure to these substances is associated with an increased risk of cancer. In rare incidences, lung cancers, especially adenocarcinoma and bronchioloalveolar cell carcinoma (a type of adenocarcinoma), develop in people whose lungs have been scarred by other lung disorders, such as tuberculosis.

Symptoms

The symptoms of lung cancer depend on its type, its location, and the way it spreads. One of the more common symptoms is a persistent cough or, in people who have a chronic cough, a change in the character of the cough. Some people cough up blood or sputum streaked with blood (hemoptysis—see page 452). Rarely, lung cancer grows into an underlying blood vessel and causes severe bleeding. Additional nonspecific symptoms of lung cancer include loss of appetite, weight loss, fatigue, chest pain, and weakness.

Complications: Lung cancer may cause wheezing by narrowing the airway. Blockage of an airway by a tumor may lead to the collapse of the part of the lung that the airway supplies, a condition called atelectasis (see page 495). Other consequences of a blocked airway are shortness of breath and pneumonia, which may result in coughing, fever, and chest pain. If the tumor grows into the chest wall, it may produce persistent, unrelenting chest pain. Fluid containing cancerous cells can accumulate in the space between the lung and the chest wall (pleural effusion—see page 518). Large amounts of fluid can lead to shortness of breath. If the cancer spreads throughout the lungs, the levels of oxygen in the blood drop and become low, causing shortness

Deaths Due to Lung Cancer

Among cancers, lung cancer is the most common cause of death in men and women. The number of deaths due to lung cancer has been decreasing in men and appears to be leveling off in women after increasing for several decades. These trends reflect a decrease in the number of smokers over the last 30 years. In 2008, more than 162,000 people are expected to have died of lung cancer—about 91,000 men and 71,000 women. This number represents about 28% of all deaths due to cancer.

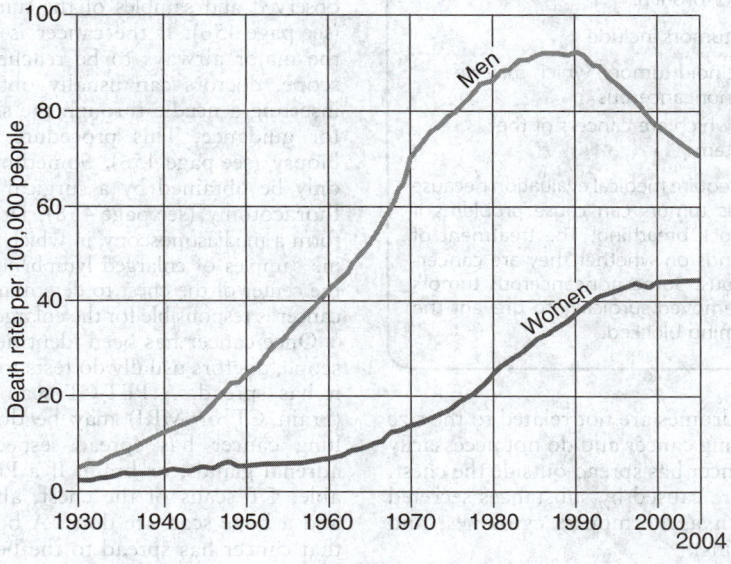

of breath and eventually enlargement of the right side of the heart and possible heart failure (cor pulmonale—see box on page 523).

Lung cancer may grow into certain nerves in the neck, causing a droopy eyelid, small pupil, sunken eye, and reduced perspiration on one side of the face—together these symptoms are called Horner's syndrome (see page 834). Cancers at the top of the lung may grow into the nerves that supply the arm, making the arm painful, numb, and weak. Tumors in this location are often called Pancoast's tumors. When the tumor grows into nerves in the center of the chest, the nerve to the voice box may become damaged, making the voice hoarse.

Lung cancer may grow into or near the esophagus, leading to difficulty swallowing or pain with swallowing.

Lung cancer may grow into the heart or in the midchest (mediastinal) region, causing abnormal heart rhythms, blockage of blood flow through the heart, or fluid in the sac surrounding the heart (pericardial sac).

The cancer may grow into or compress one of the large veins in the chest (the superior vena cava); this condition is called superior vena cava syndrome. Obstruction of the superior vena cava causes blood to back up in other veins of the upper body. The veins in the chest wall enlarge. The face, neck, and upper chest wall—including the breasts—can swell, causing pain. The condition can also produce shortness of breath, headache, distorted vision, dizziness, and drowsiness. These symptoms usually worsen when the person bends forward or lies down.

Lung cancer may also spread through the bloodstream to other parts of the body, most commonly the liver, brain, adrenal glands, spinal cord, or bones. The spread of lung cancer may occur early in the course of disease, especially with small cell lung cancer. Symptoms—such as headache, confusion, seizures, and bone pain—may develop before any lung problems become evident, making an early diagnosis more complicated.

Paraneoplastic syndromes (see box on page 1082) consist of effects that are caused by cancer but occur far from the cancer itself, such as in nerves and

Uncommon Lung Tumors

Lung tumors can be cancerous or noncancerous. Some less common noncancerous lung tumors include

- Hamartomas, which are the most common noncancerous lung tumors
- Bronchial cystadenomas, which grow in the main or smaller bronchi

Rare cancerous tumors include

- Bronchial carcinoid tumors, which may be cancerous or noncancerous
- Lymphomas, which are cancers of the lymphatic system

All lung tumors require medical evaluation because even noncancerous tumors can cause problems if they grow and block breathing. The treatment of lung tumors depends on whether they are cancerous or noncancerous. Some noncancerous tumors may need to be removed surgically to prevent the airway from becoming blocked.

muscles. These syndromes are not related to the size or location of the lung cancer and do not necessarily indicate that the cancer has spread outside the chest. These syndromes are caused by substances secreted by the cancer (such as hormones, cytokines, and various other proteins).

Diagnosis

Doctors explore the possibility of lung cancer when a person, especially a smoker, has a persistent or worsening cough or other lung symptoms (such as shortness of breath or coughed-up sputum tinged with blood). Usually, the first test is a chest x-ray, which can detect most lung tumors, although it may miss small ones. Sometimes a shadow detected on a chest x-ray done for other reasons (such as before surgery) provides doctors with the first clue, although such a shadow is not proof of cancer.

A computed tomography (CT) scan may be done next. CT scans can show characteristic patterns that help doctors make the diagnosis. They also can show small tumors that are not visible on chest x-rays and reveal whether the lymph nodes inside the chest are enlarged. Newer techniques, such as positron emission tomography (PET—see page 456) and a certain type of CT called helical (spiral) CT, are improving the ability to detect small cancers. Oncologists frequently use PET-CT scanners, which combine the PET and CT technology in one machine, to evaluate patients with suspected cancer. Magnetic resonance imaging (MRI) can also be used if the CT or PET-CT scans do not give doctors sufficient information.

A microscopic examination of lung tissue from the area that may be cancerous is usually needed to confirm the diagnosis. In rare cases, a sample of coughed-up sputum can provide enough material for an examination (called sputum cytology). Almost always, doctors need to obtain a sample of tissue directly from the tumor. One common way to obtain the tissue sample is with bronchoscopy. The person's airway is directly observed and samples of the tumor can be obtained (see page 456). If the cancer is too far away from the major airways to be reached with a bronchoscope, doctors can usually obtain a specimen by inserting a needle through the skin while using CT for guidance. This procedure is called a needle biopsy (see page 456). Sometimes, a specimen can only be obtained by a surgical procedure called a thoracotomy (see page 458). Doctors may also perform a mediastinoscopy, in which they take and examine samples of enlarged lymph nodes (a biopsy) from the center of the chest to determine if inflammation or cancer is responsible for the enlargement.

Once cancer has been identified under the microscope, doctors usually do tests to determine whether it has spread. A PET-CT scan and head imaging (brain CT or MRI) may be done to determine if lung cancer has spread, especially to the liver, adrenal glands, or brain. If a PET-CT is not available, CT scans of the chest, abdomen, and pelvis and a bone scan are done. A bone scan may show that cancer has spread to the bones. Because small cell lung cancer can spread to the bone marrow, doctors sometimes also do a bone marrow biopsy.

Cancers are categorized on how large the tumor is, whether it has spread to nearby lymph nodes, and whether it has spread to distant organs. The different categories are used to determine the stage of the cancer (see page 1083). The stage of a cancer suggests the most appropriate treatment and enables doctors to estimate the person's prognosis.

Screening: Clinical trials are underway to determine the value of screening tests to detect lung cancer in people who do not have any symptoms. These trials use chest x-rays, CT scans, sputum examinations, or all these methods to try to detect cancer when it is at an early stage. However, screening so far has not been shown to improve lung cancer detection, and therefore screening is not recommended for people who have no risk factors and no symptoms. Tests can be expensive and cause people undue worry if they produce false-positive results that incorrectly imply that a cancer is present. The opposite is also true. A screening test can give a negative result when a cancer really does exist. For these reasons, it is important for doctors to try to accurately determine a person's risk for a particular cancer before screening tests are done (see page 1081).

Prevention and Treatment

Prevention of lung cancer includes quitting smoking (see page 2096) and avoiding exposure to potentially cancer-causing substances in the work environment.

Doctors use various treatments for both small cell and non–small cell lung cancer. Surgery, chemotherapy, and radiation therapy can be used individually or in combination. The precise combination of treatments depends on the type, location, and severity of the cancer, whether the cancer has spread, and the person's overall health. For example, in some people with advanced non–small cell lung cancer, treatment includes chemotherapy and radiation therapy before, after, or instead of surgical removal. Some people with non–small cell lung cancer survive significantly longer when treated with chemotherapy, radiation therapy, or some of the newer targeted therapies. Targeted therapies include drugs, such as biologic agents that specifically target lung tumors. Recent studies have identified proteins within cancer cells and the blood vessels that nourish the cancer cells. These proteins may be involved in regulating and promoting cancer growth and metastasis. Drugs have been designed to specifically affect the abnormal protein expression and potentially kill the cancer cells or inhibit their growth. For example, doctors may give epidermal growth factor receptor (EGFR) tyrosine kinase inhibitors to people who have not responded to traditional chemotherapy regimens. Some people may receive vascular endothelial growth factor (VEGF) and VEGF receptor inhibitors in combination with standard chemotherapy regimens.

Laser therapy, in which a laser is used to remove or reduce the size of lung tumors, and photodynamic therapy, in which light is used to shrink tumors, are sometimes used. Radiofrequency ablation, in which an electrical current is used to destroy tumor cells, can sometimes be used in people who have small tumors or are unable to undergo surgery.

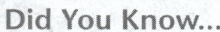

Did You Know...

Although smoking causes most cases, people who have never smoked may still get lung cancer.

Surgery: Surgery is the treatment of choice for non–small cell lung cancer that has not spread beyond the lung (early-stage disease). In general, surgery is not used for early-stage small cell lung cancer, because this aggressive cancer requires chemotherapy and radiation therapy. Surgery may not be possible if the cancer has spread beyond the lungs, if the cancer is too close to the windpipe, or if the person has other serious conditions (such as severe heart or lung disease).

Before surgery, doctors do pulmonary function tests (see page 454) to determine whether the amount of lung remaining after surgery will be able to provide enough oxygen and breathing function. If the test results indicate that removing the cancerous part of the lung will result in inadequate lung function, surgery is not possible. The amount of lung to be removed is decided by the surgeon, with the amount varying from a small part of a lung segment to an entire lung.

Although non–small cell lung cancers can be removed surgically, removal does not always result in a cure. Supplemental (adjuvant) chemotherapy after surgery can help increase the survival rate.

Occasionally, cancer that begins elsewhere (for example, in the colon) and spreads to the lungs is removed from the lungs after being removed at the source. This procedure is recommended rarely, and tests must show that the cancer has not spread to any site outside of the lungs.

Radiation Therapy: Radiation therapy is used in both non-small cell and small cell lung cancers. It may be given to people who do not want to undergo surgery, who cannot undergo surgery because they have another condition (such as severe coronary artery disease), or whose cancer has spread to nearby structures, such as the lymph nodes. Although radiation therapy is used to treat the cancer, in some people, it may only partially shrink the cancer or slow its growth. Combining chemotherapy with radiation therapy improves survival in this group. People with limited or extensive-stage small cell lung cancer who have been responding well to chemotherapy may benefit from radiation therapy to the head to prevent spread of cancer to the brain. If the cancer has already spread to the brain, radiation therapy of the brain is commonly used to reduce symptoms such as headache, confusion, and seizures. Radiation therapy is also useful for controlling the complications of lung cancer, such as coughing up of blood, bone pain, superior vena cava syndrome, and spinal cord compression.

Chemotherapy: Chemotherapy is used in both non-small cell and small cell lung cancers. In small cell lung cancer, chemotherapy, sometimes coupled with radiation therapy, is the main treatment. This approach is preferred because small cell lung cancer is aggressive and has often spread to distant parts of the body by the time of diagnosis. Chemotherapy can prolong survival in people who have extensive-stage disease. Without treatment, the median survival is only 6 to 12 weeks.

In non–small cell lung cancer, chemotherapy also prolongs survival and treats symptoms. In people with non–small cell lung cancer that has spread to other parts of the body, the median survival increases to 9 months with treatment. Targeted therapies may also improve cancer patient survival.

Other Treatments: Other treatments are often needed for people who have lung cancer. Because many people who have lung cancer have a substantial decrease in lung function whether or not they undergo treatment, oxygen therapy (see page 460) and bronchodilators (drugs that widen the airways) may aid breathing. Many people with advanced lung cancer develop such extreme pain and difficulty in breathing that they require large doses of opioids in the weeks or months before their death. Fortunately, opioids can substantially relieve pain if adequate doses are used.

Prognosis

Lung cancer has a poor prognosis. On average, people with untreated advanced non–small cell lung cancer survive 6 months. Even with treatment, people with extensive small cell lung cancer or advanced non–small cell lung cancer do especially poorly,

with a 5-year survival rate of less than 1%. Early diagnosis improves survival. People with early non–small cell lung cancer have a 5-year survival of 60 to 70%. However, people who are treated definitively for an earlier stage lung cancer and survive but continue to smoke are at high risk of developing another lung cancer.

Survivors must have regular checkups, including periodic chest x-rays and CT scans to ensure that the cancer has not returned. Usually, if the cancer returns, it occurs within the first 2 years. However, frequent monitoring is recommended for 5 years after lung cancer treatment, and then people are monitored yearly for the rest of their lives.

Because many people die of lung cancer, planning for terminal care is usually necessary. Advances in end-of-life care, particularly the recognition that anxiety and pain are common in people with incurable lung cancer and that these symptoms can be relieved by appropriate drugs, have led to an increasing number of people being able to die comfortably at home, with or without hospice services (see page 61).

Bone, Joint, and Muscle Disorders

CHAPTER

89   Biology of the Musculoskeletal System

The musculoskeletal system provides form, stability, and movement to the human body. It consists of the body's bones (which make up the skeleton), muscles, tendons, ligaments, joints, cartilage, and other connective tissue. The term "connective tissue" is used to describe the tissue that supports and binds tissues and organs together. Its chief components are elastic fibers and collagen, a protein substance.

Bones

Bone, although strong, is a constantly changing tissue that has several functions. Bones serve as rigid structures to the body and as shields to protect delicate internal organs. They provide housing for the bone marrow, where the blood cells are formed. Bones also maintain the body's reservoir of calcium. In children, some bones have areas called growth plates. Bones lengthen in these areas until the child reaches full height, at which time the growth plates close. Thereafter, bones grow in thickness rather than in length, based on the body's need for additional bone strength in certain areas.

Bones have two shapes: flat (such as the plates of the skull and the vertebrae) and tubular (such as the thighbones and arm bones, which are called long bones). All bones have essentially the same structure. The hard outer part (cortical bone) consists largely of proteins, such as collagen, and a substance called hydroxyapatite, which is composed mainly of calcium and other minerals. Hydroxyapatite is largely responsible for the strength and density of bones. The inner part of bones (trabecular bone) is softer and less dense than the hard outer part. Bone marrow is the tissue that fills the spaces in the trabecular bone. Bone marrow contains specialized cells (including stem cells) that produce blood cells. Blood vessels supply blood to the bone, and nerves surround the bone.

> **? Did You Know...**
> Bone structure adjusts throughout life in response to activity and stress (for example, weight-bearing exercise).

Bones undergo a continuous process known as remodeling (see page 544). In this process, old bone tissue is gradually replaced by new bone tissue. Every bone in the body is completely reformed about every 10 years. To maintain bone density and strength, the body requires an adequate supply of calcium, other minerals, and vitamin D and must produce the proper amounts of several hormones, such as parathyroid hormone, growth hormone, calcitonin, estrogen, and testosterone. Activity (for example, weight-bearing exercises for the legs) helps bones strengthen by remodeling. With activity and optimal amounts of hormones, vitamins, and minerals, trabecular bone develops into a complex lattice structure that is lightweight but strong.

Bones are covered by a thin membrane called the periosteum. Injury to bone transmits pain because of nerves located mostly in the periosteum. Blood enters bones through blood vessels that enter through the periosteum.

Muscles

There are three types of muscles: skeletal, smooth, and cardiac (heart). Two of these kinds—skeletal and smooth—are part of the musculoskeletal system.

Skeletal muscle is what most people think of as muscle, the type that can be contracted to move the various parts of the body. Skeletal muscles are bundles of contractile fibers that are organized in a regular pattern, so that under a microscope they appear as stripes (hence, they are also called striped or striated muscles). Skeletal muscles vary in their speeds of contraction. Skeletal muscles, which are responsible for posture and movement, are attached to bones and arranged in opposing groups around joints. For example, muscles that bend the elbow (biceps) are countered by muscles that straighten it (triceps). These countering movements are balanced. The balance makes movements smooth, which helps prevent damage to the musculoskeletal system. Skeletal muscles are controlled by the brain and are considered voluntary muscles because they operate with a person's awareness. The size and strength of skeletal muscles are maintained or increased by regular exercise. In addition, growth hormone and testosterone help muscles grow in childhood and maintain their size in adulthood.

Smooth muscles control certain bodily functions that are not readily under a person's control. Smooth muscle surrounds many arteries and contracts to adjust blood flow. It surrounds the intestines and contracts to move food and feces along the digestive tract. Smooth muscle also is controlled by the brain but not voluntarily. The triggers for contracting and relaxing smooth muscles are controlled by the body's needs, so

Inside the Knee

The knee is designed for its own protection. It is completely surrounded by a joint capsule that is flexible enough to allow movement but strong enough to hold the joint together. The capsule is lined with synovial tissue, which secretes synovial fluid to lubricate the joint. Wear-resistant cartilage covering the ends of the thighbone (femur) and shinbone (tibia) helps reduce friction during movement. Pads of cartilage (menisci) act as cushions between the two bones and help distribute body weight in the joint. Fluid-filled sacs (bursae) provide cushioning between structures such as the tibia and the tendon attached to the kneecap (patellar tendon). Five ligaments along the sides and the back of the knee reinforce the joint capsule, adding stability. The kneecap (patella) protects the front of the joint.

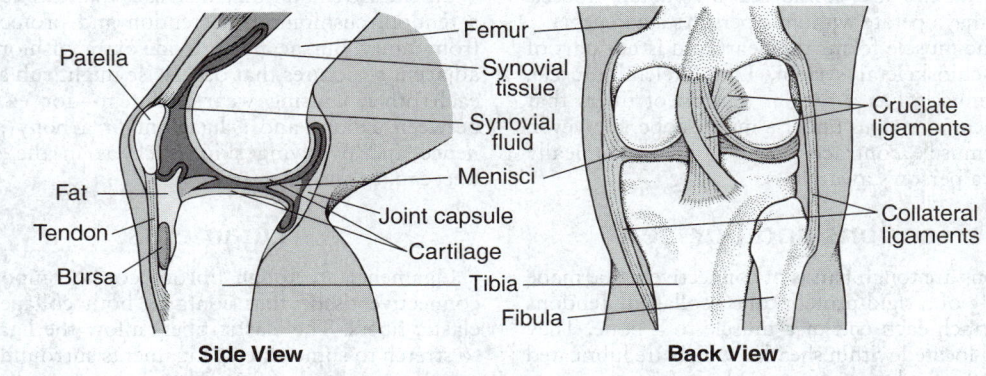

Side View **Back View**

Musculoskeletal System

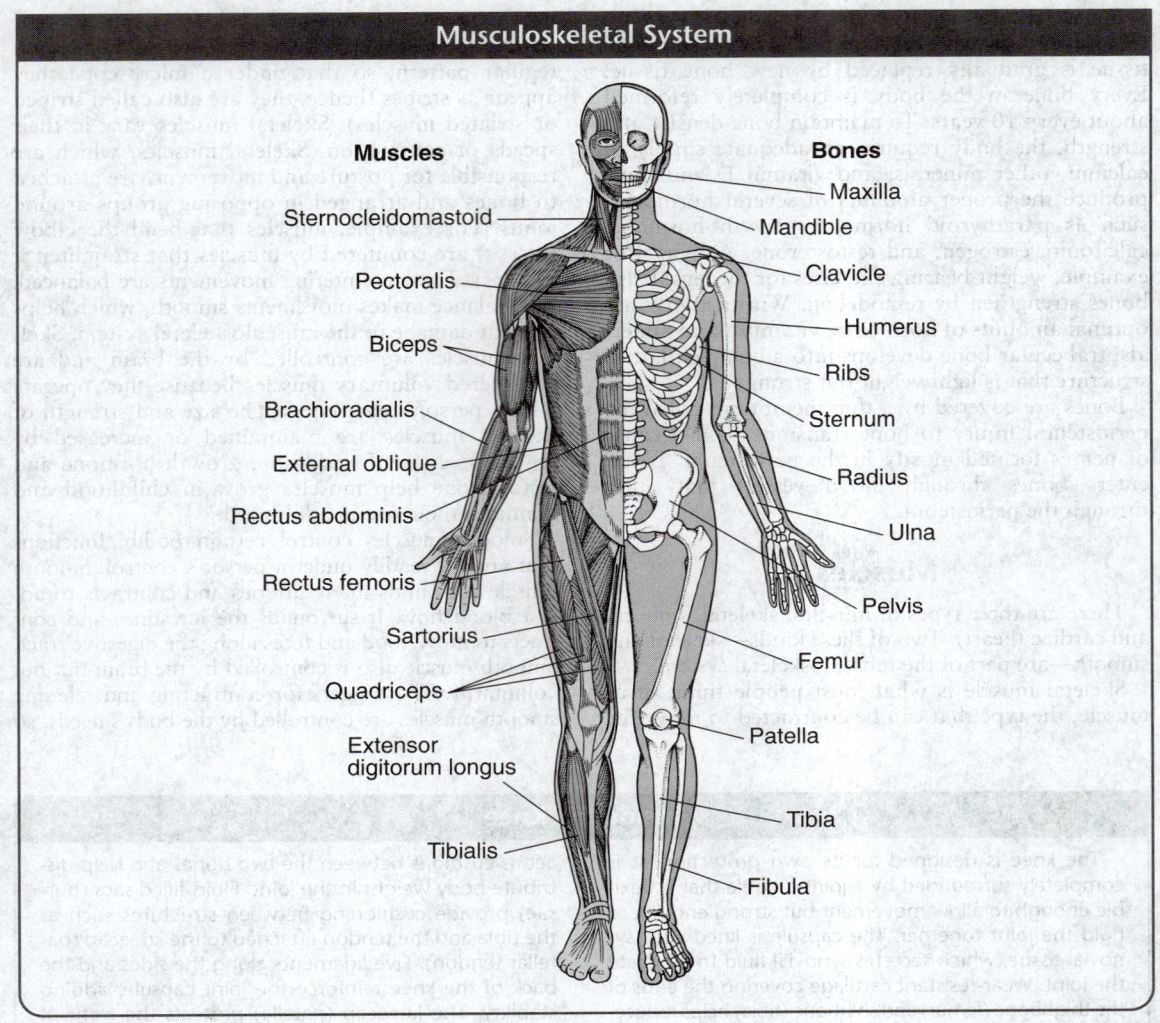

Muscles

- Sternocleidomastoid
- Pectoralis
- Biceps
- Brachioradialis
- External oblique
- Rectus abdominis
- Rectus femoris
- Sartorius
- Quadriceps
- Extensor digitorum longus
- Tibialis

Bones

- Maxilla
- Mandible
- Clavicle
- Humerus
- Ribs
- Sternum
- Radius
- Ulna
- Pelvis
- Femur
- Patella
- Tibia
- Fibula

smooth muscles are considered involuntary muscle because they operate without a person's awareness.

Cardiac muscle forms the heart and is not part of the musculoskeletal system. Like skeletal muscle, cardiac muscle has a regular pattern of fibers that also appear as stripes under a microscope. However, cardiac muscle contracts and relaxes rhythmically without a person's awareness.

Tendons and Bursae

Tendons are tough bands of connective tissue made up mostly of a rigid protein called collagen. Tendons firmly attach each end of a muscle to a bone. They are often located within sheaths, which are lubricated to allow the tendons to move without friction.

Bursae are small fluid-filled sacs that can lie under a tendon, cushioning the tendon and protecting it from injury. Bursae also provide extra cushioning to adjacent structures that otherwise might rub against each other, causing wear and tear—for example, between a bone and a ligament or a bony prominence and overlying skin (such as in the elbow, kneecap, or shoulder area).

Ligaments

Ligaments are tough fibrous cords composed of connective tissue that contains both collagen and elastic fibers. The elastic fibers allow the ligaments to stretch to some extent. Ligaments surround joints and bind them together. They help strengthen and

Musculoskeletal System

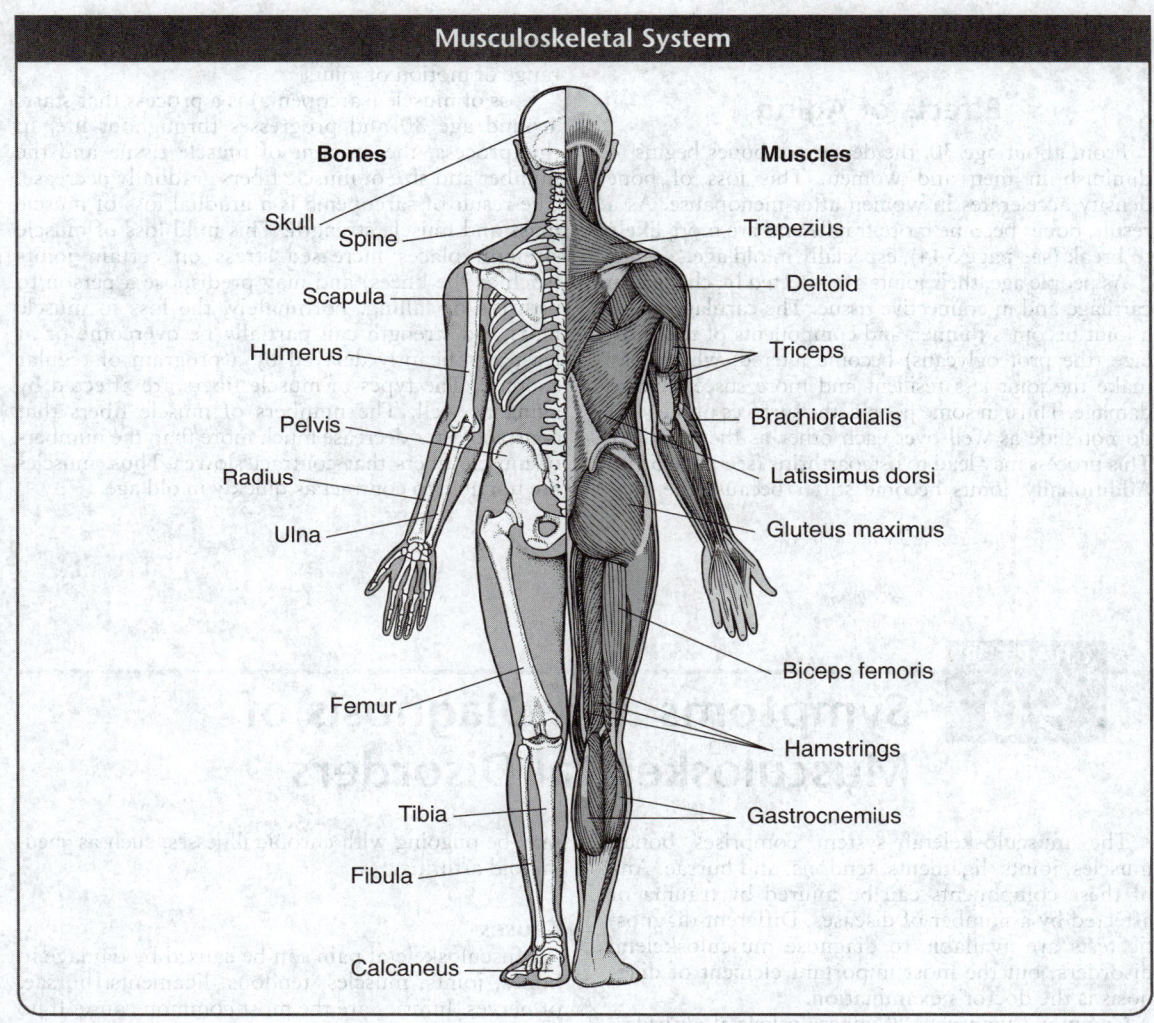

Bones

Skull
Spine
Scapula
Humerus
Pelvis
Radius
Ulna
Femur
Tibia
Fibula
Calcaneus

Muscles

Trapezius
Deltoid
Triceps
Brachioradialis
Latissimus dorsi
Gluteus maximus
Biceps femoris
Hamstrings
Gastrocnemius

stabilize joints, permitting movement only in certain directions. Ligaments also connect one bone to another (such as inside the knee).

Joints

Joints are the junction between two or more bones. Some joints do not normally move, such as those located between the plates of the skull. Other joints allow a large and complex range of motion. The configuration of a joint determines the degree and direction of possible motion. For example, the shoulder joints, which have a ball-and-socket design, allow inward and outward rotation as well as forward,

backward, and sideways motion of the arms. Hinge joints of the knees, fingers, and toes allow only bending (flexion) and straightening (extension).

The components of joints provide stability and reduce the risk of damage from constant use. In a joint, the ends of the bones are covered with cartilage—a smooth, tough, resilient, and protective tissue composed of collagen, water, and proteoglycans that reduces friction as joints move. (Collagen is a tough fibrous tissue; proteoglycans are substances that provide the cartilage's resilience.) Joints also have a lining (synovial tissue) that encloses them to form the joint capsule. Cells in the synovial tissue produce a small amount of clear fluid (synovial fluid), which provides nourishment to the cartilage and further reduces friction while facilitating movement.

Effects of Aging

From about age 30, the density of bones begins to diminish in men and women. This loss of bone density accelerates in women after menopause. As a result, bones become more fragile and are more likely to break (see page 544), especially in old age.

As people age, their joints are affected by changes in cartilage and in connective tissue. The cartilage inside a joint becomes thinner, and components of the cartilage (the proteoglycans) become altered, which may make the joint less resilient and more susceptible to damage. Thus, in some people, the surfaces of the joint do not slide as well over each other as they used to. This process may lead to osteoarthritis (see page 559). Additionally, joints become stiffer because the con-

nective tissue within ligaments and tendons becomes more rigid and brittle. This change also limits the range of motion of joints.

Loss of muscle (sarcopenia) is a process that starts around age 30 and progresses throughout life. In this process, the amount of muscle tissue and the number and size of muscle fibers gradually decrease. The result of sarcopenia is a gradual loss of muscle mass and muscle strength. This mild loss of muscle strength places increased stress on certain joints (such as the knees) and may predispose a person to arthritis or falling. Fortunately, the loss in muscle mass and strength can partially be overcome or at least significantly delayed by a program of regular exercise. The types of muscle fibers are affected by aging as well. The numbers of muscle fibers that contract faster decrease much more than the numbers of muscle fibers that contract slower. Thus, muscles are not able to contract as quickly in old age.

CHAPTER

90   Symptoms and Diagnosis of Musculoskeletal Disorders

The musculoskeletal system comprises bones, muscles, joints, ligaments, tendons, and bursae. Any of these components can be injured by trauma or affected by a number of diseases. Different diagnostic tests are available to diagnose musculoskeletal disorders, but the most important element of diagnosis is the doctor's examination.

Common symptoms of musculoskeletal disorders include pain, weakness, stiffness, joint noises, and decreased range of motion. Inflammation can cause pain, swelling, warmth, tenderness, impaired function, and sometimes redness. Inflammation can result from many different musculoskeletal disorders, including autoimmune disorders and infections. Inflammation affects a joint; fluid may accumulate inside the joint, causing swelling and decreased range of motion.

Symptoms

PAIN

Pain is the chief symptom of most musculoskeletal disorders. The pain may be mild or severe, local or widespread (diffuse). Although pain may be acute and short-lived, as is the case with most injuries, pain

may be ongoing with chronic illnesses, such as rheumatoid arthritis.

Causes

Musculoskeletal pain can be caused by damage to bones, joints, muscles, tendons, ligaments, bursae, or nerves. Injuries are the most common cause. If no injury has occurred or if pain persists for more than a few days, then another cause is often responsible.

Bone pain is usually deep, penetrating, or dull. It commonly results from injury. Other less common causes of bone pain include bone infection (osteomyelitis) and tumors.

Muscle pain is often less intense than bone pain but can be very unpleasant. For example, a muscle spasm or cramp (a sustained painful muscle contraction) in the calf is an intense pain that is commonly called a charley horse. Pain can occur when a muscle is affected by an injury, an autoimmune reaction (for example, polymyositis or dermatomyositis), loss of blood flow to the muscle, infection, or invasion by a tumor.

Tendon and ligament pain is often less intense than bone pain. It is often worse when the affected tendon or ligament is stretched or moved. Common causes of tendon pain include tendinitis, tenosynovitis, lateral and medial epicondylitis, and tendon injuries. Common causes of ligament pain include injuries (sprains).

Fibromyalgia may cause pain in the muscles, tendons, or ligaments. The pain is usually in multiple locations and may be difficult to describe precisely. Affected people usually have other symptoms.

Virtually all joint injuries and diseases produce a stiff, aching pain, often referred to as "arthritic" pain. The pain is worse when the joint is moved and may range from mild to severe. With some conditions, there may be swelling of the joint along with the pain. Joint inflammation (arthritis) is a common cause of joint pain. There are many types of arthritis, including rheumatoid and other types of inflammatory arthritis, osteoarthritis, infectious arthritis, and arthritis due to gout or pseudogout. Other causes of joint pain include autoimmune and vasculitic disorders (for example, systemic lupus erythematosus, polymyalgia rheumatica, and polyarteritis nodosa), avascular necrosis of bone, and injuries (for example, dislocations, sprains, and fractures affecting the portion of the bone inside the joint). Sometimes, pain originating in structures near the joint, such as tendons and bursae, seems to be coming from the joint.

Some musculoskeletal disorders cause pain by compressing nerves. These conditions include the "tunnel syndromes" (for example, carpal tunnel syndrome, cubital tunnel syndrome, and tarsal tunnel syndrome). The pain tends to radiate along the path supplied by the nerve and may be burning.

Bursal pain can be caused by bursitis or fibromyalgia. Usually, bursal pain is worse with movement involving the bursa. There may be swelling.

Sometimes, pain that seems to be musculoskeletal is actually caused by a disorder in another organ system. For instance, shoulder pain may be caused by a disorder affecting the spleen or gallbladder. Back pain may be caused by an abdominal aortic aneurysm. Arm pain may be caused by a heart attack (myocardial infarction). Additionally, sometimes pain that seems to be coming from one part of the musculoskeletal system actually comes from another part. For instance, knee pain in an adolescent may be caused by a disorder of the hip called slipped capital femoral epiphysis.

Evaluation and Treatment

Sometimes, the type of pain suggests where the pain has originated. For example, pain that worsens with motion suggests a musculoskeletal disorder. Pain with muscle spasm suggests that pain is caused by a muscle disorder. The site of swelling or the location of tenderness when the doctor palpates the area (for example, a joint, ligament, or bursa) often indicates the source of pain. However, often these characteristics of pain do not indicate its origin or cause. Thus, doctors usually base a specific diagnosis on the presence of other symptoms and often on the results of laboratory tests and x-rays. For example, Lyme disease often causes joint pain and a bull's eye–like skin rash; blood tests show antibodies to the bacteria that cause Lyme disease. Gout is characterized by a sudden attack of pain, swelling, and redness in the joint at the base of the big toe or other joints; tests of the joint fluid generally show the presence of uric acid crystals.

Blood tests are useful only in supporting the diagnosis made by the doctor after an examination. A diagnosis is not made or confirmed by a blood test alone. Examples of such blood tests include rheumatoid factor and antinuclear antibodies, which are used to help diagnose many of the common causes of arthritis, such as rheumatoid arthritis and systemic lupus erythematosus. Usually, such tests are recommended only if symptoms specifically suggest such a disorder or are persistent or unusually severe.

X-rays are primarily used to take images of bones; they do not show muscles, tendons and ligaments. X-rays are usually taken if the doctor suspects a fracture or, less commonly, a bone tumor or infection or to look for changes that confirm a person has a certain kind of arthritis (for example, rheumatoid arthritis or osteoarthritis).

A computed tomography (CT) scan is more sensitive than an x-ray and is often used to obtain more detail about a fracture or bone problem that was found with plain x-rays.

Unlike plain x-rays, magnetic resonance imaging (MRI) can identify abnormalities of soft tissues such as muscles, bursae, ligaments, and tendons. Thus, MRI may be used when the doctor suspects damage to a major ligament or tendon or damage to important structures inside a joint.

Pain is usually best relieved by treating its cause. In addition, the doctor may recommend analgesics such as acetaminophen, nonsteroidal anti-inflammatory drugs (NSAIDs), or, if pain is severe, opioids (see page 642). Depending on the cause, applying cold or heat or immobilizing the joint may help relieve musculoskeletal pain.

DIFFICULTY MOVING

A person may have difficulty moving all or part of the body.

Causes

Moving may be difficult because of disorders that restrict joint motion or that cause weakness. Movement may also be limited when motion causes pain. Certain nervous system abnormalities interfere with movement without causing pain or weakness. For example, Parkinson's disease causes muscle stiffness, tremor, and difficulty initiating movement.

Joint Disorders: A joint that is stiffened by scar tissue from a previous injury can have limited range and speed of motion. When a normal joint is not used, it may stiffen. For example, when a person's arm is paralyzed by a stroke or even placed in a sling for a period of time, the joints in the shoulder and elbow may develop scar tissue that freezes the joint in place if the arm is not regularly flexed and stretched. Fluid that accumulates in a joint from arthritis or an acute injury can interfere with joint motion. A piece of torn cartilage from an injury (typically in the knee) may block joint motion.

Weakness: Although many people complain of weakness when they feel tired or run down, true weakness means that full effort does not generate normal muscle contractions. Normal voluntary muscle contraction requires that the brain generate a signal that then travels through the spinal cord and nerves to reach a normally functioning muscle. Therefore, true weakness can result from injury or disease affecting the nervous system, muscles, or connections between them (neuromuscular junction).

Brain problems include strokes, injuries, tumors, and degenerative disorders (such as multiple sclerosis, which also can affect the spinal cord and nerves). Spinal cord disorders include injury, bleeding, and tumors. Spinal nerve roots can be affected by a ruptured intervertebral disk, and peripheral nerves by injury or polyneuropathy. The neuromuscular junction can be affected by myasthenia gravis, drugs such as botulinum toxin injections, and certain poisons such as organophosphates (used in nerve gas and many insecticides).

Muscle disorders causing weakness include muscular dystrophy and polymyositis. The muscle weakness that commonly occurs following immobilization (in a cast or from prolonged bed rest) and in old age is due to a reduction in muscle mass (sarcopenia) and results from lack of use. The remaining muscle mass functions normally, but there is not an adequate amount.

Weakness may be limited to one extremity or part of an extremity, as is typically the case when a single nerve, joint, or muscle is affected, or diffuse, as occurs in widespread neurologic or muscular diseases.

Pain: People with pain in the muscles, ligaments, bones, or joints tend to consciously and unconsciously limit motion. This often gives the impression of weakness even though the nervous system and muscles are able to generate movement.

Evaluation and Treatment

Doctors can often diagnose weakness based on the person's symptoms and the results of the physical examination. Doctors first try to determine whether the person can contract the muscles normally. If the person can contract the muscles normally but has trouble moving a joint, the doctor tries to move the joint for the person while the person relaxes (passive motion). If motion is painful, inflammation may be the problem. If passive motion causes little pain but is blocked, joint contracture (for example, due to scar tissue) may be the problem.

If passive motion is neither painful nor blocked, the person is giving full effort, and there is no sign of Parkinson's disease or other neurologic disorder causing difficulty initiating movement, then true muscle weakness is likely. The cause of true muscle weakness can often be determined by noting the person's symptoms, which muscles are affected, whether muscles have shrunk, and muscle tone and by testing the person's reflexes with a reflex hammer. For example, if weakness affects mainly the large muscles such as the hips, thighs, and shoulders, the cause may be a disorder producing widespread damage to muscles. If weakness affects mainly the eye muscles (causing double vision), the cause may be a disorder of the neuromuscular junction. If weakness affects mainly the fingers, hands, and feet, particularly if there is loss of sensation, the cause may be a disorder that damages many nerves (polyneuropathy). The nerves to the fingers, hands, and feet are the body's longest and thus the most vulnerable peripheral nerves. If muscles have shrunk, the disorder causing the problem has been present for months or years. If the person's reflexes are decreased or slow, the cause may be nerve damage. If reflexes are increased or more rapid than expected, the cause may be spinal cord or brain damage. The doctor checks muscle tone by testing passive movement. Muscle tone may be decreased when weakness results from a peripheral nerve disorder. Muscle tone may be increased when weakness results from a spinal cord or brain disorder.

If the cause is still not clear, other tests can help. Disorders of the brain or spinal cord are diagnosed using neuroimaging tests such as CT or MRI. To differentiate between weakness caused by damage to the peripheral nerves, muscles, and neuromuscular junction, tests such as electromyography and nerve conduction studies (see page 636) usually help. Certain other disorders (for example, low blood levels of potassium or vitamin D) are diagnosed with blood tests.

For joints that are fixed, joint flexibility can be maximized by stretching exercises and physical therapy. If the joint's range of motion is severely restricted by scar tissue, surgery may be necessary. The only way to relieve weakness is to treat the disorder causing it.

CLASSIFYING WEAKNESS

UNDERLYING PROBLEM	EXAMPLE	DESCRIPTION
Muscle disease	Muscular dystrophies	A group of inherited muscle disorders that leads to muscle weakness of varying severity
	Infections or inflammatory disorders (such as acute viral myositis or polymyositis)	Muscles tender or painful and weak
Widespread muscle damage caused by use of a drug (drug-induced myopathy)	Myopathy due to corticosteroids, statins, lithium, alcohol, clofibrate, or colchicine	Weakness that usually begins at the hips and may spread to other muscles Sometimes no pain
Low blood levels of potassium	Hypokalemic myopathy (caused by certain disorders or use of diuretics)	Intermittent periods of weakness throughout the body
Abnormal levels of thyroid hormone	High levels of thyroid hormone (hyperthyroidism) or low levels of thyroid hormone (hypothyroidism)	High or low levels of thyroid hormone producing weakness that is usually more pronounced in the shoulders and hips than in the hands and feet
Low levels of vitamin D	Osteomalacia	Pain in the back, with weakness in the legs Rarely, pain throughout the body
Disease of the neuromuscular junction	Myasthenia gravis, curare toxicity, Eaton-Lambert syndrome, insecticide poisoning, botulism, or diphtheria	Weakness or paralysis affecting all or many muscles Sometimes affecting mainly eye muscles
Damage to a single nerve (mononeuropathy)	Diabetic neuropathy or local pressure	Weakness or paralysis of muscles and loss of sensation in the area served by the injured nerve
Damage to many nerves (polyneuropathy)	Diabetes, Guillain-Barré syndrome, folate deficiency, toxins, or drugs	Weakness or paralysis of muscles and loss of sensation in the areas served by the affected nerves
Spinal nerve root damage	Ruptured disk in the spine of the neck or lower back	Pain in the neck and weakness or numbness in an arm, low back pain shooting down the leg (sciatica), and leg weakness or numbness
Degeneration of nerve cell bodies in the spinal cord	Amyotrophic lateral sclerosis	Progressive loss of muscle bulk and strength, but no loss of sensation
Spinal cord damage	Trauma to the neck or back, spinal cord tumors, spinal stenosis, multiple sclerosis, transverse myelitis, or vitamin B_{12} deficiency	Weakness or paralysis of the arms and legs below the level of injury, progressive loss of sensation below the level of injury, and back pain Problems with bowel, bladder, and sexual function
Brain damage	Strokes, tumors, head trauma, multiple sclerosis, or infections	Weakness or paralysis of muscles in the area served by the injured part of the brain, often with other symptoms of brain damage
Psychologic problems	Depression or imagined symptoms or hysteria (conversion reaction)	Complaint of whole-body weakness or paralysis with no evidence of nerve damage

JOINT STIFFNESS

Stiffness is the feeling that motion of a joint is limited or difficult. The feeling is not caused by weakness or reluctance to move the joint due to pain. Some people with stiffness are capable of moving the joint through its full range of motion. Joint stiffness usually occurs or is worse immediately after awakening or resting. Stiffness is common with arthritis. Morning stiffness commonly occurs with rheumatoid arthritis and other types of inflammatory arthritis in which stiffness typically occurs on arising and gradually lessens with activity only after an hour or two.

Doctors can sometimes diagnose the cause of stiffness by the person's symptoms and the results of a physical examination. The person is examined to make sure that the problem is not pain with motion or weakness. Because arthritis is often the cause, blood tests (for example, rheumatoid factor and antinuclear antibodies) and x-rays may be done.

Stiffness is relieved by treating the disorder causing it. Stretching, physical therapy, and taking a hot shower on arising may improve the ability to perform activities that require flexibility.

JOINT NOISES

Joint noises, such as creaks and clicks, are common in many people, but they can also occur with specific problems of the joints. For example, the base of the knee cap may creak when it is damaged by osteoarthritis, and the jaw may click in a person who has temporomandibular joint disorder. Doctors ask about the person's symptoms and perform an examination to determine whether a joint noise is a symptom of a certain disorder. Further evaluation and treatment are needed only if the evaluation suggests a significant joint problem. Joint noises themselves do not require treatment.

Diagnosis

A doctor can often diagnose a musculoskeletal disorder based on the symptoms and on the results of a physical examination. Laboratory tests, imaging tests, or other diagnostic procedures are sometimes necessary to help the doctor make or confirm a diagnosis.

Physical Examination

A doctor looks for certain things during a physical examination depending on what disorder is suspected. When evaluating bones, if a fracture is suspected (see page 1952), the doctor may notice that the affected part (such as an arm or a leg) is abnormally shaped, suggesting that the segments of bone are out of alignment. A doctor may palpate the surfaces of the bones to detect any tenderness or abnormal shape, particularly if a fracture, a tumor, or a bone infection (osteomyelitis) is suspected. Compression fractures of the spine due to osteoporosis may be very painful at first, but no abnormal shape may be evident. Abnormal bumps in bones occasionally indicate a tumor. If osteomyelitis is suspected, a doctor or nurse checks for a fever.

When a person complains of muscle weakness, the doctor checks muscles for bulk and texture and for tenderness. Muscles are also checked for twitches and involuntary movements, which may indicate a nerve disease rather than a muscle disease. Doctors look for wasting away of muscle (atrophy), which can result from damage to the muscle or its nerves or from lack of use (disuse atrophy), as sometimes occurs with prolonged bed rest. Doctors also look for muscle enlargement (hypertrophy), which normally occurs with an exercise such as weight lifting. However, when a person is ill, hypertrophy may result from one muscle working harder to compensate for the weakness of another. Muscles can also enlarge when normal muscle tissue is replaced by abnormal tissue (increasing the size but not the strength of the muscle), which occurs in amyloidosis and in certain inherited muscle disorders, such as Duchenne's muscular dystrophy.

Doctors try to establish which (if any) muscles are weak and how weak they are. The muscles can be tested systematically, usually beginning with the face and neck, then the arms, and finally the legs. Normally, a person should be able to hold the arms extended, palms up, for one minute without their sagging, turning, or shaking. Downward drift of the arm with palms turning inward is a sign of weakness. Strength is tested by pushing or pulling while the doctor pushes and pulls in the opposite direction. Strength is also tested by having the person perform certain maneuvers, such as walking on the heels and tiptoes or rising from a squatting position or getting up and down from a chair rapidly 10 times. The person is asked to look in all directions; if double vision develops, one or more eye muscles may be weak.

The doctor tests a joint's range of motion by moving the limb around a joint while the person is completely relaxed (passive movement). The doctor also checks muscle tone by testing passive movement. Resistance to such movement (passive resistance) may be decreased when the nerve leading to the muscle is damaged. Resistance to such movement may be increased when the spinal cord or brain is damaged. If a person is weak, doctors also tap the person's muscle tendon with a rubber hammer to check reflexes (see page 633). Reflexes may be slower than expected when the nerve leading to the muscle is damaged. Reflexes may be more rapid than expected when the spinal cord or brain is damaged.

Laboratory Tests

Laboratory tests are often helpful in making the diagnosis of a musculoskeletal disorder. For example, the erythrocyte sedimentation rate (ESR—a test that measures the rate at which red blood cells settle to the bottom of a test tube containing blood) is increased when inflammation is present. However, because inflammation occurs in so many conditions, the ESR alone does not establish a diagnosis. The level of creatine kinase (a normal muscle enzyme that leaks out and is released into the bloodstream when muscle is damaged) may also be tested. Levels of creatine kinase are increased when there is widespread ongoing destruction of muscle. In rheumatoid arthritis, a blood test to identify rheumatoid factor or anti-cyclic citrullinated peptide (anti-CCP) antibody is helpful in making the diagnosis. In systemic lupus erythematosus (lupus), a blood test to identify autoimmune antibodies (antinuclear antibodies) is helpful in making the diagnosis.

Laboratory tests are also often useful to help monitor the progress of treatment. For example, the ESR can be particularly useful in helping to monitor the progress of treatment in rheumatoid arthritis or polymyalgia rheumatica.

Nerve Tests

Nerve conduction studies (see page 636) help determine whether the nerves supplying the muscles are functioning normally. Electromyography (see page 636), often performed at the same time as nerve conduction studies, is a test in which electrical impulses in the muscles are recorded to help determine how well the impulses from the nerves are reaching the connection between nerves and muscles (neuromuscular junction) and, from there, the muscles. Nerve conduction studies, together with electromyography, help indicate whether there is a problem primarily in the muscles (such as myositis or muscular dystrophy); in the nervous system, which supplies the muscles (such as a stroke, spinal cord problem, or polyneuropathy); or with the neuromuscular junction (such as myasthenia gravis). Nerve conduction studies are particularly useful in diagnosis of disorders of peripheral nerves, such as polyarteritis nodosa and ulnar nerve palsy.

X-rays

X-rays (see page 2042) are most valuable for detecting abnormalities in bone and are taken to evaluate painful, deformed, or suspected abnormal areas of bone. Often, x-rays can help to diagnose fractures, tumors, injuries, infections, and deformities (such as congenital hip dysplasia). Also, sometimes x-rays are helpful in showing changes that confirm a person has a certain kind of arthritis (for example, rheumatoid arthritis or osteoarthritis). X-rays do not show soft tissues such as muscles, bursae, ligaments, tendons, or nerves. To help determine whether the joint has been damaged by injury, a doctor may use an ordinary (non-stress) x-ray or one taken with the joint under stress (stress x-ray).

Arthrography is an x-ray procedure in which a radiopaque dye is injected into a joint space to outline the structures, such as ligaments inside the joint. Arthrography can be used to view torn ligaments and fragmented cartilage in the joint. However, MRI is now generally used in preference to arthrography.

Dual-Energy X-ray Absorptiometry

The most accurate way to evaluate bone density, which is necessary when screening for or diagnosing osteoporosis, is with dual-energy x-ray absorptiometry (DEXA). In this test, low-dose x-rays are used to examine bone density at the lower spine, hip, wrist, or entire body. Measurements of bone density are very accurate at these sites. To help differentiate osteoporosis (the most common cause of an abnormal DEXA scan) from other bone disorders, doctors may need to consider the person's symptoms, medical conditions, medication use, and certain blood or urine test results as well as the DEXA results.

Computed Tomography and Magnetic Resonance Imaging

Computed tomography (CT—see page 2037) and magnetic resonance imaging (MRI—see page 2040) give much more detail than conventional x-rays and may be performed to determine the extent and exact location of damage. These tests can also be used to detect fractures that are not visible on x-rays. MRI is especially valuable for imaging muscles, ligaments, and tendons. MRI can be used if the cause of pain is thought to be a severe soft-tissue problem (for example, rupture of a major ligament or tendon or damage to important structures inside the knee joint). CT best images the bone; however, sometimes MRI is better than CT for imaging bone. The amount of time a person spends undergoing CT is much less than for MRI. MRI is more expensive than CT and, with the exception of when the open-sided units are used, many people feel claustrophobic inside the MRI unit.

Bone Scanning

Bone scanning is an imaging procedure that is occasionally used to diagnose a fracture, particularly if other tests, such as plain x-rays and CT or MRI, do not reveal the fracture. Bone scanning involves use of a radioactive substance (technetium-99m–labeled pyrophosphate) that is absorbed by any healing bone.

The technique can also be used when a bone infection or a metastasis (from a cancer elsewhere in the body) is suspected. The radioactive substance is given intravenously and is detected by a bone-scanning device, creating an image of the bone that can be viewed on a computer screen.

Joint Aspiration

Joint aspiration is used to diagnose certain joint problems. A needle is inserted into a joint space, and fluid (synovial fluid) is drawn out (aspirated) and examined under a microscope. A doctor can often make a diagnosis after analyzing the fluid. For example, a sample of synovial fluid may contain bacteria, which confirms a diagnosis of infection. Or, it may contain certain crystals, which confirms a diagnosis of gout (urate crystals) or pseudogout (calcium crystals). Usually performed in the doctor's office, this procedure is generally quick, easy, and relatively painless. The risk of joint infection is minimal.

Arthroscopy

Arthroscopy is a procedure in which a small (the diameter of a pencil) fiberoptic scope is inserted into a joint space, allowing the doctor to look inside the joint and to project the image onto a television screen. The skin incision is very small. A person receives local, spinal, or general anesthesia. During arthroscopy, doctors can take a piece of tissue for analysis (biopsy), and, if necessary, perform surgery to correct the condition. Disorders commonly found during arthroscopy include inflammation of the synovium lining the joint (synovitis); ligament, tendon, or cartilage tears; and loose pieces of bone or cartilage. Such conditions affect people with arthritis or previous joint injuries as well as athletes. All of these conditions can be repaired or removed during arthroscopy. There is a very small risk of joint infection with this procedure.

Recovery time after arthroscopic surgery is much faster than after traditional surgery. Most people do not need to stay overnight in the hospital.

CHAPTER
91   Osteoporosis

Osteoporosis is a condition in which a progressive decrease in the density of bones weakens the bones, making fractures likely.

- Aging, estrogen deficiency, low vitamin D or calcium intake, and certain disorders can decrease the amounts of the components that maintain bone density and strength.
- Fractures, particularly of the back, hip, or wrist, can occur with little or no force.
- Some people never develop symptoms, whereas others develop severe sudden pain or gradually develop aching bone pain and deformities.
- Doctors diagnose people at risk by testing their bone density.
- Osteoporosis can be prevented and treated by ensuring adequate calcium and vitamin D intake, engaging in weight-bearing exercise, and taking bisphosphonates or other drugs.

Bones contain minerals, including calcium and phosphorus, which make them hard and dense. To maintain bone density, the body requires an adequate supply of calcium and other minerals and must produce the proper amounts of several hormones, such as parathyroid hormone, growth hormone, calcitonin, estrogen, and testosterone. An adequate supply of vitamin D is also needed to absorb calcium from food and incorporate it into bones. Vitamin D is absorbed from the diet and also manufactured in the skin by sunlight (see page 929).

So that bones can adjust to the changing demands placed on them, they are continuously broken down and reformed, or remodeled (see page 535). In this process, small areas of bone tissue are removed and new bone tissue is deposited. This process is continuous. Remodeling affects the shape and density of the bones. In youth, the bones grow in width and length as the body grows. In later life, bones may sometimes enlarge in width but do not continue to grow longer.

Because more bone is formed than is broken down in the young adult years, bones progressively increase in density until about age 30, when they are at their strongest. After that, as breakdown outstrips formation, bones slowly decrease in density. If the body is unable to maintain an adequate amount of bone formation, bones continue to lose density and may become increasingly fragile, eventually resulting in osteoporosis.

Loss of Bone Density in Women

In women, bone density (or mass) progressively increases until about age 30, when bones are at their strongest. After that, bone density gradually decreases. The decrease in bone loss accelerates after menopause, which occurs on average around age 51.

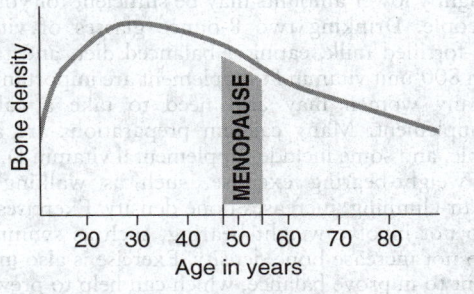

Types

About 8 million women and 2 million men in the United States have osteoporosis. There are two main types of osteoporosis: primary osteoporosis, which occurs spontaneously, and secondary osteoporosis, which is caused by another disorder or drug.

Primary Osteoporosis: More than 95% of osteoporosis in women and probably more than 80% in men is primary. Most cases occur in postmenopausal women and in older men. The terms postmenopausal, involutional, senile, and age-related osteoporosis have been used to describe this type of primary osteoporosis.

A major cause of osteoporosis is a lack of estrogen, particularly the rapid decrease that occurs at menopause. Most men over 50 have higher estrogen levels than postmenopausal women, but these also decline with aging, and low estrogen levels are associated with osteoporosis in both men and women. Estrogen deficiency increases bone breakdown and results in rapid bone loss. Bone loss is even greater if calcium intake or vitamin D levels are low. Low vitamin D levels result in calcium deficiency and increased activity of the parathyroid glands (secreting parathyroid hormone), which can also stimulate bone breakdown. For unknown reasons, bone production also decreases.

A number of other factors increase the risk of bone loss and the development of osteoporosis in women. These risk factors are probably also important in men. People who have had one fracture in which osteoporosis had been a factor are at much higher risk of having more such fractures.

Secondary Osteoporosis: Examples of disorders that may cause secondary osteoporosis are chronic kidney failure and hormonal disorders (especially Cushing's disease, hyperparathyroidism, hyperthyroidism, hypogonadism, and diabetes mellitus). Examples of drugs that may cause secondary osteoporosis are corticosteroids, barbiturates, and anticonvulsants. Excessive alcohol or caffeine consumption and cigarette smoking may worsen preexisting osteoporosis but are unlikely to cause it.

Idiopathic Osteoporosis: Idiopathic osteoporosis is a rare type of osteoporosis. The word *idiopathic* simply means that the cause is unknown. This type of osteoporosis occurs in children and young adults who have normal hormone levels, normal vitamin levels, and no obvious reason to have weak bones.

Symptoms

At first, osteoporosis causes no symptoms because bone density loss occurs very gradually. Some people never develop symptoms.

Eventually, however, bone density may decrease enough for bones to collapse or fracture, causing severe sudden pain or gradually developing aching bone pain and deformities. In long bones, such as the bones of the arms and legs, the fracture usually occurs at the ends of the bones rather than in the middle. In the bones of the spinal column (vertebrae), the fracture usually occurs in the middle to lower back. This type of bone is particularly at risk of fracture due to osteoporosis.

Vertebral crush fractures (fractures of spinal vertebrae) may occur in people who have any type of osteoporosis. These fractures are called osteoporotic fractures. The weakened vertebrae may collapse spontaneously or after a slight injury. Chronic back pain may occur because of these fractures. Usually, pain starts suddenly, stays in a particular area of the back, and worsens when a person stands or walks. The area may be tender. Usually the pain and

Risk Factors for Osteoporosis in Women

- Family members with osteoporosis
- Insufficient calcium in the diet
- Sedentary lifestyle
- White or Asian race
- Thin build
- Use of certain drugs, such as corticosteroids and excessive amounts of thyroid hormones
- Early menopause
- Cigarette smoking
- Excessive alcohol or caffeine consumption

tenderness go away gradually after a few weeks or months. If several vertebrae break, an abnormal curvature of the spine (a "dowager's hump") may develop, causing muscle strain and soreness as well as deformity.

Bones in other parts of the body may fracture, often because of a minor strain or fall. One of the most serious fractures is a hip fracture, a major cause of disability and loss of independence in older people (see page 1960). Common wrist fractures, called Colles' fractures (see page 1964), occur often, especially in people with postmenopausal osteoporosis. In addition, fractures tend to heal slowly in people who have osteoporosis.

Diagnosis

A doctor may suspect osteoporosis in the following people:

- All women age 65 or older
- Women aged 50 to 65 who have risk factors for osteoporosis
- All men and women who have had a previous osteoporotic fracture (a fracture caused by little or no force), even if the fracture occurred at a young age
- Adults age 65 or older who have unexplained back pain
- People whose bones appear thin on x-rays

Bone density testing can be used to detect or confirm suspected osteoporosis, even before a fracture occurs. A number of rapid screening techniques are available to measure density at the wrist or the heel. The most useful test, however, is dual-energy x-ray absorptiometry (DEXA), which measures bone density at the sites at which major fractures are likely to occur: the spine and hip. This test is painless and can be performed in about 5 to 15 minutes. It is useful for monitoring the response to treatment as well as for making the diagnosis.

Blood tests may be performed to measure calcium and vitamin D levels. Further testing may be needed to rule out treatable conditions that might lead to osteoporosis. If such a condition is found, the diagnosis is secondary osteoporosis.

Prevention and Treatment

Prevention is generally more successful than treatment because it is easier to prevent loss of bone density than to restore density once it has been lost. Prevention involves maintaining or increasing bone density by consuming adequate amounts of calcium and vitamin D, engaging in weight-bearing exercise, and, for some people, taking certain drugs. Treatment also involves ensuring adequate intake of cal-

cium and vitamin D and engaging in weight-bearing exercises. All people being treated need to take drugs.

Diet and Exercise: Consuming an adequate amount of calcium and vitamin D is helpful, especially before maximum bone density is reached (around age 30) but also after this time. About 1200 to 1500 milligrams of calcium and at least 800 units of vitamin D daily are recommended, although slightly lower amounts may be sufficient for younger people. Drinking two 8-ounce glasses of vitamin D-fortified milk, eating a balanced diet, and taking an 800-unit vitamin D supplement are important, but many women may also need to take a calcium supplement. Many calcium preparations are available, and some include supplemental vitamin D.

Weight-bearing exercise, such as walking and stair-climbing, increases bone density. Exercises that do not involve weight bearing, such as swimming, do not increase bone density. Exercise is also important to improve balance, which can help to prevent a fracture that may occur from falling. Curiously, in premenopausal women, high levels of exercise, such as those maintained by athletes, can actually cause a small reduction in bone density because such exercise suppresses the production of estrogen by the ovaries.

> **? Did You Know...**
>
> Most older women need to take a supplement of vitamin D that supplies 800 units per day.

Drugs: Most of the same drugs are used for prevention and treatment.

Drugs called bisphosphonates (alendronate, risedronate, ibandronate, and zoledronic acid) are useful in preventing and treating all types of osteoporosis and are usually the first drugs used. Bisphosphonates have been shown to increase bone density in the spine and hips and reduce the risk of fractures. Alendronate and risedronate can be taken by mouth (orally). Zoledronic acid can be given through a vein (intravenously). Ibandronate can be taken orally or intravenously.

An oral bisphosphonate must be swallowed with a full glass of water (6 to 8 ounces) after arising for the day, and no other food, drink, or drug should be consumed for the next 30 minutes. Food in the stomach may decrease the absorption of the drug. Because oral bisphosphonates can irritate the lining of the esophagus, the person must not lie down for at least 30 minutes after taking a dose and then must not lie down until after something has been eaten. Certain people, including those who have difficulty swallowing, gastrointestinal symptoms (for example, heartburn or nausea), and certain disorders of the esophagus or stomach, cannot take the bisphosphonates orally. These people can be given ibandronate or zoledronic acid intravenously. In addition, the following people should not take bisphosphonates:

- Women who are pregnant or nursing
- People who have low levels of calcium in the blood
- People who have severe kidney disease

It is not clear how long a person should take bisphosphonates. They can probably be taken for at least 5 years, and some have been shown to be effective for longer.

Osteonecrosis of the jaw is a condition that has occurred in some people who take bisphosphonates. In this condition, the jaw becomes damaged and infected. People who take bisphosphonates intravenously, who have cancer, or both are at highest risk. However, it is not truly clear whether bisphosphonates cause osteonecrosis of the jaw and, if they do, which particular drugs are most likely to cause it.

Calcitonin, which inhibits the breakdown of bone, is another drug used for treatment. Calcitonin seems to be less effective in reducing fracture risk than other available drugs. Calcitonin can be taken by injection or nasal spray. Its use can decrease blood levels of calcium; therefore, these levels must be monitored.

Hormonal therapy (for example, with estrogen) helps maintain bone density in women and can be used for prevention or treatment. This therapy is most effective when started within 4 to 6 years after menopause, but starting it later can still slow bone loss and reduce the risk of fractures. However, because the risks of hormonal therapy exceed its benefits for most women, hormonal therapy is usually not the treatment option used. Decisions about using estrogen replacement therapy after menopause are complex (see page 1517).

Raloxifene is an estrogen-like drug that may be less effective than estrogen in preventing and treating bone loss, but it does not have some of estrogen's negative side effects. Raloxifene is used in people who cannot or prefer not to take bisphosphonates. Raloxifene can reduce the risk of spine fractures and may reduce the risk of breast cancer.

Men do not benefit from estrogen but may benefit from testosterone replacement therapy if their testosterone level is low.

A synthetic form of parathyroid hormone called teriparatide can be injected daily in small amounts. Teriparatide increases the formation of new bone, increases bone density, and decreases the likelihood of fractures. This therapy is used in people who:

- Develop marked bone loss or fractures while being treated with a bisphosphonate
- Cannot take bisphosphonates
- Have unusually severe osteoporosis

Treatment of Fractures: Fractures resulting from osteoporosis must be treated. For hip fractures, usually part or all of the hip is replaced surgically (see page 1961). Surgery may be needed for a wrist fracture, or the wrist may need to be placed in a cast. Supportive back braces are used temporarily for people with painful vertebral crush fractures. Calcitonin can decrease the pain caused by vertebral fractures.

A collapsed vertebra can be repaired by a procedure called vertebroplasty. In this procedure, which takes about an hour for each vertebra, a material called polymethylmethacrylate (PMMA)—an acrylic bone cement—is injected into the collapsed vertebra, helping to relieve pain and reduce deformity. Kyphoplasty is a similar procedure, in which an orthopedic balloon is used to expand the vertebra back to its normal shape, before the injection of the PMMA. With vertebroplasty and kyphoplasty, deformity may be reduced in the PMMA-injected bone, but the risk of fractures in adjacent bones in the spine or ribs does not decrease and may even increase. Other risks may include cement leakage and possibly heart or lung problems.

Paget's Disease of Bone

Paget's disease of bone (osteitis deformans) is a chronic disorder of the skeleton in which areas of bone undergo abnormal turnover, resulting in areas of enlarged and softened bone.

- The breakdown and formation of bone increase, resulting in bones that are thicker, but weaker, than normal.
- Symptoms may be absent or may include bone pain, bone deformity, arthritis, and painful nerve compression.
- X-rays show the bone abnormalities.
- Pain and complications are treated, and bisphosphonates may be given.

Paget's disease can affect any bone, but the most commonly affected bones are the pelvis, thighbone (femur), skull, shin (tibia), spine (vertebrae), collarbone (clavicle), and upper arm bone (humerus).

Paget's disease rarely occurs in people younger than 40. In the United States, about 1% of people older than 40 have the disorder, and the prevalence increases with aging. However, the prevalence of the disease seems to be decreasing. Men are 50% more likely than women to develop it. Paget's disease is more common in Europe (excluding Scandinavia), Australia, and New Zealand. It is particularly common in England.

Causes

Normally, cells that break down old bone (osteoclasts) and cells that form new bone (osteoblasts) work in balance to maintain bone structure and integrity. In Paget's disease, both osteoclasts and osteoblasts become overactive in some areas of bone, and the rate at which bone is broken down and rebuilt (bone remodeling—see page 544) in these areas increases tremendously. The overactive areas enlarge but, despite being large, are structurally abnormal and weak.

The cause of Paget's disease is unknown. The disorder tends to run in families, and recent information suggests that a group of genetic defects possibly contributes. Also, some evidence suggests that a virus is involved. Even if a virus is involved, there is no evidence that the disorder is contagious.

Complications: Overgrown bone may compress nerves and other structures passing through small openings. The spinal canal may become narrow and compress the spinal cord. Osteoarthritis (see page 559) may develop in joints near the involved bone.

Rarely, heart failure develops because the increased blood flow through the affected bone puts extra stress on the heart. The affected bone becomes cancerous in fewer than 1% of people who have Paget's disease. People whose disease progresses to bone cancer (see page 553) can develop an osteosarcoma, fibrosarcoma, or chondrosarcoma.

High blood levels of calcium (hypercalcemia—see page 936) occasionally occur in bedridden older people with Paget's disease or in anyone with severe Paget's disease who becomes immobilized or dehydrated. These high levels of calcium can result in many problems, such as high blood pressure, muscle weakness, constipation, and stones in the urinary tract.

Symptoms

Paget's disease usually causes no symptoms, although bone pain, bone enlargement, or bone deformity may occur. Bone pain may be deep, aching, and occasionally severe and may worsen at night. The enlarging bones may compress nerves, causing more pain. If osteoarthritis occurs, joints become painful and stiff.

Other symptoms vary depending on which bones are affected. The skull may enlarge, and the brow and forehead may look more prominent. A person may notice this enlargement when a larger hat is needed. Enlarged skull bones may damage the inner ear (cochlea), which can cause hearing loss and dizziness. The enlarged skull bones can compress nerves, which causes headaches. The veins on the scalp may bulge, possibly because of the increased blood flow through the skull bones. The vertebrae may enlarge, weaken, and buckle, resulting in a loss of height and a hunched posture. Damaged vertebrae may pinch the nerves of the spinal cord, causing pain, numbness, tingling, weakness, or, very rarely, even paralysis in the legs. People whose hip or leg bones are affected may have bowed legs and take short, unsteady steps. Affected bones are more likely to break.

Diagnosis

Paget's disease is often discovered accidentally when x-rays or laboratory tests are performed for other reasons. Otherwise, the diagnosis may be based on the symptoms and a physical examination. The diagnosis can be confirmed by x-rays showing abnormalities characteristic of Paget's disease and by a laboratory test measuring blood levels of alkaline phosphatase, an enzyme involved in bone cell formation. A bone scan (a radionuclide test using technetium) shows which bones are affected.

Prognosis

The prognosis for people with Paget's disease is most often very good. However, the few people who develop bone cancer have a poor prognosis. People who develop other complications, such as heart failure or compression of the spinal cord, may also have a poor prognosis, unless treatment of these complications is timely and successful.

Treatment

A person who has Paget's disease needs treatment if the symptoms cause discomfort or if there is a significant risk or suggestion of complications, such as hearing loss, osteoarthritis, and deformity.

Commonly used analgesics such as acetaminophen and nonsteroidal anti-inflammatory drugs (NSAIDs) help reduce bone pain. If one leg becomes bowed and shortened, heel lifts can help make walking easier. Sometimes surgery is needed to relieve pinched nerves or to replace a joint that has become arthritic from Paget's disease.

One of several bisphosphonates—alendronate, etidronate, pamidronate, risedronate, tiludronate, or zoledronate—can be used to slow the progression of Paget's disease. Except for pamidronate and zoledronate, which are usually given by vein (intravenously), these drugs are given by mouth. These drugs are given for the following:

- Before orthopedic surgery to prevent or reduce bleeding during surgery
- To treat pain caused by Paget's disease
- To prevent or slow the progression of weakness or paralysis in people who cannot have surgery
- To attempt to prevent arthritis, further hearing loss, or further bone deformity
- To people with a blood level of alkaline phosphatase twice the normal level or higher

The newer bisphosphonates (such as zoledronate) seem to slow the progression of Paget's disease for a longer period of time.

Calcitonin is occasionally injected under the skin or into muscle. It is not as effective as the bisphosphonates and is used only when the other drugs cannot be given.

Bed rest (except for sleeping at night) should be avoided, if possible, to prevent hypercalcemia. If hypercalcemia does develop, intravenous fluids and drugs given to increase the excretion of water (diuretics—such as furosemide) are given.

Dietary intake of calcium and vitamin D (necessary for calcium absorption) should be sufficient to ensure that the incorporation of calcium into bone (bone mineralization) is adequate, because bone is being remodeled rapidly (see page 535). Otherwise, poor bone mineralization (osteomalacia) may occur.

CHAPTER

93 Osteonecrosis

Osteonecrosis (also referred to as avascular necrosis of bone, aseptic necrosis, ischemic necrosis, or osteochondritis dissecans) is the death of a segment of bone caused by an impaired blood supply.

- This disorder can be caused by an injury or can occur spontaneously.
- Typical symptoms include pain, limited range of motion of the affected joint, and, when the leg is affected, a limp.
- The diagnosis is based on symptoms and the results of x-rays and magnetic resonance imaging.
- Stopping smoking, stopping excessive alcohol use, and minimizing the use of or lowering the dose of corticosteroids reduce the risk of developing the disorder.
- Various surgical procedures can be performed if nonsurgical measures (such as rest, physical therapy, and analgesics) do not relieve symptoms.

Causes

Osteonecrosis or avascular necrosis of bone is not a specific disease but a condition in which there is death of a localized area of bone. There are two general categories of osteonecrosis: traumatic and nontraumatic.

Traumatic osteonecrosis is the most common. The most frequent cause of traumatic osteonecrosis is a displaced (separated) fracture, most often affecting the hip, which occurs in older people. A dis-

placed fracture may damage the blood vessels supplying the upper end of the thigh bone (the femoral head), resulting in death of the bone. This death of bone occurs less often in other areas of the body.

Nontraumatic osteonecrosis occurs without direct trauma or injury. This type may be caused by a disease or condition that results in the blockage of small blood vessels that supply certain areas of the bone. The areas most commonly affected are the femoral head, which is part of the hip joint; the knee; and the upper arm at the shoulder. This disorder occurs most commonly among people between the ages of 30 and 50 and often affects both hips or both shoulders. The most common causes are high doses of corticosteroids (especially when given for long periods of time) and chronic alcohol use. A number of other causes have been identified, but these occur much less often. These other causes include certain blood-clotting disorders, sickle cell disease, liver disease, tumors, Gaucher's disease, radiation therapy, and decompression sickness (which occurs in divers who surface too quickly—see page 1998). A number of disorders that are treated with high doses of corticosteroids also may be associated with osteonecrosis. In these cases, it may not be clear whether the cause is the disorder or the corticosteroids.

In about 20% of people with osteonecrosis, the cause is unknown, and these people are thus said to

Some Risk Factors for Osteonecrosis

TRAUMATIC

- Fractures and dislocations

NONTRAUMATIC

- Alcohol
- Asthma
- Blood-clotting disorders (such as systemic lupus erythematosus with antiphospholipid antibodies or high levels of blood platelets)
- Chemotherapy
- Corticosteroids
- Cushing's syndrome
- Decompression sickness
- Diabetes
- Gaucher's disease
- Gout
- High level of lipids in the blood (hyperlipidemia)
- Liver disease
- Miscellaneous conditions (such as chronic kidney disease and rare genetic mutations)
- Organ transplantation
- Pancreatitis
- Radiation
- Sickle cell disease
- Smoking
- Systemic lupus erythematosus and connective tissue disorders
- Tumors

have idiopathic osteonecrosis. If one bone has nontraumatic osteonecrosis, the same bone on the opposite side of the body also has it about 60% of the time, even if symptoms are absent.

Spontaneous osteonecrosis of the knee (SPONK) can occur in older women (occasionally men) who have no specific risk factors for the disorder. SPONK is thought to be caused by an insufficiency fracture. An insufficiency fracture is caused by normal wear and tear on bone that has been affected by osteoporosis. SPONK occurs without direct trauma or injury.

Symptoms

As osteonecrosis progresses, more and more tiny fractures may occur, particularly in bones that support weight, such as the hip. As a result, the bone usually collapses weeks or months after the blood supply is cut off. Most often pain develops gradually when the bone begins to collapse. At times, however, the onset of pain may be sudden and could be related

to increased pressure that develops in and around the affected area of bone. Regardless of how sudden, pain is increased by moving the affected bone and generally is alleviated with rest. The person avoids moving the joint to minimize pain.

If the affected bone is in the leg, standing or walking worsens the pain and a limp develops.

In osteonecrosis of the hip, pain is usually present in the groin and may extend down the thigh or into the buttocks.

SPONK causes sudden pain along the inner part of the knee. There may be tenderness in this area, and the joint often becomes swollen with excess fluid.

Osteonecrosis of the shoulder often causes fewer symptoms than osteonecrosis that occurs in other bones.

Osteoarthritis (see page 559) develops when collapse affects a large part of the bone.

Diagnosis

Because osteonecrosis is often painless at first, it may not be diagnosed in its earliest stages. Doctors suspect osteonecrosis in people who do not improve satisfactorily after sustaining certain fractures. They also suspect the disorder in people who develop unexplained pain in the hip, knee, or shoulder, particularly if these people have risk factors for osteonecrosis.

X-rays of the affected area usually show osteonecrosis unless the disorder is in its earliest stages. If x-rays appear normal, however, magnetic resonance imaging (MRI) is usually done because it is the best test for detecting osteonecrosis early, before changes appear on ordinary x-rays. The x-rays and MRI also show whether the bone has collapsed, how advanced the disorder is, and whether the joint is affected by osteoarthritis. If doctors discover nontraumatic osteonecrosis in one hip, they also examine the other hip with an x-ray or MRI.

Prevention

To minimize the risk of osteonecrosis caused by corticosteroids, doctors use these drugs only when essential, prescribe them in as low a dose as needed, and prescribe them for as short a duration as possible. To prevent osteonecrosis caused by decompression sickness, people should follow accepted rules for decompression during diving and when working in pressurized environments. Excessive alcohol use and smoking should be avoided. Various drugs (such as those that prevent blood clots, dilate blood vessels, or lower lipid levels) are being evaluated for prevention of osteonecrosis in people at high risk.

Treatment

Several nonsurgical measures are available for treating the symptoms caused by osteonecrosis.

Taking anti-inflammatory drugs or other pain relievers, minimizing activity and stress (such as weight bearing for osteonecrosis of the hip and knee), and undergoing physical therapy are ways to relieve symptoms but not cure the disorder or change its course. These measures, however, may be adequate for treatment of the shoulder, the knee, and small areas of osteonecrosis of the hip, which may eventually heal without treatment.

There are a number of surgical procedures that slow or stop progression of the disorder. These are most effective for treating early disease that has not yet progressed to bone collapse. The simplest and most common of these procedures is called core decompression, which involves taking a plug of bone out of the involved area. Core decompression often relieves pain and stimulates healing. In about 65% of people, the procedure can delay or avoid the need for total hip replacement. In younger people, core decompression may also be used even if a small amount of collapse already has taken place. The procedure is relatively simple, has a low rate of complications, and requires the use of crutches for only about 6 weeks.

Another procedure is bone grafting (transplanting bone from one site to another). For osteonecrosis of the hip, this can involve removing the dead area of bone and replacing it with more normal bone from elsewhere in the body. This graft supports the weakened area of bone and stimulates the body to form new, living bone in the affected area. An osteotomy is another procedure designed to save the affected joint. This procedure is performed particularly in the region of the hip and may be suitable for younger people in whom some degree of collapse already has occurred, which makes them poor candidates for core decompression or other procedures. Usually the osteonecrosis is in the weight-bearing area of the femoral head. Bone grafting and osteotomy are difficult procedures, however, and are not often performed in the United States. They require a person to spend several months on crutches. These procedures are done only at selected centers that have the surgical experience and facilities to achieve the best results.

A total joint replacement or other type of joint replacement procedure (arthroplasty) is the only effective procedure to relieve pain and restore mo-

Osteonecrosis of the Jaw

Osteonecrosis of the jaw (ONJ) is an oral disorder that involves exposure of the jaw bone. ONJ is usually painful, and pus may be discharged, although some people have no symptoms. The disorder may occur spontaneously or after tooth extraction, trauma, or radiation therapy to the head and neck (a disorder called osteoradionecrosis).

ONJ has recently been noticed in some people who have received high doses of bisphosphonates by vein, particularly if they have cancer or undergo oral surgery while receiving the drugs. ONJ has not been linked with the routine use of bisphosphonates taken by mouth as treatment for osteoporosis. Thus, people should still use oral bisphosphonates as prescribed. If possible, any necessary oral surgery should be done before use of bisphosphonates is begun.

Treatment typically involves scraping away some of the damaged bone, taking antibiotics by mouth, and using mouth rinses. Removing the whole affected area with surgery may worsen the condition and is not the first choice of treatment.

tion if osteonecrosis has caused significant joint collapse and osteoarthritis. About 95% of people benefit from replacement of the hip or knee. With modern techniques and devices, most joints should last more than 15 to 20 years. However, in younger people with osteonecrosis, a replacement joint may have to be revised or replaced at some later time. Therefore, some surgeons favor a more limited procedure, called surface replacement arthroplasty, to treat osteonecrosis of the hip in younger people. This procedure involves placing a metal cap over the femoral head rather than replacing the entire joint as is done in a standard total hip replacement. If the hip socket also is involved, a second metal cap is placed in the socket. It is not clear whether surface replacement arthroplasty is better than standard hip replacement, and results with these treatments are currently being evaluated. Occasionally, a partial or total replacement of the shoulder may be needed for advanced osteonecrosis that does not respond well to nonsurgical treatment.

CHAPTER 94   Bone and Joint Tumors

Bone Tumors

Bone tumors are growths of abnormal cells in bones.

- Bone tumors may be cancerous (malignant) or noncancerous (benign) and may develop within the bone or spread to the bone.
- Tumors may cause unexplained, progressively worsening bone pain, swelling, or a tendency to fracture easily.
- The diagnosis is sometimes based on the results of an imaging test (such as x-ray, computed tomography, or magnetic resonance imaging) but often requires removing a tissue sample of the tumor or bone for examination under a microscope (biopsy).

Bone tumors may be noncancerous or cancerous. A cancerous tumor may spread to other areas of the body. Also, bone tumors may be primary or metastatic. Primary tumors originate in the bone and may be noncancerous or cancerous. Metastatic tumors are cancerous tumors that originate elsewhere in the body (for example, in the breast or prostate gland) and then spread to bone. In children, most cancerous bone tumors are primary. In adults, most cancerous bone tumors are metastatic. Overall, noncancerous bone tumors are relatively common, but cancerous primary bone tumors are rare, occurring in only about 2,500 people yearly in the United States. This number excludes multiple myeloma, a cancer that affects primarily the marrow inside the bone rather than the hard bone tissue.

Symptoms

A person may sometimes have a painless lump, which may eventually become painful, but often the first symptom is bone pain. The pain can be severe (somewhat like a toothache). Pain may occur when at rest or at night and tends to progressively worsen. Sometimes a tumor, especially if cancerous, weakens a bone, causing it to fracture with little or no stress (pathologic fracture).

Diagnosis

A persistently painful joint or limb should be x-rayed. However, x-rays tend to show only that there is an abnormality suggestive of an abnormal growth or a hole in the bone, often without indicating whether a tumor is noncancerous or cancerous. However, some tumors can be identified as benign by an x-ray. For example, this identification is often possible with Paget's disease, enchondromas, bone cysts, nonossifying fibromas (fibrous growths that have no bone tissue), and fibrous dysplasia. If an x-ray is not conclusive, computed tomography (CT) and magnetic resonance imaging (MRI) often help determine the exact location and size of the tumor and give additional information as to the nature of the tumor, but these tests usually do not provide a specific diagnosis.

If cancer is suspected or is a reasonable possibility, a biopsy is usually necessary for diagnosis. For many tumors, a sample may be taken by inserting a needle into the tumor and withdrawing some cells (aspiration biopsy); however, because the needle used is very small, sometimes normal cells may be sampled and cancer cells are missed, even when cancer cells are lying right beside the normal cells. A biopsy done with a larger needle (core biopsy) is often necessary so that more tissue can be examined. Sometimes, a surgical procedure called open biopsy is necessary to obtain an adequate sample for diagnosis and can sometimes be done at the same time that surgery is done to treat the tumor.

NONCANCEROUS BONE TUMORS

Osteochondromas: Osteochondromas (osteocartilaginous exostoses), the most common type of noncancerous (benign) bone tumors, are usually recognized in people aged 10 to 20 years. These tumors are growths on the surface of a bone, which protrude as hard lumps. A person may have one or several tumors. The tendency to develop several tumors may run in families.

At some point in their lives, about 10% of people who have more than one osteochondroma (multiple osteochondromatosis) may develop a cancerous (malignant) bone tumor called a chondrosarcoma (presumably formed from an existing osteochondroma). Surgical removal is generally appropriate if one of the tumors enlarges or causes new symptoms (for example, if the tumor disturbs growth of the bone, enlarges, or presses on nearby nerves, muscles, or surrounding structures). Such people should also visit their doctor for regular examinations. However, people who have only one osteochondroma are unlikely to develop a chondrosarcoma; therefore, a single osteochondroma usually does not need to be removed unless it causes symptoms.

Enchondromas: Enchondromas may occur at any age but tend to be recognized in those aged 10 to 40 years. These tumors develop in the central part of a bone. The tumors often are discovered when x-rays are taken for other reasons and often can be diagnosed by their appearance on the x-ray. Some enchondromas may enlarge and cause pain. If an enchondroma does not cause pain and does not appear to be cancerous on x-rays or other imaging tests, it does not have to be removed or treated. However, follow-up x-rays may be taken to monitor its size. If the tumor cannot be identified with certainty on x-rays or if it causes pain, removal of a tissue sample for examination under a microscope (biopsy) may be needed to determine whether it is noncancerous or cancerous.

Chondroblastomas: Chondroblastomas are rare tumors that grow in the ends of bones. They usually occur in people aged 10 to 20 years. These tumors may cause pain, leading to their discovery. If untreated, these tumors may continue to grow and destroy bone and the joint; therefore, treatment consists of surgical removal and use of a bone graft to fill in the defect. Graft material can be bone removed from the person's own pelvis (autograft), processed bone tissue from another person (allograft), or a synthetic bone substitute. Occasionally, these tumors recur after surgery.

Chondromyxofibromas: Chondromyxofibromas are very rare tumors that occur in people younger than 30. They are usually located off to one side near the ends of the bones in the extremities (the limbs). Pain is the usual symptom. These tumors have a distinctive appearance on x-rays. Treatment consists of surgical removal, which usually provides a cure, although these tumors sometimes recur.

Osteoid Osteomas: Osteoid osteomas are very small tumors that commonly develop in people aged 10 to 35. They are most common in the arms or legs but can occur in any bone. They usually cause pain that worsens at night and is relieved by low doses of aspirin or other nonsteroidal anti-inflammatory drugs (NSAIDs). Sometimes the muscles surrounding the tumor waste away (atrophy). This condition may improve after the tumor is removed. If the tumor develops near the growth plate (the part of the bone from which growth occurs in children), bone growth can be overstimulated. This can cause the limbs to grow to unequal sizes. Bone scans using radioactive tracers help determine the exact location of the tumor. Sometimes the tumor is difficult to locate, and additional tests, such as computed tomography (CT), may be needed.

To treat the tumor permanently, usually a doctor punctures the skin and inserts a needle-like probe into the tumor, using CT as guidance for placement. A radiofrequency pulse is then applied to destroy the tumor. While this is done, the person is under general, spinal, or nerve block anesthesia (see page 2053). The prognosis is good, and pain should resolve. Surgically removing the tumor is another way to eliminate the pain permanently. Alternatively, some people prefer to take pain relievers (analgesics) indefinitely rather than undergo a procedure. The pain may eventually resolve without treatment.

Giant Cell Tumors: Giant cell tumors usually occur in people in their 20s and 30s. These tumors most commonly originate in the ends of bones and may extend into adjacent tissue. They usually cause pain. Treatment depends on the tumor's size. A tumor can be surgically removed, and the hole can be filled with bone graft or synthetic bone cement to preserve the bone's structure. Occasionally, very extensive tumors may require removal of the affected segment of bone and reconstruction of the joint. One treatment is a surgical procedure called curettage, in which the tumor is scraped out with a scoop-shaped instrument. After this treatment, about 10% of tumors recur. Giant cell tumors rarely become cancerous.

PRIMARY CANCEROUS BONE TUMORS

Multiple Myeloma: Multiple myeloma (see also page 1051) is the most common primary cancerous (malignant) bone tumor and occurs mostly in older adults. However, it is cancer that involves the bone marrow (the blood-forming tissue inside the cavity of the bone) rather than the hard tissue that makes up the bone. Thus, it is not always considered a primary bone tumor. It is more common than cancers of the hard tissue that makes up bone. Multiple myeloma may affect one or more bones, so pain may occur in one location or in several. If only one bone is involved in only one place, the condition is called a plasmacytoma. If more than one area is involved, the condition is called multiple myeloma. Treatment is complex and may include chemotherapy, radiation therapy, and sometimes surgery.

Osteosarcoma: Osteosarcoma (osteogenic sarcoma) is the second most common type of primary cancerous bone tumor but is less common than multiple myeloma. This cancer causes abnormal bone cells to grow. Although most common among people aged 10 to 25 years, osteosarcomas can occur at any age. Older people who have Paget's disease (see page 547), have undergone bone radiation, or have areas of dead bone tissue that form from sickle cell anemia and other conditions (bone infarcts) sometimes develop this type of tumor. About half of these tumors occur in or around the knee, but they can originate in any bone. They tend to spread (metastasize) to the lungs. Usually, these tumors cause pain and swelling. X-rays are taken, but removal of a tissue sample for examination under a microscope (biopsy) is needed for diagnosis.

People need a chest x-ray and a computed tomography (CT) scan to detect cancer that has metastasized to the lung and a bone scan to detect cancer that has spread to other bones.

Osteosarcomas are usually treated with a combination of chemotherapy and surgery. Usually, chemotherapy is given first. Pain often subsides during this phase of treatment. Then the tumor is surgically removed without damaging (violating) the tumor, such as by cutting it. Violating the tumor spills its cells, which can cause the cancer to recur in the same area.

About 65% of people who have this type of tumor survive for at least 5 years after diagnosis when chemotherapy is provided and the cancer has not metastasized. If chemotherapy destroys almost all of the cancer, the chance of surviving at least 5 years is greater than 90%. Because surgical procedures have improved, the affected arm or leg can usually be saved and reconstructed. In the past, the affected limb often had to be amputated.

Fibrosarcomas and Malignant Fibrous Histiocytomas: Fibrosarcomas and malignant fibrous histiocytomas affect the same age group as and are similar to osteosarcomas in appearance, location, symptoms, and prognosis. These cancerous tumors have cells that produce cancerous fibrous (connective) tissue rather than cancerous bony tissue. Treatment is similar to that of osteosarcoma.

Chondrosarcomas: Chondrosarcomas are tumors composed of cancerous cartilage cells. These tumors tend to occur in older adults. Many chondrosarcomas are slow-growing or low-grade tumors, meaning that they are less likely to spread than some other tumors. They often can be cured with surgery. However, some chondrosarcomas are high-grade tumors, which tend to metastasize. A biopsy is needed for diagnosis.

Low-grade chondrosarcomas are often removed from the bone by scraping it with a scoop-shaped instrument (curettage) and by using liquid nitrogen, phenol, or an argon beam to kill the surface tumor cells embedded in bone. Other chondrosarcomas must be completely removed surgically without damaging (violating) the tumor, which risks spreading the tumor's cells. Chondrosarcomas do not respond to chemotherapy or radiation therapy. Amputation of the arm or leg is rarely necessary. More than 75% of people who have a chondrosarcoma survive if the entire tumor is removed.

Ewing's Sarcoma of Bone: Ewing's sarcoma is a cancerous tumor that affects males more often than females and appears most commonly in people aged 10 to 25 years. Most of these tumors develop in the arms or legs, but they may develop in any bone. Pain and swelling are the most common symptoms. Tumors may become quite large, sometimes affecting the entire length of a bone. The tumor may include a large mass of soft (non-bone) tissue. Although CT and magnetic resonance imaging (MRI) can help determine the exact size of the tumor, a biopsy is needed for diagnosis. Treatment includes various combinations of surgery, chemotherapy, and radiation therapy, depending on whether surgery is practical or, if attempted, successful. Treatment can cure more than 60% of people who have Ewing's sarcoma.

Lymphoma of Bone: Lymphoma of bone (previously called reticulum cell sarcoma) is a cancerous tumor that usually affects people in their 40s and 50s. It can originate in any bone or elsewhere in the body and then spread to bone. Usually, this tumor causes pain and swelling and an accumulation of soft tissue. The damaged bone is prone to fractures. Treatment usually consists of a combination of chemotherapy and radiation therapy, which seems to be as effective as amputation or surgical removal of the tumor. Amputation is rarely necessary. If a bone seems to be prone to fracture, doctors may stabilize it surgically in an attempt to prevent fracture.

Malignant Giant Cell Tumors: Malignant giant cell tumors are rare and cancerous and are usually located at the extreme end of a long bone (arm or thigh bone). Treatment is similar to that of osteosarcomas, but the cure rate is low.

Chordomas: Chordomas are rare and cancerous and tend to occur at the ends of the spinal column, usually in the middle of the base of the spine (sacrum) or tailbone or near the base of the skull. A chordoma affecting the sacrum or tailbone causes nearly constant pain. A chordoma in the base of the skull can cause nerve problems, most commonly in those to the eye. Symptoms may exist for months to several years before diagnosis. Chordomas do not usually spread to other bones, but they may recur. Chordomas affecting the sacrum or tailbone may be cured by surgical removal. Chordomas in the base of the skull usually cannot be cured surgically but may respond to radiation therapy.

METASTATIC BONE TUMORS

- Cancers, particularly of the breast, lung, prostate gland, kidney, thyroid gland, and colon, may spread to the bone (metastasize).
- An imaging test may show the bone abnormality, or a sample of tissue may need to be removed and tested (biopsy).
- Radiation therapy, chemotherapy, or surgery may be recommended.

Prostate cancer in males and breast cancer in females are the most common cancers. Lung cancer is the most common cause of cancer death in both sexes. Metastatic bone tumors are cancers that have spread to the bone from their original site elsewhere in the body (see page 1075). Cancers most likely to spread to the bone include those of the breast, lung, prostate gland, kidney, thyroid gland, and colon. However, any cancer may eventually spread to bone. Cancer may spread to any bone, although cancers do not commonly spread to bone below the mid forearm or mid calf. When they do, most often the metastasis will be from lung or sometimes kidney cancer.

Diagnosis

A person who has or has had cancer and develops bone pain or swelling is evaluated for metastatic bone tumors. Bone scans using radioactive tracers and x-rays can help locate these tumors. Magnetic resonance imaging (MRI) or positron emission tomography (PET) is even more accurate. Occasionally, a metastatic bone tumor causes symptoms before the original cancer has been detected. Symptoms may consist of pain or a fracture where the tumor has weakened the bone (a pathologic fracture). In these situations, a biopsy usually gives clues as to the location of the original cancer, because the type of cancer tissue can often be recognized under the microscope and direct the doctor to the primary cancer (for example, lung, breast, prostate, kidney, thyroid, or colon).

Treatment

Treatment depends on the type of cancer that has spread to the bone. Some types respond to chemotherapy, some to radiation therapy, some to both, and some to neither. Radiation therapy is usually most effective. Surgery to stabilize the bone can sometimes prevent fractures. Some metastatic bone lesions require removal of part of a limb and rebuilding of the limb and joint. When the original (primary) cancer has been removed and only a single metastasis in the bone exists (especially when the metastasis develops years after the original tumor), surgical removal with reconstruction, sometimes combined with radiation therapy, chemotherapy, or both, rarely may be curative but may significantly improve the quality of life as well as the function or appearance of the limb.

One of the goals of treatment is to minimize loss of bone tissue. Loss of bone tissue can cause pain and make bones prone to fractures, which can require surgery. Bone loss can be minimized by using radiation therapy and drugs that prevent bone loss (such as bisphosphonates) before bone loss is extensive and pain occurs. If tumors cause the vertebra to collapse but not to put pressure against the spinal cord, kyphoplasty can be used. In vertebroplasty (injection alone) or kyphoplasty (use of an expanding balloon first), bone cement (methyl methacrylate) is injected into the bone to make the area expand, which can relieve pain and prevent further collapse. If the tumors appear to be at risk of collapse that could cause spinal cord damage (such as paraplegia), treatment to decompress the pressure and stabilize the spine may be recommended.

Other Bone Abnormalities

Many noncancerous (benign) bone abnormalities may resemble bone tumors but are not.

Unicameral Bone Cyst: Unicameral bone cysts occur near the parts of the bone from which growth occurs (growth plates) in the arms or legs in children. The cysts often cause nearby bones to thin, which can lead to a fracture. Cysts may heal and may disappear as the fracture heals. Most often, these cysts are treated by injection with corticosteroids, often repeatedly, processed bone putty, or synthetic bone substitutes. Cysts that are more than 2 inches (about 5 centimeters) long or wide, particularly in children, may require surgery to remove the contents of the cyst from the bone by scraping it with a scoop-shaped instrument (curettage) and transplantation of bone from one site to another (bone grafting). However, many people with these cysts respond to injections rather than invasive surgery. Regardless of treatment, the cyst remains or recurs in about 10 to 15% of people.

Fibrous Dysplasia: Fibrous dysplasia involves abnormal bone development during childhood. It may affect one bone or several bones. Birth marks and signs of early puberty (see box on page 1755) may be present; this is also called Albright's syndrome. The abnormal bone growths commonly stop developing at puberty. This condition rarely becomes cancerous (malignant). Calcitonin injections or bisphosphonates administered intravenously may help relieve the pain. A surgical procedure may correct deformities, fractures that do not heal with casting, or pain that cannot be relieved any other way.

Aneurysmal Bone Cyst: Aneurysmal bone cysts usually develop before people reach age 25, and the cause is not known. These cysts usually occur near the outer ends of the long bones (upper arm and thigh bones), but almost any bone may be affected. The cyst tends to grow slowly. A new bone shell forms around the cyst and is often wider than the original bone. Pain and swelling are common. The cyst may be present for a few weeks to a year before diagnosis.

Surgical removal of the entire cyst is the most successful treatment, but sometimes the cysts recur if they are not removed completely. Radiation should be avoided when possible because cancerous tumors occasionally develop later. However, radiation may be the treatment of choice for cysts that cannot be treated surgically and are compressing the spinal cord.

Joint Tumors

Tumors rarely affect joints unless the joints are near a bone or soft-tissue tumor. However, two conditions—synovial chondromatosis and pigmented villonodular synovitis—occur in the lining (synovium) of joints. These tumors are noncancerous (benign) but aggressive. Both conditions usually affect one joint, most often the knee and then the hip, and can cause pain and an accumulation of fluid. Treatment for both requires surgical removal of the abnormal synovium (synovectomy).

Synovial Chondromatosis: Synovial chondromatosis (previously called synovial osteochondromatosis) is a condition in which cells in the lining of the joint turn into cartilage-producing cells. These converted cells can form clumps of cartilage, which then shed into the space around the joint, forming loose bodies, each of which may be no larger than a grain of rice, and cause pain and swelling. This condition rarely becomes cancerous (malignant). Recurrence is common.

Pigmented Villonodular Synovitis: Pigmented villonodular synovitis causes the lining of the joint to become swollen and grow. This growth harms the cartilage and bone around the joint. The lining also produces extra fluid that can cause pain and swelling. The process often causes bloody fluid to appear in the joint. It usually affects one joint. A total joint replacement may be needed if the condition recurs. On rare occasions after several synovectomies, radiation therapy can be used.

CHAPTER 95   Bone and Joint Infections

Bones and the fluid and tissues of joints can become infected. Such infections include osteomyelitis and infectious arthritis.

Osteomyelitis

Osteomyelitis is a bone infection usually caused by bacteria, including mycobacteria, but is sometimes caused by fungi.

- Bacteria or fungi can infect bones by spreading through the bloodstream, spreading from nearby tissue, or directly invading the bone.
- People have pain in one part of the bone, fever, and weight loss.
- Blood tests and x-rays are done, and doctors remove a sample of bone for tests.
- Antibiotics are given for weeks, and surgery may be needed.

Osteomyelitis occurs most commonly in young children and in older people, but all age groups are at risk. Osteomyelitis is also more likely to occur in people with serious medical conditions.

When a bone becomes infected, the soft, inner part (bone marrow) often swells. As the swollen tissue presses against the rigid outer wall of the bone, the blood vessels in the bone marrow may become compressed, which reduces or cuts off the blood supply to the bone. Without an adequate blood supply, parts of the bone may die. These areas of dead bone are difficult to cure of infection because it is difficult for the body's natural infection-fighting cells and antibiotics to reach them. The infection can also spread outward from the bone to form collections of pus (abscesses) in adjacent soft tissues, such as the muscle.

Causes

Bones, which usually are well protected from infection, can become infected through three routes:

- The bloodstream (which may carry an infection from another part of the body to the bones)
- Direct invasion (infection)
- Infections in adjacent bone or soft tissues

When organisms that cause osteomyelitis spread through the bloodstream, infection usually occurs in the ends of leg and arm bones in children and in the spine (vertebrae) in adults, particularly in older people. Infections of the vertebrae are referred to as vertebral osteomyelitis. People who undergo kidney dialysis and those who inject drugs using nonsterile needles are particularly susceptible to vertebral osteomyelitis.

Bacteria or fungal spores may infect the bone directly through open fractures, during bone surgery, or from contaminated objects that pierce the bone. *Staphylococcus aureus* is the bacteria most commonly responsible. *Mycobacterium tuberculosis* (the main cause of tuberculosis) can infect the vertebrae to cause osteomyelitis.

Osteomyelitis may also occur where a piece of metal has been surgically attached to a bone, as is done to repair hip or other fractures. Also, bacteria or fungal spores may infect the bone to which an artificial joint is attached. The organisms may be carried into the area of bone surrounding the artificial joint during the operation in which the joint is installed, or the infection may occur later.

Osteomyelitis may also result from an infection in an adjacent soft tissue. The infection spreads to the bone after several days or weeks. This type of spread is particularly likely to occur in older people. Such an infection may start in an area damaged by an injury, radiation therapy, or cancer, or in a skin ulcer (particularly a foot ulcer) caused by poor circulation or diabetes. A sinus, gum, or tooth infection may spread to the skull.

Symptoms

Infections of the leg and arm bones cause fever and, sometimes days later, pain in the infected bone. The area over the bone may be sore, warm, and swollen, and movement may be painful. The person may lose weight and feel tired.

Infections of the vertebrae usually develop gradually, causing persistent back pain and tenderness when touched. Pain worsens with movement and is not relieved by resting, applying heat, or taking analgesics. Fever, usually the most obvious sign of an infection, is often absent.

When osteomyelitis results from infections in adjacent soft tissues or direct invasion by an organism, the area over the bone swells and becomes painful. Abscesses may form in the surrounding tissue. These infections may not cause fever. Infection around an infected artificial joint or limb typically causes persistent pain in that area.

Chronic osteomyelitis may develop if osteomyelitis is not treated successfully. It is a persistent infection that is very difficult to eradicate. Sometimes, chronic osteomyelitis is undetectable for a long time, causing no symptoms for months or years. More commonly, chronic osteomyelitis causes bone pain, recurring infections in the soft tissue over the bone, and constant or intermittent drainage of pus through the skin. Such drainage occurs when a passage (sinus tract) forms from the infected bone to the skin surface and pus drains through the sinus tract.

Diagnosis

Symptoms and findings during a physical examination may suggest osteomyelitis. For example, doctors may suspect osteomyelitis in a person who has persistent pain in part of a bone with or without a fever and feels tired much of the time.

Usually, the erythrocyte sedimentation rate (ESR—a test that measures the rate at which red blood cells settle to the bottom of a test tube containing blood) increases, as does the level of C-reactive protein (a protein that circulates in the blood and that dramatically increases when there is inflammation). Also, blood tests often indicate elevated levels of white blood cells. However, these blood tests are not sufficient to diagnose osteomyelitis.

An x-ray may show changes characteristic of osteomyelitis, but sometimes not until more than 3 weeks after the first symptoms occur. Computed tomography (CT) and magnetic resonance imaging (MRI) can also identify the infected area. However, these tests cannot always distinguish infections from other bone disorders. The infected area almost always appears abnormal on bone scans (images of bone made after injecting radioactive technetium), except in infants, because scans do not reliably indicate abnormalities in growing bones. White blood cell scans (images made after radioactive indium–labeled white blood cells are injected into a vein) can help distinguish between infection and other disorders in areas that are abnormal on bone scans.

To diagnose a bone infection and identify the organisms causing it, doctors may take samples of blood, pus, joint fluid, or the bone itself to test. Usually, for vertebral osteomyelitis, samples of bone tissue are removed with a needle or during surgery.

Prognosis and Prevention

The prognosis for people with osteomyelitis is usually good with early and proper treatment. However, sometimes, chronic osteomyelitis develops, and a bone abscess may recur weeks to months or even years later.

Certain people who have artificial joints or metal components attached to a bone should take preventive antibiotics before surgery, including dental surgery, because these people may be at increased risk of infection from bacteria normally present in the mouth and other parts of the body. People can ask their health care practitioner for expert, detailed recommendations regarding preventive antibiotics. People undergoing surgical or dental procedures should tell their surgeon, orthopedist, or dentist that they have an artificial joint or metal component attached to a bone so that preventive antibiotics can be taken.

Treatment

For children and adults who have recently developed bone infections through the bloodstream, antibiotics are the most effective treatment. If the bacteria causing the infection cannot be identified, then antibiotics that are effective against *Staphylococcus aureus* and many types of bacteria (broad-spectrum antibiotics) are used. Depending on the severity of the infection, antibiotics may be given by vein (intravenously) for about 4 to 8 weeks but then may be given by mouth later. Some people need months of antibiotic treatment.

If a fungal infection is identified or suspected, antifungal drugs are required for several months. If the infection is detected at an early stage, surgery is usually not necessary.

For adults who have bacterial osteomyelitis of the vertebrae, the usual treatment is antibiotics for 6 to 8 weeks. Sometimes bed rest is needed, and the person may need to wear a brace. Surgery may be needed to drain abscesses or to stabilize affected vertebrae (to prevent the vertebrae from collapsing and thereby damaging nearby nerves, the spinal cord, or blood vessels).

When osteomyelitis results from an adjacent soft-tissue infection (such as in a foot ulcer caused by poor circulation or diabetes), treatment is more complex. Usually, all the dead tissue and bone are removed surgically, and the resulting empty space is packed with healthy bone, muscle, or skin. Then the infection is treated with antibiotics.

When an abscess is present, it usually needs to be drained surgically. Surgery may also be needed for people with persistent fever and weight loss.

Usually, an artificial joint that has an infection around it is removed and replaced. Antibiotics may be given several weeks before surgery to try to eradicate the infection, so that the contaminated artificial joint can be removed and a new one can be implanted at the same time. Rarely, treatment is not successful and the infection continues, requiring surgery to fuse the joint or amputate the limb.

Infectious Arthritis

Infectious arthritis (septic arthritis) is infection in the fluid and tissues of a joint usually caused by bacteria, but sometimes caused by viruses or fungi.

- Bacteria or sometimes viruses or fungi may spread through the bloodstream or from nearby infected tissue to a joint, causing infection.
- Pain, swelling, and fever usually develop within hours or a couple of days.
- Joint fluid is withdrawn in a needle and tested.
- Antibiotics are begun immediately.

People at risk of infectious arthritis include those who have abnormal joints because of arthritis (including rheumatoid arthritis, osteoarthritis, or arthritis from injury) who develop an infection that reaches the bloodstream. For example, an older person with pneumonia and sepsis (a bloodstream infection) may fall and injure a wrist. Bleeding into the injured wrist may then result in infectious arthritis.

Infecting organisms, mainly bacteria, usually reach the joint through the bloodstream, but a joint can be infected directly if it is contaminated during surgery or by an injection or an injury. Different bacteria can infect a joint, but the bacteria most likely to cause infection depend on a person's age. Staphylococci and bacteria known as gram-negative bacilli most often infect infants and young children, whereas gonococci (bacteria that cause gonorrhea), staphylococci, and streptococci most often infect older children and adults. Occasionally, spirochetes (a type of bacteria), such as those that cause Lyme disease and syphilis, can infect joints.

Viruses—such as the human immunodeficiency virus (HIV), parvoviruses, and those that cause rubella, mumps, and hepatitis B—can infect joints in people of any age. A slowly developing chronic infectious arthritis is most often caused by *Mycobacterium tuberculosis* (the main cause of tuberculosis) or fungi.

> **? Did You Know...**
>
> People who have chronic arthritis, such as rheumatoid arthritis, and suddenly develop pain and swelling in a single joint should contact their doctor promptly because they may have an infection.

Symptoms

Infants usually have fever and pain and tend to be fussy. Generally, infants do not move the infected joint because moving or touching it is painful. Young children with knee or hip infections may refuse to walk. In older children and adults, symptoms usually begin over hours to a few days. The infected joint usually becomes red and warm, and moving or touching it is very painful. Fluid collects in the infected joint, causing it to swell and stiffen. Symptoms also include fever and chills. Less dramatic symptoms (such as less pain and a lower fever) usually occur in people with chronic infectious arthritis that is caused by mycobacteria or fungi.

The joints most commonly infected are the knee, shoulder, wrist, hip, elbow, and the joints of the fingers. Most bacterial, fungal, and mycobacterial infections affect only one joint or, occasionally, several joints. For example, the bacteria that cause Lyme disease most often infect knee joints. Gonococcal bacteria and viruses can infect a few or many joints at the same time.

Diagnosis

Usually, a sample of joint fluid is removed with a needle as soon as possible. It is examined for white blood cells and tested for bacteria and other organisms. The laboratory can almost always grow and identify the infecting bacteria from the joint fluid, unless the person has recently taken antibiotics. However, the bacteria that cause gonorrhea, Lyme disease, and syphilis are difficult to recover from joint fluid. If bacteria do grow in culture, the laboratory then tests which antibiotics would be effective.

A doctor usually orders blood tests because bacteria from joint infections often appear in the bloodstream. Sputum, spinal fluid, and urine may also be tested for bacteria to help determine the source of infection.

Prognosis and Treatment

Because an infected joint can be destroyed within days or sometimes within hours without prompt treatment, antibiotics must be started as soon as an infection is suspected, even before the laboratory has identified the infecting organism. Antibiotics that kill the most likely bacteria are given until the infecting organism is identified, usually within 48 hours of testing the joint fluid. Antibiotics are given by vein (intravenously) at first, to ensure that enough of the drug reaches the infected joint. If the antibiotics are effective against the infecting bacteria, improvement usually occurs within 48 hours. As soon as the doctor receives the laboratory results, the antibiotic may be changed depending on the sensitivity of the particular bacteria to specific antibiotics.

The doctor often removes pus with a needle to prevent its accumulation, because accumulated pus may damage a joint. If drainage with a needle is difficult (as with a hip joint) or unsuccessful, arthroscopy (a procedure using a small scope to view the interior of the joint directly—see page 544) or surgery may be needed to drain the joint. Sometimes a tube is left in place to drain the pus. Splinting the joint (to keep it from moving) can help ease pain at first, but physical therapy is also needed to prevent stiffness and permanent loss of function.

Infections caused by fungi are treated with antifungal drugs. Infections caused by mycobacteria are treated with a combination of antibiotics. Infections caused by viruses usually get better without treatment—only acetaminophen or a nonsteroidal antiinflammatory drug (NSAID) is needed for pain and fever.

<table>
<tr><td>CHAPTER
96</td><td># Joint Disorders</td></tr>
</table>

Osteoarthritis

Osteoarthritis (sometimes called degenerative arthritis, degenerative joint disease, osteoarthrosis, or hypertrophic osteoarthritis) is a chronic disorder associated with damage to the cartilage and surrounding tissues and characterized by pain, stiffness, and loss of function.

- Arthritis due to damage of joint cartilage and surrounding tissues becomes very common with aging.
- Pain, swelling, and bony overgrowth are common, as well as stiffness that follows awakening or inactivity and disappears within 30 minutes, particularly if the joint is moved.
- The diagnosis is based on symptoms and x-rays.
- Treatment includes exercises and other physical measures, drugs that reduce pain and improve function, and, for very severe changes, joint replacement or other surgery.

Osteoarthritis, the most common joint disorder, often begins in the 40s and 50s and affects almost all people to some degree by age 80. Before the age of 40, men develop osteoarthritis more often than do women, often because of injury. From age 40 to 70, women develop the disorder more often than do men. After age 70, the disorder develops in both sexes equally.

Causes

Normally, joints have such a low friction level that they are protected from wearing out, even after years of use. Osteoarthritis is caused most often by tissue damage. In an attempt to repair a damaged joint, chemicals accumulate in the joint and increase the production of the components of cartilage, such as collagen (a tough, fibrous protein in connective tissue) and proteoglycans (substances that provide

SPOTLIGHT ON AGING

Many myths about osteoarthritis persist—for example, that it is an inevitable part of aging, like gray hair and skin changes, that it results in little disability, and that treatment is not effective.

Osteoarthritis does become more common with aging. For instance, as people age, the cartilage that lines the joints tends to thin. The surfaces of a joint may not slide over each other as well as they used to, and the joint may be slightly more susceptible to injury. However, osteoarthritis is not an inevitable part of aging. It is not caused simply by the wear and tear that occurs with years of joint use. Other factors may include single or repeated injury, abnormal motion, metabolic disorders, joint infection, or another joint disorder.

Also, osteoarthritis commonly causes disability in later life. Effective treatment, such as analgesics, exercises and physical therapy, and, in some cases, surgery, is available.

Ligament damage is also common with aging. Ligaments, which bind joints together, tend to become less elastic as people age, making joints feel tight or stiff. This change results from chemical changes in the proteins that make up the ligaments. Consequently, most people become less flexible as they age. Ligaments tend to tear more easily, and when they tear, they heal more slowly. Older people should stretch before exercising to decrease the chance of ligament tears. They should also have their exercise regimen reviewed by a trainer or doctor so that exercises likely to tear ligaments can be avoided.

resilience). Next, the cartilage may swell because of water retention, become soft, and then develop cracks on the surface. Tiny cavities form in the bone beneath the cartilage, weakening the bone. The attempt of the tissues to repair the damage may lead to new growth of cartilage, bone, and other tissue. Bone can overgrow at the edges of the joint, causing bumps (osteophytes) that can be seen and felt. Ultimately, the smooth, slippery surface of the cartilage becomes rough and pitted, so that the joint can no longer move smoothly and absorb impact. All the components of the joint—bone, joint capsule (tissues that enclose most joints), synovial tissue (tissue lining the joint cavity), tendons, ligaments, and cartilage—fail in various ways, thus altering the function of the joint.

Osteoarthritis is classified as primary (or idiopathic) when the cause is not known (as in the large majority of cases). It is classified as secondary when the cause is another disease or condition, such as an infection, deformity, injury, abnormal use of a joint, metabolic disorder (for example, excess iron in the body [hemochromatosis] or excess copper in the liver [Wilson's disease]), or a disorder that damages joint cartilage (for example, rheumatoid arthritis or gout). Some people who repetitively stress one joint or a group of joints, such as foundry workers, farmers, coal miners, and bus drivers, are particularly at risk. The major risk factor for osteoarthritis of the knee comes from having an occupation that involves bending of the joint. Curiously, long-distance running does not increase the risk of developing the disorder. However, once osteoarthritis develops, this type of exercise often makes the disorder worse. Obesity may be a major factor in the development of osteoarthritis, particularly of the knee and especially in women.

Symptoms

Usually, symptoms develop gradually and affect only one or a few joints at first. Joints of the fingers, base of the thumbs, neck, lower back, big toes, hips, and knees are commonly affected. Pain, often described as a deep ache, is the first symptom and, when in the weight-bearing joints, is usually made worse by activities that involve weight bearing (such as standing. In some people, the joint may be stiff after sleep or some other inactivity, but the stiffness usually subsides within 30 minutes, particularly if the joint is moved.

As the condition causes more symptoms, the joint may become less movable and eventually may not be able to fully straighten or bend. New growth of cartilage, bone, and other tissue can enlarge the joints. The irregular cartilage surfaces cause joints to grind, grate, or crackle when they are moved. Bony growths commonly develop in the joints closest to the fingertips (called Heberden's nodes) or middle of the fingers (called Bouchard's nodes).

In some joints (such as the knee), the ligaments, which surround and support the joint, stretch so that the joint becomes unstable. Alternatively, the hip or knee may become stiff, losing its range of motion. Touching or moving the joint (particularly when standing, climbing stairs, or walking) can be very painful.

Osteoarthritis often affects the spine. Back pain is the most common symptom. Usually, damaged disks or joints in the spine cause only mild pain and stiffness. However, osteoarthritis in the neck or lower back can cause numbness, pain, and weakness in an arm or leg if the overgrowth of bone presses on nerves. The overgrowth of bone may be within the spinal canal in the lower back (lumbar spinal stenosis), pressing on nerves before they exit the canal to go to the legs. This pressure may cause

How to Live With Osteoarthritis

- Exercise affected joints gently (by exercising in a pool if possible, by using a stationary bicycle, or by walking).
- Receive acupuncture or massage at and around affected joints (these measures should preferably be done by a trained therapist).
- Apply a heating pad or a damp and warm towel to affected joints.
- Avoid gaining too much weight (so as not to place extra stress on joints), or lose weight if overweight.
- Use special equipment as necessary (for example, cane, crutches, walker, neck collar, or elastic knee support to protect joints from overuse; or a fixed seat placed in a bathtub to enable less stretching while washing).
- Wear well-supported shoes or athletic shoes.

leg pain after walking, suggesting incorrectly that the person has a reduced blood supply to the legs (intermittent claudication—see page 419). Rarely, bony growths compress the esophagus, making swallowing difficult.

Osteoarthritis may be stable for many years or may progress very rapidly, but most often it progresses slowly after symptoms develop. Many people develop some degree of disability.

Diagnosis

The doctor makes the diagnosis based on the characteristic symptoms, physical examination, and the x-ray appearance of joints (such as bone enlargement and narrowing of the joint space). By age 40, many people have some evidence of osteoarthritis on x-rays, especially in weight-bearing joints such as the hip and knee, but only half of these people have symptoms. However, x-rays are not very useful for detecting osteoarthritis early because they do not show changes in cartilage, which is where the earliest abnormalities occur. Also, changes on the x-ray often correlate poorly with symptoms. For example, an x-ray may show only a minor change in a person who has severe symptoms, or an x-ray may show numerous changes in a person who has very few, if any, symptoms.

Magnetic resonance imaging (MRI) can reveal early changes in cartilage, but it is rarely needed for the diagnosis. Also, MRI is in too short supply to justify routine use. There are no blood tests for the diagnosis of osteoarthritis, although blood tests may help rule out other disorders (such as rheumatoid arthritis—see page 563). If a joint is swollen, a

sample of the joint fluid is sometimes withdrawn using a needle and local anesthesia. Analysis of the fluid can help differentiate osteoarthritis from disorders such as infection and gout.

Treatment

Appropriate exercises—including stretching, strengthening, and postural exercises—help maintain healthy cartilage, increase a joint's range of motion, and strengthen surrounding muscles so that they can absorb stress better. Exercise can sometimes stop or even reverse osteoarthritis of the hip and knee. Stretching exercises should be performed daily. Exercise must be balanced with rest of painful joints, but immobilizing a joint is more likely to worsen the disease than relieve it. Using excessively soft chairs, recliners, mattresses, and car seats may worsen symptoms. Using car seats moved forward, straight-backed chairs with relatively high seats (such as kitchen or dining room chairs), firm mattresses, and bed boards (available at many lumber yards) and wearing wear well-supported shoes or athletic shoes are often recommended.

For osteoarthritis of the spine, specific exercises sometimes help, and back supports or braces may be needed when pain is severe. Exercises should include both muscle-strengthening as well as low-impact aerobic exercises (such as walking, swimming, and bicycle riding). If possible, people should maintain ordinary daily activities and continue to perform their normal activities, such as a hobby or job. However, physical activities may have to be adjusted to avoid bending and thus aggravating the pain of osteoarthritis.

Did You Know...

Acetaminophen is almost always preferred to nonsteroidal anti-inflammatory drugs (NSAIDs) for initial treatment of osteoarthritis because it is usually as effective and safer.

Physical therapy, often with heat therapy (see page 46), can be helpful. Range-of-motion exercises performed in warm water are helpful because heat improves muscle function by reducing stiffness and muscle spasm. Cold may be applied to reduce pain from temporary worsening in one joint. Splints or supports (such as a cane, crutch, brace, or even a walker) can protect specific joints during painful activities. Shoe inserts (orthotics) may help reduce pain caused by walking. Massage by trained therapists and deep heat treatment with diathermy or ultrasound may be useful.

Drugs are used to supplement exercise and physical therapy. Drugs, which may be used in combination or individually, do not directly alter the course of osteoarthritis. They are used to reduce symptoms and thus allow more normal daily activities. A simple pain medicine (analgesic), such as acetaminophen, may be all that is needed for mild to moderate pain. Alternatively, a nonsteroidal anti-inflammatory drug (NSAID) may be taken to lessen pain and swelling. NSAIDs reduce pain and inflammation in joints (see page 644). However, they have a higher risk of serious side effects than acetaminophen when used long term. Sometimes other types of pain medicine may be needed. For example, a cream derived from cayenne pepper—the active ingredient is capsaicin—can be applied directly to the skin over the joint.

Muscle relaxants (usually in low doses) occasionally relieve pain caused by muscles straining to support joints affected by osteoarthritis. In older people, however, they tend to cause more side effects than relief.

If a joint suddenly becomes inflamed, swollen, and painful, most of the fluid inside the joint may need to be removed and a special form of cortisone may be injected directly into the joint. This treatment may provide only short-term relief, and a joint treated with cortisone should not be used too often

or damage may result. A series of 3 to 5 weekly injections of hyaluronate (similar to a component of normal joint fluid) into the joint may provide significant pain relief in some people for prolonged periods of time (up to a year).

Several nutritional supplements (such as glucosamine sulfate and chondroitin sulfate) are being tested for potential benefit in treating osteoarthritis. So far, results are contradictory, and the potential benefit of glucosamine sulfate and chondroitin sulfate is unclear. There is less evidence that other nutritional supplements work.

Surgical treatment may help when all other treatments fail to relieve pain or improve function. Some joints, most commonly the hip (see art on page 1961) and knee (see art below), can be replaced with an artificial joint. Replacement is usually very successful, almost always improving motion and function and dramatically decreasing pain. Therefore, joint replacement should be considered when pain is unmanageable and function becomes limited. Because the artificial joint does not last forever, the procedure is often delayed as long as possible in young people so the need for repeated replacements can be minimized.

A variety of methods that restore cells inside cartilage have been used in younger people with osteoarthritis (often caused by an injury) to help heal small

Replacing a Knee

A knee joint damaged by osteoarthritis may be replaced with an artificial joint. After a general anesthetic is given, the surgeon makes an incision over the damaged knee. The knee cap (patella) may be removed, and the ends of the thigh bone (femur) and shinbone

(tibia) are smoothed so that the parts of the artificial joint (prosthesis) can be attached more easily. One part of the artificial joint is inserted into the thigh bone, the other part is inserted into the shinbone, and then the parts are cemented in place.

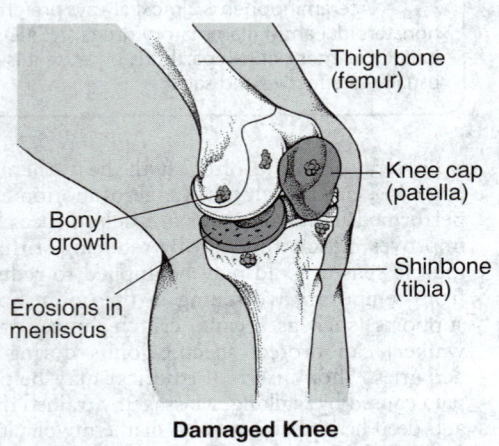

Damaged Knee

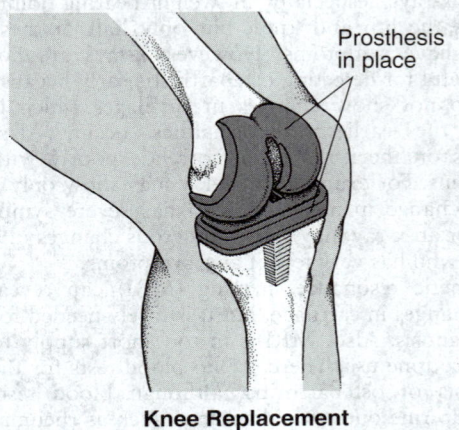

Knee Replacement

defects in cartilage. However, such methods have not yet proved valuable when cartilage defects are extensive, as commonly occurs in older people.

Rheumatoid Arthritis

Rheumatoid arthritis is an inflammatory arthritis in which joints, usually including those of the hands and feet, are inflamed, resulting in swelling, pain, and often destruction of joints.

- The immune system damages the joints and connective tissues.
- Joints (typically the small joints of the limbs) become painful and have stiffness that persists for more than 60 minutes on awakening and after inactivity.
- Fever, weakness, and damage to other organs may occur.
- Diagnosis is based mainly on symptoms but also on blood tests for rheumatoid factor and on x-rays.
- Treatment can include exercises and splinting, drugs (nonsteroidal anti-inflammatory drugs, disease-modifying antirheumatic drugs, and immunosuppressive drugs), and surgery.

Worldwide, rheumatoid arthritis develops in about 1% of the population, regardless of race or country of origin, affecting women 2 to 3 times more often than men. Usually, rheumatoid arthritis first appears between 35 years and 50 years of age, but it may occur at any age. A disorder similar to rheumatoid arthritis can occur in children. The disease is then called juvenile idiopathic arthritis, and the symptoms and prognosis are often somewhat different (see page 1829).

The exact cause of rheumatoid arthritis is not known. It is considered an autoimmune disease (see page 1124). Components of the immune system attack the soft tissue that lines the joints and can also attack connective tissue in many other parts of the body, such as the blood vessels and lungs. Eventually, the cartilage, bone, and ligaments of the joint erode, causing deformity, instability, and scarring within the joint. The joints deteriorate at a variable rate. Many factors, including genetic predisposition, may influence the pattern of the disease. Unknown environmental factors (such as viral infections) are thought to play a role.

Symptoms

People with rheumatoid arthritis may have a mild course, occasional flare-ups with long periods of remission (in which the disease is inactive), or a steadily progressive disease, which may be slow or rapid. Rheumatoid arthritis may start suddenly, with many joints becoming inflamed at the same time. More often, it starts subtly, gradually affecting different joints. Usually, the inflammation is symmetric, with joints on both sides of the body affected about equally. Typically, the small joints in the fingers, toes, hands, feet, wrists, elbows, and ankles become inflamed first. The inflamed joints are usually painful and often stiff, especially just after awakening (such stiffness generally lasts for more than 60 minutes) or after prolonged inactivity. Some people feel tired and weak, especially in the early afternoon. Rheumatoid arthritis may cause a loss of appetite with weight loss and a low-grade fever.

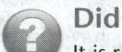

Did You Know...

It is rare for specific foods to cause flare-ups of rheumatoid arthritis.

Affected joints are tender, warm, red, and enlarged because of swelling of the soft tissue and sometimes fluid within the joint. Joints can quickly become deformed. Joints may freeze in one position so that they cannot bend or open fully. The fingers may tend to dislocate slightly from their normal position toward the little finger on each hand, causing tendons in the fingers to slip out of place.

Swollen wrists can pinch a nerve and result in numbness or tingling due to carpal tunnel syndrome (see page 601). Cysts, which may develop behind affected knees, can rupture, causing pain and swelling in the lower legs. Up to 30% of people with rheumatoid arthritis have hard bumps (called rheumatoid nodules) just under the skin, usually near sites of pressure (such as the back of the forearm near the elbow).

Rarely, rheumatoid arthritis causes an inflammation of blood vessels (vasculitis—see page 582). This condition reduces the blood supply to tissues and may cause nerve damage or leg sores (ulcers). Inflammation of the membranes that cover the lungs (pleura) or of the sac surrounding the heart (pericardium) or inflammation and scarring of the lungs or heart can lead to chest pain or shortness of breath. Some people develop swollen lymph nodes; Sjögren's syndrome, which consists of dry eyes, mouth, vagina, or a combination (see page 577); or red, painful eyes caused by inflammation (episcleritis).

Diagnosis

In addition to the important characteristic pattern of symptoms, the doctor may use the following to support the diagnosis: laboratory tests, an examination of a joint fluid sample obtained with a needle, and even a biopsy (removal of a tissue sample for examination under a microscope) of rheumatoid nodules. Characteristic changes in the joints may be seen on x-rays. Magnetic resonance imaging (MRI) seems to be more sensitive and detects joint abnormalities earlier but is not usually necessary for making the diagnosis.

Blood Tests: In 9 of 10 people who have rheumatoid arthritis, the erythrocyte sedimentation rate (ESR—a test that measures the rate at which red blood cells settle to the bottom of a test tube containing blood) is increased, which suggests that active inflammation is present. However, similar increases in the ESR occur in many other disorders. Doctors may monitor the ESR to help determine whether the disease is active.

Many people with rheumatoid arthritis have distinctive antibodies in their blood, such as rheumatoid factor, which is present in 70% of people with rheumatoid arthritis. (Rheumatoid factor also occurs in several other diseases, such as hepatitis and some other infections. Some people even have rheumatoid factor in their blood without any evidence of disease.) Usually, the higher the level of rheumatoid factor in the blood, the more severe the rheumatoid arthritis and the poorer the prognosis. The rheumatoid factor level may decrease when joints are less inflamed.

Anti-citrullinated peptide (anti-CCP) antibodies are present in 96% of people who have rheumatoid arthritis and are almost always absent in people who do not have rheumatoid arthritis. Doctors are starting to use tests for anti-CCP antibodies to help diagnose rheumatoid arthritis.

Most people have mild anemia (an insufficient number of red blood cells—see page 1031). Rarely, the white blood cell count becomes abnormally low. When a person with rheumatoid arthritis has a low white blood cell count and an enlarged spleen, the disorder is called Felty's syndrome.

Prognosis

The course of rheumatoid arthritis is unpredictable. The disorder progresses most rapidly during the first 6 years, particularly the first year, and 80% of people develop permanent joint abnormalities within 10 years. Rheumatoid arthritis may decrease life expectancy by 3 to 7 years. Heart disease, infection, gastrointestinal bleeding, drug treatment, cancer, and the underlying disease may be responsible. Rarely, rheumatoid arthritis resolves spontaneously.

Treatment relieves symptoms in 3 of 4 people; however, at least 10% are eventually severely disabled despite full treatment. Factors that tend to predict a poorer prognosis include the following:

- Being white, a woman, or both
- Having rheumatoid nodules
- Being older when the disorder begins

- Having inflammation in 20 or more joints
- Having a high ESR
- Having high levels of rheumatoid factor or anti-CCP

Treatment

Treatments include simple, conservative measures in addition to drugs and surgical treatments. Simple measures are meant to help the person's symptoms and include rest and adequate nutrition. Because disease-modifying antirheumatic drugs (DMARDs) may actually slow progression of the disease as well as relieve symptoms, they are often started soon after the diagnosis of rheumatoid arthritis is made.

Severely inflamed joints should be rested, because using them can aggravate the inflammation. Regular rest periods often help relieve pain, and sometimes a short period of bed rest helps relieve a severe flare-up in its most active, painful stage. Splints can be used to immobilize and rest one or several joints, but some systematic movement of the joints is needed to prevent adjacent muscles from weakening and joints from freezing in place.

A regular, healthy diet is generally appropriate. A diet rich in fish and plant oils but low in red meat can have small beneficial effects on the inflammation. Rarely, people have flare-ups after eating certain foods, and if so, these foods should be avoided. Many diets have been proposed but have not proven helpful. Fad diets should be avoided.

The main categories of drugs used to treat rheumatoid arthritis are the nonsteroidal anti-inflammatory drugs (NSAIDs), DMARDs, corticosteroids, and immunosuppressive drugs. Newer drugs include leflunomide, anakinra (an interleukin-1 receptor antagonist), tumor necrosis factor (TNF)–inhibiting drugs, and other drugs that modify the immune response (immunosuppressive drugs). Generally, stronger drugs have potentially serious side effects that must be looked for during treatment.

Nonsteroidal Anti-Inflammatory Drugs: NSAIDs (see page 644) are commonly used to treat the symptoms of rheumatoid arthritis. They do not prevent the damage caused by rheumatoid arthritis from progressing and thus should not be considered the primary treatment. NSAIDs can reduce the swelling in affected joints and relieve pain. Rheumatoid arthritis, unlike osteoarthritis, causes considerable inflammation. Thus, drugs that decrease inflammation, including NSAIDs, have an important advantage over drugs such as acetaminophen that reduce pain but not inflammation. However, all NSAIDs (including aspirin) cause side effects and can upset the stomach and cannot be taken by anyone who has active digestive tract (peptic) ulcers—including stomach ulcers or duodenal ulcers. Drugs called proton pump inhibitors (such as esomeprazole, lansoprazole, omeprazole, pantoprazole, and rabeprazole) can reduce the risk of stomach or duodenal ulcers. Other possible side effects of NSAIDs may include headache, confusion, worsening of high blood pressure, worsening of kidney function, and swelling. People who get hives or asthma after they take aspirin may have the same symptoms after taking other NSAIDs. NSAIDs may increase the risk of heart attacks and strokes. The risk appears to be higher if the drug is used at higher doses and for longer periods of time. The risk is higher with certain NSAIDs than others.

Aspirin is no longer used to treat rheumatoid arthritis because effective doses are often toxic.

The cyclooxygenase (COX-2) inhibitors (coxibs, such as celecoxib) are NSAIDs that act similarly to the other NSAIDs but are less likely to damage the stomach. However, if a person takes aspirin, stomach damage is almost as likely to occur as with other NSAIDs. Caution should be taken with use of coxibs and probably all NSAIDs for long periods or by people with risk factors for heart attack and stroke.

Disease-Modifying Antirheumatic Drugs (DMARDs): DMARDs, such as methotrexate, hydroxychloroquine, and sulfasalazine, slow the progression of rheumatoid arthritis and sometimes can improve the course of the disease, although most take weeks or months to have an effect. These drugs are usually added promptly after the diagnosis of rheumatoid arthritis is made. Even if pain is decreased with NSAIDs, a doctor will likely prescribe a DMARD because the disease progresses even if symptoms are absent or mild.

About 66% of people improve overall, but complete remissions are uncommon. The progression of arthritis usually slows, but pain may remain. People should be made fully aware of the risks of DMARDs and monitored carefully for evidence of toxicity.

Combinations of DMARDs may be more effective than single drugs. For example, hydroxychloroquine, sulfasalazine, and methotrexate together are more effective than methotrexate alone or the other two together. Also, combining certain immunosuppressant drugs with a DMARD is often more effective than using a single drug or certain combinations of DMARDs. For example, methotrexate can be combined with a TNF inhibitor.

Methotrexate is taken by mouth once weekly. It is anti-inflammatory at the low doses used to treat rheumatoid arthritis. It is very effective and begins to work within a few weeks, which is relatively rapid for a DMARD. If a person has liver dysfunction or diabetes and takes methotrexate, frequent doctor visits and blood tests may be warranted so that possible side effects can be detected early. The liver can scar, but this most often can be detected and reversed before major damage develops. People must refrain from drinking alcohol to minimize the risk of liver damage. Bone marrow suppression (suppression of the production of red blood cells, white blood cells, and platelets) is possible. Blood counts should be tested about every 2 months in all people taking the drug. Inflammation of the lung is rare but potentially fatal. Inflammation in the mouth and nausea can also develop. Severe relapses of arthritis can occur after methotrexate is discontinued. Folate (folic acid) tablets may decrease some of the side effects, such as mouth ulcers.

Hydroxychloroquine is given daily by mouth. Side effects, which are usually mild, include rashes, muscle aches, and eye problems. However, some eye problems can be permanent, so people taking hydroxychloroquine must have their eyes checked by an ophthalmologist before treatment begins and every 6 to 12 months during treatment. If the drug has not helped after 9 months, it is discontinued. Otherwise, hydroxychloroquine can be continued as long as necessary.

Sulfasalazine tablets can relieve symptoms and slow the development of joint damage. Sulfasalazine can also be used in people who have less severe rheumatoid arthritis or added to other drugs to boost their effectiveness. The dose is increased gradually, and improvement usually is seen within 3 months. Like the other DMARDs, it can cause stomach upset, liver problems, blood cell disorders, and rashes.

Gold compounds are not used anymore.

Corticosteroids: Corticosteroids, such as prednisone, are the most dramatically effective drugs for reducing inflammation anywhere in the body. Although corticosteroids are effective for short-term use, they may become less effective over time, and rheumatoid arthritis is usually active for years.

There is some controversy as to whether corticosteroids can slow the progression of rheumatoid arthritis. Furthermore, the long-term use of corticosteroids almost invariably leads to side effects, involving almost every organ in the body. Consequently, doctors usually reserve corticosteroids for short-term use when beginning treatment for severe symptoms (until a DMARD has taken effect) or in severe flare-ups when many joints are affected. They are also useful in treating inflammation outside of joints, for example, in the membranes covering the lungs (pleura) or in the sac surrounding the heart (pericardium). Because of the risk of side effects, the lowest effective dose is almost always used. When corticosteroids are injected into a joint, the person does not get the same side effects as when taking a

℞ DRUGS USED TO TREAT RHEUMATOID ARTHRITIS

DRUG	SOME SIDE EFFECTS	COMMENTS
Nonsteroidal anti-inflammatory drugs (NSAIDs)		
Diclofenac Ibuprofen Naproxen Many others (see table on page 646)	Upset stomach Stomach ulcers Increased blood pressure Kidney problems Possibly increased risk of heart attack and stroke	All NSAIDs treat the symptoms and decrease inflammation but do not alter the course of the disease.

Cyclooxygenase-2 (COX-2) inhibitors (coxibs), such as celecoxib	Risk of kidney problems
	Increased blood pressure
	Less risk of stomach ulcer than with
	  other NSAIDs
	Possible increased risk of heart attack
	  and stroke	

Disease-modifying antirheumatic drugs (DMARDs)		

Hydroxychloroquine	Usually mild:
	  Rashes
	  Muscle aches
	  Eye problems
		All DMARDs can slow progression of joint damage as well as gradually decrease pain and swelling.

Methotrexate	Liver disease Lung inflammation Nausea Increased susceptibility to infection Suppression of blood cell production in the bone marrow Mouth sores Decreased semen Hair loss	
Sulfasalazine	Suppression of blood cell production in the bone marrow Stomach upset Liver problems Rashes	
Corticosteroids		

Prednisone	Numerous side effects throughout the
	body with long-term use:
	  Weight gain
	  Diabetes
	  High blood pressure
	  Thinning of bones
		Prednisone can reduce inflammation quickly. It may not be useful long term because of side effects.

Immunosuppressive drugs		

Azathioprine
Cyclophosphamide
Cyclosporine
Leflunomide
	Liver disease
	An increased susceptibility to infection
	  and possibly cancer
	Suppression of blood cell production in the
	  bone marrow
	Rashes and liver disease with
	  leflunomide
		Azathioprine, cyclophosphamide, and cyclosporine are about as effective as other DMARDs but are more toxic.
		Cyclosporine does not affect the blood count but can reduce kidney function.
		Leflunomide is about as effective as methotrexate.

(continued on the following page)

℞ DRUGS USED TO TREAT RHEUMATOID ARTHRITIS (Continued)

DRUG	SOME SIDE EFFECTS	COMMENTS
Immunosuppressive drugs *(continued)*		
Adalimumab* Etanercept Infliximab	Potential risk of infection (particularly tuberculosis) or cancer Liver disease Suppression of blood cell production in the bone marrow	These drugs produce a dramatic, prompt response in most people. They can slow joint damage.
Anakinra	Pain and itching at injection site Infection Increased risk of infection and possibly cancer Suppression of blood cell production in the bone marrow	Anakinra is probably less effective than adalimumab, etanercept, and infliximab.
Rituximab	When the drug is being given: Itching at injection site Rashes Back pain High or low blood pressure Fever After the drug is given: Increased risk of infection and possibly cancer Suppression of blood cell production in the bone marrow	Rituximab is used only when people do not improve after taking a tumor necrosis factor inhibitor and methotrexate.
Abatacept	Infection Headache Upper respiratory infection Sore throat Nausea	Abatacept is used only when people do not improve after taking other drugs.

*Adalimumab, etanercept, and infliximab are tumor necrosis factor inhibitors.

corticosteroid by mouth (oral) or vein (intravenously). Corticosteroids can be injected directly into affected joints for fast, short-term relief.

People who have peptic ulcer disease, high blood pressure, infections, diabetes, and glaucoma should use oral or intravenous corticosteroids only when being closely monitored for side effects by their doctor.

Immunosuppressive Drugs: Although corticosteroids suppress the immune system, other drugs do so even more potently and are referred to as immunosuppressive drugs. Each of these drugs can slow the progression of disease and decrease the damage to bones adjacent to joints. However, by interfering with the immune system, immunosuppressive drugs may increase the risks of infection and certain cancers. Such drugs include methotrexate (which is often the first DMARD used), leflunomide, azathioprine, cyclophosphamide, cyclosporine, tumor necrosis factor (TNF) inhibitors, rituximab, and abatacept.

Immunosuppressive drugs are effective in treating severe rheumatoid arthritis. They suppress the inflammation so that corticosteroids can be avoided or given in lower doses. But immunosuppressive drugs have their own potentially toxic and serious side effects, including liver disease, an increased susceptibility to infection, the suppression of blood cell production in the bone marrow, and, with cyclophosphamide, bleeding from the bladder. In addition, azathioprine and cyclophosphamide may increase the risk of cancer. In women who are considering pregnancy, immunosuppressive drugs should be used only after discussion with a doctor.

Leflunomide is a drug with benefits that are similar to those of methotrexate but that may be less likely to cause suppression of blood cell production and lung scarring. It can be given at the same time as methotrexate. It is given daily by mouth. The major side effects are rashes, liver dysfunction, hair loss, and diarrhea.

Etanercept, infliximab, and adalimumab are TNF inhibitors and can be dramatically effective for people who do not respond sufficiently to methotrexate alone.

Corticosteroids: Uses and Side Effects

Corticosteroids are the strongest drugs available for reducing inflammation in the body. They are useful in any condition in which inflammation occurs, including rheumatoid arthritis and other connective tissue disorders, multiple sclerosis, and in emergencies such as brain swelling due to cancer, asthma attacks, and severe allergic reactions. When inflammation is severe, use of these drugs is often lifesaving.

Corticosteroids can be given by vein (especially in emergency situations), taken by mouth, or directly applied to the inflamed organ (as in inhaled versions for the lungs, in eye drops, and in a skin cream). For example, corticosteroids can be used as an inhaled preparation for treatment of asthma. They can be used as a nasal spray to treat hay fever (allergic rhinitis). They can be used as eye drops to treat eye inflammation (uveitis). They may be applied directly to an affected area for treatment of certain skin conditions such as eczema and psoriasis.

Corticosteroids are prepared synthetically to have the same action as cortisol (or cortisone), a steroid hormone produced by the outer layer (cortex) of the adrenal glands—hence the name "corticosteroid." Many synthetic corticosteroids are, however, more powerful than cortisol, and most are longer acting. Corticosteroids are chemically related to, but have different effects than, anabolic steroids (such as testosterone) that are produced by the body and sometimes abused by athletes.

Examples of corticosteroids include prednisone, dexamethasone, triamcinolone, betamethasone, beclomethasone, flunisolide, and fluticasone. All of these drugs are very strong (although strength depends on the dose used). Hydrocortisone is a milder corticosteroid that is available in over-the-counter skin creams.

Because corticosteroids reduce the body's ability to fight infections by suppressing inflammation, they are used with extreme care when infections are present. Their use may worsen high blood pressure, heart failure, diabetes, peptic ulcers, and osteoporosis. Therefore, corticosteroids are used in such conditions only when their benefit is likely to exceed their risk.

When they are taken by mouth or by injection for more than about 2 weeks, corticosteroids should not be stopped abruptly. This is because corticosteroids inhibit the production of cortisol by the adrenal glands, and this production must be given time to recover. Thus, at the end of a course of corticosteroids, the dose is gradually reduced. It is important for a person who takes corticosteroids to follow the doctor's instructions on dosage very carefully.

The long-term use of corticosteroids, particularly at higher doses and particularly when given by mouth or vein, invariably leads to many side effects, involving almost every organ in the body. Common side effects include thinning of the skin with stretch marks and bruising, high blood pressure, elevated blood sugar levels, cataracts, puffiness in the face (moon face) and abdomen, thinning of the arms and legs, poor wound healing, stunted growth in children, loss of calcium from the bones (which can lead to osteoporosis), hunger, weight gain, and mood swings. Because most of their effects are caused locally, inhaled corticosteroids and those that are applied directly to the skin have far fewer side effects than the version given by mouth or that given by vein.

Etanercept is given once or twice weekly by injection under the skin, and infliximab is given by vein every 8 weeks after loading doses. Adalimumab is injected under the skin once every 1 or 2 weeks. TNF is part of the body's immune system, so inhibition of TNF can impair the body's ability to fight infections. These drugs should be avoided in people who have active infections. Etanercept, infliximab, and adalimumab can be used with methotrexate.

Anakinra is a recombinant interleukin-1 (IL-1) receptor antagonist, which means it interrupts one of the major chemical pathways involved in inflammation. Anakinra is given as a single daily injection. Pain and itching at the injection site are the most common side effects. IL-1 is part of the immune system, so inhibiting IL-1 can impair the ability to fight infections. Anakinra can also suppress production of white blood cells. It should not be used with TNF inhibitors.

Rituximab decreases the number of B-cell lymphocytes, one of the white blood cells responsible for causing inflammation and for fighting infection. Because there is not as much evidence for the safety of rituximab as many other drugs, rituximab is usually reserved for people who do not improve enough after taking methotrexate and a TNF inhibitor. It is injected in a vein, as 2 doses, 2 weeks apart. Side effects, as with other immunosuppressive drugs, may include increased risk of infections. In addition, rituximab can cause effects while it is being given, such as rashes, nausea, back pain, itching, and high or low blood pressure.

Abatacept interferes with the communication between cells that coordinates inflammation. It is injected in the vein over several minutes. Abatacept is associated with several side effects and is used only for those who have not improved after using other drugs.

Other Treatments: Along with drugs to reduce joint inflammation, a treatment plan for rheumatoid arthritis should include nondrug therapies, such as exercise, physical or occupational therapy, and sometimes surgical treatment. Inflamed joints should be gently stretched so they do not freeze in one position. As the inflammation subsides, regular, active exercises can help, although a person should not exercise to the point of excessive tiredness (fatigue). For many people, exercise in water may be easier.

Treatment of tight joints consists of intensive exercises and occasionally the use of splints to gradually extend the joint. If drugs have not helped, surgical treatment may be needed. Surgically replacing knee or hip joints is the most effective way to restore mobility and function when the joint disease is advanced. Joints can also be removed or fused together, especially in the foot, to make walking less painful. The thumb can be fused to enable a person to grasp, and unstable vertebrae at the top of the neck can be fused to prevent them from compressing the spinal cord.

People who are disabled by rheumatoid arthritis can use several aids to accomplish daily tasks. For example, specially modified orthopedic or athletic shoes can make walking less painful, and devices such as grippers reduce the need to squeeze the hand forcefully.

Surgical repair must always be considered in terms of the total disease. For example, deformed hands and arms limit a person's ability to use crutches during rehabilitation, and seriously affected knees and feet limit the benefits of hip surgery. Reasonable objectives for each person must be determined, and ability to function must be considered. Surgical repair may be performed while the disease is active.

Joint repair with prosthetic joint replacement is indicated if damage severely limits function. Total hip and knee replacements are most consistently successful.

Other Types of Inflammatory Arthritis

Several connective tissue diseases, including the spondyloarthropathies (also called spondyloarthritides), cause prominent joint inflammation. The spondyloarthropathies affect the joints and spine. These disorders share certain characteristics. For example, they may cause back pain, inflammation of the eye (uveitis), digestive symptoms, and rashes. Some are strongly associated with the *HLA-B27* gene. Because they cause many of the same problems and share genetic characteristics, some experts think these disorders share similar causes and ways of causing symptoms. The spondyloarthropathies cause joint inflammation, similar to rheumatoid arthritis. However, in contrast to rheumatoid arthritis, rheumatoid factor (see page 564) is negative in the spondyloarthropathies (hence, they are also called the seronegative spondyloarthropathies). Among the spondyloarthropathies are psoriatic arthritis, reactive arthritis, and ankylosing spondylitis.

PSORIATIC ARTHRITIS

Psoriatic arthritis is a form of joint inflammation that occurs in some people who have psoriasis of the skin or nails.

- Joint inflammation can develop in people who have psoriasis.
- Joints commonly involved include the hips, knees, and those closest to the tips of the fingers and toes.
- The diagnosis is based on symptoms.
- Nonsteroidal anti-inflammatory drugs, methotrexate, cyclosporine, and tumor necrosis factor inhibitors (adalimumab, etanercept, and infliximab) can help.

The disease resembles rheumatoid arthritis but does not produce the antibodies characteristic of rheumatoid arthritis. Psoriatic arthritis occurs in about 5 to 40% of people with psoriasis (a skin condition causing flare-ups of red, scaly rashes and thickened, pitted nails—see page 1292). The cause of psoriatic arthritis is unknown.

Symptoms and Diagnosis

Inflammation often affects joints closest to the tips of the fingers and toes, although other joints, including the hips, knees and spine, are often affected as well. Often the joints of the upper extremities are affected more. Back pain may be present. The joints may become swollen and deformed when inflammation is chronic. Psoriatic arthritis often involves joints less symmetrically than rheumatoid arthritis and involves fewer joints. The psoriasis rash may appear before or after arthritis develops. Sometimes the rash is not noticed because it is hidden in the scalp or creases of the skin such as between the back of the buttocks and thigh. The skin and joint symptoms sometimes appear and disappear together.

The diagnosis is made by identifying the characteristic joint inflammation in a person who has arthritis and psoriasis or a family history of psoriasis. There are no tests to confirm the diagnosis, but x-rays help show the extent of joint damage.

Prognosis and Treatment

The prognosis for psoriatic arthritis is usually better than that for rheumatoid arthritis because fewer joints are affected. Nonetheless, the joints can be severely damaged.

Treatment is aimed at controlling the skin rash and relieving the joint inflammation. Several drugs that are effective in treating rheumatoid arthritis are also used to treat psoriatic arthritis, particularly nonsteroidal anti-inflammatory drugs (NSAIDs), methotrexate, cyclosporine, and tumor necrosis factor (TNF) inhibitors.

Some people take methoxsalen (psoralen) by mouth and undergo psoralen plus ultraviolet A light treatments. This combination relieves the skin symptoms and most of the joint inflammation but may not help inflammation of the spine.

REACTIVE ARTHRITIS

Reactive arthritis (sometimes called Reiter syndrome) is inflammation of the joints and tendon attachments at the joints, often related to an infection.

- Joint pain and inflammation can occur in response to an infection, usually of the genitourinary or gastrointestinal tract.
- Tendon inflammation, skin rashes, and red eye are also common.
- The diagnosis is based on symptoms.
- NSAIDs, sulfasalazine, azathioprine, and methotrexate may help treat the symptoms.

Reactive arthritis is so called because the joint inflammation seems to be a reaction to an infection originating in the gastrointestinal or genitourinary tract.

There are two forms of reactive arthritis. One form seems to occur with sexually transmitted diseases, such as a chlamydial infection, and occurs most often in men aged 20 to 40. The other form usually follows an intestinal infection such as shigellosis, salmonellosis, or a *Campylobacter* infection. Most people who have these infections do not develop reactive arthritis. People who develop reactive arthritis after exposure to these infections seem to have a genetic predisposition to this type of reaction, related in part to the same gene found in people who have ankylosing spondylitis (see page 571). There is some evidence that the chlamydia bacteria and possibly other bacteria actually spread to the joints, but the roles of the infection and the immune reaction to it are not clear.

Reactive arthritis may be accompanied by inflammation of the conjunctiva (see page 1437) and the mucous membranes (such as those of the mouth and genitals) and by a distinctive rash. This form of reactive arthritis previously was called Reiter syndrome.

Symptoms

Joint pain and inflammation may be mild or severe. Several joints are usually affected at once—especially the knees, toe joints, and areas where tendons are attached to bones, such as at the heels. Often, the large joints of the lower limbs are affected the most. Reactive arthritis often involves joints less symmetrically than rheumatoid arthritis.

Tendons may be inflamed and painful. Back pain may occur, usually when the disease is severe.

Inflammation of the urethra (the channel that carries urine from the bladder to the outside of the body) can develop, usually about 7 to 14 days after the infection. In men, inflammation of the urethra causes moderate pain and a discharge from the penis or a rash on the glans of the penis (balanitis circinata). The prostate gland may be inflamed and painful. The genital and urinary symptoms in women, if any occur, are usually mild, consisting of a slight vaginal discharge or uncomfortable urination. Other symptoms include a low-grade fever and excessive tiredness (fatigue).

The conjunctiva (the membrane that lines the eyelid and covers the eyeball) can become red and inflamed, causing itching or burning, sensitivity to light, and excessive tearing. Small and usually painless or sometimes tender sores can develop in the mouth. Occasionally, a distinctive rash of hard, thickened spots may develop on the skin, especially of the palms and soles (keratoderma blennorrhagicum). Yellow deposits may develop under the fingernails and toenails.

Rarely, heart and blood vessel complications (such as inflammation of the aorta), inflammation of the membranes covering the lungs, dysfunction of the aortic valve, and brain and spinal cord symptoms or peripheral nervous system (which includes all the nerves outside the brain and spinal cord) symptoms may develop.

In most people, the initial symptoms disappear in 3 or 4 months, but up to 50% of people experience recurring joint inflammation or other symptoms over several years. Joint and spinal deformities may develop if the symptoms persist or recur frequently. Some people who have reactive arthritis become permanently disabled.

Diagnosis

The combination of joint symptoms and a preceding infection, particularly if there are genital, urinary, skin, and eye symptoms, leads a doctor to suspect reactive arthritis. Because these symptoms may not appear simultaneously, the disease may not be diagnosed for several months. No simple laboratory tests are available to confirm the diagnosis, but x-rays are often performed to assess the status of joints. Tests may be done to exclude other disorders that can cause similar symptoms.

Treatment

When the disease affects the genitals or urinary tract, antibiotics are given to treat the infection, but treatment is not always successful and its optimal duration is not known.

Joint inflammation is usually treated with an NSAID. Sulfasalazine or drugs that suppress the immune system (such as azathioprine or methotrexate) may be used, as in rheumatoid arthritis. Physical therapy is helpful in maintaining joint mobility during the recovery phase.

Conjunctivitis and skin sores do not usually need to be treated, although severe eye inflammation (uveitis) may require corticosteroid and dilating eyedrops.

ANKYLOSING SPONDYLITIS

Ankylosing spondylitis is a disorder characterized by inflammation of the spine and large joints, resulting in stiffness and pain.

- Joint pain, back stiffness, and eye inflammation are common.
- The diagnosis is based on symptoms and x-rays.
- NSAIDs and sometimes sulfasalazine or methotrexate can help the arthritis in limbs.
- Drugs that inhibit tumor necrosis factor are very effective for spine and limb arthritis.

The disease is 3 times more common among men than women, developing most commonly between the ages of 20 and 40. Its cause is not known, but the disease tends to run in families, indicating that genetics plays a role. Ankylosing spondylitis is 10 to 20 times more common among people whose parents or siblings have it.

Symptoms

Mild to moderate flare-ups of inflammation generally alternate with periods of almost no symptoms.

The most common symptom is back pain, which varies in intensity from one episode to another and from one person to another. Pain is often worse at night and in the morning. Early morning stiffness that is relieved by activity is also very common. Pain in the lower back and the associated muscle spasms are often relieved by bending forward. Therefore, people often assume a stooped posture, which can lead to a permanent bent-over position. In others, the spine becomes noticeably straight and stiff.

Loss of appetite, low-grade fever, weight loss, excessive tiredness (fatigue), and anemia can accompany the back pain. If the joints connecting the ribs to the spine are inflamed, the pain may limit the ability to expand the chest to take a deep breath. Stiffness (fusion) of the spine can restrict the ability to expand the chest wall as well. Occasionally, pain starts in large joints, such as the hips, knees, and shoulders.

One third of the people have recurring attacks of mild eye inflammation (uveitis), which usually does not impair vision if treated promptly. In a few people,

inflammation of a heart valve results in a permanently damaged valve, or other problems can affect the heart or aorta. If damaged vertebrae press against nerves or the spinal cord, numbness, weakness, or pain can develop in the area supplied by the affected nerves. Cauda equina (horse's tail) syndrome is an occasional complication (see box on page 800). Achilles tendinitis can develop.

Diagnosis

The diagnosis is based on the pattern of symptoms and on x-rays of the spine and affected joints, which show a wearing away (erosion) of the joint between the spine and the hip bone (sacroiliac joint) and the formation of bony bridges between the vertebrae, making the spine stiff. The erythrocyte sedimentation rate (ESR), a test that measures the rate at which red blood cells settle to the bottom of a test tube containing blood, tends to be high, indicating inflammation.

Prognosis

Most people develop some disabilities but can still lead normal, productive lives. In some people, the disease is more progressive, causing severe deformities. The prognosis is discouraging for people who develop extreme stiffness of the spine.

Treatment

Treatment focuses on relieving back and joint pain, maintaining range of motion in the joints, preventing damage in other organs, and preventing or correcting spinal deformities. NSAIDs can reduce the pain and inflammation, thus enabling people to do important exercises to retain posture, including stretching and deep breathing. Sulfasalazine or methotrexate may help the pain in joints other than those of the back. The TNF inhibitors etanercept, adalimumab, or infliximab can relieve back pain and inflammation.

Corticosteroid eye drops may help in the short-term treatment of inflammation of the eyes, and an occasional corticosteroid injection may be helpful for 1 or 2 joints other than the spine. Muscle relaxants and opioid analgesics are occasionally used, but for only brief periods to relieve severe pain and muscle spasms. If hips or knees become eroded or fixed in a bent position, surgical treatment to replace the joint can relieve pain and restore function.

The long-range goals of treatment are to maintain proper posture and develop strong back muscles. Daily exercises strengthen the muscles that oppose the tendency to bend and stoop. It has been suggested that people spend some time each day—often while reading—lying on their stomach propped up on their elbows because this position extends the back and helps to keep the back flexible. Because chest wall motion can be restricted, which impairs lung function, cigarette smoking, which also impairs lung function, is strongly discouraged.

OTHER SPONDYLOARTHROPATHIES

Spondyloarthropathy can develop in association with digestive conditions (sometimes called enteropathic arthritis), such as inflammatory bowel disease, intestinal bypass surgery, or Whipple's disease. Juvenile-onset spondyloarthropathy affects the lower extremities, often affects joints on opposite sides of the body to different degrees, and begins most commonly in boys aged 7 to 16. Spondyloarthropathy can also develop in people with no characteristics of other specific spondyloarthropathy (undifferentiated spondyloarthropathy). Treatment of the arthritis of these other spondyloarthropathies is similar to that of treatment of reactive arthritis (see page 570).

Charcot's Joints

Charcot's joints (neurogenic arthropathy, neuropathic arthropathy) is progressive joint destruction, often very rapid, that develops because people cannot sense pain and thus are not aware of the early signs of joint damage.

When certain nerves are damaged, people may become unable to sense pain. A variety of disorders, such as diabetes mellitus, spinal cord disorders, and syphilis, can damage these nerves. People with nerve damage may injure a joint many times, or even fracture it, without noticing. Injuries may occur for years before the joint malfunctions. However, once it

malfunctions, the joint may be permanently destroyed within a few months.

In its early stages, Charcot's joints appear similar to osteoarthritis, because the joint is stiff and fluid accumulates in it. Usually, the joint is not painful or is less painful than would be expected considering the amount of joint damage. If the disorder progresses rapidly, the joint can become extremely painful. In these cases, the joint is usually swollen because of excess fluid and abnormal bone growth. It may look deformed because it has been fractured and ligaments have stretched, allowing the bones to slip out of place. Moving the joint may cause a coarse, grating sound because of bone fragments floating in the joint. The joint may feel like a "bag of bones."

Any joint can be affected depending on where the nerve damage is—most commonly, the knee or ankle or, in people who have diabetes, the foot. Often, only one joint is affected, and usually not more than two or three.

Doctors suspect Charcot's joints when people have a nerve disorder and joint problems. X-rays can detect joint damage, which often includes calcium deposits and abnormal bone growth. Sometimes Charcot's joints can be prevented by taking care of the feet and by avoiding injuries. Splints or special boots can sometimes help protect vulnerable joints. Treatment of the underlying nerve disorder can sometimes slow or even reverse joint damage. Diagnosing and immobilizing painless fractures and splinting unstable joints can help stop or minimize the damage. Hips and knees may be surgically repaired or replaced. However, artificial joints often loosen prematurely.

CHAPTER

97 Autoimmune Disorders of Connective Tissue

In an autoimmune disorder, antibodies or cells produced by the body attack the body's own tissues (see page 1124). Many autoimmune disorders affect connective tissue in a variety of organs. Connective tissue is the structural tissue that gives strength to joints, tendons, ligaments, and blood vessels.

In autoimmune disorders, inflammation and the immune response may result in connective tissue damage, not only in and around joints but also in other tissues, including vital organs, such as the

kidneys and organs in the gastrointestinal tract. The sac that surrounds the heart (pericardium), the membrane that covers the lungs (pleura), and even the brain can be affected. The type and severity of symptoms depend on which organs are affected.

An autoimmune disorder of connective tissue is diagnosed on the basis of its particular symptom pattern, the findings during a physical examination, and the results of laboratory tests. Sometimes the symptoms of one disease overlap with those of another so much that doctors cannot make a distinction. In this case, the disorder may be called undifferentiated connective tissue disease or an overlap disease.

Systemic Lupus Erythematosus

Systemic lupus erythematosus (disseminated lupus erythematosus or lupus) is a chronic inflammatory connective tissue disorder that can involve joints, kidneys, mucous membranes, and blood vessel walls.

- Problems in the joints, nervous system, blood, skin, kidneys, gastrointestinal tract, and other tissues and organs can develop.
- The blood count and the presence of autoimmune antibodies are tested.
- People with active lupus often need corticosteroids or other drugs that suppress the immune system.

About 70 to 90% of people who have lupus are young women in their late teens to 30s, but children (mostly girls) and older men and women can also be affected. Lupus occurs in all parts of the world but may be more common among blacks and Asians.

The cause of lupus is usually not known. Occasionally, the use of certain drugs (such as hydralazine and procainamide, which are used to treat heart conditions, and isoniazid, which is used to treat tuberculosis) can cause lupus. Drug-induced lupus usually disappears after the drug is discontinued.

The number and variety of antibodies that can appear in lupus are greater than those in any other disorder. These antibodies, which are the underlying physiologic problem in lupus, along with other unknown factors, may sometimes determine which symptoms develop. However, the levels of these antibodies may not always be proportional to the person's symptoms.

Discoid lupus erythematosus is a form of lupus that affects only the skin. In this condition, raised round rashes occur, sometimes with scarring and hair loss in affected areas. In 10% of people, manifestations of systemic lupus—for example, those affecting the joints, kidneys, and brain—may occur but are generally mild.

Symptoms

Symptoms vary greatly from person to person. Symptoms may begin suddenly with fever, resembling a sudden, severe (acute) infection. Or symptoms may develop gradually over months or years with episodes (called flare-ups) of fever, feeling unwell, or any of the symptoms discussed below alternating with periods when symptoms are absent or minimal.

Migraine-type headaches, epilepsy, or severe mental disorders (psychoses) may be the first abnormalities that are noticed. Eventually, however, symptoms may affect any organ system.

Joint Problems: Joint symptoms, ranging from intermittent joint pains (arthralgias) to sudden inflammation of multiple joints (acute polyarthritis), occur in about 90% of people and may exist for years before other symptoms appear. In long-standing disease, marked joint deformity may occur (Jaccoud's arthropathy) but is rare. However, joint inflammation is generally intermittent and usually does not damage the joints.

Skin and Mucous Membrane Problems: Skin rashes include a butterfly-like redness across the nose and cheeks (malar butterfly rash); raised bumps or patches of thin skin; and red, flat or raised areas on the face and sun-exposed areas of the neck, upper chest, and elbows. Blisters and skin ulcers are rare, although ulcers do commonly occur on mucous membranes, particularly on the roof of the mouth, on the inside of the cheeks, on the gums, and inside the nose. Generalized or patchy loss of hair (alopecia) is common during flare-ups. Mottled red areas on the sides of the palms and up the fingers; redness and swelling around the nails; and flat, reddish purple blotches between the knuckles on the inner surfaces of the fingers also may occur. Purplish spots (petechiae) may occur because of bleeding in the skin as a result of low platelet levels in the blood. Sensitivity to sunlight (photosensitivity) occurs in most people with lupus, particularly fair-skinned people.

Lung Problems: It is common for people with lupus to feel pain when breathing deeply. The pain is due to recurring inflammation of the sac around the lungs (pleurisy), with or without fluid (effusion) inside this sac. Inflammation of the lungs (lupus pneumonitis), resulting in breathlessness, is rare, although minor abnormalities in lung function are common. Life-threatening bleeding into the lungs may rarely occur. Blockage of arteries in the lung caused by the formation of blood clots (thrombosis) can also occur.

Heart Problems: People with lupus may have chest pain due to inflammation of the sac around the heart (pericarditis). More serious but rare effects on the heart are inflammation of the walls of the coronary arteries (coronary artery vasculitis), which can lead to angina (see page 406), and inflammation of the heart muscle with scarring (fibrosing myocarditis), which can lead to heart failure (see page 352). The valves of the heart can rarely be involved and may need to be surgically repaired. People are at increased risk of coronary artery disease.

Lymph Node and Spleen Problems: Widespread enlargement of the lymph nodes is common, particularly among children, young adults, and blacks of

Characteristics of Lupus

At least four of the following symptoms are usually present for a diagnosis to be made:

- Red, butterfly-shaped rash on the face, affecting the cheeks
- Typical skin rash on other parts of the body
- Sensitivity to sunlight (for example, rash or persistent burn)
- Mouth sores
- Joint inflammation (arthritis)
- Fluid around the lungs, heart, or other organs (serositis)
- Kidney dysfunction
- Low white blood cell count, low red blood cell count, or low platelet count
- Nerve or brain dysfunction
- Positive results of a blood test for antinuclear antibodies
- Positive results of a blood test for antibodies to double-stranded DNA or to phospholipids or for anti-smith antibody

all ages. Enlargement of the spleen (splenomegaly) occurs in about 10% of people. People may experience nausea, diarrhea, and vague abdominal discomfort. The occurrence of these symptoms may be the forewarning of a flare-up.

Nervous System Problems: Involvement of the brain (neuropsychiatric lupus) can cause headaches, mild impairment of thinking, personality changes, stroke, epilepsy, severe mental disorders (psychoses), or a condition in which a number of physical changes may occur in the brain, resulting in disorders such as dementia. The nerves in the body or spinal cord may also be damaged.

Kidney Problems: Kidney involvement may be minor and without symptoms or may be relentlessly progressive and fatal. The most common result of this impairment is protein in the urine that leads to swelling (edema) in the legs.

Blood Problems: The numbers of red blood cells, white blood cells, and platelets may decrease. Platelets assist in blood clotting, so if these numbers decrease greatly, bleeding may occur. Also, and for other reasons, the blood may clot too easily, which accounts for many of the problems that can affect other organs (such as strokes and blood clots to the lungs or recurrent miscarriages).

Gastrointestinal Tract Problems: Impairment of blood supply to various parts of the gastrointestinal tract may result in abdominal pain, damage to the liver or pancreas (pancreatitis), or a blockage or tear (perforation) of the gastrointestinal tract.

Pregnancy Problems: Pregnant women have a higher-than-normal risk of miscarriage and stillbirth.

Diagnosis

Doctors suspect lupus mainly on the basis of the person's symptoms and findings during a careful physical examination, particularly in a young woman. Nonetheless, because of the wide range of symptoms, distinguishing lupus from similar diseases can be difficult.

Laboratory tests can help doctors confirm the diagnosis. A blood test can detect antinuclear antibodies, which are present in almost all people who have lupus. However, these antibodies also occur in other diseases. Therefore, if antinuclear antibodies are detected, a test for antibodies to double-stranded DNA, as well as a test for other autoimmune antibodies (autoantibodies, such as anti-smith antibodies and others), are done. A high level of these DNA antibodies almost definitely means the person has lupus, but not all people who have lupus have these antibodies. Other blood tests, such as measuring the level of complement, are also performed and can help to predict the activity and course of the disease in some people. Women with lupus who have repeated miscarriages or have had problems with blood clots should be tested for antiphospholipid antibodies. This is an important test when planning contraceptive methods or pregnancy. This blood test, which detects antibodies to phospholipids, can help identify people at risk of recurrent blood clots. Women with positive antibodies to phospholipids should not take estrogen-containing oral contraceptives and should choose other methods of contraception. Blood tests can also indicate anemia, a low white blood cell count, or a low platelet count.

Laboratory tests can detect the presence of protein or red blood cells in the urine or an elevation of creatinine in the blood. These findings indicate kidney damage caused by inflammation of the filtering structure in the kidneys (glomeruli), a condition referred to as glomerulonephritis. Sometimes a kidney biopsy (removal of tissue for examination and testing) must be performed to help the doctor plan treatment. People who have lupus should be tested from time to time for kidney damage even if they have no symptoms. Testing includes blood and urine tests.

Prognosis

Lupus tends to be chronic and relapsing, often with symptom-free periods that can last for years. Flare-ups can be triggered by sun exposure, infection, surgery, or pregnancy. Flare-ups occur less often after menopause. Because many people are being diagnosed earlier than in the past and because better treatment is available, the prognosis has improved markedly over the last two decades. However, because the course of lupus is unpredictable, the prognosis varies widely. Usually, if the initial inflammation is controlled, the long-term prognosis is good. Early detection and treatment of kidney damage reduce the incidence of severe kidney disease.

Treatment

Treatment depends on which organs are affected and how active the inflammation of lupus is. The severity of the lupus is not necessarily the same as the activity of the inflammation. For example, organs may be permanently damaged and scarred from lupus that caused inflammation in the past. Such damage may be referred to as "severe," even if the lupus is not active (that is, it is not causing any inflammation or any further damage at this time). The goal of treatment is to decrease the activity of lupus—that is, to decrease inflammation, which in turn should prevent damage.

If lupus is not very active (sometimes called mild lupus), treatment may not need to be intensive. Nonsteroidal anti-inflammatory drugs (NSAIDs— see page 644) often can relieve joint pain. Hydroxychloroquine, chloroquine, or quinacrine, sometimes taken in combination, helps relieve joint and skin symptoms. Sunscreen lotions (with a sun protection factor of at least 30) should be used, especially by people who have skin rashes.

Very active lupus (sometimes called severe lupus) is treated immediately with a corticosteroid such as prednisone (see box on page 568). The dose and duration of treatment depend on which organs are affected. Sometimes an immunosuppressive drug such as azathioprine or cyclophosphamide is given to suppress the body's autoimmune attack. Mycophenolate mofetil is an alternative immunosuppressive drug. The combination of a corticosteroid and an immunosuppressive drug is most often used for severe kidney disease or nervous system disease and for vasculitis.

Once the initial inflammation is controlled, a doctor determines the dose that most effectively suppresses inflammation over the long term. Usually, the dose of prednisone is gradually decreased when symptoms are controlled and laboratory test results show improvement. Relapses or flare-ups can occur during this process. For most people who have lupus, the dose of prednisone can eventually be decreased or occasionally discontinued.

Surgical procedures and pregnancy may be more complicated for people who have lupus, and they require close medical supervision. Miscarriages and flare-ups during pregnancy are common. Pregnancy should be avoided during a flare-up, and conception should be delayed until the disease seems likely to be inactive.

People who take corticosteroids should be tested periodically and, if necessary, treated for osteoporosis (thinning of the bones), which can occur with chronic corticosteroid use. People should be monitored closely by a doctor for coronary artery disease. Other risk factors for coronary artery disease (for example, high blood pressure and high cholesterol levels) should be controlled as well as possible.

Systemic Sclerosis

Systemic sclerosis (scleroderma) is a rare, chronic disorder characterized by degenerative changes and scarring in the skin, joints, and internal organs and by blood vessel abnormalities.

- Swelling of the fingers, intermittent coolness and blue discoloration of the fingers, joints freezing in permanent (usually flexed) positions (contractures), and damage to the gastrointestinal system, lungs, heart, or kidneys may develop.
- People often have antibodies in the blood characteristic of an autoimmune disorder.
- No treatment changes the course of the disorder.
- Symptoms and organ dysfunction are treated.

The cause of systemic sclerosis is not known. The disorder is 4 times more common among women than men and is rare among children. Symptoms of systemic sclerosis may occur as part of mixed connective tissue disease, and some people with mixed connective tissue disease develop severe systemic sclerosis. Systemic sclerosis can occur in limited forms, for example, sometimes affecting just the skin or mainly only certain parts of the skin or as CREST syndrome. However, systemic sclerosis often causes damage that is widespread throughout the body (called diffuse or generalized systemic sclerosis).

Symptoms

The usual initial symptom of systemic sclerosis is swelling, then thickening and tightening of the skin at the ends of the fingers. Raynaud's syndrome, in which the fingers suddenly and temporarily become very pale and tingle or become numb, painful, or both in response to cold or emotional upset (see page 426), is also common. Fingers may become bluish. Heartburn, difficulty in swallowing, and shortness of breath are occasionally the first symptoms of systemic sclerosis. Aches and pains in several joints often accompany early symptoms. Sometimes inflammation of the muscles (polymyositis), with its accompanying muscle pain and weakness, develops.

Skin Changes: Systemic sclerosis can damage large areas of skin or only the fingers (sclerodactyly). Sometimes systemic sclerosis tends to stay restricted to the skin of the hands. Other times, the disorder progresses. The skin becomes more widely taut, shiny, and darker than usual. The skin on the face tightens, sometimes resulting in an inability to change facial expressions. Sometimes dilated blood vessels (telangiectasia often referred to as spider veins) can appear on the fingers, chest, face, lips, and tongue, and bumps composed of calcium can develop on the fingers, on other bony areas, or at the joints. Sores can develop on the fingertips and knuckles.

Joint Changes: Sometimes, a grating sound can be felt or heard as inflamed tissues move over each other, particularly at and below the knees and at the elbows and wrists. The fingers, wrists, and elbows may become stuck (forming a contracture) in flexed positions because of scarring in the skin.

Gastrointestinal System Changes: Scarring commonly damages the lower end of the esophagus (the tube connecting the mouth and stomach). The damaged esophagus can no longer propel food to the stomach efficiently. Swallowing difficulties and heartburn eventually develop in many people who have systemic sclerosis. Abnormal cell growth in the esophagus (Barrett's esophagus—see page 189) occurs in about 33% of the people, increasing their risk of esophageal blockage (stricture) due to a fibrous band or their risk of esophageal cancer. Damage to the intestines can interfere with food absorption (malabsorption) and cause weight loss.

Lung and Heart Changes: Systemic sclerosis can cause scar tissue to accumulate in the lungs, resulting in abnormal shortness of breath during exercise. The blood vessels that supply the lungs can be affected (their walls thicken), so they cannot carry as much blood. Therefore blood pressure within the arteries that supply the lungs can increase (a condition called pulmonary hypertension—see page 522). Systemic sclerosis can also cause several life-threatening heart abnormalities, including heart failure and abnormal rhythms.

Kidney Changes: Severe kidney disease can result from systemic sclerosis. The first symptom of kidney damage may be an abrupt, progressive rise in blood pressure. High blood pressure is an ominous sign, although treatment usually controls it.

CREST Syndrome: CREST syndrome, also called limited cutaneous systemic sclerosis (sclerosis) is usually a less severe form of the disorder that is less likely to cause serious internal organ damage. It is named for its symptoms: Calcium deposits in the skin and throughout the body, Raynaud's syndrome, Esophageal dysfunction, Sclerodactyly (skin damage on the fingers), and Telangiectasia (dilated blood vessels or spider veins). Skin damage is limited to the fingers. People who have CREST syndrome can develop pulmonary hypertension, which can cause heart and lung failure. The drainage system from the liver may become blocked by scar tissue (biliary cirrhosis), resulting in liver damage and jaundice.

Diagnosis

A doctor diagnoses systemic sclerosis by the characteristic changes in the skin and internal organs. The symptoms may overlap with those of several other disorders, but the whole pattern is usually distinctive. Laboratory tests alone cannot identify systemic sclerosis because test results, like the symptoms, vary greatly. However, antinuclear antibodies are present in the blood of more than 90% of people with systemic sclerosis. An antibody to centromeres (part of a chromosome) is often present in people who have CREST syndrome. A different antibody (called anti-topoisomerase) is often present in people with the more diffuse generalized form.

Prognosis

Sometimes systemic sclerosis worsens rapidly and becomes fatal. At other times, it affects only the skin for decades before affecting internal organs, although some damage to internal organs (such as the esophagus) is almost inevitable, even in CREST syndrome. The course is unpredictable. Overall, about 65% of people live for at least 10 years after the diagnosis is made. The prognosis is worst for those who have heart, lung, or, particularly, kidney damage.

Treatment

No drug can stop the progression of systemic sclerosis. However, drugs can relieve some symptoms and reduce organ damage. Nonsteroidal anti-inflammatory drugs (NSAIDs—see page 644) help relieve joint pain. If the person has weakness because of polymyositis, corticosteroids may be needed. Drugs that suppress the immune system, such as cyclophosphamide and azathioprine, may help some people whose lungs are affected. Doctors treat severe pulmonary hypertension with the drugs bosentan or epoprostenol. The person may also be given anticoagulants.

Heartburn can be relieved by eating small meals, taking antacids, and using proton pump inhibitors, which block stomach acid production. Sleeping with the head of the bed elevated often helps. Areas of the esophagus narrowed by scar tissue can be surgically widened (dilated). Tetracycline or other antibiotics can help prevent malabsorption of food caused by excessive growth (overgrowth) of bacteria in the damaged intestine. A calcium channel blocker (such as nifedipine) may relieve the symptoms of Raynaud's syndrome (see page 426) but may also increase the reflux of stomach acid. Drugs for high blood pressure, particularly angiotensin-converting enzyme (ACE) inhibitors, are useful in treating kidney disease and the rise in blood pressure.

Physical therapy and exercise can help to maintain muscle strength but cannot totally prevent joints from freezing in contractures.

Sjögren's Syndrome

Sjögren's syndrome is characterized by excessive dryness of the eyes, mouth, and other mucous membranes.

- White blood cells can infiltrate and damage glands that secrete fluids, and sometimes other organs can be damaged.
- Tests can be done to measure gland function and assess the presence of abnormal antibodies in the blood.
- Usually, measures to keep surfaces such as the eyes and mouth moist are sufficient.
- When internal organ damage is severe, corticosteroids or cyclophosphamide can be given by mouth.

Sjögren's syndrome is thought to be an autoimmune disorder, but its cause is not known. It is more common among women than men. Some people with Sjögren's syndrome also have other autoimmune disorders, such as rheumatoid arthritis, systemic lupus erythematosus, systemic sclerosis, vasculitis, mixed connective tissue disease, Hashimoto's thyroiditis, primary biliary cirrhosis, and chronic autoimmune hepatitis.

White blood cells infiltrate the glands that secrete fluids, such as the salivary glands in the mouth and the tear glands in the eyes. The white blood cells injure the glands, resulting in a dry mouth and dry eyes—the hallmark symptoms of this syndrome.

Symptoms

In some people, only the mouth or eyes are dry (a condition called sicca complex or sicca syndrome). Dryness of the eyes may severely damage the cornea, resulting in a scratchy or irritated sensation, and a lack of tears can cause permanent eye damage. Insufficient saliva in the mouth can dull taste and smell, make eating and swallowing painful, and can cause cavities. The salivary glands in the cheeks (parotids) become enlarged and slightly tender in about one third of people. The mouth may also burn, which may sometimes indicate a complicating yeast infection.

In other people, many organs are affected. Sjögren's syndrome can dry out the mucous membranes lining the digestive tract, windpipe (trachea), vulva, and vagina. Dryness of the vulva and vagina can make sexual intercourse difficult. Dryness of the trachea can cause cough. The protective sac surrounding the heart (pericardium) may be inflamed—a condition called pericarditis. Nerve, lung tissue, and other tissues may be damaged by the inflammation.

Joint inflammation (arthritis) occurs in about one third of people, affecting the same joints that rheumatoid arthritis affects, but the joint inflammation of Sjögren's syndrome tends to be milder and is usually not destructive. Lymph nodes may enlarge throughout the body. Lymphoma, a cancer of the lymphatic system, is more common among people who have Sjögren's syndrome than the general population. Skin rashes, kidney damage, Raynaud's syndrome, and vasculitis that causes damage to the peripheral nerves may occur.

Diagnosis

Although a sensation of dry mouth or dry eyes is fairly common, a sensation of dry mouth and dry eyes accompanied by joint inflammation may indicate that the person has Sjögren's syndrome. Various tests can help a doctor diagnose this disorder and differentiate it from other disorders that can cause similar symptoms.

The amount of tears produced can be estimated by placing a filter paper strip under each lower eyelid and observing how much of the strip is moistened (Schirmer's test). A person who has Sjögren's syndrome may produce less than one third of the normal amount. An ophthalmologist can test for damage to the eye's surface. More sophisticated tests to evaluate salivary gland secretion may be performed, and a doctor may order scans or the removal of tissue for examination and testing (biopsy) of the salivary glands.

Blood tests can detect abnormal antibodies, including SS-A, an antibody that is present in Sjögren's syndrome. Antinuclear antibodies (which are found in people with lupus) and rheumatoid factor (which is found in people with rheumatoid arthritis) can also be found in people with Sjögren's syndrome. The erythrocyte sedimentation rate (ESR), a test that measures the rate at which red blood cells settle to the bottom of a test tube containing blood, is elevated in about 7 of 10 people. About 1 of 3 people has a decreased number of red blood cells (anemia), and 1 in 4 people has a decreased number of certain types of white blood cells (leukopenia).

Prognosis and Treatment

The prognosis is generally good. However, if the lungs, kidneys, or lymph nodes are damaged by the antibodies, pneumonia, kidney failure, or lymphoma may result.

No cure for Sjögren's syndrome is available, but symptoms can be relieved. Dry eyes can be treated with artificial tear drops during the day and a lubricating ointment at night. A prescription eye drop containing cyclosporine can also be used.

Shields can be fitted on the sides of glasses, helping to protect the eyes from air and wind, reducing evaporation of tears. A simple surgical procedure called punctal occlusion can be performed. In this procedure, an ophthalmologist inserts small plugs into the tear ducts in the corner of the lower eyelid, so the person's tears stay on the eye longer.

A dry mouth can be moistened by continuously sipping liquids, chewing sugarless gum, or using a saliva substitute mouth rinse. Drugs that reduce the amount of saliva, such as decongestants, antidepressants, and antihistamines, should be avoided because they can worsen the dryness. The drug pilocarpine or cevimeline may help stimulate the production of saliva if the salivary glands are not too severely damaged.

Fastidious dental hygiene and frequent dental visits can minimize tooth decay and loss. Painful, swollen salivary glands can be treated with analgesics and warm compresses. Because joint symptoms are usually mild, treatment with nonsteroidal anti-inflammatory drugs (NSAIDs) and rest is often sufficient. Antimalarial drugs (such as hydroxychloroquine) can relieve joint pain, swollen lymph nodes, and skin problems. Very rarely, the drug methotrexate may be given. When symptoms resulting from damage to internal organs are severe, corticosteroids (such as prednisone) or cyclophosphamide taken by mouth can be useful.

Sjögren's syndrome that occurs along with other autoimmune diseases, such as lupus, rheumatoid arthritis, and systemic sclerosis, is referred to as secondary Sjögren's syndrome. People with secondary Sjögren's syndrome receive additional treatment for the other disease.

Polymyositis and Dermatomyositis

Polymyositis is characterized by inflammation and degeneration of the muscles. Dermatomyositis is polymyositis accompanied by skin inflammation.

- Muscle damage may cause muscle pain and difficulty lifting the arms above the shoulders, climbing stairs, or arising from a sitting position.
- Doctors check muscle enzymes in the blood and sometimes test electrical activity of muscles, perform magnetic resonance imaging (MRI) on muscles, check levels of muscle enzymes in the blood, examine a piece of muscle tissue (biopsy), or a combination.
- Oral corticosteroids are usually helpful.

These disorders result in disabling muscle weakness. The weakness typically occurs in the shoulders and hips but can affect muscles symmetrically throughout the body.

Polymyositis and dermatomyositis usually occur in adults from ages 40 to 60 or in children from ages 5 to 15 years. Women are twice as likely as men to develop either disorder. In adults, these disorders may occur alone or as part of other connective tissue disorders, such as mixed connective tissue disease.

The cause of polymyositis and dermatomyositis is unknown. Viruses or autoimmune reactions may play a role. Cancer may also trigger polymyositis and dermatomyositis. It is possible that an immune reaction against cancer may be directed against a substance in the muscles.

Symptoms

Polymyositis: In polymyositis, the symptoms are similar for people of all ages, but the disorder usually develops more abruptly in children than in adults. Symptoms, which may begin during or just after an infection, include symmetrical muscle weakness (particularly in the upper arms, hips, and thighs), joint pain (but often little muscle pain), difficulty in swallowing, fever, fatigue, and weight loss. Raynaud's syndrome (in which the fingers suddenly become very pale and tingle or become numb in response to cold or emotional upset—see page 426) occurs more commonly among people who have polymyositis along with other connective tissue disorders.

Muscle weakness may start slowly or suddenly and may worsen for weeks or months. Because muscles close to the center of the body are affected most, tasks such as lifting the arms above the shoulders, climbing stairs, and getting out of a chair can become very difficult. If the neck muscles are affected, even raising the head from a pillow may be impossible. Weakness in the shoulders or hips can confine a person to a wheelchair or bed. Muscle damage in the upper part of the esophagus can cause swallowing difficulties and regurgitation of food. The muscles of the hands, feet, and face, however, are not affected.

Joint aches and inflammation occur in about 30% of people. The pain and swelling tend to be mild.

Polymyositis usually does not affect internal organs other than the throat and esophagus. However, the lungs and heart may be affected, causing shortness of breath and a cough.

Dermatomyositis: In dermatomyositis, all the symptoms of polymyositis occur. In addition, rashes tend to appear at the same time as muscle weakness and other symptoms. A shadowy-red or purplish rash (heliotrope rash) can appear on the face with reddish purple swelling around the eyes. Another rash, which may be scaly, smooth, or raised, may appear almost anywhere on the body but is especially common on the knuckles and sides of the hands. The nail beds may redden. When the rashes fade, brownish pigmentation, scarring, shriveling, or pale depigmented patches may develop on the skin.

Diagnosis

Doctors use the following criteria to make the diagnosis of polymyositis or dermatomyositis:

- Muscle weakness at the shoulders or hips
- A characteristic rash
- Increased blood levels of certain muscle enzymes (especially creatine kinase) in the blood, indicating muscle damage
- Abnormalities in muscle electrical activity as measured by electromyography (see page 636), or on appearance on a magnetic resonance imaging (MRI) scan
- Characteristic changes in muscle tissue obtained by biopsy and observed under a microscope (the most conclusive evidence)

Laboratory tests are helpful but cannot specifically identify polymyositis or dermatomyositis. Muscle enzymes are measured repeatedly in blood samples to monitor the disorder; the levels usually fall to normal or near normal with effective treatment. Magnetic resonance imaging (MRI) may also show areas of inflammation and help the doctor select a site for biopsy. Special tests performed on muscle tissue samples may be needed to rule out other muscle disorders.

Prognosis

Within 5 years, up to 50% of people (especially children) who have received treatment experience a long remission (even apparent recovery). However, the disorder may still return at any time. About 75% of people survive at least 5 years after the diagnosis is made. This percentage is even higher among children. Adults are at risk of death from severe and progressive muscle weakness, difficulty swallowing, undernutrition, inhaling food that causes pneumonia (aspiration pneumonia), and respiratory failure, which often occurs at the same time as pneumonia. Polymyositis tends to be more severe and resistant to treatment in people whose heart or lungs are affected. In people who have cancer, it is the cancer, rather than the polymyositis, that is the cause of death.

Treatment

Modest restriction of activities when the inflammation is most intense often helps. Generally, a corticosteroid, usually prednisone, given by mouth in high doses slowly improves strength and relieves pain and swelling, controlling the disease. After about 6 to 12 weeks, when the muscle enzyme levels have returned to normal and muscle strength has returned, the dose is gradually decreased. Many adults must continue taking a low dose of prednisone or an alternative drug for many years or even indefinitely to prevent a relapse. After about a year, children may be able to stop taking the drug and stay symptom-free.

In some people, corticosteroids are not very effective or must be taken at very high doses to be effective. In some people, corticosteroids may cause muscle damage and weakness (see box on page 568). In such situations, an immunosuppressive drug (methotrexate, azathioprine, or cyclosporine) is used instead of or in addition to prednisone. When other drugs are ineffective, gamma globulin (a substance that contains large quantities of many antibodies) may be given by vein (intravenously). Other new remedies that may be effective in treating polymyositis and dermatomyositis include rituximab and a class of drugs (such as infliximab and etanercept) that inhibit a chemical called tumor necrosis factor (tumor necrosis factor inhibitors).

When polymyositis is associated with cancer, it usually does not respond well to prednisone. However, the condition usually lessens in severity if the cancer can be successfully treated.

Because people who take corticosteroids are at risk of fractures related to osteoporosis, they should be closely screened and treated for osteoporosis. Preventive measures (such as treatment of high blood pressure, high blood cholesterol levels, and osteoporosis) should be taken.

Mixed Connective Tissue Disease

Mixed connective tissue disease is a term used by some doctors to describe a disorder characterized by features of systemic lupus erythematosus, systemic sclerosis, and polymyositis.

- Raynaud's syndrome, joint pains, various skin abnormalities, weakness, and problems with internal organs can develop.
- Characteristic abnormal antibodies are usually detectable in blood.
- Treatment is similar to that of systemic lupus erythematosus, often with corticosteroids.

About 80% of people who have this disease are women. Mixed connective tissue disease affects people from ages 5 to 80. Its cause is unknown, but it seems to be an autoimmune disorder.

Symptoms

The typical symptoms are Raynaud's syndrome (in which the fingers suddenly become very pale and tingle or become numb or blue in response to cold or emotional upset—see page 426), joint inflammation (arthritis), swollen hands, muscle weakness, difficulty in swallowing, heartburn, and shortness of breath. Raynaud's syndrome may precede other symptoms by many years. Regardless of how mixed connective tissue disease starts, it tends to worsen, and symptoms spread to several parts of the body.

The hands are frequently so swollen that the fingers look like sausages. A purplish butterfly-shaped rash on the cheeks and bridge of the nose, red patches on the knuckles, a violet discoloration of the eyelids, and red spider veins on the face and hands all may appear. Skin changes similar to those in systemic sclerosis also may occur. The hair may thin.

Almost everyone with mixed connective tissue disease has aching joints. About 75% develop the swelling and pain typical of joint inflammation (arthritis). Mixed connective tissue disease damages the muscle fibers, so the muscles may feel weak and sore, especially in the shoulders and hips. Tasks such as lifting the arms above the shoulders, climbing stairs, and getting out of a chair can become very difficult.

Fluid may collect in or around the lungs. In some people, abnormal lung function is the most serious problem, causing shortness of breath during exertion.

Occasionally, the heart is weakened, leading to heart failure (see page 352). Symptoms of heart failure may include fluid retention, shortness of breath, and fatigue. The kidneys and nerves are affected in only 10% of people, and the damage is usually mild compared to the damage caused by lupus. Other symptoms may include fever, swollen lymph nodes, abdominal pain, and persistent hoarseness. Sjögren's syndrome may develop. Over time, most people develop symptoms that are more typical of lupus or systemic sclerosis.

Diagnosis

Doctors suspect mixed connective tissue disease when some symptoms from lupus, systemic sclerosis, polymyositis, or rheumatoid arthritis overlap.

Blood tests are performed to detect an antibody to ribonucleoprotein, which is present in almost all people who have mixed connective tissue disease. A high level of this antibody without the other antibodies present in lupus is characteristic of mixed connective tissue disease.

Prognosis

Despite treatment, mixed connective tissue disease worsens in about 13% of the people, causing potentially fatal complications in 6 to 12 years. The prognosis is worse for people who have mainly features of systemic sclerosis or polymyositis. Overall, 80% of people survive at least 10 years after the diagnosis is made. Symptom-free periods can last for many years with little or no continuing treatment with a corticosteroid.

Treatment

The treatment is similar to that of lupus. Corticosteroids are usually effective, especially when the disease is diagnosed early. Mild cases can be treated with aspirin or other nonsteroidal anti-inflammatory drugs (NSAIDs), hydroxychloroquine or similar drugs, or very low doses of corticosteroids. The more severe the disease, the higher the dose of corticosteroid needed. In severe cases, immunosuppressive drugs (such as azathioprine, methotrexate or cyclophosphamide) may also be needed.

In general, the more advanced the disease and the greater the organ damage, the less effective the treatment. Systemic sclerosis–like damage to the skin and esophagus is least likely to respond to treatment.

Relapsing Polychondritis

Relapsing polychondritis is characterized by episodes of painful, destructive inflammation of the cartilage and other connective tissues in many organs.

- The ears or nose may become inflamed and tender.
- Other cartilage in the body can be damaged, leading to various symptoms, such as red or painful eyes, hoarseness, cough, difficulty breathing, rashes, and pain in the breastbone.
- Blood tests are done and a piece of tissue may be removed for examination and testing (biopsy).
- If symptoms or complications are moderate or severe, corticosteroids usually help.

This disorder affects men and women equally, usually in middle age. The cause is unknown, but autoimmune reactions to cartilage are suspected.

Symptoms

Typically, one or both ears become red, swollen, and very painful. At the same time or later, a person can develop joint inflammation (arthritis), which may be mild or severe. Cartilage in any joint may be affected, and the cartilage that connects the ribs to the breastbone may become inflamed. Cartilage in the nose is also a common site of inflammation. The nose may become tender, and cartilage can collapse.

Other affected sites include the eyes, resulting in scleritis (inflammation of the white part of the eye), and the voice box (larynx) and windpipe (trachea), resulting in hoarseness, a nonproductive cough, shortness of breath, and tenderness over the Adam's apple. Rarely the cornea may develop a hole (perforate), resulting in blindness. Less often, the heart is involved, leading to heart murmurs and occasionally to heart failure. The skin may become inflamed, resulting in a variety of rashes.

Flare-ups of inflammation and pain last a few weeks, subside, then recur over a period of several years. Eventually, the supporting cartilage can be damaged, resulting in floppy ears; a sloping saddle nose; and vision, hearing, and balance problems.

People who have this disorder may die if the cartilage in their airways collapses, blocking the flow of air, or if their heart and blood vessels are severely damaged.

Diagnosis and Treatment

Relapsing polychondritis is diagnosed when a doctor observes at least three of the following symptoms developing over time:

- Inflammation of both ears
- Painful swelling in several joints
- Inflammation of the cartilage in the nose
- Inflammation of the eye
- Cartilage damage in the respiratory tract
- Hearing or balance problems

A biopsy of the affected cartilage may show characteristic abnormalities. Blood tests, such as the erythrocyte sedimentation rate (ESR), can detect evidence of chronic inflammation.

Mild relapsing polychondritis can be treated with nonsteroidal anti-inflammatory drugs (NSAIDs—see page 644) or dapsone. In more severe cases, daily doses of prednisone are given, then tapered off as the symptoms begin to lessen. Sometimes very severe cases are treated with immunosuppressive drugs such as cyclosporine, cyclophosphamide, or azathioprine. These drugs treat the symptoms but have not been shown to alter the ultimate course of the disorder.

Eosinophilic Fasciitis

Eosinophilic fasciitis is a rare disorder in which the skin of the arms and legs becomes painfully inflamed and swollen and gradually hardens.

- The connective tissue is probably damaged by an autoimmune reaction.
- Some tissue is removed for examination and testing (biopsy).
- Corticosteroids are helpful.

The word *eosinophilic* refers to the initially high blood levels of a type of white blood cell called eosinophils. The word *fasciitis* refers to inflammation of the fascia, which is the tough fibrous tissue that lies beneath the skin.

The cause of eosinophilic fasciitis is unknown. The disorder occurs mainly in men aged 40 to 50, but it may occur in women and children.

Symptoms

The usual initial symptoms are pain, swelling, and inflammation of the skin, particularly over the inside of the arms and the front of the legs. The skin of the face, chest, and abdomen may occasionally be affected also. In contrast to systemic sclerosis, the skin of the feet and hands is not affected and Raynaud's syndrome does not occur.

Symptoms may first be noticed after strenuous physical activity. Symptoms usually progress gradually. After weeks, the inflamed skin begins to harden, eventually acquiring a texture similar to an orange peel.

As the skin gradually hardens, the arms and legs become difficult to move. Eventually, the arms and legs may become stuck in unusual positions. Weight loss and fatigue are common. Muscle strength does not usually decrease, but muscle and joint pain may occur. Rarely, if the arms are involved, the person may develop carpal tunnel syndrome (see page 601).

Sometimes, the numbers of red blood cells and platelets in the bloodstream become very low, resulting in fatigue and a tendency to bleed easily.

Diagnosis

A doctor suspects eosinophilic fasciitis because of its typical symptoms. The number of eosinophils is increased in the blood, as is the erythrocyte sedimentation rate (ESR). This increase indicates inflammation.

The diagnosis is confirmed by taking a biopsy of affected skin and the tissues underneath it (the fascia). The biopsy sample must include all skin layers down to the muscle. Magnetic resonance imaging (MRI) can also help make the diagnosis but is not as conclusive as muscle biopsy.

Prognosis and Treatment

The long-term outlook is unknown.

Most people respond rapidly to high doses of corticosteroids. Treatment should be started as early as possible to prevent scarring, tissue loss (atrophy), and contractures. Corticosteroids may not reverse atrophied and scarred tissue. Doses are gradually reduced, but corticosteroids may need to be continued at low levels for 2 to 5 years. For people who cannot use corticosteroids or do not fully respond to corticosteroids, other drugs (for example, hydroxychloroquine or cyclosporine) can be tried.

Monitoring with blood tests is advised because the occasional person develops another blood disorder.

Vasculitic Disorders

Vasculitic disorders are characterized by inflammation of the blood vessels (vasculitis).

- Usually, what triggers vasculitis is unknown, but sometimes certain viruses or drugs trigger it.
- People may have general symptoms, such as fever or fatigue, followed by other symptoms depending on which organs are affected.
- Typically, a biopsy of an affected blood vessel is needed to confirm the diagnosis.
- Corticosteroids and other drugs that suppress the immune system are used to reduce inflammation and relieve symptoms.

Vasculitis can affect people of all ages, but some types are more common among certain age groups.

Usually, what triggers vasculitis is unknown. However, certain viruses, especially hepatitis viruses, and drugs sometimes trigger it. Presumably, the inflammation occurs when the immune system mistakenly identifies blood vessels or parts of a blood vessel as foreign and attacks them. Cells of the immune system, which cause inflammation, surround and infiltrate the affected blood vessels, damaging them. The damaged blood vessels may become leaky, narrow, or clogged. As a result, blood flow to the tissues supplied by the damaged vessels is disrupted. The tissues deprived of blood (ischemic areas) can be permanently damaged or die.

Vasculitis may affect arteries (large, medium-sized, or small), capillaries, veins, or a combination. It may affect a whole blood vessel or only part of it. It may affect blood vessels that supply one part of the body, such as the head or skin, or blood vessels that supply several different organs (called systemic vasculitis). Any organ system can be affected.

 Did You Know...
Blood vessels can become inflamed.

Symptoms

Symptoms may result from direct damage to the blood vessels or from indirect damage to tissues (such as nerves or organs) whose blood supply has been disrupted or reduced.

Symptoms vary, depending on the size of the affected blood vessels and the organs whose blood supply is disrupted or reduced. For example, the following may occur:

SOME DISORDERS CHARACTERIZED BY VASCULITIS		
DISORDER	**DEFINITION**	**SYMPTOMS***
Behçet's syndrome	Chronic inflammation of arteries and veins, characterized by recurring mouth sores	Recurring mouth sores Sores on the genital organs Red, painful eyes Rashes Swollen, painful joints Sometimes blood clots in arteries and veins
Churg-Strauss syndrome	Inflammation of small blood vessels (often in the lungs, sinuses, skin, nerves, and kidneys) that occurs in people with asthma or a nasal allergy	Various symptoms depending on the organ affected Cough, which sometimes brings up blood Facial pain Shortness of breath Rashes Numbness, tingling, or weakness in a limb Muscle and joint aches and pains Abdominal pain

(continued on the following page)

SOME DISORDERS CHARACTERIZED BY VASCULITIS (*Continued*)

DISORDER	DEFINITION	SYMPTOMS*
Giant cell arteritis	Inflammation of large and medium-sized arteries in the head, neck, and upper body, especially the temporal arteries (which run through the temples)	Headaches Pain in the scalp Pain in the jaws or tongue during chewing Double or blurred vision Without treatment, possibly irreversible vision loss
Henoch-Schönlein purpura	Inflammation of small blood vessels, often in the skin, intestine, and kidneys	Hard, purple spots or blotches on the skin of the lower legs Joint pains Nausea Abdominal pain Blood in the stool or urine
Microscopic polyangiitis	Inflammation of small blood vessels, usually starting in the lungs and kidneys	Shortness of breath Swelling in the legs Purplish bumps or spots on the skin Numbness, tingling, or weakness in a limb
Polyarteritis nodosa	Inflammation of medium-sized arteries	Various symptoms depending on the organ affected Muscle and joint pain Abdominal pain High blood pressure Numbness, tingling, or weakness in a limb
Takayasu's arteritis	Inflammation of the aorta, the arteries that branch off from the aorta, and the pulmonary arteries, usually in young women	Pain and fatigue in the arms or legs when they are used Dizziness Strokes High blood pressure
Wegener's granulomatosis	Inflammation of small and medium-sized blood vessels, usually in the sinuses, nose, lungs, and kidneys	Various symptoms depending on the affected organ Nosebleeds Ear infections Chronic sinusitis Cough, which sometimes brings up blood Shortness of breath Chest pain Joint and muscle aches and pain Rashes

*Many of these disorders also cause general symptoms, such as fever, fatigue, loss of appetite, and weight loss.

- **Skin:** A rash of bluish purple spots (hemorrhages) or blotches (purpura), small bumps (nodules), or sores (ulcers) on the lower legs
- **Peripheral nerves:** Numbness, tingling, or weakness in the affected limb
- **Brain:** Changes in personality, confusion, seizures, and strokes
- **Digestive tract:** Abdominal pain, diarrhea, nausea, and vomiting
- **Heart:** Angina and heart attacks
- **Kidneys:** Sometimes no symptoms or high blood pressure, retention of fluid (edema), and kidney dysfunction
- **Joints:** Joint pain or swelling

Inflammation can also cause general symptoms such as fever, night sweats, fatigue, muscle and joint aches, loss of appetite, and weight loss.

Vasculitis can also cause serious complications that require immediate treatment. For example, damaged blood vessels in the lungs, brain, or other organs may bleed (hemorrhage). Effects on the kidneys may progress rapidly, leading to kidney failure. Eye problems may result in blindness.

Diagnosis

Vasculitis is usually not suspected when symptoms first develop. Vasculitis is uncommon, and most of its symptoms are caused much more often by other disorders. Nonetheless, certain combinations of symptoms or the persistence of symptoms eventually lead doctors to suspect vasculitis. Blood and urine tests, including the following, are usually done:

- A complete blood cell count is done. If blood contains too few red blood cells (anemia), too many platelets, too many white blood cells, or a high proportion of certain kinds of white blood cells, vasculitis may be the cause. Vasculitis may cause anemia by decreasing the body's production of red blood cells or by causing internal bleeding.

- Blood is analyzed for substances produced by the body when inflammation is present. These substances include certain antibodies (such as antineutrophil cytoplasmic antibodies) and complement proteins. Antineutrophil cytoplasmic antibodies attack certain white blood cells and occur in several types of vasculitis.

- Blood tests may be done to check for infections (such as hepatitis) that may have triggered the vasculitis.

- Blood tests are done to estimate the degree of inflammation, which vasculitis usually causes. For example, how quickly red blood cells (erythrocytes) drop to the bottom of a test tube (erythrocyte sedimentation rate) is measured. A fast rate suggests inflammation. Levels of C-reactive protein (which the liver produces in response to bodywide inflammation) may be measured instead or in addition. However, inflammation has many causes other than vasculitis.

- A sample of urine is tested for red blood cells and protein. This information can help doctors determine whether the kidneys are affected.

- Blood tests may be done to measure levels of proteins that can change when vasculitis develops (total protein and albumin)

Blood and urine tests results may help in making the diagnosis but are usually not conclusive. For confirmation, a sample of the affected blood vessel is usually removed and examined under a microscope (biopsy) for signs of vasculitis. A local anesthetic is used, and the test may be done on an outpatient basis.

Other tests may be needed. For example, if the lungs seem to be affected, a chest x-ray is done. Imaging tests, such as magnetic resonance angiography, may be done to determine which blood vessels are affected. If the kidneys may be affected, blood levels of substances that increase when the kidneys are damaged (blood urea nitrogen and creatinine) are measured. Some tests may be done to rule out other disorders that can cause similar symptoms.

Prognosis

The prognosis depends on the type and severity of vasculitis and the organs that are affected. If the kidneys or heart is affected, the prognosis tends to be worse.

Treatment

Treatment depends on the type and severity of the vasculitis and the organs that are affected. But generally, treatment aims to stop the immune system from continuing to damage blood vessels.

If vital organs, such as the lungs, heart, brain, or kidneys, are affected, emergency treatment in a hospital is often necessary. Sometimes a team of specialists (experts in such fields as inflammation, lung disorders, or kidney disorders) is needed to provide care.

Mild types of vasculitis, such as those that affect only the skin, may require little treatment, possibly only close monitoring or antihistamines.

For most types of vasculitis, a corticosteroid (usually prednisone) is typically used first to reduce inflammation. Sometimes another drug that suppresses the immune system (immunosuppressant), such as azathioprine, cyclophosphamide, or methotrexate, is used with the corticosteroid (see page 567). Drugs used to treat vasculitis can have side effects. Thus, as the inflammation is being controlled, the dose of the drugs may be slowly reduced, the corticosteroid may be stopped, and less strong immunosuppressants are used. The lowest dose that can control symptoms is used. Once inflammation is controlled (called remission), all drugs may be stopped. Some people remain in remission indefinitely. In others, symptoms recur one or more times (called a relapse). If relapses occur often, people may need to take an immunosuppressant indefinitely. Some people have to take corticosteroids for a long time.

Side effects, such as decreased bone density, an increased risk of infections, cataracts, high blood pressure, weight gain, and diabetes, are more likely to occur when corticosteroids are taken for a long time. To help prevent decreased bone density, people are advised to take calcium and vitamin D supplements and are given a bisphosphonate, such as alendronate or risedronate, which help increase bone density. Bone density is measured periodically.

Immunosuppressants weaken the immune system, so the risk of developing serious infections is increased. Cyclophosphamide, one potent immunosuppressant drug, can cause bladder irritation and sometimes even bladder cancer. A complete blood count is done frequently, sometimes as often as once a week for patients who take strong immunosuppressants. Immunosuppressants may cause the number of blood cells to decrease.

People should learn as much as they can about their disorder so that they can report any important symptoms to their doctor promptly. Learning about the side effects of the drugs being used is also important. People, even when in remission, should keep in touch with their doctor because how long remission will last cannot be predicted.

Polyarteritis Nodosa

Polyarteritis nodosa is inflammation of medium-sized arteries that damages the arteries and impairs blood flow through them.

- Any organ (except the lungs) can be affected.
- Polyarteritis nodosa can be rapidly fatal or develop gradually.
- Symptoms vary depending on which organ is affected.
- Biopsy of an affected artery can confirm the diagnosis.
- Prompt treatment with a corticosteroid, another drug that suppresses the immune system, or both can delay or prevent death.

Polyarteritis nodosa most often develops during middle age, usually when people are in their 50s, but it can occur at any age. It is rare.

The cause is unknown, but it sometimes appears to be triggered by certain viral infections (such as hepatitis B) or drugs. About 1 of 5 people with polyarteritis nodosa has hepatitis B. Most often, no trigger can be identified.

Symptoms

The disorder can be mild at first but can worsen rapidly and be fatal within several months, or it can develop gradually as a chronic debilitating disease. Any organ (except the lungs) or combination of organs can be affected. Symptoms depend on which organs are affected. Occasionally, only one organ, such as the intestine or skin, is affected.

People may have general symptoms at first. They may feel generally ill and tired and have a fever. They may lose their appetite and lose weight.

Other symptoms occur when the arteries that carry blood to an organ are damaged, and the organ does not receive enough blood to function normally. Thus, symptoms vary depending on the organ that is affected:

- **Joints:** Muscle and joint pain (common) and joint inflammation (arthritis)
- **Kidneys:** High blood pressure, swelling due to water retention (edema), and decreased production of urine
- **Digestive tract:** Abdominal infection (peritonitis), severe pain, bloody diarrhea, nausea, vomiting, and tears (perforations) in the intestine
- **Heart:** Chest pain (angina) and heart attacks
- **Brain:** Headaches, seizures, and strokes
- **Nerves:** Patchy numbness, tingling, weakness, or paralysis in a hand or foot
- **Liver:** Liver damage
- **Skin:** Blue or red discoloration of the fingers or toes, rashes that are usually bumpy, purplish blotches, and occasionally skin sores

Sometimes damage to an organ is irreversible. Such organs cannot function normally. A weakened artery may rupture, causing internal bleeding. Problems, such as a heart attack, can occur long after the inflammation has been treated.

Diagnosis

Doctors suspect polyarteritis nodosa when people have a certain combination of symptoms and blood test results. For example, they may suspect it if a previously healthy middle-aged man has a fever and evidence of a certain pattern of nerve damage, such as patchy numbness, tingling, or paralysis.

To confirm the diagnosis, doctors may take a small sample of an affected blood vessel and examine it under a microscope (biopsy). If the skin, liver, or kidneys appear to be affected by vasculitis, these organs may also be biopsied. Arteriography (angiography of arteries) may be done to check for bulges (aneurysms) in the wall of affected arteries. For this test, x-rays are taken after a dye that is visible on x-rays (radiopaque dye) is injected into the arteries.

Treatment

Without treatment, polyarteritis nodosa can result in death. Prompt, appropriate treatment can delay or prevent death from this disorder. However, treatment cannot always reverse the damage already done.

Treatment depends on the severity of the disorder. Any drugs that may have triggered the disorder are stopped.

High doses of a corticosteroid, such as prednisone, can prevent polyarteritis nodosa from worsening and help people feel better. The goal is a symptom-free period (remission). Because most people need long-term treatment with a corticosteroid and because long-term treatment can have significant side effects, doctors reduce the dose once symptoms have subsided.

If the corticosteroid does not reduce the inflammation adequately, drugs that suppress the immune system (immunosuppressants), such as cyclophosphamide, may be given with the corticosteroid. Taking a corticosteroid or another immunosuppressant for a long time reduces the body's ability to fight infections. Thus, people so treated have an increased risk of infections, which may be serious or fatal if not recognized and treated promptly.

Other treatments, such as those used to control high blood pressure, are often needed to prevent damage to internal organs. Hepatitis B, if present, is treated after the inflammation has been controlled.

Giant Cell Arteritis

Giant cell (temporal) arteritis is chronic inflammation of large arteries of the head, neck, and upper body. Typically affected are the temporal arteries, which run through the temples and provide blood to part of the scalp, the jaw muscles, and salivary glands.

- The cause is unknown.
- Typically, people have a severe and often throbbing headache, pain in the scalp when they brush their hair, and pain when they chew.
- Without treatment, blindness can result.
- Symptoms and results of a physical examination suggest the diagnosis, but biopsy of the temporal artery is done to confirm it.
- Prednisone, a corticosteroid, is effective.

Giant cell arteritis typically affects people over 55. About 40 to 60% of people with giant cell arteritis also have polymyalgia rheumatica. The cause of these disorders is unknown.

Symptoms

Symptoms vary, depending on which arteries are affected. Typically, the large arteries to the head are affected, causing a severe, sometimes throbbing headache at the temples or back of the head to develop for the first time. Arteries in the temple may be tender to the touch and feel swollen and bumpy. The scalp may feel painful when the hair is brushed. Double or blurred vision, large blind spots, blindness in one eye, or other eye problems may develop. The greatest danger is permanent blindness, which can occur suddenly if the blood supply to the optic nerve is blocked. Without treatment, giant cell arteritis causes blindness in 20% of people.

Typically, the jaw and its muscles hurt and become tired soon after beginning chewing. The tongue may also hurt when eating or speaking. People may also feel tired and generally unwell. They may lose weight unintentionally and sweat more than usual.

> **Did You Know...**
>
> Combing the hair and chewing often hurt when people have giant cell arteritis.

Occasionally, blood flow to the brain is blocked, and a stroke occurs. Sometimes inflammation damages the aorta, causing its lining to tear (dissection) or a bulge (aneurysm) to form in its wall.

If polymyalgia rheumatica is also present, severe pain may occur in the neck, shoulders, and hip. These muscles may feel stiff, particularly in the early morning.

Diagnosis

Doctors suspect the diagnosis based on symptoms and results of a physical examination. Doctors feel the temples to see whether the temporal arteries feel hard, bumpy, or tender. Blood tests are done. Results can support the diagnosis. For example, anemia, a very high erythrocyte sedimentation rate (ESR), and a high level of C-reactive protein indicate inflamma-

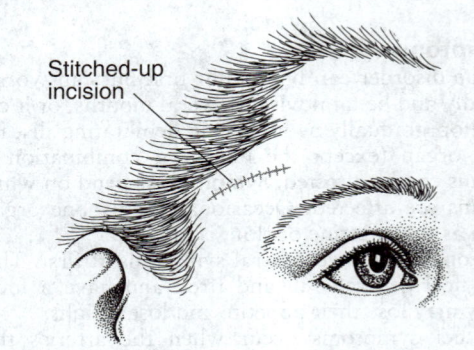

Biopsy of the Temporal Artery

A biopsy of the temporal artery is the definitive procedure for diagnosing temporal arteritis. Doppler ultrasonography is occasionally used to locate the part of the temporal artery to be biopsied. After a local anesthetic is injected, a shallow incision is made directly over the artery, and a segment of the artery at least 1 inch long is removed. The incision is then stitched up.

Stitched-up incision

tion. A biopsy of the temporal artery (in the temple) is done to confirm the diagnosis.

If giant cell arteritis is suspected in arteries other than the temporal artery, magnetic resonance angiography may be done to confirm the diagnosis.

Treatment

Treatment is started as soon as giant cell arteritis is suspected because without treatment, blindness can develop. Treatment is usually started even before a biopsy is done. Treatment does not affect the biopsy results as long as the biopsy is done within weeks after starting treatment. Prednisone, a corticosteroid, is effective. Initially, the dose is high—to stop the inflammation in the blood vessels. After several weeks, doctors gradually reduce the dose if people are improving. Some people can stop taking prednisone within a year, but many need to take very low doses for many years to control symptoms and prevent blindness.

People should take a low dose of aspirin every day to help prevent strokes.

With treatment, most people recover fully, but the disorder may recur.

POLYMYALGIA RHEUMATICA

Polymyalgia rheumatica involves inflammation of the lining of joints, causing severe pain and stiffness in the muscles of the neck, shoulders, and hips.

- The cause is unknown.
- The neck, shoulders, and hips feel stiff and painful.
- Blood tests and sometimes biopsy of a muscle help doctors make the diagnosis.
- Most people improve dramatically when they take prednisone, a corticosteroid.

Polymyalgia rheumatica occurs in people over 55. Its cause is unknown. Polymyalgia rheumatica may occur with giant cell (temporal) arteritis. Some experts think that the two disorders are variations of the same abnormal process.

Symptoms

Symptoms may develop suddenly or gradually. Severe pain and stiffness occur in the neck, shoulders, and hips. The stiffness is worse in the morning and after periods of inactivity. But muscles are not damaged or weak. People may also have a fever, feel generally unwell or depressed, and lose weight unintentionally.

Some people with polymyalgia rheumatica also have symptoms of giant cell arteritis, which can lead to blindness. Some people have mild arthritis, but if the arthritis is severe or is the main symptom, the diagnosis is more likely to be rheumatoid arthritis (see page 563).

SPOTLIGHT ON AGING

Giant cell (temporal) arteritis and polymyalgia rheumatica, which often occur together, affect people over age 55 almost exclusively. These disorders become more common as people age. They are 10 times more common among people over 80 than among those aged 50 to 59.

Giant cell arteritis typically causes a throbbing headache and problems with vision (including pain in and around the eyes). Polymyalgia rheumatica makes muscles painful and stiff. Without treatment, the pain these disorders cause, whether they occur together or separately, can make everyday living miserably difficult. Also, without prompt treatment, giant cell arteritis can cause blindness.

The main treatment of these disorders, corticosteroids, may be problematic in older people. These drugs can cause dramatic improvement and are essential for preventing blindness. However, they are more likely to have side effects in older people. People may retain fluids, their appetite may increase, and they may become confused. Blood sugar may increase, sometimes causing diabetes, and bone density may decrease. Blood pressure may increase. To reduce the risk of these effects, doctors reduce the dose of the corticosteroid and stop the drug as soon as possible.

Older people who take corticosteroids are encouraged to take measures to help maintain bone density. They can do weight-bearing exercise and take calcium and vitamin D supplements. Taking bisphosphonates (such as alendronate or risedronate) can help increase bone density.

Faithfully continuing treatment as instructed results in complete recovery for many people.

Diagnosis

Doctors base the diagnosis on symptoms and results of a physical examination and blood tests. Blood tests usually include the following:

- Erythrocyte sedimentation rate (ESR), C-reactive protein levels, or both: In people with polymyalgia rheumatica, results of both tests are usually very high, indicating active inflammation.
- Blood count: This test is done to check for anemia.
- Thyroid-stimulating hormone: This test is done to rule out hypothyroidism, which can cause weakness and sometimes pain of the shoulder and hip muscles.
- Creatine kinase: This test is done to check for muscle tissue damage (myopathy), which can cause weakness and pain of the shoulder and hip muscles.

- Rheumatoid factor: This antibody occurs in people with rheumatoid arthritis but not in those with polymyalgia rheumatica. This test helps doctors distinguish between the two.

If the diagnosis is unclear, a sample of muscle tissue may be removed and examined under a microscope (biopsy), or electromyography (see page 636) may be done to locate the source of muscle symptoms. If the cause is polymyalgia rheumatica, these test results are normal.

Treatment

Taking a low dose of prednisone, a corticosteroid, usually causes dramatic improvement. If people also have giant cell arteritis, a higher dose is needed to reduce the risk of blindness. As the symptoms subside, the dose is gradually reduced to the lowest effective one. Many people can stop taking prednisone in 1 to 4 years, although some people need to take a low dose longer.

Aspirin or other nonsteroidal anti-inflammatory drugs (NSAIDs) can help relieve pain but usually less effectively than prednisone.

Wegener's Granulomatosis

Wegener's granulomatosis often begins with inflammation of small and medium-sized blood vessels and tissues in the nose, sinuses, throat, or lungs. It may progress to inflammation of blood vessels throughout the body (generalized vasculitis).

- The cause is unknown.
- The disorder usually begins with nosebleeds, nasal congestion with crusting, sinusitis, hoarseness, wheezing, and coughing.
- Other organs may be affected, sometimes with serious complications, such as kidney failure.
- Symptoms and other findings suggest the diagnosis, but a biopsy is usually needed to confirm it.
- A corticosteroid and usually another drug that suppresses the immune system are needed to control inflammation.

Wegener's granulomatosis can occur at any age. Its cause is unknown. It resembles an infection, but no infecting organism has been identified. Collections of immune cells that cause inflammation (called granulomas) form nodules and ultimately destroy normal tissue. Various organs in the body are damaged and malfunction because the arteries that supply them with blood are damaged. Wegener's granulomatosis is often life threatening.

Symptoms

The disorder may begin suddenly or gradually. Usually, the first symptoms involve the upper respiratory tract—the nose, sinuses, ears, and windpipe (trachea). They may include the following:

- Nosebleeds, sometimes severe
- Nasal congestion with crusting in and around the nose
- Collapse of the bridge of the nose, causing it to sag
- A hole in the nasal cartilage that separates one side of the nose from the other (nasal septum)
- Sinusitis
- Hoarseness
- Middle ear infections (otitis media)
- Difficulty breathing
- Coughing (sometimes with blood)

Sometimes only the upper respiratory tract is affected for many years. People may also have a fever, feel generally unwell, and lose their appetite. Inflammation can affect the eyes, which may become swollen, red, and painful.

The disorder may progress to affect other areas of the body or may affect several organs from the beginning:

- **Lungs:** The lungs are usually affected at some point. People may feel short of breath and cough. Difficulty breathing may result from bleeding in the lungs, which requires immediate medical attention.
- **Joints:** Joints may become swollen and ache.
- **Nerves:** A limb may feel numb, tingly, or weak, or vision may be impaired. People may see double and, without treatment, may become blind.
- **Skin:** A rash or sores may appear on the skin.
- **Kidneys:** The kidneys are often affected. Kidney function may be slightly or severely impaired. Severe kidney damage causes high blood pressure and swelling due to fluid retention (edema). Life-threatening kidney failure may occur.

Anemia is common and can be severe.

Diagnosis

Wegener's granulomatosis must be diagnosed and treated early to prevent complications, including kidney disorders, lung disorders, and heart attacks.

Doctors usually suspect the diagnosis based on the distinctive pattern of symptoms. A chest x-ray is done because the lungs are usually affected. However, symptoms and chest x-rays can resemble those of several lung disorders, making the diagnosis difficult. For example, a chest x-ray may show cavities or dense areas in the lungs that look like cancer.

Although blood test results cannot specifically identify Wegener's granulomatosis, they can strongly support the diagnosis. One such test can detect antineutrophil cytoplasmic antibodies in the blood. These antibodies attack certain white blood cells and occur in several types of vasculitis. Urine tests also help support the diagnosis. People with this disorder may have blood or too much protein in their urine.

Doctors can confirm the diagnosis only by examining a small piece of tissue under a microscope (biopsy). The tissue sample may be taken from an affected area, such as the nasal passages, airways, or lungs. Skin and kidney biopsies may also be helpful.

Treatment

With treatment, symptoms usually disappear (called remission). However, in about half of treated people, symptoms return (called a relapse). Relapses may occur when treatment is stopped or many years later.

Corticosteroids are almost always used to suppress inflammation. Most people also need drugs that suppress the immune system (immunosuppressants), such as cyclophosphamide (usually used when the disorder is severe), methotrexate, or azathioprine. Most people feel better within days to weeks. But for some, improvement may take months.

During remission, the dose of the drugs is reduced. Treatment is usually continued for at least a year after the symptoms disappear. The dose of a corticosteroid can usually be gradually decreased and eventually stopped. Doses may need to be adjusted throughout the course of treatment. If symptoms worsen or recur, the dose is increased, or if drugs have been stopped, they are started again.

Because immunosuppressants weaken the immune system, the risk of developing serious infections is increased. Taking prednisone for a long time can result in weight gain, cataracts, high blood pressure, decreased bone density, diabetes, changes in mood, and difficulty sleeping. Cyclophosphamide can cause bladder irritation and sometimes bladder cancer. A complete blood count is done frequently, sometimes as often as once a week for patients who take strong immunosuppressants. Immunosuppressants may cause the number of blood cells to decrease.

People with Wegener's granulomatosis need to be closely monitored by their doctor to check whether the dose of the drugs is appropriate, whether they are having side effects from the drugs, whether they could have an infection, and, during remission, whether there is any indication of a relapse.

People should also learn as much as they can about the disorder. Thus, they can recognize signs of a relapse early. People can also learn to test their urine for blood and protein so that they can notify their doctor at the first sign of any new abnormality.

Behçet's Syndrome

Behçet's syndrome is chronic inflammation that can cause painful mouth sores, skin blisters, genital sores, and swollen joints. The eyes, blood vessels, nervous system, and digestive tract may also become inflamed.

- Typically, sores appear, disappear, and reappear in the mouth and on the genitals and skin.
- Doctors base the diagnosis on symptoms and results of a physical examination.
- Corticosteroids, other drugs that suppress the immune system, thalidomide, and colchicine are used to relieve symptoms.

Behçet's syndrome occurs worldwide but is most common in the area along the silk route from the Mediterranean to China. It is uncommon in the United States. It occurs nearly equally in men and women, typically beginning during their 20s. But it can develop at any age. The cause is unknown.

Symptoms

Almost everyone with this syndrome has recurring, painful mouth sores, similar to canker sores. Sores may appear on the tongue, gums, and lining of the mouth. Sores may also appear on the genital organs. Those on the penis, scrotum, or vulva tend to be painful. Those in the vagina may be painless.

Other symptoms appear days to years later:

- **Eyes:** Part of the eye becomes inflamed intermittently. This inflammation (relapsing iridocyclitis or uveitis—see page 1447) causes eye pain, redness, sensitivity to light, and hazy vision. Several other eye problems can occur. If untreated, blindness can develop.
- **Skin:** Skin blisters and pus-filled pimples develop in about 80% of people. A slight injury, even a puncture from a hypodermic needle, can cause small red or pus-filled bumps to form.
- **Joints:** In about half of affected people, the knees and other large joints become painful. This relatively mild inflammation (arthritis) does not progress or damage tissue.
- **Blood vessels:** Inflammation of blood vessels (vasculitis) throughout the body can cause blood clots to form and bulges (aneurysms) to develop in weakened blood vessel walls. Vasculitis can result in strokes if arteries to the brain are affected. It can cause kidney damage if arteries to the kidneys are affected. If arteries in the lungs are affected, bleeding may occur, and people may cough up blood.
- **Digestive tract:** Symptoms may range from mild discomfort to severe cramping and diarrhea.
- **Central nervous system:** Inflammation of the brain or spinal cord is less common but has serious consequences. People may have a headache first. Other symptoms include a fever and stiff neck (symptoms of meningitis), confusion, and loss of coordination. Changes in personality and memory loss may develop years later.

Symptoms can come and go unpredictably, becoming very disruptive. Symptoms or symptom-free periods (remissions) may last weeks, years, or decades. Many people eventually go into remission. Occasionally, damage to the nervous system, digestive tract, or blood vessels is fatal.

Diagnosis

The diagnosis is based on symptoms and results of a physical examination. No laboratory tests can confirm Behçet's syndrome. Doctors suspect the disorder in people, particularly young adults, who have the following:

- Recurrent mouth and genital sores
- Characteristic eye problems
- Skin bumps triggered by a slight injury

However, symptoms may resemble those of many other disorders, including reactive arthritis (previously called Reiter's syndrome), lupus (systemic lupus erythematosus), Crohn's disease, herpes, and ulcerative colitis. The diagnosis may take months to make because doctors look for a pattern of symptoms that subside and recur (remissions and relapses) to help identify the syndrome.

Blood and urine tests are done. They cannot identify the syndrome but can confirm that inflammation is present.

Treatment

There is no cure, but treatment can usually relieve specific symptoms. Which drugs are used depends on which organ is affected and how severe the disease is. For example, the following may be used:

- For inflamed eyes and skin sores: A corticosteroid (used to reduce inflammation) can be applied to the eyes or skin.
- For severe inflammation of the eyes or nervous system: Cyclosporine or azathioprine, which are drugs that suppress the immune system (immunosuppressants), may be used when eye inflammation is severe or when prednisone does not adequately control symptoms.
- For mouth and genital sores and joint pain: Colchicine (used to treat gout) can be taken by mouth to prevent new sores. Thalidomide may help mouth, genital, and skin sores heal, but the sores may recur when the drug is stopped. Etanercept, which is a tumor necrosis factor inhibitor (and thus suppresses the immune system), helps prevent new mouth and genital sores. It is given by injection.

Azathioprine may also reduce the number of mouth and genital sores, help sores heal, and reduce joint pain. Cyclophosphamide and chlorambucil are used when other drugs are ineffective or when life-threatening complications develop.

Takayasu's Arteritis

Takayasu's arteritis causes chronic inflammation, mainly of the aorta (the artery that connects directly with the heart), the arteries that branch off from it, and the pulmonary arteries.

- The cause is unknown.
- People may have general symptoms, such as fever or muscle or joint aches, followed by various symptoms, depending on which organs are affected.
- Imaging tests of the aorta, such as angiography, are done to confirm the diagnosis.
- A corticosteroid and sometimes another drug that suppresses the immune system can usually control the inflammation.

Takayasu's arteritis is rare. It affects mostly women aged 15 to 30. Its cause is unknown.

The aorta and its branches, including arteries that take blood to the head and the kidneys, become inflamed. In about half of people, the pulmonary arteries are also affected. Inflammation may cause sections of these arteries to become narrow or blocked. The walls may weaken and stretch, resulting in a bulge (aneurysm). The affected vessels cannot provide enough blood to the tissues they supply.

Symptoms

Takayasu's arteritis is a chronic disorder with symptoms that fluctuate in severity.

Sometimes the disorder begins with fevers, muscle and joint aches, loss of appetite, weight loss, and night sweats. But usually, symptoms occur when an artery narrows, reducing blood flow to part of the body, as in the following:

- **Arms or legs:** The arms and legs ache and tire easily when they are used. When walking, people may feel pain, usually in the calves—a symptom called claudication.
- **Head:** People may feel dizzy or have problems with vision. Less often, a stroke results.
- **Heart:** Sometimes blood flow to the heart is reduced, and angina or a heart attack results.
- **Kidneys:** The kidneys may malfunction, resulting in high blood pressure. High blood pressure increases the risk of kidney failure, strokes, and heart attacks.
- **Lungs:** Blood pressure in the lungs becomes very high. People feel short of breath, tire easily, and may have chest pain.

Some people do not have any symptoms. In other people, the disorder progresses, causing serious complications such as strokes, heart failure, heart attacks, kidney failure, and aneurysms.

Diagnosis

Doctors suspect the disorder based on the following, especially in young women:

- Blood pressure cannot be measured in one or both arms.
- Blood pressure is much higher or pulse is much stronger in one arm or leg than in the other.
- Blood pressure is unexpectedly high.
- A person has a disorder such as stroke, angina, heart attack, or kidney damage that has no apparent explanation and that is unexpected.

Doctors ask about symptoms, review the person's medical history, and do a complete physical examination to exclude other disorders that may cause similar symptoms.

Blood and urine tests are done. They cannot identify the disorder but may confirm that inflammation is present.

To confirm the diagnosis, doctors may use angiography—conventional, magnetic resonance, or computed tomography (CT) angiography—to evaluate the aorta and its branches. For conventional or CT angiography, a dye that can be seen on x-rays (radiopaque dye) is injected into blood vessels to outline them. Then x-rays are taken. Magnetic resonance angiography does not require the injection of a dye. These procedures can detect aneurysms and show where the arteries are narrowed.

After Takayasu's arteritis is diagnosed, regular doctor visits should be scheduled so that the doctor can check whether the disorder is progressing.

Treatment

Corticosteroids (such as prednisone) are usually used. They effectively reduce inflammation in most people. Sometimes another drug that suppresses the immune system (immunosuppressant), such as azathioprine, cyclophosphamide, mycophenolate mofetil, or methotrexate, is also used. Tumor necrosis factor inhibitors, such as infliximab and etanercept, may also be effective. However, drugs cannot control symptoms in about one fourth of people.

How long drugs should be given has not been determined. The dose of the corticosteroid is gradually reduced, and the drug is eventually stopped because these drugs, especially when used for a long time, can have serious side effects. When drugs are stopped, symptoms return in about one half of people, so the drugs may need to be restarted.

High blood pressure must be controlled to prevent complications (see page 339). Angiotensin-converting enzyme (ACE) inhibitors are often used. Taking a low dose of aspirin is usually recommended to help decrease the risk of clotting in the inflamed artery, which can lead to blockages. If an artery that supplies the heart is blocked, a heart attack can result.

If people have difficulty using their arms or walking, bypass surgery may be done to restore the blood flow to the affected limb. Other procedures to restore blood flow (such as coronary artery bypass surgery or percutaneous transluminal coronary angioplasty) may be needed, depending on the symptoms.

Churg-Strauss Syndrome

Churg-Strauss syndrome is inflammation of small blood vessels that damages organs and that usually occurs in people with a history of asthma, nasal allergies, or both.

- The cause is unknown.
- At first, people may have a runny nose or asthma for months or years or have facial pain, followed by various symptoms, depending on which organs are affected.
- Doctors base the diagnosis on symptoms and results of a physical examination, blood tests, a chest x-ray, and biopsy.
- Corticosteroids are usually effective, but if a vital organ is affected, another drug that suppresses the immune system may be used.

Churg-Strauss syndrome can occur in people of all ages. The average age at the time of diagnosis is 45 to 50. Almost all affected people have a history of asthma, nasal allergies, or both. The cause is unknown.

Inflammation may affect any organ. The nerves, sinuses, skin, joints, lungs, digestive tract, heart, and kidneys are most commonly affected. Collections of immune cells that cause inflammation (called granulomas) may form nodules in affected tissue. Granulomas can destroy normal tissue and interfere with functioning. They may also cause lumps to form under the skin.

Symptoms

At first, asthma, nasal allergies, or both may develop or worsen. People may sneeze and have a persistently runny nose and itchy eyes. Inflammation of the sinuses may cause facial pain, and polyps may develop in the nose.

People may feel generally ill and tired. They may have fevers or night sweats or lose their appetite and lose weight. Other symptoms depend on which organs are affected and may include the following:

- Muscle and joint pain
- Shortness of breath
- Cough, sometimes bringing up blood
- Chest pain

- Rashes
- Abdominal pain
- Blood in the stool
- Abnormal sensations, numbness, or weakness in a limb

Any combination of these symptoms may occur. Symptoms may occur in episodes. In subsequent episodes, people may have the same symptoms as the first episode or different ones.

Inflammation of the kidneys may not cause symptoms until the kidneys malfunction and kidney failure develops. Other complications include heart failure, heart attacks, and heart valve disorders.

Diagnosis

Early diagnosis and treatment help prevent severe organ damage.

No single test can confirm the diagnosis. The diagnosis is made by recognizing the combination of typical symptoms and results of the physical examination and other tests.

Blood tests are done. Doctors determine how many eosinophils are in the blood. These white blood cells are produced during allergic reactions, and their number increases when Churg-Strauss syndrome is present. Doctors also look for certain antibodies (antineutrophil cytoplasmic antibodies) that may be present. A chest x-ray is done to look for inflammation in the lungs. Urine tests are done to determine whether the kidneys are affected.

A sample of inflamed tissue is taken and examined under a microscope (biopsy). A biopsy can show whether the tissue contains eosinophils or granulomas. If possible, a sample is taken from the skin or muscle because the biopsy can then be done as an outpatient procedure with only a local anesthetic. Sometimes a biopsy of lung tissue is necessary. It may require hospitalization.

Treatment

Corticosteroids (such as prednisone) are usually used. These drugs can reduce inflammation. If a vital organ is affected, another drug that suppresses the immune system (immunosuppressant) is also used. Azathioprine or methotrexate may be used. Cyclophosphamide is used when the symptoms are severe.

After symptoms resolve, the dose of the drugs is gradually reduced, and after a while, the drugs may be stopped. If necessary, they can be started again. These drugs, especially when taken for a long time, can have serious side effects.

People with Churg-Strauss syndrome should learn about their disorder. Then they can recognize any new symptoms and report them immediately to the doctor.

Henoch-Schönlein Purpura

Henoch-Schönlein purpura is inflammation mainly of small vessels, usually occurring in children.

- A rash of reddish purple bumps and spots on the lower legs is usually the first symptom, followed by joint aches, digestive upset, and kidney malfunction.
- Biopsy of the affected skin can confirm the diagnosis.
- Corticosteroids can relieve joint aches and digestive upset, but occasionally, other drugs that suppress the immune system are also needed.

Henoch-Schönlein purpura usually affects children aged 3 to 15 but can occur at any age. It may develop when the immune system responds abnormally to an infection or something else. It may be triggered by upper respiratory infections, drugs, or insect bites. Blood vessels in the intestine and kidney may become inflamed.

Symptoms

A rash of small spots that look like bruises or reddish purple bumps (purpura) appear on the arms, legs, buttocks, and top of the feet. After a few days or weeks, more spots and bumps may appear, sometimes on the face or trunk. Most children also have a fever and achy, tender, and swollen joints, including the ankles, knees, hips, wrists, and elbows.

Crampy abdominal pain, nausea, vomiting, and diarrhea are common. Stools or urine may contain blood. Rarely, the intestine slides into itself, like a collapsible telescope. This complication, called intussusception, can cause sudden stomach pain and vomiting because the intestine is blocked.

Symptoms usually resolve after about 4 weeks but often recur at least once after a few weeks. Most people recover completely. Rarely, chronic kidney failure develops.

Diagnosis

Doctors suspect the disorder when the characteristic rash occurs in children. If the diagnosis is not clear, a sample from the affected skin is taken and examined under a microscope (biopsy) to look for abnormalities that can confirm the diagnosis. Urine tests are done to check for blood and excess protein, which indicate that the kidneys are affected. Blood tests are usually done to measure kidney function.

If kidney malfunction worsens, a kidney biopsy is done. It can help doctors determine how severe the problem is and what kind of recovery can be expected.

Treatment

If a drug is contributing to the disorder, it is stopped. Otherwise, treatment focuses on relieving symptoms.

It may include nonsteroidal anti-inflammatory drugs (NSAIDs) and bed rest.

Corticosteroids or other drugs, taken by mouth, may help control abdominal pain and are occasionally needed to help control severe joint pain or swelling. If the kidneys or digestive organs are severely affected, methylprednisolone (a corticosteroid), given intravenously, and cyclophosphamide (which suppresses the immune system), taken by mouth, may be used.

Microscopic Polyangiitis

Microscopic polyangiitis is inflammation of mainly small vessels throughout the body.

- People have a fever, lose weight, and have achy muscles and joints, as well as various other symptoms depending on the organs affected.
- Biopsy is done to confirm the diagnosis.
- Treatment depends on disease severity but includes corticosteroids and drugs that suppress the immune system (immunosuppressants).

Microscopic polyangiitis is rare. It can occur at any age. The cause is unknown. People with this disorder usually have abnormal antibodies called antineutrophil cytoplasmic antibodies in their blood. Some people also have hepatitis B or C.

Symptoms

Most people have a fever and lose weight. Muscles and joints often ache.

Various organs may be affected:

- **Kidneys:** The kidneys are affected in up to 90% of people. Blood may appear in the urine, but often there is no sign of kidney malfunction until it is severe. Kidney failure may develop rapidly unless diagnosis and treatment are prompt.
- **Respiratory tract:** People may have nosebleeds or facial pain due to sinusitis. If the lungs are affected, bleeding in the lungs may occur, causing people to cough up blood. The lungs may fill with fluid, and scar tissue may eventually develop. Either problem causes difficulty breathing. Bleeding in the lungs, which may occur early in the disorder, requires immediate medical attention.

- **Skin:** About one third of people have a rash of reddish purple spots and bumps, usually on the legs, feet, or buttocks. The nails may contain thin purplish lines, indicating bleeding (called splinter hemorrhages).
- **Digestive tract:** Abdominal pain, nausea, vomiting, and diarrhea may occur. Stools may contain blood.
- **Nerves:** People may have tingling, numbness, or weakness in a limb.
- **Brain:** Headache may result if the arteries to the brain are affected. Less often, bleeding in the brain (cerebral hemorrhage), stroke, or seizures occur.

Other organs are affected less often.

Diagnosis

Doctors suspect the diagnosis based on symptoms. Blood and urine tests are done. These tests cannot identify the disorder but can confirm that inflammation is present. Blood tests can also help doctors detect bleeding in the digestive tract. Blood is tested for abnormal antibodies, such as antineutrophil cytoplasmic antibodies, which attack certain white blood cells. A sample of urine is tested for red blood cells and protein. This information can help doctors determine whether the kidneys are affected.

A chest x-ray is done to determine whether the lungs are affected. The x-ray can also help doctors determine whether there is bleeding in the lungs. If there are signs of bleeding, a flexible viewing tube is inserted through the nose or mouth into the airways to directly view the lungs (bronchoscopy). This procedure can confirm the presence of bleeding.

A biopsy of affected tissue (usually the skin, lungs, or kidneys) is done to confirm the diagnosis.

Treatment

If symptoms are mild, a corticosteroid plus another drug that suppresses the immune system (immunosuppressant), such as azathioprine or methotrexate, is used. If vital organs are affected, cyclophosphamide, a stronger immunosuppressant, and a corticosteroid are used. Sometimes plasma exchange (plasmapheresis) or methylprednisolone, given intravenously, is used.

CHAPTER
99 Gout and Pseudogout

Gout and pseudogout are characterized by joint inflammation (arthritis) and pain. Both disorders are caused by deposits of crystals in the joints, although the type of crystal differs.

Gout

Gout is a disorder that results from deposits of sodium uric acid crystals, which accumulate in the joints because of high blood levels of uric acid (hyperuricemia), leading to attacks of painful joint inflammation.

- Accumulations of uric acid crystal can intermittently cause severe joint or tissue pain and inflammation.
- Doctors remove fluid from the joint and check it for uric acid crystals.
- Drugs are given to relieve inflammation and pain, prevent further attacks, and sometimes decrease blood levels of uric acid.

Gout is more common among men than women. Usually, gout develops during middle age in men and after menopause in women. Gout is rare in younger people but is often more severe in people who develop the disorder before age 30. Gout often runs in families.

Causes

Normally, uric acid, a by-product of cell nucleic acid breakdown, is present in small amounts in the blood because the body continually breaks down cells and forms new cells. Also, the body readily transforms substances in foods called purines into uric acid. Purines are part of proteins. Foods high in purines include anchovies, asparagus, consommé, herring, meat gravies and broths, mushrooms, mussels, all organ meats, sardines, and sweetbreads. Most often, the uric acid level in the blood becomes abnormally high when the kidneys cannot eliminate enough uric acid in the urine. Too much uric acid in the blood can result in uric acid crystals being formed and deposited in joints. Additionally, combining a high-purine diet with alcohol can worsen matters, because alcohol both increases the production of uric acid and interferes with its elimination by the kidneys.

Less commonly, gout may be caused by an identifiable underlying disorder and is then called secondary gout. For instance, large amounts of uric acid may be produced because of an inherited enzyme abnormality or a disease such as leukemia, in which cells multiply and are rapidly destroyed. Some types of kidney disease and certain drugs (eg, thiazide diuretics) impair the kidneys' ability to eliminate uric acid, so levels of uric acid rise.

High levels of uric acid in the blood lead to high levels of uric acid in the joints. This process may then result in the formation of uric acid crystals in the joint tissue and the fluid within the joints (synovial fluid). Gout most often affects the joints in the feet, particularly at the base of the big toe (podagra). However, it also commonly affects other areas: the ankle, instep, knee, wrist, and elbow. Gout tends to affect these cooler areas because uric acid crystals form more readily in cool than in warm areas. Rarely, gout affects the joints of the warmer, central part of the body, such as the spine, hips, or shoulders.

Symptoms

Attacks of gout (acute gouty arthritis) can occur without warning. They may be triggered by an injury, surgery, consumption of large quantities of alcohol or purine-rich food, or illness. Typically, severe pain occurs suddenly in one or more joints, often at night (probably because of the metabolic changes that occur when a person lies down). The pain becomes progressively worse and is often excruciating, particularly when the joint is moved or touched. The joint becomes inflamed—it swells and feels warm, and the skin over the joint may appear red or purplish, tight, and shiny.

Risk Factors for the Development of Gout

- Beer and alcoholic beverages
- Low dairy intake
- Certain cancers and blood disorders
- Certain drugs (such as thiazide diuretics, cyclosporine, pyrazinamide, ethambutol, nicotinic acid, and high doses of aspirin)
- Certain foods (such as anchovies, asparagus, consommé, herring, meat gravies and broths, mushrooms, mussels, all organ meats, sardines, and sweetbreads)
- Hypothyroidism
- Lead poisoning (from "moonshine" whiskey)
- Obesity
- Radiation therapy
- Chronic kidney disease
- Starvation

Other symptoms of an attack can include fever (which may reach 102° F [38.9° C]) and a general sick feeling. The first few attacks usually affect only one joint and last for a few days. The symptoms gradually disappear, joint function returns, and no symptoms appear until the next attack. However, if the disorder progresses, untreated attacks last longer, occur more frequently, and affect several joints.

After repeated attacks, gout can become severe and chronic and may lead to joint deformity.

Over time, joint motion becomes progressively restricted by damage caused by deposits of uric acid crystals in the joints and tendons. Hard lumps of uric acid crystals (tophi) are first deposited in the joint (synovial) lining or cartilage or in bone near the joints and then under the skin around joints. Tophi can also develop in the kidney and other organs, under the skin on the ears, in the tough band extending from the calf muscles to the heel (Achilles tendon), or around the elbows. They commonly develop in the fingers, hands, and feet. If untreated, tophi can burst and discharge chalky masses of uric acid crystals through the skin.

> **❓ Did You Know...**
>
> In past times, when protein was scarce, gout, which can be caused or worsened by eating too much protein, was considered a rich person's disease.

About one fifth of people who have gout develop kidney stones (urolithiasis) that are composed of uric acid (see page 299). The stones may block the urinary tract, resulting in excruciating pain and, if untreated, infection and kidney damage. In people with gout who also have another disorder that damages the kidneys (such as diabetes or high blood pressure), increasingly poor kidney function reduces the excretion of uric acid and makes the gout and its joint damage progressively worse.

Diagnosis

Doctors often diagnose gout on the basis of its distinctive symptoms and an examination of the affected joints. A high level of uric acid in the blood supports the diagnosis; however, this level is often normal, especially during an acute (sudden severe) attack. The diagnosis is confirmed when needle-shaped uric acid crystals are identified in a sample of a tophus or in joint fluid removed (joint aspiration) with a needle and viewed under a microscope with polarized light. X-rays may show joint damage and the presence of tophi (uric acid crystal tophi that displace bone and produce cysts). Gout is often similar to and sometimes misdiagnosed as another type of arthritis.

Treatment

Treatment has three goals:

- Relieve the acute attack of inflammation
- Prevent further attacks
- Prevent further deposition of uric acid in the tissues by lowering blood levels of uric acid

Relieving the Acute Attack: Nonsteroidal anti-inflammatory drugs (NSAIDs) are often effective in relieving pain and swelling in the joint (see page 644). Sometimes, additional analgesics such as oxycodone are needed to control pain. The inflamed joint may be immobilized with a splint, and ice can be applied to reduce pain.

Colchicine is the traditional, but no longer the most common, first-step treatment. Usually, joint pain begins to subside after 12 hours of treatment with colchicine and is gone within 36 to 48 hours. Colchicine is usually taken in tablet form each hour until symptoms are relieved. Colchicine can cause abdominal pain and diarrhea. It can occasionally cause more serious side effects, including damage to the bone marrow.

Corticosteroids, such as prednisone, are sometimes useful to reduce joint inflammation (including the swelling) in people who cannot tolerate the other drugs. If only one or two joints are affected, a corticosteroid suspension, such as prednisolone tebutate, can be injected using the same needle that is used to remove fluid from the joint.

Preventing Further Attacks: Avoiding alcoholic beverages, losing weight, stopping drugs that cause elevated blood levels of uric acid, and eating smaller amounts of purine-rich foods will help and rarely be all that is needed. Most people who have primary gout are overweight. As they gradually lose weight, their blood levels of uric acid often return to normal or near normal, and gout attacks subsequently cease.

Preventive daily drug treatment may be needed for people who experience repeated, severe attacks. Colchicine may be taken daily to prevent attacks or to greatly reduce their frequency. NSAIDs taken daily can also prevent attacks. However, preventing attacks does not prevent or heal existing joint damage caused by uric acid crystals because the crystals still persist in the joints, and the drugs do pose some risks for people who have kidney or liver disease.

Lowering Blood Levels of Uric Acid: A high level of uric acid in the blood causes problems for most

℞ DRUGS USED TO TREAT GOUT

DRUG	SOME SIDE EFFECTS	COMMENTS
Nonsteroidal anti-inflammatory drugs (NSAIDs)		
All NSAIDs (see table on page 646)	Upset stomach Bleeding Kidney damage High potassium levels Retention of sodium and potassium Sometimes cause swelling or high blood pressure	Used to treat an acute (sudden) attack or to prevent an attack
Antigout drug		
Colchicine	Diarrhea (occurs often) Suppression of blood cell production in the bone marrow (occurs very rarely if the drug is used properly) Muscle pain and weakness (uncommon)	Used to prevent and treat attacks
Corticosteroids		
Prednisone (taken by mouth)	Retention of sodium, with swelling or high blood pressure Multiple side effects if used long term	Used only if other treatments cannot be used, but the benefit is rapid
Prednisolone tebutate or triam-cinolone hexacetonide (taken by injection)	Pain Discomfort Joint damage with overuse Inflammation (occasionally) Infection (rarely)	Injected into the joint if only one or two joints are affected
Uricosuric drugs (drugs that increase uric acid secretion in the urine)		
Probenecid Sulfinpyrazone	Headache Nausea Vomiting Kidney stones	Can be used long-term to lower blood levels of uric acid to prevent attack
Drugs that block uric acid production		
Allopurinol	Upset stomach Skin rash Decrease in the number of white blood cells Liver damage (rare)	Can be used long-term to lower blood levels of uric acid to prevent attacks and to remove crystals in the body or stones in the kidneys

people. People who especially need their blood level of uric acid lowered include those who have the following:

- Frequent, severe attacks despite taking colchicine or NSAIDs
- Tophi
- Very high blood levels of uric acid

- Uric acid kidney stones
- Conditions that make NSAIDs or corticosteroids risky to take (such as peptic ulcer disease and chronic kidney disease)

People taking drugs to lower the blood level of uric acid should know their level, just as patients with hypertension should know their blood pressure. The goal of drug therapy is to decrease the level to 10 to 15% less than normal.

Drugs can lower blood levels of uric acid by decreasing the body's production of uric acid or increasing the excretion of uric acid in the urine. Allopurinol is most often used to lower the blood level of uric acid. This drug blocks the production of uric acid in the body and is especially helpful for people who have a high blood level of uric acid and uric acid stones or kidney damage. However, allopurinol can upset the stomach, cause a skin rash, decrease the number of white blood cells, or cause liver damage or inflammation of vessels (vasculitis). Allopurinol also can cause a gout attack when it is first taken. Because low-dose colchicine or an NSAID can decrease this risk, one of these drugs is usually given for a few months as well.

Drugs that cause excretion of uric acid in the urine (uricosuric drugs), such as probenecid or sulfinpyrazone, also can be used to lower the levels of uric acid in the blood (in people who have normal kidney function) by increasing the kidney's excretion of uric acid. Aspirin can block the effects of probenecid and sulfinpyrazone, and high doses of aspirin should not be used at the same time as either of these drugs. Low doses that protect the heart (81 milligrams daily) should be continued, because heart disease is a considerable risk in people with gout.

Although drugs that increase the excretion of uric acid in the urine (uricosuric drugs) lower the concentration of uric acid in the blood, they can increase the concentration of uric acid in the urine. Drinking plenty of fluids—at least 3 quarts a day—may help reduce the risk of uric acid stones developing in the urinary tract. Making the urine alkaline by taking acetazolamide or potassium citrate (which increases the solubility of uric acid in the urine) can further help reduce the risk of uric acid stones forming in the urinary tract. However, if the urine becomes too alkaline, crystals or stones of another and more dangerous kind—calcium oxalate—may form. When starting a uricosuric drug, there is a risk of causing a gout attack. Low-dose colchicine or an NSAID is given at the same time for a few months to decrease this risk.

Other Treatments: Most tophi on the ears, hands, or feet shrink slowly when the uric acid level becomes sufficiently low. However, extremely large tophi may have to be removed surgically.

Uric acid stones in the urinary tract can be broken up, and thereby washed out in the urine, by using ultrasound directed at the stones from outside the body (extracorporeal shock wave lithotripsy—see art on page 301).

Pseudogout

Pseudogout (calcium pyrophosphate dihydrate crystal deposition disease) is a disorder caused by deposits of calcium pyrophosphate dihydrate crystals in the cartilage and then in the fluid of the joints, leading to intermittent attacks of painful joint inflammation.

- Crystals accumulate in joints and cause varying degrees of inflammation and tissue damage.
- The diagnosis is confirmed by finding calcium pyrophosphate crystals in joint fluid.
- Treatment is with nonsteroidal anti-inflammatory drugs and sometimes injection of corticosteroids into joints.

Pseudogout usually occurs in older people and affects men and women equally.

Causes

The reason that calcium pyrophosphate dihydrate crystals deposit in the joints of some people is unknown. It may occur in people who have other diseases, such as an abnormally high calcium level in the blood caused by a high level of parathyroid hormone (hyperparathyroidism), an abnormally high iron level in the tissues (hemochromatosis), or an abnormally low magnesium level in the blood (hypomagnesemia). However, most people with pseudogout have none of these conditions. The disorder can be hereditary. The calcium crystals frequently occur in joints affected by osteoarthritis (see page 559).

Symptoms

Symptoms vary widely. Some people have attacks of painful joint inflammation, usually in the knees, wrists, or other relatively large joints. Other people have lingering, chronic pain and stiffness in joints of the arms and legs, which may be similar to rheumatoid arthritis or osteoarthritis. Sudden painful (acute) attacks are usually less severe than those of gout, but as in gout, attacks in pseudogout can cause fever. Some people have no pain between attacks, and some have no pain at any time, despite large deposits of crystals. Unlike in gout, people with pseudogout do not develop hard lumps of uric acid crystals (tophi).

Diagnosis

Doctors make the diagnosis by taking fluid from an inflamed joint through a needle (joint aspiration). Calcium pyrophosphate dihydrate crystals are found in the joint fluid. They can be distinguished from uric acid crystals (which cause gout) using a special polarized light microscope. Masses of calcium pyrophosphate crystals, unlike uric acid crystals, can be seen on an x-ray.

Prognosis and Treatment

Often, the inflamed joints heal without any residual problems, but in many people, permanent joint damage can occur, with some joints so severely destroyed that they can be confused with Charcot's joints (see page 572).

Usually, treatment can stop acute attacks and prevent new attacks but cannot reverse changes in already damaged joints. Most often, nonsteroidal anti-inflammatory drugs (NSAIDs) are used to reduce the pain and inflammation (see page 644). Colchicine can be given by mouth in daily low doses to limit the number of attacks. Sometimes, excess joint fluid is drained and a corticosteroid suspension is injected into the joint to reduce the inflammation and pain.

No specific effective long-term treatment is available; however, physical therapy (such as muscle-strengthening and range-of-motion exercises) may be helpful to maintain joint function.

CHAPTER

100 Hand Disorders

A number of different disorders may affect the hands, including ganglia, deformities, disorders related to nerves or blood vessels, injuries, and infections. Some other disorders that affect the hands are covered elsewhere in the book, including fractures, osteoarthritis, tendinitis and tenosynovitis, de Quervain's syndrome, Raynaud's syndrome, finger clubbing, and certain birth defects.

Did You Know...
Hitting a ganglion cyst with a book is not recommended.

Ganglia

Ganglia (ganglion cysts) are gelatinous swellings on the hands and wrists.

Ganglia typically occur in people between the ages of 20 and 50. Women are affected 3 times more often than are men. The most usual place for ganglia to develop is the back (dorsal aspect) of the wrist. Ganglia also develop on the front of the wrist (palmar aspect) and on the back of the finger, a few millimeters behind the cuticle (where they are also called mucous cysts).

Why ganglia develop on the wrist is not known, although they may be related to a previous injury. Ganglia on the back of the finger usually are related to arthritis of the last joint of the finger. However, in most cases, having a ganglion cyst does not mean that arthritis will develop.

Ganglia are firm, round or elliptical sac-like swellings that rise from the skin surface. They contain a clear, gelatinous, and usually sticky material. They are usually painless but occasionally cause discomfort. A doctor can readily make the diagnosis by examining the hand.

Treatment

Some ganglia disappear without treatment, so treatment may not be necessary. However, if they are unsightly, cause discomfort, or continue to increase in size, the gelatinous material inside them can (in 50% of people) be removed successfully by a doctor using a needle and a syringe. Sometimes a corticosteroid suspension is injected afterward to further ease any discomfort. The traditional method of removing a ganglion—placing the hand on a firm surface (such as a table) and hitting the ganglion with a large book—is not advisable. This method may cause injury and is unreliable. In about 50% of people, surgical removal may be necessary. After surgical removal, ganglia recur in about 5 to 15% of people.

Deformities

Hand deformities may be caused by an injury or may result from another disorder (for example, rheumatoid arthritis—see page 563). Deformities should be treated promptly, if possible. Otherwise, they tend not to respond to simple treatments, such as splinting or exercises, and often require surgery.

MALLET FINGER

Mallet finger is a deformity in which the fingertip is curled in and cannot straighten itself.

This deformity usually results from injury, which either damages the tendon or tears the tendon from the bone. It can affect one or more fingers. A doctor can make the diagnosis by examining the finger. An x-ray is usually taken to be sure that there is no fracture. The usual treatment is placing a splint on the finger with the finger straightened. The tendon may take 6 to 10 weeks to heal. Mallet finger rarely requires surgery, unless a large fragment of bone has broken off or the joint is partially dislocated.

SWAN-NECK DEFORMITY

Swan-neck deformity is a bending in (flexion) of the base of the finger, a straightening out (extension) of the middle joint, and a bending in (flexion) of the outermost joint.

The most common cause is rheumatoid arthritis. Other causes include untreated mallet finger, looseness (laxity) of the fibrous plate inside the hand at the base of the fingers or of the finger ligaments, muscle spasm affecting the hands, and misalignment in the healing of a fracture of the middle bone of the finger. Normal bending of the finger may become impossible. The deformity can therefore result in considerable disability.

True swan-neck deformity does not affect the thumb, which has one less joint than the other fingers. However, in a variant of swan-neck deformity, called duck-bill deformity, the top joint of the thumb is severely overstraightened with a bending in of the joint at the base of the thumb to form a 90° angle. If duck-bill deformity and swan-neck deformity of one or more fingers occur together, the ability to pinch can be seriously reduced.

A doctor makes the diagnosis by examining the hand and finger.

Treatment

Treatment is aimed at correcting the underlying disorder when possible. Mild deformities may be treated with finger splints (ring splints), which correct the deformity while still allowing a person to use the hand. Problems with the ability to pinch can be greatly improved by surgically realigning the joints or by fusing the thumb or finger joints together (called interphalangeal arthrodesis) into positions that allow for optimal function.

When the Fingers Are Abnormally Bent

Some disorders, such as rheumatoid arthritis, and injuries can cause the fingers to bend abnormally. In mallet finger, the fingertip is curled in and cannot straighten. In swan-neck deformity, the joint at the base of the finger bends in (flexes), the middle joint straightens out (extends), and the outermost joint bends in. In boutonnière deformity, the middle finger joint is bent inward (toward the palm), and the outermost finger joint is bent outward (away from the palm).

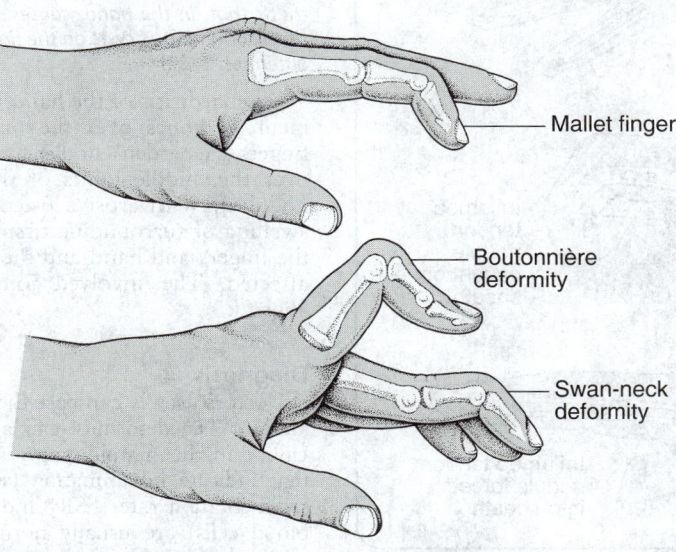

Mallet finger

Boutonnière deformity

Swan-neck deformity

What Is Trigger Finger?

In trigger finger (flexor digital tenosynovitis), a finger becomes locked in a bent position. The finger locks when one of the tendons that flex the finger becomes inflamed and swollen. Normally, the tendon moves smoothly in and out of its surrounding sheath as the finger straightens and bends. In trigger finger, the inflamed tendon can move out of the sheath as the finger bends. However, when the tendon is very swollen, it cannot easily move back in as the finger straightens, and therefore the finger locks.

Trigger finger can result from repetitive use of the hands (as may occur from using heavy gardening shears) or from inflammation (as occurs in rheumatoid arthritis). To straighten the finger, a person must force the swollen area into the sheath—causing a popping sensation similar to that felt when pulling a trigger. Splinting, moist heat, and nonsteroidal antiinflammatory drugs (NSAIDs) can help in mild cases. Sometimes a corticosteroid and a local anesthetic are injected into the tendon sheath. Surgery is commonly needed to treat chronic trigger finger.

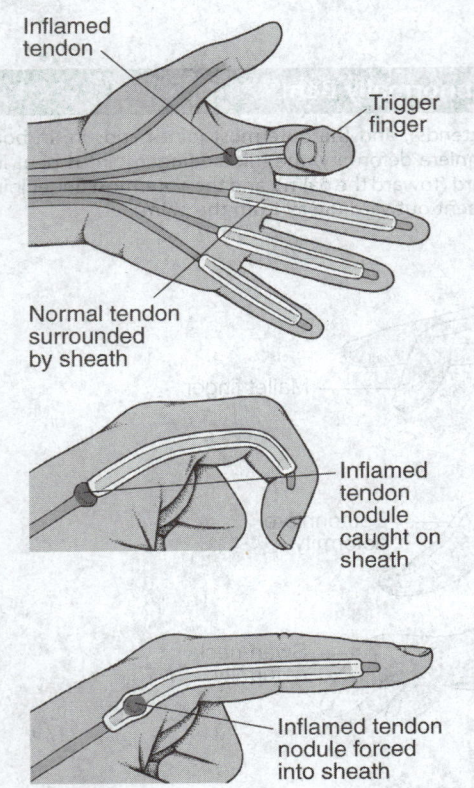

Inflamed tendon

Trigger finger

Normal tendon surrounded by sheath

Inflamed tendon nodule caught on sheath

Inflamed tendon nodule forced into sheath

BOUTONNIÈRE DEFORMITY

Boutonnière deformity (buttonhole deformity) is a deformity in which the middle finger joint is bent in a fixed position inward (toward the palm) and the outermost finger joint is bent excessively outward (away from the palm).

This disorder most often results from rheumatoid arthritis (see page 563) but can also occur from injury (such as deep cuts, joint dislocation, or fractures) or osteoarthritis (see page 559). People with rheumatoid arthritis can develop the disorder because they have long-standing inflammation of the middle joint of a finger. If the deformity is caused by an injury, the injury usually occurs at the base of a tendon (called the middle phalanx extensor tendon). As a result, the middle joint (called the proximal interphalangeal joint) becomes "buttonholed" between the outer bands of the tendon that runs to the end of the finger. The deformity can, but need not, interfere with hand function. The doctor makes the diagnosis by examining the finger.

Treatment

A boutonnière deformity caused by an extensor tendon injury can usually be corrected with a splint that keeps the middle joint fully extended for 6 weeks. When splinting is ineffective, or when boutonnière deformity is due to rheumatoid arthritis, surgery may be needed.

EROSIVE (INFLAMMATORY) OSTEOARTHRITIS

Erosive (inflammatory) osteoarthritis is a form of osteoarthritis that, in the hand, causes swelling, pain, and sometimes formation of cysts on the finger joints (particularly the outermost ones).

Osteoarthritis of the hand is apparent by enlargement of bones over the outermost joints of the fingers (Heberden's nodes) and overgrowth of bones over the middle joints of the fingers (Bouchard's nodules). With erosive osteoarthritis, there is also swelling of surrounding tissues. The joints between the fingers and hand and the wrists are usually not affected. The involved joints can become misaligned.

Diagnosis

Doctors usually can base the diagnosis on an examination. The deformity can also be seen on x-rays. Unlike in rheumatoid arthritis, results of blood tests that indicate inflammation (such as the erythrocyte sedimentation rate [ESR] and the numbers of white blood cells) are usually normal, regardless of how severe the disorder is.

Treatment

Treatment includes range-of-motion exercises in warm water to relieve pain during the exercises and to keep the joints as flexible as possible, splinting intermittently to prevent deformity, and use of analgesics or nonsteroidal anti-inflammatory drugs (NSAIDs) to relieve pain and swelling. Occasionally, a corticosteroid suspension may need to be injected into severely affected joints to relieve pain and increase range of motion. Rarely, when osteoarthritis is advanced and other treatments are not effective, the joint may need to be reconstructed or fused surgically. The hand joint that most often requires surgery for osteoarthritis is the base of the thumb.

DUPUYTREN'S CONTRACTURE

Dupuytren's contracture (palmar fibromatosis) is a progressive tightening of the bands of fibrous tissue (called fascia) inside the palms, causing a curling in of the fingers that eventually can result in a clawlike hand.

- Dupuytren's contracture develops in people who are genetically predisposed.
- Treatment involves injection of a corticosteroid into a tender nodule or, if the hand is already scarred, surgery to correct contracted (clawed) fingers.

Dupuytren's contracture is a common hereditary disorder that occurs particularly in men, especially after age 45. However, having the abnormal gene does not guarantee that someone will have the disorder. About 5% of people in the United States have Dupuytren's contracture. The disorder affects both hands in 50% of people. When only one hand is affected, the right hand is involved twice as often as the left.

Dupuytren's contracture is more common among people with diabetes, alcoholism, or epilepsy. The disorder is occasionally associated with other disorders, including thickening of fibrous tissue above the knuckles (Garrod's pads), shrinking of fascia inside the penis that leads to deviated and painful erections (penile fibromatosis [Peyronie's disease]— see page 1470), and nodules on the soles of the feet (plantar fibromatosis). However, the precise mechanism that causes the fascia of the palm to thicken and curl in is unknown.

The first symptom is usually a tender nodule in the palm (most often at the third or fourth finger). The nodule may initially cause discomfort but gradually becomes painless. Gradually, the fingers begin to curl. Eventually, the curling worsens, and the hand can become arched (clawlike). The doctor makes the diagnosis by examining the hand.

An injection of a corticosteroid suspension into the nodule may help decrease the tenderness in the area but does not delay progression of the disorder.

Surgery is usually needed when the hand cannot be placed flat on a table or when the fingers curl so much that hand function is limited. Surgery to remove the diseased fascia is difficult, because the fascia surrounds nerves, blood vessels, and tendons. Dupuytren's contracture may recur after surgery if removal of the fascia is incomplete. The disorder also may recur spontaneously, especially in people who have developed the disorder at a young age; those who have family members affected by the disorder; and those who have Garrod's pads, Peyronie's disease, or nodules on the soles of the feet.

Nerve Compression Syndromes

Carpal tunnel syndrome, cubital tunnel syndrome, and radial tunnel syndrome are nerve compression syndromes. In these disorders, something (usually bone or connective tissue) presses on a nerve, causing abnormalities of sensation, movement, or both. Symptoms include tingling, pain, loss of sensation, weakness, or a combination. The diagnosis can often be made or confirmed by electromyography and nerve conduction studies (see page 636). In these disorders, surgery may be necessary to relieve pressure on the nerve if symptoms are severe despite other treatments or if there is persistent loss of sensation or weakness.

CARPAL TUNNEL SYNDROME

Carpal tunnel syndrome is a painful compression of the median nerve as it passes through the wrist.

- The side of the hand near the thumb can tingle and become numb.
- Symptoms can usually be relieved by use of a splint or injection of a corticosteroid.

Carpal tunnel syndrome results from compression of the median nerve, which is located at the palm side of the wrist (an area called the carpal tunnel). The median nerve serves the thumb side of the hand. The compression results when swelling or bands of fibrous tissue form for a variety of reasons on the palm side of the wrist.

Causes

Carpal tunnel syndrome is common—especially among women aged 30 to 50 years—and may affect one or both hands. At slightly increased risk are people whose work requires repeated forceful movements with the wrist extended, such as using a screwdriver. Another potential factor is use of a computer keyboard that is not positioned properly. Prolonged exposure to vibrations (for example, by using certain tools) has also been claimed to cause carpal tunnel syndrome. Pregnant women and people who have diabetes, an underactive thyroid gland, gout,

Proper Keyboard Position

Using a computer keyboard that is positioned improperly can result in carpal tunnel syndrome. To prevent injury, the user should keep the wrist in a neutral position. That is, the line from the hand to the forearm should be straight. The hand may be slightly lower than the forearm. But the hand should never be higher, and the wrist should not be cocked. The keyboard should be positioned relatively low, keeping the hand slightly lower than the elbow. A wrist pad can be used to support the wrist.

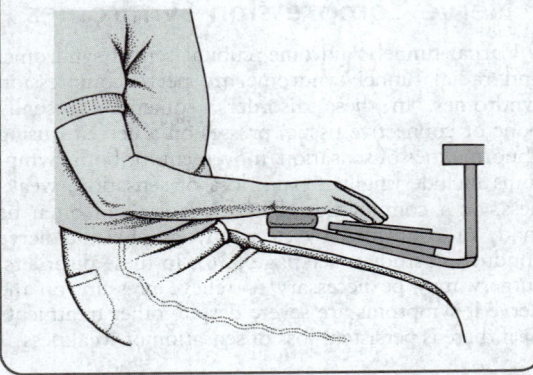

or rheumatoid arthritis are at increased risk of developing carpal tunnel syndrome. However, most cases develop for unknown reasons.

Symptoms

The symptoms, due to the nerve compression, are odd sensations, numbness, tingling, and pain in the first three fingers on the thumb side of the hand. Occasionally, there is also pain and a burning or tingling sensation in the arm. The pain may be more severe while the person is sleeping because of the way the hand is positioned. With time, the muscles in the hand on the thumb side can weaken and shrink through lack of use (atrophy).

Diagnosis

The diagnosis is made largely by examining the affected hand and wrist. A doctor may first perform nerve conduction studies (see page 636) to be certain that the problem is carpal tunnel syndrome, particularly if surgery is considered.

Treatment

Avoiding positions that overextend the wrist or put extra pressure on the median nerve, including such measures as adjusting the angle of a computer keyboard, sometimes provides some relief. Wearing wrist splints that hold the hand in a neutral position (especially at night) and taking mild analgesics often help. Treating underlying disorders (such as rheumatoid arthritis or an underactive thyroid gland) can help to relieve symptoms.

Injections of a corticosteroid suspension into the carpal tunnel occasionally bring long-lasting relief. If pain is severe or if the muscle atrophies or weakens, surgery is the best way to relieve pressure on the median nerve. A surgeon can cut away the bands of fibrous tissue that place pressure on the nerve.

CUBITAL TUNNEL SYNDROME

Cubital tunnel syndrome (ulnar neuropathy) is a disorder caused by compression of the ulnar nerve at the elbow.

The ulnar nerve passes close to the surface of the skin at the elbow ("funny bone") and is easily damaged by repeatedly leaning on the elbow, by bending the elbow for prolonged periods, or sometimes by abnormal bone growth in the area. Baseball pitchers are prone to cubital tunnel syndrome because of the extra twist of the arm required to throw a slider.

Symptoms include pain and numbness of the elbow and a pins-and-needles sensation of the ring and little fingers. Eventually, weakness of the ring and little fingers may develop. Weakness may also interfere with the ability to pinch using the thumb and index finger, because most of the small muscles in the hand are controlled by the ulnar nerve. Severe, chronic cubital tunnel syndrome can lead to muscle wasting (atrophy) and a clawlike deformity of the hand.

Nerve conduction studies (see page 636) may be needed to help pinpoint the exact area of nerve damage. People with mild cases of cubital tunnel syndrome undergo physical therapy (including a splint at night to avoid overbending the elbow) and avoid pressure over the elbow. An elbow pad worn during the day can be helpful. About 85% of people who do not respond to splinting or who have more severe cases of nerve compression may benefit from surgery, which usually consists of releasing pressure on the nerve.

RADIAL TUNNEL SYNDROME

Radial tunnel syndrome (posterior interosseous nerve syndrome) is a disorder resulting from compression of a branch of the radial nerve in the forearm or back of the arm or at the elbow.

Causes of compression of the radial nerve at the elbow include injury, ganglia, lipomas (noncancerous fatty tumors), bone tumors, and inflammation of the surrounding bursa or muscles.

Compression of the radial nerve results in cutting, piercing, or stabbing pain affecting the top of the forearm and back of the hand. Pain results when the person tries to straighten the wrist and fingers. There is no loss of sensation, because the radial nerve principally connects to muscles.

To reduce pressure on the nerve and speed healing, the person should wear a splint and avoid rotating the wrist and bending the arm at the elbow. If the wrist becomes weak and tends to droop (wristdrop), surgery may be needed to relieve pressure on the nerve.

Kienböck's Disease

Kienböck's disease is the death of bone tissue due to an impaired blood supply (avascular necrosis—see page 549) affecting the lunate bone in the hand.

The cause of this relatively unusual disease is unknown. It occurs most commonly in the dominant hand of men aged 20 to 45 years.

Symptoms generally start with wrist pain that begins gradually, in the area of the lunate bone, which is in the middle of the wrist at the base. Eventually, swelling occurs on top of the wrist, which may become stiff. The person has no recollection of injury. The disorder occurs in both hands in 10% of cases and most often occurs in workers doing heavy manual labor. Diagnosis is possible at an early stage by magnetic resonance imaging (MRI) or computed tomography (CT) and is later confirmed by x-ray.

Surgery is performed to relieve pressure on the lunate bone, for example, by lengthening or shortening bones that connect to the lunate bone. Alternative treatments attempt to reestablish the blood supply to the bone. If the lunate bone has collapsed, the wrist bones may be removed or surgically fused together as a last resort to relieve pain. Attempts to treat this disease with methods other than surgery have not been successful.

Injuries

Hand injuries cause swelling, pain, stiffness, and sometimes limited movement. The most common injuries are tears (ruptures) of ligaments or fractures of bone. When a ligament is ruptured, bones can move out of position, resulting in a dislocated joint.

Sometimes doctors can diagnose a hand injury by examining the hand. A local anesthetic may be given before the examination, which otherwise might be too painful. However, x-rays may be needed to determine whether the joint is unstable and to detect fractures. Occasionally, computed tomography (CT) or magnetic resonance imaging (MRI) is needed. Often, an untreated injury can result in a permanent deformity of the hand. Therefore, an injured hand should be immobilized so that it can heal normally. A bandage, splint, or cast may be used, depending on the injury. Surgery is sometimes necessary if bones are out of position or a joint is unstable. Hand exercises are begun as soon as possible to prevent loss of function.

Infections

Human and animal bites can cause an infection of the hands. Some other infections are felon and herpetic whitlow. Paronychia is discussed elsewhere (see page 1339).

INFECTIONS CAUSED BY BITES

The most common cause is injury to the knuckles by the teeth from a punch to the mouth. Animal bites are also common causes. Wound contamination by a number of types of bacteria can result from human and animal bites. All bite injuries are potentially dangerous and can cause significant infection.

If the skin is broken, an x-ray is often done to detect foreign bodies, which can cause or worsen infection. The injured area should be cleaned surgically, with the wound left open to drain. Antibiotics should be given to prevent joint infection (septic arthritis), which can otherwise lead to permanent destruction of the knuckle joints. Which antibiotic is effective depends on which bacteria are common in the person's community.

> **?** **Did You Know...**
> The most important measure for preventing infection of bite wounds is thorough cleaning and draining.

FELON

A felon is infection of the soft tissue (pulp) at the fingertip.

An infection of the fingertip can lead to an abscess, which creates pressure on and causes death of nearby tissues. The fingertip becomes very swollen and firm with intense throbbing pain. The doctor makes the diagnosis by examining the affected finger. If a felon is not treated promptly, the underlying bone, joint, or tendons may become infected. Treatment often requires prompt surgical drainage of the abscess, as well as antibiotics.

Common Hand Injuries

Gamekeeper's thumb is a rupture of the ligament on the palm side of the thumb, which is responsible for pinching movements. It usually results from a fall that jams the thumb backward onto a hard surface. This injury is so named because it used to be an occupational hazard of gamekeepers in England who broke the necks of rabbits with their hands. Treatment usually consists of a splint, but surgery is sometimes necessary.

Rupture of the scapholunate ligament may result from falling on an outstretched hand. Pain is felt mostly on top of the wrist. Treatment consists of surgical repair of the ligament and pinning of the bones.

Scaphoid fractures are a common type of wrist fracture. Tenderness is felt in the wrist below the thumb. Untreated scaphoid fractures often do not heal, eventually leading to arthritis of the wrist. Treatment consists of a cast or surgery. The bone may take 3 to 4 months to heal.

Dislocations may occur at the joint at the base of the thumb or other fingers or at the middle joints of the fingers. Dislocations usually result when the thumb is bent too far out or the fingers are bent too far back. Surgery is often required to correct dislocations at the base of the thumb or fingers. Dislocations of the middle joints may be treated by taping the dislocated finger to an adjacent finger. It the ligament is badly torn, a splint is used, usually for 3 weeks.

Fractures of the hook of hamate may result from striking the ground with a stick or making a divot playing golf. The lower part of the palm below the little finger is tender. The hand is put in a cast for 4 to 6 weeks, but the fracture may not fully heal. If an unhealed fracture causes pain, weakness, or numbness of the little finger, surgery to remove the unattached part of the bone may be necessary.

See page 1964 for a discussion of other hand injuries.

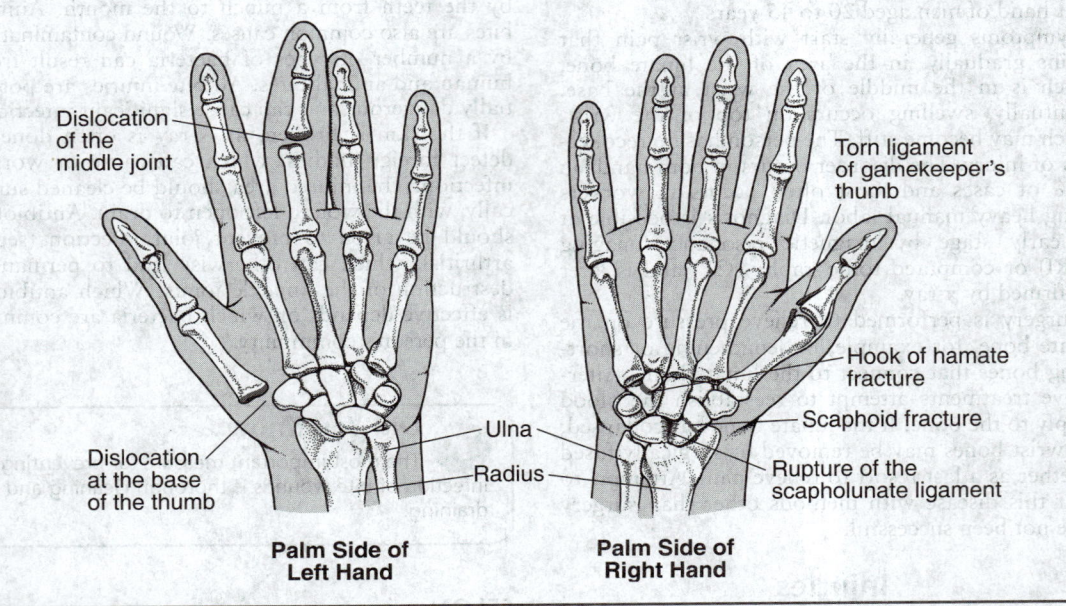

Dislocation of the middle joint
Dislocation at the base of the thumb
Ulna
Radius
Palm Side of Left Hand

Torn ligament of gamekeeper's thumb
Hook of hamate fracture
Scaphoid fracture
Rupture of the scapholunate ligament
Palm Side of Right Hand

HERPETIC WHITLOW

Herpetic whitlow is a viral infection of the fingertip.

Herpes simplex virus (similar to the one causing fever blisters) may cause an intense, painful skin infection. The fingertip is sore and swollen but is not as firm as in a felon. The appearance of tiny fluid-filled blisters (vesicles) on the fingers is diagnostic. A herpetic whitlow is often mistaken for a felon. The disorder eventually goes away without treatment. Surgery is not needed.

HAND ABSCESS

A hand abscess is an accumulation of pus affecting the hand, usually caused by a bacterial infection.

Abscesses in the hands are fairly common and usually result from injury. A superficial abscess may develop just under the skin anywhere in the hand, and nearly always results from a minor injury, such as a splinter or needle prick. Severe pain, warmth, and redness develop over the abscess, often with swelling of nearby lymph nodes in the arm. An abscess may occur in any part of the palm and spread between the metacarpal bones (the hand bones between the wrist and fingers). Such an infection may occur after the skin is ripped or the hand is punctured by something sharp. Palm abscesses may develop from an infected callus. Palm abscesses begin as intense throbbing pain with swelling and severe tenderness to touch. The swelling and pain may be greater at the top of the hand than on the palm.

Treatment involves surgically draining the pus. Antibiotics also are given.

INFECTION OF THE TENDON SHEATH

Abscesses may occur around the tendons that run along the inside of the fingers. This type of abscess is caused by an injury that penetrates one of the creases on the palm side of a finger. Pus from an untreated felon may also spread from the tip of the finger into the end of the tendon sheath. Infection and pus form around the tendon and rapidly destroy tissue. The gliding mechanism of the tendon becomes damaged, so the finger can barely move. Symptoms include swelling and pain of the finger, tenderness over the tendon sheath, and extreme pain when trying to move the finger. Swollen lymph nodes near the abscess are common. Fever is also common.

Surgical drainage of the abscess is required. Antibiotic therapy is also required.

CHAPTER

101 Foot Problems

Some foot problems start in the foot itself, for example, from a foot injury. Others result from disorders that affect many parts of the body, such as diabetes, gout, or other types of arthritis. Problems can occur in any bone, joint, muscle, tendon, or ligament of the foot. Foot fractures are fairly common (see page 1959). Nail discoloration of the foot should always be evaluated because it may be caused by certain disorders, including a fungal infection (see page 1339).

People who have diabetes or peripheral vascular disease (narrowing of the arteries that carry blood to the legs, arms, and possibly internal organs) should check their feet daily for signs of infection or ulcers and should have a doctor or foot doctor (podiatrist) check their feet at least once a year (see box on page 424).

Many foot disorders are treated by changing a person's footwear, such as wearing different shoes or using inserts or other devices (called orthotics or orthoses) that change the position or range of movement of the foot and relieve pressure on affected joints. Injections of a local anesthetic can often relieve pain and decrease muscle spasms so that joints can move more easily, and a corticosteroid may also be injected to decrease inflammation. If these treatments are not successful, sometimes surgery is needed to improve joint alignment and function and relieve pain.

Pain in the Ball of the Foot

Pain in the ball of the foot (called metatarsalgia) may have many different causes (including arthritis, poor circulation, pinching of the nerves between the toes, posture problems, and various disorders). However, most often the pain is caused by nerve damage or by an abnormality of the joints nearest the balls of the feet (metatarsal joints). Often, developing one disorder that causes pain in the ball of the foot contributes to development of another disorder that causes pain in the same location.

FREIBERG'S DISEASE

Freiberg's disease is tissue death (necrosis) of parts of the bones in the ball of the foot, usually the digit next to the big toe (the second metatarsal head).

The cause is injury to the bone, usually in pubertal girls who are growing rapidly or people in whom the bone connected to the base of the big toe is short. In both cases, the metatarsal head can be subjected to repeated stresses.

SPOTLIGHT ON AGING

With aging, many changes occur in the feet. For instance, there is typically less hair; brown coloration (pigmentation) may occur in spots or patches; and the skin may become dry. The toenails often become thicker and curved, and fungal infections of the nails occur commonly. The feet may actually enlarge in length and width because of changes in the ligaments and joints. A person with these types of changes may need to wear larger shoes. Also, feet can be damaged by a lifetime of ill-fitting shoes.

Pain is usually worse when bearing weight, particularly when pushing off of the foot, or when wearing high-heeled shoes. The joint may be swollen and stiff. Doctors examine x-rays to confirm the diagnosis. Pain may be relieved with injections of corticosteroids and by using a splint or cast. Low-heeled shoes or inserts or other devices (orthoses) that change the position or range of movement of the foot and relieve pressure on affected joints are helpful.

DAMAGE TO THE NERVES IN THE FOOT

Irritation or noncancerous (benign) growths of nerves may cause pain in the balls of the feet (interdigital nerve pain).

- Typical symptoms include a mild ache around the third or fourth toe that progresses to a burning or tingling sensation.
- The diagnosis is based on the person's history and an examination of the foot.
- Injecting a corticosteroid or sometimes applying extreme cold (cryotherapy) can help relieve symptoms.

Causes

The nerves that supply the bottom of the foot and toes (interdigital nerves) travel between the bones of the toes. Pain in the ball of the foot may be caused by irritation of the nerves or by noncancerous growths of nerve tissue (neuromas), usually between the base of the third and fourth toes (Morton's neuroma),

although these growths may occur between any of the toes. Neuromas usually develop in only one foot and are more common among women than men.

Symptoms and Diagnosis

In the early stages, a neuroma may cause only a mild ache around the third or fourth toe, occasionally accompanied by a burning or tingling sensation in the toes, particularly as the disorder progresses. These symptoms are generally more pronounced when a person wears certain types of shoes, especially those that are too narrow for the front part of the foot, including those that are pointed. As the condition progresses, a constant burning sensation may radiate to the tips of the toes, regardless of what shoes are worn. A person may also feel as if a marble or pebble is inside the ball of the foot.

Doctors diagnose the condition by considering the history of the problem and examining the foot. X-rays, magnetic resonance imaging (MRI), and ultrasound cannot accurately identify this disorder but may be helpful in ruling out other disorders that can cause similar symptoms.

Treatment

Injecting the tender spot in the foot with corticosteroids mixed with a local anesthetic and wearing proper shoes and sometimes orthoses may relieve the symptoms. Repeating the injections 2 or 3 times at intervals of 1 or 2 weeks may be necessary. Sometimes cryotherapy (application of intense cold) or injection of alcohol into the neuroma may also relieve pain. If these treatments do not help, surgical removal of the neuroma often relieves the discomfort completely but may cause permanent numbness in the area.

METATARSAL JOINT PAIN

Pain in the joints near the ball of the foot (metatarsophalangeal joint) may originate within the joints themselves.

Causes

Metatarsal joint pain commonly results from misalignment of the joint surfaces, which puts pressure on the joint lining and destroys cartilage in the joints. Mild heat and swelling may develop.

Metatarsophalangeal joint misalignment can also be caused by disorders, such as rheumatoid arthritis, that inflame the joints. In rheumatoid arthritis, hammer toes (see page 611) can develop, which can worsen joint pain and misalignment. Fat tissue, which helps cushion the joints when bearing weight, can be pushed forward under the toes, resulting in a loss of cushioning. This loss of cushioning can also damage the nerves in the ball of the foot.

Metatarsophalangeal joint pain may also result from osteoarthritis or stiffening of the joints of the ball of the foot, most often the joint at the big toe. Most people with these disorders have an abnormal motion of the foot when bearing weight and walking.

Symptoms and Diagnosis

Walking is painful. Over time, pain and stiffening can be disabling.

Doctors usually can diagnose the disorder based on the person's symptoms and an examination, although testing is done if an infection or arthritis is suspected.

Treatment

Foot orthoses that redistribute body weight away from the most severely affected joints usually provide effective treatment. Occasionally, when these measures are ineffective, surgery is needed.

SESAMOIDITIS

Sesamoiditis is pain around a small bone (the sesamoid) below the metatarsal head where it adjoins the big toe (first metatarsal head).

The cause of sesamoiditis is usually repeated injury. Sometimes the bone is fractured, or the bone or surrounding structures are inflamed. Sesamoiditis is particularly common among dancers, joggers, and those who have high-arched feet or wear high heels.

The pain of sesamoiditis is felt beneath the ball of the foot at the big toe, is usually made worse by walking, and may be worse when wearing certain shoes. The area may be warm or swollen.

The doctor bases the diagnosis on an examination of the foot. The diagnosis may be confirmed by x-rays taken to exclude a fracture of the sesamoid bone.

Simply not wearing shoes that cause pain may be sufficient. If symptoms persist, shoes with a thick sole and low heels, orthoses, or a combination can help by reducing pressure on the sesamoid bone. A nonsteroidal anti-inflammatory drug (NSAID) taken by mouth and injections of corticosteroids and a local anesthetic into the affected area can help relieve pain.

Tarsal Tunnel Syndrome

Tarsal tunnel syndrome (posterior tibial neuralgia) is pain in the ankle, foot, and toes caused by compression of or damage to the nerve supplying the heel and sole (posterior tibial nerve).

The posterior tibial nerve runs along the back of the calf, through a fibrous canal (tarsal tunnel) near the heel, and into the sole of the foot. When tissues around this nerve become inflamed, they can press on the nerve, causing pain. Disorders that can cause or contribute to tarsal tunnel syndrome include fracture, ankle swelling from heart or kidney failure, an underactive thyroid gland (hypothyroidism), and disorders such as gout or rheumatoid arthritis that inflame the joints.

Pain, the most common symptom of tarsal tunnel syndrome, usually has a burning or tingling quality. It may occur when a person stands, walks, or wears a particular type of shoe. Pain located around the ankle (usually on the inner side) and extending to the toes usually worsens during walking and is relieved by rest. Occasionally, pain also occurs during rest.

To diagnose this condition, a doctor manipulates the affected foot during a physical examination. For example, tapping the injured or compressed area just below the ankle bone often causes tingling, which may extend to the heel, arch, or toes. Nerve conduction studies (see page 636) may be useful to determine the cause or extent of the injury, especially if foot surgery is being considered.

Injections of a mixture of corticosteroids and local anesthetics into the area may relieve pain. Other treatments include wrapping the foot and placing specially constructed devices that change the position or range of movement of the foot and relieve pressure on affected joints (orthoses) in the shoe to reduce pressure on the nerve within the tarsal tunnel. When other treatments do not relieve the pain, surgery to relieve pressure on the nerve may be necessary.

Medial Plantar Nerve Entrapment

Medial plantar nerve entrapment is compression of a nerve at the inner heel (the medial plantar nerve) that causes pain, numbness, or tingling.

Symptoms include almost constant pain, whether walking or sitting. Just standing is often difficult. Burning, numbness, and tingling, which often occur when nerves are compressed, usually do not occur in medial plantar nerve entrapment.

Doctors base the diagnosis usually on the person's symptoms and the results of an examination.

Splints and other devices (foot orthoses) that change the position or range of movement of the foot and relieve pressure on affected joints to prevent irritating motion and pressure may help, as may physical therapy and application of extreme cold to the nerve (cryotherapy). If these treatments do not work, injection with an alcohol solution to deaden the nerve or surgery to free the nerve from compressive structures may help relieve pain.

Tibialis Posterior Tendinosis

Tibialis posterior tendinosis is wear and tear of a tendon that passes behind and around the inner ankle.

The usual cause is excessive ongoing strain because of a problem in how the ankle moves. Most often, the problem is that the person's arch is low and, when walking, the foot tends to turn inward because the person is overweight. Tendon dysfunction may further contribute to flattening of the arch. The tendon may tear completely, sometimes suddenly in a young person.

Early on, people have occasional pain behind the inner ankle. Over time, the pain becomes severe, and swelling occurs. Normal standing and walking become difficult. Standing on the toes is usually painful and may be impossible if the tendon is completely torn.

Doctors can often base the diagnosis on the person's symptoms and the results of an examination. However, sometimes magnetic resonance imaging (MRI) is necessary to confirm the diagnosis and to see the extent of tendon damage.

Devices that change the position or range of movement of the foot and relieve pressure on affected joints (orthoses) and ankle braces are usually enough. Complete rupture may require surgery for a person to regain normal function. Surgery is especially important in young active people with tears that develop suddenly.

Plantar Fasciosis

Plantar fasciosis is pain originating from the dense band of tissue called the plantar fascia that extends from the bottom of the heel bone to the base of the toes (ball of the foot).

- The connective tissue between the heel and ball of the foot may become damaged and painful.
- Pain is often worse when first bearing weight and is felt at the heel.
- Stretches, changing footwear, wearing devices that change the position or range of movement of the foot and relieve pressure on affected joints (orthoses) and splints, and sometimes corticosteroid injections can help.

The plantar fascia connects the bottom of the heel bones to the ball of the foot and is involved in walking and running, giving spring to the step.

Plantar fasciosis is sometimes referred to as plantar fasciitis. However, this term is not correct. The term *fasciitis* means inflammation of the fascia, but plantar fasciosis is a disorder primarily of repeated stress to the fascia rather than a disorder of inflammation. Other terms used to describe plantar fasciosis include calcaneal enthesopathy and calcaneal spur syndrome (heel spur). However, a heel spur may or may not be present. Often a small tear results from excessive strain placed on the plantar fascia. Plantar fasciosis is one of the most common causes of heel pain.

Plantar fasciosis can develop in those who have sedentary lifestyles, wear high-heeled shoes, have unusually high or low arches in the feet, or have tight calf muscles or a tight Achilles tendon (which attaches the calf muscles to the heel bone). Sedentary people are usually affected when they suddenly increase their level of activity or wear less supportive shoes. Plantar fasciosis is also common among runners and dancers because of the increased stress on the fascia, especially if the person also has poor foot posture. The development of this painful disorder occurs more often in people whose occupations involve standing or walking on hard surfaces for prolonged periods. Disorders that may cause or aggravate plantar fasciosis are obesity, rheumatoid arthritis, and other types of arthritis.

Symptoms

A person with plantar fasciosis may have pain anywhere along the course of the plantar fascia but most commonly where the fascia joins the bottom of the heel bone. The person often feels a great deal of pain after resting, particularly when placing weight on the foot first thing in the morning. The pain temporarily diminishes after the person first walks but may return later in the day. It may also begin when the person walks or runs. In this case, the pain radiates from the bottom of the heel toward the toes. Some people have burning or sticking pain along the inside border of the sole of the foot when walking.

Diagnosis

The doctor may make the diagnosis after examining the foot. Tenderness is evident where the plantar fascia enters the heel bone or at the bottom of the ball of the foot.

X-rays may reveal the presence of a heel spur protruding from the bottom front edge of the heel bone. This heel spur is a growth of extra bone produced over time by a combination of increased strain on the fascia and foot dysfunction. However, people with plantar fasciosis often do not have heel spurs, and most people with heel spurs do not have pain, so the presence of heel spurs does not necessarily confirm plantar fasciosis. Other diagnostic tests, such as magnetic resonance imaging (MRI), are rarely needed.

Treatment

To relieve the stress and pain on the fascia, the person can take shorter steps and avoid walking barefoot. Activities that involve foot impact, such as jogging, should be avoided. The person may need to lose weight. Stretching the calf muscles and foot often accelerates healing. Orthoses placed into well-fitting supportive shoes can help to cushion, elevate, and support the heel.

Other measures that may be needed include use of adhesive strapping or arch-supporting wraps, ice massage, use of nonsteroidal anti-inflammatory drugs

What Is a Heel Spur?

A heel spur is a growth of extra bone on the heel bone (calcaneus). It may form when the plantar fascia, the connective tissue extending from the bottom of the heel bone to the base of the toes, pulls excessively on the heel. The spur may be painful as it develops, but it may become less painful as the foot adjusts to it. Most spurs can be treated without surgery.

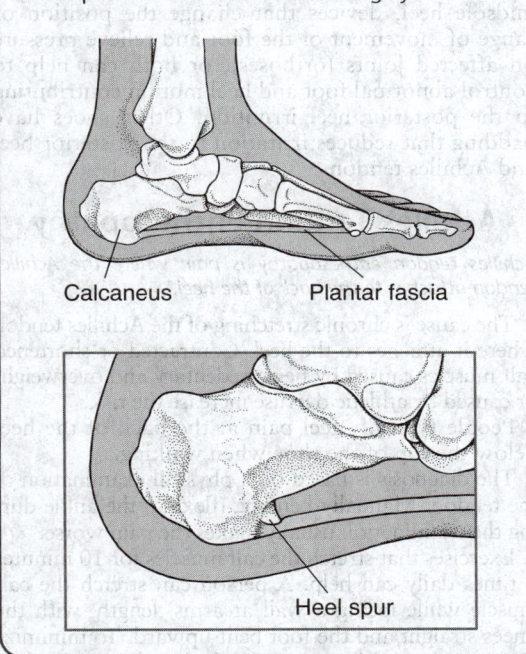

Calcaneus   Plantar fascia

Heel spur

(NSAIDs), occasional corticosteroid injections into the heel, physical therapy, and splinting at night to stretch the calf muscles and fascia during sleep. Corticosteroid injections should probably not be done more than a few times or else they might make the disorder worse. If these measures do not help sufficiently, a cast may be applied. If symptoms are still bothersome, surgery is very rarely required to attempt to partially release pressure on the fascia and remove any heel spurs.

Inferior Calcaneal Bursitis

Bursitis is painful inflammation of a bursa (a flat sac containing joint [synovial] fluid that reduces friction in areas where skin, muscles, tendons, and ligaments rub over bones). Bursitis can develop at the bottom of the heel. The heel may throb, particularly when the shoes are removed, and may be slightly warm and swollen. The diagnosis is based on a person's symptoms and examination results.

This disorder is treated by injecting a local anesthetic/corticosteroid mixture and wearing soft-soled shoes with added protective heel cushion padding.

Achilles Tendon Bursitis

Achilles tendon bursitis is inflammation of the fluid-filled sac (bursa) located either between the skin of the heel and the Achilles tendon (posterior Achilles tendon bursitis) or in front of the attachment of the Achilles tendon to the heel bone (anterior Achilles tendon bursitis, retrocalcaneal bursitis).

- Typical symptoms include swelling and warmth and a tender spot at the back of the heel.
- The diagnosis is based on symptoms, an examination, and sometimes x-rays.
- Treatment is aimed at relieving the inflammation and, depending on the location of the Achilles tendon bursitis, eliminating the pressure on the back of the heel.

The Achilles tendon is the tendon that attaches the calf muscles to the heel bone. Posterior Achilles tendon bursitis is often associated with formation of a bone prominence called Haglund's deformity or "pump bump" on the heel bone. Anterior Achilles tendon bursitis is also called Albert's disease or retromalleolar bursitis.

Posterior Achilles tendon bursitis occurs mainly in young women but can develop in men. Walking in a way that repeatedly presses the soft tissue behind the heel against the stiff back support of a shoe can cause or aggravate the bursitis. Shoes that taper sharply inward toward the posterior heel (such as high-heeled shoes) can lead to the development of this bursitis.

Any condition that puts extra strain on the Achilles tendon can cause anterior Achilles tendon bursitis. Injuries to the heel and diseases such as rheumatoid arthritis can also cause it.

Symptoms

When the bursa becomes inflamed after an injury, symptoms usually develop suddenly. When the bursa develops without an injury, symptoms may develop gradually. With both posterior and anterior Achilles tendon bursitis, symptoms usually include swelling and warmth at the back of the heel. A mildly red, swollen, tender spot develops on the back of the heel. When the inflamed bursa enlarges, it appears as a red lump under the skin of the heel and causes pain at and above the heel. If posterior Achilles tendon bursitis becomes chronic, the swelling may become hard, fluid-filled, and red or flesh-colored.

Diagnosis

The diagnosis is based on the symptoms and an examination. For anterior Achilles tendon bursitis,

Bursitis in the Heel

Normally, only one bursa is in the heel, between the Achilles tendon and the heel bone (calcaneus). This bursa may become inflamed, swollen, and painful, resulting in anterior Achilles tendon bursitis.

Abnormal pressure and foot dysfunction can cause a protective bursa to form between the Achilles tendon and the skin. This bursa may also become inflamed, swollen, and painful, resulting in posterior Achilles tendon bursitis.

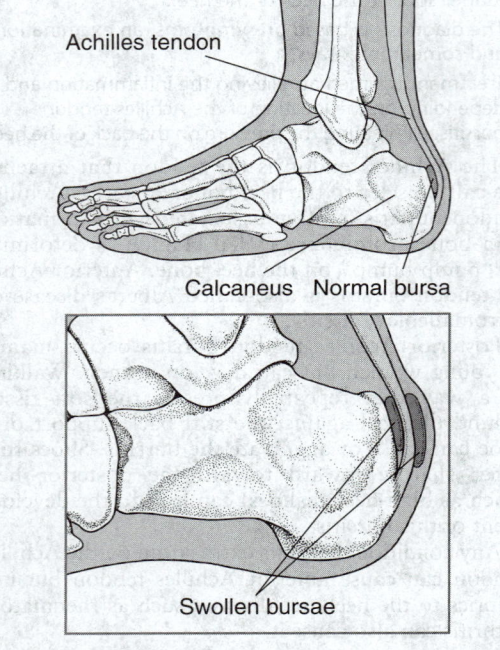

Achilles tendon

Calcaneus   Normal bursa

Swollen bursae

doctors use x-rays to rule out a fracture of the heel bone or damage to the heel bone caused by rheumatoid arthritis or another inflammatory arthritis.

Treatment

With anterior and posterior Achilles tendon bursitis, applying warm or cool compresses to the area and using nonsteroidal anti-inflammatory drugs (NSAIDs) can temporarily relieve the pain and inflammation, as can injections of a mixture of corticosteroids and local anesthetics into the inflamed bursa. The doctor is careful not to inject the mixture into the tendon. After this treatment, the person must rest. When these treatments are not effective, part of the heel bone may need to be surgically removed.

With posterior Achilles tendon bursitis, treatment is aimed at reducing the inflammation and adjusting the foot's position in the shoe to relieve pressure and motion on the back of the heel. Foam rubber or felt heel pads can be placed in the shoe to eliminate pressure by elevating the heel. Stretching the back part of the shoe or placing padding around the inflamed bursa may help. Sometimes a special shoe, such as a running shoe designed to stabilize the midsole heel, devices that change the position or range of movement of the foot and relieve pressure on affected joints (orthoses), or both can help to control abnormal foot and heel motion contributing to the posterior heel irritation. Other shoes have padding that reduces irritation to the posterior heel and Achilles tendon.

Achilles Tendon Enthesopathy

Achilles tendon enthesopathy is pain where the Achilles tendon attaches to the back of the heel.

The cause is chronic stretching of the Achilles tendon where it attaches to the heel. Contracted or shortened calf muscles caused by being sedentary and overweight or caused by athletic overuse increase the risk.

People typically feel pain at the back of the heel below the top of the shoe when walking.

The diagnosis is based on a physical examination of the tendon. Manually bending (flexing) the ankle during the examination usually makes the pain worse.

Exercises that stretch the calf muscles for 10 minutes 3 times daily can help. A person can stretch the calf muscle while facing a wall at arms' length, with the knees straight and the foot bent upward. To minimize stress to the Achilles tendon when walking, the foot and ankle should be moved actively through the ranges of motion for about a minute when rising after long periods of rest. Night splints may also be used to stretch the tendon during sleep and help prevent shortening. Heel lifts should be used temporarily to relieve pain and decrease stress on the tendon while walking.

Corns and Calluses

Corns are hard cone-shaped bumps of skin commonly found on the upper surface of the smaller toes, particularly over a joint. Calluses are somewhat rounded flat thickenings of the skin located on the under-surface of the foot.

Corns and calluses are usually caused by friction and pressure, particularly from tight or ill-fitting shoes. Hammer toe and other toe deformities are often responsible for the development of corns on the top of or at the tip of the toes. Calluses often develop under the ball of the foot because of faulty foot positioning and poor weight distribution. Symptoms include a generalized burning sensation or (at times) severe pain in a specific area. People who have diabetes and a diminished sensation to light touch and protective sensation are at increased risk of developing ulcers and an infection at the site of the callus or corn if left untreated.

Treatment usually requires removal through scraping with a scalpel. After this procedure, padding of various sorts (for example, felt or moleskin) may be applied to remove pressure from the healing area. Devices that change the position or range of movement of the foot and relieve pressure on affected joints (orthoses) or other inserts that have padding and metatarsal support pads can help to reduce pressure caused by callus build-up under the balls of the feet. Dells, which are holes cut through part of the footwear beneath the area that is painful, can also help reduce pressure and pain.

If the blood supply to the affected area is poor, surgical removal of the dead tissue may not be possible. In this case, special shoes that reduce pressure over the affected area may be necessary.

Bunion

In bunion, the joint of the base of the big toe appears to stick out (becomes prominent).

- Abnormalities in joint position or motion can distort and enlarge or seem to enlarge the joint that connects the big toe with the foot.
- Pain and swelling can affect the inner part of the joint or the entire joint.
- Changing shoes, using pads or devices that change the position or range of movement of the foot and relieve pressure on affected joints (orthoses), or a combination of measures usually helps.

A condition that is often part of the bunion is an abnormal position of the big toe or the bone to which it connects. One such condition is an abnormality in which the joint at the base of the big toe bulges outward from the inner side of the foot and the big toe points inward (toward the smaller toes). This is called hallux valgus. Other factors that contribute may include excessive turning in (pronation) of the ankles and occasionally injury. Osteoarthritis may develop, and bone spurs may form. Osteoarthritis may cause joint scarring, limiting the foot's range of motion. The joint may swell. A bursa (a painful swelling of the fluid-filled sac) can develop and become swollen and tender if tight shoes are worn.

Symptoms and Diagnosis

The first symptom may be painless enlargement of the joint or pain at the joint when wearing certain shoes. Later symptoms may include increasing enlarge-

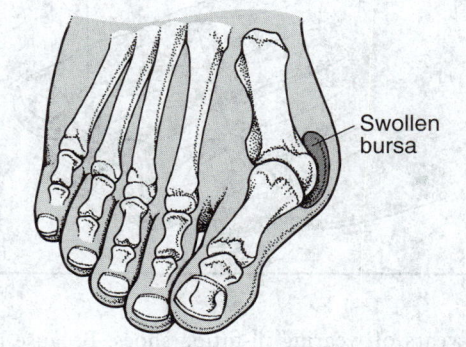

Hallux Valgus With a Bunion

A hallux valgus is a bulging out of the base of the big toe sideways, away from the foot. The end of the big toe tilts in toward the second toe. A bunion is enlargement of the base of the big toe. A bursa is a painful swelling of the fluid-filled sac at the base of the big toe. A bunion is caused by hallux valgus.

Swollen bursa

ment without pain; a painful, warm, red swelling at the inner aspect of the joint; and swelling and pain all around the joint. Joint motion may be restricted.

Doctors usually base the diagnosis on symptoms and examination findings. If the diagnosis is uncertain, x-rays are taken. If infection is suspected, doctors withdraw and analyze joint fluid. If multiple joints are affected, tests may be done to diagnose arthritis.

Treatment

Mild discomfort may significantly lessen by wearing shoes with a wide toe box. If not, bunion pads purchased in most pharmacies can shield the painful area. Orthoses can also help redistribute and relieve pressure from the affected joint. If these measures are ineffective or if the person is unwilling to wear large, wide shoes and orthoses because they are unattractive, surgery is considered. Sometimes taking nonsteroidal anti-inflammatory drugs (NSAIDs) or injecting a corticosteroid with or without an anesthetic can help relieve pain and swelling. If the joints are stiff, stretching exercises, which occasionally require injection of a local anesthetic to relieve muscle spasm, can help. Sometimes, surgery to release scar tissue and improve alignment is necessary.

Hammer Toe

Hammer toe is a toe that is in a fixed (rigid) contracted position.

Among the causes of hammer toe are a long metatarsal bone, poor foot posture, rheumatoid arthritis,

What Is Hammer Toe?

In hammer toe, the second, third, or fourth toe becomes bent and cannot be straightened without surgery.

Hammer toe

and years of wearing ill-fitting shoes. Because part of the toe is higher than normal, excessive friction may result, leading to corns and possibly ulcers on the top of the toe. Wearing shoes, particularly shoes with low and narrow toe boxes, may be painful. Doctors treat hammer toe by ensuring that the shoes are comfortable and have a wide enough toe box to avoid further irritation to the toe. Any ulcer or other skin irritation is treated. Toe pads sold in pharmacies also help by shielding the affected toes from the overlying shoe. An operation to straighten the hammer toe may be needed when other treatments do not relieve the pain and disability caused by the rigidly fixed toe.

Plantar Fibromatosis

Plantar fibromatosis is a noncancerous (benign) growth of connective tissue in the sole (the plantar fascia).

In plantar fibromatosis, bumps develop on the sole and are most obvious when the foot is bent upward against the leg. Most people also have bumps in the palms, usually located at the fourth knuckle.

Treatment is usually not worthwhile unless the bumps become large enough to cause pain when bearing weight. If so, devices that change the position or range of movement of the foot and relieve pressure on affected joints (orthoses) can help redistribute pressure away from the bumps.

CHAPTER

102 Muscular Dystrophies and Related Disorders

Muscular dystrophies are a group of inherited muscle disorders in which one or more genes needed for normal muscle function are defective, leading to muscle weakness (see page 540) of varying severity. Other inherited muscle disorders include congenital myopathies, periodic paralysis, and glycogen storage diseases. Glycogen storage diseases are a group of rare inherited disorders in which muscles cannot metabolize sugars normally (see page 1834), so they build up large stores of glycogen (a starch that is formed from sugars).

Duchenne and Becker Muscular Dystrophies

Duchenne muscular dystrophy and Becker muscular dystrophy cause weakness in the muscles closest to the torso.

- These dystrophies are caused by defects in genes responsible for muscle function, which lead to muscle weakness that develops during childhood or adolescence.

- Both dystrophies are characterized by physical weakness.
- The diagnosis is based on the results of tests done on samples of blood and a sample of muscle tissue.
- Physical therapy and sometimes prednisone or surgery provides some help.

These dystrophies are the most common muscular dystrophies and nearly always occur in boys. On average, 1 of 3,000 boys born has Duchenne muscular dystrophy, whereas on average 1 of 30,000 boys born has Becker muscular dystrophy.

The gene defect that causes Duchenne muscular dystrophy is different from the gene defect that causes Becker muscular dystrophy, but both defects involve the same gene. The gene for either of these traits is recessive and is carried on the X chromosome. Therefore, although a female can carry the defective gene, she will not develop the disease because the normal gene on one X chromosome compensates for the gene defect on the other X chromosome. However, any male who receives the defective gene will have the disease because he has only one X chromosome (see page 13).

Boys with Duchenne muscular dystrophy lack almost totally the muscle protein dystrophin, which is important for maintaining the structure of muscle cells. Boys with Becker muscular dystrophy produce dystrophin, but because the protein structure is altered, the dystrophin does not function properly.

Symptoms

In boys with Duchenne muscular dystrophy, the first symptoms are developmental delay (particularly a delay in starting to walk); difficulty walking, running, jumping, or climbing stairs; and falling. Starting between the ages of 2 years and 3 years, the gait becomes waddling, and the child has difficulty rising from the floor.

Weakness in the shoulder muscles usually follows and gets steadily worse. As the muscles weaken they also enlarge, but the abnormal muscle tissue is not strong. In boys with Duchenne muscular dystrophy, the heart muscle also gradually enlarges and weakens, causing problems with the heartbeat, which are detected by an electrocardiogram. About 33% of affected boys have mild, nonprogressive (that is, will not become worse) intellectual impairment that affects mostly verbal ability.

In boys with Duchenne muscular dystrophy, the arm and leg muscles usually contract around the joints, so that the elbows and knees cannot fully extend. Eventually, an abnormally curved spine (scoliosis) develops. By age 12, most children with the disease are confined to a wheelchair. Increasing weakness of the respiratory muscles also makes them susceptible to pneumonia and other illnesses, and most die by the age of 20.

In boys with Becker muscular dystrophy, weakness is less severe and first appears a little later, at about age 12. The pattern of weakness resembles that of Duchenne muscular dystrophy. However, very few adolescents become confined to a wheelchair. Most people survive into their 30s or 40s.

Diagnosis

Doctors suspect muscular dystrophy when a young boy becomes weak and grows weaker. An enzyme (creatine kinase) leaks out of muscle cells, causing levels of creatine kinase in the blood to be abnormally high. However, high blood levels of creatine kinase do not necessarily mean that a person has muscular dystrophy because other muscle diseases may also cause elevated levels of this enzyme. Duchenne muscular dystrophy is diagnosed when blood tests show the gene for the protein dystrophin to be absent or abnormal and when a muscle biopsy

(removal of a piece of muscle tissue for examination under a microscope) shows extremely low levels of dystrophin in the muscle. Under the microscope, the muscle generally shows dead tissue and abnormally large muscle fibers. In the late stages of Duchenne muscular dystrophy, fat and other tissues replace the dead muscle tissue. Similarly, Becker muscular dystrophy is diagnosed when blood tests show the gene for the protein dystrophin to be abnormal and a muscle biopsy shows low levels of dystrophin in the muscle, but not as low as in Duchenne muscular dystrophy.

Other tests to support the diagnosis include electrical studies of muscle function (electromyography) and nerve conduction studies (see page 636).

Families with members who have either Duchenne or Becker muscular dystrophy are advised to consult a genetic counselor for help in evaluating the risk of passing the muscular dystrophy trait on to their children. In families with a history of these disorders, doctors can perform prenatal tests on the fetus to determine if the child is likely to be affected.

Treatment

Neither Duchenne nor Becker muscular dystrophy can be cured. Physical therapy, exercise, and sometimes wearing braces help prevent the muscles from contracting permanently around joints. Sometimes surgery is needed to release tight, painful muscles. Boys need fewer calories because they are less active. They should avoid overeating.

Prednisone, a corticosteroid, taken by mouth daily, may temporarily improve strength. However, long-term use causes many side effects (see box on page 568), so it is not given to every child with muscular dystrophy. Use of prednisone is generally reserved for people whose muscle weakness has severely interfered with the normal activities of daily living. Creatine, a supplement taken by mouth, has recently been shown to improve strength. Gene therapy that would enable muscles to produce dystrophin and thereby relieve the weakness is under investigation but so far has not proved successful.

Other Forms of Muscular Dystrophy

Several uncommon forms of muscular dystrophy, all inherited, also cause progressive muscle weakness.

Emery-Dreifuss dystrophy is transmitted in various ways. Only males are affected, but females may be carriers of the gene that causes the disorder. Muscles become weak and waste away (atrophy) any time before age 20 years. The most affected muscles are those of the upper arms, lower legs, and heart. An affected heart commonly causes premature death. Heart pacemakers may help prolong life.

Facioscapulohumeral (Landouzy-Dejerine) muscular dystrophy is transmitted by an autosomal dominant gene. Therefore, a single abnormal gene is sufficient to cause the disorder, and the disorder can appear in either males or females. Symptoms usually begin between the ages of 7 and 20. The facial and shoulder muscles are always affected, so that a child has difficulty whistling, closing the eyes tightly, or raising the arms. Some people with the disease also develop a footdrop (the foot flops down). The weakness is rarely severe, and people who have Landouzy-Dejerine muscular dystrophy have a normal life expectancy.

Limb-girdle muscular dystrophies can be transmitted in various ways. They cause weakness in the muscles of either the pelvis (Leyden-Möbius muscular dystrophy) or the shoulder (Erb's muscular dystrophy). Males and females are affected equally. These inherited disorders often begin in early childhood but may not begin until adulthood. They rarely cause serious weakness.

Mitochondrial myopathies are muscle disorders inherited through faulty genes in mitochondria (the energy factories of cells, which carry their own genes). Because sperm do not contribute mitochondria during fertilization, all mitochondrial genes come from the mother (see page 11). Therefore, although they are equally likely to occur in males and females, these disorders can never be inherited from the father. These rare disorders sometimes cause increasing weakness in one or a few muscle groups, such as the eye muscles (ophthalmoplegia), and may affect other organs, such as the heart or brain. One mitochondrial myopathy is called Kearns-Sayre syndrome.

Diagnosis and Treatment

Diagnosis usually requires removing a sample of the weak muscle tissue for biopsy and either examining it under a microscope or performing chemical tests on it. Specific treatments are not available, but gene therapy is under investigation.

MYOTONIC MYOPATHIES

Myotonic myopathies are muscular dystrophies in which the muscles are not able to relax normally after contraction. Muscle weakness and spasms may also occur.

Myotonia congenita (Thomsen's disease) is a rare autosomal dominant disorder (only one affected parent is needed to pass the trait on to offspring) that affects males and females. Symptoms usually start in infancy. The hands, legs, and eyelids become very stiff because of an inability to relax the muscles. Muscle weakness, however, is usually minimal. The diagnosis is made from the child's characteristic appearance, inability to relax the grip of the hand rapidly after closing the hand, and prolonged contraction after the doctor taps a muscle. An electromyogram (a test in which electrical impulses from muscles are recorded—see page 636) is needed to confirm the diagnosis. Myotonia congenita is treated with phenytoin, quinine, procainamide, or mexiletine to relieve muscle stiffness and cramping; however, each of these drugs has undesirable side effects. Regular exercise may be beneficial. People with myotonia congenita have a normal life expectancy.

Myotonic dystrophy (Steinert's disease) is an autosomal dominant disorder affecting males and females. It is the most common muscular dystrophy among whites. Symptoms begin during adolescence or young adulthood. The disorder causes weakness and stiff muscles, especially in the hands. Drooping eyelids are also common. Symptoms can appear at any age and can range from mild to severe. People with the most severe form of the disorder have extreme muscle weakness and many other symptoms, including cataracts, small testes (in men), premature balding in the front (in men), irregular heartbeats, diabetes, and mental retardation. They usually die by age 50. Treatment with mexiletine or other drugs (for example, quinine, phenytoin, or procainamide) has been used, but these drugs do not relieve the weakness, which is the most bothersome symptom to the person. Also, each of these drugs has undesirable side effects. The only treatment for muscle weakness is supportive measures, such as ankle braces and other devices.

Congenital Myopathies

Congenital myopathies is a term used to describe a wide variety of inherited disorders of the muscles, nerves, or both, which are present at birth or infancy.

There are hundreds of congenital myopathies. The five most common types of congenital myopathy are nemaline myopathy, myotubular myopathy, central core myopathy, congenital fiber type disproportion, and multicore myopathy. Among these most common types, life span is usually normal in central core myopathy, congenital fiber type disproportion, and myotubular myopathy. However, exceptions often occur. Life span tends to be more variable in multicore myopathy and nemaline myopathy.

The diagnosis usually requires taking a sample of the weak muscle tissue for biopsy (in which a piece of tissue is removed for examination under a microscope). Specific treatments are not available, but physical therapy may help preserve function.

Periodic Paralysis

Periodic paralysis is an autosomal dominant inherited disorder (only one affected parent is needed to pass the trait on to offspring) that causes sudden attacks of weakness and paralysis. There are several forms.

- Muscles do not respond normally to stimulation, usually when the blood potassium level is too low or high.
- Weakness is intermittent, affecting mainly the limbs, and is often brought on by exercising or eating too much or too little carbohydrates.
- The diagnosis is based on the symptoms and a check of the potassium level in the blood.
- Avoiding triggers that cause attacks and taking drugs can prevent attacks effectively.

During an attack of periodic paralysis, muscles do not respond to normal nerve impulses or even to artificial stimulation with an electronic instrument. The precise form that the disorder takes varies among different families. In some families, the paralysis is related to low levels of potassium in the blood (hypokalemia). In others, the paralysis is related to high levels of potassium in the blood (hyperkalemia). In a rare form, potassium levels are normal.

Symptoms and Diagnosis

During an attack of weakness, the person remains completely awake and alert. Muscles in the eye and face are not affected. Weakness may affect only certain muscles or all four limbs.

In the hypokalemic form, attacks generally first appear before age 16 but may appear during the 20s and always by age 30. The attacks last up to 24 hours, occasionally even longer. Often, the person awakens the day after vigorous exercise with an attack of weakness. However, eating meals rich in carbohydrates (sometimes hours or even the day after) can also cause attacks. Eating carbohydrates and exer-cising vigorously drive sugar into cells. Potassium moves with the sugar, and the result is lowered potassium levels in the blood.

In the hyperkalemic form of the disorder, attacks often begin by age 10. The attacks last 15 minutes to 1 hour. Weakness tends to be less severe than in the hypokalemic form. Fasting, exercise, strenuous work, and exposure to cold may precipitate attacks.

A doctor's best clue to the diagnosis is a person's description of a typical attack. If possible, the doctor draws blood while an attack is in progress to check the level of potassium. If the levels of potassium are abnormal, doctors usually perform additional tests to be sure the abnormal levels are not from other causes. Occasionally, a doctor may give the person intravenous drugs that increase or decrease the levels of potassium in the blood to see whether an attack results.

Prevention and Treatment

Acetazolamide, a drug that alters the blood's acidity, may prevent attacks in all types of periodic paralysis. People with the hypokalemic form can take potassium chloride in an unsweetened solution while an attack is in progress. Usually symptoms improve considerably within an hour. People with the hypokalemic form should also avoid meals rich in carbohydrates and salt and avoid alcohol or strenuous exercise.

People with the hyperkalemic form can prevent attacks by eating frequent meals rich in carbohydrates and low in potassium and by avoiding fasting, strenuous activity, and exposure to cold. If an attack is severe or persistent, drugs (such as a thiazide diuretic or inhaled albuterol) can help lower the potassium level.

The muscles, bursae, tendons, and bones must be healthy and functioning correctly for the body to move normally. Muscles, which contract to produce movement, are connected to the bones by tendons. Bursae are flat sacs containing joint (synovial) fluid. They reduce friction in areas where skin, muscles, tendons, and ligaments rub over bones.

Often, muscles, bursae, and tendons are injured during sports activities (see page 1965). Injury, overuse, infection, and occasionally disease can temporarily or permanently damage these structures. Damage can cause pain, limit control over movement, and reduce the normal range of motion.

Muscle Cramps

A cramp is a sudden, brief, usually painful contraction of a muscle or group of muscles.

- Having tight calf muscles or a low blood level of electrolytes may cause painful calf cramps.
- Stretching and not consuming caffeine can help prevent muscle cramps.

Muscle cramps (also called charley horses) can occur in healthy people (usually middle-aged and older people), sometimes during rest but especially during or after vigorous exercise. They occur in younger people less often. Some people have leg cramps during sleep. These painful cramps usually affect the calf and foot muscles, causing the foot and toes to curl downward.

Having tight calf muscles is a common cause of leg cramps. Muscles become tight when they are not stretched, when people are inactive, or sometimes when fluid repeatedly accumulates (called edema) in the lower leg. Low levels of electrolytes, such as potassium, in the blood can also cause cramps. Low potassium levels may result from use of some diuretics or from other conditions that cause loss of fluids (and thus electrolytes—see page 945).

People who have hardening of the arteries in the legs (peripheral arterial disease) may develop calf pain with exertion. This pain is due to inadequate blood flow to muscles, not to a muscle contraction as with a cramp.

? Did You Know...

Stretching helps prevent cramps because it makes muscles less likely to contract spontaneously.

Prevention and Treatment

Preventing cramps is the best approach. The following measures can help:

- Not exercising immediately after eating
- Gently stretching the muscles before exercising or going to bed
- Drinking plenty of fluids (particularly sports beverages that contain potassium) after exercise
- Not consuming caffeine (for example, in coffee or chocolate)
- Not smoking
- Avoiding drugs that are stimulants, such as ephedrine or pseudoephedrine (a decongestant contained in many nonprescription products available only behind the pharmacy counter)

Stretching helps because it makes muscles and tendons more flexible and less likely to contract spontaneously. The runner's stretch is the best stretch for preventing calf cramps. A person stands with one leg forward and bent at the knee and the other leg behind with the knee straight—a lunge position. The hands can be placed on the wall for balance. Both heels remain on the floor. The knee of the front leg is bent further until a stretch is felt along the back of the other leg. The greater the distance between the two feet and the more the front knee is bent, the greater the stretch. The stretch is held for 30 seconds and repeated 5 times. Then the set of stretches is repeated on the other side.

Most of the drugs prescribed to prevent cramps from recurring (including quinine sulfate, magnesium carbonate, and benzodiazepines such as diazepam) have not proved to be effective and can have side effects. Mexiletine (used to treat abnormal heart rhythms) sometimes helps but has many side effects. Calcium supplements are safe and have few side effects, but they also have not proved to be effective.

If a cramp occurs, stretching the affected muscle often relieves the cramp. For example, for a calf cramp, the person could use a hand to pull the foot and toes upward or do the runner's stretch. Muscle pain from inadequate blood flow is relieved by rest rather than stretching.

Fibromyalgia

Fibromyalgia is characterized by poor sleep, fatigue, and widespread aching and stiffness in soft tissues, including muscles, tendons, and ligaments.

- Poor sleep, stress, strains, injury, and possibly certain personality characteristics may increase the risk of fibromyalgia.
- Pain is widespread, and certain parts of the body are tender to touch.
- Fibromyalgia is diagnosed when people feel pain in specific areas of the body and have typical symptoms.
- Improving sleep, exercising, applying heat, and getting massages usually help.

This disorder used to be called fibrositis or fibromyositis syndromes. But because inflammation (indicated by the "itis" suffix) is not present, the suffix was dropped, and the name became fibromyalgia.

Fibromyalgia is about 7 times more common among women. It usually occurs in young or middle-aged women but can also occur in men, children, and teenagers.

Fibromyalgia is not dangerous or life threatening. Nonetheless, persistent symptoms can be very disruptive.

Causes

Usually, the cause of fibromyalgia is unknown. However, certain conditions may contribute to developing the disorder. They include poor sleep, repetitive strains, an injury, and repeated exposure to dampness and cold. Mental stress may also contribute. However, stress per se may not be the problem. Rather it may be how people react to the stress. Many affected people are perfectionists or have a type A personality.

Some affected people may also have a connective tissue disorder, such as rheumatoid arthritis or systemic lupus erythematosus (lupus). Sometimes a viral or other infection (such as Lyme disease) or traumatic event can trigger fibromyalgia.

Symptoms

Most people feel a general achiness, stiffness, and pain. Symptoms can occur throughout the body. Any soft tissue (muscles, tendons, and ligaments) may be affected. But soft tissue of the neck, upper shoulders, chest, rib cage, lower back, thighs, arms, and joints are especially likely to be painful. Less often, the lower legs, hands, and feet are painful and stiff. Symptoms may occur periodically (in flare-ups) or most of the time (chronically).

Pain may be intense. It usually worsens with fatigue, straining, or overuse. Specific areas of muscle may be tender when firm fingertip pressure is applied. These areas are called tender points. During flare-ups, muscles become tight, or spasms may occur.

Many affected people do not sleep well and feel anxious, depressed, and tired. They may also have migraine or tension headaches and irritable bowel syndrome (with some combination of constipation, diarrhea, abdominal discomfort, and bloating—see page 181).

The same conditions that may contribute to the development of fibromyalgia can make symptoms worse. They include being emotionally stressed, sleeping badly, being injured, getting damp or cold, and overdoing it. Being told that symptoms are all in the head can also worsen symptoms.

Fibromyalgia tends to be chronic but may resolve on its own if stress decreases. Even with appropriate treatment, most people continue to have symptoms to some degree.

Diagnosis

The diagnosis is based on the pattern and location of the pain, as well as the presence of tender points. To detect tender points, doctors firmly press specific areas of the body to determine whether the person feels pain in one spot (a tender point). The disorder is diagnosed if people feel tenderness at 11 or more of the 18 designated tender points or if they have some tender points plus other typical symptoms.

Doctors also make sure that another disorder (such as hypothyroidism, polymyalgia rheumatica, or another muscle disorder) is not causing the symptoms, often by doing blood tests.

Fibromyalgia may be more difficult to diagnose in people who also have rheumatoid arthritis or lupus because these disorders cause some symptoms that are similar.

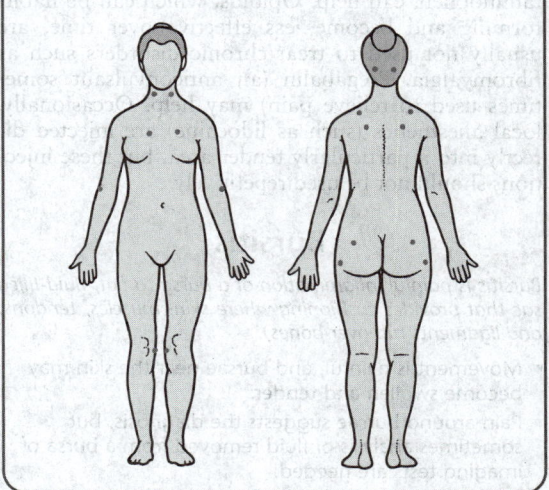

Fibromyalgia: Finding the Tender Points

Tender points are areas of tenderness that develop in people with fibromyalgia. Fibromyalgia is diagnosed when people feel pain in at least 11 of the 18 tender points or feel pain in fewer tender points but have other typical symptoms.

Treatment

People can feel better when treated appropriately. Usually, the most helpful approach includes the following:

- Reducing stress
- Stretching the affected muscles gently (holding the stretch about 30 seconds and repeating it 5 times)
- Doing exercises to improve physical conditioning (aerobic exercises) and gradually increasing the intensity (for example, by using a treadmill, exercise bicycle, or elliptical machine or by swimming)
- Applying heat to or gently massaging the affected area
- Keeping warm
- Getting enough sleep

Improving sleep is essential. For example, people should avoid caffeine and other stimulants in the evening and sleep in a quiet, dark room with comfortable bedding. They should not eat or watch TV in bed. Doctors may prescribe low doses of tricyclic antidepressants. These drugs are taken 1 or 2 hours before bedtime and used to improve sleep rather than to relieve depression. They include trazodone, amitriptyline, and nortriptyline. Cyclobenzaprine, a muscle relaxant, can also help people sleep. These drugs are usually safer than sedatives, most of which can be habit-forming. However, tricyclic antidepressants and cyclobenzaprine can have side effects, such as drowsiness and dry mouth, particularly in older people.

Aspirin or other nonsteroidal anti-inflammatory drugs (NSAIDs) are generally of limited benefit. Pain relievers, such as tramadol, propoxyphene, or acetaminophen, can help. Opioids, which can be habit-forming and become less effective over time, are usually not used to treat chronic disorders such as fibromyalgia. Pregabalin (an anticonvulsant sometimes used to relieve pain) may help. Occasionally, local anesthetics (such as lidocaine) are injected directly into a particularly tender area, but these injections should not be used repetitively.

Bursitis

Bursitis is painful inflammation of a bursa (a flat, fluid-filled sac that provides cushioning where skin, muscles, tendons, and ligaments rub over bones).

- Movement is painful, and bursae near the skin may become swollen and tender.
- Pain around bursae suggests the diagnosis, but sometimes analysis of fluid removed from a bursa or imaging tests are needed.
- Rest, splinting, nonsteroidal anti-inflammatory drugs, and sometimes corticosteroid injections usually relieve symptoms.

A bursa normally contains a small amount of fluid, which provides cushioning. Bursae reduce friction and prevent the wear and tear that can occur when one structure rubs over the other. Some bursae are located just beneath the skin (superficial). Others are located under muscles and tendons (deep). If injured or overused, a bursa may become inflamed, and extra fluid may collect in it.

Bursitis is usually caused by irritation from unusual use or overuse. It may also be caused by injury, gout, pseudogout, rheumatoid arthritis, or certain infections, especially those caused by *Staphylococcus aureus*. Often, the cause is unknown.

The shoulder is most susceptible to bursitis, but bursae in the elbows, hips (trochanteric bursitis), pelvis, knees, toes, and heels (Achilles tendon bursitis—see page 609) are commonly affected. Bursitis of the shoulder is usually caused by inflammation of tendons around the shoulder (rotator cuff tendinitis—the tendons and other structures that hold the shoulder in place are called the rotator cuff).

Symptoms

Bursitis usually causes pain and tends to limit movement, but the specific symptoms depend on the location of the inflamed bursa. For example, when a bursa in the shoulder becomes inflamed, raising the arm out from the side of the body (as when putting on a jacket) is painful and difficult. However, bursitis in the elbow may cause swelling but little or no discomfort.

Acute bursitis develops over hours or days. The inflamed area is usually painful when moved or touched. The skin over bursae located near the skin, such as those near the knee and elbow, may appear red and swollen. Acute bursitis that is caused by an infection or gout (see page 594.) may be particularly painful, and the affected area may be red and warm.

Chronic bursitis may result from repeated or persistent bouts of acute bursitis or repeated injuries. Sometimes the walls of the bursa become thick. If damaged bursae are subjected to unusual exercise or strain, inflammation tends to worsen. Long-standing pain and swelling can limit movement, making muscles weak. Flare-ups of chronic bursitis may last a few days to several weeks and frequently recur.

Diagnosis

A doctor suspects bursitis if the area around a superficial bursa is sore when touched or when certain joint movements that move or put pressure on deep bursae are painful. If a superficial bursa, particularly at the knee or elbow, is noticeably swollen, a doctor may remove a sample of fluid from the bursa with a needle. The sample is tested for causes of the inflammation, such as an infection or gout. X-rays are usually done only if bursitis is persistent or chronic.

Magnetic resonance imaging (MRI) or ultrasonography may be used to help confirm bursitis in a deep bursa.

Treatment

Acute bursitis, if not caused by an infection, is usually treated with the following:

- Rest
- Temporary immobilization of the affected joint
- Ice applied to the painful area
- Nonsteroidal anti-inflammatory drugs (NSAIDs—see page 644).

Occasionally, stronger analgesics are needed. Often, a doctor may inject a local anesthetic and a corticosteroid directly into the bursa, particularly if the shoulder is affected. This treatment frequently provides relief after a few days following the injection. The injection may have to be repeated after a few months.

People who have severe acute bursitis are occasionally given a corticosteroid, such as prednisone, by mouth for a few days. As the pain subsides, people can do specific exercises to increase the joint's range of motion.

Chronic bursitis, if not caused by an infection, is treated in a similar way, although rest and immobilization are less likely to help.

Often, physical therapy can help restore the joint's function. Exercises can help strengthen weakened muscles and reestablish the joint's full range of motion.

Infected bursae must be drained, and appropriate antibiotics, often against *Staphylococcus aureus*, are given.

Bursitis often recurs if the cause, such as gout, rheumatoid arthritis, or chronic overuse, is not treated or corrected.

Tendinitis and Tenosynovitis

Tendinitis is inflammation of a tendon. Tenosynovitis is tendinitis accompanied by inflammation of the protective covering around the tendon (tendon sheath).

- Tendons are painful, particularly when moved, and sometimes swollen.
- The diagnosis is usually based on symptoms and results of a physical examination.
- Using a splint, applying heat or cold, and taking nonsteroidal anti-inflammatory drugs can help.

Tendons are fibrous cords of tough tissue that connect muscles to bones. Some tendons are surrounded by tendon sheaths.

Tendinitis usually occurs during middle or older age, as the tendons weaken and become more susceptible to injury and inflammation. (Weakening of the tendon, called tendinopathy, usually results from many small tears that occur over time. Affected tendons may gradually or suddenly tear completely.) Tendinitis also occurs in younger people who exercise vigorously (who may develop rotator cuff tendinitis—see pages 620 and 1968) and in people who do repetitive tasks.

Certain tendons are particularly susceptible to inflammation.

- Tendons of the shoulder (rotator cuff): Inflammation of these tendons is the most common cause of shoulder pain.
- The two tendons that extend the thumb away from the hand: Inflammation of these tendons is called de Quervain's syndrome (see page 620).
- The flexor tendons that clench the fingers: Inflammation causes these tendons to get caught in their sheaths, resulting in a popping feeling (trigger finger—see art on page 600).
- The tendon above the biceps muscle in the upper arm (bicipital tendon): Pain can occur when the elbow is bent or the arm is elevated or rotated.
- Achilles tendon in the heel (see page 1974)
- The tendon that runs over the top of the foot

- Tendons near the hip bone (trochanter): Because bursae may also be affected, the term trochanteric bursitis is often used to include inflammation of these tendons.

Certain joint diseases, such as rheumatoid arthritis, systemic sclerosis, gout, diabetes, and reactive arthritis (previously called Reiter's syndrome), can cause tenosynovitis. In people with gonorrhea, especially women, gonococcal bacteria can cause tenosynovitis, usually affecting the tissues of the shoulders, wrists, fingers, hips, ankles, or feet.

Symptoms

The inflamed tendons are usually painful when moved or when pressed. Moving the joints near the tendon, even a little, may cause pain, depending on how severe the tendinitis is. Occasionally, the tendons or their sheaths swell and feel warm.

If tendinitis lasts a long time, calcium may become deposited. The area around the shoulder joint is often affected. In addition to being painful, the shoulder may feel stiff and weak. It may snap or catch when moved.

Diagnosis

Doctors can usually diagnose tendinitis based on the symptoms and results of a physical examination. Sometimes magnetic resonance imaging (MRI) or ultrasonography is helpful.

Treatment

Rest, immobilization with a splint or cast, and application of heat or cold—whichever works—are often helpful. Taking nonsteroidal anti-inflammatory drugs (NSAIDs) for 7 to 10 days can reduce the pain and inflammation.

Sometimes corticosteroids (such as betamethasone, methylprednisolone, or triamcinolone) and local anesthetics (such as lidocaine) are injected into the tendon sheath. Rarely, the injection causes pain hours later because the corticosteroid temporarily forms crystals inside the joint or sheath. This pain lasts less than 24 hours and can be treated with cold compresses and pain relievers.

Other drugs may be used, depending on the cause. For example, if gout is the cause, indomethacin or colchicine may be used.

After inflammation is controlled, exercises to increase the range of motion should be done several times a day.

Chronic, persistent tendinitis, as can occur in rheumatoid arthritis, may have to be treated surgically to remove inflamed tissues, and physical therapy may be needed after surgery. Surgery is occasionally needed to remove calcium deposits from areas of long-standing tendinitis, such as the area around the shoulder joint.

DE QUERVAIN'S SYNDROME

De Quervain's syndrome (washerwoman's sprain) is swelling and inflammation of the tendons or tendon sheaths that move the thumb outward.

This disorder usually occurs after repetitive use, particularly wringing, of the wrist. It often develops in new mothers, probably because they repeatedly pick up their baby by stretching out their arms and using only their wrists.

The main symptom is aching pain on the thumb side of the wrist and at the base of the thumb, which becomes worse with movement. The area at the base of the thumb near the wrist is also tender.

Doctors diagnose this disorder when they detect tenderness over the two tendons on the thumb side of the wrist, usually accompanied by swelling.

New mothers may be able to avoid this disorder if they use their entire arm and hold their wrists straight when they lift their baby.

Movements that cause pain should be avoided. A corticosteroid injection and a splint can help relieve symptoms. Sometimes one or two more injections, separated by several weeks, are needed.

ROTATOR CUFF TENDINITIS

Tendinitis may develop in the tendons of the muscles that help move, rotate, and hold the shoulder in place (rotator cuff).

Rotator cuff tendinitis (see also page 1968) is the most common cause of shoulder pain. It causes pain when the arm is raised (particularly between 40 and 120°) or when people dress. People often have pain during the night, especially when they lie on the affected arm.

Symptoms may occur suddenly and be severe, especially after physical activity, or they may develop more slowly and be milder.

Range-of-motion exercises, NSAIDs, and sometimes a corticosteroid injection can be used for treatment.

Baker's Cysts

Baker's cysts (popliteal cysts) are tiny sacs filled with joint (synovial) fluid that form in an extension of the joint capsule behind the knee.

A Baker's cyst results from an accumulation of trapped joint fluid, which bulges from the joint capsule behind the knee as a protruding sac. Causes of the joint fluid accumulation include rheumatoid arthritis, osteoarthritis, and overuse of the knees. Baker's cysts produce discomfort at the back of the knee. The cysts may enlarge and extend downward into the calf muscles.

A rapid increase in the amount and pressure of fluid within the cyst can cause it to rupture. The fluid released from the cyst can cause the surrounding tissues to become inflamed, resulting in symptoms that may mimic those of thrombophlebitis (see page 437). Moreover, a bulging or ruptured Baker's cyst can cause thrombophlebitis in the popliteal vein (which is located behind the knee) by pressing on the vein.

The doctor can usually make a diagnosis by asking the person specific questions about symptoms and feeling a swelling behind the knee or in the calf. Ultrasound, magnetic resonance imaging (MRI), or arthrography, can sometimes aid in the diagnosis and document how far the cyst extends.

When arthritis causes chronic knee swelling, the doctor may need to remove the fluid with a needle (a procedure called joint aspiration) and inject a long-acting corticosteroid (such as triamcinolone acetonide) to prevent the formation of a Baker's cyst. Removing the cyst surgically is an alternative if other treatments are not effective.

If the cyst has ruptured, the pain is treated with a nonsteroidal anti-inflammatory drug (NSAID). If the ruptured cyst causes thrombophlebitis in the popliteal vein, this is treated with bed rest, elevation of the leg, warm compresses, and anticoagulants. Occasionally, antibiotics are needed also.

CHAPTER

104 Biology of the Nervous System

The nervous system has two distinct parts: the central nervous system (the brain and spinal cord) and the peripheral nervous system (the nerves outside the brain and spinal cord).

The basic unit of the nervous system is the nerve cell (neuron). Nerve cells consist of a large cell body and two types of nerve fibers:

- **Axon:** One elongated extension for sending messages as electrical impulses
- **Dendrites:** Usually many branches for receiving impulses

Normally, nerves transmit impulses electrically in one direction—from the impulse-sending axon of one nerve cell to the impulse-receiving dendrites of the next nerve cell. At contact points between nerve cells (synapses), the axon secretes tiny amounts of chemical messengers (neurotransmitters). Neurotransmitters trigger the receptors on the next nerve cell's dendrites to produce a new electrical current. Different types of nerves use different neurotransmitters to convey impulses across the synapses.

The brain and spinal cord also contain support cells called glial cells. There are several types, including the following:

- **Astrocytes:** These cells help provide nutrients to nerve cells and control the chemical composition of fluids around nerve cells, enabling them to thrive.
- **Oligodendrocytes:** These cells make myelin, a fatty substance that insulates nerve axons and speeds the conduction of impulses along nerve fibers.
- **Microglia:** These cells help protect the brain against infection and help remove debris from dead cells.

Nerve cells routinely increase or decrease the number of connections they have with other nerve cells. This process may partly explain how people learn, adapt, and form memories. But the brain and spinal cord rarely produce new nerve cells. An exception is the hippocampus, an area of the brain involved in memory formation.

The nervous system is an extraordinarily complex communication system that can send and receive voluminous amounts of information simultaneously. However, the system is vulnerable to diseases and injuries. For example, nerve cells can degenerate, causing Alzheimer's, Huntington's, or Parkinson's disease. Oligodendrocytes may become inflamed, causing multiple sclerosis. Bacteria or viruses can infect the brain or

spinal cord, causing encephalitis or meningitis. A blockage in the blood supply to the brain can cause a stroke. Injuries or tumors can cause structural damage to the brain or spinal cord.

Brain

The brain's functions are both mysterious and remarkable. All thoughts, beliefs, memories, behaviors, and moods arise within the brain. The brain is the site of thinking and the control center for the rest of the body. The brain coordinates the abilities to move, touch, smell, taste, hear, and see. It enables people to form words, understand and manipulate numbers, compose and appreciate music, recognize and understand geometric shapes, communicate with others, plan ahead, and even fantasize.

The brain reviews all stimuli—from the internal organs, surface of the body, eyes, ears, nose, and mouth. It then reacts to these stimuli by correcting the position of the body, the movement of limbs, and the rate at which the internal organs function. The brain can also adjust mood and levels of consciousness and alertness.

No computer has yet come close to matching the capabilities of the human brain. However, this sophistication comes with a price. The brain needs constant nourishment. It demands an extremely large amount and continuous flow of blood and oxygen—about 20% of the blood flow from the heart. A loss of blood flow to the brain for more than about 10 seconds can cause loss of consciousness. Lack of oxygen or abnormally low sugar (glucose) levels in the blood can result in less energy for the brain and seriously injure the brain within minutes. However, the brain is defended by several mechanisms that can work to prevent these problems. For example, if blood flow to the brain decreases, the brain immediately signals the heart to beat faster and more forcefully and thus to pump more blood. If the sugar level in the blood becomes too low, the brain signals the adrenal glands to release epinephrine (adrenaline), which stimulates the liver to release stored sugar.

The brain is also protected by a thin barrier that prevents some toxic substances in the blood from reaching the brain. This barrier is called the blood-brain barrier. It exists because in the brain, unlike in most of the body, the cells that form the capillary walls are tightly sealed. (Capillaries, the smallest of the body's blood vessels, are where the exchange of

Viewing the Brain

The brain consists of the cerebrum, brain stem, and cerebellum. Each half (hemisphere) of the cerebrum is divided into lobes. Within the skull, the brain is covered by three layers of tissue called the meninges.

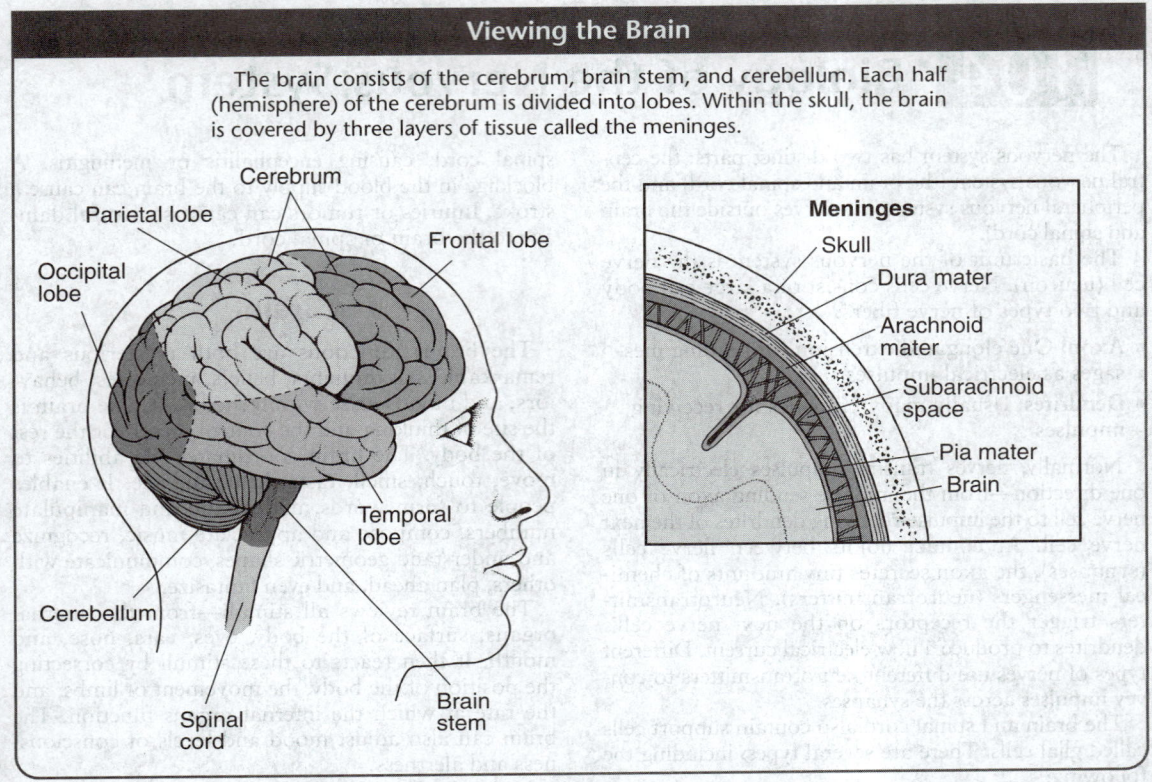

nutrients and oxygen between the blood and tissues occurs.) The blood-brain barrier limits the types of substances that can pass into the brain. For example, penicillin, many chemotherapy drugs, and most proteins cannot pass into the brain. On the other hand, substances such as alcohol, caffeine, and nicotine can pass into the brain. Certain drugs, such as antidepressants, are designed so that they can pass through the barrier. Some substances needed by the brain, such as sugar and amino acids, do not readily pass through the barrier. However, the blood-brain barrier has transport systems that move substances the brain needs across the barrier to brain tissue.

The activity of the brain results from electrical impulses generated by nerve cells (neurons), which process and store information. The impulses pass along the nerve fibers within the brain. How much and what type of brain activity occurs and where in the brain it is initiated depend on a person's level of consciousness and on the specific activity that the person is doing. The brain has three main parts: the cerebrum, the brain stem, and the cerebellum. Each has a number of smaller areas, each with specific functions.

Cerebrum: The cerebrum, the largest part of the brain, consists of dense, convoluted masses of tissue. The outer layer is the cerebral cortex (gray matter). In adults, the cerebral cortex contains most of the nerve cells in the nervous system. Underneath the cortex is the white matter, which consists mainly of nerve fibers that connect the nerve cells in the cortex with other parts of the nervous system.

The cerebrum is divided into two halves—the left and right cerebral hemispheres. The hemispheres are connected by nerve fibers that form a bridge (called the corpus callosum) through the middle of the brain. Each hemisphere is further divided into a frontal, parietal, occipital, and temporal lobe. Each lobe has specific functions, but for most activities, several areas of different lobes in both hemispheres must work together.

The **frontal lobes** have the following functions:

- Initiating many voluntary actions, ranging from looking toward an object of interest, to crossing a street, to relaxing the bladder to urinate
- Controlling learned motor skills, such as writing, playing musical instruments, and tying shoelaces

- Controlling complex intellectual processes, such as speech, thought, concentration, problem-solving, and planning for the future
- Controlling facial expressions and hand and arm gestures
- Coordinating expressions and gestures with mood and feelings

Particular areas of the frontal lobes control specific movements, typically of the opposite side of the body. In most people, the left frontal lobe controls most of the functions involved in using language.

The **parietal lobes** have the following functions:

- Interpreting sensory information from the rest of the body
- Controlling body movement
- Combining impressions of form, texture, and weight into general perceptions
- Influencing mathematical skills and language comprehension, as do adjacent areas of the temporal lobes
- Storing spatial memories that enable people to orient themselves in space (know where they are) and to maintain a sense of direction (know where they are going)
- Processing information that helps people know the position of their body parts

The **occipital lobes** have the following functions:

- Processing and interpreting vision
- Enabling people to form visual memories
- Integrating visual perceptions with the spatial information provided by the adjacent parietal lobes

The **temporal lobes** have the following functions:

- Generating memory and emotions
- Processing immediate events into recent and long-term memory
- Storing and retrieving long-term memories
- Comprehending sounds and images, thus enabling people to recognize other people and objects and to integrate hearing and speech

Large collections of nerve cells—the basal ganglia, thalamus, and hypothalamus—are located at the base of the cerebrum. The basal ganglia coordinate and smooth out movements. The thalamus generally organizes sensory messages to and from the highest levels of the brain (cerebral cortex), providing a general awareness of such sensations as pain, touch, and temperature. The hypothalamus coordinates some of the more automatic functions of the body, such as control of sleep and wakefulness, maintenance of body tem-

perature, and regulation of appetite and the balance of water within the body.

A system of nerve fibers—called the limbic system—connects the hypothalamus with other areas of the frontal and temporal lobes, including the hippocampus and amygdala. The limbic system controls the experience and expression of emotions, as well as automatic functions of the body. By producing emotions (such as fear, anger, pleasure, and sadness), the limbic system enables people to behave in ways that help them communicate and survive physical and psychologic upsets. The hippocampus is also involved in the formation and retrieval of memories. Through the limbic system, memories that are emotionally charged are easier to recall than those that are not.

> **? Did You Know...**
> The brain rarely produces new nerve cells but can do so in areas of the brain concerned with memory.

Brain Stem: The brain stem connects the cerebrum with the spinal cord. It contains a system of nerve cells and fibers (called the reticular activating system) located deep within the upper part of the brain stem. This system controls levels of consciousness and alertness.

The brain stem also automatically regulates critical body functions, such as breathing, swallowing, blood pressure, and heartbeat, and it helps adjust posture. If the entire brain stem becomes severely damaged, consciousness is lost, and these automatic body functions cease. Death soon follows.

Cerebellum: The cerebellum, which lies below the cerebrum just above the brain stem, coordinates the body's movements. With information it receives from the cerebral cortex and the basal ganglia about the position of the limbs, the cerebellum helps the limbs move smoothly and accurately. It does so by constantly adjusting muscle tone and posture. The cerebellum interacts with areas in the brain stem called vestibular nuclei, which are connected with the organs of balance (semicircular canals) in the inner ear. Together, these structures provide a sense of balance. The cerebellum also stores memories of practiced movements, enabling highly coordinated movements, such as a ballet dancer's pirouette, to be done with speed and balance.

Meninges: Both the brain and spinal cord are covered by three layers of tissue (meninges) that protect them. The thin pia mater is the innermost layer, which adheres to the brain and spinal cord. The delicate, spider web–like arachnoid mater is the middle layer. The space between the arachnoid mater and the pia

How the Spine Is Organized

A column of bones called vertebrae make up the spine (spinal column). The vertebrae protect the spinal cord, a long, fragile structure contained in the spinal canal, which runs through the center of the spine. Between the vertebrae are disks composed of cartilage, which help cushion the spine and give it some flexibility. Emerging from the spinal cord between the vertebrae are 31 pairs of spinal nerves. Each nerve emerges in two short branches (roots): one at the front (motor or anterior root) and one at the back (sensory or posterior root) of the spinal cord. The motor roots carry commands from the brain and spinal cord to other parts of the body, particularly to skeletal muscles. The sensory roots carry information to the brain from other parts of the body. The spinal cord ends about three fourths of the way down the spine, but a bundle of nerves extends beyond the cord. This bundle is called the cauda equina because it resembles a horse's tail. The cauda equina carries nerve impulses to and from the legs.

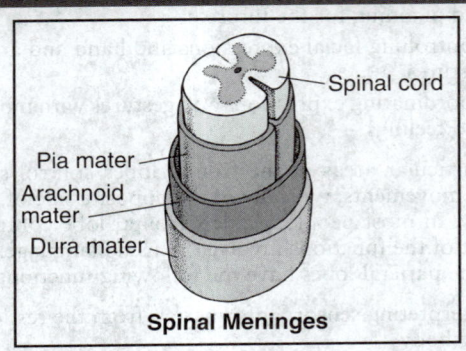

Spinal Meninges

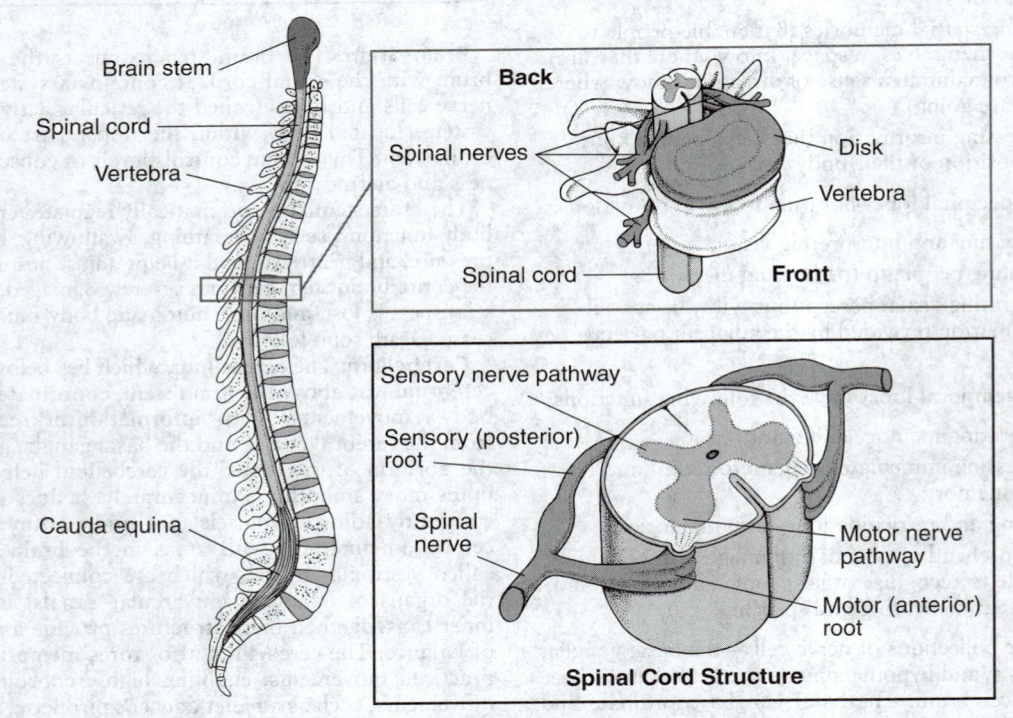

Spinal Cord Structure

mater (the subarachnoid space) is a channel for cerebrospinal fluid, which helps protect the brain and spinal cord. Cerebrospinal fluid flows over the surface of the brain between the meninges, fills internal spaces within the brain (the four ventricles), and cushions the brain against sudden jarring and minor injury. The leathery dura mater is the outermost and toughest layer. The brain and its meninges are contained in a tough, bony protective structure, the skull.

Spinal Cord

The spinal cord is a long, fragile tubelike structure that begins at the end of the brain stem and continues down almost to the bottom of the spine (spinal column). The spinal cord consists of nerves that carry incoming and outgoing messages between the brain and the rest of the body. It is also the center for reflexes, such as the knee jerk reflex (see art on page 633).

Like the brain, the spinal cord is covered by three layers of tissue (meninges). The spinal cord and meninges are contained in the spinal canal, which runs through the center of the spine. In most adults, the spine is composed of 26 individual back bones (vertebrae). Just as the skull protects the brain, vertebrae protect the spinal cord. The vertebrae are separated by disks made of cartilage, which act as cushions, reducing the forces generated by movements such as walking and jumping.

Like the brain, the spinal cord consists of gray and white matter. The butterfly-shaped center of the cord consists of gray matter. The front "wings" (called horns) contain motor nerve cells, which transmit information from the brain or spinal cord to muscles, stimulating movement. The back horns contain sensory nerve cells, which transmit sensory information from other parts of the body through the spinal cord to the brain. The surrounding white matter contains columns of nerve fibers that carry sensory information to the brain from the rest of the body (ascending tracts) and columns that carry impulses from the brain to the muscles (descending tracts).

Nerves

The peripheral nervous system consists of more than 100 billion nerve cells that run throughout the body like strings, making connections with the brain, other parts of the body, and often with each other. Peripheral nerves consist of bundles of nerve fibers. These fibers are wrapped with many layers of tissue composed of a fatty substance called myelin. These layers form the myelin sheath, which speeds the conduction of nerve impulses along the nerve fiber. Nerves conduct impulses at different speeds depending on their diameter and on the amount of myelin around them.

The peripheral nervous system has two parts: the somatic nervous system and the autonomic nervous system.

Somatic Nervous System: This system consists of nerves that connect the brain and spinal cord with

Typical Structure of a Nerve Cell

A nerve cell (neuron) consists of a large cell body and nerve fibers—one elongated extension (axon) for sending impulses and usually many branches (dendrites) for receiving impulses. Each large axon is surrounded by oligodendrocytes in the brain and spinal cord and by Schwann cells in the peripheral nervous system. The membranes of these cells consist of a fat (lipoprotein) called myelin. The membranes are wrapped tightly around the axon, forming a multilayered sheath. This myelin sheath resembles insulation, such as that around an electrical wire. Nerve impulses travel much faster in nerves with a myelin sheath than in those without one. If the myelin sheath of a nerve is damaged, nerve transmission slows or stops.

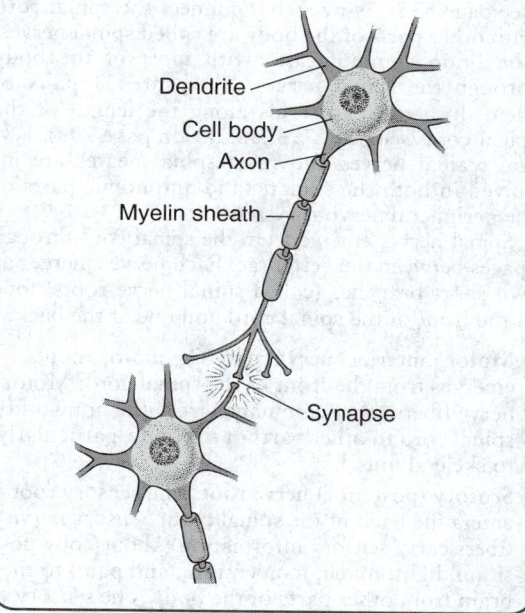

muscles controlled by conscious effort (voluntary or skeletal muscles) and with sensory receptors in the skin. (Sensory receptors are specialized endings of nerve fibers that detect information in and around the body.)

Autonomic Nervous System: This system connects the brain stem and spinal cord with internal organs and regulates internal body processes that require no conscious effort (see page 831). Examples are the rate of heart contractions, blood pressure, the rate of breathing, the amount of stomach acid secreted, and the speed at which food passes through the digestive tract. The autonomic nervous system has two divisions:

- **Sympathetic division:** Its main function is to prepare the body for stressful or emergency situations—for fight or flight.
- **Parasympathetic division:** Its main function is to prepare the body for ordinary situations.

These divisions work together, usually with one activating and the other inhibiting the actions of internal organs. For example, the sympathetic division increases pulse, blood pressure, and breathing rates, and the parasympathetic system decreases each of them.

Cranial and Spinal Nerves: Nerves that connect the brain with the eyes, ears, nose, and throat and with various parts of the head, neck, and trunk are called cranial nerves. There are 12 pairs of them (see page 835). Nerves that connect the spinal cord with other parts of the body are called spinal nerves. The brain communicates with most of the body through the spinal nerves. There are 31 pairs of them, located at intervals along the length of the spinal cord (see page 793 and art on page 797). Several cranial nerves and most spinal nerves are involved in both the somatic and autonomic parts of the peripheral nervous system.

Spinal nerves emerge from the spinal cord through spaces between the vertebrae. Each nerve emerges as two short branches (called spinal nerve roots): one at the front of the spinal cord and one at the back.

- **Motor (anterior) nerve root:** The motor root emerges from the front of the spinal cord. Motor nerve fibers carry commands from the brain and spinal cord to other parts of the body, particularly to skeletal muscles.
- **Sensory (posterior) nerve root:** The sensory root enters the back of the spinal cord. Sensory nerve fibers carry sensory information (about body position, light, touch, temperature, and pain) to the brain from other parts of the body. The sensory nerve fibers from a specific sensory nerve root carry information from a specific area of the body, called a dermatome (see art on page 796).

After leaving the spinal cord, the corresponding motor and sensory nerve roots join to form a single spinal nerve. Some of the spinal nerves form networks of interwoven nerves, called nerve plexuses. In a plexus, nerve fibers from different spinal nerves are sorted and recombined so that all fibers going to or coming from one area of a specific body part are put together into one nerve (see art on page 823). There are two major nerve plexuses: the brachial plexus, which sorts and recombines nerve fibers traveling to the arms and hands, and the lumbosacral plexus, which sorts and recombines nerve fibers going to the legs and feet.

Effects of Aging

Brain: Brain function varies normally as people pass from childhood through adulthood to old age. During childhood, the ability to think and reason steadily increases, enabling a child to learn increasingly complex skills. During most of adulthood, brain function is relatively stable. After a certain age, which varies from person to person, brain function declines. Different aspects of brain function are affected at different times:

- Short-term memory and the ability to learn new material tend to be affected relatively early.
- Verbal abilities, including vocabulary and word usage, may begin to decline at about age 70.
- Intellectual performance—the ability to process information (regardless of speed)—is usually maintained until about age 80 if no neurologic disorders are present.
- Reaction time and performance of tasks may become slower because the brain processes nerve impulses more slowly.

However, the effects of aging on brain function may be difficult to separate from the effects of various disorders that are common among older people. These disorders include depression, stroke, an underactive thyroid gland (hypothyroidism), and degenerative brain disorders such as Alzheimer's disease.

As people age, the number of nerve cells in the brain usually decreases, although the number lost varies greatly from person to person, depending on the person's health. Also, the remaining nerve cells function less well. However, the brain has certain characteristics that help compensate for these losses.

- **Redundancy:** The brain has more cells than it needs to function normally. Redundancy may help compensate for the loss of nerve cells that occurs with aging and disease.
- **Formation of new connections:** The brain actively compensates for the age-related decrease in nerve cells by making new connections between the remaining nerve cells.
- **Production of new nerve cells:** Some areas of the brain may produce new nerve cells, especially after a slight brain injury or a stroke.

Thus, people who have had a brain injury or stroke can sometimes learn new skills, as occurs during occupational therapy.

People can influence how quickly brain function declines. For example, mental and physical exercise seems to slow the loss of nerve cells in areas of the brain involved in memory. Such exercise also helps keep the remaining nerve cells functioning. On the other hand, consuming two or more drinks of alcohol a day can speed the decline in brain function.

> ### Did You Know...
> Physical and mental exercise may slow the age-related decline in brain function.
>
> Having uncontrolled high blood pressure or high cholesterol levels can speed the age-related decline in brain function.

As people age, blood flow to the brain may decrease by an average of 20%. The decrease in blood flow is greater in people who have atherosclerosis of the arteries to the brain (cerebrovascular disease). This disease is more likely to occur in people who have smoked for a long time or who have high blood pressure, high cholesterol, or high blood sugar (diabetes mellitus) that is not controlled by lifestyle changes or drugs. These people may lose brain cells prematurely, possibly impairing mental function. As a result, the risk of dementia at a relatively young age is increased.

Spinal Cord: As people age, the disks between the back bones (vertebrae) become hard and brittle, and parts of the vertebrae may overgrow. As a result, the disks lose some of their capacity to cushion, so more pressure is put on the spinal cord and on the branches of the nerves that emerge from it (spinal nerve roots). The increased pressure may injure some nerve fibers in the spinal cord. Such injury can result in decreased sensation and sometimes decreased strength and balance.

Peripheral Nerves: As people age, peripheral nerves may conduct impulses more slowly, resulting in decreased sensation, slower reflexes, and often some clumsiness. Nerve conduction slows because myelin sheaths (layers of tissues around nerves that speed conduction of impulses) degenerate. Degeneration occurs because, as people age, blood flow decreases, nearby bones overgrow and put pressure on the nerves, or both. Usually, the effect is so minimal that no change in function is noticeable unless nerves are injured by something else (for example, by diabetes).

The peripheral nervous system's response to injury is reduced. When the axon of a peripheral nerve is damaged in younger people, the nerve is able to repair itself as long as its cell body, located in or near the spinal cord, is undamaged. This self-repair process occurs more slowly and incompletely in older people, making older people more vulnerable to injury and disease.

CHAPTER 105

Diagnosis of Brain, Spinal Cord, and Nerve Disorders

A neurologic examination can detect disorders of the brain, spinal cord, and nerves in other parts of the body (peripheral nerves, which include motor and sensory nerves). This examination can also help detect muscle disorders because muscle contraction depends on stimulation by a nerve.

The two main components of a neurologic examination are the medical history and the physical examination (including mental status evaluation). If necessary, diagnostic procedures are done to confirm the diagnosis or exclude other possible disorders.

A neurologic examination differs from a psychiatric examination, which focuses on a person's behavior.

However, the two examinations overlap somewhat because abnormal behavior often provides clues about the brain's physical condition.

History

Before doing a physical examination, doctors interview the person. Doctors ask the person to describe current symptoms:

- What they are like precisely
- Where and how often they occur
- How severe they are

- How long they last
- What makes symptoms worse
- What relieves symptoms
- Whether daily activities can still be done

The person is also asked about past or present illnesses and past operations, serious illnesses in close blood relatives, allergies, and drugs currently being taken. Questions about work, social contacts, and travel may be asked to find out whether the person has been exposed to unusual infections or toxins. In addition, doctors may ask whether the person has had work-related or home-related difficulties, such as loss of a loved one, because such circumstances may affect the person's health and ability to cope with illness. Other questions are asked to identify any symptoms that the person may have overlooked or thought unimportant when describing the main problem.

Physical Examination

When a neurologic disorder is suspected, doctors usually evaluate all of the body systems during the physical examination, but they focus on the nervous system. They do a neurologic examination, which includes evaluation of mental status, cranial nerves, motor and sensory nerves, reflexes, coordination, balance, walking (gait), regulation of internal body processes (by the autonomic nervous system), and blood flow to the brain. Doctors may evaluate some areas more thoroughly than others depending on what type of disorder they suspect.

Mental Status: Doctors evaluate the following:

- Attention
- Orientation to time, place, and person
- Memory
- Various abilities, such as thinking abstractly, following commands, using language, and solving math problems
- Mood

The evaluation consists of a series of questions and tasks, such as naming objects, recalling short lists, writing sentences, and copying shapes. The person's answers are recorded and scored for accuracy. If the person reports feeling depressed, doctors ask if there have been any thoughts of suicide.

Cranial Nerves: There are 12 pairs of cranial nerves, which connect the brain with the eyes, ears, nose, face, tongue, throat, neck, upper shoulders, and some internal organs (see page 835). How many nerves doctors test depends on what type of disorder they suspect. For example, the 1st cranial nerve (the nerve of smell) is not usually tested when a muscle disorder is suspected, but it is tested in people recovering from serious head trauma (because smell is often lost). A cranial nerve may be damaged anywhere along its length as a result of injury, impaired blood flow, an autoimmune disorder, a tumor, or an infection. The exact site of the damage can often be identified by testing the functions of a particular cranial nerve.

Motor and Sensory Nerves: Motor nerves carry impulses from the brain and spinal cord to voluntary muscles (muscles controlled by conscious effort), such as muscles of the arms and legs. Weakness or paralysis of a muscle may indicate damage to the muscle itself, a motor nerve, or its connection to the muscle (synapse), the brain, or the spinal cord. Doctors look for abnormalities such as the following:

- Tremor and other involuntary muscle movements
- Muscle twitching
- Decrease in muscle size (wasting or atrophy)
- Increase in muscle size
- Increase (spasticity or rigidity) or decrease in muscle tone
- Pattern of weakness
- Dexterity

The doctor inspects the muscles for size, unusual movements, tone, strength, and dexterity. A muscle wastes away (atrophies) when the muscle or the nerves supplying it are damaged or when the muscle has not been used for months for other reasons (such as being in a cast).

Muscles may move without the person meaning them to. For example, tiny muscle twitches (fasciculations) indicate nerve damage to that muscle. Other possible involuntary movements are rhythmic movements of a body part (tremor), twitches (tics), sudden flinging of a limb (hemiballismus), quick fidgety movements (chorea), or snake-like writhing (athetosis). All of these movements suggest damage in areas of the brain (called basal ganglia) that control motor coordination.

When doctors move a person's joint passively, they note the degree of resistance to movement (muscle tone). Muscle tone that is uneven and suddenly increased (spasticity) may be due to a stroke or spinal cord injury. Muscle tone that is evenly increased (rigidity) may be due to disease of the basal ganglia, such as Parkinson's disease. Muscle tone that is severely reduced (flaccid) immediately and temporarily after a spinal cord injury produces paralysis.

Doctors test muscle strength by asking the person to push or pull against resistance or to do maneuvers that require strength, such as walking on the heels and tiptoes or rising from a chair. Sometimes

What Is a Neurologic Symptom?

Neurologic symptoms—symptoms caused by a disorder that affects part or all of the nervous system—can vary greatly because the nervous system controls so many different body functions. Symptoms can include all forms of pain, including headache and back pain. Muscles, skin sensation, the special senses (vision, taste, smell, and hearing), and other senses depend on nerves to function normally. Thus, neurologic symptoms can include muscle weakness or incoordination, abnormal sensations in the skin, and disturbances of the senses.

Neurologic disorders can interfere with sleep, making a person anxious or excited at bedtime and thus lethargic and sleepy during the day.

Neurologic symptoms may be minor (such as a foot that has fallen asleep) or life threatening (such as coma due to stroke). The characteristics and pattern of symptoms help doctors diagnose the neurologic disorder. The following are some relatively common neurologic symptoms:

PAIN

- Back pain
- Neck pain
- Headache
- Pain along a nerve pathway (as in sciatica or shingles)

MUSCLE MALFUNCTION

- Weakness
- Tremor
- Paralysis
- Involuntary movements (such as tics)
- Abnormalities in walking
- Clumsiness or poor coordination
- Muscle spasms
- Rigidity, stiffness, and spasticity
- Slowed movements

CHANGES IN SENSATION

- Numbness of the skin
- Tingling or a pins-and-needles sensation
- Hypersensitivity to light touch
- Loss of sensation for touch, cold, heat, or pain
- Loss of position sense

CHANGES IN THE SPECIAL SENSES

- Disturbances of smell and taste
- Visual hallucinations
- Partial or complete loss of vision
- Double vision
- Deafness
- Ringing or other sounds originating in the ears (tinnitus)

OTHER SYMPTOMS

- Vertigo
- Loss of balance
- Difficulty swallowing
- Slurred speech (dysarthria)

SLEEP PROBLEMS

- Difficulty falling or staying asleep
- Uncontrollable leg movements
- Falling asleep uncontrollably (as in narcolepsy) or sleeping too much

CHANGES IN CONSCIOUSNESS

- Fainting
- Confusion or delirium
- Seizures
- Coma
- Stupor

CHANGES IN COGNITION (MENTAL ABILITY)

- Difficulty understanding language or using language to speak or write (aphasia)
- Poor memory
- Difficulty with common motor skills, such as striking a match or combing one's hair, despite normal strength (apraxia)
- Inability to recognize familiar objects (agnosia)
- Inability to sustain concentration when doing a task
- Inability to distinguish right from left
- Inability to do simple arithmetic (acalculia)
- Poor visual-spatial comprehension (for example, being unable to draw a clock or becoming lost driving in a familiar neighborhood)
- Dementia (dysfunction of several cognitive functions)

MENTAL STATUS TESTING

WHAT PEOPLE MAY BE ASKED TO DO	WHAT THIS TEST INDICATES
State the current date and place, and name specific people	Orientation to time, place, and person
Repeat a short list of objects	Attention
Recall the short list of objects after 3 to 5 minutes	Immediate recall
Describe an event that happened in the last day or two	Recent memory
Describe events from the distant past	Remote memory
Interpret a proverb (such as "a rolling stone gathers no moss"), or explain a particular analogy (such as "why the brain is like a computer")	Abstract thinking
Describe feelings and opinions about the illness	Insight into illness
Name the last five presidents and the state capital	Fund of knowledge
Tell how they feel on this day and how they usually feel	Mood
Follow a simple command that involves three different body parts and requires distinguishing right from left (such as "put your right thumb in your left ear and stick out your tongue")	Language comprehension
Name simple objects and body parts, and read, write, and repeat certain phrases	Ability to use language
Without looking, identify small objects held in the hand and numbers written on the palm, and discriminate between being touched in one or two places	Ability of the brain to process and interpret complex sensory information from the hand
Copy simple and complex structures (for example, using building blocks) or finger positions, and draw a clock, cube, or house	Ability to understand spatial relationships
Brush the teeth, or take a match out of a box and strike it	Ability to perform an action
Do simple arithmetic	Ability to calculate numbers

weakness is evident when a person uses one limb more than another (for example, when swinging the arms while walking or when holding the arms up with the eyes closed). Weakness that affects the muscles of the upper arms and legs more than the hands and feet may indicate a disorder that affects all of the muscles (myopathy). Myopathies tend to affect the largest muscles first. The person may have difficulty combing hair or climbing stairs.

When the hand and feet are weaker than the upper arms and legs, the problem is often a polyneuropathy—a disorder that affects all of the nerves outside of the brain and spinal cord (peripheral nerves). Polyneuropathies tend to affect the longest nerves first (those in the hands and feet). The person may have the most trouble with fine finger movements.

When weakness is limited to one side of the body, doctors suspect a disorder affecting one side of the brain, such as a stroke. Weakness that affects the body below a certain part may be caused by a spinal cord disorder. For example, an injury to the thoracic spine causes the legs but not the arms to be paralyzed. An injury in or above the neck causes paralysis of all four limbs.

Weakness may also occur in other patterns, such as those corresponding to one or more particular peripheral nerves. Strength may decrease with repetitive activity, as occurs in myasthenia gravis.

Sensory nerves carry information from the body to the brain about such things as touch, pain, heat, cold, vibration, the position of body parts, and the shape of objects. Abnormal sensations or reduced perception of sensations may indicate damage to a sensory nerve, the spinal cord, or certain parts of the brain. Information from specific areas on the body's surface, called dermatomes (see art on page 796), is carried to a specific location (level) in the spinal cord, then to the brain. Thus, doctors may be able to pinpoint the specific level of damage to the spinal cord by identifying the areas where sensation is abnormal or lost.

The surface of the body is tested for loss of sensation. Usually, doctors concentrate on the area where the person feels numbness, tingling, or pain. A pin and a blunt object (such as the head of a safety pin) are used to see if the person can tell the difference between sharp and dull. Doctors also test the person's ability to feel gentle touch, heat, and vibration. To test position sense, doctors move the person's finger or toe up or down and ask the person to describe its position without looking.

Reflexes: A reflex is an automatic response to a stimulus. For example, the lower leg jerks when the tendon below the kneecap is gently tapped with a small rubber hammer. The pathway that a reflex follows (reflex arc) does not directly involve the brain. The pathway consists of the sensory nerve to the spinal cord, the nerve connections in the spinal cord, and the motor nerves back to the muscle. Doctors test reflexes to determine whether all parts of this pathway are functioning. The reflexes most commonly tested are the knee jerk and similar reflexes at the elbow and ankle.

The plantar reflex may help doctors diagnose abnormalities in the nerve pathways involved in the voluntary control of muscles. It is tested by firmly stroking the outer border of the sole of the foot with a key or other object that causes minor discomfort. Normally, the toes curl downward, except in infants aged 6 months or younger. Having the big toe go upward and the other toes spread out is a sign of an abnormality in the brain or spinal cord.

Testing other reflexes can provide important information. For example, doctors learn the extent of injury in a comatose person by noting whether the pupils constrict when light is shined on them (pupillary light reflex), whether the eyes blink when the cornea is touched (corneal reflex), and how the eyes move when the person's head is turned or when water is flushed into the ear canal. Seeing the anus constrict when lightly touched (anal wink) is a good sign in a person with a spinal cord injury.

Coordination, Balance, and Gait: Coordination and walking (gait) require integration of signals from sensory and motor nerves by the brain and spinal cord. To test these abilities, doctors ask a person to walk in a straight line, placing one foot in front of the other. They ask the person to use the forefinger to reach out and touch the doctor's finger, then the person's own nose, and then to repeat these actions rapidly. The person may be asked to do these actions first with the eyes open, then with the eyes closed.

For the Romberg test, the person stands still with both feet together as close as possible without losing balance. Then the eyes are closed. If balance is lost,

Reflex Arc: A No-Brainer

A reflex arc is the pathway that a nerve reflex, such as the knee jerk reflex, follows.

1. A tap on the knee stimulates sensory receptors, generating a nerve signal.
2. The signal travels along a nerve to the spinal cord.
3. In the spinal cord, the signal is transmitted from the sensory nerve to a motor nerve.
4. The motor nerve sends the signal back to a muscle in the thigh.
5. The muscle contracts, causing the lower leg to jerk upward. The entire reflex occurs without involving the brain.

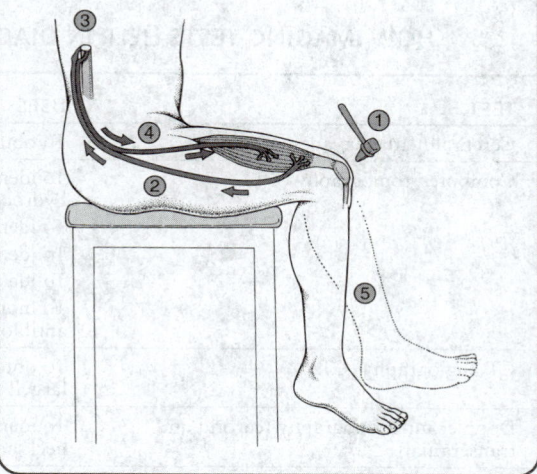

information about position from the legs is not reaching the brain, usually because the nerves or spinal cord is injured.

Autonomic Nervous System: The autonomic (involuntary) nervous system regulates internal body processes that require no conscious effort, such as blood pressure, heart rate, breathing, and temperature regulation through sweating or shivering. An abnormality of this system may cause a fall in blood pressure when a person stands up (orthostatic hypotension), reduction or absence of sweating, or sexual problems such as difficulty initiating or maintaining an erection. Doctors may do a variety of tests, such as measuring blood pressure and heart rate while the person is lying down, sitting, and standing.

Blood Flow to the Brain: A severe narrowing of the arteries to the brain reduces blood flow and increases the risk of stroke. The risk is higher for people who are older, who smoke cigarettes, or who have high blood pressure, high cholesterol levels, diabetes, or disorders of the arteries or heart. Doctors place a stethoscope on the neck (over the carotid artery) and listen for turbulent blood flow through a narrowed or irregular artery (the sound of turbulent blow flow is called a bruit). However, the best way to diagnose disorders of the arteries is to use ultrasound (called carotid duplex and transcranial ultrasonography), magnetic resonance angiography (MRA), computed tomography angiography (CTA), or cerebral angiography. Blood pressure may be measured in both arms to check for blockages in the large arteries that branch off from the aorta. Such blockages sometimes result in stroke.

Procedures

Diagnostic procedures may be needed to confirm a diagnosis suggested by the medical history and physical examination. Imaging tests such as computed tomography (CT—see page 2037), magnetic resonance imaging (MRI—see page 2040), angiography (see page 2036), positron emission tomography

HOW IMAGING TESTS HELP IN DIAGNOSING NERVOUS SYSTEM DISORDERS	
TEST	**USES**
Cerebral (catheter) angiography	To obtain detailed images of blood vessels of the brain
Computed tomography (CT)	To identify structural abnormalities (such as abscesses, tumors, and hydrocephalus) in the brain To identify bleeding or evidence of strokes in the brain To identify ruptured or herniated disks in the spine To identify spinal fractures To monitor the effects of radiation therapy on brain cancer or of antibiotics on a brain abscess
CT angiography (CTA)	To obtain detailed images of blood vessels of the brain (CTA has largely replaced cerebral angiography)
Doppler ultrasonography (carotid and transcranial)	To identify and evaluate narrowing or blockage of arteries in the neck and head and thus assess the risk of stroke
Magnetic resonance imaging (MRI)	To identify structural abnormalities (such as abscesses, tumors, and hydrocephalus) in the brain (images of brain tissue are clearer than those provided by CT, but MRI is not as readily available)
Magnetic resonance angiography (MRA)	To evaluate arteries in people who have had a stroke or TIA or in people who may have an aneurysm or arteriovenous malformation
Magnetic resonance venography (MRV)	To detect a blood clot in veins of the brain (cerebral venous thrombosis) and to monitor how treatment affects this disorder
Functional magnetic resonance imaging (fMRI)	To identify which areas of the brain are active when a task (such as reading, writing, remembering, calculating, or moving a limb) is done
Perfusion-weighted imaging (PWI) MRI	To estimate how much blood is flowing through a particular area of the brain
Diffusion-weighted imaging (DWI) MRI	To identify very early stroke and Creutzfeld-Jacob disease (CJD)
Magnetic resonance (MR) spectroscopy	To distinguish between abscesses and tumors
Positron emission tomography (PET)	To evaluate blood flow and metabolic activity in the brain To provide information about seizure disorders To help identify Alzheimer's disease, Parkinson's disease, transient ischemic attacks, and strokes

How a Spinal Tap Is Done

Cerebrospinal fluid flows through a channel (the subarachnoid space) between the middle and inner layers of tissue (meninges) that cover the brain and spinal cord—the subarachnoid space. To remove a sample of this fluid, a doctor inserts a small, hollow needle between two vertebrae in the lower spine, usually the third and fourth or the fourth and fifth lumbar vertebrae, below the point where the spinal cord ends. Usually, the person lies on the side with the knees curled to the chest. This position widens the space between the vertebrae, so that the doctor can avoid hitting the bones when the needle is inserted. Cerebrospinal fluid is allowed to drip into a test tube, and the sample is sent to a laboratory for examination.

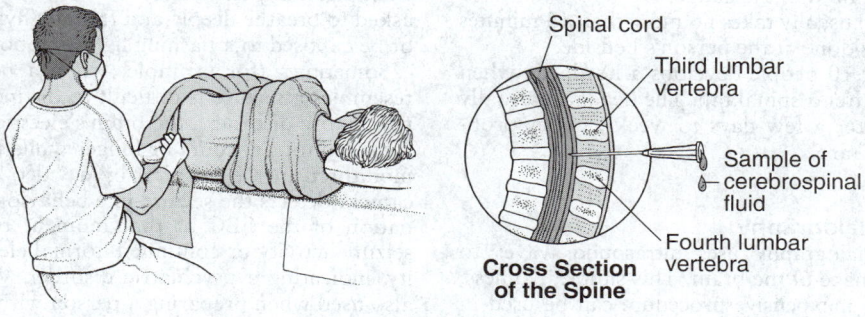

Spinal cord

Third lumbar vertebra

Sample of cerebrospinal fluid

Fourth lumbar vertebra

Cross Section of the Spine

(PET—see page 2044), and Doppler ultrasonography (see page 2044) are commonly used to diagnose neurologic disorders.

Spinal Tap

Cerebrospinal fluid flows through a channel (the subarachnoid space) between the layers of tissue (meninges) that cover the brain and spinal cord. This fluid, which surrounds the brain and spinal cord, helps cushion them against sudden jarring and minor injury.

For a spinal tap (lumbar puncture), a sample of cerebrospinal fluid is withdrawn with a needle and sent to a laboratory for examination.

The cerebrospinal fluid is checked for evidence of infections, tumors, and bleeding in the brain and spinal cord. These disorders may change the content and appearance of the cerebrospinal fluid, which normally contains few red and white blood cells and is clear and colorless. For example, the following findings suggest certain disorders:

- An increase in the number of white blood cells in the cerebrospinal fluid suggests an infection or inflammation of the brain and spinal cord.
- Cloudy fluid, due to the presence of many white blood cells, suggests meningitis (infection and inflammation of the tissues covering the brain and spinal cord) or sometimes encephalitis (infection and inflammation of the brain).

- High protein levels in the fluid may result from any injury of the brain, the spinal cord, or a spinal nerve root (the part of a spinal nerve next to the spinal cord).
- Abnormal antibodies in the fluid suggest multiple sclerosis or an infection.
- Low sugar (glucose) levels suggest meningitis or cancer.
- Blood in the fluid may indicate a brain hemorrhage.
- An increase in the fluid's pressure can result from many disorders, including brain tumors and meningitis.

Before doing a spinal tap, doctors use an ophthalmoscope to examine the optic nerve (see art on page 1422), which bulges when the pressure within the skull is increased. If the pressure is increased because of a mass (such as a tumor or abscess), a spinal tap is not done because it may suddenly reduce pressure below the brain. As a result, the brain may shift and be pressed through one of the small natural openings in the relatively rigid tissues that separate the brain into compartments (called herniation—see art on page 735). Herniation puts pressure on the brain and is potentially fatal. The medical history and neurologic examination help doctors determine whether herniation is a risk. But CT or MRI of the head is usually more accurate and is often done as a precaution before a spinal tap is done.

For a spinal tap, people typically lie on their side and draw their knees to their chest. A local anesthetic is used to numb the insertion site. Then, a needle is inserted between two vertebrae in the lower spine below the end of the spinal cord.

During a spinal tap, doctors can measure the pressure within the skull. Pressure is measured by attaching a gauge (manometer) to the needle used for the spinal tap and noting the height of the cerebrospinal fluid in the gauge.

A spinal tap usually takes no more than 15 minutes and is usually done at the person's bedside.

About 1 of 10 people develops a headache when standing up after a spinal tap. The headache usually disappears after a few days to weeks. Other problems are very rare.

Echoencephalography

Echoencephalography uses ultrasound waves to produce an image of the brain. This simple, painless, and relatively inexpensive procedure can be used in children younger than 2 years because their skull is thin enough for ultrasound waves to pass through. It can be done quickly at the bedside to detect hydrocephalus (commonly called water on the brain) or bleeding. CT and MRI have largely replaced echoencephalography because they produce much better images, especially in older children and adults.

Myelography

In myelography, x-rays of the spinal cord are taken after a radiopaque dye is injected into the cerebrospinal fluid via a spinal tap. Myelography has been largely replaced by MRI, which produces more detailed images, is simpler, and is safer. Myelography with CT is used when additional detail of the spinal canal and surrounding bone, which MRI cannot provide, is needed. Myelography with CT is also used when MRI is not available or cannot be done safely (for example, when a person has a heart pacemaker).

Electroencephalography

Electroencephalography (EEG) is a simple, painless procedure in which the brain's electrical activity is recorded as wave patterns and printed on paper or recorded in a computer (see art on page 714). EEG can help identify seizure disorders, sleep disturbances, and certain metabolic or structural disorders of the brain. For example, EEG can identify where a seizure originates and show the characteristic electrical activity associated with confusion due to liver failure (liver encephalopathy).

For the procedure, an examiner places small, round adhesive sensors (electrodes) on the person's scalp. The electrodes are connected by wires to a machine, which produces a record (tracing) of small changes in voltage detected by each electrode. These tracings constitute the electroencephalogram (the EEG).

If a seizure disorder is suspected but the initial EEG is normal, another EEG is done after using a tactic that makes seizure activity more likely. For example, the person may be deprived of sleep, be asked to breathe deeply and rapidly (hyperventilate), or be exposed to a flashing light (stroboscope).

Sometimes (for example, when a behavior that resembles a seizure is difficult to distinguish from a psychiatric disorder), the brain's electrical activity is recorded for 24 hours or longer while the person is monitored in the hospital by a video camera. The camera detects the seizure-like behavior, and examination of the EEG at that moment reveals either seizure activity or continued normal electrical activity, indicating a psychiatric disorder. Video EEG is also used when preparing a person with epilepsy for surgery to see what type of seizure results from an abnormality in the particular brain area in which the seizure originates.

Evoked Responses

Stimuli for sight, sound, and touch are used to activate specific areas of the brain, that is, to evoke responses. Based on these responses, doctors can tell how well those areas of the brain are working. For example, a flashing light stimulates the retina of the eye, the optic nerve, and the nerve pathway to the back part of the brain where vision is perceived and interpreted. EEG is used to detect electrical activity evoked by the stimuli.

Evoked responses are particularly useful in testing how well the senses are functioning in infants and children. For example, doctors can test an infant's hearing by checking for a response after a clicking sound is made at each ear. Evoked responses are also useful in identifying the effects of multiple sclerosis and other disorders on areas of the optic nerve, brain stem, and spinal cord. Such effects may or may not be detected by MRI.

Electromyography and Nerve Conduction Studies

Electromyography and nerve conduction studies help doctors determine whether muscle weakness, sensory loss, or both results from injury to the following:

- Spinal nerve root (for example, due to a ruptured disk in the spine of the neck or lower back)

- Peripheral nerve (for example, due to carpal tunnel syndrome or diabetic neuropathy)
- Connection between nerve and muscle (neuromuscular junction), for example, due to myasthenia gravis, botulism, or diphtheria
- Muscle (for example, due to polymyositis)

In **electromyography** (EMG), small needles are inserted into a muscle to record the electrical activity of the muscle when the muscle is at rest and when it is contracting. Normally, resting muscle produces no electrical activity. A slight contraction produces some electrical activity, which increases as the contraction increases. The EMG is abnormal if muscle weakness results from a problem with a spinal nerve root, peripheral nerve, muscle, or neuromuscular junction. The EMG produces a distinctive pattern of abnormalities. Unlike CT or EEG, which can be done routinely by technicians, EMG requires the expertise of a neurologist, who chooses the appropriate nerves and muscles to test and interprets the findings.

Nerve conduction studies measure the speed at which motor or sensory nerves conduct impulses. A small electrical current stimulates an impulse along the nerve being tested. The current may be delivered by several electrodes placed on the surface of the skin or by several needles inserted along the pathway of the nerve. The impulse moves along the nerve, eventually reaching the muscle and causing it to contract. By measuring the time the impulse takes to reach the muscle and the distance from the stimulating electrode or needle to the muscle, doctors can calculate the speed of nerve conduction. The nerve may be stimulated once or several times (to determine how well the neuromuscular junction is functioning). Results are abnormal only if the symptom results from a problem with a nerve or neuromuscular junction. For example,

- Slow nerve conduction may result from a nerve disorder, such as carpal tunnel syndrome (painful compression of a nerve in the wrist).
- If the muscle's response is progressively weaker after repeated stimulation, a problem with the neuromuscular junction (as occurs in myasthenia gravis) may be the cause.

Disorders that affect only the brain, spinal cord, spinal nerve roots, or the muscle do not affect the speed of nerve conduction.

CHAPTER 106 Pain

Pain is an unpleasant sensation signaling actual or possible injury.

Pain is the most common reason people visit their doctor. Pain may be sharp or dull, intermittent or constant, or throbbing or steady. Sometimes pain is very difficult to describe. Pain may be felt at a single site or over a large area. The intensity of pain can vary from mild to intolerable.

People differ remarkably in their ability to tolerate pain. One person cannot tolerate the pain of a small cut or bruise, but another person can tolerate pain caused by a major accident or knife wound with little complaint. The ability to withstand pain varies according to mood, personality, and circumstance. In a moment of excitement during an athletic match, an athlete may not notice a severe bruise but is likely to be very aware of the pain after the match, particularly if the team lost.

Acute Versus Chronic Pain: Pain may be acute or chronic. Acute pain begins suddenly and usually does not last long. Chronic pain lasts for weeks or months. Usually, pain is considered chronic if it does one of the following:

- Lasts for more than 1 month longer than expected based on the illness or injury
- Recurs off and on for months or years
- Is associated with a chronic disorder (such as cancer, arthritis, diabetes, or fibromyalgia) or an injury that does not heal

When severe, acute pain may cause anxiety, a rapid heart rate, an increased breathing rate, elevated blood pressure, sweating, and dilated pupils. Usually, chronic pain does not have these effects, but it may result in other problems, such as depression, disturbed

SPOTLIGHT ON AGING

Pain is common among older people. However, as people age, they complain less of pain. The reason may be a decrease in the body's sensitivity to pain or a more stoical attitude toward pain. Some older people mistakenly think that pain is an unavoidable part of aging and thus minimize it or do not report it.

The most common cause is a musculoskeletal disorder. However, many older people have chronic pain, which may have many causes.

Effects of pain may be more serious for older people:

- Chronic pain can make them less able to function and more dependent on other people.
- They may lose sleep and become exhausted.
- They may lose their appetite, resulting in undernutrition.
- Pain may prevent people from interacting with others and from going out. As a result, they can become isolated and depressed.
- Pain can make people less active. Lack of activity can lead to loss of muscle strength and flexibility, making activity even more difficult and increasing the risk of falls.

Older people are more likely than younger people to have side effects from pain relievers (analgesics), and some side effects are more likely to be severe. These drugs may stay in the body longer, and older people may be more sensitive to them. Many older people take several drugs, increasing the chances that a drug will interact with the analgesic, reducing the effectiveness of one of the drugs or increasing the risk of side effects.

Older people are more likely to have disorders that increase the risk of side effects from analgesics. Having a heart or blood vessel (cardiovascular) disorder or risk factors for these disorders increases the risk of heart attack, stroke, blood clots in the legs, and heart failure when NSAIDs are taken. Having a kidney disorder, heart failure, or a liver disorder makes people more vulnerable to kidney damage from NSAIDs and less able to handle the fluid retention caused by the drugs.

To reduce the risk of side effects, particularly when prescribing opioids, doctors give older people a low dose at first. The dose is increased slowly as needed, and its effects are monitored. Doctors also choose analgesics less likely to have side effects in older people. For example, acetaminophen is usually preferred to NSAIDs for treating chronic mild to moderate pain without inflammation. Certain NSAIDs (indomethacin and ketorolac) and certain opioids (such as pentazocine) are usually not given to older people because of the risk of side effects.

Nondrug treatments and support from caregivers and family members can sometimes help older people manage pain and reduce the need for analgesics.

sleep, decreased energy, a poor appetite, weight loss, decreased sex drive, and loss of interest in activities.

During treatment for chronic pain, many people experience a brief, often severe flare-up of pain. It is called breakthrough pain because it breaks through in spite of regularly scheduled pain treatment. Typically, breakthrough pain begins suddenly, lasts up to 1 hour, and feels much like the original chronic pain except it is more severe. Breakthrough pain may differ from person to person and is often unpredictable.

Chronic pain can make the nervous system more sensitive to pain. For example, chronic pain repeatedly stimulates the nerve fibers and cells that detect, send, and receive pain signals. Repeated stimulation can change the structure of nerve fibers and cells or make them more active and can thus increase pain transmission to the spinal cord and brain. As a result, pain may result from stimulation that might not ordinarily be painful, or painful stimuli may be felt as more severe.

When pain occurs repeatedly, people may anticipate it by becoming fearful and anxious. These emotions can stimulate the body to produce substances that make pain feel more intense. An example is prostaglandins, which make nerve cells more likely to respond to pain signals. Fear and anxiety can also reduce the production of substances that reduce the sensitivity of nerve cells to pain. An example is endorphins, the body's natural pain relievers. Fatigue can have the same effects on pain as fear and anxiety.

These changes in pain sensitivity partly account for pain that persists after its cause resolves and for pain that feels more severe than expected.

? Did You Know...

Chronic pain can physically change the nervous system in ways that make the pain worse and last longer.

Pain Pathways: Pain due to injury begins at special pain receptors scattered throughout the body. These pain receptors transmit signals as electrical impulses along nerves to the spinal cord and then upward to the brain. Sometimes the signal evokes a reflex response (see art on page 633). When the signal reaches the spinal cord, a signal is immediately sent back along motor nerves to the original site of the pain, triggering the muscles to contract without involving the brain. For example, when people inadvertently touch something very hot, they immediately

What Is Referred Pain?

Pain felt in one area of the body does not always represent where the problem is because the pain may be referred there from another area. For example, pain produced by a heart attack may feel as if it is coming from the arm because sensory information from the heart and the arm converge on the same nerve pathways in the spinal cord.

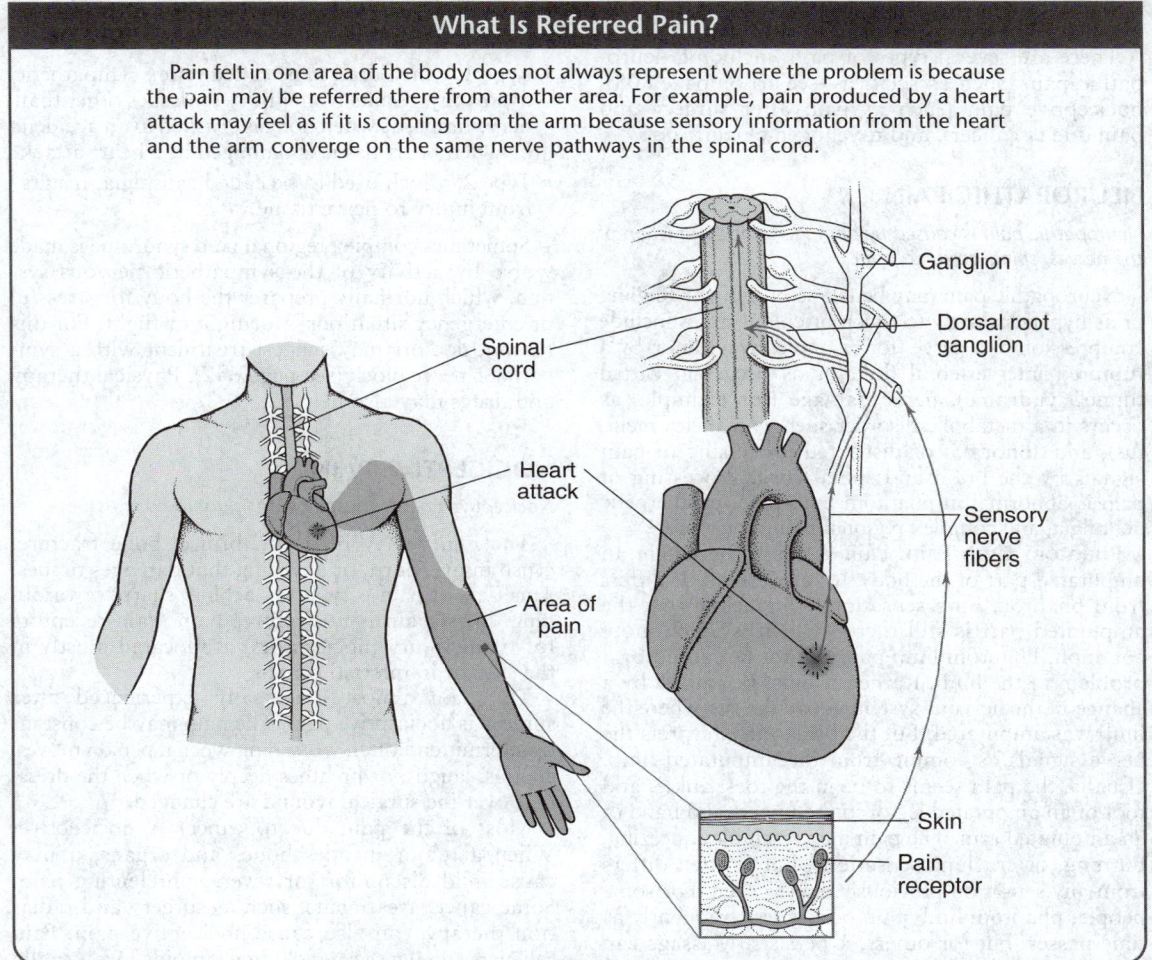

pull away. This reflex reaction helps prevent permanent damage. The pain signal is also sent to the brain. Only when the brain processes the signal and interprets it as pain do people become conscious of the pain.

Pain receptors and their nerve pathways differ in different parts of the body. For this reason, pain sensation varies with the type and location of injury. For example, pain receptors in the skin are plentiful and capable of transmitting precise information, including where an injury is located and whether the source was sharp, such as a knife wound, or dull, such as pressure, heat, or cold. In contrast, pain receptors in internal organs, such as the intestine are limited and imprecise. The intestine can be pinched, cut, or burned without generating a pain signal. However, stretching and pressure can cause severe intestinal pain, even from something as relatively harmless as a trapped gas bubble. The brain cannot identify the precise source of intestinal pain, which is difficult to locate and is likely to be felt over a large area.

Sometimes pain felt in one area of the body does not accurately represent where the problem is, because the pain is referred there from another area. Pain can be referred because signals from several areas of the body often travel through the same nerve pathways in the spinal cord and brain. For example, pain from a heart attack may be felt in the neck, jaws, arms, or abdomen. Pain from a gallbladder attack may be felt in the back of the shoulder.

Types

There are several types of pain, including neuropathic pain (such as sciatica—see art on page 808), nociceptive pain (such as pain after surgery and pain due to cancer), and psychogenic pain.

NEUROPATHIC PAIN

Neuropathic pain is caused by damage to or dysfunction of the nerves, spinal cord, or brain.

Neuropathic pain may be felt as burning or tingling or as hypersensitivity to touch or cold. Causes include compression of a nerve (for example, by a tumor, by a ruptured intervertebral disk, or as occurs in carpal tunnel syndrome), nerve damage (for example, as occurs in a metabolic disorder such as diabetes mellitus), and abnormal or disrupted processing of pain signals by the brain and spinal cord. Processing of pain is abnormal in phantom limb pain, postherpetic neuralgia, and complex regional pain syndrome.

Phantom Limb Pain: Pain seems to be felt in an amputated part of the body, usually a limb. It differs from phantom limb sensation—the feeling that the amputated part is still there—which is much more common. Phantom limb pain cannot be caused by a problem in the limb. Rather, it must be caused by a change in the nervous system above the site where the limb was amputated. But the brain misinterprets the nerve signals as coming from the amputated limb. Usually, the pain seems to be in the toes, ankle, and foot of an amputated leg or in the fingers and hand of an amputated arm. The pain may resemble squeezing, burning, or crushing sensations, but it often differs from any sensation previously experienced. For some people, phantom limb pain occurs less frequently as time passes, but for others, it persists. Massage can sometimes help, but drug therapy is sometimes necessary.

Postherpetic Neuralgia: This disorder results from herpes zoster (shingles, which causes inflammation of nerve tissue), but occurs only after shingles resolves (see box on page 1248). What causes postherpetic neuralgia is unknown. The pain is felt as a constant deep aching or burning, as a sharp and intermittent pain, or as hypersensitivity to touch or cold. The pain may be debilitating. Pain relievers and other drugs may be required, but no treatment is routinely effective.

Complex Regional Pain Syndrome: This chronic pain syndrome is defined as persistent burning pain accompanied by certain abnormalities that occur in the same area as the pain. Abnormalities include increased or decreased sweating, swelling, changes in skin color, damage to the skin, hair loss, cracked or thickened nails, muscle wasting and weakness, and bone loss. This syndrome typically occurs after an injury. There are two types:

- Type 1, which used to be called reflex sympathetic dystrophy, results from injury to tissues other than nerve tissue, as when bone is crushed in an accident or when heart tissue is damaged in a heart attack.

- Type 2, which used to be called causalgia, results from injury to nerve tissue.

Sometimes complex regional pain syndrome is made worse by activity of the sympathetic nervous system, which normally prepares the body for stressful or emergency situations—for fight or flight. For this reason, doctors may suggest treatment with a sympathetic nerve block (see page 647). Physical therapy and drugs may also help.

NOCICEPTIVE PAIN

Nociceptive pain is caused by an injury to body tissues.

The injury may be a cut, bruise, bone fracture, crush injury, burn, or anything that damages tissues. This type of pain is typically aching, sharp, or throbbing. Most pain is nociceptive pain. Pain receptors for tissue injury (nociceptors) are located mostly in the skin or in internal organs.

The pain almost universally experienced after surgery is nociceptive pain. The pain may be constant or intermittent, often worsening when a person moves, coughs, laughs, or breathes deeply or when the dressings over the surgical wound are changed.

Most of the pain due to cancer is nociceptive. When a tumor invades bones and organs, it may cause mild discomfort or severe, unrelenting pain. Some cancer treatments, such as surgery and radiation therapy, can also cause nociceptive pain. Pain relievers (analgesics), including opioids, are usually effective.

PSYCHOGENIC PAIN

Psychogenic pain is pain that is mostly related to psychologic factors.

When people have persistent pain with evidence of psychologic disturbances and without evidence of a disorder that could account for the pain or its severity, the pain may be described as psychogenic. However, psychophysiologic pain is a more accurate term because the pain results from interaction of physical and psychologic factors. Psychogenic pain is far less common than nociceptive or neuropathic pain.

Any kind of pain can be complicated by psychologic factors. Psychologic factors often contribute to chronic pain and may contribute to pain-related disability. In such cases, the pain, disability, or both usually have a physical cause, but psychologic factors exaggerate or enhance the pain, making it worse than what most people with a similar physical disorder experience. For example, people with chronic pain know it will recur and may become fearful and anxious as they anticipate the pain. These emotions make them more sensitive to pain. Sometimes doctors describe chronic pain that is worsened by psychologic factors as a chronic pain syndrome.

The fact that pain is caused or worsened by psychologic factors does not mean that it is not real. Most people who report pain are really experiencing it, even if a physical cause cannot be identified. Doctors always investigate whether a physical disorder is contributing to pain.

Pain complicated by psychologic factors requires treatment, often by a team that includes a psychologist or psychiatrist. Treatment for this type of pain varies from person to person, and doctors try to match the treatment with the person's needs. For most people who have chronic psychogenic pain, the goals of treatment are to improve comfort and physical and psychologic function. Doctors may make specific recommendations for gradually increasing physical and social activities. Drugs and nondrug treatments—such as biofeedback, relaxation training, distraction techniques, hypnosis, transcutaneous electrical nerve stimulation (TENS), and physical therapy—may be used. Psychologic counseling is often needed.

Evaluation

Neither examinations nor tests can prove that a person is in pain. Consequently, doctors ask the person about the history and characteristics of pain. The person's answers help them identify the cause and develop a treatment strategy. Questions can include the following:

- Where is the pain? What is the pain like?
- When did the pain start? Was there any injury?
- How did the pain start? Did it begin suddenly or gradually?
- Is the pain always present, or does it come and go?
- Does it occur predictably after certain activities (such as meals or physical exertion) or in certain body positions? What else makes the pain worse?
- What, if anything, helps relieve the pain?
- Does pain affect the ability to do daily activities or to interact with other people? Does it affect sleep, appetite, and bowel and bladder function? If so, how?

- Does pain affect mood and sense of well-being? Is the pain accompanied by feelings of depression or anxiety?

To evaluate the severity of pain, doctors sometimes use a scale of 0 (none) to 10 (severe) or ask the person to describe the pain as mild, moderate, severe, or excruciating. For children or for people who have difficulty communicating (for example, because of a stroke), drawings of faces in a series—from smiling to frowning and crying—can be used to determine the severity of pain.

Doctors always try to determine whether a physical disorder is causing the pain. Many chronic disorders (such as cancer, arthritis, sickle cell anemia, and inflammatory bowel disease) cause pain, as do acute disorders (such as wounds, burns, torn muscles, broken bones, sprained ligaments, appendicitis, kidney stones, and a heart attack). Doctors use specific techniques to check for sources of pain. Doctors move the person's arms and legs through their normal range of motion to see if these motions cause pain. Injury, repetitive stress, chronic pain, and other disorders can make certain areas of the body (called trigger points) become hypersensitive. Doctors touch various spots to see whether they are trigger points for pain. Different objects (such as a blunt key and a sharp pin) may be touched to the skin to check for loss of sensation or abnormal perceptions.

Doctors also consider psychologic causes. Psychologic factors (such as depression and anxiety) can worsen pain. Sometimes pain is determined to be caused mostly or completely by psychologic factors. Such pain is called psychogenic pain. Because depression and anxiety may result from chronic pain, distinguishing cause and effect may be difficult.

Doctors ask about which drugs (including over-the-counter drugs) and other treatments the person has used to treat the pain and whether they are effective.

Few people exaggerate the pain they feel. Nonetheless, doctors usually also ask questions to make sure there are no ulterior motives for reporting pain, such as time off from work with pay or extra attention from family members. Such questions are routine.

Treatment

In some cases, treating the underlying disorder eliminates or minimizes the pain. For example, setting a broken bone in a cast or giving antibiotics for an infected joint helps reduce pain. However, even if the underlying disorder can be treated, pain relievers (analgesics) may still be needed to quickly manage the pain. Doctors choose an analgesic based on the type and duration of pain and on the likely benefits and risks. Most analgesics are effective for nociceptive pain (due to ordinary injury of tissues) but are less effective for neuropathic pain (due to damage or dysfunction of the nerves, spinal cord, or brain), which often requires different drugs. For some types of pain, especially chronic pain, nondrug treatments are also important.

Analgesics fall into three categories: opioid (narcotic) analgesics, nonopioid analgesics, and adjuvant analgesics (drugs that are usually given for reasons other than pain but that sometimes relieve pain).

OPIOID ANALGESICS

Opioid analgesics (sometimes called narcotics) are the most powerful analgesics. They are the mainstay for treatment of severe acute pain (as occurs after surgery or from burns or broken bones) and chronic pain due to cancer and other serious disorders. Opioids are preferred because they are so effective in controlling pain. Using opioids to treat chronic pain not due to cancer is becoming more acceptable but is still relatively uncommon. Opioids are not appropriate for everyone.

Opioids are chemically related to morphine, a natural substance extracted from poppies, although some opioids are extracted from other plants and other opioids are produced in a laboratory.

The dose of an opioid is increased gradually, in stages, until the pain is relieved or the opioid's side effects cannot be tolerated. Older people and newborns, who are more sensitive to the effects of opioids, are usually given lower doses. Nonopioid analgesics, such as acetaminophen, are often used with opioids, sometimes in tablets that contain both drugs.

Opioids are most effective when taken every few hours, before pain becomes severe. If more pain relief is required, the dose may be increased or another drug (such as a nonsteroidal anti-inflammatory drug) may be added, as in the following situations:

- The pain temporarily worsens
- The person needs to exercise (movement can be more painful)
- A wound dressing is about to be changed

As the pain lessens, doctors reduce the dose of the opioid accordingly, and when possible, they stop the opioid and switch to a nonopioid analgesic.

Side Effects: Opioids have many side effects. Side effects are more likely to occur in people with certain disorders: kidney failure, a liver disorder, chronic obstructive pulmonary disease (COPD), dementia, or another brain disorder.

Drowsiness, constipation, nausea, vomiting, and itching are common when opioids are started.

Some people welcome the drowsiness provided by opioids, but others do not. For most people who take opioids, drowsiness disappears or decreases within a few days. If people continue to feel drowsy, they may be given stimulant drugs, such as methylphenidate, to keep them awake and alert. These drugs may be taken regularly or only before events that require alertness, such as a family gathering. For some people, drinking beverages that contain caffeine provides enough stimulation. When feeling drowsy after taking an opioid, people should avoid driving and take extra care to prevent falls and accidents. Opioids may also cause confusion, especially in older people.

Opioids often cause constipation, especially in older people. Stimulant laxatives (see page 121), such as senna, help prevent or relieve the constipation. Increasing the intake of fluids and the amount of fiber in the diet can also help. Some people need enemas.

Opioids can cause retention of urine, especially in men with benign prostatic hyperplasia. Trying to urinate a second time after a brief pause (double voiding) or applying gentle pressure on the lowest part of the abdomen (the area over the bladder) during urination may help. Sometimes a drug that relaxes muscles of the bladder (such as tamsulosin) is used.

> **? Did You Know...**
> Many people needlessly experience pain because their doctors have an unfounded fear that using opioids will lead to addiction.

Sometimes people with pain feel nauseated, and opioids can increase the nausea. Antiemetic drugs taken by mouth, suppository, or injection help prevent or relieve nausea. Some commonly used antiemetic drugs are metoclopramide, hydroxyzine, and prochlorperazine.

For most people, nausea and itching disappear or decrease within a few days. But constipation and retention of urine usually decrease much more slowly.

Taking too much of an opioid can have serious side effects, including a dangerous slowing of breathing and even coma. These effects can be reversed with naloxone, an antidote given intravenously. Nurses and family members should watch for side effects of opioids.

For most people, the same opioid dose remains effective for a long time. However, some people who take opioids repeatedly over time need higher doses because the body adapts to and thus responds

℞ OPIOID ANALGESICS

DRUG	LENGTH OF EFFECTIVENESS	COMMENTS
Morphine	By intravenous or intramuscular injection: 2 to 3 hours Immediate-release by mouth: 3 to 4 hours Controlled- and sustained-release by mouth: 8 to 24 hours	Morphine starts to work quickly. The oral form can be very effective for chronic pain. It is more likely to cause itching than other opioids.
Codeine	By mouth: 3 to 4 hours	Codeine is less potent than morphine. It is usually taken with aspirin or acetaminophen.
Fentanyl	By mouth: 3 to 4 hours By patch: up to 72 hours	Fentanyl lozenges and dissolvable tablets can be used to treat breakthrough pain. Fentanyl lozenges can also be used to relieve pain and provide sedation (before painful procedures) in children. A fentanyl patch is often used to treat chronic pain.
Hydrocodone	By mouth: 3 to 5 hours	Hydrocodone is similar to codeine in effectiveness.
Hydromorphone	By intravenous or intramuscular injection: 2 to 4 hours By mouth: 2 to 4 hours By rectal suppository: 4 hours	Hydromorphone begins to work quickly. It can be used instead of morphine and is useful for chronic pain.
Levorphanol	By intravenous or intramuscular injection: 4 hours By mouth: about 4 hours	The oral form is strong. It can be used instead of morphine.
Meperidine	By intravenous or intramuscular injection: about 3 hours By mouth: not very effective	Although meperidine can be effective for short-term use, it is not preferred for long-term use because it has side effects, such as muscle spasms, tremors, seizures, and confusion or psychosis (especially in older people).
Methadone	By mouth: 4 to 6 hours, sometimes much longer	Methadone is used for treating addiction to heroin and other opioids. It can also be used to treat chronic pain.
Oxycodone	By mouth: 3 to 4 hours	Oxycodone can be used instead of morphine to treat chronic pain. A long-acting, controlled-release formulation is available, lasting about 8 to 12 hours. The short-acting formulation is usually combined with aspirin or acetaminophen.
Oxymorphone	By intravenous or intramuscular injection: 3 to 4 hours By rectal suppository: 4 hours	Oxymorphone can be used instead of morphine to treat chronic pain. Like oxycodone, it is available in a long-acting, controlled-release formulation, lasting about 12 hours.
Pentazocine	By mouth: up to 4 hours	Pentazocine can block the pain-relieving action of other opioids. It is about as strong as codeine. The usefulness of pentazocine is limited because higher doses do not provide more pain relief and because the drug can cause confusion and anxiety, especially in older people. It is not a good choice for older people.
Propoxyphene	By mouth: 3 to 4 hours	At safe doses, propoxyphene provides little or no more pain relief than aspirin. At high doses, it is likely to have side effects. Thus, it is not often used.

less well to the drug. This phenomenon is called tolerance. Usually, the need for a higher dose means that the disorder is worsening, not that tolerance is developing.

People who take opioids for a long time usually become physically dependent on them. That is, they experience withdrawal symptoms if the drug is stopped. When opioids are stopped after long-term use, doctors reduce the dose gradually over a period of time to minimize the development of such symptoms. Physical dependence is not the same as addiction, which is characterized by a craving for the drug and compulsive, uncontrolled use of the drug despite the harm done to the user or other people. Although addiction is possible, it appears to be rare among people who take opioids to control pain and have not previously had problems with drug abuse. Too often, exaggerated concern about the addiction potential of opioids (see page 2096) leads to undertreatment of pain and needless suffering. People with severe pain should not avoid opioids, and adequate doses should be taken as needed. Doctors carefully weigh the benefits and side effects when they consider opioids for the treatment of chronic pain.

Administration: When possible, opioids are taken by mouth. When they need to be taken for a long time, they may be given through a patch placed on the skin. Opioids are given by injection when pain occurs suddenly or when people cannot take them by mouth or through a skin patch. If people are helped by an opioid but cannot tolerate its side effects, an opioid can be injected directly into the space around the spinal cord through a pump. This method gets high concentrations of the drug to the brain. For long-term pain relief, a device that slowly releases an opioid can be implanted in the space around the spinal cord.

Morphine, the prototype of these drugs, can be taken by mouth (orally) or by injection. There are three oral forms: immediate-release, controlled-release, and sustained-release. Different controlled- and sustained-release forms provide relief for 8 to 24 hours. These drugs are widely used to treat chronic pain. The immediate-release form provides short-lived relief, usually for less than 3 hours. In injected forms, 2 to 6 times less morphine is required than in oral forms because when morphine is taken by mouth, much of the drug is chemically altered (metabolized) by the liver before it reaches the bloodstream. Usually, the route used does not change the drug's effects, even though different routes use different amounts of morphine. Pain relief with injected forms is quicker than that with oral forms, but relief does not last as long.

Morphine may be injected into a vein (intravenously), into a muscle (intramuscularly), or under the skin (subcutaneously).

- Intravenously: Pain relief is almost immediate but does not last very long.
- Intramuscularly: Pain relief is less rapid but lasts somewhat longer. Intramuscular injections are painful, and pain relief is less predictable, so this route is not used often.

- Subcutaneously: Pain relief is the least rapid but lasts the longest.

Injections can be given every few hours, but repeated injections can become annoying. Alternatively, a catheter can be inserted in a vein or under the skin and connected to a continuous-infusion pump, which supplies morphine continuously. The continuous infusion can be supplemented with extra doses when needed. Sometimes a device that enables a person to release the drug by pressing a button is used. This technique is called patient-controlled analgesia. Usually, continuous infusion is used for people who have severe pain due to a serious disorder.

NONOPIOID ANALGESICS

A variety of nonopioid analgesics are available. They are often effective for mild to moderate pain. People do not become physically dependent on these drugs or tolerant of their pain-relieving effects. Aspirin and acetaminophen are available without a prescription (over-the-counter, or OTC). Several other nonopioid analgesics (such as ibuprofen, ketoprofen, and naproxen) are available OTC and by prescription, usually in higher-dose formulations, with more active ingredient per dose than OTC formulations. OTC analgesics are reasonably safe to take for short periods of time, but their labels caution against taking them for more than 7 to 10 days to treat pain. A doctor should be consulted if symptoms worsen or do not go away.

Nonsteroidal Anti-Inflammatory Drugs

Most nonopioid analgesics are classified as non-steroidal anti-inflammatory drugs (NSAIDs). NSAIDs are used to treat mild to moderate pain and may be combined with opioids to treat moderate to severe pain. NSAIDs not only relieve pain, but they also reduce the inflammation that often accompanies and worsens pain. All NSAIDs are taken by mouth. One NSAID, ketorolac, can also be given by injection into a vein (intravenously) or muscle (intramuscularly). Indomethacin can be given by suppository.

Although widely used, NSAIDs can have side effects, sometimes serious ones.

- **Problems in the digestive tract:** All NSAIDs tend to irritate the stomach's lining and cause digestive upset (such as heartburn, indigestion, nausea, bloating, diarrhea, and stomach pain), peptic ulcers, and bleeding in the digestive tract (gastrointestinal bleeding). Coxibs (COX-2 inhibitors) are less likely to irritate the stomach and cause bleeding than other NSAIDs. However, if people take a coxib and aspirin, these problems are just as likely. Taking NSAIDs with food and using antacids may help

How Nonsteroidal Anti-Inflammatory Drugs Work

Nonsteroidal anti-inflammatory drugs (NSAIDs) work in two ways:

- They reduce the sensation of pain.
- At higher doses, they reduce the inflammation that often accompanies and worsens pain.

NSAIDs have these effects because they reduce the production of hormone-like substances called prostaglandins. Different prostaglandins have different functions, such as sensitizing pain receptors to mechanical and chemical stimulation and causing blood vessels to dilate.

Most NSAIDs reduce prostaglandin production by blocking both cyclooxygenase (COX) enzymes (COX-1 and COX-2), which are crucial to the formation of prostaglandins. One type of NSAID, the coxibs (COX-2 inhibitors), tend to block mainly COX-2 enzymes.

Only COX-2 enzymes are involved in the production of prostaglandins that promote inflammation and the resulting pain. These prostaglandins are released in response to an injury—burn, break, sprain, strain, or invasion by a microorganism. The result is inflammation, which is a protective response: The blood supply to the injured area increases, bringing in fluids and white blood cells to wall off the damaged tissue and remove any invading microorganisms.

Prostaglandins that are formed through the action of COX-1 enzymes help protect the digestive tract from stomach acid and play a crucial role in blood clotting. Most NSAIDs block COX-1 enzymes and thus reduce the production of these prostaglandins. Consequently, these NSAIDs may irritate the stomach's lining and cause digestive upset, peptic ulcers, and bleeding in the digestive tract. Because coxibs block mainly COX-2 enzymes, they are less likely to cause these problems. However, coxibs block some COX-1 enzymes, so even coxibs may slightly increase the risk of these problems.

---

prevent stomach irritation. The drug misoprostol can help prevent stomach irritation and ulcers, but it can cause other problems, including diarrhea. Proton pump inhibitors (such as omeprazole) or histamine-2 (H_2) blockers (such as famotidine), which are used to treat peptic ulcers, can also help prevent stomach problems due to NSAIDs.

- **Bleeding problems:** All NSAIDs except coxibs interfere with the clotting tendency of platelets (cell-like particles in the blood that help stop bleeding when blood vessels are injured). Consequently, NSAIDs increase the risk of bleeding, especially in the digestive tract if they also irritate the stomach's lining.

- **Problems related to retaining fluids:** NSAIDs cause fluid retention and swelling in 1 to 2% of people. Regular use of NSAIDs may also increase the risk of developing a kidney disorder, sometimes resulting in kidney failure (a disorder called analgesic nephropathy).

- **Increased risk of heart and blood vessel disorders:** Recent studies suggest that with all NSAIDs except aspirin, the risk of heart attack, stroke, and blood clots in the legs may be increased. The risk appears to be higher with higher doses and longer use of the drug. The risk is also higher with some NSAIDs than with others. These problems may be related directly to the drug's effect on clotting or indirectly to a small but persistent increase in blood pressure caused by the drug.

Taking NSAIDs for a short time is unlikely to cause serious problems. If NSAIDs are taken for a long time, certain tests are done regularly. They include blood pressure measurement, blood tests (such as a complete blood count and tests to check kidney and liver function), and tests for blood in stools.

For older people, the risk of side effects due to NSAIDs, particularly indomethacin and ketorolac, is increased. For people who drink alcoholic beverages regularly and take NSAIDs, the risk of digestive upset, ulcers, and liver damage may be increased. The risk of heart attacks and stroke may be higher for people with coronary artery disease, other heart and blood vessel (cardiovascular) disorders, or risk factors for these disorders. Older people and people who have heart failure, high blood pressure, or a kidney or liver disorder require a doctor's supervision when they take NSAIDs. Some prescription heart and blood pressure drugs may not work as well when taken with these analgesics.

NSAIDs vary in how quickly they work and how long they relieve pain. Although NSAIDs are about equally effective, people respond to them differently. One person may find a particular drug to be more effective or to have fewer side effects than another.

Aspirin: Aspirin (acetylsalicylic acid) has been used for about 100 years. Aspirin is taken by mouth and provides 4 to 6 hours of moderate pain relief.

? Did You Know...

If taken for a long time, NSAIDs, including those available without a prescription, can have serious side effects.

NONSTEROIDAL ANTI-INFLAMMATORY DRUGS

TYPE	DRUG
Salicylates	Aspirin
	Choline magnesium trisalicylate
	Diflunisal
	Salsalate
Coxibs	Celecoxib
Others	Diclofenac
	Etodolac
	Fenoprofen
	Flurbiprofen
	Ibuprofen
	Indomethacin
	Ketoprofen
	Ketorolac
	Meclofenamate
	Mefenamic acid
	Meloxicam
	Nabumetone
	Naproxen
	Oxaprozin
	Piroxicam
	Sulindac
	Tolmetin

Because aspirin can irritate the stomach, it may be combined with an antacid (in a buffered product) to reduce this effect. The antacid creates an alkaline environment that helps aspirin dissolve and may reduce the time aspirin is in contact with the stomach lining. However, buffered aspirin can still irritate the stomach because aspirin also reduces the production of substances that help protect the stomach's lining. These substances are a type of prostaglandin, which are similar to hormones.

Enteric-coated aspirin is designed to pass through the stomach intact and dissolve in the small intestine, thus minimizing direct irritation of the stomach. (Enteric refers to the small intestine.) However, enteric-coated aspirin may be absorbed erratically. If food and enteric-coated aspirin are ingested at about the same time, the aspirin is not absorbed as quickly because food delays the emptying of the stomach. Consequently, pain relief is delayed.

Aspirin increases the risk of bleeding throughout the body because it makes the particles that help blood clot (platelets) less likely to do so. People who bruise easily may be especially vulnerable to this effect. Anyone who has ever had a bleeding disorder or uncontrolled high blood pressure should not take aspirin except under a doctor's supervision. People who take aspirin and anticoagulants (such as warfarin) are closely monitored to avoid life-threatening bleeding. Usually, aspirin should not be taken in the week before scheduled surgery.

Aspirin can aggravate asthma. People with nasal polyps are likely to develop wheezing if they take aspirin. A few people, who are sensitive (allergic) to aspirin, may have a severe allergic reaction (anaphylaxis), leading to a rash, itching, severe breathing problems, or shock (see page 350). Such a reaction requires immediate medical attention.

In very high doses, aspirin can have serious side effects such as abnormal breathing, fever, or confusion. One of the first signs of an overdose may be noise in the ears (tinnitus).

Most children and teenagers should not take aspirin because they could develop Reye's syndrome if they have or have just gotten over influenza or chickenpox. Although rare, Reye's syndrome can have serious consequences, including death.

Ibuprofen, Ketoprofen, and Naproxen: NSAIDs such as ibuprofen, ketoprofen, and naproxen are generally believed to be gentler on the stomach than aspirin, although few studies have compared the drugs. Like aspirin, these drugs can cause digestive upset, ulcers, and gastrointestinal bleeding. They can make asthma worse and increase blood pressure. Taking one of these drugs probably slightly increases the risk of stroke, heart attack, and blood clots in the arteries of the legs.

Although ibuprofen, ketoprofen, and naproxen generally interfere with blood clotting less than aspirin does, people should not take these drugs with anticoagulants (such as warfarin) except under a doctor's close supervision.

People who are allergic to aspirin may also be allergic to ibuprofen, ketoprofen, and naproxen. If a rash, itching, breathing problems, or shock develops, medical attention is required immediately.

Coxibs (COX-2 Inhibitors): Coxibs, such as celecoxib, differ from other NSAIDs. Other NSAIDs block two enzymes:

- COX-1, which is involved in the production of prostaglandins that protect the stomach and play a crucial role in blood clotting
- COX-2, which is involved in the production of prostaglandins that promote inflammation

Coxibs tend to block mainly COX-2 enzymes. Thus, coxibs are as effective as other NSAIDs in the treatment of pain and inflammation. But coxibs are less likely to damage the stomach and to cause nausea, bloating, heartburn, bleeding, and peptic ulcers.

They are also less likely to interfere with clotting than are other NSAIDs.

Because of these differences, coxibs may be useful for people who cannot tolerate other NSAIDs and for people who are at high risk of certain complications (such as gastrointestinal bleeding) from use of other NSAIDs. Such people include older people, people who are taking anticoagulants, those who have a history of ulcers, and those who must take an analgesic for a long time. However, blockage of COX-2 enzymes appears to make blood clots more likely to form. Thus, taking coxibs, like taking other NSAIDs, is likely to increase the risk of heart attack, stroke, and blood clots in the legs. How much the risk is increased depends on the drug used. The risk is higher when higher doses are taken and when the drug is taken for a longer time. Thus, before people who have a cardiovascular disorder (such as coronary artery disease), who have had a stroke, or who have risk factors for these disorders are given a coxib, they are told about the risk and the need to be closely monitored. Coxibs are not appropriate for people who have heart failure or who are at increased risk of heart failure (such as those who have had a heart attack).

Acetaminophen

Acetaminophen is roughly comparable to aspirin in its potential to relieve pain and lower a fever. But unlike NSAIDs, acetaminophen has virtually no useful anti-inflammatory activity, does not affect the blood's ability to clot, and has almost no adverse effects on the stomach. How acetaminophen works is not clearly understood.

Acetaminophen is taken by mouth or suppository, and its effects generally last 4 to 6 hours. Acetaminophen appears to be a very safe drug. However, high doses can lead to liver damage, which may be irreversible. People with a liver disorder should use lower doses than those usually prescribed. Whether lower doses taken for a long time can harm the liver is less certain. People who regularly consume large amounts of alcohol are probably at highest risk of liver damage from overuse of acetaminophen. People who are taking acetaminophen and stop eating because of a bad cold, influenza, or another reason may be more vulnerable to liver damage. Taking high doses for a long time may lead to kidney damage.

ADJUVANT ANALGESICS

Adjuvant analgesics are drugs that are not usually used for pain relief but may relieve pain in certain circumstances. When used to relieve pain, they are usually used with other analgesics or nondrug pain treatments.

The adjuvant analgesics most commonly used for pain are antidepressants (such as amitriptyline, bu-propion, desipramine, fluoxetine, and venlafaxine—see table on page 868), anticonvulsants (such as gabapentin and pregabalin—see table on page 716), and oral and topical local anesthetics.

Antidepressants: These drugs can potentially relieve pain in people who do not have depression. Tricyclic antidepressants may be more effective for this purpose than other antidepressants, but newer antidepressants, such as selective serotonin reuptake inhibitors (SSRIs) and selective serotonin and nor-epinephrine reuptake inhibitors (SSNRIs, such as duloxetine) are tolerated better. People may respond to one antidepressant and not to others.

Anticonvulsants: These drugs may be used to relieve neuropathic pain. Gabapentin is used most often, but many others, including carbamazepine, clonazepam, divalproex, lamotrigine, oxcarbazepine, phenytoin, pregabalin, and topiramate, may be tried. Pregabalin can be used to relieve pain caused by nerve damage due to diabetes (diabetic neuropathy) or a complication of shingles (postherpetic neuralgia). Anticonvulsants, such as divalproex, can prevent migraine headaches.

Anesthetics: Mexiletine, used to treat abnormal heart rhythms, is sometimes used to treat neuropathic pain. It is similar to local anesthetics that are placed directly on or near a sore area to help reduce pain. Doctors may inject a local anesthetic, such as lidocaine, into the skin to control pain due to an injury or even due to neuropathic pain. Local anesthetics can also be injected in nerves to block pain—a procedure called a nerve block. For example, a sympathetic nerve block involves injecting a local anesthetic into a group of nerves near the spine—in the neck for pain in the upper body or in the lower back for pain in the lower body.

Topical anesthetics, such as lidocaine applied as a lotion, ointment, or skin patch, can be used to control pain due to some conditions. These anesthetics are usually used for a short period of time. For example, gargling small amounts of an anesthetic mouthwash, limited to a few times a day, can relieve a sore throat. However, some people with chronic pain benefit from using topical anesthetics for a long time. For example, a lidocaine patch can relieve postherpetic neuralgia.

A cream containing capsaicin, a substance found in hot peppers, sometimes helps reduce the pain caused by such disorders as herpes zoster and osteoarthritis. It is most often used by people with localized pain due to arthritis. This cream must be applied several times a day.

NONDRUG PAIN TREATMENTS

In addition to drugs, many other treatments can help relieve pain. Applying cold or warm compresses directly to a painful area often helps (see page 46). Ultrasonography that provides deep heat (diathermy) may relieve the pain of osteoarthritis and muscle strain.

Some people benefit from transcutaneous electrical nerve stimulation (TENS). A gentle electric current is applied through electrodes placed on the skin's surface. TENS produces a tingling sensation without increasing muscle tension. It can be applied continuously or several times a day for 20 minutes to several hours. The timing and length of stimulation vary because each person responds differently. Often, people are taught to use the TENS device, so that they can use it as needed. TENS may be useful for chronic pain. If pain is particularly severe and other treatments are ineffective, electrodes may be implanted along the affected nerves or in the space around the spinal cord.

Occasionally, pain due to nerve damage can be treated by disrupting a nerve pathway that transmits pain signals. The pathway is disrupted by injecting a caustic substance (such as phenol) into a nerve to destroy it, by freezing the nerve (in cryotherapy), or by burning the nerve with a radiofrequency probe. These procedures may be used to treat facial pain due to trigeminal neuralgia.

Acupuncture involves inserting tiny needles into specific areas of the body (see page 2061). How acupuncture works is poorly understood, and some experts still doubt the technique's effectiveness. Some people find substantial relief with acupuncture, at least for a time.

Biofeedback and other cognitive techniques (such as relaxation training, hypnosis, and distraction techniques) can help people control, reduce, or cope with pain by changing the way they focus their attention. In one distraction technique, people may learn to visualize themselves in a calm, comforting place (such as in a hammock or on a beach) when they feel pain.

The importance of psychologic support for people in pain should not be underestimated. Friends and family members should be aware that people in pain suffer, need support, and may develop depression and anxiety, which may require psychologic counseling.

CHAPTER 107 Headaches

Headaches are a very common medical problem and a common cause of disability among men and women. Headaches interfere with the ability to work and do daily tasks. Some people have frequent headaches. Other people hardly ever have them.

Causes

Although headaches can be painful and distressing, they are rarely due to a serious condition.

Primary Headache Disorders: Most headaches are not caused by another identifiable disorder. Such headaches are called primary headache disorders. They include

- Tension-type
- Migraine
- Cluster headaches

Tension-type headaches are the most common type of headache.

Secondary Headache Disorders: Less commonly, headaches result from another disorder. Such headaches are called secondary headache disorders. Usually, disorders that cause headaches are not serious.

These disorders often affect the eyes, nose, throat, sinuses, teeth, jaws, ears, or neck and are minor or temporary. For example, a dental infection, sinus infection (sinusitis), or a problem with the joint of the jaw (temporomandibular disorder) may cause a headache.

Rarely, headaches are caused by a serious disorder, including the following:

- Brain infections, such as abscess, meningitis, and encephalitis
- Other infections, such as tuberculosis, if they affect the brain
- Brain tumors
- Accumulation of blood in the tissues that cover the brain (subdural hematoma), often due to a head injury
- Bleeding in the brain (intracerebral hemorrhage)
- Bleeding in the tissues that cover the brain (subarachnoid hemorrhage), often due to rupture of a bulge in an artery (cerebral aneurysm) or of an abnormal connection between arteries and veins (arteriovenous malformation)

- Intracranial hypertension
- Very high blood pressure (rarely)
- Breathing disorders, such as emphysema and sleep apnea
- Giant cell (temporal) arteritis

Some of these disorders, such as brain tumors, hemorrhages, hematomas, and intracranial venous hypertension, increase pressure within the skull. In their early stages, many infections, including Lyme disease and Rocky Mountain spotted fever, can cause headaches, as can influenza if severe. These infections can be serious.

Headaches commonly result from withdrawal of caffeine, withdrawal of pain relievers (analgesics) after long-term use, and use of certain drugs that widen blood vessels (such as nitroglycerin).

 Did You Know...

Headaches rarely result from a serious disorder.

If people have a sudden, excruciating (thunderclap) headache, they should seek medical attention right away.

Diagnosis

Usually, doctors can determine the type or cause of headaches on the basis of the person's medical history, the characteristics of the headache, and the results of a physical examination. Doctors ask about the characteristics of the headache: frequency, duration, location, severity, and any symptoms that accompany it. Doctors also ask what triggers the headache, what makes it worse, and what relieves it.

The following characteristics may indicate that a serious disorder is the cause of headaches, and people who experience any of them should promptly seek medical attention.

- Headaches that are increasing in frequency or severity
- Daily headaches
- A very sudden, severe headache (thunderclap headache)
- Any change in the pattern or nature of headaches
- Headaches that begin after age 50
- Headaches accompanied by symptoms such as fever, a stiff neck, changes in sensation or vision, weakness, loss of coordination, fainting, or very high blood pressure
- Headaches that cause seizures or confusion

For example, a severe headache with a fever and a stiff neck suggests meningitis—a life-threatening infection of the layers of tissues covering the brain and spinal cord (meninges). A headache that occurs very suddenly and that is more severe than any others the person has experienced may suggest a subarachnoid hemorrhage—bleeding within the meninges, which is often due to a ruptured aneurysm.

Testing: When doctors suspect a serious disorder, diagnostic tests are usually done. If a tumor, a hemorrhage, or increased pressure within the skull is suspected, computed tomography (CT) or magnetic resonance imaging (MRI) is done immediately.

If meningitis is suspected, a spinal tap (lumbar puncture—see art on page 635) is done immediately. A spinal tap may also be done if doctors suspect a subarachnoid hemorrhage or encephalitis. If doctors think that a mass (such as a tumor or abscess) may be present, CT or MRI is done before the spinal tap to determine whether a spinal tap can be done safely. A spinal tap decreases pressure below the brain. If a mass is present, the brain may shift downward and be pressed through one of the small natural openings in the tissues that separate the brain into compartments—a life-threatening disorder called herniation.

Occasionally, blood tests are done to check for a disorder such as Lyme disease. The erythrocyte sedimentation rate (ESR—the rate at which red blood cells settle to the bottom of a test tube containing a blood sample) may be determined to check for giant cell arteritis, which causes inflammation. A high ESR suggests inflammation.

Tension-Type Headaches

A tension-type headache is usually mild to moderate pain that feels like a band tightening around the head.

- Pain in other parts of the head and neck may trigger these headaches.
- Headaches may occur several or many days each month.
- Doctors base the diagnosis on symptoms and results of a physical examination, but sometimes imaging tests are done to rule out other disorders.
- Pain relievers and some drugs used to treat migraines may help, as may relaxation and stress management.

Many people occasionally have tension-type headaches. The cause is not well understood but may be related to a lower-than-normal threshold for pain. Stress may be involved. However, how stress is involved is not clearly understood, and it is not the only explanation for the symptoms. Other problems may contribute to or trigger the headaches. For example, sleep disturbances, a problem with the joint of the jaw (temporomandibular joint disorder), neck pain, or eyestrain may trigger a tension-type headache.

HOW HEADACHES DIFFER

TYPE OR CAUSE	CHARACTERISTICS*	DIAGNOSTIC TESTS
Primary (not due to another disorder)		
Cluster	The pain is severe and piercing. It affects one side of the head and is focused around the eye. The pain lasts 30 minutes to about 1 hour. People with cluster headaches cannot lie down, frequently pace, and sometimes bang their heads. Headaches occur in clusters, separated by periods when no headaches occur. They are usually not worsened by light, sounds, or smells and are not accompanied by nausea and vomiting. On the same side as the pain, the nose runs, the eye tears, the eye lid droops, and the area below the eye may swell.	Tests are the same as those for tension-type headaches.
Migraine	The pain is moderate to severe. A pulsating or throbbing pain is felt on one side or sometimes on both sides of the head. The pain lasts several hours to days. Headaches may be worsened by physical activity, light, sounds, or smells and are accompanied by nausea, vomiting, and sensitivity to sounds, light, and odors. Attacks can occur for a long period of time, then disappear for weeks, months, or years. Often, people have a sensation that a migraine is beginning. This sensation (called a prodrome) may include mood changes, loss of appetite, and nausea. Attacks may be preceded by temporary disturbances in sensation, balance, muscle coordination, speech, or vision (such as seeing flashing lights and blind spots). These disturbances are called the aura.	Tests are the same as those for tension-type headaches.
Tension-type	The pain is usually mild to moderate. It feels like tightening of a band around the head and affects the whole head. The pain lasts 30 minutes to several days. It may be worse at the end of the day. Headaches are not worsened by physical activity, light, sounds, or smells and are not accompanied by nausea and vomiting.	CT or MRI of the head is occasionally done to rule out other disorders, particularly if the headaches have developed recently or if the symptom pattern has changed.
Secondary (due to another disorder)		
Brain abscess	The pain is similar to that caused by a brain tumor. However, if an abscess ruptures, acute meningitis results, causing an intense headache and a stiff neck.	MRI or CT is done.
Brain tumor	Pain is mild to severe and may become progressively worse. It usually recurs more and more often and eventually becomes constant without relief. People often become clumsy, weak, or confused. They may vomit or have seizures.	MRI is done.
Encephalitis	Encephalitis (infection of the brain) can cause headaches. People may also have a fever. They may become very drowsy, clumsy, weak, or confused. They may vomit or have seizures. Coma can develop. Some people also have meningitis.	MRI or CT and a spinal tap are done.
Eye disorders (such as iritis, glaucoma, and papillitis)	The pain is moderate or severe and is often worse after using the eyes. It is felt at the front of the head or in or over the eyes. Vision is impaired.	An eye examination is done.

(continued on the following page)

HOW HEADACHES DIFFER (*Continued*)

TYPE OR CAUSE	CHARACTERISTICS*	DIAGNOSTIC TESTS
Giant cell (temporal) arteritis	A throbbing pain is felt on one side of the head at the temple. The scalp hurts when the hair is combed, and chewing hurts. The arteries in the temples may be enlarged. Aches and pains may occur, particularly in the shoulders, thighs, and hips. Vision may be lost.	The erythrocyte sedimentation rate (ESR) is determined, and a biopsy of the temporal artery is done.
High blood pressure (hypertension)	Extremely high blood pressure can cause headaches. The pain is throbbing, occurs in spasms, and is felt at the back or top of the head. Usually, high blood pressure does not cause headaches.	Blood pressure is measured, and blood tests and kidney function tests are done.
Intracerebral hemorrhage	The pain may be mild or severe and occurs on one or both sides. People may become very drowsy, clumsy, weak, or confused. They may vomit or have seizures. Coma can develop.	CT or MRI is done.
Meningitis	The pain is severe and constant and is felt over the whole head. It travels down the neck, making bending the neck to rest the chin on the chest difficult. People feel ill, have a fever, and vomit.	Blood tests and a spinal tap are done.
Sinus disorders	The pain is severe and may be dull or sharp. It is felt at the front of the head. It may begin suddenly and last only a short time, or it may begin gradually and be persistent. It is usually worse in the morning and less severe in the afternoon. Cold, damp weather and lying down make the pain worse. People have a runny nose, sometimes with pus or blood. They feel ill, may cough at night, and often have a fever.	CT of the sinuses or endoscopy of the nose may be done.
Subarachnoid hemorrhage	The pain is severe, constant, and widespread. It may reach its peak intensity within a few seconds. Occasionally, it is felt in and around one eye. The eyelid droops. People often describe the headache as the worst ever experienced. They may briefly lose consciousness. Some people are sleepy, confused, and hard to rouse. Others are restless. Later, the neck may become stiff, with a continuing headache and often with vomiting, dizziness, and low back pain.	MRI or CT is done. If the results are negative, a spinal tap is done.
Subdural hematoma	The pain is mild to severe and intermittent or constant. It can be felt in one spot or over the whole head and travels down the neck. People may feel sleepy or become confused or forgetful.	MRI or CT is done.
Other disorders if they affect the brain (such as cancer, cryptococcosis, sarcoidosis, syphilis, and tuberculosis)	The pain may be mild or severe and dull or sharp. It is felt over the whole head. People whose headache is caused by one of these disorders have a moderate fever and other symptoms of the disorder.	A spinal tap and MRI are done.

*One, some, or all of the characteristics listed may be present.
CT = computed tomography; MRI = magnetic resonance imaging.

Symptoms

Tension-type headaches feel like tightening of a band around the head, making the whole head ache. These headaches may be episodic or chronic.

Episodic headaches occur fewer than 15 days a month. The pain is usually mild to moderate. It may last 30 minutes to several days. These headaches typically start several hours after waking and worsen as the day progresses. They rarely awaken people from sleep.

Chronic headaches occur more than 15 days a month. Severity tends to increase as more headaches occur. The pain may vary in intensity throughout the day but is almost always present.

Unlike migraine headaches, tension-type headaches are not accompanied by nausea and vomiting and are not made worse by physical activity, light, sounds, or smells.

Some mild migraines resemble tension-type headaches.

Diagnosis

The diagnosis is based on the person's description of the headache and the results of a physical examination. Doctors ask the person about problems that may trigger the headaches.

No specific procedures can confirm the diagnosis. Sometimes computed tomography (CT) or magnetic resonance imaging (MRI) of the head is done to rule out other disorders that may be causing the headache, particularly if headaches have developed recently.

Treatment

For most mild to moderate tension-type headaches, almost any over-the-counter pain reliever (analgesic), such as aspirin, acetaminophen, or ibuprofen, can provide relief. Massaging the affected area may help relieve the pain. Most people with mild to moderate episodic headaches do not go to a health care practitioner.

Severe headaches may require stronger, prescription analgesics. Some contain opioids (narcotics), such as codeine or oxycodone (see page 642).

For some people, caffeine, an ingredient of some headache preparations, enhances the effect of analgesics. However, overuse of analgesics, caffeine (in headache preparations or caffeinated beverages), or opioids can lead to daily headaches. Such headaches, called medication overuse headaches, begin or worsen when these drugs are suddenly stopped.

If tension-type headaches are chronic, some drugs used to prevent migraine, particularly amitriptyline (a tricyclic antidepressant), can help.

Behavioral and psychologic interventions, such as relaxation and stress management techniques, may help.

Migraines

A migraine headache is a pulsating or throbbing pain that usually ranges from moderate to severe. It can affect one or both sides of the head. It is worsened by physical activity, light, sounds, or smells and is accompanied by nausea, vomiting, and sensitivity to sounds and light.

- Migraines may be triggered by lack of sleep, changes in the weather, hunger, excessive stimulation of the senses, stress, or other factors.
- Doctors base the diagnosis on typical symptoms.
- There is no cure for migraines, but drugs to stop the progression of migraines, pain relievers (analgesics), and drugs to prevent migraines can help control them.

Although migraines can start at any age, they usually begin during puberty or young adulthood. In most people, migraines recur periodically (fewer than 15 days a month). After age 50, headaches usually become significantly less severe or resolve entirely. Migraines are 3 times more common among women. In the United States, about 18% of women and 6% of men have a migraine at some time each year.

Migraine may become chronic. That is, headaches occur more than 15 days a month. These headaches often develop in people who overuse drugs to treat migraines.

Migraines tend to run in families. More than half the people who have migraines have close relatives who also have them.

Causes

Migraines occur in people whose nervous system is more sensitive than that of other people. That is, nerve cells in the brain are easily stimulated, producing electrical activity. As electrical activity spreads over the brain, various functions, such as vision, sensation, balance, muscle coordination, and speech are temporarily disturbed. These disturbances cause the symptoms that occur before the headache (called the aura). The headache occurs when the 5th cranial (trigeminal) nerve is stimulated. This nerve sends impulses (including pain impulses) from the eyes, scalp, forehead, upper eyelids, mouth, and jaw to the brain. When stimulated, the nerve may release substances that cause painful inflammation in the blood vessels of the brain (cerebral blood vessels) and the layers of tissues that cover the brain (meninges). The inflammation accounts for the throbbing headache, nausea, vomiting, and sensitivity to light and sound.

A rare subtype of migraine called familial hemiplegic migraine is associated with genetic defects on chromosomes 1, 2, and 19. The role of genes in the more common forms of migraine is under study.

Estrogen, the main female hormone, appears to trigger migraines, possibly explaining why migraines are more common among women. During puberty (when estrogen levels increase), migraines become much more common among girls than among boys. Some women have migraines just before, during, or just after menstrual periods. As menopause approaches (when estrogen levels are fluctuating), migraines become particularly difficult to control. Oral contraceptives (which contain estrogen) and estrogen therapy may make migraines worse and may increase the risk of stroke in women who have migraines with an aura. Other triggers include the following:

- Lack of sleep, including insomnia
- Changes in the weather, particularly barometric pressure
- Red wine
- Certain foods
- Hunger (as when meals are skipped)
- Excessive stimulation of the senses (for example, by flashing lights or strong odors)
- Stress

Head injuries, neck pain, or a problem with the joint of the jaw (temporomandibular joint disorder) sometimes trigger or worsen migraines.

Symptoms

In a migraine, pulsating or throbbing pain is usually felt on one side of the head, but it may occur on both sides. The pain may be moderate but is often severe and incapacitating. Physical activity, light, sounds, or smells may make the headache worse. This increased sensitivity makes many people retreat to a dark, quiet room and lie down until the headache subsides. The headache is often accompanied by nausea, sometimes with vomiting. Severe attacks can be incapacitating, disrupting family and work life.

People often have sensations warning them that an attack is about to begin. These sensations, called the prodrome, may include mood changes, loss of appetite, and nausea.

In about 25% of people, migraines are preceded by an aura. The aura involves temporary, reversible disturbances in vision, sensation, balance, muscle coordination, or speech. People may see jagged, shimmering, or flashing lights or develop a blind spot with flickering edges. Less commonly, people experience tingling sensations, loss of balance, weakness in an arm or a leg, or difficulty talking. The aura lasts minutes to an hour before and may continue after the headache begins. Some people experience an aura but have only a mild or no headache. These mild headaches are similar to tension-type headaches.

Migraine attacks may last for hours to a few days (typically 4 hours to 3 days). Usually, they subside during sleep. They may occur frequently for a long time, then disappear for many weeks, months, or even years.

> ### Did You Know...
> Only 1/4 of people have sensations that warn them that a migraine is about to begin.
>
> Taking pain relievers too often can make migraines worse.

Diagnosis

Doctors diagnose migraines when symptoms are typical and results of a physical examination (which includes a neurologic examination) are normal.

No procedure can confirm the diagnosis. If headaches have developed recently or if the pattern of symptoms has changed, computed tomography (CT) or magnetic resonance imaging (MRI) of the head may be done to exclude other disorders. For example, an imaging test may be done to check for stroke in older people who have migraines with an aura, especially when the migraine is mild or does not occur.

Prevention

When treatment does not prevent people from having frequent or incapacitating migraines, taking drugs every day to prevent migraine attacks helps. Taking preventive drugs may help people who are taking other migraine drugs too often and who need to reduce their use.

Beta-blockers, such as propranolol, are often used. The anticonvulsants topiramate and divalproex and the tricyclic antidepressant amitriptyline are also effective. The choice of a preventive drug is based on the side effects of the drug and on other disorders present. For example, people who are overweight may be given topiramate, which can promote weight loss. People with depression or insomnia may be given amitriptyline (see table on page 868).

Treatment

Migraines cannot be cured, but they can be controlled.

Doctors encourage people to keep a headache diary. In it, people write down the number and timing of attacks, possible triggers, and their response to treatment. With this information, triggers may be identified and eliminated when possible, and doctors can better plan and adjust treatment. Behavioral interventions (such as relaxation, biofeedback, and stress management) are used to control migraine attacks, especially when stress is a trigger or when people are taking too many drugs to control the migraines.

℞ DRUGS USED TO TREAT MIGRAINES

TYPE	EXAMPLES	SOME SIDE EFFECTS
Prevention		
Anticonvulsants	Divalproex Topiramate	Hair loss, stomach upset, liver dysfunction, a tendency to bleed, tremors, and weight gain (see table on page 716) With topiramate, weight loss, confusion, and depression
Beta-blockers	Atenolol Metoprolol Nadolol Propranolol Timolol	Spasm of the airways (bronchospasm), fatigue, insomnia, worsening of heart failure, and sexual dysfunction With some beta-blockers, unfavorable effects on lipid (fat) levels (see table on page 340)
Calcium channel blockers	Verapamil	Dizziness, low blood pressure, and weakness With verapamil, constipation (see table on page 341)
Tricyclic antidepressants	Amitriptyline	Drowsiness, weight gain, increased heart rate, dry mouth, confusion, and constipation (see table on page 868)
Treatment of severe migraines		
Antiemetic drugs	Metoclopramide Prochlorperazine	Low blood pressure, drowsiness, and muscle spasms
Ergot derivatives	Dihydroergotamine	Nausea, vomiting, minor muscle cramping, and, rarely, chest pain due to an inadequate blood supply to the heart muscle (angina)
Triptans (5-hydroxytryptamine [5-HT] agonists)	Almotriptan Eletriptan Naratriptan Rizatriptan Sumatriptan Zolmitriptan	Flushing, tingling, dizziness, drowsiness, nausea, a sense of pressure in the throat or chest, and, rarely, angina
Opioids	Codeine Meperidine Oxycodone	Slowing of breathing, constipation, retention of urine, drowsiness, and nausea (see table on page 643)
Treatment of mild to moderate migraines		
Analgesic	Acetaminophen	Rebound headache if the dose is increased and, occasionally, skin rash
Nonsteroidal anti-inflammatory drugs (NSAIDs)	Aspirin Indomethacin Naproxen	Worsening of headache if the dose is increased and later suddenly decreased. With indomethacin, worsening of depression, seizures, and tremors with decreased mobility and muscle stiffness and, in older people, dizziness and confusion

Some drugs stop a migraine from progressing. Some are taken to control the pain. Others are taken to prevent migraines.

When migraines are or become severe, drugs that can stop the migraine from progressing are used. They are taken as soon as people sense a migraine is beginning. They include the following:

- **Triptans** (5-hydroxytryptamine [5-HT], or serotonin, agonists) are usually used. Triptans specifically target the receptors that stimulate nerves supplying the meninges and cerebral blood vessels, where migraine symptoms originate. These drugs are most effective when taken as soon as the migraine begins.

They may be taken by mouth, inhaled, or injected under the skin.

- **Dihydroergotamine** is used to stop severe, persistent migraines.
- **Prochlorperazine**, an antiemetic, may be used when people cannot tolerate triptans or dihydroergotamine.

Because triptans and dihydroergotamine cause blood vessels to narrow (constrict), they are not recommended for people who have angina, coronary artery disease, or uncontrolled high blood pressure. If older people or people with risk factors for coronary artery disease need to take these drugs, they must be monitored closely.

If migraines are usually accompanied by nausea, a drug to relieve nausea (antiemetic) may also be taken. Antiemetics alone may stop mild or moderate migraines from progressing.

For less severe migraines, analgesics with or without caffeine can be useful. They can be taken as needed during a migraine, with or instead of a triptan.

Overuse of analgesics, caffeine (in analgesic preparations or in caffeinated beverages), or triptans can lead to daily, more severe migraines. Such headaches, called medication overuse headaches, occur when these drugs are taken more than 2 to 3 days each week. Missing or reducing a dose or taking it late may trigger or worsen a migraine.

When other treatments are ineffective in people with severe migraines, opioids may be needed (see page 643). Opioids are a last resort.

Cluster Headaches

A cluster headache causes severe pain that is felt at the temple or around the eye on one side of the head and that lasts a relatively short time (usually 30 minutes to 1 hour). Headaches usually occur regularly during a 1- to 3-month period, followed by a headache-free period of months to years.

- Excruciating pain occurs one side of the head, causing the nostril and the eye on that side to water.
- People are often restless and pace.
- Doctors base the diagnosis on symptoms.
- Oxygen, given by a face mask, or drugs are needed to treat headaches.

Cluster headaches are relatively rare, affecting about 1 to 4 of 1,000 people. Cluster headaches affect mostly men. They typically begin between the ages of 20 and 40. Drinking alcohol may trigger attacks.

Symptoms

An attack almost always starts suddenly. It may begin with itching of or a watery discharge from one nostril. Excruciating pain on the same side of the head follows and spreads around the eye. The pain reaches peak intensity within minutes and usually lasts 30 minutes to 1 hour. The pain often awakens people from sleep. People with cluster headaches, unlike those with a migraine, cannot lie down, frequently pace, and sometimes bang their heads.

After the attack, the eyelid on the same side as the headache may droop, and the pupil often constricts. The area below the eye may swell, and the eye may water. The face may be flushed. Nausea may accompany the headaches.

Attacks may occur several times a day. They usually occur regularly during a 1- to 3-month period (cluster period), occasionally longer, followed by a headache-free period of several months or even years before they recur. They usually recur at the same time of day or night. Some people do not have a headache-free interval. They have chronic cluster headaches.

Diagnosis

Diagnosis is based on the person's description of the headache and the accompanying symptoms. If the pattern of symptoms changes, magnetic resonance imaging (MRI) of the head may be done.

Treatment

Most people with cluster headaches need to take drugs to prevent recurrences. The following may be used to stop (abort) a cluster headache as it is beginning:

- Oxygen given by face mask
- A triptan or dihydroergotamine given by injection (see table on page 654)

Other drugs are given to prevent headaches:

- Prednisone, a corticosteroid given by mouth
- A local anesthetic plus a corticosteroid given by injection into the back of the head (a procedure called a nerve block)
- Drugs used to prevent migraines (such as topiramate, valproate, and verapamil)
- Lithium

Prednisone or the nerve block may be used first because they take effect more quickly. Then one of the other drugs is used for long-term prevention. Oxygen and injections of dihydroergotamine or a local anesthetic plus a corticosteroid must be given in the hospital. The other treatments can be taken at home.

Idiopathic Intracranial Hypertension

Idiopathic intracranial hypertension (benign intracranial hypertension, pseudotumor cerebri) involves increased pressure within the skull (intracranial pressure), without any evidence of a cause.

- People have daily headaches, sometimes with nausea, blurred or double vision, and noises within the skull.
- Imaging of the head is done to rule out possible causes of increased pressure, and a spinal tap is done.
- Without prompt treatment, vision can be lost.
- Weight loss, diuretics to reduce fluids in the brain, and spinal taps done periodically to reduce the pressure can help, but surgery is sometimes needed.

Idiopathic intracranial hypertension occurs in only about 1 of 100,000 people, usually in women during their reproductive years. However, among young overweight women, it is 20 times more common. As more and more people are becoming overweight, the disorder is becoming more common.

Pressure in the skull may be high in some cases because the large veins (venous sinuses) that carry blood from the brain are blocked. These changes cause blood to back up in the veins, including those that carry blood from the skull. The increased pressure does not result from tumors, infections, or blockages that prevent the fluid that surrounds the brain (cerebrospinal fluid) from draining as it normally does.

In most people, the development of idiopathic intracranial hypertension cannot be traced to any particular event. In children, this disorder sometimes develops after corticosteroids are stopped or after a child has taken large amounts of vitamin A or the antibiotic tetracycline.

Symptoms

Idiopathic intracranial hypertension usually begins with a daily or almost daily headache. At first, the headache may be mild, but it varies in intensity and may become severe. The headache may be accompanied by nausea, double or blurred vision, and pulsating noises within the skull (tinnitus). A few people do not have any symptoms.

Increased pressure within the skull may cause the optic nerve to swell near the eyeball—a condition called papilledema. Doctors can observe the swelling by looking at the back of the eye through an ophthalmoscope.

The first sign of vision problems is loss of the peripheral (side) vision. As a result, people may bump into objects for no apparent reason. Late in the disorder, vision becomes blurred. About 5% of people lose their vision, partially or completely, in one or both eyes. Once vision is lost, it may never return, even if the pressure around the brain is relieved. In some people, the disorder becomes chronic and progressively worse, increasing the risk of blindness. However, close monitoring of such people can prevent loss of vision.

The disorder recurs in about 10% of people.

Diagnosis

Doctors suspect this disorder based on symptoms and results of a physical examination. Sometimes doctors suspect it when they detect papilledema during a routine examination with an ophthalmoscope.

Then an imaging test, usually magnetic resonance imaging (MRI), is done to check for other possible causes of increased pressure within the skull. One type of MRI (called magnetic resonance venography) can provide images of the veins that carry blood from the brain. It enables doctors to determine whether these veins are narrowed. If results are normal, a spinal tap (lumbar puncture) is done to measure the pressure of the cerebrospinal fluid and to analyze the fluid. In idiopathic intracranial hypertension, the pressure of the fluid is usually increased, and the content is usually normal.

Treatment

Idiopathic intracranial hypertension often disappears without treatment within 6 months. Nonetheless, overweight people should lose weight because doing so reduces pressure within the skull. The disorder may resolve when as little as 10% or 20% of body weight is lost. However, weight reduction programs are often unsuccessful.

Drugs known to trigger the disorder, such as tetracycline, should be stopped.

Aspirin, acetaminophen, or drugs used to treat migraines may relieve the headache. Doctors may prescribe acetazolamide to help reduce the pressure. This drug is a diuretic, which helps the kidneys eliminate water in urine and thus decrease the amount of fluid in the body, including the brain.

The usefulness of doing spinal taps daily or weekly to remove cerebrospinal fluid is debated. If this treatment is used, people are closely monitored to determine whether pressure is decreasing.

People are closely monitored by an ophthalmologist so that vision problems can be recognized as soon as possible.

If vision deteriorates despite these measures, surgery to reduce pressure within the skull may be needed and may be able to save vision. In one procedure (called optic nerve sheath fenestration), slits are cut in the covering of the optic nerve behind the eyeball. These slits allow cerebrospinal fluid to escape into the tissues around the eye, where the fluid passes into veins. Alternatively, a permanent drain (shunt) can be surgically placed so that excess cerebrospinal fluid can be removed. The shunt is a piece of plastic tubing placed in the spaces within the brain or in the space just below the spinal cord in the lower back. The tubing is run under the skin, usually to the abdomen, where excess fluid can drain.

If magnetic resonance venography detects a blockage in a vein, a tube made of wire mesh (stent) may be inserted through an incision into a vein in the neck and placed in the blocked vein to hold it open.

If people are obese and other measures are ineffective, surgery to help with weight reduction (bariatric surgery, such as a gastric bypass—see page 956) may be done. If successful, it may cure the disorder.

Low-Pressure Headache

Low-pressure headaches result when cerebrospinal fluid is removed during a spinal tap (lumbar puncture) or leaks out because of a cyst or tear. Loss of this fluid, which flows around the brain, reduces pressure around the brain.

A headache commonly occurs after a spinal tap, usually hours to a day or two afterward. The procedure removes some cerebrospinal fluid. Cerebrospinal fluid flows through a channel between layers of tissue (meninges) that cover the brain and spinal cord and fills spaces within the brain. Removal of some cerebrospinal fluid reduces pressure around the brain, causing headaches, which can be severe. Young, small people are most likely to be affected.

Sometimes cerebrospinal fluid leaks because a cyst in the meninges bursts or the meninges are torn (as can occur when the head or face is injured). Rarely, a cyst may burst when people cough or sneeze.

Low-pressure headaches are intense. They occur when people sit or stand and may be relieved by lying flat. People usually also have a stiff, painful neck and may vomit.

Diagnosis

Doctors base the diagnosis on the symptoms and the situation. If people have had a spinal tap, the diagnosis is usually obvious, and testing is rarely needed. If not, imaging tests, such as magnetic resonance imaging (MRI), may be done.

Treatment

Doctors advise people who have had a spinal tap to lie flat. They are given fluids (by mouth or, if very dehydrated, intravenously), mild analgesics, and caffeine. An elastic binder may be wrapped around their abdomen. It can help increase pressure of the fluid around the brain. If the headache persists after a day of such treatment, a small amount of the person's blood can be injected in the space between the spine and the meninges in the lower back. This procedure is called an epidural blood patch. The blood plugs the hole made by the spinal tap.

A blood patch may also be effective for a leak. Surgery for a leak is rarely required.

CHAPTER

108 Dizziness and Vertigo

Dizziness is a vague term used to describe various sensations, including faintness, light-headedness, a loss of balance, a sense of spinning, a vague spaced-out feeling, and weakness. Vertigo is a specific type of dizziness. In vertigo, people feel as if they or their surroundings are moving or spinning.

Dizziness

- Dizziness may result from a disorder that affects any of the many body parts involved in balance (such as the inner ear and eyes) or from certain drugs.
- The person's description of the problem and the results of a physical examination may suggest a cause, which may lead to additional tests.
- Treatment depends on the cause and may include treatment to relieve accompanying symptoms.

Dizziness accounts for about 5 to 6% of visits to the doctor. It may occur at any age but becomes more

common as people age. It affects about 40% of people older than 40 at some time. At any age, dizziness can cause problems, particularly when doing an exacting or a dangerous task, such as driving or operating heavy machinery. People who have dizziness that persists or interferes with daily activities should see a doctor.

Doctors usually classify dizziness as

- Faintness or light-headedness
- Loss of balance
- Vertigo
- A mixture of these types
- None of these types

Dizziness may be temporary or chronic. Dizziness is considered chronic if it lasts more than a month. Chronic dizziness is more common among older people. Chronic dizziness is often difficult to classify because it often involves more than one cause and because it seems different at different times—for example, like light-headedness one time and like vertigo the next.

Did You Know...

About 95% of the time, dizziness, even if incapacitating, does not result from a serious disorder.

In older people, dizziness often does not have a single, obvious cause.

Causes

Although dizziness may be disturbing and even incapacitating, only about 5% of cases result from a serious disorder. Dizziness has many causes because many body parts work together to maintain balance. They include the inner ear, the eyes (which provide visual cues needed to maintain balance), muscles and joints, the brain (mainly the brain stem and cerebellum), and the nerves that connect all of the parts.

Each type of dizziness tends to have characteristic causes. For example, faintness and light-headedness may result from a sudden fall in blood pressure (see page 343) or from other disorders that result in an inadequate blood supply to the brain. In these disorders, the heart may be unable to pump enough to the brain, or the arteries to the brain may be blocked or narrowed.

Loss of balance may result from vision disturbances because the body depends on visual cues to maintain balance. Loss of balance may also result from musculoskeletal disorders, which cause muscle weakness and thus interfere with walking. Other causes include use of certain drugs (such as anticonvulsants and sedatives) and disorders of the inner ear.

Diagnosis

Before dizziness can be treated, doctors must determine its nature and its cause. Doctors ask the person to describe in detail the sensations felt: whether the feeling during the episode was faintness, light-headedness, loss of balance, spinning or movement of self or the surroundings (vertigo), or another sensation. The person is asked when the dizziness began, how long it lasted, what triggered or relieved it, and what other symptoms—headaches, deafness, noise in the ears (tinnitus), impaired vision, weakness, or difficulty walking—were present. Such details help pinpoint the nature of the dizziness and may suggest a cause.

One of a doctor's chief aims when performing the physical examination is to reproduce (provoke) the symptoms. A drop in blood pressure on standing up (orthostatic hypotension) is one of the most common causes of dizziness. Therefore, doctors try to provoke the fall in blood pressure by changing the person's position and seeing whether the symptoms develop when the blood pressure changes. Doctors measure blood pressure and pulse after the person has been lying down for 5 to 10 minutes, then after sitting, and again after standing up. A tilt table (see page 328) enables the doctor to perform the test more rigorously. Changes in blood pressure may be caused by dehydration, so doctors look for signs of dehydration and order laboratory tests.

The person may be asked to perform a Valsalva maneuver (breathing out vigorously against a closed mouth as if straining at stool). Such a maneuver temporarily slows the heart rate, which may reproduce the dizziness. Electrocardiography (ECG), Holter monitoring for heart rhythm abnormalities, echocardiography, and exercise stress testing may also be done to evaluate heart function.

Several tests can be used to evaluate balance and gait (see page 633), such as the Romberg test. Another test of balance has the person walking a straight line with one foot behind the other.

Vision tests are done, and the eyes may be checked for abnormal movements (such as nystagmus—(see page 662). If doctors suspect vertigo, they perform special tests to provoke the symptoms (see page 662). In addition, hearing tests can be used to detect inner ear disorders that affect both balance and hearing.

Additional diagnostic procedures may include computed tomography (CT) and magnetic resonance imaging (MRI) of the head. These procedures are especially useful if doctors suspect that the blood supply to the brain is inadequate and causing stroke-like symptoms. In addition, CT angiography, magnetic resonance angiography (MRA), or cerebral angiography (also called catheter angiography because a catheter is introduced into an artery) may show whether arteries to the brain are narrowed or blocked. CT angiography and MRA are not invasive and are generally preferred to cerebral angiography.

When other diagnostic possibilities appear unlikely or no obvious cause of dizziness is found, the doctor may inquire about a possible psychologic cause. Several tests can help doctors identify depression, somatization disorders, and other psychologic problems that may predispose the person to giddiness or a feeling of disassociation from the world. If no cause is identified, doctors reexamine the person periodically.

Treatment

Specific treatment depends on the cause identified. Getting sufficient fluids often improves orthostatic hypotension resulting from dehydration. Drugs

CLASSIFYING DIZZINESS

TYPE	DESCRIPTION	SOME POSSIBLE CAUSES
Faintness	The person feels about to black out when upright. Blood pressure drops when the person stands (orthostatic hypotension).	Dehydration Severe blood loss Blocked outflow from the heart (aortic valve stenosis) Abnormal heart rhythms Overmedicated (especially with drugs used for blood pressure control) An autonomic nervous system disorder (such as diabetic autonomic neuropathy or multiple system atrophy)
Loss of balance	The person feels unsteady and about to fall even though muscle strength is normal.	Inner ear disorders (vertigo) Cerebellar disorders (such as ataxia due to stroke or chronic alcoholism) Basal ganglia disorders (such as Parkinson's disease, Lewy body dementia, or progressive supranuclear palsy) Loss of position sense in the legs (as occurs in neuropathy or spinal cord disease) Visual disturbances (for example, caused by new glasses, double vision, or cataract surgery) Overmedication with sedatives, anticonvulsants, or other drugs Intoxication with alcohol
Vertigo	The person or the person's surroundings seem to be moving or spinning.	Benign paroxysmal positional vertigo (BPPV) Vestibular neuritis Meniere's disease Middle ear infections Migraine Motion sickness Reduced blood supply to the brain stem and cerebellum (vertebrobasilar insufficiency), as occurs during a stroke or transient ischemic attack (TIA) Multiple sclerosis Drugs toxic to the inner ear, such as aminoglycoside antibiotics, aspirin, chloroquine, cisplatin (a chemotherapy drug), furosemide (a diuretic), and quinine
Vaguely light-headed	The person feels giddy, detached from the world, or caught in a panic attack.	Abnormally rapid, deep breathing (hyperventilation with a panic attack) Anxiety disorders Depression with a feeling of disassociation from the world

(such as mineralocorticoids and midodrine) may be needed for people with orthostatic hypotension due to dysfunction of the autonomic nervous system. If the cause of dizziness is a drug, the drug is stopped or the dose reduced. Benign paroxysmal positional vertigo (BPPV) can often be relieved by a simple head-turning maneuver (Epley maneuver) done in the doctor's office (see art on page 664). If doctors suspect the symptoms are stroke-like, then risk factors are treated, such as giving antiplatelet drugs and possibly bypassing or placing a stent in a blocked artery.

Regardless of whether a cause is identified, drugs may be given to relieve accompanying symptoms (such as nausea) or to prevent blood pressure from falling.

Vertigo

Vertigo is a false sensation that the self, the surroundings, or both are moving or spinning, usually accompanied by nausea and loss of balance.

- Vertigo results from disorders that affect the inner ear or parts of the brain involved in balance.
- In addition to a sense of spinning, people may have nausea, loss of balance, hearing or vision problems, and headaches.
- Doctors can often diagnose the cause based on the person's description of the problem and results of a physical examination, but other tests are sometimes needed.
- Sometimes taking simple precautions, based on what triggers vertigo, or a drug can prevent vertigo.
- Drugs, such as the scopolamine patch, can help relieve the vertigo and nausea.

Vertigo, a type of dizziness, resembles the feeling produced by the childhood game of spinning round and round, then suddenly stopping and watching the surroundings spin. Most cases of dizziness are not vertigo.

Causes

Vertigo can be caused by disorders of body parts that are involved in maintaining balance:

- Inner ear (see page 1387)
- Brain stem and cerebellum
- Nerve tracts connecting the brain stem and cerebellum or within the brain stem

The inner ear contains structures (the semicircular canals, saccule, and utricle) that enable the body to sense position and motion. Information from these structures is sent to the brain through the vestibulocochlear nerve (8th cranial nerve, which is also involved in hearing). This information is processed in the brain stem, which adjusts posture, and the cerebellum, which coordinates movements, to provide a sense of balance.

Inner Ear Disorders: Most commonly, vertigo results from motion sickness. Motion sickness may develop in people whose inner ear is sensitive to particular motions, such as swaying or sudden stopping and starting.

Another common cause of vertigo is an abnormal collection of calcium particles in one semicircular canal of the inner ear. The resulting disorder, called benign paroxysmal positional vertigo, or BPPV, is especially common among older people. It occurs when the head is moved in certain ways.

Meniere's disease produces attacks of vertigo. The cause of Meniere's disease is thought to involve excess fluid in the inner ear (hydrops). What triggers this is unknown, but it may result from an autoimmune reaction, an allergy, an imbalance in the autonomic nervous system, a blockage to certain structures in the ear, or a viral infection.

Disorders of the vestibulocochlear nerve can cause vertigo, a hearing disorder, or both.

Other disorders that may cause vertigo by affecting the inner ear or its nerve connections include the following:

- Bacterial or viral infections, such as vestibular neuritis, herpes zoster, and mastoiditis
- Paget's disease
- Tumors, such as an auditory nerve tumor
- Inflammation of nerves

The inner ear may also be damaged by drugs, such as aminoglycoside antibiotics, aspirin, the chemotherapy drug cisplatin, the sedative phenobarbital, the anticonvulsant phenytoin, the antipsychotic chlorpromazine, and certain diuretics including furosemide. Excessive use of alcohol can cause temporary vertigo.

Disorders That Affect the Brain: A decrease in the blood supply through arteries to the brain stem, cerebellum, and back of the brain can cause vertigo. This decrease is called vertebrobasilar insufficiency because the arteries affected include the vertebral and basilar arteries. If the decreased blood supply causes temporary symptoms, a transient ischemic attack (TIA) is diagnosed. If permanent damage results, a stroke is diagnosed.

Less common disorders that cause vertigo by affecting the brain stem or cerebellum include multiple sclerosis, fractures at the base of the skull, head injuries, seizures, infections, and tumors growing in or near the base of the brain. Vertigo can sometimes be part of a migraine attack and occasionally occur without the headache.

Occasionally, vertigo is caused by disorders that suddenly increase pressure within the skull, putting pressure on the brain. These disorders include benign intracranial hypertension, brain tumors, and bleeding (hemorrhage) within the skull.

> **?** **Did You Know...**
>
> In many instances, not taking drugs to relieve vertigo is better than taking them.

Symptoms

People with vertigo have an unusual and uncomfortable sense that they, their environment, or both are spinning around. Occasionally, the person feels simply pulled to one side. The resulting loss of balance makes walking and driving difficult. Vertigo is often accompanied by the following:

- Nystagmus (the rapid jerking movement of the eyes in one direction alternating with a slower drift back

SPOTLIGHT ON AGING

As people age, some of the body parts involved in balance function less well. For example, seeing in dim light becomes more difficult, and structures in the inner ear deteriorate. The mechanisms that control blood pressure become less responsive to changes in the body's need for blood. As a result, blood pressure may fall when a person stands (causing orthostatic hypotension—see page 348) or after a meal is eaten (causing postprandial hypotension—see page 349), and the person feels faint. Usually, dizziness does not result from age-related changes alone. It is more likely to occur if a person has a disorder or takes a drug that contributes to dizziness.

Disorders that can contribute to dizziness (such as heart disorders and stroke) are more common among older people. So is pain from arthritis that affects the lower back, hips, and knees and limits walking. Older people may feel or fear being abandoned just when they are also losing their independence. Depression may cause apathy and a feeling of disassociation from the world. Also, people who are depressed often lose interest in many activities. Inactivity, regardless of cause, can accelerate osteoporosis and muscle weakness from disuse. Then, people may feel weak, unsteady, faint, and anxious when attempting to walk, fearing falls and hip fracture.

Older people are more likely to take drugs that can contribute to dizziness. These drugs include those used to treat high blood pressure, chest pain (angina), heart failure, seizures, or anxiety, as well as certain antibiotics, antihistamines, and sleep aids. Some antihistamines (such as meclizine) are used to treat vertigo. They are more likely to have side effects in older people. Thus, whenever possible, older people should avoid taking these drugs, as well as over-the-counter antihistamines and sleep aids.

Two disorders of the inner ear are common causes of dizziness in older people: benign paroxysmal positional vertigo (see page 663) and Meniere's disease (see page 1391).

In older people, chronic dizziness increases the risk of falling and fractures and decreases the ability to do daily activities. Chronic dizziness often has many causes and is thus hard to treat. When an examination does not suggest a single cause, doctors try to correct as many factors that can contribute to dizziness as possible.

If dizziness persists despite treatment, people can learn strategies to help them function better, such as the following:

- Avoiding movements that, for them, trigger dizziness, such as looking up or bending down
- Storing items at levels that are easy to reach
- Getting up slowly after sitting or lying down
- Clenching their hands and flexing their feet before standing
- Learning exercises that combine eye, head, and body movements to help prevent dizziness
- Doing physical therapy and exercises to strengthen muscles and maintain independent gait as long as possible

to the original position), which occurs repeatedly during an episode of vertigo

- Nausea, sometimes with vomiting

Vertigo may last for only a few moments or may continue for hours or even days. People who have vertigo sometimes feel better when lying down or sitting still. However, vertigo may continue even when they are not moving at all. Symptoms from an inner ear cause (for example, BPPV, Meniere's disease, or vestibular neuritis) typically improve over days to weeks, whereas symptoms caused by a disorder of the central nervous system (for example, stroke or multiple sclerosis) require weeks to months to improve.

People with Meniere's disease may have sudden, episodic attacks of vertigo. Other symptoms include the following:

- Noise in the ears (tinnitus)
- Progressive hearing loss (usually low frequency or bass sounds)
- A sense of fullness or pressure in the affected ear
- Often, severe nausea and vomiting

Episodes usually last from several minutes to several hours. At first, hearing returns to normal, but as the disease continues, hearing loss persists and worsens.

In people with a viral infection of the inner ear (vestibular neuritis), vertigo usually begins suddenly and worsens over several hours. Nausea may be intense. People with this disorder may sit very still because moving the head or eyes may trigger vomiting. Vestibular neuritis begins to subside over a period of days, but it may last weeks or even months.

Vertigo due to a brain disorder, including vertebrobasilar insufficiency, may be accompanied by the following:

- Headaches
- Slurred speech
- Double vision
- Weakness of an arm or a leg
- Uncoordinated movements
- Loss of consciousness

Vertigo due to a disorder that suddenly increases pressure within the skull may be accompanied by the following:

- Headache
- Temporary blurring of vision
- Unsteadiness when walking

Diagnosis

Doctors ask the person to describe the nature and circumstances of the sensations felt. Balance and hearing are tested.

Physical Examination: The eyes are checked for abnormal movements, such as nystagmus. Abnormal eye movements suggest a disorder affecting the inner ear or various nerve connections in the brain stem. Doctors deliberately try to induce nystagmus because the direction in which the eyes move helps doctors make the diagnosis. They can observe the direction in several ways. During an ophthalmoscopic examination, the doctor focuses on the optic disk and then covers the other eye. If the optic disk jiggles, nystagmus is present. Alternatively, the person may be given special glasses called Frenzel lenses to wear. Doctors can easily see the person's eyes through the lenses, but the person sees only a blur and cannot visually fixate on anything (visual fixation suppresses nystagmus). Sometimes, eye movements are recorded using electrodes (sensors that stick to the skin) placed around each eye (electronystagmography) or by a video camera attached to the Frenzel lenses.

Maneuvers to induce nystagmus include putting ice-cold water into the ear canal (caloric testing), rapidly shaking the person's head from side to side for 20 seconds (head shaking test), and stimulating the posterior semicircular canal by rapidly changing the position of the person's head (Dix-Hallpike maneuver). The Dix-Hallpike maneuver, which is used in the diagnosis of BPPV, is identical to the first part of the Epley maneuver (see page 664).

Testing: For many people, additional testing is not needed. When it is, computed tomography (CT) or magnetic resonance imaging (MRI) of the head can detect some of the disorders that can cause vertigo. CT can show abnormalities in bone, such as an infection of the bone behind the ear (mastoiditis), fractures at the base of the skull, erosion of bone by tumors, and abnormal bone formation as occurs in Paget's disease. MRI produces better images of the brain stem and cranial nerves than CT.

If an ear infection is suspected, doctors may take a sample of pus or fluid from the ear with a needle or swab.

If a brain infection is suspected, a spinal tap (lumbar puncture) may be done to obtain a sample of cerebrospinal fluid from the spine.

If multiple sclerosis is suspected, an MRI may be done.

If doctors suspect that the blood supply to the brain is inadequate, Doppler ultrasonography, CT angiography, magnetic resonance angiography (MRA), or catheter angiography (which uses x-rays) may be done.

Prevention and Treatment

Vertigo due to certain disorders can be prevented. For example, if vertigo is due to motion sickness, situations that cause it (such as a rocking boat) can be avoided, and fixing the eyes on an unmoving object in the distance (visual fixation) can help avert an attack or stop one that has started. A scopolamine patch can help prevent as well as treat vertigo due to motion sickness.

Drugs that may relieve vertigo and the accompanying nausea include cyclizine, dimenhydrinate, diphenhydramine, hydroxyzine, meclizine, and promethazine. These drugs can be taken by mouth. Scopolamine, taken through a skin patch (often worn behind the ear), may be used instead. It is effective for several days and may be preferred if nausea is present.

If the vertigo is severe or causes anxiety, sedatives may be useful. Most often, benzodiazepines are used. Particularly for older people, the benzodiazepines alprazolam and lorazepam are preferred because their effects do not last as long as those of other benzodiazepines.

All of these drugs may have side effects, especially in older people. Older people should avoid taking them whenever possible, but when vertigo is severe and persistent, taking a drug may be necessary but should be supervised by a doctor. Scopolamine given through a patch tends to have the fewest side effects. More often than not, vertigo is caused by BPPV in older people and can be relieved without drugs. Drugs used in the treatment of vertigo may cause agitation in infants and very young children and should not be given to them except as directed by a doctor.

Motion Sickness

Motion sickness (also known as car, sea, train, or air sickness) involves a group of symptoms, particularly nausea, caused by movement during travel.

- While traveling, people feel nauseated and dizzy and may make break into a cold sweat and start hyperventilating.
- Doctors base the diagnosis on symptoms and the situation in which they occur.
- Ways to help prevent motion sickness include keeping the gaze and head as still as possible, getting some fresh air, not reading, and not smoking or drinking alcoholic beverages before traveling.
- Eating soda crackers or sipping ginger ale may help relieve the nausea, but sometimes a drug taken by mouth, or scopolamine, given through a skin patch, is needed.

Motion sickness occurs when the parts of the inner ear that help control balance (including the semicircular canals) are stimulated too much, as can occur when motion is excessive. It can also occur when the brain receives contradictory information from its motion sensors—the eyes, the semicircular canals, and the muscle sensors (nerve endings in muscles and joints that provide information about body position). Motion sickness commonly occurs during boat travel, when the boat rolls and rocks. It may also occur in a moving car, amusement park rides, or other moving vehicles. Some people are more susceptible than others. Fear, anxiety, and poor ventilation increase the likelihood of experiencing motion sickness.

Symptoms and Diagnosis

Symptoms may begin relatively suddenly. Nausea, a vague feeling of abdominal discomfort, vertigo, headache, and fatigue usually develop. The face may become pale, and the person may break into a cold sweat. Vomiting often occurs. Other symptoms may include increased saliva production (often as a prelude to vomiting) and abnormally rapid, deep breathing (hyperventilation). Hyperventilation may cause faintness. Nausea and vomiting make the person feel weak. Prolonged vomiting can lead to low blood pressure and dehydration. However, symptoms tend to gradually subside when the motion stops or the person leaves the vehicle. Also, people who are on long trips, as on a ship, usually adapt to the motion (helped by the stabilizers used in modern ships to minimize motion) and gradually recover.

Motion sickness is diagnosed based on a description of the symptoms and the circumstances in which they occur.

Prevention and Treatment

Measures include the following:

- Using visual fixation (for example, watching the distant horizon on a rocking boat; sitting in the driver's seat and looking ahead)
- Choosing a seat where motion is felt least (such as the front seat of a car, a seat over the wings in an airplane, or the forward or middle cabin or upper deck of a ship)
- Keeping the head and body as still as possible
- Sitting face forward and in a reclining position
- Not reading
- Getting fresh air by opening a window, opening an air vent, or going to a ship's top deck
- Not drinking alcoholic beverages and not smoking (both can aggravate nausea)
- Eating small amounts of low-fat, starchy foods and not eating strong-smelling or strong-tasting foods
- Avoiding food and drink on short airplane trips, especially on small airplanes

Before traveling, people who are susceptible to motion sickness can ask their doctor to recommend an over-the-counter drug or prescribe a drug to prevent the disorder. These drugs include cyclizine, dimenhydrinate, diphenhydramine, meclizine, promethazine, and scopolamine (as a patch or as tablets). All of these drugs cause drowsiness, but they may cause agitation in infants and very young children and should not be given to them except under a doctor's supervision. Anyone who performs an activity that requires alertness or concentration, including driving, should not take a motion sickness drug. A motion sickness drug should not be taken with alcohol, sleep aids, sedatives, or other drugs that also cause drowsiness and decrease alertness.

If motion sickness develops, eating soda crackers or drinking carbonated soda, such as ginger ale, may help. Because of the nausea, scopolamine, the only drug for motion sickness that is given through a skin patch, is often more useful than other drugs, which are taken by mouth. Drugs can also be given by injection if necessary.

Benign Paroxysmal Positional Vertigo

Benign paroxysmal positional vertigo, or BPPV, is a common disorder causing short episodes of vertigo in response to changes in head position that stimulate the posterior semicircular canal of the inner ear.

- People briefly feel as it they or their surroundings are spinning when they move their head.

The Epley Maneuver: A Simple Cure for a Common Cause of Vertigo

Some people experience vertigo when they change the position of their head rapidly, as when rolling their head on the pillow, looking down to tie their shoes, or looking up to reach for an item on a high shelf. This vertigo is usually due to benign paroxysmal positional vertigo (BPPV). It occurs when tiny calcium particles are displaced from their normal location to form sludge, usually in the posterior semicircular canal (one of the canals in the inner ear). The disorder can often be cured by using the Epley maneuver to move the particles out of the canal and back to where they originated. In this maneuver, the person's body and head are moved into different positions, one after the other. Each position is maintained for about 30 seconds to allow the particles to move by gravity into a different part of the canal. To check if the maneuver worked, the person moves the head in the same way as previously caused vertigo. If vertigo does not occur, the maneuver worked. Remaining semiupright for 24 hours after the Epley maneuver, previously recommended, is no longer considered necessary.

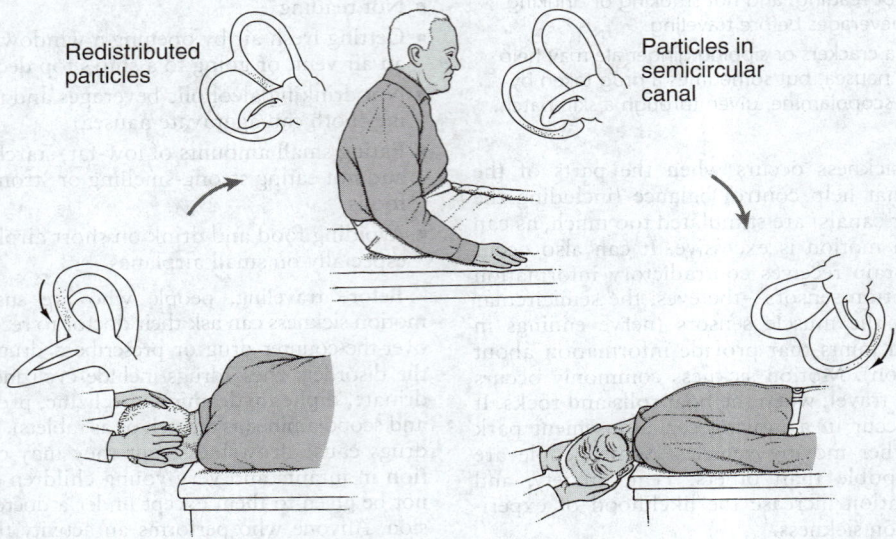

Redistributed particles

Particles in semicircular canal

Finally, the head and body are turned even more, until the nose points down at the floor. The person then sits up but keeps the head turned to the far left. Once the person is upright, the head can face forward.

First, with the person sitting, the head is turned about 45° to the right or left, depending on which side triggers the vertigo. The person then lies down with the head hanging over the edge of the examining table (or bed). The sludge triggers an exaggerated signal to the brain, resulting in vertigo.

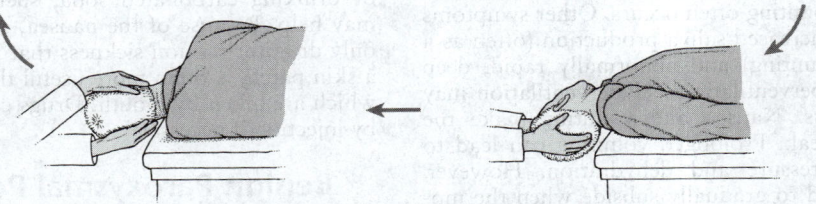

The head is turned further to the left, so that the ear is parallel to the floor.

The head is then turned to the other side at the same angle.

- People may also feel nauseated and vomit, and their eyes may move abnormally.
- Doctors base the diagnosis on symptoms and the situation in which they occur and a physical examination.
- The Epley maneuver, done once or twice, cures the disorder in most people.

Vertigo is a specific sensation of spinning. People with vertigo feel as if they, their surroundings, or both are moving or spinning.

A change in head position—typically turning the head over on the pillow on first awakening in the morning, or tipping the head backward to reach a high shelf—triggers most episodes of this disorder. BPPV usually develops when calcium particles that are normally embedded in one part of the inner ear (the utricle and saccule) are displaced and move into another part of the inner ear (the posterior semicircular canal). The inner ear contains three semicircular canals, which help with balance (see art on page 1376). The posterior canal, unlike the anterior and horizontal canals, is in the best position to receive most of the loose particles through gravity during the night. As they collect, they form a chalky sludge and may further form into a mass that exaggerates the movement of fluid in the canal when the head changes position. The result is overstimulation of nerve receptors (hair cells) inside the posterior canal, making the brain feel as if the head were moving much faster than it is. This information does not match that from the eyes and from position sensors in the joints. This mismatch results in a brief episode of vertigo. Particles may be displaced from the utricle and saccule as people age. Or, displacement may be caused by ear infections, injury, prolonged bed rest, ear surgery, head injury, or blockage of an artery to the inner ear.

This type of vertigo can be frightening, but it is usually harmless and disappears by itself. It may be accompanied by nausea, vomiting, and a specific type of nystagmus (the rapid jerking movement of the eyes in one direction alternating with a slower drift back to the original position). An episode of vertigo begins 5 to 10 seconds after the head moves and lasts less than a minute. Episodes usually subside on their own in weeks. Occasionally, they persist for months and can cause dehydration due to nausea and vomiting. No hearing loss or noise in the ears (tinnitus) occurs.

Diagnosis and Treatment

Diagnosis is based on a description of the symptoms and the circumstances in which they occur.

Usually, the test used is the Dix-Hallpike maneuver, which stimulates the posterior semicircular canal and triggers vertigo and nystagmus in people with BPPV or other types of vertigo. The person sits on the examining table with the head turned 45 degrees to the right. Then the person lies down backwards so that the head remains turned at 45 degrees and hangs over the examining table by about 20 degrees. In BPPV, there is a delay about 5 to 10 seconds before vertigo and nystagmus occur, but the delay may be as long as 30 seconds. Symptoms last 10 to 30 seconds. Maintaining the gaze on a single location (visual fixation) can shorten or even abolish nystagmus, so the maneuver is ideally done with the person wearing Frenzel lenses (which make it impossible to visually fixate on anything). If the maneuver is repeated several times, the intensity of the vertigo and nystagmus decreases (called habituation) in people who have BPPV. However, in people who have vertigo due to a brain disorder (such as stroke or multiple sclerosis), which is more serious, the Dix-Hallpike maneuver triggers symptoms immediately, the vertigo persists as long as the head is held in the same position, and habituation does not occur when the maneuver is repeated.

BPPV is easily treated. The particles simply need to be moved out of the posterior semicircular canal and back to where they came from. Doing so requires a somersault-like maneuver of the head, called the canalith repositioning maneuver or Epley maneuver. This maneuver immediately cures vertigo in about 90% of people. Repeating the maneuver cures an additional 5%. In some people, the vertigo recurs. If it does, the maneuver is repeated. People can be taught how to do the maneuver at home in case vertigo recurs. For the 5% of people who are not cured with the maneuver, drugs may be used.

Very rarely, surgery is needed. Occasionally, the horizontal canal is affected, and rolling oneself like a log can relieve the symptoms.

CHAPTER
109   Sleep Disorders

Sleep disorders are disturbances that affect the ability to fall asleep, stay asleep, or stay awake or that cause abnormal behaviors during sleep, such as night terrors or sleepwalking.

- Sleep can be disturbed by many factors, including irregular bed times, activities before bed, stress, diet, disorders, and drugs.
- Lack of sleep makes people feel sleepy, tired, and irritable during the day and interferes with functioning.
- Less often, a sleep disorder makes people unable to resist falling asleep during the day.
- A detailed description of the problem, sometimes with information from a sleep log, usually indicates the diagnosis, but sometimes testing in a sleep laboratory is needed.

Sleep is necessary for survival and good health, but why sleep is needed and exactly how it benefits people are not fully understood. Individual requirements for sleep vary widely: usually from 6 to 10 hours every day. Most people sleep at night. However, many people must sleep during the day to accommodate work schedules—a situation that can lead to sleep disorders.

How long people sleep and how rested they feel after waking can be influenced by many factors, including level of excitement or emotional distress, age, diet, and use of drugs. For example, some drugs make people sleepy, and others make sleeping difficult. Some food components or additives, such as caffeine, strong spices, and monosodium glutamate (MSG), may disturb sleep. Older people tend to fall asleep earlier, to awaken earlier, and to be less tolerant of changes in sleep habits (for example, they may be more prone to jet lag and problems related to shift work). Compared with younger adults and children, older people are more easily aroused from sleep and awaken more often during the night. Whether older people need less sleep is unclear. They probably need as much sleep as younger people but do not sleep as well as they used to, leading to daytime sleepiness and napping. Napping during the day may help compensate for poor sleep during the night, but it may also contribute to the problem.

All sleep is not the same. There are two main types of sleep: rapid eye movement (REM) sleep and nonrapid eye movement (non-REM) sleep, which has four stages. People normally cycle through the four stages of non-REM sleep, usually followed by a brief interval of REM sleep, every 90 minutes or 5 or 6 times every night.

- **Non-REM sleep:** Non-REM sleep accounts for about 75 to 80% of total sleep time in adults. Sleep progresses from stage 1 (the lightest level, when the sleeper can be awakened easily) to stage 4 (the deepest level, when the sleeper can be awakened with greater difficulty). In stage 4, blood pressure is at its lowest, and heart and breathing rates are at their slowest.
- **REM sleep:** Electrical activity in the brain is unusually high, somewhat resembling that during wakefulness. The eyes move rapidly, and muscles are paralyzed so that voluntary movement is impossible. However, some muscles may twitch involuntarily. The rate and depth of breathing increase.

The most vivid dreaming occurs during REM sleep. Most talking during sleep, night terrors, and sleepwalking occur during stages 3 and 4.

Symptoms

The most common symptoms are insomnia and excessive sleepiness during the day. People with insomnia have difficulty falling and staying asleep and wake up feeling unrefreshed. People with excessive daytime sleepiness tend to fall asleep during normal waking hours.

Some sleep disorders involve involuntary movements of the limbs or other unusual behaviors (such as nightmares) during sleep.

Other symptoms may include problems with memory, coordination, and emotions. People may perform less well in school or at their jobs. The risk of having a motor vehicle accident or developing a heart disorder is increased.

Diagnosis

Usually, sleep disorders can be diagnosed based on the medical history, including a description of the current problem, and results of a physical examination. Doctors ask for a detailed description of the problem and may ask people to keep a sleep log. In it, people record the following:

- When they go to sleep
- When they awaken in the morning
- How many times they wake up during the night
- How long they stay awake each time they wake up
- What they do before going to bed
- How they feel the next day (for example, whether they feel drowsy)

SPOTLIGHT ON AGING

Up to half of older people say that they do not sleep as well as they would like. Although causes may be the same as for younger people, age-related changes may also contribute.

As people age, they may participate in fewer activities and become less physically active, making falling sleep harder. If people have to move into a relative's home or a nursing home, they may have no control over such things as temperature and noise levels. The resulting discomfort can make sleeping more difficult.

If people go out less and spend less time outdoors, their exposure to sunlight is decreased. Exposure of the eyes to sunlight is necessary for the body to produce melatonin, a hormone that helps promote sleep. Also, the aging body produces less melatonin and growth hormone (which promotes deep sleep).

Usually, older people tend to fall asleep and wake up earlier. They may take longer to get to sleep. They also spend less time in deep sleep (which helps the body recover from daytime activities). Once asleep, they wake up more often and more easily. As a result, they feel less refreshed when they wake up, even though they may have spent a long time in bed.

Older people are more likely to have medical and emotional disorders that can interfere with sleep. Disorders interfere with sleep in several ways:

- By causing pain (as occurs in arthritis)

- By making people have to urinate more often, waking them up frequently during the night (as occurs in benign prostatic hyperplasia, diabetes, or heart failure)

- By making breathing difficult (as occurs in heart or lung disorders)

Depression, which is common among older people, also interferes with sleep.

Older people are more likely to take drugs that affect sleep. Some (such as diuretics for heart failure) increase the need to urinate and thus interrupt sleep. Other drugs make people sleepy during the day or stimulate them. Either way, sleeping at night may be harder.

Older people tend to take naps because they do not sleep well during the night. Napping may be more likely because the aging body is less able to regulate blood pressure as needed. For example, after a big meal, blood pressure decreases, and the body needs to pump relatively more blood to the head. The aging body is less able to make this adjustment. As a result, older people feel sleepy.

Generally, older people need as much sleep as they did when they were young and should not accept poor sleep as part of aging. They can take measures to improve sleep. Staying active, spending time outside, avoiding foods and beverages (such as those that contain caffeine) that can interfere with sleep, going to bed at regular times, and making sure their bedroom is conducive to sleep can help.

- Whether they take any naps, at what time, and how long they last

When the diagnosis is uncertain or when doctors suspect certain types of sleep disorders, evaluation in a sleep laboratory may be recommended. The evaluation consists of polysomnography and observation and sometimes video recording of unusual movements during an entire night's sleep. Polysomnography includes the following:

- Electroencephalography (EEG), which records the brain's electrical activity (see page 636)

- Electrocardiography (ECG), which records heart rhythm and rate

- Recording and monitoring of breathing functions

- Electro-oculography, which records eye movement during REM sleep

- Electromyography, which records muscle activity of the facial area and legs

- Oximetry, which records oxygen levels in the blood with a painless ear clip or finger clip

Insomnia

Insomnia is difficulty falling asleep or staying asleep or a disturbance in sleep quality that makes sleep seem inadequate or unrefreshing.

- People are sleepy and tired during the day and have trouble functioning.

- Doctors base the diagnosis on a detailed description of sleep habits and patterns and sometimes use testing in a sleep laboratory.

- If possible, the cause is corrected, sometimes with changes in lifestyle, but sleep aids may be needed.

Insomnia is usually a symptom that can have many different causes:

- An irregular sleep-wake schedule

Stages of the Sleep Cycle

People normally cycle through distinct stages of sleep 4 or 5 times during the night. Relatively little time is spent in stage 1 (shallow) sleep. The greatest time is spent in stage 2 sleep. Deep sleep (stages 3 and 4) occurs mostly during the first half of the night, whereas more time is spent in rapid eye movement (REM) sleep as the night progresses. Brief awakenings occur throughout the night, most of which the sleeper is typically unaware of.

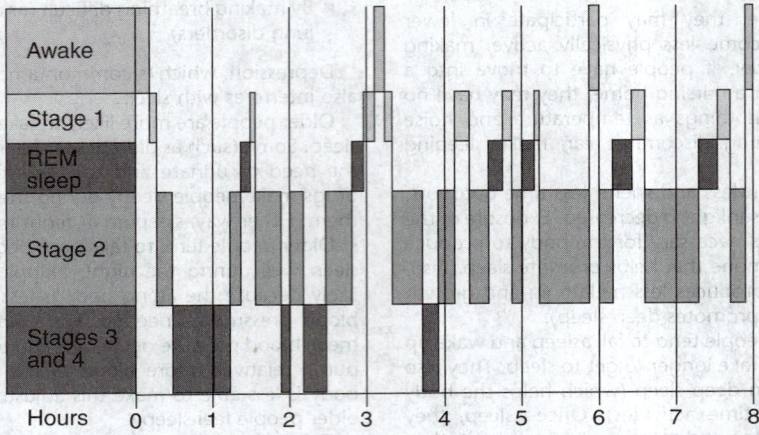

Poor sleep habits (for example, drinking a caffeinated beverage in the afternoon or evening or exercising late at night)
- Physical disorders (such as those that cause pain or make people urinate more often)
- Use or withdrawal of a drug
- Drinking large amounts of alcohol in the evening
- Emotional problems, anxiety, and stress

However, insomnia itself can be a disorder on its own. Some people have long-standing (chronic) insomnia that has little or no apparent relationship to any particular cause.

Difficulty falling and staying asleep and waking up earlier than desired are common among young and old. About 10% of adults have chronic insomnia, and about 50% have insomnia sometimes.

Because sleep patterns deteriorate as people age, older people are more likely to report insomnia than younger people. As people age, they tend to sleep less at night and to feel sleepier and to nap during the day. Stages 3 and 4 sleep, the periods of deep sleep that is most refreshing, become shorter and eventually disappear. Also, older people awaken more during all stages of sleep. Usually, these changes alone do not indicate a sleep disorder in the elderly.

There are several types of insomnia:

- **Difficulty falling asleep (sleep-onset insomnia):** Commonly, people have difficulty falling asleep when they cannot let their minds relax and they continue to think and worry. Sometimes the body is not ready for sleep at what is considered a usual time for sleep. That is, the body's internal clock is out of sync with the earth's cycle of light and dark. This problem (a type of circadian rhythm sleep disorder) is common among adolescents and young adults.

- **Difficulty staying asleep (sleep maintenance insomnia):** Older people are more likely to have difficulty staying asleep than are younger people. People with this type of insomnia fall asleep normally but wake up several hours later and cannot fall asleep again easily. Sometimes they drift in and out of a restless, unsatisfactory sleep.

- **Early morning awakening:** This type may be a sign of depression in people of any age.

Symptoms and Diagnosis

Symptoms include irritability, fatigue during the day, and problems concentrating or performing under stress.

To diagnose insomnia, doctors ask people about their sleep patterns, habits around bedtime, use of drugs (including illicit drugs), use of other substances (such as alcohol, caffeine, and tobacco), degree of psychologic stress, medical history, and level of physical activity. People may be asked to keep a sleep log. In it, they record a detailed description of the sleep

Science Wakes Up to Sleep Disorders

People with all types of sleep disorders are sent to sleep disorder specialists for evaluation, diagnosis, and treatment. Some people require testing in a sleep laboratory. The following symptoms may prompt such a referral:

- Excessive daytime sleepiness
- Long-standing (chronic) insomnia
- Dependence on sleep aids
- Pauses in breathing during sleep
- Severe snoring or choking during sleep
- Nightmares
- Sleepwalking, talking during sleep, or violent movements during sleep
- Twitching of the legs or arms during sleep
- An irresistible urge to move the legs or arms just before or during sleep

An initial evaluation by a sleep disorders specialist may include the following:

- A sleep history, often including a sleep log
- A general medical history
- A physical examination

After the initial evaluation, further testing, such as blood tests and sleep laboratory testing, may be done. Sleep laboratory testing includes overnight polysomnography and a multiple sleep latency test.

In overnight polysomnography, people spend the night in a sleep laboratory with electrodes pasted to their scalp, facial area, and chin. With this information, sleep stages can be characterized. Electrodes are also attached to other areas of the body to record heart rate and muscle activity. Other bodily functions, such as breathing pattern, are also monitored and recorded. Polysomnography is used to detect breathing disorders, epilepsy, and unusual movements and behaviors during sleep (periodic limb movement disorder and parasomnias).

In a multiple sleep latency test, people spend the day in a sleep laboratory, taking four or five naps at 2-hour intervals. This test is used to detect daytime sleepiness and to diagnose narcolepsy.

nography. For this test, brain activity, heart rate, breathing, muscle activity, and eye movements are monitored while people sleep.

Treatment

The treatment of insomnia depends on its cause and severity. If insomnia results from another disorder, treatment of that disorder may improve sleep. For most people who have insomnia, some simple changes in lifestyle, such as following a regular sleep schedule and avoiding caffeine after lunch time, can improve sleep.

When a sleep disorder interferes with normal activities and a sense of well-being, taking sleep aids (also called hypnotics) occasionally for up to a few weeks may help. Most sleep aids require a prescription. Some are available without a prescription (over-the-counter, or OTC), but an OTC sleep aid may be no safer than a prescription sleep aid, especially for older people. OTC sleep aids contain diphenhydramine or doxylamine, both antihistamines, which may have side effects, such as drowsiness or sometimes nervousness, agitation, falls, and confusion, especially in older people. OTC sleep aids should not be taken for more than 7 to 10 days. They are intended to manage an occasional sleepless night, not chronic insomnia, which could signal a serious underlying problem.

 Did You Know...

Almost half of people have insomnia at one time or another.

Taking a prescription sleep aid may be safer than taking one sold over the counter.

For people with insomnia related to a "stressed mind," the most effective and safest treatment is usually talk therapy, done by trained specialists. This approach helps people understand the problem, unlearn bad sleeping habits, and eliminate unhelpful thoughts, such as worry about losing sleep or the next day's activities. Older people who have interrupted sleep can benefit from regular bedtimes, lots of environmental light exposure during the day, regular exercise, and less napping during the day because napping may make getting a good night's sleep even harder. Many older people with insomnia do not need to take sleep aids. But if they do, they should keep in mind that these drugs can cause problems. Thus, caution is required.

People who have insomnia and depression should be evaluated by a doctor, and the depression should be treated. Treating depression often relieves the

habits, including sleep and wake times, use of naps, and any problems with sleeping.

Some people need less sleep than others, so the diagnosis of insomnia is based on individual needs.

A physical examination is done to check for disorders that can cause insomnia. Occasionally, if insomnia persists despite measures to correct it, people may be referred to a sleep disorders specialist for evaluation and sometimes tests such as polysom-

Ways to Improve Sleep

Follow a regular sleep schedule: People should go to bed at the same time each night and, more importantly, get up at the same time each morning, even on weekends and vacations.

Follow a bedtime routine: A regular pattern of activities—such as walking at a relaxed pace, listening to soft music, brushing the teeth, washing the face, and setting the alarm clock—can set the mood for sleep. This routine should be followed every night, at home or away.

Make the environment conducive to sleep: The bedroom should be kept dark, quiet, and not too warm or too cold. Loud noises can disturb sleep even when people are not awakened by them. Wearing ear plugs, using a white-noise machine or a fan, or installing heavy curtains in the bedroom (to block out outside noises) can help.

Use the bedroom primarily for sleeping: The bedroom should not be used for eating, reading, watching television, paying bills, or other activities associated with wakefulness (other than intimate activity).

Avoid substances that interfere with sleep: Food and beverages that contain alcohol or caffeine (such as coffee, tea, cola drinks, and chocolate) can interfere with sleep, as can appetite suppressants, diuretics, and nicotine (in cigarettes and nicotine patches). Caffeinated substances should not be consumed within 12 hours of bedtime. Drinking a large amount of alcohol in the evening causes early morning awakenings. Quitting smoking may help.

Use pillows: Pillows between the knees or under the waist can make people more comfortable. For people with back problems, lying on the side with a large pillow between the knees may help.

Get up: When falling asleep is difficult, getting up and doing something else in another room and coming back to bed when sleepy may be more effective than lying in bed and trying harder and harder to fall asleep.

Exercise regularly: Exercise can help people fall asleep naturally. However, exercise within 5 hours of bedtime can stimulate the heart and brain and keep people awake.

Relax: Stress and worry are major impediments to sleep. People who are not sleepy at bedtime can relax by reading or taking a warm bath. People can aim to leave their problems at the bedroom door. Avoiding too much mental stimulation during the hour or so before bedtime can help. Scheduling a "worry time" during the day to think about concerns can diminish the need to worry at bedtime.

Eat a light snack: Hunger can interfere with going to sleep. A light snack, especially if warm, can help, unless a person has gastroesophageal reflux (GERD). However, heavy meals near bedtime should be avoided. They may cause heartburn, which can interfere with sleep.

Eliminate behavior that provokes anxiety: Turn the clock away so that time is not a focus.

---

insomnia, but some antidepressants can improve sleep directly because they have sedating effects. Usually, the antidepressant relieves depression but does not improve sleep. Then doctors may prescribe a sleep aid in addition.

Melatonin (see page 2077) is sometimes used to treat insomnia, especially in older people, who may have low levels of melatonin. However, its use is controversial. Melatonin appears to be safe for short-term use (up to a few weeks), but the effects of using it for a long time are unknown. Many other medicinal herbs and dietary supplements, such as skullcap and valerian, are available in health food stores, but their effects on sleep and side effects are not well understood.

Circadian Rhythm Sleep Disorders

Circadian rhythm sleep disorders occur when people's internal sleep-wake schedule (clock) does not align with the earth's cycle of darkness (night) and light (day).

- Jet lag and shift work commonly disturb the usual rhythms of sleep and waking.
- People cannot awaken or go to sleep when they need or want to.
- Doctors base the diagnosis on symptoms, sometimes using information from a sleep log and sleep laboratory testing.
- Good sleep habits and exposure to bright light can help people readjust their sleep-wake cycle.

Circadian means around (*circa*) the day (*dies*). Circadian rhythms are the regular changes in mental and physical states that occur in about a 24-hour period—a person's internal clock. These rhythms are controlled by an area of the brain that is influenced by light (called the circadian pacemaker). After entering the eye, light stimulates cells in the back of the eye (retina) to send nerve impulses to this area. These impulses signal the brain to stop producing melatonin, a sleep-promoting hormone.

Normally, people vary in their sleep and wake times. Some (morning people or larks) prefer to sleep and wake early. Others (night people or owls) prefer to sleep and wake late. Such variations are not considered a disorder as long as people can do the following:

- Wake up when they need to do something in the morning and fall asleep the night before in time to get enough sleep before having to get up
- Sleep and wake up at the same time every day, if they want to

- Adjust to new sleep and wake times within a few days after they start a new routine

People with a circadian rhythm sleep disorder fall asleep at inappropriate times and then cannot sleep or wake up when they need or want to. Their sleep-wake cycle is disrupted.

Causes

Causes may be internal or external. Internal causes include damage to the brain (for example, due to

---

Sleep Aids: Not to Be Taken Lightly

Among the most commonly used sleep aids are sedatives, minor tranquilizers, and antianxiety drugs. Most are safe as long as a doctor supervises their use.

Most sleep aids require a doctor's prescription because they may cause problems. Many of these problems are less common with newer sleep aids.

- **Loss of effectiveness:** Once people become accustomed to a sleep aid, it may become ineffective. This effect is called tolerance.
- **Withdrawal symptoms:** If a sleep aid is taken for more than a few days, stopping it can make the original sleep problem suddenly worse (causing rebound insomnia) and can increase anxiety. Thus, doctors recommend reducing the dose slowly over a period of several weeks until the drug is stopped.
- **Habit-forming or addiction potential:** People who use sleep aids for more than a few days may feel that they cannot sleep without them. Stopping the drug makes them anxious, nervous, and irritable or causes disturbing dreams.
- **Potential for overdose:** If taken in higher than recommended doses, some of the older sleep aids can cause confusion, delirium, dangerously slow breathing, a weak pulse, blue fingernails and lips, and even death.
- **Serious side effects:** Most sleep aids, even when taken at recommended doses, are particularly risky for older people and for people with breathing problems because they tend to suppress areas of the brain that control breathing. Some can reduce daytime alertness, making driving or operating machinery hazardous. Sleep aids are especially dangerous when taken with alcohol, opioids (narcotics), antihistamines, or antidepressants because these drugs also cause daytime drowsiness and can suppress breathing. The combined effects are more dangerous. Rarely, especially if taken at higher than recommended doses or with alcohol, sleep aids have been known to cause people to walk or even drive during sleep and to cause severe allergic reactions.

Newer sleep aids can be used for longer periods of time without losing effect, becoming habit-forming, or causing withdrawal. They are also less dangerous in an overdose.

Benzodiazepines are the most commonly used sleep aids. Some benzodiazepines (such as chlordiazepoxide, diazepam, flurazepam, and nitrazepam) are longer acting than others (such as temazepam and triazolam). Doctors try to avoid prescribing long-acting benzodiazepines for older people. Older people cannot metabolize and excrete drugs as well as younger people. Thus for them, taking these drugs may be more likely to cause daytime drowsiness, slurred speech, and falls.

Other useful sleep aids are not benzodiazepines, but work at the same brain areas as the benzodiazepines. These drugs (eszopiclone, zolpidem, and zaleplon) are shorter acting than most of benzodiazepines and are less likely to lead to daytime drowsiness. Older people appear to tolerate these drugs well. There is also a longer-acting (extended-release, or ER) version of zolpidem. Ramelteon, a newer sleep aid, has the same advantages as these shorter-acting drugs. In addition, it can be used longer than benzodiazepines without losing its effectiveness or causing withdrawal symptoms. It is not habit-forming and does not appear to have overdose potential. Ramelteon affects the same area of the brain as melatonin (a hormone that helps promote sleep) and is thus called a melatonin receptor agonist.

Some **antidepressants** (most commonly trazodone) can relieve insomnia and prevent early morning awakening, but side effects, such as daytime sleepiness, can be a problem, especially for older people. Low doses are used to treat insomnia unless it is caused by depression. Then, higher doses, usually used to treat depression, are used.

Diphenhydramine and **dimenhydrinate** are two inexpensive over-the-counter antihistamines that can relieve occasional or mild sleeping problems. However, they are not the best sleep aids, and they may have side effects, including daytime sleepiness, confusion, and urinary difficulties, especially in older people.

brain infection (encephalitis), stroke, head injury, or Alzheimer's disease) and insensitivity to the cycle of night and day.

External causes include the following:

- Jet lag (especially when traveling from west to east)
- Working irregular shifts or a regular basis
- Frequently going to bed and getting up at different times
- Being confined to bed for a long time
- Blindness and not being exposed to sunlight for long periods of time
- Taking certain drugs

Sleep-wake reversals are common among people who are hospitalized because they are often awakened during the night and because their eyes are not exposed to sunlight long enough during the day.

There are several types of circadian rhythm disorders.

Jeg lag disorder is caused by rapid travel across > 2 time zones.

Shift work disorder varies in severity depending on how often shifts change, how much they change, and whether they make sleep and wake times earlier or later. Always working night or evening shifts and keeping the same bed times on days off is preferable. However, even then, daytime noise and light may interfere with sleep. Also, workers often shorten their sleep time and sleep at different times on days off to participate in social or family events.

Delayed sleep phase syndrome occurs when people consistently go to sleep and awaken late (for example, go to sleep at 3 AM and wake up at 10 AM or as late as 1 PM). This syndrome is more common among adolescents and young adults. People with this syndrome cannot fall asleep earlier even if they try.

Advanced sleep phase syndrome occurs when people consistently go to bed and awaken early. It is more common among older people. People with this syndrome cannot stay awake until later times even if they try.

Non-24-hour sleep-wake syndrome occurs when the sleep-wake cycle changes every day. Sleep and wake times vary by 1 to 2 hours each day. This syndrome is much less common and tends to occur in blind people.

Symptoms

Because people cannot sleep when they need to, they may be sleepy during the day and have difficulty concentrating, thinking clearly, and doing their usual activities. They may misuse alcohol, sleep aids, and stimulants in an effort to sleep or stay awake.

Symptoms may be worse when people change their sleep schedule frequently, as when they frequently travel across several time zones or change their shift at work. Symptoms are also worse if the change makes wake and sleep times earlier (advances the sleep cycle) because delaying sleep is easier than going to sleep earlier. The sleep cycle is advanced when people fly east or when shifts change from days to nights to evenings.

If the cause is external, the timing of other circadian body rhythms, including temperature and hormone secretion, is affected. Thus, people may feel generally unwell, irritable, nauseated, and depressed, as well as sleepy.

If the cause of the disruption can be corrected, symptoms resolve over several days as rhythms readjust. In older people, resolution may take a few weeks or months.

Diagnosis

Doctors suspect the diagnosis based on symptoms. People are usually asked to keep a sleep log and to record their sleep and wake times for a week or two. Testing in a sleep laboratory is rarely needed.

Treatment

Developing good sleep habits can help (see box on page 670).

Exposure of the eyes to bright light at appropriate times may be the most helpful strategy. Such exposure helps reset the internal clock. For example, travelers should spend time in sunlight, particularly in the morning, after they reach their destination (see page 2103). Shift workers should spend time in bright light (sunlight or artificial light) at times when they should be awake. While they are asleep, they should make the bedroom as dark and quiet as possible. Sleep masks and white-noise devices can be used. Exposure to bright light in the morning may help people with delayed sleep syndrome. Bright light in the evening may help people with advanced sleep syndrome.

Another strategy is to gradually shift the sleep-wake schedule to the one that is desired. Travelers may benefit from gradually shifting their schedule to approximate that of their destination, beginning well ahead of travel time.

If symptoms persist, sleep aids with effects that last only a short time (short-acting drugs) and drugs that stimulate the brain (such as modafinil) may help people sleep better and feel more alert during the day. However, these drugs do not adjust the body rhythms any faster.

Melatonin may help minimize the effects of jet lag and problems related to working shifts. However, its use is controversial. Melatonin appears to be safe for short-term use (up to a few weeks), but the effects of using it for a long time are unknown.

Hypersomnia and Excessive Daytime Sleepiness

Hypersomnia is a substantial increase in total sleeping time. Excessive daytime sleepiness (EDS) is the inability to stay awake and alert during the day, resulting in unintended lapses into drowsiness or sleep.

Hypersomnia, which is less common than insomnia, refers to an increase of at least 25% in total sleeping time that continues for more than a few days. EDS refers to a condition in which people are abnormally sleepy during the day. They may fall asleep while they are driving or working. In some disorders, such as narcolepsy, hypersomnia and EDS occur together in the same person. In other disorders, such as sleep deprivation, the two do not occur together.

Being unusually sleepy and falling asleep unintentionally after a period of sleep deprivation is not hypersomnia. In such cases, extra sleep is a desired response. However, hypersomnia and EDS in people who have not previously curtailed their sleep may indicate a serious disorder, such as the following:

- A brain or nerve (neurologic) disorder, including encephalitis, meningitis, and brain tumor
- A heart or lung disorder
- Liver failure
- Sleep apnea syndrome
- Narcolepsy
- Severe anxiety
- Depression, especially in people with bipolar disorder
- A disorder of the nerves that affect the muscles of legs or arms, which disrupts the refreshing quality of sleep

Chronic hypersomnia that begins during adolescence may be a symptom of narcolepsy. Hypersomnia may also result from overuse of sleep aids and other drugs that cause drowsiness.

Diagnosis

When evaluating people who have become excessively sleepy, doctors ask about their mood, sleep-wake schedule, use of drugs, and any abnormalities that occur during sleep. These abnormalities may include snoring and breathing pauses (which suggest obstructive sleep apnea), as well as grinding of teeth and kicking during sleep. Often, a sleep partner can describe the sleep abnormalities best. Doctors also do a physical examination.

Depending on other symptoms and the results of the physical examination, doctors may evaluate the heart, lungs, and liver to determine whether a disorder is causing hypersomnia. A neurologic examination may also be necessary (see page 630). It may detect impaired memory or other problems suggesting a neurologic disorder. If a neurologic disorder is suspected, computed tomography (CT) or magnetic resonance imaging (MRI) is done, and the person is referred to a neurologist. In many cases, people with hypersomnia and EDS require polysomnography with or without multiple sleep latency testing to establish the proper diagnosis.

Treatment

The treatment of hypersomnia with or without EDS depends on the underlying diagnosis. If doctors determine that the person has "idiopathic hypersomnia," that is, hypersomnia without a specific underlying cause, they often recommend proper sleep habits and regular naps. In more severe cases, stimulant drugs, such as modafinil and sometimes amphetamine, dextroamphetamine, or methylphenidate, are used to help reduce the sleepiness. If EDS and hypersomnia are caused by another condition, such as sleep apnea syndrome, a brain infection, or depression, that condition is treated.

Narcolepsy

Narcolepsy is a sleep disorder marked by excessive sleepiness during the day or recurring, uncontrollable episodes of sleep during normal waking hours, plus sudden episodes of muscle weakness (cataplexy). Sometimes sleep paralysis, vivid dreams, and hallucinations while falling asleep or waking up from sleep also occur.

- Testing in a sleep laboratory, with polysomnography and multiple sleep latency testing, is needed to confirm the diagnosis.
- Drugs are used to help keep people awake and to control other symptoms.

Narcolepsy occurs in about 1 of 2,000 people in the US and Europe. In some cases, the disorder tends to run in families, but its cause is unknown. Although narcolepsy has no serious medical consequences, it can be disabling and increases the risk of motor vehicle and other accidents. Narcolepsy persists throughout life but does not affect life expectancy.

Narcolepsy reflects, in part, abnormalities in the timing and control of rapid eye movement (REM) sleep. Many symptoms resemble what happens during REM sleep. The muscle weakness, sleep paralysis, and hallucinations of narcolepsy resemble the loss of muscle tone, paralysis, and vivid dreaming that occurs during REM sleep.

Symptoms

Symptoms usually begin during adolescence or young adulthood and persist throughout life. Only about 10% of people with narcolepsy have all the symptoms. Most people have only a few. All have excessive daytime sleepiness (EDS).

EDS has been going on for a long time, often despite long periods of excessive sleep. Many people are overcome by sudden episodes of uncontrollable sleep that can occur at any time, often without warning (called sleep attacks). Falling asleep can be resisted only temporarily. People may have many episodes or only a few in a single day. Each usually lasts a few minutes or less but may last hours. Patients typically feel refreshed upon awakening even if the sleep episode lasts a few minutes. Episodes are most likely to occur in monotonous situations, as during boring meetings or long periods of highway driving. When intentionally taking short naps, people dream vividly. Nighttime sleep may be unsatisfying and interrupted by periodic awakenings and vivid, frightening dreams.

While people are awake, during the day, a sudden episode of muscle weakness without loss of consciousness—called cataplexy—may be triggered by a sudden emotional reaction such as anger, fear, joy, laughter, or surprise. People may become limp, drop something being held, or fall to the ground. These episodes resemble the normal muscle paralysis that occurs during rapid eye movement (REM) sleep and, to a lesser degree, the experience of being "weak with laughter." Cataplexy occurs in about 3 of 4 people with narcolepsy.

Occasionally, when just falling asleep or immediately after awakening, people try to move but cannot. This experience, called sleep paralysis, can be terrifying. The touch of another person may relieve the paralysis. Otherwise, the paralysis disappears on its own after several minutes.

When just falling asleep or, less often, when awakening, people may clearly see images or hear sounds that are not there. These extremely vivid hallucinations are similar to those of normal dreaming but are more intense. Hallucinations are called hypnagogic when they occur before falling asleep or hypnopompic when they occur before awakening.

People are less able to function and concentrate. They may lose their motivation and become depressed. Family and other relationships may be hurt.

Diagnosis

Doctors cannot base the diagnosis on symptoms alone because other disorders can cause some of the same symptoms. Sleep paralysis and similar hallucinations occasionally occur in otherwise healthy adults, in people who have been sleep deprived, and in people with sleep apnea syndrome or depression. These symptoms may also occur when certain drugs are taken. Therefore, testing in a sleep laboratory is

necessary. Polysomnography is done overnight, and multiple sleep latency testing is done the next day. These tests involve monitoring and recording the activity of the brain, heart, breathing, muscles, and eyes. Various other body functions, including movement of the limbs, are also monitored and recorded.

Usually, narcolepsy does not result from abnormalities that can be detected by imaging procedures, such as computed tomography (CT) or magnetic resonance imaging (MRI).

Treatment

There is no cure for narcolepsy. However, for many people, continued treatment results in normal lives. People should also try to get enough sleep at night and take brief naps (< 30 min) at the same time every day (typically afternoon). If symptoms are mild, these measures may be all that is needed. For others, drugs that help keep people awake, such as modafinil (or sometimes dextroamphetamine or methylphenidate), are used to help reduce the sleepiness. The dose of these drugs may have to be adjusted to prevent side effects such as jitteriness, overactivity, nausea, headache, or weight loss. Doctors monitor people closely during drug treatment. Dextroamphetamine and methylphenidate are stimulants, which may cause agitation, high blood pressure, a fast heart rate, and moodiness. These drugs may also be habit-forming. Modafinil, which works in a different way, may have fewer side effects than the other drugs, although it also can be habit-forming.

Sodium oxybate, a drug taken while in bed and again during the night, can usually lessen excessive daytime sleepiness and cataplexy. Side effects include nausea, vomiting, dizziness, and sleepiness.

An antidepressant such as clomipramine or protriptyline usually helps relieve cataplexy, hallucinations, and sleep paralysis.

Periodic Limb Movement Disorder and Restless Legs Syndrome

Periodic limb movement disorder involves repetitive movements of the arms, legs, or both during sleep. Restless legs syndrome involves an irresistible urge to move and usually abnormal sensations in the legs, arms, or both when people sit still or lie down.

- In people with periodic limb movement disorders, the legs, arms, or both twitch and jerk, disrupting sleep.
- People with restless legs syndrome have trouble relaxing and sleeping because they cannot sit or lie still.
- Doctors may diagnose restless legs syndrome based on symptoms, but testing in a sleep laboratory is needed to diagnose periodic limb movement disorder.

- There is no cure, but drugs used to treat Parkinson's disease and other drugs may help control symptoms.

These disorders are more common during middle and older age. Restless legs syndrome probably affects 1 to 2% of people. It is particularly common among people older than 50. Most people with restless legs syndrome also have periodic limb movement disorder, but the reverse is not true.

What causes these disorders is unknown. But one third or more of people with restless legs syndrome have family members with the syndrome. Risk factors include a sedentary lifestyle, smoking, and obesity. Periodic leg movement disorder is common among people with narcolepsy and rapid eye movement (REM) behavior disorder. Both disorders are more likely in people who have or do the following:

- Stop taking certain drugs (including benzodiazepines such as diazepam)
- Take stimulants (such as caffeine or stimulant drugs) or certain antidepressants
- Have iron deficiency
- Have anemia
- Are pregnant
- Have a kidney or liver disorder

Symptoms

Both disorders interrupt sleep. As a result, people feel tired and sleepy during the day.

In periodic limb movement disorder, the legs or arms typically twitch and jerk every 20 to 40 seconds during sleep. People are unaware of these movements and the brief awakenings that follow. People do not have any abnormal sensations in their legs or arms.

Typically, people with restless legs syndrome have an irresistible urge to move their legs when they are sitting still or lying down. People also often feel vague but intense strange sensations in their legs, sometimes accompanied by pain. The sensations may be described as burning, creeping, or tugging or like insects crawling inside the legs. Walking or moving or stretching the legs can relieve the sensations. People may pace, constantly move their legs while they are sitting, and toss and turn in bed. Thus, people have difficulty relaxing and falling asleep. During sleep, the legs may move spontaneously and uncontrollably, often awakening the sleeper. Symptoms are more likely to occur when people are under stress. Episodes may occur occasionally, causing few problems, or several times a week, depriving people of sleep and making it difficult to concentrate and function.

Diagnosis

Doctors can often diagnose restless legs syndrome based on symptoms reported by the person or the person's bed partner. Polysomnography, including electromyography (EMG), is always done to diagnose periodic limb movement disorder. These tests are done overnight. In polysomnography, brain activity, heart rate, breathing, muscle activity, and eye movements are monitored while people sleep. People may be videotaped during an entire night's sleep to document limb movements.

If either disorder is diagnosed, blood and urine tests are done to check for disorders that can contribute, such as anemia, iron deficiency, and kidney and liver disorders.

Treatment

Avoiding caffeine, which can make symptoms worse, is recommended. Taking vitamin and mineral supplements that contain iron may help.

There is no cure for these disorders, but certain drugs can help control symptoms.

- **Drugs used to treat Parkinson's disease:** Pramipexole or ropinirole may help (see table on page 774). These drugs imitate the actions of a neurotransmitter called dopamine. They increase nerve impulses to muscles. These drugs have relatively few side effects but can cause symptoms to occur earlier in the day or to worsen when the drug's effect wears off or the drug is stopped. These drugs can also cause nausea and insomnia. Levodopa-carbidopa is sometimes used.
- **Benzodiazepines:** These drugs (such as clonazepam) cause drowsiness, helping people sleep. These drugs may improve the quality of sleep. They are taken in low doses at bedtime. Over time, they may become less effective as people become accustomed to their effects. The drugs may also make people sleepy during the day.
- **Anticonvulsants:** Gabapentin or carbamazepine (see table on page 716) is effective in some people.
- **Opioids:** An opioid such as oxycodone may be used as a last resort because they can have serious side effects, including the possibility of addiction.

Parasomnias

Parasomnias are unusual behaviors that occur during sleep.

Various unconscious and largely unremembered behaviors can occur during sleep in children and adults. Just before falling asleep, almost all people occasionally experience brief, involuntary jerks of the arms or the entire body. Occasionally, the legs jerk. Some people also experience sleep paralysis (attempting but being unable to move) or brief fleeting images or thoughts when they are just falling asleep or awakening. People may clench or grind their teeth or have nightmares. Sleepwalking, head-banging, and night terrors are more common among children and can be very distressing for their parents. Usually, children do not remember these episodes.

Night terrors are frightening episodes which result in sitting up, screaming, and flailing about. The eyes are wide open, and the heart races. Episodes usually occur during nonrapid eye movement (non-REM) stages of sleep, typically in the first few hours of the night. Night terrors are more common among children. Children should not be awakened because doing so makes them even more frightened. Although children appear to be highly distressed, they have no memory for the events or mental images after awakening and do not suffer psychologic problems as a result of these behaviors. Parents need not be overly distressed. Children usually stop having episodes when they become older. Episodes in adults are often associated with psychologic problems. Treatment with certain benzodiazepines, such as clonazepam, or tricyclic antidepressants, such as imipramine, may help. Adults may benefit from psychotherapy or drug treatment.

Nightmares are vivid, frightening dreams, followed by sudden awakening. Children and adults may have nightmares. Nightmares occur during rapid eye movement (REM) sleep. They are more likely to occur when people are under stress, have a fever, are excessively tired, or have consumed alcohol. Treatment, if necessary, focuses on the underlying problem.

Sleepwalking (somnambulism), most common in late childhood and adolescence, is walking in a semiconscious manner without being consciously aware of it. It occurs during the deepest stages of sleep. People do not dream while sleepwalking—in fact, brain activity during sleepwalking, although abnormal, is more like that of a wakeful state than of a sleeping one. Sleepwalkers may mumble repetitiously and can hurt themselves by walking into obstacles. Most sleepwalkers have no memory of sleepwalking.

No specific treatment is available, but the sleepwalker can be gently led back to bed. Leaving a light on in the bedroom or adjacent hall sometimes reduces the tendency to sleepwalk. Forcibly awakening the sleepwalker may provoke an agitated reaction and is not advised. Obstacles or breakable objects in the sleepwalker's potential path should be removed, and windows should be kept closed and locked. Benzodiazepines, particularly diazepam and clonazepam, may help.

Rapid eye movement behavior disorder involves speaking (often profanely) and sometimes making violent movements during REM sleep, usually in response to a dream. Unlike night terrors, people with rapid eye movement behavior disorder are sometimes aware of having dreamed vividly during these episodes when they wake up the next day. Violent movements may include waving the arms, punching, and kicking. The violent behavior is not intentional and is not directed at anyone. The disorder is more common among the elderly, particularly those who have disorders that cause degeneration of the brain (such as Parkinson's disease or Alzheimer's disease). People may inadvertently injure themselves or their bed partner. Also, this behavior interferes with sleep, making people tired and sleepy during the day. Doctors can often diagnose this disorder based on symptoms reported by the person or the person's bed partner. But if they cannot, polysomnography with electromyography (EMG) is usually done.

There is no cure for the disorder. But clonazepam, a benzodiazepine (which is a sedative), relieves symptoms in most people. A low dose is effective. The drug is usually continued indefinitely. Bed partners should be warned about the possibility of harm and may wish to sleep in another bed until the drug begins to work. People with the disorder should remove sharp objects and furniture from next to their bed.

Sleep Disorders in Dementia

In people with dementia (see page 688), such as Alzheimer's disease, sleep patterns are often abnormal. As dementia progresses, the time spent in light sleep increases, so people are easily awakened.

People with dementia may have disorders that contribute to sleep problems. Disorders such as arthritis, dehydration, and infections may cause pain or discomfort, interfering with sleep. Use of certain drugs or interactions between drugs may also interfere with sleep.

Treatment of the underlying disorder may help improve sleep. Naps during the day are not helpful because they may make sleeping at night more difficult. Walking outside in the sunshine, keeping the temperature in the bedroom comfortable, and not consuming beverages or foods that contain caffeine during the evening may help.

CHAPTER
110 Brain Dysfunction

Brain damage can cause many types of dysfunction. Such dysfunction ranges from complete loss of consciousness (as occurs in a coma), to disorientation and an inability to pay attention (as occurs in delirium), to impairment of one or several of the many specific functions that contribute to conscious experience. The type and severity of brain dysfunction depend on how extensive brain damage is, where the damage is, and how quickly the disorder causing it is progressing.

Brain dysfunction may be widespread (diffuse) or limited to a specific area (localized). Diffuse dysfunction is caused by disorders that affect large areas of the brain, including the following:

- Disorders that cause metabolic abnormalities, such as low levels of sugar in the blood (hypoglycemia) or low levels of oxygen in the blood (usually due to a lung or heart disorder)
- Infections, such as meningitis and encephalitis
- Very high or very low blood pressure

Diffuse brain dysfunction may also result from disorders that cause swelling of or put pressure on a large area of the brain, including the following:

- Brain abscesses
- Large brain tumors
- Severe or blunt head injuries

Certain drugs, such as opioids (narcotics), some sedatives (such as benzodiazepines and barbiturates), and antidepressants may cause diffuse brain dysfunction if people are sensitive to their effects (as older people are) or if the level of drug in the blood is too high.

Localized brain dysfunction is caused by disorders that affect a specific area of the brain, including the following:

- Brain tumors that affect a relatively small area of the brain
- Disorders that reduce the blood (and thus the oxygen) supply to a specific area, such as a stroke
- Penetrating head injuries that affect only a relatively small area of the brain
- Certain types of seizure disorders

Diffuse damage tends to affect consciousness, making people difficult to arouse (causing stupor) or impossible to arouse (causing coma). Localized damage tends to affect specific functions. However, the severity of brain dysfunction depends on the extent of brain damage as well as the location. When the cerebral cortex (the outer layer of the cerebrum, the largest part of the brain) is damaged, the degree of dysfunction is proportionate to the extent of the damage: The more extensive the damage, the more severe the dysfunction is likely to be. However, when the brain stem (which regulates critical body functions and levels of consciousness) is damaged, a relatively small amount of damage may cause complete loss of consciousness and even death.

Disorders that progress rapidly are more likely to cause noticeable symptoms of brain dysfunction than disorders that progress slowly—for example, a fast-growing brain tumor versus a slow-growing one. The brain compensates for gradual changes more easily than for rapid changes.

Three characteristics of the brain help it compensate and recover after it has been damaged:

- Redundancy: More than one area can perform the same function.
- Plasticity: Nerve cells in certain areas can change so that they can perform a different function.
- Adaptation: Areas with somewhat overlapping functions can sometimes compensate for lost functions.

Consequently, undamaged areas of the brain sometimes take over functions performed by a damaged area, contributing to recovery. However, as people age, the brain becomes less able to shift functions from one area to another. Some functions, such as vision, cannot be performed by other areas of the brain. Direct damage to areas that control such functions may have permanent effects.

Dysfunction by Location

Because different areas of the brain control specific functions (see also page 624), the location of brain damage determines the type of dysfunction that results. Which side of the brain is affected is also important because the functions of the two halves of the cerebrum (cerebral hemispheres) are not identical. Some functions of the brain are performed exclusively by one hemisphere. For example, movement and sensation on one side of the body are controlled by the hemisphere on the opposite side. Other functions are performed predominantly by one hemisphere, which is said to be dominant for that function. For example, the left hemisphere predominantly controls language in most people. This characteristic is called

When Specific Areas of the Brain Are Damaged

Different areas of the brain control specific functions. Consequently, where the brain is damaged determines which function is lost.

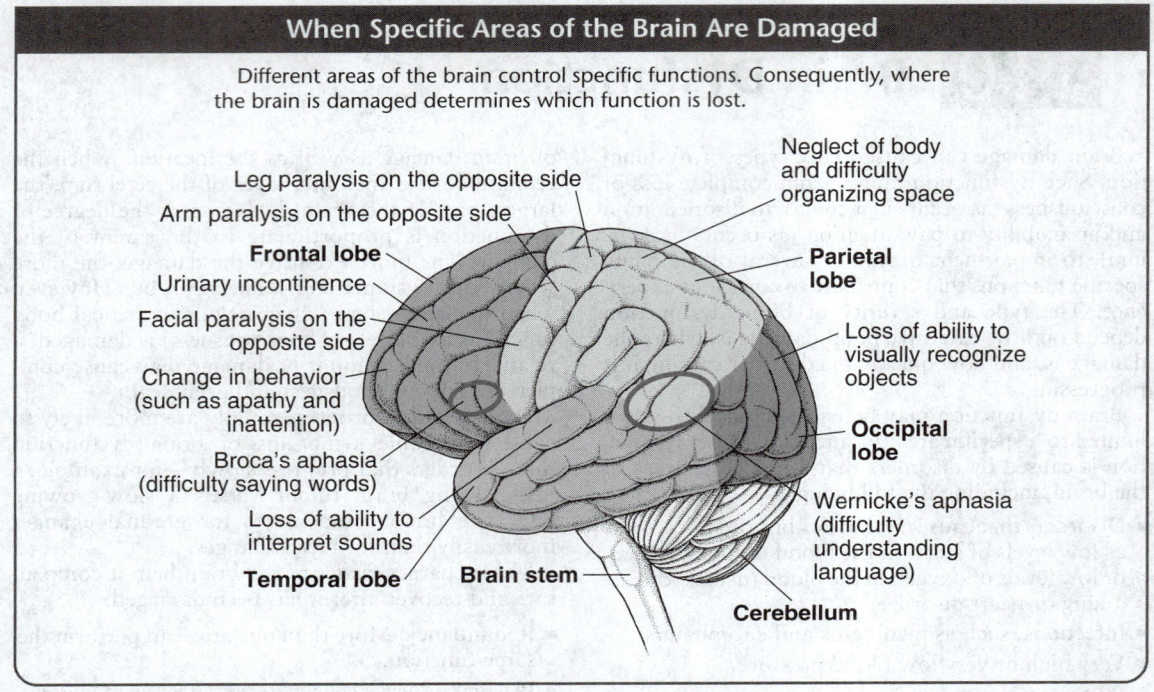

Leg paralysis on the opposite side

Arm paralysis on the opposite side

Frontal lobe

Urinary incontinence

Facial paralysis on the opposite side

Change in behavior (such as apathy and inattention)

Broca's aphasia (difficulty saying words)

Loss of ability to interpret sounds

Temporal lobe

Brain stem

Neglect of body and difficulty organizing space

Parietal lobe

Loss of ability to visually recognize objects

Occipital lobe

Wernicke's aphasia (difficulty understanding language)

Cerebellum

left-hemisphere language dominance. Damage to only one hemisphere of the brain may cause complete loss of such functions. However, most functions (such as memory) require coordination of several areas in both hemispheres. For such functions to be completely lost, both hemispheres must be damaged.

Specific patterns of dysfunction can be related to the area of the brain that has been damaged.

Frontal Lobe Damage: Generally, damage to the frontal lobes causes loss of the ability to solve problems and to plan and initiate actions, such as crossing the street or answering a complex question. But some specific impairments vary depending on which part of the frontal lobe is damaged.

If the back part of the frontal lobe (which controls voluntary movements) is damaged, weakness or paralysis can result. Because each side of the brain controls movement of the opposite side of the body, damage to the left hemisphere causes weakness on the right side of the body, and vice versa.

If the middle part is damaged, the ability to move the eyes and to perform complex movements in the correct sequence may be impaired. People may have difficulty expressing themselves in words—an impairment called Broca's (expressive) aphasia (see page 680).

If the front part is damaged, any of the following may result:

- Impaired concentration
- Reduced fluency of speech
- Apathy
- Inattentiveness
- Delayed responses to questions
- A striking lack of inhibition, including socially inappropriate behavior

People who lose their inhibitions may be inappropriately euphoric or depressed, excessively argumentative or passive, and vulgar. They may show no regard for the consequences of their behavior. They may also repeat what they say.

Parietal Lobe Damage: Damage to the front part of the parietal lobe on one side causes numbness and impairs sensation on the opposite side of the body. Affected people have difficulty identifying a sensation's location and type (pain, heat, cold, or vibration).

If the back part is damaged, people cannot tell the right from the left side (called right-left disorientation) and have problems with calculations and drawing.

If the right parietal lobe is damaged, people may be unable to do simple skilled tasks, such as combing their hair or dressing—called apraxia.

If the parietal lobe is suddenly damaged, people may ignore the serious nature of their disorder and neglect the side of the body opposite the injury or even deny its existence. Such people may become confused or delirious and unable to dress themselves or to do other ordinary tasks.

Temporal Lobe Damage: If the right temporal lobe is damaged, memory for sounds and shapes tends to be impaired. If the left temporal lobe is damaged in people with left-hemisphere language dominance, memory for words can be drastically impaired, as can the ability to understand language—an impairment called Wernicke's (receptive) aphasia. Sometimes damage to part of the temporal lobe can cause personality changes such as humorlessness, extreme religiosity, and loss of libido.

> **Did You Know...**
> Other areas of the brain can sometimes adapt and take over the functions of a damaged area.

Occipital Lobe Damage: The occipital lobe contains the main center for processing visual information. If the occipital lobe on both sides of the brain is damaged, people cannot see, even though the eyes themselves are functioning normally. This disorder is called cortical blindness. Some people with cortical blindness are unaware that they cannot see. If the front part is damaged, people have difficulty recognizing familiar objects and faces and accurately interpreting what they see.

Specific Types of Dysfunction

Many functions of the brain are performed by several areas of the brain working together (networks), not by a single area in the brain. Damage to these networks can cause aphasia, apraxia, agnosia, or amnesia.

Usually, doctors can diagnose the type of dysfunction by examining the person. They ask questions designed to evaluate specific brain functions. Imaging tests, such as computed tomography (CT) and magnetic resonance imaging (MRI), are usually needed to identify the cause of the damage.

APHASIA

Aphasia is partial or complete loss of the ability to express or understand spoken or written language. It results from damage to the areas of the brain that control language.

Testing a Person With Aphasia

Doctors can usually identify the type of aphasia based on how the person answers a few questions.

Broca's aphasia: Answers to questions are given hesitantly but are sensible.

Question: "What is this a picture of?" (dog barking)

Answer: "D—d—d—dg, eh, no...d-d... damn...p-p-pet, yeah, yeah, pet, pet, pet...b—b—...makes noise."

Wernicke's aphasia: Answers to questions are given fluently but are nonsensical.

Question: "How are you today?"

Answer: "When? Easy for my river runs black boxes wizzel abata on when boobles come."

Conduction aphasia: Language is understood and spontaneous speech is unaffected, but sentences spoken or written by others cannot be repeated.

Question: Repeat the following: "No ifs, ands, or buts about it."

Answer: "No nifs nand nor but..."

Anomia: Naming things is difficult.

Question: "What is this?" (pointing to a jacket lapel, watch band, or pen)

Answer: "What you wear, thing for time, you write with it."

- People may have difficulty reading, writing, speaking, understanding, or repeating language.
- Doctors can usually identify the problem by asking the person questions.
- Speech therapy can help many people with aphasia.

In most people, part of the left temporal lobe called Wernicke's area and part of the left frontal lobe called Broca's area control language function. Damage to any part of these small areas interferes with at least some aspect of language function. Usually, writing and speech are affected similarly. Aphasia is the most common language disorder among older people.

Aphasia usually results from disorders that do not cause progressive damage, such as a stroke, some tumors, head injury, or brain infection. In such cases, aphasia does not worsen. But if it results from a progressive disorder (such as an enlarging brain tumor), aphasia can progressively worsen.

People with aphasia have difficulty expressing or understanding language. But the nature and degree of the difficulty vary. The variety reflects the complex nature of language function. For example, aphasia may involve loss of only the ability to comprehend written words (alexia) or the ability to recall or say the names of objects (anomia). Some people with anomia cannot remember the right word at all. Others have a word in mind but cannot say it. Most people with aphasia have anomia. Or aphasia may involve only the inability to repeat words, phrases, or sentences (conduction aphasia). People with conduction aphasia understand spoken and written words and can speak fluently.

Most people with aphasia have more than one type of aphasia. One type is often more severe than the others.

Wernicke's (Receptive) Aphasia: If Wernicke's area is damaged, people have difficulty understanding spoken and written language. They usually speak fluently and with a natural rhythm, but the sentences come out as garbled, confused strings of words (sometimes referred to as word salad). They may not know that they are speaking nonsense.

Broca's (Expressive) Aphasia: If Broca's area is damaged, people may mostly understand the meaning of words and know how they want to respond. However, they have difficulty finding the words to say. Their words are forced out slowly and with great effort, sometimes interrupted by expletives. Most affected people are also unable to write words.

Complete (Global) Aphasia: If the left temporal and frontal lobes are damaged, people may be almost entirely unable to understand, speak, or write language. People may be able to utter expletives because the right side of the brain, which is more involved in emotions, is not damaged.

Treatment

Speech therapists can help people who develop aphasia after brain damage due to disorders that do not cause progressive damage (see page 56). Therapy is usually started as soon as people are able to participate, but it is helpful even when started much later. Usually, most recovery of language skills occurs during the first 3 months, but it can continue for more than 6 months.

Family members and other people who care for a person with aphasia can become frustrated. Remembering that aphasia is a physical disorder and that a person has little control over it can help.

DYSARTHRIA

Dysarthria is loss of the ability to articulate words normally.

Although dysarthria seems to be a language problem, it is really a muscular (motor) problem. It may be caused by damage to the brain stem or to the nerve fibers that connect the outer layer of the cerebrum (cerebral cortex) to the brain stem. The brain stem controls the muscles used in breathing (which help make sounds). The nerve fibers relay information needed to control and coordinate the muscles used to produce speech, including those of the lips, tongue, palate, and vocal cords.

People who have dysarthria produce sounds that approximate what they mean and that are in the correct order. Speech may be jerky, staccato, breathy, irregular, imprecise, or monotonous, depending on where the damage is. Because the ability to understand and use language is not usually affected, most people with dysarthria can read and write normally.

Speech therapy helps some people with dysarthria (see page 56).

APRAXIA

Apraxia is loss of the ability to do tasks that require remembering patterns or sequences of movements.

Apraxia, an uncommon disability, is usually caused by damage to the parietal or frontal lobes. People with apraxia cannot remember the sequence of movements needed to complete simple skilled or complex tasks. For example, buttoning a button, which consists of a series of steps, may be impossible, even though the hands are physically capable of doing the task. People with verbal (speech) apraxia cannot produce the basic sound units of speech because they cannot initiate, coordinate, or sequence the muscle movements needed to talk.

Some forms of apraxia affect only particular tasks. For example, people may lose the ability to do any one of the following: draw a picture, write a note, button a jacket, tie a shoelace, pick up a telephone receiver, or play a musical instrument.

Occupational therapy (see page 50) may help some people with apraxia learn to compensate for their losses.

AGNOSIA

Agnosia is loss of the ability to associate objects with their usual role or function.

Agnosia is relatively rare. Agnosia is caused by dysfunction in the parietal, temporal, or occipital lobes of the brain, where memories of the uses and importance of familiar objects, sights, and sounds are stored. Agnosia often develops suddenly after a head injury or stroke.

Symptoms vary depending on the lobe that is damaged:

- Parietal lobe: This type of damage usually results from a stroke. People have difficulty identifying a

Thanks for the Memories

Amnesia is a popular theme for many movies and television shows. Characters often appear with no identity and no memories of the past. They are essentially starting over, but they, for the most part, are fully equipped mentally to do so. However, this cinematic portrayal has little in common with the reality of amnesia.

In the movies: The amnesia may be unrelated to any abnormality or injury of the brain. People just forget. The reason may be unclear. Sometimes sleep seems to wipe the memory clean of the previous day's events—an improbable scenario but full of comic possibility. Or the cause may be a blow to the head, a head injury in a crash of some sort, or a psychologic trauma, such as witnessing a murder or being raped. Or memories may be removed by a special erasing device, as used in *Men in Black* or *Eternal Sunshine of the Spotless Mind*.

In reality: Amnesia usually has less glamorous causes, such as a brain infection, alcoholism, a stroke, drugs, a brain tumor, or brain surgery. Psychologic trauma occasionally causes amnesia—a disorder called dissociative amnesia. However, psychologic trauma often has the opposite effect on memory loss. People cannot forget what happened to them. They frequently replay and relive the traumatic event, even though they would rather forget it.

In the movies: People with amnesia have few if any problems with everyday activities. They may readily get a new job and make new (or new-old) friends.

In reality: Most people have great difficulty learning and retaining new information (because the brain has been damaged). As a result, they struggle with everyday activities. People have difficulty remembering names and where they are going and why. These problems cause frustration, and people with amnesia often feel very confused and get lost.

In the movies: People often go through a complete personality change. Values and behaviors are transformed. Bad people become good.

In reality: Amnesia affects personality or identity only rarely, when the specific areas of the brain that controls these functions malfunction.

In the movies: People with amnesia due a trauma have stored memories of the trauma, intact and accurate, deep in their unconscious. With the right trigger, they can replay the memories of the trauma like a video camera.

In reality: The way the brain recalls memories is dynamic. When people remember an event, they reconstruct it, pulling bits from different places in the brain. No memory, traumatic or otherwise, is ever frozen and immune from reconstruction over time.

In the movies: Amnesia can be cured mechanically. That is, amnesia caused by a blow to the head can often be reversed by another blow. Or amnesia, regardless of its cause, can be cured by looking at a familiar object or by being hypnotized.

In reality: Most of these cures are dubious. A second blow to the head is more likely to cause further damage. Hypnosis is useful only when the cause of amnesia is a traumatic event. Then, when done gently and carefully, it is often successful. Treatment and its chances of success depend on the cause.

In the movies: Memories are not really lost, just temporarily inaccessible.

In reality: Whether memories can be recovered depends on the severity and cause of the damage. Often, the damage is not severe, or the cause is temporary. In such cases, the amnesia often lasts for only minutes or hours, and most people recover their memory without treatment. However, when damage is substantial, memory often cannot be recovered.

---

familiar object (such as a key or safety pin) that is placed in the hand on the side of the body opposite the damage. However, when they look at the object, they immediately recognize and can identify it.

- Occipital lobe: People cannot recognize familiar faces or common objects, such as a spoon or a pencil, even though they can see these things. This impairment is called visual agnosia.
- Temporal lobe: People may be unable to recognize sounds even though they can hear sounds. This impairment is called auditory agnosia.

Some people with agnosia improve or recover spontaneously. Others must learn to cope with their strange disability. No specific treatment exists.

AMNESIA

Amnesia is total or partial loss of the ability to recall experiences or events that happened in the preceding few seconds, in the preceding few days, or further back in time.

Memory loss may involve events that occurred just before the cause of the amnesia (retrograde amnesia) or just after (anterograde amnesia). How far back in time memories are lost varies from a few seconds before the amnesia occurred to a few days, to further back in time, affecting remote (long-term) memories.

The brain's mechanisms for storing information and recalling it from memory are located primarily in the temporal and frontal lobes, but many areas of the brain are involved in memory. Emotions originating from the limbic system can influence the storing of memories and their retrieval. The limbic system includes part of the cerebrum and some structures deep within the brain. Areas that are responsible for alertness and awareness in the brain stem also contribute to memory. Because memory involves many interwoven brain functions, virtually any type of brain damage can result in amnesia.

How amnesia is caused is only partly understood. It may result from a head injury, disorders that reduce the supply of blood or nutrients to the brain (including strokes, seizures, and migraines), brain infection (encephalitis), brain tumors, alcoholism, severe mental stress, or use of certain drugs (such as amphotericin B or lithium).

Depending on the severity of the damage, most amnesias last for only minutes or hours, and most people recover their memory without treatment. However, if brain damage is severe, remote memories can be lost forever. A few people are never able form new memories.

Transient Global Amnesia: People suddenly but temporarily lose the ability to store new memories and to recall events that happened during the previous few hours to the previous few years. As a result, people become forgetful and confused about time, place, and sometimes the identity of other people.

This type of amnesia may be caused by temporary blockage of the arteries that supply blood to the temporal lobe. Such blockages usually result from atherosclerosis, especially in older people. Transient global amnesia may also be caused by a seizure originating in the temporal lobe. Often, the cause is unknown. In young adults, migraine headaches, which temporarily reduce blood flow to the brain, may cause transient global amnesia.

Most people with transient global amnesia have only one episode in a lifetime. About 10% have repeated episodes. Episodes usually last from 30 minutes to about 12 hours. After an episode, the confusion usually clears quickly, and total recovery is the rule, although people may not remember what happened during the episode.

Treatment depends on the cause.

Wernicke-Korsakoff Syndrome: This unusual form of amnesia may develop in alcoholics and other malnourished people, usually because of a deficiency of thiamin (vitamin B_1). The syndrome combines two disorders: an acute confusional state (Wernicke's encephalopathy—see page 2088) and an amnesia (Korsakoff's syndrome—see page 2089). Korsakoff's syndrome develops in about 80% of people with untreated Wernicke's encephalopathy.

Wernicke's encephalopathy causes loss of balance, drowsiness, a tendency to stagger, and eye movement problems in addition to confusion.

Korsakoff's syndrome may initially cause severe memory loss for recent events. More remote memory seems to be less impaired. Thus, people may be able to interact socially and converse coherently even though they cannot remember anything that happened in the preceding few days, months, or years or even in the preceding few minutes. They tend to make things up (confabulate) rather than admit that they cannot remember.

Treatment consists of thiamin and fluids given intravenously. Such treatment can correct Wernicke's encephalopathy, although recovery is usually incomplete. If untreated, Wernicke's encephalopathy can be fatal, but death rarely results in developed countries.

CHAPTER

111 Delirium and Dementia

Delirium and dementia are the most common causes of mental (cognitive) dysfunction—the inability to acquire, retain, and use knowledge normally. Although delirium and dementia may occur together, they are quite different. Delirium begins suddenly, causes fluctuations in mental function, and is usually reversible. Dementia begins gradually, is slowly progressive, and is usually irreversible. Also, the two disorders affect mental function differently. Delirium affects mainly attention. Dementia affects mainly memory. Both delirium and dementia may occur at any age but are much more common among older people because of age-related changes in the brain (see page 628).

Delirium

Delirium is a sudden, fluctuating, and usually reversible disturbance of mental function. It is characterized by inability to pay attention, disorientation, an inability to think clearly, and fluctuations in the level of alertness (consciousness).

COMPARING DELIRIUM AND DEMENTIA

FEATURE	DELIRIUM	DEMENTIA
Development	Sudden, sometimes with a definite beginning point	Slow, with an uncertain beginning point
Cause	Almost always another condition, such as an infection, dehydration, or use or stopping of certain drugs	Usually a brain disorder, such as Alzheimer's disease, vascular dementia, or Lewy body dementia
Main early symptom	Inability to pay attention	Loss of memory, especially recent events
Effect at night	Almost always worse	Often worse
Level of alertness (consciousness)	Impaired to varying degrees, can vary from being hyperalert to sluggish	Normal until late stages
Orientation to surroundings	Varies	Impaired
Effect on language	Slowed speech, often with incoherent and inappropriate language	Sometimes difficulty finding the right word
Memory	Varies	Lost, especially for recent events
Progression	Causes variations in mental function—people are alert one moment and sluggish and drowsy the next	Slowly progresses, gradually but eventually greatly impairing all mental functions
Duration	Days to weeks, sometimes longer	Almost always permanent
Need for treatment	Immediate	Needed but less urgently
Effect of treatment	Usually reverses the losses	May slow progression but cannot reverse or cure the disorder

- Many disorders and drugs can cause delirium.
- Doctors base the diagnosis on symptoms and results of a physical examination, and they use blood, urine, and imaging tests to identify the cause.
- Promptly correcting or treating the condition causing delirium usually cures it.

Delirium is an abnormal mental state, not a disease. Although the term has a specific medical definition, it is often used to describe any type of confusion. Delirium is never normal and often indicates a usually serious, newly developed problem, especially in older people. People who have delirium need immediate medical attention. If the cause of delirium is identified and corrected quickly, delirium can usually be cured.

Because delirium is a temporary condition, determining how many people have it is difficult. Delirium affects 15 to 50% of hospitalized people aged 70 or older.

Delirium may occur at any age but is more common among older people. Delirium is common among residents of nursing homes. When delirium occurs in younger people, it is usually due to drug use or a life-threatening disorder.

Causes

Development or worsening of many disorders can cause delirium. Any person can become delirious when extremely ill or taking drugs that affect brain function (psychoactive drugs). However, delirium can result from less severe conditions in older people and in people who have had a stroke or who have dementia, Parkinson's disease, or another disorder that causes nerve degeneration. In such people, delirium can result from a relatively minor illness (such as a urinary tract infection), dehydration, sensory deprivation (including being socially isolated or not having access to needed eyeglasses or hearing aids), or prolonged sleep deprivation. In some people, no cause can be identified.

Hospitalization: Being in the hospital, particularly in an intensive care unit (ICU), can contribute to or

What Is Confusion?

Confusion means different things to different people, but doctors use the term to describe people who cannot process information normally. Confused people cannot

- Follow a conversation
- Answer questions appropriately
- Understand where they are
- Make critical judgments that affect safety
- Remember important facts

Confusion has many different causes, including the use of certain drugs (prescription, over-the-counter, and illegal) and a wide variety of disorders. Delirium and dementia, though very different disorders, both cause confusion.

When a person is confused, doctors try to determine what the cause is, particularly whether it is delirium or dementia. If confusion develops or worsens suddenly, the cause may be delirium. In such cases, medical attention is needed immediately because delirium may be caused by a serious disorder. Also, treating the cause, once identified, can often reverse the delirium.

If confusion develops slowly, the cause may be dementia. Medical attention is needed but not urgently. Treatment may slow the mental decline in people with dementia but usually cannot stop the decline.

---

trigger delirium. In ICUs, people are isolated in a room that typically has no windows or clocks. Thus, people are deprived of sensory stimulation and can become disoriented. Sleep is disturbed by staff members who awaken people during the night to monitor and treat them and by loud beeping monitors, intercoms, voices in the hallway, or alarms. Furthermore, most people in ICUs have serious disorders and are treated with drugs, which can make delirium even more likely. The delirium that may result is sometimes called ICU psychosis.

Surgery: Delirium is also very common after surgery, probably because of the stress of surgery, the anesthetics used during surgery, and the pain relievers (analgesics) used after surgery.

Drugs: The most common reversible cause of delirium is drugs. In younger people, use of illegal drugs and acute intoxication with alcohol are common causes. In older people, prescription drugs are usually the cause.

Psychoactive drugs directly affect nerve cells in the brain, sometimes causing delirium. They include the following:

- Opioids (including morphine and meperidine)

- Sedatives (including benzodiazepines and sleep aids)
- Antipsychotics
- Antidepressants

Many other drugs can also cause delirium. The following are some examples:

- Drugs with anticholinergic effects (see box on page 1897), including many over-the-counter (OTC) antihistamines
- Amphetamines and cocaine, which are stimulants
- Cimetidine
- Corticosteroids
- Digoxin
- Levodopa
- Muscle relaxants

Delirium can also result from suddenly stopping a drug that has been taken for a long time—for example, a sedative (such as a benzodiazepine or barbiturate). Delirium commonly occurs in alcoholics who suddenly stop drinking alcohol (see page 2086) and in heroin users who suddenly stop using heroin.

Disorders: Abnormal blood levels of electrolytes, such as calcium, sodium, or magnesium, can interfere with the metabolic activity of nerve cells and lead to delirium. Abnormal electrolyte levels may result from use of a diuretic, dehydration, or disorders such as kidney failure and widespread cancer. An underactive thyroid gland (hypothyroidism) causes delirium with lethargy. An overactive thyroid gland (hyperthyroidism) causes delirium with hyperactivity.

In younger people, the cause of delirium is usually a condition that directly affects the brain—for example a brain infection, such as meningitis or encephalitis. In older people, the cause is usually a disorder that affects other parts of the body, such as a urinary tract infection, pneumonia, or influenza. Such infections can indirectly affect the brain.

Poisons: In younger people, ingestion of poisons, such as rubbing alcohol or antifreeze, is a common cause of delirium.

Symptoms

Delirium usually begins suddenly and progresses over hours or days. The actions of people with delirium vary but roughly resemble those of a person who is becoming progressively more intoxicated.

The hallmark of delirium is an inability to pay attention. People with delirium cannot concentrate, so they have trouble processing new information and cannot recall recent events. Thus, they do not understand what is happening around them. They become disoriented. Sudden confusion about time and often about place (where they are) may be an

SPOTLIGHT ON AGING

Delirium is more common among older people. It is a common reason that family members of older people seek help from a doctor or at a hospital. About 15 to 50% of older people experience delirium at some time during a hospital stay.

In older people, delirium can result from any condition that causes delirium in younger people. But it can also result from less severe conditions, such as the following:

- Dehydration
- A disorder that normally does not affect thinking, such as a urinary tract infection, influenza, or deficiency of thiamin or vitamin B_{12}
- Retention of urine or feces
- Sensory deprivation, as may occur when people are socially isolated or are not wearing their glasses or hearing aid
- Sleep deprivation
- Stress (any type)

Older people are much more sensitive to many drugs. In older people, drugs that affect the way the brain functions, such as sedatives, are the most common cause of delirium. However, drugs that do not affect brain function, including many over-the-counter drugs (especially antihistamines), can also cause it. Older people are more sensitive to the anticholinergic effects that many of these drugs have. One of these effects is confusion.

Why delirium occurs more often in older people is not known. One possible explanation involves acetylcholine, a neurotransmitter (a substance that enables brain cells to communicate with each other). Any stress (due to a drug, disorder, or situation) causes the level of acetylcholine to decrease, interfering with the brain's functioning. As people age, the brain produces less acetylcholine. Thus, if any condition causes the acetylcholine level to decrease further in older people, they are more likely to experience delirium.

Older people are also more likely to have other conditions that make them more susceptible to delirium, such as the following:

- Stroke
- Dementia
- Parkinson's disease
- Other disorders that cause nerve degeneration
- Use of three or more drugs
- Dehydration
- Undernutrition
- Immobility

Delirium tends to last longer in older people. It is often the first sign of another, sometimes serious disorder.

Confusion, the most obvious symptom, may be harder to recognize in older people. Younger people with delirium may be agitated, but very old people tend to become quiet and withdrawn. In such cases, recognizing delirium is even harder.

If a psychosis develops in older people, it usually indicates delirium or dementia. Psychosis due to a psychiatric disorder rarely begins during old age.

Older people are more likely to have dementia, which makes delirium harder to identify. Both cause confusion. Doctors try to distinguish the two by determining how quickly the confusion developed and what the person's previous mental function was. Doctors also ask the person a series of questions that test various aspects of thinking (mental status examination). Doctors usually treat people whose mental function suddenly worsens—even if they have dementia—as if they have delirium until proved otherwise.

Delirium and the hospitalization it usually requires can cause many other problems, such as undernutrition, dehydration, and pressure sores, which may have serious consequences in older people. Thus, older people can benefit from treatment managed by an interdisciplinary team, which includes a doctor, physical and occupational therapists, nurses, and social workers.

To help prevent delirium in an older person during a hospital stay, family members can ask hospital staff members to help—by encouraging the person to move around regularly, by placing a clock and calendar in the room, by minimizing the interruptions and noises during the night, and by making sure the person eats and drinks enough. Family members can visit and talk with the person and thus help keep the person oriented.

early sign of delirium. If delirium is severe, people may not know who they or other people are. Thinking is confused, and people with delirium ramble, sometimes becoming incoherent. Their level of awareness (consciousness) may fluctuate. That is, people may be overly alert one moment and drowsy and sluggish the next. Other symptoms also often change within minutes and tend to worsen during the evening (a phenomenon called sundowning). People with delirium often sleep restlessly or reverse their sleep-wake cycle, sleeping during the day and staying awake at night.

People may have bizarre, frightening visual hallucinations, seeing things or people that are not there. Some people develop paranoia or have delusions (false beliefs usually involving a misinterpretation of perceptions or experiences).

Personality and mood may change. Some people become so quiet and withdrawn that no one notices that they are delirious. Others become irritable, agitated, and restless and may pace. People who develop delirium after taking sedatives are likely to become very drowsy and withdrawn. Those who have taken amphetamines or who have stopped taking sedatives may become aggressive and hyperactive. Some people alternate between the two types of behavior.

Delirium can last hours, days, or even longer, depending on the severity and the cause. If the cause of delirium is not quickly identified and treated, people may become increasingly drowsy and unresponsive, requiring vigorous stimulation to be aroused (a condition called stupor—see page 701). Stupor may lead to coma or death.

> **Did You Know...**
>
> A psychosis that begins during old age usually indicates delirium or dementia.

Diagnosis

Doctors suspect delirium based on symptoms. However, mild delirium may be difficult to recognize. Doctors may not recognize delirium in hospitalized people.

Most people thought to have delirium are hospitalized to evaluate them and protect them from injuring themselves or others. Diagnostic procedures can be done quickly and safely in the hospital, and any disorders detected can be treated quickly.

Because delirium may be caused by a serious disorder (which could be rapidly fatal), doctors try to identify the cause as quickly as possible. Treating the cause, once identified, can often reverse the delirium.

Doctors first try to distinguish delirium from other disorders that affect mental function. Doctors do so by collecting as much information about the person's medical history as possible, by doing a physical examination, and by testing.

Medical History: Friends, family members, or other observers are asked for information because people with delirium are usually unable to answer. Questions include the following:

- How the confusion began (suddenly or gradually)
- How quickly it progressed
- What has the person's physical and mental health been like
- What drugs (including alcohol and illicit drugs, especially if the person is younger) and dietary supplements does the person use
- Whether any drugs have been started or stopped recently

Information may also come from medical records, the police, emergency medical personnel, or evidence such as pill bottles and certain documents. Documents such as a checkbook, recent letters, or notification of unpaid bills or missed appointments can indicate a change in mental function.

If delirium is accompanied by agitation and hallucinations, delusions, or paranoia, it must be distinguished from a psychosis due to a psychiatric disorder, such as manic-depressive illness or schizophrenia. People with a psychosis due to a psychiatric disorder do not have confusion or memory loss, and the level of consciousness does not change. A psychosis that begins during old age usually indicates delirium or dementia.

Physical Examination: During the physical examination, doctors check for signs of disorders that can cause delirium, such as infections and dehydration. A neurologic examination is also done (see page 630). People who may have delirium are given a mental status test. First, they are asked questions to determine whether the main problem is being unable to pay attention. For example, they are read a short list and asked to repeat it. Doctors must determine whether people take in (register) what is read to them. People with delirium cannot. The test also includes other questions and tasks, such as testing short-term and long-term memory, naming objects, writing sentences, and copying shapes.

Testing: Samples of blood and urine are taken and analyzed. Cultures are done to look for signs of infection. Computed tomography (CT) or magnetic resonance imaging (MRI) are usually done. Electrocardiography, pulse oximetry (using a sensor that

DELIRIUM OR PSYCHOSIS?

FEATURE	DELIRIUM	PSYCHOSIS DUE TO A PSYCHIATRIC DISORDER
Orientation	Confused about current time, date, place, or identity	Usually, aware of time, date, place, and identity
Attention	Greatly impaired	Unaffected
Memory for recent events	Lost	Retained
Ability to calculate	Unable to do simple calculations	Retained
Hallucinations	If present, mostly visual or involving touch	If present, mostly auditory
Other disorders	Often present and may be serious	History of previous psychiatric disturbances
Drug use	Often, evidence of recent drug use	Not necessarily involved

measures oxygen levels in the blood), and a chest x-ray may be used to evaluate heart and lung function.

In people with a fever or headache, a spinal tap (lumbar puncture—see art on page 635) may be done to obtain cerebrospinal fluid for analysis. Such analysis helps doctors rule out infection of or bleeding around the brain and spinal cord.

Treatment

Most people who have delirium are hospitalized. However, when the cause of delirium can be corrected readily (for example, when the cause is low blood sugar), people are observed for a short time in the emergency department and can then return home.

Once the cause is identified, it is promptly corrected or treated. For example, doctors treat infections with antibiotics, dehydration with fluids and electrolytes given intravenously, and delirium due to stopping alcohol with benzodiazepines (as well as measures to help people not start drinking alcohol again). Prompt treatment of the disorder causing delirium usually prevents permanent brain damage and may result in a complete recovery. Any drugs that may be making the delirium worse are stopped if possible.

General measures are also important. The environment is kept as quiet and calm as possible. It should be well-lit to enable people to recognize what and who is in their room and where they are. Placing clocks, calendars, and family photographs in the room can help with orientation. At every opportunity, staff and family members should reassure people and remind them of the time and place.

Procedures should be explained before and as they are done. People who need glasses or hearing aids should have access to them.

People who have delirium are prone to many problems, including dehydration, undernutrition, incontinence, falls, and pressure sores. Preventing such problems requires meticulous care. Thus, people, particularly older people, may benefit from treatment managed by an interdisciplinary team, which includes a doctor, physical and occupational therapists, nurses, and social workers.

People who are extremely agitated or who have hallucinations may injure themselves or their caregivers. The following measures can help prevent such injuries:

- Family members are encouraged to stay with the person.
- The person is put in a room near the nurses' station.
- The hospital may provide an attendant to stay with the person.
- Devices, such as intravenous lines, bladder catheters, or padded restraints, are not used if possible because they can further confuse and upset the person, increasing the risk of injury.

However, sometimes during hospitalization, padded restraints must be used—for example, to keep the person from pulling out intravenous lines and to prevent falls. Restraints are applied carefully by a staff member trained in their use, released at frequent intervals, and stopped as soon as possible, because they can upset the person and worsen agitation.

For agitation, drugs are used only after all other measures have been ineffective. Two types of drugs are usually used to control agitation, but neither is ideal:

- **Antipsychotic drugs** (see table on page 894) are most often used. However, they may prolong or worsen agitation. Newer antipsychotics, such as risperidone, are less likely to worsen agitation and have fewer side effects than older antipsychotics, such as haloperidol. But if used for a long time in people with dementia, the newer drugs may increase the risk of stroke and death.

- **Benzodiazepines** (a type of sedative—see table on page 885), such as lorazepam, usually calm people with delirium but make some people, particularly older people, more confused, drowsy, or both. Benzodiazepines are preferred when delirium is due to suddenly stopping sedatives or alcohol after heavy use for a long time. Benzodiazepines have more side effects than antipsychotics.

Doctors are careful when prescribing these drugs, particularly for older people. They use the lowest dose possible and stop the drug as soon as possible.

Prognosis

Most people recover fully if the condition causing delirium is rapidly identified and treated. Any delay greatly decreases the chance of a full recovery. Even when delirium is treated, some symptoms may persist for many weeks or months, and improvement may occur slowly. In some people, delirium evolves into chronic brain dysfunction similar to dementia.

Hospitalized people who have delirium are up to 10 times more likely to develop complications in the hospital (including death) than those who do not have delirium. Hospitalized people who have delirium, particularly older people, have a longer hospital stay, higher treatment costs, and a longer recovery time after they leave the hospital.

Dementia

Dementia is a slow, progressive decline in mental function including memory, thinking, judgment, and the ability to learn.

- Typically, symptoms include memory loss, problems using language and doing activities, personality changes, disorientation, and disruptive or inappropriate behavior.
- Symptoms progress so that people cannot function, causing them to become totally dependent on others.
- Doctors base the diagnosis on symptoms and results of a physical examination and mental status tests.

- Blood and imaging tests are used to determine the cause.
- Treatment focuses on maintaining mental function as long as possible and providing support as the person declines.

Dementia occurs primarily in people older than 65. It is very common. In the United States, at least 5 million people have dementia. It is the reason for more than 50% of admissions to nursing homes.

As people age, changes in the brain cause some decline in short-term memory and slowing in learning ability. These normal age-related changes, unlike dementia, do not affect the ability to function. Such memory loss in older people is sometimes called age-associated memory impairment. Dementia is a much more serious decline in mental ability, and one that worsens with time. People who are aging normally may misplace things or forget details, but people who have dementia may forget entire events. People who have dementia have difficulty doing normal daily tasks such as driving, cooking, and handling finances. Age-associated memory impairment is not necessarily a sign of dementia or early Alzheimer's disease.

Depression may resemble dementia, especially in older people. People with depression eat and sleep little. They complain bitterly about their memory loss but rarely forget important current events or personal matters. In contrast, people with dementia lack insight about their mental impairments and often deny memory loss. Also, people with depression regain mental function after the depression is treated. Many people have depression and dementia. In these people, treatment of depression may improve but not entirely restore mental function.

In some types of dementia (such as Alzheimer's disease), the level of acetylcholine in the brain is low. Acetylcholine is a chemical messenger (called a neurotransmitter) that helps nerve cells communicate with one another. Acetylcholine helps with memory, learning, and concentration and helps control the functioning of many organs. Other changes occur in the brain, but whether they cause or result from dementia is unclear.

Causes

Commonly, dementia occurs as a brain disorder with no other cause (called a primary brain disorder), but it can be caused by many disorders. Most commonly, dementia is Alzheimer's disease, a primary brain disorder. It accounts for 50 to 70% of cases. Other common types include vascular dementia, Lewy body dementia, and frontotemporal dementia (such as Pick's disease). People may have more than one of these dementias (a disorder called mixed dementia).

Disorders that can cause dementia include the following:

- Parkinson's disease (a common cause)
- Brain damage due to a head injury or certain tumors
- Huntington's disease
- Prion diseases, such as Creutzfeldt-Jakob disease
- Progressive supranuclear palsy
- Radiation therapy to the head

Most of the conditions that cause dementia cannot be reversed, but some can be treated and may be called reversible dementia. Treatment can often cure these dementias if the brain has not been damaged too much. If brain damage is more extensive, treatment often does not reverse the damage, but it can prevent new damage. Conditions that cause reversible dementia include the following:

- Normal-pressure hydrocephalus
- Subdural hematoma
- Human immunodeficiency virus (HIV) infection
- Deficiency of thiamin, niacin, or vitamin B_{12}
- An underactive thyroid gland (hypothyroidism)
- Brain tumors that can be removed
- Prolonged and excessive use of drugs or alcohol
- Toxins (such as lead, mercury, or other heavy metals)
- Syphilis that affects the brain
- Other infections (such as Lyme disease, viral encephalitis, and the fungal infection cryptococcosis)

A subdural hematoma (an accumulation of blood between the outer and middle layers of tissue that cover the brain) results when one or more blood vessels breaks, usually because of a head injury. Such injuries can be slight and may not be recognized.

Many disorders can worsen the symptoms of dementia. They include diabetes, chronic bronchitis, emphysema, infections, a chronic kidney disorder, liver disorders, and heart failure.

Many drugs may temporarily cause or worsen symptoms of dementia. Some of these drugs can be purchased without a prescription (over the counter). Sleep aids (which are sedatives), cold remedies, antianxiety drugs, and some antidepressants are common examples. Drinking alcohol, even in moderate amounts, may also worsen dementia, and most experts recommend that people with dementia stop drinking alcohol.

Symptoms

In people with dementia, mental function typically deteriorates over a period of 2 to 10 years. However, dementia progresses at different rates depending on the cause. In people with vascular dementia, symptoms tend to worsen in steps, worsening suddenly with each new stroke, with some improvement in between. In people with Alzheimer's disease or Lewy body dementia, symptoms tend to worsen more steadily.

The rate of progression also varies from person to person. Looking back at how fast it worsened during the previous year often gives an indication about the coming year. Symptoms may worsen when people with dementia are moved to a nursing home or other institution because people with dementia have difficulty learning and remembering new rules and routines. Problems, such as pain, shortness of breath, retention of urine, and constipation, may cause delirium with rapidly worsening confusion in people who have dementia. If these problems are corrected, people usually return to the level of functioning they had before the problem.

Symptoms of most dementias are similar. Generally, dementia causes the following:

- Memory loss
- Problems using language
- Changes in personality
- Disorientation
- Problems doing usual daily tasks
- Disruptive or inappropriate behavior

Although when symptoms occur varies, categorizing them as early, intermediate, or late symptoms helps affected people, family members, and other caregivers have some idea of what to expect. Personality changes and disruptive behavior may develop early or late. Some people with dementia have seizures, which can also occur early or late.

Early: Because dementia usually begins slowly and worsens over time, it may not be identified at first. Memory, especially for recent events, is one of the first mental functions to noticeably deteriorate. People with dementia typically have more and more difficulty doing the following:

- Finding and using the right word
- Understanding language
- Thinking abstractly, as when working with numbers
- Doing many daily tasks, such as finding their way around and remembering where they put things
- Using good judgment

Emotions may be changeable, unpredictably and rapidly switching from happiness to sadness. Changes in personality are also common. Family members may notice unusual behavior.

Some people with dementia hide their deficiencies well. They follow established routines at home and avoid complex activities such as balancing a checkbook, reading, and working. People who do not modify their lives may become frustrated with their inability to do daily tasks. They may forget to do important tasks or may do them incorrectly. For example, they may forget to pay bills or turn off the lights or stove. Early in dementia, people may be able to continue driving, but they may become confused in congested traffic and get lost more easily.

Intermediate: As dementia worsens, the existing problems worsen and expand, causing the following to become difficult or impossible:

- Remembering events from the past
- Learning and remembering new information
- Doing daily self-care tasks, such as bathing, eating, dressing, and going to the toilet
- Recognizing people and objects
- Keeping track of time and knowing where they are
- Understanding what they see and hear (leading to confusion)
- Controlling their behavior

People often get lost. They may be unable to find their own bedroom or bathroom. They can walk but are more likely to fall. In about 10% of people, this confusion leads to a psychosis, such as hallucinations, delusions, or paranoia.

As dementia progresses, driving becomes more and more difficult because it requires making quick decisions and coordinating many manual skills. People may not remember where they are going.

Personality traits may become more exaggerated. People who were always concerned with money become obsessed with it. People who were often worried become constant worriers. Some people become irritable, anxious, self-centered, inflexible, or more easily angered. Others become more passive, expressionless, depressed, indecisive, or withdrawn. If changes in their personality or mental function are mentioned, people with dementia may become hostile or agitated.

Because people are less capable of controlling their behavior, they sometimes act inappropriately or disruptively (for example, by yelling, throwing, hitting, or wandering). These actions are called behavior disorders. Several effects of dementia contribute to these actions:

- Because they have forgotten the rules of proper behavior, they may act in socially inappropriate ways. When hot, they may undress in public. When they have sexual impulses, they may masturbate in public, use off-color or lewd language, or make sexual demands.

- Because people with dementia have difficulty understanding what they see and hear, they may misinterpret an offer of help as a threat and may lash out. For example, when someone tries to help them undress, they may interpret it as an attack and try to protect themselves, sometimes by hitting.

- Because their short-term memory is impaired, they cannot remember what they are told or have done. They repeat questions and conversations, demand constant attention, or ask for things (such as meals) they have already received. They may become agitated and upset when they do not get what they ask for.

- Because they cannot express their needs clearly or at all, they may yell when in pain or wander when lonely or frightened.

Sleep patterns are often abnormal. Most people with dementia sleep an appropriate amount, but they spend less time in deep sleep. As a result, they may become restless at night. They may also have problems falling or staying asleep. If people do not exercise enough or do not participate in many activities, they may sleep too much during the day. Then they do not sleep well at night. When people with dementia cannot sleep, they may wander, yell, or call out.

Late: Eventually, people with dementia become unable to follow conversations and may become unable to speak. Memory for recent and past events is completely lost. People may not recognize close family members or even their own face in a mirror.

When dementia is advanced, the brain's ability to function is almost completely destroyed. Advanced dementia interferes with control of muscles. People cannot walk, feed themselves, or do any other daily task. They become totally dependent on others and eventually are unable to get out of bed. Eventually, people may have difficulty swallowing food without choking.

These problems increase the risk of undernutrition, pneumonia (often due to inhaling secretions or particles from the mouth), and pressure sores (because they cannot move). Death often results from an infection, such as pneumonia.

Diagnosis

Forgetfulness is usually the first sign noticed by family members or doctors. Doctors and other health care practitioners can usually diagnose dementia by asking the person and family members a series of questions, such as the following:

- What is the person's age?
- Has any family member had dementia or other types of mental dysfunction (family history)?

- When did symptoms start?
- How quickly did symptoms worsen?
- How has the person changed (for example, has the person given up hobbies and activities)?
- What drugs is the person taking (because certain drugs can cause symptoms of dementia)?
- Has the person been depressed or sad, especially if the person is older?

The person is also given a mental status test, consisting of simple questions and tasks, such as naming objects, recalling short lists, writing sentences, and copying shapes (see table on page 632). More detailed testing (called neuropsychologic testing) is sometimes needed to clarify the degree of impairment or to determine whether the person is experiencing true mental decline. This testing covers all the main areas of mental function, including mood, and usually takes 1 to 3 hours.

With information about the person's symptoms and family history and the results of mental status testing, doctors can usually diagnose dementia. They can also usually rule out delirium as the cause of symptoms. Doing so is essential because delirium can be reversed if promptly treated.

A physical examination, including a neurologic examination (see page 630), is usually done to determine whether other disorders are present. Doctors look for treatable disorders that may be causing, contributing to, or mistaken for dementia.

Blood tests are done. They include measuring blood levels of thyroid hormones to check for thyroid disorders and levels of vitamin B_{12} to check for a deficiency. Computed tomography (CT) or magnetic resonance imaging (MRI) is done to rule out abnormalities such as a brain tumor, normal-pressure hydrocephalus, a subdural hematoma, and stroke. However, some causes of the dementia (such as Alzheimer's disease) can be confirmed definitively only when a sample of brain tissue is removed and examined under a microscope. This procedure is sometimes done after death, during an autopsy.

Doctors determine whether another, unrelated physical disorder or psychiatric disorder (such as schizophrenia) is also present because treatment of these disorders may improve the general condition of people with dementia.

? Did You Know...

Dementia is a disorder, not a part of normal aging.

About half of people over 100 do not have dementia.

Treatment

For most dementias, no treatment can restore mental function. However, treating disorders that are worsening the dementia sometimes slows mental decline. For people who have dementia and depression, antidepressants (such as sertraline and paroxetine—see table on page 868) and counseling may help, at least temporarily. Abstaining from alcohol can result in long-term improvement. Drugs that may be making the dementia worse, such as sedatives and drugs that affect brain function, are stopped if possible. Pain and any other disorders or health problems (such as a urinary tract infection or constipation), whether they are related to the dementia or not, are treated. Such treatment may help maintain function in people with dementia.

Creating a safe and supportive environment can be remarkably helpful, and certain drugs can help for a while. The person with dementia, family members, other caregivers, and the health care practitioners involved should discuss and decide on the best strategy for that person.

Safety Measures: Safety is a concern. A visiting nurse or an occupational or a physical therapist can evaluate homes for safety and recommend useful changes. For example, when the light is dim, people with dementia are even more likely to misinterpret what they see, so lighting should be relatively bright. Leaving a night-light on or installing motion sensor lights may also help. Such changes can help prevent accidents (particularly falls) and help people function better.

Supportive Measures: People who have mild to intermediate dementia usually function best in familiar surroundings and can usually remain at home.

Generally, the environment should be bright, cheerful, safe, and stable and include some stimulation, such as a radio or television. The environment should be designed to help with orientation. For example, windows enable people to know generally what time of day it is. Structure and routine help people with dementia stay oriented and give them a sense of security and stability. Any change in surroundings, routines, or caregivers should be explained to people clearly and simply. Before every procedure or interaction, they should be told what is going to happen, such as a bath or a meal. Taking time to explain can help prevent a fight.

Following a daily routine for tasks such as bathing, eating, and sleeping helps people with dementia remember. Following a regular routine at bedtime may help them sleep better.

Other activities scheduled on a regular basis can help people feel independent and needed by focusing their attention on pleasurable or useful tasks.

Such activities can also help relieve depression. Activities related to interests people had before dementia are good choices. Activities should also be enjoyable and provide some stimulation but not too many choices or challenges. Physical activity relieves stress and frustration and thus can help prevent sleep problems and disruptive behavior, such as agitation and wandering. It also helps improve balance (and thus may help prevent falls) and helps keep the heart and lungs healthy. Continued mental activity, including hobbies, interest in current events, and reading, helps keep people alert and interested in life. Activities should be broken down in small parts or simplified as the dementia worsens.

Excessive stimulation should be avoided, but people should not be socially isolated. Frequent visits by staff members and familiar people encourage people to remain social. Some improvement may occur if daily routines are simplified, if expectations for people with dementia are realistic, and if they are enabled to maintain some sense of dignity and self-esteem.

Extra help may be needed. Family members can get a list of available services from health care practitioners, social or human services (listed in the telephone book), or the Internet (through Eldercare Locator). Services may include housekeeping, respite care, meals brought to the home, and daycare programs and activities designed for people with dementia. Around-the-clock-care can be arranged but is expensive.

Because dementia is usually progressive, planning for the future is essential. Long before a person with dementia needs to be moved to a more supportive and structured environment, family members should plan for this move and evaluate the options for long-term care. Such planning usually involves the efforts of a doctor, a social worker, nurses, and a lawyer, but most of the responsibility falls on family members. Decisions about moving a person with dementia to a more supportive environment involve balancing the desire to keep the person safe with the desire to maintain the person's sense of independence as long as possible. Such decisions depend on many factors, such as the following:

- Severity of the dementia
- How disruptive the person's behavior is
- Home environment
- Availability of family members and caregivers
- Financial resources
- Presence of other, unrelated disorders and physical problems

Some long-term care facilities, including assisted living facilities and nursing homes, specialize in caring for people with dementia. Staff members are trained to understand how people with dementia think and

> ## Creating a Beneficial Environment for People With Dementia
>
> People with dementia can benefit from an environment that is the following:
>
> - **Safe:** Extra safety measures are usually needed. For example, large signs can be posted as safety reminders (such as "remember to turn the stove off"), or timers can be installed on stoves or electrical equipment. Hiding car keys may help prevent accidents and placing detectors on doors may help prevent wandering. If wandering is a problem, an identification bracelet or necklace is helpful.
> - **Familiar:** People with dementia usually function best in familiar surroundings. Moving to a new home or city, rearranging furniture, or even repainting can be disruptive.
> - **Stable:** Establishing a regular routine for bathing, eating, sleeping, and other activities can give people with dementia a sense of stability. Regular contact with the same people can also help.
> - **Planned to help with orientation:** A large daily calendar, a clock with large numbers, a radio, well-lit rooms, and a night-light can help with orientation. Also, family members or caregivers can make frequent comments that remind people with dementia of where they are and what is going on.

act and how to respond to them. These facilities have routines that make the residents feel secure and provide appropriate activities that help them feel productive and involved in life. Most facilities usually have appropriate safety features. For example, signs are posted to help residents find their way, and certain doors have locks or alarms to prevent residents from wandering.

Some people with dementia worsen when they are moved from their home to a long-term care facility. However, after a short time, most people adjust and function better in the more supportive environment.

Drugs to Slow Progression: Donepezil, galantamine, rivastigmine, and memantine are used to treat Alzheimer's disease. Rivastigmine can also be used to treat dementia related to Parkinson's disease.

Donepezil, galantamine and rivastigmine are called cholinesterase inhibitors. They inhibit acetylcholinesterase, an enzyme that breaks acetylcholine down. Thus, these drugs help increase the level of acetylcholine, which helps nerve cells communicate. These drugs may temporarily improve mental function in people with dementia, but they do not slow the progression of dementia. They are most useful in early dementia, but their effectiveness varies considerably from person to person. About one third of people do not benefit. About one third improve slightly for a few months. The rest improve considerably for a longer time, but the dementia eventually progresses. If one cholinesterase inhibitor is ineffective or has side effects, another should be tried. If none is effective or all have side effects, this type of drug should be stopped. The most common side effects include nausea, vomiting, weight loss, and abdominal pain or cramps. Tacrine, the first cholinesterase inhibitor developed for treating dementia, is rarely used anymore because it can damage the liver.

Memantine, an NMDA (N-methyl-D-aspartate) antagonist, may help slow the progression of moderate to severe Alzheimer's disease. Memantine works differently from cholinesterase inhibitors and may be used with them. The combination may be more effective than a cholinesterase inhibitor alone.

Drugs to Control Behavior: If disruptive behavior develops, drugs are sometimes used. These drugs include the following:

- **Antipsychotic drugs:** These drugs (see table on page 894) are often used to control the agitation and outbursts that may accompany advanced dementia. However, these drugs tend to be effective only in people who have hallucinations, delusions, or paranoia in addition to dementia—that is, in people who have a psychosis. These drugs can also have serious side effects, such as drowsiness, shakiness, and worsening of confusion. Newer antipsychotic drugs (such as aripiprazole, olanzapine, risperidone, and quetiapine) are as effective as older antipsychotic drugs (such as haloperidol or thioridazine) but have fewer side effects. Antipsychotic drugs should be used only when there is psychosis or when other approaches do not work and when their use is essential to safety.

- **Cholinesterase inhibitors:** These drugs may help control disruptive behavior, as well as improve mental function and slow the progression of dementia.

- **Anticonvulsants:** These drugs, otherwise used to control seizures, may be used to control violent outbursts. They include carbamazepine, gabapentin, and valproate.

However, disruptive behavior is best controlled with strategies that do not include drugs and are tailored to the specific person. If drugs are used, family members should talk with the doctor about whether the drugs are really helping. Antidepressants are used only when people with dementia also have depression.

Dietary Supplements: Many dietary supplements have been tried but have generally proved of little value in treating dementia. They include lecithin, ergoloid mesylates, and cyclandelate. An extract of *Ginkgo biloba*, a dietary supplement that is marketed as a memory enhancer, may modestly benefit some people with dementia (see page 2074). However, evidence for ginkgo is inconsistent, and further study is needed. High doses may have side effects.

Vitamin B_{12} supplements are effective only in people who have vitamin B deficiency, and thyroid hormone replacement is effective only in those who have an underactive thyroid gland.

Before using any dietary supplement, people should talk with their doctor.

End-of-Life Issues: Before people with dementia become too incapacitated, decisions should be made about medical care, and financial and legal arrangements should be made. These arrangements are called advance directives. People should appoint a person who is legally authorized to make treatment decisions on their behalf (health care proxy) and discuss health care wishes with this person and their doctor (see pages 69 and 71). For example, people with dementia should decide whether they want artificial feeding or antibiotics to treat infections (such as pneumonia) when dementia is very advanced. Such issues are best discussed with all concerned long before decisions are necessary.

As dementia worsens, treatment tends to be directed at maintaining the person's comfort rather than at attempting to prolong life. Often, aggressive treatments, such as artificial feeding, increase discomfort. In contrast, less drastic treatments can relieve discomfort. These treatments include adequate control of pain, skin care (to prevent pressure sores), and attentive nursing care. Nursing care is most helpful when it is provided by one caregiver (or a few) who develops a consistent relationship with the person. A comforting, reassuring voice and soothing music may also help.

ALZHEIMER'S DISEASE

Alzheimer's disease is a progressive loss of mental function, characterized by degeneration of brain tissue, including loss of nerve cells and the development of senile plaques and neurofibrillary tangles.

- Forgetting recent events is an early sign, followed by increasing confusion, impairment of other mental functions, and problems using and understanding language and doing daily tasks.

- Symptoms progress so that people cannot function, causing them to become totally dependent on others.

Caring for Caregivers

Caring for people with dementia is stressful and demanding, and caregivers may become depressed and exhausted, often neglecting their own mental and physical health. The following measures can help caregivers:

- **Learning about how to effectively meet the needs of people with dementia and what to expect from them:** For example, caregivers need to know that scolding about making mistakes or not remembering may only make behaviors worse. Such knowledge helps prevent unnecessary distress. Caregivers can also learn how to respond to disruptive behavior and thus calm the person more quickly and sometimes prevent the behavior. Information about what to do on a daily basis may be obtained from nurses, social workers, and organizations, as well as from published and online materials.

- **Seeking help when it is needed:** Relief from the burdens of around-the-clock care of a person with dementia is often available, depending on the specific behavior and capabilities of the person and on family and community resources. Social agencies, including the social service department of the local community hospital, can help locate appropriate sources of help. Options include day-care programs, visits by home nurses, part-time or full-time housekeeping assistance, and live-in assistance. Transportation and meal services may be available. Full-time care can be very expensive, but many insurance plans cover some of the cost. Caregivers may benefit from counseling and support groups.

- **Caring for self:** Caregivers need to remember to take care of themselves. For example, engaging in physical activity can improve mood as well as health. Friends, hobbies, and activities should not be abandoned.

- Doctors base the diagnosis on symptoms and results of a physical examination, mental status tests, blood tests, and imaging tests.
- Treatment involves strategies to prolong functioning as long as possible and may include drugs to slow the progression of the disease.
- How long people live cannot be predicted, but death occurs, on average, about 7 years after the diagnosis is made.

Most dementias are Alzheimer's disease. In older people, it accounts for 50 to 70% of dementias. It is rare among people younger than 60. It becomes more common with increasing age. It affects less than 5% of people aged 60 to 74, 19% of those aged 75 to 84, but more than 30% of those older than 85. One in eight people aged 65 and over have the disease. It affects more women than men. In 2007 in the United States, over 5 million people had Alzheimer's disease.

What causes Alzheimer's disease is unknown, but genetic factors play a role: About 5 to 15% of cases run in families. Several specific gene abnormalities may be involved. Some of these abnormalities can be inherited when only one parent has the abnormal gene. That is, the abnormal gene is dominant. An affected parent has a 50% chance of passing on the abnormal gene to each child. In some of these cases, Alzheimer's disease develops before age 60.

One gene abnormality affects apolipoprotein E (apo E)—the protein part of certain lipoproteins, which transport cholesterol through the bloodstream. There are three types of apo E ($\epsilon2$, $\epsilon3$, and $\epsilon4$). People with the $\epsilon4$ type develop Alzheimer's disease more commonly and at an earlier age than other people. In contrast, people with the $\epsilon2$ type seem to be protected against Alzheimer's disease. People with the $\epsilon3$ type are neither protected nor more likely to develop the disease. (These associations have been studied primarily in whites and may not apply to other races.) However, genetic testing for apo E type cannot determine whether a specific person will develop Alzheimer's disease. Therefore, this testing is not routinely recommended.

In Alzheimer's disease, parts of the brain degenerate, destroying nerve cells and reducing the responsiveness of the remaining ones to many of the chemical messengers that transmit signals between nerve cells in the brain (neurotransmitters). The level of acetylcholine, a neurotransmitter that helps with memory, learning, and concentration, is low. Abnormalities in brain tissue consist of the following:

- Senile or neuritic plaques: Clumps of dead nerve cells containing an abnormal, insoluble protein called amyloid
- Neurofibrillary tangles: Twisted strands of insoluble proteins in the nerve cell
- Increased levels of tau: An abnormal protein that is a component of neurofibrillary tangles

Such abnormalities develop to some degree in all people as they age but are much more numerous in people with Alzheimer's disease.

Symptoms

The symptoms of Alzheimer's disease are similar to those of other dementias (see page 689). They include memory loss, changes in personality, problems using language and doing daily tasks, disorientation, and disruptive behavior. Symptoms develop gradually, so for a while, many people continue to enjoy much of what they enjoyed before developing Alzheimer's disease.

Symptoms usually begin subtly. People whose disease develops while they are still employed may not do as well in their jobs. In people who are retired and not very active, the changes may not be as noticeable.

The first sign may be forgetting recent events, although sometimes the disease begins with changes in personality. People may become emotionally unresponsive, depressed, or unusually fearful or anxious.

Early in the disease, people become less able to use good judgment and think abstractly. Speech patterns may change slightly. People may use simpler words, a general word or many words rather than a specific word, or use words incorrectly. They may be unable to find the right word.

> **? Did You Know...**
> With aging, some brain abnormalities characteristic of Alzheimer's disease develop in everyone.

People with Alzheimer's disease have difficulty interpreting visual and audio cues. Thus, they may become disoriented and confused. Such disorientation may make driving a car difficult. They may get lost on their way to the store. People may be able to function socially but may behave unusually. For example, they may forget the name of a recent visitor, and their emotions may change unpredictably and rapidly.

Many people with Alzheimer's disease often have insomnia. They have trouble falling or staying asleep. Some people become confused about day and night.

At some point, psychosis (hallucinations, delusions, or paranoia) develops in about half of people with Alzheimer's disease.

As Alzheimer's disease progresses, people have trouble remembering events in the past. They may require help with eating, dressing, bathing, and going to the toilet. Disruptive or inappropriate behavior, such as wandering, agitation, irritability, hostility, and physical aggression, is common. All sense of time and place is lost: People with Alzheimer's disease may even get lost on their way to the bathroom at home. Their increasing confusion puts them at risk of falling.

Eventually, people with Alzheimer's disease cannot walk or take care of their personal needs. They may be incontinent and unable to swallow, eat, or speak. These changes put them at risk of undernutrition, pneumonia, and pressure sores (bedsores). Memory is completely lost. Ultimately, coma and death, often due to infections, result.

Progression is unpredictable. People live, on average, about 7 years after the diagnosis is made. Most people with Alzheimer's disease who can no longer walk live no more than 6 months. However, how long people live varies widely.

Diagnosis

If dementia is diagnosed in older people and their memory has gradually deteriorated, doctors consider Alzheimer's disease the most likely cause. The diagnosis is based partly on the following:

- Symptoms, which are identified by asking the person and family members or other caregivers questions
- Results of a physical examination
- Results of mental status tests
- Results of additional tests, such as blood tests, computed tomography (CT), or magnetic resonance imaging (MRI)

Information from the additional tests helps doctors exclude other types and causes of dementia.

The diagnosis of Alzheimer's disease is confirmed only when a sample of brain tissue is removed (after death, during an autopsy) and examined under a microscope. Then, the characteristic loss of nerve cells, neurofibrillary tangles, and senile plaques containing amyloid can be seen throughout the brain, particularly in the area of the temporal lobe that is involved in forming new memories.

Analysis of spinal fluid and positron emission tomography (PET—see page 2044) have been suggested as ways to diagnose Alzheimer's disease during life. However, these tests are used so far only in research.

Treatment

Treatment involves general measures to provide safety and support, as for all dementias (see page 691).

The cholinesterase inhibitors donepezil, galantamine, and rivastigmine increase the level of the neurotransmitter acetylcholine in the brain. This level may be low. These drugs may temporarily improve cognitive function, including memory, but they do not slow the progression of the disease. About half of the people who have Alzheimer's disease benefit from these drugs. For these people, the drugs effectively turn the clock back 6 to 9 months. These drugs are most effective in people with mild to moderate disease. The most common side effects include nausea, vomiting, weight loss, and abdominal pain or cramps.

Memantine appears to slow the progression of Alzheimer's disease. Memantine can be used with a cholinesterase inhibitor.

Researchers continue to study drugs that may prevent or slow the progression of Alzheimer's disease—for example, substances that may reduce the amount of amyloid deposited. Estrogen therapy for women, nonsteroidal anti-inflammatory drugs (NSAIDs, such as ibuprofen or naproxen), and ginkgo biloba are being studied. But none has consistently proved to be effective. Moreover, estrogen appears to do more harm than good.

Vitamin E is an antioxidant that may help protect nerve cells from damage or help them function better. Vitamin E may help preserve the ability to do basic daily tasks, such as dressing and bathing, but it does not improve thinking or memory problems in people with Alzheimer's disease. When taken in reasonable amounts, vitamin E is safe and inexpensive and may slightly benefit some people. Before people take any dietary supplement, they should discuss the risks and benefits with their doctor.

Prevention

Some research tentatively suggests certain measures that may help prevent Alzheimer's disease:

- **Controlling cholesterol levels:** Some evidence suggests that having high cholesterol levels may be related to developing Alzheimer's disease. Thus, people may benefit from a diet low in saturated fats and, if needed, drugs (such as statins) to lower cholesterol and other lipids.
- **Controlling high blood pressure:** High blood pressure may damage blood vessels that carry blood to the brain and thus reduce the brain's oxygen supply, possibly disrupting connections between nerve cells.
- **Exercising:** Exercising helps the heart function better and, for unclear reasons, may help the brain function better.
- **Keeping mentally active:** People are encouraged to continue doing activities that challenge the mind, such as learning new skills, doing crossword puzzles, and reading the newspaper. These activities may promote the growth of new connections (synapses) between nerve cells and thus help delay dementia.
- **Drinking alcohol in modest amounts:** In modest amounts (not more than 3 drinks a day), alcohol may help lower cholesterol and maintain blood flow. Alcohol may even help with thinking and memory by stimulating the release of acetylcholine and causing other changes in nerve cells in the brain. However, there is no convincing evidence that people who do not drink alcohol should start to avoid Alzheimer's disease.

VASCULAR DEMENTIA

Vascular dementia is loss of mental function due to destruction of brain tissue because its blood supply is reduced or blocked. The cause is usually strokes, either a few large ones or many small ones.

- Disorders that damage blood vessels that supply the brain, usually strokes, can cause dementia.
- Symptoms tend to occur in steps, not gradually.
- Dementia is likely to be vascular dementia if people have risk factors or symptoms of a stroke.
- Eliminating the risk factors for strokes may help delay or prevent further damage.

A series of strokes may result in vascular dementia. These strokes are more common among men and usually begin after age 70. Risk factors for vascular dementia include the following:

- Having high blood pressure
- Having diabetes
- Having atherosclerosis
- Having atrial fibrillation, a type of irregular heart rhythm
- Having high levels of fats (lipids), including cholesterol
- Smoking (currently or in the past)
- Having had a stroke

High blood pressure, diabetes, and atherosclerosis damage blood vessels in the brain. Atrial fibrillation increases the risk of strokes due to blood clots from the heart. Unlike other types of dementia, vascular dementia can sometimes be prevented by correcting or eliminating the risk factors for strokes.

Strokes can destroy brain tissue by blocking the blood supply to parts of the brain. An area of brain tissue that is destroyed is called an infarct. Dementia may result from a few large strokes or many small ones. Some strokes cause little or no muscle weakness and seldom cause the paralysis that results from other strokes. They may seem minor or may not even be noticed. However, people may continue to have strokes, and after enough brain tissue is destroyed, dementia can develop. Thus, vascular dementia may develop before strokes cause severe or sometimes even noticeable symptoms.

Several terms have been used to describe vascular dementia. Some of them overlap:

- **Multi-infarct dementia:** Dementia is caused by several strokes, usually involving medium-sized blood vessels.
- **Lacunar disease:** Sometimes this term is used to describe multi-infarct dementia caused by many lacunar infarcts, which are strokes caused by blockages in small blood vessels.

- **Binswanger's dementia:** Several small blood vessels are blocked (causing lacunar infarcts) in people who have severe, poorly controlled high blood pressure and a blood vessel (vascular) disorder that affects blood vessels throughout the body.

Vascular dementia often occurs with Alzheimer's disease (as mixed dementia).

Symptoms

Unlike dementia caused by Alzheimer's disease, vascular dementia may progress in steps. Symptoms may worsen suddenly, then plateau or lessen somewhat. They then become worse months or years later when another stroke occurs. Dementia that results from many small strokes usually progresses more gradually than that due to a few large strokes. The small strokes may be so subtle that dementia may seem to develop gradually and continuously instead of in steps.

Symptoms (memory loss, difficulty planning and initiating actions or tasks, slowed thinking, and a tendency to wander) are similar to those of other dementias. However, compared with Alzheimer's disease, vascular dementia tends to cause memory loss later and to affect judgment and personality less. People have particular difficulty planning and initiating actions, slowed thinking may be noticeable.

Symptoms can vary depending on what part of the brain is destroyed. Usually, some aspects of mental function are not impaired because the strokes destroy tissue in only part of the brain. Thus, people may be more aware of their losses and more prone to depression than people with other types of dementia.

As more strokes occur and dementia progresses, people may have other symptoms due to the strokes. An arm or a leg may become weak or paralyzed. People may have difficulty speaking. For example, they may slur their speech. Vision may be blurred or partly or completely lost. Coordination may be lost, making walking unsteady. People may laugh or cry inappropriately. People may have difficulty controlling bladder function, resulting in urinary incontinence.

Death usually occurs about 5 years after symptoms begin. It is often due to a stroke or heart attack.

Diagnosis

Once dementia is diagnosed, doctors suspect vascular dementia in people who have risk factors for or symptoms of a stroke. Computed tomography (CT) or magnetic resonance imaging (MRI) may be done to check for evidence of a stroke. Results of these tests can support the diagnosis but are not definitive.

Treatment

Treatment involves general measures to provide safety and support, as for all dementias (see page 691).

Treating diabetes, high blood pressure, and high cholesterol levels can help prevent and slow or stop the progression of vascular dementia. Stopping smoking is also recommended.

There is no specific treatment for vascular dementia. Sometimes cholinesterase inhibitors and memantine, the drugs used for Alzheimer's disease, are given because some people with vascular dementia also have Alzheimer's disease. For people who have had a stroke, doctors may recommend that they take aspirin, which can reduce the risk of another stroke. People with atrial fibrillation are given warfarin, an anticoagulant, to help reduce the risk of another stroke.

LEWY BODY DEMENTIA

Lewy body dementia is progressive loss of mental function characterized by the development of Lewy bodies in nerve cells.

- Lewy bodies form throughout the brain.
- People fluctuate between alertness and drowsiness and may have difficulty drawing, as well as hallucinations, and difficulty moving that is similar to that due to Parkinson's disease.
- Diagnosis is based on symptoms.
- Strategies are used to prolong functioning as long as possible, and the drugs used to treat Alzheimer's disease may help.

Lewy body dementia is a common type of dementia, but experts disagree about its prevalence and significance. It is more common among men than among women. Lewy body dementia usually develops in people older than 60.

Microscopic changes in the brain differ from those due to Alzheimer's disease. In Lewy body dementia, abnormal round deposits of protein (called Lewy bodies) form in nerve cells. Lewy bodies result in the death of nerve cells. Lewy bodies also occur in Parkinson's disease. In Parkinson's disease, they occur only in one part of the brain (deep within the brain stem), but in Lewy body dementia, they occur throughout the outer layer of the brain (cerebral cortex). Some experts think that these two disorders are variations of the same problem. People with Alzheimer's disease may develop some Lewy bodies, although neurofibrillary tangles and senile plaques seem to be the main source of damage.

Symptoms

The symptoms of Lewy body dementia are very similar to those of Alzheimer's disease. They include memory loss, disorientation, and problems remembering, thinking, understanding, communicating, and controlling behavior. But Lewy body dementia can be distinguished by the following:

- In the early stages, mental function fluctuates, often dramatically, over a period of days to weeks but sometimes from moment to moment. One day, people may be alert and able to pay attention and converse coherently, and the next day, they may be drowsy, inattentive, and almost mute. People may stare into space for long periods.

- At first, attention and alertness may be more impaired than is memory, including memory for recent events.

- The ability to copy and draw may be impaired more severely than other brain functions.

- Psychotic symptoms, such as hallucinations, delusions, and paranoia, are more common in Lewy body dementia, and hallucinations tend to occur earlier.

In Lewy body dementia, hallucinations are usually visual ones, which are often complex and detailed. They may include recognizable animals or people. The hallucinations are often threatening. Over half of people with Lewy body dementia have complex, bizarre delusions. Instead of relieving these symptoms, antipsychotic drugs often make them and other symptoms worse or have other severe, sometimes life-threatening adverse effects (see table on page 894).

Like people who have Parkinson's disease, people with Lewy body dementia have stiff muscles, move slowly and sluggishly, shuffle when they walk, and stoop over. Balance is easily lost, making falls more likely. Tremor also develops, but it usually develops later and causes fewer problems than it does in Parkinson's disease. Problems with thinking begin within 1 year of the time that problems with muscles and movement develop.

Sleep problems are common. Many people with Lewy body dementia have rapid eye movement (REM) sleep behavior disorder. People with this disorder act out their dreams, sometimes injuring their bed partner.

The autonomic nervous system may malfunction, preventing the body from regulating internal functions, such as blood pressure and body temperature. As a result, people may faint, sweat too much or too little, have a dry mouth, or have urinary problems or constipation.

After symptoms appear, people usually live about 6 to 12 years.

Diagnosis

Doctors base the diagnosis on symptoms. Lewy body dementia is likely if mental function fluctuates in people who have visual hallucinations and symptoms of Parkinson's disease. Doctors must rule out delirium, which requires prompt treatment, because in delirium, mental function also fluctuates. Computed tomography (CT) and magnetic resonance imaging (MRI) may be done to rule out other causes of dementia.

Distinguishing Lewy body dementia from dementia due to Parkinson's disease can be difficult because symptoms are similar. Generally, Lewy body dementia is more likely if movement and muscle problems develop at the same time or shortly after the mental decline. Dementia due to Parkinson's disease is more likely if mental decline occurs after movement and muscle problems in people with Parkinson's disease.

Treatment

Treatment involves general measures to provide safety and support, as for all dementias (see page 691). There is no specific treatment for Lewy body dementia, but the same drugs used to treat Alzheimer's disease, particularly rivastigmine, may be helpful. Drugs used to treat Parkinson's disease may help relieve the symptoms of Parkinson's disease, but they may worsen confusion, hallucinations, and delusions. Antipsychotic drugs are not used if possible.

FRONTOTEMPORAL DEMENTIA

Frontotemporal dementia, which refers to a group of dementias, results from hereditary or spontaneous (occurring for unknown reasons) disorders that cause the frontal and sometimes the temporal lobe of the brain to degenerate.

- Personality, behavior, and language function are affected more and memory less than in Alzheimer's disease.

- Doctors base the diagnosis on symptoms and results of a neurologic examination and use imaging tests to assess the brain damage.

- Treatment aims to manage symptoms.

About 1 of 10 dementias is a frontotemporal dementia. Typically, the dementia develops in people younger than 65. Men and women are affected about equally. These dementias tend to run in families. Brain cells contain abnormal amounts or types of a protein called tau.

In these dementias, the frontal and temporal lobes shrink (atrophy), and nerve cells are lost. These areas of the brain are generally associated with personality and behavior. There are several types, including Pick's disease.

Pick's Disease: In this rare disorder, Pick bodies develop in nerve cells. Pick bodies contain abnormal amounts or types of tau. Pick's disease resembles Alzheimer's disease except that it affects only the frontal and temporal lobes of the brain and progresses more rapidly. Symptoms include inappropriate behavior, apathy, memory loss, carelessness, and poor personal hygiene. Death usually occurs in 2 to 10 years.

Symptoms

Frontotemporal dementias are progressive, but how quickly they progress to general dementia varies.

Generally, these dementias affect personality, behavior, and language function more and affect memory less than Alzheimer's disease does. People with a frontotemporal dementia also have difficulty thinking abstractly, paying attention, and recalling what they have been told. They are easily distracted. However, they usually remain aware of time, date, and place and are able to do their daily tasks.

In some people, muscles are affected. They may become weak and waste away (atrophy). Muscles of the head and neck are affected, making swallowing, chewing, and talking difficult.

Different types of symptoms develop, depending on which part of the frontal lobe is affected. People may have more than one type of symptom, particularly as the dementia progresses.

Changes in Personality and Behavior: Some people become uninhibited, resulting in increasingly inappropriate behavior. They may speak rudely. Their interest in sex may increase abnormally.

Behavior may become impulsive and compulsive. They may repeat the same action over and over. They may walk to the same location every day. They may compulsively pick up and manipulate random objects and put objects in their mouth. They may suck or smack their lips. They may overeat or eat only one type of food.

People neglect personal hygiene.

Problems With Language: Most people have difficulty finding words. They have increasing difficulty using and understanding language (aphasia). For some, physically producing speech (dysarthria) is difficult. Paying attention is very difficult. For some people, language problems are the only symptom for 10 or more years. For other people, other symptoms appear within a few years.

Some people cannot understand language, but they speak fluently, although what they say does not make any sense. Others have difficulty naming objects (anomia) and recognizing faces (prosopagnosia).

They speak less and less or repeat what they or others say. Eventually, they stop speaking.

Diagnosis

The diagnosis is based on symptoms, including how they developed. Family members may have to provide this information because affected people may be unaware of their symptoms. A neurologic examination and mental status tests are usually done.

Computed tomography (CT) and magnetic resonance imaging (MRI) are done to determine which parts and how much of the brain is affected and to exclude other possible causes (such as brain tumors, abscesses, or a stroke). However, CT or MRI may not detect the characteristic changes of frontotemporal dementia until late in the disorder. Positron emission tomography (PET—see page 2044) may help differentiate frontotemporal dementia from Alzheimer's disease, but PET is usually used only in research.

Treatment

There is no specific treatment. Generally, treatment focuses on managing symptoms and providing support. For example, if compulsive behavior is a problem, antipsychotic drugs may be used. Speech therapy may help people with language problems.

NORMAL-PRESSURE HYDROCEPHALUS

Normal-pressure hydrocephalus consists of difficulty walking, urinary incontinence, and dementia due to an increase in the fluid that normally surrounds the brain.

Normally, the fluid that surrounds the brain and protects it from injury (cerebrospinal fluid) is continuously produced in the spaces within the brain (ventricles), circulates in and around the brain, and is reabsorbed. Normal-pressure hydrocephalus is thought to occur when this fluid is not reabsorbed normally, causing it to accumulate. The amount of fluid in the ventricles increases and the brain is then pushed outward.

Symptoms

Usually, the main symptom is an abnormally slow, unsteady, wide-legged walk. However, in some people, the feet seem to stick to the floor (called a magnetic gait). People also have urinary incontinence and a tendency to fall.

Dementia may not develop until late in the disorder. Often, the first sign of dementia is difficulty planning, organizing, putting ideas or doing actions for a task in the right order (sequencing), thinking abstractly, and paying attention. Memory tends to be lost later.

Diagnosis

The diagnosis cannot be based on symptoms alone, particularly in older people. Other dementias can cause similar symptoms. Brain imaging (usually MRI) may detect excess cerebrospinal fluid, but this finding is also inconclusive, although it supports the diagnosis of normal-pressure hydrocephalus.

To help with the diagnosis, doctors do a spinal tap (lumbar puncture) to remove excess cerebrospinal fluid. If this procedure relieves symptoms, normal-pressure hydrocephalus is likely, and treatment is likely to be effective.

Treatment

Treatment consists of placing a piece of plastic tubing (a shunt) in the ventricles of the brain and running it under the skin, usually to the abdomen (ventriculoperitoneal shunting). Cerebrospinal fluid is then drained away from the brain. The effects of this treatment may not be evident for several hours. This procedure may significantly improve the ability to walk and function and may lessen incontinence. However, mental function improves less and in fewer people. Thus, early diagnosis is important, so that people can be treated before dementia develops.

OTHER DEMENTIAS

Dementia develops in many disorders.

Parkinson's Disease: About 40% of people with Parkinson's disease (see page 771) develop dementia, usually after age 70 and about 10 to 15 years after Parkinson's disease has been diagnosed. Dementia may be so severe that it is more disabling and causes death more often than any other effects of Parkinson's disease. People who have hallucinations and severe muscle and movement problems are most likely to develop dementia.

Symptoms may be very similar to those of Alzheimer's disease and Lewy body dementia. For example, memory is impaired, and people have difficulty processing information. People think more slowly. They may be apathetic and lack motivation. They may be moody, confused, disoriented and easily distracted.

Doctors diagnose Parkinson's disease dementia in people with Parkinson's disease when dementia develops years after motor symptoms. However, distinguishing dementia due to Parkinson's disease from Lewy body dementia can be difficult because symptoms are similar. Generally, Lewy body dementia is more likely if movement and muscle problems develop at the same time or shortly after the mental decline. Dementia due to Parkinson's disease is more likely if mental decline develops after movement and muscle problems in people with Parkinson's disease. Computed tomography (CT) and magnetic resonance imaging (MRI) may be done to rule out other causes of dementia.

Treatment involves general measures to provide safety and support, as for all dementias. Rivastigmine, a cholinesterase inhibitor, can be used to treat Parkinson's disease dementia.

Creutzfeldt-Jakob Disease: This rare disease is a prion disease that causes a rapidly progressive dementia (see page 766). Creutzfeldt-Jakob disease often leads to severe dementia and death within a year. The most common early symptoms—memory loss and confusion—may resemble those of other dementias.

Variant Creutzfeldt-Jakob disease, thought to be acquired from eating beef contaminated with prions, causes a dementia similar to that due to Creutzfeldt-Jakob disease, except the first symptoms tend to be psychiatric symptoms (such as anxiety or depression) rather than memory loss.

No treatment is available.

HIV-Associated Dementia: In the late stages of human immunodeficiency virus (HIV) infection, the virus may directly infect the brain (see page 1254). HIV damages nerve cells, causing dementia. Dementia may also result from other infections that people with HIV infection are prone to get. Unlike almost all other forms of dementia, it tends to occur in younger people.

This dementia usually begins subtly but progresses steadily over a few months or years. It usually develops after other symptoms of HIV infection. Symptoms of this dementia include slowed thinking and expression, difficulty concentrating, and apathy, but insight is not affected. Movements are slow, muscles are weak, and coordination may be impaired.

When HIV infection is diagnosed or when mental function changes in people with HIV infection, CT or MRI is done to check for a brain infection. Unless evidence suggests that pressure within the skull is increased, doctors usually do a spinal tap (lumbar puncture) to obtain a sample of cerebrospinal fluid for analysis and check for infection. Findings can support but not confirm the diagnosis of HIV-associated dementia.

Treatment with zidovudine and other drugs used to treat HIV infection sometimes produces dramatic improvement. However, because the infection is not cured, dementia may recur.

Dementia Pugilistica: This disorder, also called chronic progressive traumatic encephalopathy, may develop in people who have repeated head injuries—boxers, for example. They often develop symptoms similar to those of Parkinson's disease, and some of them also develop normal-pressure hydrocephalus.

112 Stupor and Coma

Stupor is unresponsiveness from which a person can be aroused only by vigorous, physical stimulation. Coma is unresponsiveness from which a person cannot be aroused. In coma, the person's eyes remain closed.

- The cause is usually a disorder or drug that affects large areas on both sides of the brain or specialized areas of the brain involved in maintaining consciousness.
- A physical examination, blood tests, brain imaging, and information from family and friends help doctors identify the cause.
- Possible causes are corrected, and treatments to support body functions, such as a ventilator, are provided.
- Recovery from a coma depends largely on the cause.

Normally, the brain can quickly adjust its own levels of activity and consciousness as needed. The brain makes these adjustments based on information it receives from the eyes, ears, skin, and other sensory organs. For example, the brain can decrease its metabolic activity and induce sleep.

Consciousness is controlled by the lower part of the brain (brain stem) through a system of nerve cells and fibers (the reticular activating system, also known as the ascending arousal system (see page 625). The upper part of the brain (cerebrum) helps maintain consciousness and alertness. The cerebrum is divided into two halves (cerebral hemispheres). At least one hemisphere, as well as the reticular activating system, must be functioning normally to maintain consciousness.

The brain's ability to adjust its activity and consciousness levels can be impaired in several ways:

- When people are severely deprived of sleep
- When and immediately after a seizure occurs
- When both cerebral hemispheres are suddenly and severely damaged
- When the reticular activating system malfunctions
- When blood flow or the amount of nutrients (such as oxygen or sugar) going to the brain decrease
- When toxic substances impair the brain

Periods of impaired consciousness can be short or long. The level of impairment can range from slight to severe:

- **Lethargy** is a slight reduction in alertness or clouding of consciousness. People tend to be less aware of what is happening around them and to think more slowly.

- **Obtundation,** an imprecise term, refers to a moderate reduction in alertness or clouding of consciousness.
- **Stupor** is an excessively long or deep sleeplike state. A person can be aroused from it only briefly by vigorous stimulation, such as repeated shaking, loud calling, pinching, or sticking with a pin.
- **Coma** is a state of complete unresponsiveness. A person cannot be aroused at all. A person in a deep coma lacks even the most basic responses, such as avoidance of pain, although reflexes may be present.

Causes

The various levels of impaired consciousness—lethargy, obtundation, stupor, and coma—have the same causes, of which there are many. Most commonly, the cause is a toxic substance, drug, metabolic abnormality, or another disorder that makes nerve cells throughout the brain function slowly. Some of these causes interfere with the delivery of needed substances to the brain or the body's ability to use them. Examples are a very low or high level of sugar in the blood (hypoglycemia or hyperglycemia), a very low level of oxygen in the blood, and the sudden stopping of the heart's pumping (cardiac arrest).

Disorders such as liver or kidney failure, an underactive thyroid gland (hypothyroidism), or a very low or high body temperature (hypothermia or hyperthermia) can cause many types of cells throughout the body to malfunction. Often, brain cells are affected the most.

Commonly, consciousness is impaired by drinking too much alcohol or taking too much of certain drugs, such as sedatives (see box on page 671) and opioids (narcotics—see page 642). In addition to making brain cells function slowly, alcohol and some drugs can damage brain cells indirectly. They can slow breathing so much that the oxygen level in blood becomes low enough to cause brain damage. Occasionally, taking certain antipsychotic drugs results in an unresponsive state called neuroleptic malignant syndrome (see box on page 893).

In older people, reactions to drugs, dehydration (which results in a high sodium level), and infections are common causes of impaired consciousness.

Other common causes are disorders that affect the areas of the brain that control consciousness. For example, a head injury may jar but not physically damage (stun) such areas, directly damage them, or indirectly damage them by causing bleeding

SPOTLIGHT ON AGING

Stupor and coma are particular concerns among older people for the following reasons:

- Drugs and relatively minor disorders are more likely to impair consciousness in older people, sometimes leading to stupor and coma. Drugs are a common cause of impaired consciousness, often because too much is taken. Older people may take too much when doctors prescribe a dose that is too high. Older people are more sensitive to many drugs, and a lower dose is often needed. Sometimes older people take too much of a drug by mistake. Also, older people take more drugs, increasing the risk of drug interactions. A urinary tract infection or dehydration usually has no serious effects in young adults but often impairs consciousness in older adults.

- Many disorders that are more common among older people can cause stupor or coma. They include strokes, brain tumors, bulges in weakened arteries (aneurysms) in the brain, metabolic disorders, and severe heart or lung disorders.

- If older people become less alert or less conscious of things around them, family members and friends may not notice or may assume that the change results from aging. A change in consciousness may be harder to discern in older people who have dementia or another brain disorder or who have had a stroke.

- Older people are less likely to recover from stupor or coma because the brain becomes less able to repair itself as people age.

(hemorrhage) in or around the brain. Strokes and tumors can also directly damage areas of the brain that control consciousness.

A mass in the brain, such as an accumulation of blood (hematoma), a tumor, or an abscess, can impair consciousness indirectly. A large mass can push the brain against the relatively rigid structures inside the skull, damaging brain tissue. If the areas of the brain that control consciousness are affected, stupor or coma results. The pressure may affect the entire cerebrum or the brain stem. If the pressure is high enough, the brain may be forced through a small natural opening in the relatively rigid sheets of tissue that separate the brain into compartments. This life-threatening disorder is called brain herniation (see art on page 735). Herniation can further damage brain tissue, making an already dire condition worse.

Symptoms

The brain damage or dysfunction that causes stupor and coma affects other parts of the body. The pattern of breathing is usually abnormal. People may breathe too rapidly, too slowly, too deeply, or irregularly. Or they may alternate between these abnormal patterns.

Muscles may remain contracted in unusual positions. For example, the head may be tilted back with the arms and legs extended—a position called decerebrate rigidity. The arms may be flexed—a position called decorticate rigidity. Or the entire body may be limp. Sometimes muscles contract sporadically or involuntarily.

One or both pupils of the eyes may be widened (dilated) and not react to changes in light. Or the pupils may be tiny. The eyes may not move or may move in abnormal ways.

Diagnosis

Doctors can usually tell that consciousness is impaired based on observation and examination. Doctors try to identify the level and cause of impairment because treatment differs and because impairment may progress, leading to coma and brain death. Stupor is diagnosed when vigorous, repeated attempts arouse the person only briefly. Coma is diagnosed when the person cannot be aroused at all.

People who become stuporous or comatose must be taken to the hospital immediately because either state may be caused by a life-threatening disorder. Health care practitioners try to identify the cause and provide emergency medical care at the same time.

People with disorders that put them at risk of stupor or coma (such as diabetes, which can result in a low blood sugar level) should carry medical identification or wear a Medic Alert identification bracelet or necklace. Thus, if they lose consciousness, the probable cause can be quickly identified.

Because a stuporous or comatose person cannot communicate, family members and friends must honestly provide emergency medical personnel or the doctor with any relevant information about the person, which includes the following:

- Whether the person uses drugs (prescription and recreational), alcohol, or other toxic substances and which ones are used
- Whether the person was injured before the change in consciousness
- When and how the problem began
- Whether the person has had any infections or other symptoms (such as headaches or vomiting)
- When the person last seemed normal

If a drug or toxic substance was ingested, family members or friends should give a sample of that substance or its container to the doctor. Information from the family and friends usually is valuable and is more likely to lead to the correct diagnosis than examination or testing. For example, no test can rule out all possible drug overdoses. Thus, information about empty pill containers or drug paraphernalia near the person is extremely important.

Physical Examination: Emergency medical personnel or doctors first check whether the airway is open, whether breathing is adequate, and whether blood pressure and pulse are normal. Body temperature is checked. For example, an abnormally high temperature may indicate infection, heatstroke, or an overdose of a drug that stimulates the body (such as cocaine or an amphetamine). An abnormally low temperature may indicate prolonged exposure to cold, an underactive thyroid gland, alcohol intoxication, a sedative overdose or, in older people, infection. The skin is examined for signs of injury, drug injections, illnesses, and allergic reactions, and the scalp is examined for cuts and bruises. The tongue is examined to see if it has been bitten—a finding that suggests seizures.

A neurologic examination is done as thoroughly as possible. This examination helps doctors determine how severe stupor or coma is, whether the brain stem is functioning normally, and what part of the central nervous system is damaged.

Doctors may use stimuli that cause discomfort or trigger reflexes. If the eyes open or the person grimaces or purposefully withdraws from a painful stimulus, consciousness is not severely impaired.

Doctors look for signs of brain damage or impaired brain function. For example, abnormal breathing patterns can provide clues to the depth of coma. Checking reflexes can help determine whether parts of the brain and spinal cord are malfunctioning. Unusual body positions, such as decerebrate or decorticate rigidity, may indicate substantial brain damage. Absence of reflexes and limpness of the entire body are worrisome. They may indicate widespread dysfunction in all parts of the central nervous system, including the brain stem, the cerebrum, and the nerve fibers that connect the cerebrum to the spinal cord.

The eyes also provide important clues. The position of the pupils, their size, their reaction to bright light, their ability to follow a moving object (in people who are not comatose), and the appearance of the retina are checked. If a pupil remains dilated and does not react to bright light, there may be pressure on the 3rd cranial nerve, which helps control eye movement, or on the brain stem. Such a reaction sometimes indicates a large mass in the brain causing herniation. If coma is deep and both pupils do not remain dilated but react to light, this type of a mass is unlikely. To accurately evaluate the person, doctors need to know whether the person's pupils are normally different sizes, and whether the person takes a drug to treat glaucoma, which can affect pupil size.

The person's response to certain maneuvers can provide additional information:

- Rotating the head and observing eye movements can help doctors determine whether the brain stem is functioning normally.
- Squirting cold water into one or both ears and observing eye movements can determine whether the person is really unresponsive and, if so, whether the brain stem is damaged.

Laboratory Tests: These tests provide further clues about the possible cause of stupor or coma. Blood levels of substances such as sugar, sodium, alcohol, oxygen, and carbon dioxide are measured. The red and white blood cell counts are determined. Blood tests to check liver function are done. Urine is analyzed to determine whether any commonly used or suspected toxic substances are present. The blood sugar level is also estimated using a quick test done at the person's bedside, so that a low blood sugar level can be treated immediately.

Other Tests: If no cause has been quickly identified, computed tomography (CT) or magnetic resonance imaging (MRI) of the head is done to check for a mass (such as a hematoma, a tumor, or an abscess), or for other structural brain damage.

If the cause is unclear after imaging tests or if meningitis or subarachnoid hemorrhage is possible, a spinal tap (lumbar puncture) is done to withdraw and examine a sample of cerebrospinal fluid (see art on page 635). Emergency CT or MRI of the head is often done before the spinal tap to determine whether pressure inside the skull is increased (for example, by a tumor or hemorrhage). If pressure is increased, a spinal tap could make the brain shift downward by rapidly reducing the pressure below the brain and thus, at least theoretically, cause or worsen brain herniation.

? Did You Know...

People in a locked-in state can think normally but appear unresponsive because they cannot move any part of their body except their eyes.

People in a vegetative state go to sleep and awaken normally and have eye movements but have actually lost all capacity for thought and conscious behavior.

SOME CAUSES OF STUPOR AND COMA

WHAT?	HOW?	WHAT HAPPENS?
Brain disorders		
Seizures	Seizures that recur frequently or last a long time, can ■ Overstimulate brain tissue, disrupting normal transmission of nerve impulses ■ Cause a high fever, which may make the brain malfunction or damage brain tissue Some people remain unresponsive for hours after a seizure.	Consciousness can be impaired.
Strokes	Strokes can block blood flow to parts of the brain, including to the brain stem.	If blood flow to the brain stem is blocked, consciousness may be suddenly lost, and coma can result. If blood flow to the entire brain stem is blocked and not restored within a few minutes, most or all of the brain stem is damaged, and death may result.
	Strokes may result from bleeding in the brain (intracerebral hemorrhage) or around it (subarachnoid hemorrhage). Blood can directly irritate brain tissue or increase pressure on it.	Blood can directly damage or increase pressure on brain tissue. Consciousness may be impaired, and coma may result. Even a small amount of bleeding in the brain stem can cause coma.
Tumor or abscess	A large tumor or abscess can push the brain against the relatively rigid structures inside the skull and put pressure on brain tissue, causing it to malfunction. Tumors can directly invade and damage brain tissue.	If the areas of the brain that control consciousness are affected, coma results.
Other disorders		
Cardiac arrest	In cardiac arrest, the heart stops pumping. Consequently, the brain does not receive enough blood, which carries oxygen to tissues. Brain tissue dies because it is deprived of oxygen.	Consciousness is lost within a minute or two. Nerve cells may die if cardiac arrest lasts even 4 to 5 minutes. Coma results and may soon become irreversible.
Heart or lung disorders if severe	Severe heart disorders (such as heart failure) can reduce blood flow to the brain. Severe lung disorders (such as chronic obstructive pulmonary disease, pulmonary edema, pulmonary embolism, and severe and long-lasting asthma attacks) can reduce the amount of oxygen in the blood.	With either type of disorder, the brain may not receive enough oxygen, sometimes resulting in coma.

(continued on the following page)

SOME CAUSES OF STUPOR AND COMA (*Continued*)

WHAT?	HOW?	WHAT HAPPENS?
Kidney failure Liver encephalopathy or failure	If the kidneys or liver cannot remove toxic waste products from the blood as they normally do, waste products accumulate in the blood and cause the brain to malfunction.	If coma results from chronic kidney or liver failure, it is usually reversible. If coma results from acute, severe liver failure, the brain swells because fluid accumulates in brain cells. Death often results.
Metabolic abnormalities		
Hyperglycemia	The blood sugar level is abnormally high. The blood becomes syrupy, drawing fluid from the brain.	Stupor or coma can result.
Hypoglycemia	The blood sugar level is abnormally low. The brain malfunctions or is damaged if it is deprived of sugar, which is its main source of energy.	Coma can result. Immediate treatment with glucose, given intravenously soon after coma develops, prevents permanent brain damage.
Hypernatremia	The blood sodium level is high. Hypernatremia is usually due to dehydration and can reduce the amount of water in brain cells.	An abnormal amount of water in brain cells interferes with chemical reactions there. Stupor or coma may result.
Hyponatremia	The blood sodium level is low. Hyponatremia may be due to the following: ■ Drinking too much water (for example, during college fraternity rituals) ■ Retaining too much water ■ Losing too much sodium in urine or in the digestive tract (as when diarrhea occurs) This disorder can increase the amount of water in brain cells.	An abnormal amount of water in brain cells interferes with chemical reactions there. Stupor, coma, and seizures may result.
Hypothyroidism	The thyroid gland is underactive. Untreated hypothyroidism may cause mental confusion and slowed thinking.	The confusion may progress to stupor and coma.
Infections	If brain tissue becomes infected, the brain may malfunction. Causes include infection of the brain (encephalitis) and infection of the membranes lining the brain and spinal cord (meningitis). Other infections, such as sepsis, can cause high fevers, which may make the brain malfunction or damage brain tissue.	Coma may result.
Accidents and injuries		
Asphyxiation	The brain is deprived of oxygen.	Consciousness is quickly lost, and coma and death may follow.

(continued on the following page)

SOME CAUSES OF STUPOR AND COMA (*Continued*)

WHAT?	HOW?	WHAT HAPPENS?
Head injury	Head injuries may damage the brain in the following ways: ■ Jar the brain without physically damaging it (as in a concussion) ■ Bruise the brain (as in a contusion) ■ Cut or crush brain tissue ■ Cause bleeding in or around the brain (as in an intracerebral or subarachnoid hemorrhage) Blood may directly irritate brain tissue or may accumulate as a mass (hematoma), which puts pressure on the brain (as in epidural or subdural hematoma).	Depending on the injury, coma may develop immediately or gradually over several hours.
Hyperthermia	A body temperature above 104° F (40° C), as occurs in high fevers or heatstroke, can damage the brain.	Coma can result. Nerve cells die much more quickly when body temperature is very high.
Hypothermia	A body temperature below 88° F (31.1° C) slows brain function. However, low temperatures can actually protect the brain by slowing the damage caused by lack of blood or oxygen. Also, nerve cells die much more slowly when body temperature is very low. For example, a child may fully recover after being submersed for 30 minutes in an icy lake. Being submersed that long in warm water is usually fatal.	Stupor or coma can result but usually without permanent damage if people survive. Some people recover completely.
Substances		
Alcohol	Alcohol slows brain function. Consumed in large amounts, it may affect brain tissue directly or indirectly by slowing breathing so much that the oxygen level in blood becomes low enough to cause brain damage.	A high blood alcohol level, especially when it exceeds 0.2%, can cause stupor or coma.
Carbon monoxide or similar substances inhaled in large amounts	Carbon monoxide attaches to the hemoglobin in red blood cells. It takes the place of oxygen and prevents red blood cells from carrying oxygen to tissues, including the brain.	Severe carbon monoxide poisoning can cause coma or irreversible brain damage because the brain does not receive enough oxygen.
Drugs	Many drugs even if not given in high doses can affect brain function. For example, high doses of barbiturates, opioids (including morphine), a sedative (such as diazepam), or these drugs combined with each other or with alcohol can slow brain function.	A coma can result. If treated early, this type of coma can be completely reversed.

If the cause is still unclear, electroencephalography (EEG) is done to check the brain's electrical activity. Occasionally, EEG indicates that the person is having a seizure even though the limbs are not jerking (a disorder called nonconvulsive status epilepticus).

Treatment

A rapidly deteriorating level of consciousness is a medical emergency requiring immediate treatment, sometimes even before a diagnosis is made.

People are admitted to a hospital intensive care unit, where nurses can monitor heart rate, blood pressure, temperature, and the oxygen level in the blood. Any abnormalities in these levels are immediately corrected to prevent further damage to the brain. Oxygen is often given immediately, and an intravenous line is put in place so that drugs can be given quickly. Any other disorders (such as heart or lung disorders) present are treated.

The cause is treated when possible. For example, for a low blood sugar level (hypoglycemia), glucose, a sugar, is immediately given intravenously. Giving glucose often results in instant recovery if the coma is caused by hypoglycemia. Thiamin is always given with glucose because in malnourished people (such as alcoholics), glucose alone can trigger or worsen a brain disorder called Wernicke's encephalopathy. If taking an opioid is the suspected cause, the antidote naloxone may be given. Recovery may be almost instantaneous if the opioid is the only cause of impaired consciousness.

People with deep stupor or in a coma may require a breathing tube, particularly if a feeding tube is to be inserted into the stomach. The breathing tube prevents people from inhaling stomach contents after vomiting and facilitates mechanical ventilation if their breathing is too slow or shallow. Rarely, when doctors suspect that certain toxic substances have been ingested within about 1 hour, a large tube may be inserted into the stomach so that the stomach can be pumped. Pumping the stomach is done to identify its contents and to prevent more of the substances from being absorbed. Activated charcoal may also be given through the tube or through a smaller tube inserted through the nose (nasogastric tube) to prevent further absorption of the substances.

If findings suggest that the pressure inside the skull is increased, doctors may drill a small hole in the skull and insert a pressure monitoring device into one of the fluid-filled spaces (ventricles) in the brain. If the pressure is increased, measures are taken to lower it:

- The head of the bed may be elevated.
- Diuretics or other drugs may be used to reduce fluids in the brain and rest of the body.

- A sedative may be given to control excess involuntary muscular contractions, which can increase pressure within the skull.
- Blood pressure is sometimes lowered.
- Occasionally, the skull is opened surgically, creating more room for the swollen brain and thus reducing pressure on the brain.

Long-Term Care: People in a coma require comprehensive care. They are fed through a tube inserted through the nose and into the stomach. Sometimes a tube (called a percutaneous endoscopic gastrostomy tube or PEG tube) is inserted through an incision in the abdomen directly into the stomach.

Many problems result from being unable to move, and measures to prevent them are essential. For example, lying in one position can cut off the blood supply to some areas of the body, causing skin to break down and pressure sores to form. Caretakers must turn people into different positions very frequently. Lack of movement can also lead to permanent stiffening of muscles (contractures) and make blood clots more likely to form in leg veins. To prevent these problems, physical therapists gently move the person's joints in all directions (passive range-of-motion exercises) and may splint joints in certain positions that tend to prevent contractures. Because people cannot blink, their eyes may become dry. Eye drops can help.

People who are incontinent should be kept clean from urine and stool. If the person's bladder is not functioning and urine is being retained, then doctors prefer using intermittent urinary catheterization over placing an indwelling catheter to reduce the risk of infection.

Prognosis

The likelihood of recovery can be predicted by the cause, duration, and rate of recovery from coma:

- **Overdose of a sedative:** Recovery is likely unless people stopped breathing long enough to cause brain damage.
- **A low blood sugar level:** Complete recovery is possible if the brain was not deprived of sugar for more than about 1 hour.
- **Head injury:** Substantial recovery may occur, even if the coma lasts several weeks (but not if it lasts more than 3 months).
- **Stroke:** Permanent brain damage is likely if coma lasts 6 hours or longer.
- **Cardiac arrest or oxygen deprivation:** Full recovery rarely occurs in the following cases. After 1 day, the pupils do not quickly begin to narrow

Variations in Impaired Consciousness

Vegetative state: This state results when the cerebrum, which controls thought and behavior, can no longer function, but the thalamus and brain stem, which control sleep cycles, body temperature, breathing, blood pressure, and heart rate, can function. A vegetative state occasionally develops after severe brain damage due to a head injury, oxygen deprivation, or a severe brain infection such as meningitis or encephalitis.

People in this state spontaneously open their eyes and have relatively normal sleeping and waking patterns. People can breathe, suck, chew, cough, gag, and swallow. They may even become startled in reaction to loud noises. So they may appear to be aware. However, they have lost all capacity for awareness, thought, and conscious behavior. Their apparent response to the environment is the result of reflexes. Most people in a vegetative state have obvious abnormal reflexes, including stiffening or jerking of the arms and legs.

If a vegetative state lasts for more than a few months, people are unlikely to recover consciousness. Most people who recover consciousness after a few months are severely disabled.

Minimally conscious state: In this state, people do a few things that indicate some awareness. They may reach for objects, answer "yes" whether it is appropriate or not, or follow objects with their eyes. This state may result directly from brain damage, or it may follow a vegetative state as people recover some function. A few people recover the ability to communicate and comprehend, sometimes after many years, but none recover the ability to function normally or live independently. Stimulation of deep parts of the brain and zolpidem (a sleep aid) are being studied as possible treatments. With skilled nursing care, these people can live for years.

Locked-in state: People with this rare condition are conscious and able to think but are so severely paralyzed that they can communicate only by opening and closing the eyes in response to questions. The locked-in state can be caused by strokes that affect the brain stem but not the cerebrum, or by severe paralysis of peripheral nerves, as may result from severe Guillain-Barré syndrome. People in this state cannot move their lower face, chew, swallow, speak, breathe, move their limbs, or move their eyes from side to side. Sometimes they are mistakenly thought to be unconscious. Affected people are often very depressed. Speech therapists can help develop a communication code using eye blinks. If communication can be established, affected people should make their own health care decisions. Occasionally, when the cause can be corrected, people recover certain functions.

Brain death: This condition is the most severe form of unconsciousness. The brain has permanently lost the ability to perform all vital functions, including breathing. The concept of brain death evolved partly because, with modern medicine, artificial means (such as ventilators and drugs) can maintain breathing and the heart's beating even when all brain activity stops. A brain-dead person is considered legally dead.

There are specific criteria for diagnosing brain death:

- The person does not grimace, move, or otherwise react in response to any type of stimulation.
- The eyes do not react to light.
- The person makes no attempt to breathe.

Also, doctors cannot diagnose brain death until they have corrected all treatable medical problems that could slow brain function and thus could be misdiagnosed as brain death. These problems include a very low body temperature, severe abnormalities in levels of substances (such as sugar and sodium) in the blood, overdose of a sedative, and ingestion of certain potentially toxic drugs.

After these medical problems are corrected, brain death can be diagnosed. If the diagnosis is not clear, diagnostic procedures may be done to confirm brain death. Electroencephalography (EEG—a recording of the brain's electrical activity—see page 636) shows no brain waves if a person is brain dead. Procedures may be done to show that blood is not flowing to the brain. They include angiography, single photon emission computed tomography (SPECT—which uses a radioactive molecule called a radionuclide to produce images of blood flow), and transcranial Doppler ultrasonography. Such procedures enable doctors to rapidly confirm brain death after catastrophic head injuries (as may occur in motor vehicle accidents). Also, when confirmation is quick, organ donation is possible.

After brain death is confirmed, all life support is stopped. Family members may wish to be with the person at this time. They need to be told that the limbs may move when breathing assistance is ended. These movements result from reflex muscle contractions and do not mean the person is not really brain dead.

(constrict) in response to light. After 3 days, people do not blink reflexively when the cornea is touched and do not move their limbs purposefully. After 1 week, people cannot move the limbs when asked to do so.

Sometimes doctors use evoked responses to determine whether the brain stem is functioning. This test can accurately predict a poor prognosis after only 24 hours. The brain stem is stimulated, and EEG is used to detect the response.

Results of a physical examination can also help predict prognosis. Recovery is likely if one or more of the following occur within the first days:

- Speech returns, even if it is incomprehensible.
- The eyes can follow an object.
- People can follow commands.

Children and sometimes young adults recover more fully than older people because brain cells repair themselves more quickly and completely in the young.

For people who remain in a deep coma longer than a few weeks, decisions about continued use of a ventilator, feeding tube, and drugs should be made. Family members should discuss these issues with the doctors. If people have advance medical directives (see page 69), such as a living will or durable power of attorney for health care, the directives should guide decisions about continuing care.

(see page 69)

<table>
<tr><td>CHAPTER</td></tr>
<tr><td>113</td></tr>
</table>

113 Seizure Disorders

In seizure disorders, the brain's electrical activity is periodically disturbed, resulting in some degree of temporary brain dysfunction.

- Many people have unusual sensations just before a seizure starts.
- Some seizures cause uncontrollable shaking and loss of consciousness, but more often, people simply stop moving or become unaware of what is happening.
- Doctors suspect the diagnosis based on symptoms, but imaging of the brain, blood tests, and electroencephalography (to record the brain's electrical activity) are usually needed to identify the cause.
- If needed, drugs can usually prevent seizures.

Normal brain function requires an orderly, organized, coordinated discharge of electrical impulses. Electrical impulses enable the brain to communicate with the spinal cord, nerves, and muscles as well as within itself. Seizures may result when the brain's electrical activity is disrupted.

There are two basic types of seizures:

- **Epileptic:** These seizures have no apparent cause (or trigger) and occur repeatedly. These seizures are called a "seizure disorder" or "epilepsy."
- **Nonepileptic:** These seizures are triggered (provoked) by a disorder or another condition that irritates the brain. In children, a fever can trigger a nonepileptic seizure.

Certain mental disorders can cause symptoms that resemble seizures, called psychogenic nonepileptic seizures.

About 2% of adults have a seizure at some time during their life. Two thirds of these people never have another one. Most commonly, seizure disorders begin in early childhood or in late adulthood.

Causes

Which causes are most common depend on when seizures start:

- **Before age 2:** High fevers or temporary metabolic abnormalities, such as abnormal blood levels of sugar (glucose), calcium, magnesium, vitamin B_6, or sodium, can trigger one or more seizures. Seizures do not occur once the fever or abnormality resolves. If the seizures recur without such triggers, the cause is likely to be an injury during birth, a birth defect, or a hereditary metabolic abnormality or brain disorder.
- **2 to 14 years:** Often, the cause is unknown.
- **After age 25:** A head injury, stroke, or tumor may damage the brain, causing a seizure. Alcohol withdrawal (caused by suddenly stopping drinking) is a common cause of seizures. However, in about half of people in this age group, the cause is unknown.

Seizures with no identifiable cause are called idiopathic.

Conditions that irritate the brain—such as injuries, certain drugs, sleep deprivation, infections, fever—or that deprive the brain of oxygen or fuel—such as abnormal heart rhythms, a low level of oxygen in the blood, or a very low level of sugar in the blood—can trigger a single seizure whether a person has a seizure disorder or not. A single seizure that results from such a stimulus is called a provoked seizure (and thus is a nonepileptic seizure). People with a seizure disorder are more likely to

CAUSES OF SEIZURES

CAUSE	EXAMPLES
High fever	Heatstroke Infections
Brain infections	Abscess AIDS Malaria Meningitis Rabies Syphilis Tetanus Toxoplasmosis Viral encephalitis
Metabolic disorders	High blood levels of sugar or sodium Kidney or liver failure Low blood levels of sugar, calcium, magnesium, or sodium Underactive parathyroid gland Vitamin B_6 deficiency (in newborns)
Inadequate oxygen supply to the brain	Abnormal heart rhythms Carbon monoxide poisoning Near drowning Near suffocation Stroke Vasculitis
Structural damage to the brain	Brain tumor (noncancerous or cancerous) Head injury Hydrocephalus Intracranial hemorrhage Stroke
Abnormalities present or occurring at birth	Birth defect Hereditary metabolic disorders, such as Tay-Sachs disease or phenylketonuria Injury during birth
Fluid accumulation in the brain (cerebral edema)	Eclampsia Hypertensive encephalopathy
Prescription drugs*	Buspirone (used to treat anxiety disorders) Camphor Ceftazidime (an antibiotic) Chlorpromazine (used to treat schizophrenia) Ciprofloxacin (an antibiotic) Chloroquine (used to treat malaria) Cyclosporine (used to prevent and treat rejection of organ transplants) Imipenem (an antibiotic) Indomethacin (used to relieve pain and reduce inflammation) Meperidine (used to relieve pain) Phenytoin[†] Theophylline (used to treat asthma and other airway disorders) Tricyclic antidepressants (overdose)

(continued on the following page)

CAUSES OF SEIZURES (*Continued*)

CAUSE	EXAMPLES
Recreational drugs	Amphetamines Cocaine (overdose)
Withdrawal of a drug after heavy use	Alcohol General anesthetics (used during surgery) Sedatives, including sleep aids
Exposure to toxins	Lead Strychnine

*Various drugs can cause seizures if too much is taken.
†Phenytoin, used to treat seizure disorders, can cause seizures if too much is taken.

have a seizure when they are under excess physical or emotional stress or deprived of sleep. Avoiding these conditions can help prevent seizures.

Rarely, seizures are triggered by repetitive sounds, flashing lights, video games, or even touching certain parts of the body. In such cases, the disorder is called reflex epilepsy.

Symptoms

In about 20% of people who have a seizure disorder, seizures are preceded by unusual sensations (called aura), such as the following:

- Abnormal smells or tastes
- Butterflies in the stomach
- A feeling of déjà vu
- An intense feeling that a seizure is about to begin

Almost all seizures are relatively brief, lasting from a few seconds to a few minutes. Most seizures last 1 to 2 minutes. When a seizure stops, people may have a headache, sore muscles, unusual sensations, confusion, and profound fatigue. These after-effects are called the postictal state. In some people, one side of the body is weak, and the weakness lasts longer than the seizure (a disorder called Todd's paralysis). Most people who have a seizure disorder look and behave normally between seizures.

Symptoms vary depending on which area of the brain is affected by the abnormal electrical discharge (see pages 624 and 677) as in the following:

- An intensely pleasant or unpleasant taste if the part of the cerebrum called the insula is affected
- Visual hallucinations (seeing unformed images) if the occipital lobe is affected
- Inability to speak if the area that controls speech (located in the frontal lobe) is affected

- A convulsion (jerking and spasms of muscles throughout the body) if large areas on both sides of the brain are affected

Other possible symptoms include numbness or tingling in a specific body part, brief episodes of unresponsiveness, loss of consciousness, confusion, and loss of muscle or bladder control.

Symptoms also vary depending on whether the seizure is partial or generalized. About 70% of people have only one type of seizure. The rest have two or more types.

Partial Seizures: Only one side of the brain is affected. Partial seizures may be simple or complex.

In **simple partial seizures,** abnormal electrical discharges begin in a small area of the brain and remain confined to that area. Because only a small area of the brain is affected, symptoms are related to the function controlled by that area. For example, if the small area of the brain that controls the right arm's movements (in the left frontal lobe) is affected, the right arm may begin to shake and jerk. People are completely conscious and aware of the surroundings. A simple partial seizure may progress to a complex partial seizure.

Jacksonian seizures are a type of simple partial seizures. Symptoms start in one part of the body, then spread to another. Abnormal movements may occur in the hand or foot, then move up the limb as the electrical activity spreads in the brain. People are completely aware of what is occurring during the seizure.

In **complex partial seizures,** abnormal electrical discharges begin in a small area of the temporal lobe or frontal lobe and quickly spread to other nearby areas. The seizures usually begin with an aura that lasts 1 to 2 minutes. During the aura, people start to lose touch with the surroundings. During the seizure, consciousness is impaired but not completely lost. People may do the following:

- Stare
- Chew or smack the lips involuntarily
- Move the hands, arms, and legs in strange, purposeless ways
- Utter meaningless sounds
- Not understand what other people are saying
- Resist help

Some people can converse, but their conversation lacks spontaneity, and the content is somewhat sparse. They may be confused and disoriented. This state may last for several minutes. Most people do not remember what happened during the seizure (a condition called postictal amnesia). Some people then recover fully. In others, the abnormal electrical discharge spreads to adjacent areas and to the other side of the brain, resulting in a generalized tonic-clonic seizure. Generalized seizures that result from partial seizures are called secondarily generalized seizures.

Epilepsia partialis continua is rare. Seizures occur every few seconds or minutes for days to years at a time. They typically affect an arm, a hand, or one side of the face. These seizures usually result from localized brain damage (such as scarring due to a stroke) in adults or from inflammation of the brain (as occurs in encephalitis and measles) in children.

Generalized Seizures: Large areas on both sides of the brain are affected. Generalized seizures often cause loss of consciousness and abnormal movements, usually immediately. Loss of consciousness may be brief or last a long time.

Generalized tonic-clonic seizures may be primary or secondary. Primary generalized seizures begin with abnormal discharges in a deep, central part of the brain and spread simultaneously to both sides of the brain. Secondary generalized tonic-clonic (grand mal) seizures usually begin with an abnormal electrical discharge in a small area of one side of the brain, resulting in a complex partial seizure. The discharge then quickly spreads to both sides of the brain, causing the entire brain to malfunction. In both types, consciousness is temporarily lost and a convulsion occurs when the abnormal discharges spread to both sides of the brain. In primary generalized seizures, there is no aura. During the seizure, people may do the following:

- Have severe muscle spasms and jerking throughout the body
- Fall down
- Forcefully turn their head to one side
- Clench their teeth
- Bite their tongue (often occurs)

- Drool or froth at the mouth
- Lose bladder control

The seizures usually last 1 to 2 minutes. Afterward, some people have a headache, are temporarily confused, and feel extremely tired. These symptoms may last from minutes to hours. Most people do not remember what happened during the seizure.

Absence seizures may be typical (petit mal) or atypical. Typical absence seizures usually begin in childhood, usually between the ages of 5 and 15 and do not continue into adulthood. However, adults occasionally have typical absence seizures. Unlike tonic-clonic seizures, absence seizures do not cause convulsions or other dramatic symptoms. People do not fall down, collapse, or move jerkily. Instead, they have episodes of staring with fluttering eyelids and sometimes twitching facial muscles. They are completely unaware of their surroundings. These episodes last 10 to 30 seconds. People abruptly stop what they are doing and resume it just as abruptly. They experience no after-effects and do not know that a seizure has occurred. Without treatment, many people have several seizures a day. Seizures often occur when people are sitting quietly. Seizures rarely occur during exercise. Hyperventilation can trigger a seizure.

Atypical absence seizures are less common. They last longer than typical absence seizures, jerking and other movements are more pronounced, and people are more aware of their surroundings. Most people with atypical absence seizures have neurologic abnormalities or developmental delays. Seizures usually continue into adulthood.

Atonic seizures occur primarily in children. They are characterized by a brief but complete loss of muscle tone and consciousness. They cause children to fall to the ground, sometimes resulting in injury.

Tonic seizures occur commonly during sleep. Muscle tone increases abruptly or gradually, causing muscles to stiffen. The seizures typically last only 10 to 15 seconds but can cause people, if standing, to fall to the ground. Most people do not lose consciousness. If seizures last longer, muscles may jerk a few times as the seizure ends.

Myoclonic seizures are characterized by quick jerks of one or several limbs or the trunk. The seizures are brief and do not cause loss of consciousness, but they may occur repetitively, resulting in a tonic-clonic seizure with loss of consciousness.

Infantile spasms (see page 1804) and **febrile seizures** (see page 1803) occur in children.

Juvenile myoclonic epilepsy typically begins during adolescence. Typically, seizures begin with quick jerks of both arms. About 90% of these seizures are followed by tonic-clonic seizures. Some people also have absence seizures. The seizures of juvenile myoclonic epilepsy often occur when people awaken in the morning, especially if they are sleep-deprived. Drinking alcohol also makes these seizures more likely.

Status epilepticus is the most serious seizure disorder and a medical emergency because the seizure does not stop. Electrical discharges occur throughout the brain, causing a generalized tonic-clonic seizure. Status epilepticus is diagnosed when a seizure lasts more than 5 minutes or when people do not completely regain consciousness between seizures. People have convulsions with intense muscle contractions and cannot breathe adequately. Body temperature increases. Without rapid treatment, the heart and brain can become overtaxed and permanently damaged, sometimes resulting in death.

Complications: Seizures may have serious consequences. Intense, rapid muscle contractions can cause injuries, including broken bones. Sudden loss of consciousness can cause serious injury due to falls and accidents. People may have numerous seizures without incurring serious brain damage. However, seizures that recur and cause convulsions may eventually impair intelligence.

If seizures are not well controlled, people may be unable to get a driver's license. They may have difficulty keeping a job or getting insurance. They may be socially stigmatized. As a result, their quality of life may be substantially reduced.

If seizures are not completely controlled, people are twice as likely to die as those who do not have seizures. A few people die suddenly for no apparent reason—a complication called sudden unexplained death in epilepsy.

> **? Did You Know...**
>
> Many types of seizures do not cause convulsions and loss of consciousness.
>
> Putting a spoon in the mouth of someone having a convulsion can do more harm than good.

Diagnosis

Doctors diagnose a seizure disorder when people have at least two unprovoked seizures that occur at different times. The diagnosis is based on symptoms and the observations of eyewitnesses. Symptoms that suggest a seizure include loss of consciousness, muscle spasms that shake the body, loss of bladder control, sudden confusion, and inability to pay attention. However, seizures cause such symptoms much less often than most people think. A brief loss of consciousness is more likely to be fainting (syncope—see page 344) than a seizure.

An eyewitness report of the episode can be very helpful to doctors. An eyewitness can describe exactly what happened, whereas people who have an episode usually cannot. Doctors need to have an accurate description, including the following:

- How fast the episode started
- Whether it involved abnormal muscle movements (such as spasms of the head, neck, or facial muscles), tongue biting, drooling, loss of bladder control, or muscle stiffening
- How long it lasted
- How quickly the person recovered

Although eyewitnesses may be too frightened during the seizure to remember all details, whatever they can remember can help. If possible, how long a seizure lasts should be timed with a watch or other device. Seizures that last only 1 or 2 minutes can seem to go on forever.

Doctors also need to know what people experienced before the episode: whether they had a premonition or warning that something unusual was about to happen and whether anything, such as certain sounds or flashing lights, seemed to trigger the episode. Doctors ask whether people have had a disorder that can cause seizures (such as a brain infection) or a head injury. Doctors also ask about which drugs (including alcohol) people are taking or have recently stopped. A thorough physical examination is done. It may provide clues to the cause of the symptoms.

People are usually evaluated in an emergency department. If a seizure disorder has already been diagnosed and people have completely recovered, they may be evaluated in a doctor's office.

Once a seizure is diagnosed, more tests are usually needed to identify the cause. People known to have a seizure disorder may not need additional tests. In others, blood tests are often done to measure the levels of substances such as sugar, calcium, sodium, and magnesium and to determine whether the liver and kidneys are functioning normally. A sample of urine may be analyzed to check for recreational drugs that may not be reported. Such drugs can trigger a seizure. Electrocardiography (see page 326) may be done to check for an abnormal heart rhythm. Because an abnormal heart rhythm can greatly reduce blood flow (and therefore oxygen supply) to the brain, it can trigger loss of consciousness and occasionally a seizure or symptoms that resemble a seizure.

Computed tomography (CT) is usually done promptly to check for bleeding, tumors, and other

Brain Activity During a Seizure

An electroencephalogram (an EEG) is a recording of the brain's electrical activity. The procedure is simple and painless. About 20 small adhesive electrodes are placed on the scalp, and the brain's activity is recorded under normal conditions. Then the person is exposed to various stimuli, such as bright or flashing lights, to try to provoke a seizure. During a seizure, electrical activity in the brain accelerates, producing a jagged wave pattern. Such recordings of brain waves help identify a seizure disorder. Different types of seizures have different wave patterns.

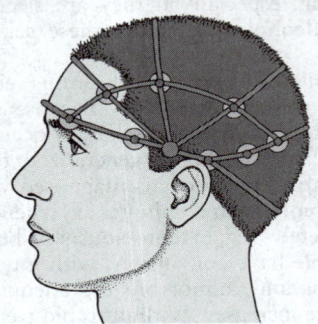

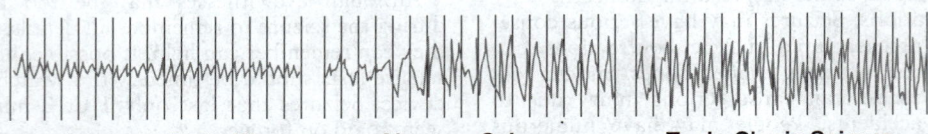

Normal Adult Brain Wave   **Absence Seizure**   **Tonic-Clonic Seizure**

structural damage to brain tissue (for example, by a stroke). If results are negative, magnetic resonance imaging (MRI) is usually done later. It provides detailed images of abnormalities and can detect most neurologic disorders.

If doctors suspect a brain infection such as meningitis or encephalitis, a spinal tap (lumbar puncture—see art on page 635) is usually done.

Electroencephalography (EEG) can help confirm the diagnosis. EEG is a painless, safe procedure that records electrical activity in the brain (see page 636). Doctors examine the recording (electroencephalogram) for evidence of abnormal electrical discharges. Because the recording time is limited, EEG can miss abnormalities, and results may be normal, even in people who have a seizure disorder. EEG is sometimes scheduled after people have been deprived of sleep for 18 to 24 hours because lack of sleep makes abnormal discharges more likely to occur.

If these tests do not identify a cause, other tests may be done. EEG may be repeated because when done a second or even a third time, it may detect the cause, which was missed the first time the test was done. If the diagnosis is still uncertain, specialized tests, such as video-EEG monitoring, can be done at an epilepsy center. For this test, people are admitted to a hospital for 2 to 7 days, and EEG is done while they are video-taped. If people are taking an anticonvulsant, it is often stopped to increase the likelihood of a seizure. If a seizure occurs, doctors compare the EEG recording with the video recording of the seizure. They may then be able to identify the type of seizure and the area of the brain where the seizure began.

Treatment

If the cause can be identified and eliminated, no additional treatment is necessary. For example, if a low blood sugar (glucose) level (hypoglycemia—see page 1014) caused the seizure, glucose is given, and the disorder causing the low level is treated. Other treatable causes include an infection, certain tumors, and an abnormal sodium level.

If people have a seizure disorder, general measures plus drugs are usually sufficient. If drugs are ineffective, surgery may be recommended.

General Measures: Exercise is recommended and social activities are encouraged. However, people who have a seizure disorder may have to make some adjustments. For example, they should eliminate or limit their consumption of alcoholic beverages and should not use recreational drugs. They should refrain from activities in which a sudden loss of consciousness could result in serious injury. For example, they should not bathe in a bathtub, climb, swim, or operate power tools. After seizures are controlled (typically for at least 6 months), they can do these activities if adequate precautions are taken. For example, they should swim only when lifeguards are present. In most states, laws prohibit people with a seizure disorder from driving until they have been free of seizures for at least 6 months to 1 year.

A family member or close friend should be trained to help if a seizure occurs. Attempting to put an object (such as a spoon) in the person's mouth to protect the person's tongue should not be tried. Such efforts can do more harm than good. The teeth may be damaged, or the person may bite the helper unintentionally as the jaw muscles contract. However, helpers should do the following during a seizure:

- Protect the person from falling
- Loosen clothing around the neck
- Place a pillow under the head

If a pillow is unavailable, helpers can put their foot or place an item of clothing under the person's head.

People who lose consciousness should be rolled onto one side to ease breathing. People who have had a seizure should not be left alone until they have awakened completely, are no longer confused, and can move about normally. Usually, their doctor should be notified.

Anticonvulsants: These drugs reduce the risk of having another seizure. Usually, they are prescribed only for people who have had more than one seizure, unless the cause has been identified and completely eliminated. They are usually not prescribed when people have had only one generalized seizure. Most anticonvulsants are taken by mouth.

Anticonvulsants can completely prevent generalized seizures in about one third of people who have them and greatly reduce the frequency of seizures in another third. Almost two thirds of people who respond to anticonvulsants can eventually stop taking them without having a relapse. However, anticonvulsants are ineffective in about 10 to 20% of people with a seizure disorder. These people are referred to a seizure center and evaluated for surgery.

There are many different types of anticonvulsants. Which one is effective depends on the type of seizure and the response to it. For most people, taking one anticonvulsant, usually the first or second one tried, controls seizures. If seizures recur, different anticonvulsants are tried. Determining which anticonvulsant is effective may take several months. Some people have to take several drugs, which increases the risk of side effects. Some anticonvulsants are not used alone but only with other anticonvulsants.

Doctors take care to determine the appropriate dose of an anticonvulsant for each person. The best dose is the smallest dose that stops all seizures while having the fewest side effects. Doctors ask people about side effects, then adjust the dose if needed.

Sometimes doctors also measure the level of anticonvulsant in the blood. Anticonvulsants should be taken just as prescribed. People who take anticonvulsants to control seizures should see a doctor regularly for dose adjustment and should always wear a Medic Alert bracelet inscribed with the type of seizure disorder and the drug being taken.

Anticonvulsants can interfere with the effectiveness of other drugs, and vice versa. Consequently, people should make sure their doctor knows all the drugs they are taking before they start taking anticonvulsants. They should also talk to their doctor and possibly their pharmacist before they start taking any other drugs, including over-the-counter drugs.

After seizures are controlled, people take the anticonvulsant until they have been seizure-free for at least 2 years. Then, the dose of the drug may be decreased gradually, and the drug eventually stopped. If a seizure recurs after the anticonvulsant is stopped, people may have to take an anticonvulsant indefinitely. Seizures usually recur within 2 years if they are going to. A recurrence is more likely in people who have had any of the following:

- A seizure disorder since childhood
- The need to take more than one anticonvulsant to be seizure-free
- Seizures while taking an anticonvulsant
- Partial or myoclonic seizures
- Abnormal EEG results within the previous year

Anticonvulsants, although very effective, may have side effects. Many cause drowsiness, but some may make children hyperactive. Blood tests are done periodically to determine whether an anticonvulsant is impairing kidney or liver function or reducing the number of blood cells. People taking anticonvulsants should be aware of possible side effects and should consult their doctor at the first sign of side effects.

For women who have a seizure disorder and are pregnant, taking an anticonvulsant increases the risk of miscarrying or of having a baby with a birth defect (see table on page 1638). However, stopping the anticonvulsant may be more harmful to the woman and the baby. Having a generalized seizure during pregnancy can injure or kill the fetus. All women who are of childbearing age and take an anticonvulsant should take folate supplements to reduce the risk of having a baby with a birth defect.

Emergency Treatment: Emergency treatment is required for status epilepticus and seizures that last more than 5 minutes. Large doses of one or more anticonvulsants are given intravenously as quickly as possible. Measures to prevent injuries are taken

℞ DRUGS USED TO TREAT SEIZURES

DRUG	USE	SOME SIDE EFFECTS
Acetazolamide	Absence seizures when other anti-convulsants are ineffective	Kidney stones, dehydration, and chemical imbalances in the blood
Carbamazepine	Generalized seizures Partial seizures	A low white blood cell count (granulocytopenia), production of too few blood cells (aplastic anemia, which can be fatal), a low platelet count (thrombocytopenia), digestive upset, inability to articulate words, lethargy, dizziness, and visual disturbances
Clonazepam	Atonic seizures Atypical absence seizures Infantile spasms Myoclonic seizures	Drowsiness, abnormal behavior, loss of coordination, and lost effectiveness of the drug after 1 to 6 months
Divalproex	Absence seizures Febrile seizures Generalized tonic-clonic seizures Infantile spasms Juvenile myoclonic epilepsy Myoclonic seizures Partial seizures	Nausea, vomiting, abdominal pain, diarrhea, temporary drowsiness, dizziness, shaking (tremor), reversible hair loss, weight gain, and liver damage
Ethosuximide	Absence seizures	Nausea, lethargy, dizziness, headache, a low white blood cell count, and a low red blood cell count
Felbamate	Atypical absence seizures Partial seizures	Headache, fatigue, liver failure, and, rarely, aplastic anemia (which can be fatal)
Fosphenytoin	Status epilepticus	Loss of coordination, drowsiness, dizziness, headache, rash, and tingling sensations
Gabapentin	Partial seizures	Drowsiness, dizziness, weight gain, and headache In children, aggressive behavior, mood swings, and hyperactivity
Lamotrigine	Generalized seizures Partial seizures	Nausea, vomiting, indigestion, headache, drowsiness, dizziness, insomnia, fatigue, loss of coordination, double vision, tremor, rash, and abnormal menstrual periods
Levetiracetam	Juvenile myoclonic epilepsy Myoclonic seizures Partial seizures Primary generalized tonic-clonic seizures	Dizziness, weakness, fatigue, loss of coordination, changes in mood and behavior, and increased risk of infection
Oxcarbazepine	Partial seizures	Headache, abdominal pain, double vision, drowsiness, dizziness, fatigue, nausea, low sodium levels in the blood, and a low white blood cell count
Phenobarbital	Generalized tonic-clonic seizures Partial seizures Status epilepticus	Drowsiness, abnormal eye movements (nystagmus), and loss of coordination In children, hyperactivity and learning difficulties
Phenytoin	Complex partial seizures Generalized tonic-clonic seizures Status epilepticus when phenytoin is given intravenously	Swollen gums, a low red blood cell count, loss of bone density, excessive hairiness (hirsutism), and swollen glands
Pregabalin	Partial seizures	Dizziness, drowsiness, loss of coordination, blurred vision, double vision, tremor, and weight gain

(continued on the following page)

℞ DRUGS USED TO TREAT SEIZURES (Continued)

DRUG	USE	SOME SIDE EFFECTS
Primidone	Generalized tonic-clonic seizures Partial seizures	Drowsiness, abnormal eye movements (nystagmus), and loss of coordination In children, hyperactivity and learning difficulties
Tiagabine	Partial seizures	Drowsiness, dizziness, confusion, abdominal pain, fatigue, nausea, and tremor
Topiramate	Atypical absence seizures Partial seizures Primarily generalized tonic-clonic seizures	Confusion, reduced concentration, difficulty finding words, fatigue, loss of appetite and weight, numbness or tingling, reduced sweating, and kidney stones
Valproate	Absence seizures Febrile seizures Generalized tonic-clonic seizures Infantile spasms Juvenile myoclonic epilepsy Myoclonic seizures Partial seizures	Nausea, vomiting, abdominal pain, diarrhea, weight gain, reversible hair loss, temporary drowsiness, shaking (tremor), and, rarely, liver damage
Zonisamide	Partial seizures	Drowsiness, fatigue, dizziness, confusion, difficulty finding words, loss of coordination, kidney stones, loss of appetite and weight, and nausea

during the prolonged seizure. People are monitored closely to make sure breathing is adequate. If it is not, a tube is inserted to help with breathing—a procedure called intubation. If seizures persist, a general anesthetic is given to stop them.

Surgery: If people continue to have seizures while taking two or more anticonvulsants or if they cannot tolerate side effects of the anticonvulsants, brain surgery may be done. These people are tested at specialized epilepsy centers to determine whether surgery can help. Tests may include the following:

- Functional MRI: To determine which areas in the brain are causing seizures
- Single-photon emission CT (SPECT): To check for areas with decreased blood flow around the time of a seizure, which may indicate which areas in the brain are causing seizures
- EEG combined with magnets used for imaging (magnetic source imaging): Also to help determine which areas in the brain are causing seizures

If a defect in the brain (such as a scar) can be identified as the cause and is confined to a small area, surgically removing that area can eliminate seizures in up to 80% of people, or it may reduce the severity and frequency of seizures. Surgically cutting the nerve fibers that connect the two sides of the brain (corpus callosum) may help people who have seizures that originate in several areas of the brain or that spread to all parts of the brain

very quickly. This procedure usually has no appreciable side effects. However, even if surgery reduces the frequency and severity of seizures, many people need to continue to take anticonvulsants. However, they can usually take lower doses or fewer drugs.

Before and after surgery, a psychologic and neurologic evaluation (see page 630) may be done to determine how well the brain is functioning.

Stimulation of the Vagus Nerve: Electrical stimulation of the 10th cranial nerve (vagus nerve) can reduce the number of partial seizures by more than one half in some people. This treatment is used when seizures continue despite use of anticonvulsants and when surgery is not a possibility.

The vagus nerve is thought to have indirect connections to areas of the brain often involved in causing seizures. A device that looks like a heart pacemaker (vagus nerve stimulator) is implanted under the left collarbone and is connected to the vagus nerve in the neck with a wire that runs under the skin. The device causes a small bulge under the skin. The operation is done on an outpatient basis and takes about 1 to 2 hours.

When people sense that a seizure is about to begin, they turn the device on with a magnet. Or, the device may be left on all the time to intermittently stimulate the vagus nerve. Vagus nerve stimulation is used in addition to anticonvulsants. Side effects include hoarseness, cough, and deepening of the voice when the nerve is stimulated.

CHAPTER
114   Stroke

A stroke occurs when an artery to the brain becomes blocked or ruptures, resulting in death of an area of brain tissue (cerebral infarction) and causing sudden symptoms.

- Most strokes are ischemic (usually due to blockage of an artery), but some are hemorrhagic (due to rupture of an artery).
- Transient ischemic attacks resemble ischemic strokes except the symptoms resolve within 1 hour.
- Symptoms occur suddenly and can include muscle weakness, paralysis, abnormal or lost sensation on one side of the body, difficulty speaking, confusion, problems with vision, dizziness, and loss of balance and coordination.
- Diagnosis is based on symptoms, but imaging and blood tests are also done.
- Recovery after a stroke depends on many factors, such as the location and amount of damage, the person's age, and the presence of other disorders.
- Controlling high blood pressure, high cholesterol levels, and high blood sugar levels and not smoking help prevent strokes.
- Treatment may include drugs to make blood less likely to clot or to break up clots and sometimes surgery.

A stroke is called a cerebrovascular disorder because it affects the brain (cerebro-) and the blood vessels (vascular).

In Western countries, strokes are the third most common cause of death and the most common cause of disabling neurologic damage. In the United States, over 600,000 people have a stroke and about 160,000 die of stroke each year. Strokes are much more common among older people than among younger adults, usually because the disorders that lead to strokes progress over time. Over two thirds of all strokes occur in people older than 65. Slightly more than 50% of all strokes occur in men, but more than 60% of deaths due to stroke occur in women, possibly because women are on average older when the stroke occurs. Blacks are more likely than whites to have a stroke and to die of it.

Types: There are two types of strokes: ischemic and hemorrhagic. About 80% of strokes are ischemic—usually due to a blocked artery, often blocked by a blood clot. Brain cells, thus deprived of their blood supply, do not receive enough oxygen and glucose (a sugar), which are carried by blood. The damage that results depends on how long brain cells are deprived of blood. If they are deprived for only a brief time, brain cells are stressed, but they may recover. If brain cells are deprived longer (but

possibly for only several minutes), brain cells die, and some functions may be lost. However, in such cases, a different area of the brain can sometimes learn how to do the functions previously done by the damaged area.

Transient ischemic attacks (TIAs), sometimes called ministrokes, are often an early warning sign of an impending ischemic stroke. They are caused by a brief interruption of the blood supply to part of the brain. Because the blood supply is restored quickly, brain tissue may not die, as it does in a stroke.

The other 20% of strokes are hemorrhagic—due to bleeding in or around the brain. In this type of stroke, a blood vessel ruptures, interfering with normal blood flow and allowing blood to leak into brain tissue. Blood that comes into direct contact with brain tissue irritates the tissue and can cause scarring, leading to seizures.

Risk Factors: The major risk factors for both types of stroke are

- Atherosclerosis (narrowing or blockage of arteries by patchy deposits of fatty material in the walls of arteries)
- High cholesterol levels
- High blood pressure
- Diabetes
- Smoking

Atherosclerosis is a more important risk factor for ischemic stroke, and high blood pressure is a more important risk factor for hemorrhagic stroke. These risk factors can be controlled to some extent.

Other risk factors include

- Having relatives who have had a stroke
- Consuming too much alcohol
- Using cocaine or amphetamines
- Having an abnormal heart rhythm called atrial fibrillation
- Having inflamed blood vessels (vasculitis)

For hemorrhagic stroke, risk factors also include using anticoagulants, having a bulge (aneurysm) in arteries within the skull, and having an abnormal connection between arteries and veins (arteriovenous malformation).

The incidence of strokes has declined in recent decades, mainly because people are more aware of the importance of controlling high blood pressure

Supplying the Brain With Blood

Blood is supplied to the brain through two pairs of large arteries:

- Internal carotid arteries, which carry blood from the heart along the front of the neck
- Vertebral arteries, which carry blood from the heart along the back of the neck

In the skull, the vertebral arteries unite to form the basilar artery (at the back of the head). The internal carotid arteries and the basilar artery divide into several branches, including the cerebral arteries. Some branches join to form a circle of arteries (circle of Willis) that connect the vertebral and internal carotid arteries. Other arteries branch off from the circle of Willis like roads from a traffic circle. The branches carry blood to all parts of the brain.

When the large arteries that supply the brain are blocked, some people have no symptoms or have only a small stroke. But others with the same sort of blockage have a massive ischemic stroke. Why? Part of the expla-nation is collateral arteries. Collateral arteries run between other arteries, providing extra connections. These arteries include the circle of Willis and connections between the arteries that branch off from the circle. Some people are born with large collateral arteries, which can protect them from strokes. Then when one artery is blocked, blood flow continues through a collateral artery, sometimes preventing a stroke. Other people are born with small collateral arteries. Small collateral arteries may be unable to pass enough blood to the affected area, so a stroke results.

The body can also protect itself against strokes by growing new arteries. When blockages develop slowly and gradually (as occurs in atherosclerosis), new arteries may grow in time to keep the affected area of the brain supplied with blood and thus prevent a stroke. If a stroke has already occurred, growing new arteries can help prevent a second stroke (but cannot reverse damage that has been done).

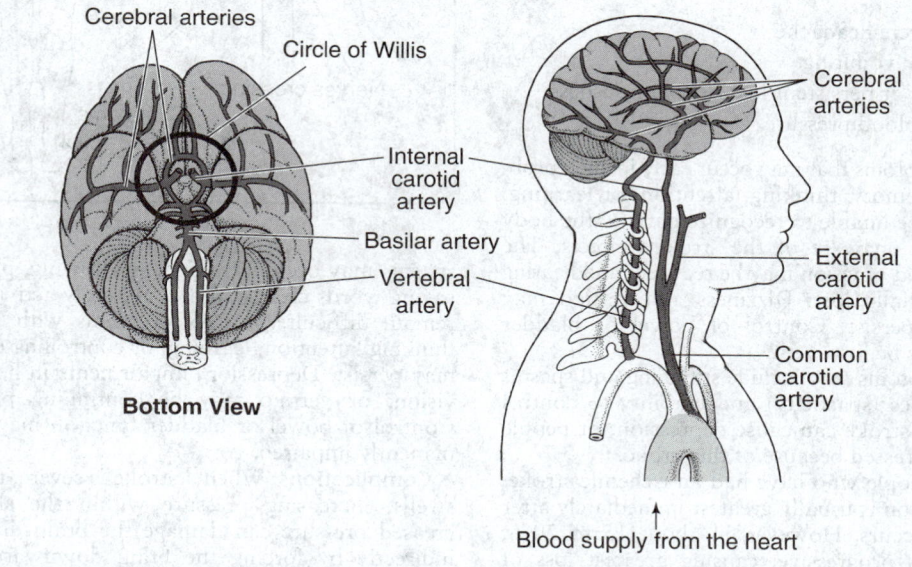

Cerebral arteries

Circle of Willis

Internal carotid artery

Basilar artery

Vertebral artery

Bottom View

Cerebral arteries

External carotid artery

Common carotid artery

Blood supply from the heart

and high cholesterol levels and stopping cigarette smoking. Controlling these factors reduces the risk of atherosclerosis.

Symptoms

Symptoms of a stroke or transient ischemic attack occur suddenly. They vary depending on the precise location of the blockage or bleeding in the brain (see page 677 and art on page 678). Each area of the brain is supplied by specific arteries. For example, if an artery supplying the area of the brain that controls the left leg's muscle movements is blocked, the leg becomes weak or paralyzed. If the area of the brain that senses touch in the right arm is damaged, sensation in the right arm is lost.

Because early treatment can help limit loss of function and sensation, everyone should know what the early symptoms of stroke are. People who have any of these symptoms should see a doctor immediately, even if the symptom goes away quickly.

Most strokes, whether ischemic or hemorrhagic, typically cause one or more of the following symptoms:

- Sudden weakness or paralysis on one side of the body (for example, half of the face, one arm or leg, or all of one side)
- Sudden loss of sensation or abnormal sensations on one side of the body
- Sudden difficulty speaking, sometimes with slurred speech
- Sudden confusion, with difficulty understanding speech
- Sudden dimness, blurring, or loss of vision, particularly in one eye
- Sudden dizziness or loss of balance and coordination, leading to falls

Symptoms of a transient ischemic attack are the same, but they usually disappear within minutes and rarely last more than 1 hour.

Symptoms of a hemorrhagic stroke may also include the following:

- Sudden severe headache
- Nausea and vomiting
- Temporary or persistent loss of consciousness
- Very high blood pressure

Other symptoms that may occur early include problems with memory, thinking, attention, or learning. People may be unable to recognize parts of the body and may be unaware of the stroke's effects. The peripheral field of vision may be reduced, and hearing may be partially lost. Dizziness and vertigo may develop or persist. Control of bowel or bladder function may be lost.

Later symptoms may include stiffening and spasms of the muscles (spasticity) and inability to control emotions. A stroke can cause depression, or people may feel depressed because of the stroke.

In most people who have had an ischemic stroke, loss of function is usually greatest immediately after the stroke occurs. However, in about 15 to 20%, the stroke is progressive, causing greatest loss of function after a day or two. In people who have had a hemorrhagic stroke, function usually is lost progressively over minutes to hours.

Over days to months, some function is usually regained because even though some brain cells die, others are only stressed and may recover. Also, certain areas of the brain can sometimes switch to the functions previously done by the damaged part—a characteristic called plasticity. However, the early effects of a stroke, including paralysis, can become permanent. Muscles that are not used usually become permanently spastic and stiff, and painful muscle

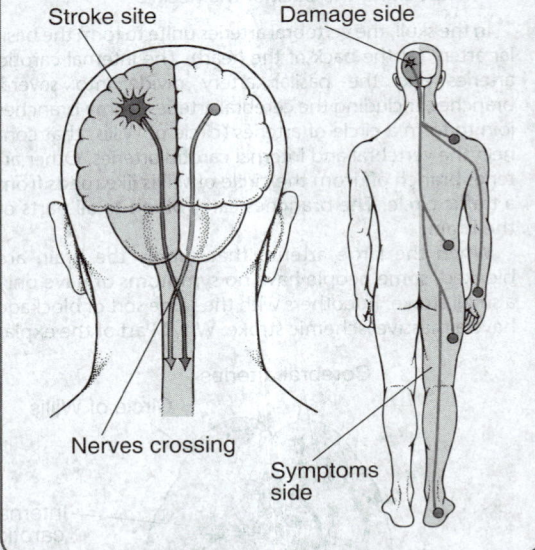

Why Strokes Affect Only One Side of the Body

Strokes usually damage only one side of the brain. Because nerves in the brain cross over to the other side of the body, symptoms appear on the side of the body opposite the damaged side of the brain.

Stroke site

Damage side

Nerves crossing

Symptoms side

spasms may occur. Walking, swallowing, physically saying words clearly, and doing daily activities may remain difficult. Various problems with memory, thinking, attention, learning, or controlling emotions may persist. Depression, impairments in hearing or vision, or vertigo may be continuing problems. Control of bowel or bladder function may be permanently impaired.

Complications: When a stroke is severe, the brain swells, increasing pressure within the skull. Increased pressure can damage the brain directly or indirectly by forcing the brain downward in the skull. The brain may be forced through the rigid structures that separate the brain into compartments, resulting in a serious problem called herniation (see art on page 735). The pressure affects the respiratory center in the lower part of the brain stem and can cause irregular breathing, loss of consciousness, coma, and death.

The symptoms caused by a stroke can lead to other problems. If swallowing is difficult, people may inhale food, fluids, or other particles from the mouth. Such inhalation (called aspiration) can cause aspiration pneumonia, which may be serious. Difficulty swallowing can also interfere with eating, resulting in undernutrition and dehydration. Not being able to move can result in pressure sores, muscle loss, and the formation of blood clots in deep veins of the legs and groin (deep vein thrombosis). Clots can break off, travel through the bloodstream, and block an artery to a lung (pulmonary embolism). If bladder control is impaired, urinary tract infections are more likely to develop.

Diagnosis

Symptoms suggest the diagnosis, but tests are needed to help doctors determine the following:

- Whether stroke has occurred
- Whether it is ischemic or hemorrhagic
- Whether immediate treatment is required

Computed tomography (CT—see page 2037) or magnetic resonance imaging (MRI—see page 2040) of the brain is done. These tests can detect most hemorrhagic strokes, except for some subarachnoid hemorrhages. These tests can also detect many ischemic strokes but sometimes not until several hours after symptoms appear. The blood sugar level is measured immediately because a low blood sugar level (hypoglycemia) can cause symptoms similar to those of stroke.

Doctors evaluate people who have had a stroke for problems that can contribute to or cause a stroke, such as infection, a low blood oxygen level, and dehydration. Tests are done as needed. People are asked about depression. The ability to swallow is evaluated, sometimes with x-rays taken after a radiopaque dye such as barium is swallowed. Depending on the type of stroke, more tests are done to identify the cause.

Prognosis

Certain factors suggest that the outcome of a stroke is likely to be poor. Strokes that cause unconsciousness or that affect a large part of the left side of the brain (which is responsible for language) may be particularly grave.

In adults who have had an ischemic stroke, problems that remain after 6 months are likely to be permanent, but children continue to improve slowly for many months. Older people fare less well than younger people. For people who already have other serious disorders (such as dementia), recovery is more limited.

If a hemorrhagic stroke is not massive and pressure within the brain is not very high, the outcome is likely to be better after than that after an ischemic stroke. Blood (in a hemorrhagic stroke) does not damage brain tissue as much as an inadequate supply of oxygen (in an ischemic stroke) does.

Prevention

Preventing strokes is preferable to treating them. The main strategy for preventing a first stroke is managing the major risk factors. High blood pressure (see page 333) and diabetes (see page 1005) should be controlled. Cholesterol levels should be measured and, if high, lowered to reduce the risk of atherosclerosis (see page 961). Smoking and use of amphetamines or cocaine should be stopped, and alcohol should be limited to no more than 2 drinks a day. Exercising regularly and, if overweight, losing weight help people control high blood pressure, diabetes, and high cholesterol levels. Having regular checkups enables a doctor to identify risk factors for stroke so that they can be managed quickly.

If people have had an ischemic stroke, taking an antiplatelet drug can reduce the risk of another ischemic stroke. Antiplatelet drugs make platelets less likely to clump and form clots, a common cause of ischemic stroke. (Platelets are tiny cell-like particles in blood that help it clot in response to damaged blood vessels.) Aspirin, one of the most effective antiplatelet drugs, is usually prescribed. One adult's tablet or 1 children's tablet (which is about one fourth the dose of an adult aspirin) is taken each day. Either dose seems to prevent strokes about equally well. Taking a combination tablet that contains a low dose of aspirin and dipyridamole (an antiplatelet drug) is slightly more effective than taking aspirin alone. Clopidogrel, another antiplatelet drug, is also slightly more effective than aspirin alone. It may be given to people who cannot tolerate aspirin. Some people are allergic to antiplatelet drugs or similar drugs and cannot take them. Also, people who have gastrointestinal bleeding should not take antiplatelet drugs.

If an ischemic stroke or a transient ischemic attack is due to blood clots originating in the heart, warfarin, an anticoagulant, may be given to inhibit blood clotting. Because taking warfarin and an antiplatelet drug or taking aspirin plus clopidogrel greatly increases the risk of bleeding, these drugs are rarely used together for stroke prevention.

Treatment

Anyone with symptoms of a stroke should seek medical attention immediately.

Doctors check the person's vital functions, such as heart rate, breathing, temperature, and blood pressure, to make sure they are adequate. If they are not, measures to correct them are taken immediately. For example, if people are in a coma or unresponsive (as may result from brain herniation), mechanical ventilation (with a breathing tube inserted through the mouth or nose) may be needed to help them breathe. If symptoms suggest that pressure within the skull is high, drugs may be given to reduce swelling in the brain, and a monitor may be put in the brain to periodically measure the pressure.

Other treatments used during the first hours depend on the type of stroke. These treatments include drugs (such as antiplatelet drugs, anticoagulants, drugs to break up clots, and drugs to control high blood pressure) and surgery to remove blood that has accumulated.

Later and ongoing treatments focus on preventing subsequent strokes, treating and preventing problems that strokes can cause, and helping people regain as much function as possible (rehabilitation).

Rehabilitation: Intensive rehabilitation can help many people overcome disabilities after a stroke (see page 53). The exercises and training of rehabilitation encourage unaffected areas of the brain to learn to perform functions that were done by the damaged area. Also, people are taught new ways to use muscles unaffected by the stroke to compensate for losses in function.

The goals of rehabilitation are the following:

- To regain as much normal function as possible
- To maintain and improve physical condition
- To help people relearn old skills and learn new ones as needed

Success depends on the area of the brain damaged and the person's general physical condition, functional and cognitive abilities before the stroke, social situation, learning ability, and attitude. Patience and perseverance are crucial. Participating actively in the rehabilitation program can help people avoid or lessen depression.

Rehabilitation is started in the hospital as soon as people are physically able—usually within 1 or 2 days of admission. After discharge from the hospital, rehabilitation can be continued on an outpatient basis, in a nursing home, in a rehabilitation center, or at home. Occupational and physical therapists can suggest ways to make life easier and the home safer for people with disabilities.

Family members and friends can contribute to a person's rehabilitation by keeping in mind what effects a stroke can have, so that they can better understand and support the person. Support groups can provide emotional encouragement and practical advice for people who have had a stroke and for those who care for them.

End-of-Life Issues

For some people who have had a stroke, quality of life is predicted to remain very poor despite treatment. For such people, care focuses on control of pain, comfort measures, and provision of fluids and nourishment. People who have had a stroke

should establish advance directives (see page 69) as soon as possible because the recurrence and progression of strokes are unpredictable. Advance directives can help a doctor determine what kind of medical care people want if they become unable to make these decisions.

Transient Ischemic Attacks

A transient ischemic attack (TIA) is a disturbance in brain function that lasts less than 1 hour and results from a temporary blockage of the brain's blood supply.

- The cause and symptoms of a TIA are the same as those of an ischemic stroke.
- TIAs differ from ischemic strokes because symptoms resolve within 1 hour.
- Symptoms suggest the diagnosis, but imaging and blood tests are also done.
- Controlling high blood pressure, high cholesterol levels, and high blood sugar levels and not smoking are recommended.
- Drugs to make blood less likely to clot and sometimes surgery (carotid endarterectomy) or angioplasty are used to reduce the risk of stroke after a TIA.

TIAs may be a warning sign of an impending ischemic stroke. People who have had a TIA are much more likely to have a stroke than those who have not. About half of these strokes occur within 1 year of the TIA, and many occur within a few days of the TIA. Recognizing a TIA and having the cause identified can help prevent a stroke.

TIAs are most common among middle-aged and older people.

TIAs differ from ischemic strokes because, after a TIA, symptoms resolve completely and quickly. Experts used to think that symptoms resolved more quickly because TIAs did not cause any permanent brain damage. That is, no brain cells died. However, most experts now think that TIAs are small ischemic strokes. That is, in TIAs, as in ischemic strokes, brain cells die. The difference is that in TIAs, the damage is usually very small.

Causes

Causes of TIAs and ischemic strokes are mostly the same. Most TIAs occur when a piece of a blood clot (thrombus) or of fatty material (atheroma, or plaque) due to atherosclerosis breaks off from the heart or from the wall of an artery, travels through the bloodstream (becoming an embolus), and lodges in an artery that supplies the brain (see page 724). Occasionally, TIAs result from a very low oxygen level in the blood, a severe deficiency of red blood cells (anemia), carbon monoxide poisoning, thickened blood (as in polycythemia), or very low blood

PREVENTING AND TREATING PROBLEMS AFTER A STROKE

PROBLEM	MEASURES
Blood clots in the legs	To prevent blood clots, doctors may give anticoagulants, such as heparin or low-molecular-weight heparin, put elastic or air-filled support stockings on the person's legs to improve blood circulation, or both. Moving the legs, which improves blood flow, can also help. People, if able, are encouraged to walk or simply move their legs (for example, extending and flexing their ankles). If people cannot move their legs, a therapist or other staff member moves their legs for them (called passive exercise).
Pressure sores	Nurses, other staff members, or caregivers should frequently turn or reposition people who are confined to a bed or wheelchair. Areas likely to develop pressure sores should be inspected every day.
Permanent shortening of muscles that limits movement (contractures)	Moving the limbs can prevent contractures. People, if able, are encouraged to move and change positions regularly. Or a therapist or other staff member moves their limbs for them and makes sure the limbs are placed in appropriate resting positions. Sometimes splints are used to keep the limbs in place.
Difficulty swallowing	People are evaluated for difficulty swallowing. If they have difficulty, care is taken to provide them with enough fluids and nourishment. Sometimes learning simple techniques (for example, how to position the head, how to breathe when swallowing) can help the person swallow safely. Tube feedings may be necessary until the ability to swallow returns.
Difficulty breathing	If people smoke, they are encouraged to stop. Therapists also teach them to do deep breathing exercises and to cough to clear the airways. Therapists may provide a handheld breathing device. If needed, oxygen is provided through a face mask or a tube inserted in the nose or in the mouth.
Urinary tract infections	If possible, a urinary catheter, which can cause urinary infections, is not used. If a catheter is needed, it is removed as soon as possible.
Discouragement and depression	Doctors discuss the effects of the stroke with affected people and their family members or other caregivers. The discussion includes the type of recovery that can be expected and ways to cope with limitations of function. People and their caregivers are put in contact with stroke support groups. Formal counseling or drugs may be necessary to treat depression.

pressure (hypotension), especially when the arteries to the brain are already narrowed (as in people with atherosclerosis).

Symptoms

Symptoms of a TIA develop suddenly. They are identical to those of an ischemic stroke (see page 725) but are temporary and reversible. They usually last less than 5 minutes and not longer than 1 hour. TIAs recur in about 5% of people with atherosclerosis. People may have several in 1 day or only two or three in several years.

Diagnosis

People who have a sudden symptom similar to any symptom of a stroke, even if it quickly resolves, should go immediately to an emergency department. Such a symptom suggests a TIA. However, other disorders, including seizures, brain tumors, migraine headaches, and abnormally low levels of sugar in the blood (hypoglycemia), cause similar symptoms, so further evaluation is needed.

If doctors suspect that a TIA has occurred, they evaluate people rapidly, usually in the hospital, because a stroke may occur soon after a TIA. Doctors check for risk factors for stroke by asking people questions, reviewing their medical history, and doing blood tests.

Imaging tests, such as computed tomography (CT) or magnetic resonance imaging (MRI), are done to check for evidence of a stroke, bleeding, and brain tumors. A specialized type of MRI, called diffusion MRI, can show areas of brain tissue that are not functioning and thus help doctors diagnose a TIA (or an ischemic stroke). However, diffusion MRI is not always available.

Other imaging tests help determine whether an artery to the brain is blocked, which artery is blocked, and how complete the blockage is. These tests provide images of the arteries that carry blood through the neck to the brain (the internal carotid arteries and the vertebral arteries) and the arteries of the brain (such as the cerebral arteries). Color Doppler ultrasonography (used only for the internal carotid arteries), magnetic resonance angiography (see page 2041), or CT angiography (see page 2039) may be done. Sometimes if the stroke is severe, cerebral angiography (using a dye injected through a catheter) is done (see page 2036).

> **? Did You Know...**
> Even if symptoms of a stroke resolve within a few minutes, people should still go to the emergency department immediately.

Treatment

Treatment of TIAs is aimed at preventing a stroke. It is the same as that after an ischemic stroke.

The first step in preventing a stroke is to control, if possible, the major risk factors for it: high blood pressure, high cholesterol levels, smoking, and diabetes. Taking an antiplatelet drug, such as aspirin, a combination tablet of low-dose aspirin plus dipyridamole, or clopidogrel, reduces the chance that clots will form and cause TIAs or ischemic strokes. (Platelets are tiny cell-like particles in the blood that help it clot in response to damaged blood vessels.)

The degree of narrowing in the carotid arteries helps doctors estimate the risk of a stroke or subsequent TIAs and thus determine the treatment. If people are thought to be at high risk (for example, if the carotid artery is narrowed at least 70%), an operation to widen the artery (called carotid endarterectomy) may be done to reduce the risk (see page 728). Carotid endarterectomy usually involves removing atheromas and clots in the internal carotid artery. However, the operation can trigger a stroke because the operation may dislodge clots or other material that can then travel through the bloodstream and block an artery. However, after the operation, the risk of stroke is lower for several years than it is when drugs are used.

In other narrowed arteries, such as the vertebral arteries, endarterectomy may not be possible because the operation is riskier to perform in these arteries than in the internal carotid arteries.

If people are not healthy enough to have surgery, angioplasty with stenting (see art on page 405) may be done. For this procedure, a thin, flexible tube (catheter) with a balloon at its tip is threaded into the narrowed artery. The balloon is then inflated for several seconds to widen the artery. To keep the artery open, doctors insert a tube made of wire mesh (a stent) into the artery.

Ischemic Stroke

An ischemic stroke is death of an area of brain tissue (cerebral infarction) resulting from an inadequate supply of blood and oxygen to the brain due to blockage of an artery.

- Ischemic stroke usually results when an artery to the brain is blocked, often by a blood clot or a fatty deposit due to atherosclerosis.
- Symptoms occur suddenly and may include muscle weakness, paralysis, lost or abnormal sensation on one side of the body, difficulty speaking, confusion, problems with vision, dizziness, and loss of balance and coordination.
- Diagnosis is usually based on symptoms and results of a physical examination, imaging tests, and blood tests.
- Treatment may include drugs to break up blood clots or to make blood less likely to clot and surgery, followed by rehabilitation.
- About one third of people recover all or most of normal function after an ischemic stroke.

Causes

An ischemic stroke typically results from blockage of an artery that supplies the brain, most commonly a branch of one of the internal carotid arteries.

Commonly, blockages are blood clots (thrombi) or pieces of fatty deposits (atheromas, or plaques) due to atherosclerosis. Such blockages often occur in the following ways:

- **By forming in and blocking an artery:** An atheroma in the wall of an artery may accumulate more fatty material and become large enough to block the artery. Or a blood clot can form and block the artery when an atheroma ruptures (see art on page 397). Clots tend to form on a ruptured atheroma because the atheroma narrows the artery and slows blood flow through it, like a clogged pipe slows the flow of water. Slow-moving blood is more likely to clot. A large clot can block enough blood flowing through the narrowed artery that brain cells supplied by that artery die.
- **By traveling to another artery:** A blood clot in the heart, a piece of an atheroma, or a blood clot in the wall of an artery can break off and travel through the bloodstream (becoming an embolus). The embolus may then lodge in an artery that supplies the brain and block blood flow there. (Embolism refers to blockage of arteries by materials that travel through the bloodstream to another part of the body.) Such blockages are more

likely to occur where arteries are already narrowed by fatty deposits.

Several conditions besides rupture of an atheroma can trigger or promote the formation of blood clots, increasing the risk of blockage by a blood clot, such as the following:

- **Heart-related problems:** Blood clots may form in the heart or on a heart valve (including artificial valves). Strokes due to such blood clots are most common among people who have recently had heart surgery and people who have a heart valve disorder or an abnormal heart rhythm (arrhythmia), especially a fast, irregular heart rhythm called atrial fibrillation.

- **Blood disorders:** Some disorders, such as an excess of red blood cells (polycythemia), make blood thick, increasing the risk of blood clots. Some disorders, such as antiphospholipid syndrome and a high homocysteine level in the blood (hyperhomocysteinemia), make blood more likely to clot.

- **Oral contraceptives:** Taking oral contraceptives, particularly those with a high estrogen dose, increases the risk of blood clots.

Another common cause of ischemic strokes is a lacunar infarction. In lacunar infarction, one of the small arteries deep in the brain becomes blocked by a mixture of fat and connective tissue—a blood clot is not the cause. This disorder is called lipohyalinosis and tends to occur in older people with diabetes or poorly controlled high blood pressure. Lipohyalinosis is different from atherosclerosis, but both disorders can cause blockage of arteries. Only a small part of the brain is damaged in lacunar infarction.

Rarely, small pieces of fat from the marrow of a broken long bone, such as a leg bone, are released into the bloodstream. These pieces can clump together and block an artery. The resulting disorder, called fat embolism syndrome, may resemble a stroke.

An ischemic stroke can also result from any disorder that reduces the amount of blood or oxygen supplied to the brain, such as severe blood loss or very low blood pressure. Occasionally, an ischemic stroke occurs when blood flow to the brain is normal but the blood does not contain enough oxygen. Disorders that reduce the oxygen content of blood include a severe deficiency of red blood cells (anemia), suffocation, and carbon monoxide poisoning. Usually, brain damage in such cases is widespread (diffuse), and coma results.

An ischemic stroke can occur if inflammation of blood vessels (vasculitis) or infection (such as herpes simplex) narrows blood vessels that supply the brain. Migraine headaches or drugs such as cocaine and amphetamines can cause spasm of the arteries, which can narrow the arteries supplying the brain and cause a stroke.

Symptoms

Usually, symptoms occur suddenly and are often most severe a few minutes after they start because most ischemic strokes begin suddenly, develop rapidly, and cause death of brain tissue within minutes to hours. Then, most strokes become stable, causing little or no further damage. Strokes that remain stable for 2 to 3 days are called completed strokes. Sudden blockage by an embolus is most likely to cause this kind of stroke.

Less commonly, symptoms develop slowly. They result from strokes that continue to worsen for several hours to a day or two, as a steadily enlarging area of brain tissue dies. Such strokes are called evolving strokes. The progression of symptoms and damage is usually interrupted by somewhat stable periods, during which the area temporarily stops enlarging or some improvement occurs. Such strokes are usually due to the formation of clots in a narrowed artery.

Many different symptoms can occur, depending on which artery is blocked and thus which part of the brain is deprived of blood and oxygen (see page 677). When the arteries that branch from the internal carotid artery (which carry blood along the front of the neck to the brain) are affected, the following are most common:

- Blindness in one eye
- Inability to see out of the same side in both eyes
- Abnormal sensations, weakness, or paralysis in one arm or leg or on one side of the body

When the arteries that branch from the vertebral arteries (which carry blood along the back of the neck to the brain) are affected, the following are most common:

- Dizziness and vertigo
- Double vision
- Generalized weakness on both sides of the body

Many other symptoms, such as difficulty speaking (for example, slurred speech), impaired consciousness (such as confusion), loss of coordination, and urinary incontinence, can occur.

Severe strokes may lead to stupor or coma. In addition, strokes, even milder ones, can cause depression or an inability to control emotions. For example, people may cry or laugh inappropriately.

If symptoms, particularly impaired consciousness, worsen during the first 2 to 3 days, the cause is often swelling due to excess fluid (edema) in the brain. Symptoms usually lessen within a few days, as the fluid is absorbed. Nonetheless, the swelling is

Clots: Causes of Ischemic Stroke

When an artery that carries blood to the brain becomes clogged or blocked, an ischemic stroke can occur. Arteries may be blocked by fatty deposits (atheromas, or plaques) due to atherosclerosis. Arteries in the neck, particularly the internal carotid arteries, are a common site for atheromas. Arteries may also be blocked by a blood clot (thrombus). Blood clots may form on an atheroma in an artery. Clots may also form in the heart of people with a heart disorder. Part of a clot may break off and travel through the bloodstream (becoming an embolus). It may then block an artery that supplies blood to the brain, such as one of the cerebral arteries.

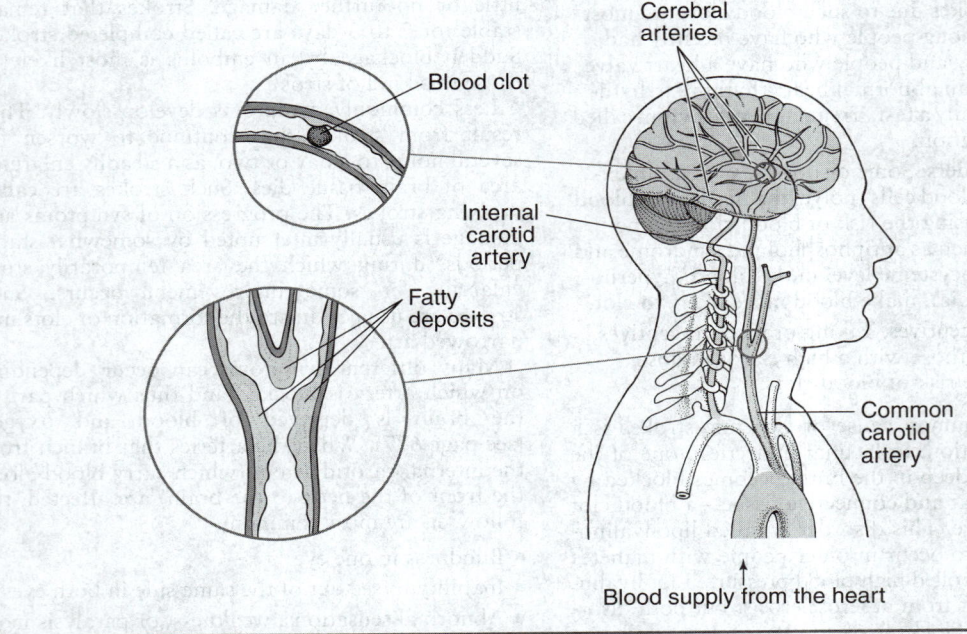

Cerebral arteries

Blood clot

Internal carotid artery

Fatty deposits

Common carotid artery

Blood supply from the heart

particularly dangerous because the skull does not expand. The resulting increase in pressure can cause the brain to shift, further impairing brain function, even if the area directly damaged by the stroke does not enlarge. If the pressure becomes very high, the brain may be forced downward in the skull, through the rigid structures that separate the brain into compartments. The resulting disorder is called herniation (see art on page 735).

Strokes can lead to other problems. If swallowing is difficult, people may not eat enough and become malnourished. Food, saliva, or vomit may be inhaled (aspirated) into the lungs, resulting in aspiration pneumonia. Being in one position too long can result in pressure sores and lead to muscle loss. Not being able to move the legs can result in the formation of blood clots in deep veins of the legs and groin (deep vein thrombosis). Clots can break off, travel through the bloodstream, and block an artery to a lung (a disorder called pulmonary embolism). People may have difficulty sleeping. The losses and problems resulting from the stroke may make people depressed.

Diagnosis

Doctors can usually diagnose an ischemic stroke based on the history of events and results of a physical examination. Doctors can usually identify which artery in the brain is blocked based on symptoms (see art on page 678). For example, weakness or paralysis of the left leg suggests blockage of the artery supplying the area on the right side of the brain that controls the left leg's muscle movements.

Computed tomography (CT) is usually done first. CT helps distinguish an ischemic stroke from a hemorrhagic stroke, a brain tumor, an abscess, and other structural abnormalities. Doctors also measure the blood sugar level to rule out a low blood sugar level (hypoglycemia), which can cause similar symptoms. If available, diffusion magnetic resonance imaging (MRI), which can detect ischemic strokes within minutes of their start, may be done next.

Identifying the precise cause of the stroke is important. If the blockage is a blood clot, another stroke is very likely unless the underlying disorder is corrected. For example, if blood clots result from an abnormal heart rhythm, treating that disorder can prevent new clots from forming and causing another stroke. Tests for causes may include the following:

- Electrocardiography (ECG) to look for abnormal heart rhythms
- Continuous ECG monitoring (done at home or in the hospital—see page 327) to record the heart rate and rhythm continuously for 24 hours (or more), which may detect abnormal heart rhythms that occur unpredictably or briefly
- Echocardiography to check the heart for blood clots, pumping or structural abnormalities, and valve disorders
- Imaging tests—color Doppler ultrasonography, magnetic resonance angiography, CT angiography, or cerebral (standard) angiography—to determine whether arteries, especially the internal carotid arteries, are blocked or narrowed
- Blood tests to check for anemia, polycythemia, blood clotting disorders, vasculitis, and some infections (such as heart valve infections and syphilis) and for risk factors such as high cholesterol levels or diabetes

Imaging tests enable doctors to determine how narrowed the carotid arteries are and thus to estimate the risk of a subsequent stroke or TIA. Such information helps determine which treatments are needed.

For cerebral angiography, a thin, flexible tube (catheter) is inserted into an artery, usually in the groin, and threaded through the aorta to an artery in the neck (see page 2036). Then, a dye is injected to outline the artery. Thus, this test is more invasive than other tests that provide images of the brain's blood supply. However, it provides more information. Cerebral angiography may be done before atheromas are removed surgically or when vasculitis is suspected.

Rarely, a spinal tap (lumbar puncture) is done—for example, after CT, when doctors still need to determine whether strokelike symptoms are due to an infection or whether a subarachnoid hemorrhage is present (see page 731). This procedure is done only if doctors are sure that the brain is not under excess pressure (usually determined by CT or MRI).

Prognosis

About 10% of people who have an ischemic stroke recover almost all normal function, and about 25% recover most of it. About 40% of people have moderate to severe impairments requiring special care, and about 10% require care in a nursing home or other long-term care facility. Some people are physically and mentally devastated and unable to move, speak, or eat normally. About 20% of people who have a stroke die in the hospital. The proportion is higher among older people. About 25% of people who recover from a stroke have another stroke within 5 years. Subsequent strokes impair function further.

During the first few days after an ischemic stroke, doctors usually cannot predict whether a person will improve or worsen. Younger people and people who start improving quickly are likely to recover more fully. About 50% of people with one-sided paralysis and most of those with less severe symptoms recover some function by the time they leave the hospital, and they can eventually take care of their basic needs. They can think clearly and walk adequately, although use of the affected arm or leg may be limited. Use of an arm is more often limited than use of a leg. Most impairments still present after 12 months are permanent.

Treatment

People who have any symptom suggesting an ischemic stroke should go to an emergency department immediately. The earlier the treatment, the better are the chances for recovery.

The first priority is to restore the person's breathing, heart rate, blood pressure (if low), and temperature to normal. An intravenous line is inserted to provide drugs and fluids when needed. If the person has a fever, it may be lowered using acetaminophen, ibuprofen, or a cooling blanket. An increase in body temperature by even a few degrees can dramatically worsen brain damage due to an ischemic stroke. Generally, doctors do not immediately treat high blood pressure unless it is very high (over 220/120 mm Hg) because, when arteries are narrowed, blood pressure must be higher than normal to push enough blood through them to the brain. However, very high blood pressure can injure the heart, kidneys, and eyes and must be lowered.

If a stroke is very severe, drugs such as mannitol may be given to reduce swelling and the increased pressure in the brain. Some people need a ventilator to breathe adequately.

Specific treatment of stroke may include drugs to break up blood clots (thrombolytic drugs), drugs to make blood less likely to clot (antiplatelet drugs and anticoagulants), and surgery, followed by rehabilitation.

Thrombolytic (Fibrinolytic) Drugs: In certain circumstances, a drug called tissue plasminogen activator (tPA) is given intravenously to break up clots and help restore blood flow to the brain. Because tPA can cause bleeding in the brain and elsewhere, it should not be given to people with certain conditions, such as the following:

- A past occurrence of a hemorrhagic stroke, a bulge (aneurysm) in an artery to the brain, other structural abnormalities in the brain, or a brain tumor
- A seizure when the stroke began
- A tendency to bleed
- Recent major surgery
- Recent bleeding (hemorrhage) in the gastrointestinal or urinary tract
- A recent head injury or other serious trauma
- A very high or very low blood sugar level
- A heart infection
- Current use of an anticoagulant (warfarin)
- A large ischemic stroke
- Blood pressure that remains high after treatment with an antihypertensive drug
- Symptoms that are resolving quickly

Before tPA is given, CT is done to rule out bleeding in the brain. To be effective and safe, tPA, given intravenously, must be started within 3 hours of the beginning of an ischemic stroke. After 3 hours, most of the damage to the brain cannot be reversed, and the risk of bleeding outweighs the possible benefit of the drug. However, pinpointing when the stroke began may be difficult. So doctors assume that the stroke began the last time a person was known to be well. For example, if a person awakens with symptoms of a stroke, doctors assume the stroke began when the person was last seen awake and well. Thus, tPA can be used in only a few people who have had a stroke.

If people arrive at the hospital 3 to 6 hours (occasionally, up to 18 hours) after the stroke began, they may be given tPA or another thrombolytic drug. But the drug must be given through a catheter instead. For this treatment, doctors make an incision in the skin, usually in the groin, and insert a catheter into an artery. The catheter is then threaded through the aorta and other arteries, to the clot. The clot is partly broken up with the catheter wire and then injected with tPA. This treatment is usually available only at specialized stroke centers.

Antiplatelet Drugs and Anticoagulants: If a thrombolytic drug cannot be used, most people are given aspirin (an antiplatelet drug) as soon as they get to the hospital. If symptoms seem to be worsening, anticoagulants such as heparin are occasionally used, but their effectiveness has not been proved. Antiplatelet drugs make platelets less likely to clump and form clots. Anticoagulants inhibit proteins in blood that help it to clot (clotting factors).

Regardless of the initial treatment, long-term treatment usually consists of aspirin or another antiplatelet drug to reduce the risk of blood clots and thus of subsequent strokes (see page 721). People who have atrial fibrillation or a heart valve disorder are given anticoagulants (such as warfarin) instead of antiplatelet drugs, which do not seem to prevent blood clots from forming in the heart. Occasionally, people at high risk of another stroke are given both aspirin and warfarin.

If people have been given a thrombolytic drug, doctors usually wait at least 24 hours before antiplatelet drugs or anticoagulants are started because these drugs add to the already increased risk of bleeding in the brain. Anticoagulants are not given to people who have uncontrolled high blood pressure or who have had a hemorrhagic stroke.

Surgery: Once an ischemic stroke is completed, surgical removal of atheromas or clots (endarterectomy) in an internal carotid artery may be done. Carotid endarterectomy can help if all of the following are present:

- The stroke resulted from narrowing of a carotid artery by more than 70%.
- Some brain tissue supplied by the affected artery still functions after the stroke.
- The person's life expectancy is at least 5 years.

In such people, carotid endarterectomy may reduce the risk of subsequent strokes. It also reestablishes the blood supply to the affected area, but it cannot restore lost function because some brain tissue is dead.

For carotid endarterectomy, a general anesthetic or a local anesthetic (to numb the neck area) may be used. If people remain awake during the operation, the surgeon can better evaluate how the brain is functioning. The surgeon makes an incision in the neck over the area of the artery that contains the blockage and an incision in the artery. The blockage is removed, and the incisions are closed. For a few days afterwards, the neck may hurt, and swallowing may be difficult. Most people can stay in the hospital 1 or 2 days. Heavy lifting should be avoided for about 3 weeks. After several weeks, people can resume their usual activities.

Carotid endarterectomy can trigger a stroke because the operation may dislodge clots or other material that can then travel through the bloodstream and block an artery. However, after the operation, the risk of stroke is lower for several years than it is when drugs are used.

In other narrowed arteries, such as the vertebral arteries, endarterectomy may not be possible because the operation is riskier to perform in these arteries than in the internal carotid arteries.

People should find a surgeon who is experienced doing this operation and who has a low rate of serious complications (such as heart attack, stroke, and death) after the operation. If people cannot find such a surgeon, the risks of endarterectomy outweigh its expected benefits.

Stents: If endarterectomy is too risky, a less invasive procedure can be done: A wire mesh tube (stent) with an umbrella filter may be placed in the carotid artery. The stent helps keep the artery open, and the filter catches blood clots and prevents them from reaching the brain and causing a stroke. The filter is similar to one used to prevent pulmonary embolism (see art on page 436). After a local anesthetic is given, a catheter is inserted through a small incision into a large artery near the groin or in the arm and is threaded to the internal carotid artery in the neck. A dye that can be seen on x-rays (radiopaque dye) is injected, and x-rays are taken so that the narrowed area can be located. After the stent and filter are placed, the catheter is removed. People remain awake for the procedure, which usually takes 1 to 2 hours. The procedure appears to be as safe as endarterectomy and is almost as effective in preventing strokes and death.

Other Treatments: Another option being studied is a tiny corkscrew-shaped device that is attached to a catheter, threaded to the clot, and used to snag the clot. The clot is then drawn out through the catheter. This treatment may be useful for people who cannot be given tPA.

Treatment of Problems Due to Strokes: Measures to prevent aspiration pneumonia (see page 471) and pressure sores (see page 1299) are started early. Heparin, injected under the skin, may be given to help prevent deep vein thrombosis (see page 433). People are closely monitored to determine whether the esophagus, bladder, and intestines are functioning. Often, other disorders such as heart failure, abnormal heart rhythms, and lung infections must be treated. High blood pressure is often treated after the stroke has been stabilized.

Because a stroke often causes mood changes, especially depression, family members or friends should inform the doctor if the person seems depressed. Depression can be treated with drug therapy and psychotherapy (see page 866).

Hemorrhagic Stroke

Hemorrhagic strokes include bleeding within the brain (intracerebral hemorrhage) and bleeding between the inner and outer layers of the tissue covering the brain (subarachnoid hemorrhage).

There are two main types of hemorrhagic strokes: intracerebral hemorrhage and subarachnoid hemorrhage. Other disorders that involve bleeding inside the skull include epidural (see page 738) and subdural (see page 739) hematomas, which are usually caused by a head injury. These disorders cause different symptoms and are not considered strokes.

INTRACEREBRAL HEMORRHAGE

An intracerebral hemorrhage is bleeding within the brain.

- Intracerebral hemorrhage usually results from chronic high blood pressure.
- The first symptom is often a severe headache.
- Diagnosis is based on symptoms and results of a physical examination and imaging tests.
- Treatment may include vitamin K, transfusions, and, rarely, surgery to remove the accumulated blood.

Intracerebral hemorrhage accounts for about 10% of all strokes but for a much higher percentage of deaths due to stroke. Among people older than 60, intracerebral hemorrhage is more common than subarachnoid hemorrhage.

Causes

Intracerebral hemorrhage most often results when chronic high blood pressure weakens a small artery, causing it to burst. Using cocaine or amphetamines can cause temporary but very high blood pressure and hemorrhage. In some older people, an abnormal protein called amyloid accumulates in arteries of the brain. This accumulation (called amyloid angiopathy) weakens the arteries and can cause hemorrhage.

Less common causes include blood vessel abnormalities present at birth, injuries, tumors, inflammation of blood vessels (vasculitis), bleeding disorders, and use of anticoagulants in doses that are too high. Bleeding disorders and use of anticoagulants increase the risk of dying from an intracerebral hemorrhage.

Symptoms

An intracerebral hemorrhage begins abruptly. In about half of the people, it begins with a severe headache, often during activity. However, in older people, the headache may be mild or absent. Symptoms suggesting brain dysfunction develop and steadily worsen as the hemorrhage expands. Some symptoms, such as weakness, paralysis, loss of sensation, and numbness, often affect only one side of the body. People may be unable to speak or become confused. Vision may be impaired or lost. The eyes may point in different directions or become paralyzed. The pupils may become abnormally large or small. Nausea, vomiting, seizures, and loss of consciousness are common and may occur within seconds to minutes.

Burst and Breaks: Causes of Hemorrhagic Stroke

When blood vessels of the brain are weak, abnormal, or under unusual pressure, a hemorrhagic stroke can occur. In hemorrhagic strokes, bleeding may occur within the brain, as an intracerebral hemorrhage. Or bleeding may occur between the inner and middle layer of tissue covering the brain (in the subarachnoid space), as a subarachnoid hemorrhage.

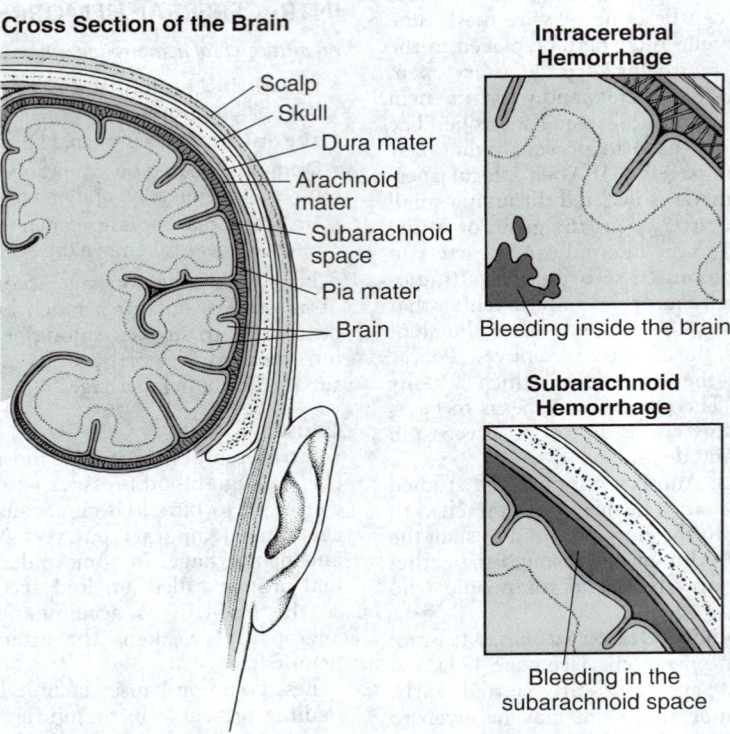

Cross Section of the Brain

- Scalp
- Skull
- Dura mater
- Arachnoid mater
- Subarachnoid space
- Pia mater
- Brain

Intracerebral Hemorrhage

Bleeding inside the brain

Subarachnoid Hemorrhage

Bleeding in the subarachnoid space

Diagnosis

Doctors can often diagnose intracerebral hemorrhages on the basis of symptoms and results of a physical examination. However, computed tomography (CT) or magnetic resonance imaging (MRI) is also done. Both tests can help doctors distinguish a hemorrhagic stroke from an ischemic stroke. The tests can also show how much brain tissue has been damaged and whether pressure is increased in other areas of the brain. The blood sugar level is measured because a low blood sugar level can cause symptoms similar to those of stroke.

Prognosis

Intracerebral hemorrhage is more likely to be fatal than ischemic stroke. The hemorrhage is usually large and catastrophic, especially in people who have chronic high blood pressure. More than half of the people who have a large hemorrhage die within a few days. Those who survive usually recover consciousness and some brain function over time. However, most do not recover all lost brain function.

Treatment

Treatment of intracerebral hemorrhage differs from that of an ischemic stroke. Anticoagulants (such as heparin and warfarin), thrombolytic drugs, and antiplatelet drugs (such as aspirin) are not given because they make bleeding worse. If people who are taking an anticoagulant have a hemorrhagic stroke, they may need a treatment that helps blood clot such as

- Vitamin K, usually given intravenously
- Transfusions of platelets

- Transfusions of blood that has had blood cells and platelets removed (fresh frozen plasma)
- Intravenous administration of a synthetic product similar to the proteins in blood that help blood to clot (clotting factors)

Surgery to remove the accumulated blood and relieve pressure within the skull, even if it may be life-saving, is rarely done because the operation itself can damage the brain. Also, removing the accumulated blood can trigger more bleeding, further damaging the brain and leading to severe disability. However, this operation may be effective for hemorrhage in the pituitary gland or in the cerebellum. In such cases, a good recovery is possible.

SUBARACHNOID HEMORRHAGE

A subarachnoid hemorrhage is bleeding into the space (subarachnoid space) between the inner layer (pia mater) and middle layer (arachnoid mater) of the tissue covering the brain (meninges).

- The most common cause is rupture of a bulge (aneurysm) in an artery.
- Usually, rupture of an artery causes a sudden, severe headache, often followed by a brief loss of consciousness.
- Computed tomography, sometimes a spinal tap, and angiography are done to confirm the diagnosis.
- Drugs are used to relieve the headache and to control blood pressure, and surgery is done to stop the bleeding.

A subarachnoid hemorrhage is a life-threatening disorder that can rapidly result in serious, permanent disabilities. It is the only type of stroke more common among women than among men.

Causes

Subarachnoid hemorrhage usually results from head injuries. However, hemorrhage due to a head injury causes different symptoms and is not considered a stroke.

Subarachnoid hemorrhage is considered a stroke only when it occurs spontaneously—that is, when the hemorrhage does not result from external forces, such as an accident or a fall. A spontaneous hemorrhage usually results from the sudden rupture of an aneurysm in a cerebral artery. Aneurysms are bulges in a weakened area of an artery's wall. Aneurysms typically occur where an artery branches. Aneurysms may be present at birth (congenital), or they may develop later, after years of high blood pressure weaken the walls of arteries. Most subarachnoid hemorrhages result from congenital aneurysms.

Less commonly, subarachnoid hemorrhage results from rupture of an abnormal connection between arteries and veins (arteriovenous malformation) in or around the brain. An arteriovenous malformation may be present at birth, but it is usually identified only if symptoms develop. Rarely, a blood clot forms on an infected heart valve, travels (becoming an embolus) to an artery that supplies the brain, and causes the artery to become inflamed. The artery may then weaken and rupture.

> **? Did You Know...**
> Almost half of people with a subarachnoid hemorrhage die before reaching the hospital.

Symptoms

Before rupturing, an aneurysm usually causes no symptoms unless it presses on a nerve or leaks small amounts of blood, usually before a large rupture (which causes headache). Then it produces warning signs, such as the following:

- Headache, which may be unusually sudden and severe (sometimes called a thunderclap headache)
- Facial or eye pain
- Double vision
- Loss of peripheral vision

The warning signs can occur minutes to weeks before the rupture. People should report any unusual headaches to a doctor immediately.

A rupture usually causes a sudden, severe headache that peaks within seconds. It is often followed by a brief loss of consciousness. Almost half of affected people die before reaching a hospital. Some people remain in a coma or unconscious. Others wake up, feeling confused and sleepy. They may also feel restless. Within hours or even minutes, people may again become sleepy and confused. They may become unresponsive and difficult to arouse. Within 24 hours, blood and cerebrospinal fluid around the brain irritate the layers of tissue covering the brain (meninges), causing a stiff neck as well as continuing headaches, often with vomiting, dizziness, and low back pain. Frequent fluctuations in the heart rate and in the breathing rate often occur, sometimes accompanied by seizures.

About 25% of people have symptoms that indicate damage to a specific part of the brain, such as the following:

- Weakness or paralysis on one side of the body (most common)
- Loss of sensation on one side of the body
- Difficulty understanding and using language (aphasia—see page 679)

Severe impairments may develop and become permanent within minutes or hours. Fever is common during the first 5 to 10 days.

A subarachnoid hemorrhage can lead to several other serious problems:

- **Hydrocephalus:** Within 24 hours, the blood from a subarachnoid hemorrhage may clot. The clotted blood may prevent the fluid surrounding the brain (cerebrospinal fluid) from draining as it normally does. As a result, blood accumulates within the brain, increasing pressure within the skull. Hydrocephalus may contribute to symptoms such as headaches, sleepiness, confusion, nausea, and vomiting and may increase the risk of coma and death.

- **Vasospasm:** About 3 to 10 days after the hemorrhage, arteries in the brain may contract (spasm), limiting blood flow to the brain. Then, brain tissues may not get enough oxygen and may die, as in ischemic stroke. Vasospasm may cause symptoms similar to those of ischemic stroke, such as weakness or loss of sensation on one side of the body, difficulty using or understanding language, vertigo, and impaired coordination.

- **A second rupture:** Sometimes a second rupture occurs, usually within a week.

Diagnosis

If people have a sudden, severe headache that peaks within seconds or that is accompanied by any symptoms suggesting a stroke, they should go immediately to the hospital. Computed tomography (CT—see page 2037) is done to check for bleeding. A spinal tap (lumbar puncture—see page 635) is done if CT is inconclusive or unavailable. It can detect any blood in the cerebrospinal fluid. A spinal tap is not done if doctors suspect that pressure within the skull is increased. Cerebral angiography (see page 2036) is done as soon as possible to confirm the diagnosis and to identify the site of the aneurysm or arteriovenous malformation causing the bleeding. Magnetic resonance angiography (see page 2041) or CT angiography (see page 2038) may be used instead.

Prognosis

About 35% of people die when they have a subarachnoid hemorrhage due to an aneurysm because it results in extensive brain damage. Another 15% die within a few weeks because of bleeding from a second rupture. People who survive for 6 months but who do not have surgery for the aneurysm have a 3% chance of another rupture each year. The outlook is better when the cause is an arteriovenous malformation. Occasionally, the hemorrhage is caused by a small defect that is not detected by cerebral angiography because the defect

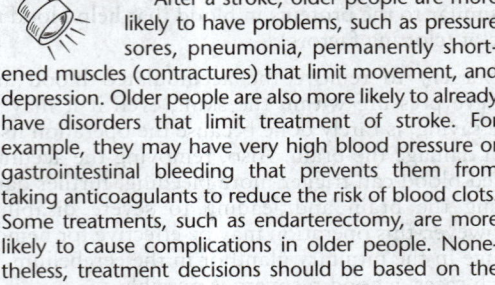

SPOTLIGHT ON AGING

After a stroke, older people are more likely to have problems, such as pressure sores, pneumonia, permanently shortened muscles (contractures) that limit movement, and depression. Older people are also more likely to already have disorders that limit treatment of stroke. For example, they may have very high blood pressure or gastrointestinal bleeding that prevents them from taking anticoagulants to reduce the risk of blood clots. Some treatments, such as endarterectomy, are more likely to cause complications in older people. Nonetheless, treatment decisions should be based on the person's health rather than on age itself.

Some disorders common among older people can interfere with their recovery after a stroke, as in the following:

- People with dementia may not understand what is required of them for rehabilitation.
- People with heart failure or another heart disorder may risk having another stroke or a heart attack triggered by exertion during rehabilitation exercises.

A good recovery is more likely when older people have a family member or caregiver to help, a living situation that facilitates independence (for example, a first-floor residence and nearby shops), and financial resources to pay for rehabilitation.

Because recovery after stroke depends on so many medical, social, financial, and lifestyle factors, rehabilitation and care for older people should be individually designed and managed by a team of health care practitioners (including nurses, psychologists, and social workers as well as a doctor or therapist). Team members can also provide information about resources and strategies to help people who have had a stroke and their caregivers with daily living.

has already sealed itself off. In such cases, the outlook is very good.

Some people recover most or all mental and physical function after a subarachnoid hemorrhage. However, many people continue to have symptoms such as weakness, paralysis, or loss of sensation on one side of the body or aphasia.

Treatment

People who may have had a subarachnoid hemorrhage are hospitalized immediately. Bed rest with no exertion is essential. Analgesics such as opioids (but not aspirin or other nonsteroidal anti-inflammatory drugs, which can worsen the bleeding) are given to control the severe headaches. Stool softeners are given to prevent straining during bowel movements. Nimodipine, a calcium channel blocker, is usually given by mouth to prevent vasospasm and subsequent ischemic stroke. Doctors take measures (such as giving drugs and adjusting the amount of intravenous fluid given) to keep blood pressure at levels low enough to avoid further hemorrhage and high enough to maintain blood flow to the damaged parts of the brain. Occasionally, a piece of plastic tubing (shunt) may be placed in the brain to drain cerebrospinal fluid away from the brain. This procedure relieves pressure and prevents hydrocephalus.

For people who have an aneurysm, a surgical procedure is done to isolate, block off, or support the walls of the weak artery and thus reduce the risk of fatal bleeding later. These procedures are difficult, and regardless of which one is used, the risk of death is high, especially for people who are in a stupor or coma. The best time for surgery is controversial and must be decided based on the person's situation. Most neurosurgeons recommend operating within 24 hours of the start of symptoms, before hydrocephalus and vasospasm develop. If surgery cannot be done this quickly, the procedure may be delayed 10 days to reduce the risks of surgery, but then bleeding is more likely to recur because the waiting period is longer.

A commonly used procedure, called neuroendovascular surgery, involves inserting coiled wires into the aneurysm. The coils are placed using a catheter that is inserted into an artery and threaded to the aneurysm. Thus, this procedure does not require that the skull be opened. By slowing blood flow through the aneurysm, the coils promote clot formation, which seals off the aneurysm and prevents it from rupturing. Neuroendovascular surgery can often be done at the same time as cerebral angiography, when the aneurysm is diagnosed.

Less commonly, a metal clip is placed across the aneurysm. This procedure prevents blood from entering the aneurysm and eliminates the risk of rupture. The clip remains in place permanently. Most clips that were placed 15 to 20 years ago are affected by the magnetic forces and can be displaced during magnetic resonance imaging (MRI). People who have these clips should inform their doctor if MRI is being considered. Newer clips are not affected by the magnetic forces.

CHAPTER

115 Head Injuries

- About half of head injuries result from motor vehicle crashes; falls, assaults, and mishaps during sports and recreational activities are also common causes.
- People with minor head injuries may have a headache or dizziness.
- People with more severe head injuries may lose consciousness or have symptoms of brain dysfunction.
- Computed tomography is used to check for severe head injuries.
- Treatment of people with severe head injuries aims to ensure that the brain gets sufficient oxygen and that pressure in the brain remains normal.

The thick, hard bones of the skull help protect the brain from injury. Also, the brain is surrounded by layers of tissue (meninges) containing cerebrospinal fluid, which cushions the brain. Consequently, most bumps and knocks on the head do not injure the brain. Head injuries that do not affect the brain are considered minor.

Head injuries that cause brain injury (traumatic brain injury, or TBI) are considered severe. In the United States, about 13 in 10,000 people sustain minor head injury, and about 3 in 10,000 sustain severe head injury each year. In the United States, head injuries are responsible for about 50,000 deaths each year, about 40% of all deaths caused by injuries of any kind. Head injuries are also responsible for about 230,000 hospitalizations. About 5.3 million people have permanent disabilities from head injury. Nearly 50% of people who have a very severe head injury die.

About half of head injuries result from motor vehicle crashes, and head injuries occur in more than 70% of severe motor vehicle crashes. Other common causes are falls in the home; physical assaults; mishaps during sports, during recreational activities, or in the workplace (for example, while operating machinery); and firearms.

Head injuries include injury to the scalp, skull fractures, concussions, bruises (contusions) and tears (lacerations) of the brain, accumulation of blood within the brain or between the brain and skull (intracranial hematoma), and damage to nerve cells throughout the brain (diffuse axonal injury). The brain can be damaged even if the skull is not fractured. Often, the degree of brain damage may be more severe than the degree of external injuries. Also, the brain may not be damaged even when external injuries are severe.

Symptoms

Minor Head Injury: A bump may appear on the head. If the scalp is cut, bleeding may be profuse, because the scalp has many blood vessels close to the skin surface. Consequently, a scalp injury may appear to be more serious than it is.

Common symptoms may include headache and the sensation of spinning or light-headedness. Some people also may have mild confusion, nausea, and, more commonly in children, vomiting. Young children may simply become irritable.

A concussion (see page 737) is a temporary, brief change in mental function without damage to the structure of the brain. Often, people lose consciousness briefly (usually a few minutes or less), but they may simply become confused or be unable to recall events and experiences (amnesia) for a brief period before or after the injury.

For some time after a concussion, people may experience headache, dizziness, fatigue, poor memory, inability to concentrate, trouble sleeping, difficulty thinking, irritability, depression, and anxiety. These symptoms are called the postconcussion syndrome.

Severe Head Injury: People may have some of the same symptoms as occur with minor head injury. Some, such as headache, may be more severe. Also, symptoms often start with a period of unconsciousness that begins at the time of impact. How long people remain unconscious varies. Some people awaken in seconds, while others do not awaken for hours or even days. On awakening, people often are drowsy, confused, restless, or agitated. They may also vomit, have seizures, or both. Balance and coordination may be impaired. Depending on which area of the brain is damaged, the ability to think, control emotions, move, feel, speak, see, hear, and remember may be impaired—sometimes permanently.

Clear fluid or blood may drain from the nose, ears, or both if a person has a fracture of the base of the skull (see page 739).

An injured brain may bleed or swell. This bleeding and swelling gradually increase the pressure on the brain because the skull cannot expand to accommodate any increase in its contents. As the pressure increases, the person's symptoms worsen and new symptoms appear. The first symptoms of increased pressure within the skull include worsening headache, impaired thinking, decreased level of consciousness, and vomiting. Later, the person may become unre-

sponsive. A pupil may widen. Eventually (usually within a day or two of injury), the increased pressure may force the brain downward, causing a herniation of the brain—an abnormal protrusion of brain tissue through a natural opening between the compartments of the brain. Herniation of the brain can cause coma or even death if too much pressure is put on the brain stem, the lower part of the brain, which controls such vital functions as heart rate and breathing.

Prognosis

Minor Head Injury: Most people recover completely, particularly if postconcussion syndrome symptoms do not develop. Postconcussion syndrome symptoms are common during the week after brain injury. They often resolve during the second week. However, sometimes symptoms persist for months or, rarely, years. People who have had a concussion seem to be more susceptible to another one, particularly if the new injury occurs before symptoms from the previous concussion have completely gone away (as may happen in an athlete who resumes playing too quickly).

Severe Head Injury: For adults who have had a severe head injury, most recovery occurs within the first 6 months, although improvement may continue for up to 2 years. Children tend to recover more fully, regardless of the injury's severity, and they continue to improve for a much longer time.

The eventual consequences of a severe head injury range from complete recovery to permanent problems or disabilities of varying degrees to death. Common long-term problems include amnesia, behavioral problems (such as anxiety, restlessness, impulsivity, lack of inhibition, or lack of motivation), sudden mood swings, sleep disturbances, and decreased intellectual function. Recovery of memory after loss of consciousness due to a severe head injury depends on how quickly consciousness is regained. People who regain consciousness in the first week are most likely to recover their memory. A seizure disorder may develop up to 4 years after a severe head injury.

The type and severity of disabilities depend on where and how badly the brain was damaged. Some functions, such as vision and control of arm and leg movements, are controlled by unique areas on one side of the brain. Damage to any of these areas usually causes impairment of the corresponding function and thus permanent disability. Undamaged areas of the brain sometimes take over functions that were lost when another area was damaged, resulting in partial recovery. However, as people age, the brain becomes less able to shift functions from one area to another. For example, language skills are handled by several parts of the brain in young children but are concentrated on one side of the brain (the left hemisphere) in adults. If the left

Herniation: The Brain Under Pressure

Bleeding or swelling in the brain can cause pressure that forces the brain downward in the skull. The result may be a herniation, in which brain tissue is forced through a small natural opening in the relatively rigid sheets of tissue that separate the brain into right and left compartments and into upper and lower compartments. (These dividers are extensions of the outer layer of tissue covering the brain, the dura mater.) Herniation compresses brain tissue and thus damages it.

The most common type of herniation is a transtentorial herniation. Part of the temporal lobe is forced through the tentorial notch—the opening in the sheet of tissue between the temporal lobe and cerebellum. The pupil of the eye may become dilated and may not constrict in response to light. A transtentorial herniation can have catastrophic consequences, including paralysis, stupor, coma, abnormal heart rhythms, disturbances or cessation of breathing, cardiac arrest, and death.

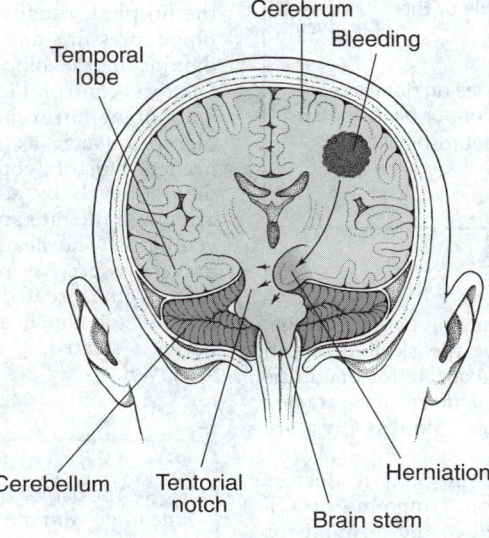

Cerebrum

Bleeding

Temporal lobe

Cerebellum   Tentorial notch

Herniation

Brain stem

hemisphere's language areas are severely damaged before age 8, the right hemisphere can assume near-normal language function. However, damage to language areas during adulthood results in permanent disability.

Rehabilitation can help people minimize the effect of most disabilities on function (see page 53).

Diagnosis and Treatment

Minor Head Injury: Diagnosis of minor head injuries is based on a person's symptoms and results of the examination. If a head injury is minor and causes no symptoms other than pain at the site of injury, mild analgesics such as acetaminophen may be used. Aspirin or any other nonsteroidal anti-inflammatory drug should not be taken because these drugs may worsen any bleeding in the brain or skull. Doctors suture lacerations and dress wounds. Someone should check the injured person every few hours during the first 24 hours after the injury to make

sure that no potentially serious symptoms develop. Children who have had a minor head injury may be allowed to sleep, but they should be awakened every few hours and checked for symptoms.

Injured people are checked for symptoms that indicate brain function could be worsening. These symptoms include persistent or increasing sleepiness and confusion, seizures, repeated vomiting, severe headache, inability to feel or move an arm or leg, inability to recognize people or the surroundings, loss of balance, problems with speaking or seeing, lack of coordination, noisy breathing, and drainage of clear fluid (cerebrospinal fluid) from the nose or ear. These symptoms may develop hours or sometimes days after the original injury. If these symptoms occur, prompt medical attention is essential.

If a head injury causes loss of consciousness, even briefly, immediate evaluation by a doctor is necessary. If doctors observe symptoms or findings that indicate possible brain injury, computed tomography

Recognizing a Serious Head Injury

Most head injuries are not serious. A serious head injury can be recognized based on certain symptoms. These symptoms indicate that brain functioning is worsening. If any of them occur in an adult or a child, medical attention should be sought immediately.

- Vomiting, paleness, irritability, or drowsiness that continues for more than 6 hours
- Loss of consciousness
- Inability to move or feel part of the body
- Inability to recognize people or the surroundings
- Inability to maintain balance
- Problems with speaking or seeing (for example, slurred speech, blurred vision, or blind spots)
- Drainage of clear fluid (cerebrospinal fluid) from the nose or ear
- Severe headache

(CT) or magnetic resonance imaging (MRI) is done, and any significant injuries of the skull or brain tissue are treated. CT is more accurate for diagnosis of skull fractures, and MRI is more accurate for certain types of brain injuries. Skull x-rays are rarely helpful.

People are admitted to the hospital if doctors suspect brain damage based on symptoms or CT findings. Children are admitted to the hospital for these reasons or if they were unconscious even briefly or had a seizure. Children are also admitted to the hospital if child abuse is suspected.

Severe Head Injury: If the injury may affect other parts of the body (for example, after a motor vehicle crash) or the person is unconscious, an ambulance should be called. When emergency personnel are moving a person who has had a severe head injury, they take great care to avoid making the injuries worse. The neck should be assumed to be broken until proved otherwise. In such cases, the person's head, neck, and spine are stabilized. Usually, the person is put in a hard neck collar, strapped to a firm board, and carefully padded to prevent movement.

When the person who may have a severe head injury reaches the hospital, doctors and nurses perform a physical examination to determine whether the injury is serious. First, they check vital signs, including heart rate, blood pressure, and breathing. A person who is not breathing adequately may need a ventilator. Doctors immediately check whether the person is oriented and able to respond to commands. They also determine how much stimulation the person needs

before opening the eyes. Doctors next assess basic brain function by checking, for example, the size of the pupils and their reaction to light, the ability to move the arms and legs, the use of language, coordination, and reflexes. CT is done to check for possible brain damage. Sometimes MRI is done in addition to CT. X-rays of the skull are usually unnecessary. They can identify skull fractures but reveal very little about brain damage. X-rays or CT scans of the neck are used when necessary to determine whether the neck is broken.

People with severe head injuries are admitted to the hospital, usually to an intensive care unit. The blood pressure and levels of oxygen and carbon dioxide in the blood are kept at desirable levels. Doctors control blood pressure by adjusting the amount of intravenous fluids given and by using diuretics (such as mannitol and furosemide) as needed. Doctors control blood oxygen and carbon dioxide levels by adjusting the amount of oxygen given and the rate and depth of breaths given by the ventilator. The head of the bed may be raised to prevent excessive pressure within the skull and brain. Pain is treated. People may need to be sedated because too much muscle activity can be harmful. Fever is treated. If seizures occur, anticonvulsants are given.

> ### ? Did You Know...
> The degree of external head injury may have little to do with the degree of brain injury.
>
> In a person with a severe head injury, the neck should not be moved because it may be broken.

A small pressure gauge may be implanted inside the skull to measure pressure within the skull and to determine how well the treatments are preventing or treating pressure elevation within the brain. Alternatively, a catheter may be inserted into one of the internal spaces (ventricles) within the brain. The ventricles contain cerebrospinal fluid, which flows over the surface of the brain between the meninges. The catheter can be used to monitor the pressure and to drain cerebrospinal fluid, reducing the pressure within the skull. Sometimes doctor need to surgically open the skull to relieve the pressure.

Cerebral Contusions and Lacerations

Cerebral contusions *are bruises on the brain, usually caused by a direct, strong blow to the head.* **Cerebral**

lacerations *are tears in brain tissue, caused by a foreign object or pushed-in bone fragment from a skull fracture.*

- Motor vehicle crashes and blows to the head are common causes of bruises and tears of brain tissue.
- Symptoms of mild or severe head injury develop.
- Computed tomography is done.
- The person is observed in the hospital and sometimes needs surgery.

Cerebral contusions and lacerations involve structural brain damage and thus are more serious than concussions. Contusions may be caused by the sudden acceleration of the brain that follows a jolt—as may be delivered by a forceful blow to the head—or by the sudden deceleration that occurs when a moving head strikes an immovable object (as in a frontal-impact motor vehicle crash). The brain can be damaged at the point of impact and on the opposite side by striking the inside of the skull. Contusions and lacerations can cause bleeding or swelling in the brain.

Contusions and lacerations may be very small, causing only minimal damage to the brain, with few symptoms or symptoms of minor head injury. However, with larger injuries, or if swelling or bleeding from a small injury is severe, people may have symptoms of severe head injury (see page 734). For example, people often are unconscious for a short time (such as a few minutes or less) or longer. When awake, people often are drowsy, confused, restless, or agitated. They may also have vomiting, seizures, or impaired balance or coordination. The ability to think, control emotions, move, feel, speak, see, hear, and remember may be impaired. A more severe injury causes swelling within the brain, damaging brain tissue further. Herniation of the brain may result, sometimes leading to coma.

Doctors do computed tomography (CT) to diagnose a contusion or laceration. If bleeding and swelling are minor, people are hospitalized and observed, usually for about a week. If bleeding is severe, doctors treat them as if they had a severe head injury (see page 736). Often people are admitted to an intensive care unit. Doctors keep the blood pressure and blood levels of oxygen and carbon dioxide at desirable levels. They may give supplemental oxygen, mechanical ventilation, pain relief, and sedation. Fever and seizures are treated.

To measure pressure in the brain, doctors may implant a pressure gauge inside the skull or insert a catheter into one of the internal spaces (ventricles) within the brain. If bleeding leads to herniation, the blood may need to be surgically removed to prevent compression of the brain. However, if removing the blood involves removing brain tissue, then brain function may eventually become impaired.

Concussion

A concussion is an injury-induced alteration in mental function or level of awareness that may involve a loss of consciousness, can occur without obvious damage to brain structures, and lasts less than 6 hours.

A person who has a concussion may temporarily feel dazed or mildly confused. Some people may not realize they have had a concussion. Consciousness may be lost for a brief time, rarely for more than 15 minutes. Memory for events just before or just after the injury may be lost.

Later, people may experience headache, the sensation of spinning, light-headedness, fatigue, poor memory, inability to concentrate, irritability, depression, and anxiety. These symptoms are called the postconcussion syndrome. People may develop impaired thinking, particularly people who had emotional problems before the concussion. Postconcussion syndrome symptoms are common during the week after concussion and commonly resolve during the second week. However, sometimes, symptoms persist for months or, rarely, years. People who have had a concussion also seem to be more susceptible to another one, particularly if the new injury occurs before symptoms from the previous concussion have completely gone away.

To diagnose a concussion, doctors need to make sure brain structures are not damaged. This is done using computed tomography (CT), magnetic resonance imaging (MRI), or both. If there is no structural brain damage, only the symptoms need be treated. For concussion, acetaminophen is given for pain. Aspirin or another nonsteroidal anti-inflammatory drug (NSAID—see page 644) should not be taken because they interfere with blood clotting and may contribute to bleeding from damaged blood vessels. Rest is the best treatment for a concussion.

Treatment for postconcussion syndrome is based on the severity of the symptoms. Rest and close observation are important. People who experience emotional difficulties may need psychotherapy. Repeated concussions may increase a person's risk in later life for dementia, Parkinson's disease, and depression. People should not return to contact sports after a concussion until all ill effects have resolved and medical evaluation has been completed.

Diffuse Axonal Injury

Diffuse axonal injury is widespread injury to axons, a part of the nerve cells in the brain.

Nerve impulses leave nerve cells through a part of the nerve cell called the axon. In diffuse axonal injury, axons throughout the brain are damaged. The usual causes include falls and motor vehicle crashes. Diffuse axonal injury may contribute to the shaken baby syndrome, in which violent shaking or throwing of a baby causes brain injury (see page 1880). As a result of diffuse axonal injury, brain cells may die, causing brain swelling, increasing pressure within the skull. Increasing pressure may compound the injury by decreasing blood supply to the brain.

Diffuse axonal injury typically causes loss of consciousness that lasts for more than 6 hours. Sometimes the person has symptoms of damage to a specific area of the brain. Increased pressure within the skull may cause coma. Computed tomography (CT) or magnetic resonance imaging (MRI) is usually done to detect diffuse axonal injury. Diffuse axonal injury is treated with the general measures used to treat all types of head injuries. Surgery is not helpful.

Intracranial Hematomas

Intracranial hematomas are accumulations of blood within the brain or between the brain and the skull.

- Intracranial hematomas form when a head injury causes blood to accumulate within the brain or between the brain and the skull.
- Symptoms may include a persistent headache, drowsiness, confusion, memory changes, paralysis on the opposite side of the body, speech or language impairment, and other symptoms depending on which area of the brain is damaged.
- Computed tomography or magnetic resonance imaging is used to detect an intracranial hematoma.
- Sometimes surgery is needed to drain blood from a hematoma.

Intracranial hematomas include

- **Epidural hematomas,** which form between the skull and the outer layer (dura mater) of tissue covering the brain (meninges)
- **Subdural hematomas,** which form between the outer layer and the middle layer (arachnoid mater—see art on page 624)
- **Intracerebral hematomas,** which form within the brain

After injury, bleeding can also occur between the arachnoid mater and the inner layer (pia mater). Bleeding in this area is called subarachnoid hemorrhage. However, because subarachnoid blood usually does not accumulate in one place, it is not considered a hematoma.

For people who are taking aspirin or anticoagulants (which increase the risk of bleeding), particularly older people, the risk of developing a hematoma after even a minor head injury is increased. Intracerebral hematomas and subarachnoid hemorrhages can also result from strokes.

Most epidural and intracerebral hematomas and many subdural hematomas develop rapidly and cause symptoms within minutes. Large hematomas press on the brain and may cause swelling and herniation of the brain. Herniation may cause loss of consciousness, coma, paralysis on one or both sides of the body, breathing difficulties, slowing of the heart, and even death.

Some hematomas, particularly subdural hematomas, may develop slowly and cause gradual confusion and memory loss, especially in older people, similar to the symptoms of dementia. People may not remember the head injury.

Diagnosis is based on results of computed tomography (CT). Treatment depends on the type and size of the hematoma and how much pressure has built up in the brain.

EPIDURAL HEMATOMAS

These hematomas are caused by bleeding from an artery or a large vein (venous sinus) located between the skull and the outer layer of tissue covering the brain. Bleeding often occurs when a skull fracture tears the blood vessel.

A severe headache may develop immediately or after several hours. The headache sometimes disappears but returns several hours later, worse than before. Deterioration in consciousness, including increasing confusion, sleepiness, paralysis, collapse, and a deep coma, can quickly follow. Some people lose consciousness after the injury, regain it, and have a period of unimpaired mental function (lucid interval) before consciousness deteriorates again.

Early diagnosis is crucial and is usually based on results of CT. Doctors treat epidural hematomas as soon as they are diagnosed, because prompt treatment is necessary to prevent permanent damage. One or more holes are drilled in the skull to drain the excess blood. The surgeon also seeks the source of the bleeding and stops the bleeding.

SUBDURAL HEMATOMAS

These hematomas are caused by bleeding from the bridging veins, located between the outer and middle layers of tissue covering the brain (meninges).

Subdural hematomas may be acute, subacute, or chronic. Rapid bleeding after a severe head injury can cause acute subdural hematomas, with symptoms that develop over minutes or a few hours, or subacute subdural hematomas, with symptoms that develop over several hours or days. Chronic subdural hematomas can develop over weeks, months, or years. By the time symptoms occur, the hematoma may be very large.

Chronic subdural hematomas are more common among alcoholics and among older people. Alcoholics, who are relatively prone to falls as well as bleeding, may ignore or forget minor to moderately severe head injuries. These injuries can lead to small subdural hematomas that may become chronic. In older people, the brain shrinks slightly, stretching the bridging veins and making them more likely to be torn if an injury, even a minor one, occurs. Also, bleeding tends to continue longer because the shrunken brain exerts less pressure on the bleeding vein, allowing more blood loss from it. After the blood is resorbed from a hematoma, the brain may not re-expand as well in older people as in younger people. As a result, a fluid-filled space (hygroma) may be left. The hygroma may refill with blood or enlarge because small vessels tear, causing repeated bleeding.

> **? Did You Know...**
> An older person with symptoms of dementia may instead have a subdural hematoma, which can be effectively treated.

Symptoms and Diagnosis

Symptoms may include a persistent headache, fluctuating drowsiness, confusion, memory changes, paralysis on the side of the body opposite the hematoma, and speech or language impairment. Other symptoms may occur depending on which area of the brain is damaged (see page 677). In infants, a subdural hematoma can cause the head to enlarge (as in hydrocephalus), because the skull is soft and pliable. Therefore, pressure within the skull increases less in infants than it does in older children and adults.

Chronic subdural hematomas are more difficult to diagnose because of the length of time between the injury and the development of symptoms. An older person with gradually developing symptoms, such as memory impairment and drowsiness, may be mistakenly thought to have dementia. CT can detect acute, subacute, and many chronic subdural hematomas. Magnetic resonance imaging (MRI) is particularly accurate for diagnosis of chronic subdural hematomas.

Treatment

Often, small subdural hematomas in adults do not require treatment because the blood is absorbed on its own. If a subdural hematoma is large and is causing symptoms such as persisting headache, fluctuating drowsiness, confusion, memory changes, and paralysis on the opposite side of the body, doctors usually drain it surgically by drilling a small hole in the skull. During surgery, a drain is usually inserted and left in place for several days, because subdural hematomas can recur. The person is moni-

tored closely for recurrences. In infants, doctors usually drain the hematoma for cosmetic if for no other reasons.

Only about 50% of people who are treated for a large acute subdural hematoma survive. People who are treated for a chronic subdural hematoma usually improve or do not worsen.

INTRACEREBRAL HEMATOMAS

These hematomas are common after a severe head injury. They are caused by a cerebral contusion. Fluid accumulation in the damaged brain (cerebral edema) is common and accounts for most deaths. CT or MRI can detect intracerebral hematomas. Because these hematomas are caused by direct damage to the brain, surgery is usually avoided because it usually does not restore brain function. Also, because the hematomas are within the brain tissue, doctors must remove the overlying brain to get at the hematoma, which also contributes to loss of brain function.

Skull Fracture

A skull fracture is a break in a bone surrounding the brain.

- Skull fracture can occur with or without brain damage.
- Symptoms may include pain, symptoms of brain damage, and, in certain fractures, fluid leaking from the nose or ears or bruises behind the ears or around the eyes.
- Computed tomography is used to diagnose skull fractures.
- Many skull fractures require no treatment.

Skull fractures can injure arteries and veins, which then bleed into the spaces around brain tissue. In people with a skull fracture, brain damage may be more severe than in people with a head injury but no fracture. However, a skull fracture often occurs without brain damage. Fractures, especially at the back and bottom (base) of the skull, can tear the meninges, the layers of tissue that cover the brain. Rarely, bacteria enter the skull through such fractures, causing infection and severe brain damage. Sometimes, pieces of the fractured skull bone press inward and damage the brain. These types of fractures are called depressed fractures. Depressed skull fractures may expose the brain to the environment and foreign material, leading to infection or the formation of abscesses (collections of pus) within the brain.

Symptoms

Certain symptoms suggest a fracture at the base of the skull:

Pockets of Blood in the Brain

A head injury can cause bleeding in the brain. It can result in a pocket of blood between the skull and the outer layer of tissue covering the brain. This pocket of blood is called an epidural hematoma. Or a pocket of blood may form between the outer and middle layers of tissue. This pocket of blood is called a subdural hematoma.

Cross Section of the Brain

- Scalp
- Skull
- Dura mater
- Arachnoid mater
- Subarachnoid space
- Pia mater
- Brain

Epidural Hematoma

Bleeding between the dura mater and the skull

Subdural Hematoma

Bleeding between the arachnoid mater and the dura mater

- Cerebrospinal fluid—the clear fluid that flows over the surface of the brain between the meninges—may leak from the nose (rhinorrhea) or ears (otorrhea).
- Blood may collect behind the eardrum, or if the eardrum is ruptured, blood may drain from the ear.
- Bruises may develop behind the ear (Battle's sign) or around the eyes (raccoon's eyes).

Blood may collect in the sinuses, which may also be fractured.

Diagnosis and Treatment

Skull fractures are usually diagnosed in people with head injury who are undergoing computed tomography (CT). CT is better than magnetic resonance imaging (MRI) for diagnosing skull fractures.

Most people with skull fractures without brain injury are admitted to the hospital and observed. People who develop seizures require anticonvulsants. Other than fractures of the base of the skull and depressed skull fractures, most skull fractures require no specific treatment.

Fractures at the Base of the Skull: People with a fracture of the base of the skull are admitted to the hospital. Bed rest and head elevation are needed until cerebrospinal fluid stops leaking. People should avoid blowing their nose because often a sinus near the nose is also fractured. If so, blowing the nose can cause air from the nose to spread to other parts of the face or head. Most meningeal tears seal up on their own within 48 hours or at least within a week after the injury. If cerebrospinal fluid continues to leak, then doctors can sometimes drain the fluid by inserting a small needle in the lower back. If fluid continues to leak, the leak is closed surgically.

> **Did You Know...**
> X-rays of the skull are rarely helpful.

Depressed Skull Fractures: In this type of fracture, one or more fragments of bone may press inward on the brain, damaging the brain. The brain may be exposed to the outside. Doctors aim to prevent infection and the formation of abscesses by removing foreign materials and dead tissue and repairing as much of the damage as possible. Doctors lift skull fragments back into position and stitch the wound closed.

Skull Fractures in Children: In infants who have a skull fracture, the membranes surrounding the brain occasionally protrude through and become trapped by the fracture, forming a fluid-filled sac called a growing fracture or leptomeningeal cyst. The sac develops over 3 to 6 weeks and may be the first evidence that the skull was fractured.

A child with a skull fracture is admitted to the hospital if

- Symptoms suggest possible brain injury.
- The child was unconscious, even briefly.
- Symptoms or CT findings suggest a fracture at the base of the skull.
- The fracture occurs in an infant.
- Child abuse is suspected.

Treatment of leptomeningeal cysts may involve observation only, since these fluid-filled sacs sometimes heal themselves. In children who develop or become at risk of developing problems such as pressure on the brain or infection, doctors surgically drain the cyst.

CHAPTER

116 Tumors of the Nervous System

A tumor is an abnormal growth, whether noncancerous (benign) or cancerous (malignant). In many parts of the body, a noncancerous tumor causes few or no problems. However, any abnormal growth or mass in the brain or spinal cord can cause considerable damage.

Some cancers elsewhere in the body cause symptoms of nervous system dysfunction even though there is no evidence that nerve tissue has been invaded. These disorders are called paraneoplastic syndromes (see box on page 1082). They can cause dementia, mood swings, seizures, incoordination, dizziness, double vision, and abnormal eye movements. The most common effect is dysfunction of peripheral nerves (polyneuropathy—see page 826), resulting in muscle weakness, numbness, and tingling.

Brain Tumors

A brain tumor is a noncancerous (benign) or cancerous (malignant) growth in the brain. It may originate in the brain or have spread (metastasized) to the brain from another part of the body.

- Symptoms may include headaches, personality changes (such as suddenly becoming depressed, anxious, or uninhibited), loss of balance, trouble concentrating, seizures, and incoordination.
- Imaging tests can often detect brain tumors, but sometimes biopsy of the tumor is needed.
- Treatment may involve surgery, radiation therapy, chemotherapy, or a combination.

Brain tumors are slightly more common among men than women. Only meningiomas, which are noncancerous, are more common among women. Brain tumors usually develop during early or middle adulthood but may develop at any age. They are becoming more common among older people.

Brain tumors may be primary or secondary. Primary brain tumors originate in the cells within or next to the brain. These tumors may be cancerous or noncancerous. Either type of brain tumor is serious because the skull is rigid, providing no room for the tumor to expand. Also, tumors may develop near parts of the brain that control vital functions. Secondary brain tumors are metastases originating in another part of the body and thus are always cancerous.

Noncancerous tumors are named for the specific cells or tissues in which they originate. For example, hemangioblastomas originate in blood vessels ("hema"

TUMORS THAT ORIGINATE IN OR NEAR THE BRAIN

TYPE OF TUMOR	ORIGIN	CANCER STATUS	PERCENTAGE OF ALL PRIMARY BRAIN TUMORS*	PEOPLE AFFECTED
Adenoma	Cells of the pituitary gland	Mostly noncancerous	10%	Adults
Astrocytoma (a type of glioma)	Cells of the tissue that supports nerve cells (glial cells)	Cancerous or noncancerous (some initially noncancerous astrocytomas become cancerous after 3–5 years, becoming anaplastic astrocytomas)	†	Children and adults
Chordoma	Embryonic cells of the spinal column	Noncancerous but invasive	Less than 1%	Children (may be present at birth) and adults
Craniopharyngioma	Embryonic cells from the pituitary gland	Mostly noncancerous	Less than 1%	Children (may be present at birth) and adults
Dermoid cysts and epidermoid tumors	Embryonic cells of the skin	Noncancerous	Less than 1%	Children and adults (dermoid cysts may be present at birth)
Ependymoma	Cells of the tissue that lines the spaces within the brain (ventricles)	Mostly noncancerous	About 1% (about 9% of childhood brain tumors)	Children
Germ cell tumors (including germinomas)	Embryonic cells near the pineal gland	Cancerous or noncancerous	1%	Children (germinomas may be present at birth)
Glioblastoma multiforme (a type of glioma)	Less differentiated forms of glial cells and oligodendrocytes	Cancerous	40%†	Adults
Hemangioblastoma	Embryonic cells that develop into blood vessels	Noncancerous	1–2%	Children and adults
Medulloblastoma	Embryonic cells of the cerebellum	Cancerous	25% of childhood brain tumors	Children (usually before puberty) and, rarely, adults
Meningioma	Cells of the layers of tissue covering the brain (meninges)	Noncancerous but may recur	20%	Adults
Oligodendroglioma (a type of glioma)	Cells that form the myelin sheath around nerve fibers in the brain (oligodendrocytes)	Usually noncancerous but sometimes becomes cancerous (becoming anaplastic oligodendroglioma)	5–10%†	Children and adults

(continued on the following page)

TUMORS THAT ORIGINATE IN OR NEAR THE BRAIN (*Continued*)				
TYPE OF TUMOR	**ORIGIN**	**CANCER STATUS**	**PERCENTAGE OF ALL PRIMARY BRAIN TUMORS***	**PEOPLE AFFECTED**
Osteoma	Bones of the skull	Noncancerous	2%	Children and adults
Osteosarcoma	Bones of the skull	Cancerous	Less than 1%	Children and adults
Pinealoma	Cells of the pineal gland	Noncancerous	Less than 1%	Children
Pituitary adenoma	Cells of the pituitary gland	Noncancerous	2%	Children and adults
Sarcoma	Connective tissue	Cancerous	1%	Children and adults

*Unless noted otherwise.
†Astrocytomas, oligodendroglioma, and glioblastoma multiforme are gliomas, which account for 65% of all primary brain tumors.

refers to blood vessels, and hemangioblasts are the cells that develop into blood vessel tissue). Some noncancerous tumors originate in cells of the embryo (embryonic cells), early in the development of the fetus. Such tumors may be present at birth.

The most common type of primary cancerous brain tumor is a glioma, which has several subtypes. Gliomas account for 65% of all primary brain tumors. However, most cancerous brain tumors are secondary—metastases from cancer that started in another part of the body.

Metastases may grow in a single part of the brain or in several different parts. Many types of cancer—including breast cancer, lung cancer, cancers of the digestive tract, malignant melanoma, leukemia, and lymphoma—can spread to the brain. Lymphomas of the brain are common among people who have AIDS and, for unknown reasons, are becoming more common among people who have a normal immune system.

Brain tumors can cause problems in the following ways:

- By directly invading and destroying brain tissue
- By directly putting pressure on nearby tissue
- By increasing pressure within the skull (intracranial pressure) because the tumor takes up space
- By causing fluids to accumulate in the brain
- By blocking normal circulation of cerebrospinal fluid through the spaces within the brain
- By causing bleeding

Symptoms

Symptoms occur whether a brain tumor is non-cancerous or cancerous. Noncancerous tumors grow slowly and may become quite large before causing symptoms.

A brain tumor can cause many different symptoms, and symptoms may occur suddenly or develop gradually. Which symptoms develop first and how they develop depend on the tumor's size, growth rate, and location. In some parts of the brain, even a small tumor can have devastating effects. In other parts of the brain, tumors can grow relatively large before any symptoms appear. As the tumor grows, it pushes and stretches but usually does not destroy nerve tissue, which can compensate for these changes very well. Thus, symptoms may not develop at first.

Many symptoms result from increased pressure within the skull. The most common is a headache (see page 648), which is often the first symptom. However, most headaches are not caused by brain tumors. A headache due to a brain tumor usually recurs more and more often as time passes. It eventually becomes constant, without relief. It is often worse when people lie down. The headache may awaken people from sleep. A gradually growing tumor causes a headache that typically is worse when people first awaken. If headaches with these characteristics start in people who have not had headaches before, a brain tumor may be the cause.

Often, increased pressure within the skull also affects mental function and mood. The personality may change. For example, people may become

Common Symptoms of Some Brain Tumors

ASTROCYTOMAS AND OLIGODENDROGLIOMAS

Some astrocytomas and oligodendrogliomas grow slowly and may initially cause only seizures. Others (anaplastic astrocytomas and anaplastic oligodendrogliomas) grow fast and are cancerous. They can cause various symptoms of brain dysfunction. Glioblastoma multiforme, a type of astrocytoma, grows so fast that it increases pressure in the brain, causing headaches and slowed thinking. If the pressure becomes high enough, drowsiness, then coma, may result.

Symptoms vary depending on the tumor's location.

- **Frontal lobes** (located behind the forehead): Tumors located here can cause weakness and personality changes. If they develop in the dominant frontal lobe (the left lobe in most people and the right lobe in some left-handers), they can cause speech disturbances.

- **Parietal lobes** (located behind the frontal lobes): Tumors located here can cause loss of or changes in sensation. Sometimes vision is partially lost in both eyes so that neither eye can see the side opposite the tumor.

- **Temporal lobes** (located above the ears): Tumors located here can cause seizures and, if they develop on the dominant side, the inability to understand and use language.

- **Occipital lobes** (toward the back of the head): Tumors located here can cause partial loss of vision in both eyes.

- **In or near the cerebellum** (above the back of the neck): Tumors located here, especially medulloblastomas in children, can cause alterations in eye movements, incoordination, unsteadiness in walking, and sometimes hearing loss and vertigo. They can block the drainage of cerebrospinal fluid, causing fluid to accumulate in the spaces within the brain (ventricles). As a result, the ventricles enlarge (a condition called hydrocephalus), and pressure within the skull increases. Symptoms include headaches, nausea, vomiting, difficulty turning the eyes upward, and lethargy. In infants, the head enlarges. Greatly increased pressure can cause herniation of the brain, which can result in coma and death.

MENINGIOMAS

Meningiomas are usually noncancerous but may recur after they are removed. They occur more often in women and usually appear in people aged 40 to 60, but they can begin growing during childhood or later life. Symptoms depend on where the tumor develops. They may include weakness or numbness, seizures, an impaired sense of smell, changes in vision, and impaired mental function. In older people, a meningioma may cause dementia.

PINEAL TUMORS

Pineal tumors usually develop during childhood and often cause early puberty. They can block the drainage of cerebrospinal fluid around the brain, leading to hydrocephalus. The most common type of pineal tumor is a germ cell tumor. Symptoms include the inability to look up and drooping eyelids.

PITUITARY GLAND TUMORS

The pituitary gland, located at the base of the skull, controls much of the body's endocrine system. Tumors of the pituitary gland (pituitary adenomas) are usually noncancerous. They may secrete abnormally large amounts of pituitary hormones or block production of hormones. When large amounts of hormones are secreted, effects vary depending on which hormone is involved.

- For growth hormone, extreme height (gigantism) or disproportionate enlargement of the head, face, hands, feet, and chest (acromegaly)
- For corticotropin, Cushing's syndrome
- For thyroid-stimulating hormone, hyperthyroidism
- For prolactin, the cessation of menstrual periods (amenorrhea) in women, production of breast milk in women who are not breastfeeding (galactorrhea), and, in men, loss of libido, erectile dysfunction, and enlargement of the breasts (gynecomastia)

Pituitary gland tumors can block hormone production by destroying the tissues in the pituitary gland that secrete hormones, eventually resulting in insufficient levels of these hormones in the body. Headaches commonly occur. If the tumor enlarges, peripheral vision in both eyes is lost.

---

withdrawn, moody, and, often, inefficient at work. They may feel drowsy, confused, and unable to think. Such symptoms are often more apparent to family members and co-workers than to the affected person. Depression and anxiety, especially if either develops suddenly, may be an early symptom of a brain tumor. People may behave bizarrely. They

may become uninhibited or behave in ways they never have before. In older people, certain brain tumors cause symptoms that may be mistaken for those of dementia (see page 689).

Other common symptoms of a brain tumor include vertigo, loss of balance, and incoordination. Later, as the pressure within the skull increases, nausea, vomiting, lethargy, increased drowsiness, intermittent fever, and even coma may occur. Vision may blur suddenly when people change positions. Some brain tumors, usually primary tumors, cause seizures.

Depending on which area of the brain is affected (see page 677), a tumor can do any of the following:

- Cause an arm, a leg, or one side of the body to become weak or paralyzed
- Impair the ability to feel heat, cold, pressure, a light touch, or sharp objects
- Make people unable to express or understand language.
- Increase or decrease the pulse and breathing rates if the tumor compresses the brain stem
- Reduce alertness
- Impair the ability to hear, smell, or see (causing such symptoms as double vision and loss of vision)

For example, a pituitary tumor may press on the nearby optic nerves (2nd cranial nerve), which are involved in vision, and thus impair peripheral vision. Any of these symptoms suggests a serious disorder and requires immediate medical attention.

If a tumor blocks the flow of cerebrospinal fluid through the spaces within the brain (ventricles), fluid may accumulate in the ventricles, causing them to enlarge (a condition called hydrocephalus). As a result, pressure within the skull increases. In addition to other symptoms of increased pressure, hydrocephalus makes turning the eyes upward difficult. In infants and very young children, the head enlarges.

If the pressure within the skull is greatly increased, the brain may be pushed downward because the skull cannot expand. Herniation of the brain (see art on page 735) may result. There are two main types:

- **Transtentorial herniation:** The upper part of the brain (cerebrum) is forced through the narrow opening (the tentorial notch) in the relatively rigid tissue that separates the cerebrum from the lower parts of the brain (cerebellum and brain stem). In people with this type of herniation, consciousness is reduced. The side of the body opposite the tumor may be paralyzed.
- **Tonsillar herniation:** A tumor that originates in the lower part of the brain pushes the lowest part of the cerebellum (cerebellar tonsils) through the opening at the base of the skull (foramen magnum). As a result, the brain stem, which controls breathing, heart rate, and blood pressure, is compressed and malfunctions. If not diagnosed and treated immediately, a tonsillar herniation rapidly results in coma and death.

People with metastases to the brain may also have symptoms related to the original cancer. For example, if the cancer originated in the lungs, people may cough up bloody mucus. With metastases, weight loss is common.

Symptoms worsen over time unless the tumor is treated. With treatment, particularly for benign tumors, some people completely recover. For others, life span is shortened, sometimes greatly. The outcome depends on the type and location of the tumor.

Diagnosis

Doctors consider the possibility of a brain tumor in people who have had a seizure for the first time or who have the characteristic symptoms. Although doctors can often detect brain dysfunction during a physical examination, other procedures are needed to diagnose a brain tumor.

Standard x-rays of the skull can detect tumors that erode bone (such as a meningioma or pituitary adenoma). However, magnetic resonance imaging (MRI) and computed tomography (CT) are more useful because they can detect all types of brain tumors. They can also show the tumor's size and exact position in great detail. When a brain tumor is detected, more diagnostic procedures are done to determine the particular kind.

Sometimes a spinal tap (lumbar puncture— (see art on page 635) is done to obtain cerebrospinal fluid for examination under a microscope. This procedure is done when doctors suspect that the tumor has invaded the layers of tissues that cover the brain (meninges), often compressing the cranial nerves, blocking the absorption of cerebrospinal fluid, or both. The procedure may also help when the diagnosis or the type of tumor is unclear. Cerebrospinal fluid may contain cancer cells. However, a spinal tap cannot be done in people who have a large tumor that is increasing pressure within the skull. In these people, removing cerebrospinal fluid during a spinal tap may cause the tumor to move, resulting in herniation of the brain.

A biopsy of the tumor (removal of a sample of the tumor for examination under a microscope) is usually needed to identify the type of tumor, including whether it is cancerous. A biopsy may be done during surgery in which all or part of the tumor is removed. If a tumor is difficult to reach, a biopsy may be done using three-dimensional needle placement (stereotactic biopsy) with CT, which enables doctors to precisely locate the tumor.

Treatment

Treatment of a brain tumor depends on its location and type. When possible, the tumor is removed surgically in a procedure called craniotomy (which involves opening the skull). Some brain tumors can be removed with little or no damage to the brain. However, many grow in an area that makes removal by traditional surgery difficult or impossible without destroying essential structures.

Traditional surgery sometimes causes brain damage that can lead to symptoms such as partial paralysis, changes in sensation, weakness, and impaired mental function. Nevertheless, removing a tumor—whether cancerous or noncancerous—is essential if its growth threatens important brain structures. Even when a cure is impossible, surgery may be useful to reduce the tumor's size, relieve symptoms, and help doctors determine whether other treatments, such as radiation therapy or chemotherapy, are warranted.

Noncancerous Tumors: Surgical removal is often safe and cures the person. However, very small tumors and tumors in older people may be left in place as long as they are not causing symptoms. Sometimes radiation therapy is given after surgery to destroy any remaining tumor cells. Radiosurgery focuses the radiation and is effective in treating noncancerous tumors such as meningiomas and acoustic neuromas. Therefore, radiosurgery often is used instead of traditional surgery for these tumors.

Cancerous Brain Tumors: Usually, a combination of surgery, radiation therapy, and chemotherapy is used. As much of the tumor as can be removed safely is removed, and then radiation therapy is begun. Radiation therapy is given over a course of several weeks. Radiosurgery is used when traditional surgery cannot be, especially for the treatment of metastases.

For very aggressive tumors, chemotherapy is given with radiation therapy. Radiation therapy plus chemotherapy rarely cures but may shrink a tumor enough to keep it under control for many months or even years.

After radiation therapy, ongoing chemotherapy is used to treat some types of cancerous brain tumors. Chemotherapy appears to be particularly effective in treating anaplastic oligodendrogliomas.

Increased Pressure Within the Skull: This extremely serious condition requires immediate medical attention. Drugs such as mannitol and corticosteroids are usually given by injection to reduce the pressure and prevent herniation. They reduce swelling around the tumor. Within days or sometimes hours, corticosteroids can often restore functions lost because of the tumor and relieve headache, even if the tumor is large.

If the tumor is blocking the flow of cerebrospinal fluid through the spaces within the brain, a device may be used to drain the cerebrospinal fluid and thus reduce the risk of herniation. The device consists of a small tube (catheter) connected to a gauge that measures the pressure within the skull. The tube is inserted through a tiny opening drilled in the skull. A local anesthetic (usually plus a sedative) or a general anesthetic may be used. The tube is removed or converted to a permanent drain (shunt) after a few days. During this time, doctors surgically remove all or part of the tumor or use radiosurgery or radiation therapy to reduce the size of the tumor and thus relieve the blockage.

Metastases: Treatment depends largely on where the cancer originated. Radiation therapy directed at the metastases in the brain is often used. Surgical removal may benefit people who have only a single metastasis. Sometimes radiosurgery is used.

Some experimental treatments, such as implantation of pellets containing chemotherapy drugs or of radioactive pellets in the tumor, are being tried.

End-of-Life Issues: People with cancerous brain tumors have a limited life expectancy and are likely to become unable to make decisions about medical care. Consequently, establishing advance directives is advisable (see page 69). Advance directives can help a doctor determine what kind of care people want if they become unable to make decisions about medical care.

Many cancer centers, especially those with hospice facilities, provide counseling and home health services.

Spinal Cord Tumors

A spinal cord tumor is a noncancerous (benign) or cancerous (malignant) growth in or around the spinal cord.

- People may have weak muscles, lose sensation in particular areas of the body, or become unable to control bowel and bladder function.
- Magnetic resonance imaging can usually detect spinal cord tumors.
- Treatment may involve surgical removal, radiation therapy, or both.

Spinal cord tumors are much less common than brain tumors. Spinal cord tumors may be primary or secondary.

Primary spinal cord tumors may be cancerous or noncancerous. They may originate in the cells within or next to the spinal cord. Only about 10% of primary spinal cord tumors originate in the cells within the spinal cord. These tumors can extend within the cord and cause a fluid-filled cavity (syrinx) to form.

The other 90% of primary spinal cord tumors originate in cells next to the spinal cord, such as those of the spinal nerve roots—the parts of spinal nerves that emerge from the spinal cord (see art on page 626). Meningiomas and neurofibromas, which originate in cells next to the cord, are the most

Understanding Tumor Treatment

Craniotomy: After part of the scalp is shaved, an incision is made through the skin. A high-speed drill and a special saw are used to remove a small piece of bone above the tumor. The tumor is located and removed using one of the following:

- A scalpel may be used to cut out the tumor.
- A laser may be used to vaporize the tumor.
- A device that emits ultrasound waves may be used to break the tumor apart, so that the pieces can be suctioned out (aspirated).

Lasers and ultrasound devices are used to remove tumors that would be difficult to cut out. Usually, the bone is then replaced, and the incision stitched closed.

Stereotactic techniques: These techniques are ways to localize tumors very precisely. Computers are used to produce a three-dimensional image. The three-dimensional image can be obtained by attaching a light-weight metal imaging frame with a series of rods to the person's skull. A local anesthetic is given, and the pins are attached to the skull, piercing the skin. The rods appear as dots on a CT scan, providing reference points, which help locate the tumor. Other devices, such as a viewing wand or compass system, do not involve attaching a frame and may be used instead. Stereotactic techniques can be used to biopsy or remove tumors or to insert implants containing a chemotherapy drug or radioactive pellets.

Radiosurgery: Radiosurgery is not really surgery because no incision is required. Focused radiation is used to destroy a tumor. Several machines, including a gamma knife and a linear accelerator, can produce this type of radiation.

When a **gamma knife** is used, an imaging frame is attached to the person's skull. The person lies on a sliding bed, and a large helmet with holes in it is placed over the frame. The head of the bed is then slid into a globe that contains radioactive cobalt. Radiation passes through the holes in the helmet and is aimed precisely at the tumor.

A **linear accelerator** circles the head of the person, who lies on a sliding bed. The linear accelerator rotates around the person and aims radiation precisely at the tumor from different angles.

Implants: After a tumor is removed and before the skull and incision are closed, wafers soaked with a chemotherapy drug may be placed in the space where the tumor was. As the wafers gradually dissolve, they release the drug to destroy any remaining cancer cells.

A thin tube (catheter) may be inserted through an incision and used to place radioactive implants directly into the tumor. The implants may be removed after a few days or months or may be left in place. Unlike people who have externally applied radiation therapy, people who have radioactive implants are radioactive for a time (that is, they give off radiation). They thus need to take precautions as advised by their doctor. After this procedure, surgery may be necessary to remove dead cancer cells.

Shunts: If a tumor causes pressure within the skull to increase, a shunt may be surgically placed. A shunt is a thin piece of tubing that is inserted into one of the spaces of the brain (ventricles) or sometimes into the space around the spine that contains cerebrospinal fluid (subarachnoid space). The other end of the tubing is threaded under the skin from the head usually to the abdominal cavity. Excess cerebrospinal fluid is drained from the brain into the abdominal cavity, where it is absorbed. The shunt contains a one-way valve that opens when there is too much fluid in the brain. Shunts may be temporary (until the tumor is removed) or permanent.

---

common primary spinal tumors. They are noncancerous.

Secondary spinal cord tumors, which are more common, are metastases of cancer originating in another part of the body and thus are always cancerous. Metastases most commonly spread to the vertebrae from cancers that originate in the lungs, breasts, prostate gland, kidneys, or thyroid gland. Metastases compress the spinal cord or nerve roots from the outside. Lymphomas may also spread to the spine and compress the spinal cord.

Symptoms

Symptoms are caused by pressure on the spinal cord and nerve roots. Pressure on the spinal cord may cause the following:

- Back pain that progressively worsens, is unrelated to activity, and is worse when people lie down
- Decreased sensation, progressive weakness, or paralysis in areas controlled by the parts of the spinal cord below the part that is compressed
- Erectile dysfunction
- Loss of bladder and bowel control

Pressure on the spinal cord may also block the blood supply to the cord, resulting in death of tissue, fluid accumulation, and swelling. Fluid accumulation may block more of the blood supply, leading to a vicious circle of damage. Symptoms due to pressure on the spinal cord can worsen quickly.

Pressure on spinal nerve roots can cause pain, numbness, tingling, weakness in areas supplied by

TUMORS THAT ORIGINATE IN OR NEAR THE SPINAL CORD

TYPE OF TUMOR	ORIGIN	CANCER STATUS	PEOPLE AFFECTED
Astrocytoma	Cells of the tissue that supports nerve cells	Cancerous or noncancerous	Children and adults
Ependymoma	Cells lining the canal in the center of the spinal cord	Noncancerous	Children and adults
Meningioma	Cells of the layers of tissue covering the spinal cord (meninges)	Noncancerous but may recur or occasionally become cancerous	Children and adults
Neurofibroma	Cells that support peripheral nerves	Usually noncancerous	Children and adults (occurs in neurofibromatosis)
Sarcoma	Cells of connective tissue in the spine	Cancerous	Children and adults
Schwannoma	Cells that form the myelin sheath around peripheral nerve fibers (Schwann cells)	Usually noncancerous	Children and adults

the compressed nerve root. Pain may radiate along the nerve whose root is compressed. If compression continues, the affected muscles may waste away. Walking may become difficult.

Diagnosis

Compression of the spinal cord by a tumor must be diagnosed and treated immediately to prevent permanent damage.

Doctors consider the possibility of a spinal cord tumor in people who have certain cancers in other parts of the body, who develop pain in a specific area of the spine, and who have certain patterns of weakness or tingling. Because the spinal cord is organized in a specific way, doctors can locate the tumor by determining which parts of the body are not functioning normally (see art on page 794).

Doctors must rule out other disorders that can affect the function of the spinal cord, such as sore back muscles, bone bruises, an inadequate blood supply to the spinal cord, fractured vertebrae, compression by a collection of pus (abscess), a blood clot, or a herniated disk.

Several procedures can help doctors diagnose a spinal cord tumor. Magnetic resonance imaging (MRI) is considered the best procedure for examining all the structures of the spinal cord and spine. When MRI is unavailable, myelography with computed tomography (CT) may be done instead. X-rays of the spine can show only changes in the bones, and many tumors do not affect the bone when they are in an early stage.

A biopsy is usually needed to diagnose the precise type of tumor, especially primary spinal cord tumors. However, a biopsy is not needed for spinal cord tumors that result from metastases if cancer has been diagnosed elsewhere in the body. Often, a biopsy requires surgery, but sometimes it can be done using a needle with CT or MRI to guide doctors as they place the needle in the tumor.

Treatment

If symptoms suggest that the tumor is compressing the spinal cord, corticosteroids (such as dexamethasone) are immediately given in high doses to reduce the swelling. Such tumors are treated as soon as possible, often surgically.

Many tumors of the spinal cord and spine can be removed surgically. If tumors cannot be removed, radiation therapy is used, sometimes after surgery to relieve the pressure on the spinal cord is done.

Recovery generally depends on how quickly treatment begins and how much damage was done. Removal of meningiomas, neurofibromas, and some other primary spinal cord tumors may be curative.

Radiation Damage

Radiation therapy is one component in the treatment of tumors of the nervous system. It is directed at the general area (such as the whole head) when people have several tumors or a tumor that does not have distinct borders. When the tumor has distinct borders, therapy can be directed specifically at the tumor.

Radiation from these treatments sometimes damages the nervous system, despite the best efforts to prevent damage (see page 1989).

Whether damage occurs and how severe it is depend on several factors:

- How much radiation is given over the entire course of treatment (total cumulative dose)
- How much radiation is given in each dose
- How long the treatments are given
- How much of the body is exposed to radiation
- How susceptible the person is

Symptoms of radiation damage can develop in the first few days (acute) or months of treatment (early-delayed) or several months or years after treatment (late-delayed). Symptoms can remain the same or worsen and can be temporary or permanent.

Acute encephalopathy can result from radiation to the brain. Fluid accumulates within the cells of the brain, causing the entire brain to swell (called cerebral edema). Symptoms include headaches, nausea, vomiting, drowsiness, and confusion. Acute encephalopathy usually begins shortly after the first or second dose of radiation is given, but sometimes it begins 2 to 4 months after radiation therapy is completed. Usually, symptoms diminish during the radiation treatments, and corticosteroids such as dexamethasone may help prevent or reduce cerebral edema.

Early-delayed radiation damage causes symptoms similar to those of acute encephalopathy. Symptoms usually diminish on their own over several days to weeks, sometimes more rapidly if corticosteroids are used.

If radiation is directed at the spine in the neck or upper back, early-delayed radiation myelopathy may develop. This disorder sometimes causes a

sensation similar to an electric shock. The sensation begins in the neck or back, usually when the neck is bent forward, and shoots down to the legs. This disorder usually resolves without treatment.

> **? Did You Know...**
>
> Radiation therapy, used to treat brain and spinal cord tumors, can damage the brain and spinal cord.

Late-delayed radiation damage causes symptoms many months or years after radiation therapy. Many children and adults who receive whole-head brain radiation therapy develop late-delayed toxicity if they survive long enough. The most common cause in children is radiation therapy to prevent leukemia or to treat a type of brain tumor called medulloblastoma (see table on page 741). Symptoms include progressively worsening dementia, memory loss, difficulty thinking, mistaken perceptions, personality changes, and, in adults, unsteadiness in walking.

After radiation therapy for tumors near the spine, late-delayed myelopathy may develop. This disorder causes weakness, loss of sensation, and sometimes the Brown-Séquard syndrome. In this syndrome, one side of the spinal cord is damaged, resulting in weakness on one side of the body and loss of pain and temperature sensation on the other side. On the weak side of the body, people may be unable to sense where their hands and feet are without looking at them (position sense). Late-delayed radiation myelopathy usually does not subside and often results in paralysis.

Nerves near the site of the radiation therapy may also be damaged. For example, radiation to a breast or lung may damage nerves in the arms, and radiation to the groin may damage nerves in the legs. Weakness or loss of sensation may result.

CHAPTER
117 Infections of the Brain and Spinal Cord

The brain and spinal cord are remarkably resistant to infection, but when they become infected, the consequences are often very serious. Infections may be caused by bacteria, viruses, fungi, or, occasionally, protozoa or parasites. Another group of brain disorders that resemble infections, called spongiform encephalopathies, are caused by prions, which are abnormal protein molecules (see page 765).

Infections usually cause inflammation. For example, infection can cause meningitis, which is inflammation of the space within the layers of tissue (meninges) that cover the brain and spinal cord. This space (the subarachnoid space) contains cerebrospinal fluid, which flows between the meninges and helps cushion the brain and spinal cord. Without treatment, bacterial meningitis spreads to the brain, causing inflammation of brain tissue (encephalitis). Viral infections can also cause encephalitis. Usually, such infections also cause meningitis. Thus, usually when bacterial meningitis or viral encephalitis develops, the resulting disorder is technically meningoencephalitis. However, infection that affects mainly the subarachnoid space and meninges is usually called meningitis, and infection that affects mainly the brain is usually called encephalitis.

In meningitis and encephalitis, inflammation occurs throughout the brain and, in meningitis, throughout the spinal cord. But sometimes infection is confined to one area (localized) as a collection of pus, called an empyema or an abscess depending on where it is located. An abscess, which resembles a boil, can form anywhere in the body, including the brain. Fungi (such as aspergilli), protozoa (such as *Toxoplasma gondii*), and parasites (such as *Taenia solium* may cause a localized brain infection similar to an abscess.

Bacteria and other infectious organisms can reach the meninges and other areas of the brain in several ways:

- By being carried by the blood
- By entering the brain directly from the outside (for example, through a skull fracture or during surgery on the brain)
- By spreading from nearby infected structures, such as the sinuses or middle ear

Acute Bacterial Meningitis

Acute bacterial meningitis is rapidly developing inflammation of the subarachnoid space (located within the layers of tissue covering the brain and spinal cord) that is caused by bacteria.

- Older children and adults develop a stiff neck, usually with a fever and headache.
- Infants and young children may have a high or low body temperature, be irritable or drowsy, or not eat well.
- Antibiotics are effective if given promptly.
- Usually, a spinal tap is done but typically after treatment is started.
- Vaccines can prevent some forms of meningitis.

The subarachnoid space is located between the middle layer (arachnoid mater) and the thin inner layer (pia mater) of tissues (called meninges) that cover the brain and spinal cord (see art on page 624). This space contains the cerebrospinal fluid, which flows through the meninges, fills internal spaces within the brain, and helps cushion the brain and spinal cord.

When bacteria invade the subarachnoid space, the immune system eventually reacts to the invaders, and immune cells gather to defend the body against them. The result is inflammation. Severe inflammation can spread to blood vessels within the brain, sometimes causing clots to form. A stroke can result. Inflammation can also cause widespread damage to brain tissue, causing swelling (edema) and small areas of bleeding. If swelling is severe, it can increase pressure within the skull (intracranial pressure), causing parts of the brain to shift. If these parts are pressed through one of the small natural openings in the tissues that separate the brain into compartments, a life-threatening disorder called brain herniation results.

Bacterial meningitis is most common among infants, children, adolescents, and people over 55. Small epidemics of one particularly dangerous type of meningitis, called meningococcal meningitis, may occur among people living in close quarters, as occurs in military barracks and college dormitories.

Meningitis may also be caused by viruses, fungi, protozoa, cancer cells, certain drugs (which trigger an allergic reaction), and irritating substances (including air and chemicals).

Causes

Different species of bacteria cause meningitis in different settings.

If meningitis is acquired outside of a hospital or nursing home (in the community), it is usually caused by *Neisseria meningitides* (which causes meningococcal meningitis) or by *Streptococcus pneumoniae*. Both species are normally present in the external environment. They also reside in the nose and upper respiratory system of some people without causing harm. Occasionally, these organisms infect the brain without an identifiable reason. In other cases, infection develops because the immune system is weakened by a disorder or by a drug that suppresses it (immunosuppressant). The following increase the risk of developing bacterial infections, including meningitis:

- Certain chronic disorders that affect the heart, lungs, liver, kidneys, joints, or the endocrine or immune system
- Use of corticosteroids or immunosuppressants, which may be used to prevent rejection of an organ transplant or to treat disorders such as cancer and autoimmune disorders

- Splenectomy (removal of the spleen)
- Chronic infections of the middle ear, nose, or sinuses
- Pneumococcal pneumonia
- Sickle cell disease

Sometimes meningitis results from a head injury. For example, a skull fracture may create an opening between the nasal sinuses and the subarachnoid space. Bacteria can travel from the sinuses through the opening and infect the meninges.

Meningitis due to *Streptococcus pneumoniae* (pneumococcal meningitis) is becoming less common because people are now routinely vaccinated against it.

Listeria monocytogenes causes bacterial meningitis in newborns, pregnant women, and people over 50. Having kidney or liver failure or taking corticosteroids or immunosuppressants increases the risk of developing meningitis due to these bacteria.

Meningitis due to *Escherichia coli* (which normally resides in the colon and in feces) or *Klebsiella bacteria* usually develops after a widespread infection of the blood (sepsis), an infection acquired in a hospital, or surgery on the brain or spinal cord. People with a weakened immune system are more likely to develop sepsis and infections in a hospital and thus to develop meningitis due to these bacteria.

Meningitis due to *Pseudomonas* bacteria is more common among people with a weakened immune system.

Meningitis due to *Staphylococcus aureus* can occur after an injury or a surgical procedure that penetrates the skull or after infection of the heart valves (causing endocarditis) by these bacteria.

Newborns, whose immune system is not completely formed, are at increased risk of developing meningitis due to *Escherichia coli* or group B streptococci.

Symptoms

In older children and adults, the following symptoms may occur early:

- Fever
- Headache
- Stiff neck (usually)

Vomiting is also common. These symptoms are sometimes preceded by a sore throat, cough, runny nose, or other symptoms suggesting a respiratory illness. The stiff neck is more than just sore. Trying to lower the chin to the chest causes pain and may be impossible. Moving the head in other directions is not as difficult.

In children up to 2 years old, some combination of the following usually occurs first:

- High or low body temperature
- Feeding problems
- Vomiting
- Irritability
- Seizures
- Sluggishness (lethargy)
- High-pitched crying

Unlike older children or adults, infants younger than 1 year may not develop a stiff neck (see page 1761).

Adults may become seriously or desperately ill within 24 hours, and children even sooner.

In meningococcal meningitis, a rash (usually red and purple spots) sometimes develops. The rash is most prominent on the trunk and lower extremities. It may be difficult to see at first if people have dark skin.

The bacterial infection causes swelling of brain tissue. In children up to 2 years old, the swelling may make the soft spots between the skull bones (fontanelles) bulge. (These soft spots enable the skull to pass through the birth canal. They harden by about age 2 years.) The swelling may block the flow of cerebrospinal fluid around the brain, causing the fluid to accumulate and put pressure on the brain (a disorder called hydrocephalus). Sometimes a collection of pus (subdural empyema) forms under the outer layer (dura mater) of the meninges.

Older children and adults can become irritable, confused, then increasingly drowsy. Drowsiness can progress to unresponsiveness that requires vigorous stimulation for arousal (stupor), coma, and death. The swelling increases pressure inside the skull and can hamper blood flow, sometimes causing symptoms of stroke, including paralysis. Some people have seizures.

In most people with meningococcal meningitis, the bloodstream and many organs are also infected—a disorder called meningococcemia. Meningococcemia can become severe within hours. As a result, areas of tissue may die, and bleeding may occur under the skin (causing red spots or purple blotches), in mucous membranes, and within the digestive tract and other organs. Without treatment, blood pressure drops, leading to shock and death. Typically, bleeding occurs within the adrenal glands, which shut down, making shock worse. This disorder, called the Waterhouse-Friderichsen syndrome, is often fatal unless treated promptly.

Sometimes meningitis develops while people are being treated for another infection (such as an ear or throat infection). Or early meningitis may be mistaken for another infection and be treated with antibiotics. In either case, the symptoms of meningitis are much milder than normal, making meningitis more difficult to recognize.

COMMON INFECTIONS THAT CAN CAUSE MENINGITIS

ORGANISM	COMMENTS
Bacterial infections	
Infection with *Escherichia coli*	Newborns, older people, and people with a weakened immune system are affected most often.
	Meningitis due to these bacteria usually develops after a widespread infection of the blood (sepsis), an infection acquired in a hospital, or surgery on the brain or spinal cord.
Infection with *Klebsiella* bacteria	Meningitis due to these bacteria usually develops after sepsis, an infection acquired in a hospital, or surgery on the brain or spinal cord, or in people with a weakened immune system.
Infection with *Listeria monocytogenes*	Newborns, people over 50, pregnant women, people with kidney or liver failure or disorders of the immune system, and people who take drugs that affect the immune system are most often affected.
	These bacteria may be present in unpasteurized milk products and on many butcher's meat counters.
Infection with *Neisseria meningitides*	Meningitis due to these bacteria (meningococcal meningitis) is highly contagious and dangerous and causes small epidemics among people living in close quarters. It can cause death within 24 hours.
Infection with group B streptococci	Newborns are affected most often.
Infection with *Streptococcus pneumoniae*	Pneumococcal meningitis occurs more often in infants, alcoholics, and people with ear infections. These bacteria also cause pneumococcal pneumonia, which increases the risk of meningitis.
Lyme disease	The bacteria that cause Lyme disease are spread by ticks. Lyme disease is common in certain areas of the northeastern United States.
	Lyme disease can affect the skin, joints, heart, brain, and spinal cord.
Rocky Mountain spotted fever	The bacteria that cause this infection are transmitted by ticks.
	The symptoms resemble those of meningitis, but the infection is not meningitis.
Syphilis	If untreated, syphilis can affect the brain, layers of tissue that cover it (meninges), or both several years after the original infection (or much earlier in people who have HIV infection or AIDS).
Tuberculosis	Immigrants from areas where tuberculosis is common (such as Asia, Africa, or Latin America), homeless people, and people with HIV infection or AIDS are affected most often.
Viral infections	
Enteroviral infections	Enteroviruses are commonly present in the digestive tract and may cause infection when hands are not washed adequately after going to the toilet. Spread among family members is common.
Herpes simplex virus type 2 infection	This virus causes genital herpes and can cause recurrent episodes of meningitis called Mollaret's meningitis.
Human immunodeficiency virus (HIV) infection	Meningitis can develop days to weeks after the initial infection.
Cytomegalovirus infection	In people with HIV infection, this virus can cause a painful meningitis that affects spinal nerves in the lower back.
Infectious mononucleosis	Rarely, this infection, caused by the Epstein-Barr virus, spreads to the meninges.

(continued on the following page)

COMMON INFECTIONS THAT CAN CAUSE MENINGITIS (*Continued*)

ORGANISM	COMMENTS
Mumps	Mumps is a common cause of meningitis worldwide but not in the United States because children are routinely vaccinated against it.
West Nile virus infection	This infection is spread by mosquitoes.
Lymphocytic choriomeningitis	Most often, this infection results from exposure to dust or food contaminated by waste products from mice and hamsters.
Fungal infections	
Cryptococcosis	People with HIV infection, AIDS, or other disorders that weaken the immune system are usually affected.
Coccidioidomycosis	This infection occurs mostly in the southwestern United States.

AIDS = acquired immunodeficiency syndrome; HIV = human immunodeficiency virus.

Diagnosis

If a child 2 years old or younger has an unexplained fever and a parent senses that the child is ill, the parent should see or call a doctor immediately, particularly if symptoms do not resolve after an adequate dose of acetaminophen. Children require immediate medical attention if they do any of the following:

- Become increasingly irritable or unusually sleepy
- Have a low body temperature
- Refuse to eat
- Have seizures
- Develop a stiff neck

Adults require immediate medical attention if they have any of the following:

- Confusion
- Stupor
- Seizures
- Some combination of fever, rash, and a stiff neck

During the physical examination, doctors look for telltale signs of meningitis, such as a stiff neck and skin rash. When doctors suspect rapidly developing meningitis, they withdraw a sample of the person's blood and send it to a laboratory, where the bacteria can be grown (cultured) overnight. If bacteria are detected, bacterial infection is confirmed. Culture also helps identify which bacteria are causing infection. Culture results can take up to 2 days. At some hospitals, new blood tests can provide the same information within a few hours.

A spinal tap (lumbar puncture—see art on page 635) is done but usually not until after tests, such as computed tomography (CT) of the brain and sometimes blood clotting tests, are done to determine whether a spinal tap is safe. CT of the head is done to check for a mass (such as a hemorrhage, tumor, or abscess), which may increase pressure within the skull. If pressure is increased, the brain may shift downward, causing brain herniation.

During a spinal tap, a thin needle is inserted between two vertebrae in the lower spine to withdraw cerebrospinal fluid. Doctors look closely at the fluid, which is normally clear but is cloudy in meningitis. The fluid's pressure is measured. Pressure is usually high in meningitis. Sugar and protein levels and the number and type of white blood cells in the fluid are determined. This information helps doctors distinguish between bacterial and viral infections. The fluid is examined under a microscope to check for and identify bacteria. If bacteria are seen, other tests are done to rapidly identify certain bacteria, such as *Neisseria meningitidis* and *Streptococcus pneumoniae*. Some of these tests can detect proteins (antigens) on the surface of bacteria and thus identify them. The polymerase chain reaction (PCR) technique, which produces many copies of a gene, may be used to identify the bacteria's unique DNA sequence.

The cerebrospinal fluid is also cultured, and after 24 hours, the resulting bacteria are tested to determine which antibiotics are effective against them (called susceptibility testing). Then, antibiotic therapy, which was already started, can be adjusted if necessary.

Until the cause of meningitis is confirmed, other tests using cerebrospinal fluid or blood samples may be done to check for viruses, fungi, cancer cells and other substances that routine tests do not identify.

Testing for herpes simplex virus, which can infect the brain (causing encephalitis), is particularly important.

Doctors also take samples of blood, urine, and mucus from the nose and throat, and in people who have a rash, they may use a small needle to remove fluid and tissue from under the skin where the rash is. These samples are cultured and examined under the microscope to see whether bacteria are present.

Treatment

Because acute bacterial meningitis can lead to death within hours, treatment is started as soon as possible, without waiting for the results of diagnostic tests and usually before a spinal tap is done. Several antibiotics are given intravenously, often in the emergency department. Doctors choose antibiotics that are effective against the bacteria most likely to be causing the infection. However, because doctors cannot identify the bacteria causing the infection based on symptoms alone, they usually choose several antibiotics that are effective against many organisms. Also, an antiviral drug that is effective against the herpesvirus that causes inflammation of the brain (encephalitis) is given. Once the infecting organism, usually a specific species of bacteria, is identified, the antibiotics are changed to ones that are most effective against that organism, and any unnecessary antibiotics and antiviral drugs are stopped.

A corticosteroid, such as dexamethasone, is given 15 minutes before or at the same time as the first antibiotic dose. The corticosteroid is continued for 2 to 4 days. Corticosteroids are given to suppress inflammation caused by fragments of bacteria, which are produced when antibiotics break bacteria apart. This inflammation causes swelling that can damage the brain. Corticosteroids can also reduce pressure within the skull and, if the adrenal glands are damaged, replace the corticosteroids normally produced by these glands.

Fluids lost because of fever, sweating, vomiting, and poor appetite are replaced. Because bacterial meningitis often affects many organs and causes serious complications, people are usually admitted to the intensive care unit.

Complications may require specific treatment.

- **Seizures:** Anticonvulsants are given (see table on page 716).
- **Shock:** Additional fluids and sometimes drugs (given intravenously) are given to increase blood pressure and treat shock (see page 350), as can occur in the Waterhouse-Friderichsen syndrome.
- **Coma:** Mechanical ventilation is used.
- **Dangerously increased pressure within the skull:** Mechanical ventilation is used to decrease the amount of carbon dioxide in the blood and thus

quickly but briefly reduce pressure in the cerebrospinal fluid. Then mannitol or a similar drug is given intravenously. Mannitol causes water in the brain to move into the bloodstream and thus reduces cerebrospinal fluid pressure within the skull. Pressure within the skull may be monitored with a gauge or a small tube (catheter) connected to a gauge. The device is inserted through a tiny opening drilled through the skull. The catheter can also be used to remove cerebrospinal fluid and thus reduce pressure when necessary.

- **Subdural empyema:** A surgeon may have to drain an empyema with a needle to ensure a successful recovery.

Prognosis

If treated early, most people recover well. But when treatment is delayed, permanent brain damage or death is more likely, especially in very young children and older people. In some people, seizures require lifelong treatment. Neurologic problems, such as permanent mental impairment, paralysis, and hearing loss, may also result.

Prevention

People with acute meningitis (particularly meningococcal meningitis) are usually placed in isolation until the infection is controlled and they can no longer spread the infection, usually for a few days or less. Vaccines for several forms of meningitis are available.

Meningococcal Meningitis: A vaccine can help prevent this type of meningitis. It is given to children 2 years old or older whose immune system is weakened. It is also recommended for the following people:

- Adolescents
- Students living in dormitories
- Military recruits
- People who may be repeatedly exposed to the bacteria

The vaccine is also used when an epidemic occurs or when there is a threat of an epidemic in a self-contained group of people (such as those living in military barracks). Family members, medical personnel, and others in close contact with people who have meningococcal meningitis should be given an antibiotic (such as rifampin or ciprofloxacin taken by mouth or ceftriaxone given by injection) as a preventive measure.

Meningitis Due to *Streptococcus pneumoniae*: A vaccine that helps protect against this infection is now routinely given to children.

SOME NONINFECTIOUS CAUSES OF MENINGITIS

TYPE	EXAMPLES
Brain disorders	Cancer that has spread to the brain from other parts of the body (such as leukemia, lymphoma, melanoma, and breast or lung cancer) Sarcoidosis Behçet's syndrome Craniopharyngioma
Drugs that affect the immune system	Azathioprine Cyclosporine Cytosine arabinoside Intravenous immune globulin OKT3 Nonsteroidal anti-inflammatory drugs (NSAIDs), such as ibuprofen, naproxen, sulindac, and tolmetin
Other drugs	Antibiotics (such as ciprofloxacin, isoniazid, penicillin, trimethoprim-sulfamethoxazole, and other sulfa drugs) Carbamazepine Phenazopyridine Ranitidine
Substances injected into the subarachnoid space*	Antibiotics Chemotherapy Dyes used in imaging procedures Anesthetics
Vaccines	Pertussis (whooping cough) Rabies Smallpox

* The space that contains cerebrospinal fluid and is located between layers of tissue covering the brain and spinal cord (meninges).

Meningitis Due to *Haemophilus influenzae*: Children are now routinely immunized with *Haemophilus influenzae* type b vaccine, which has virtually eliminated what once was the most common cause of meningitis in children.

Chronic Meningitis

Chronic meningitis is a slowly developing inflammation of the subarachnoid space (located within the layers of tissues covering the brain and spinal cord) that lasts a month or longer.

- People may have a fever, a stiff neck, a headache, double vision, or difficulty walking, or they may become confused.
- Imaging of the head and a spinal tap are required for diagnosis.
- Treatment depends on the cause.

The subarachnoid space is located between the middle layer (arachnoid mater) and the thin inner layer (pia mater) of the tissues that cover the brain and spinal cord (meninges—see art on page 624).

Chronic meningitis resembles acute bacterial meningitis, but the causes are different and the infection and inflammation develop more slowly, over weeks and months rather than hours and days. If symptoms have been present for a month or more, meningitis is described as chronic.

Causes

Chronic meningitis is usually due to infection, most commonly tuberculosis.

Infectious organisms invade the brain or the subarachnoid space and multiply slowly over weeks or months. Such organisms include the bacteria that cause tuberculosis or syphilis and fungi such as *Cryptococcus neoformans* or *Coccidioides immitis*. These fungi are more likely to cause chronic meningitis in people with a weakened immune system, such as those with human immunodeficiency virus

(HIV) infection or acquired immunodeficiency syndrome (AIDS).

Acute bacterial meningitis that has been partially treated but not eliminated by antibiotics may evolve into chronic meningitis.

Disorders that are not infections can also cause chronic meningitis. They include sarcoidosis and certain cancers, such as leukemia, lymphoma, brain tumors, and some cancers that spread (metastasize) to the brain from other parts of the body (such as breast or lung cancer).

Chemotherapy drugs that are injected directly into the subarachnoid space (such as methotrexate), drugs used to prevent rejection of a transplanted organ (such as cyclosporine and OKT3), and even nonsteroidal anti-inflammatory drugs (NSAIDs, such as ibuprofen—see page 644) can cause mild to moderate meningitis that lasts days to a few weeks. If treatments are repeated, the meningitis may last longer.

Symptoms

The symptoms of chronic meningitis are similar to those of acute bacterial meningitis, except that they develop more slowly and gradually, usually over weeks rather than days. Also, fever is often less severe.

Headache, confusion, a stiff neck, and backache are common. People may have difficulty walking. Weakness, pins-and-needles sensations, numbness, facial paralysis, and double vision are also common. Facial paralysis and double vision occur when meningitis affects the cranial nerves (which go directly from the brain to various parts of the head, neck, and trunk).

Diagnosis

Computed tomography (CT) or magnetic resonance imaging (MRI) of the head, followed by a spinal tap (lumbar puncture) with examination of the cerebrospinal fluid, can confirm the diagnosis.

By examining the cerebrospinal fluid, doctors can distinguish between chronic and acute meningitis. In chronic meningitis, the number of white blood cells in the fluid is higher than normal but is usually lower than that in acute bacterial meningitis. Also, the type of white cells is usually different. Some infectious organisms that cause chronic meningitis, such as the fungus *Cryptococcus neoformans*, are readily visible under a microscope, but many, such as the bacteria that cause tuberculosis, are not.

The cerebrospinal fluid is always sent to a laboratory, where the organism, if present, can be grown (cultured) and identified. However, culturing may take weeks. Special techniques, which may provide results more quickly, may be used to identify fungi and the bacteria that cause tuberculosis and syphilis. For example, the polymerase chain reaction (PCR) technique, which produces many copies of a gene,

may identify the unique DNA sequence of the bacteria that cause tuberculosis.

Other tests on cerebrospinal fluid are done, depending on which disorders are suspected. For example, the fluid may be analyzed for cancer cells if metastatic cancer is suspected.

Treatment

The cause of meningitis is treated. For example, chronic meningitis due to sarcoidosis is usually treated with corticosteroids (such as prednisone) for several weeks. Chronic meningitis due to cancer is treated with chemotherapy, radiation therapy, or both. The chemotherapy drug is injected directly into the subarachnoid space through an Ommaya reservoir. This device is implanted under the scalp and delivers the drug slowly, over days or weeks, through a small tube to the spaces around the brain.

Treatment of chronic meningitis due to an infection depends on the organism. Chronic meningitis due to a fungus is usually treated with antifungal drugs given intravenously or by mouth. Amphotericin B, flucytosine, and fluconazole are used most often. When the infection is particularly difficult to cure, amphotericin B is sometimes injected directly into the cerebrospinal fluid, either by repeated spinal taps or through an Ommaya reservoir. When chronic meningitis is due to *Cryptococcus neoformans* amphotericin B is usually combined with flucytosine.

Aseptic Meningitis

Aseptic meningitis is inflammation of the subarachnoid space (located within the layers of tissue covering the brain and spinal cord) that is diagnosed when standard testing does not detect bacteria.

- Viruses, often those frequently present in the digestive tract, are the most common cause.
- Headache, stiff neck, fever, and nausea may develop over days.
- A spinal tap is done, and if standard tests of cerebrospinal fluid detect inflammation but no bacteria that could cause it, aseptic meningitis is diagnosed.
- Acetaminophen and fluids can relieve symptoms, but otherwise treatment depends on the cause.

In aseptic meningitis, the space between middle and inner layers of tissues covering the brain and spinal cord (meninges) is inflamed. This space, called the subarachnoid space, forms a channel for cerebrospinal fluid, which flows over the surface of the brain and spinal cord (see art on page 624).

Causes

Aseptic meningitis is usually caused by a virus but occasionally has another cause. Unless comprehensive testing is done, the cause is often unidentified.

Viruses: Some viruses can directly infect the meninges and subarachnoid space around the brain and suddenly cause meningitis. Among the most common are

- Enteroviruses (which are often present in the digestive tract), such as echovirus and coxsackievirus
- Mosquito-borne viruses (usually West Nile virus)

Infections caused by these viruses can occur in epidemics.

Other viruses directly cause infection that occurs as isolated cases (sporadically). They include the herpes simplex virus, Epstein-Barr virus, human immunodeficiency virus (HIV), varicella-zoster virus (that causes chickenpox), and mumps virus. Mumps is a common cause of meningitis worldwide, but it is uncommon in the United States because vaccination is widespread. In Mollaret's meningitis, aseptic meningitis occurs repeatedly. It is caused by herpes simplex virus type 2, which causes most cases of genital herpes. Viruses that cause encephalitis usually also cause some degree of meningitis.

Bacteria: Sometimes aseptic meningitis is diagnosed when meningitis is caused by bacteria that are hard to identify, such as the bacteria that cause Lyme disease, syphilis, or tuberculosis.

Other Conditions: Aseptic meningitis may be caused by the following (see table on page 755):

- Fungi
- Certain noninfectious disorders
- Certain drugs, particularly drugs that affect the immune system
- Reactions to certain vaccines, such as those for pertussis (whooping cough) or rabies
- Injection of drugs or dyes (for treatment or diagnosis) in the subarachnoid space

Symptoms

Meningitis often develops after or at the same time as a flu-like illness or viral infection that causes mild symptoms. These symptoms are often general and may include fever, a general feeling of illness (malaise), cough, muscle aches, and headache.

Usually, aseptic meningitis causes symptoms that are similar to those of bacterial meningitis (fever, headache, vomiting, sluggishness, and a stiff neck). However, people do not become as ill. People may not have a fever, particularly when the cause is not an infection.

Most people recover in 1 to 2 weeks.

Diagnosis

When meningitis is suspected, a spinal tap (lumbar puncture) is usually done to obtain a sample of cerebrospinal fluid, and standard tests are done on the fluid. They include determining the number and type of white blood cells in the fluid and growing (culturing) bacteria in the fluid so that they can be identified (see page 753). Doctors diagnose aseptic meningitis when the cerebrospinal fluid contains excess white blood cells (indicating inflammation) but standard tests do not detect any bacteria that could be the cause.

Usually, standard tests do not include culturing viruses, which is technically difficult and may take many days. (An exception is enteroviruses, which can be cultured.) Instead, the polymerase chain reaction (PCR) technique is used to identify viruses (such as herpesviruses and HIV) and to measure levels of antibodies to the virus in cerebrospinal fluid and blood. Antibody levels are measured initially and 3 to 4 weeks later. Then the measurements are compared. If antibody levels increase much more in the cerebrospinal fluid than in the blood, the virus probably caused the meningitis. If the increase in cerebrospinal fluid and blood is about as same, the virus probably infected the body but did not cause the meningitis.

Treatment

The cause, if identified, is treated. For example, if the bacteria that cause Lyme disease, syphilis, or tuberculosis are identified, antibiotics specific for those bacteria are used. Cancer is treated with surgery, radiation therapy, or chemotherapy, as appropriate. If a drug is the cause, it is stopped or the dose is reduced. Most viral infections are not treated with antiviral drugs and resolve on their own. However, Mollaret's meningitis is treated with acyclovir, and cytomegalovirus infection is treated with ganciclovir.

If doctors suspect aseptic meningitis but cannot rule out bacterial meningitis at the initial examination, several antibiotics are given as if bacterial meningitis were the diagnosis. Doctors do not wait for test results. If tests do not detect any bacteria in the cerebrospinal fluid and if the fluid contains levels of sugar, protein, and white blood cells that suggest aseptic meningitis, antibiotics are stopped.

Regardless of the cause, symptoms are treated. Acetaminophen, given by mouth, and fluids, given by mouth or intravenous injection, can relieve headache and fever.

Rabies

Rabies is a viral infection of the brain that is transmitted by animals and that causes inflammation of the brain and spinal cord. Once the virus reaches the spinal cord and brain, rabies is fatal.

- The virus can be transmitted when people are bitten by an infected animal, usually a wild animal.

- Rabies can cause restlessness and confusion or paralysis.
- A skin biopsy can detect the virus.
- Infection can be prevented by immediately cleaning the wound and by injecting rabies vaccine and immune globulin.

From the point of entry (usually a bite), the rabies virus travels along nerves to the spinal cord and then to the brain, where it multiplies. From there, it travels along other nerves to the salivary glands and into the saliva. Once the rabies virus reaches the spinal cord and brain, rabies is fatal. However, the virus takes at least 10 days—usually 30 to 50 days—to reach the brain (how long depends on the bite's location). During that interval, measures can be taken to stop the virus and help prevent death.

Rabies causes an estimated 55,000 deaths worldwide each year. Most deaths occur in rural areas of Asia and Africa. In the United States, only a few people die each year.

Causes

The rabies virus is present in many species of wild and domestic animals throughout most of the world. Animals with rabies may be sick for several weeks before they die. During that time, they often spread the disease.

The rabies virus, which is present in the saliva of a rabid animal, is transmitted when the animal bites or, very rarely, licks another animal or a person. The virus cannot pass through intact skin. It can enter the body only through a puncture or another break in the skin or through the nose or mouth when many airborne droplets containing the virus are inhaled (as can occur in a cave that contains infected bats).

Many different mammals—such as dogs, cats, bats, raccoons, skunks, and foxes—can transmit rabies to people. Rabies rarely affects rodents (such as hamsters, guinea pigs, gerbils, squirrels, chipmunks, rats, and mice), rabbits, or hares. In the United States, these animals have not been known to cause rabies among people. Rabies does not affect birds and reptiles.

In the United States, vaccination has largely eliminated rabies in dogs, and the source of rabies is almost always wild animals, usually bats. In many cases, the bat bites are unnoticed. Most deaths due to rabies result from being bitten by an infected bat.

Worldwide, during the last 30 years, most people who have contracted rabies were bitten by rabid wild animals. In most countries of Latin America, Africa, Asia, and the Middle East (where vaccination of dogs is not widespread), rabies in dogs is fairly common, and dogs are responsible for most deaths due to rabies.

Symptoms

The wound from the bite may be painful or numb. Bat bites typically cause no symptoms.

Symptoms appear when the rabies virus reaches the brain or spinal cord, usually 30 to 50 days after a person is bitten. However, this interval can vary from 10 days to more than a year. The closer the bite is to the brain (for example, on the face), the more quickly symptoms appear.

Rabies may begin with a fever, headache, and a general feeling of illness (malaise). Most people become restless, confused, and uncontrollably excited. Their behavior may be bizarre. They may hallucinate and have insomnia. Saliva production greatly increases. Spasms of the muscles in the throat and larynx occur because rabies affects the area in the brain that controls swallowing, speaking, and breathing. The spasms can be excruciatingly painful. A slight breeze or an attempt to drink water can trigger the spasms. Thus, people with rabies cannot drink. For this reason, the disease is sometimes called hydrophobia (fear of water).

As the disease spreads through the brain, people become more confused and agitated. Eventually, coma and death result. The cause of death can be blockage of airways, seizures, exhaustion, or widespread paralysis.

> ### ? Did You Know...
>
> In the United States, people who are bitten by rabbits and most small rodents—such as hamsters, gerbils, squirrels, rats, and mice—almost never need a rabies vaccination.
>
> Bats are responsible for most deaths due to rabies in the United States.

In 20% of people, rabies begins with paralysis of the limb that was bitten. The paralysis then moves through the body. In these people, thinking is typically unaffected, and most of the other symptoms of rabies do not develop.

Diagnosis

Doctors suspect rabies when people have a headache, confusion, and other symptoms of the disease, especially if people have been bitten by an animal or exposed to bats (for example, if they were exploring a cave). However, many people with rabies are unaware of having been bitten by an animal or exposed to bats. A sample of skin is taken (usually from the neck) and examined under a microscope (skin biopsy) to determine whether the virus is present. Samples of saliva and urine are also exam-

Who Should Receive the Rabies Vaccine?

In the United States, the decision to give the rabies vaccine to a person who has been bitten by an animal depends on the type and status of the animal.

For people bitten by a pet dog, cat, or ferret: If the animal appears healthy and can be observed for 10 days, the vaccine is not given unless the animal develops symptoms of rabies. If the animal develops any symptom suggesting rabies, people are given vaccine immediately. Animals that develop symptoms of rabies are put to sleep (euthanized), and their brain is examined for the rabies virus. If the animal is still healthy after 10 days, it did not have rabies at the time of the bite, and vaccine is not needed.

If an animal has or appears to have rabies, the vaccine is given immediately.

If the status of an animal cannot be determined—for example, because it escaped—public health officials are consulted to determine how likely rabies is and whether the vaccine should be given.

For people bitten by skunks, raccoons, foxes, most other carnivores, or bats: Such an animal is considered rabid unless it can be tested and the results are negative. Usually, the vaccine is given immediately. Waiting to observe wild animals for 10 days is not recommended.

Because people may not notice a bat bite, they are given the vaccine if a bite seems possible. For example, if someone awakens and a bat is in the room, the vaccine is given.

For people bitten by livestock, small rodents, large rodents (such as woodchucks and beavers), rabbits, or hares: Each biting incident is considered individually, and public health officials are consulted. People who are bitten by hamsters, guinea pigs, gerbils, squirrels, chipmunks, rats, mice, other small rodents, rabbits, or hares almost never require rabies vaccination.

---

ined to check for the virus. A spinal tap (lumbar puncture) is done to obtain a sample of cerebrospinal fluid, which is also examined. A variation of the polymerase chain reaction (PCR) technique, which produces many copies of a gene, is often used to identify the bacteria's unique DNA sequence. Several samples of these fluids, taken at different times, are tested to increase the chances of detecting the virus.

Treatment

After symptoms develop, no treatment can help. The infection is virtually always fatal. Treatment involves relieving symptoms and making people as comfortable as possible.

Prevention

Before an Animal Bite: Avoiding being bitten by animals, especially wild animals, is best. Pets that are not known and wild animals should not be approached. Signs of rabies in wild animals may be subtle, but their behavior is typically abnormal, as in the following:

- Wild animals may not appear vicious, shy, or afraid when people approach them.
- Nocturnal animals (such as bats, skunks, raccoons, and foxes) are out during the day.
- Bats make unusual noises or have difficulty flying.
- Animals bite without being provoked.
- Animals are weak or agitated and vicious.

An animal that may be rabid should not be picked up to try to help it. A sick animal often bites. If an animal appears sick, people should call local health authorities, who can help remove it.

People who are likely to be exposed to the rabies virus should be given an injection of the rabies vaccine before exposure. Such people include veterinarians, laboratory workers who handle animals that may be rabid, people who live or stay more than 30 days in developing countries where rabies in dogs is widespread, and people who explore bat caves. Vaccination protects most people to some degree for the rest of their life. However, protection decreases with time, and if exposure is likely to continue, people should get a booster dose of vaccine every 2 years.

After an Animal Bite: Immediately after being bitten, people should clean the wound thoroughly with soap and water. Deep puncture wounds are flushed out with running water. Then people should see a doctor. Doctors clean the wound further with an antiseptic called benzalkonium chloride. They may trim ragged edges of the wound.

Doctors also try to determine the likelihood that rabies was transmitted. Early determination is essential because rabies can usually be prevented if appropriate measures are taken promptly.

No test can determine whether the rabies virus has been transmitted immediately after an animal bite. Thus, people who have been bitten may be given immune globulin and vaccine by injection to prevent rabies. Rabies immune globulin, which consists of antibodies to the virus, provides protection immediately but only for a short time. The rabies vaccine stimulates the body to produce antibodies to the virus. The vaccine provides protection that begins more gradually but that lasts for a much longer time.

Whether vaccine and immune globulin are needed depends on whether people have been previously immunized with rabies vaccine and what the type and status of animal are. For example, doctors determine the following:

- Whether the animal was a dog, a raccoon, or something else
- Whether it appeared sick
- Whether the attack was provoked
- Whether the animal is available for observation

If people need preventive treatment and have not been immunized previously, they are given rabies immune globulin and rabies vaccine right away (on day 0). Immune globulin is injected around the wound if possible. They are given four more injections of the vaccine on days 3, 7, 14, and 28. The injection site may be painful and swollen but usually only slightly. Serious allergic reactions are rare.

If people have already been vaccinated, the risk of developing rabies is reduced. However, the wound must be cleaned promptly, and an injection of rabies vaccine is given immediately and on day 3.

Encephalitis

Encephalitis is inflammation of the brain that occurs when a virus directly infects the brain or when a virus or something else triggers inflammation. The spinal cord may also be involved, resulting in a disorder called encephalomyelitis.

- People may have a fever, headache, or seizures, and they may feel sleepy, numb, or confused.
- Magnetic resonance imaging of the head and a spinal tap are usually done.
- Treatment involves relieving symptoms and sometimes using antiviral drugs.

Encephalitis can occur in the following ways:

- A virus directly infects the brain.
- A virus that caused an infection in the past becomes reactivated and directly damages the brain.
- A virus or vaccine triggers a reaction that makes the immune system attack brain tissue (an autoimmune reaction).

Infections that can directly lead to encephalitis can occur in epidemics or occasionally as isolated cases (sporadically).

Epidemic Encephalitis: In the United States, the most common types of epidemic encephalitis are caused by arboviruses. Arboviruses are viruses transmitted to people through the bites of arthropods, usually mosquitoes, fleas, or ticks. (Arbovirus is short for arthropod-borne virus.) The viruses are transmitted to arthropods when arthropods bite infected animals. Many species of domestic animals and birds carry these viruses.

Epidemics occur in people only periodically—when the population of mosquitoes or infected animals increases. They tend to occur when arthropods are biting—for mosquitoes and ticks, usually during warm weather. Infection spreads from arthropod to person, not from person to person.

Many arboviruses can cause encephalitis. The different types of encephalitis that result are usually named for the place the virus was discovered or the animal species that typically carries it.

In the United States, mosquitoes spread several types of encephalitis, including the following:

- **La Crosse encephalitis** is caused by the La Crosse virus (also called California virus). It is most common in the Midwest but can occur anywhere in the country. This encephalitis accounts for most cases in children. Many cases are mild and undiagnosed. Fewer than 1% of infected people die from it.
- **Eastern equine encephalitis** occurs predominantly in the eastern United States. It affects mainly young children and people older than 55. In children younger than 1 year, it can cause severe symptoms and permanent nerve or brain damage. Over half of infected people die.
- **West Nile encephalitis,** once present only in Europe and Africa, first appeared in the New York City area in 1999. It has spread throughout the United States. Several species of birds are the host for the virus. This encephalitis affects mainly older people. West Nile encephalitis develops in less than 1% of people who develop West Nile fever. About 10% of people with West Nile encephalitis die; however, those who have just West Nile fever usually recover fully.
- **St. Louis encephalitis** occurs throughout the United States but particularly in the Southeast (including Florida), Texas, and some Midwestern states. Epidemics once occurred about every 10 years but are now rare.
- **Western equine encephalitis** can occur throughout the United States but, for unknown reasons, has largely disappeared since 1988. It can affect all age groups but mainly children younger than 1 year.

In other parts of the world, encephalitis is caused by different but related arboviruses. Examples are

Venezuelan equine encephalitis and Japanese encephalitis, both spread by mosquitoes.

Sporadic Encephalitis: In the United States, sporadic encephalitis is usually caused by herpes simplex virus type 1. Herpes simplex virus causes up to one third of cases of encephalitis. It occurs at any time of the year and is fatal if not treated. Human immunodeficiency virus (HIV) causes a slowly developing brain infection, resulting in HIV-associated encephalopathy (also called HIV-associated or AIDS dementia).

Reactivation of a Previous Infection: Encephalitis can result from reactivation of herpes simplex virus type 1, varicella zoster virus (which causes chickenpox), or the virus that causes measles (which leads to a usually fatal disorder called subacute sclerosing panencephalitis years after measles occurs). After reactivated infection, brain damage can be severe.

Autoimmune Encephalitis: After certain infections or vaccines, the body's immune system sometimes attacks the layers of tissue that wrap around nerve fibers (called the myelin sheath) in the brain and spinal cord The attack occurs because proteins in myelin resemble those in the virus. As a result, nerve transmission becomes very slow. The resulting disorder, called acute disseminated encephalomyelitis, resembles multiple sclerosis except that symptoms do not come and go as they do in multiple sclerosis. The viruses most often involved include Epstein-Barr virus, cytomegalovirus, and herpes simplex virus.

Symptoms

Before symptoms of encephalitis start, people may have digestive symptoms, such as nausea, vomiting, diarrhea, or abdominal pain. Or they may feel as if they are getting a cold or the flu and have cough, fever, a sore throat, a runny nose, swollen lymph nodes, and muscle aches.

Symptoms of encephalitis include

- Fever
- Headache
- Personality changes or confusion
- Seizures
- Paralysis or numbness
- Sleepiness that can progress to coma and death

People may vomit and have a stiff neck, but these symptoms tend to be less common and less severe than when caused by meningitis.

Encephalitis due to the herpes simplex virus causes headache, fever, and flu-like symptoms at first. People also have seizures, sometimes accompanied by strange smells, vivid flashbacks, or sudden, intense emotions. As the encephalitis progresses, people become confused, have difficulty speaking and remembering, have repeated seizures, then lapse into coma.

HIV-associated encephalopathy can cause gradual personality changes, problems with coordination, and dementia.

If the spinal cord is affected, parts of the body may feel numb and weak. Which parts are affected depend on which parts of the spinal cord are affected (see art on page 794). People may have difficulty controlling bladder and bowel function. If the infection is severe, people may lose sensation, become paralyzed, and lose control of the bladder and bowels.

> **Did You Know...**
>
> Long after a case of measles or chickenpox, the virus can be reactivated and cause inflammation in the brain.

Diagnosis

Doctors suspect encephalitis based on symptoms, especially if an epidemic is in progress. Magnetic resonance imaging (MRI) can detect typical abnormalities in the brain, confirming encephalitis. If MRI is not available, computed tomography (CT) may be done. It can help doctors exclude disorders that can cause similar symptoms (such as stroke and brain tumor) and check for disorders that can make doing a spinal tap dangerous.

A spinal tap (lumbar puncture) is done to obtain a sample of cerebrospinal fluid. Usually, the spinal fluid contains white blood cells, red blood cells, or both. To identify the virus causing encephalitis, doctors take samples of blood and cerebrospinal fluid and test them for antibodies to the virus when the person is sick and later when the person is convalescing. If the increase in antibodies in cerebrospinal fluid is greater than the increase in the blood, the diagnosis is confirmed. Sometimes techniques are used to grow (culture) viruses in the cerebrospinal fluid so that they can be identified more easily. Enteroviruses can be cultured, but most other viruses cannot.

If doctors suspect that herpes simplex infection is the cause, the polymerase chain reaction (PCR) technique is usually used to identify the virus. PCR can detect the genetic material of the herpes simplex virus. Prompt identification of this virus is essential because the encephalitis it causes is serious and can be fatal. Rarely, a sample of brain tissue is removed and examined under a microscope (biopsy) to determine whether herpes simplex virus or another organism is the cause.

Treatment

If herpes simplex virus cannot be excluded, the antiviral drug acyclovir is given. Acyclovir is effective against herpes simplex and herpes zoster viruses. Usually, several antibiotics are also given in case the cause is bacteria. Cytomegalovirus encephalitis can be treated with ganciclovir.

For HIV-associated encephalopathy, a combination of drugs (see page 1261) helps the immune system function better and delays the progression of the infection and its complications, including dementia.

For other viruses and most other causes, no specific treatment is available. Treatment usually involves relieving symptoms and, when necessary, providing life support until the infection subsides—in about 1 to 2 weeks.

Lymphocytic Choriomeningitis

Lymphocytic choriomeningitis is a flu-like disorder caused by an arenavirus and often followed by meningitis. It occurs when the tissues covering the brain and spinal cord become inflamed.

- Rodents can transmit the virus to people through contaminated dust or food.
- The infection may cause no symptoms, a flu-like illness, or meningitis.
- If symptoms suggest meningitis, a spinal tap is done.
- Treatment aims to relieve symptoms.
- Most people recover completely.

The arenavirus that causes lymphocytic choriomeningitis is commonly present in rodents, especially gray house mice and hamsters. These animals are usually infected by the virus for life and excrete it in urine, feces, semen, and nasal secretions. Most often, exposure to dust or food contaminated by these waste products causes the disorder in people. The disorder usually occurs in autumn and winter when wild rodents seek shelter indoors.

Symptoms

Most people have no symptoms or very mild symptoms. Symptoms, if they develop, often occur in two phases.

First, flu-like symptoms develop 5 to 10 days after exposure to the virus. Typically, people have a fever of about 101 to 104° F (38.3 to 40° C), sometimes accompanied by shaking. People may feel generally ill (malaise), nauseated, light-headed, and weak. They may have muscle pains, a headache behind the eyes worsened by bright light, and a poor appetite. The throat may become sore. After 5 days to 3 weeks, the flu-like symptoms may subside for 1 or 2 days.

In the second phase, flu-like symptoms recur and other symptoms develop. Knuckle and finger joints may become painful and swollen, and the testes may become inflamed, swollen, and painful. People may lose their hair or vomit. Meningitis may develop, causing a headache and stiff neck, but it tends to be less severe than in acute bacterial meningitis.

Most people who develop meningitis recover completely. However, headaches and fever may recur periodically for months.

Diagnosis

At first, the disorder appears to be the flu, so usually no tests are done.

If symptoms suggest meningitis, a spinal tap (lumbar puncture) is done to obtain a sample of the cerebrospinal fluid. If lymphocytic choriomeningitis is present, the cerebrospinal fluid usually contains many white blood cells, mostly lymphocytes. A sample of blood is also obtained.

The disorder is diagnosed by identifying the virus or by detecting antibodies to the virus in blood or cerebrospinal fluid.

Treatment

No specific treatment is available. Doctors try to relieve the symptoms until the disorder subsides—in about 1 to 2 weeks.

Progressive Multifocal Leukoencephalopathy

Progressive multifocal leukoencephalopathy is a rare infection of the brain that is caused by the JC virus.

- People with a weakened immune system are most likely to get the disorder.
- People may become clumsy, have trouble speaking, and become partially blind, while mental function declines rapidly.
- Death usually occurs within 9 months.
- Imaging of the head and a spinal tap are done.
- Treating the disorder that weakened the immune system may help.

Progressive multifocal leukoencephalopathy results from infection by the JC virus (which is not related to Creutzfeldt-Jakob disease). The JC virus is often acquired during childhood. Most adults have been infected with the JC virus but do not develop the disorder. The virus appears to remain inactive until something (such as a weakened immune system) allows it to be reactivated and start to multiply. Thus, the disorder affects mainly people whose immune system has been weakened by a disorder, such as leukemia, lymphoma, or acquired immunodeficiency syndrome (AIDS), or by drugs that suppress the immune system (immunosuppressants). Such drugs may be used to prevent rejection of transplanted organs or to treat autoimmune disorders, such as systemic lupus erythematosus (lupus) or multiple sclerosis.

Symptoms

The JC virus appears to cause no symptoms until it is activated.

Symptoms may begin gradually, but they usually worsen rapidly. They vary depending on which part of the brain is infected. In about two of three people, mental function declines rapidly and progressively, causing dementia. Speaking becomes increasingly difficult. People may become partially blind. Walking may become difficult. Rarely, headaches and seizures occur. Death is common within 1 to 9 months of when symptoms start, but a few people survive longer (about 2 years).

Diagnosis

Progressively worsening symptoms in people with a weakened immune system suggest the diagnosis. Magnetic resonance imaging (MRI) of the head is done. It can usually detect abnormalities that suggest the diagnosis.

A spinal tap (lumbar puncture) is done to obtain a sample of cerebrospinal fluid. The polymerase chain reaction (PCR) technique can detect the JC virus in the cerebrospinal fluid. Sometimes the diagnosis is not confirmed until after people have died, when brain tissue can be examined.

Treatment

No treatment has proved effective. However, if the disorder that has weakened the immune system is treated, people survive longer. For example, if the cause is AIDS, highly active antiretroviral therapy is used.

If people are taking immunosuppressants, stopping the drugs may cause progressive multifocal leukoencephalopathy to subside.

Abscess of the Brain

A brain abscess is a localized collection of pus in the brain.

- An abscess may form in the brain when bacteria from an infection elsewhere in the head or in the bloodstream or from a wound enter the brain.
- Headache, sleepiness, nausea, weakness on one side of the body, or seizures may result.
- Imaging of the head is required.
- Antibiotics are given, sometimes followed by surgery.

Brain abscesses are fairly uncommon. They can result from an infection that spreads from somewhere else in the head (such as a tooth, the nose, or an ear) or that spreads from another part of the

body through the bloodstream to the brain. An abscess may form when bacteria enter after a head wound that penetrates the brain, including those that occur during brain surgery.

Many types of bacteria, including *Staphylococcus aureus* and *Bacteroides fragilis* can cause a brain abscess. *Toxoplasma gondii* (see page 1225), a protozoan, and fungi, such as aspergilli, are common causes of brain abscess in people who have a weakened immune system. The immune system may be weakened by disorders such as human immunodeficiency virus (HIV) infection, which leads to acquired immunodeficiency syndrome (AIDS), or by drugs that suppress the immune system. Such drugs may be used to prevent rejection of a transplanted organ or to treat cancer or autoimmune disorders.

Fluid collects around a brain abscess. As a result, the surrounding brain tissue swells, and pressure within the skull increases. The larger the abscess, the greater the swelling and the pressure. If the abscess leaks or breaks and the pus enters the cerebrospinal fluid, acute meningitis results.

Symptoms

A brain abscess can cause many different symptoms, depending on its location, its size, and the extent of inflammation and swelling around the abscess. People may have a headache, feel nauseated, vomit, become unusually drowsy, and then lapse into coma (which is often occurs when pressure within the brain continues to increase). Seizures may occur, one side of the body may become weak, or thinking may be impaired. Symptoms can develop over days or weeks. A fever and chills may occur at first but then disappear.

Diagnosis

The best test for diagnosing a suspected brain abscess is magnetic resonance imaging (MRI) that uses a substance called gadolinium. Gadolinium, a paramagnetic contrast agent that is injected intravenously, shows up in injured brain regions that have lost their blood-brain barrier—in other words, lost their ability to be highly selective in what molecules are permitted entry from blood into the brain. (Gadolinium is not harmful.) Alternatively, computed tomography (CT) that uses a dye visible on x-rays (radiopaque dye) can be done. MRI has higher resolution and can show early abnormalities better than CT. However, additional tests may be needed to establish the diagnosis because a brain tumor or damage due to a stroke can resemble an abscess. A specialized form of MRI, called magnetic resonance spectroscopy, can distinguish between an abscess (which contains dead or dying tissue) and a tumor (which contains living rapidly duplicating cells).

To identify the causative organism, doctors withdraw a sample of pus from the abscess with a needle. It is examined under a microscope and sent to a laboratory to grow (culture) bacteria in the fluid so that they can be identified. MRI or CT is used to guide the needle into the abscess. For this procedure (called stereotactic aspiration or biopsy), a frame is attached to the skull. The frame provides reference points that can be identified on the MRI or CT scan and enable doctors to guide the needle precisely into the abscess.

Treatment

A brain abscess is fatal unless treated with antibiotics and possibly surgery. The most commonly used antibiotics are cephalosporins (such as cefotaxime or ceftriaxone), vancomycin or nafcillin, and metronidazole. An antibiotic is usually given for 4 to 6 weeks, and MRI or CT is repeated every 2 weeks to monitor the response to treatment. If the abscess does not shrink, a surgeon may have to drain the abscess with a needle (using stereotactic techniques to guide placement of the needle) or perform open surgery to remove the entire abscess. Recovery may be quick or slow depending on how successful surgery is, how many abscesses are present, and how well the person's immune system is functioning. If people with a weakened immune system have an abscess due to *Toxoplasma gondii* or a fungus, they must take antibiotics for the rest of their life.

Doctors treat the swelling and increased pressure within the skull aggressively because these effects can permanently damage the brain. Corticosteroids, such as dexamethasone, and other drugs that reduce swelling and pressure (such as mannitol) may be used. Anticonvulsants may be given to prevent seizures.

Subdural Empyema

A subdural empyema is a collection of pus that develops under the top layer of tissue (dura mater) covering the brain, rather than in the brain itself.

A subdural empyema develops between the outer (dura mater) and middle (arachnoid mater) layers of the tissues that cover the brain (meninges).

A subdural empyema may result from a sinus infection, a severe ear infection, a head injury, surgery involving the head, or a blood infection. The same kinds of bacteria that cause brain abscesses can cause subdural empyemas. In children younger than 5 years, meningitis often accompanies a subdural empyema.

Like a brain abscess, a subdural empyema can cause headache, sleepiness, seizures, and other signs of brain dysfunction. The symptoms can evolve over several days, and without treatment, they progress rapidly to coma and death.

Diagnosis and Treatment

Use of a dye visible on x-rays (radiopaque dye also known as contrast) makes a subdural empyema visible on magnetic resonance imaging (MRI) or computed tomography (CT). A spinal tap is of little help and may be dangerous. In infants, a needle can sometimes be inserted directly into the empyema through a fontanelle (a soft spot between the skull bones) to drain the pus, relieve pressure, and help doctors make the diagnosis.

Subdural empyemas must be drained surgically. If the infection occurred because of an abnormality in the sinuses, the surgeon usually repairs the abnormality at the same time. Antibiotics are given intravenously.

Parasitic Infections

In some parts of the world, brain infections may be due to worms or other parasites. These infections are more common in developing countries and rural areas. They are less common in the United States.

Cysticercosis: This infection is caused by pork tapeworm larvae (see page 1223). It is the most common parasitic infection in the Western Hemisphere. After people eat food contaminated with cysticercus eggs, secretions in the stomach cause the eggs to hatch into larvae. The larvae enter the bloodstream and are distributed to all parts of the body, including the brain. The larvae form cysts that can cause headaches and seizures. The cysts degenerate and the larvae die, triggering inflammation, swelling, and symptoms such as headaches, seizures, personality changes, and mental impairment.

Sometimes the cysts block the flow of cerebrospinal fluid within the spaces of the brain (ventricles) putting pressure on the brain. This disorder is called hydrocephalus. Increased pressure can cause headaches, nausea, vomiting, and sleepiness.

Magnetic resonance imaging (MRI) or computed tomography (CT) can often show the cysts. But blood tests and a spinal tap (lumbar puncture) to obtain a sample of cerebrospinal fluid are often needed to confirm the diagnosis.

The infection is treated with albendazole or praziquantel. Corticosteroids are given to reduce the inflammation that occurs as the larvae die. Seizures are treated with anticonvulsants.

Occasionally, surgery is necessary to place a drain (shunt) to remove the excess cerebrospinal fluid and relieve the hydrocephalus. The shunt is a piece of plastic tubing placed in the spaces within the brain. The tubing is run under the skin, usually to the abdomen, where excess fluid can drain. Surgery to remove cysts from the brain may also be needed.

Other Infections: Echinococcosis (hydatid disease) and **coenurosis** are infections with other types of tapeworm larvae. Echinococcosis can produce large cysts in the brain. Coenurosis produces cysts, which can block the flow of fluid around the brain similar to cysticercosis.

Schistosomiasis is an infection caused by blood flukes (see page 1222).

Echinococcosis, coenurosis, and schistosomiasis can cause symptoms similar to those of cysticercosis, including seizures, headaches, personality changes, and mental impairment.

Doctors can usually diagnose these infections based on results from MRI or CT, but sometimes a spinal tap is needed. The spinal fluid may show a distinct type of inflammation with white cells called eosinophils.

These three infections are usually treated with drugs, such as albendazole, mebendazole, praziquantel, and pyrantel pamoate, but sometimes cysts must be removed surgically.

CHAPTER

118 Prion Diseases

Prion diseases (transmissible spongiform encephalopathies) are rare degenerative diseases of the brain thought to be caused by a protein that converts to an abnormal form called a prion.

Before prions were identified, diseases such as Creutzfeldt-Jakob disease and other spongiform encephalopathies were thought to be caused by viruses. Prions are much smaller than viruses and differ from viruses, bacteria, and all living cells because they do not contain any genetic material. In prion diseases, a normal protein called cellular prion protein (PrP^c) changes shape and becomes an abnormal protein molecule called scrapie prion protein (PrP^{sc})—prion. (Scrapie refers to a prion disease first observed in sheep.) The newly formed prion then converts other nearby PrP^c into prions, and the process continues. When prions reach a certain number, disease results. Prions never convert back into PrP^c.

PrP^c occurs in all cells of the body, with a high concentration in the brain. Consequently, prion diseases affect the nervous system predominantly or exclusively. When these proteins are converted into prions, they usually cause tiny bubbles to form in brain cells. Gradually, the affected cells die and the brain becomes filled with holes. When samples of brain tissue are viewed through a microscope, they somewhat resemble Swiss cheese or a sponge (hence the term "spongiform").

Prion disease may occur in families because people can inherit a mutation in the gene for PrP^c. The mutation makes PrP^c molecules more likely to convert to prions. Many different mutations exist. Each mutation generally causes different prion diseases, which, however, fit into three groups: familial Creutzfeldt-Jakob disease, fatal familial insomnia, and Gerstmann-Sträussler-Scheinker disease.

Prion diseases may occur spontaneously without any known reason. They are called sporadic and are the most common of all human prion diseases, accounting for 85 to 90% of all cases.

Prion diseases can also be acquired when prions originate from an external source, such as contaminated beef—as occurs in variant Creutzfeldt-Jakob disease (vCJD, sometimes called the human version of "mad cow disease"), implant of infected prion tissues, inoculation of prion-contaminated drugs, or use of prion-contaminated neurosurgical instruments. Other potential sources of prion disease besides cattle are elk and deer, which are affected by a prion disease called chronic wasting disease. However, no case of human prion disease has been reported from chronic wasting disease or sheep scrapie. When prions are acquired, symptoms generally develop years later. Kuru also is an acquired prion disease.

Symptoms common to most prion diseases include memory loss, confusion, loss of coordination, muscle twitches, dementia, and gait difficulty.

There is no cure for prion diseases, which are all fatal, usually within months to a few years. Treatment focuses on comfort measures and symptom relief. A number of strategies can help caregivers of people with a prion disease cope with the dementia caused by the disease (see page 691). If possible, people who have a prion disease should establish advance directives (see page 69) about what kind of medical care they want at the end of life. Family members of people who develop the hereditary form of the disease may benefit from genetic counseling.

Creutzfeldt-Jakob Disease

Creutzfeldt-Jakob disease (subacute spongiform encephalopathy) is a prion disease characterized by progressive deterioration of mental function, leading to dementia, muscle twitching (myoclonus), and staggering when walking. A variant form is acquired by eating contaminated beef.

- The disease usually occurs spontaneously but may result from eating contaminated beef or from inheriting an abnormal gene.
- At first, most people are confused and have memory problems, followed by muscle twitching and loss of coordination.
- Most people die with 6 months, although some live for 2 years or more.
- The diagnosis can usually be confirmed by electrocephalography, analysis of cerebrospinal fluid, and magnetic resonance imaging.
- There is no cure, but drugs can relieve some of the symptoms.

Sporadic Creutzfeldt-Jakob disease, the most common form, affects 1 in a million people each year throughout the world. It affects adults, mainly in their late 50s and 60s. For this form, no cause is known.

Familial CJD results from a mutation in the gene of PrP^c, which results in conversion of the normal PrP^c molecule to a disease-causing prion. Familial CJD is often inherited and usually starts at an earlier age and lasts longer.

The acquired form includes variant Creutzfeldt-Jakob disease, which is thought to be acquired from the consumption of contaminated beef or beef products. The variant form usually begins around age 30, in contrast to sporadic CJD, which usually begins around age 65. To date, the variant form has been acquired only in Europe, mainly in the United Kingdom, with the exception of two cases acquired in Saudi Arabia. Spread of the disease has been controlled by massive slaughter of cattle in the United Kingdom. Widespread surveillance for the disease in cattle has resulted in a progressively lower number of new cases in the United Kingdom.

External sources for the prion include transplantation of contaminated corneas or possibly other tissues from affected donors and brain surgery using instruments previously used to operate on a person who had CJD. Routine cleansing and sterilization procedures do not destroy prions. However, bleach is effective. Acquiring the disease this way is extremely unlikely.

Another external source is hormones derived from human pituitary glands used for treatment. For example, the disease developed in some children who were treated with growth hormone derived from human pituitary glands. These hormones are

Of Sheep and Cows

Prion diseases occur in sheep, goats, cattle, and other animals, such as minks, elk, deer, and goats. Like people with Creutzfeldt-Jakob disease, affected animals gradually become uncoordinated, then develop dementia. Scrapie, the disease in sheep, is so named because the sheep tend to scrape themselves against fence posts or other objects and tear their wool off. Mad cow disease is so named because the cattle become noticeably agitated. The disease can be transmitted from sheep to cattle by feeding cattle scrapie-infected sheep parts.

Eating contaminated beef or beef products is thought to be the cause of a new form of Creutzfeldt-Jakob disease in people. First described in 1996, this form is called variant Creutzfeldt-Jakob disease (sometimes also called the human version of "mad cow disease"). The new form differs in many ways from the usual form: It causes different changes in brain tissue (seen under a microscope), and the first symptoms tend to be psychiatric symptoms, rather than the memory loss that occurs in people who have the usual form of Creutzfeldt-Jakob disease. By early 2007, variant Creutzfeldt-Jakob disease had been diagnosed in a total of 201 people:

- 165 in the United Kingdom
- 21 in France
- 4 in Ireland
- 3 in the United States (2 acquired in the United Kingdom, 1 in Saudi Arabia)
- 2 in Holland
- 1 in Italy
- 1 in Japan (acquired in the United Kingdom)
- 1 in Canada (acquired in the United Kingdom)
- 1 in Spain
- 1 in Portugal
- 1 in Saudi Arabia

now genetically engineered rather than prepared from cadavers, so there is no longer a risk of CJD.

Three cases of CJD have been transmitted through blood transfusion. However, in all cases, the disease was acquired from donors affected by the variant form. The type of CJD acquired by medical intervention is called iatrogenic.

CJD has never been reported to be transmitted through casual or even intimate contact with people who have the disease.

Symptoms

The most common early symptoms—memory loss and confusion—may resemble those of other dementias, such as Alzheimer's disease. In some people, loss of muscle coordination occurs first. In about 10 to 20% of people, symptoms appear abruptly, starting with dizziness and double vision. In people with the variant form, the first symptoms tend to be psychiatric symptoms (such as anxiety or depression), rather than memory loss. Later symptoms are similar in both forms.

Whether symptoms develop gradually or abruptly, mental decline progresses, often producing such symptoms as neglect of personal hygiene, apathy, and irritability. Some people tire easily and become sleepy. Others cannot fall asleep.

Muscles usually begin to twitch involuntarily and quickly during the first 6 months after symptoms begin. Trembling and clumsiness may also develop, and muscle coordination is lost. Walking becomes unsteady, resulting in staggering (similar to the walk of a person who is drunk). Movements may be slow. Impairment of muscle control may result in unusual postures, such as twisting of the trunk or limbs forward and sideways. Muscles may jerk when stretched. The person may startle easily, and the resulting responses, such as jumping when a loud noise is heard, are exaggerated. Startling may trigger muscle twitching. The muscles that control breathing and coughing are usually impaired, increasing the risk of pneumonia. Vision may become blurry or dim.

The symptoms worsen, usually much more rapidly than in Alzheimer's disease, resulting in severe dementia. Most people with CJD die within 6 months after symptoms appear. About 10 to 20% of people survive for 2 years or more. People with the variant form usually survive for 1½ years. Often, the cause of death is pneumonia.

In people who have acquired the prion from an external source, no symptoms appear for months or years. In the variant form, the time interval between eating contaminated beef and onset of the disease is estimated to be 6 to 12 years.

Diagnosis and Treatment

Doctors consider CJD when mental function is deteriorating quickly, muscle twitching is present, walking is unsteady and staggering, and other dementias have been ruled out by routine testing. The variant form may be considered in people who have typical symptoms and who have eaten processed beef in the United Kingdom or in other countries at risk for mad cow disease.

Diagnosis is mainly by electroencephalography (EEG), analysis of cerebrospinal fluid, and magnetic resonance imaging (MRI). EEG is done to check for specific abnormalities in the electrical activity of the brain, which occur in 70% of people with the disease. A spinal tap is done to obtain a sample of cerebrospinal fluid, which is tested for an unusual protein called 14-3-3. This protein occurs in about 90% of people with typical CJD disease. The EEG abnormalities plus the presence of the 14-3-3 pro-

tein in cerebrospinal fluid strongly support the diagnosis of CJD. The absence of the 14-3-3 protein or the characteristic abnormalities on EEG does not rule out CJD. The definitive diagnosis is based on detecting prions in brain tissue by examination of a tissue sample under a microscope or by biochemical analysis at autopsy examination. Diagnostic brain biopsy is occasionally done, generally to rule out a treatable condition, such as inflammation of the brain or encephalitis.

Currently, CJD cannot be cured, and its progress cannot be slowed. The disease is fatal, usually within months or a few years. However, certain drugs may be given to relieve symptoms. For example, the anticonvulsant valproate and the antianxiety drug clonazepam may reduce muscle jerking.

General support and care for the person and family members are important. Day care centers and respite and long-term care may be useful. Speech and occupational therapists can help with specific problems. The CJD Foundation provides support and information

Fatal Familial Insomnia

Fatal familial insomnia is a rare prion disease that interferes with sleep and leads to deterioration of mental and motor functions. Death occurs within a few months to a few years.

Fatal insomnia includes an inherited or familial form, called fatal familial insomnia, due to a specific mutation in the PrP^c gene. The disease can also occur spontaneously, without a genetic mutation. This form is called sporadic fatal insomnia. Fatal familial insomnia and sporadic fatal insomnia differ from other prion diseases because they affect predominantly one area of the brain, the thalamus, which influences sleep.

The disease usually begins between the ages of 40 and 60 but may begin in a person's late 30s. At first, people may have minor difficulties falling asleep and occasional muscle twitching, spasms, and stiffness. Eventually, they cannot sleep. Occasionally, the sleep signs are difficult to detect. Other changes include a rapid heart rate and dementia. Death usually occurs about 7 to 36 months after symptoms begin.

The diagnosis is suggested by typical symptoms and a family history of the disease and can be confirmed by genetic testing. No treatment is available.

Gerstmann-Sträussler-Scheinker Disease

Gerstmann-Sträussler-Scheinker disease is a prion disease that causes muscle incoordination followed by slow deterioration of mental function. The disease is fatal, usually in about 5 years.

Like Creutzfeldt-Jakob disease, Gerstmann-Sträussler-Scheinker disease may occur anywhere in the world. However, it is much less common than Creutzfeldt-Jakob disease, begins earlier in life (affecting people in their 40s rather than in their late 50s and 60s), and progresses more slowly (with an average life expectancy of 5 years rather than 6 months). This disease runs in families.

Usually, the first symptoms are clumsiness and unsteadiness when walking. Muscle twitching is much less common than in Creutzfeldt-Jakob disease. Speaking becomes difficult, and dementia develops. Nystagmus (rapid movement of the eyes in one direction, followed by a slower drift back to the original position), blindness, and deafness may develop. Muscle coordination is lost. The muscles may tremble and become stiff. Usually, the muscles that control breathing and coughing are impaired, resulting in a high risk of pneumonia, which is the common cause of death.

The diagnosis is suggested by typical symptoms and a family history of the disease and can be confirmed by genetic testing. No treatment is available.

Kuru

Kuru is a prion disease that causes rapid deterioration of mental function and loss of muscle coordination. This disease used to occur in the Fore natives of the New Guinea highlands and is related to ritual endocannibalism.

Until the early 1960s, kuru was fairly common in New Guinea. Prions were probably acquired during a cannibalistic ritual accompanying the care of the dead and involving eating tissues of a dead relative as a sign of respect. Kuru probably started from the consumption of prion-contaminated tissues from a person affected by Creutzfeldt-Jakob disease. Kuru was more common among women and children because they were given the brain to eat. Many of these rituals have been abandoned, and kuru has been virtually eliminated.

Symptoms include loss of muscle coordination and difficulty walking. The limbs become stiff, and muscles twitch. Abnormal involuntary movements, such as repetitive, slow writhing or rapid jerking of the limbs and body, may develop (kuru means shivering). Emotions may switch suddenly from sadness to happiness with sudden outbursts of laughter. People with kuru become demented and eventually placid, unable to speak, and unresponsive to their surroundings.

Most people die about 3 to 24 months after symptoms appear, usually as a result of pneumonia or infection due to bedsores (pressure sores).

CHAPTER 119 Movement Disorders

Every body movement, from raising a hand to smiling, involves a complex interaction between the central nervous system (brain and spinal cord), nerves, and muscles. Damage to or malfunction of any of these components may result in a movement disorder.

Different types of movement disorders can develop, depending on the nature and location of the damage or malfunction, as in the following:

- Damage to the parts of the brain that control voluntary movement or the connections between the brain and spinal cord: Weakness or paralysis of the muscles involved in voluntary movements and exaggerated reflexes
- Damage to the basal ganglia (collections of nerve cells located at the base of the cerebrum, deep within the brain): Involuntary or decreased movements, but not weakness or changes in reflexes
- Damage to the cerebellum: Loss of coordination

Some movement disorders, such as hiccups, are temporary, usually causing little inconvenience. Others, such as Parkinson's disease, are serious and progressive, impairing the ability to speak, use the hands, walk, and maintain balance when standing.

Myoclonus

Myoclonus refers to quick, lightning-like jerks (contractions) of a muscle or a group of muscles.

Myoclonus may involve only one hand, a group of muscles in the upper arm or leg, or a group of facial muscles. Or it may involve many muscles at the same time. Hiccups are a type of myoclonus that involves only the diaphragm, the muscle that separates the chest from the abdomen.

Myoclonus may occur normally, often when a person is falling asleep. Or it may result from a disorder, such as the following:

Hiccups: Spasms of the Diaphragm

Almost everyone has had hiccups, so hiccups are hardly thought of as a movement disorder. But they are. They occur when there are spasms of the diaphragm, followed by quick, noisy closings of the glottis. (The diaphragm is the muscle that separates the chest from the abdomen and that is responsible for each breath. The glottis is the opening between the vocal cords, which closes to stop the flow of air to the lungs.) Hiccups are more likely to occur when carbon dioxide levels in the blood decrease. Such a decrease can occur when people hyperventilate.

Most bouts of hiccups have no obvious cause. They usually start in a social situation, perhaps triggered by some combination of laughing, talking, eating, and drinking. Sometimes hot or irritating food or liquids are the cause. Some less common causes of hiccups are more serious. For example, the diaphragm may become irritated because of pneumonia, chest or stomach surgery, or waste products that accumulate in the blood when the kidneys malfunction. Rarely, hiccups develop when a brain tumor or stroke interferes with the breathing center in the brain.

Hiccups usually begin suddenly and stop after several seconds or minutes, but occasionally, they persist for some time, even in healthy people. When the cause is serious, hiccups tend to persist until the cause is corrected. Hiccups due to a brain tumor or stroke may be very hard to stop and may become exhausting.

Many home remedies have been used to cure hiccups. Most involve ways to raise the level of carbon dioxide in the blood, such as the following:

- Holding the breath
- Breathing into a paper (not plastic) bag

Stimulating the vagus nerve, which runs from the brain to the stomach, may stop the hiccups. The following can stimulate this nerve:

- Drinking water quickly
- Swallowing dry bread or crushed ice
- Gently pulling on the tongue
- Gently rubbing the eyeballs

For most people with hiccups, any of these remedies work.

For persistent hiccups, treatment is needed, particularly when the cause cannot be easily corrected. Several drugs have been used with varying success. They include scopolamine, prochlorperazine, chlorpromazine, baclofen, metoclopramide, and valproate.

- Liver failure
- Kidney failure
- Cardiac arrest (when the heart's pumping stops suddenly)
- Brain damage due to a virus (viral encephalopathy)
- Metabolic disorders (such a high or low blood sugar level)
- Oxygen deprivation
- Head injuries
- Alzheimer's disease (occasionally)
- Creutzfeldt-Jakob disease
- Juvenile myoclonic epilepsy (which causes seizures)

Myoclonus can occur after a person takes high doses of certain drugs such as antihistamines, some antidepressants (such as amitriptyline), bismuth, levodopa, or opioids (narcotics).

Symptoms

Myoclonus can be mild or severe. Muscles may jerk quickly or slowly, rhythmically or not. Myoclonus may occur once in a while or frequently. It may occur spontaneously or be triggered by a stimulus, such as a sudden noise, light, or a movement. For example, reaching for an object or taking step may trigger jerks that disrupt the movement. In Creutzfeldt-Jacob disease (a rare degenerative brain disorder—see page 766), myoclonus becomes more obvious when people are suddenly startled. If myoclonus is due to a metabolic disorder, it may persist and affect muscles throughout the body, sometimes leading to seizures.

 Did You Know...

Some types of myoclonus—hiccups and the quick twitches of muscles as a person falls asleep—are normal.

Diagnosis and Treatment

The diagnosis is based on symptoms. Other tests may be done to identify the cause.

The cause is corrected if possible. For example, drugs that can cause myoclonus are stopped. A high or low blood sugar level is corrected, and kidney failure is treated with hemodialysis. If the cause cannot be corrected, valproate or levetiracetam (anticonvulsants—see table on page 716) or clonazepam (a mild sedative) sometimes helps. When given with carbidopa, the dietary supplement 5-hydroxytryptophan (which is produced by the brain) may also help.

Tremor

A tremor is an involuntary, rhythmic, shaking movement produced when muscles repeatedly contract and relax.

Everyone has a tremor to some degree. For example, when held outstretched, the hands usually tremble slightly. Such slight, rapid tremor, called physiologic tremor, is normal and reflects the precise moment-by-moment control of muscles by nerves. In most people, the tremor is too slight to be noticed.

Factors that can make a normal tremor more noticeable include stress, anxiety, fatigue, withdrawal of alcohol or certain other drugs (such as opioids), an overactive thyroid gland (hyperthyroidism), consumption of caffeine, and use of certain drugs, including theophylline and beta-adrenergic agonists such as albuterol (which are used to treat asthma), corticosteroids, and valproate (an anticonvulsant).

Types of Abnormal Tremors

There are several types of abnormal tremor. Tremors are classified according to the following:

- How fast the shaking movements are (frequency)
- How wide (amplitude) they are, ranging from fine to coarse
- How often the tremors occur
- How severe they are
- What triggers them, such as rest or movement
- What causes them

Tremors triggered by rest are called resting tremors. Tremors triggered or made worse by movement are called action tremors. Action tremors can be classified as intention tremors (triggered by aiming for a target) or postural tremors (triggered by holding a limb in one position). Causes are classified as physiologic, essential, cerebellar, or secondary. Secondary tremors are caused by disorders or drugs.

Resting Tremor: This tremor occurs when muscles are at rest, making an arm or a leg shake even when a person is completely relaxed. The tremor becomes less noticeable or disappears when the person moves the affected muscles. Resting tremors are often slow and coarse.

These tremors develop when collections of nerve cells at the base of the cerebrum (including the basal ganglia) are disturbed. Such disturbances usually result from Parkinson's disease. Antipsychotic drugs are another common cause of resting tremors.

Resting tremors may be socially embarrassing but typically do not interfere with daily activities, such as drinking a glass of water.

Intention Tremor: This tremor occurs when a person ends a purposeful movement (such as pressing a button) or aims for a target (as when reaching for an object with the hand). The person may miss the targeted object because of the tremor. Intention tremors are relatively slow and coarse.

These tremors may result from damage to the cerebellum or its connections. Thus, cerebellar tremors and intention tremors may be used synonymously. Multiple sclerosis is a common cause. Stroke, Wilson's disease, alcoholism, and overuse of sedatives or anticonvulsants can cause the cerebellum to malfunction, resulting in an intention tremor.

Postural Tremor: This tremor occurs when an arm or a leg is held in one position against gravity, as when a person holds the arms outstretched in front of the body.

If the tremor develops gradually, it is usually a physiologic or essential tremor. If a postural tremor starts more suddenly, the cause may be a toxin, a disorder (such as hyperthyroidism), withdrawal of alcohol or a drug, or use of certain drugs.

Essential Tremor: This tremor usually begins in early adulthood but can begin at any age. The tremor slowly becomes more obvious and becomes more noticeable as people age. Thus, it is sometimes incorrectly called senile tremor. It is usually rapid and fine but may be slow, coarse, or both.

Some forms of essential tremor, called benign hereditary tremor, run in families. What causes essential tremors is unknown, but these tremors (while they can be disabling if severe) do not indicate a serious disorder.

Essential tremor can affect the hands, head, and voice. Usually, the tremor stops during rest and worsens when the limbs are held in uncomfortable positions. The tremor often becomes obvious when the limbs are outstretched. For example, a tremor of the hand or wrist may become obvious when the wrist is bent upward and the fingers are spread apart. The tremor typically affects both sides of the body but may affect one side more than the other. Sometimes the head trembles and bobs, and the voice becomes shaky.

Any factor that makes normal (physiologic) tremors worse (such as stress, fatigue, or consumption of caffeine) can make essential tremors more noticeable. Drinking alcohol usually makes the tremor less noticeable.

Usually, essential tremor remains mild. However, it can be troublesome and embarrassing. It can affect handwriting and make using utensils difficult. In some people, the tremor gradually worsens over time, eventually resulting in disability.

Asterixis: Asterixis resembles a tremor but is not one. Asterixis occurs when a group of contracted muscles suddenly and temporarily goes limp. For example, when the arms and hands are outstretched, the hands suddenly drop, then resume their original position. The movements are repetitive, coarse, slow, and not rhythmic.

Asterixis commonly results from liver failure and so has been called liver flap. Asterixis may also result from kidney failure, use of certain drugs, or brain damage (encephalopathy) due to a metabolic disorder. It is often accompanied by tremors and myoclonus (see page 768).

Did You Know...

Everyone has tremors to some degree.

Simple, common-sense measures can make functioning with noticeable tremors easier.

Diagnosis

If a noticeable tremor develops, it should be evaluated by a doctor. A doctor can usually identify the type of tremor by its characteristics. The type of tremor determines which diagnostic tests are done.

- **Resting tremor:** A complete neurologic evaluation is done to check for Parkinson's disease. Computed tomography (CT) or magnetic resonance imaging (MRI) of the brain may be done.
- **Intention tremor:** An imaging procedure, such as CT or MRI, is often done to look for damage to the brain, especially the cerebellum.
- **Postural tremor:** If symptoms develop suddenly, the doctor asks about the drugs the person is taking, and tests may be done to check for other disorders, such as thyroid disorders. CT or MRI may also be done.
- **Essential tremor:** The doctor asks what drugs the person is using, whether the person is experiencing anxiety or stress, and whether an alcoholic beverage makes the tremor less noticeable. A blood test to check for hyperthyroidism is done.
- **Asterixis:** Blood tests are done to determine whether a liver, kidney, or metabolic disorder is the cause.

Treatment

For mild tremor, no treatment is needed. If tremors become bothersome, some simple measures can help:

- Grasping objects firmly and holding them close to the body to avoid dropping them
- Avoiding uncomfortable positions
- Not eating soup in public

- Using assistive devices, as instructed by an occupational therapist

Assistive devices may include rocker knives, utensils with large handles, and, particularly if the tremor is severe, button hooks, Velcro fasteners (instead of buttons or shoe laces), zipper pulls, straws, and shoe horns.

For physiologic or essential tremor, eliminating or minimizing the trigger may lessen the tremor. For example, treating hyperthyroidism may help. Drinking alcohol in moderation may lessen the tremor. However, heavy drinking followed by stopping it suddenly makes the tremor worse. If many daily activities (such as using utensils and drinking from a glass at mealtime) become difficult or if the person's work requires steady hands, drugs are used. Treatment may include a beta-blocker (such as propranolol), the anticonvulsant primidone, or both.

If due to Parkinson's disease, a resting tremor is treated as part of that disease. Drugs with anticholinergic effects such as trihexyphenidyl and benztropine usually help control the tremor.

Intention tremors are difficult to treat, but if the condition affecting the cerebellum can be corrected, the tremor may resolve. If the condition cannot be corrected, a therapist may put wrist and ankle weights on the affected limb to reduce the tremor. Or people may be taught to brace the limb during activity. These measures sometimes help.

Deep Brain Stimulation: Tiny electrodes are placed in the area of the brain involved in tremors. The electrodes deliver a painless shock to block the impulses causing tremors. Deep brain stimulation is sometimes done when drugs cannot control a severe, disabling essential tremor or a resting tremor. For essential tremors, the thalamus (a collection of nerve cells at the base of the brain) is stimulated. For resting tremors, the thalamus or subthalamic nucleus (located below the thalamus) is stimulated. Such procedures are available only at special centers.

Parkinson's Disease

Parkinson's disease is a slowly progressive degenerative disorder of the central nervous system. It is characterized by tremor when muscles are at rest (resting tremor), increased muscle tone (rigidity), slowness of voluntary movements, and difficulty maintaining balance (postural instability). Many people develop dementia.

- Parkinson's disease results from degeneration in the part of the brain that helps coordinate movements.
- Usually, the most obvious symptom is tremors that occur when muscles are relaxed.
- Muscles become stiff, movements become slow and uncoordinated, and balance is easily lost.

- Doctors base the diagnosis on symptoms.
- Changes in lifestyle, drugs (such as levodopa plus carbidopa), and sometimes surgery help lessen symptoms, but the disease is progressive, eventually causing severe disability and immobility.

Parkinson's disease affects about 1 of 250 people older than 40, about 1 of 100 people older than 65, and about 1 of 10 people older than 80. It commonly begins between the ages of 50 and 79. Rarely, Parkinson's disease occurs in children or adolescents.

When the brain initiates an impulse to move a muscle (for example, to lift an arm), the impulse passes through the basal ganglia (collections of nerve cells located deep within the brain). The basal ganglia help smooth out muscle movements and coordinate changes in posture. Like all nerve cells, those in the basal ganglia release chemical messengers (neurotransmitters) that trigger the next nerve cell in the pathway to send an impulse. A key neurotransmitter in the basal ganglia is dopamine. Its overall effect is to increase nerve impulses to muscles. In Parkinson's disease, nerve cells in part of the basal ganglia (called the substantia nigra) degenerate, reducing the production of dopamine and the number of connections between nerve cells in the basal ganglia. As a result, the basal ganglia cannot smooth out movements as they normally do, leading to tremor, loss of coordination, slow movement (bradykinesia), and a tendency to move less (hypokinesia).

> ### ❓ Did You Know...
>
> Symptoms of Parkinson's disease can be caused by many other disorders and drugs.
>
> Parkinson's disease is sometimes hard to diagnose in older people because aging causes some of the same symptoms.
>
> Early in Parkinson's disease, delaying levodopa (the most useful treatment) is sometimes the best approach.

What causes Parkinson's disease is unclear. According to one theory, Parkinson's disease may result from abnormal deposits of synuclein (a protein in the brain that helps nerve cells communicate). These deposits, called Lewy bodies, can accumulate in several regions of the brain, particularly in the substantia nigra (deep within the cerebrum) and interfere with brain function. Lewy bodies often accumulate in other parts of the brain and nervous system, suggesting that they may be involved in other disorders. In Lewy body dementia, Lewy bodies form throughout the outer layer of the brain (cerebral cortex). Lewy bodies may also be involved in Alzheimer's disease.

About 15 to 20% of affected people have relatives who have had Parkinson's disease. Thus, genetics may play a role.

Parkinsonism refers to symptoms of Parkinson's disease (such as slow movements and tremors) when they are caused by another condition. Various conditions can cause parkinsonism (see page 777).

Symptoms

Usually, Parkinson's disease begins subtly and progresses gradually. In about two thirds of people, tremors are the first symptom. In others, the first symptom is usually problems with movement or a reduced sense of smell.

Parkinson's disease typically causes the following symptoms:

- **Tremors:** Tremors are coarse and rhythmic. They usually occur in one hand while the hand is at rest (a resting tremor). The tremor is called a pill-rolling tremor because the hand moves as if it is rolling small objects around. The tremor decreases when the hand is moving purposefully and disappears completely during sleep. Emotional stress or fatigue may worsen the tremor. The tremor may eventually progress to the other hand, the arms, and the legs. A tremor may also affect the jaws, tongue, forehead, and eyelids, but not the voice. In some people, a tremor never develops.
- **Stiffness (rigidity):** Muscles become stiff, impairing movement. When the forearm is bent back or straightened out by another person, the movement may feel stiff and ratchet-like (called cogwheel rigidity).
- **Slowed movements:** Movements become slow and difficult to initiate, and people tend to move less. Thus, mobility decreases.
- **Difficulty maintaining balance and posture:** Posture becomes stooped, and balance is difficult to maintain, leading to a tendency to fall forward or backward. Because movements are slow, people often cannot move their hands quickly enough to break a fall.

Walking becomes difficult, especially taking the first step. Once started, people often shuffle, taking short steps, keeping their arms bent at the waist, and not swinging their arms. While walking, some people have difficulty stopping or turning. When the disease is advanced, some people suddenly stop walking because they feel as if their feet are glued to the ground (called freezing). Other people unintentionally and gradually quicken their steps, breaking into a stumbling run to avoid falling. This symptom is called festination.

Stiffness and decreased mobility can contribute to muscle ache and fatigue. Because the small muscles of the hands are often impaired, daily tasks, such as buttoning a shirt and tying shoelaces, become increasingly difficult. Most people with Parkinson's disease have shaky, tiny handwriting (micrographia) because initiating and sustaining each stroke of the pen is difficult. Sensation and strength are usually normal.

The face becomes less expressive (masklike) because the facial muscles that control expression do not move. This lack of expression may be mistaken for depression, or it may cause depression to be overlooked. (Depression is common among people with Parkinson's disease.) Eventually, the face can take on a blank stare with the mouth open, and the eyes may not blink often. Often, people drool or choke because muscle rigidity in the face and throat makes swallowing difficult. People with Parkinson's disease often speak softly in a monotone and may stutter because they have difficulty articulating words.

Parkinson's disease also causes other symptoms:

- Insomnia is common, often because people need to urinate frequently or because symptoms worsen during the night, making turning over in bed difficult. Rapid-eye-movement (REM) sleep behavior disorder commonly develops. In this disorder, the limbs, which normally do not move in REM sleep, may move suddenly and violently, sometimes injuring a sleep partner. Lack of sleep may contribute to depression and drowsiness during the day.

- Urination may be difficult to start and to maintain (called urinary hesitancy).

- Constipation can develop because the intestine may move its contents more slowly. Inactivity and levodopa, the main drug used to treat Parkinson's disease, can worsen constipation.

- A sudden, excessive decrease in blood pressure may occur when a person stands up (orthostatic hypotension).

- Scales (seborrheic dermatitis) develop often on the scalp and face and occasionally in other areas.

- Dementia develops in about half the people with Parkinson's disease. In many people, intellect remains normal.

Diagnosis

The diagnosis is likely if the person has fewer, slow movements and either the characteristic tremor or muscle rigidity. Mild, early disease may be difficult for doctors to diagnose because it usually begins subtly. Diagnosis is especially difficult in older people because aging can cause some of the same problems as Parkinson's disease, such as loss of balance, slow movements, muscle stiffness, and stooped posture. To exclude other causes of the symptoms, doctors ask about previous disorders, exposure to toxins, and use of drugs that could cause parkinsonism.

No tests or imaging procedures can directly confirm the diagnosis. However, computed tomography (CT) and magnetic resonance imaging (MRI) may be done to look for a structural disorder that may be causing the symptoms. Single-photon emission computed tomography (SPECT) and positron emission tomography (PET) can detect brain abnormalities typical of the disease. However, SPECT and PET are currently used only in research facilities.

If the diagnosis is unclear, doctors may give the person levodopa, a drug used to treat Parkinson's disease. If levodopa results in clear improvement, Parkinson's disease is likely.

Treatment

General measures used to treat Parkinson's disease can help people function. Many drugs (such as levodopa-carbidopa) can make movement easier and enable people with Parkinson's disease to function effectively for many years. But no drug can cure the disease. Two or more drugs may be needed. For older people, doses are often reduced. Drugs that cause or worsen symptoms, particularly antipsychotics, are avoided. If the disease is advanced and drugs are ineffective or cause severe side effects, surgery is considered.

General Measures: Various simple measures can help people with Parkinson's disease maintain mobility and independence:

- Continuing to do as many daily activities as possible
- Following a program of regular exercise
- Simplifying daily tasks—for example having buttons on clothing replaced with Velcro fasteners or buying shoes with Velcro fasteners
- Using assistive devices, such as zipper pulls and button hooks

Physical therapists (see page 48) and occupational therapists (see page 50) can help people learn how to incorporate these measures into their daily activities, as well as recommend exercises to improve muscle tone and maintain range of motion. Therapists may also recommend mechanical aids, such as wheeled walkers, to help people maintain independence.

Simple changes around the home can make it safer for people with Parkinson's disease:

- Removing throw rugs to prevent tripping

℞ DRUGS USED TO TREAT PARKINSON'S DISEASE

DRUG	SOME SIDE EFFECTS	COMMENTS
Dopamine precursor		
Levodopa (given with carbidopa)	For levodopa: Involuntary movements (of the mouth, face, and limbs), nightmares, low blood pressure when a person stands up (orthostatic hypotension), constipation, nausea, drowsiness, confusion, hallucinations, palpitations, and flushing If these drugs are suddenly stopped, neuroleptic malignant syndrome (with high fever, high blood pressure, rigidity, muscle damage, and coma), which can be life threatening	This combination is the mainstay of treatment. Carbidopa helps increase the effectiveness of levodopa and reduce its side effects. After several years, the effectiveness of the combination may lessen.
Dopamine agonists		
Bromocriptine Pramipexole Ropinirole	Drowsiness, nausea, orthostatic hypotension, involuntary movements, confusion, and hallucinations When these drugs are suddenly stopped, neuroleptic malignant syndrome	Early in the disease, these drugs may be used alone or with small doses of levodopa to possibly delay levodopa's side effects. Later in the disease, dopamine agonists are useful when the on-off effects of levodopa make it less effective.
Apomorphine	Severe nausea, vomiting, and lumps (nodules) under the skin at the injection site	This quick-acting drug is injected under the skin. It is used as rescue therapy to reverse the off effect of levodopa.
Rotigotine	Drowsiness, nausea, orthostatic hypotension, confusion, hallucinations, weight gain (possibly due to fluid retention), and sometimes irritation at the application site	This drug is available as a skin patch. It is used alone early in the disease. The patch is worn continuously for 24 hours, then removed and replaced. The patch should be placed in different locations each day to reduce the risk of skin irritation.
MAO-B inhibitors		
Rasagiline	Nausea, insomnia, drowsiness, and swelling due to fluid accumulation (edema) If people take doses that are higher than those usually used to treat Parkinson's disease and consume foods or beverages that contain tyramine (such as certain cheeses and red wine) or take certain other drugs, hypertensive crisis (a severe headache and a potentially fatal increase in blood pressure)	Rasagiline can be used alone to postpone the use of levodopa but is often given as a supplement to levodopa. At best, rasagiline is modestly effective.
Selegiline	Worsening of nausea, confusion, and involuntary movements due to levodopa	Selegiline can be used alone to postpone the use of levodopa but is often given as a supplement to levodopa. At best, selegiline is modestly effective.
COMT inhibitors		
Entacapone Tolcapone	Nausea, involuntary movements, confusion, diarrhea, back pain, and discoloration of the urine	These drugs can be used to supplement levodopa late in the disease and to extend the interval between doses of levodopa.

(continued on the following page)

℞ DRUGS USED TO TREAT PARKINSON'S DISEASE (*Continued*)

DRUG	SOME SIDE EFFECTS	COMMENTS
Anticholinergic drugs		
Benztropine Trihexyphenidyl Tricyclic antidepressants (such as amitriptyline), used if depression also needs to be treated Some antihistamines (such as diphenhydramine)	Drowsiness, confusion, dry mouth, blurred vision, dizziness, constipation, difficulty urinating, loss of bladder control, and impaired regulation of body temperature	These drugs may be given alone in the early stages of the disease or as a supplement to levodopa in the later stages. They can reduce tremor but do not affect slow movements or muscle rigidity.
Antiviral drug		
Amantadine	Nausea, dizziness, insomnia, anxiety, confusion, edema, difficulty urinating, worsening of glaucoma, and mottled discoloration of the skin due to dilated blood vessels (livedo reticularis) Rarely, when the drug is stopped or the dose is reduced, neuroleptic malignant syndrome	Amantadine is used alone in the early stages for mild disease but may become ineffective after several months. Later, it is used to supplement levodopa and to lessen involuntary movements due to levodopa.
Beta-blocker		
Propranolol	Spasm of the airways (bronchospasm), an abnormally slow heart rate (bradycardia), heart failure, possible masking of low blood sugar levels after insulin injections, impaired peripheral circulation, insomnia, fatigue, shortness of breath, depression, Raynaud's phenomenon, vivid dreams, hallucinations, and sexual dysfunction	Propranolol can be used to reduce the severity of tremors.

MAO-B = monoamine oxidase type B; COMT = catechol *O*-methyltransferase.

- Installing grab bars in bathrooms and railings in hallways and other locations to reduce the risk of falling

For constipation, the following can help:

- Consuming a high-fiber diet, including such foods as prunes and fruit juices
- Exercising
- Drinking plenty of fluids
- Using stool softeners (such as senna concentrate), supplements (such as psyllium), or stimulant laxatives (such as bisacodyl taken by mouth) to keep bowel movements regular

Difficulty swallowing may limit food intake, so the diet must be nutritious. Making an effort to sniff more deeply may improve the ability to smell, enhancing the appetite.

Levodopa-Carbidopa: Traditionally, levodopa, which is given with carbidopa, is the first drug used. These drugs, taken by mouth, are the mainstay of treatment for Parkinson's disease. However, some experts think that using levodopa early in the disease may cause side effects to develop more quickly, and people may stop responding to the drug sooner. Thus, a drug with anticholinergic effects, amantadine, or a drug that mimics the action of dopamine (a dopamine agonist) may be used first.

Levodopa reduces muscle rigidity, improves movement, and substantially reduces tremor. Taking levodopa produces dramatic improvement in people with Parkinson's disease. The drug enables many people with mild disease to return to a nearly normal level of activity and enables some people who are confined to bed to walk again. However, levodopa usually does not help people with parkinsonism (which is due to another disorder).

Levodopa is a dopamine precursor, which means that the body can convert it to dopamine. Conversion may occur in the basal ganglia, thus compensating for the decrease in dopamine production. But levodopa can also be converted to dopamine early, on its way to the brain. When levodopa is converted early, the amount of dopamine available for controlling symptoms is reduced. Also, dopamine levels in the blood increase, increasing the risk of side effects such as nausea and flushing. Giving carbidopa with levodopa prevents this early conversion of levodopa. When the two drugs are given together, a lower dose of levodopa can be used, and nausea and flushing occur less often and are less severe.

To determine the best dose of levodopa for a particular person, doctors must balance control of the disease with the development of certain side effects, which may limit the amount of levodopa the person can tolerate. These side effects include involuntary movements (of the mouth, face, and limbs), nightmares, hallucinations, and changes in blood pressure.

After taking levodopa for 5 or more years, more than half the people begin to alternate rapidly between a good response to the drug and no response—an effect called the on-off phenomenon. Within seconds, they may change from being fairly mobile to being severely impaired and immobile. The periods of mobility after each dose become shorter and may be accompanied by involuntary movements (dyskinesias) due to levodopa use, including writhing or hyperactivity. Taking lower, more frequent doses controls these effects for a while. Other options are switching to a controlled-release formulation or adding a dopamine agonist or amantadine. However, after 15 to 20 years, these effects become hard to suppress. Surgery is then considered.

Other Drugs: Other drugs are generally less effective than levodopa, but they may benefit some people, particularly if levodopa is not tolerated or is insufficient.

Dopamine agonists (such as pramipexole and ropinirole), which mimic the action of dopamine, may be useful at any stage of the disease. Another dopamine agonist, rotigotine, is available as a skin patch. Apomorphine, a quick-acting dopamine agonist injected under the skin (subcutaneously), is used to reverse the off part of levodopa's on-off phenomenon—when movement is difficult to initiate. Thus, this drug is called rescue therapy. It is usually used when people freeze in place, preventing them, for example, from walking. Affected people or another person (such as a family member) can inject the drug up to 5 times a day as needed.

Rasagiline and selegiline belong to a class of drugs called monoamine oxidase inhibitors (MAO inhibitors—see table on page 868). They prevent the breakdown of dopamine, thereby prolonging dopamine's action in the body. If taken with certain foods (such as certain cheeses), beverages (such as red wine), or drugs, MAO inhibitors can have a serious side effect called hypertensive crisis (see table on page 92). However, this effect is unlikely when Parkinson's disease is being treated because the doses used are low and the type of MAO inhibitor used (MAO type B inhibitors) is less likely to have this effect.

Entacapone prevents the breakdown of dopamine and appears to be a useful supplement to levodopa. Tolcapone works similarly to entacapone but is rarely used because it can damage the liver.

Some drugs with anticholinergic effects (see box on page 1897), such as benztropine and trihexyphenidyl, are effective in reducing the severity of a tremor and can be used in the early stages of Parkinson's disease. They can also be used in the later stages to supplement levodopa. These drugs may reduce tremor because they block the action of acetylcholine, and tremor is thought to be caused by an imbalance of acetylcholine (too much) and dopamine (too little). Other drugs with anticholinergic effects, including some antihistamines and tricyclic antidepressants, are mildly effective and may be used to supplement levodopa. However, many anticholinergic effects are troublesome, especially in older people. These effects include confusion, drowsiness, dry mouth, blurred vision, dizziness, constipation, difficulty urinating, and loss of bladder control.

Amantadine, a drug sometimes used to treat influenza, may be used alone to treat mild Parkinson's disease or as a supplement to levodopa. Amantadine probably has many effects that make it work. For example, it probably stimulates nerve cells to release dopamine.

Propranolol, a beta-blocker, may be used to reduce the severity of a tremor.

Deep Brain Stimulation: People with involuntary movements due to long-term use of levodopa may benefit from deep brain stimulation. Tiny electrodes are surgically implanted in part of the basal ganglia. By stimulating this part, deep brain stimulation often greatly reduces the involuntary movements and tremors and shortens the off part of the on-off phenomenon.

Stem Cells: Transplantation of stem cells to treat Parkinson's disease has received much publicity. Theoretically, stem cells, such as those derived from bone marrow or embryos, could be transplanted into the brain and become capable of producing dopamine. However, studies to determine whether this treatment is effective and safe in people will take many years.

Caregiver and End-of-Life Issues: Because Parkinson's disease is progressive, people eventually need help with normal daily activities, such as eating, bathing, dressing, and toileting. Caregivers can benefit from learning about the physical and psychologic effects of Parkinson's disease and about ways to enable people to function as well as possible. Because such care is tiring and stressful, caregivers may benefit from support groups.

Eventually, most people with Parkinson's disease become severely disabled and immobile. They may be unable to eat, even with assistance. Dementia develops in about half the people. Because swallowing becomes increasingly difficult, death due to aspiration pneumonia is a risk. For some people, a nursing home may be the best place for care. Before people with this disease are incapacitated, they should establish advance directives, indicating what kind of medical care they want at the end of life (see page 69).

Parkinsonism

Parkinsonism refers to symptoms of Parkinson's disease (such as slow movements and tremors) that are caused by another condition.

Various conditions can cause parkinsonism:

- Viral encephalitis, a rare brain inflammation that follows a flu-like infection
- Other degenerative disorders, such as dementia, multiple system atrophy, corticobasal ganglionic degeneration, and progressive supranuclear palsy
- Structural brain disorders, such as brain tumors and strokes
- Head injury, particularly the repeated injury that occurs in boxing (making a person punch-drunk)
- Drugs, such as antipsychotics and the antihypertensives methyldopa and reserpine
- Toxins, such as manganese, carbon monoxide, and methanol

Certain drugs and toxins interfere with or block the action of dopamine and other neurotransmitters. For example, antipsychotic drugs, used to treat paranoia and schizophrenia, block dopamine's action. Use of the substance MPTP (which was produced accidentally when illicit drug users tried to synthesize the opioid meperidine) can cause sudden, severe, irreversible parkinsonism in young people.

Symptoms

Parkinsonism causes the same symptoms as Parkinson's disease (see page 771). They include a resting tremor, stiff muscles, slow movements, and difficulty maintaining balance and walking.

The disorders that cause parkinsonism may also cause other symptoms or variations of parkinsonian symptoms, as in the following:

- Prominent memory loss due to dementia
- Symptoms of parkinsonism on only one side of the body due to certain brain tumors
- Low blood pressure and urinary problems due to multiple system atrophy
- Inability to express or understand spoken or written language (aphasia), inability to do simple skilled tasks (apraxia), and inability to associate objects with their usual role or function (agnosia) due to corticobasal ganglionic degeneration

In corticobasal ganglionic degeneration, symptoms begin after age 60. People become immobile after about 5 years, and death typically occurs after about 10 years.

Diagnosis

Doctors ask about previous disorders, exposure to toxins, and use of drugs that could cause parkinsonism. Brain imaging, such as computed tomography (CT) or magnetic resonance imaging (MRI), may be done to look for a structural disorder that may be causing the symptoms.

If the diagnosis is unclear, doctors may give the person levodopa, a drug used to treat Parkinson's disease, to rule out Parkinson's disease. If the drug results in clear improvement, Parkinson's disease is the likely cause.

Treatment

The cause is corrected or treated if possible. If a drug is the cause, stopping the drug may cure the disorder. Symptoms may lessen or disappear if the underlying disorder can be treated. The drugs used to treat Parkinson's disease (such as levodopa) are often not effective in people with parkinsonism but can sometimes offer modest improvement.

Drugs are used if symptoms are bothersome. If the cause is use of antipsychotic drugs, amantadine or a drug with anticholinergic effects, such as benztropine, may relieve symptoms.

The same general measures used to help people with Parkinson's disease maintain mobility and independence are useful (see page 773). For example, people should remain as active as possible, simplify daily tasks, use assistive devices as needed, and take measures to make the home safe (such as removing throw rugs to prevent tripping). Physical and occupational therapists can help people implement these measures. Good nutrition is also important.

Progressive Supranuclear Palsy

Progressive supranuclear palsy is characterized by muscle stiffness (rigidity), inability to move the eyes, weakness of the throat muscles, and a tendency to fall backward.

Progressive supranuclear palsy, which is much rarer than Parkinson's disease, affects many parts of the brain, particularly the basal ganglia and the brain stem. (The basal ganglia help smooth out muscle movements and coordinate changes in posture. The brain stem regulates critical body functions, such as breathing, heart rate, and swallowing, and helps adjust posture.) Brain cells in these areas degenerate, but why they do is unknown.

Symptoms usually begin in late middle age. The first symptom may be difficulty looking up without bending the neck or difficulty climbing up and down stairs. People with the disorder cannot roll their eyes downward, fix their eyes on a stationary object, or follow a moving object. They may have blurred or double vision. The upper eyelids may pull back, producing a look of astonishment. Muscles become rigid, and movements are slow. Walking is unsteady, with a tendency to fall backward. Speaking and swallowing are difficult. Other symptoms include insomnia, agitation, irritability, apathy, and rapid changes in emotion.

In the late stages, depression and dementia are common. Like Parkinson's disease, progressive supranuclear palsy results in severe muscle rigidity and disability, usually within 5 years. Usually, death, often due to infection, occurs within 10 years after symptoms begin.

The diagnosis is based on symptoms. No effective treatment exists. The drugs used to treat Parkinson's disease provide some relief.

Multiple System Atrophy

Multiple system atrophy is a progressive, fatal disorder that makes muscles stiff (rigid) and causes problems with movement, loss of coordination, and malfunction of internal body processes (such as blood pressure and bladder control).

- The parts of the brain that control movements and many internal body processes degenerate.
- Some symptoms resemble those of Parkinson's disease, but internal body processes also malfunction.
- Doctors base the diagnosis on symptoms.
- Simple measures and drugs can help lessen symptoms, but the disorder is progressive and ultimately fatal.

Multiple system atrophy usually begins when people are in their 50s. It affects about twice as many men as women. It results from degeneration of several parts of the brain and spinal cord:

- The basal ganglia (collections of nerve cells at the base of the cerebrum, deep within the brain), which help control voluntary muscle movements by balancing the actions of muscle groups that move the same muscles in opposite ways (for example, a group that bends an arm and a group that straightens the arm)
- The cerebellum, which coordinates voluntary movements (particularly complex movements done simultaneously) and helps maintain balance
- Areas that control the autonomic nervous system, which regulates involuntary body processes, such as how blood pressure changes in response to changes in posture
- Nerve cells that stimulate muscle action (motor neurons) in the cerebellum, basal ganglia, and spinal cord

The cause of the degeneration is unknown. Multiple system atrophy includes three disorders previously thought to be separate disorders:

- Olivopontocerebellar atrophy, which is characterized by symptoms similar to those of Parkinson's disease (called parkinsonism) and difficulty maintaining balance
- Striatonigral degeneration, which is very similar to Parkinson's disease except that levodopa often does not relieve symptoms
- Shy-Drager syndrome, which is characterized by parkinsonism and problems with urination, blood pressure control, and some other internal body processes

Symptoms

Multiple system atrophy is a progressive disorder. Early symptoms vary, depending on which part and how much of the brain is affected first. The disorder causes three groups of symptoms.

Parkinsonism—symptoms that resemble those of Parkinson's disease—may occur early. These symptoms result from degeneration in the basal ganglia. Muscles are stiff (rigid), and movements become slow, shaky, and difficult to initiate. When walking, people may shuffle and not swing their arms. People feel unsteady and off balance, making them more likely to fall. Posture may be stooped. Limbs may tremble jerkily, usually when they are held in one position. But people with multiple system atrophy are less likely to have tremors during rest than people with Parkinson's disease. Articulating words is difficult, and the voice may become high-pitched and quaver.

Loss of coordination may also occur early. It results from degeneration in the cerebellum. People may be unable to control movements of their arms and legs. Consequently, they have difficulty walking and take wide, irregular steps. When reaching for an item, they may reach beyond it. When sitting, they may feel unstable. People may have difficulty focusing their eyes on and following objects. Tasks that require rapidly alternating movements, such as turning a door knob or screwing in a light bulb, also become difficult.

Malfunction of internal body processes, controlled by the autonomic nervous system, may also occur early. Blood pressure may decrease dramatically when a person stands up, causing dizziness, light-headedness, or fainting—a condition called orthostatic hypotension. Blood pressure may increase when a person lies down. People may need to urinate urgently or frequently or may pass urine involuntarily (urinary incontinence). They may have difficulty emptying the bladder (urinary retention). Constipation is common. Vision becomes poor. Men may have difficulty initiating and maintaining an erection (erectile dysfunction).

Other symptoms of autonomic malfunction may occur early or late. Less sweat, tears, and saliva are produced. As a result, people may become intolerant of heat and have dry eyes and mouth. People may have difficulty swallowing and breathing. Breathing may be noisy and high-pitched. During sleep, breathing may stop repeatedly or become inadequate (sleep apnea). People may lose control of bowel movements (fecal incontinence).

Many people are confined to a wheelchair or are otherwise severely disabled within 5 years after symptoms begin. The disorder results in death 9 to 10 years after symptoms begin.

Diagnosis

The diagnosis is based on symptoms. However, symptoms may resemble those of other disorders, making the disorder difficult to diagnose.

The only sure way to diagnose multiple system atrophy is to examine brain tissue after death. Nonetheless, some tests help with the diagnosis. For example, if levodopa relieves parkinsonism, the cause is probably Parkinson's disease. Levodopa has little or no lasting effect on similar symptoms due to multiple system atrophy. Magnetic resonance imaging (MRI) of the brain may help rule out other neurologic disorders. Tests to evaluate the autonomic nervous system may be done. For example, blood pressure may be measured while the person is sitting and after the person stands to check for orthostatic hypotension. The presence of orthostatic hypotension supports the diagnosis of multiple system atrophy.

Treatment

No treatment can cure multiple system atrophy. However, a combination of simple measures and drugs may help relieve symptoms.

- Parkinsonism: Continuing to do as many daily activities as possible helps maintain muscle strength and flexibility. Stretching and exercising regularly may also help. Drugs used to treat Parkinson's disease, such as levodopa plus carbidopa or pergolide, taken by mouth, may be tried, but these drugs usually have little effect or are effective for only a few years.

- Orthostatic hypotension: Measures are taken to stabilize the sudden changes in blood pressure. Consuming more salt and water may increase the volume of blood and thus help increase blood pressure. Standing up slowly may help prevent blood pressure from decreasing too much when a person stands, as may wearing an abdominal binder or compression stockings. These garments help maintain blood pressure by promoting blood flow from the legs to the heart and thus prevent too much blood from staying (pooling) in the legs. Raising the head of the bed by about 4 inches (10 centimeters) can help prevent blood pressure from increasing too much when the person lies down. If blood pressure does increase, an antihypertensive drug (such as propranolol) may be taken at night. Fludrocortisone may be taken by mouth. It helps the body retain salt and water and thus may increase blood pressure as needed when a person stands. Other drugs, such as midodrine or pyridostigmine, taken by mouth, may also help.

- Decreased production of body fluids: If sweating is reduced or absent, people should avoid warm environments to avoid overheating the body. Good dental care and regular check-ups are essential for people with dry mouth. Artificial tears (eye drops containing substances that resemble real tears) applied every few hours may relieve dry eyes.

- Urinary retention: If needed, people can learn to insert a catheter into the bladder themselves. They insert it several times a day. It is inserted through the urethra, allowing urine in the bladder to drain out. People remove the catheter after the bladder is empty. This measure helps prevent the bladder from stretching and urinary tract infections from developing. Washing the hands, cleansing the area around the urethra, and using a sterile or clean catheter also help prevent infections. Inserting a catheter becomes more difficult as coordination deteriorates. Doctors may prescribe bethanechol, which increases the tone of bladder muscles and sometimes makes emptying the bladder easier.

- Urinary incontinence: Oxybutynin or tolterodine, taken by mouth, may be used to relax the muscles of an overactive bladder. If incontinence persists, using a catheter inserted into the bladder may help. Some people learn to insert it themselves.
- Constipation: A high-fiber diet and stool softeners are recommended. If constipation persists, enemas may be necessary.
- Erectile dysfunction: Usually, treatment consists of drugs such as sildenafil, tadalafil, or vardenafil, taken by mouth.

As the disorder progresses, people may need a breathing tube, a feeding tube (usually surgically inserted), or both. Physical, occupational, and speech therapists can teach people ways to compensate when walking, doing daily activites, and speaking become difficult. Social workers can help people find support groups and, when symptoms become disabling, home health care or hospice services.

End-of-Life Issues: Because the disorder is progressive and ultimately fatal, people should prepare advance directives soon after the disorder is diagnosed. These directives should indicate what kind of medical care people want at the end of life (see page 69).

Tics

Tics are rapid, purposeless, repetitive but not rhythmic involuntary movements that are virtually identical to one another. They can be suppressed but only for a short time and only with conscious effort.

- Tics may occur on their own or be caused by a disorder or drug.
- People feel an irresistible urge to blink, grimace, jerk their head, or move in some other way.
- Many tics disappear on their own, but if they are troublesome or severe, mild sedatives or antipsychotic drugs may help.

Tics may be simple or complex. Simple tics, such as excessive blinking, grimacing, or head jerking, may begin as nervous mannerisms. Complex tics, such as those that occur in Tourette's syndrome, often resemble fragments of normal behavior.

Tics, especially simple tics, can occur on their own. Many of these tics begin during childhood and disappear without treatment. Or tics can occur as part of another disorder, such as Huntington's disease, obsessive-compulsive disorder, some infections, or a stroke. Some drugs and toxins cause tics.

Symptoms

Before a tic occurs, people may feel an urge to do the tic. This urge is similar to the need to sneeze or scratch an itch. Tension builds up, usually in the affected body part. When people give in to the tic, they feel relief briefly.

The tic can sometimes be postponed for seconds to minutes, but usually it eventually becomes irresistible. Most people have trouble controlling tics, especially during times of emotional stress. However, some people can suppress some tics, usually with difficulty. Calling attention to a tic, particularly in children, may make the tic worse.

Treatment

For people with a simple tic (particularly children), reassurance is often best, with as little attention paid to the tic as possible.

If tics are particularly troublesome, they can be treated with drugs. For simple tics, benzodiazepines, such as clonazepam and diazepam, may help. These drugs are mild sedatives taken by mouth. Clonidine, a drug used to treat high blood pressure, occasionally helps. It blocks the action of norepinephrine, a neurotransmitter that is thought to contribute to tics. Side effects may include excessively low blood pressure.

For severe tics, antipsychotic drugs may be effective even though psychosis is not the cause of tics (see page 781). Or botulinum toxin can be injected into the aff3ected muscle, paralyzing it and thus preventing the tic.

TOURETTE'S SYNDROME

Tourette's syndrome is a hereditary disorder characterized by simple and complex muscle and vocal tics that occur frequently throughout the day for at least one year.

Tourette's syndrome is common, affecting possibly as many as 1 of 100 people. It is 3 times more common among men than among women. It often begins in early childhood. In most people, symptoms are so mild that the disorder is not recognized.

- The cause is unknown.
- The disorder often begins with simple tics, such as blinking, grimacing, or head jerking, followed by such movements as hitting and kicking and vocal outbursts, including cursing.
- Doctors base the diagnosis on symptoms.
- Drugs may not be needed, but clonidine, mild sedatives, antipsychotics, or botulinum toxin may help.

The cause is unknown but is thought to be an abnormality in dopamine or another brain neurotransmitter (a chemical messenger that nerve cells use to communicate). Genes are involved, but their precise role and the specific genes involved are unknown.

Symptoms

Tourette's syndrome often begins with simple muscle tics, such as grimacing, head jerking, and blinking. Simple tics may be only a nervous habit and may disappear with time. Such tics do not necessarily lead to Tourette's syndrome, which involves more than a simple tic. For example, people with Tourette's syndrome may repeatedly move their head from side to side, blink their eyes, open their mouth, and stretch their neck.

> **? Did You Know...**
>
> Most people with Tourette's syndrome do not randomly shout out obscenities.

The disorder may progress to bursts of complex tics, including vocal tics, hitting, kicking, and sudden, irregular, jerky breathing. Vocal tics may start as grunting, snorting, humming, or barking noises and progress to compulsive, involuntary bouts of cursing. For no apparent reason and often in the midst of conversation, some people with Tourette's syndrome may call out obscenities or words related to feces (called coprolalia). These vocal outbursts are sometimes mistakenly thought to be intentional, especially in children. Although coprolalia is a well-known feature of Tourette's syndrome, at least 85% of people with Tourette's syndrome do not have coprolalia. People may also repeat words immediately after hearing them (called echolalia).

People with Tourette's syndrome often have difficulty functioning and experience considerable anxiety in social situations. In the past, they were shunned, isolated, or even thought to be possessed by the devil. Impulsive, aggressive, and self-destructive behaviors develop in many people, and obsessive-compulsive behavior develops in about half. Children with Tourette's syndrome often have difficulty learning. Many also have attention-deficit/hyperactivity disorder. Whether Tourette's syndrome itself or the extraordinary stresses of living with the disorder cause these problems is unclear.

Diagnosis

The diagnosis is based on symptoms. Early diagnosis can help parents understand that the tics their children have are not voluntary and that punishment cannot stop the tics and may even make them worse.

Treatment

If symptoms are mild, drugs may not be needed.

Simple Tics: Doctors often first try clonidine or guanfacine. Clonidine, a drug used to treat high blood pressure, occasionally helps and is particularly useful in controlling anxiety and obsessive-compulsive behavior. Benzodiazepines, such as clonazepam and diazepam, may help. These drugs are mild sedatives taken by mouth.

Severe Symptoms: Antipsychotic drugs may be used to help suppress the tics, even though psychosis is not the cause. The lowest dose needed to make tics tolerable is used, and doses are decreased as tics lessen. Haloperidol, the most commonly used antipsychotic drug, is effective but is more likely to have side effects than other antipsychotic drugs, such as olanzapine, pimozide, and risperidone.

Side effects of antipsychotics (see table on page 894) may include symptoms similar to those of Parkinson's disease (parkinsonism), restlessness, muscle stiffness, sustained involuntary muscle contractions (dystonias), weight gain, blurred vision, sleepiness, and dulled, slowed thinking. Tardive dyskinesia, which consists of repetitive involuntary movements, may develop and persist even after the drug is stopped. Uncontrollably, the arms or legs writhe, the tongue protrudes, and the lips pucker, purse, and smack. A rare but more serious side effect called neuroleptic malignant syndrome consists of high fever, high blood pressure, muscle damage, and coma.

Injecting botulinum toxin into the muscles producing the tics may decrease the abnormal movements as well as the urge that precedes them. Botulinum, the bacterial toxin that causes botulism, is used to paralyze muscles (and to treat wrinkles).

Deep brain stimulation is considered an experimental treatment for Tourette's syndrome, but it is sometimes done in special centers when the disorder is severe and drugs have been ineffective. Electrodes are placed in the parts of the brain thought to be involved in tics.

Chorea, Athetosis, and Hemiballismus

Chorea is repetitive, brief, jerky, rapid involuntary movements that start in one part of the body and move abruptly, unpredictably, and often continuously to another part. *Athetosis* is a continuous stream of slow, flowing, writhing involuntary movements. *Hemiballismus* is a type of chorea, usually involving violent, flinging involuntary movements of one arm.

- Chorea and athetosis are usually symptoms of another disorder, although chorea may develop on its own in older people or in pregnant women.
- Chorea and athetosis usually cause slow, writhing, and dance-like, jerky movements.

- Hemiballismus is flinging movements of one side of the body, usually the arm.
- For chorea and athetosis, treating the cause may help, as may antipsychotic drugs.

Chorea and athetosis, which may occur together as choreoathetosis, are not disorders. Rather, they are symptoms that can result from several very different disorders. Chorea and athetosis result from overactivity in the basal ganglia, the part of the brain that helps smooth out and coordinate movements initiated by nerve impulses from the brain. In most forms of chorea, an excess of dopamine, the main neurotransmitter used in the basal ganglia, prevents the basal ganglia from functioning normally. Drugs and disorders that increase dopamine levels or increase the sensitivity of nerve cells to dopamine tend to worsen chorea and athetosis.

Chorea and athetosis occur in Huntington's disease, a hereditary degenerative disorder. Chorea may occur in Sydenham's chorea (also called St. Vitus' dance or Sydenham's disease), a complication of rheumatic fever (a childhood infection caused by certain streptococci). Sydenham's chorea is characterized by jerky, uncontrollable movements and can last for several months.

Chorea sometimes develops in older people for no apparent reason. This chorea, called senile chorea, tends to affect the muscles in and around the mouth. Chorea can also affect women during the first 3 months of pregnancy (a condition called chorea gravidarum), but it disappears without treatment shortly after they give birth. Rarely, a similar chorea develops in women taking oral contraceptives. Chorea can also result from lupus (systemic lupus erythematosus), overactivity of the thyroid gland (hyperthyroidism), a tumor or stroke affecting a part of the basal ganglia called the caudate nucleus, and certain drugs such as antipsychotic drugs.

Symptoms

Chorea typically involves the hands, feet, and face. The jerky movements seem to flow from one muscle to the next and may seem dancelike. The movements may merge imperceptibly into purposeful or semipurposeful acts, sometimes making the chorea hard to identify.

Athetosis usually affects the hands and feet. The slow writhing movements often alternate with holding parts of the limbs in certain positions (postures) to produce a continuous, flowing stream of movement.

Hemiballismus affects one side of the body. The arm is affected more often than the leg. It is usually caused by a stroke affecting a small area just below the basal ganglia called the subthalamic nucleus. Hemiballismus may be temporarily disabling be-cause when a person tries to move the limb, it may fling out uncontrollably.

Treatment

Chorea due to hyperthyroidism usually lessens when that disorder is treated. Sydenham's chorea and chorea caused by a stroke often gradually subside without treatment. If chorea is caused by a drug, stopping the drug may help, but the chorea does not always disappear. Pregnant women with chorea may be treated with barbiturates during the pregnancy.

Drugs that block dopamine's action may help control the abnormal movements. These drugs include antipsychotic drugs (see table on page 894), such as fluphenazine, haloperidol, and risperidone. Drugs that reduce the amount of dopamine released, such as reserpine and tetrabenazine, may also help. However, improvement may be limited.

Hemiballismus usually goes away on its own after several days, but it sometimes lasts for 6 to 8 weeks. Antipsychotic drugs may help suppress hemiballismus.

Huntington's Disease

Huntington's disease (Huntington's chorea) is a hereditary disease that begins with occasional involuntary jerking or spasms, then progresses to more pronounced involuntary movements (chorea and athetosis), mental deterioration, and death.

- Part of the brain that smooths and coordinates movements degenerates.
- Movements become slow and uncoordinated, and mental function, including self-control and memory, deteriorates.
- Doctors base the diagnosis on symptoms, family history, imaging of the brain, and gene testing.
- Drugs can help relieve the symptoms, but the disorder is progressive, ultimately ending in death.

Huntington's disease affects fewer than 1 of 10,000 people. It affects both sexes equally. The gene for Huntington's disease is dominant. Therefore, children of a person who has this disease have a 50% chance of developing it (see page 12). Symptoms usually develop subtly, beginning between the ages of 35 and 50 but can develop before adulthood. Huntington's disease is caused by gradual degeneration of small parts of the basal ganglia called the caudate nucleus and corpus striatum. The basal ganglia help smooth out and coordinate movements.

Symptoms

During the early stages of Huntington's disease, people can blend the involuntary abnormal movements into purposeful ones so that the abnormal movements are barely noticeable. However, with time,

Genetic Testing for Huntington's Disease

The genetic mutation that causes Huntington's disease is located on chromosome 4. It involves repetition of a particular section of the genetic code in the DNA.

The gene for Huntington's disease is dominant. Thus, having only one copy of the abnormal gene, inherited from one parent, is sufficient to cause the disease. Almost all people with the disease have only one copy of the abnormal gene. Children of such people have a 50% chance of inheriting the abnormal gene and thus the disease.

People who have a parent or grandparent with Huntington's disease can find out whether they have inherited the gene for the disease by taking a genetic test. For the test, a blood sample is taken and analyzed. Such people may or may not want to know whether they have inherited the gene. This issue should be discussed with an expert in genetic counseling before genetic testing.

the movements become more obvious. People may walk in a lilting or exaggeratedly jaunty way, like a puppet. They may grimace, flick the limbs, and blink more often. Movements become uncoordinated and slow. Eventually, the entire body is affected, making walking, sitting still, eating, speaking, and dressing extremely difficult.

Mental changes frequently occur before or as the abnormal movements develop. These changes are subtle at first. People may gradually become irritable and excitable. They may lose interest in their usual activities. They may be unable to control their impulses, losing their temper, having fits of despondency, or becoming promiscuous. As the disease progresses, people may behave irresponsibly and often wander aimlessly. Over years, they lose their memory and their ability to think rationally. They may become severely depressed and attempt suicide.

In advanced disease, dementia is severe, and people are confined to bed. Full-time assistance or nursing home care is needed. Death usually occurs 13 to 15 years after symptoms begin. The cause is usually pneumonia or coronary artery disease.

Diagnosis

Huntington's disease may be difficult to recognize in the early stages because symptoms are subtle. The disease may be suspected based on symptoms and a family history. Doctors should be told about relatives who have had mental problems or have been diagnosed as having a neurologic or psychiatric disorder (such as Parkinson's disease or schizophrenia) because they may have had Huntington's disease that was not diagnosed. Computed tomography (CT) or magnetic resonance imaging (MRI) is done to check for the degeneration of the basal ganglia characteristic of the disease and to rule out other disorders.

Genetic testing is done to confirm the diagnosis. Genetic testing and counseling are important for people who have a family history of the disease but no symptoms because people are likely to have children before symptoms appear. For such people, genetic counseling should precede genetic testing. They are referred to centers that have expertise in dealing with the complex ethical and psychologic issues involved.

Treatment

As soon as possible after the diagnosis is made, people with Huntington's disease should establish advance directives, indicating what kind of medical care they want at the end of life (see page 69).

No cure exists for Huntington's disease. However, drugs, such as the sedative chlorpromazine, the antipsychotic haloperidol, and the antihypertensive reserpine, can help relieve symptoms and control behavior.

Dystonia

Dystonia is characterized by involuntary sustained muscle contractions that may make people freeze in the middle of an action or make the entire body, the trunk, or another part of the body twist or turn.

- Dystonia may result from a genetic mutation, a disorder, or a drug.
- Spasms occur in the affected part of the body, distorting the position of that body part.
- The cause is corrected if possible, but drugs, such as mild sedatives, levodopa plus carbidopa, and botulinum toxin, may help.

Causes

Dystonia seems to result from overactivity in several areas of the brain—the basal ganglia, thalamus, cerebellum, and cerebral cortex. Dystonia may result from a genetic mutation (called primary dystonia) or from a disorder or drug (called secondary dystonia). Antipsychotic drugs can cause various types of dystonia, including shutting of the eyelids, twisting of the neck (spasmodic torticollis) or back, grimacing, puckering of the lips, protrusion of the tongue, and writhing of the arms or legs.

Types and Symptoms

Dystonias may affect one part (focal dystonias) or several parts (segmental dystonias) of the body.

CAUSES OF DYSTONIAS

TYPE	EXAMPLES
Disorders	Cerebral palsy
	Genetic disorders, such as generalized dystonia and dopa-responsive dystonia
	Multiple sclerosis
	A severe lack of oxygen to the brain (which may occur at birth or later in life)
	Stroke
	Toxicity due to accumulation of certain metals (such as copper in Wilson's disease)
Drugs	Antiemetics (such as metoclopramide and prochlorperazine)
	Antipsychotic drugs (such as chlorpromazine, fluphenazine, haloperidol, and thiothixene)

Sometimes they affect the whole body (generalized dystonias).

Focal and Segmental Dystonias: Dystonias that affect one or several body parts typically start in a person's 30s or 40s and affect women more often. Initially, spasms may occur randomly or only during stress. Certain movements of the affected body part may trigger the spasms, which may disappear during rest. Over days, weeks, or many years, spasms may become more frequent and may continue during rest. Eventually, the affected body part remains distorted, sometimes in a painful position. Severe disability results. The following are examples of focal and segmental dystonias:

- **Blepharospasm:** This dystonia affects mainly the eyelids. The eyelids are repeatedly and involuntarily forced shut. Occasionally, only one eye is affected at first, but ultimately, the other eye is also affected. It usually begins as excessive blinking, eye irritation, or extreme sensitivity to bright light. Many people with blepharospasm find ways to keep their eyes open, such as yawning, singing, or opening the mouth wide. These techniques become less effective as the disorder progresses. Blepharospasm can severely impair vision.

- **Spasmodic torticollis:** Torticollis specifically affects the muscles of the neck. It is one of the most common focal dystonias in adults. The cause is often unknown but, in some cases, is probably genetic. Torticollis can also be caused by drugs that block dopamine, such as haloperidol. Rarely, torticollis is present at birth (called congenital torticollis). In adults, it often begins with a pulling sensation of the neck. The head, neck, and shoulders can twist into a distorted position that persists. Early in the disorder the spasm can sometimes be suppressed with effort. Or people sometimes discover tricks that make the spasm stop temporarily. For example, they may touch their face in a particular spot (usually on the side opposite the twisting).

- **Spasmodic dysphonia:** The muscles of the vocal cords, which control speech, contract involuntarily. Speech may be impossible or may sound strained, quavery, hoarse, whispery, jerky, creaky, staccato, or garbled and be difficult to understand.

- **Occupational dystonias:** These dystonias, also called task-specific dystonias, affect one part of the body and often result from overuse. For example, golfers may have involuntary muscle spasms in the hands and wrists (called the yips). The yips may make putting nearly impossible. What is supposed to be a 3-foot putt can become a 15-foot putt when a golfer loses control because of the yips. Similarly, musicians, especially concert pianists, may have bizarre spasms of the fingers, hands, or arms that prevent them from performing. Musicians who play wind instruments may have spasms of the mouth. Persistent writer's cramp may be dystonia.

- **Meige's disease:** This dystonia combines involuntary blinking with jaw grinding and grimacing. Thus, it is also called blepharospasm-oromandibular dystonia. ("Blepharo" refers to the eyelids, "oro" refers to the mouth, and "mandibular" refers to the jaw.) It usually begins in late middle age.

Generalized Dystonias: Dystonias that affect the whole body include the following:

- **Generalized dystonia:** This rare dystonia, also called idiopathic torsion dystonia, is progressive and often hereditary. In many cases, specific genetic mutations have been identified. The gene most commonly affected is the *DYT1* gene. The resulting dystonia is called DYT1 dystonia. Involuntary movements result in sustained, often bizarre postures. Typically, symptoms begin during childhood, often with turning the foot in during walking. The dystonia may affect only the trunk or a leg but sometimes affects the whole body, ultimately confining children to a wheelchair. When this dystonia develops in adults, it usually begins in the face or arms and usually does not affect other parts of the body. Mental function is not affected.

- **Dopa-responsive dystonia:** This rare form of dystonia is hereditary. Symptoms usually begin during childhood. Typically, one leg is affected first. As a result, children tend to walk on tiptoes. Symptoms worsen at night. Walking becomes progressively more difficult, and both arms and legs are affected. However, some children have only mild symptoms, such as muscle cramps after exercise. Sometimes symptoms appear later in life and resemble those of Parkinson's disease. Movements may be slow, balance may be difficult to maintain, and a tremor may occur in the hands during rest. Symptoms lessen dramatically when people are given low doses of levodopa. If levodopa relieves the symptoms, the diagnosis is confirmed.

Treatment

Correcting or eliminating the cause of dystonia, if known, usually reduces the spasms. For example, drugs used to treat multiple sclerosis may reduce spasms related to that disease. When dystonia is due to use of an antipsychotic drug, promptly taking diphenhydramine by injection or by mouth usually stops the spasms quickly, and the antipsychotic is stopped.

For generalized dystonia, a drug with anticholinergic effects (such as trihexyphenidyl or benztropine) is most commonly used. These drugs reduce spasms by blocking specific nerve impulses involved in causing the spasms. However, anticholinergic effects also include confusion, drowsiness, dry mouth, blurred vision, dizziness, constipation, difficulty urinating, loss of bladder control, and tremor, which are troublesome, especially in older people. A benzodiazepine (a mild sedative) such as clonazepam, baclofen (a muscle relaxant), or both are also usually given. Baclofen may be given by mouth or by a pump implanted in the spinal canal. If generalized dystonia is severe or does not respond to drugs, tiny electrodes may be surgically implanted in the basal ganglia (a procedure called deep brain stimulation).

? **Did You Know...**

Drugs used to treat nausea or psychosis sometimes cause abnormal sustained muscle contractions (dystonias).

Botulinum toxin, also used to treat facial wrinkles, is used to treat some dystonias.

Some people, especially children with dopa-responsive dystonia, improve dramatically when they are treated with levodopa plus carbidopa.

If one or a few body parts are affected, botulinum toxin (a bacterial toxin used to paralyze muscles or to treat wrinkles) is injected into the overactive muscles. Botulinum weakens the muscle contraction but does not affect the nerves. These injections are particularly useful for blepharospasm and spasmodic torticollis.

Physical therapy helps some people, especially those who are treated with botulinum.

Coordination Disorders

Coordination disorders result from malfunction of the cerebellum, the part of the brain that coordinates voluntary movements.

- The cerebellum malfunctions, causing loss of coordination.
- Often, people cannot control their arms and legs, making them take wide, unsteady steps when they walk.
- Doctors base the diagnosis on symptoms, family history, and magnetic resonance imaging of the brain.
- The cause is corrected if possible, and if it cannot be, treatment focuses on relieving symptoms.

The cerebellum is the part of the brain most involved in coordinating sequences of movements. It also controls balance and posture. Anything that damages the cerebellum can lead to loss of coordination (ataxia).

Prolonged, excessive alcohol use permanently damages the cerebellum and is the leading cause of coordination disorders. Less commonly, other disorders, such as an underactive thyroid gland (hypothyroidism), vitamin E deficiency, and brain tumors, cause coordination disorders. Some hereditary disorders, such as Friedrich's ataxia, cause loss of coordination. Certain drugs (such as anticonvulsants), especially when they are given in high doses, can cause coordination disorders. In such cases, the disorder may disappear when the drug is stopped.

Symptoms

People with ataxia cannot control the position of their arms and legs or their posture. Thus, when they walk, they take wide steps and stagger and make broad, zigzag movements with their arms.

Coordination disorders can cause other abnormalities, such as the following:

- Dysmetria: People cannot control the range of body movements. For example, in attempting to reach for an object, people with dysmetria may reach beyond the object.
- Dysarthria: Speech is slurred, and fluctuations in volume cannot be controlled because speech muscles

are uncoordinated. Movement of the muscles around the mouth may be exaggerated.

- Scanning speech: People speak in a monotone with staccato-like hesitation.
- Nystagmus: When glancing at an object, the eyes may overshoot their target, and nystagmus may occur. In nystagmus, the eyes repeatedly move rapidly in one direction, then drift slowly back to their original position.
- Tremor: Damage to the cerebellum can also cause a tremor when people end a purposeful movement or try to reach a target (intention tremor) or when people try to hold their body in a certain position (postural tremor). Muscle tone may decrease.

Friedreich's Ataxia: In this progressive disorder, walking becomes unsteady between the ages of 5 and 15. Then arm movements become uncoordinated, and speech becomes slurred and hard to understand. Many children with the disorder are born with a clubfoot, curved spine (scoliosis), or both. People with Friedreich's ataxia cannot sense vibrations, cannot sense where their arms and legs are (lose their position sense), and no longer have reflexes. Mental function may deteriorate. Tremor, if present, is slight.

> **? Did You Know...**
> The most common cause of coordination disorders is prolonged, excessive alcohol use.

By their late 20s, people with this disorder may be confined to a wheelchair. Death, often due to an abnormal heart rhythm or heart failure, usually occurs by middle age.

Diagnosis and Treatment

The diagnosis is based on symptoms. Doctors also ask about relatives who have had similar symptoms (family history) and about conditions that could cause the symptoms. Magnetic resonance imaging (MRI) of the brain is usually done. Genetic testing is done if people may have a family history of coordination disorders. If possible, the cause is eliminated or treated. For example, if the coordination disorder is due to use of alcohol, alcohol is stopped. If the disorder is caused by a high dose of a drug (such as phenytoin), the dose is reduced. Some underlying disorders, such as hypothyroidism and vitamin E deficiency, can be treated. Surgery may help some people with brain tumors. For hereditary coordination disorders, there is no cure. In such cases, treatment focuses on relieving symptoms.

CAUSES OF COORDINATION DISORDERS

TYPE	EXAMPLES
Brain disorders	Birth defects of the brain
	Bleeding (hemorrhage) in the brain
	Brain tumors, particularly in children
	Head injuries (repeated)
	Strokes
Hereditary disorders	Spinocerebellar ataxias
	Friedreich's ataxia
	Ataxia-telangiectasia
Other disorders	Heatstroke or extremely high fever
	Multiple sclerosis
	Multiple system atrophy
	Underactive thyroid gland (hypothyroidism)
	Vitamin E deficiency
Drugs and toxic substances	Alcohol use (excessive and prolonged)
	Anticonvulsants such as phenytoin, particularly at high doses
	Carbon monoxide
	Heavy metals such as mercury or lead

Fragile X–Associated Tremor/ Ataxia Syndrome

Fragile X–associated tremor/ataxia syndrome is a genetic disorder that affects mostly men and causes tremor, loss of coordination, and dementia.

- The disorder results from a genetic mutation.
- In men over 50, tremors in the hands develop first, followed by loss of coordination, slowed movements, decreased facial expression, and sometimes memory loss.
- Genetic testing can confirm the diagnosis.
- Drugs used to treat Parkinson's disease can often relieve the tremors.

Fragile X–associated tremor/ataxia syndrome, a newly recognized disorder, may affect as many as 1 of 3,000 men over 50.

Fragile X-associated tremor/ataxia syndrome results from a less extensive abnormality (called a premutation) in a gene on the X chromosome (men have an X and a Y chromosome, and women have 2 X chromosomes). A more extensive (full) mutation in this gene causes fragile X syndrome (which causes mental retardation) in children. People with the premutation are considered carriers. Men with the premutation pass it to their daughters (but not to their sons). Most women with the premutation are unaffected and thus may unknowingly pass the gene on to their sons (grandsons of affected men). Children of such a woman have a 50% chance of inheriting the premutation. When the premutation is passed from mother to child, it sometimes changes into a full mutation, causing fragile X syndrome in the child.

> **? Did You Know...**
> Some cases of Alzheimer's disease or Parkinson's disease are actually a newly recognized disorder called fragile X–associated tremor/ataxia syndrome.

About 30% of men with the premutation and fewer than 5% of women with the premutation develop fragile X–associated tremor/ataxia syndrome as adults. The risk of developing the disorder increases as people age.

Symptoms

Symptoms usually develop later in life. The first symptom is often tremors in the hands, typically when people try to do a task. Other symptoms include loss of coordination, slow movements, stiffness, and decreased facial expression.

People may have problems remembering recent events and solving problems. They may think more slowly. These problems often progress to dementia. People may also have personality changes. They may become depressed, anxious, impatient, hostile, and moody.

Sensation in the feet may be lost. Internal organs may malfunction. Affected people may feel lightheaded when they stand because blood pressure does not increase as it normally does (called orthostatic hypotension). They may have to urinate more frequently. Eventually, they may lose control of the bladder and bowel movements.

After symptoms appear, people may live from about 5 to 25 years.

In women with the premutation, symptoms are usually less severe, possibly because they have another X chromosome, which seems to protect against the effects of the X chromosome with the premutation. Also, women with the premutation are more likely to have early menopause, infertility, and ovarian dysfunction than women without it.

Diagnosis and Treatment

Because this disorder is newly recognized, the diagnosis is sometimes missed or mistaken for disorders that cause similar symptoms, such as Parkinson's disease or Alzheimer's disease.

Genetic testing can confirm the diagnosis. Magnetic resonance imaging (MRI) may be done to check for characteristic abnormalities in the brain.

Grandfathers of children with fragile X syndrome should be asked whether they have symptoms suggesting fragile X–associated tremor/ataxia syndrome. Daughters and grandsons of affected men should have genetic counseling. They can be tested for the premutation so that they can make decisions about whether or not to have children and whether or not to have prenatal testing if pregnancy occurs.

Tremors can often be relieved by many of the drugs used to control tremors due to Parkinson's disease (see table on page 774).

CHAPTER

120 Multiple Sclerosis and Related Disorders

Most nerve fibers inside and outside the brain are wrapped with many layers of tissue composed of a fat (lipoprotein) called myelin. These layers form the myelin sheath. Much like the insulation around an electrical wire, the myelin sheath enables electrical impulses to be conducted along the nerve fiber with speed and accuracy. When the myelin sheath is damaged, nerves do not conduct electrical impulses normally. Sometimes the nerve fibers are also damaged.

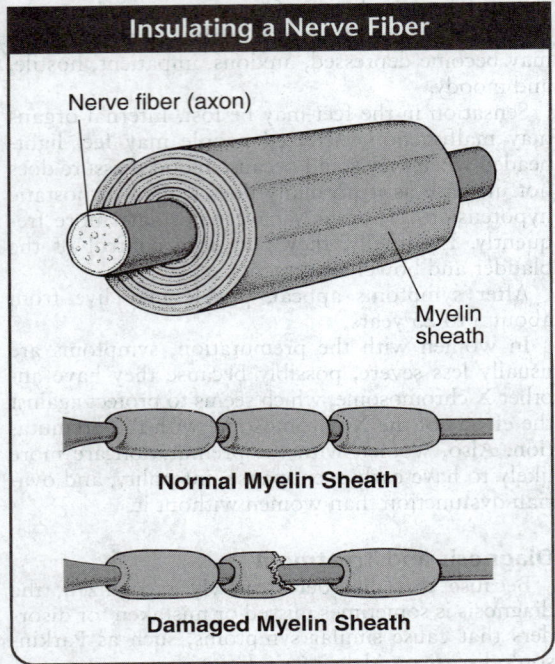

Insulating a Nerve Fiber

Nerve fiber (axon)

Myelin sheath

Normal Myelin Sheath

Damaged Myelin Sheath

When babies are born, many of their nerves lack mature myelin sheaths. As a result, their movements are jerky, uncoordinated, and awkward. As myelin sheaths develop, movements become smoother, more purposeful, and more coordinated. Myelin sheaths do not develop normally in children with certain rare hereditary diseases, such as Tay-Sachs disease, Niemann-Pick disease, Gaucher's disease, and Hurler's syndrome. These children may have permanent, often extensive, neurologic problems.

In adults, the myelin sheath can be destroyed by stroke, inflammation, immune disorders, metabolic disorders, and nutritional deficiencies (such as a lack of vitamin B_{12}). Such destruction is called demyelination. Poisons, drugs (such as the antibiotic ethambutol), and excessive use of alcohol can damage or destroy the myelin sheath. If the sheath is able to repair and regenerate itself, normal nerve function may return. However, if the sheath is severely damaged, the underlying nerve fiber can die. Because nerve fibers in the central nervous system (brain and spinal cord) rarely regenerate, such damage is irreversible.

Some disorders that cause demyelination affect mainly the central nervous system. Others affect mainly nerves in other parts of the body. Disorders that cause demyelination in the central nervous system and have no known cause are called primary demyelinating disorders. Multiple sclerosis is the most common of these disorders.

Multiple Sclerosis

In multiple sclerosis, patches of myelin and underlying nerve fibers in the eyes, brain, and spinal cord are damaged or destroyed.

- The cause is unknown but may involve an attack by the immune system against the body's own tissues (autoimmune reaction).
- Usually, periods of relatively good health alternate with episodes of worsening symptoms.
- People may have vision problems and abnormal sensations, and movements may be weak and clumsy.
- Usually, doctors base the diagnosis on symptoms and results of a physical examination and magnetic resonance imaging.
- Treatment includes corticosteroids, drugs that help keep the immune system from attacking the body, and drugs to relieve symptoms.
- Often, the disorder slowly worsens, disabling some people, but life span is unaffected unless the disorder is very severe.

The term "multiple sclerosis" refers to the many areas of scarring (sclerosis) that result from destruction of the tissues that wrap around nerves (myelin sheath). This destruction is called demyelination. Sometimes the nerve fibers that send messages (axons) are also damaged. Over time, the brain may shrink in size because axons are destroyed.

In the United States, about 400,000 people, mostly young adults, have multiple sclerosis. Most commonly, it begins between the ages of 20 and 40. It is more common among women. Most people have periods of relatively good health (remissions) alternating with periods of worsening symptoms (flare-ups or relapses). Relapses can be mild or debilitating. Recovery during remission is good but incomplete. Thus, the disorder worsens slowly over time.

Causes

The cause is unknown, but a likely explanation is that people are exposed early in life to a virus (possibly a herpesvirus or retrovirus) or some unknown substance that somehow triggers the immune system to attack the body's own tissues (autoimmune reaction—see page 1124). The autoimmune reaction results in inflammation, destruction of myelin, and damage to the myelin sheath and the underlying nerve fiber.

Heredity seems to have a role in multiple sclerosis. About 5% of people with the disorder have a brother or sister who is affected, and about 15% have a close relative who is affected. Also, multiple sclerosis is more likely to develop in people with certain genetic markers on the surface of their cells called human leukocyte antigens (see page 1099). These markers help the body to distinguish self from nonself and thus know which substances to attack.

Environment also has a role in multiple sclerosis. Where people spend the first 15 years of life affects their chance of developing multiple sclerosis. It occurs in 1 of 2,000 people who grow up in a temperate climate but in only 1 of 10,000 people who grow up in a tropical climate. Multiple sclerosis almost never occurs in people who grow up near the equator. These differences may be related to vitamin D levels. When the skin is exposed to sunlight, the body forms vitamin D. Thus, people who grow up in temperate climates may have a lower vitamin D level. People with a low level of vitamin D are more likely to develop multiple sclerosis. But how vitamin D may protect against the disorder is unknown. The climate in which later years are spent does not change the chances of developing the disorder.

Cigarette smoking also appears to increase the chances of developing the disorder. The reason is unknown.

> ### ? Did You Know...
> Nerves are covered with tissues that, like insulation around an electric wire, help the nerve conduct impulses.

Symptoms

Symptoms vary greatly, from person to person and from time to time in one person, depending on which nerve fibers are demyelinated. If nerve fibers that carry sensory information become demyelinated, problems with sensations (sensory symptoms) result. If nerve fibers that carry signals to muscles become demyelinated, problems with movement (motor symptoms) result. Symptoms often come and go, affecting one or several parts of the body. The fluctuating symptoms result from damage to myelin sheaths, followed by repair, followed by more damage. Symptoms may become more severe when people are exposed to high temperatures, such as in very warm weather, a hot bath or shower, or during a fever.

Multiple sclerosis may progress and regress unpredictably. However, there are several patterns of symptoms:

- **Relapsing-remitting pattern:** Relapses (when symptoms worsen) alternate with remissions (when symptoms are stable). Remissions may last months

COMMON SYMPTOMS OF MULTIPLE SCLEROSIS	
PART OF THE BODY	**EXAMPLES**
Nerves (affecting sensation)	Numbness Tingling A reduced sense of touch Pain or burning Itching
Eyes	Double vision Partial blindness and pain in one eye Dim or blurred vision Inability to see when looking straight ahead Uncoordinated eye movements
Genital organs	Difficulty reaching orgasm Lack of sensation in the vagina In men, impotence
Muscles and coordination	Weakness and clumsiness Difficulty walking or maintaining balance Tremor Uncoordinated movements Stiffness, unsteadiness, and unusual fatigue
Intestine and bladder	Problems controlling urination and bowel movements Constipation
Mood	Mood swings Inappropriate elation or giddiness Depression Inability to control emotions (for example, crying or laughing without reason)
Brain	Subtle or obvious mental impairment Memory loss Poor judgment Inattention
Other	Dizziness or vertigo

or years. Relapses can occur spontaneously or can be triggered by an infection such as influenza.

- **Primary progressive pattern:** The disease progresses gradually with no remissions or obvious relapses, although there may be temporary plateaus during which the disease does not progress.

- **Secondary progressive pattern:** This pattern begins with relapses alternating with remissions, followed by gradual progression of the disease.
- **Progressive relapsing pattern:** The disease progresses gradually, but progression is interrupted by sudden relapses. This pattern is rare.

Vague symptoms of demyelination in the brain sometimes begin long before the disorder is diagnosed. For example, tingling, numbness, pain, burning, and itching may occur in the arms, legs, trunk, or face. The sense of touch may be reduced. People may lose strength or dexterity in a leg or hand, which may become stiff.

Vision may become dim or blurred. Mainly, people lose the ability to see when looking straight ahead (central vision). Peripheral (side) vision is less affected. In some people, one eye becomes weaker than the other, causing double vision when looking from one side to the other. This disorder is called internuclear ophthalmoplegia. The stronger eye may move involuntarily, rapidly and repetitively moving in one direction, then slowly drifting back (a symptom called nystagmus). Partial blindness may develop in one eye, and pain occurs when the eye is moved. These symptoms result from inflammation of the optic nerve (optic neuritis). Some people with multiple sclerosis have only optic neuritis.

When the back part of the spinal cord in the neck is affected, bending the neck forward may cause an electrical shock or a tingling sensation that shoots down the back, down both legs, down one arm, or down one side of the body (a response called Lhermitte's sign). Usually, the sensation lasts only a moment and disappears when the neck is straightened. Often, it is felt as long as the neck remains bent.

As the disorder progresses, movements may become shaky, irregular, and ineffective. People may become partially or completely paralyzed. Weak muscles may contract involuntarily (called spasticity), sometimes causing painful cramps. Muscle weakness and spasticity may interfere with walking, eventually making it impossible, even with a walker or another assistive device. Speech may become slow, slurred, and hesitant.

Late in the disorder, dementia and mania (excessive elation) may develop. The nerves that control urination or bowel movements can be affected, leading to frequent and strong urges to urinate, retention of urine, constipation, and, occasionally, urinary and fecal incontinence. If relapses become more frequent, people become increasingly disabled, sometimes permanently.

Diagnosis

Because symptoms vary widely, doctors may not recognize the disorder in its early stages. Doctors suspect multiple sclerosis in younger people who suddenly develop blurred vision, double vision, or movement problems and abnormal sensations in various unrelated parts of the body. Fluctuating symptoms and a pattern of relapses and remissions support the diagnosis.

When doctors suspect multiple sclerosis, they thoroughly evaluate the nervous system during a physical examination (see page 630). They examine the back of the eye (retina) with an ophthalmoscope (see art on page 1422). The optic disk (the spot where the optic nerve joins the retina) may be inflamed or unusually pale, indicating inflammation of the optic nerve.

Magnetic resonance imaging (MRI) is the best imaging test for detecting multiple sclerosis. It usually detects areas of demyelination in the brain and spinal cord. Before MRI, doctors may inject gadolinium, a paramagnetic contrast agent, into the bloodstream. Gadolinium helps distinguish areas of recent demyelination and active inflammation from areas of long-standing demyelination.

The diagnosis may be clear based on the physical examination and MRI. If not, other tests are done to obtain additional information:

- **Spinal tap (lumbar puncture):** A sample of cerebrospinal fluid is removed (see page 635). The protein content of the fluid may be higher than normal. The concentration of antibodies may be high, and a specific pattern of antibodies is detected in up to 90% of people with multiple sclerosis.
- **Evoked responses:** For this test, sensory stimuli, such as flashing lights, are used to activate certain areas of the brain, and the brain's electrical responses are recorded (see page 636). In people with multiple sclerosis, the brain's response to stimuli may be slow because signal conduction along demyelinated nerve fibers is impaired. This test can also detect slight damage to the optic nerve.

Other tests can help doctors distinguish multiple sclerosis from disorders that cause similar symptoms, such as AIDS, vasculitis, arthritis of the neck, Guillain-Barré syndrome, hereditary ataxias, lupus, Lyme disease, rupture of a spinal disk, syphilis, and a cyst in the spinal cord (syringomyelia). For example, blood tests may be done to rule out Lyme disease, syphilis, and lupus, and imaging tests can help rule out arthritis of the neck, rupture of a spinal disk, and syringomyelia.

Prognosis

What effects multiple sclerosis has and how quickly it progresses vary greatly and unpredictably. Remissions can last months up to 10 years or more. However, some people, particularly men who develop the disorder during middle age, have frequent attacks and are rapidly incapacitated. Nonetheless, about 75% of people who have multiple sclerosis never need a wheelchair, and for about 40%, normal activities are not disrupted. Unless the disorder is very severe, life span is usually unaffected.

> **? Did You Know...**
>
> Spending the first 15 years of life in a temperate (rather than tropical) climate increases the risk of multiple sclerosis.
>
> Three fourths of people with multiple sclerosis never need a wheelchair.

Treatment

No treatment for multiple sclerosis is uniformly effective. Corticosteroids are most commonly used. They probably work by suppressing the immune system. They are given for short periods to relieve immediate symptoms. For example, prednisone may be taken by mouth, or methylprednisolone may be given intravenously. Although corticosteroids may shorten relapses and slow the progression of multiple sclerosis, they do not stop its progression.

Corticosteroids are rarely used for a long time because they can have many side effects, such as increased susceptibility to infection, diabetes, weight gain, fatigue, decreased bone density (osteoporosis), and ulcers. Corticosteroids are started and stopped as needed.

Other drugs that help keep the immune system from attacking myelin sheaths are usually used. They include the following:

- Interferon-beta injections reduce the frequency of relapses and may help prevent or delay disability.
- Glatiramer acetate injections may have similar benefits for people with early mild multiple sclerosis.
- Mitoxantrone, a chemotherapy drug, can reduce the frequency of relapses and slow the progression of the disorder. It is given for only up to 2 years and only when other drugs do not work because it can eventually lead to heart damage.
- Natalizumab is an antibody given intravenously as an infusion once a month. It is more effective than other drugs in reducing the number of relapses and preventing further damage in the brain. However, natalizumab may increase the risk of a rare, fatal infection of the brain and spinal cord (progressive multifocal leukoencephalopathy). Natalizumab is used only by specially trained doctors, and people who take it must be checked periodically for signs of progressive multifocal leukoencephalopathy.
- Immune globulin, given intravenously once a month, occasionally helps when other drugs have been ineffective.

Plasmapheresis is recommended by some experts for severe relapses not controlled by corticosteroids. However, the benefits of plasmapheresis have not been established. For this treatment, blood is withdrawn, abnormal antibodies are removed from it, and the blood is returned to the person (see box on page 1030).

Other drugs can be used to relieve or control specific symptoms:

- Muscle spasms: The muscle relaxants baclofen or tizanidine
- Urinary incontinence: Oxybutynin, bethanechol, or tamsulosin
- Pain due to abnormalities in nerves: The anticonvulsant gabapentin or sometimes tricyclic antidepressants (such as amitriptyline), the anticonvulsant carbamazepine, or opioids
- Tremors: The beta-blocker propranolol
- Fatigue: Amantadine (used to treat Parkinson's disease) or, less often, modafinil (used to treat excessive sleepiness)
- Depression: Antidepressants such as sertraline or amitriptyline, counseling, or both

People with multiple sclerosis can often maintain an active lifestyle, although they may tire easily and may not be able to keep up with a demanding schedule. Regular exercise such as riding a stationary bicycle, walking, swimming, or stretching reduces spasticity and helps maintain cardiovascular, muscular, and psychologic health. Physical therapy can help with maintaining balance, the ability to walk, and range of motion and can help reduce spasticity and weakness. People should walk on their own for as long as possible. Doing so improves their quality of life and helps prevent depression. Avoiding high temperatures—for example, by not taking hot baths or showers—can help because heat can worsen symptoms. People who smoke should stop. Taking vitamin D supplements helps prevent osteoporosis or slow its progression and may help slow the progression of multiple sclerosis.

People with urine retention can learn to catheterize themselves and empty the bladder, and those with constipation can take stool softeners or laxatives regularly. People who become weak and unable to move easily may develop pressure sores, so they and their caregivers must take extra care to prevent the sores.

If people are disabled, occupational therapists and social workers can help with rehabilitation.

Other Primary Demyelinating Diseases

Acute Disseminated Encephalomyelitis: Also called parainfectious or postinfectious encephalomyelitis, this rare type of inflammation leads to demyelination of nerves in the brain and spinal cord. (Demyelination is the destruction of the tissues that wrap around nerves, called the myelin sheath.)

This disorder usually develops after a viral infection. Acute disseminated encephalomyelitis is thought to be a misguided immune reaction triggered by the virus. In the United States, this disorder usually results from some types of influenza, hepatitis A or B, or infection with enteroviruses, Epstein-Barr virus, or human immunodeficiency virus (HIV). Measles, chickenpox, and rubella used to be common causes before childhood vaccination became widespread.

Typically, the inflammation develops 1 to 3 weeks after the viral illness begins. It can be treated with corticosteroids given intravenously. Guillain-Barré syndrome (see page 828) seems to be a similar disorder of the peripheral nerves.

Adrenoleukodystrophy and Adrenomyeloneuropathy: Both are rare hereditary metabolic disorders. Adrenoleukodystrophy affects young boys, usually between the ages of 4 and 8. A milder, more slowly developing form of the disorder can begin in adults in their 20s or 30s. Adrenomyeloneuropathy affects adolescent boys.

In these disorders, widespread demyelination is accompanied by adrenal gland dysfunction. Boys have behavioral problems and problems with hearing and vision. Eventually, mental deterioration, involuntary and uncoordinated muscle contractions (spasticity), and blindness occur.

No cure for either disorder is known. Dietary supplements with glycerol trioleate and glycerol trierucate (known as Lorenzo's oil) have not been shown to slow the progression of the disease. Bone marrow transplantation is an experimental treatment.

Leber's Hereditary Optic Neuropathy: This disorder causes demyelination leading to partial blindness. The disorder is more common among men. Usually, symptoms begin between the ages of 15 and 35. This disorder is inherited through the mother, and the defective genes seem to be located in mitochondria (structures in cells that provide energy for the cell).

No treatments are available. But limiting consumption of alcohol, which may affect the mitochondria, and not using tobacco products may help.

Tropical Spastic Paraparesis: Also called HTLV-associated myelopathy (see page 806), this disorder causes demyelination in the spinal cord and results from infection with the human T-cell lymphotropic virus (HTLV). The disorder worsens over several years. Gradually, the legs become weak and muscle spasms occur—a condition called spastic weakness. Frequent, strong urges to urinate, urinary incontinence, and bowel dysfunction also develop.

No cure is available, but corticosteroids may help, as may interferon-beta or immune globulin given intravenously (these drugs help prevent the immune system from attacking myelin sheaths). Muscle relaxants such as baclofen or tizanidine help relieve spasms.

Neuromyelitis Optica: Also called Devic disease, this disorder causes symptoms similar to those of multiple sclerosis and used to be considered a variant of multiple sclerosis. However, neuromyelitis optica typically affects only the eyes and the spinal cord, and multiple sclerosis also affects the brain.

Neuromyelitis optica causes inflammation of the optic nerve (optic neuritis). One or both eyes may be affected. The disorder causes episodes of eye pain and dim, blurred, or lost vision. Days to weeks (sometimes years) later, the limbs are affected. People may temporarily lose sensation, and the arms and legs may become weak and sometimes paralyzed. People may be unable to control bladder and bowel function.

In some people, the part of the spinal cord that controls breathing is inflamed, leading to difficulty breathing, which is life threatening.

The disorder progresses differently in each person. As the disorder progresses, people may have brief, frequent, painful muscle spasms. Eventually, blindness, loss of sensation and muscle weakness in the limbs, and bladder and bowel dysfunction may become permanent.

To diagnose the disorder, doctors evaluate the nervous system (neurologic examination) during a physical examination (see page 630). The optic nerve is examined with an ophthalmoscope (see art on page 1422). Tests include magnetic resonance imaging (MRI) and a blood test to detect specific antibodies in people with neuromyelitis optica.

There is no cure. However treatments can stop episodes, control symptoms, and prevent episodes from recurring. A corticosteroid (such as methylprednisolone) and a drug that suppresses the immune system (an immunosuppressant, such as azathioprine) are often used to stop and prevent episodes. Rituximab, a relatively new drug, may be used to reduce the number of abnormal antibodies and to control disorder. Plasma exchange (plasmapheresis) may help people who do not respond to corticosteroids. For this treatment, blood is removed, then abnormal antibodies are removed, and the blood is returned to the person.

Treatment of symptoms is similar to that for multiple sclerosis (see page 791). Baclofen or tizanidine may relieve muscle spasms.

CHAPTER
121 Spinal Cord Disorders

- Causes of spinal cord disorders include injuries, infections, a blocked blood supply, and compression by a fractured bone or a tumor.
- Typically, muscles are weak or paralyzed, sensation is abnormal or lost, and controlling bladder and bowel function may be difficult.
- Doctors base the diagnosis on symptoms and results of a physical examination and imaging tests, such as magnetic resonance imaging.
- The condition causing the spinal cord disorder is corrected if possible.
- Often, rehabilitation is needed to recover as much function as possible.

The spinal cord is the main pathway of communication between the brain and the rest of the body. It is a long, fragile, tubelike structure that extends downward from the base of the brain. The cord is protected by the back bones (vertebrae) of the spine (spinal column). The vertebrae are separated and cushioned by disks made of cartilage.

The spine is divided into four sections, and each section is referred to by a letter.

- Cervical (C): Neck
- Thoracic (T): Chest
- Lumbar (L): Lower back
- Sacral (S): Pelvis

Within each section of the spine, the vertebrae are numbered beginning at the top. These labels (letter plus a number) are used to indicate locations (levels) in the spinal cord.

Along the length of the spinal cord, 31 pairs of spinal nerves emerge through spaces between the vertebrae. Each spinal nerve runs from a specific vertebra in the spinal cord to a specific area of the body. Based on this fact, the skin's surface has been divided into areas called dermatomes. A dermatome is an area of skin whose sensory nerves all come from a single spinal nerve root. Loss of sensation in a particular dermatome enables doctors to locate where the spinal cord is damaged.

A spinal nerve has two nerve roots. The only exception is the first spinal nerve, which has no sensory root. The root in the front (the motor or anterior root) contains nerve fibers that carry impulses (signals) from the spinal cord to muscles to stimulate muscle movement (contraction). The root in the back (the sensory or posterior root) contains nerve fibers that carry sensory information about touch, position, pain, and temperature from the body to the spinal cord.

The spinal cord ends in the lower back (around L1 or L2), but the lower spinal nerve roots continue, forming a bundle that resembles a horse's tail (called the cauda equina).

The spinal cord is highly organized (see art on page 626). The center of the cord consists of gray matter shaped like a butterfly. The front "wings" (anterior or motor horns) contain nerve cells that carry signals from the brain or spinal cord through the motor root to muscles. The back (posterior or sensory) horns contain nerve cells that receive signals about pain, temperature, and other sensory information through the sensory root from nerve cells outside the spinal cord.

The outer part of the spinal cord consists of white matter that contains pathways of nerve fibers (called tracts or columns). Each tract carries a specific type of nerve signal either going to the brain (ascending tracts) or from the brain (descending tracts).

Causes

Some spinal cord disorders originate outside the cord. They include injuries, most infections (see page 749), blockage of the blood supply, and compression. The spinal cord may be compressed by bone (which may result from cervical spondylosis or a fracture), an accumulation of blood (hematoma), a tumor, a localized collection of pus (abscess), or a ruptured or herniated disk.

> **? Did You Know...**
> Doctors can often tell where the spinal cord is damaged based on symptoms and results of a physical examination.

Less commonly, spinal cord disorders originate in the cord. They include fluid-filled cavities (syrinxes), inflammation (as occurs in acute transverse myelitis), tumors, abscesses, bleeding (hemorrhage), infection with the human immunodeficiency virus (HIV), multiple sclerosis, and syphilis.

Symptoms

Because of the way the spinal cord functions and is organized, damage to the cord often produces specific

Where Is the Spinal Cord Damaged?

The spine (spinal column) contains the spinal cord, which is divided into four sections: cervical (neck), thoracic (chest), lumbar (lower back), and sacral (pelvis). Each section is referred to by a letter (C, T, L, or S). The vertebrae in each section of the spine are numbered beginning at the top. For example, the first vertebra in the cervical spine is labeled C1, the second in the cervical spine is C2, the second in the thoracic spine is T2, the fourth in the lumbar spine is L4, and so forth. These labels are also used to identify specific locations (called levels) in the spinal cord.

Nerves run from a specific level of the spinal cord to a specific area of the body. By noting where a person has weakness, paralysis, sensory loss, or other loss of function, a neurologist can determine where the spinal cord is damaged.

Effects of Spinal Injury

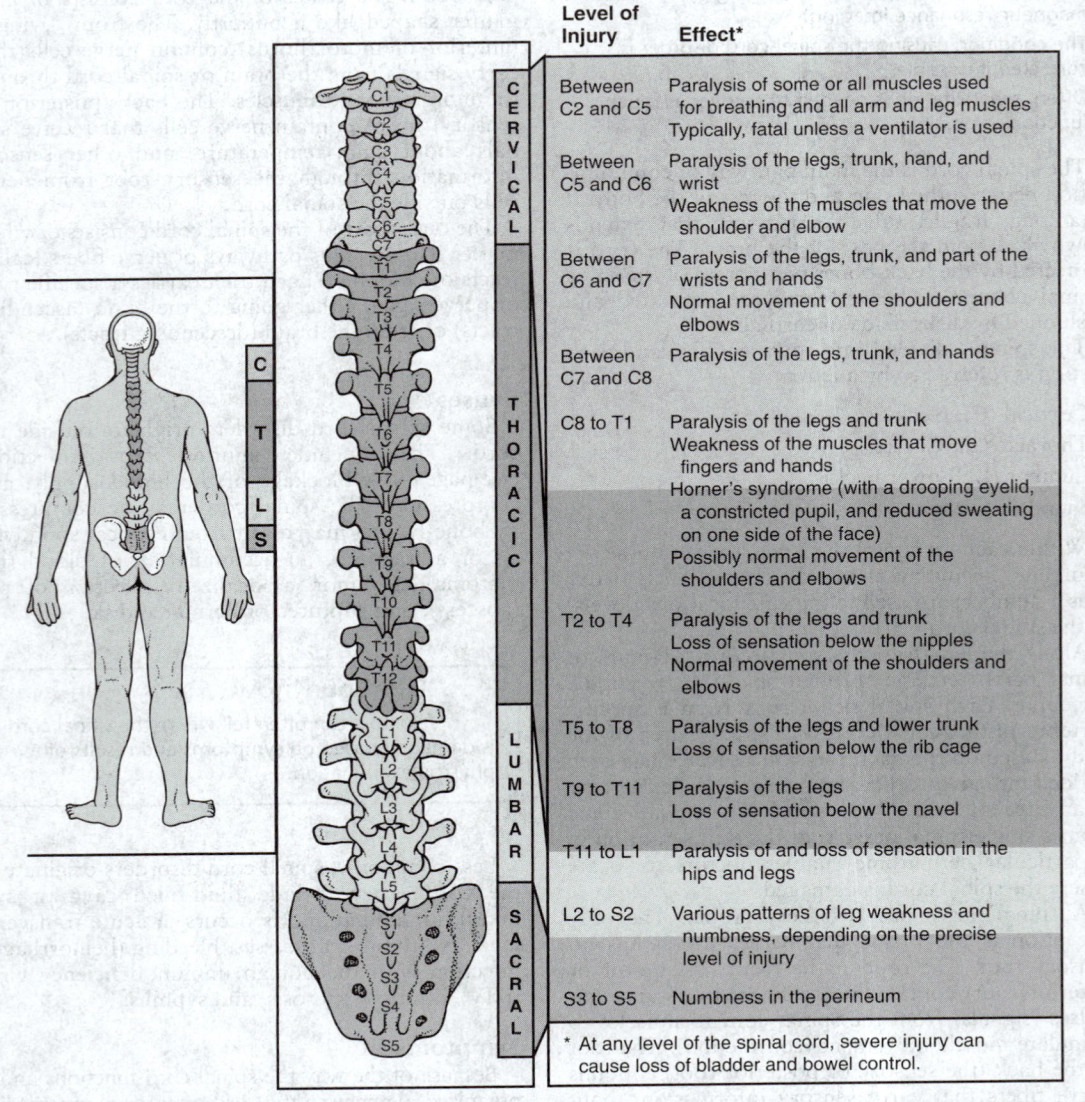

Level of Injury	Effect*
Between C2 and C5	Paralysis of some or all muscles used for breathing and all arm and leg muscles Typically, fatal unless a ventilator is used
Between C5 and C6	Paralysis of the legs, trunk, hand, and wrist Weakness of the muscles that move the shoulder and elbow
Between C6 and C7	Paralysis of the legs, trunk, and part of the wrists and hands Normal movement of the shoulders and elbows
Between C7 and C8	Paralysis of the legs, trunk, and hands
C8 to T1	Paralysis of the legs and trunk Weakness of the muscles that move fingers and hands Horner's syndrome (with a drooping eyelid, a constricted pupil, and reduced sweating on one side of the face) Possibly normal movement of the shoulders and elbows
T2 to T4	Paralysis of the legs and trunk Loss of sensation below the nipples Normal movement of the shoulders and elbows
T5 to T8	Paralysis of the legs and lower trunk Loss of sensation below the rib cage
T9 to T11	Paralysis of the legs Loss of sensation below the navel
T11 to L1	Paralysis of and loss of sensation in the hips and legs
L2 to S2	Various patterns of leg weakness and numbness, depending on the precise level of injury
S3 to S5	Numbness in the perineum

* At any level of the spinal cord, severe injury can cause loss of bladder and bowel control.

patterns of symptoms based on where the damage occurred. The following may occur in various patterns:

- Weakness
- Loss of sensation (such as the ability to feel a light touch, pain, temperature, or vibration)
- Changes in reflexes
- Loss of bladder control (urinary incontinence)
- Loss of bowel control (fecal incontinence)
- Erectile dysfunction
- Paralysis
- Back pain

By identifying which functions are lost, doctors can tell which part of the spinal cord (such as the front, back, or entire cord) is damaged. By identifying the specific location of symptoms (for example, which muscles are paralyzed and which parts of the body lack sensation), doctors can determine exactly where the spinal cord is damaged (that is, the specific level of damage).

Functions may be completely or partially lost. Functions controlled by areas above the damage are not affected.

When weakness or paralysis occurs, muscles often go limp (flaccid), losing their tone. But some disorders (such as injuries and hereditary spastic paraparesis) can cause paralysis with muscle spasms (called spastic paralysis). Spasms can occur because signals from the brain cannot pass through the damaged area to help control some reflexes. As a result, the reflexes become more pronounced over days to weeks. Then, the muscles controlled by the reflex may tighten, feel hard, and twitch uncontrollably from time to time.

> ### Did You Know...
> Nerves from the lowest parts of the spinal cord go to the anus, not to the feet.

Diagnosis

Often, doctors can recognize a spinal cord disorder based on its characteristic pattern of symptoms. Doctors always do a physical examination, which provides clues to the diagnosis. An imaging test is done to confirm the diagnosis and determine the cause.

Magnetic resonance imaging (MRI) is the most accurate imaging test for spinal cord disorders. MRI shows the spinal cord, as well as abnormalities in the soft tissues around the cord (such as abscesses, hematomas, tumors, and ruptured disks) and in

bone (such as tumors, fractures, and cervical spondylosis). If MRI is not available, myelography with computed tomography (CT) is used. For myelography, a radiopaque dye is injected into the fluid around the spinal cord, and x-rays are taken. It is not as accurate or as safe as MRI.

>
> ### Did You Know...
> People who suddenly lose sensation, experience weakness in one or more limbs, or develop incontinence should see a doctor immediately.

Treatment

If symptoms of spinal cord dysfunction (such as paralysis or loss of sensation) suddenly occur, people should see a doctor immediately. Sometimes doing so can prevent permanent nerve damage or paralysis. If possible, the cause is treated or corrected. However, such treatment is often impossible or unsuccessful.

People who are paralyzed or confined to bed because of a spinal cord disorder require skilled nursing care to prevent complications, which include the following:

- Pressure sores: Nurses inspect the person's skin daily, keep the skin dry and clean, and turn the person frequently (see page 1300). When necessary, a special bed called a Stryker frame is used. It can be turned to shift pressure on the body from front to back and from side to side.
- Urinary problems: If a person is immobile and cannot use a toilet, a urinary catheter may be needed. To help reduce the risk of a urinary tract infection, nurses use sterile techniques when the catheter is inserted and apply antimicrobial ointments or solutions daily.
- Pneumonia: To reduce the risk of pneumonia, therapists and nurses may teach the person deep breathing exercises. They may also place the person at an angle to help drain secretions that accumulate in the lungs (postural drainage) or suction secretions out.
- Blood clots: Anticoagulant drugs, such as heparin or low molecular weight heparin, may be given by injection. If a person cannot take anticoagulants (for example, because of a bleeding disorder or stomach ulcers), a filter, sometimes called an umbrella (see art on page 436), is inserted into the inferior vena cava (the large vein that carries blood from the abdomen to the heart). The filter traps blood clots that have broken loose from leg veins before they reach the heart.

Dermatomes

The surface of the skin is divided into specific areas, called dermatomes. A dermatome is an area of skin whose sensory nerves all come from a single spinal nerve root.

Spinal roots come in pairs—one of each pair on each side of the body. There are 8 pairs of sensory nerve roots for the 7 cervical vertebrae. Each of the 12 thoracic, 5 lumbar, and 5 sacral vertebrae has one pair of spinal nerve roots. In addition, at the end of the spinal cord, there is a pair of coccygeal nerve roots, which supply a small area of the skin around the tailbone (coccyx). There are dermatomes for each of these nerve roots.

Sensory information from a specific dermatome is carried by sensory nerve fibers to the spinal nerve root of a specific vertebra. For example, sensory information from a strip of skin along the lower back, the outside of the thigh, the inside of the lower leg, and the heel is carried by sensory nerve fibers of the sciatic nerve to the fifth lumbar vertebra (L5) nerve root.

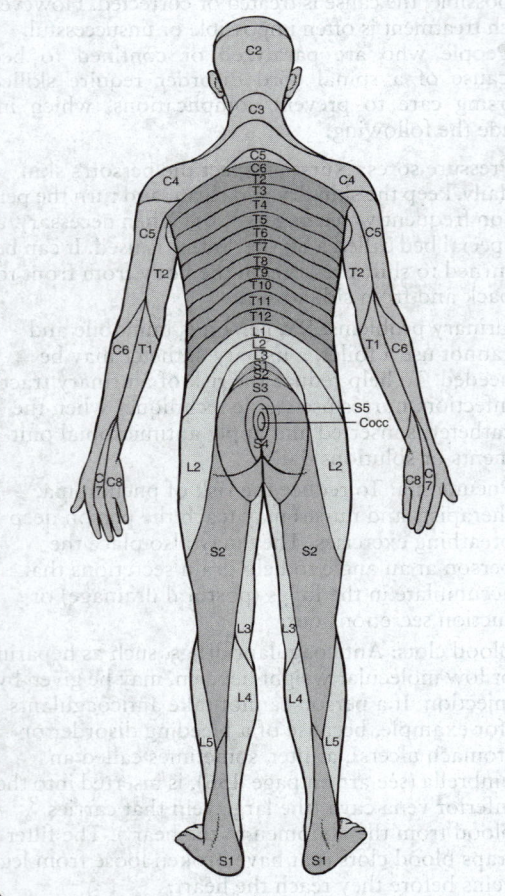

Extensive loss of body functions can be devastating, causing depression and loss of self-esteem. Formal counseling can be very helpful. Learning exactly what has happened and what to expect in the near and distant future helps people cope with the loss and prepare them for rehabilitation.

Rehabilitation: Rehabilitation helps people recover as much function as possible. The best care is provided by a team that includes nurses, physical and occupational therapists (see page 53), a social worker, a nutritionist, a psychologist, and a counselor, as well as the person and family members. A nurse may teach the person ways to manage bladder and bowel dysfunction, such as how to insert a catheter, when to use laxatives, or how to stimulate bowel movements using a finger.

Physical therapy involves exercises for muscle strengthening and stretching. People may learn how to use assistive devices such as braces, a walker, or a wheelchair and how to manage muscle spasms. Occupational therapy helps people relearn how to do their daily tasks and helps them improve dexterity and coordination. They learn special techniques to help compensate for lost functions. Therapists or counselors help some people make the adjustments needed to return to work and to hobbies and activities. People are taught ways to deal with sexual dysfunction. Sex is still possible for many people, even though sensation is usually lost.

Emotional support from family members and close friends is important.

Injuries of the Spinal Cord and Vertebrae

- Most spinal cord injuries result from motor vehicle accidents.
- Symptoms, such as loss of sensation and loss of muscle control, may be temporary or permanent.
- Magnetic resonance imaging or computed tomography is the best way to identify the injury.
- Treatment involves immobilization of the spine, drugs to relieve symptoms, sometimes surgery, and usually rehabilitation.

Injuries may affect the spinal cord or the roots of the spinal nerves, which pass through the spaces between the back bones (vertebrae) of the spine. The bundle of nerves that extend downward from the spinal cord (cauda equina) may also be injured. Injuries of the spinal cord include the following:

- Jarring by a blunt injury (such as a fall or a collision)
- Pressure (compression) by broken bones, swelling, or an accumulation of blood (hematoma)
- Partial or complete tears (severing)

To and From and Up and Down the Spinal Cord

Spinal nerves carry nerve impulses to and from the spinal cord through two nerve roots:

- **Motor (anterior) root:** Located toward the front, this root carries impulses from the spinal cord to muscles to stimulate muscle movement.
- **Sensory (posterior) root:** Located toward the back, this root carries sensory information about touch, position, pain, and temperature from the body to the spinal cord.

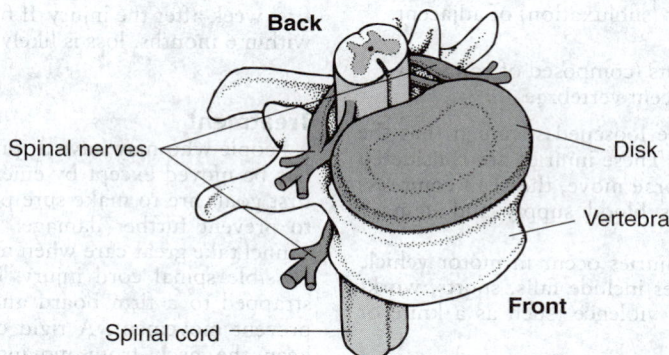

In the center of the spinal cord, a butterfly-shaped area of gray matter helps relay impulses to and from spinal nerves. Its "wings" are called horns.

- **Motor (anterior) horns:** These horns contain nerve cells that carry signals from the brain or spinal cord through the motor root to muscles.
- **Posterior (sensory) horns:** These horns contain nerve cells that receive signals about pain, temperature, and other sensory information through the sensory root from nerve cells outside the spinal cord.

Impulses travel up (to the brain) or down (from the brain) the spinal cord through distinct pathways (tracts). Each tract carries a different type of nerve signal either going to or from the brain. The following are examples:

- **Lateral spinothalamic tract:** Signals about pain and temperature, received by the sensory horn, travel through this tract to the brain.
- **Dorsal columns:** Signals about the position of the arms and legs, received by the sensory horn, travel through these tracts to the brain.
- **Corticospinal tracts:** Signals to move a muscle travel from the brain through these tracts to the motor horn, which routes them to the muscle.

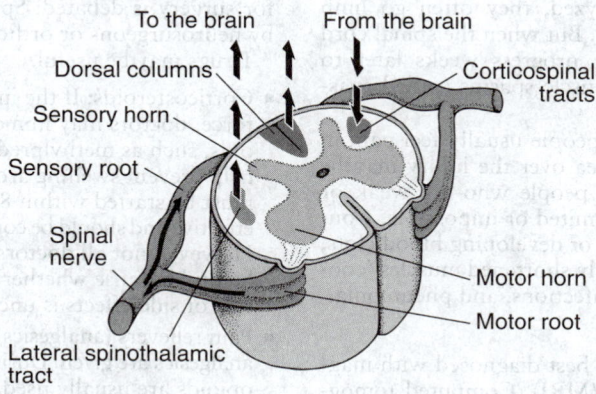

Because the spinal cord is surrounded and protected by the spine, injuries of the spine or its connective tissue (such as disks and ligaments—see art on page 807) can also injure the spinal cord. Such injuries include the following:

- Fractures
- Complete separation (dislocation) of adjacent vertebrae
- Partial misalignment (subluxation) of adjacent vertebrae
- Loosened attachments (composed of connective tissue) between adjacent vertebrae

Attachments may be loosened so much that the vertebrae move freely. These injuries are considered unstable. When vertebrae move, they can compress the spinal cord or its blood supply and damage spinal nerve roots.

Most spinal cord injuries occur in motor vehicle accidents. Other causes include falls, sports, work-related accidents, and violence (such as a knife or gunshot wound).

Symptoms

If the spinal cord is injured, the nerves at and below the site of the injury malfunction, causing loss of muscle control and loss of sensation.

Loss of muscle control or sensation may be temporary or permanent, partial or total, depending on the severity of the injury. An injury that severs the cord or destroys nerve pathways in the spinal cord causes permanent loss, but a blunt injury that jars the cord may cause temporary loss, which can last days, weeks, or months. Sometimes swelling causes symptoms that suggest an injury more severe than it is, but the symptoms usually lessen as the swelling subsides.

Partial loss of muscle control results in muscle weakness. Paralysis usually refers to complete loss. When muscles are paralyzed, they often go limp (flaccid), losing their tone. But when the spinal cord is injured, paralysis may progress weeks later to involuntary, prolonged muscle spasms (called spastic paralysis).

If the spine is injured, people usually feel pain in the neck or back. The area over the injury may be tender to the touch. For people who are weak or paralyzed, movement is limited or impossible. Consequently, they are at risk of developing blood clots, pressure sores, permanently shortened muscles (contractures), urinary tract infections, and pneumonia.

Diagnosis

Spinal cord injuries are best diagnosed with magnetic resonance imaging (MRI). Computed tomography (CT) is an alternative.

Injuries of the spine (affecting bone) are diagnosed most accurately with CT. However, x-rays are sometimes done first because they may be more readily available than CT.

Prognosis

Recovery is more likely if paralysis is partial and if movement or sensation starts to return during the first week after the injury. If function is not regained within 6 months, loss is likely to be permanent.

Treatment

People who may have a spinal cord injury should not be moved except by emergency personnel. The first goals are to make sure people can breathe and to prevent further damage. Thus, emergency personnel take great care when moving a person with a possible spinal cord injury. Usually, the person is strapped to a firm board and carefully padded to prevent movement. A rigid collar may be used to keep the neck from moving. When the spine is severely damaged, the vertebrae may no longer be held in place or may be broken, making the spine unstable. Thus, even slight movement of the injured person can cause the spine to shift, putting pressure on the spinal cord. Pressure on the cord increases the risk of permanent paralysis.

Surgery is needed to remove blood and bone fragments if they have accumulated around the spinal cord. If the spine is unstable, people are kept immobile until the bone and other tissues have had time to heal. Sometimes a surgeon implants steel rods to stabilize the spine so that it cannot move and cause additional injury. If an injury causes only partial loss of function, surgery done soon after the injury may enable people to recover more function and become mobile sooner. However, the best time for surgery is debated. Spinal surgery may be done by neurosurgeons or orthopedic surgeons.

Drugs may be useful.

- Corticosteroids: If the injury is caused by a blunt force, doctors may immediately give corticosteroids, such as methylprednisolone, by injection to help prevent swelling around the injury. The drugs must be started within 8 hours of the injury to be effective and should be continued for about 24 hours. However, not all doctors think corticosteroids are helpful because whether the benefit outweighs the risk of side effects is unclear.
- Pain relievers (analgesics): If the injury causes pain, analgesics are given. During the first hours and days, opioids are usually used. Milder analgesics, such as acetaminophen or ibuprofen, may be used later.

- Muscle relaxants: If muscle spasms develop, muscle relaxants, such as baclofen or tizanidine, may be used.

Experimental treatments to stimulate growth of spinal nerves are being studied. For example, a certain type of white blood cell (macrophage) can be extracted from, then injected into the injured person. Experimental drugs can be injected into the space around the spinal cord (epidurally) or taken by mouth. Using stem cells is another possibility, but this treatment requires much more study.

Rehabilitation, including physical and occupational therapy, can help people recover more quickly or more completely (see page 53).

Compression of the Spinal Cord

Injuries and disorders can put pressure on the spinal cord, causing back pain, tingling, muscle weakness, and other symptoms.

- The spinal cord may be compressed by bone, blood (hematomas), pus (abscesses), tumors, or a ruptured or herniated disk.
- Symptoms, such as back pain, abnormal sensations, muscle weakness, or impaired bladder and bowel control, may be mild or severe.
- Doctors base the diagnosis on symptoms and the results of a physical examination, magnetic resonance imaging, or another imaging test.
- Depending on the cause, surgery or a corticosteroid drug is used to relieve the pressure.

Normally, the spinal cord is protected by the spine, but certain injuries and disorders may put pressure (compress) on the spinal cord, disrupting its normal function. These injuries and disorders may also compress the roots of spinal nerves, which pass through the spaces between the back bones (vertebrae), or the bundle of nerves that extend downward from the spinal cord (cauda equina).

The spinal cord may be compressed suddenly, causing symptoms in minutes or over a few hours or days, or slowly, causing symptoms that worsen over many weeks or months.

Causes

The spinal cord may be compressed by the following:

- Bone: If the back bones (vertebrae) are broken (fractured), are dislocated, or grow abnormally (as occurs in cervical spondylosis), they may compress the spinal cord. Vertebrae that are weakened by cancer or osteoporosis may break after a slight or even no injury.
- Connective tissue: Connective tissue, such as ligaments, can compress the spinal cord after a severe spinal injury.
- An accumulation of blood (hematoma): Blood may accumulate in or around the spinal cord. The most common cause of a spinal hematoma is an injury, but many other conditions can cause hematomas. They include abnormal connections between blood vessels (arteriovenous malformations), tumors, bleeding disorders, and use of anticoagulants (which interfere with blood clotting) or thrombolytic drugs (which break up blood clots).
- Tumors: Cancer that has spread (metastasized) to the spine or the space around the spinal cord is a common cause of compression. Rarely, a tumor within the spine causes compression.
- A localized collection of pus (abscess): Less commonly, pus accumulates in or around the spinal cord and compresses it.
- A ruptured or herniated disk: A herniated disk can compress spinal nerve roots (the part of spinal nerves next to the spinal cord) and occasionally the spinal cord itself.

Sometimes the cauda equina syndrome results in compression of the spinal cord.

Sudden compression usually results from an injury, which often causes a fracture or dislocation of a vertebra. Gradual compression may result from cancer or cervical spondylosis, but bones weakened gradually (for example, by cancer or osteoporosis) may suddenly fracture, which can suddenly worsen compression. Hematomas, abscesses, and ruptured disks can cause sudden compression but often cause compression gradually over days to weeks. The most common cause of slowly developing compression (over months to years) is cervical spondylosis (degeneration of disks and vertebrae in the neck—see page 801).

Symptoms

Slight compression may cause mild symptoms if it disrupts only some nerve impulses going up and down the spinal cord. These symptoms may include discomfort or pain in the back, slight muscle weakness, tingling, other changes in sensation, and, in men, difficulty initiating and maintaining an erection (erectile dysfunction). Pain may radiate down a leg, sometimes to the foot. If the cause is cancer, an abscess, or a hematoma, the back may be tender to the touch in the affected area. Sometimes sensation is lost. Reflexes, including the urge to urinate, may

What Is the Cauda Equina Syndrome?

A bundle of nerves extends downward from the bottom of the spinal cord, through the lower vertebrae and over the sacrum (the bone at the base of the spine). This bundle is called the cauda equina, which means horse's tail in Latin, because that is what the bundle looks like. The cauda equina may be compressed by a ruptured or herniated disk, a tumor, an abscess, damage due to an injury, or swelling due to inflammation (as occurs in ankylosing spondylitis). The symptoms that result are called the cauda equina syndrome.

Pain is felt in the lower back, but sensation is reduced in the buttocks, thighs, bladder, and rectum—the area of the body that would touch a saddle. Thus, this condition is called saddle anesthesia. Sensation and muscle control may be impaired in the lower legs. Other symptoms may occur:

- Reduced sexual response, including erectile dysfunction in men
- Retention of urine
- Loss of bladder control (urinary incontinence)
- Loss of bowel control (fecal incontinence)
- Loss of reflexes in the ankle

People who have the cauda equina syndrome require immediate medical attention. Surgery to relieve the compression must be done as soon as possible. Corticosteroids may be given to reduce swelling.

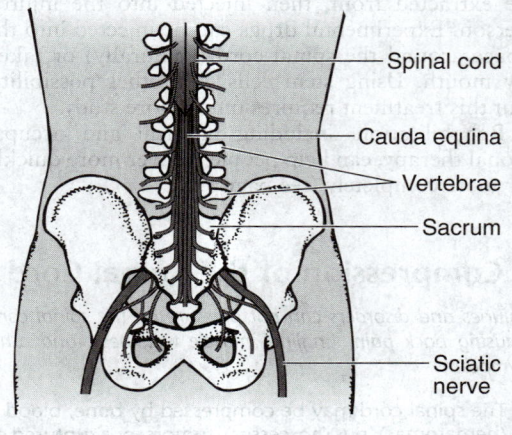

Spinal cord

Cauda equina

Vertebrae

Sacrum

Sciatic nerve

be exaggerated, sometimes causing muscle spasms and increased sweating. If compression increases, symptoms may worsen.

Substantial compression may block most nerve impulses, causing severe muscle weakness, numbness, retention of urine, and loss of bladder and bowel control. If all nerve impulses are blocked, paralysis and complete loss of sensation result. A beltlike band of discomfort may be felt at the level of spinal cord compression. Once compression begins to cause symptoms, the damage usually worsens from minimal to substantial unpredictably but rapidly in a few hours to a few days.

Diagnosis

People with symptoms suggesting spinal cord compression require immediate medical attention because prompt diagnosis and treatment may reverse or lessen loss of function.

Because the spinal cord is organized in a specific way, doctors can determine which part of the spinal cord is affected based on the symptoms and results of a physical examination. For example, if the legs (but not the arms) are weak and numb and bladder and bowel functions are impaired, the spine may be damaged at the midchest (thoracic) level. The location of pain or tenderness along the spine also helps doctors determine the site of the damage.

Magnetic resonance imaging (MRI) is done immediately. Or if MRI is unavailable, myelography (x-ray of the spinal column after injection of a radiopaque dye) with computed tomography (CT) is done. These tests usually show where the spinal cord is compressed and may indicate the cause. MRI or myelography with CT can detect a fracture or dislocation of a vertebra, a herniated disk, an abnormal bone growth, an area of bleeding, an abscess, or a tumor. During myelography, a spinal tap (lumbar puncture) is done to inject a small amount of radiopaque dye into the space around the cord. Thus, doctors can determine whether compression completely blocks the normal flow of cerebrospinal fluid through this space.

If the cause is thought to be a fracture or dislocation due to injury, x-rays may also be taken. They provide information quickly, enabling doctors to quickly evaluate the problem.

The cause of the compression is confirmed during surgery to relieve the pressure on the spinal cord.

If surgery is not done immediately and if MRI or myelography with CT detects an unidentifiable abnormal mass causing compression, a biopsy is done instead of surgery to identify it. Guided by CT, doctors insert a needle into the abnormal mass.

Treatment

If loss of function is partial or very recent (usually when compression occurs suddenly), the compression must be relieved immediately. When compression is detected and treated quickly, before nerve pathways are destroyed, treatment can prevent permanent damage to the spinal cord, and function is usually completely recovered. Surgery is typically needed to relieve compression. Surgery may also be needed to insert steel rods and thus stabilize the spine.

Other treatment varies depending on the cause.

For certain disorders, high doses of corticosteroids, such as dexamethasone or methylprednisolone, are given intravenously as soon as possible. These disorders include tumors if the cause is unknown and possibly blunt injuries. Corticosteroids can reduce swelling in or around the spinal cord, which may be contributing to compression. If an abscess causes symptoms of spinal cord dysfunction (such as paralysis and loss of bowel or bladder control), a neurosurgeon surgically removes the abscess as soon as possible. Antibiotics are also given. If symptoms of spinal cord dysfunction have not developed, drawing the pus out through a needle, giving antibiotics, or both may be all that is needed.

If the cause is a hematoma, the accumulated blood is surgically drained immediately. People who have a bleeding disorder or who are taking anticoagulants are given injections of vitamin K and transfusions of plasma to eliminate or reduce the tendency to bleed.

If the cause is cancer, treatment usually includes surgery, radiation therapy, or both.

Cervical Spondylosis

Cervical spondylosis is degeneration of the disks and vertebrae in the neck, putting pressure on (compressing) the spinal cord in the neck.

- Osteoarthritis is the usual cause.
- The first symptoms are often an unsteady, jerky walk and pain and loss of flexibility in the neck.
- Magnetic resonance imaging or computed tomography can confirm the diagnosis.
- Treatment includes a soft neck collar, nonsteroidal anti-inflammatory drugs, muscle relaxants, and sometimes surgery.

Cervical spondylosis usually affects middle-aged and older people. It is the most common cause of spinal cord dysfunction among people older than 55.

As people age, osteoarthritis becomes more common. It causes vertebrae in the neck to degenerate.

When bone in the vertebrae attempts to repair itself, it overgrows, producing abnormal outgrowths of bone (spurs) and narrowing the spinal canal in the neck. (The spinal canal is the passageway that runs through the center of the spine and contains the spinal cord.) The disks between vertebrae also degenerate, decreasing the cushioning that otherwise protects the spinal cord. As a result, the spinal cord may be compressed, causing dysfunction. Some people are born with a narrow spinal canal. In them, compression due to spondylosis may be more severe.

Often, the spinal nerve roots (the part of spinal nerves located next to the cord (see art on page 626) are also compressed.

Occasionally in people with osteoarthritis, flexing the neck causes one vertebra to slip over the vertebra next to it (a disorder called spondylolisthesis). As a result, the spinal canal is suddenly narrowed, and each time the neck moves, the spinal cord is slightly but repeatedly injured.

? Did You Know...

Cervical spondylosis is the most common cause of spinal cord problems in people over 55.

Symptoms

Symptoms may result from compression of the spinal cord, the spinal nerve roots, or both.

If the spinal cord is compressed, a change in walking is usually the first sign. Leg movements may become jerky (spastic), and walking becomes unsteady. Sensation may be decreased in the feet and hands. The neck may be painful and become less flexible. Reflexes may be increased, sometimes causing muscle spasms, particularly in the legs. Coughing, sneezing, and other movements of the neck may worsen symptoms. Sometimes the hands are affected more than the legs and feet. If severe, compression may impair bladder and bowel function.

If spinal nerve roots are compressed, the neck is usually painful, and the pain often radiates to the head, shoulders, or arms. Muscles in one or both arms may become weak and waste away, making the arms limp. Reflexes in the arms may be decreased.

Diagnosis

Doctors suspect cervical spondylosis based on symptoms, especially in older people or in people who have osteoarthritis. Magnetic resonance imaging (MRI) or computed tomography (CT) can confirm the diagnosis. MRI provides much more information because it shows the spinal cord and roots. CT does not. However, both procedures show where the spinal canal is narrowed, how compressed the spinal cord is, and which spinal nerve roots may be affected.

Treatment

Without treatment, symptoms of spinal cord dysfunction due to cervical spondylosis sometimes lessen or stabilize, but they may worsen.

Initially, especially if only nerve roots are compressed, a soft neck collar, nonsteroidal anti-inflammatory drugs (NSAIDs) such as ibuprofen, and muscle relaxants such as methocarbamol may provide relief.

If the spinal cord is compressed, surgery is usually needed. An incision may be made through the front of the neck (anterior cervical fusion) or back of the neck (posterior laminectomy). Part of the affected vertebrae is removed to make more room for the spinal cord. Bone spurs, if present, are removed, and the spine may be stabilized by fusing the vertebrae together. As a rule, surgery does not reverse the existing nerve damage, but it prevents additional nerve damage. The earlier the surgery, the better is the outcome.

Because the spine may be unstable after surgery, people may need to wear a rigid brace to hold the head still while healing occurs.

If muscle spasms occur, baclofen, a muscle relaxant, helps relieve them.

Syrinx

A syrinx is a fluid-filled cavity that develops in the spinal cord (called a syringomyelia), in the brain stem (called a syringobulbia), or in both.

- Syrinxes may be present at birth or develop later because of an injury or a tumor.
- People become less sensitive to pain and temperature and experience weakness in the hands and legs, or they may have vertigo and problems with eye movements, taste, and speech.
- Magnetic resonance imaging with a contrast agent can detect a syrinx.
- Surgery to drain the syrinx may be done, but it may not correct the problem.

Syrinxes are rare. In about half of the people who have a syrinx, it is present at birth, and then for poorly understood reasons, it enlarges during the teen or young adult years. Often, children who have a syrinx at birth also have other structural abnormalities of the brain, spinal cord, or junction between the skull and spine. Usually, syrinxes that develop later in life are due to injuries or tumors. About 30% of tumors that originate in the spinal cord eventually produce a syrinx.

Syrinxes that grow in the spinal cord press on it from within. They tend to first affect nerve fibers that carry information about pain and temperature from the body to the brain. Later, they affect fibers that carry signals from the brain to stimulate muscle movement. Syrinxes can occur anywhere along the length of the spinal cord. But they often begin in the neck and may extend downward to affect the entire cord. Syrinxes that extend into or begin in the lower part of the brain stem may compress pathways of the spinal cord and cranial nerves (which lead directly from the brain to other parts of the head and neck).

Symptoms

Symptoms usually begin subtly between adolescence and about age 45.

Syrinxes in the neck often make people less sensitive to pain and temperature, particularly in the arms, upper back, lower neck, and hands. Thus, cuts and burns on the arms and hands are common. People may not recognize this decreased sensitivity for years. As a syrinx expands and lengthens, it can cause weakness and atrophy, usually beginning in the hands and later causing weakness and spasms in the legs. Symptoms may be more severe on one side of the body.

Syrinxes in the brain stem can cause vertigo, nystagmus (rapid movement of the eyes in one direction followed by a slower drift back to the original position), loss of sensation in the face (on one or both sides), loss of taste, difficulty speaking, hoarseness, difficulty swallowing, and weakness and wasting away (atrophy) of the tongue.

Diagnosis

Doctors may suspect a syrinx in a young child or teenager who has typical symptoms. Magnetic resonance imaging (MRI) with a paramagnetic contrast agent, such as gadolinium, can outline the syrinx (and a tumor if present).

Treatment

A neurosurgeon may make a hole in a syrinx to drain it and prevent it from expanding, but surgery does not always correct the problem. Even if the syrinx is drained, the nervous system may already be damaged irreversibly. Symptoms may not be relieved, or the syrinx may recur.

Disorders that contributed to or caused the syrinx (such as structural abnormalities or spinal tumors) are corrected when possible.

Hereditary Spastic Paraparesis

Hereditary spastic paraparesis is a rare hereditary disorder that causes gradual weakness with muscle spasms (spastic weakness) in the legs.

- People have exaggerated reflexes, cramps, and spasms, making walking difficult.
- Doctors look for other family members who have the disorder, rule out disorders that can cause similar symptoms, and may do genetic tests.
- Treatment includes physical therapy, exercise, and drugs to reduce spasticity.

Hereditary (familial) spastic paraparesis affects both sexes and may begin at any age. It affects about 3 of 100,000 people. Usually, the gene for this disorder is dominant (see page 12). Therefore, children of a person with the disorder have a 50% chance of developing it. This disorder has several forms. All forms cause degeneration of the nerve pathways that carry signals from the brain down the spinal cord (to muscles). More than one area of the spinal cord may be affected.

Symptoms

Symptoms may begin at any age—from age 1 to old age—depending on the form.

Reflexes become exaggerated, and leg cramps, twitches, and spasms occur, making leg movements stiff and jerky (called a spastic gait). Walking gradually becomes more difficult. People may stumble or trip because they tend to walk on their tiptoes with the feet turned inwards. Shoes are often worn down in the area over the big toe. Fatigue is common. In some people, muscles in the arms also become weak and stiff.

Usually, symptoms continue to slowly worsen, but sometimes they level off after adolescence. Life span is not affected.

About 10% of people with the disorder have other abnormalities due to damage of the brain, spinal cord, or nerves. For example, they may have eye problems, lack of muscle control, hearing loss, mental retardation, dementia, and peripheral nerve disorders.

Diagnosis

The disorder is diagnosed by excluding other disorders that cause similar symptoms (such as multiple sclerosis and spinal cord compression) and by determining whether other family members have hereditary spastic paraparesis. Blood tests (genetic testing) are sometimes done to check for the genes that cause the disorder.

Treatment

Treatment focuses on relieving symptoms. Physical therapy and exercise can help maintain mobility and muscle strength, improve range of motion and endurance, reduce fatigue, and prevent cramps and spasms.

Baclofen is the drug of choice to reduce spasticity. Alternatively, botulinum toxin, clonazepam, dantrolene, diazepam, or tizanidine may be used. Some people benefit from using splints, a cane, or crutches. A few people require a wheelchair.

Acute Transverse Myelitis

Acute transverse myelitis is inflammation that affects the spinal cord across its entire width (transversely) and thus blocks transmission of nerve impulses traveling up or down the spinal cord.

- The disorder may develop in people who have certain disorders, such as multiple sclerosis, Lyme disease, or lupus, or who take certain drugs.
- People have sudden back pain and feel a band of tightness around the affected area, sometimes followed by severe symptoms, such as paralysis.
- Magnetic resonance imaging may help doctors make the diagnosis, but a spinal tap may be needed.
- About one third of people recover, about one third continue to have some problems, and about one third recover very little.
- The cause is treated if possible, or treatment may involve corticosteroids or sometimes plasma exchange.

In the United States, acute transverse myelitis is estimated to occur in about 1,400 people each year. Also, about 33,000 people are thought to have some type of disability due to the disorder. The entire width of one or more areas of the spinal cord, usually in the chest (thoracic area), becomes inflamed.

What triggers acute transverse myelitis is unknown, but it may result from an autoimmune reaction (when the immune system misinterprets the body's tissues as foreign and attacks them). The disorder may develop during the following:

- Multiple sclerosis (most commonly)
- Neuromyelitis optica, a disorder that can also cause visual problems and may come and go
- Certain bacterial infections (such as Lyme disease, syphilis, or tuberculosis)
- Inflammation of blood vessels (vasculitis), including systemic lupus erythematosus (lupus)

- Viral meningoencephalitis (an infection of the brain and its surrounding tissues)
- Use of certain antiparasitic or antifungal drugs
- Intravenous injection of heroin or amphetamines

It sometimes develops after mild viral infections or a vaccination.

Symptoms

Usually, symptoms begin suddenly with pain in the back and a bandlike tightness around the affected area of the body (such as the chest or abdomen). Within hours to a few days, tingling, numbness, and muscle weakness develop in the feet and move upward. Urinating becomes difficult, although some people feel an urgent need to urinate (urgency). Symptoms may worsen over several more days and may become severe, resulting in paralysis, loss of sensation, retention of urine, and loss of bladder and bowel control. The degree of disability depends on the location (level) of the inflammation in the spinal cord and the severity of the inflammation.

Diagnosis

Symptoms suggest the diagnosis. But doctors must distinguish acute transverse myelitis from other disorders that cause similar symptoms, such as Guillain-Barré syndrome, spinal cord compression, or blockage of the blood supply to the spinal cord. Magnetic resonance imaging (MRI) is done first. If MRI does not detect spinal cord compression, a spinal tap (lumbar puncture) is done to obtain a sample of spinal cord fluid (see page 635). If acute transverse myelitis is present, the number of certain white blood cells and the protein level in the fluid is increased. If the disorder is advanced, MRI typically shows swelling of the spinal cord due to inflammation.

Tests, such as a chest x-ray and blood tests, are also done to look for the cause. Doctors may also ask people about use of drugs.

Prognosis

Occasionally, the disorder recurs in people with multiple sclerosis or lupus. Multiple sclerosis eventually develops in about 10 to 20% of people who have transverse myelitis with no identified cause.

Generally, the more quickly the disorder progresses, the worse the outlook. Severe pain suggests worse inflammation. The outcome is split evenly:

- About one third of people recover.
- About one third continue to have some muscle weakness and urinary problems (urgency or loss of bladder control).

- About one third recover very little, remaining confined to a wheelchair or bed, continuing to have bladder and bowel problems, and requiring help with daily activities.

Treatment

If transverse myelitis is caused by another disorder, that disorder is treated.

If the cause cannot be identified, high doses of corticosteroids such as prednisone are often given to suppress the immune system, which may be involved in acute transverse myelitis. Plasma exchange—removal of a large amount of plasma (the liquid part of blood) plus plasma transfusions—may also be done. However, whether these treatments are useful is unclear.

Symptoms are treated.

Blockage of the Spinal Cord's Blood Supply

Blockage of an artery carrying blood to the spinal cord prevents the cord from getting blood and thus oxygen. As a result, tissues can die (called infarction).

- Causes include severe atherosclerosis, inflammation of blood vessels, and blood clots.
- Sudden back pain with pain radiating from the affected area is followed by muscle weakness and inability to feel heat, cold, or pain in the affected areas and sometimes paralysis.
- Magnetic resonance imaging or myelography is usually done.
- Treatment focuses on correcting the cause if possible or on relieving symptoms.
- Spinal cord dysfunction and paralysis are usually permanent.

Like all tissues in the body, the spinal cord requires a constant supply of oxygenated blood. Only a few arteries, which are branches of the aorta, supply blood to the front part of the spinal cord. But this blood accounts for three fourths of the blood the spinal cord receives. Thus, blockage of any one of these arteries can be disastrous. Such a blockage occasionally results from the following:

- Severe atherosclerosis of the aorta
- Separation of the layers of the aorta's wall (aortic dissection)
- Inflammation of blood vessels (vasculitis), such as polyarteritis nodosa
- A blood clot that breaks off from the wall of the heart and travels through the bloodstream (becoming an embolus)
- Surgery to repair a bulge (aneurysm) in the abdominal aorta

Symptoms

The first symptoms are usually sudden back pain and pain that radiates along the nerves branching from the affected area of the spinal cord. The pain is followed by muscle weakness, and people cannot feel heat, cold, or pain in areas controlled by the part of the spinal cord below the level of the blockage. People immediately notice symptoms, which may lessen slightly over time. If the blood supply to the front of the spinal cord is greatly reduced, the legs are numb and paralyzed. But sensations transmitted through the back of the cord—including touch, the ability to feel vibration, and the ability to sense where the limbs are without looking at them (position sense)—remain intact. The back of the cord receives blood from other sources.

Weakness and paralysis can lead to the development of pressure sores and breathing difficulties. Bladder and bowel function may be impaired, as may sexual function.

Diagnosis

The diagnosis is usually based on symptoms. Magnetic resonance imaging (MRI) or, if MRI is unavailable, myelography (see page 636) is done. These tests can help doctors rule out other disorders that cause similar symptoms. A spinal tap (lumbar puncture—see page 635) may be done to rule out transverse myelitis as the cause of symptoms. Angiography can confirm that an artery to the front of the spinal cord is blocked, but it is usually unnecessary.

Treatment

When possible, the cause (such as aortic dissection or polyarteritis nodosa) is treated, but otherwise, treatment focuses on relieving symptoms because paralysis and spinal cord dysfunction are usually permanent.

Because some sensations are lost and paralysis may develop, preventing pressure sores from forming is important. Therapy to help fluids drain from the lungs (such as deep breathing exercises, postural drainage, and suctioning) may be necessary. Physical and occupational therapy (see page 53) can help preserve muscle function. Because bladder function is usually impaired, a catheter is needed to drain urine. This treatment prevents the bladder from enlarging and forming bulges that weaken it.

Subacute Combined Degeneration

Subacute combined degeneration is progressive degeneration of the spinal cord due to vitamin B$_{12}$ deficiency.

- Nerve fibers that control movement and sensation are damaged.
- People have general weakness, tingling and numbness in the hands and feet, and stiff limbs and may become irritable, drowsy, and confused.
- Blood tests can confirm vitamin B$_{12}$ deficiency.
- Vitamin B$_{12}$, if promptly given by injection or by mouth, usually results in complete recovery.

This disorder affects about 1 of 10,000 people, usually those older than 40. It is due to a deficiency of vitamin B$_{12}$, which usually also causes pernicious anemia. Usually, the deficiency is not related to diet but to the body's inability to absorb vitamin B$_{12}$.

Vitamin B$_{12}$ is necessary for the formation and maintenance of a fatty sheath (myelin sheath) that surrounds some nerve cells and that speeds transmission of nerve signals. In subacute combined degeneration, the sheath is damaged, causing sensory and motor nerve fibers from the spinal cord to degenerate. The brain, nerves of the eyes, and peripheral nerves are sometimes also damaged.

Symptoms

The disorder begins with a general feeling of weakness. Tingling, a pins-and-needles sensation, and numbness are felt in both hands and feet. These sensations tend to be constant and to gradually worsen. People may not be able to feel vibrations and may lose the sense of where their limbs are (position sense). The limbs feel stiff, movements become clumsy, and walking may become difficult. Reflexes may be decreased, increased, or absent. Vision may be reduced.

People who have this disorder may become irritable, apathetic, drowsy, suspicious, and confused. Their emotions may change rapidly and unpredictably. Rarely, dementia develops.

Diagnosis and Treatment

Blood tests to measure levels of vitamin B$_{12}$ can confirm the deficiency.

Recovery is more likely if the disorder is treated early. When treated within a few weeks after symptoms appear, most people recover completely. If treatment is delayed, the progression of symptoms may be slowed or stopped, but full recovery of lost function is less likely.

Most people are immediately given injections of vitamin B$_{12}$, which are continued indefinitely to prevent symptoms from recurring. Large doses of vitamin B$_{12}$ taken by mouth can be used if the deficiency is mild and symptoms of nerve damage have not developed.

Tropical Spastic Paraparesis/ HTLV-1–Associated Myelopathy

Tropical spastic paraparesis/HTLV-1–associated myelopathy is a slowly progressive disorder of the spinal cord caused by the human T-lymphotrophic virus 1 (HTLV-1).

- The virus is spread through sexual contact, use of illicit intravenous drugs, exposure to blood, or breastfeeding.
- People have weakness, stiffness, and muscle spasms in the legs, making walking difficult, and many have urinary incontinence.
- To diagnose the disorder, doctors ask about possible exposure to the virus and do magnetic resonance imaging and a spinal tap.
- Drugs, such as corticosteroids, may help, and spasms are treated with muscle relaxants.

The human T-lymphotrophic virus 1 (HTLV-1) virus is similar to the human immunodeficiency virus (HIV), the virus that causes AIDS. The HTLV-1 virus can cause certain kinds of leukemia and lymphoma (cancers of the white blood cells). This virus is transmitted through sexual contact, use of illicit intravenous drugs, or exposure to blood. It can be transmitted from mother to child through breastfeeding. It is most common among prostitutes, IV drug users, people undergoing hemodialysis, and people from certain areas such as those near the equator, southern Japan, and parts of South America. A similar disorder can result from infection with a similar virus, human T-lymphotrophic virus 2 (HTLV-2).

The virus resides in white blood cells. Because the spinal fluid contains white blood cells, the spinal cord can be damaged. Damage to the spinal cord results more from the body's reaction to the virus than from the virus itself.

Symptoms

The muscles in both legs gradually become weak. People may not be able to feel vibrations and may lose the sense of where their feet and toes are (position sense). Their limbs feel stiff, movements become clumsy, and walking may become difficult. Muscle spasms in the legs are common, as is urinary incontinence. The disorder usually progresses over several years.

Diagnosis

The diagnosis is usually based on symptoms and the person's risk of being exposed to the virus. Thus, a doctor may ask people about their sexual contacts and use of illicit intravenous drugs. Magnetic resonance imaging (MRI) of the spinal cord is done. Samples of blood and spinal fluid, obtained by a spinal tap (lumbar puncture), are tested for parts of the virus or antibodies to the virus.

Treatment

Interferon-alpha, immune globulin (given intravenously), and corticosteroids (such as methylprednisolone, given by mouth) may help, although their usefulness has not been established. Spasms can be treated with muscle relaxants such as baclofen or tizanidine.

CHAPTER

122 Low Back and Neck Pain

Low back and neck pain are among the most common reasons for health care visits. The pain usually results from problems with the spine, including the bones of the spine (vertebrae) and the muscles and ligaments that support it. Occasionally, low back or neck pain results from another disorder, such as a stomach ulcer, pneumonia, premenstrual syndrome, or infection of the prostate gland. Some disorders cause only low back or neck pain. Others can cause both.

Low Back Pain

- Common causes include sprains and strains, osteoarthritis, osteoporosis, a ruptured or herniated disk, fibromyalgia, and, in older people, spinal stenosis.

- Pain may be intermittent or constant, superficial or deep, or dull or sharp, depending on the cause.
- Doctors base the diagnosis on symptoms, results of a physical examination, and sometimes x-rays or other imaging tests.
- Exercising regularly is the best way to prevent low back pain.
- For most low back pain, avoiding activities that stress the back, taking pain relievers, and applying ice or heat are often all that is needed.

Low back pain is very common and becomes more common as people age. It is very costly in terms of healthcare payments, disability payments, and missed work. Thus, although low back pain rarely results from life-threatening disorders, it is a

A Herniated Disk

The tough covering of a disk in the spine can tear (rupture), causing pain. The soft, jelly-like interior may then bulge out (herniate) through the covering, causing more pain. Pain occurs because the bulge puts pressure on the spinal nerve root next to it. Sometimes the nerve root becomes inflamed or is damaged.

More than 80% of herniated disks occur in the lower back. They are most common among people aged 30 to 50 years. Between these ages, the covering weakens. The interior, which is under high pressure, may squeeze through a tear or a weakened spot in the covering and bulge out. After age 50, the interior of the disk begins to harden, making a herniation less likely.

A disk may herniate because of a sudden, traumatic injury or repeated minor injuries. Being overweight or lifting heavy objects, particularly lifting incorrectly, increases the risk.

Often, herniated disks cause no symptoms, but they may cause slight to debilitating pain. Movement intensifies the pain.

Where the pain occurs depends on which disk is herniated and which spinal nerve root is affected. The pain may be felt along the pathway of the nerve compressed by the herniated disk. For example, a herniated disk commonly causes sciatica—pain along the sciatic nerve.

A herniated disk can also cause numbness and muscle weakness. If the pressure on the nerve root is great, the legs may be paralyzed. If the cauda equina (the bundle of nerves extending from the bottom of the cord) is affected, control of bladder and bowels can be lost. If these serious symptoms develop, medical attention is required immediately.

Most people recover without any treatment, usually within 3 months, but often much faster. Applying cold (such as ice packs) or heat (such as a heating pad) or using over-the-counter analgesics may help relieve the pain. Sometimes surgery to remove part or all the disk and part of a vertebra is necessary. In 10 to 20% of people who have surgery for sciatica due to a herniated disk, another disk ruptures.

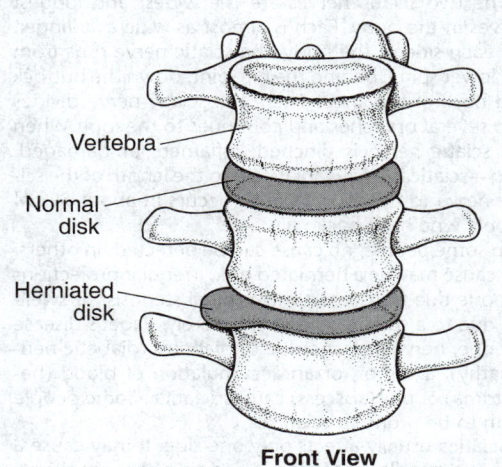

Front View

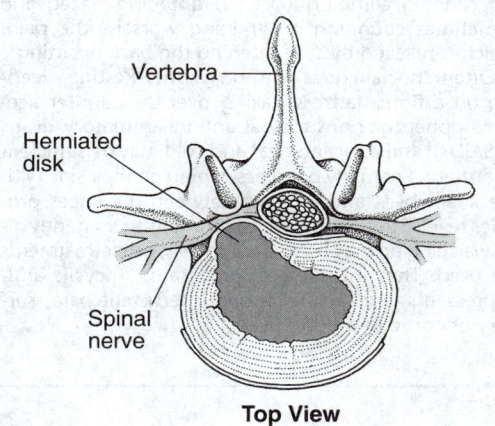

Top View

significant health problem. However, the number of back injuries in the workplace is decreasing, perhaps because awareness of the problem has increased and preventive measures have improved.

The spine (spinal column) consists of the back bones (vertebrae), which are separated and cushioned by shock-absorbing disks made of cartilage. The vertebrae are also covered by a thin layer of cartilage. They are held in place by ligaments and muscles, which include the following:

- Two iliopsoas muscles, which run along both sides of the spine

- Two erector spinae muscles, which run along the length of the spine behind it
- Many short paraspinal muscles, which run between the vertebrae

These muscles help stabilize the spine. The abdominal muscles, which run from the bottom of the rib cage to the pelvis, also help stabilize the spine by supporting the abdominal contents.

Enclosed in the spine is the spinal cord (see page 627 and 793). Along the length of the spinal cord, the spinal nerves emerge through spaces between the vertebrae to connect with nerves

What Is Sciatica?

The two sciatic nerves are the widest and longest nerves in the body. Each is almost as wide as a finger. On each side of the body, the sciatic nerve runs from the lower spine, behind the hip joint, down the buttock and back of the knee. There the sciatic nerve divides into several branches and continues to the foot. When the sciatic nerve is pinched, inflamed, or damaged, pain—sciatica—may radiate along the length of the sciatic nerve to the foot. Sciatica occurs in about 5% of people who have back pain.

In some people, no cause can be detected. In others, the cause may be a herniated disk, irregular projections of bone due to osteoarthritis, spinal stenosis, or swelling due to a sprained ligament. Rarely, Paget's disease of bone, nerve damage due to diabetes (diabetic neuropathy), a tumor, or an accumulation of blood (hematoma) or pus (abscess) causes sciatica. Some people seem to be prone to sciatica.

Sciatica usually affects only one side. It may cause a pins-and-needles sensation, a nagging ache, or shooting pain. Numbness may be felt in the leg or foot. Walking, running, climbing stairs, straightening the leg, and sometimes coughing or straining worsens the pain, which is relieved by straightening the back or sitting.

Often, the pain goes away on its own. Resting, sleeping on a firm mattress, taking over-the-counter acetaminophen or nonsteroidal anti-inflammatory drugs (NSAIDs), and applying heat and cold may be sufficient treatment. For many people, sleeping on their side with the knees bent and a pillow between the knees provides relief. Stretching the hamstring muscles gently after warming up may help. Occasionally, other treatments are used. They include anticonvulsants, tricyclic antidepressants, and, for severe and persistent pain, surgery or corticosteroids.

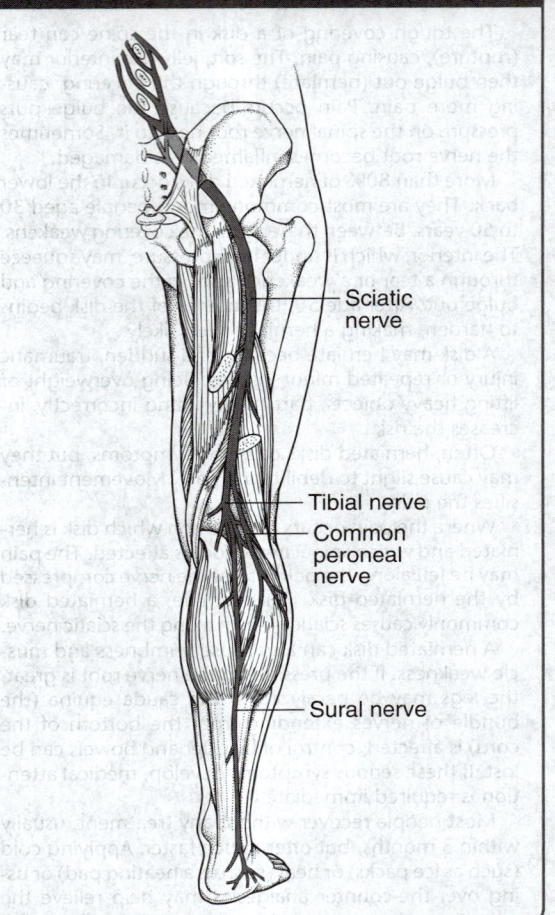

Sciatic nerve

Tibial nerve

Common peroneal nerve

Sural nerve

---

throughout the body. The part of the spinal nerve nearest the spinal cord is called the spinal nerve root. Because of their position, spinal nerve roots can be compressed when the spine is injured, resulting in pain.

The lower (lumbar) spine consists of five vertebrae. It connects the chest to the pelvis and legs, providing mobility—for turning, twisting, and bending. It also provides strength—for standing, walking, and lifting. Thus, the lower back is involved in almost all activities of daily living. Low back pain can limit many activities and reduce the quality of life.

Causes

Low back pain has many causes, although often no specific cause can be identified.

Muscle strains and ligament sprains are the most common causes. Strains and sprains may result from lifting, exercising, or moving in an unexpected way (such as when falling or when in a car accident). When due to exercise, injury to the lower back is sometimes called weight lifter's back (lumbar strain). Weight lifter's back may be caused not only by snatching a heavy weight from the ground in weight lifting but also by pushing against an opposing lineman in football, suddenly turning to dribble after a rebound in basketball, swinging a bat in baseball, or swinging a club in golf. The lower back is more likely to be injured when a person's physical conditioning is poor and the supporting muscles of the back are weak. Having poor posture, lifting incorrectly, being overweight, and being tired also contribute.

Osteoarthritis (degenerative arthritis) causes the cartilage that covers and protects the vertebrae to deteriorate. This disorder is thought to be due, at least in part, to the wear and tear of years of use. People who repetitively stress one joint or a group of joints are more likely to develop osteoarthritis. The disks between the vertebrae deteriorate, narrowing the spaces between them and often compressing spinal nerve roots. Irregular projections of bone (spurs) may develop on the vertebrae and compress spinal nerve roots. All of these changes can cause low back pain as well as stiffness.

In **osteoporosis**, bone density decreases, making the bones more likely to fracture. The vertebrae are particularly susceptible to the effects of osteoporosis. Osteoporosis often results in crush (compression) fractures (which sometimes cause sudden, severe back pain) and compression of spinal nerve roots (which may cause chronic back pain). However, most fractures due to osteoporosis occur in the upper and middle back and cause upper and middle rather than low back pain.

A **ruptured or herniated disk** can cause low back pain. A disk has a tough covering and a soft, jelly-like interior. If a disk is suddenly squeezed by the vertebrae above and below it (as when lifting a heavy object), the covering may tear (rupture), causing pain. The interior of the disk can squeeze through the tear in the covering, so that part of the interior bulges out (herniates). This bulge can compress, irritate, and even damage the spinal nerve root next to it, causing more pain. A ruptured or herniated disk also commonly causes sciatica.

In **ankylosing spondylitis**, the spine and large joints are inflamed, resulting in stiffness and back pain. This disorder is more common among men, usually starting between the ages of 20 and 40.

Spinal stenosis is narrowing of the spinal canal (the passageway that runs through the center of the spine and contains the spinal cord). It is a common cause of low back pain in older people. Spinal stenosis also develops in middle-aged people who were born with a narrow spinal canal. It is caused by such disorders as osteoarthritis, spondylolisthesis, rheumatoid arthritis, ankylosing spondylitis, and Paget's disease of the bone. Spinal stenosis may cause sciatica as well as low back pain.

Fibromyalgia is a common cause of low back pain. This disorder causes chronic widespread (diffuse) pain in muscles, tendons, ligaments, and other soft tissues (see page 616). It is most common among women aged 20 to 50.

Referred pain (see box on page 639) sometimes causes low back pain. Referred pain originates in another part of the body, such as the lungs, kidneys, uterus, prostate gland, or organs of the digestive tract but is felt in the lower back. For example, low back pain can be caused by premenstrual syndrome, a prostate infection, pancreatitis, a severe peptic ulcer, an abdominal aortic aneurysm, pelvic inflammatory disease, or ectopic pregnancy.

Compression of the spinal cord, a serious disorder, can cause low back pain (see page 799). Compression may result from a severe injury, a herniated disk, accumulation of blood (hematoma), an abscess, or a tumor.

Spondylolisthesis is partial displacement of a vertebra in the lower back. It usually occurs in people who have a birth defect (spondylolysis) that weakens part of the vertebrae. Usually, during adolescence, a minor injury causes a part of the vertebra to fracture. The vertebra then slips forward over the one below it. If it slips far, pain can result.

Other less common causes of low back pain include shingles, cancer that has spread to the spine from other organs (such as the breasts, lungs, prostate gland, or kidneys), bone cancer (multiple myeloma), infections (such as an abscess in the spinal cord or a bone infection), Paget's disease of bone, and birth defects (such as scoliosis).

Stress may contribute to low back pain, but how it does so is unclear. Heavy physical labor, obesity, smoking, and lack of exercise also contribute to low back pain.

Symptoms

Low back pain varies depending on the cause and type of pain. It may be

- Intermittent or constant
- Superficial or deep
- Dull and aching, throbbing, or sharp and stabbing

Back pain may interfere with sleep.

Types of low back pain include the following:

Local Pain: Pain occurs in a specific area of the lower back. It is usually due to sprains and strains. Sudden pain may be felt when the injury occurs. Local pain can often be relieved by changes in position or by light activity followed by stretching. Intense physical activity or prolonged inactivity (such as bed rest) tends to make it worse. Local pain may be constant and aching or, at times, intermittent and sharp. The lower back may be sore when touched. Muscle spasms may occur because the body moves in unusual ways as it tries to avoid the

Did You Know...

Strengthening abdominal muscles, as well as back muscles, helps prevent low back pain.

movements that trigger pain. Usually, local pain resolves gradually over days to weeks.

Pain Due to Compression of a Spinal Nerve Root: A nerve root may be compressed by disorders such as a herniated disk, osteoarthritis, spinal stenosis, or Paget's disease of bone. The pain often occurs within minutes or hours of lifting a very heavy weight, but it may occur spontaneously. It tends to be a dull ache sometimes accompanied by a sharp, intense radiating pain. The pain can radiate to different parts of the body, depending on which nerve root is affected. Commonly, the pain extends from the lower back into the buttock and down the leg past the knee on the affected side, indicating sciatica. Coughing, sneezing, straining, or bending over while keeping the legs straight can trigger the sharp, radiating pain. The pain varies by cause:

- Herniated disk: The pain is worsened by walking a distance.
- Spinal stenosis: The pain is typically increased by straightening the back (as when walking) and is relieved by bending the spine forward (as when leaning forward).
- Compression fracture due to osteoporosis: The pain may start suddenly, stay in a particular area of the back, and worsen when a person stands or walks. The area near the fracture may be tender.

Usually, the pain and tenderness disappear gradually after a few weeks or months. If pressure on the nerve root is great or if the spinal cord is also compressed, the pain may be accompanied by muscle weakness in the leg, a pins-and-needles sensation, or even loss of sensation and loss of bladder and bowel control.

Referred Pain: Back pain that originates in other organs tends to be deep, aching, constant, and relatively widespread, but it can vary. Typically, movement does not affect it, unlike pain from back disorders, and it may worsen at night.

Other Types: Some disorders cause typical types of pain:

- Infection or cancer: Pain is constant and progressively worsens. It is unrelieved by rest.
- Ankylosing spondylitis: The pain is accompanied by stiffness that is worse just after a person wakes up.
- Fibromyalgia: Pain occurs throughout the body or moves from part to part. Muscles ache, feel stiff, and may be tender to the touch. The pain may be throbbing, aching, or stabbing. Fibromyalgia is often accompanied by poor sleep.

Diagnosis

Doctors ask the person about the pain:

- What the pain is like

- What relieves or worsens it
- When and how it started
- Whether other symptoms are also present

Doctors also do a physical examination, focusing on the spine and including evaluation of the nervous system (a neurologic examination). As part of the physical examination, doctors may ask the person to move in certain ways to determine the type of pain. For example, they may ask the person to lie flat, then lift the leg without bending the knee.

With information about the pain, the person's medical history, and results of a physical examination, doctors may be able to identify the cause. Usually, no other tests are needed because most back pain results from strains and sprains and resolves within 6 weeks. If another cause is suspected or if back pain persists, other tests are often needed.

X-rays of the lower back can help detect degenerative changes due to osteoarthritis, compression fractures due to osteoporosis, and scoliosis. However, magnetic resonance imaging (MRI) or computed tomography (CT) provides clearer images and can confirm or exclude the diagnosis of a herniated disk, spinal stenosis, or cancer. These tests can also indicate whether degenerative changes due to osteoarthritis are responsible for compressing nerves. If compression of the spinal cord is suspected, MRI is done immediately. Rarely, when results of MRI are unclear, myelography (see page 636) with CT is required. Occasionally, electromyography and nerve conduction studies (see page 636) are done to confirm the location of nerve damage.

Prevention

The most effective way to prevent low back pain is to exercise regularly. Aerobic exercise and specific muscle-strengthening and stretching exercises can help.

Aerobic exercise, such as swimming and walking, improves general fitness and generally strengthens muscles. Specific exercises to strengthen and stretch the muscles in the abdomen, buttocks, and back can help stabilize the spine and decrease strain on the disks that cushion the spine and the ligaments that hold it in place.

Muscle-strengthening exercises include pelvic tilts and abdominal curls. Stretching exercises include the sitting leg stretch, knee-to-chest stretch, and hip and quadriceps stretch. Stretching exercises can increase back pain in some people and therefore should be done carefully. As a general rule, any exercise that causes or increases back pain should be stopped. Exercises should be repeated until the muscles feel mildly but not completely fatigued.

Exercises to Prevent Low Back Pain

Pelvic Tilts

Lie on the back with the knees bent, the heels on the floor, and the weight on the heels. Press the small of the back against the floor, contract the buttocks (raising them about half an inch from the floor), and contract the abdominal muscles. Hold this position for a count of 10. Repeat 20 times.

Abdominal Curls

Lie on the back with the knees bent and feet on the floor. Place the hands across the chest. Contract the abdominal muscles, slowly raising the shoulders about 10 inches from the floor while keeping the head back (the chin should not touch the chest). Then release the abdominal muscles, slowly lowering the shoulders. Do 3 sets of 10.

Knee-to-Chest Stretch

Lie flat on the back. Place both hands behind one knee and bring it to the chest. Hold for a count of 10. Slowly lower that leg and repeat with the other leg. Do this exercise 10 times.

Sitting Leg Stretch

Sit on the floor with the knees straight but slightly flexed (not locked) and the legs as far apart as possible. Place both hands on the same knee. Slowly slide both hands toward the ankle. Stop if pain is felt and go no farther than a position that can be held comfortably for 10 seconds. Slowly return to a sitting position. Repeat with the other leg. Do this exercise 10 times for each leg.

Hip and Quadriceps Stretch

Stand with one foot on the floor and the knee of the other leg bent at about a 90° angle. Grasp the front of the ankle of the bent leg with the hand on the same side. (The other hand may be placed on the back of a chair or on the wall for balance.) Keeping the knees together, press the foot against the hand and away from the body. Hold for a count of 10. Repeat with the other leg. Do this exercise 10 times.

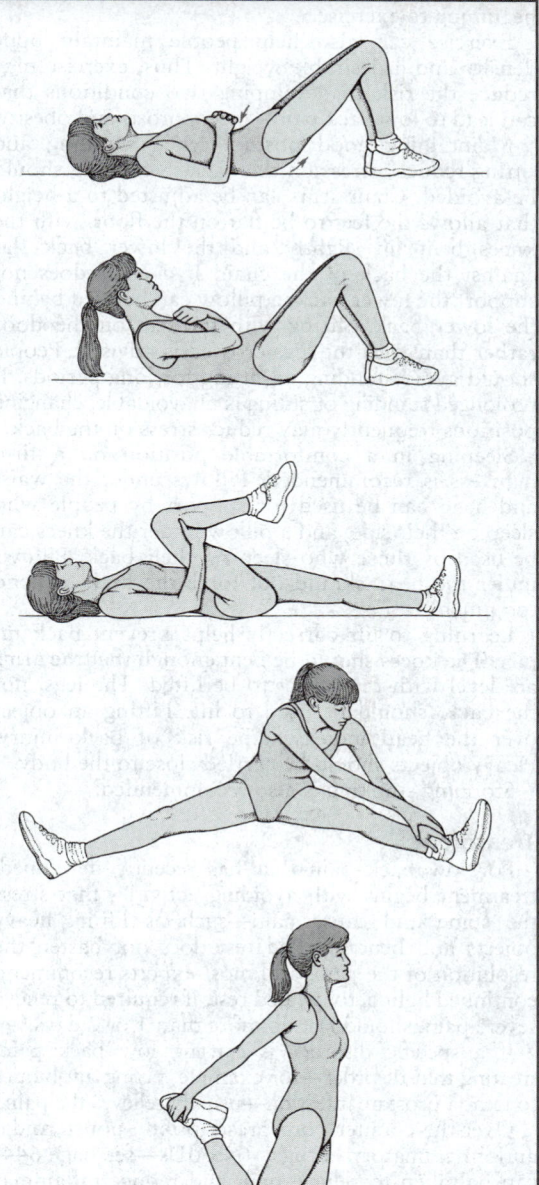

Breathing during each exercise is important. People who have back pain should consult a doctor before beginning to exercise.

Exercise can also help people maintain bone density and a desirable weight. Thus, exercise may reduce the risk of developing two conditions that can lead to low back pain—osteoporosis and obesity.

Maintaining good posture when standing and sitting reduces stress on the back. Slouching should be avoided. Chair seats can be adjusted to a height that allows the feet to be flat on the floor, with the knees bent up slightly and the lower back flat against the back of the chair. If a chair does not support the lower back, a pillow can be used behind the lower back. Sitting with the feet on the floor rather than with the legs crossed is advised. People should avoid standing or sitting for long periods. If prolonged standing or sitting is unavoidable, changing positions frequently may reduce stress on the back.

Sleeping in a comfortable position on a firm mattress is recommended. Pillows under the waist and head can be used for support by people who sleep on their side, and a pillow under the knees can be used by those who sleep on their back. Pillows under the head should not force the neck to bend too much.

Learning to lift correctly helps prevent back injury. The knees should be bent enough that the arms are level with the object to be lifted. The legs, not the back, should be used to lift. Lifting an object over the head increases the risk of back injury. Heavy objects should be carried close to the body.

Stopping smoking is also recommended.

Treatment

For low back pain that has recently developed, treatment begins with avoiding activities that stress the spine and cause pain—such as lifting heavy objects and bending. Bed rest does not hasten the resolution of the pain, and most experts recommend continued light activity. Bed rest, if required to relieve severe pain, should last no more than 1 or 2 days.

If a specific disorder is causing low back pain, treating that disorder—for example, giving antibiotics to treat a prostate infection—usually relieves the pain.

Over-the-counter or prescription nonsteroidal anti-inflammatory drugs (NSAIDs—see page 644) can be taken to relieve pain and reduce inflammation. If inflammation is not contributing to the pain (and it usually does not), acetaminophen is typically recommended for pain relief instead of an NSAID. Acetaminophen is slightly safer than NSAIDS.

Muscle relaxants, such as carisoprodol, cyclobenzaprine, diazepam, metaxalone, or methocarbamol, are sometimes given to relieve muscle spasms, but their usefulness is controversial. These drugs are not recommended for older people, who are more likely to have side effects.

Application of heat or cold and massage may help (see page 46). Usually, traction is not useful. Spinal manipulation, done by chiropractors or some other doctors (such as osteopathic doctors), may hasten the resolution of pain due to muscle spasm, strains, or sprains. However, it may have risks for people with osteoporosis or a herniated disk. Some reports suggest that acupuncture may have similar benefits, but others suggest little or no benefit.

After the pain has subsided, light activity, as recommended by a doctor or physical therapist, can speed healing and recovery. Specific exercises to strengthen and stretch the back and to strengthen the abdominal muscles are usually recommended to help prevent low back pain from becoming chronic or recurring. Other preventive measures (maintaining good posture, using a firm mattress with appropriately placed pillows, lifting correctly, and stopping smoking) should be continued or started. In response to these measures, most episodes of back pain resolve in several days to 2 weeks. Regardless of treatment, 80 to 90% of such episodes resolve within 6 weeks.

Treatment of Chronic Pain: If low back pain is chronic, additional measures are needed. Aerobic exercise may help, and weight reduction, if necessary, is advised. If the pain is severe, acetaminophen or NSAIDs may not provide sufficient pain relief, and opioid analgesics (see page 642) may be required. If these analgesics are ineffective, other treatments can be considered.

Transcutaneous electrical nerve stimulation (TENS) may be used (see page 648). The TENS device produces a gentle tingling sensation by generating a low oscillating current. A therapist applies the device to the painful area several times a day for 20 minutes to several hours at a time, depending on the severity of the pain. People are sometimes taught to use the device themselves.

Sometimes a corticosteroid (such as dexamethasone or methylprednisolone) plus a local anesthetic (such as lidocaine) is periodically injected into the epidural space—between the spine and the outer layer of tissue covering the spinal cord. These epidural injections are more effective for sciatica than for lumbar spinal stenosis. However, they are usually effective only for several days to weeks. Their main use is to relieve pain enough that an exercise program, which can provide long-term pain relief, can be started.

If a disorder causes severe and constant pain, serious symptoms, or sciatica lasts 6 months or more, surgery may be necessary. If a herniated disk is causing relentless sciatica, weakness, loss of sensation, or loss of bladder and bowel control, surgi-

DISORDERS THAT CAUSE ONLY NECK PAIN

DISORDERS	DESCRIPTION	SOME CAUSES	SYMPTOMS
Atlantoaxial subluxation	The first and second vertebrae are misaligned.	Traumatic injury (which is the most common cause and is usually immediately fatal) Rheumatoid arthritis	People have vague neck pain, and the spinal cord may be compressed, sometimes intermittently. Rarely, compression is fatal.
Cervical spondylosis (see page 801)	In the neck, the vertebrae and the disks between them degenerate. As a result, the nerves that emerge through the vertebrae may be pinched. Sometimes the spinal canal is narrowed (cervical spinal stenosis) and the spinal cord is compressed.	Osteoarthritis (usually)	Pain occurs in the structures around the neck. The pain may extend (radiate) down the nerve, sometimes to the shoulders and upper back. Spinal cord compression may cause weakness and tingling in the hands and feet.
Temporomandibular joint disorders (see page 1367)	Problems occur in the joint of the jawbone. Women are more commonly affected, usually during their early 20s or their 40s.	Muscle tension Internal joint derangement (the disk inside the joint is abnormally placed) Arthritis Ankylosis (fusion of joint bones) Hypermobility (looseness of the jaw joint)	The neck near the jaw may be stiff and painful. Chewing may make the pain may worse.
Spasmodic torticollis (see page 784)	The neck muscles contract, causing the head to tilt and rotate into abnormal positions.	Unknown (often) Certain drugs, including antipsychotic drugs Possibly inherited	Contractions may be painful. They may be sustained or occur in spasms, causing jerky movements of the head. Symptoms may begin at any age but usually begin between ages 20 and 60, most often between ages 30 and 50.

cal removal of the disk (diskectomy) and part of the vertebra (laminectomy) may be necessary. A general anesthetic is usually required. The hospital stay after surgical removal of a disk is usually 1 or 2 days. Often, microsurgical techniques, with a small incision and a local anesthetic, can be used. Hospitalization is not required. However, when the incision is small, the surgeon may not be able to see and therefore may not remove all fragments of the herniated disk. After either procedure, most people can resume all of their activities after a few weeks. More than 90% of people recover fully.

For severe spinal stenosis, a large part of the vertebra may be surgically removed to widen the spinal canal. A general anesthetic is usually required. The hospital stay is usually 4 or 5 days. People may need 3 to 4 months before they can resume all of their activities. About two thirds of people have a good or full recovery. For most of the rest, symptoms are prevented from worsening.

When the spine is unstable because of degeneration due to osteoarthritis, vertebrae may be fused together. However, fusion decreases mobility and may put additional stress on the rest of the spine.

Neck Pain

■ Neck pain usually results from strains and sprains.

- Pain from the neck may shoot down an arm or cause a headache.
- Doctors base the diagnosis on symptoms, results of a physical examination, and sometimes x-rays or other imaging tests.
- Treatment includes taking pain relievers, applying ice or heat, wearing a neck collar, and learning how to stand, sit, and sleep to avoid straining the neck.

The neck's flexibility makes it susceptible to wear and tear and to injuries that overstretch it, such as whiplash. Also, the neck has the critical job of holding up the head. Poor posture makes that job more difficult. Thus, neck pain, like back pain, is common, and it becomes more common as people age.

The spine contains the spinal cord (see pages 627 and 793). Along the length of the spinal cord, spinal nerves emerge through spaces between the vertebrae to connect with nerves throughout the body. The part of the spinal nerve nearest the spinal cord (spinal nerve root) can be compressed when the spine is injured, resulting in pain. The part of the spine in the neck (cervical spine) consists of seven back bones (vertebrae), which are separated by disks.

The neck also contains muscles and ligaments to support the spine.

Causes

Most of the disorders that can cause low back pain can also cause neck pain, and most involve the spine, the tissues that support it, or both. The most common causes are muscle strains and ligament strains. Other causes include injuries, arthritis, a ruptured or herniated disk, meningitis, and fibromyalgia.

Some disorders cause neck pain but not back pain.

Other disorders that can cause neck pain include a tear in a neck artery's lining (dissection), a blockage or tumor in the esophagus, infections (such as a bone infection), and inflammation of the esophagus or thyroid gland.

Sometimes neck pain is referred pain (see box on page 639), which originates in another part of the body. Referred neck pain may result from angina or a heart attack.

Symptoms

The neck may be tender, stiff, or both as well as painful. Pain may be worsened by movement. The pain may extend to the shoulders and upper back or may cause a headache. If a nerve is compressed, the pain may shoot down an arm. People may also feel tingling, numbness, or weakness in the arms or sometimes the legs. If the spinal cord is compressed, people may lose control of bladder and bowel functions (incontinence). Other symptoms occur depending on the disorder.

Diagnosis

Doctors can often base the diagnosis on a description of symptoms, risk factors (which may suggest a cause), and results of a physical examination, which includes evaluation of the nervous system (neurologic examination). As part of the physical examination, doctors may move or ask the person to move the neck in all directions to check its range of motion and to determine whether movement makes the pain worse.

X-rays can help identify some disorders, but magnetic resonance imaging (MRI) or computed tomography (CT) may be needed at some point to confirm the diagnosis. If spinal cord compression is suspected, MRI is done immediately. Other tests may also be needed. They include blood tests to check for infection or inflammation and electromyography and nerve conduction studies to determine whether the cause is related to muscles or nerves (see page 636).

Treatment

Treatment depends on the cause. But often, taking over-the-counter analgesics, such as acetaminophen or nonsteroidal anti-inflammatory drugs (NSAIDs), can relieve the pain. If inflammation is not contributing to the pain, acetaminophen is usually recommended instead of NSAIDs because it is thought to be safer. Ice or heat may also help (see page 46). People are taught how to stand, sit, and sleep in ways that do not strain the neck.

Doctors may recommend wearing a soft neck collar and using contour pillow for 10 to 14 days to help relieve pain and muscle spasms. People with unstable atlantoaxial subluxation may need to wear a rigid collar. Doctors or physical therapists may also suggest stretching exercises.

If more pain relief is needed, doctors may prescribe analgesics. Muscle relaxants, such as carisoprodol, cyclobenzaprine, diazepam, metaxalone, or methocarbamol, are sometimes used, but their usefulness is controversial. Muscle relaxants are not recommended for older people, who are more likely to have side effects.

For spasmodic torticollis, physical therapy or massage can sometimes temporarily stop the contractions. Drugs (including the anticonvulsant carbamazepine and some mild sedatives such as clonazepam), taken by mouth or injected, can usually relieve the pain. But drugs control contractions in only up to one third of people. If the pain is severe or if posture is distorted, botulinum toxin (a bacterial toxin used to paralyze muscles) may be injected into the affected muscles.

For shingles, antiviral drugs may shorten the duration of the symptoms, and wet compresses on the blisters may help relieve pain.

If the spinal cord or a spinal nerve is compressed or if the neck is unstable, surgery is usually needed.

123 Peripheral Nerve Disorders

The peripheral nervous system refers to the parts of nervous system outside the central nervous system, that is, those outside the brain and spinal cord. The nerves that connect the head, face, eyes, nose, muscles, and ears to the brain (cranial nerves—see page 835) and the nerves that connect the spinal cord to the rest of the body, including the 31 pairs of spinal nerves, are part of the peripheral nervous system. This system also includes more than 100 billion nerve cells that run throughout the body.

Dysfunction of peripheral nerves may result from damage to any part of the nerve:

- Axon (the part that sends messages)
- Body of the nerve cell
- Myelin sheath (the membranes that surround the axon, enabling nerve impulses to travel quickly—see art on page 788).

If motor nerves (which stimulate muscle action) are damaged, muscles may weaken or become paralyzed. If sensory nerves (which carry sensory information) are damaged, abnormal sensations may be felt or sensation may be lost. Some peripheral nerve disorders are progressive and fatal.

Muscle Stimulation Disorders

Muscle stimulation (motor neuron) disorders are characterized by progressive deterioration of the nerves and other structures involved in muscle movement. These disorders develop when motor nerves do not stimulate muscles normally.

- Amyotrophic lateral sclerosis is the most common of these disorders.
- Typically, muscles are weak and waste away, and movements become stiff, clumsy, and awkward.
- Doctors base the diagnosis on results of electromyography, magnetic resonance imaging, and blood tests.
- There is no specific treatment or cure, but drugs can help lessen symptoms.

For normal muscle function, muscle tissue and nerve connections between the brain and muscle must be normal. In muscle stimulation disorders (motor neuron disorders), motor nerves do not stimulate muscles normally. As a result, muscles weaken, waste away (atrophy), and can become completely paralyzed even though the muscles themselves are not the cause of the problem.

Muscle stimulation disorders include amyotrophic lateral sclerosis (the most common), primary lateral sclerosis, progressive pseudobulbar palsy, progressive muscular atrophy, progressive bulbar palsy, and postpolio syndrome. These disorders are more common among men and usually develop in people who are in their 50s. The cause is usually unknown. About 10% of people who have a muscle stimulation disorder have a hereditary type and thus have family members who also have the disorder.

In all of these disorders, the parts of the nervous system involved in muscle movement—including motor nerves in the spinal cord and in other parts of the body and parts of the brain—progressively deteriorate, causing muscle weakness that can progress to paralysis. However, in each disorder, a different part of the nervous system is affected. Consequently, each disorder has different effects. For example, some affect the mouth and throat first, and others affect a hand or foot first or most severely.

Symptoms

Muscles are affected, but people do not have pain or any changes in sensation. Depression is common.

Amyotrophic Lateral Sclerosis (Lou Gehrig's Disease): This progressive disorder begins with weakness, often in the hands and less frequently in the feet or mouth and throat. Weakness may progress more on one side of the body than on the other and usually proceeds up the arm or leg. Cramps are also common and may occur before the weakness, but no changes in sensation occur. People may lose weight and feel unusually tired.

Over time, weakness increases. Muscles twitch and become tight, followed by muscle spasms (spasticity). Tremors may appear. Controlling facial expressions may become difficult. Weakening of muscles in the throat may lead to difficulty speaking (dysarthria) and swallowing (dysphagia). Excess

Using the Brain to Move a Muscle

Moving a muscle usually involves communication between the muscle and the brain through nerves. The impetus to move a muscle may originate with the senses. For example, special nerve endings in the skin (sensory receptors) enable people to sense pain, as when they step on a sharp rock, or to sense temperature, as when they pick up a very hot cup of coffee. This information is sent to the brain, and the brain may send a message to the muscle about how to respond. This type of exchange involves two complex nerve pathways: the sensory nerve pathway to the brain and the motor nerve pathway to the muscle.

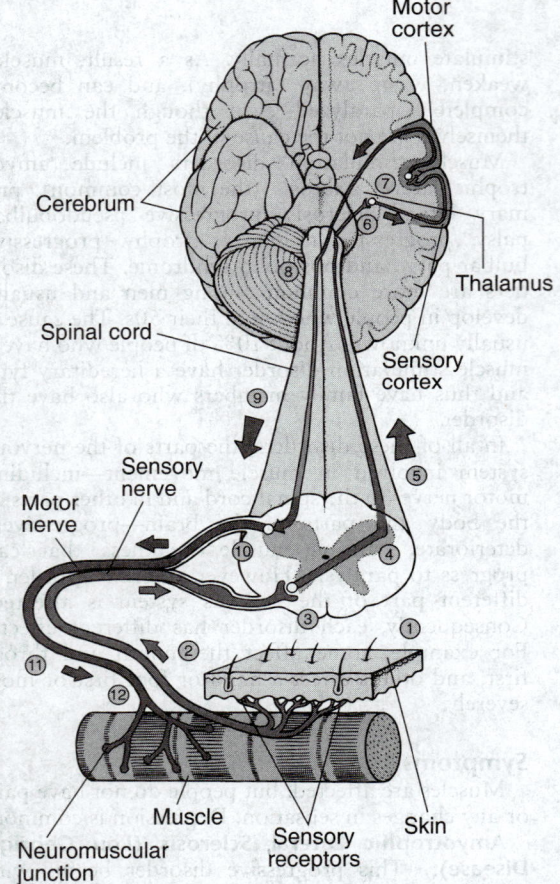

1. If sensory receptors in the skin detect pain or a change in temperature, they transmit an impulse (signal), which ultimately reaches the brain.
2. The impulse travels along a sensory nerve to the spinal cord.
3. The impulse crosses a synapse (the junction between two nerve cells) between the sensory nerve and a nerve cell in the spinal cord.
4. The impulse crosses from the nerve cell in the spinal cord to the opposite side of the spinal cord.
5. The impulse is sent up the spinal cord and through the brain stem to the thalamus, which is a sensory processing center deep in the brain.
6. The impulse crosses a synapse in the thalamus to nerve fibers that carry the impulse to the sensory cortex of the cerebrum (the area that recieves and interprets information from sensory receptors).
7. The sensory cortex perceives the impulse. A person may then decide to initiate movement, which triggers the motor cortex (the area that plans, controls, and executes voluntary movements) to generate an impulse.
8. The nerve carrying the impulse crosses to the opposite side at the base of the brain.
9. The impulse is sent down the spinal cord.
10. The impulse crosses a synapse between the nerve fibers in the spinal cord and a motor nerve, which is located in the spinal cord.
11. The impulse travels out of the spinal cord along the length of the motor nerve.
12. At the neuromuscular junction, the impulse crosses from the motor nerve to the motor end plate on the muscle, where it stimulates muscle movement.

saliva is produced, sometimes causing drooling. As the disorder progresses, people may be unable to control emotional responses and may laugh or cry inappropriately.

Eventually, the muscles involved in breathing may weaken, leading to breathing problems. Some people need a ventilator to breathe.

How rapidly amyotrophic lateral sclerosis progresses varies. About 50% of people with the disorder die within 3 years of the first symptoms, 10% live 10 years or more, and a few people survive as long as 30 years.

Primary Lateral Sclerosis and Progressive Pseudobulbar Palsy: These disorders are rare, slowly progressive variants of amyotrophic lateral sclerosis. Primary lateral sclerosis affects mainly the arms and legs, and progressive pseudobulbar palsy affects mainly the muscles of the face, jaw, and throat. In both disorders, severe stiffness accompanies muscle weakness. Emotions may be changeable: People with progressive pseudobulbar palsy may switch from happiness to sadness quickly and without reason. Inappropriate emotional outbursts are common. Many years later, muscles begin to twitch and waste away. The disorders usually progress for several years before total disability results.

Progressive Muscular Atrophy: This disorder can develop at any age. It is similar to amyotrophic lateral sclerosis, but it progresses more slowly, spasticity does not occur, and muscle weakness is less severe. Involuntary contractions or twitching of muscle fibers may be the earliest symptoms. The hands are usually affected first, followed by the arms, shoulders, and legs. Eventually, the whole body is affected. Many people with this disorder survive 25 years or longer.

Progressive Bulbar Palsy: In this disorder, the nerves controlling the muscles of chewing, swallowing, and talking are affected, making these functions increasingly difficult. The voice may have a nasal tone. In some people, emotions are changeable. Because swallowing is difficult, food or saliva is often inhaled (aspirated) into the lungs, causing choking or gagging and increasing the risk of pneumonia. Death, which is often due to pneumonia, usually occurs 1 to 3 years after the disorder begins.

Postpolio Syndrome: In some people who have had polio, muscles may become tired, painful, and weak 15 years or more after recovery from polio. Sometimes muscle tissue also wastes away, suggesting a reactivation of the polio infection. However, in most people who have had polio, such symptoms are not due to postpolio syndrome but to the development of a new disorder, such as diabetes, a slipped (herniated) disk, or osteoarthritis.

Diagnosis

Doctors suspect one of these disorders in adults who have progressive muscle weakness without pain or loss of sensation. Doctors ask people which parts of the body are affected, when the disorder started, what symptoms appeared first, and how the symptoms changed over time. This information gives them clues about the cause of symptoms.

Muscle weakness can have many causes (see table on page 541), so diagnostic tests, such as the following, are needed to help narrow the possibilities:

- Magnetic resonance imaging (MRI) of the brain and sometimes the spinal cord is done to check for abnormalities that may cause similar symptoms.

- Electromyography (see page 636), which involves stimulating muscles and recording their electrical activity, can help determine whether the problem is in nerves or muscles.

- Nerve conduction studies, which measures how fast nerves transmit impulses, may also be done. The speed of impulses is not affected until late in these disorders, so if impulses are unexpectedly slow, the cause of symptoms may be another disorder.

- Blood tests are done to check for other disorders (such as infections and metabolic disorders) that do not affect the nerves but can cause weakness.

Treatment

Muscle stimulation disorders have no specific treatment or cure. Care provided by a team of several types of health care practitioners (multidisciplinary team) helps people cope with progressive disability. Physical therapy helps people maintain muscle strength and helps prevent shortening of muscles (contractures). Nurses or other caregivers must feed people with swallowing difficulties carefully to prevent choking. Some people must be fed through a tube inserted through the abdominal wall into the stomach (gastrostomy tube).

Baclofen may help make muscles less spastic, and phenytoin or quinine may help decrease cramps. Drugs with anticholinergic effects, such as amitriptyline (an antidepressant), may be used because of one of its anticholinergic effects—reducing saliva formation. Amitriptyline or fluvoxamine (also an antidepressant) may help people who have changeable emotions or depression.

In some people with amyotrophic lateral sclerosis, riluzole, a drug that protects nerve cells, can prolong life. It is taken by mouth.

If pain develops as the disorder progresses (for example, it may become painful to sit in one spot without being able to shift position), opioids and benzodiazepines, which are mild sedatives, may be used.

In a few people with progressive bulbar palsy, surgery to improve swallowing helps.

Because amyotrophic lateral sclerosis and progressive bulbar palsy are progressive and incurable, people with one of these disorders are advised to establish advanced directives that specify what kind of care they want at the end of life (see page 69).

Neuromuscular Junction Disorders

Nerves connect with muscles at the neuromuscular junction. There, the ends of nerve fibers connect to special sites on the muscle's membrane called motor end plates. These plates contain receptors

Overactive Nerves: Two Syndromes

Sometimes nerves repeatedly send electrical impulses to muscles, resulting in overstimulation. Overstimulation is thought to be a factor in Stiff-person syndrome and Isaac's syndrome.

Stiff-person syndrome: This syndrome is more common among women and often occurs in people with diabetes or certain kinds of cancer, including Hodgkin lymphoma (Hodgkin's disease).

The cause may be an autoimmune reaction—when the body produces antibodies that attack its own tissues. Antibodies to an enzyme called glutamic acid decarboxylase are present, but whether they cause the symptoms is unknown.

Muscles of the trunk, abdomen, and legs gradually become stiffer and enlarge. Muscles of the arms, head, and neck are affected less.

The sedative diazepam can consistently relieve the muscle stiffness. Plasmapheresis, in which toxic substances are filtered from the blood, is sometimes tried but often without success. Without treatment, the disorder progresses, leading to disability and stiffness throughout the body.

Isaac's syndrome: This rare disorder has no known cause. It often occurs in people with cancer.

Muscles, particularly those in the arms and legs, continually twitch, moving like a bag of worms. This symptom is called myokymia. The hands and feet may intermittently have spasms and cramps. Muscle stiffness is common. Sweating may be increased.

Symptoms can be relieved by carbamazepine or phenytoin, both of which are anticonvulsants.

---

that enable the muscle to respond to acetylcholine, a chemical messenger (neurotransmitter) released by the nerve to transmit a nerve impulse across the neuromuscular junction. After a nerve stimulates a muscle at this junction, an electrical impulse flows through the muscle, causing it to contract.

Did You Know...

Nerve gases used in chemical warfare interfere with communication between nerves and muscles.

Disorders in which the neuromuscular junction malfunctions include myasthenia gravis, botulism, and Eaton-Lambert syndrome. In addition, many drugs (including very high doses of some antibiotics), certain insecticides (organophosphates), curare (an extract from plants formerly placed on the tip of some poison darts and used to paralyze and kill), and the nerve gases used in chemical warfare can cause the neuromuscular junction to malfunction. Some of these substances prevent the normal breakdown of acetylcholine after the nerve impulse has been transmitted to the muscle.

MYASTHENIA GRAVIS

Myasthenia gravis is an autoimmune disorder that impairs communication between nerves and muscles, resulting in episodes of muscle weakness.

- Myasthenia gravis may result from malfunction of the immune system.
- People usually have drooping eyelids and double vision, and muscles become unusually tired and weak after exercise.
- Response to a drug given intravenously helps doctors determine whether people may have myasthenia gravis.
- Electromyography, blood tests, and imaging tests are needed to confirm the diagnosis.
- Some drugs can improve muscle strength rapidly, and others can slow progression of the disorder.

Myasthenia gravis is more common among women. It usually develops in women between the ages of 20 and 40. However, the disorder may affect men or women at any age. Rarely, it begins during childhood.

In myasthenia gravis, the immune system produces antibodies that attack one type of receptor on the muscle side of the neuromuscular junction—the receptors that respond to the neurotransmitter acetylcholine. As a result, communication between the nerve cell and the muscle is disrupted. What causes the body to attack its own acetylcholine receptors—an autoimmune reaction—is unknown. According to one theory, malfunction of the thymus gland may be involved. In the thymus gland, certain cells of the immune system learn how to differentiate between the body and foreign substances. The thymus gland also contains muscle cells (myocytes) with acetylcholine receptors. For unknown reasons, the thymus gland may instruct the immune system cells to produce antibodies that attack the acetylcholine receptors. People may inherit a predisposition to this autoimmune abnormality. About 65% of people who have myasthenia gravis have an enlarged thymus gland, and about 10% have a tumor of the thymus gland (thymoma). About half of thymomas are cancerous (malignant). Some people with the disorder do not have antibodies to acetylcholine receptors but have antibodies to an enzyme involved in the formation of the neuromuscular junction instead. These people may require different treatment.

The disorder may be triggered by infections, surgery, or use of certain drugs, such as nifedipine or verapamil (used to treat high blood pressure), quinine (used to treat malaria), and procainamide (used to treat abnormal heart rhythms).

Neonatal myasthenia develops in 12% of babies born to women who have myasthenia gravis. Antibodies against acetylcholine receptors, which circulate in the blood, may pass from a pregnant woman through the placenta to the fetus. In such cases, the baby has muscle weakness that disappears several days to a few weeks after birth. The remaining 88% of babies are not affected.

Symptoms

Episodes of worsened symptoms (exacerbations) are common. At other times, symptoms may be minimal or absent.

The most common symptoms are

- Weak, drooping eyelids
- Weak eye muscles, which cause double vision
- Excessive weakness of affected muscles after they are used

The weakness disappears when the muscles are rested but recurs when they are used again.

In 40% of people with myasthenia gravis, the eye muscles are affected first, but 85% eventually have this problem. In 15% of people, only the eye muscles are affected, but in most people, the whole body is affected. Difficulty speaking and swallowing and weakness of the arms and legs are common. Hand grip may alternate between weak and normal. This fluctuating grip is called milkmaid's grip. Neck muscles may become weak. Sensation is not affected.

When people with myasthenia gravis use a muscle repetitively, the muscle usually becomes weak. For example, people who once could use a hammer well become weak after hammering for several minutes. However, muscle weakness varies in intensity from hour to hour and from day to day, and the course of the disease varies widely.

About 15% of people have severe episodes (called myasthenia crisis), sometimes triggered by an infection. The arms and legs may become extremely weak, but even then, they do not lose sensation. In some people, the muscles needed for breathing weaken. This condition is life threatening.

Diagnosis

Doctors suspect myasthenia gravis in people with episodes of weakness, especially when the eye or facial muscles are affected or when weakness increases with use of the affected muscles and disappears with rest. Because acetylcholine receptors are damaged, drugs that increase levels of acetylcholine can be used to help confirm the diagnosis. Edrophonium, injected intravenously, is most commonly used. People are asked to exercise the affected muscle until it tires. Then they are given the drug. If it temporarily and quickly improves muscle strength, myasthenia gravis is a possible diagnosis.

Other diagnostic tests are needed to confirm the diagnosis. They include electromyography (stimulating muscles, then recording their electrical activity) and blood tests to detect antibodies to acetylcholine receptors and sometimes the other antibodies present in people with the disorder. Blood tests are also done to check for other disorders. Computed tomography (CT) or magnetic resonance imaging (MRI) of the chest is done to assess the thymus gland and to determine whether a thymoma is present.

Treatment

Drugs may be used to help improve strength quickly or to suppress the autoimmune reaction and slow progression of the disorder.

Drugs that increase the amount of acetylcholine, such as pyridostigmine (taken by mouth), may improve muscle strength. Long-acting capsules are available for nighttime use to help people who experience severe weakness or difficulty swallowing when they awaken in the morning. Doctors must periodically adjust the dose, which may have to be increased during episodes of weakness. However, doses that are too high can cause weakness that is difficult to distinguish from that caused by the disorder. Also, the effectiveness of these drugs may decrease with long-term use. Increasing weakness, which may be due to a decrease in the drug's effectiveness, must be evaluated by a doctor with expertise in treating myasthenia gravis.

Common side effects of pyridostigmine include abdominal cramps and diarrhea. Drugs that slow the activity of the digestive tract, such as atropine or propantheline, may be needed to counteract these effects.

To suppress the autoimmune reaction, doctors may also prescribe a corticosteroid, such as prednisone, or an immunosuppressant, such as cyclosporine or azathioprine. These drugs are taken by mouth. Most people need to take a corticosteroid indefinitely. When the corticosteroid is started, symptoms may worsen initially, but improvement occurs within a few months. The dose is then reduced to the minimum that is effective. Corticosteroids, when taken for a long time, can have moderate or severe side effects. Thus, azathioprine may be given so that the corticosteroid can be stopped or its dose reduced. With azathioprine, improvement takes about 18 months.

Immune globulin (a solution containing many different antibodies collected from a group of donors) may be given intravenously once a day for 5 days.

Over two thirds of people improve in 1 to 2 weeks, and effects may last 1 to 2 months.

When drugs do not provide relief or when a myasthenic crisis occurs, plasmapheresis (see box on page 1030) may be used. In plasmapheresis, toxic substances (in this case, abnormal antibodies) are filtered from the blood.

If a thymoma is present, the thymus gland must be surgically removed to prevent the thymoma from spreading. If no thymoma is present, the benefit of removing the thymus gland is uncertain.

BOTULISM

Botulism is an uncommon, life-threatening poisoning caused by toxins produced by the bacterium Clostridium botulinum.

- Botulism toxins, usually consumed in food, can weaken or paralyze muscles.
- Botulism may begin with dry mouth, double vision, and inability to focus the eyes or with gastric distress.
- Doctors examine samples of blood, stool, or tissue from the wound, and electromyography may be done.
- Careful food preparation and storage help prevent botulism.
- An antitoxin is used to prevent or slow the effects of the toxin.

Botulism is usually foodborne.

The toxins that cause botulism, which are very potent poisons, can severely impair nerve function. Because these toxins damage nerves, they are called neurotoxins. Botulism toxins paralyze muscles by inhibiting the release of the neurotransmitter acetylcholine from nerves. In very small doses, the toxin can be used to relieve muscle spasms and to reduce wrinkles.

Causes

The bacterium *Clostridium botulinum* forms reproductive cells called spores. Like seeds, spores can exist in a dormant state for many years, and they are highly resistant to destruction. When moisture and nutrients are present and oxygen is absent (as in the intestine or sealed jars or cans), the spores start to grow and produce toxins. Some toxins produced by *Clostridium botulinum* are not destroyed by the intestine's protective enzymes.

Clostridium botulinum is common in the environment, and spores can be transported by air. Many cases of botulism result from ingesting or inhaling small amounts of soil or dust. Spores can also enter the body through the eyes or a break in the skin.

There are several different forms of botulism.

Foodborne botulism occurs when food contaminated with the toxins is eaten. The most common sources of foodborne botulism are home-canned foods, particularly foods with a low acid content, such as asparagus, green beans, beets, and corn. Other sources include chopped garlic in oil, chili peppers, tomatoes, foil-wrapped baked potatoes that have been left at room temperature too long, and home-canned or fermented fish. However, about 10% of outbreaks result from eating commercially prepared foods, most commonly, vegetables, fish, fruits, and condiments (such as salsa). Less commonly, beef, milk products, pork, poultry, and other foods cause botulism.

Wound botulism occurs when *Clostridium botulinum* contaminates a wound or is introduced into other tissues. Inside the wound, the bacteria produce toxins that are absorbed into the bloodstream. Injecting drugs with needles that are not sterilized can cause this type of botulism, as can injecting contaminated heroin into a muscle or under the skin (skin popping).

Infant botulism develops in infants who eat food containing spores of the bacteria rather than toxins. The spores then grow in the infant's intestine, where they produce toxins. The cause of most cases is unknown, but some cases have been linked to the ingestion of honey. Infant botulism occurs most commonly among infants younger than 6 months.

> **? Did You Know...**
>
> The toxin that causes botulism can be used to treat uncontrollable muscle spasms and to reduce wrinkles.
>
> Injecting illicit drugs increases the risk of botulism.

Symptoms

Symptoms of foodborne botulism develop suddenly, usually 18 to 36 hours after toxins enter the body, although symptoms can start as soon as 4 hours or as late as 8 days after ingesting the toxins. The more toxin ingested, the sooner people become sick. Usually, people who become sick within 24 hours of eating contaminated food are the most severely affected.

The first symptoms of foodborne or wound botulism commonly include dry mouth, double vision, drooping eyelids, and an inability to focus on nearby objects. The pupils of the eyes do not constrict normally when exposed to light during an eye examination. However, in foodborne botulism, the first symptoms are often nausea, vomiting, stomach cramps, and diarrhea. People who have wound botulism do not have any digestive symptoms.

Nerve damage by the toxins affects muscle strength but not sensation. Muscle tone in the face may be lost. Speaking and swallowing become difficult. Because swallowing is difficult, food or saliva is often inhaled (aspirated) into the lungs, causing choking or gagging and increasing the risk of pneumonia. Some people become constipated. The muscles of the arms and legs and the muscles involved in breathing become progressively weaker as symptoms gradually move down the body. Breathing problems may be life threatening. The mind usually remains clear.

In about 90% of infants with infant botulism, constipation is the first symptom. Then the muscles become paralyzed, beginning in the face and head and eventually reaching the arms, legs, and muscles involved in breathing. Eyelids droop, crying is weak, infants are less able to suck, and their face loses its expression. Problems range from being tired and feeding slowly to losing a substantial amount of muscle tone and having difficulty breathing. When infants lose muscle tone, they may feel abnormally limp.

Diagnosis

Doctors suspect botulism based on symptoms. However, other disorders can cause similar symptoms, so additional information is needed.

Electromyography (stimulating muscles and recording their electrical activity—see page 636) may be useful. In most cases of botulism, it shows abnormal muscle responses after electrical stimulation.

For foodborne botulism, a likely food source provides a clue. For example, when botulism occurs in two or more people who ate the same food prepared in the same place, the diagnosis is clearer. The diagnosis is confirmed when the toxins are detected in the blood or when the bacteria are detected in a culture of stool. Toxins may also be identified in food that the person ate.

For wound botulism, doctors ask whether people have had an injury that broke the skin. Doctors may inspect the skin for puncture marks suggesting use of an illicit drug. The diagnosis is confirmed when the toxins are detected in the blood or when the bacteria are detected in a culture of tissue from the wound.

Detecting the bacteria or the toxins in a sample of an infant's stool confirms the diagnosis of infant botulism.

Sometimes determining whether botulism developed from a wound or from food is impossible.

Prevention

The spores of *Clostridium botulinum* are highly resistant to heat and may survive boiling for several hours. However, the toxins are readily destroyed by heat. Stored foods can cause botulism if they were inadequately cooked before they were stored. The bacteria can produce some toxins at temperatures as low as 37.4° F (3° C), a typical refrigerator temperature, so refrigerating food does not automatically make it safe.

Did You Know...

Infants should not be fed honey.

The following measures can help prevent foodborne botulism:

- Cooking food at 176° F (79.9° C) for 30 minutes, which almost always destroys toxins
- Boiling home-canned food for 10 minutes, which destroys the toxins
- Discarding canned foods that are discolored or smell spoiled
- Discarding cans that are swollen or leaking
- Refrigerating oils infused with garlic or herbs
- Keeping potatoes that have been baked in aluminum foil hot until served
- Not feeding children younger than 2 years honey, which may contain *Clostridium botulinum* spores

If people are unsure whether a can should be discarded, they can check it when they start to open it. Before making the first puncture, they can place a few drops of water in the spot to be punctured. If water is expelled rather than sucked into the can when the can is punctured, the can is contaminated and should be discarded.

Any food that may be contaminated should be disposed of carefully. Even tiny amounts of toxins ingested, inhaled, or absorbed through the eye or a break in the skin can cause serious illness. Skin contact should be avoided as much as possible, and hands should be washed immediately after handling the food.

If a wound becomes infected, promptly seeking medical attention can reduce the risk of wound botulism.

Researchers and other people who work with the bacteria or its toxin are immunized.

Treatment

People who may have botulism should go to the hospital immediately. Laboratory tests to confirm the diagnosis are done, but treatment often cannot be delayed until the results are known. To help eliminate any unabsorbed toxin, doctors may give activated charcoal by mouth or through a tube inserted into the stomach.

Vital signs (pulse, breathing rate, blood pressure, and temperature) are measured often. If breathing problems begin, people are transferred to an intensive care unit and may be temporarily placed on a ventilator. Such treatment has reduced the percentage of deaths due to botulism from about 70% in the early 1900s to less than 10%.

A substance that blocks the action of the toxins (antitoxin) is given as soon as possible after botulism has been diagnosed. It is most likely to help if given within 72 hours of when symptoms begin. The antitoxin may slow or stop further physical deterioration, so that the body can heal itself over a period of months. However, the antitoxin cannot undo damage already done. Also, some people have a serious allergic (anaphylactic) reaction to the antitoxin, which is derived from horse serum, or develop serum sickness (see box on page 2018). The antitoxin is not recommended for infant botulism, but use of a botulism immune globulin (derived from the blood of people immunized against botulism) in infants is being studied. People may need to be fed through an intravenous tube. Infants may need to be fed through a thin plastic feeding tube (a nasogastric tube) passed through the nose and down the throat.

Some people who recover from botulism feel tired and are short of breath for years afterward. They may need long-term physical therapy.

EATON-LAMBERT SYNDROME

Eaton-Lambert syndrome is an autoimmune disorder that causes weakness.

Eaton-Lambert syndrome is caused by antibodies that interfere with the release of acetylcholine rather than attack acetylcholine receptors (as occurs in myasthenia gravis—see page 818). Eaton-Lambert syndrome usually precedes, occurs with, or develops after certain cancers, especially lung cancer.

Eaton-Lambert syndrome causes muscle weakness, but persistent use of a muscle causes an increase rather than a decrease in strength (as occurs in myasthenia gravis). People also tire easily. The mouth is dry, the eyelid droops, and the upper arms and thighs are painful. Men may have erectile dysfunction.

Symptoms suggest the diagnosis, but electromyography (stimulating muscles, then recording their electrical activity) is needed to confirm the diagnosis.

Treating cancer, if present, sometimes relieves symptoms due to Eaton-Lambert syndrome. Guanidine, a drug that increases the release of acetylcholine, often lessens symptoms but may inhibit the bone marrow's production of blood cells and impair liver function. Corticosteroids and plasmapheresis (filtering of toxic substances, including abnormal antibodies, from the blood) help some people.

Plexus Disorders

The networks of interwoven nerve fibers from different spinal nerves (plexuses) may be damaged by injury, tumors, collections of blood, or autoimmune reactions.

- Pain, weakness, and loss of sensation occur in all or part of an arm or a leg.
- Electromyography and evoked responses help doctors locate the damage, and magnetic resonance imaging helps locate the damage and identify the cause.
- Sometimes treating the disorder causing the problem improves nerve function.

A plexus is like an electrical junction box, which distributes wires to different parts of a house. In a plexus, nerve fibers from different spinal nerves (which connect the spinal cord to the rest of the body) are sorted. The fibers are recombined so that all fibers going to a specific body part are put together in one nerve. Damage to nerves in the major plexuses causes problems in the arms or legs that these nerves supply. The major plexuses are the brachial plexus, which is located in the neck and shoulders and distributes nerves throughout the arms, and the lumbosacral plexus, which is located in the lower back and pelvis and distributes nerves to the pelvis and legs.

Causes

The most common causes of damage are physical injury and cancer. An accident that pulls the arm or severely bends the arm at the shoulder may damage the brachial plexus (located near the shoulder). In newborns, the brachial plexus can be damaged during birth if the delivery requires pulling or other maneuvers. A fall can injure the lumbosacral plexus (located near the hip).

A cancer growing in the upper part of the lung can invade and destroy the brachial plexus. Or a cancer of the intestine, bladder, or prostate can invade the lumbosacral plexus. Other masses, such as a noncancerous (benign) tumor, an abscess, or a collection of blood (hematoma), may cause plexus disorders by putting pressure on a plexus.

Radiation therapy for breast cancer or diabetes, which can damage nerves throughout the body, may also damage nerves in a plexus.

Acute brachial neuritis (sudden malfunction of the brachial plexus) is probably caused by an autoimmune reaction—when the body produces antibodies that attack its own tissues. This disorder occurs primarily in men. It typically occurs in young adults but can occur at any age.

Symptoms

Malfunction of the brachial plexus causes pain, weakness, and loss of sensation in an arm. All or

Nerve Junction Boxes: The Plexuses

Much like the electrical junction box in a house, a nerve plexus is a network of interwoven nerves. Nerve fibers from different spinal nerves are sorted and recombined in plexuses, so that all fibers going to a specific body part are put together in one nerve. Four nerve plexuses are located in the trunk of the body:

- The cervical plexus provides nerve connections to the head, neck, and shoulder.
- The brachial plexus provides connections to the chest, shoulders, upper arms, forearms, and hands.
- The lumbar plexus provides connections to the back, abdomen, groin, thighs, knees, and calves.
- The sacral plexus provides connections to the pelvis, buttocks, genitals, thighs, calves, and feet.

Because the lumbar and sacral plexuses are interconnected, they are sometimes referred to as the lumbosacral plexus. The spinal nerves in the chest do not join a plexus. They are the intercostal nerves, which are located between the ribs.

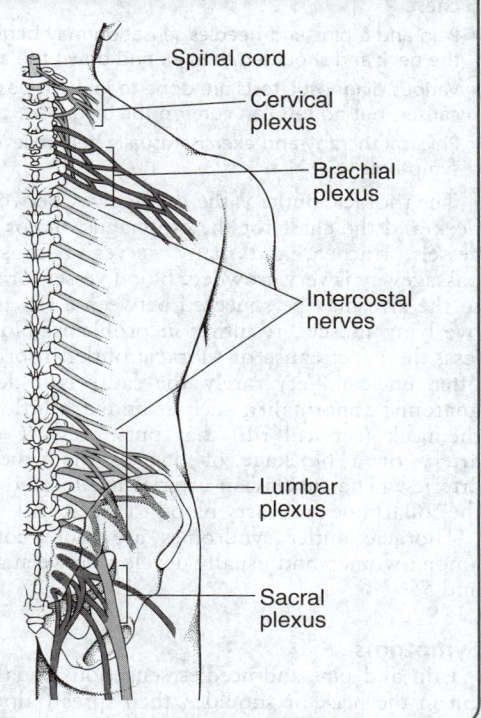

Spinal cord

Cervical plexus

Brachial plexus

Intercostal nerves

Lumbar plexus

Sacral plexus

part of the arm (such as the forearm or biceps) may be affected. If the cause is an injury, recovery tends to occur slowly, over several months, although some severe injuries cause permanent weakness.

Acute brachial neuritis causes severe pain in the upper arms and shoulders. Usually, the arm becomes weak and reflexes are impaired as the pain resolves. Weakness develops within 3 to 10 days. Then people typically regain their strength over the next few months.

Malfunction of the lumbosacral plexus causes pain in the lower back and leg as well as weakness and loss of sensation in all or part of a leg (such as the foot or calf). Recovery depends on the cause.

Diagnosis

Doctors suspect that a plexus is involved when symptoms are located in a part of the body supplied by a specific plexus. The location of the symptoms indicates which plexus is affected.

Electromyography and nerve conduction studies can also help locate the damage (see page 636). Magnetic resonance imaging (MRI) can help deter-

mine whether a cancer, another mass, or an injury is causing the plexus disorder.

Treatment

Treatment depends on the cause. Cancer near the plexus may be treated with radiation therapy, chemotherapy, or both. Occasionally, a cancer or another mass that is damaging the plexus must be removed surgically.

If diabetes is the cause, controlling blood sugar levels can help.

Doctors sometimes prescribe corticosteroids for acute brachial neuritis and other plexus disorders thought to be caused by an autoimmune reaction, but these drugs have no proven benefit. When an injury is the cause, time for healing may be all that is needed, but sometimes surgery is required.

Thoracic Outlet Syndromes

Thoracic outlet syndromes are a group of disorders caused by pressure on nerves as they pass between the neck and chest. These disorders cause pain and pins-and-needles sensations (paresthesias) in the hand, shoulder, and arm.

- Nerves and blood vessels may be squeezed as they go through the tight passageway from the neck to the chest.
- Pain and a pins-and-needles sensation may begin in the neck and shoulder, then extend down the arm.
- Various diagnostic tests are done to look for possible causes, but no test can confirm the diagnosis.
- Physical therapy and exercise usually help relieve symptoms.

The thoracic outlet is the passageway between the neck and the chest for the esophagus, major blood vessels, trachea, and many nerves. Because this passageway is very crowded, blood vessels or nerves to the arm may be squeezed between a rib and the overlying muscle, resulting in problems. Nonetheless, the exact cause of thoracic outlet disorders is often unclear. Very rarely, the cause is a clear-cut anatomic abnormality, such as an extra little rib in the neck (cervical rib) that puts pressure on an artery or a blockage of one of the subclavian arteries. (The subclavian arteries are located under the collarbone and carry blood to the arms.)

Thoracic outlet syndromes are more common among women and usually develop between age 35 and 55.

Symptoms

Pain and pins-and-needles sensations usually begin in the neck or shoulder, then spread along the inner surface of the arm into the hand and sometimes down the side of the torso.

If pressure is put on one of the subclavian arteries, the hand, arm, and shoulder on the affected side may swell, or the overlying skin may look bluish because the oxygen supply is inadequate (a condition called cyanosis). Sometimes the pressure is severe enough to cause Raynaud's syndrome, in which the fingers become pale or blue and often numb when exposed to cold. In severe cases, the pressure may cause gangrene in the fingers.

Diagnosis

Doctors base the diagnosis on symptoms and results of a physical examination and several diagnostic tests. Nerve conduction studies and electromyography (see page 636) may detect abnormalities characteristic of thoracic outlet syndrome. Through a stethoscope placed on the collar bone or near the top of the armpit, doctors may hear sounds indicating abnormal blood flow (bruits) in a compressed artery. Angiography of the arteries in the arm (brachial arteries) may be done to detect abnormal blood flow. In this test, x-rays are taken after a dye that is visible on x-rays (radiopaque dye) is injected into the bloodstream. Magnetic resonance imaging (MRI) may be done to look for anatomic abnormalities. However, none of these tests can definitively confirm or rule out the diagnosis of thoracic outlet syndrome.

Treatment

For most people with symptoms of thoracic outlet syndrome, physical therapy and exercise result in improvement. Nonsteroidal anti-inflammatory drugs (NSAIDs) and antidepressants given in low doses may also help.

Surgery may be needed if an anatomic abnormality or blockage of the subclavian artery is confirmed or if symptoms continue to progress. However, because a definitive diagnosis is difficult to make and because symptoms often persist after surgery, most doctors try to avoid surgery.

Mononeuropathy

Mononeuropathy is damage to a single peripheral nerve.

- Pressure on a nerve for a long time can damage it.
- The affected area may tingle, feel prickly, or be numb, and the affected muscle may be weak.
- Usually, the diagnosis is based on symptoms and results of a physical examination.
- Modifying or stopping the activity that caused the problem and taking pain relievers usually help, but sometimes physical therapy or surgery is needed.

Causes

Physical injury is the most common cause of a mononeuropathy. Injury is commonly caused by the following:

- Prolonged pressure on a nerve that runs close to the surface of the body near a prominent bone, such as a nerve in an elbow, a shoulder, a wrist, or a knee (as may occur during a long, sound sleep, especially in alcoholics)
- Pressure from a misfitting cast or from crutches that fit poorly or that are used incorrectly
- Pressure from staying in a cramped position for a long time, as when gardening or when playing cards with the elbows resting on a table

Injury may result from pressure that occurs when people cannot move for long periods, as when they are under anesthesia for surgery, are confined to bed (particularly older people), or are paralyzed. Less commonly, injury results from the following:

- Accidents
- Prolonged exposure to cold or heat
- Radiation therapy for cancer
- Repeated injuries, such as those due to tight gripping of small tools or to excessive vibration from an air hammer

- Infections, such as leprosy or Lyme disease
- A collection of blood (hematoma)
- Cancer, which may directly invade a nerve
- Some toxic substances and some drugs

If the pressure on the nerve is mild, people may feel only pins-and needles-sensations without any weakness. For example, people may hit their elbow (funny bone), or a foot may fall asleep. These episodes can be considered temporary mononeuropathies.

Nerves that run close to the body's surface near a bone are more vulnerable to injury. Examples are the median nerve in the wrist (resulting in carpal tunnel syndrome—see page 601), the ulnar nerve in the elbow, the radial nerve in the upper arm, and the peroneal nerve near the knee.

> **❓ Did You Know...**
>
> Using crutches that are the wrong height can damage a nerve and make the hand and wrist weak.

Symptoms

Abnormal sensations, including pins-and-needles or loss of sensation, occur in the area supplied by the injured nerve. Pain and weakness may or may not be present.

Carpal Tunnel Syndrome: The median nerve passes through a narrow passageway at the wrist. Pressure on this nerve causes pain and abnormal sensations in the fingers, the palm side of the hand and wrist, and sometimes the arm and shoulder (see page 601).

Ulnar Nerve Palsy: The ulnar nerve passes close to the surface of the skin at the elbow. The nerve is easily damaged by repeatedly leaning on the elbow or by hitting the elbow (funny bone). Sometimes the nerve is damaged by an abnormal bone growth in the area. Usually, people feel a tingling, pins-and-needles sensation. Ulnar nerve palsy results from more severe injury and makes the muscles in the hand weak. Severe, chronic ulnar nerve palsy can cause muscles to waste away (atrophy), resulting in a clawhand deformity (the fingers are frozen in a bent position because the muscles become tight). Avoiding pressure on the elbow is recommended.

Radial Nerve Palsy: The radial nerve passes along the underside of the bone in the upper arm. Prolonged pressure on this nerve results in radial nerve palsy. This disorder is sometimes called Saturday night palsy because it occurs in people who drink heavily (often during weekends) and then sleep soundly with an arm draped over the back of a

---

> ### When the Foot's Asleep
>
> A sleeping foot can be considered a temporary neuropathy. The foot falls asleep when pressure is put on the nerve (usually the peroneal nerve but sometimes the sciatic nerve) supplying it. Pressure interferes with the blood supply to the nerve, making the nerve give off abnormal signals (a pins-and-needles sensation), called a paresthesia. Relieving the pressure, for example, by moving around, restores the nerve's blood supply. As a result, the nerve can function normally, and the pins-and-needles sensation stops.

chair or under their partner's head. If crutches fit incorrectly and press on the inside of the arm near the armpit, they can cause this disorder. The nerve damage weakens the wrist and fingers so that the wrist may flop into a bent position with the fingers curved (a condition called wristdrop). Occasionally, the back of the hand may lose feeling. Usually, radial nerve palsy resolves once the pressure is relieved.

Peroneal Nerve Palsy: The peroneal nerve passes close to the surface of the skin on the outer, lower part of the knee. Pressure on this nerve results in peroneal nerve palsy. This disorder weakens the muscles that lift the foot, so that the foot cannot be flexed upward (a condition called footdrop). It is most common among thin people who are confined to bed, people who are incorrectly strapped into a wheelchair, and people (especially thin people) who habitually cross their legs for long periods of time. Avoiding pressure on the nerve—for example, by not crossing the legs—usually relieves the symptoms.

Diagnosis

Usually, doctors can diagnose mononeuropathies based on symptoms and results of a physical examination, including feeling (palpating) the affected muscle when it is moving to check for weakness. Sometimes electromyography and nerve conduction studies are done to rule out other possible causes, to determine where the nerve is damaged, or to determine how severe the disorder is.

Treatment

If the cause is a disorder, it is treated. For example, a tumor may be surgically removed.

Usually, when temporary pressure is the cause, the following can help relieve symptoms:

- Resting
- Not putting pressure on the nerve

- Placing heat on the affected area
- Taking nonsteroidal anti-inflammatory drugs (NSAIDs), such as ibuprofen, to reduce inflammation

Some people with carpal tunnel syndrome benefit from corticosteroid injections.

Braces or splints are often used to prevent shortening of muscles (contractures) until the symptoms resolve. Surgery may be done to relieve pressure on a nerve if the disorder progresses despite other treatments.

For severe, chronic ulnar nerve palsy, physical therapy helps prevent tightening of muscles. Surgical repair is often unsuccessful.

Multiple Mononeuropathy

Multiple mononeuropathy (mononeuritis multiplex) is the simultaneous malfunction of two or more peripheral nerves in separate areas of the body. It causes abnormal sensations and weakness.

Multiple mononeuropathy typically affects only a few nerves, often in different areas of the body. In contrast, polyneuropathy affects many nerves, usually in about the same areas on both sides of the body. However, if multiple mononeuropathy involves many nerves, it may be difficult to distinguish from polyneuropathy.

Several disorders can cause multiple mononeuropathy, and each disorder produces characteristic symptoms. Diabetes is probably the most common cause, although diabetes more commonly causes polyneuropathy. Other common causes of multiple mononeuropathy include polyarteritis nodosa, lupus (systemic lupus erythematosus), Sjögren's syndrome, rheumatoid arthritis, sarcoidosis, amyloidosis, and infections (such as Lyme disease and HIV infection). Multiple mononeuropathy may result from direct invasion of the nerve by bacteria, as occurs in leprosy. A disorder may affect the nerves all at once or affect them progressively, a few at a time.

People have pain, weakness, abnormal sensations, or a combination of symptoms in the areas supplied by the affected nerves. Symptoms often begin on one side of the body. When diabetes is the cause, muscles of the eyes and thighs are often affected.

Doctors base the diagnosis on symptoms and results of a physical examination, but electromyography and nerve conduction tests are usually done to confirm the diagnosis.

Treatment depends on the cause.

Polyneuropathy

Polyneuropathy is the simultaneous malfunction of many peripheral nerves throughout the body.

- Infections, toxins, drugs, cancers, nutritional deficiencies, and disorders can cause many peripheral nerves to malfunction.
- Sensation, strength, or both may be impaired, often in the feet or hands before the arms, legs, or trunk.
- Doctors base the diagnosis on results of electromyography, nerve conduction studies, and blood and urine tests.
- If treating the underlying disorder does not relieve symptoms, physical therapy, drugs, and other measures may help.

Polyneuropathy may be acute (beginning suddenly) or chronic (developing gradually, often over months or years).

Causes

Acute polyneuropathy has many causes:

- Infections involving a toxin produced by bacteria, as occurs in diphtheria
- An autoimmune reaction (when the body attacks its own tissues), as occurs in Guillain-Barré syndrome
- Toxic substances, including heavy metals such as lead and mercury
- Drugs, including the anticonvulsant phenytoin, some antibiotics (such as chloramphenicol, nitrofurantoin, and sulfonamides), some chemotherapy drugs (such as vinblastine and vincristine), and some sedatives (such as barbital and hexobarbital)
- Cancer, such as multiple myeloma, which damages nerves by directly invading or putting pressure on them or by triggering an autoimmune reaction

The cause of chronic polyneuropathy is often unknown. Causes include the following:

- Diabetes
- Excessive use of alcohol
- Nutritional deficiencies (such as thiamin deficiency), an uncommon cause in the United States, except among alcoholics who are malnourished
- Anemia due to vitamin B_{12} deficiency (pernicious anemia)
- An underactive thyroid gland (hypothyroidism)
- Liver failure
- Kidney failure
- Certain cancers, such as lung cancer
- Vitamin B_6 (pyridoxine) taken in excessive amounts

The most common form of chronic polyneuropathy usually results from poor control of blood sugar levels in people with diabetes (see page 1007) but may result from excessive use of alcohol.

Diabetic neuropathy refers to the several forms of polyneuropathy that diabetes can cause. (Diabetes can also cause mononeuropathy or multiple mononeuropathy, which leads to weakness, typically of the eye or thigh muscles.)

In some people, the cause is hereditary.

Depending on the cause, polyneuropathies may affect motor nerves (which control muscle movement), sensory (which transmit sensory information), cranial nerves (which connect the head, face, eyes, nose, muscles, and ears to the brain), or a combination.

Symptoms

Acute polyneuropathy (for example, as occurs in Guillain-Barré syndrome) begins suddenly in both legs and progresses rapidly upward to the arms. Symptoms include weakness and a pins-and-needles sensation or loss of sensation. The muscles that control breathing may be affected, resulting in respiratory failure.

In the most common form of chronic polyneuropathy, only sensation is affected. Usually, the feet are affected first, but sometimes the hands are. A pins-and-needles sensation, numbness, burning pain, and loss of vibration sense and position sense (knowing where the arms and legs are) are prominent symptoms. Because position sense is lost, walking and even standing become unsteady. Consequently, muscles may not be used. Eventually, they may weaken and waste away.

Diabetic neuropathy commonly causes painful tingling or burning sensations in the hands and feet—a condition called distal polyneuropathy. Pain is often worse at night and may be aggravated by touch or by a change in temperature. People may lose the senses of temperature and pain, so they often burn themselves and develop open sores caused by prolonged pressure or other injuries. Without pain as a warning of too much stress, joints are susceptible to injuries. This type of injury is called Charcot's joints (see page 572).

Polyneuropathy often affects the nerves of the autonomic nervous system, which controls involuntary functions in the body (such as blood pressure, heart rate, digestion, salivation, and urination). Typical symptoms are constipation, loss of bowel or bladder control (leading to fecal or urinary incontinence), sexual dysfunction, and fluctuating blood pressure—most notably a sudden fall in blood pressure when a person stands up (orthostatic hypotension). The skin may become pale and dry, and sweating may be reduced.

People who have a hereditary form may have hammer toes, high arches, and a curved spine (scoliosis). Abnormalities in sensation and muscle weakness may be mild. Affected people may not notice these symptoms or may consider them unimportant.

How completely people recover depends on the cause of polyneuropathy.

Diagnosis

Doctors usually recognize polyneuropathy by the symptoms. A physical examination and tests such as electromyography and nerve conduction studies (see page 636) can provide additional information about absent or reduced sensation in the feet.

After polyneuropathy is diagnosed, its cause, which may be treatable, must be identified. Doctors ask whether other symptoms are present and how quickly the symptoms developed. Blood and urine tests may detect a disorder that is causing polyneuropathy—for example, diabetes, kidney failure, or an underactive thyroid gland. Infrequently, a nerve biopsy is necessary.

Sometimes polyneuropathy affecting the hands and feet is the first indication that people have diabetes. Sometimes, when extensive testing detects no obvious cause, the cause is an inherited neuropathy that affects other family members so mildly that the disorder was never suspected.

Treatment

Specific treatment depends on the cause, as for the following:

- **Excessive amounts of vitamin B_6:** If the vitamin is stopped, polyneuropathy may resolve.

- **Diabetes:** Careful control of blood sugar levels may slow progression of the disorder and occasionally relieves symptoms. Transplantation of cells that produce insulin (islet cells—see page 1133), located in the pancreas, sometimes results in a cure.

- **Multiple myeloma or liver or kidney failure:** Treatment of these disorders may result in slow recovery.

- **Cancer:** Surgically removing the cancer may be necessary to relieve pressure on the nerve.

- **An underactive thyroid gland:** Thyroid hormone is given.

- **Autoimmune disorders:** Treatments include plasmapheresis (filtering of toxic substances, including abnormal antibodies, from the blood), immune globulin given intravenously, corticosteroids, and drugs that suppress the immune system (immunosuppressants).

If the cause cannot be corrected, treatment focuses on relieving pain and problems related to muscle weakness. Physical therapy sometimes reduces muscle stiffness and can prevent shortening of muscles (contractures). Physical and occupational therapists can recommend useful assistive devices. Some drugs that are usually not considered pain relievers can lessen pain due to nerve damage. They include the antidepressant amitriptyline, the anti-convulsant gabapentin, and mexiletine (used to treat abnormal heart rhythms). Lidocaine, an anesthetic applied as a lotion, an ointment, or a skin patch, may also help.

GUILLAIN-BARRÉ SYNDROME

Guillain-Barré syndrome (acute inflammatory demyelinating polyneuropathy) is a form of polyneuropathy that causes one episode of increasing muscle weakness. The episode lasts 8 weeks or less.

- An autoimmune reaction may damage the myelin sheath around nerves.
- Usually, weakness begins in both legs and moves up the body.
- Electromyography and nerve conduction studies can help confirm the diagnosis.
- Plasmapheresis or immune globulin given intravenously may speed recovery.

The presumed cause is an autoimmune reaction: The body's immune system attacks the myelin sheath, which surrounds the axon of many nerves and enables nerve impulses to travel quickly. In about 80% of people with this syndrome, symptoms begin about 5 days to 3 weeks after a mild infection (such as a *Campylobacter* infection, mononucleosis, or another viral infection), surgery, or an immunization.

Symptoms

Symptoms usually begin in both legs, then progress upward to the arms. Occasionally, symptoms begin in the arms or head and progress downward. Symptoms include weakness and a pins-and-needles sensation or loss of sensation. Weakness is more prominent than abnormal sensation. Reflexes are decreased or absent. In 90% of people who have Guillain-Barré syndrome, weakness is most severe within 3 weeks. In 5 to 10%, the muscles that control breathing become so weak that a ventilator is needed. Because the facial and swallowing muscles become weak, a few people need to be fed intravenously or through a tube placed directly through the abdominal wall into the stomach (gastrostomy tube).

If the disorder is very severe, internal functions controlled by the autonomic nervous system may be impaired. For example, blood pressure may fluctuate widely, heart rhythm may become abnormal, and severe constipation may develop.

In a variant called Miller-Fisher syndrome, only a few symptoms develop: Eye movements become paralyzed, walking becomes difficult, and normal reflexes disappear.

Diagnosis

Doctors suspect the diagnosis based on the pattern of symptoms. Tests are done to confirm the diagnosis. People are usually admitted to the hospital to have the tests because the syndrome can worsen rapidly and impair the muscles involved in breathing.

Analysis of cerebrospinal fluid obtained by a spinal tap (lumbar puncture—see art on page 635), electromyography, nerve conduction studies, and blood tests can help doctors exclude other possible causes of severe weakness, such as transverse myelitis and spinal cord injuries. A combination of high protein levels and no inflammatory cells in the cerebrospinal fluid and characteristic results from electromyography strongly suggest Guillain-Barré syndrome.

Prognosis

Damage stops progressing within 8 weeks. Without treatment, most people improve slowly over several months. However, with early treatment, people can improve very quickly—in days or weeks. About 30% of adults and even more children with the disorder have residual weakness 3 years after the syndrome began. On average, less than 2% of people die.

After improving initially, 3 to 10% of people develop a disorder called chronic inflammatory demyelinating polyneuropathy (see page 829).

Treatment

Guillain-Barré syndrome can worsen rapidly and is a medical emergency. People who develop this syndrome should be hospitalized immediately. Establishing the diagnosis is crucial because the sooner appropriate treatment is started, the better the chance of a good outcome.

In the hospital, people are closely monitored so that breathing can be assisted with a ventilator if necessary. Nurses take precautions to prevent pressure sores and injuries by providing soft mattresses and by turning the people with severe weakness every 2 hours. If weakness is less severe, physical therapy is started to help preserve joint and muscle function. Heat therapy may be used first to relieve pain and thus make physical therapy more comfortable.

Plasmapheresis (filtering of toxic substances, including antibodies to the myelin sheath) from the blood—see box on page 1030) or immune globulin given intravenously is the treatment of choice. These treatments are relatively safe, shorten the hospital stay, speed recover, and reduce the risk of death and permanent disability.

Corticosteroids do not help and may worsen the syndrome.

CHRONIC INFLAMMATORY DEMYELINATING POLYNEUROPATHY

Chronic inflammatory demyelinating polyneuropathy (chronic acquired demyelinating polyneuropathy, or chronic relapsing polyneuropathy) is a form of polyneuropathy that, like Guillain-Barré syndrome, causes increasing muscle weakness, but the weakness lasts longer than 8 weeks.

Chronic inflammatory demyelinating polyneuropathy develops in 3 to 10% of people with Guillain-Barré syndrome.

Weakness and abnormal sensations (numbness and pins-and-needles) last longer than 8 weeks. Weakness can worsen continually or come and go. Reflexes are decreased or absent. In most people with this disorder, blood pressure fluctuates less, abnormal heart rhythms occur less often, and other internal functions are less impaired than in people with Guillain-Barré syndrome. Also, weakness may be more irregular, affecting the two sides of the body differently, and weakness may progress more slowly.

Diagnosis and Treatment

Doctors suspect the diagnosis based on symptoms. Electromyography, nerve conduction studies, and a spinal tap to obtain cerebrospinal fluid are done to confirm the diagnosis. Rarely, a biopsy of the nerve is needed.

Corticosteroids such as prednisone can relieve symptoms. Immunosuppressants such as azathioprine may also be used. However, if chronic inflammatory demyelinating polyneuropathy is severe or progresses rapidly, plasmapheresis or immune globulin given intravenously may be preferred to corticosteroids. People may need treatment for months or years.

Hereditary Neuropathies

Hereditary neuropathies affect the peripheral nerves, causing subtle symptoms that worsen gradually.

Hereditary neuropathies may affect only motor nerves (motor neuropathies), only sensory nerves (sensory neuropathies), or both sensory and motor nerves (sensorimotor neuropathies). Some hereditary neuropathies are relatively common but often are not recognized. Hereditary sensory neuropathies are especially rare. These neuropathies tend to impair the ability to sense pain and temperature.

The genes responsible for many of these neuropathies have been identified. They include some forms of Charcot-Marie-Tooth disease, Refsum's disease (see box on page 1839), porphyria (see page 975), Fabry's disease (see page 1840), and hereditary neuropathy with liability to pressure palsies (see page 830).

CHARCOT-MARIE-TOOTH DISEASE

Charcot-Marie-Tooth disease (peroneal muscular atrophy) is a hereditary neuropathy in which the muscles of the lower legs become weak and waste away (atrophy).

Charcot-Marie-Tooth disease is the most common hereditary neuropathy, affecting 1 of 2,500 people. It is a sensorimotor neuropathy. That is, it affects motor nerves (which stimulate muscle action) and sensory nerves (which carry sensory information).

There are 2 main types and several subtypes of the disease. In some types, axons (the part of the nerve that sends messages) die because the myelin sheath surrounding them is damaged or destroyed (demyelinated). In other types, axons die even though the sheath is not damaged. Most types of the disease are inherited as an autosomal (not sex-linked) dominant trait. That is, only one gene from one parent is required for the disease to develop.

Symptoms

Symptoms vary by type of the disease.

Type 1: Symptoms begin in middle childhood. Weakness begins in the lower legs. It causes an inability to flex the foot (footdrop) and wasting away of the calf muscles (stork leg deformity). Later, hand muscles begin to waste away. The hands and feet become unable to sense vibration, pain, and temperature, and this loss of sensation gradually moves up the limbs.

In milder subtypes of type 1, high arches and hammer toes may be the only symptoms. In one subtype, males have severe symptoms, and females have mild symptoms or may be unaffected.

The disease progresses slowly and does not affect life span.

Type 2: The neuropathy progresses more slowly and causes somewhat similar symptoms, often beginning during the teenage years.

Diagnosis and Treatment

The distribution of weakness, the age at which the disease began, the family history, the presence of foot deformities (high arches and hammer toes), and the results of nerve conduction studies help doctors identify the different types of Charcot-Marie-Tooth disease and distinguish them from other causes of neuropathy. Genetic testing and counseling for Charcot-Marie-Tooth disease is available.

No treatment can stop the progression of the disease. Wearing braces helps correct footdrop, and sometimes orthopedic surgery is needed to stabilize the foot. Physical therapy (to strengthen muscles) and occupational therapy may be helpful.

HEREDITARY NEUROPATHY WITH LIABILITY TO PRESSURE PALSIES

Hereditary neuropathy with liability to pressure palsies is a hereditary disorder in which nerves become very sensitive to pressure, injury, and use.

In this neuropathy, nerves are susceptible to damage resulting from relatively slight pressure or injury or from repetitive use. Usually, this neuropathy starts during adolescence or young adulthood, but it may start at any age. It affects both sexes equally. It is inherited as an autosomal (not sex-linked) dominant trait (see page 12).

Peroneal nerve palsy with footdrop, ulnar nerve palsy, and carpal tunnel syndrome commonly develop. Numbness or weakness occurs periodically in the affected area. Symptoms vary from unnoticeable and mild to severe and incapacitating. Episodes may last several minutes to months.

Doctors may have difficulty diagnosing this neuropathy because the symptoms come and go. Electromyography and genetic testing help establish the diagnosis. Rarely, biopsy of a nerve is required.

Activities that cause symptoms should be avoided or modified. Supports, such as wrist splints and elbow pads, can reduce pressure, prevent reinjury, and allow the nerve to repair itself over time. Rarely, surgery is needed.

About half of the people who have symptoms recover completely within days to months. In people who do not recover completely, symptoms are rarely severe.

Spinal Muscular Atrophies

Spinal muscular atrophies are hereditary disorders in which nerve cells in the spinal cord and brain stem degenerate, causing progressive muscle weakness and wasting.

- These disorders are inherited.
- The four main types cause various degrees of muscle weakness and wasting.
- Depending on the type, people may be confined to a wheelchair, and life span may be shortened.
- The diagnosis, suggested by symptoms, is based on family history, tests of muscle and nerve function, and sometimes blood tests to detect the defective gene.
- There is no cure, but physical therapy and use of braces can help.

The disorders are usually inherited as a recessive autosomal (not sex-linked) trait. That is, two genes are required, one from each parent (see page 12). These disorders may also affect the central nervous system. There are four main types of spinal muscular atrophy.

Symptoms

Symptoms of the four main types first appear during infancy and childhood.

In acute (type I) spinal muscular atrophy (Werdnig-Hoffmann disease), muscle weakness is usually apparent at or within a few days of birth. It is virtually always apparent by age 6 months. Infants lack muscle tone and reflexes and have difficulty sucking, swallowing, and eventually breathing. Death occurs in 95% of children within the first year and in all by age 4 years, usually due to respiratory failure.

In children with intermediate (type II) spinal muscular atrophy, weakness typically develops between age 6 and 15 months. Fewer than one fourth of them learn to sit. None can crawl or walk. Muscles are weak, and swallowing may be difficult. Most children are confined to a wheelchair by age 2 to 3 years. The disorder is often fatal in early life, usually because of respiratory problems. But some children survive with permanent weakness that does not continue to worsen. These children often have severe curvature of the spine (scoliosis).

Chronic (type III) spinal muscular atrophy (Wohlfart-Kugelberg-Welander disease) begins in children between age 15 months and 19 years and worsens slowly. Consequently, people with this disorder usually live longer than those with type I or II spinal muscular atrophy. Some of them have a normal life span. Weakness and wasting of muscles begin in the hips and thighs and later spread to the arms, feet, and hands.

Type IV spinal muscular atrophy first appears during adulthood, usually between age 30 and 60 years. Muscles, mainly in the hips, thighs, and shoulders, become weak and waste away.

Diagnosis and Treatment

Doctors usually test for these rare disorders when unexplained weakness and muscle wasting occur in young children. Because these disorders are inherited, a family history may help doctors make the diagnosis. Electromyography and nerve conduction studies (see page 636) help confirm the diagnosis. The specific defective gene has been identified for some of the types and can be detected by blood tests. Occasionally, biopsy of a muscle is done. If there is a family history of one of the disorders, amniocentesis can be done to help determine whether an unborn child has the defective gene.

No specific treatments are available. Physical therapy and wearing braces can sometimes help. Physical and occupational therapists can provide adaptive devices to enable children to feed themselves, write, or use a computer.

124 Autonomic Nervous System Disorders

The autonomic nervous system regulates certain body processes, such as blood pressure and the rate of breathing. This system works automatically (autonomously), without a person's conscious effort.

Disorders of the autonomic nervous system can affect any body part or process. Autonomic disorders may result from other disorders that damage autonomic nerves (such as diabetes), or they may occur on their own. Autonomic disorders may be reversible or progressive.

Anatomy: The autonomic nervous system is the part of the nervous system that supplies the internal organs, including the blood vessels, stomach, intestine, liver, kidneys, bladder, genitals, lungs, pupils and muscles of the eye, heart, and sweat, salivary, and digestive glands (see also page 627).

The autonomic nervous system has two main divisions: the sympathetic and the parasympathetic. After the autonomic nervous system receives information about the body and external environment, it responds by stimulating body processes, usually through the sympathetic division, or inhibiting them, usually through the parasympathetic division.

An autonomic nerve pathway involves two nerve cells. One cell is located in the brain stem or spinal cord. It is connected by nerve fibers to the other cell, which is located in a cluster of nerve cells (called an autonomic ganglion). Nerve fibers from these ganglia connect with internal organs. Most of the ganglia for the sympathetic division are located just outside the spinal cord on both sides of it. The ganglia for the parasympathetic division are located near or in the internal organs.

Function: The autonomic nervous system controls blood pressure, heart and breathing rates, body temperature, digestion, metabolism (thus affecting body weight), the balance of water and electrolytes (such as sodium and calcium), the production of body fluids (saliva, sweat, and tears), urination, defecation, sexual response, and other processes.

Many organs are controlled primarily by either the sympathetic or the parasympathetic division. Sometimes the two divisions have opposite effects on the same organ. For example, the sympathetic division increases blood pressure, and the parasympathetic division decreases it. Overall, the two divisions work together to ensure that the body responds appropriately to different situations.

Generally, the sympathetic division prepares the body for stressful or emergency situations—fight or flight. Thus, it increases heart rate and the force of heart contractions and widens (dilates) the airways to make breathing easier. It causes the body to release stored energy. Muscular strength is increased. This division also causes palms to sweat, pupils to dilate, and hair to stand on end. It slows body processes that are less important in emergencies, such as digestion and urination.

The parasympathetic division controls body process during ordinary situations. Generally, it conserves and restores. It slows the heart rate and decreases blood pressure. It stimulates the gastrointestinal tract to process food and eliminate waste. Energy from the processed food is used to restore and build tissues.

Both the sympathetic and parasympathetic divisions are involved in sexual activity, as are the parts of the nervous system that control voluntary actions and transmit sensation from the skin (somatic nervous system).

Two chemical messengers (neurotransmitters), acetylcholine and norepinephrine, are used to communicate within the autonomic nervous system. Nerve fibers that secrete acetylcholine are called cholinergic fibers. Fibers that secrete norepinephrine are called adrenergic fibers. Generally, acetylcholine has parasympathetic (inhibiting) effects and norepinephrine has sympathetic (stimulating) effects. However, acetylcholine has some sympathetic effects. For example, it sometimes stimulates sweating or makes the hair stand on end.

Symptoms

In men, difficulty initiating and maintaining an erection (erectile dysfunction) can be an early symptom of an autonomic disorder. Autonomic disorders commonly cause dizziness or light-headedness due to an excessive decrease in blood pressure when a person stands (orthostatic hypotension).

People may sweat less or not at all and thus become intolerant of heat. The eyes and mouth may be dry.

After eating, a person with an autonomic disorder may feel prematurely full or even vomit because the stomach empties very slowly (gastroparesis). Some people pass urine involuntarily (urinary incontinence), often because the bladder is overactive. Other people have difficulty emptying the bladder (urine retention) because the bladder is underactive. Constipation may occur, or control of bowel movements may be lost.

The pupils may not dilate and narrow (constrict) as light changes.

Diagnosis

Doctors can check for signs of autonomic disorders during the physical examination. They measure blood pressure and heart rate while a person is lying down or sitting and after the person stands. They examine the pupils for abnormal responses or lack of response to changes in light.

Other tests can provide additional information. Tilt table testing may be done to check blood pressure and heart rate responses to changes in position (see page 328). Blood pressure is measured after the person, who is lying flat on a pivoting table, is tilted into an upright position. Blood pressure is also measured continuously while the person performs a Valsalva maneuver (forcefully trying to exhale without letting air escape, as during a bowel movement). Electrocardiography is done to determine whether the heart rate changes as it normally does during deep breathing and the Valsalva maneuver.

Sweat testing is also done. For this test, the sweat glands are stimulated by electrodes that are filled with acetylcholine and placed on the legs and wrist. Then, the volume of sweat is measured to determine whether sweat production is normal. A slight burning sensation may be felt during the test. In another test (thermoregulatory sweat test), a dye is applied to the skin, and a person is placed in a closed, heated compartment to stimulate sweating. Sweat causes the dye to change color. As a result, doctors can identify which areas of the body sweat too much or too little.

Other tests may be done to check for disorders that can cause the autonomic disorder.

Treatment

Disorders that may be contributing to the autonomic disorder are treated. If no other disorders are present or if such disorders cannot be treated, the focus is on relieving symptoms.

Simple measures can help relieve some symptoms:

- **Orthostatic hypotension:** People are advised to elevate the head of the bed by about 4 inches (10 centimeters) and to stand up slowly. Wearing a compression or support garment, such as an abdominal binder or compression stockings, may help. Consuming more salt and water helps maintain blood volume and thus blood pressure. Sometimes drugs (midodrine, pyridostigmine, or fludrocortisone taken by mouth) are used.

- **Decreased or absent sweating:** If sweating is reduced or absent, avoiding warm environments is useful.

- **Urinary retention:** If urinary retention is caused by inability of the bladder to contract normally, people can be taught to insert a catheter into the bladder themselves. They insert it several times a day and remove it after the bladder is empty. Bethanechol can be used to increase bladder tone and thus ease bladder emptying.

- **Constipation:** A high-fiber diet and stool softeners are recommended. If constipation persists, enemas may be necessary.

- **Erectile dysfunction:** Usually, treatment consists of drugs such as sildenafil, tadalafil, or vardenafil taken by mouth.

Autonomic Neuropathies

Autonomic neuropathies are disorders affecting the peripheral nerves that particularly damage the nerves that automatically (without conscious effort) regulate body processes (autonomic nerves).

- Causes include diabetes, amyloidosis, autoimmune disorders, cancer, excessive alcohol consumption, and certain drugs.
- People may feel light-headed when they stand and have urination problems, constipation, vomiting, and men may have erectile dysfunction.
- Doctors do a physical examination and various tests to check for autonomic malfunction and possible causes.
- The cause is corrected or treated if possible.

The nervous system has central and peripheral parts. The central nervous system includes the brain and spinal cord. The peripheral nervous system includes the nerves that connect the body's tissues with the brain and spinal cord. Peripheral nerves include autonomic nerves, which automatically (unconsciously) regulate body processes. Peripheral nerves also include somatic nerves, the nerves that connect with muscles under voluntary (conscious) control or with sensory receptors in the skin.

Autonomic neuropathies are a type of peripheral neuropathy, a disorder in which peripheral nerves are damaged throughout the body. In autonomic neuropathies, there is much more damage to the autonomic nerves than to the somatic nerves.

Causes

Common causes include diabetes, amyloidosis (accumulation of an abnormal protein in tissues), and autoimmune disorders (when the immune system misinterprets the body's tissues as foreign and attacks them). Viral infections may trigger an autoimmune reaction that results in destruction of autonomic nerves. Some of the antibodies produced by the

℞ SOME DRUGS USED TO TREAT SYMPTOMS OF AUTONOMIC DISORDERS

SYMPTOM	DRUG	DRUG'S EFFECT
Constipation	Fiber supplements (such as bran or psyllium) Stool softeners (such as docusate, lactulose, or polyethylene glycol)	Fiber supplements add bulk to the stool and thus stimulate the natural contractions of the intestine. Fiber supplements and stool softeners help move food through the intestine more quickly.
Fullness in the stomach	Metoclopramide	This drug stimulates contractions in the gastrointestinal tract and thus helps move food through it more quickly.
Erectile dysfunction	Sildenafil Tadalafil Vardenafil	These drugs increase the frequency, rigidity, and duration of erections.
Orthostatic hypotension	Fludrocortisone	This drug helps the body retain salt and thus helps maintain blood volume and blood pressure.
	Midodrine	This drug causes small arteries (arterioles) to constrict and thus helps maintain blood pressure.
	Pyridostigmine	This drug causes arterioles to constrict only when people stand and thus helps maintain blood pressure when people stand but does not increase blood pressure when they are lying or sitting down.
Urinary incontinence	Oxybutynin Tolterodine	These drugs relax the muscles of an overactive bladder.
Urine retention	Bethanechol	This drug stimulates contractions of the bladder and thus helps the bladder empty.

immune system attack acetylcholine receptors (the part of nerve cells that enables them to respond to acetylcholine). Acetylcholine is one of the chemical messengers (neurotransmitters) used to communicate within the autonomic nervous system. A similar reaction often occurs in Guillain-Barré syndrome. Other causes include cancer, drugs, excessive alcohol consumption, and toxins.

Symptoms

A common symptom is an excessive decrease in blood pressure when the person stands (orthostatic hypotension). As a result, the person feels lightheaded or as if about to faint. Men may have difficulty initiating and maintaining an erection (erectile dysfunction). Some people involuntarily pass urine (urinary incontinence), often because the bladder is overactive. Other people have difficult emptying the bladder (urine retention) because the bladder is underactive. After eating, some people feel prematurely full or even vomit because the stomach empties slowly (gastroparesis). Severe constipation may occur.

When somatic nerves are damaged, people may lose sensation or feel a tingling (pins-and-needles) sensation in the hands and feet, or muscles may become weak.

Diagnosis and Treatment

A physical examination and certain tests are done to check for signs of autonomic disorders and possible causes (such as diabetes or amyloidosis). Blood tests are done to check for antibodies to acetylcholine receptors, which indicate an autoimmune reaction. About one half of people with an autonomic neuropathy due to an autoimmune reaction have these antibodies.

The cause, if identified, is treated. Neuropathies due to an autoimmune reaction are sometimes treated with drugs that lessen the reaction, such as azathioprine, cyclophosphamide, or prednisone. If symptoms are severe, immune globulin (a solution containing many different antibodies collected from a group of donors) may be given intravenously, or plasma exchange (plasmapheresis) may be done. In plasmapheresis, blood is withdrawn, filtered to remove abnormal antibodies, then returned to the person.

Horner's Syndrome

In Horner's syndrome, on one side of the face, the eyelid droops, the pupil is small (constricted), and sweating is decreased. The cause is disruption of the nerve fibers that connect the eye and the brain.

- Horner's syndrome may occur on its own or result from a disorder that disrupts nerve fibers connecting the eyes and brain.
- The upper eyelid droops, the pupil remains small, and the affected side of the face may sweat less.
- Doctors test the pupil to see whether it can widen, and may do imaging tests to look for a cause.
- The cause, if identified, is treated.

Horner's syndrome can develop in people of any age.

Causes

Some of the nerve fibers that connect the eyes and brain take a circuitous route. From the brain, they go down the spinal cord. They exit the spinal cord in the chest, then go back up the neck beside the carotid artery, through the skull, and into the eye. If these nerve fibers are disrupted anywhere along their pathway, Horner's syndrome results. Horner's syndrome may occur on its own or be caused by another disorder. For example, it can be caused by disorders of the head, brain, neck, or spinal cord, such as lung cancer, other tumors, swollen lymph glands in the neck (cervical adenopathy), dissection of the aorta or carotid artery, a thoracic aortic aneurysm, and injuries. Horner's syndrome may be present at birth (congenital).

Symptoms

Horner's syndrome affects the eye on the same side as the disrupted nerve fibers. Symptoms include a drooping upper eyelid (ptosis) and a constricted pupil (miosis). The affected side of the face may sweat less than normal or not at all, and rarely, it appears flushed. In the congenital form, the iris of the affected eye remains blue-gray as it is at birth.

Diagnosis and Treatment

The disorder is suspected based on symptoms. To confirm the diagnosis, doctors may apply eye drops that contain small amounts of cocaine to the affected eye. If the pupil does not widen (dilate) after 30 minutes, Horner's syndrome is diagnosed. Doctors may apply other drugs to the eye later. How the pupil reacts to them indicates the general location of the damage. Magnetic resonance imaging (MRI) or computed tomography (CT) of the brain, spinal cord, chest, or neck is often needed to look for tumors and other serious disorders.

The cause, if identified, is treated. However, there is no specific treatment for Horner's syndrome.

Often, no treatment is necessary because, typically, the eyelid only droops very slightly.

Pure Autonomic Failure

Pure autonomic failure is dysfunction of many of the processes controlled by the autonomic nervous system, such as blood pressure. It is not fatal.

- The cause is usually unknown but sometimes is an autoimmune disorder.
- Blood pressure may decrease when people stand, and they may sweat less and may have eye problems, retain urine, become constipated, or lose control of bowel movements.
- Doctors do a physical examination and tests to look for signs of autonomic malfunction.
- Treatment focuses on relieving symptoms.

In pure autonomic failure (previously called idiopathic orthostatic hypotension or Bradbury-Eggleston syndrome), many processes regulated by the autonomic nervous system malfunction. They malfunction because nerve cells that are part of autonomic pathways are lost. The affected cells are located in clusters (called autonomic ganglia) on either side of the spinal cord or near or in internal organs. The brain and spinal cord are not affected. The peripheral nerves other than the autonomic ganglia are also unaffected. Pure autonomic failure affects more women and tends to begin in a person's 40s or 50s. It does not lead to death.

The cause is usually unknown. Sometimes the cause is an autoimmune disorder, which occurs when the immune system misinterprets the body's tissues (in this case, a part called the A3 acetylcholine receptor) as foreign and attacks them.

The most common symptom is an excessive decrease in blood pressure when a person stands (orthostatic hypotension). People may sweat less and become intolerant of heat. The pupils may not widen (dilate) and narrow (constrict) normally. Vision may be blurred. People may have difficulty emptying the bladder (urine retention). They may be constipated or lose control of bowel movements. Men may have difficulty initiating and maintaining an erection (erectile dysfunction).

Diagnosis and Treatment

Doctors check for signs of autonomic dysfunction during the physical examination and with tests. For example, doctors measure levels of norepinephrine, one of the chemical messengers (neurotransmitters) used by nerve cells to communicate with each other. No test can confirm the diagnosis, so doctors diagnose this disorder by excluding other disorders.

There is no specific treatment, so the focus is on relieving symptoms (see page 832).

CHAPTER 125 Cranial Nerve Disorders

Twelve pairs of nerves—the cranial nerves—lead directly from the brain to various parts of the head, neck, and trunk. Some of the cranial nerves are involved in the special senses (such as seeing, hearing, and taste), and others control muscles in the face or regulate glands. The nerves are named and numbered (according to their location, from the front of the brain to the back).

A cranial nerve disorder may affect the connections between cranial nerve centers within the brain. An example is internuclear ophthalmoplegia. Or, a disorder may affect only one cranial nerve. Examples are trigeminal neuralgia, Bell's palsy, hemifacial spasm, and glossopharyngeal neuralgia.

> **? Did You Know...**
>
> Some cranial nerve disorders cause problems with eye movement.
>
> Others cause brief, intermittent attacks of excruciating facial pain.

Symptoms depend on which nerves are damaged. For example, damage often occurs to nerves that control eye movement. If both eyes have trouble moving in the same direction, people may not be able to look in that direction. If only one eye can look in a certain direction, people may have double vision (two images seen side by side) when they look in that direction.

When doctors suspect a cranial nerve disorder, they test the function of a cranial nerve by asking the person to do simple tasks, such as to follow a moving target with the eyes.

Internuclear Ophthalmoplegia

Internuclear ophthalmoplegia is impairment of horizontal eye movements caused by damage to certain connections between nerve centers in the brain stem.

In internuclear ophthalmoplegia, the nerve fibers that coordinate both eyes in horizontal movements—looking from side to side—are damaged. These fibers connect collections of nerve cells (centers or nuclei) that the 3rd cranial nerve (oculomotor nerve) and the 6th cranial nerve (abducens nerve) originate from. In older people, the disorder usually results from a stroke, and only one eye is affected. In younger people, it usually results from multiple sclerosis, and both eyes are often affected. Less common causes include Lyme disease, tumors, and toxicity due to a drug (such as tricyclic antidepressants).

Horizontal eye movements are impaired, but vertical ones are not. The affected eye cannot turn inward, but it can turn outward. When a person looks to the side opposite the affected eye, the following happens:

- The affected eye, which should turn inward, cannot move past the midline. That is, the affected eye looks straight ahead.
- As the other eye turns outward, it often makes involuntary, repetitive fluttering movements called nystagmus. That is, the eye rapidly moves in one direction, then slowly drifts in the other direction.

People with internuclear ophthalmoplegia may have double vision.

One-and-a-half syndrome results when the disorder that causes internuclear ophthalmoplegia also damages the center that coordinates and controls horizontal eye movements (horizontal gaze center). When the person tries to look the either side, the affected eye remains motionless in the middle. The other eye can turn outward but not inward. As in internuclear ophthalmoplegia, vertical eye movements are not affected.

In internuclear ophthalmoplegia and one-and-a-half syndrome, the eyes can turn inward when the person looks inward (as when focusing on a nearby object) even though the eyes cannot turn inward when the person looks to the side.

For internuclear ophthalmoplegia or one-and-a-half syndrome, treatment and outlook (whether the disorder abates or eventually resolves) depends on the disorder that caused it.

Conjugate Gaze Palsies

In conjugate gaze palsies, the two eyes cannot move in one direction (side to side, up, or down) at the same time.

Conjugate gaze palsies affect horizontal gaze (looking to the side) most often. Upward gaze is affected less often, and downward gaze is affected even less often. People may notice that they cannot look in certain directions.

There are no specific treatments.

Viewing the Cranial Nerves

Twelve pairs of cranial nerves emerge from the underside of the brain, pass through openings in the skull, and lead to parts of the head, neck, and trunk.

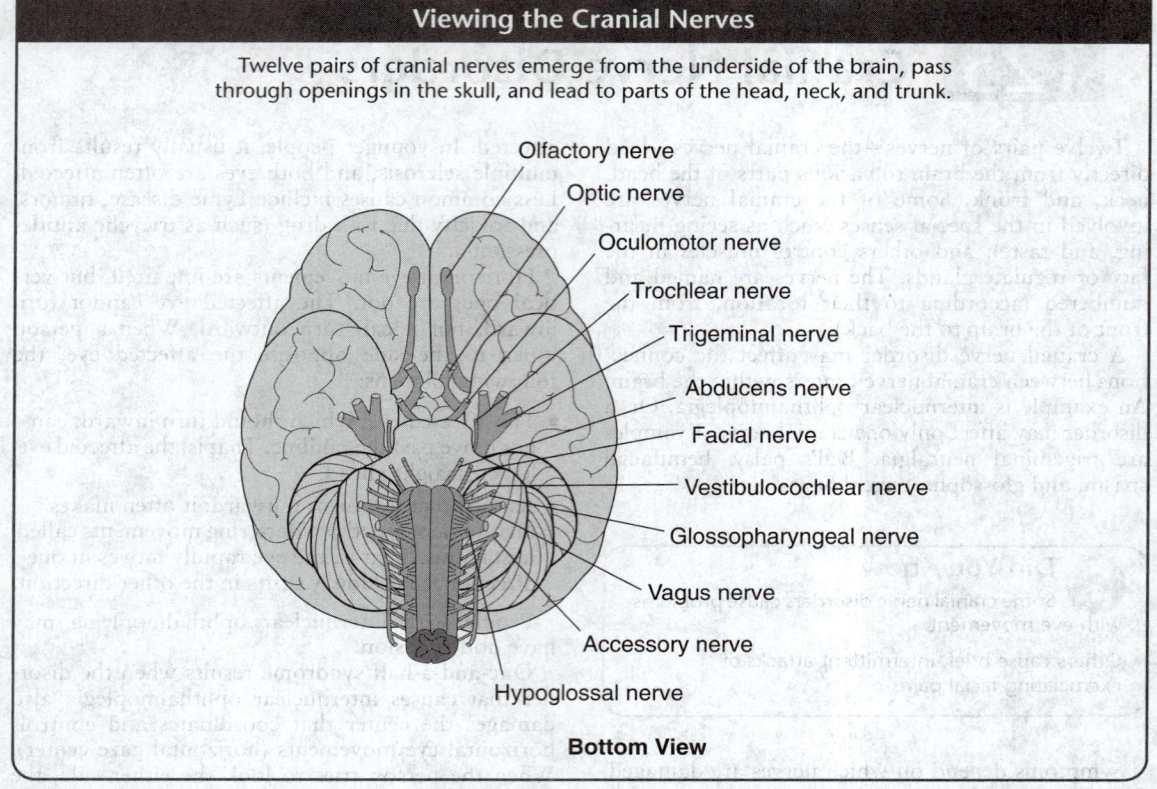

Olfactory nerve
Optic nerve
Oculomotor nerve
Trochlear nerve
Trigeminal nerve
Abducens nerve
Facial nerve
Vestibulocochlear nerve
Glossopharyngeal nerve
Vagus nerve
Accessory nerve
Hypoglossal nerve

Bottom View

Horizontal Gaze Palsy: The most common cause is damage to the brain stem, often by a stroke. Often, the palsy is complete and severe. That is, the eyes cannot move to the side at all. Palsies can also be caused by damage to the front part of the cerebrum, usually by a stroke. The resulting palsy may not be as severe as that caused by damage to the brain stem, and symptoms often lessen with time.

Vertical Gaze Palsy: Vertical gaze decreases gradually with aging, but vertical gaze palsy is more severe than age-related changes. Usually, upward gaze is affected. The most common cause is damage to the top part of the brain stem (midbrain), usually by a stroke or tumor.

The pupils are usually large (dilated). In response to light, they may constrict more slowly and less completely than normal. When people attempt to look up, the eyes rapid move in one direction, then slowly drift in the other direction. These involuntary, fluttering eye movements are called nystagmus.

If downward gaze but not upward gaze is impaired, the cause is usually progressive supranuclear palsy (see page 778).

Palsies of Cranial Nerves That Control Eye Movement

These disorders involve paralysis of cranial nerves that control eye movement (the 3rd, 4th, or 6th nerves), impairing the ability to move the eyes. How eye movement is affected depends on which nerve is affected.

The eye is moved by three pairs of muscles, controlled by the 3rd, 4th, and 6th cranial nerves. These muscles move the eye up and down, right and left, and diagonally. People may have double vision when they look in certain directions.

THIRD CRANIAL NERVE (OCULOMOTOR NERVE) PALSY

A palsy of the 3rd cranial nerve can be caused by brain disorders—such as a head injury, a bulge (aneurysm) in an artery supplying the brain, a hemorrhage, or a tumor—or by diabetes.

Symptoms

The affected eye turns outward when the unaffected eye looks straight ahead, causing double vision. The affected eye can move only to the middle when looking inward and cannot move up and down. Because the 3rd cranial nerve also raises the eyelids and controls the pupils, the eyelid droops, and the pupil may be widened (dilated). It may not narrow (constrict) in response to light.

The disorder causing the palsy may worsen, resulting in a serious, life-threatening condition. For example, a severe headache may occur suddenly, or a person may become increasingly drowsy or less responsive. In such cases, the cause may be a ruptured aneurysm, which then bleeds. Dilation of and lack of response to light (fixation) by both pupils indicates deep coma and possibly brain death (see box on page 708).

Diagnosis and Treatment

The diagnosis is based on results of a neurologic examination and computed tomography (CT) or magnetic resonance imaging (MRI). If the pupil is affected or if symptoms suggest a serious underlying disorder, CT is done immediately. If a ruptured aneurysm is suspected and CT does not detect blood, a spinal tap (lumbar puncture—see art on page 635), magnetic resonance angiography, CT angiography, or cerebral angiography is done.

Treatment depends on the cause. Emergency treatment is required if a life-threatening disorder is the cause.

FOURTH CRANIAL NERVE (TROCHLEAR NERVE) PALSY

Often, the cause cannot be identified. The most common identified cause is a head injury, often due to a motorcycle accident. Occasionally, diabetes causes this palsy. Rarely, the cause is a tumor, an aneurysm, or multiple sclerosis.

One or both eyes may be affected. The affected eye cannot turn inward and down. As a result, people see double images, one above and slightly to the side of the other. Thus, going down stairs, which requires looking inward and down, is difficult. However, tilting the head to the side opposite the affected muscle can compensate and eliminate the double images. This position can eliminate the double images because people use eye muscles that are unaffected by the palsy to focus both eyes on an object.

> **? Did You Know...**
>
> Palsy of the 4th cranial nerve causes double vision, but tilting the head to one side eliminates it.

Usually, the diagnosis is suspected if a person has characteristic abnormal eye movements. CT or MRI may be done.

The disorder causing the palsy, if identified, is treated. Eye exercises may help. Sometimes surgery is necessary to eliminate double vision.

SIXTH CRANIAL NERVE (ABDUCENS NERVE) PALSY

Many disorders can cause this palsy:

- Head injuries
- Tumors
- Multiple sclerosis
- Aneurysms
- Brain infections, such as meningitis, a brain abscess or a parasitic infection
- Complications of an ear or eye infection
- Blockage of an artery supplying the nerve, as can result from diabetes, a stroke, a transient ischemic attack, or vasculitis
- Wernicke's encephalopathy (commonly due to chronic alcoholism)
- Benign intracranial hypertension (pseudotumor cerebri—see page 655)
- Respiratory infections (in children)

Some of these disorders put pressure on the nerve by causing nearby swelling or by increasing pressure within the skull. Others interfere with blood flow to the nerve.

If this palsy occurs alone (without other cranial nerve palsies), its cause is often never identified.

Symptoms

The affected eye cannot turn fully outward and may turn inward when people look straight ahead. Double vision occurs when people look toward the side of the affected eye. Other symptoms depend on the cause. They include severe headache, accumulation of fluid (edema) in the conjunctiva, numbness in the face and mouth, loss of vision, and inability to move the eye in other directions.

Diagnosis and Treatment

Usually, doctors can easily identify a 6th cranial nerve palsy, but the cause is less obvious. An ophthalmoscope is used to look into the eye and check for evidence of tumors, increased pressure, and abnormalities in blood vessels. CT or, preferably, MRI is done to exclude tumors and other abnormalities. If the results are unclear, a spinal tap (lumbar puncture) is done to determine whether pressure within the skull is increased and whether a tumor or swelling due to an infection is compressing the nerve. If symptoms suggest vasculitis, blood is withdrawn to check for signs of inflammation, such as certain abnormal antibodies (antinuclear

TESTING CRANIAL NERVES

CRANIAL NERVE NUMBER	NAME	FUNCTION	TEST
1st	Olfactory	Smell	The ability to smell is tested by asking the person to identify items with very specific odors (such as soap, coffee, and cloves) placed under the nose. Each nostril is tested separately.
2nd	Optic	Vision	The ability to see is tested by asking the person to read an eye chart. Peripheral vision is tested by asking the person to detect objects or movement from the corners of the eyes.
		Detection of light	The ability to detect light is tested by shining a bright light (as from a flashlight) into each pupil in a darkened room.
3rd	Oculomotor	Eye movement upward, downward, and inward	The ability to move each eye up, down, and inward is tested by asking the person to follow a target moved by the examiner.
		Narrowing (constriction) or widening (dilation) of the pupil in response to changes in light	The pupils' response to light is checked by shining a bright light (as from a flashlight) into each pupil in a darkened room.
		Raises the eyelids	The upper eyelid is checked for drooping (ptosis).
4th	Trochlear	Eye movement downward and inward	The ability to move each eye down and inward is tested by asking the person to follow a target moved by the examiner.
5th	Trigeminal	Facial sensation	Sensation in areas of the face is tested using a pin and a wisp of cotton. The blink reflex is tested by touching the cornea of the eye with a cotton wisp.
		Chewing	Strength and movement of muscles that control the jaw are tested by asking the person to clench the teeth and open the jaw against resistance.
6th	Abducens	Eye movement outward	The ability to move each eye outward beyond the midline is tested by asking the person to look to the side.
7th	Facial	Facial expression, taste in the front two thirds of the tongue, and production of saliva and tears	The ability to move the face is tested by asking the person to smile, to open the mouth and show the teeth, and to close the eyes tightly. Taste is tested using substances that are sweet (sugar), sour (lemon juice), salty (salt), and bitter (aspirin, quinine, or aloes).
8th	Auditory (vestibulocochlear)	Hearing	Hearing is tested with a tuning fork or with headphones that play tones of different frequencies (pitches) and loudness (audiometry).
		Balance	Balance is tested by asking the person to walk a straight line.

(continued on the following page)

TESTING CRANIAL NERVES (*Continued*)			
CRANIAL NERVE NUMBER	NAME	FUNCTION	TEST
9th	Glossopharyngeal	Swallowing, gag reflex, and speech	Because the 9th and 10th cranial nerves control similar functions, they are tested together.
10th	Vagus	Swallowing, gag reflex, and speech Control of muscle in internal organs (including the heart)	The person is asked to swallow. The person is asked to say "ah-h-h" to check movement of the palate (roof of the mouth) and uvula (the small, soft projection that hangs down at the back of throat). The back of the throat may be touched with a tongue blade, which evokes the gag reflex in most people. The person is asked to speak to determine whether the voice sounds nasal.
11th	Accessory	Neck turning and shoulder shrugging	The person is asked to turn the head and to shrug the shoulders against resistance provided by the examiner.
12th	Hypoglossal	Tongue movement	The person is asked to stick out the tongue, which is observed for deviation to one side or the other.

antibodies and rheumatoid factor) in the blood and an abnormal erythrocyte sedimentation rate (ESR—how quickly red blood cells settle to the bottom of a test tube containing blood). After all tests are done, the cause may remain unknown.

Treatment depends on the cause. When the cause is treated, the palsy usually resolves. Palsies with no identifiable cause usually resolve without treatment within 2 months, as do those due to a blocked blood vessel.

Trigeminal Neuralgia

Trigeminal neuralgia (tic douloureux) is severe facial pain due to malfunction of the 5th cranial nerve (trigeminal nerve). This nerve carries sensory information from the face to the brain and controls the muscles involved in chewing.

- The cause is usually unknown but sometimes is an abnormally positioned artery that compresses the trigeminal nerve.
- People have repeated short, lightning-like bursts of excruciating stabbing pain in the lower part of the face.
- Doctors base the diagnosis on the characteristic pain.
- Certain anticonvulsants or antidepressants, baclofen, or a local anesthetic may relieve the pain, but surgery is sometimes needed.

Trigeminal neuralgia usually occurs in middle-aged and older people, although it can affect adults of all ages. It is more common among women.

In most cases, the cause is unknown. A common known cause is an abnormally positioned artery that compresses the trigeminal nerve near where it exits the brain. Occasionally in younger people, trigeminal neuralgia results from nerve damage due to multiple sclerosis. Rarely, trigeminal neuralgia results from damage due to herpes zoster (a viral infection) or compression by a tumor.

Symptoms

The pain can occur spontaneously but is often triggered by touching a particular spot (called a trigger point) on the face, lips, or tongue or by an action such as brushing the teeth or chewing. Repeated short, lightning-like bursts of excruciating stabbing pain can be felt in any part of the lower portion of the face but are most often felt in the cheek next to the nose or in the jaw.

Usually, only one side of the face is affected. The pain usually lasts seconds but may last up to 2 minutes. Recurring as often as 100 times a day, the pain can be incapacitating. Because the pain is intense, people tend to wince, and thus the disorder is sometimes called a tic. The disorder commonly resolves on its own, but bouts of the disorder often recur after a long pain-free interval.

Diagnosis

Although no specific test exists for identifying trigeminal neuralgia, its characteristic pain usually makes it easy for doctors to diagnose. However, doctors must distinguish trigeminal neuralgia from other possible causes of facial pain, such as disorders of the jaw, teeth, or sinuses and trigeminal neuropathy (which is often due to compression of the trigeminal nerve caused by a tumor, stroke, an aneurysm, or multiple sclerosis). Trigeminal neuropathy can be distinguished because it causes loss of sensation and often weakness in parts of the face and trigeminal neuralgia does not.

Treatment

Because the bouts of pain are brief and recurrent, typical analgesics are not usually helpful, but other drugs, especially certain anticonvulsants (which stabilize nerve membranes), may help. The anticonvulsant carbamazepine is usually tried first. Gabapentin or phenytoin, also anticonvulsants, may be prescribed if carbamazepine is ineffective or has intolerable side effects. Baclofen (a drug used to reduce muscle spasms) or a tricyclic antidepressant (such as amitriptyline—see table on page 868) may be used instead. A local anesthetic may be injected into or around the nerve (a nerve block) to provide temporary pain relief.

If the pain continues to be severe, surgery may be done. If the cause is an abnormally positioned artery, a surgeon separates the artery from the nerve and places a small sponge between them. This procedure (called vascular decompression) usually relieves the pain for many years. If the cause is a tumor, the tumor can be surgically removed.

If people have pain unrelieved by drugs and surgery seems too risky, a test can be done to determine whether other procedures would help. For the test, alcohol is injected into the nerve to temporarily block its function. If alcohol relieves the pain, disrupting the nerve may relieve the pain, sometimes permanently. The nerve may be cut surgically or with a radiofrequency probe (using heat) or gamma knife (using radiation), or it may be destroyed by injecting a drug such as glycerol into it. However, these treatments are used as a last resort. They often provide only temporary relief—for months to a few years—and afterward, discomfort in the face returns and is even more severe.

Bell's Palsy

Bell's palsy is sudden weakness or paralysis of muscles on one side of the face due to malfunction of the 7th cranial nerve (facial nerve). This nerve moves the facial muscles, stimulates the salivary and tear glands, and enables the front part of the tongue to detect tastes.

- The disorder may result from a herpes simplex viral infection.
- People may feel pain behind the ear, then one side of the face may become weak or completely paralyzed.
- Doctors usually base the diagnosis on symptoms.
- Corticosteroids may be used to reduce swelling of the nerve.
- With or without treatment, most people recover completely within several months.

Bell's palsy affects about 23 of 100,000 people at some time. Bell's palsy may result from herpes simplex virus type 1, which causes herpes mouth infections. But the cause is sometimes unknown. Lyme disease can cause facial nerve paralysis, which is similar to Bell's palsy. In blacks, sarcoidosis (see page 511) is a common cause of facial nerve paralysis.

Symptoms

Pain behind the ear may be the first symptom. It may develop several hours or even a day or two before the facial muscles weaken. Facial weakness occurs suddenly. The effect ranges from mild weakness to complete paralysis. By 48 hours, the weakness is as severe as it will be. Only one side of the face is affected. It becomes flat and expressionless. However, people often feel as though the face is twisted because the muscles on the unaffected side tend to pull the face to that side every time they make a facial expression. Wrinkling the forehead, blinking, and grimacing may be difficult or impossible. For most people, the face feels numb or heavy, even though sensation remains normal.

Closing the eye on the affected side may be difficult. People may be unable to close the eye completely, and they blink less frequently. The eye also tends to turn upward when it is closed.

> **Did You Know...**
>
> Bell's palsy is often caused by the same virus that causes herpes mouth infections.
>
> Lyme disease can cause facial nerve paralysis, similar to Bell's palsy.

Bell's palsy may interfere with the production of saliva and tears. People may have dry eyes and mouth, or they may drool. Because fewer tears are produced and the eye blinks less often (blinking helps moisten the eye's surface), the eye becomes dry, resulting in pain and eye damage. Eye damage is usually minor but can be serious if the eye is not moistened and protected another way. People may be unable to taste with the front part of the tongue on the affected side. The ear on the affected side may perceive sounds as abnormally loud (a condition called hyperacusis) because the muscle that stretches the eardrum is paralyzed. This muscle is located in the middle ear.

Occasionally, as the facial nerve heals, it forms abnormal connections, resulting in unexpected movements of some facial muscles or in watering of the eyes ("crocodile tears") during salivation. Because the facial muscles are not used for a long time, permanent tightening of the muscles (contractures) occasionally occurs.

Diagnosis

There is no specific test for Bell's palsy, but it can usually be diagnosed based on symptoms. Bell's palsy (and other types of facial nerve paralysis) can be distinguished from a stroke because a stroke usually causes weakness only in the lower part of the face rather than in the entire face. People who have had a stroke can close the eyes tightly and wrinkle the brow. Also, a stroke typically causes weakness of an arm and a leg.

Doctors can distinguish Bell's palsy from other, rare disorders that cause facial nerve paralysis (such as tumors, infections, and skull fractures) because the other disorders cause different symptoms and symptoms usually develop slowly. Usually, doctors can exclude these disorders on the basis of the person's history and results of x-rays, magnetic resonance imaging (MRI), or computed tomography (CT). A blood test may be done to check for Lyme disease, and a blood test and a chest x-ray may be done to check for sarcoidosis.

Treatment and Prognosis

An antiviral drug that is effective against herpes simplex virus (such as acyclovir, famciclovir, or valacyclovir) is usually given by mouth even when the cause is unknown. These drugs prevent the virus, if present, from replicating. If symptoms have been present less than 48 hours, a corticosteroid, such as prednisone, is given by mouth to reduce swelling of the nerve. Taking a corticosteroid may slightly speed and improve the recovery of movement.

If the eye cannot close completely, it must be protected from dryness to reduce the risk of eye damage. Eye drops consisting of artificial tears or a salt (saline) solution are applied to the eye until it can close completely. People may need to wear an eye patch some of the time, particularly during sleep. Rarely, in severe cases, the upper and lower eyelids are sewn together.

When facial paralysis is partial, most people recover completely within several months whether they are treated or not. When the paralysis is total, the outcome varies. Tests (nerve conduction studies and electromyography—see page 636) can be done to help predict the likelihood of recovery. Many people do not recover completely. The facial muscles may remain weak, causing the face to droop.

Hemifacial Spasm

Hemifacial spasm is painless involuntary twitching of one side of the face due to malfunction of the 7th cranial nerve (facial nerve). This nerve moves the facial muscles, stimulates the salivary and tear glands, and enables the front part of the tongue to detect tastes.

Hemifacial spasm affects men and women but is more common among middle-aged and older women.

The spasms may be caused by an abnormally positioned artery or loop of an artery that compresses the 7th cranial nerve where it exits the brain stem.

Muscles on one side of the face twitch involuntarily, usually beginning with the eyelid, then spreading to the cheek and mouth. Twitching may be intermittent at first but may become almost continuous. The disorder is essentially painless but can be embarrassing.

The diagnosis is made when doctors see the spasms. Magnetic resonance imaging (MRI) should be done to check for a tumor, other structural abnormalities, and evidence of multiple sclerosis. Usually, MRI can detect the abnormal loop of artery pressing against the nerve.

Botulinum toxin is the drug of choice. It is injected into the affected muscles. The same drugs used to treat trigeminal neuralgia—carbamazepine, gabapentin, phenytoin, baclofen, and tricyclic antidepressants (see table on page 868)—may help. If drug treatment is unsuccessful, surgery may be done to separate the abnormal artery from the nerve by placing a small sponge between them (see art on page 842).

Glossopharyngeal Neuralgia

Glossopharyngeal neuralgia consists of recurring attacks of severe pain in the back of the throat, the area near the tonsils, the back of the tongue, and part of the ear. The pain is due to malfunction of the 9th cranial nerve (glossopharyngeal nerve), which moves the muscles of the throat and carries information from the throat, tonsils, and tongue to the brain.

■ The cause is usually unknown but sometimes is an abnormally positioned artery that compresses the glossopharyngeal nerve.

Taking the Pressure Off a Nerve

When pain results from an abnormally positioned artery pressing on a cranial nerve, the pain can be relieved by a surgical procedure called vascular decompression. This procedure may be done to treat trigeminal neuralgia, hemifacial spasms, or glossopharyngeal neuralgia.

If the trigeminal nerve is compressed, an area on the back of the head is shaved, and an incision is made. The surgeon cuts a small hole in the skull and lifts the edge of the brain to expose the nerve. Then the surgeon separates the artery from the nerve and places a small sponge between them. A general anesthetic is required, but the risk of side effects from the procedure is small. Side effects include facial numbness, facial weakness, double vision, infection, bleeding, alterations in hearing and balance, and paralysis. Usually, this procedure relieves the pain, but in about 15% of people, pain recurs.

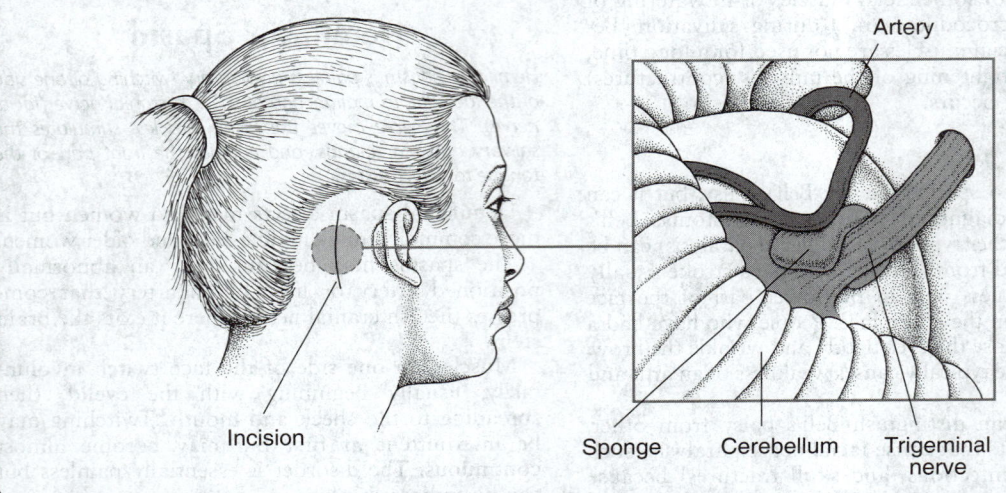

- People have brief attacks of excruciating pain, affecting one side of the tongue or throat and sometimes an ear.
- Doctors diagnose the disorder if a local anesthetic applied to the back of the throat eliminates the pain.
- Certain anticonvulsants or antidepressants, baclofen, or a local anesthetic may relieve the pain, but surgery is sometimes needed.

Glossopharyngeal neuralgia, a rare disorder, usually begins after age 40 and occurs more often in men. Often, its cause is unknown. But sometimes glossopharyngeal neuralgia results from an abnormally positioned artery that compresses the glossopharyngeal nerve near where it exits the brain stem. Rarely, the cause is a tumor in the brain or neck.

Symptoms

Attacks are brief and occur intermittently, but they cause excruciating pain. Attacks may be triggered by a particular action, such as chewing, swallowing, talking, coughing, or sneezing. The pain usually begins at the back of the tongue or back of the throat. Sometimes pain spreads to the ear. The pain may last several seconds to a few minutes and usually affects only one side of the throat and tongue. In 1 to 2% of people, the heartbeat is affected. It slows so much that it stops temporarily, causing fainting.

Diagnosis and Treatment

Glossopharyngeal neuralgia is distinguished from trigeminal neuralgia (which causes similar pain) based on the pain's location or results of a specific test. For the test, a doctor touches the back of the throat with a cotton-tipped applicator. If pain results, the doctor applies a local anesthetic to the back of the throat. If the anesthetic eliminates the pain, the glossopharyngeal neuralgia is diagnosed. Magnetic resonance imaging (MRI) is done to check for tumors.

The same drugs used to treat trigeminal neuralgia—carbamazepine, gabapentin, phenytoin, baclofen, and tricyclic antidepressants (see table on page 868)—may help. If these drugs are ineffective, applying a local anesthetic (such as cocaine) to the back of the throat may provide temporary relief. However, for permanent relief, surgery may be needed. The glossopharyngeal nerve is separated from the artery that is compressing it by placing a small sponge between them.

Hypoglossal Nerve Disorders

Disorders of the 12th cranial nerve (hypoglossal nerve) cause weakness or wasting (atrophy) of the tongue on the affected side. This nerve moves the tongue.

Causes include a tumor or bone abnormality at the base of the skull, a stroke, infection of the brain stem, or an injury to the neck, such as that due to surgical removal of a blockage from an artery in the neck (endarterectomy). Amyotrophic lateral sclerosis (Lou Gehrig's disease) can also damage the hypoglossal nerve.

The tongue becomes weak on the affected side and eventually wastes away (atrophies). As a result, people have difficulty speaking, chewing, and swallowing. Damage due to amyotrophic lateral sclerosis causes tiny, subtle twitching movements (fasciculations) on the surface of the tongue.

Magnetic resonance imaging (MRI) is usually done to look for a tumor or evidence of a stroke. A spinal tap (lumbar puncture) may be necessary if cancer or infection is possible. Treatment depends on the cause.

Mental Health Disorders

126 Overview of Mental Health Care

Mental health (psychiatric or psychologic) disorders involve disturbances in thinking, emotion, or behavior. Small disturbances in these aspects of life are common, but when such disturbances interfere with daily life, they are considered mental illness or a mental health disorder. The effects of mental illness may be long-lasting or temporary. These disorders are caused by complex interactions between physical, psychologic, social, cultural, and hereditary influences.

Mental Illness in Society

About 30 to 50% of adults will experience a mental illness at some point in their lives. More than 50% of these people experience moderate to severe symptoms. In fact, 4 of the 10 leading causes of disability among people aged 5 and older are mental health disorders, with depression being the number one cause of all illnesses that cause disability. Unfortunately, despite this high prevalence of mental illness, only about 20% of people who have a mental illness receive professional help.

Although tremendous advances have been made in the understanding and treatment of mental illnesses, the stigma surrounding them persists. For example, people with mental illness may be blamed for their illness or viewed as lazy or irresponsible. Mental illness may be seen as less real or legitimate than physical illness, leading to reluctance on the part of policy makers and insurance companies to pay for treatment. Parents may be blamed for causing mental illness in their children. The public may shun people with mental illness and avoid living near them, working with them, and socializing with them.

Currently, mental illness is thought to be caused by a complex interaction of genetics and environment. Chemical messengers in the brain called neurotransmitters appear to be disordered in some mental illnesses. By providing images of brain dysfunction, brain imaging techniques, such as magnetic resonance imaging (MRI) and positron emission tomography (PET), have shown that many mental health disorders have a physical component. Research has shown that there is a hereditary component to many mental health disorders. Often, a mental health disorder occurs when people whose genetic make-up makes them vulnerable to such disorders experience extra stress in their family or social life or at work.

Mental illness cannot always be clearly differentiated from normal behavior. Distinguishing normal bereavement from depression, for example, may be difficult in the face of a significant loss, such as the death of a spouse or child. Likewise, a diagnosis of anxiety disorder in relation to a person's worry and stress regarding work is somewhat arbitrary, because most people experience these feelings at some time. The line between a person's having certain personality traits and having a personality disorder can be blurry. Mental illness and mental health, therefore, are best thought of as a continuum. Any dividing line is usually based on how long symptoms last, how much people change from their usual self, and how severely symptoms affect their life.

Deinstitutionalization

A movement in recent decades to bring mentally ill people out of institutions has been made possible by the development of effective drugs, along with some change in attitude about the mentally ill. With the deinstitutionalization movement, greater emphasis has been placed on viewing mentally ill people as members of families and communities.

Research has demonstrated that certain interactions between families and patients can improve or worsen mental illness. Therefore, family therapy techniques that dramatically prevent the chronically mentally ill from needing to be reinstitutionalized have been developed. Today, the family of a mentally ill person is more involved than ever as an ally in treatment. The family doctor also plays an important role in rehabilitating a mentally ill person into the community. In addition, mentally ill people who must be hospitalized are less likely to be isolated and restrained than in the past, and they are often discharged early into day treatment centers. These settings are less expensive because fewer staff members are needed, the emphasis is on group therapy rather than individual therapy, and people sleep at home or in halfway houses.

However, the deinstitutionalization movement has had its share of problems. Because mentally ill people who are not a danger to themselves or society can no longer be institutionalized or treated against their will, many have become homeless or ended up in the prison system. Although these legal measures protect people's civil rights, they make it more difficult to provide needed treatment to many mentally ill people, some of whom may be extremely irrational when untreated. Homelessness also has an effect on society.

Social Support

Everyone requires a social network to satisfy the human need to be cared for, accepted, and emotionally supported, particularly in times of stress. Research has demonstrated that strong social support may significantly improve recovery from both physical and mental illnesses. Changes in society have diminished the traditional support once offered by neighbors and families. As an alternative, self-help groups and mutual aid groups have sprung up throughout the country.

Some self-help groups, such as Alcoholics Anonymous and Narcotics Anonymous, focus on addictive behavior. Others act as advocates for certain segments of the population, such as the handicapped and older people. Still others, such as the National Alliance for the Mentally Ill, provide support for family members of people who have a severe mental illness.

Classification and Diagnosis of Mental Illness

In 1952, the American Psychiatric Association first published the *Diagnostic and Statistical Manual of Mental Disorders (DSM-I)*, marking the first attempt to approach the diagnosis of mental illness through standardized definitions and criteria. The latest edition, *DSM-IV-TR*, published in 2000, provides a classification system that attempts to separate mental illnesses into diagnostic categories based on descriptions of symptoms (that is, what people say and do as a reflection of how they think and feel) and on the course of the illness. Newer revisions of the DSM are expected to describe mental disorders along a continuous spectrum of symptoms, rather than classifying them by categories.

The *International Classification of Disease, 10th Revision, Clinical Modification (ICD-10-CM)*, a book published by the World Health Organization, uses diagnostic categories similar to those in the *DSM-IV-TR*. This similarity suggests that diagnoses of specific mental illnesses are becoming more standard and consistent throughout the world.

Advances have been made in diagnostic methods. Several brain imaging techniques are available. They include computed tomography (CT—see page 2037), magnetic resonance imaging (MRI—see page 2040), and positron emission tomography (PET), a type of scan that measures blood flow to specific areas of the brain (see page 2044). These imaging techniques are being used to map brain structure and function in people with normal and abnormal behavior, and they give scientists greater understanding of how the brain functions in people with and without mental illness. Research that has differentiated one mental health disorder from another has led to greater precision in diagnosis.

Treatment of Mental Illness

Extraordinary advances have been made in the treatment of mental illness. Understanding what causes some mental health disorders helps doctors tailor treatment to those disorders. As a result, many mental health disorders can now be treated nearly as successfully as physical disorders.

Most treatment methods for mental health disorders can be categorized as either somatic or psychotherapeutic. Somatic treatments include drug therapy and electroconvulsive therapy. Psychotherapeutic treatments include individual, group, or family and marital psychotherapy; behavior therapy techniques (such as relaxation training or exposure therapy); and hypnotherapy. Most studies suggest that for major mental health disorders, a treatment approach involving both drugs and psychotherapy is more effective than either treatment method used alone.

Psychiatrists are not the only mental health care practitioners trained to treat mental illness. Others include clinical psychologists, social workers, nurses, and some pastoral counselors. However, psychiatrists (and psychiatric nurse practitioners in some states) are the only mental health care practitioners licensed to prescribe drugs. Other mental health care practitioners practice psychotherapy primarily. Many primary care doctors and other non-mental health care doctors also prescribe drugs to treat mental health disorders.

Drug Therapy

A number of psychoactive drugs are highly effective and widely used by psychiatrists and other medical doctors. These drugs are often categorized according to the disorder for which they are primarily prescribed. For example, antidepressants are used to treat depression.

Selective serotonin reuptake inhibitors (SSRIs), such as fluoxetine, sertraline, and citalopram, are the newest and most widely used class of antidepressants. Other classes of antidepressants include the serotonin-norepinephrine reuptake inhibitors (SNRIs), such as venlafaxine or duloxetine, and the norepinephrine/dopamine drugs, such as bupropion.

Antipsychotic drugs, such as chlorpromazine, haloperidol, and thiothixene, are helpful in treating psychotic disorders such as schizophrenia. Newer antipsychotic drugs (commonly called atypicals), such as risperidone, olanzapine, quetiapine, ziprasidone, and aripiprazole, are now commonly used as first-line therapy. For patients who do not respond to traditional and atypical antipsychotics, clozapine is increasingly used.

SSRIs and antianxiety drugs, such as clonazepam, lorazepam, and diazepam, as well as antidepressants, are used to treat anxiety disorders, such as panic

TYPES OF MENTAL HEALTH CARE PRACTITIONERS

PRACTITIONER	TRAINING	EXPERTISE
Psychiatrist	Medical doctor with 4 or more years of psychiatric training after graduation from medical school	Can prescribe drugs, perform electroconvulsive therapy, and admit people to the hospital May only practice psychotherapy, only prescribe drugs, or do both
Psychologist	Practitioner who has a master's or doctoral degree but not a medical degree. Many have postdoctoral training and most have training to administer psychologic tests that are helpful in diagnosis	May conduct psychotherapy but cannot perform physical examinations, prescribe drugs (in most states), or admit people to the hospital
Psychiatric social worker	A practitioner with specialized training in certain aspects of psychotherapy, such as family and marital therapy or individual psychotherapy. Often trained to interface with the social service systems in the state. May have a master's degree and sometimes a doctorate as well	Cannot perform physical examinations or prescribe drugs
Advanced practice psychiatric nurse	Registered nurse with a master's degree or higher, and training in behavioral health	May practice psychotherapy independently in some states and may prescribe drugs under the supervision of a doctor
Psychoanalyst	May be a psychiatrist, psychologist, or social worker who has many years of training in the practice of psychoanalysis (a type of intensive psychotherapy involving several sessions a week and designed to explore unconscious patterns of thought, feeling, and behavior)	Conducts psychoanalysis and, if also a psychiatrist, may prescribe drugs and admit people to hospitals

disorder and phobias. Mood stabilizers, such as lithium, carbamazepine, and valproate, have been used to treat manic-depressive illness (bipolar disorder).

Electroconvulsive Therapy

With electroconvulsive therapy, electrodes are attached to the head, and while the person is sedated, a series of electrical shocks are delivered to the brain to induce a brief seizure. This therapy has consistently been shown to be the most effective treatment for severe depression. Many people treated with electroconvulsive therapy experience temporary memory loss. However, contrary to its portrayal in the media, electroconvulsive therapy is safe and rarely causes any other complications. The modern use of anesthetics and muscle relaxants has greatly reduced any risk. Other forms of brain stimulation, such as repetitive transcranial magnetic stimulation (rTMS) and vagal nerve stimulation, are under study and may be beneficial for people with severe depression that does not respond to drugs or psychotherapy.

Psychotherapy

In recent years, significant advances have been made in the field of psychotherapy. Psychotherapy, sometimes referred to as "talk therapy," works on the assumption that the cure for a person's suffering lies within that person and that this cure can be facilitated through a trusting, supportive relationship with a psychotherapist. By creating an empathetic and accepting atmosphere, the therapist often is able to help the person identify the source of the problems and consider alternatives for dealing with them. The emotional awareness and insight that the person gains through psychotherapy often results in a change in attitude and behavior that allows the person to live a fuller and more satisfying life.

Psychotherapy is appropriate in a wide range of conditions. Even people who do not have a mental health disorder may find psychotherapy helpful in coping with such problems as employment difficulties, bereavement, or chronic illness in the family. Group psychotherapy, couples therapy, and family therapy are also widely used.

Most mental health practitioners practice one of six types of psychotherapy: supportive psychotherapy, psychoanalysis, psychodynamic psychotherapy, cognitive therapy, behavioral therapy, or interpersonal therapy.

Supportive psychotherapy, which is most commonly used, relies on the empathetic and supportive relationship between the person and the therapist. It encourages expression of feelings, the therapist provides help with problem solving. Problem-focused psychotherapy, a form of supportive therapy, may be conducted successfully by primary care doctors.

Psychoanalysis is the oldest form of psychotherapy and was developed by Sigmund Freud in the first part of the 20th century. The person typically lies on a couch in the therapist's office 4 or 5 times a week and attempts to say whatever comes to mind, a practice called free association. Much of the focus is on understanding how past patterns of relationships repeat themselves in the present. The relationship between the person and the therapist is a key part of this focus. An understanding of how the past affects the present helps the person develop new and more adaptive ways of functioning in relationships and in work settings.

Psychodynamic psychotherapy, like psychoanalysis, emphasizes the identification of unconscious patterns in current thoughts, feelings, and behaviors. However, the person is usually sitting instead of lying on a couch and attends only 1 to 3 sessions per week. In addition, less emphasis is placed on the relationship between the person and therapist.

Cognitive therapy helps people identify distortions in thinking and understand how these distortions lead to problems in their lives. The premise is that how people feel and behave is determined by how they interpret experiences. Through the identification of core beliefs and assumptions, people learn to think in different ways about their experiences, reducing symptoms and resulting in improvement in behavior and feelings.

Behavioral therapy is related to cognitive therapy. Sometimes a combination of the two, known as cognitive-behavioral therapy, is used. The theoretical basis of behavioral therapy is learning theory, which holds that abnormal behaviors are due to faulty learning. Behavioral therapy involves a number of interventions that are designed to help the person unlearn maladaptive behaviors while learning adaptive behaviors. Exposure therapy, often used to treat phobias, is one example of a behavioral therapy (see box on page 858).

Interpersonal therapy was initially conceived as a brief psychologic treatment for depression and is designed to improve the quality of a depressed person's relationships. It focuses on unresolved grief, conflicts that arise when people fill roles that differ from their expectations (such as when a woman enters a relationship expecting to be a stay-at-home mother and finds that she must also be the major provider for the family), social role transitions (such as going from being an active worker to being retired), and difficulty communicating with others. The therapist teaches the person to improve aspects of interpersonal relationships, such as overcoming social isolation and responding in a less habitual way to others.

CHAPTER

127   Somatoform Disorders

Somatoform disorders include several mental health disorders. In some, people report physical symptoms or concerns that suggest but are not fully explained by a physical disorder. In one, people are preoccupied with a slight or nonexistent defect in appearance. These symptoms or concerns are considered disorders if they cause significant distress or interfere with daily functioning.

Somatoform disorder refers to what many people used to call a psychosomatic disorder. In somatoform disorders, the physical symptoms cannot be fully ex-

plained by any underlying physical disorder. People with a somatoform disorder are not faking. They sincerely believe that they have a serious physical problem.

The somatoform disorders include body dysmorphic disorder, conversion disorder, hypochondriasis, somatization disorder, and pain disorder (see page 640). Children are also affected (see page 1872). Treatment varies according to which somatoform disorder a person has.

Munchausen Syndrome: Faking Illness for Attention

Munchausen syndrome is not a somatoform disorder, but its features are somewhat similar. That is, mental health problems underlie physical symptoms. The key difference is that people with Munchausen syndrome consciously fake the symptoms of a physical disorder. They repeatedly fabricate illnesses and often wander from hospital to hospital for treatment.

However, Munchausen syndrome is more complex than simple dishonest fabrication and simulation of symptoms. The disorder is associated with severe emotional problems. People with the disorder are usually quite intelligent and resourceful. They not only know how to mimic diseases but also have sophisticated knowledge of medical practices. They can manipulate their care so that they are hospitalized and subjected to intense testing and treatment, including major operations. Their deceits are conscious, but their motivation and quest for attention are largely unconscious.

Munchausen by proxy is a bizarre variant of Munchausen syndrome. In it, a caregiver (often a parent) intentionally produces or feigns symptoms in someone in their care (often a child). The caregiver falsifies the child's medical history and may injure the child with drugs or add blood or bacterial contaminants to urine specimens. All is done in an effort to fake disease. The motivation for such behavior appears to be a psychologic need to experience the role of a sick person through a substitute (proxy). People with this disorder also have a pathologic need for attention and an intense relationship with the child.

Body Dysmorphic Disorder

In body dysmorphic disorder, a preoccupation with a nonexistent or slight defect in appearance results in significant distress or impaired functioning.

- People typically spend hours a day worrying about their perceived defect, which may involve any body part.
- Doctors diagnose the disorder when concerns about appearance cause significant distress or interfere with functioning.
- Certain antidepressants and cognitive-behavioral therapy may help.

People with body dysmorphic disorder believe they have a flaw or defect in their physical appearance that in reality is nonexistent or slight. The disorder usually begins during adolescence. It is believed to occur in men and women about equally or somewhat more frequently in women.

? Did You Know...

People may be so concerned about a nonexistent or slight defect in their appearance that they avoid going out in public.

Symptoms

Symptoms may develop gradually or abruptly, vary in intensity, and tend to persist unless appropriately treated. Concerns commonly involve the face or head but may involve any body part or several parts and may change from one body part to another. For example, people may be concerned about hair thinning, acne, wrinkles, scars, color of complexion, or excessive facial or body hair. Or people may focus on the shape or size of a body part, such as the nose, eyes, ears, mouth, breasts, legs, or buttocks. Some men with normal or even athletic builds think that they are puny and obsessively try to gain weight and muscle; this is called muscle dysmorphia.

Most people with body dysmorphic disorder have difficulty controlling their preoccupation and spend hours each day worrying about their perceived defect. Many people check themselves often in mirrors, others avoid mirrors, and still others alternate between the two behaviors. Many people compulsively and excessively groom themselves, pick at their skin, seek reassurance, and change their clothes. Most try to camouflage their nonexistent or slight defect—for example, by growing a beard to hide perceived scars or by wearing a hat to cover slightly thinning hair. Many have cosmetic medical (most often, dermatologic), dental, or surgical treatment, sometimes repeatedly, to correct their perceived defect. Such treatment is usually unsuccessful and may intensify their preoccupation. Men with muscle dysmorphia may take anabolic steroids such as testosterone.

Because people with body dysmorphic disorder feel self-conscious about their appearance, they may avoid going out in public, including going to work, school, and social events. Some with severe symptoms leave their homes only at night, and others not at all. This behavior can result in social isolation. Distress and dysfunction caused by the disorder can lead to repeated hospitalization and suicidal behavior.

Diagnosis and Treatment

Because many people with body dysmorphic disorder are too embarrassed and ashamed to reveal their symptoms, the disorder may go undiagnosed for years. It is distinguished from normal concerns about appearance because the preoccupations are time-consuming and cause significant distress or impair functioning.

Treatment with serotonin reuptake inhibitors, a class of antidepressants, is often effective. Cognitive-behavioral therapy that specifically focuses on this disorder may also lessen symptoms.

Conversion Disorder

In conversion disorder, physical symptoms that resemble those of a neurologic disorder develop. The symptoms are triggered by mental factors such as conflicts or other stresses.

- An arm or leg may be paralyzed, or people may lose their sense of touch, sight, or hearing.
- Many physical examinations and tests are usually done to make sure symptoms do not result from a physical disorder.
- Reassurance from a supportive, trusted doctor is important; hypnosis and cognitive-behavioral therapy may also help.

Conversion disorder, once referred to as hysteria, is thought to be caused by mental factors, such as stress and conflict, which people with this disorder experience as (convert into) physical symptoms. Although conversion disorder tends to develop during late child-hood to early adulthood, it may appear at any age. The disorder appears to be more common among women.

Symptoms

The symptoms—such as paralysis of an arm or leg or loss of sensation in a part of the body—suggest nervous system dysfunction. Other symptoms may include seizures and loss of one of the special senses, such as vision or hearing.

Often, symptoms begin after some distressing social or psychologic event.

People may have only one episode in their lifetime or episodes that occur sporadically. Usually, the episodes are brief. Most people with conversion symptoms who are hospitalized improve within 2 weeks. However, in 20 to 25% of people, symptoms recur within a year and, for some people, become chronic.

Diagnosis

The diagnosis tends to be initially difficult for a doctor to make because people believe that the symptoms stem from a physical problem and may resist being seen by a psychiatrist or other mental health practitioner. Also, doctors take great care to be certain no physical disorder is causing the symptoms. Thus, the diagnosis is usually considered only after extensive physical examinations and tests fail to detect a physical disorder that can fully account for the symptoms.

Mind and Body

How the mind and body interact to influence health has long been discussed. The term *psychosomatic* expresses this interaction. Paired with *disorder*, the term was once used to refer to physical symptoms that appear to be caused or worsened by mental factors, rather than by a physical disorder. Now, the term *somatoform disorders* is used to refer to these disorders. The term does not imply that physical symptoms are imagined or are being faked (as in Munchausen syndrome). People with a psychosomatic disorder actually experience the symptoms.

The mind and body interact in many other ways.

Social and mental stress can aggravate many physical disorders, including diabetes mellitus, coronary artery disease, and asthma. Such stress can trigger, worsen, or prolong physical symptoms.

Stress can cause physical symptoms even when no physical disorder is present. Sometimes physical symptoms result from the body's automatic response to emotional stress, as when heart rate and blood pressure increase in response to fear.

Sometimes a physical symptom appears to be a metaphor for an emotional experience, as when people with a "broken heart" have chest pain. Or a physical symptom may reflect identification with another person's pain. For example, people may have chest pain after a family member or friend has had a heart attack.

Physical symptoms can evolve from stress or mental symptoms in anyone, including people who do not have a serious underlying mental health disorder. Such physical symptoms are often mild and transient. They can be difficult for a doctor to diagnose, and various diagnostic tests may be required to eliminate the possibility of an underlying physical disorder.

Mental factors can also influence the course of a disorder. For example, people with high blood pressure may deny having it or deny its seriousness. Denial is a defense mechanism that helps reduce anxiety. However, denial may prevent people from following their treatment plan. For example, they may not take their prescribed drugs, thus worsening their disorder.

Conversely, a physical disorder can influence or lead to a mental condition. For example, people with a life-threatening, recurring, or chronic physical disorder may become depressed. The depression, in turn, may worsen the effects of the physical disorder.

Treatment

A supportive, trustful doctor-patient relationship is essential. The most helpful approach may involve collaboration of a primary care doctor with a psychiatrist and a doctor from another field, such as a neurologist or internist. As the doctor evaluates a possible physical disorder and reassures the person that the symptoms do not indicate a serious underlying disease, the person may begin to feel better, and the symptoms may fade.

The following treatments may help:

- Hypnosis may help by enabling people to control how stress and other mental states affect their bodily functions.
- Narcoanalysis is a rarely used procedure similar to hypnosis except that people are given a sedative to make them drowsy.
- Psychotherapy, including cognitive-behavioral therapy, is effective for some people.

Any coexisting psychiatric disorders (such as depression) should be treated.

Hypochondriasis

In hypochondriasis, people are preoccupied with the fear of having a serious disease or are preoccupied with the belief that they actually have a disease. These feelings are usually based on a misinterpretation of normal bodily sensations or minor physical symptoms.

- People believe that signs of normal body functions, such as a grumbling in the intestines or sweating, indicate a serious physical disorder.
- Even though a thorough medical evaluation determines that no physical or other mental disorder can account for the symptoms, people remain preoccupied with their concerns.
- A supportive, trustful relationship with a doctor may help, but referral to a psychiatrist is often needed.

Hypochondriasis begins most commonly during early adulthood and appears to affect both sexes equally.

Symptoms

People misinterpret normal bodily functions or minor physical symptoms that are not related to any abnormality or disorder. These symptoms may include abdominal bloating, rumbling in the abdomen, awareness of the heartbeat, sweating, pain, and fatigue. People may describe their symptoms in minute detail. They think that the symptoms indicate a serious physical disorder. For example, they may think headaches indicate a brain tumor. The symptoms cause them great distress. As people become increasingly concerned with health issues, personal relationships and work performance often suffer.

Examination and reassurance by a doctor do not relieve the concerns of people with hypochondriasis.

They tend to believe that the doctor has somehow failed to find the underlying disorder.

Some people with hypochondriasis also have depression or anxiety.

Hypochondriasis often persists, lasting years. In some people, it comes and goes. Some people recover completely.

Diagnosis

Hypochondriasis is suspected when healthy people with minor symptoms are preoccupied with the significance of the symptoms and do not respond to reassurance after a thorough medical evaluation.

The diagnosis of hypochondriasis is confirmed if the situation persists for at least 6 months despite a medical evaluation and a doctor's reassurance and if the symptoms cannot be attributed to depression or another mental health disorder.

Treatment

Treatment can be difficult because people with hypochondriasis believe that something inside the body is seriously wrong. Reassurance does not relieve these concerns. However, a supportive, trustful relationship with a caring doctor is beneficial, especially if regular visits are scheduled. If symptoms are not adequately relieved, people may benefit from referral to a psychiatrist or another mental health practitioner for further evaluation and treatment, with continuing care by the primary doctor.

Treatment with serotonin reuptake inhibitors, a class of antidepressants, may be effective. Cognitive-behavioral therapy may also relieve symptoms.

Somatization Disorder

Somatization disorder is a chronic, severe disorder characterized by many recurring physical symptoms that cannot be fully explained by a physical disorder. These symptoms include some combination of pain and digestive, sexual, and neurologic symptoms.

- People typically have many symptoms (such as headache, nausea, diarrhea, constipation, and fatigue) over a period of several years.
- They seek treatment for their physical complaints, and many physical examinations and tests may be done to make sure symptoms do not result from a physical disorder.
- Having a supportive, trustful relationship with a doctor can be very helpful; cognitive-behavioral therapy can also help.

Somatization disorder often runs in families and occurs predominantly in women. Male relatives of women with the disorder tend to have a high incidence of antisocial personality (see page 881) and substance-related disorders. Many people with somatization disorder also have symptoms of depression and anxiety, a personality disorder, and excessive dependence on others (see page 882).

? **Did You Know...**
People with a somatization disorder are not faking their symptoms.

The physical symptoms in somatization disorders may reflect a plea for help and attention and a desire to be cared for. The symptoms may also have other purposes, such as enabling people to avoid the responsibilities of adulthood. However, symptoms are not intentionally produced or feigned. The symptoms tend to be uncomfortable and prevent people from engaging in many enjoyable pursuits.

Symptoms

Symptoms first appear during adolescence or early adulthood (before age 30). People have many physical complaints, which they may describe as "unbearable," "beyond description," or "the worst imaginable."

Any part of the body may be affected. Specific symptoms and their frequency vary among different cultures. Typical symptoms include headaches, nausea and vomiting, abdominal pain, diarrhea or constipation, painful menstrual periods, fatigue, fainting, pain during intercourse, and loss of sexual desire. Men frequently complain of erectile or other sexual dysfunction. Anxiety and depression also occur.

People with somatization disorder demand help and emotional support and may become angry when they feel their needs are not being met. Often dissatisfied with their medical care, they may go from doctor to doctor, seeking medical tests and treatment.

Diagnosis

People with somatization disorder are not aware that their basic problem is psychologic, so they press their doctors for diagnostic tests and treatments. Doctors usually conduct many physical examinations and tests to determine whether a physical disorder adequately explains the symptoms. Referrals to specialists for consultations are common, even for people who have developed a reasonably satisfactory relationship with one doctor.

Once a doctor determines that the problem is psychologic, somatization disorder can be distinguished from similar mental health disorders by its many symptoms and their tendency to persist over a period of years.

Prognosis

Somatization disorder tends to fluctuate in severity but may persist throughout life. Symptoms are rarely completely relieved for any length of time. Some people become more depressed after many years. Suicide is a risk.

Treatment

Treatment is difficult. Psychotherapy, particularly cognitive-behavioral therapy, may help. Drugs may lessen symptoms of coexisting mental disorders such as depression.

Usually, people with this disorder are best helped by a supportive, trustful relationship with a doctor who coordinates their health care, offers symptomatic relief, sees them regularly, and protects them from unnecessary diagnostic or therapeutic procedures. However, the doctor must remain alert to the possibility that these people may develop an actual physical disorder that requires evaluation and treatment.

CHAPTER 128 Anxiety Disorders

Anxiety disorders involve a state of distressing chronic but fluctuating nervousness that is inappropriately severe for the person's circumstances.

- Anxiety disorders can make people sweat, feel short of breath or dizzy, have a rapid heartbeat, tremble, and avoid certain situations.
- These disorders are usually diagnosed using specific established criteria.
- Drugs, psychotherapy, or both can substantially help most people.

Anxiety is a normal response to a threat or to psychologic stress and is experienced occasionally by everyone. Normal anxiety has its root in fear and serves an important survival function. When someone is faced with a dangerous situation, anxiety induces the fight-or-flight response. With this response, a variety of physical changes, such as increased blood flow to the heart and muscles, provide the body with the necessary energy and strength to deal with life-threatening situations, such as running from an aggressive animal or fighting off an attacker. However, when anxiety

How Anxiety Affects Performance

The effects of anxiety on performance can be shown on a curve. As the level of anxiety increases, performance efficiency increases proportionately, but only up to a point. As anxiety increases further, performance efficiency decreases. Before the peak of the curve, anxiety is considered adaptive because it helps people prepare for a crisis and improve their functioning. Beyond the peak of the curve, anxiety is considered maladaptive because it produces distress and impairs functioning.

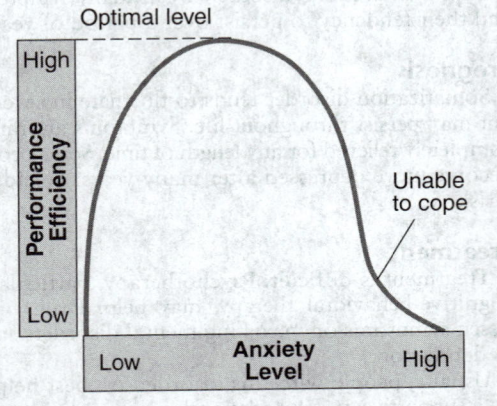

occurs at inappropriate times, occurs frequently, or is so intense and long-lasting that it interferes with a person's normal activities, it is considered a disorder.

Anxiety disorders are more common than any other category of mental health disorder and are believed to affect about 15% of adults in the United States. However, anxiety disorders often are not recognized by people who have them or by health care practitioners and consequently are seldom treated.

Causes

The causes of anxiety disorders are not fully known, but both physical and psychologic factors are involved. Because anxiety disorders are prevalent in some families, heredity probably plays a role. Anxiety is viewed at a psychologic level as a response to environmental stresses, such as the breakup of a significant relationship or exposure to a life-threatening disaster. When a person's response to stresses is inappropriate or a person is overwhelmed by events, an anxiety disorder can arise. For example, some people find speaking before a group exhilarating. But others dread it, becoming anxious with symptoms such as sweating, fear, rapid heart rate, and tremor. Such people may avoid speaking even in a small group.

Anxiety disorders may also be caused by a physical disorder or the use of a drug. For example, an overactive thyroid or adrenal gland can cause anxiety, as can a tumor called a pheochromocytoma. Drugs that can cause anxiety include corticosteroids, cocaine, amphetamines, ephedrine, and sometimes caffeine if too much is consumed. Withdrawal from alcohol or certain sedatives can also cause symptoms of an anxiety disorder. In older people, dementia may be the most common cause of anxiety.

Symptoms

Anxiety can arise suddenly, as in panic, or gradually over minutes, hours, or days. Anxiety can last for any length of time, from a few seconds to years. It ranges in intensity from barely noticeable qualms to a full-blown panic attack (see page 857), which may cause shortness of breath, dizziness, an increased heart rate, and trembling (tremor).

Anxiety disorders can be so distressing and interfere so much with a person's life that they can lead to depression (see page 863). People who have an anxiety disorder (except for certain very specific phobias, such as fear of spiders) are at least twice as likely to have depression as those without an anxiety disorder. Sometimes depression develops first and an anxiety disorder develops later.

Diagnosis

The diagnosis of an anxiety disorder is based largely on symptoms. The ability to tolerate anxiety varies, and determining what constitutes abnormal anxiety can be difficult. Doctors usually use specific established criteria, based mainly on symptoms and exclusion of other causes of symptoms.

Doctors ask whether family members have had similar symptoms. A family history of an anxiety disorder (except posttraumatic stress disorder, which results from a specific event) may help doctors make the diagnosis. Doctors also do a physical examination. Blood and other tests may be done to check for disorders that can cause anxiety.

 Did You Know...

Anxiety disorders are the most common type of mental health disorder.

People with an anxiety disorder are more likely than other people to have depression.

Treatment

Accurate diagnosis is important because treatment varies from one anxiety disorder to another. Additionally, anxiety disorders must be distinguished from

℞ ANTIANXIETY DRUGS

DRUG	USES	SOME SIDE EFFECTS	COMMENTS
Benzodiazepines			
Alprazolam Chlordiazepoxide Clonazepam Clorazepate Diazepam Lorazepam Oxazepam	Generalized anxiety disorder Panic disorder Phobic disorders	Sleepiness, impaired coordination, and slowed reaction time May lead to drug dependence	Most commonly used type of antianxiety drug Promote mental and physical relaxation by reducing nerve activity in the brain Begin to work quickly, sometimes within an hour Should not be used by people who are dependent on alcohol
Buspirone			
	Generalized anxiety disorder	Dizziness and headache	Does not cause drowsiness or interact with alcohol Does not lead to drug dependence May take several weeks to start working
Antidepressants*			
Selective serotonin reuptake inhibitors (such as paroxetine) Norepinephrine/ serotonin reuptake inhibitors (such as duloxetine and venlafaxine) Monoamine oxidase inhibitors Tricyclic antidepressants (such as clomipramine)	Generalized anxiety disorder Panic disorder Phobic disorders Obsessive-compulsive disorder Posttraumatic stress disorder	See table on page 868	See table on page 868

*Not all of the antidepressants listed work for all of the uses that are listed.

anxiety that occurs in many other mental health disorders, which involve different treatment approaches. Depending on the anxiety disorder, drug therapy or psychotherapy (such as behavioral therapy), alone or in combination, can significantly relieve the distress and dysfunction for most people.

Generalized Anxiety Disorder

Generalized anxiety disorder consists of excessive, usually daily, nervousness and worry (lasting 6 months or longer) about many activities or events.

- Anxieties are general in nature and may shift from topic to topic.
- For this disorder to be diagnosed, several other symptoms (such as difficulty concentrating) must accompany the anxiety.
- Treatment involves a combination of drugs (usually antianxiety drugs and sometimes antidepressants) and counseling.

Generalized anxiety disorder is common. About 3% of adults have it during any 12-month period. Women are twice as likely as men to have the disorder. It often begins in childhood or adolescence (see page 1869) but may start at any age. For most people, the disorder fluctuates, worsening at times (especially during times of stress), and persists over many years.

Symptoms and Diagnosis

People with generalized anxiety disorder constantly feel worried or distressed and have difficulty controlling these feelings. The severity, frequency, or duration of the worries is disproportionately greater than the situation warrants. Worries are general in nature and often shift from one topic to another over time. Common worries include work responsibilities, money, health, safety, car repairs, and chores.

For a doctor to diagnose generalized anxiety disorder, a person must experience worry or anxiety and three or more of the following symptoms:

- Restlessness
- Easy fatigue
- Difficulty concentrating
- Irritability
- Muscle tension
- Disturbed sleep

Treatment

The disorder is best managed with a combination of some form of counseling and drug therapy. Counseling can address the root causes of anxiety and provide ways to cope.

Antianxiety drugs such as benzodiazepines are usually prescribed. However, because long-term use of benzodiazepines can lead to drug dependence (see page 2091), the drug, if stopped, must be tapered off slowly rather than stopped abruptly. The relief that benzodiazepines bring usually outweighs any mild side effects and the possibility of drug dependence.

Buspirone is another antianxiety drug effective for some people with generalized anxiety disorder. Its use does not lead to drug dependence. However, buspirone may take 2 weeks or longer to start working, in contrast to benzodiazepines, which begin to work within an hour.

Some antidepressants, such as venlafaxine, paroxetine, and other selective serotonin reuptake inhibitors, are also effective for treatment of generalized anxiety disorder. These antidepressants start to relieve anxiety quickly, sometimes after a few days. Initially, people may be given a benzodiazepine and an antidepressant. When the antidepressant starts working, the dose of benzodiazepine is decreased, then stopped.

Herbal products such as kava (see page 2076) and valerian (see page 2078) may have antianxiety effects, although their effectiveness and safety for treating anxiety disorders such as generalized anxiety disorder require further study.

Cognitive-behavioral therapy has been shown to be beneficial for generalized anxiety disorder. With this therapy, people learn to recognize where their thinking is distorted, to control their distorted thinking, and to modify their behavior accordingly. Relaxation, yoga, meditation, exercise, and biofeedback techniques may also be of some help (see page 2063).

Anxiety Induced by Physical Disorders or Drugs

Anxiety can be caused by a physical disorder or the use or discontinuation of a drug. Physical disorders that can cause anxiety include the following:

- Brain and nerve (neurologic) disorders, such as head injuries, brain infections, and some inner ear disorders
- Heart disorders, such as heart failure and abnormal heart rhythms (arrhythmias)
- Hormonal (endocrine) disorders, such as an overactive adrenal or thyroid gland
- Lung (respiratory) disorders, such as asthma and chronic obstructive pulmonary disease (COPD)

Even fever can cause anxiety.

Drugs that can induce anxiety include the following:

- Alcohol
- Stimulants
- Caffeine
- Cocaine
- Many prescription drugs, such as theophylline (used, for example, to treat asthma)
- Some over-the-counter weight-loss products, such as those containing the herbal product guarana, caffeine, or both

Drugs that can induce anxiety when stopped include benzodiazepines.

Anxiety may occur in dying people as a result of fear of death, pain, and difficulty breathing (see page 63).

Treatment

A doctor aims to correct the causes rather than treat the secondary anxiety symptoms. Anxiety should subside after the medical disorder is treated or the drug has been stopped long enough for any withdrawal symptoms to abate.

If anxiety remains, antianxiety drugs or psychotherapy (such as behavioral therapy) is used. For people who are dying, strong pain relievers (analgesics) with potent antianxiety effects, such as morphine, are often appropriate. No dying person should have to experience intense anxiety.

Panic Attacks and Panic Disorder

Panic is acute, short-lived, extreme anxiety with accompanying physical symptoms.

- Panic attacks can cause such symptoms as chest pain, choking, dizziness, nausea, and shortness of breath.
- Doctors base the diagnosis on the person's description of attacks and fears of future attacks.
- Treatment may include antidepressants, antianxiety drugs, exposure therapy, cognitive-behavioral therapy, and supportive psychotherapy.

Panic attacks may occur in any anxiety disorder, usually in response to a specific situation tied to the main characteristic of the disorder. For example, a person with a phobia of snakes may panic when encountering a snake. However, situational panic attacks differ from the spontaneous, unprovoked ones that define a person's problem as panic disorder.

Panic attacks are common, occurring in at least 10% of adults each year. Women are 2 to 3 times more likely than men to have panic attacks and panic disorder. Most people recover from panic attacks without treatment, but a few develop panic disorder. Panic disorder is present in 2 to 3% of the population during any 12-month period. Panic disorder usually begins in late adolescence (see page 1869) or early adulthood.

Symptoms

A panic attack involves the sudden appearance of at least four of the following symptoms:

- Chest pain or discomfort
- Choking
- Dizziness, unsteadiness, or faintness
- Fear of dying
- Fear of going crazy or of losing control
- Feelings of unreality, strangeness, or detachment from the environment
- Flushes or chills
- Nausea, stomachache, or diarrhea
- Numbness or tingling sensations
- Palpitations or accelerated heart rate
- Shortness of breath or a sense of being smothered
- Sweating
- Trembling or shaking

Symptoms peak within 10 minutes and usually dissipate within minutes, leaving little for a doctor to observe except the person's fear of another terrifying attack. Because panic attacks sometimes are unexpected or occur for no apparent reason, especially when people experience them as part of panic disorder, people who have them frequently anticipate and worry about another attack—a condition called anticipatory anxiety—and try to avoid places where they have previously panicked.

Because symptoms of a panic attack involve many vital organs, people often worry that they have a dangerous medical problem involving the heart, lungs, or brain. Thus, they may seek help from a doctor or hospital emergency department. If the correct diagnosis of panic attack is not made, they may have the additional worry that a serious medical problem has been overlooked. Although panic attacks are uncomfortable—at times extremely so—they are not dangerous.

Panic disorder is diagnosed when people experience at least two unprovoked and unexpected panic attacks, which are followed by at least 1 month of fear that another attack will occur. The frequency of attacks can vary greatly. Some people have weekly or even daily attacks that occur for months, whereas others have several daily attacks followed by weeks or months without attacks.

> **Did You Know...**
> Although panic attacks cause symptoms involving the heart and other vital organs, they are not dangerous.

Treatment

Some people recover without formal treatment. For others, panic disorder waxes and wanes over years.

People with panic disorder are more receptive to treatment if they understand that the disorder involves both physical and psychologic processes and that treatment must address both. Drug therapy and behavioral therapy can generally control the symptoms.

Drugs: Drugs that are used to treat panic disorder include antidepressants and antianxiety drugs such as benzodiazepines. Most types of antidepressants—tricyclic antidepressants, monoamine oxidase inhibitors (MAOIs) serotonin reuptake inhibitors (SSRIs), and serotonin/norepinephrine reuptake inhibitors (SNRIs)—are effective (see table on page 868). Benzodiazepines work faster than antidepressants but can cause drug dependence (see page 2091) and are probably more likely to cause sleepiness, impaired coordination, and slowed reaction time. SSRIs are the preferred drugs because they are as effective as the other drugs but usually have fewer side effects. For example, they are much less likely to cause sleepiness, and they do not cause drug dependence, although if stopped abruptly most SSRIs (and SNRIs) can cause uncomfortable withdrawal symptoms that can last a week or more. Initially, people may be given a benzodiazepine

What Is Exposure Therapy?

Unlike systematic desensitization, which pairs relaxation with gradual exposure to the sources of anxiety, exposure therapy purposefully permits anxiety to occur (although sometimes it does not occur). By being repeatedly exposed to the feared object or situation, either literally or using imagination, people experience the anxiety over and over until the feared stimulus eventually loses its effect. This process is called habituation.

Two variants of exposure therapy are flooding and graduated exposure.

- **Flooding** exposes people to the anxiety-producing stimulus for as long as 1 or 2 hours.
- **Graduated exposure** gives people a greater degree of control over the length and frequency of exposures.

Both types of exposure treatment may use the most feared stimulus first, unlike systematic desensitization, which begins with the least feared stimulus.

and an antidepressant. When the antidepressant starts working, the dose of benzodiazepine is decreased, then stopped.

When a drug is effective, it prevents or greatly reduces the number of panic attacks. A drug may have to be taken for a long time because panic attacks often return once the drug is stopped.

Psychotherapy: Exposure therapy, a type of behavioral therapy in which people are exposed repeatedly to whatever triggers a panic attack, often helps to diminish the fear. Exposure therapy is repeated until people become very comfortable with the anxiety-provoking situation. In addition, people who are afraid that they will faint during a panic attack can practice an exercise in which they spin in a chair or breathe quickly (hyperventilate) until they feel faint. This exercise teaches them that they will not actually faint during a panic attack. Practicing slow, shallow breathing (respiratory control) helps many people who tend to hyperventilate.

Cognitive-behavioral therapy also may help. People are taught the following:

- Not to avoid situations that cause panic attacks
- To recognize when their fears are unfounded
- To respond instead with slow, controlled breathing or other techniques that promote relaxation

Supportive psychotherapy, which includes education and counseling, is beneficial because a therapist can provide general information about the disorder, its treatment, realistic hope for improvement, and the support that comes from a trusting relationship with a doctor.

Phobic Disorders

Phobias involve persistent, unrealistic, intense anxiety about and fear of certain situations, circumstances, or objects.

- The anxiety caused by a phobic disorder can interfere with daily living because people avoid certain activities and situations.
- The diagnosis is usually obvious based on symptoms.
- Treatment may include exposure therapy, cognitive-behavioral therapy, and drugs (such as antidepressants and, for specific phobias, benzodiazepines).

People who have a phobia avoid situations that trigger their anxiety and fear, or they endure them with great distress. However, they recognize that their anxiety is excessive and therefore are aware that they have a problem.

AGORAPHOBIA

Agoraphobia is anxiety about being trapped in situations or places with no way to escape easily if anxiety or panic develops, often resulting in avoidance.

Agoraphobia is diagnosed in about 4% of women and 2% of men during any 12-month period. Most people with this disorder develop it in their early 20s. Agoraphobia rarely develops after age 40.

Although agoraphobia literally means "fear of the marketplace," the term more specifically describes the fear of being trapped, often in a busy place filled with people, without a graceful and easy way to leave if anxiety becomes severe. Typical situations that are difficult for people with agoraphobia include the following:

- Standing in line at a bank or supermarket
- Sitting in the middle of a long row in a theater or classroom
- Riding on a bus or airplane

Some people develop agoraphobia after experiencing a panic attack in one of these situations. Other people simply feel uncomfortable in these settings and may never, or only later, develop panic attacks. Agoraphobia often interferes with daily living, sometimes so drastically that it makes people housebound.

Treatment

If agoraphobia is not treated, it usually waxes and wanes in severity and may even disappear without formal treatment, possibly because the person has conducted some personal form of behavioral therapy.

Exposure therapy, a type of behavioral therapy in which people are exposed repeatedly to the anxiety-provoking situation, is the best treatment for agoraphobia. This therapy helps more than 90% of people who practice it faithfully. Cognitive-behavioral therapy may also help. With this therapy, people learn to recognize when their thinking is distorted, to control the distorted thinking, and to modify their behavior accordingly. Substances that depress the central nervous system (brain and spinal cord), such as alcohol or large doses of antianxiety drugs, may interfere with behavioral therapy and are often tapered off before therapy is begun.

If people with agoraphobia are deeply depressed or have panic attacks, they may need to take an antidepressant.

SOCIAL PHOBIA

Social phobia (social anxiety disorder) is fear of and anxiety about exposure to certain social or performance situations, often resulting in avoidance.

Humans are social animals, and their ability to relate comfortably in social situations affects many important aspects of their lives, including family, education, work, leisure, dating, and mating.

Although some anxiety in social situations is normal, people with social phobia have so much anxiety that they either avoid social situations or endure them with distress. About 13% of people have social phobia sometime in their life. The disorder affects about 9% of women and 7% of men during any 12-month period. Men are more likely than women to have the most severe form of social anxiety, avoidant personality disorder (see page 882). Some people are shy by nature and, early in life, show timidness that later develops into social phobia. Others first experience anxiety in social situations around the time of puberty (see page 1871).

People with social phobia are concerned that their performance or actions will seem inappropriate. Often they worry that their anxiety will be obvious—that they will sweat, blush, vomit, or tremble or that their voice will quaver. They also worry that they will lose their train of thought or that they will not be able to find the words to express themselves.

Some social phobias are tied to specific performance situations, producing anxiety only when the people must perform a particular activity in public. The same activity performed alone produces no anxiety. Situations that commonly trigger anxiety among people with social phobia include the following:

- Public speaking
- Performing publicly, such as reading in church or playing a musical instrument
- Eating with others
- Signing a document before witnesses
- Using a public bathroom

A more general type of social phobia is characterized by anxiety in many social situations.

In both types of social phobia, people's anxiety comes from the belief that if their performance falls short of expectations, they will feel embarrassed and humiliated.

Treatment

Social phobia often persists if left untreated, causing many people to avoid activities that they would otherwise like to do.

Exposure therapy, a type of behavioral therapy in which people are exposed repeatedly to the

SOME COMMON PHOBIAS*	
PHOBIA	**DEFINITION**
Acrophobia	Fear of heights
Amathophobia	Fear of dust
Astraphobia	Fear of thunder and lightning
Aviophobia	Fear of flying
Belonephobia	Fear of needles, pins, or other sharp objects
Brontophobia	Fear of thunder
Claustrophobia	Fear of confined spaces
Eurotophobia	Fear of female genitals
Gephyrophobia	Fear of crossing bridges
Hydrophobia	Fear of water
Odontiatophobia	Fear of dentists
Phartophobia	Fear of passing gas in a public place
Phasmophobia	Fear of ghosts
Phobophobia	Fear of having fears or developing a phobia
Spargarophobia	Fear of asparagus
Triskaidekaphobia	Fear of all things associated with the number thirteen
Trypanophobia	Fear of injections
Zoophobia	Fear of animals (usually spiders, snakes, or mice)

* There are over 500 named phobias, listed at the Phobia List web site. Most are extremely rare.

anxiety-provoking situation, is effective. But arranging for exposure to last long enough to allow people to get used to the anxiety-provoking situation and grow comfortable in that situation may not be easy. For example, people who are afraid of speaking in front of their boss may not be able to arrange a series of speaking sessions in front of that boss. Substitute situations may help, such as joining Toastmasters (an organization for those who have anxiety about speaking in front of an audience) or reading a book to nursing home residents. Cognitive-behavioral therapy may also help (see page 858).

Antidepressants, such as selective serotonin reuptake inhibitors (SSRIs) and monoamine oxidase inhibitors (MAOIs), and antianxiety drugs can often help people with social phobia. Many people use alcohol as a social lubricant, but for some people, alcohol abuse and dependence can result. Beta-blockers are commonly used to reduce the increased heart rate, trembling, and sweating experienced by people who are distressed by performing in public, but these drugs do not treat the underlying anxiety.

SPECIFIC PHOBIAS

A specific phobia is an irrational fear of specific objects or situations.

Specific phobias, as a group, are among the most common anxiety disorders, but are often less troubling than other anxiety disorders. During any 12-month period, about 13% of women and 4% of men have a specific phobia.

Some specific phobias cause little inconvenience, while others severely interfere with functioning. For example, a city dweller who is afraid of snakes may have no trouble avoiding them. However, a city dweller who fears small, closed places such as elevators may encounter them frequently.

Some specific phobias, such as fear of large animals, the dark, or strangers, begin early in life. Many such phobias stop as people get older. Other phobias, such as fear of rodents, insects, storms, water, heights, flying, or enclosed places, typically develop later in life.

At least 5% of people are to some degree phobic about blood, injections, or injury. These people can actually faint because of a decrease in heart rate and blood pressure, which does not happen with other phobias and anxiety disorders. Many people with other phobias and anxiety disorders hyperventilate. Hyperventilating can cause them to feel as though they might faint, although they virtually never faint.

Treatment

People can often cope with a specific phobia by avoiding the feared object or situation. When treatment is needed, exposure therapy is the treatment of choice.

A therapist can help ensure that the therapy is carried out correctly, although it can be done without a therapist. Even people with a phobia of blood or needles respond well to exposure therapy. For example, people who faint while blood is drawn can have a needle brought close to a vein and then removed when the heart rate begins to slow down. Repeating this process allows the heart rate to return to normal. Eventually, people should be able to have blood drawn without fainting.

Drug therapy is not very useful in helping people overcome specific phobias. However, benzodiazepines (antianxiety drugs) may give people short-term control over a phobia, such as the fear of flying.

Obsessive-Compulsive Disorder

Obsessive-compulsive disorder is characterized by recurring, unwanted, anxiety-provoking, intrusive ideas, images, or impulses (obsessions) that may even seem silly, weird, nasty, or horrible to the person experiencing them. The person also has urges (compulsions) to do something that will relieve the discomfort caused by the obsessions.

- Most obsessive-compulsive behavior is related to concerns about harm or risk.
- Treatment may include exposure therapy (with prevention of compulsive rituals) and antidepressants.

Obsessive-compulsive disorder occurs about equally in men and women and affects about 2% of the population. Children are also affected (see page 1869).

The obsessions are usually related to a sense of harm, risk, or danger. Common obsessions include the following:

- Concerns about contamination (for example, worrying that touching doorknobs will cause disease)
- Doubts (for example, worrying that the front door was not locked)
- Fear of loss
- Fear of becoming aggressive and physically injuring someone

More than 95% of people with obsessive-compulsive disorder feel a compulsion to perform rituals—repetitive, purposeful, intentional acts. Rituals used to control an obsession include the following:

- Washing or cleaning to be rid of contamination
- Checking to allay doubt (for example, checking to make sure a door is locked)
- Hoarding to prevent loss
- Avoiding the people who might become objects of aggression

Most rituals, such as excessive hand washing or repeated checking to make sure a door has been locked, can be observed. Other rituals, such as repetitive counting or quietly mumbling statements intended to diminish danger, cannot be observed. Obsessions are not always accompanied by compulsions.

Most people with obsessive-compulsive disorder are aware that their obsessive thoughts do not reflect actual risks and that their compulsive behaviors are ineffective. Obsessive-compulsive disorder, therefore, differs from psychotic disorders, in which people lose contact with reality. Obsessive-compulsive disorder also differs from obsessive-compulsive personality disorder (see page 882), in which specific personality traits are defined (for example, being a perfectionist). People with obsessive-compulsive disorder are aware that their compulsive behaviors are excessive to the point of being bizarre, and they are afraid they will be embarrassed or stigmatized. Thus, they often perform their rituals secretly, even though the rituals may occupy several hours each day.

About one third of people with obsessive-compulsive disorder are depressed at the time the disorder is diagnosed. Altogether, two thirds become depressed at some point.

> **? Did You Know...**
>
> Most people with obsessive-compulsive disorder know that their obsessions and compulsions are irrational.

Treatment

Exposure therapy is effective in treating obsessive-compulsive disorder. Exposure therapy involves repeatedly exposing people to the situations or people that trigger obsessions, rituals, or discomfort but not letting them perform the compulsive ritual. Discomfort or anxiety gradually diminishes during repeated exposure as people learn that rituals are unnecessary for decreasing discomfort. The improvement usually persists for years, probably because people who have mastered this self-help approach continue to practice it as a way of life without much effort after formal treatment has ended.

Selective serotonin reuptake inhibitors (such as fluoxetine) and clomipramine, a tricyclic antidepressant, are effective. Many experts believe that a combination of exposure therapy and drug therapy is the best treatment.

Psychodynamic psychotherapy and psychoanalysis have generally not been effective for people with obsessive-compulsive disorder.

Posttraumatic Stress Disorder

Posttraumatic stress disorder (PTSD) is characterized by recurrent, intrusive recollections of an overwhelming traumatic event.

- Events that threaten death or serious injury can cause intense, long-lasting distress.
- Affected people may relive the event, have nightmares, and avoid anything that reminds them of the event.
- Treatment may include psychotherapy (supportive and exposure therapy) and antidepressants.

Experiencing or witnessing traumatic events that threaten death or serious injury can affect people long after the experience is over. Intense fear, helplessness, or horror experienced during the traumatic event can haunt a person.

Events that can lead to posttraumatic stress disorder include the following:

- Engaging in combat
- Experiencing or witnessing sexual or physical assault
- Being affected by a disaster, either natural (for example, a hurricane) or man-made (for example, a severe automobile accident)

Sometimes symptoms do not begin until many months or even years after the traumatic event took place. If posttraumatic stress disorder has been present for 3 months or longer, it is considered chronic.

Posttraumatic stress disorder affects at least 8% of people sometime during their life, including childhood (see page 1870). Many people who undergo or witness traumatic events, such as combat veterans and victims of rape or other violent acts, experience posttraumatic stress disorder.

Symptoms

In posttraumatic stress disorder, people have frequent, unwanted memories replaying the traumatic event. Nightmares are common. Sometimes events are relived as if happening (flashbacks). Intense distress often occurs when people are exposed to an event or situation that reminds them of the original trauma. Examples of such reminders are anniversaries of the traumatic event, seeing a gun after being pistol-whipped during a robbery, and being in a small boat after a near-drowning accident.

People persistently avoid things that are reminders of the trauma. They may also attempt to avoid thoughts, feelings, or conversations about the traumatic event and avoid activities, situations, or people who serve as reminders. Avoidance may also include memory loss (amnesia) for a particular aspect of the traumatic event. People have a numbing or deadening of emotional responsiveness and symptoms of increased arousal (such as difficulty falling asleep, being vigilant for warning signs of risk, or being easily startled). Symptoms of depression are common, and people show less interest in previously enjoyed activities. Feelings of guilt are also common. For example, they may feel guilty that they survived when other people did not.

Treatment

Treatment involves psychotherapy (including exposure therapy) and drug therapy. Because of the often intense anxiety associated with traumatic memories, supportive psychotherapy plays an especially important role in treatment. The therapist is openly empathic and sympathetic in recognizing the psychologic pain. The therapist reassures people that their response is valid but encourages them to face their memories (as a form of exposure therapy). They are also taught ways to control anxiety, which help modulate and integrate the painful memories into their personality.

Insight-oriented psychotherapy can help people who feel guilty understand why they are punishing themselves and help rid them of guilty feelings.

Antidepressants appear to provide some benefit. Selective serotonin reuptake inhibitors (SSRIs), tricyclic antidepressants, and monoamine oxidase inhibitors (MAOIs) are especially helpful.

Chronic posttraumatic stress disorder may not disappear but often becomes less intense over time even without treatment. Nevertheless, some people remain severely handicapped by the disorder.

Acute Stress Disorder

Acute stress disorder is a brief period of intrusive recollections occurring shortly after an overwhelming traumatic event. It is similar to posttraumatic stress disorder, except that it begins within 4 weeks of the traumatic event and lasts only 2 days to 4 weeks.

People with acute stress disorder have been exposed to a terrifying event. They mentally reexperience the traumatic event, avoid things that remind them of it, and have increased anxiety. They also have three or more of the following symptoms:

- A sense of numbing, detachment, or lack of emotional responsiveness
- Reduced awareness of surroundings (for example, being dazed)
- A feeling that things are not real
- A feeling that they are not real
- An inability to remember an important part of the traumatic event

The number of people with acute stress disorder is unknown. The likelihood of developing acute stress disorder is greater when traumatic events are severe.

Treatment

Many people recover from acute stress disorder once they are removed from the traumatic situation and given appropriate support in the form of understanding, empathy for their distress, and an opportunity to describe what happened and their reaction to it. Some people benefit from describing their experience several times.

CHAPTER

129 Mood Disorders

Mood disorders are mental health disorders involving emotional disturbances consisting of long periods of excessive sadness (depression) or excessive joyousness or elation (mania). Depression and mania represent the two extremes, or poles, of mood disorders.

Mood disorders are sometimes called affective disorders. *Affect* (emphasis on the first syllable) means emotional state as revealed through facial expressions and gestures.

Sadness and joy are part of the normal experience of everyday life and differ from the depression and mania that characterize mood disorders. Sadness is a natural response to loss, defeat, disappointment, trauma, or catastrophe. Sadness may be psychologically beneficial because it enables people to withdraw from offensive or unpleasant situations, which may aid recovery.

Grief or bereavement is the most common of the normal reactions to a loss or separation, such as the death of a loved one, divorce, or romantic disappointment. Usually, bereavement and loss do not cause persistent, incapacitating depression except in people predisposed to mood disorders.

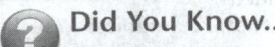 **Did You Know...**

In the United States, about one of six people have depression severe enough to require medical attention.

Joyousness or elation, usually linked to success and achievement, can sometimes be a defense against depression or a denial of the pain of loss. People who are dying sometimes have brief periods of elation and restless activity, and some recently bereaved people may even become elated rather

What Is Seasonal Affective Disorder?

Many people report feeling sadder in late autumn and winter, blaming this tendency on the shortening of daylight hours and colder temperatures. However, some people develop a more intense sadness known as seasonal affective disorder, which is a type of depression. Seasonal affective disorder (also called autumn-winter depression) is characterized by recurring episodes of depression that usually begin in October or November and end by February or March. The disorder is more common in extreme northern and southern latitudes, where the winter season is typically longer and harsher. It is believed that seasonal affective disorder may be caused by longer secretion of melatonin (a hormone produced by the pineal gland, which is located in the middle of the brain) that normally occurs at night.

Symptoms include lethargy, decreased interest in and withdrawal from usual activities, oversleeping, and overeating. In spring, the symptoms steadily resolve. However, in some people, spring triggers a rapid swing to symptoms that are almost the opposite of those experienced during the winter. These symptoms (called spring-summer hypomania) include increased energy and involvement in activities, decreased need for sleep, and decreased appetite.

Phototherapy is the most effective treatment. People are placed in a closed room that is bathed in high levels of artificial light (light levels in a normally-lit room are not adequate). The light is controlled to mimic the season that the therapist is trying to create: longer days for summer and shorter days for winter.

---

than grieve normally. In people predisposed to mood disorders, these reactions may be the prelude to mania.

A mood disorder is diagnosed when sadness or elation is overly intense and continues beyond what would be expected for a particular event. Unlike normal emotional reactions, depression and mania greatly impair the ability to function physically, socially, and at work.

Some mood disorders involve mainly depression. Depression is termed a unipolar disorder. Other mood disorders, termed bipolar disorders, involve episodes of depression alternating with episodes of mania. Mania without depression (called unipolar mania) is very rare.

About 17% of the U.S. population experience depression severe enough to require medical attention. Of these people, one third have long-lasting (chronic) depression, and many of the remainder continue to have episodes of depression separated by periods of normal mood (recurring depression). Nearly 4% of the U.S. population have a bipolar disorder.

Depression

The disorder depression is a feeling of sadness intense enough to interfere with functioning. It may follow a recent loss or other sad event but is out of proportion to that event and lasts beyond an appropriate length of time.

- Heredity, side effects of drugs, emotionally distressing events, imbalances in the body, and other factors can contribute to depression.
- Depression can make people sad and sluggish or anxious and fearful.
- Doctors base the diagnosis on symptoms.
- Antidepressants, psychotherapy, and sometimes electroconvulsive therapy can help.

After anxiety, depression is the most common mental health disorder. About 30% of people who visit a primary care practitioner have symptoms of depression. However, only some of these people have major depression. People who become depressed typically do so in their mid teens, 20s, or 30s, although depression can begin at almost any age, including during childhood (see page 1863). People born in the latter part of the 20th century seem to have higher rates of depression and suicide than those of previous generations, in part because rates of substance abuse have increased.

An episode of depression, if untreated, typically lasts about 6 months but sometimes lasts for 2 years or more. Episodes tend to recur several times over a lifetime.

Causes

The exact cause of depression is unclear, but a number of factors may make depression more likely. They include a family tendency (heredity), side effects of certain drugs, and emotionally distressing events, particularly those involving a loss. Depression does not reflect a weakness of character and may not reflect a personality disorder, childhood trauma, or poor parenting. Depression may arise or worsen without any apparent or significant life stresses.

Genetic abnormalities may contribute. They can affect the function of substances that help nerve cells communicate (neurotransmitters). Serotonin, dopamine and norepinephrine are neurotransmitters that may be involved in depression.

Social class, race, and culture do not appear to affect the chance that people will experience depression during their lifetime. However, a person's sex does: Women are twice as likely as men to experience depression, although the reasons are not entirely

SOME CAUSES OF DEPRESSION

CONDITION	EXAMPLES
Brain and nervous system disorders	Brain tumors Dementia (in early stages) Head injury Multiple sclerosis Parkinson's disease Sleep apnea Stroke Seizures that affect the temporal lobe (complex partial seizures)
Cancers	Abdominal cancers (ovary or colon) Cancer spreading throughout the body (metastatic) Cancer of the pancreas
Connective tissue disorders	Systemic lupus erythematosus (lupus)
Hormonal disorders	Addison's disease Cushing's syndrome Diabetes High levels of parathyroid hormone Low and high levels of thyroid hormone Low levels of pituitary hormones (hypopituitarism)
Infections	AIDS Influenza Mononucleosis Syphilis (late stage) Tuberculosis Viral hepatitis Viral pneumonia
Nutritional disorders	Pellagra (vitamin B_6 deficiency) Pernicious anemia (vitamin B_{12} deficiency)
Drugs	Alcohol Amphetamine withdrawal Amphotericin B Antipsychotic drugs Beta-blockers (some) Cimetidine Contraceptives (oral) Corticosteroids Cycloserine Hormone (estrogen) therapy Interferon Mercury Methyldopa Metoclopramide Reserpine Thallium Vinblastine Vincristine

clear. Of physical factors, hormones are the ones most involved. Changes in hormone levels, which can cause mood changes shortly before menstruation and after childbirth, might play some role in women. In women, levels of enzymes that affect mood may be higher. Abnormal thyroid function, which is fairly common among women, may also be a factor.

People with transient depression become temporarily depressed in reaction to certain situations:

- Holidays (holiday blues)
- Meaningful anniversaries, such as the anniversary of a loved one's death
- Before menstrual periods (premenstrual syndrome, or if the depression is more serious, premenstrual dysphoric disorder)
- During the first 2 weeks after giving birth (baby blues or, if the depression is more serious, postpartum depression)

Such reactions are normal and do not lead to severe, lasting depression except in people predisposed to depression. Depression may occur with or be caused by a number of physical disorders. Physical disorders may cause depression directly (as when a thyroid disorder affects hormone levels) or indirectly (as when rheumatoid arthritis causes pain and disability). Often, a physical disorder both directly and indirectly causes depression. For example, AIDS may cause depression directly if the human immunodeficiency virus (HIV), which causes AIDS, damages the brain. AIDS may cause depression indirectly by having an overall negative effect on the person's life.

The use of some prescription drugs can cause depression. For unknown reasons, corticosteroids often cause depression when the body produces them in large amounts as part of a disorder (as in Cushing's syndrome), but they tend to cause hypomania or, rarely, mania when they are given as a drug. Sometimes stopping a drug can cause depression.

A number of mental health disorders can predispose a person to depression. They include certain anxiety disorders, alcoholism, other substance abuse disorders, and schizophrenia. People who have had depression are more likely to have it again.

Symptoms

Symptoms typically develop gradually over days or weeks and can vary greatly. For example, a person who is becoming depressed may appear sluggish and sad or irritable and anxious.

Many people with depression cannot experience emotions—including grief, joy, and pleasure—in a normal way; in the extreme, the world appears to have become colorless and lifeless. Depressed people may be preoccupied with intense feelings of guilt and self-denigration and may not be able to concentrate. They may experience feelings of despair, loneliness, and low self-esteem. They are often indecisive and withdrawn, feel progressively helpless and hopeless, and think about death and suicide.

Symptoms can vary depending on the type of depression.

- **Catatonic depression:** People are very withdrawn. Thinking, speech, and general activity may slow down so much that all voluntary activities stop. They may not take care of their children or pets or even feed themselves. Some people mimic others' speech (echolalia) or movements (echopraxia).
- **Melancholic depression:** People do not receive pleasure from activities they usually enjoy. They appear sluggish, sad, and withdrawn. They speak little, stop eating, and lose weight. Their face may show no emotions. They may feel excessively or inappropriately guilty.
- **Psychotic depression:** People have false beliefs (delusions), often of having committed unpardonable sins or crimes, of having incurable or shameful disorders, or of being watched or persecuted. People may have hallucinations, usually of voices accusing them of various misdeeds or condemning them to death. A few imagine that they see coffins or deceased relatives.
- **Atypical depression:** People with this type appear anxious and fearful (especially in the evening). They have an increased appetite, resulting in weight gain, and although initially unable to sleep, they sleep for increasingly longer periods. They tend to cheer up in response to positive events but are excessively sensitive to perceived criticism or rejection. Some people become agitated. They are very restless—wringing their hands and talking continuously.

Most depressed people have difficulty falling asleep and awaken repeatedly, particularly early in the morning. Poor appetite and weight loss sometimes lead to emaciation, and in women, menstrual periods may stop. However, overeating and weight gain are common in people with mild depression.

Some depressed people complain of having a physical illness, with various aches and pains. Some fear calamity or the possibility of becoming insane. Others think they have an incurable or shameful illness, such as cancer or a sexually transmitted disease, and think they are infecting other people.

Suicide: Thoughts of death are among the most serious symptoms of depression. Many depressed people want to die or feel they are so worthless that they should die. As many as 15% of untreated depressed people end their life by suicide. A suicide threat is an emergency (see page 873). When people threaten to kill themselves, a doctor may hospitalize them so that they can be supervised until treatment reduces the risk of suicide. The risk is especially high in the following situations:

- When depression is not treated or is inadequately treated.
- When treatment is started (when people are becoming more active mentally and physically but their mood is still dark)
- When people continue to feel excessively sad even while returning to normal activities
- When people have a significant anniversary
- When people alternate between depression and mania (bipolar disorder—see page 870)
- When people feel very anxious
- When people are drinking alcohol or taking recreational or illicit drugs

Substance Abuse: People with depression are more likely to abuse alcohol or other recreational drugs in an attempt to help them sleep or feel less anxious. However, depression causes alcoholism and drug abuse less often than was once thought. People are also more likely to smoke heavily and to neglect their health. Thus, the risk of developing or worsening other disorders, such as chronic obstructive pulmonary disease, is increased.

> **? Did You Know...**
>
> Depression involves more than feeling sad all the time. People may feel worthless and guilty, lose interest in their normal pleasures, have sleep disorders, or lose or gain weight.

Dysthymia: In some depressed people, symptoms are mild, but the disorder lasts for years, often decades. This type of depression, called dysthymia, often begins during adolescence and involves distinct changes in personality. People with dysthymia are gloomy, pessimistic, skeptical, humorless, or incapable of having fun. They are passive, lack energy, and keep to themselves. They constantly complain and are quick to criticize others and reproach themselves. They are preoccupied with inadequacy, failure, and negative events, sometimes to the point of morbid enjoyment of their own failures.

Diagnosis

A doctor is usually able to diagnose depression based on symptoms. A previous history of depression or a family history of depression helps confirm the diagnosis. Excessive worrying, panic attacks, and obsessions are common in depression and may lead the doctor to incorrectly think that the person has an anxiety disorder.

In older people, depression may be difficult to notice, especially if they do not work or have little social interaction. Also, depression may be mistaken for dementia because it can cause similar symptoms. However, symptoms of dementia due to depression resolve when depression is treated. Symptoms of dementia do not.

Standardized questionnaires are used to help identify depression and determine how severe it is. Two such questionnaires are the Hamilton Depression Rating Scale, conducted verbally by an interviewer, and the Beck Depression Inventory, a self-administered questionnaire. Doctors also ask people whether they have any thoughts or plans to harm themselves. Such thoughts indicate that depression is severe.

No test can confirm depression. However, laboratory tests may help a doctor determine whether depression is caused by an endocrine or other physical disorder. For example, blood tests are usually done to detect a thyroid disorder or vitamin deficiency. In younger people, tests may be done to detect drug abuse. A thorough neurologic examination is done to check for Parkinson's disease, which causes some of the same symptoms. People who have severely disturbed sleep may need to have testing (polysomnography—see box on page 669) to distinguish sleep disorders from depression.

Prognosis and Treatment

If untreated, depression may last about 6 months to several years. Although mild symptoms persist in many people, functioning tends to return to normal. However, most people with depression have repeated episodes, averaging 4 to 5 times over a lifetime.

Most people with depression do not require hospitalization. However, some people should be hospitalized, especially if they are contemplating suicide or have attempted it, are frail because of weight loss, or are at risk of heart problems because of severe agitation.

Drug therapy is the cornerstone of treatment. Other treatments include psychotherapy and electroconvulsive therapy. Sometimes a combination of therapies is used. Depression can usually be treated successfully. If a cause (such as a drug or another disorder) can be identified, it is corrected first, but drugs to treat depression may also be needed.

Drug Therapy: Several types of antidepressants—selective serotonin reuptake inhibitors (SSRIs), heterocyclic antidepressants, monoamine oxidase inhibitors

SPOTLIGHT ON AGING

Depression affects about 1 of every 6 older people. Some older people have had depression earlier in their lives. Others develop it for the first time during old age.

Some causes of depression may be more common among older people. For example, older people may be more likely to experience emotionally distressing events that involve a loss, such as the death of a loved one, the ending of a significant relationship, or a loss of familiar surroundings, as when moving away from a familiar neighborhood. Other sources of stress, such as reduced income, a worsening chronic illness, a gradual loss of independence, or social isolation, may also contribute.

Disorders that can lead to depression are common among older people. Such disorders include cancer, heart attack, heart failure, thyroid disorders, stroke, dementia, and Parkinson's disease.

In older people, depression can cause symptoms that resemble those of dementia: slower thinking, decreased concentration, confusion, and difficulty remembering. Depression can so resemble dementia that it is sometimes called dementia of depression or pseudodementia. However, doctors can distinguish depression from dementia because the symptoms resolve when depression is treated. Symptoms of dementia do not.

Depression is often difficult to diagnose among older people for several reasons:

- The symptoms may be less noticeable because older people may not work or may have less social interaction.
- Some people believe that depression is a weakness and are reluctant to tell anyone that they are experiencing sadness or other symptoms.
- The absence of emotion may be interpreted as indifference rather than depression.
- Family members and friends may regard a depressed person's symptoms simply as evidence that the person is getting older.
- The symptoms may be attributed to another disorder, such as dementia.

Because depression may be difficult to identify, many doctors routinely ask older people questions about their mood. Family members should be alert for subtle changes in personality, especially lack of enthusiasm and spontaneity, loss of sense of humor, and new forgetfulness.

Selective serotonin reuptake inhibitors (SSRIs) are the antidepressants used most often for older people who are depressed. They are less likely to have side effects. Citalopram and escitalopram are particularly useful.

(MAOIs), and several new types—are available, as well as psychostimulants. Most must be taken regularly for at least several weeks before they begin to work. The chances that any given antidepressant will work for a particular person are about 65%. Side effects vary with each type of drug. Sometimes when treatment with one drug does not relieve depression, a combination of antidepressant drugs is prescribed.

Selective serotonin reuptake inhibitors (SSRIs) are now the most commonly used class of antidepressants. SSRIs are effective in treating depression and dysthymia as well as other mental health disorders that often coexist with depression. Although SSRIs can cause nausea, diarrhea, tremor, weight loss, and headache, these side effects are usually mild or go away with continued use. Most people tolerate the side effects of SSRIs better than the side effects of heterocyclic antidepressants. SSRIs are less likely to adversely affect the heart than heterocyclic antidepressants. However, a few people may seem more agitated, depressed, and anxious the first week after they start SSRIs or the dose is increased. Some people, especially younger children and adolescents, become increasingly suicidal if these symptoms are

not detected and rapidly treated. People taking SSRIs and their loved ones should be warned of this possibility and instructed to call their doctor if symptoms worsen with treatment. However, because people with untreated depression sometimes commit suicide, people and their doctors must balance this risk against the risk of drug treatment. Also, with long-term use, SSRIs may have additional side effects, such as weight gain and sexual dysfunction (in one third of people). Abruptly stopping some of the SSRIs may result in a discontinuation syndrome that includes dizziness, anxiety, irritability, nausea, and flu-like symptoms.

Newer antidepressants are as effective and safe as SSRIs and have similar side effects. These drugs include

- Norepinephrine-dopamine reuptake inhibitors
- Serotonin modulators
- Serotonin-norepinephrine reuptake inhibitors

As may occur with SSRIs, the risk of suicide may be temporarily increased when these drugs are first started, and abruptly stopping serotonin-norepinephrine reuptake inhibitors may result in a discontinuation syndrome.

R︎x DRUGS USED TO TREAT DEPRESSION

DRUG	SOME SIDE EFFECTS	COMMENTS
Heterocyclic (including tricyclic) antidepressants		
Amitriptyline Amoxapine Clomipramine Desipramine Doxepin Imipramine Maprotiline Nortriptyline Protriptyline Trimipramine	Drowsiness, weight gain, increased heart rate, decreased blood pressure, dry mouth, confusion, blurred vision, constipation, difficulty starting to urinate, and delayed orgasm With clomipramine and maprotiline, seizures	Side effects are usually more pronounced in older people. Overdosage can cause serious, potentially life-threatening toxicity.
Selective serotonin reuptake inhibitors (SSRIs)		
Citalopram Escitalopram Fluoxetine Fluvoxamine Paroxetine Sertraline	Sexual dysfunction (primarily, delayed orgasm but also loss of desire in some people), nausea, diarrhea, headache, weight loss (short-term), weight gain (long-term), discontinuation syndrome,* forgetfulness, blunting of emotions, and easy bruising	SSRIs are the most commonly used class of antidepressants. They are also effective for dysthymia, generalized anxiety disorder, obsessive-compulsive disorder, panic disorder, phobic disorder, posttraumatic stress disorder, premenstrual dysphoric disorder, and bulimia. Toxicity due to overdosage is less serious than that with other antidepressants.
Monoamine oxidase inhibitors (MAOIs)		
Isocarboxazid Phenelzine Selegiline Tranylcypromine	Insomnia, nausea, weight gain, sexual dysfunction (loss of desire and delayed orgasm), pins-and-needles sensation, dizziness, insomnia, lowered blood pressure (particularly when a person stands), and severe high blood pressure	People who take these drugs must follow dietary restrictions and avoid using certain drugs. Selegiline is available as a patch. With the patch, people do not have to follow the dietary restrictions unless the patch contains a high dose.
Psychostimulants		
Dextroamphetamine Methylphenidate	Nervousness, tremor, insomnia, and dry mouth	These drugs are usually used with antidepressants. Used alone, they are usually ineffective as antidepressants.
Serotonin modulators (5-HT$_2$ blockers)		
Mirtazapine	Drowsiness and weight gain	Mirtazapine does not cause nausea or sexual dysfunction.
Nefazodone	Mild drowsiness and, rarely, serious liver problems	Nefazodone produces restful sleep.
Trazodone	Prolonged drowsiness, painful and persistent erection (priapism), and an excessive decrease in blood pressure when a person stands	
Serotonin-norepinephrine reuptake inhibitors		
Duloxetine Venlafaxine	Nausea, dry mouth, discontinuation syndrome,* and, if high doses are taken, an increase in blood pressure	Most of the side effects can be prevented or minimized when low doses are used and when changes in dosages are made slowly.

(continued on the following page)

℞ DRUGS USED TO TREAT DEPRESSION (*Continued*)

DRUG	SOME SIDE EFFECTS	COMMENTS
Norepinephrine-dopamine reuptake inhibitors		
Bupropion	Headache, agitation, discontinuation syndrome,* high blood pressure in a few people, and rarely seizures	Bupropion is useful for depressed people who also have attention-deficit/hyperactivity disorder or cocaine dependence and those trying to stop smoking. Bupropion does not cause sexual dysfunction.

*Discontinuation syndrome consists of dizziness, anxiety, irritability, nausea, and flu-like symptoms that occur when a drug is stopped abruptly.

Heterocyclic (including tricyclic) antidepressants, once the mainstay of treatment, are now used infrequently because they have more side effects than other antidepressants. They often cause drowsiness and lead to weight gain. They can also cause an increase in heart rate and a decrease in blood pressure when a person stands. Other side effects include blurred vision, dry mouth, confusion, constipation, and difficulty starting to urinate. These other side effects, called anticholinergic effects, are often more severe in older people (see box on page 1897). Abruptly stopping heterocyclic antidepressants, as with SSRIs, may result in a discontinuation syndrome.

Monoamine oxidase inhibitors (MAOIs) may be effective but are rarely prescribed except when other antidepressants have not worked. People who use MAOIs must adhere to a number of dietary restrictions and take special precautions to avoid a serious reaction involving a sudden, severe rise in blood pressure with a severe, throbbing headache (hypertensive crisis). This crisis can cause a stroke. Precautions include

- Not eating foods or beverages that contain tyramine, such as beer on tap, red wines (including sherry), liqueurs, overripe foods, salami, aged cheeses, fava or broad beans, yeast extracts (marmite), canned figs, raisins, yogurt, cheese, sour cream, pickled herring, caviar, liver, extensively tenderized meats, and soy sauce
- Not taking pseudoephedrine, contained in many over-the-counter cough and cold remedies
- Not taking dextromethorphan (a cough suppressant), reserpine (an antihypertensive drug), or meperidine (an analgesic)
- Carrying an antidote, such as chlorpromazine tablets, at all times and, if a severe, throbbing headache occurs, taking the antidote at once and going to the nearest emergency room

People who take MAOIs should also avoid taking other types of antidepressants, including heterocyclic antidepressants, SSRIs, bupropion, and serotonin modulators (mirtazapine, nefazodone, and venlafaxine). Taking an MAOI with another antidepressant can cause a dangerously high body temperature, breakdown of muscle, kidney failure, and seizures. These effects, called neuroleptic malignant syndrome, can be fatal (see box on page 893).

Psychostimulants, such as dextroamphetamine and methylphenidate, as well as other drugs, are sometimes used, often with antidepressants.

St. John's wort, an herbal dietary supplement, is sometimes used to relieve mild depression, although its effectiveness is not proven. Due to potentially harmful interactions between St. John's wort and many prescription drugs, people interested in taking this herbal supplement need to discuss possible drug interactions with their doctor (see page 2078).

Psychotherapy: Psychotherapy alone may be just as effective as drug therapy for mild depression. When used with drugs, it can be useful for severe depression.

Individual or group psychotherapy can help people with depression gradually resume former responsibilities and adapt to the normal pressures of life, building on the improvement caused by antidepressants. Interpersonal psychotherapy can provide supportive guidance to people while they adjust to changes in life roles. Cognitive-behavioral therapy can help change hopelessness and negative thinking.

Electroconvulsive Therapy: Electroconvulsive therapy is sometimes used to treat people with severe depression, particularly people who are psychotic, threatening to commit suicide, or refusing to eat. It is also used to treat depression during pregnancy when drugs are ineffective. This type of therapy is usually very effective and can relieve depression quickly, unlike most antidepressants, which can take up to several weeks. The speed with which it takes effect can save lives.

For electroconvulsive therapy, electrodes are placed on the head, and an electrical current is applied to induce a seizure in the brain. For reasons that are not understood, the seizure relieves depression. Usually, at least five to seven treatments, one treatment every other day, are given. Because the electrical current can cause muscle contractions and pain, general anesthesia is required during treatments. Electroconvulsive therapy may cause some temporary memory loss and, rarely, permanent memory loss.

Bipolar Disorder

In bipolar disorder (formerly called manic-depressive illness), episodes of depression alternate with episodes of mania or a less severe form of mania called hypomania. Mania is characterized by excessive physical activity and feelings of elation that are greatly out of proportion to the situation.

- Heredity probably plays a part in bipolar disorder.
- Episodes of depression and mania may occur separately or together.
- Periods of excessive sadness and loss of interest in life alternate with periods of elation, extreme energy, and often irritability, with periods of relatively normal mood in between.
- Doctors base the diagnosis on the pattern of symptoms.
- Drugs that stabilize mood, such as lithium and certain antiseizure drugs, and sometimes psychotherapy can help.

Bipolar disorder is so named because it includes the two extremes, or poles, of mood disorders—depression and mania. It affects slightly less than 4% of the U.S. population to some degree. Bipolar disorder affects men and women equally. However, women are more likely to have symptoms of depression, and men are more likely to have symptoms of mania. Bipolar disorder usually begins in a person's teens, 20s, or 30s and rarely earlier (see page 1864).

Bipolar disorders are classified as

- **Bipolar I disorder:** People have had at least one manic episode and usually depressive episodes
- **Bipolar II disorder:** People have had major depressive episodes, at least minor manic (hypomanic) episode, but no full manic episodes

---

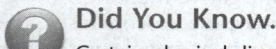

? Did You Know...

Certain physical disorders and drugs can cause symptoms of bipolar disorder.

People experiencing mania often think they are in their best form.

Causes

Hereditary is thought to be involved in the development of bipolar disorder. Abnormal levels of certain substances the body produces, such as the neurotransmitters norepinephrine or serotonin, may be involved. (Neurotransmitters are substances that nerve cells use to communicate.)

Bipolar disorder sometimes begins after a stressful event, or such an event triggers another episode. However, no cause-and-effect relationship has been proved.

The symptoms of bipolar disorder—depression and mania—can occur in certain disorders, such as high levels of thyroid hormone (hyperthyroidism). Also, episodes may be triggered by drugs, such as cocaine and amphetamines.

Symptoms

In bipolar disorder, episodes of symptoms alternate with virtually symptom-free periods (remissions). Episodes last anywhere from a few weeks to 3 to 6 mo. Cycles—time from onset of one episode to that of the next—vary in length. Some people have infrequent episodes, perhaps only a few over a lifetime, whereas others have four or more episodes each year (called rapid cycling). Despite this large variation, the cycle time for each person is relatively consistent.

Episodes consist of depression, mania, or less severe mania (hypomania). Only a minority of people alternate back and forth between mania and depression with each cycle. In most, one or the other predominates to some extent.

Depression: Depression in bipolar disorder resembles depression that occurs alone (see page 863). People feel excessively sad and lose interest in their activities. They think and move slowly and may sleep more than usual. They may be overwhelmed with feelings of hopelessness and guilt.

Mania: Episodes of mania end more abruptly than those of depression and are typically shorter, lasting a week or longer. People feel exuberant, energetic, and elated or irritable. They may also feel overly confident, act or dress extravagantly, sleep little, and talk more than usual. Their thoughts race. They are easily distracted and constantly shift from one theme or endeavor to another. They pursue one activity (such as business endeavors, gambling, or dangerous sexual behavior) after another, without thinking about the consequences (such as loss of money or injury). However, people tend to think that they are in their best mental state.

People lack insight into their condition. This lack plus their huge capacity for activity can make them impatient, intrusive, meddlesome, and aggressively irritable when crossed. As a result, they may have problems with social relationships and may feel that they are being treated unjustly or are being persecuted. Some people have hallucinations, hearing and seeing things that are not there.

Manic psychosis is an extreme form of mania. People have psychotic symptoms that resemble

SOME CAUSES OF MANIA

CONDITION	EXAMPLES
Brain and nervous system disorders	Brain tumors Head injury Huntington's disease Multiple sclerosis Seizures that affect the temporal lobe (complex partial seizures) Stroke Sydenham's disease
Connective tissue disorders	Systemic lupus erythematosus (lupus)
Infections	AIDS Encephalitis Influenza Syphilis (late stage)
Hormonal disorders	High levels of thyroid hormones (hyperthyroidism)
Drugs	Amphetamines Antidepressants (most) Antidepressant withdrawal Bromocriptine Cocaine Corticosteroids Levodopa Methylphenidate

schizophrenia (see page 889). They may have extremely grandiose delusions, such as of being Jesus. Others may feel persecuted, such as being pursued by the FBI. Activity level increases markedly; patients may race about and scream, swear, or sing. Mental and physical activity may be so frenzied that there is a complete loss of coherent thinking and behavior (delirious mania), causing extreme exhaustion. People so affected require immediate treatment.

Hypomania: Hypomania is not as severe as mania. People feel cheerful, need little sleep, and are mentally and physically active. For some people, hypomania is a productive time. They have a lot of energy, feel creative and confident, and often function well in social situations. However, people in this mental state often make commitments that they cannot keep or start projects that they do not finish. They are easily distracted and easily irritated, sometimes resulting in angry outbursts. They rapidly change moods. People with hypomania may recognize such effects and be bothered by them, as are the people around them.

Mixed Episodes: When depression and mania or hypomania occur in one episode, people may mo-

mentarily become tearful in the middle of elation, or their thoughts may start racing in the middle of depression. Often, people go to bed depressed and wake early in the morning and feel elated and energetic. At least one of three people with bipolar disorder has mixed episodes.

Diagnosis

The diagnosis is based on the distinctive pattern of symptoms. However, people with mania may not accurately report their symptoms because they do not think anything is wrong with them. So doctors often have to obtain information from family members. Doctors also ask people whether they have any thoughts about suicide.

Doctors review the drugs being taken to check whether any could contribute to the symptoms. Doctors may also check for signs of other disorders that may be contributing to symptoms. For example, they may do blood tests to check for hyperthyroidism.

Doctors determine whether people are experiencing an episode of mania or depression so that the correct treatment can be given.

Treatment

For severe mania or depression, hospitalization is often required. For less severe mania, hospitalization may be needed during periods of overactivity to protect people and their family members from disastrous financial activities or sexual behavior. Most people with hypomania can be treated as outpatients. People with rapid recycling are more difficult to treat. Without treatment, bipolar disorder recurs in almost all people.

Treatment may include drugs to stabilize mood (mood stabilizers, such as lithium and some anticonvulsants), antipsychotic drugs, and certain antidepressants, as well as psychotherapy. Electroconvulsive therapy is sometimes used when mood stabilizers do not relieve depression. Phototherapy may be used when moods are related to the seasons.

Lithium: Lithium can lessen the symptoms of mania and depression. Lithium helps prevent mood swings in many people. Because lithium takes 4 to 10 days to work, a drug that works more rapidly, such as an anticonvulsant or a newer (second-generation) antipsychotic drug, is often given to control excited thought and activity.

Lithium can have side effects. It can cause tremors, muscle twitching, nausea, vomiting, diarrhea, thirst, excessive urination, and weight gain. It often worsens a person's acne or psoriasis. However, these side effects are usually temporary and are often lessened or relieved when doctors adjust the dose. Sometimes lithium must be stopped because of side effects, which then resolve. Doctors monitor the level of lithium in the blood with regular blood tests because if levels are too high, side effects are more likely. Long-term use of lithium can cause hypothyroidism and rarely can impair kidney function. Therefore, thyroid and kidney function must be monitored with regular blood tests.

A very high level of lithium in the blood can cause persistent headaches, mental confusion, drowsiness, seizures, and abnormal heart rhythms. Side effects are more likely to occur in older people and people with impaired kidney function. Women who are trying to become pregnant must stop taking lithium because, rarely, lithium can cause heart defects in a developing fetus.

Anticonvulsants: The anticonvulsants carbamazepine, oxcarbazepine, and valproate may be used to treat mania when it first occurs or to treat mania and depression when they occur together (mixed state). Unlike lithium, these drugs do not damage the kidneys. However, carbamazepine can greatly reduce the number of red and white blood cells. Rarely, valproate damages the liver (primarily in children) or severely damages the pancreas. With close monitoring by a doctor, these problems can be caught in time. Carbamazepine and valproate can be useful, especially when people have not responded to other treatments. Oxcarbazepine has fewer side effects.

Lamotrigine is sometimes used, especially during episodes of depression. Lamotrigine can cause a serious rash. Rarely, the rash becomes the life-threatening Stevens-Johnson syndrome (see page 1290). People who are taking lamotrigine should watch for any new rash or flu-like symptoms and report these symptoms to the doctor.

Antipsychotics: Sudden manic episodes are increasingly treated with second-generation antipsychotics because they act quickly and the risk of serious side effects is less than that with other drugs used to treat bipolar disorder. These drugs include aripiprazole, olanzapine, quetiapine, risperidone, and ziprasidone.

Long-term side effects may include weight gain and the metabolic syndrome. Metabolic syndrome (see page 960) is excess fat in the abdomen with reduced sensitivity to insulin's effects (insulin resistance), a high blood sugar level, abnormal cholesterol levels, and high blood pressure. The risk of this syndrome may be lower with aripiprazole and ziprasidone.

Antidepressants: All antidepressants can cause swings from depression to hypomania or mania, sometimes rapidly. Therefore, these drugs are used only for short periods and usually are given along with a mood-stabilizing drug. Their effect on mood is closely monitored. At the first sign of a swing to hypomania or mania, the antidepressant is stopped.

Psychotherapy: Psychotherapy is often recommended for people taking mood-stabilizing drugs, mostly to help them take their treatment as directed. Group therapy often helps people and their partners or relatives understand bipolar disorder and its effects. Individual psychotherapy may help people learn how to better cope with problems of daily living.

Education: Learning about the effects of the drugs used to treat the disorder can help people take them as directed. People may resist taking the drugs because they believe that these drugs make them less alert and creative. However, decreased creativity is relatively uncommon because mood stabilizers usually enable people to function better at work and school and in relationships and artistic pursuits.

People should learn how to recognize symptoms as soon as they start, as well as learn ways to help prevent symptoms. For example, avoiding stimulants (such as caffeine and nicotine) and alcohol can help, as can getting enough sleep.

Doctors or therapists may talk to people about the consequences of their actions. For example, if people are inclined to sexual excesses, they are given information about how their actions can affect their marriage and about health risks of promiscuity, particularly AIDS. If people tend to be financially extravagant, they may be advised to turn their finances over to a trusted family member.

Cyclothymic Disorder

In cyclothymic disorder, relatively mild and short episodes of elation (hypomania) alternate with mild and short episodes of sadness (depression).

Cyclothymic disorder resembles bipolar disorder but is less severe. The episodes of elation and sadness are less intense, typically last for only a few days, and recur fairly often at irregular intervals. This disorder may develop into bipolar disorder or may continue as extreme moodiness.

Having cyclothymic disorder may contribute to success in business, leadership, achievement, and artistic creativity. However, it may also cause uneven work and school records, frequent change of residence, repeated romantic breakups or marital failure, and alcohol and drug abuse.

Treatment

People need to learn how to live with the extremes of their temperamental inclinations. However, living with cyclothymic disorder is not easy because interpersonal relationships are often stormy. Getting a job with flexible hours or, for people with artistic inclinations, pursuing a career in the arts may make it easier.

A drug that stabilizes mood (such as lithium or an anticonvulsant) may be used if the disorder makes functioning difficult. People may tolerate the anticonvulsant divalproex better than lithium. Antidepressants are not used unless depression is severe and has lasted a long time because they can cause rapid switching from one mood to the other (rapid cycling).

Support groups can help by providing a forum to share commons experiences and feelings.

CHAPTER

130 Suicidal Behavior

Suicidal behavior includes three types of self-destructive acts: completed suicide, attempted suicide, and suicide gestures. Thoughts and plans about suicide are called suicide ideation.

- Suicide usually results from the interaction of many factors, usually including depression.
- Some methods, such as guns, are more likely to result in death, but choice of a less lethal method does not necessarily mean that the intent was less serious.
- Any suicide threat or suicide attempt must be taken seriously, and help and support should be provided.
- Telephone and email hot lines are available for people who are considering suicide.

Suicidal behavior includes the following:

- Completed suicide: An intentional act of self-harm that results in death.
- Attempted suicide: An act of self-harm that is intended to result in death but does not. Frequently, suicide attempts involve at least some ambivalence about wishing to die and may be a cry for help.
- Suicide gesture: An act of self-harm that is unlikely to result in death. For example, people may scratch their wrists only superficially or take an overdose of vitamins.

Suicide gestures and thoughts and plans about suicide (suicide ideation) may reflect pleas for help from people who still wish to live and should not be dismissed lightly. Information about the frequency of suicide comes mainly from death certificates and inquest reports and probably underestimates the true rate. Even so, suicidal behavior is an all-too-common health problem. Suicidal behavior occurs in people of all ages and of both sexes. Suicide is the 3rd leading cause of death among young people aged 10 to 24 and the 11th leading cause of death overall in the United States. Men older than 70 have the highest rate of completed suicides. But suicide attempts are more common before middle age. Attempted suicide is particularly common among adolescent girls and single men in their 30s. Across all age groups, women attempt suicide twice as often as men, but men are four times more likely to die in their attempts. Suicidal behavior in children and adolescents is discussed in Chapter 287 (see page 1865).

> **? Did You Know...**
> Suicide is the 3rd leading cause of death among young people, but the rate of completed suicides is highest among men over 70.

Risk Factors for Suicide

- Over age 65
- Male
- Painful or disabling illness
- Living alone
- Debt or poverty
- Bereavement or loss
- Humiliation or disgrace
- Depression, especially when accompanied by psychosis or anxiety
- Persistent sadness even when other symptoms of depression are lessening
- A history of drug or alcohol abuse
- A history of prior suicide attempts
- A history of suicide in family members
- Traumatic childhood experiences, including physical or sexual abuse
- Preoccupation with and talk about suicide
- Well-defined plans for suicide

People who have been separated, divorced or widowed are more likely to attempt suicide. Rates of attempted and completed suicide are higher among those who live alone. Having a family member who has attempted suicide may increase the risk as well.

Whites are more likely to attempt suicide than other ethnic groups. Black women attempt suicide nearly as often as white women but are less likely to die in their attempts.

Suicide is less common among people who are in a secure relationship than among single people. It is also less common among practicing members of most religious groups, particularly Roman Catholics.

Causes

Suicidal behaviors usually result from the interaction of several factors. The most common is depression (see page 863). Depression is involved in over 50% of attempted suicides. Marital problems, unhappy or ended love affairs, disputes with parents (among adolescents), or the recent loss of a loved one (particularly among older people) may trigger the depression. Often, one factor, such as a disruption of an important relationship, is the last straw in a series of upsetting circumstances. About one in six people who kill themselves leaves a suicide note, which sometimes provides clues as to why.

People with certain general medical disorders may become depressed and attempt suicide. Most disorders associated with increased suicide rates either directly affect the nervous system and brain (such as AIDS, dementia, or temporal lobe epilepsy) or involve treatments that can cause depression (such as certain drugs used to treat high blood pressure). The risk of suicide may be higher if depression includes anxiety or features of psychosis, such as false beliefs (delusions), than if it does not.

People who have traumatic childhood experiences, including abuse, are more likely to attempt suicide, perhaps because they are at higher risk of becoming depressed.

Depression may be intensified by the use of alcohol, which, in turn, makes suicidal behavior more likely. Alcohol also reduces self-control. About 30% of people who attempt suicide drink alcohol before the attempt. Because alcoholism, particularly binge drinking, often causes deep feelings of remorse during dry periods, alcoholics are suicide-prone even when sober.

Other mental health disorders besides depression also put people at risk of suicide. People with schizophrenia (see page 889) and other psychotic disorders may hear voices (auditory hallucinations) commanding them to kill themselves. People with borderline personality disorder (see page 882) or antisocial personality disorder (see page 881), especially those with a history of violent behavior, may use suicide gestures or attempted suicide as a means of getting back at someone or of making a statement.

Antidepressants and the Risk of Suicide: The risk of suicide attempts is greatest in the month before starting antidepressant treatment, and the risk of death by suicide is no higher in the month when antidepressants are started than in subsequent months. However, some antidepressants slightly increase suicidal thoughts and behaviors (but not completed suicide), so people taking antidepressants should be carefully monitored for suicidal risk.

Because of recent public health warnings about the possible association between taking antidepressants and an increased risk of suicide, doctors have been prescribing antidepressants less often for children and young people. However, during this same time, suicide rates among young people have increased by 14%. Thus, it is possible that by discouraging drug treatment of depression, these warnings may have resulted in more, not fewer, deaths by suicide. Many doctors think that the best approach is to treat depression but to clearly warn people and their family members to watch for worsening symptoms or suicidal thoughts and, if they occur, to immediately call a doctor or to seek care at a hospital.

Methods

The choice of method is often influenced by cultural factors and availability. It may or may not reflect the seriousness of intent. Some methods (such as jumping from a tall building) make survival virtually impossible, whereas other methods (such as overdosing on drugs) make rescue possible. However, even if a person uses a method that proves not to be fatal, the intent may have been just as serious as that of a person whose method was fatal.

? Did You Know...

Taking antidepressants has been linked with an increased risk of suicide or suicidal thoughts, but not taking antidepressants may increase the risk even more.

Although most men and women who kill themselves use guns, more than twice as many men commit suicide this way.

Suicide attempts most often involve drug overdose and self-poisoning. Violent methods, such as shooting and hanging, are uncommon among suicide attempts because they usually result in death.

For completed suicides in the United States, guns are most frequently used by both men (74%) and women (31%). The second most common method is hanging for men and drug overdose for women.

Prevention

Although some attempted or completed suicides come as a shock even to family members and friends, many people give clear warnings. Any suicide threat or suicide attempt should be regarded as a plea for help and must be taken seriously. If the threat or attempt is ignored, a life may be lost.

If a person is threatening or has already attempted suicide, the police should be contacted immediately so that emergency services can arrive as soon as possible. Until help arrives, the person should be spoken to in a calm, supportive manner.

A doctor may hospitalize people who have threatened or attempted suicide. Even if they do not agree to hospitalization, most states allow a doctor to hospitalize people against their wishes if the doctor believes that they are at high risk of harming themselves or other people.

Impact of Suicide

Any suicidal act has a marked emotional effect on all involved. Family, friends, and doctors may feel guilt, shame, and remorse at not having prevented the suicide. They may also feel anger toward the person. Eventually, they may realize that they could not have prevented the suicide.

Sometimes a grief counselor or a self-help group, such as Survivors of Suicide, can help family and friends deal with their feelings of guilt and sorrow. The primary care doctor or local mental health services (for example, at the county or state level) can often help locate these resources. In addition, national organizations, such as the American Foundation for Suicide Prevention, often maintain directories of local support groups. Resources are also available on the Internet.

The effect of attempted suicide is similar. However, family members and friends have the opportunity to resolve their feelings by responding appropriately to the person's cry for help.

Assisted Suicide

Assisted suicide refers to the help given by health care practitioners, family members, or friends to people who wish to end their life. Assisted suicide is very controversial because it reverses the doctor's usual goal, which is to preserve life.

Assisted suicide is illegal in all states except Oregon. In the rest of the United States, doctors can provide treatment intended to minimize physical and emotional suffering, but they cannot intentionally hasten death.

Suicide Intervention: Crisis Hot Lines

People threatening suicide are in crisis, and suicide prevention centers, located around the country, provide 24-hour telephone hot lines for such people. (E-mail hot lines on the Internet are also available.) Suicide prevention centers are staffed by specially trained volunteers.

When potentially suicidal people call a hot line, a volunteer seeks to establish a relationship with them, reminding them of their identity (for example, by using their name repeatedly). The volunteer may offer constructive help for the problem that brought on the crisis and encourage them to take positive action to resolve it.

The volunteer may remind them that they have family members and friends who care and want to help. Finally, the volunteer may try to facilitate emergency face-to-face professional help for them.

Sometimes people call a hot line to say that they have already committed a suicidal act (for example, taken a drug overdose or turned on the gas) or are in the process of doing so. In such cases, the volunteer tries to obtain their address. If that is not possible, another volunteer contacts the police to trace the call and attempt a rescue. If possible, people are kept talking on the telephone until the police arrive.

CHAPTER
131   Eating Disorders

Eating disorders are grouped into three categories:

- **Anorexia nervosa:** Refusing to maintain a minimally normal body weight, with or without bingeing and purging
- **Bulimia nervosa:** Bingeing and purging without weight loss
- **Binge eating disorder:** Bingeing without purging

Bingeing is the rapid consumption of a much larger amount of food than most people would eat in a similar time under similar circumstances. Binges are accompanied by a feeling of loss of control. Purging is self-induced vomiting or misuse of laxatives or enemas.

Eating disorders are more common among women, especially younger women, than among men.

Anorexia Nervosa

Anorexia nervosa is characterized by a relentless pursuit of thinness, a distorted body image, an extreme fear of obesity, refusal to maintain a minimally normal body weight, and, in women, the absence of menstrual periods.

- Anorexia nervosa usually begins during adolescence and is more common among females.
- People with anorexia constantly diet despite continued weight loss, are obsessed with food, and deny that they have a problem.
- Severe or rapid weight loss can have life-threatening consequences.
- Doctors base the diagnosis on symptoms and do a physical examination and tests to check for adverse effects of excessive weight loss.
- Cognitive-behavioral therapy, usually for 1 to 2 years, can help.

Hereditary and social factors play a role in the development of anorexia nervosa. The desire to be thin pervades Western society, and obesity is considered unattractive, unhealthy, and undesirable. Even before adolescence, children are aware of these attitudes, and more than half of preadolescent girls diet or take other measures to control their weight. Yet only a small percentage of these girls develop anorexia nervosa. Other factors, such as psychologic susceptibility, probably predispose certain people to develop anorexia nervosa. In areas with a genuine food shortage, anorexia nervosa is rare.

The disorder usually begins during adolescence, occasionally earlier, and less commonly during adulthood. Anorexia nervosa affects primarily people in middle and upper socioeconomic classes. In Western society, the number of people who have this disorder seems to be increasing. About 0.9% of females have severe anorexia nervosa, compared with only about 0.3% of males. However, mild cases may not be identified.

> **? Did You Know...**
> Between one third and one half of people with anorexia nervosa binge and then purge.

Symptoms

Anorexia nervosa may be mild and transient or severe and persistent.

The first indications of the impending disorder may be a subtle increased concern with diet and body weight. Such concerns seem out of place because most people who have anorexia nervosa are already thin. Preoccupation and anxiety about weight intensify as people become thinner. Even when emaciated, people claim to feel fat, deny that anything is wrong, do not complain about weight loss, and usually resist treatment.

Anorexia means lack of appetite, but people who have anorexia nervosa are actually hungry and preoccupied with food. They study diets and count calories. They hoard, conceal, and deliberately waste food. They collect recipes and prepare elaborate meals for others.

About 30 to 50% of people who have anorexia nervosa binge and then purge by vomiting or taking laxatives. The others simply restrict the amount of food they eat. They also frequently lie about how much they have eaten and conceal their vomiting and their peculiar dietary habits. Many people also take diuretics (drugs that cause the kidneys to excrete more water) to treat perceived bloating and in an effort to lose weight.

Women with anorexia nervosa stop having menstrual periods, sometimes before losing much weight. Women and men may lose interest in sex. Typically, they have a low heart rate, low blood pressure, a low body temperature, and fine soft hair or excess body and facial hair. Tissues swell because fluid accumulates (called edema). People commonly report bloating, abdominal distress, and constipation. Self-induced vomiting can erode tooth enamel, enlarge the salivary glands in the cheeks (parotid glands), and inflame the esophagus. Depression is common.

Even when people become very thin, they tend to remain active, often exercising excessively to control their weight. Until they become emaciated, they have few symptoms of nutritional deficiencies.

Hormonal changes resulting from anorexia nervosa include markedly reduced levels of estrogen (in women) and thyroid hormone and increased levels of cortisol. If people become severely malnourished, every major organ system in the body is likely to be affected. Bone density may decrease, increasing the risk of osteoporosis.

Rapid or severe weight loss can cause life-threatening problems. Problems with the heart and with fluids and electrolytes (sodium, potassium, chloride) are the most dangerous:

- The heart gets weaker and pumps less blood through the body.
- Heart rhythm may become abnormal.
- People may become dehydrated and prone to fainting.
- The blood may become alkaline (a condition called metabolic alkalosis (see page 974).
- Potassium levels in the blood may decrease.

Vomiting and taking laxatives and diuretics can worsen the situation. Sudden death, probably due to abnormal heart rhythms, may occur.

Diagnosis

Because people do not think they have a problem, they resist evaluation and treatment. Usually, they are brought to the doctor's office by family members, or they come because of another disorder. Doctors measure height and weight. Doctors also ask people how they feel about their body and weight and whether they have other symptoms. Doctors may use questionnaires developed to detect eating disorders. If people have the following, anorexia is likely:

- A low body weight, with a body mass index (BMI) of less than 17.5
- Fear of obesity
- Denial of illness
- Absence of menstrual periods in women

Doctors also do a physical examination and blood and urine tests to check for effects of weight loss and undernutrition. A bone density test may be done to check for loss of bone density. Electrocardiography (ECG) may be done to check for abnormal heart rhythms.

> **Did You Know...**
> Without treatment, nearly 10% of people with severe anorexia nervosa die.

Recognizing Anorexia

People who have anorexia usually deny they have a problem and try to conceal their unusual eating habits rather than seek help. Because many people who have anorexia are meticulous, compulsive, and intelligent, with very high standards for achievement and success, they are often able to conceal the disorder until it is severe. Thus, family members and friends may be unaware of the disorder until it has become severe. Because anorexia has serious, sometimes life-threatening complications, family members and friends of someone who often diets or is excessively concerned about weight need to know how to recognize the disorder.

People with anorexia often do the following:

- Complain about being fat although they are very thin
- Deny being thin
- Think about food all the time
- Measure their food
- Hoard, conceal, or deliberately waste food
- Prepare elaborate meals for others
- Skip meals
- Pretend to eat or lie about how much they have eaten
- Exercise compulsively
- Dress in bulky clothing or many layers
- Weigh themselves several times a day
- Base their self-esteem on how thin they are

Prognosis

Without treatment, nearly 10% of people with severe anorexia die. When symptoms are mild and unrecognized, people rarely die. With treatment, about one half of people regain most or all of the weight they lost, and hormonal and other physical problems due to the disorder resolve. About one fourth improve some, gaining some weight back, but they may periodically return to their former eating habits (relapse). The remaining one fourth have frequent relapses and continue to have physical and mental problems due to the disorder.

Treatment

When weight loss has been rapid or severe—for example, to more than 25% below the ideal body weight—restoring body weight quickly is crucial. People with anorexia may need to be hospitalized to ensure that they consume enough calories and nutrients. Although eating food is the best treatment, people rarely need to be fed through a tube inserted through their nose and down their throat into their stomach (nasogastric tube). Doctors also check for problems due to anorexia nervosa, and any problems are treated. For example, if bone density has been lost, people are given calcium and vitamin D supplements and sometimes a bisphosphonate, such as alendronate, ibandronate, or risedronate. During hospitalization, psychiatric and nutritional counseling are provided. Hospitalization also helps by taking people out of their normal circumstances and disrupting their dysfunctional eating habits and behaviors. Thus, it may reverse a downhill course.

However, most people are treated as outpatients. Cognitive-behavioral therapy is usually used. Typically, therapy is needed for 1 year if people have regained the lost weight and up to 2 years if people are still underweight. This therapy is more effective for adolescents who have had the disorder for less than 6 months. Therapy is particularly important because most people with anorexia do not wish to be treated or to regain weight. Family therapy is useful with adolescents. It can improve interactions among family members and teach parents to help the affected adolescent regain the lost weight.

Treatment also involves seeing a doctor regularly for check-ups. It may involve a nutritionist, who may provide specific meal plans or information about the calories needed to restore weight to a normal level.

There are no specific drugs to treat anorexia nervosa. However, newer antipsychotic drugs, such as olanzapine, may help people gain weight and relieve their excessive fear of being fat. Selective serotonin reuptake inhibitors (a type of antidepressant), such as fluoxetine, may help prevent people who have regained weight from losing it again. They are particularly useful for people who also have depression.

Bulimia Nervosa

Bulimia nervosa is characterized by the repeated rapid consumption of large amounts of food (bingeing), followed by attempts to rid the body of the excess food consumed (purging).

- People eat large amounts of food, then induce vomiting, use laxatives, diet, or vigorously exercise to compensate.
- Doctors suspect the diagnosis when people are overly concerned about their weight and their weight fluctuates a lot.
- Cognitive-behavioral therapy, a selective serotonin reuptake inhibitor (a type of antidepressant), or both may be used to treat the disorder.

As in anorexia nervosa, bulimia nervosa is influenced by hereditary and social factors. Also as in anorexia nervosa, most people who have bulimia

nervosa are young women, are deeply concerned about body shape and weight, and belong to the middle or upper socioeconomic classes. Bulimia nervosa affects mainly adolescents and young adults, occurring in 1.6% of females and 0.5% of males.

Symptoms

People repeatedly eat in binges. That is, they eat large amounts of food within a relatively short period of time, often within 2 hours. Emotional stress often triggers the binge-purge cycle, which usually is done in secret. Bingeing, which is accompanied by a feeling of a loss of control, usually includes eating when not hungry and eating to the point of pain. People tend to consume high-calorie foods, such as ice cream and cake. The amount of food consumed varies and sometimes involves thousands of calories. Binges may occur as often as several times a day.

> ### ? Did You Know...
>
> People with bulimia tend to feel very remorseful or guilty about their behavior.
>
> People with bulimia may have scars on their knuckles from using their fingers to induce vomiting.

In an attempt to counteract the effects of the excess food, people use various means to purge:

- Vomiting
- Taking laxatives
- Rigorously dieting or fasting
- Overexercising
- Any combination of the above

Many also take diuretics to treat perceived bloating. However, unlike in anorexia nervosa, the body weight of people with bulimia nervosa tends to fluctuate around normal.

Self-induced vomiting can erode tooth enamel, enlarge the salivary glands in the cheeks (parotid glands), and inflame the esophagus. Vomiting and purging can lower potassium levels in the blood, causing abnormal heart rhythms. Sudden death can result from an abnormal heart rhythm in people who repeatedly take large quantities of ipecac to induce vomiting. Rarely, people who have this disorder eat so much during a binge that their stomach ruptures or their esophagus tears, leading to life-threatening complications.

Compared with people who have anorexia nervosa, those who have bulimia nervosa tend to be more aware of their behavior and to feel remorseful or guilty about it. They are more likely to admit their concerns to a doctor or other confidant. Generally, people with bulimia nervosa are more outgoing. They also are more prone to impulsive behavior, drug or alcohol abuse, and depression.

Diagnosis

Bulimia nervosa is suspected when people, particularly young women, express marked concern about weight gain and have wide fluctuations in weight, especially if there is evidence of excessive laxative use (such as diarrhea and abdominal cramps). Doctors also check for other clues:

- Swollen salivary glands in the cheeks
- Scars on the knuckles from using the fingers to induce vomiting
- Erosion of tooth enamel from stomach acid
- A low level of potassium detected by a blood test

Technically, the diagnosis is confirmed when people describe binge-purge behavior and report having two or more binge-eating episodes a week for at least 3 months. But doctors may diagnose the disorder without this information when symptoms strongly suggest it.

Treatment

The two most effective approaches to treatment are cognitive-behavioral therapy and drug therapy. Treatment may be most effective when both are used.

In cognitive-behavioral therapy, dysfunctional thoughts are identified and examined, and people are helped to give them up. People meet with a therapist once or twice a week over a period of 4 to 5 months, for a total of about 16 to 20 sessions. Cognitive-behavioral therapy reduces the frequency of bingeing in about two thirds of people with bulimia and stops bingeing altogether in about one third. People who have had this therapy continue to reduce or refrain from bingeing for at least 1 year.

Selective serotonin reuptake inhibitors, a type of antidepressant, are somewhat effective and best used with cognitive-behavioral therapy in the treatment of bulimia nervosa. However, when the drugs are stopped, bingeing frequently recurs.

Binge Eating Disorder

Binge eating disorder is characterized by the consumption of large amounts of food with a feeling of loss of control (bingeing). Bingeing is not followed by attempts to rid the body of the excess food consumed (purging).

- Binge eating disorder is more common among people who are obese.
- People eat large amounts rapidly, do not purge, and are very distressed by their behavior.

- Doctors base the diagnosis on people's description of their behavior.
- Weight-loss programs and the weight-loss drug sibutramine may help control weight, cognitive-behavioral therapy may help control the binges, and a selective serotonin reuptake inhibitor (a type of antidepressant) may do both.

Overall, about 3.5% of women and 2% of men have binge eating disorder. But the disorder becomes more common with increasing body weight. In some weight reduction programs, 30% of obese people have the disorder.

Most people with binge eating disorder are obese, and the disorder contributes to their consumption of excessive calories. In contrast, most people with bulimia nervosa have a normal or near-normal weight, and most people with anorexia nervosa are thin. People with binge eating disorder are older than those with anorexia nervosa or bulimia nervosa, and nearly half are men.

> ### ? Did You Know...
> Nearly half of the people with binge eating disorder are men.
>
> About half of obese people with binge eating disorder are depressed.

Symptoms

People eat a much larger amount of food than most people would eat in a similar time under similar circumstances. During and after a binge, people feel as if they lost control. Bingeing occurs in episodes, as opposed to constant overeating. They may also do the following:

- Eat much more rapidly than normal
- Eat until they feel uncomfortably full
- Eat large amounts of food when they do not feel hungry
- Eat alone because they are embarrassed
- Feel disgusted, depressed, or guilty after overeating

People with binge eating disorder are distressed by it, especially if they are trying to lose weight. Among people who are obese, about 50% of those with the disorder are depressed compared with fewer than 5% of those without the disorder.

Diagnosis

Technically, the diagnosis is confirmed when people report binges on 2 days a week for at least 6 months with a feeling of no control over eating. But doctors may diagnose the disorder without this information when people's description of their behavior and symptoms strongly suggest it.

Treatment

Most people are treated in conventional behavioral weight reduction programs. Although these programs pay little attention to binge eating specifically, people tend to accept this because they are usually more concerned about their weight than about their binge eating. Conventional weight reduction programs are effective in not only producing weight loss but also in helping control binge eating. Binge eating apparently does not limit weight loss in these programs.

The following treatments may help:

- **Cognitive-behavioral therapy** can help control binge eating but has little effect on body weight.

- **Sibutramine**, a weight-loss drug, helps people lose weight and slightly reduces the number of binges.

- **Selective serotonin reuptake inhibitors** (a type of antidepressant), such as fluoxetine, can control binge eating and weight, but stopping the drug is frequently followed by a return to binge eating.

- **Self-help groups** that follow the principles of Alcoholics Anonymous (such as Overeaters Anonymous and Food Addicts Anonymous) are widespread, but their effectiveness is uncertain.

- **Surgery** may be done to treat obesity, but its effects on binge eating are unclear.

CHAPTER 132   Personality Disorders

Personality disorders are patterns of perceiving, reacting, and relating to other people and events that are relatively inflexible and that impair a person's ability to function socially.

- Behavior may be odd or eccentric, dramatic or erratic, or anxious or inhibited.
- Doctors consider the diagnosis when inappropriate thinking or behavior is repeated despite negative consequences.
- Drugs do not change people's personality traits, but psychotherapy may help people recognize their problem and change their socially undesirable behaviors.

Everyone has characteristic patterns of perceiving and relating to other people and events (personality traits). That is, people tend to cope with stresses in an individual but consistent way. For example, some people respond to a troubling situation by seeking someone else's help; others prefer to deal with problems on their own. Some people minimize problems; others exaggerate them. Regardless of their usual style, however, mentally healthy people are likely to try an alternative approach if their first response is ineffective.

In contrast, people with a personality disorder are rigid and tend to respond inappropriately to problems, to the point that relationships with family members, friends, and coworkers are affected. These maladaptive responses usually begin in adolescence or early adulthood and do not change over time. Personality disorders vary in severity. They are usually mild and rarely severe.

Most people with a personality disorder are distressed about their life and have problems with relationships at work or in social situations. Many people also have mood, anxiety, substance abuse, or eating disorders.

People with a personality disorder are unaware that their thought or behavior patterns are inappropriate; thus, they tend not to seek help on their own. Instead, they may be referred by their friends, family members, or a social agency because their behavior is causing difficulty for others. When they seek help on their own, usually because of the life stresses created by their personality disorder or because of troubling symptoms (for example, anxiety, depression, or substance abuse), they tend to believe their problems are caused by other people or by circumstances beyond their control.

Until fairly recently, many psychiatrists and psychologists felt that treatment did not help people with a personality disorder. However, specific types of psychotherapy (talk therapy), sometimes with drugs, have now been shown to help many people. Choosing an experienced, understanding therapist is essential.

Personality disorders are grouped into three clusters. Cluster A personality disorders involve odd or eccentric behavior; cluster B, dramatic or erratic behavior; and cluster C, anxious or inhibited behavior.

Cluster A: Odd or Eccentric Behavior

Paranoid Personality: People with a paranoid personality are distrustful and suspicious of others. Based on little or no evidence, they suspect that others are out to harm them and usually find hostile or malicious motives behind other people's actions. Thus, people with a paranoid personality may take actions that they feel are justifiable retaliation but that others find baffling. This behavior often leads to rejection by others, which seems to justify their original feelings. They are generally cold and distant in their relationships.

People with a paranoid personality often take legal action against others, especially if they feel righteously indignant. They are unable to see their own role in a conflict. They usually work in relative isolation and may be highly efficient and conscientious.

Sometimes people who already feel alienated because of a defect or handicap (such as deafness) are more likely to suspect that other people have negative ideas or attitudes toward them. Such heightened suspicion, however, is not evidence of a paranoid personality unless it involves wrongly attributing malice to others.

Schizoid Personality: People with a schizoid personality are introverted, withdrawn, and solitary. They are emotionally cold and socially distant. They are most often absorbed with their own thoughts and feelings and are fearful of closeness and intimacy with others. They talk little, are given to daydreaming, and prefer theoretical speculation to practical action. Fantasizing is a common coping (defense) mechanism.

Schizotypal Personality: People with a schizotypal personality, like those with a schizoid personality, are socially and emotionally detached. In addition, they display oddities of thinking, perceiving, and communicating similar to those of people with schizophrenia (see page 889). Although schizotypal personality is sometimes present in people with schizophrenia before they become ill, most adults with a schizotypal personality do not develop schizophrenia.

Some people with a schizotypal personality show signs of magical thinking—that is, they believe that their thoughts or actions can control something or someone. For example, people may believe that they can harm others by thinking angry thoughts. People with a schizotypal personality may also have paranoid ideas.

Cluster B: Dramatic or Erratic Behavior

Histrionic (Hysterical) Personality: People with a histrionic personality conspicuously seek attention, are dramatic and excessively emotional, and are overly concerned with appearance. Their lively, expressive manner results in easily established but often superficial and transient relationships. Their expression of emotions often seems exaggerated, childish, and contrived to evoke sympathy or attention (often erotic or sexual) from others.

People with a histrionic personality are prone to sexually provocative behavior or to sexualizing nonsexual relationships. However, they may not really want a sexual relationship; rather, their seductive

Consequences of Personality Disorders
■ People with a personality disorder are at high risk of behaviors that can lead to physical illness (such as alcohol or drug addiction), self-destructive behavior, reckless sexual behavior, hypochondriasis, and clashes with society's values.
■ They may have inconsistent, detached, overemotional, abusive, or irresponsible styles of parenting, leading to medical and psychiatric problems in their children.
■ They are vulnerable to mental breakdowns (a period of crisis when a person has difficulty performing even routine mental tasks) as a result of stress.
■ They may develop a mental health disorder. The type (for example, anxiety, depression, or psychosis) depends in part on the type of personality disorder.
■ They are less likely to follow a prescribed treatment regimen. Even when they follow the regimen, they are usually less responsive to drugs than most people are.
■ They often have a poor relationship with their doctor because they refuse to take responsibility for their behavior or they feel overly distrustful, deserving, or needy. The doctor may then start to blame, distrust, and ultimately reject the person.

behavior often masks their wish to be dependent and protected. Some people with a histrionic personality also are hypochondriacal and exaggerate their physical problems to get the attention they need.

Narcissistic Personality: People with a narcissistic personality have a sense of superiority, a need for admiration, and a lack of empathy. They have an exaggerated belief in their own value or importance, which is what therapists call grandiosity. They may be extremely sensitive to failure, defeat, or criticism. When confronted by a failure to fulfill their high opinion of themselves, they can easily become enraged or severely depressed. Because they believe themselves to be superior in their relationships with other people, they expect to be admired and often suspect that others envy them. They believe they are entitled to having their needs met without waiting, so they exploit others, whose needs or beliefs they deem to be less important. Their behavior is usually offensive to others, who view them as being self-centered, arrogant, or selfish. This personality disorder typically occurs in high achievers, although it may also occur in people with few achievements.

Antisocial Personality: People with an antisocial personality (previously called psychopathic or sociopathic personality), most of whom are male, show callous disregard for the rights and feelings of others. Dishonesty and deceit permeate their relationships. They exploit others for material gain or personal gratification (unlike narcissistic people, who exploit others because they think their superiority justifies it).

Characteristically, people with an antisocial personality act out their conflicts impulsively and irresponsibly. They tolerate frustration poorly, and sometimes they are hostile or violent. Often they do not anticipate the negative consequences of their antisocial behaviors and, despite the problems or harm they cause others, do not feel remorse or guilt. Rather, they glibly rationalize their behavior or blame it on others. Frustration and punishment do not motivate them to modify their behaviors or improve their judgment and foresight but, rather, usually confirm their harshly unsentimental view of the world.

People with an antisocial personality are prone to alcoholism, drug addiction, sexual deviation, promiscuity, and imprisonment. They are likely to fail at their jobs and move from one area to another. They often have a family history of antisocial behavior, substance abuse, divorce, and physical abuse. As children, many were emotionally neglected and physically abused. People with an antisocial personality have a shorter life expectancy than the general population. The disorder tends to diminish or stabilize with age.

Borderline Personality: People with a borderline personality, most of whom are women, are unstable in their self-image, moods, behavior, and interpersonal relationships. Their thought processes are more disturbed than those of people with an antisocial personality, and their aggression is more often turned against the self. They are angrier, more impulsive, and more confused about their identity than are people with a histrionic personality. Borderline personality becomes evident in early adulthood but becomes less common in older age groups.

People with a borderline personality often report being neglected or abused as children. Consequently, they feel empty, angry, and deserving of nurturing. They have far more dramatic and intense interpersonal relationships than people with cluster A personality disorders. When they fear being abandoned by a caring person, they tend to express inappropriate and intense anger. People with a borderline personality tend to see events and relationships as black or white, good or evil, but never neutral.

When people with a borderline personality feel abandoned and alone, they may wonder whether they actually exist (that is, they do not feel real). They can become desperately impulsive, engaging in reckless promiscuity, substance abuse, or self-mutilation. At times they are so out of touch with reality that they have brief episodes of psychotic thinking, paranoia, and hallucinations.

People with a borderline personality commonly visit primary care doctors. Borderline personality is also the most common personality disorder treated by therapists, because people with the disorder relentlessly seek someone to care for them. However, after repeated crises, vague unfounded complaints, and failures to comply with therapeutic recommendations, caretakers—including doctors—often become very frustrated with them and view them erroneously as people who prefer complaining to helping themselves.

Cluster C: Anxious or Inhibited Behavior

Avoidant Personality: People with an avoidant personality are overly sensitive to rejection, and they fear starting relationships or anything new. They have a strong desire for affection and acceptance but avoid intimate relationships and social situations for fear of disappointment and criticism. Unlike those with a schizoid personality, they are openly distressed by their isolation and inability to relate comfortably to others. Unlike those with a borderline personality, they do not respond to rejection with anger; instead, they withdraw and appear shy and timid. Avoidant personality is similar to generalized social phobia (see page 859).

 Did You Know...

People with a personality disorder do not know that there is anything wrong with their thinking or behavior.

Dependent Personality: People with a dependent personality routinely surrender major decisions and responsibilities to others and permit the needs of those they depend on to supersede their own. They lack self-confidence and feel intensely insecure about their ability to take care of themselves. They often protest that they cannot make decisions and do not know what to do or how to do it. This behavior is due partly to a reluctance to express their views for fear of offending the people they need and partly to a belief that others are more capable. People with other personality disorders often have traits of a dependent personality, but the dependent traits are usually hidden by the more dominant traits of the other disorder. Sometimes adults with a prolonged illness or physical handicap develop a dependent personality.

Obsessive-Compulsive Personality: People with an obsessive-compulsive personality are preoccupied with orderliness, perfectionism, and control. They are reliable, dependable, orderly, and methodical, but their inflexibility makes them unable to adapt to change.

Because they are cautious and weigh all aspects of a problem, they have difficulty making decisions. They take their responsibilities seriously, but because they cannot tolerate mistakes or imperfection, they often have trouble completing tasks. Unlike the mental health disorder called obsessive-compulsive disorder (see page 860), obsessive-compulsive personality does not involve repeated, unwanted obsessions and ritualistic behavior.

People with an obsessive-compulsive personality are often high achievers, especially in the sciences and other intellectually demanding fields that require order and attention to detail. However, their responsibilities make them so anxious that they can rarely enjoy their successes. They are uncomfortable with their feelings, with relationships, and with situations in which they lack control or must rely on others or in which events are unpredictable.

Other Personality Types

Some personality types are not classified as disorders.

Passive-Aggressive (Negativistic) Personality: People with a passive-aggressive personality behave in ways that appear inept or passive. However, these behaviors are actually ways to avoid responsibility or to control or punish others. People with a passive-aggressive personality often procrastinate, perform tasks inefficiently, or claim an implausible disability. Frequently, they agree to perform tasks they do not want to perform and then subtly undermine completion of the tasks. Such behavior usually enables them to deny or conceal hostility or disagreements.

Cyclothymic Personality: People with cyclothymic personality alternate between high-spirited buoyancy and gloomy pessimism. Each mood lasts weeks or longer. Mood changes occur regularly and without any identifiable external cause. Many gifted and creative people have this personality type (see also page 873).

Depressive Personality: This personality type is characterized by chronic moroseness, worry, and self-consciousness. People have a pessimistic outlook, which impairs their initiative and disheartens others. To them, satisfaction seems undeserved and sinful. They may unconsciously believe their suffering is a badge of merit needed to earn the love or admiration of others.

Diagnosis

A doctor bases the diagnosis of a personality disorder on a person's history, specifically, on repetition of maladaptive thought or behavior patterns. These patterns tend to become apparent because the person tenaciously resists changing them despite their negative consequences. In addition, a doctor is likely to notice the person's immature and maladaptive use of mental coping mechanisms, which interferes with their daily functioning. A doctor may also talk with people who interact with the person.

Treatment

Relief of anxiety, depression, and other distressing symptoms (if present) is the first goal. Drug therapy can help. Drugs such as selective serotonin reuptake inhibitors (SSRIs) can help both depression and impulsivity. Anticonvulsant drugs can help reduce impulsive, angry outbursts. Other drugs such as risperidone have been helpful with both depression and feelings of depersonalization in people with borderline personality. Reducing environmental stress can also quickly relieve symptoms.

However, drug therapy does not generally affect the personality traits themselves. Because these traits take many years to develop, treatment of the maladaptive traits may take many years as well. No short-term treatment can cure a personality disorder, although some changes may be accomplished faster than others. Behavioral changes can occur within a year; interpersonal changes take longer. For example, for people with a dependent personality, a behavioral change might be to stop stating that they cannot make decisions; the interpersonal change might be to interact with coworkers or family members in such a way that they actually seek out or at least accept some decision-making responsibilities.

Although treatments differ according to the type of personality disorder, some general principles apply to all treatments. Because people with a personality disorder usually do not see a problem with their own behavior, they must be confronted with the harmful consequences of their maladaptive thoughts and behaviors. Thus, a therapist needs to repeatedly point out the undesirable consequences of their thought and behavior patterns. Sometimes the therapist finds it necessary to set limits on behavior (for example, people might be told that they cannot raise their voice in anger). The involvement of family members is helpful and often essential because they can act in ways that either reinforce or diminish the problematic behavior or thoughts. Group and family therapy, group living in designated residential settings, and participation in therapeutic social clubs or self-help groups can all be valuable in helping to change socially undesirable behaviors.

Because personality disorders are particularly difficult to treat, choosing a therapist with experience, enthusiasm, and an understanding of the person's areas of emotional sensitivity and usual ways of coping is important. Kindness and direction alone do not change personality disorders. Psychotherapy is the cornerstone of most treatments and usually must continue for more than a year to change a person's maladaptive behavior or interpersonal patterns.

COMMON COPING MECHANISMS

MECHANISM	DEFINITION	RESULT	PERSONALITY DISORDERS INVOLVED
Projection	Attributing one's own feelings or thoughts to others	Leads to prejudice, suspiciousness, and excessive worrying about external dangers	Typical of paranoid and schizotypal personalities Used by people with borderline, antisocial, or narcissistic personality when under acute stress
Splitting	Use of black-or-white, all-or-nothing thinking to divide people into groups of idealized all-good saviors and vilified all-bad evildoers	Allows a person to avoid the discomfort of having both loving and hateful feelings for the same person as well as feelings of uncertainty and helplessness	Typical of borderline personality
Acting out	A direct behavioral expression of an unconscious wish or impulse that enables a person to avoid thinking about a painful situation or experiencing a painful emotion	Leads to acts that are often irresponsible, reckless, and foolish Includes many delinquent, promiscuous, and substance-abusing acts, which can become so habitual that the person remains unaware and dismissive of the feelings that initiated the acts	Very common in people with antisocial or borderline personality
Turning aggression against self	Expressing the angry feelings one has toward others by hurting one's self directly (for example, through self-mutilation) or indirectly (for example, in body dysmorphic disorder) When indirect, it is called passive aggression	Includes failures and illnesses that affect others more than oneself and silly, provocative clowning	Dramatic in people with borderline personality
Fantasizing	Use of imaginary relationships and private belief systems to resolve conflict and to escape from painful realities, such as loneliness	Is associated with eccentricity, avoidance of interpersonal intimacy, and avoidance of involvement with the outside world	Used by people with an avoidant or schizoid personality, who, in contrast to people with psychoses, do not believe and thus do not act on their fantasies
Hypochondriasis	Use of health complaints to gain attention	Provides a person with nurturing attention from others May be a passive expression of anger toward others	Used by people with dependent, histrionic, or borderline personality

In the context of an intimate, cooperative doctor-patient relationship, people can begin to understand the sources of their distress and recognize their maladaptive behavior. Psychotherapy can help them more clearly recognize the attitudes and behaviors that lead to interpersonal problems, such as dependency, distrust, arrogance, and manipulativeness.

For maladaptive behaviors, such as recklessness, social isolation, lack of assertiveness, or temper outbursts, group therapy and behavior modification, sometimes within a day hospital or residential setting, are effective. These behaviors can be changed in months. Participation in self-help groups or family therapy can also help change maladaptive behaviors.

Dialectical behavioral therapy is effective for borderline personality disorder. This therapy involves weekly individual psychotherapy and group therapy as well as telephone contact with therapists between scheduled sessions. It aims to help people understand their behaviors and teach them problem solving and adaptive behaviors. Psychodynamic therapy is also effective for people with borderline or avoidant personality disorder. These therapies help people with a personality disorder think about the effects their behaviors have on others. For some people with personality disorders, primarily those that involve maladaptive attitudes, expectations, and beliefs (such as narcissistic or obsessive-compulsive personality), psychoanalysis (see page 849) is recommended and is usually continued for at least 3 years.

CHAPTER 133 Dissociative Disorders

Occasionally everyone has minor problems integrating their memories, perceptions, identity, and consciousness. For example, people may drive somewhere and then realize that they do not remember the drive. They may not remember it because they are absorbed—with personal concerns, a program on the radio, or a conversation with a passenger—or are just daydreaming. Such problems, referred to as normal dissociation, typically do not disrupt everyday activities.

In contrast, people with a dissociative disorder may totally forget a series of their activities that occurred over minutes, hours, or sometimes much longer. They may sense they are missing a period of time. Dissociation thus disrupts the continuity of self and the recollection of life events. Dissociative disorders involve the following:

- Poorly integrated memory (dissociative amnesia)
- Fragmentation of identity and memory (dissociative fugue or dissociative identity disorder)
- Disruption of the experience and perception of self (depersonalization disorder)

> **? Did You Know...**
> A minor blow to the head cannot cause people to suddenly forget who they are and everything they know.

Dissociative disorders are usually triggered by overwhelming stress or trauma. For example, people may have been abused or mistreated during childhood. They may have experienced or witnessed traumatic events, such as accidents or disasters. Or they may experience inner conflict so intolerable that their mind is forced to separate incompatible or unacceptable information and feelings from conscious thought.

Depersonalization Disorder

Depersonalization disorder involves a persistent or recurring feeling of being detached from one's body or mental processes (depersonalization) and a feeling of being an outside observer of one's life.

- The disorder is usually triggered by life-threatening danger or other severe stress.
- Feelings of detachment from self may occur periodically or continuously.
- After tests are done to rule out other possible causes, psychologic testing helps to diagnose the disorder.
- Psychotherapy and cognitive-behavioral therapy help some people.

Feeling temporarily detached (depersonalized) is the third most common psychologic symptom (after anxiety and depression). This feeling often occurs after people experience life-threatening danger, take certain drugs (for example, marijuana, hallucinogens, ketamine, Ecstasy), become very tired, or are deprived of sleep or sensory stimulation (as may occur when they are in an intensive care unit). Depersonalization disorder occurs in about 2% of the population.

Symptoms

People feel detached from their body, mind, feelings, or sensations. People may say they feel unreal, like an automaton, or as if they were in a dream or in some other way detached from the world. People may describe themselves as the "walking dead." The symptoms almost always cause great discomfort. Some people find them intolerable.

Symptoms are often persistent. Symptoms recur in episodes in about one third of people and occur continuously in about two thirds. Episodic symptoms sometimes become continuous.

People often have great difficulty describing their symptoms and may fear or believe that they are going crazy. However, people always remain aware that their unreal experiences are not real but rather are just the way that they feel. This awareness is what separates depersonalization disorder from a psychotic disorder. People with a psychotic disorder always lack such insight.

Diagnosis

Doctors suspect the disorder based on symptoms. A physical examination and sometimes other tests are done to rule out other disorders that could cause the symptoms, including other mental health disorders and substance abuse. Tests may include magnetic resonance imaging (MRI), electroencephalography (EEG), and urine tests to check for drugs. Psychologic tests and special structured interviews and questionnaires can also help doctors with the diagnosis.

Treatment and Prognosis

Depersonalization disorder often disappears without treatment. People are treated only if the disorder persists, recurs, or causes distress. Psychodynamic psychotherapy and cognitive-behavioral therapy have been effective for some people. Depersonalization disorder is often associated with or triggered by other mental health disorders, which require treatment. Any stresses associated with the beginning of the depersonalization disorder must also be addressed.

Techniques that can help include the following:

- Cognitive techniques can help block obsessive thinking about the unreal state of being.
- Behavioral techniques can help people become absorbed in tasks that distract them from the depersonalization.
- Grounding techniques use the five senses (hearing, touch, smell, taste, and sight) to help people feel more connected to themselves and the world. For example, loud music is played or a piece of ice is put in the hand. These sensations are difficult to ignore, making people aware of themselves in the present moment.
- Psychodynamic techniques focus on helping people to work through intolerable conflicts and their associated feelings, which are dissociated from consciousness.

Some degree of relief is usually achieved with treatment. Complete recovery is possible for many people, especially those whose symptoms occur in connection with stresses that can be dealt with during treatment. Other people do not respond well to treatment, although they may gradually improve on their own. A few remain unresponsive to all treatments. Antianxiety drugs and antidepressants sometimes help, particularly if people also have anxiety or depression.

Dissociative Amnesia

Dissociative amnesia is amnesia caused by trauma or stress, resulting in an inability to recall important personal information.

- People have gaps in their memory, which may span a few minutes to years.
- After tests are done to rule out other possible causes, psychologic testing helps identify the disorder.
- Memory retrieval techniques, including hypnosis and drug-facilitated interviews, are used to fill in the memory gaps.
- Psychotherapy is needed to help people deal with the experiences that triggered the disorder.

Amnesia is the total or partial inability to recall recent experiences or ones from the distant past. When amnesia is caused by a psychologic rather than a physical disturbance, it is called dissociative amnesia.

In dissociative amnesia, the lost memory usually involves information that is normally part of routine conscious awareness or autobiographic memory— who one is, where one went, to whom one spoke, and what one did, said, thought, and felt. Often, it is information about traumatic or stressful events. Sometimes the information, though forgotten, continues to influence behavior.

The disorder is most common among young adults, usually people who have been involved in wars, accidents, or natural disasters. It may also block memories of sexual abuse during childhood. Dissociative amnesia can persist for some time after a traumatic event. Sometimes, people appear to spontaneously recover memories. Unless confirmed by another person, it is often unclear whether such recovered memories reflect real events from the past.

Symptoms

The most common symptom is memory loss. Shortly after loss of memory, some people seem confused. Many people are somewhat depressed or very distressed by their amnesia. Most people have one or more gaps in their memory. Gaps usually span a few minutes to a few hours or days but may span years or even an entire life. Most people are aware that they have lost some time. However, some become aware of lost time only later, when memories reappear or they are confronted with evidence of things that they have done but do not recall. Some people forget some but not all events over a period of time. Others cannot recall their entire previous life or forget things as they occur.

Diagnosis

Doctors carefully review the person's symptoms and do a physical examination to exclude physical causes of amnesia. Tests, including magnetic resonance imaging

(MRI), electroencephalography (EEG), and blood tests for toxins and drugs, are sometimes needed to exclude physical causes. A psychologic examination is also done. Special psychologic tests often help doctors better characterize and understand the person's dissociative experiences and thus develop a treatment plan.

> **Did You Know...**
> When doctors use techniques to help people remember, they must be very careful not to do or say anything that could create a false memory.

Treatment and Prognosis

Doctors begin treatment by helping people feel safe and secure. If the missing memories are not spontaneously recalled or if the need to recall the memories is urgent, memory retrieval techniques are often successful. Using hypnosis or drug-facilitated interviews (interviews conducted after a sedative such as a barbiturate or benzodiazepine is given intravenously), doctors question people about the past. Doctors use hypnosis and drug-facilitated interviews to reduce the anxiety associated with the period for which there are gaps in memory and to penetrate or bypass the defenses people have created to protect themselves from recalling painful experiences or conflicts. However, doctors must be careful not to suggest what should be recalled or to cause extreme anxiety. Furthermore, memories recalled through such techniques may not be accurate and may require confirmation from another person or source. Therefore, before hypnosis or a drug-facilitated interview, doctors inform people that memories retrieved with these techniques may or may not be accurate and ask for consent to proceed.

Filling in the memory gap to the greatest extent possible helps restore continuity to personal identity and sense of self. Once amnesia has resolved, continued psychotherapy helps people understand the trauma or conflicts that caused the disorder, find ways to resolve them, and move on with their life.

Most people recover what appears to be their missing memories and resolve the conflicts that caused the amnesia. However, some people never break through the barriers that prevent them from reconstructing their missing past.

Dissociative Fugue

Dissociative fugue involves one or more episodes of sudden, unexpected, but purposeful travel from home during which people cannot remember some or all of their past life, including who they are (their identity). These episodes are called fugues.

■ Unbearable stress or a traumatic event may trigger dissociative fugue.

■ When in a fugue, people disappear from their usual routine and may assume a new identity, forgetting all or some of their usual life.

■ Usually, doctors make the diagnosis by reviewing the history and collecting information about the circumstances before travel, the travel itself, and the establishment of an alternate life.

■ Usually, fugues last only hours or days, then resolve on their own.

■ Memory retrieval techniques, including hypnosis and drug-facilitated interviews, may be tried but may be unsuccessful.

Dissociative fugue affects about 2 of 1,000 people in the United States. It is much more common among people who have been in wars, accidents, or natural disasters.

Causes

Dissociative fugue is usually triggered by severe trauma, such as wars, accidents, natural disasters, or sexual abuse during childhood.

Dissociative fugue is often mistaken for malingering because both conditions may give people an excuse to avoid their responsibilities (as in an intolerable marriage), to avoid accountability for their actions, or to reduce their exposure to a known hazard, such as a battle. However, dissociative fugue, unlike malingering, occurs spontaneously and is not faked.

Many fugues seem to represent disguised wish fulfillment (for example, an escape from overwhelming stresses, such as divorce or financial ruin). Other fugues are related to feelings of rejection or separation, or they may develop as an alternative to suicidal or homicidal impulses.

Symptoms

A fugue may last from hours to weeks, months, or occasionally even longer. People in a fugue state, having lost their customary identity, usually disappear from their usual haunts, leaving their family and job. If the fugue is brief, they may appear simply to have missed some work or come home late. If the fugue lasts several days or longer, people may travel far from home and begin a new job with a new identity, unaware of any change in their life.

During the fugue, they may appear normal and attract no attention. However, at some point, they may become aware of the memory loss or confused about their identity. If they are confused, they may come to the attention of medical or legal authorities. During the fugue, people often have no symptoms or are only mildly confused. However, when the fugue ends, they may experience depression, discomfort, grief, shame, intense conflict, and suicidal or aggressive impulses.

Diagnosis

A doctor may suspect dissociative fugue when people seem confused about their identity or are puzzled about their past or when confrontations challenge their new identity or absence of one. The doctor carefully reviews symptoms and does a physical examination to exclude physical disorders that may contribute to or cause memory loss. A psychologic examination is also done.

Sometimes dissociative fugue cannot be diagnosed until people abruptly return to their pre-fugue identity and are distressed to find themselves in unfamiliar circumstances. The diagnosis is usually made retroactively when a doctor reviews the history and collects information that documents the circumstances before people left home, the travel itself, and the establishment of an alternate life.

> **? Did You Know...**
> Dissociative fugue is often mistaken for malingering because it enables people to escape their responsibilities or undesirable or dangerous situations, such as a bad marriage or a battle.

Treatment

Most fugues last for hours or days, then disappear on their own.

Treatment, when needed, may include hypnosis or drug-facilitated interviews (interviews conducted after a sedative is given intravenously to relax people). However, efforts to restore memories of what happened during the fugue itself are usually unsuccessful.

A therapist may help people explore their patterns of handling the types of situations, conflicts, and moods that triggered the fugue to prevent subsequent fugues.

Dissociative Identity Disorder

In dissociative identity disorder, formerly called multiple personality disorder, two or more identities alternate within the same person.

- Extreme stress during childhood may prevent some children from integrating their experiences into one cohesive identify.
- People have several personalities that may or may not know about and interact with each other, as well as many other symptoms, including severe headaches, memory gaps, and a tendency toward self-harm.
- A thorough psychologic interview and special questionnaires, sometimes facilitated by hypnosis or sedatives, help doctors diagnose the disorder.
- Extensive psychotherapy may help people integrate their personalties or at least help the personalities cooperate.

About 1% of people may have dissociative identity disorder.

Causes

Dissociative identity disorder appears to be caused by the interaction of several factors. They include the following:

- Overwhelming stress
- An ability to separate memories, perceptions, or identity from conscious awareness
- Abnormal psychologic development
- Insufficient protection and nurturing during childhood

As children develop, they must learn to integrate complicated and different types of information and experiences into a cohesive, complex identity. Children who are abused or experience a major loss or trauma may go through phases when they keep different emotions and perceptions of themselves and others separate. This separation may lead to the development of multiple personalities. However, most of these vulnerable children are sufficiently protected and soothed by adults, so dissociative identity disorder does not develop.

Symptoms

People with dissociative identity disorder often describe an array of symptoms that can resemble those of other mental health disorders as well as those of many physical disorders. For example, they often develop severe headaches or other aches and pains and may experience sexual dysfunction. Different groups of symptoms occur at different times. Some of these symptoms may indicate that another disorder is present, but some may reflect the intrusion of past experiences into the present. For example, sadness may indicate coexisting depression, but it also may indicate that one of the personalities is reliving emotions associated with past misfortunes.

People are prone to injuring themselves. Substance abuse, episodes of self-mutilation, and suicide attempts are common. Some people remain deeply attached to the people who have abused them.

Some of a person's personalities are aware of important personal information of which other personalities are unaware. Some personalities appear to know and interact with one another in an elaborate inner world. For example, personality A may be aware of personality B and know what B does, as if observing B's behavior. Personality B may or may not be aware of personality A, and so on with other personalities present.

The switching of personalities and the lack of awareness of the behavior of the other personalities often make life chaotic. Because the personalities often interact with each other, affected people may report hearing internal conversations among the personalities or hearing the voices of other personalities commenting on their behavior or addressing them.

Affected people experience distortion of time, with time lapses and amnesia. After an episode of amnesia, they may discover objects or samples of handwriting that they cannot account for or recognize. They may also find themselves in different places from where they last remember being and have no idea why or how they got there. They may not be able to recall things they have done or account for changes in their behavior. Often, they refer to themselves as "we," "he," or "she" and may not know why. Most people cannot recall much about the first 3 to 5 years of life, but people with dissociative identity disorder may not recall much about the period between the ages of 6 and 11 as well.

People with the disorder may feel detached from themselves (depersonalization) and experience familiar people and surroundings as if they were unfamiliar, strange, or unreal (derealization). They are often concerned about issues of control, both self-control and the perceived control over others.

Dissociative identity disorder is chronic and potentially disabling or fatal, although many people function very well and lead creative and productive lives.

Diagnosis

Doctors conduct a thorough psychologic interview and use special questionnaires developed to help identify dissociative identity disorder. A medical examination may be needed to determine whether people have a physical disorder that would explain certain symptoms.

Interviews may need to be long and involve careful use of hypnosis or a sedative given intravenously to relax the person (a drug-facilitated interview).

The sedative may allow doctors to encounter other personalities or make the person more likely to reveal information about a forgotten period of time. However, some doctors feel that hypnosis and drug-facilitated interviews should not be used because the techniques themselves may cause symptoms of dissociative identity disorder.

Prognosis

Some symptoms may come and go spontaneously, but dissociative identity disorder does not clear up on its own. How well people recover depends on the symptoms and features they have. For example, people who have other serious mental health disorders, who do not function well in life, or who remain deeply attached to their abusers do less well. They may require treatment longer, and treatment is less successful.

Treatment

The goal of treatment is usually to integrate the personalities into a single personality. However, integration is not always possible. In these situations, the goal is to achieve a harmonious interaction among the personalities that allows more normal functioning.

Drug therapy can relieve some specific coexisting symptoms, such as anxiety or depression, but does not affect the disorder itself.

Psychotherapy is often long, arduous, and emotionally painful. People may experience many emotional crises from the actions of the personalities and from the despair that may occur when traumatic memories are recalled during therapy. Several periods of psychiatric hospitalization may be necessary to help people through difficult times and to come to grips with particularly painful memories. Generally, two or more psychotherapy sessions a week for at least 3 to 6 years are necessary.

CHAPTER

134 Schizophrenia and Delusional Disorder

Schizophrenia and delusional disorder are distinct disorders that may share certain features, such as paranoia, suspiciousness, and unrealistic thinking. However, schizophrenia is associated with psychosis—a loss of contact with reality—and with a decline in general functioning. In contrast, in delusional disorder, contact with reality is preserved except for the very specific and focused unrealistic thinking in the delusions, and functioning is much less impaired. In addition, schizophrenia is relatively common, whereas delusional disorder is rare.

Schizophrenia

Schizophrenia is a mental disorder characterized by loss of contact with reality (psychosis), hallucinations (usually, hearing voices), firmly held false beliefs (delusions), abnormal thinking, a restricted range of emotions (flattened affect), diminished motivation, and disturbed work and social functioning.

- Schizophrenia is probably caused by hereditary and environmental factors.
- People may have a variety of symptoms, ranging from bizarre behavior and rambling, disorganized speech to loss of emotions and little or no speech to inability to concentrate and remember.
- Doctors diagnose schizophrenia based on symptoms after they do tests to rule out other possible causes.
- How well people do depends largely on whether they take the prescribed drugs as directed.
- Treatment involves antipsychotic drugs, rehabilitation and community support activities, and psychotherapy.

Schizophrenia is a major health problem throughout the world. The disorder typically strikes young people at the very time they are establishing their independence and can result in lifelong disability and stigma. In terms of personal and economic costs, schizophrenia has been described as among the worst disorders afflicting humankind.

Schizophrenia is the 9th leading cause of disability worldwide. It affects about 1% of the population. Schizophrenia affects men and women equally. In the United States, schizophrenia accounts for about 1 of every 5 Social Security disability days and 2.5% of all health care expenditures. Schizophrenia is more common than Alzheimer's disease and multiple sclerosis.

Determining when schizophrenia begins (onset) is often difficult because unfamiliarity with symptoms may delay medical care for several years. The average age at onset is 18 for men and 25 for women. Onset during childhood or early adolescence is uncommon (see page 1862). Onset is also uncommon late in life.

> **❓ Did You Know...**
>
> Schizophrenia is more common than Alzheimer's disease and multiple sclerosis.
>
> Various disorders, including thyroid disorders, brain tumors, seizure disorders, and other mental health disorders, can cause symptoms similar to those of schizophrenia.

Deterioration in social functioning can lead to substance abuse, poverty, and homelessness. People with untreated schizophrenia may lose contact with their families and friends and often find themselves living on the streets of large cities.

Causes

What precisely causes schizophrenia is not known, but current research suggests a combination of hereditary and environmental factors. Fundamentally, however, it is a biologic problem (involving changes in the brain), not one caused by poor parenting or a mentally unhealthy environment. People who have a parent or sibling with schizophrenia have about a 10% risk of developing the disorder, compared with a 1% risk among the general population. An identical twin whose co-twin has schizophrenia has about a 50% risk of developing schizophrenia. These statistics suggest that heredity is involved.

Other causes may include problems that occurred before, during, or after birth, such as influenza in the mother during the 2nd trimester of pregnancy, oxygen deprivation at birth, a low birth weight, and incompatibility of the mother's and infant's blood type.

Symptoms

The onset of schizophrenia may be sudden, over a period of days or weeks, or slow and insidious, over a period of years. Although the severity and types of symptoms vary among different people with schizophrenia, the symptoms are usually sufficiently severe as to interfere with the ability to work, interact with people, and care for oneself. In some people with schizophrenia, mental function declines, leading to an impaired ability to pay attention, think in the abstract, and solve problems. The severity of mental impairment largely determines overall disability in people with schizophrenia.

Symptoms may be triggered or worsened by environmental stresses, such as stressful life events. Drug use, including use of marijuana, may trigger or worsen symptoms as well.

Categories: Overall, the symptoms of schizophrenia fall into four major categories:

- Positive symptoms
- Negative symptoms
- Disorganization
- Cognitive impairment

People may have symptoms from one, two, or all categories.

Positive symptoms involve an excess or a distortion of normal functions. They include the following:

- **Delusions** are false beliefs that usually involve a misinterpretation of perceptions or experiences. For example, people with schizophrenia may have persecutory delusions, believing that they are being tormented, followed, tricked, or spied on. They may have delusions of reference, believing that passages from books, newspapers, or song lyrics are directed specifically at them. They may have delusions of thought withdrawal or thought insertion, believing that others can read their mind, that their thoughts are being transmitted to others, or that thoughts and impulses are being imposed on them by outside forces.

- **Hallucinations** of sound, sight, smell, taste, or touch may occur, although hallucinations of sound (auditory hallucinations) are by far the most common. People may hear voices in their head commenting on their behavior, conversing with one another, or making critical and abusive comments.

Negative symptoms involve a decrease in or loss of normal functions. They include the following:

- **Blunted affect** refers to a flattening of emotions. The face may appear immobile. People make little or no eye contact and lack emotional expressiveness. Events that would normally make them laugh or cry produce no response.
- **Poverty of speech** refers to a decreased amount of speech. Answers to questions may be terse, perhaps one or two words, creating the impression of an inner emptiness.
- **Anhedonia** refers to a diminished capacity to experience pleasure. People may take little interest in previous activities and spend more time in purposeless ones.
- **Asociality** refers to a lack of interest in relationships with other people. These negative symptoms are often associated with a general loss of motivation, sense of purpose, and goals.

Disorganization involves thought disorders and bizarre behavior:

- **Thought disorder** refers to disorganized thinking, which becomes apparent when speech is rambling or shifts from one topic to another. Speech may be mildly disorganized or completely incoherent and incomprehensible.
- **Bizarre behavior** may take the form of childlike silliness, agitation, or inappropriate appearance, hygiene, or conduct. Catatonia is an extreme form of bizarre behavior in which people maintain a rigid posture and resist efforts to be moved or, in contrast, display purposeless and unstimulated motor activity.

Cognitive impairment refers to difficulty concentrating, remembering, organizing, planning, and problem solving. Some people are unable to concentrate sufficiently to read, follow the story line of a movie or television show, or follow directions. Others are unable to ignore distractions or remain focused on a task. Consequently, work that involves attention to detail, involvement in complicated procedures, and decision making may be impossible.

Disorders That Resemble Schizophrenia

General medical and neurologic conditions such as thyroid disorders, brain tumors, seizure disorders, kidney failure, toxic reactions to drugs, and vitamin deficiencies can sometimes cause symptoms similar to those of schizophrenia. In addition, a number of mental disorders share features of schizophrenia.

- **Brief psychotic disorder:** Symptoms of this disorder resemble those of schizophrenia but last only for 1 day to 1 month. This time-limited disorder often occurs in people with a preexisting personality disorder or in people who have experienced a severe stress, such as loss of a loved one.
- **Schizophreniform disorder:** The schizophrenia-like symptoms characteristic of this disorder last for 1 to 6 months. This disorder may resolve or may progress to manic-depressive illness or schizophrenia.
- **Schizoaffective disorder:** This disorder is characterized by the presence of mood symptoms, such as depression or mania, plus more typical symptoms of schizophrenia.
- **Schizotypal personality disorder:** This personality disorder (see page 881) may share symptoms of schizophrenia, but they are generally not severe enough to meet the criteria for psychosis. People with this disorder tend to be shy and to isolate themselves and may be mildly suspicious and have other disturbances in thinking. Genetic studies indicate that schizotypal personality disorder may be a mild form of schizophrenia.

Subtypes of Schizophrenia: Some researchers believe schizophrenia is a single disorder, but others believe it is a syndrome (a collection of symptoms) based on numerous underlying disorders. Subtypes of schizophrenia have been proposed in an effort to classify people into more distinct groups. However, the subtype in a particular person may change over time. Subtypes include the following:

- **Paranoid:** People are preoccupied with delusions or auditory hallucinations. Disorganized speech and inappropriate emotions are less prominent.
- **Disorganized:** Speech and behavior are disorganized, and people do not express emotions or have inappropriate emotions.
- **Catatonic:** Symptoms are mainly physical. They include immobility, excessive motor activity, and assumption of bizarre postures.

- **Undifferentiated:** People have a mixture of symptoms from the other subtypes: delusions and hallucinations, thought disorder and bizarre behavior, and negative symptoms.
- **Residual:** People have had a clear history of prominent schizophrenia symptoms that are followed by a long period of mild negative symptoms.

Diagnosis

No definitive test exists to diagnose schizophrenia. A doctor makes the diagnosis based on a comprehensive assessment of a person's history and symptoms. Schizophrenia is diagnosed when symptoms persist for at least 6 months and cause significant deterioration in work, school, or social functioning. Information from family members, friends, or teachers is often important in establishing when the disorder began.

Laboratory tests are often done to rule out substance abuse or an underlying medical, neurologic, or hormonal disorder that can have features of psychosis. Examples of such disorders include brain tumors, temporal lobe epilepsy, thyroid disorders, autoimmune disorders, Huntington's disease, liver disorders, and side effects of drugs. Testing for drug abuse is sometimes done.

People with schizophrenia have brain abnormalities that may be seen on a computed tomography (CT) or magnetic resonance imaging (MRI) scan. However, the abnormalities are not specific enough to help in diagnosing schizophrenia.

> **Did You Know...**
> About 10% of people with schizophrenia commit suicide.

Prognosis

For people with schizophrenia, the prognosis depends largely on adherence to drug treatment. Without drug treatment, 70 to 80% of people have another episode within the first year after diagnosis. Drugs taken continuously can reduce this percentage to about 20 to 30% and can lessen the severity of symptoms significantly in most people. After discharge from a hospital, people who do not take prescribed drugs are very likely to be readmitted within the year. Taking drugs as directed dramatically reduces the likelihood of being readmitted.

Despite the proven benefit of drug therapy, half of people with schizophrenia do not take their prescribed drugs. Some do not recognize their illness and resist taking drugs. Others stop taking their drugs because of unpleasant side effects. Memory problems, disorganization, or simply a lack of money prevents others from taking their drugs.

Adherence is most likely to improve when specific barriers are addressed. If side effects of drugs are a major problem, a change to a different drug may help. A consistent, trusting relationship with a doctor or other therapist helps some people with schizophrenia to accept their illness more readily and recognize the need for adhering to prescribed treatment.

Over longer periods, the prognosis varies. In general, one third of people achieve significant and lasting improvement, one third achieve some improvement with intermittent relapses and residual disabilities, and one third experience severe and permanent incapacity. Factors associated with a better prognosis include the following:

- Sudden onset of the disorder
- Older age at onset
- A good level of skills and accomplishments before becoming ill
- Presence of positive rather than negative symptoms

Factors associated with a poor prognosis include the following:

- Younger age at onset
- Poor social and vocational functioning before becoming ill
- A family history of schizophrenia
- Presence of negative rather than positive symptoms

About 10% of people with schizophrenia commit suicide.

Treatment

Generally, treatment aims

- To reduce the severity of psychotic symptoms
- To prevent the recurrence of symptomatic episodes and the associated deterioration in functioning
- To provide support and thus enable people to function at the highest level possible

Antipsychotic drugs, rehabilitation and community support activities, and psychotherapy are the major components of treatment.

Antipsychotic Drugs: Drugs can be effective in reducing or eliminating symptoms, such as delusions, hallucinations, and disorganized thinking. After the immediate symptoms have cleared, the continued use of antipsychotic drugs substantially reduces the probability of future episodes. However, antipsychotic drugs have significant side effects, which can include drowsiness, muscle stiffness, tremors, weight gain, and motor restlessness. Antipsychotic drugs may also cause tardive dyskinesia, an involuntary movement disorder most often characterized by puckering of the lips and tongue or

What Is Neuroleptic Malignant Syndrome?

Neuroleptic malignant syndrome is unresponsiveness caused by use of certain antipsychotic drugs. It develops in up to 3% of people who are treated with antipsychotic drugs, usually within the first few weeks of treatment. The syndrome is most common among men who, because they are agitated, are given rapidly increased doses of the drugs or high doses initially.

Symptoms include muscle rigidity, a dangerously high temperature, a fast heart rate, a fast breathing rate, high blood pressure, and coma. Damaged muscles release the protein myoglobin, which is excreted in the urine. Myoglobin turns the urine brown. This condition (myoglobinuria) can result in kidney damage or even kidney failure.

People with this syndrome are usually treated in an intensive care unit. The antipsychotic drug is stopped, fever is controlled (usually by wetting people and blowing air on them and by placing special cooling blankets on them). People are also given a muscle relaxant (such as bromocriptine or dantrolene). Giving sodium bicarbonate intravenously helps prevent myoglobulinuria by making the urine alkaline.

Almost 30% of people with this syndrome die, but most of the rest recover completely. After recovery, up to 30% of people develop the syndrome again if they are given the same antipsychotic drug.

writhing of the arms or legs. Tardive dyskinesia may not go away even after the drug is stopped. For tardive dyskinesia that persists, there is no effective treatment. A rare but potentially fatal side effect of antipsychotic drugs is neuroleptic malignant syndrome. It is characterized by muscle rigidity, fever, high blood pressure, and changes in mental function (such as confusion and lethargy).

Some newer antipsychotic drugs, termed second-generation antipsychotic drugs, have fewer side effects. However, these drugs seem to cause significant weight gain. They also increase the risk of the metabolic syndrome (see page 960). In this syndrome, fat accumulates in the abdomen, blood levels of triglycerides (a fat) are elevated, levels of high density cholesterol (HDL, the "good" cholesterol) are low, and blood pressure is high. Also, insulin is less effective (called insulin resistance), increasing the risk of diabetes. These drugs may relieve positive symptoms (such as hallucinations), negative symptoms (such as lack of emotion), and cognitive impairment (such as reduced mental functioning and attention span) to a greater extent than the older antipsychotic drugs, although some doctors question these differences.

Clozapine, the first of the second-generation antipsychotic drugs, is effective in up to half of people who do not respond to other antipsychotic drugs. However, clozapine can have serious side effects, such as seizures or potentially fatal suppression of bone marrow activity (which includes making blood cells). Thus, it is usually used only for people who have not responded to other antipsychotic drugs. People who take clozapine must have their white blood cell count measured weekly, at least for the first 6 months, so that clozapine can be stopped at the first indication that the number of white blood cells is decreasing.

Rehabilitation and Community Support Activities: Community support activities, such as on-the-job coaching, are directed at teaching the skills needed to survive in the community. These skills enable people with schizophrenia to work, shop, care for themselves, manage a household, and get along with others. Hospitalization may be needed during severe relapses, and involuntary hospitalization may be needed if people pose a danger to themselves or others. However, the general goal is to have people live in the community. To achieve this goal, some people need to live in a supervised apartment or group home where someone can ensure that drugs are taken as prescribed.

A few people with schizophrenia are unable to live independently, either because they have severe, persistent symptoms or because they lack the skills necessary to live in the community. They usually require full-time care in a safe and supportive setting.

Psychotherapy: Generally, psychotherapy aims to establish a collaborative relationship between people, their family members, and doctor. That way people may learn to understand and manage their disorder, to take antipsychotic drugs as prescribed, and to manage stresses that can aggravate the disorder. A good doctor-patient relationship is often a major determinant of whether treatment is successful. Psychotherapy reduces the severity of symptoms in some people and helps prevent relapse in others.

Delusional Disorder

Delusional disorder is characterized by one or more false beliefs that persist for at least 1 month.

- The false beliefs tend to be ordinary things that could occur, such as being deceived by a spouse.
- This disorder may develop in people with a paranoid personality disorder.
- Doctors base the diagnosis mainly on the person's history after they rule out other possible causes.
- People usually remain functional and employed.
- A good doctor-patient relationship is essential to treatment.

Delusional disorder usually first affects people in middle or late adult life. Delusions tend to be nonbizarre and involve situations that could conceivably occur in real life, such as being followed, poisoned, infected, loved at a distance, or deceived by a spouse or lover. Several subtypes of delusional disorder are recognized:

Erotomanic: People believe that another person is in love with them. Efforts to contact the object of the delusion through telephone calls, letters, or even surveillance and stalking may be common. Behavior related to the delusion may cause conflict with the law.

Grandiose: People are convinced that they have some great talent or have made some important discovery.

Jealous: People are convinced that a spouse or lover is unfaithful. This belief is based on incorrect inferences supported by dubious evidence. Under such circumstances, physical assault may be a significant danger.

Persecutory: People believe that they are being plotted against, spied on, maligned, or harassed. People may repeatedly attempt to obtain justice by appealing to courts and other government agencies. Rarely, violence may be resorted to in retaliation for imagined persecution.

Somatic: People are preoccupied with a bodily function or attribute, such as an imagined physical deformity or odor. The delusion can also take the form of an imagined general medical condition, such as a parasitic infection.

℞ ANTIPSYCHOTIC DRUGS

DRUG	SOME SIDE EFFECTS	COMMENTS
Older antipsychotic drugs		
Chlorpromazine Fluphenazine Haloperidol Loxapine Mesoridazine Molindone Perphenazine Pimozide Thioridazine Thiothixene Trifluoperazine	Dry mouth Blurred vision Seizures Increased heart rate and decreased blood pressure Constipation Sudden but often reversible tremor and muscle stiffness that may progress to rigidity Uncontrolled movements of the face and arms (tardive dyskinesia) Muscle rigidity, fever, high blood pressure, and changes in mental function (neuroleptic malignant syndrome)	Side effects are much more likely in older people and in people with impaired balance or serious medical disorders. Long-acting injectable forms of haloperidol and perphenazine are available. Eye examination and electrocardiography (ECG) are recommended while people are taking thioridazine.
Newer antipsychotic drugs		
Aripiprazole Clozapine Olanzapine Paliperidone Quetiapine Risperidone Ziprasidone	Drowsiness and weight gain (most common), which can be substantial Possibly an increased risk of accumulation of fat in the abdomen, abnormal cholesterol levels in the blood, high blood pressure, and resistance to the effects of insulin (metabolic syndrome)	Newer antipsychotic drugs are less likely to cause tremor, muscle stiffness, uncontrolled movements (including tardive dyskinesia), and neuroleptic malignant syndrome, but these effects may occur. A long-acting injectable form of risperidone is available. Clozapine is used much less often because it can cause bone marrow suppression, a reduced white blood cell count, and seizures. However, it is often effective in people who are not responsive to other drugs. Clozapine and olanzapine are most likely to cause weight gain, and aripiprazole is the least likely. Ziprasidone does not cause weight gain but may lead to abnormalities on an electrocardiogram.

Antipsychotic Drugs: How Do They Work?

Antipsychotic drugs appear to be most effective in treating hallucinations, delusions, disorganized thinking, and aggression. Although antipsychotic drugs are most commonly prescribed for schizophrenia, they appear to be effective in treating these symptoms whether they result from schizophrenia, mania, dementia, or use of a substance such as amphetamines.

Antipsychotic drugs work by influencing how information is transmitted between individual brain cells. The adult brain is made up of more than 10 billion nerve cells called neurons. Each neuron in the brain has a single long fiber called an axon, which transmits information to other neurons. Like wires connected in a vast telephone switchboard, each neuron makes contact with several thousand other neurons.

Information travels down a cell's axon as an electrical impulse. When the impulse reaches the end of the axon, a tiny amount of a chemical called a neurotransmitter is released to pass information on to the next cell down the line.

A receptor on the receiving cell detects the neurotransmitter, which causes the receiving cell to generate a new impulse.

Symptoms of psychosis appear to be caused by excessive activity of cells sensitive to the neurotransmitter dopamine. Therefore, antipsychotic drugs work by blocking receptors so that communication between groups of cells is reduced.

How well different antipsychotic drugs block different types of neurotransmitters varies. Every effective antipsychotic drug known blocks dopamine receptors. The new antipsychotic drugs (clozapine, olanzapine, quetiapine, risperidone, and ziprasidone) also block serotonin receptors. Experts thought that this property might make these drugs more effective. However, recent brain imaging studies have not supported this view. Clozapine, which blocks many other receptors, is clearly the most effective drug for psychotic symptoms. But it is underused because of its side effects and the need for monitoring with blood tests.

Symptoms

A delusional disorder may arise from a preexisting paranoid personality disorder (see page 880). Beginning in early adulthood, people with a paranoid personality disorder have a pervasive distrust and suspiciousness of others and their motives. Early symptoms of delusional disorder may include feeling exploited, being preoccupied with the loyalty or trustworthiness of friends, reading threatening meanings into benign remarks or events, bearing grudges for a long time, and responding readily to perceived slights.

Diagnosis

After ruling out other specific conditions that are associated with delusions, a doctor bases the diagnosis largely on the person's history. The doctor must assess the degree of dangerousness, particularly the extent to which the people are willing to act on their delusions.

Prognosis and Treatment

Delusional disorder does not usually cause severe impairment. However, people may become progressively more involved with their delusion. Most people are able to remain employed.

A good doctor-patient relationship helps. Hospitalization may be needed if the doctor believes that people are dangerous.

Antipsychotic drugs are not generally used but are sometimes effective in suppressing symptoms. A long-term treatment goal is to shift the person's focus away from the delusion to a more constructive and gratifying area, although this goal is frequently difficult to achieve.

CHAPTER

135 Sexuality

Sexuality is a normal part of human experience. However, the types of sexual behavior that are considered normal vary greatly within and among different cultures. In fact, defining "normal" sexuality may be impossible. There are wide variations in people's sexual behavior, including the frequency of or need for sexual release. Some people desire sexual activity several times a day, but others are satisfied with infrequent activity (for example, a few times a year).

Although younger people are often reluctant to view older people as sexually interested, most older people remain interested in sex and report satisfying sex lives well into old age. Problems with sexual function, such as erectile dysfunction in men (see page 1483) and pain during sexual intercourse (dyspareunia), painful spasm of vaginal muscles (vaginismus), or problems with orgasm in women (see page 1505), affect people of all ages. However, such problems tend to be more common among older people. Many of these problems can be effectively treated with drugs (most notably those for erectile dysfunction).

A person's attitude toward sexual behavior is influenced greatly by parents. If a parent has a forbidding, puritanical rejection of physical affection, including touching, children may be less able to enjoy sex and develop healthy intimate relationships as adults. Parents can damage their children's ability to develop sexual and emotional intimacy by doing the following:

- Being emotional distant
- Punishing children too severely
- Being overtly seductive and exploiting children sexually
- Being verbally and physically hostile
- Rejecting children
- Being cruel

Societal attitudes about sexuality change with time, as illustrated by the following:

Masturbation: Once regarded as a perversion and even a cause of mental disease, masturbation is now recognized as a normal sexual activity throughout life. About 97% of males and 80% of females have masturbated. In general, males masturbate more frequently than females. Many people continue to masturbate even when they are involved in a sexually gratifying relationship. Although masturbation is normal and is often recommended as a safe sex option, it may cause guilt and psychologic suffering that stems from the disapproving attitudes of other people. These feelings can result in considerable distress and can even affect sexual performance.

Homosexuality: As with masturbation, homosexuality, once considered abnormal by the medical profession, has not been considered a disorder for more than three decades. It is widely recognized as a sexual orientation that is present from childhood. An estimated 4 to 5% of adults are involved exclusively in homosexual relationships throughout their lives, and an additional 2 to 5% of people periodically engage in sex with someone of the same sex (bisexuality). Adolescents may experiment with same-sex play, but this experimentation does not necessarily indicate an enduring interest in homosexual or bisexual activity as adults (see page 1753).

Homosexuals discover that they are attracted to people of the same sex, just as heterosexuals discover that they are attracted to people of the opposite sex. The attraction appears to be the result of biologic and environmental influences and is not a matter of choice. Therefore, the popular term "sexual preference" makes little sense in matters of sexual orientation, whether the orientation is heterosexual or homosexual.

Most homosexuals adjust well to their sexual orientation, although they must overcome widespread societal disapproval and prejudice. This adjustment may take a long time and may be associated with substantial psychologic stress. Many homosexual men and women experience bigotry in social situations and in the workplace, adding to their stress. Discrimination based on sexual orientation (or perceived sexual orientation) remains widespread, although it is illegal in the United States.

Frequent Sexual Activity With Different Partners: For some heterosexuals and homosexuals, frequent sexual activity with different partners is a common practice throughout life. This behavior may serve as a reason to seek professional counseling because having many sex partners is linked to the transmission of certain diseases (such as HIV infection, herpes simplex, hepatitis, syphilis, gonorrhea, and cervical cancer) and may also signify difficulty in forming meaningful, lasting relationships.

Extramarital Sex: In the United States, most people engage in sexual activity before they are married or while they are not married. This behavior is part of the trend toward more sexual freedom in developed countries. However, most cultures discourage married people from engaging in sex with someone other than their spouse. However, this behavior occurs frequently despite social disapproval. One objective problem that results is the possible spread of sexually transmitted diseases to unsuspecting spouses.

Gender Identity

Gender identity is how people see themselves, whether masculine, feminine, or somewhere in-between. Gender role is how people present themselves in public in terms of gender. It includes the way people dress, speak, wear their hair, in fact everything that people say and do that indicates masculinity or femininity. For most people, gender identity is consistent with their anatomic sex and their gender role (as when a man has an inner sense of masculinity and publicly acts in masculine ways).

Gender identity is well established by early childhood (18 to 24 months of age). During childhood, boys come to know they are boys, and girls come to know they are girls. Children sometimes prefer activities considered to be more appropriate for the other sex.

However, this preference does not mean that a young girl who, for example, likes to play baseball and wrestle has a gender identity problem, as long as she sees herself as and is content with being female. Similarly, a boy who plays with dolls and prefers cooking to sports or to rough types of play does not have a gender identity problem as long as he identifies himself as and is comfortable with being male. Young boys often pass through phases where they play with girls' toys or clothes, but few of them have problems with gender identity as adults.

 Did You Know...

Many young boys go through a phase of playing with girls' toys.

Children born with genitals that are not clearly male or female (see page 1718) usually do not have a gender identity problem if they are decisively reared as one sex or the other, even if they are raised in the gender role that is opposite to their biologic sex pattern. There have been some highly publicized cases, however, in which this approach has failed.

Gender Identity Disorders and Transsexualism

Gender identity disorders involve a significant discrepancy between a person's anatomic sex and the inner sense of self as masculine, feminine, mixed, or neutral. Transsexualism is the most extreme form of gender identity disorder.

- Children focus on activities typically associated with the other sex and have negative feelings about their genitals.
- Doctors base the diagnosis on symptoms indicating a strong preference to be the other sex.
- People who feel a strong need to live as the other sex may be helped by counseling, hormone therapy, and sometimes irreversible genital surgery.

People with a gender identity disorder believe that they are victims of a biologic accident and that they are cruelly imprisoned in a body incompatible with their gender identity. That is, people who are biologically male feel like women trapped in a man's body, and vice versa. For transsexuals, the incompatibility felt is complete, severe, disturbing, and long-standing. Transsexualism appears to occur in about 1 of 11,900 male and 1 of 30,000 female births.

Most transsexuals are biologic males who identify themselves as females, sometimes early in childhood, and regard their genitals and masculine features with repugnance. However, most children with gender identity problems do not become transsexual adults.

Rarely, transsexuals are people who were born with genitals that are not clearly male or female (ambiguous genitals) or who have a genetic abnormality, such as Turner's syndrome or Klinefelter's syndrome. However, when children are clearly and consistently considered and reared as either boys or girls, even when genitals are ambiguous, most of them have a clear sense of their gender identity.

Symptoms

Problems with gender identity usually develop by age 2. Children who have these problems may do the following:

- Prefer cross-dressing
- Insist that they are of the other sex
- Intensely and persistently desire to participate in games and activities associated with the other sex
- Have negative feelings toward their genitals

For example, a young girl may insist she will grow a penis and become a boy; she may stand to urinate. A boy may sit to urinate and wish to be rid of his penis and testes. For boys with a gender identity disorder, distress at the physical changes of puberty is often followed by a request for treatment that will make their body more like a woman's.

Although most transsexuals began having gender identity problems in early childhood, sometimes gender identity disorders first become apparent during adulthood. People, usually men, may be cross-dressers first and not acknowledge their identification with the other sex until later in life. Some of these men marry or join the military as a way to escape or deny their feelings of wanting to be the other sex. Once they accept these feelings, many publicly adopt a convincing feminine gender role. Others experience problems, such as depression and suicidal behavior.

Most boys with a gender identity disorder do not grow up to have the disorder as adults, but many are homosexual or bisexual in their sexual orientation.

Diagnosis

Most children with a gender identity disorder are not evaluated until they are 6 to 9 years old.

With children, a doctor bases the diagnosis on whether they have the following:

- A strong, persistent desire to be or insistence that they are the other sex
- A strong, persistent sense of discomfort about their sex or belief that they were born the wrong sex
- Significant distress or problems functioning caused by these feelings

With adolescents and adults, a doctor bases the diagnosis on whether they do the following:

- Express a desire to be the other sex frequently
- Try to pass as the other sex
- Want to live or be treated as the other sex
- Believe that they feel and react like the other sex

Treatment

Cross-gender behavior in adults, such as cross-dressing, may not require treatment if people do not have psychologic distress or trouble functioning in society.

Transsexuals may seek psychologic help, either to assist them in coping with the difficulties of living in a body that they do not feel comfortable with or to help them through a gender transition. Many transsexuals appear to be helped most by a combination of counseling, hormone therapy, electrolysis, and sometimes genital surgery (which is irreversible).

Some transsexuals with a milder form of gender identity disorder are satisfied with changing their gender role by working, living, and dressing in society as a member of the opposite sex. This approach may include obtaining identification (such as a driver's license) that helps them work and live in society as the opposite sex. They may never seek to alter their anatomy in any way. Many of these people, who are sometimes referred to as "transgenderists," meet no criteria for a mental health disorder.

> **? Did You Know...**
>
> Children with a gender identity disorder may insist that they are the opposite sex.

Other transsexuals, in addition to adopting the behavior, dress, and mannerisms of the opposite sex, appropriately receive hormone treatments to change their secondary sex characteristics. In biologic males, use of the female hormone estrogen causes breast growth and other body changes, such as wasting of the genitals (genital atrophy) and the inability to maintain an erection. In biologic females, use of the male hormone testosterone causes such changes as growth of facial hair, deepening of the voice, and changes in body odor and distribution of body fat.

Still other transsexuals request sex reassignment surgery. For biologic males, surgery involves removal of the penis and testes and creation of an artificial vagina. For biologic females, surgery involves removal of the breasts and the internal reproductive organs (uterus and ovaries), closure of the vagina, and creation of an artificial penis. For both sexes, surgery is preceded by use of the appropriate sex hormone (estrogen in male-to-female transformation and testosterone in female-to-male transformation), and a real-life experience living in the opposite gender role for at least 1 year.

Although transsexuals who have sex reassignment surgery cannot procreate, many are able to have satisfactory sexual relations. The ability to achieve orgasm is often retained after surgery, and some people report feeling comfortable sexually for the first time. However, few transsexuals endure the sex reassignment process for the sole purpose of being able to function sexually as the opposite sex. Confirmation of their inner sense of gender identity is the usual motivation.

Paraphilias

Paraphilias are frequent, intense, sexually arousing fantasies or behaviors that involve inanimate objects, children or nonconsenting adults, or suffering or humiliation of oneself or the partner.

Sexual arousal may depend on one of the above. Once these arousal patterns are established, usually in late childhood or near puberty, they are often lifelong.

Some degree of variety in sexual activity is very common in healthy adult sexual relationships and fantasies. When people mutually agree to engage in them, noninjurious sexual behaviors of an unusual nature may be part of a loving and caring relationship. When taken to the extreme, however, such sexual behaviors are paraphilias—psychosexual disorders that seriously impair the capacity for affectionate, reciprocal sexual activity. Partners of people with a paraphilia may feel like an object or as if they are unimportant or unnecessary in the sexual relationship. Paraphilias cause significant distress and interfere with functioning. Distress may result from other people's reactions or from guilt about doing something socially unacceptable.

The most common paraphilias are transvestic fetishism, pedophilia, exhibitionism, and voyeurism. Others include sexual masochism and sadism. Most people with paraphilias are men, and many have more than one type of paraphilia. Some of them also have a severe personality disorder, such as an antisocial or narcissistic personality. Some paraphilias are against the law.

FETISHISM

Fetishism is use of a physical object (the fetish) as the preferred way to produce sexual arousal.

People with fetishes may become sexually stimulated and gratified by wearing another person's undergarments, wearing rubber or leather, or holding, rubbing, or smelling objects, such as high-heeled shoes. People with this disorder may not be able to function sexually without their fetish. The fetish may replace typical sexual activity with a partner or may be integrated into sexual activity with a willing partner.

Transvestic Fetishism: In transvestic fetishism (cross-dressing), men prefer to wear women's clothing, or, far less commonly, women prefer to wear men's clothing. However, they do not wish to change their sex, as transsexuals do. Cross-dressing may not hurt a couple's sexual relationship, although if a partner is not cooperative, transvestites may feel anxious, depressed, and guilty and ashamed about their desire.

Transvestic fetishism is considered a mental health disorder only if it causes distress, interferes with functioning, or involves daredevil behavior likely to lead to injury, loss of a job, or imprisonment. Transvestites also cross-dress for reasons other than sexual stimulation—for example, to reduce anxiety, to relax, or, in the case of male transvestites, to experiment with the feminine side of their otherwise male personalities. Some men who appear to be transvestites only in their teens and twenties develop gender identity disorder later in life and may seek to change their body through hormones and genital surgery.

Only a few transvestites seek medical care. They may be motivated by an unhappy spouse or by worry about how the cross-dressing is affecting their social life and work. Some seek medical care for other problems, such as substance abuse or depression. Treatment involves psychotherapy to help them accept themselves and control behaviors that could cause problems.

PEDOPHILIA

Pedophilia is a preference for sexual activity with young children.

In Western societies, pedophilia is defined as sexual fantasy about or sexual relations with a prepubertal child younger than 13 by a person 16 or older. Some pedophiles are attracted only to children, often of a specific age range or developmental stage. Others are attracted to both children and adults. Pedophiles may be attracted to young boys, young girls, or both, but most pedophiles prefer children of the opposite sex. Usually, the adult is known to the child and may be a family member, stepparent, or a person with authority (such as a teacher). Looking or general touching seems more common than touching the genitals or having sexual intercourse.

Although state laws vary in the United States, the law generally considers a person older than 18 to be committing statutory rape if the victim is 16 or younger. Statutory rape cases often do not meet the definition of pedophilia, highlighting the somewhat arbitrary nature of selecting a specific age cutoff point in a medical or legal definition. In many other countries and cultures, children as young as 12 can legally marry, further complicating the definition of pedophilia and statutory rape.

Pedophilia is much more common among men than among women. Both boys and girls can be victims, although more reported cases involve girls. Pedophiles may focus only on children within their families (incest), or they may prey on children in the community. Force or coercion may be used to engage children sexually, and threats (for example, to harm the child or the child's pets) may be invoked to prevent the child from telling anyone.

Many pedophiles have or develop substance abuse or dependence and depression. They often come from dysfunctional families, and marital conflict is common.

Treatment

Pedophilia can be treated with long-term psychotherapy and drugs that alter the sex drive and reduce testosterone levels. Results vary. Outcome is best when participation is voluntary and the person receives training in social skills and treatment of other problems, such as drug abuse or depression. Treatment that is sought only after criminal apprehension and legal action may be less effective. Simple incarceration, even long-term, does not change pedophilic desires or fantasies. However, some incarcerated pedophiles who are committed to long-term, monitored treatment (usually including drugs) can refrain from pedophilic activity and be reintegrated into society.

For drug treatment, doctors in the United States usually use the drug medroxyprogesterone acetate, which is injected into a muscle. This drug (a progestin) is similar to the female hormone progesterone. Alternatives are drugs such as leuprolide and goserelin that stop the pituitary gland from signaling the testicles to produce testosterone. It is not clear how useful these drugs are in women who are pedophiles.

EXHIBITIONISM

Exhibitionism involves exposing the genitals in order to become sexually excited or having a strong desire to be observed by other people during sexual activity.

Exhibitionists (usually males) expose their genitals, usually to unsuspecting strangers, and become sexually excited when doing so. They may be aware of their need to surprise, shock, or impress the unwilling observer. The victim is almost always a woman or a child of either sex. Actual sexual contact is almost never sought, so exhibitionists rarely commit rape. Exhibitionism usually starts when people are in their mid 20s. Most exhibitionists are married, but the marriage is often troubled.

About 30% of male sex offenders who are arrested are exhibitionists. They tend to persist in their behavior. About 20 to 50% are re-arrested.

Exposure of genitals to unsuspecting strangers for sexual excitement is rare among women. Women have other venues to expose themselves: dressing provocatively (which is increasingly accepted as normal) and appearing in various media and entertainment venues. Participation in these venues may not constitute a mental health disorder.

For some people, exhibitionism is expressed as a strong desire to have other people watch their sexual acts. Such people want to be seen by a consenting audience, rather than to surprise people. People with this form of exhibitionism may make pornographic films or become adult entertainers. They are rarely troubled by their desire and thus may not have a mental health disorder.

Treatment

Treatment usually begins after exhibitionists are arrested. It includes psychotherapy, support groups, and antidepressants called selective serotonin reuptake inhibitors (SSRIs). If these drugs are ineffective, drugs that alter the sex drive and reduce testosterone levels may be used. People must give their informed consent to the use of these drugs, and doctors periodically do blood tests to monitor the drug's effects on liver function and serum testosterone levels.

VOYEURISM

Voyeurism involves becoming sexually aroused by watching someone who is disrobing, naked, or engaged in sexual activity.

In voyeurism, it is the act of observing (peeping) that is arousing, not sexual activity with the observed person. Voyeurs do not seek sexual contact with the people being observed. When voyeurs observe unsuspecting people, they may have problems with the law.

Voyeurism usually begins during adolescence or early adulthood. Some degree of voyeurism is common, more among boys and men but increasingly among women. Society often regards mild forms of this behavior as normal when involving consenting adults. Viewing sexually explicit pictures and shows, now widely available in private on the Internet, is not considered voyeurism because it lacks the element of secret observation, which is the hallmark of voyeurism.

As a disorder, voyeurism is much more common among men. When voyeurism is a disorder, voyeurs spend a lot of time seeking out viewing opportunities. It may become the preferred method of sexual activity and consume countless hours of watching.

Treatment

When voyeurs are arrested, treatment usually begins. It includes therapy, support groups, and antidepressants called selective serotonin reuptake inhibitors (SSRIs). If these drugs are ineffective, drugs that alter the sex drive and reduce testosterone levels may be used. People must give their informed consent to the use of these drugs, and doctors periodically do blood tests to monitor the drug's effects on liver function and serum testosterone levels.

SEXUAL MASOCHISM AND SADISM

Sexual masochism involves acts in which a person experiences sexual excitement from being humiliated, beaten, bound, or otherwise abused. Sexual sadism involves acts in which a person experiences sexual excitement from inflicting physical or psychologic suffering on another person.

Some amount of sadism and masochism is commonly play-acted in healthy sexual relationships, and mutually compatible partners often seek one another out. For example, the use of silk handkerchiefs for simulated bondage and mild spanking during sexual activity are common practices between consenting partners and are not considered sadomasochistic.

Most sadists interact with a consenting partner (who may have sexual masochism). In these relationships, the humiliation and beating are simply acted out, with participants knowing that it is a game and carefully avoiding actual humiliation or injury. Fantasies of total control and dominance are often important, and sadists may bind and gag their partner in elaborate ways.

In contrast, the disorder of sexual masochism or of sexual sadism takes these acts to an extreme or involves nonconsenting victims (and thus constitutes a crime). Some acts result in severe bodily or psychologic harm and even death. For example, masochistic sexual activity may involve asphyxiophilia, in which the person is partially choked or strangled (by a partner or by self-application of a noose around the neck). A temporary decrease in oxygen to the brain at the point of orgasm is sought as an enhancement to sexual release, but the practice may accidentally result in death.

Treatment of masochism and sadism is usually ineffective.

Disorders of Nutrition and Metabolism

136 Overview of Nutrition

Nutrition is the process of consuming, absorbing, and using nutrients needed by the body for growth, development, and maintenance of life.

To receive adequate, appropriate nutrition, people need to consume a healthy diet, which consists of a variety of nutrients—the substances in foods that nourish the body. A healthy diet enables people to maintain a desirable body weight and composition (the percentage of fat and muscle in the body) and to do their daily physical and mental activities.

If people consume too much food, obesity may result. If they consume large amounts of certain nutrients, usually vitamins or minerals, harmful effects (toxicity) may occur. If people do not consume enough nutrients, a nutritional deficiency disorder may result.

To determine whether people are consuming a proper amount of nutrients, doctors ask them about their eating habits and diet and do a physical examination to assess the composition and functioning of the body. Height and weight are measured, and body mass index (BMI) is calculated. BMI is calculated by dividing weight (in kilograms) by the square of the height (in meters). A BMI between 19 and 24 is usually considered normal for men and women.

Body composition, including the percentage of body fat, is sometimes estimated by measuring skinfold thickness or doing bioelectrical impedance analysis. More accurate ways to determine this percentage include weighing people under water (hydrostatic weighing) and doing a dual-energy x-ray absorptiometry (DEXA) scan, but these methods are seldom used.

Levels of many nutrients can be measured in blood and sometimes in tissues. For example, measuring the level of albumin, the main protein in blood, may help determine whether people are deficient in protein. Nutrient levels decrease when nutrition is inadequate.

Components of the Diet: Generally, nutrients are divided into two classes:

- **Macronutrients:** Macronutrients are required daily in large quantities. They include proteins, fats, carbohydrates, some minerals, and water.

- **Micronutrients:** Micronutrients are required daily in small quantities—in milligrams (one thousandth of a gram) to micrograms (one millionth of a gram). They include vitamins and certain minerals that enable the body to use macronutrients. These minerals are called trace minerals because the body needs only very small amounts.

Fat Versus Lean: Body Composition

Maintaining an appropriate weight is important for physical and psychologic health. A standardized height-weight table can be used as a guide. But body mass index (BMI) is more reliable.

A less obvious but important consideration is how much of the body is fat and how much is muscle (body composition). There are several ways to determine body composition:

Hydrostatic weighing: People are weighed underwater in a small pool. Bone and muscle are denser than water, so people with a high percentage of lean tissue weigh more in water and people with a high percentage of fat weigh less. Although this method is considered the most accurate, it requires special equipment, considerable time, and expertise to do.

Skinfold thickness: Body composition can be estimated by measuring the amount of fat under the skin (skinfold thickness). A fold of skin on the back of the left upper arm (triceps skinfold) is pulled away from the arm

and measured with a caliper. A skinfold measurement of about $1/2$ inch in men and about 1 inch in women is considered normal. This measurement plus the circumference of the left upper arm can be used to estimate the amount of skeletal muscle in the body (lean body mass).

Bioelectric impedance analysis: This test measures the resistance of body tissues to the flow of an undetectable low-voltage electrical current. Typically, people stand barefoot on metal footplates, and the electrical current is sent up one foot and down the other. Body fat and bone resist the flow much more than muscle tissue does. By measuring the resistance to the current, doctors can estimate the percentage of body fat. This test takes only about 1 minute.

Dual-energy x-ray absorptiometry (DEXA): This imaging procedure accurately determines the amount and distribution of body fat. DEXA uses a very low dose of radiation and is safe. However, it is too expensive to use routinely.

WHO IS OVERWEIGHT?

	NORMAL*	OVERWEIGHT	OBESE		EXTREMELY OBESE	
BMI	19–24	25–29	30–34	35–39	40–47	48–54
HEIGHT† (INCHES)	BODY WEIGHT† (POUNDS)					
60–61	97–127	128–153	153–180	179–206	204–248	245–285
62–63	104–135	136–163	164–191	191–220	218–265	262–304
64–65	110–144	145–174	174–204	204–234	232–282	279–324
66–67	118–153	155–185	186–217	216–249	247–299	297–344
68–69	125–162	164–196	197–230	230–263	262–318	315–365
70–71	132–172	174–208	209–243	243–279	278–338	334–386
72–73	140–182	184–219	221–257	258–295	294–355	353–408
74–75	148–192	194–232	233–272	272–311	311–375	373–431
76	156–197	205–238	246–279	287–320	328–385	394–443

*BMIs lower than those listed as normal are considered underweight.
†Calculations are done using height in meters and weight in kilograms. Height is without shoes. Weight is without clothes.
BMI = body mass index.

Water is required in amounts of 1 milliliter for each calorie of energy expended or about 2.6 quarts (2,500 milliliters) a day. The requirement for water can be met by the water naturally contained in many foods, and by drinking fruit or vegetable juices and caffeine-free coffee or tea as well as water. Alcoholic beverages and caffeinated coffee, tea, and sodas may make people urinate more, so they are less useful.

Foods consumed in the daily diet contain as many as 100,000 substances. But only 300 are classified as nutrients, and only 45 are classified as essential nutrients: vitamins, minerals, some amino acids (components of protein), and some fatty acids (components of fats). Essential nutrients cannot be synthesized by the body and must be consumed in the diet.

Foods contain many other useful components, including fibers (such as cellulose, pectins, and gums). Foods also contain additives (such as preservatives, emulsifiers, antioxidants, and stabilizers), which improve the production, processing, storage, and packaging of foods (see page 908).

Carbohydrates, Proteins, and Fats

Carbohydrates, proteins, and fats supply 90% of the dry weight of the diet and 100% of its energy.

All three provide energy (measured in calories), but the amount of energy in 1 gram (1/28 ounce) differs: 4 calories in a gram of carbohydrate or protein and 9 calories in a gram of fat. These nutrients also differ in how quickly they supply energy. Carbohydrates are the quickest, and fats are the slowest.

Carbohydrates, proteins, and fats are digested in the intestine, where they are broken down into their basic units: carbohydrates into sugars, proteins into amino acids, and fats into fatty acids and glycerol. The body uses these basic units to build substances it needs for growth, maintenance, and activity (including other carbohydrates, proteins, and fats).

Carbohydrates

Depending on the size of the molecule, carbohydrates may be simple or complex.

■ **Simple carbohydrates:** Various forms of sugar, such as glucose and sucrose (table sugar), are simple carbohydrates. They are small molecules, so they can be broken down and absorbed by the body quickly and are the quickest source of energy. They quickly increase the level of blood glucose (blood sugar). Fruits, dairy products, honey, and maple syrup contain large amounts of simple carbohydrates, which provide the sweet taste in most candies and cakes.

■ **Complex carbohydrates:** These carbohydrates are composed of long strings of simple carbohydrates. Because complex carbohydrates are larger molecules than simple carbohydrates, they must be broken down into simple carbohydrates before they can be absorbed. Thus, they tend to provide energy to the body more slowly than simple carbohydrates but still more quickly than protein or fat. Because they are digested more slowly than simple carbohydrates, they are less likely to be converted to fat. They also increase blood sugar levels more slowly and to lower levels than simple carbohydrates but for a longer time. Complex carbohydrates include starches and fibers, which occur in wheat products (such as breads and pastas), other grains (such as rye and corn), beans, and root vegetables (such as potatoes).

Carbohydrates may be refined or unrefined. Refined means that the food is highly processed. The fiber and bran, as well as many of the vitamins and minerals they contain, have been stripped away. Thus, the body processes these carbohydrates quickly, and they provide little nutrition although they contain about the same number of calories. Refined products are often enriched, meaning vitamins and minerals have been added back to increase their nutritional value. A diet high in simple or refined carbohydrates tends to increase the risk of obesity and diabetes.

If people consume more carbohydrates than they need at the time, the body stores some of these carbohydrates within cells (as glycogen) and converts the rest to fat. Glycogen is a complex carbohydrate that the body can easily and rapidly convert to energy. Glycogen is stored in the liver and the muscles. Muscles use glycogen for energy during periods of intense exercise. The amount of carbohydrates stored as glycogen can provide almost a day's worth of calories. A few other body tissues store carbohydrates as complex carbohydrates that cannot be used to provide energy.

Most authorities recommend that about 50 to 55% of total daily calories should consist of carbohydrates.

Glycemic Index: The glycemic index of a carbohydrate represents how quickly its consumption increases blood sugar levels. Values range from 1 (the slowest) to 100 (the fastest, the index of pure glucose). However, how quickly the level actually increases also depends on what other foods are ingested at the same time and other factors.

The glycemic index tends to be lower for complex carbohydrates than for simple carbohydrates, but there are exceptions. For example, fructose (the sugar in fruits) has little effect on blood sugar.

The following also influence a food's glycemic index:

■ **Processing:** Processed, refined, or finely ground foods tend to have a higher glycemic index.

■ **Type of starch:** Different types of starch are absorbed differently. For example, potato starch is digested and absorbed into the bloodstream relatively quickly. Barley is digested and absorbed much more slowly.

GLYCEMIC INDEX OF SOME FOODS

CATEGORY	FOOD	INDEX
Beans	Kidney	33
	Red lentils	27
	Soy	14
Bread	Pumpernickel	49
	White	69
	Whole wheat	72
Cereals	All bran	54
	Corn flakes	83
	Oatmeal	53
	Puffed rice	90
	Shredded wheat	70
Dairy	Milk, ice cream, yogurt	34–38
Fruit	Apple	38
	Banana	61
	Orange	43
	Orange juice	49
	Strawberries	32
Grains	Barley	22
	Brown rice	66
	White rice	72
Pasta	—	38
Potatoes	Instant mashed (white)	86
	Mashed (white)	72
	Sweet	50
Snacks	Corn chips	72
	Oatmeal cookies	57
	Potato chips	56
Sugar	Fructose	22
	Glucose	100
	Honey	91
	Refined sugar	64

- **Fiber content:** The more fiber a food has, the harder it is to digest. As a result, sugar is absorbed more slowly into the bloodstream.

- **Ripeness of fruit:** The riper the fruit, the more sugar it contains, and the higher its glycemic index.

- **Fat or acid content:** The more fat or acid a food contains, the more slowly it is digested and the more slowly its sugars are absorbed into the bloodstream.

- **Preparation:** How a food is prepared can influence how quickly it is absorbed into the bloodstream. Generally, cooking or grinding a food increases its glycemic index because these processes make food easier to digest and absorb.

- **Other factors:** The way the body processes food varies from person to person, affecting how quickly carbohydrates are converted to sugar and absorbed. How well a food is chewed and how quickly it is swallowed also have an effect.

The glycemic index is thought to be important because carbohydrates that increase blood sugar levels quickly (those with a high glycemic index) also quickly increase insulin levels. The increase in insulin may result in low blood sugar levels (hypoglycemia) and hunger, which tends to lead to consuming excess calories and gaining weight. Carbohydrates with a low glycemic index do not increase insulin levels so much. As a result, people feel satiated longer after eating. Consuming carbohydrates with a low glycemic index also tends to result in more healthful cholesterol levels and reduces the risk of obesity and diabetes mellitus and, in people with diabetes, the risk of complications due to diabetes.

In spite of the association between foods with a low glycemic index and improved health, using the index to choose foods does not automatically lead to a healthy diet. For example, the glycemic index of potato chips and some candy bars—not healthful choices—is lower than that of some healthful foods, such as brown rice. Some foods with a high glycemic index contain valuable vitamins and minerals. Thus, this index should be used only as a general guide to food choices.

Glycemic Load: The glycemic index indicates only how quickly carbohydrates in a food are absorbed into the bloodstream. It does not include how much carbohydrate a food contains, which is also important. Glycemic load, a relatively new term, includes the glycemic index and the amount of carbohydrate in a food. A food, such as carrots, bananas, watermelon, or whole-wheat bread, may have a high glycemic index but contain relatively little carbohydrate and thus have a low glycemic load. Such foods have little effect on the blood sugar level.

Proteins

Proteins consist of units called amino acids, strung together in complex formations. Because proteins are complex molecules, the body takes longer to break them down. As a result, they are a much slower and longer-lasting source of energy than carbohydrates.

There are 20 amino acids. The body synthesizes some of them from components within the body, but it cannot synthesize 9 of the amino acids—called essential amino acids. They must be consumed in the diet. Everyone needs 8 of these amino acids: isoleucine, leucine, lysine, methionine, phenylalanine, threonine, tryptophan, and valine. Infants also need a 9th one, histidine. The percentage of protein the body can use to synthesize essential amino acids varies from protein to protein. The body can use 100% of the protein in egg and a high percentage of the proteins in milk and meats.

The body needs proteins to maintain and replace tissues and to function and grow. If the body is getting enough calories, it does not use protein for energy. If more protein is consumed than is needed, the body breaks the protein down and stores its components as fat.

The body contains large amounts of protein. Protein, the main building block in the body, is the primary component of most cells. For example, muscle, connective tissues, and skin are all built of protein.

Adults need to eat about 60 grams of protein per day (0.8 grams per kilogram of weight or 10 to 15% of total calories). Adults who are trying to build muscle need slightly more. Children also need more because they are growing.

Fats

Fats are complex molecules composed of fatty acids and glycerol. The body needs fats for growth and energy. It also uses them to synthesize hormones and other substances needed for the body's activities (such as prostaglandins). Fats are the slowest source of energy but the most energy-efficient form of food. Each gram of fat supplies the body with about 9 calories, more than twice that supplied by proteins or carbohydrates. Because fats are such an efficient form of energy, the body stores any excess energy as fat. The body deposits excess fat in the abdomen (omental fat) and under the skin (subcutaneous fat) to use when it needs more energy. The body may also deposit excess fat in blood vessels and within organs, where it can block blood flow and damage organs, often causing serious disorders.

Fatty Acids: When the body needs fatty acids, it can make (synthesize) certain ones. Others, called essential fatty acids, cannot be synthesized and must be consumed in the diet. The essential fatty acids make up about 7% of the fat consumed in a normal diet and about 3% of total calories (about 8 grams). They include linoleic acid and linolenic acid, which are present in certain vegetable oils. Eicosapentaenoic acid and docosahexaenoic acid, which are fatty acids essential for brain development, can be synthesized from linolenic acid. However, they also are present in certain marine fish oils, which are a more efficient source.

Linoleic acid and arachidonic acid are omega-6 fatty acids. Linolenic acid, eicosapentaenoic acid, and docosahexaenoic acid are omega-3 fatty acids. A diet rich in omega-3 fatty acids may reduce the risk of coronary artery disease. Lake trout and certain deep-sea fish contain large amounts of omega-3 fatty acids. In the United States, people tend to consume enough omega-6 fatty acids, which occur in the oils used in many processed foods, but not enough omega-3 fatty acids.

Kinds of Fat: There are different kinds of fat: monounsaturated, polyunsaturated, and saturated (see box on page 403). In general, saturated fats are more likely to increase cholesterol levels and increase the risk of atherosclerosis. Foods derived from animals commonly contain saturated fats, which tend to be solid at room temperature. Fats derived from plants commonly contain monounsaturated or polyunsaturated fatty acids, which tend to be liquid at room temperature. Palm and coconut oil are exceptions. They contain more saturated fats than other plant oils.

Trans fats (trans fatty acids) are a different category of fat. They are man-made, formed by adding hydrogen atoms (hydrogenation) to monounsaturated or polyunsaturated fatty acids. Fats may be partially or fully hydrogenated (or saturated with hydrogen atoms). In the United States, the main dietary source of trans fats is partially hydrogenated vegetable oils, present in many commercially prepared foods. Consuming trans fats may adversely affect cholesterol levels in the body and may contribute to the risk of atherosclerosis.

Fat in the Diet: Authorities generally recommend that fat be limited to less than 30% of daily total calories (or fewer than 90 grams per day) and that saturated fats and trans fats should be limited to less than 10%. When possible, monounsaturated fats and polyunsaturated fats, particularly omega-3 fats, should be substituted for saturated fats and trans fats. People with high cholesterol levels may need to reduce their total fat intake even more. When fat intake is reduced to 10% or less of daily total calories, cholesterol levels tend to decrease dramatically.

Vitamins and Minerals

Vitamins and minerals are essential nutrients. That is, they cannot be synthesized by the body and so must be consumed in the diet.

Vitamins are classified as water soluble—vitamin C and the eight members of the vitamin B complex—or fat soluble—vitamins A, D, E, and K (see page 917). Only vitamins A, E, and B_{12} are stored to any large extent in the body.

Some minerals are required in fairly large quantities (about 1 or 2 grams a day) and are considered

WHERE'S THE FAT?	
TYPE OF FAT	**SOURCE**
Monounsaturated	Avocado, olive, and peanut oils Peanut butter
Polyunsaturated	Canola, corn, soybean, sunflower, and many other liquid vegetable oils
Saturated	Meats, particularly beef Full-fat dairy products such as whole milk, butter, and cheese Coconut and palm oils Artificially hydrogenated vegetable oils
Omega-3 fatty acids	Flaxseed Lake trout and certain deep-sea fish, such as mackerel, salmon, herring, and tuna Green leafy vegetables Walnuts
Omega-6 fatty acids	Vegetable oils (including sunflower, safflower, corn, cottonseed, and soybean oils) Fish oils Egg yolks
Trans fats	Commercially baked foods, such as cookies, crackers, and doughnuts Some french fries and other fried foods Margarine Shortening Potato chips

COMPARING SOLUBLE AND INSOLUBLE FIBER

TYPE OF FIBER	SOURCES	FUNCTIONS
Soluble	Apples Barley Beans Citrus fruits Lentils Oat bran Oatmeal Pectin (from fruit) Psyllium Rice bran Strawberries	Helps moderate the changes in blood sugar and insulin levels that occur after eating a meal Helps reduce cholesterol levels May reduce the risk of coronary artery disease
Insoluble	Apples Brown rice Pears Prunes Many vegetables, including cabbage, root vegetables, and zucchini Whole grains and whole-grain breads and pastas	Provides bulk to feces and thus helps food move through the digestive tract, preventing constipation Helps eliminate cancer-causing substances produced by the bacteria in the large intestine Reduces pressure in the intestine, helping prevent diverticular disease Is helpful in losing weight because the body processes it slowly

macronutrients (see page 932). They include calcium, chloride, magnesium, phosphorus (occurring mainly as phosphate in the body), potassium, and sodium. Minerals required in small amounts (trace minerals) are considered micronutrients. They include chromium, copper, fluoride, iodine, iron, manganese, molybdenum, selenium, and zinc. Except for chromium, all of these minerals are incorporated into enzymes or hormones required in metabolism. Chromium helps the body keep blood sugar levels normal. Trace minerals such as arsenic, cobalt, fluoride, nickel, silicon, and vanadium, which may be essential in animal nutrition, have not been established as requirements in human nutrition. Fluoride helps stabilize the mineral content of bones and teeth by forming a stable compound with calcium and thus helps prevent tooth decay. All trace minerals are toxic at high levels, and some (arsenic, nickel, and chromium) can cause cancer.

Some vitamins (such as vitamins C and E) and minerals (such as selenium) act as antioxidants, as do other substances in fruits and vegetables (such as beta-carotene). Antioxidants protect cells against damage by free radicals, which are by-products of the normal activity of cells. Free radicals readily participate in chemical reactions—some useful to the body and some not—and are thought to contribute to such disorders as heart and blood vessel disorders and cancer. People who eat enough fruits and vegetables, which are rich in antioxidants, are less likely to develop heart and blood vessel disorders and certain cancers. However, whether these benefits are due to antioxidants, other substances in the fruits and vegetables, or other factors is not known.

Getting enough vitamins and minerals from foods is usually preferable to getting them from supplements. Foods, unlike supplements, contain other substances necessary for good health. However, always eating a healthy, well-balanced diet may be difficult. So taking a multivitamin that contains the recommended daily allowances for vitamins and minerals is a good idea, particularly when a healthy diet may not be possible.

Fiber

Some foods contain fiber, which is a tough complex carbohydrate. Fiber may be partly soluble: It dissolves in water, and the body may be able to digest some of it. Or it may be insoluble: It does not dissolve in water, and the body cannot digest it. Eating too much insoluble fiber can interfere with absorption of certain vitamins and minerals.

Authorities generally recommend that about 30 grams of fiber be consumed daily. In the United States, the average amount of fiber consumed daily is about 12 grams because people tend to eat products made with highly refined wheat flour and do not eat many fruits and vegetables. An average serving of fruit, a vegetable, or cereal contains 2 to 4 grams of fiber. Meat and dairy foods do not contain fiber.

> **? Did You Know...**
>
> Eating a lot of insoluble fiber (in such foods as brown rice, prunes, and many vegetables) can reduce the absorption of certain vitamins and minerals.

Food Additives and Contaminants

Additives: Substances, such as preservatives, emulsifiers, antioxidants, and stabilizers, are often added to a food to do the following:

- Enable it to be processed more easily
- Preserve it longer and reduce spoilage
- Prevent contamination by microorganisms and thus prevent food-borne disorders
- Improve taste, add color, or enhance its aroma, making it more appealing

In commercially prepared foods, the amount of additives that can be included is limited to that shown to be safe by laboratory tests. However, weighing the benefits of additives against the risks is often complex. For example, nitrite, which is used in cured meats, not only improves flavor but also inhibits the growth of bacteria that cause botulism. However, nitrite converts to nitrosamines, which can cause cancer in animals. On the other hand, the amount of nitrite added to cured meat is small compared with the amount of nitrates that occurs naturally in food and that is converted to nitrite by the salivary glands.

Rarely, some additives (such as sulfites) cause allergic reactions. Sulfites, which occur naturally in wines, are added to such foods as dried fruit and dried potatoes as a preservative.

Contaminants: Foods may be contaminated because the air, water, and soil are polluted, for example, by heavy metals (such as lead, cadmium, and mercury) or PCBs (polychlorinated biphenyls). PCBs used to be used as coolants and in many other products and are now present in the air, soil, and water in many places. Foods may be contaminated by pesticides, packaging

materials, or during cooking or processing. Foods may also be contaminated by drugs (such as antibiotics and growth hormone) that are given to animals.

Sometimes limited amounts of contaminants are allowed in foods because the contaminants cannot be completely eliminated without damaging the foods. Common contaminants include

- Pesticides
- Heavy metals
- Nitrates (in green leafy vegetables)
- Aflatoxins, produced by molds (in nuts and milk)
- Growth-promoting hormones (in dairy products and meat)

Levels that have not caused illness or other problems in people are considered safe. However, determining whether a small amount of a contaminant has caused a problem is very difficult. Thus, safe levels are often determined by general agreement rather than by hard evidence. Whether problems can result from consuming a small amount of some contaminants over a long time is unclear, although with very tiny amounts such problems are unlikely. If problems occur, they probably affect only a few people.

Foods may contain animal hairs, animal feces, and insect parts in such tiny amounts that removal is impossible.

Calories

A calorie is a measure of energy. Foods have calories. That is, foods supply the body with energy, which is released when foods are broken down during digestion. Energy enables cells to do all of their functions, including building proteins and other substances needed by the body. The energy can be used immediately or stored for use later.

When the supply of energy—the number of calories consumed in foods—exceeds the body's immediate needs, the body stores the excess energy. Most excess energy is stored as fat. Some is stored as carbohydrates, usually in the liver and muscles. As a result, weight is gained. An excess of only 200 calories per day for 10 days is likely to result in a weight gain of nearly 1/2 pound, mostly as fat.

> **? Did You Know...**
>
> After the first few pounds are lost, weight loss slows down when the body has burned all its stored carbohydrates and starts burning stored fat.

When too few calories are consumed for the body's needs, the body begins to use carbohydrates stored in

How Are Calories in Foods Measured?

Food labels contain the number of calories per serving. But how is this number determined? The answer is surprisingly simple: The food is burned. A sample of the food is placed in an insulated, oxygen-filled chamber that is surrounded by water. This chamber is called a bomb calorimeter. The sample is burned completely. The heat from the burning increases the temperature of the water, which is measured and which indicates the number of calories in the food. For example, if water temperature increases by 20 degrees, the food contains 20 calories. This method of measuring calories is called direct calorimetry.

the liver and muscle. Because the body mobilizes stored carbohydrates quickly and because water is usually excreted as carbohydrates are mobilized, weight loss tends to be fast initially. However, the small amount of stored carbohydrates provides energy for only a short time. Next, the body uses stored fat. Because fat contains more energy per pound, weight loss is slower as the body uses fat for energy. However, the amount of fat stored is much larger and can, in most people, provide energy for a long time. Only during prolonged, severe shortages of energy, does the body break down protein. If normally nourished people experience total starvation (when no food is consumed), death occurs in 8 to 12 weeks.

Energy requirements vary markedly from about 1,000 to more than 4,000 calories a day depending on age, sex, weight, physical activity, disorders present, and the rate at which people burn calories (metabolic rate). However, typically, the number of calories needed per day to maintain body weight is about

- 1,600 for sedentary women, young children, and older adults
- 2,000 for older children, active adult women, and sedentary men
- 2,400 for active adolescent boys and young men

The division of caloric intake by a 24-hour period (daily intake) is arbitrary. Also, the needs of the body vary depending on its activity at any particular time. Vigorous activity, especially aerobic exercise, increases needs substantially, and a lack of activity decreases needs.

Nutritional Requirements

General guidelines for a healthy diet have been developed even though daily nutritional requirements, including those for essential nutrients, vary depending

on age, sex, height, weight, physical activity, and the rate at which the body burns calories (metabolic rate). Recommended dietary allowances for protein, vitamins (see table on page 918), and minerals (see table on page 934) are periodically published by The Food and Nutrition Board of the National Academy of Sciences–National Research Council and the U.S. Department of Agriculture. These allowances are intended to meet the needs of healthy people.

The U.S. Department of Agriculture also provides an interactive tool at www.mypyramid.gov. It enables people to enter information about themselves (their age, sex, activity level, and foods usually eaten) so that they can evaluate their diet and get recommendations about healthful foods and portion sizes that can help them reach and maintain a healthy weight. The amount of food needed each day from each food group varies depending on the person's energy needs.

In general, authorities recommend that fat intake be reduced to about 30% of calories or less and the intake of fruits, vegetables, and cereals be higher than most Americans eat. Drinking enough fluids is also important.

Diets

A diet is whatever a person eats, regardless of the goal—whether it is losing weight, gaining weight, reducing fat intake, avoiding carbohydrates, or having no particular goal. However, the term is often used to imply a goal of losing weight, which is an obsession for many people.

Standard healthy diets for children and adults are based on the needs of average people who have certain characteristics:

- They do not need to lose or gain weight.
- They do not need to restrict any component of the diet because of disorders, risk, or advanced age.
- They expend average amounts of energy through exercise or other vigorous activities.

Thus, for a particular person, a healthy diet may vary substantially from what is recommended in standard diets. For example, special diets are required by people who have diabetes, certain kidney or liver disorders, coronary artery disease, high cholesterol levels, osteoporosis, diverticular disease, chronic constipation, or food sensitivities. There are special dietary recommendations for young children, but little guidance is available for other age groups, such as older people.

WEIGHT LOSS DIETS

Weight loss requires consuming fewer calories than the body uses. Losing ½ pound of fat by dieting

SPOTLIGHT ON AGING

The best diet for older people has not been determined. However, older people may benefit from changing some aspects of their diet, based on the way the body changes as it ages. No changes are required for some nutrients such as carbohydrates and fats.

- **Calories:** As people age, they tend to be less active and thus use less energy, making it easier to gain weight. If they try to consume fewer calories to avoid weight gain, they may not get all the nutrients needed— particularly vitamins and minerals. If older people stay physically active, their need for calories may not change.

- **Protein:** As people age, they tend to lose muscle. If older people do not consume enough protein, they may lose even more muscle. For older people who have problems eating (for example, because of difficulty swallowing or dental disorders), protein can be consumed in foods that are easier to chew than meat, such as fish, dairy products, eggs, peanut butter, beans, and soy products.

- **Fiber:** Eating enough fiber can help counter the slowing of the digestive tract that occurs as people age. Older people should eat 8 to 12 servings of high-fiber foods daily. Getting fiber from foods is best, but fiber supplements, such as psyllium, may be needed.

- **Vitamins and minerals:** Older people may need to take supplements of specific vitamins and minerals in addition to a multivitamin. Calcium, vitamin D, and vitamin B_{12} are examples. Getting enough calcium and vitamin D from the diet is difficult. These nutrients are needed to maintain strong bones, which are particularly important for older people. Some older people do not absorb enough vitamin B_{12} even though they consume enough in foods because the stomach and intestine become less able to remove vitamin B_{12} from food or to absorb it. Older people with this problem can absorb vitamin B_{12} better when it is given as a supplement.

- **Water:** As people age, they are more likely to become dehydrated because their ability to sense thirst decreases. Thus, older people need to make a conscious effort to drink enough fluids rather than wait until they feel thirsty.

- Older people are more likely to have disorders or take drugs that can change the body's nutritional needs or the body's ability to meet those needs. Disorders and drugs can decrease appetite or interfere with the absorption of nutrients. When older people see their doctor, they should ask their doctor whether the disorders they have or the drugs they take affect nutrition in any way.

requires 10 days of consuming 200 fewer calories or 5 to 7 days of consuming 400 fewer calories per day than the body uses. One pound of body fat stores about 3,500 calories.

Most conservative weight loss diets involve consuming at least 1,200 to 1,400 calories a day. When rapid weight loss is needed, fewer than 1,200 calories may be consumed, but only for a short time. Such diets often have too little of essential nutrients, such as protein, iron, and calcium. Consuming fewer than 800 calories does not increase the amount of weight lost and is harder to tolerate.

To be healthy, weight loss diets should provide about the same volume of food (by including more fiber and fluids) as the normal diet. They should also be low in saturated fat and sugar and include essential nutrients, including antioxidants. The following general guidelines may help people lose weight:

- **Reading food labels:** People learn what nutrients and how many calories food, including beverages, contains. Then, people can plan their diet more effectively.

- **Counting calories:** People keep track of the number of calories they eat. This strategy helps people control calorie intake.

- **Choosing nutrient-rich, low-calorie foods:** When fewer calories are consumed, getting the needed nutrients—particularly vitamins and minerals—is more difficult. So people should choose foods that contain many nutrients but not many calories. Whole-grain cereals and whole-grain breads that are fortified with vitamins are good choices. Fruits and vegetables that are deeply colored (such as strawberries, peaches, broccoli, spinach, and squash) tend to contain more nutrients than those that are less deeply colored.

- **Eating small meals frequently:** This strategy can help with weight loss for several reasons. Insulin levels usually increase after eating, and more insulin is produced when many calories are consumed, especially when the meal is rich in carbohydrates. High insulin levels promote the deposition of fat and increase appetite. Eating small, frequent meals prevents insulin levels from increasing, thus discouraging fat deposition and helping suppress appetite.

- **Eating certain types of foods at certain times of the day:** For example, fast-energy foods, such as carbohydrates, are best eaten when the body needs a large supply of energy—that is, in the morning and during vigorous exercise. The body's need for energy is lowest at night, so avoiding carbohydrates in the evening may help.

- **Using sugar and fat substitutes:** Such substitutes and foods that contain them can sometimes help people reduce calorie intake. However, in some cases, sugar substitutes have effects on metabolism that slow the rate of weight loss.

- **Exercising:** Combining increased exercise with dieting greatly enhances weight loss because exercise increases the number of calories the body uses. For example, vigorous walking burns about 4 calories per minute, so that 1 hour of brisk walking per day burns about 240 calories. Running is even better, burning about 6 to 8 calories per minute.

> **? Did You Know...**
> Regardless of the weight loss diet followed, people must consume fewer calories than the body uses to lose weight.

Many people follow a specific diet to lose weight. **High Protein–Low Carbohydrate Diets:** Diets high in protein and low in simple carbohydrates have become popular as a way to lose weight. Most of these diets usually also restrict fat because each gram of fat supplies so many calories. However, some high protein–low carbohydrate diets, such as the Atkins diet, do not restrict fat.

The theory behind these diets is that slower-burning energy sources—protein and fat—provide a steady supply of energy and thus are less likely to lead to weight gain. In addition, people tend to feel full longer after eating protein than after eating carbohydrates because carbohydrates empty from the stomach quickly and are digested quickly. Carbohydrates also stimulate insulin production, which promotes fat deposition and increases appetite. However, the reason that these diets cause weight loss appears to be that people tire of the foods allowed by the diet and thus consume fewer calories.

Experts disagree about whether avoiding foods with a high glycemic index helps with weight loss, particularly in low-carbohydrate diets, or not. The effect of the glycemic index is less important when only a small percentage of total calories is carbohydrates. In a low-carbohydrate diet, the difference between how fast the carbohydrates in various foods (with their different glycemic indexes) are digested is sometimes so small that it makes little difference to most dieters. Avoiding foods with a high glycemic index also sometimes eliminates foods with valuable vitamins and minerals. Experts also disagree on how important the glycemic load (the glycemic index plus the amount of carbohydrate in a food) is for weight loss.

Some experts do not recommend following a high-protein diet for a long time. Some evidence suggests that over years, very high protein diets impair kidney function and may contribute to the decrease in kidney function that occurs in older people. People with certain kidney and liver disorders should not consume a high-protein diet. High-protein diets can speed the body's processing of certain drugs and thus may affect how well the drug works.

Very low carbohydrate diets (of less than 100 grams a day) can lead to the accumulation of keto acids (ketosis). When people do not consume enough energy for the body's needs, the body breaks down fats. As part of this process, the body produces keto acids. In small amounts, keto acids are easily excreted by the kidneys without causing symptoms. However, in large amounts, they can cause nausea, fatigue, bad breath, and even more serious symptoms, such as dizziness (due to dehydration) and abnormal heart rhythms (due to electrolyte imbalances). People following a low-carbohydrate diet (or any other weight loss diet) should drink large amounts of water to help flush keto acids from the body.

Low-carbohydrate diets tend to cause large amounts of weight to be lost during the first week or so, as the body converts stored carbohydrates (glycogen) to energy. As glycogen is broken down, the body also excretes large amounts of water, adding to the weight loss. However, once the body begins to use stored fat for energy, weight loss slows. People following a low-carbohydrate diet may substitute fats for the carbohydrates they are avoiding. In such cases, the diet may be so high in fat that the total caloric intake exceeds what the body uses. In such cases, weight loss stops after glycogen is used up.

Low-Fat Diets: Fat supplies a large number of calories per gram and is more readily deposited as body fat than are proteins and carbohydrates. Reducing the amount of fat rather than the amount of protein or carbohydrate may be an easier way to reduce total caloric intake because a small reduction in fat saves so many calories. A reduction of only 10 grams of fat per day saves about 90 calories. However, the best reason for reducing the amount of fat in the diet is to lower cholesterol levels in the blood (see page 961). Lowering cholesterol levels benefits most dieters because weight increases their risk of atherosclerosis, which can lead to heart attacks or stroke. Because lowering cholesterol levels can help prevent or delay atherosclerosis, a low-fat diet tends to be the best weight loss diet for overall health.

High-Fiber Diets: Fiber indirectly helps with weight loss in several ways:

- It provides bulk, which makes people feel full faster.
- It slows the rate at which the stomach empties so people feel full longer.
- It requires more chewing, forcing people to eat more slowly and perhaps less.

High-fiber foods, such as fruits and vegetables, wheat bread, and beans, are filling without providing many calories. Eating more high-fiber foods may enable people to eat fewer less filling, high-calorie foods, such as high-fat foods. However, fiber supplements, such as guar gum and cellulose, are not effective for weight loss.

Liquid Diets: Many people use liquid diets to lose weight, mainly because they are convenient. However, the contents of such liquids vary, and many are unlikely to be of much help in losing weight. Some commercially available liquid diets are well-balanced, with appropriate proportions of protein, carbohydrates, and fat plus supplemental vitamins and minerals. But others contain a large proportion of carbohydrates, producing a sweet and tasty drink,

and are not necessarily low in calories. Such liquid diets are more useful as a supplement to other foods for people who are trying to gain weight.

Usually, a commercial liquid-diet serving (a drink) contains 220 calories, and a drink is consumed 4 times a day instead of meals. Such diets are effective for short-term weight loss. For long-term weight loss, two or three meals are replaced with a liquid-diet drink. The remaining one or two meals should be low-fat, low-calorie, and nutritious.

An alternative to commercial diets is the all-milk diet. This diet is simple and inexpensive and may be useful for short-term weight loss.

Grapefruit Diet: One popular fad diet involves consuming large amounts of grapefruit and grapefruit juice. The theory behind this diet is that grapefruit contains an enzyme that helps burn fat, but this theory has never been proved.

Although grapefruits are a healthful food—containing no fat, little sodium, and large amounts of vitamin C, beta-carotene (at least in pink grapefruits), and fiber—a diet based primarily on one fruit is nutritionally unsound. A grapefruit diet may help some people reduce total caloric intake, but it does not supply a balance of nutrients, which is needed for good health. Furthermore, eating grapefruit alters the levels of several drugs in the blood (see table on page 92), and eating large amounts of grapefruit often causes diarrhea.

Food-Combining and Food-Cycling Diets: These fad diets are based on a theory that eating certain

SOME FAD DIETS

TYPE OF DIET	WEIGHT LOSS APPROACH	DISADVANTAGES
Atkins	High-protein Low-carbohydrate 2,000 calories a day	Is particularly high in fat and cholesterol
Beverly Hills	Low-fat Low-protein High-carbohydrate	Is deficient in protein, iron, calcium, zinc, and vitamin B_{12}
Pritikin	Low-fat Low-protein High-carbohydrate	Unpalatable and less likely to be followed because it is so low-fat
Rice	Low-fat Low-protein High-carbohydrate	Is deficient in protein, iron, calcium, zinc, and vitamin B_{12}
Richard Simmons	Low-calorie (900 calories a day)	Causes deficiencies in iron, calcium, protein, and vitamins A, thiamin (B_1), riboflavin (B_2), and niacin (B_3) if it is followed a long time

kinds of foods at different times promotes weight loss. An example is the Beverly Hills Diet, which recommends cycling different foods, usually over a 6-week period. For part of the time, people eat nothing but fruits. Later, people eat only breads, then only protein, then only fats. No scientific evidence supports this approach to weight loss, and the diet is intrinsically unhealthful.

Fad Diets: There are many fad diets, including some of the above. Many fad diets promise quick weight loss and do not provide any scientific evidence of their effectiveness. Some require extreme reductions in the number of calories consumed. Others rely on supplements alleged to help burn fat. Still others are based on eating a single type of food. These diets have not been shown to lead to sustained weight loss, and many are dangerous. They provide inadequate amounts of essential nutrients and, over time, can lead to serious metabolic disturbances, such as loss of bone density and strength (including osteoporosis), problems with menstruation, abnormal heart rhythms, high cholesterol levels, kidney stones, and worsening of gout.

Undernutrition

Undernutrition is a deficiency of calories or of one or more essential nutrients.

Undernutrition is usually thought of as a deficiency primarily of calories (that is, overall food consumption) or of protein. Deficiencies of vitamins and minerals are usually considered separate disorders. However, when calories are deficient, vitamins and minerals are likely to be also. Undernutrition, which is often used interchangeably with malnutrition, is actually a type of malnutrition. Malnutrition is an imbalance between the nutrients the body needs and the nutrients it gets. Thus, malnutrition also includes overnutrition (consumption of too many calories or too much of any specific nutrient—protein, fat, vitamin, mineral, or other dietary supplement).

In developed countries, undernutrition is usually far less common than overnutrition. However, undernutrition does occur, especially in people who are very poor, such as the homeless, and in those who have psychiatric disorders. Also, people who are very ill may be unable to eat enough food because they have lost their appetite or because their body's need for nutrients is greatly increased. Infants, children, and adolescents are at risk of undernutrition because they are growing and thus need a lot of calories and nutrients.

Undernutrition also occurs in older people. About 1 of 7 older people who live in the community consume fewer than 1,000 calories a day—not enough for adequate nutrition. As many as half of older people in hospitals and long-term care facilities do not consume enough calories.

When not enough calories are consumed, the body first breaks down its own fat and uses it for calories—much like burning the furniture to keep a house warm. After fat stores are used up, the body may break down its other tissues, such as muscle and tissues in internal organs, leading to serious problems, including death.

A severe deficiency of protein and calories (called protein-energy undernutrition or protein-energy malnutrition) results when people do not consume enough protein and calories for a long time.

In developing countries, protein-energy undernutrition often occurs in children. It contributes to death in more than half of children who die (for example, by increasing the risk of developing life-threatening infections and, if they develop, increasing their severity). However, this disorder can affect anyone, regardless of age, if food supplies are inadequate. Protein-energy undernutrition has two main forms:

> **? Did You Know...**
>
> About 1 of 7 older people who live in the community and about half of older people in long-term care facilities have undernutrition.
>
> Drinking too much alcohol can cause undernutrition.

Marasmus: Marasmus is a severe deficiency of calories and protein. It tends to develop in infants and very young children. It typically results in weight loss and dehydration. Breastfeeding usually protects against marasmus.

Starvation is the most extreme form of marasmus (and undernutrition). It results from a partial or total lack of essential nutrients for a long time.

HOW STARVATION AFFECTS THE BODY

BODY AREA AFFECTED	EFFECTS
Digestive system	Decreased production of stomach acid Shrinking of the stomach Frequent, often fatal, diarrhea
Cardiovascular system (heart and blood vessels)	Reduced heart size, reduced amount of blood pumped, slow heart rate, and low blood pressure Ultimately, heart failure
Respiratory system	Slow breathing and reduced lung capacity Ultimately, respiratory failure
Reproductive system	Reduced size of ovaries and testes Loss of sex drive (libido) Cessation of menstrual periods
Nervous system	Apathy and irritability In children, mental retardation (sometimes) Mental dysfunction, particularly in older people
Muscles	Reduced muscle size and strength, impairing the ability to exercise or work
Blood	Anemia
Metabolism (body processes to convert food into energy or to synthesize needed substances)	Low body temperature (hypothermia) Fluid accumulation in the arms, legs, and abdomen Disappearance of fat
Skin and hair	Thin, dry, inelastic skin Dry, sparse hair that falls out easily
Immune system	Impaired ability to fight infections and repair wounds

Kwashiorkor: Kwashiorkor is a severe deficiency more of protein than of calories. Kwashiorkor is less common than marasmus. The term is derived from an African word meaning "first child-second child" because a first-born child often develops kwashiorkor when the second child is born and replaces the first-born child at the mother's breast. Because children tend to develop kwashiorkor after they are weaned, they are usually older than those who have marasmus. Kwashiorkor tends to be confined to certain areas of the world where staple foods and foods used to wean babies are deficient in protein even though they provide enough calories as carbohydrates. Examples of such foods are yams, cassava, rice, sweet potatoes, and green bananas. However, anyone can develop kwashiorkor if their diet consists mainly of carbohydrates. People with kwashiorkor retain fluid, making them appear puffy and swollen. If kwashiorkor is severe, the abdomen may protrude.

Causes

Undernutrition may result from the following:

- Lack of access to food
- Disorders or drugs that interfere with the intake, metabolism or absorption of nutrients
- A greatly increased need for calories

Taking certain drugs may contribute to undernutrition. Many drugs decrease appetite. Examples are drugs used to treat high blood pressure (such as diuretics), heart failure (such as digoxin), or cancer (such as cisplatin). Some drugs cause nausea, which decreases appetite. Others (such as thyroxine and theophylline) increase metabolism, and still others may interfere with the absorption of certain nutrients in the intestine. Also, stopping certain drugs (such as antianxiety drugs and antipsychotics) or alcohol may lead to weight loss.

Drinking too much alcohol, which has calories but little nutritional value, decreases the appetite. Because alcohol damages the liver, it can also interfere with the absorption and use of nutrients. Smoking dulls taste and smell, making food less appealing. Smoking also seems to cause other changes in the body that contribute to a low body weight. For example, smoking stimulates the sympathetic nervous system, which increases the body's use of energy.

In older people, many factors, including age-related changes in the body, work together to cause undernutrition.

Symptoms

The most obvious sign of a calorie deficiency is loss of body fat (adipose tissue).

If the calorie deficiency is severe, adults can lose up to half of their body weight, and children can lose even more. Bones protrude, and the skin becomes thin, dry, inelastic, pale, and cold. Eventually, fat in the face is lost, causing the cheeks to look hollow and the eyes to seem sunken. The hair becomes dry and sparse, falling out easily. Severe wasting away of muscle and fat tissue is called cachexia. Cachexia is thought to result from excess production of substances called cytokines, which are produced by the immune system in response to a disorder, such as cancer or AIDS.

Other symptoms include fatigue, an inability to stay warm, diarrhea, loss of appetite, irritability, and apathy, sometimes leading to unresponsiveness (stupor). People feel weak, unable to do their normal activities. The number of some types of white blood cells decreases, resembling what happens in people who have AIDS. As a result, the immune system is weakened, increasing the risk of infections. If the calorie deficiency continues for a long time, liver, heart, and respiratory failure may develop. Total starvation (when no food is consumed) is fatal in 8 to 12 weeks.

In children who are severely undernourished, behavioral development may be markedly slow, and mental retardation may occur. Undernutrition, even when treated, may have long-lasting effects in children. Impairments in mental function and digestive problems may persist, sometimes throughout life. With treatment, most adults recover fully.

Diagnosis

Doctors can usually diagnose severe, long-standing undernutrition based on the person's appearance. They also ask questions about diet, weight loss, the ability to shop for and prepare food, the presence of other disorders, and the use of drugs. These questions may help confirm the diagnosis,

---

Causes of Undernutrition

LACK OF ACCESS TO FOOD

- Poverty
- Famine
- Inability to obtain food (for example, due to lack of transportation or physical impairment)
- Voluntary restriction of calories (as for a strict reducing diet or a fast)

DISORDERS THAT INTERFERE WITH THE INTAKE, METABOLISM, OR ABSORPTION OF NUTRIENTS

- Vomiting
- Diarrhea
- AIDS
- Cancer
- Diabetes
- Kidney failure
- Malabsorption disorders
- Inflammatory bowel disorders (such as Crohn's disease and ulcerative colitis)
- Liver disorders
- Anorexia nervosa
- Depression
- Alcoholism
- Drug abuse

DRUGS THAT INTERFERE WITH THE INTAKE, METABOLISM, OR ABSORPTION OF NUTRIENTS

- Drugs used to treat anxiety, high blood pressure, heart failure, an underactive thyroid gland, asthma, and cancer

CONDITIONS THAT GREATLY INCREASE THE NEED FOR CALORIES

- Injury, such as burns
- Surgery
- An overactive thyroid gland (hyperthyroidism)
- Infections that are widespread or severe
- High fever
- Demanding exercise, such as rehabilitation or training for athletic competition
- Pregnancy and breastfeeding
- Growth and development in infants, children, and adolescents

---

particularly when undernutrition is less obvious, and identify a cause. Identifying the cause is particularly important in children.

Blood tests may be done to measure the level of albumin (which decreases when people do not consume enough protein) and the number of certain types of white blood cells. A physical examination, x-rays, and skin tests may be done to determine the severity and effects of undernutrition. If doctors suspect the cause is another disorder, other tests may be done to help identify the cause.

Treatment

For most people, treatment involves gradually increasing the number of calories consumed. Eating several small, nutritious meals each day is the best way. For people who have been starving, foods are reintroduced carefully. People who have difficulty digesting solid food may need liquid supplements. If undernutrition is severe, people may need to be hospitalized. Multivitamin supplements are also given.

Nutrients are given by mouth whenever possible. If they cannot be given by mouth, nutrients may be given through a tube inserted into the digestive tract or into a vein (intravenously).

Tube Feeding: This method may be used to feed people whose digestive tract is functioning normally but who cannot eat enough to meet their nutritional needs (such as people with severe burns) or who cannot swallow (such as some people who have had a stroke). For tube feeding, a thin plastic tube (a

SPOTLIGHT ON AGING

Undernutrition in older people is serious because it increases the risk and severity of fractures, problems after surgery, pressure sores, and infections.

Older people are at risk of undernutrition for many reasons:

Age-related changes in the body: In the aging body, production of and sensitivity to hormones (such as growth hormone, insulin, and androgens) change. As a result, the percentage of fat in the body increases. How the body produces and uses energy also changes. Older people tend to feel full sooner and have less of an appetite. Thus, they may eat less. They may also eat less because the ability to taste and smell decreases, reducing the enjoyment of food. The ability to absorb some nutrients is reduced.

Some older people produce less saliva, resulting in dental problems and difficulty swallowing.

Disorders: Many disorders that contribute to undernutrition are common among older people. Depression can cause loss of appetite. A stroke or tremors may make chewing, swallowing, or preparing food difficult. Arthritis or other physical impairments, which reduce the ability to move, may make shopping for and preparing food more difficult. Malabsorption disorders interfere with the absorption of nutrients. Cancer can reduce the appetite and increase the body's need for calories. People with dementia may forget to eat and so lose weight. People with advanced dementia cannot feed themselves and may resist attempts by others to feed them. Dental problems (such as ill-fitting dentures or gum disease) may make chewing and thus digesting food more difficult. Anorexia nervosa that has been present for a long time may be made worse by an event late in life, such as death of a partner or fear of aging.

Drugs: Many of the drugs used to treat disorders common among older people (such as depression, cancer, heart failure, and high blood pressure) can contribute to undernutrition. Drugs can increase the body's need for nutrients, change how the body uses nutrients, or decrease the appetite. Some drugs have side effects that interfere with eating, such as nausea, diarrhea, and constipation.

Living situation: Older people who live alone may be less motivated to prepare and eat meals. They may have limited funds, causing them to buy cheap, less nutritious food or less total food. They may be physically unable or afraid to go out to buy food or may not have transportation to a grocery store.

- They may be confused and unable to say when they are hungry or what they would like to eat.
- They may be unable to choose foods they like.
- They may be unable to feed themselves.
- If they eat slowly, especially if they need to be fed by a staff member, the staff member may not allow enough time to feed them adequately.

Older people who are hospitalized sometimes have the same problems.

Prevention and treatment: Older people can be encouraged to eat more, and food can be made more appealing. For example, strongly flavored or favorite foods, rather than low-salt or low-fat foods, can be served. Older people who need help with feeding should be given more help. Depression and other disorders, if present, should be treated. For older people living in institutions, making the dining room more attractive and giving them more time to eat may enable them to eat more.

nasogastric tube) is passed through the nose and down the throat until it reaches the stomach or small intestine. If tube feeding is needed for a long time, the tube can be inserted directly into the stomach or small intestine through a small incision in the abdomen.

Food given through a tube (enteral nutrition) should contain all the nutrients a person needs. Special solutions, including some for people with specific needs (such as restriction of fluid intake), are available. Or, solid foods may be processed and given through a nasogastric tube. Tube feedings may be given slowly and continuously or in a larger amount (called a bolus) every few hours.

Tube feeding causes many problems, and the problems may be life threatening:

- Inhalation (aspiration) of food into the lungs: For older people, aspiration is the most common problem caused by tube feeding. Aspiration of food can lead to pneumonia. Food is less likely to be aspirated when the head of the bed is elevated for 1 to 2 hours after tube feeding, reducing the risk of spitting food up (regurgitation), and when the solution is given slowly.

- Diarrhea and abdominal discomfort: Changing the solution or giving it more slowly may lessen these problems.

- Irritation of tissues: The tube may irritate and erode tissues of the nose, throat, or esophagus. If tissues become irritated, the feeding tube can usually be removed, and feedings can be continued using a different type of tube.

Intravenous Feeding: This method is used when the digestive tract cannot adequately absorb nutrients (for example, in people with a malabsorption disorder). It is also used when the digestive tract must be temporarily kept free of food (for example, in people with ulcerative colitis or severe pancreatitis). Food given intravenously (parenteral nutrition) can supply part of a person's nutritional requirements (partial parenteral nutrition) or all of them (total parenteral nutrition). Because total parenteral nutrition requires a large intravenous tube (cathe-

ter), it is inserted into a large vein, such as the subclavian vein, located under the collarbone.

Intravenous feeding can also cause problems:

- Infection: Infection is a constant risk because the catheter is usually left in place for a long time and the solutions that pass through it contain a lot of glucose—a sugar—which promotes the growth of bacteria. People receiving total parenteral nutrition are closely monitored for signs of infection.

- Too much water (volume overload): Giving too much water can cause fluid to collect in the lungs, making breathing difficult. Thus, doctors monitor the person's weight and the amount of urine excreted regularly. They can sometimes reduce the risk by calculating the amount of water required before starting feedings.

- Nutritional imbalances and deficiencies: Rarely, deficiencies of certain vitamins and minerals occur. Doctors measure the blood levels of dissolved minerals (electrolytes), sugar (glucose), and urea (a measure of kidney function) to identify certain nutritional imbalances. They can then adjust the solution accordingly. They periodically monitor the levels.

- Decreased bone density: In some people, total parenteral nutrition causes bone density to decrease. The reason is unknown, and the best treatment is to temporarily or permanently stop this type of feeding.

- Liver problems: Total parenteral nutrition can cause liver malfunction, most commonly in premature infants. Blood tests are done to monitor liver function.

- Gallbladder problems: Gallstones may develop. Treatment involves adjusting the solution, stopping feedings for a few hours a day, and, if possible, providing food by mouth or feeding tube.

Drugs: People who are very undernourished are sometimes given drugs to increase appetite, such as dronabinol or megestrol, or drugs to increase muscle mass, such as growth hormone or an anabolic steroid (for example, nandrolone or testosterone).

138 Vitamins

Vitamins are a vital part of a healthy diet. The recommended dietary allowance (RDA)—the amount most healthy people need each day to remain healthy—has been determined for most vitamins. A

safe upper limit (tolerable upper intake level) has been determined for some vitamins. Intake above this limit increases the risk of a harmful effect (toxicity).

Consuming too little of a vitamin can cause a nutritional disorder. However, people who eat a variety of foods are unlikely to develop most vitamin deficiencies.

Deficiency of vitamin D is an exception. It is common among certain groups of people (such as older people) even if they eat a variety of foods. For other vitamins,

VITAMINS				
VITAMIN	**GOOD SOURCES**	**MAIN FUNCTIONS**	**RECOMMENDED DIETARY ALLOWANCE**	**SAFE UPPER LIMIT**
Biotin	Liver, kidneys, egg yolks, milk, fish, dried yeast, cauliflower, nuts, and legumes	Required for the metabolism of carbohydrates and fatty acids	30 micrograms (but no RDA has been established)	—
Folate (folic acid)	Fresh green leafy vegetables, asparagus, broccoli, fruits (especially citrus), liver, other organ meats, dried yeast, and enriched breads, pastas, and cereals (Note: Extensive cooking destroys 50–95% of the folate in food.)	Required for the formation of red blood cells, for DNA and RNA synthesis, and for normal development of the nervous system in a fetus	400 micrograms 600 micrograms for pregnant women 500 micrograms for breastfeeding women	1,000 micrograms
Niacin (nicotinic acid or nicotinamide)	Dried yeast, liver, meat, fish, legumes, and whole-grain or enriched cereal products	Required for the metabolism of carbohydrates, fats, and many other substances	14 milligrams for women 16 milligrams for men	35 milligrams
Pantothenic acid	Liver, beef, egg yolks, yeast, potatoes, broccoli, and whole grains	Required for the metabolism of carbohydrates and fats	5 milligrams (but no RDA has been established)	—
Riboflavin (vitamin B_2)	Milk, cheese, liver, meat, fish, eggs, and enriched cereals	Required for the metabolism of carbohydrates and amino acids and for healthy mucous membranes, such as those lining the mouth	1.1 milligrams for women 1.3 milligrams for men 1.4 milligrams for pregnant women 1.6 milligrams for breastfeeding women	—
Thiamin (vitamin B_1)	Dried yeast, whole grains, meat (especially pork and liver), enriched cereals, nuts, legumes, and potatoes	Required for the metabolism of carbohydrates and for normal nerve and heart function	1.1 milligrams for women 1.2 milligrams for men 1.4 milligrams for pregnant or breastfeeding women	—
Vitamin A (retinol)	As vitamin A: Fish liver oils, liver, egg yolks, butter, cream, and fortified milk As carotenoids (converted to vitamin A in the body), such as beta-carotene: Dark green and yellow-orange vegetables, and yellow-orange fruits	Required to form light-sensitive nerve cells (photoreceptors) in the retina, helping maintain night vision Helps maintain the health of the skin, cornea, and lining of the lungs, intestine, and urinary tract Helps protect against infections	700 micrograms for women 900 micrograms for men 770 micrograms for pregnant women 1,200 micrograms for breastfeeding women	3,000 micrograms

(continued on the following page)

VITAMINS (*Continued*)

VITAMIN	GOOD SOURCES	MAIN FUNCTIONS	RECOMMENDED DIETARY ALLOWANCE	SAFE UPPER LIMIT
Vitamin B_6	Dried yeast, liver, other organ meats, whole-grain cereals, fish, and legumes	Required for the metabolism of amino acids and fatty acids, for normal nerve function, for the formation of red blood cells, and for healthy skin	1.3 milligrams 1.5 milligrams for women older than 50 1.7 milligrams for men older than 50 1.9 milligrams for pregnant women 2.0 milligrams for breastfeeding women	100 milligrams
Vitamin B_{12} (cobalamins)	Meats (especially beef, pork, liver, and other organ meats), eggs, fortified cereals, milk, clams, oysters, salmon, and tuna	Required for the formation and maturation of red blood cells, for nerve function, and for DNA synthesis	2.4 micrograms 2.6 micrograms for pregnant women 2.8 micrograms for breastfeeding women	—
Vitamin C (ascorbic acid)	Citrus fruits, tomatoes, potatoes, broccoli, strawberries, and sweet peppers	Required for the formation, growth, and repair of bone, skin, and connective tissue; for healing of wounds and burns; and for normal function of blood vessels Acts as an antioxidant, protecting cells against damage by free radicals Helps the body absorb iron	75 milligrams for women 90 milligrams for men 85 milligrams for pregnant women 120 milligrams for breastfeeding women 35 milligrams more for smokers	2,000 milligrams
Vitamin D	Formed in the skin when the skin is exposed to direct sunlight Fortified milk, fatty fish, fish liver oils, and egg yolks	Promotes the absorption of calcium and phosphorus from the intestine Required for bone formation, growth, and repair. Strengthens the immune system and reduces the risk of autoimmune disorders	200 IU for people aged 50 and younger 400 IU for people aged 51 to 70 600 IU for people older than 70	2,000 IU
Vitamin E	Vegetable oil, margarine, nuts, and wheat germ	Acts as an antioxidant, protecting cells against damage by free radicals	15 milligrams (22 IU of natural or 33 IU of synthetic) 19 milligrams for breastfeeding women	1,000 milligrams
Vitamin K	Green leafy vegetables (such as collards, spinach, and kale) and soybean and canola oils	Helps in the formation of blood clotting factors and thus is necessary for normal blood clotting Required for healthy bones and other tissues	90 micrograms for women 120 micrograms for men	—

IU = international unit; DNA = deoxyribonucleic acid; RNA = ribonucleic acid.

deficiency can develop if people follow a restrictive diet that does not contain enough of a particular vitamin. For example, vegans, who consume no animal products, may become deficient in vitamin B_{12}, which is available in animal products. Consuming large amounts (megadoses) of certain vitamins (usually as supplements) without medical supervision may also have harmful effects.

Vitamins are called essential micronutrients because the body requires them but only in small amounts.

Some vitamins—A, D, E, and K—are fat soluble. Other vitamins—B vitamins and vitamin C—are water soluble. B vitamins include biotin, folate (folic acid), niacin, pantothenic acid, riboflavin (vitamin B_2), thiamin (vitamin B_1), and vitamins B_6 (pyridox-ine) and B_{12} (cobalamins). Deficiency of biotin or pantothenic acid almost never occurs.

The body does not store most vitamins. Therefore, people must consume them regularly. Vitamins A, B_{12}, and D are stored in significant amounts, mainly in the liver.

Disorders that impair the intestine's absorption of food (called malabsorption disorders) can cause vitamin deficiencies. Some disorders impair the absorption of fats. These disorders can reduce the absorption of fat-soluble vitamins—A, D, E, and K—and increase the risk of a deficiency. Such disorders include chronic diarrhea, Crohn's disease, cystic fibrosis, pancreatitis, and blockage of the bile ducts.

> **Did You Know...**
> Consuming very large doses of vitamins can be harmful.

Liver disorders and alcoholism can interfere with the processing (metabolism) or storage of vitamins. In a few people, hereditary disorders impair the way the body handles vitamins and thus cause a deficiency.

Drugs can also contribute to deficiency of a vitamin. They may interfere with absorption, metabolism, or storage of a vitamin.

Folate

Folate (folic acid), with vitamin B_{12}, is necessary for the formation of normal red blood cells and the synthesis of DNA (deoxyribonucleic acid), which is the genetic material of cells. Folate is also necessary for normal development of a fetus's nervous system. A low intake of folate may increase the risk of bone fractures in older adults. Whether folate supplementation can improve cognitive function in older adults remains unclear.

In the United States, folate is added to enrich foods made from grains. Folate in supplements or in enriched foods is easier for the body to absorb than the folate that occurs naturally in food.

FOLATE DEFICIENCY

- Not eating enough raw leafy vegetables and citrus fruits can cause folate deficiency.
- Anemia can develop, causing fatigue, paleness, irritability, shortness of breath, and dizziness.
- A severe deficiency may result in a red and sore tongue, a reduced sense of taste, weight loss, depression,

---

Vitamins: Fat Versus Water Soluble

Vitamins are classified as fat soluble:

- Vitamin A
- Vitamin D
- Vitamin E
- Vitamin K

or water soluble:

- B vitamins
- Vitamin C

This difference affects nutrition in several ways.

Fat-soluble vitamins: These vitamins dissolve in fats (lipids). They are stored in the liver and in fatty tissues. If too much of the fat-soluble vitamins A or D are consumed, they can accumulate and may have harmful effects.

Because fats in foods help the body absorb fat-soluble vitamins, a low-fat diet may result in a deficiency. Some disorders interfere with absorption of fats and thus of fat-soluble vitamins. Examples are chronic diarrhea, Crohn's disease, cystic fibrosis, pancreatitis, and blockage of the bile ducts. Some drugs, such as mineral oil, have the same effect. Fat-soluble vitamins dissolve in mineral oil, which the body does not absorb. So when people take mineral oil, it carries these vitamins unabsorbed out of the body.

Cooking does not destroy fat-soluble vitamins.

Water-soluble vitamins: These vitamins dissolve in water. They are eliminated in urine and tend to be eliminated from the body more quickly than fat-soluble vitamins. Water-soluble vitamins are more likely to be destroyed when food is stored and prepared. Refrigerating fresh produce, storing milk and grains out of strong light, and using the cooking water from vegetables to prepare soups can help prevent the loss of the vitamins.

SOME DRUGS THAT CAUSE VITAMIN DEFICIENCY

DRUG	VITAMIN	DRUG	VITAMIN
Alcohol	Folate Thiamin Vitamin B_6	Hydralazine	Vitamin B_6
		Levodopa	Vitamin B_6
Antacids	Vitamin B_{12}	Mineral oil (long-term use)	Folate Vitamin D Vitamin E Vitamin K
Antibiotics, such as isoniazid, tetracycline, and trimethoprim-sulfamethoxazole	B vitamins Folate Vitamin K		
		Metformin	Folate Vitamin B_{12}
Anticoagulants, such as warfarin	Vitamin E Vitamin K	Nitrous oxide (repeated exposure)	Vitamin B_{12}
Anticonvulsants, such as phenytoin and phenobarbital	Biotin Folate Vitamin B_6 Vitamin D Vitamin K	Oral contraceptives	Folate Thiamin Vitamin B_6
		Penicillamine	Vitamin B_6
Antipsychotic drugs	Riboflavin Vitamin D	Phenothiazines	Riboflavin
		Primidone	Folate Vitamin D
Barbiturates such as phenobarbital	Folate Riboflavin Vitamin D	Rifampin	Vitamin D Vitamin K
Chemotherapy drugs, such as methotrexate	Folate	Sulfasalazine	Folate
Cholestyramine	Many vitamins	Thiazide diuretics	Riboflavin
Corticosteroids	Vitamin C Vitamin D	Triamterene	Folate
Cycloserine	Vitamin B_6	Tricyclic antidepressants, such as amitriptyline and imipramine	Riboflavin

tingling or loss of sensation in the hands and feet, muscle weakness, loss of reflexes, difficulty walking, confusion, and dementia.

- The diagnosis is based on blood tests.
- Folate supplements taken by mouth usually correct the deficiency.

Because the body stores only a small amount of folate, a diet lacking in folate leads to a deficiency within a few months. Folate deficiency is common because many people do not eat enough raw leafy vegetables or citrus fruits. Also, prolonged cooking destroys much of the folate in food. Common causes of deficiency include undernutrition and alcoholism, particularly when combined. Alcohol consumed in large amounts interferes with the absorption and processing (metabolism) of folate. Malabsorption disorders interfere with absorption of folate. Certain anticonvulsants (such as phenytoin and phenobarbital) and drugs used to treat ulcerative colitis (such as sulfasalazine) decrease the absorption of this vitamin. Methotrexate (used to treat cancer and rheumatoid arthritis), triamterene (used to treat high blood pressure), metformin (used to treat diabetes), and trimethoprim-sulfamethoxazole (an antibiotic) interfere with the metabolism of folate.

Women who are pregnant or breastfeeding and people undergoing dialysis may develop this deficiency because their need for folate is increased.

Folate deficiency causes an anemia similar to that due to vitamin B_{12} deficiency.

Symptoms

Anemia develops gradually and may be more severe than symptoms suggest. Fatigue may be the first symptom. In addition to the general symptoms of anemia (such as paleness, irritability, shortness of breath, and dizziness), folate deficiency, if severe, may result in a red and sore tongue, a reduced sense of taste, weight loss, and depression. If a pregnant woman has folate deficiency, her infant may have a birth defect of the spinal cord or brain (neural tube defect).

Did You Know...

Cooking can destroy most of the folate in foods.

If a pregnant woman has folate deficiency, her fetus may have a birth defect of the brain or spinal cord.

Diagnosis

If a blood test detects large red blood cells in people who have anemia or who are undernourished, doctors measure the folate level in a blood sample. A low level indicates this deficiency. Doctors also measure the vitamin B_{12} level to rule out vitamin B_{12} deficiency because this deficiency can also result in anemia and large red blood cells.

Prevention and Treatment

As a preventive measure, people who are taking drugs that interfere with the absorption or metabolism of folate should take a folate supplement. Women who are pregnant or who could become pregnant should take folate supplements to reduce the risk of having an infant with a birth defect. Women who have had a baby with a neural tube defect are often prescribed higher doses of folate. Folate supplementation has not been proven to reduce cardiovascular disease but may reduce strokes.

Treatment consists of taking daily doses of a folate supplement by mouth.

FOLATE EXCESS

Folate is generally not toxic. If people with vitamin B_{12} deficiency take very high doses of folate, doctors may be delayed in recognizing the nerve damage due to vitamin B_{12} deficiency. Because the diagnosis is delayed, nerve damage may be more severe and more difficult to treat.

Niacin

Niacin (nicotinic acid) is essential for the metabolism of carbohydrates, fats, and many other substances in the body. Foods rich in tryptophan (an amino acid), such as dairy products, can compensate for not consuming enough niacin in the diet because the body can convert tryptophan to niacin.

Niacin is sometimes used in two ways: as a synonym for nicotinic acid and as a broader term that includes nicotinamide and nicotinic acid, two forms of this B vitamin.

NIACIN DEFICIENCY

- A distinctive dark red rash appears on the hands, feet, calves, neck, and face, and the tongue and mouth turn bright red.
- People have digestive tract problems, fatigue, insomnia, apathy, and later confusion and memory loss.
- The diagnosis is based on the diet history, symptoms, and sometimes urine tests.
- High doses of nicotinamide or nicotinic acid, taken by mouth, can correct the deficiency.

Niacin deficiency is uncommon in developed countries. It causes a disorder called pellagra, which affects the skin, digestive tract, and brain. Pellagra develops only if tryptophan is also deficient because the body can convert tryptophan to niacin. People who live in areas where maize (Indian corn) is the main food source are at risk of developing pellagra because maize is low in niacin and tryptophan. Furthermore, the niacin in maize cannot be absorbed in the intestine unless the maize is treated with alkali (as it is when tortillas are prepared). Pellagra may be a seasonal disorder, appearing each spring and lasting through the summer, when the diet consists mainly of maize products.

Alcoholics and other undernourished people are at risk of developing pellagra. Inadequate intake of iron, riboflavin, and vitamin B_6 increases the risk of niacin deficiency. Niacin deficiency may also occur when the antibiotic isoniazid is taken for a long time. Pellagra develops in people who have Hartnup disease, a rare hereditary disorder in which tryptophan absorption is impaired (see page 287).

Symptoms

Typically, people develop a symmetric, dark red rash that resembles a sunburn and becomes worse when it is exposed to sunlight (a condition called photosensitivity). The location of the rash is distinctive: on the hands (like gloves), on the feet and calves (like boots), around the neck (like a necklace), and on the face forming a butterfly shape. Skin abnormalities are persistent, and the affected areas may become brown and scaly.

The whole digestive tract is affected. The tongue and mouth may become inflamed and bright red. The tongue may swell, the mouth may burn, and sores may develop on both. The throat and esophagus may also burn. Other symptoms include nausea, vomiting, abdominal discomfort, constipation, and diarrhea (which may be bloody).

Later, fatigue, insomnia, and apathy develop. Malfunction of the brain (encephalopathy) usually follows. It is characterized by confusion, disorientation, hallucinations, and memory loss.

Diagnosis and Treatment

The diagnosis is based on the diet history and symptoms. Measuring a by-product of niacin in urine can help establish the diagnosis, but this test is not always available. The diagnosis is confirmed if nicotinamide relieves symptoms.

Pellagra is treated with daily doses of niacin taken by mouth. Supplements of other B vitamins are also taken.

NIACIN EXCESS

Nicotinic acid (but not nicotinamide) in high doses may be prescribed to lower high cholesterol and triglyceride (lipid) levels in the blood. Such doses can cause flushing, itching, gout, and liver damage (rarely) and increase the level of sugar (glucose) in the blood. Most side effects can be minimized by starting with a relatively low dose and gradually increasing the dose. Taking aspirin before taking nicotinic acid and taking nicotinic acid after meals also help. If the side effects of nicotinic acid are intolerable, the dose may be decreased, other (especially extended-release) formulations may be tried, or niacin may be stopped and another lipid-lowering drug substituted (see table on page 967).

Riboflavin

Riboflavin (vitamin B_2) is essential for the metabolism of carbohydrates (to produce energy) and amino acids. It also helps keep mucous membranes (such as those lining the mouth) healthy. Riboflavin is not toxic.

RIBOFLAVIN DEFICIENCY

- People have painful cracks in the corners of the mouth and on the lips, scaly patches on the head, and a magenta mouth and tongue.
- The diagnosis is based on symptoms, urine tests, and response to riboflavin supplements.
- High doses of riboflavin supplements, usually taken by mouth, can correct the deficiency.

Riboflavin deficiency usually occurs with deficiencies of other B vitamins. It usually results from not consuming enough protein and calories. Chronic disorders (such as recurrent diarrhea, liver disorders, and

chronic alcoholism) and malabsorption disorders increase the risk of riboflavin deficiency, as can hemodialysis and peritoneal dialysis—procedures that filter the blood (see page 265).

Symptoms

Symptoms may vary. Painful cracks form in the corners of the mouth and on the lips. The mouth and tongue are sore, and the tongue may turn magenta. Red, greasy, scaly (seborrheic) patches may appear around the nose, between the nose and the lips, on the ears and eyelids, and in the genital area.

Diagnosis and Treatment

The diagnosis is based on symptoms and evidence of general undernutrition (see page 915). The diagnosis is confirmed by measuring riboflavin excreted in urine or by giving riboflavin supplements, which relieve symptoms if deficiency is the cause.

As a preventive measure, people who are undergoing hemodialysis or peritoneal dialysis or who have a malabsorption disorder should take riboflavin supplements.

High doses of riboflavin are taken by mouth until symptoms resolve. If this treatment is ineffective, riboflavin can be given by injection into a muscle. Supplements of other B vitamins are also taken.

Thiamin

Thiamin (vitamin B_1) is widely available in the diet. It is essential for the metabolism of carbohydrates (to produce energy) and for normal nerve and heart function. Thiamin is not toxic.

THIAMIN DEFICIENCY

- A diet consisting mainly of white flour, white sugar, and other highly processed carbohydrates can cause thiamin deficiency.
- At first, people have vague symptoms such as fatigue and irritability, but a severe deficiency (beriberi) can affect the nerves, muscles, heart, and brain.
- The diagnosis is based on symptoms.
- Thiamin supplements, usually taken by mouth, can correct the deficiency.

Thiamin deficiency often occurs with other B vitamin deficiencies. It may result from a deficiency in the diet. People whose diet consists mainly of highly processed carbohydrates (such as polished white rice, white flour, and white sugar) are at risk of thiamin deficiency. Polishing rice removes almost all of the vitamins. Alcoholics, who often substitute alcohol for food and thus do not consume enough thiamin, are at high risk of developing this deficiency.

Thiamin deficiency may also result from disorders or conditions that increase the body's need for thiamin. Examples are thyroid disorders, pregnancy, breastfeeding, and fever. Liver disorders may interfere with the processing (metabolism) of the vitamin.

Symptoms

Early symptoms are vague. They include fatigue, irritability, poor memory, loss of appetite, sleep disturbances, abdominal discomfort, and weight loss. Eventually, a severe thiamin deficiency (beriberi) may develop, characterized by nerve, heart, and brain abnormalities. Different forms of beriberi cause different symptoms.

Dry Beriberi: Nerve and muscle abnormalities develop. Symptoms include a prickling (pins-and-needles) sensation in the toes, a burning sensation in the feet that is particularly severe at night, and leg cramps and pain. Muscles may become weak and waste away (atrophy).

Wet Beriberi: Heart abnormalities develop. The heart pumps more blood and beats faster. Blood vessels widen (dilate), making the skin warm and moist. Because the heart cannot continue to work at this level, heart failure eventually develops. As a result, fluid accumulates in the legs (as edema) and in the lungs (as congestion), and blood pressure may fall, leading to shock and death.

Brain Abnormalities: Thiamin deficiency causes brain abnormalities primarily in alcoholics. Brain abnormalities may first cause symptoms after an alcoholic binge by suddenly worsening a long-standing deficiency. Brain abnormalities can also cause symptoms after an alcoholic is given carbohydrates intravenously. Symptoms occur because these extra carbohydrates further increase thiamin requirements. These brain abnormalities are called the Wernicke-Korsakoff syndrome (see page 682), which has two parts:

- **Wernicke's encephalopathy** causes confusion, difficulty walking, and eye problems, including involuntary eye movements (nystagmus) and partial paralysis of the eyes. If Wernicke's encephalopathy is not promptly treated, symptoms may worsen, resulting in coma and even death.

- **Korsakoff's psychosis** causes memory loss for recent events, confusion, and a tendency to make up facts to fill in gaps in memories (confabulation).

Infantile Beriberi: This form occurs in infants (usually by age 3 to 4 wk) who are breastfed by a mother who has a thiamin deficiency. In these infants, heart failure may occur suddenly. They may lose their voice (aphonia) to some degree, and they may not have certain reflexes.

Diagnosis and Treatment

The diagnosis is based on symptoms. Tests to confirm the diagnosis are not readily available. Blood tests to measure electrolyte levels are usually done to exclude other possible causes. The diagnosis is confirmed if thiamin supplements relieve symptoms.

All forms of the deficiency are treated with thiamin supplements. They are usually given by mouth. They are given intravenously if symptoms are severe.

Wernicke-Korsakoff syndrome, a medical emergency, is treated with high doses of thiamin given intravenously or by injection into a muscle (intramuscularly) for several days. Use of alcohol should be stopped. When people who may be alcoholics must be fed intravenously, they are given thiamin supplements first to prevent the syndrome from developing or worsening.

With treatment, most people recover completely. In some people with Wernicke-Korsakoff syndrome, some brain damage is permanent. Symptoms of beriberi may recur years after apparent recovery.

Vitamin A

Vitamin A (retinol) is necessary for the function of light-sensitive nerve cells (photoreceptors) in the eye's retina. It also helps keep the skin and the lining of the lungs, intestine, and urinary tract healthy and protects against infections. Carotenoids, such as beta-carotene, are pigments in vegetables that give them their yellow, orange or red color. Once consumed, carotenoids are slowly converted to vitamin A in the body. Carotenoids are best absorbed from cooked or homogenized vegetables served with some fat or oil.

Drugs related to vitamin A (retinoids) are used to treat severe acne and psoriasis and are being investigated for the treatment of certain types of cancer.

VITAMIN A DEFICIENCY

- Night blindness is an early symptom.
- Blindness can eventually develop.
- The eyes, skin, and other tissues become dry and damaged, and infections develop more often.
- The diagnosis is based on symptoms and blood tests.
- Taking high doses of vitamin A for several days corrects the deficiency.

Vitamin A deficiency is common in areas of the world where people do not eat enough of certain foods:

- Animal and fish liver
- Orange, yellow, and green vegetables
- Eggs
- Fortified milk products

For example, the deficiency occurs in southern and eastern Asia, where rice is the main food. Disorders that impair the intestine's absorption of fats can reduce the absorption of vitamin A and increase the risk of vitamin A deficiency. Surgery on the intestine or pancreas can have the same effect. Liver disorders can interfere with the storage of vitamin A. Most multiple vitamins contain little or no vitamin A.

Did You Know...

Many multiple vitamins contain little or no vitamin A.

Symptoms

An early symptom of vitamin A deficiency is night blindness, which is caused by a disorder of the retina. Soon thereafter, the whites (conjunctiva) and corneas of the eyes may become dry—a condition called xerophthalmia. Xerophthalmia is particularly common among children who have a severe deficiency of calories (energy) or protein which includes an inadequate intake of vitamin A. Foamy deposits (Bitot's spots) may appear in the whites of the eyes. The dry cornea may soften and ulcerate, and blindness may result. Vitamin A deficiency is a common cause of blindness in developing countries.

The skin becomes dry and scaly, and the lining of the lungs, intestine, and urinary tract thicken and stiffen. The immune system does not function normally, making infections more likely, particularly in infants and children.

Children's growth and development may be slowed.

Diagnosis and Treatment

The diagnosis is based on symptoms and a low level of vitamin A in the blood.

If people have conditions that put them at risk of developing this deficiency, they should take vitamin A supplements.

People who have the deficiency are given high doses of vitamin A for several days. Infants should not be given high doses repeatedly because such doses can be toxic. If symptoms persist after 2 months, doctors usually check for a disorder that impairs fat absorption.

VITAMIN A EXCESS

- Consuming too much vitamin A causes hair loss, cracked lips, dry skin, weakened bones, headaches, and increased pressure in the brain.
- The diagnosis is based on symptoms and blood tests.

- Most people recover completely when they stop taking vitamin A supplements.

Too much vitamin A can cause toxicity. For example, taking daily doses 10 times the RDA (recommended daily allowance) or greater for a period of months can cause toxicity. Special formulations of high dose vitamin A may be taken to treat severe acne or other skin disorders. A smaller dose can cause toxicity in infants, sometimes within a few weeks. Sometimes children accidentally take a very high dose, and toxicity occurs quickly.

Carotenoids can be consumed in foods without causing toxicity because their conversion to vitamin A is very slow. However, when large amounts are consumed, the skin turns a deep yellow (carotenosis), especially on the palms and soles. High-dose supplements of beta-carotene may increase the risk of cancer.

Symptoms, Diagnosis, and Treatment

Consuming too much vitamin A over a period of time can cause coarse hair, partial loss of hair (including the eyebrows), cracked lips, and dry, rough skin, which may peel. Later symptoms include severe headaches, increased pressure within the brain (intracranial pressure), and general weakness. Bone and joint pain are common, especially among children. Fractures may occur easily, especially in older people. Children may lose their appetite and not grow and develop normally. The liver and spleen may enlarge.

Did You Know...

In infants or children, very high doses of vitamin A can have harmful effects.

Taking very high doses of vitamin A or isotretinoin (a drug derived from vitamin A) during pregnancy can cause birth defects.

Consuming very large amounts of vitamin A all at once can cause drowsiness, irritability, headache, nausea, and vomiting within hours, followed by peeling of the skin. Pressure within the brain is increased, particularly in children, and vomiting occurs. Coma and death may occur unless vitamin A consumption is stopped.

Taking isotretinoin (a vitamin A derivative used to treat severe acne) during pregnancy may cause birth defects. Women who are or who may become pregnant should not consume vitamin A in amounts above the safe upper limit (3,000 micrograms) because birth defects are a risk.

The diagnosis of vitamin A excess is based on symptoms and a high level of vitamin A in the blood.

Treatment involves stopping vitamin A supplements. Most people recover completely.

Vitamin B_6

Vitamin B_6 (pyridoxine) is essential for the metabolism of carbohydrates, amino acids, and fats (lipids), as well as for normal nerve function and for the formation of red blood cells. It also helps keep the skin healthy.

VITAMIN B_6 DEFICIENCY

- Many foods contain vitamin B_6, but extensive processing can remove the vitamin.
- People may have seizures, a scaly rash, a red tongue, cracks in the corners of the mouth, or a pins-and-needles sensation in the hands and feet.
- The diagnosis is based on symptoms, the presence of possible causes, and response to vitamin B_6 supplements.
- Vitamin B_6 supplements, taken by mouth, can correct the deficiency.

Because vitamin B_6 is present in many foods, the deficiency rarely results from inadequate intake. However, such a deficiency can occur because extensive processing can remove vitamin B_6 from foods. The deficiency often results from malabsorption disorders, alcoholism, or use of drugs that deplete vitamin B_6 stored in the body. These drugs include the antibiotic isoniazid, the antihypertensive hydralazine, and penicillamine (used to treat such disorders as rheumatoid arthritis and Wilson's disease).

Vitamin B_6 deficiency can cause seizures, particularly in infants. Anticonvulsants may be ineffective in treating these seizures. In adults, the deficiency can cause inflammation of the skin (dermatitis) and a red, greasy, scaly rash. The hands and feet may feel numb and prickling—like pins and needles. The tongue may become sore and red, and cracks may form in the corners of the mouth. People may become confused, irritable, and depressed. Because vitamin B_6 is needed to form red blood cells, deficiency can cause anemia.

The diagnosis is based on the symptoms, the presence of conditions that can cause the deficiency, and response to vitamin B_6 supplements. Blood tests to confirm the diagnosis are not readily available.

Causes are corrected when possible. People who have the deficiency or who are taking a drug that depletes vitamin B_6 in the body should take vitamin B_6 supplements by mouth.

VITAMIN B_6 EXCESS

Vitamin B_6 in very high doses may be prescribed for such disorders as carpal tunnel syndrome, premenstrual syndrome, and nerve damage (neuropathy), although there is little evidence of benefit. Taking such high doses may cause pain and numbness in the feet and legs. People may be unable to tell where their arms and legs are (position sense) and to feel vibrations. Thus, walking becomes difficult.

The diagnosis is based on symptoms and a history of taking high doses of vitamin B_6. Treatment involves stopping vitamin B_6 supplements. Recovery from this disorder may be slow, and people may continue to have some difficulty walking.

> **? Did You Know...**
>
> High doses of vitamin B_6 supplements probably do not help people with carpal tunnel syndrome, premenstrual syndrome, and nerve damage and can have harmful effects.

Vitamin B_{12}

Vitamin B_{12} (cobalamins), with folate, is necessary for the formation and maturation of red blood cells and the synthesis of DNA (deoxyribonucleic acid), which is the genetic material of cells. Vitamin B_{12} is also necessary for normal nerve function. Unlike most other vitamins, B_{12} is stored in substantial amounts, mainly in the liver, until it is needed by the body. Usually, the body's stores of this vitamin would take about 3 to 5 years to exhaust.

People should not take high doses of vitamin B_{12} as a cure-all, but otherwise the vitamin does not appear to be toxic.

VITAMIN B_{12} DEFICIENCY

- Anemia develops, causing paleness, weakness, fatigue, and, if severe, shortness of breath and dizziness.
- A severe deficiency may cause tingling or loss of sensation in the hands and feet, muscle weakness, loss of reflexes, difficulty walking, confusion, and dementia.
- The diagnosis is based on blood tests.
- When high doses of vitamin B_{12} supplements are taken, most symptoms resolve.
- Symptoms due to nerve damage, such as neuropathy or dementia in older people, may persist.

Vitamin B_{12} occurs in foods that come from animals. Normally, vitamin B_{12} is readily absorbed in the last part of the small intestine (ileum), which leads to the large intestine. However, to be absorbed, the vitamin must combine with intrinsic factor, a protein produced in the stomach. Without intrinsic factor, vitamin B_{12} moves through the intestine and is excreted in stool.

Because vitamin B_{12} is necessary for the formation of mature blood cells, deficiency of this vitamin can result in anemia. The anemia is characterized by abnormally large red blood cells (macrocytes) and white blood cells with abnormal nuclei. Anemia may not develop until 3 to 5 years after the deficiency begins because a large amount of vitamin B_{12} is stored in the liver.

Vitamin B_{12} deficiency can cause nerve damage (neuropathy) even when no anemia develops, particularly in people older than 60.

Causes

Vitamin B_{12} deficiency can result when people do not consume enough vitamin B_{12} or when the body does not absorb or store enough of the vitamin.

Inadequate Consumption: Vitamin B_{12} deficiency develops in people who do not consume any animal products (vegans) unless they take supplements. If a vegan mother breastfeeds her infant, the infant is at risk of vitamin B_{12} deficiency.

Inadequate Absorption: The most common cause of vitamin B_{12} deficiency is inadequate absorption. The following conditions can cause absorption to be inadequate:

- Overgrowth of bacteria in part of the small intestine
- Malabsorption disorders
- Inflammatory bowel disease
- Fish tapeworm infection
- Surgery that removes the part of the small intestine where vitamin B_{12} is absorbed
- Drugs such as antacids and metformin (used to treat diabetes)
- Lack of intrinsic factor
- Decreased stomach acidity (common among older people)

Intrinsic factor may be lacking because abnormal antibodies, produced by an overactive immune system, attack and destroy the stomach cells that produce intrinsic factor—an autoimmune reaction. Intrinsic factor may be lacking because the part of the stomach where it is produced was surgically removed. Vitamin B_{12} deficiency due to lack of intrinsic factor causes a type of anemia called pernicious anemia.

Among older people, absorption may be inadequate because stomach acidity is decreased. Decreased stomach acidity reduces the body's ability to remove vitamin B_{12} from the protein in meat. The vitamin B_{12} found in vitamin supplements, however, can continue to be well absorbed even in people with decreased stomach acid.

Inadequate Storage: Liver disorders may interfere with the storage of vitamin B_{12}.

Symptoms

Anemia due to vitamin B_{12} deficiency develops gradually, allowing the body to adapt somewhat. Consequently, symptoms may be mild even when anemia is severe. Symptoms of anemia are paleness, weakness, and fatigue. If severe, anemia causes shortness of breath, dizziness, and a rapid heart rate. Occasionally, the spleen and liver enlarge. Younger adults who have pernicious anemia (due to lack of intrinsic factor) are more likely to develop stomach and other gastrointestinal cancers.

In people with nerve damage, the legs are affected earlier and more often than the arms. Tingling is felt in the feet and hands, and sensation in the legs, feet, and hands is lost. People become less able to tell where their arms and legs are (position sense) and to feel vibrations. Mild to moderate muscle weakness develops, and reflexes may be lost. Walking becomes difficult. Some people become confused, irritable, and mildly depressed. Advanced vitamin B_{12} deficiency may lead to delirium, paranoia, and impaired mental function, including dementia.

Diagnosis

Usually, vitamin B_{12} deficiency is suspected when routine blood tests detect large red blood cells. If the deficiency is suspected, the level of vitamin B_{12} in the blood is measured. Usually, doctors also measure the blood level of folate to rule out folate deficiency, which can also result in large red blood cells.

If vitamin B_{12} deficiency is confirmed in an older person, no other tests are done because the cause, such as low stomach acidity, is usually not serious. In a younger person, other tests, including other blood tests, may be done to determine the cause. These tests (including the Schilling test) usually focus on intrinsic factor. Endoscopy (use of a flexible viewing tube to directly examine a body cavity) may be done to check for destruction of stomach cells that produce intrinsic factor.

Prevention and Treatment

Giving infants of vegan mothers vitamin B_{12} supplements from birth helps prevent the deficiency.

Older people with vitamin B_{12} deficiency benefit from taking vitamin B_{12} supplements because the deficiency usually results from difficulty absorbing the vitamin from meat. They can absorb the vitamin more easily from supplements than from meat.

Treatment of vitamin B_{12} deficiency or pernicious anemia consists of high doses of vitamin B_{12} supplements. If people have the deficiency but no symptoms, the vitamin may be taken by mouth. Blood tests are done periodically to make sure the vitamin B_{12} level returns to and remains normal. People who have symptoms due to nerve damage are usually given vitamin B_{12} by injection into a muscle. Injections, which may be self-administered, are given daily or weekly for several weeks until the vitamin B_{12} level returns to normal. Then injections are given once a month indefinitely, unless the disorder causing it can be corrected. Anemia usually resolves in about 6 weeks. But severe symptoms due to nerve damage—for example, dementia in older people—may not resolve.

Vitamin C

Vitamin C (ascorbic acid) is essential for the formation, growth, and repair of bone, skin, and connective tissue (which binds other tissues and organs together and includes tendons, ligaments, and blood vessels). Vitamin C helps maintain healthy teeth and gums. It helps the body absorb iron, which is needed to make red blood cells. Vitamin C also helps burns and wounds heal. Like vitamin E, vitamin C is an antioxidant: It protects cells against damage by free radicals, which are by-products of normal cell activity that participate in chemical reactions. Some of these reactions can be harmful.

VITAMIN C DEFICIENCY

- Not eating enough fresh fruits and vegetables can cause the deficiency.
- People feel tired, weak, and irritable.
- Severe deficiency, called scurvy, causes bruising, gum and dental problems, dry hair and skin, and anemia.
- The diagnosis is based on symptoms and sometimes blood tests.
- Increasing consumption of fresh fruits and vegetables or taking supplements by mouth usually corrects the deficiency.

In adults, vitamin C deficiency usually results from a diet low in vitamin C. For example, vitamin C deficiency may result from a diet deficient in fresh fruits and vegetables. Also, cooking can destroy some of the vitamin C in food. Pregnancy, breast-feeding, disorders that cause a high fever or inflammation, surgery, and burns can significantly increase the body's requirements for vitamin C and the risk of vitamin C deficiency. Smoking increases the vitamin C requirement by 30%.

Scurvy: Severe vitamin C deficiency causes scurvy. Scurvy in infants is rare because breast milk usually supplies enough vitamin C and infant formulas are fortified with the vitamin. Scurvy is rare in the United States but may occur in alcoholics and older people who are malnourished.

Did You Know...

Cooking can destroy some of the vitamin C in foods.

Pregnancy, breastfeeding, fever, surgery, and smoking greatly increase the body's requirements for vitamin C.

Symptoms

Adults feel tired, weak, and irritable if their diet is low in vitamin C. They may lose weight and have vague muscle and joint aches.

The symptoms of scurvy develop after a few months of deficiency. Bleeding may occur under the skin (particularly around hair follicles or as bruises), around the gums, and into the joints. The gums become swollen, purple, and spongy. The teeth eventually loosen. The hair becomes dry and brittle, and the skin becomes dry, rough, and scaly. Anemia may develop. Infections may develop, and wounds do not heal.

Infants may be irritable, have pain when they move, and lose their appetite. Infants do not gain weight as they normally do. In infants and children, bone growth is impaired, and bleeding and anemia may occur.

Diagnosis and Treatment

The diagnosis of scurvy is based on symptoms. Measuring the vitamin C level in blood can help establish the diagnosis, but this test is not always available. In children, x-rays are done to check for impaired bone growth.

The deficiency can be prevented by consuming the recommended amounts of fresh fruits and vegetables or by taking the recommended amount of vitamin C in daily supplements. Smokers require more.

Scurvy is treated with high doses of daily vitamin C supplements. Most symptoms disappear after 1 to 2 weeks. Vitamin C plus iron supplements can cure the anemia.

VITAMIN C EXCESS

Some people take high doses of vitamin C because it is an antioxidant, which protects cells against damage by free radicals. Free radicals are thought to contribute to many disorders, such as atherosclerosis, cancer, lung disorders, the common cold, eye cataracts, and memory loss. Whether taking high doses of vitamin C protects against or has any beneficial effect on these disorders is unclear. Evidence of a protective effect against cataracts is strongest.

High doses (up to the safe upper limit—2,000 milligrams a day) of vitamin C are usually not toxic to healthy adults. Occasionally, higher doses cause nausea or diarrhea and interfere with the interpretation of some blood test results.

Vitamin D

Two forms of vitamin D are important for nutrition:

- **Vitamin D₂ (ergocalciferol):** This form is synthesized from plants and yeast precursors. It is also the form used in very high dose supplements.

- **Vitamin D₃ (cholecalciferol):** This form is the most active form of vitamin D. It is formed in the skin when the skin is exposed to direct sunlight. The most common food source is fortified foods, mainly cereals and dairy products. Vitamin D₃ is also present in fish liver oils and fatty fish. Human breast milk contains only small amounts of vitamin D.

Vitamin D is stored mainly in the liver. Vitamin D₂ and D₃ are not active in the body. Both forms must be processed (metabolized) by the liver and kidneys into an active form called calcitriol. This active form promotes absorption of calcium and phosphorus from the intestine. Calcium and phosphorus, which are minerals, are incorporated into bones to make them strong and dense (a process called mineralization). Thus, vitamin D is necessary for the formation, growth, and repair of bones. Vitamin D also enhances immune function and improves muscle strength. Requirements for vitamin D increase as people age.

VITAMIN D DEFICIENCY

- The most common cause is lack of exposure to sunlight, but certain disorders can also cause the deficiency.

- Without enough vitamin D, muscle and bone weakness and pain occur.

- Infants develop rickets: The skull is soft, bones grow abnormally, and infants are slow to sit and crawl.

- Blood tests and sometimes x-rays are done to confirm the diagnosis.

- From birth, breastfed infants should be given vitamin D supplements because breast milk contains little vitamin D

- Vitamin D supplements taken by mouth or given by injection usually result in a complete recovery.

Vitamin D deficiency is common. Most commonly, it occurs when the skin is not exposed to enough sunlight. Almost no one consumes enough vitamin D from foods to prevent vitamin D deficiency when exposure to sunlight is inadequate.

In vitamin D deficiency, calcium and phosphate levels in the blood decrease because vitamin D is necessary for absorption of these minerals. Because not enough calcium and phosphate are available to maintain healthy bones, vitamin D deficiency may result in a bone disorder called rickets in children or osteomalacia in adults. In a pregnant woman, vitamin D deficiency causes the deficiency in the fetus, and the newborn has a high risk of rickets. Occasionally, the deficiency is severe enough to cause osteomalacia in the woman. Vitamin D deficiency makes osteoporosis worse. To try to increase the low calcium level in blood caused by vitamin D deficiency, the body may produce more parathyroid hormone. However, as the parathyroid hormone level becomes high (a condition called hyperparathyroidism), the hormone draws calcium out of bone to increase the calcium level in blood. Thus, bones are weakened.

> ### ? Did You Know...
>
> Lack of exposure to sunlight can cause vitamin D deficiency.
>
> Most older people need vitamin D supplements.

Causes

The most common cause is inadequate exposure to sunlight. Thus, vitamin D deficiency occurs mainly among people who do not spend much time outdoors: older people and people who live in an institution such as a nursing home. The deficiency can also occur in the winter at northern and southern latitudes or in people who keep their bodies covered, such as Muslim women. Because breast milk contains only small amounts of vitamin D, breastfed infants who are not exposed to enough sunlight are at risk of the deficiency and rickets.

When the skin is exposed to enough sunlight, the body usually forms enough vitamin D. However, certain circumstances increase the risk of vitamin D deficiency even when there is exposure to sunlight:

- The skin forms less vitamin D in response to sunlight in certain groups of people. They include people with darker skin (particularly blacks), older people, and people who use sunscreen.

- The body may not be able to absorb enough vitamin D from foods. In malabsorption disorders, people cannot absorb fats normally (see page 163). They also cannot absorb vitamin

D because it is a fat-soluble vitamin, which is normally absorbed with fats in the small intestine.

- The body may not be able to convert vitamin D to an active form. Certain kidney and liver disorders and several rare hereditary disorders interfere with this conversion, as do certain drugs, such as some anticonvulsants and rifampin.

Symptoms

Vitamin D deficiency can cause muscle aches, weakness, and bone pain in people of all ages. Muscle spasms, which are caused by a low calcium level, may be the first sign of rickets in infants.

In young infants who have rickets, the entire skull may be soft. Older infants may be slow to sit and crawl, and the spaces between the skull bones (fontanelles) may be slow to close. In children aged 1 to 4 years, bone growth may be abnormal, causing an abnormal curve in the spine and bowlegs or knock-knees. These children may be slow to walk. For older children and adolescents, walking is painful. The pelvic bones may flatten, narrowing the birth canal in adolescent girls. In adults, the bones, particularly the spine, pelvis, and leg bones, weaken. Affected areas may be painful to touch, and fractures may occur.

In older people, bone fractures may result from only slight jarring or a minor fall.

Diagnosis

Doctors suspect vitamin D deficiency when people report an inadequate diet or exposure to sunlight. Doctors also suspect the deficiency in older adults, especially in those with decreased bone density (for example, with osteoporosis) or broken bones. Blood tests to measure vitamin D can confirm the deficiency. X-rays may also be taken. The diagnosis of rickets or osteomalacia is based on symptoms, the characteristic appearance of bones on x-rays, and a low level of vitamin D in the blood.

Prevention and Treatment

Many people need to take vitamin D supplements. Getting enough exposure to sunlight may be difficult, especially because the skin also needs to be protected from sun damage. The diet rarely contains enough vitamin D to compensate for lack of sunlight. Many multiple vitamins contain little or no vitamin D, so most people need to take vitamin D supplements. These supplements are particularly important for people who are at risk (such as people who are older, housebound, or living in long-term care facilities). Commercially available liquid milk (but not cheese or yogurt) is fortified in the United States and Canada. Many other countries do not fortify milk with vitamin D. Breakfast cereals may also be fortified.

SPOTLIGHT ON AGING

Older people are likely to develop vitamin D deficiency for several reasons:

- Their requirements are higher than those of younger persons.
- They tend to spend less time outdoors, or stay indoors more in the winter, and thus are not exposed to enough sunlight.
- They may not be exposed to enough sunlight because they are housebound, live in long-term care facilities, or need to stay in the hospital for a long time.
- When exposed to sunlight, their skin does not form as much vitamin D.
- They consume so little vitamin D in their diet that even taking vitamin D supplements in low doses (such as 400 units per day) does not prevent the deficiency.
- They may have disorders or take drugs that interfere with the processing of vitamin D.

New studies suggest that older adults may need more vitamin D than the current recommended dietary allowance or even the recommended upper limits. In fact, they may need 1,000 to 2,000 IU (or more) daily, but taking such high amounts should be done only after consulting a doctor. Older people who take high amounts of vitamin D supplements need to have periodic blood tests to check their levels of calcium, vitamin D, and parathyroid hormone.

In breastfed infants, starting vitamin D supplements at birth is particularly important because breast milk contains little vitamin D. Commercial infant formulas contain enough vitamin D.

Treatment involves taking high doses of vitamin D by mouth or by injection daily or weekly for 1 to 2 months or longer. If muscle spasms are present or calcium is thought to be deficient, calcium supplements are also given. If phosphate is deficient, phosphate supplements are given. Usually, this treatment leads to a complete recovery. People with a chronic liver or kidney disorder may require special formulations of vitamin D supplements.

VITAMIN D EXCESS

Taking very high daily doses of vitamin D—for example, 50 or more times the recommended daily allowance (RDA)—over several months can cause toxicity and a high calcium level in the blood (hypercalcemia—see page 936).

Early symptoms are loss of appetite, nausea, and vomiting, followed by excessive thirst, weakness, nervousness, and high blood pressure. Because the calcium level is high, calcium may be deposited throughout the body, particularly in the kidneys, blood vessels, lungs, and heart. The kidneys may be permanently damaged and malfunction, resulting in kidney failure.

Vitamin D excess is usually diagnosed when blood tests detect a high calcium level in a person who takes high doses of vitamin D. The diagnosis is confirmed by measuring the level of vitamin D in the blood.

Treatment consists of the following:

- Stopping vitamin D supplements
- Following a low-calcium diet for a while to offset the effects of a high calcium level in the body
- Taking drugs (such as corticosteroids or bisphosphonates) to suppress the release of calcium from the bones

Vitamin E

Vitamin E (tocopherol) is an antioxidant: It protects cells against damage by free radicals, which are by-products of normal cell activity that participate in chemical reactions. Some of these reactions can be harmful. Many people take vitamin E supplements to help prevent certain disorders. Vitamin E supplements do not protect against heart and blood vessel disorders. Whether they protect against Alzheimer's disease, tardive dyskinesia (repetitive involuntary movements of the mouth, tongue, arms, or legs), and prostate cancer among smokers is controversial.

VITAMIN E DEFICIENCY

- The deficiency may cause impaired reflexes and coordination, difficulty walking, and weak muscles.
- Premature infants with the deficiency may develop a serious form of anemia.
- The diagnosis is based on symptoms and results of a physical examination.
- Taking vitamin E supplements corrects the deficiency.

A very low fat diet lacks vitamin E because vegetable oils are the main source of this vitamin. Disorders that impair fat absorption can also reduce the absorption of vitamin E and increase the risk of vitamin E deficiency. Newborns have a relatively low reserve of vitamin E because only small amounts of vitamin E cross the placenta. Thus, newborns are at increased risk of a vitamin E deficiency. Adults have large amounts of vitamin E stored in fat tissue. In the United States and other developed countries, vitamin E deficiency is rare among older children and adults.

Symptoms, Diagnosis, and Treatment

Symptoms may include slow reflexes, difficulty walking, loss of coordination, loss of position sense (knowing where the limbs are without looking at them), and muscle weakness. Vitamin E deficiency can cause a form of anemia in which red blood cells rupture (hemolytic anemia). Premature infants who have a vitamin E deficiency are at risk of this serious disorder. In premature infants, bleeding (hemorrhage) may occur within the brain, and blood vessels in the eyes may grow abnormally (a disorder called retinopathy of prematurity—see page 1699). Affected newborns also have weak muscles.

Diagnosis is based on symptoms, the presence of conditions that increase risk, and results of a physical examination. Blood tests to measure the level of vitamin E are not readily available.

Treatment involves taking vitamin E supplements by mouth. Premature newborns may be given supplements to prevent disorders from developing. Most full-term newborns do not need supplements because they get enough vitamin E in breast milk or commercial formulas.

 Did You Know...
A very low fat diet may be low in vitamin E.

VITAMIN E EXCESS

Many adults take relatively large amounts of vitamin E for months to years without any apparent harm. However, high doses of vitamin E may increase the risk of bleeding (including bleeding within the brain, causing stroke), particularly for adults who are also taking an anticoagulant (especially warfarin). Occasionally, adults who take very high doses develop muscle weakness, fatigue, nausea, and diarrhea.

The diagnosis is based on the person's history of using vitamin E supplements and symptoms.

Treatment involves stopping vitamin E supplements. If necessary, vitamin K, which helps blood clot, is given to stop bleeding.

Vitamin K

Vitamin K has two forms:

- **Phylloquinone:** This form occurs in plants and is consumed in the diet. It is absorbed better when it is consumed with fat. Phylloquinone is not toxic.
- **Menaquinone:** This form is produced by bacteria in the intestine, but only small amounts of it can be absorbed. In some countries, this form is used for supplementation.

Vitamin K is necessary for the synthesis of the proteins that help control bleeding (clotting factors) and thus for the normal clotting of blood. It is also needed for healthy bones and other tissues.

VITAMIN K DEFICIENCY

- Bleeding, the main symptom, can be life threatening in newborns.
- Blood tests to check coagulation can confirm the diagnosis.
- All newborns should be given a vitamin K injection.
- Vitamin K supplements taken by mouth or injected under the skin can correct the deficiency.

Vitamin K deficiency can result from lack of vitamin K in the diet or from disorders that impair fat absorption and that thus reduce the absorption of vitamin K. Taking large amounts of mineral oil may reduce the absorption of vitamin K. Vitamin K deficiency can develop in people who take certain drugs, including anticonvulsants and some antibiotics. Doctors frequently prescribe vitamin K antagonists (anticoagulants such as warfarin) to people who are at high risk for harmful blood clots, such as those with deep vein thrombosis (DVT), pulmonary embolism, or irregular heart rhythms (such as atrial fibrillation).

Newborns are prone to vitamin K deficiency because only small amounts of vitamin K cross the placenta and because, during the first few days after birth, their intestine does not contain bacteria to produce vitamin K. The deficiency can cause hemorrhagic disease of the newborn, characterized by a tendency to bleed. A vitamin K injection is usually given to newborns to protect them from this disease. Breastfed infants who have not received this injection at birth are especially susceptible to vitamin K deficiency because breast milk contains only small amounts of vitamin K. Hemorrhagic disease is more likely in infants who are breastfed or who have a disorder that impairs fat absorption or a liver disorder. Formulas for infants contain vitamin K.

> **? Did You Know...**
>
> Newborns are at risk of vitamin K deficiency because they receive only a little vitamin K before birth and they have not yet acquired the bacteria that produce the vitamin.

Symptoms

The main symptom is bleeding (hemorrhage)—into the skin (causing bruises), from the nose, from a wound, in the stomach, or in the intestine. Sometimes bleeding in the stomach causes vomiting with blood. Blood may be seen in the urine or stool. In newborns, life-threatening bleeding within or around the brain may occur. Having a liver disorder increases the risk of bleeding because proteins that help blood clot (clotting factors) are made in the liver. Vitamin K deficiency may also weaken bones.

Diagnosis and Treatment

Doctors suspect vitamin K deficiency when abnormal bleeding occurs in people with conditions that put them at risk. Blood tests to measure how well blood clots are done to help confirm the diagnosis. Knowing how much vitamin K people consume helps doctors interpret results of the blood test.

A vitamin K injection in the muscle is recommended for all newborns to reduce the risk of bleeding within the brain after delivery. Otherwise, vitamin K is usually taken by mouth or given by injection under the skin. If a drug is the cause, the dose of the drug is adjusted or extra vitamin K is given.

People who have vitamin K deficiency and a severe liver disorder may also need blood transfusions to replenish the clotting factors. A damaged liver may be unable to synthesize clotting factors even after vitamin K injections are given.

CHAPTER

139 Minerals and Electrolytes

Minerals are necessary for the normal functioning of the body's cells. The body needs large quantities of calcium, chloride, magnesium, phosphate, potassium, and sodium. These minerals are called macrominerals. Bone, muscle, heart, and brain function depends on these minerals. The body needs small quantities of chromium, copper, fluoride, iodine, iron, manganese, molybdenum, selenium, and zinc. These minerals are called trace minerals. Except for

chromium, all trace minerals are incorporated into enzymes or hormones required in body processes (metabolism). Chromium helps the body keep blood sugar levels normal. All trace minerals are harmful if too much is ingested.

Minerals are an essential part of a healthy diet. The recommended dietary allowance (RDA)—the amount most healthy people need each day to remain healthy—has been determined for most minerals. People who have a disorder may need more or less than this amount.

Consuming too little or too much of certain minerals can cause a nutritional disorder. People who eat a balanced diet containing a variety of foods are unlikely to develop a nutritional disorder or a major mineral deficiency, except for calcium, iodine, or iron deficiency. However, people who follow restrictive diets may not consume enough of a particular mineral (or vitamin). For example, vegetarians, including those who eat eggs and dairy products, are at risk of iron deficiency. Infants are more likely to develop deficiencies because they are growing rapidly (thus requiring large amounts of nutrients).

Consuming large amounts (megadoses) of mineral supplements without medical supervision may have harmful (toxic) effects.

Electrolytes: Some minerals—especially the macrominerals—are important as electrolytes. The body uses electrolytes to help regulate nerve and muscle function and to maintain acid-base balance (see page 972) and fluid balance.

To function normally, the body must keep fluid levels from varying too much in the areas of the body that contain fluid (called compartments). The three main compartments are

- Fluid within cells
- Fluid in the space around cells
- Blood

Electrolytes, particularly sodium, help the body maintain normal fluid levels in these compartments (called fluid balance), because how much fluid a compartment contains depends on the concentration of electrolytes in it. If the electrolyte concentration is high, fluid moves into that compartment. If the electrolyte concentration is low, fluid moves out of that compartment. To adjust fluid levels, the body can actively move electrolytes in or out of cells. Thus, having electrolytes in the right concentrations (called electrolyte balance) is important in maintaining fluid balance among the compartments.

The kidneys help maintain electrolyte concentrations by filtering electrolytes from blood, returning some electrolytes, and excreting any excess into the urine. Thus, the kidneys help maintain a balance between daily consumption and excretion.

If the balance of electrolytes is disturbed, disorders can develop. An electrolyte imbalance can result from the following:

- Becoming dehydrated
- Taking certain drugs
- Having certain heart, kidney, or liver disorders
- Being given intravenous fluids or feedings in inappropriate amounts

Diagnosis

Doctors can detect many common nutritional disorders or an electrolyte imbalance by measuring the levels of minerals in a sample of blood or urine.

Calcium

About 99% of the body's calcium is stored in the bones, but cells (particularly muscle cells) and blood also contain calcium. Calcium is essential for the following:

- Formation of bone and teeth
- Muscle contraction
- Normal functioning of many enzymes
- Blood clotting
- Normal heart rhythm

The body precisely controls the amount of calcium in cells and blood. The body moves calcium out of bones into blood as needed to maintain a steady level of calcium in the blood. If people do not consume enough calcium, too much calcium is mobilized from the bones, weakening them. Osteoporosis can result. To maintain a normal level of calcium in blood without weakening the bones, people need to consume at least 1,000 to 1,500 milligrams of calcium a day. The level of calcium in blood is regulated primarily by two hormones: parathyroid hormone and calcitonin.

Parathyroid hormone is produced by the four parathyroid glands, located around the thyroid gland in the neck. When the calcium level in blood decreases, the parathyroid glands produce more parathyroid hormone. When the calcium level in blood increases, the parathyroid glands produce less hormone. Parathyroid hormone does the following:

- Stimulates bones to release calcium into blood
- Causes the kidneys to excrete less calcium in urine
- Stimulates the digestive tract to absorb more calcium
- Causes the kidneys to activate vitamin D, which enables the digestive tract to absorb more calcium

Calcitonin is produced by cells of the thyroid gland. It lowers the calcium level in blood by slowing the breakdown of bone, but only slightly.

HYPOCALCEMIA

In hypocalcemia, the calcium level in blood is too low.

- A low calcium level may result from a problem with the parathyroid glands, as well as from diet, kidney disorders, or certain drugs.

MINERALS

MINERAL	GOOD SOURCES	MAIN FUNCTIONS	RECOMMENDED DIETARY ALLOWANCE FOR ADULTS	SAFE UPPER LIMIT
Calcium	Milk and milk products, meat, fish eaten with the bones (such as sardines), eggs, fortified cereal products, beans, fruits, and vegetables	Required for the formation of bone and teeth, for blood clotting, for normal muscle function, for the normal functioning of many enzymes, and for normal heart rhythm	1,000 milligrams 1,200 milligrams for people over 50	2,500 milligrams
Chloride	Salt, beef, pork, sardines, cheese, green olives, corn bread, potato chips, sauerkraut, and processed or canned foods (usually as salt)	Involved in electrolyte balance	1,000 milligrams	—
Chromium	Liver, processed meats, whole-grain cereals, and nuts	Enables insulin to function (insulin controls blood sugar levels) Helps in the processing (metabolism) and storage of carbohydrates, protein, and fat	35 micrograms for men aged 50 and younger 25 micrograms for women aged 50 and younger 30 micrograms for men over 50 20 micrograms for women over 50	—
Copper	Organ meats, shellfish, cocoa, mushrooms, nuts, dried legumes, dried fruits, peas, tomato products, and whole-grain cereals	Is a component of many enzymes that are necessary for energy production, for antioxidant action*, and for formation of the hormone epinephrine, red blood cells, bone, and connective tissue	900 micrograms	10,000 micrograms
Fluoride	Seafood, tea, and fluoridated water	Required for the formation of bone and teeth	3 milligrams for women 4 milligrams for men	10 milligrams
Iodine	Seafood, iodized salt, eggs, cheese, and drinking water (in amounts that vary by the iodine content of local soil)	Required for the formation of thyroid hormones	150 micrograms	1,100 micrograms
Iron	As heme† iron: Beef, poultry, fish, kidneys, and liver As nonheme iron: Soybean flour, beans, molasses, spinach, clams, and fortified grains and cereals	Required for the formation of many enzymes in the body Is an important component of muscle cells and of hemoglobin, which enables red blood cells to carry oxygen and deliver it to the body's tissues	8 milligrams for women over 50 and for men 18 milligrams for women aged 50 and younger (premenopause) 27 milligrams for pregnant women 9 milligrams for breastfeeding women	45 milligrams

(continued on the following page)

MINERALS (*Continued*)

MINERAL	GOOD SOURCES	MAIN FUNCTIONS	RECOMMENDED DIETARY ALLOWANCE FOR ADULTS	SAFE UPPER LIMIT
Magnesium	Leafy green vegetables, nuts, cereal grains, beans, and tomato paste	Required for the formation of bone and teeth, for normal nerve and muscle function, and for the activation of enzymes	320 milligrams for women 420 milligrams for men	—
Manganese	Whole-grain cereals, pineapple, nuts, tea, beans, and tomato paste	Required for the formation of bone and the formation and activation of certain enzymes	2.3 milligrams for men 1.8 milligrams for women	6 to 11 milligrams
Molybdenum	Milk, legumes, whole-grain breads and cereals, and dark green vegetables	Required for metabolism of nitrogen, the activation of certain enzymes, and normal cell function Helps break down sulfites (present in foods naturally and added as preservatives)	45 micrograms	1,100 to 2,000 micrograms
Phosphorus	Dairy products, meat, poultry, fish, cereals, nuts, and legumes	Required for the formation of bone and teeth and for energy production Used to form nucleic acids, including DNA (deoxyribonucleic acid)	700 milligrams	4,000 milligrams
Potassium	Whole and skim milk, bananas, tomatoes, oranges, melons, potatoes, sweet potatoes, prunes, raisins, spinach, turnip greens, collard greens, kale, other green leafy vegetables, most peas and beans, and salt substitutes (potassium chloride)	Required for normal nerve and muscle function Involved in electrolyte balance	3.5 grams	—
Selenium	Meats, seafood, nuts, and cereals (depending on the selenium content of soil where grains were grown)	Acts as an antioxidant* with vitamin E Required for thyroid gland function	55 micrograms	400 micrograms
Sodium	Salt, beef, pork, sardines, cheese, green olives, corn bread, potato chips, sauerkraut, and processed or canned foods (usually as salt)	Required for normal nerve and muscle function Helps the body maintain a normal electrolyte and fluid balance	1,000 milligrams	2,400 milligrams
Zinc	Meat, liver, oysters, seafood, peanuts, fortified cereals, and whole grains (depending on the zinc content of soil where grains were grown)	Used to form many enzymes and insulin Required for healthy skin, healing of wounds, and growth	15 milligrams	—

*Antioxidants protect cells against damage due to reactive by-products of normal cell activity called free radicals.
†The body absorbs heme iron better than nonheme iron.

- As hypocalcemia progresses, people may become confused, depressed, and forgetful and have tingling in their fingers and feet as well as stiff, achy muscles.
- Usually, the disorder is detected by routine blood tests.
- Calcium and vitamin D supplements may be used.

About 40% of the calcium in blood is attached (bound) to proteins in blood, mainly albumin. Protein-bound calcium acts as a reserve but has no active function in the body. Only unbound calcium affects the body's functions. Thus, hypocalcemia causes problems only when the level of unbound calcium is low. Unbound calcium has an electrical (ionic) charge, so it is called ionized calcium.

Causes

Hypocalcemia most commonly results when too much calcium is lost in urine or when not enough calcium is moved from bones into the blood. Causes of hypocalcemia include the following:

- A low level of parathyroid hormone (hypoparathyroidism), as can occur when the parathyroid glands are damaged during thyroid gland surgery
- Lack of response to a normal level of parathyroid hormone (pseudohypoparathyroidism)
- No parathyroid glands at birth
- A low level of magnesium (hypomagnesemia), which reduces the activity of parathyroid hormone
- Vitamin D deficiency (due to inadequate consumption or inadequate exposure to sunlight)
- Kidney dysfunction (a common cause), which results in more calcium excreted in urine and makes the kidneys less able to activate vitamin D
- Inadequate consumption of calcium
- Disorders that decrease calcium absorption
- Pancreatitis
- Certain drugs, including rifampin (an antibiotic), anticonvulsants (such as phenytoin and phenobarbital), bisphosphonates (such as alendronate, ibandronate, risedronate, and zoledronic acid), calcitonin, chloroquine, corticosteroids, and plicamycin

Symptoms

The calcium level in blood can be moderately low without causing any symptoms. Over time, hypocalcemia can affect the brain and cause neurologic or psychologic symptoms, such as confusion, memory loss, delirium, depression, and hallucinations. These symptoms disappear if the calcium level is restored.

An extremely low calcium level may cause tingling (often in the lips, tongue, fingers, and feet), muscle aches, spasms of the muscles in the throat (leading to difficulty breathing), stiffening and spasms of muscles (tetany), seizures, and abnormal heart rhythms.

Diagnosis

Hypocalcemia is often detected by routine blood tests before symptoms become obvious. Doctors measure the total calcium level (which includes calcium bound to albumin) and the albumin level in blood to determine whether the level of unbound calcium is low.

Blood tests are done to evaluate kidney function and to measure magnesium, phosphate, parathyroid hormone, and vitamin D levels. Other substances in blood may be measured to help determine the cause.

Treatment

Calcium supplements, given by mouth, are often all that is needed to treat hypocalcemia. If a cause is identified, treating the disorder causing hypocalcemia or changing drugs may restore the calcium level.

Once symptoms appear, calcium is usually given intravenously. Taking vitamin D supplements helps increase the absorption of calcium from the digestive tract. Thiazide diuretics may be given to decrease the excretion of calcium by the kidneys, particularly when hypocalcemia is caused by hypoparathyroidism.

HYPERCALCEMIA

In hypercalcemia, the level of calcium in blood is too high.

- A high calcium level may result from a problem with the parathyroid glands, as well as from diet, cancer, or disorders affecting bone.
- At first, people have digestive problems, feel thirsty, and may urinate a lot, but if severe, the disorder can be life threatening.
- Usually, the disorder is detected by routine blood tests.
- Drinking lots of fluids may be sufficient, but diuretics may increase calcium excretion and drugs can be used to slow the release of calcium from bone if needed.

Causes

Causes include the following:

- **Hyperparathyroidism:** One or more of the four parathyroid glands secrete too much parathyroid hormone, which helps control the amount of calcium in blood.
- **Too much calcium:** Occasionally, hypercalcemia develops in people with peptic ulcers if they drink a lot of milk and take calcium-containing antacids for relief. The resulting disorder is called the milk-alkali syndrome.
- **Too much vitamin D:** If people take very high daily doses of vitamin D over several months, the

amount of calcium absorbed from the digestive tract increases substantially.

- **Cancer:** Cells in kidney, lung, and ovary cancers may secrete large amounts of a protein that, like parathyroid hormone, increases the calcium level in blood. These effects are considered a paraneoplastic syndrome (see box on page 1082). Calcium can also be released into blood when cancer spreads (metastasizes) to bone and destroys bone cells. Such bone destruction occurs most commonly with prostate, breast, and lung cancers. Multiple myeloma (a cancer involving bone marrow) can also lead to the destruction of bone and result in hypercalcemia. Other cancers can increase the calcium level in blood by means not yet fully understood.

- **Bone disorders:** If bone is broken down (resorbed) or destroyed, calcium is released into the blood, sometimes causing hypercalcemia. In Paget's disease, bone is broken down, but the calcium level in blood is usually normal. However, the calcium level can become too high if people with Paget's disease become dehydrated or spend too much time sitting or lying down—when the bones are not bearing weight.

- **Inactivity:** Rarely, people who are immobilized, such as paraplegics, quadriplegics, or people who must remain in bed for a long time, develop hypercalcemia because calcium in bone is released into the blood when bones do not bear weight for long periods of time.

 Did You Know...

Lack of mobility can make the calcium level high because bones weaken and release calcium into the blood.

Symptoms and Diagnosis

Hypercalcemia often causes no symptoms. The earliest symptoms are usually constipation, nausea, vomiting, abdominal pain, and loss of appetite. People may excrete abnormally large amounts of urine, resulting in dehydration and increased thirst.

Very severe hypercalcemia often causes brain dysfunction with confusion, emotional disturbances, delirium, hallucinations, and coma. Muscle weakness may occur, and abnormal heart rhythms and death can follow. Long-term or severe hypercalcemia commonly results in kidney stones containing calcium. Less commonly, kidney failure develops, but it usually resolves with treatment. However, if enough calcium accumulates within the kidneys, damage is irreversible.

What Is Hyperparathyroidism?

The parathyroid glands release parathyroid hormone, which increases the absorption of calcium from the digestive tract and causes bones to release stored calcium. If the parathyroid glands release too much parathyroid hormone, hyperparathyroidism results. People with hyperparathyroidism have too much calcium and a normal or low level of phosphate in their blood. Parathyroid hormone causes the kidneys to excrete more phosphate, but it also causes the bones to release phosphate into the blood. The balance between these two effects determines whether the phosphate level remains normal or decreases.

Primary hyperparathyroidism: An abnormality causes the release of too much parathyroid hormone. In about 90% of people with primary hyperparathyroidism, the abnormality is a noncancerous tumor (adenoma) in one of the parathyroid glands. In the remaining 10%, the glands simply enlarge and produce too much hormone. Rarely, cancers of the parathyroid glands cause hyperparathyroidism.

Primary hyperparathyroidism is more common among women than among men. It is more likely to develop in older people and in people who have received radiation therapy to the neck. Sometimes it occurs as part of the syndrome of multiple endocrine neoplasia, a rare hereditary disorder (see page 1016).

Primary hyperparathyroidism is usually treated by surgically removing one or more of the parathyroid glands. The goal is to remove all parathyroid tissue that is producing excess hormone. Surgery is successful in almost 90% of cases.

Secondary hyperparathyroidism: Excess parathyroid hormone is released in response to a large decrease in the calcium level in blood, as can occur in chronic kidney disease and vitamin D deficiency. Treatment depends on the cause.

Hypercalcemia is usually detected during routine blood tests.

Treatment

If hypercalcemia is not severe, correcting the cause is often sufficient. If people have mild hypercalcemia or conditions that can cause hypercalcemia and if their kidney function is normal, they are usually advised to drink plenty of fluids. Fluids stimulate the kidneys to excrete calcium and help prevent dehydration.

If the calcium level is very high or if symptoms of brain dysfunction or muscle weakness appear, fluids and diuretics are given intravenously as long as kidney function is normal. Dialysis is a highly effective, safe, reliable treatment, but it is usually used only for people with severe hypercalcemia that cannot be treated by other methods.

Several other drugs (including bisphosphonates, calcitonin, corticosteroids, and, rarely, plicamycin) can be used to treat hypercalcemia. These drugs work primarily by slowing the release of calcium from bone.

Hypercalcemia caused by cancer is particularly difficult to treat. If the cancer cannot be controlled, hypercalcemia usually returns despite the best treatment.

Chromium

Chromium enables insulin (which controls blood sugar levels) to function and helps in the processing (metabolism) and storage of carbohydrates, protein, and fat. Only a small amount of the chromium in food is absorbed. Chromium is absorbed better when eaten with foods that contain vitamin C and niacin. Supplements do not enhance muscle size or strength in men.

Deficiency: Chromium deficiency is rare in developed countries. Children who are undernourished may have chromium deficiency and grow poorly. Several conditions can reduce the amount of chromium in the body:

- A diet high in simple sugars, which causes more chromium to be excreted in urine
- Infections
- Exercise if strenuous
- Pregnancy and breastfeeding
- Injuries
- Intravenous feeding (total parenteral nutrition) for a long time

Symptoms may include weight loss, confusion, impaired coordination, and a reduced response to sugar (glucose) in blood, increasing the risk of diabetes. Treatment may involve chromium supplements.

Excess: Small amounts of chromium taken by mouth are not harmful. In the workplace, people may be exposed to a different, toxic form of chromium. This form results from industrial pollution. This form may irritate the skin, cartilage of the nose, lungs, and digestive tract and may cause lung cancer.

Copper

Most of the copper in the body is located in the liver, bones, and muscle, but traces of copper occur in all tissues of the body. The liver excretes excess copper into the bile for elimination from the body.

Copper is a component of many enzymes, including ones that are necessary for the following:

- Energy production
- Formation of the hormone epinephrine
- Formation of red blood cells, bone, or connective tissue (which binds other tissues and organs together)
- Antioxidant action (to help protect cells against damage by free radicals, which are reactive by-products of normal cell activity)

WILSON'S DISEASE

In Wilson's disease, a rare hereditary disorder, the liver does not excrete excess copper into the bile as it normally does, resulting in accumulation of copper in the liver and liver damage.

- Copper accumulates in the liver, brain, eyes, and other organs.
- People with Wilson's disease may have tremors, difficulty speaking and swallowing, problems with coordination, personality changes, or hepatitis.
- Blood tests and eye examinations help confirm the diagnosis.
- People must take drugs to remove copper and must avoid foods high in copper for the rest of their life.

Because the liver does not excrete excess copper, copper accumulates in the liver and damages it, causing cirrhosis. The damaged liver releases copper directly into the blood, and copper is carried to other organs, such as the brain, kidneys, and eyes, where it also accumulates.

Symptoms

Symptoms usually begin between ages 6 and 30. In almost half of affected people, the first symptoms result from brain damage. They include tremors, difficulty speaking and swallowing, drooling, incoordination, involuntary jerky movements (chorea), personality changes, and even psychosis (such as schizophrenia or manic-depressive illness). In most of the other people, the first symptoms result from liver damage, which causes hepatitis and eventually cirrhosis.

The cornea of the eyes may contain outer gold or greenish gold rings (Kayser-Fleischer rings) caused by copper that accumulates there. People may have anemia because red blood cells rupture (causing hemolytic anemia). Women may have no menstrual periods or repeated miscarriages.

Diagnosis

Doctors suspect Wilson's disease based on symptoms, such as unexplained hepatitis, tremors, and personality changes. The following tests help confirm the diagnosis:

- Slit-lamp examination of the eyes for Kayser-Fleischer rings
- Blood tests to measure levels of copper and copper proteins
- Measurement of copper excreted in the urine
- If the diagnosis is still unclear, a liver biopsy

If children have a family history of the disease, tests are done after about age 1 year. Tests done earlier are likely to miss the disease.

Treatment

Drugs that bind with copper, such as penicillamine, taken by mouth, are used to remove the accumulated copper. People also need to follow a diet that is low in copper. Foods to avoid include beef liver, cashews, black-eyed peas, vegetable juice, shellfish, mushrooms, and cocoa. For the rest of their life, people with Wilson's disease must take penicillamine, another similar drug, or zinc supplements. These drugs help prevent copper from reaccumulating. Without lifelong treatment, Wilson's disease is fatal.

People who do not take the drugs as directed, especially younger people, may develop liver failure. Liver transplantation can cure the disease.

? **Did You Know...**

Greenish gold rings around the outer rim of the corneas of the eyes may be a sign of Wilson's disease.

COPPER DEFICIENCY

Copper deficiency is rare among healthy people. It occurs most commonly among infants who are premature, who are recovering from severe undernutrition, or who have persistent diarrhea. A severe disorder that impairs absorption of nutrients (such as celiac disease, Crohn's disease, cystic fibrosis, or tropical sprue) or weight-loss (bariatric) surgery may cause this deficiency. Consumption of too much zinc can reduce the absorption of copper, causing a deficiency. Some male infants inherit a genetic abnormality that causes copper deficiency. This disorder is called Menkes syndrome.

Symptoms of copper deficiency include fatigue, anemia, and a decreased number of white blood cells. Sometimes osteoporosis develops or nerves are damaged. Nerve damage can cause tingling and loss of sensation in the feet and hands. Muscles may feel weak. Some people become confused, irritable, and mildly depressed. Coordination is impaired.

Menkes syndrome causes severe mental retardation, vomiting, and diarrhea. The skin lacks pigment, and the hair is sparse, steely, or kinky. Bones may be weak and malformed, and arteries are fragile, sometimes rupturing.

Copper deficiency is usually diagnosed based on symptoms and on blood tests that detect low levels of copper and ceruloplasmin (a copper-carrying protein).

The cause is treated, and a copper supplement is given by mouth. For infants with Menkes syndrome, copper is injected under the skin (subcutaneously).

COPPER EXCESS

Consumption of excess copper is rare. People may consume small amounts of excess copper in acidic food or beverages that have been in copper vessels, tubing, or valves a long time. Consuming even relatively small amounts of copper may cause nausea, vomiting, and diarrhea. Large amounts, usually consumed by people intending to commit suicide, can damage the kidneys, inhibit urine production, and cause anemia due to the rupture of red blood cells (hemolytic anemia) and even death. Rarely, liver damage or cirrhosis occurs in children. It probably results from drinking milk that has been boiled or stored in corroded copper or brass vessels.

Doctors measure copper and ceruloplasmin levels in blood or urine. However, a liver biopsy is usually required for diagnosis unless large amounts of copper were consumed.

If large amounts of copper were consumed, the stomach is pumped, and dimercaprol is injected into a muscle. Then drugs that bind with copper, such as penicillamine, are given to remove excess copper. Occasionally, death occurs despite treatment. Children with liver damage are treated with penicillamine.

Fluoride

In the body, most fluoride is contained in bones and teeth. Fluoride is necessary for the formation and health of bones and teeth.

FLUORIDE DEFICIENCY

Fluoride deficiency can lead to tooth decay and possibly osteoporosis. Consuming enough fluoride can prevent tooth decay and may strengthen bones. The addition of fluoride (fluoridation) to drinking water that is low in fluoride or the use of fluoride supplements significantly reduces the risk of tooth decay. In areas where drinking water is not fluoridated, children may be given fluoride by mouth.

FLUORIDE EXCESS

People who live in areas where the drinking water has a naturally high fluoride level may consume too much fluoride—causing a condition called fluorosis. Fluoride accumulates in teeth, particularly permanent teeth. Chalky white, irregular patches appear on the surface of the tooth enamel. The patches become stained yellow or brown, causing the enamel to appear mottled. The teeth may also become pitted. These defects appear to affect appearance only and may even make the enamel more resistant to cavities. Fluoride also accumulates in bones. Rarely, consuming too much fluoride for a long time results in dense but weak bones, abnormal bone growths (spurs) on the spine, and crippling due to calcium accumulation (calcification) in ligaments.

The diagnosis is based on symptoms.

Treatment involves reducing fluoride consumption. For example, if people live in areas with high fluoride levels in the water, they should not drink fluoridated water or take fluoride supplements. Children should always be instructed not to swallow fluoridated toothpaste.

Iodine

The thyroid gland contains most of the iodine in the body. Iodine in the thyroid gland is necessary for the formation of thyroid hormones. Iodine occurs in seawater. A small amount of iodine enters the atmosphere and, through rain, enters ground water and soil near the sea. In many areas, including the United States, table salt is fortified with iodine (in its combination form iodide) to help make sure people consume enough.

IODINE DEFICIENCY

Iodine deficiency is rare in areas where iodine is added to table salt. However, the deficiency is common worldwide. People living far from the sea and at higher altitudes are at particular risk of iodine deficiency because their environment, unlike that near the sea, contains little, if any, iodine.

When iodine is deficient, the thyroid gland enlarges, forming a goiter, as it attempts to capture more iodine for the production of thyroid hormones. The thyroid gland becomes underactive and produces too little thyroid hormones (hypothyroidism —see page 995). The person's IQ may be decreased. Fertility is reduced. In adults, hypothyroidism may cause puffy skin, a hoarse voice, impaired mental function, dry and scaly skin, sparse and coarse hair, intolerance to cold, and weight gain.

If pregnant women have iodine deficiency, the risk of miscarriage and stillbirth is increased. The fetus may grow slowly, and the brain may develop abnormally. Unless affected babies are treated soon after birth, mental retardation with short stature (cretin-ism) develops. Babies may have birth defects or hypothyroidism.

> **? Did You Know...**
>
> Lack of iodine during pregnancy increases the risk of miscarriage, stillbirth, and mental retardation and birth defects in the baby.

Diagnosis and Treatment

Iodine deficiency is diagnosed based on blood tests indicating low levels of thyroid hormones or a high level of thyroid-stimulating hormone (TSH) or on the presence of a goiter (only in adults). The amount of iodine in urine is measured. The lower the amount, the more severe the deficiency. Imaging tests, such as ultrasonography or thyroid scanning, may be done to measure the thyroid gland and to evaluate any abnormalities.

Treatment consists of iodine supplements, taken by mouth. Infants may also require supplements of thyroid hormone, sometimes throughout life.

IODINE EXCESS

Excess consumption of iodine is uncommon. It usually results from taking iodine supplements to treat a prolonged iodine deficiency. Sometimes people who live near the sea consume too much iodine because they eat a lot of seafood and seaweed and drink water that is high in iodine, as is common in northern Japan.

Consuming too much usually does not affect thyroid function, but sometimes does. It may cause the thyroid gland to become overactive and produce excess thyroid hormones (hyperthyroidism—see page 992). As a result, the thyroid gland enlarges, forming a goiter. (Goiters can also form when the thyroid gland is underactive.) If people consume very large amounts of iodine, they may have a brassy taste in their mouth and produce more saliva. Iodine can irritate the digestive tract and cause a rash.

Consuming too much iodine may also make the thyroid gland become underactive (hypothyroidism), especially if the thyroid gland had been underactive previously (for example, in people with Hashimoto's thyroiditis—see page 996).

Diagnosis and Treatment

Doctors suspect hyperthyroidism or hypothyroidism due to excess iodine based on symptoms, particularly in people who report taking iodine supplements, who live near the sea, or who consume a lot of seaweed or seafood. Blood tests to determine levels of thyroid hormones and thyroid-stimulating hormone (TSH) are done. Imaging tests may also be done.

People are advised to use salt that is not fortified with iodine and to reduce their consumption of foods that contain iodine. If people have hypothyroidism due to consuming too much iodine, consuming less iodine often cures the disorder, but some people must take thyroid hormones for the rest of their life.

Iron

Much of the iron in the body is contained in hemoglobin. Hemoglobin is the component of red blood cells that enables them to carry oxygen and deliver it to the body's tissues. Iron also is an important component of muscle cells. It is also necessary for the formation of many enzymes in the body.

The body recycles iron: When red blood cells die, the iron in them is returned to the bone marrow to be used again in new red blood cells. A small amount of iron is lost each day, mainly in cells shed from the lining of the intestine. This amount is usually replaced by the 1 to 2 milligrams of iron absorbed from food each day.

Food contains two types of iron:

- **Heme iron:** Animal products contain heme iron. It is absorbed much better than nonheme iron.
- **Nonheme iron:** Most foods and iron supplements contain nonheme iron. It accounts for more than 85% of iron in the average diet. However, less than 20% of nonheme iron that is consumed is absorbed into the body. Nonheme iron is absorbed better when it is consumed with animal protein and with vitamin C.

IRON DEFICIENCY

- Iron deficiency usually results from loss of blood in adults but, in children and pregnant women, may result from an inadequate diet.
- Anemia develops, making people appear pale and feel weak and tired.
- Doctors base the diagnosis on symptoms and blood test results.
- Doctors look for a source of bleeding, and if one is identified, they treat it.
- Iron supplements, usually taken by mouth, are often needed.

Iron deficiency is one of the most common mineral deficiencies in the world. It causes anemia in men, women, and children.

In adults, iron deficiency is most commonly caused by loss of blood. In premenopausal women, monthly menstrual bleeding may cause the deficiency. In men and postmenopausal women, iron deficiency usually indicates bleeding, most often in the digestive tract—

for example, from a bleeding ulcer or a polyp in the colon. Chronic bleeding due to colon cancer is a serious cause in middle-aged and older people.

Iron deficiency may result from an inadequate diet, primarily in infants and small children, who need more iron because they are growing. Adolescent girls who do not eat meat are at risk of developing iron deficiency because they are growing and starting to menstruate. Pregnant women are at risk of this deficiency because the growing fetus requires large amounts of iron.

Symptoms

When iron reserves in the body are exhausted, anemia develops (see page 1035). Anemia causes paleness, weakness, and fatigue. People usually do not notice how pale they are because it happens so gradually. Concentration and learning ability may be impaired. When severe, anemia may cause shortness of breath, dizziness, and a rapid heart rate. Occasionally, severe anemia causes chest pain and heart failure. Menstrual periods may stop.

In addition to anemia, iron deficiency may cause pica (a craving for nonfoods such as ice, dirt, or pure starch), spoon nails (thin, concave fingernails), and leg cramps at night. Rarely, iron deficiency causes a thin membrane to grow across part of the esophagus, making swallowing difficult.

Diagnosis

Iron deficiency is diagnosed based on symptoms and blood test results. Results include a low level of hemoglobin (which contains iron), a low hematocrit (the percentage of blood volume that is red blood cells), a low number of red blood cells, and the presence of abnormally small red blood cells. Blood tests also include the following:

- **Transferrin:** Transferrin is the protein that carries iron in blood when iron is not inside red blood cells. If the percentage of iron in transferrin is less than 10%, iron deficiency is likely.
- **Ferritin:** Ferritin is a protein that stores iron. Iron deficiency is confirmed if the ferritin level is low.

However, the ferritin level may be normal or high when iron deficiency is present if people have inflammation, an infection, cancer, or liver damage.

Occasionally, a bone marrow examination is needed to make the diagnosis. A sample of bone marrow cells is removed, usually from the hipbone, through a needle and examined under a microscope to determine the iron content.

Treatment

Because the most common cause of iron deficiency in adults is excessive bleeding, doctors first look for a source of bleeding. If the source is excessive menstrual bleeding, drugs, such as oral contraceptives (birth control pills), may be needed to control it. Surgery may be needed to repair a bleeding ulcer or remove a polyp in the colon. A blood transfusion may be necessary if the anemia is severe.

Normal dietary intake of iron may not be sufficient to replace lost iron (because less than 20% of iron in a typical diet is absorbed into the body). Thus, most people with iron deficiency need to take iron supplements by mouth usually once or twice a day. Iron in supplements is absorbed best when taken on an empty stomach, 30 minutes before meals or 2 hours after meals, particularly if the meals include foods that reduce the absorption of iron (such as vegetable fibers, phytates, bran, coffee, and tea). However, taking iron supplements on an empty stomach can cause indigestion and constipation. So some people must take the supplements with meals. Antacids and calcium supplements can also reduce iron absorption. Consuming vitamin C in juices or taking it as a supplement enhances iron absorption, as does eating small amounts of meat, which contains the more easily absorbed form of iron (heme iron). Iron supplements almost always turn stools black—a harmless side effect.

Rarely, iron is given by injection. Injections are necessary for people who cannot tolerate tablets or for a few people who cannot absorb enough iron from the digestive tract.

Correcting iron deficiency anemia usually takes 3 to 6 weeks, even after the bleeding has stopped. After the anemia is corrected, an iron supplement should be taken for 6 months to replenish the body's reserves. Blood tests are usually done periodically to determine whether people are receiving enough iron and to check for continued bleeding.

Women who are not menstruating and men should not take iron supplements or multiple vitamins with iron unless they are specifically instructed to do so by a doctor. Taking such supplements can make diagnosing bleeding from the intestine difficult. Such bleeding may be due to serious disorders, including colon cancer.

Because a developing fetus requires iron, iron supplements are recommended for most pregnant women. Most babies, particularly those who are premature or who have a low birth weight, need an iron supplement. It is given as an iron-fortified formula or, to breastfed babies, as a separate liquid supplement.

IRON EXCESS

Excess iron can accumulate in the body. Causes include the following:

- Repeated blood transfusions
- Iron therapy given in excessive amounts or for too long
- Chronic alcoholism
- An overdose of iron
- A hereditary disorder called hemochromatosis

Excess iron consumed all at once causes vomiting, diarrhea, and damage to the intestine and other organs. Excess iron consumed over a period of time may damage coronary arteries.

Often, deferoxamine is given intravenously. This drug binds with iron and carries it out of the body in urine. Hemachromatosis is treated with bloodletting (phlebotomy).

HEMOCHROMATOSIS

In hemochromatosis, a hereditary disorder, too much iron is absorbed, resulting in the accumulation of iron in the body.

- Iron can accumulate and damage any part of the body.
- People may develop symptoms of cirrhosis or diabetes or simply feel tired.
- Blood tests identify people who require genetic testing, which can confirm the disorder.
- Bloodletting, done periodically, can prevent further damage.

In the United States, over 1 million people have hemochromatosis. The disorder is potentially fatal but usually treatable. The gene associated with hemochromatosis has been identified.

Symptoms

Usually, symptoms develop gradually, often not appearing until middle age or later. In women, symptoms usually start after menopause because the loss of iron during menstrual bleeding and the increased requirement for iron during pregnancy compensate to some degree.

Symptoms vary because iron accumulation can damage any part of the body, including the brain, liver, pancreas, lungs, or heart. The first symptoms, particularly in men, may be those of cirrhosis (due to liver damage) or those of diabetes (due to pancreas damage). Or, the first symptoms, particularly in women, may be vague and affect the whole body. Fatigue is an example. Liver dysfunction is the most common problem. The following problems can also occur:

- Bronze-colored skin
- Heart failure (occasionally)
- Joint pains
- Increased risk of liver cancer
- Infertility
- An underactive thyroid gland (hypothyroidism)
- Chronic fatigue

In many men, levels of male hormones decrease. Erectile dysfunction (impotence) may occur. Hemochromatosis can worsen neurologic disorders that are already present.

Diagnosis

Identifying hemochromatosis based on symptoms may be difficult. However, blood tests to measure the levels of iron and two other substances can identify people who should be further evaluated. These substances are ferritin, a protein that stores iron, and the iron in transferrin, the protein that carries iron in blood when iron is not inside red blood cells. If the ferritin level and percentage of iron in transferrin are high, genetic testing is usually done to confirm the diagnosis. A liver biopsy may be necessary to determine whether the liver has been damaged.

Genetic testing is recommended for people with hemochromatosis and all of their first-degree relatives (siblings, parents, and children).

Treatment

Usually, bloodletting (phlebotomy) is the best treatment. It prevents additional organ damage but does not reverse existing damage. Bloodletting is done once or sometimes twice a week. Each time, about 500 milliliters (1 pint) of blood is removed until the iron level and percentage of iron in transferrin are normal. Bloodletting is then done periodically to keep these substances at normal levels.

With early diagnosis and treatment of hemochromatosis, a long, healthy life is possible.

Magnesium

Bone contains most of the body's magnesium. Blood contains very little. Magnesium is necessary for the formation of bone and teeth and for normal nerve and muscle function. Many enzymes in the body depend on magnesium to function normally. The body obtains magnesium from foods and excretes it in urine and stool.

HYPOMAGNESEMIA

In hypomagnesemia, the level of magnesium in blood is too low.

Usually, the level becomes low because people consume less (most often, because of starvation) or because the intestine cannot absorb nutrients normally (called malabsorption). But sometimes hypomagnesemia develops because the kidneys or intestine excrete too much magnesium. Hypomagnesemia may result from the following:

- Consuming large amounts of alcohol (common), which reduces consumption of food (and thus magnesium) and increases excretion of magnesium

- Protracted diarrhea (common), which increases excretion
- High levels of aldosterone, antidiuretic hormone, or thyroid hormones, which increase excretion
- Drugs that increase excretion, including diuretics, the antifungal drug amphotericin B, and the chemotherapy drug cisplatin
- Breastfeeding, which increases requirements for magnesium

Hypomagnesemia may cause nausea, vomiting, sleepiness, weakness, personality changes, muscle spasms, tremors, and loss of appetite. If severe, hypomagnesemia can cause seizures, especially in children.

The diagnosis is usually based on blood tests indicating that the magnesium level is low.

Magnesium is given by mouth when the deficiency causes symptoms or persists. All alcoholics are given magnesium. If a very low magnesium level is causing severe symptoms or if people cannot take magnesium by mouth, magnesium is given by injection into a muscle or vein.

HYPERMAGNESEMIA

In hypermagnesemia, the level of magnesium in blood is too high.

Hypermagnesemia usually develops only when people with kidney failure are given magnesium salts or take drugs that contain magnesium (such as some antacids or laxatives).

Hypermagnesemia may cause weakness, low blood pressure, and impaired breathing. When hypermagnesemia is severe, the heart can stop beating.

The diagnosis is based on blood tests indicating that the magnesium level is high.

People with severe hypermagnesemia are given calcium gluconate intravenously. Diuretics (particularly if given intravenously) can increase the kidneys' excretion of magnesium. However, if the kidneys are not functioning well (as is typical) or if hypermagnesemia is severe, dialysis is usually needed.

Molybdenum

Molybdenum is required for processing (metabolizing) nitrogen, activating certain enzymes, and enabling cells to function normally. Molybdenum also helps break down sulfites (which occur in foods naturally and are added as preservatives).

Molybdenum deficiency is rare. It may result from genetic disorders or inadequate consumption. Symptoms seem to vary. They may include mental retardation, seizures, increased heart and breathing rates, headache, nausea, vomiting, and coma.

Molybdenum excess is even more rare. It may cause swollen, painful joints and abnormalities of the digestive tract, liver, and kidneys.

Phosphate

In the body, almost all phosphorus is combined with oxygen, forming phosphate. Bone contains about 85% of the body's phosphate. The rest is located primarily inside cells, where it is involved in energy production.

Phosphate is necessary for the formation of bone and teeth. Phosphate is also used as a building block for several important substances, including those used by the cell for energy, cell membranes, and DNA (deoxyribonucleic acid). The body obtains phosphate from foods and excretes it in urine and stool.

HYPOPHOSPHATEMIA

In hypophosphatemia, the level of phosphate in blood is too low.

The phosphate level in blood may become low over time, resulting in chronic hypophosphatemia. Chronic hypophosphatemia usually develops because too much phosphate is excreted. Causes include the following:

- Hyperparathyroidism
- Chronic diarrhea
- Impaired kidney function or hemodialysis
- An underactive thyroid gland (hypothyroidism)
- Use of diuretics for a long time
- Use of large amounts of aluminum-containing antacids for a long time
- Use of large amounts of theophylline (used to treat asthma)

The phosphate level in blood can suddenly fall dangerously low in people recovering from the following conditions because the body uses large amounts of phosphate during recovery:

- Severe undernutrition (including starvation)
- Diabetic ketoacidosis
- Severe alcoholism
- Severe burns

This may result in an irregular heart rhythm and even death.

> **? Did You Know...**
> Some people who survived concentration camps died because their already low phosphate level suddenly fell when they began eating a normal diet, a phenomenon called refeeding syndrome.

Symptoms occur only when the phosphate level in blood becomes very low. Muscle weakness develops, followed by stupor, coma, and death. In mild chronic hypophosphatemia, the bones can weaken, resulting in bone pain and fractures. People may become weak and lose their appetite.

Diagnosis and Treatment

The diagnosis is based on blood tests indicating that the phosphate level is low. Doctors do other tests to identify the cause if it is not readily apparent.

Any drugs that can reduce the phosphate level are stopped. If hypophosphatemia is mild and causes no symptoms, drinking low-fat or skim milk, which provides a large amount of phosphate, may help. Or people can take phosphate by mouth, but doing so usually causes diarrhea. If hypophosphatemia is very severe or if phosphate cannot be taken by mouth, phosphate may be given intravenously.

HYPERPHOSPHATEMIA

In hyperphosphatemia, the level of phosphate in blood is too high.

Hyperphosphatemia is rare except in people with severe kidney dysfunction. In these people, the kidneys do not excrete enough phosphate. Dialysis, often used to treat them, is not very effective at removing phosphate and thus does not reduce the risk of hyperphosphatemia.

Less commonly, hyperphosphatemia develops in people with the following:

- A low level of parathyroid hormone (hypoparathyroidism)
- Lack of response to a normal level of parathyroid hormone (pseudohypoparathyroidism)
- Diabetic ketoacidosis
- Crush injuries
- Destruction of muscle tissue (rhabdomyolysis)
- Severe bodywide infections
- Large amounts of phosphate taken by mouth or given in an enema

Most people with hyperphosphatemia do not have symptoms. However, in people with severe kidney dysfunction, calcium combines with phosphate to form crystals (calcify) in the walls of the blood vessels and heart. Severe arteriosclerosis (hardening of the arteries) can result, leading to strokes, heart attacks, and poor circulation. Crystals can also form in the skin, where they cause severe itching.

Diagnosis and Treatment

The diagnosis is based on blood tests indicating that the phosphate level is high.

Hyperphosphatemia in people with kidney dysfunction is treated by reducing consumption of phosphate and reducing absorption of phosphate from the digestive tract. Foods that are high in phosphate should be avoided. Drugs that bind with phosphate, such as sevelamer and calcium compounds, should be taken with meals as prescribed by a doctor. By binding with phosphate, these drugs make it harder to absorb, and more phosphate is excreted. Sevelamer is often used for people undergoing dialysis because calcium compounds can make calcium-phosphate crystals more likely to form in tissues.

Potassium

Most of the body's potassium is located inside the cells. Potassium is necessary for the normal functioning of cells, nerves, and muscles.

The body must maintain the potassium level in blood within a narrow range. A potassium level that is too high or too low can have serious consequences, such as an abnormal heart rhythm or even stopping of the heart (cardiac arrest). The body can use the potassium stored within cells to help maintain a constant level of potassium in blood.

The body maintains the right level of potassium by matching the amount of potassium consumed with the amount lost. Potassium is consumed in food and drinks that contain electrolytes (including potassium) and lost primarily in urine. Some potassium is also lost through the digestive tract and in sweat. Healthy kidneys can adjust the excretion of potassium to match changes in consumption.

Some drugs and certain conditions affect the movement of potassium into and out of cells, which greatly influences the potassium level in blood.

HYPOKALEMIA

In hypokalemia, the level of potassium in blood is too low.

- A low potassium level has many causes but usually results from vomiting, diarrhea, adrenal gland disorders, or use of diuretics.
- A low potassium level can make muscles feel weak, cramp, twitch, or even become paralyzed, and abnormal heart rhythms may develop.
- The diagnosis is based on blood tests to measure the potassium level.
- Usually, eating foods rich in potassium or taking potassium supplements by mouth is all that is needed.

Typically, the potassium level becomes low because too much is lost from the digestive tract. Sometimes too much potassium is excreted in urine, usually because of diuretics that cause the kidneys to excrete excess sodium, water, and potassium. In many adrenal disorders, such as Cushing's syndrome (see page 1001), the adrenal glands produce too much aldosterone, a hormone that causes the kidneys to excrete large amounts of potassium.

Certain drugs cause more potassium to move from blood into cells and can result in hypokalemia. However, these drugs usually cause temporary hypokalemia, unless another condition is also causing potassium to be lost.

Hypokalemia is rarely caused by consuming too little because many foods contain potassium.

WHAT MAKES THE POTASSIUM LEVEL DECREASE?

CAUSE	DISORDERS	DRUGS OR OTHER CIRCUMSTANCES
Increased loss from the digestive tract (most common)	Vomiting Diarrhea	Laxatives if used a long time
Increased excretion in urine	Cushing's syndrome Aldosteronism due to a tumor in the adrenal glands A low level of magnesium (hypomagnesemia) Gitelman's syndrome Liddle syndrome Bartter syndrome Fanconi syndrome	Diuretics (commonly) Licorice (natural) if consumed in large amounts Tobacco chewing (certain types)
Increased movement from blood into cells	An overactive thyroid gland (hyperthyroidism)	Insulin Some drugs used to treat asthma: albuterol, terbutaline, and theophylline

WHAT MAKES THE POTASSIUM LEVEL INCREASE?

CAUSE	DISORDERS	DRUGS OR OTHER CIRCUMSTANCES
Increased consumption	—	A diet containing potassium-rich foods Potassium supplements Intravenous treatments that contain potassium, such as total parenteral nutrition and blood transfusions
Decreased excretion in urine	Kidney failure	Aliskiren Angiotensin-converting enzyme (ACE) inhibitors Angiotensin-receptor blockers Cyclosporine (used to prevent rejection of organ transplants) Diuretics that help the kidneys conserve potassium, such as eplerenone, spironolactone, and triamterene Nonsteroidal anti-inflammatory drugs Tacrolimus (used to prevent rejection of organ transplants)
Release of potassium from cells	Burns if severe Crush injuries (involving the destruction of large amounts of muscle tissue) Diabetes Metabolic acidosis	Cancer chemotherapy Crack cocaine overdose Exercise if strenuous and prolonged

Symptoms and Diagnosis

A slight decrease in the potassium level in blood usually causes no symptoms. A larger decrease can cause muscle weakness, cramping, twitches, and even paralysis. Abnormal heart rhythms may develop. They may develop even when the decrease is slight if people already have a heart disorder or take the heart drug digoxin.

The diagnosis is made by measuring the potassium level in the blood. Doctors then try to identify what is causing the decrease. The cause may be clear based on the person's symptoms (such as vomiting) or use of drugs or other substances. If the cause is not clear, doctors measure how much potassium is excreted in urine to determine whether excess excretion is the cause.

Treatment

If a disorder is causing hypokalemia, it is treated.

Usually, potassium can be replaced by eating potassium-rich foods or by taking potassium supplements by mouth. Because potassium can irritate the digestive tract, supplements should be taken in small doses with food several times a day rather than in a single large dose. Special types of potassium supplements, such as wax-impregnated or microencapsulated potassium chloride, are much less likely to irritate the digestive tract.

Potassium is given intravenously in the following situations:

- The potassium level is dangerously low.
- Supplements taken by mouth are ineffective.
- People continue to lose too much potassium to be replaced using supplements taken by mouth.
- The low level causes abnormal heart rhythms.

Most people who take diuretics do not need to take potassium supplements. Nevertheless, doctors periodically check the potassium level in blood so that the drug regimen can be changed if necessary. Alternatively, diuretics that help the kidneys conserve potassium (potassium-sparing diuretics), such as amiloride, eplerenone, spironolactone, or triamterene can be used, but only if the kidneys are functioning normally.

HYPERKALEMIA

In hyperkalemia, the level of potassium in blood is too high.

- A high potassium level has many causes, including kidney disorders, drugs that affect kidney function, and consumption of too much supplemental potassium.
- Usually, hyperkalemia must be severe before it causes symptoms, mainly abnormal heart rhythms.

- Doctors usually detect hyperkalemia when blood tests or electrocardiography is done for other reasons.
- Treatment includes reducing consumption of potassium, stopping drugs that may cause hyperkalemia, and using drugs to increase potassium excretion.

Usually, hyperkalemia results from several simultaneous problems, including the following:

- Kidney disorders (such as kidney failure) that prevent the kidneys from excreting enough potassium
- Drugs that prevent the kidneys from excreting normal amounts of potassium (a common cause of mild hyperkalemia)
- A diet high in potassium
- Treatments that contain potassium

The most common cause of mild hyperkalemia is the use of drugs that decrease blood flow to the kidneys or prevent the kidneys from excreting normal amounts of potassium. Kidney failure can cause severe hyperkalemia on its own. Addison's disease can also cause hyperkalemia.

Hyperkalemia can develop after a large amount of potassium is released from the cells. The rapid movement of potassium from cells into blood can overwhelm the kidneys and result in life-threatening hyperkalemia.

Symptoms and Diagnosis

Mild hyperkalemia causes few, if any, symptoms. When hyperkalemia becomes more severe, it can cause abnormal heart rhythms. If the level is very high, the heart can stop beating.

Usually, hyperkalemia is first detected when routine blood tests are done or when a doctor notices certain changes on an electrocardiogram. To identify the cause, doctors determine which drugs people are taking and do blood tests to check kidney function.

Treatment

For mild hyperkalemia, reducing consumption of potassium or stopping drugs that prevent the kidneys from excreting potassium may be all that is needed. If the kidneys are functioning, a diuretic may be given to increase potassium excretion. If needed, a resin that absorbs potassium from the digestive tract and passes out of the body in the stool can be given by mouth or enema.

For moderate to severe hyperkalemia, the potassium level must be reduced immediately. Calcium is given intravenously to protect the heart but does not lower the potassium level. Then insulin and glucose are given. They move potassium from blood into cells, thus lowering the potassium level in blood. Albuterol (used mainly to treat asthma) may be given to help lower the potassium level. It is inhaled.

If these measures do not work or if people have kidney failure, dialysis may be necessary to remove the excess potassium.

Selenium

Selenium occurs in all tissues. Selenium works with vitamin E as an antioxidant. It helps protect cells against damage by free radicals, which are reactive by-products of normal cell activity. Selenium may help protect against some cancers. Selenium is also necessary for the thyroid gland to function normally.

SELENIUM DEFICIENCY

Selenium deficiency is rare, even in New Zealand and Finland, where selenium intake is much lower than in the United States and Canada. In certain areas of China, where selenium intake is even lower, people with selenium deficiency are more likely to develop Keshan disease, a viral disease that affects mainly children and young women. Keshan disease damages the walls of the heart, resulting in cardiomyopathy.

In selenium deficiency, antioxidants are lacking in the heart and muscles. As a result, cardiomyopathy and muscle weakness may occur.

Doctors suspect selenium deficiency based on the person's circumstances and symptoms. Treatment with a selenium supplement may result in a complete recovery. Taking selenium supplements can prevent but not cure cardiomyopathy due to Keshan disease.

SELENIUM EXCESS

Taking more than 1 milligram of a nonprescription selenium supplement each day can have harmful effects. Symptoms include nausea, vomiting, diarrhea, hair loss, abnormal nails, a rash, fatigue, and nerve damage. The breath may smell like garlic.

The diagnosis is based on symptoms, particularly rapid hair loss. Treatment involves reducing selenium consumption.

Sodium

Most of the body's sodium is located in blood and in the fluid around cells. Sodium helps the body keep fluids in a normal balance (see page 969). Sodium plays a key role in normal nerve and muscle function.

The body obtains sodium through food and drink and loses it primarily in sweat and urine. Healthy kidneys maintain a consistent level of sodium in the body by adjusting the amount excreted in the urine. When sodium consumption and loss are not in balance, the total amount of sodium in the body is affected.

Controlling Blood Volume: The total amount of sodium affects the amount of fluid in blood and around cells. The body continually monitors blood volume and sodium (and other electrolyte) concentrations. When either becomes too high, sensors in the heart, blood vessels, and kidneys detect the increases and stimulate the kidneys to increase sodium excretion, thus returning blood volume to normal. When blood volume or sodium concentration becomes too low, those sensors trigger mechanisms to increase blood volume. These mechanisms include the following:

- The kidneys stimulate the adrenal glands to secrete the hormone aldosterone. Aldosterone causes the kidneys to retain sodium and to excrete potassium. When sodium is retained, less urine is produced, eventually causing blood volume to increase.
- The pituitary gland secretes antidiuretic hormone. Antidiuretic hormone causes the kidneys to conserve fluid. Then blood volume increases.

HYPONATREMIA

In hyponatremia, the level of sodium in blood is too low.

- A low sodium level has many causes, including consumption of too many fluids, kidney failure, heart failure, cirrhosis, and use of diuretics.
- At first, people become sluggish and confused, and if hyponatremia worsens, they may have muscle twitches and seizures and become progressively unresponsive.
- The diagnosis is based on blood tests to measure the sodium level.
- Restricting fluids and stopping use of diuretics can help, but severe hyponatremia is an emergency requiring use of drugs, intravenous fluids, or both.

Causes

Hyponatremia occurs when the body contains too little sodium for the amount of fluid it contains. The body may have too much, too little, or about a normal amount of fluid. In all cases, however, sodium is diluted. For example, people with severe vomiting or diarrhea lose sodium. If they replace their fluid losses with water, sodium is diluted. Disorders, such as cirrhosis and heart failure, can cause the body to retain sodium and fluid. Often the body retains more fluid than sodium, which means the sodium is diluted.

Symptoms

The brain is particularly sensitive to changes in the sodium level in blood. Therefore, symptoms of brain dysfunction, such as sluggishness (lethargy) and confusion, occur first. If the sodium level in blood falls quickly, symptoms tend to develop rapidly and be more severe. Older people are more likely to have severe symptoms.

As hyponatremia becomes more severe, muscle twitching and seizures may occur. People may be-

Causes of Hyponatremia
■ Addison's disease (underactive adrenal glands)
■ Blockage of the small intestine
■ Burns if severe
■ Cirrhosis (formation of scar tissue in the liver)
■ Consumption of too much water, as occurs in some psychiatric disorders
■ Diarrhea
■ Drugs such as barbiturates, carbamazepine, chlorpropamide, clofibrate, diuretics (most common), opioids, tolbutamide, and vincristine
■ Heart failure
■ Hypothyroidism
■ Kidney disorders
■ Pancreatitis
■ Peritonitis (inflammation of the abdominal cavity)
■ Syndrome of inappropriate secretion of antidiuretic hormone (SIADH)
■ Vomiting

come unresponsive, aroused only by vigorous stimulation (stupor), and eventually cannot be aroused (coma). Death may follow.

Diagnosis and Treatment

Hyponatremia is diagnosed by measuring the sodium level in blood. Determining the cause is more complex. Doctors consider the person's circumstances, including other disorders present and drugs taken. Blood and urine tests are done to evaluate the amount of fluid in the body, the concentration of blood, and content of urine.

Mild hyponatremia can be treated by restricting fluid intake to less than 1 quart per day. If a diuretic is the cause, it is reduced or stopped. If the cause is a disorder, it is treated. Occasionally, people are given a sodium solution intravenously, a diuretic to increase excretion of fluid, or both, usually slowly, over several days. These treatments can correct the sodium level.

Severe hyponatremia is an emergency. To treat it, doctors slowly increase the level of sodium in blood with drugs, intravenous fluids, or sometimes both. Increasing the level too rapidly can result in severe and often permanent brain damage.

SYNDROME OF INAPPROPRIATE SECRETION OF ANTIDIURETIC HORMONE

Syndrome of inappropriate secretion of antidiuretic hormone (SIADH) develops when too much antidiuretic hormone is released by the pituitary gland, causing the body to retain fluid and lower the sodium level by dilution.

Antidiuretic hormone (also called vasopressin) helps regulate the amount of water in the body by controlling how much water is excreted by the kidneys. High levels of antidiuretic hormone decrease water excretion by the kidneys. The pituitary gland produces and releases antidiuretic hormone when the blood volume or blood pressure goes down or when levels of electrolytes (such as sodium) become too high.

Pain, stress, exercise, a low blood sugar level, and certain disorders of the heart, thyroid gland, kidneys, or adrenal glands can stimulate the release of antidiuretic hormone from the pituitary gland, as can the following drugs:

- Chlorpropamide (which lowers the blood sugar level)
- Carbamazepine (an anticonvulsant)
- Vincristine (a chemotherapy drug)
- Clofibrate (which lowers cholesterol levels)
- Antipsychotic drugs
- Aspirin, ibuprofen, and many other nonprescription pain relievers (analgesics)
- Vasopressin (synthetic antidiuretic hormone) and oxytocin (both drugs help the body conserve fluids)

Secretion of antidiuretic hormone is termed inappropriate if it occurs even though blood volume and blood pressure are normal or high, electrolyte concentrations are low, and other triggers of antidiuretic hormone release are not present. When antidiuretic hormone is released in these situations, the sodium level in blood decreases, and the body retains too much fluid.

SIADH is common among older people and is fairly common among people who are hospitalized.

Many conditions increase the risk of developing SIADH. SIADH may result when antidiuretic hormone is produced outside the pituitary gland, as occurs in some lung and other cancers.

Symptoms of SIADH tend to be those of the low sodium level in blood (hyponatremia) that accompanies it (see page 948).

Diagnosis and Treatment

Doctors suspect SIADH based on a person's circumstances and symptoms. Blood and urine tests are done to measure the sodium and potassium levels and to determine how concentrated the blood and urine are (osmolality). Doctors also rule out other possible causes of excess antidiuretic hormone (such as pain, stress, drugs, or cancer). Once SIADH is diagnosed, doctors try to identify the cause and determine how well the pituitary gland is functioning.

Doctors restrict fluid intake and treat the cause if possible. If the sodium level in blood continues to

WHAT CAUSES SIADH?	
TYPE OF DISORDER	**EXAMPLES**
Brain or nervous system	Abscesses in the brain
	Bleeding (hemorrhage) within the layers of tissue covering the brain
	Encephalitis (inflammation of the brain)
	Guillain-Barré syndrome
	Head injury
	Hypothalamus disorders, including tumors (rare)
	Meningitis
	Strokes
	Tumors
Lung	Acute respiratory failure
	Pneumonia
	Tuberculosis
Cancers	Brain cancer
	Lung cancer
	Lymphoma
	Pancreatic cancer
	Cancer of the small intestine
Other	Surgery
	Undernutrition

SIADH = syndrome of inappropriate secretion of antidiuretic hormone.

decrease or does not increase despite restriction of fluid intake, drugs that decrease the effect of antidiuretic hormone on the kidneys (such as demeclocycline or thiazide diuretics) may be used.

HYPERNATREMIA

In hypernatremia, the level of sodium in blood is too high.

- Hypernatremia has many causes, but dehydration is most common, including not drinking enough fluids, diarrhea, kidney dysfunction, and diuretics.
- Mainly, people are thirsty, and they may become confused or have muscles twitches and seizures.
- Blood tests are done to measure the sodium level.
- Usually, fluids are given intravenously to slowly reduce the sodium level in the blood.

In hypernatremia, the body contains too little water for the amount of sodium. The sodium level in blood becomes abnormally high when water loss exceeds sodium loss, as typically occurs in dehydration.

SPOTLIGHT ON AGING

As people age, the body is less able to balance fluid and sodium for several reasons:

- **Decreased thirst:** As people age, they sense thirst less quickly or less intensely and thus may not drink fluids when needed.
- **Changes in the kidneys:** The kidneys may function less well. As a result, more fluid may be excreted in urine, and the kidneys may become less able to concentrate urine.
- **Less fluid in the body:** The older body contains less fluid. Only 45% of body weight is fluid in healthy older people, compared with 60% in younger people. This change means that a slight loss of fluid and sodium, as can result from a fever or even breathing rapidly, can have more serious consequences.
- **Inability to obtain water:** Some older people have physical problems that prevent them from getting something to drink when they want or need it. Others may have dementia, which may prevent them from realizing they are thirsty or from saying so. These people may have to depend on other people to provide them with water.

In older people, a low sodium level in blood (hyponatremia) usually results from retaining too much water, as occurs in heart failure. Older people who are given fluids intravenously during hospitalization or before surgery are at high risk of developing hyponatremia. Using liquid nutritional supplements, which are often low in sodium, is another cause of hyponatremia in older people.

A high sodium level in blood (hypernatremia), which is common among older people, usually results from dehydration, which is typically caused by loss of fluid, not consuming enough fluid, or both.

Disorders that increase the risk of sodium-fluid imbalance, such as heart failure and kidney disorders, are common among older people.

Taking a diuretic (which forces the kidneys to excrete more water) increases the risk of hypernatremia further—especially when the weather is hot or when older people become ill and do not drink enough water. Taking a certain type of diuretic (thiazide diuretics, such as hydrochlorothiazide), particularly if the kidneys are not functioning normally, can result in a dangerously low sodium level. Severe symptoms can develop within a few weeks after the drug is started.

Symptoms of hyponatremia or hypernatremia are usually more severe in older people. For example, hyponatremia can result in delirium, causing confusion, agitation, or lethargy.

Usually, hypernatremia results from dehydration (see page 970). For example, people may lose body fluids and become dehydrated from drinking too little, vomiting, diarrhea, diuretic use, or excessive sweating. People with diabetes mellitus and high blood sugar may have excessive urine volumes, causing dehydration. Diabetes insipidus (which causes excessive urine volume without high blood sugar—see page 986) and kidney disorders can also cause dehydration. Rarely adrenal gland disorders can cause hyponatremia without dehydration. Hypernatremia is most common among older people.

Hypernatremia typically causes thirst. The most serious symptoms of hypernatremia result from brain dysfunction. Severe hypernatremia can lead to confusion, muscle twitching, seizures, coma, and death.

Diagnosis and Treatment

The diagnosis is based on blood tests indicating that the sodium level is high.

Hypernatremia is treated by replacing fluids. In all but the mildest cases, dilute fluids (containing water and a small amount of sodium in carefully adjusted concentrations) are given intravenously. The sodium level in blood is reduced very slowly because reducing the level too rapidly can cause permanent brain damage.

Zinc

Zinc is widely distributed in the body—in bones, teeth, hair, skin, liver, muscle, white blood cells, and testes. It is a component of more than 100 enzymes, including those involved in the formation of RNA (ribonucleic acid) and DNA (deoxyribonucleic acid).

The level of zinc in the body depends on the amount of zinc consumed in the diet. Zinc is necessary for healthy skin, healing of wounds, and growth. Much of the zinc consumed in the diet is not absorbed.

ZINC DEFICIENCY

- Zinc deficiency has many causes, including diet, various disorders, alcoholism, and diuretics.
- People lose their appetite and hair and may feel sluggish and irritable.
- Measuring the zinc level in blood is available but is not a good test for zinc status.
- Zinc supplements taken by mouth can cure the deficiency.

Many conditions can increase the risk of developing zinc deficiency.

In acrodermatitis enteropathica, a rare hereditary disorder, zinc cannot be absorbed. This disorder may result in diarrhea, hair loss, and zinc deficiency.

Symptoms

Early symptoms include a loss of appetite and, in infants and children, slowed growth and development. People may lose their hair in patches. They may feel sluggish and irritable. Taste and smell may be impaired. Rashes may develop. In men, sperm production may be reduced. The body's immune system may be impaired, and wounds may heal more slowly and less completely.

If pregnant women have zinc deficiency, the baby may have birth defects and may weigh less than expected at birth.

In acrodermatitis enteropathica, symptoms usually appear when an affected infant is weaned.

> **? Did You Know...**
>
> Lack of zinc can weaken the immune system and make wounds heal more slowly.
>
> Zinc deficiency is common among older people who live in institutions and people who are homebound.

Diagnosis and Treatment

Doctors suspect zinc deficiency based on the person's circumstances, symptoms, and response to zinc supplements. Blood and urine tests do not accurately measure zinc status.

Zinc supplements are taken by mouth until symptoms disappear.

ZINC EXCESS

People rarely consume too much zinc. Usually, zinc excess results from consuming acidic foods or beverages

WHAT CAN CAUSE ZINC DEFICIENCY?

CAUSE	EXAMPLES
Diet	Dietary deficiency of zinc is uncommon in developed countries
Disorders	Alcoholism Bloodstream infection (sepsis) Chronic kidney disease Diabetes mellitus Disorders that impair absorption (malabsorption) Liver disorders Lung cancer Pancreatic disorders
Injuries	Burns if severe
Treatments	Diuretics Intravenous feedings for a long time

packaged in a zinc-coated (galvanized) container. In certain industries, inhaling zinc oxide fumes can result in zinc excess.

People may have a metallic taste in the mouth, as well as nausea, vomiting, and diarrhea. Consuming 1 gram or more—about 70 times the recommended daily allowance (RDA)—daily may be fatal. Inhaling zinc oxide fumes can cause rapid breathing, sweating, fever, and metallic mouth taste—a disorder called metal fume fever. Consuming too much zinc for a long time can reduce the absorption of copper, cause anemia, and impair the immune system.

Doctors suspect the diagnosis based on the person's circumstances and symptoms.

Treatment involves reducing zinc consumption. People with metal fume fever usually recover after being in a zinc-free environment for 12 to 24 hours.

CHAPTER

140 Obesity and the Metabolic Syndrome

Obesity

Obesity is the accumulation of excessive body fat.

- Obesity usually results from consuming too many calories and not burning enough calories in physical activity.

- Being obese increases the risk of many disorders, such as diabetes, high blood pressure, heart disease, and certain cancers, and can result in early death.

- Increasing activity and reducing caloric intake are essential to treating obesity, but some people also need to take drugs.

- Losing as little of 5 to 10% of body weight can help lessen weight-related problems, such as diabetes, high blood pressure, and high cholesterol levels.
- People who are very obese and who have serious weight-related problems may benefit from weight-loss surgery.

The body mass index (BMI) is used to define overweight and obesity. BMI is weight (in kilograms) divided by height (in meters squared). Overweight is usually defined as a BMI of 25 to 29.9. Obesity is defined as a BMI of 30 or higher. Obesity is considered to be severe if BMI is 40 or higher.

Obesity has become increasingly common throughout the world. In the United States, obesity has increased dramatically: 34% of adults are obese, and over 17% of children and adolescents are overweight or obese. Obesity is much easier to prevent than treat. Once people gain excess weight, the body resists losing weight. For example, when people diet or reduce the number of calories they consume, the body compensates by increasing appetite and reducing the number of calories burned during rest.

Causes

Obesity can result from certain disorders, but the increase in obesity results largely from environmental changes that have increased the availability of high-calorie foods and reduced the opportunity for physical activity.

Excess calories are stored in the body as fat. The number of calories needed varies from person to person, depending on age, sex, activity level, and metabolic rate. A person's resting (basal) metabolic rate—the amount of calories the body burns while at rest—is determined mostly by how much muscle (lean) tissue a person has. The more muscle people have, the higher their metabolic rate.

Physical Inactivity: In developed countries, lack of physical activity contributes greatly to the increase in obesity. Opportunities for physical activity have been engineered away by technological advances, such as elevators, cars, and remote controls. More time is spent doing sedentary activities such as using the computer, watching television, and playing video games. Also, people's jobs have become more sedentary as office or desk jobs have replaced manual labor. Sedentary people use fewer calories than more active people and thus require fewer calories in the diet. If caloric intake is not reduced accordingly, people gain weight.

Diet: The diet in developed countries is energy dense. That is, it consists of foods that have a large number of calories in a given amount (volume). Foods contain more processed carbohydrates (such as high-fructose corn syrup), more fat, and less fiber. Fats, by nature, are energy dense. A gram of fat has 9 calories, but carbohydrates and proteins have 4 calories per gram.

Convenience foods, such as energy-dense snacks offered at vending machines and fast food restaurants, contribute to the increase in obesity. High-calorie beverages, including soda, juices, coffee drinks, and alcohol, also contribute significantly. For example, a 12-ounce soda or bottle of beer has 150 calories; a 12-ounce coffee beverage or fruit smoothie can have 500 or more calories. An additional 500 calories per day results in a weight gain of 1 pound per week.

Genes: Obesity tends to run in families. However, families share not only genes but also environment, and separating the two influences is difficult. Genes can affect how quickly the body burns calories at rest and during exercise. They can also affect appetite and thus how much food is consumed.

Many genes influence weight, but each gene has only a very small effect. Obesity rarely results when only one gene is abnormal.

Mutations in the following genes are relatively common:

- Gene for the melanocortin 4 receptor: Receptors are structures on the surface of cells that inhibit or produce an action in the cell when certain substances (such as chemical messengers) bind with them. Melanocortin 4 receptors are located mainly in the brain. They help the body regulate its use of energy. A mutation in this gene may account for obesity in 1 to 4% of children.
- *Ob* gene: This gene controls the production of leptin, a hormone made by fat cells. Leptin travels to the brain and interacts with receptors in the hypothalamus (the part of the brain that helps regulate appetite). The message carried by leptin is to decrease food intake and increase the amount of calories (energy) burned. A mutation in the *ob* gene prevents leptin production and results in severe obesity in a very small number of children. In these cases, administration of leptin reduces weight to a normal amount.

Background: Certain characteristics can increase the risk of becoming overweight or obese. They include the following:

- Certain racial and ethnic backgrounds, such as African Americans, Hispanics, and Pacific Islanders
- A lower socioeconomic group
- A lower education level
- Obesity during childhood (see page 1756), which tends to persist into adulthood.

Pregnancy and Menopause: Gaining weight during pregnancy is normal and necessary. However, pregnancy can be the beginning of weight problems if women do not return to their prepregnancy weight. Having several children close together may com-

DETERMINING BODY MASS INDEX

HEIGHT	WEIGHT (POUNDS)																
	100	**110**	**120**	**130**	**140**	**150**	**160**	**170**	**180**	**190**	**200**	**210**	**220**	**230**	**240**	**250**	**260**
4'10"	21	23	25	27	29	31	33	36	38	40	42	44	46	48	50	52	54
4'11"	20	22	24	26	28	30	32	34	36	38	40	42	45	47	49	51	53
5'0"	20	21	23	25	27	29	31	33	35	37	39	41	43	45	47	49	51
5'1"	19	21	23	25	26	28	30	32	34	36	38	40	42	43	45	47	49
5'2"	18	20	22	24	26	27	29	31	33	35	37	38	40	43	44	46	48
5'3"	18	19	21	23	25	27	28	30	32	34	35	37	39	41	43	44	46
5'4"	17	19	21	22	24	26	27	29	31	33	34	36	38	39	41	43	45
5'5"	17	18	20	22	23	25	27	28	30	32	33	35	37	38	40	42	43
5'6"	16	18	19	21	23	24	26	27	29	31	32	34	36	37	39	40	42
5'7"	16	17	19	20	22	23	25	27	28	30	31	33	34	36	38	39	41
5'8"	15	17	18	20	21	23	24	26	27	29	30	32	33	35	36	38	40
5'9"	15	16	18	19	21	22	24	25	27	28	30	31	32	34	35	37	38
5'10"	14	16	17	19	20	22	23	24	26	27	29	30	32	33	34	36	37
5'11"	14	15	17	18	20	21	22	24	25	26	28	29	31	32	33	35	36
6'0"	13	15	16	18	19	20	22	23	24	26	27	28	30	31	33	34	35
6'1"	13	15	16	17	18	20	21	22	24	25	26	28	29	30	32	33	34
6'2"	12	14	15	17	18	19	21	22	23	24	26	27	28	30	31	32	33
6'3"	12	14	15	16	17	19	20	21	22	24	25	26	27	29	30	31	33
6'4"	12	13	15	16	17	18	19	21	22	23	24	26	27	28	29	30	32
6'5"	12	13	14	15	17	18	19	20	21	23	24	25	26	27	29	30	31
6'6"	12	13	14	15	16	17	19	20	21	22	23	24	25	27	28	29	30

Underweight: Less than 17.9
Normal: 18 to 24.9 (18 to 22.9 for Asians)
Overweight: 25 to 29.9 (23 to 29.9 for Asians)
Obese, moderate: 30 to 40
Obese, severe: More than 40

pound the problem. Breastfeeding can help women return to their prepregnancy weight.

After menopause, many women gain weight. This weight gain may result from reduced activity. Hormonal changes may cause fat to be redistributed and accumulate around the waist. Fat in this location increases the risk of health problems (see page 960).

Aging: As people age, body composition may change as muscle tissue decreases. The result is a higher percentage of body fat and a lower basal metabolic rate (because muscle burns more calories).

Lifestyle: Sleep deprivation or lack of sleep (usually considered less than 6 to 8 hours per night) can result in weight gain. Sleeplessness results in hormonal changes that increase appetite and cravings for energy-dense foods.

Stopping smoking usually results in weight gain. Nicotine decreases appetite and increases the metabolic rate. When nicotine is stopped, people may eat more food and their metabolic rate decreases, so that fewer calories are burned. As a result, body weight may increase by 5 to 10%.

Hormones: Hormonal disorders rarely cause obesity. The following are among the most common examples:

- Cushing's syndrome is caused by excessive levels of cortisol in the body. The syndrome can result from a benign tumor in the pituitary gland (pituitary adenoma) or from a tumor in the adrenal gland or elsewhere, such as in the lungs. Cushing's syndrome typically causes fat to accumulate in the face, making it look full (called moon face), and behind the neck (called a buffalo hump).

- Polycystic ovary syndrome (see page 1528) affects about 5 to 10% of women. Affected women tend to be overweight or obese. Levels of testosterone and other male hormones are increased, causing fat to accumulate in the waist and abdomen, which is more harmful than the fat that is distributed throughout the body.

Eating Disorders: Two eating disorders are associated with obesity:

- **Binge eating disorder** is characterized by binging, by eating large amounts of food during a short amount of time, and usually by a feeling of guilt or remorse or sense of being out of control. Most affected people do not "purge" (for example, by vomiting or using laxatives or diuretics). The disorder is diagnosed when bingeing episodes occur at least twice a week for 6 or more months (see page 879).

- **Night-eating syndrome** involves not eating much during the day, consuming a lot of food or calories in the evening, and awakening to eat in the middle of the night.

Drugs: Many drugs used to treat common disorders promote weight gain. These drugs include those used to treat psychiatric disorders including depression, those used to treat seizures, some antihypertensives (such as beta-blockers), corticosteroids, and some drugs used to treat diabetes mellitus.

Symptoms

The most obvious and only true symptom of obesity is a change in overall appearance. However, being obese also increases the risk of many health problems. Virtually every organ system can be affected. These weight-related health problems can cause symptoms, such as shortness of breath, difficulty breathing during activity, snoring, skin abnormalities including acne, and joint and back pain.

Obesity increases the risk of the following:

- High cholesterol levels
- High blood pressure
- Metabolic syndrome
- Coronary artery disease
- Heart failure
- Diabetes or a high blood sugar level (insulin resistance or prediabetes)
- Cancer of the breast, uterus, ovaries, colon, prostate, kidneys, or pancreas
- Gallstones and other gallbladder disorders
- A low testosterone level, erectile dysfunction, and reduced fertility in men
- Menstrual disorders, infertility, and increased risk of miscarriage in women
- Skin abnormalities, including acne and facial hair in women
- Varicose veins
- Fatty liver, hepatitis, and cirrhosis
- Blood clots (deep vein thrombosis and pulmonary embolism)
- Asthma
- Obstructive sleep apnea
- Kidney disorders, including nephrotic syndrome
- Arthritis, gout, low back pain, and other joint disorders
- Depression and anxiety

Obesity doubles or triples the risk of early death. The more severe the obesity, the higher the risk. In the United States, 300,000 deaths a year are attributed to obesity.

Diagnosis

Obesity is diagnosed by determining the BMI (see page 952). The BMI does not distinguish between lean and fat tissue. Thus, some people have a high BMI because they have excess muscle (for example, if they are body builders), but they are not considered obese. Conversely, some people have a normal weight but a high percentage of body fat, which is unhealthy. Therefore, body composition, especially percentage of body fat, is also important. Body composition can be measured using dual-energy x-ray absorptiometry (DEXA), which is also used to check for bone loss, or bioelectric impedance, which can be done in a doctor's office.

Waist circumference is measured. This measurement helps identify and quantify abdominal (visceral) obesity, which is fat that accumulates in the midsection (see page 960). Abdominal obesity is much more harmful than fat that is distributed throughout the body under the skin (subcutaneous fat).

Treatment

The main treatment for obesity is changing lifestyle, which includes changes in diet, increased physical activity, and behavioral modification to help with weight loss and maintenance. Some people may also need to take drugs or to have weight-loss (bariatric) surgery.

Successful weight loss requires motivation and a sense of readiness. People who are most successful have realistic goals and recognize that healthy weight loss can be achieved only with lifelong lifestyle changes rather than a magic bullet or fad diet that cannot be sustained. Seeking the support of health care practitioners such as dieticians or physicians can be beneficial. Programs that require regular contact increase accountability and can increase success rate. Some examples include Overeaters Anonymous (OA), Take Off Pounds Sensibly (TOPS), community-based and work-site programs, and organized commercial programs such as Weight Watchers. Typically, weekly meetings are conducted by counselors and supplemented by instructional and guidance materials.

Dietary Change: Healthy eating for weight loss requires reducing the number of calories consumed and choosing a wide range of foods that provide good nutrition. Reducing the number of calories consumed by 500 to 1,000 calories a day results in weight loss of 1 to 2 pounds per week, which is a healthy rate of weight loss. This approach usually means consuming 1,200 to 1,500 calories a day. Weight can be lost more rapidly with a very low calorie diet, but such diets should be supervised by a doctor. The following changes in diet are recommended:

- Eating 5 or more servings of fruits and vegetables a day
- Eating lean protein—for example, fish or chicken breast or vegetable protein, such as soy
- Switching to no-fat dairy products
- Eating whole grains
- Eliminating high-calorie beverages
- Limiting consumption of restaurant and fast food
- Switching from harmful fats, such as saturated fat and trans fat, to good fats, such as monounsaturated fats (found in olive and canola oils) and polyunsaturated fats (in deep-sea fish and vegetable oils) and limiting the amount of fat consumed.

Saturated and trans fats not only contribute to weight gain and obesity but can be harmful by leading to abnormal cholesterol levels and an increased risk of coronary artery disease.

Physical Activity: Increasing physical activity is essential to healthy weight loss and weight maintenance. Physical activity includes not only exercise (that is, structured physical activity) but also lifestyle activities, such as taking the stairs instead of the elevator, gardening, and walking instead of driving when possible. Lifestyle activities can burn a considerable number of calories. Also, physical activity helps people maintain weight loss. People who do not exercise while dieting are more likely to regain the weight they lose.

As a general guide, people need to walk at least 150 minutes each week to promote health and to maintain weight. For weight loss, 60 to 90 minutes of physical activity per day is needed. Aerobic exercise, such as jogging, walking briskly (3 to 4 miles an hour), biking, singles tennis, skating, and cross-country skiing, burn more calories than less active exercises (see page 43). For example, vigorous walking burns about 4 calories per minute, so that 1 hour of brisk walking per day burns about 240 calories. Running burns about 6 to 8 calories per minute.

To get the most benefit from exercise, people should do strength training (with weights or another form of resistance) every 48 to 72 hours, about 3 days of the week. Strength training increases the amount of muscle tissue, which increases the metabolic rate, so that the body burns more calories when at rest.

Behavioral Modification: Ultimately, for weight loss to be effective and long-lasting, people must change their behavior. Weight-loss programs that help people change their behavior are the most effective. Some of the skills involved in behavioral modification include problem solving, stress management, and self-monitoring.

> **? Did You Know...**
> Losing as little as 5 to 10% of body weight can greatly reduce weight-related health risks.

Drugs: For people who are obese or overweight and have weight-related disorders, drugs can be useful. Drugs are most effective when used with changes in diet, increased physical activity, and structured programs that include behavioral modification. Some weight-loss drugs are intended to be used for a short time. Others are intended to be used for a long time. Seven weight-loss drugs are currently available by prescription: orlistat, sibutramine, phentermine, benzphetamine, diethylpropion, mazindol, and phendimetrazine.

Orlistat limits the breakdown and absorption of fats in the intestine, producing, in effect, a low-fat diet. It is also currently available over the counter. It can cause bloating, gas and loose stools. Orlistat can interfere with the absorption of the fat-soluble vitamins: A, D, E, and K. If not enough vitamin D is absorbed, some people develop osteoporosis and bone fractures. People who take orlistat should take a vitamin supplement that contains these nutrients. The supplement should be taken at least 2 hours before or after taking orlistat.

SPOTLIGHT ON AGING

In the United States, the percentage of older people who are obese has been increasing. Obesity in older people is a concern because excess weight increases the risk of certain health problems that tend to become more common as people age: diabetes, cancer, abnormal levels of fats (lipids) in the blood (dyslipidemia), high blood pressure, heart failure, coronary artery disease, and joint disorders.

Several age-related changes contribute to gaining weight:

- **Decreased physical activity:** Some reasons for decreased activity are related to aging. They include retirement, loss of capacity for exercise, development of disorders that make movement painful (such as arthritis), and problems with balance. Other factors may also limit physical activity. For example, people may not want to walk because there are no sidewalks, there is too much traffic, or the neighborhood seems unsafe.

- **Loss of muscle tissue:** Muscle tissue is lost partly because levels of growth hormone and sex hormones (estrogen in women and testosterone in men) decrease. But the main reason older people lose lean tissue is physical inactivity. The less muscle tissue people have, the fewer calories

their body burns when resting and the easier it is to gain weight.

- **Increased body fat:** When the amount of muscle tissue decreases, the percentage of fat in the body increases. Fat tissue burns fewer calories. Also, the higher percentage of fat means that older people with a normal body mass index (BMI), which is based only on weight and height, may have a higher risk of weight-related health problems than expected. Waist circumference predicts health risks better than BMI in older people.

- **Shifting of body fat to the waist:** With aging, body fat tends to shift to the waist. Fat that accumulates around the waist and abdomen (as opposed to the hips and thighs) increases the risk of health problems.

Older people are at greater risk of undernutrition than younger people. Therefore, when they try to lose weight, they should be sure to consume a healthy and balanced diet. Whether weight loss in older people has health risks is controversial. Doctors help older people devise weight-loss strategies based on their individual circumstances. Treatment may include diet, exercise, drugs, and surgery. In older people, weight loss is best supervised by a doctor.

Sibutramine, phentermine, benzphetamine, diethylpropion, mazindol, and phendimetrazine are believed to reduce appetite by affecting chemical messengers in the part of the brain that controls appetite. Some of these drugs may also increase the metabolic rate so that more calories are burned.

The combination of fenfluramine and phentermine (often called fen-phen) was the most effective drug treatment. However, fenfluramine was removed from the market because heart valve problems occurred in people who took this combination.

Some nonprescription diet aids, including medicinal herbs, claim to enhance weight loss by increasing metabolism or by increasing a feeling of fullness. These supplements have not been shown to be effective and may contain harmful additives or stimulants, such as ephedra, and should be avoided.

Many new drugs for the treatment of obesity are being developed and will probably change the way obesity is treated in the future.

BARIATRIC SURGERY

Bariatric surgery alters the stomach, intestine, or both to produce weight loss.

In the United States, more than 200,000 people have bariatric surgery each year. This number accounts for almost two thirds of the total number of bariatric procedures done worldwide. These procedures result in substantial weight loss. People may lose half or even more of their excess weight and as much as 80 to 160 pounds. Weight loss is rapid at first, and then slows gradually over a period of about 2 years. Weight loss is often maintained for years. The loss greatly reduces the severity and risk of weight-related medical problems (such as high blood pressure and diabetes). It improves mood, self-esteem, body image, activity level, and ability to work and interact with other people.

When obesity is severe (BMI of more than 40), surgery is the treatment of choice. Surgery is also appropriate when people with a BMI of more than 35 have serious weight-related health problems, such as diabetes, high blood pressure, sleep apnea, or heart failure.

To qualify for surgery, people also need to do the following:

- Understand its risks and effects
- Be motivated to follow the changes in diet and lifestyle required after surgery
- Have tried other methods of losing weight
- Be physically and mentally able to undergo surgery

Whether bariatric surgery is appropriate for people younger than 18 or older than 65 is controversial.

Banding the Stomach

For this procedure, an adjustable band is placed around the upper part of the stomach. It enables people to adjust the size of the passageway for food through the stomach.

After a small incision is made in the abdomen, a viewing tube (laparoscope) is inserted. While looking through the laparoscope, the surgeon places the band around the upper part of the stomach. On the inside of the band is an inflatable ring, which is connected to tubing with a small port at the other end. The port is placed just under the skin. A special needle can be inserted into the port through the skin. The needle is used to insert a salt water (saline) solution into the band or to remove it. Thus, the passageway can be made smaller or larger. When the passageway is smaller, the upper part of the stomach fills faster, causing people to feel "full" more quickly and thus eat less.

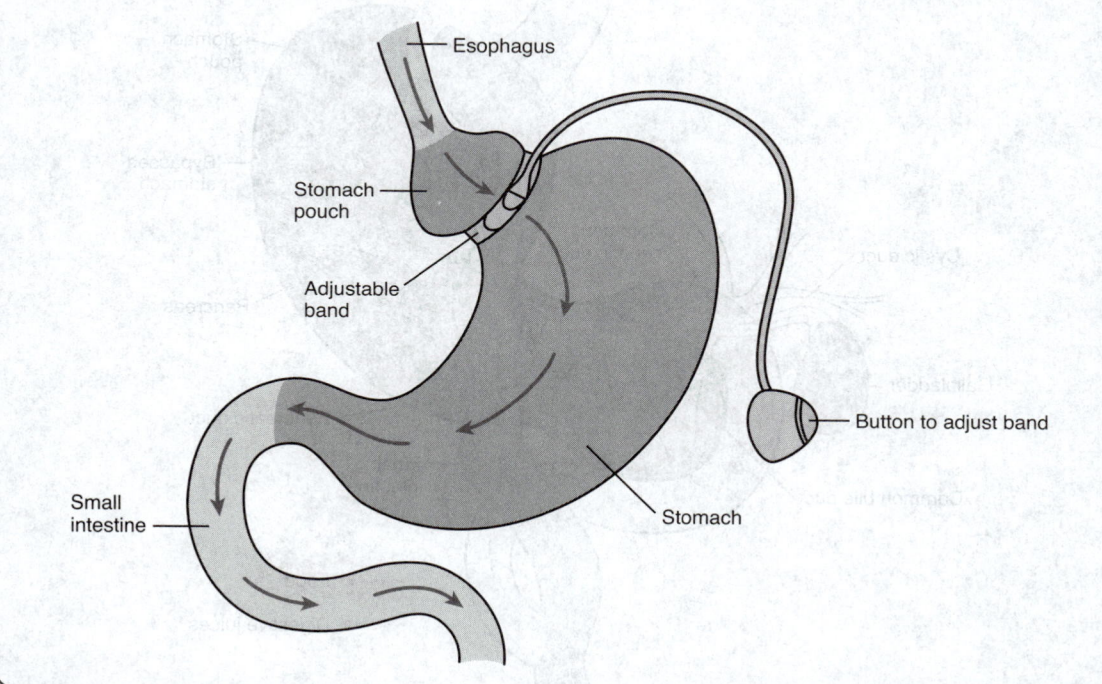

Types

Bariatric surgery is often done using a flexible viewing tube (laparoscope) inserted into a small incision (about 1 inch long) just below the navel. This technique is called laparoscopy. Four to six other surgical instruments are then inserted into the abdomen through similar small incisions. Whether laparoscopy can be used depends on the type of procedure and the person's size. If laparoscopy cannot be used, surgery involves a larger abdominal incision (called open abdominal surgery). Compared with open abdominal surgery, laparoscopy is much less invasive and recovery is much more rapid.

Bariatric surgery may restrict the amount of food people can eat, reduce the amount of food absorbed, or both.

Procedures That Restrict: These procedures include adjustable gastric banding and vertical banded gastroplasty. By restricting the amount of food that people can eat, these procedures make people feel "full" sooner.

Adjustable gastric banding can be done using a laparoscope. A band (sometimes called a lap band) is placed at the upper end of the stomach to divide the stomach into a small upper part and a larger lower part. Food passes through the band on its way to the intestine, but the band slows that passage. Connected to the band is a piece of tubing with a device that allows access at the other end (a port). The port is placed just under the skin so that the tightness of the band can be adjusted after surgery. Fluid can be injected through the port into the band to expand it

Bypassing Part of the Digestive Tract

For this procedure, part of the stomach is detached from the rest, creating a small pouch. The pouch is connected to a lower part of the small intestine by a piece of small intestine—an arrangement that resembles a Y. As a result, parts of the stomach and small intestine are bypassed. However, digestive juices (bile acids and pancreatic enzymes) can still mix with food, enabling the body to absorb vitamins and minerals and reducing the risk of nutritional deficiencies.

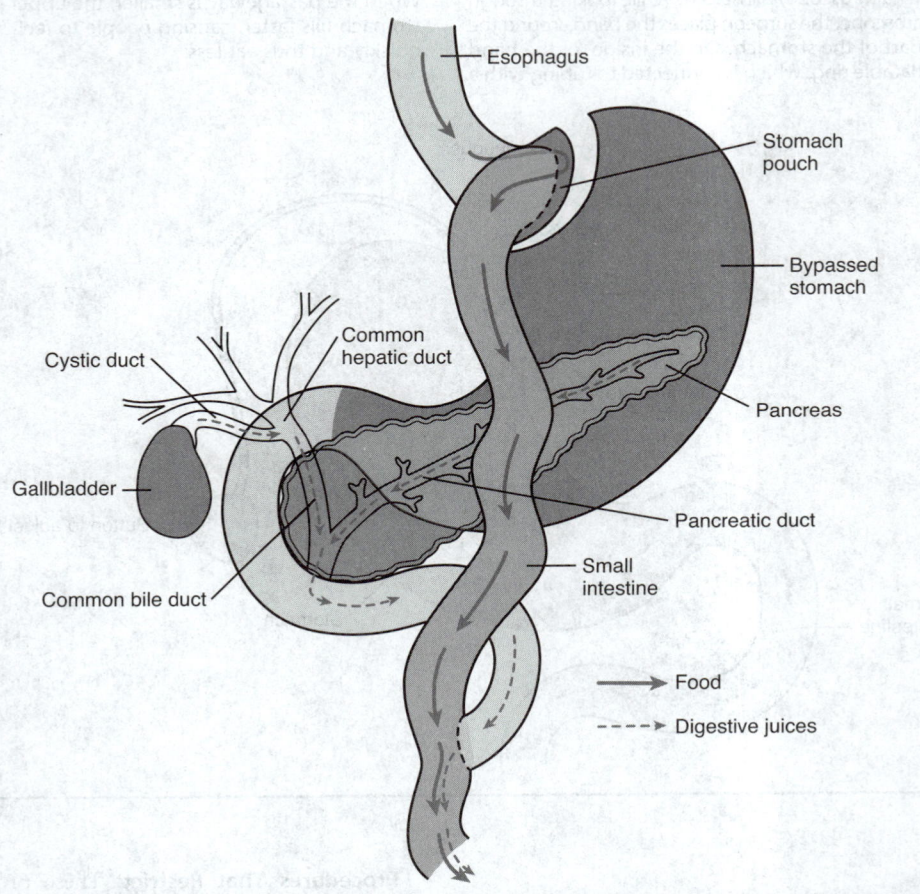

and make the passageway through the stomach smaller. Or fluid can be removed from the band to shrink it and make the passageway larger. When the passageway is smaller, the upper part of the stomach fills more quickly, sending a message to the brain that the stomach is full. As a result, people eat smaller meals and lose substantial amounts of weight over time.

Vertical banded gastroplasty is no longer commonly done. For this procedure, staples are placed vertically down the stomach along about two thirds of its length. Thus, the top two thirds is divided, with one part smaller than the other. A nonadjust-able plastic band is placed at the bottom of the staple line, where the divided parts of the stomach join. Food from the esophagus enters the smaller part, and the band restricts and thus delays the movement of food through the stomach. As a result, people cannot eat as much, and they feel full sooner.

Procedures That Reduce Absorption: These procedures include Roux-en-Y gastric bypass and biliopancreatic diversion with a duodenal switch. These procedures reroute food so that it bypasses parts of the stomach and small intestine, where it is normally absorbed. Thus, less food is absorbed. These procedures also restrict the movement of food through the digestive system.

Roux-en-Y gastric bypass accounts for most of the bariatric procedures in the United States, although banding is becoming more popular. Roux-en-Y gastric bypass can often be done through a laparoscope. The part of the stomach next to the esophagus is detached from the rest, creating a small pouch. As a result, the amount of food that can be eaten at one time is drastically reduced. A section of small intestine is used to connect the pouch to a lower part of the small intestine (this arrangement resembles a Y—hence the name). The opening between them is made narrow to further restrict the movement of food. This connection bypasses the lower part of the stomach and upper part of the small intestine, where much of the absorption occurs. However, it allows digestive juices (bile acids and pancreatic enzymes) to mix with the food. This mixing, which is necessary for food to be absorbed, enables vitamins and minerals to be digested and then absorbed and thus reduces the risk of nutritional deficiencies. Most people stay in the hospital overnight or longer.

For many people who have had a gastric bypass, eating foods high in fat and refined sugar can cause dumping syndrome. Symptoms include indigestion, nausea, diarrhea, abdominal pain, sweating, light-headedness, and weakness. Dumping syndrome occurs when undigested food from the stomach moves into the small intestine too quickly. This syndrome usually stops occurring after a short time.

Biliopancreatic diversion with a duodenal switch is rarely used. Part of the stomach is removed. In contrast to the Roux-en-Y bypass, the part of the stomach that is left connects normally to the esophagus and the small intestine. Also, the valve between the stomach and small intestine is left intact and can function normally. Thus, the stomach empties normally. The small intestine is divided. The part that connects with the stomach (duodenum) is cut and attached to the lower part (ileum), bypassing much of the small intestine. As a result, digestive juices (bile acids and pancreatic enzymes) cannot mix with food as well, and absorption is reduced. Nutritional deficiencies often result.

Evaluation

Before surgery, people are evaluated to determine whether they are able to withstand the stress of surgery. A physical examination and tests are done. Tests may include the following:

- Tests that are routinely done before surgery to check how well vital organs are functioning
- Blood tests, including liver function tests, blood sugar levels, and lipid levels (after fasting)

- Ultrasonography of the abdomen, including the gallbladder
- Echocardiography (ultrasonography of the heart)
- Pulmonary function tests
- Evaluation of the digestive tract (with ultrasonography or endoscopy)
- Thyroid function tests
- Sleep evaluation (including polysomnography) and testing for sleep apnea

Psychiatric and nutritional evaluations are also done. People should tell their doctor about any drugs or medicinal herbs they are taking. Some drugs, including anticoagulants (such as warfarin) and aspirin, may be stopped before surgery.

After Surgery

After surgery, pain relievers are prescribed.

For the first 2 weeks, the diet is liquids only. People are asked to drink small amounts frequently throughout the day. They should drink as much fluid as prescribed and should take a liquid protein supplement. For the next 2 weeks, people should consume a soft diet. After 4 weeks, they can start eating solid foods. The following can help people avoid digestive problems and discomfort:

- Taking small bites of food
- Chewing food thoroughly
- Avoiding high-fat and high-sugar foods, such as "fast food," cakes, and cookies
- Eating only small amounts at each meal

Usually, people can resume taking their routine drugs after surgery, but tablets may have to be crushed.

People should start walking or doing leg exercises the day after surgery. To avoid blood clots, they should not stay in bed for long periods of time. They can return to their usual activities after about 1 week and to their usual exercises (such as aerobics and strength training) after a few weeks. They should consult their doctor before doing any heavy lifting and manual labor.

Possible Problems: Most people lose their appetite after surgery. People experience pain, and some have nausea and vomiting. Constipation is common. Drinking more fluids and not staying in bed too long at a time can help relieve constipation.

Serious complications, such as problems with the incision, infections, and lung problems, can occur after any operation (see page 2056). In addition, the following complications can occur after bariatric surgery. However, when surgery is done at specialized centers, they occur in fewer than 10% of people. Most can be treated.

After Bariatric Surgery: When to Call the Doctor

After bariatric surgery, some symptoms are common and do not indicate a problem. However, the following symptoms require a call or visit to the doctor:

- Signs of infection at the incision site, such as redness, severe pain, swelling, a bad odor, or oozing
- Separation of stitched edges of the incision
- Continued or increasing abdominal pain
- Persistent fever or chills
- Vomiting
- Persistent bleeding
- Abnormal beating of the heart
- Diarrhea
- Dark, tarry, foul-smelling stools
- Shortness of breath
- Sweating
- Sudden paleness
- Persistent chest pain

- **Blockage of the intestine:** In about 2 to 4% of people, the intestine becomes blocked because it becomes twisted or scar tissue forms. A blockage can develop weeks to months to years after surgery. Symptoms include severe abdominal pain, nausea, and vomiting.
- **Leakage:** In about 1% of people, the new connection between the stomach and intestine leaks. Leakage usually occurs within 2 weeks of surgery. As a result, the stomach's contents can leak into the abdominal cavity and cause a serious infection (peritonitis). Symptoms include a fast heart rate, abdominal pain, fever, shortness of breath, and a general sick feeling.
- **Bleeding:** Bleeding may occur at the connection between the stomach and intestine, elsewhere in the digestive tract, or in the abdominal cavity. People may vomit blood or have bloody diarrhea or dark, tarry stools.
- **Gallstones:** Many people who successfully follow a diet aimed at quick weight loss develop gallstones. To reduce this risk after bariatric surgery, people are given supplemental bile salts, but these supplements do not always prevent gallstones. About 7% of people who have bariatric surgery need to have their gallbladder removed later.
- **Nutritional deficiencies:** If people do not make a concentrated effort to eat enough protein, a protein deficiency may develop. Vitamins and minerals (such as vitamins B_{12} and D, calcium, and iron) may not be absorbed as well after the surgery. Taking supplements, including a multivitamin, can help.
- **Death:** Up to 0.5% of people die after surgery. Usually, the cause is a blood clot that travels to the lungs or a severe infection from leakage of one of the connections in the stomach or intestines along with a preexisting heart or lung disorder. Risk is higher for older people and for people who have had open surgery or who are very obese.

Follow Up: Visits to the doctor are scheduled every 4 to 6 weeks during the first several months after surgery—the time when weight loss is most rapid. Then visits are scheduled every 6 to 12 months. Weight and blood pressure are measured, and eating habits are discussed. People should report any problems they are having. Blood tests are done at each visit.

Metabolic Syndrome

Metabolic syndrome (also called syndrome X or insulin resistance syndrome) is characterized by excess abdominal fat, resistance to the effects of insulin (insulin resistance), abnormal levels of fats in the blood, and high blood pressure.

- Excess abdominal fat increases the risk of high blood pressure, coronary artery disease, and type 2 diabetes.
- Doctors measure waist circumference, blood pressure, and fasting blood sugar and fat (lipid) levels.
- Changes in eating habits, exercise, behavioral techniques, and drugs may be used to help people lose weight.
- Diabetes, high blood pressure, and abnormal fat levels are treated.

In developed countries, metabolic syndrome is a serious problem. In the United States, more than 40% of people over 50 may have it. Even children and adolescents can develop metabolic syndrome, but how many have it is unknown.

Metabolic syndrome is more likely to develop when people store excess fat around the abdomen (apple-shaped) rather than around the hips (pear-shaped). The following people tend to store excess fat in the abdomen:

- Most men
- Women after menopause

Storing excess fat in the abdomen increases the risk of the following:

- Coronary artery disease
- High blood pressure
- Type 2 diabetes

- Abnormal levels of fats (lipids), including cholesterol, in the blood (dyslipidemia)
- Fatty liver
- Gout
- Polycystic ovary syndrome (in women)
- Chronic kidney disease

Metabolic syndrome itself causes no symptoms.

Diagnosis

Waist circumference should be measured in all people because even people who are not overweight or appear lean can store excess fat in the abdomen. The greater the waist circumference, the higher the risk of metabolic syndrome and its complications. Risk is substantially increased if waist circumference is more than the following:

- 31 inches (80 centimeters) in white or Asian women
- 37 inches (94 centimeters) in white men
- 33 inches (85 centimeters) in Asian men

If waist circumference is high, doctors should measure blood pressure and blood sugar and fat levels after fasting. These levels are often both abnormal. The metabolic syndrome is diagnosed when the waist circumference is more than 40 inches (102 centimeters) in men or more than 35 inches (88 centimeters) in women (indicating excess fat in the abdomen) and when people have or are being treated for two or more of the following:

- A fasting blood sugar level of more than 100 mg/dL (milligrams per deciliter)
- Blood pressure of more than 130/80 mm Hg (millimeters of mercury)
- A fasting blood triglyceride (a fat) level of more than 150 mg/dL
- A high density lipoprotein (HDL—the good) cholesterol level of 40 mg/dL or less for men or 50 mg/dL or less for women

Treatment

The initial treatment involves changes in diet and exercise. Each part of the syndrome should also be treated with drugs if necessary. If people have diabetes or a high blood sugar level, drugs that increase the body's sensitivity to insulin, such as metformin or a thiazolidinedione drug (for example, rosiglitazone or pioglitazone), may help. Also, exercise is important for people with diabetes because it enables the body to use blood sugar more efficiently and can often help lower the blood sugar level. High blood pressure and abnormal fat levels in blood are also treated. Drugs to lower blood pressure (antihypertensives) or to lower lipid levels are used if needed. Other risk factors for coronary artery disease, if present, should be controlled. For example, smokers are advised to stop smoking.

CHAPTER 141 Cholesterol Disorders

Cholesterol and triglycerides are important fats (lipids) in the blood. Cholesterol is an essential component of cell membranes, brain and nerve cells, and bile, which helps the body absorb fats and fat-soluble vitamins. The body uses cholesterol to make vitamin D and various hormones, such as estrogen, testosterone, and cortisol. The body can produce all the cholesterol that it needs, but it also obtains cholesterol from food. Triglycerides, which are contained in fat cells, can be broken down, then used to provide energy for the body's metabolic processes, including growth. Triglycerides are produced in the intestine and liver from smaller fats called fatty acids. Some types of fatty acids are made by the body, but others must be obtained from food (see page 906).

Fats, such as cholesterol and triglycerides, cannot circulate freely in the blood, because blood is mostly water. To be able to circulate in blood, cholesterol and triglycerides are packaged with proteins and other substances to form particles called lipoproteins.

There are different types of lipoproteins. Each type has a different purpose and is broken down and excreted in a slightly different way. Lipoproteins include chylomicrons, very low density lipoproteins (VLDL), low-density lipoproteins (LDL), and high-density lipoproteins (HDL). Cholesterol transported by LDL is called LDL cholesterol, and cholesterol transported by HDL is called HDL cholesterol.

The body can regulate lipoprotein levels (and therefore lipid levels) by increasing or decreasing the production rate of lipoproteins. The body can also regulate

LIPOPROTEINS: LIPID CARRIERS

TYPE	ORIGIN	LIPID CONTENT	FUNCTION
Chylomicrons	Formed from fats in food processed by the intestine	Mostly triglycerides	Transports digested fats (as triglycerides) to muscle and fat cells
Very low density lipoprotein (VLDL)	Formed in the liver	More than 1/2 triglycerides About 1/4 cholesterol	Transports triglycerides from the liver to fat cells
Low-density lipoprotein (LDL)	Formed from VLDL after it delivers triglycerides to fat cells	More than 1/2 cholesterol Less than 1/10 triglycerides	Transports cholesterol to various cells
High-density lipoprotein (HDL)	Formed in the liver and small intestine	About 1/4 cholesterol About 1/20 triglycerides	Removes cholesterol from tissues in the body and transports it to the liver

how quickly lipoproteins enter and are removed from the bloodstream.

Levels of cholesterol and triglycerides vary considerably from day to day. From one measurement to the next, cholesterol levels can vary by about 10%, and triglyceride levels can vary by up to 25%.

Lipid levels may become abnormal because of changes that occur with aging, various disorders (including some hereditary ones), use of certain drugs, or lifestyle (such as consuming a high-fat diet, being physically inactive, or being overweight).

Abnormal levels of lipids (especially cholesterol) can lead to long-term problems, such as atherosclerosis. Generally, a high total cholesterol level (which includes LDL, HDL, and VLDL cholesterol) or a high level of LDL (the "bad") cholesterol increases the risk of atherosclerosis and thus the risk of heart attack and stroke. However, not all types of cholesterol increase this risk. A high level of HDL (the "good") cholesterol may decrease risk, and conversely, a low level of HDL cholesterol increases risk. The effect of triglyceride levels on the risk of heart attack is less clear-cut. But very high levels of triglycerides (higher than 500 milligrams per deciliter of blood, or mg/dL) can increase the risk of pancreatitis. For people older than 20, levels of total cholesterol, triglycerides, LDL cholesterol, and HDL cholesterol after fasting should be measured at least once every 5 years. Collectively, these measurements are called the fasting lipoprotein profile.

Dyslipidemia

Dyslipidemia is abnormal levels of lipids (cholesterol, triglycerides, or both) carried by lipoproteins in the blood. This term includes hyperlipoproteinemia (hyperlipidemia), which refers to abnormally high levels of total cholesterol, low density lipoprotein (LDL)—the bad—cholesterol, or triglycerides, as well as an abnormally low level of high density lipoprotein (HDL)—the good—cholesterol.

- Lifestyle, genetics, disorders, drugs, or a combination can contribute.
- Atherosclerosis can result, causing angina, heart attacks, strokes, and peripheral arterial disease.
- Doctors measure levels of triglycerides and the various types of cholesterol in blood.
- Exercise, dietary changes, and drugs can be effective.

Levels of lipoproteins and therefore lipids, particularly low density lipoprotein (LDL) cholesterol, increase slightly as people age. Levels are normally slightly higher in men than in women, but levels increase in women after menopause. The increase in levels of lipoproteins that occurs with age can result in dyslipidemia and increase the risk of atherosclerosis.

A high level of high density lipoprotein (HDL)—the good—cholesterol is beneficial and is not considered a disorder. A level that is too low is considered dyslipidemia and increases the risk of atherosclerosis (see page 396).

Factors that increase the risk of dyslipidemia include the following:

- Having close relatives who have had dyslipidemia (having a family history of the disorder)
- Being overweight
- Consuming a diet high in saturated fats and cholesterol
- Being physically inactive
- Consuming large amounts of alcohol

Some people are more sensitive to the effects of diet than others, but most people are affected to some degree. One person can eat large amounts of animal fat, and the total cholesterol level does not rise above desirable levels. Another person can follow a strict low-fat diet, and the total cholesterol does not fall below a high level. This difference seems to be mostly genetically determined. A person's genetic makeup influences the rate at which the body makes, uses, and disposes of these fats. Also, body type does not always predict levels of cholesterol. Some overweight people have low cholesterol levels, and some thin people have high levels. Eating excess calories can result in high triglyceride levels, as can consuming large amounts of alcohol.

Some disorders, including some hereditary disorders (see page 966), cause lipid levels to increase. Diabetes that is poorly controlled or kidney failure can cause total cholesterol levels or triglyceride levels to increase. Some liver disorders and an underactive thyroid gland (hypothyroidism) can cause the total cholesterol level to increase.

Use of drugs such as estrogens (taken by mouth), oral contraceptives, corticosteroids, retinoids, thiazide diuretics (to some extent), and possibly antiviral drugs used to treat human immunodeficiency virus (HIV) infection and AIDS can cause triglyceride levels to increase.

Cigarette smoking, poorly controlled diabetes, or kidney disorders (such as nephrotic syndrome) may contribute to a low HDL cholesterol level. Drugs such as beta-blockers and anabolic steroids can lower the HDL cholesterol level.

DESIRABLE LIPID LEVELS IN ADULTS

LIPID	GOAL (mg/dL)*
Total cholesterol	Less than 200 mg/dL
Low-density lipoprotein (LDL) cholesterol	Less than 100 mg/dL
High-density lipoprotein (HDL) cholesterol	More than 40 mg/dL
Triglycerides	Less than 150 mg/dL

*mg/dL = milligrams per deciliter of blood.

? Did You Know...

Margarines made primarily from liquid oil (squeeze or tub margarines) and those that contain plant stanols or sterols, unlike stick margarines, are healthier substitutes for butter.

Symptoms

High lipid levels in the blood usually cause no symptoms. Occasionally, when levels are particularly high, fat is deposited in the skin and tendons and forms bumps called xanthomas. Very high triglyceride levels can cause the liver or spleen to enlarge and may increase the risk of developing pancreatitis. Pancreatitis can cause severe abdominal pain and is occasionally fatal.

The risk of developing atherosclerosis increases as the total cholesterol level increases, even if the level is not high enough to be considered dyslipidemia. Atherosclerosis can affect the arteries that supply blood to the heart (causing coronary artery disease), those that supply blood to the brain (causing cerebrovascular disease), and those that supply the rest of the body (causing peripheral arterial disease). Therefore, having a high total cholesterol level also increases the risk of having a heart attack or stroke. Having a low total cholesterol level is generally considered better than having a high one. However, having a very low cholesterol level may not be healthy either (see page 968). For adults, a total cholesterol level of less than 200 mg/dL is desirable. In parts of the world (such as China and Japan) where the average cholesterol level is 150 mg/dL, coronary artery disease is less common than it is in countries such as the United States. The risk of a heart attack more than doubles when the total cholesterol level approaches 300 mg/dL.

The total cholesterol level is only a general guide to the risk of atherosclerosis. Levels of the components of total cholesterol—particularly LDL and HDL cholesterol—are more important. A high level of LDL (bad) cholesterol increases the risk. A high level of HDL (good) cholesterol decreases the risk, and a low level of HDL cholesterol (defined as less than 40 mg/dL) increases the risk. Experts consider an LDL cholesterol level of less than 100 mg/dL optimal.

Whether high triglyceride levels increase the risk of a heart attack or stroke is uncertain. Triglyceride levels higher than 150 mg/dL are considered abnormal, but high levels do not appear to increase risk for everyone. For people with high triglyceride levels, the risk of heart attack or stroke is increased if they also have a low HDL cholesterol level, diabetes, kidney disease, or many close relatives who have had atherosclerosis (family history).

Diagnosis

Levels of total cholesterol, LDL cholesterol, HDL cholesterol, and triglycerides—the lipid profile—are measured in a blood sample. The lipid profile should

LIMITING FAT AND CHOLESTEROL IN THE DIET

TYPE OF FAT	RECOMMENDED AMOUNTS	FOOD SOURCES
Saturated	7–10% of total calories Less than 7% for people who have high lipid levels or coronary artery disease	Meats Nonskim dairy products, such as whole milk, cheese, and butter Artificially hydrogenated vegetable oils
Polyunsaturated	Up to 10% of total calories	
Monounsaturated	Up to 20% of total calories	Canola oil Olive oil Nuts Avocado
Cholesterol	Less than 0.3 grams (300 milligrams) a day Less than 0.2 grams (200 milligrams) a day for people with high lipid levels or coronary artery disease	Egg yolks Organ meats, such as liver Meat Poultry Fish and other seafood Nonskim dairy products

be measured in all adults 20 years and older, and the measurement should be repeated every 5 years. Because consuming food or beverages may cause triglyceride levels to increase temporarily, people must fast at least 12 hours before the blood sample is taken.

When lipid levels in the blood are very high, special blood tests are done to identify the specific underlying disorder. Specific disorders include several hereditary disorders (hereditary dyslipidemias), which produce different lipid abnormalities and have different risks.

Treatment

Usually, the best treatment for people is to lose weight if they are overweight, stop smoking if they smoke, decrease the total amount of fat and cholesterol in their diet, increase physical activity, and then, if necessary, take a lipid-lowering drug.

A diet low in fats and cholesterol can lower the LDL cholesterol level. Experts recommend limiting calories from fat to no more than 25 to 35% of the total calories consumed over several days.

The type of fat consumed is also important (see box on page 403). Fats may be saturated, polyunsaturated, or monounsaturated. Saturated fats increase cholesterol levels more than other forms of fat. Saturated fats should provide no more than 7 to 10% of total calories consumed each day. Polyunsaturated fats (which include omega-3 fats and omega-6 fats) and monounsaturated fats may help

decrease levels of triglycerides and LDL cholesterol in the blood. The fat content of most foods is included on the label of the container.

Large amounts of saturated fats occur in meats, egg yolks, full-fat dairy products, some nuts (such as macadamia nuts), and coconut. Vegetable oils contain smaller amounts of saturated fat, but only some vegetable oils are truly low in saturated fats.

Margarine, which is produced from polyunsaturated vegetable oils, was once thought to be a healthier substitute for butter, which is high in saturated fat (about 60%). However, some margarines (and some processed foods) contain trans fats, which may increase LDL (bad) cholesterol levels and lower HDL (good) cholesterol levels. Margarines made primarily from liquid oil (squeeze or tub margarines) contain less saturated fat than butter, contain no cholesterol, and contain fewer trans fats than stick margarines. Margarines that contain plant stanols or sterols can slightly lower total and LDL cholesterol levels.

Eating lots of fruits, vegetables, and grains, which are naturally low in fat and contain no cholesterol, is recommended. Also recommended are foods rich in soluble fiber, which binds fats in the intestine and helps lower the cholesterol level. Such foods include oat bran, oatmeal, beans, peas, rice bran, barley, citrus fruits, strawberries, and apple pulp. Psyllium, usually taken to relieve constipation, can also lower the cholesterol level.

A PRACTICAL APPROACH TO A LOW-CHOLESTEROL, LOW-SATURATED FAT DIET

FOOD CATEGORY	FOODS TO REDUCE	FOODS TO CHOOSE
Meats and meat products	Fatty cuts of beef, lamb, and pork Spareribs Organ meats, such as liver Regular cold cuts Sausage Hot dogs	Fish Chicken and turkey (without the skin) Lean cuts of beef, lamb, pork, and veal
Dairy products and eggs	Whole milk Evaporated or condensed whole milk Cream Half-and-half	Nonfat (skim) milk ½% fat milk 1% fat milk
	Most nondairy creamers	Buttermilk
	Whipped toppings	Low or nonfat whipped toppings
	Whole-milk yogurt	Nonfat or low-fat yogurt
	Whole-milk cottage cheese Cheeses (such as blue, Roquefort, Camembert, cheddar, and Swiss) Cream cheese	Low-fat cottage cheese Low-fat cheeses
	Sour cream	Low or nonfat sour cream
	Ice cream	Sherbet, sorbet, and frozen low-fat yogurt
	Butter and butter-margarine mixtures	Less solid forms of margarines made from liquid vegetable oils (packaged in a tub or squeeze bottle) Olive oil Canola oil Margarine products containing a plant sterol or stanol
	Egg yolks (to less than 3 a week)	Cholesterol-free egg substitutes Egg whites (2 whole egg whites can be substituted for 1 egg in recipes)
Commercial baked goods	Pies Cakes Doughnuts Croissants Pastries Muffins Biscuits High-fat crackers High-fat cookies Egg noodles Breads made with several eggs	Homemade baked goods made with unsaturated oils Angel food cake Low-fat cookies and crackers Whole-grain* (oatmeal, bran, rye, and multigrain) breads and cereals

(continued on the following page)

A PRACTICAL APPROACH TO A LOW-CHOLESTEROL, LOW-SATURATED FAT DIET (*Continued*)

FOOD CATEGORY	FOODS TO REDUCE	FOODS TO CHOOSE
Saturated fats and oils	Chocolate	Cocoa powder Carob Nonfat chocolate syrup
	Coconut oil Palm oil Lard Bacon	Unsaturated vegetable oils: canola, olive, corn, safflower, sesame, soybean, and sunflower
Dressings	Dressings made with egg yolk	Low-fat mayonnaise and salad dressings made with liquid oils
Fruits and vegetables	Fruits and vegetables prepared in butter, saturated fats, cream, or sauces made with saturated fat	Fresh, frozen, canned, and dried fruits or vegetables*
	Coconut	Seeds and nuts*

*Fruits, vegetables, grains, seeds, and nuts contain no cholesterol, and most contain little or no saturated fat.

Regular physical activity can help lower the LDL cholesterol level and increase the HDL cholesterol level. An example is walking briskly for 30 to 45 minutes 3 to 4 times a week.

Treatment with lipid-lowering drugs depends not only on the lipid levels but also on whether coronary artery disease, diabetes, or other major risk factors for coronary artery disease (see page 402) are present. For people who have coronary artery disease or diabetes, the goal for the LDL cholesterol level is 100 mg/dL or less. Consequently, such people usually require lipid-lowering drugs. For people who do not have coronary artery disease or diabetes but have two or more other risk factors for coronary artery disease, the goal is 130 mg/dL or less. For those with one or no risk factors, the goal is 160 mg/dL or less.

There are different types of lipid-lowering drugs: bile acid binders, fibric acid derivatives, niacin (a lipoprotein synthesis inhibitor), cholesterol absorption inhibitors, supplements of omega-3 fats, and statins. Each type lowers lipid levels by a different mechanism. Consequently, the different types of drugs have different side effects and may affect lipid levels differently. Following a low-fat diet when drugs are used is recommended.

Lipid-lowering drugs do more than lower lipid levels—they can also prevent coronary artery disease. In addition, niacin and statins have been shown to reduce the risk of early death.

> **? Did You Know...**
> Eating oat bran, oatmeal, beans, peas, rice bran, barley, citrus fruits, strawberries, and apple pulp can help lower cholesterol.

HEREDITARY DYSLIPIDEMIAS

Cholesterol and triglyceride levels are highest in people with hereditary dyslipidemias, which interfere with the body's metabolism and elimination of lipids. People can also inherit a tendency for HDL cholesterol to be unusually low. Consequences of hereditary dyslipidemias can include premature atherosclerosis, which can lead to angina or heart attacks. Peripheral arterial disease is also a consequence, often causing decreased blood flow to the legs, with pain during walking (claudication—see page 419). Stroke is another possible consequence.

In **lipoprotein lipase deficiency** and **apolipoprotein CII deficiency,** rare disorders caused by the lack of certain proteins needed for the removal of triglyceride containing particles, the body cannot remove chylomicrons from the bloodstream, resulting in very high triglyceride levels. Without treatment, levels are often considerably higher than 1,000 mg/dL. Symptoms appear during childhood and young adulthood. They include recurring bouts of abdominal

℞ LIPID-LOWERING DRUGS

TYPE	MECHANISM OF ACTION	INDICATIONS	SOME SIDE EFFECTS
Bile acid binders			
Cholestyramine Colesevelam Colestipol	Bind bile acids in the intestine, causing the acids to be excreted rather than used to make bile and causing the liver to remove more LDL cholesterol from the bloodstream to make bile	High LDL cholesterol	Abdominal pain Binding of some other drugs (reducing their effectiveness) Bloating Constipation Nausea Increase in triglyceride level (slight)
Cholesterol absorption inhibitor			
Ezetimibe	Decreases cholesterol absorption in the small intestine	High LDL cholesterol	Few serious side effects Face and lip swelling (rare) Loose stools Muscle aches
Fibric acid derivatives			
Bezafibrate* Ciprofibrate* Fenofibrate Gemfibrozil	Increase the breakdown of lipids and speed the removal of VLDL from the bloodstream May decrease VLDL production by the liver	High triglycerides Low HDL cholesterol Dysbetalipoproteinemia Possibly high VLDL cholesterol	Abdominal pain Bloating Diarrhea Gallstones High liver enzyme levels Muscle aches due to inflammation (myositis) Nausea Rash
Lipoprotein synthesis inhibitor			
Niacin	Slows removal of HDL Lowers triglyceride levels At high doses, decreases production rate of VLDL, which is used to synthesize LDL	High triglycerides Low HDL cholesterol High LDL and VLDL cholesterol Dysbetalipoproteinemia	Digestive upset Flushing Gout High blood sugar level (hyperglycemia) High liver enzyme levels Itching Ulcers
Statins (HMG-CoA reductase inhibitors)			
Atorvastatin Fluvastatin Lovastatin Pravastatin Rosuvastatin Simvastatin	Block the synthesis of cholesterol, increasing the removal of LDL from the bloodstream	High LDL cholesterol, triglycerides, or both	Bloating Constipation (mild) Fatigue Headache Loose stools Rarely, high liver enzyme levels Rarely, muscle aches due to inflammation (myositis) or degeneration (rhabdomyolysis)
Fat supplements			
Omega-3 fatty acids	Lower levels of triglycerides May decrease production of VLDL	High triglycerides	Belching Diarrhea Weight gain if taken in addition to other fats (instead of as substitutes)

HDL = high density lipoprotein; HMG-CoA = 3-hydroxy-3-methylglutaryl coenzyme A; LDL = low density lipoprotein.

*Not available in the United States.

pain, an enlarged liver and spleen, and pinkish yellow bumps in the skin on the elbows, knees, buttocks, back, front of the legs, and back of the arms. These bumps, called eruptive xanthomas, are deposits of fat. Eating fats worsens symptoms. Although this disorder does not lead to atherosclerosis, it can cause pancreatitis, which is occasionally fatal. People who have this disorder must avoid eating fats of all types—saturated, unsaturated, and polyunsaturated.

In **familial hypercholesterolemia,** the total cholesterol level is high. This severe disorder affects about 1 of 500 people. People may have inherited one abnormal gene or they may have inherited two abnormal genes, one from each parent. People who have two abnormal genes (homozygotes) are more severely affected than people who have only one abnormal gene (heterozygotes). Affected people may have fatty deposits (xanthomas) in the tendons at the heels, knees, elbows, and fingers. Rarely, xanthomas appear by age 10. Familial hypercholesterolemia can result in rapidly progressive atherosclerosis and early death due to coronary artery disease. Children with two abnormal genes may have a heart attack or angina by age 20, and men with one abnormal gene often develop coronary artery disease between ages 30 and 50. Women with one abnormal gene are also at increased risk, but the risk starts later.

Treatment begins with following a diet that is low in saturated fats and cholesterol. When applicable, losing weight, stopping smoking, and increasing physical activity are advised. One or more lipid-lowering drugs are usually needed. Some people benefit from a liver transplant.

In **familial combined hyperlipidemia,** the levels of cholesterol, triglycerides, or both may be high. This disorder affects about 1 to 2% of people. The lipid levels typically become abnormal after age 30 but sometimes at a younger age, especially in people who are overweight, who have a diet that is very high in fat, or who have metabolic syndrome (see page 960).

Treatment involves limiting intake of fat, cholesterol, and sugar as well as exercising and, when applicable, losing weight. Many people with this disorder need to take lipid-lowering drugs.

In **familial dysbetalipoproteinemia,** levels of VLDL and total cholesterol and triglycerides are high. These levels are high because an unusual form of VLDL accumulates in the blood. Fatty deposits (xanthomas) may form in the skin over the elbows and knees and in the palms, where they can cause yellow creases. This uncommon disorder results in the early development of severe atherosclerosis. By middle age, atherosclerosis often produces blockages in the coronary and peripheral arteries.

Treatment involves achieving and maintaining recommended body weight and limiting intake of cholesterol, saturated fats, and carbohydrates. A lipid-lowering drug is usually needed. With treatment, lipid levels can be improved, the progression of atherosclerosis may be slowed, and the fatty deposits in the skin may become smaller or disappear.

In **familial hypertriglyceridemia,** triglyceride levels are high. This disorder affects about 1% of people. In some families affected by this disorder, atherosclerosis tends to develop at a young age, but in others, it does not. When applicable, losing weight and limiting alcohol consumption often lower triglyceride levels to normal. If these measures are ineffective, use of a lipid-lowering drug can help. For people who also have diabetes, good control of the diabetes is important.

In people who have a **genetic disorder that causes high triglycerides** (such as familial hypertriglyceridemia or familial combined hyperlipidemia), certain disorders and substances can increase triglycerides to extremely high levels. Examples of disorders include poorly controlled diabetes and kidney dysfunction. Examples of substances include excessive alcohol consumption and use of certain drugs that increase triglyceride levels. Symptoms can include fatty deposits (eruptive xanthomas) in the skin on the front of the legs and back of the arms, an enlarged spleen and liver, abdominal pain, and a decreased sensitivity to touch due to nerve damage. This disorder can cause pancreatitis, which is occasionally fatal. Limiting fat intake (to less than 50 grams a day) can help prevent nerve damage and pancreatitis. Losing weight and not drinking alcohol can also help. Lipid-lowering drugs may be effective.

In **hypoalphalipoproteinemia,** the HDL cholesterol level is low. A low HDL cholesterol level is often inherited. Many different genetic abnormalities can cause the low HDL level.

Hypolipoproteinemia

Hypolipoproteinemia is abnormally low levels of lipids in the blood.

- Low lipid levels may result from rare genetic abnormalities or other disorders.
- People with these genetic abnormalities may have fatty stools, grow poorly, and be mentally retarded.
- Some genetic abnormalities are treated with supplements of fats, vitamin E, and other vitamins.

Having low lipid levels rarely causes a problem, but it may indicate the presence of another disorder. For example, a low cholesterol level may indicate an overactive thyroid gland (hyperthyroidism), anemia, undernutrition, cancer, chronic infection, or impaired absorption of foods from the digestive tract (malabsorption). Therefore, doctors may suggest further evaluation when the total cholesterol is less than 120 milligrams per deciliter of blood (mg/dL) or when the low-density lipoprotein (LDL) cholesterol is less than 50 mg/dL. A few rare hereditary disorders, such as abetalipoproteinemia and hypoalphalipoproteinemia, result in lipid levels low enough to have serious consequences.

In **abetalipoproteinemia,** virtually no LDL cholesterol is present, and the body cannot make chylomicrons. As a result, the absorption of fat and fat-soluble vitamins is greatly impaired. Symptoms first develop during infancy. Growth is poor. Bowel movements contain excess fat (a condition called steatorrhea), which can make the stools oily, foul smelling, and more likely to float in water. The retina of the eye degenerates, causing blindness (this condition is similar to retinitis pigmentosa). The central nervous system may be damaged, resulting in loss of coordination (ataxia) and mental retardation. Although abetalipoproteinemia cannot be cured, taking massive doses of vitamin E may delay the development of or slow the damage to the central nervous system.

In **hypobetalipoproteinemia,** the LDL cholesterol level is very low. Usually, there are no symptoms and no treatment is required. In the most severe form of hypobetalipoproteinemia, almost no LDL cholesterol is present. If family members have the disorder, the diagnosis is more likely. Symptoms and treatment are similar to those of abetalipoproteinemia.

In **chylomicron retention disease,** a hereditary disorder, the body cannot make chylomicrons. Affected infants tend to develop symptoms similar to those of abetalipoproteinemia. Treatment is supplements of fats and vitamins A, D, E, and K.

CHAPTER 142 Water Balance

Water accounts for about one half to two thirds of an average person's weight. Fat tissue has a lower percentage of water and women tend to have more fat, so the percentage of water in the average woman is lower (52 to 55%) than it is in the average man (60%). The percentage of water is also lower in older people and in obese people. The percentage of water is higher (70%) at birth and in early childhood. A 150-pound (68-kilogram) man has about 10 gallons (38 liters) of water in his body: 6 to 7 gallons (23 to 27 liters) inside the cells, 2 gallons (about 7 liters) in the space around the cells, and slightly less than 1 gallon (4 liters, or about 8% of the total amount of water) in the bloodstream. The body regulates the amount of water in each of these areas. Water is moved as needed to keep the amount in each area relatively constant, thus enabling the body to function normally.

Water intake must balance water loss. To maintain water balance—and to protect against dehydration, the development of kidney stones, and other medical problems—healthy adults should drink at least 1½ to 2 quarts (about 2 liters) of fluids a day. Drinking too much is usually better than drinking too little, because excreting excess water is much easier for the body than conserving water. However, when the kidneys are functioning normally, the body can handle wide variations in fluid intake.

The body obtains water primarily by absorbing it from the digestive tract. Additionally, a small amount of water is produced when the body processes (metabolizes) certain nutrients.

The body loses water primarily by excreting it in urine from the kidneys. Depending on the body's needs, the kidneys may excrete less than a pint or up to several gallons of urine a day. Additionally, about 1½ pints (a little less than a liter) of water are lost daily when water evaporates from the skin and is breathed out by the lungs. Profuse sweating—which may be caused by vigorous exercise, hot weather, or a fever—can dramatically increase the amount of water lost through evaporation. Normally, little water is lost from the digestive tract. However, prolonged vomiting or severe diarrhea can result in the loss of a gallon or more a day.

Usually, people can drink enough fluids to compensate for excess water loss. However, people who have severe vomiting or diarrhea may feel too ill to drink enough fluids to compensate for water loss, and dehydration may result. Also, confusion, restricted mobility, or loss of consciousness can prevent people from being able to drink enough fluids.

A Careful Balancing Act

In the body, several mechanisms work together to maintain water balance. One of the most important is thirst. When the body needs water, nerve centers deep within the brain are stimulated, resulting in the sensation of thirst. The sensation becomes stronger as the body's need for water increases, motivating a person to drink the needed fluids. When the body has excess water, thirst is suppressed.

Another mechanism for maintaining water balance involves the pituitary gland (located at the base of the brain) and the kidneys. When the body is low in water, the pituitary gland secretes antidiuretic hormone (also called vasopressin) into the bloodstream. Antidiuretic hormone stimulates the kidneys to conserve water and excrete less urine. When the body has excess water, the pituitary gland secretes little antidiuretic hormone, enabling the kidneys to excrete excess water in the urine.

The body can move water from one area to another as needed. When water loss is severe, the amount of water in the bloodstream decreases, so the body moves water from inside the cells to the bloodstream until it can be replaced through increased intake of fluids. When the body has excess water, the amount of water in the bloodstream increases, so the body moves water from the bloodstream into and around the cells. In this way, blood volume and blood pressure can be kept relatively constant.

Mineral salts (electrolytes), such as sodium and potassium, are dissolved in the water in the body. Water balance and electrolyte balance (see page 933) are closely linked. The body works to keep the total amount of water and the levels of electrolytes in the bloodstream constant. For example, when the sodium level becomes too high, thirst develops, leading to an increased intake of fluids. In addition, a hormone secreted by the brain in response to thirst causes the kidneys to excrete less urine. The combined effect is an increased amount of water in the bloodstream. As a result, sodium is diluted and the balance of sodium and water is restored. When the sodium level becomes too low, the kidneys excrete more urine, which decreases the amount of water in the bloodstream, again restoring the balance.

Dehydration

Dehydration is a deficiency of water in the body.

- Vomiting, diarrhea, excessive sweating, and use of diuretics may cause dehydration.

- People feel thirsty, and as dehydration worsens, they may sweat less and excrete less urine.
- If dehydration is severe, people may be confused or feel light-headed.
- Treatment is restoring lost water and electrolytes, usually by drinking but sometimes with intravenous fluids.

Dehydration occurs when the body loses more water than it takes in. Vomiting, diarrhea, the use of diuretics (drugs that increase urine excretion), profuse sweating (for example, during heat waves, particularly with prolonged exertion), and decreased water intake can lead to dehydration.

Dehydration is particularly common among older people, because their thirst center may not function as well as that in younger people. Therefore, some older people may not recognize that they are becoming dehydrated. Certain disorders such as diabetes mellitus (see page 1005), diabetes insipidus (see page 986), and Addison's disease (see page 999) can increase the excretion of urine and thereby lead to dehydration.

Dehydration is also common in infants and children because the amount of fluid lost during diarrhea or vomiting may represent a larger proportion of their body fluids than in older children and adults (see page 1733).

Symptoms and Diagnosis

At first, dehydration stimulates the thirst center of the brain, causing people to drink more fluids. If water intake cannot keep up with water loss, dehydration becomes more severe. Sweating decreases, and less urine is excreted. Water moves from inside the cells to the bloodstream to maintain the needed amount of blood (blood volume) and blood pressure. If dehydration continues, tissues of the body

SPOTLIGHT ON AGING

Older people are particularly susceptible to dehydration. In older people, common causes of dehydration include confusion and disorders that make obtaining fluids difficult (usually because of restricted mobility). Additionally, older people sense thirst more slowly and less intensely than younger people do, so those who are otherwise well may not drink enough fluids. Also, older people have a higher percentage of body fat. Because fat tissue contains less water than lean tissue, the total amount of water in the body tends to decrease with age. Also, because the kidneys excrete excess water less well, older people develop overhydration more easily than younger people.

begin to dry out, and cells begin to shrivel and malfunction. Symptoms of mild to moderate dehydration include thirst, reduced sweating, reduced skin elasticity, reduced urine production, and dry mouth. With severe dehydration, blood pressure can fall, causing light-headedness or faintness, particularly upon standing (a condition called orthostatic hypotension). If dehydration continues, shock and severe damage to internal organs, such as the kidneys, liver, and brain, occur. Brain cells are particularly susceptible to more severe levels of dehydration. Consequently, confusion is one of the best indicators that dehydration has become severe. Very severe dehydration can lead to coma.

Dehydration can often be diagnosed because of the symptoms and the results of an examination. But sometimes doctors do blood tests for people who appear seriously ill or who take certain drugs or have certain disorders. Dehydration normally causes the sodium level in the bloodstream to increase (see page 948). The reason is that although the common causes of dehydration (such as profuse sweating, vomiting, and diarrhea) result in a loss of electrolytes (especially sodium and potassium), even more water is lost, so the concentration of sodium in the blood rises.

Prevention

Prevention is better than cure. Adults should drink at least 6 glasses of fluids daily (including fluid from eating foods high in water content, such as fruits and vegetables). Fluid intake should be increased on hot days and during or after prolonged exercise. Exercise, fever, and hot weather increase the body's need for water. Flavored sports drinks have been formulated to replace electrolytes lost during vigorous exercise. These drinks can be used to prevent dehydration. Before exercising, people with heart or kidney disorders should consult their doctors about how to safely replace fluids.

Treatment

For treating mild dehydration, drinking plenty of water may be all that is needed. With moderate and severe dehydration, lost electrolytes (especially sodium and potassium) must be replaced. Oral rehydration solutions that contain appropriate amounts of electrolytes are available without a prescription. These solutions work well to treat mild dehydration, especially that caused by vomiting or diarrhea in children (see box on page 1733). Sports drinks do not necessarily contain enough electrolytes to be an adequate substitute for these solutions.

More severe dehydration requires treatment by doctors with intravenous solutions containing sodium chloride. The intravenous solution is given rapidly at first and then more slowly as the physical condition improves.

Treatment is also directed at the cause of dehydration. For example, when people have diarrhea, drugs to control or stop the diarrhea may be necessary.

Overhydration

Overhydration is an excess of water in the body.

- People can have overhydration if they drink too much or if they have a disorder that decreases the body's ability to excrete water.
- Often, no symptoms occur, but people may become confused or have seizures.
- Fluid intake is restricted and diuretics may be given.

Overhydration occurs when the body takes in more water than it loses. Overhydration can occur, for example, when athletes drink excessive amounts of water or sports drinks to avoid dehydration, or when people drink much more water than their body needs because of a psychiatric disorder called psychogenic polydipsia. The result is too much water and not enough sodium. Thus, overhydration generally results in low sodium levels in the blood (hyponatremia—see page 948), which can be dangerous. However, drinking large amounts of water usually does not cause overhydration if the pituitary gland, kidneys, liver, and heart are functioning normally. To exceed the body's ability to excrete water, a young adult with normal kidney function would have to drink more than 6 gallons of water a day on a regular basis.

> **? Did You Know...**
> Drinking too much fluid can be harmful, even in healthy people.

Overhydration is much more common among people whose kidneys do not excrete urine normally—for example, among people with a disorder of the heart, kidneys, or liver. Overhydration may also result from the syndrome of inappropriate secretion of antidiuretic hormone (see page 948). In this syndrome, the pituitary gland secretes too much antidiuretic hormone, stimulating the kidneys to conserve water when that is not needed. Premature infants may become overhydrated if they receive too large an amount of intravenous fluids.

Brain cells are particularly susceptible to overhydration and to low sodium levels in the blood. When overhydration occurs slowly, brain cells have time to adapt, so few symptoms occur. When overhydration occurs quickly, confusion, seizures, or coma may develop.

Doctors try to distinguish between overhydration and excess blood volume. With overhydration and normal blood volume, the excess water usually moves into the cells, and tissue swelling (edema) does not occur. With overhydration and excess blood volume, an excess amount of sodium prevents the excess water from moving into the cells. Instead, the excess water accumulates around the cells, resulting in edema in the chest, abdomen, and lower legs.

Treatment

Regardless of the cause of overhydration, fluid intake usually must be restricted (but only as ad-vised by doctors). Drinking less than a quart of fluids a day usually results in improvement over several days. If overhydration occurs because of heart, liver, or kidney disease, restricting the intake of sodium (sodium causes the body to retain water) is also helpful.

Sometimes, doctors prescribe a drug to increase sodium and water excretion in the urine (diuretic). In general, diuretics are more useful when overhy-dration is accompanied by excess blood volume.

CHAPTER

143   Acid-Base Balance

An important property of blood is its degree of acidity or alkalinity. Body acidity increases when the level of acidic compounds in the body rises (through increased intake or production, or decreased elimina-tion) or when the level of basic (alkaline) compounds in the body falls (through decreased intake or produc-tion, or increased elimination). Body alkalinity in-creases with the reverse of these processes. The body's balance between acidity and alkalinity is referred to as acid-base balance. The acidity or alkalinity of any solution, including blood, is indicated on the pH scale.

The blood's acid-base balance is precisely controlled, because even a minor deviation from the normal range can severely affect many organs. The body uses different mechanisms to control the blood's acid-base balance.

Role of the Lungs: One mechanism the body uses to control blood pH involves the release of carbon dioxide from the lungs. Carbon dioxide, which is mildly acidic, is a waste product of the metabolism of oxygen (which all cells need) and, as such, is constantly produced by cells. As with all waste products, carbon dioxide gets excreted into the

blood. The blood carries carbon dioxide to the lungs, where it is exhaled. As carbon dioxide accu-mulates in the blood, the pH of the blood decreases (acidity increases). The brain regulates the amount of carbon dioxide that is exhaled by controlling the speed and depth of breathing. The amount of carbon dioxide exhaled, and consequently the pH of the blood, increases as breathing becomes faster and deeper. By adjusting the speed and depth of breath-ing, the brain and lungs are able to regulate the blood pH minute by minute.

Role of the Kidneys: The kidneys are also able to affect blood pH by excreting excess acids or bases. The kidneys have some ability to alter the amount of acid or base that is excreted, but because the kidneys make these adjustments more slowly than the lungs do, this compensation generally takes several days.

Buffer Systems: Yet another mechanism for con-trolling blood pH involves the use of buffer systems, which guard against sudden shifts in acidity and alkalinity. The pH buffer systems are combinations of the body's own naturally occurring weak acids and weak bases. These weak acids and bases exist in balance under normal pH conditions. The pH buffer systems work chemically to minimize changes in the pH of a solution by adjusting the proportion of acid and base. The most important pH buffer system in the blood involves carbonic acid (a weak acid formed from the carbon dioxide dissolved in blood) and bicarbonate ions (the corresponding weak base).

Acidosis and Alkalosis: There are two abnormali-ties of acid-base balance.

- Acidosis: The blood has too much acid (or too little base), resulting in a decrease in blood pH.

What Is the Blood pH?

Acidity and alkalinity are expressed on the pH scale, which ranges from 0 (strongly acidic) to 14 (strongly basic, or alkaline). A pH of 7.0, in the middle of this scale, is neutral. Blood is normally slightly basic, with a pH range of 7.35 to 7.45. To function properly, the body maintains the pH of blood close to 7.40.

- Alkalosis: The blood has too much base (or too little acid), resulting in an increase in blood pH.

Acidosis and alkalosis are not diseases but rather are the result of a wide variety of disorders. The presence of acidosis or alkalosis provides an important clue to doctors that a serious problem exists.

Acidosis and alkalosis are categorized as metabolic or respiratory, depending on their primary cause. Metabolic acidosis and metabolic alkalosis are caused by an imbalance in the production of acids or bases and their excretion by the kidneys. Respiratory acidosis and respiratory alkalosis are caused primarily by changes in carbon dioxide exhalation due to lung or breathing disorders.

Acidosis

Acidosis is excessive blood acidity caused by an overabundance of acid in the blood or a loss of bicarbonate from the blood (metabolic acidosis), or by a buildup of carbon dioxide in the blood that results from poor lung function or slow breathing (respiratory acidosis).

- Blood acidity increases when people ingest substances that contain or produce acid or when the lungs do not expel enough carbon dioxide.
- People with metabolic acidosis have nausea, vomiting, and fatigue and may breathe faster and deeper than normal.
- People with respiratory acidosis have headache and confusion, and breathing may appear shallow, slow or both.
- Tests on blood samples show there is too much acid.
- Doctors treat the cause of the acidosis.

If an increase in acid overwhelms the body's pH buffering systems, the blood will become acidic. As blood pH drops, the parts of the brain that regulate breathing are stimulated to produce faster and deeper breathing. Breathing faster and deeper increases the amount of carbon dioxide exhaled.

The kidneys also try to compensate by excreting more acid in the urine. However, both mechanisms can be overwhelmed if the body continues to produce too much acid, leading to severe acidosis and eventually coma.

Causes

Metabolic acidosis develops when the amount of acid in the body is increased through ingestion of a substance that is, or can be broken down (metabolized) to, an acid—such as wood alcohol (methanol), antifreeze (ethylene glycol), or large doses of aspirin (acetylsalicylic acid). Metabolic acidosis can also occur as a result of abnormal metabolism. The body produces excess acid in the advanced stages of

---

Major Causes of Metabolic Acidosis and Metabolic Alkalosis

METABOLIC ACIDOSIS

- Diabetic ketoacidosis (buildup of ketones)
- Drugs and substances such as acetazolamide, alcohol, aspirin, and iron
- Lactic acidosis (buildup of lactic acid as occurs in shock)
- Loss of bases, such as bicarbonate, through the digestive tract from diarrhea, an ileostomy, or a colostomy
- Kidney failure
- Poisons such as carbon monoxide, cyanide, ethylene glycol, and methanol
- Renal tubular acidosis (a form of kidney malfunction)

METABOLIC ALKALOSIS

- Loss of acid from vomiting or drainage of the stomach
- Overactive adrenal gland (Cushing's syndrome)
- Use of diuretics (thiazides, furosemide, ethacrynic acid)

---

shock and in poorly controlled type 1 diabetes mellitus. Even the production of normal amounts of acid may lead to acidosis when the kidneys are not functioning normally and are therefore not able to excrete sufficient amounts of acid in the urine.

Respiratory acidosis develops when the lungs do not expel carbon dioxide adequately, a problem that can occur in diseases that severely affect the lungs (such as emphysema, chronic bronchitis, severe pneumonia, pulmonary edema, and asthma). Respiratory acidosis can also develop when diseases of the brain or of the nerves or muscles of the chest impair breathing. In addition, people can develop respiratory acidosis when their breathing is slowed due to oversedation from opioids (narcotics) or strong drugs that induce sleep (sedatives).

Symptoms

People with mild metabolic acidosis may have no symptoms but usually experience nausea, vomiting, and fatigue. Breathing becomes deeper and slightly faster (as the body tries to correct the acidosis by expelling more carbon dioxide). As the acidosis worsens, people begin to feel extremely weak and drowsy and may feel confused and increasingly

Major Causes of Respiratory Acidosis and Alkalosis

RESPIRATORY ACIDOSIS

- Lung disorders, such as emphysema, chronic bronchitis, severe asthma, pneumonia, or pulmonary edema
- Sleep-disordered breathing
- Diseases of the nerves or muscles of the chest that impair breathing, such as Guillain-Barré syndrome or amyotrophic lateral sclerosis
- Overdose of drugs such as alcohol, opioids, and strong sedatives

RESPIRATORY ALKALOSIS

- Anxiety
- Aspirin overdose (early stages)
- Fever
- Low levels of oxygen in the blood
- Pain

buterol) may help people who have lung diseases such as asthma and emphysema. People who have severely impaired breathing or lung function, for whatever reason, may need mechanical ventilation to aid breathing (see page 527).

Acidosis may also be treated directly. If the acidosis is mild, the administration of intravenous fluids may be all that is needed. Rarely, when acidosis is very severe, bicarbonate may be given intravenously. However, bicarbonate provides only temporary relief and may cause harm—for instance, by overloading the body with sodium and water.

Alkalosis

Alkalosis is excessive blood alkalinity caused by an overabundance of bicarbonate in the blood or a loss of acid from the blood (metabolic alkalosis), or by a low level of carbon dioxide in the blood that results from rapid or deep breathing (respiratory alkalosis).

- People may have irritability, muscle twitching, or muscle cramps, or even muscle spasms.
- Blood is tested to diagnose alkalosis.
- Metabolic alkalosis is treated by replacing water and electrolytes.
- Respiratory alkalosis is treated by slowing breathing.

nauseated. Eventually, blood pressure can fall, leading to shock, coma, and death.

The first symptoms of respiratory acidosis may be headache and drowsiness. Drowsiness may progress to stupor and coma. Stupor and coma can develop within moments if breathing stops or is severely impaired, or over hours if breathing is less dramatically impaired.

Diagnosis

The diagnosis of acidosis generally requires the measurement of blood pH in a sample of arterial blood, usually taken from the radial artery in the wrist. Arterial blood is used because venous blood contains high levels of bicarbonate and thus is generally not as accurate a measure of the body's pH status.

To learn more about the cause of the acidosis, doctors also measure the levels of carbon dioxide and bicarbonate in the blood. Additional blood tests may be done to help determine the cause.

Treatment

The treatment of metabolic acidosis depends primarily on the cause. For instance, treatment may be needed to control diabetes with insulin or to remove the toxic substance from the blood in cases of poisoning.

The treatment of respiratory acidosis aims at improving the function of the lungs. Drugs that open the airways (bronchodilators, such as al-

Metabolic alkalosis develops when the body loses too much acid or gains too much base. For example, stomach acid is lost during periods of prolonged vomiting or when stomach acids are suctioned with a stomach tube (as is sometimes done in hospitals). In rare cases, metabolic alkalosis develops in a person who has ingested too much base from substances such as baking soda (bicarbonate of soda). In addition, metabolic alkalosis can develop when excessive loss of sodium or potassium affects the kidneys' ability to control the blood's acid-base balance. For instance, loss of potassium sufficient to cause metabolic alkalosis may result from an overactive adrenal gland or the use of diuretics.

Respiratory alkalosis develops when rapid, deep breathing (hyperventilation) causes too much carbon dioxide to be expelled from the bloodstream. The most common cause of hyperventilation, and thus respiratory alkalosis, is anxiety. Other causes of hyperventilation and consequent respiratory alkalosis include pain, low levels of oxygen in the blood, fever, and aspirin overdose (which can also cause metabolic acidosis—see page 973).

Symptoms and Diagnosis

Alkalosis may cause irritability, muscle twitching, muscle cramps, or no symptoms at all. If the alkalosis is severe, prolonged contraction and spasms of muscles (tetany) can develop.

A sample of blood usually taken from an artery shows that the blood is alkaline.

Treatment

Doctors usually treat metabolic alkalosis by replacing water and electrolytes (sodium and potassium) while treating the cause. Occasionally, when metabolic alkalosis is very severe, dilute acid is given intravenously.

With respiratory alkalosis, usually the only treatment needed is slowing down the rate of breathing. When respiratory alkalosis is caused by anxiety, a conscious effort to slow breathing may make the condition disappear. If pain is causing the person to breathe rapidly, relieving the pain usually suffices. Breathing into a paper (not a plastic) bag may help raise the carbon dioxide level in the blood as the person breathes carbon dioxide back in after breathing it out.

CHAPTER 144 Porphyrias

Porphyrias are a group of disorders caused by deficiencies of enzymes involved in the production of heme.

Heme is a chemical compound that contains iron and gives blood its red color. Heme is the key component of several important proteins in the body. One of the proteins is hemoglobin, which enables red blood cells to carry oxygen.

Heme is produced in the bone marrow and liver through a complex process regulated by eight different enzymes. The enzymes work one after another in separate steps that take the starting compound through several different intermediate compounds (heme precursors, also called porphyrins), finally producing heme. If there is a deficiency in one of these enzymes, certain heme precursors may accumulate. They may accumulate in the bone marrow or liver, appear in excess in the blood, and get excreted in the urine or stool. The accumulated heme precursors cause symptoms. The specific heme precursors that accumulate and the symptoms that develop depend on which enzyme is deficient.

Porphyrias are a number of different disorders, each caused by a deficiency in one of the heme production enzymes. Each enzyme deficiency is caused by damage to the gene (a mutation) responsible for the production of the enzyme in question. The damaged gene is almost always inherited from one of the parents or, rarely, both.

Porphyrias are commonly divided into two types:

- Acute
- Cutaneous

Acute porphyrias cause intermittent attacks of abdominal, mental, and neurologic symptoms. These attacks are typically triggered by prescription drugs (including oral contraceptives), alcohol, exposure to organic solvents, and other factors such as fasting, infections, or stress. The most common acute porphyria is acute intermittent porphyria. Others include variegate porphyria, hereditary coproporphyria, and the extremely rare delta-aminolevulinic acid dehydratase-deficiency porphyria. Some acute porphyrias also cause skin (cutaneous) symptoms.

Cutaneous porphyrias cause symptoms involving the skin, usually when the skin is exposed to sunlight. In these porphyrias, certain porphyrins are deposited in the skin. When exposed to light and oxygen, these porphyrins generate a charged, unstable form of oxygen capable of damaging the skin. The skin becomes fragile and blistered. The most common cutaneous porphyria is porphyria cutanea tarda. Others include erythropoietic protoporphyria, and the extremely rare hepatoerythropoietic porphyria and congenital erythropoietic porphyria.

Classifying Porphyrias

Porphyrias can be classified in several ways. Classification according to the specific enzyme deficiency is the most accurate. A simpler classification system distinguishes porphyrias that cause neurologic, mental, and abdominal symptoms (acute porphyrias) from those that cause skin photosensitivity (cutaneous porphyrias). A third classification system is based on whether the excess precursors originate primarily in the liver (hepatic porphyrias) or primarily in the bone marrow (erythropoietic porphyrias). Some porphyrias are classified into more than one of these categories.

Investigating the Family

In order to avoid exposure to substances that can precipitate acute porphyria, people need to know whether they carry the gene for a deficient enzyme. A child whose parent has an enzyme deficiency that can cause an acute porphyria should be tested well before puberty. The genes in the child's blood sample are analyzed for the enzyme. Older family members of a person with an enzyme deficiency should also be tested to confirm or reject the possibility that they are predisposed to developing an acute porphyria.

In many of the porphyrias of both types, the urine may take on a red or reddish brown discoloration. Sometimes the discoloration appears only after the urine has stood in light for about 30 minutes.

Porphyria Cutanea Tarda

Porphyria cutanea tarda is the most common porphyria and causes blistering and fragility of skin exposed to sunlight.

- People have chronically recurring blisters on the sun-exposed areas of their bodies.
- Doctors test urine and stool samples for high levels of porphyrins.
- Removing blood (phlebotomy), giving chloroquine, or both are helpful.

Porphyria cutanea tarda occurs throughout the world. As far as is known, one form of this porphyria is the only one that can occur in people who do not have an inherited deficiency of an enzyme involved in heme production.

Porphyria cutanea tarda results from underactivity of the enzyme uroporphyrinogen decarboxylase, which leads to accumulation of porphyrins in the liver. Skin damage occurs because of overproduction of porphyrins in the liver being transported by the blood to the skin.

Porphyria cutanea tarda has several common precipitating factors. These factors include excess iron in the liver, moderate or heavy alcohol use, taking estrogens, and infection with hepatitis C virus. Infection with the human immunodeficiency virus (HIV) is a less common precipitating factor. These factors are thought to interact with iron and oxygen in the liver and thereby inhibit or damage the enzyme uroporphyrinogen decarboxylase.

In about 80% of people with porphyria cutanea tarda, the disorder does not appear to be hereditary and is called sporadic. In the remaining 20%, the disorder is hereditary and is called familial.

Symptoms and Diagnosis

People with porphyria cutanea tarda experience chronic, recurring blisters of various sizes on sun-exposed areas such as the arms, face, and especially the backs of the hands. Crusting and scarring follow the blisters and take a long time to heal. The skin, especially on the hands, is also sensitive to minor injury. Hair growth on the face and other sun-exposed areas may increase. Liver damage usually occurs, and cirrhosis and even liver cancer may eventually develop.

To diagnose porphyria cutanea tarda, doctors test urine and stool for unusually high levels of porphyrins. The specific porphyrins that are increased provide a pattern that allows doctors to distinguish porphyria cutanea tarda from other porphyrias.

Treatment

Porphyria cutanea tarda is the most readily treated porphyria. Avoiding alcohol and other precipitating factors is beneficial.

A procedure called phlebotomy, in which a pint (almost half a liter) of blood is removed, is the most widely recommended treatment. With phlebotomy, the excess iron is gradually removed, the activity of uroporphyrinogen decarboxylase in the liver returns toward normal, and porphyrin levels in the liver and blood fall gradually. The skin symptoms resolve, and the skin eventually returns to normal. Phlebotomy sessions are stopped when people become slightly iron deficient. Anemia may develop if too many phlebotomy sessions are done or if sessions are done too frequently.

Very low doses of chloroquine or hydroxychloroquine are also effective in treating porphyria cutanea tarda. These drugs remove excess porphyrins from the liver. However, doses that are too high cause porphyrins to be removed too rapidly, resulting in a temporary worsening of the disorder and damage to the liver.

Combining phlebotomy and chloroquine treatments accelerates improvement.

For women taking estrogen, doctors stop the estrogen therapy (because it is a precipitating factor of the porphyria) until phlebotomy has been completed and porphyrin levels are normal. The estrogen is then restarted and seldom causes a recurrence of the porphyria.

Acute Intermittent Porphyria

Acute intermittent porphyria, which causes abdominal pain and neurologic symptoms, is the most common acute porphyria.

- Many people never experience symptoms.
- Symptoms may include acute onset of vomiting, abdominal or back pain, weakness in arms or legs, and mental symptoms.
- Laboratory tests are done on urine samples taken during the attack.
- Maintaining good nutrition and avoiding alcohol and drugs that trigger attacks are important.
- Attacks are treated by giving heme and sometimes glucose.

Acute intermittent porphyria occurs in people of all ethnic groups but may be more common in people from Northern Europe. In most countries, it is the most common of the acute porphyrias. People first experience sudden onset of neurologic symptoms. Attacks are more common in women than in men and occur only very rarely before puberty.

Acute intermittent porphyria is due to a deficiency of the enzyme porphobilinogen deaminase (also known as hydroxymethylbilane synthase) that leads to accumulation of the heme precursors delta-aminolevulinic acid and porphobilinogen initially in the liver. The disorder is inherited due to a single abnormal gene from one parent. The normal gene from the other parent keeps the deficient enzyme at half-normal levels, which is sufficient to produce normal amounts of heme. Very rarely, the disorder is inherited from both parents (and therefore two abnormal genes are present). Symptoms may then appear in childhood and include developmental abnormalities.

Most people with a deficiency of porphobilinogen deaminase never develop symptoms. In some people, however, certain factors can precipitate symptoms, producing an attack. Many drugs (including barbiturates, anticonvulsants, and sulfonamide antibiotics) can bring on an attack. Sex hormones, such as progesterone and related steroids, can precipitate symptoms, as can low-calorie and low-carbohydrate diets, ingestion of alcohol, and exposure to organic solvents (for example, in dry cleaning fluids or paints). Mental stress or an infection is sometimes implicated. Usually a combination of factors is involved. Sometimes the factors that cause an attack cannot be identified.

Symptoms

Many people never experience symptoms. Symptoms occur as attacks usually lasting a few days but occasionally longer. Such attacks usually first appear after puberty. In some women, attacks develop during the second half of the menstrual cycle.

Abdominal pain is the most common symptom. The pain can be so severe that doctors may mistak-

enly think that abdominal surgery is needed. Gastrointestinal symptoms include nausea, vomiting, and constipation or diarrhea. The bladder may be affected, making urination difficult and sometimes resulting in an overly full bladder. A rapid heart rate, high blood pressure, sweating, and restlessness are also common during attacks. Interference with sleep is typical. High blood pressure can continue after the attack. Mental symptoms are common, from irritation, restlessness, insomnia, and agitation to tiredness and depression.

Most of these symptoms, including the gastrointestinal ones, result from effects on the nervous system. Nerves that control muscles can be affected, leading to weakness, usually beginning in the shoulders and arms. The weakness can progress to virtually all the muscles, including those involved in breathing. Tremors and seizures may develop. Irregular heart rhythm is a dangerous complication during an attack. Recovery from symptoms may occur within a few days, although complete recovery from severe muscle weakness may take several months or years. Attacks are rarely fatal. However, in a few people, attacks are disabling.

Long-term complications of acute porphyria may include high blood pressure, kidney failure, and liver tumors.

Diagnosis

The severe gastrointestinal and neurologic symptoms resemble those of many more common disorders. Laboratory tests done on samples of urine taken during an attack show increased levels of two heme precursors (delta-aminolevulinic acid and porphobilinogen). Levels of these precursors are very high during attacks and remain high in people who have repeated attacks. The precursors can form porphyrins, which are reddish. These porphyrins turn the urine red to red-brown. The color is especially evident after the urine specimen is exposed to light.

Relatives without symptoms can be identified as carriers of the disorder by measuring porphobilinogen deaminase in red blood cells or sometimes by DNA testing. Diagnosis before birth is also possible but usually is not needed because most affected people never get symptoms.

Prevention and Treatment

Attacks of acute intermittent porphyria can be prevented by maintaining good nutrition and avoiding alcohol and the drugs that can provoke them. Crash diets to lose weight rapidly should be avoided. Heme can be given by vein to prevent attacks. Premenstrual attacks in women can be prevented with one of the gonadotropin-releasing hormone agonists used to treat endometriosis (see page 1531), although this treatment should only be directed by doctors who are experts in treating porphyria.

People who have attacks of acute intermittent porphyria are often hospitalized for treatment of severe symptoms. People with severe attacks are treated with heme given intravenously. Blood and urine levels of delta-aminolevulinic acid and porphobilinogen are promptly lowered and symptoms subside, usually within several days. If treatment is delayed, recovery takes longer, and some nerve damage may be permanent.

Glucose given intravenously or a diet high in carbohydrates can also be beneficial, particularly in people whose attacks are brought on by a low-calorie or low-carbohydrate diet, but these measures are less effective than heme. Pain can be controlled with drugs (such as opioids).

Nausea, vomiting, anxiety, and restlessness are treated with a phenothiazine for a short time. Insomnia may be treated with chloral hydrate or low doses of a benzodiazepine but not a barbiturate. An overly full bladder may be treated by draining the urine with a catheter.

Doctors ensure that people do not take any of the drugs known to precipitate an attack, and—if possible—address other factors that may have contributed to the attack. Treatment of seizures is problematic, because almost any anticonvulsant would worsen an attack. Beta-blockers may be used to treat rapid heart rate and high blood pressure.

Erythropoietic Protoporphyria

Erythropoietic protoporphyria is a condition characterized by photosensitivity.

- The heme precursor protoporphyrin accumulates in the bone marrow and red blood cells.
- People have severe skin pain and swelling soon after exposure to sunlight.
- Doctors test blood to look for elevated levels of protoporphyrin.
- People should avoid exposure to sunlight.
- Sometimes, beta-carotene can help protect the skin.

Erythropoietic protoporphyria is uncommon. It usually appears in childhood.

In erythropoietic protoporphyria, a deficiency of the enzyme ferrochelatase leads to accumulation of the heme precursor protoporphyrin in the bone marrow, red blood cells, blood plasma, skin, and eventually liver. The enzyme deficiency is inherited from one parent, but in order to develop the disorder people must also inherit a slightly abnormal gene for the enzyme from the other parent.

Accumulation of protoporphyrin in the skin results in extreme sensitivity to sunlight and severe pain after exposure. The sunlight activates the protoporphyrin molecules, which damage the surrounding tissue. Accumulation of protoporphyrins in the liver can cause liver damage. Protoporphyrins excreted in the bile can lead to bile stones.

Symptoms and Diagnosis

Symptoms usually start in childhood. Severe skin pain and swelling develop soon after exposure to sunlight. Because blistering and scarring do not occur, doctors usually do not recognize the disorder. Gallstones cause characteristic abdominal pain (see page 243). Liver damage may lead to increasing liver failure, with jaundice, abdominal pain, and enlargement of the spleen.

Porphyrin levels in urine are not usually increased. The diagnosis is therefore made when increased levels of protoporphyrin are detected in red blood cells.

> **Did You Know...**
> Young children often cannot describe their symptoms, so doctors and parents may have difficulty connecting their discomfort to sun exposure.

Prevention and Treatment

Extreme care should be taken to avoid exposure to sunlight. Accidental sun exposure is given the same treatment as sunburn (see page 1327). Beta-carotene, when taken in sufficient amounts to cause a slight protective yellowing of the skin, makes many people more tolerant of sunlight. However, sunlight should still be avoided. People who develop gallstones that contain protoporphyrin may need to have them surgically removed. Porphyrin accumulation in red blood cells and the condition of the liver should be monitored yearly by testing blood, urine, and stool samples. Liver damage, if severe, may necessitate liver transplantation.

Hormonal Disorders

CHAPTER

145 Biology of the Endocrine System

The endocrine system consists of a group of glands and organs that regulate and control various body functions by producing and secreting hormones. The glands of the endocrine system do not have ducts but rather release their hormones directly into theë bloodstream. While the individual organs that comprise the endocrine system have different and often unrelated functions, they are traditionally grouped together, although this organization may not have much significance for nondoctors.

Doctors who specialize in disorders of the endocrine system are known as endocrinologists. Many endocrinologists further subspecialize in the functions and disorders of specific glands.

Endocrine Glands

The major glands of the endocrine system, each of which produces one or more specific hormones, are the hypothalamus, the pituitary gland, the thyroid gland, the parathyroid glands, the islets of the pancreas, the adrenal glands, the testes in men, and the ovaries in women. During pregnancy, the placenta also acts as an endocrine gland in addition to its other functions.

Not all organs that secrete hormones or hormone-like substances are considered part of the endocrine system. For example, the kidneys produce the hormone renin to help control blood pressure and the hormone erythropoietin to stimulate the bone marrow to produce red blood cells. In addition, the gastrointestinal system produces a variety of hormones that control digestion, affect insulin secretion from the pancreas, and alter behaviors, such as those associated with hunger. Fat (adipose) tissue also produces hormones that regulate metabolism and appetite. Additionally, the term "gland" does not mean that the organ is part of the endocrine system. For example, sweat glands, glands in mucus membranes, and mammary glands secrete substances other than hormones.

Endocrine Function

The main function of endocrine glands is to secrete hormones directly into the bloodstream. Hormones are chemical substances that affect the activity of another part of the body (target site). In essence, hormones serve as messengers, controlling and coordinating activities throughout the body.

Upon reaching a target site, a hormone binds to a receptor, much like a key fits into a lock. Once the hormone locks into its receptor, it transmits a message that causes the target site to take a specific action. Hormone receptors may be within the nucleus or on the surface of the cell.

Ultimately, hormones control the function of entire organs, affecting such diverse processes as growth and development, reproduction, and sexual characteristics. Hormones also influence the way the body uses and stores energy and control the volume of fluid and the levels of salts and sugar in the blood. Very small amounts of hormones can trigger very large responses in the body.

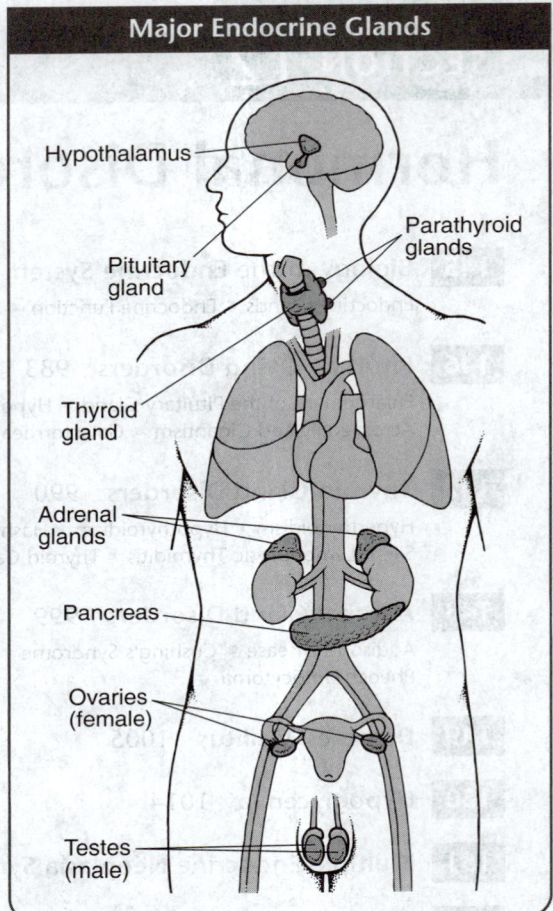

Major Endocrine Glands

Hypothalamus

Pituitary gland

Parathyroid glands

Thyroid gland

Adrenal glands

Pancreas

Ovaries (female)

Testes (male)

Although hormones circulate throughout the body, each type of hormone influences only certain organs and tissues. Some hormones affect only one or two organs, whereas others have influence throughout the body. For example, thyroid-stimulating hormone, produced in the pituitary gland, affects only the thyroid gland. In contrast, thyroid hormone, produced in the thyroid gland, affects cells throughout the body and is involved in such important functions as regulating growth of cells, controlling the heart rate, and affecting the speed at which calories are burned. Insulin, secreted by the islet cells of the pancreas, affects the processing (metabolism) of glucose, protein, and fat throughout the body.

Most hormones are proteins. Others are steroids, which are fatty substances derived from cholesterol.

MAJOR HORMONES

WHERE HORMONE IS PRODUCED	HORMONE	FUNCTION
Pituitary gland	Antidiuretic hormone (vasopressin)	Causes kidneys to retain water and, along with aldosterone, helps control blood pressure
	Corticotropin (ACTH)	Controls the production and secretion of hormones by the adrenal glands
	Growth hormone	Controls growth and development Promotes protein production
	Luteinizing hormone and follicle-stimulating hormone	Control reproductive functions, including the production of sperm and semen, egg maturation, and menstrual cycles Control male and female sexual characteristics (including hair distribution, muscle formation, skin texture and thickness, voice, and perhaps even personality traits)
	Oxytocin	Causes muscles of the uterus and milk ducts in the breast to contract
	Prolactin	Starts and maintains milk production in the ductal glands of the breast (mammary glands)
	Thyroid-stimulating hormone	Stimulates the production and secretion of hormones by the thyroid gland
Parathyroid glands	Parathyroid hormone	Controls bone formation and the excretion of calcium and phosphorus
Thyroid gland	Thyroid hormone	Regulates the rate at which the body functions (metabolic rate)
	Calcitonin	In people, has unclear function but in other species, regulates calcium balance
Adrenal glands	Aldosterone	Helps regulate salt and water balance by retaining salt and water and excreting potassium
	Cortisol	Has widespread effects throughout the body Especially has anti-inflammatory action Maintains blood sugar level, blood pressure, and muscle strength Helps control salt and water balance
	Dehydroepiandrosterone (DHEA)	Has effects on bone, mood, and the immune system
	Epinephrine and norepinephrine	Stimulate the heart, lungs, blood vessels, and nervous system
Pancreas	Glucagon	Raises the blood sugar level
	Insulin	Lowers the blood sugar level Affects the processing (metabolism) of sugar, protein, and fat throughout the body
Kidneys	Erythropoietin	Stimulates red blood cell production
	Renin	Controls blood pressure
Ovaries	Estrogen	Controls the development of female sex characteristics and the reproductive system
	Progesterone	Prepares the lining of the uterus for implantation of a fertilized egg and readies the mammary glands to secrete milk

(continued on the following page)

MAJOR HORMONES (*Continued*)		
WHERE HORMONE IS PRODUCED	**HORMONE**	**FUNCTION**
Testes	Testosterone	Controls the development of male sex characteristics and the reproductive system
Digestive tract	Cholecystokinin	Controls gallbladder contractions that cause bile to enter the intestine Stimulates release of digestive enzymes from the pancreas
	Glucagon-like peptide	Increases **insulin** release from the pancreas
	Ghrelin	Controls growth hormone release from the pituitary gland Causes sensation of hunger
Adipose (fat) tissue	Resistin	Blocks the effects of **insulin** on muscle
	Leptin	Controls appetite
Placenta	Chorionic gonadotropin	Stimulates ovaries to continue to release progesterone during early pregnancy
	Estrogen and progesterone	Keep uterus receptive to fetus and placenta during pregnancy

Endocrine Controls

To control endocrine functions, the secretion of each hormone must be regulated within precise limits. The body is normally able to sense whether more or less of a given hormone is needed.

Many endocrine glands are controlled by the interplay of hormonal signals between the hypothalamus, located in the brain, and the pituitary gland, which sits at the base of the brain. This interplay is referred to as the hypothalamic-pituitary axis. The hypothalamus secretes several hormones that control the pituitary gland. The pituitary, sometimes called the master gland, in turn controls the functions of many other endocrine glands (see page 983). The pituitary controls the rate at which it secretes hormones through a feedback loop in which the blood levels of other endocrine hormones signal the pituitary to slow down or speed up.

Many other factors can control endocrine function. For example, a baby sucking on its mother's nipple stimulates her pituitary gland to secrete prolactin and oxytocin, hormones that stimulate breast milk production and flow. Rising blood sugar levels stimulate the islet cells of the pancreas to produce insulin. Part of the nervous system stimulates the adrenal gland to produce epinephrine.

Endocrine Disorders

Endocrine disorders involve either too much or too little hormone secretion. Disorders may result from a problem in the gland itself or because the hypothalamic-pituitary axis provides too much or too little stimulation. Depending on the type of cell they originate in, tumors can produce excess hormones or squeeze out normal glandular tissue, decreasing hormone production. Sometimes the body's immune system (see page 1124) attacks an endocrine gland, decreasing hormone production.

Doctors usually measure levels of hormones in the blood to tell how an endocrine gland is functioning. Sometimes blood levels alone do not give enough information about endocrine gland function, so doctors measure hormone levels after giving a stimulus (such as a sugar-containing drink, a drug, or a hormone that can trigger hormone release) or after having the patient take an action (such as fasting).

Effects of Aging

Levels of most hormones decrease with aging, but some hormones remain at levels typical of those in younger adults, and some even increase. Even when hormone levels do not decline, endocrine function generally declines with age because hormone receptors become less sensitive. Although such decreased function suggests that hormone replacement therapy might be beneficial in older people, such therapy generally does not appear to reverse aging or prolong life and, in some cases (such as estrogen replacement in older women), is potentially harmful. However, ongoing research is examining the beneficial effects of providing some hormones to older people.

CHAPTER

146 Pituitary Gland Disorders

The pituitary is a pea-sized gland that is housed within a bony structure (sella turcica) at the base of the brain. The sella turcica protects the pituitary but allows very little room for expansion.

The pituitary controls the function of most other endocrine glands and is therefore sometimes called the master gland. In turn, the pituitary is controlled in large part by the hypothalamus, a region of the brain that lies just above the pituitary. By detecting the levels of hormones produced by glands under the pituitary's control (target glands), the hypothalamus or the pituitary can determine how much stimulation the target glands need.

The pituitary has two distinct parts: the front (anterior) lobe, which accounts for 80% of the pituitary gland's weight, and the back (posterior) lobe. The lobes are connected to the hypothalamus by a stalk that contains blood vessels and nerve cell projections (nerve fibers, or axons). The hypothalamus controls the anterior lobe by releasing hormones through the connecting blood vessels. It controls the posterior lobe through nerve impulses.

The **anterior lobe** of the pituitary produces and releases (secretes) six main hormones:

- Growth hormone, which regulates growth and physical development and has important effects on body shape by stimulating muscle formation and reducing fat tissue
- Thyroid-stimulating hormone, which stimulates the thyroid gland to produce thyroid hormones
- Adrenocorticotropic hormone (ACTH, also called corticotropin), which stimulates the adrenal glands to produce cortisol and other hormones
- Follicle-stimulating hormone and luteinizing hormone (the gonadotropins), which stimulate the testes to produce sperm, the ovaries to produce eggs, and the sex organs to produce sex hormones (testosterone and estrogen)
- Prolactin, which stimulates the mammary glands of the breasts to produce milk

The anterior lobe also produces several other hormones, including one that causes the skin to darken (beta-melanocyte–stimulating hormone) and ones that inhibit pain sensations and help control the immune system (endorphins).

The **posterior lobe** of the pituitary produces only two hormones: antidiuretic hormone and oxytocin. Antidiuretic hormone (also called vasopressin) regulates the amount of water excreted by the kidneys and is therefore important in maintaining water balance in the body (see page 969). Oxytocin causes the uterus to contract during childbirth and immediately after delivery to prevent excessive bleeding. Oxytocin also stimulates contractions of the milk ducts in the breast, which move milk to the nipple (the let-down) in lactating women.

The hormones produced by the pituitary are not all produced continuously. Most are released in bursts every 1 to 3 hours, with alternating periods of activity and inactivity. Some of the hormones, such as ACTH, growth hormone, and prolactin, follow a circadian rhythm: The levels rise and fall predictably during the day, usually peaking just before awakening and dropping to their lowest levels just before sleep. The levels of other hormones vary according to other factors. For example, in women, the levels of luteinizing hormone and follicle-stimulating hormone, which control reproductive functions, vary during the menstrual cycle.

The pituitary gland can malfunction in several ways, usually as a result of developing a noncancerous tumor (adenoma). The tumor may overproduce one or more pituitary hormones, or the tumor may press on the normal pituitary cells, causing underproduction of one or more pituitary hormones. The tumor may also cause enlargement of the pituitary gland, with or without disturbing hormone production. Sometimes there is overproduction of one hormone by a pituitary tumor and underproduction of another at the same time due to pressure. Too little or too much of a pituitary hormone results in a wide variety of symptoms.

Doctors can diagnose pituitary gland malfunction using several tests. Imaging tests, such as a computed tomography (CT) or magnetic resonance imaging (MRI) scan, can show whether the pituitary has enlarged or shrunk. Such scans can usually determine whether a tumor exists in the gland.

Doctors can measure the levels of pituitary hormones, usually by a simple blood test. Doctors select which pituitary hormone levels they want to measure depending on the person's symptoms. Sometimes, levels of pituitary hormones are not easy to interpret because the levels vary greatly during the day and according to the body's needs. For these hormones, measuring a random blood sample does not provide useful information.

For some of those hormones, doctors give a substance that would normally affect hormone production and then they measure the level of the hormone. For example, if a doctor injects insulin, the

Pituitary: The Master Gland

The pituitary, a pea-sized gland at the base of the brain, produces a number of hormones. Each of these hormones affects a specific part of the body (a target organ or tissue). Because the pituitary controls the function of most other endocrine glands, it is often called the master gland.

Hormone	Target Organ or Tissue
Adrenocorticotropic hormone (ACTH)	Adrenal glands
Antidiuretic hormone	Kidneys
Beta-melanocyte–stimulating hormone	Skin
Endorphins	Brain and immune system
Enkephalins	Brain
Follicle-stimulating hormone	Ovaries or testes
Growth hormone	Muscles and bones
Luteinizing hormone	Ovaries or testes
Oxytocin	Uterus and mammary glands
Prolactin	Mammary glands
Thyroid-stimulating hormone	Thyroid gland

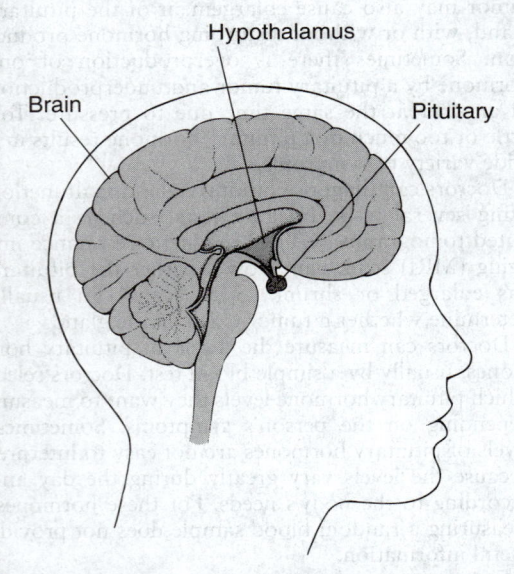

levels of ACTH, growth hormone, and prolactin should increase. Rather than measuring growth hormone levels directly, doctors often measure another hormone, insulin-like growth factor 1 (IGF-1). Growth hormone is produced in bursts and its levels quickly fall, but IGF-1 levels reflect the overall daily production of growth hormone. For all of these reasons, interpreting the results of blood tests for pituitary hormones is complex.

Enlargement of the Pituitary Gland

Enlargement of the pituitary gland is usually due to a tumor but may be due to bleeding into the gland or involvement by some other disease, such as tuberculosis or sarcoidosis. An enlarged pituitary gland may produce symptoms such as headaches. Because the growing gland often presses on the optic nerve, which passes above the pituitary gland, loss of vision may occur. Vision loss often initially affects only the upper, outermost fields of vision in both eyes. Underproduction or overproduction of pituitary hormones may also occur. Treatment depends on the cause of the enlargement.

Hypopituitarism

Hypopituitarism is an underactive pituitary gland that results in deficiency of one or more pituitary hormones.

- Hypopituitarism can be caused by several factors, including certain inflammatory diseases, a tumor of the pituitary gland, or an insufficient blood supply to the pituitary gland.

- Symptoms depend on what hormone is deficient and may include short height, infertility, intolerance to cold, fatigue, and an inability to produce breast milk.

- The diagnosis is based on measuring the blood levels of hormones produced by the pituitary gland and on imaging tests performed on the pituitary gland.

- Treatment focuses on replacing deficient hormones with synthetic ones but sometimes includes surgical removal or irradiation of any pituitary tumors.

Hypopituitarism, an uncommon disorder, can be caused by a number of factors, including a pituitary tumor or an insufficient blood supply to the pituitary gland.

Symptoms and Complications

Although symptoms sometimes begin suddenly and dramatically, they usually begin gradually and may go unrecognized for a long time. Symptoms depend on which pituitary hormones are deficient. In some cases, the pituitary gland's production of a single hormone decreases. More typically, the levels of several hormones decrease at the same time (panhypopituitarism). Production of growth hormone, luteinizing hormone, and follicle-stimulating hormone often decreases before that of thyroid-stimulating hormone and adrenocorticotropic hormone.

Growth Hormone Deficiency: A lack of growth hormone typically leads to poor overall growth and short height (dwarfism) if it occurs in childhood. In adults, growth hormone deficiency does not affect height, because the bones have finished growing, but it can cause increased fat and reduced muscle tissue, thinning of bones, and reduced energy and quality of life.

Deficiency of Gonadotropins (Follicle-Stimulating Hormone and Luteinizing Hormone): In premenopausal women, deficiencies of these hormones cause menstrual periods to stop (amenorrhea), infertility, vaginal dryness, and loss of some female sexual characteristics. In men, deficiencies of these hormones result in wasting away (atrophy) of the testes, decreased sperm production and consequent infertility, and loss of some male sexual characteristics. Deficiencies of luteinizing hormone and follicle-stimulating hormone can also occur in Kallmann's syndrome, in which people may also have a cleft lip or palate, are color-blind, and are unable to sense smells.

Thyroid-Stimulating Hormone Deficiency: Thyroid-stimulating hormone deficiency leads to an underactive thyroid gland (hypothyroidism), which results in such symptoms as confusion, intolerance to cold, weight gain, constipation, and dry skin (see page 995). Most cases of hypothyroidism, however, are due to a problem originating in the thyroid gland itself, not to low levels of pituitary hormones.

Adrenocorticotropic Hormone Deficiency: Adrenocorticotropic hormone (ACTH) deficiency leads to an underactive adr enal gland, which results in fatigue, low blood pressure, low levels of sugar in the blood, and low tolerance for stress. This is the most serious pituitary hormone deficiency. If the body is unable to make any ACTH, the person may die.

Prolactin Deficiency: Prolactin deficiency reduces or eliminates a woman's ability to produce breast milk after childbirth. One cause of low prolactin levels and deficiency of other pituitary hormones is Sheehan's syndrome, a rare complication of childbirth. Sheehan's syndrome typically develops because of excessive blood loss and shock during childbirth, which results in partial destruction of the pituitary gland. Symptoms include fatigue, loss of pubic and underarm hair, and inability to produce breast milk. Prolactin deficiency has no known ill effects in men.

What Causes an Underactive Pituitary?

CAUSES AFFECTING PRIMARILY THE PITUITARY

- Pituitary tumors
- Inadequate blood supply to the pituitary (due to severe bleeding, blood clots, anemia, or other conditions)
- Infections and inflammatory diseases
- Sarcoidosis or amyloidosis (unusual diseases)
- Irradiation (as for a brain tumor)
- Surgical removal of pituitary tissue
- Autoimmune disease

CAUSES AFFECTING PRIMARILY THE HYPOTHALAMUS, WHICH THEN AFFECTS THE PITUITARY

- Tumors of the hypothalamus
- Inflammatory diseases
- Head injuries
- Surgical damage to the pituitary or to the blood vessels or nerves leading to it

---

Diagnosis

Because the pituitary gland stimulates other glands, a deficiency in pituitary hormones often reduces the amount of hormones those other glands produce. Therefore, a doctor considers the possibility of pituitary malfunction when investigating a deficiency in another gland, such as the thyroid or adrenal gland. When symptoms suggest that several glands are underactive, a doctor may suspect hypopituitarism or a polyglandular deficiency syndrome.

An evaluation usually begins by measuring levels of the hormones that the pituitary gland produces and at the same time measuring levels of the hormone produced by the target organ. For example, a person with hypothyroidism due to failure of the pituitary gland has low levels of thyroid hormone and low or inappropriately normal levels of thyroid-stimulating hormone, which is produced by the pituitary gland. In contrast, a person with hypothyroidism due to failure of the thyroid gland itself has low levels of thyroid hormone and high levels of thyroid-stimulating hormone.

Growth hormone production by the pituitary is difficult to evaluate because no test accurately measures it. The body produces growth hormone in several bursts each day, and the hormone is quickly used. Thus, the blood level at any given moment does not indicate whether production is normal over the course of a day. Instead, doctors measure

Polyglandular Deficiency Syndromes

Polyglandular deficiency syndromes are hereditary disorders in which several endocrine glands malfunction simultaneously. The actual cause of the malfunction may be related to an autoimmune reaction in which the body's immune defenses mistakenly attack the body's own cells. Polyglandular deficiency syndromes are classified into three types:

Type 1: In this type, which develops in children, the parathyroid and adrenal glands are underactive, which can lead to diabetes, hepatitis, malabsorption of nutrients and weight loss, and hair loss. Affected children are prone to chronic yeast infections as well.

Type 2: In this type, which develops in adults, the adrenal and thyroid glands are underactive, although the thyroid gland sometimes becomes overactive. People with type 2 polyglandular deficiency also develop diabetes.

Type 3: This type is very similar to type 2, except that the adrenal glands remain normal.

the levels of insulin-like growth factor 1 (IGF-1) in the blood. Production of IGF-1 is controlled by growth hormone, and the level of IGF-1 tends to change slowly in proportion to the overall amount of growth hormone produced by the pituitary. In infants and young children, doctors may instead measure levels of a similar substance, IGF-binding protein type 3.

Because the levels of luteinizing hormone and follicle-stimulating hormone fluctuate with the menstrual cycle, their measurement in women may be difficult to interpret. However, in postmenopausal women who are not taking estrogen, luteinizing hormone and follicle-stimulating hormone levels normally are high.

Production of ACTH is usually measured by assessing the response of its target hormone (cortisol) to stimuli, such as a low level of sugar in the blood after an insulin injection. If the level of cortisol does not change and the level of ACTH in the blood is normal or low, a deficiency of ACTH production is confirmed.

Once hypopituitarism is established by blood tests, the pituitary gland is usually evaluated with a computed tomography (CT) or magnetic resonance imaging (MRI) scan to identify structural problems. CT or MRI scans help reveal individual (localized) areas of abnormal tissue growth as well as general enlargement or shrinkage of the pituitary gland. The blood vessels that supply the pituitary can be examined with cerebral angiography (see page 2036).

Treatment

When possible, treatment is aimed at removing the cause of the pituitary hormone deficiency, such as a tumor. Surgical removal of a tumor is often the most appropriate first treatment, and removal also usually reduces any pressure symptoms and vision problems caused by the tumor. For all but the largest tumors, surgery can usually be done through the nose (transphenoidal).

Supervoltage or proton beam irradiation of the pituitary gland can be used to destroy a tumor. Large tumors and those that have extended beyond the sella turcica may be impossible to remove with surgery alone. If so, doctors use supervoltage irradiation after surgery to kill the remaining tumor cells. Irradiation of the pituitary gland tends to cause a slow loss of pituitary function. The loss may be partial or complete. Therefore, the function of the target glands is generally evaluated every 3 to 6 months for the first year and yearly thereafter. Tumors that produce prolactin can be treated with drugs that act like dopamine, such as bromocriptine or cabergoline. These drugs shrink the tumor while also lowering prolactin levels.

When it is not possible to remove the cause of the hormone deficiency, such as an insufficient blood supply to the pituitary gland, treatment focuses on replacing the deficient hormones, usually by replacing the target hormones. For example, people deficient in thyroid-stimulating hormone are given thyroid hormone. Those deficient in ACTH are given adrenocortical hormones such as hydrocortisone. Those deficient in luteinizing hormone and follicle-stimulating hormone are given estrogen, progesterone, or testosterone.

Growth hormone is the one pituitary hormone that is replaced. Growth hormone treatment must be given by injection. When given to children who have growth hormone deficiency before the growth plates in their bones close, replacement growth hormone prevents them from being exceptionally short. Growth hormone is now also being used to treat some adults with growth hormone deficiency to improve body composition, increase bone density, and enhance quality of life.

Central Diabetes Insipidus

Central diabetes insipidus is a lack of antidiuretic hormone that causes excessive production of very dilute urine (polyuria).

- Central diabetes insipidus has several causes, including a brain tumor, tuberculosis, a brain injury or surgery, and some forms of other diseases.
- The main symptoms are excessive thirst and excessive urine production.
- The diagnosis is based on urine tests, blood tests, and a water deprivation test.

- People with central diabetes insipidus usually are given the drugs vasopressin or desmopressin as a nasal spray.

Causes

Central diabetes insipidus usually results from the decreased production of antidiuretic hormone (vasopressin), the hormone that helps regulate the amount of water in the body (see box on page 970). Antidiuretic hormone is unique in that it is produced in the hypothalamus but is then stored and released into the bloodstream by the pituitary gland.

Central diabetes insipidus may be caused by insufficient production of antidiuretic hormone by the hypothalamus. Alternatively, the disorder may be caused by failure of the pituitary gland to release antidiuretic hormone into the bloodstream. Other causes of central diabetes insipidus include damage done during surgery on the hypothalamus or pituitary gland; a brain injury, particularly a fracture of the base of the skull; a tumor; sarcoidosis or tuberculosis; an aneurysm (a bulge in the wall of an artery) or blockage in the arteries leading to the brain; some forms of encephalitis or meningitis; and the rare disease Langerhans' cell histiocytosis. Another type of diabetes insipidus, nephrogenic diabetes insipidus, may be caused by abnormalities in the kidneys (see page 285).

Symptoms and Diagnosis

Symptoms may begin gradually or suddenly at any age. Often the only symptoms are excessive thirst and excessive urine production. A person may drink huge amounts of fluid—4 to 40 quarts (3 to 30 liters) a day—to compensate for the fluid lost in urine. Ice-cold water is often the preferred drink. When compensation is not possible, dehydration can quickly follow, resulting in low blood pressure and shock. The person continues to urinate large quantities of dilute urine, and this excessive urination is particularly noticeable during the night.

Doctors suspect diabetes insipidus in people who produce large amounts of urine. They first test the urine for sugar to rule out diabetes mellitus. Blood tests show abnormal levels of many electrolytes, including a high level of sodium. The best test is a water deprivation test, in which urine production, blood electrolyte levels, and weight are measured regularly for a period of about 12 hours, during which the person is not allowed to drink. A doctor monitors the person's condition throughout the course of the test. At the end of the 12 hours—or sooner if the person's blood pressure falls or heart rate increases or if he loses more than 5% of his body weight—the doctor stops the test and injects antidiuretic hormone. The diagnosis of central diabetes insipidus is confirmed if, in response to antidiuretic hormone, the person's excessive urination

stops, the urine becomes more concentrated, the blood pressure rises, and the heart beats more normally. The diagnosis of nephrogenic diabetes insipidus is made if, after the injection, the excessive urination continues, the urine remains dilute, and blood pressure and heart rate do not change.

Treatment

Vasopressin or desmopressin (a modified form of vasopressin) may be taken as a nasal spray several times a day. The dose is adjusted to maintain the body's water balance and a normal urine output. Taking too much of these drugs can lead to fluid retention, swelling, and other problems. People with central diabetes insipidus who are undergoing surgery or are unconscious are generally given injections of vasopressin.

Sometimes central diabetes insipidus can be controlled with drugs that stimulate production of antidiuretic hormone, such as chlorpropamide, carbamazepine, clofibrate, and thiazide diuretics. These drugs are unlikely to relieve symptoms completely in people whose diabetes insipidus is severe.

Acromegaly and Gigantism

Overproduction of growth hormone causes excessive growth. In children, the condition is called gigantism. In adults, it is called acromegaly.

- Excessive growth hormone is almost always caused by a noncancerous (benign) pituitary tumor.
- Children develop great stature; adults develop deformed bones but do not grow taller.
- Heart failure, weakness, and vision problems are common.
- The diagnosis is based on blood tests and x-rays of the skull and hands.
- Other imaging tests are done to look for the cause.
- A combination of surgery, radiation therapy, and drug therapy is used to treat the overproduction of growth hormone.

Growth hormone stimulates the growth of bones, muscles, and many internal organs. Excessive growth hormone, therefore, leads to abnormally robust growth of all of these tissues. Overproduction of growth hormone is almost always caused by a noncancerous (benign) pituitary tumor (adenoma). Certain rare tumors of the pancreas and lungs also can produce hormones that stimulate the pituitary to produce excessive amounts of growth hormone, with similar consequences.

Symptoms

If excessive growth hormone production starts before the growth plates have closed (that is, in children), the condition produces gigantism. The long bones grow enormously. A person grows to unusually great stature, and the arms and legs lengthen. Puberty may be delayed, and the genitals may not develop fully.

In most cases, excessive production of growth hormone begins between the ages of 30 and 50, long after the growth plates of the bones have closed. Increased growth hormone in adults produces acromegaly, in which the bones become deformed rather than elongated. Because changes occur slowly, they are usually not recognized for years.

The person's facial features become coarse, and the hands and feet swell. Larger rings, gloves, shoes, and hats are needed. Overgrowth of the jawbone (mandible) can cause the jaw to protrude (prognathism). Cartilage in the voice box (larynx) may thicken, making the voice deep and husky. The ribs may thicken, creating a barrel chest. Joint pain is common; after many years, crippling degenerative arthritis may occur.

In both gigantism and acromegaly, the tongue may enlarge and become more furrowed. Coarse body hair, which typically darkens, increases as the skin thickens. The sebaceous and sweat glands in the skin enlarge, producing excessive perspiration and often an offensive body odor. The heart usually enlarges, and its function may be so severely impaired that heart failure occurs. Sometimes a person feels disturbing sensations and weakness in the arms and legs as enlarging tissues compress the nerves. Nerves that carry messages from the eyes to the brain may also be compressed, causing loss of vision, particularly in the outer visual fields. The pressure on the brain may also cause severe headaches.

Nearly all women with acromegaly have irregular menstrual cycles. Some women produce breast milk even though they are not breastfeeding (galactorrhea) because of either too much growth hormone or a related increase in prolactin. About one third of men who have acromegaly develop erectile dysfunction. There is also an increased likelihood of developing diabetes mellitus, high blood pressure (hypertension), heart failure, sleep apnea, and certain tumors, particularly affecting the large intestine, which may become cancerous. Life expectancy is reduced in people with untreated acromegaly.

Diagnosis

In children, rapid growth may not seem abnormal at first. Eventually, however, the abnormality of the extreme growth becomes clear.

In adults, because the changes induced by high levels of growth hormone occur slowly, acromegaly often is not diagnosed until many years after the first symptoms appear. Serial photographs (those taken over many years) may help a doctor establish the diagnosis. An x-ray of the skull may show thickening of the bones and enlargement of the nasal sinuses. X-rays of the hands show thickening of the bones under the fingertips and swelling of the tissue around the bones. Blood sugar levels and blood pressure may be high.

The diagnosis is confirmed by blood tests, which usually show high levels of both growth hormone and insulin-like growth factor 1 (IGF-1). Because growth hormone is released in short bursts and the levels of growth hormone often fluctuate dramatically even in people without acromegaly, a single high level of growth hormone in the blood is insufficient to make the diagnosis. Doctors must give something that would normally suppress growth hormone levels, most commonly a glucose drink (the oral glucose tolerance test), and show that normal suppression does not occur. This test is not necessary when the clinical features of acromegaly are obvious, the IGF-1 level is high, or a tumor is seen in the pituitary on scanning.

 Did You Know...
A woman with acromegaly can produce breast milk even if she is not breastfeeding.

A computed tomography (CT) or magnetic resonance imaging (MRI) scan is usually done to look for abnormal growths in the pituitary gland. Because acromegaly is usually present for some years before being diagnosed, a tumor is seen on these scans in most people.

Treatment

Stopping or reducing the overproduction of growth hormone is not easy; thus, doctors may need to use a combination of surgery, radiation therapy, and drug therapy.

Surgery by an experienced surgeon is currently regarded as the best first treatment for most people with acromegaly caused by a tumor. It results in an immediate reduction in tumor size and growth hormone production, most often without causing deficiency of other pituitary hormones. Unfortunately, tumors are often large by the time they are found, and surgery alone does not usually produce a cure. Radiation therapy is often used as a follow-up treatment, particularly if a substantial amount of the tumor remains after surgery and acromegaly persists.

Radiation therapy involves the use of supervoltage irradiation, which is less traumatic than surgery. This treatment may take several years to have its full effect, however, and often results in later deficiencies of other pituitary hormones, as normal tissue is often also affected. More directed radiation therapy, such as stereotactic radiosurgery, is being tried to speed results and spare the normal pituitary tissue.

Drug therapy can also be used to lower growth hormone levels. Occasionally, bromocriptine and other drugs that act like dopamine are of some benefit. The most effective drugs, however, are those that are forms of somatostatin, the hormone that normally blocks growth hormone production and secretion. These drugs include octreotide and its newer long-acting analogs, which only have to be given about once a month. These drugs are effective in controlling acromegaly in many people as long as they continue to be taken (they do not provide a cure). Their use has been limited by the need to inject them and by their high cost. This may change as such drugs become longer acting and more readily available. Several new growth hormone blocker drugs, such as pegvisomant, are now available and may be useful for people who do not respond to somatostatin-type drugs.

Galactorrhea

Galactorrhea is the production of breast milk in men or in women who are not breastfeeding.

- The most common cause of galactorrhea is a tumor in the pituitary gland.
- Galactorrhea can cause unexpected milk production and infertility in both men and women.
- The diagnosis is based on measuring the blood levels of the hormone prolactin.
- Imaging tests may be done to look for a cause.
- When drugs alone do not stop prolactin production or shrink the tumor, surgery and sometimes radiation therapy may be done.

In both sexes, the most common cause of galactorrhea is a prolactin-secreting tumor (prolactinoma) in the pituitary gland. Prolactinomas usually are very small when first diagnosed. They tend to be larger in men than in women, probably because they come to attention later. Overproduction of prolactin and the development of galactorrhea may also be induced by drugs, including phenothiazines, certain drugs given for high blood pressure (especially methyldopa), opioids, and birth control pills. There are other causes of galactorrhea that do not involve high levels of prolactin, such as an underactive thyroid gland (hypothyroidism).

Symptoms

Although unexpected breast milk production may be the only symptom of a prolactinoma, many women

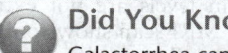

Did You Know...

Galactorrhea can occur in both women and men.

also stop menstruating (amenorrhea) or have less frequent menstrual periods. Women with prolactinomas often have low levels of estrogen, which can produce vaginal dryness, and thus discomfort with sexual intercourse. About two thirds of men with prolactinomas lose interest in sex (reduced libido) and have erectile dysfunction. A high prolactin level can cause infertility in both men and women.

When a prolactinoma is large, it may press on the nerves of the brain that are located just above the pituitary gland, causing the person to have headaches or to become blind in specific visual fields (see box on page 1460).

Diagnosis

The diagnosis is usually suspected in women when menstrual periods are reduced or absent or when breast milk is unexpectedly produced. It is also suspected in men with reduced libido and decreased levels of testosterone in the blood who are producing breast milk. It is confirmed by finding a high level of prolactin in the blood. Computed tomography (CT) or magnetic resonance imaging (MRI) scans are done to search for a prolactinoma. If no tumor is detected and there is no other apparent cause of the high prolactin level (such as a drug), a pituitary tumor is still the most likely cause, particularly in women. In this case, the tumor is probably too small to be seen on the scan.

If a prolactinoma is large on imaging studies, an ophthalmologist tests the person's visual fields for possible effects on vision.

Treatment

Drugs can be given to stimulate dopamine, the chemical in the brain that blocks prolactin production. They include bromocriptine and cabergoline. These drugs are taken by mouth and are effective only as long as they are used. They seldom result in cure of the tumor. In most people, they lower prolactin levels enough to restore menstrual periods (in women), stop galactorrhea, and increase estrogen levels in women and testosterone levels in men, and they are often able to restore fertility. They also usually shrink the tumor and improve any vision problems. Surgery is also effective for treating small prolactinomas but is not usually used first because drug treatment is safe, effective, and easy to use.

When a person's prolactin levels are not extraordinarily high and a CT or MRI scan shows only a small prolactinoma or none at all, a doctor may not recommend treatment. This is probably appropriate in women who are not having problems getting pregnant as a result of the high prolactin level, whose menstrual periods remain regular, and who are not troubled by galactorrhea, and in men whose testosterone level is not low. Low estrogen levels usually accompany amenorrhea and increase the risk of osteoporosis in women. Low testosterone levels increase the risk of osteoporosis in men.

To overcome the effects of low estrogen levels caused by a prolactinoma, estrogen or oral contraceptives that contain estrogen may be given to women with small prolactinomas who do not want to become pregnant. Although estrogen treatment has not been shown to stimulate the growth of small prolactinomas, most experts recommend a CT or MRI scan every year for at least 2 years to be sure the tumor is not enlarging substantially.

Doctors generally treat people who have larger tumors with drugs to stimulate dopamine (dopamine agonists—for example, bromocriptine or cabergoline) or with surgery. If drugs reduce the prolactin levels and symptoms disappear, surgery may not be necessary. These drugs are generally safe, but heart valve fibrosis and leakage have been reported recently when they were used to treat Parkinson's disease in much higher doses than they are used to treat increased prolactin levels. Even when surgery is necessary, dopamine agonists may be prescribed to help shrink the tumor before the operation. They are often given after surgery, because a large prolactin-secreting tumor is unlikely to be cured with surgery. Occasionally, prolactinomas subside so the dopamine agonists can be stopped without the prolactin level rising again. This is more common with small tumors and after pregnancy.

Radiation therapy is sometimes needed, as for other pituitary tumors, when the tumor does not respond to medical or surgical treatment.

Empty Sella Syndrome

In empty sella syndrome, the sella turcica (the bony structure at the base of the brain that houses the pituitary gland) enlarges, but the pituitary remains normal-sized or shrinks.

People with empty sella syndrome have a defect in the tissue barrier that normally keeps the cerebrospinal fluid around the brain separate from the sella turcica. As a result, cerebrospinal fluid puts increased pressure on the pituitary gland and the walls of the sella turcica. The sella turcica may enlarge, and the pituitary gland may shrink.

Empty sella syndrome occurs most often in middle-aged women who are overweight and who have high blood pressure. Less commonly, the condition occurs after pituitary surgery, radiation therapy, or infarction (death) of a pituitary tumor.

The empty sella syndrome may produce no symptoms at all and seldom produces serious symptoms. About half of those affected have headaches, and some people have high blood pressure as well. In rare cases, there is leaking of the cerebrospinal fluid from the nose or problems with vision.

The empty sella syndrome can be diagnosed by computed tomography (CT) or magnetic resonance imaging (MRI) scanning. Pituitary function is checked to rule out hormone excess or deficiency, but it is almost always normal.

Treatment is indicated only for overproduction or underproduction of pituitary hormones and is seldom needed.

CHAPTER 147 Thyroid Gland Disorders

The thyroid is a small gland, measuring about 2 inches (5 centimeters) across, that lies just under the skin below the Adam's apple in the neck. The two halves (lobes) of the gland are connected in the middle (called the isthmus), giving the thyroid gland the shape of a bow tie. Normally, the thyroid gland cannot be seen and can barely be felt. If it becomes enlarged (goiter), doctors can feel it easily, and a prominent bulge may appear below or to the sides of the Adam's apple.

The thyroid gland secretes thyroid hormones, which control the speed at which the body's chemical functions proceed (metabolic rate). Thyroid hormones influence the metabolic rate in two ways: by stimulating almost every tissue in the body to produce proteins and by increasing the amount of oxygen that cells use. Thyroid hormones affect many vital body functions: the heart rate, the respiratory rate, the rate at which calories are burned, skin maintenance, growth, heat production, fertility, and digestion.

The two thyroid hormones are T_4 (thyroxine) and T_3 (triiodothyronine). T_4, the major hormone produced by the thyroid gland, has only a slight, if any, effect on speeding up the body's metabolic rate. Instead, T_4 is converted into T_3, the more active hormone. The conversion of T_4 to T_3 occurs in the liver and other tissues. Many factors control the conversion of T_4 to T_3, including the body's needs from moment to moment and the presence or absence of illnesses. Most of the T_4 and T_3 in the bloodstream is carried bound to a protein called thyroxine-binding globulin. Only a little of the T_4 and T_3 are circulating free in the blood. However, it is this free hormone that is active. When the free hormone is used by the body, some of the bound hormone is released from the binding protein.

To produce thyroid hormones, the thyroid gland needs iodine, an element contained in food and water. The thyroid gland traps iodine and processes it into thyroid hormones. As thyroid hormones are used, some of the iodine contained in the hormones is released, returns to the thyroid gland, and is recycled to produce more thyroid hormones. Oddly, the thyroid gland releases slightly less of the thyroid hormones if it is exposed to high levels of iodine transported to it in the blood.

The body has a complex mechanism for adjusting the level of thyroid hormones. First, the hypothalamus, located just above the pituitary gland in the brain,

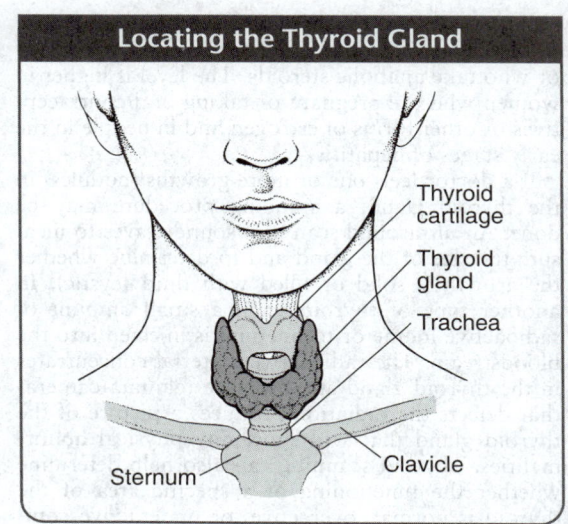

Locating the Thyroid Gland

- Thyroid cartilage
- Thyroid gland
- Trachea
- Sternum
- Clavicle

secretes thyrotropin-releasing hormone, which causes the pituitary gland to produce thyroid-stimulating hormone (TSH). Just as the name suggests, TSH stimulates the thyroid gland to produce thyroid hormones. The pituitary gland slows or speeds the release of TSH, depending on whether the levels of thyroid hormones circulating in the blood are getting too high or too low.

The thyroid gland also produces the hormone calcitonin, which may contribute to bone strength by helping calcium to be incorporated into bone.

Diagnostic Tests

To determine how well the thyroid gland is functioning, doctors usually measure the levels of TSH, T_4, and T_3 in the blood.

Usually the TSH level is the best indicator of thyroid function. Because this hormone stimulates the thyroid gland, blood levels of TSH are high when the thyroid gland is underactive (and thus needs more stimulation) and low when the thyroid gland is overactive (and thus needs less stimulation). However, in rare cases in which the pituitary gland is not functioning normally, the level of TSH does not accurately reflect thyroid gland function.

When doctors measure the levels of thyroid hormones T_4 and T_3 in the blood, they usually measure both the bound and free forms of each hormone (total T_4 and total T_3). However, if the level of thyroxine-binding globulin is abnormal, the total thyroid hormone levels can be misinterpreted, so doctors sometimes measure the level of free hormones in the blood. The level of thyroxine-binding

SPOTLIGHT ON AGING

Aging itself has only minor effects on the thyroid gland and thyroid hormones. As people get older, the thyroid gland shrinks and shifts lower in the neck. The level of T_3 may fall slightly, but the speed of vital functions changes very little. However, thyroid disorders become more common with aging.

Disorders that affect thyroid function, particularly hyperthyroidism and hypothyroidism, can be thought of as great masqueraders in older people. These disorders often cause symptoms that are easily mistaken for symptoms of other conditions or even as signs of getting old. Increased or decreased thyroid function can dramatically worsen the way an older person feels and can greatly diminish the ability to carry out daily activities. For these reasons, the great masqueraders must be unmasked and recognized for what they are so that they can be effectively treated.

Screening older people for hyperthyroidism and hypothyroidism is helpful. Many experts recommend measuring the level of thyroid-stimulating hormone in the blood every year in people over 65.

globulin is lower in people who have kidney disease or diseases that reduce protein synthesis by the liver or who take anabolic steroids. The level is higher in women who are pregnant or taking oral contraceptives or other forms of estrogen and in people in the early stages of hepatitis.

If a doctor feels one or more growths (nodules) in the thyroid gland, a scanning procedure may be done. An ultrasound scan uses sound waves to measure the size of the gland and to determine whether the growth is solid or filled with fluid (cystic). In another type of thyroid scan, a small amount of radioactive iodine or technetium is injected into the bloodstream. The radioactive material concentrates in the thyroid gland and a device (gamma camera) that detects the radiation produces a picture of the thyroid gland that will show any physical abnormalities. Thyroid scanning can also help determine whether the functioning of a specific area of the thyroid is normal, overactive, or underactive compared with the rest of the gland.

Additional testing may be necessary in rare cases in which doctors cannot determine whether the problem lies in the thyroid or in the pituitary gland.

If cancer of the thyroid gland is suspected, doctors use a small needle to obtain a sample of thyroid tissue for study (a biopsy). When medullary thyroid cancer is suspected, blood levels of calcitonin are measured, because these cancers always secrete calcitonin.

Hyperthyroidism

Hyperthyroidism is overactivity of the thyroid gland that leads to high levels of thyroid hormones and speeding up of vital body functions.

- Graves' disease is the most common cause of hyperthyroidism.
- Heart rate and blood pressure may increase, heart rhythms may be abnormal, and people may sweat excessively, feel nervous and anxious, have difficulty sleeping, and lose weight without trying.
- Blood tests can confirm the diagnosis.
- Usually, propylthiouracil or methimazole can control hyperthyroidism.

Hyperthyroidism affects about 1% of people in the United States. It can occur at any age but is more common in women during menopause and after childbirth.

Causes

Hyperthyroidism has several causes, including Graves' disease, thyroiditis, inflammation from toxic substances or radiation exposure, toxic thyroid nodules, and overstimulation due to an overactive pituitary gland.

Euthyroid Sick Syndrome

In euthyroid sick syndrome, thyroid test results are abnormal even though the thyroid gland is functioning normally.

Euthyroid sick syndrome commonly occurs in people who have a severe illness other than thyroid disease. When people are sick or malnourished or have had surgery, the thyroid hormone T_4 is not converted normally to the active T_3 hormone. Large amounts of reverse T_3, an inactive thyroid hormone, accumulate. Despite this abnormal conversion, the thyroid gland continues to function and to control the body's metabolic rate normally. Because no problem exists with the thyroid gland, no treatment is needed. Laboratory tests show normal results once the underlying illness resolves.

Graves' disease, the most common cause of hyperthyroidism, is an autoimmune disorder caused by an abnormal protein (antibody) in the blood that stimulates the thyroid to produce and secrete excess thyroid hormones into the blood. This cause of hyperthyroidism is often hereditary, especially in women, and almost always leads to a diffusely enlarged thyroid.

Thyroiditis is inflammation of the thyroid gland. In subacute thyroiditis, silent lymphocytic thyroiditis, and, much less often, Hashimoto's thyroiditis, hyperthyroidism occurs as stored hormones are released from the inflamed gland. Hypothyroidism usually follows because the levels of stored hormones are depleted. Finally, the gland usually returns to normal function.

Inflammation from toxic substances or radiation exposure, like the three main types of thyroiditis, can also cause hyperthyroidism.

A toxic (hyperfunctional) thyroid nodule (adenoma) is an area of abnormal local tissue growth within the thyroid gland. This abnormal tissue produces thyroid hormones even without stimulation by thyroid-stimulating hormone (TSH). Thus, a nodule escapes the mechanisms that normally control the thyroid gland and produces thyroid hormones in large quantities. Toxic multinodular goiter (Plummer's disease), in which there are many nodules, is uncommon in adolescents and young adults and tends to become more common with aging.

Drugs and iodine can cause hyperthyroidism. Drugs include amiodarone, interferon-alpha, and, rarely, lithium. Excess iodine, as may occur in people taking certain expectorants, or iodine-containing contrast agents for x-ray studies may cause hyperthyroidism.

An overactive pituitary gland can produce too much TSH, which in turn leads to overproduction of thyroid hormones. However, this is an extremely rare cause of hyperthyroidism.

Symptoms

Most people with hyperthyroidism have an enlarged thyroid gland (goiter). The entire gland may be enlarged, or nodules may develop within certain areas. The gland may be tender and painful.

Symptoms of hyperthyroidism, regardless of the cause, reflect the speeding up of body functions: increased heart rate and blood pressure, abnormal heart rhythms (arrhythmias), excessive sweating, hand tremors (shakiness), nervousness and anxiety, difficulty sleeping (insomnia), weight loss despite increased appetite, increased activity level despite fatigue and weakness, and frequent bowel movements, occasionally with diarrhea. Older people with hyperthyroidism may not develop these characteristic symptoms but have what is sometimes called apathetic or masked hyperthyroidism, in which they become weak, sleepy, confused, withdrawn, and depressed. Hyperthyroidism can cause changes in the eyes. A person with hyperthyroidism may appear to be staring.

If the cause of hyperthyroidism is Graves' disease, eye symptoms include puffiness around the eyes, increased tear formation, irritation, and unusual sensitivity to light. Two distinctive additional symptoms may occur: bulging eyes (proptosis—see page 1464) and double vision (diplopia—see page 1418). The eyes bulge outward because of inflammation in the orbits behind the eyes. The muscles that move the eyes become inflamed and unable to function properly, making it difficult or impossible to move the eyes normally or to coordinate eye movements, resulting in double vision. The eyelids may not close completely, exposing the eyes to injury from foreign particles and dryness. These eye changes may begin before any other symptoms of hyperthyroidism, providing an early clue to Graves' disease, but most often occur when other symptoms of hyperthyroidism are noticed. Eye symptoms may even appear or worsen after the excessive thyroid hormone secretion has been treated and controlled.

When Graves' disease affects the eyes, there may also be thickening of the skin, usually over the shins, which has the texture of an orange-peel. The thickened area may be itchy and red and feels hard when pressed with a finger. As with deposits behind the eyes, this problem may begin before or after other symptoms of hyperthyroidism are noticed.

Diagnosis

Doctors usually suspect hyperthyroidism on the basis of the symptoms. Blood tests are used to

SPOTLIGHT ON AGING

Hyperthyroidism affects about the same percentage of older people as younger people—about 1%. However, hyperthyroidism is often more serious among older people because they tend to have other disorders as well.

Hyperthyroidism in older people often results from Graves' disease. Almost as often, hyperthyroidism is caused by the gradual growth of many small lumps in the thyroid gland (toxic thyroid nodules). Some drugs can cause hyperthyroidism as well. The most common is amiodarone, a drug used to treat heart disease but which may stimulate or damage the thyroid gland.

Hyperthyroidism can produce many vague symptoms that can be attributed to other conditions. Typically, symptoms differ between older and younger people. Among older people, the most common symptoms are weight loss and fatigue. The heart rate may or may not be increased, and the eyes usually do not bulge. Older people are also more likely to have abnormal heart rhythms (such as atrial fibrillation), other heart problems (such as angina and heart failure), and constipation. Occasionally, older people sweat profusely, become nervous and anxious, and have hand tremors and frequent bowel movements or diarrhea.

confirm the diagnosis. Often, testing begins with measurement of TSH. If the thyroid gland is overactive, the level of TSH is low. However, in rare cases in which the pituitary gland is overactive, the level of TSH is normal or high. If the level of TSH in the serum is low, doctors measure the levels of the thyroid hormones in the blood. If there is a question of whether Graves' disease is the cause, doctors check a sample of blood for the presence of antithyroid antibodies. More specific antibodies can be measured, but such a test is rarely needed.

If a toxic thyroid nodule is suspected as the cause, a thyroid scan will show whether the nodule is overactive, that is, whether it is producing excess hormones. Such a scan may also help doctors in their evaluation of Graves' disease: In a person with Graves' disease, the scan shows the entire gland to be overactive, not just one area. In thyroiditis, the scan shows low activity.

Prognosis and Treatment

Treatment of hyperthyroidism depends on the cause. In most cases, the problem causing hyperthyroidism can be cured, or the symptoms can be eliminated or greatly reduced. If left untreated, however, hyperthyroidism places undue stress on the heart and many other organs.

Beta-blockers such as propranolol help control many of the symptoms of hyperthyroidism. These drugs can slow a fast heart rate, reduce tremors, and control anxiety. Doctors therefore find beta-blockers particularly useful for people with extreme hyperthyroidism and for people with bothersome or dangerous symptoms that have not responded to other treatments. However, beta-blockers do not reduce excess thyroid hormone production. Therefore, other treatments are added to bring hormone production to normal levels.

Propylthiouracil and methimazole are the drugs most commonly used to treat hyperthyroidism; they work by decreasing the gland's production of thyroid hormones. Each drug is taken by mouth, beginning with high doses that are later adjusted according to blood test results. These drugs can usually control thyroid function in 6 to 12 weeks. Larger doses of these drugs may work more quickly but increase the risk of side effects. Pregnant women who take propylthiouracil or methimazole are closely monitored, because these drugs cross the placenta and can induce goiter or hypothyroidism in the fetus. Carbimazole, a drug that is widely used in Europe, is converted into methimazole in the body.

Iodine, given by mouth, is sometimes used to treat hyperthyroidism. It is reserved for those in whom rapid treatment is needed. It may also be used to control hyperthyroidism until the person can have surgery to remove the thyroid. It is not used long-term.

Did You Know...

People who receive radioactive iodine should not go near infants and young children for 2 to 4 days.

Radioactive iodine may be given by mouth to destroy part of the thyroid gland. Very little radioactivity is introduced to the body as a whole, but a great deal is delivered to the thyroid gland because the thyroid gland takes up the iodine and concentrates it. Hospitalization is rarely necessary. After treatment, the person should probably not be near infants and young children for 2 to 4 days. No special precautions are needed in the workplace. There are no precautions needed for sleeping with a partner. Pregnancy should be avoided for about 6 months. People who have had radioactive iodine treatment may set off radiation alarms at airports and sometimes other places for several weeks after treatment and, therefore, should carry a doctor's note describing their treatment if they travel on public transportation.

Thyroid Storm

Thyroid storm, which is sudden extreme overactivity of the thyroid gland, is a life-threatening emergency. All body functions are accelerated to dangerously high levels. Severe strain on the heart can lead to a life-threatening irregular heartbeat (arrhythmia), extremely fast pulse, and shock. Thyroid storm may also cause fever, extreme weakness, restlessness, mood swings, confusion, altered consciousness (even coma), and an enlarged liver with mild jaundice (a yellowish discoloration of the skin and the whites of the eyes).

Thyroid storm is generally caused by untreated or inadequately treated hyperthyroidism and can be triggered by infection, injury, surgery, poorly controlled diabetes, pregnancy or labor, or other stresses. Also, thyroid storm can occur when drugs being used to treat thyroid problems are stopped. It is rare in children.

Some doctors try to adjust the dose of radioactive iodine to destroy only enough of the thyroid gland to bring its hormone production back to normal, without reducing thyroid function too much. Other doctors use a larger dose to completely destroy the thyroid. Most of the time, people who undergo this treatment must take thyroid hormone replacement therapy for the rest of their life (see page 996). Although concerns have been raised that radioactive iodine may cause cancer, an increased risk of cancer in people who have had radioactive iodine treatment has never been confirmed. Radioactive iodine is not given to pregnant or nursing women, because it crosses the placenta and enters the milk and may destroy the fetus's or breastfed infant's thyroid gland.

Surgical removal of the thyroid gland, called thyroidectomy, is a treatment option for young people with hyperthyroidism. Surgery is also an option for people who have a very large goiter as well as for those who are allergic to or who develop severe side effects from the drugs used to treat hyperthyroidism. Hyperthyroidism is permanently controlled in more than 90% of people who choose this option. Hypothyroidism often occurs after surgery, and people then have to take replacement thyroid hormone for the rest of their lives. Rare complications of surgery include paralysis of the vocal cords and damage to the parathyroid glands (the tiny glands behind the thyroid gland that control calcium levels in the blood).

In Graves' disease, additional treatment may be needed for the eye and skin symptoms. Eye symp-

℞ DRUGS USED TO TREAT HYPERTHYROIDISM

DRUG	SOME SIDE EFFECTS	COMMENTS
Thionamides		
Carbimazole	Allergic reactions (usually rashes)	Decrease the production of thyroid
Methimazole	Nausea	hormones
Propylthiouracil	Loss of taste	
	Infection (rare) due to a low white blood cell count	
	Liver dysfunction	
	Joint aching	
Nonmetallic element		
Iodine	Rash	Decreases the production and release of thyroid hormones
Radioactive isotope		
Radioactive iodine	Hypothyroidism	Destroys the thyroid gland
Beta-blockers		
Atenolol	In people with respiratory disease, may cause wheezing	Block many of the stimulating effects of excess thyroid hormones on other organs
Metoprolol	Can worsen peripheral vascular disease	
Propranolol	Can cause depression	
	May reduce blood pressure (hypotension)	

toms may be helped by elevating the head of the bed, by applying eye drops, by sleeping with the eyelids taped shut, and, occasionally, by taking diuretics (drugs that hasten fluid excretion). Double vision may be helped by using eyeglass prisms. Finally, corticosteroids taken by mouth, x-ray treatment to the orbits, or eye surgery may be needed if the eyes are severely affected. Corticosteroid creams or ointments can help relieve the itching and hardness of the abnormal skin. Often the problem disappears without treatment months or years later.

Hypothyroidism

Hypothyroidism is underactivity of the thyroid gland that leads to inadequate production of thyroid hormones and a slowing of vital body functions.

- Facial expressions become dull, the voice is hoarse, speech is slow, eyelids droop, and the eyes and face become puffy.
- Usually only one blood test is needed to confirm the diagnosis.
- People with hypothyroidism need to take thyroid hormone for the rest of their life.

Hypothyroidism is common, especially among older people, particularly women; it affects about 10% of older women. It can, however, occur at any age. Very severe hypothyroidism is called myxedema.

Causes

Hypothyroidism has several causes.

Primary hypothyroidism results from a disorder of the thyroid gland itself. The most common cause is Hashimoto's thyroiditis (see page 996). As the thyroid is gradually destroyed, hypothyroidism develops.

Subacute thyroiditis and silent lymphocytic thyroiditis can both cause transient hypothyroidism. The hypothyroidism is transient because the thyroid is not destroyed.

Hypothyroidism can develop after treatment of hyperthyroidism or thyroid cancer because use of radioactive iodine or drugs that interfere with the body's ability to make thyroid hormones or surgical removal of the thyroid gland leads to a lack of thyroid hormone production.

A chronic lack of iodine in the diet is the most common cause of hypothyroidism in many developing countries. However, iodine deficiency is a rare cause of hypothyroidism in the United States because iodine is added to table salt and is also used to sterilize the udders of dairy cattle and thus is present in dairy products. Rarer causes of hypothyroidism include some inherited disorders in which an abnormality of

SPOTLIGHT ON AGING

More than 10% of older people have some degree of hypothyroidism. Women are affected about twice as often as men. Typical symptoms, such as weight gain, muscle cramps, tingling, and the inability to tolerate cold, are less common among older people. When such symptoms do occur among older people, they are less obvious. Older people may also have less typical symptoms. For example, they may lose weight, become confused, and have a decreased appetite, joint stiffness, joint and muscle pains, weakness, and a tendency to fall.

Because symptoms in older people can be different, are often subtle and vague, and are common among older people who do not have hypothyroidism, doctors may not recognize these symptoms as being caused by hypothyroidism. A screening test, in which blood levels of thyroid-stimulating hormone are measured, is important. The test should be done every year in people over 65.

the enzymes in thyroid cells prevents the gland from making or secreting enough thyroid hormones.

In secondary hypothyroidism, which is much rarer than primary, the pituitary gland fails to secrete enough thyroid-stimulating hormone (TSH), which is necessary for normal stimulation of the thyroid.

Symptoms

Insufficient thyroid hormones cause body functions to slow. Symptoms are subtle and develop gradually. They may be mistaken for depression, especially among older people. Facial expressions become dull, the voice is hoarse and speech is slow, eyelids droop, and the eyes and face become puffy. Many people with hypothyroidism gain weight, become constipated, and are unable to tolerate cold. The hair becomes sparse, coarse, and dry, and the skin becomes coarse, dry, scaly, and thick. Some people develop carpal tunnel syndrome, which makes the hands tingle or hurt (see page 601). The pulse may slow, the palms and soles may appear slightly orange (carotenemia), and the side parts of the eyebrows slowly fall out. Some people, especially older people, may appear confused, forgetful, or demented—signs that can easily be mistaken for Alzheimer's disease or other forms of dementia.

If untreated, hypothyroidism can eventually cause anemia, a low body temperature, and heart failure. This situation may progress to confusion, stupor, or coma (myxedema coma), a life-threatening complication in which breathing slows, seizures occur, and blood flow to the brain decreases. Myxedema coma can be triggered in a person with hypothyroidism by physical stresses, such as exposure to the cold, as well as by an infection, injury, surgery, and drugs such as sedatives that depress brain function.

Diagnosis

Usually hypothyroidism can be diagnosed with one simple blood test: the measurement of TSH. Many experts suggest that the test be done at least every other year in people older than 55, because hypothyroidism is so common among older people yet so difficult, in its mild stages, for doctors to distinguish from other disorders that affect people in this age group.

In those rare cases of hypothyroidism caused by inadequate secretion of TSH, a second blood test is needed. This blood test measures the level of the thyroid hormone T_4 (thyroxine) that is not bound by protein (free). A low level confirms the diagnosis of hypothyroidism.

Treatment

Treatment involves replacing thyroid hormone using one of several oral preparations. The preferred form of hormone replacement is synthetic T_4. Another form, desiccated (dried) thyroid, is obtained from the thyroid glands of animals. In general, desiccated thyroid is less satisfactory than synthetic T_4 because the content of thyroid hormones in the tablets may vary. In emergencies, such as myxedema coma, doctors may give synthetic T_4, T_3 (triiodothyronine), or both intravenously.

Treatment begins with small doses of thyroid hormone, because too large a dose can cause serious side effects, although large doses may be necessary. The starting dose and the rate of increase are especially small in older people, who are often most at risk of side effects. The dose is gradually increased until the levels of thyroid-stimulating hormone in the person's blood return to normal. During pregnancy, doses usually need to be increased.

Hashimoto's Thyroiditis

Hashimoto's thyroiditis (autoimmune thyroiditis) is chronic, autoimmune inflammation of the thyroid.

- Hashimoto's thyroiditis results when the body attacks the cells of the thyroid gland—an autoimmune reaction.
- Usually, people feel tired and cannot tolerate cold.
- The diagnosis is based on results of a physical examination and blood test.
- Most people develop hypothyroidism and need to take thyroid hormone for the rest of their life.

Hashimoto's thyroiditis is the most common type of thyroiditis and the most common cause of hypothyroidism. For unknown reasons, the body turns against itself (an autoimmune reaction—see page 1124). The thyroid is invaded by white blood cells, and antibodies are created that attack the thyroid gland. In about 50% of people with Hashimoto's thyroiditis, the thyroid is underactive initially. In most of the rest, the thyroid is normal at first (although in a small number of people, the gland initially becomes overactive), after which it usually becomes underactive.

Some people with Hashimoto's thyroiditis have other endocrine disorders, such as diabetes, an underactive adrenal gland, or underactive parathyroid glands, and other autoimmune diseases, such as pernicious anemia, rheumatoid arthritis, Sjögren's syndrome, or systemic lupus erythematosus (lupus).

Hashimoto's thyroiditis is most common among women, particularly older women, and tends to run in families. The condition occurs more frequently among people with certain chromosomal abnormalities, including Down, Turner's, and Klinefelter's syndromes.

Symptoms

Hashimoto's thyroiditis often begins with a painless, firm enlargement of the thyroid gland or a feeling of fullness in the neck. The gland usually has a rubbery texture and sometimes feels lumpy. If the thyroid is underactive, people may feel tired and intolerant of cold and have other symptoms of hypothyroidism (see page 996). The few who have an overactive thyroid (thyrotoxicosis) initially may have palpitations, nervousness and intolerance of heat.

Diagnosis

Doctors measure blood levels of thyroid hormones T_4 and T_3 and thyroid-stimulating hormone to determine how the gland is functioning. However, the diagnosis is based on a physical examination and the results of a blood test to determine whether the person has antithyroid antibodies, which attack the thyroid gland.

Treatment

No specific treatment is available for Hashimoto's thyroiditis.

Most people eventually develop hypothyroidism and then must take thyroid hormone replacement therapy for the rest of their lives. Thyroid hormone may also be useful in reducing the size of the enlarged thyroid gland. People with Hashimoto's thyroiditis should avoid excess iodine (which can cause hypothyroidism) from natural sources, such as kelp tablets and seaweed.

Subacute Thyroiditis

Subacute thyroiditis (granulomatous thyroiditis) is acute inflammation of the thyroid, probably caused by a virus.

Subacute thyroiditis usually begins suddenly. In this disorder, inflammation causes the thyroid gland to release excessive amounts of thyroid hormones, resulting in hyperthyroidism, almost always followed by transient hypothyroidism and finally normal thyroid function.

Subacute thyroiditis often follows a viral illness and begins with what many people call a sore throat but actually proves to be neck pain localized to the thyroid. Many people with subacute thyroiditis feel extremely tired. The thyroid gland becomes increasingly tender, and the person usually develops a low-grade fever (99 to 101° F [37 to 38° C]). The pain may shift from one side of the neck to the other, spread to the jaw and ears, and hurt more when the head is turned or when the person swallows. Subacute thyroiditis is often mistaken at first for a dental problem or a throat or ear infection.

Most people recover completely from this type of thyroiditis. Generally the thyroiditis resolves by itself within a few months, but sometimes it comes back or, more rarely, damages enough of the thyroid gland to cause permanent hypothyroidism.

Aspirin or other nonsteroidal anti-inflammatory drugs (NSAIDs) can relieve the pain and inflammation. In severe cases, doctors may recommend corticosteroids, such as prednisone, which are gradually decreased over 6 to 8 weeks. When corticosteroids are discontinued abruptly or too early, symptoms often return in full force. When symptoms of hyperthyroidism are severe, a beta-blocker may be recommended.

Silent Lymphocytic Thyroiditis

Silent lymphocytic thyroiditis (postpartum thyroiditis) is painless, autoimmune inflammation of the thyroid that typically develops after childbirth and goes away on its own.

Silent lymphocytic thyroiditis occurs most often among women, typically one to three months after childbirth, and causes the thyroid to become enlarged without becoming tender. The disorder recurs with each subsequent pregnancy.

For several weeks to several months, people have hyperthyroidism followed by hypothyroidism before eventually recovering normal thyroid function.

Hyperthyroidism may require treatment for a few weeks, often with a beta-blocker such as atenolol. During the period of hypothyroidism, the person may need to take thyroid hormone, usually for no longer than about 12 months. However, hypothyroidism becomes permanent in about 10% of people with subacute painless thyroiditis, and these people must take thyroid hormone for the rest of their lives.

Thyroid Cancer

The cause of thyroid cancer is not known, but the thyroid gland is very sensitive to radiation. Thyroid cancer is more common among people who were treated with radiation to the head, neck, or chest, most often for noncancerous (benign) conditions, when they were children (although radiation treatment for noncancerous conditions is no longer used).

Thyroid Nodules: Rather than causing the whole thyroid gland to enlarge, a cancer usually causes small growths (nodules) to develop within the thyroid. However, most thyroid nodules are not cancerous (malignant). A nodule is more likely to be cancerous if it

- Is solid rather than filled with fluid (cystic)
- Is not producing thyroid hormone
- Is hard
- Is growing quickly
- Occurs in a man

A painless lump in the neck is usually the first sign of thyroid cancer. When doctors find a nodule in the thyroid gland, they request several tests. The first tests are generally measurement of the blood levels of thyroid-stimulating hormone (TSH), thyroid hormones T_4 (thyroxine, or tetraiodothyronine) and T_3 (triiodothyronine), and sometimes thyroid antibodies. If these tests show hyperthyroidism is present, a thyroid scan is done to determine whether the nodule is producing thyroid hormones. Nodules that are producing hormones ("hot" nodules) are almost never cancerous. If the tests do not indicate hyperthyroidism or Hashimoto's thyroiditis, or if the nodules are not "hot," doctors usually do a fine-needle biopsy. In a fine-needle biopsy, a sample of the nodule is removed through a small needle and then examined under a microscope. This procedure is not very painful, is carried out in the doctor's office, and may involve the use of a local anesthetic as well as ultrasound to guide needle placement. An ultrasound scan may be done to determine how large the nodule is, whether it is solid or filled with fluid, and whether other nodules are present.

Types of Cancer

Papillary Cancer: Papillary cancer is the most common type, accounting for 70 to 80% of all thyroid cancers. About 2 to 3 times as many women as men have papillary cancer. Papillary cancer is more common in young people but grows and spreads more quickly in older people. People who have received radiation treatment to the neck, usually for a noncan-

cerous condition in infancy or childhood or for some other cancer in adulthood, are at greater risk of developing papillary cancer.

Papillary cancer grows within the thyroid gland but sometimes spreads (metastasizes) to nearby lymph nodes. If left untreated, papillary cancer may spread to more distant sites.

Papillary cancer is almost always curable. Nodules smaller than 1 centimeter are removed along with the thyroid tissue immediately surrounding them, although many experts recommend removing the entire thyroid gland. For larger nodules, most or all of the thyroid gland is usually removed. Radioactive iodine is often given to destroy any remaining thyroid tissue or cancer. Thyroid hormone is also given in large doses to suppress the growth of any remaining thyroid tissue.

Follicular Cancer: Follicular cancer accounts for about 15% of all thyroid cancers and is more common among older people. Follicular cancer is also more common in women than in men.

Much more aggressive than papillary cancer, follicular cancer tends to spread (metastasize) through the bloodstream, spreading cancerous cells to various parts of the body.

Treatment for follicular cancer requires surgically removing as much of the thyroid gland as possible and destroying any remaining thyroid tissue, including the metastases, if present, with radioactive iodine. It is usually curable, but less so than papillary cancer.

Anaplastic Cancer: Anaplastic cancer accounts for less than 5% of thyroid cancers and is most common among older women. This cancer grows very quickly and usually causes a large growth in the neck. It also tends to spread throughout the body.

About 80% of people with anaplastic cancer die within 1 year, even with treatment. However, treatment with chemotherapy and radiation therapy before and after surgery has resulted in some cures. Radioactive iodine is not helpful in the treatment of this type of cancer.

Medullary Cancer: Medullary cancer is a rare cancer that begins in the thyroid gland but in a different type of cell than that which produces thyroid hormone. The origin of this cancer is the C-cell, which is normally dispersed throughout the thyroid and secretes the hormone calcitonin. The cancer produces excessive amounts of calcitonin. Because medullary thyroid cancer can also produce other hormones, it can cause unusual symptoms.

This cancer tends to spread (metastasize) through the lymphatic vessels to the lymph nodes and through the blood to the liver, lungs, and bones. Medullary cancer can develop along with other types of endocrine cancers in what is called multiple endocrine neoplasia syndrome (see page 1016).

Treatment requires surgically removing the thyroid gland. Additional surgery may be needed to determine whether the cancer has spread to the lymph nodes. More than two thirds of people whose medullary thyroid cancer is part of multiple endocrine neoplasia syndrome are cured. When medullary thyroid cancer occurs alone, the chances of survival are not as good.

148 Adrenal Gland Disorders

The body has two adrenal glands, one near the top of each kidney. The inner part (medulla) of the adrenal glands secretes hormones, such as adrenaline (epinephrine), that help control blood pressure, heart rate, sweating, and other activities also regulated by the sympathetic nervous system. The outer part (cortex) secretes different hormones, including corticosteroids (cortisone-like hormones, such as cortisol) and mineralocorticoids (particularly aldosterone, which controls blood pressure and the levels of salt and potassium in the body). The adrenal glands also play a role in stimulating the production of androgens (testosterone and similar hormones).

The adrenal glands are controlled in part by the brain. The hypothalamus, a small area of the brain involved in hormonal regulation, produces corticotropin-releasing hormone and antidiuretic hormone. These two hormones trigger the pituitary gland to secrete corticotropin (also known as adrenocorticotropic hormone or ACTH), which stimulates the adrenal glands to produce corticosteroids. The renin-angiotensin-aldosterone system, regulated mostly by the kidneys, causes the adrenal glands to produce more or less aldosterone.

The body controls the levels of corticosteroids according to need. The levels tend to be much higher in the early morning than later in the day. When the body is stressed, from illness or otherwise, the levels of corticosteroids increase dramatically.

Addison's Disease

In Addison's disease, the adrenal glands are underactive, resulting in a deficiency of adrenal hormones.

- Addison's disease may be caused by an autoimmune reaction, cancer, an infection, or some other disease.
- A person with Addison's disease feels weak, tired, and dizzy when standing up after sitting or lying down and may develop dark skin patches.
- Doctors measure sodium and potassium in the blood and measure cortisol and corticotropin levels to make the diagnosis.

- People are given corticosteroids and fluids.

Addison's disease can start at any age and affects males and females about equally. In 70% of people with Addison's disease, the cause is not precisely known, but the adrenal glands are affected by an autoimmune reaction (see page 1124) in which the body's immune system attacks and destroys the adrenal cortex. In the other 30%, the adrenal glands are destroyed by cancer, an infection such as tuberculosis, or another identifiable disease. In infants and children, Addison's disease may be due to a genetic abnormality of the adrenal glands.

Secondary adrenal insufficiency is a term given to a disorder that resembles Addison's disease. In this disorder, the adrenal glands are underactive because the pituitary gland is not stimulating them, not because the adrenal glands have been destroyed or have otherwise directly failed.

When the adrenal glands become underactive, they tend to produce inadequate amounts of all of the adrenal hormones. Thus, Addison's disease affects the balance of water, sodium, and potassium in the body, as well as the body's ability to control blood pressure and react to stress. In addition, loss of androgens, such as dehydroepiandrosterone (DHEA), may cause a loss of body hair in women. In men, testosterone from the testes more than makes up for this loss. DHEA may have additional effects that do not relate to androgens.

When the adrenal glands are destroyed by infection or cancer, the adrenal medulla and thus the source of epinephrine is lost. However, this loss does not cause symptoms.

A deficiency of aldosterone in particular causes the body to excrete large amounts of sodium and retain potassium, leading to low levels of sodium and high levels of potassium in the blood. The kidneys are not able to concentrate urine, so when a person with Addison's disease drinks too much water or loses too much sodium, the level of sodium in the blood falls. Inability to concentrate urine ultimately causes the person to urinate excessively and become dehydrated. Severe dehydration and a

A Close Look at the Adrenal Glands

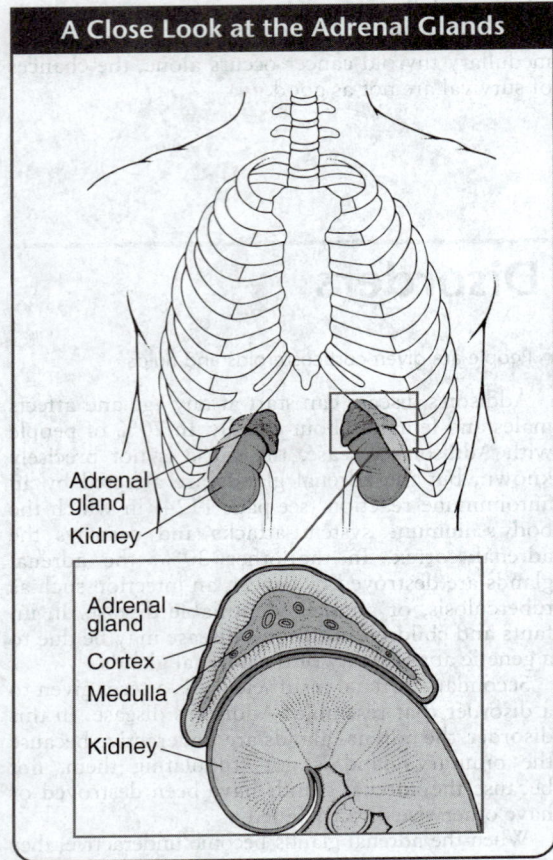

Adrenal gland
Kidney

Adrenal gland
Cortex
Medulla
Kidney

low sodium level reduce blood volume and can culminate in shock.

Corticosteroid deficiency leads to an extreme sensitivity to insulin so that the level of sugar in the blood may fall dangerously low (hypoglycemia). The deficiency prevents the body from manufacturing carbohydrates from protein, fighting infections properly, and controlling inflammation. Muscles weaken, and even the heart can become weak and unable to pump blood adequately. In addition, the blood pressure may become dangerously low.

People with Addison's disease are not able to produce additional corticosteroids when they are stressed. They therefore are susceptible to serious symptoms and complications when confronted with illness, extreme fatigue, severe injury, surgery, or, possibly, severe psychologic stress.

In Addison's disease, the pituitary gland produces more corticotropin in an attempt to stimulate the adrenal glands. Corticotropin also stimulates mela-

nin production, so the skin and the lining of the mouth often develop a dark pigmentation.

Symptoms

Soon after developing Addison's disease, a person feels weak, tired, and dizzy when standing up after sitting or lying down. These problems may develop gradually and insidiously. People with Addison's disease develop patches of dark skin. The darkness may seem like tanning, but it appears on areas not even exposed to the sun. Even people with dark skin can develop excessive pigmentation, although the change may be harder to recognize. Black freckles may develop over the forehead, face, and shoulders, and a bluish black discoloration may develop around the nipples, lips, mouth, rectum, scrotum, or vagina.

Most people lose weight, become dehydrated, have no appetite, and develop muscle aches, nausea, vomiting, and diarrhea. Many become unable to tolerate cold. Unless the disease is severe, symptoms tend to become apparent only during times of stress. Periods of hypoglycemia, with nervousness and extreme hunger for salty foods, can occur, particularly in children.

If Addison's disease is not treated, severe abdominal pains, profound weakness, extremely low blood pressure, kidney failure, and shock may occur (adrenal crisis). An adrenal crisis often occurs if the body is subjected to stress, such as an accident, injury, surgery, or severe infection. Death may quickly follow.

Diagnosis

Because the symptoms may start slowly and subtly, and because no single laboratory test may give definitive results in the early stages, doctors often do not suspect Addison's disease at the outset. Sometimes a major stress makes the symptoms more obvious and precipitates a crisis.

Blood tests may show low sodium and high potassium levels and usually indicate that the kidneys are not working well. Doctors who suspects Addison's disease measure cortisol levels, which may be low, and corticotropin levels, which may be high. However, doctors may need to confirm the diagnosis by measuring cortisol levels before and after an injection of corticotropin. If cortisol levels are low, further tests are needed to determine if the problem is Addison's disease or secondary adrenal insufficiency.

Treatment

Regardless of the cause, Addison's disease can be life threatening and must be treated with corticosteroids and intravenous fluids. Usually, treatment can be started with hydrocortisone or prednisone (a synthetic corticosteroid) taken by mouth. However, people who are severely ill may be given cortisol intravenously or intramuscularly at first and then hydrocortisone tablets. Because the body normally produces most cortisol in the morning, replacement hydrocortisone should also be taken in divided doses, with the largest dose in the morning. Hydrocortisone will need to be taken every day for the rest of the person's life. Larger doses of hydrocortisone are needed when the body is stressed, especially from an illness, and may need to be given by injection if the person has severe diarrhea or vomiting.

Most people also need to take fludrocortisone tablets every day to help restore the body's normal excretion of sodium and potassium. Supplemental testosterone is not usually needed, although there is some evidence that replacement with DHEA improves the quality of life. Although treatment must be continued for life, the outlook is excellent.

Cushing's Syndrome

In Cushing's syndrome, the level of corticosteroids is excessive, usually from overproduction by the adrenal glands.

- Cushing's syndrome usually results from a tumor that causes the adrenal glands to produce excessive corticosteroids.
- People with Cushing's syndrome usually develop excessive fat throughout the torso and have a large, round face.
- Doctors measure the level of cortisol to detect Cushing's syndrome.
- Surgery or radiation therapy is often needed to remove a tumor.

The adrenal glands may overproduce corticosteroids because of a problem in the adrenal glands or because of too much stimulation from the pituitary gland. An abnormality in the pituitary gland, such as a tumor, can cause the pituitary to produce large amounts of corticotropin, the hormone that controls the production of corticosteroids from the adrenal glands. Tumors outside the pituitary gland, such as small-cell lung cancer, can produce corticotropin as well (a condition called ectopic corticotropin syndrome). Corticotropin may also be produced by a tumor called a carcinoid, which may occur almost anywhere in the body.

Sometimes a noncancerous tumor (adenoma) develops in the adrenal glands, which causes them to overproduce corticosteroids. Adrenal adenomas are extremely common. Half of all people have them by the age of 70. Only a small fraction of adenomas produce excess hormone, however. Cancerous tumors of the adrenal glands are very rare.

Cushing's syndrome can also develop in people who must take large doses of corticosteroids be-

---

Suppression of Adrenal Function by Corticosteroids

In people who take large doses of corticosteroids, such as prednisone, the function of the adrenal glands can become suppressed. This suppression occurs because large doses of corticosteroids prevent the hypothalamus and pituitary gland from producing the hormones that normally stimulate adrenal function. If the person abruptly stops taking corticosteroids, the body cannot restore adrenal function quickly enough, and temporary adrenal insufficiency (a condition similar to Addison's disease) results. Also, when stress occurs, the body is not able to stimulate production of the additional corticosteroids that are needed.

Therefore, doctors never stop the use of corticosteroids abruptly if people have been taking them for more than 2 or 3 weeks. Instead, doctors gradually reduce (taper) the dose over weeks and sometimes months. Also, the dose may need to be increased in people who become ill or otherwise severely stressed while taking corticosteroids. Corticosteroid use may need to be resumed in people who become ill or otherwise severely stressed within weeks of having the corticosteroid tapered and stopped.

---

cause of a serious medical condition. Those who must take large doses have the same symptoms as those who produce too much of the hormone. The symptoms can occasionally occur even if the corticosteroids are inhaled, as for asthma, or are used topically for a skin condition.

Symptoms

Corticosteroids alter the amount and distribution of body fat. Excessive fat develops throughout the torso and may be particularly noticeable at the top of the back. A person with Cushing's syndrome usually has a large, round face (moon face). The arms and legs are usually slender in proportion to the thickened trunk. Muscles lose their bulk, leading to weakness. The skin becomes thin, bruises easily, and heals poorly when bruised or cut. Purple streaks that look like stretch marks may develop over the abdomen. People with Cushing's syndrome tend to tire easily.

High corticosteroid levels over time raise the blood pressure, weaken bones (osteoporosis), and diminish resistance to infections. The risk of developing kidney stones and diabetes is increased, and mental disturbances, including depression and hallucinations, may occur. Women usually have an irregular menstrual cycle. Children with Cushing's syndrome grow slowly

What Is Nelson's Syndrome?

People who have both their adrenal glands removed as treatment for Cushing's disease may develop Nelson's syndrome. In this disorder, a pituitary tumor develops, producing large amounts of corticotropin and other hormones that stimulate melanocytes, leading to darkening of the skin. The enlarging pituitary tumor may compress nearby structures in the brain, producing headaches and defects in vision.

Some experts believe that this compression may be prevented, at least in some people, by radiation therapy to the pituitary gland. If necessary, Nelson's syndrome can be treated with radiation therapy or surgical removal of the pituitary gland.

and remain short. In some people, the adrenal glands also produce large amounts of androgens (testosterone and similar hormones), leading to increased facial and body hair in women and balding.

Diagnosis

When doctors suspect Cushing's syndrome, they measure the level of cortisol, the main corticosteroid hormone, in the blood. Normally, cortisol levels are high in the morning and lower late in the day. In people who have Cushing's syndrome, cortisol levels are very high throughout the day.

If the cortisol levels are high, doctors may recommend a dexamethasone suppression test. Dexamethasone suppresses the pituitary gland and should lead to suppression of cortisol secretion by the adrenal glands. If Cushing's syndrome is caused by too much pituitary stimulation, the level of cortisol will fall to some extent, although not as much as in people who do not have Cushing's syndrome. If Cushing's syndrome has another cause, the level of cortisol will remain high. A high corticotropin level further suggests overstimulation of the adrenal gland.

Imaging tests may be needed to determine the exact cause, including a computed tomography (CT) or magnetic resonance imaging (MRI) scan of the pituitary or adrenal glands and a chest x-ray or CT scan of the lungs. However, these tests may occasionally fail to find the tumor.

When overproduction of corticotropin is thought to be the cause, blood samples may be taken from the veins that drain the pituitary to see if that is the source.

Treatment

Treatment depends on whether the problem is in the adrenal glands, the pituitary gland, or elsewhere. Surgery or radiation therapy may be needed to remove or destroy a pituitary tumor. Tumors of the adrenal gland

(usually adenomas) can often be removed surgically. Both adrenal glands may have to be removed if these treatments are not effective or if no tumor is present. People who have both adrenal glands removed, and many people who have part of their adrenal glands removed, must take corticosteroids for life. Tumors outside the pituitary and adrenal glands that secrete excess hormones are usually surgically removed. Certain drugs, such as metyrapone or ketoconazole, can lower cortisol levels and can be used while awaiting more definitive treatment such as surgery.

Virilization

Virilization is the development of exaggerated masculine characteristics, usually in women, often as a result of the adrenal glands overproducing androgens (testosterone and similar hormones).

- Virilization is caused by excess production of androgens usually because of enlargement of the adrenal gland or a tumor.
- Symptoms include excess facial and body hair, baldness, acne, deepening of the voice, increased muscularity, and an increased sex drive.
- The body changes make it easy for doctors to recognize virilization, and the dexamethasone suppression test can help doctors determine the cause.
- The adrenal gland that contains the tumor is surgically removed, although sometimes drugs can reduce the excess hormone production.

The most common cause of virilization is an enlargement of the hormone-producing portions of the adrenal cortex (adrenal hyperplasia). Sometimes the cause is a hormone-producing tumor (adenoma or cancer) in the gland. Occasionally, virilization occurs when a cancer outside the adrenal gland produces androgens. Athletes who take large amounts of androgens (anabolic steroids—see page 2090) to increase their muscle bulk may develop symptoms of virilization. Cystic enlargement of the ovaries may cause virilization, but such cases are almost always mild. Sometimes an abnormality in an enzyme (a protein) in the adrenal glands can also produce virilization.

Symptoms and Diagnosis

Symptoms of virilization include excess facial and body hair (hirsutism), baldness, acne, deepening of the voice, increased muscularity, and an increased sex drive. In women, the uterus shrinks, the clitoris enlarges, the breasts become smaller, and normal menstruation stops.

The combination of body changes makes virilization relatively easy for doctors to recognize. A test can determine the level of androgens in the blood. If the level is very high, a dexamethasone suppression test can help determine if the problem is coming from the adrenal glands and whether the problem is an adenoma or adrenal hyperplasia. If the problem is adrenal hyperplasia, dexamethasone prevents the adrenal glands from producing androgens. If the problem is an adenoma or cancer, dexamethasone reduces androgen production only partially or not at all. Doctors may also order a computed tomography (CT) or magnetic resonance imaging (MRI) scan to obtain a view of the adrenal glands.

Treatment

Androgen-producing adenomas and adrenal cancers are usually treated by surgically removing the adrenal gland that contains the tumor. For adrenal hyperplasia, small amounts of corticosteroids, such as dexamethasone, generally reduce the production of androgens. The mild virilization caused by cystic ovaries may need no treatment. It can be treated with drugs that lower the free testosterone levels, such as oral contraceptives, or that block the effects of testosterone.

Hyperaldosteronism

In hyperaldosteronism, overproduction of aldosterone leads to fluid retention and increased blood pressure, weakness, and, rarely, periods of paralysis.

- Hyperaldosteronism can be caused by a tumor in the adrenal gland or may be a response to some diseases.
- High aldosterone levels can cause high blood pressure and low potassium levels; low potassium levels may cause weakness, tingling, muscle spasms, and periods of temporary paralysis.
- Doctors measure the levels of sodium, potassium, and aldosterone in the blood.
- Sometimes, a tumor is removed, or people take drugs that block the action of aldosterone.

Aldosterone, a hormone produced and secreted by the adrenal glands, signals the kidneys to excrete less sodium and more potassium. Aldosterone production is regulated partly by corticotropin (secreted by the pituitary gland) and partly through the renin-angiotensin-aldosterone system (see box on page 334). Renin, an enzyme produced in the kidneys, controls the activation of the hormone angiotensin, which stimulates the adrenal glands to produce aldosterone.

Hyperaldosteronism can be caused by a tumor (usually a noncancerous adenoma) in the adrenal gland (a condition called Conn's syndrome), although sometimes both glands are involved and are overactive. Sometimes hyperaldosteronism is a response to certain diseases, such as very high blood pressure (hypertension) or narrowing of one of the arteries to the kidneys.

> ### Eating Real Licorice
>
> Eating large amounts of real licorice can produce all the symptoms of hyperaldosteronism. Real licorice contains a chemical that can act like aldosterone. However, most candy sold as licorice contains little or no real licorice.

Symptoms and Diagnosis

High aldosterone levels can lead to low potassium levels. Low potassium levels often produce no symptoms but may lead to weakness, tingling, muscle spasms, and periods of temporary paralysis. Some people become extremely thirsty and urinate frequently.

Doctors who suspects hyperaldosteronism first tests the levels of sodium and potassium in the blood. Doctors may also measure aldosterone levels. If they are high, spironolactone or eplerenone, drugs that block the action of aldosterone, may be given to see if the levels of sodium and potassium return to normal. In Conn's syndrome, the levels of renin are also very low.

When too much aldosterone is being produced, doctors examine the adrenal glands for a noncancerous tumor (adenoma). Computed tomography (CT) or magnetic resonance imaging (MRI) can be helpful, but sometimes blood samples from each of the adrenals must be tested to determine the source of the hormone.

Treatment

If a tumor is found, it can usually be surgically removed. When the tumor is removed, blood pressure returns to normal, and other symptoms disappear about 70% of the time. If no tumor is found and both glands are overactive, partial removal of the adrenal glands may not control high blood pressure, and complete removal will produce Addison's disease, requiring treatment for life. However, spironolactone or eplerenone can usually control the symptoms, and drugs for high blood pressure are readily available. Rarely do both adrenal glands have to be removed.

Pheochromocytoma

A pheochromocytoma is a tumor that usually originates from the adrenal glands' chromaffin cells, causing overproduction of catecholamines, powerful hormones that induce high blood pressure and other symptoms.

- High blood pressure is the most important symptom, but a fast and pounding pulse, excessive sweating, light-headedness when standing, rapid breathing, severe headaches, and many other symptoms may also occur.

- Doctors measure the levels of catecholamines in the blood and use imaging tests to try to find the tumor.
- Usually, the best treatment is to remove the pheochromocytoma.

Most pheochromocytomas grow within the adrenal glands. About 10% grow in chromaffin cells outside the adrenal glands. Only 5% of pheochromocytomas that grow within the adrenal glands are cancerous, but this percentage is higher for those outside the adrenal glands. Pheochromocytomas may occur in men or women at any age, but they are most common in people between the ages of 30 and 60.

Some people who develop pheochromocytomas have a rare inherited condition, called multiple endocrine neoplasia, that makes them prone to tumors in the thyroid, parathyroid, and adrenal glands (see page 1016). Pheochromocytomas may also develop in people who have von Hippel–Lindau disease and in those who have neurofibromatosis (von Recklinghausen's disease) or other genetic diseases.

Symptoms

Pheochromocytomas may be quite small. However, even a small pheochromocytoma can produce large amounts of potent catecholamines. Catecholamines are hormones such as adrenaline (epinephrine), norepinephrine, and dopamine, which tend to greatly increase blood pressure, heart rate, and other symptoms usually associated with life-threatening situations.

The most prominent symptom of a pheochromocytoma is high blood pressure, which may be very severe. Other symptoms include a fast and pounding heart rate, excessive sweating, light-headedness when standing, rapid breathing, cold and clammy skin, severe headaches, chest and stomach pain, nausea, vomiting, visual disturbances, tingling fingers, constipation, and an odd sense of impending doom. When these symptoms appear suddenly and forcefully, they can feel like a panic attack. In half of the people, symptoms come and go, sometimes triggered by pressure on the tumor, massage, drugs (especially anesthetics and beta-blocking drugs), emotional trauma, and, on rare occasions, the simple act of urination. However, many people may have these symptoms as manifestations of an anxiety state, not a glandular disorder.

Diagnosis

Doctors may not suspect a pheochromocytoma, because almost half of the people have no symptoms other than persistent high blood pressure. However, when high blood pressure occurs in a young person, comes and goes, or accompanies other symptoms of pheochromocytoma, doctors may request certain laboratory tests. For example, the level of certain catecholamines or products created when these catecholamines are broken down may be measured in blood or urine samples. Because of high blood pressure and other symptoms, doctors may prescribe a beta-blocker before knowing that the cause is a pheochromocytoma. Beta-blockers can make high blood pressure worse in people with pheochromocytoma. This paradoxical reaction often makes the diagnosis of pheochromocytoma clear.

If the level of catecholamines is high, a computed tomography (CT) or magnetic resonance imaging (MRI) scan can help locate the pheochromocytoma. A test using injected radioactive chemicals that tend to accumulate in pheochromocytomas is also useful. A scan is then performed to see where the radioactive chemicals are.

Treatment

Usually the best treatment is to remove the pheochromocytoma. Surgery is often delayed, however, until doctors can bring the tumor's secretion of catecholamines under control with drugs, because having high levels of catecholamines can be dangerous during surgery. Phenoxybenzamine is generally given to stop hormone secretion. Once this step is accomplished, a beta-blocker can safely be given to further control symptoms.

If the pheochromocytoma is cancerous and has spread, chemotherapy with cyclophosphamide, vincristine, and dacarbazine may help slow the tumor's growth. Treatment with a radioisotope known as metaiodobenzylguanidine (MIBG) that targets the tumor tissue can also be highly effective. The dangerous effects of the excess catecholamines secreted by the tumor can almost always be blocked by continuing to take phenoxybenzamine or a similar drug and beta-blockers.

Diabetes Mellitus

Diabetes mellitus is a disorder in which blood sugar (glucose) levels are abnormally high because the body does not produce enough insulin to meet its needs.

- Urination and thirst are increased, and people lose weight when they are not trying to.
- Diabetes damages the nerves and causes problems with sensation.
- Diabetes damages blood vessels and increases the risk of heart attack, stroke, and kidney failure.
- Doctors diagnose diabetes by measuring blood sugar levels.
- People with diabetes need to follow a low-sugar, low-fat diet, exercise, and usually take drugs.

Insulin, a hormone released from the pancreas, controls the amount of sugar in the blood. When people eat or drink, food is broken down into materials, including the simple sugar glucose, that the body needs to function. Sugar is absorbed into the bloodstream and stimulates the pancreas to produce insulin. Insulin allows sugar to move from the blood into the cells. Once inside the cells, it is converted to energy, which is either used immediately or stored as fat or glycogen until it is needed.

The levels of sugar in the blood vary normally throughout the day. They rise after a meal and return to normal within about 2 hours after eating. Once the levels of sugar in the blood return to normal, insulin production decreases. The variation in blood sugar levels is usually within a narrow range, about 70 to 110 milligrams per deciliter (mg/dL) of blood. If people eat a large amount of carbohydrates, the levels may increase more. People older than 65 years tend to have slightly higher levels, especially after eating.

If the body does not produce enough insulin to move the sugar into the cells, the resulting high levels of sugar in the blood and the inadequate amount of sugar in the cells together produce the symptoms and complications of diabetes.

Doctors often use the full name diabetes mellitus, rather than diabetes alone, to distinguish this disorder from diabetes insipidus, a relatively rare disorder that does not affect blood sugar levels (see page 986).

Types

Prediabetes: Prediabetes is a condition in which blood sugar levels are too high to be considered normal but not high enough to be labeled diabetes. People have prediabetes if their fasting blood sugar level is between 101 mg/dL and 126 mg/dL or if their blood sugar level 2 hours after a glucose tolerance test is between 140 mg/dL and 200 mg/dL. Identifying people with prediabetes is important because the condition carries a higher risk for future diabetes as well as heart disease. Decreasing body weight by 5 to 10% through diet and exercise can significantly reduce the risk of developing future diabetes.

Type 1: In type 1 diabetes (formerly called insulin-dependent diabetes or juvenile-onset diabetes), more than 90% of the insulin-producing cells of the pancreas are permanently destroyed. The pancreas, therefore, produces little or no insulin. Only about 10% of all people with diabetes have type 1 disease. Most people who have type 1 diabetes develop the disease before age 30.

Scientists believe that an environmental factor—possibly a viral infection or a nutritional factor in childhood or early adulthood—causes the immune system to destroy the insulin-producing cells of the pancreas. A genetic predisposition may make some people more susceptible to the environmental factor.

Type 2: In type 2 diabetes (formerly called non-insulin-dependent diabetes or adult-onset diabetes), the pancreas continues to produce insulin, sometimes even at higher-than-normal levels. However, the body develops resistance to the effects of insulin, so there is not enough insulin to meet the body's needs.

Type 2 diabetes was once rare in children and adolescents but has recently become more common. However, it usually begins in people older than 30 and becomes progressively more common with age. About 15% of people older than 70 have type 2 diabetes. People of certain racial and ethnic backgrounds are at increased risk of developing type 2 diabetes: blacks, Native Americans, and Hispanics who live in the United States have a twofold to threefold increased risk. Type 2 diabetes also tends to run in families.

Obesity is the chief risk factor for developing type 2 diabetes, and 80 to 90% of people with this disorder are overweight or obese. Because obesity causes insulin resistance, obese people need very large amounts of insulin to maintain normal blood sugar levels.

Certain disorders and drugs can affect the way the body uses insulin and can lead to type 2 diabetes. High levels of corticosteroids (from Cushing's disease or from taking corticosteroid drugs) and pregnancy (gestational diabetes—see page 1630) are the most common causes of altered insulin use. Diabetes also may occur in people with excess production of growth hormone (acromegaly) and in people with certain hormone-secreting tumors. Severe or recurring pancreatitis and other disorders that directly damage the pancreas can lead to diabetes.

Symptoms

The two types of diabetes have very similar symptoms. The first symptoms are related to the direct effects of high blood sugar levels. When the blood sugar level rises above 160 to 180 mg/dL, sugar spills into the urine. When the level of sugar in the urine rises even higher, the kidneys excrete additional water to dilute the large amount of sugar. Because the kidneys produce excessive urine, people with diabetes urinate large volumes frequently (polyuria). The excessive urination creates abnormal thirst (polydipsia). Because excessive calories are lost in the urine, people lose weight. To compensate, people often feel excessively hungry. Other symptoms include blurred vision, drowsiness, nausea, and decreased endurance during exercise.

Type 1: In people with type 1 diabetes, the symptoms often begin abruptly and dramatically. A condition called **diabetic ketoacidosis** may quickly develop. Without insulin, most cells cannot use the sugar that is in the blood. Cells still need energy to survive, and they switch to a back-up mechanism to obtain energy. Fat cells begin to break down, producing compounds called ketones. Ketones provide some energy to cells but also make the blood too acidic (ketoacidosis). The initial symptoms of diabetic ketoacidosis include excessive thirst and urination, weight loss, nausea, vomiting, fatigue, and—particularly in children—abdominal pain. Breathing tends to become deep and rapid as the body attempts to correct the blood's acidity (see page 973). The breath smells like nail polish remover, the smell of the ketones escaping into the breath. Without treatment, diabetic ketoacidosis can progress to coma and death, sometimes within a few hours.

Type 2: People with type 2 diabetes may not have any symptoms for years or decades before they are diagnosed. Symptoms may be subtle. Increased urination and thirst are mild at first and gradually worsen over weeks or months. Eventually, people feel extremely fatigued, are likely to develop blurred vision, and may become dehydrated.

Sometimes during the early stages of diabetes, the blood sugar level is abnormally low, a condition called hypoglycemia (see page 1014).

Because people with type 2 diabetes produce some insulin, ketoacidosis does not usually develop. However, the blood sugar levels can become extremely high (often exceeding 1,000 mg/dL). Such high levels often happen as the result of some superimposed stress, such as an infection or drug use. When the blood sugar levels get very high, people may develop severe dehydration, which may lead to mental confusion, drowsiness, and seizures, a condition called **nonketotic hyperglycemic-hyperosmolar coma.**

Complications

People with diabetes may experience many serious, long-term complications. Some of these complications begin within months of the onset of diabetes, although most tend to develop after a few years. Most of the complications are progressive. The more strictly people with diabetes are able to control the levels of sugar in the blood, the less likely it is that these complications will develop or become worse.

> **? Did You Know...**
>
> People who can strictly control their blood sugar levels may be able to minimize or delay diabetes complications.

Most complications are the result of problems with blood vessels. High sugar levels over a long time cause narrowing of both the small and large blood vessels. The narrowing reduces blood flow to many parts of the body, leading to problems. There are several causes of blood vessel narrowing. Complex sugar-based substances build up in the walls of small blood vessels, causing them to thicken and leak. Poor control of blood sugar levels also tends to cause the levels of fatty substances in the blood to rise, resulting in atherosclerosis (see page 396) and decreased blood flow in the larger blood vessels. Atherosclerosis is between 2 and 6 times more common in people with diabetes than in people who do not have diabetes and tends to occur at younger ages.

Over time, elevated levels of sugar in the blood and poor circulation can harm the heart, brain, legs, eyes, kidneys, nerves, and skin, resulting in angina, heart failure, strokes, leg cramps on walking (claudication), poor vision, kidney failure, damage to nerves (neuropathy), and skin breakdown. Heart attacks and strokes are more common among people with diabetes.

Poor circulation to the skin can lead to ulcers and infections and causes wounds to heal slowly. People with diabetes are particularly likely to have ulcers and infections of the feet and legs. Too often, these wounds heal slowly or not at all, and amputation of the foot or part of the leg may be needed.

People with diabetes often develop bacterial and fungal infections, typically of the skin. When the levels of sugar in the blood are high, white blood cells cannot effectively fight infections. Any infection that develops tends to be more severe.

Damage to the blood vessels of the eye can cause loss of vision (diabetic retinopathy—see page 1457). Laser surgery can seal the leaking blood vessels of the eye and prevent permanent damage to the retina. Therefore, people with diabetes should have yearly eye examinations to check for damage.

The kidneys can malfunction, resulting in kidney failure that may require dialysis or kidney transplantation. Doctors usually check the urine of people with diabetes for abnormally high levels of protein (albumin), which is an early sign of kidney damage. At the earliest sign of kidney complications, people are often given angiotensin-converting enzyme (ACE) inhibitors, drugs that slow the progression of kidney damage.

Damage to nerves can manifest in several ways. If a single nerve malfunctions, an arm or leg may suddenly become weak. If the nerves to the hands, legs, and feet become damaged (diabetic polyneuropathy), sensation may become abnormal, and tingling or burning pain and weakness in the arms and legs may develop (see page 826). Damage to the nerves of the skin makes repeated injuries more likely because people cannot sense changes in pressure or temperature.

Diagnosis

The diagnosis of diabetes is made when people have abnormally high levels of sugar in the blood. Blood sugar levels are often checked during a routine physical examination. Checking the levels of sugar in the blood annually is particularly important in older people, because diabetes is so common in later life. People may have diabetes, particularly type 2 diabetes, and not know it. Doctors may also check blood sugar levels in people who have symptoms of diabetes such as increased thirst, urination, or hunger. Doctors may also check blood sugar levels in people who have disorders that can be complications of diabetes, such as frequent infections, foot ulcers, and yeast infections.

To measure the blood sugar levels, a blood sample is usually taken after people have fasted overnight. However, it is possible to take blood samples after people have eaten. Some elevation of blood sugar levels after eating is normal, but even after a meal the levels should not be very high. Fasting blood sugar levels should never be higher than 126 mg/dL. Even after eating, blood sugar levels should not be higher than 200 mg/dL.

Doctors can also measure the level of a protein in the blood, hemoglobin A_{1C} (also called glycosylated or glycolated or hemoglobin). Glycosylated hemoglobin forms when the blood has been exposed to high blood sugar levels over a period of time. Doctors do not usually use this test to diagnose diabetes, but the test can help confirm the diagnosis when blood sugar

---

The Foot in Diabetes

Diabetes causes many changes in the body. The following changes in the feet are common and difficult to treat.

- Damage to the nerves (neuropathy) affects sensation to the feet, so that pain is not felt. Irritation and other forms of injury may go unnoticed. An injury may wear through the skin before any pain is felt.

- Changes in sensation alter the way people with diabetes carry weight on their feet, concentrating weight in certain areas so that calluses form. Calluses (and dry skin) increase the risk of skin breakdown.

- Diabetes can cause poor circulation in the feet, making ulcers more likely to form when the skin is damaged and making the ulcers slower to heal.

Because diabetes can affect the body's ability to fight infections, a foot ulcer, once it forms, easily becomes infected. Because of neuropathy, people may not feel discomfort from the infection until it becomes serious and difficult to treat, leading to gangrene. People with diabetes are more than 30 times more likely to require amputation of a foot or leg than are people without diabetes.

Foot care is critical (see box on page 424). The feet should be protected from injury, and the skin should be kept moist with a good moisturizer. Shoes should fit properly and not cause areas of irritation. Shoes should have appropriate cushioning to spread out the pressure caused by standing. Going barefoot is ill advised. Regular care from a podiatrist, such as having toenails cut and calluses removed, may also be helpful. Also, sensation and blood flow to the feet should be regularly evaluated by doctors.

---

levels are not extremely high. The test demonstrates long-term trends in blood sugar levels.

Another kind of blood test, an oral glucose tolerance test, may be done in certain situations, such as in routine screening of pregnant women for gestational diabetes (see page 1630) or in older people who have symptoms of diabetes but normal glucose levels when fasting. However, it is not routinely used for testing for diabetes, including in pregnant women at very low risk. In this test, people fast, have a blood sample taken to determine the fasting blood sugar level, and then drink a special solution containing a large, standard amount of glucose. More blood samples are then taken over the next 2 to 3 hours and are tested to

LONG-TERM COMPLICATIONS OF DIABETES

TISSUE OR ORGAN AFFECTED	EFFECTS	COMPLICATIONS
Blood vessels	Fatty material (atherosclerotic plaque) builds up and blocks large or medium-sized arteries in the heart, brain, legs, and penis. The walls of small blood vessels are damaged so that the vessels do not transfer oxygen to tissues normally, and the vessels may leak.	Poor circulation causes wounds to heal poorly and can lead to heart disorders, strokes, gangrene of the feet and hands, erectile dysfunction (impotence), and infections.
Eyes	The small blood vessels of the retina are damaged.	Decreased vision and, ultimately, blindness occur.
Kidneys	Blood vessels in the kidneys thicken. Protein leaks into urine. Blood is not filtered normally.	The kidneys malfunction, and ultimately, kidney failure occurs.
Nerves	Nerves are damaged because glucose is not metabolized normally and because the blood supply is inadequate.	Legs suddenly or gradually weaken. People have reduced sensation, tingling, and pain in their hands and feet.
Autonomic nervous system	The nerves that control blood pressure and digestive processes are damaged.	Swings in blood pressure occur. Swallowing becomes difficult. Digestive function is altered, and sometimes bouts of diarrhea occur. Erectile dysfunction develops.
Skin	Blood flow to the skin is reduced, and sensation is decreased, resulting in repeated injury.	Sores and deep infections (diabetic ulcers) develop. Healing is poor.
Blood	White blood cell function is impaired.	People become more susceptible to infections, especially of the urinary tract and skin.
Connective tissue	Glucose is not metabolized normally, causing tissues to thicken or contract.	Carpal tunnel syndrome and Dupuytren's contracture develop.

determine whether the level of sugar in the blood rises abnormally high.

Treatment

Treatment of diabetes involves diet, exercise, education, and, for most people, drugs. If people with diabetes strictly control blood sugar levels, complications are less likely to develop. The goal of diabetes treatment, therefore, is to keep blood sugar levels within the normal range as much as possible. Treatment of high blood pressure and cholesterol levels can prevent some of the complications of diabetes as well. A low dose of aspirin taken daily is also helpful.

People with diabetes benefit greatly from learning about the disorder, understanding how diet and exercise affect their blood sugar levels, and knowing how to avoid complications. A nurse trained in diabetes education can provide information about managing diet, exercising, monitoring blood sugar levels, and taking drugs.

People with diabetes should always carry or wear medical identification (such as a bracelet or tag) to alert health care practitioners to the presence of diabetes. This information allows health care practitioners to start life-saving treatment quickly, especially in the case of injury or altered mental status.

Diet management is very important in people with both types of diabetes. Doctors recommend a healthy, balanced diet and efforts to maintain a healthy weight. Some people benefit from meeting with a dietitian to develop an optimal eating plan.

People with type 1 diabetes who are able to maintain a healthy weight may be able to avoid the need for large doses of insulin. People with type 2 diabetes may be able to avoid the need for all drugs by achieving and maintaining a healthy weight. Some people who have been unsuccessful in losing weight through diet and exercise may take drugs to help them lose weight or may even undergo stomach reduction surgery.

In general, people with diabetes should not eat much sweet food. They should also try to eat meals on a regular schedule. Long periods between eating should be avoided. People with diabetes also tend to have high levels of cholesterol in the blood, so limiting the amount of saturated fat in the diet is important. Drugs may also be needed to help control the level of cholesterol in the blood.

> ### ? Did You Know...
> Many people have type 2 diabetes and are not aware of it.

Appropriate amounts of exercise can also help people control their weight and maintain blood sugar levels within the normal range. Because blood sugar levels go down during exercise, people must be alert for symptoms of low blood sugar. Some people need to eat a small amount of food with sugar during prolonged exercise, decrease their insulin dose, or both. People with diabetes should stop smoking and consume only moderate amounts of alcohol (up to one drink per day for women and two for men).

Diabetic ketoacidosis is a medical emergency, because it can cause coma and death. Hospitalization, usually in an intensive care unit, is necessary. Large amounts of fluids are given intravenously along with electrolytes, such as sodium, potassium, chloride, and phosphate, to replace those fluids and electrolytes lost through excessive urination. Insulin is generally given intravenously so that it works quickly and the dose can be adjusted frequently. Blood levels of sugar, ketones, and electrolytes are measured every few hours. Doctors also measure the blood's acid level. Sometimes, additional treatments are needed to correct a high acid level. However, controlling the levels of sugar in the blood and replacing electrolytes usually allow the body to restore the normal acid-base balance.

Nonketotic hyperglycemic-hyperosmolar coma is treated much like diabetic ketoacidosis. Fluids and electrolytes must be replaced. The levels of sugar in the blood must be restored to normal levels gradually to avoid sudden shifts of fluid into the brain. The blood sugar levels tend to be more easily controlled than in diabetic ketoacidosis, and blood acidity problems are not severe.

Insulin Replacement Therapy

People with type 1 diabetes almost always require insulin therapy, and many people with type 2 diabetes require it as well. Insulin is injected. It currently cannot be taken by mouth because insulin is destroyed in the stomach. A nasal spray form of insulin was available but has been discontinued. New forms of insulin, such as forms that can be taken by mouth or applied to the skin, are being tested.

Insulin is injected under the skin into the fat layer, usually in the arm, thigh, or abdominal wall. Small syringes with very thin needles make the injections nearly painless. An air pump device that blows the insulin under the skin can be used for people who cannot tolerate needles. An insulin pen, which contains a cartridge that holds the insulin, is a convenient way for many people to carry insulin, especially for people who take several injections a day outside the home. Another device is an insulin pump, which pumps insulin continuously from a reservoir through a small needle left in the skin. Additional doses of insulin can be released at programmed times, or release can be triggered as needed. The pump more closely mimics the way the body normally produces insulin. For some people, the pump offers an added degree of control, whereas others find wearing the pump annoying or develop sores at the needle site.

Insulin is available in three basic forms, divided by speed of onset and duration of action:

- **Rapid-acting insulin,** such as regular insulin, is fast and short acting. Regular insulin reaches its maximum activity in 2 to 4 hours and works for 6 to 8 hours. Lispro, aspart, and glulisine insulins, special types of regular insulin, are the fastest of all, reaching maximum activity in about 1 hour and working for 3 to 5 hours. Rapid-acting insulin is often used by people who take several daily injections and is injected 15 to 20 minutes before meals or just after eating.

- **Intermediate-acting insulin** (such as insulin zinc suspension, lente, or isophane insulin suspension) starts to work in 1 to 3 hours, reaches its maximum activity in 6 to 10 hours, and works for 18 to 26 hours. This type of insulin may be used in the morning to provide coverage for the first part of the day or in the evening to provide coverage during the night.

- **Long-acting insulin** (such as extended insulin zinc suspension, ultra-lente, or glargine) has very little effect in the first few hours but provides coverage for 20 to 36 hours depending on which of these types is used.

Insulin preparations are stable at room temperature for months, allowing them to be carried, brought to work, or taken on a trip. Insulin should not, however, be exposed to extreme temperatures.

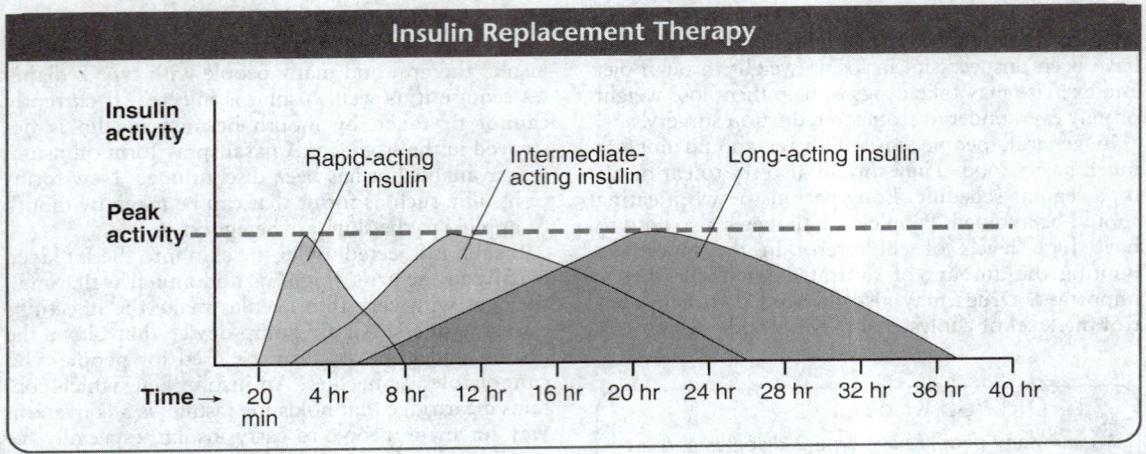

Insulin Replacement Therapy

The choice of insulin is complex. The following factors are considered before deciding which insulin is best:

- How willing and able people are to monitor their blood sugar levels and adjust the insulin dosage
- How varied daily activity is
- How adept people are at learning about and understanding the disorder
- How stable blood sugar levels are during the day and from day to day

The easiest regimen to follow is a single daily injection of an intermediate-acting insulin. However, such a regimen provides the least control over blood sugar levels and is, therefore, rarely the best approach. Stricter control may be achieved by combining two insulins—a rapid-acting and an intermediate-acting insulin—in one morning dose. This combination requires more skill, but it offers people greater opportunity to adjust the blood sugar levels. A second injection of one insulin or both may be taken at dinner or at bedtime. Strictest control is usually achieved by injecting a rapid-acting and an intermediate-acting insulin in the morning and evening along with several additional injections of rapid-acting insulin during the day. Adjustments can be made as insulin needs change. Measuring blood sugar levels at various times during the day helps determine the adjustment. Although this regimen requires the most knowledge of the disorder and attention to the details of treatment, it is considered the best option for most people who are treated with insulin, especially people with type 1 diabetes.

Some people, especially older people, take the same amount of insulin every day. Other people adjust the amount of insulin every day. Other people adjust the insulin dose daily depending on their diet, exercise, and blood sugar patterns. In addition, insulin needs may change if people gain or lose weight or experience emotional stress or illness, especially infection.

Over time, some people develop resistance to insulin. Because the injected insulin is not exactly like the insulin the body manufactures, the body can produce antibodies to the insulin. Although this is less common with newer insulin preparations, these antibodies may interfere with the insulin's activity, requiring very large doses.

Insulin injections can affect the skin and underlying tissues. An allergic reaction, which occurs rarely, produces pain and burning, followed by redness, itchiness, and swelling around the injection site for several hours. More commonly, the injections either cause fat deposits, making the skin look lumpy, or destroy fat, causing indentation of the skin. Many people rotate the injection sites, for example, using the thigh one day, the stomach another, and an arm the next, to avoid these problems.

Oral Antihyperglycemic Drugs

Oral antihyperglycemic drugs can often lower blood sugar levels adequately in people with type 2 diabetes. However, they are not effective in type 1 diabetes. There are several types. Sulfonylureas (for example, glyburide) and meglitinides (for example, repaglinide) stimulate the pancreas to produce more insulin (insulin secretagogues). Biguanides (for example, metformin) and thiazolidinediones (for example, rosiglitazone) do not affect the release of insulin but increase the body's response to it (insulin sensitizers). Doctors may prescribe one of these drugs alone or with a sulfonylurea drug. Another class of drug is the glucosidase inhibitors, such as acarbose, which work by delaying absorption of glucose in the intestine.

Oral antihyperglycemic drugs are usually prescribed for people with type 2 diabetes if diet and exercise fail to lower the levels of sugar in the blood adequately. The drugs are sometimes taken only once a day, in the morning, although some people need two or three doses. More than one type of oral drug may be used if one is not adequate. If oral antihyperglycemic drugs cannot control blood sugar levels well enough, insulin injections alone or in combination with the oral drugs may be needed.

Monitoring Treatment

Monitoring blood sugar levels is an essential part of diabetes care. People with diabetes must adjust their diet, exercise, and take drugs to control blood sugar levels. Monitoring blood sugar levels provides the information needed to make those adjustments. Waiting until symptoms of low or high blood sugar levels develop is a recipe for disaster.

Many things cause blood sugar levels to change:

- Diet
- Exercise
- Stress
- Illness
- Drug
- Time of day

The blood sugar levels may jump after people eat foods they did not realize were high in carbohydrates. Exercise may cause the levels of sugar in the blood to fall low, requiring that additional sugar be eaten. Emotional stress, an infection, and many drugs tend to increase blood sugar levels. Blood sugar levels increase in many people in the early morning hours because of the normal release of hormones (growth hormone and corticosteroids), a reaction called the dawn phenomenon. And blood sugar may shoot too high if the body releases sugar in response to low blood sugar levels (Somogyi effect).

Blood sugar levels can be measured easily at home or anywhere. Most blood sugar monitoring devices use a drop of blood obtained by pricking the tip of the finger with a small lancet. The lancet holds a tiny needle that can be jabbed into the finger or placed in a spring-loaded device that easily and quickly pierces the skin. Most people find the pricking nearly painless. Then, a drop of blood is placed on a reagent strip. In response to sugar, the reagent strip undergoes some chemical changes. A machine reads the changes in the test strip and reports the result on a digital display. Most of these machines time the reaction and read the result automatically. Some devices allow the blood sample to be obtained from other sites, such as the palm, forearm, upper arm, thigh, or calf. The machines are smaller than a deck of cards.

A newer device reads blood sugar through the skin without needing a sample of blood. The device is worn like a wristwatch and can measure the level of sugar in the blood every 15 minutes. Alarms on the device can be set to sound when blood sugar levels drop too low or climb too high. Disadvantages of this device are that it must be calibrated periodically with a blood test, it may irritate the skin, and it is somewhat large. Other devices can monitor glucose continuously. However, these devices are not routinely used, as they are expensive and have not been shown to be better than glucose meters. In certain circumstances, these devices are less reliable, such as in severe hypoglycemia.

Most people with diabetes should keep a record of their blood sugar levels and report them to their doctor or nurse for advice in adjusting the dose of insulin or the oral antihyperglycemic drug. Many people can learn to adjust the insulin dose on their own as necessary.

Although urine can also be tested for the presence of sugar, checking urine is not a good way to monitor treatment or adjust therapy. Urine testing can be misleading because the amount of sugar in the urine may not reflect the current level of sugar in the blood. Blood sugar levels can get very low or reasonably high without any change in the sugar levels in the urine.

Doctors can monitor treatment using a blood test called hemoglobin A_{1C}. When the blood sugar levels are high, changes occur in hemoglobin, the protein that carries oxygen in the blood. These changes are in direct proportion to the blood sugar levels over an extended period. Thus, unlike the blood sugar measurement, which reveals the level at a particular moment, the hemoglobin A_{1C} measurement demonstrates whether the blood sugar levels have been controlled over the previous few months. People with diabetes aim for a hemoglobin A_{1C} level of less than 7%. Achieving this level is difficult, but the lower the hemoglobin A_{1C} level, the less likely people are to have complications. Levels above 9% show poor control, and levels above 12% show very poor control. Most doctors who specialize in diabetes care recommend that hemoglobin A_{1C} be measured every 3 to 6 months. Fructosamine, an amino acid that has bonded with glucose, is also useful for measuring blood sugar control over a period of a few weeks.

Monitoring and Preventing Complications

At the time of diagnosis and then at least yearly, people are monitored for the presence of diabetes complications, such as kidney, eye, and nerve damage. Worsening of complications can be prevented

℞ ORAL ANTIHYPERGLYCEMIC DRUGS

DRUG	NUMBER OF DAILY DOSES	SOME SIDE EFFECTS
Biguanides		
Metformin	2 to 3	Diarrhea
Extended-release metformin	1 to 2	Increased acidity of body fluids (rare)
		Liver failure (rare)
Sulfonylureas		
Acetohexamide	1 to 2	Weight gain
Chlorpropamide	1	Low sodium in blood (hyponatremia) with chlorpropamide
Glimepiride	1	
Glipizide	1 to 2	
Glyburide	1 to 2	
Micronized glyburide	1 to 2	
Tolazamide	1 to 2	
Tolbutamide	1 to 2	
Meglitinides		
Nateglinide	3	Minimal weight gain
Repaglinide	3	
Thiazolidinediones		
Pioglitazone	1	Weight gain
		Fluid retention (edema)
Rosiglitazone	1 to 2	Weight gain
		Fluid retention
		Possible increase in heart attacks
Alpha-glucosidase inhibitors		
Acarbose	3	Diarrhea
Miglitol	3	Abdominal pain
		Bloating
Dipeptidyl peptidase-4 inhibitor		
Sitagliptin	1	Headache
		Diarrhea
		Lung infections
Glucagon-like peptide agonist		
Exenatide	2	Nausea
		Vomiting
Amylin analog		
Pramlintide	3	Nausea
		Low blood sugar levels

or delayed by strict blood sugar control or by early drug treatment. Risk factors for heart problems, such as increased blood pressure and high choles-terol levels, are evaluated at each doctor visit and are treated with drugs if necessary. Another common problem in people with diabetes is gum disease

SPOTLIGHT ON AGING

Older people need to follow the same general principles of diabetes management—education, diet, exercise, and drugs—as younger people. However, risking hypoglycemia by strictly controlling blood sugar levels may not be beneficial for people with a short life expectancy, such as those with advanced cancer. Also, managing diabetes can be more difficult for older people. Poor eyesight may make it hard for them to read glucose meters and dose scales on insulin syringes. They may have problems manipulating the syringe because they have arthritis or Parkinson's disease or have had a stroke. When older people have hypoglycemia, their symptoms may be less obvious. If they have hypoglycemia but have difficulty communicating, dementia or both, they may not be able to let anyone know they are having symptoms.

Education: In addition to learning about diabetes itself, older people may have to learn how to fit management of diabetes in with their management of other disorders. Learning about how to avoid complications, such as dehydration, skin breakdown, and circulation problems, and to manage factors that can contribute to diabetes, such as high blood pressure and high cholesterol levels, is especially important. Such problems become more common as people age, whether they have diabetes or not.

Diet: Many older people have difficulty following a healthy, balanced diet that can control blood sugar levels and weight. Changing long-held food preferences and dietary habits may be hard. Some older people have other disorders that can be affected by diet and may not understand how to integrate the dietary recommendations for their various disorders.

Some older people cannot control what they eat because someone else is cooking for them at home or in a nursing home or other institution. When people with diabetes do not do their own cooking, the people who shop and prepare meals for them must also understand the diet that is needed. Older people and their caregivers usually benefit from meeting with a dietitian to develop a healthy, feasible eating plan.

Exercise: Older people may have a difficult time adding exercise to their daily life, particularly if they have not been active or if they have a disorder that limits their movement, such as arthritis. However, they may be able to add exercise to their usual routine. For example, they can walk instead of drive or climb the stairs instead of take the elevator. Also, many community organizations offer exercise programs designed for older people.

Drugs: Taking the drugs used to treat diabetes, particularly insulin, may be difficult for some older people. For those with vision problems or other problems that make accurately filling a syringe difficult, a caregiver can prepare the syringes ahead of time and store them in the refrigerator. People whose insulin dose is stable may purchase pre-filled syringes. Prefilled insulin pen devices may be easier for people with physical limitations. Some of these devices have large numbers and easy-to-turn dials.

Monitoring blood sugar levels: Poor vision, limited manual dexterity due to arthritis, tremor, or stroke, or other physical limitations may make monitoring blood sugar levels more difficult for older people. However, special monitors are available. Some have large numerical displays that are easier to read. Some provide audible instructions and results. Some monitors read blood sugar levels through the skin and do not require a blood sample. People can consult a diabetes educator to determine which meter is most appropriate.

Complications of treatment: The most common complication of treating high blood sugar levels is low blood sugar levels. The risk is greatest for older people who are frail, who are sick enough to require frequent hospital admissions, or who are taking several drugs. Of all available drugs to treat diabetes, long-acting sulfonylurea drugs are most likely to cause low blood sugar levels in older people. When they take these drugs, they are also more likely to have serious symptoms, such as fainting and falling, and to have diffculty thinking or using parts of the body due to low blood sugar levels.

(gingivitis), and regular visits to the dentist for cleaning and preventive care are important.

Hypoglycemia: Keeping blood sugar levels from getting too high is difficult. The main difficulty with trying to strictly control the levels of sugar in the blood is that low blood sugar levels (hypoglycemia) may occur (see page 1014). Recognizing the presence of low blood sugar is important because treatment of hypoglycemia is an emergency. Symptoms may include hunger pangs, racing heart beat, shakiness, sweating,

and inability to think clearly. Sugar must get into the body within minutes to prevent permanent harm and relieve symptoms. Most of the time, people can eat sugar. Almost any form of sugar will do, although glucose works more quickly than table sugar (typical table sugar is sucrose). Many people with diabetes carry glucose tablets or foil packets of a glucose-containing liquid. Other options are to drink a glass of milk (which contains lactose, a type of sugar), sugar water, or fruit juice or to eat a piece of cake, some fruit, or another sweet food. In more serious situations, it may be necessary for emergency medical practitioners to inject glucose into a vein.

Another treatment for hypoglycemia involves the use of glucagon. Glucagon can be injected into the muscle and causes the liver to release large amounts of glucose within minutes. Small transportable kits containing a syringe filled with glucagon are available for people with diabetes to use in emergency situations.

Experimental Treatments

Experimental treatments are also showing promise for the treatment of type 1 diabetes. In one such treatment, insulin-producing cells are transplanted into body organs. This procedure is not yet routinely done, however, because immunosuppressant drugs must be given to prevent the body from rejecting the transplanted cells. Newer techniques may make suppression of the immune system unnecessary.

150 Hypoglycemia

Hypoglycemia is abnormally low levels of sugar (glucose) in the blood.

- Hypoglycemia can be caused by drugs taken to control diabetes, fasting, some severe diseases, reactions to carbohydrates, a tumor in the pancreas, and some types of stomach surgery.
- A fall in blood sugar causes symptoms such as sweating, fatigue, and weakness, whereas severe hypoglycemia causes symptoms such as confusion, seizures, and coma.
- The diagnosis for a person who has diabetes is based on finding low sugar levels in the blood while the person is experiencing symptoms.
- Symptoms of hypoglycemia are treated by consuming sugar in any form.
- Doses of drugs that cause symptoms may need to be decreased.

Normally, the body maintains the levels of sugar in the blood within a range of about 70 to 110 milligrams per deciliter (mg/dL) of blood. In hypoglycemia, the sugar levels in the blood become too low. In diabetes mellitus, the sugar levels in the blood become too high, a condition called hyperglycemia. Although diabetes is characterized by high levels of sugar in the blood, many people with diabetes periodically experience hypoglycemia due to side effects of diabetes treatment. Hypoglycemia is uncommon among people without diabetes.

Low levels of sugar in the blood interfere with the function of many organ systems. The brain is particularly sensitive to low sugar levels, because sugar is the brain's major energy source. If the sugar levels in the blood fall far below their usual range, the brain responds by stimulating the adrenal glands to release epinephrine (adrenaline) and cortisol, the pancreas to release glucagon, and the pituitary gland to release growth hormone, all of which cause the liver to release sugar into the blood.

Causes

Drugs: Most cases of hypoglycemia occur in people with diabetes and are caused by the insulin or other drugs (for example, sulfonylureas) they take to lower the levels of sugar in their blood. People with diabetes sometimes call the hypoglycemia that can occur after taking insulin an "insulin reaction" or "being shaky." Insulin reactions are more common when intense efforts are made to keep the sugar levels in the blood as close to normal as possible. People with diabetes who reduce food intake to lose weight or who develop kidney failure are more likely to have hypoglycemia. Older people are more susceptible than younger people to hypoglycemia resulting from sulfonylurea drugs.

If, after taking a dose of a drug for diabetes, a person eats less than usual or is more physically active than normal, the drug may lower the level of sugar in the blood too much. People who have had severe diabetes for a long time are particularly prone to hypoglycemia in these situations because they may not produce enough glucagon or epinephrine. The amounts of glucagon and epinephrine that are released are often too low to counteract a low level of sugar in the blood.

Many drugs other than those for diabetes, most notably pentamidine, used to treat a form of pneumonia that occurs most often as part of AIDS, and quinine, used to treat muscle cramps, occasionally cause hypoglycemia.

An uncommon type of drug-related hypoglycemia sometimes occurs in people who secretly take insulin or other drugs as part of a psychologic disorder such as Munchausen syndrome (see box on page 850).

Fasting: In otherwise healthy people, prolonged fasting (even up to several days) and prolonged strenuous exercise (even after a period of fasting) are unlikely to cause hypoglycemia.

However, there are several diseases or conditions in which the body fails to maintain adequate levels of sugar in the blood after a period without food (fasting hypoglycemia). In people who drink heavily without eating, alcohol can block the release of stored sugar from the liver. In people with liver disease, such as viral hepatitis, cirrhosis, or cancer, the liver may not store sufficient sugar. Infants and children who have an abnormality of the enzyme systems that control sugar use also may have fasting hypoglycemia.

A rare cause of fasting hypoglycemia is a tumor in the pancreas that produces large amounts of insulin. In some people, an autoimmune disorder lowers sugar levels in the blood by changing insulin secretion or by some other means. Disorders that lower hormone production by the pituitary and adrenal glands (most notably Addison's disease) can cause hypoglycemia. Other severe diseases, such as kidney or heart failure, cancer, and shock, may also cause hypoglycemia, particularly in a person who is also being treated for diabetes.

Reaction to Eating: Hypoglycemia can occur after a person eats a meal containing a large amount of carbohydrates if, for some reason, the body produces more insulin than is needed. However, this type of reaction is probably rare. In some cases, people with normal blood sugar levels experience symptoms that can be confused with hypoglycemia.

? Did You Know...

Sometimes people who are hypoglycemic are mistakenly thought to be drunk.

After certain types of stomach surgery, such as removal of part of the stomach, sugars are absorbed very quickly, stimulating excess insulin production, which then may cause hypoglycemia. Problems with digestion of some sugars (fructose and galactose) and amino acids (leucine) may also cause hypoglycemia if an affected person eats foods containing those substances.

Symptoms

The symptoms of hypoglycemia rarely develop until the level of sugar in the blood falls below 60 milligrams per deciliter of blood. Some people develop symptoms at slightly higher levels, especially when blood sugar levels fall quickly, and some do not develop symptoms until the sugar levels in their blood are much lower.

The body first responds to a fall in the level of sugar in the blood by releasing epinephrine from the adrenal glands. Epinephrine stimulates the release of sugar from body stores but also causes symptoms similar to those of an anxiety attack: sweating, nervousness, shaking, faintness, palpitations, and hunger. More severe hypoglycemia reduces the sugar supply to the brain, causing dizziness, fatigue, weakness, headaches, inability to concentrate, confusion, inappropriate behavior that can be mistaken for drunkenness, slurred speech, blurred vision, seizures, and coma. Severe and prolonged hypoglycemia may permanently damage the brain. Symptoms can begin slowly or suddenly, progressing from mild discomfort to severe confusion or panic within minutes. Sometimes, people who have had diabetes for many years (especially if tightly controlled) are no longer able to sense the early symptoms of hypoglycemia, and faintness or even coma may develop without any other warning.

In a person with an insulin-producing pancreatic tumor, symptoms are likely to occur early in the morning after an overnight fast, especially if the sugar stores in the blood are further depleted by exercise before breakfast. At first, people with a tumor usually have only occasional episodes of hypoglycemia, but over months or years, episodes may become more frequent and severe.

Diagnosis

In someone who is known to have diabetes, a doctor may suspect hypoglycemia when symptoms are described. The diagnosis may be confirmed when low sugar levels in the blood are measured while the person is experiencing symptoms.

In an otherwise healthy person who does not have diabetes, a doctor is usually able to recognize hypoglycemia based on the symptoms, medical history, a physical examination, and simple tests.

Doctors first measure the level of sugar in the blood. A low sugar level in the blood found at the time a person is experiencing typical symptoms of hypoglycemia confirms the diagnosis in a person without diabetes, especially if the relationship between a low sugar level in the blood and symptoms is demonstrated more than once. If symptoms are relieved as the sugar levels in the blood rise within a few minutes of ingesting sugar, the diagnosis is supported.

When the relationship between a person's symptoms and the level of sugar in the blood remains unclear in a person who does not have diabetes, additional tests may be needed. Often, the next step is measurement of the sugar level in the blood after a night of fasting in a hospital or other closely supervised setting. More extensive tests may also be needed.

If use of a drug such as pentamidine or quinine is thought to be the cause of hypoglycemia, the drug is stopped and blood sugar levels are measured to determine if they increase. If the cause remains unclear, other laboratory tests may be needed.

If an insulin-producing tumor is suspected, measurements of insulin levels in the blood during fasting (sometimes up to 72 hours) may be needed. If the insulin measurements suggest a tumor, the doctor will try to locate it before treatment.

Treatment

People prone to hypoglycemia should carry or wear medical identification to inform health care practitioners of their condition.

Symptoms: The symptoms of hypoglycemia are relieved within minutes of consuming sugar in any form, such as candy, glucose tablets or a sweet drink, such as a glass of fruit juice. People with recurring episodes of hypoglycemia, especially those with diabetes, often prefer to carry glucose tablets because the tablets take effect quickly and provide a consistent amount of sugar. People with hypoglycemia, whether or not they have diabetes, may benefit from consuming sugar followed by a food that provides longer-lasting carbohydrates (such as bread or crackers). When hypoglycemia is severe or prolonged and taking sugar by mouth is not possi-

ble, doctors quickly give sugar intravenously to prevent brain damage.

People who are known to be at risk of episodes of severe hypoglycemia may keep glucagon on hand for emergencies. Glucagon administration stimulates the liver to release large amounts of sugar. It is given by injection and generally restores blood sugar to an adequate level within 5 to 15 minutes. Glucagon kits are easy to use, and family members can be trained to administer the glucagon.

Cause: If a drug is causing hypoglycemia, the dose is adjusted or the drug is changed. Insulin-producing tumors should be removed surgically. However, because these tumors are small and difficult to locate, a specialist should perform the surgery. Before surgery, the person may be given a drug such as octreotide or diazoxide to control symptoms. Sometimes more than one tumor is present, and if the surgeon does not find them all, a second operation may be necessary.

People who do not have diabetes but are prone to hypoglycemia often can avoid episodes by eating frequent small meals rather than the usual three meals a day. Limiting intake of carbohydrates, especially simple sugars, is sometimes advocated to prevent "reactive hypoglycemia" (after a meal) but is of unclear benefit.

CHAPTER

151 Multiple Endocrine Neoplasia Syndromes

Multiple endocrine neoplasia syndromes are rare, inherited conditions in which several endocrine glands develop non-cancerous (benign) or cancerous (malignant) tumors or grow excessively without forming tumors.

- Multiple endocrine neoplasia syndromes are caused by gene mutations, so they tend to run in families.
- Symptoms vary depending on which glands are affected.
- Genetic screening tests can be done to detect disease in family members of people who have multiple endocrine neoplasia syndromes.
- No cure is available, but doctors treat the changes in each gland as they occur with surgery or with drugs to control excess hormone production.

Multiple endocrine neoplasia syndromes can appear in infants or in people as old as age 70. Almost all the multiple endocrine neoplasia syndromes are inherited.

Multiple endocrine neoplasia syndromes occur in three patterns, called types 1, 2A, and 2B, although

the types occasionally overlap. The tumors and the abnormally large glands often produce excess hormones. Although tumors or abnormal growth may occur in more than one gland at the same time, changes often take place over time.

Multiple endocrine neoplasia syndromes are caused by inherited genetic mutations. A single gene responsible for type 1 disease has been identified. Abnormalities in a different gene have been identified in people with types 2A and 2B disease.

Types

Type 1 Disease: People with multiple endocrine neoplasia type 1 develop tumors, or excessive growth and activity, of two or more of the following glands:

- The parathyroid glands (the small glands located next to the thyroid gland)
- The pancreas

- The pituitary gland
- The thyroid gland (less often affected)
- The adrenal glands (less often affected)

Almost all people with type 1 disease have tumors of the parathyroid glands; most of the tumors are noncancerous, but they cause the glands to produce too much parathyroid hormone (hyperparathyroidism—see box on page 937). The excess parathyroid hormone usually raises the levels of calcium in the blood, sometimes leading to kidney stones.

Most people with type 1 disease also develop tumors of the hormone-producing cells (islet cells) of the pancreas. Some of these tumors produce high levels of insulin and, consequently, low levels of sugar in the blood (hypoglycemia), especially if the person has not eaten for several hours. More than half of islet cell tumors produce excessive gastrin, which stimulates the stomach to overproduce acid. People with tumors that produce gastrin generally develop peptic ulcers that often bleed, perforate, and leak stomach contents into the abdomen, or obstruct the stomach. The high acid levels commonly interfere with the activity of enzymes from the pancreas, resulting in diarrhea and fatty, smelly stools (steatorrhea). The remaining islet cell tumors may produce other hormones, such as vasoactive intestinal polypeptide, which can cause severe diarrhea and lead to dehydration. Some islet cell tumors produce no hormones at all.

Some of the islet cell tumors are cancerous and able to spread (metastasize) to other areas of the body. Cancerous islet cell tumors tend to grow more slowly than other types of cancer that develop in the pancreas.

Most people with type 1 disease develop pituitary gland tumors. Some of these tumors produce the hormone prolactin, leading to menstrual abnormalities and sometimes breast secretions in women and erectile dysfunction (impotence) in men. Other tumors produce growth hormone, leading to acromegaly (see page 987). A small percentage of pituitary tumors produce corticotropin, which overstimulates the adrenal glands, leading to high levels of corticosteroid hormones and Cushing's syndrome (see page 1001). A few pituitary tumors produce no hormones at all. Some pituitary tumors cause headaches, impaired vision, and decreased pituitary gland function by pressing against nearby parts of the brain.

In some people with type 1 disease, tumors or excessive growth and activity of the thyroid and adrenal glands develop. A small percentage of people develop a different type of tumor, known as carcinoid tumors (see page 1018). Some people also develop soft, noncancerous fatty growths just below the skin (lipomas).

Type 2A Disease: People with multiple endocrine neoplasia type 2A develop tumors or excessive growth and activity in two or three of the following glands:

- The thyroid gland
- The adrenal glands
- The parathyroid glands

Occasionally an itchy skin condition called cutaneous lichen amyloidosis also occurs in people with type 2A disease.

Almost everyone with type 2A disease develops medullary thyroid cancer (see page 998). About 50% develop certain tumors of the adrenal glands (pheochromocytomas—see page 1003), which usually raise blood pressure because of the epinephrine and other substances they produce. The high blood pressure may be intermittent or constant and is often very severe.

Some people with type 2A disease have overactive parathyroid glands and therefore have increased levels of calcium in the blood, which may lead to kidney stones. In others, the parathyroid glands increase in size without producing large amounts of parathyroid hormone, so these people do not have problems related to high calcium levels.

Type 2B Disease: Multiple endocrine neoplasia type 2B can consist of medullary thyroid cancer, pheochromocytomas, and growths around nerves (neuromas). Some people with type 2B disease have no family history of it. In these people the disease is the result of a new gene defect (genetic mutation).

The medullary thyroid cancer that occurs in type 2B disease tends to develop at an early age and has been found in infants as young as 3 months of age. The medullary thyroid tumors in type 2B disease grow faster and spread more rapidly than those in type 2A disease.

Most people with type 2B disease develop neuromas in their mucous membranes. The neuromas appear as glistening bumps around the lips, tongue, and lining of the mouth. Neuromas may also occur on the eyelids and glistening surfaces of the eyes, including the conjunctiva and cornea. The eyelids and lips may thicken.

Digestive tract abnormalities cause constipation and diarrhea. Occasionally, the colon develops large, dilated loops (megacolon). These abnormalities probably result from neuromas growing on the intestinal nerves.

People with type 2B disease often develop spinal abnormalities, especially curvature of the spine. They may also have abnormalities of the bones of the feet and thighs. Many people have long limbs and loose joints. Some of these abnormalities are similar to those that occur in Marfan syndrome (see page 1827).

CONDITIONS THAT OCCUR WITH SPECIFIC TYPES OF MULTIPLE ENDOCRINE NEOPLASIA SYNDROMES

CONDITION	MEN 1	MEN 2A	MEN 2B
Parathyroid gland tumors	≥ 90%	10–20%	—
Pancreatic tumors	60–70%	—	—
Pituitary gland tumors	15–42%	—	—
Thyroid gland tumors (specifically medullary carcinoma)	—	> 90%	> 90%
Pheochromocytoma (tumor of the adrenal glands)	—	50%	60%
Neuromas on mucous membranes	—	—	Almost 100%
Bodily changes similar to those in people with Marfan syndrome	—	—	Almost 100%

MEN = Multiple endocrine neoplasia.

Diagnosis

Tests are available to identify the genetic abnormality present in each of the multiple endocrine neoplasia syndromes. Doctors usually do these genetic tests in people who have one of the tumors associated with multiple endocrine neoplasia and in family members of people already diagnosed with one of the syndromes. Screening of family members is particularly important because about half of the children of people with a multiple endocrine neoplasia syndrome inherit the disease.

Treatment

No cure is known for any of the multiple endocrine neoplasia syndromes. Doctors treat the changes in each gland individually. A tumor is treated by removing it surgically when possible. If removal is not possible (and before removal), doctors give drugs to correct the hormone imbalance caused by gland overactivity. An excessively large and overactive gland without a tumor is treated with drugs to counteract the effects of gland overactivity.

Because medullary thyroid cancer is ultimately fatal if untreated, doctors will most likely recommend preventive surgical removal of the thyroid gland if genetic testing has revealed evidence of type 2A or type 2B disease, even if the diagnosis of medullary thyroid cancer has not been made before the surgery. Unlike other types of thyroid cancer, this aggressive type of thyroid cancer cannot be treated with radioactive iodine. Once the thyroid is removed, people must take thyroid hormone for the rest of their life. Pheochromocytomas must be removed surgically after the person's blood pressure has been controlled with appropriate drugs.

CHAPTER
152 Carcinoid Tumors

Carcinoid tumors are noncancerous (benign) or cancerous (malignant) growths that sometimes produce excessive amounts of hormone-like substances, resulting in the carcinoid syndrome.

- People with carcinoid tumors may have cramping pain and changes in bowel movements.
- People with carcinoid syndrome usually have flushing and sometimes diarrhea.

- Doctors measure the amount of a serotonin byproduct in a person's urine.
- Imaging tests are needed to determine tumor location.
- Sometimes tumors are removed surgically.
- People may need to take drugs to control symptoms.

Carcinoid tumors usually originate in hormone-producing cells that line the small intestine or other cells of the digestive tract. They can also occur in the pancreas, testes, ovaries, or lungs. Carcinoid tumors can produce an excess of hormone-like substances, such as serotonin, bradykinin, histamine, and prostaglandins. Excess levels of these substances can sometimes result in a diverse set of symptoms called carcinoid syndrome. Carcinoid tumors use the amino acid tryptophan to produce the excess serotonin. Because tryptophan is normally used to make niacin (vitamin B_3), people may develop a niacin deficiency, causing the disease pellagra (see page 922).

When carcinoid tumors occur in the digestive tract or pancreas, the substances they produce are released into a blood vessel that flows directly to the liver (portal vein), where enzymes destroy them. Therefore, carcinoid tumors that originate in the digestive tract generally do not produce symptoms unless the tumors have spread to the liver.

If the tumors have spread to the liver, the liver is unable to process the substances before they begin circulating throughout the body. Depending on which substances are being released by the tumors, the person will have the various symptoms of carcinoid syndrome. Carcinoid tumors of the lungs, testes, and ovaries also cause symptoms because the substances they produce bypass the liver and circulate widely in the bloodstream.

Symptoms

Most people with carcinoid tumors have symptoms similar to those of other intestinal tumors, mainly cramping pain and changes in bowel movements as a result of obstruction.

Carcinoid Syndrome: Fewer than 10% of people with carcinoid tumors develop symptoms of carcinoid syndrome, although this percentage varies depending on where the tumor is located. Uncomfortable flushing, typically of the head and neck, is the most common and often the earliest symptom of carcinoid syndrome. Flushing, the result of blood vessel dilation, is often triggered by emotions, by eating, or by drinking alcohol or hot liquids. The flushing may be followed by periods when the skin is bluish (cyanosis). Excessive contraction of the intestine may result in abdominal cramping and diarrhea. The intestine may not be able to absorb nutrients properly, resulting in undernutrition and fatty, foul-smelling stools.

Heart damage may occur, resulting in swelling of the feet and legs (edema). Wheezing and shortness of breath may result from obstructed airflow in the lungs. Some people with carcinoid syndrome lose interest in sex, and some men have erectile dysfunction.

Diagnosis

When symptoms lead a doctor to suspect a carcinoid tumor, the diagnosis can often be confirmed by measuring the amount of 5-hydroxyindoleacetic acid (5-HIAA)—one of the chemical by-products of serotonin—in the person's urine, which is collected over a 24-hour period. For at least 3 days before undergoing this test, the person refrains from eating foods that are rich in serotonin—bananas, tomatoes, plums, avocados, pineapples, eggplants, and walnuts. Certain drugs, including guaifenesin (found in many cough syrups), methocarbamol (a muscle relaxant), and phenothiazines (antipsychotics), also interfere with test results.

Different tests are used to locate carcinoid tumors. These tests include computed tomography (CT), magnetic resonance imaging (MRI), and arteriography. Sometimes exploratory surgery is needed to locate the tumor.

Radionuclide scanning is another useful test. Most carcinoid tumors have receptors for the hormone somatostatin. Doctors can therefore inject a radioactive form of somatostatin into the blood and use radionuclide scanning to locate a carcinoid tumor and determine if it has spread. About 90% of tumors can be located using this technique. MRI or CT can be helpful in confirming whether the tumor has spread to the liver.

Treatment

When a carcinoid tumor is restricted to a specific area, such as the appendix, small intestine, rectum, or lungs, surgical removal may cure the disease. If the tumor has spread to the liver, surgery rarely cures the disease but may help relieve symptoms. The tumors grow so slowly that even people whose tumors have spread often survive for 10 to 15 years.

Neither radiation therapy nor chemotherapy is effective in curing carcinoid tumors. However, combinations of certain chemotherapy drugs (streptozocin with fluorouracil and sometimes doxorubicin) may relieve symptoms. A drug called octreotide can also relieve symptoms, and tamoxifen and interferon-alpha may reduce the tumor's growth. Phenothiazines, cimetidine, and phentolamine are used to control flushing in people with carcinoid syndrome. Prednisone is sometimes given to people with carcinoid tumors of the lung who have episodes of severe flushing. Diarrhea may be controlled with codeine, tincture of opium, diphenoxylate, or cyproheptadine. Pellagra may be prevented by drugs that block the production of serotonin, such as methyldopa and phenoxybenzamine.

Blood Disorders

CHAPTER
153   Biology of Blood

Blood is a complex mixture of plasma (the liquid component), white blood cells, red blood cells, and platelets. The body contains about 5 to 6 quarts (about 5 liters) of blood. Once blood is pumped out of the heart, it takes 20 to 30 seconds to make a complete trip through the circulation and return to the heart.

Blood performs various essential functions as it circulates through the body. It delivers oxygen and essential nutrients (such as fats, sugars, minerals, and vitamins) to the body's tissues. It carries carbon dioxide to the lungs and other waste products to the kidneys for elimination from the body. It transports hormones (chemical messengers) to allow various parts of the body to communicate with each other. Also, it carries components that fight infection and stop bleeding.

Components of Blood

Plasma

Plasma is the liquid component of blood, in which the red blood cells, white blood cells, and platelets are suspended. It constitutes more than half of the blood's volume and consists mostly of water that contains dissolved salts (electrolytes) and proteins. The major protein in plasma is albumin. Albumin helps keep fluid from leaking out of blood vessels and into tissues, and albumin binds to and carries substances such as hormones and certain drugs. Other proteins in plasma include antibodies (immunoglobulins), which actively defend the body against viruses, bacteria, fungi, and cancer cells, and clotting factors, which control bleeding.

Plasma has other functions. It acts as a reservoir that can either replenish insufficient water or absorb excess water from tissues. When body tissues need additional liquid, water from plasma is the first resource to meet that need. Plasma also prevents blood vessels from collapsing and clogging and helps maintain blood pressure and circulation throughout the body simply by filling blood vessels and flowing through them continuously. Plasma circulation also plays a role in regulating body temperature by carrying heat generated in core body tissues through areas that lose heat more readily, such as the arms, legs, and head.

Red Blood Cells

Red blood cells (also called erythrocytes) make up about 40% of the blood's volume. Red blood cells contain hemoglobin, a protein that gives blood its red color and enables it to carry oxygen from the lungs and deliver it to all body tissues. Oxygen is used by cells to produce energy that the body needs, leaving carbon dioxide as a waste product. Red blood cells carry carbon dioxide away from the tissues and back to the lungs. When the number of red blood cells is too low (anemia), blood carries less oxygen, and fatigue and weakness develop. When the number of red blood cells is too high (polycythemia), blood can become too thick, which may cause the blood to clot more easily and increase the risk of heart attacks and strokes.

White Blood Cells

White blood cells (also called leukocytes) are fewer in number than red blood cells, with a ratio of about 1 white blood cell to every 600 to 700 red blood cells. White blood cells are responsible primarily for defending the body against infection. There are five main types of white blood cells.

Neutrophils, the most numerous type, help protect the body against infections by killing and ingesting bacteria and fungi and by ingesting foreign debris.

Lymphocytes consist of three main types: T lymphocytes and natural killer cells, which both help protect against viral infections and can detect and destroy some cancer cells, and B lymphocytes, which develop into cells that produce antibodies.

Monocytes ingest dead or damaged cells and help defend against many infectious organisms.

Eosinophils kill parasites, destroy cancer cells, and are involved in allergic responses.

Basophils also participate in allergic responses.

Some white blood cells flow smoothly through the bloodstream, but many adhere to blood vessel walls or even penetrate the vessel walls to enter other tissues. When white blood cells reach the site of an infection or other problem, they release substances that attract more white blood cells. The white blood cells function like an army, dispersed throughout the body but ready at a moment's notice to gather and fight off an invading organism. White blood cells accomplish this by engulfing and digesting organisms and by producing antibodies that attach to organisms so that they can be more easily destroyed (see page 1102).

When the number of white blood cells is too low (leukopenia), infections are more likely to occur. A higher than normal number of white blood cells (leukocytosis) may not directly cause symptoms, but the high number of cells can be an indication of a disease such as an infection or leukemia.

Platelets

Platelets (also called thrombocytes) are cell-like particles that are smaller than red or white blood cells. Platelets are fewer in number than red blood cells, with a ratio of about 1 platelet to every 20 red blood cells. Platelets help in the clotting process by gathering at a bleeding site and clumping together to form a plug that helps seal the blood vessel. At the same time, they release substances that help promote further clotting. When the number of platelets is too low (thrombocytopenia), bruising and abnormal bleeding become more likely. When the number of platelets is too high (thrombocythemia), blood may clot excessively, producing a stroke or heart attack.

Formation of Blood Cells

Red blood cells, most white blood cells, and platelets are produced in the bone marrow, the soft fatty tissue inside bone cavities. Two types of white blood cells, T and B lymphocytes, are also produced in the lymph nodes and spleen, and T lymphocytes are produced and mature in the thymus gland.

Within the bone marrow, all blood cells originate from a single type of unspecialized cell called a stem cell. When a stem cell divides, it first becomes an immature red blood cell, white blood cell, or platelet-producing cell. The immature cell then divides, matures further, and ultimately becomes a mature red blood cell, white blood cell, or platelet.

The rate of blood cell production is controlled by the body's needs. Normal blood cells last for a limited time (ranging from a few hours to a few days for white blood cells, to about 10 days for platelets, to about 120 days for red blood cells) and must be replaced constantly. Certain conditions may trigger additional production of blood cells. When the oxygen content of body tissues is low or the number of red blood cells decreases, the kidneys produce and release erythropoietin, a hormone that stimulates the bone marrow to produce more red blood cells. The bone marrow produces and releases more white blood cells in response to infections. It produces and releases more platelets in response to bleeding.

Effects of Aging

Aging has some effect on bone marrow and blood cells. The amount of fat in the marrow increases with age, which means there is less cell-producing marrow. While this decrease generally does not cause problems, it may when the body experiences an increased demand for blood cells: the marrow of an older person may be less able to meet those increased demands. Anemia is the most common result.

154 Symptoms and Diagnosis of Blood Disorders

Disorders that affect the cells in the blood (blood cells) or proteins in the blood clotting or immune systems are called blood disorders or hematologic disorders. Laboratory tests to detect blood disorders generally begin with examination of the blood, which is easily obtained from a vein with a needle and syringe or sometimes from the fingertip by a needle prick. However, evaluation may require examination of the bone marrow, because that is where blood cells develop.

Symptoms

Symptoms of blood disorders are often vague and nonspecific, that is, they could indicate a disorder of almost any part of the body. However, although no single symptom unmistakably indicates a blood disorder, certain groups of symptoms suggest the possibility. Such groups of symptoms most commonly relate to decreases in blood cells, such as a reduced number of red blood cells (anemia), a reduced number of white blood cells (leukopenia), or a reduced number of platelets (thrombocytopenia). For example, a person who has fatigue, weakness, and shortness of breath may have anemia. A person who has fever and infection may have too few white blood cells. A person who bleeds or bruises easily may have too few platelets.

Occasionally, symptoms may relate to increased numbers of blood cells. For example, people with thickened (more viscous) blood due to increased numbers of red blood cells (polycythemia) or white blood cells may experience symptoms such as shortness of breath, headaches, dizziness, and confusion. Blood can also become thickened because of an increased production of immune-related proteins, as in multiple myeloma.

Finally, disorders of substances (factors) responsible for normal blood clotting may result in insufficient blood clotting (manifesting as excessive bruising or bleeding or as small red or purple spots on the skin) or in the formation of abnormal blood clots (producing warm, painful areas in the legs or sudden shortness of breath, chest pain, or both). These problems may arise because the body does not produce enough of these factors, the factors are abnormal, or the body is using up the factors too quickly.

Diagnosis

Laboratory Blood Tests

Doctors depend on many different laboratory tests of blood samples to diagnose and monitor diseases. Because the liquid portion of the blood (plasma) carries so many substances essential to the body's functioning, blood tests can be used to find out what is happening in many parts of the body.

Testing blood is easier than obtaining a tissue sample from a specific organ. For example, thyroid function can be evaluated more easily by measuring the level of thyroid hormones in the blood than by directly sampling the thyroid. Likewise, measuring liver enzymes and proteins in the blood (see box on page 212) is easier than sampling the liver. However, certain blood tests are used to measure the components and function of the blood itself. These are the tests that are mostly used to diagnose blood disorders.

Complete Blood Count: The most commonly performed blood test is the complete blood count (CBC), which is an evaluation of all the cellular components (red blood cells, white blood cells, and platelets). Automated machines perform this test in less than 1 minute on a small drop of blood. The CBC is supplemented in some instances by examination of blood cells under a microscope.

The CBC determines the number of red blood cells and the amount of hemoglobin (the oxygen-carrying protein in red blood cells) in the blood. In addition, the average size, degree of variability of size, and hemoglobin content of red blood cells is assessed by a CBC and can alert laboratory workers to the presence of abnormal red blood cells (which may then be further characterized by microscopic examination). Abnormal red blood cells may be fragmented or shaped like teardrops, crescents, needles, or a variety of other forms. Knowing the specific shape and size of red blood cells can help a doctor diagnose a particular cause of anemia. For example, sickle-shaped cells are characteristic of sickle cell disease, small cells containing insufficient amounts of hemoglobin are likely due to iron deficiency anemia, and large oval cells suggest anemia due to a deficiency of folate (folic acid) or vitamin B_{12}.

The CBC also determines the number of white blood cells. The specific types of white blood cells (see page 1022) can be counted (differential white blood cell count) when a doctor needs more information. If the total number of white blood cells or the number of one of the specific types of white blood cells is above or below normal, the doctor can examine these cells under a microscope. The microscopic examination can identify features that are characteristic of certain diseases. For example, large numbers of white blood cells that have a very immature appearance (blasts) may indicate leukemia (cancer of the white blood cells).

Platelets are usually also counted as part of a CBC. The number of platelets is an important measure of the blood's protective mechanisms for stopping bleeding (clotting). A high number of platelets (thrombocytosis or thrombocythemia) can lead to blood clots in small blood vessels, especially those in the heart or brain. In some disorders, a high number of platelets may paradoxically result in excess bleeding.

Reticulocyte Count: The reticulocyte count measures the number of newly formed (young) red blood cells (reticulocytes) in a specified volume of blood. Reticulocytes normally make up about 1% of the total number of red blood cells. When the body needs more red blood cells, as in anemia, the bone marrow normally responds by producing more reticulocytes. Thus, the reticulocyte count is a measure of the capacity of the bone marrow to make new red blood cells.

Special Tests of Blood Cells: Once a doctor determines that something is wrong with one or more of the cell types in the blood, many additional tests are available to shed more light on the problem. Doctors can measure the proportion of the different types of white blood cells and can determine subtypes of these cells by assessing certain markers on the surface of the cells. Tests are available to measure the ability of white blood cells to fight infection, to assess the functioning of platelets and their ability to clot, and to measure the contents of red blood cells to help determine the cause of anemia or why the cells are not functioning properly. Most of these tests are done on samples of blood, but some require a sample from the bone marrow.

Clotting Tests: One measure of the body's ability to stop bleeding is the count of the number of platelets.

COMPLETE BLOOD COUNT (CBC)

TEST	WHAT IT MEASURES	NORMAL VALUES
Hemoglobin	Amount of this oxygen-carrying protein within red blood cells	Men: 12.7 to 13.7 grams per deciliter Women: 11.5 to 12.2 grams per deciliter
Hematocrit	Proportion of total blood volume made up of red blood cells	Men: 42 to 50% Women: 36 to 45%
Mean corpuscular volume	Average volume of individual red blood cells	86 to 98 femtoliters
Mean corpuscular hemoglobin concentration	Average concentration of hemoglobin within red blood cells	33.4 to 35.5 grams per deciliter
White blood cell count	Number of white blood cells in a specified volume of blood	4,500 to 10,500 per microliter
Differential white blood cell count	Percentages of the different types of white blood cells	Segmented neutrophils: 34 to 75% Band neutrophils: 0 to 8% Lymphocytes: 12 to 50% Monocytes: 2 to 9% Eosinophils: 0 to 5% Basophils: 0 to 3%
Platelet count	Number of platelets in a specified volume of blood	140,000 to 450,000 per microliter

Sometimes doctors need to test how well the platelets function. Other tests can measure the overall function of the many proteins needed for normal blood clotting (clotting factors). The most common of these tests are the prothrombin time (PT) and the partial thromboplastin time (PTT). The levels of individual clotting factors can also be determined.

Proteins and Other Substances: Some blood cells produce proteins that can be measured in the blood or urine. Doctors may measure these proteins to determine if the cells are abnormal. For example, a blood disorder in which certain red blood cells, called plasma cells, become cancerous produces unusual proteins (Bence Jones proteins) that can be measured in blood and urine. Certain abnormal white blood cells produce unusual antibodies.

Erythropoietin is a protein made in the kidneys that stimulates the bone marrow to produce red blood cells. The level of this protein and several others that affect red blood cell production can be measured in the blood. Levels of iron and certain vitamins that are necessary for the production of healthy blood cells also can be measured.

Other Blood Tests: Specialized blood tests can be used to determine whether uncommon blood disorders are present. For example, on rare occasions, doctors must measure the total volume of blood or the total number of certain blood cells in the body. These measurements can be done using radioactive isotopes that mix in the blood or attach to blood cells.

Blood Typing: Blood type, which is determined by the presence of certain proteins on the surface of red blood cells, can be identified by measuring the reaction of a small sample of a person's blood to certain antibodies. Blood typing requires evaluation of both the plasma and red blood cells. Blood typing must be done before blood can be transfused (see box on page 1027).

Bone Marrow Examination

Sometimes a sample of bone marrow must be examined to determine why blood cells are abnormal or why there are too few or too many of any kind of blood cell. A doctor can take two different types of bone marrow samples: a bone marrow aspirate and a bone marrow core biopsy. Both types are usually taken from the hipbone (iliac crest), although aspirates are rarely taken from the breastbone (sternum). In very young children, bone marrow samples are occasionally taken from one of the bones in the lower leg (tibia).

When both types of samples are needed, they are taken at the same time. After the skin and tissue over the bone are numbed with a local anesthetic, the sharp needle of a syringe is inserted into the

Taking a Bone Marrow Sample

Bone marrow samples are usually taken from the hipbone (iliac crest). The person may lie on one side, facing away from the doctor, with the knee of the top leg bent. After numbing the skin and tissue over the bone with a local anesthetic, the doctor inserts a needle into the bone and withdraws the marrow.

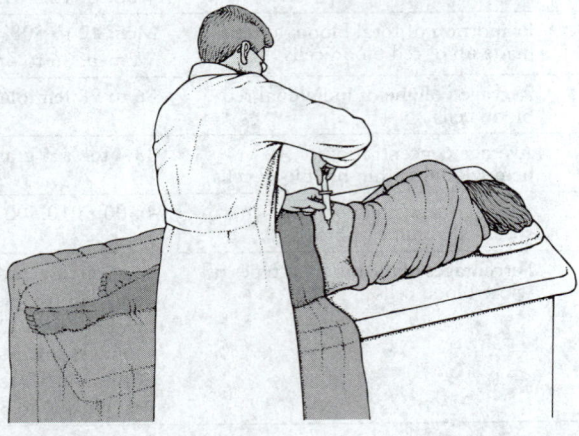

bone. For a bone marrow aspirate, the doctor pulls back on the plunger of the syringe and draws out a small amount of the soft bone marrow, which can be spread on a slide and examined under a microscope. Special tests, such as cultures for bacteria, fungi, or viruses, chromosomal analysis, and analysis of cell surface proteins (flow cytometry), can be performed on the sample. Although the aspirate often provides enough information for a diagnosis to be made, the process of drawing the marrow into the syringe breaks up the fragile bone marrow. As a result, determining the original arrangement of the cells is difficult.

When the exact anatomic relationships of cells must be determined and the structure of the tissues evaluated, the doctor also performs a core biopsy. A small core of intact bone marrow is removed with an internal coring device. This core is preserved and sliced into thin sections that are examined under a microscope.

A bone marrow sampling generally involves a slight jolt of pain, followed by minimal discomfort. The procedure takes a few minutes.

CHAPTER 155 Blood Transfusion

A blood transfusion is the transfer of blood or a blood component from one person (a donor) to another (a recipient).

In the United States, about 29 million blood transfusions are given every year. Transfusions are given to increase the blood's ability to carry oxygen, restore the body's blood volume, improve immunity, and correct clotting problems. Accident victims, people undergoing surgery, and people receiving treatment for cancers (such as leukemia) or other diseases (such as the blood diseases sickle cell anemia and thalassemia) are typical recipients.

The Food and Drug Administration (FDA) strictly regulates the collection, storage, and transportation of blood and its components. These regulations were developed to protect both the donor and the recipient. Additional standards are upheld by many state and local health authorities, as well as by organizations such as the American Red Cross and the American Association of Blood Banks. Because of these regulations, giving and receiving blood is very safe. However, transfusions still pose risks for the recipient, such as allergic reactions, fever and chills, excess blood volume, and bacterial and viral infections. Even though the chance of contracting AIDS, hepatitis, or other infections from transfusions is remote, doctors are well aware of these risks and order transfusions only when there is no alternative.

Donation Process

Donating blood is very safe. The entire process of donating whole blood (that is, blood with all component cells) takes about 1 hour. Blood donors must be at least 17 years old and weigh at least 110 pounds. In addition, they must be in good health: their pulse, blood pressure, and temperature are measured, and a blood sample is tested to check for anemia. They are asked a series of questions about their health, factors that might affect their health, and countries they have visited.

Did You Know...

There are very few disorders that disqualify people from giving blood.

Most people who are deferred from giving blood are eligible to donate at a later time.

Doctors test donated blood for many infectious diseases, so the chance a person will get a disease from donated blood is rare.

Conditions that permanently disqualify a person from donating blood include hepatitis B or C, heart disease, certain types of cancer (leukemia, lymphoma, and any type of cancer that has recurred after treatment or that has ever been treated with chemotherapy drugs), severe asthma, bleeding disorders, possible exposure to prion diseases (such as variant Creutzfeldt-Jakob disease—see page 766), AIDS, and possible exposure to the human immunodeficiency virus (HIV, the virus that causes AIDS) due to high-risk behaviors (see page 1254). Conditions that temporarily disqualify a person include malaria (if it has been less than 3 years since the person last experienced symptoms), cancer that has been treated with surgery or radiation (if it has been less than 5 years since the person last received treatment), pregnancy,

Blood Typing

Blood is classified by type. A person's blood type is determined by the presence or absence of certain proteins (Rh factor and blood group antigens A and B) on the surface of red blood cells.

The four main blood types are A, B, AB, and O, and for each type, the blood is either Rh-positive or Rh-negative. For example, a person with O-negative blood has red blood cells that lack both A and B antigens and the Rh factor. A person with AB-positive blood has red blood cells that have A and B antigens and the Rh factor. Some blood types are far more common than others. The most common blood types in the United States are O-positive and A-positive, followed by B-positive, O-negative, A-negative, AB-positive, B-negative, and AB-negative.

A blood transfusion is safest when the blood type of the transfused blood precisely matches the recipient's blood type. Therefore, before a transfusion, blood banks do a test called a "type and cross-match" on the donor's and the recipient's blood. This test minimizes the chance of a dangerous or possibly fatal reaction.

However, in an emergency, anyone can receive type O red blood cells. Thus, people with type O blood are known as universal donors. People with type AB blood can receive red blood cells from any blood type and are thus known as universal recipients. Recipients whose blood is Rh-negative must receive blood from Rh-negative donors, but recipients whose blood is Rh-positive may receive Rh-positive or Rh-negative blood.

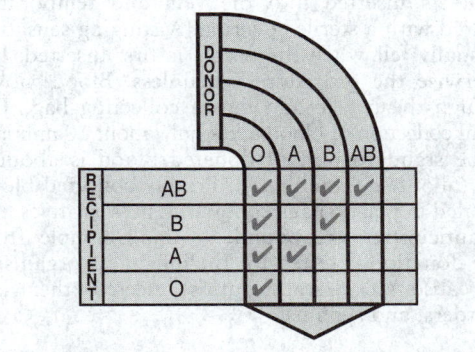

recent major surgery, poorly controlled high blood pressure, low blood pressure, anemia, the use of certain drugs, exposure to some forms of hepatitis, and a recent blood transfusion.

Generally, donors are not allowed to give blood more than once every 56 days. The practice of paying donors for blood has almost disappeared,

Testing Donated Blood for Infections

Blood transfusions can transmit infectious organisms carried in the donor's blood. That is why health officials have restricted blood donor eligibility and made blood testing thorough. All blood donations are tested for infection with the organisms that cause viral hepatitis, AIDS, selected other viral disorders (such as West Nile virus), Chagas' disease, and syphilis.

VIRAL HEPATITIS

Donated blood is tested for infection with the viruses that cause the types of viral hepatitis (types B and C) that are transmitted by blood transfusions. These tests cannot identify all cases of infected blood, but with the rigorous testing and donor screening procedures, a transfusion poses almost no risk of transmitting hepatitis C. The current risk is 1 infection for every 1,500,000 units of blood transfused. Hepatitis B remains the most common potentially serious disorder transmitted by blood transfusions, with a current risk of about 1 infection for every 137,000 units of blood transfused.

AIDS

In the United States, donated blood is tested for the human immunodeficiency virus (HIV), the cause of AIDS. The test is not 100% accurate, but potential donors are interviewed as part of the screening process. Interviewers ask about risk factors for AIDS—for instance, whether the potential donors or their sex partners have injected drugs or had sex with a man who has male sex partners. Because of the blood test and the screening interview, the risk of contracting HIV infection through a blood transfusion is extremely low—1 in 2,000,000 according to recent estimates.

SYPHILIS

Blood transfusions rarely transmit syphilis. Not only are blood donors screened and donations tested for the organism that causes syphilis, but the donated blood is also refrigerated at low temperatures, which kills the infectious organisms.

---

because it encouraged needy people to present themselves as donors and then sometimes to deny having any conditions that would disqualify them.

A person who is deemed eligible to donate blood sits in a reclining chair or lies on a cot. A health care worker examines the inside surface of the person's elbow and determines which vein to use. After the area immediately surrounding the vein is cleaned, a needle is inserted into the vein and temporarily secured with a sterile covering. A stinging sensation is usually felt when the needle is first inserted, but otherwise the procedure is painless. Blood moves through the needle and into a collecting bag. The actual collection of blood takes only about 10 minutes.

The standard unit of donated blood is about 1 pint (about 450 milliliters). Freshly collected blood is sealed in plastic bags containing preservatives and an anticlotting compound. A small sample from each donation is tested for the infectious organisms that cause AIDS, viral hepatitis, selected other viral disorders, and syphilis.

Types of Transfusions

Most blood donations are divided (fractionated) into their components: red blood cells, platelets, clotting factors, plasma, antibodies (immunoglobulins), and white blood cells. Depending on the situation, people may receive only the cells from blood, only the clotting factors from blood, or some other blood component. Transfusing only selected blood compo-

nents allows the treatment to be specific, reduces the risks of side effects, and can efficiently use the different components from a single unit of blood to treat several people.

Red Blood Cells: Packed red blood cells, the most commonly transfused blood component, can restore the blood's oxygen-carrying capacity. This component may be given to a person who is bleeding or who has severe anemia. The red blood cells are separated from the fluid component of the blood (plasma) and from the other cellular and cell-like components. This step concentrates the red blood cells so that they occupy less space, thus the term "packed." Red blood cells can be refrigerated for up to 42 days. In special circumstances—for instance, to preserve a rare type of blood—red blood cells can be frozen for up to 10 years.

Platelets: Platelets can help restore the blood's clotting ability. They are usually given to people with too few platelets (thrombocytopenia), which may result in severe and spontaneous bleeding. Platelets can be stored for only 5 to 7 days.

Blood Clotting Factors: Blood clotting factors are proteins found in blood plasma that normally work with platelets to help the blood clot. Clotting factors may be obtained from plasma or manufactured. Manufactured proteins are called recombinant factor concentrates. Without clotting factors, bleeding would not stop after an injury. Individual concentrated blood clotting factors can be given to people who have an inherited bleeding disorder, such as hemophilia or von Willebrand's disease, and to those who are unable to produce enough clotting factors (usually because of severe infection or liver disease).

Plasma: Plasma, the fluid component of the blood, contains many proteins, including blood clotting factors. Plasma is used for bleeding disorders in which the missing clotting factor is unknown or when the specific clotting factor is not available. Plasma also is used when bleeding is caused by insufficient production of all or many of the different clotting factors, as a result of liver failure or severe infection. Plasma that is frozen right after it is separated from the cells of donor blood (fresh frozen plasma) can be stored for up to 1 year.

Antibodies: Antibodies (immunoglobulins), the disease-fighting components of blood, are sometimes given to provide temporary immunity to people who have been exposed to an infectious disease or who have low antibody levels. Infections for which antibodies are available include chickenpox, hepatitis, rabies, and tetanus. Antibodies are produced from treated plasma donations.

White Blood Cells: White blood cells are transfused to treat life-threatening infections in people who have a greatly reduced number of white blood cells or whose white blood cells are functioning abnormally. The use of white blood cell transfusions is rare, because improved antibiotics and the use of cytokine growth factors have greatly reduced the need for such transfusions. White blood cells are obtained by hemapheresis and can be stored for up to 24 hours.

Blood Substitutes: Blood substitutes that use certain chemicals or specially treated solutions of hemoglobin (a protein that allows red blood cells to carry oxygen) to carry and deliver oxygen to tissues are being developed. These solutions can be stored at room temperature for up to 2 years, making them attractive for transport to the site of trauma or to the battlefield. However, further research is needed before these blood substitutes become available for routine use.

Special Donation Procedures

Plateletpheresis: In plateletpheresis, a donor gives only platelets rather than whole blood. Whole blood is drawn from the donor, and a machine that separates the blood into its components selectively removes the platelets and returns the rest of the blood to the donor. Because donors get most of their blood back, they can safely give 8 to 10 times as many platelets during one of these procedures as they would give in a single donation of whole blood. Collecting platelets from a donor takes about 1 to 2 hours, compared with collecting whole blood, which takes about 10 minutes.

Autologous Transfusion: In an autologous transfusion, donors are recipients of their own blood. For example, in the weeks before undergoing elective surgery, a person may donate several units of blood to be transfused if needed during or after the surgical procedure. The person takes iron pills after donating the blood to help the body replenish the lost blood cells before surgery. Also, during some types of surgery and in certain kinds of injuries, blood that is lost can be collected and immediately given back to the person (intraoperative blood salvage). An autologous transfusion is the safest type of blood transfusion, because it eliminates the risks of incompatibility and blood-borne disease.

> **? Did You Know...**
> Doctors can specify what type of blood cells are given during a transfusion so that people get only those cells that are needed to treat their disorder.

Directed or Designated Donation: Family members or friends can donate blood specifically for one another if the recipient's and donor's blood types and Rh factors are compatible. For some recipients, knowing who donated the blood is comforting, although a donation from a family member or friend is not necessarily safer than one from an unrelated person. Blood from a family member is tested as are all blood samples and then treated with radiation to prevent graft-versus-host disease, which, although rare, occurs more often when the recipient and donor are related.

Stem Cell Pheresis: In stem cell pheresis, a donor gives only stem cells (undifferentiated cells that can develop into any type of cell) rather than whole blood. Prior to the donation procedure, the donor receives an injection of a special type of protein (growth factor) that stimulates the bone marrow to release stem cells into the bloodstream. Whole blood is drawn from the donor, and a machine that separates the blood into its components selectively removes the stem cells and returns the rest of the blood to the donor. Stem cell donors must be compatible with recipients by lymphocyte type (human leukocyte antigen, or HLA), a type of protein found on certain cells, rather than blood type. Stem cells are sometimes used to treat people with leukemia, lymphoma, or other cancers of the blood. This procedure is called stem cell transplantation. The recipient's own stem cells can be obtained, or donated stem cells can be given.

Controlling Diseases by Purifying the Blood

In hemapheresis, blood is removed from a person and then returned after fluid, substances in the fluid, blood cells, or platelets are removed or reduced in quantity. Sometimes this process is used to obtain needed blood cells or platelets from a donor (for example, stem cell pheresis or plateletpheresis). This process is also used to purify blood by removing harmful substances or excessive numbers of blood cells or platelets in people with serious illnesses who have not responded to other treatments. To be helpful for purifying blood, hemapheresis must remove the undesirable substance or blood cell faster than the body produces it.

The two most common types of hemapheresis that are used to purify blood are plasmapheresis and cytapheresis.

In plasmapheresis, harmful substances are removed from the plasma. Plasmapheresis is used to treat such disorders as myasthenia gravis and Guillain-Barré syndrome (neurologic disorders that cause muscle weakness), Goodpasture's syndrome (an autoimmune disorder involving bleeding in the lungs and kidney failure), pemphigus vulgaris (severe, sometimes fatal, blistering of the skin), cryoglobulinemia (a type of abnormal antibody formation), and thrombotic thrombocytopenic purpura (a rare clotting disorder).

In cytapheresis, excess numbers of certain blood cells are removed. Cytapheresis can be used to treat polycythemia (an excess of red blood cells), certain types of leukemia (a type of cancer in which there are excess white blood cells), and thrombocythemia (an excess of platelets).

Hemapheresis is repeated only as often as necessary because the large fluid shifts between blood vessels and tissues that occur as blood is removed and returned may cause complications in people who are already ill. Hemapheresis can help control some diseases but generally does not cure them.

Precautions and Adverse Reactions

To minimize the chance of an adverse reaction during a transfusion, health care practitioners take several precautions. Before starting the transfusion, usually a few hours or even a few days beforehand, a technician mixes a drop of the donor's blood with the recipient's to make sure they are compatible. This procedure is called cross-matching.

After double-checking labels on the bags of blood that are about to be given to ensure the units are intended for that recipient, the health care practitioner gives the blood to the recipient slowly, generally over 1 to 2 hours for each unit of blood. Because most adverse reactions occur during the first 15 minutes of the transfusion, the recipient is closely observed at first. After that, a nurse checks on the recipient periodically and must stop the transfusion if an adverse reaction occurs.

Most transfusions are safe and successful; however, mild reactions occur occasionally, and severe and even fatal reactions, rarely. The most common reactions are fever and allergic reactions (hypersensitivity), which occur in about 1 to 2% of transfusions. Symptoms of an allergic reaction include itching, a widespread rash, swelling, dizziness, and headache. Less common symptoms are breathing difficulties, wheezing, and muscle spasms. Rarely, an allergic reaction is severe enough to cause low blood pressure and shock. Another rare reaction, called transfusion-related acute lung injury, or TRALI, is caused by antibodies in the donor's plasma. This reaction, which is more common when the donor is a woman who has been pregnant, may cause serious breathing difficulties. More general use of male donor plasma has decreased the number of people who have this reaction.

Treatments are available that allow transfusions to be given to people who previously had allergic reactions to them. People who have allergic reactions to donated blood may have to be given washed red blood cells. Washing the red blood cells removes components of the donor blood that may cause allergic reactions. More commonly, the transfused blood is filtered to reduce the number of white blood cells (a process called leukocyte reduction). Leukocyte reduction is usually done by placing a special filter in the tubing through which the transfusion is flowing. Alternatively, the blood may be filtered before it is stored.

Despite careful typing and cross-matching of blood, mismatches due to subtle differences between donor and recipient blood (and, very rarely, errors) can still occur that cause the transfused red blood cells to be destroyed shortly after the transfusion (a hemolytic reaction). Usually, this reaction starts as general discomfort or anxiety during or immediately after the transfusion. Sometimes breathing difficulty, chest pressure, flushing, and severe back pain develop. Very rarely, the reactions become more severe and even fatal. A doctor can confirm that a hemolytic reaction is destroying red blood cells by checking to see whether hemoglobin released from these cells is in the person's blood and urine.

Transfusion recipients can become overloaded with fluid. Recipients who have heart disease are most vulnerable, so their transfusions are given more slowly and they are monitored closely.

Graft-versus-host disease is an unusual complication that affects primarily people whose immune system is impaired by drugs or disease. In this disease, the recipient's (host's) tissues are attacked by the donated white blood cells (the graft). The symptoms include fever, rash, low blood pressure, low blood counts, tissue destruction, and shock. These reactions can be fatal but are eliminated by treating with radiation those blood products that are intended for people with a weakened immune system.

156 Anemia

Anemia is a condition in which the number of red blood cells or the amount of hemoglobin (the protein that carries oxygen in them) is low.

Red blood cells contain hemoglobin, a protein that enables them to carry oxygen from the lungs and deliver it to all parts of the body. When the number of red blood cells is reduced or the amount of hemoglobin in them is low, the blood cannot carry an adequate supply of oxygen. An inadequate supply of oxygen in the tissues produces the symptoms of anemia.

Causes

The causes of anemia are numerous, but most can be grouped within three major mechanisms that produce anemia:

- Blood loss (excessive bleeding)
- Inadequate production of red blood cells
- Excessive destruction of red blood cells

Anemia may be caused by excessive bleeding. Bleeding may be sudden, as may occur in an injury or during surgery. Often, bleeding is gradual and repetitive, typically from abnormalities in the digestive or urinary tract or heavy menstrual periods. Chronic bleeding typically leads to low levels of iron, which leads to worsening anemia.

Anemia may also result when the body does not produce enough red blood cells. Many nutrients are needed for red blood cell production. The most critical are iron, vitamin B_{12}, and folate (folic acid), but the body also needs trace amounts of vitamin C, riboflavin, and copper, as well as a proper balance of hormones, especially erythropoietin (a hormone that stimulates red blood cell production). Without these nutrients and hormones, production of red blood cells is slow and inadequate, or the red blood cells may be deformed and unable to carry oxygen adequately. Chronic disease also may affect red blood cell production. In some circumstances, the bone marrow space may be invaded and replaced (for example, by leukemia, lymphoma, or metastatic cancer), resulting in decreased production of red blood cells.

Anemia may also result when too many red blood cells are destroyed. Normally, red blood cells live about 120 days. Scavenger cells in the bone marrow, spleen, and liver detect and destroy red blood cells that are near or beyond their usual life span. If red blood cells are destroyed prematurely (hemolysis), the bone marrow tries to compensate by producing new cells faster. When destruction of red blood cells exceeds their production, hemolytic anemia results. Hemolytic anemia is relatively uncommon compared with the anemia caused by excessive bleeding and decreased red blood cell production.

Symptoms and Diagnosis

Symptoms vary depending on the severity of the anemia and how rapidly it develops. Some people with mild anemia, particularly when it develops slowly, have no symptoms at all. Other people may experience symptoms only with physical exertion. More severe anemia may produce symptoms even when people are resting. Symptoms are more severe when mild or severe anemia develops rapidly, such as with bleeding that occurs when a blood vessel ruptures.

Mild anemia often causes fatigue, weakness, and paleness. In addition to these symptoms, more severe anemia may produce faintness, dizziness, increased thirst, sweating, a weak and rapid pulse, and rapid breathing. Severe anemia may produce painful lower leg cramps during exercise, shortness of breath, and chest pain, especially if people already have impaired blood circulation in the legs or certain types of lung or heart disease.

COMMON CAUSES OF ANEMIA

MECHANISM	EXAMPLES
Chronic excessive bleeding	Bladder tumors Cancer in the digestive tract Heavy menstrual bleeding Hemorrhoids Kidney tumors Nosebleeds Polyps in the digestive tract Ulcers in the stomach or small intestine
Sudden excessive bleeding	Injuries Childbirth A ruptured blood vessel Surgery
Decreased red blood cell production	Aplastic anemia Chronic disorders Folate deficiency Iron deficiency Leukemia Lymphoma Metastatic cancer Myelodysplasia (abnormalities in bone marrow tissue) Myelofibrosis Multiple myeloma Vitamin B_{12} deficiency Vitamin C deficiency
Increased red blood cell destruction	Autoimmune reactions against red blood cells An enlarged spleen Glucose-6-phosphate dehydrogenase (G6PD) deficiency Hemoglobin C disease Hemoglobin E disease Hemoglobin S-C disease Hereditary elliptocytosis Hereditary spherocytosis Mechanical damage to red blood cells Paroxysmal nocturnal hemoglobinuria Sickle cell disease Thalassemia

Sometimes anemia is detected before people notice symptoms, when routine blood tests are done.

Low levels of hemoglobin and a low hematocrit (the percentage of red blood cells in the total blood volume) found in a blood sample confirm the anemia. Other tests, such as examining a blood sample under a microscope and less often examining a sample taken from the bone marrow, help determine the cause of the anemia.

Anemia Due to Excessive Bleeding

Anemia from excessive bleeding results when loss of red blood cells through bleeding exceeds production of new red blood cells.

- When blood loss is rapid, blood pressure falls, and people may be dizzy.
- When blood loss occurs gradually, people may be tired, short of breath, and pale.

- Stool, urine, and imaging tests may be needed to determine the source of bleeding.
- The cause of bleeding is corrected, and transfusions and iron supplements are given if needed.

Excessive bleeding is the most common cause of anemia. When blood is lost, the body quickly pulls water from tissues outside the bloodstream in an attempt to keep the blood vessels filled. As a result, the blood is diluted, and the hematocrit (the percentage of red blood cells in the total blood volume) is reduced. Eventually, increased production of red blood cells by the bone marrow may correct the anemia. However, over time, bleeding reduces the amount of iron in the body, so that the bone marrow is not able to increase production of new red blood cells to replace those lost.

Rapid Blood Loss: The symptoms may be severe initially, especially if anemia develops rapidly from a sudden loss of blood, such as from an injury, surgery, childbirth, or a ruptured blood vessel. Losing large amounts of blood suddenly can create two problems:

- Blood pressure falls because the amount of fluid left in the blood vessels is insufficient.
- The body's oxygen supply is drastically reduced because the number of oxygen-carrying red blood cells has decreased so quickly.

Either problem may lead to a heart attack, stroke, or death.

Chronic Blood Loss: Far more common than a sudden loss of blood is chronic (long-term) bleeding, which may occur from various parts of the body. Although large amounts of bleeding, such as that from nosebleeds and hemorrhoids, are obvious, small amounts of bleeding may not be noticed. For example, a small amount of blood may not be visible in the stool. This type of blood loss is described as occult. If a small amount of bleeding continues for a long time, a significant amount of blood may be lost. Such gradual bleeding may occur with common disorders, such as ulcers in the stomach or small intestine and diverticulosis, polyps, or cancers in the large intestine. Other sources of chronic bleeding include kidney or bladder tumors, which may cause blood to be lost in the urine, and heavy menstrual bleeding.

Symptoms and Diagnosis

Symptoms are similar to those of other types of anemia and vary from mild to severe, depending on how much blood is lost and how rapidly. When the blood loss is rapid—over several hours or less—loss of just one third of the blood volume can be fatal. Dizziness upon sitting or standing after a period of lying down (orthostatic hypotension) is common

SPOTLIGHT ON AGING

Many disorders that cause anemia, especially cancer, tend to be more common among older people. Thus, many older people develop anemia. Iron deficiency anemia, usually due to abnormal bleeding, is the most common anemia among older people.

Symptoms of anemia are basically the same in older people as in younger people. However, older people may not look pale. Also, even when anemia is mild, older people are more likely to become confused, depressed, agitated, or listless than younger people. They may also become unsteady and have difficulty walking. These problems can interfere with being able to live independently. However, some older people with mild anemia have no symptoms at all, particularly when anemia develops gradually, as it often does in older people.

In older people, anemia caused by vitamin B_{12} deficiency may be mistaken for dementia because this type of anemia may affect the nerves and mental function.

Having anemia may shorten the life expectancy of older people. Thus, identifying the cause and correcting it are particularly important.

when blood loss is rapid. When the blood loss is slower—over several weeks or longer—loss of up to two thirds of the blood volume may cause only fatigue and weakness or no symptoms at all, if the person drinks enough fluids.

Other symptoms may occur from the bleeding or the disorder that causes the bleeding. People may notice black, tarry stools if they have bleeding from the stomach or small intestine. Bleeding from the kidney or bladder may cause red or brown urine. Women may notice long, heavy menstrual periods. Some disorders that cause chronic bleeding, such as stomach ulcers, produce discomfort. Other disorders, such as diverticulosis and intestinal cancers and polyps at an early stage, cause no symptoms.

Doctors do blood tests to detect anemia when people describe symptoms of anemia, have noticed bleeding, or both. Stool and urine are tested for blood in an effort to identify the source of bleeding. Imaging tests or endoscopy may be needed to identify the source of bleeding.

Treatment

For large or rapid blood loss, the source of bleeding must be found and the bleeding stopped. Transfusion of red blood cells may be needed.

With slow or small blood loss, the body may produce enough red blood cells to correct the

MORE ABOUT SOME CAUSES OF ANEMIA

CAUSE	MECHANISM	TREATMENT	COMMENTS
Enlarged spleen	An enlarged spleen traps and destroys too many red blood cells.	The disorder that caused the spleen to enlarge is treated. Sometimes the spleen must be removed surgically.	Symptoms tend to be mild. Often, an enlarged spleen also traps platelets and white blood cells, thus reducing their number in the bloodstream.
Mechanical damage to red blood cells	Abnormalities in blood vessels (such as an aneurysm), an artificial or damaged heart valve, or extremely high blood pressure can break normal red blood cells apart.	The cause of the damage is identified and corrected.	The kidneys eventually filter the damaged red blood cells out of the blood but may be damaged by them. The spleen also filters the damaged red cells out of the blood.
Paroxysmal nocturnal hemoglobinuria	The immune system destroys red blood cells. Hemoglobin from these damaged cells is concentrated in urine during the night, resulting in dark, reddish urine in the morning.	Corticosteroids and a new antibody drug, eculizumab, help relieve symptoms, but the only cure is allogeneic bone marrow transplantation. People with blood clots may need to take an anticoagulant. Bone marrow transplantation may be needed.	People may have severe stomach cramps and clotting in the large veins of the abdomen and legs. Symptoms often occur in episodes (paroxysmally).
Hereditary spherocytosis	Red blood cells become misshapen and rigid, getting trapped and destroyed in the spleen.	Treatment is usually not needed, but severe anemia may require removal of the spleen.	This hereditary disorder can also cause bone abnormalities, such as a tower-shaped skull.
Hereditary elliptocytosis	Red blood cells are oval or elliptical in shape rather than the normal disk shape.	Severe anemia may require removal of the spleen.	The anemia is usually mild and requires no treatment.
Glucose-6-phosphate dehydrogenase (G6PD) deficiency	The G6PD enzyme is missing from red blood cell membranes. Without this enzyme, red blood cells are more likely to break apart when the person is stressed by triggers such as fever, infection, diabetic crisis, or certain drugs such as aspirin and sulfa drugs.	Anemia can be prevented by preventing or avoiding things that trigger it.	This hereditary disorder almost always affects males. About 10% of black males and a smaller percentage of white people of Mediterranean origin have the disorder.

anemia without the need for blood transfusions. Because iron, which is required to produce red blood cells, is lost during bleeding, most people who have anemia from bleeding need to take iron supplements, usually tablets, for several months.

Iron Deficiency Anemia

Iron deficiency anemia results from low or depleted stores of iron, which is needed to produce red blood cells.

- Excessive bleeding is the most common cause.
- People may be weak, short of breath, and pale.
- Blood tests can detect low levels of iron.
- Iron supplements are used to restore iron levels.

Iron deficiency anemia usually develops slowly, because it may take several months for the body's iron reserves to be used up. As the iron reserves are decreasing, the bone marrow gradually produces fewer red blood cells. When the reserves are depleted, the red blood cells are not only fewer in number but also abnormally small.

Iron deficiency is one of the most common causes of anemia, and blood loss is the most common cause of iron deficiency in adults. In men and postmenopausal women, iron deficiency usually indicates bleeding in the digestive tract. In premenopausal women, menstrual bleeding is the most common cause of iron deficiency. Iron deficiency may also result from too little iron in the diet (see page 941), especially in infants, young children, adolescent girls, and pregnant women.

> **? Did You Know...**
> In the United States, anemia rarely results from consuming too little iron because supplemental iron is added to many foods.

Symptoms and Diagnosis

Symptoms of iron deficiency anemia tend to develop gradually and are similar to symptoms produced by other types of anemia. Many people with iron deficiency anemia have pica. People with pica have a craving to ingest something, most commonly ice but sometimes a substance that is not food, such as dirt, clay, or chalk.

Once doctors diagnose anemia, tests for iron deficiency are often done. With iron deficiency, the red blood cells tend to be small and pale. Blood levels of iron and transferrin (the protein that carries iron when it is not inside red blood cells) are measured and compared. The most accurate test for iron deficiency is a measurement of the blood level of ferritin (a protein that stores iron). A low level of

ferritin indicates iron deficiency. However, sometimes ferritin levels are misleading because they can be falsely elevated (and thus appear normal) by liver damage, inflammation, infection, or cancer. In this case, doctors may measure the level of a protein on the surface of cells that binds to transferrin (transferrin receptor).

Treatment

Because excessive bleeding is the most common cause of iron deficiency, the first step is to locate its source.

Normal dietary iron intake usually cannot compensate for iron loss from chronic bleeding, and the body has a very small iron reserve. Consequently, lost iron must be replaced by taking iron supplements.

Correcting iron deficiency anemia with iron supplements usually takes 3 to 6 weeks, even after the bleeding has stopped. Iron supplements are usually taken by mouth. An iron supplement is absorbed best when taken 30 minutes before breakfast with a source of vitamin C (either orange juice or a vitamin C supplement). Iron supplements are typically continued for 6 months after the blood counts return to normal to fully replenish the body's reserves. Blood tests are done periodically to ensure that the iron supply is sufficient. Treating the iron deficiency treats pica.

Vitamin Deficiency Anemia

Vitamin deficiency anemia results from low or depleted levels of vitamin B_{12} or folate (folic acid).

- People may be weak, short of breath, and pale.
- Nerves may also malfunction.
- Blood tests can detect abnormal cells that indicate vitamin deficiency anemia.
- The deficient vitamin is replaced.

Vitamin B_{12} deficiency and folate (folic acid) deficiency cause megaloblastic anemia. In megaloblastic anemia, the bone marrow produces red cells that are large and abnormal (megaloblasts).

Deficiency of vitamin B_{12} (see page 926) or folate (see page 920) most often develops due to a lack of these vitamins in the diet or an inability to absorb these vitamins from the digestive tract. Deficiency of these vitamins is sometimes caused by drugs used to treat cancer, such as methotrexate, hydroxyurea, fluorouracil, and cytarabine. A form of vitamin B_{12} deficiency called pernicious anemia results from an inability to absorb vitamin B_{12} from the diet.

Symptoms and Diagnosis

Symptoms of anemia due to vitamin B_{12} or folate deficiency develop slowly and are similar to symptoms

Aplastic Anemia: When the Bone Marrow Shuts Down

When the bone marrow cells that develop into mature blood cells and platelets (stem cells) are damaged or suppressed, the bone marrow can shut down. This bone marrow failure is called aplastic anemia. A common cause of aplastic anemia is an autoimmune disorder, in which the immune system suppresses bone marrow stem cells. Other causes include infection with parvovirus, radiation exposure, toxins (such as benzene), chemotherapy drugs, and other drugs (such as chloramphenicol).

The bone marrow failure leads to too few red blood cells (anemia), too few white blood cells (leukopenia), and too few platelets (thrombocytopenia). The anemia causes fatigue, weakness, and paleness. The leukopenia causes increased susceptibility to infection. The thrombocytopenia causes easy bruising and bleeding. In some people, only red blood cell production is affected (resulting in a condition called pure red blood cell aphasia). When parvovirus infection is the cause, only red blood cell production is likely to be affected. Aplastic anemia is diagnosed when microscopic examination of a sample of bone marrow (bone marrow biopsy) reveals a sharp decrease in the number of stem cells and in the maturation of blood cells.

People with severe aplastic anemia quickly die unless immediately treated. Transfusions of red blood cells, platelets, and substances called growth factors may temporarily increase the numbers of red blood cells, white blood cells, and platelets. Stem cell or bone marrow transplantation can cure aplastic anemia in younger and middle-aged people. Older adults and people without a suitable bone marrow donor often respond to treatment with corticosteroids and drugs that suppress the immune system.

---

produced by other types of anemia. Vitamin B_{12} deficiency can also cause nerves to malfunction, causing tingling, loss of sensation, and muscle weakness (see page 926).

Once anemia has been diagnosed, tests are done to determine if a deficiency of vitamin B_{12} or folate is the cause. Anemia due to vitamin B_{12} or folate deficiency is suspected when megaloblasts are seen in a blood sample that is examined under a microscope. Changes in white blood cells and platelets also can be detected, especially when people have had megaloblastic anemia for a long time.

The blood levels of vitamin B_{12} and folate are measured, and other tests may be done to determine the cause of the vitamin deficiency.

Treatment

The treatment of anemia due to vitamin B_{12} or folate deficiency consists of replacing the deficient vitamin.

Commonly, vitamin B_{12} is administered by injection. At first, injections are given daily or weekly for several weeks until the blood levels of vitamin B_{12} return to normal. Then injections are given once a month. Vitamin B_{12} can also be taken daily as a nose spray, a tablet placed under the tongue, or a tablet that is swallowed. Generally, intramuscular injections of vitamin B_{12} are necessary to correct pernicious anemia. People who have anemia due to vitamin B_{12} deficiency usually must take vitamin B_{12} supplements for life.

Folate can be taken as one tablet daily. People who have trouble absorbing folate take supplements for life.

Anemia of Chronic Disease

In anemia of chronic disease, some chronic disorder slows the production of red blood cells, the result of production of proteins called cytokines that interfere with the production of red blood cells.

Chronic disease often leads to anemia, especially in older adults. Conditions such as infections, inflammation, and cancer particularly suppress production of red blood cells in the bone marrow. Since the suppression is usually not severe, anemia develops slowly and is evident only after time. Problems with how the body uses iron contribute to anemia of chronic disease. Because the bone marrow is unable to use stored iron to create new red blood cells, this type of anemia is often called iron-reutilization anemia.

Because this type of anemia develops slowly and is generally mild, it usually produces few or no symptoms. When symptoms do occur, they usually result from the disease causing the anemia rather than from the anemia itself. There are no specific laboratory tests, so the diagnosis is typically made by excluding other causes.

Because no specific treatment exists for this type of anemia, doctors treat the disorder causing it. Taking additional iron or vitamins does not help. On the rare occasion that the anemia becomes severe, transfusions may help. Alternatively, erythropoietin or darbepoietin, drugs that stimulate the bone marrow to produce red blood cells, may be given.

Autoimmune Hemolytic Anemia

Autoimmune hemolytic anemia is a group of disorders characterized by a malfunction of the immune system that produces autoantibodies, which attack red blood cells as if they were substances foreign to the body.

- Some people have no symptoms, and other people are tired, short of breath, and pale.
- Severe disease may cause jaundice or abdominal discomfort and fullness.
- Blood tests are used to detect anemia and determine the cause of the autoimmune reaction.
- Some people need corticosteroids or drugs that suppress the immune system.

Autoimmune hemolytic anemia is an uncommon group of disorders that can occur at any age. These disorders affect women more often than men. About half of the time, the cause of autoimmune hemolytic anemia cannot be determined (idiopathic autoimmune hemolytic anemia). Autoimmune hemolytic anemia can also be caused by or occur with another disorder, such as systemic lupus erythematosus (lupus), and rarely it follows the use of certain drugs, such as penicillin.

Destruction of red blood cells by autoantibodies may occur suddenly, or it may develop gradually. In some people, the destruction may stop after a period of time. In other people, red blood cell destruction persists and becomes chronic. There are two main types of autoimmune hemolytic anemia: warm antibody hemolytic anemia and cold antibody hemolytic anemia. In the warm antibody type, the autoantibodies attach to and destroy red blood cells at temperatures equal to or in excess of normal body temperature. In the cold antibody type, the autoantibodies become most active and attack red blood cells only at temperatures well below normal body temperature.

Symptoms

Some people with autoimmune hemolytic anemia may have no symptoms, especially when the destruction of red blood cells is mild and develops gradually. Others have symptoms similar to those that occur with other types of anemia, especially when the destruction is more severe or rapid. When severe or rapid destruction of red blood cells occurs, mild jaundice may also develop. When destruction persists for a few months or longer, the spleen may enlarge, resulting in a sense of abdominal fullness and, occasionally, discomfort.

When the cause of autoimmune hemolytic anemia is another disease, symptoms of the underlying disorder, such as swollen and tender lymph nodes and fever, may dominate.

Diagnosis

Once doctors diagnose anemia, increased destruction of red blood cells is suspected when a blood test shows an increase in the number of red blood cells that are immature (reticulocytes). Alternatively, a blood test may show an increased amount of a substance called bilirubin and a decreased amount of a protein called haptoglobin.

Autoimmune hemolytic anemia as the cause is confirmed when blood tests detect increased amounts of certain antibodies, either attached to red blood cells (direct antiglobulin or direct Coombs' test) or in the liquid portion of the blood (indirect antiglobulin or indirect Coombs' test). Other tests sometimes help determine the cause of the autoimmune reaction that is destroying red blood cells.

Treatment

If symptoms are mild or if destruction of red blood cells seems to be slowing on its own, no treatment is needed. If red blood cell destruction is increasing, a corticosteroid such as prednisone is usually the first choice for treatment. High doses are used at first, followed by a gradual reduction of the dose over many weeks or months. When people do not respond to corticosteroids or when the corticosteroid causes intolerable side effects, surgery to remove the spleen (splenectomy) is often the next treatment. The spleen is removed because it is one of the places where antibody-coated red blood cells are destroyed. When destruction of red blood cells persists after removal of the spleen or when surgery cannot be done, immunosuppressive drugs, such as cyclophosphamide or azathioprine, are used.

When red blood cell destruction is severe, blood transfusions are sometimes needed, but they do not treat the cause of the anemia and provide only temporary relief.

Sickle Cell Disease

Sickle cell disease is an inherited condition characterized by sickle (crescent)-shaped red blood cells and chronic anemia caused by excessive destruction of red blood cells.

- People usually have anemia and jaundice.
- Worsening anemia, fever, and shortness of breath with pain in the long bones, abdomen, and chest indicate sickle cell crisis.
- A special blood test called electrophoresis can be used to determine whether people have sickle cell disease.
- Avoiding activities that may cause crises and treating infections and other disorders quickly can help prevent crises.

Sickle cell disease affects blacks almost exclusively. About 10% of blacks in the United States have one copy of the gene for sickle cell disease (that is, they have sickle cell trait). People who have sickle cell trait do not develop sickle cell disease,

Red Blood Cell Shapes

Normal red blood cells are flexible and disk-shaped, thicker at the edges than in the middle. In several hereditary disorders, red blood cells become spherical (in hereditary spherocytosis), oval (in hereditary elliptocytosis), or sickle-shaped (in sickle cell disease).

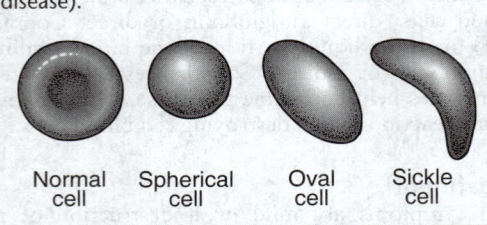

| Normal cell | Spherical cell | Oval cell | Sickle cell |

although rarely they may notice blood in their urine. About 0.3% of blacks have two copies of the gene. These people develop the disease.

In sickle cell disease, the red blood cells contain an abnormal form of hemoglobin (the protein that carries oxygen). The abnormal form of hemoglobin is called hemoglobin S. When red blood cells contain a large amount of hemoglobin S, they can become deformed into a sickle-shape. Not every red blood cell is sickle-shaped. The sickle-shaped cells become more numerous when people have infections or low levels of oxygen in the blood.

The sickle cells are fragile and break apart easily. Because the sickle cells are stiff, they have difficulty traveling through the smallest blood vessels, causing blocked blood flow, and reduced oxygen supply. The blocked blood flow can cause pain and, over time, cause damage to the spleen, kidneys, brain, bones, and other organs. Kidney failure and heart failure may occur.

Symptoms and Complications

People who have sickle cell disease always have some degree of anemia and mild jaundice. Some people have few other symptoms. Others have severe, recurring symptoms that cause enormous disability and early death. Sickle cell trait usually does not cause any problems, but rarely, people die suddenly while undergoing very strenuous exercise that causes severe dehydration, such as during military or athletic training.

Sickle Cell Crisis: Anything that reduces the amount of oxygen in the blood, such as vigorous exercise, mountain climbing, flying at high altitudes without sufficient oxygen, or an illness, may bring on a sickle cell crisis. A sickle cell crisis may consist of a sudden worsening of anemia, pain (often in the abdomen or long bones of the arms and legs), fever, and sometimes shortness of breath. Abdominal pain may be severe, and vomiting may occur.

In children, sickle cell crisis may take the form of a chest syndrome, characterized by severe chest pain and difficulty breathing. The exact cause of the chest syndrome is unknown but may be related to or produced by an infection or a blocked blood vessel resulting from a blood clot or an embolus (a piece of a blood clot that has broken off and lodged in a blood vessel).

Complications: Most people who have sickle cell disease develop an enlarged spleen during childhood. By the time the person reaches adolescence, the spleen is often so badly injured that it shrinks and no longer functions. Because the spleen helps fight infection, people with sickle cell disease are more likely to develop pneumococcal pneumonia and other infections. Viral infections, in particular, can decrease blood cell production, so anemia becomes more severe.

The liver can become progressively larger throughout life, and gallstones often form from the pigment of broken-apart red blood cells.

The heart usually enlarges, and heart murmurs are common.

Children who have sickle cell disease often have a relatively short torso but long arms, legs, fingers, and toes. Changes in the bones and bone marrow may cause bone pain, especially in the hands and feet. Episodes of joint pain with fever may occur, and the hip joint may become so damaged that it eventually needs to be replaced.

Poor circulation to the skin may cause sores on the legs, especially at the ankles. Young men may develop persistent, often painful erections (priapism). Episodes of priapism may permanently damage the penis so that the man can no longer have erections. Blocked blood vessels may cause strokes that damage the nervous system. In older people, lung and kidney function may deteriorate.

Diagnosis

Doctors recognize anemia, stomach and bone pain, and nausea in a young black person as signs of a sickle cell crisis. When doctors suspect sickle cell disease, they do blood tests. Sickle-shaped red blood cells and fragments of destroyed red blood cells can be seen in a blood sample examined under a microscope. Another blood test called hemoglobin electrophoresis is also done. In electrophoresis, an electrical current is used to separate the different types of hemoglobin and thus detect abnormal hemoglobin.

Screening: Blood tests are done on relatives of people with the disorder because they also may have sickle cell disease or trait. Discovering the trait in people may be important for family planning, to determine their risk of having a child with sickle cell disease.

Newborns are routinely screened with a blood test. Newer tests can be done during early pregnancy to screen the fetus and allow prenatal counseling (see page 1611) for couples who are at risk of having a child with sickle cell disease. Fetal cells obtained through amniocentesis or chorionic villus sampling are tested for the presence of the sickle cell gene.

Treatment

Because sickle cell disease is rarely cured, treatment is aimed at preventing crises, controlling the anemia, and relieving symptoms. People who have this disease should try to avoid activities that reduce the amount of oxygen in their blood and should seek prompt medical attention for even minor illnesses, such as viral infections. Because people are at increased risk of infection, they should receive pneumococcal and *Haemophilus influenzae* vaccines.

Sickle cell crisis may require hospitalization. People are given fluid intravenously and drugs to relieve pain. Blood transfusions and oxygen may be given if doctors suspect that anemia is severe enough to pose a risk of stroke, heart attack, or lung damage. Conditions that may have caused the crisis, such as an infection, are treated.

Drugs can help control sickle cell disease. Hydroxyurea increases the production of a form of hemoglobin found predominantly in fetuses, which decreases the number of red blood cells becoming sickle-shaped. Therefore, it reduces the frequency of sickle cell crises.

Bone marrow or stem cells from a family member or other donor who does not have the sickle cell gene may be transplanted in a person with the disease. Although such transplantation may be curative, it is risky, and recipients must take drugs that suppress the immune system for the rest of their life.

Gene therapy, a technique in which normal genes are implanted in precursor cells (cells that produce blood cells), is being studied.

Hemoglobin C, S-C, and E Diseases

Hemoglobin C, S-C, and E diseases are inherited conditions characterized by abnormally shaped red blood cells and chronic anemia that is caused by excessive destruction of red blood cells.

Hemoglobin C, S, and E are abnormal forms of hemoglobin (the protein in red blood cells that carries oxygen). These abnormal forms of hemoglobin result from inheriting an abnormal gene.

Hemoglobin C disease occurs mostly in blacks. One copy of the gene that causes hemoglobin C disease is present in 2 to 3% of blacks in the United States. However, people must inherit two copies of the abnormal gene to develop the disease. In general, symptoms are few. Anemia varies in severity. People who have this disease, particularly children, may have episodes of abdominal and joint pain, an enlarged spleen, and mild jaundice, but they do not have severe crises, as occur in sickle cell disease.

Hemoglobin S-C disease occurs in people who have one copy of the gene for sickle cell disease and one copy of the gene for hemoglobin C disease. Hemoglobin S-C disease is more common than hemoglobin C disease, and its symptoms are similar to those of sickle cell disease but milder.

Hemoglobin E disease affects primarily people from Southeast Asia. This disease produces anemia but none of the other symptoms that occur in sickle cell disease and hemoglobin C disease. Diagnosis is by a blood test called hemoglobin electrophoresis. Treatment varies depending on the severity of symptoms but can include some of the same treatments that are used in people with sickle cell disease.

Thalassemias

Thalassemias are a group of inherited disorders resulting from an imbalance in the production of one of the four chains of amino acids that make up hemoglobin (the oxygen-carrying protein found in red blood cells).

- Symptoms depend on the type of thalassemia.
- Some people have jaundice, skin ulcers, and abdominal fullness or discomfort.
- Diagnosis usually requires special hemoglobin tests.
- Mild thalassemia may not require treatment, but severe thalassemia may require bone marrow transplantation.

Hemoglobin is made up of two pairs of globin chains. Normally, adults have one pair of alpha chains and one pair of beta chains. Sometimes one or more of these chains is abnormal. Thalassemias are categorized according to the amino acid chain affected. The two main types are alpha-thalassemia (the alpha globin chain is affected) and beta-thalassemia (the beta globin chain is affected). Alpha-thalassemia is most common in blacks (25% carry at least one copy of the defective gene), and beta-thalassemia is most common in people from the Mediterranean area and Southeast Asia. Thalassemias are also categorized according to whether people have one copy of the defective gene (thalassemia minor) or two copies of the defective gene (thalassemia major).

All thalassemias have similar symptoms, but they vary in severity. In alpha-thalassemia minor and beta-thalassemia minor, people have mild anemia with no symptoms. In alpha-thalassemia major, people have moderate or severe symptoms of anemia, including fatigue, shortness of breath, paleness, and an enlarged spleen.

In beta-thalassemia major, people have severe symptoms of anemia, and they may also have jaundice, skin ulcers, and gallstones. People may also have an enlarged spleen, which leads to a feeling of fullness and abdominal discomfort. Over-active bone marrow may cause some bones, especially those in the head and face, to thicken and enlarge. The long bones in the arms and legs may weaken and fracture easily.

Children who have beta-thalassemia major may grow more slowly and reach puberty later than they normally would. Because iron absorption may be increased and frequent blood transfusions (providing even more iron) are needed, excessive iron may accumulate and be deposited in the heart muscle, eventually causing iron overload disease and heart failure and early death.

Thalassemias are more difficult to diagnose than other hemoglobin disorders. Testing a drop of blood by electrophoresis is helpful but may be inconclusive, especially for alpha-thalassemia. Therefore, the diagnosis is usually based on special hemoglobin tests and determination of hereditary patterns.

Most people who have a mild thalassemia do not need treatment, but people who have a severe form may need bone marrow transplantation. Gene therapy, in which normal genes are inserted in the person, is being studied but to date has been unsuccessful.

CHAPTER 157   Bleeding and Clotting Disorders

Hemostasis is the body's way of stopping injured blood vessels from bleeding. Hemostasis includes clotting of the blood. Too much clotting can block blood vessels that are not bleeding; consequently, the body has control mechanisms to limit clotting and dissolve clots that are no longer needed. An abnormality in any part of this system that controls bleeding can lead to excessive bleeding or excessive clotting, both of which can be dangerous. When clotting is poor, even a slight injury to a blood vessel may lead to major blood loss. When clotting is uncontrolled, small blood vessels in critical places can become clogged with clots. Clogged vessels in the brain can cause strokes; clogged vessels leading to the heart can cause heart attacks; and pieces of clots from veins in the legs, pelvis, or abdomen can travel through the bloodstream to the lungs and block major arteries there (pulmonary embolism).

Hemostasis involves three major processes: narrowing (constriction) of blood vessels, activity of platelets, and activity of blood clotting factors.

An injured blood vessel constricts so that blood flows out more slowly and clotting can start. At the same time, the accumulating pool of blood outside the blood vessel (a hematoma) presses against the vessel, helping prevent further bleeding. As soon as a blood vessel wall is damaged, a series of reactions activates platelets so that they stick to the injured area. The "glue" that holds platelets to the blood vessel wall is von Willebrand factor, a protein produced by the cells of the vessel wall. The proteins collagen and thrombin act at the site of the injury to induce platelets to stick together. As platelets accumulate at the site, they form a mesh that plugs the injury. The platelets change shape from round to spiny, and they release proteins and other substances that entrap more platelets and clotting proteins in the enlarging plug that becomes a blood clot.

Formation of a clot also involves activation of a sequence of blood clotting factors that generate thrombin. Thrombin converts fibrinogen, a blood clotting factor that is normally dissolved in blood, into long strands of fibrin that radiate from the clumped platelets and form a net that entraps more platelets and blood cells. The fibrin strands add bulk to the developing clot and help hold it in place to keep the vessel wall plugged.

The reactions that result in the formation of a blood clot are balanced by other reactions that stop the clotting process and dissolve clots after the blood vessel has healed. Without this control system, minor blood vessel injuries could trigger widespread clotting throughout the body—which actually happens in some diseases.

Blood Clots: Plugging the Breaks

When an injury causes a blood vessel wall to break, platelets are activated. They change shape from round to spiny, stick to the broken vessel wall and each other, and begin to plug the break. They also interact with other blood proteins to form fibrin. Fibrin strands form a net that entraps more platelets and blood cells, producing a clot that plugs the break.

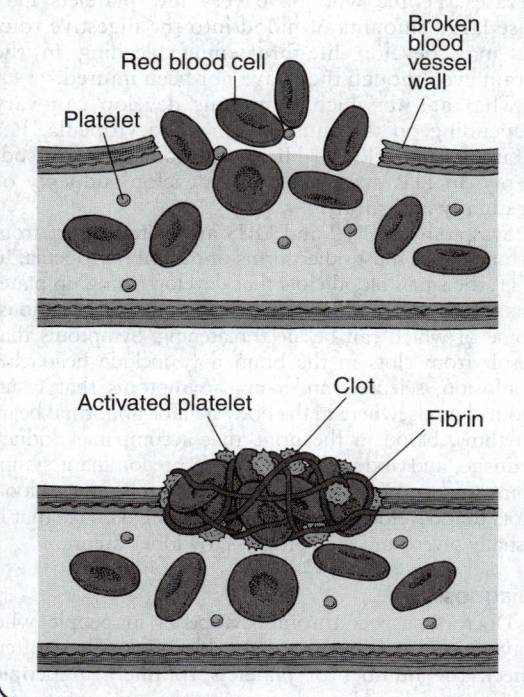

Hereditary Hemorrhagic Telangiectasia

Hereditary hemorrhagic telangiectasia (Rendu-Osler-Weber disease) is a hereditary disorder in which blood vessels are malformed, making them fragile and prone to bleeding.

Blood vessels under the skin may break and bleed, causing small, red-to-violet discolorations, especially on the face, lips, lining of the mouth and nose, and tips of the fingers and toes. Severe nosebleeds may also occur. Small blood vessels in the digestive and urinary tracts, as well as in the brain and spinal cord, may also be affected, causing bleeding in these sites.

Treatment is aimed at stopping an occurrence of bleeding. Treatment may involve applying pressure, using a topical drug that narrows blood vessels (astringent), or using a laser beam to destroy the leaking blood vessel. Severe bleeding may require more invasive techniques. Bleeding almost always recurs, resulting in iron deficiency anemia; consequently, people with hereditary hemorrhagic telangiectasia need to take iron supplements. Some people may also need to take drugs that inhibit the formation of fibrin.

Thrombocytopenia

Thrombocytopenia is a deficiency of platelets (thrombocytes).

- Thrombocytopenia occurs when the bone marrow makes too few platelets or when too many platelets are destroyed.
- Bleeding in the skin and bruising occur.
- Blood tests are used to make the diagnosis and determine the cause.
- Sometimes platelet transfusions are needed.

The blood usually contains about 140,000 to 440,000 platelets per microliter. Bleeding can occur with relatively minor trauma when the platelet count falls below about 50,000 platelets per microliter of blood. The most serious risk of bleeding, however, generally does not occur until the platelet count falls below 10,000 to 20,000 platelets per microliter. At these very low levels, bleeding may occur without any injury.

Causes

Many diseases can cause thrombocytopenia. Thrombocytopenia can occur when the bone marrow does not produce enough platelets, as happens in leukemia and some anemias. Infection with the human immunodeficiency virus (HIV), the virus that causes AIDS, often results in thrombocytopenia. Platelets can become entrapped in an enlarged spleen, as happens in myelofibrosis and Gaucher's disease, reducing the number of platelets in the bloodstream. Massive blood transfusions can dilute the concentration of platelets in the blood. Finally, the body may use or destroy too many platelets, as occurs in many disorders, three of the most notable being idiopathic thrombocytopenic purpura, thrombotic thrombocytopenic purpura, and hemolytic-uremic syndrome.

Idiopathic Thrombocytopenic Purpura (ITP): ITP is a disease in which antibodies form and destroy the body's platelets. Why the antibodies form is not known. Although the bone marrow increases platelet production to compensate for the destruction, the supply cannot keep up with the demand.

Thrombotic Thrombocytopenic Purpura (TTP): TTP is a rare disease in which small blood clots form suddenly throughout the body. The blood clots mean that an abnormally high number of platelets are being used, which leads to a sharp decrease in the number of platelets in the bloodstream.

Causes of Thrombocytopenia

BONE MARROW DOES NOT PRODUCE ENOUGH PLATELETS

- Leukemia
- Lymphoma
- Aplastic anemia
- Heavy alcohol consumption
- Megaloblastic anemias, including vitamin B_{12} and folate deficiency anemias
- Some bone marrow disorders

PLATELETS BECOME ENTRAPPED IN AN ENLARGED SPLEEN

- Cirrhosis with congestive splenomegaly
- Myelofibrosis
- Gaucher's disease

PLATELETS BECOME DILUTED

- Massive blood replacement or exchange transfusion with stored blood containing too few platelets
- Cardiopulmonary bypass surgery

USE OR DESTRUCTION OF PLATELETS INCREASES

- Idiopathic thrombocytopenic purpura
- HIV infection
- Drugs such as heparin, quinidine, quinine, sulfa-containing antibiotics, some oral drugs for diabetes, gold salts, and rifampin
- Conditions involving disseminated intravascular coagulation within blood vessels, as can occur with obstetric complications, cancer, blood poisoning (septicemia) from gram-negative bacteria, and traumatic brain damage
- Thrombotic thrombocytopenic purpura
- Hemolytic-uremic syndrome
- Paroxysmal nocturnal hemoglobinuria

Hemolytic-Uremic Syndrome (HUS): HUS is a disorder related to TTP in which the number of platelets suddenly decreases, red blood cells are destroyed, and the kidneys stop functioning. HUS is rare but can occur with certain bacterial infections (particularly intestinal infections with *Escherichia coli* O157:H7 or some strains of *Shigella dysenteriae*) and with the use of some drugs (including quinine, cyclosporine, and mitomycin C). The syndrome is most common in infants, young children, and women who are pregnant or have just given birth, although it can occur in older children, adults, and women who are not pregnant.

Symptoms and Complications

Bleeding in the skin may be the first sign of a low platelet count. Many tiny red dots (petechiae) often appear in the skin on the lower legs, and minor injuries may cause small scattered bruises. The gums may bleed, and blood may appear in the stool or urine. Menstrual periods may be unusually heavy. Bleeding may be hard to stop.

Bleeding worsens as the number of platelets decreases. People who have very few platelets may lose large amounts of blood into the digestive tract or may develop life-threatening bleeding in the brain even though they have not been injured.

The rate at which symptoms develop can vary depending on the cause of thrombocytopenia. For example, in TTP and HUS, symptoms develop suddenly. In ITP, symptoms may develop suddenly or gradually and subtly.

Symptoms in TTP and HUS are quite distinct from symptoms of most other forms of thrombocytopenia. In TTP, the small blood clots that develop (using up platelets) cause a wide range of symptoms and complications, some of which can be life threatening. Symptoms that result from clots in the brain may include headache, confusion, seizures, and coma. Symptoms that result from clots elsewhere in the body include abnormal heart rhythms, blood in the urine that accompanies kidney damage, and abdominal pain. The predominant symptoms and complications of HUS are related to blood clots that develop in the kidneys, causing damage that is usually severe and may progress to kidney failure.

Diagnosis

Doctors suspect thrombocytopenia in people who have abnormal bruising and bleeding. They often check the number of platelets routinely in people who have disorders that cause thrombocytopenia. Sometimes they discover thrombocytopenia when blood tests are performed for other reasons in people who have no bruising or bleeding.

Determining the cause of thrombocytopenia is critical to treating the condition. Certain symptoms may help determine the cause. For example, people usually have a fever when thrombocytopenia results from an infection. In contrast, they usually do not have a fever when the cause is ITP, TTP, or HUS. An enlarged spleen, which a doctor may be able to feel during a physical examination, suggests that the spleen is trapping platelets and that thrombocytopenia results from a disorder that causes the spleen to enlarge. HUS is diagnosed when poor kidney function is identified by blood tests that show high levels of urea nitrogen and creatinine.

A sample of blood may be examined under a microscope, or the platelet count may be measured with an electronic counter to determine the severity of thrombocytopenia and provide clues to its cause. A sample of bone marrow removed and examined under a microscope (bone marrow aspiration and biopsy—see page 1025) may be needed to provide information about platelet production.

Treatment

People who have a very low platelet count are often treated in a hospital or advised to stay in bed to avoid accidental injury. When bleeding is severe, platelets may be transfused.

Addressing the underlying cause can often treat the thrombocytopenia. Thrombocytopenia caused by a drug usually is corrected by discontinuing the drug. The effects produced by antibodies that destroy platelets in ITP can be blocked temporarily with a corticosteroid (for example, prednisone) or intravenous immune globulin, allowing the number of platelets to increase. Danazol may have similar effects as prednisone. Drugs that suppress the immune system, including cyclophosphamide and sometimes azathioprine, may reduce the formation of antibodies. Most adults (but not children) with ITP eventually require surgical removal of the spleen (splenectomy) to increase the number of platelets. People with TTP are often treated with plasma transfusions along with plasmapheresis (see box on page 1030). The two procedures together are called plasma exchange.

Complications that require long-term treatment can result from some causes of thrombocytopenia. For example, the number of platelets usually increases as people recover from HUS. However, lifelong dialysis or kidney transplantation may be needed if the kidney failure persists.

Von Willebrand's Disease

Von Willebrand's disease is a hereditary deficiency or abnormality of the blood protein von Willebrand factor, which affects platelet function.

The von Willebrand factor is found in plasma, platelets, and the walls of blood vessels. When the factor is missing or defective, platelets cannot adhere to the vessel wall at the site of an injury. As a result, bleeding does not stop as quickly as it should.

Symptoms and Diagnosis

Often, a person with von Willebrand's disease has a parent who has a history of bleeding problems. Typically, a child bruises easily or bleeds excessively after a cut, tooth extraction, or surgery. A young woman may have increased menstrual bleeding. Bleeding may worsen at times. On the other hand, hormonal changes, stress, pregnancy, inflammation, and infections may stimulate the body to increase production of the von Willebrand factor and tempo-

Drugs and Blood Clots: A Complicated Relationship

The relationship between drugs and the body's ability to control bleeding (hemostasis) is complicated. The body's ability to form blood clots is vital to hemostasis, but too much clotting increases the risk of a heart attack, stroke, or pulmonary embolism. Many drugs, either intentionally or unintentionally, affect the body's ability to form blood clots.

Some people are at high risk of forming blood clots and are intentionally given drugs to decrease the risk. Drugs may be given that reduce the stickiness of platelets, so that they will not clump together to block a blood vessel. Aspirin, ticlopidine, clopidogrel, abciximab, and tirofiban are examples of drugs that interfere with the activity of platelets.

Other people at risk of forming blood clots may be given an anticoagulant, a drug that inhibits the action of blood proteins called clotting factors. Although often called "blood thinners," anticoagulants do not really thin the blood. Commonly used anticoagulants are warfarin, given by mouth, and heparin, given by injection. People who take these drugs must be under close medical supervision. Doctors monitor the effects of these drugs with blood tests that measure the time it takes for a clot to form, and they adjust the dose on the basis of test results. Doses that are too low may not prevent clots, while doses that are too high may cause severe bleeding. Another type of anticoagulant, low-molecular-weight heparin, does not require as much supervision. Lepirudin, bivalirudin, and argatroban are newer types of anticoagulants that directly act on thrombin, a protein that helps induce clotting.

If a person already has a blood clot, a thrombolytic (fibrinolytic) drug can be given to help dissolve the clot. Thrombolytic drugs, which include streptokinase and tissue plasminogen activator, are sometimes used to treat heart attacks and strokes caused by blood clots. These drugs may save lives, but they can also put the person at risk of severe bleeding. Surprisingly, heparin, a drug given to reduce the risk of clot formation, sometimes has an unintended activating effect on platelets that increases the risk of clotting (heparin-induced thrombocytopenia).

Estrogen, alone or in oral contraceptives, can have the unintended effect of causing excessive clot formation. Certain drugs used to treat cancer (chemotherapy drugs), such as asparaginase, can also increase the risk of clotting.

rarily improve the capacity of platelets to stick to the blood vessel wall and stop bleeding.

Laboratory tests typically show that the time it takes for blood to clot is abnormally long. Bleeding time is the amount of time that elapses before bleeding stops after a small cut is made on the forearm. Doctors may order tests that measure the amount of von Willebrand factor in the blood. Because the von Willebrand factor is the protein that carries an important clotting factor (factor VIII) in the blood, the level of factor VIII in the blood may also be decreased.

Treatment

Many people with von Willebrand's disease never need treatment. If excessive bleeding occurs, a transfusion of concentrated blood clotting factors containing von Willebrand factor may be given. For some mild forms of the disease, drug treatment with desmopressin may be given to increase the amount of the von Willebrand factor long enough for surgery or dental procedures to be performed without transfusions.

Hemophilia

Hemophilia is a bleeding disorder caused by a deficiency in one of two blood clotting factors: factor VIII or factor IX.

- Several different gene abnormalities can cause the disorder.
- People bleed unexpectedly or after minor injuries.
- Blood tests are needed for diagnosis.
- Transfusions are given to replace missing clotting factors.

There are two forms of hemophilia. Hemophilia A, which accounts for about 80% of all cases, is a deficiency in clotting factor VIII. Hemophilia B is a deficiency in clotting factor IX. The bleeding patterns and consequences of these two types of hemophilia are similar.

Deficiency of clotting factor XI also causes a hereditary bleeding disorder. About 50% of cases of factor XI deficiency occur among people of Eastern European Jewish ancestry. Factor XI deficiency affects both males and females and may cause bleeding after injury or surgery. Spontaneous bleeding episodes are usually less frequent and milder than in hemophilia A or B.

Hemophilia is caused by several different gene abnormalities. They are sex-linked, which means that the gene abnormalities are inherited through the mother and that nearly everyone with hemophilia is male.

Symptoms and Complications

The severity of the symptoms depends on how a particular gene abnormality affects the blood clotting activity of factor VIII or IX. People whose clotting activity is 5 to 25% of normal have very mild hemophilia that may go undiagnosed; however, these people may bleed more than expected after surgery, dental extractions, or a major injury. People whose blood clotting activity is 1 to 5% of normal may have only mild hemophilia. They have few unprovoked bleeding episodes, but surgery or injury may cause uncontrolled and fatal bleeding. When the clotting activity is less than 1% of normal, hemophilia is severe. Serious episodes of bleeding occur and recur for no apparent reason.

In severe hemophilia, the first bleeding episode often occurs during or immediately after delivery. The infant may develop a collection of blood under the scalp (cephalhematoma) or may bleed excessively during circumcision. A bleeding episode generally occurs before 18 months of age and may follow a minor injury. A child who has hemophilia bruises easily. Even an injection into a muscle can cause bleeding that results in a large bruise and hematoma. Recurring bleeding into the joints and muscles can lead to crippling deformities. Bleeding can swell the base of the tongue until it blocks the airway, making breathing difficult. A slight bump on the head can trigger substantial bleeding in the brain or between the brain and the skull, causing brain damage and death.

 Did You Know...
Hemophilia can affect both males and females.

Diagnosis and Treatment

A doctor may suspect hemophilia in a child (especially a boy) who bleeds without an apparent cause or bleeds more than expected after injury. A blood test can determine whether the person's clotting is abnormally slow. If it is, further blood tests can confirm the diagnosis of hemophilia and can determine its type and severity.

People who have hemophilia should avoid situations that might provoke bleeding and should avoid drugs (for example, aspirin) that interfere with the function of platelets. They should be conscientious about dental care so that they will not need to have teeth extracted. If people who have milder forms of hemophilia need to have dental or other surgery, the drugs aminocaproic acid or desmopressin may be given to improve temporarily the body's ability to control bleeding so that transfusions can be avoided.

Often, treatment involves transfusions to replace the deficient clotting factor. These factors are normally present in the liquid component of blood (plasma). Clotting factors may be obtained from donated blood by concentrating or purifying them from plasma products, or they may be produced using special technological procedures as highly purified recombinant factor concentrates. Recombinant forms of both factor VIII and IX are available; because they are not obtained from human donors, they do not have the risk of infection that is present with factors derived from donated blood. The dose, frequency, and duration of therapy are determined by the site and severity of the bleeding problem. Clotting factors may also be used to prevent bleeding before surgery or at the first sign of bleeding.

Some people with hemophilia develop antibodies to transfused clotting factors, which destroy the factors. As a result, factor replacement therapy becomes less effective. If antibodies are detected in the blood of a person with hemophilia, the dosage of the recombinant factor or plasma concentrates may be increased, or different types of clotting factors or drugs to reduce the antibody levels may be needed.

Thrombophilia

Thrombophilia is a disorder in which the blood clots easily or excessively.

- Inherited and acquired disorders can increase blood clotting.
- Clots cause legs or arms to swell.
- Blood levels of proteins that control clotting are measured.
- People may need anticoagulants.

Most disorders that cause thrombophilia increase the risk of blood clot formation in veins; a few increase the risk of clot formation in both arteries and veins.

Causes

Some of the disorders that cause thrombophilia are inherited. Many of these result from changes in the amount or function of certain proteins in the blood that control clotting. For example, activated protein C resistance (Factor V Leiden mutation); a specific mutation in the prothrombin gene (prothrombin 20210 mutation); and a deficiency of protein C, protein S, or antithrombin all cause an increase in the production of fibrin, an important protein involved in clot formation. Hyperhomocysteinemia, an increase in the amount of homocysteine (a type of amino acid) in the blood, may increase the risk of clotting in veins and arteries.

Other disorders that cause thrombophilia are acquired after birth. These disorders include disseminated intravascular coagulation (often associated with cancer) and antiphospholipid antibody (anticardiolipin) syndrome (including the presence of the lupus "anticoagulant"), which increase the risk of clotting because of overactivation of blood clotting factors.

Other factors may increase the risk of clotting along with thrombophilia. Many involve conditions that result in a person's not moving around sufficiently, causing blood to pool in the veins. Examples include paralysis, prolonged sitting (especially in confined spaces as in a car or airplane), prolonged bed rest, recent surgery, and heart attack. Heart failure, a condition in which the blood is not pumped sufficiently through the bloodstream, is a risk factor. Conditions that result in increased pressure on veins, including obesity and pregnancy, also increase risk.

Symptoms and Complications

Most of the inherited disorders do not begin to cause an increased risk of clotting until young adulthood, although clots can form at any age. Many people with inherited disorders develop a deep vein clot (deep vein thrombosis) in the legs, which can result in leg swelling. Formation of a deep leg clot may be followed by pulmonary embolism. After several deep vein clots have occurred, more serious swelling and skin discoloration may develop (chronic deep vein insufficiency). Sometimes, clots form in superficial leg veins, causing pain and redness (superficial thrombophlebitis). Less commonly, clots may form in arm veins, abdominal veins, and veins inside the skull. Hyperhomocysteinemia and the antiphospholipid syndrome may result in venous or arterial clots. When clots obstruct blood flow in arteries, tissues lose their blood supply and may be damaged or destroyed.

Diagnosis and Treatment

A person who has had at least two separate instances of a blood clot without an apparent predisposing factor may have an inherited thrombophilia disorder. An inherited disorder may also be suspected if a person with an initial blood clot has a family history of blood clots. A young healthy person who develops an initial clot for no apparent reason may have an inherited disorder.

Blood tests that measure the amount or activity of different proteins that control clotting are used to identify specific inherited disorders that cause thrombophilia. These tests are usually more accurate when performed after a blood clot has been treated.

The inherited disorders that cause thrombophilia are incurable. People who have had two or more clots are especially likely to be advised to take the anticoagulant warfarin for the rest of their lives. When a person has had only one clot, warfarin or heparin to prevent future clots may be used only when the person is at higher risk for clot formation, including during a period of prolonged bed rest.

People with hyperhomocysteinemia may be advised to take vitamin supplements with folate (folic acid), vitamin B$_6$ (pyridoxine), and vitamin B$_{12}$ (cobalamin), which can reduce homocysteine levels. However, it is unclear whether these supplements also reduce clot formation.

Disseminated Intravascular Coagulation

Disseminated intravascular coagulation is a condition in which small blood clots develop throughout the bloodstream, blocking small blood vessels. The increased clotting depletes the platelets and clotting factors needed to control bleeding, causing excessive bleeding.

- There are a number of possible causes, including infection and surgery.
- Excessive clotting is followed by excessive bleeding.
- The number of clotting factors in the blood is measured.
- The underlying disorder is treated.

Disseminated intravascular coagulation (DIC) begins with excessive clotting. The excessive clotting is usually stimulated by a substance that enters the blood as part of a disease (such as an infection or certain cancers) or as a complication of childbirth, retention of a dead fetus, or surgery. People who have a severe head injury or who have been bitten by a poisonous snake are also at risk. As the clotting factors and platelets are depleted, excessive bleeding occurs.

Symptoms and Diagnosis

DIC that develops suddenly usually causes bleeding, which may be very severe. If the condition follows surgery or childbirth, bleeding may be uncontrollable. Bleeding may occur at the site of an intravenous injection or in the brain, digestive tract, skin, muscles, or cavities of the body.

If DIC develops more slowly, as in people with cancer, then clots in veins are more common than bleeding.

Blood tests may show that the number of platelets in a blood sample has dropped and that the blood is taking a long time to clot. The diagnosis of DIC is confirmed if test results show diminished amounts of clotting factors and large quantities of proteins that are produced when clots are broken up by the body (fibrin degradation products).

Treatment

The underlying cause must be identified and corrected, whether it is an obstetric problem, an infection, or a cancer. The clotting problems subside when the cause is corrected.

DIC that develops suddenly is life threatening and is treated as an emergency. Platelets and clotting factors are transfused to replace those depleted and to stop bleeding. Heparin may be used to slow the clotting in people who have more chronic, milder DIC in which clotting is more of a problem than bleeding.

CHAPTER

158 White Blood Cell Disorders

White blood cells (leukocytes) are an important part of the body's defense against infectious organisms and foreign substances. To defend the body adequately, a sufficient number of white blood cells must receive a message that an infectious organism or foreign substance has invaded the body, get to where they are needed, and then kill and digest the harmful organism or substance (see page 1099 and art on page 1100).

Like all blood cells, white blood cells are produced in the bone marrow. They develop from stem (precursor) cells that mature over time into one of the five major types of white blood cells—neutrophils, lymphocytes, monocytes, eosinophils, and basophils.

Normally, people produce about 100 billion white blood cells a day. The number of white blood cells in a given volume of blood is expressed as cells per microliter of blood. The total white blood cell count normally ranges between 4,000 and 11,000 cells per microliter. The proportion of each of the five major types of white blood cells and the total number of cells of each type can also be determined in a given volume of blood.

Too few or too many white blood cells indicates a disorder. Leukopenia, a decrease in the number of white blood cells to fewer than 4,000 cells per microliter of blood, makes people more susceptible to infections. Leukocytosis, an increase in the number of white blood cells to more than 11,000 cells per microliter of blood, may result from the normal response of the body to help fight an infection. However, an increase in the number of white blood cells can also result when the regulation of white blood cell development is disrupted and immature or abnormal cells are released into the blood.

Some white blood cell disorders involve only one of the five types of white blood cells. Other disorders may involve a few types together or all five types. Disorders of neutrophils and disorders of lymphocytes are the most common. Disorders that involve monocytes and eosinophils are less common, and disorders involving basophils are rare.

Neutropenia

Neutropenia is an abnormally low number of neutrophils in the blood.

- Neutropenia significantly increases the risk of life-threatening infection.
- Neutropenia is often caused by cancer chemotherapy or radiation therapy.
- Doctors suspect neutropenia in people who have frequent or unusual infections.
- A blood sample is used to make the diagnosis of neutropenia, and a sample of bone marrow is needed if the cause is not obvious.
- Treatment depends on the cause and severity of the disorder.

Neutrophils serve as the major defense of the body against acute bacterial and certain fungal infections. Neutrophils usually constitute about 45 to 75% of all white blood cells in the bloodstream. When the neutrophil count falls below 1,000 cells per microliter of blood, the risk of infection increases somewhat; when it falls below 500 cells per microliter, the risk of infection increases greatly. Without the key defense provided by neutrophils, people have problems controlling infections and are at risk of dying from an infection.

Causes

Neutropenia can develop if neutrophils are used up or destroyed in the bloodstream faster than the bone marrow can make new ones. With some bacterial infections, some allergic disorders, and some drug treatments, neutrophils are destroyed faster than they are produced. People with an autoimmune disease can make antibodies that destroy neutrophils and result in neutropenia. People with an enlarged spleen (see page 1072) may have a low neutrophil count because the enlarged spleen traps and destroys neutrophils.

Neutropenia can also develop if the production of neutrophils in the bone marrow is reduced, as can occur in some people with cancer, viral infections such as influenza, bacterial infections such as tuberculosis, myelofibrosis, or deficiencies of vitamin B_{12} or folate (folic acid). People who have received radiation therapy that involves the bone marrow may also develop neutropenia. Many drugs, including phenytoin, chloramphenicol, sulfa drugs, and many drugs used in cancer treatment (chemotherapy), as well as certain toxins (benzene and insecticides) can also impair the bone marrow's ability to produce neutrophils.

> **? Did You Know...**
>
> Because neutropenia has no symptoms, doctors often do not suspect the disorder unless people have frequent or unusual infections.

Production of neutrophils in the bone marrow is also affected by a severe disorder called aplastic anemia (in which the bone marrow may shut down production of all blood cells—see box on page 1036). Certain rare hereditary diseases also cause the number of neutrophils to decrease.

Symptoms and Diagnosis

Neutropenia can develop suddenly over a few hours or days (acute neutropenia), or it can develop gradually and last for months or years (chronic neutropenia). Because neutropenia itself has no specific symptoms, it is usually diagnosed when an infection occurs. In acute neutropenia, people can develop fever and painful sores (ulcers) around the mouth and anus. Bacterial pneumonia and other severe infections can follow. In chronic neutropenia, the course may be less severe if the number of neutrophils is not extremely low, and the course can occasionally be intermittent (cyclic neutropenia).

When people have frequent or unusual infections, doctors suspect neutropenia and order a complete blood cell count to make the diagnosis. A low neutrophil count indicates neutropenia. In many cases, the neutropenia is expected and the cause is known, as in people receiving chemotherapy or radiation therapy. When the cause is not known, it must be determined.

Doctors usually take a sample of bone marrow through a needle (see page 1025). The bone marrow sample is examined under a microscope to determine whether it looks normal, has a normal number of neutrophil stem cells, and shows normal development of neutrophils. By determining whether the number of stem cells is decreased and whether these cells are maturing normally, doctors may be able to determine whether the problem lies in faulty production of the cells or whether too many cells are being used or destroyed in the bloodstream. Sometimes, the bone marrow examination indicates that other diseases, such as leukemia or other cancers, or infections, such as tuberculosis, are affecting the bone marrow.

Treatment

The treatment of neutropenia depends on its cause and severity. Drugs that may cause neutropenia are stopped whenever possible, and exposures to suspected toxins are avoided. Sometimes the bone marrow recovers by itself without treatment. The neutropenia accompanying viral infections (such as influenza) may be transient and resolve after the infection has cleared. People who have mild neutropenia generally have no symptoms and may not need treatment.

People who have severe neutropenia can rapidly succumb to infection because their bodies lack the means to fight invading organisms. When these people develop infections, they are generally hospitalized and immediately given strong antibiotics, even before the cause and exact location of the infection are identified. Fever, the symptom that usually indicates infection in people who have neutropenia, is an important sign that immediate medical attention is needed.

Growth factors called colony-stimulating factors, which stimulate the production of white blood cells, are sometimes helpful. Corticosteroids may help if the neutropenia is caused by an autoimmune reaction. Antithymocyte globulin or other types of therapy that suppress the activity of the immune system may be used when a disorder such as aplastic anemia is present. Removing an enlarged spleen may cure the neutropenia resulting from hypersplenism.

When neutropenia is caused by another disorder (such as tuberculosis or leukemia or other cancers), treatment of the underlying disorder may resolve the neutropenia. Bone marrow (or stem cell) transplantation is not used to treat neutropenia per se, but it may be recommended to treat certain serious causes of neutropenia, such as aplastic anemia or leukemia.

Neutrophilic Leukocytosis

Neutrophilic leukocytosis is an abnormally high number of neutrophils in the blood.

Neutrophils help the body fight infections and heal injuries. Neutrophils may increase in response to a number of conditions or disorders. In many instances, the increased number of neutrophils is a necessary reaction by the body, as it tries to heal or ward off an invading microorganism or foreign substance. Infections by bacteria, viruses, fungi, and parasites may all increase the number of neutrophils in the blood. The number may rise in people who have an injury, such as a hip fracture or burn. Inflammatory disorders, including autoimmune disorders such as rheumatoid arthritis, can cause an increase in the number and activity of neutrophils. Some drugs, such as corticosteroids, also lead to an increased number of neutro-

phils in the blood. Myelocytic leukemias can lead to an increased number of immature or mature neutrophils in the blood.

Doctors may do blood tests, including a complete blood count, if people have symptoms, such as prolonged fever, weight loss, or fatigue. If doctors discover an increased number of neutrophils, a blood sample is viewed under a microscope to determine if immature neutrophils (myeloblasts) are leaving the bone marrow and entering the bloodstream. Immature neutrophils in the bloodstream may indicate the presence of a disorder in the bone marrow, such as leukemia. When immature neutrophils are found in the bloodstream, doctors usually take a sample of bone marrow (bone marrow biopsy—see page 1025).

An increased number of mature neutrophils in the blood is not usually a problem in itself. Therefore, doctors focus on treating the condition or disorder that caused the number of neutrophils to increase.

Lymphocytopenia

Lymphocytopenia is an abnormally low number of lymphocytes in the blood.

- Many disorders can decrease the number of lymphocytes in the blood, but AIDS and malnutrition are the most common.
- People may have no symptoms, or they may have fever and other symptoms of an infection.
- A blood sample is used to make the diagnosis of lymphocytopenia, but a sample of bone marrow or lymph node may be needed to determine the cause.
- Doctors treat the cause of lymphocytopenia.
- Some people are given gamma globulin, and some benefit from stem cell transplantation.

Lymphocytes usually constitute 20 to 40% of all white blood cells in the bloodstream. The lymphocyte count is normally above 1,500 cells per microliter of blood in adults and above 3,000 cells per microliter of blood in children. A reduction in the number of lymphocytes may not cause a significant decrease in the total number of white blood cells.

Various disorders and conditions, including infection with human immunodeficiency virus (HIV)—the virus that causes AIDS, can decrease the number of lymphocytes in the blood. Also, the number of lymphocytes can decrease briefly during starvation, times of severe stress, and during use of corticosteroids (such as prednisone), chemotherapy for cancer, and radiation therapy. Severe reduction in lymphocytes can occur in certain hereditary disorders (the hereditary immunodeficiency disorders—see page 1104).

There are three types of lymphocytes: B lymphocytes, T lymphocytes, and natural killer cells, all of which have important functions in the immune system. Too

Some Causes of Lymphocytopenia

- AIDS
- Cancer (leukemias, lymphomas, Hodgkin lymphoma)
- Chronic infections (such as miliary tuberculosis)
- Hereditary disorders (certain agammaglobulinemias, DiGeorge anomaly, Wiskott-Aldrich syndrome, severe combined immunodeficiency syndrome, and ataxia-telangiectasia)
- Rheumatoid arthritis
- Some viral infections
- Systemic lupus erythematosus (lupus)

few B lymphocytes can lead to a decrease in the number of plasma cells and reduced antibody production. People who have too few T lymphocytes or too few natural killer cells have problems controlling certain infections, especially viral, fungal, and parasitic infections. Severe lymphocyte deficiencies can result in uncontrolled infections that can be fatal.

Symptoms and Diagnosis

Mild lymphocytopenia may cause no symptoms and is usually detected by chance when a complete blood cell count is done for other reasons. Drastically reduced numbers of lymphocytes lead to infections with bacteria, viruses, fungi, and parasites.

When the numbers of lymphocytes are drastically reduced, doctors usually take a sample of bone marrow to examine under a microscope (bone marrow biopsy). The number of specific types of lymphocytes (T lymphocytes, B lymphocytes, and natural killer cells) can also be determined in the blood. A decrease in certain types of lymphocytes may help doctors diagnose some diseases, such as AIDS or certain hereditary immunodeficiency disorders.

Treatment

Treatment depends mainly on the cause. Lymphocytopenia caused by a drug usually begins to resolve within days after a person stops taking the drug. If the lymphocytopenia is the result of AIDS, combination therapy with at least three antiviral agents of different classes can increase the number of T lymphocytes and improve survival.

Did You Know...

AIDS and undernutrition are the most common causes of lymphocytopenia.

Gamma globulin (a substance rich in antibodies) may be given to help prevent infections in people with too few B lymphocytes (who therefore have a deficiency of antibody production). People with a hereditary immunodeficiency may benefit from bone marrow (stem cell) transplantation. If an infection develops, a specific antibiotic, antifungal, antiviral, or antiparasitic drug directed against the infective organism is given.

Lymphocytic Leukocytosis

Lymphocytic leukocytosis is an abnormally high number of lymphocytes in the blood.

The number of lymphocytes can increase in response to infections, especially by viruses. Some bacterial infections, such as tuberculosis, may also increase the number. Certain types of cancer, such as lymphomas and acute or chronic lymphocytic leukemia, may produce an increase in the number of lymphocytes, in part by releasing immature lymphocytes (lymphoblasts) or the lymphoma cells into the bloodstream. Graves' disease and Crohn's disease may also result in an increase in the number of lymphocytes in the bloodstream.

When the number of lymphocytes increases, symptoms may result from the infection or other disease that has caused the number of lymphocytes to increase, rather than from the increase in lymphocytes per se. When an infection is suspected, doctors may do blood tests. When doctors discover an increased number of lymphocytes, a blood sample is examined under a microscope to determine if the lymphocytes in the bloodstream appear activated (as occurs in response to viral infections) or if they appear immature or abnormal (as occurs in certain leukemias or lymphomas).

Treatment for lymphocytic leukocytosis depends on the cause.

Monocyte Disorders

Monocytes help other white blood cells remove dead or damaged tissues, destroy cancer cells, and regulate immunity against foreign substances. Monocytes are produced in the bone marrow and then enter the bloodstream, where they account for about 1 to 10% of the circulating leukocytes (200 to 600 monocytes per microliter of blood). After a few hours in the bloodstream, they migrate to tissues (such as spleen, liver, lung, and bone marrow tissue), where they mature into macrophages, the main scavenger cells of the immune system. Genetic abnormalities that affect the function of monocytes and macrophages and cause buildup of debris within the cells result in the lipid storage diseases (such as Gaucher's disease—see page 1839—and Niemann-Pick disease—see page 1840).

An increased number of monocytes in the blood (monocytosis) occurs in response to chronic infections, in autoimmune disorders, in blood disorders, and in cancers. A proliferation of macrophages in tissues can occur in response to infections, sarcoidosis (see page 511), and Langerhans' cell histiocytosis (granulomatosis—see page 509).

A low number of monocytes in the blood (monocytopenia) can occur in response to the release of toxins into the blood by certain types of bacteria (endotoxemia), as well as in people receiving chemotherapy or corticosteroids.

Eosinophilic Disorders

Eosinophils usually account for less than 7% of the circulating leukocytes (100 to 500 eosinophils per microliter of blood). These cells have a role in the protective immunity against certain parasites but also contribute to the inflammation that occurs in allergic disorders.

An increased number of eosinophils in the blood (eosinophilia) usually indicates the response of the body to abnormal cells, parasites, or substances that cause an allergic reaction (allergens).

A low number of eosinophils in the blood (eosinopenia) can occur with Cushing's syndrome, stress reactions, and treatment with corticosteroids but does not usually cause problems because other parts of the immune system compensate adequately.

Idiopathic hypereosinophilic syndrome is a disorder in which the number of eosinophils increases to more than 1,500 cells per microliter of blood for more than 6 months without an obvious cause.

People of any age can develop idiopathic hypereosinophilic syndrome, but it is more common in men older than 50. The increased number of eosinophils can damage the heart, lungs, liver, skin, and nervous system. For example, the heart can become inflamed in a condition called Löffler's endocarditis, leading to formation of blood clots, heart failure, heart attacks, or malfunctioning heart valves.

Symptoms may include weight loss, fevers, night sweats, fatigue, cough, chest pain, swelling, stomachache, rashes, pain, weakness, confusion, and coma. Additional symptoms of this syndrome depend on which organs are damaged. The syndrome is suspected when repeated blood tests reveal that the number of eosinophils is persistently increased in people who have these symptoms. The diagnosis is confirmed when doctors determine that the eosinophilia is not caused by a parasitic infection, an allergic reaction, or another diagnosable disorder.

Without treatment, generally more than 80% of the people who have this syndrome die within 2 years, but with treatment, more than 80% survive. Heart damage is the principal cause of death. Some people need no treatment other than close observation for 3 to 6 months, but most need drug treatment with prednisone or hydroxyurea. Some people with idiopathic hypereosinophilic syndrome have an acquired abnormality of a gene that regulates cell growth. This type of hypereosinophilia can respond to treatment with imatinib, a drug used to treat cancer. If these drugs fail, various other drugs may be used, and they can be combined with a procedure to remove eosinophils from the blood (leukapheresis).

Basophilic Disorders

Basophils account for less than 3% of the circulating leukocytes (0 to 300 basophils per microliter of blood). These cells have some role in immune surveillance and wound repair. Basophils can release histamine and other mediators and play a role in the initiation of allergic reactions. A decrease in the number of basophils (basopenia) can occur as a response to thyrotoxicosis, acute hypersensitivity reactions, and infections. An increase in the number of basophils (basophilia) can occur in people with hypothyroidism. In the myeloproliferative disorders (for example, polycythemia vera and myelofibrosis), a marked increase in the number of basophils can occur.

CHAPTER 159   Plasma Cell Disorders

Plasma cell disorders (plasma cell dyscrasias) are uncommon. They begin when a single group (clone) of plasma cells multiplies excessively and produces a large quantity of a single type of antibody (immunoglobulin). Plasma cells develop from B lymphocytes, a type of white blood cell that normally produces antibodies, which help the body fight infection. Plasma cells are present mainly in bone marrow and lymph nodes. Every plasma cell divides repeatedly to form a clone, composed of many identical cells. The cells of a clone produce only one specific type of antibody. Because thousands of different clones exist, the body can produce a vast number of different antibodies (see page 1103) to fight the body's frequent exposure to infectious microorganisms.

In plasma cell disorders, one clone of plasma cells multiplies uncontrollably. As a result, this clone produces vast amounts of a single antibody (monoclonal antibody) known as the M-protein. In some cases (such as with monoclonal gammopathies), the antibody produced is incomplete, consisting of only light chains or heavy chains (functional antibodies normally consist of two pairs of two different chains called a light chain and heavy chain). These abnormal plasma cells and the antibodies they produce are limited to one type, and levels of other types of antibodies that help fight infections fall. Thus, people with plasma cell disorders are often at higher risk of infections. The ever-increasing number of abnormal plasma cells also invades and damages various tissues and organs, and the antibody produced by the clone of plasma cells can sometimes damage vital organs, especially the kidneys and bones.

Plasma cell disorders include monoclonal gammopathies of undetermined significance, multiple myeloma, macroglobulinemia, and heavy chain diseases. These disorders are more common among older people.

Monoclonal Gammopathies of Undetermined Significance

A monoclonal gammopathy of undetermined significance is a buildup of monoclonal antibodies produced by abnormal but noncancerous plasma cells.

In general, monoclonal gammopathies of undetermined significance occur in more than 5% of people older than 70, but they do not cause significant health problems. These disorders do not usually cause symptoms, so they are almost always discovered by chance when laboratory tests are done for other purposes, such as to measure protein in the blood. However, the monoclonal antibody can bind to nerves and lead to numbness, tingling, and weakness. People with these disorders also are more likely to have bone loss and fractures.

The M-protein levels in people with a monoclonal gammopathy of undetermined significance often remain stable for years—25 years in some people—and do not require treatment. However, if evaluation shows evidence of significant loss of bone density (osteopenia or osteoporosis), doctors may recommend treatment with bisphosphonates.

For unknown reasons, in about one quarter of people with these disorders, there is a progression to a cancer, such as multiple myeloma, macroglobulinemia, or B-cell lymphoma, often after many years. This progression cannot be prevented. People with a monoclonal gammopathy of undetermined significance are usually monitored with a physical examination and blood and sometimes urine tests about twice a year, to determine if a progression to cancer is beginning to occur. If progression is detected early, symptoms and complications of the cancer may be prevented or treated sooner.

Multiple Myeloma

Multiple myeloma is a cancer of plasma cells in which abnormal plasma cells multiply uncontrollably in the bone marrow and occasionally in other parts of the body.

- People often have bone pain and fractures, and they may also have kidney problems, immunocompromise, weakness, and confusion.
- Diagnosis is made by measuring the amounts of different types of antibodies in blood and urine and confirmed by a bone marrow biopsy.
- Chemotherapy drugs and corticosteroids are often used for treatment.

Typically, multiple myeloma occurs in people at least 60 years of age. Although its cause is not certain, the increased occurrence of multiple myeloma among close relatives indicates that heredity plays a role. Exposure to radiation is thought to be a possible cause, as is exposure to benzene and other solvents.

Normally, plasma cells make up less than 1% of the cells in the bone marrow. In multiple myeloma, typically the majority of bone marrow elements are cancerous plasma cells. The overabundance of these cancerous plasma cells in the bone marrow leads to the increased production of proteins that suppress the development of other normal bone marrow elements, including white blood cells, red blood cells, and platelets (cell-like particles that help the body form blood clots). In addition, the abnormal plasma cells almost always produce a large amount of a single type of antibody accompanied by a markedly reduced amount of all other types of normal antibodies.

Often, collections of cancerous plasma cells develop into tumors that lead to loss of bone, most commonly in the pelvic bones, spine, ribs, and skull. Infrequently, these tumors develop in areas other than bone, particularly in the lungs, liver, and kidneys.

Symptoms

Because plasma cell tumors often invade bone, bone pain, often in the back, ribs, and hips, may occur. Other symptoms result from the complications.

Complications: Fractures may occur if loss of bone density (osteoporosis) from plasma cell tumors weakens bones.

In addition, calcium released from the bones may result in abnormally high levels of calcium in the blood, possibly causing constipation, increased frequency of urination, kidney problems, weakness, and confusion.

The reduced production of red blood cells often leads to anemia, which causes fatigue, weakness, and pallor and may lead to heart problems. Decreased production of white blood cells leads to repeated infections, which may cause fever and chills. Decreased platelet production impairs the blood's ability to clot and results in easy bruising or bleeding.

Pieces of monoclonal antibodies, known as light chains, frequently end up in the collecting system of the kidneys, sometimes permanently damaging them by interfering with their filtering function and leading to kidney failure. The light chain pieces of the antibody in the urine (or blood) are called Bence Jones proteins. The increased number of growing cancerous cells can lead to the overproduction and excretion of uric acid in the urine, which can lead to kidney stones. Deposits of certain types of antibody pieces in the kidneys or other organs can lead to amyloidosis (see page 2107), another serious disorder found in a small number of people with multiple myeloma.

In rare instances, multiple myeloma interferes with blood flow to the skin, fingers, toes, nose, kidneys, and brain because the blood thickens (hyperviscosity syndrome—see page 1054).

Diagnosis

Multiple myeloma may be discovered even before people have symptoms, when laboratory tests done for another reason show elevated protein levels in the blood or protein in the urine, or an x-ray done for another reason shows specific areas of bone loss. Bone loss may be widespread or more often appear as isolated punched-out areas in bones.

Multiple myeloma is sometimes suspected because of symptoms, such as back pain or bone pain in other sites, fatigue, fevers, and bruising. Blood tests done to investigate such symptoms may reveal that a person has anemia, a decreased white blood cell count, a decreased platelet count, or kidney failure.

The most useful laboratory tests are blood and urine protein electrophoresis and immunoelectrophoresis. They detect and identify an overabundance of a single type of antibody found in most people who have multiple myeloma. Doctors also measure the different types of antibodies, especially IgG, IgA, and IgM.

Calcium levels are usually measured as well. A urine specimen collected over a 24-hour period is analyzed for the amount and types of protein in it. Bence Jones proteins are found in the urine of half of the people who have multiple myeloma.

A bone marrow aspirate and biopsy (see page 1025) are done to confirm the diagnosis. In people with multiple myeloma, these specimens show a large number of plasma cells abnormally arranged in sheets and clusters. Individual cells also may appear abnormal.

In addition, other blood tests are useful in determining the overall outlook for the person. Higher levels of beta$_2$-microglobulin and lower levels of albumin in the person's blood when the disease is diagnosed usually indicate the likelihood of a shortened survival and are likely to affect treatment decisions.

Treatment and Prognosis

Multiple myeloma remains incurable despite recent remarkable advances in therapy. Treatment is aimed at preventing or relieving symptoms and complications, destroying abnormal plasma cells, and slowing progression of the disorder.

The most consistently helpful group of drugs for multiple myeloma is corticosteroids, such as prednisone, methylprednisolone, or dexamethasone, although many new drugs are showing great promise. In addition, chemotherapy slows the progression of multiple myeloma by killing the abnormal plasma cells. Because chemotherapy kills normal cells as well as abnormal ones, the blood cells are monitored and the dose is adjusted if the number of normal white blood cells and platelets decreases too much. Melphalan, and less often cyclophosphamide, are the chemotherapy drugs most often added to corticosteroids. Doxorubicin and newer chemically related drugs are also effective. Nearly one third of people respond to treatment with thalidomide or bortezomib, but giving these drugs together with chemotherapy drugs or corticosteroids increases their effectiveness. A newer drug that is related to thalidomide, lenalidomide, also is effective in treating multiple myeloma, especially in people in whom myeloma is difficult to treat or recurs. Combining lenalidomide with corticosteroids improves its effectiveness.

> **? Did You Know...**
> Because multiple myeloma is such a serious disorder, doctors use thalidomide, even though it can cause birth defects, but very strict precautions are needed.

Many new combinations of treatment are being used. One involves several months of conventional chemotherapy followed by high-dose chemotherapy. Because this high-dose treatment is also toxic to normal blood cells made in the bone marrow, stem cells (unspecialized cells that transform into immature blood cells, which eventually mature to become red blood cells, white blood cells, and platelets) are collected from the person's blood before the high-dose chemotherapy is administered. These stem cells are then returned (transplanted) to the person after the high-dose treatment (see page 1133). Generally, this procedure is reserved for people who are younger than 70.

Strong analgesics and radiation therapy directed at the affected bones can help relieve bone pain, which can be severe. Radiation therapy may also prevent the development of fractures. However, radiation therapy may damage bone marrow function, which can impact the ability of the patient to be treated with anti-myeloma drugs. Monthly intravenous administration of pamidronate (a bisphosphonate—a drug that slows loss of bone density) and the more potent drug zoledronic acid can reduce the development of bony complications, and most people with multiple myeloma receive these drugs as part of their treatment forever. People are encouraged to take calcium and vitamin D supplements as long as they do not have high levels of calcium in their blood, and doctors encourage them to stay active because these actions help prevent bone loss. Prolonged bed rest tends to accelerate bone loss and makes the bones more vulnerable to fractures. Most people can enjoy a normal lifestyle that includes most activities. Drinking plenty of fluids dilutes the urine and helps prevent dehydration, which can make kidney failure more likely.

People who have signs of infection—fever, chills, cough productive of sputum, or reddened areas of the skin—should seek medical attention promptly because they may need antibiotics. People also may be at risk of infections with the herpes zoster virus, especially when they are treated with specific anti-myeloma drugs such as bortezomib. An oral antiviral drug called acyclovir taken long-term may help prevent herpes infections. People who have severe anemia may need transfusions of red blood cells. Erythropoietin or darbepoietin, drugs that stimulate red blood cell formation, may adequately treat the anemia in some people. High levels of calcium in the blood can be treated with intravenous fluids and often require intravenous bisphosphonates. People who have high levels of uric acid in the blood or widespread disease may benefit from allopurinol, a drug that blocks the body's production of uric acid.

Currently, no cure is available for multiple myeloma, but most people respond to treatment. Recently, the number of effective treatments has increased, and as a result, the average survival has nearly doubled. But survival time varies widely depending on certain features, such as kidney problems, blood levels of certain proteins including beta$_2$-microglobulin and serum albumin, and genetic characteristics, at the time of diagnosis and the response to treatment. Importantly, bisphosphonates to reduce bony complications, substances that stimulate the production of blood cells (growth factors) to increase the number of red and white blood cells, and better pain relievers have also greatly improved the quality of life. Occasionally, people who survive for many years after successful treatment of multiple myeloma develop leukemia or irreversible loss of bone marrow function. These late complications may result from chemotherapy and often lead to severe anemia and an increased susceptibility to infections and bleeding.

Because multiple myeloma is ultimately fatal, people with multiple myeloma are likely to benefit from discussions of end-of-life care that involve their doctors and appropriate family and friends. Points for discussion may include advance directives (see page 69), the use of feeding tubes, and pain relief (see page 61).

Macroglobulinemia

Macroglobulinemia (Waldenström's macroglobulinemia) is a plasma cell cancer in which a single clone of plasma cells produces excessive amounts of a certain type of large antibody (IgM) called macroglobulins.

- Although many people have no symptoms, some people have abnormal bleeding, recurring bacterial infections, and bone fractures from severe osteoporosis.

- Blood tests are needed to make the diagnosis.
- Macroglobulinemia is not curable, but progression can be slowed with chemotherapy drugs.

Men are affected by macroglobulinemia more often than women, and the average age at which the disorder appears is 65 years. Its cause is unknown.

Symptoms and Complications

Many people who have macroglobulinemia have no symptoms, and the disorder is discovered by chance when an elevated level of blood proteins is found during routine blood tests. Others have symptoms resulting from interference with blood flow to the skin, fingers, toes, nose, and brain that occurs when the large quantity of macroglobulins thickens the blood (hyperviscosity syndrome). These symptoms include bleeding from the skin and mucous membranes (such as the lining of the mouth, nose, and digestive tract), fatigue, weakness, headache, confusion, dizziness, and even coma. The thickened blood also may aggravate heart conditions and cause increased pressure in the brain. Tiny blood vessels in the back of the eyes can become filled with blood and may bleed, resulting in damage to the retina and impaired eyesight.

People who have macroglobulinemia may also have swollen lymph nodes and an enlarged liver and spleen due to infiltration by cancerous plasma cells. Recurring bacterial infections resulting from inadequate production of normal antibodies may cause fever and chills. Anemia, which may result in weakness and fatigue, occurs when cancerous plasma cells prevent normal blood-forming cells in the bone marrow from being produced. Infiltration of bones by cancerous plasma cells may cause loss of bone density (osteoporosis), which can weaken bones and increase the risk of fractures.

Some people develop a condition called cryoglobulinemia. Cryoglobulinemia involves the development of antibodies that clog up the blood vessels in cold temperatures.

Diagnosis

Blood tests are done when macroglobulinemia is suspected. The three most useful tests are serum protein electrophoresis, measurement of immunoglobulins, and immunoelectrophoresis.

Doctors may do other laboratory tests as well. For example, doctors may check a blood sample to determine if the numbers of red and white blood cells and platelets are normal. In addition, serum viscosity, which is a test to check the thickness of the blood, is often done. Blood clotting test results may be abnormal, and other tests may detect cryoglobulins. An examination of a urine sample may

What Is Cryoglobulinemia?

Cryoglobulins are abnormal antibodies produced by plasma cells and dissolved in the blood. When cooled below normal body temperature, cryoglobulins form large collections of solid particles (precipitates). When warmed to normal body temperature, they re-dissolve.

The formation of cryoglobulins (cryoglobulinemia) is uncommon. In most instances, people who form cryoglobulins have an underlying disorder as the cause. These disorders include cancers such as macroglobulinemia and chronic lymphocytic leukemia, autoimmune disorders such as systemic lupus erythematosus (lupus), and infections by such organisms as hepatitis C virus. Rarely, a cause for the formation of cryoglobulins cannot be found.

Precipitates of cryoglobulins can trigger inflammation of blood vessels (vasculitis), which causes various symptoms, such as bruises, joint aches, and weakness. People with cryoglobulinemia may also be very sensitive to cold or develop Raynaud's syndrome, in which the hands and feet become very painful and turn white when chilled. The vasculitis may damage the liver and kidneys. Damage may progress to liver failure and kidney failure in some people and can be fatal.

Avoiding cold temperatures helps prevent vasculitis. Treating the underlying disorder may reduce the formation of cryoglobulins. For example, using interferon-alpha to treat hepatitis C virus infection helps to reduce formation of cryoglobulins. Plasmapheresis may help, especially when combined with interferon.

show Bence Jones proteins (pieces of abnormal antibodies). A bone marrow biopsy may reveal an increased number of lymphocytes and plasma cells, which helps confirm the diagnosis of macroglobulinemia, and the appearance of these cells helps differentiate this disorder from multiple myeloma.

X-rays may show a loss of bone density (osteoporosis). Computed tomography (CT) scans may reveal an enlarged spleen, liver, or lymph nodes.

Treatment and Prognosis

Although chemotherapy, usually with chlorambucil or fludarabine, can slow the growth of abnormal plasma cells, the disorder remains incurable. Other drugs, such as melphalan or cyclophosphamide, are sometimes used, alone or in combination. Drugs that work differently from the chemotherapy drugs may be helpful. The monoclonal antibody rituximab is effective at slowing the growth of the abnormal plasma cells. Thalidomide and the newer drugs lenalidomide and bortezomib, are being used with some success, especially when they are used with corticosteroids.

A person whose blood is thickened must be treated promptly with plasmapheresis, a procedure in which blood is withdrawn, the abnormal antibodies are removed from it, and the red blood cells are returned to the person (see box on page 1030). However, only a small number of people with macroglobulinemia require this procedure.

The disease remains incurable, but most patients survive more than 5 years.

Heavy Chain Diseases

Heavy chain diseases are plasma cell cancers in which a clone of plasma cells produces a large quantity of pieces of abnormal antibodies called heavy chains.

Heavy chain diseases are categorized according to the type of heavy chain produced: alpha, gamma, or mu.

Alpha heavy chain disease affects mainly younger adults of Middle Eastern or Mediterranean ancestry.

Infiltration of the intestinal tract wall by cancerous plasma cells often prevents proper absorption of nutrients from food (malabsorption), resulting in severe diarrhea and weight loss. Alpha heavy chain disease progresses rapidly, and half of the affected people die within 1 year. Treatment with cyclophosphamide, prednisone (a corticosteroid), and antibiotics may slow the progression of the disease or lead to a remission.

Gamma heavy chain disease affects mainly older adults. Some people with gamma heavy chain disease have no symptoms. Infiltration of the bone marrow by cancerous plasma cells causes other people to have symptoms of recurring infections, such as repeated episodes of fever and chills associated with a decreased number of white blood cells, and fatigue and weakness associated with severe anemia. Cancerous plasma cells may also enlarge the liver and spleen. People with symptoms may respond to chemotherapy drugs, corticosteroids, and radiation therapy.

Mu heavy chain disease, the rarest of the three heavy chain diseases, may cause enlargement of the liver and spleen as well as enlargement of the lymph nodes in the abdomen. Length of survival and response to chemotherapy drugs vary widely.

CHAPTER

160 Leukemias

Leukemias are cancers of white blood cells or of cells that develop into white blood cells.

White blood cells develop from stem cells in the bone marrow. Sometimes the development goes awry, and pieces of chromosomes get rearranged. The resulting abnormal chromosomes interfere with normal control of cell division, so that affected cells multiply uncontrollably and become cancerous (malignant), resulting in leukemia. Leukemia cells ultimately occupy the bone marrow, replacing or suppressing the function of cells that develop into normal blood cells. This interference with normal bone marrow cell function can lead to inadequate numbers of red blood cells (causing anemia), white blood cells (increasing the risk of infection), and platelets (increasing the risk of bleeding). Leukemia cells may also invade other organs, including the liver, spleen, lymph nodes, testes, and brain.

Leukemias are grouped into four main types:

- Acute lymphocytic leukemia
- Acute myelocytic leukemia
- Chronic lymphocytic leukemia
- Chronic myelocytic leukemia

The types are defined according to how quickly they progress and the type and characteristics of the white blood cells that become cancerous. Acute leukemias progress rapidly and consist of immature cells. Chronic leukemias progress slowly and consist of more mature cells. Lymphocytic leukemias develop from cancerous changes in lymphocytes or in cells that normally produce lymphocytes. Myelocytic (myeloid) leukemias develop from cancerous changes in cells that normally produce neutrophils, basophils, eosinophils, and monocytes.

Causes

The cause of most types of leukemia is not known. Exposure to radiation, to some types of chemotherapy, or to certain chemicals (such as benzene) increases the risk of developing some types of leukemia, although leukemia develops only in a very small number of such people. Certain hereditary disorders, such as Down syndrome and Fanconi's syndrome, increase the risk as well. In some people, leukemia is caused by certain abnormalities of the chromosomes. A virus known as human T lymphotropic virus 1 (HTLV-1), which is similar to the virus that causes AIDS, is strongly suspected of causing a rare type of lymphocytic leukemia called adult T-cell leukemia. Infection with the Epstein-Barr virus has been associated with an aggressive form of lymphocytic leukemia called Burkitt's leukemia.

Treatment

Many leukemias can be effectively treated, and some can be cured. When leukemia is under control, people are said to be in remission. If leukemia cells appear again, people are said to have a relapse. For some people in relapse, quality of life eventually deteriorates, and the potential benefit for further treatment may be extremely limited. Keeping people comfortable may become more important than trying to modestly prolong life. Affected people and their family members must be involved in these decisions. Much can be done to provide compassionate care, relieve symptoms (see page 61), and maintain dignity.

Acute Lymphocytic Leukemia

Acute lymphocytic (lymphoblastic) leukemia is a life-threatening disease in which the cells that normally develop into lymphocytes become cancerous and rapidly replace normal cells in the bone marrow.

- People may have symptoms, such as fever, weakness, and paleness, because they have too few normal blood cells.
- Blood tests and a bone marrow biopsy are usually done.
- Chemotherapy is given and is often effective.

Acute lymphocytic leukemia (ALL) occurs in people of all ages but is the most common cancer in children, accounting for 25% of all cancers in children younger than 15 years. ALL most often affects young children between the ages of 2 and 5 years. Among adults, it is somewhat more common in people older than 45.

In ALL, very immature leukemia cells accumulate in the bone marrow, destroying and replacing cells that produce normal blood cells. The leukemia cells are also carried in the bloodstream to the liver, spleen, lymph nodes, brain, and testes, where they may continue to grow and divide. They can irritate the layers of tissue covering the brain and spinal cord, causing inflammation (meningitis), and can cause anemia, liver and kidney failure, and other organ damage.

Symptoms and Diagnosis

Early symptoms result from the inability of the bone marrow to produce enough normal blood

cells. Fever and excessive sweating, which may indicate infection, result from too few normal white blood cells. Weakness, fatigue, and paleness, which indicate anemia, result from too few red blood cells. Easy bruising and bleeding, sometimes in the form of nosebleeds or bleeding gums, result from too few platelets. Leukemia cells in the brain may cause headaches, vomiting, and irritability, and leukemia cells in the bone marrow may cause bone and joint pain. A sense of fullness in the abdomen and sometimes pain can result when leukemia cells enlarge the liver and spleen.

> **? Did You Know...**
> Nearly 80% of children with acute lymphocytic leukemia are cured.

Blood tests, such as a complete blood count (see page 1024), can provide the first evidence of ALL. The total number of white blood cells may be decreased, normal, or increased, but the number of red blood cells and platelets is almost always decreased. In addition, very immature white blood cells (blasts) are present in blood samples examined under a microscope. A bone marrow biopsy (see page 1025) is almost always done to confirm the diagnosis and to distinguish ALL from other types of leukemia.

Prognosis

Before treatment was available, most people who had ALL died within 4 months of the diagnosis. Now, nearly 80% of children and 30 to 40% of adults with ALL are cured. For most people, the first course of chemotherapy brings the disease under control (complete remission). Children between the ages of 3 and 7 have the best prognosis. Children younger than 2 and older adults fare least well. The white blood cell count and particular chromosome abnormalities in the leukemia cells also influence outcome.

Treatment

Chemotherapy is highly effective and is administered in phases. The goal of initial treatment (induction chemotherapy) is to achieve remission by destroying leukemia cells so that normal cells can once again grow in the bone marrow. People may need to stay in the hospital for a few days or weeks, depending on how quickly the bone marrow recovers. Blood and platelet transfusions may be necessary to treat anemia and to prevent bleeding, and antibiotics may be needed to treat bacterial infections. Intravenous fluids and therapy with a drug called allopurinol may also be used to help rid the body of harmful substances, such as uric acid, that are released when leukemia cells are destroyed.

One of several combinations of drugs is used, and doses are repeated for several days or weeks. One combination consists of prednisone (a corticosteroid) taken by mouth and weekly doses of vincristine (a chemotherapy drug) given with an anthracycline drug (usually daunorubicin), asparaginase, and sometimes cyclophosphamide, given intravenously. Other drugs are being investigated.

For treatment of leukemia cells in the layers of tissue covering the brain and spinal cord (the meninges), methotrexate, cytosine arabinoside, or both are usually injected directly into the cerebrospinal fluid. This chemotherapy may be given in combination with radiation therapy to the brain. Even when there is little evidence that the leukemia has spread to the brain, a similar type of treatment is usually given as a preventive measure because of the high likelihood of spread to the meninges.

A few weeks after the initial, intensive treatment, additional treatment (consolidation chemotherapy) is given to destroy any remaining leukemia cells. Additional chemotherapy drugs, or the same drugs as were used during the induction phase, may be used a few times over a period of several weeks. Further treatment (maintenance chemotherapy), which usually consists of fewer drugs, sometimes at lower doses, may continue for 2 to 3 years. For some people who are at high risk of relapse because of particular chromosomal changes found in their cells, stem cell transplantation (see page 1133) during the first remission is often recommended.

Leukemia cells may begin to appear again (a condition termed relapse), often in the blood, bone marrow, brain, or testes. Reappearance in the bone marrow is particularly serious. Chemotherapy is given again, and although most people respond to treatment, the disease has a strong tendency to come back, especially in children younger than 2 and in adults. When leukemia cells reappear in the brain, chemotherapy drugs are injected into the cerebrospinal fluid 1 or 2 times a week. When leukemia cells reappear in the testes, radiation therapy is given along with chemotherapy.

For people who have relapsed, high doses of chemotherapy drugs along with allogeneic stem cell transplantation offers the best chance of cure. But transplantation can be done only if stem cells can b obtained from a person who has a compatible tissue type (HLA-matched). The donor is usually a sibling, but cells from matched, unrelated donors (or occasionally partially matched cells from family members or unrelated donors, as well as umbilical stem cells) are sometimes used. Stem cell transplantation is rarely used for people older than 65, because it is much less likely to be successful and side effects are much more likely to be fatal.

After relapse, additional treatment for people who are unable to undergo stem cell transplantation is often poorly tolerated and ineffective, frequently causing people to feel much sicker. However, remissions can occur. End-of-life care should be considered for people who do not respond to treatment (see page 57).

Acute Myelocytic Leukemia

Acute myelocytic (myeloid, myelogenous, myeloblastic, myelomonocytic) leukemia is a life-threatening disease in which the cells that normally develop into neutrophils, basophils, eosinophils, and monocytes become cancerous and rapidly replace normal cells in the bone marrow.

- People may be tired or pale, easily susceptible to infection and fever, and bruise or bleed easily.
- Blood tests and bone marrow examination are needed for diagnosis.
- Treatment includes chemotherapy to achieve remission plus additional chemotherapy to avoid relapse.

Acute myelocytic leukemia (AML) is the most common type of leukemia among adults, although it affects people of all ages.

In AML, immature leukemia cells rapidly accumulate in the bone marrow, destroying and replacing cells that produce normal blood cells. The leukemia cells are released into the bloodstream and are transported to other organs, where they continue to grow and divide. They can form small masses (chloromas) in or just under the skin or gums or in the eyes.

Acute promyelocytic leukemia is a subtype of AML. In this subtype, chromosomal changes in promyelocytes—cells that are at an early stage in the development into mature neutrophils—prevent binding and activity of vitamin A. Without vitamin A activity, normal cell maturation is disrupted, and abnormal promyelocytes accumulate.

Symptoms and Diagnosis

The first symptoms of AML are very similar to those of acute lymphocytic leukemia (see page 1056). Although meningitis occurs less often than in acute lymphocytic leukemia, AML cells can cause inflammation of the layers of tissue covering the brain and spinal cord (meninges).

The diagnosis of AML is also similar to that of acute lymphocytic leukemia. A bone marrow biopsy (see page 1025) is almost always done to confirm the diagnosis and to distinguish AML from other types of leukemia.

Myelodysplastic Syndromes

In myelodysplastic syndromes, a line of identical cells (clone) develops and occupies the bone marrow. These abnormal cells do not grow and mature normally. The cells also interfere with normal bone marrow function, resulting in deficits of red blood cells, white blood cells, and platelets. In some people, red blood cell production is predominantly affected. Myelodysplastic syndromes occur most often in people older than 50 years. Men are more than twice as likely as women to be affected.

The cause is usually not known. However, in some people, exposure of bone marrow to radiation therapy or certain types of chemotherapy drugs may play a role.

Symptoms develop very slowly. Fatigue, weakness, and other symptoms of anemia are common. Fever due to infections may develop if the number of white blood cells decreases. Easy bruising and abnormal bleeding can result if the number of platelets drops.

A myelodysplastic syndrome may be suspected when people have unexplained persistent anemia, but diagnosis requires a bone marrow biopsy.

People with myelodysplastic syndromes often need transfusions of red blood cells. Platelets are transfused only if people have uncontrolled bleeding or if surgery is needed and the number of platelets is low. People who have very low numbers of neutrophils—the white blood cells that fight infection—may benefit from intermittent injections of a special type of protein called a colony-stimulating factor.

The drugs azacitidine and deoxyazacitidine can reduce the need for transfusions and prolong survival, but they do not cure myelodysplastic syndromes. Allogeneic stem cell transplantation cures a few people.

Although myelodysplastic syndromes are thought to be a type of leukemia, they progress gradually, over a period of several months to years. In 10 to 30% of people, a myelodysplastic syndrome transforms into acute myelocytic leukemia (AML). Treatment with chemotherapy during the early stages of a myelodysplastic syndrome does not help prevent transformation to AML. If transformation to AML occurs, chemotherapy may be helpful, but the AML is unlikely to be curable.

Prognosis

Without treatment, most people with AML die within a few weeks to months of the diagnosis. With therapy, between 20% and 40% of people survive at least 5 years, without any relapse. Because relapses almost always occur within the first 5 years after initial treatment, most people who remain leukemia-free after 5 years are considered cured. People who have the poorest prognosis are those older than 60, those who develop AML after undergoing chemotherapy and radiation therapy for other cancers, and those whose leukemia evolved slowly after a period of months to years of abnormal blood counts.

Treatment

Treatment is aimed at bringing about prompt remission—the destruction of all leukemia cells. However, AML responds to fewer drugs than does acute lymphocytic leukemia. In addition, treatment often makes people sicker before they get better, because the treatment suppresses bone marrow activity, resulting in fewer white blood cells, particularly neutrophils. Having too few neutrophils makes infection likely. Meticulous care is taken to prevent infections, and any that occur are promptly treated. Red blood cell and platelet transfusions are invariably also needed.

The first course of drug treatment (induction chemotherapy) generally includes cytarabine for 7 days by a continuous infusion and daunorubicin (or idarubicin or mitoxantrone) for 3 days.

Once AML is in remission, people usually receive a few courses of additional chemotherapy (consolidation chemotherapy) a few weeks or months after the initial treatment to help ensure that as many leukemia cells as possible are destroyed. A preventive treatment to the brain usually is not needed, and long-term lower-dose chemotherapy (as is used in acute lymphocytic leukemia) has not been shown to improve survival.

People who have not responded to treatment and younger people who are in remission but who are likely to have a high rate of relapse (generally identified by certain chromosomal abnormalities) may be given high doses of chemotherapy drugs followed by stem cell transplantation (see page 1133).

When relapse occurs, additional chemotherapy for people unable to undergo stem cell transplantation is less effective and often poorly tolerated. Another course of chemotherapy is most effective in younger people and in people whose initial remission lasted more than 1 year. Doctors take many factors into consideration when determining the advisability of additional intensive chemotherapy for people with AML in relapse. A newer drug, gemtuzumab ozogamicin, which combines an antibody with a chemotherapy drug as an attempt to specifically "target" the leukemia cells, is effective in some people after relapse has occurred. The long-term benefits of the drug have not been determined.

People with acute promyelocytic leukemia can be treated with a type of vitamin A called all-*trans*-retinoic acid. Results are best when chemotherapy is used also; currently more than 70% of people with acute promyelocytic leukemia can be cured. Arsenic chemical compounds are also uniquely effective in this subtype of AML.

Chronic Lymphocytic Leukemia

Chronic lymphocytic leukemia is a disease in which mature lymphocytes become cancerous and gradually replace normal cells in lymph nodes.

- People may have no symptoms, or they may have general symptoms such as tiredness.
- People may also have enlarged lymph nodes and a sense of abdominal fullness.
- Blood tests and examination of a bone marrow sample are needed for diagnosis.
- Treatment includes chemotherapy drugs, monoclonal antibodies, and sometimes radiation therapy.

More than three fourths of the people who have chronic lymphocytic leukemia (CLL) are older than 60, and the disease does not occur in children. This type of leukemia affects men 2 to 3 times more often than women. CLL is the most common type of leukemia in North America and Europe. It is rare in Japan and Southeast Asia, which indicates that heredity plays some role in its development.

The number of cancerous mature lymphocytes increases first in the blood and lymph nodes. They then spread to the liver and spleen, both of which begin to enlarge. Cancerous lymphocytes also invade the bone marrow, where they crowd out normal cells, resulting in a decreased number of red blood cells and a decreased number of normal white blood cells and platelets in the blood. The level of antibodies, proteins that help fight infections, also decreases. The immune system, which ordinarily defends the body against foreign organisms and substances, sometimes becomes misguided, reacting to and destroying normal body tissues. This misguided activity can sometimes result in the destruction of red blood cells and platelets.

In the great majority of cases, CLL is a disorder of B lymphocytes (B cells—see page 1102). There are other types of CLL other than B-cell CLL. Hairy cell leukemia, a slow-growing uncommon type of B-cell leukemia, produces a large number of abnormal white blood cells with distinctive hairlike projections that are visible under a microscope. T-cell leukemia (leukemia of T lymphocytes) is much less common than B-cell leukemia. Sézary syndrome is a rare type of T-cell leukemia in which cancerous T lymphocytes that start as a skin cancer called mycosis fungoides (see box on page 1064) grow and divide more rapidly and enter the bloodstream, becoming leukemia cells.

Symptoms and Diagnosis

In early stages of CLL, most people have no symptoms, and the disease is diagnosed only because of an increased white blood cell count. Later symptoms may include enlarged lymph nodes, fatigue, loss of appetite, weight loss, shortness of breath when exercising, and a sense of abdominal fullness resulting from an enlarged spleen.

As CLL progresses, people may appear pale and bruise easily. Bacterial, viral, and fungal infections generally do not occur until late in the course of the disease.

Sometimes the disease is discovered accidentally when blood counts ordered for some other reason show an increased number of lymphocytes. A bone marrow biopsy is usually not needed to confirm the diagnosis because specialized tests to characterize the lymphocytes can be done on the cells in the blood. Blood tests also may show that the numbers of red blood cells, platelets, and antibodies are low.

 Did You Know...

Chronic lymphocytic leukemia does not occur in children.

Prognosis

Most types of CLL progress slowly. Doctors determine how far the disease has progressed (staging) to predict the survival time. Staging is based on factors such as the number of lymphocytes in the blood and bone marrow, size of the spleen and liver, presence or absence of anemia, and platelet count.

People who have B-cell leukemia often survive 10 to 20 years or longer after the diagnosis is made and usually do not need treatment in the early stages. People who are anemic or who have a low number of platelets need more immediate treatment and have a less favorable prognosis. Usually, death occurs because the bone marrow can no longer produce a sufficient number of normal cells to carry oxygen, fight infections, and prevent bleeding. The prognosis for people who have T-cell leukemia is usually worse.

For reasons probably related to changes in the immune system, people who have CLL are more likely to develop other cancers, such as skin or lung cancers. CLL can also transform into a more aggressive type of cancer of the lymphatic system (lymphoma).

Treatment

Because CLL progresses slowly, many people do not need treatment for years—until the number of lymphocytes begins to increase, the lymph nodes begin to enlarge, or the number of red blood cells or platelets decreases.

Drugs, which include corticosteroids, chemotherapy drugs, and monoclonal antibodies, used to treat the leukemia itself help relieve symptoms and shrink enlarged lymph nodes and spleen but do not cure the disease. For B-cell CLL, initial drug treatment includes alkylating drugs such as chlorambucil, which kill cancer cells by interacting with their DNA, or a drug called fludarabine, which interferes with the cell's ability to make DNA. Either treatment can control CLL for months to many years and can be used again with success when the leukemia regrows. Sometimes fludarabine is given together with a chemotherapy drug and a monoclonal antibody. This combination therapy often is successful in inducing remission. Eventually CLL becomes resistant to these drugs, and sometimes treatments with other drugs or monoclonal antibodies (such as rituximab or alemtuzumab) are considered. For hairy cell leukemia, 2-chlorodeoxyadenosine and deoxycoformycin are highly effective and can control the disease for more than 15 years.

Anemia due to a decreased number of red blood cells is treated with blood transfusions and occasionally with injections of erythropoietin or darbepoietin (drugs that stimulate red blood cell formation). Low platelet counts are treated with platelet transfusions, and infections are treated with antibiotics. Radiation therapy is used to shrink enlarged lymph nodes or an enlarged liver or spleen if the enlargement is causing discomfort and chemotherapy is ineffective.

Chronic Myelocytic Leukemia

Chronic myelocytic (myeloid, myelogenous, granulocytic) leukemia is a disease in which cells that normally would develop into neutrophils, basophils, eosinophils, and monocytes become cancerous.

- People pass through a phase in which they have nonspecific symptoms such as tiredness, anorexia, and weight loss.
- As the disease progresses, the lymph nodes and spleen enlarge, and people may also be pale and bruise or bleed easily.
- Blood tests, bone marrow examination, and chromosome analysis are needed for diagnosis.
- Treatment is with imatinib or with high doses of chemotherapy drugs followed by stem cell transplantation.

Chronic myelocytic leukemia (CML) may affect people of any age and of either sex but is uncommon in children younger than 10 years. The disease most commonly develops in adults between the ages of 40 and 60. The cause usually is a rearrangement of two particular chromosomes into what is called the Philadelphia chromosome. The Philadelphia chromosome produces an abnormal enzyme (tyrosine kinase), which is responsible for the abnormal growth pattern of the white blood cells in CML.

In CML, most of the leukemia cells are produced in the bone marrow, but some are produced in the spleen and liver. In contrast to the acute leukemias, in which large numbers of immature white blood cells (blasts) are present, the chronic stage of CML is characterized by marked increases in the numbers of normal-appearing white blood cells and sometimes platelets. During the course of the disease, more and more leukemia cells fill the bone marrow and others enter the bloodstream.

Eventually the leukemia cells undergo more changes, and the disease progresses to an accelerated phase and then inevitably to blast crisis. In blast crisis, only immature leukemia cells are produced, a sign that the disease has become much worse. Massive enlargement of the spleen is common in blast crisis, as well as fever and weight loss.

Symptoms and Diagnosis

Early on, in its chronic stage, CML may produce no symptoms. However, some people become fatigued and weak, lose their appetite, lose weight, develop a fever or night sweats, and notice a sensation of being full—which is usually caused by an enlarged spleen. As the disease progresses to blast crisis, people become sicker because the number of red blood cells and platelets decreases, leading to paleness, bruising, and bleeding.

The diagnosis of CML is suspected based on the results of a simple blood test. The test may show an abnormally high white blood cell count. In blood samples examined under a microscope, less mature white blood cells, normally found only in bone marrow, are seen.

Tests that analyze chromosomes (cytogenetics or molecular genetics) are needed to confirm the diagnosis by detecting the Philadelphia chromosome.

Prognosis and Treatment

Although most treatments do not cure the disease, they do slow its progress. The drug imatinib and similar newer drugs block the abnormal enzyme produced by the Philadelphia chromosome. These drugs are more effective than other treatments and cause only minor side effects. With imatinib therapy, taken by mouth, survival is over 90% at 5 years past diagnosis.

Stem cell transplantation (see page 1133) combined with high doses of chemotherapy drugs may cure CML. However, only certain people can have transplantation. Stem cells must come from a donor who has a compatible tissue type, usually a sibling. Transplantation is most effective during the early stage of the disease and is considerably less effective if the CML is rapidly progressing or there is a blast crisis.

People in a blast crisis live only a few months without treatment. Treatment with imatinib plus chemotherapy drugs sometimes extends survival to 12 months or more. There are also older chemotherapy regimens that can be given to people who relapse after receiving imatinib or who have CML without a Philadelphia chromosome. The main drugs used are busulfan, hydroxyurea, and interferon. None of these drugs prolongs survival, but they may help relieve symptoms.

CHAPTER
161 Lymphomas

Lymphomas are cancers of lymphocytes, which reside in the lymphatic system and in blood-forming organs.

Lymphomas are cancers of a specific type of white blood cells known as lymphocytes. These cells help fight infections. Lymphomas can develop from either B or T lymphocytes. T lymphocytes are important in regulating the immune system and in fighting viral infections. B lymphocytes produce antibodies.

Lymphocytes move about to all parts of the body through the bloodstream and through a network of tubular channels called lymphatic vessels (see art on page 1098). Scattered throughout the network of lymphatic vessels are lymph nodes, which house collections of lymphocytes. Lymphocytes that become cancerous (lymphoma cells) may remain confined to a single lymph node or may spread to the bone marrow, the spleen, or virtually any other organ.

The two major types of lymphoma are Hodgkin lymphoma, previously known as Hodgkin's disease, and non-Hodgkin lymphoma. Non-Hodgkin lymphomas are more common than Hodgkin lymphoma. Burkitt's lymphoma and mycosis fungoides are subtypes of non-Hodgkin lymphomas.

Hodgkin Lymphoma

Hodgkin lymphoma is a type of lymphoma distinguished by the presence of a particular kind of cancer cell called a Reed-Sternberg cell.

- The cause is unknown.
- Lymph nodes enlarge but are not painful.
- Other symptoms, such as muscle weakness, fever, and shortness of breath, develop depending on where the cancer cells are growing.
- A lymph node biopsy is needed for diagnosis.

- Chemotherapy and radiation therapy are used for treatment.
- Most people are cured.

In the United States, about 8,000 new cases of Hodgkin lymphoma occur every year. The disease is more common in males than in females—about three men are affected for every two women. Hodgkin lymphoma rarely occurs before age 10. It is most common in people between the ages of 15 and 40 and in people older than 50.

The cause of Hodgkin lymphoma is unknown. There is strong evidence that, in some people, Epstein-Barr virus infection causes B lymphocytes to become cancerous and transform into Reed-Sternberg cells. Although there are some families in which more than one person has Hodgkin lymphoma, it is not contagious.

Symptoms

People with Hodgkin lymphoma usually become aware of one or more enlarged lymph nodes, most often in the neck but sometimes in the armpit or groin. Although usually painless, sometimes the enlarged lymph nodes may be painful for a few hours after a person drinks alcoholic beverages.

People with Hodgkin lymphoma sometimes experience fever, night sweats, and weight loss. They can also have itching and fatigue. Some people have Pel-Ebstein fever, an unusual pattern of high temperature for several days alternating with normal or below-normal temperature for days or weeks. Other symptoms may develop, depending on where the cancerous cells are growing. For example, enlargement of lymph nodes in the chest may partially narrow and irritate airways, resulting in a cough, chest discomfort, or shortness of breath. Enlargement of the spleen or lymph nodes in the abdomen may cause discomfort in the abdomen.

SYMPTOMS OF HODGKIN LYMPHOMA

SYMPTOMS*	CAUSE
Weakness and shortness of breath, resulting from too few red blood cells (anemia) Infection and fever, resulting from too few white blood cells Bleeding, resulting from too few platelets Possibly bone pain	Lymphoma cells are invading the bone marrow.
Loss of muscle strength Hoarseness	Enlarged lymph nodes are compressing nerves in the spinal cord or nerves to the vocal cords.
Jaundice	Lymphoma cells are blocking the flow of bile from the liver.
Swelling of the face, neck, and arms (superior vena cava syndrome)	Enlarged lymph nodes are blocking the flow of blood returning from the head to the heart.
Swelling of legs and feet (edema)	Lymphoma cells are blocking the flow of lymph fluid from the legs.
Cough and shortness of breath	Lymphoma cells are invading the lungs.
Decreased ability to fight infection and increased susceptibility to fungal and viral infections	Lymphoma cells are continuing to spread.

*Some of these symptoms may occur for more than one reason.

Diagnosis

Doctors suspect Hodgkin lymphoma when a person with no apparent infection develops persistent and painless enlargement of lymph nodes that lasts for several weeks. The suspicion is stronger when lymph node enlargement is accompanied by fever, night sweats, and weight loss. Rapid and painful enlargement of lymph nodes—which may occur when a person has a cold or infection—is not typical of Hodgkin lymphoma. Sometimes enlarged lymph nodes deep within the chest or abdomen are found unexpectedly on a chest x-ray or computed tomography (CT) scan done for another reason.

Abnormalities in blood cell counts and other blood tests may provide supportive evidence. However, to make the diagnosis, doctors must perform a biopsy of an affected lymph node to see if it is abnormal and if Reed-Sternberg cells are present. Reed-Sternberg cells are large cancerous cells that have more than one nucleus. Their distinctive appearance can be seen when a biopsy specimen of lymph node tissue is examined under a microscope.

The type of biopsy depends on which node is enlarged and how much tissue is needed. Doctors must remove enough tissue to be able to distinguish Hodgkin lymphoma from other disorders that can cause lymph node enlargement, including non-Hodgkin lymphomas, infections, or other cancers.

The best way to obtain enough tissue is with an excisional biopsy. A small incision is made to remove a piece of the lymph node. Occasionally, when an enlarged lymph node is close to the body's surface, a sufficient amount of tissue can be obtained by inserting a hollow needle through the skin and into the lymph node (needle biopsy). When an enlarged lymph node is deep inside the abdomen or chest, surgery may be needed to obtain a piece of tissue.

Staging

Before treatment is started, doctors must determine how extensively the lymphoma has spread—the stage of the disease. The choice of treatment and the prognosis are based on the stage. An initial examination may detect only a single enlarged lymph node, but procedures to find if and where the lymphoma has spread (staging) may detect considerably more disease.

The disease is classified into four stages based on the extent of its spread (I, II, III, IV; the higher the number, the more the lymphoma has spread). The four stages are subdivided, based on the absence (A) or presence (B) of one or more of the following symptoms:

- Unexplained fever (more than 100° F [about 37.5° C] for 3 consecutive days)

STAGES OF HODGKIN LYMPHOMA

STAGE	EXTENT OF SPREAD	LIKELIHOOD OF CURE*
I	Limited to one lymph node region†	More than 80%
II	Involves two or more lymph node regions on the same side of the diaphragm, above or below it (for example, some enlarged nodes in the neck and some in the armpit)	More than 80%
III	Involves lymph node regions above and below the diaphragm (for example, some enlarged nodes in the neck and some in the groin)	70 to 80%
IV	Involves other parts of the body (such as the bone marrow, lungs, or liver), as well as lymph nodes	More than 50%

*Survival for 5 years with no further disease.
†A lymph node region is an area of the body with groups of lymph nodes that drain lymph fluid.

- Night sweats
- Unexplained loss of more than 10% of body weight in the preceding 6 months

For example, a person with a stage II lymphoma who has experienced night sweats is said to have stage IIB Hodgkin lymphoma.

Several procedures are used to stage or assess Hodgkin lymphoma. Basic blood tests, including tests of liver and kidney function, along with chest x-rays and computed tomography (CT) scans of the chest, abdomen, and pelvis are standard. CT scans are quite accurate in detecting enlarged lymph nodes or spread of the lymphoma to the liver and other organs.

Positron emission tomography (PET) scanning is the most sensitive technique for determining the stage of Hodgkin lymphoma and for evaluating the person's response to treatment. Because living tissue can be identified on a PET scan, doctors can use this imaging technique to distinguish scar tissue from active Hodgkin lymphoma after the person has undergone treatment (although PET scanning is not always accurate because inflammation can appear on PET scans). Most people with Hodgkin lymphoma do not need surgery to determine whether the disorder has spread to the abdomen, because all people receive chemotherapy, which treats the lymphoma no matter where it is located.

Treatment and Prognosis

With chemotherapy, with or without radiation therapy, most people who have Hodgkin lymphoma can be cured.

Chemotherapy is used for all stages of disease. Doctors usually use more than one chemotherapy drug. Several combinations may be used. Involved field radiation therapy (radiation therapy delivered only to the affected areas of the body, avoiding exposing unaffected areas to radiation) may be added after chemotherapy. Treatments are usually given on an outpatient basis over about 4 weeks.

More than 80% of people with stage I or stage II disease are cured with chemotherapy followed by involved field radiation therapy. The cure rate of people with stage III disease ranges from 70 to 80%. Cure rates for people with stage IV disease, while not as high, are above 50%.

Although chemotherapy greatly improves the chances for a cure, side effects can be serious. The drugs may cause temporary or permanent infertility, an increased risk of infection, potential damage to other organs, such as the heart or lungs, and reversible hair loss. After radiation therapy, there is an increased risk of cancer, such as lung, breast, or stomach cancer, occurring 10 or more years after treatment in organs that were in the radiation field. Non-Hodgkin lymphomas may develop in some people many years after successful treatment for Hodgkin lymphoma, regardless of the treatment used.

A person who has a remission (the disease under control) after initial treatment but then relapses (lymphoma cells reappear) may still be cured with second-line treatment. The cure rate for people who relapse is at least 50%. Among people who relapse in the first 12 months after initial treatment, cure rates are somewhat lower, whereas the rates for people who relapse later tend to be somewhat

Unusual Non-Hodgkin Lymphomas

Mycosis fungoides is a rare, persistent, very slow-growing non-Hodgkin lymphoma. Most people who develop it are older than 50. It originates from mature T lymphocytes (T cells) and first affects the skin. Mycosis fungoides starts so subtly and grows so slowly that it may not be noticed initially. It causes a long-lasting, itchy rash—sometimes a small area of thickened, itchy skin that later develops nodules and slowly spreads. In some people, it develops into a form of leukemia (Sézary syndrome). In other people, it progresses to the lymph nodes and internal organs. Even with a biopsy, doctors have trouble diagnosing this disease in its early stages. However, later in the course of the disease, a biopsy shows lymphoma cells in the skin.

The thickened areas of skin are treated with a form of radiation called electron beam or with sunlight and corticosteroids applied to the skin. Nitrogen mustard applied directly to the skin can help reduce the itching and size of the affected areas. Interferon drugs can also reduce symptoms. If the disease spreads to lymph nodes and other organs, chemotherapy may be needed. On average, people live 7 to 10 years after the diagnosis is made, but survival varies widely depending on how far the cancer has spread. Treatment does not cure the disease but slows it down even further.

Burkitt's lymphoma is a very fast-growing non-Hodgkin lymphoma that originates from B lymphocytes (B cells). Burkitt's lymphoma can develop at any age, but it is most common in children and young adults, particularly males. Unlike other lymphomas, Burkitt's lymphoma has a specific geographic distribution: It is most common in central Africa and rare in the United States. Infection with Epstein-Barr virus is associated with Burkitt's lymphoma. It is more common in people who have AIDS.

Burkitt's lymphoma grows and spreads quickly, often to the bone marrow, blood, and central nervous system. When it spreads, weakness and fatigue often develop. Large numbers of lymphoma cells may accumulate in the lymph nodes and organs of the abdomen, causing swelling. Lymphoma cells may invade the small intestine, resulting in blockage or bleeding. The neck and jaw may swell, sometimes painfully. To make the diagnosis, doctors do a biopsy of the abnormal tissue and order procedures to stage the disease.

Without treatment, Burkitt's lymphoma is rapidly fatal. Rarely, surgery may be needed to remove parts of the intestine that are blocked or bleeding or have ruptured. Intensive chemotherapy, which includes chemotherapy to the fluid surrounding the brain and spinal cord to prevent spread to these areas, can cure 70 to 80% of people.

higher. People who relapse after initial treatment generally are treated with a "salvage" chemotherapy regimen followed by high-dose chemotherapy. Autologous stem cell transplantation, which involves using the person's own stem cells (see page 1933), may be done after high-dose chemotherapy. High-dose chemotherapy with stem cell transplantation is generally a safe procedure, with less than a 1 to 2% risk of death related to the treatment.

Non-Hodgkin Lymphomas

Non-Hodgkin lymphomas are a diverse group of cancers that develop in B or T lymphocytes.

- Often, lymph nodes in the neck, under the arms, or in the groin enlarge rapidly and painlessly.
- People may have pain or shortness of breath or other symptoms when enlarged lymph nodes press on organs.
- A lymph node biopsy is needed for diagnosis.
- Treatment may involve radiation therapy, chemotherapy, monoclonal antibodies, or a combination.
- Most people are cured or survive for many years.

This group of cancers is actually more than 20 different diseases, which have distinct appearances under the microscope, different cell patterns, and different clinical courses. Most non-Hodgkin lymphomas (85%) are from B cells. Less than 15% develop from T cells. Non-Hodgkin lymphoma is more common than Hodgkin lymphoma. In the United States, about 65,000 new cases are diagnosed every year, and the number of new cases is increasing, especially among older people and people whose immune system is not functioning normally. People who have had organ transplants and some people who have been infected with the human immunodeficiency virus (HIV) are at risk of developing non-Hodgkin lymphoma.

Although the cause of non-Hodgkin lymphomas is not known, evidence strongly supports a role for viruses in some of the less common types. A rare type of rapidly progressive non-Hodgkin lymphoma, which occurs in southern Japan and the Caribbean, may result from infection with human T-cell lymphotropic virus 1 (HTLV-1), a retrovirus similar to HIV. The Epstein-Barr virus is associated with many cases of Burkitt's lymphoma, another type of non-Hodgkin lymphoma.

SYMPTOMS OF NON-HODGKIN LYMPHOMA

SYMPTOMS	CAUSE
Difficulty breathing Swelling of the face	Lymph nodes in the chest are enlarged.
Loss of appetite Severe constipation Abdominal pain or distention	Lymph nodes in the abdomen are enlarged.
Progressive swelling of the legs	Lymph vessels in the groin or abdomen are blocked.
Weight loss Diarrhea Flatulence Bloating and cramping (indicating malabsorption—nutrients are not absorbed normally into the blood)	Lymphoma cells are invading the small intestine.
Shortness of breath Chest pain Cough (indicating fluid accumulation around the lungs, called pleural effusion)	Lymph vessels in the chest are blocked.
Thickened, dark, itchy areas of skin	Lymphoma cells are infiltrating the skin.
Weight loss Fever Night sweats	The disease is spreading throughout the body.
Fatigue Shortness of breath Pale skin (indicating anemia, or too few red blood cells)	One or more of the following occurs: ■ Bleeding into the digestive tract ■ Destruction of red blood cells by an enlarged spleen or by abnormal antibodies ■ Invasion and destruction of bone marrow by lymphoma cells ■ Inability of the bone marrow, damaged by treatment (drugs or radiation therapy), to produce enough red blood cells
Susceptibility to severe bacterial infections	Lymphoma cells are invading the bone marrow and lymph nodes, reducing antibody production.

Symptoms

The first symptom is often rapid and usually painless enlargement of lymph nodes in the neck, under the arms, or in the groin. Enlarged lymph nodes within the chest may press against airways, causing cough and difficulty in breathing. Deep lymph nodes within the abdomen may press against various organs, causing loss of appetite, constipation, abdominal pain, or progressive swelling of the legs.

Since some lymphomas can appear in the bloodstream and bone marrow, people can develop symptoms related to too few red blood cells, white blood cells, or platelets. Too few red blood cells can cause anemia, leading to fatigue, shortness of breath, and pale skin. Too few white blood cells can lead to infections. Too few platelets may lead to increased bruising or bleeding. Non-Hodgkin lymphomas also commonly invade the bone marrow, digestive tract, skin, and occasionally the nervous system, causing various symptoms. Some people have persistent fever without an evident cause, the so-called fever of unknown origin. This type of fever commonly reflects an advanced stage of disease.

In children, the first symptoms—anemia, rashes, and neurologic symptoms, such as weakness and abnormal sensation—are likely to be caused by infiltration of lymphoma cells into the bone marrow, blood, skin, intestine, brain, and spinal cord. Lymph nodes that become enlarged are usually deep ones, leading to the following:

- Accumulation of fluid around the lungs, which causes difficulty in breathing
- Pressure on the intestine, which causes loss of appetite or vomiting
- Blocked lymph vessels, which causes fluid retention, most noticeably in the arms and legs

Diagnosis and Classification

Doctors do a biopsy of an enlarged lymph node to diagnose non-Hodgkin lymphomas and to distinguish them from Hodgkin lymphoma and other disorders that cause enlarged lymph nodes.

Although more than 20 different disorders can be called non-Hodgkin lymphomas, doctors sometimes group them into two broad categories.

Indolent lymphomas are characterized by

- A long survival period (many years)
- Rapid response to many treatments
- Lack of cure when standard therapies are used

Aggressive lymphomas are characterized by

- Rapid progression without therapy
- High rates of cure with standard chemotherapy

Although non-Hodgkin lymphomas are usually diseases of middle-aged and older people, children and young adults may develop lymphomas, and lymphomas that develop in children and young adults are commonly aggressive subtypes.

Staging

Many people with non-Hodgkin lymphomas have disease that has spread at the time of diagnosis. In only 10 to 30% of people, the disease is limited to one region. People with these lymphomas undergo similar staging procedures as people with Hodgkin lymphoma (see page 1062). In addition, a bone marrow biopsy is almost always done.

Treatment and Prognosis

For some people with indolent lymphomas, treatment is not needed. Almost everyone else benefits from treatment. For people with aggressive lymphomas, cure is possible. For people with indolent lymphomas, treatment, when needed, extends life and relieves symptoms for many years. The likelihood of a cure or long-term survival depends on the type of non-Hodgkin lymphoma and the stage when treatment starts. It is somewhat of a paradox that indolent lymphomas usually respond readily to treatment by going into remission (in which the disease is under control), often followed by long-term survival, but the disease usually is not cured. In contrast, aggressive non-Hodgkin lymphomas, which usually require

very intensive treatment to achieve remission, have a good chance of being cured.

Stage I and II Non-Hodgkin Lymphomas: People with indolent lymphomas who have very limited disease (stages I and II) are often treated with radiation therapy limited to the site of the lymphoma and adjacent areas. With this approach, most people do not have a disease recurrence in the irradiated area. Non-Hodgkin lymphomas can recur elsewhere in the body as long as 10 years after treatment, so people require long-term monitoring. People with aggressive lymphomas at a very early stage need to be treated with combination chemotherapy and sometimes radiation therapy. With this approach, 70 to 90% of people are cured.

> **? Did You Know...**
>
> Non-Hodgkin lymphomas are actually a group of more than 20 different diseases.

Stage III and IV Non-Hodgkin Lymphomas: Almost all people with indolent lymphomas have stage III or IV disease. They do not always require treatment initially, but they are monitored for evidence of lymphoma progression, which could signal a need for therapy, sometimes years after the initial diagnosis. There is no evidence that early treatment extends survival in people with indolent lymphomas at more advanced stages. If the disease begins to progress, there are many treatment choices.

It is not known which treatment option is best initially, so the choice of treatment is influenced by the extent of disease and the person's symptoms. Treatment may include therapy with monoclonal antibodies (rituximab) alone or chemotherapy with or without rituximab. These antibodies are given intravenously. Sometimes, the monoclonal antibodies are modified so that they can carry radioactive particles or toxic chemicals directly to the cancer cells in different parts of the body. Treatment usually produces a remission. The average length of remission ranges from 2 years to more than 5 years. When rituximab is combined with chemotherapy, the results of remission are better. The roles of maintenance chemotherapy (chemotherapy given after the initial treatment to help prevent relapse) and combined chemotherapy plus radioimmunotherapy are being studied.

A decision about treatment after a relapse (in which lymphoma cells reappear) depends on the extent of the disease and the symptoms. If non-Hodgkin lymphoma relapses, a type of radiation therapy called radioimmunotherapy is an option. After an initial relapse, remissions tend to become shorter.

For people with aggressive stage III or IV non-Hodgkin lymphomas, combinations of chemotherapy drugs are given promptly, often together with rituximab. Many potentially effective combinations of chemotherapy drugs are available. Combinations of chemotherapy drugs are often given names created by using single letters from each of the drugs that are included. For example, one of the oldest and still one of the most commonly used combinations is known as CHOP (cyclophosphamide, [hydroxy]doxorubicin, vincristine [Oncovin], and prednisone). Rituximab has been shown to improve the outcome of CHOP and is now routinely added to the combination (R-CHOP). More than 70% of people with aggressive non-Hodgkin lymphomas at an advanced stage are cured with R-CHOP chemotherapy. Newer combinations of drugs are being studied. Chemotherapy, which often causes different types of blood cells to decrease in number, is sometimes better tolerated if special proteins (called growth factors) are also given to stimulate growth and development of blood cells.

Relapse: Chemotherapy at usual doses is of very limited value when relapse occurs. Many people who have a relapse of an aggressive lymphoma receive high doses of chemotherapy drugs combined with autologous stem cell transplantation, involving the person's own stem cells (see page 1133). With this type of treatment, up to 50% of people may be cured. Sometimes stem cells from a sibling or even an unrelated donor (allogeneic transplant) can be used, but this type of transplantation has a greater risk of complications.

CHAPTER

162 Myeloproliferative Disorders

In myeloproliferative disorders (myelo = bone marrow, proliferative = rapid multiplication), the blood-producing cells in the bone marrow (precursor cells) develop and reproduce excessively or are crowded out by an overgrowth of fibrous tissue. Typically, these disorders are acquired and not inherited, although rarely there are families in which several members have these disorders. It is likely that family members inherit a predisposition to the disorder rather than the disorder itself.

Three major myeloproliferative disorders are polycythemia vera, myelofibrosis, and thrombocythemia. The proliferation of blood-producing cells is always noncancerous (benign) when it begins. However, in a small number of people, a myeloproliferative disorder progresses or transforms to a cancerous (malignant) condition, such as leukemia.

Polycythemia Vera

Polycythemia vera (primary polycythemia) is a disorder of the blood-producing cells of the bone marrow that results in overproduction of red blood cells.

- The cause is not known.
- People may feel tired and weak, light-headed, or short of breath.
- Blood tests are done for diagnosis.
- Phlebotomy is done to remove excess red blood cells.

In polycythemia vera, the excess of red blood cells increases the volume of blood and makes it thicker, so that it flows less easily through small blood vessels. Sometimes the spleen and liver also produce excess blood cells.

Polycythemia vera occurs in about 2 in every 100,000 people. The average age at which the disorder is diagnosed is 60, and it rarely occurs in people younger than 20. More men than women develop polycythemia vera. The cause is not known.

Symptoms and Complications

Often, people with polycythemia vera have no symptoms for years. The earliest symptoms usually are weakness, tiredness, headache, light-headedness, shortness of breath, and night sweats. Vision may be distorted, and people may have blind spots or see flashes of light. Bleeding from the gums and more bleeding than would be expected from small cuts are common. The skin, especially the face, may look red. People may itch all over, particularly after bathing or showering. Burning sensations in the hands and feet or, more rarely, bone pain may be felt.

Sometimes the first symptoms are from a blood clot. A clot may form in almost any blood vessel, including those of the arms, legs, heart (causing a heart attack), brain (causing a stroke), or lungs. Blood clots may also block blood vessels that drain blood from the liver (Budd-Chiari syndrome).

MAJOR MYELOPROLIFERATIVE DISORDERS

DISORDER	BONE MARROW CHARACTERISTICS	BLOOD CHARACTERISTICS
Polycythemia vera	Increased number of cells that produce the circulating blood cells	Increased number of red blood cells Often, increased number of platelets and white blood cells
Myelofibrosis	Excess fibrous tissue	Increased number of immature red and white blood cells Misshapen red blood cells Decreased overall number of red blood cells (anemia) The numbers of white blood cells and platelets often eventually decrease, but in some people they increase
Thrombocythemia	Increased number of cells that produce platelets (megakaryocytes)	Increased number of platelets

In some people, the number of platelets (cell-like particles that help the body form blood clots) in the bloodstream increases. The liver and spleen may enlarge as both organs begin to produce blood cells. The spleen also enlarges as it removes red blood cells from the circulation. As the liver and spleen enlarge, a sense of fullness in the abdomen may develop. Pain can suddenly become intense should a blood clot develop in blood vessels of the liver or spleen.

The excess of red blood cells may be associated with other complications, including stomach ulcers, gout, and kidney stones. Rarely, polycythemia vera progresses to leukemia.

Diagnosis

Polycythemia vera may be discovered through routine blood tests done for another reason, even before people have any symptoms. The level of the protein that carries oxygen in red blood cells (hemoglobin) and the percentage of red blood cells in the total blood volume (the hematocrit) are abnormally high. The number of platelets and white blood cells may also be increased.

Most doctors consider a high hematocrit result to be an indication of polycythemia vera. However, the diagnosis cannot be based solely on the hematocrit result. Therefore, to help make the diagnosis, a test that uses radioactively labeled red blood cells to determine the total number of red blood cells in the body (red blood cell mass) is sometimes done.

Once the increased red blood cell mass (polycythemia) is discovered, doctors must determine whether it is polycythemia vera or polycythemia caused by some other condition (secondary polycythemia). The medical history may help differentiate between polycythemia vera and secondary polycythemia, but sometimes doctors must investigate further.

Blood levels of erythropoietin, a hormone that stimulates the bone marrow to produce red blood cells, also may be measured. Levels of erythropoietin are extremely low in polycythemia vera, but they are often, but not always, normal or high in secondary polycythemia. Rarely, cysts in the liver or kidneys and tumors in the kidneys or brain produce erythropoietin; people with these conditions have high levels of erythropoietin and may develop secondary polycythemia.

Removal of a sample of bone marrow for examination under a microscope (bone marrow biopsy—see page 1025) can also be helpful to diagnose polycythemia vera.

Prognosis and Treatment

Without treatment, about half of the people who have polycythemia vera with symptoms die in less than 2 years. With treatment, they live an average of 15 to 20 years.

Treatment does not cure polycythemia vera, but it does control it and can decrease the likelihood of complications, such as the formation of blood clots. The aim of treatment is to decrease the number of red blood cells. Usually, blood is removed from the body in a procedure called phlebotomy, similar to the way blood is removed when donating blood. A

What Are the Other Types of Polycythemia?

Polycythemia vera (which literally translates as "true polycythemia") is also known as a type of primary polycythemia. Primary means that the polycythemia is not caused by another disorder.

Congenital polycythemias are present at birth, usually caused by an inherited genetic disorder. Diagnosis is typically made when symptoms begin at an early age or when there is a family history. Certain blood tests can also help with the diagnosis, as well as identifying the specific genetic disorder.

Secondary polycythemia is caused by oxygen deprivation, which can result, for example, from smoking, severe lung disease, or heart disease. In secondary polycythemia, a high concentration of red blood cells results from an actual increase in the erythropoietin level in the blood. People who spend long periods of time in circumstances low in oxygen, such as people who live at high altitude, sometimes develop polycythemia but do not have polycythemia vera (see box on page 2005).

Secondary polycythemia may be treated with oxygen. Smokers are advised to quit and are offered treatments to assist quitting. Any underlying disorder that is causing the oxygen deprivation and secondary polycythemia is treated as effectively as possible. Phlebotomy is used to lower the number of red blood cells.

In **relative polycythemia,** a high concentration of red blood cells results from abnormally low levels of fluid (plasma). The low plasma level can result from burns, vomiting, diarrhea, drinking an inadequate amount of fluids, and the use of drugs that speed elimination of salt and water by the kidneys (diuretics). Relative polycythemia is treated by giving fluids by mouth or intravenously and by treating any underlying conditions that are contributing to the low plasma level.

pint of blood is removed every other day until the hematocrit reaches a normal level. Then blood is removed every few months as needed to maintain the hematocrit at a normal level.

Because phlebotomy may increase the number of platelets and does not reduce the size of an enlarged liver or spleen, people who undergo phlebotomy may need drugs to suppress production of red blood cells and platelets. Hydroxyurea, a chemotherapy drug, is frequently given, but when used for many years there is concern that it may increase the risk of transformation to leukemia, although this risk has not been proven. Alternative drugs for lowering the

number of platelets, such as interferon-alpha and anagrelide, are sometimes used in younger people who may need treatment for long periods. Some people are given radioactive phosphorus intravenously, but doctors restrict this type of treatment to people older than 70 because of the potential for transformation to leukemia. Baby aspirin has been proven to decrease the risk of blood clots.

Other drugs can help control some of the symptoms. For example, antihistamines can help relieve itching, and aspirin can relieve burning sensations in the hands and feet as well as bone pain.

Myelofibrosis

Myelofibrosis is a disorder in which fibrous tissue replaces the blood-producing cells in the bone marrow, resulting in abnormally shaped red blood cells, anemia, and an enlarged spleen.

- Myelofibrosis may occur on its own or as a result of other blood disorders.
- People may feel tired and weak, have frequent infections, and bleed easily.
- Blood tests and a bone marrow biopsy are done for diagnosis.
- Drugs and other treatments lessen the severity of anemia, increase red blood cell production, and fight infections.
- Sometimes stem cell transplantation is used.

In normal bone marrow, cells called fibroblasts produce fibrous (connective) tissue that supports the blood-producing cells. In myelofibrosis, the fibroblasts produce too much fibrous tissue, which crowds out the blood-producing cells. Consequently, red blood cell production decreases, fewer red blood cells are released into the bloodstream, and anemia develops, becoming progressively more severe. In addition, many of these red blood cells are immature or misshapen. Variable numbers of immature white blood cells and platelets also may be present in the blood. As myelofibrosis progresses, the number of white blood cells may increase or decrease, and the number of platelets typically decreases.

Myelofibrosis is rare, affecting fewer than 2 of 100,000 people in the United States. It occurs with a peak incidence at age 76.

Myelofibrosis may develop on its own (in which case it is also called idiopathic myelofibrosis or agnogenic myeloid metaplasia) or may accompany other blood disorders, such as chronic myelocytic leukemia, polycythemia vera, thrombocythemia, multiple myeloma, lymphoma, and myelodysplasia. It may also occur in people with tuberculosis, pulmonary hypertension, systemic lupus erythematosus (lupus), and systemic sclerosis (scleroderma) and in people in whom a cancer has spread to the bones.

Symptoms, Complications, and Diagnosis

Often, myelofibrosis produces no symptoms for years. However, in some people it rapidly leads to anemia, low levels of platelets in the blood, or leukemia. Eventually, anemia becomes severe enough to cause weakness, tiredness, weight loss, and a general feeling of illness (malaise). Fever and night sweats may occur. With the reduced number of white blood cells, the body is at risk for infections, so people often have frequent infections. With the reduced number of platelets, the body is at risk for bleeding.

The liver and spleen often enlarge as they try to take over some of the job of making blood cells. The spleen also destroys abnormal red cells and platelets made in the bone marrow. The destruction of so many red blood cells and platelets contributes to the spleen enlargement. Enlargement of the liver and spleen may cause pain in the abdomen and may lead to abnormally high blood pressure in certain veins (portal hypertension—see page 217) and bleeding from varicose veins in the esophagus (esophageal varices—see page 217).

Anemia and the misshapen, immature red blood cells, seen in blood samples viewed under a microscope, suggest myelofibrosis. However, a bone marrow biopsy (see page 1025) is needed to confirm the diagnosis.

Prognosis and Treatment

Because myelofibrosis generally progresses slowly, people who have it may live for 10 years or longer, but outcomes are determined by how well the bone marrow functions. Occasionally, the disorder worsens rapidly. Treatment aims to delay the progression of the disorder and to relieve complications. However, only stem cell transplantation can cure the disorder.

The combination of androgen (a male sex hormone) and prednisone temporarily lessens the severity of the anemia in about one third of people with myelofibrosis. In a few people, red blood cell production can be stimulated with erythropoietin or darbepoietin, drugs that stimulate the bone marrow to produce red blood cells. In other people, blood transfusions are needed to treat the anemia. Bacterial infections are treated with antibiotics.

Hydroxyurea, a chemotherapy drug, or interferon-alpha, a drug that affects the immune system, may decrease the size of the liver or spleen, but either drug may worsen the anemia. Rarely, the spleen becomes extremely large and painful and may have to be removed. Removal of the spleen may increase the number of red blood cells and reduce the need for transfusions.

Stem cell (bone marrow) transplantation is sometimes offered to people who are in otherwise good health and who have an appropriate matched donor (see page 1133). A transplant is the only treatment available that may cure myelofibrosis, but it also has significant risks.

Thrombocythemia

Thrombocythemia (primary thrombocythemia) is a disorder in which excess platelets are produced, leading to abnormal blood clotting or bleeding.

- The cause is not known.
- The hands and feet may tingle, and the fingertips may feel cold.
- Routine blood tests usually provide a diagnosis, but sometimes a bone marrow biopsy is needed.
- Treatments that suppress symptoms and decrease platelet production are given.

Platelets (thrombocytes) are normally produced in the bone marrow by cells called megakaryocytes. In thrombocythemia, megakaryocytes increase in number and produce too many platelets.

Thrombocythemia affects about 2 to 3 of 100,000 people. It usually occurs in people older than 50 and more frequently in women. The cause of thrombocythemia is unknown.

Symptoms

Often, thrombocythemia does not produce symptoms. However, an excess of platelets can cause blood clots to form spontaneously, blocking the flow of blood through blood vessels, especially smaller ones but also in large vessels, including vessels in the brain, liver, and heart. Older people with thrombocythemia are much more likely to form clots than are younger people.

Other Causes of a High Platelet Count

When the cause of thrombocythemia is known, the disorder is called secondary thrombocythemia. Bleeding, removal of the spleen, infections, rheumatoid arthritis, certain cancers, premature destruction of red blood cells (hemolysis), iron deficiency, and sarcoidosis can cause secondary thrombocythemia.

People with secondary thrombocythemia may have no symptoms related to the high number of platelets. Symptoms of the underlying condition usually dominate. When symptoms from a high number of platelets do occur, they are similar to those of primary thrombocythemia. Secondary thrombocythemia is diagnosed—and distinguished from primary thrombocythemia—when people with high platelet counts have a condition that readily accounts for the high number of platelets.

Treatment is aimed at the cause. If the treatment is successful, the platelet count usually returns to normal.

Symptoms are due to the blockage of blood vessels and may include tingling and other abnormal sensations in the hands and feet (paresthesias), cold fingertips, chest pain, vision changes, headaches, weakness, and dizziness. Bleeding, usually mild, may occur, often consisting of nosebleeds, easy bruising, slight oozing from the gums, or bleeding in the digestive tract. The spleen and liver may enlarge.

Diagnosis

Doctors make a diagnosis of thrombocythemia on the basis of the symptoms or after finding increased platelets during routine screening of the blood. Blood tests may be used to confirm the diagnosis. In addition, microscopic examination of the blood may reveal abnormally large platelets, clumps of platelets, and fragments of megakaryocytes.

To distinguish primary thrombocythemia, whose cause is unknown, from secondary thrombocythemia, which has a known cause, doctors look for signs of other conditions that could increase the platelet count. Removal of a sample of bone marrow for examination under a microscope (bone marrow biopsy—see page 1025) is sometimes helpful and can exclude chronic myelocytic leukemia as a cause of an increased platelet count.

Treatment

Thrombocythemia may require treatment with a drug that decreases platelet production. Such drugs include hydroxyurea, anagrelide, and interferon-alpha. Treatment with one of these drugs is typically

> ## SPOTLIGHT ON AGING
>
> Thrombocythemia is more likely to occur in older people. They are also more likely to have blockages of crucial large blood vessels, such as those in the heart and brain, because older people are more likely to have conditions, such as atherosclerosis, that also may result in blood vessel blockage.
>
> Older people are given the same drugs as younger people. They are able to tolerate the side effects fairly well. However, because older people may have other disorders and decreased marrow reserve, they may not be able to tolerate any therapy as well as younger people.

started when clotting complications develop. The age of the person, the other risks present, and previous history of forming blood clots (thrombosis) determine the need for such treatment. The drug is continued until the platelet count falls into a safe range. The dose must be adjusted to maintain an adequate number of platelets and other circulating cells. Small doses of aspirin, which makes platelets less sticky and impairs clotting, may also be used.

If drug treatment does not slow platelet production quickly enough, it may be combined with or replaced by plateletpheresis, a procedure reserved for emergency situations. In this procedure, blood is withdrawn, platelets are removed from it, and the platelet-depleted blood is returned to the person.

CHAPTER 163 Spleen Disorders

The spleen, a spongy, soft organ about as big as a person's fist, is located in the upper left part of the abdomen, just under the rib cage. The splenic artery brings blood to the spleen from the heart. Blood leaves the spleen through the splenic vein, which drains into a larger vein (the portal vein) that carries the blood to the liver. The spleen has a covering of fibrous tissue (the splenic capsule) that supports its blood vessels and lymphatic vessels.

The spleen is made up of two basic types of tissue: the white pulp and the red pulp, each with different functions. The white pulp is part of the infection-fighting (immune) system. It produces white blood cells called lymphocytes, which in turn produce antibodies (specialized proteins that protect against invasion by foreign substances). The red pulp filters the blood, removing unwanted material. The red pulp contains other white blood cells called phagocytes that ingest microorganisms, such as bacteria, fungi, and viruses. It also monitors red blood cells, destroying those that are abnormal or too old or damaged to function properly. In addition, the red pulp serves as a reservoir for different elements of the blood, especially white blood cells and platelets (cell-like particles involved in clotting). However, releasing these elements is a minor function of the red pulp.

Viewing the Spleen

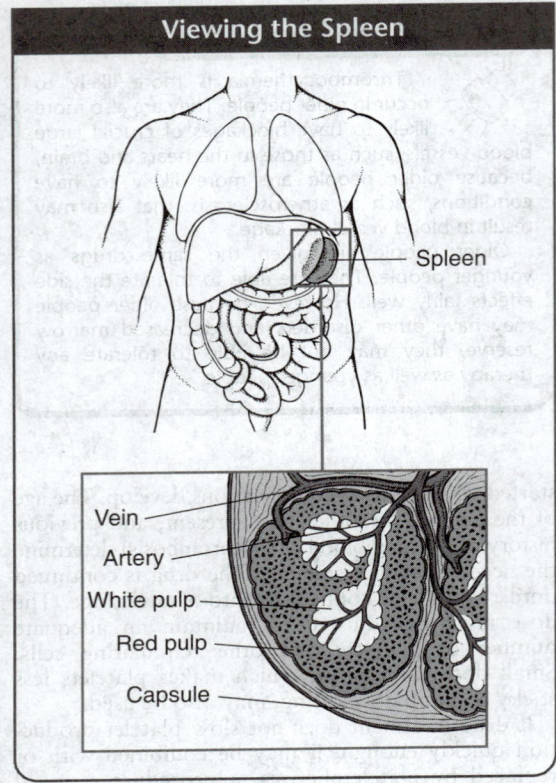

People can live without a spleen. Sometimes the spleen must be removed surgically (splenectomy) because of irreparable damage (for example, due to an injury sustained in a car crash). When the spleen is removed, the body loses some of its ability to produce protective antibodies and to remove unwanted microorganisms from the blood. As a result, the body's ability to fight infections is impaired. People who do not have a spleen are at particularly high risk of infections because of the spleen's role in fighting certain kinds of bacteria, such as *Streptococcus pneumoniae, Neisseria meningitidis,* and *Haemophilus influenzae.* Because of this risk, people receive vaccinations to help protect them from infection with these organisms. Yearly vaccinations against influenza are also recommended after a splenectomy. Some people take antibiotics to prevent infections, particularly when they have another disorder (such as sickle cell disease or cancer) that increases the risk of developing life-threatening infections.

Despite these problems, however, the spleen is not critical to survival. Other organs (primarily the liver) compensate for the loss by increasing their infection-fighting ability and by monitoring for and removing red blood cells that are abnormal, too old, or damaged.

Enlarged Spleen

- Many disorders, including infections, anemias, and cancers, can cause an enlarged spleen.
- Symptoms are usually not very specific but can include fullness or pain in the upper left abdomen or back.
- Usually doctors can feel an enlarged spleen, but x-rays and other imaging tests may be used to determine how large the spleen is.
- Treating the disorder that is causing the spleen to enlarge usually takes care of the problem, but sometimes the spleen must be removed.

An enlarged spleen (splenomegaly) is not a disease in itself but the result of an underlying disorder. Many disorders can make the spleen enlarge. To pinpoint the cause, doctors must consider disorders ranging from chronic infections to blood cancers.

When the spleen enlarges, it traps and stores an excessive number of blood cells and platelets (hypersplenism), thereby reducing the number of blood cells and platelets in the bloodstream. This process creates a vicious circle: the more cells and platelets the spleen traps, the larger it grows; the larger it grows, the more cells and platelets it traps. Eventually, the greatly enlarged spleen also traps normal red blood cells, destroying them along with the abnormal ones. In addition, excessive numbers of blood cells and platelets can clog the spleen, interfering with its functioning.

An enlarged spleen may outgrow its own blood supply. When parts of the spleen do not get enough blood, they may become damaged, causing them to bleed or die.

Symptoms

An enlarged spleen does not cause many symptoms, and the symptoms that it does cause may be mistaken for many other medical conditions. Because the enlarged spleen lies next to the stomach and sometimes presses against it, people may feel full after eating a small snack or even without eating. People may also have abdominal or back pain in the area of the spleen. The pain may spread to the left shoulder, especially if parts of the spleen do not get enough blood and start to die.

> **? Did You Know...**
> An enlarged spleen is not a disease itself but a result of an underlying disorder.

When the spleen removes too many blood cells and platelets from the bloodstream, a variety of problems may develop. These problems include anemia as a result of too few red blood cells, frequent infections as a result of too few white blood cells, and the tendency to bleed as a result of too few platelets.

Diagnosis

Doctors may suspect that the spleen is enlarged when people complain of fullness or pain in the upper left portion of the abdomen or back. Usually, doctors can feel an enlarged spleen during a physical examination. An x-ray of the abdomen may also show that the spleen is enlarged. In some cases, ultrasonography or computed tomography (CT) is needed to determine how large the spleen is and whether it is pressing on other organs. Magnetic resonance imaging (MRI) provides similar information and also traces blood flow through the spleen. Other specialized scanning devices use mildly radioactive particles to assess the spleen's size and function and to determine whether it is accumulating or destroying large numbers of blood cells.

Blood tests show decreased numbers of red blood cells, white blood cells, and platelets. When blood cells are examined under a microscope, their shape and size may provide clues to the cause of the spleen enlargement. An examination of bone marrow (see page 1025) may show cancer of the blood cells (such as leukemia or lymphoma) or an accumulation of unwanted substances (such as occurs in storage diseases). Blood protein measurement can determine whether other conditions are present that can cause the spleen to enlarge, such as amyloidosis, sarcoidosis, malaria, kala-azar, brucellosis, and tuberculosis. Liver function tests help determine whether the liver is also diseased.

Doctors cannot easily remove a sample of the spleen for examination because inserting a needle or cutting spleen tissue may cause uncontrollable bleeding. If an enlarged spleen is removed during surgery to diagnose or treat certain diseases, the spleen is sent to a laboratory, where the cause of enlargement can usually be determined.

Treatment

When possible, doctors treat the underlying disorder that caused the enlarged spleen. Surgical removal of the spleen (splenectomy) may be necessary but can cause problems, including an increased susceptibility to infections. However, the risks are worth taking in certain critical situations:

- When the spleen destroys red blood cells so rapidly that severe anemia develops
- When the spleen so depletes stores of white blood cells that infection is likely
- When the spleen so depletes stores of platelets that bleeding is likely
- When the spleen is so large that it causes pain or puts pressure on other organs
- When the spleen is so large that parts of it bleed or die

As an alternative to surgery, radiation therapy can sometimes be used to shrink the spleen.

Causes of an Enlarged Spleen

INFECTIONS

- Brucellosis
- Hepatitis
- Infectious mononucleosis
- Kala-azar
- Malaria
- Psittacosis
- Subacute bacterial endocarditis
- Syphilis
- Tuberculosis

ANEMIAS

- Hereditary elliptocytosis
- Hereditary spherocytosis
- Sickle cell disease (mainly in children)
- Thalassemia

BLOOD CANCERS AND MYELOPROLIFERATIVE DISORDERS

- Hodgkin lymphoma and other lymphomas
- Leukemia
- Myelofibrosis
- Polycythemia vera

STORAGE DISEASES

- Gaucher's disease
- Hand-Schüller-Christian disease
- Letterer-Siwe disease
- Niemann-Pick disease
- Wolman's disease

OTHER CAUSES

- Amyloidosis
- Blood clot in a vein from the spleen or to the liver
- Cirrhosis
- Cysts in the spleen
- External pressure on veins from the spleen or to the liver
- Felty's syndrome
- Sarcoidosis
- Systemic lupus erythematosus (lupus)

Spleen Injury

- An injured spleen is usually painful.
- Imaging tests such as ultrasonography or computed tomography are used to diagnose an injured spleen.

■ Blood transfusions are often needed to treat a spleen injury, and sometimes surgery to remove or repair the spleen is done.

Because of the spleen's position in the abdomen, a severe blow to the stomach area can damage the spleen, tearing its covering, the tissue inside, or both. The tears range from small ones that stop bleeding spontaneously to very large ones that cause potentially fatal hemorrhage. Sometimes a collection of blood (hematoma) forms under the covering of the spleen or deep within it.

Injury to the spleen is the most common serious complication of abdominal injury resulting from car crashes, falls from a height, athletic mishaps, and beatings. Sometimes other abdominal organs also are damaged.

When the spleen is injured, blood is released into the abdomen. The amount of bleeding depends on the size of the injury. A hematoma of the spleen may rupture in the first few days after injury, although rupture sometimes does not occur for months.

Symptoms

An injured or ruptured spleen makes the abdomen painful and tender. Blood in the abdomen acts as an irritant and causes pain. The pain is in the left side of the abdomen just below the rib cage. Sometimes the pain is felt in the left shoulder. The abdominal muscles contract reflexively and feel rigid. If enough blood leaks out, blood pressure falls and people feel light-headed, have blurred vision and confusion, and lose consciousness (fainting).

Diagnosis

Doctors usually do ultrasonography or a computed tomography (CT) scan of the abdomen if they suspect an injury to the spleen. Rarely, if doctors suspect a severe hemorrhage, surgery is done immediately to make a diagnosis and control the bleeding. People with severe bleeding also are given intravenous fluids and sometimes blood transfusions.

Treatment

Doctors used to always remove a damaged spleen. However, removing the spleen can cause later problems, including an increased susceptibility to infections. Doctors now realize that most small and many moderate-sized injuries to the spleen can heal without surgery, although blood transfusions are sometimes required and people must be treated in the hospital. When surgery is necessary, usually the entire spleen is removed (splenectomy), but sometimes surgeons are able to repair a small tear.

After a splenectomy, certain precautions are needed to prevent infections (see page 1072).

Cancer

CHAPTER
164 Overview of Cancer

A cancer is an abnormal growth of cells (usually derived from a single cell). The cells have lost normal control mechanisms and thus are able to expand continuously, invade adjacent tissues, migrate to distant parts of the body, and promote the growth of new blood vessels from which the cells derive nutrients. Cancerous (malignant) cells can develop from any tissue within the body.

As cancerous cells grow and multiply, they form a mass of cancerous tissue—called a tumor—that invades and destroys normal adjacent tissues. The term tumor refers to an abnormal growth or mass. Tumors can be cancerous or noncancerous. Cancerous cells from the primary (initial) site can spread throughout the body (metastasize).

Types of Cancer

Cancerous tissues (malignancies) can be divided into those of the blood and blood-forming tissues (leukemias and lymphomas) and "solid" tumors, often termed cancer. Cancers can be carcinomas or sarcomas.

Leukemias and **lymphomas** are cancers of the blood and blood-forming tissues and cells of the immune system. They often harm the body by crowding out normal blood cells in the bone marrow and bloodstream, so that normal functioning cells are gradually replaced by cancerous blood cells. They expand lymph nodes, producing large masses in the armpit, groin, abdomen, or chest.

Carcinomas are cancers of epithelial cells, which are cells that cover the surface of the body, produce hormones, and make up glands. Examples of carcinomas are cancer of the skin, lung, colon, stomach, breast, prostate, and thyroid gland. Typically, carcinomas occur more often in older than in younger people.

Sarcomas are cancers of mesodermal cells, which are the cells that form muscles and connective tissue. Examples of sarcomas are leiomyosarcoma (cancer of smooth muscle that is found in the wall of digestive organs) and osteosarcoma (bone cancer). Typically, sarcomas occur more often in younger than in older people.

Development and Spread

Cancerous cells develop from healthy cells in a complex process called malignant transformation.

Initiation: The first step in cancer development is initiation, in which a change in the cell's genetic material primes the cell to become cancerous. The change in the cell's genetic material may occur spontaneously or be brought on by an agent that causes cancer (a carcinogen). Carcinogens include many chemicals, tobacco, viruses, radiation, and sunlight. However, not all cells are equally susceptible to carcinogens. A genetic flaw in a cell may make it more susceptible. Even chronic physical irritation may make a cell more susceptible to carcinogens.

Promotion: The second and final step in the development of cancer is promotion. Agents that cause promotion, or promoters, may be substances in the environment or even some drugs (such as barbiturates). Unlike carcinogens, promoters do not cause cancer by themselves. Instead, promoters allow a cell that has undergone initiation to become cancerous. Promotion has no effect on cells that have not undergone initiation. Thus, several factors, often the combination of a susceptible cell and a carcinogen, are needed to cause cancer.

MOST COMMON CANCERS IN MEN AND WOMEN*

GROUP	CANCER
Men	Prostate
	Lung
	Colon and rectum
	Bladder
	Non-Hodgkin lymphoma
Women	Breast
	Lung
	Colon and rectum
	Uterus
	Non-Hodgkin lymphoma

* In decreasing order of frequency. The order is based on statistics from the American Cancer Society. Skin cancer is probably the most common cancer in both men and women, but only one type of skin cancer—melanoma—is required to be reported, so how common other types are is less clear. Thus, skin cancer figures are incomplete and are therefore generally excluded from statistics.

Talking About Cancer

Aggressiveness: The degree to which (or speed at which) a tumor grows and spreads.

Anaplasia: A lack of differentiation. Thus, an anaplastic cancer is highly undifferentiated and usually very aggressive.

Benign: Noncancerous. Thus, a benign tumor is unable to spread to adjacent tissues or to metastasize.

Carcinogen: An agent that causes cancer.

Carcinoma-in-situ: Cancerous cells that are still contained within the tissue where they have started to grow and that have not yet become invasive or spread to other parts of the body.

Cure: Complete elimination of the cancer with the result that the specific cancer will not grow back.

Differentiation: The extent to which the cancerous cells resemble normal cells—less resemblance means the cancer is less differentiated and more aggressive.

Invasion: The capacity of a cancer to infiltrate and destroy surrounding tissue.

Malignant: Cancerous.

Metastasis: Cancerous cells that have spread to a completely new location.

Neoplasm: General term for a tumor, whether cancerous or noncancerous.

Recurrence (relapse): Cancerous cells return after treatment, either in the primary location or as metastases (spread).

Remission: Absence of all evidence of a cancer after treatment.

Survival rate: The percentage of people who survive for a given time period after treatment (for example, the 5-year survival rate is the percentage of people who survive 5 years).

Tumor: An abnormal growth or mass.

Some carcinogens are sufficiently powerful to be able to cause cancer without the need for promotion. For example, ionizing radiation (which is used in x-rays and is produced in nuclear power plants and atomic bomb explosions) can cause various cancers, particularly sarcomas, leukemia, thyroid cancer, and breast cancer.

Spread: Cancer can grow directly into surrounding tissue or spread to tissues or organs, nearby or distant. Cancer can spread through the lymphatic system. This type of spread is typical of carcinomas. For example, breast cancer usually spreads first to the nearby lymph nodes, and only later does it spread to distant sites. Cancer can also spread via the bloodstream. This type of spread is typical of sarcomas.

? Did You Know...

The -oma ending on the name of a cell type describes cancer cells of a particular type. For example, a meningioma is a cancer that develops in the covering of the brain or spinal cord (the meninges), and a hepatoma is a cancer that starts in the liver.

Risk Factors for Cancer

Many genetic and environmental factors increase the risk of developing cancer. However, not all people who are exposed to carcinogens or who have other risk factors develop cancer.

Family History and Genetic Factors: Some families have a significantly higher risk of developing certain cancers. Sometimes the increased risk is due to a single gene, and sometimes it is due to several genes interacting together. Environmental factors—common to the family—may alter this genetic interaction and produce cancer.

An extra or abnormal chromosome may increase the risk of cancer. For example, people with Down syndrome, who have three instead of the usual two copies of chromosome 21, have a 12 to 20 times higher risk of developing acute leukemia.

Age: Some cancers, such as Wilms' tumor, retinoblastoma, and neuroblastoma, occur almost exclusively in children. Why these cancers occur in the young is not well understood, but probably the cancers result from mutations that are inherited or that occur during fetal development. However, most cancers are more common in older people. In the United States, more than 60% of cancers occur in people older than 65. The increased cancer rate is probably due to a combination of increased and prolonged exposure to carcinogens and weakening of the body's immune system.

Environmental Factors: Numerous environmental factors increase the risk of developing cancer.

Tobacco smoke contains carcinogens that substantially increase the risk of developing cancers of the lungs, mouth, throat, esophagus, kidneys, and bladder.

Pollution in the air, whether from industrial waste or cigarette smoke, can increase the cancer risk. Many chemicals are known to cause cancer, and many others are suspected of doing so. For example, asbestos exposure may cause lung cancer and mesothelioma (cancer of the pleura), especially in smokers. Exposure to pesticides is associated with a higher risk of some types of cancer (for example, leukemia and non-Hodgkin lymphoma). The time between exposure to the chemicals and development of the cancer may be many years.

Exposure to radiation is a risk factor in the development of cancer. Extended exposure to ultraviolet radiation, primarily from sunlight, causes skin cancer. Ionizing radiation is particularly carcinogenic. Exposure to the radioactive gas radon, which is released from soil, increases the risk of lung cancer. Normally, radon disperses rapidly into the atmosphere and produces no harm. However, when a building is placed on soil with a high radon content, radon can accumulate within the building, sometimes producing sufficiently high levels in the air to cause harm. Radon is breathed into the lungs, where it may eventually cause lung cancer. In exposed people who also smoke, the risk of lung cancer is further increased.

Many other substances have been investigated as possible causes of cancer, but more study is needed to identify those chemicals that increase the risk of cancer.

Geography: The risk of cancer varies according to where people live, although the reasons for the geographic differences are often complex and poorly understood. This geographic variation in cancer risk is probably multifactorial: a combination of genetics, diet, and environment.

Genes That Cause Cancer

Abnormalities (mutations) affecting critical genes are believed to contribute to the development of cancer. These genes produce proteins that regulate growth and alter cell division and other basic cell properties.

Gene mutations causing cancer may result from the damaging effects of chemicals, sunlight, drugs, viruses, or other environmental agents. In some families, these abnormal cancer-causing genes are inherited.

The two major categories of genes involved with cancer are oncogenes and tumor suppressor genes.

Oncogenes are mutated forms of genes that in their normal state regulate cell growth. If they become overactive and signal cells to divide when these cells should not, cancer may develop. The mutation of oncogenes is not entirely understood, but many factors may contribute, including x-rays; sunlight; toxins at work, in the air, or in chemicals (for example, in tobacco smoke); and infectious agents (for example, certain viruses).

Tumor suppressor genes normally suppress the development of cancers by coding for proteins that repair damaged DNA and suppress growth. Cancer is more likely when DNA damage impairs tumor suppressor gene function, allowing affected cells to divide continuously.

SOME CARCINOGENS

CARCINOGEN	TYPE OF CANCER
Environmental and industrial	
Arsenic	Lung
Asbestos	Lung
	Pleura
Aromatic amines	Bladder
Benzene	Leukemia
Chromates	Lung
Diesel exhaust	Lung
Ionizing radiation	Leukemia
Nickel	Lung
	Nasal sinuses
Pesticides	Lung
Radon	Lung
Ultraviolet radiation	Skin
Vinyl chloride	Liver
Associated with lifestyle	
Betel nuts	Mouth
	Throat
Tobacco	Bladder
	Esophagus
	Kidney
	Lung
	Mouth
	Throat
Used in medicine	
Chemotherapy drugs (such as topoisomerase inhibitors)	Bladder
	Leukemia
Diethylstilbestrol	Breast (in women who took the drug and in women exposed before birth)
	Cervix (when exposed before birth)
	Vagina (when exposed before birth)
Oxymetholone	Liver
Radiation therapy	Sarcomas

For example, the risk of colon and breast cancers is low in Japan, yet in Japanese people who immigrate to the United States, the risk increases and eventually equals that of the rest of the American population. In contrast, the Japanese have extremely high rates of stomach cancer. When these people immigrate to the United States and eat a Western diet, the risk declines to that of the United States, although the decline may not be evident until the next generation.

Diet: Substances consumed in the diet can increase the risk of cancer. For instance, a diet high in fat has been linked to an increased risk of colon, breast, and possibly prostate cancer. People who drink large amounts of alcohol are at much higher risk of developing esophageal cancer. A diet high in smoked and pickled foods or in barbecued meats increases the risk of developing stomach cancer. People who are overweight or obese have a higher risk of cancer of the breast, lining of the uterus (endometrium), colon, kidneys, and esophagus.

Drugs and Medical Treatments: Certain drugs and medical treatments may increase the risk of developing cancer. For example, estrogens in oral contraceptives may slightly increase the risk of breast cancer, but this risk decreases over time. The hormones estrogen and progestin that may be given to women during menopause (hormone replacement therapy) also increase the risk of breast cancer. Diethylstilbestrol (DES) increases the risk of breast cancer in women who took the drug and in daughters of these women who were exposed before birth. Long-term use of anabolic steroids may slightly increase the risk of liver and prostate cancer. Treatment of cancer with chemotherapy drugs and with radiation therapy may increase the risk of people developing a second cancer years later.

Infections: Several viruses are known to cause cancer in humans, and several others are suspected of causing cancer. The human papillomavirus (HPV, which causes genital warts) is one cause of cervical cancer in women. Hepatitis B virus or hepatitis C virus can cause liver cancer. Some human retroviruses cause lymphomas and other cancers of the blood system. Some viruses produce types of cancer in certain countries but not in others. For instance, the Epstein-Barr virus causes Burkitt's lymphoma (a type of cancer) in Africa and cancers of the nose and pharynx in China.

Some bacteria also may cause cancer. *Helicobacter pylori*, which causes stomach ulcers, can increase the risk of stomach cancer and lymphomas.

Some parasites can cause cancer. *Schistosoma haematobium* can cause chronic inflammation and scarring of the bladder, which may lead to cancer.

Another type of parasite, *Opisthorchis sinensis*, has been linked to cancer of the pancreas and bile ducts.

Inflammatory Disorders: Inflammatory disorders often increase the risk of cancer. Such disorders include ulcerative colitis (which can result in colon cancer).

Defenses Against Cancer

Even when a cell becomes cancerous, the immune system is thought to be able to recognize it as abnormal and destroy it before it replicates or spreads. Cancer is more likely to progress in people whose immune system is altered or impaired, as in people with AIDS, people receiving immunosuppressive drugs, people with certain autoimmune disorders, and older people, in whom the immune system works less well than in younger people. However, even when the immune system is functioning normally, cancer can escape the immune system's protective surveillance.

Tumor Antigens: An antigen is a foreign substance recognized and targeted for destruction by the body's immune system (see page 1095). Antigens are found on the surface of all cells, but normally the immune system does not react to a person's own cells. When a cell becomes cancerous, new antigens—unfamiliar to the immune system—appear on the cell's surface. The immune system may regard these new antigens, called tumor antigens, as foreign and may be able to contain or destroy the cancerous cells. This is the mechanism by which the body destroys abnormal cells and is often able to destroy cancerous cells before they can become established. However, even a fully functioning immune system cannot always destroy all cancerous cells. And, once cancerous cells reproduce and form a mass of cancerous cells (a cancerous tumor), the body's immune system is highly unlikely to be able to destroy it.

Tumor antigens have been identified in several types of cancer, including malignant melanoma. Vaccines made from tumor antigens might be able to prevent or treat cancer by stimulating the immune system. Such vaccines are an area of great research interest.

Certain tumor antigens can be detected with blood tests. These antigens are sometimes called **tumor markers.** Measurements of some of these tumor markers can be used to evaluate people's response to treatment (see table on page 1085). However, except for the marker prostate specific antigen (PSA), tumor markers are not very helpful as screening tests in people who have no symptoms of cancer.

CHAPTER

165 Symptoms and Diagnosis of Cancer

Cancer can produce many different symptoms, some subtle and some not at all subtle. Some symptoms develop early in the course of cancer and are therefore important warning signs that should be evaluated by a doctor. Other symptoms develop only after the cancer progresses and are therefore not helpful in the early detection of cancer. Still other symptoms, such as nausea, loss of appetite, fatigue, and vomiting, may be the result of the cancer or its treatment, may be warning signs, or may even result from conditions other than cancer. Some symptoms occur with many or almost all cancers, and others are specific to the type of cancer and where it is growing.

Screening programs allow early detection and diagnosis of cancer. The earlier cancer is diagnosed, the more effective treatment is likely to be.

Symptoms

At first, cancer, as a tiny mass of cells, produces no symptoms whatsoever. As a cancer grows, its physical presence can affect nearby tissues. Also, some cancers secrete certain substances or trigger immune reactions that cause symptoms in other parts of the body that are not near to the cancer (paraneoplastic syndromes).

Cancer affects nearby tissues by growing into or pushing on them, thus irritating or compressing them. Irritation typically causes pain. Compression may keep tissues from performing their normal functions. For example, a bladder cancer or a cancerous lymph node in the abdomen may compress the tube (ureter) connecting a kidney with the bladder, blocking the flow of urine. A lung cancer may block

Warning Signs of Cancer

Because cancer is more likely to be cured if less advanced when treatment is begun, it is critical that cancer be discovered early. Some symptoms may give early warning of cancer and should, therefore, trigger a person to seek medical care. Fortunately, most of these symptoms are usually caused by far less serious conditions. Nonetheless, the development of any of the warning signs of cancer should not be ignored.

Some of the warning signs are general. That is, they are vague changes that do not help pinpoint any particular cancer. Still, their presence can help direct doctors to do the physical examinations and laboratory tests necessary to exclude or confirm a diagnosis. Other symptoms are much more specific and steer doctors to a particular kind of cancer or location. Some warning signs of cancer are

- Weight loss
- Fatigue
- Night sweats
- Loss of appetite
- New, persistent pain
- Recurrent nausea or vomiting
- Blood in urine
- Blood in stool (either visible or detectable by special tests)
- Sudden depression
- A recent change in bowel habits (constipation or diarrhea)
- Recurrent fever
- Chronic cough
- Changes in the size or color of a mole or changes in a skin ulcer that does not heal
- Enlarged lymph nodes

airflow through one segment of a lung, causing partial lung collapse and predisposing to infection. Cancer anywhere may compress a blood vessel, shutting off blood flow or causing bleeding. When cancer grows in an area with a lot of space, such as in the wall of the large intestine, it may not cause any symptoms until it becomes quite large. In contrast, a cancer growing in a more restricted space, such as on a vocal cord, may cause symptoms (such as hoarseness) when it is relatively small. If a cancer spreads (metastasizes) to other parts of the body, the same local effects of irritation and compression eventually occur, but in the new location, so the symptoms may be quite different. Cancers that involve the membrane covering the lungs (pleura) or the baglike structure that surrounds the

heart (pericardium) often ooze fluid, which collects around those organs; large fluid collections can interfere with breathing or the pumping of the heart.

Pain

Cancers are typically painless at first. As they grow, the first symptom is often a mild discomfort, which may steadily worsen into increasingly severe pain as the cancer enlarges. The pain may result from the cancer compressing or eroding into nerves or other structures. However, not all cancers cause severe pain. Similarly, lack of pain does not guarantee that a cancer is not growing or spreading.

Bleeding

At first, a cancer may bleed slightly because its cells are not well attached to each other and its blood vessels are fragile. Later, as the cancer enlarges and invades surrounding tissues, it may grow into a nearby blood vessel, causing bleeding. The bleeding may be slight and undetectable or detectable only with testing. Such is often the case in early-stage colon cancer. Or, particularly with advanced cancer, the bleeding may be more significant, even massive and life threatening.

The site of the cancer determines the site of the bleeding. Cancer anywhere along the gastrointestinal tract can cause bleeding in the stool. Cancer anywhere along the urinary tract can cause bleeding in the urine. Other cancers can bleed into internal areas of the body. Bleeding into the lungs can cause the person to cough up blood.

Weight Loss and Fatigue

Commonly, a person with cancer experiences weight loss and fatigue, which can worsen as the cancer progresses. Some people notice weight loss despite a good appetite. Others lose their appetite and may even become nauseated by food or have difficulty swallowing. They may become very thin; the loss of underlying fat is particularly noticeable in the face. People with advanced cancer are often very tired and sleep many hours a day. If anemia develops, these people may find that they feel tired or become short of breath with even slight activity.

Swollen Lymph Nodes

As a cancer begins to spread around the body, it may first spread to nearby lymph nodes, which become swollen. The swollen lymph nodes may be painless or tender, and they may feel hard or rubbery. They may be freely moveable, or if the cancer is more advanced, they may be stuck to the skin above, to the deeper layers of tissue below, or to each other.

SOME COMPLICATIONS OF CANCER

COMPLICATION	DESCRIPTION
Cardiac tamponade	Fluid accumulates in the baglike structure surrounding the heart (pericardium, or pericardial sac). This fluid puts pressure on the heart and interferes with its ability to pump blood. Fluid can accumulate when a cancer invades the pericardium and irritates it.
Pleural effusion	Fluid accumulates in the baglike structure around the lungs (pleural sac), causing shortness of breath.
Superior vena cava syndrome	Cancer partially or completely blocks the vein (superior vena cava) that drains blood from the upper part of the body into the heart. Blockage of the superior vena cava causes the veins in the upper part of the chest and neck to swell, resulting in swelling of the face, neck, and upper part of the chest.
Spinal cord compression	Cancer compresses the spinal cord or the spinal cord nerves, resulting in pain and loss of function (such as urinary or fecal incontinence). The longer the compression of the spinal cord or spinal cord nerves persists, the less likely normal nerve function will return when the compression is relieved.
Brain dysfunction	The brain functions abnormally as a result of a cancer growing within it, either as a primary brain cancer or more commonly as a metastasis from a cancer elsewhere in the body. Many different symptoms can occur, including confusion, drowsiness, agitation, headaches, abnormal vision, abnormal sensations, weakness, nausea, vomiting, and seizures.
Bleeding	Cancer grows into and erodes nearby blood vessels. Serious, even fatal, bleeding can result from cancers in areas containing many large blood vessels, such as the neck and chest.

Depression

Cancer often results in depression. Depression can be related to the symptoms of the illness, a fear of dying, or a loss of independence. Additionally, some cancers may produce substances that directly cause depression by affecting the brain.

Neurologic and Muscular Symptoms

Cancer can grow into or compress nerves, causing any of several neurologic and muscular symptoms, including a change in sensation (such as tingling sensations) or muscle weakness. When a cancer grows in the brain, symptoms may be hard to pinpoint but can include confusion, dizziness, headaches, nausea, changes in vision, and seizures. Neurologic symptoms may also be part of a paraneoplastic syndrome.

Respiratory Symptoms

Cancer can compress or block structures, such as the airways in the lungs, causing shortness of breath, cough, or pneumonia. Shortness of breath can also occur when the cancer causes a large pleural effusion, bleeding into the lungs, or anemia.

Diagnosis

Cancer is suspected based on a person's symptoms, the results of a physical examination, and sometimes the results of screening tests. Occasionally, x-rays obtained for other reasons, such as an injury, show abnormalities that might be cancer. Confirmation that cancer is present requires other tests (termed diagnostic tests). After cancer is diagnosed, it is staged. Staging is a way of describing how advanced the cancer has become, including such criteria as how big it is and whether it has spread to neighboring tissues or more distantly to lymph nodes or other organs.

SCREENING

Screening tests serve to detect the *possibility* that a cancer is present before symptoms occur. Screening tests usually are not definitive; results are confirmed or disproved with further examinations and tests. Diagnostic tests are performed once a doctor suspects that a person has cancer.

Although screening tests can help save lives, they can be costly and sometimes have psychologic or

What Are Paraneoplastic Syndromes?

Paraneoplastic syndromes occur when a cancer produces one or more substances that circulate in the bloodstream to cause symptoms at sites distant from the tumor. These substances can affect the function of other tissues and organs, resulting in a variety of symptoms. Paraneoplastic syndromes may affect many different organ systems, including the nervous system and the endocrine (hormone) system, causing such problems as low blood sugar, diarrhea, or high blood pressure.

General syndromes such as the development of fever, night sweats, and loss of weight and appetite can be experienced by many people with cancer. Most of the syndromes discussed below are uncommon, and most cancer patients do not experience these more specific paraneoplastic syndromes.

Neurologic syndromes: Polyneuropathy is a dysfunction of peripheral nerves, resulting in weakness, loss of sensation, and reduced reflexes. Subacute sensory neuropathy is a rare form of polyneuropathy that sometimes develops before the cancer is diagnosed. It causes a disabling loss of sensation and incoordination but little weakness.

Paraneoplastic cerebellar degeneration occurs rarely in patients with breast cancer, ovarian cancer, small cell carcinoma of the lung, or other solid tumors. This disorder may be caused by an autoantibody (an antibody that attacks the body's own tissues) that destroys the cerebellum. Symptoms can include unsteadiness in walking, incoordination of the arms and legs, difficulty speaking, dizziness, and double vision. Symptoms may appear before the cancer is detected.

Uncontrollable eye movements (opsoclonus) and quick contractions of the arms and legs (myoclonus) can occur in some children with neuroblastoma.

Subacute motor neuronopathy occurs in some people with Hodgkin and non-Hodgkin lymphoma. The nerve cells of the spinal cord are affected, weakening the arms and legs.

Eaton-Lambert syndrome occurs in some people with small cell carcinoma of the lung. This syndrome is characterized by extreme muscle weakness caused by lack of proper activation of the muscle by the nerve.

Thymoma is a rare tumor that can be associated with myasthenia gravis, a syndrome of weakness resulting from antibodies that damage the nerve connections in muscle tissue.

Endocrine syndromes: Small cell carcinoma of the lung may secrete a substance that stimulates the adrenal gland to produce increased hormone levels, which can cause weakness, weight gain, and high blood pressure (Cushing's syndrome). Small cell carcinoma of the lung may also produce antidiuretic hormone, causing water retention, decreased sodium levels, weakness, confusion, and seizures in some people.

Very high calcium levels in the blood (hypercalcemic syndrome) may occur in people with solid tumors or leukemias. This can occur when the cancer secretes a hormone-like substance in the blood that causes release of calcium from bone. High calcium levels may also result if the cancer directly invades bone, thereby releasing calcium into the bloodstream. As a result of the high calcium levels in the blood, the person develops confusion, which can progress to coma and even death.

Excessive production of other hormones can cause carcinoid syndrome—flushing, wheezing, diarrhea, and heart valve problems.

Other syndromes: Polymyositis is muscle weakness and soreness resulting from muscle inflammation. When polymyositis is accompanied by skin inflammation, the condition is called dermatomyositis.

Hypertrophic osteoarthropathy can occur in people with lung cancer. This syndrome alters the shape of the fingers and toes and can cause painful swelling of some joints.

---

physical repercussions. Screening tests can produce false-positive results—results that suggest a cancer is present when it actually is not. False-positive results can create undue psychologic stress and can lead to other tests that are expensive and risky. Screening tests can also produce false-negative results—results that show no hint of a cancer that is actually present. False-negative results can lull people into a false sense of security. For these reasons, there are only a small number of screening tests that are considered reliable enough for doctors to use routinely.

Doctors determine whether a particular person is at special risk for cancer—because of age, sex, family history, previous history, or lifestyle—before they choose to perform screening tests. The American Cancer Society has provided cancer screening guidelines that are widely used. Other groups have also developed screening guidelines. Sometimes recommendations vary among different groups, depending on how the groups' experts weigh the relative strength and importance of available scientific evidence.

In women, two of the most widely used screening tests are the Papanicolaou (Pap) test to detect cervical cancer and mammography to detect breast cancer. Both screening tests have been successful in reducing the death rates from these cancers in certain age groups.

In men, prostate-specific antigen (PSA) levels in the blood may be used to screen for prostate cancer. PSA levels are high in men with prostate cancer, but levels also are elevated in men with noncancerous (benign) enlargement of the prostate. As such, the main drawback to its use as a screening test is the large number of false-positive results, which generally lead to more invasive tests. Whether the PSA test should be used routinely to screen for prostate cancer is unresolved, with varying recommendations from different groups. Men over 50 should discuss the PSA test with their doctor.

A common screening test for colon cancer involves checking the stool for blood that cannot be seen by the naked eye (occult blood). Finding occult blood in the stool is an indication that something is wrong somewhere in the gastrointestinal tract. The problem may be cancer, although many other disorders, such as ulcers, hemorrhoids, diverticulosis (small pouches in the colon wall), and abnormal blood vessels in the intestinal walls, can also cause small amounts of blood to leak into the stool. In addition, taking an aspirin or another nonsteroidal anti-inflammatory drug (NSAID) or even eating red meat can temporarily produce a positive result. Positive results on the most commonly used test can occasionally be caused by consuming certain raw fruits and vegetables (turnips, cauliflower, broccoli, melons, radishes, and parsnips). Some people with blood in the stool may have negative test results because they have consumed vitamin C. Newer screening tests for occult blood that use a different technique are much less susceptible to such errors but are somewhat more costly. Outpatient procedures such as sigmoidoscopy and colonoscopy are also often used for colon cancer screening.

Some screening tests can be done at home. For example, monthly breast self-examinations may help women detect breast cancer. Periodically examining the testes may help men detect testicular cancer, one of the most curable forms of cancer, especially when diagnosed early. Checking the mouth for sores may help detect mouth cancer in an early stage.

Tumor markers are substances secreted into the bloodstream by certain tumors. It was first thought that measuring levels of these markers would be an excellent way to screen asymptomatic people for cancer. However, tumor markers are often present to some extent in the blood of people who do not have cancer. Finding a tumor marker does not necessarily mean a person has cancer, and tumor markers have a very limited role in cancer screening.

DIAGNOSTIC TESTS AND STAGING

Diagnosis

Usually, when a doctor first suspects cancer, some type of imaging study, such as x-ray (see page 2042), ultrasonography (see page 2044), or computed tomography (CT—see page 2037), is performed. For example, a person with chronic cough and weight loss might have a chest x-ray; a person with recurrent headaches and trouble seeing might have a CT scan or magnetic resonance imaging (MRI—see page 2040) of their head. Although these tests can show the presence, location, and size of an abnormal mass, they cannot confirm that cancer is the cause. Cancer is confirmed by finding cancer cells on microscopic examination of samples from the suspected area. Usually, the sample must be a piece of tissue, although sometimes examination of the blood is adequate (such as in leukemia). Obtaining a tissue sample is termed a biopsy. Biopsies can be performed by cutting out a small piece of tissue with a scalpel, but very commonly the sample is obtained using a hollow needle. Such tests are commonly done without the need for an overnight hospital stay (outpatient procedure). Doctors often use ultrasonography or a CT scan to guide the needle to the right location. Because biopsies can be painful, the person is usually given a local anesthetic to numb the area.

In people with findings on examination or imaging tests that suggest cancer, measuring blood levels of tumor markers may provide additional evidence for or against the diagnosis of cancer. In people who have been diagnosed with certain types of cancer, tumor markers may be useful to monitor the effectiveness of treatment and to detect possible recurrence of the cancer. For some cancers, the level of a tumor marker drops following treatment and increases if the cancer recurs.

Staging

When cancer is diagnosed, staging tests help determine how extensive the cancer is in terms of its location, size, growth into nearby structures, and spread to other parts of the body. People with cancer sometimes become impatient and anxious during staging tests, wishing for a prompt start of treatment. However, staging allows doctors to determine the most appropriate treatment as well as help to determine prognosis.

Staging may use scans or other imaging tests, such as x-ray, CT, MRI, bone scintigraphy, or positron emission tomography (PET). The choice of staging test(s) depends on the type of cancer. CT is used to detect cancer in many parts of the body, including the brain and lungs and parts of the abdomen, including the adrenal glands, lymph

CANCER SCREENING RECOMMENDATIONS*

PROCEDURE	FREQUENCY
Skin cancer	
Physical examination	Should be part of a routine checkup May be needed more frequently by people at high risk of developing skin cancer
Whole-body photography	Not routinely needed; may be helpful for people with multiple moles or in whom examination of the skin is difficult
Lung cancer	
Chest x-ray	Not recommended on a routine basis
Sputum cytology	Not recommended on a routine basis
Low-dose spiral computed tomography	Not recommended on a routine basis, but is under investigation
Rectal and colon cancer	
Stool examination for occult blood	Yearly after age 50[†]
Sigmoidoscopic or colonoscopic examination	Every 5 years beginning at age 50 (sigmoidoscopy)[†] Every 10 years beginning at age 50 (colonoscopy)
Prostate cancer	
Rectal examination	Yearly after age 50
Blood test for prostate-specific antigen	Yearly after age 50
Cervical cancer	
Papanicolaou (Pap) test	Annual regular Pap test (or newer liquid-based Pap test every 2 years) beginning between ages 18 and 21. Some women 70 years of age or older who have had 3 or more normal Pap tests in a row may choose to stop having cervical cancer screening. For women over 30, some doctors recommend testing every 3 years with a conventional Pap test plus the human papillomavirus DNA test
Breast cancer	
Breast self-examination	Consideration of monthly self-examinations after age 20
Breast physical examination by health care provider	Every 3 years between ages 20 and 39, then yearly
Mammography	Yearly, starting at age 40

*Recommendations for screening are influenced by many factors. These screening recommendations, based primarily on those of the American Cancer Society, are for asymptomatic people with an average risk of cancer. For people with a higher risk, such as those with a strong family history of certain cancers or those who have had a previous cancer, screening may be recommended more frequently or to start at a younger age. Screening tests other than those listed here may also be recommended. Furthermore, other organizations, such as the U.S. Preventive Services Task Force, may have slightly different recommendations. A person's physician can help the person decide when to begin screening and which tests should be used.

†The combination of yearly stool examination for occult blood and sigmoidoscopy every 5 years is preferred over either of these options alone.

nodes, liver, and spleen. MRI is of particular value in detecting cancers of the brain, bone, and spinal cord.

Biopsies are often needed for staging and can sometimes be done together with the initial surgical treatment of a cancer. For example, during a laparotomy (an abdominal operation) to remove colon cancer, a surgeon removes nearby lymph nodes to check for spread of the cancer. During surgery for breast

SELECTED TUMOR MARKERS*

TUMOR MARKER	DESCRIPTION	COMMENT ABOUT TESTING
Alpha-fetoprotein (AFP)	Elevated AFP levels often are found in the blood of people with liver cancer (hepatoma). In addition, elevated AFP is often found in people with certain cancers of the ovary or testis.	Testing can be useful in diagnosing these cancers and in monitoring treatment.
Beta-human chorionic gonadotropin (β-HCG)	This hormone is produced during pregnancy but also occurs in women who have a cancer originating in the placenta and in men with various types of testicular cancer.	Testing can be useful in diagnosing such cancers and in monitoring treatment.
Beta$_2$ (β$_2$)-microglobulin	Levels may be elevated in people with multiple myeloma or other cancers of blood cells.	This test cannot be recommended for cancer screening.
Calcitonin	Calcitonin is produced by certain cells in the thyroid gland (C cells). Blood levels are elevated in medullary thyroid cancer.	This test may be used to monitor response to treatment of medullary thyroid cancer.
Carbohydrate antigen 125 (CA-125)	Levels may be elevated in women with a variety of gynecologic diseases, including ovarian cancer.	This test is not recommended for routine cancer screening.
Carbohydrate antigen 19-9 (CA 19-9)	Levels may be elevated in people with cancers of the digestive tract, particularly pancreatic cancer.	This test cannot be recommended for cancer screening.
Carbohydrate antigen 27.29 (CA27.29)	Levels may be elevated in people with breast cancer.	This test cannot be recommended for cancer screening.
Carcinoembryonic antigen (CEA)	Levels may be elevated in the blood of people with cancer of the colon. Blood levels may also be elevated in patients with other cancers or noncancerous conditions.	After surgery for colon cancer, testing can be useful in monitoring treatment and detecting recurrence.
Lactate dehydrogenase	Levels can be elevated for a variety of reasons.	This test cannot be recommended for cancer screening. However, it is useful in assessing prognosis and monitoring treatment, particularly for people with testicular cancer, melanomas, or lymphomas.
Prostate-specific antigen (PSA)	Levels are elevated in men with noncancerous (benign) enlargement of the prostate and often are considerably higher in men with prostate cancer. What constitutes a meaningfully abnormal level is somewhat uncertain, but men with an elevated PSA level should be evaluated further by a doctor.	Testing can be useful in screening for cancer and in monitoring its treatment.
Thyroglobulin	Elevated blood levels may occur in people with thyroid cancer or benign thyroid conditions.	This test cannot be recommended for routine screening but may be helpful for monitoring response to treatment of thyroid cancer.

*Because tumor markers can also be produced by noncancerous tissue, doctors generally do not use them to screen healthy people. Exceptions may include PSA for prostate cancer and AFP for people at risk of hepatoma. In families with inherited medullary thyroid cancer, a rare condition, calcitonin blood levels also may be a useful screening test.

cancer, the surgeon biopsies or removes lymph nodes located in the armpit to determine whether the breast cancer has spread there. This information, along with features of the primary tumor, helps the doctor determine whether further treatment is needed. When staging is based only on initial biopsy results, physical examination, and imaging, the stage is referred to as clinical. When the doctor uses results of a surgical procedure or additional biopsies, the stage is referred to as pathologic. The clinical and pathologic stage may differ.

In addition to imaging tests, doctors often obtain blood tests to see if the cancer has begun to affect the liver, bone, or kidneys.

166 Prevention and Treatment of Cancer

There are many different types of cancer, and people have different risks for the different cancers. Therefore, no set of prevention strategies is effective in every person. However, some general strategies do reduce risk of cancer in many people. Treatment also varies by type of cancer and the characteristics of the person being treated.

Prevention

Reducing the risk of certain cancers may be possible through dietary (see page 1093) and other lifestyle changes. How risk can be reduced depends on the specific cancer. Tobacco use is directly associated with one third of all cancers. Not smoking and avoiding exposure to tobacco smoke can greatly reduce the risk of lung, kidney, bladder, and head and neck cancer. Avoiding the use of smokeless tobacco (snuff, chew) decreases the risk of cancer of the mouth and tongue.

Other lifestyle changes reduce the risk of several types of cancer. Decreasing alcohol intake can reduce the risk of head and neck, liver, and esophageal cancer. A reduced intake of fat in the diet appears to decrease the risk of breast and colon cancer. Avoiding sun exposure (especially during the middle of the day) can reduce the risk of skin cancer. Covering exposed skin and using sunscreen lotion with a high sun protection factor (SPF) against ultraviolet light also help reduce the risk of skin cancer. Use of aspirin and other nonsteroidal anti-inflammatory drugs (NSAIDs) reduces the risk of colorectal cancer. Papanicolaou (Pap) tests can help prevent cervical cancers by detecting precancerous changes in cells of the cervix.

Vaccination can prevent certain types of cancer that are caused by viruses. Cervical cancer is caused by infections with certain strains of sexually transmitted human papillomavirus (HPV). Vaccination against HPV before the first sexual encounter (see page 1148) can largely prevent cervical cancer. HPV infection may also increase the risk of anal cancer and some forms of head and neck cancer. As another example, infection with hepatitis B virus increases the risk of liver cancer; vaccination against hepatitis B virus can help prevent this type of cancer.

Preventing Cancer

According to the American Cancer Society, the risk of developing certain cancers may be reduced by making lifestyle changes.

MEASURES KNOWN TO REDUCE THE RISK OF CANCER:

- Avoiding smoking or exposure to tobacco smoke
- Avoiding occupational carcinogens (for example, asbestos)
- Avoiding prolonged exposure to sunlight without sunscreen protection
- Avoiding excessive alcohol intake
- Avoiding use of hormone therapy (for example, estrogen and progesterone) for symptoms of menopause

MEASURES THAT MAY REDUCE THE RISK OF CANCER:

- Limiting intake of high-fat foods, particularly from animal sources (for example, high-fat meats and whole-fat dairy products)
- Increasing intake of fruits and vegetables
- Being physically active
- Keeping weight below the obese level

Early detection of cancerous or precancerous growths can save lives. For women 40 years of age or older, having yearly mammograms can help detect breast cancers while they are still curable. For people 50 years of age or older, having a colonoscopy (inspection of the large intestine through a flexible viewing tube) every few years can detect polyps and early cancers of the colon.

Treatment Principles

Treating cancer is one of the most complex aspects of medical care. It involves a team that encompasses many types of doctors working together (for example, primary care doctors, gynecologists, medical oncologists, surgeons, radiotherapists, and pathologists) and many other types of health care practitioners (for example, nurses, physiotherapists, social workers, and pharmacists).

Treatment decisions take into account many factors, including the likelihood of cure or of prolonging life when cure is not possible, the effect of treatment on symptoms, the side effects of treatment, and the person's wishes. People undergoing cancer treatment hope for the best outcome and the longest survival with the highest quality of life. However, people must understand the risks involved with treatment. They should discuss their wishes regarding medical care with all of their doctors and should participate in decisions about treatment (see page 69).

When the diagnosis of cancer is first made, the main goals of treatment are to remove the cancer if possible (through a single treatment or through a combination of surgery, radiation therapy, or chemotherapy). Chemotherapy is usually the only way to treat any cancer cells that have spread (metastasized) beyond the original (primary) site. Using combinations of chemotherapy drugs may help eliminate the original cancer and, at the same time, eliminate cancer cells elsewhere in the body, even when there is no sign of those cells.

Even when a cure is impossible, symptoms resulting from the cancer can often be relieved with treatment that improves the quality of life (palliative therapy). For example, if a tumor cannot be removed surgically, radiation to the tumor may shrink it, temporarily reducing pain and symptoms in the immediate vicinity of the tumor (local symptoms).

As treatments become more complex, specific approaches to care, called treatment protocols, have been developed to ensure that people receive the safest and most effective care. Treatment protocols ensure that people receive a standard approach derived from careful scientific experiments. Protocols are typically developed and refined through clinical trials. A clinical trial allows doctors to compare new drugs and treatment combinations with standard treatments to determine whether new treatments are more effective. Often, people with cancer are offered the opportunity to participate in such a trial, but not all people with cancer are eligible (see page 2026).

Surgery

Surgery is a traditional form of cancer treatment. It is the most effective in eliminating most types of cancer before it has spread to lymph nodes or distant sites (metastasized). Surgery may be used alone or in combination with other treatments, such as radiation therapy and chemotherapy. If the cancer has not metastasized, surgery may cure the person. However, it is not always possible to be sure before surgery whether the cancer has or has not spread. During surgery, doctors often remove lymph nodes near the tumor to see if the cancer has spread to them. If so, the person may be at a high risk of having the cancer recur and may need chemotherapy or radiation after surgery to prevent a recurrence.

Surgery is not the main treatment once a cancer has metastasized. However, surgery is sometimes used to reduce tumor size (a procedure called debulking), so that radiation therapy and chemotherapy may be more effective, or to relieve symptoms such as severe pain or intestinal obstruction. Surgically removing metastases rarely results in a cure because finding all the tumors is difficult. Tumors that remain usually continue to grow. However, in certain cancers that have a very small number of metastases, particularly to the liver, brain, or lung, surgical removal of the metastases can be beneficial.

Surgery is not the preferred treatment for all early-stage cancers. Some cancers occur in inaccessible sites. In other instances, removing the cancer might require removing a necessary organ, or surgery might impair the organ's function. In such cases, radiation treatment with or without chemotherapy may be preferable.

Radiation Therapy

Radiation is a form of intense energy generated by a radioactive substance, such as cobalt, or by specialized equipment, such as an atomic particle (linear) accelerator.

Radiation preferentially kills cells that divide rapidly and cells that have difficulty repairing their DNA (nuclear material). Cancer cells divide more

Response to Treatment

While being treated for cancer, the person is assessed to see how the cancer is responding to therapy. When a cancer disappears for any length of time after treatment, a person is said to have had a **complete response (remission).**

The most successful treatment produces a **cure.** A cure means that all evidence of cancer disappears and does not return over a long period of observation. With some forms of cancer, doctors consider people cured if they remain disease-free for 5 years or longer. With other forms, a longer period is required.

With a **partial response,** the size of a tumor (usually determined by x-rays) is reduced by more than half, although it remains visible on x-ray. With a partial response, the person usually has fewer symptoms and may have a prolonged life, although the cancer eventually grows back.

In some people, treatment does not lead to a complete or partial response, but the cancer may not grow or spread and the person may experience no new symptoms for an extended period of time. This response is also considered beneficial. In the least successful experience, the tumor continues to increase in size or new sites of disease appear despite treatment.

Sometimes a cancer completely disappears but returns later **(relapse).** The interval between these two events is called the **disease-free interval.** The interval from diagnosis of cancer to the time of death is the **total survival time.** In people who have a partial response, the duration of response is measured from the time of the partial response to the time when the cancer begins to enlarge or spread again.

Some types of cancer, such as breast cancers or lymphomas (tumors of the lymph nodes), respond well to chemotherapy or radiation therapy and are termed **responsive.** Other cancers, such as melanoma (a skin cancer) or malignant brain tumors, respond to chemotherapy or radiation therapy in only a few people and are termed **resistant.** Tumors of the intestinal tract and lungs often respond to chemotherapy at first but become resistant later despite continued treatment.

Some cancers produce proteins that are detectable in the bloodstream. These substances are termed **tumor markers.** An example is prostate-specific antigen (PSA), levels of which increase in men with prostate cancer. Most tumor markers are not specific enough to be useful in screening (detecting a cancer before a person develops symptoms) because a number of disorders other than cancer can cause these substances to appear in the blood. However, tumor markers (such as CA 125 for ovarian cancer) can help doctors assess a person's response to treatment. If the tumor marker was present before treatment but no longer appears in a blood sample after treatment, the treatment has probably been successful. If the tumor marker disappears after treatment but later reappears, the cancer has probably returned.

---

often than normal cells and often cannot repair damage done to them by radiation. Therefore, cancer cells are more likely than most normal cells to be killed by radiation. Nonetheless, cancer cells differ in how easily they are killed by radiation; some cells are very resistant and cannot be effectively treated with radiation.

Types of Radiation Therapy

In its most common form, radiation therapy uses an external beam of gamma radiation generated by a linear accelerator. Less commonly, electron or proton beam radiation is used. Proton beam radiation, which can be focused on a very specific area, effectively treats certain cancers in areas in which damage to normal tissue is a particular concern, such as the eye, brain, or spinal cord. All types of external beam radiation are focused on the particular area or organ of the body that contains the cancer. To avoid overexposing normal tissue, several beam paths are used and surrounding tissues are shielded as much as possible. New technologies of focusing external beam radiation, called intensity modulated radiation therapy (IMRT), help protect surrounding tissues and allow a higher dose of radiation to be delivered to cancer cells.

External beam radiation therapy is given as a series of equally divided doses over a prolonged period of time. This method increases the lethal effects of the radiation on cancer cells while decreasing the toxic effects on normal cells. Toxic effects are decreased because normal cells can repair themselves quickly between doses while cancer cells cannot. Typically, a person receives daily doses of radiation over a period of 6 to 8 weeks. To ensure that the same area is treated each time, the person is precisely positioned using foam casts or other devices.

In other radiation therapy strategies, a radioactive substance may be injected into a vein to travel to the cancer (for example, radioactive iodine, which is used in treatment of thyroid cancer). Another technique uses small pellets ("seeds") of radioactive material placed directly into the cancer (for example, radioactive palladium used for prostate cancer). These implants provide intense radiation to the cancer, but little radiation reaches surrounding tissues. Implants contain short-lived radioactive substances that stop producing radiation after a period of time.

More recently, radioactive substances have been attached to proteins called monoclonal antibodies, which seek out cancer cells and attach to them. The radioactive material attached to the antibody concentrates at the cancer cells and destroys them.

Uses

Radiation therapy plays a key role in curing many cancers, including Hodgkin lymphoma, early-stage non-Hodgkin lymphoma, squamous cell cancer of the head and neck, seminoma (a testicular cancer), prostate cancer, early-stage breast cancer, some forms of non–small cell lung cancer, and medulloblastoma (a brain or spinal cord tumor). For early-stage cancers of the windpipe (larynx) and prostate, the rate of cure is essentially the same with radiation therapy as with surgery. Sometimes, radiation therapy is combined with other forms of treatment. Certain kinds of chemotherapy drugs, such as cisplatin, enhance the effectiveness of radiation therapy, and these drugs may be given with radiation treatments.

Radiation therapy can reduce symptoms when a cure is not possible, as for bone metastases in multiple myeloma and painful tumors in people with advanced lung, esophageal, head and neck, and stomach cancers. By temporarily shrinking the tumors, radiation therapy can relieve symptoms caused by spread of cancer to bone or brain.

Side Effects

Unfortunately, radiation can damage normal tissues near the tumor. Side effects depend on how large an area is being treated, what dose is given, and how close the tumor is to sensitive tissues. Sensitive tissues are those in which cells normally divide rapidly, such as skin, bone marrow, hair follicles, and the lining of the mouth, esophagus, and intestine. Radiation can also damage the ovaries or testes. Doctors try to accurately target the radiation therapy to prevent excessive damage to normal cells.

Symptoms depend on the area receiving radiation and may include fatigue, mouth sores, skin problems (redness, itching, peeling), painful swallowing, lung inflammation (pneumonitis), hepatitis, gastrointestinal problems (nausea, loss of appetite, vomiting, diarrhea), urinary problems (increased frequency, burning with urination), and low blood count. Radiation to head and neck tumors often causes damage to the overlying skin as well as the lining of the mouth and throat. Doctors try to identify and treat such symptoms as early as possible so the person remains comfortable and can continue with treatments.

Chemotherapy

Chemotherapy involves the use of drugs to destroy cancer cells. Although an ideal drug would destroy cancer cells without harming normal cells, most drugs are not that selective. Instead, drugs are designed to inflict greater damage on cancer cells than on normal cells, typically by using drugs that affect a cell's ability to grow. Uncontrolled and rapid growth is characteristic of cancer cells. However, because normal cells also need to grow, and some grow quite rapidly (such as those in the bone marrow and those lining the mouth and intestine), all chemotherapy drugs affect normal cells and cause side effects.

One new approach to limiting side effects and increasing effectiveness uses a variety of "molecularly targeted" drugs. These drugs kill cancer cells by attacking specific pathways and processes vital to the cancer cells' survival and growth. For example, cancer cells need blood vessels to provide nutrients and oxygen. Some drugs can block blood vessel formation to cancer cells or the master signaling pathways that control cell growth. Imatinib, the first such drug, is highly effective in chronic myelocytic leukemia and certain cancers of the digestive tract. Erlotinib and gefitinib target receptors located on the surface of cells in non–small cell lung cancer. Molecularly targeted drugs have proven useful in treating many other cancers, including breast and kidney cancers.

Not all cancers respond to chemotherapy. The type of cancer determines which drugs are used, in what combination, and at what dose. Chemotherapy may be used as the sole treatment or combined with radiation therapy, surgery, or both.

High-Dose Chemotherapy: In an attempt to increase the antitumor effects of cancer drugs, the dose may be increased and the time between cycles of therapy may be decreased (dose-dense chemotherapy). Dose-dense chemotherapy, with shortened rest periods, is routinely used in breast cancer treatment. High-dose chemotherapy is often used for treatment of people whose cancer has recurred after standard dose therapy, particularly for people with myeloma, lymphoma, and leukemia. However, high-dose chemotherapy can cause life-threatening injury to the bone marrow. Therefore, high-dose chemotherapy is commonly combined with bone marrow rescue strategies. In bone marrow rescue, bone marrow cells are harvested before the chemotherapy and returned to the person after chemotherapy. In some cases, stem cells can be isolated from the bloodstream rather than from the bone marrow and can be infused back into the person after chemotherapy to restore bone marrow function.

℞ CHEMOTHERAPY DRUGS

EXAMPLES	HOW THE DRUG WORKS	SOME SIDE EFFECTS
Alkylating agents		
Cyclophosphamide Chlorambucil Melphalan	Form a chemical bond with DNA, causing breaks in DNA and errors in replication of DNA	Suppress bone marrow Injure lining of stomach Cause hair loss May decrease fertility Suppress the immune system May cause leukemia
Antimetabolites		
Methotrexate Cytarabine Fludarabine 6-Mercaptopurine 5-Fluorouracil	Block synthesis of DNA	Same as for alkylating agents Do not increase risk of leukemia
Antimitotics		
Vincristine Paclitaxel Vinorelbine Docetaxel	Block division of cancer cells	Same as for alkylating agents Also can cause nerve damage Do not cause leukemia
Topoisomerase inhibitors		
Doxorubicin Irinotecan	Prevent DNA synthesis and repair through blockage of enzymes called topoisomerases	Same as for alkylating agents Doxorubicin can cause heart damage
Platinum derivatives		
Cisplatin Carboplatin Oxaliplatin	Form bonds with DNA, causing breaks	Same as for alkylating agents Also can cause nerve and kidney damage and hearing loss
Hormonal therapy		
Tamoxifen	Blocks estrogen action (in breast cancer)	Can cause endometrial cancer, blood clots, and hot flashes
Aromatase inhibitors		
Bicalutamide	Blocks androgen action (in prostate cancer)	Can cause erectile dysfunction (impotence) and diarrhea
Anastrozole Exemestane Letrozole	Block estrogen formation	Can cause bone loss (osteoporosis) and menopausal symptoms
Signaling inhibitors		
Imatinib	Blocks signal for cell division in chronic myelocytic leukemia	Can cause abnormal liver function test results and fluid retention
Gefitinib Erlotinib	Blocks epidermal growth factor receptor	Can cause rash and diarrhea
Monoclonal antibodies		
Rituximab	Induces cell death through binding to cell surface receptors on lymphocyte-derived tumors	Can cause an allergic reaction

(continued on the following page)

℞ CHEMOTHERAPY DRUGS (Continued)

EXAMPLES	HOW THE DRUG WORKS	SOME SIDE EFFECTS
Monoclonal antibodies (continued)		
Trastuzumab	Blocks growth factor receptors on breast cancer cells	Can cause heart failure
Gemtuzumab ozogamicin	Contains a specific antibody that attaches to a receptor found on leukemic cells and then delivers a toxic dose of its chemotherapeutic component to the leukemic cells	Can cause prolonged platelet suppression, which increases the risk of bleeding
Biologic response modifier		
Interferon-alpha	Unknown	Can cause fever, chills, bone marrow suppression, thyroid deficiency, and hepatitis
Differentiating agents		
Tretinoin	Induces differentiation and death of leukemic cells	Can cause severe difficulty with breathing (respiratory distress)
Arsenic trioxide	Induces differentiation and death of leukemic cells	Causes abnormal heart rhythms and a rash
Agents that block blood vessel formation (antiangiogenic agents)		
Bevacizumab	Blocks vascular endothelial growth factor (VEGF)	Can cause high blood pressure, protein loss in urine, bleeding, clotting, and intestinal perforation
Sorafinib Sunitinib	Block VEGF receptors	Can cause high blood pressure and protein loss in urine

Side Effects

Chemotherapy commonly causes nausea, vomiting, loss of appetite, weight loss, fatigue, and low blood cell counts that lead to anemia and increased risk of infections. With chemotherapy, people often lose their hair, but other side effects vary according to the type of drug.

Nausea and Vomiting: These symptoms can usually be prevented or relieved with drugs (antiemetics). Nausea may also be reduced by eating small meals and by avoiding foods that are high in fiber, that produce gas, or that are very hot or very cold.

Low Blood Cell Counts: Cytopenia, a deficiency of one or more types of blood cell, can develop because of the toxic effects chemotherapy drugs have on bone marrow (where blood cells are made). For example, a person may develop abnormally low numbers of red blood cells (anemia), white blood cells (neutropenia or leukopenia), or platelets (thrombocytopenia). If anemia is severe, specific growth factors, such as erythropoietin or darbepoietin, can be given to increase red blood cell formation, or packed red blood cells can be transfused. If thrombocytopenia is severe, platelets can be transfused to lower the risk of bleeding.

A person with neutropenia is at increased risk of developing an infection. A fever higher than 100.4° F in a person with neutropenia is treated as an emergency. Such a person must be evaluated for infection and may require antibiotics and even hospitalization. White blood cells are rarely transfused because, when transfused, they survive only a few hours and produce many side effects. Instead, certain substances (such as granulocyte-colony stimulating factor) can be administered to stimulate white blood cell production.

Other Common Side Effects: Many people develop inflammation or even sores of the mucous membranes, such as the lining of the mouth. Mouth sores are painful and can make eating difficult. Various oral solutions (usually containing an antacid, an antihistamine, and a local anesthetic) can reduce the discomfort. On rare occasions, people need nutritional support by a feeding tube that is placed directly into the stomach or small intestine or even by vein. A variety of drugs can reduce the diarrhea caused by radiation therapy to the abdomen.

Organ Damage and Other Cancers: Sometimes drugs may damage other organs, such as the lungs, heart, or liver. For example, anthracyclines cause heart damage when used in high total doses.

People treated with chemotherapy, particularly alkylating agents, may have an increased risk of developing leukemia several years after treatment. Some drugs, especially alkylating agents, cause infertility in some women and in most men who receive these treatments.

Immunotherapy

Immunotherapy is used to stimulate the body's immune system against cancer. For example, vaccines composed of antigens derived from tumor cells can boost the body's production of antibodies or immune cells (T lymphocytes). Extracts of weakened tuberculosis bacteria, which are known to boost the immune response, have been successful when instilled into the bladder to prevent recurrence of bladder tumors.

Monoclonal antibody therapy involves the use of experimentally produced antibodies to target specific proteins on the surface of cancer cells. Trastuzumab is one such antibody, which attacks the HER-2/*neu* receptor present on the surface of cancer cells in 25% of women with breast cancer. Trastuzumab enhances the effect of chemotherapy drugs. Rituximab is highly effective in treating lymphomas and chronic lymphocytic leukemia. Rituximab linked to a radioactive isotope can be used to deliver radiation directly to lymphoma cells. Gemtuzumab ozogamicin, a combined antibody and drug, is effective in some people with acute myelocytic leukemia.

Biologic response modifiers improve the immune system's ability to find and destroy cancer cells, such as by stimulating normal cells to produce chemical messengers (mediators). Interferon (of which there are several types) is the best-known and most widely used biologic response modifier. Almost all human cells produce interferon naturally, but it can also be made through biotechnology. Although its precise mechanisms of action are not totally clear, interferon has a role in the treatment of several cancers, such as Kaposi's sarcoma and malignant melanoma. Interleukin 2, which is produced by certain white blood cells, also can be helpful in renal cell carcinoma and metastatic melanoma.

Combination Therapy

Chemotherapy drugs are most effective when given in combination (combination chemotherapy). The rationale for combination chemotherapy is to use drugs that work by different mechanisms of action, thereby decreasing the likelihood that resistant cancer cells will develop. When drugs with different effects are combined, each drug can be used at its optimal dose, without intolerable side effects.

For some cancers, the best approach is a combination of surgery, radiation therapy, and chemotherapy. Surgery or radiation therapy treats cancer that is confined locally, while chemotherapy also kills the cancer cells that have spread to distant sites. Sometimes radiation therapy or chemotherapy is given before surgery to shrink a tumor, thereby improving the opportunity for complete surgical removal. Radiation therapy and low-dose chemotherapy after surgery help to destroy any remaining cancer cells. The stage of the cancer often determines whether single therapy or a combination is needed. For example, early-stage breast cancer may be treated with surgery alone or surgery combined with radiation therapy, chemotherapy, or with all three treatments, depending on the size of the tumor and the risk of recurrence. Locally advanced breast cancer is usually treated with chemotherapy, radiation therapy, and surgery.

Sometimes combination chemotherapy is used not to cure but to reduce symptoms and prolong life. Combination chemotherapy can be useful for people with advanced cancers that are not suitable for radiation therapy or surgical treatment (for example, those with unresectable non–small cell lung cancer, esophageal cancer, or bladder cancer).

Alternative Medicine

Some people turn to alternative medicine, including certain medicinal herbs (see page 2067), to treat their cancer, instead of or in addition to standard treatment. However, most types of alternative medicine have not been subjected to careful scientific studies. Thus, very little is known about the effectiveness of alternative medicine in treating cancer.

Although benefits of alternative medicine for cancer have not been scientifically proven, there is significant potential for harm because

- The alternative medicine may be toxic.
- The alternative medicine may interact with standard treatment, such as chemotherapy, thus reducing its effectiveness.
- The alternative medicine may be costly, reducing the person's ability to afford standard treatment.
- If alternative medicine is used instead of standard treatment, the person will not obtain the proven benefits of standard treatment.

People using alternative medicine should inform their doctor. Hiding the use of alternative medicine could be harmful.

Diet and Cancer

Many studies have tried to determine whether eating specific foods increases or decreases a person's risk of getting cancer. Unfortunately, different studies sometimes have conflicting results, so it is hard to know what effect foods or dietary supplements have on cancer risk. Some foods and supplements have been studied more than others, and the American Cancer Society has tried to summarize what is currently known.

Antioxidants: Antioxidants, such as vitamin C, vitamin E, and beta-carotene (vitamin A), are part of a well-balanced diet. However, whether taking supplements containing these antioxidants decreases the risk of cancer is not known. There is some evidence that taking high doses of beta-carotene supplements may increase the risk of certain types of cancer.

Bioengineered Foods: Genes from different plants or from certain microorganisms are added to the genes of some plants to increase the plants' hardiness or resistance to pests or to improve them in some other way. No current evidence demonstrates that bioengineered foods have any effect on cancer risk.

Calcium: High calcium intake, especially through calcium supplements, may increase the risk of prostate cancer.

Coffee: Although some older studies appeared to show a link between coffee consumption and cancer risk, more recent studies have not shown any connection.

Saturated Fats: Saturated fats may increase cancer risk. Of more importance, however, is that foods that contain high levels of saturated fats also contain many calories and may contribute to obesity, which is a risk factor for cancer.

Fiber: There is little evidence that eating a diet that is high in fiber reduces cancer risk.

Fish and Omega-3 Fatty Acids: Some studies in animals have shown that omega-3 fatty acids may slow cancer progression, but similar results have not been obtained in people.

Fluoride: Studies have not shown an increased risk of cancer in people who drink fluoridated water or who use toothpastes or undergo dental fluoride treatments.

Folate: Folate taken daily may decrease the risk of colon cancer.

Food Additives: Food additives must be approved by the Food and Drug Administration before they are included in foods, so new additives undergo extensive testing. So far, no evidence shows that the levels of additives found in food products increase the risk of cancer.

Garlic: Whether garlic is effective in reducing the risk of cancer is not yet known.

Irradiated Foods: Radiation, which is sometimes used to kill microorganisms in food, does not appear to increase cancer risk.

Lycopene: Some studies suggest that lycopene, which is found mainly in tomatoes, may reduce the risk of some cancers.

Processed Meats: People who eat large amounts of processed meats may be at risk for stomach cancer. Some investigators attribute this finding to nitrates, which are in luncheon meats, hams, and hot dogs. This connection is unproved. Eating meats processed by salting or smoking may increase exposure to potential cancer-causing substances.

Meats Cooked at High Temperatures: Eating meat cooked at high temperatures, for example by grilling or broiling, may increase cancer risk.

Organic Food: Whether eating foods grown with organic methods reduces cancer risk is not yet known.

Pesticides: There is no evidence that pesticide residue found in small amounts on foods increases the risk of cancer.

Saccharin: Saccharin does not cause cancers in people.

Salt: Diets containing large amounts of food that has been preserved by pickling or salting may increase the risk of stomach and throat cancer. No studies have found a similar risk for a small or moderate amount of salt for flavor.

Selenium: Some studies suggest that selenium protects against some types of cancer.

Soy: Studies do not yet show that soy supplements reduce cancer risk.

Tea: Tea has not been shown to reduce cancer risk.

Vitamin D: Vitamin D may have some benefit in reducing the risk of prostate cancer.

Immune Disorders

CHAPTER
167 Biology of the Immune System

The immune system is designed to defend the body against foreign or dangerous cells or substances that invade it. Such invaders include microorganisms (commonly called germs, such as bacteria, viruses, and fungi), parasites (such as worms), cancer cells, and even transplanted organs and tissues (see page 1128). To defend the body against these invaders, the immune system must be able to distinguish between what belongs in the body (self) and what does not (nonself or foreign). Any substances that are identi-fied as nonself, particularly if they are perceived as dangerous (for example, if they can cause disease), stimulate an immune response in the body. Such substances are called antigens.

Antigens may be contained within or on bacteria, viruses, other microorganisms, or cancer cells. Antigens may also exist on their own—for example, as food molecules or pollen. A normal immune response consists of recognizing a potentially harmful foreign antigen, activating and mobilizing forces to defend against it, and attacking it. If the immune system malfunctions and mistakes self for nonself, it may attack the body's own tissues, causing an autoimmune disorder, such as rheumatoid arthritis, thyroiditis, or systemic lupus erythematosus (lupus).

Disorders of the immune system occur when

- The body generates an immune response against itself (an autoimmune disorder—see page 1124).
- The body cannot generate appropriate immune responses against invading microorganisms (an immunodeficiency disorder—see page 1104).
- An excessive immune response to often harmless foreign antigens damages normal tissues (an allergic reaction—see page 1112).

Lines of Defense

The body has a series of defenses. Defenses include physical barriers, white blood cells, and antibodies and other chemical substances.

Physical Barriers: The first line of defense against invaders is mechanical or physical barriers:

- The skin
- The cornea of the eyes
- Membranes lining the respiratory, digestive, urinary, and reproductive tracts

As long as these barriers remain unbroken, many invaders cannot enter the body. If a barrier is broken—for example, if extensive burns damage the skin—the risk of infection is increased. In addition, the barriers are defended by secretions containing enzymes that can destroy bacteria. Examples are sweat, tears in the eyes, mucus in the respiratory and digestive tracts, and secretions in the vagina.

Cells: The next line of defense involves certain white blood cells (leukocytes) that travel through the bloodstream and into tissues, searching for and attacking microorganisms and other invaders. This defense has two parts: innate and acquired immunity.

Innate (natural) immunity does not require a previous encounter with a microorganism or other invader to work effectively. It responds to invaders immediately, without needing to learn to recognize them. Several types of white blood cells are involved:

- Phagocytes ingest invaders.
- Natural killer cells are formed ready to kill cells that are infected with certain viruses and cancer cells.
- Professional antigen-presenting cells help T cells (T lymphocytes) recognize invaders.
- Some white blood cells release substances involved in inflammation and allergic reactions, such as histamine. These cells often act on their own to destroy invaders.

In acquired (adaptive or specific) immunity, lymphocytes (B cells and T cells) encounter an invader, learn how to attack it, and remember the specific invader so that they can attack it even more efficiently the next time they encounter it. Specific immunity takes time to develop after the initial encounter with a new invader because the lymphocytes must adapt to it. Thereafter, response is quick. B cells and T cells work together to destroy invaders. Some of these cells do not directly destroy invaders but instead enable other white blood cells to recognize and destroy invaders.

Substances: Innate immunity and acquired immunity interact, influencing each other directly or through substances that attract or activate other cells of the immune system (immune cells)—as part of the mobilization step in defense. These substances include cytokines (which are the messengers of the immune system), antibodies, and complement proteins (which form the complement system). These substances are not contained in cells but are dissolved in a body fluid, such as plasma (the liquid part of blood).

Some of these substances, including some cytokines, promote inflammation. Inflammation, with redness and swelling, occurs because the substances attract immune cells to the affected tissue and, to get the immune cells there, more blood flows to the tissue and more fluids enter the tissue. The purpose of inflammation is to contain the infection so that it does not spread. Then other substances produced by the immune system help the inflammation resolve and damaged tissues heal. Although inflammation may be bothersome, it indicates that the immune system is doing its job. However, excessive or long-term (chronic) inflammation can be harmful.

Organs: The immune system includes several organs in addition to cells dispersed throughout the body. These organs are classified as primary or secondary lymphoid organs.

The **primary lymphoid organs** are the sites where white blood cells are produced:

- The bone marrow produces all the different types of white blood cells, including neutrophils, eosinophils, basophils, monocytes, B cells, and the cells that develop into (precursors) T cells.
- In the thymus, T cells are produced and trained to recognize foreign antigens and to ignore the body's own antigens. (T cells are critical for specific immunity.)

When needed to defend the body, the white blood cells are mobilized, mainly from the bone marrow. They then move into the bloodstream and travel to wherever they are needed.

Understanding the Immune System

Antibody (immunoglobulin): A protein that is produced by B cells and that interacts with a specific antigen.

Antigen: Any substance that the immune system recognizes and that can stimulate an immune response.

B cell (B lymphocyte): A white blood cell that produces antibodies specific to the antigen that stimulated their production.

Basophil: A white blood cell that releases histamine (a substance involved in allergic reactions) and that produces substances to attract other white blood cells (neutrophils and eosinophils) to a trouble spot.

Cell: The smallest unit of a living organism, composed of a nucleus and cytoplasm surrounded by a membrane.

Chemotaxis: The process of using a chemical substance to attract cells to a particular site.

Complement system: A group of proteins that are involved in a series of reactions (cascade) designed to defend the body and that have various immune functions, such as killing bacteria and other foreign cells, making foreign cells easier for macrophages to identify and ingest, attracting macrophages and neutrophils to a trouble spot, and enhancing the effectiveness of antibodies.

Cytokines: Proteins secreted by cells that act as the immune system's messengers and that help regulate an immune response.

Dendritic cell: A cell that is derived from white blood cells, resides in tissues, and helps T cells recognize foreign antigens.

Eosinophil: A white blood cell that kills bacteria, that kills other foreign cells too big to ingest, that may help immobilize and kill parasites, that participates in allergic reactions, and that helps destroy cancer cells.

Helper T cell: A white blood cell that helps B cells recognize and produce antibodies against foreign antigens, that helps killer T cells become active, and that stimulates macrophages.

Histocompatibility: Literally, compatibility of tissue. Determined by human leukocyte antigens and used to determine whether a transplanted tissue or organ will be accepted by the recipient.

Human leukocyte antigens (HLA): A group of molecules that are located on the surface of cells and that are unique in each organism, enabling the body to distinguish self from nonself. Also called the major histocompatibility complex.

Immune complex: Antibody attached to an antigen.

Immune response: The reaction of the immune system to an antigen.

Immunoglobulin: An antibody molecule.

Interleukin: A type of messenger (cytokine) secreted by some white blood cells to affect other white blood cells.

Killer (cytotoxic) T cell: A T cell that attaches to foreign or abnormal cells and kills them.

Leukocyte: A white blood cell, such as a monocyte, a neutrophil, an eosinophil, a basophil, or a lymphocyte.

Lymphocyte: The white blood cell responsible for specific immunity, including producing antibodies (by B cells), distinguishing self from nonself (by T cells), and killing infected cells and cancer cells (killer T cells).

Macrophage: A large cell that develops from a white blood cell called a monocyte, that ingests bacteria and other foreign cells, and that helps T cells identify microorganisms and other foreign substances.

Major histocompatibility complex (MHC): A synonym for human leukocyte antigens.

Mast cell: A cell in tissues that releases histamine and other substances involved in inflammatory and allergic reactions.

Molecule: A group of atoms chemically combined to form a unique chemical substance.

Natural killer cell: A type of white blood cell that is naturally able to kill abnormal cells, such as certain infected cells and cancer cells (that is, it does not have to learn that the cells are abnormal).

Neutrophil: A white blood cell that ingests and kills bacteria and other foreign cells.

Phagocyte: A cell that ingests and kills or destroys invading microorganisms, other cells, and cell fragments.

Phagocytosis: The process of a cell engulfing and ingesting an invading microorganism, another cell, or a cell fragment.

Receptor: A molecule on a cell's surface or inside the cell that allows only molecules that fit precisely in it—as a key fits in its lock—to attach to it.

Regulatory (suppressor) T cell: A white blood cell that helps end an immune response.

T cell (T lymphocyte): A white blood cell that is involved in specific immunity and that may be one of three types: helper, killer (cytotoxic), or regulatory.

Lymphatic System: Helping Defend Against Infection

The lymphatic system is a vital part of the immune system, along with the thymus, bone marrow, spleen, tonsils, appendix, and Peyer's patches in the small intestine.

The lymphatic system is a network of lymph nodes connected by lymphatic vessels. This system transports lymph throughout the body.

Lymph is formed from fluid that seeps through the thin walls of capillaries into the body's tissues. This fluid contains oxygen, proteins, and other nutrients that nourish the tissues. Some of this fluid reenters the capillaries and some of it enters the lymphatic vessels (becoming lymph). Small lymphatic vessels connect to larger ones and eventually form the thoracic duct. The thoracic duct is the largest lymphatic vessel. It joins with the subclavian vein and thus returns lymph to the bloodstream. The fluid also transports foreign substances (such as bacteria), cancer cells, and dead or damaged cells that may be present in tissues into the lymphatic vessels. Lymph also contains many white blood cells.

All substances transported by the lymph pass through at least one lymph node, where foreign substances can be filtered out and destroyed before fluid is returned to the bloodstream. In the lymph nodes, white blood cells can collect, interact with each other and antigens, and generate immune responses to foreign substances. Lymph nodes contain a mesh of tissue that is tightly packed with B cells, T cells, dendritic cells, and macrophages. Harmful microorganisms are filtered through the mesh, then identified and attacked by B cells and T cells.

Lymph nodes are often clustered in areas where the lymphatic vessels branch off, such as the neck, armpits, and groin.

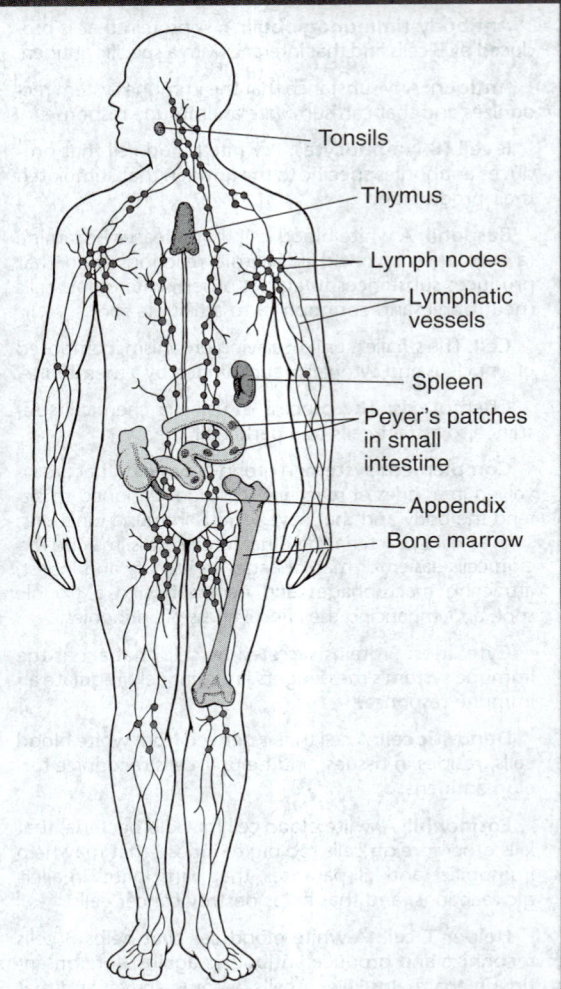

- Tonsils
- Thymus
- Lymph nodes
- Lymphatic vessels
- Spleen
- Peyer's patches in small intestine
- Appendix
- Bone marrow

The **secondary lymphoid organs** include the spleen, lymph nodes, tonsils, appendix, and Peyer's patches in the small intestine. These organs trap microorganisms and other foreign substances and provide a place for mature cells of the immune system to collect, interact with each other and with the foreign substances, and generate a specific immune response.

The lymph nodes are strategically placed in the body and are connected by an extensive network of lymphatic vessels, which act as the immune system's circulatory system. The lymphatic system transports microorganisms, other foreign substances, cancer cells, and dead or damaged cells from the tissues to the lymph nodes (which filter out and destroy these substances and cells), and then to the bloodstream.

Lymph nodes are one of the first places that cancer cells can spread. Thus, doctors often evaluate lymph nodes to determine whether a cancer has spread. Cancer cells in a lymph node can cause the node to swell. Lymph nodes can also swell after an infection because immune responses to infections are generated in lymph nodes. Sometimes, bacteria that are carried to a lymph node are not killed and cause an infection in the lymph node (lymphadenitis).

Plan of Action

A successful immune response to invaders requires recognition, activation and mobilization, regulation, and resolution.

Recognition: To be able to destroy invaders, the immune system must first recognize them. That is, the immune system must be able to distinguish what is nonself (foreign) from what is self. The immune system can make this distinction because all cells have identification molecules on their surface. Microorganisms are recognized because the identification molecules on their surface are foreign. In people, identification molecules are called human leukocyte antigens (HLA) or the major histocompatibility complex (MHC). HLA molecules are called antigens because they can provoke an immune response in another person (normally, they do not provoke an immune response in the person who has them). Each person has an almost unique combination of human leukocyte antigens. Each person's immune system normally recognizes this unique combination as self. A cell with molecules on its surface that are not identical to those on the body's own cells is identified as being foreign. The immune system then attacks that cell. Such a cell may be a microorganism, a cell from transplanted tissue, or one of the body's cells that has been infected by an invading microorganism or altered by cancer.

Some white blood cells—B cells (B lymphocytes)—can recognize invaders directly. But others—T cells (T lymphocytes)—need help from other cells of the immune system (called antigen-presenting cells). These cells ingest an invader and break it into fragments. The antigen fragments from the invader are combined with HLA molecules as they are assembled in the antigen-presenting cell and moved to the cell's surface. T cells that come into contact with the antigen-presenting cell then learn to recognize the invader's antigen fragments. T cells are then activated and can begin fighting the invaders that have that antigen.

Activation and Mobilization: White blood cells are activated when they recognize invaders. For example, when the antigen-presenting cell presents antigen fragments bound to HLA to a T cell, the T cell attaches to the fragments and is activated. B cells can be activated directly by invaders. Once activated, white blood cells ingest or kill the invader or do both. Usually, more than one type of white blood cell is needed to kill an invader.

Immune cells, such as macrophages and activated T cells, release substances that attract other immune cells to the trouble spot, thus mobilizing defenses. The invader itself may release substances that attract immune cells.

Regulation: The immune response must be regulated to prevent extensive damage to the body. Regulatory (suppressor) T cells help control the response by secreting cytokines (chemical messengers of the immune system) that inhibit immune responses.

Resolution: Resolution involves confining the invader and eliminating it from the body. After the invader is eliminated, most white blood cells self-destruct and are ingested. Those that are spared are called memory cells. The body retains memory cells, which are part of acquired immunity, to remember specific invaders and respond more vigorously to them at the next encounter.

Innate Immunity

Innate (natural) immunity is so named because it is present at birth and does not have to be learned through exposure to an invader. It thus provides an immediate response to foreign cells. However, its components treat all foreign substances in much the same way. They recognize only a limited number of identifying substances (antigens) on foreign cells, although these antigens are present on many different cells. Innate immunity has no memory of the encounters and does not provide any lasting protection against future infection.

The white blood cells involved in innate immunity are

- Monocytes (which develop into macrophages)
- Neutrophils
- Eosinophils
- Basophils
- Natural killer cells

Each type has a different function. The complement system and cytokines also participate in innate immunity.

Macrophages

Macrophages develop from a type of white blood cell called monocytes after monocytes move from the bloodstream to the tissues. Monocytes move to the tissues when infection occurs. There, over a period of about 8 hours, monocytes enlarge greatly and produce granules within themselves, becoming macrophages. The granules are filled with enzymes and other substances that help kill and digest bacteria and other foreign cells. Macrophages stay in the tissues. They ingest bacteria, foreign cells, and damaged and dead cells. (The process of a cell ingesting a microorganism, another cell, or cell fragments is called phagocytosis, and cells that ingest are called phagocytes.)

How T Cells Recognize Antigens

T cells are part of the immune surveillance system. They travel through the bloodstream and lymphatic system. When they reach the lymph nodes or another secondary lymphoid organ, they look for foreign substances (antigens) in the body. However, a T cell cannot recognize an antigen unless it has been processed and presented to the T cell by another white blood cell, called an antigen-presenting cell. Antigen-presenting cells consist of dendritic cells (which are the most effective), macrophages, and B cells.

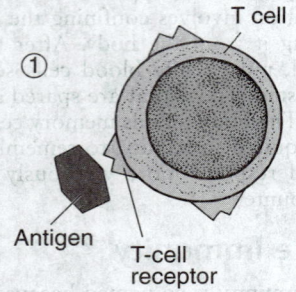

① T cell, Antigen, T-cell receptor

1. By itself, a T cell cannot recognize an antigen circulating in the body because the antigen does not fit into the T-cell receptor, a special molecule that is located on the T cell's surface.

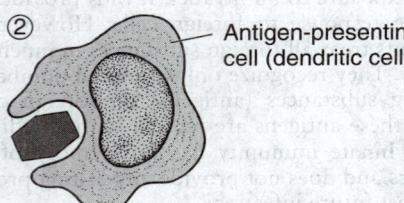

② Antigen-presenting cell (dendritic cell)

2. A cell that can process antigens, such as a dendritic cell, ingests the antigen.

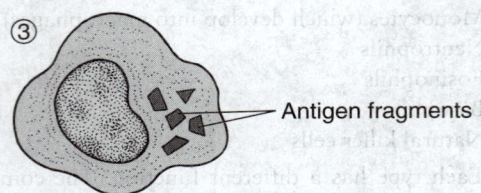

③ Antigen fragments

3. Enzymes in the antigen-presenting cell break the antigen into fragments.

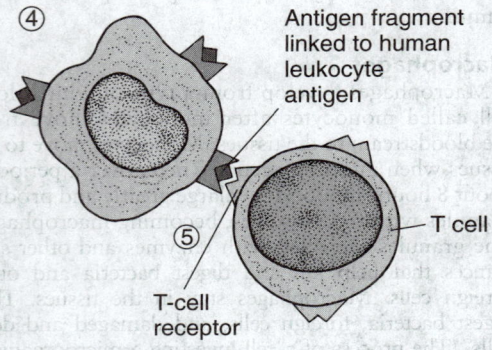

④ Antigen fragment linked to human leukocyte antigen

⑤ T cell, T-cell receptor

4. Some antigen fragments are combined with human leukocyte antigen (HLA) molecules as they are assembled inside the antigen-presenting cell. Then the HLA molecules with the antigen fragments are transported to the cell's surface.

5. The T-cell receptor can recognize the antigen fragment when it is attached to and presented by an HLA molecule. The T-cell receptor attaches to the part of the HLA molecule presenting the antigen fragment, fitting in it as a key fits in a lock. The T cell is then activated and can begin fighting the invaders who have that antigen.

Macrophages secrete substances that attract other white blood cells to the site of the infection. They also help T cells recognize invaders and thus participate in acquired immunity.

Neutrophils

Neutrophils, the most common type of white blood cell in the bloodstream, are among the first immune cells to defend against infection. They ingest bacteria and other foreign cells. Neutrophils contain granules that release enzymes to help kill and digest these cells.

Neutrophils circulate in the bloodstream and must be signaled to leave the bloodstream and enter tissues. The signal often comes from the bacteria themselves, from complement proteins, or from damaged tissue, all of which produce substances that attract neutrophils to a trouble spot. (The process of attracting cells is called chemotaxis.)

Neutrophils also release substances that produce fibers in the surrounding tissue. These fibers may trap bacteria, thus keeping them from spreading and making them easier to destroy.

Eosinophils

Eosinophils can ingest bacteria but also target foreign cells that are too large to ingest. Eosinophils contain granules that release enzymes and other toxic substances when foreign cells are encountered. These substances make holes in the target cell's membranes.

Eosinophils circulate in the bloodstream. However, they are less active against bacteria than are neutrophils and macrophages. Their main function may be to attach to and thus help immobilize and kill parasites.

Eosinophils help destroy cancer cells. They also produce chemicals involved in inflammation and allergic reactions (see page 1112). People with allergies, parasitic infections, or asthma often have more eosinophils in the bloodstream than people without these disorders.

Basophils

Basophils do not ingest foreign cells. They contain granules filled with histamine, a substance involved in allergic reactions. When basophils encounter allergens (antigens that cause allergic reactions), they release histamine. Histamine increases blood flow to damaged tissues. Basophils also produce substances that attract neutrophils and eosinophils to a trouble spot.

Natural Killer Cells

Natural killer cells are called "natural" killers because they are ready to kill as soon as they are formed. Natural killer cells attach to foreign cells and release enzymes and other substances that damage the outer membranes of the foreign cells. Natural killer cells kill certain microorganisms, cancer cells, and cells infected by viruses. Thus, natural killer cells are important in the initial defense against viral infections.

Also, natural killer cells produce cytokines that regulate some of the functions of T cells, B cells, and macrophages.

Dendritic Cells

Dendritic cells reside in the skin, lymph nodes, and tissues throughout the body. Most dendritic cells ingest and break antigens into fragments (called antigen processing), enabling helper T cells to recognize the antigen. Dendritic cells present antigen fragments to T cells in the lymph nodes.

Another type of dendritic cell, the follicular dendritic cell, presents unprocessed (intact) antigen that has been linked with antibody (antibody-antigen complex) to B cells.

After T and B cells are presented with the antigen, they become activated.

Complement System

The complement system consists of more than 30 proteins that act in a sequence: One protein activates another and so on. This sequence is called the complement cascade. Complement proteins have many functions in acquired immunity as well as innate:

- Killing bacteria directly
- Helping destroy bacteria by attaching to them and thus making the bacteria easier for neutrophils and macrophages to identify and ingest
- Attracting macrophages and neutrophils to a trouble spot
- Causing bacteria to clump together
- Neutralizing viruses
- Helping immune cells remember specific invaders
- Promoting antibody formation
- Enhancing the effectiveness of antibodies
- Helping the body eliminate immune complexes, which consist of an antibody attached to a foreign substance (antigen), and dead cells

Cytokines

Cytokines are the messengers of the immune system. White blood cells and certain other cells of the immune system produce cytokines when an antigen is detected.

There are many different cytokines, which affect different parts of the immune system. Some stimulate activity. They stimulate certain white blood cells to become more effective killers and to attract other white blood cells to a trouble spot. Other cytokines inhibit activity, helping end an immune response. Some cytokines, called interferons, interfere with the reproduction (replication) of viruses. Cytokines also participate in specific immunity.

Acquired Immunity

Acquired (adaptive or specific) immunity is not present at birth. It is learned. As a person's immune system encounters foreign substances (antigens), the components of acquired immunity learn the best way to attack each antigen and begin to develop a memory for that antigen. Acquired immunity is also called specific immunity because it tailors its attack to a specific antigen previously encountered. Its hallmarks are its ability to learn, adapt, and remember. Acquired immunity takes time to develop after initial exposure to a new antigen. However, because a memory is formed, subsequent responses to a previously encountered antigen are more effective and more rapid than those generated by innate immunity.

Lymphocytes are the type of white blood cell responsible for acquired immunity. Typically, an acquired immune response begins when antibodies, produced by B cells (B lymphocytes), encounter antigen. Dendritic cells, cytokines, and the complement system (which enhances the effectiveness of antibodies) are also involved.

Lymphocytes

Lymphocytes enable the body to remember antigens and to distinguish self from nonself (foreign). Lymphocytes circulate in the bloodstream and lymphatic system and move into tissues as needed.

The immune system can remember every antigen encountered because, after an encounter, some lymphocytes develop into memory cells. These cells live a long time—for years or even decades. When these cells encounter an antigen for the second time, they recognize it immediately and respond quickly, vigorously, and specifically to that particular antigen. This specific immune response is the reason that people do not contract chickenpox or measles more than once and that vaccination can prevent certain disorders.

Lymphocytes may be T cells or B cells.

T Cells: T cells are produced in the thymus. There, they learn how to distinguish self from nonself. Only the T cells that ignore self antigen molecules are allowed to mature and leave the thymus. Without this training process, T cells could attack the body's cells and tissues.

Mature T cells are stored in secondary lymphoid organs (lymph nodes, spleen, tonsils, appendix, and Peyer's patches in the small intestine). These cells circulate in the bloodstream and the lymphatic system. After they first encounter a foreign or abnormal cell, they are activated and search for those particular cells.

There are different types of T cells:

- **Killer (cytotoxic) T cells** attach to particular foreign or abnormal (for example, infected) cells because they have encountered them before. Killer T cells may kill these cells by making holes in their cell membrane and injecting enzymes into the cells or by binding with certain sites on their surface called death receptors. This binding triggers reactions within the foreign or abnormal cell that lead to death.

- **Helper T cells** help other immune cells. Some helper T cells help B cells produce antibodies against foreign antigens. Others help activate killer T cells to kill foreign or abnormal cells or help activate macrophages enabling them to ingest foreign or abnormal cells more efficiently.

- **Suppressor (regulatory) T cells** produce substances that help end the immune response or sometimes prevent certain harmful responses from occurring.

Sometimes T cells—for reasons that are not completely understood—do not distinguish self from nonself. This malfunction can result in an autoimmune disorder, in which the body attacks its own tissues (see page 1124).

B Cells: B cells are formed in the bone marrow. B cells have particular sites (receptors) on their surface where antigens can attach.

The B-cell response to antigens has two stages:

- Primary immune response: When B cells first encounter an antigen, the antigen attaches to a receptor, stimulating the B cells. Some B cells change into memory cells, which remember that specific antigen, and others change into plasma cells. Helper T cells help B cells in this process. Plasma cells produce antibodies that are specific to the antigen that stimulated their production. After the first encounter with an antigen, production of enough of the specific antibody takes several days. Thus, the primary immune response is slow.

- Secondary immune response: But thereafter, whenever B cells encounter the antigen again, memory B cells very rapidly recognize the antigen, multiply, change into plasma cells, and produce antibodies. This response is quick and very effective.

Antibodies

When a B cell encounters an antigen, it is stimulated to mature into a plasma cell or a memory B cell. Plasma cells then release antibodies (also called immunoglobulins, or Ig). Antibodies protect the body in the following ways:

- Helping cells ingest antigens (cells that ingest antigens are called phagocytes)
- Inactivating toxic substances produced by bacteria
- Attacking bacteria and viruses directly
- Activating the complement system, which has many immune functions

Antibodies are essential for fighting off certain types of bacterial and fungal infections. They can also help fight viruses.

Each antibody molecule has two parts. One part varies. It is specialized to attach to a specific antigen. The other part is one of five structures, which determines the antibody's class—IgM, IgG, IgA, IgE, or IgD. This part is the same within each class and determines the function of the antibody.

IgM: This class of antibody is produced when a particular antigen is encountered for the first time. The response triggered by the first encounter with an antigen is the primary immune response. IgM then attaches to the antigen, activating the complement system and making the antigen easier to ingest.

Normally, IgM is present in the bloodstream but not in the tissues.

IgG: IgG, the most prevalent class of antibody, is produced in greater amounts when a particular antigen is encountered again. More antibody is produced in this response, called the secondary immune response, than in the primary immune response. The secondary immune response is also faster and the antibodies produced—mainly IgG—are more effective. IgG protects against bacteria, viruses, fungi, and toxic substances.

IgG is present in the bloodstream and tissues. It is the only class of antibody that crosses the placenta from mother to fetus. The mother's IgG protects the fetus and infant until the infant's immune system can produce its own antibodies. Also, IgG is the most common class of antibody used in treatment.

IgA: These antibodies help defend against the invasion of microorganisms through body surfaces lined with a mucous membrane, including those of the nose, eyes, lungs, and digestive tract. IgA is present in the bloodstream, in secretions produced by mucous membranes, and in colostrum (the fluid produced by the breasts during the first few days after delivery, before breast milk is produced).

IgE: These antibodies trigger immediate allergic reactions (see page 1112). IgE binds to basophils (a type of white blood cell) in the bloodstream and mast cells

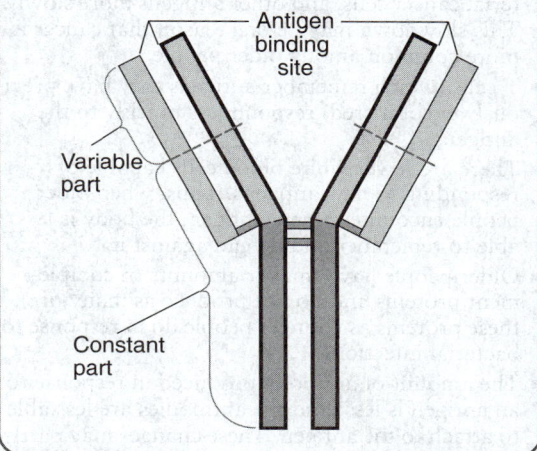

Basic Y Structure of Antibodies

An antibody molecule is basically shaped like a Y. The molecule has two parts:

- Variable part: This part varies from antibody to antibody, depending on which antigen the antibody targets. The antigen attaches to the variable part.
- Constant part: This part can be one of five structures, which determines the antibody's class—IgM, IgG, IgA, IgE, or IgD. This part is the same within each class.

Antigen binding site

Variable part

Constant part

in tissues. When basophils or mast cells with IgE bound to them encounter allergens (antigens that cause allergic reactions), they release substances (such as histamine) that cause inflammation and damage surrounding tissues. Thus, IgE is the only class of antibody that often seems to do more harm than good. However, IgE helps defend against certain parasitic infections that are common in some developing countries.

Small amounts of IgE are present in the bloodstream and mucus of the digestive system. These amounts are higher in people with asthma, hay fever, other allergic disorders, and parasitic infections.

IgD: IgD is present mainly on the surface of immature B cells. It helps these cells mature. Small amounts of these antibodies are present in the bloodstream. Their function in the bloodstream, if any, is not well understood.

Effects of Aging

The immune system changes throughout life. At birth, specific immunity is not fully developed.

However, newborns have some antibodies, which crossed the placenta from the mother during pregnancy. These antibodies protect newborns against infections until their own immune system fully develops. Breastfed newborns also receive antibodies from the mother in breast milk.

As people age, the immune system becomes less effective in the following ways:

- The immune system becomes less able to distinguish self from nonself (that is, antigens). As a result, autoimmune disorders become more common.
- Macrophages (which ingest antigens) destroy bacteria, cancer cells, and other antigens more slowly. This slowdown may be one reason that cancer is more common among older people.
- T cells (which remember antigens they have previously encountered) respond less quickly to the antigens.
- There are fewer white blood cells capable of responding to new antigens. Thus, when older people encounter a new antigen, the body is less able to remember and defend against it.
- Older people have smaller amounts of complement proteins and do not produce as many of these proteins as younger people do in response to bacterial infections.
- The amount of antibody produced in response to an antigen is less, and the antibodies are less able to attach to the antigen. These changes may partly explain why pneumonia, influenza, infectious endocarditis, and tetanus are more common among older people and result in death more often. These

> ## Strategies for Attack
>
> Different types of invading microorganisms are attacked and destroyed in different ways. Some microorganisms are directly recognized, ingested, and destroyed by cells that ingest such invaders (phagocytes), such as neutrophils and macrophages. However, phagocytes cannot directly recognize certain bacteria because the bacteria are enclosed in a capsule. In these cases, B cells have to help phagocytes with recognition. B cells produce antibodies against the antigens in the bacteria's capsule. The antibodies attach to the capsule. The phagocyte can then recognize the bacteria.
>
> Some microorganisms cannot be completely eliminated. To defend against these microorganisms, the immune system builds a wall around them. The wall is formed when phagocytes, particularly macrophages, adhere to each other. The wall around the microorganisms is called a granuloma. Some bacteria thus imprisoned may survive in the body indefinitely. If the immune system is weakened (even 50 or 60 years later), the walls of the granuloma may crumble, and the bacteria may start to multiply, causing symptoms.

changes may also partly explain why vaccines are less effective in older people.

These changes in immune function may contribute to the greater susceptibility of older people to some infections and cancers.

---

168 Immunodeficiency Disorders

Immunodeficiency disorders involve malfunction of the immune system, resulting in infections that develop and recur more frequently, are more severe, and last longer than usual.

- Immunodeficiency disorders usually result from use of a drug or from a long-lasting serious disorder (such as cancer) but occasionally are inherited.
- People usually have frequent, unusual, or unusually severe infections.
- Doctors suspect immunodeficiency based on symptoms and do blood tests to identify the particular disorder.

- People are given antibiotics to prevent and treat infections.
- Immune globulin may be given if antibodies (immunoglobulins) are missing.
- If the disorder is severe, stem cell transplantation may be done.

Immunodeficiency disorders impair the immune system's ability to defend the body against foreign or abnormal cells that invade or attack it (such as bacteria, viruses, fungi, and cancer cells). As a result, unusual bacterial, viral, or fungal infections and rare cancers may develop.

SOME CONGENITAL IMMUNODEFICIENCY DISORDERS

CLASSIFICATION	DISORDER
Problems with B cells (lymphocytes) and their production of antibodies	Common variable immunodeficiency Deficiency of a specific antibody (immunoglobulin), such as IgA deficiency Transient hypogammaglobulinemia of infancy X-linked agammaglobulinemia
Problems with T cells (lymphocytes)	Chronic mucocutaneous candidiasis DiGeorge syndrome X-linked lymphoproliferative syndrome
Problems with B and T cells	Ataxia-telangiectasia Hyperimmunoglobulinemia E syndrome Severe combined immunodeficiency Wiskott-Aldrich syndrome
Problems with the movement or killing activity of phagocytes	Chédiak-Higashi syndrome (rare) Chronic granulomatous disease Leukocyte adhesion defects
Problems with complement proteins	Complement component 1 (C1) inhibitor deficiency (hereditary angioedema) C3 deficiency C6 deficiency C7 deficiency C8 deficiency

There are two types of immunodeficiency disorders:

- **Congenital (primary):** These disorders are present at birth and are usually hereditary. They typically become evident during infancy or childhood. There are more than 200 congenital immunodeficiency disorders. All are relatively rare.

- **Acquired (secondary):** These disorders develop later in life and often result from use of a drug or from another disorder, such as diabetes or human immunodeficiency virus (HIV) infection. They are more common than congenital immunodeficiency disorders.

Some immunodeficiency disorders shorten life span. Others persist throughout life but do not affect life span, and a few resolve with or without treatment.

Causes

Congenital Immunodeficiency: These disorders are caused by a genetic abnormality, which is often X-linked (see page 13). That is, only boys are affected. As a result, about 60% of people with congenital immunodeficiency disorders are male.

Congenital immunodeficiency disorders are classified by which part of the immune system (see page 1095) is affected:

- B cells (lymphocytes), a type of white blood cell that produces antibodies (immunoglobulins)
- T cells (lymphocytes), a type of white blood cell that helps identify and destroy foreign or abnormal cells
- B and T cells
- Phagocytes (cells that ingest and kill microorganisms)
- Complement proteins (proteins with various immune functions, such as killing bacteria and other foreign cells and making foreign cells easier for other immune cells to identify and ingest—see page 1101)

The affected component of the immune system may be missing, reduced in number, or abnormal and malfunctioning. Problems with B cells are the most common congenital immunodeficiency disorders, accounting for more than half.

Acquired Immunodeficiency Disorders: These most commonly result from drugs (mainly immunosuppressants, which are used to treat serious disorders).

Immunosuppressants are used to intentionally suppress the immune system. For example, some are used to prevent rejection of a transplanted organ or tissue (see table on page 1130). Corticosteroids, a type of immunosuppressant, are used to suppress inflammation due to various disorders, such as rheumatoid arthritis. However, immunosuppressants also suppress the body's ability to fight infections and perhaps to destroy cancer cells. Chemotherapy and radiation therapy can also suppress the immune system, sometimes leading to immunodeficiency disorders.

Immunodeficiency disorders may result from almost any prolonged serious disorder. For example, diabetes can result in an immunodeficiency disorder because white blood cells do not function well when the blood sugar level is high. Human immunodeficiency virus (HIV) infection results in acquired immunodeficiency syndrome (AIDS), the most common severe acquired immunodeficiency disorder.

Undernutrition—whether of all nutrients or only one—can impair the immune system. When undernutrition causes weight to decrease to less than 80% of recommended weight, the immune system is often impaired. A decrease to less than 70% usually results in severe impairment.

Symptoms

People with an immunodeficiency disorder tend to have one infection after another. Usually, respiratory infections develop first and recur often. Most people eventually develop severe bacterial infections that persist, recur, or lead to complications. For example, sore throats and head colds may progress to pneumonia. However, having many colds does not suggest an immunodeficiency disorder.

Infections of the skin and the membranes lining the mouth, eyes, and digestive tract are common. Thrush, a fungal infection of the mouth, may be an early sign of an immunodeficiency disorder. Sores may form in the mouth. Ear infections and skin infections by bacteria or viruses are also common. Bacterial infections (for example, with staphylococci) may cause pus-filled sores to form (pyoderma). Warts (caused by viruses) may form.

Many people lose weight.

Infants or young children may have chronic diarrhea and may not grow and develop as expected (called failure to thrive). The earlier symptoms begin in children, the more severe the immunodeficiency.

Other symptoms vary depending on the severity and duration of the infections.

Diagnosis

Doctors must first suspect that an immunodeficiency exists. Then they do tests to identify the specific immune system abnormality.

Doctors suspect immunodeficiency when a severe or an unusual infection recurs often or when an organism that normally does not cause severe infection (such as *Pneumocystis* or cytomegalovirus) causes severe infection. The results of a physical examination may also suggest immunodeficiency. Rashes, hair loss, chronic cough, weight loss, and an enlarged liver and spleen are often present. Lymph nodes and tonsils may be extremely small in some forms of immunodeficiency, whereas in other types the lymph nodes may be swollen. Certain symptoms may suggest a particular disorder to doctors.

To help identify the type of immunodeficiency disorder, doctors ask at what age the person began to have recurring or unusual infections. Infections in infants younger than 6 months usually indicate an abnormality in T cells. Infections in older children usually indicate an abnormality in B cells and antibody production. The type of infection may also help doctors identify the type of immunodeficiency disorder.

Doctors ask the person about risk factors, such as diabetes, use of certain drugs, exposure to toxic substances, and the possibility of having close relatives with immunodeficiency disorders (family history). The person is asked about past and current sexual activity and use of intravenous drugs to determine whether HIV infection could be the cause (see page 1254).

Tests: Laboratory tests are needed to confirm the diagnosis of immunodeficiency and to identify the type of immunodeficiency disorder. A blood sample is taken and analyzed to determine the total number of white blood cells and the percentages of each main type of white blood cell. The white blood cells are examined under a microscope for abnormalities. Antibody levels, the number of red blood cells and platelets, and the levels of complement proteins are determined. If any results are abnormal, additional tests are usually done.

Skin tests may be done if the immunodeficiency is thought to be due to a T-cell abnormality. The skin test resembles the tuberculin skin test, which is used to screen for tuberculosis. Small amounts of proteins from common infectious organisms such as yeast are injected under the skin. If a reaction (redness, warmth, and swelling) occurs within 48 hours, the T cells are functioning normally. No reaction suggests a T-cell abnormality.

People whose families are known to carry a gene for a hereditary immunodeficiency disorder may wish to have genetic testing to learn whether they carry the gene for the disorder and their chances of having an affected child. Talking with a genetic counselor before testing is helpful. Several immuno-

DRUGS THAT CAN CAUSE IMMUNODEFICIENCY

TYPE	EXAMPLES
Anticonvulsants	Carbamazepine Phenytoin Valproate
Immunosuppressants	Azathioprine Cyclosporine Mycophenolate mofetil Sirolimus Tacrolimus
Corticosteroids	Methylprednisolone Prednisone
Chemotherapy drugs	Alemtuzumab Busulfan Cyclophosphamide Melphalan
Monoclonal antibodies (substances that target and suppress specific parts of the immune system)	Muromonab (OKT3)

deficiency disorders, such as X-linked agammaglobulinemia, Wiskott-Aldrich syndrome, severe combined immunodeficiency, and chronic granulomatous disease, can be detected in a fetus by testing a sample of the fluid around the fetus (amniotic fluid) or the fetus's blood (prenatal testing). Such testing may be recommended for people with a family history of an immunodeficiency disorder when the mutation has been identified in the family.

Prevention and Treatment

Some of the disorders that can cause immunodeficiency disorders can be prevented or treated. The following are examples:

- HIV infection: Following safe sex guidelines and not sharing needles to inject drugs can reduce the spread of this infection.
- Cancer: Successful treatment usually restores the function of the immune system unless people need to continue taking immunosuppressants.
- Diabetes: Good control of blood sugar levels can help white blood cells function better and thus prevent infections.

Strategies for preventing and treating infections depend on the type of immunodeficiency disorder.

For example, people who have an immunodeficiency disorder due to a deficiency of antibodies are at risk of bacterial infections. The following can help reduce the risk:

- Being treated periodically with immune globulin (antibodies obtained from the blood of people with a normal immune system) given intravenously
- Practicing good personal hygiene (including conscientious dental care)
- Not eating undercooked food
- Drinking only bottled water
- Avoiding contact with people who have infections

DISORDERS THAT CAN CAUSE IMMUNODEFICIENCY

TYPE	EXAMPLES
Blood	Aplastic anemia Leukemia Myelofibrosis Sickle cell disease
Cancer	Brain cancer Intestinal cancer Lung cancer
Chromosomal	Down syndrome
Infections	Cytomegalovirus infections Epstein-Barr virus infections Human immunodeficiency virus (HIV) infection Measles Varicella
Hormonal	Diabetes mellitus
Kidney	Build up of toxic substances in the blood (uremia) Nephrotic syndrome
Liver	Hepatitis
Musculoskeletal	Rheumatoid arthritis Systemic lupus erythematosus (lupus)
Spleen	Removal of spleen
Other	Alcoholism Burns Undernutrition

Antibiotics are given as soon as a fever or another sign of an infection develops and before surgical and dental procedures, which may introduce bacteria into the bloodstream.

If an immunodeficiency disorder increases the risk of viral infections (as immunodeficiency due to a T-cell abnormality does), antiviral drugs, such as amantadine for influenza or acyclovir for herpes or chickenpox, are promptly given at the first sign of infection. Such treatment may be lifesaving.

If a disorder (such as severe combined immunodeficiency) increases the risk of developing serious infections or particular infections, people may be given antibiotics in advance to prevent these infections.

If the immunodeficiency disorder does not prevent antibody production, people are vaccinated. However, people who have a B- or T-cell abnormality are given only killed viral and bacterial vaccines rather than live vaccines. Live viruses may cause an infection in such people. Live vaccines include rotavirus vaccines, oral poliovirus vaccine, measles-mumps-rubella vaccine, chickenpox (varicella) vaccine, and bacille Calmette-Guérin (BCG) vaccine. An influenza vaccine given once a year is recommended for people who can produce antibodies and for their immediate family members.

Stem cell transplantation (see page 1133) can correct some immunodeficiency disorders, particularly severe combined immunodeficiency. Stem cells are usually obtained from bone marrow but occasionally from blood (including umbilical cord blood). Stem cell transplantation, which is available at some major medical centers, is usually reserved for severe disorders.

Transplantation of thymus tissue is sometimes helpful. Gene therapy for a few congenital immunodeficiency disorders has been successful, but it is not widely used because leukemia is sometimes a risk.

Ataxia-Telangiectasia

Ataxia-telangiectasia is a hereditary disorder characterized by incoordination, dilated capillaries, and increased susceptibility to infections.

The increased susceptibility to infections in people with ataxia-telangiectasia results from malfunction of B and T cells (lymphocytes), which help the body defend itself against microorganisms and abnormal cells. Often, levels of certain types (classes) of antibodies (immunoglobulins)—IgA and IgE—are also low. Sinus and respiratory infections recur, often leading to pneumonia and chronic lung disorders such as bronchitis. The risk of cancer, especially leukemia, brain tumors, and stomach cancer, is increased.

This disorder also causes abnormalities in the cerebellum (the part of the brain that coordinates the body's movements), which are unrelated to the immunodeficiency disorder. Incoordination (ataxia) results, usually when children begin to walk, but it may be delayed until age 4. Speech becomes slurred, and muscles progressively weaken, leading to severe disability. Mental retardation may develop and progress. Between the ages of 1 and 6, capillaries in the skin and eyes become dilated and visible. The dilated capillaries (telangiectasia), called spider veins, are usually most obvious on the eyeballs and ears. The endocrine system may be affected, resulting in small testes (in boys), infertility, and diabetes.

Doctors suspect the diagnosis based on symptoms. Blood tests to measure the levels of IgA and genetic tests can help confirm the diagnosis.

Antibiotics and immune globulin (to provide the missing immunoglobulins) help prevent infections but do not relieve the other problems. Ataxia-telangiectasia usually progresses to paralysis, dementia, and death, typically by age 30.

Chronic Granulomatous Disease

Chronic granulomatous disease is a hereditary immunodeficiency disorder in which phagocytes (a type of white blood cell) malfunction.

Normally, phagocytes (neutrophils, eosinophils, monocytes, and macrophages) ingest and kill microorganisms. In chronic granulomatous disease, phagocytes can ingest but cannot produce the substances (such as hydrogen peroxide and superoxide) that kill certain bacteria and fungi. This disorder usually affects boys.

Symptoms usually first appear during early childhood but sometimes not until adolescence. Chronic infections occur in the skin, lungs, lymph nodes, mouth, nose, and intestines. Pockets of pus (abscesses) can develop around the anus and in the lungs, bones, and liver. The lymph nodes tend to fill with bacteria and enlarge. The skin over the lymph nodes may break down. As a result, the abscess drains. The liver and spleen enlarge. Children may grow slowly.

To diagnose the disorder, doctors take a sample of blood and send it to a laboratory, which measures the activity of phagocytes in response to microorganisms.

Antibiotics are given regularly and indefinitely to prevent infection. Interferon-gamma, injected 3 times a week, can reduce the number and severity of infections. Antifungal drugs are also given regularly if people have had even one fungal infection. Stem cell transplantation has been successful in some people but, because it has risks, is usually recommended only if people have a brother or sister who has the exact same tissue type and who can donate the cells.

Chronic Mucocutaneous Candidiasis

Chronic mucocutaneous candidiasis is a hereditary immunodeficiency disorder due to malfunction of T cells (lymphocytes).

Because T cells malfunction, the body is less able to fight fungal infections, including infection with *Candida* (candidiasis—see page 1232), a yeast. The ability to fight other infections is not reduced.

Candidal infections develop and persist, usually beginning during infancy but sometimes during early adulthood. The fungus may cause mouth infections (thrush) and infections of the scalp, skin, and nails. Membranes lining the mouth, eyelids, digestive tract, and vagina may also be infected. In infants, the first symptoms are often thrush that is difficult to treat, diaper rash, or both. Severity varies. The disorder may affect one nail or cause a disfiguring rash that covers the face and scalp. The rash is crusted and thick and may ooze. On the scalp, the rash may cause hair to fall out. Many people also have endocrine disorders, such as underactive parathyroid glands (hypoparathyroidism) and underactive adrenal glands (Addison's disease), as well as hepatitis and autoimmune disorders, such as Graves' disease.

Doctors suspect this infection when people have the characteristic rash. The diagnosis can be confirmed by examining a sample from the infected area under a microscope and identifying the yeast.

Usually, the infections can be controlled with an antifungal drug applied to the skin. If infections persist, they can be effectively treated with fluconazole or another similar antifungal drug taken by mouth. Drugs may have to be taken for a long time. Usually, this disorder is chronic but does not affect life span.

Common Variable Immunodeficiency

Common variable immunodeficiency is a congenital immunodeficiency disorder characterized by very low antibody (immunoglobulin) levels despite a normal number of B cells (lymphocytes).

Common variable immunodeficiency usually develops between the ages of 10 and 20, sometimes earlier and sometimes later. The number of B cells is normal, but the cells do not mature and thus cannot produce immunoglobulins. In some people with this disorder, T cells (lymphocytes) also malfunction.

Recurring lung infections, particularly pneumonia, are common. People may develop a chronic cough, cough up blood, or have difficulty breathing.

Autoimmune disorders, including Addison's disease, thyroiditis, and rheumatoid arthritis, often develop. Diarrhea may occur, and food may not be absorbed well from the digestive tract. The spleen may enlarge. Stomach cancer and lymphoma develop in 10% of people.

Doctors suspect the disorder if typical symptoms occur in people who have several family members with autoimmune disorders. Blood tests are done to measure immunoglobulin levels.

Infusions of immune globulin (to provide the missing immunoglobulins) are given throughout life, and antibiotics are promptly given to treat infections. Autoimmune disorders are treated as needed with rituximab (a monoclonal antibody also used to treat lymphomas and rheumatoid arthritis) or a corticosteroid. Life span may be shortened.

DiGeorge Syndrome

DiGeorge syndrome is a congenital immunodeficiency disorder in which the thymus gland is absent or underdeveloped at birth.

Usually, DiGeorge syndrome is due to a chromosomal abnormality, but it does not usually run in families. Boys and girls are equally affected. The fetus does not develop normally, and abnormalities often occur in the following:

- **Heart:** Children are often born with a congenital heart disorder.
- **Parathyroid gland:** Children are usually born with underdeveloped or no parathyroid glands (which help regulate calcium levels in the blood). As a result, calcium levels are low, leading to muscle spasms (tetany). Spasms usually start within 48 hours after birth.
- **Face:** Typically, children have unusual facial features, with low-set ears, a small jawbone that recedes, and wide-set eyes. They may have a split in the roof of the mouth (cleft palate).
- **Thymus gland:** The thymus gland is necessary for the normal development of T cells. Consequently, the number of T cells is low, limiting their ability to fight many infections. Infections begin soon after birth and recur often. However, how well T cells function varies considerably. Also, T cells may spontaneously start functioning better.

Doctors suspect the diagnosis based on symptoms. Blood tests are done to determine the total number of blood cells and the number of T and B cells and to evaluate how well T cells and the parathyroid glands are functioning. A chest x-ray may be taken to check the size of the thymus gland. Chromosomal tests may be done to look for abnormalities.

For children who have some T cells, the immune system may function adequately without treatment. Infections that develop are treated promptly. For children who have very few or no T cells, the disorder is fatal unless transplantation of thymus tissue is done. Such transplantation can cure the immunodeficiency. Before the thymus tissue is transplanted, it is placed in a culture dish and treated to eliminate mature T cells. These cells may identify the recipient's tissue as foreign and attack it, causing graft-versus-host disease.

Calcium and vitamin D supplements are given by mouth to prevent muscle spasms. Sometimes the heart disease is worse than the immunodeficiency, and surgery to prevent severe heart failure or death may be needed. The prognosis usually depends on the severity of the heart disorder.

Hyperimmunoglobulinemia E Syndrome

Hyperimmunoglobulinemia E syndrome (hyper-IgE syndrome, or Buckley syndrome) is a hereditary immunodeficiency disorder characterized by early onset of recurrent boils and pneumonia but with very high levels of immunoglobulin E (IgE) and normal levels of other types (classes) of antibodies (immunoglobulins).

In hyper-IgE syndrome, the number of B and T cells (lymphocytes) is normal. The syndrome is caused by a mutation in a particular gene.

Symptoms usually begin during infancy. In most infants, pockets of pus (abscesses) form in the skin, joints, lungs, or other organs. The abscesses are usually caused by infections with staphylococcal bacteria, and they recur frequently. Lung infections may develop leaving giant cysts after the pneumonia has resolved. An itchy dermatitis develops. Bones are weak, resulting in many fractures. Facial features may be coarse. Loss of baby teeth is delayed.

The diagnosis is suspected based on recurrent boils and pneumonia at a young age and confirmed by blood tests that detect a high level of IgE. Genetic tests can be done to check for the abnormal gene.

Antibiotics, such as dicloxacillin or cephalexin, are given continuously to prevent staphylococcal infections. Life span depends on the severity of the lung infections.

Selective Immunoglobulin Deficiency

Selective immunoglobulin deficiency is a congenital immunodeficiency disorder resulting in a low level of one type (class) of antibody (immunoglobulin), even though the levels of other immunoglobulins are normal.

There are several classes of immunoglobulins. Each class helps protect the body from infection in a different way (see page 1103). The level of any class may be low, but the most commonly affected class is immunoglobulin A (IgA).

Selective IgA Deficiency: This disorder usually persists throughout life. The disorder sometimes results from a chromosomal abnormality. If people have a genetic makeup that makes them susceptible, the deficiency may result from taking phenytoin (an anticonvulsant), sulfasalazine (an antibiotic), or gold compounds or penicillamine (used to treat rheumatoid arthritis). The deficiency also occurs in family members of people with common variable immunodeficiency.

Most people with selective IgA deficiency have few or no symptoms. Others develop chronic lung infections, sinusitis, allergies, chronic diarrhea, or autoimmune disorders, such as inflammatory bowel disease or systemic lupus erythematosus (lupus). A few people develop common variable immunodeficiency.

If given standard blood transfusions or immune globulin infusions (both of which normally contain IgA), some people with selective IgA deficiency produce antibodies against IgA. The next time such people are given a blood transfusion or immune globulin, they may have a severe allergic (anaphylactic) reaction (see page 1123). They should wear a medical identification bracelet or tag to alert doctors to take precautions against such reactions.

Some people improve spontaneously. Life span is usually unaffected unless an autoimmune disorder or common variable immunodeficiency develops.

Doctors suspect the deficiency in people with many infections, especially if they are taking drugs that can cause it or if they have other associated disorders. Blood tests to measure immunoglobulin levels are done to confirm the diagnosis.

Usually, no treatment of selective IgA deficiency is needed. Antibiotics are given to people who have recurring infections. Selective IgA deficiency that results from taking a drug may resolve if the drug is stopped, but this does not happen very often.

Severe Combined Immunodeficiency

Severe combined immunodeficiency is a congenital immunodeficiency disorder resulting in low levels of antibodies (immunoglobulins) and no T cells (lymphocytes).

Severe combined immunodeficiency is the most serious immunodeficiency disorder. It can be caused by several different genetic defects. All forms are hereditary. One form of the disorder is due to a deficiency of the enzyme adenosine deaminase.

Because there are no T cells, B cells cannot produce immunoglobulins, so immunoglobulin levels are low.

Most infants with severe combined immunodeficiency develop pneumonia, thrush, and diarrhea, usually by age 6 months. More serious infections, including *Pneumocystis* pneumonia, can also develop. As a result, infants do not grow and develop normally. They may have peeling rashes, and all affected infants have a severely underdeveloped thymus gland. If not treated, these children usually die before age 1 year.

Diagnosis and Treatment

Symptoms suggest the disorder. Blood tests are done to measure the number of B and T cells and immunoglobulin levels and to evaluate how well B and T cells are functioning.

People with this disorder are kept in a protected environment to prevent exposure to possible infections. In the past, children with this disorder were kept in strict isolation, sometimes in a plastic tent, leading to the disorder being called bubble boy syndrome.

Treatment with antibiotics and immune globulin helps but does not protect against severe viral infections. The only effective treatment is transplantation of bone marrow stem cells from an unaffected sibling with the exact same tissue type or from a parent with a half-matched tissue type. If transplantation is done by age 3 months, 96% of infants survive.

If adenosine deaminase is deficient and transplantation is not possible, replacement of that enzyme, given by injection, can be partially effective.

Gene therapy may be effective, depending on which form of severe combined immunodeficiency is present. Gene therapy consists of removing some white blood cells from the infant's bone marrow, inserting a normal gene into the cells, and returning the cells to the infant. However, in one form of severe combined immunodeficiency, leukemia is a risk after such treatments.

Spleen Disorders and Immunodeficiency

The spleen is crucial to the function of the immune system. The spleen filters the blood, removing and destroying bacteria and other infectious organisms in the bloodstream. It also produces antibodies (immunoglobulins). For people whose spleen is absent at birth or has been damaged or removed because of disease, the risk of developing severe bacterial infections is increased.

People who do not have a spleen are given pneumococcal and meningococcal vaccines in addition to the usual childhood vaccines. People who have a spleen disorder or no spleen are given antibiotics at the first sign of infection. Children who do not have a spleen should take antibiotics, usually penicillin or ampicillin, continuously until at least age 5 to prevent an infection in the bloodstream. If they have an immunodeficiency disorder, they may take these antibiotics indefinitely.

Transient Hypogammaglobulinemia of Infancy

In transient hypogammaglobulinemia of infancy, production of normal amounts of antibodies (immunoglobulins) in infants is delayed.

At birth, the immune system is not fully developed. Most of the immunoglobulins in infants are those produced by the mother and transferred via the placenta before birth. Immunoglobulins from the mother protect infants against infection until infants start to produce their own, usually by age 6 months. About the same time, levels of immunoglobulins from the mother start to decrease. In infants with transient hypogammaglobulinemia of infancy, production of normal amounts of immunoglobulins is delayed. As a result, immunoglobulin levels become low starting at age 3 to 6 months and return to normal at about age 12 to 36 months. The condition rarely leads to serious infections and is not thought to be a true immunodeficiency.

This condition is more common among premature infants because they receive fewer immunoglobulins from the mother. Although the condition is present at birth, it is not hereditary.

Blood tests are done to measure levels of immunoglobulins and to evaluate immunoglobulin production in response to vaccines. Most infants with the disorder produce normal amounts of antibodies in response to the vaccines they are given and to infectious organisms they are exposed to. Therefore, they do not have a problem with infections and need no treatment. However, some infants, particularly those born prematurely, have frequent infections. These infants may be given antibiotics to prevent infections from developing. This disorder usually resolves without treatment.

Wiskott-Aldrich Syndrome

Wiskott-Aldrich syndrome is a hereditary immunodeficiency disorder characterized by abnormal antibody (immunoglobulin) production, T-cell (lymphocyte) malfunction, a low platelet count, and eczema.

Wiskott-Aldrich syndrome affects only boys. It results from a mutation in a gene that codes for a protein needed by T and B cells to function. Thus, these cells malfunction. B cells do not produce immunoglobulins normally. Platelets (cell particles that help blood clot) are small and malformed. The spleen removes and destroys them, causing the platelet count to be low.

Because the number of platelets is low, bleeding problems, usually bloody diarrhea, may be the first symptom. Eczema also develops at an early age. Susceptibility to infections, particularly of the respiratory tract, is increased because immunoglobulin levels are low and T cells malfunction. The risk of developing cancers such as lymphoma and leukemia is increased.

Blood tests help doctors diagnose the disorder. The total number of white blood cells and the percentages of the different types are determined, as is the number of platelets. Platelets are examined to check for abnormalities. Levels of immunoglobulins are measured. Doctors also determine how well the patients make antibodies in response to vaccines and other substances that usually trigger an immune response (antigens). Genetic testing may be done to identify the mutation.

Stem cell transplantation is necessary to preserve life. Without it, most boys with this disorder die by age 15. Surgical removal of the spleen may relieve the bleeding problems. Antibiotics are given continuously to prevent infections, and immune globulin is given to provide the missing antibodies.

X-Linked Agammaglobulinemia

X-linked agammaglobulinemia (Bruton's disease) is a hereditary immunodeficiency disorder due to an abnormality in the X chromosome. It results in few or no B cells (lymphocytes) and very low levels of antibodies (immunoglobulins).

X-linked agammaglobulinemia affects only boys. For about the first 6 months after birth, immunoglobulins from the mother protect against infection. At about age 6 months, levels of these immunoglobulins start to decrease, and affected infants start having recurring infections of the ears, sinuses, and lungs, usually due to bacteria such as pneumococci, streptococci, and *Haemophilus* bacteria. Some unusual viral infections of the brain may develop. The tonsils are very small, and lymph nodes do not develop.

Blood tests are done to measure immunoglobulin and antibody levels and the number of B cells.

Infusions of immune globulin are given throughout life to provide the missing antibodies and thus help prevent infections. Antibiotics are promptly given to treat bacterial infections and may be given continuously. Despite these measures, chronic sinus and lung infections often develop. With treatment, life span is often unaffected, unless brain infections develop.

CHAPTER

169 Allergic Reactions

Allergic reactions (hypersensitivity reactions) are inappropriate responses of the immune system to a normally harmless substance.

- Usually, allergies make the eyes water and itch, the nose run, the skin itch, rashes develop, and people sneeze.
- Some symptoms, called anaphylactic reactions, are life threatening.
- Symptoms suggest the diagnosis, and skin tests can help identify the allergy trigger.
- People who have had severe reactions should always carry a self-injecting syringe of epinephrine and antihistamines.
- Avoiding the trigger is best, but if it is impossible, allergy shots can sometimes desensitize the person.
- Severe reactions require emergency treatment in the hospital.

Normally, the immune system—which includes antibodies, white blood cells, mast cells, complement proteins, and other substances—defends the body against foreign substances (called antigens). However, in susceptible people, the immune system can overreact when exposed to certain chemicals (allergens) in the environment, foods, or drugs, which are harmless in most people. The result is an allergic reaction. Some people are allergic to only one substance. Others are allergic to many. About one third of the people in the United States have an allergy.

Allergens may cause an allergic reaction when they land on the skin or in the eye, are inhaled, are eaten, or are injected. An allergic reaction can occur in several ways:

- As part of a seasonal allergy (such as hay fever), caused by exposure to such substances as grass or ragweed pollen
- Triggered by taking a drug (see page 93)
- Triggered by eating certain foods
- Triggered by breathing in dust or animal dander

In many allergic reactions, the immune system, when first exposed to an allergen, produces a type of antibody called immunoglobulin E (IgE). IgE binds to a type of white blood cell called basophils in the bloodstream and to a similar type of cell called mast cells in the tissues. The first exposure may make people sensitive to the allergen but does not cause symptoms. When sensitized people subsequently encounter the allergen, the basophils and mast cells with IgE on their surface release substances (such as histamine, prostaglandins, and leukotrienes) that cause swelling or inflammation in the surrounding tissues. Such substances begin a cascade of reactions that continue to irritate and harm tissues. These reactions range from mild to severe.

Symptoms

Most allergic reactions are mild, consisting of watery and itchy eyes, a runny nose, itchy skin, and some sneezing. Rashes (including hives) are common and often itch. Hives are small, pale, slightly elevated areas of swelling (wheals) that are surrounded by a red area. Swelling may occur in larger areas under the skin. Swelling is caused by fluids leaking from blood vessels (angioedema—see page 1122). Depending on which areas of the body are affected, angioedema may be serious. Allergies may trigger attacks of asthma.

Certain allergic reactions, called anaphylactic reactions (see page 1123), can be life threatening. The airways can narrow (constrict), causing wheezing, and the lining of the throat and airways may swell, interfering with breathing. Blood vessels can widen (dilate), causing a dangerous fall in blood pressure.

Diagnosis

Doctors first determine whether a reaction is allergic. They may ask whether the person has close relatives with allergies because a reaction is more likely to be allergic in such cases. Blood tests are usually done to detect a type of white blood cell called eosinophils. Eosinophils are produced in large numbers when an allergic reaction occurs.

Because each allergic reaction is triggered by a specific allergen, the main goal of diagnosis is to identify that allergen. Often, the person and doctor can identify the allergen based on when the allergy started and when and how often the reaction occurs (for example, during certain seasons or after eating certain foods).

Skin tests (see also page 1278) are the most useful way to identify specific allergens. Usually, a skin prick test is done first. Dilute solutions are made from extracts of pollens (from trees, grasses, weeds, or fungal spores), dust, animal dander, insect venom, foods, and some drugs. A drop of each solution is placed on the person's skin, which is then pricked with a needle. If the person is allergic to one or more of these substances, the person has a wheal and flare reaction:

- A pale, slightly elevated swelling—the wheal—appears at the pinprick site within 15 to 20 minutes.
- The wheal is surrounded by a well-defined red area—the flare.
- The resulting area is about 1/2 inch (about 1.3 centimeters) in diameter.

The skin prick test can identify most allergens. If no allergen is identified, a tiny amount of each solution can be injected into the person's skin (intradermal test). This type of skin test is more likely to detect a reaction to an allergen. Antihistamines should not be taken before skin tests because they may suppress a reaction to the tests.

The radioallergosorbent test (RAST) is used when skin tests cannot be used—for example, when a skin rash is widespread. This test measures blood levels of different types of IgE that are specific to particular allergens. If a large amount of one type of IgE is detected, the immune system is mounting an allergic reaction against that allergen. Thus, this test helps doctors identify the allergen. People may be asked to stop taking certain drugs a few days to a week before the test. These drugs, which include over-the-counter and prescription antihistamines, tricyclic antidepressants, and monoamine oxidase inhibitors (also antidepressants), can interfere with test results. People who are taking beta-blockers are not tested.

Prevention

Environmental Measures: Avoiding an allergen, if possible, is the best approach. Avoiding an allergen may involve the following:

- Stopping a drug
- Keeping a pet out of the house
- Installing high-efficiency air filters
- Not eating a particular food
- For people with severe seasonal allergies, possibly moving to an area that does not have the allergen
- Removing items that collect dust, such as upholstered furniture and carpets
- Covering mattresses and pillows with finely woven fabrics that cannot be penetrated by dust mites and allergen particles
- Using synthetic-fiber pillows
- Washing bed sheets, pillowcases, and blankets in hot water frequently
- Using dehumidifiers in basements and other damp rooms
- Treating homes with heat-steam

Allergen Immunotherapy: Because some allergens, especially airborne allergens, cannot be avoided, allergen immunotherapy (also called desensitization), usually allergy shots or injections, can be given to desensitize people to the allergen. With allergen immunotherapy, allergic reactions can be prevented or reduced in number or severity. However, allergen immunotherapy is not always effective. Some people and some allergies tend to respond better than others.

Immunotherapy is used most often for allergies to pollens, house dust mites, molds, and venom of stinging insects. When people are allergic to unavoidable allergens, such as insect venom, immunotherapy helps prevent anaphylactic reactions (see page 1123). Sometimes it is used for allergies to animal dander, but such treatment is unlikely to be useful. Immunotherapy for food allergies is usually not advised because it can cause severe reactions and is less effective. Also, foods can usually be avoided.

Immunotherapy is not used when the allergen, such as penicillin and other drugs, can be avoided. However, if people need to take a drug that they are allergic to, immunotherapy, closely monitored by a doctor, can be done to desensitize them.

In immunotherapy, tiny amounts of the allergen are usually injected under the skin. The dose is gradually increased until a dose adequate to control symptoms (maintenance dose) is reached. A gradual increase is necessary because exposure to a high dose of the allergen too soon can cause an allergic reaction. Injections are usually given once or twice a week until the maintenance dose is reached. Then injections are usually given every 2 to 6 weeks. The procedure is most effective when maintenance injections are continued throughout the year, even for seasonal allergies.

Alternatively, high doses of the allergen may be placed under the tongue (sublingual) and held there for a few minutes, then swallowed. The dose is gradually increased, as for injections. The sublingual technique is relatively new, and how often the dose should be given has not been established. It ranges from every day to 3 times a week.

Allergen immunotherapy may take 3 to 4 years to complete.

Because immunotherapy injections occasionally cause dangerous allergic reactions, people remain in the doctor's office for at least 30 minutes afterward. If they have mild reactions to immunotherapy (such as sneezing, coughing, flushing, tingling sensations, itching, chest tightness, wheezing, and hives), a drug—usually an antihistamine, such as diphenhydramine or loratadine—may help. For more severe reactions, epinephrine (adrenaline) is injected.

Treatment

Avoiding the allergen is the best way to treat as well as prevent allergies. If mild symptoms occur, antihistamines are often all that is needed. If they are ineffective, other drugs, such as mast cell stabilizers and corticosteroids may help. Nonsteroidal anti-inflammatory drugs (NSAIDs) are not useful. Severe symptoms, such as those involving the airways (including anaphylactic reactions), require emergency treatment.

Pregnant women with allergies should avoid allergens in order to control their symptoms whenever possible. If symptoms are severe, then pregnant women should use inhaled antihistamines rather than oral antihistamines unless they cannot obtain adequate relief. Breastfeeding women should also try to avoid antihistamines, but if they are necessary then inhaled antihistamines are preferred to oral antihistamines. If oral antihistamines are essential for controlling symptoms, they should be taken immediately after feeding the baby.

Antihistamines: The drugs most commonly used to relieve the symptoms of allergies are antihistamines. Antihistamines block the effects of histamine rather than stop its production. Taking antihistamines partially relieves the runny nose, watery eyes, and itching and reduces the swelling due to hives or mild angioedema. But antihistamines do not ease breathing when airways are constricted.

Antihistamines are available as tablets, capsules, or liquid solutions to be taken by mouth or as nasal sprays, eye drops, or lotions or creams. Which is used depends on the type of allergic reaction. Some antihistamines are available without a prescription (over-the-counter), and some require a prescription.

Antihistamines have anticholinergic effects, such as drowsiness, dry mouth, blurred vision, constipation, difficulty with urination, confusion, and lightheadedness (particularly after a person stands up), as well as drowsiness. Often, prescription antihistamines have fewer of these effects.

Some antihistamines are more likely to cause drowsiness (sedation) than others. Sedating antihistamines are widely available over the counter. People should not take sedating antihistamines if they are going to drive, operate heavy equipment, or do other activities that require alertness. Sedating antihistamines should not be given to children under 2 years of age because they may have serious or life-threatening side effects. Over-the-counter antihistamines are also a particular problem for older people (see box on page 1897) and for people with glaucoma, benign prostatic hyperplasia, or dementia because of the drugs' anticholinergic effects. In general, doctors use antihistamines cautiously in people with cardiovascular disease.

℞ SOME ANTIHISTAMINES

DRUG	DEGREE OF ANTICHOLINERGIC EFFECTS*	DEGREE OF DROWSINESS†
Nonprescription		
Brompheniramine	Moderate	Some
Cetirizine	Few to none	Little to none in most people and moderate in some people
Chlorpheniramine	Moderate	Some
Clemastine	Strong	Moderate
Desloratadine	Few to none	Little to none
Diphenhydramine	Strong	Extreme
Loratadine	Few to none	Little to none
Prescription‡		
Azatadine	Moderate	Moderate
Azelastine	Few to none	Some
Cyproheptadine	Moderate	Some
Dexchlorpheniramine	Moderate	Some
Fexofenadine	Few to none	Little to none
Hydroxyzine	Moderate	Extreme
Levocetirizine	Few to none	Little to none
Promethazine	Strong	Extreme

*Anticholinergic effects include dry mouth, blurred vision, constipation, difficulty with urination, confusion, and light-headedness (particularly after a person stands up). Older people are particularly susceptible to these effects.

†The degree of drowsiness varies, depending on the dose, other active ingredients in the formulation (as in decongestants), and the person.

‡Some formerly prescription-only antihistamines are now also available over the counter.

Not everyone reacts the same way to antihistamines. For example, Asians seem to be less susceptible to the sedative effects of diphenhydramine than are people of Western European origin. Also, antihistamines cause the opposite (paradoxical) reaction in some people, making them feel nervous, restless, and agitated.

Mast Cell Stabilizers: Mast cell stabilizers inhibit mast cells from releasing histamines and other substances that cause swelling and inflammation. These drugs include cromolyn and nedocromil. They are taken when antihistamines and other drugs are not effective or have bothersome side effects. These drugs may help control allergic symptoms.

Cromolyn is available by prescription for use with an inhaler or nebulizer (which delivers the drug in aerosol form to the lungs), as eye drops, or in forms to be taken by mouth. It is available without a prescription as a nasal spray. Cromolyn usually affects only the areas where it is applied, such as the back of the throat, lungs, eyes, or nose. When taken by mouth, cromolyn is not absorbed into the bloodstream, but it can relieve the digestive symptoms of mastocytosis (see page 1120).

Nedocromil is available by prescription as eye drops.

Corticosteroids: When antihistamines and mast cell stabilizers cannot control allergy symptoms, a corticosteroid may help. Corticosteroids can be taken as a nasal spray to treat nasal symptoms or through an inhaler, usually to treat asthma. Doctors prescribe a corticosteroid (such as prednisone) to be taken by mouth only when symptoms are very severe or widespread and all other treatments are ineffective. If taken by mouth for more than 3 to 4 weeks, corticosteroids have many, sometimes serious side effects (see box on page 568). Therefore, corticosteroids taken by mouth are used for as short a time as possible.

Creams and ointments that contain corticosteroids can help relieve the itching associated with allergic skin rashes. One corticosteroid, hydrocortisone, is available over the counter.

Other Drugs: Leukotriene modifiers, such as montelukast, are anti-inflammatory drugs used to treat mild persistent asthma and seasonal allergic rhinitis. They inhibit leukotrienes, which contribute to inflammation and cause airways to constrict.

Omalizumab is a monoclonal antibody (which is a manufactured [synthetic] antibody designed to interact with a specific substance). Omalizumab binds to IgE, an antibody that is produced in large amounts during an allergic reaction, and prevents the IgE from binding to mast cells and basophils and triggering an allergic reaction. Omalizumab may be used to treat allergic rhinitis or persistent or severe asthma when other treatments are ineffective. When it is used, the dose of a corticosteroid can be reduced. It is given by injection under the skin (subcutaneously).

Emergency Treatment: Severe allergic reactions, such as an anaphylactic reaction, require prompt emergency treatment. People who have severe allergic reactions should always carry a self-injecting syringe of epinephrine. Many of these people also carry antihistamine tablets. If a severe reaction occurs, these treatments should be used as quickly as possible. Usually, the combination of epinephrine and an antihistamine stops the reaction. Nonetheless, people who have had a severe allergic reaction should go to the hospital emergency department, where they can be closely monitored and treatment can be repeated or adjusted as needed.

Seasonal Allergies

Seasonal allergies result from exposure to airborne substances (such as pollens) that appear only during certain times of the year.

- Seasonal allergies cause itchy skin, a runny nose, watery and bloodshot eyes, and sneezing.
- Symptoms and their seasonal appearance usually suggest the diagnosis, and skin tests can help identify the allergy trigger.
- Antihistamines, decongestants, and corticosteroid nasal sprays help relieve symptoms.

Seasonal allergies (commonly called hay fever) are common. They occur only during certain times of the year—particularly the spring, summer, or fall—depending on what a person is allergic to. Symptoms involve primarily the membrane lining the nose, causing allergic rhinitis, or the membrane lining the eyelids and covering the whites of the eyes (conjunctiva), causing allergic conjunctivitis (see page 1440).

The term hay fever is somewhat misleading because symptoms do not occur only in the summer when hay is traditionally gathered and never include fever. Hay fever is usually a reaction to pollens and grasses. The pollens that cause hay fever vary by season:

- Spring: Usually trees (such as oak, elm, maple, alder, birch, juniper, and olive)
- Summer: Grasses (such as Bermuda, timothy, sweet vernal, orchard, and Johnson grass) and weeds (such as Russian thistle and English plantain)
- Fall: Ragweed

Also, different parts of the country have very different pollen seasons. In the western United States, mountain cedar (a juniper) is one of the main sources of tree pollen from December to March. In the arid Southwest, grasses pollinate for much longer, and in the fall, pollen from weeds, such as sagebrush and Russian thistle, can cause hay fever. People may react to one or more pollens, so their pollen allergy season may be from early spring to late fall. Seasonal allergy is also caused by mold spores, which can be airborne for long periods of time during the spring, summer, and fall.

Allergic conjunctivitis may result when airborne substances, such as pollens, contact the eyes directly.

Symptoms

Hay fever can make the nose, roof of the mouth, back of the throat, and eyes itch. Itching may start gradually or abruptly. The nose runs, producing a clear watery discharge, and may become stuffed up. In children, the stuffy nose may lead to an ear infection. The lining of the nose may become swollen and bluish red.

The sinuses may also become stuffed up, causing headaches. Sneezing is common.

The eyes may water, sometimes profusely, and itch. The whites of the eyes may become red, and the eyelids may become red and swollen. Wearing contact lenses can irritate the eyes further.

Other symptoms include coughing, wheezing, and irritability. A few people become depressed, lose their appetite, and have problems sleeping.

The severity of symptoms varies with the seasons. Many people who have allergic rhinitis also have asthma (which results in wheezing), possibly caused by the same allergens that contribute to allergic rhinitis and conjunctivitis.

Diagnosis

The diagnosis is based on symptoms plus the circumstances in which they occur—that is, whether they occur only during certain seasons. This information can also help doctors identify the allergen.

The nasal discharge may be examined to see whether it contains eosinophils (a type of white blood cell produced in large numbers during an allergic reaction). Skin tests can help confirm the diagnosis and identify the allergen (see page 1113).

Treatment

Nasal Symptoms: Antihistamines are usually used first (see page 1114). Sometimes a decongestant, such as pseudoephedrine, is taken by mouth with the antihistamine to help relieve a stuffy nose. Many antihistamine-decongestant combinations are available as a single tablet. However, people with high blood pressure should not take a decongestant unless a doctor recommends it and monitors its use. Nonprescription decongestant nose drops or sprays should not be used for more than a few days at a time because using them continually for a week or more may worsen or prolong nasal congestion. This reaction is called a rebound effect, which may eventually result in chronic congestion. Antihistamines may also have other side effects, particularly anticholinergic effects. They include sleepiness, dry mouth, blurred vision, constipation, difficulty with urination, confusion, and light-headedness.

A corticosteroid nasal spray is also effective. This spray may be prescribed instead of or in addition to antihistamines. Most of these sprays have few side effects, although they can cause nosebleeds and a sore nose.

Other drugs are sometimes useful. Cromolyn is available by prescription as a nasal spray and may help relieve a runny nose. To be effective, it must be used regularly. Azelastine (an antihistamine) and ipratropium, both available by prescription as nasal sprays, may be effective. But these drugs can have anticholinergic effects similar to those of antihistamines taken by mouth, especially drowsiness.

Montelukast, a leukotriene modifier, reduces inflammation and helps relieve a runny nose. But how it is best used has not been established. Omalizumab may be used when other treatments are ineffective. This drug binds to immunoglobulin E (IgE), an antibody produced in large amounts during an allergic reaction. Both montelukast and omalizumab are available by prescription.

Regularly flushing out the sinuses with a warm water and salt (saline) solution may help loosen and wash out mucus and hydrates the nasal lining. This technique is called sinus irrigation.

When these treatments are ineffective, a corticosteroid may be taken by mouth or by injection for a short time (usually for fewer than 10 days). If taken by mouth or injection for a long time, corticosteroids can have serious side effects.

Eye Symptoms: Bathing the eyes with plain eyewashes (such as artificial tears) can help reduce irritation. Any substance that may be causing the allergic reaction should be avoided. Contact lenses should not be worn during episodes of conjunctivitis.

Eye drops containing antihistamines and a drug that causes blood vessels to narrow (a vasoconstrictor) are often effective. These eye drops are available without a prescription. However, they may be less effective and have more side effects than prescription eye drops (see page 1440). Eye drops containing cromolyn, available by prescription, are used to prevent rather than relieve allergic conjunctivitis. They can be used when exposure to the allergen is anticipated. If symptoms are very severe, eye drops containing corticosteroids, available by prescription, may be used. During treatment with corticosteroid eye drops, the eyes should be checked regularly for increased pressure and infection by an ophthalmologist.

Allergen Immunotherapy: If other treatments are ineffective, allergen immunotherapy helps some people (see page 1114). Immunotherapy is needed in the following situations:

- When symptoms are severe
- When the allergen cannot be avoided
- When the drugs usually used to treat allergic rhinitis or conjunctivitis cannot control symptoms
- If asthma develops

Allergen immunotherapy for hay fever should be started after the pollen season to prepare for the next season. Immunotherapy has more side effects when started during pollen season because the allergens have stimulated the immune system. Immunotherapy is most effective when continued year-round.

Year-Round Allergies

Year-round (perennial) allergies result from exposure to airborne substances (such as house dust) that are present throughout the year.

- The nose is congested, itchy, and sometimes runny, and the mouth and throat are itchy.
- The symptoms and activities that trigger the allergy usually suggest the diagnosis.
- Avoiding the allergen is best, but drugs, such as antihistamines, can help relieve symptoms.

Perennial allergies may occur at any time of year—unrelated to the season—or may last year-round. Perennial allergies are often a reaction to house dust. House dust may contain mold and fungal spores, fibers of fabric, animal dander, dust mites, and bits of insects. Substances in and on cockroaches are often the cause of allergic symptoms. These substances are present in houses year-round but may cause more severe symptoms during the cold months when more time is spent indoors.

Usually, perennial allergies cause nasal symptoms (allergic rhinitis) but not eye symptoms (allergic conjunctivitis). However, allergic conjunctivitis can result when certain substances are purposely or inadvertently placed in the eyes. These substances include drugs used to treat eye disorders, cosmetics such as eyeliner and face powder, and hair dye. The cleaning solutions for contact lenses can cause a chemical allergic reaction.

Did You Know...
Cockroaches are often to blame for allergies.

Symptoms and Diagnosis

The most obvious symptom is a chronically stuffy nose. The nose runs, producing a clear watery discharge. The nose, roof of the mouth, and back of the throat may itch. Itching may start gradually or abruptly. Sneezing is common.

The eustachian tube, which connects the middle ear and the back of the nose, may become swollen. As a result, hearing can be impaired, especially in children. Children may also develop chronic ear infections. Some people have recurring sinus infections (chronic sinusitis) and growths inside the nose (nasal polyps). When affected, the eyes may become red and itch. The whites of the eyes may become red, and the eyelids may become red and swollen.

Many people who have a perennial allergy also have asthma, possibly caused by the same allergens that contribute to the allergic rhinitis and allergic conjunctivitis.

Diagnosis is based on symptoms plus the circumstances in which they occur—that is, in response to certain activities, such as petting a cat.

Prevention

Avoiding the allergen, if possible, is recommended, thus preventing the development of symptoms.

If people are allergic to house dust, some changes in the environment can prevent or lessen symptoms:

- Removing items that collect dust, such as knick-knacks, magazines, and books
- Replacing upholstered furniture or vacuuming it frequently
- Replacing draperies and shades with blinds
- Removing carpets or replacing them with throw rugs
- Covering mattresses and pillows with finely woven fabrics that cannot be penetrated by dust mites and allergen particles

- Using synthetic-fiber pillows
- Frequently dusting and wet-mopping rooms
- Using air conditioners and dehumidifiers to reduce the high indoor humidity that encourages the breeding of dust mites
- Installing high-efficiency air filters

If a person is allergic to animal dander, the family pet may be limited to certain rooms of the house or, if possible, kept out of the house. Washing the pet weekly can also help.

Treatment

Drug treatment is similar to that for seasonal allergies. It includes antihistamines, nasal decongestants, and corticosteroid nasal sprays.

For people with chronic sinusitis and nasal polyps, surgery is sometimes needed to improve sinus drainage and remove infected material or to remove the polyps. Before and after surgery, regularly flushing out the sinuses with a warm water and salt (saline) solution may be helpful. This technique is called sinus irrigation.

Food Allergy

A food allergy is an allergic reaction to a particular food.

- Food allergies are commonly triggered by certain nuts, peanuts, shellfish, fish, milk, eggs, wheat, and soybeans.
- Symptoms vary by age and may include rashes, wheezing, a runny nose, and, occasionally in adults, more serious symptoms.
- Skin prick tests, blood tests, and an elimination diet help doctors identify the food triggering the allergy.
- The only effective treatment is to eliminate the food from the diet.

Many different foods can cause allergic reactions. Allergic reactions to foods may be severe and sometimes include an anaphylactic reaction (see page 1123).

Food allergies may start during infancy. They are most common among children whose parents have food allergies, allergic rhinitis, or allergic asthma. Infants and young children with food allergies tend to be allergic to the most common allergic triggers (allergens), such as those in eggs, milk, wheat, peanuts, and soybeans. To prevent such allergies from developing, many parents avoid exposing their young children to these foods. However, new evidence calls this approach into question, and more study is needed. Older children and adults tend to be allergic to nuts and seafood. Children may outgrow a food allergy. Thus, food allergies are less common among adults. However, if adults have food allergies, the allergies tend to persist throughout life.

Food allergies are sometimes blamed for such disorders as hyperactivity in children, chronic fatigue, arthritis, poor athletic performance, and depression. However, these associations have not been substantiated.

Some reactions to food are not an allergic reaction. For example, food intolerance differs from a food allergy because it does not involve the immune system. Instead, it involves a reaction in the digestive tract that results in digestive upset. For example, some people lack an enzyme necessary for digesting the sugar in milk (lactose—see page 165). Other reactions to a food may result from contamination or deterioration of the food.

In some people, food additives can cause a reaction that resembles but is not an allergic reaction. For example, monosodium glutamate (MSG—see box on page 153), some preservatives (such as metabisulfite), and dyes (such as tartrazine, a yellow dye used in candies, soft drinks, and other foods) can cause symptoms such as asthma and hives. Similarly, eating certain foods, such as cheese, wine, and chocolate, triggers migraine headaches in some people.

Symptoms

In infants, the first symptom of a food allergy may be a rash such as eczema (atopic dermatitis) or a rash that resembles hives. The rash may be accompanied by nausea, vomiting, and diarrhea. By about age 1 year, the rash tends to develop less often, but children may wheeze, feel short of breath, or get a runny nose when they eat the food that triggers their allergy. By about age 10, food allergies—most commonly to milk and less commonly to eggs and peanuts—tend to subside. Allergies to airborne substances, such as allergic asthma and hay fever, may develop as food allergies subside.

In adults, food allergies cause itching in the mouth, hives, eczema, and, occasionally, a runny nose and asthma. For some adults with a food allergy, eating a tiny amount of the food may trigger a severe reaction. A rash may cover the entire body, the throat may swell, and the airways may narrow, making breathing difficult. Occasionally, this reaction is severe and becomes life threatening—an anaphylactic reaction.

For some people, allergic reactions to food (especially wheat or celery) occur only if they exercise immediately after eating the food. In a few people, eating certain foods triggers or worsens a migraine headache.

Diagnosis

Doctors suspect a food allergy based primarily on the person's history. If a food allergy is suspected, skin prick tests with extracts from various foods may be done. A drop of each extract is placed on the person's skin, which is then pricked with a needle. A skin reaction to a food tested does not necessarily mean that a person is allergic to that food, but no skin reaction means that an allergy to that food is unlikely. Alternatively, a radioallergosorbent test (RAST) may be done. A sample of blood is withdrawn, and doctors measure how much immunoglobulin E (IgE), a type of antibody, binds to various allergens. If the level of IgE against any of these allergens is abnormally high, that allergen is probably triggering the allergy.

If either test identifies a particular food, an oral challenge test may be done to confirm the diagnosis. In this test, the person is given another food, such as milk or applesauce, in two batches: one with the suspected food in it and one without the suspected food in it. Then the doctor observes as the person eats the food:

- If no symptoms develop after the suspected food is eaten, the person is not allergic to the food.
- If symptoms develop after the suspected food is eaten and not after the other food is eaten, the person is probably allergic to the suspected food.

Another way to identify the food allergy is an elimination diet. The person stops eating all foods that may be causing the symptoms for about 1 week. The doctor provides the diet the person is to follow. Only the foods or fluids specified in the diet may be eaten, and only pure products should be used. Following such a diet is not easy because many food products have ingredients that are not obvious or expected. For example, many rye breads contain some wheat flour. Eating in restaurants is not advisable because the person and the doctor need to know the ingredients of every meal eaten. If no symptoms occur, foods are added back one at a time. Each added food is given for several days or until symptoms appear, and thus the allergen is identified. Or the doctor may ask the person to eat a small amount of a food in the office. The doctor then observes the person's reaction to the food.

> **? Did You Know...**
> People with severe food allergies should always carry antihistamines and an epinephrine syringe in case they have a severe reaction.

Treatment

People with food allergies must eliminate the foods that trigger their allergies from their diet.

Desensitization by first eliminating the food, then eating small amounts of the food or placing drops of food extracts under the tongue is not effective.

Antihistamines are useful only for relieving hives and swelling. Cromolyn, taken by mouth, can also relieve symptoms. This form of cromolyn is available only by prescription.

People with severe food allergies often carry antihistamines to take immediately if a reaction starts. They should also carry a self-injecting syringe of epinephrine to use when needed for severe reactions.

Mastocytosis

Mastocytosis is an uncommon abnormal accumulation of mast cells in the skin and sometimes in various other parts of the body.

- People may have itchy spots and bumps, flushing, digestive upset, and sometimes bone pain.
- Symptoms suggest the diagnosis, and a biopsy of the skin or bone marrow can confirm it.
- If mastocytosis affects only the skin, it may resolve without treatment, but if it affects other parts of the body, it cannot be cured.
- Antihistamines help relieve itching, and histamine-2 (H_2) blockers help relieve digestive upset.

Mastocytosis is rare. It differs from typical allergic reactions because it is chronic rather than episodic. Mastocytosis develops when mast cells increase in number and accumulate in tissues over a period of years. Mast cells, a component of the immune system, produce histamine, a substance involved in allergic reactions and the production of stomach acid. Because the number of mast cells increases, levels of histamine increase. What causes the disorder is unclear.

Mastocytosis may affect primarily the skin (called cutaneous mastocytosis) or other parts of the body (called systemic mastocytosis).

- **Cutaneous mastocytosis:** This form usually occurs in children. Occasionally, mast cells accumulate only as a single mass in the skin (mastocytoma), typically before age 6 months. More commonly, mast cells congregate in many areas of the skin, forming small reddish brown spots or bumps (called urticaria pigmentosa). Urticaria pigmentosa only rarely progresses to systemic mastocytosis in children but may do so more often in adults.
- **Systemic mastocytosis:** This form usually occurs in adults. Mast cells accumulate in the skin, stomach, intestine, liver, spleen, lymph nodes, and bone marrow (where blood cells are produced). Organs may continue to function, with little disruption. But if many mast cells accumulate in the bone marrow, too few blood cells are produced, and serious blood disorders, such as leukemia, can

---

Anaphylactoid Versus Anaphylactic

Anaphylactoid reactions resemble anaphylactic reactions. However, anaphylactoid reactions, unlike anaphylactic reactions, may occur after the first exposure to a substance. For example, anaphylactoid reactions may occur after the first injection of certain drugs, such as polymyxin, pentamidine, opioids, or the radiopaque dyes sometimes used with x-ray procedures. Also, anaphylactoid reactions are not allergic reactions because immunoglobulin E (IgE), the class of antibodies involved in allergic reactions, does not cause them. Rather, the reaction is caused directly by the substance.

Aspirin and other nonsteroidal anti-inflammatory drugs (NSAIDs) can cause anaphylactoid reactions in some people, particularly those with year-round allergic rhinitis and nasal polyps. Dyes that can be seen on x-ray (radiopaque dyes) are a common cause. Other triggers include blood transfusions and exercise.

If possible, doctors avoid using radiopaque dyes in people who have anaphylactoid reactions to such dyes. However, some disorders cannot be diagnosed without dyes. In such cases, doctors use dyes that are less likely to cause reactions. In addition, drugs that block anaphylactoid reactions, such as prednisone, diphenhydramine, or ephedrine, are usually given before the dye is injected.

---

develop. If many mast cells accumulate in organs, the organs malfunction. The resulting problems can be life threatening.

Symptoms

A single mastocytoma does not cause symptoms. Spots and bumps may itch, particularly if they are rubbed or scratched. Itching may be worsened by changes in temperature, contact with clothing or other materials, or use of some drugs (including nonsteroidal anti-inflammatory drugs). Consuming hot beverages, spicy foods, or alcohol or exercising may also make itching worse. Rubbing or scratching the spots may result in hives and make the skin turn red.

Flushing is common. Peptic ulcers may develop because too much histamine is produced, stimulating secretion of excess stomach acid. Ulcers can cause stomach pain. Nausea, vomiting, and chronic diarrhea may also occur. The abdomen may enlarge if the liver and spleen malfunction, causing fluid to accumulate. If bone marrow is affected, bone pain can result.

Widespread reactions, including anaphylactic reactions, may occur. With systemic mastocytosis, the widespread reactions tend to be severe. They include anaphylactoid reactions, which cause fainting and a life-threatening drop in blood pressure (shock). Anaphylactoid reactions resemble anaphylactic reactions, but no allergen triggers them.

Systemic mastocytosis may affect the bone marrow, and up to 30% of adults with systemic mastocytosis develop cancers, particularly myelocytic leukemias. In these people, life expectancy may be shortened.

Diagnosis

Doctors suspect the diagnosis based on symptoms, particularly spots that, when scratched, result in hives and redness. A biopsy can confirm the diagnosis. Usually, a sample of skin tissue is removed and examined under a microscope for mast cells. Sometimes a sample is taken from the bone marrow. Blood tests to measure levels of chemical substances related to mast cells are done. High levels support the diagnosis of systemic mastocytosis.

Treatment

A mastocytoma usually disappears spontaneously. Itching may be treated with antihistamines. For children, no other treatment is needed. If adults have itching and rashes, ultraviolet light and corticosteroid creams may be applied to the skin.

Systemic mastocytosis cannot be cured, but symptoms can be controlled with antihistamines and histamine-2 (H_2) blockers, which reduce acid production in the stomach (see table on page 143). Cromolyn given by mouth can relieve digestive problems and bone pain. Aspirin can relieve flushing but may make other symptoms worse. Children are not given aspirin because Reye's syndrome is a risk.

If systemic mastocytosis is aggressive, interferon-alpha, injected under the skin once a week, may reduce the disorder's effects on bone marrow. Corticosteroids (such as prednisone), taken by mouth, may also be used but only for a short time. When taken by mouth for more than 3 to 4 weeks, they can have many, sometimes serious side effects.

If many mast cells accumulate in the spleen, the spleen may be removed. If leukemia develops, chemotherapy drugs (such as daunomycin, etoposide, and mercaptopurine) may help.

A self-injecting syringe of epinephrine should always be carried for prompt emergency treatment of anaphylactic reactions.

Physical Allergy

A physical allergy is an allergic reaction triggered by a physical stimulus.

A physical allergy differs from other allergic reactions because the trigger is a physical stimulus. Physical stimuli include the following:

- Cold
- Sunlight
- Heat or other stimuli that cause sweating (such as emotional stress or exercise)
- Vibration
- Minor injuries (such as those due to scratching)
- Physical pressure

For some people, symptoms occur only in response to a physical stimulus. For some people who have other allergies, a physical stimulus makes symptoms worse.

What causes this type of allergic reaction is not understood. One theory suggests that the physical stimulus changes a protein in the skin. The immune system mistakes this protein for a foreign substance and attacks it. Sensitivity to sunlight (photosensitivity) is an example. Ultraviolet light changes proteins in the skin, which the body then identifies as foreign and attacks. Photosensitivity is sometimes triggered by the use of drugs (such as antibiotics), some cosmetics (such as skin creams, lotions, and oils), or other substances.

A few people who are sensitive to cold have abnormal proteins (called cryoglobulins or cryofibrinogen) in the blood. Sometimes the presence of these proteins indicates a serious disorder such as cancer, a connective tissue disorder, or chronic infection.

Symptoms

Itching, skin blotches, hives, and swelling of tissues under the skin (angioedema) are the most common symptoms. The symptoms tend to develop within minutes of exposure to the physical stimulus.

When people who are sensitive to heat are exposed to heat or engage in any activity that causes sweating, they may develop small, intensely itchy hives that are surrounded by a ring of redness—a condition called cholinergic urticaria.

When people who are sensitive to cold are exposed to cold, they may develop hives, asthma, a runny nose, nasal stuffiness, or angioedema. Rarely, a widespread anaphylactic reaction occurs.

Diagnosis and Treatment

The diagnosis is based on symptoms and the circumstances in which they occur. To diagnose reactions caused by cold, doctors place an ice cube on the skin for 4 minutes, remove the ice cube, then watch for the development of a hive. People may be advised not to use cosmetics and skin creams, lotions, and oils for a while to help determine whether one of these substances may be worsening the allergy.

The best treatment is to avoid the stimulus that causes the physical allergy. For example, people who are very sensitive to sunlight should use a sunscreen and avoid exposure to the sun as much as possible.

An antihistamine can usually relieve itching. The most effective treatments are cyproheptadine for hives caused by cold and hydroxyzine for hives caused by heat or emotional stress.

Exercise-Induced Allergic Reactions

Exercise-induced allergic reactions occur during or after exercise.

Exercise can trigger the following:

- **Asthma:** Exercise often triggers an asthma attack in people who have asthma, but some people have asthma only when they exercise. Exercise may trigger or worsen asthma because breathing fast cools and dries the airways, and as the airways warm again, they narrow. Exercise-induced asthma is more likely to occur when the air is cold and dry. The chest feels tight. People may wheeze, cough, and have difficulty breathing.

- **Anaphylactic reactions:** Rarely, vigorous exercise triggers a widespread, potentially severe allergic (anaphylactic) reaction. In some people, this reaction occurs only if they eat a specific food before exercising. Breathing becomes difficult or blood pressure falls, leading to dizziness and collapse. An anaphylactic reaction can be life threatening.

Typically, symptoms triggered by exercise—asthma or an anaphylactic reaction—occur after 5 to 10 minutes of vigorous exercise. Often, symptoms begin after exercise has stopped.

Diagnosis

The diagnosis is based on the symptoms and their relationship to exercise. An exercise challenge test can also help doctors make the diagnosis. For this test, lung function is measured before and after exercise on a treadmill or stationary bicycle (see page 475).

Treatment

For people with exercise-induced asthma, the goal of treatment is to be able to exercise without symptoms. Becoming more physically fit may make symptoms less likely to develop during exercise. Inhaling a beta-adrenergic drug (such as those used to treat asthma—see table on page 479) about 15 minutes before starting to exercise often helps prevent reactions. Cromolyn, usually taken through an inhaler, may be helpful.

For people with asthma, taking the drugs usually used to control asthma often prevents symptoms from developing during exercise. For some people with asthma, taking drugs to treat asthma and gradually increasing the intensity and duration of exercise enables them to tolerate exercise.

People who have had an exercise-induced anaphylactic reaction should avoid the form of exercise that triggered the attack. If eating a specific food before exercise triggers symptoms, they should not eat the food before exercise. A self-injecting syringe of epinephrine should always be carried for prompt emergency treatment. Exercising with other people is recommended.

Hives and Angioedema

Hives, also called urticaria, is a skin reaction characterized by pale, slightly elevated swellings (wheals) that are surrounded by a red area and have clearly defined borders. Angioedema is swelling of larger areas of tissue under the skin, sometimes affecting the face and throat.

- Common triggers include insect bites or stings and foods such as eggs, shellfish, peanuts, and nuts.
- Hives may itch, and angioedema may involve swelling in the face, throat, and airways.
- Seeing a doctor is particularly important when insect bites or stings trigger a reaction.
- Antihistamines can relieve mild symptoms, but if angioedema makes swallowing or breathing difficult, prompt emergency treatment is needed.

Hives and angioedema, which may occur together, can be severe. Common triggers are drugs, insect stings or bites, allergy injections (allergen immunotherapy), and certain foods—particularly eggs, fish, shellfish, nuts, and fruits. Eating even a tiny amount of some foods can suddenly result in hives or angioedema. But with other foods (such as strawberries), these reactions occur only after a large amount is eaten. Also, hives sometimes follow viral infections such as hepatitis, infectious mononucleosis, and German measles.

Hives or angioedema can be chronic, recurring over weeks or months. In most cases, no specific cause is identified. The cause may be habitual, unintentional intake of a substance, such as penicillin in milk or a preservative or dye in foods. Hives often occur in people with an autoimmune thyroid disorder. Use of certain drugs, such as aspirin or other nonsteroidal anti-inflammatory drugs (NSAIDs—see page 644), can also cause chronic hives or angioedema. Chronic angioedema that occurs without hives may be hereditary angioedema.

Symptoms

Hives usually begin with itching. Then wheals quickly develop. The wheals usually remain small (less than ½ inch [about 1.3 centimeters] across). Wheals that are larger (up to 4 inches [about 10.2 centimeters] across) may look like rings of redness with a pale center. Typically, crops of hives come and go. One spot may remain for several hours, then disappear, and later, another may appear elsewhere. After the hive disappears, the skin usually looks completely normal.

Angioedema may affect part or all of the hands, feet, eyelids, tongue, lips, or genitals. Sometimes the membranes lining the mouth, throat, and airways swell, making breathing difficult.

Diagnosis

The cause is often obvious, and tests are seldom needed because the reactions usually resolve and do not recur. In children, when hives appear suddenly, disappear quickly, and do not recur, an examination by a doctor is usually unnecessary because the cause is usually a viral infection.

If the cause is a bee sting, people should see a doctor. Then they can obtain advice about treatment if another bee sting occurs. When angioedema or hives recur without an obvious cause, an examination by a doctor is recommended.

Treatment

Usually, if hives appear suddenly, they subside without any treatment within days and sometimes within minutes. If the cause is obvious, people should avoid it if possible. If the cause is not obvious, people should stop taking all nonessential drugs until the hives subside.

For hives and mild angioedema, taking antihistamines partially relieves the itching and reduces the swelling. Corticosteroids, taken by mouth, are prescribed only for severe symptoms when all other treatments are ineffective, and they are given for as short a time as possible. When taken by mouth for more than 3 to 4 weeks, they have many, sometimes serious side effects (see box on page 568). Corticosteroid creams do not help.

In about half of the people with chronic hives, the hives disappear without treatment within 2 years. For some adults, the antidepressant doxepin, which is also a potent antihistamine, helps relieve chronic hives.

If severe angioedema results in difficulty swallowing or breathing or in collapse, prompt emergency treatment is necessary. People who have these reactions should always carry a self-injecting syringe of epinephrine and antihistamine tablets to be used immediately if a reaction occurs. After a severe allergic reaction, such people should go to the hospital emergency department, where they can be checked and treated as needed.

Hereditary Angioedema: Not an Allergy

Hereditary angioedema looks much like the angioedema of an allergic reaction. However, the cause is different. Hereditary angioedema is a genetic disorder due to a deficiency or malfunction of C1 inhibitor. C1 inhibitor is part of the complement system, which is part of the immune system. In this disorder, an injury, a viral infection, or stress (such as that due to anticipating a dental or surgical procedure) may trigger attacks of swelling (angioedema).

Areas of the skin and tissue under the skin may swell, as may the membranes lining the mouth, throat, windpipe, and digestive tract. Typically, the swollen areas are painful, not itchy. Hives do not appear. Nausea, vomiting, and cramps are common. Swelling in the windpipe can interfere with breathing.

Diagnosis and Treatment

Doctors diagnose the disorder by measuring C1 inhibitor levels or activity in a sample of blood.

The drug aminocaproic acid can sometimes relieve the swelling. Epinephrine, antihistamines, and corticosteroids are often given, although there is no proof that these drugs are effective. If a sudden attack interferes with breathing, the airway must be opened—for example, by inserting a breathing tube in the windpipe.

Certain treatments may help prevent subsequent attacks. For example, before a dental or surgical procedure, people with hereditary angioedema may be given a transfusion of fresh plasma to increase levels of C1 inhibitor in the blood. However, there are concerns that this treatment could trigger an attack.

For long-term prevention, anabolic steroids (androgens) taken by mouth, such as stanozolol or danazol, can stimulate the body to produce more C1 inhibitor. Because these drugs can have masculinizing side effects, the dose is reduced as soon and as much as possible when these drugs are given to women.

Anaphylactic Reactions

Anaphylactic reactions (anaphylaxis) are sudden, widespread, potentially severe and life-threatening allergic reactions.

- These reactions begin with a feeling of uneasiness, followed by tingling sensations and dizziness.
- People then rapidly develop severe symptoms, including generalized itching and hives, wheezing and difficulty breathing, fainting, or a combination of these and other allergy symptoms.
- These reactions can quickly become life threatening.
- Avoiding the trigger is the best approach.
- Affected people should always carry antihistamines and a self-injecting syringe of epinephrine.
- Anaphylactic reactions require emergency treatment.

Anaphylactic reactions are most commonly caused by the following:

- Drugs (such as penicillin)
- Insect stings
- Certain foods (particularly eggs, seafood, and nuts)
- Allergy injections (allergen immunotherapy)
- Latex

But they can be caused by any allergen. Like other allergic reactions, an anaphylactic reaction does not usually occur after the first exposure to an allergen but may occur after a subsequent exposure. However, many people do not recall a first exposure. Any allergen that causes an anaphylactic reaction in a person is likely to cause that reaction with subsequent exposures, unless measures are taken to prevent it.

Symptoms and Diagnosis

Anaphylactic reactions begin within 1 to 15 minutes of exposure to the allergen. Rarely, reactions begin after 1 hour. Symptoms vary, but people usually have the same symptoms each time.

The heart beats quickly. People may feel uneasy and become agitated. Blood pressure may fall, causing fainting. Other symptoms include tingling (pins-and-needles) sensations, dizziness, itchy and flushed skin, throbbing in the ears, coughing, a runny nose, sneezing, hives, and swelling of tissue under the skin (angioedema). Breathing may become difficult and wheezing may occur because the windpipe (upper airway) constricts or becomes swollen. People may have nausea, vomiting, abdominal cramps, and diarrhea.

An anaphylactic reaction may progress so rapidly that it leads to collapse, cessation of breathing, seizures, and loss of consciousness within 1 to 2 minutes.

The reaction may be fatal unless emergency treatment is given immediately.

The diagnosis is based on symptoms. Because symptoms can quickly become life threatening, no tests are done.

Prevention and Treatment

Avoiding the allergen is the best prevention. People who are allergic to certain unavoidable allergens (such as insect stings) may benefit from long-term allergen immunotherapy (see page 1114).

People who have these reactions should always carry a self-injecting syringe of epinephrine and antihistamine tablets for prompt treatment. If they encounter a trigger (for example, if they are stung by an insect) or if they start to develop symptoms, they should immediately inject themselves and take the antihistamines. Usually, this treatment stops the reaction. Nonetheless, after a severe allergic reaction and immediately after injecting themselves, such people should go to the hospital emergency department, where they can be closely monitored and treatment can be adjusted as needed. People should also wear a Medic Alert bracelet with their allergies listed.

In emergencies, doctors give epinephrine by injection under the skin, into a muscle, or into a vein. If breathing is severely impaired, a breathing tube may be inserted into the windpipe (trachea) through the person's mouth or nose (intubation) or through a small incision in the skin over the trachea. If blood pressure is very low, fluids are given intravenously, sometimes with drugs that cause blood vessels to narrow (vasoconstrictors). Antihistamines (such as diphenhydramine) and histamine-2 (H_2) blockers (such as cimetidine) are given intravenously until symptoms disappear. Beta-agonists that are inhaled (such as albuterol) are given to widen the airways and help with breathing.

CHAPTER

170 Autoimmune Disorders

An autoimmune disorder is a malfunction of the body's immune system that causes the body to attack its own tissues.

- Autoimmune disorders can be triggered in many ways.
- Symptoms vary depending on which disorder develops and which part of the body is affected.
- Several blood tests are usually needed to confirm the presence of an autoimmune disorder.

- Autoimmune disorders are treated with drugs that suppress the activity of the immune system.

The immune system defends the body against what it perceives to be foreign or dangerous substances (see page 1096). Such substances include microorganisms, parasites (such as worms), cancer cells, and even transplanted organs and tissues. Substances that can stimulate an immune response are called antigens. Antigens are molecules that may be contained within cells or on the surface of cells (such as bacteria, viruses, or cancer cells). Some antigens, such as pollen or food molecules, exist on their own.

Even cells in a person's own tissues can have antigens. But, normally, the immune system reacts only to antigens from foreign or dangerous substances, not to antigens from a person's own tissues. However, the immune system sometimes malfunctions, interpreting the body's own tissues as foreign and producing antibodies (called autoantibodies) or immune cells that target and attack particular cells or tissues of the body. This response is called an autoimmune reaction. It results in inflammation and tissue damage. Such effects may constitute an autoimmune disorder, but some people produce such small amounts of autoantibodies that an autoimmune disorder does not occur.

Some of the more common autoimmune disorders include rheumatoid arthritis, systemic lupus erythematosus (lupus), and vasculitis, among others. Additional diseases that are believed to be due to autoimmunity include glomerulonephritis, Addison's disease, mixed connective tissue disease, polymyositis, Sjögren's syndrome, progressive systemic sclerosis, and some cases of infertility.

Causes

Autoimmune reactions can be triggered in several ways:

- A substance in the body that is normally confined to a specific area (and thus is hidden from the immune system) is released into the bloodstream. For example, a blow to the eye can cause the fluid in the eyeball to be released into the bloodstream. The fluid stimulates the immune system to recognize the eye as foreign and attack it.

- A normal body substance is altered, for example, by a virus, a drug, sunlight, or radiation. The altered substance may appear foreign to the immune system. For example, a virus can infect and thus alter cells in the body. The virus-infected cells stimulate the immune system to attack.

- A foreign substance that resembles a natural body substance may enter the body. The immune system may inadvertently target the similar body substance as well as the foreign substance. For example, the bacteria that cause strep throat have some antigens that are similar to those in human heart cells. Rarely, the immune system may attack a person's heart after strep throat (this reaction is part of rheumatic fever).

- The cells that control antibody production—for example, B lymphocytes (a type of white blood cell)—may malfunction and produce abnormal antibodies that attack some of the body's cells.

Heredity may be involved in some autoimmune disorders. Susceptibility to the disorder, rather than the disorder itself, may be inherited. In susceptible people, a trigger, such as a viral infection or tissue damage, may cause the disorder to develop. Hormonal factors may also be involved, because many autoimmune disorders are more common among women.

Symptoms and Diagnosis

Autoimmune disorders may cause a fever. However, symptoms vary depending on the disorder and the part of the body affected. Some autoimmune disorders affect certain types of tissue throughout the body—for example, blood vessels, cartilage, or skin. Other autoimmune disorders affect a particular organ. Virtually any organ, including the kidneys, lungs, heart, and brain, can be affected. The resulting inflammation and tissue damage can cause pain, deformed joints, weakness, jaundice, itching, difficulty breathing, accumulation of fluid (edema), delirium, and even death.

Blood tests that indicate the presence of inflammation may suggest an autoimmune disorder. For example, the erythrocyte sedimentation rate (ESR) is often increased, because proteins that are produced in response to inflammation interfere with the ability of red blood cells (erythrocytes) to remain suspended in blood. Frequently, the number of red blood cells is decreased (anemia) because inflammation decreases their production.

However, inflammation has many causes, many of which are not autoimmune. Thus, doctors often obtain blood tests to detect different antibodies that can occur in people who have particular autoimmune disorders. Examples of these antibodies are antinuclear antibodies, which are typically present in systemic lupus erythematosus, and rheumatoid factor or anti-cyclic citrullinated peptide (anti-CCP) antibodies, which are typically present in rheumatoid arthritis. But even these antibodies may sometimes occur in people who do not have an autoimmune disorder, so doctors usually use a combination of test results and the person's signs and symptoms to decide whether an autoimmune disorder is present.

Treatment

Treatment involves control of the autoimmune reaction by suppressing the immune system. However, many of the drugs used to control the autoimmune reaction also interfere with the body's ability to fight disease, especially infections.

SOME AUTOIMMUNE DISORDERS

DISORDER	MAIN TISSUES AFFECTED	CONSEQUENCES
Autoimmune hemolytic anemia	Red blood cells	Anemia (decreased number of red blood cells) develops, causing fatigue, weakness, and light-headedness. The spleen may enlarge. The anemia can be severe and even fatal.
Bullous pemphigoid	Skin	Large blisters, surrounded by red, swollen areas, form on the skin. Itching is common. With treatment, the prognosis is good.
Goodpasture's syndrome	Lungs and kidneys	Symptoms, such as shortness of breath, coughing up blood, fatigue, swelling, and itching, may develop. The prognosis is good if treatment begins before severe lung or kidney damage occurs.
Graves' disease	Thyroid gland	The thyroid gland is stimulated and enlarged, resulting in high levels of thyroid hormones (hyperthyroidism). Symptoms may include a rapid heart rate, intolerance of heat, tremor, weight loss, and nervousness. With treatment, the prognosis is good.
Hashimoto's thyroiditis	Thyroid gland	The thyroid gland is inflamed and damaged, resulting in low levels of thyroid hormones (hypothyroidism). Symptoms may include weight gain, coarse skin, intolerance to cold, and drowsiness. Lifelong treatment with thyroid hormone is necessary and usually relieves the symptoms completely.
Multiple sclerosis	Brain and spinal cord	The covering of affected nerve cells is damaged. As a result, the cells cannot conduct nerve signals normally. Symptoms may include weakness, abnormal sensations, vertigo, problems with vision, muscle spasms, and incontinence. Symptoms vary over time and may come and go. The prognosis varies.
Myasthenia gravis	The connection between nerves and muscles (neuromuscular junction)	Muscles, particularly those of the eyes, weaken and tire easily, but the weakness varies in intensity. The pattern of progression varies widely. Drugs can usually control the symptoms.
Pemphigus	Skin	Large blisters form on the skin. The disorder can be life threatening.
Pernicious anemia	Certain cells in the stomach's lining	Damage to cells in the stomach's lining makes absorbing vitamin B_{12} difficult. (Vitamin B_{12} is necessary for the production of mature blood cells and the maintenance of nerve cells.) Anemia results, often causing fatigue, weakness, and light-headedness. Nerves can be damaged, resulting in weakness and loss of sensation. Without treatment, the spinal cord may be damaged, eventually contributing to loss of sensation, weakness, and incontinence. The risk of stomach cancer is increased. Otherwise, with treatment, the prognosis is good.
Rheumatoid arthritis	Joints or other tissues, such as lung, nerve, skin, and heart tissue	Many symptoms are possible. They include fever, fatigue, joint pain, joint stiffness, deformed joints, shortness of breath, loss of sensation, weakness, rashes, chest pain, and swellings under the skin. The prognosis varies.

(continued on the following page)

SOME AUTOIMMUNE DISORDERS (*Continued*)

DISORDER	MAIN TISSUES AFFECTED	CONSEQUENCES
Systemic lupus erythematosus (lupus)	Joints, kidneys, skin, lungs, heart, brain, and blood cells	The joints, although inflamed, do not become deformed. Symptoms of anemia, such as fatigue, weakness, and light-headedness, and those of kidney, lung, or heart disorders, such as fatigue, shortness of breath, itching, and chest pain, may occur. A rash may develop. The prognosis varies widely, but most people can lead an active life despite occasional flare-ups of the disorder.
Type 1 diabetes mellitus	Beta cells of the pancreas (which produce insulin)	Symptoms may include excessive thirst, urination, and appetite, as well as various long-term complications. Lifelong treatment with insulin is needed, even if the destruction of pancreatic cells stops, because not enough pancreatic cells remain to produce enough insulin. The prognosis varies greatly and tends to be worse when the disease is severe and lasts a long time.
Vasculitis	Blood vessels	Vasculitis can affect blood vessels in one part of the body (such as the nerves, head, skin, kidneys, lungs, or intestine) or several parts. There are several types. Symptoms (such as rashes, abdominal pain, weight loss, difficulty breathing, cough, chest pain, headache, loss of vision, and symptoms of nerve damage or kidney failure) depend on which part of the body is affected. The prognosis depends on the cause and how much tissue is damaged. Usually, the prognosis is much better with treatment.

❓ Did You Know...

Antigens, substances that can trigger an immune response, can even exist on a person's own cells.

Autoimmune disorders or susceptibility to autoimmune disorders may be inherited.

Virtually any organ can be affected by an autoimmune disorder.

Drugs that suppress the immune system (immunosuppressants), such as azathioprine, chlorambucil, cyclophosphamide, cyclosporine, mycophenolate, and methotrexate, are often given, usually by mouth and often for a long time (see table on page 1130). However, these drugs suppress not only the autoimmune reaction but also the body's ability to defend itself against foreign substances, including microorganisms that cause infection and cancer cells. Consequently, the risk of certain infections and cancers increases.

Often, corticosteroids, such as prednisone, are given, usually by mouth. These drugs relieve inflammation as well as suppress the immune system. Corticosteroids given for a long time have many side effects (see box on page 568). When possible, corticosteroids are used for a short time—when the disorder begins or when symptoms worsen. However, cortico-steroids must sometimes be used indefinitely.

Certain autoimmune disorders (for example, multiple sclerosis and thyroid disorders) are also treated with drugs other than immunosuppressants and corticosteroids. Treatment to relieve symptoms may also be needed.

Etanercept, infliximab, and adalimumab block the action of tumor necrosis factor (TNF), a substance that can cause inflammation in the body. These drugs are very effective in treating rheumatoid arthritis, but they may be harmful if used to treat certain other autoimmune disorders, such as multiple sclerosis. These drugs can also increase the risk of infection and certain cancers.

Certain new drugs specifically target white blood cells. White blood cells help defend the body against infection but also participate in autoimmune reactions. Abatacept blocks the activation of one kind of white blood cell (T cell) and is used in rheumatoid arthritis. Rituximab, first used against certain white blood cell cancers, works by depleting certain white blood cells (B lymphocytes) from the body. It is effective in rheumatoid arthritis and is under evaluation in a variety of autoimmune disorders. Other agents directed against white blood cells are being developed.

Plasmapheresis is used to treat a few autoimmune disorders. Blood is withdrawn and filtered to remove the abnormal antibodies. Then the filtered blood is returned to the person.

Some autoimmune disorders resolve as inexplicably as they began. However, most autoimmune disorders are chronic. Drugs are often required throughout life to control symptoms. The prognosis varies depending on the disorder.

CHAPTER

171 Transplantation

Transplantation is the removal of living, functioning cells, tissues, or organs from the body and then their transfer back into the same body or into a different body.

The most common type of transplantation is a blood transfusion (see page 1026). Blood transfusions are used to treat millions of people each year. More typically, transplantation refers to the transfer of organs (solid organ transplants) or tissues.

Organ transplantation, unlike blood transfusion, involves major surgery, the use of drugs to suppress the immune system (immunosuppressants), and the possibility of transplant rejection and serious complications, including death. However, for people whose vital organs have failed, organ transplantation may offer the only chance of survival.

Donors

A tissue or organ donor can be a living person or a person who has recently died (deceased donor).

Tissues and organs from living donors are preferable because they are usually healthier. Stem cells (from bone marrow or blood) and kidneys are the tissues most often donated by living donors. Usually, a kidney can be safely donated because the body has two kidneys and can function well with only one. Living donors can also donate a part of the liver or a lung. Organs from living donors are usually transplanted within minutes of being removed. In the United States, being paid to donate an organ is illegal, but reimbursement for cells and tissues is allowed.

Some organs, such as the heart, obviously cannot be taken from living donors. Organs from deceased donors usually come from people who previously agreed to donate organs. In many states, people can indicate their willingness to donate organs on their driver's license, although family members are also consulted even when donor status is indicated on the license. Permission for donation also may be obtained from the deceased's closest family member when the deceased's wishes are unknown. Deceased donors can be otherwise healthy people who have been in a major accident, as well as those who died of a medical disorder. Doctors do not take the potential for organ donation into account when deciding whether to recommend withdrawal of life support from people who are terminally ill or who are brain dead (see box on page 708).

One donor can provide several people with transplants. For example, one donor could provide two corneas, a pancreas, two kidneys, two liver segments, two lungs, and a heart. When people die, organs deteriorate quickly. Some organs last only a few hours outside the body. Other organs, if kept cold, can last a few days.

In the United States, a national organization (United Network for Organ Sharing) matches donors and recipients for transplantation through the use of a computer database. The database includes all people who are on a waiting list for a transplant, along with their tissue type. When organs become available, that information is entered and a match is made, allowing transplantation to occur with minimal delay.

> **? Did You Know...**
> Some people with medical disorders can still become organ donors. Doctors evaluate the condition of the organs after a person dies and then decide whether they can be used.

Pretransplantation Screening

Because transplantation is somewhat risky and donor organs are scarce, potential recipients are screened for factors that may affect the likelihood of success.

Tissue Matching: The immune system normally attacks foreign tissue (see page 1096), including transplants. This reaction is called rejection. Rejection is triggered when the immune system recognizes certain molecules on the surface of a cell as foreign. These cell-surface molecules are called antigens.

For blood transfusions, rejection is relatively easily avoided because red blood cells have only three main antigens on their surface. These antigens determine the blood type and are called A, B, and Rh. Doctors test to make sure that antigens in the donor blood and the recipient blood are a complete match.

For organ transplantation, however, many antigens are involved. These antigens are called human leukocyte antigens (HLA) and occur on the surface of every cell in the body. Each person has unique HLA, which determines the tissue type. Ideally, the donor's tissue type exactly matches the recipient's tissue type. However, a perfect HLA match is extremely rare, and some people are too ill to wait for a highly compatible donor. In these cases, doctors sometimes use donor tissue that is not an exact match but that is a close match. A close HLA match between the donor and recipient reduces the frequency and severity of rejection and improves the long-term outcome. With the use of immunosuppressants, the success of transplantation is less affected by the degree of matching.

Before transplantation, the recipient's blood is screened for antibodies against the tissues of the donor. The body may have produced such antibodies in response to a blood transfusion, a previous transplant, or a pregnancy. If these antibodies are present, transplantation is not possible because immediate, severe rejection will occur. Although some procedures and drugs are available to remove the antibodies, there is less experience with these techniques and they are not widely used.

Medical Screening: Some disorders, in particular cancers and infections, can be transmitted during transplantation. Doctors screen donors for cancer by thoroughly reviewing their medical history and carefully inspecting the organ in the operating room at the time of organ recovery. Organs containing cancers are obviously not used for transplant. The decision to use organs from donors who previously had cancer in another organ is made based on the likelihood that tumor cells persist or may have spread to the organ being transplanted.

Most bacterial infections are evident to doctors based on the donor's overall health and have often been diagnosed and treated even before the decision to donate. If treatment has been adequate, organ transplantation is safe, although the recipient may receive additional antibiotic treatment. To prevent transmission of viral infections, which are often not

so obvious, doctors usually test the donor's blood. Viral infections for which blood tests are done include cytomegalovirus (CMV), Epstein-Barr virus (EBV), hepatitis B and C viruses, human immunodeficiency virus (HIV), and human T-cell lymphotropic virus (HTLV). Some viral infections in the donor, such as HIV and HTLV, mean that transplantation cannot be done. Other viral infections, such as CMV and EBV, do not prevent transplantation, but the recipient must take antiviral drugs afterwards.

Because organ transplant recipients are given immunosuppressants in high doses at the time of transplant, recipients who have active infections or cancers cannot undergo transplant until these conditions are controlled or cured. Many immunosuppressants are also unsafe for fetuses, so pregnant women cannot undergo transplant. However, some women who have received a transplant may be able to get pregnant and have healthy babies once the function of their transplanted organ is stable and their immunosuppressants can be specially adjusted.

People with poor overall health, other medical problems in addition to single organ failure, and certain viral infections are less likely to do well with a transplant. The decision to transplant is individualized to the person's specific circumstances.

Psychosocial Screening: The lifelong regimen of drugs, treatments, and follow-up visits required to keep a transplanted organ functioning is quite demanding, and not all people are willing or able to comply. In addition to nurses and doctors, psychiatrists and social workers are involved to help people and their families understand the long-term commitment and difficulties involved in accepting a transplant. Everybody's input is important in determining whether organ transplantation is right for a person.

Suppression of the Immune System

Even if tissue types are closely matched, transplanted organs, unlike transfused blood, are usually rejected unless measures are taken to prevent rejection. Rejection results in destruction of the transplanted organ and can cause fever, chills, nausea, fatigue, and sudden changes in blood pressure. Rejection, if it occurs, usually begins soon after transplantation but can occur after weeks, months, or even years. Rejection can be mild and easily controlled or severe, worsening despite treatment.

Rejection can usually be controlled with drugs that suppress the immune system and the body's ability to recognize and destroy foreign substances. With the use of these immunosuppressants, the transplanted organ is more likely to survive. Immunosuppressants must be taken indefinitely. High doses are usually necessary only during the first few weeks after transplantation or during an episode of rejection. After

℞ DRUGS USED TO PREVENT TRANSPLANT REJECTION

DRUG	POSSIBLE SIDE EFFECTS	COMMENTS
Corticosteroids (potent anti-inflammatory drugs that suppress the immune system as a whole)		
Dexamethasone Prednisolone Prednisone	Excess hair on the face Facial puffiness Fragile skin High blood sugar levels (as occur in diabetes mellitus) Muscle weakness Osteoporosis Stomach ulcers Water retention	Given by vein in high doses at the time of transplantation Gradual reduction of the dose to a maintenance dose given by mouth, usually indefinitely
Polyclonal immunoglobulins (antibodies directed toward specialized cells of the immune system)		
Antilymphocyte globulin Antithymocyte globulin	Severe allergic (anaphylactic) reactions with fever and chills, usually occurring only after the first or second dose Reaction to the foreign proteins in the drug with fever, rash, and joint pain (serum sickness)	Given by vein Used at the time of transplantation or for rejection episodes
Monoclonal antibodies (antibodies that target lymphocytes)		
Basiliximab Daclizumab Infliximab Muromonab (OTK3)	Drug tolerance (the drug becomes less effective for subsequent rejection episodes) Fever Irritation of the digestive tract Joint pain Muscle pain Seizures Severe allergic (anaphylactic) reactions Shaking (rigors)	Given by vein Used at the time of transplantation or for rejection episodes Severe side effects usually only after the first few doses
Calcineurin inhibitors (drugs that prevent activation and expansion of the immune system)		
Cyclosporine	Excessive hairiness (hirsutism) Gum enlargement High blood pressure Increased risk of cancer Kidney damage Liver damage Tremor	Given by mouth Used as maintenance immunosuppression in people who have received a solid organ transplant
Tacrolimus	Diarrhea Headache Heart enlargement High blood pressure Increased risk of lymphoma Insomnia Kidney damage Liver damage Nausea Tremor	Given by mouth Used as maintenance immunosuppression in people who have received a solid organ transplant
Rapamycins (drugs that prevent proliferation of lymphocytes)		
Everolimus Sirolimus	Anemia Diarrhea High blood pressure Increased cholesterol levels Increased risk of lymphoma Joint pain Low potassium levels Rash	Given by mouth Used with corticosteroids or calcineurin inhibitors in people who have received a kidney or liver transplant Everolimus usually given to people who have received a heart transplant

(continued on the following page)

℞ DRUGS USED TO PREVENT TRANSPLANT REJECTION (*Continued*)

DRUG	POSSIBLE SIDE EFFECTS	COMMENTS
Mitotic inhibitors (drugs that suppress cell division and thus the production of white blood cells)		
Azathioprine	Hepatitis (rare) Increased risk of infection Low white blood cell count Nausea Tendency to bleed Tiredness Vomiting	Given by mouth Used as maintenance immunosuppression in people who have received a solid organ transplant
Mycophenolate mofetil	Blood infection (sepsis) Diarrhea Increased risk of lymphoma Nausea Vomiting	Given by mouth Used as maintenance immunosuppression in people who have received a solid organ transplant

that, smaller doses can usually prevent rejection (maintenance immunosuppression). A further reduction of immunosuppression may be required if recipients suffer from serious infections or side effects, but reducing the dose of the immunosuppressant increases the risk of rejection. At the first sign of rejection, doctors increase the dose of the immunosuppressant, change the type of immunosuppressant, or add an additional immunosuppressant.

Complications: Although immunosuppressants suppress the immune system's reaction to the transplanted organ, they also reduce the ability of the immune system to fight infections and to destroy cancer cells. Thus, transplant recipients are at increased risk of developing infections and certain cancers.

Recipients may get the same infections that any person recovering from surgery would. Such infections include those of the surgical site or the transplanted organ, pneumonia, or urinary infections. People also are at risk for unusual (opportunistic) infections that affect mainly people with weakened immune systems. Such infections may be caused by bacteria (for example, *Listeria* or *Nocardia*), viruses (for example, CMV or EBV), fungi (for example, *Pneumocystis* or *Aspergillus*), or parasites (for example, *Toxoplasma*).

Cancers due to immunosuppression include certain skin cancers, lymphoma, cervical cancer, and Kaposi's sarcoma.

Kidney Transplantation

For people of all ages who have irreversible kidney failure, kidney transplantation is a lifesaving alternative to dialysis. In the United States, more than 17,000 kidneys are transplanted each year. Over 95% of kidneys from living donors are functioning 1 year after transplantation. Three percent to 5% of these kidneys stop functioning each year after the first. About 82 to 91% of kidneys from deceased donors are functioning 1 year after transplantation. Five percent to 8% of these kidneys stop functioning each year after the first. Transplanted kidneys sometimes function for more than 30 years. People with successful kidney transplants can usually lead normal, active lives.

About two thirds of transplanted kidneys come from deceased donors. The kidneys are removed, cooled, and transported quickly to a medical center for transplantation to a person who has a compatible blood and tissue type and who does not make antibodies to the tissues of the donor.

Kidney transplantation is a major operation. The donated kidney is placed in the pelvis through an incision and is attached to the recipient's blood vessels and bladder. Usually, the nonfunctioning kidneys are left in place. Occasionally, they are removed because they are causing uncontrollable high blood pressure or are infected.

Despite the use of immunosuppressants, one or more episodes of rejection may occur after transplantation. Acute rejection can be accompanied by fever, decreased urine production with weight gain, pain and swelling of the kidney, and elevated blood pressure. Blood tests show deteriorating kidney function. Because these symptoms can also occur with infections or drug toxicity, the diagnosis of rejection can be confirmed with a needle biopsy of the kidney.

Acute rejection occurs within 3 to 4 months of transplantation. It can usually be controlled with high doses of immunosuppressants or antibody therapy given for a short time. Sometimes, using a different drug for maintenance immunosuppression helps control rejection.

Chronic rejection that develops over many months to years is relatively common and causes kidney function to gradually deteriorate. If rejection cannot be controlled, the kidney will fail and dialysis must be started again. The rejected kidney may be left in place unless fever, tenderness, blood in the urine, or high blood pressure persists. The chance of success with second transplants is almost as good as that with first transplants.

Compared with the general population, kidney transplant recipients are 10 to 15 times more likely to develop cancer, probably because the immune system helps defend the body against cancer as well as infections. Cancer of the lymphatic system (lymphoma) is 30 times more common among kidney transplant recipients than the general population, but lymphoma is still uncommon. Skin cancer is common.

Liver Transplantation

Liver transplantation is the only option for people whose liver no longer functions. A whole liver can be obtained only from a person who has died, but a living donor can provide a part of the liver. A donated liver can be stored for 8 to 15 hours. Many people die while waiting for a suitable liver, but 85 to 90% of liver transplant recipients survive for at least 1 year. Most recipients are people whose liver has been destroyed by primary biliary cirrhosis, hepatitis, or drug toxicity (such as high doses of acetaminophen). People whose liver has been destroyed by alcoholism can receive a transplant if they stop drinking. Liver transplantation is also done for some people who have liver cancer that is not too far advanced. About 86% of patients who receive a transplant to treat cancer are still alive after 1 year. Although viral hepatitis and autoimmune disorders tend to recur in the transplanted liver, survival is still good.

The damaged liver is removed through an incision in the abdomen, and the new liver is connected to the recipient's blood vessels and bile ducts. Usually, blood transfusions are required. Typically, the operation lasts 4½ hours or more, and the hospital stay is 7 to 12 days.

Liver transplants are rejected somewhat less vigorously than transplants of other organs, such as the kidney and heart. Nonetheless, immunosuppressants must be taken after transplantation. If the recipient develops an enlarged liver, nausea, pain, fever, jaundice, or abnormal liver function (detected by blood tests), doctors may do a biopsy using a needle. Biopsy results help doctors determine whether the liver is being rejected and whether immunosuppressant therapy should be adjusted.

Heart Transplantation

Heart transplantation is reserved for people who have severe heart failure and who cannot be treated effectively with drugs or other forms of surgery. In some medical centers, heart machines can keep people alive for weeks or months until a compatible heart can be found. Also, newly developed, implantable artificial hearts are being used to tide people over until a heart is available or, in some experimental situations, to be used as a long-term replacement. Nonetheless, many people die while waiting.

About 95% of people who have had a heart transplant are substantially better able to exercise and carry out daily activities than they were before the transplantation. About 85% of heart transplant recipients survive for at least 1 year.

Through an incision in the chest, most of the damaged heart is removed, but the back walls of the upper heart chambers (atria) are left. The donated heart is then attached to what remains of the recipient's heart. The procedure takes about 3 to 5 hours. The hospital stay after this operation is usually 7 to 14 days.

Immunosuppressants must be taken to prevent rejection of a transplanted heart. Rejection, if it occurs, usually causes fever, weakness, and a rapid or other abnormal heart rhythm. With rejection, the transplanted heart may not function well, causing low blood pressure and fluid accumulation in the legs and sometimes the abdomen, resulting in swelling—a condition called edema. Fluid may also accumulate in the lungs. If rejection is mild, no symptoms may occur, but electrocardiography (ECG) may detect changes in the heart's electrical activity.

If doctors suspect rejection, they usually do a biopsy. A catheter is inserted through an incision in the neck into a vein and is threaded to the heart. A device at the end of the catheter is used to remove a small piece of heart tissue, which is examined under a microscope. Doctors also routinely do biopsies once a year to look for rejection that has not yet caused symptoms.

Nearly half of all deaths that occur after heart transplantation are due to infections. About one fourth of people who have a heart transplant develop atherosclerosis in the coronary arteries.

Lung and Heart-Lung Transplantation

Lung transplants are done for people whose lungs no longer function. Most recipients are people who have severe chronic obstructive pulmonary disease, idiopathic pulmonary fibrosis, cystic fibrosis, α_1-antitrypsin deficiency, and primary pulmonary hypertension. Usually, one lung is transplanted, but two lungs can be transplanted. When a lung disorder has also damaged the heart, one or both lungs and a heart may be transplanted at the same time. Because preserving a lung for transplantation is difficult, lung transplantation must be done as soon as possible after a lung has been obtained.

Lung transplants can come from a living donor or from someone who has recently died. A living donor cannot donate more than one entire lung and usually donates only one lobe. A person who has died can provide both lungs or the heart and lungs.

Through an incision in the chest, the recipient's lung or lungs are removed and replaced with those of the donor. The blood vessels to and from the lung (pulmonary artery and pulmonary vein) and the main airway (bronchus) are connected to the transplanted lung or lungs. The operation takes 4 to 8 hours for one lung and 6 to 12 hours for two lungs. A heart and lung may be transplanted at the same time. The hospital stay after these operations is usually 7 to 14 days.

About 70% of people who receive a lung transplant survive for at least 1 year. The risk of infection is high because the lungs are continually exposed to air, which contains bacteria and other microorganisms that can cause disease. The site at which the airway is attached sometimes heals poorly. Scar tissue may form, narrowing the airway, reducing air flow, and causing shortness of breath. Treatment of this complication consists of widening (dilating) the airway—for example, by placing a stent (a wire-mesh tube) in the airway to hold it open.

Rejection of a lung transplant can be difficult to detect, evaluate, and treat. More than 80% of people who receive a lung transplant develop some symptoms of rejection within a month of transplantation. Symptoms include fever, shortness of breath, and weakness. Weakness develops because the transplanted lung cannot provide enough oxygen to supply the body. Later, scar tissue may form in the small airways and gradually block them, possibly indicating gradual rejection.

Pancreas Transplantation

Pancreas transplantation is done for people with diabetes whose pancreas cannot make any insulin. It is a major operation, requiring a long incision in the abdomen and a general anesthetic. The recipient's pancreas is not removed. Typically, the operation takes about 3 hours and the hospital stay is 1 to 3 weeks.

More than 80% of people with diabetes who receive a pancreas transplant have normal blood sugar levels afterward and no longer need insulin,

but they trade this for the need to take immunosuppressants, with the risk of infections and other side effects. Because injectable insulin is a safe and reasonably effective treatment for diabetes, pancreas transplantation is usually done only in certain diabetic people. People who are most likely to benefit include those who repeatedly have life-threatening low blood sugar levels from use of insulin, and those who also need a kidney transplant. People who need a kidney transplant need to have their abdomen opened and to take immunosuppressants anyway, so they incur few additional risks if they receive a pancreas transplant at the same time.

PANCREATIC ISLET CELL TRANSPLANTATION

The cells in the pancreas that produce insulin are called islet cells. Islet cells may be separated from the pancreas of a deceased donor. The islet cells are then transplanted by injecting them into a vein that goes to the liver. The islet cells lodge in the small blood vessels of the liver, where they can live and produce insulin. Sometimes two or three infusions are done, requiring two or three deceased donors.

Some people must have their pancreas removed because of disorders such as chronic pancreatitis (see page 161). Such people will then become diabetic even if they were not diabetic previously. After the pancreas is removed, doctors can sometimes harvest the islet cells from the person's own pancreas. These islet cells can then be transplanted back into the person's body (autologous transplantation). Because the cells are the person's own, immunosuppressants are not needed.

Transplanting islet cells is simpler and safer than a pancreas transplant, and about 75% of people who receive an islet cell transplant no longer need insulin. However, the long-term success of islet cell transplantation is not yet proved.

Stem Cell Transplantation

Stem cells are unspecialized cells from which other more specialized cells can be derived. Stem cells obtained from embryos and fetuses are thought to be best because they are more likely to survive transplantation than those obtained from children or adults. However, adults also have some kinds of stem cells. Stem cells for different kinds of blood cells can be obtained from the bone marrow (bone marrow transplantation) or, in small numbers, from the blood.

Stem cell transplantation can be used as part of the treatment for blood disorders such as leukemia, certain types of lymphoma (including Hodgkin lymphoma), aplastic anemia, thalassemia, sickle cell anemia, and some congenital metabolic or immunodeficiency disorders (such as chronic granulomatous disease). Certain types of stem cells can also be used as transplants for people whose bone marrow has been destroyed by high doses of chemotherapy or radiation therapy used to treat some cancers. Stem cell transplantation may some day become useful for treating other disorders, such as Parkinson's disease and Alzheimer's disease, in which the transplanted stem cells can become brain cells.

Stem cells may be the person's own cells (autologous transplantation) or those of a donor (allogeneic transplantation). When the person's own stem cells are used, they are collected before chemotherapy or radiation therapy because these treatments can damage stem cells. They are injected back into the body after the treatment.

For bone marrow transplantation, the donor is usually given a general anesthetic. Doctors then remove marrow from the donor's hip bone with a syringe. Removal of bone marrow takes about 1 hour.

Sometimes stem cells from adults are obtained from blood during an outpatient procedure. First, the donor is given a drug that causes the bone marrow to release more stem cells into the bloodstream. Then blood is removed through a catheter inserted in one arm and is circulated through a machine that removes stem cells. The rest of the blood is returned to the person through a catheter inserted in the other arm. Usually, about six 2- to 4-hour sessions during a period of 1 to 2 weeks are required to obtain enough stem cells. Stem cells can be preserved for later use by freezing them.

Stem cells are injected into the recipient's vein. The injected stem cells migrate to and begin to multiply in the recipient's bones and produce blood cells.

Stem cell transplantation is risky because the recipient's white blood cells have been destroyed or reduced in number by chemotherapy or radiation therapy. As a result, the risk of infection is very high for about 2 to 3 weeks—until the donated stem cells can produce enough white blood cells to protect against infections.

Another problem is that the new bone marrow obtained from another person may produce cells that attack the recipient's cells, causing graft-versus-host disease (see page 1031). Furthermore, the original disorder may recur.

The risk of infection can be reduced by keeping the recipient in isolation for a period of time (until the transplanted cells begin to produce white blood cells). During this time, everyone entering the room must wear masks and gowns and wash their hands thoroughly. Antibodies isolated from the donor's blood may be given intravenously to the recipient to

---

What Are Stem Cells?

Stem cells are undifferentiated cells that have the potential to become one of 200 types of cells in the body, including blood, nerve, muscle, heart, glandular, and skin cells. Some stem cells can be triggered to become any kind of cell in the body. Others are already partially differentiated and can only become, for example, any kind of nerve cell. Stem cells divide, producing more stem cells, until they are triggered to specialize. Then as they continue to divide, they become more and more specialized until they lose the ability to be anything but one kind of cell.

Researchers hope to use stem cells to repair or replace cells or tissues damaged or destroyed by such disorders as Alzheimer's disease, Parkinson's disease, diabetes, and spinal injuries by triggering the genes that cause the stem cells to specialize. Researchers are so far able to obtain stem cells from four sources:

Embryos: During in vitro fertilization, sperm from the man and several eggs from the woman are placed in a culture dish. The sperm fertilizes the egg and the resulting cell divides, forming an embryo. Several of the healthiest-looking embryos are placed in the woman's uterus. The rest are discarded or frozen to be used later if needed. Stem cells can be obtained from the embryos that are not used. Because the embryos then lose the ability to grow into a complete human being, the use of stem cells from embryos is controversial, but researchers think that these stem cells have the most potential for producing different kinds of cells and for surviving after transplantation.

Fetuses: After 8 weeks of development, an embryo is called a fetus. Stem cells can be obtained from fetuses that have been miscarried or aborted.

Umbilical Cord: Stem cells can be obtained from the blood in the umbilical cord or placenta after a baby is born. These stem cells can produce only blood cells and have been used for transplantation only in recent years.

Children and Adults: The bone marrow and blood of children and adults contain stem cells. These stem cells can produce only blood cells. These stem cells are most often used for transplantation.

---

help protect against infection. Growth factors, which stimulate the production of blood cells, can help reduce the risk of infection and graft-versus-host disease.

Recipients of a stem cell transplant usually remain in the hospital for 1 to 2 months. After discharge from the hospital, follow-up visits are necessary at regular intervals. Most people need at least 1 year to recover.

Corneal Transplants and Why They Usually Work

Corneal transplantation is a common and highly successful type of transplantation. A scarred or cloudy cornea can be replaced with a clear, healthy one. Doctors using a surgical microscope carry out the procedure in about 1 hour. Donated corneas come from people who have recently died. A general or local anesthetic is used. The donated cornea is cut to the right size, the damaged cornea is removed, and the donated cornea is sewn in place. The recipient usually stays in the hospital 1 or 2 nights but may go home the same day.

A cornea is rarely rejected because it does not have its own blood supply. It receives oxygen and other nutrients from nearby tissues and fluid. The components of the immune system that initiate rejection in response to a foreign substance—certain white blood cells and antibodies—are carried in the bloodstream. Thus, these cells and antibodies do not reach the transplanted cornea, do not encounter the foreign tissue there, and do not initiate rejection. Tissues with a rich blood supply are much more likely to be rejected.

Transplantation of Other Organs

Skin grafts can be used in people who have lost large areas of skin—for example, because of extensive burns. Skin grafting is most successful when healthy skin is removed from one part of the body and grafted to another part. When such grafting is not possible, skin from a donor or even from animals (such as pigs) can be used as a temporary measure. Such grafts last only a short time, but they can provide temporary protection until normal skin grows to replace them. The amount of skin available for grafting may be increased by growing small pieces of the person's skin in a tissue culture or by making many tiny cuts in the grafted skin, so that it can be stretched to cover a much larger area.

Cartilage may be transplanted successfully without the use of immunosuppressants. The body's immune system attacks transplanted cartilage much less vigorously than other tissues. In children, cartilage is usually used to repair defects in the ears or nose. In adults, it can be used to repair joints damaged by injury and occasionally by arthritis.

Corneas, the transparent domes on the surface of the eyes, can usually be transplanted successfully without the use of immunosuppressants.

Bone from one part of the body can be used to replace bone in another part. Bone transplanted from one person to another survives only a short time. However, it stimulates growth of new bone, stabilizes the area until new bone can form, and provides a framework for new bone to fill in.

Transplantation of the small intestine may be used when the intestine does not absorb nutrients because of a disorder or has had to be removed because of a disorder or injury, and other forms of nutrition have failed. Intestinal transplants are particularly prone to both infection and rejection, and less than 80% last for more than 1 year. Because the small intestine contains a large amount of lymphatic tissue, the new intestinal tissue may produce cells that attack the recipient's cells, causing graft-versus-host disease.

Parkinson's disease can be treated by transplanting tissue from a person's adrenal glands to that person's brain. Alternatively, brain tissue from aborted fetuses can be used. Both procedures can relieve symptoms. However, the ethics of using tissue from aborted fetuses is controversial.

Thymus glands from aborted or miscarried fetuses can be transplanted into children who are born without a thymus gland (a disorder called DiGeorge syndrome). When the thymus gland is missing, the immune system is impaired, because white blood cells, which are a vital part of the immune system's defense against foreign substances, mature in the thymus gland. Transplantation of a thymus gland restores the impaired immune system in these children. However, the new thymus may produce cells that attack the recipient's cells, causing graft-versus-host disease.

Rarely, transplantation of limbs and faces from one person to another has been attempted, but this technique is experimental.

Reattaching a Body Part

If fingers, hands, and arms are relatively undamaged after being severed from the body, they can sometimes be reattached successfully. Reattachment of legs is less successful. The severed part is kept clean and is put in a plastic bag and placed on ice until it can be used. Prompt reattachment is crucial so that the blood supply to the severed part can be restored.

SECTION 16

Infections

1137

CHAPTER
172   Biology of Infectious Disease

Microorganisms are tiny living creatures, such as bacteria and viruses. Microorganisms are present everywhere. Despite their overwhelming abundance, relatively few of the thousands of species of microorganisms invade, multiply, and cause disease in people.

Many microorganisms live on the skin and in the mouth, upper airways, intestine, and genitals (particularly the vagina) without causing disease. Whether a microorganism lives as a harmless companion to a person or invades and causes disease depends on the nature of the microorganism and on the state of the person's natural defenses.

Resident Flora

Healthy people live in harmony with most microorganisms that establish themselves on (colonize) the body. The microorganisms that usually occupy a particular body site are called the resident flora. Microorganisms that colonize people for hours to weeks but do not establish themselves permanently are called transient flora.

The resident flora at each site includes several different types of microorganisms. Some sites are normally colonized by several hundred different types of microorganisms. Environmental factors—such as diet, sanitary conditions, air pollution, and hygienic habits—influence what species make up a person's resident flora. If disturbed, for example by washing or use of antibiotics, the resident flora usually promptly reestablishes itself.

Rather than causing disease, the resident flora often protects the body against disease-causing organisms. However, under certain conditions, microorganisms that are part of a person's resident flora may cause disease. Such conditions include the use of antibiotics and a weakened immune system (as occurs in people with AIDS or cancer, people taking corticosteroids, and those receiving chemotherapy). When antibiotics used to treat an infection kill a large proportion of certain types of bacteria of the resident flora, other resident bacteria or fungi can grow unchecked. For example, a vaginal yeast infection may occur in women taking antibiotics for a bladder infection.

Development of Infection

Infectious diseases are usually caused by microorganisms that invade the body and multiply. Invasion by most microorganisms begins when they adhere to cells in a person's body. Adherence is a very specific process, involving "lock-and-key" connections between the microorganism and cells in the body. Whether the microorganism remains near the invasion site or spreads to other sites depends on such factors as whether it produces toxins, enzymes, or other substances.

Some microorganisms that invade the body produce toxins. For example, *Clostridium tetani* in an infected wound produces a toxin that causes tetanus. Some diseases are caused by toxins produced

TYPES OF INFECTIOUS ORGANISMS

TYPE	DESCRIPTION	EXAMPLES	SOME DISORDERS THAT CAN RESULT
Bacteria	Bacteria are microscopic, single-celled organisms.	*Streptococcus pyogenes* *Escherichia coli*	Strep throat Urinary tract infections
Viruses	Viruses are small infectious organisms—much smaller than a fungus or bacterium. They cannot reproduce on their own. They must invade a living cell and use that cell's machinery to reproduce.	Varicella zoster Rhinovirus	Chickenpox and shingles The common cold
Fungi	Fungi are neither plants nor animals. Their size ranges from microscopic to easily seen with the naked eye. They include yeasts, molds, and mushrooms.	*Candida albicans* *Tinea pedis*	Vaginal yeast infections Athlete's foot
Parasites	Parasites are organisms that survive by living inside another, usually much larger organism (the host). They include worms and single-celled animals (protozoa).	*Enterobius vermicularis* (a pinworm) *Plasmodium falciparum*	Itching around the anus Malaria

by microorganisms outside the body. Food poisoning caused by staphylococci is one example. Most toxins contain components that bind specifically with molecules on certain cells (target cells). Toxins play a central role in such diseases as tetanus, toxic shock syndrome, botulism, anthrax, and cholera.

After invading the body, microorganisms must multiply to cause infection. After multiplication begins, one of three things can happen:

- Microorganisms continue to multiply and overwhelm the body's defenses.
- A state of balance is achieved, causing chronic infection.
- The body—with or without medical treatment—destroys and eliminates the invading microorganism.

Many disease-causing microorganisms have properties that increase the severity of the diseases they cause (virulence) and help them resist the body's defense mechanisms. For example, some bacteria produce enzymes that break down tissue, allowing the infection to spread faster.

Some microorganisms have ways of blocking the body's defense mechanisms, such as the following:

- Interfering with the body's production of antibodies or T cells (a type of white blood cell), which are specifically armed to attack the microorganisms
- Being enclosed in protective outer coats (capsules) that prevent white blood cells from ingesting the microorganisms. (The fungus *Cryptococcus* actually

develops a thicker capsule after it enters the lungs for the specific purpose of resisting the body's defenses.)

- Resisting being split open (lysed) by substances circulating in the bloodstream
- Producing substances that counter the effects of antibiotics

Microorganisms that do not at first have ways of blocking the body's defenses sometimes develop them over time. For example, some microorganisms exposed to penicillin become resistant to that drug.

Defenses Against Infection

Physical barriers and the immune system defend the body against organisms that can cause infection. Physical barriers include the skin, mucous membranes, tears, earwax, mucus, and stomach acid. Also, the normal flow of urine washes out microorganisms that enter the urinary tract. The immune system uses white blood cells and antibodies to identify and eliminate organisms that get through the body's physical barriers (see page 1096).

Physical Barriers

Usually, the skin prevents invasion by microorganisms unless it is damaged—for example, by an injury, insect bite, or burn. Other effective physical barriers are the mucous membranes, such as the

Identifying an Infectious Organism

Usually, doctors need to know which specific microorganism is causing a disease. Many different microorganisms can cause a given disease (for example, pneumonia can be caused by viruses, bacteria, or fungi), and the treatment is different for each organism.

There are many ways to identify microorganisms.

Examination under a microscope: Despite the development of rapid identification systems, direct microscopic examination of samples taken from the site of infection is often the most rapid method of identifying microorganisms that cause disease. Chemical stains are usually applied to make the microorganisms easier to see. The size and shape of the microorganisms and their stained color can help distinguish between different types. However, the microorganisms must be of sufficient size and number to be seen with a regular microscope. For example, viruses are too small to be seen with a regular microscope.

Culture: Usually, microorganisms are too few or too small to see, so they may be grown in the laboratory until there are enough to be identified with chemical tests. The process of growing the organism is called a culture. Many microorganisms, such as the bacteria that cause gonorrhea or strep throat, can be grown this way.

Cultures can also be used to test the sensitivity of microorganisms to various antibiotics. This testing can help a doctor determine which drug to use in treating an infected person. This strategy is particularly important because microorganisms are constantly developing resistance to antibiotics that were previously effective.

Tests that detect antibodies: Some microorganisms, such as the bacteria that cause syphilis and the human immunodeficiency virus (HIV), are very difficult to culture. These infections, and many others, can be identified by finding antibodies to the microorganisms in the infected person's blood or body fluids (for example, cerebrospinal fluid).

Antibody-based tests are used to identify many infections, but they are not always reliable. These tests may not become positive for several days or weeks after people become ill. Also, these tests may indicate infection when none is present because they detect antibodies from a previous infection. Antibodies often stay in the body for many years after an infection has gone away.

Nucleic acid amplification tests: These tests, such as the polymerase chain reaction (PCR), identify pieces of the microorganism's genetic material (DNA), which are present only when the organism is present.

These tests are done only when a doctor already suspects a particular disease. Therefore, a doctor's understanding of all the features of a disease, including symptoms, physical examination results, and risk factors, is essential for diagnosing an infection.

---

linings of the mouth, nose, and eyelids. Typically, mucous membranes are coated with secretions that fight microorganisms. For example, the mucous membranes of the eyes are bathed in tears, which contain an enzyme called lysozyme that attacks bacteria and helps protect the eyes from infection.

The airways filter out particles that are present in the air that is breathed in. The walls of the passages in the nose and airways are coated with mucus. Microorganisms in the air become stuck to the mucus, which is coughed up or blown out of the nose. Mucus removal is aided by the coordinated beating of tiny hairlike projections (cilia) that line the airways. The cilia sweep the mucus up the airways, away from the lungs.

The digestive tract has a series of effective barriers, including stomach acid, pancreatic enzymes, bile, and intestinal secretions. The contractions of the intestine (peristalsis) and the normal shedding of cells lining the intestine help remove harmful microorganisms.

The bladder is protected by the urethra, the tube that drains urine from the body. In males older than 6 months, the urethra is long enough that bacteria are seldom able to pass through it to reach the bladder, unless the bacteria are unintentionally placed there by catheters or surgical instruments. In females, the urethra is shorter, occasionally allowing external bacteria to pass into the bladder. The flushing effect as the bladder empties is another defense mechanism in both sexes. The vagina is protected by its normal acidic environment.

The Blood

One way the body defends against infection is by increasing the number of certain types of white blood cells (neutrophils and monocytes), which engulf and destroy invading microorganisms. The increase can occur within several hours, largely because white blood cells are released from the bone marrow, where they are made. The number of neutrophils increases first. If an infection persists, the number of monocytes increases. The blood carries white blood cells to sites of infection. The number of eosinophils, another type of white blood cell, increases in allergic reactions and many parasitic infections, but usually not in bacterial infections.

Certain infections, such as typhoid fever, actually lead to a decrease in the white blood cell count. How these infections cause the decrease is not known.

Inflammation

Any injury, including an invasion by microorganisms, causes inflammation in the affected area. Inflammation,

Biological Warfare and Terrorism

Biological warfare is the use of microbiological agents for hostile purposes. Such use is contrary to international law and has rarely occurred during formal warfare in modern history, despite the extensive preparations and stockpiling of biological agents by most major powers during the 20th century. It is uncertain whether other countries or dissident groups have biologic warfare capability. For a variety of reasons (including uncertain military efficacy and the threat of massive retaliation), experts consider the use of biological agents in formal warfare unlikely. However, biological agents are thought by some people to be an ideal weapon for terrorists. These agents may be delivered clandestinely, and they have delayed effects, allowing the user to remain undetected.

Potential biological agents include anthrax, botulinum toxin, brucellosis, encephalitis viruses, hemorrhagic fever viruses (Ebola and Marburg), plague, tularemia, and smallpox. Each of these is potentially fatal and, except for anthrax and botulinum toxin, can be passed from person to person.

Anthrax spores are relatively easy to prepare and, unlike most other agents, can be spread through the air, creating the potential for distribution by airplane. Theoretically, 1 kilogram of anthrax could kill 10,000 people, although technical difficulties with preparing the spores in a sufficiently fine powder would probably limit actual deaths to a fraction of this number.

Despite these theoretical concerns, the only successful terrorist use of anthrax—multiple pieces of contaminated mail delivered to a variety of locations in the United States in 2001—resulted in only a handful of deaths and a small number of serious infections (22 total cases). More people were contaminated with anthrax spores without developing illness, possibly because of extensive use of the antibiotic ciprofloxacin. However, there was extreme public anxiety related to these incidents.

The number of false threats of anthrax reported was very large. In 1999, the FBI received an average of one false report of anthrax use per day. Even more false reports, both hoaxes and reports by alarmed citizens mistaking harmless material for anthrax, were reported after the 2001 anthrax attack.

The only other successful use of a biological agent by a terror group in the United States occurred in 1984. In this event, 751 people developed diarrhea resulting from the intentional contamination of a salad bar with *Salmonella* in Oregon. The bacteria were introduced by a religious cult trying to influence the results of a local election. No one died, and the election was not affected.

Defense against bioterrorism involves several factors:

- Intelligence information to disrupt the terrorists before they can use the weapons
- Early detection
- Availability of protective antibiotics
- Immunization of selected populations (such as the military)

---

a complex reaction, results from many different conditions. Through release of different substances from the damaged tissue, inflammation directs the body's defenses to do the following:

- Wall off the area
- Attack and kill any invaders
- Dispose of dead and damaged tissue
- Begin the process of repair

However, inflammation may not be able to overcome large numbers of microorganisms.

During inflammation, the blood supply increases. An infected area near the surface of the body becomes red and warm. The walls of blood vessels become more porous, allowing fluid and white blood cells to pass into the affected tissue. The increase in fluid causes the inflamed tissue to swell. The white blood cells attack the invading microorganisms and release substances that continue the process of inflammation. Other substances trigger clotting in the tiny vessels (capillaries) in the inflamed area, which delays the spread of the infecting microorganisms and their

toxins. Many of the substances produced during inflammation stimulate the nerves, causing pain. Reactions to the substances released during inflammation include the chills, fever, and muscle aches that commonly accompany infection.

Infection From Medical Devices

Usually, people think of infection as occurring when microorganisms invade the body and adhere to specific cells. But microorganisms can also adhere to medical devices (such as catheters, artificial joints, and artificial heart valves) that are placed in the body.

Microorganisms may be present on the device when it is inserted if the device was accidentally contaminated. Or infecting organisms from another site may spread through the bloodstream and lodge on an already implanted device. Because implanted material has no natural defenses, the microorganisms can easily grow and spread, causing disease.

Some Causes of Fever

- Infection
- Cancer
- An allergic reaction
- Hormone disorders, such as pheochromocytoma or hyperthyroidism
- Connective tissue disorders, such as rheumatoid arthritis, systemic lupus erythematosus (lupus), and giant cell arteritis
- Excessive exercise, especially in hot weather
- Excessive exposure to the sun, especially in hot weather
- Certain drugs, including anesthetics, antipsychotics, tumor necrosis factor inhibitors (used to treat rheumatoid arthritis), drugs with anticholinergic effects, and overdoses of aspirin
- Damage to the hypothalamus (the part of the brain that controls temperature), as may result from a head injury or a tumor

Immune Response

When an infection develops, the immune system responds by producing several substances and agents that are designed to attack the specific invading microorganisms (see page 1099). For example, the immune system may create killer T cells (a type of white blood cell) that can recognize and kill the invading microorganism. Also, the immune system produces antibodies that are specific to the invading microorganism. Antibodies attach to and immobilize microorganisms—killing them outright or helping the neutrophils target and kill them.

Fever

Body temperature increases as a protective response to infection and injury. The elevated body temperature (fever) enhances the body's defense mechanisms, although it can cause discomfort. However, certain people (such as alcoholics, the very old, and the very young) may experience a drop in temperature in response to severe infection.

Temperature is considered elevated when it is higher than 100° F (37.8° C) as measured by an oral thermometer. Although 98.6° F (37° C) is considered normal temperature, body temperature varies throughout the day. It is lowest in the early morning and highest in the late afternoon—sometimes reaching 99.9° F (37.7° C).

A part of the brain called the hypothalamus controls body temperature. Fever results from an actual resetting of the hypothalamus's thermostat. The body raises its temperature to a higher level by moving (shunting) blood from the skin surface to the interior of the body, thus reducing heat loss. Shivering (chills) may occur to increase heat production through muscle contraction. The body's efforts to conserve and produce heat continue until blood reaches the hypothalamus at the new, higher temperature. The new, higher temperature is then maintained. Later, when the thermostat is reset to its normal level, the body eliminates excess heat through sweating and shunting of blood to the skin.

Fever does not stay at a constant temperature. Sometimes temperature peaks every day and then returns to normal. Alternatively, temperature varies but does not return to normal—called remittent fever. Doctors no longer think that the pattern of rise and fall of fever is very important in diagnosis.

Substances that cause fever are called pyrogens. Pyrogens can come from inside or outside the body. Microorganisms and the substances they produce (such as toxins) are examples of pyrogens formed outside the body. Pyrogens formed inside the body are usually produced by monocytes and macrophages (types of white blood cells). Pyrogens from outside the body cause fever by stimulating the body to release its own pyrogens. However, infection is not the sole cause of fever. Fever may also result from inflammation, cancer, or an allergic reaction.

Usually, fever has an obvious cause, which is often—but not always—an infection (such as influenza, pneumonia, or a urinary tract infection). Usually, a doctor can easily diagnose the infection with a brief history, physical examination, and occasionally a few simple tests, such as a chest x-ray and urine tests. However, sometimes the cause is not readily discernible.

If fever continues for several days and has no obvious cause, a more detailed investigation is required. There are many potential causes of such a fever. Common causes in adults include infections, diseases caused by antibodies produced by the body against its own tissues (autoimmune disorders), and undetected cancer (especially leukemia or lymphoma).

To determine the cause of a fever, a doctor begins by asking a person about present and previous symptoms and disorders, drugs currently being taken, exposure to infections, and recent travel. The pattern of the fever usually does not help with the diagnosis. However, there are some exceptions: A fever that recurs every other day or every third day is typical of malaria.

Recent travel (especially overseas) may give clues to the cause of a fever because some infections occur only in certain areas. For example, coccidioidomycosis (a fungal infection) occurs almost exclusively in the southwestern United States. A history of exposure to certain materials or animals is also important. For example, people who work in a meatpacking plant are more likely to develop brucellosis.

After asking questions, the doctor does a thorough physical examination to find a source of infection or evidence of disease. Blood and other body fluids may be sent to the laboratory to try to grow the microorganism in a culture. Other blood tests can be used to detect antibodies against specific microorganisms. An increase in the white blood cell count usually indicates infection. The differential count (the proportion of different types of white blood cells) gives further clues. For example, an increase in neutrophils suggests a relatively new bacterial infection. An increase in eosinophils suggests the presence of parasites, such as tapeworms or roundworms.

A **fever of unknown origin** may be diagnosed when people have a fever of at least 101° F (38.3° C) for several weeks and extensive investigation does not reveal a cause. In such cases, the cause may be an unusual chronic infection or something other than infection, such as a connective tissue disorder, cancer, or another disorder. Ultrasonography, computed tomography (CT), or magnetic resonance imaging (MRI) may help a doctor diagnose the cause. Injection of white blood cells labeled with a radioactive marker can be used to identify areas of infection or inflammation. If these test results are negative, the doctor may need to obtain a biopsy specimen from the liver, bone marrow, or another site of suspected infection. The specimen is then examined under a microscope and cultured.

Because fever helps the body defend against infection and because fever itself is not dangerous (unless it is higher than about 106° F [41.1° C]), there is some debate as to whether fever should be routinely treated. However, people with a high fever generally feel much better when the fever is treated.

Drugs used to lower body temperature are called antipyretics. The most effective and widely used antipyretics are acetaminophen and nonsteroidal anti-inflammatory drugs (NSAIDs), such as aspirin and ibuprofen. However, aspirin should not be given to children and teenagers to treat a fever because it increases the risk of Reye's syndrome (see box on page 1769), which can be fatal.

Prevention of Infection

Several measures help protect people against infection. Hand washing is an effective way of preventing the spread of infectious microorganisms from one person to another. Hand washing is particularly important for people who handle food or who have frequent physical contact with other people. People visiting hospital patients who are seriously ill may

SPOTLIGHT ON AGING

Infections are more likely and usually more severe in older people than in younger people for several reasons:

- Aging reduces the immune system's effectiveness (see page 1103).
- Many long-term (chronic) disorders that are common among older people—such as chronic obstructive pulmonary disease, cancer, and diabetes mellitus—also increase the risk of infection.
- Older people are more likely to be in a hospital or a nursing home, where the risk of acquiring a serious infection is greater. In hospitals, the widespread use of antibiotics allows antibiotic-resistant organisms to thrive, and infections with these microorganisms are often more difficult to treat than infections acquired at home.

be asked to wash their hands and put on a gown, mask, and gloves before entering the patient's room.

Sometimes, to prevent an infection, antibiotics are given to people who do not yet have an infection. This preventive measure is called prophylaxis. Many healthy people who undergo certain types of surgery—particularly abdominal surgery and organ transplantation—require prophylactic antibiotics.

Vaccination can also prevent infections (see page 1144). People who are at increased risk of developing infections (especially infants, children, older people, and people with AIDS) should receive all the vaccinations necessary to reduce this risk.

Infections in People With Impaired Defenses

Many disorders, drugs, and other treatments can cause a breakdown in the body's natural defenses. Such a breakdown can lead to infections, which can even be caused by microorganisms that normally live harmlessly on or in the body. A breakdown can result from the following:

- Extensive burns: Risk of infection is increased because damaged skin cannot prevent invasion by harmful microorganisms.
- Medical procedures: During a procedure, foreign material may be introduced into the body, increasing the risk of infection. Such procedures include insertion of a catheter into the urinary tract or a blood vessel and insertion of a tube into the windpipe.

- Drugs that suppress the immune system: These drugs include cancer chemotherapy drugs, drugs used to prevent rejection after an organ transplant (such as azathioprine, methotrexate, and cyclosporine), and corticosteroids (such as prednisone).
- Radiation treatments: Such treatments may suppress the immune system, particularly when bone marrow is exposed to radiation.

- AIDS: The ability to fight certain infections decreases dramatically in people with AIDS, especially late in the disease (see page 1254). People with AIDS are at particular risk of opportunistic infections (infections by microorganisms that generally do not cause infection in people with a healthy immune system). People with AIDS also become more severely ill from many common infections.

CHAPTER
173 Immunization

Immunization enables the body to better defend itself against diseases caused by certain bacteria or viruses. Immunization may occur on its own (when people are exposed to bacteria or viruses), or doctors may provide it. When people are immunized against a disease, they do not get the disease or get only a mild form of it.

There are two types of immunization: active and passive.

In **active immunization**, vaccines are used to stimulate the body's natural defense mechanisms. Vaccines are preparations that contain one of the following:

- Noninfectious fragments of bacteria or viruses
- A usually harmful substance (toxin) that is produced by a bacteria but has been modified to be harmless—called a toxoid
- Weakened (attenuated), live whole organisms that do not cause infection

The body's immune system responds to a vaccine by producing substances (such as antibodies and white blood cells) that recognize and attack the specific bacteria or virus contained in the vaccine. Then whenever the person is exposed to the specific bacteria or virus, the body automatically produces these antibodies and other substances. The process of giving a vaccine is called vaccination, although many doctors use the more general term immunization.

In **passive immunization**, antibodies against a specific infectious organism are given directly to a person. These antibodies are obtained from several sources:

- The blood (serum) of animals (usually horses) that have been exposed to a particular organism or toxin and have developed immunity
- Blood collected from a large group of people—called pooled human immune globulin

- People known to have antibodies to a particular disease (that is, people who have been immunized or who are recovering from the disease)—called hyperimmune globulin—because these people have higher levels of antibodies in their blood
- Antibody-producing cells (usually taken from mice) grown in a laboratory

Passive immunization is used for people whose immune system does not respond adequately to an infection or for people who acquire an infection before they can be vaccinated (for example, after exposure to the rabies virus). Passive immunization can also be used to prevent disease when people are likely to be exposed and do not have time to get or complete a vaccination series. For example, a solution containing gamma globulin (a common type of antibody) is used to help prevent hepatitis in people who travel to certain parts of the world. Passive immunization lasts for only a few days or weeks, until the body eliminates the injected antibodies.

> **Did You Know...**
> Some vaccines contain a weakened but living form of the virus that they protect against.

Vaccines and antibodies are usually given by injection into a muscle (intramuscularly) or under the skin (subcutaneously). Antibodies are sometimes injected into a vein (intravenously).

Vaccines available today are highly reliable, and most people tolerate them well. They rarely have side effects, but they do not work in everyone.

Some vaccines are given routinely—for example, the tetanus toxoid is given to adults, preferably every 10 years. Some vaccines are routinely given to children.

Other vaccines are usually given mainly to specific groups of people. For example, the yellow fever vaccine is given only to people traveling to certain parts of Africa and South America. Still other vaccines are given after possible exposure to a specific disease. For example, the rabies vaccine may be given to a person who has been bitten by a dog.

Common Vaccinations

Children typically are given a number of vaccines according to a standard schedule (see art on page 1685). If vaccines are missed, most can be given later, according to a catch-up schedule. Adults may also be advised to receive certain vaccines. When advising adults about vaccination, a doctor considers the person's age, health history, childhood vaccinations, occupation, geographic location, travel plans, and other factors. Because vaccines are widely used in the United States, many diseases, once common, are now rare or well controlled.

More than one vaccine may be given at a time. They may be given in one combination vaccine or in individual injections at different injection sites.

Vaccines usually cause no problems, although mild side effects, such as soreness or redness at the injection site, may occur. There has been concern about the safety of thimerosal (a mercury-based preservative in some vaccines) in infants, but there is no evidence of harm. In particular, there is no convincing evidence that vaccines containing thimerosal are related to the development of autism. Nevertheless, most manufacturers have developed thimerosal-free vaccines for use in infants. Information about vaccines that currently contain low levels of mercury or thimerosal is available at the Institute for Vaccine Safety web site.

The only reason for not being vaccinated is a serious allergic reaction (such as an anaphylactic reaction) to the vaccine or to one of its components. However, some vaccines, usually ones that contain live virus, should not be used or should be delayed in people with certain conditions:

- A weakened immune system due to a disorder, such as AIDS, or to drugs that suppress the immune system (immunosuppressants), including corticosteroids
- Pregnancy
- Some progressive nervous system disorders, such as Guillain-Barré syndrome

Diphtheria-Tetanus-Pertussis

The diphtheria, tetanus, and pertussis vaccine is a combination vaccine that protects against these three diseases:

- Diphtheria usually causes inflammation of the throat and mucous membranes of the mouth. However, the bacteria that cause diphtheria produce a toxin that can damage the heart, kidneys, and

PROTECTING CHILDREN THROUGH VACCINES	
DISEASE	**WHEN DO VACCINATIONS TYPICALLY START**
Chickenpox (varicella)	Age 12–15 months
Diphtheria	Age 2 months
Haemophilus influenzae type b infections (such as meningitis)	Age 2 months
Hepatitis A	Age 12–18 months
Hepatitis B	Birth
Human papillomavirus (for girls)	Age 11 years
Influenza	Age 6 months
Measles	Age 12–15 months
Meningococcal meningitis	Age 11–12 years / Age 2 years for children at high risk
Mumps	Age 12–15 months
Pertussis	Age 2 months
Pneumococcal infections	Age 2 months
Polio	Age 2 months
Rotavirus	Age 2 months
Rubella (German measles)	Age 12–15 months
Tetanus	Age 2 months

nervous system. Diphtheria was once a leading cause of death in children.
- Tetanus causes severe muscle spasms, which result from a toxin produced by bacteria. The bacteria usually enter the body through a wound.
- Pertussis (whooping cough) is a very contagious respiratory infection that is particularly dangerous to children younger than 2 years old and to people who have a weakened immune system.

The vaccine has two forms: DTaP for children under 7 years and Tdap for adolescents and adults. Tdap has lower doses of diphtheria and pertussis vaccine, indicated by the lower case *d* and *p*.

Administration: The vaccine is given as an injection into a muscle. Five injections are given: typically at

PROTECTING ADULTS THROUGH VACCINES

DISEASE*	WHO SHOULD BE VACCINATED
Anthrax	People who may be exposed to anthrax, such as the following: ■ Some military personnel ■ Some laboratory workers
Chickenpox (varicella)	All adults who have not had the vaccine or the disease
Diphtheria	All adults (usually as a combination vaccine with tetanus and pertussis)
Haemophilus influenzae type b infections (such as meningitis)	Adults at increased risk, such as the following: ■ People who do not have a functioning spleen ■ People who have a weakened immune system (such as those with AIDS) ■ People who have had radiation therapy or chemotherapy for cancer ■ People taking corticosteroids for a long time
Hepatitis A	Adults at increased risk, such as the following: ■ Travelers to areas where the disease is common ■ Military personnel ■ People who inject illegal drugs, especially those who share needles ■ Male homosexuals ■ People who have a chronic liver disorder ■ People who are treated with blood clotting factors
Hepatitis B	Adults at increased risk, such as the following: ■ Health care workers ■ Travelers to areas where the disease is common ■ People with a chronic liver disorder ■ People who undergo dialysis ■ People who inject illegal drugs, especially those who share needles ■ People who have multiple sex partners ■ Male homosexuals ■ Sex partners and household contacts of people known to be carriers of hepatitis B
Human papillomavirus	All females aged 11–26 years
Influenza	Adults over 50 Anyone who requests vaccination, particularly those at increased risk, such as the following: ■ Health care workers ■ People with a chronic disorder such as diabetes, asthma, or a heart disorder ■ People with a weakened immune system ■ Residents of long-term care facilities
Measles	All adults who have not had the infection or two doses of the vaccine, usually given as a combination vaccine with mumps and rubella
Meningococcal meningitis	People at increased risk, such as the following: ■ People who do not have a functioning spleen ■ Adolescents entering high school if they have not already been vaccinated ■ All college students living in dormitories and military recruits if they have not already been vaccinated ■ Travelers to areas where the disease is common
Mumps	All adults who have not had the infection or two doses of the vaccine, usually given as a combination vaccine with measles and rubella

(continued on the following page)

PROTECTING ADULTS THROUGH VACCINES (*Continued*)

DISESAE*	WHO SHOULD BE VACCINATED
Pertussis (whooping cough)	All adults (usually given as a combination vaccine with tetanus and diphtheria)
Pneumococcal infections (such as meningitis and pneumonia)	Adults at increased risk, such as the following: ■ People over 65 ■ People with a chronic disorder, especially a heart or lung disorder ■ People with spinal fluid leakage ■ People with a weakened immune system ■ People who do not have a functioning spleen ■ Alcoholics
Polio	Adults at increased risk, such as travelers to areas where polio is common
Rabies	People who have been bitten by certain animals
Rubella (German measles)	All adults who have not had the infection or two doses of the vaccine, usually given as a combination vaccine with measles and mumps
Shingles (herpes zoster)	People over 60
Smallpox	Not currently recommended except for military personnel
Tetanus	All adults (boosters every 10 years after the primary series, which is usually given during childhood as a combination vaccine with diphtheria and tetanus)
Tuberculosis (bacille Calmette-Guérin, or BCG)	Not usually used in the United States
Typhoid	People traveling to areas where the disease is common
Yellow fever	People traveling to certain parts of Africa and South America, where the disease is common

*Vaccines are available In the United States for these diseases.

age 2 months, 4 months, 6 months, 15 to 18 months, and 4 to 6 years. Because pertussis is becoming more common among adults, a booster is recommended at age 11 to 12 years to be followed by a tetanus-diphtheria booster every 10 years. Adults who missed the series of vaccinations given during childhood should get it as adults.

Side Effects: The injection site may become sore, swollen, and red. Serious side effects are rare. They include high fever, inconsolable crying, seizures, and a severe allergic reaction. Serious side effects usually result from the pertussis part of the vaccine. If they occur, the pertussis vaccine is not used again. A vaccine against diphtheria and tetanus may be used instead to complete the vaccination series. The vaccine is not repeated if seizures occur 3 to 7 days after the vaccine is given.

Haemophilus influenzae Type b

The *Haemophilus influenzae* type b (Hib) vaccine helps protect against bacterial infections due to Hib, such as pneumonia and meningitis. These infections may be serious in children. Use of the vaccine has decreased the incidence of serious infections in children by 99%. These infections are uncommon in adults.

Different formulations of the vaccine are available.

Administration: The vaccine is given as an injection into a muscle. Doses are given at age 2 months and 4 months or at age 2 months, 4 months, and 6 months, depending on which formulation is used. In either case, a final dose is given at age 12 to 15 months (for a total of three or four doses). All children should be vaccinated. Adults at increased risk of these infections (such as those with a weakened immune system) may benefit from this vaccination.

Side Effects: Occasionally, the injection site becomes sore, swollen, and red.

Hepatitis A

The hepatitis A vaccine helps protect against hepatitis A. Typically, hepatitis A is less serious than hepatitis B. Hepatitis A often causes no symptoms, although it can cause fever, nausea, vomiting, and jaundice. Hepatitis A does not lead to chronic hepatitis. Use of the vaccine has reduced the number of people who become infected.

Administration: The hepatitis A vaccine is given as an injection into a muscle. Two doses are given to all children: typically at age 12 to 18 months and 6 to 12 months later. It is also recommended for adults at increased risk of the infection.

Side Effects: Sometimes the injection site is sore. No serious side effects have been reported.

Hepatitis B

The hepatitis B vaccine helps protect against hepatitis B. Generally, hepatitis B is more serious than hepatitis A and is occasionally fatal. Symptoms can be mild or severe. They include decreased appetite, nausea, and fatigue. In 5 to 10% of people, hepatitis B becomes chronic.

Administration: The vaccine is typically given in a series of three injections into a muscle. However, if people who have been vaccinated are exposed to the virus, a doctor measures their antibody levels against hepatitis B. If the antibody levels are low, they may need another injection of hepatitis B vaccine.

Vaccination is recommended for all children and adults, especially for adults at high risk of exposure to the hepatitis B virus.

Side Effects: Occasionally, the injection site becomes sore, and a mild fever develops. People with a history of severe allergic reaction to baker's yeast, which is used in the production of the vaccine, should not be given the vaccine.

Herpes Zoster

The herpes zoster vaccine helps reduce the risk of shingles (herpes zoster) and the residual pain it can cause (postherpetic neuralgia). The herpes zoster virus is the same virus that causes chickenpox. After chickenpox resolves, the virus remains in the body. It can be reactivated years later and cause shingles, which is a painful rash, usually on only one part of the body. The rash resolves after several weeks, but postherpetic neuralgia can last for months or years.

The vaccine is similar to the varicella vaccine and contains live virus.

Administration: The vaccine is given in one dose as an injection under the skin. It can be given to people over 60.

Side Effects: Rarely, the injection site becomes sore.

Human Papillomavirus

The human papillomavirus (HPV) vaccine helps protect against cervical cancer and genital warts, which are caused by the human papillomavirus.

Administration: The vaccine is given as an injection into a muscle in three doses: initially, then at 2 and 6 months after the first dose. It is recommended for girls aged 11 to 13 years but can be given up to age 26.

Side Effects: The injection site sometimes becomes sore, swollen, and red. No serious side effects have been reported.

Influenza

The influenza virus vaccine helps protect against influenza. There are two types of influenza virus, type A and type B, and many different strains within each type. The strains of virus that cause influenza outbreaks change each year. Thus, a new vaccine is needed each year.

Influenza can be mild, causing fever, aches, and fatigue, but it can be serious, sometimes causing death—usually in children under age 1 year or in people over 65.

Administration: The vaccine is given as a single injection into the muscle. The vaccine is recommended for children aged 6 to 59 months, people over 50, and others who are at increased risk. Also, the vaccine is usually given to anyone who requests it.

Influenza vaccine is available as an injection or a nasal spray. The nasal spray, which contains live virus, is recommended only for healthy people who are aged 2 to 49 and not pregnant.

Influenza epidemics usually begin in late December or midwinter. Therefore, the best time to get the vaccine is in September or October. A vaccine against avian influenza has been developed in case the virus becomes able to spread from person to person.

> **? Did You Know...**
> People with an egg allergy may have an allergic reaction to the influenza vaccine because it is made from viruses grown in eggs.

Side Effects: Occasionally, the injection site becomes sore. Very rarely, the vaccine causes Guillain-Barré syndrome, a progressive nerve disorder. The nasal spray sometimes causes a runny nose and sore throat. People who have a severe allergy to eggs may have a severe allergic reaction to the vaccine because the vaccine is made from viruses grown in eggs.

Measles, Mumps, and Rubella

The measles, mumps, and rubella (MMR) vaccine is a combination vaccine that helps protect against these three viral infections:

- Measles causes a rash, fever, and cough. It affects mainly children. In healthy children, it is rarely serious.

However, it can lead to brain damage or pneumonia and is occasionally fatal.

- Mumps causes the salivary glands to swell and become painful. Mumps can affect the testes, brain, and pancreas, especially in adults. Mumps is more serious in adults.
- Rubella (German measles) causes a runny nose, swollen lymph nodes, and a rash with a light reddening of the skin, especially the face. In adults, it may cause joint pain. If pregnant women get rubella, they may miscarry, the fetus may die, or the baby may have birth defects.

Administration: The vaccine is given as an injection under the skin. Two doses are given: at age 12 to 15 months and typically at age 4 to 6 years. If people born after 1956 have never had any one of these infections and have not received two doses of the vaccine, they should be given at least one dose of the vaccine. Adults who are likely to be exposed to these diseases (such as those beginning college, joining the military, working in schools or child care centers, or traveling internationally) should get a second dose of the vaccine.

Pregnant women and people who are have had serious allergic reactions to gelatin or to the antibiotic neomycin should not be vaccinated.

There are individual vaccines for measles, mumps, or rubella. However, a combination vaccine that helps protect against all three is usually used. The combination vaccine is recommended because anyone who needs protection against one of these infections usually also needs protection against the other two.

Side Effects: Some people have mild side effects, such as a fever, a general feeling of illness (malaise), and a rash. Joints may become temporarily stiff and painful, usually in teenage girls and women.

Meningococcal Infections

The meningococcal vaccine protects against infections caused by the bacteria, *Neisseria meningitidis*, which can lead to meningitis or death. These bacteria are the leading cause of bacterial meningitis in children and the second leading cause of bacterial meningitis in adults. The infection can cause the following symptoms:

- Initially, fever, nausea, headache, and leg pain
- Later, a rash, decreased blood pressure, and cold hands and feet
- Progression from feeling well to being very sick within hours

Administration: The vaccine is given in one dose as an injection under the skin or into a muscle. Two formulations are available in the United States: the polysaccharide vaccine for children aged 2 to 10 years and the conjugate vaccine for people aged 11 years or older.

The meningococcal vaccine is recommended for all children at age 11 to 12 years. It is also recommended for the following:

- Children aged 2 to 10 years if they have a weakened immune system, sickle cell disease, or a chronic infection
- Adolescents entering high school if they have not already been vaccinated
- All college students living in dormitories and military recruits if they have not already been vaccinated
- Travelers to areas where the disease is common
- Adults who do not have a functioning spleen

Side Effects: The injection site may become sore, swollen, and red. A few people have a mild fever and fatigue. Guillain-Barré syndrome developed in a few people after they were vaccinated with the conjugate vaccine. Thus, this vaccine should not be given to people who have had this syndrome.

Pneumococcal Infection

Pneumococcal vaccines help protect against bacterial infections caused by *Streptococcus pneumoniae*, such as ear infections, sinusitis, pneumonia, and meningitis.

Administration: Two formulations of the pneumococcal vaccine are available. The conjugate vaccine is given typically at age 2 months, 4 months, 6 months, and 12 to 15 months. The polysaccharide vaccine is given to older children at high risk of developing pneumonia or another pneumococcal infection in two doses: at age 24 months and 3 to 5 years later. The polysaccharide vaccine is also recommended for older children and adults who are at high risk of developing these infections.

The polysaccharide vaccine is effective in about two of three adults, although it is less effective in debilitated older people. It is more effective in preventing some of the serious complications of pneumococcal pneumonia than in preventing the pneumonia itself. Although one injection of the vaccine may provide lifetime protection, people at high risk are advised to be vaccinated again after 5 years.

Side Effects: Occasionally, the injection site becomes painful and red. Other side effects include fever, irritability, drowsiness, loss of appetite, and vomiting.

Polio

The polio vaccine protects against polio, a very contagious viral infection that affects the nerves. Polio can cause permanent muscle weakness, paralysis, and sometimes death.

Smallpox: A Vaccine in the Wings

The smallpox vaccine has not been routinely given in the United States for 30 years because the disease has been eliminated. Because the vaccine's protective effects wear off after about 10 years, most people are now susceptible to smallpox.

Recent fears about the possible use of smallpox by terrorists have led to the suggestion that smallpox vaccination resume. If smallpox vaccination is resumed, it is likely to be recommended only for people in the area of a smallpox outbreak. Military personnel are now vaccinated, and enough smallpox vaccine has been prepared to vaccinate everyone in the United States if needed.

The vaccine is generally safe, although serious adverse effects occur in about 100 of every million previously unvaccinated people, and death occurs in 1 per million. The risk of serious adverse effects and death is lower in previously vaccinated people.

The vaccine is most effective when given very early after exposure. However, the vaccine may also be beneficial if given in the first days after symptoms appear. There is no treatment for smallpox.

Two formulations are available. One contains killed virus and is injected. The other contains live, weakened virus and is taken by mouth. The live-virus vaccine is no longer available in the United States because it causes polio in about 1 of every 2.4 million people who receive the vaccine.

Administration: The vaccine is given in four doses: at age 2 months, 4 months, 6 to 18 months, and 4 to 6 years. Because polio is now so rare in the United States, unvaccinated people over 18 years are not given the vaccine unless they are traveling to an area where polio is common.

Side Effects: People who have allergies to the antibiotics streptomycin, neomycin, or polymyxin B may have an allergic reaction to the vaccine. The vaccine may contain small amounts of these antibiotics.

Rotavirus

The rotavirus vaccine helps protect against gastroenteritis, which causes vomiting, diarrhea, and, if symptoms persist, dehydration.

Administration: This vaccine is part of the recommended vaccination schedule for children. Three doses are given: at age 2 months, 4 months, and 6 months.

Side Effects: No severe side effects have been reported, but mild, temporary diarrhea occurs in 1 to 3% of children within 7 days of receiving the vaccine.

Tetanus

The tetanus vaccine protects against the toxin produced by the tetanus bacteria, not the bacteria itself. Typically, the bacteria enter the body through a wound and begin to grow and produce the toxin. The toxin causes severe muscle spasms and can be fatal. Therefore, vaccination is particularly important.

Administration: The vaccine is typically given during childhood, as part of the diphtheria, tetanus, and pertussis vaccine (see page 1145). The combination vaccine is given in five injections, followed by a booster that contains the same amount of tetanus vaccine but a smaller amount of diphtheria and pertussis vaccine. The booster is given at age 11 to 12 years. Because immunity against pertussis is decreasing, people aged 16 to 64 should receive this booster if they have not received it previously. A booster of the tetanus vaccine is recommended every 10 years thereafter. Also, people sometimes need to be vaccinated after an injury.

Side Effects: Sometimes the injection site is sore, swollen, and red. Serious side effects are rare and include severe allergic reactions.

Varicella

The varicella vaccine helps protect against chickenpox (varicella), a very contagious infection caused by the varicella-zoster virus. It causes an itchy rash that looks like small blisters with a red base. In some people, the brain, lungs, heart, and joints become infected. The virus remains in the body. If it is reactivated, it can cause shingles years later.

Administration: Vaccination against varicella is part of the routine vaccination schedule recommended for children. The vaccine is given as an injection under the skin. Two doses are given: at age 12 to 15 months and at age 4 to 6 years. It is also recommended for all adolescents and adults who have not had the vaccine or the disease. It is given to them in two doses 4 to 8 weeks apart.

Because the vaccine contains live virus, it is not given to pregnant women, people with a weakened immune system, or people with cancer of the bone marrow or lymphatic system.

Side Effects: The vaccine is safe, and side effects are mild. In fewer than one fourth of the people who get the vaccine, the injection site becomes painful, swollen, and red. Very occasionally, a chickenpox-like rash develops.

Taking aspirin and related drugs (salicylates) after vaccination can cause Reye's syndrome in children under 16 years old. Thus, such children should not be given these drugs for 6 weeks after vaccination.

Vaccination Before Foreign Travel

Residents of the United States may be required to receive specific vaccines before traveling to areas that have infectious diseases not normally found in the United States (see table on page 2101). Recommendations change frequently in response to disease outbreaks. The Centers for Disease Control and Prevention (CDC) provide the most up-to-date information on vaccination requirements in their Travelers' Health section.

---

174 Bacterial Infections

Bacteria are microscopic, single-celled organisms. There are thousands of different kinds, and they live in every conceivable environment all over the world. They live in soil, seawater, and deep within the earth's crust. Some bacteria have been reported even to live in radioactive waste. Some bacteria live in the bodies of people and animals—on the skin and in the airways, mouth, and digestive, reproductive, and urinary tracts—often without causing any harm.

Only a few kinds of bacteria cause disease. They are called pathogens. Sometimes bacteria that normally reside harmlessly in the body cause disease. Bacteria can cause disease by producing harmful substances (toxins), invading tissues, or doing both.

Classification

Bacteria can be classified in several ways:

- **Scientific names:** Bacteria, like other living things, are classified by genus (based on having one or several similar characteristics) and, within the genus, by species. Their scientific name is genus followed by species (for example, *Clostridium botulinum*). Within a species, there may be different types, called strains. Strains differ in genetic makeup and chemical components. Sometimes certain drugs and vaccines are effective only against certain strains.

- **Staining:** Bacteria may be classified by the color they turn after certain chemicals (stains) are applied to them. A commonly used stain is the Gram stain. Some bacteria stain blue. They are called gram-positive. Others stain pink. They are called gram-negative. Gram-positive and gram-negative bacteria stain differently because their cell walls are different. They also cause different types of infections, and different types of antibiotics are effective against them.

- **Shapes:** All bacteria may be classified as one of three basic shapes: spheres (cocci), rods (bacilli), and spirals or helixes (spirochetes).

- **Need for oxygen:** Bacteria are also classified by whether they need oxygen to live and grow. Those that need oxygen are called aerobes. Those that have trouble living or growing when oxygen is present are called anaerobes. Some bacteria, called facultative bacteria, can live and grow with or without oxygen.

Bacterial Defenses

Bacteria have many ways of defending themselves.

Biofilm: Some bacteria secrete a substance that helps them attach to other bacteria, cells, or objects. This substance combines with the bacteria to form a sticky layer called biofilm. For example, certain bacteria form a biofilm on teeth (called dental plaque). The biofilm traps food particles, which the bacteria process and use, and in this process, they probably cause tooth decay. Biofilms also help protect bacteria from antibiotics.

Capsules: Some bacteria are enclosed in a protective capsule. This capsule helps prevent white blood cells, which fight infection, from ingesting the bacteria. Such bacteria are described as encapsulated.

Outer Membrane: Under the capsule, gram-negative bacteria have an outer membrane that protects them against certain antibiotics. When disrupted, this membrane releases toxic substances called endotoxins. Endotoxins contribute to the severity of symptoms during infections with gram-negative bacteria.

Spores: Some bacteria produce spores, which are an inactive (dormant) form. Spores can enable bacteria to survive when environmental conditions are difficult. When conditions are favorable, each spore germinates into an active bacterium.

Flagella: Flagella are long, thin filaments that protrude from the cell surface and enable bacteria to move. Bacteria without flagella cannot move on their own.

Antibiotic Resistance: Bacteria develop resistance to drugs because they acquire genes from other bacteria that have become resistant or because their genes mutate. For example, soon after the drug penicillin

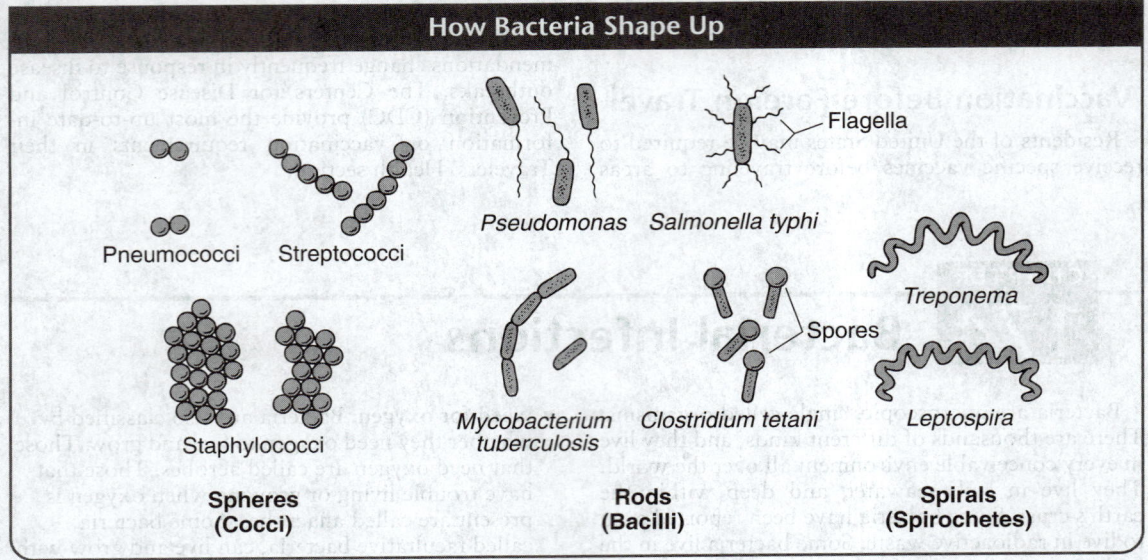

How Bacteria Shape Up

Pneumococci   Streptococci

Pseudomonas   *Salmonella typhi*   — Flagella

Staphylococci

Mycobacterium tuberculosis   *Clostridium tetani* — Spores

Treponema

Leptospira

Spheres (Cocci)   **Rods (Bacilli)**   **Spirals (Spirochetes)**

was introduced in the mid-1940s, a few individual *Staphylococcus aureus* bacteria acquired genes that made penicillin ineffective against them. The strains that possessed these special genes had a survival advantage when penicillin was commonly used to treat infections. Strains of *Staphylococcus aureus* that lacked these new genes were killed by penicillin, allowing the remaining penicillin-resistant bacteria to reproduce and over time become dominant. Chemists then altered the penicillin molecule, making a different but similar drug, methicillin, which could kill the penicillin-resistant bacteria. Soon after methicillin was introduced, strains of *Staphylococcus aureus* developed genes that made them resistant to methicillin and related drugs. These strains are called methicillin-resistant *Staphylococcus aureus* (MRSA). The genes that encode for drug resistance can be passed to following generations of bacteria or sometimes even to other species of bacteria.

The more often antibiotics are used, the more likely resistant bacteria are to develop. Therefore, doctors try to use antibiotics only when they are necessary. Giving antibiotics to people who probably do not have a bacterial infection, such as those who have cough and cold symptoms, does not make people better but does help create resistant bacteria. Because antibiotics have been so widely used (and misused), many bacteria are resistant to certain antibiotics.

Resistant bacteria can spread from person to person. Because international travel is so common, resistant bacteria can spread to many parts of the world in a short time. Spread of these bacteria in hospitals is a particular concern. Resistant bacteria are common in hospitals because antibiotics are so often necessary and hospital personnel and visitors may spread the bacteria if they do not strictly follow appropriate sanitary procedures. Also, many hospitalized patients have a weakened immune system, making them more susceptible to infection.

? Did You Know...

Botulinum toxin, produced by clostridial bacteria, can cause food poisoning and muscle paralysis but can also be used to reduce wrinkles and to treat muscle spasms.

Resistant bacteria can also spread to people from animals. Resistant bacteria are common among farm animals because antibiotics are often routinely given to healthy animals to prevent infections that can impair growth or cause illness.

Actinomycosis

Actinomycosis is a chronic infection caused mainly by Actinomyces israelii, anaerobic bacteria that normally reside on the enamel of teeth, gums, tonsils, and membranes lining the intestines and vagina.

- Infection occurs only when tissue is broken, enabling the bacteria to enter deeper tissues.

- Abscesses form in various areas, such as the intestine or face, causing pain, fever, and other symptoms.
- Symptoms suggest the diagnosis, and doctors confirm it by taking x-rays and identifying the bacteria in a sample of infected tissue.
- Abscesses are drained, and antibiotics are given.
- With treatment, most people recover fully.

These bacteria cause infection only when the surface of the tissue on which they reside is broken, enabling them to enter other, deeper tissues, which have no defenses against them. As the infection spreads, scar tissue and abnormal channels (called fistulas or tracts) form. After months to years, fistulas may eventually reach the skin and allow pus to drain. Pockets of pus (abscesses) may develop in the chest, abdomen, face, or neck.

Men are affected most often, but actinomycosis occasionally develops in women who use an intrauterine device (IUD).

Symptoms

Actinomycosis has several forms. All cause abscesses.

Abdominal: The bacteria infect the intestine, usually the area near the appendix, and the lining of the abdominal cavity (peritoneum). Chronic abdominal pain, fever, vomiting, diarrhea or constipation, and severe weight loss are common symptoms. Fistulas may form from the interior of the abdomen to the skin above it and between the intestine and other organs.

Pelvic: The bacteria spread to the uterus, usually from an IUD that has been in place for years. Abscesses and scar tissue may form in the fallopian tubes, ovaries, and nearby organs such as the bladder and ureters. Fistulas may form between these organs. Symptoms include chronic abdominal or pelvic pain, fever, weight loss, and vaginal bleeding and discharge.

Cervicofacial: Usually, small, hard, sometimes painful swellings develop in the mouth and on the face, neck, or skin below the jaw (lumpy jaw). These swellings may soften and discharge pus that contains small, round, yellowish granules. The infection may extend to the cheek, tongue, throat, salivary glands, skull, bones of the neck (cervical vertebrae) and face, brain, or the space within the tissues covering the brain (meninges).

Thoracic: This form affects the chest (thorax). People have chronic chest pain and fever. They lose weight and cough, sometimes bringing up sputum. People probably become infected when they inhale fluids that contain bacteria from their mouth. Abscesses may form in the lungs and eventually spread to the membrane between the lungs and chest wall (pleura). There, abscesses cause irritation (pleuritis), and infected fluid collects (called an empyema). Fistulas may form, enabling the infection to spread to the ribs, skin of the chest, and spine.

Generalized: Rarely, the bacteria are carried in the bloodstream to infect other organs, such as the brain, lungs, liver, kidneys, and heart valves.

Diagnosis

Doctors suspect the infection in people who have typical symptoms. Then, x-rays are taken, and samples of pus or tissue are obtained and checked for *Actinomyces israelii*. Often, a needle is inserted through the skin to take a sample from an abscess or infected tissue. Sometimes computed tomography (CT) or ultrasonography is used to help doctors place the needle in the infected area. Sometimes surgery is necessary to remove a sample.

Characteristic x-ray findings and identification of the bacteria in a sample confirm the diagnosis.

Treatment

Treatment consists of draining abscesses with a needle (usually inserted through the skin) and giving high doses of antibiotics such as penicillin or tetracycline. Antibiotics may be needed for as long as 6 to 12 months.

Bacteria in the Body

The body normally contains several hundred different species of bacteria but many trillions of individual bacteria. The bacteria outnumber the cells of the body by about 10 to 1. Most of these bacteria reside on the skin and teeth, in the spaces between teeth and gums, and in the mucous membranes that line the throat, intestine, and vagina. The species differ at each site, reflecting the different environment at each site. Many of them are anaerobes—that is, they do not require oxygen.

Usually, these anaerobes do not cause disease. Many have useful functions, such as helping break down food in the intestine. However, these bacteria can cause disease if the mucous membranes are damaged. Then, bacteria can enter tissues that are usually off-limits to them and that have no defenses against them. The bacteria may infect nearby structures (such as the sinuses, middle ear, lungs, brain, abdomen, pelvis, and skin) or enter the bloodstream and spread.

What Are Clostridia?

Clostridia are bacteria that normally reside in the intestine of 3 to 8% of healthy adults and even more newborns. Clostridia also reside in animals, soil, and decaying vegetation. These bacteria do not require oxygen to live. That is, they are anaerobes.

Clostridia cause disease in different ways, depending on the species:

- They may produce a toxin in food, which is then consumed, as occurs in foodborne botulism.
- They may produce a toxin after they are in the body if circumstances enable them to multiply excessively (overgrow), as occurs in tetanus, *Clostridium perfringens* food poisoning, and a type of antibiotic-associated diarrhea and colitis called *Clostridium difficile*–induced diarrhea and colitis.
- They may produce a toxin and invade tissue, causing infection, as occurs in gas gangrene.

Clostridia can infect the gallbladder, colon, and female reproductive organs. Rarely, one species, *Clostridium sordellii*, causes toxic shock syndrome in women who have infections of the reproductive organs.

Clostridia may also spread to the blood (causing bacteremia). Widespread bacteremia (sepsis) can cause fever and serious symptoms such as low blood pressure, jaundice, and anemia. Sepsis can develop after a clostridial infection and be rapidly fatal.

Foodborne botulism can develop when people eat food that contains botulinum toxin, produced by *Clostridium botulinum*. Usually, botulism results from eating uncooked or undercooked food because heat (cooking) destroys the toxin. Botulinum toxin enters the bloodstream from the small intestine and is carried to nerves. This toxin prevents nerves from sending impulses to muscles. About 18 to 36 hours after consuming the toxin, people become tired and dizzy. Their mouth becomes dry. They may feel nauseated and vomit. The abdomen may swell (distend), and constipation may develop. Muscles of the face become slack or paralyzed, causing the eyelids and face to droop and vision to blur. Swallowing and talking become difficult. The muscle weakness then spreads to the upper torso and downward. The muscles involved in breathing may weaken—a problem that may become life threatening.

Clostridium perfringens **food poisoning** can develop when people eat food (usually beef) that contains bacteria (rather than the bacteria's toxin). The bacteria develop from spores, which are inactive (dormant) forms of the bacteria that can survive the heat of cooking. If food that contains spores is not eaten soon after it is cooked, the spores develop into bacteria, which then multiply in the food. If the food is served without adequate reheating, the bacteria are consumed. They multiply in the small intestine and produce a toxin that causes watery diarrhea and abdominal cramping. This type of food poisoning is usually mild but can cause serious problems in older people. Rarely, certain strains of these bacteria produce a toxin that damages the intestine and causes an infection called necrotizing enteritis, which is often fatal.

Clostridium difficile–**induced diarrhea and colitis** (inflammation of the colon) can develop after antibiotics are taken to treat an infection (see page 176). Antibiotics may destroy some of the bacteria that normally reside in the intestine. If enough are destroyed, *Clostridium difficile* may overgrow. These bacteria may already be present in the intestine. Or people may get them from other people, pets, or the environment. Being very young or very old, staying in a hospital or nursing home, or having one or more severe disorders increases the risk of this disorder. When the bacteria overgrow, they release two toxins. One causes the intestine to produce fluids and abnormal membranes to form. The other damages the lining of the large intestine.

CT or magnetic resonance imaging (MRI) may be used to determine whether abscesses are resolving. Surgery, with or without antibiotics, may be necessary, particularly if the infection affects critical areas such as the spine.

If actinomycosis is diagnosed early and treated appropriately, most people recover fully.

Anthrax

Anthrax is a potentially fatal infection with Bacillus anthracis, *which may affect the skin, the lungs, or, rarely, the digestive (gastrointestinal) tract.*

- Infection in people usually results from skin contact but can result from inhaling spores or eating contaminated meat.

- Symptoms include bumps and blisters (after skin contact), difficulty breathing and chest pain (after inhaling spores), and abdominal pain and bloody diarrhea (after eating contaminated meat).
- Symptoms suggest the infection, and identifying the bacteria in samples taken from infected tissue confirms the diagnosis.
- People at high risk of being exposed to anthrax are vaccinated.
- Antibiotics must be given soon after exposure to reduce the risk of dying.

Anthrax can occur in wild and domestic animals that graze, such as cattle, sheep, and goats. Anthrax bacteria produce spores that can live for years in soil. Grazing animals become infected when they have contact with or consume the spores. Usually, anthrax is transmitted to people when they have contact with infected animals or animal products (such as wool, hides, and hair). Spores may remain in animal products for decades and are not easily killed by cold or heat. Even minimal contact is likely to result in infection. Although infection in people usually occurs through the skin, it can also result from inhaling spores or eating contaminated, undercooked meat. Anthrax cannot spread from person to person.

Anthrax is a potential biological weapon because anthrax spores can be spread through the air and inhaled.

Anthrax bacteria produce several toxins, which cause many of the symptoms.

Symptoms

Symptoms vary depending on how the infection is acquired: through the skin, through inhalation, or through the gastrointestinal tract.

Skin Anthrax: More than 95% of cases involve the skin. A painless, itchy, red-brown bump appears 1 to 12 days after exposure. The bump forms a blister, which eventually breaks open and forms a black scab (eschar), with swelling around it. Nearby lymph nodes may swell, and people may feel ill—sometimes with muscle aches, headache, fever, nausea, and vomiting. About 20% of untreated people die, but with treatment, death is rare.

Inhalation Anthrax (Woolsorter's Disease): This form is the most serious. It results from inhaling anthrax spores. Spores may stay in the lungs for weeks but eventually enter white blood cells, where they germinate, and the resulting bacteria multiply and spread to lymph nodes in the chest. The bacteria produce toxins that make the lymph nodes swell, break down, and bleed, spreading the infection to nearby structures. Infected fluid accumulates in the space between the lungs and the chest wall.

Symptoms develop 1 to 43 days after exposure. Initially, they are vague and similar to those of influenza, with mild muscle aches, a low fever, chest discomfort, and a dry cough. After a few days, breathing suddenly becomes very difficult, and people have chest pain and a high fever with sweating. Blood pressure rapidly becomes dangerously low (causing shock), followed by coma. These severe symptoms probably result from a massive release of toxins. Infection of the brain and the fluid around the meninges (an infection called meningoencephalitis) frequently develops. Many people die 24 to 36 hours after severe symptoms start, even with early treatment. Without treatment, all people with inhalation anthrax die. In the 2001 outbreak in the United States, 5 of the 11 people treated for inhalation anthrax died.

Gastrointestinal Anthrax: Gastrointestinal anthrax is rare. When people eat contaminated meat, the bacteria grow in the mouth, throat, or intestine and release toxins that cause extensive bleeding and tissue death. People have a fever, a sore throat, a swollen neck, abdominal pain, and bloody diarrhea. They also vomit blood. At least half of untreated people with gastrointestinal anthrax die. With treatment, about half of people die.

? Did You Know...

Anthrax spores are not easily killed by cold or heat and can survive for decades.

Over 1.25 million people have received the anthrax vaccine without having a serious adverse reaction.

Diagnosis

Doctors suspect skin anthrax based on its typical appearance. Knowing that people have had contact with animals or animal products or were in an area where other people developed anthrax supports the diagnosis. If inhalation anthrax is suspected, chest x-ray and computed tomography (CT) are done.

Samples from infected skin, fluids around the lungs, or stool are removed and examined with a microscope or cultured (enabling bacteria, if present, to multiply). Anthrax bacteria, if present, can be readily identified. If people have inhalation anthrax, doctors may also take samples of the sputum or blood or do a spinal tap (lumbar puncture) to obtain a sample of the fluid that surrounds the brain and spinal cord (cerebrospinal fluid). The samples are examined and analyzed. Blood tests may be done to check for fragments of the bacteria's genetic material or antibodies to the toxins produced by the bacteria.

Prevention and Treatment

A vaccine against anthrax can be given to people at high risk of infection. Because of anthrax's potential as a biological weapon, most members of the armed forces have been vaccinated. To be effective, the vaccine must be given in six doses. Despite widely publicized anxiety, over 1.25 million people have received the anthrax vaccine without having serious adverse reactions.

People who are exposed to anthrax may be given an antibiotic by mouth, usually ciprofloxacin or doxycycline or, if they cannot take these antibiotics, amoxicillin. The antibiotic is continued for 60 days to prevent the infection from developing. People may not need to take the antibiotic as long if they are also given several doses of anthrax vaccine.

OTHER BACTERIAL INFECTIONS

SOURCE	SYMPTOMS	TREATMENT	COMMENTS
Brucellosis (*Brucella* bacteria)			
Domestic animals, deer, elk, and buffalo Unpasteurized contaminated milk and other dairy products	Fever that may return repeatedly for months to years, night sweats, loss of appetite, weight loss, low back pain, bone and joint pain, and depression	Doxycycline, given by mouth, plus streptomycin, injected daily	Risk is increased for travelers who consume unpasteurized milk or cheese in areas where brucellosis is common and for laboratory workers, meat packers, veterinarians, farmers, and livestock producers, who may handle infected animal tissue. Sometimes infection develops in the back bones (vertebrae), long bones, joints, or heart valves. The bacteria can be spread through the air (in an aerosol) and thus could be used in biological warfare.
Cat-scratch disease (*Bartonella henselae*)			
Domestic cats	At the site of a cat scratch, a red blister that ruptures and forms a crust Swelling of nearby lymph nodes, which become tender and fill with pus, sometimes after the scratch has healed Occasionally, drainage of pus from the lymph nodes to the skin	Application of heat, pain relievers, and sometimes azithromycin	Most domestic cats throughout the world are infected, but most show no signs of illness. Cat-scratch disease usually resolves on its own. But if the immune system is weakened, as occurs in people with human immunodeficiency virus (HIV) infection or AIDS, infection can spread throughout the body and be fatal without treatment. Such people can avoid the infection by avoiding domestic cats.
Erysipeloid (*Erysipelothrix rhusiopathiae*)			
Puncture wound or scrape that occurs while handling animal matter (such as infected carcasses or fish)	At the site of injury, a purplish red, hard area, which may itch and burn	Penicillin or erythromycin	Risk is increased for butchers, farmers, cooks, and fishermen. Rarely, the bacteria spread through the bloodstream and infect the joints or heart valves.

(continued on the following page)

OTHER BACTERIAL INFECTIONS (*Continued*)

SOURCE	SYMPTOMS	TREATMENT	COMMENTS
Gonorrhea (*Neisseria gonorrhoeae*)			
Sexual contact with infected people	A discharge from the urethra or vagina and pain during urination	A single injection of ceftriaxone into a muscle	Occasionally, these bacteria spread through the bloodstream and infect the skin or joints. About half of affected people also have a chlamydial infection that must be treated simultaneously with azithromycin or doxycycline.
Relapsing fever (*Borrelia* species)			
Body lice and soft-bodied ticks, often carried by rats	Sudden chills followed by a high fever (fevers come and go at 1- to 2-week intervals) Severe headache, red eyes, a dry cough, vomiting, muscle and joint pain, a reddish rash on the trunk and limbs, jaundice, an enlarged liver and spleen, and an irregular heart rhythm	Tetracycline, erythromycin, doxycycline, or penicillin	In the United States, tick-borne infection usually occurs only in the western mountain states, and louse-borne infection is rare. Campers may be bitten by infected ticks. Complications can include a tendency to bleed, eye inflammation (iridocyclitis), and, in pregnant women, miscarriage. Within 2 hours after the first dose of the antibiotic, a dangerous reaction (Jarisch-Herxheimer reaction) may occur, causing sweating, shaking chills, fever, and a fall in blood pressure.

The longer treatment is delayed, the greater the risk of death. Thus, treatment is usually started as soon as anthrax is first suspected:

- Skin anthrax is treated with ciprofloxacin or doxycycline given by mouth.
- Inhalation or gastrointestinal anthrax is treated with a combination of antibiotics, including intravenous ciprofloxacin or doxycycline plus clindamycin, with or without rifampin. Corticosteroids may help relieve symptoms of inhalational anthrax.

Bejel, Yaws, and Pinta

Bejel, yaws (frambesia), and pinta are infections caused by bacteria (called treponemal spirochetes) that are closely related to Treponema pallidum, *which causes the sexually transmitted disease syphilis.*

- These very contagious infections are usually spread in areas where hygiene is poor.
- Bejel causes mouth sores and destructive lumps in bone, yaws causes skin sores and disfiguring growths on the legs and around the nose and mouth, and pinta causes itchy patches on the skin.
- Doctors diagnose these infections when people have typical symptoms and have spent time in areas where the infections are common.
- One injection of penicillin kills the bacteria.

Bejel, yaws, and pinta are treponematoses, as is syphilis. Unlike syphilis, these infections are transmitted by nonsexual contact—chiefly between children living in conditions of poor hygiene. Bejel may be spread when eating utensils are shared.

Bejel occurs mainly in the hot arid countries of the eastern Mediterranean region and Saharan West Africa. Yaws occurs in humid equatorial countries. Pinta is common among the natives of Mexico, Central America, and South America. Bejel, yaws, and pinta rarely occur in the United States, except among immigrants from areas of the world where these diseases are common.

Symptoms

Yaws and pinta, like syphilis, begin with skin symptoms. Bejel begins with mouth sores. These symptoms subside, and after a period with few or no symptoms, new symptoms develop.

Bejel affects the mucous membranes of the mouth, then the skin and bones. The initial mouth sore may not be noticed. Moist patches then develop in the mouth. They resolve over a period of months to years. During this time, people have few or no symptoms. Then, lumps develop in long bones, mainly leg bones, and in the tissues around the mouth, nose, and roof of the mouth (palate). These lumps destroy tissue, causing bones to be deformed and disfiguring the face.

Yaws also affects the skin and bones. Several weeks after exposure to *Treponema*, yaws begins as a slightly raised sore at the site of infection, usually on a leg. The sore heals, but soft nodules (granulomas) form, then break open on the face, arms, legs, and buttocks. The granulomas heal slowly and may recur. Painful open sores on the soles of the feet (crab yaws) may develop, making walking difficult. Later, areas of the shinbones may be destroyed, and many other destructive, disfiguring growths (gangosa), especially around the nose, mouth, and palate, may develop.

Pinta affects only the skin. It begins as flat, itchy, reddened areas on the hands, feet, legs, arms, face, or neck. After several months, slate-blue patches develop in the same areas on both sides of the body. They develop where bones are close to skin, for example, on the elbow. Later, the patches lose their color. The affected skin on the palms and soles may thicken.

Diagnosis

Doctors make the diagnosis when typical symptoms appear in people who live in or have visited an area where such infections are common. Because the bacteria that cause these infections and the bacteria that cause syphilis are so similar, people who have one of these infections test positive for syphilis.

Treatment

A single injection of penicillin kills the bacteria. Then, the skin can heal. However, some scarring may remain, particularly if a lot of tissue has been destroyed.

People who are allergic to penicillin are given tetracycline if they are 8 years old or older or erythromycin if they are pregnant or under 8 years old. These drugs are given by mouth.

Because the infections are very contagious, public health officials try to identify and treat infected people and their close contacts.

Campylobacter Infections

Several species of Campylobacter *(most commonly* Campylobacter jejuni*) can infect the digestive tract, often causing diarrhea.*

- People can be infected when they consume contaminated food or drink or have contact with infected people or animals.
- These infections cause diarrhea, abdominal pain, and fever.
- Identifying the bacteria in a stool sample confirms the diagnosis.
- For some people, replacing lost fluids is all that is needed, but if symptoms are severe, antibiotics are also needed.

Campylobacter bacteria normally inhabit the digestive tract of many farm animals (including cattle, sheep, pigs, and fowl). The feces of these animals may contaminate water in lakes and streams. Meat (usually poultry) and unpasteurized milk may also be contaminated. People may be infected in several ways:

- Eating or drinking contaminated (untreated) water, unpasteurized milk, undercooked meat (usually poultry), or food prepared on kitchen surfaces touched by contaminated meat
- Contact with an infected person (particularly oral-anal sexual contact)
- Contact with an infected animal

Campylobacter bacteria cause inflammation of the colon (colitis) that results in fever and diarrhea. These bacteria are a common cause of infectious diarrhea in the United States and among people who travel to countries where food or water may be contaminated. Infections are most commonly caused by *Campylobacter jejuni*.

Symptoms

Symptoms usually develop 2 to 5 days after exposure and continue for about 1 week. Symptoms of *Campylobacter* colitis include diarrhea, abdominal pain, and cramps, which may be severe. The diarrhea may be bloody and can be accompanied by nausea, vomiting, and fever ranging from 100 to 104° F (38 to 40° C).

In some people with colitis, the bloodstream is temporarily infected (called bacteremia). This infection usually causes no symptoms or complications. However, the bloodstream is repeatedly or continuously infected in a few people. This type of bacteremia usually develops in people with a disorder that weakens the immune system, such as AIDS, diabetes, or cancer. This infection causes a long-lasting or recurring fever. Other symptoms develop as the bloodstream carries the infection to other structures, such as the following:

- The space within the tissues covering the brain and spinal cord (causing meningitis)
- Bones (causing osteomyelitis)
- Joints (causing infectious arthritis)
- Rarely, heart valves (causing endocarditis)

Guillain-Barré syndrome (see page 828) develops in about 1 of 1,000 of people with *Campylobacter* colitis. Guillain-Barré syndrome causes weakness or paralysis. Most people recover, but muscles may be greatly weakened. People may have difficulty breathing and need to use a mechanical ventilator. Weakness does not always completely resolve. *Campylobacter* colitis is thought to trigger about 20 to 40% of all cases of Guillain-Barré syndrome.

Weeks to months after the diarrhea resolves, reactive arthritis may develop. Usually, the disorder causes inflammation and pain in the knees, hips, and Achilles tendon.

Diagnosis

Doctors may take a sample of stool and send it to a laboratory to grow (culture) the bacteria. However, stool is not always tested. Stool cultures take days to complete, and doctors do not usually need to know which bacteria caused the diarrhea to effectively treat it. If the bacteria are identified, they are tested to see which antibiotics are effective (a process called susceptibility testing).

If doctors suspect that the bloodstream is infected, they take a sample of blood to be cultured.

Treatment

Many people get better in a week or so without specific treatment. Some people require extra fluids intravenously or by mouth. People who have a high fever, bloody or severe diarrhea, or worsening symptoms may need to take azithromycin for 3 days or erythromycin for 5 days. Both drugs are taken by mouth. If the bloodstream is infected, antibiotics such as imipenem, gentamicin, or azithromycin are required for 2 to 4 weeks.

Cholera

Cholera is a serious infection of the intestine that is caused by the bacteria Vibrio cholerae *and that causes severe diarrhea.*

- People are infected when they consume contaminated food, often seafood, or water.
- Cholera is rare except in areas where sanitation is inadequate.
- People have watery diarrhea and vomit, usually with no fever.
- Identifying the bacteria in a stool sample confirms the diagnosis.
- Replacing lost fluids and giving antibiotics treat the infection effectively.

Several species of *Vibrio* bacteria cause diarrhea (see page 149). The most serious illness, cholera, is caused by *Vibrio cholerae.* Cholera may occur in large outbreaks.

Vibrio cholerae normally lives in aquatic environments along the coast. People acquire the infection by consuming contaminated water, seafood, or other foods. Once infected, people excrete the bacteria in stool. Thus, the infection can spread rapidly, particularly in areas where human waste is untreated.

Once common throughout the world, cholera is now largely confined to developing countries in the tropics and subtropics. It is common (endemic) in parts of Asia, the Middle East, Africa, and South and Central America. Small outbreaks have occurred in Europe, Japan, and Australia. In the United States, cholera can occur along the coast of the Gulf of Mexico.

In endemic areas, outbreaks usually occur when war or civil unrest disrupts public sanitation services. Infection is most common during warm months and among children. In newly affected areas, outbreaks may occur during any season and affect all ages equally.

For infection to develop, many bacteria must be consumed. Then, there may be too many for stomach acid to kill, and some bacteria can reach the small intestine, where they grow and produce a toxin. The toxin causes the small intestine to secrete enormous amounts of salt and water. The body loses this fluid as watery diarrhea. It is the loss of water and salt that causes death. The bacteria remain in the small intestine and do not invade tissues.

Because stomach acid kills the bacteria, people who produce less stomach acid are more likely to get cholera. Such people include young children, older people, and people taking drugs that reduce stomach acid, including proton pump inhibitors (such as omeprazole) and histamine-2 (H_2) blockers (such as ranitidine). People living in endemic areas gradually acquire some immunity.

Symptoms

Most infected people have no symptoms. When symptoms occur, they begin 1 to 3 days after exposure, usually with sudden, painless, watery diarrhea and vomiting. Usually, fever is absent.

? **Did You Know...**
Without treatment, more than one half of people with severe cholera die.

Diarrhea and vomiting may be mild to severe. In severe infections, more than 1 quart of water and salts is lost per hour. The stool looks gray and has flecks of mucus in it. Within hours, dehydration can become severe, causing intense thirst, muscle cramps, and weakness. Very little urine is produced. The eyes may become sunken, and the skin on the fingers may become very wrinkled. If dehydration is not treated, loss of water and salts can lead to kidney failure, shock, coma, and death.

In people who survive, symptoms usually subside in 3 to 6 days. Most people are free of the bacteria in 2 weeks. The bacteria remain in a few people indefinitely without causing symptoms. Such people are called carriers.

Diagnosis

Doctors take a sample of stool or use a swab to obtain a sample from the rectum. It is sent to a laboratory where bacteria can be grown (cultured). Identifying *Vibrio cholerae* in the sample confirms the diagnosis.

Blood and urine tests to evaluate dehydration and kidney function are done.

Prevention

Purification of water supplies and appropriate disposal of human waste are essential. Other precautions include using boiled or chlorinated water and avoiding uncooked vegetables and undercooked fish and shellfish. Shellfish tend to carry other forms of *Vibrio* as well.

Several vaccines for cholera are available outside the United States. These vaccines provide only partial protection for a limited time and therefore are not generally recommended. New vaccines are currently being tested.

Treatment

Rapid replacement of lost body water and salts is lifesaving. Most people can be treated effectively with a solution given by mouth. These solutions are designed to replace the fluids the body has lost. For severely dehydrated people who cannot drink, a salt solution is given intravenously. In epidemics, if the intravenous solution is not available, people are sometimes given a salt solution through a tube inserted through the nose into the stomach. After enough fluids are replaced to relieve symptoms, people should

drink at least enough of the salt solution to replace the fluids they have lost through diarrhea and vomiting. Solid foods can be eaten after vomiting stops and appetite returns.

People are usually given an antibiotic to reduce the severity of diarrhea and make it stop sooner. Also, people who take an antibiotic are slightly less likely to spread the infection during an outbreak. Tetracycline or doxycycline is effective in adults, unless the bacteria in the area are resistant to tetracycline. Then, ciprofloxacin can be used. Because tetracycline and doxycycline discolor the teeth in children under 8 years old, azithromycin, erythromycin, or trimethoprim-sulfamethoxazole is used instead.

More than 50% of untreated people with severe cholera die. Less than 1% of people who receive prompt, adequate fluid replacement die.

Gas Gangrene

Gas gangrene (clostridial myonecrosis) is a life-threatening infection of muscle tissue caused mainly by the anaerobic bacteria Clostridium perfringens *and several other species of clostridia.*

- Gas gangrene can develop after certain types of surgery or injuries.
- Blisters with gas bubbles form near the infected area, and the heartbeat and breathing become rapid.
- Symptoms suggest the diagnosis, and imaging tests or culture of a sample taken from infected tissue is usually done.
- Treatment involves high doses of antibiotics and surgical removal of dead or infected tissue.

Gas gangrene is a fast-spreading clostridial infection of muscle tissue that, if untreated, quickly leads to death. The bacteria produce gas that becomes trapped in the infected tissue. Several thousand cases occur in the United States every year. Gas gangrene usually develops after injuries or surgery. High-risk injuries include wounds that

- Are deep and severe
- Involve muscle
- Are contaminated with dirt, decaying vegetable matter, or the person's stool
- Contain crushed or dead tissue

High-risk surgery includes operations on the colon or gallbladder.

Gas gangrene can occur when there is no injury or surgery—usually in people with colon cancer. People with open fractures and frostbite are also susceptible to gas gangrene. Gas gangrene may develop when a contaminated needle is used to inject an illegal drug into a muscle.

Symptoms

Gas gangrene causes severe pain in the infected area. Initially, the area is swollen and pale but eventually turns red, then bronze, and finally blackish green. Large blisters often form. Gas bubbles may be visible within the blister or may be felt under the skin, usually after the infection progresses. Fluids draining from the wound smell rotten (putrid).

People quickly become sweaty and very anxious. They may vomit. Heart rate and breathing often become rapid. In some people, the skin turns yellow, indicating jaundice. These effects are caused by toxins produced by the bacteria. Typically, people remain alert until late in the illness, when dangerously low blood pressure (shock) and coma develop. Kidney failure and death rapidly follow.

Without treatment, death occurs within 48 hours. Even with treatment, about one of eight people with an infected limb and about two of three people with infection in the torso die.

Diagnosis

The initial diagnosis is based on symptoms and results of a physical examination. X-rays are taken to check for gas bubbles in muscle tissue, or computed tomography (CT) or magnetic resonance imaging (MRI) is done to check for signs of muscle involvement. These findings support the diagnosis. However, gas bubbles may also occur in other anaerobic infections.

Fluids from the wound are examined under a microscope to check for clostridia, and cultures are done to confirm their presence. However, not all people with clostridia have gas gangrene. Confirmation of the diagnosis may require exploratory surgery or removal of a tissue sample for examination under a microscope (biopsy) to check for characteristic changes in muscle.

Prevention and Treatment

Doctors do the following to prevent gas gangrene:

- Clean wounds thoroughly
- Remove foreign objects and dead tissue from wounds
- Give antibiotics intravenously before, during, and after abdominal surgery to prevent infection

No vaccine can prevent clostridial infection.

If gas gangrene is suspected, treatment must begin immediately. High doses of antibiotics, typically penicillin and clindamycin, are given, and all dead and infected tissue is removed surgically. About one of five people with gas gangrene in a limb requires amputation. Treatment in a high-pressure oxygen (hyperbaric oxygen) chamber is of uncertain value, and such chambers are not always readily available.

Klebsiella, Enterobacter, and *Serratia* Infections

Klebsiella, Enterobacter, and Serratia are closely related gram-negative bacteria that occasionally infect people in hospitals or in long-term care facilities.

- These bacteria may infect the urinary or respiratory tract, intravenous catheters used to give drugs or fluids, burns, wounds made during surgery, or the bloodstream.
- Identifying the bacteria in a sample taken from infected tissue confirms the diagnosis.
- If the infection is acquired in the community, antibiotics can cure it, but if it is acquired in a health care facility, it is difficult to treat because bacteria tend to be resistant.

Klebsiella bacteria reside in the intestine of up to one third of healthy people. *Enterobacter* and *Serratia* bacteria usually reside outside the body, often in hospitals and long-term care facilities. People in such places can become infected.

These bacteria may infect different areas:

- Urinary or respiratory tract
- Catheters inserted into a vein (intravenous catheter), used to administer drugs or fluids
- Burns
- Wounds made during surgery
- Bloodstream

Rarely, *Klebsiella* bacteria cause pneumonia in people who live outside a health care facility (in the community), usually in alcoholics, older people, people with diabetes, or people with a weakened immune system. Typically, this severe infection causes cough, bringing up a sticky, dark brown or dark red sputum, and collections of pus (abscesses) in the lung or in the membrane between the lungs and chest wall (empyema).

One species of *Klebsiella* can cause inflammation of the colon (colitis) after antibiotics are taken. This disorder is called antibiotic-associated colitis. The antibiotics kill bacteria that normally reside in the intestine. Then *Klebsiella* bacteria are able to multiply and cause problems. However, this type of colitis usually results from toxins produced by *Clostridium difficile* (see page 176).

Diagnosis

Doctors suspect one of these infections in people at high risk of getting one, such as people who live in a long-term care facility or in a place when there was an outbreak. To confirm the diagnosis, doctors take a sample of sputum, lung secretions (obtained through a bronchoscope), blood, urine, or infected tissue. The sample is stained with Gram stain, cultured, and examined under a microscope. These bacteria can be readily identified.

Other tests depend on the type of infection. They may include imaging tests, such as ultrasonography, x-rays, and computed tomography (CT).

Bacteria identified in samples are tested to determine which antibiotics are likely to be effective (a process called susceptibility testing).

Treatment

If *Klebsiella* pneumonia is acquired in the community, antibiotics, usually a cephalosporin (such as ceftriaxone) or fluoroquinolone (such as levofloxacin), given intravenously, can cure it.

If an infection with any of these three bacteria is acquired in a health care facility, the infection is difficult to treat because bacteria acquired in such facilities are usually resistant to many antibiotics.

Escherichia coli Infections

Escherichia coli (E. coli) *is a group of gram-negative bacteria that normally reside in the intestine of healthy people, but some strains can cause infection.*

- People develop intestinal *E. coli* infections by eating contaminated food, touching infected animals, or swallowing contaminated water in a pool.
- Intestinal infections can cause diarrhea, sometimes severe or bloody, and abdominal pain.
- Antibiotics can effectively treat *E. coli* infections outside the digestive tract and most intestinal infections but are not used to treat intestinal infections by one strain of these bacteria.

Some strains of *E. coli* normally inhabit the digestive tract of healthy people. However, some strains of *E. coli* cause infection in the digestive tract and in other parts of the body, most commonly the urinary tract. *E. coli* is the most common cause of bladder infection in women. These bacteria can also cause infection of the prostate gland (prostatitis), gallbladder infection, infections that develop after appendicitis and diverticulitis, wound infections (including wounds made during surgery), infections in pressure sores, foot infections in people with diabetes, pneumonia, meningitis in newborns, and bloodstream infections. Many *E. coli* infections affecting areas outside the digestive tract develop in people who are debilitated, who are staying in a health care facility, or who have taken antibiotics.

One strain produces a toxin that causes brief watery diarrhea. This disorder (called traveler's diarrhea—see page 152) usually occurs in travelers who consume contaminated food or water in areas where water is not adequately purified.

Another strain (*E. coli* O157:H7) produces a toxin that damages the colon and causes inflammation (colitis). People are usually infected with this strain by doing the following:

- Eating contaminated ground beef that is not cooked thoroughly (one of the most common sources)
- Going to a petting zoo and touching animals that carry the bacteria in their digestive tract
- Eating ready-to-eat food (such as produce at salad bars) that was washed with contaminated water or contaminated by cattle manure
- Swallowing inadequately chlorinated water that has been contaminated by the stool of infected people in swimming or wading pools

Inadequate hygiene, particularly common among young children in diapers, can easily spread the bacteria from person to person.

Symptoms

Symptoms depend on the part of the body affected and the strain of *E. coli* causing the infection.

In infections due to *E. coli* O157:H7, diarrhea begins about 3 days after exposure. Diarrhea becomes bloody about 1 to 3 days later. (This disease is sometimes called hemorrhagic colitis.) People usually have severe abdominal pain and diarrhea many times a day. They also often feel an urge to defecate but may not be able to. Most people do not have a fever. Because the infection is easily spread, people must often be hospitalized and isolated.

The diarrhea resolves on its own in 85% of people. However, in about 15% of children and fewer older people, red blood cells are destroyed and kidney failure occurs about 1 week after symptoms begin. This complication (called hemolytic-uremic syndrome—see page 1042) is a common cause of chronic kidney disease in children.

 Did You Know...

E. coli is the most common cause of bladder infection in women.

Diagnosis

Samples of blood, stool, sometimes urine, or other infected material are taken and sent to a laboratory to grow (culture) the bacteria. Identifying the bacteria in the sample confirms the diagnosis. If the bacteria are identified, they may be tested to see which antibiotics are effective (a process called susceptibility testing).

If *E. coli* O157:H7 is detected, blood tests must be done frequently to check for hemolytic-uremic syndrome.

Treatment

For traveler's diarrhea, loperamide can be given to slow movement of food through the intestine and thus help control diarrhea. Antibiotics (such as azithromycin, ciprofloxacin, or rifaximin) can also be given to end symptoms more quickly.

Many people with diarrhea due to *E. coli* O157:H7 need to be given fluids containing salts intravenously. This infection is not treated with loperamide or antibiotics. Antibiotics may make diarrhea worse and increase the risk of hemolytic-uremic syndrome. If hemolytic-uremic syndrome develops, people are admitted to an intensive care unit and may require hemodialysis.

Many other *E. coli* infections, usually bladder or other urinary tract infections, are treated with antibiotics, such as trimethoprim-sulfamethoxazole or a fluoroquinolone. However, many bacteria, particularly those acquired in a health care facility, are resistant to these antibiotics. For more serious infections, antibiotics that are effective against many different bacteria (broad-spectrum antibiotics) may be used. Several antibiotics may be used together until doctors get the test results indicating which antibiotics are likely to be effective.

Haemophilus influenzae Infections

Haemophilus influenzae can cause infection in the respiratory tract, which can spread to other organs.

- Infection is spread through sneezing, coughing, or touching.
- The bacteria can cause middle ear infections, sinusitis, and more serious infections, including meningitis and epiglottitis.
- Identifying the bacteria in a sample taken from infected tissue confirms the diagnosis.
- Children are routinely given a vaccine that effectively prevents infections due to *Haemophilus influenzae* type b.
- Infections are treated with antibiotics given by mouth or, for serious infections, intravenously.

Many species of *Haemophilus* normally reside in the upper airways of children and adults and rarely cause disease. One species causes chancroid, a sexually transmitted disease. Other species cause infections of heart valves (endocarditis) and, rarely, collections of pus (abscesses) in the brain, lungs, and liver. The species responsible for the most infections is *Haemophilus influenzae*.

Haemophilus influenzae can cause infections in children and sometimes in adults who have a chronic lung disorder or a weakened immune system. Infection is spread by sneezing, coughing, or touching infected people. One type of *Haemophilus influenzae*, called type b, is more likely to cause serious infections.

In children, *Haemophilus influenzae* type b (Hib) can spread through the bloodstream (causing bacteremia)

and infect the joints, bones, lungs, skin of the face and neck, eyes, urinary tract, and other organs. The bacteria may cause two severe, often fatal infections: meningitis and epiglottitis (infection of the flap of tissue over the voice box). Some strains cause infection of the middle ear in children, the sinuses in children and adults, and the lungs in adults, especially those with chronic obstructive pulmonary disease (COPD) or AIDS.

Symptoms and Diagnosis

Symptoms vary depending on the part of the body affected.

To diagnose the infection, doctors take a sample of blood, pus, or other body fluids and send it to a laboratory to grow (culture) the bacteria. If people have symptoms of meningitis, doctors do a spinal tap (lumbar puncture) to obtain a sample of the fluid that surrounds the brain and spinal cord (cerebrospinal fluid). Identifying the bacteria in a sample confirms the diagnosis.

Prevention and Treatment

Children are routinely vaccinated against *Haemophilus influenzae* type b. The vaccine is very effective, especially in preventing meningitis, epiglottitis, and bacteremia.

Treatment of meningitis must begin as soon as possible. An antibiotic—usually, ceftriaxone or cefotaxime—is given intravenously. Corticosteroids may help prevent brain damage.

Epiglottitis must also be treated as soon as possible. People may need help breathing. An artificial airway, such as a breathing tube, may be inserted, or rarely, an opening may be made in the windpipe (a procedure called tracheostomy). The antibiotic rifampin is used because it can eradicate the bacteria from the throat. People are given this antibiotic before they are discharged from the hospital.

If the household of a person with a serious *Haemophilus influenzae* type b infection includes a child who is under 4 years old and is not fully immunized against *Haemophilus influenzae* type b, the child should be vaccinated. Also, all members of the household, except pregnant women, should be given an antibiotic, such as rifampin, by mouth to prevent infection.

Other *Haemophilus influenzae* infections are treated with various antibiotics given by mouth. They include amoxicillin-clavulanate, azithromycin, cephalosporins, clarithromycin, fluoroquinolones, and trimethoprim-sulfamethoxazole.

Leptospirosis

Leptospirosis is a potentially serious disorder caused by Leptospira *bacteria.*

- Most people are infected through contact with contaminated soil or water during outdoor activities.
- Fever, headache, and other symptoms occur in two phases, separated by a few days.
- A severe, potentially fatal form damages many organs, including the liver and kidneys.
- Detecting antibodies against the bacteria in blood or identifying the bacteria in a sample taken from infected tissue confirms the diagnosis.
- Antibiotics and sometimes fluids containing salts are given, but people with the severe form may require transfusions and hemodialysis.

Leptospirosis occurs in many wild and domestic animals. Some animals act as carriers and pass the bacteria in their urine. Others become ill and die. People acquire these infections directly through infected animals or indirectly through soil or water contaminated by urine from an infected animal.

Leptospirosis is an occupational disease of farmers and sewer and slaughterhouse workers. However, most people become infected during outdoor activities when they come in contact with contaminated soil or water, particularly while swimming or wading. The 40 to 100 infections reported every year in the United States occur mainly in the late summer and early fall. Because mild leptospirosis typically causes vague, flu-like symptoms that go away on their own, many infections are probably unreported.

Symptoms

In about 90% of infected people, symptoms are mild. In the rest, the disorder involves many organs. This potentially fatal form of leptospirosis is called Weil's syndrome.

Leptospirosis usually occurs in two phases:

- **First phase:** About 2 to 20 days after infection occurs, fever, headache, nausea, vomiting, severe muscle aches in the calves and back, and chills occur suddenly. The eyes usually become very red on the third or fourth day. Some people cough, occasionally bringing up blood, and have chest pain. Most people recover within 1 week.
- **Second (immune) phase:** In some people, symptoms recur a few days later. They result from inflammation caused by the immune system as it eliminates the bacteria from the body. The fever returns, and the space within the tissues covering the brain and spinal cord (meninges) often becomes inflamed. This inflammation (meningitis) causes a stiff neck and headache.

Weil's Syndrome: This form can occur during the second phase. It causes jaundice (yellowish discoloration of the skin and whites of the eyes), kidney failure, and a tendency to bleed. People may have nosebleeds or cough up blood, or bleeding may occur within tissues in the skin, lungs, and, less commonly, digestive tract. Anemia can develop. Several organs such as the heart, lungs, and kidneys may stop functioning.

Most people who do not develop jaundice recover. About 5 to 10% of people with jaundice (which indicates liver damage) die. The death rate is probably higher in people with Weil's syndrome and people over 60. If leptospirosis develops during early pregnancy, the risk of miscarriage is increased.

Diagnosis

To confirm the diagnosis, doctors take a sample of blood and urine. These samples are analyzed. If people have symptoms of meningitis, doctors do a spinal tap (lumbar puncture) to obtain a sample of the fluid that surrounds the brain and spinal cord (cerebrospinal fluid). Usually, several samples are taken over several weeks. These samples are sent to a laboratory to grow (culture) the bacteria.

Identifying the bacteria in cultures or, more commonly, detecting antibodies against the bacteria in blood confirms the diagnosis.

Prevention and Treatment

The antibiotic doxycycline can prevent leptospirosis. It is given to people who were exposed to the bacteria at the same time as people who have been infected.

Mild infections are treated with antibiotics such as amoxicillin or doxycycline, given by mouth. For severe infections, antibiotics such as penicillin, doxycycline, or erythromycin may be given intravenously. Fluids containing salts may also be given. People with the infection do not have to be isolated, but care must be taken when handling and disposing of their urine.

People with Weil's syndrome may need blood transfusions and hemodialysis.

Listeriosis

Listeriosis is infection caused by the gram-positive bacteria Listeria monocytogenes.

- People may consume the bacteria in commercially prepared foods that require no further cooking.
- People have fever, chills, and muscle aches plus nausea, vomiting, and diarrhea.
- Identifying the bacteria in a sample of blood or cerebrospinal fluid confirms the diagnosis.
- Antibiotics can cure the infection.

Listeria monocytogenes resides in the intestine of many animals worldwide. Most cases of listeriosis result from eating contaminated food. The bacteria grow in food at refrigerator temperatures and survive in the freezer. Pasteurization of dairy products destroys the bacteria unless many bacteria are present. Adequate cooking or reheating of food kills the bacteria. However, they can reside in food-filled cracks and inaccessible areas in commercial food preparation facilities and recontaminate food. If the food requires no further cooking once purchased, the bacteria that remain are consumed with the food. They can grow in a refrigerated, packaged, ready-to-eat product without changing the food's taste or smell. Foods involved in previous outbreaks of listerosis include soft cheeses (such as Latin American white cheeses, feta, Brie, and Camembert), delicatessen salads (such as cole slaw), unpasteurized milk, cold cuts, turkey franks, other hot dogs, shrimp, and undercooked chicken.

The bacteria sometimes enter the bloodstream from the intestine and spread, causing invasive listeriosis. Bacteria may spread to the space within the tissues covering the brain and spinal cord (causing meningitis), the eyes, heart valves (causing endocarditis), or, in pregnant women, the uterus. Collections of pus (abscesses) may form in the brain and spinal cord. In the United States, invasive listeriosis develops in only about 2,500 people each year but is fatal in 20 to 30%. It is more common among pregnant women, newborns, people aged 60 or older, and people with a weakened immune system, such as those with human immunodeficiency (HIV) infection. About one third of cases occur in pregnant women.

> **? Did You Know...**
> Pregnant women are particularly susceptible to listeriosis, which can harm the fetus.

Symptoms

People typically have chills, fever, and muscle aches (resembling the flu), with nausea, vomiting, and diarrhea. Usually, symptoms resolve in 5 to 10 days.

If invasive listeriosis develops, symptoms vary depending on the area infected. If meningitis develops, people have a headache and a stiff neck. They may become confused and lose their balance. If the uterus or placenta is infected in a pregnant woman, spontaneous abortion or stillbirth may result. Or the newborn may have a bloodstream infection (sepsis) or meningitis. About one half of newborns infected near or at the end of the pregnancy die.

Diagnosis

A sample of blood is withdrawn. If people have symptoms of meningitis, a spinal tap (lumbar puncture) is done to obtain a sample of the fluid that surrounds the brain and spinal cord (cerebrospinal fluid). The samples are sent to a laboratory to grow (culture) the bacteria. Identifying the bacteria in the sample confirms the diagnosis.

Treatment

The antibiotic ampicillin or, for people who are allergic to penicillin, trimethoprim-sulfamethoxazole usually cures listeriosis. These antibiotics are given intravenously. If the heart valves are infected, a second antibiotic (such as gentamicin) may be given at the same time.

Eye infections can be treated with erythromycin, given by mouth, or trimethoprim-sulfamethoxazole, given intravenously.

Lyme Disease

Lyme disease is caused by the bacteria Borrelia burgdorferi, *which is usually transmitted to people by deer ticks.*

- Most people are infected when they go outdoors in wooded areas where the disease is common.
- Typically, a large, red spot appears at the site of the bite and slowly enlarges, often surrounded by several red rings.
- Untreated, the disease can cause fever, muscle aches, swollen joints, and eventually problems related to brain and nerve malfunction.
- The diagnosis is based on typical symptoms, opportunity for exposure, and blood tests to detect antibodies to the bacteria.
- Taking antibiotics usually cures the disease, but some symptoms, such as joint pain, may persist.

Lyme disease was recognized and named in 1975 when a cluster of cases occurred in Lyme, Connecticut. It is now the most common insect-borne infection in the United States. It occurs in 49 states. About 80% of the cases occur along the northeastern coast from Massachusetts to Maryland. Most of the remaining reported cases occur in Wisconsin, Minnesota, and the coastal regions of northern California and Oregon. Lyme disease also occurs in Europe, China, Japan, Australia, and the former Soviet Union.

Usually, people get Lyme disease in the summer and early fall. Children and young adults who live in wooded areas are most often infected.

The bacteria that cause Lyme disease are transmitted by the deer tick (*Ixodes*), so named because the adult ticks often feed on the blood of deer. Young deer ticks (larvae and nymphs) feed on the blood of rodents, particularly the white-footed mouse, which is a carrier of Lyme disease bacteria. Ticks are usually in the nymph stage when they infect people. Deer do not carry or transmit Lyme disease bacteria. They are only a source of blood for adult ticks.

Preventing Tick Bites

People can reduce their chances of picking up or being bitten by a tick by doing the following:

- Staying on paths and trails when walking in wooded areas
- Walking in the center of trails to avoid brushing up against bushes and weeds
- Not sitting on the ground or on stone walls
- Wearing long-sleeved shirts
- Wearing long pants and tucking them into boots or socks
- Wearing light-colored clothing, which makes ticks easier to see
- Applying an insect repellent containing diethyltoluamide (DEET) to the skin
- Applying an insect repellent containing permethrin to clothing

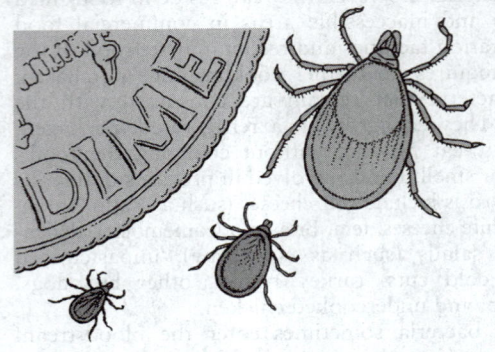

Actual size

Deer tick (nymph)   Deer tick (adult)   Dog tick (adult)

Usually, Lyme disease is transmitted by young deer ticks (nymphs), which are very small, much smaller than dog ticks. So people who may have been exposed to ticks should check the whole body very carefully, especially hairy areas, every day. Inspection is effective because ticks must be attached for more than a day to transmit Lyme disease.

To remove a tick, people should use fine-pointed tweezers to grasp the tick by the head or mouthparts right where they enter the skin and should gradually pull the tick straight off. The tick's body should not be grasped or squeezed. Petroleum jelly, alcohol, lit matches, or any other irritants should not be used.

The bacteria that cause Lyme disease are transmitted to people when an infected tick bites and stays attached for one or two days. Brief periods of attachment rarely transmit disease. At first, the bacteria multiply at the site of the tick bite. After 3 to 32 days, the bacteria migrate from the site of the bite into the surrounding skin, causing a rash (erythema migrans). The bacteria enter the bloodstream and spread to other organs, such as the skin in other areas of the body and the heart, nervous system, and joints.

? Did You Know...

Usually, people get Lyme disease only if a tick remains attached to them for at least a day.

Symptoms

Lyme disease has three stages: early localized, early disseminated (widespread), and late. The early and late stages are usually separated by a period without symptoms.

Early-Localized Stage: Typically, a large, raised, red spot (erythema migrans) appears at the site of the bite, usually on the thigh, buttock, or trunk or in the armpit. Usually, the spot slowly expands to a diameter of 6 inches (15 centimeters), often clearing in the center, resulting in several concentric red rings. Although erythema migrans does not itch or hurt, it may be warm to the touch. The spot usually disappears after about 3 to 4 weeks. About 25% of infected people never develop—or at least never notice—the characteristic red spot.

Early-Disseminated Stage: This stage begins when the bacteria spread through the body. Fatigue, chills, fever, headaches, stiff neck, muscle aches, and painful, swollen joints are common. In nearly half of people, more, usually smaller erythema migrans spots appear on other parts of the body. Less commonly, people have a backache, nausea, vomiting, sore throat, swollen lymph nodes, and an enlarged spleen. Although most symptoms come and go, feelings of illness and fatigue may persist for weeks. These symptoms are often mistaken for influenza or common viral infections, especially if erythema migrans is not present.

Sometimes more serious symptoms develop. The nervous system is affected in about 15% of people. The most common problems are headache, stiff neck, meningitis, and Bell's palsy, which causes weakness on one or occasionally both sides of the face. These problems may last for months. Nerve pain and weakness may develop in other areas and persist longer. About 8% of infected people have irregular heartbeats (arrhythmias) and inflammation of heart tissue (myocarditis) and the sac around the heart (pericarditis) with chest pain. Irregular heartbeats may cause palpitations, light-headedness, or fainting.

Late Stage: If the initial infection is untreated, other problems develop months to years later. Arthritis develops in more than half of people, usually within several months. Swelling and pain typically recur in a few large joints, especially the knee, for several years. The knees are commonly more swollen than painful, often hot to the touch, and, rarely, red. Cysts may develop and rupture behind the knees, suddenly increasing the pain. In about 10% of people with arthritis, knee problems last longer than 6 months.

A few people develop abnormalities related to brain and nerve malfunction. Mood, speech, memory, and sleep may be affected. Some people have numbness or shooting pains in the back, legs, and arms.

Diagnosis

The diagnosis is usually based on typical symptoms (particularly erythema migrans), opportunity for exposure (living in or visiting an area where Lyme disease is common), and test results.

Usually, doctors use tests that measure antibodies to the bacteria in blood. However, antibodies may be absent if the test is done during the first several weeks of infection or if antibiotics are given before antibodies develop. Antibodies develop in more than 95% of people who have had the infection for at least a month, particularly if they have not taken antibiotics. Once antibodies develop, they persist permanently. Thus, antibodies may be present after Lyme disease has resolved.

Interpreting the results of blood tests is difficult. The uncertainty causes several problems. For example, in areas where Lyme disease is common, many people who have painful joints, trouble concentrating, or persistent fatigue worry that they have late-stage Lyme disease, even though they never had a rash or any other symptoms of early-stage Lyme disease. Usually, Lyme disease is not the cause. But they may have antibodies for the bacteria because they were infected years before and the antibodies persist indefinitely. Thus, if a doctor treats people based solely on results of antibody tests, many

people who do not have Lyme disease are treated with long, useless courses of antibiotics.

Cultures are not helpful because *Borrelia burgdorferi* is difficult to grow in the laboratory.

Sometimes doctors insert a needle into a joint to take a sample of joint fluid or do a spinal tap (lumbar puncture) to take a sample of the fluid that surrounds the brain and spinal cord (cerebrospinal fluid). Fragments of the bacteria's genetic material may be present.

Treatment

If people are bitten by a tick but have no rash or other symptoms, antibiotics are usually used only if they can be given within 72 hours after an engorged tick is found attached. These people may be given one dose of doxycycline by mouth to prevent Lyme disease from developing.

Although all stages of Lyme disease respond to antibiotics, early treatment is more likely to prevent complications. Antibiotics such as doxycycline, amoxicillin, cefuroxime, or azithromycin, taken by mouth for 2 weeks, are effective during the early stages of the disease. They can also help treat a type of arrhythmia called first-degree heart block and probably Bell's palsy. Doxycycline is not given to children under 9 years old or to pregnant women.

For arthritis, antibiotics such as amoxicillin or doxycycline are given by mouth for 30 to 60 days, or ceftriaxone or penicillin is given intravenously for 2 to 4 weeks.

For most neurologic abnormalities (except possibly Bell's palsy) and more severe (third-degree) heart block, ceftriaxone or penicillin is given intravenously for 2 to 4 weeks.

Antibiotics eradicate the bacteria and, in most people, relieve arthritis. However, arthritis sometimes persists even after all the bacteria are gone because inflammation continues. Nonsteroidal anti-inflammatory drugs (NSAIDs), such as aspirin or ibuprofen, may relieve the pain of swollen joints. Fluid that collects in affected joints may be drained. Using crutches may help.

Antibiotics do not appear to relieve the chronic fatigue.

A vaccine that was only moderately effective against Lyme disease was removed from the market because it was not widely used.

Meningococcal Infections

Meningococcal infections are caused by Neisseria meningitidis *(meningococci) and include meningitis and bloodstream infections.*

■ Infection is spread by direct contact with nasal and throat secretions.

- People feel generally ill and have other, often serious symptoms, depending on the area infected.
- Identifying the bacteria in a sample taken from infected tissue confirms the diagnosis.
- Antibiotics and fluids must be given intravenously as soon as possible.

More than 90% of meningococcal infections are infections of the space within the tissues covering the brain and spinal cord (meningitis—see page 750) or of the bloodstream (sepsis—see page 1186). Infections of the lungs, joints, and heart are less common.

In temperate climates, most meningococcal infections occur during winter and spring. Local outbreaks can occur, most often in sub-Saharan Africa between Senegal and Ethiopia. This area is known as the meningitis belt.

Meningococci reside in the throat and nose of some people without causing symptoms. Such people are called carriers. People often become carriers after outbreaks. Infection usually occurs in people who have been exposed to meningococci rather than in carriers. Infection is spread by direct contact with nasal and throat secretions.

Children aged 6 months to 3 years are most commonly infected. Infections are also common among adolescents, military recruits, college freshmen living in dormitories, people with certain immune system disorders, and microbiologists working with meningococci.

Symptoms

Most people feel very ill.

Meningitis can cause fever, headache, red rash, and a stiff neck and, in infants, feeding problems, a weak cry, and sluggishness.

Bloodstream infections may cause a rash of red or purple spots. A severe infection may cause low blood pressure, a tendency to bleed, and dysfunction (failure) of many organs (such as the kidneys and liver).

Overall, 10 to 15% of people who are treated die of meningococcal infections. More than half of people with severe bloodstream infections die. Of people who recover, 10 to 20% have serious complications, such as permanent hearing loss, mental retardation, or loss of fingers or toes.

Rarely, infection develops more slowly and causes more gradual, mild symptoms.

Diagnosis

Doctors suspect meningococcal infection in people who have typical symptoms, particularly if symptoms occur during an outbreak. To confirm the diagnosis, they take samples of blood or other infected tissues or do a spinal tap (lumbar puncture) to obtain a sample of the fluid that surrounds the brain and spinal cord (cerebrospinal fluid). The samples are examined under a microscope to check for and identify bacteria. The samples are also sent to a laboratory, where the bacteria can be grown (cultured) and identified. The polymerase chain reaction (PCR) technique, which produces many copies of a gene, may be used to identify the bacteria's unique genetic material (DNA).

The bacteria may also be tested to determine which antibiotics are effective (a process called susceptibility testing).

Prevention

A meningococcal vaccine is available in the United States. Vaccination is recommended for the following:

- People living in an area affected by an epidemic (to control the epidemic)
- Military recruits
- All children aged 11 to 19 years
- College students who live in dormitories or who are freshmen
- Travelers to areas where these infections are common, such as sub-Saharan Africa during the dry season from December to June and Saudi Arabia to attend the Hajj
- People who work with meningococci in laboratories or industry
- People who are aged 2 years and older and have an immune system disorder, particularly those whose spleen has been removed or damaged (as can occur in people with sickle cell disease)

Family members, medical personnel, and other people in close contact with people who have a meningococcal infection should be given an antibiotic by mouth (such as a few doses of rifampin or one dose of ciprofloxacin or levofloxacin) or by injection (such as one dose of ceftriaxone) to prevent infection from developing. Meningococcal vaccine is also given (in addition to antibiotics) to people in close contact with a person who has a meningococcal infection.

Treatment

People are usually admitted to an intensive care unit and given antibiotics and fluids intravenously as soon as possible. Corticosteroids may be given to children or adults who have meningitis.

Plague

Plague is a severe infection caused by the gram-negative bacteria Yersinia pestis.

- The bacteria are spread by the rat flea.

- Depending on the form, plague can cause fever, chills, swollen lymph nodes, headache, a rapid heartbeat, cough, difficulty breathing, vomiting, and diarrhea.
- Identifying the bacteria in samples of blood, sputum, or pus from lymph nodes confirms the diagnosis.
- Antibiotics can reduce the risk of death, and isolating infected people helps prevent spread of plague.

In the past, massive plague epidemics, such as the black death of the Middle Ages, killed many people. The main contributing factors were large numbers of rodents, urban crowding, and poor sanitation. Plague now occurs mostly in rural areas. In the United States, more than 90% of infections occur in southwestern states such as Arizona, California, Colorado, and New Mexico, particularly among campers. Each year, plague affects about 10 to 15 people in the United States and 1,000 to 3,000 people worldwide.

The bacteria that cause plague usually infect wild rodents, such as rats and prairie dogs. The bacteria are spread by the rat flea. When wild rats die, the fleas may move to rats that live close to people, then to household pets, especially cats. The rat fleas may then bite people and transmit infection. Rarely, the infection is spread from person to person by coughing or sneezing. The bacteria lodge in the lungs and cause a type of pneumonia (pneumonic plague). Spread between people usually happens only when people live with or care for a person with pneumonic plague.

Plague can also be acquired by handling infected animals (for example, by hunters) or eating undercooked meat from infected animals.

Plague bacteria is a potential biological weapon. The bacteria can be spread through the air and inhaled. The size of the airborne particle determines where the bacteria lodge in the respiratory tract. Small particles lodge in the lungs, causing pneumonic plague.

Symptoms

Plague has several forms: bubonic, pestis minor, pneumonic, or septicemic. Symptoms vary depending on the form of plague.

Bubonic plague is the most common form. Symptoms may appear a few hours to 12 days after exposure (typically, after 2 to 5 days). Chills and fever of up to 106° F (41° C) occur suddenly. The heartbeat becomes rapid and weak, and blood pressure may drop. Many people become delirious. Shortly before the fever or at the same time, lymph nodes in the groin, armpits, or neck usually swell. They are firm, red, warm, and very tender. During the second week, pus may drain from the lymph nodes. The liver and spleen may enlarge. More than 60% of untreated people die, usually between the third and fifth day.

Pestis minor is a mild form of bubonic plague. Its symptoms—swollen lymph nodes, fever, headache, and exhaustion—disappear within a week.

Pneumonic plague is infection of the lungs. Symptoms begin abruptly 2 or 3 days after exposure to the bacteria. People have a high fever, chills, a rapid heartbeat, and often a severe headache. Within 24 hours, they develop a cough that brings up clear sputum, which soon becomes flecked with blood. Then the sputum becomes pink or bright red (resembling raspberry syrup) and foamy. Breathing is rapid and labored. Most untreated people die within 48 hours after symptoms start.

Septicemic plague is infection that spreads into the blood. About 40% of people have nausea, vomiting, diarrhea, and abdominal pain. Without treatment, many organs malfunction, often causing death.

Diagnosis

To diagnose plague, doctors take samples of blood, sputum, or pus from lymph nodes. Samples are examined under a microscope and sent to a laboratory to grow (culture) bacteria. The blood sample is also tested for antibodies to the bacteria. Tests that rapidly detect the bacteria or its genetic material (DNA), such as polymerase chain reaction (PCR), may be done.

Prevention

Controlling rodents and using repellents to prevent fleabites can help. The vaccine against plague is no longer available in the United States. People who are traveling to locations with a plague outbreak may take an antibiotic such as doxycycline, trimethoprim-sulfamethoxazole, or ciprofloxacin.

Treatment

Treatment begins immediately and reduces the risk of death to less than 15%. Streptomycin is given by injection for 7 to 10 days. Other antibiotics such as gentamicin, doxycycline, and ciprofloxacin are also effective.

People with pneumonic plague must be isolated so that they do not spread the bacteria through the air—called respiratory isolation. It includes the following:

- Limiting access to the room
- Requiring people who work within about 6½ feet (2 meters) of the infected person to wear a mask, eye protection, a gown, and gloves

Anyone who has had unprotected contact with a person or animal (such as a domestic cat) with pneumonic plague must take doxycycline or ciprofloxacin for 7 days.

Pneumococcal Infections

Pneumococcal infections are caused by the gram-positive bacteria Streptococcus pneumoniae *(pneumococcus).*

- Bacteria are dispersed in the air when infected people cough or sneeze.
- The most common infections are pneumonia, meningitis, sinusitis, and middle ear infection (otitis media).
- These infections usually cause fever and a general feeling of illness, with other symptoms depending on which part of the body is infected.
- Diagnosis may be based on symptoms, x-ray findings, or identification of the bacteria in samples of infected material.
- Young children are routinely vaccinated against these infections, and vaccination is recommended for all people at high risk.
- Penicillin or another antibiotic is usually effective treatment.

Pneumococci commonly reside in the upper respiratory tract of healthy people, their natural host, particularly during the winter and early spring. The bacteria spread to other people when they inhale infected droplets dispersed by sneezing or coughing. Spread is more likely among self-contained groups of people, such as people who live, stay, or work in nursing homes, prisons, military bases, shelters for the homeless, or day care centers.

Certain conditions make people more likely to develop these infections, and vaccination is recommended for such people. Older people, even if healthy, tend to have more severe symptoms and complications when they get a pneumococcal infection.

Most pneumococcal infections occur in the lungs (pneumonia), middle ear (otitis media, which is common among children), or sinuses (sinusitis). Pneumonia may develop after influenza, which damages the lining of the respiratory tract.

The bacteria may also spread to and through the bloodstream (causing bacteremia). Infections may occur in the space within the tissues covering the brain and spinal cord (meningitis) or, less often, in heart valves, bones, joints, or the abdominal cavity.

Symptoms and Diagnosis

Symptoms vary depending on the site of the infection.

Pneumococcal Pneumonia: Often, symptoms begin suddenly. People have fever, chills, a general feeling of illness (malaise), shortness of breath, and a cough. The cough brings up sputum that becomes rust-colored.

Commonly, sharp, stabbing chest pains occur on one side. Deep breathing and coughing make the pains worse. This pain is called pleurisy.

Chest x-rays are taken to look for signs of pneumonia. Doctors take a sample of sputum and examine it under a microscope. A sample of sputum, pus, or blood may be sent to a laboratory to grow (culture) bacteria. However, these tests do not always enable doctors to identify the bacteria.

Pneumococcal Meningitis: People have fever, headache, and a general feeling of illness (malaise). Moving the neck becomes painful and difficult, but this problem is not always obvious early in the disease. Infants may only be reluctant to eat and be irritable or sluggish.

The diagnosis requires a spinal tap (lumbar puncture) to obtain a sample of the fluid that surrounds the brain and spinal cord (cerebrospinal fluid). The sample is checked for signs of infection, such as white blood cells and bacteria.

Pneumococcal Otitis Media: These infections cause ear pain and a red, bulging eardrum or pus behind the eardrum.

The diagnosis is usually based on symptoms and results of a physical examination. Cultures and other diagnostic tests are usually not done.

Prevention

Two types of pneumococcal vaccines are available.

Conjugate vaccine is the only one that works in children under 2 years old. It is routinely given to children starting at age 2 months but can be started at age 6 weeks. Three doses are given at 2-month intervals, followed by a fourth dose, usually at age 12 to 15 months (see box on page 1685). Because of this vaccine, serious pneumococcal infections—pneumonia, otitis media, and meningitis—are much less common among children.

Nonconjugate polysaccharide vaccine is recommended for people who are at high risk of pneumococcal infections or complications after a pneumococcal infection. These people include the following:

- All adults aged 65 years or older
- Native Alaskans and American Indians
- People with a chronic disorder such as certain heart or lung disorders (except asthma), kidney failure, nephrotic syndrome, liver dysfunction (including cirrhosis), sickle cell disease, diabetes, or leakage of spinal fluid
- Alcoholics
- People with a disorder that weakens the immune system, such as some cancers and human immunodeficiency virus (HIV) infection
- People who take corticosteroids or drugs to suppress the immune system, such as those used to prevent rejection of an organ transplant or to treat cancer
- People who do not have a functioning spleen

The nonconjugate vaccine is effective against many more types of pneumococci than the conjugate vaccine. Thus, children at high risk, such as those with sickle cell anemia or AIDS, are given one dose of the nonconjugate vaccine at age 2 years (but at least 2 months after the last dose of conjugate vaccine), even if they have had the conjugate vaccine.

Treatment

Penicillin (or the related drugs, ampicillin and amoxicillin) is used for most pneumococcal infections. It is usually taken by mouth but, if the infection is severe, may be given intravenously.

Pneumococci that are resistant to penicillin are becoming more common. Thus, other antibiotics, such as ceftriaxone, cefotaxime, fluoroquinolones, or vancomycin, are often used.

Pseudomonas Infections

Pseudomonas infections are caused by any of several types of the gram-negative bacteria Pseudomonas, *especially* Pseudomonas aeruginosa.

- Infections range from mild external ones (affecting the ear or hair follicles) to serious internal infections (affecting the lungs, bloodstream, or heart valves).
- Symptoms vary depending on which area of the body is infected.
- Identifying the bacteria in a sample taken from infected tissue confirms the diagnosis.
- Antibiotics are applied externally for external infections or given intravenously for more serious, internal infections.

Pseudomonas bacteria, including *Pseudomonas aeruginosa*, are present throughout the world in soil and water. These bacteria favor moist areas, such as sinks, toilets, inadequately chlorinated swimming pools and hot tubs, and outdated or inactivated antiseptic solutions. These bacteria may temporarily reside in the skin, ears, and intestine of healthy people.

Pseudomonas aeruginosa infections range from minor external infections to serious, life-threatening disorders. Infections occur more often and tend to be more severe in people who

- Are weakened (debilitated) by certain severe disorders
- Have diabetes or cystic fibrosis
- Are hospitalized
- Have a disorder that weakens the immune system, such as human immunodeficiency virus (HIV) infection
- Take drugs that suppress the immune system, such as those used to treat cancer or to prevent rejection of transplanted organs

These bacteria can infect the blood, skin, bones, ears, eyes, urinary tract, heart valves, and lungs, as well as wounds (such as burns, injuries, or wounds made during surgery). Use of medical devices, such as catheters inserted into the bladder or a vein, breathing tubes, and mechanical ventilators, increase the risk of *Pseudomonas aeruginosa* infections. These infections are commonly acquired in hospitals.

Symptoms

Pseudomonas aeruginosa causes several different infections.

Swimmer's ear (external otitis) is a mild external infection that can occur in otherwise healthy people. Water containing the bacteria can enter the ear during swimming. Swimmer's ear causes pain and a discharge from the ear (see page 1385).

Hot-tub folliculitis is another mild external infection. Hair roots (follicles) become infected in people who use hot tubs or whirlpools, particularly if the hot tubs and whirlpools are inadequately chlorinated. Spending a lot of time in the water softens the follicles, making them easier for bacteria to invade. An itchy skin rash consisting of tiny pimples develops. Pimples may have a drop of pus in their center.

Malignant external otitis is a deep ear infection. It is most common among people with diabetes. Tissues become swollen and inflamed, partly or completely closing the ear canal. Symptoms may include fever, loss of hearing, inflammation of tissues around the infected ear, severe ear pain, a foul-smelling discharge from the ear, and nerve damage.

Eye infections due to these bacteria may damage the cornea, often permanently. Enzymes produced by the bacteria can rapidly destroy the eye. Infections may result from contamination of contact lenses or contact lens solution.

Soft-tissue infections include those in muscle, tendons, ligaments, fat, and skin. These infections can occur in deep puncture wounds, especially in the feet of children who are wearing sneakers and step on a nail. These bacteria can also infect pressure sores, burns, and wounds due to injuries or surgery. When these bacteria grow in soiled dressings, the dressings turn green and smell like newly mowed grass.

Severe pneumonia can develop in hospitalized people, especially those who need to use a breathing tube and a mechanical ventilator.

Urinary tract infections usually develop after a procedure involving the urinary tract is done, when the urinary tract is blocked, or when a catheter must remain in the bladder a long time.

Bloodstream infections (**bacteremia**) often result when the following occur:

- Bacteria enter the bloodstream from an infected organ (such as the urinary tract).
- A contaminated illegal drug is injected into a vein.
- A contaminated needle or syringe is used to inject illegal drugs.

Sometimes the source of the bacteria is unknown, as may occur in people who have too few white blood cells after cancer chemotherapy. Purple-black spots surrounded by a red rim on the skin often develop in the armpits and groin. Without treatment, infection can lead to shock and death.

Bone and joint infections usually occur in the spine and the joint between the collar bone and breastbone. The bacteria usually spread to bones and joints from the bloodstream but may spread from nearby soft tissues that have been infected after an injury or surgery.

Heart valve infections are rare. They usually occur in people who inject intravenous drugs and in people with artificial heart valves. The bacteria usually spread to heart valves from the bloodstream.

Diagnosis

Doctors diagnose *Pseudomonas aeruginosa* infections by taking a sample of blood or other body fluids and growing the bacteria in cultures. Tests to determine which antibiotics are likely to be effective (susceptibility tests) are also done.

Prevention and Treatment

To prevent swimmer's ear, people who have had it should irrigate their ears with an acetic acid solution before and after swimming. Acetic acid drops with or without corticosteroids are usually effective for treatment.

Hot-tub folliculitis usually resolves without treatment.

Eye infections are treated with highly concentrated antibiotic drops, applied frequently at first. Sometimes antibiotics must be injected directly into the eye.

Serious *Pseudomonas aeruginosa* infections are difficult to treat. Malignant external otitis, internal infections (such as pneumonia or heart valve infection), and blood infections require weeks of antibiotics given intravenously. Usually, a combination of antibiotics is required because many strains, particularly those acquired in health care facilities, are resistant to many antibiotics. Doctors choose an antibiotic that is usually effective in their geographic area. They may change the antibiotics after test results indicate which antibiotics are likely to be effective.

For heart valve infections, open-heart surgery to replace the valve plus antibiotic therapy is usually needed (see box on page 381).

Salmonella Infections

Salmonella infections are caused by the gram-negative bacteria Salmonella.

- People are usually infected when they eat contaminated food, such as undercooked chicken or eggs.
- The bacteria usually infect the digestive tract but can travel through the bloodstream and infect other parts of the body.
- People have nausea and crampy abdominal pain, followed by watery diarrhea, fever, and vomiting.
- Identifying the bacteria in a sample, usually of stool, confirms the diagnosis.
- Lost fluids are replaced, and antibiotics are usually not helpful for salmonellal intestinal infections.

Two species of *Salmonella* cause typhoid fever: *Salmonella typhi* and *Salmonella paratyphi*. *Salmonella typhi* resides only in people. *Salmonella paratyphi* resides mainly in people but sometimes in domestic animals. Other species of *Salmonella* normally reside in the digestive tract of many wild and domestic animals, such as cattle, sheep, pigs, fowl, and reptiles (including snakes, lizards, and turtles). Many of these can cause infections in people. One species, *Salmonella enteritidis*, causes most *Salmonella* infections in the United States.

Salmonella bacteria are excreted in the feces of infected animals and people, leading to contamination. In the United States during the 1970s, many infections were spread by pet turtles, so their sale was prohibited, resulting in fewer infections. Recently, the legal and illegal sale of pet reptiles has increased. Up to 90% of pet reptiles are infected with *Salmonella*.

People are infected usually by eating undercooked poultry or eggs but sometimes by eating undercooked beef and pork, unpasteurized dairy products, or contaminated seafood or fresh produce. *Salmonella* bacteria can infect the ovaries of hens and thus infect the egg before the egg is laid. Other foods may be contaminated by animal feces (for example, in slaughterhouses) or by infected food handlers who do not adequately wash their hands after using a toilet.

Because stomach acid tends to destroy *Salmonella*, a large number of these bacteria must be consumed for infection to develop, unless people have a deficiency of stomach acid. Such a deficiency may occur in children under 1 year old, in older people, and in people taking antacids or drugs that inhibit stomach acid production, including histamine-2 (H_2) blockers (such as ranitidine) or proton pump inhibitors (such as omeprazole).

The bacteria cause inflammation of the intestine (gastroenteritis) and thus are a common cause of diarrhea. Sometimes the bacteria enter the bloodstream (causing bacteremia) and spread, causing infections or collections of pus (abscesses) at distant sites, such as the bones, joints, urinary tract, and lungs. Bacteria may collect and cause infection on artificial (prosthetic) joints or heart valves, on a blood vessel graft, or on tumors. The lining of arteries, usually the aorta (the largest artery in the body), may be infected. Abscesses and infected arteries can cause chronic bacteremia. The infection is more likely to spread through the bloodstream in the following:

- Infants
- Older people
- People with disorders that affect red blood cells such as sickle cell anemia or malaria
- People with a disorder that weakens the immune system, such as human immunodeficiency virus (HIV) infection
- People who take drugs that suppress the immune system, such as those used to treat cancer or prevent rejection of an organ transplant

Symptoms

When the intestine is infected, symptoms usually start 12 to 48 hours after the bacteria are ingested. Nausea and crampy abdominal pain occur, soon followed by watery diarrhea, fever, and vomiting. Symptoms resolve within a week. Long after symptoms are gone, a few people continue to excrete the bacteria in their stool. Such people are called carriers.

Up to about 30% of adults develop reactive arthritis weeks to months after diarrhea stops. This disorder causes pain and swelling, usually in the hips, knees, and Achilles tendon (which connects the heel bone and calf muscle).

Other symptoms may develop if bacteremia develops and infection spreads. For example, if a bone is infected, the area over it is often tender or painful. If a heart valve is infected, people may feel short of breath. If the aorta is infected, the back and abdomen may be painful.

> ### ? Did You Know...
> In the United States, up to 90% of pet reptiles are infected with *Salmonella*.

Diagnosis

Doctors take a sample of stool, pus, or blood or use a swab to obtain a sample from the rectum. The sample is sent to a laboratory where bacteria can be grown (cultured). Identifying the bacteria in the sample confirms the diagnosis.

Treatment

The intestinal infection is treated with fluids given by mouth or, for severe infection, intravenously.

Antibiotics do not shorten recovery time and may result in bacteria being excreted in the stool longer. Therefore, antibiotics are usually not given. However, people at risk of bacteremia and people with implanted devices or materials (such as an artificial joint or heart valve or a blood vessel graft) are given antibiotics. They may be given ciprofloxacin or azithromycin for 1 week. Antibiotics are given to people who continue to excrete the bacteria in the stool after symptoms are gone.

People with bacteremia are given ciprofloxacin or ceftriaxone intravenously for 2 weeks.

Abscesses are drained surgically, and antibiotics are given for 4 weeks.

If the aorta, a heart valve, or other areas (such as joints) are infected, surgery is usually required, and antibiotics are given for weeks or months.

TYPHOID FEVER

Typhoid fever (enteric fever) is caused by the bacteria Salmonella typhi *or the related bacteria,* Salmonella paratyphi.

- Typhoid fever can be spread by consuming food or water contaminated with the stool or urine of an infected person.
- People have flu-like symptoms, sometimes followed by delirium, cough, exhaustion, occasionally rash, and diarrhea.
- Samples of blood, stool, other body fluids, or tissues are sent to a laboratory to grow (culture) the bacteria.
- To prevent infection, people traveling to areas where typhoid fever is common should be vaccinated and, when there, should avoid certain foods and not drink unbottled water.
- Infected people with or without symptoms are treated with antibiotics.

Typhoid fever is common in developing countries (mostly in the Indian subcontinent, the Philippines, and Latin America) where sanitary conditions are poor. Most cases in the United States are acquired while traveling in these countries.

Salmonella typhi is present only in people. People who are infected excrete the bacteria in stool and, rarely, in urine. A few infected people develop chronic infection of the gallbladder or urinary tract. They continue to excrete the bacteria in stool or urine, even though they no longer have any symptoms. Such people are called carriers. Thus, they do not know they can spread the infection. During the early 20th century, one such woman, a cook named Mary Mallon, spread typhoid fever to many people and became known as Typhoid Mary.

The bacteria may contaminate food or drink when hands are inadequately washed after defecation or urination. Water supplies may be contaminated when sewage is inadequately treated. Flies may spread the bacteria directly from stool to food.

Like all *Salmonella* bacteria, many of these bacteria must be consumed for infection to develop, unless the immune system is impaired or people have a deficiency of stomach acid.

The bacteria spread from the digestive tract to the bloodstream (causing bacteremia) and may infect distant organs such as the liver, spleen, gallbladder, lungs (causing pneumonia), joints (causing infectious arthritis), kidneys (causing pyelonephritis), heart valves (causing endocarditis), genital tract, the space within the tissues covering the brain and spinal cord (causing meningitis), and bone (causing osteomyelitis).

> **? Did You Know...**
>
> Mary Mallon, so-called Typhoid Mary, was a cook who spread typhoid fever to many people during the early 20th century.

Symptoms

Typically, a flu-like illness begins about 8 to 14 days (up to 30 days) after infection. People may have a fever, headache, muscle and joint pains, abdominal pains, and a dry cough. They may lose their appetite. After a few days, the temperature peaks at about 103° to 104° F (39° to 40° C). Often the heartbeat is slow, and people feel exhausted and sometimes become delirious. During the second week, a rash of flat, rose-colored spots develops in about 10% of people. People may be constipated at first, but after 2 weeks, diarrhea may occur. In less than 5% of people, the intestine is torn (perforated) or bleeds. If infection spreads to other organs, symptoms of those infections may also develop.

Without treatment, people may have fever for 3 to 4 weeks. Up to 20% may relapse after initial recovery, and up to 20% may die. Most people who die are malnourished, very young, or very old. Stupor (unresponsiveness that requires vigorous stimulation to be aroused), coma, and shock are signs of severe infection and a poor prognosis.

Diagnosis

To confirm the diagnosis, doctors take samples of blood, stool, other body fluids, or tissues and send them to a laboratory where the bacteria can be grown (cultured). The samples are examined and tested to determine whether the bacteria are present.

Prevention

People who travel to areas where typhoid fever is common should avoid eating raw vegetables and other foods served or stored at room temperature. Generally, people can safely consume foods that are served very hot immediately after cooking, bottled or canned beverages that are sealed, hot tea or coffee, and fruit that they have peeled themselves. People should assume that ice and water (unless it is boiled or chlorinated before use) are unsafe. Sealed bottled water should be used for brushing teeth.

A vaccine given by mouth and a polysaccharide vaccine given by injection can help prevent typhoid fever. Both vaccines have few side effects. Vaccination is recommended for

- Travelers to regions where typhoid fever is common
- People who live in a household with carriers
- Laboratory workers who work with the bacteria

People are usually protected for at least 2 years after vaccination by injection and for 5 years after taking the vaccine by mouth. However, they can be infected if many bacteria are ingested. In the United States, 75% of cases of typhoid fever occur in travelers who were not vaccinated or who did not keep their vaccinations up to date.

Treatment

When antibiotics are used, fever lasts only 3 to 5 days, rather than 3 to 4 weeks, and the risk of death is reduced to less than 1%. Complete recovery may take weeks or months.

The antibiotic chloramphenicol is used worldwide. However, it can damage cells in bone marrow that make blood cells. Also, *Salmonella typhi* bacteria are becoming increasingly resistant to it. Thus, other antibiotics (such as ceftriaxone, ciprofloxacin, or azithromycin) are often used. People who are delirious, comatose, or in shock may also be given corticosteroids.

In 10 to 20% of people given antibiotics, the infection recurs, typically about 1 week after treatment is stopped. This infection is milder than the initial illness and is treated the same way.

Carriers must report to the local health department and are prohibited from working with food. Taking antibiotics for 4 to 6 weeks may eradicate the bacteria in many carriers. However, if carriers have abnormalities of the biliary or urinary tract (for example, kidney or gallbladder stones), surgery to correct these abnormalities is needed before bacteria can be eradicated.

Shigellosis

Shigellosis is infection that is caused by the gram-negative bacteria Shigella *and that results in watery diarrhea or dysentery (the frequent and often painful passage of small amounts of stool that contains blood, pus, and mucus).*

- The bacteria are excreted in stool and can be easily spread when hygiene or sanitation is inadequate.
- People may have watery diarrhea, sometimes leading to severe dehydration.
- Identifying the bacteria in a sample of stool can confirm the diagnosis.
- For people with shigellosis and people who care for them, meticulous hygiene is necessary to avoid spreading the infection.
- Fluids are given by mouth or, if the infection is severe, intravenously.
- Antibiotics are used.

Shigella bacteria are a common cause of dysentery throughout the world. Probably about a quarter of a million people in the United States develop shigellosis each year.

Because stomach acid does not easily destroy these bacteria, ingesting even a small number of them causes infection. In the large intestine, the bacteria cause inflammation and are then excreted in stool. As a result, infection spreads easily from person to person when hands are soiled. Infection is also spread through the following:

- Oral-anal sex
- Food contaminated by infected food handlers who do not wash their hands with soap after using a toilet
- Water contaminated with human waste
- Swimming and wading pools that are inadequately chlorinated

Infection easily spreads among people who live together. Outbreaks also occur in places that are overcrowded and have inadequate sanitation, such as

- Day-care centers for children
- Long-term care facilities
- Refugee camps
- Institutions for the intellectually disabled (mentally retarded)
- Cruise ships
- Military camps
- Developing countries

Children are more likely to become infected and to have severe symptoms, such as seizures.

There are four species of *Shigella*. All cause diarrhea. However, one—*Shigella dysenteriae*—is more likely to cause severe diarrhea, dysentery, and complications.

Symptoms

Mild infections cause low-grade fever (about 100.4 to 102° F [38 to 38.9° C]) and watery diarrhea 1 to 2 days after people ingest the bacteria. Abdominal cramps and a frequent urge to defecate are common with more severe infections. Severe infections may cause low-grade or moderate fever and watery diarrhea that progresses to dysentery. In dysentery, bowel movements are frequent and contain blood, pus, and mucus.

Children, particularly young children, are most likely to have severe complications:

- High fever (up to 106° F [41° C]), sometimes with delirium
- Severe dehydration with weight loss
- Up to 20 bowel movements a day
- With severe diarrhea, protrusion of part of the rectum out of the body (rectal prolapse)
- Rarely, marked swelling of the intestine and tearing (perforation) of the large intestine
- Hemolytic-uremic syndrome if the infection is due to *Shigella dysenteriae*

Severe dehydration can lead to shock and death, mainly in chronically ill, malnourished, or debilitated children and in older people. In hemolytic-uremic syndrome, red blood cells are destroyed, causing anemia with fatigue, weakness, and lightheadedness. Blood clots abnormally, causing the kidneys to stop functioning. Seizures or strokes can also occur.

Some adults develop eye inflammation, painful urination, and reactive arthritis (see page 570) weeks to months after the diarrhea.

Diagnosis

A doctor suspects shigellosis based on the typical symptoms of pain, fever, and watery or bloody diarrhea in people who are likely to have been exposed to the bacteria. To confirm the diagnosis, doctors may take a sample of stool and send it to a laboratory to grow (culture) the bacteria.

Prevention

Prevention includes the following:

- Infected people should not prepare food for others.
- After using the toilet, infected people should wash their hands, and someone should clean and disinfect the toilet before it is used again.
- People caring for people with shigellosis should wash their hands with soap and water, particularly before they touch other people or handle food.
- Infected children with symptoms should not have contact with uninfected children.
- Diapers of infected children should be disposed of in a sealed garbage can, and the area used to

change diapers should be wiped with disinfectant after each use.

- Stool that contaminates clothing and bedclothes of infected people should be flushed away in running water, and the soiled clothing and bedclothes should be washed in a washing machine using the hot water cycle. When finished, surfaces of the sink, toilet, and washing machine should be wiped down with a disinfectant, such as diluted chlorine bleach.

Currently, no vaccine is available.

Treatment

Water and salts lost because of diarrhea are replaced, usually by mouth. Symptoms typically resolve within 4 to 8 days. Antibiotics are not routinely required for mild infections.

Severe infections may last 3 to 6 weeks and require hospitalization so that fluids containing salts can be given intravenously and complications, such as hemolytic-uremic syndrome, can be treated. Antibiotics, such as azithromycin, ciprofloxacin, or trimethoprim-sulfamethoxazole, are given, particularly when people are very young or very old, when the infection is severe, or when the infection is likely to spread to other people. Antibiotics reduce the severity of symptoms and the length of time the bacteria are excreted in stool.

Drugs to stop diarrhea (such as diphenoxylate or loperamide) may prolong the infection and should not be used.

Staphylococcus aureus Infections

Staphylococcus aureus *is the most dangerous of all of the many common staphylococcal bacteria.*

- These bacteria are spread by having direct contact with an infected person, by using a contaminated object, or by inhaling infected droplets dispersed by sneezing or coughing.
- Skin infections are common, but the bacteria can spread through the bloodstream and infect distant organs.
- Skin infections may cause blisters, abscesses, and redness and swelling in the infected area.
- The diagnosis is based on the appearance of the skin or identification of the bacteria in a sample of the infected material.
- Thoroughly washing the hands can help prevent spread of infection.
- Antibiotics are chosen based on whether they are likely to be effective against the strain causing the infection.

Staphylococcus aureus is present in the nose of adults (temporarily in 60% and permanently in 20 to 30%) and sometimes on the skin. People who have the bacteria but do not have any symptoms caused by the bacteria are called carriers. People most likely to be carriers include those whose skin is repeatedly punctured or broken, such as the following:

- People who have diabetes mellitus and have to regularly inject insulin
- People who inject illegal drugs
- People who are being treated with hemodialysis or chronic ambulatory peritoneal dialysis
- People with skin infections, AIDS, or previous staphylococcal bloodstream infections

People can move the bacteria from their nose to other body parts with their hands, sometimes leading to infection. Carriers can develop infection if they have surgery, are treated with hemodialysis or chronic ambulatory peritoneal dialysis, or have AIDS.

The bacteria can spread from person to person by direct contact, through contaminated objects (such as telephones, door knobs, television remote controls, or elevator buttons), or, less often, by inhalation of infected droplets dispersed by sneezing or coughing.

Staphylococcus aureus infections range from mild to life threatening. The bacteria tend to infect the skin (see page 1315), often causing abscesses. However, the bacteria can travel through the bloodstream (causing bacteremia) and infect almost any site in the body, particularly heart valves (endocarditis—see page 386) and bones (osteomyelitis—see page 556). The bacteria also tend to accumulate on medical devices in the body, such as artificial heart valves or joints, heart pacemakers, and tubes (catheters) inserted through the skin into blood vessels.

Certain staphylococcal infections are more likely in certain situations:

- **Endocarditis:** When people inject illegal drugs, have an infected blood vessel catheter, or have an artificial heart valve
- **Osteomyelitis:** If *Staphylococcus aureus* spreads to the bone from infection in the bloodstream or from infection in adjacent soft tissue, as may occur in deep pressure sores or foot sores due to diabetes
- **Lung infection (pneumonia):** When people have had influenza (particularly) or a bloodstream infection or when they are hospitalized because they need tracheal intubation and mechanical ventilation (see page 527)

There are many strains of *Staphylococcus aureus*. Some strains produce toxins that can cause the symptoms of staphylococcal food poisoning (see page 151), toxic shock syndrome (see page 1182), and scalded skin syndrome (see page 1319).

Many strains have developed resistance to the effects of antibiotics. If carriers take antibiotics, the antibiotics kill the strains that are not resistant, leaving mainly the resistant strains. These bacteria may then multiply, and if they cause infection, the infection is more difficult to treat. Whether the bacteria are resistant and which antibiotics they resist often depend on where people got the infection: in a hospital or other health care facility or outside of such a facility (in the community).

Methicillin-Resistant *Staphylococcus aureus* (MRSA): Because antibiotics are widely used in hospitals, hospital staff members commonly carry resistant strains. When people are infected in a health care facility, the bacteria are usually resistant to several types of antibiotics, including all antibiotics that are related to penicillin (called beta-lactam antibiotics). Strains of bacteria that are resistant to beta-lactam antibiotics are called methicillin-resistant *Staphylococcus aureus* (MRSA). MRSA strains are common if infection is acquired in a health care facility, and more and more infections acquired in the community, including mild abscesses and skin infections, are caused by MRSA strains.

> **? Did You Know...**
>
> Staphylococcal infections may be difficult to treat because many of the bacteria have developed resistance to antibiotics.

Symptoms

Skin infections due to *Staphylococcus aureus* can include the following:

- **Folliculitis** is the least serious. A hair root (follicle) is infected, causing a slightly painful, tiny pimple at the base of a hair.
- **Impetigo** consists of shallow, fluid-filled blisters that rupture, leaving honey-colored crusts. Impetigo may itch or hurt.
- **Abscesses (boils or furuncles)** are warm, painful collections of pus just below the skin.
- **Cellulitis** is infection of skin and the tissue just under it. Cellulitis spreads, causing pain and redness.
- **Toxic epidermal necrolysis** and, in newborns, scalded skin syndrome are serious infections. Both lead to large-scale peeling of skin.

All staphylococcal skin infections are very contagious.

Breast infections (mastitis), which may include cellulitis and abscesses, can develop 1 to 4 weeks after delivery. The area around the nipple is red and painful. Abscesses often release large numbers of bacteria into the mother's milk. The bacteria may then infect the nursing infant.

Pneumonia often causes a high fever, shortness of breath, and a cough with sputum that may be tinged with blood. Lung abscesses may develop. They sometimes enlarge and involve the membranes around the lungs (causing pleurisy) and sometimes cause pus to collect (called an empyema). These problems make breathing even more difficult.

Bloodstream infection is a common cause of death in people with severe burns. Symptoms typically include a persistent high fever and sometimes shock.

Endocarditis can quickly damage heart valves, leading to heart failure (with difficulty breathing) and possibly death.

Osteomyelitis causes chills, fever, and bone pain. The skin and soft tissues over the infected bone become red and swollen, and fluid may accumulate in nearby joints.

Diagnosis

Skin infections are usually diagnosed based on their appearance. Other infections require samples of blood or infected fluids, which are sent to a laboratory to grow (culture) the bacteria. Laboratory results confirm the diagnosis and determine which antibiotics can kill the staphylococci (called susceptibility testing).

If a doctor suspects osteomyelitis, x-rays, computed tomography (CT), magnetic resonance imaging (MRI), or a combination is also done. These tests can show where the damage is and help determine how severe it is.

Prevention

People can help prevent the spread of these bacteria by always thoroughly washing their hands with soap and water or with antibacterial hand sanitizer gels. The bacteria can be eliminated from the nose by applying the antibiotic mupirocin inside the nostrils. However, because overusing mupirocin can lead to mupirocin resistance, this antibiotic is used only when people are likely to get an infection. For example, it is given to people before certain operations or to people who live in a household in which the skin infection is spreading.

Treatment

Infections due to *Staphylococcus aureus* are treated with antibiotics. Doctors try to determine whether the bacteria are resistant to antibiotics and, if so, to which antibiotics.

Infection that is acquired in a hospital is treated with antibiotics that are effective against methicillin-resistant *Staphylococcus aureus* (MRSA): ceftobiprole, vancomycin, linezolid, quinupristin plus dalfopristin, or daptomycin. If results of testing later indicate that the strain is susceptible to methicillin and the person is not allergic to penicillin, a drug related to methicillin, such as nafcillin, is used. Depending on how severe the infection is, antibiotics may be given for weeks.

MRSA infection can be acquired outside of a health care facility. The community-acquired MRSA strains are usually susceptible to other antibiotics, such as trimethoprim-sulfamethoxazole, clindamycin, minocycline, or doxycycline, as well as to the antibiotics used to treat MRSA infections acquired in the hospital. Mild skin infections due to MRSA, such as folliculitis, are usually treated with an ointment, such as one that contains bacitracin, neomycin, and polymyxin B (available without a prescription) or mupirocin (available by prescription only). If more than an ointment is required, antibiotics effective against MRSA are given by mouth or intravenously. Which antibiotic is used depends on the severity of the infection and the results of susceptibility testing.

If an infection involves bone or foreign material in the body (such as heart pacemakers, artificial heart valves and joints, and blood vessel grafts), rifampin is sometimes added to the antibiotic regimen. Usually, infected bone and foreign material has to be removed surgically to cure the infection.

Abscesses, if present, are usually drained.

OTHER STAPHYLOCOCCAL INFECTIONS

Staphylococcus aureus produces an enzyme called coagulase. Other species of staphylococci do not and thus are called coagulase-negative staphylococci. These bacteria normally reside in the skin of all healthy people.

These bacteria, although less dangerous than *Staphylococcus aureus*, can cause serious infections, usually when acquired in a hospital. The bacteria may infect catheters inserted through the skin into a blood vessel or implanted medical devices (such as pacemakers or artificial heart valves and joints).

These bacteria are often resistant to many antibiotics. Vancomycin, which is effective against many resistant bacteria, is used, sometimes with rifampin. Medical devices, if infected, often must be removed.

Streptococcal Infections

Streptococcal infections are caused by any one of several species of Streptococcus.

- Different groups of these bacteria are spread in different ways—for example, through coughing or sneezing, through contact with infected wounds or sores, or during vaginal delivery (from mother to child).
- These infections affect various areas of the body, including the throat, middle ear, sinuses, lungs, skin, tissue under the skin, heart valves, and bloodstream.
- Symptoms may include red and painful swollen tissues, scabby sores, sore (strep) throat, and a rash, depending on the area affected.
- Doctors may be able to diagnose the infection based on symptoms and can confirm the diagnosis by identifying the bacteria in a sample of infected tissue, sometimes supplemented with imaging tests.
- Antibiotics are given by mouth or, for serious infections, intravenously.

Many species of streptococci live harmlessly in and on the body. Some species that can cause infection are also present in some healthy people but cause no symptoms. These people are called carriers.

Types of Streptococci: The species that cause disease are divided into groups based on their appearance when grown in the laboratory and on their different chemical components. Each group tends to produce specific infections. Groups include group A, group B, and viridans.

Spread: Group A streptococci, as well as *Streptococcus pneumoniae*, are spread through inhalation of droplets of secretions from the nose or throat, dispersed when an infected person coughs or sneezes, or through contact with infected wounds or sores on the skin. Usually, the bacteria are not spread through casual contact, but they may spread in crowded environments such as dormitories, schools, and military barracks. After 24 hours of antibiotic treatment, people no longer can spread the bacteria to others.

Group B streptococci can be spread to newborns through vaginal secretions during vaginal delivery.

Viridans streptococci inhabit the mouth of healthy people but can invade the bloodstream, especially in people with periodontal inflammation, and infect heart valves (causing endocarditis).

> **? Did You Know...**
> The bacteria that cause a particularly dangerous streptococcal infection called necrotizing fasciitis are sometimes described as flesh eating.

Symptoms

Symptoms vary, depending on where the infection is:

STREPTOCOCCI AND SOME DISORDERS THEY CAUSE

SPECIES	CIRCUMSTANCES	DISORDERS
Group A		
Streptococcus pyogenes	Ears, nose, and throat	Middle ear infection (otitis media) Sinusitis Sore throat (pharyngitis, called strep throat)
	Skin	Cellulitis (infection of tissues just under the skin) Erysipelas (a superficial form of cellulitis) Impetigo (a skin infection) Wound infections
	Other	Infection of heart valves (endocarditis) Necrotizing fasciitis Pleurisy Pneumonia Scarlet fever (no longer common) Streptococcal toxic shock syndrome
	Disorders that develop after streptococcal infections	Glomerulonephritis (kidney inflammation) Rheumatic fever
Group B		
Streptococcus agalactiae	In adults, especially those with diabetes mellitus	Abscesses Cellulitis Wound infections
	In newborns	Bloodstream infections (sepsis) Meningitis Pneumonia
	In women after delivery of a baby	Bloodstream infections Infection of the uterus (endometritis)
Viridans		
Various species	—	Dental cavities Infection of heart valves (endocarditis) that have been damaged by a disorder such as a congenital heart disorder or rheumatic fever
Streptococcus pneumoniae	—	Meningitis Middle ear infection (otitis media) Pneumonia acquired outside of health care facilities (in the community) Sinusitis

- **Cellulitis:** The infected skin becomes red, and the tissue under it swells, causing pain.

- **Impetigo:** Usually, scabby, yellow-crusted sores form (see page 1317).

- **Necrotizing fasciitis:** The connective tissue that covers muscle (fascia) is infected. People have sudden chills, fever, and severe pain and tenderness in the affected area. The skin may appear normal until infection is severe (see page 1318).

- **Strep throat (pharyngitis):** This infection usually occurs in children 5 to 15 years old. Children under 3 years old seldom get strep throat. Symptoms often appear suddenly. The throat becomes sore. Children may also have chills, fever, headache, nausea, vomiting, and a general feeling of illness (malaise). The throat is beefy red, and the tonsils are swollen, with or without patches of pus. Lymph nodes in the neck are usually enlarged and tender. However, children under 3 years old may not have these symptoms. They may have only a runny nose. If people with a sore throat have a cough, red eyes, hoarseness, diarrhea, or a stuffy nose, the cause is probably a viral infection, not a streptococcal infection.

- **Scarlet fever:** A rash appears first on the face, then spreads to the trunk and limbs. The rash feels like coarse sandpaper. The rash is worse in skinfolds, such as the crease between the legs and the trunk. As the rash fades, the skin peels. Red bumps develop on the tongue, which is coated with a yellowish white film. The film then peels, and the tongue appears beefy red (strawberry tongue).

Diagnosis

Doctors suspect strep throat based on the following:

- Fever
- Enlarged and tender lymph nodes in the neck
- Pus in or on the tonsils
- Absence of cough

The main reason for diagnosing strep throat is to reduce the chance of developing complications, such as infection of the sinuses, middle ear, or mastoid bone or rheumatic fever, by using antibiotics. However, because symptoms of group A strep throat are often similar to those of throat infection due to a virus, testing with a throat culture or another test is necessary to confirm the diagnosis. Several diagnostic tests (called rapid tests) can be completed in minutes. For these tests, a swab is used to take a sample from the throat. If these results indicate infection (positive results), the diagnosis of strep throat is confirmed, and a throat culture, which takes longer to process, is not needed. However, results of rapid tests sometimes indicate no infection when infection is present (called false-negative results). If results are negative in children and adolescents, culture is needed. A sample taken from the throat with a swab is sent to a laboratory so that group A streptococci, if present, can be grown (cultured) overnight. In adults, negative results do not require confirmation by culture because the incidence of streptococcal infection and risk of rheumatic fever in adults is so low.

If group A streptococci are identified, they may be tested to see which antibiotics are effective (a process called susceptibility testing).

Cellulitis and impetigo can often be diagnosed based on symptoms, although culture of a sample taken from impetigo sores can often help doctors identify other microorganisms that may be the cause, such as *Staphylococcus aureus*.

To diagnose necrotizing fasciitis, doctors frequently use x-rays, computed tomography (CT), or magnetic resonance imaging (MRI) and culture. Exploratory surgery is often required to confirm the diagnosis.

Treatment

Strep throat usually resolves within 1 to 2 weeks, even without treatment. Antibiotics reduce the severity of symptoms but shorten their duration by only about 1 day. Nevertheless, antibiotics are given to help prevent the spread of the infection to the middle ear, sinuses, and mastoid bone, as well as to prevent spread to other people. Antibiotic therapy also helps prevent rheumatic fever, although it may not prevent kidney inflammation (glomerulonephritis). Usually, antibiotics need not be started immediately. Waiting up to 9 days for culture results before starting antibiotics does not increase the risk of rheumatic fever. An exception is when a family member has or has had rheumatic fever. Then, every streptococcal infection in any family member should be treated as soon as possible.

Usually, penicillin or amoxicillin is given by mouth for 10 days. One injection of a long-acting penicillin (benzathine) can be given instead. People who cannot take penicillin can be given erythromycin, clarithromycin, or clindamycin by mouth for 10 days or azithromycin for 5 days. Usually, the bacteria that cause strep throat are not resistant to penicillin. In the United States, about 5 to 10% of these bacteria are resistant to erythromycin and related drugs (azithromycin and clarithromycin), but in some countries, more than 10% are resistant.

Fever, headache, and sore throat can be treated with acetaminophen or nonsteroidal anti-inflammatory drugs (NSAIDs), which reduce pain and fever. Neither bed rest nor isolation is necessary.

Serious streptococcal infections (such as necrotizing fasciitis, endocarditis, and severe cellulitis) require penicillin, given intravenously, sometimes with other antibiotics. In necrotizing fasciitis, dead, infected tissue must be surgically removed.

Tetanus

Tetanus (lockjaw) results from a toxin produced by the anaerobic bacteria Clostridium tetani. The toxin makes muscles become rigid and contract involuntarily (spasm).

- Tetanus is rare in the United States but is common in developing countries.
- Diagnosis is based on symptoms
- Vaccination and wound care can prevent tetanus.
- Treatment focuses on treating symptoms until they resolve.

AFTER A WOUND: WHO NEEDS A TETANUS SHOT?

Number of previous vaccinations	CLEAN, MINOR WOUNDS		DEEP OR DIRTY WOUNDS*	
	Tetanus vaccine†	Tetanus immune globulin	Tetanus vaccine	Tetanus immune globulin
Uncertain or fewer than 3	Yes	No	Yes	Yes
3 or more‡	Yes, if it is more than 10 years since the last dose	No	Yes, if it is more than 5 years since the last dose	No

*Included are wounds contaminated with dirt, stool, or saliva, as well as puncture wounds, wounds involving loss of tissue, wounds caused by a penetrating object or crushing, burns, and frostbite.

†Which form of the tetanus vaccine is used depends on the person's age. For people 7 years old or older, tetanus and diphtheria toxoid (Td) vaccine is used. Children younger than 7 years old are given diphtheria, tetanus, and acellular pertussis vaccine (DTaP). Children who cannot be given pertussis vaccine (for example, those who have a seizure or certain other brain or nerve disorders) are given diphtheria and tetanus vaccine (DT)

‡If only three injections of tetanus vaccine have been received, a fourth dose should be given.

Although rare in the United States, tetanus kills up to 500,000 people each year, mainly in developing countries.

Clostridium tetani is present in soil and animal feces. Tetanus bacteria may enter the body through wounds contaminated with soil or feces (especially if the wound is not adequately cleaned) and skin punctures by nonsterile needles (such as those used to inject illegal drugs or to tattoo or do body piercing). Sometimes the injury is so small that people do not even go to a doctor. Injuries that involve dead skin (such as burns, frostbite, gangrene, or crush injuries) are more likely to cause tetanus. When oxygen is absent in dead tissue, tetanus spores reproduce and produce a toxin that travels through the body and prevents nerves from sending signals to other nerves. Occasionally, tetanus results when the uterus is damaged during an induced abortion or childbirth. In developing countries, soil contamination of the stump of the umbilical cord can cause tetanus in newborns.

Vaccination during childhood plus booster doses every 10 years during adulthood can prevent tetanus. Thus, the infection occurs mainly in people who have not been vaccinated or not kept their vaccinations up to date. This situation is more common in developing countries. In the United States, tetanus is a risk for people who inject drugs. The risk is also higher for older people but usually only if they have never been vaccinated.

Symptoms

Symptoms usually begin about 5 to 10 days after the injury. Muscles contract involuntarily (spasm) and become rigid. Spasms usually begin in the jaw (causing lockjaw) and throat (making swallowing difficult), followed by the neck, shoulder, face, and then the abdomen and limbs. Back muscles contract, making the back arch. Spasms of sphincter muscles can lead to constipation and difficulty urinating. People may have a rapid heart beat, profuse sweating, and a high fever. Slight disturbances—such as noise, a draft, or the bed being jarred—can trigger painful muscle spasms throughout the body. Such spasms may interfere with breathing, sometimes so much that people turn blue. Rarely, muscle spasms may be limited to muscle groups near the wound. Such localized tetanus may persist for weeks. Even when the illness is severe, people remain fully conscious.

Worldwide, about 50% of people who have tetanus die. But in the United States, only about 10 to 15% die if the disorder is treated appropriately. People who inject drugs, the very young, and the very old are more likely to die of tetanus.

Did You Know...

Promptly and thoroughly cleaning dirty wounds can help prevent tetanus.

Diagnosis

A doctor suspects tetanus when certain muscles (commonly, jaw and back muscles) become rigid or spasms occur, particularly in people who have a wound. The bacteria can sometimes be grown (cultured) from a sample taken from the wound. Detecting the bacteria in cultures confirms the diagnosis, but tetanus is possible even if no bacteria are detected.

Prevention

Preventing tetanus is far better than treating tetanus. Tetanus rarely develops in people who have completed a primary series of tetanus vaccinations (three or more injections into a muscle) and had vaccinations every 10 years, as recommended. The tetanus vaccine stimulates the body to produce antibodies that neutralize the toxin. But neutralization can take weeks. In young children, the tetanus vaccine is given as part of a series that includes the diphtheria and pertussis (whooping cough) vaccines. Adults who have completed the primary series of tetanus vaccination should get tetanus boosters every 10 years.

When people are injured, they can help prevent tetanus by promptly and thoroughly cleaning wounds. People who have wounds may be given tetanus vaccine to prevent tetanus from developing. Because the vaccine takes weeks to be effective, tetanus immune globulin is sometimes given in addition. It provides antibodies that neutralize the toxin immediately.

Treatment

People with tetanus are admitted to an intensive care unit. The room is kept quiet to prevent disturbances that could trigger muscle spasms. Wounds are cleaned thoroughly, and dead tissue and foreign material are removed.

Antibiotics (usually metronidazole) are given intravenously to kill the bacteria and thus stop the production of toxin. However, antibiotics have no effect on toxin that has already been produced. Tetanus immune globulin is usually given to neutralize the toxin already produced. Tetanus vaccine is given unless vaccinations are known to be up to date.

Sedatives, such as the benzodiazepine diazepam, may be given to control muscle spasms, to help relax rigid muscles, and to relieve pain and anxiety. If muscle rigidity interferes with breathing, an opening may be made in the windpipe (called tracheostomy). Sometimes mechanical ventilation is also needed. If swallowing is difficult, nutrition and fluids are given intravenously or, less often, through a tube inserted through the nose and into the stomach.

After people recover, they are given the full series of vaccinations to prevent future episodes of tetanus.

Toxic Shock Syndrome

Toxic shock syndrome is a group of rapidly progressive and severe symptoms that include fever, rash, dangerously low blood pressure, and failure of several organs. It is caused by toxins produced by Staphylococcus aureus *or group A* streptococci.

- Using superabsorbent tampons or having an infection caused by *Staphylococcus aureus* or group A streptococci increases the risk of this syndrome.
- The syndrome can be fatal, particularly when caused by streptococci.
- Changing tampons frequently and not using superabsorbent tampons can help reduce the risk of the syndrome.
- Treatment focuses on relieving symptoms and preventing production of more toxin.

Toxic shock syndrome results from toxins produced by *Staphylococcus aureus* or group A streptococci. It may occur when *Staphylococcus aureus* infects tissue (for example, in a wound) or is simply growing on a tampon (especially the superabsorbent type) in the vagina. Exactly why superabsorbent tampons increase the risk of this syndrome is unknown. Leaving a diaphragm in the vagina for more than 24 hours also increases the risk slightly. This syndrome may also occur in the following situations:

- When a surgical incision is infected, even when the infection seems minor
- When the uterus becomes infected after delivery of a baby
- After nose surgery if bandages are used to pack the nose
- In otherwise healthy people who have a group A streptococcal tissue infection, usually of the skin

Symptoms

If staphylococci or streptococci are the cause, symptoms develop suddenly and worsen rapidly over a few days. People may have a high fever, a red and sore throat, red eyes, diarrhea, and muscle aches. A rash that resembles sunburn covers the entire body, including the palms and soles. Then, the skin peels. Blood pressure falls to dangerously low levels, and people become delirious. Fluid accumulates in tissues, causing swelling (edema). Blood does not clot normally, making bleeding more likely and more severe. Several organs such as the kidneys, liver, heart, and lungs may malfunction or stop functioning.

In streptococcal toxic shock syndrome, the wound is painful. Gangrene may develop around the wound.

When streptococci are involved, up to 70% of people die. When staphylococci are involved, 5% of people die if the syndrome is related to menstruation, and 15% die if it is not. If people survive, recovery is usually complete.

When the source is a tampon infected by staphylococci, the syndrome may recur, usually within 4 months of the first episode. Occasionally, the syndrome recurs more than once. Each episode tends to be milder. To reduce the risk of recurrences, women who have had the syndrome should not use tampons or diaphragms.

Diagnosis

The diagnosis is usually based on the symptoms and results of a physical examination and routine blood tests. Samples of blood and infected tissue are sent to a laboratory where bacteria can be grown (cultured).

Prevention

Women who use tampons can take several measures to prevent infection:

- Not using superabsorbent tampons
- Using the least absorbent tampons needed
- Alternating use of tampons and pads
- Changing tampons every 4 to 8 hours

Otherwise, there are no recommendations for preventing toxic shock syndrome.

Treatment

If toxic shock syndrome is suspected, people are hospitalized, usually in an intensive care unit. Fluids that contain salts and often drugs to increase blood pressure to normal levels are given intravenously. Many people need help with breathing, usually with a mechanical ventilator. Tampons, diaphragms, and other foreign objects are removed from the vagina promptly. Antibiotics and, for severe cases, immune globulin (which can neutralize the toxin) are given intravenously. Areas that could contain the bacteria, such as surgical wounds and the vagina, are flushed out with water (irrigated).

If wounds are infected, surgery may be needed to clean them out further, to remove infected tissue, or sometimes, if gangrene has developed, to remove a limb.

Tularemia

Tularemia (rabbit fever, deer fly fever) is infection that is caused by the bacteria Francisella tularensis, *which is acquired from wild animals, usually rabbits.*

- Handling carcasses, being bitten by a tick, inhaling infected sprayed particles, and eating or drinking infected material can cause infection.
- Symptoms can include fever, sores, and swollen lymph nodes.

- Cultures of tissue samples or blood help doctors make the diagnosis.
- Injections of antibiotics are almost always effective.
- Preventing tick bites, handling carcasses carefully, and disinfecting water can reduce the risk of tularemia.

Francisella tularensis is normally present in animals, especially rodents, rabbits, and hares. People may be infected by doing the following:

- Handling infected animal carcasses (as when hunters skin rabbits or when butchers, farmers, fur handlers, and laboratory workers handle animals or animal products)
- Being bitten by an infected tick, deerfly, or other insect, usually during the summer (particularly for children)
- Eating or drinking contaminated food (such as undercooked rabbit meat) or water
- Inhaling airborne particles that contain the bacteria (as when grass is mowed or brush is cut or when people are working with the bacteria in a laboratory)

Francisella tularensis is a potential biological weapon. It can be spread through the air and be inhaled. The size of the airborne particles determines where they lodge in the respiratory tract. Small particles lodge in air sacs of the lungs and cause pneumonia.

Tularemia is not spread from person to person.

Symptoms

Different types of tularemia affect different parts of the body and thus cause different symptoms. Symptoms usually appear 3 to 5 days after exposure to the bacteria but can take up to 14 days.

Sores may develop near the scratch or bite that started the infection. Lymph nodes near the infected area may swell and become painful. A fever up to 104° F (40° C) may appear suddenly, with chills, drenching sweats, and muscle aches. People may have a general feeling of illness (malaise) and feel nauseated. They may vomit and lose weight. A rash may appear at any time. Sometimes pus collects, forming an abscess.

Overall, without treatment, 5 to 15% of people with tularemia die. However, with certain types of tularemia (typhoidal or pneumonic), 30 to 60% die. With appropriate treatment, fewer than 1% die. Death usually results from overwhelming infection, pneumonia, meningitis, or infection of the lining of the abdominal cavity (peritonitis).

Relapses are uncommon but can occur if treatment is inadequate. People who have had tularemia are immune to reinfection.

Types of Tularemia

There are several types of tularemia.

Ulceroglandular: This type is the most common. Open painful sores develop where the bacteria entered the skin: through a break in the skin, usually on the hands and fingers, or a tick bite, usually in the groin, armpit, or trunk. The bacteria travel to nearby lymph nodes, making them swollen and painful. Occasionally, the skin around the lymph nodes breaks down, and pus may drain from them.

Glandular: The lymph nodes become swollen and painful, but sores do not form.

Oculoglandular: An eye becomes painful, swollen, and red, and pus often oozes from it. Nearby lymph nodes become swollen and painful. This type probably results from touching the eye with a contaminated finger or from having infected fluid splashed into the eye.

Oropharyngeal: The throat (pharynx) is sore, and lymph nodes in the neck are swollen. Some people also have abdominal pain, nausea, vomiting, and diarrhea. This type is usually caused by eating undercooked contaminated meat.

Typhoidal: Chills, high fever, and abdominal pain develop, but no sores form and lymph nodes do not swell. This type develops when the bloodstream is infected. Sometimes the source of infection is unknown.

Pneumonic: The lungs are infected. People may have a dry cough, be short of breath, and have chest pain. This type is caused by inhaling the bacteria or spread of the bacteria through the bloodstream to the lungs. This type develops in 10 to 15% of people with ulceroglandular tularemia and in 50% of people with typhoidal tularemia.

Diagnosis

A doctor suspects tularemia in people who develop sudden fever, swollen lymph nodes, and characteristic sores after having been exposed to ticks or deer flies or after having even slight contact with a wild mammal (especially a rabbit).

Samples of infected material, such as blood, fluids from a lymph node, pus from sores, or sputum, are taken. They are sent to a laboratory where the bacteria can be grown (cultured). Blood may also be tested for antibodies to the bacteria.

Prevention

If people are visiting areas where tularemia is common, they should do all of the following:

- Apply insect repellent containing 25 to 30% diethyltoluamide (DEET) to exposed skin
- Wear clothing treated with a repellent containing permethrin
- Stay on paths and trails when walking in wooded areas
- Walk in the center of trails to avoid brushing against bushes and weeds
- Wear long pants and tuck them into socks and boots
- Thoroughly search their clothing, themselves, family members, and pets for ticks
- Not drink or bathe, swim or work in untreated water, which may be contaminated

Promptly searching for ticks can help prevent the infection because transmission of infection usually requires that ticks be attached for 4 or more hours. If found, ticks should be removed immediately (see box on page 1166).

When handling rabbits and rodents, people should wear protective clothing (such as rubber gloves and face masks) because bacteria may be present. Wild birds and game should be thoroughly cooked before they are eaten.

A vaccine is available, but it is given only to people whose occupation puts them at risk, mainly laboratory workers. After exposure to the bacteria (for example, after a laboratory accident), people are given doxycycline or ciprofloxacin to prevent the infection from developing.

Treatment

People who have tularemia do not need to be isolated. Tularemia is usually treated with injections of gentamicin or streptomycin for 7 to 14 days. Other antibiotics, including fluoroquinolones (such as ciprofloxacin and levofloxacin) and tetracyclines (such as minocycline and doxycycline), are also effective.

Rarely, large abscesses must be drained surgically. Applying warm compresses to an affected eye, wearing dark glasses, and using prescription eye drops may help. People with intense headaches are usually treated with opioids, such as oxycodone.

Bacteremia, Sepsis, and Septic Shock

Bacteremia, sepsis, and septic shock are related:

- **Bacteremia:** Bacteria are present in the bloodstream. Bacteremia can result from a serious infection or from something as harmless as vigorous toothbrushing. Most often, only a small number of bacteria are present, and they are removed by the body on its own. In such cases, most people have no symptoms. However, occasionally, bacteremia leads to infections, sepsis, or both.

- **Sepsis:** Bacteremia or another infection triggers a serious bodywide response (sepsis), which typically includes fever, weakness, a rapid heart rate, a rapid breathing rate, and an increased number of white blood cells.

- **Septic shock:** Sepsis that causes dangerously low blood pressure (shock) is septic shock. As a result, internal organs typically receive too little blood, causing them to malfunction. Septic shock is life threatening.

Bacteremia

Bacteremia is the presence of bacteria in the bloodstream (see also page 1761).

- Bacteremia may result from ordinary activities (such as toothbrushing), dental or medical procedures, or from infections (such as pneumonia or a urinary tract infection).

- Having an artificial joint or heart valve or having heart valve abnormalities increases the risk that bacteremia will persist or cause problems.

- Bacteremia usually causes no symptoms, but sometimes bacteria accumulate in certain tissues or organs and cause serious infections.

- People at high risk of complications from bacteremia are given antibiotics before certain dental and medical procedures.

Usually, bacteremia, particularly if it occurs during ordinary activities, does not cause infections because bacteria typically are present only in small numbers and are rapidly removed from the bloodstream by the immune system. However, if bacteria are present long enough and in large enough numbers, particularly in people who have a weakened immune system, bacteremia can lead to other infections and sometimes trigger a serious bodywide response called sepsis.

Bacteria that are not removed by the immune system may accumulate in various places throughout the body, causing infections there, as in the following:

- Tissues that cover the brain (meningitis)
- The sac around the heart (pericarditis)
- The cells lining the heart valves and the heart (endocarditis)
- Bones (osteomyelitis)
- Joints (infectious arthritis)

In bacteremia, bacteria tend to lodge and collect on structures, such as abnormal heart valves, and any artificial material present in the body, such as intravenous catheters and artificial (prosthetic) joints and heart valves. These collections (colonies) of bacteria may remain attached to the sites and continuously or periodically release bacteria into the bloodstream.

Causes

Ordinary activities sometimes cause bacteremia in healthy people. For example, vigorous toothbrushing can cause bacteremia because bacteria living on the gums around the teeth are forced into the bloodstream. Bacteria may also enter the bloodstream from the intestine during digestion. Bacteremia that occurs during ordinary activities rarely leads to infections.

Dental or medical procedures can lead to bacteremia. During dental procedures (as during tooth cleaning by a dental hygienist), bacteria living on the gums may become dislodged and enter the bloodstream. Bacteremia may also occur when catheters are inserted into the bladder or tubes are inserted into the digestive or urinary tract. Bacteria may be present at the site of insertion (such as the bladder or intestine). So even though sterile techniques are used, these procedures may move bacteria into the bloodstream. Surgical treatment of infected wounds, abscesses, and pressure sores can dislodge bacteria from the infected site, causing bacteremia.

In some bacterial infections, such as pneumonia and skin abscesses, bacteria may periodically enter the bloodstream, causing bacteremia. Many common childhood bacterial infections cause bacteremia.

Injecting recreational drugs can cause bacteremia because the needles used are usually contaminated with bacteria.

Symptoms and Diagnosis

Usually, bacteremia that results from ordinary events such as dental procedures causes no symptoms. Bacteremia due to other conditions sometimes causes fever. If people with bacteremia have a fever, a rapid heart rate, and rapid breathing, sepsis is likely.

If bacteremia is suspected, doctors usually do blood tests to try to grow (culture) the bacteria in the laboratory.

Prevention and Treatment

People who are at high risk of complications due to bacteremia (such as those who have an artificial heart valve or joint or certain heart valve abnormalities) are often given antibiotics before procedures that can cause bacteremia:

- Dental procedures
- Surgical treatment of infected wounds
- Insertion of bladder catheters

Antibiotics help prevent bacteremia and thus infections and sepsis from developing.

If an infection or sepsis develops, it is treated.

Sepsis and Septic Shock

Sepsis is a serious bodywide response to bacteremia or another infection. Septic shock is life-threatening low blood pressure (shock) due to sepsis.

- Usually, sepsis results from certain bacterial infections, often acquired in a hospital.
- Having certain conditions, such as a weakened immune system, certain chronic disorders, an artificial joint or heart valve, and certain heart valve abnormalities, increases the risk.
- At first, people have a high (or sometimes low) body temperature, sometimes with shaking chills and weakness.
- As sepsis worsens, the heart beats rapidly, breathing becomes rapid, people become confused, and blood pressure drops.
- Doctors suspect the diagnosis based on symptoms and confirm it by detecting bacteria in a sample of blood, urine, or other material.
- Antibiotics are given immediately, and people with septic shock are given oxygen and fluids and sometimes drugs to increase blood pressure.

Usually, the body's response to infection is limited to the specific area infected. But in sepsis, the response to infection occurs throughout the body—called a systemic response. This response includes an abnormally high temperature (fever) or low temperature (hypothermia) plus one or more of the following:

- Rapid heart rate
- Rapid breathing rate
- An abnormally high or low number of white blood cells

As sepsis worsens, organs begin to malfunction and blood pressure may decrease. Sepsis is considered severe if organs malfunction. Septic shock is diagnosed when blood pressure remains low despite intensive treatment. In the United States, about 90,000 people, usually those who are hospitalized, die of septic shock each year.

Sepsis occurs when toxins produced by the bacteria cause cells in the body to release substances that trigger inflammation (cytokines). Although cytokines help the immune system fight infection, they can have harmful effects:

- They can cause the blood vessels to widen (dilate), decreasing blood pressure.
- They can cause blood to clot in tiny blood vessels inside organs.

These effects lead to a series of harmful complications:

- Blood flow decreases to vital organs (such as the kidneys, heart, and brain).
- The heart attempts to compensate by working harder, increasing the heart rate and the amount of blood pumped. Eventually, the bacterial toxins and the increased work of pumping weaken the heart. As a result, the heart pumps less blood, and vital organs receive even less blood.
- When tissues do not receive enough blood, they release excess lactic acid (a waste product) into the bloodstream, making the blood more acidic.

All of these effects result in a vicious circle of worsening organ malfunction:

- The kidneys excrete little or no urine, and metabolic waste products (such as urea nitrogen) accumulate in the blood.
- The walls of blood vessels may leak, allowing fluid to escape from the bloodstream into tissues and cause swelling.
- Lung function worsens because blood vessels in the lungs leak fluid, which accumulates, making breathing difficult.

Blood clots continue to form, using up the proteins in blood that make up clots (clotting factors). Then, excessive bleeding may occur.

Causes

Most often, sepsis is caused by infection with certain kinds of bacteria, usually acquired in a hospital. Rarely, fungi, such as *Candida*, cause sepsis. Infections that can lead to sepsis begin most commonly in the lungs, abdomen, or urinary tract. In most people, these infections do not lead to sepsis. However, sometimes bacteria spread into the bloodstream (a condition called bacteremia). Sepsis may then develop. If the initial infection involves a collection of pus (abscess), the risk of bacteremia and sepsis is increased. Occasionally, sepsis is triggered by toxins released by bacteria, rather than from bacteria entering the bloodstream (bacteremia).

Risk Factors

The risk of sepsis is increased in people with conditions that reduce their ability to fight serious infections. These conditions include the following:

- Being a newborn
- Being over 35
- Being pregnant
- Having certain chronic disorders such as diabetes or cirrhosis
- Having a weakened immune system—due to use of drugs that suppress the immune system (such as chemotherapy drugs or corticosteroids) or due to certain disorders (such as cancer, AIDS, and immune disorders)

The risk is also increased in people who are more likely to have bacteria enter their bloodstream. Such people include those who have a medical device inserted into the body (such as a catheter inserted into a vein or the urinary tract, drainage tubes, or breathing tubes). When medical devices are inserted, they can move bacteria into the body. Bacteria may also collect on the surface of such devices, making infection and sepsis more likely. The longer the device is left in place, the greater the risk.

Other conditions also increase the risk of sepsis:

- Injecting recreational drugs: The drugs and needles used are rarely sterile. Each injection may cause bacteremia to varying degrees. People who use these drugs are also at risk of disorders that can weaken the immune system (such as AIDS).
- Having an artificial (prosthetic) joint or heart valve or certain heart valve abnormalities: Bacteria tend to lodge and collect on these structures. The bacteria may continuously or periodically be released into the bloodstream.
- Having an infection that persists despite treatment with antibiotics: Some bacteria that cause infections and sepsis are resistant to antibiotics. Antibiotics do not eradicate the resistant bacteria. Thus, if an infection persists in people who are taking antibiotics, it is more likely to be caused by bacteria that are resistant to antibiotics and that can cause sepsis.

Symptoms

Most people have a fever, but some have a low body temperature. People may have shaking chills and feel weak. Other symptoms may also be present depending on the type and location of the initial infection. Breathing, heart rate, or both may be rapid.

As sepsis worsens, people become confused and less alert. The skin becomes warm and flushed. The pulse is rapid and pounding, and people breathe rapidly. People urinate less often and in smaller amounts, and blood pressure decreases. Later, body temperature often falls below normal, and breathing becomes very difficult. The skin may become cool and mottled or blue because blood flow is reduced. Reduced blood flow may cause tissue, including tissue in vital organs (such as the intestine), to die, resulting in gangrene.

When septic shock develops, blood pressure is low despite treatment.

With treatment, the risk of death is about 15% for people with sepsis and 40% or more for people with septic shock.

Diagnosis

Doctors usually suspect sepsis when a person who has an infection suddenly develops a very high or low temperature, a rapid heart or breathing rate, or low blood pressure. To confirm the diagnosis, doctors look for bacteria in the bloodstream (bacteremia), evidence of another infection that could be causing sepsis, and an abnormal number of white blood cells in a blood sample.

Samples of blood are taken to try to grow (culture) the bacteria in the laboratory—a process that takes 1 to 3 days. However, if people have been taking antibiotics for their initial infection, bacteria may be present but not grow in the culture. Sometimes catheters are removed from the body, and the tips are cut off and sent for culture. Finding bacteria in a catheter that had contact with the blood indicates that bacteria are probably in the bloodstream.

To check for other infections that may cause sepsis, doctors take samples of fluids or tissue, such as urine, cerebrospinal fluid, tissue from wounds, or sputum coughed up from the lungs. These samples are cultured and checked for bacteria. Imaging tests may also be done.

Other tests are done to look for signs of organ malfunction and other complications of sepsis. They may include the following:

- Blood tests to measure levels of lactic acid and other metabolic waste products, which may be high, and the number of platelets (cells that help the blood clot), which may be low
- Blood tests or a sensor placed on a finger (pulse oximetry) to measure oxygen levels and thus evaluate how well the lungs and blood vessels are functioning
- Electrocardiography (ECG) to look for abnormalities in heart rhythm and thus determine whether the blood supply to the heart is adequate
- Other tests to determine whether shock results from sepsis or another problem

Treatment

Sepsis and septic shock must be treated immediately with antibiotics—even before test results confirm the diagnosis. A delay in antibiotic treatment greatly decreases the chances of survival. People with symptoms of septic shock are immediately admitted to an intensive care unit for treatment.

When choosing the initial antibiotics, doctors consider which bacteria are most likely to be present, which depends on where the infection started. Often, two or three antibiotics are given together to increase the chances of killing the bacteria, particularly when the source of the bacteria is unknown. Later, when the test results are available, doctors can substitute the antibiotic that is most effective against the specific bacteria causing the infection.

If present, abscesses are drained, and catheters or other medical devices that may have started the infection are removed. Surgery may be done to remove dead tissue.

Severe sepsis or septic shock can be treated with drotrecogin alfa (activated protein C). This drug is an artificially produced human protein that prevents inflammation and blood clotting. It may reduce the risk of death due to severe sepsis or septic shock.

People with septic shock are also given large amounts of fluid intravenously to increase the amount of fluid in the bloodstream and thus increase blood pressure. Drugs, such as dopamine or norepinephrine (which cause blood vessels to narrow), may be needed to increase blood flow to the brain, heart, and other organs. Oxygen is given through a mask, through nasal prongs, or, if a breathing (endotracheal) tube has been inserted, through that tube. If needed, a mechanical ventilator is used to help with breathing.

CHAPTER 176 Antibiotics

- Although doctors try to use antibiotics for specific bacterial infections, they sometimes start antibiotics without waiting for tests that identify the specific bacteria.
- Bacteria can develop resistance to the effects of antibiotics.
- Taking antibiotics as directed, even after symptoms disappear, is essential to curing the infection and to preventing the development of resistance in bacteria.
- Antibiotics can have side effects, such as upset stomach, diarrhea, and, in women, vaginal yeast infections.
- Some people are allergic to certain antibiotics.

Antibiotics (antibacterials) are drugs derived wholly or partially from bacteria or molds and are used to treat bacterial infections. They are ineffective against viral infections (see page 1236) and fungal infections (see page 1229). Antibiotics either kill microorganisms or stop them from reproducing, allowing the body's natural defenses to eliminate them.

Selecting an Antibiotic

Each antibiotic is effective only against certain bacteria. In selecting an antibiotic to treat a person with an infection, doctors estimate which bacteria are likely to be the cause. For example, some infections are caused only by certain types of bacteria. If one antibiotic is predictably effective against all of these bacteria, further testing is not needed. If infections may be caused by many different types of bacteria or by bacteria that are not predictably susceptible to antibiotics, a laboratory is asked to identify the infecting bacteria from samples of blood, urine, or tissue taken from the person (see box on page 1140). The infecting bacteria are then tested for susceptibility to a variety of antibiotics. Results of these tests usually take a day or two and thus cannot guide the initial choice of antibiotic.

Antibiotics that are effective in the laboratory do not necessarily work in an infected person. The effectiveness of the treatment depends on how well the drug is absorbed into the bloodstream, how much of the drug reaches the sites of infection in the body, and how quickly the body eliminates the drug. These factors may vary from person to person, depending on other drugs being taken, other disorders present, and the person's age. In selecting an antibiotic, doctors also consider the nature and seriousness of the infection, the drug's possible side effects, the possibility of allergies or other serious reactions to the drug, and the cost of the drug.

Combinations of antibiotics may be needed to treat the following:

- Severe infections, particularly during the first days when the bacteria's susceptibility to antibiotics is not known
- Certain infections caused by bacteria that rapidly develop resistance to a single antibiotic
- Infections caused by more than one type of bacteria if each type is susceptible to a different antibiotic

Antibiotic Resistance

Bacteria, like all living organisms, change over time in response to environmental challenges. Because of the widespread use and misuse of antibiotics, bacteria

SPOTLIGHT ON AGING

When doctors prescribe antibiotics for older people, they may start with a lower dose than usual because the kidneys tend to function less well as people age. In such cases, the kidneys may not be able to eliminate antibiotics from the body as effectively, increasing the risk of side effects.

Doctors also consider the following:

- What other drugs the person is taking because older people tend to take many drugs and drug interactions are a risk
- Whether the antibiotic regimen is complex and hard to follow
- Whether the person has family members or caregivers who can help the person take the antibiotic as prescribed
- Whether the person lives in a nursing home because different bacteria may cause infections in such situations

are constantly exposed to these drugs. Although many bacteria die when exposed to antibiotics, some develop resistance to the drugs' effects. For example, 50 years ago, *Staphylococcus aureus* (a common cause of skin infections) was very sensitive to penicillin. But over time, strains of this bacteria developed an enzyme able to break down penicillin, making the drug ineffective. Researchers responded by developing a form of penicillin that the enzyme could not break down, but after a few years, the bacteria adapted and became resistant to this modified penicillin. Other bacteria have also developed resistance to antibiotics.

Medical research continues to develop drugs to combat bacteria. But patients and doctors can help prevent the development of resistance in bacteria. Taking antibiotics only when necessary can help. That is, people should take antibiotics only for infections caused by bacteria, not for those caused by viruses such as a cold or the flu. Also, taking antibiotics for the complete time prescribed helps limit the development of resistance.

Taking Antibiotics

For severe bacterial infections, antibiotics are usually first given by injection (usually into a vein but sometimes into a muscle). When the infection is controlled, antibiotics can then be taken by mouth. For less severe infections, antibiotics can be given by mouth from the start.

Antibiotics need to be taken until the infecting bacteria are eliminated from the body, which may

be days after the symptoms disappear. So people must take antibiotics for the entire time prescribed whether they have symptoms or not. Antibiotics are rarely given for fewer than 5 days. (An exception is certain uncomplicated urinary tract infections.) Stopping treatment too soon can result in a return of the infection or the development of antibiotic-resistant bacteria.

A doctor, nurse, or pharmacist can explain how the prescribed antibiotic should be taken and what side effects it may have. Some antibiotics must be taken on an empty stomach. Others may be taken with food. Metronidazole, a common antibiotic, causes an unpleasant reaction with alcohol. Also, some antibiotics can interact with other drugs people may be taking, possibly reducing the effectiveness or increasing the side effects of the antibiotic or the other drugs. Some antibiotics make the skin sensitive to sunlight.

Antibiotics are sometimes used to prevent infections (called prophylaxis). Antibiotics may be given to people who have been exposed to a person with meningitis to prevent meningitis from developing. Some people with abnormal or artificial heart valves take antibiotics before dental and surgical procedures to prevent bacteria from infecting the damaged or artificial valves (such procedures can allow bacteria to enter the body). People undergoing surgery with a high risk of introducing infection (such as major orthopedic or intestinal surgery) may be given antibiotics immediately before the operation. To be effective and to avoid the development of resistance in bacteria, doctors give preventive antibiotics for only a short time. Antibiotics may also be given to people who have a weakened immune system, such as people with leukemia, people taking chemotherapy for cancer, or people with AIDS, because such people are particularly susceptible to serious infections. They may need to take the antibiotics for a long time.

Did You Know...

If a virus is causing the infection, taking antibiotics is useless and can contribute to the development of resistance in bacteria.

Home Antibiotic Therapy

Usually, antibiotics are given by mouth, and the length of treatment does not cause hardship. However, some infections—such as those involving bone (osteomyelitis) or the heart (endocarditis)—require antibiotics to be given intravenously for a long time, often 4 to 6 weeks. If people have no other conditions that need treatment in the hospital and are feeling relatively well, intravenous (IV) antibiotics may be given at home.

R͓x ANTIBIOTICS

DRUG	COMMON USES	SOME SIDE EFFECTS
Aminoglycosides		
Amikacin Gentamicin Kanamycin Neomycin Netilmicin Streptomycin Tobramycin	Infections caused by gram-negative bacteria, such as *Escherichia coli* and *Klebsiella* species	Hearing loss Dizziness Kidney damage
Carbapenems		
Ertapenem Doripenem Imipenem-cilastatin Meropenem	Gangrene, sepsis, pneumonia, abdominal and urinary infections, infections due to susceptible bacteria resistant to other antibiotics, and (except for ertapenem) *Pseudomonas* infections	Seizures (especially with imipenem) Confusion
Cephalosporins, 1st generation		
Cefadroxil Cefazolin Cephalexin	Mainly skin and soft-tissue infections	Gastrointestinal upset and diarrhea Nausea Allergic reactions
Cephalosporins, 2nd generation		
Cefaclor Cefoxitin Cefprozil Cefuroxime Loracarbef	Some respiratory and, for cefoxitin, abdominal infections	Gastrointestinal upset and diarrhea Nausea Allergic reactions
Cephalosporins, 3rd generation		
Cefdinir Cefditoren Cefixime Cefoperazone Cefotaxime Cefpodoxime Ceftazidime Ceftibuten Ceftizoxime Ceftriaxone	Given by mouth: Broad coverage of many bacteria for people with mild-to-moderate infections, including skin and soft-tissue infections Given by injection: Serious infections (such as meningitis or infections acquired in a hospital)	Gastrointestinal upset and diarrhea Nausea Allergic reactions
Cephalosporins, 4th generation		
Cefepime	Serious infections (including *Pseudomonas* infections), particularly in people with a weakened immune system and infections due to susceptible bacteria that are resistant to other antibiotics	Gastrointestinal upset and diarrhea Nausea Allergic reactions
Cephalosporins, 5th generation		
Ceftobiprole	Complicated skin infections (including foot infections in people with diabetes) due to susceptible bacteria, such as *Escherichia coli*, *Pseudomonas aeruginosa*, and methicillin-resistant *Staphylococcus aureus* (MRSA)	

(continued on the following page)

℞ ANTIBIOTICS (Continued)

DRUG	COMMON USES	SOME SIDE EFFECTS
Fluoroquinolones		
Ciprofloxacin Levofloxacin Lomefloxacin Moxifloxacin Norfloxacin Ofloxacin Trovafloxacin	Sepsis, urinary tract infections, bacterial prostatitis, bacterial diarrhea, and gonorrhea	Nausea (rare) Nervousness, tremors, and seizures Inflammation or rupture of tendons Abnormal heart rhythms (arrhythmias) Antibiotic-associated diarrhea and inflammation of the colon (colitis) With trovafloxacin, sometimes fatal liver damage
Glycylcycline		
Tigecycline	Complicated abdominal infections and complicated skin infections due to susceptible bacteria, such as *Escherichia coli, Staphylococcus aureus* (including those resistant to methicillin), and anaerobes	Gastrointestinal upset Sensitivity to sunlight Permanent staining of teeth in the fetus if used late in pregnancy or in children under 8 years of age
Macrolides		
Azithromycin Clarithromycin Dirithromycin Erythromycin Troleandomycin	Streptococcal infections, syphilis, respiratory infections, mycoplasmal infections, and Lyme disease	Nausea, vomiting, and diarrhea (especially at higher doses) Jaundice Abnormal heart rhythms
Monobactam		
Aztreonam	Infections caused by gram-negative bacteria	Allergic reactions Can be used in patients allergic to antibiotics such as penicillins, cephalosporins, and carbapenems
Penicillins		
Amoxicillin Ampicillin Carbenicillin Cloxacillin Dicloxacillin Nafcillin Oxacillin Penicillin G Penicillin V Piperacillin Ticarcillin	Wide range of infections, including streptococcal infections, syphilis, and Lyme disease	Nausea, vomiting, and diarrhea Allergy with serious anaphylactic reactions Brain and kidney damage (rare)
Polypeptides*		
Bacitracin Colistin Polymyxin B	Ear, eye, skin, or bladder infections Usually applied directly to the skin, and rarely given by injection	Kidney and nerve damage (when given by injection)
Sulfonamides		
Mafenide Sulfacetamide Sulfamethizole Sulfasalazine Sulfisoxazole Trimethoprim-sulfamethoxazole	Urinary tract infections (except sulfasalazine, sulfacetamide, and mafenide) For mafenide, only topically for burns	Nausea, vomiting, and diarrhea Allergy (including skin rashes) Crystals in urine (rare) Decrease in white blood cell and platelet counts Sensitivity to sunlight Possibly increased tendency to bleed if used with warfarin

(continued on the following page)

℞ ANTIBIOTICS (Continued)

DRUG	COMMON USES	SOME SIDE EFFECTS
Tetracyclines		
Demeclocycline Doxycycline Minocycline Oxytetracycline Tetracycline	Syphilis, chlamydial infections, Lyme disease, mycoplasmal infections, and rickettsial infections	Gastrointestinal upset Sensitivity to sunlight Staining of teeth in the fetus if used late in pregnancy or in children under 8 years of age
Miscellaneous antibiotics		
Chloramphenicol	Typhoid, other salmonellal infections, and meningitis	Severe decrease in white blood cell count (rare)
Clindamycin	Streptococcal and staphylococcal infections, respiratory infections, and lung abscess	Antibiotic-associated diarrhea and inflammation of the colon (colitis)
Daptomycin	Complicated skin infections, bloodstream infections, and certain heart valve infections (endocarditis) due to susceptible bacteria, including methicillin-resistant *Staphylococcus aureus* (MRSA) Not used when infection involves the lungs	Gastrointestinal upset Muscle pain and weakness
Ethambutol	Tuberculosis	Vision disturbances
Fosfomycin	Bladder infections	Diarrhea
Isoniazid	Tuberculosis	Nausea and vomiting Jaundice
Linezolid	Serious infections caused by gram-positive bacteria that are resistant to many other antibiotics	Nausea Headache Diarrhea Anemia and low white blood cell and platelet counts Numbness and tingling in the hands and feet (peripheral neuropathy) Visual disturbances Confusion, agitation, tremors or coma in some people who also use selective serotonin-reuptake inhibitors (SSRIs)
Metronidazole	Vaginitis caused by *Trichomonas* or *Gardnerella* species and pelvic and abdominal infections	Nausea Headache (especially if the drug is taken with alcohol) Metallic taste Numbness and tingling in the hands and feet (peripheral neuropathy) Dark urine
Nitrofurantoin	Urinary tract infections	Nausea and vomiting Allergy
Pyrazinamide	Tuberculosis	Liver dysfunction Gout (occasionally)

(continued on the following page)

Rx ANTIBIOTICS (Continued)

DRUG	COMMON USES	SOME SIDE EFFECTS
Quinupristin-dalfopristin	Serious infections caused by gram-positive bacteria that are resistant to other antibiotics	Aching muscles and joints
Rifampin	Tuberculosis and leprosy	Rash Liver dysfunction Red-orange saliva, sweat, tears, and urine
Spectinomycin	Gonorrhea	Allergy Fever
Telithromycin	Mild to moderate community-acquired pneumonia	Visual disturbances Liver damage (possibly fatal) Worsening of symptoms in people with myasthenia gravis (possibly fatal)
Vancomycin	Serious infections, especially those due to MRSA, *Enterococcus*, or bacteria resistant to other antibiotics	Flushing, itching Allergic reactions Decrease in white blood cell and platelet counts

*Polypeptide antibiotics are usually applied directly to the skin or eye and are rarely given by injection.

When antibiotics have to be given a long time, the short IV catheters that are inserted into a small vein in the arm or hand (such as those used in most routine hospital procedures) may not be desirable. These catheters last only up to 3 days. Instead, a special type of IV catheter may be inserted into a large central vein, usually in the neck or chest.

Some devices for infusing antibiotics are simple enough that people and their family members can learn to operate them on their own. In other cases, a visiting nurse must come to the home to give each dose. In either situation, people are carefully supervised to make sure the antibiotic is being given correctly and to watch for possible complications and side effects.

If antibiotics are given at home through an IV catheter, the risk of developing an infection at the site where the catheter is inserted and in the bloodstream is increased. Pain, redness, and pus at the catheter insertion site or chills and fever (even without problems at the insertion site) may indicate a catheter-related infection.

Side Effects and Allergic Reactions

Common side effects of antibiotics include upset stomach, diarrhea, and, in women, vaginal yeast infections. Some side effects are more severe and, depending on the antibiotic, may impair the function of the kidneys, liver, bone marrow, or other organs. Blood tests are sometimes used to check for effects on kidney and other organ function.

Some people who take antibiotics, especially cephalosporins, clindamycin, or fluoroquinolones, develop colitis, an inflammation of the large intestine. This type of colitis results from toxins produced by the bacteria *Clostridium difficile*, which is resistant to many antibiotics and which grows in the intestines unchecked when other normal bacteria in the intestine are killed by the antibiotics (see page 176).

Antibiotics can also cause allergic reactions. Mild allergic reactions consist of an itchy rash or slight wheezing. Severe allergic reactions (anaphylaxis) can be life-threatening and usually include swelling of the throat, inability to breathe, and low blood pressure.

Many people tell their doctor that they are allergic to an antibiotic when they have only experienced side effects that are not allergy-related. The distinction is important because people who are allergic to an antibiotic should not be given that drug or an antibiotic closely related to it. However, people who have experienced only minor side effects can usually take related drugs or even continue taking the same drug. Doctors can determine the significance of any unpleasant reaction people have to an antibiotic.

177 Tuberculosis

Tuberculosis is a contagious infection caused by the airborne bacteria Mycobacterium tuberculosis.

- Tuberculosis is spread only when people breathe air contaminated by a person who has active disease.
- Cough is the most common symptom, but people may also have night sweats, feel generally unwell, and, if tuberculosis affects other organs, have various other symptoms.
- The diagnosis usually involves a tuberculin skin test or a blood test, a chest x-ray, and examination and culture of a sputum sample.
- Two or more antibiotics are always given to reduce the chances of bacterial resistance.
- Early diagnosis and treatment plus isolation of people with active disease until they have responded to treatment help prevent tuberculosis from spreading.

Tuberculosis usually affects the lungs, although it can affect almost any organ in the body. Other related bacteria (called mycobacteria), such as *Mycobacterium bovis* or *Mycobacterium africanum*, can occasionally cause a similar disease.

Tuberculosis has been a serious public health problem for a long time. In the 1800s, the disease caused more than 30% of all deaths in Europe. With the advent of antituberculosis antibiotics in the late 1940s, the battle against tuberculosis seemed to be won. However—because of factors such as inadequate public health resources, reduced immune response due to AIDS, the development of drug resistance, and extreme poverty in many parts of the world—tuberculosis continues to be a deadly disease worldwide, as the following statistics from 2006 show:

- There were 9.2 million new cases of symptomatic tuberculosis and 3 million deaths from the disease. The number of new cases varies widely by country, age, race, sex, and socioeconomic status.
- Of the 9.2 million new cases, about 3 million occurred in Africa, 3 million in Southeast Asia, and about 2 million in the Western Pacific region.
- India and China reported the largest total number of new cases, but South Africa had the highest rate of new cases in the world, with 940 new cases per 100,000 people.

About one third of all the people in the world are thought to have a dormant (latent) tuberculosis infection, although only about 5 to 10% of these infections progress to active tuberculosis.

In the United States, the rate of new cases has decreased 10-fold since 1953 (when national reporting for tuberculosis first began). In 2007, 13,293 cases (about 4.4 cases per 100,000 people) were reported. However, there is a wide range of incidence, from 10.2 per 100,000 people in Washington, DC to 0.4 per 100,000 in Wyoming. Over half of new cases occurred in people born outside the United States in areas where tuberculosis is relatively common (such as Africa, Southeast Asia, or Latin America). In the United States, US-born blacks, the homeless, people in jails and prisons, and other disenfranchised minorities are much more likely to be infected. The rate of new cases among these high-risk groups is likely to be almost as high as that in areas of the world where tuberculosis is relatively common.

> **Did You Know...**
> Tuberculosis caused 3 million deaths worldwide in 2006.

In developing countries, tuberculosis is a disease of young adults. In the United States and other developed countries, tuberculosis has traditionally been more common among older people. More cases have occurred among older people because they were more likely to have acquired the infection in an era when tuberculosis was more common. Moreover, the body's immune system weakens as people age, allowing inactive (dormant) bacteria to become reactivated. However, the incidence of tuberculosis among older people is declining because fewer people in each generation entering old age have inactive (latent) infection. Because the number of new cases among people born outside the United States is increasing, the age profile of tuberculosis infection in the United States is getting younger.

How Infection Develops

With most infectious diseases (such as strep throat or pneumonia), people become sick right after the microorganism enters the body and are noticeably ill within 1 or 2 weeks. Tuberculosis does not follow this pattern.

Stages of Infection: There are several stages:

- Primary infection
- Latent infection
- Active disease

Diseases Resembling Tuberculosis

Many types of mycobacteria (a group of bacteria that includes tuberculosis bacteria) exist. Many of them can cause infections with symptoms similar to those of tuberculosis.

The most common are a group known as *Mycobacterium avium complex* (MAC). Although these mycobacteria are common, they usually cause infection only in people with a weakened immune system or with lungs that have been damaged by smoking for a long time, an old tuberculosis infection, bronchitis, emphysema, or other disorders. Similar to tuberculosis, a MAC infection affects primarily the lungs but may also affect the lymph nodes, bones, skin, and other tissues. Unlike tuberculosis, a MAC infection cannot be passed from one person to another.

The infection usually develops slowly. The first symptoms include coughing and spitting up mucus. As the infection progresses, people may regularly spit up blood and have trouble breathing. A chest x-ray may or may not show an infection. Laboratory analysis of sputum taken from the infected person is needed to distinguish the infection from tuberculosis.

In people with AIDS or other disorders that weaken the immune system, a MAC infection can spread throughout the body. Symptoms include a fever, anemia, blood disorders, diarrhea, and stomach pain.

MAC infection of the lymph nodes may develop in children, typically those aged 1 to 5 years. The infection is usually caused by eating soil or drinking water that is contaminated with the mycobacteria. Antibiotics are usually not necessary to cure the infection. Instead, the infected lymph nodes may be surgically removed.

MAC infections used to be very difficult to treat because the bacteria were resistant to most of the antibiotics effective against tuberculosis. However, newer antibiotics, such as clarithromycin and azithromycin (which do not work in tuberculosis), are effective against MAC when they are used with ethambutol and rifabutin.

Other mycobacteria grow in swimming pools and even in home aquariums. These mycobacteria can cause skin infections, which may clear up without treatment. However, people with chronic infections usually need treatment with tetracycline, clarithromycin, or another antibiotic for 3 to 6 months.

Another type of mycobacteria, *Mycobacterium fortuitum*, can infect wounds and artificial body parts, such as a mechanical heart valve or a breast implant. Antibiotics and surgical removal of the infected areas usually cure the infection.

Except for very young children and people with a weakened immune system, few people become sick immediately after tuberculosis bacteria enter their body (this stage is called primary infection). In most cases, tuberculosis bacteria that enter the lungs are immediately killed by the body's defenses. Bacteria that survive are engulfed by white blood cells called macrophages. The engulfed bacteria can remain alive inside these cells in a dormant state for many years, walled off inside collections of cells that form tiny scars (this stage is called latent infection). In 90 to 95% of cases, the bacteria never cause any further problems, but in about 5 to 10% of infected people, they eventually start to multiply and cause active disease. At this stage, infected people actually become sick and can spread the disease.

More than half the time, dormant bacteria reactivate within the first 2 years after the primary infection, but they may not reactivate for a very long time, even decades. Usually, doctors do not know why the dormant bacteria reactivate, but reactivation is more likely to occur when the person's immune system becomes impaired—for example, from very advanced age, infection with the human immunodeficiency virus (HIV), the use of corticosteroids, or the use of some of the new prescription anti-inflammatory drugs such as adalimumab, etanercept, and infliximab.

Like many infectious diseases, tuberculosis spreads more quickly and is much more dangerous in people who have a weakened immune system. For such people, tuberculosis can be life threatening. In the United States, about 10% of people with tuberculosis die of the disease or a related condition. In parts of the world where tuberculosis is common, the mortality is much higher.

Transmission of Infection: *Mycobacterium tuberculosis* can live only in people. These bacteria are not normally carried by animals, insects, soil, or other nonliving objects. People can be infected with tuberculosis only from a person who has active disease. Touching someone who has the disease does not spread it because the bacteria are spread almost exclusively through the air. *Mycobacterium bovis*, which can live in animals, is an exception. In developing countries, children become infected with it by drinking unpasteurized milk from infected cattle. In developed countries, this type of tuberculosis is no longer a problem because cattle are tested for tuberculosis and milk is pasteurized.

People with active tuberculosis in their lungs often contaminate the air with bacteria when they cough, sneeze, or even speak. These bacteria can stay in the air for several hours. If another person breathes them in, that person may become infected.

? Did You Know...

People with active tuberculosis often contaminate the air when they cough, sneeze, or even talk.

Thus, people who have contact with a person who has active tuberculosis (such as family members or health care practitioners who treat such a person) are at increased risk of getting the infection. People who have latent infection or tuberculosis that is not in their lungs do not expel bacteria into the air and cannot spread the infection.

Progression and Spread of Infection: The progression of tuberculosis from latent infection to active disease varies greatly. Progression to active disease is far more likely and much faster in people with HIV infection and other conditions (including use of drugs) that weaken the immune system. If people with AIDS become infected with *Mycobacterium tuberculosis*, they have a 5 to 10% chance of developing active disease each year. In contrast, people who have latent tuberculosis but do not have AIDS have only a 5 to 10% chance of developing active disease during their lifetime.

In people with a fully functioning immune system, active tuberculosis is usually limited to the lungs (pulmonary tuberculosis). Tuberculosis that affects other parts of the body (extrapulmonary tuberculosis) comes from pulmonary tuberculosis that has spread

from the lungs through the blood. As in the lungs, the infection may not cause disease, but the bacteria may remain dormant in a very small scar. Dormant bacteria in these scars can reactivate later in life, leading to symptoms related to the organs involved.

In pregnant women, tuberculosis bacteria may spread to the fetus and cause disease (called congenital tuberculosis). However, such cases are extremely uncommon.

Symptoms and Complications

Pulmonary Tuberculosis: Cough is the most common symptom of tuberculosis. Because the disease develops slowly, infected people at first may blame the cough on smoking, a recent episode of flu, the common cold, or asthma. The cough may produce a small amount of green or yellow sputum in the morning. Eventually, the sputum may be streaked with blood, although large amounts of blood are rare.

People may awaken in the night and be drenched with a cold sweat, with or without fever. Sometimes there is so much sweat that people have to change nightclothes or even the bed sheets. However, tuberculosis does not always cause night sweats, and many other conditions can cause night sweats.

People also feel generally unwell, with decreased energy and appetite. Weight loss often occurs after they have been ill for a while.

Rapidly developing shortness of breath plus chest pain may signal the presence of air (pneumothorax—see page 520) or fluid (pleural effusion) in the space

TUBERCULOSIS: A DISEASE OF MANY ORGANS

SITE OF INFECTION	SYMPTOMS OR COMPLICATIONS
Abdominal cavity	Fatigue, swelling, slight tenderness, and appendicitis-like pain
Bladder	Painful urination and blood in urine
Bones (mainly in children)	Swelling and minimal pain
Brain	Fever, headache, nausea, drowsiness, and, if untreated, coma and brain damage
Pericardium (the membrane around the heart)	Fever, enlarged neck veins, and shortness of breath
Joints	Arthritis-like symptoms
Kidneys	Kidney damage and infection around the kidneys
Lymph nodes	Painless, red, and swollen lymph nodes, which may drain pus
Reproductive organs in men	Lump in the scrotum
Reproductive organs in women	Sterility
Spine	Pain, leading to collapsed vertebrae and leg paralysis

between the lungs and the chest wall (see page 518). About one third of tuberculosis infections first show up as pleural effusion. Eventually, many people with untreated tuberculosis develop shortness of breath as the infection spreads in the lungs.

Extrapulmonary Tuberculosis: The kidneys and lymph nodes are probably the most common sites for tuberculosis that develops outside the lungs. Tuberculosis can also affect the bones, brain, abdominal cavity, membrane around the heart (pericardium), joints (especially weight-bearing joints, such as the hips and knees), and reproductive organs. Tuberculosis in these areas can be difficult to diagnose.

Symptoms of extrapulmonary tuberculosis are vague, usually with fatigue, poor appetite, intermittent fevers, sweats, and possibly weight loss. Sometimes the infection causes pain, discomfort, a collection of pus (abscess), or other symptoms, depending on the area involved:

■ **Lymph nodes:** In a new tuberculosis infection, the bacteria may travel from the lungs to the lymph nodes that drain the lungs. If the body's natural defenses can control the infection, it goes no further, and the bacteria become dormant. However, very young children have weaker defenses, and in them, these lymph nodes may become large enough to compress the bronchial tubes, causing a brassy cough and possibly a collapsed lung. Occasionally, bacteria spread up the lymph vessels to the lymph nodes in the neck. An infection in lymph nodes in the neck may break through the skin and discharge pus.

■ **Brain:** Tuberculosis that infects the tissues covering the brain (tuberculous meningitis) is life threatening. In the United States and other developed countries, tuberculous meningitis most commonly occurs among older people or people with a weakened immune system. In developing countries, tuberculous meningitis is most common among children from birth to age 5. Symptoms include fever, constant headache, neck stiffness, nausea, and drowsiness that can lead to coma. Tuberculosis may also infect the brain itself, forming a mass called a tuberculoma. The tuberculoma may cause symptoms such as headaches, seizures, or muscle weakness.

■ **Pericardium:** In tuberculous pericarditis, the pericardium thickens and sometimes leaks fluid into the space between the pericardium and the heart. These effects limit the heart's ability to pump and cause swollen neck veins and difficulty breathing. In parts of the world where tuberculosis is common, tuberculous pericarditis is a common cause of heart failure.

■ **Intestine:** Intestinal tuberculosis occurs mainly in developing countries. This infection may not cause any symptoms but can cause abnormal swelling of tissues in the abdomen. This swelling may be mistaken for cancer.

Diagnosis

Sometimes the first indication of tuberculosis is an abnormal chest x-ray or a positive tuberculin skin test (also known as a Mantoux test or PPD for purified protein derivative). These tests are often done as routine screening tests. For example, skin tests are done routinely for people who are at risk of tuberculosis because they

■ Live or work with people who have active disease (as an annual test)

■ Have just emigrated from areas where tuberculosis is common

■ Are starting to take a drug that may weaken the immune system and reactivate latent tuberculosis if present

When people have symptoms that suggest tuberculosis, the following may be done:

■ Chest x-ray

■ Tuberculin skin test

■ Examination and culture of a sputum sample

■ Blood tests

The sputum sample is examined under a microscope to look for tuberculosis bacteria and is used to grow the bacteria in a culture. Microscopic examination provides results much faster than a culture but is less accurate. It detects only about half the cases of tuberculosis identified by culture. However, traditional cultures do not provide results for many weeks because tuberculosis bacteria grow slowly. For this reason, treatment of people who may have tuberculosis is often begun while doctors wait for results of sputum examination and culture. A widely available culture test can routinely identify *Mycobacterium tuberculosis* growth within 21 days.

Newly available blood tests can confirm the presence of *Mycobacterium tuberculosis* within 24 hours. These tests appear to be at least as accurate as the tuberculin skin test, possibly more accurate. Other new tests can detect and identify genetic material of the bacteria in sputum in a few days. Genetic tests can also rapidly identify bacteria that are resistant to the usual drugs used to treat tuberculosis and thus can help doctors choose effective treatment. New tests that detect tuberculosis bacteria in sputum or urine are being developed.

Chest x-ray findings in tuberculosis often resemble those in other disorders, so the diagnosis may depend on the results of the tuberculin skin test and examination of sputum for *Mycobacterium tuberculosis*. Although a

Skin and Blood Tests for Tuberculosis

A tuberculin skin test is done by injecting a small amount of protein derived from tuberculosis bacteria between the layers of the skin, usually on the forearm. About 2 days later, the injection site is checked. Swelling that feels firm to the touch and is larger than a certain size indicates a positive result. Redness around the site without swelling is not positive. Some people who are very ill or who have a weakened immune system may not respond to the skin test even if they are infected with tuberculosis.

In the two new blood tests that detect tuberculosis infection, a sample of blood is mixed with synthetic proteins similar to those produced by the tuberculosis bacteria. If people are infected with tuberculosis bacteria, their white blood cells produce certain substances (interferons) in response to the synthetic proteins. The blood is then checked for the presence of interferons to determine whether tuberculosis infection is present. Sometimes the results are not conclusive. These tests may be more useful for people with a weakened immune system.

A positive blood or skin test indicates infection, but not necessarily active disease. Also, occasionally, people with active tuberculosis may have a negative tuberculosis blood or skin test.

---

tuberculin skin test is one of the most useful tests for diagnosing tuberculosis, it indicates only that an infection by the bacteria has occurred some time in the past. It does not indicate whether the infection is currently active. Results may also indicate tuberculosis when it is not present (false-positive results) because people have an infection with one of the close, generally harmless relatives of tuberculosis (see box on page 1195) or have been recently vaccinated against tuberculosis. The new blood tests are not influenced by recent vaccination against the disease. However, like the tuberculin skin test, these tests indicate infection only—not whether the disease is active.

A sample of sputum is usually adequate, but occasionally a doctor needs to obtain a sample of lung fluid or tissue to make the diagnosis. An instrument called a bronchoscope is inserted through the mouth or nostril and into the airways. It is used to inspect the bronchial tubes and to obtain a sample of lung fluid or tissue. This procedure is most often done when other disorders, such as lung cancer, are suspected.

When symptoms suggest tuberculous meningitis, a doctor may need to do a spinal tap (lumbar puncture) to obtain a sample of spinal fluid for analysis. Because tuberculosis bacteria are hard to find in spinal fluid and because cultures usually take weeks, the polymerase chain reaction (PCR) technique may be used. It produces many copies of a gene, making identification of the bacteria's DNA easier. Although test results are available quickly, doctors usually begin antibiotic therapy if they have any suspicion of tuberculous meningitis. Early treatment can prevent death and minimize brain damage.

Treatment

A number of antibiotics are effective against tuberculosis. But because tuberculosis bacteria are very slow-growing, antibiotics must be taken for a long time—usually for 6 months or longer. Treatment must be continued long after people feel completely well. Otherwise, the disease tends to recur because it was not fully eliminated.

Most people find it difficult to remember to take their drugs every day for such a long time. Other people, for various reasons, stop treatment as soon as they feel better. Because of these problems, many experts recommend that people with tuberculosis receive their drugs from a health care worker, who watches them take the pills. This approach is called directly observed therapy (DOT). Because DOT ensures that people take every dose, the drugs are often given for a shorter time and are usually given just 2 or 3 times per week.

Two or more antibiotics that work in different ways are always given because treatment with only one drug can leave behind a few bacteria resistant to that drug. With most other bacteria, a few bacteria would not be enough to cause a relapse, but people treated with only one drug soon develop tuberculosis resistant to that drug. A third and fourth drug are usually used during the initial, intensive phase of treatment to shorten the duration of treatment and to ensure success even if drug resistance exists at the outset.

The most commonly used antibiotics are isoniazid, rifampin, pyrazinamide, and ethambutol. Streptomycin is sometimes added to this regimen. All of these drugs have side effects, but 95% of people with tuberculosis are cured with these drugs and do not experience any serious side effects.

There are many different combinations and dose schedules for these drugs. Isoniazid, rifampin, and pyrazinamide may be contained in the same capsule, reducing the number of pills people have to take each day and reducing the chance of developing drug resistance. Unlike other antibiotics, those used to treat tuberculosis are usually taken all together, once a day.

Surgery to remove a portion of the lung is seldom needed if people faithfully follow the drug treatment plan. However, surgery is sometimes needed to treat very drug-resistant infections and to drain pus that has accumulated. When tuberculous pericarditis causes significant restriction of the heart's motion, the pericardium may need to be removed surgically. A tuberculoma in the brain may need to be surgically removed.

? **Did You Know...**

Treatment of tuberculosis must be continued long after people feel well.

Prevention

Prevention has two aspects: stopping the spread of infection and treating early infection before it becomes active disease.

Stopping the Spread: Because tuberculosis bacteria are airborne, good ventilation with fresh air lowers the concentration of bacteria and limits their spread. Also, germicidal ultraviolet lamps can be used to kill airborne tuberculosis bacteria in buildings where people at risk are gathered, such as homeless shelters, jails, and hospital and emergency department waiting areas. Health care workers who handle samples of infected tissue or interact with people who may be infected wear special masks, called respirators, to help protect them. No precautions are needed if people have no symptoms even if their skin or blood test for tuberculosis is positive.

People with active tuberculosis can help reduce the spread of bacteria by coughing into a tissue. Also, they should remain in isolation until they are responding to treatment and no longer coughing. After only a few days to weeks of treatment with the correct antibiotics, people are less likely to spread the disease. They usually do not need to be isolated for longer than 2 weeks. However, if infected people live or work with people who are at high risk (such as young children or people with AIDS), repeated analyses of sputum samples may be needed to determine when the danger of spreading the infection is past. Also, people who continue to cough during treatment, do not take their drugs as instructed, or have drug-resistant tuberculosis may need to be isolated longer so that they do not spread the disease.

Treating Early Infection: Because tuberculosis is spread only by people with active disease, early recognition and treatment of active disease is one of the best ways to stop it from spreading. People who have a positive tuberculin skin or blood test should be treated even if they are not yet ill. The antibiotic isoniazid is very effective at stopping the infection before it becomes active disease. It is given daily for 6 to 9 months. For some people, rifampin alone may be prescribed daily for 4 months. In some countries, isoniazid and rifampin are used together for 3 months.

Preventive therapy definitely benefits younger people who have a positive tuberculin skin test. It also is likely to help older people at high risk of tuberculosis (for example, if their skin or blood test recently changed from negative to positive, if they have been recently exposed, or if they have a weakened immune system). For older people with long-standing latent infection, the risk of toxicity from the antibiotics may be greater than the risk of developing tuberculosis. In such cases, doctors often consult an expert in the subject before they decide whether to use preventive therapy.

If people with a positive skin or blood test become infected with HIV, the risk of developing active infection is very high. Similarly, the risk is also high if people who have a latent infection take corticosteroids or other drugs that suppress the immune system (including some of the newer anti-inflammatory drugs). Such people usually need treatment of latent tuberculosis infection.

In much of the developing world, a vaccine called bacille Calmette-Guérin (BCG) is used to prevent development of serious complications, such as meningitis, in people who are at high risk of becoming infected with *Mycobacterium tuberculosis*. The value of BCG is debated, and the vaccine continues to be used only in countries where the likelihood of contracting tuberculosis is very high. The vaccine may have a

---

What Is Miliary Tuberculosis?

A potentially life-threatening type of tuberculosis may result when a large number of the bacteria spread throughout the body by way of the bloodstream, often in people with a weakened immune system. This infection is called miliary tuberculosis because the millions of tiny spots that form in the lungs are the size of millet, the small round seeds in bird food.

Symptoms can be vague and difficult to identify. They include weight loss, fever, chills, weakness, general discomfort, and difficulty breathing. Infection of the bone marrow may cause severe anemia and other blood abnormalities, suggesting leukemia. If bacteria are intermittently released into the bloodstream from a hidden lesion, people may have a fever that comes and goes and may gradually lose weight, wasting away.

DRUGS USED TO TREAT TUBERCULOSIS

DRUG	ROUTE	SIDE EFFECTS
Isoniazid	By mouth	Liver injury in 1 person in 10,000, resulting in nausea, vomiting, and jaundice Sometimes numbness in the limbs
Rifampin	By mouth	Liver injury, particularly when rifampin is combined with isoniazid (but the effects go away when people stop the drug) Reddish orange discoloration of urine, tears, and sweat
Pyrazinamide	By mouth	Liver injury and sometimes gout
Ethambutol	By mouth	Sometimes blurred vision and decreased color perception (because the drug affects the optic nerve)
Streptomycin	By injection into a muscle	Dizziness and slight hearing loss (due to damage to nerves of the inner ear)

role in protecting health care workers and others exposed to tuberculosis that is resistant to two or more drugs. Research is under way to develop a more effective vaccine. About 10% of people who have received BCG at birth have a positive reaction to the tuberculin skin test 15 years later, even if they are not infected with tuberculosis bacteria. However, people vaccinated at birth often incorrectly attribute a positive skin test later in life to the BCG vaccine. In most countries, tuberculosis is stigmatized, and many people are reluctant to believe that they have even latent infection, much less active disease. The newer tuberculosis blood tests are not affected by BCG vaccination.

CHAPTER

178 Leprosy

Leprosy (Hansen's disease) is a chronic infection caused by the bacteria Mycobacterium leprae. *It results in damage primarily to the peripheral nerves (the nerves outside the brain and spinal cord), skin, testes, eyes, and mucous membranes of the nose.*

- Leprosy ranges from mild (with one or a few skin areas affected) to severe (with many skin areas affected and damage to many organs).
- Rashes and bumps appear, the affected areas become numb, and muscles may become weak.
- The diagnosis is suggested by symptoms and confirmed by a biopsy of the affected tissue.
- Antibiotics can stop leprosy from progressing but cannot reverse any nerve damage or deformity.

Because without treatment, people with leprosy are visibly disfigured and often have significant disability, they have long been feared and shunned by others. Although leprosy is not highly contagious, rarely causes death, and can be effectively treated with antibiotics, it still causes anxiety. As a result, people with leprosy and their family members often have psychologic and social problems.

During 2007, over 250,000 new cases were reported. About 90% of these cases occurred in the following eight countries (listed from the most cases to the least): India, Brazil, Indonesia, Congo, Bangladesh, Nigeria, Nepal, and Ethiopia. In 2006, 137 new cases were reported in the United States. Cases occurred in 30 states, but over half occurred in six states: California, Florida, Louisiana, Massachusetts, New York, and Texas. Almost all cases of leprosy in the United States involve people who emigrated from developing countries.

Leprosy can develop at any age but appears to develop most often in people aged 5 to 15 years or over 30.

How leprosy is spread is unclear. However, it may be passed from person to person through droplets expelled from the nose and mouth of an infected person and breathed in or touched by an uninfected person. But even after contact with the bacteria, most people do not contract leprosy. About half of the people with leprosy probably contracted it through close, long-term contact with an infected person.

Casual and short-term contact does not seem to spread the disease. Leprosy cannot be contracted by simply touching someone with the disease, as is commonly believed. Health care workers often work for many years with people who have leprosy without contracting the disease. Armadillos are the only confirmed source other than people, although other animal and environmental sources may exist.

About 95% of people who are infected with *Mycobacterium leprae* do not develop leprosy because their immune system fights off the infection. People who develop leprosy may have genes that make them susceptible to the infection once they are exposed.

Classification: Leprosy can be categorized by the type and number of skin areas affected. People with 5 or fewer affected skin areas have a type of leprosy called paucibacillary. No bacteria can be detected on samples from those areas. People with 6 or more affected areas have a type of leprosy called multibacillary. Bacteria may or may not be detected on samples from those areas.

Leprosy can also be classified as tuberculoid, lepromatous, or borderline based on the symptoms people have and other findings. People with tuberculoid leprosy typically have few skin areas affected (paucibacillary), and the disease is milder, less common, and less contagious. People with lepromatous or borderline leprosy typically have more skin areas affected (multibacillary), and the disease is more severe, common, and contagious.

In both classifications, the type of leprosy determines how well people fare in the long term, what complications are likely, and how long antibiotic treatment is needed.

Symptoms

Because the bacteria that cause leprosy multiply very slowly, symptoms usually do not begin until at least 1 year after people have been infected. On average, symptoms appear 5 to 7 years after infection. Once symptoms begin, they progress slowly.

Leprosy affects mainly the skin and peripheral nerves. Characteristic rashes and bumps develop. Infection of the nerves makes the skin numb or the muscles weak in areas controlled by the infected nerves.

Specific symptoms vary depending on the type of leprosy.

- **Tuberculoid leprosy:** A rash appears, consisting of one or a few flat, whitish areas. Areas affected by this rash are numb because the bacteria damage the underlying nerves.
- **Lepromatous leprosy:** Many small bumps or larger raised rashes of variable size and shape appear on the skin. There are more areas of numbness than in tuberculoid leprosy, and certain muscle groups may be weak. Much of the skin and many areas of the body, including the kidneys, nose, and testes, may be affected.

- **Borderline leprosy:** Features of both tuberculoid and lepromatous leprosy are present. Without treatment, borderline leprosy may become less severe and more like the tuberculoid form, or it may worsen and become more like the lepromatous form.

The most severe symptoms result from infection of the peripheral nerves, which causes deterioration of the sense of touch and a corresponding inability to feel pain and temperature. People with peripheral nerve damage may unknowingly burn, cut, or otherwise harm themselves. Repeated damage may eventually lead to loss of fingers and toes. Also, damage to peripheral nerves may cause muscle weakness that can result in deformities. For example, the fingers may be weakened, causing them to curve inward (like a claw). Muscles may become too weak to flex the foot—a condition called footdrop. Infected nerves may enlarge so that during a physical examination, doctors can feel them.

Skin infection can lead to areas of swelling and lumps, which can be particularly disfiguring on the face.

Other areas of the body may be affected:

- **Feet:** Sores may also develop on the soles of the feet, making walking painful.
- **Nose:** Damage to the nasal passages can result in a chronically stuffy nose and nosebleeds and, if untreated, complete erosion of the nose.
- **Eyes:** Damage to the eyes may lead to glaucoma or blindness.
- **Sexual function:** Men with lepromatous leprosy may have erectile dysfunction (impotence) and become infertile. The infection can reduce the amount of testosterone and sperm produced by the testes.
- **Kidneys:** The kidneys may malfunction. In severe cases, kidney failure may occur.

During the course of untreated or even treated leprosy, the immune system may produce inflammatory reactions. These reactions can cause fever and inflammation of the skin, peripheral nerves, and, less commonly, the lymph nodes, joints, testes, kidneys, liver, and eyes. The skin around bumps may swell and become red and painful, and the bumps may form open sores. People may have a fever and swollen lymph glands.

Diagnosis

Symptoms (such as distinctive rashes that do not disappear, enlarged nerves, loss of the sense of touch, and deformities that result from muscle weakness) provide strong clues to the diagnosis of leprosy.

Examination of a sample of infected skin tissue under a microscope (biopsy) confirms the diagnosis. Because leprosy bacteria do not grow in the laboratory, culture of tissue samples is not useful. Blood tests to measure antibodies to the bacteria have limited usefulness because antibodies are not always present.

Did You Know...

Leprosy is not easily spread.

If leprosy is severe, people may have to take antibiotics for the rest of their life.

Prevention

Because leprosy is not very contagious, risk of spread is low. Only the untreated lepromatous form is contagious, although even then the infection is not easily spread. Once treatment has begun, leprosy cannot be spread. Avoiding contact with bodily fluids from and the rash on infected people is the best prevention. The BCG (bacille Calmette-Guérin) vaccine, used to prevent tuberculosis, provides some protection against leprosy, but it is not often used to prevent leprosy.

Treatment

Antibiotics can stop the progression of leprosy but do not reverse any nerve damage or deformity. Thus, early detection and treatment are vitally important. Because some leprosy bacteria are resistant to certain antibiotics, doctors prescribe more than one drug. The drugs chosen depend on the type of leprosy:

- Multibacillary: The standard combination of drugs is dapsone, rifampin, and clofazimine. People take rifampin and clofazimine once a month under a health care practitioner's supervision. They take dapsone plus clofazimine once a day on their own. This regimen is continued for 12 to 24 months, depending on the severity of the disease.
- Paucibacillary: People take rifampin once a month with supervision and dapsone once a day without supervision for 6 months. People who have only a single affected skin area are given a single dose of rifampin, ofloxacin, and minocycline.

Dapsone is relatively inexpensive and generally safe to use. It occasionally causes allergic rashes and anemia. Rifampin, which is more expensive, is even more effective than dapsone. Its most serious side effects are damage to the liver and flu-like symptoms. Clofazimine is extremely safe. The main side effect is temporary skin pigmentation.

Because the bacteria are difficult to eradicate, antibiotics must be continued for a long time. Depending on the severity of the infection and the doctor's judgment, treatment continues from 6 months to many years. Some doctors recommend lifelong treatment with dapsone for people with lepromatous leprosy.

CHAPTER

179 Rickettsial and Related Infections

Rickettsial infections and related infections (such as ehrlichiosis and Q fever) are caused by an unusual type of bacteria that can live only in another organism.

- Most of these infections are spread through ticks, mites, fleas, or lice.
- A fever, a severe headache, and usually a rash develop, and people feel generally ill.
- Symptoms suggest the diagnosis, and doctors use special cultures and blood tests to confirm it.
- Antibiotics are given as soon as doctors suspect one of these infections.

Rickettsiae are an unusual type of bacteria that cause several diseases, including Rocky Mountain spotted fever and epidemic typhus. Rickettsiae differ from most other bacteria in that they can live and multiply only inside the cells of another organism (host) and cannot survive on their own in the environment. *Ehrlichia* bacteria and *Coxiella burnetii* bacteria are similar to rickettsiae and cause similar diseases.

People are the main host for some species of these bacteria. However, for most species, animals are the usual host. These animals are called the reservoir of infection. Animals in the reservoir may or may not be ill from the infection. Rickettsiae are usually spread to people through the bites of ticks, mites, fleas, or lice that previously fed on an infected animal. These organisms are called vectors because they convey (transmit) organisms that cause disease. Q fever, caused by *Coxiella burnetii*, can be spread through the air or in food. Each species of rickettsiae and related bacteria has its own hosts and vectors.

In people, rickettsiae infect the cells lining small blood vessels, causing the blood vessels to become inflamed or blocked or to bleed into the surrounding tissue. Where this damage occurs and how the body responds determine which symptoms develop.

Symptoms

Different rickettsial infections tend to cause similar symptoms:

- Fever
- Severe headache
- A characteristic rash
- A general feeling of illness (malaise)

Because the rash often does not appear for several days, early rickettsial infection is often mistaken for a common viral infection, such as influenza.

As severe rickettsial diseases progress, people typically experience confusion and severe weakness—often with cough, difficulty breathing, and sometimes vomiting and diarrhea. In some people, the liver or spleen enlarges, the kidneys malfunction, and blood pressure falls dangerously low. Death can result.

Diagnosis

Because rickettsiae are transmitted by ticks, mites, fleas, and lice, a history of a bite from one or more of these vectors is a helpful clue—particularly in geographic areas where rickettsial infection is common. However, many people do not recall such a bite.

Often, doctors cannot confirm a rickettsial infection quickly because rickettsiae cannot be identified using commonly available laboratory tests. Special cultures and blood tests for rickettsiae are not routinely available and take so long to process that people usually need to be treated before test results are available. Doctors base their decision to treat on the person's symptoms and the likelihood of possible exposure.

Useful tests include immunofluorescence assay and polymerase chain reaction (PCR) testing, which use a sample from the rash or blood. These tests make the bacteria easier to identify. Immunofluorescence assays label foreign substances produced by the bacteria (antigens) with a fluorescent dye that makes them easier to detect. PCR increases the amount of the bacteria's DNA.

Treatment

Rickettsial infections respond promptly to early treatment with the antibiotics doxycycline (preferred), chloramphenicol, or tetracycline. These antibiotics are given by mouth unless people are very sick. In such cases, antibiotics are given intravenously. Most people noticeably improve in 1 or 2 days, and fever usually disappears in 2 to 3 days. People take the antibiotic for a minimum of 1 week—longer if the fever persists. When treatment begins late, improvement is slower and the fever lasts longer. If the infection is untreated or if treatment is begun too late, death can occur, especially in people with epidemic typhus or Rocky Mountain spotted fever.

Ciprofloxacin and other similar antibiotics may be used to treat some rickettsial infections.

Rocky Mountain Spotted Fever

Rocky Mountain spotted fever (spotted fever, tick fever, tick typhus) is a rickettsial infection that is transmitted by dog ticks and wood ticks. It causes a rash, headache, and high fever.

- People become infected when a tick carrying the infection bites them.
- A severe headache, chills, extreme exhaustion, and muscle pains develop, followed a few days later by a rash.
- Avoiding tick bites is the best way to prevent the infection.
- People are given antibiotics immediately if they have been bitten by a tick and have typical symptoms.

Rocky Mountain spotted fever (RMSF) is caused by the bacteria *Rickettsia rickettsii* and is probably the most common rickettsial infection in the United States. It was first recognized in the Rocky Mountain states but occurs throughout most of the continental United States. It is most common in the Midwest and on the southern Atlantic seaboard. It also occurs in Central and South America. The infection occurs mainly from March to September, when adult ticks are active and people are likely to be in tick-infested areas. In the southern states, the disease may occur throughout the year. People who spend a lot of time in tick-infested areas—such as children younger than 15—have an increased risk of infection.

Ticks acquire rickettsiae by feeding on infected mammals. Infected female ticks can also transmit rickettsiae to their offspring. Infection is spread to people through bites by wood ticks or dog ticks. Rickettsial infection is probably not transmitted directly from person to person.

Rickettsiae live and multiply in the cells lining blood vessels. Blood vessels in and under the skin and in the brain, lungs, heart, kidneys, liver, and spleen are commonly infected. Small infected blood vessels may become blocked by blood clots.

> **? Did You Know...**
> Almost three fourths of people with symptoms remember having a tick bite.

Symptoms

Typically, symptoms include a severe headache, chills, extreme exhaustion (prostration), and muscle pains. Symptoms begin suddenly 3 to 12 days after a tick bite. The more quickly symptoms begin, the more severe the infection. A high fever develops within several days and, in severe infections, persists for 1 to 3 weeks. A hacking, dry cough may also develop. Nausea and vomiting are common.

SOME RICKETTSIAL AND RELATED INFECTIONS

INFECTION	INFECTING ORGANISM	HOST	AREAS WHERE INFECTION OCCURS	DESCRIPTION
Epidemic typhus	*Rickettsia prowazekii*, transmitted by lice	People	Throughout the world (uncommon in the United States, but occasionally occurs in homeless people)	After an incubation of 7 to 14 days, symptoms begin suddenly, with fever, headache, and extreme fatigue (prostration). A rash appears on the 4th to 6th day. Untreated, the infection may be fatal, especially in people older than 50.
Murine typhus	*Rickettsia typhi*, transmitted by fleas	Cats, rodents, and opossums	Throughout the world	Symptoms are very similar to those of epidemic typhus but are less severe. People also have shaking chills.
Scrub typhus	*Rickettsia tsutsugamushi*, transmitted by mites and mite larvae (chiggers)	Rodents	Asiatic-Pacific area, bounded by Japan, India, Australia, and Thailand	After an incubation of 6 to 21 days, symptoms begin suddenly, with fever, chills, headache, and swollen lymph nodes. A black scab may develop at the site of the chigger bite. A rash appears on the 5th to 8th day.
Rickettsialpox	*Rickettsia akari*, transmitted by mites and chiggers	Rodents	First observed in New York City Other areas of the United States and Russia, Korea, and Africa	About 1 week before the fever develops, a small buttonlike sore (ulcer) with a black center appears on the skin. Fever comes and goes, lasts about a week, and is accompanied by chills, profuse sweating, headache, sensitivity to the sun, and muscle pains.
Q fever	*Coxiella burnetii*, transmitted by inhaling infected droplets containing the bacteria or by consuming contaminated raw milk	Sheep, cattle, and goats	Throughout the world	After an incubation of 9 to 28 days, symptoms begin suddenly, with fever, severe headache, chills, extreme weakness, muscle aches, loss of appetite, sweating, an unproductive cough, chest pain, and inflammation of the airways (pneumonitis), but no rash.

On about the fourth day of the fever, a rash appears on the wrists and ankles and rapidly extends to the palms, soles, forearms, neck, face, armpits, buttocks, and trunk. At first, the rash is flat and pink but later darkens and becomes slightly raised. It does not itch. Warm water—for example, in a bath—makes the rash more evident. In about 4 days, small purplish areas (petechiae) develop because of bleeding in the skin. A sore may form where these areas merge.

As this infection progresses, it may cause other symptoms:

- Restlessness, insomnia, delirium, or sometimes coma if the blood vessels in the brain are affected
- Abdominal pain
- Inflammation of the airways (pneumonitis) and pneumonia
- Heart damage
- Anemia
- Severe low blood pressure and death (uncommonly, when the infection is severe)

Prevention

There is no vaccine against this infection, so avoiding tick bites is the best prevention (see box on page 1166). The following measures can help:

- Tucking trousers into boots or socks and applying insecticide that contains permethrin to clothing limits tick access to skin.
- Tick repellents such as DEET (diethyltoluamide) may be applied to the skin. These repellents are effective but, rarely, cause toxic reactions, such as seizures, in small children.
- Searching frequently for ticks helps prevent infection because the tick must be attached for 24 hours on average to transmit infection.
- Attached ticks should be removed carefully with tweezers. The head of the tick should be grasped as close to the skin as possible. Care must be taken when removing a tick because rickettsiae may be transmitted if an infected tick that is engorged with blood is crushed while being removed.

Treatment

Doctors immediately prescribe antibiotics if they suspect the infection based on symptoms and the potential for exposure to infected ticks—even if laboratory test results are not yet available. Early treatment with antibiotics has reduced the death rate from about 20% to 5%.

Doxycycline (preferred), chloramphenicol, and tetracycline are effective. They are given by mouth when the infection is mild and intravenously when it is more severe. However, a doctor usually does not prescribe antibiotics for people who have had a tick bite but have no symptoms. Instead, the doctor may ask them to immediately report symptoms.

Ehrlichioses

Ehrlichioses are tick-borne infections that cause fever, chills, headache, and a general feeling of illness (malaise). These symptoms begin suddenly.

Ehrlichia bacteria, like rickettsiae, can live only inside the cells of an animal or a person. However, unlike rickettsiae, *Ehrlichia* bacteria inhabit white blood cells (such as granulocytes and monocytes). Different species inhabit different types of white blood cells.

Ehrlichioses are most common in the southeastern and south central United States. They also occur in Europe. They are most likely to develop between spring and late fall, when ticks are most active. Infection is spread to people through tick bites, sometimes resulting from contact with animals that carry the brown dog tick or deer tick.

Symptoms

Symptoms usually begin 1 to 2 weeks after a tick bite. The first symptoms are fever, chills, severe headache, body aches, and malaise. As the infection progresses, other symptoms may develop:

- Vomiting
- Diarrhea
- Seizures
- Confusion
- Coma
- Cough
- Difficulty breathing

Skin rash is much less common than in rickettsial infections. Death is uncommon but can occur in people with a weakened immune system or who are not treated soon enough.

Diagnosis and Treatment

Doctors do blood tests, which may detect a low white blood cell count, a low platelet count (thrombocytopenia), and abnormal blood clotting. But these findings occur in many other disorders. Blood tests to check for antibodies to these bacteria may be helpful, but results are usually not positive until several weeks after the illness begins. Polymerase chain reaction (PCR) testing may be more useful. It increases the amount of the bacteria's DNA and thus makes the bacteria easier to identify. Sometimes white blood cells contain characteristic spots (morulae) that can be seen under a microscope. The presence of morulae confirms the diagnosis of ehrlichiosis.

If people who may have been exposed to infected ticks have typical symptoms, treatment is usually started based on the person's symptoms before test results are available. Doxycycline, chloramphenicol, and tetracycline are all effective. When treatment is started early, most people respond rapidly and well. A delay in treatment may lead to serious complications, including death in 2 to 5% of people.

180 Parasitic Infections

- Parasitic infections are more common in rural or developing areas than in developed areas.
- In developed areas, these infections may occur in immigrants or in people with a weakened immune system.
- Parasites usually enter the body through the mouth or skin.
- Doctors diagnose the infection by taking samples of blood, stool, urine, phlegm or other infected tissue and examining or sending them to a laboratory for analysis.
- Travelers to areas where food, drink, and water may be contaminated are advised to cook it, boil it, peel it, or forget it.

A parasite is an organism that lives on or inside another organism (the host) and harms the host.

Parasitic infections are common in rural or developing areas of Africa, Asia, and Latin America and less common in developed areas. A person who visits such an area can unknowingly acquire a parasitic infection, and a doctor may not readily diagnose the infection when the person returns home. In developed areas, parasitic infections may also affect immigrants and people with a weakened immune system (such as those who have AIDS or who take drugs that suppress the immune system). The infections may occur in places with poor sanitation and unhygienic practices (as occurs in some mental institutions and day care centers).

Parasites usually enter the body through the mouth or skin. Parasites that enter through the mouth are swallowed and can remain in the intestine or burrow through the intestinal wall and invade other organs. Parasites that enter through the skin bore directly through the skin or are introduced through the bites of infected insects (called vectors because they convey or transmit organisms that cause disease). Some parasites enter through the soles of the feet when a person walks barefoot or through the skin when a person swims or bathes in water containing the parasites. Rarely, parasites are spread through blood transfusions, through injections with a needle previously used by an infected person, or from a pregnant woman to her fetus.

Parasites that infect people include protozoa (such as amebas), which consist of only one cell, and worms (helminths, such as hookworms and tapeworms), which are larger and consist of many cells and have internal organs. Protozoa, which reproduce by cell division, can reproduce inside people. Helminths, in contrast, produce eggs or larvae that develop in the environment before they become capable of infecting people. Development in the environment may involve another animal (an intermediate host). Some protozoa (such as those that cause malaria) and some helminths (such as those that cause river blindness) have complex life cycles and are transmitted by insect vectors.

Diagnosis

Doctors suspect a parasitic infection in people who have typical symptoms and who live or have traveled to an area where sanitation is poor or where such an infection is known to occur. Laboratory analysis of specimens, including special tests to identify proteins released by the parasite (antigen testing), may be needed. Samples of blood, stool, urine, or phlegm (sputum) may be taken. The doctor may also take a sample of tissue that may contain the parasite. For example, a biopsy may be done to obtain a sample of lung or intestinal tissue. A sample of skin may be snipped. Several samples and repeated examinations may be necessary to find the parasite.

If parasites live in the intestinal tract, their eggs or cysts (a dormant form of the parasite) may be found in the person's stool when a sample is examined under a microscope. Or parasites may be identified by testing the stool for proteins or other materials that they release. Antibiotics, laxatives, and antacids should not be used until after the stool sample has been collected. These drugs can reduce the number of parasites enough to make seeing the parasites in a stool sample difficult or impossible.

Prevention

In areas of the world where food, drink, and water may be contaminated with parasites, wise advice for travelers is to avoid drinking tap water and to "cook it, boil it, peel it, or forget it." Because some parasites survive freezing, ice cubes can sometimes transmit disease unless the cubes are made from purified water. Information about precautions needed in specific areas is available from the Centers for Disease Control and Prevention.

Amebiasis

Amebiasis is an infection of the large intestine and sometimes the liver and other organs that is caused by the single-celled protozoan parasite Entamoeba histolytica, *an ameba.*

- The amebas may be spread from person to person or through food or water.

- People may have no symptoms or may have diarrhea, cramping abdominal pain, tenderness in the upper abdomen, and fever.

- Doctors base the diagnosis on analysis of a stool sample and, if needed, other tests, such as colonoscopy or ultrasonography.

- People are given a drug that kills the amebas, followed by a drug that kills the dormant form of the amebas.

Amebiasis is relatively common in areas of Africa, the Indian subcontinent, and Latin America where sanitation is poor. In the United States, it is most likely to occur in immigrants and, less commonly, in people who have traveled to developing countries.

Entamoeba histolytica exists in two forms: as an active parasite (trophozoite) and as a dormant parasite (cyst). Infection begins when cysts are swallowed. The cysts hatch, releasing trophozoites that multiply and can cause ulcers in the lining of the intestine. Occasionally, they spread to the liver or other parts of the body. Some trophozoites become cysts, which are excreted in stool (feces) along with trophozoites. Outside the body, the fragile trophozoites die, but the hardy cysts survive.

Cysts can be spread directly from person to person or indirectly through food or water.

In places with poor sanitation, amebiasis is acquired by ingesting food or water that is contaminated with feces. Fruits and vegetables may be contaminated when grown in soil fertilized by human feces, washed in polluted water, or prepared by someone who is infected. Amebiasis may occur and spread in places with adequate sanitation if infected people are incontinent or hygiene is poor (for example, in day care centers or mental institutions). Amebiasis can also be spread through certain sexual practices (such as oral-anal sex).

Symptoms

Many infected people have few or no symptoms. Symptoms that may occur include increased gas (flatulence), cramping abdominal pain, and intermittent diarrhea, constipation, or both. In severe cases, the abdomen is tender when touched, and the stool contains mucus and blood. The person may also have a fever. Diarrhea may lead to dehydration. Wasting of the body (emaciation) and anemia can occur in people with chronic infection. Sometimes a large lump (ameboma) forms and blocks the intestine. Occasionally, trophozoites cause tearing (perforation) of the intestinal wall, resulting in severe abdominal pain and an abdominal infection (peritonitis) that requires immediate medical attention.

In some people, the amebas spread to the liver where they can cause an abscess. Symptoms include fever, sweats, chills, weakness, nausea, vomiting, weight loss, and pain or discomfort in the right upper abdomen over the liver. Rarely, amebas spread to other organs (including the lungs or brain). The skin may also become infected, especially around the buttocks, genitals, or wounds caused by abdominal surgery or injury.

Diagnosis

To diagnose amebiasis, a doctor collects stool samples for analysis. The best approach is to test the stool for a protein released by the amebas (antigen testing). Microscopic examination is often inconclusive. Three to six stool samples may be needed to find the amebas, and even when they are seen, they cannot be distinguished from other amebas such as *Entamoeba dispar*, which look the same but are genetically different and do not cause disease. A flexible viewing tube (colonoscope) may be used to look inside the large intestine and to obtain a tissue sample if ulcers or other signs of infection are found there.

When amebas spread to sites outside the intestine (such as the liver), they may no longer be present in the stool. Ultrasonography, computed tomography (CT), or magnetic resonance imaging (MRI) can be done to confirm an abscess in the liver, but these tests do not indicate the cause. Blood tests are then done to check for antibodies to the amebas. Or, if doctors suspect that a liver abscess is due to amebas, they often simply start a drug that kills amebas (an amebicide). If the person improves, the diagnosis is probably amebiasis.

Treatment

If amebiasis is suspected and the person has symptoms, an amebicide—either metronidazole or tinidazole—is used. Tinidazole, given in a single dose, has fewer side effects than metronidazole, which

OTHER PARASITES

GEOGRAPHIC AREA	SOURCE	COMMON SYMPTOMS	DIAGNOSIS	TREATMENT
Dog heartworm (*Dirofilaria* species)				
Worldwide (but rare in people)	Larvae are transmitted to people through the bite of infected mosquitoes.	Usually, no symptoms Occasionally, chest pain, cough, and blood in phlegm (sputum) Rarely, nodules under the skin, swelling of the face or eyelid, and a change in vision	Biopsy of lung tissue	None needed
Dwarf tapeworm (*Hymenolepis nana*)				
Worldwide	Eggs may be ingested in food or water contaminated by human feces or may be transferred to the mouth after contact with infected people. Or infected insects, such as fleas and beetles, may be ingested accidentally (for example, in insect-infested grains).	Nausea, vomiting, diarrhea, abdominal discomfort, and weight loss in children with a severe infection	Stool tests	Praziquantel
***Echinococcus* species (a tapeworm)**				
Areas of the world where sheep or cattle are raised, as in the Mediterranean, Middle East, Australia, South Africa, and South America, and in areas of Canada, Alaska, California, and Midwestern United States	Eggs excreted in the feces of infected dogs or wild carnivores may be transferred from the hands to the mouth after touching the animal's fur or be ingested in contaminated food.	Abdominal pain and jaundice if the liver is involved Chest pain and coughing up blood or the contents of cysts if the lungs are involved Hives or a severe life-threatening allergic reaction (anaphylaxis)	CT, ultrasonography, or MRI of the liver Sometimes withdrawal of fluid from a cyst in the liver Chest x-ray or CT of the lungs	Albendazole alone or with surgical removal of cysts *or* Drainage of the cyst with a needle guided by ultrasonography, followed by injection, then removal of a salt solution to kill the parasites in the cyst (percutaneous aspiration-injection-reaspiration)

(continued on the following page)

OTHER PARASITES (*Continued*)

GEOGRAPHIC AREA	SOURCE	COMMON SYMPTOMS	DIAGNOSIS	TREATMENT
Intestinal flukes				
Most common in the Far East	Flukes on aquatic plants (such as water chestnuts) or in raw or undercooked freshwater fish are ingested.	Usually no symptoms, but with severe infections, abdominal pain, diarrhea, and fever	Stool tests	Praziquantel
Liver flukes (*Clonorchis sinensis*)				
The Far East	Fluke cysts are ingested in raw, dried, salted, or pickled freshwater fish.	Abdominal pain, jaundice, diarrhea, and, years later, cancer of the biliary tract	Stool tests and sometimes colonoscopy	Praziquantel If the biliary tract is blocked, surgery
***Loa loa* (a filarial worm)**				
Rain forest belt of western and central Africa	Larvae are transmitted to people through the bite of infected tabanid flies (such as horseflies and deerflies).	Itchy, red areas of swelling (most commonly on the wrists and ankles) and awareness of worms passing across the eye but no eye damage	Blood tests	Diethylcarbamazine (DEC)
Lung flukes (*Paragonimus westermani*)				
Most common in the Far East	Cysts in raw, pickled, or undercooked freshwater crabs and crayfish are ingested.	Difficulty breathing, cough, chest pain, and coughing up blood	Sputum or stool tests, chest x-ray or chest CT, and blood tests	Praziquantel
Sheep liver fluke (*Fasciola hepatica*)				
Areas of the world where sheep or cattle are raised, including Bolivia, Peru, Portugal, France, Iran, Egypt, and Asia	Flukes on watercress or other water plants contaminated by sheep or cattle feces are ingested.	Abdominal pain, fever, fatigue, vague discomfort (malaise), and weight loss due to liver damage	Stool tests and CT, ultrasonography, or MRI of the liver	Bithionol or triclabendazole
***Strongyloides stercoralis*, or threadworm (a roundworm)**				
Moist subtropics and tropics and the southeastern United States	Larvae in stool (feces) contaminate the soil and enter through the skin, usually the feet.	Abdominal pain, diarrhea, nausea, vomiting, hives or a rash that changes location, wheezing, and asthma	Stool tests, blood tests, and sometimes colonoscopy If infection is severe and widespread, sputum testing	Ivermectin or albendazole

(continued on the following page)

OTHER PARASITES (*Continued*)				
GEOGRAPHIC AREA	**SOURCE**	**COMMON SYMPTOMS**	**DIAGNOSIS**	**TREATMENT**
Trypanosoma brucei gambiense, mainly in West Africa, and *Trypanosoma brucei rhodesiense*, mainly in East Africa (protozoa that cause African sleeping sickness)				
Parts of equatorial Africa	Protozoa are injected through the skin when tsetse flies bite.	Painful bump at the bite site, followed by fever, headache, rash, enlarged lymph nodes, and, eventually (when the brain and spinal fluid are infected), sleepiness, difficulty walking, coma, and, if untreated, ultimately death (the infection progresses over many months in West African disease but within weeks in East African disease)	Blood tests and spinal tap	West African sleeping sickness: Eflornithine or the same drugs used to treat East African sleeping sickness

East African sleeping sickness: Suramin, pentamidine, or melarsoprol (if the brain and spinal fluid are infected) |
| *Trypanosoma cruzi* (protozoa that cause Chagas' disease) | | | | |
| North, Central, and South America | While biting a person, Triatomine bugs (kissing or assassin bugs) defecate, depositing the protozoa in their feces. The protozoa enter through the bug's bite wound, penetrate mucous membranes, or are rubbed into the eyes. The protozoa are sometimes transmitted through blood transfusions or organ transplants or from a pregnant woman to her fetus. | Initially, rash or swelling at the point of entry, swelling around one eye, generalized weakness, and rare but potentially fatal heart or brain infection

Years later, long-term heart and gastrointestinal problems | Blood tests | Nifurtimox (United States) or benznidazole (Latin America) |

(continued on the following page)

OTHER PARASITES *(Continued)*				
GEOGRAPHIC AREA	**SOURCE**	**COMMON SYMPTOMS**	**DIAGNOSIS**	**TREATMENT**
Wuchereria bancrofti, Brugia malayi, and *Brugia timori* (worms that cause lymphatic filariasis)				
Tropical and subtropical areas worldwide	Larvae are transmitted to people through the bite of infected mosquitoes.	Fever, swollen lymph nodes in the groin and armpits, swelling and pain in the groin and limbs, and bacterial infections	Blood tests, including for *Wuchereria bancrofti* only, and antigen testing	Diethylcarbamazine (DEC) alone or with doxycycline Antibiotics to treat coexisting bacterial skin infections Local measures (such as elevation and an elastic bandage) to reduce swelling (edema)

CT = computed tomography; MRI = magnetic resonance imaging.

requires several doses. Drinking alcohol within a few days of taking metronidazole or tinidazole may result in nausea, vomiting, flushing, and headaches.

Neither metronidazole nor tinidazole always kills cysts that are in the large intestine. A second drug (such as paromomycin, iodoquinol, or diloxanide) is used to kill these cysts and thus prevent a relapse. One of these drugs can be used alone to treat people who do not have symptoms but have the amebas in their stool.

People who are dehydrated are given fluids.

Amebic Infections Due to Free-Living Amebas

Free-living amebas are protozoa that live in soil or water and do not need to live in people or animals. Although they rarely cause human infection, certain types of these amebas can cause serious, life-threatening diseases. The most common diseases caused by free-living amebas are primary amebic meningoencephalitis, granulomatous amebic encephalitis, and amebic keratitis.

PRIMARY AMEBIC MENINGOENCEPHALITIS

Primary amebic meningoencephalitis is a rare, usually fatal infection of the central nervous system (brain and spinal cord) caused by Naegleria fowleri.

The amebas that cause this infection live in fresh, often stagnant water throughout the world. When people, usually children or young adults, swim in contaminated water, the amebas can enter the central nervous system through the mucous membranes of the nose. When they reach the brain, they cause inflammation, tissue death, and bleeding.

Symptoms begin within 1 to 2 weeks. Sometimes the first symptom is a change in smell or taste. Later, people have a headache, a stiff neck, sensitivity to light, nausea, and vomiting. They may become confused and sleepy and may have seizures. The infection can progress rapidly, causing death within 10 days.

Doctors suspect the infection in people who have symptoms and have been swimming recently in fresh water, but the diagnosis is difficult to confirm. A spinal tap (lumbar puncture) is done to obtain a sample of cerebrospinal fluid. This test can exclude other possible causes of meningitis and brain infection, but doctors are not always able to find the amebas in the sample.

Because few people survive, determining the best treatment is difficult. A few antifungal drugs and antibiotics may help. Amphotericin B may be injected into a vein (intravenously) or into the space around the spinal canal (intrathecally). Sometimes miconazole, rifampin, or sulfisoxazole, taken by mouth, is also given. Miconazole may be given intrathecally.

GRANULOMATOUS AMEBIC ENCEPHALITIS

Granulomatous amebic encephalitis is a rare, usually fatal infection of the central nervous system caused by Acanthamoeba *species or* Balamuthia mandrillaris. *It usually occurs in people with a weakened immune system or generally poor health.*

The amebas that cause this infection live in water, soil, and dust throughout the world. Many people are exposed, but few are infected. It usually occurs in people whose immune system is weakened or whose general health is poor. Amebas probably enter through the skin or lungs and spread to the brain through the bloodstream.

Symptoms begin gradually. People may have a low-grade fever, blurred vision, changes in personality, and problems with speaking, coordination, or vision. One side of the body or face may become paralyzed. Sores may develop on the skin. Headache and seizures are common. Most infected people die, usually 7 to 120 days after symptoms begin.

Computed tomography (CT) and a spinal tap are usually done. These tests help exclude other possible causes but usually cannot confirm the diagnosis. Sores typically contain amebas and, if present, are biopsied. The diagnosis is often made after death.

Some antifungal drugs and antibiotics may be used. Dibromopropamidine, pentamidine, or propamidine seems most useful. Others may include amphotericin B, flucrocytosine, itraconazole, ketoconazole, miconazole, neomycin, paromomycin, or trimethoprim-sulfamethoxazole.

AMEBIC KERATITIS

Amebic keratitis is infection of the cornea caused by Acanthamoeba *species. It usually occurs in people who wear contact lenses.*

Amebic keratitis may be progressively destructive. Most (85%) infected people wear contact lenses. Infection is more likely if lenses are worn during swimming or if the lens cleaning solution used is unsterile. Some infections develop after the cornea is scraped.

Typically, painful sores develop on the cornea. Symptoms include eye redness, excess tear production, sensation of a foreign body, and pain when the eyes are exposed to bright light. Vision is usually impaired.

For diagnosis, doctors take a sample of tissue from the cornea.

Early, superficial infection can be treated more easily. If sores are superficial, doctors use a cotton-tipped applicator to remove infected and damaged cells. A combination of two or more antimicrobial drugs, such as polyhexamethylene biguanide (used to disinfect contact lenses) plus propamidine (applied topically), works best. They are applied hourly for the first 3 days. Other drugs applied topically (such as the antifungal drugs clotrimazole or fluconazole or the antibiotic chlorhexidine) are sometimes also used. Fluconazole or itraconazole may be taken by mouth, particularly if the infection is severe. Treatment is intensive the first month, then gradually decreased

as healing occurs. Treatment often lasts 6 to 12 months. If treatment is stopped too soon, the infection is likely to recur. Surgery to repair the cornea (keratoplasty) is rarely needed unless diagnosis and treatment are delayed.

Ascariasis

Ascariasis is infection caused by Ascaris lumbricoides, *an intestinal roundworm.*

- People acquire the infection by swallowing the roundworm eggs, usually in food.
- People may have no symptoms or may have fever, coughing, wheezing, abdominal cramps, nausea, and vomiting.
- Children with a heavy infection may not grow normally, or worms can block the intestine, resulting in severe pain and vomiting.
- Doctors usually diagnose the infection by identifying the eggs or worms in a stool sample.
- People are treated with antiparasitic drugs such as albendazole.

Ascariasis is the most common roundworm infection in people, occurring in over 1.4 billion people worldwide. The infection is common in areas with poor sanitation and often occurs in tropical or subtropical areas. In the United States, ascariasis occurs most often in immigrants and in people who have lived abroad in areas where hygiene is poor, but occasionally it occurs among people who have not traveled.

Infection begins when a person swallows *Ascaris* eggs, often in contaminated food. Food is contaminated through contact with soil that has been contaminated by human stool (feces) containing the eggs. *Ascaris* eggs are hardy and can survive in the soil for years.

> **? Did You Know...**
> More than 1.4 billion people worldwide have a roundworm infection called ascariasis.

Once swallowed, *Ascaris* eggs hatch and release larvae in the intestine. Each larva migrates through the wall of the small intestine and is carried through the lymphatic vessels and bloodstream to the lungs. Once inside the lungs, the larva passes into the air sacs (alveoli), moves up the respiratory tract and into the throat, and is swallowed. The larva matures in the small intestine, where it remains as an adult worm. This process takes 2 to 3 months. Adult worms range from 6 to 20 inches in length and from 1/10 to 2/10 inch in diameter. They live 1 to 2 years. Eggs laid by the adult worms are excreted in stool, develop in the soil, and begin the cycle of infection again when they are ingested.

Symptoms and Diagnosis

Many people who have ascariasis do not develop symptoms. However, the migration of larvae through the lungs can cause fever, coughing, wheezing, and sometimes blood in phlegm (sputum). A large number of worms in the intestine can cause abdominal cramps and, occasionally, a blockage of the intestine, most commonly in children living in areas with poor sanitation. A blockage can cause nausea, vomiting, abdominal swelling (distention), and abdominal pain. Sometimes adult worms migrate to the mouth or nose, are vomited up, or passed in the stool—situations that can be psychologically distressing. Adult worms occasionally block the opening into the appendix, biliary tract, or pancreatic duct, producing severe abdominal pain. Infected children may not grow or gain weight normally.

Ascariasis is diagnosed by identifying eggs or adult worms in a stool sample or, rarely, by seeing adult worms that have migrated to the throat or nose. If computed tomography (CT) or ultrasonography is done for other reasons, adult worms may be seen. Rarely, the effects of larvae migrating through the lungs can be seen on a chest x-ray.

Prevention and Treatment

The best strategies for preventing ascariasis include using adequate sanitation and avoiding uncooked and unwashed foods, particularly in areas where human feces is used as fertilizer.

To treat a person with ascariasis, a doctor prescribes albendazole, mebendazole, or pyrantel pamoate. However, because these drugs may harm the fetus, they should not be taken by pregnant women.

Babesiosis

Babesiosis is infection of red blood cells caused by the single-celled protozoan parasite Babesia.

Babesiosis is transmitted by the same type of deer ticks (family Ixodidae) that transmits Lyme disease. This infection is common among animals but is relatively uncommon among people. In the United States, *Babesia microti* infects people on the offshore islands or coastal regions of Massachusetts, Connecticut, New York, and New Jersey. Cases also occur in Wisconsin, Georgia, and California. Other *Babesia* species infect people in other areas of the world.

Babesia live inside red blood cells and eventually destroy them. Some people, especially healthy people younger than 40, do not have noticeable symptoms. Other people have fever, headache, muscle and joint aches, and fatigue. Anemia may result from the breakdown of red blood cells. The liver and spleen often enlarge.

The risk of severe disease and death is highest for people whose spleen has been removed or who take drugs or have disorders that weaken the immune system (particularly AIDS). In these people, babesiosis may resemble malaria (causing a high fever, anemia, dark urine, jaundice, and kidney failure).

To diagnose babesiosis, a doctor usually examines a blood sample under a microscope.

Usually, no treatment is needed for a mild infection in healthy people with a functioning spleen because the infection typically disappears on its own. People with symptoms are treated with atovaquone plus azithromycin or quinine plus clindamycin. Atovaquone and azithromycin have fewer side effects. In areas where deer ticks are common, people can reduce the risk of getting the infection by taking precautions against ticks (see box on page 1166).

Cryptosporidiosis

Cryptosporidiosis is an intestinal infection caused by Cryptosporidium, *a protozoan.*

- People acquire the infection by consuming contaminated water or food or by having contact with contaminated people or objects.

- Abdominal cramping and watery diarrhea may begin suddenly, sometimes accompanied by nausea, vomiting, fever, and weakness.

- Doctors diagnose the infection by examining or analyzing a stool sample for signs of the parasite.

- Adequate sanitation and hand washing can help prevent spread of the infection, as can boiling water before drinking it.

- Healthy people often recover on their own, but people with a weakened immune system require treatment with drugs.

Cryptosporidium parasites infect people and many kinds of animals throughout the world. The infection is acquired by ingesting parasites in water or food contaminated by human or animal feces or by having contact with soil, a person, or an item that has been contaminated with the parasite. Cryptosporidiosis is a common cause of diarrhea among children living in developing areas where sanitation is poor. It occasionally occurs among travelers to such areas. People with a weakened immune system, particularly those with AIDS, are prone to cryptosporidiosis and are more likely to have severe, persistent disease.

The eggs (oocysts) of *Cryptosporidium* are very hardy and are frequently present in surface water in the United States. The parasite is not killed by freezing or by the usual levels of chlorine in swimming pools or drinking water.

Symptoms and Diagnosis

Symptoms may begin abruptly 7 to 10 days after infection and consist mainly of abdominal cramps and profuse, watery diarrhea. Nausea, vomiting, loss of appetite, fever, and weakness may also occur. In people with a weakened immune system, symptoms may begin gradually, and the diarrhea can vary from mild to severe (as much as 3 to 4 gallons of watery stool per day in people with AIDS).

To diagnose cryptosporidiosis, a doctor sends a stool sample to be tested for a protein released by the parasite (antigen testing). Another approach is to examine stool under a microscope, but several stool samples may be needed to find the parasite.

> **? Did You Know...**
> People with a healthy immune system typically do not need treatment for cryptosporidiosis.

Prevention and Treatment

Prevention involves adequate sanitation and hand washing, particularly in health care facilities and day care centers and after contact with soil, animals, or infected people. When public health departments discover a localized outbreak of the disease, they typically advise people to boil drinking water (including water for toothbrushing and food washing), to eat only cooked foods, and to avoid unpasteurized milk and juice. Tap water filters that use reverse osmosis or have the words "absolute 1 micron" or "tested and certified by NSF Standard 53 for cyst removal/reduction" are effective. Other types of filters may not be.

People with a healthy immune system typically recover on their own. Nitazoxanide is given to children to speed recovery and may be useful for healthy adults. However, it is usually ineffective in people who have AIDS and thus have a weakened immune system. If possible, the problem with the immune system should be treated. If people take drugs that suppress the immune system (immunosuppressants), the drugs should be stopped, or their doses decreased if possible. Unless the immune system problem is corrected, diarrhea may continue throughout life. In people with AIDS, antiretroviral drugs can improve immune function and relieve diarrhea caused by *Cryptosporidium parvum*, but such people may remain permanently infected. People with severe diarrhea may require treatment with fluids, given by mouth or by vein, and antidiarrheal drugs such as loperamide. However, loperamide may not help people with AIDS.

Dracunculiasis

Dracunculiasis is infection caused by the roundworm Dracunculus medinensis.

- People become infected by drinking water containing tiny crustaceans infected with the roundworm.
- A blister forms, with swelling, redness, and pain in the area around it, and the joints near the blister may be damaged.
- Doctors diagnose the infection when they see the worm at the blister.
- Drinking only water that has been filtered, boiled, or chlorinated helps prevent the infection.
- The worm is removed by slowly rolling it on a stick or surgically.

The infection occurs mainly in a narrow belt across several countries in southern Africa and in Yemen and only during certain seasons.

People become infected by drinking water containing tiny infected crustaceans, which are intermediate hosts for the worms. After ingestion, the crustaceans die and release the larvae, which penetrate the wall of the intestine. Larvae mature into adult worms in about 1 year. After mating, female worms move through tissues under the skin, usually to the feet. There, they create an opening to the skin so that when they release larvae, the larvae can leave the body, enter water, and find the crustacean host. If the larvae do not reach the skin, they die and disintegrate or harden (calcify) under the skin.

Symptoms and Diagnosis

Symptoms st-art when the worm breaks through the skin. A blister forms at the opening. The area around the blister itches, burns, and is inflamed—swollen, red, and painful. Materials released by the worm may cause an allergic reaction, which can result in difficulty breathing, vomiting, and an itchy rash. Symptoms subside and the blister heals after the adult worm leaves the body. In about 50% of people, bacterial infections develop around the opening for the worm. Sometimes joints and tendons near the blister are damaged.

Diagnosis is obvious when the adult worm appears at the blister. X-rays may be taken to locate calcified worms.

Prevention and Treatment

Filtering drinking water through a piece of cheesecloth, boiling water, and drinking only chlorinated water help prevent dracunculiasis.

Usually, the adult worm is slowly removed over days to weeks by rolling it on a stick. The worm can be surgically removed after a local anesthetic is used, but in many areas, this method is unavailable.

Metronidazole is sometimes used to treat concurrent bacterial infection and reduce inflammation.

Giardiasis

Giardiasis is an infection of the small intestine caused by the single-celled protozoan parasite Giardia lamblia.

- People may have abdominal cramping, gas, belching, diarrhea, and nausea and feel vaguely tired.
- People acquire the infection by drinking contaminated water or by having contact with contaminated stool.
- Doctors diagnose the infection by testing or examining a stool sample.
- Hikers should boil fresh water before drinking it.
- Infected people are treated with an antiparasitic drug, such as tinidazole.

Giardiasis occurs worldwide and is the most common parasitic infection of the intestine in the United States. *Giardia* protozoa are a common contaminant of fresh water, including many lakes and streams—even ones that appear clean. Poorly filtered municipal water supply systems contribute to some outbreaks. Most people acquire the infection from drinking contaminated water, but direct person-to-person transmission of cysts passed in the stool also occurs—typically between children or sex partners. Giardiasis is more common among children in day care centers, people who practice oral-anal sex, and people who have traveled to developing countries. Backpackers and hikers who drink untreated water from streams and lakes are also at risk. Wild animals can harbor the parasite.

Symptoms and Diagnosis

Some infected people have no symptoms. In other people, symptoms appear about 1 to 2 weeks after infection. Symptoms typically include abdominal cramps, gas (flatulence), belching, and watery, foul-smelling diarrhea. Nausea may come and go. People may feel tired and vaguely uncomfortable and lose their appetite. If untreated, the diarrhea may persist for weeks. A few people develop diarrhea that persists longer. These people may not absorb enough nutrients from food, resulting in significant weight loss. Occasionally, chronic giardiasis prevents children from growing as expected (a condition called failure to thrive).

The symptoms often suggest the diagnosis. The easiest way to make the diagnosis is by testing the stool for proteins (antigens) released by *Giardia lamblia*. Microscopic examination of stool samples or secretions taken from the small intestine may also detect the parasite. However, because people who have been infected for a long time tend to excrete the parasites at unpredictable intervals, repeated microscopic examinations of stool are often needed.

Prevention and Treatment

Boiling water kills the parasite and is the safest way for hikers to ensure that surface water is safe to drink. Wells, reservoirs, and swimming pools can sometimes be disinfected using iodine or chlorine. This method is less reliable because it varies depending on how cloudy or muddy the water is (turbidity), what its temperature is, and how often it is disinfected. The amount of chlorine routinely used in drinking water may be insufficient to kill the cysts. Some handheld filtration devices can remove cysts from water, but whether a particular filter system is effective is not always known.

 Did You Know...

Giardiasis is the most common parasitic intestinal infection in the United States.

Infected people who have symptoms can be treated with tinidazole, metronidazole, or nitazoxanide, taken by mouth. Treating infected people who do not have symptoms might help reduce the spread of the infection but is impractical and expensive. Tinidazole, taken in a single dose, has fewer side effects than metronidazole, which requires several doses. Drinking alcohol within a few days of taking tinidazole or metronidazole may cause nausea, vomiting, flushing, and headaches. Nitazoxanide is available in liquid form, which is useful for children, and as tablets. It has few side effects.

Pregnant women should not take metronidazole or tinidazole. The safety of nitazoxanide during pregnancy has not been assessed. Consequently, the treatment of pregnant women is delayed if possible until after pregnancy. If symptoms are severe and treatment cannot be delayed, paromomycin can be used.

Hookworm Infection

Hookworm infection (ancylostomiasis) is an infection of the intestines caused by either Ancylostoma duodenale *or* Necator americanus.

- People can become infected when walking barefoot because hookworm larvae can penetrate the skin.
- At first, people have an itchy rash where the larvae penetrate the skin, then fever, coughing, and wheezing or abdominal pain, loss of appetite, and diarrhea.
- Doctors diagnose the infection by identifying hookworm eggs in a stool sample.
- The infection is treated with antiparasitic drugs such as albendazole.

About 1.3 billion people are infected with hookworms, which are intestinal roundworms. The infection is most common in tropical areas where

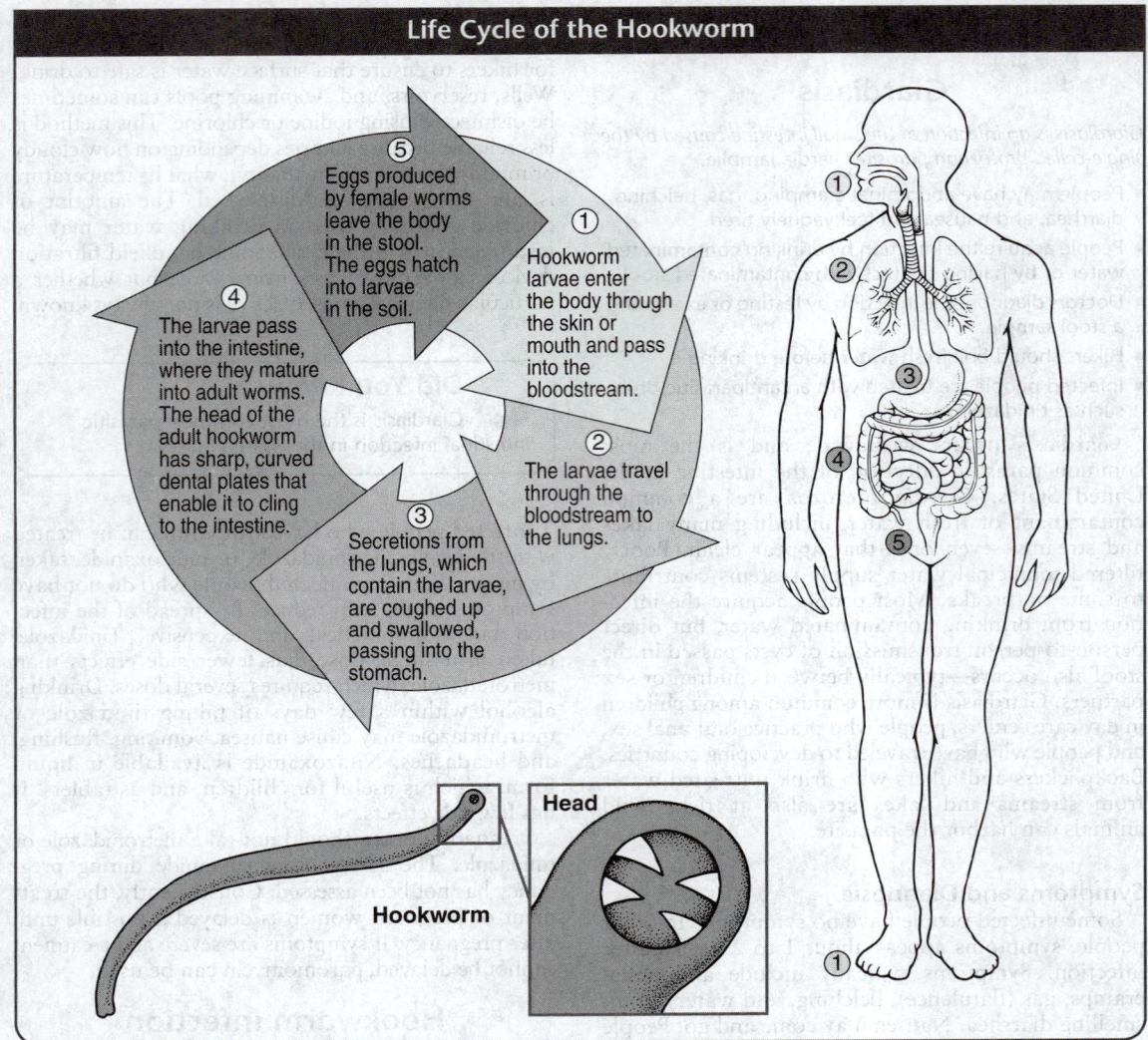

Life Cycle of the Hookworm

⑤ Eggs produced by female worms leave the body in the stool. The eggs hatch into larvae in the soil.

① Hookworm larvae enter the body through the skin or mouth and pass into the bloodstream.

② The larvae travel through the bloodstream to the lungs.

③ Secretions from the lungs, which contain the larvae, are coughed up and swallowed, passing into the stomach.

④ The larvae pass into the intestine, where they mature into adult worms. The head of the adult hookworm has sharp, curved dental plates that enable it to cling to the intestine.

Head

Hookworm

---

sanitation is poor. Hookworms thrive in warm, moist places. Two species of hookworm cause infection in people: *Ancylostoma duodenale* and *Necator americanus*. Both species are present in tropical areas of Africa, Asia, India, and China. *Ancylostoma duodenale* is present in the Middle East, North Africa, southern Europe, and Japan. *Necator americanus* is present in Central and South America. It once was common in the southern part of the United States but is now rare there.

Eggs are passed in stool and hatch in the soil after they incubate for 1 to 2 days. Larvae emerge and

live in the soil. When fully developed, the larvae can penetrate the skin. A person can become infected by walking barefoot or sitting in contaminated soil. Once larvae enter the body, they move through the lymphatic vessels and the bloodstream to the lungs. The larvae pass into the air spaces of the lungs and move up the respiratory tract. They are coughed up into the throat and swallowed. About a week after penetrating the skin, they reach the intestine. Once inside the intestine, the larvae develop into adults. They attach themselves by their mouth to the lining of the upper small intestine, where they suck blood and produce substances that keep blood from clotting.

Symptoms and Diagnosis

Many people with hookworm infection do not have symptoms. However at the start of infection, an itchy, red, raised rash (ground itch) may develop where the larvae penetrate the skin. The movement of the larvae through the lungs can cause fever, coughing, and wheezing. When adult worms first attach in the intestine, they can cause pain in the upper abdomen, loss of appetite, diarrhea, and weight loss. Over time, anemia develops as blood is lost and people become iron deficient. Children with severe anemia may not grow normally. Severe anemia may also cause heart failure and widespread tissue swelling.

The diagnosis is made by identifying hookworm eggs in a sample of stool. Stool should be examined within several hours after defecation. Blood tests for anemia and nutritional deficiencies, particularly iron, are also done.

Treatment

A doctor prescribes albendazole, mebendazole, or pyrantel pamoate, taken by mouth. Because of possible adverse effects to the fetus, these drugs cannot be taken by pregnant women. Iron supplements are given to people with anemia.

Leishmaniasis

Leishmaniasis is caused by several species of Leishmania *protozoa. Leishmaniasis includes disorders that affect internal organs and those that affect the skin and sometimes mucous membranes of the nose and mouth.*

- The protozoa are usually spread through the bite of infected sand flies.
- Symptoms may be mild symptoms or include bouts of fever, vomiting, diarrhea, and fatigue or sores that may cause scars or severe disfigurement.
- Doctors diagnose the infection by analyzing samples of infected tissue or doing blood tests.
- Using insect repellents and bed nets and clothing treated with insecticides helps prevent sand fly bites.
- Drugs used to treat the infection depend on the species of protozoa and the geographic location.

Tiny infected sand flies spread the protozoa when they bite people or animals, such as dogs or rodents. Rarely, infection is spread in blood transfusions, through injections with a needle previously used by an infected person, from mother to child at birth, or through sexual contact.

The form that affects internal organs (**visceral leishmaniasis, or kala-azar**) occurs in India, Africa (particularly the Sudan), Central Asia, the area around the Mediterranean, South and Central America, and infrequently China. Parasites spread from the skin to the lymph nodes, spleen, liver, and bone marrow. The form that affects the skin (**cutaneous leishmaniasis**) occurs in southern Europe, Asia, Africa, Mexico, and Central and South America. Outbreaks have occurred among US military personnel training in Panama or serving in Iraq or Afghanistan. Occasionally, travelers to affected areas develop the disorder. People with a weakened immune system, particularly those with AIDS, are more susceptible to leishmaniasis.

Symptoms and Diagnosis

Usually, symptoms of visceral leishmaniasis are mild and may not be noticed. The disorder progresses in a minority of infected people. In them, symptoms typically develop gradually over weeks to months. People may have irregular bouts of fever. They may lose weight, vomit, have diarrhea, and be generally tired. The liver, spleen, and lymph nodes enlarge. The number of blood cells decreases, causing anemia and making people more susceptible to other infections. Without treatment, 80 to 90% of people who develop symptoms die within 1 to 2 years. After treatment, skin sores develop in some people and may last a few months to several years.

In cutaneous leishmaniasis, the first symptom is a bump at the site of a sand fly bite. It appears after several weeks or months and contains protozoa. As the infection spreads, more bumps may appear. The initial bump slowly enlarges and becomes an open sore, which may ooze or form a scab. The sores are painless and cause no other symptoms unless another infection develops in them. The sores typically heal on their own after several months but may persist for years. They leave scars similar to those due to burns. Scars may be permanent. Sometimes after the skin sores heal, sores appear on mucous membranes in the nose and mouth. The first sign may be a stuffy nose or nosebleeds. These sores may cause severe disfigurement. Occasionally, sores appear on skin all over the body, causing a condition that resembles leprosy.

In people with AIDS, leishmaniasis often recurs.

Doctors diagnose leishmaniasis by taking a sample of the infected tissue. The samples may be analyzed to determine whether the protozoa they contain can infect the mucous membranes. Blood tests can be used to confirm visceral leishmaniasis in people with symptoms.

Prevention and Treatment

Prevention begins with treating infected people and trying to prevent sand fly bites. People who are treated are less susceptible to reinfection by the same species of *Leishmania*. Insect repellents containing DEET (diethyltoluamide) provide protection. Insect screens, bed nets, and clothing are more effective if treated with insecticides such as permethrin or pyrethrum because the tiny flies can pass through them otherwise.

Drugs used to treat the infection depend on the species and the geographic location.

For visceral leishmaniasis, liposomal amphotericin B given by vein is the drug of choice in the United States and other developed countries. Amphotericin B deoxycholate is also effective but has more side effects. In Latin America and Africa, drugs that contain antimony (such as sodium stibogluconate or meglumine antimonate) are often used. These drugs may cause nausea, vomiting, fatigue, and heart problems (which require stopping the drug). If the protozoa are resistant to drugs that contain antimony (common in India), miltefosine, which is not available in the United States, can be used. Transfusions or antibiotics to treat concurrent bacterial infections may be needed. Adequate nutrition is also important because undernutrition can worsen the disorder.

Treatment of cutaneous leishmaniasis depends on the extent of the disease and the possibility of spread to mucous membranes. Antimony drugs are often used, particularly if spread to mucous membranes is possible. Other drugs used include fluconazole or itraconazole, usually taken by mouth, and paromomycin ointment. Widespread sores are difficult to treat. Reconstructive surgery may be needed if the nose or face is disfigured, but surgery should be delayed 6 to 12 months after treatment, when the risk of recurrence is less likely.

Malaria

Malaria is infection of red blood cells with one of four species of Plasmodium, *a protozoan.*

- Usually, malaria is spread through the bite of an infected female mosquito.
- People have a shaking chill, followed by a fever, and may have a headache, body aches, and nausea and feel tired.
- One type of malaria causes serious symptoms, such as delirium, confusion, seizures, coma, severe breathing problems, kidney failure, and sometimes death.
- Doctors diagnose the infection by identifying the protozoa in a sample of blood.
- Eliminating mosquito breeding areas, killing larvae in standing water, preventing mosquito bites, and taking preventive drugs before traveling to affected areas can help.
- Antimalarial drugs such as chloroquine are used to treat the infection.

Malaria is spread by the bite of an infected female mosquito. Very rarely, the disease is transmitted from an infected mother to her fetus, through transfusion of contaminated blood, or through injection with a needle previously used by a person with malaria. The four species of malaria parasites that infect people are *Plasmodium falciparum*, *Plasmodium vivax*, *Plasmodium ovale*, and *Plasmodium malariae*.

Although drugs and insecticides have made malaria rare in the United States and in most developed countries, the disease remains common and deadly in other areas. Worldwide, about 300 to 500 million people are infected with malaria, and 1 to 2 million deaths occur each year. Most of these deaths occur in children who are younger than 5 years and live in Africa. In the United States and other developed countries, malaria may occur in immigrants, visitors from the tropics, or North American travelers returning from tropical areas.

The cycle of malarial infection begins when a female mosquito bites a person with malaria. The mosquito ingests blood that contains reproductive cells of the parasite. Once inside the mosquito, the parasite reproduces, develops, and migrates to the mosquito's salivary gland. When the mosquito bites another person, parasites are injected along with the mosquito's saliva. Inside the newly infected person, the parasites move to the liver and multiply again. They typically mature over an average of 1 to 3 weeks, then leave the liver and invade the person's red blood cells. The parasites multiply yet again inside the red blood cells, eventually causing the infected cells to rupture, releasing parasites to invade other red blood cells.

Plasmodium vivax and *Plasmodium ovale* can remain in the liver in a dormant form that periodically releases mature parasites into the bloodstream, causing recurring attacks of symptoms. The dormant form is not killed by many antimalarial drugs. *Plasmodium falciparum* and *Plasmodium malariae* do not persist in the liver. However, mature forms of *Plasmodium malariae* can persist in the bloodstream for months or even years before they cause symptoms.

Symptoms and Complications

After infection occurs, symptoms usually appear within a few weeks to several months, but they may not occur until years later. The initial symptoms of all forms of malaria are similar. As the infected red blood cells rupture and release parasites, a person typically develops a shaking chill followed by a fever that can exceed 104° F (40° C). Fatigue and vague discomfort (malaise), headache, body aches, and nausea are common. The fever typically falls after several hours, and heavy sweating and extreme fatigue follow. Fevers occur unpredictably at first, but with time, they may become periodic. Fevers occur at 48-hour intervals with *Plasmodium vivax* and

Plasmodium ovale and at 72-hour intervals with *Plasmodium malariae*. The fevers caused by *Plasmodium falciparum* are often not periodic, but sometimes occur at 48-hour intervals.

As the infection progresses, the spleen enlarges, and anemia may become severe. Jaundice may develop. The level of sugar (glucose) in the blood can fall in people infected with *Plasmodium falciparum*. The level may be life-threateningly low in people who have a large number of parasites in their blood—particularly if they are treated with the drug quinine.

Falciparum Malaria: This infection, caused by *Plasmodium falciparum*, is the most dangerous form of malaria and can be fatal. In falciparum malaria, infected red blood cells stick to the walls of small blood vessels and clog them, damaging many organs—particularly the brain (cerebral malaria), lungs, kidneys, and gastrointestinal tract. Cerebral malaria is a particularly dangerous complication that can cause a high fever, headache, drowsiness, delirium, confusion, seizures, and coma. It most commonly occurs in infants, young children, pregnant women, and people who have never been exposed to malaria and who travel to high-risk areas. In falciparum malaria, fluid can accumulate in the lungs and cause severe breathing problems. Damage to several organs can cause a fall in blood pressure. Other symptoms include diarrhea, kidney failure, and jaundice.

> ### ? Did You Know...
>
> Each year, about 300 to 500 million people throughout the world are infected with malaria, and 1 to 2 million people die.
>
> Symptoms of malaria sometimes do not appear until years after the initial infection.

Blackwater fever is an uncommon complication of falciparum malaria. It is caused by the rupture of large numbers of red blood cells, which releases blood pigment (hemoglobin) into the bloodstream. The released hemoglobin is excreted in the urine, which turns the urine dark. Kidney damage may be severe enough to require dialysis. Blackwater fever is more likely to develop in people who have taken quinine for treatment.

Diagnosis

A doctor suspects malaria when a person develops fever and other characteristic symptoms during or after travel to an area where malaria is present.

Periodic fever develops in less than half of American travelers with malaria but, when present, suggests the diagnosis. Identification of parasites by microscopic examination of a blood sample confirms the diagnosis. More than one sample may be needed. Laboratories try to identify the species of *Plasmodium* found in the sample because the treatment, complications, and prognosis vary depending on the species involved. *Plasmodium falciparum* infection is an emergency and requires immediate evaluation and treatment.

Prevention

Mosquito control measures, which include eliminating breeding areas and killing larvae in the standing water where they live, are very important. Also, people who live in or travel to areas where malaria is prevalent can take precautions to limit mosquito exposure:

- Using insecticide (permethrin or pyrethrum) sprays in homes and outbuildings
- Placing screens on doors and windows
- Using permethrin-impregnated mosquito netting over beds
- Applying mosquito repellents containing DEET (diethyltoluamide) on exposed areas of the skin
- Wearing long pants and long-sleeved shirts, particularly between dusk and dawn, to protect against mosquito bites
- If mosquito exposure is likely to be long or involve many mosquitoes, spraying permethrin on clothing before it is worn

Drugs: Drugs should be taken to prevent malaria during travel in areas where it is prevalent. The preventive drug is started before travel begins, continued throughout the stay, and extended for a time (which varies for each drug) after the person leaves the high-risk area. Preventive drugs reduce but do not eliminate the risk of malaria. Several drugs can be used to prevent (and treat) malaria. Drug resistance is a serious problem, particularly with the dangerous *Plasmodium falciparum*. The prevalence of drug-resistant strains varies in different parts of the world. Thus for prevention, the choice of drug varies by geographic location. Information about travel to specific sites is available from the Centers for Disease Control and Prevention.

Chloroquine is the preferred drug for prevention of malaria in Mexico, areas of Central America west of the Panama Canal, Haiti, the Dominican Republic, and some areas of the Middle East. Strains of *Plasmodium falciparum* that are resistant to chloroquine are present in most other areas of the world where malaria occurs. In those areas, doxycycline, the combination atovaquone-proguanil, or mefloquine is effective. The use of mefloquine has decreased in recent years because of infrequent, but potentially severe, psychiatric side effects. It is also ineffective or less effective for prevention of *Plasmodium falciparum* in some areas of Southeast Asia (and occasionally elsewhere).

Vaccines for preventing malaria are still in the experimental stage.

Treatment

For treatment, the choice of drug is based on the infecting species of *Plasmodium*. Chloroquine is the drug of choice in areas where *Plasmodium* species have not developed resistance to it. Primaquine is added to kill persistent parasites in the liver of people infected with *Plasmodium vivax* or *Plasmodium ovale*. Before primaquine is given, a blood test is done to look for a relatively common enzyme deficiency—glucose-6-phosphate dehydrogenase (G6PD) deficiency. In people with G6PD deficiency, primaquine may cause their red blood cells to break down.

Malaria in areas with known chloroquine resistance can be treated with quinine plus doxycycline or, if uncomplicated, with atovaquone-proguanil. Atovaquone-proguanil has fewer side effects than quinine. Mefloquine can be used in higher doses than those recommended for prevention, but side effects are common. If the person cannot take drugs by mouth, quinidine may be given intravenously, but the person must be monitored in the hospital because intravenous quinidine can cause low blood pressure and abnormal heart rhythms.

A number of artemisinin drugs (such as artemether), which are typically given with a second antimalarial drug to prevent recurrence, are now widely used to treat *Plasmodium falciparum* malaria in Southeast Asia and China and are being increasingly used in Africa and elsewhere. A combination of artemether and lumefantrine is widely used. Artemisinin drugs act rapidly and are generally well tolerated.

Travelers who develop a fever while they are in areas where malaria is prevalent should be examined by a doctor immediately. If medical care is not available, self-treatment for presumed malaria with atovaquone-proguanil is sometimes recommended until medical evaluation is possible. This approach should be discussed with a doctor before traveling.

Chloroquine is relatively safe for adults, children, and pregnant women. It has a bitter taste and can cause intestinal symptoms, such as abdominal pain, loss of appetite, nausea, and diarrhea. The drug must be kept away from children because overdoses can be fatal.

Doxycycline can cause intestinal symptoms, vaginal yeast infections in women, and severe sunburn in a small percentage of people. People should take it with a full glass of liquid and should not lie down for several hours to ensure that the drug reaches the stomach. If the drug does not reach the stomach, it can cause irritation of the esophagus and cause severe pain. Doxycycline should not be used in pregnant women or in children younger than 8 years old because it can permanently stain the fetus's or the children's teeth.

Mefloquine causes vivid dreams. Occasionally, it can also have severe psychologic side effects. It can cause seizures in people with a seizure disorder and affect the heart in people taking certain drugs for heart disorders. Thus, mefloquine is avoided in people who are known to have a seizure disorder or psychiatric problems or who take certain drugs for heart disorders. People who are taking the drug, especially if they are traveling, should ask for written information about the side effects.

Atovaquone-proguanil is the best tolerated of the drugs used to prevent and treat malaria, but it occasionally causes a rash or intestinal symptoms.

Quinine often causes headache, nausea, vomiting, visual disturbances, and ringing in the ears. This combination of symptoms is called cinchonism. Quinine may also cause a low blood sugar level in people infected with *Plasmodium falciparum*.

Artemisinin drugs are derived from a Chinese medicinal herb for malaria, quinghaosu, which comes from the wormwood plant. The route of administration varies. Some are given by mouth, and others are given by injection or suppository. Side effects are uncommon and include abdominal pain, diarrhea, and drug fever.

Antimalarial drugs may harm a fetus. Thus, an expert should be consulted if a pregnant woman is treated.

After beginning treatment, most people improve within 24 to 48 hours, but with falciparum malaria, fever can persist for 5 days.

Microsporidiosis

Microsporidiosis is infection caused by Microsporidia *protozoa.*

- This infection usually causes symptoms only in people with a weakened immune system, such as people with AIDS.
- Symptoms vary but include chronic diarrhea in people with AIDS, abdominal pain, fever, weight loss, a persistent cough, headache, nasal congestion, and eye irritation.
- Doctors diagnose the infection by identifying the protozoa in a sample of the infected tissue.
- Antiparasitic drugs can control but not eliminate the infection.

Several species of *Microsporidia* cause infection in people, but symptoms occur mainly in those with

AIDS or other disorders that weaken the immune system. These protozoa may infect the intestine, biliary tract, cornea, muscles, respiratory tract, urinary tract, and, occasionally, the brain. The infection may spread throughout the body.

Microsporidia spread through spores, which can be ingested or inhaled or enter through the eye. They may spread from person to person or through contact with an animal. Inside the body, the spores pierce a cell and inject it with material that becomes spores. The cell eventually ruptures, releasing the spores. The spores then spread throughout the body, causing inflammation, or are excreted in the breath, stool, or urine.

Symptoms and Diagnosis

Symptoms vary depending on which species causes the infection and how well a person's immune system is working. People with a normal immune system typically have no symptoms, but microsporidiosis can cause chronic diarrhea in people with AIDS. Other symptoms may include abdominal pain, jaundice, fever, weight loss, a persistent cough, pain in the side (flank), muscle aches, headache, nasal congestion, and eye irritation with redness. Vision may be blurred. If infection is severe, blindness may result.

To diagnose microsporidiosis, doctors examine a sample of the affected tissue under a microscope, usually using special techniques to make the protozoa more visible. Samples of stool, urine, blood, sputum, cerebrospinal fluid (taken by spinal tap), cornea (taken by scraping), or other tissue (taken by biopsy) may be needed.

Treatment

If the immune system is normal, treatment is rarely needed. If it is not, albendazole or fumagillin, taken by mouth, may help control but does not eliminate the infection. Eye drops containing albendazole and fumagillin may relieve eye symptoms. If they do not, surgery to repair the cornea (keratoplasty) may be required. In people with AIDS, antiretroviral drugs can lessen symptoms.

Onchocerciasis

Onchocerciasis (river blindness) is infection with the round-worm Onchocerca volvulus.

- The infection is spread through the bite of female blackflies, which breed in streams.
- The infection may cause only intense itching but sometimes causes a rash, swollen lymph nodes, impaired vision, or complete blindness.
- Usually, doctors diagnose the infection by identifying a prelarval form of the worm in a skin sample.

- Administration of ivermectin twice a year in areas where the infection in common helps control the infection.

Worldwide, about 18 million people have onchocerciasis. About 270,000 of them are blind, and 500,000 are visually impaired. Onchocerciasis is a leading cause of blindness in the developing world. Onchocerciasis is most common in tropical and southern (sub-Saharan) areas of Africa. It occasionally occurs in Yemen, southern Mexico, Guatemala, Ecuador, Colombia, Venezuela, and Brazil (along the Amazon).

Onchocerciasis is spread though the bite of female blackflies that breed in swiftly flowing streams (hence, the term river blindness). The cycle of infection begins when a blackfly bites an infected person and is infected with prelarval forms of the worm called microfilariae. They develop into larvae in the fly. When the fly bites another person, larvae are passed into that person's skin. The larvae move under the skin and form lumps (nodules), where they develop into adult worms in 12 to 18 months. Adult female worms may live up to 15 years in these nodules. After mating, mature female worms produce eggs, which develop into microfilariae that leave the worm. A worm may produce 1,000 microfilariae each day. Thousands of microfilariae move through the tissues of the skin and eyes and are responsible for the disease.

Usually, many bites are necessary before the infection causes symptoms. Thus, the infection is much less likely to develop in visitors to affected areas.

Because the infection is transmitted near rivers, many people avoid those areas. Not being able to live or to work near a river affects their ability to raise crops. Thus, onchocerciasis can contribute to food shortages in some areas.

Symptoms and Diagnosis

Symptoms occur when the microfilariae die. Their death can cause intense itching, which may be the only symptom. A rash with redness may develop. Over time, the skin may thicken, roughen, and wrinkle. It may lose its pigment in patchy spots. Lymph nodes, including those in the genital area, may become inflamed and swollen. Nodules containing adult worms may be seen or felt under the skin.

Effects on vision range from mild impairment (blurring) to complete blindness. The eye may become inflamed and appear red. Exposure to bright light may cause pain. Without treatment, the cornea may become completely opaque and may scar—the cause of blindness. Other structures in the eye, including the iris, pupil, and retina, may be affected. The optic nerve may become inflamed and degenerate. Blindness can result in a decreased life span.

Usually, a sample of skin is snipped and examined for microfilariae. This method is painful. Alternatives are to test blood, but these tests are not always reliable or available. Microfilariae may also be seen in the eye using a slit lamp. Nodules can be removed and checked for adult worms, but this procedure is rarely necessary.

> **? Did You Know...**
> Onchocerciasis, or river blindness, is a leading cause of blindness in the developing world.

Prevention and Treatment

Theoretically, avoiding fly-infested areas, wearing protective clothing, and liberally using insect repellents may help reduce the risk of infection. Ivermectin given once or twice a year dramatically reduces the number of microfilariae, prevents the development of further disease, and helps control the infection in people who are repeatedly exposed to it.

For treatment, ivermectin is given as a single dose by mouth and is repeated every 6 to 12 months until symptoms are gone. Ivermectin kills microfilariae, reducing the number of microfilariae in the skin and eyes, and reduces production of microfilariae for several months. It does not appear to kill adult worms. Side effects are usually mild. In the past, nodules were surgically removed, but this treatment has been replaced by ivermectin.

Pinworm Infection

Pinworm infection (enterobiasis) is caused by the intestinal roundworm Enterobius vermicularis *and usually affects children.*

- People acquire the infection when they swallow eggs of the roundworm.
- Often, people have no symptoms other than itching around the anus.
- The infection can be diagnosed by finding the eggs or sometimes the adult pinworm around the anus.
- An antiparasitic drug such as albendazole, given once at diagnosis and once 2 weeks later, cures the infection.

Pinworm infection is the most common roundworm infection in children in the United States.

Infection occurs after pinworm eggs (ova) are swallowed. The eggs develop into larvae in the small intestine, then move to the large intestine. There, the larvae mature within 2 to 6 weeks, and the adult worms mate. After the eggs develop, the adult female worm moves to the rectum and exits through the anus to lay eggs. The eggs are deposited in a sticky, gelatinous substance that sticks to the skin around the anus. From there, eggs can be transferred to fingernails, clothing, bedding, toys, or food. Eggs can survive outside the body up to 3 weeks at normal room temperature. Eggs are often introduced into the mouth from fingers or from contaminated food. Children may reinfect themselves by transferring eggs from the area around their anus to their mouth. Children who suck their thumbs are at increased risk of infection, as are adults who live with children or who practice oral-anal sex.

> **? Did You Know...**
> Pinworm infection is the most common roundworm infection in children in the United States.

Symptoms and Diagnosis

Many children who carry pinworms have no symptoms. However, in some, the area around the anus itches because the eggs and the sticky substance around them irritate the skin. With scratching, the skin can become raw and infected with bacteria. In girls, pinworms may cause vaginal itching and irritation.

The diagnosis is made by finding the eggs or, less commonly, adult pinworms around the anus. Eggs can be obtained by patting the skinfolds around the anus with the sticky side of a strip of transparent tape. Eggs should be obtained in the early morning before the child defecates or wipes the area. The tape can be taken to the doctor for microscopic examination. The best way to search for adult pinworms is to examine the child's anus about 1 to 2 hours after the child has been put to bed for the night. The worms are white and hair-thin, but they wiggle and are visible to the naked eye.

Treatment

A single dose of albendazole, mebendazole, or pyrantel pamoate, repeated after 2 weeks, cures pinworm infection. Despite successful drug treatment, reintroduction of infection is common. Thus, some doctors recommend treating the entire family. Clothing, bedding, and toys should be washed frequently, and the environment should be vacuumed to try to eliminate eggs. Anti-itching creams or ointments applied directly to the area around the anus may relieve symptoms.

Schistosomiasis

Schistosomiasis (bilharziasis) is infection caused by flatworms (flukes), called schistosomes.

- People acquire the infection by swimming or bathing in fresh water that is contaminated with the flatworms.
- The infection may cause an itchy rash (swimmer's itch), then sometimes after several weeks, fever, chills, muscle aches, fatigue, nausea, abdominal pain, and other symptoms, depending on which organ is affected.
- Doctors confirm the diagnosis by identifying eggs in a sample of stool or urine.
- The infection is treated with praziquantel.

Schistosomiasis affects over 200 million people in tropical and subtropical regions of South America, Africa, and Asia. Five *Schistosoma* species cause most of the cases of schistosomiasis in people:

- *Schistosoma hematobium* infects the urinary tract (including the bladder).
- *Schistosoma mansoni, Schistosoma japonicum, Schistosoma mekongi,* and *Schistosoma intercalatum* infect the intestine and liver. *Schistosoma mansoni* is widespread in Africa and is the only schistosome in the Western Hemisphere.

Schistosomiasis is acquired by swimming, wading, or bathing in fresh water that is contaminated with the free-swimming stage of the parasite. Schistosomes multiply inside specific types of water-dwelling snails, from which they are released to swim free in the water. If they encounter a person's skin, they burrow in and move through the bloodstream to the lungs, where they mature into adult flukes. The adults pass through the bloodstream to their final home in small veins in the bladder or intestine, where they may remain for years. The adult flukes lay large numbers of eggs in the walls of the intestine or bladder. The eggs cause local tissue damage and inflammation, which results in ulcers, bleeding, and scar tissue formation. Some eggs pass into the stool (feces) or urine. If urine or stool of infected people enters fresh water, the eggs hatch, and the parasite enters snails to begin the cycle again.

Schistosoma mansoni and *Schistosoma japonicum* typically lodge in small veins of the intestine. Some eggs flow from there through the bloodstream to the liver. The resulting liver inflammation can lead to scarring and increased pressure in the vein that carries blood between the intestinal tract and the liver (the portal vein). High blood pressure in the portal vein (portal hypertension) can cause enlargement of the spleen and bleeding from veins in the esophagus.

The eggs of *Schistosoma hematobium* typically lodge in the bladder, sometimes causing ulcers, bleeding into the urine, and scarring. Chronic *Schistosoma hematobium* infection increases the risk of bladder cancer.

All types of schistosomiasis can affect other organs (such as the lungs, spinal cord, and brain). Eggs that reach the lungs can result in inflammation and increased blood pressure in the arteries of the lungs (pulmonary hypertension).

Symptoms and Diagnosis

When schistosomes first penetrate the skin, an itchy rash (swimmer's itch) may develop. About 4 to 8 weeks later (when the adult flukes begin laying eggs), fever, chills, muscle aches, fatigue, vague discomfort (malaise), nausea, and abdominal pain may develop. Lymph nodes may temporarily enlarge, then return to normal. This group of late symptoms is called Katayama fever.

Other symptoms depend on the organs affected:

- If blood vessels of the intestine are chronically infected: Abdominal discomfort, pain, and bleeding (seen in the stool), which may result in anemia
- If the liver is affected and pressure in the portal vein is high: An enlarged liver and spleen or vomiting large amounts of blood
- If the bladder is chronically infected: Painful, frequent urination, bloody urine, and an increased risk of bladder cancer
- If the urinary tract is chronically infected: Inflammation and eventual scarring that can block the ureters
- If the brain or spinal cord is chronically infected (rare): Seizures or muscle weakness

Travelers and immigrants from areas where schistosomiasis is common should be asked whether they have swum or waded in fresh water. A doctor can confirm the diagnosis by examining samples of stool or urine for eggs. Usually, several samples are needed. Blood tests can be done to determine whether someone has been infected with *Schistosoma mansoni* or another species, but the tests do not indicate how severe the infection is or how long the person has had it. Occasionally, a doctor takes a sample of intestinal or bladder tissue to be examined under a microscope for eggs. Ultrasonography can be used to assess the severity of schistosomiasis in the urinary tract or liver.

Prevention and Treatment

Schistosomiasis is best prevented by avoiding swimming, bathing, or wading in fresh water in areas known to contain schistosomes. For treatment, 2 or 3 doses of praziquantel are taken by mouth over 1 day.

Tapeworm Infection

Tapeworm infection of the intestine occurs when people eat raw, contaminated pork, beef, or freshwater fish.

- People acquire tapeworms by eating undercooked meat or freshwater fish that contain tapeworm cysts.
- Tapeworms in the intestine usually cause no symptoms but may cause abdominal discomfort, diarrhea, and loss of appetite.
- Tapeworms that cause cysts to form in the body produce various symptoms, such as headaches, seizures, and confusion.
- Doctors diagnose the infection by finding worm segments or eggs in a stool sample or, for cysts elsewhere in the body, by doing imaging or blood tests.
- Thoroughly cooking meat and freshwater fish can help prevent the infection.
- Antiparasitic drugs such as praziquantel may be used to treat the infection, and corticosteroids may be used to relieve symptoms.

Several species of tapeworms, such as *Taenia saginata* (beef tapeworm), *Taenia solium* (pork tapeworm), and *Diphyllobothrium latum* (fish tapeworm), can cause infection in people.

The pork and beef tapeworms are large, flat worms that live in the intestine and can grow 15 to 30 feet in length. Egg-bearing sections of the worm (proglottids) are passed in the stool. If untreated human waste is released into the environment, the eggs may be ingested by intermediate hosts, such as pigs, cattle, or (in the case of fish tapeworms) small crustaceans, which are in turn ingested by fish. The eggs hatch into larvae in the intermediate host. The larvae invade the intestinal wall and are carried through the bloodstream to skeletal muscle and other tissues, where they form cysts. People acquire the parasite by eating the cysts in raw or undercooked meat or certain types of freshwater fish. The cysts hatch and develop into adult worms, which latch onto the intestinal wall. The worms then grow in length and begin producing eggs.

Did You Know...

Tapeworms can grow to be 15 to 30 feet long.

With the pork tapeworm only, people who ingest the eggs can become an intermediate host (people cannot be intermediate hosts for other tapeworms). They may swallow the pork tapeworm eggs in food or water contaminated with human feces, or they may transfer the eggs to their mouth after contact with an infected person or with contaminated clothing and furniture. Or eggs may reach the stomach if

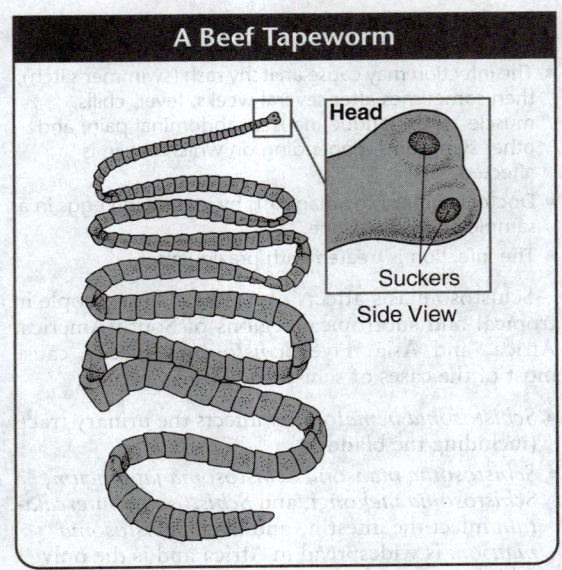

A Beef Tapeworm

Head

Suckers

Side View

proglottids are regurgitated from the intestine. As in animal intermediate hosts, the eggs develop into larvae. The larvae penetrate the intestinal wall and travel to the brain (see page 764), muscles, other organs, or tissue under the skin, where they form cysts (cysticerci). In people, this form of the disease is called cysticercosis.

Symptoms and Diagnosis

Although tapeworms in the intestine usually cause no symptoms, some people experience upper abdominal discomfort, diarrhea, and loss of appetite. Occasionally, people with a tapeworm can feel a piece of the worm move out through the anus or see part of the ribbon-like tapeworm in stool. The fish tapeworm can cause anemia because it absorbs vitamin B_{12}, which is necessary for red blood cells to mature.

Cysts in the brain and the tissues covering the brain (meninges) in people with cysticercosis can result in headaches, seizures, confusion, or other neurologic symptoms. Rarely, cysts develop in the eyes, sometimes causing blindness, or in the spinal cord, sometimes causing muscle weakness or paralysis.

A doctor diagnoses intestinal tapeworm infection by finding worm segments or eggs in a stool sample. In people with cysticercosis, cysts in the brain or other tissues can be seen using computed tomography (CT) or magnetic resonance imaging (MRI). Blood tests for antibodies to the pork tapeworm may also be helpful.

Prevention and Treatment

The first line of defense against tapeworms is thoroughly cooking meat and freshwater fish to a temperature of more than 135° F (57° C). Prolonged freezing can also kill cysts. Thus, freshwater fish should not be served as sushi and should be eaten only after it has been cooked, properly frozen, or cured in brine. Smoking and drying do not kill cysts. Another line of defense is careful evaluation of meat and fish by trained inspectors. Cysts are visible in infected meat. Adequate treatment of human waste interrupts the life cycle and thus helps prevent cysticercosis.

A person with an intestinal tapeworm is treated with a single oral dose of praziquantel. Cysticercosis is usually not treated unless it involves the brain. If the infected person has symptoms, corticosteroids such as prednisone are given to reduce inflammation.

Depending on various factors, such as symptoms and the number and location of cysts in the brain, antiparasitic drugs (such as albendazole or praziquantel) may be given with corticosteroids. These drugs are not used for cysts in the eye or spinal cord because they can elicit severe, locally damaging inflammatory responses.

Toxocariasis

Toxocariasis (visceral larva migrans) is infection caused by larvae of the roundworms Toxocara canis *or* Toxocara cati.

- Young children can acquire the infection when they eat soil contaminated with animal feces that contain the roundworm eggs.
- Most often, the infection causes fever, cough or wheezing, and an enlarged liver, but it may cause vision problems.
- Doctors confirm the diagnosis by identifying antibodies to the roundworm in a sample of blood.
- Regularly deworming dogs and cats can help prevent the infection.
- Treatment is usually unnecessary but may include antiparasitic drugs and corticosteroids.

Toxocariasis occurs mainly in young children, who acquire *Toxocara* eggs by ingesting soil contaminated by the feces of dogs, cats, or other animals that carry the parasite. Sandboxes, where dogs and cats often defecate, pose a particular hazard for exposure to the eggs. Children frequently transfer the eggs from their hands to their mouth and may eat the contaminated sand. Occasionally, adults ingest eggs picked up from contaminated soil, other surfaces, or hands and become infected. Adults and children who have a craving for nonfoods, such as soil or clay (a condition called pica),

are at particular risk. After the eggs are swallowed, larvae hatch in the intestine. The larvae penetrate the intestinal wall and spread through the bloodstream. Almost any tissue of the body may be affected, but the liver and lungs are most commonly involved. The larvae can remain alive for many months, causing damage by moving through tissues and stimulating inflammation. The larvae do not mature to adulthood in people. They require an intermediate host for maturation: dogs, cats, or other animals.

Symptoms and Diagnosis

Symptoms may start within several weeks after eggs are ingested. Fever, cough or wheezing, and liver enlargement are the most common. Some people have a skin rash, spleen enlargement, or recurring pneumonia. When larvae infect the eyes, inflammation and decreased vision may result.

A doctor may suspect toxocariasis in a person who has an enlarged liver, inflammation of the lungs, a fever, and high levels of eosinophils (a type of white blood cell). The diagnosis is confirmed by identifying *Toxocara* antibodies in the blood. Rarely, a sample of liver or other tissue is obtained and examined (biopsied) for evidence of larvae or inflammation resulting from their presence.

Prevention and Treatment

Prevention involves deworming dogs and cats regularly. Covering sandboxes when not in use prevents animals from defecating in them. Pica and clay eating should be discouraged.

In most people with toxocariasis, the infection resolves on its own, and treatment is unnecessary. Albendazole or mebendazole plus corticosteroids are given when symptoms are severe or the eyes are infected. Occasionally, laser photocoagulation (application of an intense beam of light) is used to kill larvae in the eyes.

Toxoplasmosis

Toxoplasmosis is infection caused by the single-celled protozoan parasite Toxoplasma gondii.

- People acquire the infection by transferring the parasite's eggs from a contaminated object to the mouth or by eating contaminated food.
- Infected pregnant women may transmit the parasite to the fetus, sometimes causing a miscarriage, stillbirth, or serious problems in the baby.
- Usually, only people with a weakened immune system have symptoms, which may include weakness on one side of the body, confusion, coma, trouble breathing, or organ malfunction.

- Doctors usually diagnose the infection by doing blood tests that detect antibodies against the parasite.
- Cooking meat thoroughly or freezing it and washing the hands thoroughly after handling raw meat, soil, or cat litter help prevent spread of the infection.
- Most people do not require treatment, but adults with symptoms and infants with the infection are treated with sulfadiazine plus pyrimethamine and leukovorin.

Toxoplasma gondii is present worldwide wherever there are cats. The parasite infects a large number of animals as well as people. Many people in the United States have been infected, although few ever develop symptoms. Severe infection usually develops only in fetuses and people with an immune system weakened by AIDS, cancer, or drugs used to suppress rejection of an organ transplant (immunosuppressants).

Although the parasite can grow in the tissues of many animals, it produces eggs (oocysts) only in cells lining the intestine of cats. Eggs are shed in a cat's stool and can survive for up to 18 months in the soil.

People may acquire the infection by transferring *Toxoplasma* eggs from contaminated soil or other objects to their mouth or by eating contaminated food. Occasionally, animals such as pigs acquire toxoplasmosis from eating material contaminated with *Toxoplasma* eggs. People can become infected by eating raw or undercooked meat from infected animals. Rarely, the parasite is transmitted through blood transfusions or by an organ transplanted from an infected person.

A woman who acquires the infection during pregnancy can transfer *Toxoplasma gondii* to her fetus through the placenta. The result may be a miscarriage, stillbirth, or a baby born with congenital toxoplasmosis (see table on page 1707). A woman who was infected before the pregnancy does not pass the parasite on to her fetus.

People with a weakened immune system, primarily those who have AIDS or cancer or who take drugs to suppress rejection of an organ transplant, are especially at risk of toxoplasmosis. Symptoms usually develop in these people when a previously acquired *Toxoplasma* infection is reactivated but can develop when an organ is transplanted from an infected person. The infection usually affects the brain, but it may affect the eye or spread throughout the body (disseminate). In people with a weakened immune system due to AIDS, cancer, or immunosuppressants taken after organ transplantation or for other reasons, toxoplasmosis is very serious and may be fatal if untreated.

Symptoms

Most people with a healthy immune system have few symptoms and recover fully.

Children born with congenital toxoplasmosis may be severely ill and die shortly after birth, or they may have no symptoms until months or years later. Some never become ill. Typical symptoms in newborns can include inflammation of the eyes (chorioretinitis), which can result in blindness, as well as enlargement of the liver and spleen, jaundice, rash, easy bruising, seizures, a large or small head, and intellectual disability (mental retardation).

Toxoplasmosis acquired after birth seldom causes symptoms in people with a healthy immune system. When symptoms occur, they are usually mild and include swollen but painless lymph nodes, intermittent low fevers, a vague ill feeling, and sometimes a sore throat. Some people develop only chorioretinitis, with blurred vision, eye pain, and sensitivity to light. Chorioretinitis usually results from reactivation of congenital toxoplasmosis.

Symptoms of toxoplasmosis in people with a weakened immune system depend on the site of infection. Toxoplasmosis of the brain (encephalitis) causes symptoms such as weakness on one side of the body, trouble speaking, headache, confusion, seizures, and coma. Acute disseminated toxoplasmosis can cause a rash, high fever, chills, trouble breathing, and fatigue. In some people, infection causes inflammation of the liver (hepatitis), lungs (pneumonitis), or heart (myocarditis). The affected organ may stop functioning adequately (called organ failure). These types of toxoplasmosis can be life threatening.

> **? Did You Know...**
> Eggs of the toxoplasmosis parasite can grow only in the intestine of cats.

Diagnosis

The diagnosis is usually based on blood tests that detect antibodies against the parasite. However, if the person's immune system is impaired by AIDS, the blood test may be falsely negative. To determine whether a fetus has been infected, a doctor usually takes a sample of the fluid around the fetus (amniotic fluid) to be analyzed. If toxoplasmosis of the brain is suspected, computed tomography (CT) or magnetic resonance imaging (MRI) of the brain is done. Less commonly, a piece of infected tissue is removed and examined under a microscope (biopsied) to identify parasites or characteristic proteins (antigens) released by the parasite.

Prevention and Treatment

Pregnant women should avoid contact with cats. If contact is unavoidable, pregnant women should at least avoid cleaning cat litter boxes or wear gloves when doing so. Meat should be cooked thoroughly, to a temperature of 165 to 170° F (74 to 77° C), and hands should be washed thoroughly after handling raw meat, soil, or cat litter. Freezing to a temperature of 9° F (13° C) or below also destroys the parasite.

Potential organ donors should be tested. Trimethoprim-sulfamethoxazole, which is given to transplant recipients and people with AIDS to prevent *Pneumocystis* pneumonia, usually also prevents development of symptomatic toxoplasmosis infections. The combination of pyrimethamine and dapsone or atovaquone with or without pyrimethamine are alternatives for people who do not tolerate sulfonamides. Leucovorin is given with pyrimethamine to protect the bone marrow from pyrimethamine's toxic effects. The use of highly active antiretroviral therapy can reduce the risk of toxoplasmosis in people with AIDS.

Infected adults without symptoms and with a healthy immune system do not require treatment. Adults with symptoms and infants with congenital toxoplasmosis are treated with sulfadiazine plus pyrimethamine and leukovorin. Higher doses of pyrimethamine are typically used in people with AIDS or other conditions that weaken the immune system. If people cannot take sulfadiazine, clindamycin can be used with pyrimethamine instead. In addition to these drugs, people with chorioretinitis are given prednisone or another corticosteroid to reduce inflammation. Women who acquire toxoplasmosis during pregnancy may be treated with spiramycin to prevent transmission to the fetus.

In people with AIDS, toxoplasmosis tends to recur, so drugs are often continued indefinitely.

Trichinosis

Trichinosis is infection caused by the roundworm Trichinella spiralis.

- People acquire the infection by eating undercooked contaminated meat.
- At first, people have nausea, diarrhea, abdominal cramps, then muscle pain, weakness, fever, headache, and sometimes inflammation of other organs.
- Several weeks after the initial infection, a blood test to detect antibodies to the roundworm can confirm the diagnosis.
- Thoroughly cooking or freezing meats can kill the roundworm.
- Antiparasitic drugs such as albendazole can eliminate the worms from the intestine, but bed rest and analgesics are needed to relieve muscle pain.

Trichinella larvae live in the muscle tissue of animals, typically pigs, wild bears, walruses, horses, and many carnivores. People develop trichinosis if they eat uncooked or poorly cooked meat from an animal that carries the parasite. In most people, infections result from eating pork, particularly in regions where pigs are fed uncooked meat scraps and garbage, or eating meat from wild boar, bear, or walrus. Trichinosis is now rare in the United States.

When a person eats meat containing live *Trichinella* cysts, the cyst wall is digested, releasing larvae that quickly mature to adulthood and mate in the intestine. After the male worms mate, they die and thus play no further role in infection. The females burrow into the intestinal wall and, by the seventh day, begin to produce larvae.

Production of larvae continues for about 4 to 6 weeks. Then, the female worm dies or is excreted from the body. The larvae are carried through the body through the lymphatic vessels and bloodstream. The larvae penetrate muscles, causing inflammation. In 1 to 2 months, they form cysts that can live for years in the body.

Certain muscles, such as those in the tongue, around the eyes, and between the ribs, are most often infected. Larvae that reach the heart muscle are often killed by the intense inflammatory reaction they provoke.

Symptoms

Symptoms vary, depending on the stage of infection, number of invading larvae, tissues invaded, and general physical condition of the person. Many people have no symptoms. Symptoms occur in two stages.

- **Stage 1:** Intestinal infection develops 1 to 2 days after eating contaminated meat. Symptoms include nausea, diarrhea, abdominal cramps, and a slight fever.
- **Stage 2:** Symptoms from the larval invasion of muscles usually start after about 7 to 15 days. Symptoms include muscle pain and tenderness, weakness, fever, headache, and swelling of the face, particularly around the eyes. The pain is often most pronounced in the muscles used to breathe, speak, chew, and swallow. A skin rash that does not itch may develop. In some people, the whites of the eyes become red, and their eyes hurt and become sensitive to bright light.

If many larvae are present, the heart, brain, and lungs may become inflamed. Heart failure, abnormal heart rhythms, seizures, and severe breathing problems may result. Death can occur but is rare.

Without treatment, most symptoms disappear by the third month of infection, although vague muscle pain and fatigue can persist longer.

Diagnosis

Unlike most other worm infections, trichinosis cannot be diagnosed by microscopic examination of the stool. Blood tests for antibodies to *Trichinella spiralis* are fairly reliable, but they are not positive until 2 to 3 weeks after symptoms start. If the results are negative, a doctor usually bases an initial diagnosis of trichinosis on symptoms and the presence of elevated levels of eosinophils (a type of white blood cell) in a blood sample. The antibody test is repeated several weeks later to confirm the diagnosis. A biopsy of muscle tissue (in which a sample of tissue is removed and examined under a microscope), done after the second week of infection, may reveal larvae or cysts but is seldom necessary.

Prevention and Treatment

Trichinosis is prevented by thoroughly cooking meats, especially pork and pork products, to a temperature of 160° F (71° C). Alternatively, larvae can usually be killed by freezing meat at 5° F (−15° C) for 3 weeks or at −20° F (−29° C) for 6 days. However, larvae of worms that infect arctic mammals can survive these temperatures. Smoking or salting does not reliably kill the larvae. Also, pigs should not be fed uncooked meat products.

Mebendazole or albendazole, taken by mouth, eliminates the worms from the intestine but has little effect on the cysts in muscle. Bed rest and analgesics help relieve muscle pain. Corticosteroids (such as prednisone) may be prescribed to reduce inflammation in severe infection. Most people with trichinosis recover fully.

Whipworm Infection

Whipworm infection (trichuriasis) is an intestinal infection caused by the roundworm Trichuris trichiura.

- People acquire the infection by eating foods contaminated with soil that contains the roundworm eggs or by swallowing eggs picked up from contaminated soil.
- People may have no symptoms or may have abdominal pain, loss of appetite, diarrhea, bleeding from the intestine, or anemia, depending on the severity of the infection.
- Doctors usually diagnose the infection by identifying eggs in a stool sample.

- Adequate sanitation and good personal hygiene help prevent spread of the infection.
- An antiparasitic drug such as albendazole is used to treat the infection.

Trichuriasis is a common infection, occurring mainly in the subtropics and tropics, where poor sanitation and a warm, moist climate provide the conditions needed for *Trichuris* eggs to incubate in the soil. About 1 billion people are infected worldwide.

People acquire the parasite by swallowing food contaminated by soil that contains eggs or by transferring eggs from their hands to their mouth after contact with contaminated soil. Children may swallow contaminated soil. The larvae hatch in the small intestine, migrate to the large intestine, and embed their heads in the intestinal lining. Each larva grows into a worm that is about 4½ inches long and may live for 7 to 10 years. Eggs are excreted in the stool.

Symptoms and Diagnosis

Mild infections often cause no symptoms. Abdominal pain, loss of appetite, and diarrhea occur when a large number of worms are present in the colon. People with an extremely large number of worms, especially children, may have chronic diarrhea, weight loss, bleeding from the intestine, and anemia. Occasionally, a massive infection causes the rectum to protrude through the anus (rectal prolapse).

A doctor bases a diagnosis of trichuriasis on seeing the typical barrel-shaped eggs in stool samples examined under a microscope or occasionally by observing adult worms during a colonoscopy.

Prevention and Treatment

Prevention depends on adequate sanitation (particularly sanitary toilet facilities) and good personal hygiene. Hands should be washed before handling food, and unwashed fruits and vegetables should be avoided.

Mebendazole or albendazole, taken by mouth, is used to treat the infection. Sometimes a single dose of albendazole is adequate, but if infection is heavy, it is used daily for three days. Neither mebendazole nor albendazole is given to pregnant women because they can harm the fetus.

CHAPTER
181 Fungal Infections

- Because fungal spores are often present in the air or in the soil, fungal infections usually begin in the lungs or on the skin.
- Fungal infections are rarely serious unless the immune system is weakened, usually by drugs or disorders.
- Fungal infections usually progress slowly.
- Antifungal drugs may be applied directly to the infected site or, if the infection is serious, taken by mouth or injected.

Fungi are neither plants nor animals. They were once thought to be plants but are now classified as their own kingdom. Some fungi, including yeasts such as *Candida* and molds such as aspergilli, can be seen only through a microscope. Others, including bread molds and mushrooms, can be seen with the naked eye. Fungi can grow in a round shape (as yeasts) or in long, thin threads (hyphae). Some fungi go through both forms during their life cycle.

Some fungi reproduce by spreading microscopic spores. These spores are often present in the air, where they can be inhaled or come into contact with the surfaces of the body, primarily the skin. Consequently, fungal infections usually begin in the lungs or on the skin. Of the wide variety of spores that land on the skin or are inhaled into the lungs, most do not cause infection. Except for some superficial skin infections, fungal infections are rarely passed from one person to another. Typically, if the immune system is normal, fungal infections do not spread to organs deep in the body.

> 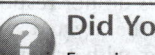 **Did You Know...**
> Fungi are their own kingdom—neither plants nor animals.

Certain types of fungi (such as *Candida*) are normally present on body surfaces or in the intestine. Although normally harmless, these fungi sometimes cause localized infections of the skin and nails (see page 1320), vagina (see page 1540), mouth (see pages 1320 and 1364), or sinuses (see box on page 1399). Fungi seldom cause serious harm, except in people who have a weakened immune system or who have foreign material, including medical devices (such as an intravenous catheter or an artificial joint or heart valve), in their body.

Sometimes the normal balances that keep fungi in check are upset and infections occur. For example, the bacteria normally present in the digestive tract and vagina limit the growth of certain fungi in those areas. When people take antibiotics, the helpful bacteria can be killed, allowing the fungi to grow unchecked. The resulting overgrowth of fungi can cause symptoms, which are usually mild. As the bacteria grow back, the balance is restored, and the problem usually resolves.

Some fungal infections—histoplasmosis, blastomycosis, coccidioidomycosis, and paracoccidioidomycosis—can be serious in otherwise healthy people. The fungi that cause these infections exist in the environment in various parts of the world. Therefore, some fungal infections are more common in certain geographic areas. For example, in the United States, coccidioidomycosis occurs almost exclusively in the Southwest. Histoplasmosis is especially common in the Ohio and Mississippi River valleys. Blastomycosis is particularly common in the eastern and central United States (and in Africa).

Because many fungal infections develop slowly, months or years may pass before people seek medical attention. But in people with a weakened immune system, fungal infections can be very aggressive, spreading quickly to other organs and often leading to death. The immune system may be weakened by taking drugs that suppress the immune system (immunosuppressants), such as chemotherapy drugs or drugs used to prevent rejection of an organ transplant, or by having a disorder, such as AIDS.

Several drugs effective against fungal infections are available, but the structure and chemical makeup of fungi make them difficult to kill. Antifungal drugs may be applied directly to a fungal infection of the skin or other surface, such as the vagina or inside of the mouth. Antifungal drugs may also be taken by mouth or injected when needed to treat more serious infections. For serious infections, several months of treatment are often needed.

Aspergillosis

Aspergillosis is infection, usually of the lungs, caused by the fungus Aspergillus.

- A ball of fungus fibers, blood clots, and white blood cells may form in the lungs or sinuses.
- People may have no symptoms or may cough up blood or have a fever, chest pain, and difficulty breathing.
- If fungi spread to the liver or kidneys, these organs may malfunction.

- Diagnosis usually involves an x-ray or computed tomography and, if possible, culture of a sample of infected material.
- Antifungal drugs are used, and sometimes surgery is needed to remove the fungi.

Aspergilli are very common and frequently occur in compost heaps, air vents, and airborne dust. Inhalation of *Aspergillus* spores is the primary cause of aspergillosis. Aspergillosis has several forms:

- **Pulmonary aspergilloma:** Aspergillosis usually develops in open spaces in the body, such as cavities in the lungs caused by preexisting lung disorders. The infection may also develop in the ear canals and sinuses. In the sinuses and lungs, aspergillosis develops as a ball (aspergilloma) composed of a tangled mass of fungus fibers, blood clots, and white blood cells. The ball gradually enlarges, destroying lung tissue in the process, but usually does not spread to other areas.
- **Invasive aspergillosis:** Less often, aspergillosis becomes very aggressive and rapidly spreads throughout the lungs and often through the bloodstream to the brain, heart, liver, and kidneys. This rapid spread occurs mainly in people with a weakened immune system.
- **Allergic bronchopulmonary aspergillosis:** Some people who have asthma or cystic fibrosis develop a chronic allergic reaction with cough, wheezing and fever if *Aspergillus* colonizes the lining of their airways (see page 516).

Symptoms

A fungus ball in the lungs may cause no symptoms and may be discovered only when a chest x-ray is taken for other reasons. Or it may cause repeated coughing up of blood and, rarely, severe, even fatal bleeding. A rapidly invasive infection in the lungs often causes cough, fever, chest pain, and difficulty breathing. Without treatment, this form of invasive aspergillosis is fatal.

Aspergillosis that spreads to other organs makes people very ill. Symptoms include fever, chills, shock, delirium, and blood clots. Kidney failure, liver failure (causing jaundice), and breathing difficulties may develop. Death can occur quickly.

Aspergillosis of the ear canal causes itching and occasionally pain. Fluid draining overnight from the ear may leave a stain on the pillow. Aspergillosis of the sinuses causes a feeling of congestion and sometimes pain or discharge.

Diagnosis

Doctors suspect the diagnosis based on symptoms. An x-ray or computed tomography (CT) of the infected area also provides clues for making the diagnosis.

Whenever possible, doctors send a sample of infected material to a laboratory to grow (culture), examine, and confirm identification of the fungus. A viewing tube (bronchoscope or rhinoscope) may be used to obtain this material from the lungs or sinuses.

Treatment

Aspergillosis that affects only a sinus or a single area in the lung requires treatment but does not pose an immediate danger because it progresses slowly. However, if the infection is widespread or if people appear seriously ill, treatment is started immediately.

Invasive aspergillosis is treated with antifungal drugs, such as amphotericin B or voriconazole. However, some forms of *Aspergillus* do not respond to these drugs and may need to be treated with caspofungin, a newer antifungal drug, with or without the other drugs.

Doctors treat aspergillosis in the ear canal by scraping out the fungus and applying drops of antifungal drugs. Collections of fungi in the sinuses must usually be removed surgically. If fungus balls in the lungs grow near large blood vessels, they may also need to be removed surgically because they may invade the blood vessel and cause bleeding.

Risk Factors for Developing Fungal Infections

USE OF DRUGS THAT SUPPRESS THE IMMUNE SYSTEM

- Cancer chemotherapy drugs
- Corticosteroids
- Drugs to prevent rejection of an organ transplant, such as azathioprine, methotrexate, and cyclosporine

DISORDERS

- AIDS
- Burns, if extensive
- Diabetes
- Hodgkin lymphoma or other lymphomas
- Kidney failure
- Lung disorders, such as emphysema
- Leukemia

Blastomycosis

Blastomycosis (North American blastomycosis, Gilchrist's disease) is infection, mainly of the lungs, caused by the fungus Blastomyces dermatitidis.

- People have a fever, chills, and drenching sweats and sometimes chest pain, difficulty breathing, and a cough.

℞ DRUGS FOR SERIOUS FUNGAL INFECTIONS

DRUG	COMMON USES	SOME SIDE EFFECTS
Amphotericin B	Wide variety of fungal infections	Chills, fever, headache, vomiting, lowered potassium levels in blood, kidney damage, and anemia
Anidulafungin Caspofungin Micafungin	*Aspergillus*, candidal, and possibly other infections	Fever, nausea, and inflammation of veins
Fluconazole	Candidal and other fungal infections, including cryptococcal	Liver inflammation (hepatitis) but less than that with ketoconazole
Flucytosine	Candidal and cryptococcal infections	Bone marrow and kidney damage
Itraconazole	Candidal and other fungal infections	Nausea, diarrhea, and liver inflammation but less than that with ketoconazole Erratic absorption of the drug from the intestine
Ketoconazole	Candidal and other fungal infections	Nausea and vomiting, blocked production of testosterone and cortisol, and liver inflammation
Posaconazole	*Aspergillus*, candidal, and many other fungal infections	Nausea, vomiting, and rarely liver inflammation
Voriconazole	*Aspergillus* and candidal infections	Visual disturbances that are reversible

- The infection may spread to the skin, bones, reproductive and urinary tracts, and tissues covering the brain, causing swelling, pain, and other symptoms.
- A sample of infected sputum or tissues is removed and sent for culture.
- Antifungal drugs must be taken for months.

Spores of *Blastomyces* probably enter the body through the airways when the spores are inhaled. Thus, blastomycosis affects primarily the lungs, but the fungi occasionally spread through the bloodstream to other areas of the body, including the skin.

Most infections occur in the United States, chiefly in the Southeast and the Mississippi River valley, where the fungus lives in the soil near river beds. Infections have also occurred in widely scattered areas of Africa. Men aged 20 to 40 years are most commonly infected. Unlike most fungal infections, blastomycosis is not more common among people with AIDS.

Symptoms

Blastomycosis of the lungs begins gradually with a fever, chills, and drenching sweats. Chest pain, difficulty breathing, and a cough that may or may not bring up sputum may also develop. The lung infection usually progresses slowly, but people sometimes get better without treatment.

When blastomycosis spreads, it can affect many areas of the body, but the skin, bones, and reproductive and urinary tracts (including the prostate gland) are the most common sites. Skin infection begins as very small, raised bumps (papules), which may contain pus. Raised, warty patches then develop, surrounded by tiny, painless collections of pus (abscesses). Tissues over infected bones may become swollen and painful. In men, the coiled tube on top of testes (epididymis) may swell, causing pain, or infection of the prostate gland (prostatitis) may cause discomfort.

Occasionally, fungi spread to the tissues that cover the brain and spinal cord (meninges), causing fungal meningitis. This infection can cause headache and confusion.

Diagnosis and Treatment

A doctor diagnoses blastomycosis by sending a sample of sputum or infected tissue to a laboratory to be examined under a microscope and cultured.

Blastomycosis may be treated with amphotericin B, given intravenously, or itraconazole or voriconazole, given by mouth. With treatment, people begin to feel better fairly quickly, but the drug must be continued for months. Without treatment, blastomycosis slowly worsens and leads to death.

Candidiasis

Candidiasis (candidosis, moniliasis, yeast infection) is infection caused by several species of Candida, *especially* Candida albicans.

- The most common type of candidiasis is a superficial infection of the mouth, vagina, or skin that causes white or red patches and itching, irritation, or both.
- People whose immune system is weakened may have serious infections of the esophagus and other internal organs.
- A sample of infected material is examined under a microscope and sent for culture.
- Antifungal drugs may be applied to the surface or taken by mouth, but serious infections require drugs given by vein.

Candida is normally present on the skin, in the intestinal tract, and, in women, in the genital area. Usually, *Candida* in these areas does not cause problems. However, the fungi sometimes cause infection of the skin (see page 1320), the mucous membranes of the mouth (see pages 1320 and 1364), or vagina (see page 1540). Such infections can develop in people with a healthy immune system, but they are more common or persistent in people with diabetes, cancer, or AIDS and in pregnant women. Candidiasis is also common among people who are taking antibiotics because the antibiotics kill the bacteria that normally compete with *Candida*, allowing *Candida* to grow unchecked.

Some people, mainly those with a weakened immune system, develop candidiasis that spreads through the bloodstream (called candidemia) to other parts of the body, such as the heart valves, spleen, kidneys, and eyes. Without treatment, this infection progresses.

Symptoms

Infection of the mouth (thrush or trench mouth) causes the following:

- Creamy, white, painful patches inside the mouth
- Cracking at the corners of the mouth (cheilitis)
- A red, painful, smooth tongue

Patches in the esophagus cause pain during swallowing.

When the skin is infected, a burning rash develops. Some types of diaper rash are caused by *Candida*.

If the infection spreads to other parts of the body, it is more serious. It can cause fever, a heart murmur, enlargement of the spleen, dangerously low blood pressure (shock), and decreased urine production. An infection of the retina and inner parts of the eye can cause blindness. If the infection is severe, several organs may stop functioning, and death can occur.

Diagnosis

Many candidal infections are apparent from the symptoms alone. To confirm the diagnosis, a doctor must identify the fungi in a sample viewed under a microscope. Samples of blood or other infected tissues may be sent to a laboratory to be cultured and examined to identify the fungi.

Treatment

Candidiasis that occurs only on the skin or in the mouth or vagina can be treated with antifungal drugs (such as clotrimazole and nystatin) that are applied directly to the affected area. A doctor may prescribe the antifungal drug fluconazole to be taken by mouth.

Candidiasis that has spread throughout the body is usually treated with amphotericin B given intravenously. Other antifungal drugs—fluconazole and related drugs (posaconazole and voriconazole) or caspofungin and related drugs (micafungin and anidulafungin)—are also effective.

Candidiasis is more serious and less responsive to treatment in people with certain disorders, such as diabetes. In people with diabetes, controlling blood sugar levels facilitates cure of the infection.

Coccidioidomycosis

Coccidioidomycosis (San Joaquin fever, valley fever) is infection, usually of the lungs, caused by the fungus Coccidioides immitis.

- The infection is caused by inhaling spores of the fungus.
- If mild, the lung infection causes flu-like symptoms and sometimes shortness of breath, but the infection may worsen and spread throughout the body, causing various symptoms.
- The diagnosis can be confirmed by identifying the fungi in samples of infected materials examined under a microscope or cultured.
- Antifungal drugs, given by mouth or intravenously, must be taken for years, sometimes for life.

The spores of *Coccidioides* are present in soil in the southwestern United States, Central America, and South America. Farmers and others who work with or are exposed to disturbed soil are most likely to inhale the spores and become infected. People who become infected while traveling may not develop symptoms until after they go home.

Coccidioidomycosis occurs in two forms:

- Mild lung infection (acute primary coccidioidomycosis): The infection disappears without treatment. It accounts for about half of cases.
- Severe, progressive infection (progressive coccidioidomycosis): The infection spreads throughout

the body and is often fatal. It is more common among men and among blacks, Filipinos, and Native Americans. This form is more likely to occur when the immune system is weakened—by disorders (particularly AIDS) or by drugs that suppress the immune system (immunosuppressants).

> **? Did You Know...**
>
> An allergic reaction to the *Coccidioides* fungus usually means that people are effectively fighting off the infection.

Symptoms

Most people with acute primary coccidioidomycosis have no symptoms. If symptoms develop, they appear 1 to 3 weeks after people are infected. Symptoms are usually mild and often flu-like. They include a cough, fever, chills, chest pain, and sometimes shortness of breath. The cough may produce sputum and occasionally blood. Some people develop desert rheumatism, which includes inflammation of the surface of the eye (conjunctivitis) and joints (arthritis) and formation of skin nodules (erythema nodosum). These effects, which can be painful, are allergic reactions to the fungus and usually imply that people are fighting off the fungus effectively.

The progressive form is uncommon and may develop weeks, months, or even years after the initial infection. Symptoms include mild fever and loss of appetite, weight, and strength. The lung infection may worsen, causing increased shortness of breath. The infection may also spread from the lungs to the bones, joints, liver, spleen, and kidneys. Joints may become swollen and painful. The fungi can also infect the brain and the tissues covering the brain (meninges), causing meningitis. This infection is often chronic, causing headaches, confusion, loss of balance, double vision, and other problems. Untreated meningitis is always fatal.

Diagnosis

A doctor may suspect coccidioidomycosis if people develop symptoms after living in or recently traveling through an area where the infection is common. Chest x-rays usually show abnormalities. But to identify the fungi and thus confirm the diagnosis, doctors may examine samples of blood, sputum, pus, or other infected tissue under a microscope or send them to a laboratory to be cultured.

Treatment

Acute primary coccidioidomycosis typically goes away without treatment, and recovery is usually complete. However, some doctors prefer to treat coccidioidomycosis if it affects the lungs.

For the progressive form, fluconazole is given by mouth, or amphotericin B is given intravenously. Alternatively, the doctor may treat the infection with voriconazole or posaconazole.

If meningitis develops, amphotericin B or fluconazole is given intravenously. In addition, amphotericin B may be injected directly into the spinal fluid.

Although drug treatment can be effective in localized infections (for example, in the skin, bones, or joints), relapses often occur after treatment is stopped. Treatment must therefore be continued for years, often for life.

Allergic symptoms often require treatment, such as corticosteroids.

Cryptococcosis

Cryptococcosis is infection caused by the fungus Cryptococcus neoformans.

- People may have no symptoms or may have headache and confusion, a cough and an achy chest, or a rash, depending on where the infection is.
- The diagnosis is based on culture and examination of tissue and fluid samples.
- Antifungal drugs are given by mouth or, if the infection is severe, intravenously.

Cryptococcus occurs primarily in soil that is contaminated with pigeon droppings. The fungus is present around the world, but infection was relatively rare until the AIDS epidemic began. The fungus sometimes infects people with Hodgkin lymphoma or sarcoidosis and those who are receiving long-term corticosteroid treatment. However, cryptococcosis can also develop in people with a normal immune system.

Cryptococcosis occurs mainly in the following:

- Tissues covering the brain and spinal cord (meninges), resulting in meningitis
- Lungs
- Skin

Other organs are sometimes involved.

Symptoms and Diagnosis

Cryptococcosis usually causes mild and vague symptoms. Other symptoms occur depending on where the infection is:

- **Meningitis:** Headache and confusion
- **Lung infection:** No symptoms in some people, a cough or an aching chest in others, and, if the infection is severe, difficulty breathing
- **Skin infection:** A rash, consisting of bumps (sometimes filled with pus) or open sores

To diagnose the infection, a doctor takes samples of tissue and body fluids to be cultured and examined. Blood and spinal fluid may be tested for certain substances released by *Cryptococcus*.

Treatment

People with a functioning immune system who have *Cryptococcus* in only a small part of their lungs usually do not require any treatment. However, people with a lung infection are often treated with fluconazole, given by mouth, to shorten the duration of their illness. For meningitis, amphotericin B and flucytosine are given intravenously, followed by fluconazole given by mouth. For a skin infection, people are usually given fluconazole by mouth or, if the infection is severe, amphotericin B intravenously.

People with a weakened immune system may be given fluconazole, amphotericin B, sometimes flucytosine, or a combination. If people with AIDS develop cryptococcosis, they usually need to take an antifungal drug, usually fluconazole, for the rest of their life. However, they may be able to stop the antifungal drug if their CD4 count (the number of one type of white blood cell) increases and stays high enough for at least 6 months.

Histoplasmosis

Histoplasmosis is infection caused by the fungus Histoplasma capsulatum. *It occurs mainly in the lungs but can sometimes spread throughout the body.*

- The infection is caused by inhaling spores of the fungus.
- Most people do not have symptoms, but some feel sick and have a fever and cough, sometimes with difficulty breathing.
- Sometimes the infection spreads, causing the liver, spleen and lymph nodes to enlarge and damaging other organs.
- The diagnosis is based on culture and examination of tissue and fluid samples.
- Whether treatment with antifungal drugs is needed depends on the severity of the infection.

The spores of *Histoplasma* are present in the soil and are particularly common in the eastern and Midwestern United States, along the Ohio and Mississippi river valleys. Farmers and others who work with soil are most likely to inhale the spores. Severe infection can result when large numbers of spores are inhaled. People with human immunodeficiency virus (HIV) infection are more likely to develop histoplasmosis, especially the form that spreads through the bloodstream to other parts of the body, such as the liver, spleen, lymph nodes, adrenal glands, digestive system, and bone marrow.

Symptoms

Most people with histoplasmosis do not develop any symptoms. However, the following three forms cause symptoms, as do some rare forms.

Acute Pulmonary Histoplasmosis: Symptoms usually appear 3 to 21 days after people inhale the spores. People may feel sick, have a fever and a cough, and feel as though they have the flu. Symptoms usually disappear without treatment in 2 weeks and rarely last longer than 6 weeks.

This form is very rarely fatal but can become serious in people with a weakened immune system (such as those with AIDS).

Progressive Disseminated Histoplasmosis: This form does not normally affect healthy adults. It usually occurs in infants or very young children and in people with a weakened immune system. Symptoms are vague at first. People may experience fatigue, weakness, and a general feeling of illness (malaise). Symptoms may worsen very slowly or extremely rapidly. The liver, spleen, and lymph nodes may enlarge. Less commonly, the infection causes ulcers to form in the mouth and intestines. Rarely, the adrenal glands are damaged, causing Addison's disease (see page 999).

Without treatment, this form is fatal in 90% of people. Even with treatment, death may occur rapidly in people with AIDS.

Chronic Cavitary Histoplasmosis: This lung infection develops gradually over several weeks, causing a cough and increased difficulty breathing. Symptoms include weight loss, a mild fever, and a general feeling of illness (malaise).

Most people recover without treatment within 2 to 6 months. However, breathing difficulties may gradually worsen, and some people cough up blood, sometimes in large amounts. Lung tissue is destroyed, and scar tissue forms. Lung damage or bacterial invasion of the lungs may eventually cause death.

Diagnosis

To make the diagnosis, a doctor obtains samples of the sputum, bone marrow, urine, or blood. Samples may also be taken from the liver, lymph nodes, or any mouth ulcers that are present. These samples are sent to a laboratory for culture and examination. Urine and blood may be tested for proteins (antigens) released by the fungus.

For some rare forms of the infection, the help of infectious disease specialists is required for diagnosis (and treatment).

Treatment

People with acute pulmonary histoplasmosis rarely require drug treatment. However, fluconazole or itraconazole is often prescribed to shorten the duration of the illness.

People with progressive disseminated histoplasmosis need treatment and often respond well to amphotericin B given intravenously or to itraconazole (or other related drugs) given by mouth. If people with AIDS develop histoplasmosis, they may need to take an antifungal drug, usually itraconazole, for the rest of their life. However, they may be able to stop the antifungal drug treatment if their CD4 count (the number of one type of white blood cell) increases and stays high enough for at least 6 months.

In chronic cavitary histoplasmosis, itraconazole or, for more serious infections, amphotericin B may eliminate the fungus. However, treatment cannot reverse the destruction caused by the infection. Thus, most people continue to have breathing problems, similar to those caused by chronic obstructive pulmonary disease. Therefore, treatment should begin as soon as possible to limit lung damage.

Mucormycosis

Mucormycosis (zygomycosis) is infection caused by Mucorales molds.

- The infection is caused by inhaling spores produced by the mold.
- The infection causes pain, fever, and sometimes cough and can destroy structures in the face.
- Doctors diagnose the infection by identifying the fungus in tissue samples.
- Most people are given high doses of amphotericin B intravenously, and surgery is done to remove infected and dead tissue.

Mucormycosis is caused by inhaling spores produced by *Mucorales* molds. These molds are common in the environment and include many common bread molds. People probably breathe in the spores of these molds all the time. However, most of these molds do not cause infection.

This infection most commonly affects the nose, sinuses, eyes, and brain—a form called rhinocerebral mucormycosis. This severe and potentially fatal infection typically affects people whose immune system is weakened by a disorder, such as undernutrition or uncontrolled diabetes. The other common site of infection is the lungs. Rarely, the skin and digestive system are infected.

Symptoms

Symptoms of rhinocerebral mucormycosis include pain, fever, and infection of the eye socket (orbital cellulitis) with bulging of the affected eye (proptosis). Pus is discharged from the nose. The roof of the mouth (palate), the facial bones surrounding the eye socket or sinuses, or the divider between the nostrils (septum) may be destroyed by the infection. Infection in the brain may cause seizures, partial paralysis, and coma.

Mucormycosis in the lungs causes fever, cough, and sometimes difficulty breathing.

The fungus tends to invade arteries. As a result, blood clots form and tissue dies. The fungus grows uncontrolled in the dead tissue, which becomes black. The surrounding area may bleed.

Diagnosis

Because symptoms of mucormycosis can resemble those of other infections, a doctor may not be able to diagnose it immediately. Usually, the diagnosis is made when a doctor identifies the fungus in cultures of samples of infected tissue.

 Did You Know...

Without early diagnosis and treatment, mucormycosis can damage the face so badly that the required surgery results in disfigurement.

Treatment

Most people with mucormycosis are treated with high doses of amphotericin B given intravenously. People with uncontrolled diabetes are given insulin to lower blood sugar levels.

Infected tissue and especially dead tissue must be removed by surgery. Early diagnosis and treatment of this infection are important to avoid death or extensive surgery, which often causes disfigurement.

Mucormycosis is very serious. Even when as much infected and dead tissue as possible is removed and antifungal drugs are used appropriately, many people with this infection die.

Paracoccidioidomycosis

Paracoccidioidomycosis (South American blastomycosis) is infection caused by the fungus Paracoccidioides brasiliensis.

Paracoccidioidomycosis usually involves the skin, mouth, throat, and lymph nodes, although it sometimes appears in the lungs, liver, or spleen. It is very common in South and Central America but rare in the United States. It infects people after they inhale the spores, which grow in the soil. Men aged 20 to 50 are typically affected.

Symptoms

Infected lymph nodes become swollen and may drain pus, but there is little pain. The lymph nodes most commonly infected are those in the neck and under the arms. Painful ulcers may form in the mouth. If the lungs are affected, people may have a cough and difficulty breathing. The liver and spleen may enlarge.

Symptoms last a long time but are rarely fatal.

Diagnosis and Treatment

To diagnose the infection, a doctor takes tissue samples for examination under a microscope and for culture.

The antifungal drug itraconazole is the treatment of choice. Amphotericin B is also effective, but because of its side effects, it is reserved for very severe cases.

Sporotrichosis

Sporotrichosis is infection caused by the fungus Sporothrix schenckii.

- The infection develops when the fungi enter the body through a puncture wound.
- Usually, the skin and lymph nodes are infected, resulting in bumps on the skin and swollen lymph nodes.
- Rarely, the lungs, joints, or other parts of the body are infected.
- Diagnosis requires culture and identification of the fungus in a sample of infected tissue.
- Itraconazole is used to treat most infections, but amphotericin B is required for bodywide infections.

Sporothrix fungi typically grow on rosebushes, barberry bushes, sphagnum moss, and other mulches. In contrast to many other fungal infections, *Sporothrix* fungi enter the body through a puncture wound to the skin. Most often, farmers, gardeners, and horticulturists are infected.

Sporotrichosis affects mainly the skin and nearby lymphatic vessels. Very rarely, bones, joints, lungs, or other tissues are infected.

Symptoms and Diagnosis

An infection of the skin typically starts on a finger as a small, nontender bump (nodule) that slowly enlarges and forms a sore. Over the next several days or weeks, the infection spreads through the lymphatic vessels of the finger, hand, and arm to the lymph nodes, forming nodules and sores along the way. Even at this stage, there is little or no pain. Usually, people have no other symptoms. This infection is seldom fatal.

An infection in the lungs may cause pneumonia, with a slight chest pain and cough. Lung infection usually occurs in people who have another lung disorder, such as emphysema. Joint infection causes swelling and makes movement painful. Rarely, an infection develops in other areas and can spread throughout the body. Such infections are life threatening.

The characteristic nodules and sores may lead a doctor to suspect sporotrichosis. The diagnosis is confirmed by growing (culturing) and identifying *Sporothrix* in samples of infected tissue.

Treatment

Skin infections are treated with itraconazole given by mouth. Potassium iodide, given by mouth, may be prescribed instead, but it is not as effective and, in most people, has side effects (such as a rash, a runny nose, and inflammation of the eyes, mouth, and throat).

Lung and bone infections may also be treated with itraconazole. For bodywide infections, amphotericin B is given intravenously.

CHAPTER

182   Viral Infections

- People may get viruses by swallowing or inhaling them, being bitten by insects or parasites, or through sexual contact.
- Most commonly, viral infections involve the nose, throat, and upper airways.
- Doctors may base the diagnosis on symptoms, blood tests and cultures, or examination of infected tissues.
- Antiviral drugs may interfere with the reproduction of viruses or strengthen the immune response to the viral infection.

A virus is a small infectious organism—much smaller than a fungus or bacterium—that must invade a living cell to reproduce (replicate). The virus attaches to a cell (called the host cell), enters it, and releases its DNA or RNA inside the cell. The virus's DNA or RNA is the genetic material containing the information needed to replicate the virus. The virus's genetic material takes control of the cell and forces it to replicate the virus. The infected cell usually dies because the virus keeps it from performing its normal functions. When it dies, the cell releases new viruses, which go on to infect other cells.

Some viruses do not kill the cells they infect but instead alter the cell's functions. Sometimes the infected cell loses control over normal cell division and becomes cancerous. Some viruses leave their genetic material in the host cell, where the material remains dormant for an extended time (latent infection). When the cell is disturbed, the virus may begin replicating again and cause disease.

Viruses usually infect one particular type of cell. For example, cold viruses infect only cells of the upper respiratory tract. Additionally, most viruses infect only a few species of plants or animals. Some infect only people. Many viruses commonly infect infants and children (see page 1768).

Viruses are spread (transmitted) in various ways. Some are swallowed, some are inhaled, and some are spread by the bites of insects and parasites (for example, mosquitoes and ticks). Some are spread sexually.

Defenses: The body has a number of defenses against viruses. Physical barriers, such as the skin, discourage easy entry. Infected cells also make interferons, substances that can make uninfected cells more resistant to infection by many viruses.

When a virus enters the body, it triggers the body's immune defenses. These defenses begin with white blood cells, such as lymphocytes and monocytes, which learn to attack and destroy the virus or the cells it has infected (see page 1096). If the body survives the virus attack, some of the white blood cells remember the invader and are able to respond more quickly and effectively to a subsequent infection by the same virus. This response is called immunity. Immunity can also be produced by getting a vaccine.

> **Did You Know...**
>
> A virus takes control of the cell it infects and forces it to make more viruses.

Types of Viral Infections: Probably the most common viral infections are those of the nose, throat, and upper airways (upper respiratory infections). These infections include sore throat, sinusitis, and the common cold. Influenza is a viral respiratory infection. In small children, viruses also commonly cause croup and inflammation of the windpipe (laryngotracheobronchitis) or other airways deeper inside the lungs (bronchiolitis—see page 1786). Respiratory infections are more likely to cause severe symptoms in infants, older people, and people with a lung or heart disorder.

Some viruses (such as rabies, West Nile virus, and several different encephalitis viruses) infect the nervous

VIRUSES AND CANCER: A LINK*

VIRUS	CANCER
Epstein-Barr virus	Burkitt's lymphoma
	Certain nose and throat cancers
	B-cell lymphomas in people with a weakened immune system (such as those with AIDS)
Hepatitis B and C viruses	Liver cancer
Herpesvirus 8	Kaposi's sarcoma in people with AIDS
	Non-Hodgkin lymphoma in people with AIDS
Human papillomavirus	Cervical cancer

*Some viruses alter the DNA of their host cells in a way that helps cancer develop. Only a few viruses are known to cause cancer, but there may be others.

system (see page 749). Viral infections also develop in the skin, sometimes resulting in warts or other blemishes (see page 1324).

Other common viral infections are caused by herpesviruses. Eight different herpesviruses infect people. Three of them—herpes simplex virus type 1, herpes simplex virus type 2, and varicella-zoster virus—cause infections that produce blisters on the skin or mucus membranes. Another herpesvirus, Epstein-Barr virus, causes infectious mononucleosis. Cytomegalovirus is a cause of serious infections in newborns and in people with a weakened immune system. It can also cause symptoms similar to infectious mononucleosis in people with a healthy immune system. Human herpesviruses 6 and 7 cause a childhood infection called roseola infantum (see page 1781). Human herpesvirus 8 has been implicated as a cause of cancer (Kaposi's sarcoma) in people with AIDS.

All of the herpesviruses cause lifelong infection because the virus remains within its host cell in a dormant (latent) state. Sometimes the virus reactivates and produces further episodes of disease. Reactivation may occur rapidly or many years after the initial infection.

Diagnosis

Common viral infections may be diagnosed based on symptoms. For infections that occur in epidemics

℞ ANTIVIRAL DRUGS

DRUG	COMMON USES	SOME SIDE EFFECTS
Acyclovir	Genital herpes Herpes zoster (shingles) Chickenpox	Few serious side effects Nausea Vomiting Diarrhea Headache Rashes Kidney damage (rare) Confusion (rare)
Amantadine	Influenza A	Nausea or loss of appetite Nervousness Light-headedness Unsteadiness Sleeplessness Confusion
Cidofovir	Cytomegalovirus infections	Kidney damage Low white blood cell count
Famciclovir	Genital herpes Herpes zoster (shingles) Chickenpox	Few serious side effects (similar to acyclovir)
Foscarnet	Cytomegalovirus infections Herpes simplex virus infections	Kidney damage Electrolyte disturbances Seizures
Ganciclovir	Cytomegalovirus infections	Low white blood cell count Anemia
Interferon-alpha	Hepatitis B and C	Flu-like symptoms Depression Low white blood cell count Anemia Low platelet count
Oseltamivir	Influenza A and B	Nausea and vomiting Dizziness
Penciclovir (cream)	Cold sores	Few side effects Headache Mild burning or stinging at the site of application
Ribavirin	Respiratory syncytial virus infection in children Hepatitis C	Breakdown of red blood cells, causing anemia
Rimantadine	Influenza A	Similar to amantadine, but usually milder and less common
Trifluridine (eye drops)	Herpes simplex infection of the cornea (keratitis)	Stinging of the eyes Swelling of the eyelids
Valacyclovir	Genital herpes Herpes zoster (shingles) Chickenpox	Few serious side effects (similar to acyclovir)
Valganciclovir	Cytomegalovirus infections	Low white blood cell count Anemia Low platelet count Gastrointestinal symptoms (such as nausea, vomiting, diarrhea, or abdominal pain)
Vidarabine (ointment)	Herpes simplex keratitis	Few side effects Irritation of the eyes Sensitivity to light
Zanamivir (inhaled powder)	Influenza A and B	Irritation of the airway

(such as influenza), the presence of other similar cases may help doctors identify a particular infection. For other infections, blood tests and cultures (growing microorganisms in the laboratory from samples of blood, body fluid, or other material taken from an infected area) may be done. Blood may be tested for antibodies to viruses or for antigens (proteins on or in viruses that trigger the body's defenses). Polymerase chain reaction (PCR) techniques may be used to make many copies of the viral genetic material, enabling doctors to rapidly and accurately identify the virus. Tests are sometimes done quickly— for instance, when the infection is a serious threat to public health or when symptoms are severe. A sample of blood or other tissues is sometimes examined with an electron microscope, which provides high magnification with clear resolution.

Treatment

Drugs that combat viral infections are called antiviral drugs. Many antiviral drugs work by interfering with replication of viruses. Most drugs used to treat human immunodeficiency virus (HIV) infection (see page 1261) work this way. Because viruses are tiny and replicate inside cells using the cells' own metabolic functions, there are only a limited number of metabolic functions that antiviral drugs can target. In contrast, bacteria are relatively large organisms, commonly reproduce by themselves outside of cells, and have many metabolic functions that antibacterial drugs (antibiotics) can target. Therefore, antiviral drugs are much more difficult to develop than antibacterial drugs. Antiviral drugs can be toxic to human cells. Viruses can develop resistance to antiviral drugs.

Other antiviral drugs strengthen the immune response to the viral infection. These drugs include several types of interferons, immunoglobulins, and vaccines. Interferon drugs are replicas of naturally occurring substances that slow or stop viral replication. Immune globulin is a sterilized solution of antibodies (also called immunoglobulins) collected from a group of people. Vaccines are materials that help prevent infection by stimulating the body's natural defense mechanisms. Many immune globulins and vaccines are given before exposure to a virus to prevent infection. Some immune globulins and some vaccines, such as those for rabies and hepatitis B, are also used after exposure to the virus to help prevent infection from developing or reduce the severity of infection. Immune globulins may also help treat some established infections and prevent infection after future exposures to the virus.

Most antiviral drugs can be given by mouth. Some can also be given by injection into a vein (intravenously) or muscle (intramuscularly). Some are applied as ointments, creams, or eye drops or are inhaled as a powder.

Antibiotics are not effective against viral infections, but if a person has a bacterial infection in addition to a viral infection, an antibiotic is often necessary.

Common Cold

The common cold is a viral infection of the lining of the nose, sinuses, throat, and large airways.

- Usually, colds are spread when a person's hands come in contact with nasal secretions from an infected person.
- Colds often start with a scratchy or sore throat or discomfort in the nose, followed by sneezing, a runny nose, a cough, and a general feeling of illness.
- Doctors base the diagnosis on symptoms.
- Good hygiene, including frequent hand washing, is the best way to prevent colds.
- Rest, decongestants, antihistamines, cough syrups, and nonsteroidal anti-inflammatory drugs can help relieve symptoms.

Common colds are among the most common illnesses. Many different viruses cause colds, but rhinoviruses (of which there are 100 subtypes) are implicated more often than others. Colds caused by rhinoviruses occur more commonly in the spring and fall. Different viruses cause colds during other times of the year.

Colds spread mainly when people's hands come in contact with nasal secretions from an infected person. These secretions contain cold viruses. When people then touch their mouth, nose, or eyes, the viruses gain entry to the body and cause a cold. Less often, colds are spread when people breathe air containing droplets that were coughed or sneezed out by an infected person. A cold is most contagious during the first 1 or 2 days after symptoms develop. Becoming chilled does not cause colds, nor does it increase a person's susceptibility to infection. General health and eating habits also do not seem to affect susceptibility to infection, nor does having an abnormality of the nose or throat (such as enlarged tonsils or adenoids).

Symptoms and Diagnosis

Symptoms start 1 to 3 days after infection. Usually, the first symptom is a scratchy or sore throat or discomfort in the nose. Later, people start sneezing, have a runny nose, and feel mildly ill. Fever is not common, but a mild fever may occur at the beginning of the cold. At first, secretions from the nose are watery and clear and can be annoyingly plentiful, but eventually, they become thicker, opaque, yellow-green, and less plentiful. Many people also develop a mild cough. Symptoms usually disappear in 4 to 10 days, although the cough often lasts into the second week.

Complications may prolong the disease. Rhinovirus infection often triggers asthma attacks in people with asthma. Some people develop bacterial infections of the middle ear (otitis media) or sinuses. These infections develop because congestion in the nose blocks the normal drainage of those areas, allowing bacteria to grow in collections of blocked secretions. Other people develop bacterial infections of the lower airways (secondary bronchitis or pneumonia).

Doctors are usually able to diagnose a cold based on the typical symptoms. A high fever, severe headache, rash, difficulty breathing, or chest pain suggests that the infection is not a simple cold. Laboratory tests are not usually needed to diagnose a cold. If complications are suspected, doctors may order blood tests and x-rays.

Did You Know...

Colds seldom cause a fever.
Antibiotics are useless in treating colds.

Prevention

Because so many different viruses cause colds and because each virus changes slightly over time, an effective vaccine has not yet been developed. The best preventive measure is practicing good hygiene. Because many cold viruses are spread through contact with the secretions of an infected person, people with cold symptoms and people in their household and office should wash their hands frequently. Sneezing and coughing should be done into tissues, which should be carefully disposed of. When possible, people with symptoms should sleep in a separate room. People who are coughing or sneezing because of a cold should not go to work or school where they might infect others. Cleaning shared objects and surfaces with a disinfectant can also help reduce the spread of common cold viruses.

Despite their popularity, echinacea and high-dose vitamin C (up to 2,000 milligrams per day) have not been shown to prevent colds.

Treatment

People with a cold should stay warm and comfortable and try to avoid spreading the infection to others. Anyone with a fever or severe symptoms should rest at home. Drinking fluids and inhaling steam or mist from a vaporizer may help to keep secretions loose and easier to expel.

Currently available antiviral drugs are not effective against colds. Antibiotics do not help people with colds, even when the nose or cough produces thick or colored mucus.

Echinacea (see page 2073), zinc preparations, and vitamin C have been suggested as treatment. Some small studies have shown them to be effective. Others have shown them to be ineffective. But no well-designed, large clinical studies have confirmed their effectiveness. Thus, most experts do not recommend them as treatment.

Several popular nonprescription (over-the-counter) remedies help relieve cold symptoms. Because they do not cure the infection, which usually resolves after a week regardless of treatments tried, doctors feel that their use is optional, depending on how bad the person feels. Several different types of drugs are used:

- Decongestants, which help open clogged nasal passages
- Antihistamines, which help dry a runny nose
- Cough syrups, which may make coughing easier by thinning secretions or which suppresses cough

These drugs are most often sold as combinations but can also be obtained individually. For relieving nasal congestion, inhaled decongestants are better than forms taken by mouth. However, using inhaled forms for more than 3 to 5 days, then stopping, may make congestion worse than it was originally. Ipratropium, a nasal spray available only by prescription, helps dry a runny nose. Older antihistamines, such as chlorpheniramine, can cause drowsiness. Newer antihistamines, available only by prescription, are less likely to cause drowsiness but are ineffective for treating the common cold.

Nonsteroidal anti-inflammatory drugs (NSAIDs), such as aspirin, ibuprofen, and naproxen, can relieve aches and pains and reduce fever, as can acetaminophen. Aspirin is generally not recommended for children because in children, it increases the risk of Reye's syndrome. Cough suppressants are not routinely recommended because coughing is a good way to clear secretions and debris from the airways during a viral infection. However, a severe cough that interferes with sleep or causes great discomfort can be treated with a cough suppressant.

Influenza

Influenza (flu) is infection of the lungs and airways with one of the influenza viruses.

- The virus is spread by inhaling droplets coughed or sneezed out by an infected person or by having direct contact with an infected person's nasal secretions.
- Influenza often starts with chills, followed by a fever, muscle aches, headache, a sore throat, a cough, a runny nose, and a general feeling of illness.

℞ NONPRESCRIPTION COLD REMEDIES

ACTION	DRUG	SOME SIDE EFFECTS
Analgesics/antipyretics		
Relieve aches and pains and reduce fever	Acetaminophen	Minimal
	Aspirin	Stomach irritation Risk of Reye's syndrome in children
	Ibuprofen	Stomach irritation
	Naproxen	Stomach irritation
Antihistamines		
Open nasal passages and help relieve sneezing	Brompheniramine Chlorpheniramine Clemastine Diphenhydramine	Drowsiness, dry mouth, and, in older people, blurred vision, difficulty urinating, constipation, light-headedness when they stand, and confusion
Cough suppressants		
May help reduce cough	Benzonatate	Confusion and stomach upset
	Codeine	Constipation, drowsiness, difficulty urinating, and stomach upset
	Dextromethorphan	Minimal, but at high doses, confusion, nervousness, and irritability
Decongestants, nasal sprays		
Open clogged nasal passages	Naphazoline Oxymetazoline Phenylephrine Xylometazoline	Rebound congestion (worse congestion when the drug wears off) if the drug is used for more than a few days
Decongestant, oral		
Dries runny nose	Pseudoephedrine	Palpitations, high blood pressure, nervousness, and insomnia
Expectorant		
May help loosen mucus	Guaifenesin	Minimal, but at high doses, headache and stomach upset

- People can often diagnose influenza themselves based on symptoms, but sometimes samples of blood or respiratory secretions must be analyzed to identify the virus.
- An annual influenza vaccination is the best way to prevent influenza.
- Resting, drinking plenty of fluids, and avoiding exertion can help, as can taking pain relievers, decongestants, and sometimes antiviral drugs.

Every year, throughout the world, widespread outbreaks of influenza occur during late fall or early winter. Influenza occurs in epidemics, in which many people get sick all at once. Influenza epidemics may occur in two waves: first in schoolchildren and the people who live with them and, second, in people who are confined to home or live in long-term care facilities, mainly older people. In each epidemic, usually only one strain of influenza virus is responsible for the disease. The name of a strain often reflects where it was first found: a location (for example, Hong Kong flu) or an animal (for example, swine flu).

There are two types of influenza virus, type A and type B, and many different strains within each type. About 95% of influenza cases are caused by influenza virus type A. The illnesses produced by the different types and strains are similar. The strain of influenza virus causing outbreaks is always changing, so each year the influenza virus is a little different from the previous year's. It often changes enough that previously effective vaccines no longer work.

Influenza is distinctly different from the common cold. It is caused by a different virus and produces symptoms that are more severe. Also, influenza affects cells much deeper down in the respiratory tract.

The influenza virus is spread by inhaling droplets that have been coughed or sneezed out by an infected person or by having direct contact with an infected person's nasal secretions. Handling household articles that have been in contact with an infected person or an infected person's secretions may sometimes spread the disease.

Symptoms and Diagnosis

Symptoms start 1 to 4 days after infection and can begin suddenly. Chills or a chilly sensation is often the first indication. Fever is common during the first few days, sometimes reaching 102 to 103° F (about 39° C). Many people feel so ill, weak, and tired that they remain in bed for days. They have aches and pains throughout the body, particularly in the back and legs. Headache is often severe, with aching around and behind the eyes. Bright light may make the headache worse.

At first, respiratory symptoms may be relatively mild. They may include a scratchy sore throat, a burning sensation in the chest, a dry cough, and a runny nose. Later, the cough can become severe and bring up phlegm (sputum). The skin may be warm and flushed, especially on the face. The mouth and throat may redden, the eyes may water, and the whites of the eyes may become bloodshot. People, especially children, may have nausea and vomiting. A few people lose their sense of smell for a few days or weeks. Rarely, the loss is permanent.

Most symptoms subside after 2 or 3 days. However, fever sometimes lasts up to 5 days. Cough, weakness, sweating, and fatigue may persist for several days or occasionally weeks. Mild airway irritation, which can result in a decrease in how long or hard a person can exercise, or slight wheezing may take 6 to 8 weeks to completely resolve.

The most common complication of influenza is pneumonia, which can be viral, bacterial, or both. In viral pneumonia, the influenza virus itself spreads into the lungs. In bacterial pneumonia, unrelated bacteria (such as pneumococci or staphylococci) attack the person's weakened defenses. With either, people may have a worsened cough, difficulty breathing, persistent or recurring fever, and sometimes blood or pus in the sputum. Pneumonia is more common among older people and among people with a heart or lung disorder. In long-term care facilities, as many as 7% of older people who develop influenza have to be hospitalized, and 1 to 4% die. Younger people with a chronic disorder are also at risk of developing severe complications.

Because most people are familiar with the symptoms of influenza and because influenza occurs in epidemics, it is often correctly diagnosed by the person who has it or by family members. The severity of symptoms and the presence of a high fever and body aches help distinguish influenza from a cold, especially when the illness occurs during an influenza outbreak. It is more difficult to correctly identify influenza by symptoms alone when no outbreak is occurring.

Tests on samples of blood or respiratory secretions can be used to identify the influenza virus. Such tests are done mainly when people appear very ill or when a doctor suspects another cause for the symptoms. Some tests can be done in the doctor's office.

Prevention

Annual vaccination is the best way to avoid getting influenza. Influenza vaccines contain inactivated (killed) influenza virus or pieces of the virus and are given by injection. A newer vaccine, inhaled as a nasal spray, contains weakened live viruses. This vaccine is used only in healthy people aged 5 to 49 years. Influenza vaccines usually protect against three different strains of influenza virus. Different vaccines may be given every year to keep up with changes in the virus. Doctors try to predict the strain of virus that will attack each year based on the strain of virus that predominated during the previous influenza season and the strain causing disease in other parts of the world.

Vaccination is useful for most people but is particularly important for people who are likely to become very ill if infected. These people include the young (particularly those younger than 24 months), those older than 65, those with a weakened immune system, and those with a chronic disorder such as diabetes or a lung, heart, or kidney disorder. In older people who live in long-term care facilities, the vaccine is less likely to prevent influenza, but it reduces the chances of developing pneumonia and of dying. Other than occasional soreness at the injection site, side effects from the vaccine are rare.

In the United States, vaccination takes place during the fall so that levels of antibodies are highest during the peak influenza months: November through March. For most people, about 2 weeks is needed for the vaccination to provide protection.

Several antiviral drugs can be used to prevent infection with the influenza virus. Doctors may prescribe these drugs when people have had a clear, recent exposure to someone with influenza. These drugs are also given to people who have conditions that make vaccination ineffective or dangerous. The drugs are used during epidemics of influenza to protect unvaccinated people who are at high risk of complications of influenza: older people and people with a chronic disorder.

Amantadine and rimantadine are older antiviral drugs that provide protection against influenza type A but not influenza type B. These drugs can cause stomach upset, nervousness, sleeplessness, and others, especially in older people and in people with a brain or kidney disorder. Rimantadine tends to have fewer side effects than amantadine. Another drawback of both amantadine and rimantadine is that the influenza virus rapidly develops resistance to them. During the 2005 to 2006 influenza season, concerns about resistance prompted the Centers for Disease Control and Prevention to discourage the use of these drugs for prevention and treatment. Two newer drugs, oseltamivir and zanamivir, can prevent infection with influenza virus type A or type B. These drugs have minimal side effects.

Treatment

The main treatment for influenza is to rest adequately, drink plenty of fluids, and avoid exertion. Normal activities may resume 24 to 48 hours after the body temperature returns to normal, but most people take several more days to recover. People may treat fever and aches with acetaminophen or nonsteroidal anti-inflammatory drugs (NSAIDs), such as aspirin or ibuprofen. Because of the risk of Reye's syndrome, children should not be given aspirin. Acetaminophen and ibuprofen can be used in children if needed. Other measures as listed for the common cold, such as nasal decongestants and steam inhalation, may help relieve symptoms.

The same antiviral drugs that prevent infection (amantadine, rimantadine, oseltamivir, and zanamivir) are also helpful in treating people who have influenza. However, these drugs work only if taken in the first day or two after symptoms begin, and they shorten the duration of fever and respiratory symptoms only by a day or so. Nevertheless, these drugs are very effective in some people. Most doctors recommend zanamivir or oseltamivir, which are effective against influenza type A and type B. If a bacterial infection develops, antibiotics are added.

BIRD FLU

Bird flu (avian influenza) is an infection with strains of influenza that normally occur in wild birds and sometimes pigs.

Bird flu is caused by several strains of influenza A that normally infect wild birds. The infection can be easily spread to domestic birds and sometimes pigs. However, it rarely spreads from animals to people.

Preventing Influenza With a Vaccine

WHO SHOULD GET THE INFLUENZA VACCINE

- Anyone 50 years of age or older
- Children 6 months to 5 years of age
- Residents of long-term care facilities
- Adults and children who are 6 months of age or older and who have diabetes, a chronic heart or lung disorder, kidney failure, certain blood disorders, or a weakened immune system
- Family members and caregivers of people in the above groups
- Family members and caregivers of children less than 6 months of age
- Doctors and health care workers
- All pregnant women
- Children who are younger than 18 years of age and regularly take aspirin (who are at risk of Reye's syndrome if they develop influenza)

WHO SHOULD NOT GET THE INFLUENZA VACCINE

- People with a severe allergy to eggs
- People who have had a severe reaction to an influenza vaccination in the past
- People who have had Guillain-Barré syndrome
- People who currently have a disorder that causes fever (other than a mild cold)

Most people who have been infected with bird flu have had close contact with an infected bird. Human infection with the avian flu strain H5N1 first occurred in Hong Kong, then in Vietnam, Indonesia, Cambodia, China, Thailand, Turkey, Azerbaijan, Djibouti, Egypt, and Iraq. There have been 230 cases between 2003 and the middle of 2006. Other strains of avian influenza have caused eye infections (conjunctivitis) and respiratory disorders in poultry workers in Canada and the Netherlands.

People infected with the current strain of bird flu (H5N1) cannot spread the infection to other people. Experts are concerned mainly that the genetic material of the virus could change (mutate) and enable the virus to spread from person to person. Then, bird flu could spread rapidly and widely, causing a major worldwide epidemic (pandemic).

Symptoms vary depending on which strain of the virus is the cause. People may have extreme difficulty breathing and flu-like symptoms (such as fever, cough, sore throat, and muscle aches). Some people have conjunctivitis or pneumonia. The risk of death has been high: 30% in one outbreak and almost 80% in another.

People who have flu-like symptoms and have had contact with birds in an area where birds are known to carry the infection should contact a doctor. The doctor can send a sample taken by swabbing the nose or throat.

Spread is contained by identifying and destroying infected flocks of domestic birds. Infected people are given oseltamivir or zanamivir, which are usually effective. Amantadine and rimantadine are ineffective against many strains of the bird flu virus. A vaccine for bird flu is being developed.

H1N1 SWINE FLU

H1N1 swine flu is a flu infection caused by a new strain of influenza A virus.

Pigs (swine) can develop influenza. Most often, pigs are infected by strains of influenza that are slightly different from those that infect people. These strains very rarely spread to people, and when they do, they very rarely then spread from person to person. The H1N1 swine flu virus is a combination of swine, bird (avian), and human influenza viruses. H1N1 swine flu spreads easily from person to person, just like ordinary flu. People cannot get H1N1 swine flu from eating pork, and almost never get it from contact with pigs.

In 2009, H1N1 swine flu became a category 6 pandemic. This category indicates the widest spread of disease but does not indicate the severity of the disease. Because the H1N1 virus is new in people, some details about how it affects people are not yet clear. But symptoms are typically flu-like. They include fever, cough, sore throat, body aches, headache, chills, runny nose, and fatigue. Nausea, vomiting, and diarrhea are also common.

In most people, symptoms seem to develop from 1 to 5 days after exposure to the virus and continue for up to another week. People can spread the infection for about 8 days, from the day before symptoms appear until symptoms are gone. Symptoms are usually mild but can become severe, leading to pneumonia or respiratory failure. The infection can make chronic disorders (such as heart and lung disorders and diabetes) worse and, during pregnancy, can cause complications (such as miscarriage or premature birth). Also at high risk are people with kidney or liver disorders or a weakened immune system due to drugs or disorders such as AIDS. Severe complications can develop and progress rapidly—in some countries, even in young, healthy people.

Doctors may take samples of secretions from the nose and mouth. A test that can confirm H1N1 infection can be done.

People with flu-like symptoms should stay home, cover their mouth and nose with a tissue when sneezing or coughing, and wash their hands frequently.

People who have been in close contact with someone who has swine flu may be given antiviral drugs. There is currently no vaccine for swine flu, but doctors are working on one.

People should see a doctor immediately if they have severe vomiting, shortness of breath, chest or abdominal pain, or sudden dizziness or confusion. Children should be taken to a doctor immediately if they have blue lips or skin, are not drinking enough fluids, are breathing rapidly or with difficulty, are unusually drowsy or irritable (including not wanting to be held), or have a fever with a rash. People at high risk of severe complications should contact a doctor if even mild symptoms develop, as should children under 5 years old and pregnant women. If a fever and a worse cough develop after flu-like symptoms disappear in any person, a doctor's attention is required.

Treatment focuses on relieving symptoms. For example, acetaminophen can relieve fever and aches. Getting enough rest and drinking plenty of fluids can help. The antiviral drugs oseltamivir or zanamivir may be used if people are at risk of complications or have severe symptoms. These drugs are most effective when started within 48 hours after symptoms appear. In the United States, most people have recovered from H1N1 swine influenza fully without taking these drugs.

Severe Acute Respiratory Syndrome

Severe acute respiratory syndrome is a respiratory illness caused by a coronavirus.

Severe acute respiratory syndrome (SARS) was first detected in China in late 2002. A worldwide outbreak occurred, resulting in almost 8,500 cases in 29 countries, including Canada and the United States, by mid 2003. As of mid 2006, no cases had been reported worldwide since 2004.

Symptoms and Diagnosis

Symptoms begin about 2 to 10 days after contact with the virus. The first symptoms resemble those of other more common infections and include fever, headache, chills, and muscle aches. Runny nose and sore throat are unusual. About 3 to 7 days later, a dry cough and difficulty breathing may develop. Most people recover within 1 to 2 weeks. However, about 10 to 20% develop severe difficulty breathing, resulting in insufficient oxygen in the blood. About half of these people need assistance with breathing. However, few people in the United States have had symptoms this severe.

About 10% of infected people die. Death is due to extreme difficulty breathing.

SARS is suspected only if people who may have been exposed to an infected person have a fever plus a cough or difficulty breathing. If a doctor suspects SARS, a chest x-ray is usually taken. The doctor may take a swab of secretions from the person's nose and throat to try to identify the virus. A sample of sputum may also be examined.

Prevention and Treatment

Travel advice from the Centers for Disease Control and Prevention (CDC) should be heeded. Wearing a mask is not recommended except for people who are in close contact with someone who may have SARS. People exposed to someone who may have SARS (such as family members, airline personnel, or health care workers) should be alert for symptoms of the infection. If they have no symptoms, they may attend work, school, and other activities as usual. If they develop fever, headache, chills, muscle aches, cough, or difficulty breathing, they should avoid face-to-face contact with other people and see a doctor.

If doctors think a person may have SARS, the person is isolated in a room with a ventilation system that limits the spread of microorganisms in the air.

Doctors may try treating SARS with antiviral drugs, such as oseltamivir and ribavirin, and corticosteroids. However, there is no evidence that these or any other drugs are effective. The virus eventually disappears. People with mild symptoms need no specific treatment. Those with moderate difficulty breathing may need to be given oxygen through plastic nasal prongs or a face mask. Those with severe difficulty breathing may need mechanical ventilation to aid breathing.

Herpes Simplex Virus Infections

Herpes simplex virus infection causes recurring episodes of small, painful, fluid-filled blisters on the skin, mouth, lips (cold sores), eyes, or genitals.

- This very contagious infection is spread by direct contact with sores or sometimes with the affected area when no sores are present.
- Herpes causes blisters or sores in the mouth or on the genitals and, often with the first infection, a fever and general feeling of illness.
- The virus sometimes infects other parts of the body, including the eyes and brain.
- Usually, doctors easily recognize the sores caused by herpes, but sometimes analysis of material from a sore, blood tests, or biopsy of a sore is necessary.
- No drug can eradicate the infection, but antiviral drugs can help relieve symptoms and help symptoms resolve a little sooner.

There are two types of herpes simplex virus (HSV): HSV-1 and HSV-2. HSV-1 is the usual cause of cold sores on the lips (herpes labialis) and sores on the cornea of the eye (herpes simplex keratitis—(see page 1444)). HSV-2 is the usual cause of genital herpes. This distinction is not absolute: genital infections are sometimes caused by HSV-1. Infection can also ccur in other parts of the body such as the brain (a serious illness) or gastrointestinal tract. Widespread infection may occur in newborns or in people with a weakened immune system.

HSV is very contagious and can be spread by direct contact with sores and sometimes by contact with the oral and genital areas of people who have chronic HSV infection and who are between episodes of sores.

HSV infections produce an eruption of tiny blisters. The first eruption is called primary herpes. After the eruption of blisters subsides, the virus remains in a dormant (latent) state inside the collection of nerve cells (ganglia) near the spinal cord that supply the nerve fibers to the infected area. Periodically, the virus reactivates, begins growing again, and travels through the nerve fibers back to the skin—causing eruptions of blisters in the same area of skin as the earlier infection. Sometimes the virus is present on the skin or mucous membranes even when no blisters can be seen.

The virus may reactivate many times. Reactivation of a latent oral or genital HSV infection may be triggered by a fever, menstruation, emotional stress, or suppression of the immune system (for example, by a drug taken to prevent rejection of an organ transplant). An episode of cold sores can develop after physical trauma, such as a dental procedure or overexposure of the lips to sunlight. Often, the trigger is unknown.

Symptoms and Complications

An eruption of tiny blisters appears on the skin or on the mucous membranes, such as those lining the eyes, vagina, cervix, or inside of the mouth. The skin around the blisters is often red.

Oral Infection: The first oral infection with HSV usually causes many painful sores inside the mouth (herpetic gingivostomatitis). In addition, people usually feel sick and have a fever, a headache, and body aches. The mouth sores last 10 to 14 days and are often very severe, making eating and drinking extremely uncomfortable. In some first oral infections, swollen gums are the only symptom. Occasionally, no symptoms develop. Herpetic gingivostomatitis most commonly develops in children.

Unlike the first oral infection, recurrences usually produce only a single sore. The sore is called a cold sore or fever blister (so named because they are often triggered by colds or fevers). Other triggers include sunburn on the lips, certain foods, anxiety, certain dental procedures, and any condition that reduces the body's resistance to infection. If people have a cold sore, they should postpone dental visits until the sore heals.

Cold sores typically develop on the lips. Before a cold sore appears, people usually feel a tingling at the site, lasting from minutes to a few hours, followed by redness and swelling. Usually, fluid-filled blisters form and break open, leaving sores. The sores quickly form a scab. After about a week, the scab falls off and the episode ends. Less often, tingling and redness occur without blister formation. Sometimes small clusters of sores develop on the gums or the roof of the mouth. These sores also last about a week and then go away.

> **? Did You Know...**
> Usually, when cold sores recur, only one develops at a time.

Genital Infection: The first genital HSV infection (genital herpes) can be severe and prolonged, with painful blisters in the genital area. Fever and a general feeling of illness (malaise) are common, and some people have burning during urination, difficulty urinating, or pain during defecation. Some people have no symptoms.

Recurrences of genital herpes begin with symptoms (including local tingling, discomfort, itching, or aching in the groin) that precede the blisters by several hours to 2 to 3 days. Painful blisters surrounded by a reddish rim appear on the skin or mucous membranes of the genitals. The blisters quickly break open, leaving sores. Blisters may also appear on the thighs or buttocks or around the anus. In women, blisters may develop on the vulva. These blisters are usually obvious and very painful. Internal blisters may develop in the vagina or on the cervix. They are less painful and are not visible. A typical episode of recurring genital herpes lasts a week.

Bacteria sometimes infect genital sores due to HSV infection. Such sores may appear more irritated or have a thick or foul-smelling discharge

Other Infections and Complications: In people with a weakened immune system, recurrences of oral or genital herpes can result in progressive, gradually enlarging sores that take weeks to heal. The infection may progress inside the body, moving down into the esophagus and lungs or up into the colon. Ulcers in the esophagus cause pain during swallowing, and lung infection causes pneumonia with cough and shortness of breath.

Sometimes HSV-1 or HSV-2 enters through a break in the skin of a finger, causing a swollen, painful, red fingertip (herpetic whitlow). Health care workers who are exposed to saliva or other body secretions (such as dentists) when not wearing gloves are most commonly affected.

HSV-1 can infect the cornea of the eye. This infection (called herpes simplex keratitis) causes a painful sore, tearing, sensitivity to light, and blurred vision. Over time, particularly without treatment, the cornea can become cloudy, causing a significant loss of vision and requiring corneal transplantation.

Infants or adults with a skin disorder called atopic eczema (see page 1286) can develop a potentially fatal HSV infection in the area of skin that has the eczema (eczema herpeticum). Therefore, people with atopic eczema should avoid being near anyone with an active herpes infection.

HSV can infect the brain. This infection (called herpes encephalitis) begins with confusion, fever, and seizures and can be fatal.

Infrequently, a pregnant woman can transmit HSV infection to her baby (called neonatal herpes). Transmission usually occurs at birth, when the baby comes into contact with infected secretions in the birth canal. Rarely, HSV is transmitted to the fetus during pregnancy. Transmission during birth is more likely when the mother has recently acquired the herpes infection and when the mother has visible herpes sores in the vaginal area, although babies may become infected from mothers who have no apparent sores. When acquired at birth, the infection appears between the 1st and 4th week of life. Newborns with HSV infection become very ill. They may have widespread disease, brain infection, or skin infection. Without treatment, two thirds die, and even with treatment, many have brain damage.

Diagnosis

HSV infection is usually easy for doctors to recognize. If unsure, doctors may use a swab to take a sample of material from the sore and send the swab to a laboratory to grow (culture) and identify the virus. Sometimes doctors examine material scraped from the blisters under a microscope. Although the virus itself cannot be seen, scrapings sometimes contain enlarged infected cells (giant cells) that are characteristic of infection by a herpes-type virus. Blood tests to identify antibodies to HSV and biopsy of the sores can also be helpful. Certain blood tests can distinguish between HSV-1 infection and HSV-2 infection. This information helps doctors determine the risk of transmission, for example, to sex partners.

If a brain infection is suspected, magnetic resonance imaging (MRI) or computed tomography (CT) of the brain, and a spinal tap (lumbar puncture) to obtain a sample of cerebrospinal fluid may be done.

Treatment

Antiviral Drugs: No current antiviral treatments can eradicate HSV infection, and treatment of a first oral or genital infection does not prevent chronic infection of nerves. However, during recurrences, antiviral drugs, such as acyclovir, valacyclovir, or famciclovir, may relieve discomfort slightly and help symptoms resolve a day or two sooner. Treatment is most effective if started early, usually within a few hours after symptoms start—preferably at the first sign of tingling or discomfort, before blisters appear. For people who have frequent, painful attacks, the number of outbreaks can be reduced by continuous therapy (suppression) with antiviral drugs. Antiviral drugs are available by prescription only.

Penciclovir cream, applied every 2 hours during waking hours, can shorten the healing time and duration of symptoms of a cold sore by about a day. Nonprescription creams containing docosanol (applied 5 times a day) may provide some relief. Acyclovir, valacyclovir, or famciclovir taken by mouth for a few days may be the most effective treatment.

Severe HSV infections, including herpes encephalitis and infections in newborns, are treated with acyclovir given intravenously. If the virus becomes resistant to acyclovir, foscarnet can be given.

People with herpes simplex keratitis are usually given trifluridine eye drops. An ophthalmologist should supervise treatment.

Other Treatments: For people who have minimal discomfort, the only treatment needed for recurring herpes of the lips or genitals is to keep the infected area clean by gentle washing with soap and water. Applying ice may be soothing and reduce swelling.

Applying prescription or nonprescription topical anesthetics, such as tetracaine cream or benzocaine ointment, may help relieve pain. If the mouth contains many sores, the mouth can be rinsed with lidocaine, which should not be swallowed. Topical anesthetics should be used only about once every few hours. If used more often, these drugs can have harmful side effects.

Pain relievers may be taken for pain.

Prevention: People should avoid activities and foods known to trigger recurrences. For example, they should avoid exposure to sunlight as much as possible.

Because HSV infection is contagious, people with infection of the lips should avoid kissing as soon as they feel the first tingling (or, if no tingling is felt, when a blister appears) until the sore has completely healed. They should not share a drinking glass and, if possible, should not touch their lips. They should also avoid oral sex. People with genital herpes should use condoms at all times. Even when there are no visible blisters and no symptoms, the virus may be present on the genitals and can be spread to sex partners. Vaccines for the prevention of HSV infections are being developed.

Shingles

Shingles (herpes zoster) is infection that results from reactivation of the varicella-zoster virus, the virus that causes chickenpox.

- What causes the virus to reactivate is usually unknown, but sometimes reactivation occurs when a disorder or drugs weakens the immune system.
- Shingles causes a painful skin eruption of fluid-filled blisters and sometimes results in chronic pain in the affected area.
- Doctors diagnose shingles when typical blisters appear on a strip of skin.
- The chickenpox vaccine and the shingles vaccine for people over 60 can help prevent shingles.
- Antiviral drugs, if started before blisters appear, can help relieve symptoms and help them resolve sooner, but pain relievers, including opioids, are often needed.

Chickenpox and shingles are caused by the varicella-zoster virus (another member of the herpesvirus family). Chickenpox is the initial infection (see page 1772), and shingles is a reactivation of the virus, usually years later. During chickenpox, the virus spreads in the bloodstream and infects collections of nerve cells (ganglia) of the spinal or cranial nerves. The virus remains in the ganglia in a dormant (latent) state. The virus may never cause symptoms again, or it may reactivate many years later. When it reactivates, the virus travels down the nerve fibers to the skin, where it creates painful sores resembling those of chickenpox. This outbreak of sores (shingles) almost always appears on a strip of the skin over the infected nerve fibers and only on one side of the body. This strip of skin, the area supplied by nerve fibers from a single spinal nerve, is called a dermatome (see art on page 796). Adjacent dermatomes may also be infected.

Unlike HSV infections, which can recur many times, there is usually only one outbreak of shingles in a person's lifetime. However, people with a weakened immune system may have shingles more than once. They may also have unusual sores, sores on many dermatomes, or sores on both sides of the body.

Shingles may develop at any age but is most common after age 50. Most often, the reason for reactivation is unknown. However, reactivation sometimes occurs when the immune system is weakened by another disorder, such as AIDS or Hodgkin lymphoma, or by use of drugs that suppress the immune system (for example to prevent rejection of a transplanted organ). The occurrence of shingles does not usually mean that the person has another serious disease.

Symptoms and Complications

During the 2 or 3 days before shingles develops, some people feel ill and have chills, a fever, nausea, diarrhea, or difficulty urinating. Others experience pain, a tingling sensation, or itching in a strip of skin on one side of the body. Clusters of small, fluid-filled blisters surrounded by a small red area then develop on this strip of skin. The blisters occur only on the limited area of skin supplied by the

What Is Postherpetic Neuralgia?

Chronic pain in areas of skin supplied by nerves infected with herpes zoster is called postherpetic neuralgia. Exactly why the pain occurs is not well understood. However, it does not indicate that the virus is actively reproducing (replicating).

The pain may be constant or intermittent, and it may worsen at night or in response to heat or cold. Sometimes the pain is incapacitating.

Postherpetic neuralgia occurs most often in older people: 25 to 50% of people who are older than 50 years and who have had shingles also have some postherpetic neuralgia. However, only about 10% of all people with shingles develop postherpetic neuralgia. Few have severe pain.

In most instances, the pain subsides within 1 to 3 months. But in 10 to 20% of people, the pain persists for more than 1 year. It rarely persists more than 10 years.

Mild pain requires no specific treatment other than nonprescription pain-relieving drugs (such as acetaminophen) or creams (such as capsaicin). Although a number of treatments for severe postherpetic neuralgia have been tried, no treatment is routinely successful. Doctors may prescribe certain anticonvulsants (such as gabapentin and pregabalin), certain antidepressants (such as amitriptyline), or topical lidocaine ointment. Opioids are sometimes needed. Direct injection of a corticosteroid into the cerebrospinal fluid is done rarely and may be helpful.

infected nerve fibers. Most often, blisters appear on the trunk, usually on only one side. However, a few blisters may also appear elsewhere. The affected area is usually sensitive to any stimulus, including light touch, and may be very painful. Symptoms are usually less severe in children than in adults.

The blisters begin to dry and form a scab about 5 days after they appear. Until scabs appear, the blisters contain varicella-zoster virus, which, if spread to susceptible people, can cause chickenpox. Blisters that cover large areas of skin or persist for more than 2 weeks usually indicate that the immune system is not functioning normally.

The affected skin, especially in older people and in people with a weakened immune system, may become infected by bacteria. Scratching the blisters increases this risk. Bacterial infections increase the risk of scarring.

One episode of shingles gives most people lifelong immunity from further attacks. Fewer than 4% of people have more than one episode. Scarring or hyperpigmentation of the skin, which can be extensive, may occur, but most people recover without lasting effects. A few people, more commonly older people, continue to have chronic pain in the area (postherpetic neuralgia).

Involvement of the part of the facial nerve leading to the eye can be serious, and if it is not treated adequately, vision may be affected. The part of the facial nerve leading to the ear may also be affected, sometimes causing pain, partial paralysis of the face, and hearing loss.

Diagnosis

People who suspect they have shingles should see a doctor right away because to be effective, treatment must be started early. Doctors ask them to precisely describe the location of the pain. Pain in a vague band on one side of the body suggests shingles. If

characteristic blisters appear in the typical pattern (on a strip of skin representing a dermatome), the diagnosis is clear. Rarely, doctors take a sample from the blisters to be analyzed or do a skin biopsy to confirm the diagnosis.

Prevention and Treatment

Preventing chickenpox by vaccinating children with the varicella vaccine is recommended. Adults who are not immune should also be vaccinated. Vaccination is particularly important for such people if they have frequent contact with children, live or work in places where infections can be spread (including college dormitories, barracks, and institutions such as prisons and nursing homes), have close contact with people with immune system problems, or travel overseas. Adults are considered to be immune and not need vaccination if they have ever had chickenpox or shingles, if a laboratory test done on a blood sample shows they have immunity, or if they were born before 1980 (except for women who may become pregnant and for health care workers). The vaccine sometimes has side effects, which are usually minor. However, rarely, the vaccine itself causes a mild form of shingles. The vaccine should not be given during pregnancy or to people with a weakened immune system (for example, people who have leukemia).

Another vaccine, developed to prevent shingles, can be given to healthy people older than 60, regardless of whether they have had a history of shingles. This vaccine decreases the chance of getting shingles by one half and decreases the chance of getting postherpetic neuralgia by two thirds. If shingles develops in people who have been vaccinated, it is less severe than in those who have not been vaccinated.

Several antiviral drugs are effective in treating shingles. Oral antiviral drugs such as famciclovir, valacyclovir, and acyclovir are often given, particularly to older people and to people with a weakened immune system. The drugs should be started as soon as shingles is suspected, before blisters appear if possible. The drugs are likely to be ineffective if started more than 3 days after blisters appear. These drugs do not cure the disease, but they can help relieve and shorten the duration of symptoms. Some doctors recommend taking corticosteroids in addition, but it is not clear whether this approach helps. If an eye or ear is involved, the appropriate specialist (ophthalmologist or otolaryngologist) should be consulted.

Wet compresses are soothing, but pain-relieving drugs are often required. Nonsteroidal anti-inflammatory drugs (NSAIDs) or acetaminophen may be tried, but oral opioid analgesics are often necessary (see page 642). To prevent bacterial infections from developing, people with shingles should keep the affected skin clean and dry and should not scratch the blisters.

Epstein-Barr Virus Infection

Epstein-Barr virus causes a number of diseases, including infectious mononucleosis.

- The infection is spread through kissing or other close contact with an infected person.
- Symptoms vary, but the most common are extreme fatigue, fever, sore throat, and swollen lymph nodes.
- A blood test is done to confirm the diagnosis.
- Acetaminophen or nonsteroidal anti-inflammatory drugs can relieve fever and pain.

Infection with the Epstein-Barr virus (EBV) is very common. In the United States, about 50% of all children 5 years of age and nearly 95% of adults have had an EBV infection. Most of these infections cause symptoms similar to those of a cold or other mild viral infections. Sometimes adolescents and young adults develop different and more severe symptoms from EBV infection. This disease is called infectious mononucleosis. Infectious mononucleosis is named for the large numbers of white blood cells (mononuclear cells) in the bloodstream. Adolescents and young adults usually catch infectious mononucleosis by kissing or having other close contact with someone infected with EBV.

After the initial infection, EBV remains in the body, mainly in white blood cells, for life. Infected people shed the virus periodically in their saliva. They are most likely to infect others during shedding, which usually causes no symptoms.

Rarely, EBV contributes to the development of several uncommon types of cancer, such as Burkitt's lymphoma and certain cancers of the nose and throat. It is thought that specific viral genes alter the growth cycle of infected cells and cause them to become cancerous. EBV does not cause chronic fatigue syndrome (see page 2109), as was once suspected.

Symptoms and Complications

EBV can cause a number of different symptoms, depending on the strain of the virus and several other, poorly understood factors. In most children younger than 5, the infection causes no symptoms. In adolescents and adults, it may or may not cause symptoms. The usual time between infection and the appearance of symptoms is thought to be 30 to 50 days. This interval is called the incubation period.

The four main symptoms of infectious mononucleosis are

- Extreme fatigue
- Fever
- Sore throat
- Swollen lymph nodes

Not everyone has all four symptoms. Usually, the infection begins with a general feeling of illness (malaise) and fatigue that last several days to a week. These vague symptoms are followed by fever, sore throat, and swollen lymph nodes. The fever usually peaks at about 103° F (about 39° C) in the afternoon or early evening. The throat is often very sore, and puslike material may be present at the back of the throat. Most commonly, the lymph nodes of the neck are swollen, but any lymph node may be swollen. In some people, the only symptom is swollen lymph nodes. Fatigue is usually most pronounced during the first 2 to 3 weeks and may last 6 weeks or more.

The spleen is enlarged in about 50% of people with infectious mononucleosis. In most infected people, an enlarged spleen causes few if any symptoms, but it may rupture, particularly if injured. The liver may also enlarge slightly. Less commonly, jaundice and swelling around the eyes occur. Skin rashes develop infrequently. However, people with an EBV infection who take the antibiotic ampicillin usually develop a rash. Other very rare complications include seizures, nerve damage, behavioral abnormalities, inflammation of the brain (encephalitis) or tissues covering the brain (meningitis), anemia, and blockage of airways by the swollen lymph nodes.

How long symptoms last varies. After about 2 weeks, symptoms subside, and most people can resume their usual activities. However, fatigue may persist for several more weeks and, occasionally, for months or longer.

Diagnosis

The symptoms of infectious mononucleosis also occur in many other viral and bacterial infections. Therefore, infectious mononucleosis is often unrecognized. Usually, a simple blood test known as a heterophil antibody or a monospot test is done to confirm the diagnosis. Sometimes early in the infection or in young children, the monospot test is negative, and other specific antibody blood tests are necessary to confirm the diagnosis.

Often, a complete blood count is also done. Finding many characteristic mononuclear white blood cells (atypical lymphocytes) may be the first clue that the diagnosis is infectious mononucleosis.

Treatment

There is no specific treatment. People with infectious mononucleosis may be as active as they want. However, because of the risk of rupturing the spleen, heavy lifting and contact sports should be avoided for 1 month, even if the spleen is not noticeably enlarged. Before such activities are resumed, doctors may wish to confirm that the spleen has returned to normal size.

Acetaminophen or nonsteroidal anti-inflammatory drugs (NSAIDs, such as aspirin or ibuprofen) can relieve fever and pain. However, aspirin should not be given to children because of the risk of Reye's syndrome, which can be fatal. Some complications, such as severe swelling of the airways, may be treated with corticosteroids. Currently available antiviral drugs have little effect on the symptoms of infectious mononucleosis and should not be used.

Cytomegalovirus Infection

Cytomegalovirus infection is a common herpesvirus infection with a wide range of symptoms: from no symptoms to fever and fatigue (resembling infectious mononucleosis) to severe symptoms involving the eyes, brain, or other internal organs.

- This virus is easily spread through sexual and nonsexual contact with body secretions.
- Most people have no symptoms, but some feel ill and have a fever, and people with a weakened immune system or an infected fetus can have serious symptoms, including blindness.
- Doctors may diagnose the infection by culturing a sample of infected body fluid, such as urine.
- Often, no treatment is required, but if the infection is severe, antiviral drugs may be used.

Infection with cytomegalovirus (CMV), a herpesvirus, is very common. Blood tests show that 60 to 90% of adults have had a CMV infection at some time. Usually, this infection causes no symptoms. Serious infections typically develop only in infants infected before birth (see table on page 1705) and in people with a weakened immune system—for example, people with AIDS or those who have received an organ transplant. People who have received an organ transplant are particularly susceptible to CMV infection because they are given drugs that suppress the immune system (immunosuppressants) to prevent rejection of the transplant.

CMV spreads very easily. Infected people may shed the virus in their urine or saliva for months. The virus is also excreted in cervical mucus, semen, stool, and breast milk. Thus, the virus is spread through sexual and nonsexual contact. CMV infection may develop in people who receive a transfusion of infected blood or an infected organ transplant.

CMV may cause symptoms soon after infection. It can remain dormant in various tissues for life. Various stimuli can reactivate the dormant CMV, resulting in disease.

Symptoms

Most people infected with CMV have no symptoms. A few infected people feel ill and have a fever. CMV infection in adolescents and young adults can cause an illness with symptoms of fever and fatigue that resembles infectious mononucleosis. If a person receives a transfusion of blood containing CMV, fever and sometimes liver inflammation may develop 2 to 4 weeks later.

If a person with a severely weakened immune system becomes infected with CMV, the infection may be severe, sometimes resulting in serious disease or death. In people with AIDS, CMV infection is a common viral complication. The virus tends to infect the retina of the eye. This infection (CMV retinitis) can cause blindness. Infection of the brain (encephalitis), pneumonia, or painful ulcers of the intestine or esophagus may also develop.

If a pregnant woman transmits CMV to the fetus, miscarriage, stillbirth, or death of the newborn may result. Death is caused by bleeding, anemia, or extensive damage to the liver or brain. Newborns who survive may have hearing loss and intellectual disability (mental retardation).

Diagnosis and Treatment

CMV infection may develop gradually and not be recognized immediately. Diagnosis is often unnecessary in healthy adults and children because treatment is unnecessary. However, doctors always consider the possibility of CMV infection in people who have a weakened immune system and an eye, a brain, or a gastrointestinal infection. CMV infection is also suspected in newborns who have a fever or who seem sick.

Once CMV infection is suspected, a doctor conducts tests to detect the virus in body fluids or tissues. In newborns, the diagnosis is usually made by culturing the urine. In people with a weakened immune system, doctors may be able to identify the virus in a sample of blood, other body fluids, or lung or other tissues. Blood tests to estimate how many viruses are present may be done. CMV retinitis can be identified by an ophthalmologist, who examines internal eye structures to check for characteristic abnormalities using an ophthalmoscope.

Mild CMV infection is usually not treated. It subsides on its own. When the infection threatens life or eyesight, an antiviral drug (valganciclovir, ganciclovir, cidofovir, foscarnet, or a combination) may be given. For people with CMV retinitis, a small device containing sustained-release ganciclovir can be implanted in the eye. Occasionally, ganciclovir or foscarnet is injected directly into the eye. These drugs have serious side effects and may not cure the infection. However, treatment slows the disease's progression and preserves sight. If CMV infection occurs in people whose immune system is temporarily weakened or suppressed (by a disorder or drug), the infection usually subsides without treatment when the immune system recovers or the drug is stopped.

People who have had an organ transplant are often given antiviral drugs (such as ganciclovir, valganciclovir, or valacyclovir) to prevent CMV infection.

Hemorrhagic Fevers

Hemorrhagic fevers are serious viral infections characterized by bleeding.

- These infections may be spread through contact with skin or body fluids of an infected person, through the droppings or urine of infected rodents, or when contaminated food is eaten.
- Symptoms may include fever, muscle and body aches, headache, and vomiting, as well as bleeding from the mouth, nose, or internal organs.
- To confirm the diagnosis, doctors do blood tests or sometimes examine infected tissue under a microscope.
- Treatment includes giving fluids and other treatments to maintain body functions.

Several groups of viruses, including filoviruses and arenaviruses, can cause fever and other symptoms that are accompanied by bleeding (hemorrhagic fever). Bleeding occurs because the viruses make the blood vessels leak. These infections occur primarily in parts of Africa and South America and are often fatal.

Ebola Virus and Marburg Virus: These two dangerous African viruses are classified as filoviruses. The original source of these viruses in nature (the host) is not known. However, the first infections of people with Marburg virus were thought to come from monkeys. To date, no infections of people have occurred in the United States.

Both viruses can be spread from person to person through contact with skin, body fluids such as blood, or other infected body tissues. Family members and health care workers are most likely to be infected.

Symptoms begin 2 to 21 days (usually 5 to 10 days) after exposure. They include fever, muscle aches, headache, vomiting, diarrhea, cough, rash, and swollen glands. Bleeding under the skin can be seen as purplish spots or patches, and the gums, nose, rectum, or internal organs may bleed, as may puncture wounds. Ebola or Marburg viral infections may cause delirium, coma, and low blood pressure and are often fatal. From 25 to 90% of infected people die. Ebola infection is more likely to be fatal.

Doctors suspect one of these infections in people who bleed easily, have typical symptoms (fever, low blood pressure, delirium, or coma), and have recently traveled to areas where the infections are common. Blood tests to identify the virus help confirm the diagnosis. Samples of blood or infected tissue, especially liver tissue, may be examined under a microscope.

No vaccine is available, but one is being studied. The only treatment for these infections is general supportive care, which includes giving fluids intravenously and other treatments to maintain body functions. Recovery takes a long time. Strict isolation is necessary to prevent further spread. These viruses have not yet spread to large regions, but such spread is always a concern.

Lassa Fever and South American Hemorrhagic Fevers: Caused by arenaviruses, these infections spread from rodents or their urine or droppings to people, usually when contaminated food is eaten. They can spread from person to person through contact with body fluids (such as saliva, urine, feces, or blood). Lassa fever occurs mainly in West Africa. The South American fevers are confined mostly to Bolivia and Argentina.

The infections cause fever, a general feeling of illness (malaise), chest pain, diffuse body aches, and vomiting. Bleeding from the mouth, nose, stomach, and intestinal tract is common in South American hemorrhagic fevers. Overt bleeding is less common in Lassa fever. But bleeding sometimes occurs from puncture wounds, the gums, or the nose and often occurs under the skin (seen as small purplish spots). When death occurs, it usually results from shock caused by widespread leakage of fluid from blood vessels. These infections are often fatal. About 2% to 20% of people with Lassa fever die. In women who are pregnant or have just had a baby, the death rate is higher (up to 92%).

These infections are suspected when people who may have been exposed to the virus have characteristic symptoms. The diagnosis is confirmed by blood tests to identify the virus or antibodies to the virus.

Strict isolation is required to prevent spread to health care workers and family members. An experimental vaccine is effective against some South American hemorrhagic fevers. Treatment is supportive care, which includes giving fluids and electrolytes if needed. The antiviral drug ribavirin does not cure the infection but reduces the risk of death in people with Lassa fever. It may also be beneficial in South American hemorrhagic fevers.

Hantavirus Infection

Hantavirus infection is a viral disease that is spread from rodents to people.

- The virus is spread through contact with infected rodents or their droppings.
- The infection starts with sudden fever, headache, muscle aches, and sometimes abdominal symptoms, which may be followed by a cough and shortness of breath or by a rash and kidney problems.
- Blood tests to identify the virus can confirm the diagnosis.
- Oxygen and drugs to stabilize blood pressure are used if the lungs are affected, and dialysis may be needed if the kidneys are affected.

Hantaviruses infect various species of rodents throughout the world. The virus is present in the urine, feces, and saliva of the rodents. The infection is spread when people have contact with rodents or their droppings or possibly when they inhale virus particles in places with large amounts of rodent droppings. Some evidence suggests that rarely, the virus spreads from person to person. Hantavirus infections are becoming more common.

There are several strains of hantavirus. Some strains affect the lungs, causing hantavirus pulmonary syndrome. Other strains affect the kidneys, causing hemorrhagic fever with renal syndrome. However, many symptoms of the two infections are the same. The pulmonary syndrome was first recognized in the southwestern United States in 1993. Since then, about 450 cases have occurred in the United States, most in the western states. Cases have also occurred in several Central and South American countries. The renal syndrome occurs primarily in parts of Europe and Korea.

Symptoms

Symptoms begin with sudden fever, headache, and muscle aches, typically about 1 to 5 weeks after exposure to the rodent droppings or urine. People may also have abdominal pain, diarrhea, or vomiting.

These symptoms continue for several days (usually for about 4 but sometimes up to 15 days). People with the pulmonary syndrome then develop a cough and shortness of breath, which may become severe within hours. This syndrome causes death in about 50 to 75% of people.

In some people with the renal syndrome, the infection is mild and does not cause symptoms. In others, vague symptoms last for 3 or 4 days. Then in most people, the face becomes red, resembling a sunburn, and is covered with hives. A rash may develop on the trunk. Very low blood pressure (shock) develops in a few people. Kidney failure develops, and urine production may stop (called anuria). In some people, symptoms are mild, and they recover completely. In others, symptoms become severe, with death occurring in 6 to 15%.

Diagnosis and Treatment

Diagnosis is suspected when people who may have been exposed to the virus have characteristic symptoms. Blood tests to identify the virus can confirm the diagnosis.

Treatment is mostly supportive. For the pulmonary syndrome, oxygen and drugs to stabilize blood pressure appear to be most crucial to recovery. For the renal syndrome, dialysis may be needed and can be lifesaving, and ribavirin, given intravenously, may help reduce the severity of symptoms and the risk of death. Most people recover in 3 to 6 weeks but recovery may take up to 6 months.

Yellow Fever

Yellow fever is a mosquito-borne viral disease that occurs mainly in the tropics.

Yellow fever is caused by a flavivirus. Mosquitoes are responsible for spreading yellow fever. Yellow fever is one of the most recognized and historically important viral infections. In the past, major epidemics of yellow fever caused tens of thousands of deaths. Once common in tropical and temperate zones around the world, the disease now occurs only in the tropical areas of Central Africa and Central and South America.

Some infected people do not have symptoms. The first symptoms are headache, muscle aches, chills, and mild fever, which begin suddenly. Nausea, vomiting, constipation, extreme fatigue, and restlessness are common. All of these symptoms subside after a few days. Some people then recover, but others develop a high fever, nausea, vomiting, and severe generalized pain a few hours or days after the initial symptoms subside. The skin turns yellow (jaundice) because the liver is infected. Often, there is bleeding from the nose, mouth, and gastrointestinal tract. People may become confused and apathetic. Some people develop very low blood pressure (shock). Severe infection can cause seizures, malfunction of several organs, and coma. Up to 10% of people with severe symptoms die.

Doctors suspect yellow fever when people living in an area where the infection is common have typical symptoms. It is diagnosed by growing (culturing) the virus or by detecting antibodies to the virus in the blood.

Avoiding mosquito bites is key to prevention. A vaccine that is 95% effective at preventing yellow fever is available. Many countries require vaccination for travelers coming into their country from areas where yellow fever occurs.

Treatment involves supportive care, including drugs to treat or prevent bleeding. There is no specific treatment for the infection.

Dengue Fever

Dengue fever is a mosquito-borne viral infection that causes fever, generalized body aches, and, if severe, external and internal bleeding.

Dengue fever is common in the tropics and subtropics worldwide. It is most common in Southeast Asia but is becoming more common in Central and South America. The infection is caused by a flavivirus and is spread by mosquitoes.

Dengue fever varies in severity. Children typically have mild symptoms such as a low fever, fatigue, runny nose, and cough. Symptoms are more severe in adults and include fever, headache, and severe generalized body aches, particularly in the back, legs, and joints. These aches are often so painful that the disease has been called breakbone fever. Lymph nodes are swollen, and a rash may appear on the face. Symptoms last for 2 or 3 days, then subside. They usually recur, and a rash appears on the limbs and spreads to the trunk. The palms may be bright red, swollen, and itchy. Some people, mainly children, develop bleeding from the nose, mouth, and gastrointestinal tract (dengue hemorrhagic fever)—usually after a second infection with a dengue virus. Sometimes the blood vessels leak fluid into the lungs, causing difficulty breathing. Dengue fever is occasionally fatal.

Doctors suspect dengue fever when typical symptoms occur in people who live or have traveled in an area where the infection is common. It is usually diagnosed by blood tests for antibodies to the virus.

Treatment focuses on relieving symptoms. There is no specific treatment, but an experimental vaccine to prevent dengue fever is being tested.

Smallpox

Smallpox (variola) is a highly contagious, very deadly disease caused by the smallpox virus.

- People can acquire the infection by breathing air exhaled or coughed out by an infected person.

- People have a fever, headache, backache, and rash, sometimes with severe abdominal pain, and they feel very ill.
- The diagnosis is confirmed when the virus is identified in a sample taken from the rash.
- Vaccination within the first few days of exposure can prevent the disease or limit its severity.
- Treatment involves fluids, relief of symptoms, and treatments to maintain blood pressure and help with breathing.

The smallpox virus can exist only in people—not in animals. There are two main forms. The severe form is the most common and is the one of concern. The other form is much less common and much less severe.

Over 200 years ago, a vaccine against smallpox (the first vaccine ever) was developed. The vaccine proved very effective and was given to people throughout the world. The last case of smallpox was reported in 1977. In 1980, the World Health Organization (WHO) declared the disease eliminated and recommended stopping vaccination.

Because the vaccine's protective effects gradually wear off, nearly all people—even those previously vaccinated—are now susceptible to smallpox (see box on page 1150). This lack of protection is a concern only because samples of the virus have been stored, and some people worry that terrorist groups could obtain the virus and release it into the population. The resulting epidemic would be devastating. The virus is stored at two research facilities, one in the United States and one in Russia.

The smallpox virus spreads directly from person to person and is acquired by breathing air contaminated with droplets of moisture breathed or coughed out by an infected person. Contact with clothing or bed linens used by an infected person can also spread the disease. Smallpox usually spreads to people who have close personal contact with an infected person. A large outbreak in a school or workplace would be uncommon. The virus survives no more than 2 days in the environment—less if temperature and humidity are high.

Symptoms and Diagnosis

Symptoms usually begin 7 to 17 days after infection. Infected people develop fever, headache, and backache and feel extremely ill. They may have severe abdominal pain and become delirious. After 2 or 3 days, a rash of flat, red spots develops on the face and arms and inside the mouth, spreading shortly thereafter to the trunk and legs. People are contagious only after the rash has started and are most contagious for the first 7 to 10 days after the rash appears. After 1 or 2 days, the spots turn into blisters, which fill with pus (forming pustules). After

8 or 9 days, the pustules become crusted. About 30% of people with smallpox die, usually in the second week of the disease. Some of the survivors are left with large, disfiguring scars.

A doctor suspects smallpox when people have the disease's characteristic spots—particularly when there is an outbreak of the disease. The diagnosis can be confirmed by identifying the smallpox virus in a sample that is taken from the blisters or pustules and examined under a microscope or sent to a laboratory for the virus to be grown (cultured) and analyzed.

> **? Did You Know...**
> Nearly everyone, even people who were previously vaccinated, is now susceptible to smallpox.

Prevention and Treatment

Prevention is the best response to the threat of smallpox. Vaccination within the first few days of exposure can prevent the disease or limit its severity. People with symptoms suggesting smallpox need to be isolated to prevent spread of the infection. Contacts of these people need not be isolated because they cannot spread the infection unless they become sick and develop a rash. However, contacts are watched closely and isolated at the first sign of infection.

Vaccination is dangerous for some people, especially those with a weakened immune system. Rarely, even some healthy people have adverse reactions to smallpox vaccination. Adverse reactions are less common in previously vaccinated people than in those who have never received the vaccine. About 1 in every million previously unvaccinated healthy people and 1 in every 4 million previously vaccinated healthy people die from the vaccine. Vaccination before exposure is recommended only for people at high risk of exposure, mainly laboratory technicians and health care workers who handle the vaccine and related materials. After exposure, vaccination can reduce the severity of symptoms. Vaccination up to 4 days after exposure is beneficial but is most effective when given soon after exposure.

Treatment of smallpox is supportive. It includes fluids, symptom relief, assistance with breathing (for example, with a face mask to supply oxygen), and treatments to maintain blood pressure.

CHAPTER

183 Human Immunodeficiency Virus Infection

- Human immunodeficiency virus (HIV) is transmitted through contact with a body fluid that contains the virus.
- HIV destroys certain types of white blood cells, weakening the body's defenses against infections and cancers.
- When people are first infected, symptoms of fever, rashes, swollen lymph nodes, and fatigue may last a few days to several weeks.
- Many infected people remain well for more than a decade, but within about 10 years, about half of people become ill and develop AIDS, defined by the presence of serious infections and cancers. Eventually, most untreated people develop AIDS.
- Blood tests to check for HIV antibody and to measure the amount of HIV virus can confirm the diagnosis.
- Antiretroviral drugs, usually two or three taken together, can slow the replication of HIV but cannot kill HIV.

HIV infections may be caused by one of two retroviruses, HIV-1 or HIV-2. HIV-1 has caused a worldwide epidemic, but HIV-2 tends to be limited to West Africa.

HIV progressively destroys some types of white blood cells called $CD4^+$ lymphocytes. Lymphocytes help defend the body against foreign cells, infectious organisms, and cancer (see page 1102). Thus, when HIV destroys $CD4^+$ lymphocytes, people become susceptible to attack by many other infectious organisms. Many of the complications of HIV infection, including death, usually result from these other infections and not from HIV infection directly.

Acquired immunodeficiency syndrome (AIDS) is the most severe form of HIV infection. HIV infection is considered to be AIDS when at least one serious complicating illness develops or the number (count) of $CD4^+$ lymphocytes decreases substantially.

HIV-1 originated in West-Central Africa in the first half of the 20th century when a closely related chimpanzee virus first infected people. HIV-1 spread globally in the 1970s, and AIDS was first recognized in 1981. In North America as of December 2007, about 1.3 million people had HIV infection, and about 46,000 to 56,000 new infections and 21,000 deaths occur each year. Worldwide, about 33.2 million people are estimated to be infected. There are about 2.5 million new infections and 2.1 million deaths each year. Most (95%) occur in developing countries. One half occur in women, and one in seven occur in children under 15 years old. In parts of Africa, more than 30% of people between the ages of 15 and 45 are infected, threatening to dramatically reduce the life expectancy of a whole generation.

Transmission of Infection

The transmission of HIV requires contact with a body fluid that contains the virus or infected cells. HIV can appear in nearly any body fluid, but transmission occurs mainly through blood, semen, vaginal secretions, and breast milk. Although tears, urine, and saliva may contain low concentrations of HIV, transmission through these fluids is extremely rare, if it occurs at all. HIV is not transmitted by casual contact (such as touching, holding, or dry kissing) or by close, nonsexual contact at work, school, or home. No case of HIV transmission has been traced to the coughing or sneezing of an infected person or to a mosquito bite. Transmission from an infected doctor or dentist to a patient is extremely rare.

HIV is transmitted in the following ways:

- Sexual contact with an infected person, when the mucous membrane lining the mouth, vagina, penis, or rectum is exposed to contaminated body fluids (as occurs during unprotected sexual intercourse)
- Injection or infusion of contaminated blood, as can occur with blood transfusions, the sharing of needles, or an accidental prick with an HIV-contaminated needle
- Transfer from an infected mother to a child before birth, during birth, or after birth through the mother's milk

Susceptibility to HIV infection increases when the skin or a mucous membrane is torn or damaged—even minimally—as can happen during vigorous vaginal or anal sexual intercourse. Sexual transmission of HIV is more likely if either partner has herpes, syphilis, or another sexually transmitted disease (STD) that causes breaks in the skin or inflammation of the genitals. However, HIV can be transmitted even

> ### ? Did You Know...
>
> No instance of HIV transmission through coughing, sneezing, or a mosquito bite has been documented.

> ### What Is a Retrovirus?
>
> The human immunodeficiency virus (HIV) is a retrovirus, which, like many other viruses, stores its genetic information as RNA rather than as DNA (most other living things use DNA). When HIV enters a human cell, it releases its RNA, and an enzyme called reverse transcriptase makes a DNA copy of the HIV RNA. The resulting HIV DNA is integrated into the infected cell's DNA. This process is the reverse of that used by human cells, which make an RNA copy of DNA. Thus, HIV is called a retrovirus, referring to the reversed (backward) process. Other RNA viruses (such as polio, influenza, or measles), unlike retroviruses, do not make DNA copies after they invade cells. They simply make RNA copies of their original RNA.
>
> Each time an HIV-infected cell divides, it makes a new copy of the integrated HIV DNA as well as its own genes. The HIV DNA copy is either
>
> - **Inactive (latent):** The virus is present but does no damage.
> - **Activated:** The virus takes over the functions of the infected cell, causing it to produce and release many new HIV copies, which then invade other cells.

if neither partner has another STD or obvious breaks in the skin. HIV transmission can also occur during oral sex, although it is less common than during vaginal or anal intercourse.

In the United States, Europe, and Australia, HIV has been transmitted mainly through male homosexual contact and the sharing of needles among injecting drug users, but transmission through heterosexual contact has been rapidly increasing. HIV transmission in Africa, the Caribbean, and Asia occurs primarily between heterosexuals, and HIV infection occurs equally among men and women. In the United States, about 30% of adults who have HIV infection are women. Before 1992, most American women with HIV were infected by injecting drugs with contaminated needles, but now most are infected through sexual contact.

A health care worker who is accidentally pricked with an HIV-contaminated needle has about a 1 in 300 chance of contracting HIV. The risk increases if the needle penetrates deeply or if the needle contains HIV-contaminated blood (as with a needle used to draw blood) rather than simply being coated with blood (as with a needle used to inject a drug or stitch a cut). Infected fluid splashing into the mouth or eyes has less than a 1 in 1,000 chance of causing infection. Taking a combination of antiretroviral

WHAT IS THE RISK OF HIV TRANSMISSION DURING SEXUAL ACTIVITIES?

RISK	ACTIVITY
None (unless sores are present)	Dry kissing Body-to-body rubbing and massage Use of inserted sexual devices that are not shared with others Stimulation of the genitals by a partner if there is no contact with semen or vaginal fluids Bathing or showering together Contact with feces or urine if the skin is intact
Theoretical (extremely low risk unless sores are present)	Wet kissing Oral sex done to a male (fellatio) if ejaculation does not occur and a condom is used Oral sex done to a female (cunnilingus) if a barrier is used Oral-anal contact Vaginal or anal penetration by a hand with or without a glove Use of inserted sexual devices that are shared but are disinfected
Low	Oral sex done to an infected male with or without ingestion of semen if a condom is not used or is used incorrectly (risk is less if oral sex is done to an uninfected male by an infected person) Oral sex done to a female if no barrier is used Vaginal or anal intercourse if a condom is used correctly (for example, using only water-based lubricants and not spilling any semen) Use of inserted sexual devices that are shared but are not disinfected
High	Vaginal or anal intercourse with or without ejaculation if a condom is not used or is used incorrectly

drugs as soon after exposure as possible appears to reduce, but not eliminate, the risk of becoming infected from an accident in a health care setting and is recommended.

People with hemophilia used to require frequent infusions of whole blood or other blood products, and many became infected because the blood products they received were contaminated with HIV. AIDS became the leading cause of death among these people. However, since 1985 in most developed countries, all blood collected for transfusion is tested for HIV, and when possible, some blood products are treated with heat to eliminate the risk of HIV infection. The current risk of HIV infection from a single blood transfusion (which is carefully screened for HIV and other bloodborne viruses in most developed countries) is estimated to be less than 1 in 600,000.

Mothers and Children: HIV infection in a large number of women of childbearing age has led to an increase in HIV infection among children (see page 1774). In about 30 to 50% of pregnancies involving women who are infected with HIV and are not treated, HIV is transmitted to the fetus through the placenta or at birth during passage through the birth canal. Infants also can acquire HIV through breast milk. The risk from breastfeeding depends on the duration of breastfeeding but may be as high as 75%.

Drug treatment of infected pregnant women during the 2nd and 3rd trimesters of pregnancy along with drugs given by vein during delivery can reduce the risk of transmission by about two thirds or more. Cesarean delivery and treating the mother at delivery and the baby for several weeks after birth with drugs also reduce the risk. Infected mothers should not breastfeed if they live in countries where formula feeding is safe and affordable. However, in countries where infectious diseases and undernutrition are common causes of infant deaths and where safe, affordable infant formula is not available, the World Health Organization recommends that mothers breastfeed. In such cases, the protection from potentially fatal infections provided by breastfeeding may counterbalance the risk of HIV transmission.

Mechanism of Infection

Once in the body, HIV attaches to several types of white blood cells. The most important are certain

Simplified Life Cycle of the Human Immunodeficiency Virus

Like all viruses, human immunodeficiency virus (HIV) reproduces (replicates) using the genetic machinery of the cell it infects, usually a CD4+ lymphocyte.

1. HIV first attaches to and penetrates its target cell.
2. HIV releases RNA, the genetic code of the virus, into the cell. For the virus to replicate, its RNA must be converted to DNA. The RNA is converted by an enzyme called reverse transcriptase. HIV mutates easily at this point because reverse transcriptase is prone to errors during the conversion of viral RNA to DNA.
3. The viral DNA enters the cell's nucleus.
4. With the help of an enzyme called integrase, the viral DNA becomes integrated with the cell's DNA.
5. The DNA of the infected cell now produces RNA as well as proteins that are needed to assemble a new HIV.

6. A new virus is assembled from RNA and short pieces of protein.
7. The virus pushes (buds) through the membrane of the cell, wrapping itself in a fragment of the cell membrane and pinching off from the infected cell.
8. To be able to infect other cells, the budded virus must mature. It becomes mature when another HIV enzyme (HIV protease) cuts structural proteins in the virus, causing them to rearrange.

Drugs used to treat HIV infection were developed based on the life cycle of HIV. These drugs inhibit the three enzymes (reverse transcriptase, integrase, and protease) that the virus uses to replicate or attach to and enter cells.

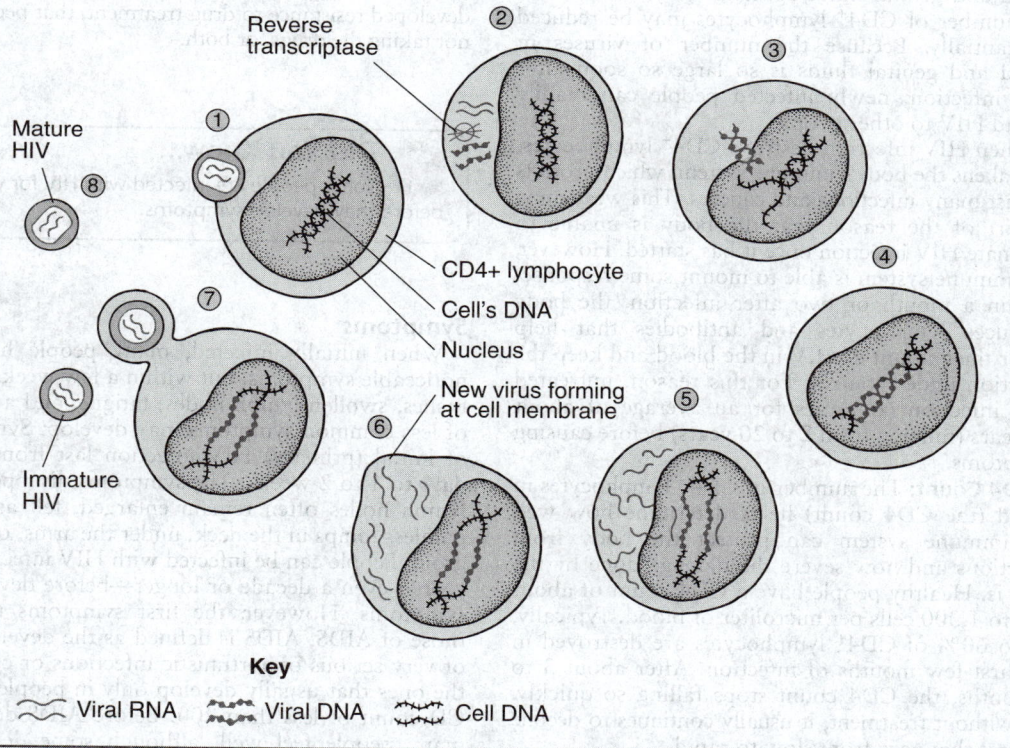

Key

〰 Viral RNA   〰 Viral DNA   〰 Cell DNA

helper T lymphocytes. Helper T activate and coordinate other cells of the immune system. On their surface, these lymphocytes have a receptor called CD4, which enables HIV to attach to them. Thus, these helper are designated as CD4$^+$.

HIV stores its genetic information as ribonucleic acid (RNA). Once inside a CD4$^+$, the virus uses an enzyme called reverse transcriptase to make a copy of its RNA, but the copy is made as deoxyribonucleic acid (DNA). HIV mutates easily at this point because reverse transcriptase is prone to making errors during the conversion of viral RNA to DNA. These mutations make HIV more difficult to control—by the body's immune system and by drugs.

The viral DNA copy is incorporated into the DNA of the infected lymphocyte. The lymphocyte's own genetic machinery then reproduces (replicates) the virus. Eventually, the lymphocyte is destroyed. The thousands of new viruses produced by each infected cell infect other lymphocytes and can destroy them as well. Within a few days or weeks, the blood and genital fluids contain many viruses, and the number of CD4$^+$ lymphocytes may be reduced substantially. Because the number of viruses in blood and genital fluids is so large so soon after HIV infection, newly infected people can readily spread HIV to other people.

When HIV infection destroys CD4$^+$ lymphocytes, it weakens the body's immune system, which protects against many infections and cancers. This weakening is part of the reason that the body is unable to eliminate HIV infection once it has started. However, the immune system is able to mount some response. Within a month or two after infection, the body produces lymphocytes and antibodies that help lower the amount of HIV in the blood and keep the infection under control. For this reason, untreated HIV infection continues for an average of about 10 years (ranging from 2 to 20 years) before causing symptoms.

CD4 Count: The number of CD4$^+$ lymphocytes in blood (the CD4 count) helps determine how well the immune system can protect the body from infections and how severe the damage done by the HIV is. Healthy people have a CD4 count of about 800 to 1,300 cells per microliter of blood. Typically, 40 to 60% of CD4$^+$ lymphocytes are destroyed in the first few months of infection. After about 3 to 6 months, the CD4 count stops falling so quickly, but without treatment, it usually continues to decline at rates that vary from slow to rapid.

If the CD4 count falls below about 200 cells per microliter of blood, the immune system becomes less able to fight certain infections (such as the fungal infection that causes *Pneumocystis jiroveci* pneumonia). These infections do not usually appear in people with a healthy immune system. Such infections are called opportunistic infections because they take advantage of a weakened immune system. A count below about 50 cells per microliter of blood is particularly dangerous because additional opportunistic infections that can rapidly cause severe weight loss, blindness, or death commonly occur.

Viral Load: The amount of HIV in the blood (specifically, the number of copies of HIV RNA) is called the viral load. Viral load represents how quickly HIV is replicating. When people are first infected, the viral load increases rapidly. Then, even without treatment, it drops to a lower level, which remains fairly constant, called the set point. This level varies widely from person to person. Viral load also indicates how contagious the infection is and how fast the infection is likely to worsen.

During successful treatment, the viral load decreases to a very low or undetectable level. However, inactive (latent) HIV is still present within cells, and if treatment is stopped, HIV starts replicating. An increase in the viral load during treatment indicates that the HIV has developed resistance to drug treatment, that people are not taking the drugs, or both.

? Did You Know...

Some people are infected with HIV for years before they develop symptoms.

Symptoms

When initially infected, many people have no noticeable symptoms, but within a few weeks, fever, rashes, swollen lymph nodes, fatigue, and a variety of less common symptoms may develop. Symptoms of initial (primary) HIV infection last from a few days to 1 to 2 weeks. The symptoms disappear, but lymph nodes often remain enlarged, felt as small, painless lumps in the neck, under the arms, or in the groin. People can be infected with HIV infection for years—even a decade or longer—before developing symptoms. However, the first symptoms may be those of AIDS. AIDS is defined as the development of very serious opportunistic infections or cancer—the ones that usually develop only in people with a CD count of less than 200. Before AIDS develops, many people feel well, although some develop a variety of vague symptoms such as weight loss, fatigue, recurring fever or diarrhea, anemia, and thrush (a fungal infection of the mouth or vagina).

Symptoms of AIDS are usually those of the specific opportunistic infections and cancers that develop. For

COMMON OPPORTUNISTIC INFECTIONS ASSOCIATED WITH AIDS

INFECTION	DESCRIPTION	SYMPTOMS
Candidal esophagitis	A yeast infection of the esophagus	Painful swallowing and burning in the chest
Pneumocystis jiroveci pneumonia	An infection of the lungs with the fungus *Pneumocystis jiroveci*	Difficulty breathing, cough, and fever
Toxoplasmosis	Infection with the parasite *Toxoplasma gondii*, usually in the brain	Headache, confusion, lethargy, and seizures
Tuberculosis	Infection of the lungs and sometimes other organs with tuberculosis bacteria	Cough, fevers, night sweats, weight loss, and chest pain
Mycobacterium avium complex infection	Infection of the intestine or lungs with bacteria that resemble tuberculosis bacteria	Fever, weight loss, diarrhea, and cough
Cryptosporidiosis	Infection of the intestine with the parasite *Cryptosporidium*	Diarrhea, abdominal pain, and weight loss
Cryptococcal meningitis	Infection of the lining of the brain with the yeast *Cryptococcus*	Headache, fever, and confusion
Cytomegalovirus infection	Infection of the eyes or intestinal tract with cytomegalovirus	Eye: Clouding of vision or blindness Intestinal tract: Diarrhea and weight loss
Progressive multifocal leukoencephalopathy	Infection of the brain with the JC virus	Weakness on one side of the body and loss of coordination or balance

example, people may have white patches in their mouth due to thrush or pain and rash due to herpes zoster.

However, HIV can also cause symptoms when it directly infects parts of the body:

- **Brain:** Memory loss, difficulty thinking and concentrating, or both, eventually resulting in dementia, as well as weakness, tremor, or difficulty walking
- **Kidneys:** Swelling in the legs and face, fatigue, and changes in urination (more common in blacks than in whites), but often not until the infection is severe
- **Heart:** Shortness of breath, cough, wheezing, and fatigue (uncommon)
- **Genital organs:** Decreased levels of sex hormones, which, for men, leads to a decreased interest in sex (common)

HIV is probably directly responsible for a substantial loss of weight (AIDS wasting) in some people. Wasting in people with AIDS may also be caused by a series of infections or by an untreated, persistent digestive tract infection.

Kaposi's sarcoma, a cancer caused by another sexually transmitted type of herpesvirus (see page 1336), appears as painless, red to purple, raised patches on the skin. It affects many people with AIDS, especially homosexual men. Cancers of the immune system (lymphomas, typically non-Hodgkin lymphoma) may develop, sometimes first appearing in the brain. When the brain is affected, these cancers can cause weakness of an arm or a leg, headache, confusion, or personality changes. Having AIDS increases the risk of other cancers. Homosexual men are prone to developing cancer of the rectum due to the same human papillomaviruses (HPV) that cause cancer of the cervix in women.

Usually, death is caused by the cumulative effects of opportunistic infections or cancers, wasting, and dementia.

Diagnosis

Doctors usually ask about risk factors for HIV infection, such as occupational exposure, high-risk sexual activities, and use of injecting street drugs, and about symptoms, such as fatigue, rashes, and weight loss. They do a physical examination to check for signs of opportunistic infections, such as swollen lymph nodes and white patches inside the mouth (indicating thrush). Early diagnosis is important because it may help infected people live longer, be healthier, and be less likely to transmit HIV to other people.

If doctors suspect HIV infection, simple, accurate, screening tests that detect antibodies to HIV are done. Tests may be done on a blood sample in the laboratory or on a blood or saliva sample in the doctor's office. If screening test results are positive, they are confirmed by a more accurate, specific test such as the Western blot. Often, these tests are not positive in the first weeks up to 2 months after initial HIV infection because antibodies to HIV are not yet being produced. Tests include the following:

- **Enzyme-linked immunosorbent assay (ELISA):** This screening test is often used to detect HIV antibodies, but it requires complex equipment.

- **Newer rapid screening tests:** These tests are being increasingly used to detect antibodies because they are quicker and simpler than ELISA, can be done more in almost any setting, and provide immediate results.

- **Western blot:** This test is usually done to confirm the diagnosis when screening test results are positive. It is more difficult to do than screening tests but is more accurate.

Other tests, such as tests to measure viral load or P24 antigen, detect HIV in the blood sooner after infection than tests that detect antibodies to HIV. However, the P24 antigen test has difficulty detecting low levels of the antigen.

Anyone who is concerned about being infected with HIV can request to be tested. Such testing is confidential.

If HIV infection is diagnosed, blood tests should be done regularly to measure the CD4 count and viral load. When the CD4 count is low, serious infections are more likely to develop and to make people ill. Viral load helps predict how fast the CD4 count is likely to decrease over the next few years. These two measurements help doctors determine when to start antiretroviral drugs, what effects treatment is likely to have, and whether other drugs may be needed to prevent complicating infections. With successful treatment, the viral load falls to very low levels within weeks, and the CD4 count begins a long, slow recovery toward normal levels.

Doctors may do other tests to check for disorders that commonly occur in people with HIV infection. For example, a bone marrow examination may be done to check for disorders (such as lymphomas)

Strategies for Preventing the Transmission of HIV

- Abstain from sexual activity.
- Use a latex condom for each act of intercourse with an infected partner or a partner whose HIV status is unknown (vaginal spermicides and sponges do not protect against HIV infection).
- If engaging in oral sex, withdraw before ejaculation.
- For newly monogamous couples, get tested for HIV infection and other sexually transmitted diseases (STDs) before engaging in unprotected sexual intercourse.
- Never share needles or syringes.
- Wear rubber gloves (preferably latex) when touching body fluids of a person who might be infected with HIV.
- If accidentally exposed to fluids containing HIV (for example, after a needlestick), seek treatment with antiretroviral drugs to prevent infection.

---

that affect the production of blood cells in the bone marrow. A spinal tap (lumbar puncture) or computed tomography (CT) or magnetic resonance imaging (MRI) of the head may be done to check for disorders that affect the brain or spinal cord.

AIDS is diagnosed when the CD4 count falls below 200 cells per microliter of blood or when extreme wasting or certain serious opportunistic infections or cancers develop.

Prevention

Transmission of HIV through its most common routes—sexual contact or sharing of needles—is almost completely preventable. However, the measures required for prevention—sexual abstinence or condom use (see box on page 1265) and access to clean needles—are sometimes personally or socially unpopular. Many people have difficulty changing their addictive or sexual behaviors, so they continue to put themselves at risk of HIV infection. Also, safe sex practices are not foolproof. For example, condoms can leak or break.

Vaccines for preventing HIV infection or slowing the progression of AIDS in people who are already infected have so far been elusive. Research continues, but in recent clinical trials, several promising vaccines have not proved useful.

Other measures can help. Circumcision of men, an inexpensive, safe procedure, appears to reduce the risk of infection by about half.

Because HIV is not transmitted through the air or by casual contact (such as touching, holding, or dry kissing), hospitals and clinics do not isolate HIV-infected people unless they have another contagious infection. Surfaces contaminated with HIV can easily be cleaned and disinfected because HIV is inactivated by heat and by common disinfectants such as hydrogen peroxide and alcohol. People who are likely to come into contact with blood or other body fluids at their job should wear protective latex gloves, masks, and eye shields. These universal precautions apply to body fluids from all people, not just those from people with HIV, for two reasons: People with HIV may not know that they are infected, and other viruses can be transmitted by body fluids.

People who have been exposed to HIV from a blood splash, needlestick, or sexual contact may reduce the chance of infection by taking anti-HIV drugs (antiretroviral drugs) for a short time. These drugs must be started as soon as possible after the exposure. Taking two or three drugs for 4 weeks is currently recommended. Because the risk of infection varies, doctors and infected people make decisions about preventive treatment individually, based on the type of exposure.

> **? Did You Know...**
> Drugs used to treat HIV infection help only if people take the drugs consistently and for the rest of their life.

Treatment

Antiretroviral Drugs: Several classes of drugs are used to treat HIV infection. All of the drugs, called antiretroviral drugs, block the activity of one of the enzymes HIV needs to replicate inside human cells. These drugs include the following:

- **Reverse transcriptase inhibitors:** These drugs prevent HIV reverse transcriptase from converting HIV RNA into DNA. There are three types of these drugs: nucleoside, nucleotide, and non-nucleoside.

- **Protease inhibitors:** These drugs prevent protease from activating certain proteins inside newly produced viruses. The result is immature, defective viruses that do not infect new cells.

- **Fusion inhibitors:** These drugs prevent HIV from entering cells. To enter a human cell, HIV must bind to a CD4 receptor and one other receptor, such as the CCR-5 receptor. One type of fusion inhibitor, CCR-5 inhibitors, blocks this receptor, preventing HIV from entering human cells.

- **Integrase inhibitors:** These drugs prevent HIV DNA from being integrated into human DNA.

These drugs prevent the virus from replicating. If replication is sufficiently slowed, the destruction of $CD4^+$ lymphocytes by HIV is decreased dramatically and the CD4 count begins to increase. As a result, much of the damage to the immune system caused by HIV can be reversed. Doctors can detect this reversal by measuring the CD4 count, which begins to return toward normal levels.

HIV invariably develops resistance to any of these drugs when they are used alone. Resistance develops after a few days to several months of use, depending on the drug and the virus. HIV varies because of mutations that occur when it replicates. Treatment is most effective when at least two or three drugs are given in combination—usually one of the following combinations:

- Three reverse transcriptase inhibitors (two nucleoside plus one non-nucleoside)
- Two nucleoside reverse transcriptase inhibitors plus one or two protease inhibitors

These combinations of drugs are often referred to as highly active antiretroviral therapy (HAART). HAART is used because

- Combinations are more powerful than single drugs in reducing levels of HIV in the blood.
- Combinations help prevent the development of drug resistance.
- Some HIV drugs (such as ritonavir) boost the blood levels of other HIV drugs (including most protease inhibitors) by slowing their removal from the body.

HAART can delay or prevent AIDS in HIV-infected people, thus extending their life.

Combinations of antiretroviral drugs have unpleasant and serious side effects. Metabolism of fats may be disturbed, probably primarily by protease inhibitors. Fat slowly accumulates in the abdomen (called central obesity) and breasts of women and is lost from the face, arms, and legs. Blood levels of cholesterol and triglycerides (two types of fat in the blood) are increased, increasing the risk of heart attacks and strokes. Many drugs cause rashes (skin reactions). Some skin reactions can be very dangerous, especially if the drug causing the reaction is nevirapine.

Nucleoside reverse transcriptase inhibitors damage mitochondria, which help the cell generate energy. Side effects include anemia, foot pain caused by nerve damage (neuropathy), liver damage that uncommonly progresses to severe liver failure, and heart damage that can result in heart failure. Individual drugs differ in their tendency to cause these problems. Careful monitoring and changes of drugs can usually prevent serious problems.

When HAART is successful, it can cause the immune reconstitution inflammatory syndrome. In

℞ DRUGS FOR HIV INFECTION

DRUG*	SOME SIDE EFFECTS†
Fusion inhibitors	
Enfuvirtide	Painful rash at the injection site and allergic (hypersensitivity) reactions (including rash, fever, chills, nausea, and low blood pressure)
Maraviroc (a CCR-5 inhibitor)	Inadequate blood flow (ischemia) to the heart or heart attacks
Integrase inhibitors	
Raltegravir	None
Non-nucleoside reverse transcriptase inhibitors	
All of these drugs	Rash (occasionally severe or life threatening) and liver dysfunction
Delavirdine	Side effects of the drug class
Efavirenz	Dizziness, sleepiness, nightmares, confusion, agitation, forgetfulness, and euphoria
Etravirine	Side effects of the drug class
Nevirapine	Side effects of the drug class
Nucleoside and nucleotide reverse transcriptase inhibitors	
All of these drugs	Lactic acidosis (buildup of lactic acid, a waste product of metabolism) and liver damage
Abacavir	Fever, rash (occasionally severe or life threatening), loss of appetite, nausea, vomiting, and a low white blood count
Didanosine (ddI)	Peripheral nerve damage, inflammation of the pancreas, nausea, and diarrhea
Emtricitabine	Headache, nausea, diarrhea, and darkening of the skin (hyperpigmentation), especially on the palms and soles
Lamivudine (3TC)	Headache, fatigue, and peripheral nerve damage
Stavudine (d4T)	Peripheral nerve damage and loss of fat in the face, arms, and legs
Tenofovir	Mild to moderate diarrhea, nausea, vomiting, kidney damage, and flatulence
Zalcitabine (ddC)	Peripheral nerve damage, pancreas inflammation, and mouth sores
Zidovudine (AZT)	Anemia, susceptibility to infection (resulting from bone marrow damage), headache, insomnia, weakness, and muscle aches
Protease inhibitors	
All of these drugs	Nausea, vomiting, diarrhea, abdominal discomfort, increased levels of blood sugar and cholesterol (common), increased abdominal fat, liver dysfunction, nail discoloration and deformity (ingrown nails), and a bleeding tendency (in people with hemophilia, bleeding)
Amprenavir	Rash
Darunavir	Headache, coldlike symptoms, severe rash, and fever
Fosamprenavir	Rash
Indinavir	Kidney stones
Lopinavir	Mouth tingling and altered taste
Nelfinavir	Side effects of the drug class
Ritonavir	Mouth tingling and altered taste
Saquinavir	Side effects of the drug class
Tipranavir	Liver inflammation

*All drugs, except enfuvirtide, are taken by mouth.

†Side effects listed for the class of drug can occur when any drug in that class is used.

this syndrome, symptoms of various infections worsen because immune responses improve (are reconstituted), increasing inflammation (see page 1140), or sometimes because parts of dead viruses persist, triggering immune responses.

Drug treatment is beneficial only if the drugs are taken on schedule. Missed doses allow the virus to replicate and develop resistance. No treatments can eliminate the virus from the body, although the HIV level often decreases so much that it cannot be detected. An undetectable level is the goal of treatment. If treatment is stopped, the HIV level increases, and the CD4 count begins to fall.

The best time to start drug treatment is unclear. The benefit of starting treatment in people who are not very sick and whose CD4 count is still near normal is also unclear. However, people with a low CD4 count (below 200) or a high viral load should be treated, even if they have no symptoms. Before starting a treatment regimen, they are taught about the necessity of taking drugs as directed, not skipping any doses, and taking the drugs for the rest of their life. Taking the drugs as directed for a life time may be difficult because the drugs have many significant and unpleasant side effects and are very expensive. Because taking HIV drugs irregularly often leads to drug resistance, health care practitioners try to make sure that people are both willing and able to adhere to the treatment regimen.

Prevention of Opportunistic Infections: If the CD4 count is low, drugs to prevent opportunistic infections are routinely prescribed.

- If the CD4 count drops below 200 cells per microliter of blood, the antibiotic trimethoprim-sulfamethoxazole is given to prevent *Pneumocystis jiroveci* pneumonia. This antibiotic also prevents toxoplasmosis, which can cause localized damage to the brain.

- If the CD4 count drops below 50 cells per microliter of blood, azithromycin taken weekly or clarithromycin or rifabutin taken daily may prevent *Mycobacterium avium* complex infections.

- People recovering from cryptococcal meningitis or those who have thrush, an infection of the mouth, esophagus, or vagina with the fungus *Candida* may be given the antifungal drug fluconazole for long periods.

- People with recurring herpes simplex infections of the mouth, lips, genitals, or rectum may require

prolonged treatment with an antiviral drug (such as acyclovir) to prevent recurrences.

Other Drugs: Other drugs may help with the weakness and weight loss associated with AIDS. Megestrol and dronabinol (a marijuana derivative) stimulate appetite. Many people with AIDS claim that natural marijuana is even more effective, and use of marijuana for this purpose has been legalized in a few states. Anabolic steroids (such as testosterone) can help people regain muscle tissue. If testosterone levels are reduced in men, testosterone injections or patches on the skin can increase the levels.

Prognosis

Exposure to HIV does not always lead to infection, and some people who have had repeated exposures over many years remain uninfected. Moreover, many infected people remain well for more than a decade. A few HIV-infected, untreated people have remained well for over 20 years. Why some people become ill so much sooner than others is not fully understood, but a number of genetic factors appear to influence both susceptibility to infection and progression to AIDS after infection.

If infected people are not treated, AIDS develops in many, as follows:

- For the first several years after infection: 1 to 2% each year
- Each year thereafter: 5%
- Within 10 to 11 years: 50%
- Eventually: More than 95%, possibly all if they live long enough

Early in the AIDS epidemic, most people with AIDS experienced a rapid decline in their quality of life after they were first hospitalized for the infection. Many spent much of their remaining time in the hospital and died within 2 years of developing AIDS. However, with current therapy, AIDS has become more manageable. Many people live for years after AIDS is diagnosed, and they continue to lead productive, active lives. Nevertheless, illness due to infections and the expense and side effects of drugs may reduce quality of life. If people cannot tolerate or take drugs consistently, AIDS progresses. Cure is not yet possible, although intensive research for a cure continues.

184 Sexually Transmitted Diseases

Sexually transmitted (venereal) diseases are infections that are typically, but not exclusively, passed from person to person through sexual contact.

- Sexually transmitted diseases may be caused by bacteria, viruses, or protozoa.
- Some infections can be spread through kissing or close body contact.
- Some infections may spread to other parts of the body, sometimes with serious consequences.
- Using condoms can help prevent these infections.

Sexual intercourse provides an easy opportunity for organisms to spread (be transmitted) from one person to another because it involves close contact and transfer of genital and other body fluids. Sexually transmitted diseases (STDs) are relatively common. For example, an estimated 360,000 cases of gonorrhea

and over 1 million chlamydial infections are reported, and even more probably occur every year in the United States—making them the two most common STDs.

Causes

Many infectious organisms—from tiny viruses, bacteria, and parasites to visible insects (such as lice)—can be spread through sexual contact. Some hepatitis and *Salmonella* infections (which causes diarrhea) can be transmitted during sexual activity, but they are often spread in other ways. Thus, they are not typically considered STDs.

Transmission: Although STDs usually result from having vaginal, oral, or anal sex with an infected partner, genital penetration is not necessary to spread an infection. Some STDs can be spread in other ways, including

- Kissing or close body contact—for pubic lice infestation, scabies, and molluscum contagiosum
- From mother to child before or during birth—for syphilis, herpes, chlamydial infection, gonorrhea, human immunodeficiency virus (HIV) infection, and human papillomavirus (HPV) infection
- Breastfeeding—for HIV infection
- Contaminated medical instruments—for HIV infection

Symptoms

Symptoms vary greatly, but the first symptoms usually involve the area where the organisms entered the body. For example, sores may form in the genital area or mouth. There may be a discharge from the penis or the vagina, and urination may be painful.

Complications: When STDs are not diagnosed and treated promptly, some organisms can spread through the bloodstream and infect internal organs, sometimes causing serious, even life-threatening problems. Such problems include heart and brain infections due to syphilis, AIDS due to HIV, and cervical cancer due to HPV.

In women, some organisms that enter the vagina can move up the vagina to the cervix (the lower part of the uterus), enter the uterus, and reach the fallopian tubes and sometimes the ovaries (see art on page 1492). Damage to the uterus and fallopian tubes can result in infertility or a mislocated (ectopic) pregnancy. The infection may spread to the membrane that lines the abdominal cavity (peritoneum),

TYPES OF SEXUALLY TRANSMITTED DISEASES

TYPE	DISEASE
Bacterial	Chancroid
	Chlamydial urethritis and cervicitis
	Gonorrhea
	Granuloma inguinale
	Lymphogranuloma venereum
	Syphilis
Viral	Genital herpes simplex (see page 1245)
	Genital warts (caused by the human papillomavirus)
	Molluscum contagiosum (see page 1325)
	Human immunodeficiency virus (HIV) infection or AIDS (see page 1254)
Parasitic (protozoan)	Trichomoniasis
Insect	Pubic lice infestation
	Scabies (due to burrowing mites)

causing peritonitis. These infections are considered pelvic inflammatory disease (see page 1541).

In men, organisms that enter through the penis may infect the tube that carries urine from the bladder through the penis (urethra). Complications that can result from chronic infection of the urethra include the following:

- Tightening of the foreskin, so that it cannot be pulled over the head of the penis
- Narrowing of the urethra, blocking the flow of urine
- Development of an abnormal channel (fistula) between the urethra and the skin of the penis

Occasionally in men, organisms spread up the urethra through the tube that carries sperm from the testis (ejaculatory duct and vas deferens) to infect the epididymis (the coiled tube on top of each testis—see art on page 1466).

In both sexes, some STDs can cause persistent swelling of the genital tissues or infection of the rectum (proctitis).

Diagnosis

Doctors often suspect an STD based on symptoms. To identify the organism involved and thus confirm the diagnosis, doctors may take a sample of blood, urine, or discharge from the vagina or penis and examine it. The sample may be sent to a laboratory for the organisms to be grown (cultured) to aid in identification. Sometimes genetic testing is required to identify the organism's unique genetic material. Other tests vary depending on the STD suspected.

Prevention

The following can help prevent STDs:

- Regular and correct use of condoms
- Avoidance of unsafe sex practices, such as frequently changing sex partners or having sexual intercourse with partners who have other sex partners or with prostitutes
- Circumcision (which can reduce the spread of HIV from women to men)
- Prompt diagnosis and treatment of STDs (to prevent spread to other people)
- Identification followed by counseling or treatment of the sexual contacts of infected people

The only vaccines available are those for HPV infection and hepatitis A and B.

Treatment

Most STDs can be effectively treated with drugs. However, some new strains of bacteria and viruses,

---

How to Use a Condom

- Use a new condom for each act of sexual intercourse.
- Use the correct size condom.
- Carefully handle the condom to avoid damaging it with fingernails, teeth, or other sharp objects.
- Put the condom on after the penis is erect and before any genital contact with the partner.
- Place the rolled condom over the tip of the erect penis.
- Leave 1/2 inch at the tip of the condom to collect semen.
- With one hand, squeeze trapped air out of the tip of the condom.
- If uncircumcised, pull the foreskin back before unrolling the condom.
- With the other hand, roll the condom over the penis to its base and smooth out any air bubbles.
- Make sure that lubrication is adequate during intercourse.
- With latex condoms, use only water-based lubricants. Oil-based lubricants (such as petroleum jelly, shortening, mineral oil, massage oils, body lotions, and cooking oil) can weaken latex and cause the condom to break.
- Hold the condom firmly against the base of the penis during withdrawal, and withdraw the penis while it is still erect to prevent slippage.

---

such as HIV, have become resistant to some drugs, making treatment more difficult. As new drugs are developed and more people are treated, resistance to drugs is likely to increase (see page 1188).

People who are being treated for a bacterial STD should abstain from sexual intercourse until the infection has been eliminated from them and their sex partners. Thus, sex partners should be tested and treated simultaneously.

Viral STDs, especially herpes, hepatitis B and C, and HIV infection, usually persist for life. Antiviral drugs can control but not yet cure all of these infections, except hepatitis C, which can be cured in some people after prolonged treatment.

Chancroid

Chancroid is a sexually transmitted disease caused by the bacteria Haemophilus ducreyi, *which causes painful genital sores.*

In developed countries, chancroid is rare, but it is a common cause of genital ulcers throughout much of the developing world, where it may be acquired by men from prostitutes. Because chancroid causes genital sores, people who have it are more likely to become infected with and to spread human immunodeficiency virus (HIV).

Symptoms

Symptoms begin 3 to 7 days after infection. Small, painful blisters form on the genitals or around the anus and rapidly rupture to form shallow sores. These sores may enlarge and run together. The lymph nodes in the groin may become tender, enlarged, and matted together, forming collections of pus (abscesses) called buboes. The skin over the abscess may become red and shiny and may break down and discharge pus from the lymph nodes onto the skin. Sores may form in other areas of the skin.

Diagnosis and Treatment

Doctors suspect chancroid in people with genital sores that have no obvious cause. Tests for chancroid are not readily available, but blood tests may be done to exclude other causes.

Several antibiotics are effective for chancroid. The following may be used:

- Ceftriaxone in a single injection
- Azithromycin taken by mouth in a single dose
- Ciprofloxacin taken by mouth for 3 days
- Erythromycin taken by mouth for 7 days

Chlamydial and Other Infections

Chlamydial infections include sexually transmitted diseases of the urethra and cervix that are caused by the bacteria Chlamydia trachomatis. *Less commonly, other bacteria, such as* Ureaplasma *and mycoplasmas, cause infection of the urethra.*

- Symptoms include a discharge from the penis or vagina and painful or more frequent urination.
- If unnoticed or untreated in women, these infections can result in infertility, miscarriage, and an increased risk of a mislocated pregnancy.
- DNA tests of a sample of the discharge or of urine can detect chlamydial infection.
- Antibiotics can cure the infection, and sex partners should be treated at the same time.

Several bacteria can cause diseases that resemble gonorrhea. These bacteria include *Chlamydia trachomatis, Trichomonas vaginalis, Ureaplasma,* and several types of mycoplasmas. Laboratories can identify chlamydiae but have difficulty identifying the other bacteria. So the infections caused by these other bacteria are called nongonococcal, nonchlamydial infections, usually of the urethra (urethritis).

Chlamydial infection is the most commonly reported sexually transmitted disease (STD). In the United States, over 1 million cases were reported in 2006. Because the infection frequently causes no symptoms, the number of infected people may be 4 times higher. In men, chlamydiae cause about half of the urethral infections not caused by gonorrhea. Most of the remaining urethral infections in men are probably caused by *Ureaplasma urealyticum* or mycoplasmas. In women, chlamydiae account for virtually all of the cervical infections (cervicitis) that produce pus and that are not caused by gonorrhea. Sometimes both sexes have gonorrhea and chlamydial infection at the same time.

Symptoms

In men, symptoms of chlamydial urethritis start 7 to 28 days after the infection is acquired during intercourse. Typically, men feel a mild burning sensation in their urethra during urination and may have a clear or cloudy discharge from the penis. The discharge is usually less thick than the discharge in gonorrhea. The discharge may be small, and symptoms mild. However, early in the morning, the opening of the penis is often red and stuck together with dried secretions. Occasionally, the infection begins more dramatically—with a frequent urge to urinate, painful urination, and a discharge of pus from the urethra.

Many women with chlamydial cervicitis have few or no symptoms. But some have frequent urges to urinate, painful urination, and secretions of yellow mucus and pus from the vagina.

Complications: If the infection spreads up women's reproductive tract, it may infect the tubes that connect the ovaries to the uterus (fallopian tubes). This infection, called salpingitis or pelvic inflammatory disease, causes severe lower abdominal pain. In some women, the lining of the abdominal cavity (peritoneum) becomes inflamed. This inflammation, called peritonitis, causes more severe pain in the lower abdomen and sometimes in the area around the liver, in the right upper abdomen.

If the anus is infected, people may have rectal pain or tenderness and a yellow discharge of pus and mucus from the rectum.

Chlamydiae may be transferred to the eye, causing infection of the conjunctiva (conjunctivitis).

Chlamydial genital infections occasionally cause a joint inflammation called reactive arthritis (previously called Reiter's syndrome—see page 570). Reactive arthritis typically affects several joints at once. The lower limbs are affected most often. The inflammation seems to be an immune reaction to the genital infection rather than spread of the infection to the joints. Symptoms typically begin 1 to 3 weeks after the initial chlamydial infection.

If chlamydial urethritis is not treated, symptoms usually disappear in 4 to 6 weeks. However, if untreated, a chlamydial infection can cause complications, especially in women who have been infected a long time. Complications include chronic abdominal pain and scarring of the fallopian tubes. The scarring can cause infertility and a mislocated (ectopic) pregnancy (see page 1644).

In men, chlamydial infections may cause epididymitis, which causes painful swelling of the scrotum on one or both sides (see page 1472). Other bacteria from the intestine also contribute to these complications probably by infecting areas that have been damaged by chlamydiae.

> **? Did You Know...**
>
> Chlamydial infections are the most common sexually transmitted disease.
>
> Because chlamydial infection and gonorrhea often occur together, people with one of them are routinely treated for both.

Diagnosis

Doctors suspect these infections based on symptoms, such as a discharge from the penis or cervix. In most cases, doctors diagnose chlamydial infections by doing tests that detect the bacteria's unique genetic material (DNA or RNA). Usually, a sample of the discharge from the penis or cervix is used. For some types of these tests, a urine sample can be used. Thus, people can avoid the discomfort of having a swab inserted into the penis or having a pelvic examination to obtain a sample.

Gonorrhea, which is often also present, can be diagnosed using the same sample. Specific tests for genital infections with *Ureaplasma* and mycoplasmas are not usually done. These infections are sometimes diagnosed in people with characteristic symptoms after gonorrhea and chlamydial infections are ruled out.

Screening: Because chlamydial infection is so common and because many infected women have no symptoms, these tests are recommended for sexually active women aged 15 to 25 to screen for STDs.

Treatment

Chlamydial, ureaplasmal, and mycoplasmal infections are treated with a single dose of azithromycin or with doxycycline or levofloxacin taken by mouth for 7 days. At the same time, an antibiotic such as ceftriaxone, injected into a muscle, is given to treat gonorrhea because the symptoms of the two infections are similar and because many people have

Possible Complications of Chlamydial and Ureaplasmal Infections

IN MEN

- Infection of the epididymis
- Narrowing (stricture) of the urethra

IN WOMEN

- Infection of the fallopian tubes (salpingitis)
- Infection of the membrane that lines the abdominal cavity (peritonitis)
- Infection of the surface of the liver

IN MEN AND WOMEN

- Infection of the membrane that covers part of the eye (conjunctivitis)

IN NEWBORNS

- Conjunctivitis
- Pneumonia

both infections at the same time. Pregnant women are given azithromycin instead of tetracycline or doxycycline, which must be avoided during pregnancy. If symptoms persist or return, treatment is repeated for a longer period.

Infected people should abstain from sexual intercourse until they have completed treatment to avoid infecting their sex partners. Sex partners should be treated simultaneously if possible and should abstain from sexual intercourse until they complete treatment. The risk of another chlamydial infection or another STD within 3 to 4 months is high enough that people should be screened again at that time.

Genital Warts

Genital warts (condylomata acuminata) are growths in or around the vagina, penis, or rectum caused by the human papillomavirus, which is sexually transmitted.

- Some types of human papillomavirus (HPV) cause visible genital warts, and other types cause less visible warts that increase the risk of cancer.
- Genital warts grow rapidly and sometimes cause burning pain.
- Doctors identify visible warts based on their appearance, and they examine the cervix and anus to check for less visible warts.
- Vaccines can prevent most types of HPV infection that can cause cancer.
- Visible warts can usually be removed with a laser or by freezing (cryotherapy) or surgery, but sometimes drugs are applied to the warts.

In the United States, about 1.4 million people have genital warts, which are caused by HPV. An estimated 24 million people have an HPV infection, and 5.5 million are infected each year. About 50% of women have been infected at least once by age 50. Most infections go away within 1 to 2 years, but some persist. Persistent infection can increase the risk of certain types of cancer.

There are over 70 known types of HPV. Some types cause common skin warts. Other types cause different types of genital infections:

- **External (easily seen) genital warts:** These warts are caused by certain types of HPV, especially types 6 and 11. These types are transmitted sexually and infect the genital and rectal areas.

- **Internal (less visible) genital warts:** Other HPV types, especially types 16 and 18, infect the genital area but do not cause easily visible warts. They cause tiny flat warts on the cervix or in the anus, which may be visible only with a magnifying instrument called a colposcope. These less visible spots usually cause no symptoms, but the HPV types that cause them increase the risk of developing cervical, bladder, and rectal cancer and therefore should be treated.

HPV can also be spread during oral sex, causing infections of the mouth and increasing the risk of oral cancer.

> **? Did You Know...**
> Some types of the virus that causes genital warts can also cause cancer.

Symptoms

In men, warts usually occur on the penis, especially under the foreskin in uncircumcised men, or in the urethra. In women, genital warts occur on the vulva, vaginal wall, cervix, and skin around the vaginal area. Genital warts may develop in the area around the anus and in the rectum, especially in people who engage in anal sex. Warts cause no symptoms in many people but cause occasional burning pain in some.

The warts usually appear 1 to 6 months after infection with HPV, beginning as tiny, soft, moist, pink or gray growths. They grow rapidly and become rough, irregular bumps, which sometimes grow out from the skin on narrow stalks. Their rough surfaces make them look like a small cauliflower. Warts often grow in clusters.

Warts may grow more rapidly and spread in pregnant women and in people who have a weakened immune system, such as those who have human immunodeficiency virus (HIV) infection.

Diagnosis

Genital warts usually can be diagnosed based on their appearance. If warts look unusual, bleed, become open sores (ulcerate), or persist after treatment, they should be removed surgically and examined under a microscope to check for cancer.

If women have warts on the cervix, a Papanicolaou (Pap) test is done to rule out other abnormalities (such as cervical cancer—see page 1575). If genital warts are diagnosed, women should have a Pap test and colposcopy of the vagina and cervix (using a magnifying instrument) twice a year so that any abnormalities can be identified and treated promptly.

Colposcopy is done to check for less visible warts on the cervix or in the anus. A stain may be applied to the area so that warts can be seen more easily. A sample taken from a wart may be analyzed using tests, such as the polymerase chain reaction (PCR). This test produces many copies of a gene, which may enable doctors to identify HPV's unique genetic material (DNA). These tests help confirm the diagnosis and enable doctors to identify the type of HPV.

Prevention

A vaccine for HPV is available that protects against the two types of HPV (types 6 and 11) that cause about 80% of genital warts. This vaccine also protects against the two types of HPV (types 16 and 18) that are believed to cause the majority (about 70%) of cervical cancers. The HPV vaccine has been recommended for girls and women 9 to 26 years old for prevention of initial infection. Three doses are given, preferably at age 11 to 12 years. The vaccine should be administered before the onset of sexual activity, but girls and women who are sexually active should still be vaccinated. The vaccine's role in preventing HPV in boys and men has not been established.

Because of the location of these warts, condoms do not fully protect against infection.

Treatment

If the immune system is healthy, it often eventually controls HPV and eliminates the warts and the virus, even without treatment. HPV infection is gone after 8 months in half of people and lasts longer than 2 years in fewer than 10%. If people with genital warts have a weakened immune system, treatment is required, and the warts often return.

No treatment for external warts is completely satisfactory, and some treatments are uncomfortable and leave scars. External genital warts may be removed with a laser or by freezing (cryotherapy) or surgery. A local or general anesthetic is used.

Alternatively, podophyllin toxin, imiquimod, or trichloroacetic acid can be applied directly to the warts. However, this approach requires many applications over weeks to months, may burn the surrounding skin, and is frequently ineffective. After treatment, the area may be painful. Imiquimod cream causes less burning but may be less effective. The warts may return after apparently successful treatment.

For warts in the urethra, a viewing tube (endoscope) with surgical attachments may be the most effective way to remove them. It requires a general anesthetic. Or drugs, such as thiotepa inserted into the urethra or the chemotherapy drug 5-fluorouracil injected into the wart, are often effective. Interferon-alpha injections into the wart or into a muscle are somewhat effective, but they must be given several times a week for many weeks and are expensive.

All sex partners should be examined for warts and other STDs and treated, if necessary. Sex partners should also have regular examinations to check for HPV infection.

Gonorrhea

Gonorrhea is a sexually transmitted disease caused by the bacteria Neisseria gonorrhoeae, *which infect the lining of the urethra, cervix, rectum, and throat or the membranes that cover the front part of the eye (conjunctiva and cornea).*

- Gonorrhea is usually spread through sexual contact.
- People have a discharge from the penis or vagina and may need to urinate more frequently and urgently.
- Rarely, gonorrhea infects the joints, skin, or heart.
- Microscopic examination and culture of a sample of the discharge or DNA tests of urine can detect the infection.
- Antibiotics can cure the infection.

In the United States, the number of gonorrhea cases reported each year has decreased by 75% since it peaked at nearly 900,000 in 1985. However, the number appears to have leveled off for about the last 10 years, with about 360,000 cases reported in 2006.

Gonorrhea is almost always spread through sexual contact. After one episode of vaginal intercourse with an infected person, the chance of spread from women to men is about 20%. The chance of spread from men to women may be higher. If pregnant women are infected, the bacteria can spread to the eyes of the fetus during birth. However, in most developed countries, infection is prevented because all newborns are routinely treated after delivery with medicated eye ointment.

Many people with gonorrhea have other sexually transmitted diseases (STDs), such as chlamydial infection, syphilis, or human immunodeficiency virus (HIV) infection.

Did You Know...

If pregnant women have gonorrhea, the eyes of the fetus may become infected, so newborns are routinely treated to prevent this infection.

Symptoms

In men, symptoms begin within about 3 to 10 days after infection. Usually, gonorrhea causes symptoms only at the sites of initial infection. In some people, infection spreads through the bloodstream to other parts of the body, especially to the skin, joints, or both.

Men feel mild discomfort in the urethra, followed a few hours later by mild to severe pain during urination, a yellow-green discharge of pus from the penis, and a frequent urge to urinate. The opening at the tip of the penis may become red and swollen. The bacteria sometimes spread to the epididymis (the coiled tube on top of each testis), which swells and feels tender to the touch.

About 10 to 20% of infected women have minimal or no symptoms. Thus, the infection may be detected only during routine screening or after diagnosis of the infection in their male partner. Symptoms typically do not begin until at least 10 days after infection. Some women feel only mild discomfort in the genital area and have a puslike discharge from the vagina. However, other women have more severe symptoms, such as a frequent urge to urinate, pain during urination, and fever because the urethra may also be infected.

Bacteria commonly spread up the genital tract and infect the tubes that connect the ovaries to the uterus (fallopian tubes). This infection, called salpingitis or pelvic inflammatory disease, causes severe lower abdominal pain, especially during intercourse. In some women, the lining of the abdominal cavity (peritoneum) becomes inflamed. This inflammation, called peritonitis, causes severe pain in the entire abdomen. Infection in the abdomen may concentrate around the liver. This infection, called perihepatitis or Fitz-Hugh-Curtis syndrome, causes pain in the upper right part of the abdomen. Women who have had pelvic inflammatory disease have an increased risk of infertility and mislocated (ectopic) pregnancies.

Anal sex with an infected partner may result in gonorrhea of the rectum, which makes bowel movements painful. Other symptoms include constipation, itching, bleeding, and a discharge from the rectum. The area around the anus may become red and raw, and stool may be coated with mucus and pus. When a doctor examines the rectum with a viewing tube (anoscope), mucus and pus may be visible on the wall of the rectum.

Oral sex with an infected partner may result in gonorrhea of the throat (gonococcal pharyngitis). Usually, the infection causes no symptoms uncommonly a sore throat.

If infected fluids come into contact with the eyes, gonococcal conjunctivitis may develop, causing swelling of the eyelids and a discharge of pus from the eyes. In adults, often only one eye is infected. Newborns usually have infection in both eyes. Blindness may result if the infection is not treated early.

Gonorrhea in children usually results from sexual abuse. In girls, the genital area (vulva) may be irritated, red, and swollen, and they may have a discharge from the vagina. If the urethra is infected, children, mainly boys, may have pain during urination.

Rarely, the infection spreads through the bloodstream to other parts of the body, especially the skin and joints. Joints become swollen, tender, and extremely painful, limiting movement. The skin over infected joints may be red and warm. If the bloodstream is infected, people may have a fever, feel generally ill, and develop arthritis in one or more joints. Red spots may appear on the skin. This infection is called disseminated gonococcal infection or arthritis-dermatitis syndrome.

Joint, bloodstream, and heart infections can be treated, but recovery from arthritis may be slow.

Diagnosis

In more than 90% of infected men, gonorrhea may be diagnosed within an hour by identifying the bacteria (gonococci) in samples of the discharge examined under a microscope. The sample is usually obtained by inserting a small swab a few centimeters into the urethra. However, identifying bacteria in a sample of discharge from the cervix is more difficult. The bacteria can be seen in only about half of infected women.

The sample of discharge is also sent to a laboratory for tests. Such tests are very reliable in both sexes but take longer than a microscopic examination. If a doctor suspects an infection of the throat, rectum, or bloodstream, samples from these areas are sent for culture (to be grown in a laboratory).

Other highly sensitive tests can be done to detect the DNA of gonococci and of chlamydia (which are often also present). Laboratories can test for both infections in a single specimen. For some of these tests, urine samples can be used. Thus, these tests are convenient for screening men and women who have no symptoms or who are unwilling to have fluid samples taken from their genitals.

Because many people have more than one STD, doctors may test samples of blood and genital fluids for other STDs, such as syphilis and HIV infection.

If a joint is red and swollen, doctors draw fluid from the joint using a needle. The fluid is sent for culture and other tests.

Treatment

A single injection of a cephalosporin antibiotic, such as ceftriaxone, into a muscle or a single dose of cefixime taken by mouth, cures most people. Some antibiotics (such as penicillin, ciprofloxacin, levofloxacin, and ofloxacin) are no longer used because many strains of gonococci have developed resistance to them. Usually, people with gonorrhea are also given antibiotics to kill chlamydiae because people are often infected with both. A single dose of azithromycin is most commonly used. A single high dose of azithromycin can cure both gonorrhea and chlamydial infection if people are allergic to cephalosporins, but the required dose often causes stomach upset.

If gonorrhea has spread through the bloodstream, people are usually treated in the hospital and given antibiotics intravenously.

If symptoms recur or persist after treatment, doctors may take samples for culture to make sure people are cured and do tests to determine whether the gonococci are resistant to the antibiotics used.

People with gonorrhea should abstain from sexual activity until treatment is completed to avoid infecting sex partners. All sex partners who have had sexual contact with infected people in the past 60 days should be tested for gonorrhea and other STDs and, if the tests are positive, should be treated. People who were exposed to gonorrhea within 2 weeks are treated for it without waiting for test results.

Granuloma Inguinale

Granuloma inguinale is a rare sexually transmitted disease that is caused by the bacteria Calymmatobacterium granulomatis *and that leads to chronic inflammation and scarring of the genitals.*

Granuloma inguinale is extremely rare in developed countries but still occurs in Papua New Guinea, Australia, southern Africa, and parts of Brazil and India.

Symptoms

Symptoms usually begin 1 to 12 weeks after infection. The first symptom is a painless, red nodule that slowly enlarges into a round, raised lump. The lump then breaks down to form a sore near the site of the initial infection:

- Penis, scrotum, groin, and thighs in men
- Vulva, vagina, and surrounding skin in women
- Face in both sexes
- Anus and buttocks in people who have anal intercourse

Sores may spread to other areas. They heal slowly and cause scarring. Occasionally, the infection spreads through the bloodstream to the bones, joints, or liver.

Diagnosis and Treatment

Diagnosis is suspected in people who live in areas where the infection occurs and who have sores typical of the infection. To confirm the diagnosis, doctors take a sample of fluid scraped from the sore and examine it under a microscope.

Trimethoprim-sulfamethoxazole or doxycycline taken by mouth for at least 3 weeks is effective.

Lymphogranuloma Venereum

Lymphogranuloma venereum is a sexually transmitted disease that is caused by Chlamydia trachomatis *and that causes painful, swollen lymph glands in the groin and sometimes infection of the rectum.*

Lymphogranuloma venereum is caused by types of *Chlamydia trachomatis* other than those that usually cause infection of the urethra (urethritis) and cervix (cervicitis). The infection occurs mostly in tropical and subtropical areas and is rare in the United State. In Western Europe, this infection has become a common cause of rectal infection (proctitis) in homosexual men.

Symptoms begin 3 or more days after infection. A small, painless, fluid-filled blister develops, usually on the penis or in the vagina. Typically, the blister becomes a sore that quickly heals and is often unnoticed. Then, lymph nodes in the groin on one or both sides may swell and become tender. The enlarged, tender lymph nodes (called buboes) attach to the deeper tissues and the overlying skin, which becomes inflamed. If infection lasts a long time or recurs, lymphatic vessels (which drain fluids from tissues) may be blocked, causing genital tissues to swell. Rectal infection may cause scarring, which can narrow the rectum.

Lymphogranuloma venereum is suspected based on its characteristic symptoms. The diagnosis can be confirmed by a blood test that identifies antibodies against *Chlamydia trachomatis*.

If given early in the infection, doxycycline, erythromycin, or tetracycline, taken by mouth for 3 weeks, cures the infection, but swelling may persist if lymphatic vessels are irreversibly damaged.

Syphilis

Syphilis is a sexually transmitted disease caused by the bacteria Treponema pallidum.

- Syphilis can occur in three stages of symptoms, separated by periods of apparent good health.

- It begins with a painless sore at the infection site and, in the second stage, causes a rash, fever, fatigue, and loss of appetite.

- If untreated, syphilis can damage the heart, brain, spinal cord, and other organs.

- Doctors usually do two types of blood tests—one to screen for and one to confirm the infection.

- Penicillin can eliminate the infection, but people can be reinfected.

In the United States, the annual number of people with symptoms diagnosed for the first time peaked in 1990, when there were about 50,000 cases. Only about 6,000 such cases were reported in 2000, but the number went up to about 9,700 in 2006. Most people with syphilis are men, often homosexual men, living in cities. The percentage of blacks infected is 3 times that of other ethnic or racial groups.

Syphilis causes symptoms in three stages (primary, secondary, and tertiary), separated by periods when no symptoms occur (latent stages).

Syphilis is highly contagious during the primary and secondary stages. Infection is usually spread through sexual contact. A single sexual encounter with a person who has early-stage syphilis results in infection about one third of the time. The bacteria enter the body through mucous membranes, such as those in the vagina or mouth, or through the skin. Within hours, the bacteria reach nearby lymph nodes, then spread throughout the body through the bloodstream.

Syphilis can also be spread in other ways. It can infect a fetus during pregnancy (see table on page 1706), causing birth defects and other problems. It can also be spread through contact with skin. However, the bacteria cannot survive long outside the human body.

People with syphilis often have other infections, including other sexually transmitted diseases (STDs).

Symptoms

Each stage of symptoms (primary, secondary, and tertiary) is progressively worse. If not treated, syphilis can persist without symptoms for many years and may damage the heart or brain, possibly leading to death. If detected and treated early, syphilis can be cured, and there is no permanent damage.

Primary Stage: A painless sore (called a chancre) appears at the infection site—typically the penis, vulva, or vagina. A chancre may also appear on the anus, rectum, lips, tongue, throat, cervix, fingers, or other parts of the body. Usually only one chancre develops, but occasionally several develop. Symptoms usually start 3 to 4 weeks after infection but may start from 1 to 13 weeks later.

The chancre begins as a small red raised area, which soon turns into a painless open, deep sore. The chancre does not bleed and is hard to the touch.

Lymph nodes in the groin usually swell and are also painless. About half of infected women and one third of infected men are unaware of the chancre because it causes few symptoms. Chancres in the rectum or mouth, usually occurring in homosexual men, are often unnoticed. The chancre usually heals in 3 to 12 weeks. Then, people appear to be completely healthy.

Secondary Stage: The bacteria spread in the bloodstream, causing a widespread rash, swollen lymph nodes, and, less commonly, symptoms in other organs. The rash typically appears 6 to 12 weeks after infection. About one fourth of infected people still have a chancre at this time. Usually, the rash does not itch or hurt. It varies in appearance. Unlike rashes caused by most other diseases, this rash commonly appears on the palms or soles. It may be short-lived or may last for months. Even without treatment, the rash eventually resolves, but it may recur weeks or months later. If a rash develops on the scalp, hair may fall out in patches, making it appear moth-eaten.

> ### ? Did You Know...
>
> A single sexual encounter with a person who has syphilis results in infection about one third of the time.
>
> About half of the women and one third of the men who have the initial sore of syphilis do not notice it.

Raised bumps called papules (condylomata lata) may develop in moist areas of the skin, such as the armpits, genital area, and anus. These painful papules are very infectious. They may break open and weep. As they resolve, they flatten and turn a dull pink or gray. Mouth sores develop in more than 80% of people.

Secondary-stage syphilis can cause fever, fatigue, loss of appetite, and weight loss. About 50% of people have enlarged lymph nodes throughout the body, and in about 10%, the eyes become inflamed. About 10% of people have inflamed bones and joints that ache. In some people, the skin and whites of the eyes turn yellow (called jaundice) because hepatitis develops. Some have headaches or problems with hearing or vision because the brain, inner ears, or eyes are infected.

Latent Stage: After the secondary stage, people recover and have no symptoms for a time, which may last from years to decades. During this time, the infection is inactive (latent) and is not contagious. However, the bacteria are still present, and tests for

syphilis are positive. The latent stage is classified as early (if the initial infection occurred within the previous 12 months) or late (if the initial infection occurred more than 12 months previously).

Tertiary (Third) Stage: Symptoms range from mild to devastating. Tertiary syphilis has three main forms: benign tertiary syphilis, cardiovascular syphilis, and neurosyphilis.

Benign tertiary syphilis usually develops 3 to 10 years after the initial infection. It is rare today. Soft, rubbery growths called gummas appear on the skin, most commonly on the scalp, face, upper trunk, and legs. They also often develop in the liver or bones, but they can develop in virtually any organ. They may break down, forming an open sore. If untreated, gummas destroy the tissue around them. In bone, they usually cause deep, penetrating pain. Gummas grow slowly, heal gradually, and leave scars.

Cardiovascular syphilis usually appears 10 to 25 years after the initial infection. The bacteria infect the heart and the blood vessels connected to it, including the aorta (the largest artery in the body). The following may result:

- The wall of the aorta may weaken, forming a bulge (aneurysm). The aneurysm may press on the windpipe or other structures in the chest, causing difficulty breathing, a cough, and hoarseness.
- The valve leading from the heart to the aorta (aortic valve) may leak.
- The arteries that carry blood to the heart (coronary arteries) may narrow.

These problems can cause chest pain, heart failure, and death.

Neurosyphilis (which affects the brain and spinal cord) occurs during the first 5 to 10 years after infection. It develops in about 5% of all people with untreated syphilis. It occurs in the following forms:

- **Meningovascular:** The arteries of the brain or spinal cord become inflamed, causing a chronic form of meningitis. At first, people may have a headache and a stiff neck. They may feel dizzy, have difficulty concentrating and remembering things, and have insomnia. Vision may be blurred. Muscles in the arms, shoulders, and eventually legs may become weak or even paralyzed. This form can cause strokes.
- **Paretic:** This form usually begins when people are in their 40s or 50s. The first symptoms are gradual changes in behavior. For example, people may become less careful about personal hygiene, and their moods may change abruptly. They may become irritable and more and more confused. They may have delusions of grandeur. Headaches, insomnia, difficulty concentrating, poor judg-

ment, and fatigue are common. Tremors may occur in the mouth, tongue, outstretched hands, or whole body. Usually, dementia eventually results.

- **Tabetic (tabes dorsalis):** The spinal cord progressively deteriorates. Symptoms begin gradually, typically with an intense, stabbing pain in the legs that comes and goes irregularly. Walking becomes unsteady. People may feel like they are walking on foam rubber. People usually become thin. Erectile dysfunction is common. Eventually, people have difficulty controlling urination (incontinence) and may become paralyzed.

Diagnosis

Health care practitioners suspect primary syphilis if people have a typical chancre. They suspect secondary syphilis if people have a typical rash on the palms and soles. Laboratory tests are needed to confirm the diagnosis. Two types of blood tests are used:

- **A screening test,** such as the Venereal Disease Research Laboratory (VDRL) or the rapid plasma reagin (RPR) test, is done first. Screening tests are inexpensive and easy to do. But they may need to be repeated because for 3 to 6 weeks after the initial infection, results can be negative even though syphilis is present. Such results are called false-negative. Screening test results are sometimes positive when syphilis is not present (false-positive) because another disorder is present.

- **A confirmatory test** must usually be done to confirm a positive screening test. This blood test measures antibodies specific to the bacteria that cause syphilis, *Treponema pallidum.* Results of confirmatory tests may also be false-negative during the first few weeks after initial infections and thus may need to be repeated.

Screening test results may become negative after successful treatment, but the confirmatory test results stay positive indefinitely.

In the primary or secondary stages, syphilis may also be diagnosed using darkfield microscopy. A sample of fluid is taken from a skin or mouth sore and examined using a specially equipped light microscope. The bacteria appear bright against a dark background, making them easier to identify.

In the latent stage, antibody tests of blood and spinal fluid are used to diagnose syphilis.

In the tertiary stage, the diagnosis is based on symptoms and antibody test results. Depending on which symptoms are present, other tests are done. For example, a chest x-ray may be taken or another imaging test may be done to check for an aneurysm in the aorta. If neurosyphilis is suspected, a spinal tap (lumbar puncture) is needed to obtain spinal fluid, which is tested for antibodies to the bacteria.

Treatment

Penicillin given by injection is the best antibiotic for primary, secondary, and early latent syphilis. For primary and secondary stages of syphilis, one dose of a long-acting penicillin is all that is needed. However, some people need another dose 1 week later. For late latent stage and some forms of the tertiary stage, three doses are given, separated by 1 week.

If syphilis affects the eyes, inner ears, or brain, penicillin may be given intravenously every 4 hours for 10 to 14 days. People who are allergic to penicillin may be given other antibiotics such as ceftriaxone (given by injection daily for 10 days) or doxycycline (taken by mouth for 14 days).

Because people with primary or secondary syphilis can pass the infection to others, they must avoid sexual contact until they and their sex partners have completed treatment. If people have primary-stage syphilis, all their sex partners of the previous 3 months are at risk of being infected. If they have secondary-stage syphilis, all sex partners of the previous year are at risk. Such sex partners require a blood test for antibodies to the bacteria. If test results are positive, the sex partners need to be treated. Some doctors simply treat all sex partners without waiting for test results.

More than half of people with syphilis in an early stage, especially those with secondary-stage syphilis, develop a reaction 2 to 12 hours after the first treatment. This reaction, called a Jarisch-Herxheimer reaction, causes fever, headache, sweating, shaking chills, and a temporary worsening of the sores caused by syphilis. Doctors sometimes mistake this reaction for an allergic reaction to penicillin. Rarely, people with neurosyphilis have seizures or become paralyzed. Symptoms of this reaction usually subside within 24 hours and rarely cause permanent damage.

After treatment, examinations and blood tests are done periodically until no infection is detected. If treatment of primary, secondary, or latent-stage syphilis is successful, most people have no more symptoms. But treatment of tertiary-stage syphilis cannot reverse any damage done to organs, such as the brain or heart. People with such damage usually do not improve after treatment. People who have been cured of syphilis do not become immune to it and can be infected again.

Trichomoniasis

Trichomoniasis is a sexually transmitted infection of the vagina or urethra that is caused by the protozoa Trichomonas vaginalis *and that causes vaginal irritation and discharge.*

- Women may have a greenish yellow, frothy, fishy-smelling vaginal discharge with irritation and soreness in the genital area.

- Men are less likely to have symptoms but may have a frothy, puslike discharge from the penis, and urination may be painful and frequent.
- Examination of a sample of the discharge under a microscope usually enables doctors to identify the infection.
- A single dose of an antibiotic cures most women, but most men need to take an antibiotic for 7 days.

Trichomonas vaginalis commonly causes a sexually transmitted disease (STD) of the vagina in women and an STD of the urinary tract in men and women. Women are much more likely to develop symptoms. About 20% of women develop trichomoniasis of the vagina (trichomonas vaginitis) during their reproductive years (see page 1539). Many people with trichomoniasis also have gonorrhea or other STDs.

Symptoms

In women, the infection usually starts with a greenish yellow, frothy, fishy-smelling vaginal discharge. In some women, the discharge is slight. The vulva may be irritated and sore, and sexual intercourse may be painful. In severe cases, the vulva and surrounding skin may be inflamed, and the labia swollen. Urination may be painful or frequent, as occurs in a bladder infection. Urinary and vaginal symptoms may occur alone or together.

Most men with trichomoniasis of the urethra have no or only mild symptoms, but they can still infect their sex partners. Some men have a frothy, puslike discharge from the penis, pain during urination, and an urge to urinate frequently, usually early in the morning. Rarely, the epididymis (the coiled tube on top of each testis) and prostate gland are infected.

 Did You Know...

About 1 of 5 women develop trichomoniasis of the vagina.

Most men with trichomoniasis have no symptoms, but they can still infect their sex partners.

Diagnosis

Doctors suspect trichomoniasis in women with vaginal infections, in men with urethral infections, and in their sex partners.

The organism is much more difficult to detect in men than in women. In women, the diagnosis can usually be made quickly by examining a sample of the vaginal discharge with a microscope and identifying the organism. If results are unclear, the sample is cultured

for several days. In men, a sample of the discharge from the end of the penis (obtained in the morning, before urination) may be examined under a microscope and sent to the laboratory for culture. Occasionally, microscopic examination of the urine detects *Trichomonas*, but identification is more likely if a urine culture is done.

Tests for other STDs are usually also done because many people with trichomoniasis also have gonorrhea or a chlamydial infection.

Treatment

A single dose of metronidazole or tinidazole (which are antibiotics), taken by mouth, cures up to 95% of infected women. However, their sex partners must be treated simultaneously, or women may be reinfected. Whether single-dose treatment is effective in men is unclear. But men are usually cured after taking the antibiotic for 7 days.

If taken with alcohol, metronidazole may cause nausea and flushing of the skin. The drug may also cause a metallic taste in the mouth, nausea, or a decrease in the number of white blood cells. Women who take the drug may be more susceptible to vaginal yeast infections (vaginal candidiasis). Metronidazole is best avoided during pregnancy, at least during the first 3 months.

Infected people should abstain from sexual intercourse until the infection is cured, or they can infect their partners.

Other Sexually Transmitted Diseases

Some bacteria (*Shigella*, *Campylobacter*, and *Salmonella*), viruses (hepatitis A, B, and C), and parasites (*Giardia* and some amebas) are sometimes transmitted during sexual intercourse, although they are typically transmitted in other ways. These organisms, except for hepatitis B and C viruses, typically infect the digestive tract and are acquired when people consume contaminated food or water. In the digestive system, the organisms multiply and are excreted from the body in the feces. They can be spread through contact with the anus or feces of an infected person—for example, during anal sex.

Symptoms vary depending on the organism. They may include diarrhea, fever, abdominal pain or bloating, nausea, vomiting, and jaundice.

Infections recur frequently, especially in homosexual men with many sex partners. Some infections cause no symptoms but may have serious long-term complications, such as chronic hepatitis B or C.

SECTION 17

Skin Disorders

CHAPTER
185 Biology of the Skin

The skin is the body's largest organ. It serves many important functions, including regulating body temperature, maintaining water and electrolyte balance, and sensing painful and pleasant stimuli. The skin keeps vital chemicals and nutrients in the body while providing a barrier against dangerous substances from entering the body and provides a shield from the harmful effects of ultraviolet radiation emitted by the sun. In addition, skin color, texture, and folds help mark people as individuals. Anything that interferes with skin function or causes changes in appearance can have important consequences for physical and mental health.

Structure and Function

The skin has three layers—the epidermis, dermis, and fat layer (also called the subcutaneous layer). Each layer performs specific tasks.

Epidermis: The epidermis is the relatively thin, tough, outer layer of the skin. Most of the cells in the epidermis are keratinocytes. They originate from cells in the deepest layer of the epidermis called the basal layer. New keratinocytes slowly migrate up toward the surface of the epidermis. Once the keratinocytes reach the skin surface, they are gradually shed and are replaced by younger cells pushed up from below.

The outermost portion of the epidermis, known as the stratum corneum, is relatively waterproof and, when undamaged, prevents most bacteria, viruses, and other foreign substances from entering the body. The epidermis (along with other layers of the skin) also protects the internal organs, muscles, nerves, and blood vessels against trauma. In certain areas of the body that require greater protection (such as the palms of the hands and the soles of the feet), the outer keratin layer of the epidermis (stratum corneum) is much thicker.

Scattered throughout the basal layer of the epidermis are cells called melanocytes, which produce the pigment melanin, one of the main contributors to skin color. Melanin's primary function, however, is to filter out ultraviolet radiation from sunlight (see page 1326), which can damage DNA, resulting in numerous harmful effects, including skin cancer.

Getting Under the Skin

The skin has three layers. Beneath the surface of the skin are nerves, nerve endings, glands, hair follicles, and blood vessels.

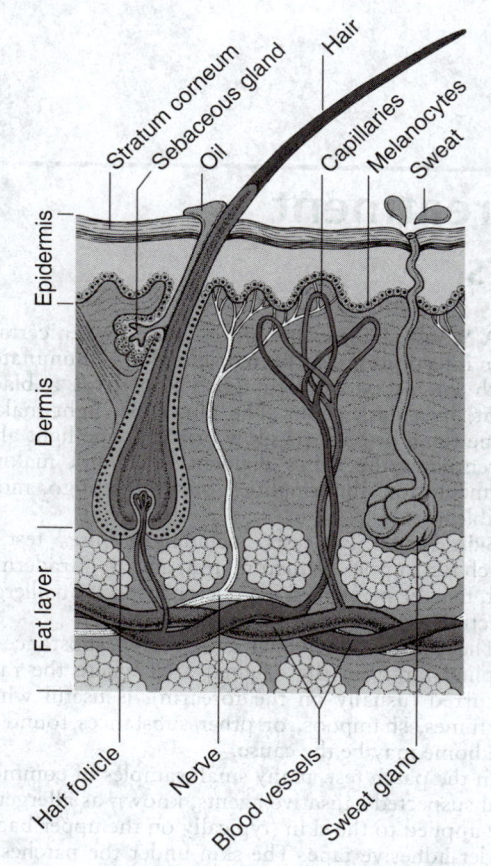

nerve endings than others. For example, the fingertips and toes contain many nerves and are extremely sensitive to touch.

The sweat glands produce sweat in response to heat and stress. Sweat is composed of water, salt, and other chemicals. As sweat evaporates off the skin, it helps cool the body. Specialized sweat glands in the armpits and the genital region (apocrine sweat glands) secrete a thick, oily sweat that produces a characteristic body odor when the sweat is digested by the skin bacteria in those areas.

The sebaceous glands secrete sebum into hair follicles. Sebum is an oil, that keeps the skin moist and soft and acts as a barrier against foreign substances.

The hair follicles produce the various types of hair found throughout the body. Hair not only contributes to a person's appearance but has a number of important physical roles, including regulating body temperature, providing protection from injury, and enhancing sensation. A portion of the follicle also contains stem cells capable of regrowing damaged epidermis.

The blood vessels of the dermis provide nutrients to the skin and help regulate body temperature. Heat makes the blood vessels enlarge (dilate), allowing large amounts of blood to circulate near the skin surface, where the heat can be released. Cold makes the blood vessels narrow (constrict), retaining the body's heat.

Over different parts of the body, the number of nerve endings, sweat glands and sebaceous glands, hair follicles, and blood vessels varies. The top of the head, for example, has many hair follicles, whereas the soles of the feet have none.

Fat Layer: Below the dermis lies a layer of fat that helps insulate the body from heat and cold, provides protective padding, and serves as an energy storage area. The fat is contained in living cells, called fat cells, held together by fibrous tissue. The fat layer varies in thickness, from a fraction of an inch on the eyelids to several inches on the abdomen and buttocks in some people.

Effects of Aging

Aging results in thinning of the dermis and epidermis. The underlying fat can be lost as well. The decrease in volume and overall effectiveness of all three skin layers results in a number of important medical and cosmetic effects. The skin loses some of its elasticity and becomes drier due to decreased production of essential oils such as sebum. The number of nerve endings in the skin decreases, so sensation is diminished. The number of sweat glands and blood vessels decreases as well, reducing the skin's ability to respond to heat exposure. The number of melanocytes tends to decrease with aging,

The epidermis also contains Langerhans' cells, which are part of the skin's immune system. Although these cells help detect foreign substances and defend the body against infection, they also play a role in the development of skin allergies.

Dermis: The dermis, the skin's next layer, is a thick layer of fibrous and elastic tissue (made mostly of collagen, elastin, and fibrillin) that gives the skin its flexibility and strength. The dermis contains nerve endings, sweat glands and oil (sebaceous) glands, hair follicles, and blood vessels.

The nerve endings sense pain, touch, pressure, and temperature. Some areas of the skin contain more so the skin has less protection against ultraviolet radiation. All of these changes make the skin more susceptible to damage and slower to heal.

Sun damage produces most of the skin changes that people commonly associate with aging (see page 1326). Long-term exposure to the ultraviolet radiation in sunlight is responsible for fine and coarse wrinkles, irregular pigmentation, brown and red spots, and the rough texture of sun-exposed skin.

CHAPTER

186 Diagnosis and Treatment of Skin Disorders

Many problems that appear on the skin are limited to the skin. Sometimes, however, the skin provides clues to a disorder that affects the entire body. Consequently, doctors often must consider many possible diseases when evaluating skin problems. They may need to order blood tests or other laboratory tests to look for an internal disease in people who come to them with a skin problem.

Diagnosis

Doctors can identify many skin disorders simply by looking at the skin. Revealing characteristics include size, shape, color, and location of the abnormality as well as the presence or absence of other symptoms or signs. To check the distribution of a skin problem, the doctor usually asks the person to undress completely, even though the person may have noticed an abnormality on only a small area of skin.

Sometimes, a biopsy, in which a small piece of skin is removed for examination under a microscope, must be performed. For this simple procedure, the doctor generally numbs a small area of skin with a local anesthetic and, using a small knife (scalpel), scissors, razor blade (shave biopsy), or round cutter (punch biopsy), removes a piece of skin the size of which is determined by the type of lesion, its location, and the type of tests to be performed.

When an infection (such as from fungi, bacteria, viruses, or mites) is suspected, a doctor may scrape off some material from the skin and examine it under a microscope (skin scraping), sometimes after applying special chemicals or stains. The material can also be sent to a laboratory, where the specimen is placed in a culture medium (a substance that allows microorganisms to grow). If the specimen contains bacteria, fungi, or viruses, they will often grow in the culture and can then be identified.

A Wood's light examination is used when certain skin infections are suspected. The skin is illuminated with an ultraviolet light (also known as a black light) in a dark room. The ultraviolet light makes some fungi or bacteria glow brightly. The light also accentuates the skin's pigment (melanin), making pigmentation abnormalities, such as vitiligo, more visible.

Skin Tests: Skin tests, including a "use" test, a patch test, a prick (puncture) test, and an intradermal test, may be performed if a doctor suspects an allergic reaction as the cause of a rash.

The use test, in which a suspected substance is applied far from the original area where the rash occurred (usually on the forearm), is useful when perfumes, shampoos, or other substances found in the home may be the cause.

In the patch test, many small samples of common and suspected causative agents, known as allergens, are applied to the skin (typically on the upper back) under adhesive tape. The skin under the patches is evaluated first after 48 hours, when the patches are removed, and then again at 96 hours. It often takes the skin several days to produce a visible reaction. If the substance produces a characteristic red, usually itchy rash, the person is probably allergic to it. Sometimes the substances produce an irritation that is not a true allergic reaction.

In the prick test, a drop of an extract of the suspected substance is placed on the skin. Then, the drop is pricked or punctured with a needle to introduce a very tiny amount of the substance into the skin. The skin is then observed for redness, hives, or both, which usually occur within 30 minutes.

In the intradermal test, tiny amounts of a substance are injected under the skin. The area is then watched for redness and swelling, which indicate an allergic reaction.

Medical Names for Marks and Growths on the Skin

Atrophic skin: Thinning of the skin that results in a depression and often has a wrinkled "cigarette paper" appearance.

Bulla: A fluid-filled spot (vesicle) larger than 1/5 inch (5 millimeters) in diameter.

Crust (scab): Dried blood, pus, or skin fluids on the surface of the skin. A crust can form wherever the skin has been damaged.

Cyst: A hollow lump in the skin that has a wall. The central hollow area may contain fluid or solid material.

Erosion: Loss of part or all of the top layers (epidermis) of the skin. Erosions occur when infection, pressure, irritation, or temperature has damaged the skin. They heal without scarring.

Excoriation: A hollowed-out or linear crusted area caused by scratching, rubbing, or picking at the skin.

Lesion: A general term for any abnormal mark or growth on the skin.

Lichenification: Thickened skin that has accentuated skinfolds or creases that appear as deep grooves and wrinkles. Lichenification is produced by prolonged scratching or rubbing.

Macule: A flat, discolored spot of any shape about 1/5 inch (5 millimeters) or less in diameter. Freckles, flat moles, port-wine stains, and many rashes are macular. A patch is a large macule.

Nodule: A solid raised area—deeper and easier to feel than a papule—that is usually round. A nodule sometimes appears to form below the surface of the skin and press upward.

Papule: A solid bump about 1/5 inch (5 millimeters) or less in diameter. Warts, insect bites, skin tags, and some skin cancers are papules.

Plaque: A flat, raised area or group of small bumps (papules) typically more than 1/5 inch (5 millimeters) in diameter.

Pustule: A fluid-filled spot (vesicle) containing pus.

Scales: Areas of heaped-up, dead epidermal cells, producing a flaky, dry patch. Scales occur with psoriasis, seborrheic dermatitis, and many other disorders.

Scar: An area where normal skin has been replaced by fibrous (scar-forming) tissue. Scars form after destruction of some part of the dermis.

Telangiectasia: Dilated blood vessels near the surface of the skin that often have a twisted appearance and that whiten (blanch) when pressure is applied.

Ulcer: Similar to an erosion, only deeper, penetrating at least part of the dermis. The causes are the same as for erosions. They heal with scarring.

Vesicle: A small, fluid-filled spot 1/5 inch (5 millimeters) or smaller in diameter. A bulla is a vesicle larger than 5 millimeters in diameter. Herpes zoster (shingles), chickenpox, burns, allergic reactions, and irritations form vesicles and bullae.

Wheal (hive): Swelling in the skin that produces an elevated, soft, spongy area that appears relatively suddenly and then almost always disappears within 24 hours. Wheals are common allergic reactions to drugs, insect bites, or something that touches the skin.

Although rare, prick and intradermal tests can cause a severe allergic reaction, known as anaphylaxis, which can be life threatening. Therefore, these types of tests should be performed only by a trained health care practitioner.

Treatment

Topical drugs (drugs applied directly to the skin) are a mainstay of treating skin disorders. Systemic drugs are taken by mouth or given by injection and are distributed throughout the body. Rarely, when a high concentration of a drug is needed at the affected area, a doctor injects the drug just under the skin (intradermal injection).

Topical Preparations

The active ingredient, or drug, in a topical preparation is mixed with an inactive ingredient (vehicle). The vehicle determines the consistency of the product (for example, thick and greasy or light and watery) and whether the active ingredient remains on the surface or penetrates the skin. Depending on the vehicle used, the same drug can be placed in an ointment, cream, lotion, solution, gel, oil, foam, or powder. In addition, many preparations are available in different strengths (concentrations).

Ointments (such as petroleum jelly) are oily and contain very little water. They are messy, greasy, and difficult to wash off. Ointments are most appropriate when the skin needs lubrication or moisture. Ointments are usually better than creams at delivering active ingredients into the skin. A given concentration of a drug is more potent in an ointment than in a cream. Ointments are less irritating than creams and much less irritating than gels, lotions, and solutions for open wounds such as erosions or ulcers.

Creams, the most commonly used preparations, are emulsions of oil in water, meaning they are primarily water with an oil component. (An ointment is the opposite, some water mixed mostly with oil.) Creams are easy to apply and appear to vanish when rubbed into the skin. They are relatively non-irritating.

Lotions are similar to creams but contain more water. They are actually suspensions of finely dispersed, powdered material in a base of water or oil and water. They are less effective than ointments, creams, and gels at delivering drugs and are considered of lower potency for a given drug concentration. Lotions have a number of beneficial effects. They are easy to apply to hairy skin, and they are particularly useful for cooling or drying inflamed or oozing lesions, such as those caused by contact dermatitis, athlete's foot (tinea pedis), and jock itch (tinea cruris).

Baths and soaks are used when treatment must be applied to large areas of the body. This technique is most often used in the form of sitz baths for over-the-counter (OTC) treatments of mild skin problems such as hemorrhoids. Baths are not often used to apply potent prescription drugs because of difficulties controlling the amount of drug delivered.

Solutions are liquids in which a drug is dissolved. The most commonly used liquids are alcohol, propylene glycol, polyethylene glycol, and plain water. Solutions are convenient to apply but tend to dry rather than moisturize the skin. However, this drying effect is useful for wet, oozing (weeping) skin disorders. Depending on the vehicle used, solutions can be irritating to the skin, particularly when those containing alcohol and propylene glycol are applied to open wounds.

Powders are dried forms of substances that are used to protect areas where skin rubs against skin—for instance, between the toes or buttocks, in the armpits or groin, or under the breasts. Powders are used on skin that has been softened and damaged by moisture (macerated). They may be mixed with active drugs such as antifungals.

Gels are water- or alcohol-based substances thickened without oil or fat. The skin does not absorb gels as well as it absorbs preparations containing oil or fat. Gels tend to be quite irritating on open wounds and diseased skin.

Types of Topical Drugs

Topical drugs can be divided into several overlapping categories: cleansing agents, protective agents, moisturizing agents, drying agents, anti-itch agents, anti-inflammatory agents, anti-infective agents, and keratolytics.

Cleansing Agents: The principal cleansing agents are soaps, detergents, and solvents (a liquid substance capable of dissolving other substances). Soap is the most popular cleanser, but detergents are used as well. Certain soaps dry the skin; others have a creamy base that is less drying.

Because baby shampoos are excellent cleansing agents and are usually gentle to the skin, they are good for cleansing wounds, cuts, and abrasions. Also, people who have psoriasis, eczema, and other scaling diseases can use baby shampoos to wash away dead scaly skin. Oozing lesions, however, should generally be cleansed only with water and gentle soaps because detergents and harsher soaps can irritate the area.

Many chemicals are added to cleansing agents. For example, some soaps have antibacterial substances added to them. Antibacterial soap does not improve hygiene or prevent disease, and routine use may disrupt the normal balance of bacteria on the skin. Antidandruff shampoos and lotions may contain zinc dipyrithione, selenium sulfide, or tar extracts to help treat flaking skin, eczema, and psoriasis of the scalp.

Water is the main solvent for cleansing. Other solvents include petroleum jelly, which can cleanse the skin of material that cannot be dissolved with soap and water, such as tar. Small amounts of alcohol can safely be used to cleanse the skin before injections or blood drawing. Alcohol gels are useful for routine hand hygiene when handwashing is not possible. Other solvents, such as acetone (nail polish remover), gasoline, and paint thinner, are rarely used for skin cleansing. These solvents dissolve the skin's natural oils, causing significant drying and irritation. They may also be absorbed through the skin, resulting in poisoning.

Protective Agents: Many different kinds of preparations help protect the skin. Oils and ointments supply an oil-based barrier that can help protect scraped or irritated skin and retain moisture. Powders may protect skin that rubs against skin or clothing. Synthetic hydrocolloid dressings protect pressure sores (bedsores, decubitus ulcers) and other areas of raw skin. Sunscreens and sunblocks reflect, absorb, or filter out harmful ultraviolet light.

Moisturizing Agents: Moisturizers (emollients) restore and help maintain water and oils in the skin. The best time to apply a moisturizer is when the skin is already moistened—immediately after a bath or shower, for instance. Moisturizers typically contain glycerin, mineral oil, or petrolatum and are available as lotions, creams, ointments, and bath oils. Some stronger moisturizers contain compounds such as urea, lactic acid, and glycolic acid.

Drying Agents: Excessive moisture in areas where skin rubs against skin can cause irritation and skin breakdown (maceration), particularly in body folds where the environment tends to be warmer and moister. The areas most commonly affected are between the toes or buttocks, in the armpits or groin, and under the breasts and abdominal skin folds. These warm moist areas also provide fertile breeding grounds for infections, especially with fungi and bacteria.

Talcum powder is the most commonly used drying agent. Talc absorbs moisture from the skin surface. Most of the many talc preparations vary only in their scents and packaging. Cornstarch is another good drying agent. Talc is usually preferred, except for babies, because babies can accidentally inhale the powder, and cornstarch is less dangerous to breathe than talc.

Solutions containing aluminum salts are drying agents commonly found in OTC antiperspirants. Prescription doses of aluminum salts are available to treat excessive sweating.

Astringents are liquid drying agents that narrow blood vessels. The most commonly used astringent solutions contain aluminum acetate (Burow's solution or Domeboro's solution). Usually applied with dressings or as soaks, astringents are used to treat infectious eczema, oozing skin lesions, and pressure sores. Witch hazel is also a popular OTC astringent.

Anti-Itch Agents: Skin disease is often accompanied by itching. Itching and mild pain can sometimes be controlled with soothing agents such as chamomile, eucalyptus, camphor, menthol, zinc oxide, talc, glycerin, and calamine. These are available as OTC preparations.

Antihistamines, which block certain types of allergic reactions, are sometimes included in topical preparations to relieve the itching associated with allergic reactions. Doxepin is an effective topical antihistamine for many conditions. However, the antihistamine diphenhydramine (common in many nonprescription topical preparations) can trigger an allergic reaction when applied to the skin and is usually not recommended. Taking antihistamines by mouth does not seem to produce this type of reaction, so oral rather than topical antihistamines are preferred to relieve itching.

Anti-Inflammatory Agents: Corticosteroids are the main topical drugs used to relieve inflammation (swelling, itching, and redness) of the skin. Corticosteroids are most effective for rashes caused by allergic or inflammatory reactions to things such as poison ivy, metals, cloth, drugs, eczema, and many others. Because they lower resistance to bacterial and fungal infections and inhibit wound healing, corticosteroids usually should not be used on infected areas or wounds. For acne-like disorders, topical corticosteroids tend to not work very well and sometimes instead induce an acne-like eruption. Corticosteroids are sometimes mixed with antifungal drugs to help reduce redness and itching while simultaneously eradicating the fungus.

Topical corticosteroids are sold as lotions, creams, ointments, solutions, foams, oils, and gels. Creams are most effective if rubbed in gently until they vanish. In general, ointments are the most potent. The type and concentration of corticosteroid in the preparation determines the overall strength. Hydrocortisone is available in concentrations of up to 1% without a prescription; concentrations of 0.5% or less offer little benefit. Stronger corticosteroid preparations require a prescription. Doctors usually prescribe potent

corticosteroids first, then less potent corticosteroids as the disorder improves. Generally, topical corticosteroids are applied 2 to 3 times a day in a thin layer, but high-potency formulations may be applied only once a day.

Corticosteroids should be used with caution on areas where the skin is thin, such as the face, and on areas of natural occlusion, such as the armpits and groin. Doctors usually use low-potency corticosteroids on these sensitive areas for no more than a few days to a week (see box on page 568). Prolonged use (more than 1 month) in any area can cause skin breakdown, stretch marks, acne-like eruptions, and sometimes an allergic skin reaction (contact dermatitis) to the corticosteroid itself. Perioral dermatitis (a red, bumpy rash around the mouth, chin, and sometimes the eyes) occurs more commonly with mid-potency or high-potency formulations used on the face and less commonly with mild formulations. High-potency formulations may inhibit adrenal gland functions when used in children, when used over large areas of skin, or when used for long periods of time, especially if used under occlusive dressings.

When a stronger dose of topical corticosteroid is needed for one spot or a small area that does not respond to treatment, a doctor may inject the corticosteroid just under the skin or occasionally apply plastic tape infused with the corticosteroid flurandrenolide. Another way to deliver a strong dose is to apply a thin plastic film, such as household plastic wrap, over the topical corticosteroid (occlusive dressing). The plastic film increases the drug's absorption and effectiveness and is usually left on overnight. Such dressings are usually reserved for disorders such as severe psoriasis and eczema. Risks of using corticosteroids under an occlusive dressing include development of prickly heat (miliaria), skin thinning (atrophy), stretch marks (striae), dilated red blood vessels on the surface of the skin (telangiectasias), and bacterial or fungal infections.

Several allegedly anti-inflammatory herbal products are commonly used in commercial products, although their effectiveness has not been well established. Herbal and "natural" products are often not standardized and commonly cause allergic and irritant reactions of the skin. Among the most popular are chamomile and calendula.

Tar Preparations: Tar preparations, which are byproducts of coal manufacturing, slow skin cell division and are useful in treating disorders that cause excess skin production (scaling) such as psoriasis. Side effects include irritation, inflammation of follicles (folliculitis), staining of clothes and furniture, and sensitivity to sunlight (photosensitization). They should not be used on infected skin.

Anti-Infective Agents: Viruses, bacteria, fungi, and parasites can all infect the skin. By far, the best way to prevent such infections is by carefully washing the skin with soap and water. Stronger disinfecting agents are commonly used by nurses and doctors to disinfect their hands to prevent spreading infections to patients. Antibacterial preparations or "preps" are used on the skin before surgery to lower the number of bacteria on the skin and thereby prevent postoperative infections. Once a skin infection has occurred, it may be treated with topical or systemic drugs depending on the severity and type of infection diagnosed or suspected. Topical anti-infective agents include antibiotics, antifungals, and insecticides.

Topical antibiotics have few uses. Clindamycin and erythromycin are sometimes used as primary or additional treatment for acne. Mupirocin can be used to treat impetigo (a staphylococcal infection of the skin). Nonprescription antibiotics such as bacitracin and polymyxin are often used in postoperative care of a skin biopsy site and to prevent infection in scrapes, minor burns, and abrasions. Although considered generally quite safe, topical antibiotics do have some side effects. For example, neomycin (a common ingredient in nonprescription antibiotic ointments) frequently causes an allergic reaction.

Topical antifungals work quite well for treating a wide variety of fungal infections of the skin (such as ringworm and athlete's foot). However, these topical drugs work poorly for treating fungal infections of the nails. Typically, nail infections are treated with oral antifungals (usually terbinafine), but relapse is very common even when oral drugs are taken.

Insecticides (such as permethrin and malathion) are used to treat lice infestations and scabies.

Non-antibiotic topical antiseptics include iodine solutions (such as povidone iodine and clioquinol), gentian violet, silver preparations (such as silver nitrate and silver sulfadiazine), and zinc pyrithione. Iodine is used to prepare the skin for surgery. Gentian violet is used when an inexpensive and chemically and physically stable antiseptic, antimicrobial, or both is needed. Silver preparations (such as silver sulfadiazine) are effective in treating burns and ulcers and have strong antimicrobial properties; several wound dressings are infused with silver. Zinc pyrithione is an antifungal and a common ingredient in shampoos that treat dandruff caused by an overgrowth of a common skin fungus. Healing wounds should usually not be treated with topical antiseptics other than silver because they are irritating and tend to kill fragile regrowth (granulation tissue).

Keratolytics: Keratolytics are agents that soften skin cells and ease the flaking and peeling process. Examples include salicylic acid and urea.

Salicylic acid in varying concentrations is used to treat psoriasis, seborrheic dermatitis, acne, and warts. Side effects are common and include burning, irritation, and systemic toxicity if large areas of skin are covered. Salicylic acid should rarely be used in children and infants.

Urea can be used to moisturize, sooth itching, and reduce scaling. It is commonly used to treat excessive skin build up on the soles of the feet (plantar keratodermas and calluses), keratosis pilaris (dry bumps on thighs and back of arms in people with allergies), and severe dry skin (ichthyosis). Side effects are irritation and burning. Urea should not be applied to large areas of skin.

Dressings

Dressings protect open wounds, facilitate healing, increase drug absorption, and protect clothing. Dressings are nonocclusive (air can reach the wound) or occlusive (wounds are covered and sealed from contact with air).

Nonocclusive Dressings: The most common nonocclusive dressings are gauze dressings. They maximally allow air to reach the wound and allow the wound to dry. Nonocclusive dressings wetted with solution, usually saline, are used to help cleanse and remove (debride) thickened, crusted, or dead tissue. The dressings are applied wet and removed after the solution has evaporated (wet-to-dry dressings). The dried materials stick to the dressing.

Occlusive Dressings: Occlusive dressings increase the absorption, potency, and effectiveness (and side effects) of topical drugs. Transparent impermeable films such as polyethylene (plastic household wrap) or flexible, transparent, semi-permeable dressings are the most common types of occlusive dressings. Hydrocolloid dressings are used to speed the healing of skin ulcers. Zinc oxide gelatin (Unna's paste boot) is an effective occlusive dressing for skin inflammation and ulcers of the lower legs (which can occur in stasis dermatitis). Occlusive dressings are sometimes recommended for treating severe psoriasis, atopic dermatitis, skin lesions of lupus erythematosus, and chronic hand dermatitis, among other conditions.

Other occlusive dressings are used to protect and help heal burns. Doctors have recently discovered that other types of open wounds also heal faster and more completely when kept moist and under an occlusive dressing. These dressings help maintain a proper level of moisture and provide a framework on which new skin can regrow. Such dressings include sophisticated commercial products as well as plain petroleum jelly or an antibiotic ointment under a bandage.

Itching and rashes may develop as the result of infection or irritation or from a reaction of the immune system. Some rashes occur mostly in children (see page 1734), whereas others almost always occur in adults. Sometimes an immune reaction is triggered by substances a person touches or eats, but many times doctors do not know why the immune system reacts to produce a rash.

The diagnosis of most noninfectious rashes is based on the appearance of the rash. The cause of a rash cannot be determined by blood tests, and tests of any kind are rarely performed. However, persistent rashes, particularly those that do not respond to treatment, may lead the doctor to perform a skin biopsy, in which a small piece of skin is surgically removed for examination under a microscope. Also, if the doctor suspects a contact allergy as the cause, skin tests may be performed (see page 1278).

Itching

Itching (pruritus) is a sensation that instinctively demands scratching.

- Skin disorders, certain diseases, drugs, pregnancy, dry skin, contact with irritants, and scratching can cause itching.
- Typical symptoms include dry skin, flaking, scaling, and visible insect bites.
- The diagnosis is based on symptoms, allergy skin testing, blood tests, stoppage of drugs, or sometimes a biopsy or skin scraping.
- Brief bathing in lukewarm water, moisturizers, antihistamines, corticosteroid creams, and certain types of drugs can relieve itching.

Itching may be caused by a skin disorder or by a disease that affects the whole body (systemic disease). Skin disorders that cause severe itching include infestations with parasites (such as scabies, mites, or lice), insect bites, hives, atopic dermatitis, and allergic dermatitis and contact dermatitis. These disorders usually also produce a rash. Systemic diseases that can cause itching include liver disease, kidney failure, lymphomas, leukemias and other blood disorders, and, occasionally, thyroid disease, diabetes, and cancer. However, itching from these diseases usually does not result in a rash.

Many drugs can cause itching, including barbiturates, morphine, and aspirin, as well as any drug to which a person has an allergy.

Itching is also common during the later months of pregnancy. Usually, pregnancy-related itching does not indicate any abnormality, but it can result from mild liver problems.

Often, contact with wool clothing or irritants, such as solvents or cosmetics, causes itching. Dry skin (xerosis), which is especially common among older people, can cause severe, widespread itching. Dry skin also can result from cold weather or prolonged exposure to water. Hot baths typically worsen itching.

The act of scratching can itself irritate the skin and lead to more itching, creating an itching-scratching-itching cycle. Vigorous scratching may cause redness and deep scrapes in the skin. In some people, even gentle scratching causes raised, red streaks that can itch intensely. Prolonged scratching and rubbing can thicken and scar the skin.

Diagnosis

Doctors try to determine the cause of itching to eliminate it. Often, the cause is obvious, such as an insect bite or poison ivy. Itching that lasts longer than a few days or that comes and goes frequently without an obvious cause usually requires testing. If an allergy is suspected, skin tests may be performed (see pages 1113 and 1278). If a systemic disease is suspected, blood tests are usually performed to check liver function, kidney function, and blood sugar levels. The number of eosinophils, a type of white blood cell, may be checked as well, because a high number may indicate an allergic reaction. Sometimes, the doctor may have a person discontinue one or more drugs to see whether the itching is relieved. A biopsy, in which a small piece of skin is surgically removed for examination under a microscope, or skin scraping (see page 1278) may help identify the cause, including an infectious one.

Treatment

For itching of any cause, bathing should be kept brief and preferably in cool or lukewarm water with very little or no soap. The skin should be patted dry gently rather than rubbed vigorously. Many people with itching benefit from an over-the-counter moisturizing cream applied right after bathing. The moisturizer should be odorless and colorless, because additives that provide color or scent may irritate the skin and may even cause itching. Fingernails, especially children's, should be kept short to minimize abrasions from scratching. Coating the affected area with soothing compounds, such as menthol, camphor, chamomile, eucalyptus, or calamine, also may help.

When the Skin Is Dry

Normal skin owes its soft, pliable texture to its water content. To help protect against water loss, the outer layer of skin contains oil, which slows evaporation and holds moisture in the deeper layers of skin. If the oil is depleted, the skin becomes dry.

Dry skin (xerosis) is common, especially among people past middle age. Common causes are cold weather and frequent bathing. Bathing washes away surface oils, allowing the skin to dry out. Dry skin may become irritated and often itches—sometimes it sloughs off in small flakes and scales. Scaling most often affects the lower legs. Rubbing or scratching dry skin can lead to infection and scarring.

A form of severe dry skin is called ichthyosis. Ichthyosis can be an inherited disorder or can result from a number of other medical problems, such as an underactive thyroid gland, lymphoma, and AIDS.

The key to treating simple dry skin is keeping the skin moist. Taking fewer baths allows protective oils to remain on the skin. Moisturizing ointments or creams containing petroleum jelly, mineral oil, or glycerin also can hold water in the skin. Harsh soaps, detergents, and the perfumes in some moisturizers irritate the skin and may further dry it.

When scaling is a problem, solutions or creams containing salicylic or lactic acid or urea may help remove the scales. For some forms of severe ichthyosis, creams containing substances related to vitamin A, such as tretinoin, help the skin shed excessive scales.

Taking antihistamines by mouth may decrease itching. Some antihistamines, such as hydroxyzine and diphenhydramine, usually cause sleepiness and dry mouth and are mainly used at bedtime. Other antihistamines, such as loratadine and cetirizine, usually do not cause sleepiness. Generally, creams containing antihistamines (such as diphenhydramine) should not be used, because they themselves can cause an allergic reaction.

Corticosteroid creams decrease inflammation and control itching and may be used when itching is limited to a small area. Itching from some conditions, such as poison ivy, may require high-strength corticosteroid creams. However, only mild corticosteroids, such as 1% hydrocortisone, should be applied to the face, because stronger corticosteroids may thin the sensitive skin in this area. Also, powerful corticosteroid creams applied over large areas or for a long time can cause serious medical problems, especially in infants, because these drugs are absorbed into the bloodstream. Corticosteroids taken by mouth are sometimes used when large areas of the body are involved.

Specific treatments may be needed. For example, when fungal, parasitic, or bacterial infections cause itching, topical or systemic drugs may be required. Topical drugs are applied directly to the affected area of the skin. Systemic drugs are taken by mouth or are injected and are distributed throughout the body.

Dermatitis

Dermatitis (eczema) is inflammation of the upper layers of the skin, causing itching, blisters, redness, swelling, and often oozing, scabbing, and scaling.

- Known causes include contact with a particular substance, certain drugs, varicose veins, constant scratching, and fungal infection.
- Typical symptoms include a red itchy rash, blisters, pimples, open sores, oozing, crusting, and scaling.
- The diagnosis is typically based on symptoms and confirmed by results of patch tests or skin samples or the presence of suspected drugs, irritants, or infection.
- Avoiding known irritants and allergens reduces the risk of dermatitis.
- Treatment depends on the cause and the specific symptoms.

Dermatitis is a broad term covering many different disorders that all result in a red, itchy rash. The term eczema is sometimes used for dermatitis. Some types of dermatitis affect only specific parts of the body, whereas others can occur anywhere. Some types of dermatitis have a known cause, whereas others do not. However, dermatitis is always the skin's way of reacting to severe dryness, scratching, an irritating substance, or an allergen. Typically, that substance comes in direct contact with the skin, but sometimes the substance is swallowed. In all cases, continuous scratching and rubbing may eventually lead to thickening and hardening of the skin.

Dermatitis may be a brief reaction to a substance. In such cases, it may cause symptoms, such as itching and redness, for just a few hours or for only a day or two. Chronic dermatitis persists over a period of time. The hands and feet are particularly vulnerable to chronic dermatitis, because the hands are in frequent contact with many foreign substances and the feet are in the warm, moist conditions created by socks and shoes that favor fungal growth.

Chronic dermatitis may represent a contact, fungal, or other dermatitis that has been inadequately diagnosed or treated, or it may be one of several chronic skin disorders of unknown origin. Because chronic dermatitis produces cracks and blisters in the skin, any type of chronic dermatitis may lead to bacterial infection.

CONTACT DERMATITIS

Contact dermatitis is skin inflammation caused by direct contact with a particular substance. The rash is very itchy, is confined to a specific area, and often has clearly defined boundaries.

Substances can cause skin inflammation by one of two mechanisms—irritation (irritant contact dermatitis) or allergic reaction (allergic contact dermatitis).

Irritant contact dermatitis, which accounts for 80% of all cases of contact dermatitis, occurs when a chemical substance causes direct damage to the skin; symptoms are more painful than itchy. Typical irritating substances are acids, alkalis (such as drain cleaners), solvents (such as acetone in nail polish remover), strong soaps, and plants (such as poinsettias and peppers). Some of these chemicals cause skin changes within a few minutes, whereas others require longer exposure. People vary in the sensitivity of their skin to irritants. Even very mild soaps and detergents may irritate the skin of some people after frequent or prolonged contact.

Allergic contact dermatitis is a reaction by the body's immune system to a substance contacting the skin. Sometimes a person can be sensitized by only one exposure, and other times sensitization occurs only after many exposures to a substance. After a person is sensitized, the next exposure causes itching and dermatitis within 4 to 24 hours, although some people, particularly older people, do not develop a reaction for 3 to 4 days.

Thousands of substances can result in allergic contact dermatitis. The most common include substances found in plants such as poison ivy, rubber (latex), antibiotics, fragrances, preservatives, and some metals (such as nickel and cobalt). About 10% of women are allergic to nickel, a common component of jewelry. People may use (or be exposed to) substances for years without a problem, then suddenly develop an allergic reaction. Even ointments, creams, and lotions used to treat dermatitis can cause such a reaction. People may also develop dermatitis from many of the materials they touch while at work (occupational dermatitis).

Sometimes contact dermatitis results only after a person touches certain substances and then exposes the skin to sunlight (photoallergic or phototoxic contact dermatitis). Such substances include sunscreens, aftershave lotions, certain perfumes, antibiotics, coal tar, and oils.

Symptoms and Diagnosis

Regardless of cause or type, contact dermatitis results in itching and a rash. The itching is usually severe, but the rash varies from a mild, short-lived

---

Common Causes of Allergic Contact Dermatitis

Cosmetics: Hair-removing chemicals, hair dyes, nail polish, nail polish remover, deodorants, moisturizers, aftershave lotions, perfumes, sunscreens

Metal compound (in jewelry): Nickel

Plants: Poison ivy, poison oak, poison sumac, ragweed, primrose, thistle

Drugs in skin creams: Antibiotics (sulfonamides, neomycin), antihistamines (diphenhydramine, promethazine), anesthetics (benzocaine), antiseptics (thimerosal), stabilizers

Chemicals used in clothing manufacturing: Tanning agents in shoes; rubber accelerators and antioxidants in gloves, shoes, undergarments, other apparel

---

redness to severe swelling and large blisters. Most commonly, the rash contains tiny blisters. The rash develops only in areas contacted by the substance. However, the rash appears earlier in thin, sensitive areas of skin, and later in areas of thicker skin or on skin that had less contact with the substance, giving the impression that the rash has spread. Touching the rash or blister fluid cannot spread contact dermatitis to other people or to other parts of the body that did not make contact with the substance.

Determining the cause of contact dermatitis is not always easy. The person's occupation, hobbies, household duties, vacations, clothing, topical drug use, cosmetics, and household members' activities must be considered. Most people are unaware of all the substances that touch their skin. Often, the location of the initial rash is an important clue, particularly if it occurs under an item of clothing or jewelry or only in areas exposed to sunlight. However, many substances that people touch with their hands are unknowingly transferred to the face, where the more sensitive facial skin may react even if the hands do not.

The "use test," in which a suspected substance is applied far from the original area of contact dermatitis (usually on the forearm), is useful when perfumes, shampoos, or other substances used in the home are suspected.

If a doctor suspects contact dermatitis and a process of elimination does not pinpoint the cause, patch testing can be performed. For this test, small patches containing substances that commonly cause dermatitis are placed on the skin for 1 to 2 days to see whether a rash develops beneath one of them. Although useful, patch testing is complicated. People may be sensitive to many substances, and the substance they react to on a patch may not be the cause of their dermatitis. A doctor must decide which substances to test based on what a person might have been exposed to.

Poison Ivy Dermatitis

About 50 to 70% of people are sensitive to the plant oil urushiol contained in poison ivy, poison oak, and poison sumac. Similar oils are also present in the shells of cashew nuts; the leaves, sap, and fruit skin of the mango; and Japanese lacquer. Once a person has been sensitized by contact with these oils, subsequent exposure produces a contact dermatitis.

The oils are quickly absorbed into the skin but may remain active on clothing, tools, and pet fur for long periods of time. Smoke from burning plants also contains the oil and may cause a reaction in certain people. Sensitivity to poison ivy tends to run in families.

Symptoms begin 8 to 48 hours after contact and consist of intense itching, a red rash, and multiple blisters, which may be tiny or very large. Typically, the blisters occur in a straight line following the track where the plant brushed along the skin. The rash may appear at different times in different locations either because of repeat contact with contaminated clothing and other objects or because some parts of the skin are more sensitive than others. The blister fluid itself is not contagious. The itching and rash last for 2 to 3 weeks.

Recognition and avoidance of contact with the plants is the best prevention. A number of commercial barrier creams and lotions can be applied before exposure to minimize, but not completely prevent, absorption of oil by the skin. The oil can soak through latex rubber gloves. Washing the skin with soap and water prevents absorption of the oil if done immediately. Stronger solvents, such as acetone, alcohol, and various commercial products, are probably no more effective. Desensitization with various shots or pills or by eating poison ivy leaves is not effective.

Treatment helps relieve symptoms but does not shorten the duration of the rash. The most effective treatment is with corticosteroids. Small areas of rash are treated with strong topical corticosteroids (drugs applied to the skin), such as triamcinolone, clobetasol, or diflorasone—except on the face and genitals, where only mild corticosteroids, such as 1% hydrocortisone, should be applied. People with large areas of rash or significant facial swelling are given high-dose corticosteroids taken by mouth. Cool compresses wet with water or aluminum acetate may be used on large blistered areas. Antihistamines given by mouth may help with itching. Lotions and creams containing antihistamines are seldom used.

Prevention and Treatment

Contact dermatitis can be prevented by avoiding contact with the causative substance. If contact does occur, the material should be washed off immediately with soap and water. If circumstances risk ongoing exposure, gloves and protective clothing may be helpful. Barrier creams are also available that can block certain substances, such as poison ivy and epoxy resins, from contacting the skin. Desensitization with injections or tablets of the causative substance is not effective in preventing contact dermatitis.

Treatment is not effective until there is no further contact with the substance causing the problem. Once the substance is removed, the redness usually disappears after a week. Blisters may continue to ooze and form crusts, but they soon dry. Residual scaling, itching, and temporary thickening of the skin may last for days or weeks.

Itching can be relieved with a number of topical drugs or drugs taken by mouth (see page 1283). In addition, small areas of dermatitis can be soothed by applying pieces of gauze or thin cloth dipped in cool water or aluminum acetate (Burow's solution) several times a day for an hour. Larger areas may be treated with short, cool tub baths with or without colloidal oatmeal. The doctor may drain fluid from a large blister, but the blister is not removed.

ATOPIC DERMATITIS

Atopic dermatitis is chronic, itchy inflammation of the upper layers of the skin that often develops in people who have hay fever or asthma and in people who have family members with these conditions.

Atopic dermatitis is one of the most common skin diseases, affecting between 9% and 30% of children or adolescents in the United States. Almost 66% of people with the disorder develop it before age 1, and 90% by age 5. In half of these people, the disorder will be gone by the adolescent years, whereas in others it is lifelong.

Doctors do not know what causes atopic dermatitis, but people who have it usually have many allergic disorders, particularly asthma, hay fever, and food allergies. The relationship between the dermatitis and these disorders is not clear because atopic dermatitis is not an allergy to a particular substance. Atopic dermatitis is not contagious.

Many conditions can make atopic dermatitis worse, including emotional stress, changes in temperature or humidity, bacterial skin infections, and contact with irritating clothing (especially wool). In some infants, food allergies may provoke atopic dermatitis.

Symptoms

Infants may develop red, oozing, crusted rashes on the face, scalp, diaper area, hands, arms, feet, or legs.

Large areas of the body may be affected. In older children and adults, the rash often occurs (and recurs) in only one or a few spots, especially on the hands, upper arms, in front of the elbows, or behind the knees.

Although the color, intensity, and location of the rash vary, the rash always itches. The itching often leads to uncontrollable scratching, triggering a cycle of itching-scratching-itching that makes the problem worse. Scratching and rubbing can also tear the skin, leaving an opening for bacteria to enter and cause infections.

In people with atopic dermatitis, infection with the herpes simplex virus, which in other people usually affects a small area with tiny, slightly painful blisters (see page 1245), may produce a serious illness with widespread dermatitis, blistering, and high fever (eczema herpeticum).

Diagnosis and Treatment

A doctor makes the diagnosis based on the typical pattern of the rash and often on whether other family members have allergies.

No cure exists, but itching can be relieved with topical drugs or drugs taken by mouth (see page 1283). Certain other measures can help. Avoiding contact with substances known to irritate the skin or foods that the person is sensitive to can prevent a rash. The skin should be kept moist, either with commercial moisturizers or with petroleum jelly or vegetable oil. Moisturizers are best applied immediately after bathing, while the skin is damp.

Specific treatments include applying a corticosteroid ointment or cream. To limit the use of corticosteroids in people being treated for long periods, doctors sometimes replace the corticosteroids with petroleum jelly for a week or more at a time. Ointments or creams containing an immune system–modulating drug, such as tacrolimus or pimecrolimus, also are helpful and can limit the need for long-term corticosteroid use. Some doctors prescribe such drugs first. Corticosteroid tablets are a last resort for people with stubborn cases.

Phototherapy (exposure to ultraviolet light) may help adults (see box on page 1294). This treatment is rarely recommended for children because of its potential long-term side effects, including skin cancer and cataracts.

For severe cases, the immune system can be suppressed with cyclosporine, azathioprine, or mycophenolate mofetil taken by mouth, or injections of interferon-gamma.

SEBORRHEIC DERMATITIS

Seborrheic dermatitis is chronic inflammation that causes yellow, greasy scales to form on the scalp and face and occasionally on other areas.

The cause is unknown. Seborrheic dermatitis occurs most often in infants, usually within the first 3 months of life, and in those aged 30 to 70 years. The disorder is more common among men, often runs in families, and is worse in cold weather. A form of seborrheic dermatitis also occurs in as many as 85% of people with AIDS.

Symptoms

Seborrheic dermatitis usually begins gradually, causing dry or greasy scaling of the scalp (dandruff), sometimes with itching but without hair loss. In more severe cases, yellowish to reddish scaly pimples appear along the hairline, behind the ears, in the ear canal, on the eyebrows, on the bridge of the nose, around the nose, on the chest, and on the upper back. In infants younger than 1 month of age, seborrheic dermatitis may produce a thick, yellow, crusted scalp rash (cradle cap) and sometimes yellow scaling behind the ears and red pimples on the face. Frequently, a stubborn diaper rash accompanies the scalp rash. Older children and adults may develop a thick, tenacious, scaly rash with large flakes of skin.

Treatment

The scalp can be treated with a shampoo containing pyrithione zinc, selenium sulfide, an antifungal drug, salicylic acid and sulfur, or tar. The person usually uses the medicated shampoo every other day until the dermatitis is controlled and then twice weekly. Ketoconazole cream is often effective as well. In adults, thick crusts and scales, if present, can be loosened with overnight application of corticosteroids or salicylic acid under a shower cap.

Often, treatment must be continued for many weeks. If the dermatitis returns after the treatment is discontinued, treatment can be restarted. Topical corticosteroids are also used on the head and other affected areas. On the face, only mild corticosteroids, such as 1% hydrocortisone, should be used. Even mild corticosteroids must be used cautiously, because long-term use can thin the skin and cause other problems.

In infants and young children who have a thick scaly rash on the scalp, 2% salicylic acid in mineral oil can be rubbed gently into the rash with a soft toothbrush at bedtime. The scalp can also be shampooed daily with mild baby shampoo, and 1% hydrocortisone cream can be rubbed into the scalp.

NUMMULAR DERMATITIS

Nummular dermatitis is a persistent, usually itchy, rash and inflammation characterized by coin-shaped spots, often with tiny blisters, scabs, and scales.

The cause is unknown. Nummular dermatitis usually affects middle-aged people, occurs along with dry skin, and is most common in winter. However, the rash may come and go without any apparent reason.

The round spots start as itchy patches of pimples and blisters that later ooze and form crusts. The rash may be widespread. Often, spots are more obvious on the backs of the arms or legs and on the buttocks, but they also appear on the torso.

Most people benefit from skin moisturizers. Other treatments include antibiotics taken by mouth, corticosteroid creams and injections, and phototherapy (exposure to ultraviolet light). All treatments, however, are often unsatisfactory.

GENERALIZED EXFOLIATIVE DERMATITIS

Generalized exfoliative dermatitis (erythroderma) is severe inflammation that causes the entire skin surface to become red, cracked, and covered with scales.

Certain drugs (especially penicillins, sulfonamides, isoniazid, phenytoin, and barbiturates) may cause this disorder. In some cases, it is a complication of other skin diseases, such as atopic dermatitis, psoriasis, and contact dermatitis. Certain lymphomas (cancers of the lymph nodes) may also cause generalized exfoliative dermatitis. In many cases, the cause is unknown.

Symptoms and Diagnosis

Exfoliative dermatitis may start rapidly or slowly. At first the entire skin surface becomes red and shiny. Then the skin becomes scaly, thickened, and sometimes crusted. Sometimes the hair and nails fall out. Some people have itching and swollen lymph nodes. Although many people have a fever, they may feel cold and have chills because so much heat is lost through the damaged skin. Large amounts of fluid and protein may seep out, and the damaged skin is a poor barrier against infection.

Because symptoms of exfoliative dermatitis are similar to those of skin infection, doctors send samples of skin and blood to the laboratory to exclude infection as a cause.

Treatment

Early diagnosis and treatment are important in preventing infection from developing in the affected skin and in keeping fluid and protein loss from becoming life threatening.

People with severe exfoliative dermatitis often need to be hospitalized and given antibiotics (for infection), intravenous fluids (to replace the fluids lost through the skin), and nutritional supplements. Care may include the use of drugs and heated blankets to control body temperature. Cool baths followed by applications of petroleum jelly and gauze may help protect the skin. Corticosteroids (such as prednisone) given by mouth or intravenously are used only when other measures are unsuccessful or the disease worsens. Any drug or chemical that could be causing the dermatitis should be eliminated. If lymphoma is causing the dermatitis, treatment of the lymphoma is helpful.

STASIS DERMATITIS

Stasis dermatitis is inflammation on the lower legs from pooling of blood and fluid.

Stasis dermatitis tends to occur in people who have varicose (dilated, twisted) veins (see page 437) and swelling (edema). It usually occurs on the ankles but may spread upward to the knees. At first, the skin becomes reddened and mildly scaly. Over several weeks or months, the skin turns dark brown. Eventually, areas of the skin may break down and form an open sore (ulcer), typically near the ankle. Ulcers sometimes become infected with bacteria. Stasis dermatitis makes the legs feel itchy and swollen, but not painful. Ulcers are usually painful.

Treatment

Long-term treatment is aimed at keeping blood from pooling in the veins around the ankles. When sitting, the person should elevate the legs above the level of the heart. Properly fitted prescription support hose (compression stockings) also prevent pooling of blood and decrease swelling. Department store "support" stockings are not adequate.

For dermatitis of recent onset, soothing compresses, such as gauze pads soaked in tap water or aluminum acetate (Burow's solution), may make the skin feel better and can help prevent infection by keeping the skin clean. If the disorder worsens, as evidenced by increased warmth, redness, small ulcers, or pus, a more absorbent dressing can be used. Corticosteroid creams are also helpful and are often combined with zinc oxide paste and applied in a thin layer. Corticosteroids should not be applied directly to an ulcer because this will interfere with healing.

When a person has large or extensive ulcers, special moisture-containing hydrocolloid or hydrogel dressings may be used. Antibiotics are used only when the skin is already infected. Sometimes, skin from elsewhere on the body may be grafted to cover very large ulcers.

Some people may need an Unna's paste boot, which is a woven stretch wrap filled with a gelatin paste that contains zinc. The wrap is applied to the ankle and lower leg where it hardens, similar to but softer than a cast. The boot limits swelling and helps protect the skin from irritation, and the paste helps heal the skin. At first the boot is changed every 2 or 3 days, but later it is left on for a week at a time. After the ulcer heals, an elastic support should be applied before the person rises in the morning. Regardless of the dressing used, reduction of swelling (usually with compression) is essential for healing.

In stasis dermatitis, the skin is easily irritated. Antibiotic creams, first-aid (anesthetic) creams, alcohol, witch hazel, lanolin, or other chemicals should not be used because they can make the disorder worse.

LOCALIZED SCRATCH DERMATITIS

Localized scratch dermatitis (lichen simplex chronicus, neurodermatitis) is chronic, itchy inflammation of the top layer of the skin.

Localized scratch dermatitis is caused by chronic scratching of an area of skin. The act of scratching triggers more itching, beginning a vicious circle of itching-scratching-itching. Sometimes the scratching begins for no apparent reason. Other times scratching starts because of a contact dermatitis, parasitic infestation, or other condition, but the person continues to scratch long after the inciting cause is gone. Doctors do not know why this happens, but psychologic factors may play a role. The disorder does not seem to be allergic. More women than men have localized scratch dermatitis, and it is common among Asians and Native Americans. It usually develops between the ages of 20 and 50.

Symptoms and Diagnosis

Localized scratch dermatitis can occur anywhere on the body, including the anus (pruritus ani—see page 183) and the vagina (pruritus vulvae—see page 1500), but is most common on the head, arms, and legs. In the early stages, the skin looks normal, but it itches. Later, dryness, scaling, and dark patches develop as a result of the scratching and rubbing.

Doctors try to discover any possible underlying allergies or diseases that may be causing the initial itching. When the disorder occurs around the anus or vagina, the doctor may investigate the possibility of pinworms, trichomoniasis, hemorrhoids, local discharges, fungal infections, warts, contact dermatitis, or psoriasis as the cause.

Treatment

For the disorder to clear up, the person must stop all scratching and rubbing of the area. Standard treatments for itching should be followed (see page 1283). Applying surgical tape saturated with a corticosteroid (applied in the morning and replaced in the evening) helps relieve itching and inflammation and protects the skin from scratching. The doctor may inject longer-acting corticosteroids under the skin to control the itching.

When this disorder develops around the anus or vagina, the best treatment is a corticosteroid cream. Zinc oxide paste may be applied over the cream to protect the area. This paste can be removed with mineral oil.

PERIORAL DERMATITIS

Perioral dermatitis is a red, bumpy rash around the mouth and on the chin that resembles acne or rosacea.

The disorder, whose cause is unknown, mainly affects women between the ages of 20 and 60. Perioral dermatitis is distinguished from acne by the lack of blackheads and whiteheads (comedones). Perioral dermatitis can be hard to separate from rosacea, but symptoms, including tiny blisters and skin scaling, can help make the distinction. Other symptoms of rosacea must be present for that diagnosis to be made instead of perioral dermatitis.

Treatment is with tetracyclines or other antibiotics taken by mouth. If these antibiotics do not clear up the rash and the disorder is particularly severe, isotretinoin, an acne drug, may help. Corticosteroids and some oily cosmetics, especially moisturizers, tend to worsen the disorder.

POMPHOLYX

Pompholyx is a chronic dermatitis characterized by itchy blisters on the palms and sides of the fingers and sometimes on the soles of the feet.

Pompholyx is sometimes called dyshidrosis, which means "abnormal sweating," but the disorder has nothing to do with sweating. Doctors do not know what causes pompholyx, but fungal infection, contact dermatitis, or stress may be a factor as well as some ingested substances such as nickel, chromium, and cobalt. It is more common among adolescents and young adults.

The blisters are often scaly, red, and oozing. Pompholyx comes and goes in attacks that last 2 to 3 weeks. Pompholyx takes weeks to go away on its own. Wet compresses with potassium permanganate or aluminum acetate (Burow's solution) may help the blisters resolve. Strong topical corticosteroids, tacrolimus, or pimecrolimus may help itching and inflammation. Pompholyx can also be treated with antibiotics taken by mouth and with phototherapy.

Drug Rashes

Drug rashes are a side effect of a drug that manifests as a skin reaction.

- Drug rashes usually are caused by an allergic reaction to a drug.

- Typical symptoms include mild redness, peeling, hives, and others, such as a runny nose and watery eyes.
- Every drug a person takes is stopped to figure out which one is causing the rash.
- Most drug rashes resolve with the withdrawal of the drug; however, serious reactions require injections of epinephrine, diphenhydramine, and a corticosteroid.

Most drug rashes result from an allergic reaction to the drug (see page 96). The drug does not have to be applied to the skin to cause a drug rash. Sometimes a person can be sensitized to a drug by one exposure, and other times sensitization occurs only after many exposures to a substance. Later exposure to the drug may trigger an allergic reaction, such as a rash.

Sometimes a rash develops directly without involving an allergic reaction. For example, corticosteroids and lithium produce a rash that looks like acne, and anticoagulants (blood thinners) may cause bruising when blood leaks under the skin. Other important nonallergic rashes that may result from drugs are those that occur in Stevens-Johnson syndrome, toxic epidermal necrolysis, and erythema nodosum.

Certain drugs make the skin particularly sensitive to the effects of sunlight (photosensitivity). These drugs include certain antipsychotics, tetracycline, sulfa antibiotics, chlorothiazide, and some artificial sweeteners. No rash appears when the drug is taken, but later exposure to the sun produces a reddened area of skin that is sometimes itchy or that appears grayish blue.

Symptoms

Drug rashes vary in severity from mild redness with tiny bumps over a small area to peeling of the entire skin. Rashes may appear suddenly within minutes after a person takes a drug, or they may be delayed for hours or days. People with an allergic rash often have other allergic symptoms—runny nose, watery eyes, wheezing, and even collapse from dangerously low blood pressure. Hives are very itchy (see page 1122), whereas other drug rashes itch little, if at all.

Diagnosis and Treatment

Figuring out whether a drug is responsible may be difficult because a rash can result from only a minute amount of a drug, it can erupt long after a person has taken a drug, and it can persist for weeks or months after a person has discontinued a drug. Every drug a person has taken is suspect, including those bought without a prescription—even eye drops, nose drops, and suppositories are possible causes. Sometimes the only way to determine which drug is causing a rash is to have the person discontinue all but life-sustaining drugs. Whenever possible, chemically unrelated drugs are substituted. If there are no such substitutes, the person starts taking the drugs again one at a time to see which one causes the reaction. However, this method can be hazardous if the person has had a severe allergic reaction to the drug. Skin testing is not helpful, except when penicillin is the suspected drug.

Most drug reactions disappear when the responsible drug is discontinued. Standard itching treatments are used as needed (see page 1283). Serious allergic eruptions, particularly those accompanied by significant symptoms such as wheezing or difficulty breathing, are treated with injections of epinephrine, diphenhydramine, and a corticosteroid.

Stevens-Johnson Syndrome and Toxic Epidermal Necrolysis

Stevens-Johnson syndrome and toxic epidermal necrolysis are two forms of the same life-threatening skin disease that cause rash, skin peeling, and sores on the mucous membranes.

- Stevens-Johnson syndrome and toxic epidermal necrolysis usually are caused by drugs or a bacterial infection.
- Typical symptoms for both diseases include fever, body aches, a flat red rash, blisters that break out on the mucous membranes, and small areas of peeling skin (Stevens-Johnson syndrome) or large areas of peeling skin (toxic epidermal necrolysis).
- Affected people are hospitalized in a burn unit, given fluids and sometimes corticosteroids and antibiotics, and all suspected drugs are stopped.

In Stevens-Johnson syndrome, a person has blistering of mucous membranes, typically in the mouth, eyes, and vagina, and patchy areas of rash. In toxic epidermal necrolysis, there is a similar blistering of mucous membranes, but in addition the entire top layer of the skin (the epidermis) peels off in sheets from large areas of the body. Both disorders can be life threatening.

Nearly all cases are caused by a reaction to a drug, most often sulfa antibiotics; barbiturates; anticonvulsants, such as phenytoin and carbamazepine; certain nonsteroidal anti-inflammatory drugs (NSAIDs); or allopurinol. Some cases are caused by a bacterial infection. Occasionally, a cause cannot be identified. The disorder occurs in all age groups but is more common among older people, probably because older people tend to use more drugs. The disorder is also more likely to occur in people with AIDS.

Symptoms

Stevens-Johnson syndrome and toxic epidermal necrolysis usually begin with fever, headache, cough, and body aches. Then a flat red rash breaks out on the face and trunk, often spreading later to the rest of the body in an irregular pattern. The areas of rash enlarge and spread, often forming blisters in their center. The skin of the blisters is very loose and easy to rub off. In Stevens-Johnson syndrome, less than 10% of the body surface is affected. In toxic epidermal necrolysis, large areas of skin peel off, often with just a gentle touch or pull. In many people with toxic epidermal necrolysis, 30% or more of the body surface peels away. The affected areas of skin are painful, and the person feels very ill with chills and fever. In some people, the hair and nails fall out. The active stage of rash and skin loss can last between 1 day and 14 days.

In both disorders, blisters break out on the mucous membranes lining the mouth, throat, anus, genitals, and eyes. The damage to the lining of the mouth makes eating difficult, and closing the mouth may be painful, so the person may drool. The eyes may become very painful, swell, and become so filled with pus that they seal shut. The corneas can become scarred. The opening through which urine passes (urethra) may also be affected, making urination difficult and painful. Sometimes the mucous membranes of the digestive and respiratory tracts are involved, resulting in diarrhea and difficulty breathing.

The skin loss in toxic epidermal necrolysis is similar to a severe burn and is equally life threatening. Huge amounts of fluids and salts can seep from the large, raw, damaged areas. A person who has this disorder is very susceptible to organ failure and infection at the sites of damaged, exposed tissues. Such infections are the most common cause of death in people with this disorder.

Treatment

People with Stevens-Johnson syndrome or toxic epidermal necrolysis are hospitalized. Any drugs suspected of causing the disorder are immediately discontinued. When possible, people are treated in a burn unit and given scrupulous care to avoid infection. If the person survives, the skin grows back on its own, and unlike burns, skin grafts are not needed. Fluids and salts, which are lost through the damaged skin, are replaced intravenously.

Use of corticosteroids to treat the disorder is controversial. Some doctors believe that giving large doses within the first few days is beneficial, whereas others believe that corticosteroids should not be used. These drugs suppress the immune system, which increases the potential for serious infection. If infection develops, doctors give antibiotics immediately.

In many cases, doctors give intravenous human immunoglobulin to treat toxic epidermal necrolysis. This substance helps to prevent further immune damage to the skin and further progression of blistering.

Erythema Multiforme

Erythema multiforme is a recurring disorder characterized by patches of red, raised skin that often look like targets and usually are distributed symmetrically over the body.

- Erythema multiforme can be caused by a reaction to an infection with herpes simplex virus.
- Typical symptoms include red patches with purple-gray centers (target lesions) that suddenly appear on arms, legs, face, palms, and soles and on the body.
- The diagnosis is based on symptoms.
- This disorder resolves without treatment, but symptoms can be treated with corticosteroids, lidocaine, and sometimes acyclovir.

Most cases are caused by a reaction to infection with the herpes simplex virus (see page 1245). This viral infection is apparent as visible cold sores in about two thirds of people before the erythema multiforme appears. Doctors are not sure whether other infectious diseases cause a few cases of erythema multiforme. Doctors are unsure exactly how herpes simplex causes this disorder, but a type of immune reaction is suspected.

Symptoms

Usually, erythema multiforme appears suddenly, with reddened patches erupting on the arms, legs, and face. Sometimes the rash is also present on the palms or soles. The red patches are distributed equally on both sides of the body. These red patches often develop red concentric rings with purple-gray centers ("target" or "iris" lesions) and small blisters. The reddened areas usually are symptomless, although they sometimes itch mildly. Painful blisters often form on the lips and lining of the mouth but not the eyes.

Attacks of erythema multiforme may last 2 to 4 weeks. Some people have only one attack, but some have recurrences an average of 6 times a year for almost 10 years. Recurrences are more common in the spring and can probably be triggered by sunlight. The frequency of recurrence usually decreases with time.

Diagnosis and Treatment

Doctors diagnose erythema multiforme by its characteristic appearance. However, Stevens-Johnson syndrome (see page 1290) may at first look very similar to erythema multiforme, so doctors monitor the person carefully until the diagnosis is clear.

Erythema multiforme resolves on its own. If itching is bothersome, standard treatments may be used. Corticosteroids given by mouth may be helpful. If painful mouth blisters make eating difficult, a topical anesthetic (an anesthetic applied to the skin), such as lidocaine, may be applied. If oral intake is still poor, nutrition and fluids are given intravenously. People with frequent recurrences may benefit from an antiviral drug, such as acyclovir, given at the first sign of an outbreak.

Erythema Nodosum

Erythema nodosum is an inflammatory disorder that produces tender red bumps (nodules) under the skin, most often over the shins but occasionally on the arms and other areas.

- Erythema nodosum usually is caused by another disease, drug sensitivity, or bacterial, fungal, or viral infection.
- Typical symptoms include fever, joint pain, and characteristic painful red bumps and bruises on the person's shins.
- The diagnosis is based on symptoms and supported by results of a chest x-ray, blood tests, and a biopsy.
- People stop taking suspected drugs; underlying infections are treated with antibiotics; and pain is relieved by bed rest, nonsteroidal anti-inflammatory drugs, and sometimes an injection of a corticosteroid.

Quite often, erythema nodosum is a symptom of some other disease or of sensitivity to a drug. Young adults, particularly women, are most prone to the disorder, which may recur for months or years. Bacterial, fungal, or viral infections may also cause erythema nodosum.

Streptococcal infection is one of the most common causes of erythema nodosum, particularly in children. Sarcoidosis, ulcerative colitis, and various drugs, such as sulfa antibiotics and oral contraceptives, are other common causes. Numerous other infections and several types of cancer are also thought to cause the eruption.

Erythema nodosum nodules usually appear on the shins and resemble raised bumps and bruises that gradually change from pink to bluish brown. Fever and joint pain are common. Lymph nodes in the chest occasionally become enlarged and are detected with a chest x-ray. The painful nodules are usually the telltale sign for the doctor. Evaluation includes chest x-ray, blood tests, and skin biopsy, in which a small piece of skin is surgically removed for examination under a microscope.

Treatment

Drugs that might be causing erythema nodosum are discontinued, and any underlying infections are treated. If the disorder is caused by a streptococcal infection, a person may have to take antibiotics, such as penicillin, or a cephalosporin.

The nodules may go away in 3 to 6 weeks without treatment. Bed rest and nonsteroidal anti-inflammatory drugs (NSAIDs) may help relieve the pain caused by the nodules. Individual nodules may also be treated by injecting them with a corticosteroid. When a person has many nodules, corticosteroid or potassium iodide tablets sometimes are prescribed to speed relief of pain.

Granuloma Annulare

Granuloma annulare is a chronic, harmless skin disorder of unknown cause in which small, firm, raised bumps form a ring with normal or slightly sunken skin in the center.

The bumps are red, violet, or flesh-colored, and a person may have one ring or several. The bumps usually cause no pain or itching and they most often form on the feet, legs, hands, or fingers of children and adults. In a few people, clusters of granuloma annulare bumps erupt when the skin is exposed to the sun.

Most often, granuloma annulare heals without any treatment. Corticosteroid creams under waterproof bandages, surgical tape saturated with a corticosteroid, or injected corticosteroids may help clear up the rash. People with large affected areas often benefit from treatment that combines phototherapy (exposure to ultraviolet light) with the use of psoralens (drugs that make the skin more sensitive to the effects of ultraviolet light). This treatment is called PUVA (psoralens plus ultraviolet A).

Psoriasis

Psoriasis is a chronic, recurring disease that causes one or more raised, red patches that have silvery scales and a distinct border between the patch and normal skin.

- A problem with the immune system may play a role.
- Characteristic scales appear on various parts of the body in large or small patches.
- This disease is treated with a combination of exposure to ultraviolet light (phototherapy) and drugs applied to the skin and taken by mouth.

The patches of psoriasis occur because of an abnormally high rate of growth of skin cells. The reason for the rapid cell growth is unknown, but a problem with the immune system is thought to play a role. The disorder often runs in families. Psoriasis is common and affects about 1 to 5% of the population worldwide. Light-skinned people are at greater risk, whereas blacks are less likely to get the disease.

Symptoms

Psoriasis begins most often in people aged 10 to 40, although people in all age groups are susceptible.

It usually starts as one or more small patches on the scalp, elbows, knees, back, or buttocks. The first patches may clear up after a few months or remain, sometimes growing together to form larger patches. Some people never have more than one or two small patches, and others have patches covering large areas of the body. Thick patches or patches on the palms of the hands, soles of the feet, or skinfolds of the genitals are more likely to itch or hurt, but many times the person has no symptoms. Although the patches do not cause extreme physical discomfort, they are very obvious and often embarrassing to the person. The psychologic distress caused by psoriasis can be severe. Many people with psoriasis may also have deformed, thickened, and pitted nails.

Psoriasis persists throughout life but may come and go. Symptoms are often diminished during the summer when the skin is exposed to bright sunlight. Some people may go for years between occurrences. Psoriasis may flare up for no apparent reason or as a result of a variety of circumstances. Flare-ups often result from conditions that irritate the skin, such as minor injuries and severe sunburn. Sometimes flare-ups follow infections, such as colds and strep throat. Flare-ups are more common in the winter and after stressful situations. Many drugs, such as antimalarial drugs, lithium, and beta-blockers, can also cause psoriasis to flare up.

Some uncommon types of psoriasis can have more serious effects. Psoriatic arthritis produces joint pain and swelling (see page 569). Erythrodermic psoriasis causes all of the skin on the body to become red and scaly. This form of psoriasis is serious because, like a burn, it keeps the skin from serving as a protective barrier against injury and infection. In another uncommon form of psoriasis, pustular psoriasis, large and small pus-filled blisters (pustules) form on the palms of the hands and soles of the feet. Sometimes, these pustules are scattered on the body.

Treatment

Many drugs are available to treat psoriasis. Most often, a combination of drugs is used, depending on the severity and extent of the person's symptoms.

Topical Drugs: Topical drugs (drugs applied to the skin) are used most commonly. Nearly everyone with psoriasis benefits from skin moisturizers (emollients). Other topical agents include corticosteroids, often used together with calcipotriene, a vitamin D derivative, or coal tar or pine tar. Tazarotene or anthralin may also be used. Very thick patches can be thinned with ointments containing salicylic acid, which make the other drugs more effective. Many of these drugs are irritating to the skin, and doctors must find which ones work best for each person.

Phototherapy: Phototherapy (exposure to ultraviolet light) also can help clear up psoriasis for several months at a time. Phototherapy is often used in combination with various topical drugs, particularly when large areas of skin are involved. Traditionally, treatment has been with phototherapy combined with the use of psoralens (drugs that make the skin more sensitive to the effects of ultraviolet light). This treatment is called PUVA (psoralens plus ultraviolet A). Some doctors are now using narrow-band ultraviolet B (UVB) treatments, which are equally effective but avoid the need to use psoralens and the side effects they cause, such as extreme sensitivity to sunshine.

Oral Drugs: For serious forms of psoriasis and psoriatic arthritis, drugs taken by mouth are used. These drugs include cyclosporine, methotrexate, and acitretin. Cyclosporine is an immunosuppressant drug that may cause high blood pressure and damage the kidneys. Methotrexate interferes with the growth and multiplication of skin cells. Doctors use methotrexate to treat people whose psoriasis does not respond to other forms of therapy. Liver damage and impaired immunity are possible side effects. Acitretin is particularly effective in treating pustular psoriasis but often raises fat (lipid) levels in the blood and might cause problems with the liver and bones. It can also cause birth defects and should not be taken by a woman who might become pregnant.

Pityriasis Rosea

Pityriasis rosea is a mild disease that causes the formation of many small patches of scaly, rose-colored, inflamed skin.

- Pityriasis rosea may be caused by a viral infection.
- The most common symptoms are itching, an initial large, tan- or rose-colored circular patch, followed by multiple patches that appear on the torso.
- The diagnosis is based on symptoms.
- This disease usually resolves with no treatment, and itching that is not severe may be alleviated with artificial or natural sunlight.

The cause of pityriasis rosea is not certain but a viral infection may be involved. However, the disorder is not thought to be contagious. It can develop at any age but is most common among young adults. Pityriasis rosea affects women more often and usually appears during spring and autumn.

Symptoms

Pityriasis rosea causes a rose-red or light-tan patch of skin about 1 to 4 inches (2 to 10 centimeters) in diameter that doctors call a herald or mother patch. This round or oval area usually develops on the torso. Sometimes the patch appears without any previous symptoms, but some people have a vague feeling of illness, loss of appetite, fever, and joint pain a few days before the patch appears. In 7 to 14 days, many similar but smaller patches appear on other parts of the body. These secondary patches are most common on the torso, especially along and radiating

---

Phototherapy: Using Ultraviolet Light to Treat Skin Disorders

For many years, people have known that exposure to sunlight is helpful for certain skin disorders. Doctors now know that one component of sunlight—ultraviolet (UV) light—is responsible for this effect. UV light has many different effects on skin cells, including altering the amounts and kinds of chemicals they make and causing the death of certain cells that can be involved in skin diseases. The use of UV light to treat disease is called phototherapy. Psoriasis and atopic dermatitis are the disorders most commonly treated with phototherapy.

Because natural sunlight exposure varies in intensity and is not practical for a large part of the year in certain climates, phototherapy is nearly always performed with artificial UV light. Treatments are given in a doctor's office or in a specialized treatment center. UV light, which is invisible to the human eye, is classified as A, B, or C, depending on its wavelength. Ultraviolet A (UVA) penetrates deeper into the skin than ultraviolet B (UVB). UVA or UVB is chosen based on the type and severity of the

person's disorder Ultraviolet C is not used in phototherapy. Some lights produce only certain specific wavelengths of UVA or UVB (narrow-band therapy), which are used to treat specific disorders. Narrow-band therapy helps limit the sunburning associated with phototherapy.

Phototherapy is sometimes combined with the use of psoralens. Psoralens are drugs that may be taken by mouth before treatment with UV light. Psoralens sensitize the skin to the effects of UV light, allowing shorter, less intense exposure. The combination of psoralens plus UVA is known as PUVA therapy.

Side effects of phototherapy include pain and reddening similar to sunburn with prolonged exposure to UV light. UV light exposure also increases the long-term risk of skin cancer, although the risk is small for brief courses of treatment. Psoralens often cause nausea. In addition, because psoralens enter the lens of the eye, UV-resistant sunglasses must be worn for at least 12 hours after undergoing PUVA therapy.

---

from the spine. Most people with pityriasis rosea have some itching, and in some people the itching can be severe.

Diagnosis and Treatment

A doctor usually makes the diagnosis based on the appearance of the rash, particularly the herald patch. Usually the rash goes away in 4 to 5 weeks without treatment, although sometimes it lasts for 2 months or more. Both artificial and natural sunlight may speed clearing and relieve the itching. Other standard treatments for itching may be used as needed (see page 1283). Corticosteroids taken by mouth are necessary only for very severe itching.

Rosacea

Rosacea (acne rosacea) is a persistent skin disorder that produces redness, tiny pimples, and noticeable blood vessels, usually on the central area of the face.

- The cause is unknown.
- Typical symptoms include redness, small visible blood vessels, and small pimples that appear on the cheeks and nose.
- The diagnosis is based on symptoms and on the person's age when symptoms first appear.
- Worsening of rosacea can be prevented by avoiding certain foods, alcohol, caffeine, and exposure to sunlight, extremes of temperature, wind, and cosmetics.
- Treatment includes antibiotics taken by mouth or applied to the skin and antifungal or other medicated creams.

The cause of rosacea is not known. The disorder usually appears during or after middle age—age of onset helps distinguish it from acne. Rosacea is most common among people of Celtic or Northern European descent who have fair complexions but it does affect and is probably under-recognized in darker-skinned people. Although usually easy for doctors to recognize, rosacea sometimes looks like acne and certain other skin disorders. It is often called adult acne.

The skin over the cheeks and nose becomes red, often with small pimples. The skin may appear thin and frail, with small blood vessels visible just below the surface. The skin around the nose may thicken, making it look red and bulbous (rhinophyma).

Treatment

People with rosacea should avoid foods that cause the blood vessels in the skin to dilate—for example, spicy foods, alcohol, coffee, and other caffeinated beverages. Other triggers include sunlight, emotional stress, cold or hot weather, exercise, wind, cosmetics, and hot baths or hot drinks.

Certain antibiotics taken by mouth relieve rosacea. Tetracyclines are usually most effective and produce the fewest side effects. Antibiotics that are applied to the skin, such as metronidazole, clindamycin, and erythromycin, are also effective. In rare cases, antifungal creams, such as ketoconazole or terbinafine cream, are used. Topical azelaic acid gel also can be an effective treatment for rosacea.

Isotretinoin is effective when taken by mouth or when applied to the skin. Corticosteroids applied to the skin tend to make rosacea worse. Severe rhinophyma is unlikely to improve completely with drugs. Therefore, a person with this disorder may need surgery or laser treatment (see box on page 1331).

Lichen Planus

Lichen planus, a recurring itchy disease, starts as a rash of small, discrete red or purple bumps that then combine and become rough, scaly patches.

- The cause may be a reaction to certain drugs, chemicals, or infectious organisms.
- Typical symptoms include an itchy rash made of red or purple bumps that form into scaly patches appearing on different parts of the body and sometimes in the mouth.
- This disease can last for more than 1 year, and it can recur.
- Drugs or chemicals that may be causing lichen planus should be avoided.
- Lichen planus usually resolves without treatment, but symptoms may be treated with corticosteroids, exposure to ultraviolet light, or lidocaine-containing mouthwashes.

The cause of lichen planus is not known, but it may be a reaction by the immune system to a variety of drugs (especially gold, bismuth, arsenic, quinine, quinidine, and quinacrine), chemicals (especially certain chemicals used to develop color photographs), and infectious organisms. The disorder itself is not infectious.

Symptoms

The rash of lichen planus almost always itches, sometimes severely. The bumps are usually violet and have angular borders. When light is directed at the bumps from the side, the bumps display a distinctive sheen. New bumps may form wherever scratching or a mild skin injury occurs. Sometimes a dark discoloration remains after the rash heals.

Usually, the rash is evenly distributed on both sides of the body—most commonly on the torso, on the inner surfaces of the wrists, on the legs, on the head of the penis, and in the vagina. About half of those who get lichen planus also develop mouth sores. The face is less often affected. On the legs, the rash may become especially large, thick, and scaly. The rash sometimes results in patchy baldness on the scalp.

Lichen planus in the mouth usually results in a bluish white patch that forms in lines. This type of mouth patch often does not hurt, and the person may not know it is there. Sometimes painful sores form in the mouth, which often interfere with eating and drinking.

Prognosis and Treatment

Lichen planus usually clears up by itself after 1 or 2 years, although it sometimes lasts longer, especially when the mouth is involved. Symptoms recur in about 20% of people. Prolonged treatment may be needed during outbreaks of the rash. However, between outbreaks, no treatment is needed. People with mouth sores have a slightly increased risk of oral cancer, but the rash on the skin does not turn cancerous.

Drugs or chemicals that may be causing lichen planus should be avoided, and standard treatments can be used to relieve itching (see page 1283). Corticosteroids may be injected into the bumps, applied to the skin, or taken by mouth, sometimes with other drugs, such as acitretin or cyclosporine. Phototherapy (exposure to ultraviolet light) combined with the use of psoralens (drugs that make the skin more sensitive to the effects of ultraviolet light) may also be helpful. This treatment is called PUVA (psoralens plus ultraviolet A). For painful mouth sores, a mouthwash containing lidocaine, an anesthetic, may be used before meals to form a pain-killing coating.

Keratosis Pilaris

Keratosis pilaris is a common disorder in which dead cells shed from the upper layer of skin plug the openings of hair follicles.

The cause is not known, although heredity probably plays a role. Also, people with atopic dermatitis are more likely to have keratosis pilaris.

The plugs or bumps that occur in keratosis pilaris make the skin feel rough (like chicken skin) and dry. Sometimes the plugs resemble small pimples. Generally, these plugs do not itch or hurt and cause only cosmetic problems. The upper arms, thighs, and buttocks are most commonly affected. The face may break out as well, particularly in children. Plugs are more likely to develop in cold weather and to clear up in the summer.

Treatment is not needed unless the person is bothered by the appearance of the disorder. Skin moisturizers are the main treatment. Creams with salicylic acid, lactic acid, or tretinoin can also be used. Keratosis pilaris is likely to come back when treatment is stopped.

188 Acne

Acne is a common skin condition causing pimples on the face and upper torso.

- Acne is caused by a buildup of dead skin cells, bacteria, and dried sebum that blocks the hair follicles in the skin.
- Pimples, cysts, and sometimes abscesses form on the skin, usually on the face, chest, shoulders, or back.
- To diagnose acne, doctors examine the skin.
- Common treatments include topical antibiotics for mild acne, oral antibiotics for moderate acne, and oral isotretinoin for severe acne.

Acne is caused by an interaction between hormones, skin oils, and bacteria, which results in inflammation of hair follicles. Acne is characterized by pimples, cysts, and sometimes abscesses. Both cysts and abscesses are pus-filled pockets, but abscesses are somewhat larger and deeper.

Sebaceous glands, which secrete an oily substance (sebum), lie in the dermis, the middle layer of skin. These glands are attached to the hair follicles. Sebum, along with dead skin cells, passes up from the sebaceous gland and hair follicle and out to the surface of the skin through the pores.

Acne results when a collection of dried sebum, dead skin cells, and bacteria clogs the hair follicles, blocking the sebum from leaving through the pores. If the blockage is incomplete, a blackhead (open comedone) develops; if the blockage is complete, a whitehead (closed comedone) develops. The blocked sebum-filled hair follicle promotes overgrowth of the bacterium *Propionibacterium acnes*, which is normally present in the hair follicle. This bacterium breaks down the sebum into substances that irritate the skin. The resulting inflammation produces the skin eruptions that are commonly known as acne pimples. Deeper inflammation produces cysts and sometimes an abscess.

Acne occurs mainly during puberty, when the sebaceous glands are stimulated by increased hormone levels, especially the androgens (such as testosterone), resulting in excessive sebum production. By a person's early to mid-20s, hormone production stabilizes and acne usually disappears. Other conditions that involve hormonal changes can affect the occurrence of acne as well. For example, acne may occur with each menstrual period in young women and may clear up or substantially worsen during pregnancy. The use of certain drugs, particularly corticosteroids and anabolic steroids, can cause acne by stimulating the sebaceous glands. Certain cosmetics may worsen acne by clogging the pores.

Because acne naturally varies in severity for most people—sometimes worsening, sometimes improving—pinpointing the factors that may produce an outbreak is difficult. Acne is often worse in the winter and better in the summer, perhaps because of sunlight's anti-inflammatory effect. There is no relationship, however, between acne and specific foods or sexual activity.

Symptoms

Most acne occurs on the face but is also common on the shoulders, back, and upper chest. Anabolic steroid use typically causes acne on the shoulders and upper back.

There are three levels of acne severity: mild, moderate, and severe. Yet even mild acne can be vexing, especially to adolescents, who see each pimple as a major cosmetic challenge.

People with **mild acne** develop only a few (less than 20) noninflamed blackheads or whiteheads, or a moderate number of small, mildly irritated pimples. Blackheads appear as small flesh-colored bumps with tiny, dark dots at their center. Whiteheads have a similar appearance but lack the dark dots. Pimples are mildly uncomfortable and have a white center surrounded by a small area of reddened skin.

People with **moderate acne** have more comedones and pimples and sometimes larger, more inflamed pimples (pustules).

People with **severe (deep, or cystic) acne** have numerous large, red, painful pus-filled lumps (nodules) that sometimes even join together under the skin into giant, oozing abscesses.

Scarring: Mild acne usually does not leave scars. However, squeezing pimples or trying to open them in other ways increases inflammation and the depth of injury to the skin, making scarring more likely. The nodules and abscesses of severe acne often rupture and, after healing, typically leave scars. Scars may be tiny, deep holes (ice pick scars); wider pits of varying depth; or large, irregular indentations. Acne scars last a lifetime and, for some people, are cosmetically significant and a source of psychologic stress.

Treatment

General care of acne is very simple. Affected areas should be gently washed once or twice a day with a mild soap. Antibacterial or abrasive soaps, alcohol pads, and heavy frequent scrubbing provide no added benefit and may further irritate the skin. Cosmetics should be water-based; very greasy products

Comparing Mild Acne and Severe Acne

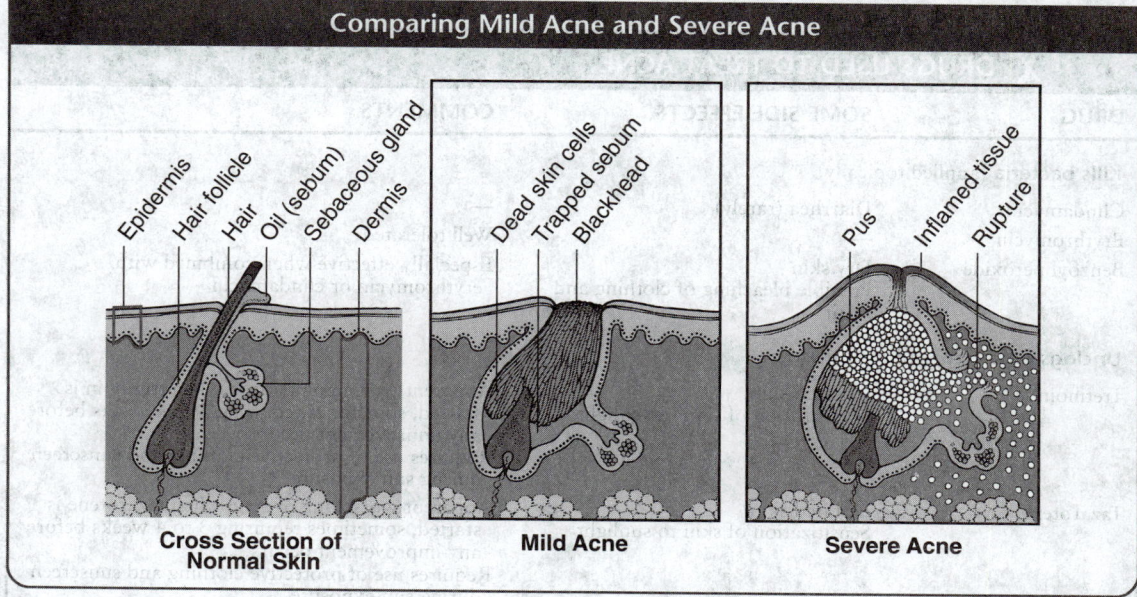

Cross Section of Normal Skin

Epidermis · Hair follicle · Hair · Oil (sebum) · Sebaceous gland · Dermis

Mild Acne

Dead skin cells · Trapped sebum · Blackhead

Severe Acne

Pus · Inflamed tissue · Rupture

can worsen acne. Although there are no restrictions on specific foods (for example, pizza or chocolate), a healthy, balanced diet should be followed (see page 909).

Beyond these routine measures, acne treatment depends on the severity of the condition. Mild acne requires the simplest treatment that poses the fewest risks of side effects. More severe acne or acne that does not respond to preliminary treatment requires additional treatment. A treatment plan should always include education, support, and the most practical option for the person.

Mild Acne: Drugs used to treat mild acne are applied to the skin (topical drugs). They work by either killing bacteria (antibacterials) or drying up or unclogging the pores.

The two most commonly prescribed antibacterials are the antibiotics clindamycin and erythromycin. Benzoyl peroxide, another effective antibacterial, is available with or without a prescription.

Older nonprescription creams that contain salicylic acid, resorcinol, or sulfur work by drying out the pimples and causing slight peeling. These drugs, however, are less effective than antibiotics or benzoyl peroxide.

If topical antibacterials fail, doctors use other topical prescription drugs that help unclog the pores. The most common such drug is tretinoin. Tretinoin is very effective but is irritating to the skin and makes it more sensitive to sunlight. Doctors therefore use this drug cautiously, starting with low concentrations and infrequent applications, which can be gradually increased. Benzoyl peroxide inactivates tretinoin, so the two must not be applied together. Newer prescription drugs with effects similar to tretinoin include adapalene, azelaic acid, and tazarotene. Blackheads and whiteheads can be removed by a doctor. A large pimple may be opened with a sterile needle. Other instruments, such as a loop extractor, can also be used to drain plugged pores and pimples.

? Did You Know...

Vigorous washing and scrubbing may irritate the skin and can make acne worse.

Moderate Acne: Moderate acne is usually treated with antibiotics given by mouth. Typical antibiotics include tetracycline, doxycycline, minocycline, and erythromycin. Doctors often combine a topical treatment and an oral antibiotic. People may need to take antibiotics for weeks, months, or even years to prevent a recurrence. Women who take antibiotics for a long time sometimes develop vaginal yeast infections that may require treatment.

℞ DRUGS USED TO TREAT ACNE

DRUG	SOME SIDE EFFECTS	COMMENTS
Kills bacteria (applied topically)		
Clindamycin	Diarrhea (rarely)	—
Erythromycin	—	Well tolerated
Benzoyl peroxide	Dry skin Possible bleaching of clothing and hair	Especially effective when combined with erythromycin or clindamycin
Unclogs pores (applied topically)		
Tretinoin	Irritated skin Sensitization of skin to sunlight	Apparent worsening of acne when tretinoin is started, sometimes requiring 3 to 4 weeks before any improvement occurs Requires use of protective clothing and sunscreen during sun exposure
Tazarotene	Irritated skin Sensitization of skin to sunlight	Apparent worsening of acne when tazarotene is started, sometimes requiring 3 to 4 weeks before any improvement occurs Requires use of protective clothing and sunscreen during sun exposure
Adapalene	Some redness, burning, and increased sun sensitivity	As effective as tretinoin but less irritating Requires use of protective clothing and sunscreen during sun exposure
Azelaic acid	May lighten skin	Minimally irritating May be used by itself or with tretinoin Should be used cautiously in people with darker skin because of skin-lightening effects
Kills bacteria (taken by mouth)		
Tetracycline	Possible sensitization of skin to sunlight	Inexpensive and safe, but must be taken on an empty stomach Requires use of protective clothing and sunscreen during sun exposure
Doxycycline	Possible sensitization of skin to sunlight	Requires use of protective clothing and sunscreen during sun exposure
Minocycline	Headache Dizziness Skin discoloration	Most effective antibiotic
Erythromycin	Stomach upset	Frequently, development of bacterial resistance to erythromycin
Unclogs pores (taken by mouth)		
Isotretinoin	Possible harm to a developing fetus Possible effect on blood cells, the liver, and fat (triglyceride and cholesterol) levels Dry eyes, chapped lips, and drying of the mucous membranes Pain or stiffness of large joints and lower back with high dosages Associated with depression, suicidal thoughts, attempted suicide, and (rarely) completed suicide	For sexually active women, requires a pregnancy test before they start isotretinoin and at monthly intervals while they are taking the drug, plus use of two forms of contraception or sexual abstinence, beginning 1 month before they start the drug and continuing while they take it and for 1 month after they stop taking it Requires blood tests to check whether the drug is affecting blood cells, the liver, or fat levels

Severe Acne: For the most severe acne, when antibiotics do not work, oral isotretinoin is the best treatment. Isotretinoin, which is related to the topical drug tretinoin, is the only drug that can potentially cure acne. However, isotretinoin can have very serious side effects. *Isotretinoin can harm a developing fetus, and women taking it must use strict contraceptive measures so they do not become pregnant.* Other, less serious side effects may occur as well. Therapy generally continues for 20 weeks. If more therapy is needed, it should not be restarted for at least 4 months.

Other acne treatments are useful for specific people. For example, a woman with severe acne that worsens with her menstrual period may be helped by taking oral contraceptives. This treatment takes 2 to 4 months to produce results.

Doctors sometimes treat large, inflamed nodules or abscesses by injecting corticosteroids into them.

Occasionally, a doctor cuts open a nodule or abscess to drain it.

Treatment of severe acne scars depends on their shape, depth, and location. Individual scars of any depth may be cut out and the skin sewn back together. Wide indented scars can be improved cosmetically in a procedure called subcision, in which small cuts are made under the skin to release the scar tissue. This procedure often allows the skin to resume its normal contours. Multiple shallow scars may be treated with chemical peels or laser resurfacing (see box on page 1331). Dermabrasion, a procedure in which the skin surface is rubbed with an abrasive metal instrument to remove the top layer, also may help remove small scars. Sometimes scars are injected with various substances such as collagen, fat, or a variety of synthetic materials. These substances may raise the scarred area to make it level with the rest of the skin.

CHAPTER

189 Pressure Sores

Pressure sores (bedsores, decubitus ulcers, pressure ulcers) are areas of skin damage resulting from a lack of blood flow due to pressure.

- Sores often result from pressure but may also result from pulling on the skin or friction, particularly over bony areas.
- The diagnosis is usually based on a physical examination.
- Treatment includes cleansing, removal of pressure from the affected area, special dressings, and, sometimes, surgery.

Pressure sores can occur in people of any age who are bedridden, chairbound, or unable to reposition themselves. They are more common among older people. They tend to occur over bony projections where pressure on skin can be concentrated, such as over the hip bones, tailbone, heels, ankles, and elbows. They occur where there is pressure on the skin from a bed, wheelchair, cast, splint, or other hard object. Pressure sores lengthen the time spent in hospitals or nursing homes and increase the cost of care. Pressure sores can be life threatening if they are untreated or if underlying health conditions prevent them from healing.

Causes

Causes that contribute to the development of pressure sores include

- Pressure
- Traction
- Friction
- Moisture
- Inadequate nutrition

Pressure on skin, especially when over bony areas, reduces or cuts off blood flow to the skin. If blood flow is cut off for more than 1 or 2 hours, the skin dies, beginning with its outer layer (epidermis). The dead skin breaks down and forms an open sore (ulcer). Most people do not develop pressure sores because they constantly shift position without thinking, even when they are asleep. However, some people cannot move normally and are therefore at greater risk of developing pressure sores. They include people who are paralyzed, comatose, very weak, sedated, or restrained. Paralyzed and comatose people are at particular risk because they also may be unable to move or feel pain (pain normally motivates people to move or to ask to be moved).

Traction also reduces blood flow to the skin. Traction occurs when the skin is stretched by being wedged against something or when it sticks to something, often bed linens. When the skin is stretched, the effect is much like pressure.

Common Sites for Pressure Sores

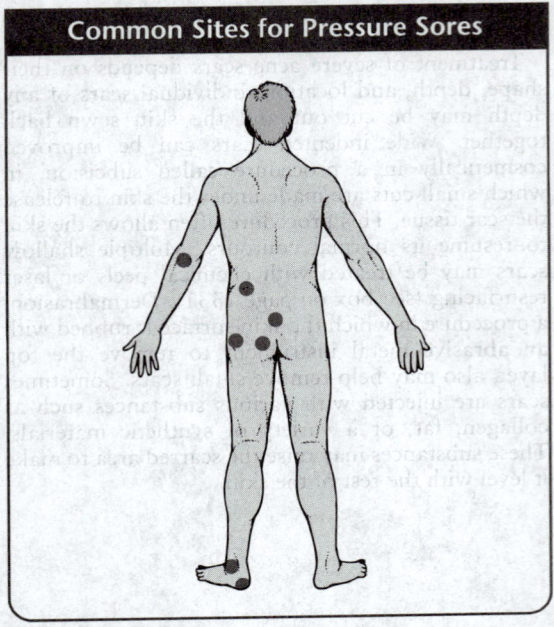

Friction can lead to or worsen pressure sores. Repeated friction may wear away the top layers of skin. Such skin friction may occur if people are pulled repeatedly across a bed.

Moisture can increase skin friction and weaken or damage the protective outer layer of skin if the skin is exposed to it a long time. For example, the skin may be in prolonged contact with perspiration, urine, or feces.

Inadequate nutrition increases the risk of developing pressure sores and slows the healing process of sores that do develop. Malnourished people may not have enough body fat to pad the skin and bones or to keep the blood vessels from being squeezed shut. Also, skin repair is impaired in people whose diets are deficient in protein, vitamin C, or zinc.

Symptoms

For most people, pressure sores cause some pain and itching. However, in people whose senses are dulled, even severe sores may be painless.

Pressure sores are categorized into four stages according to the severity of damage:

- Stage I: Redness and inflammation
- Stage II: Some shallow skin loss, including abrasions, blisters, or both
- Stage III: Full-thickness skin loss down to the layer of fat

- Stage IV: Full-thickness skin loss with exposure of underlying muscle, tendon, or bone

Pressure sores do not always progress from mild to severe stages. Sometimes the first noticeable sign is a late-stage sore.

If pressure sores become infected, they may have an unpleasant odor. Pus may be visible in or around the sore. The area around the pressure sore may become red or feel warm, and pain may worsen if the infection spreads to the surrounding skin (causing cellulitis). Infection delays healing of shallow sores and can be life threatening in deeper sores. Infection can even penetrate the bone (osteomyelitis), requiring weeks of treatment with antibiotics. In the most severe cases, infection can spread into the bloodstream (sepsis), causing fever or shaking chills.

Diagnosis

Doctors can usually diagnose pressure sores by doing a physical examination. A doctor or nurse usually measures the size and depth of a sore to determine its stage and plan treatment.

If the damage is severe, radionuclide bone scanning or gadolinium-enhanced MRI (magnetic resonance imaging) may be done to check whether infection has spread from the sore to bone—a disorder called osteomyelitis. To diagnose osteomyelitis, doctors may need to take a small sample (biopsy) of bone to see if bacteria grow from it (culture).

> **? Did You Know...**
>
> Inadequate nutrition increases the chances of developing pressure sores and slows the healing of sores that do develop.
>
> Repositioning people who cannot move themselves at least every 1 to 2 hours can help prevent pressure sores.

Prevention

Prevention is the best strategy for dealing with pressure sores. In most cases, pressure sores can be prevented by meticulous attention from all caregivers, including nurses, nurses' aides, and family members. Close daily inspection of a bedridden or chairbound person's skin can detect early redness or discoloration. Any sign of redness or discoloration at pressure areas is a signal that the person needs to be repositioned and kept from lying or sitting on the discolored area until it returns to normal.

Because shifting position is necessary to keep the blood flowing to the skin, oversedation should be avoided and activity encouraged. People who cannot move themselves should be repositioned every 2 hours if they are in bed and every hour if they are in a chair—more often if possible. The skin must be kept clean and dry because moisture increases the risk of developing pressure sores. Dry skin is less likely to stick to fabrics and cause friction or traction. For people confined to bed, sheets should be changed frequently to make sure they are clean and dry. Applying noncaking body powder to skin in areas where two parts of the body press against each other (such as the buttocks and groin) can help keep the skin in these areas dry.

Bony projections (such as heels and elbows) can be protected with soft materials, such as foam wedges and heel protectors. Donut-shaped devices and sheepskins should be avoided as they only shift pressure or friction from one vulnerable site to another. Special beds, mattresses, and seat cushions can be used to reduce pressure in people who are wheelchair-bound or bedridden. These products can reduce pressure and offer extra relief. A doctor or nurse can recommend the most appropriate mattress surface or seat cushion. It is important to remember that none of these devices eliminate pressure completely or are a substitute for frequent repositioning.

Treatment

Treating a pressure sore is much more difficult than preventing one. The main goals of treatment are to relieve pressure on the sores, keep them clean and free of infection, and provide adequate nutrition. Adequate nutrition is important in helping pressure sores heal and in preventing new sores from forming. A well-balanced, high-protein diet is recommended as well as a daily high-potency vitamin and mineral supplement. Supplemental vitamin C and zinc may help with healing as well. Electrical stimulation, heat therapy, massage therapy, and hyperbaric oxygen therapy have not proven helpful.

In the earliest stage, pressure sores usually heal by themselves once pressure is removed. When the skin is broken, a doctor or nurse considers the location and condition of the pressure sore when recommending a dressing. Film (see-through) dressings help protect early-stage pressure sores and allow them to heal more quickly. Hydrocolloid (oxygen- and moisture-retaining) patches protect, keep the skin appropriately moist, and provide a healthy environment for deep sores. Other types of dressings may be used for deeper sores, those that ooze a lot of fluids, and those that are infected.

If the sore appears infected or oozes, rinsing with saline and dabbing gently with a gauze pad are

SPOTLIGHT ON AGING

Aging itself does not cause pressure sores. But it causes changes in tissues that make pressure sores more likely to develop. As people age, the outer layers of the skin thin. Many older people have less fat and muscle, which help absorb pressure. The number of blood vessels decreases, and blood vessels rupture more easily. All wounds, including pressure sores, heal more slowly.

Certain conditions make pressure sores more likely to develop:

- Being unable to move normally because of a disorder such as stroke
- Having to stay in bed for a long time, for example, because of surgery
- Being excessively sleepy (such people are less likely to change position or ask someone to reposition them)
- Losing sensation because of nerve damage (such people do not feel discomfort or pain, which would prompt them to change positions)
- Becoming less responsive to what is happening in and around them, including their own discomfort or pain, because of a disorder such as dementia

helpful. A doctor may need to remove (debride) dead tissue with a scalpel or a chemical solution. Removal of dead tissue is usually painless, because pain is not felt in dead tissue. Some pain may be felt because healthy tissue is nearby. Health care practitioners may flood (irrigate) the sore, particularly its deep crevices, with a sterile solution to help clean away hidden debris.

Sometimes a bed that circulates air (an air-fluidized bed) is used in hospitals and nursing homes. This special bed helps reduce or redistribute pressure on the body.

Deep pressure sores are difficult to treat. Sometimes they require skin and muscle flaps, in which healthy, thicker tissue with a good blood supply is surgically repositioned to cover the damaged area. This type of surgery is not always successful, however, especially for frail older people who are malnourished. Often, when infections develop deep within a sore, antibiotics are given. When bones beneath a sore become infected, the bone infection (osteomyelitis—see page 556) is extremely difficult to cure and may spread through the bloodstream, requiring many weeks of treatment with an antibiotic.

CHAPTER
190 Sweating Disorders

Sweat is made by sweat glands in the skin and carried to the skin's surface by ducts. Sweating helps keep the body cool. Thus, people sweat more when it is warm. They also sweat when they are nervous, under stress, or exercising.

Sweat is composed mostly of water, but it also contains salt (mostly sodium chloride) and other chemicals. When a person sweats a lot, the lost salt and water must be replaced.

Prickly Heat

Prickly heat (miliaria) is an itchy skin rash caused by trapped sweat.

Prickly heat develops when the narrow ducts carrying sweat to the skin surface get clogged. The trapped sweat causes inflammation, which produces irritation (prickling), itching, and a rash of very tiny blisters. Prickly heat also can appear as large, reddened areas of skin.

Prickly heat is most common in warm, humid climates, but overdressed people in cool climates can also develop prickly heat. It tends to occur on areas of the body where skin touches skin, such as under the breasts, on the inner thighs, and under the arms.

What Causes Prickly Heat?

Prickly heat results when sweat glands are blocked and ruptured, and sweat is trapped below the skin.

Normal Sweat Gland Duct　　**Clogged Sweat Gland Duct**

Clog

Duct

Sweat gland

The condition is controlled by keeping the skin cool and dry. Use of powders and antiperspirants often helps. Conditions that increase sweating should be avoided, thus an air-conditioned environment is ideal.

Once the rash develops, corticosteroid creams or lotions are used, sometimes with a bit of menthol added. However, these topical treatments are not as effective as keeping the skin cool and dry.

Excessive Sweating

People with excessive sweating (hyperhidrosis) sweat profusely, and some sweat almost constantly. Although people with a fever or those exposed to very warm environments sweat, people with excessive sweating tend to sweat even without these circumstances. Excessive sweating may affect the entire surface of the skin, but often it is limited to the palms of the hands, soles of the feet, armpits, or genital area.

Usually, no specific cause is found. However, a number of disorders can cause excessive sweating.

People who sweat excessively are frequently anxious about their condition, and it may lead to social withdrawal. This anxiety may make the sweating worse.

Severe, chronic wetness can make the affected area white, wrinkled, and cracked. Sometimes the area becomes red and inflamed. The area may emit a foul odor (bromhidrosis) due to the breakdown of sweat by bacteria and yeasts that normally live on the skin. Clothing may also become soaked with sweat.

Treatment

Excessive sweating can be controlled to some degree with commercial antiperspirants. However, stronger treatment is often needed, especially for the palms, soles, armpits, or genital area. Applying an aluminum chloride solution at night may help—prescription and nonprescription strengths of this drug are available. A person first dries the sweaty area and then applies the solution. If the response is inadequate, a plastic film can be applied over the solution to enhance its effectiveness. In the morning, the person removes the film and washes the area. If the solution irritates the skin, the plastic film should be left off. Some people need two applications daily; this regimen usually gives relief in a week. Then an application once or twice a week is sufficient to maintain relief.

SOME CAUSES OF EXCESSIVE SWEATING

TYPE	EXAMPLES
Hormonal (endocrine) disorders	An overactive thyroid gland (hyperthyroidism), low blood sugar levels, certain pituitary gland disorders
Drugs	Antidepressants, aspirin and other nonsteroidal anti-inflammatory drugs, some drugs for diabetes, caffeine, theophylline. Withdrawal from opioids
Nervous system disorders	Injuries, dysfunction of the autonomic nervous system, damage to certain nerves by cancer
Cancer*	Lymphoma, leukemia
Infections*	Tuberculosis, heart infection (endocarditis), severe fungal infections of the entire body
Other	Carcinoid syndrome, pregnancy, menopause, anxiety

* Causes primarily night sweats.

A solution of methenamine also may help. Tap water iontophoresis, a process in which a weak electrical current is applied to the sweaty area, is sometimes used. Drugs taken by mouth, such as phenoxybenzamine and propantheline, sometimes control sweating, and injections of botulinum toxin A into the affected area diminish sweating. If drugs are not effective, a more drastic measure to control severe sweating involves surgically cutting the nerves leading to the sweat glands. Excessive sweating limited to the armpits is sometimes treated by liposuction to remove the sweat glands.

For people in whom odor is a problem, cleansing twice daily with soap and water usually removes the bacteria and yeast that cause odor. In some people, a few days of washing with an antiseptic soap, which may be combined with use of antibacterial creams containing clindamycin or erythromycin, may be necessary. Shaving the hair in the armpits may also help control odor. Clothing should be washed often as well.

Diminished Sweating

Some people sweat too little (a condition called hypohidrosis). Diminished sweating is usually limited to a specific area of the body. It can be caused by a skin injury (such as from trauma, radiation, infection [such as leprosy], or inflammation) or by a connective tissue disorder (such as systemic sclerosis, systemic lupus erythematosus, or Sjögren's syndrome) that wastes away the sweat glands. Diminished sweating also may be caused by drugs, especially those that have anticholinergic effects (see box on page 1897). Nerve damage caused by diabetes (diabetic neuropathy) can also cause diminished sweating, as can a variety of syndromes existing at or before birth. Sometimes, people who have very severe heatstroke stop sweating.

A doctor makes the diagnosis by observing the person. If there is diminished sweating over a large portion of the body, the person may overheat, and cooling measures (such as air-conditioning and wearing wet garments) are the best treatment.

CHAPTER 191 Hair Disorders

Hair originates in the hair follicles. These follicles are located in the dermis, the skin layer just below the surface layer and above the subcutaneous fat. Hair follicles are present everywhere on the surface of the body except the lips, palms of the hands, and soles of the feet. New hair is made in the hair matrix at the base of the hair follicle. Living cells in the hair matrix multiply and push upward. These cells rapidly dehydrate, die, and compact into a dense, hard mass that forms the hair shaft. The hair shaft, which is made up of dead protein, is covered by a delicate covering (cuticle) composed of platelike scales.

Hair is colored by the pigment melanin, which is also responsible for skin color. Human hair colors come from two types of melanin: eumelanin in black or brown hair and pheomelanin in auburn or blond hair.

Hair grows in cycles. Each cycle consists of a long growing phase followed by a brief transitional phase and then a short resting phase. At the end of the resting phase, the hair falls out and a new hair starts growing in the follicle, beginning the cycle again. Eyebrows and eyelashes have a growing phase of 1 to 6 months. Scalp hairs have a growing phase of 2 to 6 years. Normally, about 100 scalp hairs reach the end of the resting phase each day and fall out.

Hair growth is regulated by male hormones (androgens, such as testosterone and dihydrotestosterone), which are present in both men and women, although in different amounts. Testosterone stimulates hair growth in the pubic area and underarms. Dihydrotestosterone stimulates hair growth in the beard area and hair loss at the scalp.

Hair disorders include excessive hairiness (hirsutism and hypertrichosis), hair loss (alopecia), and ingrown beard hairs (pseudofolliculitis barbae). Most disorders are not serious or life threatening, but they are often perceived as major cosmetic issues that require treatment.

Hirsutism and Hypertrichosis

Hirsutism is the excessive growth of thick or dark hair in women in locations that are more typical of male hair patterns (for example, mustache, beard, central chest, shoulders, lower abdomen, back, and inner thighs). Hypertrichosis is an increase in hair growth anywhere on the body in men and women.

- Overproduction of male hormones because of tumors or the use of certain drugs can cause hirsutism.
- In women, excess hair caused by overproduction of male hormones may be accompanied by acne, a deepened voice, and male-pattern hair loss.
- Doctors review the person's current drug use, changes in physique, family history, and hormone levels.
- Treatment may include hormonal therapy and hair removal.

Hirsutism is excessive thick or dark hair in women in locations on the body where men usually have more hair, such as the mustache and beard areas, central chest, shoulders, lower abdomen, back, and inner thighs. Whether hair growth is considered excessive may differ depending on ethnic background, cultural interpretation, and individual opinion. Men vary significantly in amount of body hair, but they rarely seek medical evaluation for large amounts of body hair. **Hypertrichosis** is simply an increase in the amount of hair growth anywhere on the body. Hypertrichosis may be generalized or localized.

Causes

A person's age, sex, racial and ethnic origin, as well as hereditary factors, determine the amount of body hair. Rarely, excess hair is present at birth because of a hereditary disorder. Usually, excess hair develops later in life.

Hirsutism: Hirsutism most often is the result of

- A familial tendency, particularly among people of Mediterranean or Middle Eastern ancestry
- Polycystic ovary syndrome (see page 1528)

Sometimes, excess hair is caused by tumors or other disorders of the pituitary gland, adrenal glands, or ovaries that cause levels of male hormones (androgens) to increase abnormally. Anabolic steroids, which may be abused by female athletes and bodybuilders, are androgens. Excess androgens in women also may cause enlarged muscles, acne, a deepened voice, male-pattern hair loss, and an enlarged clitoris. Menstrual periods may become irregular or stop. These changes are called virilization.

> **? Did You Know...**
> Shaving does not increase the thickness of hair or the rate of hair growth.

Hypertrichosis: Hypertrichosis is usually caused by a body-wide (systemic) illness or a drug. Illnesses include the following:

- Dermatomyositis
- General systemic illness (such as advanced HIV infection)
- Hypothyroidism or other endocrine disorders
- Undernutrition
- Porphyria cutanea tarda
- Some central nervous system disorders

Drug causes of hypertrichosis include minoxidil, phenytoin, cyclosporine, and anabolic steroids.

Diagnosis

Because some excess hair results from medical disorders, doctors must distinguish excess hair that is the result of an underlying medical problem from hair growth that is simply a cosmetic concern.

Doctors first look for other symptoms of virilization or features of Cushing's syndrome (see page 1001), such as a large, round face and a pad of fat between the shoulders. Doctors also ask about excess hair in family members, review the person's drug use (including illicit use of anabolic steroids), and look for an underlying medical condition.

Unless the cause of the excess hair is clearly the use of a particular drug, women should have blood tests to measure various hormone levels, as well as ultrasonography or computed tomography (CT) scanning to check for a tumor of the adrenal glands or ovaries.

Treatment

Doctors treat any specific cause of excess hair. Drugs that may be the cause are stopped or changed if possible. Treatment for the excess hair itself is unnecessary unless people find the hair cosmetically objectionable.

Hormonal Treatments: When androgen excess is the cause, two types of hormonal drugs can be used.

- Oral contraceptives reduce ovarian androgen production.
- Antiandrogenic drugs block the effects of testosterone.

Antiandrogenic drugs, such as spironolactone, flutamide, and finasteride, may cause birth defects, so they are usually used together with oral contraceptives.

Hair Removal: Hair removal methods may be temporary or permanent.

Temporary hair removal methods include shaving or clipping the hair. Shaving does not increase the thickness of hair or rate of hair growth. Other common temporary hair removal measures include plucking, waxing, and use of a depilatory (a liquid or cream preparation), which chemically removes hair at the skin surface.

Permanent hair removal requires that the hair follicles be destroyed. Electrolysis, in which an electric needle is inserted into each hair follicle, destroys the hair follicles by heat and electrical current. Multiple treatments are often necessary, and many follicles often survive the procedure, allowing hair regrowth. Laser treatments also may permanently reduce unwanted hair (see box on page 1331). However, while multiple laser treatments may permanently destroy many hair follicles, some hair eventually grows back.

As an alternative to hair removal, eflornithine cream substantially slows hair growth in many people and may decrease the need to manually remove hair. Hair bleach may mask excess hair by lightening it, rendering it less noticeable.

Alopecia

Alopecia is the loss of hair on the head or on any other part of the body.

- Hair loss may occur because of changes in hormone levels, the use of certain drugs, stress, and some skin disorders.
- Doctors diagnose the type of hair loss by examining the hair and skin.
- Treatments include minoxidil, finasteride, hair transplantation, wigs, and corticosteroids.

Hair loss that occurs on the head is generally called baldness. Hair loss is often of great concern to people for cosmetic reasons, but it can also be a sign of a body-wide (systemic) illness.

Causes

Hair grows in cycles. Each cycle consists of a long growing phase (anagen), a brief transitional phase (catagen), and a short resting phase (telogen). At the end of the resting phase, the hair falls out, and the cycle begins again as a new hair starts growing in the follicle. Normally, about 100 scalp hairs reach the end of resting phase each day and fall out. When many more than 100 hairs per day go into resting phase, hair loss (telogen effluvium) may occur. A disruption of the growing phase causing loss of hairs is called anagen effluvium.

The **most common cause** of hair loss is

- Androgenetic alopecia

Other common causes of hair loss are

- Drugs (including chemotherapeutic agents)
- Infections (including fungal infections)
- Systemic illnesses (particularly those that cause high fever, systemic lupus erythematosus, endocrine disorders, and nutritional deficiencies)

Other factors include heredity, aging, and local skin conditions.

Androgenetic Alopecia: This form of alopecia eventually affects about half of all men (male-pattern hair loss) and women (female-pattern hair loss). The hormone dihydrotestosterone plays a major role, along with heredity. The hair loss can begin at any age, even during the teenage years.

In men, hair loss usually begins at the forehead or on the top of the head toward the back. Some men lose only some hair and have only a receding hairline or a small bald spot in the back. Others, especially men whose hair loss begins at a young age, lose all of the hair on the top of the head but retain hair on the sides and back of the scalp. This pattern is referred to as male-pattern hair loss.

> **Did You Know...**
> About 100 scalp hairs normally fall out each day.

In women, hair loss begins on the top of the head and is usually a thinning of the hair rather than a complete loss of hair. The hairline typically stays intact. This pattern is referred to as female-pattern hair loss.

Losing Hair

In men, hair is usually first lost at the forehead or on the top of the head toward the back. This is called male-pattern hair loss.

In women, hair is usually first lost on the top of the head. Typically, the hair thins rather than is completely lost, and the hairline stays intact. This pattern is called female-pattern hair loss.

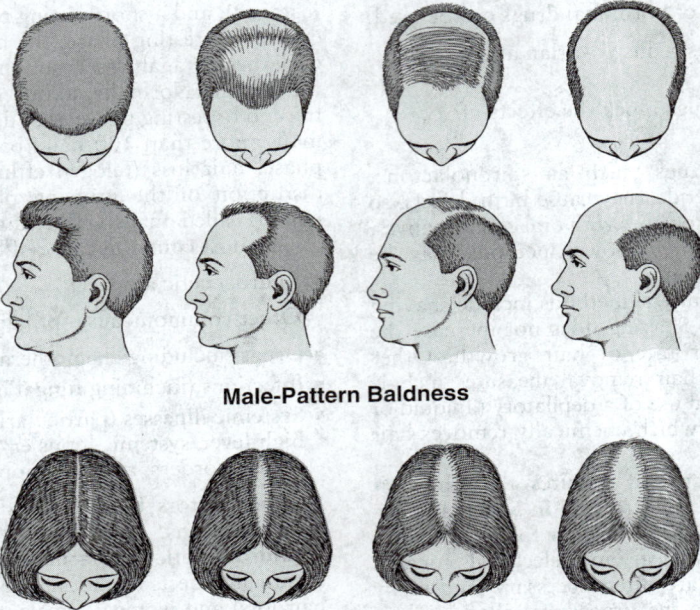

Male-Pattern Baldness

Female-Pattern Baldness

Anagen Effluvium: Anagen effluvium is hair loss caused by exposure to drugs or other chemicals that disrupt the growing phase (anagen) of hair. Examples include chemotherapy drugs, certain poisons (such as boric acid, mercury, and thallium), and radiation.

Telogen Effluvium: Telogen effluvium is hair loss caused by physical or psychologic stress that increases the number of hairs that go into resting phase (telogen). Sudden weight loss, severe illness (particularly one that involves a high fever), or surgery may cause hair loss. Some drugs—including chemotherapy drugs, blood pressure drugs, lithium, anticonvulsants, oral contraceptives, anticoagulants, ACE inhibitors, vitamin A, and retinoids—can also cause the condition. Telogen effluvium may also result from an underactive or overactive thyroid gland or pituitary gland and commonly occurs after pregnancy and menopause.

The hair typically falls out 3 or 4 months after the event that caused the stress. Usually, the hair loss is temporary, and the hair grows back.

Alopecia Areata: In this common skin disorder, round, irregular patches of hair are suddenly lost. The margins of the patches have characteristic short, broken hairs, which resemble exclamation points. The cause is believed to be an autoimmune reaction in which the body's immune defenses mistakenly attack the hair follicles. Alopecia areata is not the result of another disease, but some people may also have a thyroid disorder or vitiligo (a skin pigment disorder).

The site of hair loss is usually the scalp or beard. Rarely, all body hair is lost, a condition called alopecia universalis. Alopecia areata occurs in both sexes and at all ages but is most common in children and young adults. The hair usually grows back in several months. In people with widespread hair loss, regrowth is less likely.

Hair Pulling (Trichotillomania): This disorder is the habitual pulling out of normal hair. The habit is most common in children but may occur in adults.

The hair pulling may not be noticed for a long time, causing confusion for doctors and parents who mistakenly think that an illness such as alopecia areata or a fungal infection is causing the hair loss.

Traction Alopecia: This disorder is hair loss caused by tight braids, rollers or ponytails that pull constantly on hair. Hair loss most often occurs at the hairline of the forehead and temples.

Scarring Alopecia: Scarring alopecia is the result of destruction of the hair follicle causing it to be replaced by scar tissue. Diseases that cause scarring alopecia include systemic lupus erythematosus, lichen planus, persistent bacterial or fungal infections, and skin cancer. The skin may also be damaged from burns, other physical injuries, and radiation therapy.

Diagnosis

Doctors diagnose male-pattern or female-pattern hair loss based on its typical appearance. Determining the cause of other types of hair loss simply by observation is sometimes difficult. Doctors usually gently pull or pluck out a few hairs and examine the hair shafts under a microscope. Less often, doctors do a biopsy of the skin (see page 1278). A biopsy helps determine if the hair follicles are normal. If they are not normal, the biopsy may indicate possible causes. If the doctors' examination finds signs of hormonal irregularities or other serious illness, blood tests to identify those disorders may be needed.

Treatment

Male-pattern and female-pattern hair loss can sometimes be treated effectively with drugs.

Minoxidil may prevent further hair loss and increase hair growth when applied directly to the scalp twice a day. Finasteride works by blocking the effects of male hormones on the hair follicles and is taken by mouth daily. Improvement may occur after either of these drugs is taken for several months. The most important effect of these drugs may be to prevent further hair loss. The effects last only as long as the drugs are taken. Finasteride is not used for women who have hair loss.

Hair transplantation is a more permanent solution, in which hair follicles are removed from one part of the scalp and transplanted to the bald area. In a newer hair transplantation technique, only one or two hairs are transplanted at a time. Although this technique is more time consuming, it does not require removal of large plugs of skin and allows the implants to be oriented in the same direction as the natural hair.

Telogen effluvium or anagen effluvium generally resolves after the inciting event or exposure to chemicals ends. Because the hair loss is usually temporary, wigs often offer the best treatment. A person undergoing chemotherapy should consult a wig maker even before therapy begins so that an appropriate wig can be ready when needed.

Alopecia areata can be treated with corticosteroids. For small bald patches, corticosteroids are typically injected under the skin of the bald patch, and minoxidil may be applied topically as well. For larger patches, corticosteroids are sometimes taken by mouth. Another treatment for alopecia areata involves applying irritating chemicals, such as anthralin or other substances to the scalp to induce a mild allergic reaction or irritation. The irritation sometimes promotes hair growth.

Scarring alopecia is particularly difficult to treat. When possible, the cause of the scarring is treated, but after an area is fully scarred, hair will not grow back.

Ingrown Beard Hairs

Ingrown beard hairs (pseudofolliculitis barbae) is inflammation caused by hairs that curl so that the tips puncture the skin.

This hair disorder most often occurs with the curly hairs of the beard, especially in black men. Each ingrown hair results in a tiny, mildly painful pimple with a barely visible hair curling into the center.

Doctors diagnose the condition by its typical appearance.

Treatment involves teasing the tips of any ingrown hairs out of the skin with the point of a needle or sharp scalpel. If there is much inflammation, doctors sometimes give hydrocortisone or antibiotic cream.

The best preventive treatment is to stop shaving and grow the beard. When the hairs are longer, they do not curl back and puncture the skin.

A man who does not want a beard can use a depilatory (a liquid or cream preparation that removes unwanted hair), although it often irritates the skin. Also, hair can be permanently removed with electrolysis or with laser treatment (see box on page 1331). People who must shave should wet the beard first and should shave in the same direction in which the hair grows. People should avoid shaving closely with multiple razor strokes. Applying eflornithine cream may help by slowing hair growth.

CHAPTER
192 Pigment Disorders

Various shades and colors of human skin are created by the brown pigment, melanin. Without melanin, the skin would be pale white with varying shades of pink caused by the blood flowing through it. Fair-skinned people produce very little melanin, darker-skinned people produce moderate amounts, and very dark-skinned people produce the most. People with albinism have little or no melanin.

Melanin is produced by special cells (melanocytes) that are interspersed among the other cells in the top layer of the skin, the epidermis. After melanin is produced, it spreads into other nearby skin cells.

When exposed to sunlight, melanocytes produce increased amounts of melanin, causing the skin to darken, or tan. In some fair-skinned people, certain melanocytes produce more melanin than others in response to sunlight. This uneven melanin production results in spots of pigmentation known as freckles. A tendency to freckle runs in families. Increased amounts of melanin can be produced in response to hormonal changes, such as those that may take place in Addison's disease, in pregnancy, or with oral contraceptive use. Some cases of skin darkening, however, are not related to increased melanin at all, but rather to abnormal pigments that make their way into the skin. Diseases such as hemochromatosis or hemosiderosis or some drugs that are applied to the skin, swallowed, or injected can cause skin darkening. A buildup of bilirubin (the main pigment in bile) causes the skin to turn yellow (jaundice).

An abnormally low amount of melanin (hypopigmentation) may affect large areas of the body or small patches. Decreased melanin usually results from a previous injury to the skin, such as a blister, ulcer, burn, or skin infection. Sometimes pigment loss results from an inflammatory condition of the skin or, in rare instances, is hereditary.

Albinism

Albinism is a rare hereditary disorder in which little or no melanin is formed.

Albinism occurs in people of all races and throughout the world.

Albinism is easily recognized by its typical appearance. People with albinism have white hair, pale skin, and pink or pale blue eyes. The genetic disorder causing albinism also results in abnormal vision and, often, in involuntary eye movements (nystagmus).

 Did You Know...
Albinism occurs in people of all races.

Because melanin protects the skin from the sun, people with albinism are very prone to sunburn and skin cancer. Even a few minutes of bright sunlight can cause serious burns.

There is no cure for albinism. People with the disorder can minimize or prevent problems by doing the following:

- Staying out of direct sunlight
- Wearing sunglasses with UV (ultraviolet) protection and clothing that protects from the sun
- Applying sunscreen that blocks UVA and UVB light with a sun protection factor (SPF) rating of at least 30 (see page 1327)

Clothing, even when it covers the body, varies in how well it protects against UV light. Generally, the tighter the weave and the heavier the weight, the more protection a fabric provides.

Vitiligo

Vitiligo is a disorder in which a localized loss of melanocytes causes patches of skin to turn white.

- Patches of whitened skin are present on various parts of the body.
- Doctors usually base the diagnosis on the appearance of the skin.
- Corticosteroid creams or phototherapy plus light-sensitizing drugs may darken the skin, or, if needed, skin grafts may be used.

The cause of vitiligo is unknown, but it may involve an attack by the immune system on the cells that produce the skin pigment melanin (melanocytes). Vitiligo tends to run in families and may occur with certain other diseases. Vitiligo is associated with autoimmune disorders, thyroid disease being the most common. The relationship between the disorders is unclear; however, people with diabetes, Addison's disease, and pernicious anemia also are somewhat more likely to develop vitiligo. The disorder may occur after physical trauma or sunburn.

Although vitiligo does not pose a medical problem, it may cause considerable psychologic distress.

Symptoms

In some people, one or two well-defined patches of vitiligo appear. In other people, patches appear over a large part of the body. The changes are most striking in people with dark skin. Commonly affected areas are the face, elbows, knees, hands, shins, and genitals. The affected skin is extremely prone to sunburn. The areas of skin affected by vitiligo also produce white hair because melanocytes are lost from the hair follicles.

Diagnosis

Vitiligo is recognized by its typical appearance. A Wood's light examination is often done to help distinguish vitiligo from other causes of lightened skin (see page 1278). Other tests, including skin biopsies, are rarely necessary.

Treatment

No cure is known for vitiligo, although skin color may return spontaneously. Treatment may be helpful. Small patches sometimes darken when treated with strong corticosteroid creams. Drugs such as tacrolimus or pimecrolimus may be applied to the face, where strong corticosteroid creams may cause side effects. Some people simply use bronzers, skin stains, or makeup to darken the area. Because many people still have a few melanocytes in the patches of vitiligo, exposure to ultraviolet (UV) light in a doctor's office (phototherapy) restimulates pigment production in more than half of them (see box on page 1294). In particular, psoralens (drugs that make the skin more sensitive to light) combined with ultraviolet A light (PUVA) or narrow-band ultraviolet B light treatment without psoralens can be given. However, phototherapy takes months to be effective and may need to be continued indefinitely.

Areas that do not respond to phototherapy may be treated with various skin-grafting techniques and even transplantation of melanocytes grown from unaffected areas of the person's skin. All affected areas of skin should be protected from the sun with clothing and sunscreen.

Some people who have very large areas of vitiligo sometimes prefer to bleach the pigment out of the unaffected skin to achieve an even color. Bleaching is done with repeated applications of hydroquinone cream to the skin for weeks to years. The effects of bleaching are irreversible.

SPOTLIGHT ON AGING

Lentigines (commonly called liver spots or age spots) are flat, tan to brown oval spots on the skin. Lentigines commonly result from spending a lot of time in the sun. They appear most frequently on areas that are exposed to the sun, such as the face and back of the hands. Lentigines that result from sun exposure are called solar lentigines. They tend to increase in number as people age. Thus, these spots are more common with advancing age. Lentigines are noncancerous, but people who have them may be at higher risk for melanoma.

Doctors can remove them with freezing treatments (cryotherapy) or laser therapy. Bleaching agents such as hydroquinone are not effective.

Some lentigines that are not related to exposure to sunlight (nonsolar lentigines) sometimes occur in people with certain rare hereditary disorders, such as Peutz-Jeghers syndrome (characterized by many lentigines on the lips and polyps in the stomach and intestine), xeroderma pigmentosum, and Leopard syndrome.

Melasma

Melasma causes dark brown patches of pigmentation to appear on sun-exposed areas, usually the face.

Melasma tends to appear during pregnancy (mask of pregnancy) and in women who take oral contraceptives, although it can occur in anyone. The disorder is most common in sunny climates and among people with darker skin.

Irregular, patchy areas of dark color appear on the skin, usually on both sides of the face. The pigmentation most often occurs in the center of the face and on the cheeks, forehead, upper lip, and nose. Sometimes people have the patches only on the sides of the face. Rarely, melasma appears on the forearms. The patches do not itch or hurt and are only of cosmetic significance.

If the skin is protected from the sun, melasma often fades after pregnancy or when an oral contraceptive is stopped. People with melasma can use sunscreens on the dark patches and avoid sun exposure to prevent the condition from getting worse. Skin-bleaching creams containing hydroquinone and retinoic acid can help lighten the dark patches.

CHAPTER 193

Blistering Diseases

A blister (bulla) is a bubble of fluid that forms beneath a thin layer of dead skin. The fluid is a mixture of water and proteins that oozes from injured tissue. Blisters most commonly form in response to a specific injury, such as a burn or irritation, and usually involve only the topmost layers of skin. These blisters heal quickly, usually without leaving a scar. Blisters that develop as part of a systemic (bodywide) disease may start in the deeper layers of the skin and cover widespread areas. These blisters heal more slowly and may leave scars.

Many diseases and injuries can cause blistering, but three autoimmune diseases—bullous pemphigoid, dermatitis herpetiformis, and pemphigus vulgaris—are among the most serious. In an autoimmune disease, the body's immune system, which normally protects the body against foreign invaders, mistakenly attacks the body's own cells (see page 1124)—in this case, the skin.

Bullous Pemphigoid

Bullous pemphigoid is an autoimmune disease that causes blistering of the skin.

- Bullous pemphigoid occurs when the immune system attacks the skin and causes blistering.
- People develop large, itchy blisters with areas of inflamed skin.
- Doctors can diagnose bullous pemphigoid by examining skin samples under a microscope and checking for certain antibody deposits.
- Treatment involves corticosteroids and drugs that suppress the immune system.

Bullous pemphigoid tends to occur mainly in older people. It is a less serious disease than pemphigus, is rarely fatal, and does not result in widespread peeling of skin. It can involve a large portion of the skin, however, and can be very uncomfortable, with itchiness often the first sign of the disease.

In bullous pemphigoid, the immune system forms antibodies directed against the skin, resulting in large, tense, very itchy blisters surrounded by areas of red, inflamed skin. Blisters in the mouth are uncommon and are not severe. The areas of skin that are not blistered appear normal.

Diagnosis and Treatment

Doctors usually recognize bullous pemphigoid by its characteristic blisters. However, it is not always easy to distinguish it from pemphigus vulgaris and other blistering conditions, such as severe poison ivy. Bullous pemphigoid is diagnosed with certainty by examining a sample of skin under a microscope (skin biopsy). Doctors differentiate bullous pemphigoid from pemphigus vulgaris by noting the layers of skin involved and the particular appearance of antibody deposits.

Mild bullous pemphigoid sometimes resolves without treatment, but resolution usually takes months or years. Therefore, most people receive drug therapy. Nearly everyone responds quickly to high-dose corticosteroids, which are gradually reduced (tapered) after several weeks. The combination of nicotinamide and minocycline or tetracycline is sometimes successful. Sometimes azathioprine or cyclophosphamide is given as well for more severe disease. Immunoglobulin given intravenously is a safe, promising new treatment, especially for people who do not respond to conventional drug therapy. Although some local skin care may be needed, most people do not require hospitalization or intensive skin care treatment.

Dermatitis Herpetiformis

Dermatitis herpetiformis is an autoimmune disease causing clusters of intensely itchy small blisters and hivelike swellings.

- In dermatitis herpetiformis, glutens in wheat, rye, and barley products cause the immune system to attack the skin.
- People have small, itchy blisters and hivelike eruptions on various areas of the body.
- Doctors diagnose dermatitis herpetiformis by examining skin samples under a microscope.
- People usually respond to treatment with dapsone and a gluten-free diet.

Despite its name, dermatitis herpetiformis has nothing to do with the herpesvirus. In people with dermatitis herpetiformis, glutens (proteins) in wheat, rye, and barley products somehow activate the immune system, which attacks parts of the skin and causes the rash and itching. People with dermatitis herpetiformis often have celiac sprue (see page 165), which is an intestinal disorder caused by sensitivity to gluten, although they may not have symptoms from the celiac sprue. People also have a higher incidence of other autoimmune diseases, such as thyroiditis, systemic lupus erythematosus, sarcoidosis, and diabetes. People with dermatitis herpetiformis occasionally develop lymphoma in the intestines.

Small blisters usually develop gradually, mostly on the elbows, knees, buttocks, lower back, and back of the head. Sometimes blisters break out on the face and neck. Itching and burning are likely to be severe. Anti-inflammatory drugs, such as ibuprofen, may worsen the rash.

> **? Did You Know...**
> Dermatitis herpetiformis is not related to the herpesvirus.

Diagnosis and Treatment

The diagnosis is based on a skin biopsy, in which doctors find particular kinds and patterns of antibodies in the skin samples.

The blisters do not go away without treatment. People are usually placed on a gluten-free diet (a diet that is free of wheat, rye, and barley). The drug dapsone, taken by mouth, almost always provides relief in 1 to 2 days but requires that blood counts be checked regularly. Once the disease has been brought under control with drugs and the person has followed a strict gluten-free diet for 6 months or longer, drug treatment usually can be discontinued. However, some people can never stop taking the drug. In most people, any reexposure to gluten, however small, triggers another outbreak. A gluten-free diet may prevent the development of intestinal lymphoma.

Pemphigus Vulgaris

Pemphigus vulgaris is a rare, severe autoimmune disease in which blisters of varying sizes break out on the skin, the lining of the mouth, the genitals, and other mucous membranes.

- Pemphigus vulgaris occurs when the immune system mistakenly attacks proteins in the upper layers of the skin.
- People experience severe blistering in the mouth and on other areas of the body, and sometimes sheets of skin peel off.
- Doctors can diagnose pemphigus vulgaris by examining skin samples under a microscope.
- Treatment usually involves corticosteroids or drugs that suppress the immune system.

Pemphigus develops most often in middle-aged or older people. It rarely develops in children. In this disease, the immune system produces antibodies that attack specific proteins that connect the epidermal cells (the cells in the top layer of skin) to each other. When these connections are disrupted, the cells separate from each other and from the lower layers

of the skin, and blisters form. Similar-appearing blisters occur with a less dangerous skin disorder, bullous pemphigoid.

Symptoms

The major symptom of pemphigus vulgaris is the development of clear, soft, usually painless (but sometimes itchy and tender) blisters of various sizes. In addition, the top layer of skin may detach from the lower layers in response to slight pinching or rubbing, causing it to peel off in sheets and to leave painful erosions.

The blisters often first appear in the mouth and soon rupture, forming painful sores (ulcers). More blisters and ulcers may follow until the entire lining of the mouth is affected, causing difficulty swallowing. Blisters form on the skin as well. These blisters then rupture, leaving raw, painful, crusted wounds. The person feels generally ill. Blisters may be widespread, and once ruptured, they may become infected. When severe, pemphigus vulgaris is as harmful as a serious burn. Similar to a burn, the damaged skin oozes large amounts of fluid and is prone to infection by many types of bacteria.

> **? Did You Know...**
> Pemphigus vulgaris is usually fatal without treatment, but 90% of people survive if they receive treatment.

Diagnosis and Treatment

Doctors usually recognize pemphigus vulgaris by its characteristic blisters, but the disorder is diagnosed with certainty by examining a sample of skin under a microscope (skin biopsy). Sometimes doctors use special chemical stains that allow antibody deposits to be seen under the microscope. Doctors differentiate pemphigus vulgaris from bullous pemphigoid by noting the layers of skin involved and the particular appearance of antibody deposits.

Without treatment, pemphigus vulgaris is usually fatal. With treatment, 90% of people survive. High doses of corticosteroids are the mainstay of treatment. If the disease is controlled, the dose of corticosteroids is gradually reduced (tapered). If the person does not respond to treatment or the disease flares up as the dose is tapered, an immunosuppressant, such as azathioprine, cyclophosphamide, or rituximab, is also given. People with severe pemphigus vulgaris may also undergo plasmapheresis, a process in which antibodies are filtered from the blood (see box on page 1030).

Immune globulin given intravenously is a new, safe and effective treatment for severe pemphigus vulgaris. Some people respond well enough to discontinue drug therapy, whereas others must continue taking low doses of the drugs for long periods.

In a hospital, the raw skin surfaces require extraordinary care, similar to the care given to people with severe burns. Antibiotics may be needed to treat infections in ruptured blisters. Dressings, sometimes coated with petroleum jelly, can protect raw, oozing areas.

CHAPTER 194 Parasitic Skin Infections

Most skin parasites are tiny insects or worms that burrow into the skin and make their home there. Some parasites live in the skin for part of their life cycle; others, for their entire life cycle. Parasitic skin infections frequently cause severe itching and inflammation.

Scabies

Scabies is a mite infestation of the skin that produces tiny reddish bumps and severe itching.

- Scabies usually spreads from person to person through physical contact.
- People with scabies have severe itching, even though there are typically few mites on the body.
- Doctors diagnose scabies by examining the itchy areas and sometimes by looking at skin scrapings under a microscope.
- Treatments include permethrin or lindane applied to the skin and ivermectin taken by mouth.

Scabies is caused by the itch mite *Sarcoptes scabiei.* The female itch mite tunnels in the topmost layer of the skin and deposits her eggs in burrows. Young mites (larvae) then hatch in a few days. The infestation causes intense itching, probably from an allergic reaction to the mites.

The infestation spreads easily from person to person on physical contact, often spreading through an entire household. In rare cases, mites may be spread on clothing, bedding, and other shared objects, but their survival is brief, and normal laundering destroys them.

Symptoms and Diagnosis

The hallmark of scabies is intense itching, which is usually worse at night. The burrows of the mites are often visible as very thin lines up to ½ inch (about 1 centimeter) long, sometimes with a tiny bump at one end. Sometimes, only tiny bumps are seen, many of which are scratched open because of the itching. The burrows can be anywhere on the body except the face. Common sites are the webs between the fingers and toes, the wrists, ankles, buttocks, nipples, and, in males, the genitals. Over time, the burrows may become difficult to see because they are obscured by inflammation induced by scratching. People with a weakened immune system may develop severe infestations, which produce large areas of thickened, crusted skin.

Usually, itching and the appearance of burrows are all that are needed to make a diagnosis of scabies. However, doctors can confirm the presence of mites, eggs, or mite feces by taking a scraping from the bumps or burrows and looking at it under a microscope.

Treatment

Scabies can be cured by applying a cream containing 5% permethrin, which is left on the skin overnight and then washed off. For older children and adults, lindane lotion is an alternative. With either drug, a second treatment is required a week later. Ivermectin taken by mouth in two doses given a week apart also is effective and is especially helpful for severe infestations in people with a weakened immune system.

Even after successful treatment, itching may persist for 2 to 4 weeks because of a continued allergic reaction to the mite bodies, which remain in the skin for a while. The itching can be treated with mild corticosteroid cream and antihistamines taken by mouth (see page 1284). Occasionally, the skin irritation and deep scratches lead to a bacterial infection, which may require antibiotics given by mouth.

Family members and people who have had close physical contact, such as sexual contact, with a person with scabies should be treated as well. Clothing and bedding used during the preceding few days should be washed in hot water and dried in a hot dryer or dry cleaned.

Lice Infestation

Lice infestation (pediculosis) is a skin infestation by tiny wingless insects.

- Lice spread most frequently through person-to-person contact.
- People with lice usually have severe itching.
- Lice and their eggs can be found by looking through hair on the head or other parts of the body.
- Treatment usually involves shampoos, creams, or lotions.
- Some people require an antiparasitic drug taken by mouth.

Lice are barely visible wingless insects that live by sucking blood. They spread easily from person to person by body contact and shared clothing and other personal items. Three species of lice inhabit different parts of the body.

Head lice infest the scalp hair. The infestation is spread by personal contact and possibly by shared combs, brushes, hats, and other personal items. Head lice are a common scourge of school children of all social strata. Head lice are less common among blacks. There is no association between head lice and poor hygiene or low socioeconomic status.

Body lice usually infest people who have poor hygiene and those living in close quarters or crowded institutions. They live in the seams of garments that are in contact with the skin. Body lice are spread by sharing contaminated clothing and bedding. Unlike head lice, body lice sometimes transmit serious diseases such as typhus, trench fever, and relapsing fever.

Pubic lice ("crabs"), which primarily infest the genital area, are typically spread during sexual contact. These lice may infest the chest hair, underarm hair, beard hair, eyebrows, and eyelashes as well.

Symptoms and Diagnosis

Lice infestation usually causes severe itching in the infested area. Intense scratching often breaks the skin, which can lead to bacterial infections. Children may hardly notice head lice or may have only a vague scalp irritation.

Head lice can be found by moving a fine-tooth detection comb through wet hair from the scalp outward. Lice themselves are sometimes hard to find, but their eggs are easier to see. Female lice lay shiny grayish white eggs (nits) that can be seen as tiny globules firmly stuck to hairs near their base. With chronic scalp infestations, the nits grow out with the hair and therefore can be found some distance from the scalp, depending on the duration of the infestation.

Nits are distinguished from other foreign material present on hair shafts by the fact that they are so strongly attached. Adult body lice and their eggs also may be found in the seams of clothing worn close to the skin. Public lice can be found by close inspection.

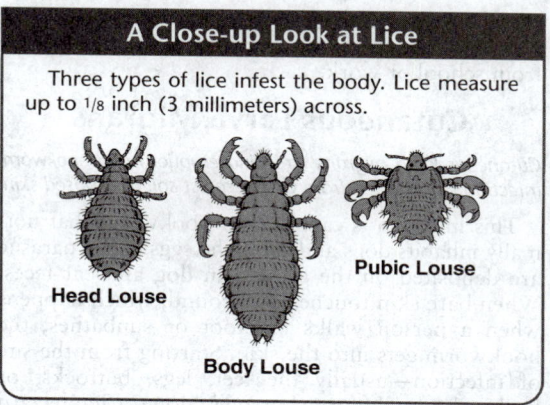

A Close-up Look at Lice

Three types of lice infest the body. Lice measure up to 1/8 inch (3 millimeters) across.

Head Louse

Body Louse

Pubic Louse

Treatment

Several effective prescription and nonprescription drugs are available to treat lice. Nonprescription shampoos and creams containing pyrethrins plus piperonyl butoxide are applied for 10 minutes and are then rinsed out. Prescription permethrin (a synthetic form of pyrethrin), applied as a liquid or as a cream, is also effective. Lindane—a prescription drug that can be applied as a lotion or shampoo—also cures lice infestation but is not as effective as the other preparations and is not recommended for young children because of possible neurologic side effects. Prescription malathion is highly effective at killing both adult lice and eggs, but it is not considered a first line of treatment because it is flammable, has an unpleasant odor, and must remain on the skin for 8 to 12 hours. All louse treatments are repeated in 7 to 10 days to kill newly hatched lice. Lice have started to become resistant to drugs and may be hard to kill. One dose of the drug ivermectin is usually given by mouth if lice resist standard treatment.

Most drug treatments also kill nits but do not remove them. Dead nits do not have to be removed, but drugs do not always kill all nits. Because it is not possible to distinguish between living and dead nits, doctors recommend removing them. Nonetheless, a very small percentage of children with nits in their scalp actually have live lice. Removal requires a fine-tooth comb—which is often packaged with the medication—and careful searching (hence the term "nit-picking"). Because the nits are so strongly stuck to the hair, several nonprescription preparations are available to loosen them. Nits are carried away from the scalp as the hair grows. If there are no nits within 1/4 inch of the scalp, the person does not have any live lice. The nits of body lice are destroyed simply by throwing away infested clothing or decontaminating it by thorough laundering or dry cleaning. For head lice, doctors do not have good evidence whether it is necessary to clean or throw away people's personal items or to exclude people from school or work.

Cutaneous Larva Migrans

Cutaneous larva migrans (creeping eruption) is a hookworm infection transmitted from warm, moist soil to exposed skin.

This infection is caused by a hookworm that normally inhabits dogs and cats. The eggs of the parasite are deposited on the ground in dog and cat feces. When bare skin touches the ground, which happens when a person walks barefoot or sunbathes, the hookworm gets into the skin. Starting from the site of infection—usually the feet, legs, buttocks, or back—the hookworm burrows along a haphazard tract, leaving a winding, threadlike, raised, red rash. The eruption itches intensely.

A liquid preparation of thiabendazole applied to the affected area effectively treats the infection. Albendazole or ivermectin given by mouth also is effective.

Cutaneous Myiasis

Cutaneous myiasis is skin infestation by the larvae (maggots) of certain fly species.

There are three main types of skin infestation by fly larvae:

- Furuncular (pimple- or boil-like) myiasis
- Wound myiasis
- Migratory myiasis

The disorders vary depending on the species of fly involved. Infestation usually occurs in tropical countries. People in the United States who have myiasis usually have recently arrived from or visited a tropical country.

Furuncular Myiasis: Many of the common sources are known as bot flies. The most well-known species of flies that cause furuncular myiasis come from South and Central America and sub-Saharan and tropical Africa. Many of the flies do not lay eggs on humans. Instead, the flies lay their eggs on other insects (such as mosquitoes) or on objects (such as drying laundry) that may come into contact with people's skin. Eggs hatch into larvae, which burrow into the skin and develop into mature larvae. The mature larvae are up to 1/2 to 1 inch (about 1.3 to 2.5 centimeters) long, depending on the species. If people are not treated, the larvae eventually emerge from the skin and drop to the ground to continue their life cycle.

Typical symptoms include itching, a sensation of movement, and sometimes sharp, stabbing pain. At first, people have a small red bump that may resemble a common insect bite or a beginning pimple (furuncle). Later, the bump enlarges, and a small opening may be visible at the center. The opening may drain clear, yellowish fluid, and sometimes a small portion of the larva is visible.

Because larvae require oxygen, blocking the skin opening may cause them to leave or at least come closer to the surface. When they are closer to the surface, it is easier to pull them out. To block the skin opening, some people apply petroleum jelly, nail polish, or even bacon or a paste of tobacco. Larvae that die before being removed are harder to get out and often cause an intense inflammatory reaction. Another option for removal is squeezing the skin. Sometimes doctors inject a local anesthetic, make a small incision, and pull the larva out with forceps. The drug ivermectin, given by mouth or applied to the skin, also may kill the larva or cause it to leave.

Wound Myiasis: Open wounds, typically in homeless people, alcoholics, and others in poor social circumstances, may become infested with fly larvae. The most common flies are green or black blowflies. Unlike the maggots of common houseflies, most larvae that cause wound myiasis invade healthy as well as dead tissue. Doctors remove the larvae by flushing the wounds and pulling the larvae out. Doctors also cut away any dead tissue.

Migratory Myiasis: The most common sources are flies that typically infest horses and cattle. People can become infested if they have contact with infested animals. Less often, the flies lay eggs directly on people. Larvae do not stay in one spot. They burrow under the skin, causing itchy lesions that may be mistaken for cutaneous larva migrans (see above). The treatment is the same as for furuncular myiasis.

CHAPTER
195 Bacterial Skin Infections

The skin provides a remarkably good barrier against bacterial infections. Although many bacteria come in contact with or reside on the skin, they are normally unable to establish an infection. When bacterial skin infections do occur, they can range in size from a tiny spot to the entire body surface. They can range in seriousness as well, from harmless to life threatening.

Many types of bacteria can infect the skin. The most common are *Staphylococcus* and *Streptococcus*. Skin infections caused by less common bacteria may develop in people while hospitalized or living in a nursing home, while gardening, or while swimming in a pond, lake, or ocean.

Some people are at particular risk of contracting skin infections. For example, people with diabetes are likely to have poor blood flow, especially to the hands and feet, and the high levels of sugar in their blood decrease the ability of white blood cells to fight infections. People with human immunodeficiency virus (HIV) or AIDS or other immune disorders and those undergoing chemotherapy are at higher risk as well, because they have a weakened immune system. Skin that is inflamed or damaged by sunburn, scratching, or other trauma is more likely to be infected. In fact, any break in the skin predisposes a person to infection.

Prevention involves keeping the skin undamaged and clean. When the skin is cut or scraped, the injury should be washed with soap and water and covered with a sterile bandage. Antibiotic creams and ointments may be applied to open areas to keep the tissue moist and to try to prevent bacterial invasion. If an infection develops, small areas may be treated with antibiotic creams. Larger areas require antibiotics taken by mouth or given by injection. Abscesses (pus-filled pockets) should be cut open by the doctor and allowed to drain, and any dead tissue must be surgically removed.

Cellulitis

Cellulitis is a spreading bacterial infection of the skin and the tissues immediately beneath the skin.

- Redness, pain, and tenderness are felt over an area of skin, and some people have a fever, chills, and other more serious symptoms.
- Antibiotics are needed to treat the infection.

Cellulitis may be caused by many different bacteria. The most common are those of the *Streptococcus* species. Streptococci spread rapidly in the skin because they produce enzymes that hinder the ability of the tissue to confine the infection. *Staphylococcus* bacteria can also cause cellulitis, as can many other bacteria, especially after bites by humans or animals or after injuries in water or dirt.

Bacteria usually enter through small breaks in the epidermis that result from scrapes, punctures, burns, and skin disorders. Areas of the skin that become swollen with fluid (edema) are especially vulnerable. Cellulitis is more common in people with poor blood circulation (chronic venous insufficiency). However, cellulitis can also occur in skin that is not obviously injured.

Symptoms

Cellulitis most commonly develops on the legs but may occur anywhere. The first symptoms are redness, pain, and tenderness over an area of skin. These symptoms are caused both by the bacteria themselves and by the body's attempts to fight the infection. The infected skin becomes hot and swollen and may look slightly pitted, like an orange peel. Fluid-filled blisters, which may be small (vesicles) or large (bullae), sometimes appear on the infected skin. The borders of the affected area are not distinct, except in a form of cellulitis called erysipelas.

Most people with cellulitis feel only mildly ill, but some may have a fever, chills, rapid heart rate, headache, low blood pressure, and confusion.

As the infection spreads, nearby lymph nodes may become enlarged and tender (lymphadenitis), and the lymphatic vessels may become inflamed (lymphangitis—see page 1318). Sometimes, bacteria spread through the blood (bacteremia—see page 1185), which can cause more serious illness.

When cellulitis affects the same site repeatedly, especially the leg, lymphatic vessels may be damaged, causing permanent swelling of the affected tissue.

Diagnosis and Treatment

A doctor usually diagnoses cellulitis based on its appearance and symptoms. Laboratory identification of the bacteria from blood, pus, or tissue specimens usually is not necessary unless a person is seriously ill or the infection is not responding to drug therapy. Sometimes, doctors need to perform tests to differentiate cellulitis from a blood clot in the deep veins of the leg (deep vein thrombosis—see page 433), because the symptoms of these disorders are similar.

Prompt treatment with antibiotics can prevent the infection from spreading rapidly and reaching the blood and internal organs. Antibiotics that are effective against both streptococci and staphylococci (such as dicloxacillin or cephalexin) are used. People with mild cellulitis may take antibiotics by mouth. Those with rapidly spreading cellulitis, high fever, or other evidence of serious infection often receive intravenous antibiotics (such as oxacillin or nafcillin). Also, the affected part of the body, when possible, is kept immobile and elevated to help reduce swelling. Cool, wet dressings applied to the infected area may relieve discomfort.

Symptoms of cellulitis usually disappear after a few days of antibiotic therapy. However, symptoms often get worse before they get better probably because, with the death of the bacteria, substances that cause tissue damage are released. When this occurs, the body continues to react even though the bacteria are dead. Antibiotics are continued for 10 days or longer even though the symptoms may disappear earlier.

Erysipelas

Erysipelas is a superficial form of cellulitis typically caused by streptococci.

Erysipelas causes a painful, red, raised patch on the skin. The edges have a distinct border and do not blend into the nearby normal skin. The patch feels warm and firm to the touch. It occurs most frequently on the legs and face. People often have a high fever, chills, and a general feeling of illness (malaise).

Doctors base the diagnosis on the characteristic appearance of the rash.

Antibiotics given by mouth, such as penicillin, can cure the infection. For a severe infection, intravenous penicillin is needed. Cold packs and drugs for pain may relieve discomfort. Fungal foot infections may be an entry site for infection and may require treatment with antifungal drugs to prevent recurrence.

Erythrasma

Erythrasma is infection of the top layers of the skin caused by the bacterium Corynebacterium minutissimum.

Erythrasma affects mostly adults, especially those with diabetes and those living in the tropics. Erythrasma often appears in areas where skin touches skin, such as the webs of the toes, and genital area—especially in men, where the thighs touch the scrotum. The armpits, skin folds under the breasts or on the abdomen, and the area between the vaginal opening and the anus (perineum) are prone to this infection, particularly among those with diabetes and among obese middle-aged women. The infection can produce irregularly shaped pink or brown patches that may later turn into fine scales. In some people, the infection spreads to the torso and anal area.

Although erythrasma may be confused with a fungal infection, doctors can easily diagnose erythrasma because skin infected with *Corynebacterium* glows coral-red under an ultraviolet light.

An antibiotic given by mouth, such as erythromycin or tetracycline, can eliminate the infection. Antibacterial soaps, such as chlorhexidine, may also help. Topical drugs such as erythromycin and clindamycin are also effective. Antifungal creams such as miconazole may be helpful if yeast or fungus is present in the affected areas as well. Erythrasma may recur, necessitating a second treatment.

Folliculitis and Skin Abscesses

Folliculitis and skin abscesses are pus-filled pockets in the skin resulting from bacterial infection. They may be superficial or deep, affecting just hair follicules or deeper structures within the skin.

Folliculitis is a type of skin abscess that involves the hair follicle. Abscesses may appear both on the skin surface and within the deeper structures of the skin without always involving a hair follicle. Most abscesses are caused by *Staphylococcus aureus* bacteria (see page 1176) and appear to be pus-filled pockets on the skin surface. Recently, a strain of *Staphylococcus* has appeared that is resistant to previously effective antibiotics. This strain is called methicillin-resistant *Staphylococcus aureus* (MRSA). Sometimes the bacteria enter the skin through a hair follicle, small scrape, or puncture, although often there is no obvious point of entry. People who have poor hygiene or chronic skin diseases or whose nasal passages contain *Staphylococcus* are more likely to have episodes of folliculitis or skin abscesses. A weakened immune system, obesity, old age, and possibly diabetes are also common risk factors. Some people may have recurring episodes of infection for unknown reasons.

Doctors may try to eliminate *Staphylococcus* from people prone to recurring infections by instructing them to wash the entire body with antibacterial soap, apply antibiotic ointment inside the nose, and take antibiotics by mouth.

Folliculitis: Folliculitis is an infection of a hair follicle. It looks like a tiny white pimple at the base of a hair. There may be only one infected follicle or many. Each infected follicle is slightly painful, but the person otherwise does not feel sick.

Some people develop folliculitis after exposure to a poorly chlorinated hot tub or whirlpool. This condition, sometimes called "hot-tub folliculitis" or "hot-tub dermatitis," is caused by the bacterium *Pseudomonas aeruginosa*. It begins anytime from 6 hours to 5 days after the exposure. Areas of skin covered by a bathing suit, such as the torso and buttocks, are the most common sites.

Sometimes stiff hairs in the beard area curl and reenter the skin (ingrown hair) after shaving, causing irritation without substantial infection. This type of folliculitis is called pseudofolliculitis barbae (see page 1307).

Folliculitis is treated with antibacterial cleansers or topical antibiotics. Large areas of folliculitis may require antibiotics taken by mouth. Hot-tub folliculitis goes away in a week without any treatment. However, adequate chlorination of the hot tub is necessary to prevent recurrences and to protect others from infection. Folliculitis caused by ingrown hairs is treated by a number of methods with varying success. For severe, recurring problems, doctors may take a bacterial culture (a sample of pus is sent to a laboratory and placed in a culture medium that allows microorganisms to grow). The results of the culture are used to guide choice of antibiotic. The person may need to temporarily stop shaving.

Skin Abscesses: Skin abscesses, also called boils, are warm, painful, pus-filled pockets of infection below the skin surface that may occur on any body surface. Abscesses may be one to several inches in diameter. Furuncles are smaller, more superficial abscesses that by definition involve a hair follicle and the surrounding tissue. Carbuncles are multiple furuncles that are connected to one another below the skin surface. If not treated, abscesses often come to a head and rupture, discharging a creamy white or pink fluid. Bacteria may spread from the abscess to infect the surrounding tissue and lymph nodes. The person may have a fever and feel generally sick.

A skin abscess may go away with application of warm compresses. Otherwise, a doctor treats an abscess by cutting it open and draining the pus. After draining the abscess, a doctor makes sure all of the pus has been removed by washing out the pocket with a sterile salt solution. Sometimes the drained abscess is packed with gauze, which is removed 24 to 48 hours later. If the abscess is completely drained, antibiotics usually are not needed. However, if the abscess is on the middle or upper part of the face, antibiotics that kill staphylococci, such as dicloxacillin and cephalexin, may be used because of the risk that the infection will spread to the brain. Antibiotics also are needed if the infection has spread or if the person has a weakened immune system.

People who have recurrent skin abscesses can wash their skin with liquid soap that contains special antiseptics, or they can take antibiotics for 1 to 2 months.

Hidradenitis Suppurativa

Hidradenitis suppurativa is inflammation of the apocrine sweat glands, resulting in painful accumulations of pus under the skin.

Hidradenitis suppurativa develops in some people after puberty because the apocrine sweat glands (the specialized sweat glands under the arms, in the genital area, around the anus, and under the breasts) are chronically blocked. Doctors do not know why the blockage occurs, but it is not related to the use of deodorants or powders or to underarm shaving. The blockage causes the glands to swell and rupture, frequently leading to infection by various bacteria. The abscesses (pus-filled pockets) that result are painful and foul smelling and tend to recur. After several recurrences, the skin in the area becomes thick and scarred.

Hidradenitis suppurativa resembles common skin abscesses. A doctor makes the diagnosis based on the location of the abscesses and on the fact that they recur often.

For people with mild cases, a doctor injects corticosteroids into the area and prescribes antibiotics, such as tetracycline or erythromycin, to be taken by mouth. Clindamycin applied topically is also effective. In some cases, a doctor cuts open the abscesses to drain the pus. For severe cases, isotretinoin, an anti-inflammatory drug, may be given by mouth. Laser treatment has also been used. In severe cases, cutting out the involved area followed by skin grafting may be necessary.

Impetigo

Impetigo is a skin infection, caused by Staphylococcus aureus, Streptococcus pyogenes, *or both, that leads to the formation of scabby, yellow-crusted sores and, sometimes, small blisters filled with yellow fluid.*

Impetigo is common. It affects mostly children. Impetigo can occur anywhere on the body but most commonly occurs on the face, arms, and legs. The blisters that may form (bullous impetigo) can vary from pea-sized to large rings and can last for days to weeks. Impetigo often affects normal skin but may follow an injury or a condition that causes a break in the skin, such as a fungal infection, sunburn, or an insect bite. Poor hygiene and a moist environment are also risk factors. Some people have *Staphylococcus* bacteria living in their nose without causing disease (they are considered nasal carriers). These nasal bacteria may cause repeat infection in the person and sometimes in others.

Impetigo is itchy and slightly painful. The itching often leads to extensive scratching, particularly in children, which serves to spread the infection. Impetigo is very contagious—both to other areas of the person's own skin and to other people. Impetigo typically causes clusters of sores to rupture and develop a honey-colored crust over the sores. Bullous impetigo is similar except that the sores typically enlarge rapidly to form blisters. The blisters burst and expose larger bases, which become covered with honey-colored varnish or crust.

Doctors base the diagnosis on the appearance of the rash. In people who have repeated infections, a swab of the nose is taken and sent to the laboratory to determine whether they are a nasal carrier of staphylococci.

The infected area should be washed gently with soap and water several times a day to remove any crusts. Small areas are treated with topical antibiotics. If large areas are involved, an antibiotic taken by mouth may be needed. People who are nasal carriers are treated with topical antibiotics applied to the nasal passages.

Lymphadenitis

Lymphadenitis is inflammation of one or more lymph nodes, which usually become swollen and tender.

Lymphadenitis almost always results from an infection, which may be caused by bacteria, viruses, protozoa, rickettsiae, or fungi. Typically, the infection spreads to a lymph node from a skin, ear, nose, or eye infection or from such infections as infectious mononucleosis, cytomegalovirus infection, streptococcal infection, tuberculosis, or syphilis. The infection may affect many lymph nodes or only those in one area of the body.

Symptoms and Diagnosis

Infected lymph nodes enlarge and are usually tender and painful. Sometimes, the skin over the infected nodes looks red and feels warm. The person may have a fever. Occasionally, pockets of pus (abscesses) develop. Enlarged lymph nodes that do not cause pain, tenderness, or redness may indicate a serious different disorder, such as lymphoma, tuberculosis, or Hodgkin lymphoma. Such lymph nodes require a doctor's attention.

Usually, lymphadenitis can be diagnosed on the basis of symptoms, and its cause is an obvious nearby infection. When the cause cannot be identified easily, a biopsy (removal and examination of a tissue sample under a microscope) and a culture (a sample is sent to a laboratory and placed in a culture medium that allows microorganisms to grow) may be needed to confirm the diagnosis and to identify the organism causing the infection.

Treatment

Treatment depends on the organism causing the infection. For a bacterial infection, an antibiotic is usually given intravenously or by mouth. Warm compresses may help relieve the pain in inflamed lymph nodes. Usually, once the infection has been treated, the lymph nodes slowly shrink, and the pain subsides. Sometimes the enlarged nodes remain firm but no longer feel tender. Abscesses must be drained surgically.

Lymphangitis

Lymphangitis is inflammation of one or more lymphatic vessels, usually caused by a streptococcal infection.

Streptococci bacteria usually enter the lymphatic vessels (part of the body's immune system—see art on page 1098) from a scrape or wound in an arm or a leg. Often, a streptococcal infection in the skin and the tissues just beneath the skin (cellulitis—see page 1315) spreads to the lymph vessels. Occasionally, staphylococci or other bacteria are the cause.

Red, irregular, warm, tender streaks develop on the skin in the affected arm or leg. The streaks usually stretch from the infected area toward a group of lymph nodes, such as those in the groin or armpit. The lymph nodes become enlarged and feel tender.

Common symptoms include a fever, chills, a rapid heart rate, and a headache. Sometimes these symptoms occur before the red streaks appear. The spread of the infection from the lymph system into the bloodstream can cause infection throughout the body, often with startling speed. The skin or tissues over the infected lymph vessel become inflamed. Rarely, skin ulcers develop. Sometimes, bacteria enter the bloodstream (bacteremia).

The diagnosis of lymphangitis is based on its typical appearance. A blood test usually shows that the number of white blood cells has increased to fight the infection. Doctors have difficulty identifying the organisms causing the infection unless the organisms have spread through the bloodstream or pus can be taken from a wound in the affected area.

Most people recover quickly with antibiotics that kill staphylococci and streptococci, such as dicloxacillin, nafcillin, or oxacillin.

Necrotizing Skin Infections

Necrotizing skin infections, including necrotizing cellulitis and necrotizing fasciitis, are severe forms of cellulitis characterized by death of infected tissue (necrosis).

- The infected skin is red, warm to the touch, and sometimes swollen, and gas bubbles may form under the skin.
- The person usually feels very ill and has a high fever.
- Treatment involves removing dead skin, which sometimes requires extensive surgery, and giving intravenous antibiotics.

Most skin infections do not result in the death of skin and nearby tissues. Sometimes, however, bacterial infection can cause small blood vessels in the infected area to clot. This clotting causes the tissue fed by these vessels to die from lack of blood. Because the body's immune defenses that travel through the bloodstream (such as white blood cells and antibodies) can no longer reach this area, the infection spreads rapidly and may be difficult to control. Death can occur, even with appropriate treatment.

Some necrotizing skin infections spread deep in the skin along the surface of the muscle (fascia) and are termed necrotizing fasciitis. Other necrotizing skin infections spread on the outer layers of skin and are termed necrotizing cellulitis. Several different bacteria, such as *Streptococcus* and *Clostridia*, may cause necrotizing skin infections, although in many people the infection is caused by a combination of bacteria. The streptococcal infection in particular has been termed "flesh-eating disease" by the lay press, although it differs little from the others.

Some necrotizing skin infections begin at puncture wounds or lacerations, particularly wounds contaminated with dirt and debris. Other infections begin in surgical incisions or even healthy skin. Sometimes people with diverticulitis, intestinal perforation, or tumors of the intestine develop necrotizing infections of the abdominal wall, genital area, or thighs. These infections occur when certain bacteria escape from the intestine and spread to the skin. The bacteria may initially create an abscess in the abdominal cavity and spread directly outward to the skin, or they may spread through the bloodstream to the skin and other organs.

Symptoms and Diagnosis

Symptoms often begin just as for cellulitis (see page 1315). The skin may look pale at first, but quickly becomes red or bronze and warm to the touch, and sometimes becomes swollen. Later, the skin turns violet, often with the development of large fluid-filled blisters (bullae). The fluid from these blisters is brown, watery, and sometimes foul smelling. Areas of dead skin turn black (gangrene). Some types of infection, including those caused by *Clostridia* and mixed bacteria, produce gas (see page 1160). The gas creates bubbles under the skin and sometimes in the blisters themselves, causing the skin to feel crackly when pressed. Initially the infected area is painful, but as the skin dies, the nerves stop working and the area loses sensation.

The person usually feels very ill and has a high fever, a rapid heart rate, and mental deterioration ranging from confusion to unconsciousness. Blood pressure may fall because of toxins secreted by the bacteria and the body's response to the infection (septic shock—see page 1186).

A doctor makes a diagnosis of necrotizing skin infection based on its appearance, particularly the presence of gas bubbles under the skin. X-rays may show gas under the skin as well. The specific bacteria involved are identified by laboratory analysis of infected fluid and tissue samples. However, treatment must begin before a doctor can be certain which bacteria are causing the infection.

Prognosis and Treatment

The overall death rate is about 30%. Older people, those who have other medical disorders, and those in whom the disease has reached an advanced stage have a poorer outcome. A delay in diagnosis and treatment and insufficient surgical removal of dead tissue worsen the prognosis.

The treatment for necrotizing fasciitis is surgical removal of the dead tissue plus intravenous antibiotic therapy. Large amounts of skin, tissue, and muscle must often be removed, and in some cases, an affected arm or leg may have to be amputated. Some doctors recommend treatment in a high-pressure (hyperbaric) oxygen chamber, but it is not clear how much this helps.

Staphylococcal Scalded Skin Syndrome

Staphylococcal scalded skin syndrome is a reaction to a staphylococcal skin infection in which the skin blisters and peels off as though burned.

- In addition to the blistered, peeling skin, the person has fever, chills, and weakness.
- The diagnosis is based on the appearance of the skin, but sometimes a biopsy is done.
- Treatment involves antibiotics given intravenously.

Certain types of staphylococci bacteria secrete toxic substances that cause the top layer of the epidermis to split from the rest of the skin. Because the toxin spreads throughout the body, staphylococcal infection of a small area of skin may result in peeling over the entire body. Staphylococcal scalded skin syndrome occurs almost exclusively in infants and children under the age of 6. It rarely occurs in older people except for those with kidney failure or a weakened immune system. Like other staphylococcal infections, staphylococcal scalded skin syndrome is contagious.

Symptoms

Symptoms begin with an isolated, crusted infection that may look like impetigo (see page 1317). In newborns, the infection may appear in the diaper area or around the stump of the umbilical cord. In older children, the face is the typical site of infection. In adults, the infection may begin anywhere. In all people with this disorder, scarlet-colored areas appear around the crusted area within a day of the beginning of infection. These areas may be painful. The skin may be extremely tender and have a wrinkled tissue paper–like consistency. Then, other large areas of skin distant from the initial infection redden and develop blisters that break easily.

The top layer of the skin then begins peeling off, often in large sheets, with even slight touching or gentle pushing. The peeled areas look scalded. Within another 1 to 2 days, the entire skin surface may be involved, and the person becomes very ill with a fever, chills, and weakness. With the loss of the protective skin barrier, other bacteria and infective organisms can easily penetrate the body, causing what doctors call superinfections. Also, critical amounts of fluid can be lost because of oozing and evaporation, resulting in dehydration.

Diagnosis and Treatment

A diagnosis is made by the appearance of skin peeling after an apparent staphylococcal infection. If no signs of staphylococcal infection are observed, doctors often perform a biopsy, in which a small piece of skin is removed and sent to the laboratory to be tested. Swabs taken from the nose, the thin mucous membrane that covers the eyes (conjunctiva), the throat, and the nasal passages and upper throat (nasopharynx) are sent to the laboratory to be cultured for bacteria.

Treatment is with antibiotics for at least a week. Local wound care with topical emollients soothes the skin and protects it from drying out.

CHAPTER 196 Fungal Skin Infections

Fungi usually make their homes in moist areas of the body where skin surfaces meet: between the toes, in the genital area, and under the breasts. Many fungi that infect the skin (dermatophytes) live only in the topmost layer of the epidermis (stratum corneum) and do not penetrate deeper. Obese people are more likely to get these infections because they have excessive skinfolds. People with diabetes tend to be more susceptible to fungal infections as well.

Strangely, fungal infections on one part of the body can cause rashes on other parts of the body that are not infected. For example, a fungal infection on the foot may cause an itchy, bumpy rash on the fingers. These eruptions (dermatophytids, or id reactions) are allergic reactions to the fungus. They do not result from touching the infected area.

Doctors may suspect a fungal infection when they see a red, irritated, or scaly rash in one of the commonly affected areas. They can usually confirm the diagnosis by scraping off a small amount of skin and having it examined under a microscope or placed in a culture medium where the specific fungus can grow and be identified (see page 1278).

Candidiasis

Candidiasis (yeast infection, moniliasis) is infection by the yeast Candida.

- Candidiasis tends to occur in moist areas of the skin.
- Candidiasis may cause rashes, scaling, itching, and swelling.
- Doctors examine the affected areas and view skin samples under a microscope or in a culture.

- Antifungal creams or antifungal drugs given by mouth usually cure candidiasis.

Candida yeast is a normal resident of the mouth, digestive tract, and vagina that usually causes no harm. Under certain conditions, however, *Candida* can overgrow on mucous membranes and moist areas of the skin. Typical areas affected are the lining of the mouth, the groin, the armpits, the skin under the breasts in women, and the skinfolds of the stomach. Conditions that enable *Candida* to infect the skin include the following:

- Hot, humid weather
- Tight, synthetic underclothing
- Poor hygiene
- Inflammatory diseases (such as psoriasis) that occur in skinfolds
- Use of antibiotics or corticosteroids and other drugs that suppress the immune system
- Disorders such as diabetes or a weakened immune system

People taking antibiotics may develop candidiasis because the antibiotics kill the bacteria that normally reside on the body, allowing *Candida* to grow unchecked. Corticosteroids or immunosuppressive therapy after organ transplantation can also lower the body's defenses against candidiasis. Inhaled corticosteroids, often used by people with asthma, sometimes produce candidiasis of the mouth. Pregnant women, people receiving cancer therapy drugs, obese people, and people with diabetes also are more likely to be infected by *Candida*.

In some people (usually people with a weakened immune system), *Candida* invades deeper tissues as well as the blood, causing life-threatening systemic candidiasis (see page 1232).

Symptoms

Symptoms vary, depending on the location of the infection.

Infections in skinfolds (intertriginous infections) or in the navel usually cause a bright red rash, sometimes with softening and breakdown of skin. Small pustules may appear, especially at the edges of the rash, and the rash may itch intensely or burn. A candidal rash around the anus may be raw, white or red, and itchy. Babies may develop a candidal rash in the diaper area (see page 1735).

Vaginal candidiasis (vulvovaginitis, yeast infection—see page 1540) is common, especially in women who are pregnant, have diabetes, or are taking antibiotics. Symptoms of these infections include a white or yellow cheeselike discharge from the vagina and burning, itching, and redness along the walls and external area of the vagina.

Penile candidiasis most often affects men with diabetes, uncircumcised men, or men whose female sex partners have vaginal candidiasis. Sometimes the rash may not cause any symptoms, but usually, the infection produces a red, raw, itching, burning or sometimes painful rash on the head of the penis and sometimes the scrotum.

Thrush is candidiasis inside the mouth (see also page 1232). The creamy white patches typical of thrush cling to the tongue and sides of the mouth and may be painful. The patches cannot be scraped off easily with a finger or blunt object. Thrush in otherwise healthy children is not unusual, but in adults it may signal a weakened immune system, possibly caused by cancer, diabetes, or AIDS. The use of antibiotics that kill off competing bacteria increases the chances of getting thrush.

Perlèche is candidiasis at the corners of the mouth, which causes cracks and tiny fissures. It may stem from chronic lip licking, thumb sucking, ill-fitting dentures, or other conditions that make the corners of the mouth moist enough that yeast can grow.

Candidal paronychia is candidiasis in the nail beds, which causes painful redness and swelling (see page 1339). This disorder typically occurs in people with diabetes or a weakened immune system or in otherwise healthy people whose hands are subjected to frequent wetting or washing.

Diagnosis and Treatment

Usually, doctors can identify candidiasis by observing its distinctive rash or the thick, white, pasty residue it generates. To confirm the diagnosis, doctors may scrape off some of the skin or residue with a scalpel or tongue depressor. The sample is then examined under a microscope or placed in a culture medium (a substance that allows microorganisms to grow) to identify the specific fungus (see page 1278).

Generally, candidiasis of the skin is easily cured with creams containing miconazole, clotrimazole, oxiconazole, ketoconazole, econazole, ciclopirox, or nystatin. The cream is usually applied twice daily for 7 to 10 days. Corticosteroid creams are sometimes used with antifungal creams because they quickly reduce itching and pain (although they do not help cure the infection itself and, used alone, worsen the infection). Candidiasis that does not respond to antifungal creams and liquids may be treated with gentian violet, a purple dye that is painted on the infected area to kill the yeast.

Keeping the skin dry helps clear up the infection and prevents it from returning. Talcum powder helps keep the surface area dry, and talcum powder with nystatin may further help prevent a recurrence.

Different treatments are prescribed for vaginal yeast infections, thrush, and nail infections.

Ringworm

Ringworm (tinea) is a fungal skin infection caused by several different fungi and generally classified by its location on the body.

- The fungi that cause ringworm infections tend to spread in moist areas of the skin.
- Symptoms include rashes, scaling, and itching.
- Doctors usually examine the affected area and view a skin sample under a microscope or in a culture.
- Antifungal drugs applied directly to the affected areas or taken by mouth usually cure the infection.

Despite its name, ringworm infection does not involve worms. The name arose because of the ring-shaped skin patches created by the infection. Symptoms vary depending on the location of the infection. Doctors can frequently identify a ringworm infection by its appearance. Most often, there is little or no inflammation and the infected areas are mildly itchy with a scaling, slightly raised border. These patches can come and go intermittently. Areas of the body that are most commonly affected include the head, skin, and nails (infections called tinea unguium and onychomycosis—see page 1339). Treatment varies by site but always involves topical or oral antifungal drugs.

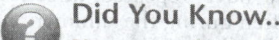

? Did You Know...
Ringworm infection is caused by fungi, not by worms.

ATHLETE'S FOOT

Athelete's foot (tinea pedis) is a fungal infection of the feet.

Tinea pedis is a common fungal infection that usually appears during warm weather. The infection may spread from person to person in communal showers and bathrooms or in other moist areas where infected people walk barefoot. People who wear tight shoes are also at risk. The infection is usually caused by *Trichophyton* or *Epidermophyton.* These fungi most commonly grow in the warm, moist areas between the toes. The fungus can produce mild scaling with or without redness and itching. The scaling may involve a small area or the entire sole of the foot. Sometimes scaling is severe, with breakdown and painful cracking (fissuring) of the skin. Fluid-filled blisters can also form. Because the fungus may cause the skin to crack, athlete's foot can lead to bacterial infection (see page 1315), especially in older people and in people with inadequate blood flow to the feet.

Diagnosis is usually obvious to doctors based on their clinical examination and review of risk factors.

Treatment

The safest treatment is using topical antifungal drugs, but recurrence is common and treatment must often be prolonged. Oral antifungal drugs such as itraconazole and terbinafine are usually most effective but may have side effects. Use of a topical antifungal at the same time may reduce recurrences.

Reducing moisture on the feet and in footwear helps prevent recurrences. Wearing open-toe shoes or shoes that "breathe" and frequently changing socks are important, especially during warm weather. Spaces between toes should be thoroughly towel-dried after bathing. Applying antifungal powders (eg, miconazole), gentian violet, Burow's solution (5% aluminum subacetate) soaks, or 20 to 25% aluminum chloride hexahydrate powder helps keep the feet dry.

JOCK ITCH

Jock itch (tinea cruris) is a fungal infection of the groin.

Tinea cruris is much more common in men than in women and develops most frequently in warm weather. The infection begins in the skinfolds of the genital area and can spread to the upper inner thighs. Usually the scrotum is not involved (unlike in yeast infection). The rash has a scaly, pink border. Jock itch can be quite itchy and may be painful. A susceptible person may have repeated infections. Flare-ups occur more often during the summer.

The diagnosis is usually obvious to doctors based on a physical examination. Treatment involves antifungal cream or lotion. Oral antifungal drugs may be needed in people who have inflammatory or widespread infections or infections that do not heal with use of topical drugs.

SCALP RINGWORM

Scalp ringworm (tinea capitis) is a fungal infection of the scalp.

Tinea capitis is primarily caused by *Trichophyton.* Scalp ringworm is highly contagious and is common among children (see page 1735). It may produce a pink scaly rash that may be somewhat itchy, or it may produce a patch of hair loss without a rash. Less commonly, it can cause a painful, inflamed, swollen patch on the scalp that sometimes oozes pus (a kerion). A kerion is caused by an allergic reaction to the fungus and may result in scarring hair loss.

Diagnosis

Tinea capitis is diagnosed by physical examination and by the doctor examining a sample of hair or scale from the scalp under a microscope. The sample is prepared with a special solution that helps identify the type of fungus causing the infection.

Treatment

In children, treatment involves an antifungal drug called griseofulvin taken orally for 6 to 8 weeks. An antifungal cream should be applied to the scalp to prevent spread, especially to other children, until the tinea capitis is cured. Selenium sulfide 2.5% shampoo should also be used at least twice a week. Children may attend school during treatment.

In adults, treatment is with the oral antifungal drug terbinafine or itraconazole. How long treatment is needed depends on the drug used. For severely inflamed areas and for a kerion, doctors may prescribe a short course of prednisone to lessen symptoms and perhaps reduce the chance of scarring.

BODY RINGWORM

Body ringworm (tinea corporis) is a fungal infection of the face, trunk, arms, and legs.

Tinea corporis may be caused by *Trichophyton, Microsporum,* or *Epidermophyton.* The infection generally produces round patches with pink scaly borders and clear areas in the center. Sometimes the rash is itchy. Body ringworm can develop anywhere on the skin and can spread rapidly to other parts of the body or to other people with whom there is close bodily contact. Diagnosis is usually by physical examination.

Treatment

Tinea corporis is treated with a topical antifungal cream, lotion, or gel applied twice a day and continued for 7 to 10 days after the rash completely disappears. If

Topical Antifungal Drugs

- Amorolfine
- Butenafine
- Ciclopirox
- Clotrimazole
- Econazole
- Haloprogin
- Ketoconazole
- Miconazole
- Naftifine
- Nystatin (for *Candida* only)
- Oxiconazole
- Selenium sulfide (shampoo for tinea versicolor)
- Sulconazole
- Terbinafine
- Terconazole
- Tioconazole
- Tolnaftate
- Undecylenate

the cream is discontinued too soon, the infection may not be eradicated, and the rash will return. Several days may pass before antifungal creams reduce symptoms. Corticosteroid creams are often used to help relieve itching for the first few days. Low-dose hydrocortisone is available over the counter. More potent corticosteroids require a prescription and may be used in addition to an antifungal cream. If the ringworm infection oozes, a bacterial infection also may have developed. Such an infection may require treatment with antibiotics, either applied to the skin or taken by mouth.

Extensive and resistant infections can occur in people infected with *Trichophyton rubrum* and in people with debilitating systemic (body-wide) diseases. For such people, the most effective therapy is an oral drug, such as itraconazole or terbinafine, taken for 2 to 3 weeks.

BEARD RINGWORM

Beard ringworm (tinea barbae) is a fungal infection of the beard area most often caused by Trichophyton mentagrophytes *or* Trichophyton verrucosum.

Tinea barbae usually involves superficial circular patches, but deeper infection may occur. An inflammatory kerion may also develop, which can result in scarring hair loss. Tinea barbae is rare. Most skin infections in the beard area are caused by bacteria, not fungi. Doctors diagnose the infection by examining a sample of skin under a microscope.

Treatment is with an antifungal drug, such as griseofulvin, terbinafine, or itraconazole, taken by mouth. If the area is severely inflamed, doctors may add a short course of prednisone to lessen symptoms and perhaps reduce the chance of scarring.

Tinea Versicolor

Tinea versicolor (pityriasis versicolor) is a fungal infection of the topmost layer of the skin causing scaly, discolored patches.

The infection, caused by the yeast *Malassezia furfur*, is quite common, especially in young adults.

Tinea versicolor rarely causes pain or itching, but it prevents areas of the skin from tanning, producing patches that are lighter in color than surrounding skin. People with naturally dark skin may notice lighter patches. People with naturally fair skin may get darker or lighter patches. The patches are often on the chest or back and may scale slightly. Over time, small areas can join to form large patches.

Diagnosis

Doctors can diagnose tinea versicolor by its appearance. Doctors may use an ultraviolet light to show the infection more clearly or may examine scrapings from the infected area under a microscope to confirm the diagnosis.

Treatment

Topical antifungal cream such as ketoconazole may be used, as well as terbinafine solution spray. Prescription selenium sulfide shampoo is effective if applied full-strength to the affected areas (including the scalp) at bedtime, left on overnight, and washed off in the morning. Treatment is usually continued for 3 or 4 nights. Alternatively, the shampoo can be applied for 10 minutes a day for 10 days. Prescription ketoconazole shampoo is also effective. It is applied and washed off in 5 minutes. It is used as a single application or daily for 3 days.

Antifungal drugs taken by mouth, such as itraconazole, ketoconazole, or fluconazole, are sometimes used to treat widespread, resistant infection (see table on page 1231). However, because these drugs may cause unwanted side effects, topical drugs are usually preferred.

The skin may not regain its normal pigmentation for many months after the infection is gone. Tinea versicolor commonly comes back after successful treatment because the fungus that causes it normally lives on the skin. Therefore, many doctors recommend use of 2.5% selenium sulfide shampoo or ketoconazole shampoo monthly or every other month to prevent recurrences. Pyrithione zinc soap may also be used regularly to prevent recurrence.

197 Viral Skin Infections

Many viral infections—such as measles, chickenpox, and rubella—cause rashes, spots, or sores on the skin, as well as other symptoms. Herpesviruses often cause rashes and sores (see page 1245). However, in two common viral infections, warts and molluscum contagiosum, the virus remains solely within the skin and does not spread to other parts of the body.

Warts

Warts (verrucae) are small skin growths caused by any of 100 or more related human papillomaviruses.

- Raised or flat growths appear on any part of the skin.
- Most warts are painless.
- Doctors identify warts by sight or rarely do a biopsy.
- Warts that do not go away by themselves can be removed with chemicals or frozen, burned, or cut off.

Warts can develop at any age but are most common among children and least common among older people. People may have one or two warts or hundreds. Because prolonged or repeated contact is necessary for the virus to spread, warts are most often spread from one area of the body to another, but they can spread also from one person to another. Sexual contact is often sufficient to spread genital warts (see page 1267).

Most warts are harmless, although they may be quite bothersome. The exceptions are certain types of genital warts that sometimes cause cervical cancer in women.

Symptoms

Warts are classified by their location and shape. Some warts grow in clusters (mosaic warts), but others appear as isolated, single growths. Warts are painless, except for plantar warts.

Common Warts: Common warts (also called verrucae vulgaris), which almost everyone gets, are firm growths that usually have a rough surface. They are round or irregularly shaped; are gray, yellow, or brown; and are usually less than 1/2 inch (about 1 centimeter) across. Generally, they appear on areas that are frequently injured, such as the knees, face, fingers, elbows, and around the nails (periungual warts). Common warts may spread to surrounding skin.

Plantar Warts: These warts develop on the sole of the foot, where they are usually flattened by the pressure of walking and are surrounded by thickened skin. They tend to be hard and flat, with a rough surface and well-defined boundaries. They can be very painful when standing or walking, which puts pressure on the warts. Warts may appear on the top of the foot or on the toes, where they are usually raised and fleshier. Warts are often gray or brown and have a small black center. Unlike corns and calluses, plantar warts tend to bleed from many tiny spots, like pinpoints, when a doctor shaves or cuts the surface away with a knife. There can also be clusters of smaller warts, called mosaic warts.

Periungual Warts: Periungual warts are thickened, cauliflower-like growths around the nails. The nail may lose its cuticle, and other skin infections can develop around the nail. These warts are more common among people who bite their nails.

Filiform Warts: These warts are long, narrow, small growths that usually appear on the eyelids, face, neck, or lips.

Flat Warts: Flat warts, which are more common among children and young adults, usually appear in groups as smooth yellow-brown, pink, or flesh-colored spots, most frequently on the face and tops of the hands. The beard area in men and the legs in women are also common locations for flat warts, where they may be spread by shaving.

Genital Warts: Also called venereal warts or condylomata acuminata, genital warts occur on the penis, anus, vulva, vagina, and cervix. They are irregular, bumpy growths often with the texture of a small cauliflower (see page 1267).

> **? Did You Know...**
> Warts are most often spread from one part of the body to another, but they can spread also from one person to another.

Diagnosis

Doctors recognize warts by their typical appearance. Growths on the skin that cannot be definitely identified may need to be removed for examination under a microscope (biopsy).

Treatment

Many warts, particularly common warts, disappear on their own within a year or two. Because warts rarely leave a scar when they heal spontaneously, they do not need to be treated unless they cause pain or psychologic distress. Genital warts are more likely to persist and are more contagious, so doctors often remove them or treat them with drugs. All types of warts may recur after removal. Plantar warts are the most difficult to cure.

In general, warts can be removed with the following:

- **Chemicals:** Typical chemicals used include salicylic acid, trichloroacetic acid, cantharidin, and podophyllin. Flat warts are often treated with peeling agents such as retinoic or salicylic acid. 5-Fluorouracil cream or solution may also be used. Imiquimod, a new cream for the treatment of genital warts, is sometimes used to treat other warts. Some chemicals can be applied by the person, but others must be applied by a doctor. Most of these chemicals can burn normal skin, so when they are applied at home, directions must be followed carefully. Chemicals usually require multiple applications over several weeks to months. The wart is scraped either at home or in the office to remove dead tissue before each treatment.

- **Freezing (cryotherapy):** Freezing is safe. It does not usually require that the area be numbed but may be too painful for children to tolerate. Warts may be frozen with various commercial freezing probes or with liquid nitrogen sprayed on or applied with a cotton swab. Cryotherapy is often used for plantar warts and warts under the fingernails. Multiple treatments at monthly intervals are often required, especially for large warts.

- **Burning and cutting:** These methods are effective but are more painful and usually leave a scar. A laser or electrical current is used to burn warts off. A pulsed dye laser is also effective but, like freezing, usually requires multiple treatments (see box on page 1331).

Molluscum Contagiosum

Molluscum contagiosum is infection of the skin by a poxvirus that causes flesh-colored or white smooth, waxy bumps.

The bumps are usually less than ¼ inch (about 0.5 centimeters) in diameter and have a tiny dimple in the center. The virus that causes molluscum is contagious. It spreads by direct skin contact and is common among children. Genital lesions are often transmitted sexually in adults.

Molluscum contagiosum can infect almost any part of the skin. The bumps usually are not itchy or painful and may be discovered only coincidentally during a physical examination. However, the bumps can become very inflamed (resembling a boil) and itchy as the body fights off the virus. This inflammation may indicate that the bumps will soon disappear.

Most growths disappear spontaneously in 1 to 2 years, but they can remain for 2 to 3 years. No treatment is needed unless they are disfiguring or otherwise bothersome. The growths can be treated by freezing or removing their core with a needle or sharp scraping instrument (curette). Sometimes doctors apply trichloroacetic acid or cantharidin to the bumps. Other doctors prescribe retinoic acid or imiquimod cream, which is applied for weeks or months.

CHAPTER

198 Sunlight and Skin Damage

The skin shields the rest of the body from the sun's rays.

Ultraviolet Light: Ultraviolet (UV) light, although invisible to the human eye, is the component of sunlight that has the most effect on skin. UV light is classified into three types, ultraviolet A (UVA), ultraviolet B (UVB), and ultraviolet C (UVC), depending on its wavelength.

UV light in small amounts is beneficial because it helps the body produce vitamin D. However, larger amounts of UV light damage deoxyribonucleic acid (DNA—the body's genetic material) and alter the amounts and kinds of chemicals that the skin cells make. These changes are responsible for the damaging effects of UV light, including burning, premature skin aging, wrinkling, and skin cancer. Although UVA penetrates deeper into the skin, UVB is responsible for more of the damaging effects of UV light.

The amount of UV light reaching the earth's surface is increasing, especially in the northern latitudes. This increase is attributable to depletion of the protective ozone layer high in the atmosphere. Ozone, a naturally occurring chemical, blocks much UV light from reaching the surface of the earth. Chemical reactions between ozone and chlorofluorocarbons (chemicals in refrigerants and spray can propellants) are depleting the amount of ozone in the protective ozone layer. The amount of UV light reaching the earth's surface also varies depending on other factors. UV light is more intense between 10 AM and 3 PM, in the

Actinic Keratoses: Precancerous Growths

Actinic keratoses (solar keratoses) are precancerous growths caused by long-term sun exposure. These growths are usually pink or red and appear as flaky, scaly areas. They may also be light gray or brown and feel hard, rough, or gritty. The surrounding skin often appears thin.

Actinic keratoses usually can be removed by freezing them with liquid nitrogen (cryotherapy). However, if a person has too many growths, a liquid or cream containing fluorouracil may be applied. Often, during such treatment, the skin temporarily looks worse because fluorouracil causes redness, scaling, and burning of the keratoses and of the surrounding sun-damaged skin. A relatively new drug, imiquimod, is useful in treating actinic keratoses because it helps the immune system to recognize and destroy cancerous skin growths.

summer, and at higher altitudes. Smoke and smog filter out much UV light, but UV rays may pass through light clouds, fog, and about 1 foot of clear water.

Natural Protection: The skin undergoes certain changes when exposed to UV light to protect against damage. The epidermis (the skin's uppermost layer) thickens, blocking UV light. The melanocytes (pigment-producing skin cells) make increased amounts of melanin, which darkens the skin, resulting in a tan. Melanin absorbs the energy of UV light and helps prevent the light from damaging skin cells and penetrating deeper into the tissues.

Sensitivity to sunlight varies according to the amount of melanin in the skin. Darker-skinned people have more melanin and therefore greater protection against the sun's harmful effects, although they are still vulnerable to some extent. The amount of melanin present in a person's skin depends on heredity as well as on the amount of recent sun exposure. Some people are able to produce large amounts of melanin in response to UV light, whereas others produce very little. People with albinism (see page 1308) are born being able to make little or no melanin at all.

Sunlight and Skin Damage: Exposure to sunlight prematurely ages the skin. Exposure to UV light is responsible for the wrinkles, both fine and coarse; irregular pigmentation; redness; and leathery, rough texture of sun-exposed skin. Although fair-skinned people are most vulnerable, anyone's skin will change with enough exposure.

The more sun exposure people have, the higher their risk of skin cancers, including squamous cell carcinoma, basal cell carcinoma, and malignant melanoma (see page 1335).

Treatment: The key to minimizing the damaging effects of the sun is avoiding further sun exposure. Damage that is already done is difficult to reverse. Moisturizing creams and makeup help hide wrinkles. Chemical peels, alpha-hydroxy acids, tretinoin creams, and laser skin resurfacing may improve the appearance of thin wrinkles and irregular pigmentation. Deep wrinkles and substantial skin damage, however, require significant treatment to be reversed.

Sunburn

- Brief overexposure to ultraviolet light causes sunburn.
- Sunburn causes painful reddened skin and sometimes causes blisters, fever, and chills.
- People can prevent sunburn by avoiding excessive sun exposure and by using sunscreens.
- Cold water compresses, moisturizers, and nonsteroidal anti-inflammatory drugs ease pain until the sunburn heals.

Sunburn results from a brief (acute) overexposure to ultraviolet (UV) light. The amount of sun exposure required to produce a burn varies with each person's pigmentation and ability to produce more melanin.

Sunburn results in painful reddened skin. Severe sunburn may produce swelling and blisters. Symptoms may begin as soon as 1 hour after exposure and typically reach their peak within 3 days. Some severely sunburned people develop a fever, chills, and weakness and on rare occasions even may go into shock (characterized by very low blood pressure, fainting, and profound weakness). Several days after a sunburn, people with naturally fair skin may have peeling in the burned area, usually accompanied by itching. These peeled areas are even more sensitive to sunburn for several weeks. People who have had severe sunburns when young are at greater risk of skin cancer in later years even if they have not had long-term sun exposure.

 Did You Know...

People can get sunburned even on cloudy days because clouds do not filter ultraviolet light.

Even sunscreens that are waterproof or water-resistant need to be reapplied after swimming.

Prevention

Avoidance: The best—and most obvious—way to prevent sun damage is to stay out of strong, direct sunlight. If sun exposure is unavoidable, the person should seek shade as soon as possible, cover up in UV-protective clothing, and wear sunscreen, a hat, and UV-protective sunglasses. Many materials are capable of filtering or blocking UV radiation, but many are not. Clothing, ordinary window glass, smoke, and smog filter out most of the damaging rays. However, water is not a good filter. UVA and UVB light can penetrate a foot (about 30 centimeters) of clear water. Clouds and fog are also not good filters of UV light—a person can get sunburned on a cloudy or foggy day. Snow, water, and sand reflect sunlight, magnifying the amount of UV light that reaches the skin. People also burn more quickly at high altitudes, where the thin air allows more burning UV light to reach the skin.

Sunscreens: Before exposure to strong direct sunlight, a person should apply a sunscreen, an ointment or cream containing chemicals that protect the skin by filtering out UV light. Older sunscreens tended to filter only UVB light, but many newer sunscreens are now "full spectrum" and effectively filter UVA light as well.

Sunscreens contain substances, such as para-aminobenzoic acid (PABA) and benzophenone, which absorb UV light. Because PABA does not immediately bind strongly to the skin, sunscreens containing PABA must be applied 30 minutes before going out in the sun or into the water. PABA may irritate the skin or cause an allergic reaction in some people. Many sunscreens contain both PABA and benzophenone or other chemicals. These combination sunscreens provide protection from a broader range of UV light. Many sunscreens claim to be either waterproof or water-resistant, but most of these nonetheless require more frequent application among people who are swimming or sweating.

Other sunscreens, called sunblocks, contain physical barriers such as zinc oxide or titanium dioxide. These thick, white ointments block almost all sunlight from the skin and can be used on small, sensitive areas, such as the nose and lips. Some cosmetics contain zinc oxide or titanium dioxide. Newer-formulated sunblocks have a more pleasing thickness and color, which allow them to be combined with other traditional chemical blockers thereby providing even more sun protection to a given formulation.

In the United States, sunscreens are rated by their sun protection factor (SPF) number—the higher the SPF number, the greater the protection. Sunscreens rated between 2 and 12 provide some protection; those rated between 13 and 29 provide good protection; those rated 30 and above provide maximum protection. The SPF, however, only quantifies the protection against UVB exposure; there is no scale for UVA protection.

Treatment

Cold tap water compresses can soothe raw, hot areas, as can skin moisturizers without anesthetics or perfumes that might irritate or sensitize the skin.

Are Tans Healthy?

In a word—no. Although a suntan is often considered an emblem of good health and of an active, athletic life, tanning for its own sake has no health benefit and is actually a health hazard. Any exposure to ultraviolet A or B (UVA or UVB) light can alter or damage the skin. Long-term exposure to natural sunlight causes skin damage and increases the risk of skin cancer. Exposure to the artificial sunlight used in tanning salons is harmful as well. The UVA lights used in these establishments cause the same long-term effects as exposure to UVB light, such as wrinkling and mottled pigmentation (photoaging) and skin cancer. Quite simply, there is no safe tan.

Self-tanning, or sunless, lotions do not really tan the skin but, rather, stain it. They therefore provide a safe way to achieve a tanned look without risking dangerous exposure to ultraviolet rays. However, because they do not increase melanin production, self-tanning lotions do not offer protection from the sun. Therefore, sunscreens should still be used during exposure to sunlight. Results with the use of self-tanning lotions may vary, depending on a person's skin type, the formulation used, and the manner in which the lotion is applied.

Nonsteroidal anti-inflammatory drugs (NSAIDs—see page 644) help relieve pain and inflammation. Ointments or lotions containing local anesthetics (eg, benzocaine) temporarily relieve pain but should be avoided because they occasionally trigger an allergic reaction. Corticosteroid tablets also may help relieve the inflammation but are used only for the most serious burns. Specific antibiotic burn creams are required only for severe blistering. Most sunburn blisters break on their own and do not need to be popped and drained. Sunburned skin rarely becomes infected, but if an infection develops, healing may be delayed. A doctor can determine the severity of an infection and prescribe antibiotics if necessary.

Sunburned skin begins healing by itself within several days, but complete healing may take weeks. After burned skin peels, the newly exposed layers are thin and initially very sensitive to sunlight and must be protected for several weeks.

Photosensitivity Reactions

- Sunlight can trigger immune reactions.
- People develop itchy eruptions or areas of redness and inflammation on patches of sun-exposed skin.
- These reactions typically resolve without treatment.

Some Substances That Sensitize the Skin to Sunlight

ANTIANXIETY DRUGS

- Alprazolam
- Chlordiazepoxide

ANTIBIOTICS

- Fluoroquinolones
- Sulfonamides
- Tetracyclines
- Trimethoprim

ANTIDEPRESSANTS

- Tricyclic antidepressants

ANTIFUNGAL DRUGS (taken by mouth)

- Griseofulvin

ANTIHYPERGLYCEMICS

- Sulfonylureas

ANTIMALARIAL DRUGS

- Chloroquine
- Quinine

ANTIPSYCHOTICS

- Phenothiazines

DIURETICS

- Furosemide
- Thiazides

CHEMOTHERAPY DRUGS

- Dacarbazine
- Fluorouracil
- Methotrexate
- Vinblastine

DRUGS USED TO TREAT ACNE (taken by mouth)

- Isotretinoin

HEART DRUGS

- Amiodarone
- Quinidine

SKIN PREPARATIONS

- Antibacterials (chlorhexidine, hexachlorophene)
- Antifungal drugs
- Coal tar
- Fragrances
- Sunscreens

Photosensitivity, sometimes referred to as a sun allergy, is an immune system reaction that is triggered by sunlight. Photosensitivity reactions include solar urticaria, chemical photosensitization, and polymorphous light eruption and are usually characterized by an itchy eruption on patches of sun-exposed skin. People may inherit a tendency to these reactions. Certain diseases, such as systemic lupus erythematosus and some porphyrias, also may cause the skin to break out in response to sunlight.

Solar Urticaria: Hives (large, itchy red bumps) that develop after only a few minutes of exposure to sunlight are called solar urticaria. The hives appear within 10 minutes of sun exposure and generally last for only a few hours. A person can be prone to developing solar urticaria for a very long time, sometimes indefinitely. People with large affected areas sometimes have headaches and feel dizzy, weak, and nauseated.

Chemical Photosensitivity: In chemical photosensitivity, people develop redness, inflammation, and sometimes brown or blue discoloration in areas of skin that have been exposed to sunlight for a brief period. This reaction differs from sunburn in that it occurs only after the person has taken certain drugs (such as tetracycline) or chemicals or has applied them to the skin (such as perfume or aftershave). These substances make some people's skin more sensitive to the effects of ultraviolet (UV) light. Some people develop hives with itching, which indicates a type of drug allergy that is triggered by sunlight.

Polymorphous Light Eruption: This eruption is an unusual reaction to sunlight, the cause of which is not understood. It is one of the most common sun-related skin problems and is most common among women and among people from northern climates who are not regularly exposed to the sun. The eruption appears as multiple red bumps and irregular red patches on sun-exposed skin. These patches, which are itchy, generally appear between 30 minutes and several hours after sun exposure; however, new patches may develop many hours or several days later. The bumps and patches usually go away within several days to a week. Typically, people with this condition who continue to go out in the sun gradually become less sensitive to the effects of sunlight.

Diagnosis

There are no specific tests for photosensitivity reactions. A doctor suspects a photosensitivity reaction when a rash appears only in areas exposed to sunlight. A close review of any diseases, drugs taken by mouth, or substances applied to the skin (such as drugs or cosmetics) may help a doctor pinpoint the cause of the photosensitivity reaction. Doctors may perform tests to rule out diseases, such as systemic lupus erythematosus, that are known to make someone susceptible to such reactions.

Prevention and Treatment

A person with sensitivity to sunlight from any cause should wear protective clothes, avoid sunlight as much as possible, and use sunscreens. If possible, any drugs or chemicals that could cause photosensitivity should be discontinued after consulting with a doctor.

People with polymorphous light eruption or lupus photosensitivity sometimes benefit from treatment with corticosteroids applied to the skin or hydroxychloroquine or corticosteroids taken by mouth. Occasionally, people can be desensitized to the effects of sunlight by gradually increasing their exposure to UV light.

Noncancerous Skin Growths

Cells of the skin and underlying tissue may accumulate and cause growths. Growths may be raised or flat and range in color from dark brown or black to flesh-colored to red. They may be present at birth or develop later.

When the growth is controlled and the cells do not spread to other parts of the body, the skin growth (tumor) is noncancerous (benign). When the growth is uncontrolled, the tumor is cancerous (malignant), and the cells invade normal tissue and even spread (metastasize) to other parts of the body. Noncancerous skin growths are often more of a cosmetic problem than anything else.

Doctors do not know what causes most noncancerous skin growths. Some growths, however, are known to be caused by viruses (for example, warts), systemic (bodywide) disease (for example, xanthelasmas or xanthomas caused by excess fats in the blood), and environmental factors (for example, moles or milia stimulated by sunlight).

Moles

Moles (nevi) are small, usually dark, skin growths that develop from pigment-producing cells in the skin (melanocytes).

- Most people have some moles, but the tendency to develop atypical moles is hereditary.
- Moles and atypical moles that change drastically should be biopsied for possible melanoma.
- Most noncancerous moles do not require treatment, but moles that are uncomfortable or a cosmetic concern can be removed with a scalpel and local anesthetic.

Moles vary in size from small dots to more than 1 inch (about 2.5 centimeters) in diameter. Almost everyone has a few moles, and many people have large numbers of them. Moles may be flat or raised, smooth or rough (wartlike), and may have hairs growing from them. Although they are usually brown or dark brown,

some moles are flesh-colored or yellow-brown. They may be red at first but often darken.

Moles commonly develop in childhood or adolescence, although in some people they continue to develop throughout life. Moles respond to changes in hormone levels in women and may first appear, enlarge, or darken during pregnancy. Once formed, moles remain for a lifetime and get less pigmented and more raised or fleshy with time. In fair-skinned people, moles occur more commonly on sun-exposed areas of the skin.

Moles usually are easily recognized by their typical appearance. They do not itch or hurt, and they are not a form of cancer. However, moles sometimes develop into or resemble melanoma, a cancerous growth of melanocytes (see page 1335). In fact, many melanomas begin in moles, so a mole that looks suspicious should be removed and examined under a microscope.

The following changes in a mole are warnings of melanoma:

- Enlargement, especially with an irregular border
- Darkening
- Inflammation
- Spotty color changes
- Bleeding
- Broken skin
- Itching
- Pain

People with more than 10 or 20 moles have a somewhat increased risk of melanoma. They should self-monitor for changes in their moles and also have them examined periodically as part of their primary care. If a mole proves to be cancerous, additional surgery may be needed to remove the skin surrounding it.

Most moles, however, are harmless and do not require removal. Depending on their appearance and location, some moles may even be considered beauty marks. Normal moles that are unattractive or located where clothing can irritate them can be removed by a doctor using a scalpel and a local anesthetic.

> **? Did You Know...**
> Among women, moles may appear, enlarge, or darken during pregnancy.

Atypical Moles (Dysplastic Nevi): Atypical moles tend to be multicolored and have irregular shapes and borders or increased size in comparison with normal moles. The tendency to grow atypical moles is hereditary. People with even a few atypical moles have a slightly increased risk of developing melanoma. This risk increases greatly if the person has close family members with melanoma.

People with atypical moles—particularly those with a family history of melanoma—must look for any changes that might indicate melanoma. They should have their skin checked at least yearly by a dermatologist to look for changes in the color or size of a mole. To help monitor such changes, dermatologists often use full-body color photographs. Atypical moles that change should be removed.

Sunlight accelerates the development of and changes in atypical moles. Even moderate sun exposure during childhood may be harmful and increase the risk of developing melanoma decades later. Therefore, people with atypical moles should avoid sun exposure. When in the sun, they should always use a sunscreen or sunblock with a high sun protection factor (SPF) rating to help shield against cancer-producing ultraviolet (UV) rays (see page 1327).

Skin Tags

Skin tags are soft, small, flesh-colored or slightly darker skin growths that develop mostly on the neck, in the armpits, or in the groin area.

Usually, skin tags cause no trouble, but they may be unattractive, and clothing or nearby skin may rub and irritate them so that they bleed or hurt. A doctor can easily remove skin tags with scissors or a scalpel or with an electric needle.

Lipomas

Lipomas are soft deposits of body fat that grow under the skin, causing round or oval lumps.

A lipoma appears as a smooth, soft bump under the skin. Lipomas range in firmness, some feeling rather hard. The skin over the lipoma has a normal appearance. Lipomas rarely grow more than 3 inches (about 7.5 centimeters) across. They can develop anywhere on the body but are particularly common on the forearms, torso, and back of the neck. Lipomas are more common in women than in men. Some people have only one, but other people develop many lipomas. Lipomas rarely cause problems, although they may occasionally be painful.

Usually, a doctor can easily recognize lipomas, and no tests are required for diagnosis. Lipomas are not a form of cancer, and they rarely become cancerous. If a lipoma begins to change in any way, a doctor may do a biopsy (removal of a tissue sample for examination under a microscope). Treatment usually is not required, but bothersome lipomas may be removed by surgery or by liposuction (removal of fat with a suction device).

Dermatofibromas

Dermatofibromas are small red-to-brown bumps (nodules) that result from an accumulation of collagen, which is a protein made by the cells (fibroblasts) that populate the soft tissue under the skin.

Dermatofibromas are common and usually appear as single firm bumps, often on the legs, and particularly in women. Some people develop many dermatofibromas. The cause is unknown. Dermatofibromas are harmless and usually do not cause any symptoms, except for occasional pain or itching. Usually, dermatofibromas are not treated unless they become bothersome or enlarge. A doctor can remove them with a scalpel.

Growths and Malformations of the Vessels

Growths and malformations of the vessels (angiomas) are collections of abnormally dense blood or lymph vessels, usually located in and below the skin, that cause red or purple discolorations.

- Many growths and malformations of the vessels appear at birth or shortly afterward.
- Doctors usually diagnose these growths and malformations by clinical examination.
- Treatment depends on the type of growth or malformation present.

Growths and malformations of the vessels include hemangiomas, port-wine stains, lymphangiomas, pyogenic granulomas, and spider angiomas (nevus araneus). Some appear at birth or soon afterward, and may be referred to as birthmarks. These different growths and malformations are usually recognized by their appearance, so biopsies are rarely necessary.

Using Lasers to Treat Skin Problems

A laser is a device that produces an intense beam of light that has one particular color (wavelength). Laser light does not affect human tissue until it is absorbed. Whether tissue absorbs laser light depends on the tissue and the color of the light. For example, blood vessels absorb yellow, blue, and green light best, so lasers of these colors are used to selectively target blood vessels in the treatment of vascular growths. Other colors are used to target different conditions. Laser beams may be continuous or briefly pulsed in individual flashes. The pulse duration helps determine the effect of the laser beam.

Laser treatments are sometimes combined with photodynamic therapy, in which certain light-absorbing chemicals are applied to the skin or given intravenously. When these chemicals are struck by laser light, they absorb the laser energy and help destroy tumors.

Blood vessel growths, such as hemangiomas, and malformations, such as port-wine stains, are commonly treated with laser therapy. Laser therapy is also used to remove unwanted hair, tattoos, skin discoloration, scars from acne or sun damage, and cancerous tumors.

Up to one third of all newborns have some type of growth or malformation of the vessels (vascular birthmark), most of which disappear by themselves.

HEMANGIOMAS

Hemangiomas are abnormal overgrowths of blood vessels that can appear as red or purple lumps in the skin and on other parts of the body.

Hemangiomas of infancy develop soon after birth and tend to enlarge rapidly during the first 6 to 18 months of life. After this, they begin to shrink. About three quarters of hemangiomas disappear by age 7, although the skin that remains is often slightly discolored or scarred. Hemangiomas also develop during middle age and later, especially on the trunk.

Hemangiomas of Infancy: These grow within and under the skin. They cause the skin to bulge and may be purple or, if they are very deep, flesh-colored. Most deep hemangiomas grow between 1/4 and 2 inches (0.5 and 5 centimeters) across, although sometimes they grow much larger. More than half occur on the head and neck. Sometimes, hemangiomas develop in organs, such as the liver (see page 239).

Hemangiomas of infancy do not cause pain but occasionally break open (ulcerate) and bleed. Hemangiomas around the eye may grow large enough to block vision, which can lead to permanent vision loss if uncorrected. Hemangiomas may also block the nose or throat, which can obstruct breathing.

Because hemangiomas of infancy usually go away on their own, doctors may not treat them when they first appear unless they grow rapidly, obstruct vision or breathing, ulcerate, or are cosmetically distressing.

When treatment is required, doctors prescribe oral or injectable corticosteroids or laser treatments. Surgical removal is usually not recommended because the vast majority of lesions go away on their own with less scarring when left alone. For older children in whom the hemangioma has shrunk to the greatest degree, surgery may improve the appearance of the skin.

Superficial Hemangiomas: Superficial hemangiomas (cherry angiomas or strawberry hemangiomas) are very common. They usually appear as raised, red, blood vessel growths on the torso and can number from a few to dozens. Superficial hemangiomas are harmless; if they are bothersome, a doctor can remove them with an electric needle or scalpel.

PORT-WINE STAIN

Port-wine stain (capillary malformation, nevus flammeus) is a flat pink, red, or purplish discoloration present at birth due to malformed blood vessels.

Port-wine stains are harmless, permanent discolorations. However, their cosmetic appearance may be psychologically bothersome or even devastating. They appear as smooth, flat pink, red, or purple patches of skin. Port-wine stains may be small or may cover large areas of the body. Stains that appear on the nape of the neck of newborns have been referred to as stork bites. Rarely, facial port-wine stains appear as part of the Sturge-Weber syndrome, a rare congenital disorder that can be associated with neurologic problems such as seizures and mental retardation (intellectual disability).

Small port-wine stains can be covered with cosmetic cover-up cream. If a stain is bothersome, its appearance can be greatly improved with laser therapy.

LYMPHANGIOMAS

Lymphangiomas (lymphatic malformations) are skin bumps caused by a collection of enlarged lymph vessels—the channels that carry lymph (a clear fluid related to blood) throughout the body.

Lymphangiomas are uncommon but usually appear between birth and age 2. They may be tiny bumps or large, deforming growths. Lymphangiomas do not itch or hurt and are not a form of cancer. Most lymphangiomas are yellowish tan, but a few are reddish. When injured or punctured, they release a colorless fluid.

Treatment is not usually needed. Removal by surgery is usually not successful since lymphangiomas grow deep and wide beneath the surface.

PYOGENIC GRANULOMAS

Pyogenic granulomas are scarlet or reddish-brown slightly raised areas caused by increased growth of capillaries (the smallest blood vessels) and swelling of the surrounding tissue.

The condition develops rapidly, usually after injury to the skin (the injury is sometimes not noticed). For unknown reasons, pyogenic granulomas may also develop during pregnancy, appearing even on the gums (pregnancy tumors). Pyogenic granulomas appear as 1/4- to 1/2-inch (about 0.5- to 1.5-centimeter) growths that rise from the surface of the skin. They do not hurt, but they bleed easily when bumped or scratched because they consist almost entirely of capillaries.

Pyogenic granulomas sometimes disappear by themselves, but if they persist, a doctor usually removes them surgically or with an electric needle (electrocoagulation). A sample of tissue may be sent to a laboratory to ensure that the growth is not a type of skin cancer. Sometimes pyogenic granulomas recur after treatment.

SPIDER ANGIOMAS

Spider angiomas (also called nevus araneus, spider nevus, or vascular spiders) are small, bright red spots consisting of a central dilated blood vessel surrounded by slender dilated capillaries that resemble spider legs.

Spider angiomas on the face are commonly seen in fair-skinned people. In most people, there is no known cause, but people with cirrhosis often develop many spider angiomas, as do many women who are pregnant or who are using oral contraceptives. Spider angiomas are not present at birth.

Spider angiomas are usually less than 1/4 inch (about 0.5 centimeters) across. They are harmless and cause no symptoms but may be of cosmetic concern. Spider angiomas that develop during pregnancy or oral contraceptive use usually disappear on their own 6 to 9 months after childbirth or after discontinuing oral contraceptive use. If treatment is desired for cosmetic reasons, a doctor can destroy the central blood vessel with laser therapy or with an electric needle.

Seborrheic Keratoses

Seborrheic keratoses (seborrheic warts) are warty, flesh-colored, brown, or black growths that can appear anywhere on the skin.

These harmless growths are very common in middle-aged and older people. Some people have scores of lesions. Although these growths can appear anywhere, they most often appear on the torso and the temples.

Seborrheic keratoses are round or oval and vary in size from less than 1/4 inch (0.5 centimeters) to several inches. They appear to be stuck on the skin and usually have a warty and waxy or scaly surface. These growths develop slowly. They are not cancerous and do not become so. Dark brown keratoses with irregular pigment may sometimes be mistaken for atypical moles or melanomas.

Treatment is not needed unless the keratoses become irritated or itchy or are cosmetically undesirable. They are best removed by freezing them with liquid nitrogen or by using an electric needle.

Keratoacanthomas

Keratoacanthomas are round, firm, usually flesh-colored or slightly reddish growths that have a central crater that is scaly or crusted.

Keratoacanthomas appear most commonly on the face, forearm, and back of the hand and grow quickly. In 1 or 2 months, they can grow into lumps up to 1 inch (about 2.5 centimeters) wide, after which they usually begin to shrink. They usually disappear within 6 months, often leaving a scar.

Most doctors consider keratoacanthomas to be a form of squamous cell carcinoma, a type of skin cancer (see page 1334). Therefore, doctors often recommend they be treated after performing a biopsy, in which a piece of skin is removed and examined under a microscope. Keratoacanthomas are usually cut out or scraped (curetted).

Keloids

Keloids are smooth, shiny, flesh-colored, raised growths of scar-like tissue that form over areas of injury or surgical wounds.

Keloids are an extreme overgrowth of scar tissue. They may form in the months after an injury. They may be raised as much as 1/4 inch (about 0.5 centimeters) or more above the surface of the skin. Keloids may form in any injury, even those resulting from acne. They are more common in blacks than in whites and typically develop on the chest, shoulders, back, and, sometimes, face and earlobes. Keloids do not hurt, but they may itch or be sensitive to touch.

Keloids respond poorly to therapy, but monthly injections of corticosteroids may flatten them somewhat. A doctor may try surgical or laser removal, but new, larger keloids often form in the scar resulting from the treatment; corticosteroid injections before and after surgery may reduce this risk. Silicone patches or pressure garments applied to keloids are helpful in flattening them.

Epidermal Cysts

An epidermal cyst is a common slow-growing bump due to an enlarging sac under the skin that accumulates a cheesy substance composed of skin secretions.

Epidermal cysts, often incorrectly referred to as sebaceous cysts, are flesh-colored and range from 1/2

to 2 inches (about 1 to 5 centimeters) across. They often have an enlarged pore overlying them. They can appear anywhere but are most common on the back, head, and neck. They tend to be firm and easy to move within the skin. Epidermal cysts are not painful unless they become infected or inflamed.

Large epidermal cysts are removed surgically after an anesthetic is injected to numb the area. The thin sac wall must be removed completely or the cyst will grow back. Cysts that have burst under the skin often cause tenderness and swelling and need to be cut open to drain. Tiny cysts that are bothersome can be lanced and drained.

CHAPTER 200 Skin Cancers

Skin cancer is the most common form of cancer in the United States. The three main types of skin cancer—basal cell carcinoma, squamous cell carcinoma, and melanoma—are caused, at least in part, by long-term sun exposure. Lymphoma can also develop in the skin (see box on page 1064). Fair-skinned people are particularly susceptible to developing most forms of skin cancer because they produce less melanin. Melanin, the protective pigment in the outer layer of skin (epidermis), helps protect from ultraviolet (UV) light. However, skin cancer also can develop in dark-skinned people and in people whose skin has not had significant sun exposure. Most skin cancers are curable, especially when treated at an early stage. Therefore, any unusual skin growth that persists for more than a few weeks is best examined by a doctor.

Doctors treat most skin cancers by removing them surgically. Usually, the scar that is left after surgery is small. Larger or more invasive cancer may require removal of a significant amount of skin, which may have to be replaced with a skin graft (see page 1135).

Screening: Although people should notify their doctor of any unusual or changed skin marks, doctors do not know whether routine yearly skin examinations to screen for skin cancer would reduce the number of deaths from skin cancer.

Prevention: Because many skin cancers seem to be related to UV exposure, doctors recommend a number of measures to limit UV exposure.

- Avoid the sun (for example, seek shade, minimize outdoor activities between 10 AM and 3 PM, when

the sun's rays are strongest, and avoid sunbathing and the use of tanning beds)
- Wear protective clothing (eg, long-sleeved shirt, pants, broad-brimmed hat)
- Use sunscreen (at least SPF 30 with UVA protection, used as directed), but sunscreen should not be used in order to prolong sun exposure.

However, current evidence is inadequate to determine whether these measures reduce the chances of people getting or dying from melanoma. In people with a history of nonmelanoma skin cancers (that is, basal cell carcinoma or squamous cell carcinoma), sun protection does decrease the risk of developing new cancers.

> **? Did You Know...**
> Most skin cancers are caused, at least in part, by spending a lot of time in the sun.

Basal Cell Carcinoma

Basal cell carcinoma is a cancer that originates in cells of the outer layer of skin (epidermis).

- Usually, a small, shiny bump appears on the skin and enlarges slowly.
- The bumps may break open and form a scab, sometimes with bleeding, or become flat, resembling a scar.

- Although this cancer can often be identified by sight, doctors usually do a biopsy.
- The cancer is removed, and chemotherapy drugs may also be applied to the skin.

Basal cells are found in the lowest layer of the epidermis. Although basal cell carcinoma may not originate in the basal cells, the disease is so named because the cancer cells resemble basal cells. Basal cell carcinoma is the most common human cancer. More than 800,000 people develop this type of cancer in the United States each year. Basal cell carcinoma usually develops on skin surfaces that are exposed to sunlight, commonly on the head or neck.

The tumors usually begin as small, shiny, firm, raised growths (papules) that enlarge very slowly, sometimes so slowly that they go unnoticed as new growths. However, the growth rate varies greatly from tumor to tumor, with some growing as much as 1/2 inch (about 1 centimeter) in a year.

Basal cell carcinomas can vary greatly in their appearance. Some are raised bumps that may break open and form scabs in the center. Some are flat pale or red patches that look somewhat like scars. The border of the cancer is sometimes thickened and pearly white. The cancer may alternately bleed and form a scab and heal, leading a person to falsely think that it is a sore rather than a cancer.

Basal cell carcinomas rarely spread (metastasize) to distant parts of the body. Instead, they invade and slowly destroy surrounding tissues. When basal cell carcinomas grow near the eye, mouth, bone, or brain, the consequences of invasion can be serious and can lead to death. Yet, for most people, the tumors simply grow slowly into the skin.

Diagnosis, Treatment, and Prevention

Doctors often can recognize a basal cell carcinoma simply by looking at it, but a biopsy is the standard procedure for confirming the diagnosis (see page 1278).

Doctors remove the cancer in the office by scraping and burning it with an electric needle (curettage and electrodesiccation) or by cutting it out. Also, certain chemotherapy drugs may be applied to the skin. A technique called Mohs microscopically controlled surgery may be required for some basal cell carcinomas that regrow or occur in certain areas, such as around the nose and eyes. Rarely, radiation treatment is used.

Treatment is nearly always successful, and basal cell carcinoma is rarely fatal. However, almost 25% of people with a history of basal cell carcinoma develop a new basal cell cancer within 5 years. Thus, anyone with one basal cell carcinoma should have a yearly skin examination.

Because basal cell carcinoma is often caused by sun exposure, people can help prevent this cancer by staying out of the sun and using protective clothing and sunscreen. In addition, any skin change that persists for more than a few weeks should be evaluated by a doctor.

Squamous Cell Carcinoma

Squamous cell carcinoma is cancer that originates in the squamous cells (keratinocytes).

- Thick, scaly growths appear on the skin and do not heal.
- To diagnose the cancer, doctors do a biopsy.
- Treatment with surgery, chemotherapy drugs applied to the skin, and sometimes radiation therapy can usually cure the cancer unless it has spread.
- If the cancer spreads to other parts of the body, it can be fatal.

Squamous cells (keratinocytes) are the main structural cells of the epidermis (the outer layer of skin). Squamous cell carcinoma usually develops on sun-exposed areas but may grow anywhere on the skin or in the mouth, where sun exposure is minimal. It may develop on normal skin but is more likely to develop in precancerous skin growths caused by previous sun exposure (actinic keratoses—see box on page 1326). Squamous cell carcinoma is characterized by its thick, scaly, irregular appearance. Fair-skinned people are much more susceptible to squamous cell carcinoma than darker-skinned people. This type of cancer is also more likely to develop in chronic sores—such as chronic skin ulcers—or in skin that has been scarred, particularly by burns.

Squamous cell carcinoma begins as a red area with a scaly, crusted surface that does not heal. As it grows, the tumor may become somewhat raised and firm, sometimes with a wartlike surface. Eventually, the cancer becomes an open sore and grows into the underlying tissue.

Most squamous cell carcinomas affect only the area around them, penetrating into nearby tissues. However, some spread (metastasize) to distant parts of the body and can be fatal. Those that occur near the ears, lips, and in scars are more likely to spread.

Bowen's Disease: This is an early form of squamous cell carcinoma that is confined to the epidermis and has not yet invaded the deeper layers of the skin. The affected skin is red-brown and scaly or crusted and flat, sometimes looking like a patch of psoriasis or dermatitis or a fungal infection (ringworm).

Diagnosis, Treatment, and Prevention

When doctors suspect squamous cell carcinoma, they do a biopsy to differentiate this skin cancer from similar-looking diseases.

Doctors treat squamous cell carcinoma and Bowen's disease by scraping and burning the tumor with an

Mohs Microscopically Controlled Surgery

Because skin cancer cells often have spread beyond the edges of the visible patch on the skin, doctors sometimes use a special surgical technique to make sure they remove all of the cancer. In this technique, called Mohs microscopically controlled surgery or Mohs micrographic surgery, doctors first remove the visible tumor and then begin cutting away the edges of the wound bit by bit. During surgery, doctors examine pieces of tissue to look for cancer cells. Tissue removal from the area continues until the samples no longer contain cancer cells. This procedure enables doctors to limit the amount of tissue removed and thus is especially useful for cancers near such important sites as the eye.

After removing all of the cancer, doctors decide how best to replace the skin that has been cut away. They may use a skin graft (see page 1135) to bring the edges of the remaining skin together with sutures. Or they may place dressings on top of the wound and let the skin heal on its own.

Mohs surgery reduces recurrence rates for skin cancers. This surgery is useful for basal cell and squamous cell cancer but is rarely used for melanoma.

---

electric needle (curettage and electrodesiccation), by cutting the tumor out, or by applying chemotherapy drugs to the skin. A technique called Mohs microscopically controlled surgery may be used. Sometimes radiation treatments are used. These treatments are usually effective, and most people survive.

Squamous cell carcinoma that has spread to other parts of the body can be fatal. It is treated with radiation or chemotherapy, but treatment may not be effective.

Because squamous cell carcinoma is often caused by sun exposure, doctors recommend that people stay out of the sun and use protective clothing and sunscreen, starting in early childhood.

Melanoma

Melanoma is a cancer that originates in the pigment-producing cells of the skin (melanocytes).

- Melanomas can begin on normal skin or in existing moles.
- They may be irregular, flat or raised brown patches of skin with spots of different colors or firm black or gray lumps.
- To diagnose melanoma, doctors do a biopsy.
- Melanomas are removed, and if they have spread, chemotherapy drugs are used.

Melanocytes are the pigmented cells in the skin that give skin its distinctive color. Sunlight stimulates melanocytes to produce more melanin (the pigment that darkens the skin) and increases the risk of melanoma.

Melanoma can begin as a new, small, pigmented skin growth on normal skin, most often on sun-exposed areas, or it may develop from preexisting pigmented moles (see page 1329). Sometimes melanoma runs in families. Melanoma readily spreads (metastasizes) to distant parts of the body, where it continues to grow and destroy tissue.

Melanomas can vary in appearance. Some are flat, irregular brown patches containing small black spots. Others are raised brown patches with red, white, black, or blue spots. Sometimes melanoma appears as a firm black or gray lump.

Diagnosis

A new mole or changes in a mole—such as enlargement (especially with an irregular border), darkening, inflammation, spotty color changes, bleeding, broken skin, itching, and pain—are warnings of possible melanoma. If these or other findings lead doctors to suspect melanoma, they do a biopsy. They remove the entire growth if it is small or only part of it if it is large. The tissue is then examined under a microscope to determine whether the growth is a melanoma and, if so, whether all the cancer has been removed.

Most darkly pigmented growths that are sent for biopsy are not melanoma but, rather, simple moles. Nonetheless, removing a harmless mole is preferable to allowing a cancer to grow. Some growths are neither simple moles nor melanomas, but something in between. These growths, called atypical moles (dysplastic nevi), sometimes turn into melanoma later.

Treatment

The less a melanoma has grown into the skin, the greater the chance that surgery will cure it. Almost 100% of the earliest, most shallow melanomas are cured by surgery. Thus, doctors treat melanomas by cutting them out, taking a border of almost ½ inch (1 centimeter) of skin around the tumor. However, melanomas that have grown deeper than about 1/32 inch (about 1 millimeter) into the skin have a greater chance to have spread (metastasized) through the lymphatic and blood vessels. Melanomas that have spread are often fatal.

Chemotherapy is used to treat melanomas that have spread, but few are cured. Some of the people treated live for less than 9 months. However, the course of the disease varies greatly and depends in part on the strength of the body's immune defenses.

Warning Signs of Melanoma

- Enlarging pigmented (especially black or deep blue) spot or mole
- Changes in color of an existing mole, especially the spread of red, white, brown, or blue pigmentation to surrounding skin
- Changes in characteristics of skin over the pigmented spot, such as changes in size or shape
- Bleeding or breaking open (ulceration) of an existing mole

Some people survive in apparent good health for several years despite the spread of the melanoma. New and experimental treatments such as interleukin-2 and vaccines, which stimulate the body to attack the melanoma cells, have yielded promising results.

 Did You Know...

If diagnosed early, surgery can cure almost 100% of shallow melanomas.

Prevention

Because melanoma is often caused by long-term sun exposure, doctors recommend that people stay out of the sun and use protective clothing and sunscreen, starting in early childhood. However, doctors do not know how effective these measures are in preventing melanoma.

Anyone who has had a melanoma is at risk of developing other melanomas. Therefore, such people need yearly skin examinations. People who have many moles should have total body skin examinations at least once a year. In people without risk factors, doctors do not know whether routine yearly skin examinations reduce the number of deaths from melanoma.

Kaposi's Sarcoma

Kaposi's sarcoma is a cancer that produces multiple flat pink, brown, or purple patches or bumps on the skin. It is caused by herpesvirus type 8.

- One or a few spots may appear on the toes or a leg, or spots may appear anywhere on the body, then spread to other areas, including internal organs.
- Although this cancer can often be identified by sight, doctors usually also do a biopsy.
- Spots may be removed or treated with radiation therapy, but if the cancer is aggressive, treatment includes chemotherapy drugs or interferon-alpha.

Kaposi's sarcoma occurs in several distinct groups of people and acts differently in each group. It occurs in the following:

- Older men, usually of Mediterranean or Jewish heritage
- Children and young adults from certain parts of Africa
- People receiving immunosuppressants after organ transplantation
- People with AIDS (which accounts for most of the cases in the United States)

Symptoms

In older men, Kaposi's sarcoma usually appears as a single purple or dark brown spot on the toes or a leg. The cancer may grow to several inches or more as a deeply colored, flat or slightly raised area that tends to bleed and break open. Several additional spots may appear on the leg, but the cancer rarely spreads to other parts of the body and is almost never fatal.

In the other groups, Kaposi's sarcoma is more aggressive. Similar appearing spots develop, but they are often multiple and may occur anywhere on the body. Within several months, the spots spread to other parts of the body, often including the mouth, where they cause pain with eating. They may also develop in lymph nodes and internal organs, especially the digestive tract, where they can cause diarrhea and internal bleeding that leads to blood in the stool.

 Did You Know...

In the United States, most cases of Kaposi's sarcoma occur in people with AIDS.

Diagnosis and Treatment

Doctors usually recognize Kaposi's sarcoma by its appearance. A biopsy is usually done to confirm the diagnosis.

Older men with slow-growing Kaposi's sarcoma in one or two spots may have the tumors removed surgically or by freezing. People with multiple spots usually receive radiation therapy. Some people with very few spots and no other symptoms may choose to receive no treatment unless the condition spreads.

People who have the more aggressive form, but whose immune system is normal, often respond to interferon-alpha or chemotherapy drugs.

In people taking immunosuppressants, the tumors sometimes disappear when immunosuppressants are stopped. However, if these drugs must be continued because of the person's underlying condition, chemotherapy and radiation therapy are used. These treatment methods are less successful than in people with a healthy immune system.

In people with AIDS, treatment with chemotherapy and radiation has not been very successful. However, intensive treatment with AIDS drugs helps, provided that people's immune system improves because of the treatment. In general, treating Kaposi's sarcoma does not appear to prolong the lives of people with AIDS.

Paget's Disease of the Nipple

Paget's disease of the nipple is a rare type of skin cancer that originates in glands in or under the skin.

The term Paget's disease also refers to an unrelated metabolic bone disease (see page 547). These distinct diseases should not be confused with each other.

Paget's disease occurs mainly on the nipple and results from a cancer of the breast milk ducts that has spread to the skin of the nipple. Both men and women are affected. The underlying cancer may or may not be felt by the person or the doctor. Sometimes Paget's disease develops in areas other than the breast (extramammary Paget's disease). It can develop in the genital area or around the anus as the result of a cancer originating in underlying sweat glands or even in nearby structures such as the genitals, intestines, or urinary tract.

The skin in Paget's disease appears red, oozing, and crusting. It looks like an inflamed reddened patch of skin (dermatitis) as may result from many other possible causes. Itching and pain are common. Because Paget's disease looks very much like common dermatitis, a biopsy is necessary to make the diagnosis.

Paget's disease of the nipple is managed like other types of breast cancer (see page 1557). Paget's disease outside the breast area is treated by surgically removing the entire growth.

CHAPTER 201 Nail Disorders

The nail unit is made up of the nail plate and the surrounding structures. These structures include the nail bed, which underlies the nail and forms the attachment of the nail to the finger; the nail matrix, which is located at the base of the nail and is the site of nail growth; the cuticle, which connects the top of the nail plate to the skin behind it; and the nail folds (the folds of hard skin) at the sides of the nail plate, which is where the skin and nail meet.

> **? Did You Know...**
> Some babies are born without nails, a condition called anonychia.

Causes

Many disorders can affect the nails. These disorders can affect any portion of the nail unit and can impact the appearance of the nail plate itself. Nail disorders can result from

- Infections
- Injuries
- Internal diseases (such as certain lung diseases, which can cause yellow nail syndrome)
- Structural problems (such as an ingrown toenail)

Deformities and Discoloration

About 50% of nail deformities are caused by a fungal infection (see page 1339). The remainder result from various causes, including trauma, psoriasis, lichen planus, and occasionally cancer. Drugs, infections, and diseases can cause discoloration of the nails (chromonychia). For example, infection with *Pseudomonas* bacteria can cause a yellow-green discoloration (see page 1340).

The doctor can often make a diagnosis by examination. However, to confirm the diagnosis, the doctor may need to take fungal scrapings and perform a culture (the process of growing the organisms in a laboratory). If the nail's appearance does not improve with treatment of the underlying disorder, manicurists may be able to hide deformities with appropriate trimming and polishes.

Birth Deformities: Some babies are born without nails (anonychia). In nail-patella syndrome (see page 273), nails are missing or are small with pitting and ridges. Darier's disease causes red and white streaks on the nails and V-shaped notches to form on the tips of the nails.

Deformities Associated With Disease: Sometimes, diseases that involve other organs can cause changes in the nails as well.

- In Plummer-Vinson syndrome (see page 136), many people have concave, spoon-shaped nails (koilonychia).

- People with iron deficiency may also have spoon-shaped nails.
- Kidney failure may cause the bottom half of the nails to turn white and the top half of the nails to turn pink or appear pigmented (half-and-half nails).
- Cirrhosis may cause the nails to turn white, although the very top part of the nails may remain pinker (Terry's nail). Low levels of the blood protein called albumin (which may occur in people with cirrhosis) may cause horizontal white lines to form on the nails.
- Some lung diseases may cause yellow nail syndrome, in which nails become thick, over-curved, and yellow or yellow-green in color.
- Lymphedema, an accumulation of lymphatic fluid in tissues, also can cause yellow nail syndrome.
- People who have human immunodeficiency virus (HIV) infection, hyperthyroidism, or Cushing's syndrome may have melanonychia striata.

Deformities Associated With Skin Diseases: Sometimes, skin diseases also affect the nail unit and may change the appearance of the nails. Some drugs given to treat skin diseases can change the nail plate. For example, retinoids, such as isotretinoin and etretinate, can cause dryness and brittleness of the nails.

- In psoriasis, nails may have irregular pits (tiny depressions in the surface of the nail), oil spots (yellow-brown spots under the nail), separation of the nail plate from its bed (onycholysis), and thickening and crumbling of the nail plate.
- Lichen planus of the nail bed causes scarring with early nail ridging and splitting, later leading to pterygium formation. Pterygium of the nail is scarring from the base of the nail outward in a V formation, which leads to loss of the nail.
- People with alopecia areata, a disorder in which round, irregular patches of hair are suddenly lost, may have regular nail pits that form a pattern.
- Trachyonychia—rough, opaque nails—may occur with alopecia areata, lichen planus, atopic dermatitis, and psoriasis. Trachyonychia most frequently occurs in children.

Drugs: Different drugs lead to discoloration of the nail, which usually gets better after the drug is stopped and the nail grows out.

- Chemotherapy drugs such as bleomycin may cause a darkening (hyperpigmentation) of the nail plate. Horizontal (transverse) pigmented or white bands may also be seen in people treated with certain chemotherapy drugs.
- Chloroquine, a drug used in the treatment of parasitic infections and certain types of autoimmune diseases, can cause the nail bed to turn blue-black.

SPOTLIGHT ON AGING

With aging, nails become dry and brittle and flat or concave instead of convex. They may develop ridges along their length. Nail color may change to yellow or gray. Brittle nails may split.

Toenails require special attention in older people and in people with diabetes or peripheral vascular disease. Such people may have poor sensation in their feet, which increases the risk of injury when they try to trim their nails. A foot doctor (podiatrist) can help care for their nails to prevent local breakdown and secondary infections.

- Silver, which can be absorbed after occupational exposure or through taking dietary supplements containing colloidal silver protein, can cause the nails to turn a dark blue-gray.
- Drugs that contain gold, which is sometimes used in the treatment of rheumatoid arthritis, can turn nails light or dark brown.
- Minocycline, an antibiotic, can cause blue discoloration.
- Zidovudine (AZT), a drug used to treat HIV infection, may cause brown-black longitudinal streaks. However, these streaks can also be present in people who have AIDS but are not receiving AZT.
- Severe arsenic poisoning can cause horizontal white lines to form on the nails.

Melanonychia Striata: Melanonychia striata are brown-black lines in the nail plate caused by the brown pigment melanin. The lines extend from the base of the nail to its tip. In dark-skinned people, these lines may be normal and require no treatment. Similar pigment changes can also be caused by moles or skin cancer around or under the nail, so doctors need to evaluate the surrounding skin.

Onychogryphosis: Onychogryphosis is a disorder in which the nail, most often on the big toe, becomes thickened and takes on an extremely curved, hooked appearance (ram's horn nail). The curved hooked nail may injure an adjoining toe and is caused by one side of the nail growing faster than the other. This disorder involves damage to the nail bed, which is most often caused by repetitive injury (such as by ill-fitting shoes), but may also occur in disorders such as psoriasis. Onychogryphosis is common in older people. The nails should be kept trimmed, and injury to nearby toes can be prevented by placing lamb's wool between the toes. Footwear or stockings that gather at the toes should be avoided.

Onycholysis: Onycholysis is separation of the nail plate from the nail bed or complete nail plate loss. It can occur from trauma (as in prolonged hiking or skiing with ill-fitting footgear); from overzealous nail cleaning; with diseases such as psoriasis and thyrotoxicosis; or from exposure to certain chemicals or drugs. Drugs that cause onycholysis include doxorubicin, bleomycin, captopril, 5-fluorouricil, and retinoids. Other drugs, including tetracyclines, psoralens, fluoroquinolones, and quinine, may cause onycholysis most often when the nails are exposed to sunlight (photo-onycholysis).

People with onycholysis are at risk of infection with yeast and fungus. Keeping the nail dry and applying antifungal preparations to the nail unit can help. Partial onycholysis may occur in people with a fungal infection.

Onychotillomania: People with this disorder pick at and tear their nails. The most common manifestation is the habit-tic deformity, in which the person frequently picks at or rubs the central cuticle with a neighboring finger. This is most often seen on the thumb and leads to a washboard-like appearance in the center of the nail plate. Onychotillomania can also cause bleeding beneath the nails (subungual hemorrhage), infection in the nail unit, and even complete loss of the nail plate.

Infections

Infections may involve the nail itself, the bed under the nail, or the skin around the nail. Most nail infections are fungal (onychomycosis), but bacterial and viral infections can occur. Bacterial infections may occur in the cuticle or nail folds (paronychia).

ONYCHOMYCOSIS

Onychomycosis is a fungal infection of the nails.

About 10% of people have onychomycosis, which most often affects the toenails rather than the fingernails. The fungus can be acquired through contact with an infected person or contact with a surface such as a bathroom floor where the fungus is present. The fungus commonly occurs as part of an infection called athlete's foot (see page 1322). Older people, people who have diabetes, and people with poor circulation to the feet are particularly prone to fungal infections.

Symptoms

Infected nails have an abnormal appearance but are not itchy or painful. In mild infections, the nails have patches of white or yellow discoloration. A chalky, white scale may slowly spread beneath the nail's surface. In more severe infections, the nails thicken and appear deformed and discolored. They may detach from the nail bed. Usually, debris from the infected nail collects under its free edge.

Diagnosis and Treatment

A doctor usually makes the diagnosis based on the appearance of the nails. To confirm the diagnosis, the doctor may need to examine a sample of the nail debris under a microscope and culture it to determine which fungus is causing the infection.

Fungal infections are difficult to cure, so treatment depends on how severe or bothersome the symptoms are. If treatment is desired, the doctor may prescribe itraconazole or terbinafine taken by mouth. Although these drugs are taken for a long time (about 3 months), they remain bound to the nail plate and continue to be effective after use of the drug is stopped. Ciclopirox, an antifungal drug that is placed in a nail lacquer, is not very effective when used alone but can improve the cure rate when used in addition to drugs taken by mouth, particularly in resistant infections. Ciclopirox can be of some help to people who cannot take oral drugs for other health reasons.

To limit the possibility of a relapse, the nails should be kept trimmed short, the feet should be dried after bathing, absorbent socks should be worn, and antifungal foot powder may be used. Old shoes may harbor a high density of fungal spores and, if possible, should not be worn.

PARONYCHIA

Paronychia is infection of the cuticle.

Paronychia is usually acute, but chronic cases can occur. In acute paronychia, bacteria (usually *Staphylococcus aureus* or streptococci) enter through a break in the skin resulting from a hangnail, trauma to a nail fold (the fold of hard skin overlapping the sides of a nail), loss of the cuticle, or chronic irritation (such as that from water and detergents). Paronychia is more common in people who bite or suck their fingers. In toes, infection often begins at an ingrown toenail (see page 1340).

Paronychia develops along the nail margin (the sides and base of the nail fold). Over the course of hours to days, people with paronychia develop pain, warmth, redness, and swelling. Pus usually accumulates under the skin along the nail margin and sometimes beneath the nail. Rarely, mainly in people who have diabetes or other disorders that cause poor circulation, infection penetrates deep into the finger or toe and can threaten the digit or, in extreme cases, the limb.

The doctor makes the diagnosis by examining the affected finger or toe. In its earliest stage, paronychia may be treated with an antibiotic taken by mouth (such as dicloxacillin, cephalexin, or clindamycin) and frequent warm soaks to increase the blood flow. If pus accumulates, it must be drained. The doctor numbs the finger or toe with a local anesthetic (such as lidocaine) and lifts up the nail fold with an instrument. Cutting the skin is usually unnecessary. A thin gauze wick is inserted for 24 to 48 hours to allow the area to drain.

CHRONIC PARONYCHIA

Chronic paronychia is recurrent or persistent inflammation of the nail fold, typically of the fingers.

Chronic paronychia occurs almost always in people whose hands are chronically wet (for example, dishwashers, bartenders, and housekeepers), particularly if they have diabetes or an impaired immune system. The yeast *Candida* is often present, but its role in causing chronic paronychia is unclear because eliminating the yeast completely does not always cure the condition. Chronic paronychia may be the result of an irritant skin inflammation (dermatitis) in addition to colonization with *Candida*.

The nail fold is painful and red as in acute paronychia, but pus usually does not accumulate. Often there is loss of the cuticle and separation of the nail fold from the nail plate. A space then forms that allows irritants and microorganisms to enter. The nail can become distorted.

The doctor makes the diagnosis by examining the affected finger.

Keeping the hands dry and protected can help the cuticle reform and close the space between the nail fold and nail plate. Gloves or barrier creams are used if water contact is necessary. Corticosteroid creams applied to the nail may be helpful. Antifungal treatments are helpful only in reducing fungal organisms. Applying a solution of thymol in ethanol several times a day to the space formed by loss of the cuticle aids in keeping the space dry and free of microorganisms.

GREEN NAIL SYNDROME

Green nail syndrome is infection with Pseudomonas, *a type of bacteria.*

Green nail syndrome is caused by an infection with *Pseudomonas*, species. It usually develops in people who have onycholysis and whose hands are often in water. The nail in the area of onycholysis becomes greenish in color. The area can be treated by soaking in a 1% acetic acid solution twice a day or by trimming back the nail and treating the area with an antibiotic solution.

VERRUCA VULGARIS

Verruca vulgaris is common warts.

Verruca vulgaris is caused by infection with human papillomavirus and frequently infects the cuticle and sometimes the area beneath the nail. Nail biting (onychophagia) can spread this infection. Warts in these areas are especially difficult to treat. Freezing (cryotherapy) with liquid nitrogen may be effective.

Ingrown Toenail

An ingrown toenail is a condition in which the edges of the nail grow into the surrounding skin.

An ingrown nail can result when a deformed toenail grows improperly into the skin or when the skin around the nail grows abnormally fast and engulfs part of the nail. Wearing narrow, ill-fitting shoes and trimming the nail into a curve with short edges rather than straight across can cause or worsen ingrown toenails.

Ingrown nails may produce no symptoms at first but eventually may become painful, especially when pressure is applied to the ingrown area. The area is usually red and may be warm. If not treated, the area is prone to infection. Once infected, the area becomes more painful, red, and swollen. Pus may accumulate under the skin next to the nail (an infection of the cuticle called paronychia) and drain (see page 1339).

For mildly ingrown toenails, the doctor can gently lift the edge of the nail out from under the surrounding skin and place sterile cotton under the nail until the swelling goes away. If an ingrown nail requires further attention, the doctor usually numbs the area with a local anesthetic (such as lidocaine), then cuts away and removes the ingrown section of nail. The inflammation can then subside, and the ingrown nail usually does not recur.

Trauma

Even minor trauma to the finger may cause changes in the nail. The nail may develop a small spot of white discoloration that starts at the injury location and grows up with the nail.

Severe damage to the nail bed, particularly from a crush injury, often results in permanent nail deformity. To reduce the risk of a permanent nail deformity, the injury should be repaired immediately (which requires removal of the nail).

Subungual Hematoma: Blood often collects under the nail (subungual hematoma) immediately after an injury (usually a direct blow, such as with a hammer). The blood appears as a purple-black spot beneath part or all of the nail and causes a great deal of pain. The doctor can release the blood and relieve the pain by making a small hole in the nail plate. Usually the doctor uses a heated wire (electrocautery device) to burn the hole. This procedure is painless and takes only a few seconds.

Because the blood has separated the nail from its bed, the nail usually falls off after several weeks, unless the hematoma is small. A new nail grows below the existing nail and replaces it when fully grown in.

A tumor beneath the nail can cause a similar purple-black spot, although such a spot appears slowly and not within minutes of an injury. However, any small hematomas should be watched to make sure that they grow out with the nail. Growing out with the nail distinguishes hematomas from tumors because tumors remain in the same spot under the nail.

Tumors

Benign and malignant tumors can affect the nail unit, causing a deformity. These tumors include noncancerous myxoid cysts, pyogenic granulomas, glomus tumors, Bowen's disease (an early form of skin cancer), squamous cell carcinoma, and malignant melanoma. When doctors suspect cancer, they perform a biopsy and may recommend complete removal of the tumor as soon as possible.

Hutchinson's sign—a black discoloration of the area around the nail, including the lunula (half-moon at the base of the nail), cuticle, and nail fold (the fold of hard skin overlapping the sides of the nail)—may mean there is cancer in the nail bed. When this sign is present, doctors perform a biopsy and begin treatment as quickly as possible.

Mouth and Dental Disorders

CHAPTER

202 Biology of the Mouth

The mouth is the entrance to both the digestive and the respiratory systems. The inside of the mouth is lined with mucous membranes. When healthy, the lining of the mouth (oral mucosa) is reddish pink; the gums are paler pink and fit snugly around the teeth.

The roof of the mouth (palate) is divided into two parts. The front part has ridges and is hard (hard palate). The back part is relatively smooth and soft (soft palate). The moist mucous membranes lining the mouth continue outside, forming the pink and shiny portion of the lips, which meets the skin of the face at the vermilion border. The lip mucosa, although moistened by saliva, is prone to drying.

At the back of the mouth hangs a narrow muscular structure called the uvula, which can be seen when a

1343

A View of the Mouth

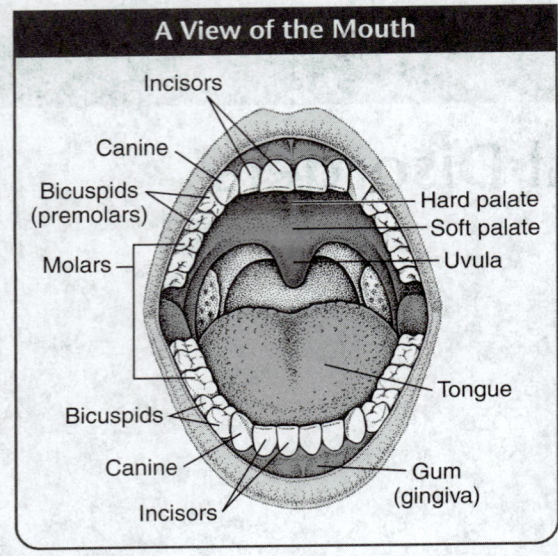

Incisors
Canine
Bicuspids (premolars)
Molars
Bicuspids
Canine
Incisors

Hard palate
Soft palate
Uvula
Tongue
Gum (gingiva)

food is eaten, the flow of saliva washes away bacteria that can cause tooth decay (cavities) and other disorders. Saliva helps keep the lining of the mouth healthy and prevents loss of minerals from teeth. It not only neutralizes acids produced by bacteria but also contains many substances (such as antibodies and enzymes) that kill bacteria, yeasts, and viruses.

A tooth is divided into the crown, which is the part above the gum line, and the root, which is the part below the gum line. The crown is covered with shiny white enamel, which protects the tooth. Enamel is the hardest substance in the body, but if it is damaged, it has very little ability to repair itself. Under the enamel is dentin, which is similar to bone but is harder. Dentin surrounds the central (pulp) chamber, which contains blood vessels, nerves, and connective tissue.

The blood vessels and nerves enter the pulp chamber through the root canals, which are also surrounded by dentin. In the root, dentin is covered by cementum, a thin bonelike substance. Cementum is surrounded by a membrane (periodontal ligament) that cushions the tooth and attaches the cementum layer, and thereby the whole tooth, firmly to the jaw.

People have two sets of natural teeth: baby (deciduous) teeth and adult (permanent) teeth. There are 20 baby teeth: one pair each of upper and lower central (front) incisors, lateral incisors, canines (cuspids), first molars, and second molars. There are 32 permanent teeth: one pair each of upper and lower central incisors, lateral incisors, canines, bicuspids (premolars), second bicuspids, first molars, second molars, and third molars (wisdom teeth). Wisdom teeth, however, vary—not everyone gets all four wisdom teeth, and some people do not get any wisdom teeth. The wisdom teeth are the last permanent teeth to come in, typically between the ages of 17 and 21.

There is a broad range of normal times for teeth to push through the gum tissue (erupt) into the mouth. For baby teeth, the central incisors are the first teeth to erupt, occurring at about 6 months of age. These are followed by the lateral incisors, first baby molars, canines, and, finally, second baby molars. By about 2½ years of age, all the baby teeth can usually be seen in the child's mouth. Each of these baby teeth will be pushed out by a permanent tooth, starting at about age 6. The permanent 6-year molars come into the mouth just behind the last baby molars and, therefore, do not replace any teeth. This lack of replacement is also true for the permanent second and third molars.

person says "Ahh." The uvula hangs from the back of the soft palate, which separates the back of the nose from the back of the mouth. Normally, the uvula hangs vertically. Its nerve supply comes from the vagus (10th cranial) nerve.

On the floor of the mouth lies the tongue, which is used to taste and mix food. The tongue is not normally smooth. It is covered with tiny projections (papillae) that contain taste buds, which sense the taste of food. The sense of taste is relatively simple, distinguishing only sweet, sour, salty, and bitter. Sweet and salty taste receptors are located at and near the tip; sour, on the sides; and bitter, on the most posterior (back) part of the tongue. Smell is sensed by olfactory receptors high in the nose. The sense of smell is much more complex than that of taste, distinguishing many subtle variations. The senses of taste and smell work together to enable people to recognize and appreciate flavors (see art on page 1400).

The salivary glands produce saliva. There are three major pairs of salivary glands: parotid, submandibular, and sublingual. Besides the major salivary glands, many tiny salivary glands are distributed throughout the mouth. Saliva passes from the glands into the mouth through small tubes (ducts).

Saliva serves several purposes. Saliva aids in chewing and eating by gathering food into lumps so that food can slide out of the mouth and down the esophagus and by dissolving foods so that they can more easily be tasted. Saliva also coats food particles with digestive enzymes and begins digestion. After

In rare cases, a child is born with a tooth (a natal tooth), or a baby tooth erupts in the mouth within a month of birth (a neonatal tooth). These teeth are usually baby lower incisors, but they may be extra

Color Changes in the Mouth

White areas can appear anywhere in the mouth and often are simply food debris that can be wiped away. However, because more persistent white areas can be an early sign of mouth cancer, they should always be evaluated by a dentist or doctor. White areas can indicate many other conditions besides cancer, such as a white spongy patch (a hereditary condition called white sponge nevus), a white line running along the inside of the cheek opposite the teeth (linea alba), and a grayish white area of the mucosa (leukoedema).

The mouth may have dark blue or black areas due to silver amalgam from a dental filling, graphite from falling with a pencil in the mouth, or a mole. Heavy cigarette smoking can lead to dark brown or black discoloration called smoker's melanosis. Ingesting lead or drugs that contain silver can lead to a gray discoloration of the gums. Minocycline, an antibiotic, discolors bone, which may show through near the teeth as gray or brown. Children's teeth darken noticeably and permanently after even short-term use of tetracyclines (a class of antibiotic) by the mother during the second half of pregnancy or by the child during tooth development (specifically calcification of the crowns, which lasts until age 9). Brown areas in the mouth can also be hereditary. For example, darkly pigmented areas are particularly common among dark-skinned and Mediterranean people.

Sometimes color changes in the mouth are a sign of a bodywide disease:

- Anemia may cause the lining of the mouth to be pale instead of the normal healthy reddish pink.
- Measles, a viral disease, can cause spots to form inside the cheeks. These spots, called Koplik's spots, resemble tiny grains of white sand surrounded by a red ring.
- Addison's disease and cancer (such as malignant melanoma) can cause color changes as well.
- In a person with AIDS, purplish patches caused by Kaposi sarcoma may appear on the palate.
- Small red spots on the palate can be a sign of a blood disorder or infectious mononucleosis.

(supernumerary) teeth. These teeth are removed only if they interfere with nursing or if they become exceedingly loose, which may pose a risk of choking.

In many children, the permanent lower incisors come in behind each other, resembling a cluster of grapes. Lack of space due to crowding or rotated permanent teeth may be the problem, and early orthodontic therapy (braces) may be necessary. Thumb or finger sucking may also affect the position of teeth, sometimes requiring early orthodontic therapy.

Effects of Aging

With aging, the taste buds become less sensitive, so older people may add abundant seasonings (particularly salt) or may find their food tastes bland. Older people may also have disorders or take drugs that affect their ability to taste. Such disorders include infections in the mouth, nose, or sinuses; gum disease; oral cancer; and chronic liver or kidney disease. Drugs affecting taste include some of those for high blood pressure (such as captopril), high cholesterol (such as the statins), and depression.

Many older people retain their teeth, especially people who do not develop cavities or periodontal disease, a destructive disease of the gums and supporting structures caused by the long-term accumulation of bacteria. Some older people lose some or all of their teeth and need partial or full dentures. Tooth loss is the major reason that older people cannot chew as well and thus may not consume enough nutrients.

Tooth enamel tends to wear away with aging, making the teeth vulnerable to damage and decay. Periodontal disease, however, is the major cause of tooth loss. Periodontal disease is more likely to occur in people with poor oral hygiene, in people who smoke, and in people with certain disorders, such as diabetes mellitus, poor nutrition, leukemia, or AIDS.

A modest decrease in saliva production occurs with aging. Decreased salivary flow increases the likelihood of tooth decay. Some experts also believe that it may make the lining of the esophagus more susceptible to injury.

203 Lip and Tongue Disorders

The lips and tongue may undergo changes in size, color, and surface. Some of these changes may indicate a medical problem. Other changes are harmless. For example, with aging, the lips may grow thinner. Also, the side of the tongue may enlarge (bump out) where teeth are missing.

Lip Disorders

Swelling: An allergic reaction can make the lips swell. The reaction may be caused by sensitivity to certain foods or beverages, drugs, lipstick, or airborne irritants. When a cause can be identified and then eliminated, the lips usually return to normal. But frequently, the cause of the swelling remains a mystery. A condition called hereditary angioedema may cause recurring bouts of swelling. Nonhereditary conditions—such as erythema multiforme, sunburn, cold and dry weather, or trauma—may also cause the lips to swell.

Treatment depends on the cause. A corticosteroid ointment is sometimes used to reduce swelling caused by an allergic reaction. Occasionally, excess lip tissue may be removed surgically to improve appearance.

Inflammation: With inflammation of the lips (cheilitis), the corners of the mouth may become painful, irritated, red, cracked, and scaly. Cheilitis may result from a deficiency of vitamin B_2 in the diet, but this deficiency is rare in the United States and can be treated by taking supplements of this vitamin.

Most commonly, skinfolds and irritated skin (angular cheilitis) may develop in the corners of the mouth if a person has dentures that do not separate the jaws adequately. Treatment consists of replacing the dentures, which helps reduce the folds at the corners of the mouth.

Discoloration: Freckles and irregularly shaped brownish areas (melanotic macules) are common around the lips and may last for many years. These marks are not cause for concern. Multiple, small, scattered brownish black spots may be a sign of a hereditary disease called Peutz-Jeghers syndrome, in which polyps form in the stomach and intestines (see page 192). Kawasaki disease, a disease of unknown cause that usually occurs in infants and children 8 years old or younger, can cause dryness and cracking of the lips and reddening of the lining of the mouth (see box on page 1772).

Sores: A raised area or a sore with hard edges on the lip may be a form of skin cancer (see pages 1333 and 1353). Other sores may develop as symptoms of other medical conditions, such as oral herpes simplex virus infection (cold sores—see page 1245) or syphilis (see page 1271). Still others, such as keratoacanthoma, have no known cause.

Sun Damage: Sun damage may make the lips, especially the lower lip, hard and dry. Red speckles or a white filmy look signal damage that increases the chance of subsequent cancer. This type of damage can be reduced by covering the lips with a lip balm containing sunscreen or by shielding the face from the sun's harmful rays with a wide-brimmed hat.

Tongue Disorders

Injury: Traumatic injury is the most common cause of tongue discomfort. The tongue has many nerve endings for pain and touch and is more sensitive to pain than most other parts of the body. The tongue is frequently bitten accidentally but heals quickly. A sharp, broken filling or tooth can do considerable damage to this delicate tissue.

"Hairiness": An overgrowth of the normal projections on the top of the tongue (villi) can give it a hairy appearance. The tongue may also appear hairy after a fever, after antibiotic treatment, or when peroxide mouthwash is used too often. These "hairs" on the top of the tongue should not be confused with hairy leukoplakia. Hairy leukoplakia forms on the side of the tongue and is characteristic of AIDS.

Discoloration: The tongue's villi may become discolored if a person smokes or chews tobacco, eats certain foods, or has colored bacteria growing on the tongue. The top of the tongue may look black if a person takes bismuth preparations for an upset stomach. Brushing the tongue with a toothbrush or scraping it with a tongue scraper can remove such discoloration.

Iron deficiency anemia may make the tongue look pale and smooth. Pernicious anemia, which is caused by a deficiency of vitamin B_{12}, may also make the tongue look pale and smooth. The first sign of scarlet fever may be a change from the tongue's normal color to a strawberry, and then raspberry, color. A strawberry-red tongue in a young child may also be a sign of Kawasaki disease. A smooth red tongue and painful mouth may indicate pellagra, a type of undernutrition caused by a deficiency of niacin (vitamin B_3) in the diet. A red tongue may also be inflamed (glossitis)—the tongue is red, painful, and swollen.

Burning Mouth Syndrome

Burning mouth syndrome (also called oral dysesthesia) occurs most commonly in women after menopause. The most commonly affected part of the mouth is the tongue (pain in the tongue is termed glossodynia). A painful burning sensation may affect the entire mouth (particularly the tongue, lips, and roof of the mouth [palate]) or just the tongue. The sensation may be continuous or intermittent and may gradually increase throughout the day. Symptoms that commonly accompany the burning sensation include a dry mouth, thirst, and altered taste. Possible consequences include changes in eating habits, irritability, depression, and avoidance of other people.

Burning mouth syndrome is not the same as the temporary discomfort that many people experience after eating irritating or acidic foods. Burning mouth syndrome is poorly understood. It probably represents a number of different conditions with different causes but a common symptom.

A common cause is the use of antibiotics, which alters the balance of bacteria in the mouth, leading to an overgrowth of the fungus Candida (a condition called thrush). Ill-fitting dentures and allergies to dental materials may be causes as well.

Overuse of mouth rinses and sprays may lead to burning tongue syndrome, as can anything that leads to a dry mouth, such as alcohol or tobacco use, and many drugs. Sensitivities to certain foods and food additives, particularly sorbic acid and benzoic acid (which are food preservatives), propylene glycol (used as a moisturizing agent in foods, drugs, and cosmetics), chicle (in some chewing gums), and cinnamon, may play some role. Deficiencies of vitamins, including B_{12}, folate, and B complex, can cause burning mouth syndrome. Iron deficiency has also been implicated.

The condition is easy for doctors to diagnose but difficult to treat. Frequent drinks of water or use of chewing gum may help keep the mouth moist. Antidepressants, such as nortriptyline, or antianxiety drugs, such as clonazepam, are sometimes helpful, although these drugs may make the symptoms worse by causing dry mouth. Sometimes symptoms disappear without treatment but may return later.

Whitish patches, similar to those sometimes found inside the cheeks, may accompany fever, dehydration, the second stage of syphilis, thrush, lichen planus, leukoplakia, or mouth breathing.

In geographic tongue, some areas of the tongue are white or yellow and rough, whereas others are red and smooth. The areas of discoloration move around over a period of weeks to years. The condition is usually painless, and no treatment is needed.

Sores and Bumps: Sores on the tongue can be caused by allergic reactions, oral herpes simplex virus infection, canker sores, tuberculosis, bacterial infections, or early-stage syphilis. Sores can also be caused by allergies or other immune system disorders.

Although small bumps on both sides of the tongue are usually harmless, a bump on only one side may be cancerous. Unexplained red or white areas, sores, or lumps (particularly when hard) on the tongue—especially if painless—may be signs of cancer and should be examined by a doctor or dentist (see page 1353). Most oral cancers grow on the sides of the tongue or on the floor of the mouth. Cancer almost never appears on the top of the tongue, except when the cancer occurs after untreated syphilis.

Discomfort: Tongue discomfort can result from irritation by certain foods, especially acidic ones (for example, pineapple), or by certain ingredients in toothpaste, mouthwash, candy, or gum. Some drugs can cause tongue discomfort, as can injury and infection. A common infection causing tongue discomfort is thrush (candidiasis—see page 1320), in which an overgrowth of fungi forms a white film that covers the tongue. Intense pain of the entire mouth can be caused by burning mouth syndrome.

Usually, it is a process of elimination to find out just what is causing the discomfort. Tongue discomfort not caused by an infection is usually treated by eliminating the cause. For example, the person may try changing brands of toothpaste, stop eating irritating foods, or have a sharp or broken tooth repaired by a dentist. Warm salt-water rinses may help. Thrush can be treated with an antifungal drug, such as nystatin or fluconazole.

204 Salivary Gland Disorders

- Salivary glands that malfunction or swell can decrease saliva production.
- Decreased saliva causes dry mouth and tooth decay.
- Saliva flow can be measured, or doctors may biopsy salivary gland tissue.
- Sometimes blockages can be removed, but some people need to use saliva substitutes.

There are three major pairs of salivary glands in the mouth. The largest pair of salivary glands, called the parotid glands, lies just behind the angle of the jaw, below and in front of the ears. Two smaller pairs, the sublingual glands and the submandibular glands, lie deep in the floor of the mouth. In addition to these major glands, many tiny salivary glands are distributed throughout the mouth. All of the glands produce saliva, which aids in breaking down food as part of the digestive process.

Other than cancer (see page 1353), two major types of disorders affect the salivary glands: one that results in salivary gland malfunction, whereby not enough saliva is produced, and one that results in salivary gland swelling. When the flow of saliva is insufficient or almost nonexistent, the mouth feels dry. This condition is called dry mouth (xerostomia).

Salivary Gland Malfunction: Certain diseases and disorders, as well as certain drugs, can cause the salivary glands to malfunction and thus decrease saliva production.

Diseases include Parkinson's disease, human immunodeficiency virus (HIV) infection, Sjögren's syndrome, depression, and chronic pain. Drugs that decrease saliva production include certain antidepressants, antihistamines, antipsychotics, sedatives, methyldopa, and diuretics.

The salivary glands often malfunction after a person has had chemotherapy or head and neck radiation for the treatment of cancer. Dry mouth due to radiation is usually permanent, especially if the radiation dose is high; that due to chemotherapy is usually temporary.

However, not all cases of dry mouth are caused by salivary gland malfunction. Drinking too little liquid and breathing through the mouth can dry the mouth. Anxiety or stress can also result in a dry mouth. The mouth may also dry somewhat as a person ages, although this is probably due to the greater likelihood of taking a drug that causes dry mouth than to the aging process itself.

Because saliva offers considerable natural protection against tooth decay, an inadequate amount of saliva leads to more cavities—especially in the roots of teeth. Dry mouth, if severe, can also lead to difficulty speaking and swallowing.

In rare cases, the salivary glands produce too much saliva. Increased saliva production is usually very brief and occurs in response to eating certain foods, such as sour foods. Sometimes even thinking about eating these foods can increase saliva production.

Salivary Gland Swelling: Salivary gland swelling can occur when one of the ducts that carry saliva from the salivary gland to the mouth is blocked. Pain may occur, especially during eating.

The most common cause of blockage is a stone. Salivary gland stones are most common in adults; 25% of those with stones have more than one. A stone can form from salts contained in the saliva. Blockage makes saliva back up inside the duct, causing the salivary gland to swell. A blocked duct and gland filled with stagnant saliva may become infected with bacteria. A typical symptom of a blocked salivary duct is swelling that worsens just before mealtime or particularly when a person eats a pickle (a sour pickle's taste stimulates saliva flow, but if the duct is blocked, the saliva has no place to go and the gland swells).

Mumps, certain bacterial infections, and other diseases (such as AIDS, Sjögren's syndrome, diabetes mellitus, and sarcoidosis) may be accompanied by

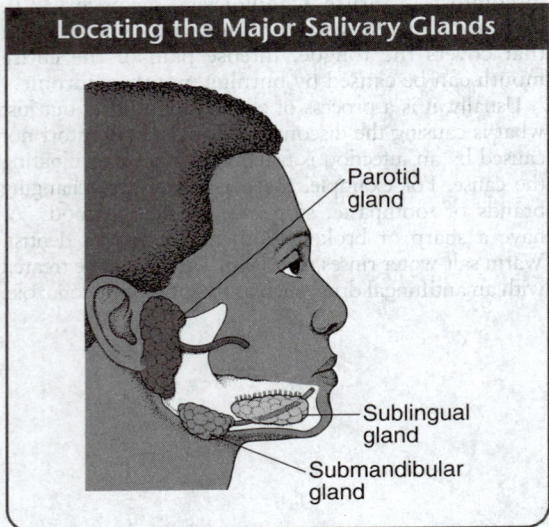

Locating the Major Salivary Glands

Parotid gland

Sublingual gland

Submandibular gland

swelling of the major salivary glands. Swelling also can result from cancerous or noncancerous tumors in the salivary glands. Swelling resulting from a tumor is usually firmer than that caused by an infection. If the tumor is cancerous, the gland may feel stone-hard and may be fixed firmly to surrounding tissues (see page 1353). Most noncancerous tumors are moveable.

An injury to the lower lip—for instance, from accidental biting—may harm any of the minor salivary glands found there and block the flow of saliva. As a result, an affected gland may swell and form a small, soft lump (mucocele) that appears bluish. The lump usually disappears by itself within a few weeks.

Diagnosis and Treatment

There are no good quantitative tests to diagnose salivary gland malfunction. However, the salivary glands can be squeezed ("milked"), and the ducts observed for saliva flow.

Swelling due to blockage of a salivary duct is diagnosed because of the relationship of pain to mealtimes. To diagnose other causes of swelling, a dentist or doctor may perform a biopsy to obtain a sample of salivary gland tissue and examine it under a microscope.

If a salivary duct is blocked by a stone, a dentist can sometimes push the stone out by pressing on both sides of the duct. If that fails, a fine-wire–like instrument can be used to pull out the stone. As a last resort, the stone can be removed surgically.

A mucocele that does not disappear on its own can be removed surgically if it becomes bothersome. Similarly, both noncancerous and cancerous salivary

SPOTLIGHT ON AGING

Many older people have a dry mouth. Although aging itself affects moisture in the mouth only slightly, it does make people more susceptible to conditions that dry the mouth, and older people are more likely to take drugs that may dry the mouth.

For many people, a dry mouth is only an occasional annoyance. For others, it is a persistent problem that interferes with tasting, chewing, swallowing, speaking, and wearing dentures. Persistent dry mouth increases the risk of tooth decay and periodontal disease. Persistent dry mouth is usually a symptom of a disorder or a side effect of a drug.

gland tumors can usually be removed surgically. Treatment of other causes of salivary gland swelling varies with the cause.

Anyone who has a disorder or who is taking a drug that dries the mouth must follow a meticulous oral hygiene routine (brushing, flossing, and fluoride rinses), avoid sugars, and undergo dental examinations, cleanings, and fluoride treatments every 3 to 4 months.

When no specific treatment is available, saliva substitutes are marginally helpful. One drug that does help some people is pilocarpine, but the drug is often ineffective if the salivary glands have been damaged by radiation.

CHAPTER

205 Mouth Sores

- Infections, irritants, and inflammation can cause noncancerous mouth sores.
- These sores cause pain.
- People can use anesthetic mouth rinses to relieve pain.
- Sometimes a laser or silver nitrate is used to treat sores.

Mouth sores vary in appearance and size and can affect any part of the mouth, inside and outside. Some sores may be raised, usually filled with fluid (in which case they are called vesicles or bullae, depending on size), whereas others may be ulcers. An ulcer is a hole that forms in the lining of the mouth when the top layer of cells breaks down and

the underlying tissue shows through. An ulcer appears white because of the dead cells and food debris inside the hole.

Causes

There are many types and causes of mouth sores. Because the normal flow of saliva helps protect the lining of the mouth, any condition that decreases saliva production makes mouth sores more likely. Any sore that lasts for 10 days or more must be examined by a dentist or doctor to ensure that it is not cancerous or precancerous (see page 1352).

Injury or Irritation: Any type of damage to the mouth, for instance, when the inside of the cheek is accidentally bitten or scraped by jagged teeth or poor-fitting dentures, can cause blisters (vesicles or bullae) or ulcers to form in the mouth. Typically, the surface of a blister breaks down quickly (ruptures), forming an ulcer. Noncancerous ulcers are always painful until healing is well under way.

Many foods, drugs, and chemicals can be irritating or trigger a type of allergic reaction, causing mouth sores. Acidic foods may be particularly irritating, as can certain ingredients in common substances such as toothpaste, mouthwash, candy, and gum. The most common drugs causing mouth sores include certain cancer chemotherapy drugs and drugs containing gold.

Infection: Viruses are the most common infectious causes of mouth sores. Cold sores of the lip and, less commonly, ulcers on the palate, caused by the herpes simplex virus (see page 1245), are perhaps the most well known. Herpes zoster, the virus responsible for chickenpox as well as the painful skin disorder called shingles (see page 1247), can cause multiple sores to form on one side of the mouth. These sores are the result of a flare-up of the virus, which, just like herpes simplex virus, never leaves the body. Herpes zoster is treated much like severe herpes simplex, but occasionally the mouth may remain painful for months or years or even permanently after the sores have healed.

A bacterial infection can lead to sores and swelling in the mouth. Infections may be caused by an overgrowth of organisms normally present in the mouth or by newly introduced organisms. Bacterial infections from teeth or gums can spread to form a pus-filled pocket of infection (abscess) or cause widespread inflammation (cellulitis). Bacterial infections that spread from decayed lower teeth to the floor of the mouth can cause a very severe infection underneath the tongue called Ludwig's angina. The swelling caused by this infection may force the tongue upward and block the airway. Infections from an upper tooth can spread to the brain.

Syphilis may produce a red, painless sore (chancre) that develops in the mouth or on the lips during the early stage of infection (see page 1271). The sore usually heals after several weeks. About 4 to 10 weeks later, a white area (mucous patch) may form on the lip or inside the mouth if the syphilis has not been treated. Both the chancre and the mucous patch are highly contagious, and kissing may spread the disease during these stages. In late-stage syphilis, a hole (gumma) may appear in the palate or tongue. The disease is not contagious at this stage.

Inflammatory Disorders: Behçet's syndrome, an inflammatory disease affecting many organs, includ-

? Did You Know...

A mouth sore that lasts more than 10 days should be checked by a doctor or dentist.

ing the eyes, genitals, skin, joints, blood vessels, brain, and gastrointestinal tract (see page 589), can cause recurring, painful mouth sores. Stevens-Johnson syndrome, a type of allergic reaction, causes skin blisters and mouth sores. Some people with inflammatory bowel disease also develop mouth sores. People with severe celiac sprue, which is caused by an intolerance to gluten (a component of wheat and some other grains), often develop mouth sores. Lichen planus, a skin disease, can rarely cause mouth sores as well, although most of the time these sores are not as uncomfortable as those on the skin (see page 1295). Pemphigus vulgaris (see page 1311) and bullous pemphigoid (see page 1310), both skin diseases, can also cause blisters to form in the mouth.

Other Causes: Canker sores are one of the most common causes of mouth sores. Their cause is unknown.

An uncommon condition called necrotizing sialometaplasia may begin after an injury to the mouth. In this condition, a large, gaping sore up to 1 inch (about 2½ centimeters) in diameter forms on the roof of the mouth within 1 or 2 days of an injury. Despite its unsettling appearance, necrotizing sialometaplasia is relatively painless and heals without treatment in 1 to 3 months. A doctor may distinguish the condition from oral cancer based on the symptoms (cancer would take a long time to reach the same size and by then would be painful) and sometimes by performing a biopsy (removing a tissue sample for examination under a microscope).

Treatment

Doctors treat the cause, if known. Frequent, gentle toothbrushing with a soft brush may help keep sores from becoming infected.

Pain can be helped by avoiding acidic or highly salty foods and any other substances that are irritating. An anesthetic such as dyclonine or lidocaine may be used as a mouth rinse. However, because these mouth rinses numb the mouth and throat and thus may make swallowing difficult, children using them should be watched to ensure that they do not choke on their food. Lidocaine in a thicker preparation (viscous lidocaine) can also be swabbed directly on the mouth sore. Sucralfate and aluminum-magnesium antacids can be soothing when applied alone, but many doctors mix them with a combination of lidocaine, diphenhydramine (an antihistamine), and kaolin to form a rinse. Amlexanox paste is another alternative.

Once doctors are sure that the sore is not caused by an infection, they may prescribe a corticosteroid gel to be applied to each sore.

Some mouth sores can be treated with a low-powered laser, which relieves pain immediately and prevents sores from returning. Chemically burning the sore with a small stick coated with silver nitrate may similarly relieve pain but is not as effective as a laser.

Recurrent Aphthous Stomatitis

Recurrent aphthous stomatitis (canker sores, aphthous ulcers) is small, painful sores inside the mouth that typically begin in childhood and recur frequently.

- Mouth injury, stress, and some foods may trigger an attack.
- People feel burning pain, and a day or so later an ulcer develops on the soft tissue of the mouth.
- Doctors make the diagnosis because of the pain and the appearance of the ulcers.
- Treatment is with mouth rinses and sometimes corticosteroids.

Recurrent aphthous stomatitis (RAS) is very common. The cause is unknown, but the disorder tends to run in families. Many factors seem to predispose to or trigger attacks. Such factors include injury to the mouth; stress (for example, a college student may get canker sores during final exam week); and certain foods, particularly chocolate, coffee, peanuts, eggs, cereals, almonds, strawberries, cheese, and tomatoes. People with AIDS often have large canker sores that persist for weeks.

People who have RAS get canker sores repeatedly. Some have only one or two sores a few times a year. Others have almost continuous outbreaks. For unknown reasons, pregnant women, people who are taking oral contraceptives, and people who are using tobacco products are less likely to develop sores.

Symptoms and Diagnosis

Symptoms usually begin with pain or burning, followed in 1 to 2 days by an ulcer. There is never a blister. Pain is severe—far more so than would be expected from something so small—and lasts 4 to 7 days. The ulcers almost always form on soft, loose tissue such as that on the inside of the lip or cheek, on the tongue, on the floor of the mouth, on the soft palate, or in the throat. Ulcers appear as shallow, round or oval spots with a yellow-gray center and a red border. Most ulcers are small, less than 1/2 inch (1 1/4 centimeters) in diameter, and often appear in clusters of two or three. They usually disappear by themselves within 10 days and do not leave scars. Larger ulcers are less common. They are irregularly shaped, can take many weeks to heal, and frequently leave scars.

People with a severe outbreak may also have a fever, swollen lymph nodes in the neck, and a generally run-down feeling.

A doctor or dentist identifies RAS by its appearance and the pain it causes.

Treatment

Treatment consists of relieving the pain with the same general measures used for other mouth sores. In addition, doctors often recommend chlorhexidine mouth rinses. If there are many ulcers, doctors sometimes also recommend a corticosteroid such as dexamethasone applied as a rinse. If there are fewer ulcers, doctors recommend other corticosteroids such as fluocinonide or clobetasol applied as an ointment or mixed in a protective carboxymethylcellulose paste. People who have repeated outbreaks of canker sores may start using the mouth rinse as soon as they feel a sore developing. If the corticosteroids that are applied directly to the affected areas do not work, prednisone tablets may be taken by mouth. However, before prescribing a corticosteroid, a doctor ensures that the person does not also have oral herpes simplex infection, which can be further spread by corticosteroids. Corticosteroid rinses and tablets are absorbed by the body more than are corticosteroids given in gel form, so the side effects may be a concern (see box on page 568). Sometimes stronger immune-suppressing drugs are needed.

Mouth Growths

Noncancerous (benign) growths, precancerous (dysplastic) changes, and cancerous (malignant) growths can originate in any type of tissue in and around the mouth, including bone, muscle, and nerve. Most commonly, growths form on the lips, the sides of the tongue, the floor of the mouth, and the back portion of the roof of the mouth (soft palate). Among people who use chewing tobacco and snuff, the insides of the cheeks and lips are common sites of cancer. Rarely, cancers found in the mouth region have spread there from other parts of the body, such as the lungs, breast, or prostate.

Noncancerous Growths

- Mouth growths may be lumps, warts, bony growths, or cysts.
- Some growths cause pain or irritation.
- Some growths need to be removed surgically.

A variety of growths that are noncancerous may occur in and around the mouth. A lump or raised area on the gums (gingiva) is not a cause for alarm. Such a lump may be caused by a gum or tooth abscess or by irritation. Noncancerous growths due to irritation are relatively common and, if necessary, can be removed by surgery. In 10 to 40% of people, noncancerous growths on the gums recur because the irritant remains. Occasionally such irritation, particularly if it persists over a long period of time, can lead to cancer. Because any unusual growths in or around the mouth can be cancer, the growths should be checked by a doctor or dentist without delay.

Ordinary warts (verrucae vulgaris) can infect the mouth if a person sucks or chews one that is growing on a finger. A different type of wart—a genital wart (see page 1268)—may be transmitted through oral sex. A doctor may remove an ordinary wart using one of several methods (see page 1325). Genital warts can be removed by several methods, but they tend to recur.

A slow-growing projection of bone (torus) may form in the middle of the roof of the mouth or on the lower jaw by the side of the tongue. This hard growth is both common and harmless. It appears during puberty and persists throughout life. Even a large growth can be left alone unless it gets scraped during eating or the person needs a denture that will cover the area. However, multiple bony growths in the mouth may indicate Gardner's syndrome, a hereditary disorder of the digestive tract that includes colon cancer (see page 192).

Keratoacanthomas are noncancerous growths that form on the lips and other sun-exposed areas, such as the face, forearms, and hands. A keratoacanthoma usually reaches its full size of 1/2 to 1 inch (about 1¼ to 2½ centimeters) or more in diameter within 1 or 2 months, then begins to shrink after another few months and eventually disappears without treatment.

Many kinds of cysts (hollow, fluid-filled swellings) cause jaw pain and swelling. Often, they are next to an impacted wisdom tooth, and even though they are not cancerous, they can destroy considerable areas of the jawbone as they expand. Certain types of cysts are more likely to recur after surgical removal. Various types of cysts may also develop in the floor of the mouth. Often, these cysts are surgically removed because they make swallowing uncomfortable or because they are unattractive.

Odontomas are overgrowths of tooth-forming cells that look like small, misshapen extra teeth. In children, they may get in the way of normal teeth coming in. In adults, they may push teeth out of alignment. They are usually removed surgically.

Most (75 to 80%) tumors of the salivary glands are noncancerous, slow-growing, and painless. They usually occur as a single, soft, movable lump beneath normal skin or under the lining (mucosa) of the inside of the cheek. Occasionally, when hollow and fluid-filled, they are firm. The most common type (called a mixed tumor or pleomorphic adenoma) occurs mainly in women older than 40. This type can become cancerous and is removed surgically. Unless completely removed, this type of tumor is likely to grow back. Other types of noncancerous tumors are also removed surgically but are much less likely to become cancerous or to grow back once removed.

Precancerous Changes

White, red, or mixed white-red areas that are not easily wiped away, persist for more than 2 weeks, and are not definable as some other condition may be precancerous. The same risk factors are involved in precancerous changes as in cancerous growths, and precancerous changes may become cancerous if not removed.

Leukoplakia is a flat white spot that may develop when the moist lining of the mouth (oral mucosa) is irritated for a long period. The injured spot appears white because it has a thickened layer of keratin—the same material that covers the skin and normally is less abundant in the lining of the mouth.

Erythroplakia is a red and flat or worn away area that results when the lining of the mouth thins. The area appears red because the underlying capillaries are more visible. Erythroplakia is a much more ominous predictor of oral cancer than leukoplakia.

Cancerous Growths

- Cancer can occur on the roof or floor of the mouth, the tongue, the lips, or the tonsils.
- Oral cancers may look like open sores or discolored areas in the mouth.
- Doctors do biopsies and possibly x-rays to diagnose oral cancers.
- Treatment is usually with surgery and radiation therapy.

Each year, cancer of the mouth (oral cancer) develops in 30,000 people in the United States and causes 8,000 deaths, mostly in people older than 50. Oral cancer represents more than 2% of all cancers and 1.5% of all cancer-related deaths—a high rate considering the size of the mouth in relation to the rest of the body.

Because early detection vastly improves the likelihood of cure, screening for oral cancer should be an integral part of medical and dental examinations. Cancerous growths less than 1/2 inch (about 1 1/4 centimeters) across usually can be cured. Unfortunately, most oral cancers are not diagnosed until they are larger and have spread to the lymph nodes under the jaw and in the neck. Because of delayed detection, 25% of oral cancers are fatal.

Risk Factors

A hereditary factor, although not yet well understood, makes certain people more susceptible to developing oral cancer. The two greatest controllable risk factors for developing oral cancer are tobacco and alcohol use. Tobacco use—including smoking cigarettes (particularly more than 2 packs per day), cigars, or pipes; chewing tobacco; and dipping snuff—accounts for 80 to 90% of all oral cancers. Cigars and cigarettes are equally dangerous as risk factors in the development of oral cancer, followed in descending order by chewing tobacco and pipe smoking.

Chronic or heavy alcohol use (particularly more than 6 drinks per day) increases the risk of oral cancer. The combination of tobacco and alcohol is more likely to cause cancer than either one alone. There is some evidence that the alcohol contained in mouthwash can contribute to oral cancer. Therefore, people who smoke and drink alcohol should choose a mouthwash that contains the lowest concentration of alcohol (which is stated on the label).

People who have had oral cancer are at risk of recurrence. Hereditary predisposition may contribute to recurrence, as may the radiation used to treat the cancer. People who continue to use tobacco and alcohol after developing oral cancer have more than twice the chance as the rest of the population (30% versus 12%) of developing a second oral cancer.

Certain strains of the human papillomavirus (HPV) also predispose people to oral cancer. These viruses cause genital warts (see page 1267) and may infect the mouth during oral sex.

Other factors that add to the risk of oral cancer include repeated irritation from the sharp edges of broken teeth, fillings, or dental prostheses (such as dentures). Syphilis, if untreated for many years, may give rise to tongue cancer. This syphilis-induced cancer is the only cancer that forms on the top of the tongue. Sun damage and use of tobacco products can cause cancer of the lip.

About two thirds of oral cancers occur in men, but increased tobacco use among women over the past few decades is gradually closing the gender gap. As with most cancers, risk increases with age.

Types of Oral Cancer

Squamous cell carcinoma is the most common type of oral cancer. About 40% of squamous cell carcinomas begin on the floor of the mouth or on the side or bottom of the tongue, and another 40% occur on the lower lip. The remainder begin on the roof of the mouth or the tonsils. These cancers form a hard lump or a firm-bordered sore (ulcer) that may bleed intermittently. Affected areas may appear white, red, or mixed white and red and can be smooth or raised. Another type of cancer is called verrucous (warty) carcinoma, which appears as a white grooved surface on the lining of the mouth (mucosa).

Other types of cancer, such as malignant melanoma (see page 1335) and Kaposi's sarcoma (see page 1336), are less common. Malignant melanoma is usually associated with a history of sunburns and occurs on the surface of the skin. However, it occasionally occurs in the mouth, most commonly on the roof of the mouth, usually as a result of spread from a skin site. A malignant melanoma often has uneven, irregularly shaped borders and ranges in color from dark blue or brown to black. Its color may be spotty, however, or even speckled. As with most cancers, it occasionally bleeds. Kaposi's sarcoma is a cancer of the blood vessels near the skin and in the lining of the mouth and throat. In people with AIDS, when Kaposi's sarcoma occurs in the mouth, it usually occurs on the roof of the mouth. The tumor is usually blue or purple and is slightly raised.

Cancers of the salivary glands are much less common than noncancerous growths. The most common salivary gland cancer is mucoepidermoid carcinoma, which typically forms in a small minor salivary gland on the roof of the mouth. It may also occur as a lump in one of the large (major) salivary glands, either under or behind the lower jaw.

Cancers of the jawbone include osteosarcoma and metastatic tumors (those that have spread to the jaw from another part of the body).

> ### ? Did You Know...
> The greatest controllable risk factors for oral cancer are tobacco use and alcohol use.

Symptoms

Oral cancers are usually painless for a considerable length of time but eventually do cause pain. Pain usually starts when the cancer erodes into nearby nerves. When pain from cancer of the tongue or roof of the mouth begins, it usually occurs with swallowing, as with a sore throat.

The early growth of salivary gland tumors may or may not be painful. When these tumors do become painful, the pain may be worsened by food, which stimulates the secretion of saliva. Cancer of the jawbone often causes pain and a numb or pins-and-needles sensation (paresthesia), somewhat like the feeling of a dental anesthetic wearing off. Cancer of the lip or cheek may first become painful when the enlarged tissue is inadvertently bitten.

Squamous cell carcinomas often look like open sores (ulcers) and tend to grow into the underlying tissues. Cancers of the lip and other parts of the mouth often feel rock hard and are attached to the underlying tissues. Most noncancerous lumps in these areas are freely movable. A person who chews tobacco or uses snuff may develop white, ridged bumps on the insides of the cheeks that can develop into verrucous (warty) carcinoma. However, squamous cell carcinoma is much more common. Oral cancers tend to grow fast and feel hard. Cancer beginning in the small salivary glands commonly appears as a small swelling.

Discolored areas on the gums, tongue, or lining of the mouth may be signs of cancer. An area in the mouth that has recently become brown or darkly discolored may be a melanoma. Sometimes a brown, flat, freckle-like area (smoker's patch) develops at the site where a cigarette or pipe is habitually held between the lips.

Diagnosis

Oral cancers are suspected because of their appearance and, later, their symptoms. Doctors must distinguish a melanoma from normal pigmentation or from discoloration due to other causes. However, only a biopsy (removal of a tissue specimen for examination under a microscope) can determine whether a suspicious area is cancerous.

X-rays cannot always distinguish jaw cancers from cysts, noncancerous bone growths, or cancers that have spread from elsewhere in the body. However, x-rays may show the irregular borders of jaw cancer and can show the loss of parts of neighboring teeth, which is characteristic of a rapidly growing cancer.

Prognosis

Cancers originating in or around the mouth can spread to nearby lymph nodes, which become hard and swollen. Spread of cancers to more distant parts of the body is uncommon with squamous cell carcinoma but is more likely with osteosarcoma and is very likely with malignant melanoma, which can reach organs such as the brain.

The cure rate for squamous cell carcinoma is high if the entire cancer and the surrounding normal tissue are removed before the cancer has spread to the lymph nodes. On average, 68% of people survive at least 5 years after the diagnosis. However, if the cancer has spread to lymph nodes, the 5-year survival rate is only 25%. Regrettably, cure rates for squamous cell carcinoma have not improved much over the past several decades. However, verrucous carcinoma is rarely fatal because it develops late in life and grows slowly. The 5-year survival rate for malignant melanoma that has spread is only 5 to 10%.

Prevention

Diligent, routine examination of the mouth is the best strategy for finding cancerous and noncancerous growths. Avoiding excessive alcohol and tobacco use can greatly reduce the risk of most oral cancers. Smoothing rough edges from broken teeth or fillings is another preventive measure. Staying out of the sun reduces the risk of lip cancer. If sun damage covers a large area of the lip, a lip shave, in which the entire outer surface is removed using either surgery or a laser, may prevent a progression to cancer.

Treatment

For squamous cell carcinoma and most other types of oral cancer, the mainstays of treatment are surgery and radiation therapy. These two treatments are often used together, particularly for larger cancers. For malignant melanoma, surgery is the main approach because the cancer usually does not respond to radiation therapy.

During surgery, the extent of the cancer can be determined (staging). The lymph nodes under and behind the jaw and along the neck may be removed. Consequently, surgery for oral cancers can be disfiguring and psychologically traumatic. Newer methods are being used, however, to minimize disfigurement. In the case of the lips, the Mohs technique—a method of determining the extent of disease during different phases of surgery by examining each slice of tissue under a microscope after its removal—minimizes disfigurement, as does the use of lasers to destroy cancer cells. Reconstructive surgery can improve function and restore normal appearance after the disease is controlled. Missing teeth and jaw parts can be replaced with prosthetic devices.

A person with oral cancer may receive radiation therapy after surgery or just radiation therapy. Although radiation may not always be curative, especially if the cancer is extensive, it is sometimes used to shrink the cancer and thus relieve symptoms (palliation). Radiation therapy often destroys the salivary glands and leaves the person's mouth dry, which can lead to cavities and other dental problems. If the salivary glands have not been destroyed, saliva production usually recovers several weeks after the radiation treatment is completed. Because

jawbones exposed to radiation do not heal well, dental problems should be completely treated before radiation is given. Any teeth likely to become problematic are removed, and time is allowed for healing before radiation.

Chemotherapy has been shown to have little value in the treatment of most oral cancers except to relieve symptoms. For people who cannot be treated with surgery or radiation therapy, the drugs cisplatin, fluorouracil, bleomycin, and methotrexate relieve pain and shrink tumors but usually do not cure the cancer.

Good dental hygiene is critical for people who have had radiation therapy for oral cancer because the mouth heals poorly if dental surgery, such as tooth extractions, is ever needed. Such hygiene includes regular examinations and thorough home care, including daily home fluoride applications. If the person eventually has a tooth pulled, hyperbaric oxygen therapy may help the jaw heal without the loss of bone and surrounding soft tissue in the area that receives the radiation (osteoradionecrosis).

CHAPTER

207 Tooth Disorders

Common tooth disorders include cavities (caused by tooth decay), pulpitis, periapical abscess, impacted teeth, and malocclusion. Fractured, loosened, and knocked-out teeth are considered urgent dental problems (see page 1371), as are some toothaches. Tooth decay, which often leads to toothache and tooth loss, can be largely prevented with good oral hygiene, which helps remove plaque and prevent tartar buildup.

Plaque is a filmlike substance composed of bacteria, saliva, food debris, and dead cells. Plaque is continually being deposited on teeth, day and night. It occurs in everyone. Because plaque can encourage growth of the kind of bacteria that leads to tooth decay, it needs to be removed by daily brushing and flossing.

Tartar (calculus) is hardened (calcified) plaque that forms a white covering at the base of the teeth, particularly the tongue side of the front lower teeth and the cheek side of the upper molars (the teeth at the back of the mouth). Because tartar is formed from plaque, daily brushing to remove plaque can significantly reduce the buildup of tartar. However, once tartar has formed, it can be adequately removed only by a dentist or dental hygienist.

Although a healthy mouth can be maintained with meticulous brushing and flossing, limiting sugar intake and using fluoridated water also help reduce the risk of tooth decay.

Symptoms

Pain affecting an individual tooth (toothache) is probably the most recognized symptom of a tooth disorder. A tooth may be painful all the time or only under certain circumstances, as when chewing or when tapped by a dental instrument. Pain in a tooth suggests tooth decay or gum disease. However, pain may also result when roots are exposed, when people chew too forcefully or grind their teeth (bruxism), or when a tooth is fractured. Sinus congestion can cause similar symptoms of pain in the area of the upper teeth.

Worn-down or loose teeth can be a symptom of gum disease or bruxism, a disorder characterized by frequent clenching or grinding of the teeth. Bruxism occurs mostly during sleep, so that the person is unaware of it, but it may also occur during the day. People who have bruxism must concentrate on not clenching or grinding their teeth during the day.

THE LANGUAGE OF DENTISTS	
WHAT MOST PEOPLE CALL IT	**WHAT DENTISTS CALL IT**
Adult tooth	Permanent tooth
Baby tooth	Deciduous tooth
Back teeth	Molars and premolars
Bite	Occlusion
Braces	Orthodontic bands and wires or appliances
Cap	Crown
Cavities	Caries
Cleaning	Prophylaxis
Eye teeth	Canines or cuspids
Filling	Restoration
Front teeth	Incisors and canines
Gums	Gingivae
Gum disease	Periodontal disease, periodontitis, or gingivitis
Harelip	Cleft lip
Laughing gas	Nitrous oxide
Lower jaw	Mandible
Plate	Complete or partial denture (removable)
Roof of the mouth	Palate
Side teeth	Bicuspids or premolars
Silver filling	Amalgam restoration
Tartar	Calculus
Uneven bite	Malocclusion
Upper jaw	Maxilla

Attrition refers to the worn surfaces of the teeth where grinding of food occurs. Attrition may make chewing less effective.

Abnormally shaped teeth can be a symptom of genetic diseases, hormonal disorders, or infections acquired before birth. Teeth can be misshapen due to fractures or chipping caused by trauma to the mouth.

Abnormal tooth color is not the same as the darkening or yellowing of teeth that occurs as people grow older or expose their teeth to staining substances, such as coffee, tea, and cigarette smoke. Graying of a tooth may be a symptom of a previous infection within the tooth that has seriously damaged the pulp, which is the living center of the tooth. The same may occur when a permanent tooth replaces an infected baby tooth. Permanent discoloration of the teeth may occur if people took tetracycline before age 9 years or if their mothers took tetracycline during pregnancy. Excess fluoride ingestion during childhood can cause mottling of the outer surface of the tooth (the enamel).

Abnormal tooth enamel (enamel is the hard outer surface of teeth) may be due to a diet containing insufficient vitamin D. Abnormal enamel may also be the result of a childhood infection (such as measles or chickenpox) occurring when the permanent teeth were forming. Abnormal enamel may also be due to repeated vomiting, as occurs in bulimia nervosa, because the stomach acid dissolves the surface of the teeth. Swimmers who spend a lot of time in chlorinated pools can lose tooth enamel, as can people who work with acids. Damaged tooth enamel can allow bacteria to more easily invade the tooth and form a cavity.

Cavities

Cavities (dental caries) are decayed areas in the teeth, the result of a process that gradually dissolves a tooth's hard outer surface (enamel) and progresses toward the interior.

- Bacteria and debris build up on tooth surfaces, and the bacteria produce acids that cause decay.
- Tooth pain occurs after decay reaches the inside of the tooth.
- Dentists can detect cavities by examining the teeth and taking x-rays periodically.
- Good oral hygiene and regular dental care plus a healthy diet can help prevent cavities.
- Fluoride treatments can help cavities in the enamel heal, but for deeper cavities, dentists must drill out the decay and fill the resulting space.

Along with the common cold and gum disease, cavities are among the most common human afflictions. If cavities are not properly treated by a dentist, they continue to enlarge. Ultimately, an untreated cavity can lead to tooth loss.

Risk Factors: There are many risk factors for cavities:

- Defects in the tooth surface
- Sugary or acidic foods
- Too little fluoride in the teeth
- Reduced saliva flow

For tooth decay to develop, a tooth must be susceptible, acid-producing bacteria must be present, and nutrients must be available for the bacteria to thrive. A susceptible tooth has relatively little protective fluoride incorporated into the enamel or has pronounced pits, grooves, or fissures that retain plaque. Poor oral hygiene that allows plaque and tartar to accumulate can accelerate this process. Although the mouth contains large numbers of bacteria, only certain types generate acid, which causes decay. The most common decay-causing bacteria are *Streptococcus mutans*.

The nutrients that decay-causing bacteria need come from the person's diet. When infants are put to bed with a bottle, their teeth have prolonged contact with the formula or milk, which increases the likelihood of decay. Large amounts of sugar in the diet also provide food for the bacteria.

Acid in the diet (for example, in cola beverages, which contain phosphoric acid) accelerates tooth decay.

Reduced saliva flow due to drugs or disorders (such as Sjögren's syndrome) places people at greater risk of tooth decay. Older people often take drugs that reduce saliva flow, increasing their risk of cavities.

Some people have especially active decay-causing bacteria in their mouth. A parent (almost always the mother) may pass these bacteria to a child through kissing or sharing eating utensils. The bacteria flourish in the child's mouth after the first teeth come in and can then cause cavities. So, a tendency toward tooth decay that runs in families does not necessarily reflect poor oral hygiene or bad eating habits.

Gum recession also makes cavities more likely to develop because it can expose the roots of teeth. Then bacteria can access the inner layers of the tooth more easily. Gum recession makes older people prone to root cavities.

Progression of Tooth Decay: Decay in the enamel progresses slowly. After penetrating into the second layer of the tooth—the somewhat softer, less resistant dentin—decay spreads more rapidly and moves toward the pulp, the innermost part of the tooth, which contains the nerves and blood supply. Although a cavity may take 2 or 3 years to penetrate the enamel, it can travel from the dentin to the pulp—a much greater distance—in as little as a year. Thus, root decay that starts in the dentin can destroy a lot of tooth structure in a short time.

Smooth surface decay, the most preventable and reversible type, grows the slowest. In smooth surface decay, a cavity begins as a white spot where bacteria dissolve the calcium of the enamel. Smooth surface decay between the permanent teeth usually begins between the ages of 20 and 30.

Pit and fissure decay, which usually starts during the teen years in the permanent teeth, forms in the narrow grooves on the chewing surface and on the cheek side of the back teeth. Decay at these locations progresses rapidly. Many people cannot adequately

SPOTLIGHT ON AGING

Only a generation ago, most people expected to go through old age with false teeth or no teeth at all. This expectation has changed greatly during the last several decades. Although nearly half of people 85 or older have none of their natural teeth, the likelihood of losing teeth with aging is steadily decreasing. There are several reasons for this change: improved nutrition, better access to dental care, and better treatment for tooth decay and periodontal disease.

When teeth are lost, chewing is greatly hindered, and speaking becomes a challenge. The face looks dramatically different without the support teeth normally provide for the lips, cheeks, nose, and chin.

People who have lost some or all of their teeth can still eat, but they tend to eat soft foods. Soft foods tend to be relatively high in carbohydrates and low in protein, vitamins, and minerals. Foods that are high in protein, vitamins, and minerals, such as meats, poultry, grains, and fresh fruits and vegetables, tend to be harder to chew. Consequently, older people who eat mainly soft foods may become undernourished.

Partial or full dentures are useful for people who have lost nearly all or all of their teeth. Dentists carefully construct dentures so that they fit well and look natural. Typically, constructing dentures takes several months and involves a sequence of carefully planned steps. Once they have dentures, people should see their dentist at least once a year. The shape of the mouth can change over time or as weight is lost or gained, in which case the dentures may have to be refitted.

Dentures can improve appearance and speech, but they are far from a perfect solution. They restore less than 20% of the chewing ability provided by natural teeth. Dentures can also cause discomfort and interfere with tasting. Some people find dentures embarrassing.

Dentures must be kept clean. They should be removed after each meal and cleaned with toothpaste or baking soda on a toothbrush or denture brush. Also, the mouth should be cleaned to remove food debris. Dentures should be removed before going to sleep, cleaned carefully, and kept in a safe place. Soaking dentures overnight in a cleaning solution can be helpful but is not necessary if dentures are cleaned well with a toothbrush.

clean these cavity-prone areas because the grooves are narrower than the bristles of a toothbrush.

Root decay begins on the root surface covering (cementum) that has been exposed by receding gums, usually in people past middle age. This type

Types of Cavities

The illustration on the left shows a tooth with no cavities. The illustration on the right shows a tooth with the three types of cavities.

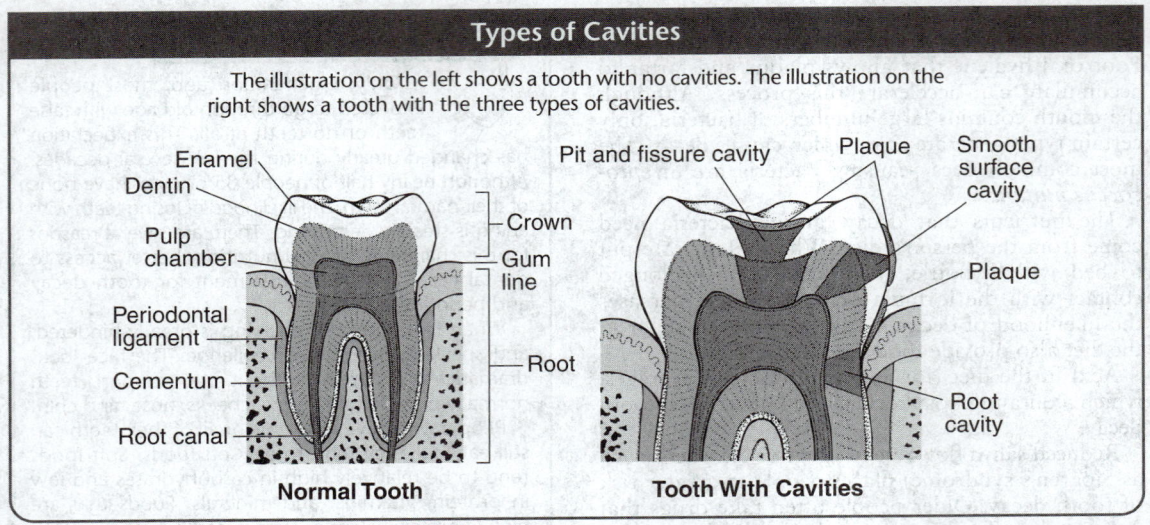

Normal Tooth Enamel, Dentin, Pulp chamber, Periodontal ligament, Cementum, Root canal, Crown, Gum line, Root

Tooth With Cavities Pit and fissure cavity, Plaque, Smooth surface cavity, Plaque, Root cavity

of decay often results from difficulty cleaning the root areas, a lack of adequate saliva flow, a diet high in sugar, or a combination of these factors. Root decay can be the most difficult type of tooth decay to prevent and treat.

> **? Did You Know...**
> Parents can pass decay-causing bacteria to their children through kissing or sharing eating utensils.

Symptoms

Whether tooth decay causes pain depends on which part of the tooth is affected and how deeply the decay extends. A cavity in the enamel causes no pain. The pain starts when the decay reaches the dentin. People may feel pain only when drinking something cold or eating candy. This indicates that the pulp is still healthy. If the cavity is treated at this stage, dentists can restore the tooth, and most likely no further pain or chewing difficulties will develop.

A cavity that gets close to or actually reaches the pulp causes irreversible damage. Pain lingers even after a stimulus (such as cold water) is removed. The tooth may hurt even without stimulation (spontaneous toothache).

If irreversible damage to the pulp occurs and the pulp subsequently dies, the pain may stop temporarily. The tooth then may become sensitive when

people bite or when the tongue or a finger presses on it because the area at the end of the root has become inflamed or because infection has developed at the root. Infection may produce a collection of pus (abscess—see page 1361), which causes constant pain that is worse when people bite.

Diagnosis

If a cavity is treated before it starts to hurt, the chance of damage to the pulp is reduced, and more of the tooth structure is saved. To detect cavities early, a dentist inquires about pain, examines the teeth, probes the teeth with dental instruments, and may take x-rays. People should have a dental examination every 6 to 12 months. Not every examination includes x-rays. Depending on the dentist's assessment of a person's teeth, x-rays may be taken every 12 to 36 months.

Prevention

Several general strategies are key to preventing cavities:

- Good oral hygiene and regular dental care
- Healthy diet
- Fluoride (in water, toothpaste, or both)
- Sometimes sealants and antibacterial therapy

Oral Hygiene: Good oral hygiene, which involves brushing before or after breakfast and before bedtime and flossing daily to remove plaque, can effectively control smooth surface decay. Brushing helps prevent cavities from forming on the top and sides of the teeth, and flossing gets between the teeth where a brush cannot reach.

Electric and ultrasonic toothbrushes are excellent, but an ordinary toothbrush, used properly, is quite sufficient. Normally, proper brushing takes only about 3 minutes. Floss is gently moved back and forth between the teeth, then wrapped around the tooth and root surfaces in a "C" shape at the gum line. When the floss is moved with a vertical sliding motion, it can remove plaque and food debris.

Initially, plaque is quite soft, and removing it with a soft-bristled toothbrush and dental floss at least once every 24 hours makes decay unlikely. Once plaque begins to harden, a process that begins after about 72 hours, removing it becomes more difficult.

Diet: Although all carbohydrates can cause tooth decay to some degree, the biggest culprits are sugars. All simple sugars, including table sugar (sucrose) and the sugars in honey (levulose and dextrose), fruit (fructose), and milk (lactose), have the same effect on the teeth. Whenever sugar comes in contact with plaque, *Streptococcus mutans* bacteria in the plaque produce acid. The amount of sugar eaten is of little consequence. The amount of time the sugar stays in contact with the teeth is what matters. Thus, sipping a sugary soft drink over an hour is more damaging than eating a candy bar in 5 minutes, even though the candy bar may contain more sugar.

People who tend to develop cavities should eat sweet snacks less often. Rinsing the mouth after eating a snack removes some of the sugar, but brushing the teeth is more effective. Drinking artificially sweetened soft drinks also helps, although diet colas contain acid that can promote tooth decay. Drinking tea or coffee without sugar also can help people avoid cavities, particularly on exposed root surfaces.

> **? Did You Know...**
>
> Over half the people in the United States have drinking water that contains enough fluoride to reduce tooth decay.

Fluoride: Fluoride can make the teeth, particularly the enamel, more resistant to the acid that helps cause cavities. Fluoride taken internally is effective while the teeth are growing and hardening—until about age 11. Water fluoridation is the most efficient way to supply children with fluoride, and over half of the United States population now has drinking water with enough fluoride to reduce tooth decay. However, if a water supply has too much fluoride, the teeth can become spotted or discolored (fluorosis). If a child's water supply does not have enough fluoride, doctors or dentists can prescribe sodium fluoride drops or tablets. Dentists may apply fluoride directly to the teeth of people of any age if they are prone to tooth decay. Fluoridated toothpaste and concentrated mouth rinses containing fluoride are beneficial for adults as well as children.

Sealants: Sealants protect hard-to-reach pits and fissures (grooves), particularly on the back teeth. After thoroughly cleaning the area to be sealed, dentists roughen the enamel with an acid solution to help the sealant adhere to the teeth. Dentists then place a liquid plastic in and over the pits and fissures of the teeth. When the liquid hardens, it forms such an effective barrier that any bacteria inside a pit or fissure stop producing acid because food can no longer reach them. About 90% of the sealant remains after 1 year and 60% after 10 years. The occasional need for repair or replacement of sealants can be assessed at periodic dental examinations.

Antibacterial Therapy: People who are very prone to tooth decay may need antibacterial therapy. Dentists first remove decayed areas and seal all pits and fissures in the teeth. Then dentists prescribe a powerful mouth rinse (chlorhexidine) for several weeks to kill off the bacteria in any remaining plaque. The hope is that less harmful bacteria will replace the cavity-causing bacteria. To keep bacteria under control, people may use daily home fluoride rinses and chew gum containing xylitol (a sweetener that inhibits the bacteria in plaque).

Treatment

If decay is halted before it reaches the dentin, the enamel can actually repair itself (remineralization) if people use fluoride. Fluoride treatment requires use of prescription-strength fluoride-containing mouthwash. Once decay reaches the dentin, dentists drill out the decayed material inside the tooth and then fill the resulting space with a filling (restoration). Treating the decay at an early stage helps maintain the strength of the tooth and limits the chance of damage to the pulp.

Fillings: Fillings are made of various materials and may be put inside the tooth or around it. Silver amalgam (a combination of mercury, silver, copper, tin, and, occasionally, zinc, palladium, or indium) is most commonly used for fillings in back teeth, where strength is important and the silver color is relatively inconspicuous. Silver amalgam is relatively inexpensive and lasts an average of 14 years. However, the amalgam can last for more than 40 years if it is carefully placed using a rubber dam and the person's oral hygiene is good. The minute amount of mercury that escapes from silver amalgam is too small to affect health. Gold fillings (inlays and onlays) are excellent but are more expensive. Also, at least two dental visits are required to permanently place them.

Crowns, Bridges, and Implants

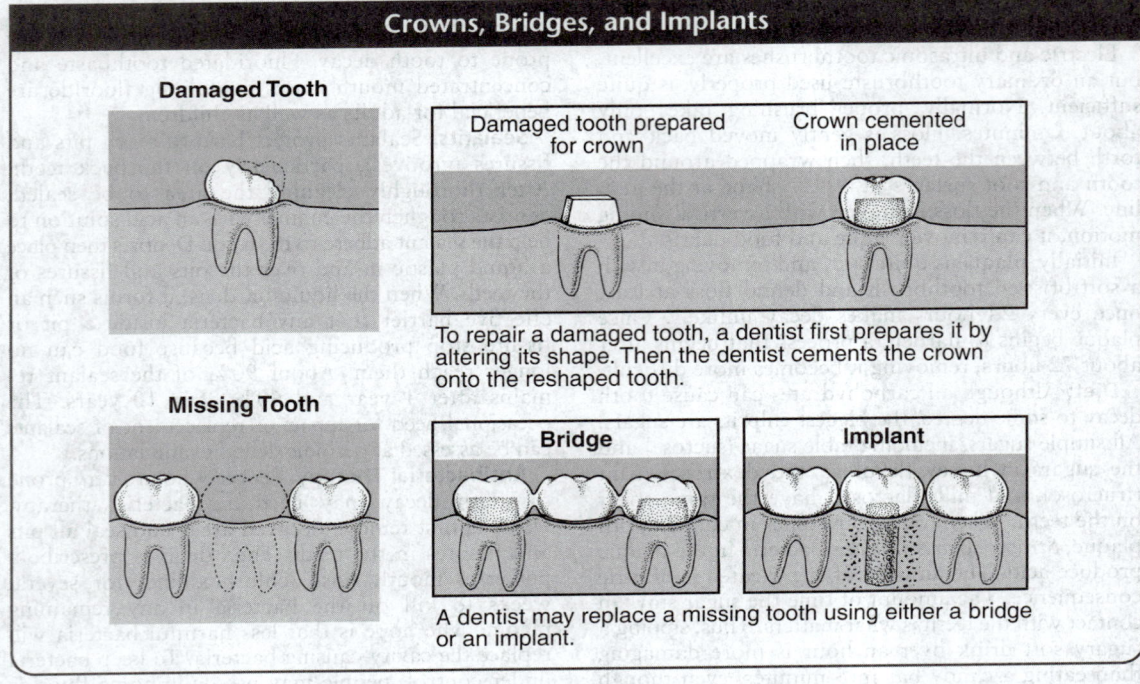

Damaged Tooth

Damaged tooth prepared for crown

Crown cemented in place

To repair a damaged tooth, a dentist first prepares it by altering its shape. Then the dentist cements the crown onto the reshaped tooth.

Missing Tooth

Bridge

Implant

A dentist may replace a missing tooth using either a bridge or an implant.

Composite resins and porcelain fillings are used in the front teeth, where silver would be conspicuous. Increasingly, these fillings are also being used in back teeth. Although they have the advantage of being the color of the teeth, they are more expensive than silver amalgam and may not last as long, particularly in the back teeth, which take the full force of chewing.

Glass ionomer, a tooth-colored filling, is formulated to release fluoride once in place, a benefit for people especially prone to tooth decay. Glass ionomer is also used to restore areas damaged by overzealous brushing.

Root Canal Treatment and Tooth Extraction: When tooth decay advances far enough to permanently harm the pulp, the only way to eliminate pain is to remove the pulp by root canal (endodontic) treatment or tooth removal (extraction).

If a tooth is extracted, it should be evaluated for replacement as soon as possible. Otherwise, neighboring teeth may change position and alter the person's bite.

Bridges, Crowns, and Implants: The replacement for an extracted tooth may be a bridge—a fixed partial denture in which teeth on either side of the missing tooth are covered with crowns—or a removable partial denture. Also, implants may be

used to replace missing teeth in people who have sufficient healthy bone in their jaw. Implants are metal fixtures inserted into the jawbone. The metal is a special alloy to which bone cells can attach. After a period of time, usually 4 months, the implant becomes solid with the bone, and a post is attached. Then an artificial tooth (crown) is attached to the post. The resulting tooth can handle the force of normal chewing. Implants are considered more desirable now because they do not decay and they offer a fixed solution to removable bridges.

A crown is a cap (restoration) that fits over a tooth. Getting a properly shaped crown usually takes two visits to the dentist, although sometimes more visits are needed. On the first visit, dentists prepare the tooth by tapering it slightly, take an impression of the prepared tooth, and put a temporary crown on it. A permanent crown is then made in a dental prosthetics laboratory, using the impression. On the next visit, the temporary crown is removed, and the final crown is permanently cemented onto the prepared tooth.

Usually, crowns are made of an alloy of gold or another metal. A porcelain coating can be used to mask the color of the metal. Crowns also may be made entirely of porcelain, although porcelain is harder and more abrasive than tooth enamel and may cause wear on the opposing tooth. Also, crowns made entirely of porcelain or similar material have a slightly greater tendency to break than do those made of metal.

Pulpitis

Pulpitis is painful inflammation of the tooth pulp, the innermost part of the tooth that contains the nerves and blood supply.

The most common cause of pulpitis is tooth decay, and the second most common cause is injury. Mild inflammation, if relieved, may not damage the tooth permanently. Severe inflammation may cause the pulp to die.

Symptoms and Diagnosis

Pulpitis can cause intense tooth pain. To determine if the pulp is healthy enough to save, dentists can do certain tests. For example, dentists can apply a hot or cold stimulus. If pain persists after the stimulus is removed or if pain occurs spontaneously, the pulp may not be healthy enough to save.

Dentists may also use an electric pulp tester, which indicates whether the pulp is alive but not whether it is healthy. If the person feels the small electrical charge delivered to the tooth, the pulp is alive. Sensitivity to tapping on a tooth often means that inflammation has spread to the surrounding tissues.

Treatment

The inflammation stops when the cause is treated. When pulpitis is detected early, a temporary filling containing a sedative can eliminate the pain. This filling can be left in place for 6 to 8 weeks and then replaced with a permanent filling. Often a permanent filling can be put in immediately.

When pulp damage is extensive and cannot be reversed, the only way dentists can stop the pain is by removing the pulp by root canal treatment or tooth removal (extraction).

Periapical Abscess

A periapical abscess is a collection of pus, usually from an infection that has spread from a tooth to the surrounding tissues.

The body attacks an infection with large numbers of white blood cells. Pus is the accumulation of these white blood cells, dead tissue, and bacteria. Usually, pus from a tooth infection spreads from the root tip through the bone into the gums so the gums swell near the root of the tooth. The swelling from the pus is often the cause of intense pain. Depending on the location of the tooth, the infection may spread further into soft tissues (cellulitis), causing swelling in the jaw, into the floor of the mouth, or in the area of the cheeks. Eventually, the tissue may break open, allowing the pus to drain.

Root Canal Treatment for a Badly Damaged Tooth

1. The tooth is numbed (anesthetized).
2. A rubber dam is placed around the tooth to isolate it from bacteria in the rest of the mouth.
3. A hole is drilled through the chewing surface of a back tooth or the tongue side of a front tooth.
4. Fine instruments are passed through the hole into the pulp canal space, and all the remaining pulp is removed.
5. The canal is smoothed and tapered from the opening to the end of the root.
6. The canal is sealed with a filling.

Dentists treat an abscess by draining the pus, which requires oral surgery or root canal treatment. Antibiotics help eliminate the infection, but removing the diseased pulp and draining the pus are more important.

Impacted Teeth

Impacted teeth are teeth that are unable to emerge (erupt) properly from the gum.

Impaction is usually caused by the overcrowding of teeth, which leaves insufficient room for a new tooth to emerge. Impaction can occur when a baby tooth is lost before the new tooth is ready to emerge, which allows the remaining teeth to drift into the space reserved for the new tooth. However, most teeth that become impacted are wisdom teeth because they are the last permanent teeth to come in and the jaw lacks enough room to accommodate them.

Impacted teeth are likely to become infected and are of little use in chewing, so they are usually removed. Often the removal can be done in the dentist's office with the person remaining awake, with use of a local anesthetic or with sedation to calm the person. Sometimes the surgery is done in a hospital with the person asleep, with use of a general anesthetic.

Malocclusion

Malocclusion is an abnormal alignment of the teeth or upper and lower jaws that prevents the teeth from meeting properly.

- If teeth are out of alignment, abnormal pressure is put on them, making them more likely to loosen or fracture.
- Malocclusion may make biting, chewing, or speaking difficult.
- Braces or retainers can usually realign teeth, but sometimes surgery is needed.

Occlusion refers to the alignment of the teeth and the way in which the upper and lower teeth fit together.

A Brighter Smile Through Cosmetic Dentistry

Cosmetic dentistry can dramatically improve a person's appearance. The techniques used avoid the time involved with orthodontic therapy and the loss of tooth structure necessitated by crowns and bridges.

Bonding involves the attachment of tooth-colored fillings to natural teeth with minimal tooth preparation. Bonding is a conservative way to restore fractured or chipped teeth, to close spaces between the teeth, or to cover a portion of the tooth to change the shade, color, or shape. A mild acid solution is used to clean and mildly roughen the tooth surface so that a tooth-colored resin (generally made of a special type of plastic called a composite) can adhere to this surface. Bonding allows dentists to improve the appearance of the teeth without removing large amounts of tooth structure.

Porcelain veneers are similar to bonding, but they use tooth-colored porcelain instead of composite to mask discoloration or change the shape of the teeth. The process requires two visits. An impression is made after the teeth are prepared. Porcelain veneers are then made in a dental prosthetic laboratory. The veneers are bonded to the teeth using a thin resin cement.

Bleaching, or tooth whitening, is a process used by dentists to lighten teeth. The effectiveness of bleaching varies according to the original color of the teeth. Products used for home bleaching usually contain a peroxide gel that is placed into a custom-made closely fitting mouth-guard–like tray that holds the solution near the teeth. The bleaching agent is placed into the mouth for a few hours per day or even overnight for 2 to 4 weeks, depending on the concentration of the bleaching agent. Bleaching can also be done in a dentist's office, in which the process is much quicker. The most common side effect of bleaching is tooth sensitivity. Bleaching may not be effective for people whose teeth are darkened or discolored because of cavities, because of a side effect of some drugs or diseases, or because of a tooth that has died.

Ideally, the upper teeth fit slightly over the lower teeth. Proper alignment of teeth prevents undue force from being placed on just a few teeth and keeps the lips, cheeks, and tongue away from the biting surfaces. If the teeth are maloccluded (out of alignment), undue strain is placed on some of the teeth, which may fracture portions of the crown or loosen the teeth.

Causes

A common cause of malocclusion is disproportion between jaw size and tooth size or between the size of the upper and lower jaws. These differences can result in the overcrowding of teeth and in an abnormal bite. Another cause is loss of one or more teeth. When a tooth is lost, nearby teeth tend to drift into the newly available space, moving them out of alignment. Less common causes of malocclusion include misalignment of a jaw fracture, thumb sucking beyond the age of 4, tumors of the mouth or jaw, and improper fitting of crowns, fillings, retainers, or braces. Malocclusion may have a hereditary component.

Symptoms and Diagnosis

Malocclusion usually causes no symptoms at first. Eventually, though, it may result in a loosening or fracture of misaligned teeth because of the strain placed on them. Severe malocclusions may also cause difficulty or discomfort when biting or chewing, as well as speech difficulties. Malocclusions that prevent full access for proper oral hygiene may increase the risk of gum disease and cavities.

Malocclusion can be diagnosed by the dentist during a dental examination.

Prevention and Treatment

After loss or removal of a tooth or teeth (for example, to make way for other permanent teeth), movement of remaining teeth can be prevented with braces or other orthodontic appliances. Once the teeth are properly aligned and the braces are removed, the person is usually required to continue wearing a retainer at night for 2 to 3 years to maintain the position of the teeth.

Malocclusion can be corrected in a number of ways. Teeth can be realigned by applying a continuous mild force through the use of an orthodontic appliance, such as braces (wires and springs carried by brackets that are fixed to the teeth with dental adhesive) or a retainer (a removable brace combining wires and a plastic plate that snaps into the roof of the mouth). For some minor malocclusions, orthodontic therapy can be done with appliances that are barely visible. Occasionally, when an orthodontic appliance alone is not sufficient, jaw surgery may be necessary. Other methods of treating malocclusion include selective grinding of some teeth or building them up with the use of crowns or other dental restorations.

Periodontal Diseases

Periodontal diseases inflame and destroy the structures surrounding and supporting the teeth, primarily the gums, the jawbones, and the outer layer of the tooth root.

Periodontal diseases are caused mainly by accumulation of bacteria. They are more likely to occur in people with poor oral hygiene, in people who smoke, and in people with certain diseases and disorders, such as diabetes mellitus, poor nutrition, leukemia, and AIDS.

Gingivitis

Gingivitis is inflammation of the gums (gingivae).

- Gingivitis results most often from inadequate brushing and flossing but may result from medical disorders or the use of certain drugs.
- The gums are red and swollen and bleed easily.
- Good oral hygiene, frequent professional cleanings, adequate nutrition, and mouthwashes usually help.

Gingivitis is an extremely common disease in which the gums become red and swollen and bleed easily. Gingivitis causes little pain in its early stages and thus may not be noticed. However, gingivitis that is left untreated may progress to periodontitis, a more severe gum disease that can result in tooth loss.

> **? Did You Know...**
> During pregnancy, gingivitis may develop or worsen because pregnant women may unintentionally neglect oral hygiene because of fatigue or morning sickness.

Plaque-Induced Gingivitis

Inadequate brushing and flossing is by far the most common cause of gingivitis. Without adequate brushing, plaque (a filmlike substance made up primarily of bacteria) remains along the gum line of the teeth. Plaque also accumulates in faulty fillings and around the teeth next to poorly cleaned partial dentures, bridges, and orthodontic appliances. When plaque stays on the teeth for more than 72 hours, it hardens into tartar (calculus), which cannot be completely removed by brushing and flossing.

The gums appear red rather than a healthy pink. They swell and become movable instead of being firm and tight against the teeth. The gums may bleed easily, especially while brushing or eating.

Plaque-induced gingivitis can be prevented with good oral hygiene—the daily use of a toothbrush and dental floss. Some mouthwashes also help control plaque. After tartar forms, it can be removed only by a dentist or dental hygienist. Depending on how fast tartar forms, people may need professional cleanings every 3 to 12 months. People with poor oral hygiene, medical conditions that can lead to gingivitis, or a tendency to develop plaque may need professional cleanings more often. Because of their excellent blood supply, gums quickly become healthy again after tartar and plaque are removed, as long as people brush and floss carefully.

Drug-Induced Gingivitis

Some drugs can cause an overgrowth of gum tissue, so that removing plaque becomes more difficult, and gingivitis often develops. Phenytoin (taken to control seizures), cyclosporine (taken by people who have had organ transplants), and calcium channel blockers such as nifedipine (taken to control blood pressure and heart rhythm abnormalities) can cause such an overgrowth. Also, oral or injectable contraceptives can aggravate gingivitis, as can exposure to lead or bismuth (which is used extensively in cosmetics) or to other heavy metals such as nickel (used in jewelry).

Medical conditions that might cause or worsen gingivitis should be treated or controlled. If people must take a drug that causes gum tissue overgrowth, the excess gum tissue may need to be removed surgically. However, meticulous oral hygiene at home and frequent cleanings by a dentist or dental hygienist may slow the rate of tissue growth and eliminate the need for surgery.

Gingivitis Due to Vitamin Deficiency

Vitamin deficiencies, in rare cases, can cause gingivitis. Vitamin C deficiency (scurvy) can lead to inflamed, bleeding gums. Niacin deficiency (pellagra) also causes inflamed, bleeding gums and a predisposition to certain mouth infections, such as thrush, or to inflammation of the tongue (glossitis).

Vitamin C and niacin deficiencies can be treated with vitamin C and niacin supplements, plus a diet that includes more fresh fruits and vegetables.

Gingivitis Due to Infections

Viral infections can cause gingivitis. Acute herpetic gingivostomatitis is a painful viral infection of the gums and other parts of the mouth caused by the herpes virus (see page 1245). The infection turns the gums bright red and causes many small white or yellow sores to form inside the mouth.

Acute herpetic gingivostomatitis usually gets better in 2 weeks without treatment. Intensive cleaning does not help, so a person should brush gently while the infection is still painful. Dentists may recommend an anesthetic mouth rinse to relieve discomfort while eating and drinking.

Fungal infections can cause gingivitis as well. Fungi commonly grow in the mouth in very small amounts. Use of antibiotics or a change in overall health can increase the number of fungi in the mouth. Thrush (candidiasis) is a fungal infection in which the overgrowth of fungi, particularly *Candida albicans*, forms a white film that irritates the gums. This film can also coat the tongue and corners of the mouth and leaves a bleeding surface if wiped away (see page 1232).

Thrush can be treated with an antifungal drug, such as nystatin, in the form of a mouth rinse or a lozenge designed to dissolve slowly in the mouth. Good oral hygiene (proper brushing and flossing) and treatment of underlying dental problems, such as ill-fitting dentures, can also help. Dentures can be soaked overnight in nystatin solution as well.

Gingivitis Due to Pregnancy

Pregnancy can worsen mild gingivitis, primarily because of hormonal changes. Some pregnant women may unknowingly contribute to the problem by neglecting oral hygiene because they feel nauseated in the morning (morning sickness). Also, during pregnancy, a minor irritation, often the buildup of tartar, may cause a lumplike overgrowth of gum tissue, called a pregnancy tumor. The bloated tissue bleeds easily if injured and may interfere with eating.

If pregnant women are neglecting oral hygiene because of morning sickness, dentists can suggest ways to keep the teeth and gums clean without exacerbating the nausea. Gentle brushing without toothpaste or even salt water rinses after brushing can help. A bothersome pregnancy tumor can be surgically removed. However, such tumors tend to recur until, and even after, the pregnancy ends.

Gingivitis Due to Menopause

Menopause can cause desquamative gingivitis, a poorly understood, painful condition that occurs most commonly in postmenopausal women. In this condition, the outer layers of the gums separate from the underlying tissue, exposing nerve endings. The gums become so loose that the outer layers can be rubbed away with a cotton swab or blown off with a dentist's air syringe.

If desquamative gingivitis develops during menopause, hormone replacement therapy may help. Otherwise, dentists may prescribe a corticosteroid rinse or a corticosteroid paste that is applied directly to the gums.

Gingivitis Due to Leukemia

Leukemia can cause gingivitis. In fact, gingivitis is the first sign of disease in about 25% of children with leukemia. An infiltration of leukemia cells into the gums causes the gingivitis, and a reduced ability to fight infections worsens it. The gums appear red and bleed easily. Often, the bleeding continues for several minutes or more because blood does not clot normally in people with leukemia.

A person with gingivitis due to leukemia can prevent bleeding by gently wiping the teeth and gums with a gauze pad or sponge instead of brushing and flossing. Dentists can prescribe chlorhexidine mouth rinse to control plaque and prevent mouth infections. When the leukemia is in remission (when evidence of the cancer disappears), good dental care can restore the gums to health.

Gingivitis Due to an Impacted Tooth

Gingivitis can develop in the gums surrounding the crown of an impacted tooth (a tooth that has not fully emerged). In this condition, called pericoronitis, the gum swells over the tooth that has not fully emerged. The flap of gum over the partially emerged tooth can trap fluids, bits of food, and bacteria.

Pericoronitis most commonly occurs with wisdom teeth, particularly the lower wisdom teeth. If the upper wisdom tooth emerges before the lower one, it may bite on this flap, increasing the irritation. Infections can develop and spread to the throat or cheek.

When people have pericoronitis, dentists may flush under the flap of gum to rinse out the debris and bacteria. If x-rays show that a lower tooth is not likely to emerge completely, dentists may remove the upper tooth and prescribe antibiotics for a few days before removing the lower one. Sometimes dentists remove the lower tooth immediately.

Periodontitis

Periodontitis (pyorrhea) is a severe form of gingivitis in which the inflammation of the gums extends to the supporting structures of the tooth.

- Plaque and tartar build up between the teeth and gums, then spread to the bone under the teeth.
- The gums swell and bleed, the breath smells bad, and teeth become loose.

- Doctors take x-rays and measure the depth of pockets in the gums to determine how severe periodontitis is.
- Repeated professional cleanings and sometimes dental surgery and antibiotics are needed.

Periodontitis is one of the main causes of tooth loss in adults and is the main cause in older people. Infection erodes the bone that holds the teeth in place. The erosion weakens the attachments and loosens the teeth. An affected tooth may eventually fall out or need to be pulled (extracted).

> **? Did You Know...**
> Periodontitis is the main cause of tooth loss in older people.

Causes

Most periodontitis results from a long-term accumulation of plaque and tartar on the teeth and the gums. Pockets form between the teeth and gums and extend downward between the root of the tooth and the underlying bone. These pockets collect plaque in an oxygen-free environment, which promotes the growth of aggressive forms of bacteria. If the disease continues, eventually so much bone is lost that the tooth may become painfully loose.

The rate at which periodontitis develops differs considerably, even among people with similar amounts of tartar. That is because plaque contains different types and numbers of bacteria and because people have different responses to the bacteria. Periodontitis may produce bursts of destructive activity that lasts for months followed by periods when the disease apparently causes no further damage.

Many diseases and disorders—including diabetes mellitus, Down syndrome, Crohn's disease, leukopenia, and AIDS—can predispose a person to periodontitis. In people with AIDS, periodontitis progresses quickly.

Symptoms and Diagnosis

The early symptoms of periodontitis are bleeding, red gums, and bad breath (halitosis). Dentists measure the depth of the pockets in the gums with a thin probe, and x-rays show how much bone has been lost. As more and more bone is lost, the teeth loosen and shift position. Frequently, the front teeth tilt outward. Periodontitis usually does not cause pain until the teeth loosen enough to move while chewing or until an abscess (a collection of pus) forms.

Treatment

Unlike gingivitis, which usually disappears with good self-care, periodontitis requires repeat professional care. People using good oral hygiene can clean only 1/12 inch

Periodontitis: From Plaque to Tooth Loss

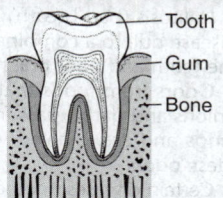

Healthy gums and bone hold the tooth firmly in place.

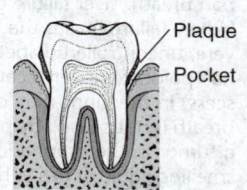

Plaque buildup irritates the gums, and they become inflamed. In time, the gums pull away from the tooth, creating a pocket that fills with more plaque.

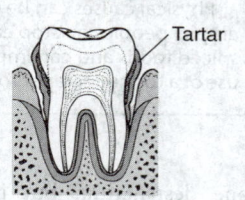

The pockets get deeper, and the plaque hardens into tartar. More plaque accumulates on top.

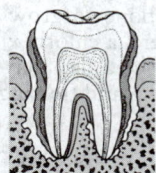

Tartar moves down to the root of the tooth and eventually destroys the bone supporting the tooth. Without this support, the tooth loosens and falls out.

(2 to 3 millimeters) below the gum line. Dentists can clean pockets up to 1/5 inch (4 to 5 millimeters) deep using scaling and root planing, which thoroughly remove tartar and the diseased root surface. For pockets of 1/4 inch (5 millimeters) or more, surgery is often required. Dentists or periodontists may access the tooth below the gum line surgically (periodontal flap surgery) to thoroughly clean the teeth and correct bone defects caused by the infection. Dentists or periodontists may also remove part of the infected and separated gum (a gingivectomy) so that the rest of the gum can reattach tightly to the teeth and people can then remove the plaque at home.

Dentists may prescribe antibiotics (such as amoxicillin or metronidazole), especially if an abscess has developed. Dentists may also insert antibiotic-impregnated materials (filaments or gels) into deep gum pockets, so that high concentrations of the drug can reach the diseased area. Periodontal abscesses cause a burst of

Understanding Halitosis

Halitosis (bad breath) is most often caused by gum disease due to a combination of food lodged between the teeth and poor oral hygiene.

Odors from foods that contain volatile oils, such as onions and garlic, pass from the bloodstream into the lungs and are exhaled. Oral hygiene cannot remove these odors.

Certain diseases in other areas of the body also cause bad breath. Liver failure gives the breath a mousy odor, kidney failure makes the breath smell like urine, and severe, uncontrolled diabetes makes the breath smell like nail polish remover (acetone). A collection of pus (abscess) in the lungs may cause very severe halitosis. Bad breath is not caused by poor digestion. However, rarely, a tumor in the esophagus or stomach may cause foul-smelling liquid or gas to be regurgitated into the mouth.

Physical causes can be corrected or removed. For example, people can stop eating garlic, onions, and other spiced foods and can improve their oral hygiene. Daily use of a tongue scraper to clean the top and back of the tongue is effective. Many deodorant mouthwashes and sprays are available. One of the best active ingredients in these products is chlorophyll. The effects of most of these products, however, do not last more than a couple of hours.

Imagined halitosis: Halitosis that is imagined is called psychogenic halitosis. People believe that their breath smells bad when it actually does not. This problem may occur in people who tend to exaggerate normal body sensations. Sometimes psychogenic halitosis is caused by a serious mental disorder, such as schizophrenia. People with obsessive thoughts may have an overwhelming sense of feeling dirty. People with paranoia may have the delusion that their organs are rotting. Such people may believe that their breath smells bad.

Some people with psychogenic halitosis may be helped by having a doctor or dentist assure them that they do not have bad breath. If the problem continues, they may benefit from seeing a psychotherapist.

---

bone destruction, but immediate treatment with surgery and antibiotics may allow much of the damaged bone to grow back. If the mouth is sore after surgery, a chlorhexidine mouth rinse used for 1 minute twice a day may be temporarily substituted for brushing and flossing.

Trench Mouth

Trench mouth (Vincent's infection, acute necrotizing ulcerative gingivitis) is a painful, noncontagious infection of the gums, causing pain, fever, and sometimes fatigue.

- If the normal bacteria in the mouth overgrow, the gums can become infected.
- The gums hurt, and people have extremely bad breath.
- A professional cleaning, sometimes followed by hydrogen peroxide rinses and antibiotics, plus good oral hygiene are effective.

The term trench mouth comes from World War I, when many soldiers in the trenches developed the infection. Trench mouth is now rare, although minor gum infections probably occur relatively commonly. The severe form usually affects only people with an impaired immune system.

The infection is caused by an abnormal overgrowth of the bacteria that normally exist harmlessly in the mouth. Poor oral hygiene usually contributes to the development of trench mouth, as do physical or emotional stress, poor diet, and lack of sleep. The infection occurs most often in people who have gingivitis and experience a stressful event. Trench mouth is far more common among smokers than among nonsmokers.

Usually, trench mouth begins abruptly with painful gums, an uneasy feeling, and fatigue. The breath smells extremely foul. The tips of the gums between the teeth erode and become covered with a gray layer of dead tissue. The gums bleed easily, and eating and swallowing cause pain. Often, the lymph nodes under the jaw swell, and a mild fever develops.

Diagnosis and Treatment

Because the breath smells so foul, doctors sometimes suspect the diagnosis immediately, as soon as they come into contact with affected people.

Treatment begins with a gentle, thorough professional cleaning. Rinsing several times a day with a hydrogen peroxide solution (ordinary drugstore hydrogen peroxide mixed half-and-half with water) may be recommended instead of brushing for the first few days because of the sensitivity of the gums. Antibiotics (such as amoxicillin, erythromycin, or tetracycline) may be given as well. The infection responds very well to good oral hygiene (daily brushing and flossing).

Gum Recession

Gum recession is the loss of gum tissue from the base of a tooth with exposure of the root surface.

Recession usually occurs in response to overaggressive brushing but can also result from injury or the natural aging process in thin, delicate gum tissue. Most people have some slight recession.

Recession may make the teeth very sensitive to cold, to sweet foods, or to touch. It may be accompanied by bone loss and may make the teeth more vulnerable to root cavities.

Treatment is needed when the gums or teeth are sensitive or when plaque accumulates and is difficult to remove. Treatment involves a grafting procedure, in which soft tissue is removed from the roof of the mouth or from donor tissues and stitched to the area.

CHAPTER 209 Temporomandibular Disorders

- Temporomandibular disorders are caused by problems with the jaw muscles or joints or the fibrous tissue connecting them.
- People may have headaches and tenderness of the chewing muscles or may hear clicking of the joints.
- Doctors or dentists can usually diagnose these disorders with a physical examination, but sometimes an imaging test is needed.
- Treatment usually involves splint therapy and pain relief.

The temporomandibular joints are the connections between the temporal bones of the skull and the lower jawbone (mandible). There are two temporomandibular joints, one on each side of the face just in front of the ears. Ligaments, tendons, and muscles support the joints and are responsible for jaw movement.

The temporomandibular joint is one of the most complicated joints in the body: It opens and closes like a hinge and slides forward, backward, and from side to side. During chewing, it may sustain an enormous amount of pressure depending on the position and health of the upper and lower teeth, which act much like a doorstop for the joints during closing. The temporomandibular joint contains a piece of special cartilage called a disk. The disk keeps the skull and the lower jawbone from rubbing against each other.

Temporomandibular disorders, previously called TMJ disorders (temporomandibular joint disorders), are most common among women in their early 20s and between the ages of 40 and 50. In rare cases, babies are born with temporomandibular joint abnormalities. Temporomandibular disorders include problems with the joints, the muscles, and the bands of fibrous tissue that connect them (fascia).

Causes

Most often, the cause of a temporomandibular disorder is a combination of muscle tension and anatomic problems within the joints. Sometimes, there is a psychologic component as well. Specific causes include muscle pain and tightness, internal joint derangement, arthritis, ankylosis, and hypermobility.

Muscle Pain and Tightness: Muscle pain and tightness around the jaw (myofascial pain syndrome) come mainly from muscle overuse, often brought on by problems of misalignment of the upper and lower sets of teeth, missing teeth, injury to the head or neck, or even toothache. Pain is also caused by trying to open the jaw too widely. Muscle pain and tightness can also result from clenching or grinding the teeth (bruxism) at night due to psychologic or sleep-related stress. Clenching and grinding while asleep exert far more force than clenching and grinding while awake.

Internal Joint Derangement: In the most common form of internal joint derangement, the disk inside the joint lies in front of (anterior to) its normal position. Internal joint derangement can occur with or without reduction. Reduction means the parts of a joint have returned to their normal positions. Disk displacement with reduction is more common than displacement without reduction and occurs in about one third of the adult population. In derangement with reduction, the disk lies in front of its normal position only when the mouth is closed. As the mouth opens and the jaw slides forward, the disk slips back into its normal position. As the mouth closes, the disk slips forward again. In internal joint derangement without reduction, the disk never slips back into its normal position, and the degree to which the mouth can be opened is limited.

Arthritis: Arthritis in a temporomandibular joint may result from osteoarthritis, rheumatoid arthritis, infectious arthritis, or injury, particularly injury that causes bleeding into the joint. Such injuries are fairly common among children who are struck on the side of the chin.

Osteoarthritis, a type of arthritis in which the cartilage of the joints degenerates (see page 559), is

Locating the Temporomandibular Joint

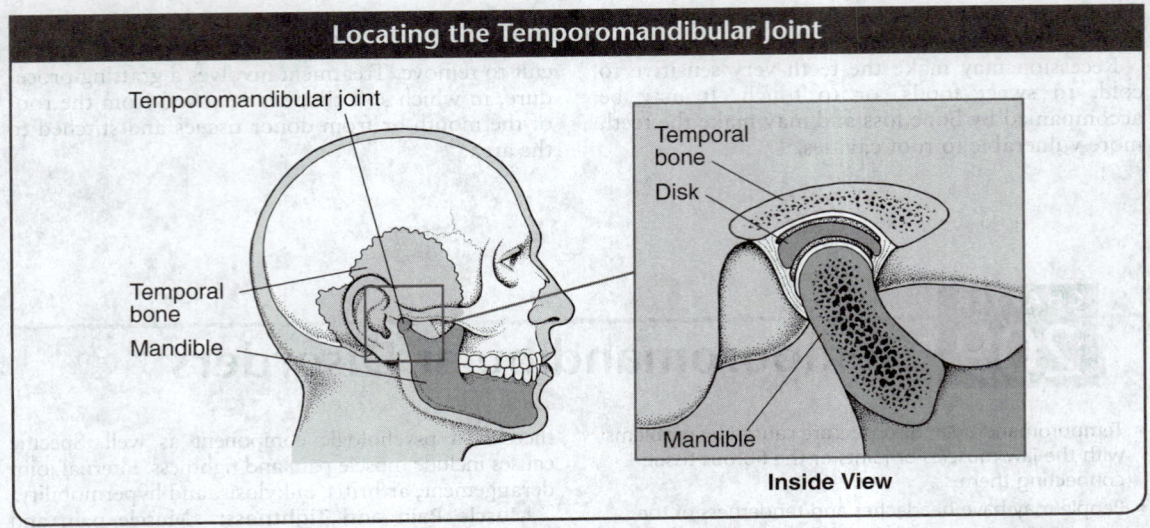

Temporomandibular joint

Temporal bone

Mandible

Temporal bone

Disk

Mandible

Inside View

most common among older people. The cartilage in the temporomandibular joints is not as strong as the cartilage in other joints. Osteoarthritis occurs mainly when the disk is missing or has developed holes.

Rheumatoid arthritis, a disease in which the body attacks its own cells (an autoimmune disease), causing inflammation (see page 563), affects the temporomandibular joint in about 17% of people with this type of arthritis. The temporomandibular joint generally is the last joint to be affected by rheumatoid arthritis.

Infectious arthritis is caused by an infection that has spread from an adjoining area of the head or neck or that has been carried by the bloodstream from another part of the body (see page 558).

Ankylosis: Ankylosis is loss of joint movement resulting from fusion of bones within the joint or from calcification (the deposit of calcium into body tissues) of the ligaments around it.

Hypermobility: Hypermobility (looseness of the jaw) results when the ligaments that hold the joint together become stretched. In hypermobility, dislocation is usually caused by the shape of the joints, ligament looseness (laxity), and muscle tension. It may be caused by trying to open the mouth too wide or by being struck on the jaw.

Symptoms

Symptoms of temporomandibular disorders include headaches, tenderness of the chewing muscles, and clicking or locking of the joints. Sometimes the pain seems to occur near the joint rather than in it. Temporomandibular disorders may be the reason for recurring headaches that do not respond to

usual medical treatment. Other symptoms include pain or stiffness in the neck radiating to the arms, dizziness, earaches or stuffiness in the ears, and disrupted sleep.

People with temporomandibular disorders often have difficulty opening their mouth wide. For example, most people without temporomandibular disorders can place the tips of their index, middle, and ring fingers held vertically in the space between the upper and lower front teeth without forcing. For people with temporomandibular disorders (with the exception of hypermobility), this space usually is markedly smaller.

Muscle Pain and Tightness: People with muscle pain usually have very little pain in the joint itself. Rather, they feel pain and tightness on the sides of the face upon awakening or after stressful periods during the day. Nighttime clenching and grinding of the teeth may cause a person to awaken with a headache, which may slowly diminish over the day. As the jaw opens, it may move slightly (deviate) to one side or the other. The chewing muscles are typically tender to the touch.

Internal Joint Derangement: Internal joint derangement related to anterior disk displacement *with* reduction usually causes a clicking or popping sound in the joint when the mouth opens wide or the jaw shifts from side to side. In many people, these joint sounds are the only symptoms. However, some people experience pain, particularly when chewing hard foods. In a small percentage of people who have missing teeth and who grind their teeth, these sounds progress to locking of the joints.

Internal joint derangement related to anterior disk displacement *without* reduction usually causes symptoms of pain and makes it difficult for people to open their mouth wide, as is typical of most temporomandibular disorders. After 6 to 12 months, the pain may decrease, but the limited degree to which the mouth can be opened generally persists.

Arthritis: With osteoarthritis, because it occurs mainly when the disk is missing or has developed holes, the person feels a grating sensation in the temporomandibular joints when opening and closing the mouth. When osteoarthritis is severe, the top of the jawbone flattens out, and the person cannot open the mouth wide. The jaw may also shift toward the affected side, and the person may be unable to move it back.

Rheumatoid arthritis usually affects both temporomandibular joints about equally, which is rarely the case in other types of temporomandibular disorders. When rheumatoid arthritis is severe, especially in young people, the top of the jawbone may degenerate and shorten. This damage can lead to sudden misalignment of many or all of the upper and lower teeth. If the damage is severe, the jawbone may eventually fuse to the skull (ankylosis).

Ankylosis: Typically, calcification (the deposit of calcium into body tissues) of the ligaments around the joint (extraarticular ankylosis) is not painful, but the mouth can open only about 1 inch (about 2½ centimeters) or less. Fusion of bones within the joint (intraarticular ankylosis) causes pain and more severely limits jaw movement.

Hypermobility: In a person with hypermobility, the jaw may slip forward completely out of its socket (dislocate), causing pain and an inability to close the mouth. Dislocation may occur suddenly and repeatedly.

Diagnosis

A dentist or doctor almost always diagnoses a temporomandibular disorder based solely on a person's medical history and on a physical examination. Part of the examination involves gently pressing on the side of the face or placing the little finger in the person's ear and gently pressing forward while the person opens and closes the jaw. Also, the doctor gently presses on the chewing muscles to detect pain or tenderness and notes whether the jaw slides when the person bites.

When a doctor suspects internal joint derangement, further tests can be done. Magnetic resonance imaging (MRI) is now the gold standard with which doctors assess whether internal joint derangement has occurred or why a person is not responding to treatment. Doctors occasionally use electromyography (see page 636), which analyzes muscle activity, to monitor treatment and, less commonly, to make a diagnosis. Laboratory tests are rarely useful.

A doctor suspects osteoarthritis when a creaking sound is heard when the person opens the mouth (crepitus). X-rays and a computed tomography (CT) scan can confirm the diagnosis. Infectious arthritis may be suspected when the area over and around the temporomandibular joint is inflamed and when movement of the joint is painful and limited. Infection in another part of the body serves as a clue as well. To confirm the diagnosis of infectious arthritis, the doctor may insert a needle into the temporomandibular joint and withdraw fluid (aspiration), which is then analyzed for bacteria.

If hypermobility is the cause, the person generally can open the mouth wider than the breadth of three fingers. The jaw may be chronically dislocated. If ankylosis is the cause, the jaw's range of motion tends to be markedly reduced.

Treatment

Treatment varies considerably according to the cause. Two common treatments are splint therapy and analgesics to relieve pain.

Muscle Pain and Tightness: Splint therapy usually is the main treatment for jaw muscle pain and tightness. For people who realize that they clench or grind their teeth, splint therapy can help them break the habit. A thin plastic splint is made to fit over either the upper or the lower set of teeth and is adjusted to give the person an even bite. The splint, usually worn at night (a nightguard), reduces grinding, allowing the jaw muscles to rest and recover. For pain during the day, a splint allows the jaw muscles to remain relaxed and the bite to be stable, thereby reducing discomfort. The splint can also prevent damage to teeth that are under exceptional stress from the grinding. Day splints are worn only until symptoms subside, usually less than 8 weeks. Longer use may be warranted depending on the severity of symptoms.

Physical therapy may also be prescribed. Physical therapy may involve ultrasound treatment, electromyographic biofeedback (in which the person learns to relax the muscles), spray and stretch exercises (in which the jaw is stretched open with a passive jaw motion device after the skin over the painful area has been sprayed with a refrigerant or numbed with ice), or friction massage. Transcutaneous electrical nerve stimulation (TENS) also may help. Stress management, sometimes along with electromyographic biofeedback, often brings dramatic improvement.

Drug therapy may also be helpful. For instance, muscle-relaxing drugs, such as cyclobenzaprine, may be prescribed to ease tightness and pain, particularly while the person waits for a splint to be made.

Physical Therapy for Jaw Muscles

- Ultrasound is a method of delivering deep heat to painful areas. When warmed by the ultrasound, the blood vessels dilate, and the blood can more quickly carry away the accumulated lactic acid, a muscle waste product that may cause pain.
- Electromyographic biofeedback monitors muscle activity with a gauge. The person attempts to relax the entire body or a specific muscle while watching the gauge. In this way, the person learns to control or relax particular muscles.
- Spray and stretch exercises involve spraying a skin refrigerant over the cheek and temple, so the jaw muscles can be stretched.
- Friction massage consists of rubbing a rough towel over the cheek and temple to increase circulation and speed lactic acid removal.
- Transcutaneous electrical nerve stimulation (TENS) involves using a device that stimulates the nerve fibers that do not transmit pain. The resulting impulses are thought to block the painful impulses that the person has been feeling.

However, these drugs are not a cure, generally are not recommended for older people, and are prescribed for only a short time, usually for a month or less. Analgesics such as aspirin or other nonsteroidal anti-inflammatory drugs (NSAIDs) also relieve pain. A prescription for opioid analgesics is usually not given because treatment may be needed for some time and these drugs can be addictive. Sleep aids (sedatives) may be used occasionally and for a short time to help people who have trouble sleeping because of the pain. Botulinum toxin injected into the muscle has recently been used successfully to relieve muscle spasms.

Regardless of the type of treatment, most people experience significant relief within about 3 months. If the symptoms are not severe, many people recover without treatment within 2 to 3 years.

Internal Joint Derangement: In internal joint derangement with or without reduction, treatment is needed only if a person has jaw pain or trouble moving the jaw. If a person seeks treatment right after symptoms develop, a dentist or doctor may be able to manually move the disk back into its normal position. If a person has had the disorder for fewer than 3 months, a splint may be applied to hold the lower jaw forward. This splint keeps the disk in position, permitting the supporting ligaments to tighten. Over 2 to 4 months, the splint is adjusted to allow the jaw to return back to its normal position, with the expectation that the disk will remain in place.

A person with internal joint derangement with or without reduction should avoid opening the mouth wide—for instance, when yawning or biting into a thick sandwich—because injured joints are not as protected in these activities as a normal jaw would be. People with this disorder are advised to cut food into small pieces and to eat food that is easy to chew.

Sometimes the slipped disk becomes stuck in front of the temporomandibular joint, preventing the jaw from opening fully. The disk must then be manually moved out of position to allow the joint to move fully. Passive jaw motion devices, which stretch the jaw, have been used to slowly increase jaw motion. These devices are used several times a day. One such device is a threaded screw-type instrument that is placed between the front teeth and turned, much like a car jack, to gradually create a wider opening. If such a device is not available, then a doctor may use a stack of tongue depressors placed between the front teeth, with an additional tongue depressor being added to the middle of the stack.

If internal joint derangement cannot be treated by nonsurgical means, an oral-maxillofacial surgeon may need to reshape the disk and sew it back into place. However, the need for traditional surgery is relatively rare since the introduction of procedures such as arthroscopy (see page 544). All surgical procedures are used in combination with splint therapy.

Arthritis: A person with osteoarthritis in a temporomandibular joint needs to rest the jaw as much as possible, use a splint or other device to control muscle tightness, and take an analgesic (such as aspirin, acetaminophen, or another nonsteroidal anti-inflammatory drug) for pain. The pain usually goes away in 6 months with or without treatment. Even without treatment, most of the symptoms subside, probably because the band of tissue behind the disk becomes scarred and functions like the original disk. Usually, jaw movement is sufficient for normal activities, though the jaw may not open as wide as it used to.

Rheumatoid arthritis of the temporomandibular joint is treated with the drugs used for rheumatoid arthritis of any joint (see table on page 566). Maintaining joint mobility and preventing fusion of the joint are particularly important. Usually, the best way to accomplish these goals is by exercising the jaw under a physical therapist's direction. To relieve symptoms, particularly muscle tightness, the person wears a splint at night. A splint that does not restrict jaw movement is used. If joint fusion freezes the jaw, the person may need surgery and, in rare cases, an artificial joint to restore jaw mobility.

Infectious arthritis is treated with antibiotics. Penicillin is usually the antibiotic used initially, until test results determine the type of bacteria present and thus the best antibiotic to use. Pus in the joint, if present, may be removed with a needle.

Ankylosis: Occasionally, stretching exercises help people with calcification, but people with calcification or bone fusion usually need surgery to restore jaw movement.

Hypermobility: Prevention and treatment of dislocation resulting from hypermobility are the same as those for other causes of a dislocated jaw (see page 1372). When dislocation occurs, a helper is sometimes needed to snap the jaw back into position. Many people who experience repeated dislocations, however, learn how to maneuver the joint back into place themselves by consciously relaxing the muscles and lightly shifting the lower jaw until it pops back into place. Surgery to tighten the ligaments of the temporomandibular joint is sometimes necessary to prevent recurrent dislocations.

(see page 1372)

CHAPTER 210 Urgent Dental Problems

Certain dental problems require prompt treatment to relieve discomfort and minimize damage to the structures of the mouth. Such urgent dental problems include

- Toothaches
- Fractured, loosened, and knocked-out teeth
- Jaw fractures
- A dislocated jaw
- Infections
- Certain complications that can develop after dental treatment

Toothaches

Most toothaches are caused by cavities (tooth decay). Some toothaches are caused by a tooth abscess or by inflammation of the gum around the crown of a tooth (pericoronitis). Much less commonly, toothaches result from inflammation of the nasal sinuses (sinusitis).

If several upper teeth hurt when a person is chewing or is bending down (for instance, to tie a shoe), the cause is probably sinusitis—especially if the toothache develops while the person has or recently has had a cold. Additional symptoms suggesting sinusitis are headache and tenderness and swelling of the skin above the affected sinus.

Fractured, Loosened, or Knocked-Out Teeth

The upper front teeth are prone to injury and fracture. A person who has brief, sharp pain while chewing or while eating something cold may have an incomplete fracture of a tooth. As long as the fracture is incomplete and part of the tooth has not split off, the dentist can often correct the problem with a simple filling. More extensive fractures may require a crown, with or without root canal treatment.

If a tooth is not sensitive to air after an injury, most likely only the hard outer surface (enamel) has been damaged. Even if the enamel has been slightly chipped, immediate treatment is not required. Fractures of the intermediate layer of the tooth (dentin) are usually painful when exposed to air and food, so people with such fractures seek dental care quickly. If the fracture affects the innermost part of the tooth (pulp), a red spot and often some blood will appear in the fracture. Root canal treatment may be needed to remove the remaining injured pulp before it causes severe pain.

If an injury loosens a tooth in the socket or if the surrounding gum tissue bleeds a great deal, a person should see a dentist immediately. Seriously loosened baby (deciduous) teeth in the front of the mouth are often removed to prevent harm to existing permanent teeth without losing space for the permanent teeth that are yet to erupt.

> **? Did You Know...**
> A container of milk can be used to transport a knocked-out tooth to the dentist.

Knocked-out (avulsed) baby teeth should not be reimplanted because reimplanting these teeth may damage permanent tooth buds. However, a knocked-out permanent tooth requires immediate treatment. The tooth should be rinsed off and placed back in its socket. If that is not possible, the tooth should be wrapped in a moistened paper

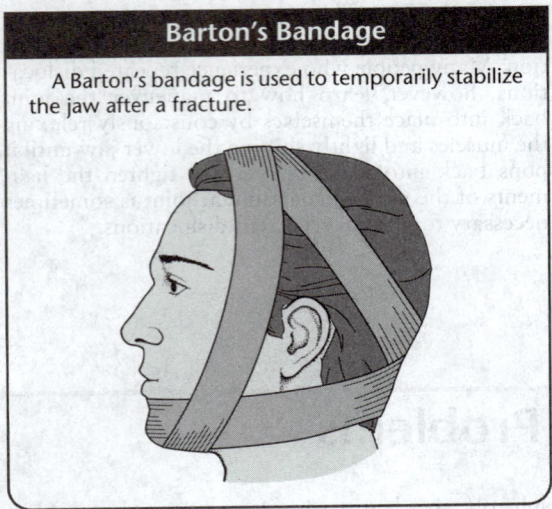

Barton's Bandage

A Barton's bandage is used to temporarily stabilize the jaw after a fracture.

towel or placed in a glass of milk (the milk provides a good medium for sustaining the tooth). In either case, the injured person and the tooth should be taken immediately to the nearest dentist.

If a tooth is reimplanted within 30 minutes, the likelihood that it will stay healthy is good. After 30 minutes, the longer the tooth is out of the socket, the worse the chance for long-term success. The dentist usually splints the tooth to the surrounding teeth for 7 to 10 days. If the bone around the tooth also has been fractured, the tooth may have to be splinted for 6 to 10 weeks. Reimplanted teeth eventually need root canal treatment.

Jaw Fracture

The term "jaw fracture" usually refers to fracture of the lower jaw (mandible). A fractured jaw causes pain and usually changes the way the teeth fit together. Often, the mouth cannot be opened wide, or it shifts to one side when opening or closing.

Fractures of the upper jaw (maxilla) are usually considered facial fractures. These may cause double vision (because the muscles of the eye attach nearby), numbness in the skin below the eye (because of injuries to nerves), or an irregularity in the cheekbone that can be felt when running a finger along it.

Any injury forceful enough to fracture the jaw may also injure the spine in the neck or cause a concussion or bleeding within the skull. Jaw fractures cause swelling, which rarely becomes severe enough to block the airway. Sometimes a fracture extends through a tooth or its socket (called an open fracture), creating an opening into the mouth that can allow oral bacteria to infect the jaw bone.

If people suspect their jaw is fractured, they should hold the jaw still with the teeth together. Emergency personnel may wrap a bandage under the jaw and over the top of the head several times (Barton's bandage). When wrapping the bandage, people must be careful not to cut off breathing.

At the hospital, neck x-rays are often taken to rule out spinal damage.

The upper and lower jaws may be wired together for up to 6 weeks to allow the bone to heal. During this time, people are only able to drink liquids through a straw. Alternatively, many jaw fractures can be repaired surgically with a plate (a piece of metal that is screwed into the bone on each side of the fracture). If a plate is used, the jaws are immobilized for only a few days, after which people should eat only soft foods for several weeks. In children, some jaw fractures are not immobilized. Instead, initial treatment allows restricted motion, and normal activity resumes in a few weeks. Antibiotics are usually given to people with an open fracture.

Jaw Dislocation

A dislocated jaw (dislocated mandible) generally is very painful. The mouth cannot be closed, and the jaw may be twisted to one side. A dislocated jaw is typically caused by the following:

- Opening the mouth excessively wide (such as during yawning, vomiting, or a prolonged dental procedure)
- An injury

Dislocation is likely to occur in people who have had previous dislocations or who have looseness of the jaw (hypermobility), which may result from a temporomandibular disorder.

A doctor or dentist typically maneuvers the jaw back into place by hand (manual reduction).

Once the jaw is back in place, people are cautioned to avoid opening the mouth wide for at least 6 weeks. For those who have had more than one dislocation, surgery may be needed to reduce the risk of further dislocations. For instance, the ligaments connecting the jaw to the skull (at the temporomandibular joint) can be shortened, thereby tightening the joint.

Problems After Dental Treatment

Swelling is common after certain dental procedures, particularly tooth extractions and periodontal surgery. Holding an ice pack—or better yet, a plastic bag of frozen peas or corn (which adapts to facial contours)—to the cheek can prevent much of the swelling. Ice therapy can be used for the first

Putting a Dislocated Jaw Back in Place

After wrapping their fingers with gauze, doctors or dentists place their thumbs inside the mouth on the lower back teeth. They place their other fingers around the bottom of the lower jaw. They press down on the back teeth and push the chin up until the jawbone returns to its normal location.

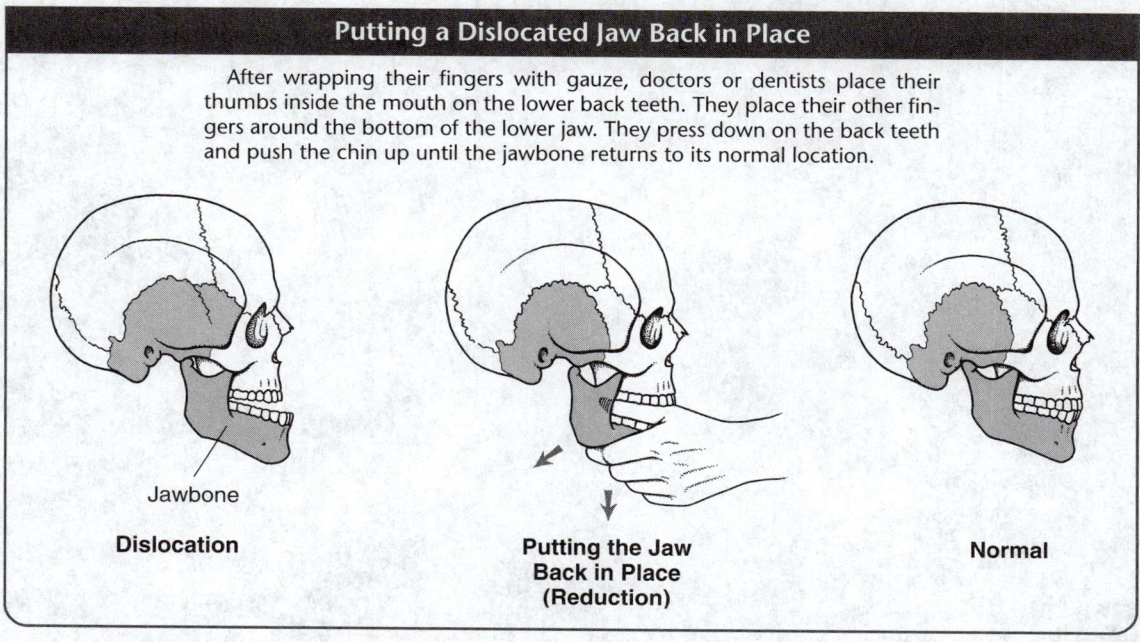

Jawbone

Dislocation

Putting the Jaw Back in Place (Reduction)

Normal

18 hours. Cold should be held on the cheek for 25-minute periods and then removed for 5-minute periods. If swelling persists or increases after 3 days or if pain is severe, an infection may have developed, and the person should contact the dentist.

Dry Socket: A dry socket (exposure of the bone in the socket, causing delayed healing) may develop after a lower back tooth has been removed and the normal blood clot in the socket is lost. Typically, discomfort lessens for 2 or 3 days after the extraction and then suddenly worsens, sometimes accompanied by an earache. Although the condition goes away by itself after 1 to 2 weeks, a dentist can place a dressing soaked with an anesthetic in the socket to eliminate the pain. The dentist replaces the dressing every day or two for about a week.

Bleeding: Bleeding after oral surgery is common. Bleeding in the mouth may appear worse than it is because a small amount of blood may mix with saliva. Usually, the bleeding can be stopped by keeping steady pressure on the surgical site for the first hour, normally by having the person bite down on a piece of gauze. If bleeding continues, the area can be wiped clean, and another piece of gauze or a moistened tea bag can be held against the area with steady biting pressure. Keeping the gauze or tea bag steadily in place for at least an hour is important. Most problems with bleeding

occur because the person frequently removes the pack to see if the bleeding has stopped. If bleeding continues for more than a few hours, the dentist should be notified.

People who regularly take an anticoagulant (a drug that prevents clots) or aspirin (even if they take only one aspirin every few days) should mention it to the dentist a week before surgery because these drugs increase the tendency to bleed. The dentist and the person's doctor may adjust the drug dosage or temporarily stop the drug.

Osteonecrosis of the Jaw: In this disorder (see box on page 551), prolonged exposure of bone through the gum tissue usually causes pain, but osteonecrosis of the jaw may also be accompanied by loose teeth, infection, or a discharge of pus. The disorder may occur after

- Tooth extraction
- An injury
- Radiation therapy to the head and neck (osteoradionecrosis)

Or osteonecrosis of the jaw may occur spontaneously. This disorder has developed in some people who were given high intravenous doses of bisphosphonates (certain drugs used to treat osteoporosis), particularly people requiring oral surgery while receiving the drugs.

Ear, Nose, and Throat Disorders

CHAPTER
211 Biology of the Ears, Nose, and Throat

The ears, nose, and throat have two things in common: they are located near each other and have separate but related functions. The ears and nose are sensory organs—necessary for the senses of hearing, balance, and smell. The throat mainly functions as a pathway through which food and fluids travel to the esophagus and air passes to the lungs. Primary care doctors often diagnose and treat disorders involving these organs, but doctors called otolaryngologists specialize in them.

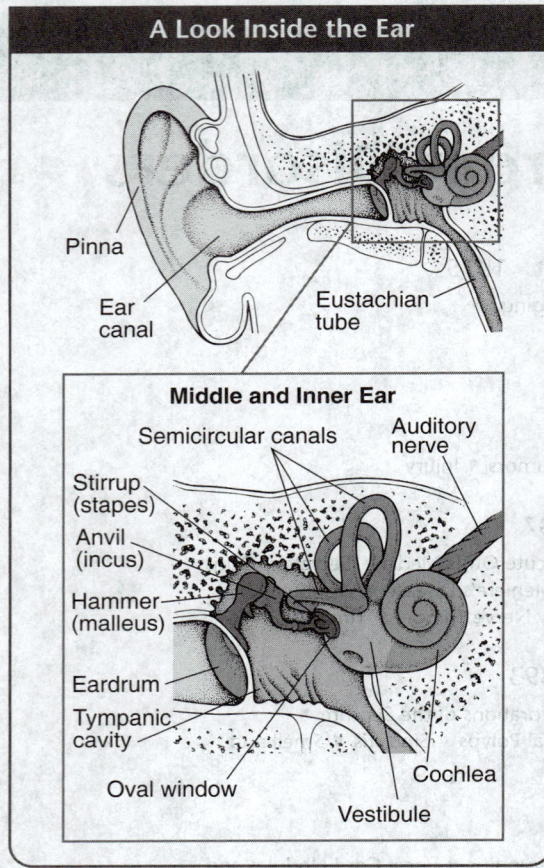

A Look Inside the Ear

- Pinna
- Ear canal
- Eustachian tube

Middle and Inner Ear

- Semicircular canals
- Auditory nerve
- Stirrup (stapes)
- Anvil (incus)
- Hammer (malleus)
- Eardrum
- Tympanic cavity
- Oval window
- Cochlea
- Vestibule

Ears

The ear, which is the organ of hearing and balance, consists of the outer, middle, and inner ear. The outer, middle, and inner ear function together to convert sound waves into nerve impulses that travel to the brain, where they are perceived as sound. The inner ear also helps to maintain balance.

Outer Ear

The outer ear consists of the external part of the ear (pinna or auricle) and the ear canal (external auditory meatus). The pinna consists of cartilage covered by skin and is shaped to capture sound waves and funnel them through the ear canal to the eardrum (tympanic membrane), a thin membrane that separates the outer ear from the middle ear.

Middle Ear

The middle ear consists of the eardrum and a small air-filled chamber containing a chain of three tiny bones (ossicles) that connect the eardrum to the inner ear. The ossicles are named for their shapes. The hammer (malleus) is attached to the eardrum. The anvil (incus) is the middle bone between the hammer and the stirrup (stapes), which is attached to the oval window, a thin membrane at the entrance to the inner ear. Vibrations of the eardrum are amplified mechanically by the ossicles and transmitted to the oval window.

The middle ear also contains two tiny muscles. The tensor tympani muscle is attached to the hammer and helps to tune and protect the ear. The stapedius muscle is attached to the stirrup and oval window. This muscle contracts in response to a loud noise, making the chain of ossicles more rigid so that less sound is transmitted. This response, called the acoustic reflex, helps protect the delicate inner ear from sound damage.

The eustachian tube, a small tube that connects the middle ear with the back of the nose, allows outside air to enter the middle ear. This tube, which opens when a person swallows, helps maintain equal air pressure on both sides of the eardrum and prevents fluid from accumulating in the middle ear. If air pressure is not equal, the eardrum may bulge or retract, which can be uncomfortable and distort hearing. Swallowing or voluntary "popping" of the ears can relieve pressure on the eardrum caused by sudden changes in air pressure, as often occurs when flying in an airplane. The eustachian tube's connection with the middle ear explains why upper respiratory infections (such as the common cold), which inflame and block the eustachian tube, can lead to middle ear infections or changes in middle ear pressure, resulting in pain.

Inner Ear

The inner ear (labyrinth) is a complex structure consisting of two major parts: the cochlea, the organ of hearing; and the vestibular system, the organ of balance. The vestibular system consists of the saccule and the utricle, which determine position sense, and the semicircular canals, which help maintain balance.

The cochlea, a hollow tube coiled in the shape of a snail's shell, is filled with fluid. Within the cochlea is the organ of Corti, which consists, in part, of about 20,000 specialized cells, called hair cells. These cells have small hairlike projections (cilia) that extend into the fluid. Sound vibrations transmitted from the ossicles in the middle ear to the oval window in the inner ear cause the fluid and cilia to vibrate. Hair cells in different parts of the cochlea vibrate in response to different sound frequencies and convert the vibrations into nerve impulses. The nerve impulses are transmitted along fibers of the cochlear nerve to the brain. The round window is a small, membrane-covered opening between the fluid-filled cochlea and the middle ear. This window helps dampen the pressure caused by sound waves in the cochlea.

Despite the protective effect of the acoustic reflex, loud noise can damage and destroy hair cells. Once a hair cell is destroyed, it does not seem to regrow. Continued exposure to loud noise causes progressive damage, eventually resulting in hearing loss and sometimes noise or ringing in the ears (tinnitus).

The semicircular canals are three fluid-filled tubes at right angles to one another. Movement of the head causes the fluid in the canals to move. Depending on the direction the head moves, the fluid movement will be greater in one of the canals than in the others. The canals contain hair cells that respond to this movement of fluid. The hair cells initiate nerve impulses that tell the brain which way the head is moving, so that appropriate action can be taken to maintain balance.

If the semicircular canals malfunction, as may occur in an upper respiratory infection and other conditions both temporary and permanent, the person's sense of balance may be lost or a whirling sensation (vertigo) may develop.

Nose and Sinuses

The nose is the organ of smell and a main passageway for air into and out of the lungs. The nose warms, moistens, and cleans air before it enters the lungs. The bones of the face around the nose contain hollow spaces called paranasal sinuses. There are four groups of paranasal sinuses: the maxillary, ethmoid, frontal, and sphenoid sinuses (see art on page 1398). Sinuses reduce the weight of the facial bones and skull while maintaining bone strength and shape. The air-filled spaces of the nose and sinuses also add resonance to the voice.

The supporting structure of the upper part of the external nose consists of bone, while the lower part consists of cartilage. Inside the nose is the nasal cavity, which is divided into two passages by the nasal septum. The nasal septum is composed of both bone and cartilage and extends from the nostrils to the back of the throat. Bones called nasal conchae project into the nasal cavity, forming a series of folds (turbinates). These folds greatly increase the surface area of the nasal cavity. Polyps may develop between the folds, often in people with asthma, allergies, or cystic fibrosis and in those using aspirin for long periods.

Lining the nasal cavity is a mucous membrane rich with blood vessels. The increased surface area and the many blood vessels enable the nose to warm and humidify incoming air quickly. Cells in the mucous membrane produce mucus and have tiny hairlike projections (cilia). Usually, the mucus traps incoming dirt particles, which are then moved by the cilia toward the front of the nose or down the throat to be removed from the airway. This action helps clean the air before it goes to the lungs. Sneezing automatically clears the nasal passages in response to irritation, just as coughing clears the lungs.

Like the nasal cavity, the sinuses are lined with a mucous membrane composed of cells that produce mucus and have cilia. Incoming dirt particles are trapped by the mucus, then moved by the cilia into the nasal cavity, through small sinus openings (ostia). Because these openings are so small, the drainage can easily be blocked by conditions such as colds or allergies, which cause swelling of the mucous membranes. Blockage of normal sinus drainage leads to sinus inflammation and infection (sinusitis).

One of the most important functions of the nose is its role in the sense of smell. Smell receptor cells are located in the upper part of the nasal cavity. These cells are special nerve cells that have cilia. The cilia of each cell are sensitive to different chemicals and, when stimulated, create a nerve impulse that is sent to the nerve cells of the olfactory bulb, which lies inside the skull just above the nose. The olfactory nerves

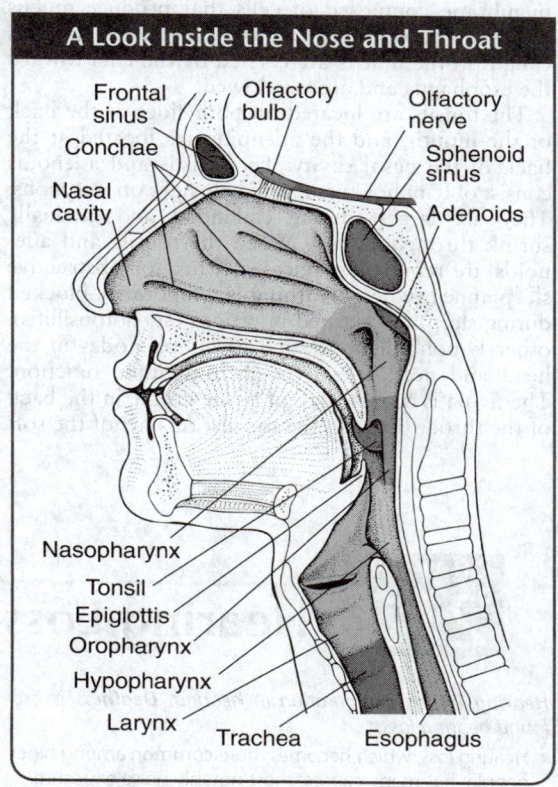

A Look Inside the Nose and Throat

- Frontal sinus
- Olfactory bulb
- Olfactory nerve
- Conchae
- Sphenoid sinus
- Nasal cavity
- Adenoids
- Nasopharynx
- Tonsil
- Epiglottis
- Oropharynx
- Hypopharynx
- Larynx
- Trachea
- Esophagus

carry the nerve impulse from the olfactory bulb directly to the brain, where it is perceived as a smell.

The sense of smell, which is not fully understood, is much more sophisticated than the sense of taste. Distinct smells are far more numerous than tastes. The subjective sense of taste while eating (flavor) involves taste and smell (see art on page 1400) as well as texture and temperature. This is why food seems somewhat tasteless when a person has a decreased sense of smell, as may occur when the person has a cold. Because the smell receptors are located in the upper part of the nose, normal breathing does not draw much air over them. Sniffing, however, increases the flow of air over the smell receptor cells, greatly increasing their exposure to odors.

Throat

The throat (pharynx) is located behind the mouth, below the nasal cavity, and above the esophagus and windpipe (trachea). It consists of an upper part (nasopharynx), a middle part (oropharynx), and a lower part (hypopharynx). The throat is a muscular passageway through which food is carried to the esophagus and air is carried to the lungs. Like the nose and mouth, the throat is lined with a mucous membrane composed of cells that produce mucus and have hairlike projections (cilia). Dirt particles caught in the mucus are carried by the cilia toward the esophagus and are swallowed.

The tonsils are located on both sides of the back of the mouth, and the adenoids are located at the back of the nasal cavity. The tonsils and adenoids consist of lymphoid tissue and help fight off infections. They are largest during childhood and gradually shrink throughout life. When the tonsils and adenoids are removed surgically, either for obstructive sleep apnea (when breathing is temporarily blocked during sleep) or repeated infections (adenotonsillitis), other lymphoid tissue such as lymph nodes in the head and neck take over their immune function. The uvula is a small flap of tissue visible in the back of the throat between the tonsils. As part of the soft palate, the uvula helps prevent food and fluids from entering the nasal cavity during swallowing and assists in the formation of certain sounds during speech. A long uvula may cause snoring and occasionally contributes to sleep apnea.

At the top of the trachea is the voice box (larynx), which contains the vocal cords and is primarily responsible for producing the sound of the voice. When relaxed, the vocal cords form a V-shaped opening that air can pass through freely. When contracted, they vibrate as air from the lungs passes over them, generating sounds that can be modified by the tongue, nose, and mouth to produce speech.

The epiglottis is a stiff flap of cartilage located above and in front of the larynx. During swallowing, the epiglottis covers the opening to the larynx to prevent food and fluids from entering the trachea. Thus, the epiglottis protects the lungs.

Effects of Aging

Aging greatly affects the function of the ears, nose, and throat. The effects of aging result from many factors such as wear and tear, noise, and the cumulative effect of infections, as well as the effect of substances such as drugs, alcohol, and tobacco.

A progressive loss of hearing, especially for higher-pitched sounds, is common (presbycusis). This change can alter a person's ability to understand speech. Vestibular imbalance and ringing in the ears (tinnitus) are also more common among older people but are not normal. Changes occur because some structures in the ear that help with hearing or balance deteriorate slightly. Hearing aids can help people with hearing loss hear better.

The sense of smell may decline with age, making tastes less distinct. Changes in the voice also occur with age. The tissues in the larynx may stiffen, affecting the pitch and quality of the voice and causing hoarseness. Changes in the tissues of the throat (pharynx) may lead to the leakage of food or fluids into the trachea during swallowing (aspiration). If persistent or severe, aspiration may cause pneumonia.

CHAPTER

212 Hearing Loss and Deafness

Hearing loss is deterioration in hearing. *Deafness* is profound hearing loss.

- Hearing loss, which becomes more common among older people, has many causes, most notably noise exposure.

- Audiometry defines the extent and characteristics of hearing loss.

- Most hearing loss is not treatable except with hearing aids and, rarely, surgery.

More than 28 million people in the United States are deaf or have hearing loss. Older people are the most affected: 30 to 40% of people aged 65 and older have significant hearing loss. Children also develop hearing loss (see page 1813), which can be detrimental to language and social development. Every year, about 1 of 5,000 people develops sudden deafness. Sudden deafness is severe hearing loss, usually in only one ear, that develops over a period of a few hours or less.

Many people with hearing loss also develop ringing in the ears (tinnitus). Sometimes people notice the ringing sound before they fully recognize their hearing loss.

Causes

Hearing loss has many causes. The most common cause is exposure to noise. Usually damage results after long-term exposure to loud noise, but even brief exposure to extremely loud noise can permanently harm hearing. Listening to loud music through headphones has become a common cause of hearing loss, even as industrial exposure to loud noise has been reduced. Head trauma can lead to hearing loss, especially in young children.

Hearing loss may be caused by a mechanical problem in the external ear canal or middle ear that blocks the conduction of sound (conductive hearing loss). Blockage of the external ear canal can be due to something as mundane as an accumulation of wax or something as uncommon as a tumor. The most common cause of conductive hearing loss in the middle ear, especially in children, is an accumulation of fluid. Fluid can accumulate as a result of ear infections or conditions, such as allergies or tumors, that block the eustachian tube, which drains the middle ear.

Hearing loss also may be caused by damage to the sensory structures (hair cells) of the inner ear, auditory nerve, or auditory nerve pathways in the brain (sensorineural hearing loss). These sensory structures may be damaged by drugs, infections, tumors, and skull injuries. Hearing loss can be a mixture of conductive and sensorineural loss.

Age: Age-related hearing loss is called presbycusis. As some people age, structures of the ear become less elastic and undergo other changes that make them less able to respond to sound waves, contributing to hearing loss. In many people, exposure to noise over many years worsens the changes caused by aging. Age-related hearing loss begins early, starting some time after age 20. However, it progresses very slowly, and most people do not notice any changes until well after age 50.

Age-related hearing loss first affects the highest pitches (frequencies) and only later affects lower

Causes of Hearing Loss

CONDUCTIVE HEARING LOSS

- Cholesteatoma (noncancerous tumor in the middle ear caused by an ear infection)
- Chronic middle ear fluid (otitis media with effusion)
- Middle ear infection (otitis media)
- Obstruction of external ear canal (for example, with wax, a tumor, or pus from an infection)
- Otosclerosis (bony overgrowth of the ossicles)
- Perforated eardrum

SENSORINEURAL HEARING LOSS

- Aging
- Brain tumors
- Certain drugs
- Childhood infections (mumps, meningitis)
- Congenital infection (toxoplasmosis, rubella, cytomegalovirus, herpes, syphilis)
- Congenital abnormality
- Demyelinating diseases (diseases that destroy the myelin sheath covering nerves)
- Genetic
- Loud noise
- Meniere's disease
- Sudden pressure changes caused by flying, diving, and strenuous exercise
- Viral infection of the inner ear (labyrinthitis)

pitches. Loss of the ability to hear high-pitched sounds often makes it more difficult to understand speech. Although the loudness of speech seems normal to the person, certain consonant sounds—such as the sound of letters C, D, K, P, S, and T—become hard to distinguish, so that many people with hearing loss think the speaker is mumbling. Words can be misinterpreted. For example, a person may hear "bone" when the speaker said "stone." Some people complain more that others are not speaking clearly rather than that they cannot hear well. Women and children, whose voices tend to be higher in pitch than those of men, are particularly difficult to understand. Many people also notice a change in the vibrancy of certain musical sounds, such as those of violins and flutes.

Otosclerosis: In otosclerosis, a hereditary disorder, the bone surrounding the middle and inner ear grows excessively. This exuberant growth immobilizes the stirrup (the ear bone attached to the inner ear) so that it cannot transmit sounds properly. Otosclerosis

SPOTLIGHT ON AGING

Even mild hearing loss makes understanding speech difficult. As a result, an older person with mild hearing loss may avoid conversations. Understanding speech may be particularly difficult if there is background noise or more than one person is talking, such as in a restaurant or at a family gathering. Constantly asking others to talk louder can frustrate both the listener and the speaker. People with hearing loss may misunderstand a question and give an apparently bizarre answer, leading others to believe they are confused. They may misjudge the loudness of their own speech and thus shout, discouraging others from conversing with them. Thus, hearing loss can lead to social isolation, inactivity, loss of social support, and depression. In a person with dementia, hearing loss can make communicating even more difficult.

tends to run in families and may develop in someone who had measles as a child. Hearing loss first becomes evident in late adolescence or early adulthood. About 10% of adults have some evidence of otosclerosis, but only about 1% develops hearing loss as a result.

Noise: About 30 million people in the United States are exposed to levels of noise that can cause hearing loss. Noise destroys the hair cells in the inner ear. Although people vary greatly in their sensitivity to loud noise, everyone loses some hearing if exposed to sufficiently loud noise long enough.

Both the loudness and duration of exposure are important—the louder the noise, the less time it takes to cause hearing loss. Extremely loud noise can cause hearing loss with even a single, brief exposure. Although brief exposure to loud noise usually causes only temporary hearing loss lasting a few hours to a day or so (called a temporary threshold shift), loss can be permanent, especially when the person is exposed many times. The person may have tinnitus (see page 1392) and problems comprehending speech. When a person experiences these symptoms, it is a warning that a sound is too loud and must be avoided.

Common sources of potentially damaging noise include highly amplified music, power tools, heavy machinery, and many types of powered vehicles, such as snowmobiles. Many people are exposed to injurious levels of noise during the course of their jobs, and hearing loss is a significant occupational hazard for many people. Explosions and gunfire also damage hearing.

Ear Infections: Young children commonly have some degree of conductive hearing loss after an ear infection (otitis media), because infection may lead to accumulation of fluid (effusion) in the middle ear. Most children regain normal hearing in 3 to 4 weeks after the infection resolves, but a few have persistent hearing loss. Chronic, long-standing infections of the middle ear often result in both conductive and sensorineural losses. Hearing loss is more likely to occur in children who have recurring ear infections.

Autoimmune Disorders: Autoimmune disorders sometimes cause hearing loss. For example, hearing loss may occur in people who have rheumatoid arthritis, systemic lupus erythematosus, and polyarteritis nodosa. A fluctuating hearing loss, which may be progressive, occurs in both ears. The cause is an attack by the immune system on the cells of the cochlea.

Drugs: Drugs sometimes cause hearing loss. Intravenous antibiotics in the aminoglycoside family are the drugs most commonly implicated, particularly when given in high doses. Some people have a rare hereditary disorder that makes them extremely susceptible to hearing loss caused by aminoglycosides. Other drugs include vancomycin, quinine, and the cancer chemotherapy drugs cisplatin and nitrogen mustard. Hearing loss can be caused by aspirin (salicylate), but hearing can come back when the drug is discontinued.

Sudden Deafness: Sudden deafness is deafness that occurs within minutes or over a few hours. It may be caused by something as trivial as wax accumulation or may be caused by head trauma, sudden changes in pressure (as occurs in airplanes), or internal pressure changes caused by severe straining (as may occur with weight lifting). Some infections, drugs, and disorders of the blood vessels to the ear can cause it as well.

Tumors: Hearing loss that is more severe in one ear may be caused by a noncancerous (benign) tumor. Such tumors include a vestibular schwannoma (more commonly termed an acoustic neuroma) and a meningioma. The hearing loss may be accompanied by tinnitus, difficulty with balance, and facial numbness or weakness.

Diagnosis

Doctors should screen for hearing problems during regular checkups, but hearing loss generally needs to be evaluated by an otolaryngologist—a doctor who specializes in the care of the ear. An audiologist is a trained professional who tests hearing and performs hearing evaluation tests that measure the degree of hearing loss and the particular sound frequencies that are impaired. If hearing loss is present, other tests help determine how much the hearing loss affects the person's ability to understand speech and whether the hearing loss is sensorineural, conductive, or mixed. Some hearing tests also help identify possible causes of hearing loss. Although many hearing tests require the person's active participation, some do not.

Sudden deafness is an emergency that requires immediate evaluation by a specialist. Blood tests are performed, and, rarely, exploratory surgery is necessary.

First, a doctor examines the ears. Using a hand-held otoscope, the doctor looks to make sure the ear canal is completely open. The otoscope also allows the doctor to see the eardrum, which helps determine whether a middle-ear infection is present or whether fluid has accumulated behind the eardrum. Sometimes doctors screen for hearing loss using a hand-held tone generator. Some combination of the following tests is usually needed to better understand the hearing loss, determine its cause, and direct treatment.

Audiometry is the first step in hearing testing. In this test, a person wears headphones that play tones of different frequency (pitch) and loudness into one ear or the other. The person signals when a tone is heard, usually by raising the corresponding hand. For each pitch, the test identifies the quietest tone the person can hear in each ear. The results are presented in comparison to what is considered normal hearing. Because loud tones presented to one ear may also be heard by the other ear, a sound other than the test tone (usually white noise) is presented to the ear not being tested.

Speech threshold audiometry measures how loudly words have to be spoken to be understood. A person listens to a series of two-syllable, equally accented words (spondees), such as "railroad," "stairway," and "baseball," presented at different volumes. The volume at which the person can correctly repeat half of the words (spondee threshold) is recorded.

Discrimination, the ability to hear differences between words that sound similar, is tested by presenting pairs of similar one-syllable words. The percentage of words correctly repeated is the discrimination score. People with a conductive hearing loss usually have a normal discrimination score, although at a higher volume. People with sensorineural hearing loss often have abnormal discrimination at all volumes.

Tympanometry tests how well sound can pass through the eardrum and middle ear. This test does not require the active participation of the person being tested and is commonly used in children. A device containing a microphone and a sound source is placed snugly in the ear canal, and sound waves are bounced off the eardrum as the device varies the pressure in the ear canal. Abnormal tympanometry results suggest a conductive type of hearing loss.

The **Rinne tuning fork test** is a screening test that helps distinguish between conductive and senso-

rineural hearing loss. This test compares how well a person hears sounds conducted by air with how well the person hears sounds conducted by the skull bones. To test hearing by air conduction, the tuning fork is placed near the ear. To test hearing by bone conduction, the base of a vibrating tuning fork is placed against the head so the sound bypasses the middle ear and goes directly to the nerve cells of the inner ear. If hearing by air conduction is reduced but hearing by bone conduction is normal, the hearing loss is conductive. If both air and bone conduction hearing are reduced, the hearing loss is sensorineural or mixed. People with sensorineural hearing loss may need further evaluation to look for other conditions, such as Meniere's disease or brain tumors.

Measurement of Loudness

Loudness is measured on a logarithmic scale. This means that an increase of 10 decibels (dB) represents a 10-fold increase in sound intensity and a doubling of the perceived loudness. Thus, 20 dB is 100 times the intensity of 0 dB and seems 4 times as loud; 30 dB is 1,000 times the intensity of 0 dB and seems 8 times as loud.

Decibels	Example
0	Faintest sound heard by human ear
30	Whisper, quiet library
60	Normal conversation, sewing machine, typewriter
90	Lawnmower, shop tools, truck traffic (8 hours per day is the maximum exposure without protection*)
100	Chainsaw, pneumatic drill, snowmobile (2 hours per day is the maximum exposure without protection)
115	Sandblasting, loud rock concert, automobile horn (15 minutes per day is the maximum exposure without protection)
140	Gun muzzle blast, jet engine (noise causes pain, and even brief exposure injures unprotected ears; injury may occur even with hearing protectors)
180	Rocket launching pad

*Mandatory federal standard, but protection is recommended for sound levels above 85 dB.

Auditory brain stem response is a test that measures nerve impulses in the brain stem resulting from sound signals in the ears. The information helps determine what kind of signals the brain is receiving from the ears. Test results are abnormal in people with some sensorineural types of hearing loss and in people with many types of brain tumors. Auditory brain stem response is used to test infants and also can be used to monitor certain brain functions in people who are comatose or undergoing brain surgery.

Electrocochleography measures the activity of the cochlea and the auditory nerve by means of an electrode placed on, or through, the eardrum. This test and the auditory brain stem response can be used to measure hearing in people who cannot or will not respond voluntarily to sound. For example, these tests are used to find out whether infants and very young children have profound hearing loss (deafness) and whether a person is faking or exaggerating hearing loss (psychogenic hypacusis).

Otoacoustic emissions testing uses sound to stimulate the inner ear (cochlea). The ear itself then generates a very low-intensity sound that matches the stimulus. These cochlear emissions are recorded using sophisticated electronics and are used routinely in many nurseries to screen newborns for congenital hearing loss. This test is also used in adults to help determine the reason for a hearing loss.

Other tests can measure the ability to interpret and understand distorted speech, understand a message presented to one ear when a competing message is presented to the other ear, fuse incomplete messages to each ear into a meaningful message, and determine where a sound is coming from when it is presented to both ears at the same time. Depending on the person's symptoms and the results of the hearing tests, some people need computed tomography (CT) or magnetic resonance imaging (MRI) to look for tumors invading structures of the ear or blocking the eustachian tube.

Prevention and Treatment

Age-related hearing loss and many other causes of hearing loss are not preventable. However, many measures can be taken to help prevent noise-induced hearing loss, such as limiting exposure to loud noise, reducing noise levels whenever possible, and staying away from the source of the noise. The volume of music played through headphones should always be kept at a reasonable level. The louder the noise, the less time a person should spend near it. For occupational or firearm exposure, the use of hearing protectors, such as plastic or foam rubber plugs in the ear canals or glycerin-filled muffs over the ears, is essential. Plastic plugs can also be used in other loud environments.

Treatment of hearing loss depends on the cause. When the cause is obstruction of the canal from debris or wax, a doctor can vacuum (wash) the canal or recommend over-the-counter drops that dissolve ear wax. When the cause is fluid in the middle ear, children and adults may need to have a small tube placed in the eardrum (tympanostomy—see art on page 1810). The tube helps prevent fluid from accumulating. Some children also need to have their adenoids removed (adenoidectomy), which helps keep the eustachian tubes open. Hearing loss caused by autoimmune disorders and sudden hearing loss are treated with corticosteroids, such as prednisone.

Damage to the eardrums or the bones in the middle ear may require reconstructive surgery. For some people with otosclerosis, hearing may be restored by removing the stirrup surgically and replacing it with an artificial one. Brain tumors causing hearing loss may, in some cases, be removed and the hearing preserved.

Most other causes of hearing loss have no cure. In these cases, treatment involves compensating for the hearing loss as much as possible. Most people with moderate to severe loss use hearing aids. Those with severe to profound loss are greatly helped by a cochlear implant.

Hearing Aids: Sound amplification with a hearing aid helps people who have either conductive or sensorineural hearing loss. Unfortunately, a hearing aid does not restore hearing to normal. A hearing aid should, however, significantly improve a person's ability to communicate and enjoy sounds.

Many people are reluctant to wear hearing aids because of social stigma. Doctors should discuss such issues and encourage people to meet with an audiologist to evaluate the array of different hearing aid designs available. Some older people and those with arthritis or neurologic problems find it difficult to manipulate the smallest hearing aids and should consider slightly larger devices.

All hearing aids have a microphone to pick up sounds, a battery-powered amplifier to increase their volume, and a means of transmitting the sound to the person. Most hearing aids transmit the sounds through a small speaker placed in the ear canal. Other hearing aids, which require surgical implantation, transmit sounds directly to the bones of the middle ear (ossicles) or the skull instead of through a speaker. Hearing aids differ in how big the components are and where they are located. As a general rule, larger hearing aids are more noticeable and less attractive but are easier to adjust. Larger hearing aids can often accommodate features that are not available in small ones.

Hearing aids have different electronic characteristics that are chosen to suit the person's particular

Hearing Aids: Amplifying the Sound

The behind-the-ear hearing aid is the most powerful but least attractive hearing aid. The in-the-ear hearing aid is the best choice for severe hearing loss. It is easy to adjust but is difficult to use with telephones. The in-the-canal hearing aid is used for mild to moderate hearing loss. This aid is relatively inconspicuous but is difficult to use with telephones. The completely-in-the-canal hearing aid is used for mild to moderate hearing loss. This aid has good sound, is nearly invisible, and can be easily used with telephones. It is removed by pulling on a small string. However, it is the most expensive and hard to adjust.

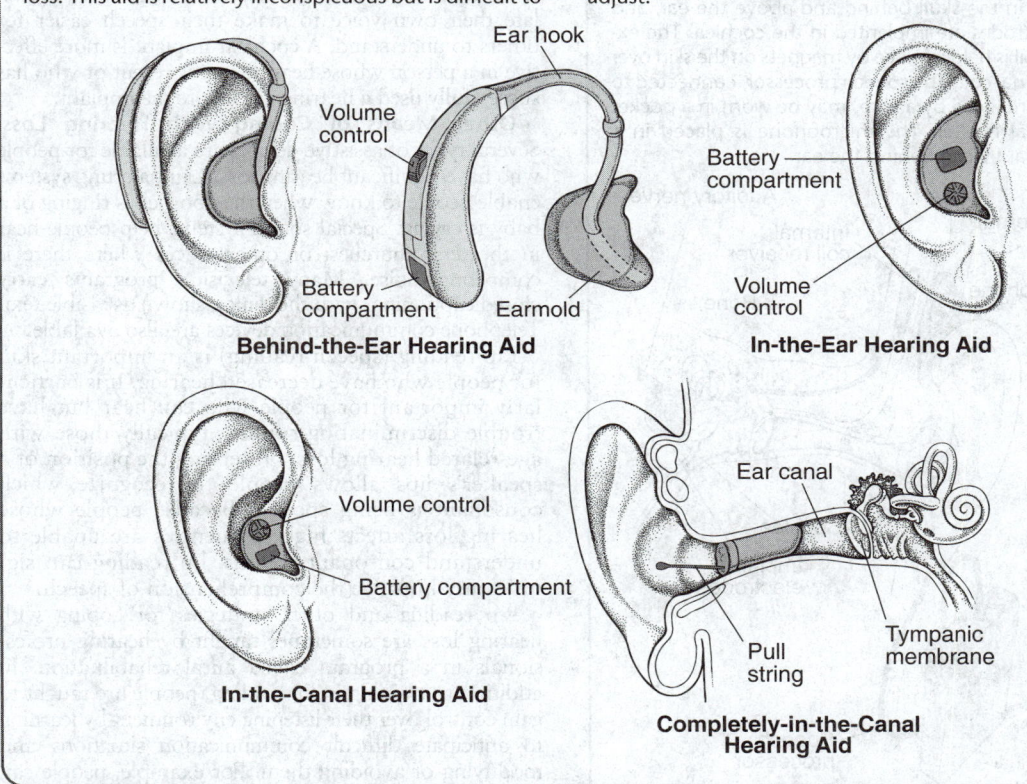

Behind-the-Ear Hearing Aid

In-the-Ear Hearing Aid

In-the-Canal Hearing Aid

Completely-in-the-Canal Hearing Aid

type of hearing loss. For example, people whose hearing loss affects mainly higher frequencies do not benefit from simple amplification, which merely makes the mumbled speech they hear sound louder. Hearing aids that selectively amplify the high frequencies markedly improve speech recognition. Other hearing aids contain vents in the ear mold, which facilitate the passage of high-frequency sound waves into the ear. Many hearing aids use digital sound processing with multiple frequency channels so that the amplification can even more precisely match the person's hearing loss. People who cannot tolerate loud sounds may need hearing aids with special electronic circuitry, which keeps the maximum volume of sound at a tolerable level.

Telephone use can be difficult for people with hearing aids. With typical hearing aids, placing the ear next to the phone handle causes squealing. Some hearing aids have a phone coil. With the flip of a switch the microphone is turned off, and the phone coil links electromagnetically to the magnet in the phone handle. As long as the hearing aid has the proper features, this setup can be arranged by the phone company with simple changes to the phone. Hearing aids with complex features tend to be the most expensive but are often essential to meet hearing needs.

Cochlear Implants: Most profoundly deaf people who cannot hear sounds even with a hearing aid benefit from a cochlear implant. Cochlear implants provide electrical signals directly into the auditory

Cochlear Implant: Aid for the Severely to Profoundly Deaf

A cochlear implant, a type of hearing aid for severely to profoundly deaf people, consists of an internal coil, electrodes, an external coil, a speech processor, and a microphone. The internal coil is surgically implanted in the skull behind and above the ear, and the electrodes are implanted in the cochlea. The external coil is held in place by magnets on the skin over the internal coil. The speech processor, connected to the external coil by a wire, may be worn in a pocket or special holster. The microphone is placed in a hearing aid worn behind the ear.

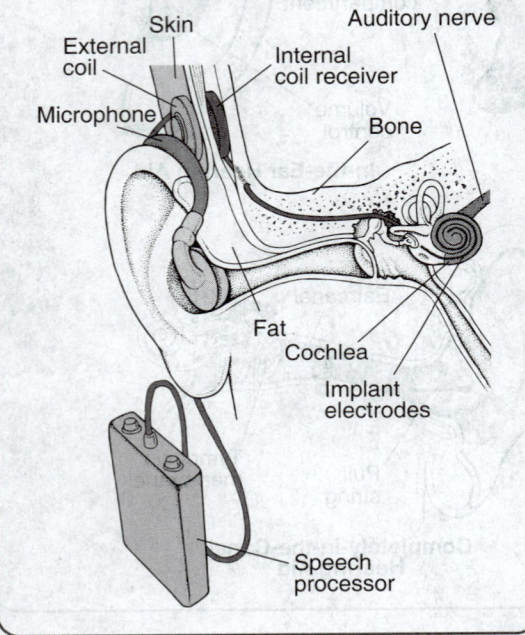

A cochlear implant does not transmit sounds as well as a normal cochlea but does provide substantial benefit to the hearing impaired. It helps people read lips. Most implantees can distinguish words without reading lips and also use the telephone.

A cochlear implant also helps deaf people hear and distinguish environmental and warning signals, such as doorbells, telephones, and alarms. It helps them modulate their own voice to make their speech easier for others to understand. A cochlear implant is more effective in a person whose hearing loss is recent or who has successfully used a hearing aid before the implant.

Other Means of Coping With Hearing Loss: Several types of assistive devices are available for people who have significant hearing loss. Light alerting systems enable people to know when the doorbell is ringing or a baby is crying. Special sound systems help people hear in theaters, churches, or other places where there is competing noise. Many television programs carry closed captioning, with the dialog shown as visible text. Telephone communication devices are also available.

Lip reading (speech reading) is an important skill for people who have decreased hearing. It is particularly important for people who can hear but have trouble discriminating sounds, typically those with age-related hearing loss. Observing the position of a speaker's lips allows people to recognize which consonant is being spoken. Because people whose hearing loss affects high frequencies are unable to understand consonant sounds, lip reading can significantly improve the comprehension of speech.

Lip reading and other strategies for coping with hearing loss are sometimes taught by hearing professionals in a program called aural rehabilitation. In addition to training in lip reading, people are taught to gain control over their listening environment by learning to anticipate difficult communication situations and modifying or avoiding them. For example, people can visit a restaurant during off-peak hours, when it is quieter. They can ask for a booth, which blocks out some extraneous sounds. They can request that specials of the day be written rather than spoken. In direct conversations, people may ask the speaker to face them. At the beginning of a telephone conversation, people can identify themselves as being hearing-impaired.

People with profound hearing loss often communicate using sign language. American Sign Language (ASL) is the version most widely used in the United States. Other forms include Signed English, Signing Exact English, and Cued Speech.

nerve by means of multiple electrodes inserted into the cochlea, which is the inner ear structure containing the auditory nerve. An external microphone and processor pick up sound signals and convert them to electrical impulses. The impulses are transmitted electromagnetically by an external coil through the skin to an internal coil, which connects to the electrodes. The electrodes stimulate the auditory nerve.

CHAPTER 213 Outer Ear Disorders

The outer ear consists of the external part of the ear (pinna or auricle) and the ear canal (external auditory meatus—see art on page 1376). Disorders of the outer ear include blockages, infections (external otitis and perichondritis), eczema, and tumors. The outer ear is also prone to certain types of injury.

Blockages

Earwax (cerumen) may block the ear canal. Even large amounts of earwax often cause no symptoms. Symptoms can range from itching to a loss of hearing. A doctor may remove the earwax by gently flushing out the ear canal with warm water (irrigation). However, if a person has had a perforated eardrum, irrigation is not used because water can enter the middle ear and may cause a middle ear infection. Similarly, irrigation is not used if there is any discharge from the ear, because the discharge may be coming from a perforated eardrum. In these situations, a doctor may remove earwax with an earwax curette, an instrument with a loop at the end, or a vacuum device.

Certain solvents help soften earwax, but they usually must be followed by irrigation, because the solvent rarely dissolves all of the earwax. People should not attempt removal at home with cotton swabs, bobby pins, pencils, or any other implements. Such attempts usually just pack the earwax in more and can damage the eardrum. Soap and water on a washcloth provide adequate external ear hygiene.

Other blockages can occur when people, particularly children, put foreign objects, such as beads, erasers, and beans, into the ear canal. Usually, a doctor removes such objects with a blunt hook or small vacuum device. Sometimes metal and glass beads can be flushed out by irrigation, but water causes some objects, such as beans, to swell, complicating removal. Objects that are deep in the canal are more difficult to remove because of the risk of injury to the eardrum. A general anesthetic is used when a child does not cooperate or when removal is particularly difficult.

Insects, particularly cockroaches, may also block the ear canal. To kill the insect, a doctor fills the canal with mineral oil or thickened lidocaine, a numbing agent. This measure also provides immediate pain relief and enables the doctor to remove the insect.

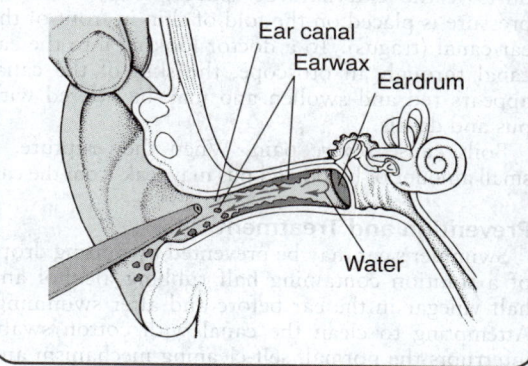

Irrigating the Ear Canal

The tip of a water-filled syringe is placed just inside the ear canal, and a stream of warm water is gently directed into the canal to remove earwax. This procedure should be performed by a doctor or a nurse.

Ear canal
Earwax
Eardrum
Water

External Otitis

External otitis is infection of the ear canal.

- External otitis is caused by bacteria or, rarely, fungi.
- Typical symptoms are itching, pain, and discharge.
- A doctor looks in the ear with an otoscope (a device for viewing the canal and eardrum) for redness, swelling, and pus.
- Debris removal, ear drops, and pain relievers are the most common forms of treatment.

External otitis may affect the entire canal, as in generalized external otitis, or just one small area, as when pus accumulates in a boil (furuncle) or pimple.

Causes

A variety of bacteria or, rarely, fungi can cause generalized external otitis. Certain people, including those who have allergies, psoriasis, eczema, or scalp dermatitis, are particularly prone to external otitis. Injuring the ear canal while cleaning it or getting water or irritants, such as hair spray or hair dye, in the canal often leads to external otitis. External otitis is particularly common after swimming, in which case it is sometimes called **swimmer's ear**. Earplugs and hearing aids make external otitis more likely, particularly if these devices are not properly cleaned.

Symptoms and Diagnosis

Symptoms of generalized external otitis are itching and pain. Sometimes an unpleasant-smelling white or yellow discharge drains from the ear. The ear canal may have no swelling or slight swelling, or, in severe cases, it may be swollen completely closed. If the ear canal swells or fills with pus and debris, hearing is impaired. Usually, the canal is tender and hurts if the external ear (pinna) is pulled or if pressure is placed on the fold of skin in front of the ear canal (tragus). To a doctor looking into the ear canal through an otoscope, the skin of the canal appears red and swollen and may be littered with pus and debris.

Boils cause severe pain. When they rupture, a small amount of blood and pus may leak from the ear.

Prevention and Treatment

Swimmer's ear may be prevented by putting drops of a solution containing half rubbing alcohol and half vinegar in the ear before and after swimming. Attempting to clean the canal with cotton swabs interrupts the normal, self-cleaning mechanism and can push debris toward the eardrum, where it accumulates. Also, these actions may cause minor damage that predisposes to external otitis.

To treat generalized external otitis from any cause, a doctor first removes the infected debris from the canal with suction or dry cotton wipes. After the ear canal is cleared, hearing often returns to normal. Usually, a person is given ear drops containing vinegar and drops containing a corticosteroid such as hydrocortisone to use several times a day for up to a week. Vinegar is helpful because bacteria do not grow as well once the normal acidity of the ear canal is restored. With moderate or severe infection, antibiotic drops also are prescribed. If the ear canal is very swollen, a doctor inserts a small wick in the canal to allow the drops to penetrate.

Analgesics such as acetaminophen or codeine may help reduce pain for the first 24 to 48 hours, until the inflammation begins to subside. An infection that has spread beyond the ear canal (cellulitis—see page 1315) may be treated with an antibiotic given by mouth.

Treatment of boils depends on how advanced the infection is. In an early stage of infection, a heating pad can be applied for a short time and analgesics can be given to help relieve pain. The heat may also help speed healing. A boil that has come to a head is cut open to drain the pus. An antibiotic is then applied directly to the area or given by mouth.

MALIGNANT EXTERNAL OTITIS

Malignant external otitis is infection of the external ear that has spread to involve the skull bone containing part of the ear canal, the middle ear, and the inner ear (temporal bone).

Malignant external otitis occurs mainly in people with weakened immune systems and in older people with diabetes. Infection of the external ear, usually caused by the bacteria *Pseudomonas*, spreads into the temporal bone, causing severe, life-threatening infection.

People have severe earache, a foul-smelling discharge from the ear, and usually decreased hearing.

The diagnosis is based on computed tomography (CT) scan results. Often doctors need to take a small piece of tissue from the ear canal to make sure that the symptoms are not the result of cancer.

Malignant external otitis is treated with a 6-week course of antibiotics given by vein.

Perichondritis

Perichondritis is infection of the tissue surrounding the cartilage of the earlobe (pinna), ear canal, or both.

Injury, burns, insect bites, ear piercing, or a boil on the ear may cause perichondritis. The infection also tends to occur in people whose immune system is weakened and in people who have diabetes. The first symptoms are redness, pain, and swelling of the earlobe. The person may have a fever. Pus accumulates between the cartilage and the layer of connective tissue around it (perichondrium). Sometimes the pus cuts off the blood supply to the cartilage, destroying it and leading eventually to a deformed ear. Although destructive and long-lasting, perichondritis tends to cause only mild discomfort.

A doctor makes an incision to drain the pus, allowing blood to reach the cartilage again. Antibiotics are given by mouth for milder infections and by vein for severe infections. The choice of antibiotic depends on how severe the infection is and which bacteria are causing it.

Tumors

Tumors of the ear may be noncancerous (benign) or cancerous (malignant). Most ear tumors are found when people see them or when a doctor looks in the ear because people notice their hearing seems decreased.

Noncancerous tumors may develop in the ear canal, blocking it and causing hearing loss and a buildup of earwax. Such tumors include small sacs filled with skin secretions (sebaceous cysts), osteomas (bone tumors), and growths of excess scar tissue after an injury (keloids). The most effective treatment is surgical removal of the tumor. After treatment, hearing usually returns to normal.

Basal cell and squamous cell cancers (see page 1333) are common skin cancers that often develop on the external ear after repeated and prolonged exposure to the sun. When these cancers first appear, they can be successfully treated by removing them surgically or by applying radiation therapy. More advanced cancers may require surgical removal of a larger area of the external ear.

Ceruminoma (cancer of the cells that produce earwax) develops in the outer third of the ear canal and can spread. Ceruminomas have nothing to do with earwax buildup. Treatment consists of removing the cancer and the surrounding tissue surgically.

Injury

A number of different injuries can affect the outer ear. A blunt blow to the external ear can cause bruising between the cartilage and the layer of connective tissue around it (perichondrium). When blood collects in this area, the external ear becomes swollen and purple. The collected blood (hematoma) can cut off the blood supply to the cartilage, allowing that portion of the cartilage to die, leading in time to a deformed ear. This deformity, called a cauliflower ear, is common among wrestlers, boxers, and rugby players.

A doctor cuts open the hematoma and removes the blood with suction. After the hematoma is empty, the doctor applies a compression dressing, which is left on for 3 to 7 days to keep the hematoma from coming back. The dressing keeps the skin and perichondrium in their normal positions, allowing blood to reach the cartilage again.

If a cut (laceration) goes all the way through the ear, the area is cleaned thoroughly, the skin is sewn back together, and a dressing is applied to protect the area and allow the cartilage to heal. The cartilage is not sewn.

A forceful blow to the jaw may fracture the bones surrounding the ear canal and distort the canal's shape, often narrowing it. The shape can be corrected surgically.

CHAPTER

214 Middle and Inner Ear Disorders

The middle ear consists of the eardrum (tympanic membrane) and an air-filled chamber containing a chain of three bones (ossicles) that connect the eardrum to the inner ear (see page 1376). The fluid-filled inner ear (labyrinth) consists of two major parts: the organ of hearing (cochlea) and the organ of balance (vestibular system, which consists of the semicircular canals, the saccule, and the utricle). The middle ear acts as an amplifier of sound, whereas the inner ear acts as a transducer, changing mechanical sound waves into an electrical signal that is sent to the brain via the nerve of hearing (statoacoustic nerve). Middle and inner ear disorders cause many of the same symptoms, and a disorder of the middle ear may affect the inner ear and vice versa.

Eardrum Perforation

A perforation is a hole in the eardrum.

- Eardrum perforations are often caused by middle ear infections.
- Perforation causes sudden ear pain, sometimes with bleeding from the ear, hearing loss, or noise in the ear.
- Doctors can see the perforation with an otoscope.
- Usually the eardrum heals on its own, but sometimes surgical repair is needed.

A middle ear infection (otitis media) is the most common cause of eardrum perforation. The eardrum can also be perforated by a sudden change in pressure—either an increase, such as that caused by an explosion, a slap, or diving underwater; or a decrease, such as occurs while flying in an airplane. Another cause is burns from heat or chemicals. The eardrum may also be perforated (punctured) by objects placed in the ear, such as a cotton-tipped swab, or by objects entering the ear accidentally, such as a low-hanging twig or a thrown pencil. An object that penetrates the eardrum can dislocate or fracture the chain of small bones (ossicles) that connect the eardrum to the inner ear. Pieces of the broken ossicles or the object itself may even penetrate the inner ear. A blocked eustachian tube, which connects the middle ear and the back of the nose, may lead to the perforation because of severe imbalance of pressure (barotrauma).

Symptoms and Diagnosis

Perforation of the eardrum causes sudden severe pain, sometimes followed by bleeding from the ear, hearing loss, and noise in the ear (tinnitus—see page 1392). The hearing loss is more severe if the chain of ossicles has been disrupted or the inner ear has been injured. Injury to the inner ear may also cause vertigo (a whirling sensation). Pus may begin to drain from the ear in 24 to 48 hours, particularly if water or other foreign material enters the middle ear. A doctor diagnoses eardrum perforation by looking in the ear with a special instrument called an otoscope. Sometimes formal hearing tests are performed.

Treatment

The ear is kept dry. An antibiotic given by mouth may be used if the ear becomes infected. Ear drops may be given for contaminated injuries. Usually, the eardrum heals without further treatment, but if it does not heal within 2 months, surgery to repair the eardrum (tympanoplasty) may be needed. People with a severe injury, particularly one accompanied by marked hearing loss, severe vertigo, or both, may need to have more immediate surgery. If a perforation is not repaired, the person may develop a smoldering infection—chronic otitis media—in the middle ear.

A persistent conductive hearing loss (see page 1379) occurring after perforation of the eardrum suggests a disruption or fixation of the ossicles, which may be repaired surgically. A sensorineural hearing loss or vertigo that persists for more than a few hours after the injury suggests that something has injured or penetrated the inner ear.

Barotrauma

Barotrauma (barotitis media or aerotitis media) is damage to the middle ear caused by unequal air pressure on the two sides of the eardrum.

The eardrum separates the ear canal and the middle ear. If air pressure in the ear canal from outside air and air pressure in the middle ear are unequal, the eardrum can be damaged. Normally, the eustachian tube, which connects the middle ear and the back of the nose, helps maintain equal pressure on both sides of the eardrum by allowing outside air to enter the middle ear. When outside air pressure changes suddenly—for example, during the ascent or descent of an airplane or a deep-sea dive (see page 1996)—air must move through the eustachian tube to equalize the pressure in the middle ear.

If the eustachian tube is partly or completely blocked because of scarring, a tumor, an infection, the common cold, or an allergy, air cannot move in and out of the middle ear. The resulting pressure difference may bruise the eardrum or even cause it to rupture and bleed. If the pressure difference is very great, the oval window (the entrance into the inner ear from the middle ear) may rupture, allowing fluid from the inner ear to leak into the middle ear. Hearing loss or vertigo occurring during descent in a deep-sea dive suggests that such leakage is taking place. The same symptoms occurring during ascent suggest that an air bubble has formed in the inner ear.

Prevention and Treatment

When sudden changes in pressure cause a sense of fullness or pain in the ear, often the pressure in the middle ear can be equalized and the discomfort can be relieved by several maneuvers. If outside pressure is decreasing, as in a plane ascending, the person should try breathing with the mouth open, chewing gum, or swallowing. Any of these measures may open the eustachian tube and allow air out of the middle ear. If outside pressure is increasing, as in a plane descending or a diver going deeper underwater, the person should pinch the nose shut, hold the mouth closed, and try to blow gently out through the nose. This will force air through the blocked eustachian tube. People who have an infection or an allergy affecting the nose and throat may experience discomfort when they fly in a plane or dive. However, if flying is necessary, a decongestant, such as phenylephrine nose drops or nasal spray, relieves congestion and helps open the eustachian tubes, equalizing pressure on the eardrums. Diving should be avoided until the infection or allergy is controlled.

Infectious Myringitis

Infectious myringitis is infection of the eardrum by a virus or bacteria.

Myringitis is caused by a variety of viruses and bacteria. The bacteria *Mycoplasma* is a common cause. The eardrum becomes inflamed, and small, fluid-filled blisters (vesicles) form on its surface. Blisters may also be present in otitis media; however, in myringitis, there is no pus or fluid in the middle ear.

Pain begins suddenly and lasts for 24 to 48 hours. There may be some hearing loss.

Doctors diagnose myringitis by looking at the eardrum with an otoscope. Because it is difficult to tell whether the infection is viral or bacterial, most people are treated with antibiotics and analgesics. A doctor may need to rupture the vesicles with a small blade to relieve the pain.

Acute Otitis Media

Acute otitis media is a bacterial or viral infection of the middle ear.

The Eustachian Tube: Keeping Air Pressure Equal

The eustachian tube helps maintain equal air pressure on both sides of the eardrum by allowing outside air to enter the middle ear. If the eustachian tube is blocked, air cannot reach the middle ear, so the pressure there decreases. When air pressure is lower in the middle ear than in the ear canal, the eardrum bulges inward. The pressure difference can cause pain and can bruise or rupture the eardrum.

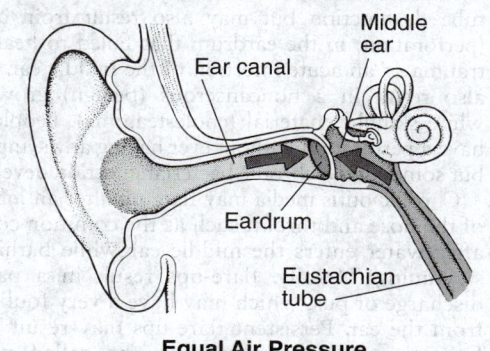

Equal Air Pressure

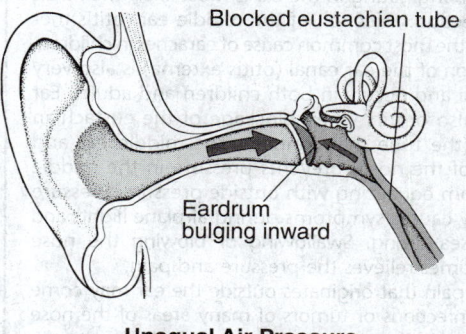

Unequal Air Pressure

Acute otitis media results from infection by viruses or bacteria, often as a complication of the common cold or of allergies. Acute otitis media is more common among children than adults (see page 1809). Symptoms and treatment are similar in adults and older children.

The infected ear is painful, with a red, bulging eardrum. Most people with acute otitis media get better without treatment. However, because it is hard to predict whose symptoms will not lessen, some doctors treat all people with antibiotics, such as amoxicillin. Other doctors give antibiotics only if the illness is severe or if symptoms do not lessen after 72 hours. Pain relief is important. Acetaminophen or nonsteroidal anti-inflammatory drugs (NSAIDs) can relieve pain. Decongestants containing phenylephrine may help adults (but not children), and antihistamines are useful for people who have allergies but not for those with colds.

If a person has severe or persistent pain and fever, and the eardrum is bulging, a doctor may perform a myringotomy, in which an opening is made through the eardrum to allow fluid to drain from the middle ear. The opening, which does not affect hearing, usually heals without treatment. People who have repeated bouts of otitis media may need to have drainage tubes (tympanostomy tubes) placed in their eardrums (see art on page 1810).

Secretory Otitis Media

Secretory otitis media is an accumulation of fluid in the middle ear.

- Secretory otitis media occurs when acute otitis media has not completely resolved or allergies cause blockage of the eustachian tube.
- People may have fullness and some temporary hearing loss in the affected ear.
- Doctors examine the ear and use tympanometry to diagnose this disorder.
- Doctors may need to make an opening in the eardrum to let fluid drain.

Secretory (serous) otitis media can develop from acute otitis media that has not completely cleared or from a blocked eustachian tube (which connects the middle ear and the back of the nose). Allergies are a common cause of eustachian tube blockage. Secretory otitis media can occur at any age but is particularly common among children (see page 1810).

Normally, pressure in the middle ear is equalized 3 or 4 times a minute as the eustachian tube opens during swallowing. If the eustachian tube is blocked, pressure in the middle ear tends to decrease as oxygen is absorbed into the bloodstream from the middle ear. As the pressure decreases, fluid accumulates in the middle ear, reducing the eardrum's ability to move. Usually, although not always, the fluid contains some bacteria, but symptoms of active infection (such as redness, pain, and pus) are rare. People usually notice a fullness in the affected ear and may hear a popping or crackling sound when they swallow. Some hearing loss commonly develops.

A doctor examines the ear to make the diagnosis. Tympanometry (see page 1381) helps determine whether fluid is in the middle ear.

When the Ear Aches

An earache is pain that seems to originate in the ear. The actual source of pain may be within the ear or in nearby structures that share the same nerves to the brain. This type of pain is called referred pain.

Pain originating in the ear is most likely the result of infection. Infection of the middle ear (otitis media) is the most common cause of earaches in children. Infection of the ear canal (otitis externa) is also very painful and occurs in both children and adults. Ear pain also occurs when blockage of the eustachian tube (the tube that connects the middle ear and back of the nose) prevents pressure in the middle ear from equalizing with outside pressure. Pressure mainly causes symptoms during airplane flights and undersea diving. Swallowing or blowing the nose sometimes relieves the pressure and pain.

Ear pain that originates outside the ear may come from infections or tumors of many areas of the nose and throat. If a person with an earache has no apparent ear disorder, doctors look for problems with the nose, sinuses, teeth, gums, jaw joint (temporomandibular joint), tongue, tonsils, throat (pharynx), voice box (larynx), windpipe (trachea), esophagus, and salivary glands in the cheek (parotid glands). Sometimes, the first symptom of cancer in any of these structures is pain that feels like an earache.

Treatment

Decongestants, such as phenylephrine and ephedrine, and, in people with allergies, antihistamines can be taken to reduce nasal congestion but do not help the secretory otitis media. Antibiotics are not helpful. Low pressure in the middle ear can be temporarily increased by forcing air past the blockage in the eustachian tube. To do this, the person breathes out with the mouth closed and the nostrils pinched shut.

If symptoms become chronic (lasting more than 3 months), a doctor may perform a myringotomy, in which an opening is made through the eardrum to allow fluid to drain from the middle ear. A tiny drainage tube (tympanostomy tube—see art on page 1810) can be inserted into the opening in the eardrum to help fluid drain and allow air to enter the middle ear.

Chronic Otitis Media

Chronic otitis media is a long-standing infection of the middle ear.

- Chronic otitis media is caused by a cholesteatoma or by an eardrum perforation that has not healed.

- A flare up may occur after an ear infection or after water enters the middle ear.
- The person may have a persistent discharge of foul-smelling pus.
- Doctors clean the ear canal and give eardrops.

Chronic otitis media is usually caused by eustachian tube dysfunction but may also result from a hole (perforation) in the eardrum that failed to heal after trauma or an acute infection of the middle ear. It can also result in a noncancerous (benign) growth of white skinlike material (cholesteatoma). People may have a perforation without ever having any symptoms, but sometimes a chronic bacterial infection develops.

Chronic otitis media may flare up after an infection of the nose and throat, such as the common cold, or after water enters the middle ear while bathing or swimming. Usually, flare-ups result in a painless discharge of pus, which may have a very foul smell, from the ear. Persistent flare-ups may result in the formation of protruding growths called polyps, which extend from the middle ear through the perforation and into the ear canal. Persistent infection can destroy parts of the ossicles—the small bones in the middle ear that connect the eardrum to the inner ear and conduct sounds from the outer ear to the inner ear—causing conductive hearing loss (see page 1379). Other serious complications include inflammation of the inner ear, facial paralysis, and brain infections. Some people with chronic otitis media develop a cholesteatoma in the middle ear. A cholesteatoma, which destroys bone, greatly increases the likelihood of other serious complications.

A doctor diagnoses chronic otitis media when pus or skinlike material accumulates in a hole or in a pocket in the eardrum that often drains.

Treatment

When chronic otitis media flares up, a doctor thoroughly cleans the ear canal and middle ear with suction and dry cotton wipes, then prescribes a solution of acetic acid with hydrocortisone or antibiotic ear drops. Water must be kept out of the ear when a perforation is present.

Usually, the eardrum can be repaired by a procedure called tympanoplasty. If the ossicular chain has been disrupted, it may be repaired at the same time. A cholesteatoma must be removed surgically. Otherwise, serious complications can develop.

Mastoiditis

Mastoiditis is a bacterial infection in the mastoid process, the prominent bone behind the ear.

This disorder usually occurs when untreated or inadequately treated acute otitis media spreads from the middle ear into the surrounding bone—the mastoid process.

Usually, symptoms appear days to weeks after acute otitis media develops, as the spreading infection destroys the inner part of the mastoid process. A collection of pus (abscess) may form in the bone. The skin covering the mastoid process may become red, swollen, and tender, and the external ear is pushed sideways and down. Other symptoms are fever, pain around and within the ear, and a creamy, profuse discharge from the ear. The pain tends to be persistent and throbbing. Hearing loss can become progressively worse.

Computed tomography (CT) shows that the air cells (spaces in bone that normally contain air) in the mastoid process are filled with fluid. As mastoiditis progresses, the spaces enlarge. Inadequately treated mastoiditis can result in deafness, blood poisoning (sepsis), infection of the tissues covering the brain (meningitis), brain abscess, or death.

Treatment is with antibiotics given by vein. A sample of ear discharge is examined to identify the organism causing the infection and to determine the antibiotics most likely to eliminate the bacteria. Antibiotics may be given by mouth once the person starts to recover and are continued for at least 2 weeks. If an abscess has formed in the bone, surgical drainage (mastoidectomy) is required.

Meniere's Disease

Meniere's disease is a disorder characterized by recurring attacks of disabling vertigo (a whirling sensation), hearing loss, and noise in the ear (tinnitus).

- Symptoms include sudden, unprovoked attacks of severe, disabling vertigo, nausea, and vomiting.
- Doctors usually perform hearing tests and sometimes magnetic resonance imaging.
- A low-salt diet and a diuretic may lower the frequency of attacks.
- Drugs such as meclizine, lorazepam, or scopolamine may help relieve vertigo.

Meniere's disease (also called endolymphatic hydrops) is thought to be caused by an imbalance in the fluid that is normally present in the inner ear. This fluid is continually being secreted and reabsorbed, maintaining a constant amount. Either an increase in production of inner ear fluid or a decrease in its reabsorption results in an imbalance of fluid. Why either happens is not known.

Symptoms include sudden, unprovoked attacks of severe, disabling vertigo, nausea, and vomiting. These symptoms usually last for 2 to 3 hours but can (rarely) last up to 24 hours. Periodically, a person may feel a fullness or pressure in the affected ear. Hearing tends to fluctuate but progressively worsens over the years. Tinnitus, which may be constant or intermittent, may be worse before, during, or after an attack of vertigo. Both hearing loss and tinnitus usually affect only one ear.

In one form of Meniere's disease, hearing loss and tinnitus precede the first attack of vertigo by months or years. After the attacks of vertigo begin, hearing may improve.

Diagnosis and Treatment

A doctor suspects Meniere's disease because of the typical symptoms of vertigo with tinnitus and hearing loss in one ear. Doctors usually perform hearing tests and sometimes magnetic resonance imaging (MRI) to look for other causes. A low-salt diet and a diuretic (a drug that increases the excretion of urine) may lower the frequency of attacks in some people. When attacks do occur, vertigo may be relieved temporarily with drugs given by mouth, such as meclizine, lorazepam, or scopolamine. Scopolamine is also available in skin patches. Nausea and vomiting may be relieved by suppositories containing the drug prochlorperazine.

Several procedures are available for people who are disabled by frequent attacks of vertigo despite drug treatment. The procedures aim to either reduce fluid pressure in the inner ear or destroy inner ear balance function. The endolymphatic shunt procedure, in which a thin sheet of flexible plastic material is placed in the inner ear, is the least destructive of these procedures. To destroy inner ear balance function, a solution of gentamicin can be injected through the eardrum into the middle ear. Gentamicin selectively destroys balance function before affecting hearing, but hearing loss is still a risk. The risk of hearing loss is lower if doctors inject the gentamicin only once and wait several weeks before repeating if necessary. Cutting the vestibular nerve permanently destroys inner ear balance, while preserving hearing, and is successful 95% of the time in controlling vertigo. This procedure is usually performed on people whose symptoms do not lessen after an endolymphatic shunt or on people who never want to experience another spell of vertigo. Finally, when vertigo is disabling and hearing has deteriorated in the involved ear, the semicircular canals can be drilled away in a procedure called a labyrinthectomy.

None of the surgical procedures that treat vertigo are useful in treating the hearing loss that often accompanies Meniere's disease.

Vestibular Neuronitis

Vestibular neuronitis is a disorder characterized by a sudden severe attack of vertigo (a whirling sensation), caused by inflammation of the nerve to the semicircular canals.

Vestibular neuronitis is probably caused by a virus. It may occur as a single, isolated attack of vertigo lasting several days, although many people have additional attacks of milder vertigo for several weeks thereafter. The first attack of vertigo is usually the most severe. The attack, which is accompanied by nausea and vomiting, lasts for 7 to 10 days. The eyes flicker involuntarily away from the affected side (a sign called nystagmus). Each subsequent attack is shorter and less severe than the previous one and typically occurs only when the head is in certain positions. Hearing is usually not affected.

The diagnosis involves hearing tests and tests for nystagmus (see page 662). Magnetic resonance imaging (MRI) of the head may be performed to make sure the symptoms are not caused by another disorder, such as a tumor.

Treatment of vertigo is the same as for Meniere's disease and consists of drugs such as meclizine, lorazepam, or scopolamine. Nausea and vomiting may be relieved by suppositories containing the drug prochlorperazine. If vomiting continues for a long time, a person may need to be given fluids and electrolytes intravenously. The disorder eventually goes away without treatment.

Temporal Bone Fracture

The temporal bone (the skull bone containing part of the ear canal, the middle ear, and the inner ear) can be fractured by a blow to the head.

Temporal bone fractures frequently rupture the eardrum and may also damage the ossicles (the chain of small bones that connects the eardrum to the inner ear) and the cochlea (the organ of hearing).

Symptoms include facial paralysis on the side of the fracture and profound hearing loss, which may be conductive, sensorineural, or both (see page 1379). People may have bleeding from the ear, blood behind the eardrum, or patchy bruising of the skin behind the ear. Sometimes, cerebrospinal fluid leaks from the brain through the fracture and appears as clear fluid draining from the ear or nose. Leakage of this fluid indicates that the brain is exposed to infection.

Diagnosis is made with computed tomography (CT). Treatment usually requires an antibiotic given intravenously to prevent infection of the tissues covering the brain (meningitis). Sometimes, persistent facial paralysis caused by pressure on the facial nerve can be relieved by surgery. Damage to the eardrum and structures of the middle ear is repaired surgically weeks or months later if necessary.

Auditory Nerve Tumors

An auditory nerve tumor (acoustic neuroma, acoustic neurinoma, vestibular schwannoma, eighth nerve tumor) is a

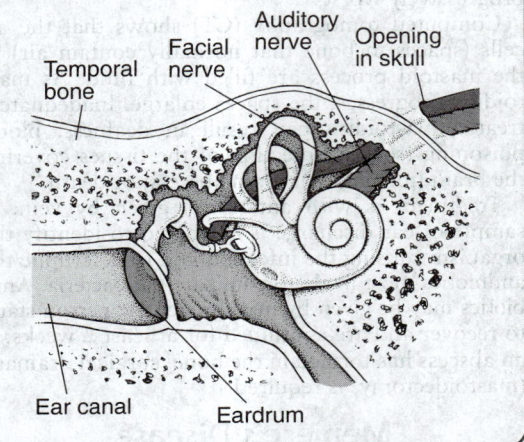

How Ear Disorders Affect the Facial Nerve

Because the facial nerve winds through the ear, disorders of the middle and inner ear can affect it. For example, herpes zoster of the ear may affect the facial nerve as well as the auditory nerve. The facial nerve then swells and presses against the opening in the skull that it passes through. The pressure on this nerve can cause temporary or permanent facial paralysis. Treatment depends on the disorder causing the problem.

noncancerous (benign) tumor that originates in the cells that wrap around the auditory nerve (Schwann cells).

Auditory nerve tumors usually grow from the vestibular (balance) nerve. Early symptoms include noise in the ear (tinnitus), hearing loss, and imbalance or unsteadiness when the person turns quickly. If the tumor grows larger and compresses other parts of the brain, such as the facial nerve or the trigeminal nerve, weakness and numbness of the face may result. Early diagnosis is based on a magnetic resonance imaging (MRI) scan and hearing tests.

Tumors are removed by surgery, which may be performed with a microscope (microsurgery) to avoid damaging the facial nerve.

Tinnitus

Tinnitus is noise originating in the ear rather than in the environment.

- Tinnitus can be a symptom of ear damage, an ear infection, eustachian tube blockage, or hearing loss.
- People have a ringing or buzzing in the ears, especially in quiet environments.

- Hearing tests and imaging tests are used to try to find the cause.
- People may use hearing aids or tinnitus maskers to decrease the sound.

Tinnitus is a symptom and not a specific disease. It is very common—10 to 15% of people experience some degree of tinnitus.

More than 75% of ear-related problems include tinnitus as a symptom, including injury caused by loud noises or explosions, ear infections, a blocked ear canal or eustachian tube (which connects the middle ear and the back of the nose), otosclerosis (a type of hearing loss), tumors of the middle ear, and Meniere's disease. Certain drugs (such as aminoglycoside antibiotics and high doses of aspirin) also may cause tinnitus.

Tinnitus may also occur with disorders outside the ears, including anemia, heart and blood vessel disorders such as hypertension and arteriosclerosis, an underactive thyroid gland (hypothyroidism), and head injury. Tinnitus that is only in one ear or that pulsates is a more serious sign. A pulsating sound may result from certain tumors, a blocked artery, an aneurysm, or other blood vessel disorders.

The noise heard by people with tinnitus may be a buzzing, ringing, roaring, whistling, or hissing sound. Some people hear more complex sounds that vary over time. These sounds are more noticeable in a quiet environment and when the person is not concentrating on something else. Thus, tinnitus tends to be most disturbing to people when they are trying to sleep. However, the experience of tinnitus is highly individual. Some people are very disturbed by their symptoms, whereas others find them quite bearable.

Diagnosis and Treatment

Because a person who has tinnitus usually has some hearing loss, thorough hearing tests are performed as well as magnetic resonance imaging (MRI) of the head and computed tomography (CT) of the temporal bone (the skull bone that contains part of the ear canal, the middle ear, and the inner ear).

Attempts to identify and treat the disorder causing tinnitus are often unsuccessful. Various techniques can help make tinnitus tolerable, although the ability to tolerate it varies from person to person. Often a hearing aid helps suppress tinnitus. Many people find relief by playing background music to mask the tinnitus. Some people use a tinnitus masker, a device worn like a hearing aid that produces a constant level of neutral sounds. For the profoundly deaf, an implant in the cochlea (the organ of hearing) may reduce tinnitus.

CHAPTER 215   Nose, Sinus, and Taste Disorders

The upper part of the nose consists mostly of bone. The lower part of the nose gains its support from cartilage. Inside the nose is a hollow cavity (nasal cavity), which is divided into two passages by a thin sheet of cartilage and bone called the nasal septum. The bones of the face contain the paranasal sinuses, which are hollow cavities that open into the nasal cavity (see page 1377).

Because of its prominent position, the nose is especially vulnerable to injury, including fractures. Infections, nosebleeds, and polyps also can affect the nose. The mucous membrane of the nose may become inflamed (rhinitis). This inflammation may spread to the lining of the sinuses (rhinosinusitis).

Fractures of the Nose

- Typically, a broken nose bleeds, hurts, and swells.
- To diagnose a broken nose, a doctor looks at and feels the bridge of the nose.

- Doctors sometimes need to push the broken pieces of bone back into place.

The bones of the nose are broken (fractured) more often than any other facial bone. When nasal bones break, the mucous membrane lining the nose usually tears, resulting in a nosebleed. Most commonly, the bridge of the nose is pushed to one side. Sometimes, the cartilage of the nasal septum can break. If blood collects under the mucous membrane that lines the cartilage of the nasal septum (septal hematoma), the cartilage may die. The dead cartilage may disintegrate, resulting in a saddle nose deformity, in which the bridge of the nose sags in the middle.

Diagnosis

A person whose nose bleeds, hurts, and is swollen and tender after a blunt injury may have a broken nose. Applying ice packs every 2 hours for 15 minutes at a time, taking pain relievers (such as acetaminophen or ibuprofen), and sleeping with the head elevated help limit pain and swelling. However, medical attention is needed.

The mucous membrane and other soft tissues swell quickly, making the break difficult for a doctor to find, so the evaluation needs to be done either very quickly (within the first few hours) or later after the swelling has started to subside but before the bones become fixed in their new position. Ordinarily, a doctor diagnoses a broken nose by gently feeling the bridge of the nose for irregularities in shape and alignment, unusual movement of bones, the rough sensation of broken bones moving against one another, and tenderness. X-rays of the nose may not be as accurate as the doctor's eyes and fingers for determining proper bone alignment.

> **? Did You Know...**
> Doctors rarely do x-rays on people who may have broken their nose.

Treatment

Doctors usually wait 3 to 5 days after an injury for the swelling to go down before they push the broken pieces of bone back into place (called reduction). Waiting makes it easier for doctors to see and feel when the pieces are perfectly aligned. Many nasal fractures are in a good position and do not have to be reduced.

First, doctors give adults a local anesthetic, which numbs the area. Children are given a general anesthetic, which causes temporary unconsciousness. Before reducing the fracture, any blood that has collected in the septum is drained through a small incision in the mucous membrane of the septum to prevent the destruction of the cartilage. By pressing with their fingers, doctors manipulate the bones into their normal position. The nose is then stabilized with an external splint. Internal packing (stenting) may also be used. Antibiotics are given while the packing is in place to decrease the risk of infection. Nasal bone fractures heal in about 6 weeks. Fractures of the septum are difficult to set and often require surgery later.

Deviated Septum

Usually, the nasal septum is straight, lying about in the middle of the two nostrils. Occasionally, it may be bent (deviated) because of a birth defect or injury and positioned so that one nostril is much smaller than the other. Most people have some minor deviation of the septum so that one nostril is tighter than the other. A minor deviation usually causes no symptoms and requires no treatment.

However, if severe, a deviation may block one side of the nose, making a person prone to inflammation of the sinuses (sinusitis), particularly if the deviated septum blocks drainage from a sinus into the nasal cavity. Also, a deviated septum may make a person prone to nosebleeds because of the drying effect of airflow over the deviation. Other symptoms may include facial pain, headaches, and noisy night breathing. A deviated septum that causes breathing problems can be surgically repaired.

Perforations of the Septum

Ulcers and holes (perforations) in the nasal septum may occur as a result of nasal surgery; repeated injury such as that resulting from picking the nose; cosmetic piercing; exposure to toxins (such as acids, chromium, phosphorus, and copper vapor); chronic nasal spray use (including corticosteroids and over-the-counter phenylephrine or oxymetazoline sprays); oxygen inhaled through the nose; or diseases such as tuberculosis, leprosy, Wegener's granulomatosis, and syphilis. Frequent use of cocaine snorted through the nose causes ulcerations and perforations because it decreases blood flow.

Symptoms may include crusting around the nostrils and repeated nosebleeds. People who have small perforations in the septum may make a whistling sound when they breathe.

Bacitracin ointment or mupirocin ointment reduces the crusting, as may saline nasal spray. Doctors can sometimes surgically repair perforations using a person's own tissue from another part of the nose or with an artificial membrane made of a soft, pliable plastic. Most perforations do not need to be repaired unless bleeding or crusting is a major problem.

Nosebleeds

- Nose picking and injuries are the most common causes of nosebleeds.
- People typically bleed from the front part of the nose.
- Avoiding nose picking, humidifying the air during the winter, and, for some people, moistening the front of the nasal septum with petroleum jelly are ways to prevent nosebleeds.
- If pinching the sides of the nose together does not stop the bleeding, people should seek medical attention.

Nosebleeds (epistaxis) have a variety of causes, the most common of which are nose picking and injury. The cold, dry air of winter also makes nosebleeds more likely. People who take aspirin or other drugs that interfere with the blood's ability to clot (anticoagulants) commonly develop nosebleeds. Some people get them rather often, and others rarely get them.

Bleeding usually comes from the front part of the nasal septum, which contains many blood vessels. There may be just a trickle of blood or a strong stream. Most nosebleeds are more frightening than serious. However, bleeding from the back part of the nose (posterior nosebleed, an uncommon occurrence) is more dangerous and difficult to treat.

> **? Did You Know...**
> Although many older people with nosebleeds have high blood pressure, blood pressure is rarely the cause of nosebleeds.

Prevention and Treatment

Important steps to prevent nosebleeds include avoiding picking the nose, humidifying the air during the winter, and, for some people, moistening the front of the nasal septum with saline gel or petroleum jelly.

Bleeding usually can be controlled at home by pinching the sides of the nose together for 10 minutes. It is important to hold the nose with a firm pinch and not let go even once during the 10 minutes. Other home techniques, such as ice packs to the nose, wads of tissue paper in the nostrils, and placing the head in various positions, are not effective.

If the pinch technique does not stop the bleeding, the person should see a doctor. The doctor packs the bleeding nostril with a piece of cotton saturated with a drug that causes blood vessels in the nose to narrow (constrict), such as phenylephrine. A local anesthetic, such as lidocaine, numbs the nose so the doctor can look in the nose and find the bleeding site. For minor bleeds, often nothing more is done. For more severe or recurring bleeding, sometimes the doctor seals (cauterizes) the bleeding source with a chemical (silver nitrate) or electrocautery (cauterization using an electrical current to produce heat). Another treatment is to place a long absorbent sponge in the nostril. The sponge swells in contact with moisture and compresses the bleeding site. The sponge is removed after 2 to 4 days. Rarely, the doctor may need to pack the entire nasal cavity on one side with a long strip of gauze. Nasal packing is usually removed after 3 days.

In some people, particularly those who are older and have narrowing of the arteries (arteriosclerosis), the bleeding source is sometimes further back in the nose (posterior nosebleed). Bleeding in this area is very difficult to stop and can be life threatening. For a posterior nosebleed, the pinch technique does not stop the bleeding, which then runs down the throat instead of out the nose. For a posterior nosebleed, doctors may place a specially shaped balloon in the nose and inflate it to compress the bleeding site. However, this and other types of nasal packing are very uncomfortable and interfere with the person's breathing. Doctors usually give people sedatives by vein before placing this kind of balloon and packing. Also, people who have had this type of packing are admitted to the hospital and given oxygen and antibiotics to prevent an infection of the sinuses. Because of the discomfort and breathing risks associated with nasal packing, doctors sometimes cauterize or clip the bleeding vessel while looking in the nose through a small visualizing device (endoscope). Occasionally, doctors, guided by x-ray techniques, can pass a small catheter through the person's blood vessels to the bleeding site and inject material to block the bleeding vessel.

Nasal Vestibulitis

Nasal vestibulitis is infection of the area just inside the opening of each nostril (the nasal vestibule).

Minor infections at the opening of the nose may result in pimples at the base of nasal hairs (folliculitis) and sometimes crusts around the nostrils. The cause is usually the bacteria *Staphylococcus*. The infection may result from nose picking or excessive nose blowing and causes annoying crusts and bleeding when the crusts slough off. Bacitracin ointment or mupirocin ointment usually cures these infections.

More serious infections result in boils (furuncles) in the nasal vestibule. Boils may develop into a spreading infection under the skin (cellulitis) at the tip of the nose. A doctor becomes concerned about infections in this part of the face because veins lead from there to the brain. A life-threatening condition called cavernous sinus thrombosis can develop if the bacteria spread to the brain through these veins (see box on page 1463).

A person with nasal vestibulitis usually takes an antibiotic by mouth and applies moist hot cloths 3 times a day for about 15 to 20 minutes at a time. A doctor may need to surgically drain large boils or those that do not respond to antibiotic therapy.

Rhinitis

Rhinitis is inflammation and swelling of the mucous membrane of the nose, characterized by a runny nose and stuffiness and usually caused by the common cold (see page 1239) or an allergy (see page 1116).

- Colds and allergies are the most common causes of rhinitis.
- Symptoms of rhinitis include a runny nose, sneezing, and stuffiness.
- Typically, the diagnosis is based on the symptoms.
- The various forms of rhinitis are treated in various ways, such as with antibiotics, antihistamines, surgery, allergy shots, and avoidance of irritants.

The nose is the most commonly infected part of the upper airways. Rhinitis may be acute (short-lived) or chronic (long-standing). Acute rhinitis commonly results from viral infections but may also be a result of allergies or other causes. Chronic rhinitis usually occurs with chronic sinusitis (chronic rhinosinusitis).

Acute Viral Rhinitis: Acute viral rhinitis (the common cold) can be caused by a variety of viruses. Symptoms consist of runny nose, sneezing, congestion, postnasal drip, cough, and a low-grade fever. Stuffiness can be relieved by taking decongestants such as phenylephrine as a nasal spray or pseudoephedrine by mouth. These drugs, available over the counter, cause the blood vessels of the nasal mucous membrane to narrow (constrict). Nasal sprays should be used for only 3 or 4 days because after that period of time, when the effects of the drugs wear off, the mucous membrane often swells even more than before. This phenomenon is called rebound congestion. Antihistamines help control runny nose but cause drowsiness and other problems, especially in older people (see box on page 1897). Antibiotics are not effective for acute viral rhinitis.

Allergic Rhinitis: Allergic rhinitis is caused by a reaction of the body's immune system to an environmental trigger. The most common environmental triggers include dust, molds, pollens, grasses, trees, and animals. Symptoms include itching, sneezing, runny nose, stuffiness, and itchy, watery eyes. A doctor may diagnose allergic rhinitis based on a person's history of symptoms. Often, the person has a family history of allergies. More detailed information may be obtained from blood tests or skin testing.

Avoiding the substance that triggers the allergy prevents symptoms but is often not possible. Nasal corticosteroid sprays decrease nasal inflammation caused by many sources and are relatively safe for long-term use. Antihistamines help prevent the allergic reaction and thus symptoms. Antihistamines dry the mucous membrane of the nose but many of them also cause sleepiness and other problems, especially in older people. Newer ones require a prescription but do not have these side effects. Allergy shots (desensitization) help to build long-term tolerance to specific environmental triggers, but they may take months or years to become fully effective. Antibiotics do not relieve the symptoms of allergic rhinitis.

Chronic Rhinitis: Chronic rhinitis is usually an extension of rhinitis caused by inflammation or an infection. However, it also may occur with diseases such as syphilis, tuberculosis, rhinoscleroma (a skin disease characterized by very hard, flattened tissues that first appear on the nose), rhinosporidiosis (an infection in the nose characterized by bleeding polyps), leishmaniasis, blastomycosis, histoplasmosis, and leprosy—all of which are characterized by the formation of inflamed lesions (granulomas) and the destruction of soft tissue, cartilage, and bone. Chronic rhinitis causes nasal obstruction, pus-filled discharge from the nose, and frequent bleeding.

Both low humidity and airborne irritants can result in chronic rhinitis. Decongestants may relieve symptoms. Any underlying bacterial infection requires a culture (examination of microorganisms grown from a sample to identify infection with bacteria or fungi) or biopsy (removal of a tissue sample for identification under a microscope) and appropriate treatment.

Atrophic Rhinitis: Atrophic rhinitis is a form of chronic rhinitis in which the mucous membrane thins (atrophies) and hardens, causing the nasal passages to widen (dilate) and dry out. This atrophy often occurs in older people. The cells normally found in the mucous membrane of the nose—cells that secrete mucus and have hairlike projections to move dirt particles out—are replaced by cells like those normally found in the skin. The disorder can develop in someone who had sinus surgery in which a significant amount of intranasal structures and mucous membranes were removed. A prolonged bacterial infection of the lining of the nose is also a factor.

Crusts form inside the nose, and an offensive odor develops. People may have recurring severe nosebleeds and can lose their sense of smell (anosmia).

Treatment is aimed at reducing the crusting, eliminating the odor, and reducing infections. Topical antibiotics, such as bacitracin applied inside the nose, kill bacteria. Estrogens and vitamins A and D sprayed into the nose or taken by mouth may reduce crusting by promoting mucosal secretions. Other antibiotics, given by mouth or by vein, may also be helpful. Surgery to narrow the nasal passages may reduce crusting because the decreased airflow prevents drying of the thinned mucous membrane.

Vasomotor Rhinitis: Vasomotor rhinitis is a form of chronic rhinitis. Nasal stuffiness, sneezing, and a runny nose—common allergic symptoms—occur when allergies do not seem to be present. In some people, the nose reacts strongly to irritants (such as dust and pollen), perfumes, and pollution. The disorder comes and goes but is worsened by dry air. The swollen mucous membrane varies from bright red to purple. Sometimes, people also have slight inflammation of the sinuses. When persistent, endoscopy of the nose or computed tomography (CT—see page 2037) of the sinuses may be needed. If inflammation of the sinus is not severe, treatment is aimed at relieving symptoms. Avoiding smoke and irritants and using a humidified central heating system or vaporizer to increase humidity may be beneficial.

Polyp Formation in the Nose

Polyps usually develop in the area where the sinuses open into the nasal cavity. Polyps may block drainage from the sinuses. Fluid may accumulate in the blocked sinuses, causing a sinus infection.

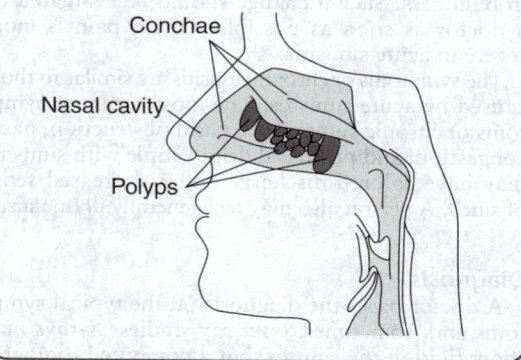

Conchae

Nasal cavity

Polyps

Nasal Polyps

Nasal polyps are fleshy outgrowths of the mucous membrane of the nose.

- Nasal polyps are more likely to develop in people who have allergies or asthma.
- Some of the symptoms caused by polyps are nasal obstruction and congestion.
- Doctors usually diagnose nasal polyps based on their characteristic appearance.
- Corticosteroids can shrink or eliminate polyps, but sometimes polyps must be removed surgically.

Polyps are common teardrop-shaped growths that form around the openings to the sinus cavities. A mature polyp resembles a peeled, seedless grape. Unlike polyps in the colon or bladder, polyps in the nose are not tumors and do not suggest an increased risk of cancer. They are merely a reflection of inflammation, although there may be a family history of the problem. The doctor may perform a biopsy of the polyp to ensure that it is not a cancer.

Polyps may develop during infections and may disappear after the infection subsides, or they may begin slowly and persist. Many people are not aware that they have nasal polyps, although they may have sneezing, nasal congestion, obstruction, drainage of fluid down the throat (postnasal drip), facial pain, excessive discharge from the nose, loss of smell (anosmia), reduced ability to smell (hyposmia), itching around the eyes, and chronic infections.

People with nasal polyps may be seriously allergic to aspirin and other nonsteroidal anti-inflammatory drugs (NSAIDs—see page 644). People with nasal polyps can

develop sinus infections if the polyps block drainage from the sinuses. Many develop asthma as well. Nasal polyps also can form if a foreign body is in the nose.

Corticosteroids in the form of nasal sprays or oral tablets may shrink or eliminate polyps. Endoscopic surgery or oral corticosteroids are needed if polyps block the airways or cause frequent sinus infections. Polyps tend to grow back unless the underlying irritation, allergy, or infection is controlled. Using an aerosol corticosteroid spray may slow or prevent recurrences. However, a doctor may need to examine the person periodically with nasal endoscopy (looking in the nose with a small rigid or flexible viewing tube) to evaluate and treat persistent or recurring problems.

Sinusitis

Sinusitis is inflammation of the sinuses, most commonly caused by a viral or bacterial infection or by an allergy.

- Some of the most common symptoms of sinusitis are pain, tenderness, nasal congestion, and headache.
- The diagnosis is based on symptoms, but sometimes x-rays or other imaging tests are needed.
- Antibiotics can eliminate the underlying infection.

Sinusitis is one of the most common medical conditions. About 10 to 15 million people each year develop symptoms of sinusitis. Sinusitis may occur in any of the four groups of sinuses: maxillary, ethmoid, frontal, or sphenoid. Sinusitis nearly always occurs in conjunction with inflammation of the nasal passages (rhinitis), and some doctors refer to the disorder as rhinosinusitis. It may be acute (short-lived) or chronic (long-standing).

Acute Sinusitis: Sinusitis is defined as acute if it is totally resolved in less than 30 days. Acute sinusitis may be caused by a variety of bacteria and often develops after something blocks the openings to the sinuses. Such blockage commonly results from a viral infection of the upper airways, such as the common cold. During a cold, the swollen mucous membranes of the nasal cavity tend to block the openings of the sinuses. Air in the sinuses is absorbed into the bloodstream, and the pressure inside the sinuses decreases, causing pain and drawing fluid into the sinuses. This fluid is a breeding ground for bacteria. White blood cells and more fluid enter the sinuses to fight the bacteria. This influx increases the pressure and causes more pain.

Allergies also cause mucous membrane swelling, which blocks the openings to the sinuses. Additionally, people with a deviated septum are more prone to obstructed sinuses.

Chronic Sinusitis: Sinusitis is defined as chronic if it has been ongoing for more than 8 to 12 weeks. Doctors do not understand exactly what causes

Locating the Sinuses

The sinuses are hollow cavities in the bones around the nose. The two frontal sinuses are located just above the eyebrows. The two maxillary sinuses are located in the cheekbones, and the two groups of ethmoid sinuses are located on either side of the nasal cavity. The two sphenoid sinuses (not shown) are located behind the ethmoid sinuses.

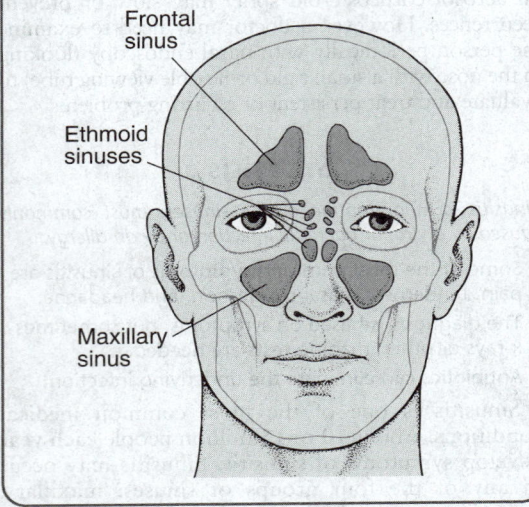

Frontal sinus

Ethmoid sinuses

Maxillary sinus

chronic sinusitis, but it may follow a viral infection, a severe allergy, or exposure to an environmental pollutant. Often the person has a family history, and a genetic predisposition seems to be a factor. If the person has a bacterial or fungal infection, the inflammation is much worse. Occasionally, chronic sinusitis of the maxillary sinus results when an upper tooth abscess spreads into the sinus above.

Symptoms

Acute sinusitis usually results in pain, tenderness, congestion and obstruction in the nose, reduced ability to smell (hyposmia), bad breath (halitosis), a productive cough (especially at night), and swelling over the affected sinus. Maxillary sinusitis causes pain over the cheeks just below the eyes, toothache, and headache. Frontal sinusitis causes headache over the forehead. Ethmoid sinusitis causes pain behind and between the eyes, a bacterial infection of the skin around the eye socket (periorbital cellulitis), tearing, and headache (often described as splitting) over the forehead. Sphenoid sinusitis causes pain that does not occur in well-defined areas and may be felt in the front or back of the head.

In acute sinusitis, yellow or green pus may be discharged from the nose. Fever and chills also can occur, but their presence may suggest that the infection has spread beyond the sinuses. Any change in vision or swelling around the eye is a very serious condition that can quickly—within minutes to hours—result in blindness. Such a change should be evaluated by a doctor as soon as possible. Often, pain is more severe in acute sinusitis.

The symptoms of chronic sinusitis are similar to those caused by acute sinusitis. The most common symptoms of chronic sinusitis are nasal obstruction, nasal congestion, and postnasal drip. People with sinusitis may have colored discharge and a decreased sense of smell. A person also may feel generally ill (malaise).

Diagnosis

A doctor bases the diagnosis on the typical symptoms and, sometimes, on x-ray studies. X-rays may show fluid in the sinuses, but a computed tomography (CT) scan is better able to determine the extent and severity of sinusitis. If a person has maxillary sinusitis, the teeth may be x-rayed to check for tooth abscesses. Sometimes a doctor passes a thin viewing scope (endoscope) into the nose to inspect the sinus openings and to obtain samples of fluid for culture. This procedure, which requires a local anesthetic (to numb the area), can be done in the doctor's office.

Sinusitis in children is suspected when a pus-filled discharge from the nose persists for more than 10 days along with extreme tiredness (fatigue) and cough. Pain or discomfort in the face may be present. Fever is uncommon. When examining the nose, a doctor sees pus-filled drainage. A CT scan can confirm the diagnosis.

Treatment

Treatment of acute sinusitis is aimed at improving sinus drainage and curing the infection. Steam inhalation; hot, wet towels over the affected sinuses; and hot beverages may help relieve the tightened or constricted blood vessels and promote drainage. Nasal sprays, such as phenylephrine, which cause blood vessels to narrow (constrict), can be used for a limited time. Similar drugs, such as pseudoephedrine, taken by mouth are not as effective. For acute sinusitis, antibiotics such as amoxicillin or trimethoprim/sulfamethoxazole are given.

People who have chronic sinusitis take antibiotics, such as amoxicillin/clavulanate or cefuroxime, for a longer period of time. When antibiotics are not effective, surgery may be performed either to wash out the sinus and obtain material for culture or to improve sinus drainage, which allows the inflammation to resolve.

Smell and Taste Disorders

- Smell may be lost temporarily when a person smokes or has a cold or seasonal allergy.
- Smell may be lost permanently after a head injury.
- People may lose their sense of taste if they have a condition that causes a very dry mouth.
- Doctors can test smell by using common fragrant substances.
- Taste is tested by using sweet, salty, sour, and bitter substances.
- Infections are treated with antibiotics, and blockages are removed, but sometimes the ability to smell is not restored.

Because disorders of smell and taste are rarely life threatening, they may not receive close medical attention. Yet, these disorders can be frustrating because they can affect the ability to enjoy food and drink and to appreciate pleasant aromas. They can also interfere with the ability to notice potentially harmful chemicals and gases and thus may have serious consequences. Occasionally, impairment of smell and taste is due to a serious disorder, such as a tumor.

Smell and taste are closely linked. The taste buds of the tongue identify taste, and the nerves in the nose identify smell. Both sensations are communicated to the brain, which integrates the information so that flavors can be recognized and appreciated. Some tastes—such as salty, bitter, sweet, and sour—can be recognized without the sense of smell. However, more complex flavors (such as raspberry) require both taste and smell sensations to be recognized.

A reduced ability to smell (hyposmia) and loss of smell (anosmia) are the most common disorders of smell and taste. Because distinguishing one flavor from another is based largely on smell, people often first notice that their ability to smell is reduced when their food seems tasteless.

Causes

Smell: The ability to smell can be affected by changes in the nose, in the nerves leading from the nose to the brain, or in the brain. For example, if nasal passages are stuffed up from a common cold, the ability to smell may be reduced because odors are prevented from reaching the smell receptors (specialized nerve cells in the mucous membrane lining the nose). Because the ability to smell affects taste, food often does not taste right to people with colds. Smell receptors can be temporarily damaged by the influenza (flu) virus. Some people cannot

Fungal Sinus Infections

A variety of fungi that are normally found throughout the environment can be present in the nose and sinuses of most healthy people. In certain situations, however, fungi can cause significant nasal and sinus inflammation.

Fungus balls are overgrowths of fungi in otherwise healthy people. Symptoms include sinus pain, pressure, nasal congestion, drainage of fluids, and chronic infections. Surgery is needed to open the affected sinus and remove the fungal debris.

Allergic fungal sinusitis is a disorder in which fungi cause a reaction characterized by marked nasal congestion and the formation of nasal and sinus polyps. The polyps obstruct the nose and the openings to the sinuses and cause chronic inflammation. The polyps and inflammation often involve only one side of the nose. Surgery is typically required to open up the sinuses and to remove the fungal debris. Long-term reatment is also required with corticosteroids, antibiotics, and, sometimes, antifungal drugs applied directly to the area or taken by mouth. These drugs reduce the inflammation and eliminate the fungus. However, even after prolonged treatment, the disorder is very likely to recur.

Invasive fungal sinusitis is a very serious disorder that develops most often in people whose immune system is impaired by chemotherapy or by diseases such as poorly controlled diabetes, leukemia, lymphoma, multiple myeloma, or AIDS. It may spread rapidly. Symptoms include pain, fever, and discharge of pus from the nose. The fungus may spread to the eye socket, causing a bulging of the affected eye (proptosis) and blindness. A doctor bases the diagnosis on the results of a biopsy (removal of a tissue sample for identification under a microscope). Treatment is with surgery and antifungal drugs given by vein. Doctors also must control the underlying disease and stimulate a weakened immune system because these infections can cause death.

smell or taste for several days or even weeks after a bout of the flu, and rarely, loss of smell or taste becomes permanent. Polyps, tumors, other infections in the nose, seasonal allergies (allergic rhinitis), and smoking (tobacco) may interfere with the ability to smell. Occasionally, serious infections of the nasal sinuses or radiation therapy for cancer causes a loss of smell or taste that lasts for months or even becomes permanent. These conditions can damage or destroy smell receptors.

A common cause of permanent loss of smell is a head injury, as may occur in a car accident. Permanent loss of smell results when fibers of the olfactory

How People Sense Flavors

To distinguish most flavors, the brain needs information about both smell and taste. These sensations are communicated to the brain from the nose and mouth. Several areas of the brain integrate the information, enabling people to recognize and appreciate flavors.

A small area on the mucous membrane that lines the nose (the olfactory epithelium) contains specialized nerve cells called smell receptors. These receptors have hairlike projections (cilia) that detect odors. Airborne molecules entering the nasal passage stimulate the cilia, triggering a nerve impulse in nearby nerve fibers. The fibers extend upward through the bone that forms the roof of the nasal cavity (cribriform plate) and connect to enlargements of nerve cells (olfactory bulbs). These bulbs form the cranial nerves of smell (olfactory nerves). The impulse travels through the olfactory bulbs, along the olfactory nerves, to the brain. The brain interprets the impulse as a distinct odor. Also, the area of the brain where memories of odors are stored—the smell and taste center in the middle part of the temporal lobe—is stimulated. The memories enable a person to distinguish and identify many different odors experienced over a lifetime.

Thousands of tiny taste buds cover most of the tongue's surface. A taste bud contains several types of taste receptors with cilia. Each type detects one of the five basic tastes: sweet, salty, sour, bitter, or savory (also called umami, the taste of monosodium glutamate). These tastes can be detected all over the tongue, but certain areas are more sensitive for each taste. Sweetness is most easily identified by the tip of the tongue, whereas saltiness is best appreciated at the front sides of the tongue. Sourness is best perceived along the sides of the tongue, and bitter sensations are readily detected in the back one third of the tongue. Food placed in the mouth stimulates the cilia, triggering a nerve impulse in nearby nerve fibers, which are connected to the cranial nerves of taste (the facial and glossopharyngeal nerves). The impulse travels along these cranial nerves to the brain, which interprets the combination of impulses from the different types of taste receptors as a distinct taste. Sensory information about the food's smell, taste, texture, and temperature is processed by the brain to produce a distinct flavor when food enters the mouth and is chewed.

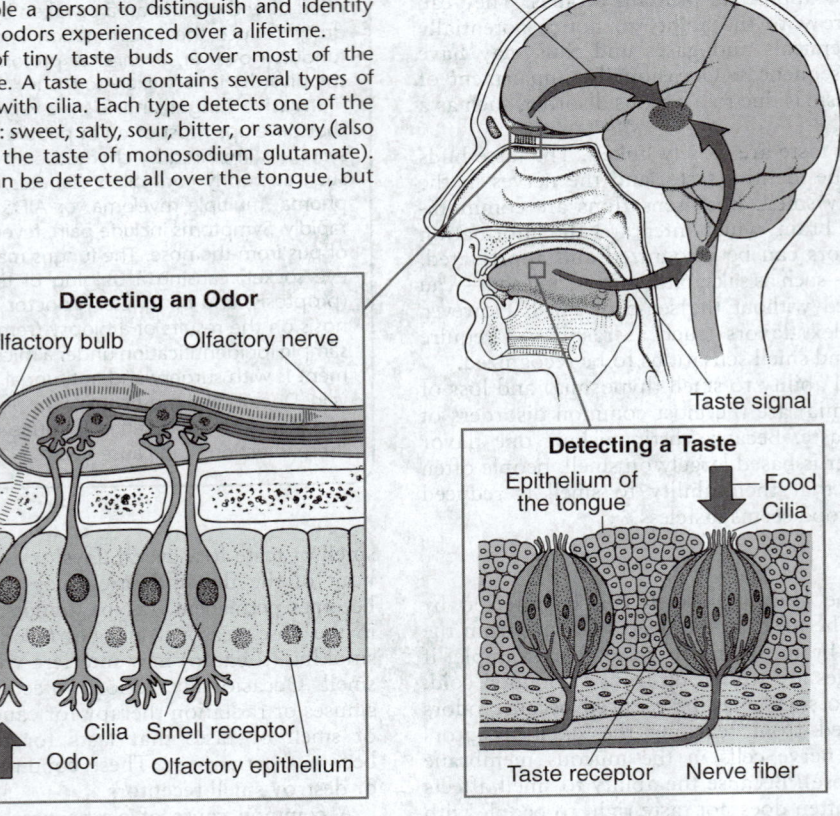

Smell signal

Smell and taste center

Taste signal

Detecting an Odor

Olfactory bulb   Olfactory nerve

Cilia   Smell receptor

Odor   Olfactory epithelium

Detecting a Taste

Epithelium of the tongue   Food

Cilia

Taste receptor   Nerve fiber

nerves—the pair of cranial nerves that connect smell receptors to the brain—are damaged or sheared at the roof of the nasal cavity. The roof of the nasal cavity is formed by a bone (cribriform plate) that separates the brain from the nasal cavity. Damage to the olfactory nerves can also result from fractures of the cribriform plate or from infections (such as abscesses) or tumors near this bone.

Alzheimer's disease and some other degenerative brain disorders can also damage the olfactory nerves, commonly causing of loss of smell. A very few people are born without a sense of smell.

Oversensitivity to smell (hyperosmia) is much less common than loss of smell. Pregnant women commonly become oversensitive to smell. Hyperosmia can also be psychosomatic. Psychosomatic hyperosmia is more likely to develop in people who have a histrionic personality (characterized by conspicuous seeking of attention with dramatic behavior—see page 881).

Some disorders can distort the sense of smell, making innocuous odors smell disagreeable (a condition called dysosmia). These disorders include the following:

- Infections in the sinuses
- Partial damage to the olfactory nerves
- Poor dental hygiene
- Mouth infections
- Depression
- Viral hepatitis, which may cause dysosmia that results in nausea triggered by otherwise inoffensive odors

Seizures originating in the part of the brain where memories of smell are stored—the middle part of the temporal lobe—may produce a brief, false sensation of vivid, unpleasant smells (olfactory hallucinations). These smells are part of the intense feeling that a seizure is about to begin (called an aura) and do not indicate a smell disorder. Brain infections due to herpesviruses (herpes encephalitis) may also cause olfactory hallucinations.

> **Did You Know...**
>
> Occasionally, smell and taste disorders are due to a serious disorder, such as a tumor.
>
> Because the ability to smell and taste decreases with aging, older people may eat less and become undernourished.

Taste: A reduction in the ability to taste (hypogeusia) or loss of taste (ageusia) usually results from conditions that affect the tongue, usually by causing a very dry mouth. Such conditions include Sjögren's syndrome, heavy smoking (especially pipe smoking), radiation

SPOTLIGHT ON AGING

After age 50, the ability to smell and to taste gradually begins to decrease. The membranes lining the nose become thinner and drier, and the nerves involved in smell deteriorate. Older people can still detect strong smells, but detecting subtle smells is more difficult.

As people age, the number of taste buds also decreases, and those that are left become less sensitive. These changes tend to reduce the ability to taste sweet and salt more than the ability to taste sour and bitter. Thus, many foods start to taste bitter.

Because smell and taste are diminished as people age, many foods taste bland. The mouth tends to be dry more often, further reducing the ability to taste and smell. Also, many older people have a disorder or take drugs that contribute to dry mouth. Because of these changes, older people may eat less. Then, they may not get the nutrition they need, and if they already have a disorder, their condition may worsen.

therapy to the head and neck, dehydration, and use of drugs (including antihistamines and the antidepressant amitriptyline). Nutritional deficiencies, such as decreased zinc, copper, and nickel levels, can alter both taste and smell.

In Bell's palsy, the sense of taste is often impaired on the front two thirds of one side of the tongue (the side affected by the palsy). But this loss may not be noticed because taste is normal or increased in the rest of the tongue. Burns to the tongue may temporarily destroy taste buds. Neurologic disorders, including depression and seizures, may impair taste.

A distortion of taste (dysgeusia) may be caused by inflammation of the gums (gingivitis) and by many of the same conditions that result in loss of taste or smell, including depression and seizures. Taste may be distorted by some drugs, such as the following:

- Antibiotics
- Anticonvulsants
- Antidepressants
- Certain chemotherapy drugs
- Diuretics
- Drugs used to treat arthritis
- Thyroid drugs

Diagnosis

To test smell, doctors hold common fragrant substances (such as soap, a vanilla bean, coffee, and cloves) under the person's nose, one nostril at a time. The person is then asked to identify the smell. Smell can also be tested more formally using standardized commercial smell test kits. Taste can be tested using substances that are sweet (sugar), sour (lemon juice), salty (salt), and bitter (aspirin, quinine, or aloes).

Doctors and dentists check the mouth and nasal passages for abnormalities, including infection and dryness. If the cause is not apparent, computed tomography (CT) or magnetic resonance imaging (MRI) of the head is needed to look for structural abnormalities (such as a tumor, an abscess, or a fracture) near the cribriform plate.

Treatment

Treatment depends on the cause of a smell or taste disorder. For example, sinus infections and irritation may be treated with steam inhalation, nasal sprays, antibiotics, and sometimes surgery (see page 1398). Nutritional deficiencies need to be corrected. Tumors are surgically removed or treated with radiation, but such treatment usually does not restore the sense of smell. Polyps in the nose are removed, sometimes restoring the ability to smell. People who smoke tobacco should stop. Other recommendations may include the following:

- Changing or stopping a drug
- Sucking on candy to keep the mouth moist
- Improving dental hygiene
- Waiting several weeks to see if the cause of the problem (such as the flu) disappears

Rarely, zinc supplements, which can be purchased without a prescription, are effective, especially for distortion of smell or for reduction or distortion of taste when no cause has been identified.

CHAPTER
216 Throat Disorders

Disorders of the throat (pharynx) and voice box (larynx) may represent short-lived (acute) inflammation and infections, persistent (chronic) inflammation, or abnormal growths. Specific disorders include vocal cord polyps and nodules, contact ulcers, vocal cord paralysis, laryngoceles, laryngeal papillomas (see page 1815), and cancer (see page 1406).

Throat infections (pharyngitis) are particularly common among children, although adults may be affected as well. Causes, symptoms, and treatment are similar in both groups (see page 1811), except that in adults (and sexually abused children), gonorrhea, a sexually transmitted disease, may affect the throat.

Tonsillar Cellulitis and Abscess

Tonsillar cellulitis is a bacterial infection of the tissues around the tonsils. A tonsillar abscess is a collection of pus behind the tonsils.

- Sometimes, bacteria that infect the throat spread deep into surrounding tissues.
- Typical symptoms include sore throat, pain when swallowing, fever, swelling, and redness.
- The diagnosis is based on examination of the throat and sometimes the results of imaging studies.
- Antibiotics help eliminate the infection.
- An abscess is drained with a needle or through a small incision.

Sometimes, bacteria (usually streptococci and staphylococci) that infect the throat can spread deeper into the surrounding tissues. This condition is called cellulitis. If the bacteria grow unchecked, a collection of pus (abscess) may form. Abscesses may form next to the tonsils (peritonsillar) or in the side of the throat (parapharyngeal). Tonsillar cellulitis and tonsillar abscesses are most common among adolescents and young adults.

Symptoms

With tonsillar cellulitis or a tonsillar abscess, swallowing causes severe pain that often radiates into the ear. People have a severe sore throat, feel ill, have a fever, and may tilt their head toward the side of the abscess to help relieve pain. Spasms of the chewing muscles make opening the mouth difficult (trismus). Cellulitis causes general redness and swelling above the tonsil and on the soft palate. An abscess pushes the tonsil forward, and the uvula (the small, soft projection that hangs down at the back of the throat) is swollen and can be pushed to the side opposite the abscess. Other common symptoms include a "hot potato" voice (speaking as if a hot object is in the mouth), drooling, and severe bad breath (halitosis).

Diagnosis and Treatment

A doctor makes the diagnosis by viewing the throat. Tests are not usually performed, but if the doctor is not sure whether an abscess is present, computed tomography (CT) or ultrasonography can be used to identify one. Sometimes if an abscess is suspected, the doctor inserts a needle into the area and tries to draw out pus.

Antibiotics, such as penicillin or clindamycin, are given by vein. If no abscess is present, the antibiotic usually starts to clear the infection within 48 hours. If an abscess is present, a doctor must insert a needle in it or cut into it to drain the pus. The area is first numbed with an anesthetic spray or injection. Treatment with antibiotics is continued by mouth.

Peritonsillar abscesses tend to recur. Recurrences can be prevented by removing the tonsils (tonsillectomy—see page 1813), which is usually performed 4 to 6 weeks after the infection has subsided or earlier if the infection is not controlled with antibiotics.

Epiglottitis

Epiglottitis is a bacterial infection of the epiglottis.

- Epiglottitis may block the windpipe (trachea) and be fatal.
- The main symptoms are severe sore throat and noisy, difficult breathing.
- Doctors make the diagnosis by looking at the epiglottis in the operating room with a flexible light.
- The *Haemophilus influenzae* type B (Hib) vaccine can prevent epiglottitis caused by these bacteria.
- Antibiotics are given to eliminate the infection, and a breathing tube is inserted to keep the airway from swelling shut.

The epiglottis is a small flap of stiff tissue that closes the entrance to the voice box (larynx) and trachea during swallowing. Sometimes, the epiglottis becomes infected with bacteria, usually *Haemophilus influenzae* type B. *Haemophilus influenzae*–related epiglottitis was most common among children, but routine vaccination against *Haemophilus* has almost eliminated this infection in children. Now more cases of epiglottitis occur in adults. However, children may get epiglottitis caused by other bacteria, and unvaccinated children can be infected by *Haemophilus*.

The swelling caused by this infection may block the airway and lead to difficulty breathing and death. Because children have a smaller airway than adults, epiglottitis is more dangerous in children (see page 1764) but can also be fatal in adults.

Symptoms are severe throat pain, difficulty swallowing, fever, drooling, and a muffled voice. Because the infection is in the epiglottis, the back of the throat often does not appear infected. As swelling of the epiglottis starts to narrow the airway, the person first begins to make a squeaking noise when breathing in (stridor) and then has progressively worse trouble breathing. The condition progresses rapidly.

A doctor suspects the diagnosis based on the person's symptoms. If an adult is not having stridor or any trouble breathing, the doctor may look down the throat with a mirror or take x-rays, which often show the swollen epiglottis. Sometimes the doctor looks down the throat with a thin, flexible viewing tube inserted through the nose (nasopharyngeal laryngoscopy). Children are more likely to have sudden, complete blockage of their airway, particularly when their throat is examined. To minimize this danger, doctors usually examine the throat and epiglottis only in the operating room and do not send children for x-rays.

Epiglottitis caused by *Haemophilus influenzae* type B can be effectively prevented with the *Haemophilus influenzae* type B (Hib) vaccine.

A person without difficulty breathing is given antibiotics and is hospitalized and closely observed in an intensive care unit. If the person has difficulty breathing, doctors insert a plastic breathing tube through the mouth or nose into the trachea (endotracheal intubation). The tube keeps the airway from swelling shut. Sometimes the airway is so swollen that the doctor cannot insert a tube this way and must cut open the front of the neck and insert the tube directly into the trachea (tracheotomy or cricothyroidotomy).

Laryngitis

Laryngitis is inflammation of the voice box (larynx).

- A virus is usually what causes the inflammation.
- Typical symptoms include hoarseness and loss of voice.
- The diagnosis is based on symptoms and changes of the voice.
- Usually, resting the voice and avoiding any irritants are adequate treatment.

The most common cause of short-lived (acute) laryngitis is a viral infection of the upper airways, such as the common cold. Laryngitis also may accompany bronchitis or any other inflammation or infection of the upper airways. Excessive use of the voice, an allergic reaction, and inhalation of irritants such as cigarette smoke can cause acute or persistent (chronic) laryngitis. Bacterial infections of the vocal cords are extremely rare.

Chronic laryngitis, in which symptoms last longer than 3 weeks, may be caused by gastroesophageal reflux, and less commonly by lingering bronchitis. People with bulimia who vomit frequently may develop laryngitis.

Symptoms are an unnatural change of voice, such as hoarseness, or even loss of voice that develops within hours to a day or so. The throat may tickle or feel raw, and a person may have a constant urge to clear the throat. Symptoms vary with the severity of the inflammation. Fever, a general feeling of illness (malaise), difficulty in swallowing, and a sore throat may occur in severe infections.

A diagnosis is based on the typical symptoms and voice changes. Sometimes a doctor looks down the throat with a mirror or a thin, flexible viewing tube, which shows some reddening and sometimes some swelling of the lining of the larynx. Because cancer of the larynx may cause hoarseness, a person whose symptoms persist more than a few weeks should be evaluated for cancer (see page 1406).

Treatment of viral laryngitis depends on the symptoms. Resting the voice (by not speaking), taking cough suppressants, drinking extra fluids, and inhaling steam relieve symptoms and help healing. Whispering, however, may irritate the larynx even more. Stopping smoking and treating bronchitis, if present, may alleviate laryngitis. An antibiotic is given only for infection caused by bacteria. Depending on the possible cause, specific treatments to control gastroesophageal reflux, bulimia, or drug-induced laryngitis may be helpful.

Vocal Cord Nodules and Polyps

Vocal cord nodules and polyps are noncancerous (benign) growths that cause hoarseness and a breathy voice.

Vocal cord polyps are often the result of an acute injury (such as from shouting at a football game) and typically occur on only one vocal cord. Vocal cord nodules occur on both vocal cords and result mainly from abuse of the voice (habitual yelling, singing, or shouting or using an unnaturally low frequency).

Symptoms include chronic hoarseness and a breathy voice, which tend to develop over days to weeks. A doctor makes the diagnosis by examining the vocal cords with a thin, flexible viewing tube. Sometimes the doctor removes a small piece of tissue for examination under a microscope (biopsy) to make sure the growth is not cancerous (malignant).

Treatment is to avoid whatever is irritating the larynx and rest the voice. If abuse of the voice is the cause, voice therapy conducted by a speech therapist may be needed to teach the person how to speak or sing without straining the vocal cords. Most nodules go away with this treatment, but most polyps must be surgically removed to restore the person's normal voice.

Vocal Cord Contact Ulcers

Vocal cord contact ulcers are raw sores on the mucous membrane covering the cartilage to which the vocal cords are attached.

Vocal cord contact ulcers are usually caused by abusing the voice with forceful speech, particularly as a person starts to speak. These ulcers typically occur in singers, teachers, preachers, sales representatives, lawyers, and other people whose occupation requires them to talk or otherwise use their voice a lot. Backflow (gastroesophageal reflux) of stomach acid also may cause vocal cord contact ulcers.

Symptoms include mild pain while speaking or swallowing and varying degrees of hoarseness. A doctor makes the diagnosis by examining the vocal cords with a thin, flexible viewing tube. Occasionally, a small tissue sample is removed and examined under a microscope (biopsy) to make sure that the ulcers are not cancerous (malignant) and are not caused by tuberculosis.

> **? Did You Know...**
> Gastroesophageal reflux can cause ulcers to grow near the vocal cords.

Treatment involves resting the voice by talking as little as possible for at least 6 weeks so that the ulcers can heal. To avoid recurrences, people who develop vocal cord contact ulcers need voice therapy to learn how to use the voice properly. A speech therapist can provide such instruction.

If the person has gastroesophageal reflux, treatment includes taking antacids, not eating within 2 hours of retiring for the night, and keeping the head elevated while sleeping. Antibiotics also can help prevent bacterial infections while the ulcers are healing.

Vocal Cord Paralysis

Vocal cord paralysis is the inability to move the muscles that control the vocal cords.

- Paralysis can be caused by tumors, injuries, or nerve damage caused by infection or toxins.
- Typical symptoms include voice changes and possible difficulty breathing.
- The diagnosis is based on examination of the voice box (larynx), bronchial tubes, or esophagus.
- Several procedures can help keep the airway from closing.

Vocal cord paralysis may affect one or both vocal cords. Females are affected more often than males. Paralysis can result from brain disorders, such as brain tumors, strokes, and demyelinating diseases, or damage to the nerves that lead to the larynx. Nerve damage may be caused by noncancerous (benign)

Vocal Cord Problems

When relaxed, the vocal cords normally form a V-shaped opening that allows air to pass freely through to the trachea. The cords open when air is drawn into the lungs (inspiration) and close during swallowing or speech.

Holding a mirror in the back of a person's mouth, a specially trained doctor can often see the vocal cords and check for problems, such as contact ulcers, polyps, nodules, paralysis, and cancer. All of these problems affect the voice. Paralysis may affect one (one-sided) or both vocal cords (two-sided—not shown).

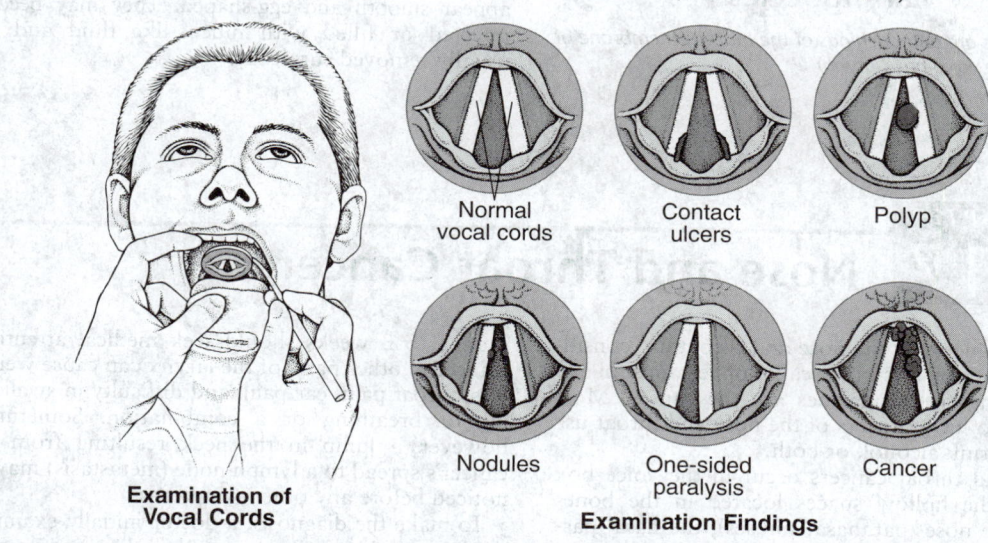

Normal vocal cords

Contact ulcers

Polyp

Nodules

One-sided paralysis

Cancer

Examination of Vocal Cords

Examination Findings

and cancerous (malignant) tumors; injury; a viral infection of the nerves; Lyme disease; or neurotoxins (substances that poison or destroy nerve tissue), such as lead, mercury, arsenic, or the toxins produced in diphtheria.

Symptoms and Diagnosis

Vocal cord paralysis may affect speaking, breathing, and swallowing. Paralysis may allow food and fluids to be inhaled into the windpipe (trachea) and lungs. If only one vocal cord is paralyzed, the voice is hoarse and breathy. Usually, the airway is not obstructed because the normal cord on the other side opens sufficiently. When both vocal cords are paralyzed, the voice is reduced in strength but otherwise sounds normal. However, the space between the paralyzed cords is very small, and the airway is inadequate so that even moderate exercise causes difficulty in breathing and a harsh, high-pitched sound with each breath.

A doctor tries to find the cause of the paralysis. Examination of the larynx, bronchial tubes, or

esophagus with a thin, flexible viewing tube may be performed. Magnetic resonance imaging (MRI) or computed tomography (CT) of the head, neck, chest, and thyroid gland and x-rays of the esophagus also may be needed.

Treatment

If only one side is paralyzed, an operation can be done to move the paralyzed vocal cord to the best position for more normal speech. The operation may involve inserting an adjustable spacer near the paralyzed cord or injecting a substance into the paralyzed cord to move the cords closer together.

When both sides are paralyzed, keeping the airway open adequately is difficult. A tracheostomy (surgery to create an opening into the trachea through the neck) may be needed. The tracheostomy opening may be permanent or may be used only when the person has an upper respiratory tract infection. In another procedure, called an arytenoidectomy, the vocal cords are permanently separated, thus widening the airway. However, this procedure may worsen voice quality. Laser removal of part of one or both vocal cords is preferred to arytenoidectomy and helps widen the airway. If performed correctly, laser removal can preserve satisfactory voice quality and eliminate the need for a tracheostomy.

Laryngoceles

Laryngoceles are outpouchings of the mucous membrane of a part of the voice box (larynx).

Laryngoceles may bulge inward, resulting in hoarseness and airway obstruction, or outward, causing a visible lump in the neck. Laryngoceles are filled with air and can be expanded when a person breathes out forcefully with the mouth closed and the nostrils pinched shut. Laryngoceles tend to occur in musicians who play wind instruments.

On a computed tomography (CT) scan, laryngoceles appear smooth and egg-shaped. They may become infected or filled with mucus-like fluid and are usually removed surgically.

CHAPTER 217 Nose and Throat Cancers

Often, cancers of the nose and throat are considered together by doctors because of certain similarities. Among the similarities are the causes. Most people who have cancers of the nose and throat use tobacco, drink alcohol, or both.

Nose and throat cancers occur in the voice box (larynx), the hollow spaces located in the bones around the nose (paranasal sinuses), the nasal passages and upper throat (nasopharynx), and the tonsils. Cancer of the mouth is very similar to nose and throat cancers in a number of ways (see page 1353). Because these cancers can cause death, a person with nose and throat cancer that has not responded to treatment should make all necessary plans. The person should have frank discussions with the doctor about wishes for medical care and end-of-life care (see page 69).

Laryngeal Cancer

- People may be hoarse or have a lump in the neck or difficulty breathing or swallowing.
- A biopsy is needed for diagnosis.
- The prognosis depends on how advanced the cancer is.
- Treatment is usually with surgery and radiation therapy, but sometimes chemotherapy is also used.

Cancer of the voice box (larynx), a common area of cancer within the head and neck, occurs more often in men than in women. It is linked to cigarette smoking and alcohol consumption.

Symptoms and Diagnosis

This cancer commonly originates on the vocal cords or the surrounding structures and often causes hoarseness. A person who has been hoarse for more

than 2 to 3 weeks should seek medical attention. Cancer in other parts of the larynx can cause weight loss, throat pain, ear pain, and difficulty in swallowing or breathing or a combination. Sometimes, however, a lump in the neck resulting from the cancer's spread to a lymph node (metastasis) may be noticed before any other symptoms.

To make the diagnosis, a doctor initially examines the larynx with a mirror or with a thin viewing tube used for direct viewing of the larynx (laryngoscope) and removes a tissue sample for examination under a microscope (biopsy). A biopsy is most often performed in the operating room with the person under general anesthesia. Occasionally, it may be performed in the doctor's office, after a topical anesthetic has been applied. If cancer is present, people also may undergo a computed tomography (CT) scan of the neck and a chest x-ray or CT scan of the chest. A positron emission tomography (PET) scan also may be done.

? Did You Know?
A person who has been hoarse for more than 2 to 3 weeks should be checked by a doctor.

Staging and Prognosis

Staging is a way for doctors to describe how advanced the cancer has become, taking into account both the size and spread (metastasis) of the cancer (see page 1083). Staging helps the doctor guide therapy and assess prognosis. Cancer of the larynx is staged according to the size and location of the original tumor, the number and size of metastases to

Speech Without Vocal Cords

Speech requires a source of sound waves (vibrations) and a means of shaping those vibrations into words. The vocal cords normally provide the vibrations, which are then shaped into words by the tongue, palate, and lips. People whose vocal cords have been removed can regain their voice if a new source of sound vibrations can be provided, because their tongue, palate, and lips remain able to shape these new vibrations into words. There are three ways that people with no larynx can produce sound vibrations: esophageal speech, an electrolarynx, or a tracheoesophageal fistula (TEF). In all 3 techniques, sound is articulated into speech by the throat (pharynx), palate, tongue, teeth, and lips.

For esophageal speech, a person is taught to swallow air into the esophagus and gradually expel the air, as in a belch, to produce a sound. Esophageal speech is difficult for the person to learn and may be hard for other people to understand, but it requires no surgery or mechanical accessories.

An electrolarynx is a battery-powered vibrating device that acts as a sound source when held against the neck. It produces an artificial, mechanical sound. An electrolarynx is easier to use and understand than esophageal speech, but it requires batteries and must be carried with the person. Although it carries a great deal of social stigma for many people, an electrolarynx is functional immediately with little or no training.

A TEF is a one-way valve surgically inserted between the windpipe (trachea) and the esophagus. The valve diverts air into the esophagus while the person exhales, producing a sound. TEF requires significant practice and training but eventually can produce easy and fluent speech in many people. The valve may stay in place for many months, but it requires daily cleaning. If the valve malfunctions, secretions, fluids, and food may accidentally enter the windpipe. Some types of valves require the person to block the opening in the windpipe with a finger to operate the valve, while others can be operated hands-free.

Treatment

Treatment depends on the stage and the precise location of the cancer within the larynx. For early-stage cancer, doctors may use either surgery or radiation therapy. Usually, radiation is aimed not only at the cancer but also at the lymph nodes on both sides of the neck, because many of these cancers spread to those lymph nodes. When the vocal cords are affected, radiation therapy may be preferred over surgery because it may preserve a more normal voice. However, for very early-stage cancers of the larynx, microsurgery, sometimes performed with a laser, provides identical cure rates with equal preservation of the voice and can be completed in a single treatment. Using an endoscope to remove a laryngeal tumor has gained in popularity and is a viable alternative to radiation for larger tumors as well.

Tumors larger than 3/4 inch (about 2 centimeters) and those that have invaded bone or cartilage are usually treated with combination therapy. One combination consists of surgery to remove part or all of the larynx and vocal cords (partial or total laryngectomy) followed by radiation therapy. Radiation therapy is also commonly combined with chemotherapy as the primary treatment for advanced laryngeal cancers. This treatment provides cure rates equivalent to the surgery and radiation combination, and the voice is preserved in a significant number of people. However, surgery still may be required to remove any cancer that remains after this treatment. If the cancer is too advanced for surgery or radiation therapy, chemotherapy can help reduce the pain and the size of the tumor but is unlikely to provide a cure.

Treatment almost always has significant side effects. Surgery often affects swallowing and speaking. In such cases, rehabilitation is necessary. Using an endoscope to remove cancer reduces side effects on swallowing and speech when compared to surgery done through a neck incision. A number of methods have been developed that allow people without vocal cords to speak, often with good results. Depending on the specific tissue removed, reconstructive surgery may be performed. Radiation may cause skin changes (such as inflammation, itching, and loss of hair), scarring, loss of taste, and dry mouth, and, occasionally, destruction of normal tissues. People whose teeth will be exposed to the radiation treatments must have dental problems corrected and any unhealthy teeth removed, because radiation makes any subsequent dental work more likely to fail, and severe infections of the jawbone may occur. Chemotherapy typically causes a variety of side effects, depending on the drug used. These side effects may include nausea, vomiting, hearing loss, and infections.

the lymph nodes in the neck, and evidence of metastases in distant parts of the body. Stage I cancer is the least advanced, and stage IV is the most advanced.

The larger the cancer and the more it has spread, the worse the prognosis. If the tumor also has invaded muscle, bone, or cartilage, cure is less likely. About 85 to 95% of people with small cancers that have not spread anywhere survive for 5 years, compared with fewer than 50% of those who have cancer that has spread to the local lymph nodes. For people who have metastases beyond the local lymph nodes, the chance of surviving longer than 2 years is poor.

Paranasal Sinus Cancer

Cancer of the paranasal sinuses occurs mainly in the maxillary and ethmoid sinuses (see art on page 1398). Although rare in the United States, these cancers are more common in Japan and among the Bantu people of South Africa. Doctors are not sure what causes these cancers, but they are more common among people who regularly inhale certain types of wood and metal dust. Doctors do not think chronic sinusitis causes these cancers.

Because the sinuses provide room for the cancer to grow, most people do not develop symptoms until the cancer is well advanced. Symptoms, including pain, a sensation of nasal obstruction, double vision, nosebleeds, and loosened teeth in the jawbone underneath the affected sinus, result from the pressure of the cancer on nearby structures.

Doctors treat cancer of the sinuses with a combination of surgery and radiation therapy. Recent advances in surgical techniques have allowed doctors to remove the tumors completely, spare uninvolved parts of the face, such as the eye, and reconstruct the area with much better appearance. The earlier the cancer is treated, the better the prognosis. However, survival is generally poor. Only about 10 to 20% of people live more than 5 years.

Nasopharyngeal Cancer

- People often have a sensation of fullness or pain in the ears and may have hearing loss.
- A biopsy is needed for diagnosis, and imaging tests are done to evaluate the extent of the cancer.
- Treatment involves radiation therapy, chemotherapy, and sometimes surgery.

Cancer of the nasal passages and upper throat (nasopharynx) may occur in people of any age group. Although rare in North America, cancer of the nasopharynx is one of the most common cancers in Asia. This cancer is also more common among Chinese people who immigrated to North America than other Americans. It is less common among American-born Chinese than their immigrant parents or grandparents.

The Epstein-Barr virus, which causes infectious mononucleosis, plays a role in the development of nasopharyngeal cancer. There is also a hereditary predisposition. In addition, children and young adults who eat large amounts of salted fish (especially people with a poor intake of vitamins) are more likely to develop nasopharyngeal cancer.

Often, the first symptom is persistent blockage of the nose or eustachian tubes, which causes a sensation of fullness or pain in the ears and may cause hearing

Finding a Lump in the Neck

A doctor may discover an abnormal lump in the neck of a person who has no other symptoms. Most lumps are enlarged lymph nodes, which may enlarge because of a nearby infection, such as of the throat. However, an enlarged lymph node may also be caused by cancer, either a cancer of the lymph node (lymphoma) or a cancer that has spread to the lymph node from elsewhere in the body (metastasis). Lymph nodes in the neck are a common site for the spread of cancer from many parts of the body. Painless lumps are somewhat more worrisome than painful ones. Any lump that stays more than a few days should be evaluated by a doctor.

A doctor first examines the ears, nose, throat (pharynx), voice box (larynx), tonsils, base of the tongue, and thyroid and salivary glands. This examination often includes looking down the throat with a mirror or a thin flexible viewing tube. If there is no obvious source of infection or a visible cancerous spot, further tests are needed. The initial test is often a needle biopsy of the enlarged lymph node but may be computed tomography (CT) or magnetic resonance imaging (MRI) of the head and neck. Children, in whom lumps are caused most often by infection, are usually first given a trial of antibiotics.

To look for cancer originating in other parts of the body, doctors usually obtain x-rays of the upper digestive tract, a thyroid scan, and a CT scan of the chest. Direct examination of the larynx (laryngoscopy), lungs (bronchoscopy), and esophagus (esophagoscopy) may be needed.

When cancer cells are found in an enlarged lymph node and there are no signs of cancer anywhere else, the entire lymph node containing the cancer cells is removed along with additional lymph nodes and fatty tissue within the neck. If the tumor is large enough, doctors may also remove the internal jugular vein, along with nearby muscles and nerves. Radiation therapy is often given as well.

loss, particularly in one ear. If a eustachian tube is blocked, fluid may accumulate in the middle ear. A person also may have a discharge of pus and blood from the nose, swollen lymph nodes, and nosebleeds. Rarely, part of the face or an eye becomes paralyzed. Often, the cancer spreads to lymph nodes in the neck.

A doctor diagnoses the cancer by performing a biopsy of the tumor, in which a sample of tissue is removed and examined under a microscope. Computed tomography (CT) of the base of the skull and magnetic resonance imaging (MRI) of the head and neck are performed to evaluate the extent of the cancer. A positron emission tomography (PET) scan also commonly is done to assess the extent of the cancer.

The tumor is treated with radiation therapy and chemotherapy. If the tumor is large or persists, surgery may be needed, although these tumors are often not amenable to surgical removal. Overall, 35% of the people survive for at least 5 years after diagnosis. Early treatment improves prognosis significantly.

Tonsillar Cancer

- Tonsillar cancer is strongly linked to smoking and alcohol consumption.
- People usually have a sore throat and sometimes a lump in the neck.
- A biopsy is needed for diagnosis, and other tests are done to evaluate the extent of the cancer.
- Treatment involves radiation therapy, surgery, and chemotherapy.

Cancer of the tonsils occurs predominantly in men. It is strongly linked to smoking and alcohol consumption. Recent evidence suggests that human papillomavirus (HPV) is associated with tonsil cancer as well. People who have HPV-related tumors and who are non-smokers seem to have better survival rates. This cancer often spreads to the lymph nodes in the neck. Cancer of the tonsils occurs most often in people between the ages of 50 and 70.

A sore throat is often the first symptom. Pain usually radiates to the ear on the same side as the affected tonsil. Sometimes, however, a lump in the neck resulting from the cancer's spread to a lymph node (metastasis) may be noticed before any other symptoms. A doctor diagnoses the cancer by performing a biopsy of the tonsil, in which a sample of tissue is removed for examination under a microscope. Evaluation usually includes laryngoscopy (examination of the larynx), bronchoscopy (examination of the lungs), and esophagoscopy (examination of the esophagus). These areas are evaluated because of the high risk of additional cancers being present (up to 10%). A chest x-ray is done, and a computed tomography (CT) scan of the head and neck usually is also done.

About 50% of the people survive for at least 5 years after diagnosis, although the exact number depends on the stage of the cancer at the time of treatment.

Treatment typically includes radiation therapy, surgery, and chemotherapy. Small tumors may be treated with surgery alone or radiation therapy. Large tumors commonly are treated with a combination of chemotherapy and radiation therapy. Surgery may be needed for tumors that do not respond to the combination. Surgery may involve removal of the tumor, lymph nodes in the neck, and part of the jaw. There have been notable advances in the reconstruction used after surgery to remove the cancer, resulting in significant improvements in function and appearance.

Eye Disorders

CHAPTER
218 Biology of the Eyes

The structures and functions of the eyes are complex. Each eye constantly adjusts the amount of light it lets in, focuses on objects near and far, and produces continuous images that are instantly transmitted to the brain.

Structure and Function

The orbit is the bony cavity that contains the eyeball, muscles, nerves, and blood vessels, as well as the structures that produce and drain tears. Each orbit is a pear-shaped structure that is formed by several bones.

The eye has a relatively tough white outer layer (sclera or white of the eye). Near the front of the eye, the sclera is covered by a thin mucous membrane (conjunctiva), which runs to the edge of the cornea and also covers the moist back surface of the eyelids.

Light enters the eye through the cornea, a transparent dome on the front surface of the eye. The cornea serves as a protective covering for the front of the eye and also helps focus light on the retina at the back of the eye. After passing through the cornea, light travels through the pupil (the black dot in the middle of the iris), which is actually a hole through the iris. The iris—the circular, colored area of the eye—controls the amount of light that enters the eye so that the pupil dilates (enlarges) and constricts (shrinks) like the aperture of a camera lens. The iris allows more light into the eye when the environment is dark and allows less light into the eye when the environment is bright. The size of the pupil is controlled by the action of the pupillary sphincter muscle and dilator muscle.

Behind the iris sits the lens. By changing its shape, the lens focuses light onto the retina. Through the action of small muscles (called the ciliary muscles), the lens becomes thicker to focus on nearby objects and thinner to focus on distant objects.

The retina contains the cells that sense light (photoreceptors) and the blood vessels that nourish them. The most sensitive part of the retina is a small area called the macula, which has millions of tightly packed photoreceptors. The high density of photoreceptors in the macula makes the visual image detailed, just as high-resolution film has more tightly packed grains. Each photoreceptor is linked to a nerve fiber. The nerve fibers from the photoreceptors are bundled together to form the optic nerve. The optic disk, the first part of the optic nerve, is at the back of the eye. The photoreceptors in the retina convert the image into electrical impulses, which are carried to the brain by the optic nerve.

There are two main types of photoreceptor: cones and rods. Cones are responsible for sharp, detailed central vision and color vision and are clustered mainly in the macula. The rods are responsible for night and peripheral (side) vision. Rods are more numerous than cones and much more sensitive to

An Inside Look at the Eye

Posterior chamber · Vitreous humor · Anterior chamber · Optic nerve · Pupil · Lens · Cornea · Iris · Macula · Ciliary muscle · Retina · Conjunctiva · Sclera

Tracing the Visual Pathways

Nerve signals travel from each eye along the corresponding optic nerve and other nerve fibers (called the visual pathway) to the back of the brain, where vision is sensed and interpreted. The two optic nerves meet at the optic chiasm, which is an area behind the eyes immediately in front of the pituitary gland and just below the front portion of the brain (cerebrum). There, the optic nerve from each eye divides, and half of the nerve fibers from each side cross to the other side and continue to the back of the brain. Thus, the right side of the brain receives information through both optic nerves for the left field of vision, and the left side of the brain receives information through both optic nerves for the right field of vision. The middle of these fields of vision overlaps. It is seen by both eyes (called binocular vision).

An object is seen from slightly different angles by each eye so the information the brain receives from each eye is different, although it overlaps. The brain integrates the information to produce a complete picture.

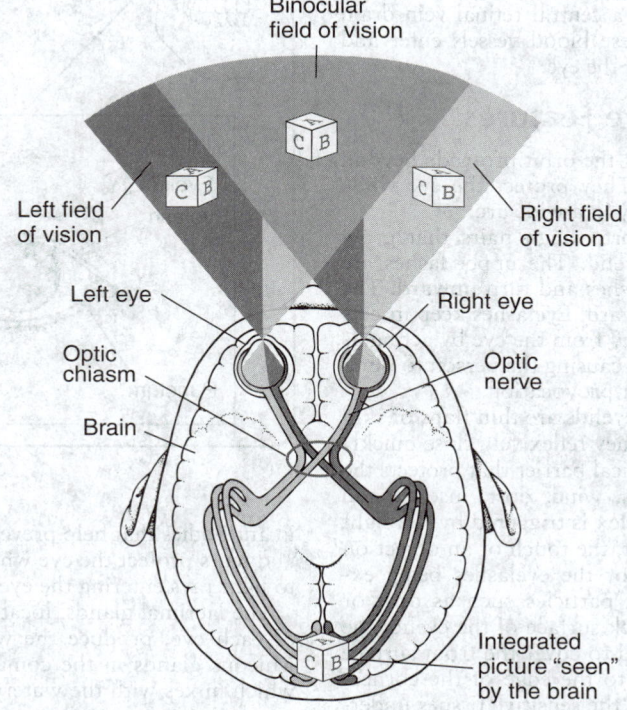

light, but they do not register color. Rods are grouped mainly in the peripheral areas of the retina and do not contribute to detailed central vision as the cones do.

The eyeball is divided into two sections, each of which is filled with fluid. The front section (anterior segment) extends from the inside of the cornea to the front surface of the lens. It is filled with a fluid called the aqueous humor, which nourishes the internal structures. The back section (posterior segment) extends from the back surface of the lens to the retina. It contains a jellylike fluid called the vitreous humor. The pressure generated by these fluids fills out the eyeball and helps maintain its shape.

The anterior segment itself is divided into two chambers. The front (anterior) chamber extends from the cornea to the iris. The back (posterior) chamber extends from the iris to the lens. Normally, the aqueous humor is produced in the posterior chamber, flows slowly through the pupil into the anterior chamber, and then drains out of the eyeball through outflow channels located where the iris meets the cornea.

Muscles, Nerves, and Blood Vessels

Several muscles working together move the eye, allowing people to look in different directions without moving their head. Each eye muscle is stimulated by a specific cranial nerve (see page 835). The optic nerve (a cranial nerve), which carries impulses from the retina to the brain, as well as other cranial nerves, which transmit impulses to each eye muscle, travel through the orbit.

An ophthalmic artery and a central retinal artery (an artery that branches off of the ophthalmic artery) provide blood to each eye. Similarly, ophthalmic veins (vortex veins) and a central retinal vein drain blood from the eye. These blood vessels enter and leave through the back of the eye.

Protective Features

The bony structures of the orbit protrude beyond the surface of the eye. They protect the eye while allowing it to move freely in a wide arc.

The eyelashes are short, tough hairs that grow from the edge of the eyelid. The upper lashes are longer than the lower lashes and turn upward. The lower lashes turn downward. Eyelashes keep insects and foreign particles away from the eye by acting as a physical barrier and by causing the person to blink reflexively at the slightest provocation.

The upper and lower eyelids are thin flaps of skin that can cover the eye. They reflexively close quickly (blink) to form a mechanical barrier that protects the eye from foreign objects, wind, dust, insects, and very bright light. The reflex is triggered by the sight of an approaching object, the touch of an object on the surface of the eye, or the eyelashes being exposed to wind or small particles such as dust or insects. On the moist back surface of the eyelid, the conjunctiva loops around to cover the front surface of the eyeball, right up to the edge of the cornea. The conjunctiva protects the sensitive tissues underneath it.

When blinked, the eyelids help spread tears over the surface of the eye. Tears consist of a salty fluid that continuously bathes the surface of the eye to keep it moist and transfers oxygen and nutrients to the cornea, which lacks the blood vessels that supply these substances to other tissues. When closed, the eyelids help trap the moisture against the surface of the eye. Small glands at the edge of the upper and lower eyelids secrete an oily substance that contributes to the tear film and keeps tears from evaporating. Tears keep the surface of the eye moist. Without such moisture, the normally transparent cornea can become dried, injured, infected, and opaque. Tears also trap and sweep away small particles that enter the eye. Moreover, tears are rich

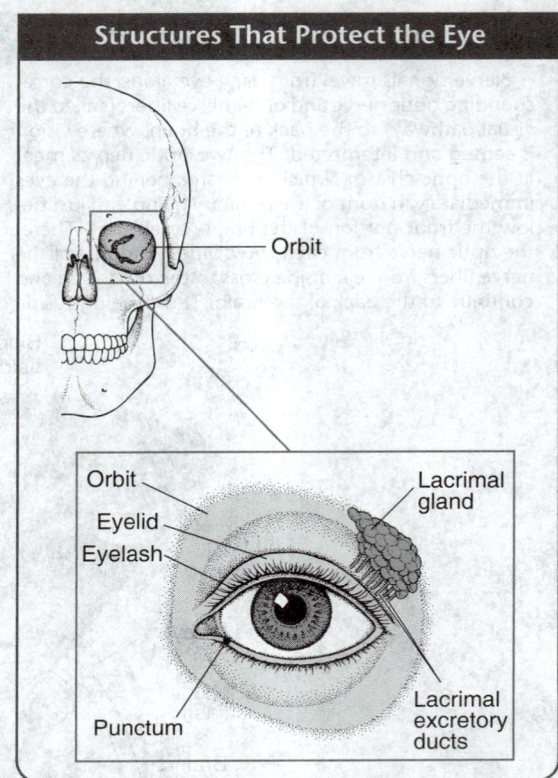

Structures That Protect the Eye

Orbit

Orbit
Eyelid
Eyelash
Punctum
Lacrimal gland
Lacrimal excretory ducts

in antibodies that help prevent infection. The eyelids and tears protect the eye while allowing clear access to light rays entering the eye.

The lacrimal glands, located at the top outer edge of each eye, produce the watery portion of tears. Mucous glands in the conjunctiva produce mucus, which mixes with the watery portion of the tears to create a more protective tear film. Tears drain from each eye into the nose through one of the two nasolacrimal ducts. Each of these ducts has openings at the edge of the upper and lower eyelids near the nose, called the punctum.

Effects of Aging

In middle age, the lens of the eye becomes less flexible and less able to thicken, and thus less able to focus on nearby objects, a condition called presbyopia. Reading glasses, or bifocal lenses, can help compensate for this problem.

In old age, changes to the sclera (the white of the eyes) include yellowing or browning due to many years of exposure to ultraviolet light, wind, and dust; random splotches of pigment (more common among people with a dark complexion); and a bluish hue due to increased transparency of the sclera.

The number of mucous cells in the conjunctiva may decrease with age. Tear production may also decrease with age, so that fewer tears are available to keep the surface of the eye moist. Both of these changes explain why older people are more likely to have dry eyes.

Arcus senilis (a deposit of calcium and cholesterol salts) appears as a gray-white ring at the edge of the cornea. It is common among people older than 60. Arcus senilis does not affect vision.

Some diseases of the retina are more likely to occur in old age, including macular degeneration, diabetic retinopathy, and retinal detachment. Other eye diseases, such as cataracts, also become common.

The muscles that squeeze the eyelids shut decrease in strength with age. This decrease in strength, combined with gravity and age-related looseness of the eyelids, sometimes results in the lower eyelid falling away from the eyeball, a condition called ectropion. In some older people, the fat around the orbit shrinks, causing the eyeball to sink into the orbit. Because of lax tissues in the eyelids, the orbital fat can also bulge forward into the eyelids making them appear constantly puffy.

The muscles that work to regulate the size of the pupils weaken with age. The pupils become smaller, react more sluggishly to light, and dilate more slowly in the dark. Therefore, people older than 60 may find that objects are not as bright, that they are dazzled initially when going outdoors (or when facing oncoming cars during night driving), and that they have difficulty going from a brightly lit environment to a darker one. These changes may be particularly bothersome when combined with the effects of a cataract.

Other changes in eye function also occur as people age. The sharpness of vision (acuity) is reduced despite use of the best glasses, especially in people who have a cataract, macular degeneration, or advanced glaucoma. The amount of light that reaches the back of the retina is reduced, increasing the need for brighter illumination and for greater contrast between objects and the background. Older people may also see increased numbers of floating black spots (floaters). Floaters usually do not significantly interfere with vision.

Symptoms and Diagnosis of Eye Disorders

Eye symptoms may involve changes in vision, changes in the appearance of the eye, or an abnormal sensation in the eye. Eye symptoms typically develop as a result of a problem in the eye but occasionally indicate a problem elsewhere in the body. For example, changes in vision may indicate a problem in the brain. Sometimes eye symptoms develop as part of an illness that affects several organ systems.

A person who experiences eye symptoms should be checked by a doctor. However, some eye diseases cause few or no symptoms in their early stages, so the eyes should be checked regularly (every 1 to 2 years or more frequently if there is an eye condition) by an ophthalmologist (a physician and surgeon who specializes in the diagnosis and treatment of eye diseases) or by an optometrist (a non-physician who specializes in refraction problems).

A person with eye or vision problems describes the location and duration of the symptoms, and then the doctor examines the eye, the area around it, and possibly other parts of the body, depending on the suspected cause. An eye examination usually includes refraction, a visual field testing, ophthalmoscopy, a slit-lamp examination, and tonometry.

Symptoms

CHANGES IN VISION

Changes in vision may involve loss of vision or distortion of vision. People often describe either type of change as blurring of vision.

Loss of Vision

Loss of vision is a complete or nearly complete absence of sight. People with loss of vision may see nothing whatsoever, or they may be able to distinguish light from dark and may even be able to detect vague shapes. Loss of vision may involve part or all of the visual field of one or both eyes and may be sudden or gradual, temporary or permanent. People usually notice sudden loss of vision immediately. However, gradual loss may not be noticed and may not be discovered for some time—perhaps not until a car accident or other event prompts a thorough vision examination.

Complete loss of vision may occur in one or both eyes. Common causes include blockage of the blood supply to the retina, diabetes, disorders that damage the optic nerve, glaucoma, cataracts, macular degeneration, injuries, and, in certain areas of the world, infections. Occasionally, complete or partial loss of vision occurs temporarily. This temporary loss of vision can be caused by a transient ischemic attack (sometimes called a mini stroke).

Many types of loss of vision involve only part of the visual field (visual field defects). For example, a stroke or tumor that affects the left side of the brain could result in an inability to see all or part of the right side of the visual field in both eyes (affected people can still see normally on the other side in both eyes). Another type of visual field defect results in an inability to see the outside part of the visual field in either eye (affected people can still see normally in the middle part of the visual field in both eyes). This pattern of visual field loss can be caused by a problem such as a tumor or aneurysm near the pituitary gland (which lies just below the brain, behind a cross-over of the optic nerve fibers). Some people lose the ability to see things in the

When the Visual Pathways Are Damaged

Nerve signals travel along the optic nerve from each eye. The two optic nerves meet at the optic chiasm. There, the optic nerve from each eye divides, and half of the nerve fibers from each side cross to the other side. Because of this arrangement, the brain receives information via both optic nerves for the left visual field and for the right visual field. Damage to an eye or the visual pathway causes different types of vision loss depending on where the damage occurs.

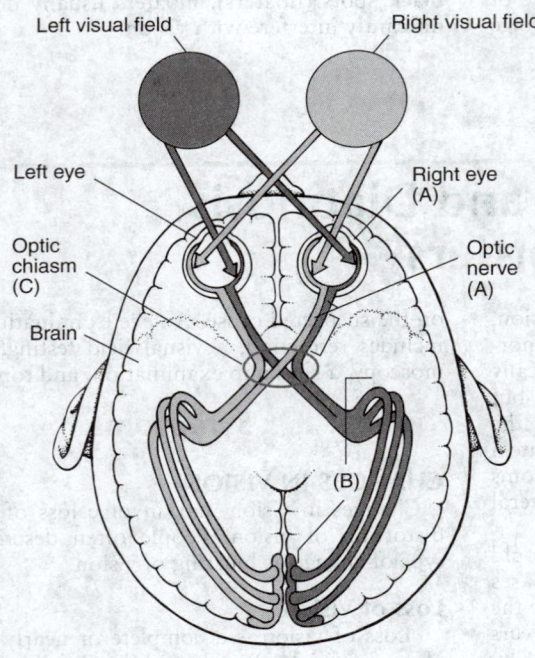

Left visual field

Right visual field

Left eye

Right eye (A)

Optic chiasm (C)

Optic nerve (A)

Brain

(B)

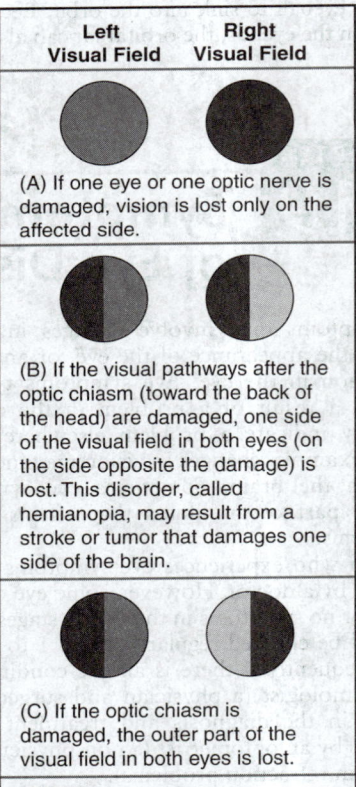

Left Visual Field	Right Visual Field

(A) If one eye or one optic nerve is damaged, vision is lost only on the affected side.

(B) If the visual pathways after the optic chiasm (toward the back of the head) are damaged, one side of the visual field in both eyes (on the side opposite the damage) is lost. This disorder, called hemianopia, may result from a stroke or tumor that damages one side of the brain.

(C) If the optic chiasm is damaged, the outer part of the visual field in both eyes is lost.

⬤ = Visual field lost.

How and Why Blindness Develops

Anything that blocks the passage of light from the environment to the back of the eye or disrupts the transmission of nerve impulses from the back of the eye to the brain will interfere with vision. Legal blindness is defined as a visual acuity of 20/200 or worse in the better eye, even after correction with eyeglasses or contact lenses, or a visual field restricted to less than 20° in the better eye. Many people who are considered legally blind can distinguish shapes and shadows but not normal detail.

Blindness can occur under the following circumstances:

LIGHT CANNOT REACH THE RETINA

- Damage to the cornea caused by infections such as trachoma, leprosy, or onchocerciasis, which results in an opaque corneal scar
- Damage to the cornea caused by vitamin A deficiency, which causes dry eyes (keratomalacia) and results in an opaque corneal scar
- Damage to the cornea caused by a severe injury that results in an opaque corneal scar
- A cataract, which causes loss of clarity of the lens

LIGHT RAYS DO NOT FOCUS ON THE RETINA PROPERLY

- Severe focusing (refraction) errors that are not fully correctible with eyeglasses or contact lenses

THE RETINA CANNOT SENSE LIGHT RAYS NORMALLY

- Detached retina
- Diabetes mellitus
- Macular degeneration
- Retinitis pigmentosa
- Inadequate blood supply to the retina, usually due to a blockage of the retinal artery or vein, which may be caused by inflammation of the blood vessel wall (such as that caused by temporal arteritis), or due to a blood clot that travels to the eye from somewhere else (such as from the carotid artery in the neck)
- Cytomegalovirus infection of the retina in people who have AIDS

NERVE IMPULSES FROM THE RETINA ARE NOT TRANSMITTED TO THE BRAIN NORMALLY

- Disorders affecting the optic nerve or its pathways inside the brain, such as brain tumors, strokes, infections, and multiple sclerosis
- Glaucoma
- Inflammation of the optic nerve (optic neuritis)

THE BRAIN CANNOT INTERPRET INFORMATION SENT BY THE EYE

- Disorders that affect the areas of the brain that interpret visual impulses (visual cortex), such as strokes and tumors

center of their visual field, but they retain their side or peripheral vision (where things are seen out of the "corner" of the eye). This type of defect can be caused by macular degeneration and certain disorders that damage the optic nerve. Smaller, irregular patches of vision may be lost as a result of disorders that damage the retina, such as diabetic retinopathy, hypertensive retinopathy, and retinal detachment. Loss of peripheral vision in all directions, so that the only remaining vision is in the middle of the field (tunnel vision), can be caused by glaucoma and certain retinal disorders (for example, retinitis pigmentosa).

The cause of vision loss can often be determined by the person's symptoms and the results of an examination, which usually includes refraction, visual field testing, ophthalmoscopy, slit-lamp examination, and tonometry. Additional examination and tests are done based on what disorders doctors suspect.

The disorder causing vision loss is treated. Depending on the cause, however, there may be no effective treatment.

Distortion of Vision

Distortion of vision is an inability to see clearly and correctly. This distortion may involve a poor focus due to refractive error, lack of depth perception, double vision, glare or halos, flashes of light, or floaters. It may also involve color blindness.

Refractive Error: Refractive error is an inability of the eye to properly focus an image onto the retina. It causes objects to appear blurred. Refractive error usually results from a mismatch between the focusing power of the cornea or lens and the length of the eye. Such a mismatch causes images to be focused slightly in front of or behind the retina. If only distant objects are blurred, the person is nearsighted (myopic). If only nearby objects are blurred, the person is farsighted (hyperopic). With myopia and hyperopia, objects tend to be blurred throughout the visual field, and the degree of blurring tends to be related to the distance between the eye and the object. Upon reaching middle age, most people—even those with previously excellent vision—develop difficulty focusing on nearby objects (presbyopia).

What Is Astigmatism?

Astigmatism is an irregularity in the curvature (curved differently in different directions) of the cornea or lens that causes light traveling in different planes to be focused differently. For example, vertical lines may be in focus when horizontal lines are not (or vice versa). The irregularity can be in any plane, however, and is often different in each eye. A person with astigmatism (each eye should be tested separately) tends to see certain lines more boldly (that is, in better focus) than the others. Astigmatism is correctible with prescription eyeglasses or contact lenses. It often occurs together with nearsightedness or farsightedness.

The diagram below is of a standard chart used to test for astigmatism in one eye at a time.

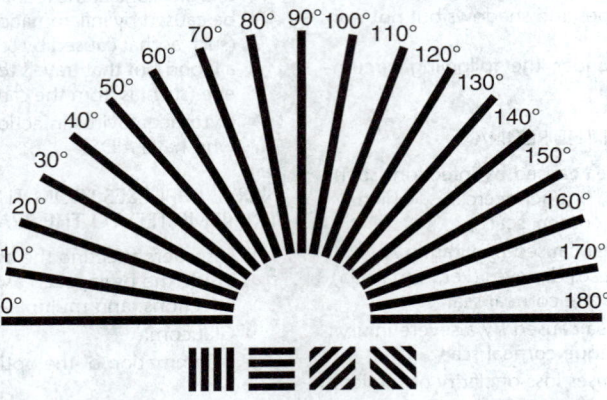

Astigmatism is another type of refractive error. Astigmatism results when the cornea is irregularly curved. For example, this curvature might result in horizontal lines being in focus but vertical lines being blurred. The irregular curvature can occur in any direction and can be different in each eye. Astigmatism can occur together with nearsightedness or farsightedness.

Refractive error is treated with corrective lenses (glasses or contact lenses) or refractive surgery such as laser in situ keratomileusis (LASIK). A person may need more than one type of corrective lens (for example, one to see distant objects and another to see nearby objects, as in bifocals). The blurred vision from refractive error can usually be fully corrected.

Impaired Depth Perception: Depth perception is the ability to determine the relative position of objects in space. People with impaired depth perception may have difficulty distinguishing which of two objects is closer.

The retina, being a two-dimensional surface like a piece of film in a camera, can only produce a two-dimensional image. The brain integrates the two-dimensional images from each eye to create a sense of three dimensions (stereopsis). Stereopsis allows people intuitively to perceive depth. Disorders in which the eyes do not align properly (such as strabismus) can interfere with stereopsis.

However, unlike stereopsis, some depth perception clues can be detected with only one eye. These clues include relative size, overlap, relative motion, movement parallax, and haziness and texture. For example, a car that looks larger, overlaps another, or moves faster across our field of vision is closer. Movement parallax means that when the head is shifted from side to side closer objects appear to move faster and farther across the field of vision. Objects that are farther away tend to appear hazy (because of the atmosphere), and their surface texture is less apparent. Most of these clues require knowledge of the normal size and appearance of the objects.

Double Vision (Diplopia): Double vision is seeing two images of one object. Double vision almost always occurs only when both eyes are open. This type of double vision is typically due to poor alignment of the eyes, usually caused by weakness in one or more of the muscles (or nerves) that control eye movements. This weakness results in cross-eyes (strabismus—see page 1818). Other causes include fatigue, alcohol intoxication, multiple sclerosis, and injury. The sudden appearance of double vision may indicate a serious disorder of the brain or nervous system, such as a tumor, aneurysm, or stroke. Rarely, double vision occurs when only one eye is open. Possible causes include cataracts, irregular astigmatism, displacement of the lens of the eye, and retinal detachment.

People are evaluated to determine whether double vision occurs with only one eye open (indicating a problem in the affected eye) or when both eyes are open (indicating a problem with eye movements). If double vision occurs only with both eyes open, doctors pay special attention to how well the eye muscles move the eyeball. The person is asked to move both eyes in all directions without moving the head. The doctor may also cover one of the eyes with a red lens or use prisms to help identify weakness in the muscles that control eye movements.

Treatment is directed at the disorder causing double vision.

Glare and Halos: Some people experience glare ("star bursts") or halos around bright lights, especially when driving at night. Such symptoms are more common in older people and in those who have had certain types of refractive surgery or who have certain types of cataracts. Glare and halos can also occur in people whose pupils are widely dilated (for example, those who have been given eye drops for an examination). When the pupil is widely dilated, light is able to pass through the peripheral part of the lens of the eye, where it is bent differently from light passing through the more central parts of the lens and therefore causes glare.

An eye examination is done. Sometimes symptoms can be relieved by treating the cause (for example, a cataract). Otherwise, people should take precautionary measures, such as minimizing driving at night or after receiving eye drops for an examination and avoiding looking directly at oncoming headlights while driving.

Night Blindness: Older people frequently have difficulty seeing in low light. This is sometimes referred to as night blindness. Most commonly night blindness results from a cataract, although night blindness is a feature in certain forms of retinal degeneration, such as retinitis pigmentosa. The eyes of some older people dilate slowly and take longer to adjust to low light. An eye examination should focus on detection of cataracts and should include an ophthalmoscopy. The cause is treated. Improving household lighting, particularly in the kitchen and around steps and other areas in which falls can occur, may improve safety.

Flashing Lights: Some people experience bright flashes of light, flickering lights, or streaks of light. This visual sensation most commonly results from shifting of the jellylike substance that fills the back of the eye (vitreous humor) or less commonly from a detached retina or a migraine headache. Before a migraine headache, some people temporarily see jagged, zigzag-like, bright, shimmery lines. Flashes

---

What Causes Color Blindness?

Color blindness (dyschromatopsia) affects how people perceive certain colors. It is usually present from birth and is nearly always due to an X-linked recessive gene, which means that almost all affected people are men. Women, who are not usually affected themselves, can pass the gene for color blindness on to their children.

Most cases of color blindness are due to a relative deficiency or abnormality of one of the types of light-sensing retinal cells (photoreceptors). Red-green color blindness, the most common form, is one example. Blue-yellow color blindness, however, may be caused by optic nerve disease and is usually due to acquired rather than inherited disease. Color blindness is also sometimes due to a problem with how the brain interprets color (rather than a problem with the eyes).

A person may be tested for color blindness if it is known that a family member has the abnormality. Some people may be tested because they notice they have difficulty with matching colors. Other people may be unaware of any problem until they are tested for a job or need a license (such as for piloting an airplane) that requires them to be able to distinguish colors.

---

of light can also result from a blow to the back of the head ("seeing stars"), probably because of stimulation of the part of the brain where vision is interpreted. An eye examination should concentrate on an ophthalmoscopy. A detached retina or migraine headache is treated. Otherwise, treatment may be unnecessary.

Floaters: Floating spots (floaters) are dark specks that appear to move in front of the eye. They are fast-moving or slow-moving clumps of the microscopic fibers that make up the vitreous humor. Floaters become increasingly common with age. Floaters rarely affect vision and are generally considered normal. However, a sudden increase in the number of floaters (especially in association with flashing lights) may indicate a serious problem, such as a detached retina. A person with these symptoms should be urgently evaluated by an ophthalmologist. If a detached retina is detected, it is treated.

Color Blindness: People who have color blindness (dyschromatopsia) are unable to perceive certain colors, or they may perceive certain colors with different intensity than do people with normal color vision. For instance, in the most common form of color blindness (red-green color blindness), people are less able to distinguish dark or pastel green or red or both. Often, the changes are subtle, and many people are unaware they have color blindness. People are often tested for color blindness if someone else in the family has the disorder or if a doctor suspects a problem with the nerve that carries information from the retina to the brain (optic nerve). Color blindness cannot be treated. At traffic lights, people with red-green color blindness should be guided by cues other than the color of the light.

CHANGES IN THE APPEARANCE OF THE EYES

Red Eye

The most common change in appearance is a red eye. Redness is usually due to dilation of blood vessels in the eye, usually in the thin membrane that covers the insides of the eyelids (conjunctiva), but sometimes in other eye structures such as the white of the eye (sclera), the connective tissue layer between the sclera and the conjunctiva (episclera), or the circular, colored area of the eye (iris) and nearby structures (uveal tract). Dilation is the result of inflammation, which can have many causes.

Many conditions dilate the blood vessels in the conjunctiva, including fatigue, allergies, infections, abrasions or ulcers of the cornea, and foreign bodies in the eye.

Conditions that inflame the sclera, episclera, and uveal tract include episcleritis, scleritis, and acute closed-angle glaucoma. These conditions usually also cause eye pain.

Sometimes redness is caused by bleeding of vessels in the conjunctiva. A forceful cough or a direct blow can cause a blood vessel in the conjunctiva to burst, resulting in a solid, bright red patch of blood on the sclera. Sometimes the bleeding turns the whole sclera bright red. With an allergy or a bacterial infection, the eyelids and other tissue around the eye may also become red, swollen, or both.

An eye examination usually reveals the cause of red eye, particularly if a slit-lamp examination is done. The cause is treated. Doctors do not usually recommend using eye drops, such as tetrahydrozoline, that simply shrink the dilated blood vessels.

Dark Spots

Dark (pigmented) spots can appear on the iris or conjunctiva. Some are present at birth, and others may appear with age. Although often insignificant, any dark spot that grows should be evaluated by an ophthalmologist to ensure that it is not cancer.

Pupil Size

Normally, both pupils (the black area in the middle of the iris) are the same size. Pupils become large (dilate) in the dark and become small (constrict) in bright light. Although some people have much larger pupils than others, large or small pupils by themselves do not necessarily indicate a problem or abnormality. The pupils tend to become smaller with age. Constricted or dilated pupils may be caused by certain drugs used to treat eye diseases. Pupil constriction may be caused by opioid drugs, such as morphine. Pupil dilation may be caused by amphetamines, antihistamines, cocaine, and marijuana. Small, irregularly shaped pupils may be caused by syphilis.

Unequal pupils (one large and one small) may be caused by conditions that affect one eye differently than the other. Such conditions may include injury or inflammation of the eye, injury of the nerves that control the pupil, head injury, brain tumors, and using eye drops in only one eye. Rarely, a person is born with pupils of different sizes.

During a complete eye examination, doctors shine light into each pupil, which causes them to constrict. No treatment is needed to modify pupil size.

Inflammation Around the Eye

The eyelids and tissues around the eyes may become swollen, red, or both as a result of allergy, infection, or other inflammation. Disorders can involve the eyelids (as in a chalazion, stye, or blepharitis), tear ducts (as in dacryocystitis), or sinuses. The roots of the eyelashes may become infected, sometimes resulting in the eyelashes falling out. Allergies or infections may also lead to abnormal secretions from the eyes, which may harden (crusting) and cause difficulty in opening the eyes when waking.

An eye examination, including a slit-lamp examination, is usually done. If infection is suspected, a culture (the process of growing a sample of the eye cells in a laboratory) may be needed. Doctors sometimes need to determine whether the sinuses are infected, which may require imaging studies such as a computed tomography (CT) scan. The cause is treated.

Other Changes

The sclera become yellow, as does the skin, in people who have jaundice (see page 214). The eyelids may droop (ptosis). Ptosis may occur in people who have myasthenia gravis (see page 818) and disorders that cause nerve damage. Sometimes the eyes are unusually wide open and prominent, usually because they are being pushed forward (exophthalmos). Exophthalmos can occur in people who have Graves' disease (see page 992).

People with these symptoms require an eye examination and a general medical evaluation. Treatment is directed at the cause.

ABNORMAL EYE SENSATION

Eye Pain

Pain may occur around the eye, in the eye, or behind the eye. Sharp eye pain that worsens with blinking or that is accompanied by a sensation of "something in the eye" is often caused by a corneal disorder, such as an abrasion, foreign body, ulcer, or infection. Severe, deep, aching pain in the eye may be caused by acute closed-angle glaucoma, especially if accompanied by significantly blurred vision, a red eye, and a "steamy" appearing cornea. A deep, boring pain in the eye can be a symptom of scleritis, a potentially serious inflammation of the thick fibrous coat of the eye, or uveitis, an inflammation of the inner structures of the eye. In some of these disorders, pain is worse with exposure to light (photophobia).

Light Sensitivity

Sensitivity to bright light occurs normally during extremely sunny conditions or when coming out of a dark environment into bright sunlight. Such sensitivity can also be caused by drugs used to dilate the pupils (mydriatics). However, pain resulting from bright light (photophobia) can be a symptom of a migraine headache or a number of eye disorders, for example, those that involve inflammation or infection within the front part of the eye (uveitis), a corneal disorder (such as keratitis), or an eye injury. It may also be due to meningitis (which is also typically accompanied by a severe headache and neck stiffness—see page 750).

Doctors first try to differentiate light sensitivity from photophobia. The cause of light sensitivity or photophobia can usually be determined by the person's symptoms and an eye examination. A slit-lamp examination is particularly useful for detecting disorders that cause photophobia. Light sensitivity and photophobia can be minimized by protecting the eyes from light (for example, by wearing sunglasses). When photophobia is the result of inflammation within the eye, dilating eye drops can help to relieve pain.

Itching

Itching may result from allergy and is usually accompanied by watering of the eyes (tearing). Inflammation of the eyelids (blepharitis) and dry eyes may also cause itching. Much less commonly, itching may result from infection or infestation with lice or other parasites. Abnormalities that cause itching can usually be diagnosed by a slit-lamp examination. Until the cause of itching is relieved, applying a cool washcloth may provide some relief.

Dryness

The sensation of dryness of the eyes can be caused by a variety of conditions, including inadequate tear production, accelerated tear evaporation, or, less commonly, refractive surgery, vitamin A deficiency, or Sjögren's syndrome. Dry eyes may also be a result of aging.

Tear production may be measured, particularly if Sjögren's syndrome is suspected. Doctors may also try to determine whether tears evaporate too quickly. They place a tiny amount of yellow dye (fluorescein) in an open eye and measure how long it takes for tears to evaporate. During the day, dry eyes can be relieved with the use of eye drops that substitute for a person's tears (artificial tears). At night, an ointment can be used before bed to relieve morning dryness.

Diagnosis

Diagnosis of eye disorders is initially based on the symptoms that the person is experiencing, the appearance of the eyes, and the results of an examination. A variety of tests can be carried out to confirm a problem or to determine the extent or severity of the disorder. Each eye is tested separately.

Refraction

Refraction is the procedure by which focusing error is assessed. Problems with visual acuity (sharpness of vision) that result from refractive errors, such as nearsightedness, farsightedness, astigmatism, and presbyopia, are diagnosed by refraction. Acuity is usually measured on a scale that compares a person's vision at 20 feet (about 6 meters) with that of someone who has perfect vision. Thus, a person who has 20/20 vision sees objects that are 20 feet away with the same clarity as a person with normal vision, but a person who has 20/200 vision sees at 20 feet only as clearly as a person with perfect vision sees at 200 feet (about 61 meters). One important visual acuity test uses the **Snellen chart** (eye chart), which is a large card or lighted box that displays rows of letters in smaller and smaller sizes. The chart is read from a standard distance. The degree of visual acuity is determined by the size of the row of letters that the person can read. For those who are unable to read, a modified chart can be used in which the letters are represented by an upper case "E," which is rotated randomly. The person is asked to describe the way the "E" is facing.

Automated refraction is done with machines that determine the refractive error of the eye by measuring how light is changed when it enters the eye. The person sits in front of the autorefractor, a beam of light is emitted from the device, and the eye's response is measured. The machine uses this information to calculate the lens prescription needed to correct the person's refractive error. This measurement takes only a few seconds.

A **phoropter** is the device commonly used, in conjunction with a Snellen chart, to determine the best corrective lenses for a person being assessed for eyeglasses or contact lenses. The phoropter contains a complete range of corrective lenses, allowing the person to compare different levels of correction while viewing the chart. Typically, the eye doctor uses the phoropter to refine the information obtained from the autorefractor before prescribing lenses.

Visual Field Testing

The visual field is the entire area of vision that is seen out of each eye, including the corners (peripheral vision). The visual field may be tested as a routine part of an eye examination. It may also be tested in detail if people notice specific changes in vision, for example, if they keep bumping into objects on one side. The simplest way to test peripheral vision is for a doctor to face the person and gradually move a finger in toward the center of vision from above, below, left, and right. The person tells the doctor when the moving finger is first detected. The person must fix his vision on the doctor's face (and not look for the finger) for the result of the test to be valid. The eye not being tested is closed.

The visual field may be measured in greater detail with a tangent screen or a Goldmann perimeter. With these tests, the person stares at the center of a black screen or a hollow, white, spherical device (which resembles a small satellite dish). An object or a light is moved slowly from the periphery toward the center of vision from many different directions. The person indicates when light is first seen out of the corner of the eye. A mark is made on the screen or perimeter indicating where the person can see, thus allowing recognition of blind spots. Visual fields can be measured using computerized automated perimetry. Here, the person stares at the center of a large shallow bowl and presses a button whenever a flash of light is seen.

The Amsler grid is used to test the central area of vision. The grid consists of a black card covered with a white grid and with a white dot in its center. The person notes any distortion in the lines of the grid while staring at the white dot. Each eye is tested at a normal reading distance and while wearing reading glasses, if the person normally uses them. If an area of the grid cannot be seen, an abnormal blind spot may exist. Beyond the area tested by the Amsler grid, there is a normal, small blind spot where the optic nerve leaves the eye; however, people are not aware of it. Wavy lines suggest a possible problem with the macula. The test is simple enough to be used at home and is useful for monitoring macular degeneration.

Color Vision Testing

A variety of tests can be used to detect a reduced ability to perceive certain colors (color blindness). Ishihara plates, which are most commonly used, are patterns of small, colored circles crowded together on a white background to form a large circle. The small circles are usually arranged so that people with normal color vision see a particular number. Those who have color blindness see another number or no number, depending on the type of color blindness.

What Is an Ophthalmoscope?

An ophthalmoscope is an instrument that enables a doctor to examine the inside of a person's eye. The instrument has an angled mirror, various lenses, and a light source. With it, a doctor can see the retina, the optic nerve, the retinal veins and arteries, and certain problems that can affect the vitreous humor (the jellylike substance in the eye).

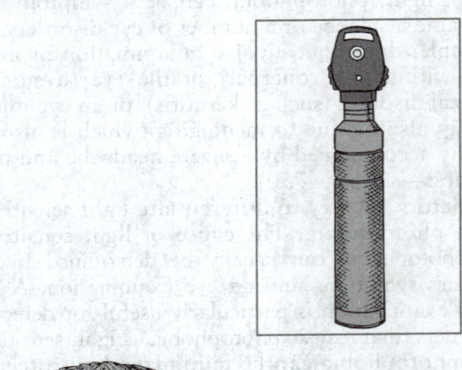

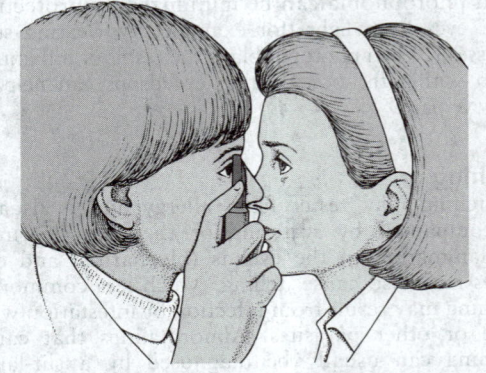

Ophthalmoscopic Examination

Ophthalmoscopy

A direct ophthalmoscope is a handheld device like a small flashlight with magnifying lenses that shines a light into the eye to enable a doctor to examine the cornea, lens, vitreous humor (the jellylike substance that fills the back of the eye), retina, optic nerve, and the retinal veins and arteries. The person looks straight ahead as the beam of light is shone into the eye. Often, eye drops are given to dilate (enlarge) the pupil, which allows the doctor to have a better view. Ophthalmoscopy is painless, but if eye drops are used to dilate the pupils, vision may be temporarily blurred, and the person will be more sensitive to light for a few hours afterward.

Ophthalmoscopy is a standard part of every regular eye examination. Ophthalmoscopy is used to detect not only changes in the retina due to eye disease but also changes in the eyes due to certain diseases affecting other parts of the body. For instance, it is used to detect the changes that occur in the retinal blood vessels in people who have high blood pressure, arteriosclerosis, and diabetes mellitus. Ophthalmoscopy may also provide a clue to elevated pressure within the brain, which results in a swelling (pushing-out) of the normally cupped optic disk (papilledema). Tumors on the retina can be seen with ophthalmoscopy. Macular degeneration can be diagnosed with ophthalmoscopy as well.

Sometimes the doctor uses an instrument called an indirect ophthalmoscope, in which a binocular device is placed on the doctor's head and a handheld lens is used in front of the person's eye to focus the image inside the eye. This method gives a three-dimensional view, allowing a better view of objects that have depth, including a detached retina. It also allows a brighter light source to be used, which is important if the interior of the eye is cloudy, for instance, because of a cataract. The indirect ophthalmoscope also allows a much wider field of view than a direct ophthalmoscope, so that the doctor can examine more of the retina.

Slit-Lamp Examination

The slit lamp is a table-mounted binocular microscope that shines a light into the eye to allow the doctor to examine the entire eye under high magnification. The slit lamp has better optics than the direct ophthalmoscope, providing magnification and a three-dimensional view, which allows measurement of depth. Often, eye drops are used to dilate the pupils so that the doctor can view even more of the eye, including the lens, vitreous humor, retina, and optic nerve. Sometimes, in people who have or might have glaucoma, an additional lens is placed on or held in front of the eye to allow examination

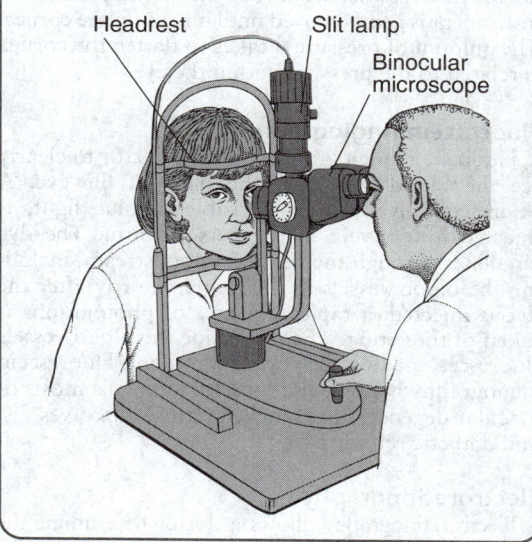

What Is a Slit Lamp?

A slit lamp is an instrument that enables a doctor to examine the entire eye under high magnification and that allows measurement of depth. The slit lamp focuses a bright light into the eye.

Headrest   Slit lamp

Binocular microscope

of the angle between the iris and the front part of the eye (inside surface of the cornea). This examination is called gonioscopy.

Tonometry

With tonometry, the pressure of the aqueous humor within the eye can be measured. The aqueous humor is the fluid in the front part of the eye between the cornea and the iris. Normal pressure within the eye is 8 to 21 millimeters of mercury (mm Hg). Pressure in the eye is measured to detect certain types of glaucoma and monitor its treatment.

The noncontact (air-puff) tonometer can be used to screen for elevated pressure in the eye. This device is not highly accurate, but it is useful in identifying people who may need further testing. A small puff of air is blown against the cornea, which causes the person to blink but is not uncomfortable. The puff of air flattens the cornea, and the device measures the time (in thousandths of a second) it takes to do so. It takes less time for the puff of air to flatten the cornea in an eye with normal pressure than it does an eye in which pressure is elevated.

Portable, handheld instruments are also used for tonometry. Eye drops that numb the eye are given, then the instrument is gently placed on the cornea, and a pressure reading is obtained. Portable tonometers can be used in the emergency department or a doctor's office to quickly detect increased pressure in the eye.

Applanation tonometry is a more accurate method. The applanation tonometer is usually attached to a slit lamp. After numbing the eye with drops, the doctor observes the eye through a slit lamp while the instrument is gently moved until it rests on the cornea. The amount of pressure it takes to flatten the cornea is related to the pressure within the eye.

Fluorescein Angiography

Fluorescein angiography allows a doctor to clearly see the blood vessels at the back of the eye. A fluorescent dye, which is visible in blue light, is injected into a vein in the person's arm. The dye circulates through the person's bloodstream, including the blood vessels in the retina. Shortly after the dye is injected, a rapid sequence of photographs is taken of the retina. The dye inside the blood vessels fluoresces, making the vessels stand out. Fluorescein angiography is particularly useful in the diagnosis of macular degeneration, blocked retinal blood vessels, and diabetic retinopathy.

Electroretinography

Electroretinography allows a doctor to examine the function of the light-sensing cells (photoreceptors) in the retina by measuring the response of the retina to flashes of light. Eye drops numb the eye and dilate the pupil. A recording electrode in the form of a contact lens is then placed on the cornea, and another electrode is placed on the skin of the face nearby. The eyes are then propped open. The room is darkened, and the person stares at a flashing light. The electrical activity generated by the retina in response to the flashes of light is recorded by the electrodes. Electroretinography is particularly useful

for evaluating diseases, such as retinitis pigmentosa, in which the photoreceptors are affected.

Ultrasonography

The eye can be examined by ultrasonography (see page 2044). A probe is placed gently against the closed eyelid and painlessly bounces sound waves off the eyeball. The reflected sound waves produce a two-dimensional image of the inside of the eye. Ultrasonography is useful when an ophthalmoscope or slit lamp cannot view the retina because the inside of the eye is cloudy or something is blocking the line of sight. Ultrasonography can be used to determine the nature of abnormal structures, such as a tumor, inside the eye. Ultrasonography also can be used to examine blood vessels supplying the eye (Doppler ultrasonography) and to determine the thickness of the cornea (pachymetry).

Pachymetry

Pachymetry (measuring the thickness of the cornea) is very important in refractive eye surgery, such as laser in situ keratomileusis (LASIK).

Pachymetry is usually done by using ultrasonography. For ultrasound pachymetry, the eye is numbed with drops, and an ultrasound probe is placed gently onto the surface of the cornea. Optical pachymetry methods do not require numbing eye drops because the instruments do not touch the eye.

Computed Tomography and Magnetic Resonance Imaging

These imaging techniques (see also pages 2037 and 2040) can be used to provide detailed information about the structures inside the eye and the bony structure that surrounds the eye (the orbit). Computed tomography is particularly useful for locating foreign bodies inside the eye.

CHAPTER

220   Refractive Disorders

In refractive disorders, the eye focuses light rays incorrectly on the retina, causing blurred vision.

- The shape of the eye or cornea or age-related stiffness of the lens may decrease the focusing power of the eye.
- Objects may appear blurry when far away, near, or both.
- An ophthalmologist (medical doctor who specializes in diagnosing and treating eye diseases and performing eye

surgery) or optometrist (a nonphysician who specializes in refractive errors) determines how best to correct refraction.

- Glasses, contact lenses, or refractive surgery can correct vision.

The eye normally creates a clear image because the cornea and lens bend (refract) incoming light rays to focus them on the retina. The shape of the

Understanding Refraction

Normally, the cornea and lens bend (refract) incoming light rays to focus them on the retina. When there is a refractive error, the cornea and lens cannot focus light rays on the retina. Refractive errors can be corrected by eyeglasses or contact lenses.

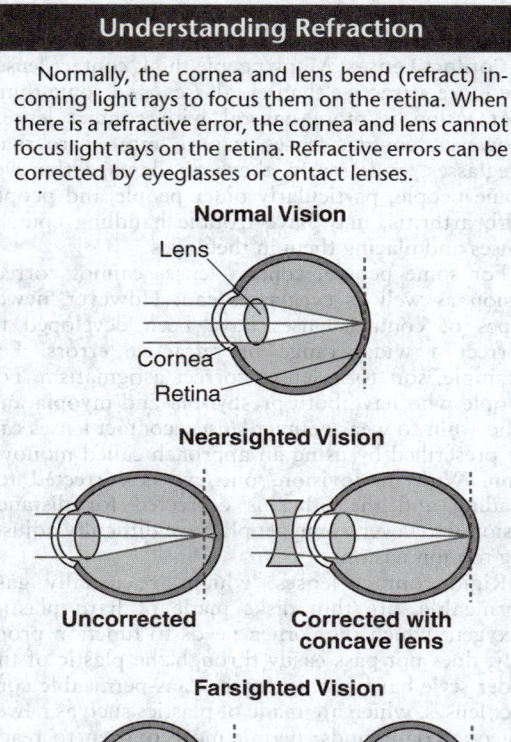

Normal Vision

Lens

Cornea

Retina

Nearsighted Vision

Uncorrected

Corrected with concave lens

Farsighted Vision

Uncorrected

Corrected with convex lens

cornea is fixed, but the lens changes shape to focus on objects at various distances from the eye. By becoming more rounded, the lens allows near objects to be focused. By becoming flatter, the lens allows objects farther away to be focused. When the cornea and lens cannot focus the image of an object sharply on the retina, it is called a refractive error.

Causes

The lens and cornea may not bend light rays to focus them on the retina correctly for several reasons. The eyeball may be too large for the refractive power of the cornea and lens. Because of this, light is focused in front of (rather than directly on) the retina, and the person has trouble clearly seeing distant objects. This is called nearsightedness (myopia). In some people, the eyeball is too small for the refractive power of the cornea and lens, so light is focused behind the retina. This is called farsightedness (hyperopia). People who are farsighted have trouble clearly seeing anything close and far as they get older. Some people have an imperfectly shaped cornea (not perfectly round or spherical), which may cause objects to appear blurred at any distance. This is called astigmatism (see box on page 1418). Sometimes people have a significant difference between the refractive errors of the eyes. This is called anisometropia.

As people reach their early 40s, the lens becomes increasingly stiff. The lens does not change shape easily, so it cannot focus on nearby objects, a condition called presbyopia. If a person has had a lens removed to treat cataracts (see page 1445) but has not had a lens implant, objects look blurred from any distance. The absence of a lens (as a result of birth defect, eye injury, or eye surgery for cataract) is called aphakia.

Symptoms and Diagnosis

A person who has a refractive error may notice that vision is blurred. For example, a child who becomes nearsighted may have difficulty seeing the chalkboard in school.

Everyone should have regular eye examinations by a family doctor, internist, ophthalmologist, or optometrist. A Snellen eye chart is used to determine sharpness of vision (visual acuity). Visual acuity is measured in relation to what a person with normal (unimpaired) vision sees. For example, a person with 20/60 vision sees at 20 feet (about 6 meters) what a person with normal vision sees at 60 feet (about 18 meters). In other words, the person must be 20 feet away to read letters that a person with normal vision can read from 60 feet away. Although refractive errors usually occur in otherwise healthy eyes, testing generally also includes assessments unrelated to refractive error, such as a test of the visual fields (see page 1422) and eye movements. The eyes are tested together and individually.

Treatment

The usual treatment for refractive errors is to wear corrective lenses. However, certain surgical procedures and laser treatments that change the shape of the cornea also can correct refractive errors.

? Did You Know...

Vision corrected by rigid contact lenses is usually sharper than vision corrected by soft contact lenses.

The best way to reduce the risk of infection is to not sleep in contact lenses.

What Are Low-Vision Aids?

Aids for coping with vision loss (referred to as low-vision aids) can be an enormous help to people with only partial vision. Low-vision aids for reading, writing, watching television, and engaging in outdoor activities include the following:

- Large-print books
- Large-numbered telephones, clocks, watches, and thermometers
- Closed-circuit television to magnify objects
- Electronic "talking" clocks and other "talking" devices
- Computer programs that can scan text and then produce larger text or read the text out loud
- Light filters to improve contrast
- Color-coded pill boxes
- Handheld magnifying glasses
- Glare-reducing sunglasses
- Handheld binoculars

Eye doctors working with other health care practitioners can usually evaluate how vision loss affects a person. They can then recommend a combination of low-vision aids that they believe would best help the person carry out daily tasks.

Corrective Lenses

Refractive errors can be corrected with glass or plastic lenses mounted in a frame (eyeglasses) or with a small piece of plastic floating on the cornea (contact lens). Good vision correction is possible with both eyeglasses and contact lenses. For most people, the choice is a matter of appearance, convenience, cost, and comfort.

Eyeglasses: Plastic lenses for eyeglasses are lighter but tend to scratch. Glass lenses are more durable but are more likely to break. Plastic lenses are more commonly used because they are thinner and can also be coated with a substance that helps them resist scratches. Both glass and plastic lenses can be tinted or treated with a chemical that darkens them automatically when exposed to light. Lenses can also be coated to reduce the amount of potentially damaging ultraviolet light that reaches the eye.

Bifocals contain two lenses—an upper lens that corrects the view of distant objects and a lower lens that corrects the view of nearby objects, as in reading. However, people also need to focus at middle distances, such as when viewing a computer screen. Trifocals meet this need by adding a lens for middle distance. Continuously variable lenses (progressive add lenses) also permit focusing at middle distances and

have a cosmetic advantage in that there is no line or sharp division between the regions of the eyeglass lens.

Contact Lenses: Many people think contact lenses are more attractive than eyeglasses, and some think that vision is more natural with contact lenses. However, contact lenses require more care than eyeglasses, and, rarely, they can damage the eye. Some people, particularly older people and people with arthritis, may have trouble handling contact lenses and placing them in their eyes.

For some people, contact lenses cannot correct vision as well as eyeglasses can. However, newer types of contact lenses have been developed to correct a wider range of refractive errors. For example, soft toric lenses correct astigmatism. For people who have both presbyopia and myopia and who want to wear contact lenses, contact lenses can be prescribed by using an approach called monovision. With monovision, one eye is corrected for reading and the other is corrected for distance vision. However, some people have difficulty adjusting to monovision.

Rigid contact lenses, which are usually gas-permeable, are thin disks made of hard plastic. Oxygen, which the cornea needs to function properly, does not pass easily through the plastic of the older style hard contact lenses. Gas-permeable contact lenses, which are made of plastics such as newer silicone compounds, permit more oxygen to reach the cornea. Rigid contact lenses can be used to correct irregularities in the cornea (astigmatism).

Rigid contact lenses usually require some time for the eye to adapt to their presence and need to be worn for up to a week before they feel comfortable for a prolonged period. The contact lenses are worn for a gradually increasing number of hours each day. Although rigid contact lenses may be uncomfortable at first, they should not be painful. Pain indicates an improper fit. Vision with rigid contact lenses is usually sharper than vision with soft contact lenses.

Soft hydrophilic (water-absorbing) contact lenses are made of flexible plastic. They are larger than rigid contact lenses and cover the entire cornea. Not all soft contact lenses allow oxygen to reach the cornea easily.

Because they are larger, soft contact lenses are easier to handle than are rigid contact lenses. They are also less likely than rigid contact lenses to fall out or to allow dust and other particles to get trapped underneath. In addition, soft contact lenses are usually comfortable from the first wearing. Soft contact lenses require scrupulous care to prevent problems, because the risk of infection is higher with soft contact lenses than with rigid contact lenses.

Most contact lenses must be removed and cleaned every day (daily wear). Most contact lenses must be disinfected each night and cleaned of protein and calcium deposits. Some require weekly treatment with an enzyme. They are not disposable. Some contact lenses are disposable. They do not require cleaning, enzyme treatment, or disinfecting if used only for one day. Some lenses are used for 1 to 4 weeks and then thrown away. Some regular or disposable soft contact lenses are designed so that they may be kept in the eye during sleep for a number of days (extended wear). Most can be kept in place for up to 7 days, but newer contact lenses are available that can be kept in place for up to 30 days. However, the risk of infection is higher with contact lenses that are worn overnight.

Wearing contact lenses poses a risk of serious, vision-threatening, painful complications, including the formation of ulcers on the cornea. Ulcers can be caused by an infection, which can lead to a loss of vision (see page 1442). The risks can be greatly reduced by following the instructions of the eye doctor and the manufacturer and by using common sense.

The risk of serious infections increases when swimming with contact lenses and if contact lenses are cleaned with homemade saline solution, saliva, tap water, or distilled water. Sleeping while wearing any type of contact lens also increases the risk of serious infections. The risk of infection increases for every night a person sleeps in soft contact lenses. The best way to reduce the risk of infection is to not sleep in contact lenses. If a person experiences discomfort, excessive watering of the eye, vision changes, or eye redness, the contact lenses should be removed immediately. If the symptoms do not resolve quickly, the person should contact an eye doctor.

Surgery for Refractive Errors

Surgical and laser procedures (refractive surgery) can be used to correct nearsightedness, farsightedness, and astigmatism. These procedures are used to reshape the cornea so that it is better able to focus light on the retina. The goal of refractive surgery is to decrease dependence on eyeglasses or contact lenses. Before deciding on such a procedure, people should have a thorough discussion with an ophthalmologist and should carefully consider their own needs and expectations, along with the risks and benefits.

The best candidates for refractive surgery are people who cannot tolerate contact lenses and those who enjoy activities, such as swimming or skiing, which are difficult to do with eyeglasses or contact lenses. Many people undergo this surgery for convenience and cosmetic purposes. However, refractive surgery is not recommended for all people with

SPOTLIGHT ON AGING

Most commonly, vision loss among older people is due to clouding of the lens of the eye (cataracts) or to damage to the optic nerve (as occurs in glaucoma) or the retina (as occurs in age-related macular degeneration and diabetic retinopathy). A less common cause of vision loss is blockage of the blood supply to the eye. Eyelid disorders mostly change the appearance of the eye and do not usually cause vision loss, but they can cause discomfort.

Whatever the reason for vision loss, any vision change can compromise an older person's quality of life and, indirectly, health. For example, poor eyesight may contribute to a car crash or to a fall. Loss of vision can be especially devastating to older people coping with other problems as well, such as poor balance and hearing loss. In such cases, vision loss can contribute to significant injury and can impair a person's ability to do daily activities.

refractive errors. For example, people whose eyeglass or contact lens prescription has changed in the past year and those with autoimmune diseases or connective tissue diseases, with a cone-shaped cornea (keratoconus), with severe dry eyes, who are taking certain drugs (for example, isotretinoin or amiodarone), and with a few exceptions, people younger than 18 years of age, usually should not have laser refractive surgery.

The doctor determines the exact refractive error (eyeglass prescription) before surgery. The eyes are thoroughly examined, and special attention is paid to the surface cells of the cornea (including whether the cornea has a loose or well-anchored surface), the shape and thickness of the cornea (using pachymetry—see page 1424), the pupil size in light and dark, the intraocular pressure, the optic nerve, and the retina. Refractive surgical procedures are generally brief and cause little discomfort. Eye drops are used to numb the eye. Because the eye is not held still, the person must not move the eye during the procedure. Usually, a person can go home soon after the procedure.

After refractive surgery, most people have distance vision that is good enough to do most things well (for example, driving or going to the movies), although not everyone has perfect 20/20 vision without eyeglasses after the procedure. About 95% of people do not need corrective lenses for distance vision. The people most likely to have 20/20 distance vision after surgery are those who have weak eyeglass prescriptions before refractive surgery. Even if they do not wear eyeglasses for distance vision, most people older than 40 still need to wear eyeglasses for reading after refractive surgery.

Complications may include overcorrection, undercorrection, excessive inflammation, infection, double vision, sensitivity to bright light, glare and halos around lights, difficulty with seeing or driving at night, wrinkling of the cornea, and deposition of cells or other material in the cornea. Rarely, even with eyeglasses, a person may have worse vision after refractive surgery. Because treating undercorrection is usually easier than treating overcorrection, surgeons prefer not to overcorrect. If undercorrection or overcorrection occurs, further correction can usually be done.

Laser in Situ Keratomileusis (LASIK): LASIK, the most common refractive surgical procedure, is used to correct nearsightedness, farsightedness, and astigmatism. In LASIK, a very thin flap is created in the central part of the cornea with a laser or a cutting device called a microkeratome. The flap is lifted, and pulses from an excimer laser vaporize tiny amounts of corneal tissue under the flap to reshape the cornea. The flap is then laid back in place and heals over several days. LASIK causes little discomfort during and after surgery. Vision improvement is rapid, and many people are able to go back to work within 1 to 3 days. People who have any conditions that preclude refractive surgery, as well as those who have thin corneas or a loose corneal surface, may not be good candidates for LASIK.

Photorefractive Keratectomy (PRK): This procedure also uses an excimer laser to reshape the cornea. It is used primarily to correct moderate nearsightedness, astigmatism, and farsightedness. Unlike LASIK, no flap is created. The cells on the surface of the cornea are removed at the start of the procedure. As in LASIK, computer-controlled pulses of highly focused ultraviolet light remove small amounts of the cornea and thus change its shape to better focus light onto the retina and improve vision without eyeglasses. This procedure usually takes less than 1 minute per eye. Although there is more discomfort and longer healing time than with LASIK (because the removed surface cells need to grow back), PRK can be done on people who cannot have LASIK, such as those with loose corneal surface cells or thin corneas.

Other Refractive Surgery: Other techniques are available that may have advantages over or different risks than LASIK and PRK. For people who are very nearsighted, a plastic lens can be placed inside the eye, in front of or behind the iris (phakic intraocular lens implantation). Sometimes the natural lens is removed, and the plastic lens is placed behind the iris (clear lensectomy with intraocular lens implantation). Clear lensectomy with intraocular lens implantation may be better for people with hyperopia and who need reading glasses (presbyopia). Because these techniques make an opening into the eye, there is a very small risk (but significantly higher than for LASIK) of severe infection inside the eye. Other risks of phakic intraocular lens implantation include cataract formation, glaucoma, and swelling of the cornea over time. Clear lensectomy should usually be avoided in young people who are very nearsighted because they have an increased risk of retinal detachment.

Intracorneal ring segments (INTACS) are used for people with mild nearsightedness without astigmatism. Small plastic arcs are implanted into the middle layer of the cornea near its outer edge. Because no tissue is removed during the procedure, the intracorneal ring segment procedure can be reversed by removing the small plastic arcs. Risks include astigmatism, undercorrection, overcorrection, infection, glare, and seeing halos.

Conductive keratoplasty (CK) is used for people with mild farsightedness without astigmatism or for people that only need to wear reading glasses (presbyopia). It is a quick surgical procedure that does not involve any cutting. Rather, several small laser spots are placed in the cornea. The laser spots cause contraction of the cornea in a ring pattern and change the shape of the cornea. There are few risks, but some people lose some of the effect over time, and a few develop astigmatism.

Astigmatic keratotomy is used to correct naturally occurring astigmatism and astigmatism that occurs after cataract surgery or corneal transplantation. In this procedure, the surgeon makes one or two curved or straight deep cuts in the surface or outer part of the cornea parallel to the edge of the cornea. These cuts change the shape of the cornea to help lessen the corneal irregularities of astigmatism.

221 Injuries to the Eye

The structure of the face and eyes is well suited for protecting the eyes from injury. The eyeball is set into the orbit, a socket surrounded by a strong, bony ridge. The eyelids close quickly to form a barrier to foreign objects, and the eye can tolerate minor impact without damage. Because of these protective features, many eye injuries do not affect the eyeball and are thus not dangerous, even though extensive bruising and swelling to surrounding structures may make them look worse than they are. However, injury occasionally damages the eye so severely that vision is affected and sometimes completely lost. In rare instances, the eye must be removed.

Causes

Common causes of eye injury include domestic or industrial accidents (for instance, from using a hammer or liquid chemicals or cleaners), assault, car battery explosions, sports injuries (including air-gun or paint pellet-gun injuries), and motor vehicle collisions (including air-bag injuries). Exposure to strong ultraviolet light, as from a welding arc or bright sunlight reflected off snow, can injure the transparent dome on the front surface of the eye (cornea—see page 1441).

Evaluation

A person with an eye injury should be examined by a doctor. Glasses (if worn) should be brought so that the person's vision can be assessed with their normal correction—this can help the doctor know whether any abnormal vision is a new problem or an old one. The eye examination may include a slit-lamp examination (see page 1423) and ophthalmoscopy (see page 1423). The slit lamp contains a light, an adjustable binocular magnifying instrument, and a table that adjusts the position of these components. A slit-lamp examination assesses mainly the front of the eye, particularly the eye surface and eyelid. Ophthalmoscopy assesses mainly the back of the eye. Often, ophthalmoscopy is done after the eye is dilated with eye drops such as cyclopentolate and phenylephrine. After dilation, more of the eye can be seen, particularly the retina.

If the injury is serious, particularly if the vision is affected, the doctor who first examines the person arranges for an ophthalmologist (a medical doctor who specializes in eye disorders) to evaluate and treat the person.

Blunt Injuries to the Eye

A blunt impact may damage the structures at the front of the eye (the eyelid, conjunctiva, sclera, cornea, iris, and lens) and those at the back of the eye (retina and optic nerve). Such an impact may also break (fracture) the bones that surround the eye. Blunt trauma occasionally also results in cuts (lacerations) to the tissues of the eye.

Injured eyes may be very swollen and difficult to open. Still, doctors need to open the eyes to examine them and make sure there is no injury that will affect vision. The eyes almost always can be opened gently, although instruments may be needed to do so.

BLACK EYE

In the first 24 hours after a blunt eye injury, blood may leak into the skin of the eyelid and surrounding areas, causing swelling and a bruise (contusion), commonly called a black eye. The blood usually drains toward the bottom of the eye after a day or two, resulting in swelling and discoloration just below the lower eyelid. Black eyes themselves have no effect on vision, although other eye injuries that accompany them may be serious.

Black eyes resolve without treatment after a few days or weeks. During the first 24 to 48 hours, ice packs may help reduce swelling and ease the pain of a black eye, followed by warm compresses to aid absorption of the blood. Nonsteroidal anti-inflammatory drugs (such as aspirin or ibuprofen) or acetaminophen can be given if the pain is significant.

SUBCONJUNCTIVAL HEMORRHAGE

A blood vessel on the conjunctiva (the thin layer of tissue that covers most of the eye's surface) may break, causing a solid red patch of blood on the white of the eye. Sometimes the whole white of the eye appears red. The blood lies under the conjunctiva (subconjunctival hemorrhage) and is superficial. Therefore, although the blood may look alarming, it is minor and resolves without treatment. The red area may become slightly green and then yellow within a few days. All traces of the blood typically disappear within 1 to 2 weeks. A subconjunctival hemorrhage often occurs together with a black eye.

HYPHEMA

A hyphema (anterior chamber hemorrhage) is bleeding into the front chamber (the fluid-filled space between the clear cornea and the colored iris—see art on page 1412) of the eye. Additional bleeding may occur up to several days after the injury. A hyphema may result in permanent, partial, or complete loss of vision. Vision loss may be caused by increased pressure within the eye (glaucoma), by blood staining the cornea, or both.

People with hyphema often have blurred vision and pain when exposed to bright light. If the hyphema is large enough, a layer of blood is visible behind the lower part of the cornea when the person is upright. However, the layer may be so small that it can be seen only with magnification.

Treatment

A person with a hyphema should be examined by an ophthalmologist (a medical doctor who specializes in eye disorders) as soon as possible. Treatment usually involves bed rest with the head of the bed elevated to encourage the blood to settle. Eye drops are given to dilate the pupil (such as atropine) and to reduce inflammation within the eye (usually corticosteroids). A protective shield (either a commercial product or the bottom part of a paper cup) is taped over the eye to prevent further injury. Pressure within the eye is measured at least once daily for the first few days. If the pressure is elevated, the ophthalmologist may give eye drops such as those used to treat acute glaucoma. Aspirin and other nonsteroidal anti-inflammatory drugs, which can predispose to bleeding, should be avoided for several weeks. Because a hyphema increases the life-long risk of developing glaucoma, people who have had a hyphema should have their eyes examined every year.

RETINAL DETACHMENT

Blunt injury may cause part of the retina or the entire retina to tear or to separate (detach) from its underlying surface at the back of the eyeball (see page 1454). Usually, only part of the retina is detached (often the outside, or peripheral, part of the retina), but if treatment does not occur soon, more of the retina can detach.

Initially, retinal detachment may create images of irregular dark floating shapes (floaters) or flashes of light. Parts of vision may be blurred or lost, usually side (peripheral) vision. If more of the retina detaches, more vision is blurred or lost.

A person with these symptoms needs to see a doctor as soon as possible. The diagnosis is made by an ophthalmologist, who examines the back of the eye with a bright light (ophthalmoscopy) after the eye has been dilated. Sometimes an ultrasound examination is done. An ophthalmologist can sometimes reattach a detached retina or prevent the injury from

worsening by using various treatments such as surgery, lasers, or freezing therapy (cryopexy).

OTHER BLUNT INJURIES TO THE EYEBALL

Other injuries that can occur after a blunt force include bleeding in the back section of the eye (vitreous hemorrhage), tearing of the iris, and displacement (dislocation) of the lens. Usually, the force required to cause these injuries is high. Affected people tend to have obvious, severe eye injuries with many abnormalities. All affected people have impaired vision. Examination by an ophthalmologist and treatment should occur as soon as possible.

Fractures of the Orbit

- Pain and swelling develop, and double vision or decreased vision may occur.
- Computed tomography is usually done.
- Sometimes the fracture is repaired surgically.

A severe blow to the face can fracture any of several bones that form the orbit. Occasionally, the eyeball itself also is damaged.

Blowout Fracture: Sometimes the eye is struck in such a way that the force of the blow is received by the eyeball and not blocked by the strong bones around the eye (as when struck by a small object such as a golf ball). In this case, the pressure on the eyeball is transmitted to the walls of the orbit. This pressure can fracture the most fragile part of the orbit, which is typically the part underneath the eyeball (orbital floor). This is known as a blowout fracture. Fractures can also occur to the sides (walls) and roof of the orbit. Sometimes part of the eye or the muscles attached to it are forced through the fractured bone and become trapped.

Blowout fractures sometimes cause double vision, a sunken eyeball, an eyeball that is stuck looking downward, a decreased sensitivity to touch and pain around the cheek and upper lip (caused by injury to the nerves below the orbit), or an accumulation of air in the tissues under the skin (subcutaneous emphysema). Double vision can occur if one of the muscles that move the eye is trapped in the fracture. The trapped muscle prevents the eye from aiming itself at the object the other eye is looking at. Subcutaneous emphysema occurs if a fracture of the orbital floor allows air from the nose or sinuses to enter the tissues around the eye, particularly when people blow their nose.

Symptoms

Fractures are painful, and the area swells because blood and fluid accumulate. The accumulated blood usually causes the swollen area to appear blue or purple (a black eye). Sometimes the nose bleeds.

Vision may be impaired if the eyelids are swollen shut, or on rare occasions if the eyeball is damaged or if blood from torn blood vessels accumulates behind the eyeball (retrobulbar hematoma) and puts pressure on the nerve leading to the brain (optic nerve).

Diagnosis and Treatment

Diagnosis is suspected based on the symptoms and results of a physical examination. A doctor who suspects an orbital fracture performs a computed tomography (CT) scan, which shows any fractures, collections of blood, and displaced or trapped tissue.

People who have an orbital fracture should avoid blowing their nose, which may produce swelling by causing the air they blow out to collect under the skin around the eye. Using a nasal spray that constricts blood vessels (topical vasoconstrictor) for 2 to 3 days may help minimize nosebleeds. Applying ice as for other fractures and injuries can help decrease pain and swelling. Keeping the head elevated above the level of the heart may also help prevent further swelling. Analgesics can help control pain. Surgical repair of the facial bones is usually necessary if a blowout fracture traps muscles or soft tissues of the orbit and causes double vision or nerve injury or makes the eyeball sunken or if symptoms do not go away in 2 weeks. After ensuring that the fracture has not damaged a vital structure, the surgeon restores the bones to their proper position, sometimes using implants, a thin plastic sheet, or a bone graft to connect the broken parts and assist healing.

Lacerated Eyeball

Most cuts (lacerations) around the eyes affect the eyelids rather than the eyeball. Of those that affect the eyeball, many are superficial and minor. However, some cuts go through the white of the eye (sclera) or the transparent dome on the front surface of the eye (cornea), penetrating the eye's interior. Such cuts are considered a rupture of the eyeball (globe). The globe also can be ruptured by a blunt force. Such lacerations can seriously damage the structures necessary for vision. They also predispose to infection within the eye (endophthalmitis).

Most people with a ruptured globe can barely see. The eye is often obviously distorted, and the pupil may be shaped like a teardrop. Sometimes fluid leaks out of the eye.

Diagnosis and Treatment

An immediate evaluation by an ophthalmologist (a medical doctor who specializes in eye disorders) is required. Surgical repair is often necessary, except for some injuries that affect only the thin mucous membrane that covers the cornea (conjunctiva). Even before surgery, antibiotics are given to reduce the chance of infection within the eye. Antibiotics are given intravenously (by vein). Ointments should be avoided. A protective shield (either a commercial product or the bottom part of a paper cup) is taped over the eye to avoid unintentional pressure that could force the contents of the eye through the laceration. If necessary, vomiting can be controlled with drugs that treat nausea. Eye drops are given to dilate the pupil, which can help prevent scar tissue from forming on the colored part of the eye (iris) and may reduce the ache and sensitivity to light that often occur after an injury. Drugs for pain are given by vein or, if surgical repair is not needed, by mouth.

Even after all possible medical and surgical treatment, a serious injury may result in partial or total loss of vision. Very rarely, after a severe eyeball laceration (or eye surgery), the uninjured eye becomes inflamed (sympathetic ophthalmia), which may result in partial loss of vision or even blindness if left untreated. Often, corticosteroid drops, pills, and injections can effectively prevent this reaction. Doctors often remove an irreversibly damaged eye to prevent sympathetic ophthalmia.

Eyelid Lacerations

If the skin around the eye or on the eyelid has been cut, stitches may be needed. When possible, stitches near the edge of the eyelid should be placed by an ophthalmologist (a medical doctor who specializes in eye disorders) to ensure that no deformities develop that will affect the way the eyelids close. An injury that causes the eyelid to droop or affects the tear ducts (ducts that drain tears off of the eye) also should be repaired by an ophthalmologist. The tear ducts are in parts of both the lower and upper eyelids nearest the nose.

Corneal Abrasions and Foreign Bodies

The most common eye injuries involve the surface of the transparent dome on the front surface of the eye (cornea). They include scratches (abrasions) and foreign bodies. Foreign bodies in the cornea leave abrasions behind after they are removed. Most of these injuries are minor.

Causes

Particles are common causes of corneal abrasions. Particles can be dispersed via explosions, wind, or working with tools (for example, hammering or drilling). Tree branches or falling debris can also cause corneal abrasions. Another common source of abrasions is contact lenses. Poorly fitting lenses, lenses worn when the eyes are dry, lenses that have been incompletely cleaned and that have particles attached to them, lenses left in the eyes too long, lenses left in inappropriately during sleep, and forceful or inept removal of lenses can result in scratches on the surface of the eyes. Most corneal abrasions heal without developing infections (such as conjunctivitis and corneal ulcers), but those contaminated with soil or vegetable matter (for example, an injury caused by a tree branch) are more likely to become infected.

Symptoms

Corneal abrasions and foreign bodies usually cause pain, tearing, and a feeling that there is something in the eye. They may also cause redness (due to bleeding from blood vessels on the surface of the eye) or, occasionally, swelling of the eye and eyelid. Vision may become blurred. Light may be a source of irritation or may cause the muscle that constricts the pupil to undergo a painful spasm.

Injuries that penetrate the eye may cause similar symptoms. If a foreign object penetrates the inside of the eye, fluid may gush out.

Diagnosis and Treatment

Prompt diagnosis and appropriate treatment can help prevent infection. The diagnosis is based on the person's symptoms, the circumstances of the injury, and the examination.

The surface of the eye is usually numbed with an anesthetic drop (such as proparacaine). An eye drop containing a dye (fluorescein) that glows under special lighting makes surface objects more visible and reveals abrasions. Using a slit lamp (see page 1423) or other magnifying instrument, the doctor then removes any remaining foreign objects. Often the foreign object can be lifted out with a moist sterile cotton swab or flushed out with sterile water (irrigation). If the person is able to stare without moving the eye, foreign objects that cannot be dislodged easily with a swab can often be removed painlessly with a needle or a special instrument. When metal foreign bodies are removed, they can leave a ring of rust, which may need to be removed with a low-speed rotary sterile burr (a small surgical tool with a tiny, rotating, grinding and drilling surface). Sometimes a foreign body is trapped under the upper eyelid. The eyelid must be flipped over (a painless procedure) to remove the foreign body.

Corneal abrasions are treated similarly whether or not a foreign body was removed. Usually, an antibiotic ointment that tends to destroy *Pseudomonas* bacteria (such as ciprofloxacin ointment) is given for a few days to prevent infection. Large abrasions may require additional treatment: The pupil is kept dilated with cycloplegic eye drops (such as cyclopentolate or homatropine). These drops prevent painful spasm of the muscles that constrict the pupil. Pain can be treated with oral drugs such as acetaminophen or acetaminophen with oxycodone. Anesthetics that are applied directly to the eye, although they relieve pain effectively, should not be used after evaluation and treatment because they can impair healing. Eye patches may increase the risk of infection and usually are not used, particularly for abrasions that result from a contact lens or an object that may be contaminated with soil or vegetable matter.

Fortunately, the surface cells of the eye regenerate rapidly. Even large abrasions tend to heal in 1 to 3 days. A contact lens should not be worn for 5 days after the abrasion heals. A follow-up examination by an ophthalmologist 1 or 2 days after the injury is wise.

Protective eyewear (safety glasses) can help prevent many injuries.

INTRAOCULAR FOREIGN BODIES

Rarely, a foreign body penetrates the eye, causing an intraocular (inside the eye) foreign body. A serious infection can develop.

Causes

Explosions can cause intraocular foreign bodies. So can anything with a metal-on-metal mechanism. Explosions and certain tool mechanisms often cause small particles to fly in a person's face. For example, using high-speed machines (such as drills, grinders, and saws) or hammering a nail or other metal object with a hammer can produce white-hot particles of metal that resemble sparks. Any of these white-hot particles can enter the unprotected eye and become embedded deep within it.

Foreign bodies that penetrate the inside of the eye can infect the inside of the eye (endophthalmitis).

Symptoms and Diagnosis

During the first hours after injury, symptoms of intraocular foreign bodies may be similar to those of corneal abrasions and foreign bodies. However, people with intraocular foreign bodies may also have a noticeable loss of vision. Fluid may leak from the eye, but if the foreign body is small, the leak may be so small that the person is not aware of it. Also, pain may increase after the first several hours.

When a foreign object has penetrated the eye, an ophthalmologist should examine the person as soon as possible. The eye is examined as for corneal abrasions and foreign bodies by using eye drops that contain a dye that glows under special lighting (fluorescein) and a slit lamp (see page 1423). The dye and slit lamp make visible any small leaks of fluid from the eye and puncture marks. Any foreign bodies outside of the eyeball are removed. If an intraocular foreign body is suspected after the examination, an imaging study such as computed tomography (CT) is done.

Prevention and Treatment

People with certain occupations or hobbies, particularly those that use grinders, drills, saws, or hammers, should wear protective eyewear (such as face shields, safety glasses, or goggles) to help prevent intraocular foreign bodies and other eye injuries.

Antibiotics such as ceftazidime and vancomycin are given intravenously. A protective shield (such as a commercially prepared shield or the bottom part of a paper cup) is taped over the eye to avoid unintentional pressure that could further damage the eye. An ophthalmologist should remove the foreign body as soon as possible. Prompt removal reduces the risk of infection. Sometimes a surgical procedure is needed to remove the foreign body.

Chemical Burns to the Eye

The eyelids close quickly in a reflex reaction to protect the eyes from harm. However, irritating or harmful chemicals still sometimes get onto the surface of the eye, causing burns. The most dangerous chemical burns involve strong acids or alkali. Alkali substances include lye (caustic soda), which is found in many drain cleaners. Burns may involve liquids, which splash, or, less commonly, powdered material, which can blow into the eyes.

Severe chemical burns of the transparent dome on the front surface of the eye (cornea), especially alkali injuries, can lead to scarring, perforation of the eye, and blindness. Burns to the eye are very painful. Because the pain is so great, a person tends to keep the eyelids closed. Closed eyelids keep the substance against the eye for a prolonged period, which may worsen the damage.

Treatment

A chemical burn of the eye is treated immediately, even before medical personnel arrive. The eye is opened and flushed (irrigated) with water or saline. With burns caused by strong acids or alkali or other severely caustic substances, the eye should be irrigated continuously for 30 to 120 minutes. Irrigation can be continued where it began, in an ambulance, or in a hospital. Because pain may make it difficult for the person to keep the injured eye open, another person may have to hold the eyelid open while the eye is irrigated. If possible, the water or saline should be at room temperature. A doctor or other health care practitioner can instill an anesthetic drop in the eye to make it much easier to keep the injured eye open.

After irrigation, the doctor examines the surface of the eye and the inside of the eyelid and removes any substance still embedded in the tissue. The inside of the eyelid is also swabbed to remove any tiny particles that may not be visible. A doctor may instill a drop of a drug (such as homatropine) that dilates the pupil, relaxing the muscles of the colored part of the eye (iris) and preventing them from having painful spasms. Although anesthetic eye drops relieve pain, they also slow healing and are avoided after the initial irrigation. If the cornea is burned, an antibiotic ointment (such as ciprofloxacin) is put in the eye. Pain can be treated with acetaminophen or, if very severe, acetaminophen with oxycodone.

Severe burns need to be treated by an ophthalmologist (a medical doctor who specializes in diagnosing and treating eye diseases and performing eye surgery) within 24 hours to preserve vision and prevent major complications, such as damage to the cornea and iris, perforation of the eye, and deformities of the eyelid. Corticosteroid drops (such as prednisolone) may also be given by an ophthalmologist for a limited period of time. Severe burns require frequent eye examinations.

Wearing safety glasses or a face shield when handling potentially hazardous chemicals is essential to help prevent chemical burns.

Traumatic Iritis and Chemical Iritis

Iritis (also known as iridocyclitis or uveitis) is inflammation of the pigmented inside lining of the eye (uvea), iris, or both.

Iritis can develop after blunt eye trauma or a chemical burn, typically within 3 days. However, iritis can also develop without injury.

Symptoms may include tearing, redness of the eye, and a painful ache in the eye. Usually people have some blurred vision or pain when exposed to bright light (photophobia).

A doctor bases the diagnosis on the person's history, symptoms, and the results of a slit-lamp examination (see page 1423).

Iritis is treated by instilling into the eye a drug that dilates the pupil. The drug relaxes the muscles of the colored part of the eye (iris), which spasm painfully. These drugs are called cycloplegics and include cyclopentolate and homatropine. Corticosteroid eye drops (such as prednisolone) are often used to shorten symptom duration. Cycloplegics and corticosteroids are usually adequate to relieve pain, but if necessary, the person can also take acetaminophen.

CHAPTER
222

Eyelid and Tearing Disorders

The eyelids play a key role in protecting the eyes. They sweep away debris when the eyes close and help spread moisture (tears) over the surface of the eyes when they open. The eyelids provide a mechanical barrier against injury by closing rapidly when needed.

An abnormality of the tear (lacrimal) glands can lead to insufficient tear production or to a deficiency in the composition of the tears themselves. Without adequate or normal tear production, the eyes can dry and may be unable to normally fight infections from airborne particles, fingertips, or surrounding skin. Abnormal tear production may be due to a problem within the tear glands (lacrimal glands) and ducts (lacrimal excretory ducts, which carry tears into the eye) or due to a body-wide (systemic) disease that affects the tear glands, such as Sjögren's syndrome (see page 577).

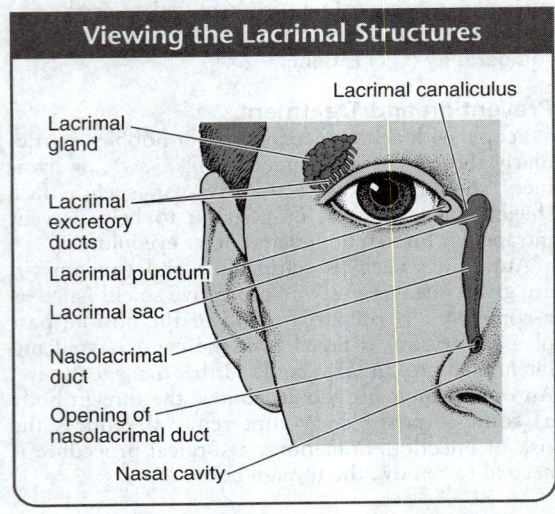

Viewing the Lacrimal Structures

- Lacrimal canaliculus
- Lacrimal gland
- Lacrimal excretory ducts
- Lacrimal punctum
- Lacrimal sac
- Nasolacrimal duct
- Opening of nasolacrimal duct
- Nasal cavity

Blepharitis

Blepharitis is inflammation of the edges of the eyelids, possibly with thickening scales, crusts, shallow ulcers, or redness and swelling at the edges of the eyelids.

- The inflammation is caused by certain infections, allergic reactions, and some skin conditions.
- The eyelids become irritated, red, and swollen and may burn and itch.
- Usually the diagnosis is based on symptoms and the appearance of the eyelids.
- Any underlying disorders are treated, and sometimes antibiotic ointments, artificial tears, or both are given.

Causes

Disorders that may cause blepharitis include staphylococcal infection of the eyelids or the ducts of the deeper glands that open at the edges of the eyelids, certain viral infections, and allergic reactions (to pollens or sometimes to eye drops). Skin conditions such as seborrheic dermatitis (see page 1287) and rosacea (see page 1294) affect the face including the eyelids, leading to inflammation and blepharitis. Sometimes the inflammation has no known cause.

Symptoms

Blepharitis may cause the feeling that something is in the eye. The eyes and eyelids may itch and burn, and the edges of the eyelids may become red. The eyes may become watery and sensitive to bright light. The eyelids may swell, and some of the eyelashes may fall out. Sometimes, small abscesses containing

pus (pustules) develop in the sacs at the base of the eyelashes and eventually form shallow ulcers (ulcerative blepharitis). A crust may form and stick tenaciously to the edges of the eyelids. When the crust is removed, the surface may bleed. During sleep, secretions dry and make the eyelids stick together.

Blepharitis tends to recur and stubbornly resist treatment. It is inconvenient and unattractive but usually does not damage the cornea or result in loss of vision. Occasionally, ulcerative blepharitis can result in a loss of the eyelashes, scarring of the eyelid margins, and, rarely, even inflammation affecting the cornea.

Diagnosis

Diagnosis is usually based on the symptoms and the appearance of the eyelids. A doctor may use a slit lamp (see art on page 1423) to examine the eyelids more closely. Occasionally, a sample of material is taken from the edges of the eyelids and is cultured to identify the type of bacteria responsible and the antibiotics to which they are susceptible.

Treatment

Artificial tears and eye lubricant ointments (for use overnight) may help. The causative problem is treated when possible. For example, an eye drop that seems to be the cause can be stopped. Warm compresses placed over the closed eyelid may relieve symptoms and speed resolution. For blepharitis caused by seborrheic dermatitis, treatment usually includes keeping the eyelids clean by gently scrubbing the edges of the eyelids each day with a wash cloth or cotton swab dipped in a dilute solution of baby shampoo (2 to 3 drops in ½ cup of warm water). For inflamed oil glands at the edge of the eyelids, warm compresses may relieve inflammation, easing the itching and burning. Occasionally, a doctor may prescribe an antibiotic ointment, such as bacitracin plus polymyxin B ointment, gentamicin ointment, erythromycin ointment, or sulfacetamide ointment, or an antibiotic taken by mouth, such as doxycycline. When seborrheic dermatitis is the cause, the face and scalp must be treated as well (see page 1287). If rosacea is the cause, it also can be treated (see page 1294).

Canaliculitis

Canaliculitis is infection of the lacrimal canaliculus, also called the lacrimal duct (see art on page 1434).

Canaliculitis may cause tearing, discharge, red eye, and mild tenderness. Redness and tenderness are most prominent at the side of the eye near the nose. The symptoms can resemble those of dacryocystitis. An ophthalmologist (a medical doctor who specializes in diagnosing and treating eye diseases and performing eye surgery) can often irrigate the infected duct with an antibiotic solution. People should then apply warm compresses and use antibiotic eye drops. Occasionally, the infection requires surgical treatment.

Chalazion

A chalazion is an enlargement of an oil gland deep in the eyelid caused by an obstruction of the gland's opening.

At first, a chalazion looks and feels like a stye: swollen eyelid, mild pain, and irritation. However,

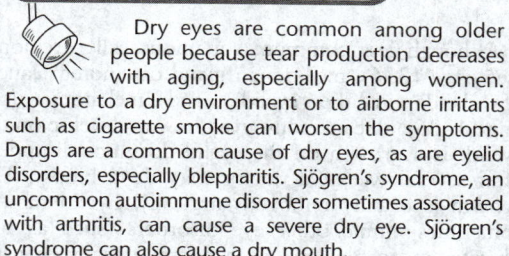

SPOTLIGHT ON AGING

Dry eyes are common among older people because tear production decreases with aging, especially among women. Exposure to a dry environment or to airborne irritants such as cigarette smoke can worsen the symptoms. Drugs are a common cause of dry eyes, as are eyelid disorders, especially blepharitis. Sjögren's syndrome, an uncommon autoimmune disorder sometimes associated with arthritis, can cause a severe dry eye. Sjögren's syndrome can also cause a dry mouth.

Using Eye Drops and Eye Ointments

The person receiving the drop or ointment should lean back and look up. With a clean forefinger, the lower eyelid is gently pulled down to create a pocket. Eye drops are then dropped into the pocket, not directly onto the eye. When using eye ointments, a small strip of ointment is placed in the pocket. Blinking distributes the drop or ointment over the eye.

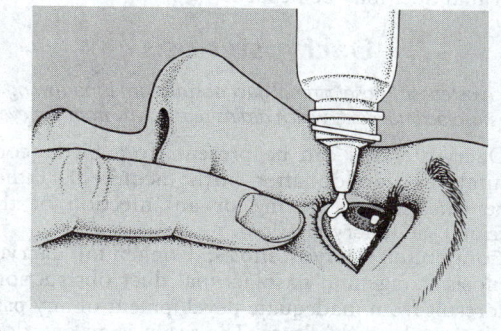

these symptoms disappear after 1 or 2 days, leaving a round, painless swelling in the eyelid that grows slowly for the first week. Occasionally, the swelling continues to grow and may press on the eyeball and cause slight blurring. A red or gray area may develop on the underside of the eyelid.

Most chalazions disappear without treatment within 2 to 8 weeks. If hot compresses are applied several times a day, chalazions may disappear sooner. If they remain after this time or if they cause vision changes, a doctor can drain them or inject a corticosteroid. Antibiotics are usually not an effective means of treatment.

Dacryocystitis

Dacryocystitis is infection of the lacrimal sac.

The lacrimal sac is a small chamber into which tears drain. The usual cause of dacryocystitis is a blockage of the nasolacrimal duct, which leads from the lacrimal sac into the nose. Dacryocystitis may occur suddenly (acute) or be longstanding (chronic). In acute infection, the area around the lacrimal sac is painful, red, and swollen. The eye may become red and watery and may ooze pus. Slight pressure applied to the lacrimal sac may push pus through the lacrimal punctum, the opening at the inner corner of the eye, near the nose.

Often the infection is mild. Sometimes, the infection is severe and can cause fever. Sometimes an abscess may form, which can rupture through the skin, creating a passage for drainage.

An acute infection is usually treated with an antibiotic taken by mouth. If a fever is present or if the infection is severe, antibiotics given by vein may be required. Applying warm compresses to the area several times a day also helps. If an abscess develops, minor surgery may be done to open and drain it. For chronic infections, especially if recurrent, more extensive surgery to bypass the blocked nasolacrimal duct may be needed.

Dacryostenosis

Dacryostenosis (nasolacrimal duct obstruction) is narrowing of the nasolacrimal duct, which drains tears away from the eye.

Dacryostenosis can be present from birth (congenital) or develop after birth (acquired). Either type can lead to tearing or an infection of the lacrimal sac (dacryocystitis).

Congenital Dacryostenosis: Congenital dacryostenosis (congenital nasolacrimal duct obstruction) can result from inadequate development of any part of the nasolacrimal ducts. The result is an overflow of tears that run down the cheek (epiphora) or persistent crusting. One or both eyes can be affected. The problem is usually first noticed in 3- to 12-week-old infants. This type of blockage usually disappears without treatment by the age of 6 to 9 months, as the nasolacrimal system develops. Sometimes the blockage resolves faster when parents gently massage the area above the duct with a fingertip.

If the blockage does not clear up, an ear, nose, and throat specialist (otorhinolaryngologist) or an eye specialist (ophthalmologist) may have to open the nasolacrimal duct with a small probe, which is usually inserted through the duct opening (lacrimal punctum) at the corner of the eyelid.

Acquired Dacryostenosis: Acquired dacryostenosis is often a result of age-related narrowing of the duct but can also occur from scarring after an injury or surgery. Simply inserting a probe as is done with congenital dacryostenosis is generally not effective. If dacryostenosis causes persistent, bothersome tearing or repeated episodes of infection, surgery may be needed.

Entropion and Ectropion

Entropion is a condition in which the eyelid is turned inward (inverted), causing the eyelashes to rub against the eyeball. Ectropion is a condition in which the eyelid is turned outward (everted) so that its edge does not touch the eyeball.

Normally, the upper and lower eyelids close tightly, protecting the eye from damage and preventing tear evaporation. If the edge of one eyelid turns inward (entropion), the eyelashes rub against the eye, which can lead to ulcer formation and scarring of the cornea. If the edge of one eyelid turns outward (ectropion), the two eyelids cannot meet properly, and tears are not spread over the eyeball. These conditions are more common among older people (generally the result of tissue relaxation with aging), among those with eye changes caused by infection, surgery, or trauma, and among those who have blepharospasm (see page 784).

Both entropion and ectropion can irritate the eyes, causing a feeling that something is in the eye, watering, and redness. Artificial tears and eye lubricant ointments (for use overnight) can be used to keep the eye moist and soothe the irritation. Entropion and ectropion can be treated surgically—for instance, to preserve sight if damage to the eyes (such as corneal ulcer with entropion) is likely or has occurred, for comfort, or for cosmetic reasons.

Eyelid Tumors

Noncancerous (benign) and cancerous (malignant) growths can form on the eyelids. One of the most common types of benign tumor is xanthelasma, a yellow-white, flat growth that consists of fatty material. Because xanthelasmas may indicate elevated cholesterol levels, especially in young people, a doctor may check the person's cholesterol level by taking a blood sample. Xanthelasmas need not be removed unless their appearance becomes bothersome.

Basal cell carcinoma (see page 1333) is a type of skin cancer that frequently occurs at the eyelid margins, at the inner corner of the eyes, and on the upper cheeks. A doctor bases the diagnosis on the results of a biopsy (removal of a tissue sample for examination under a microscope). The growth is usually removed surgically.

> **? Did You Know...**
>
> A growth on the eyelid that persists for weeks should be removed and examined under a microscope (biopsied) to exclude cancer.

Although less common, squamous cell carcinoma (see page 1334), meibomian gland carcinoma (cancer of glands in the eyelid), and melanoma (see page 1335), all cancerous growths, can develop on the eyelid. If a growth on the eyelid does not disappear after several weeks, a doctor may do a biopsy. The growth is usually removed surgically. Eyelid tumors sometimes mimic other eye disorders (such as blepharitis and chalazion), so a doctor usually biopsies any growths that do not respond to initial treatments.

Stye

A stye (hordeolum) is a rapidly developing infection of one or more of the tiny glands at the edge of the eyelid or underneath the eyelid that sometimes develops a small abscess.

- The infection is usually caused by one of the *Staphylococcus* bacteria.
- The edge of the eyelid becomes red, tender, painful, and swollen.
- Treatment involves repeated hot compresses.
- Internal styes may have to be drained by a doctor.

A stye is usually caused by a staphylococcal infection. Sometimes the person also has blepharitis (see page 1434). A person may have one or two styes in a lifetime, but some people develop them repeatedly. Rarely, a stye develops in one of the deeper glands of the eyelid (an internal stye).

Symptoms

A stye usually begins with redness, tenderness, and pain at the edge of the eyelid. Then a small, round, tender, swollen area forms. The eye may water, become sensitive to bright light, and feel as though something is in it. Usually, only a small area of the eyelid is swollen, but sometimes the entire eyelid swells. Often a tiny, yellowish spot develops at the center of the swollen area, usually at the edge of the eyelid. The stye tends to rupture after 2 to 4 days, releasing a small amount of pus and ending the problem.

With an internal stye, pain and other symptoms are usually more severe than with an external stye. Pain, redness, and swelling tend to occur underneath the eyelid. Occasionally, inflammation is severe and may be accompanied by fever or chills.

Treatment

Although antibiotics are sometimes used to treat styes, they usually do not really help much. The best treatment is to apply hot compresses for 5 to 10 minutes 2 to 3 times a day. The warmth helps the stye come to a head, rupture, and drain. Because an internal stye rarely ruptures by itself, a doctor may have to open it to drain the pus. Internal styes tend to recur.

Trichiasis

Trichiasis is misalignment of eyelashes, which rub against the eyeball, in a person who does not have entropion.

The cause of trichiasis is usually unknown. The eye becomes red and irritated, has a foreign body sensation, and develops tearing and sensitivity and sometimes pain when exposed to light. If the condition persists, scarring can occur. A doctor bases the diagnosis on the symptoms and an examination. Trichiasis differs from entropion in that the eyelid position is normal. An eye doctor can remove the eyelashes with forceps. If eyelashes grow back, other methods can be used to remove them, such as electrolysis or cryosurgery (use of extreme cold to destroy the hair follicle).

CHAPTER 223

Conjunctival and Scleral Disorders

The conjunctiva is the thin, transparent lining that covers the back of the eyelid and loops back to cover the sclera (the white of the eye), right up to the edge of the cornea (see art on page 1412). The conjunctiva helps protect the eye by keeping small foreign objects and infection-causing microorganisms out and by contributing to the maintenance of the tear film.

The most common disorder of the conjunctiva is inflammation (conjunctivitis). There are many causes of inflammation, including infections by bacteria (including chlamydia), viruses, or fungi; allergic reactions; chemicals or foreign bodies in the eye; and overexposure to sunlight. Conjunctivitis tends to be relatively short-lived, although it sometimes lasts for months or years. Long-standing conjunctivitis is often caused by chronic irritation of the eye that occurs when an eyelid is turned outward (ectropion) or inward (entropion), by some eye drops, or by chronic dryness. Whatever the cause, people with conjunctivitis typically have similar symptoms, such as redness, itching or irritation, discharge, and, sometimes, slightly blurred vision.

The sclera is the tough, white, outer coat of the eyeball. The sclera provides the eyeball with structural strength and protects against penetration and rupture. Rarely, the sclera becomes inflamed (scleritis).

Infectious Conjunctivitis

Infectious conjunctivitis is inflammation of the conjunctiva usually caused by viruses or bacteria.

What Is Pinkeye?

Although most eye inflammations result in a pink discoloration of the eye (because of dilated blood vessels in the conjunctiva), doctors usually use the term pinkeye for conjunctivitis caused by infection with a bacteria or virus. One of the most severe forms of pinkeye is the result of infection with several particular strains of adenovirus. This infection, epidemic keratoconjunctivitis, is extremely contagious and often results in large outbreaks within a community or school. The infection is spread through contact with infected secretions. Such contact may take place person-to-person or through contaminated objects, possibly including doctors' instruments.

The symptoms of this infection are similar to other types of viral conjunctivitis—redness, irritation, sensitivity to light, and thin, watery discharge. Many people develop a swollen lymph node in front of the ear on the affected side. These symptoms typically last from 1 to 3 weeks. Some people have blurred vision, which may last for weeks or months before resolving.

Epidemic keratoconjunctivitis resolves completely without specific treatment. Doctors sometimes give corticosteroid drops to people with very blurred vision or severe sensitivity to light. Good hygiene, particularly hand washing, is needed to minimize the spread of the infection. Separate towels, washcloths, and bedding help minimize the spread to other members of the household. People generally stay home from work or school for several days or, in severe cases, even weeks.

- Bacteria and viruses can infect the conjunctiva.
- Redness, irritation, tearing or discharge, and sensitivity to light are common.
- Good hygiene helps prevent the infection from spreading.
- Antibiotic eye drops are often given.

A variety of microorganisms may infect the conjunctiva. The most common organisms are viral, particularly those from the group known as adenoviruses. Bacterial infections are less frequent. Both viral and bacterial conjunctivitis are quite contagious, easily passing from one person to another, or from a person's infected eye to the uninfected eye. Fungal infections are rare and occur mainly in people who use corticosteroid eye drops for a long time or have eye injuries involving vegetable matter. Newborns are particularly susceptible to eye infections, which they acquire from organisms in the mother's birth canal (neonatal conjunctivitis—see table on page 1705).

Inclusion conjunctivitis is a particularly long-lasting form of conjunctivitis caused by certain strains of the bacterium *Chlamydia trachomatis*. Inclusion conjunctivitis usually spreads by contact with genital secretions from a person who has a genital chlamydial infection. Trachoma (see page 1439) is another type of conjunctivitis caused by *Chlamydia trachomatis*. Another type of conjunctivitis is caused by *Neisseria gonorrhoeae* (gonorrhea), a sexually transmitted disease that also may spread to the eye.

Severe infections may scar the conjunctiva, causing abnormalities in the tear film. Sometimes, severe conjunctival infections spread to the cornea (the transparent part of the eye).

Symptoms

When infected, the eye sometimes feels irritated, and bright light may cause discomfort. The conjunctiva becomes pink from dilated blood vessels, and a discharge appears in the eye. Often the discharge causes the person's eyes to stick shut, particularly overnight. This discharge may also cause the vision to blur. Vision improves when the discharge is blinked away. If the cornea is infected, vision also blurs but does not improve with blinking. Very rarely, severe infections that have scarred the conjunctiva lead to long-term vision difficulties.

Viral conjunctivitis differs from bacterial conjunctivitis in the following ways:

- Eye discharge tends to be watery in viral conjunctivitis and thicker white or yellow in bacterial conjunctivitis.
- An upper respiratory infection increases the likelihood of a viral cause.
- A lymph node in front of the ear may be swollen and painful in viral conjunctivitis but is usually not in bacterial conjunctivitis.

These factors, however, cannot always accurately differentiate viral conjunctivitis from bacterial conjunctivitis.

People with inclusion conjunctivitis or with conjunctivitis caused by gonorrhea often have symptoms of a genital infection, such as penile or vaginal discharge and burning during urination.

Diagnosis

Doctors diagnose infectious conjunctivitis by its symptoms and appearance. The eye is usually closely examined with a slit lamp (an instrument that magnifies the surface of the eye). Samples of infected secretions may be sent to a laboratory to identify the infecting organism by a culture. However, doctors usually do this only when the symptoms are severe or recurrent or when chlamydia or *Neisseria gonorrhea* is thought to be the cause.

Prognosis and Treatment

Most people with infectious conjunctivitis eventually get better without treatment. However, some infections, particularly those caused by some bacteria, may last a long time if not treated. Inclusion conjunctivitis may persist for months if not treated.

If discharge accumulates on the eyelid, people should gently wash the eyelid (with the eye closed) with tap water and a clean washcloth. Warm or cool compresses sometimes soothe the feeling of irritation. Because infective (bacterial or viral) conjunctivitis is highly contagious, people should wash their hands before and after cleaning the eye or applying drugs. Also, a person should be careful not to touch the infected eye and then touch the other eye. Towels and washcloths used to clean the eye should be kept separate from other towels and washcloths. People with infectious conjunctivitis generally stay home from work or school for a few days, just as they would with a cold. In the most severe cases of viral conjunctivitis, people sometimes stay home for weeks.

Antibiotics are helpful only in bacterial conjunctivitis. However, because it is difficult to distinguish between bacterial and viral infection, doctors sometimes prescribe antibiotics for everyone with conjunctivitis. Antibiotic eye drops or ointments, such as ciprofloxacin or trimethoprim-polymyxin, which are effective against many types of bacteria, are used for 7 to 10 days. Drops are applied 4 times daily. Ointments last longer and are applied every 6 hours but blur vision.

Inclusion conjunctivitis requires antibiotics, such as azithromycin, doxycycline, or erythromycin, which are taken by mouth. Gonococcal conjunctivitis may be treated with an injection of ceftriaxone. Corticosteroid eye drops may be needed in some people with severe adenoviral conjunctivitis, particularly in those in whom inflammation of the eye is interfering with important daily activities. Antiviral drops are not helpful for most conjunctivitis caused by viruses, with some exceptions. For example, a person with viral conjunctivitis caused by herpes may apply antiviral drugs to the eyes (trifluridine eye drops) or take them by mouth (acyclovir).

Trachoma

Trachoma (also called granular conjunctivitis or Egyptian ophthalmia) is a prolonged infection of the conjunctiva caused by the bacterium Chlamydia trachomatis.

- *Chlamydia trachomatis* can infect the eye, usually in children who live in lesser-developed, hot, dry countries.
- Eye redness, watering, irritation, and, if severe, scarring and loss of vision may develop.
- Antibiotics are usually effective.

Trachoma results from infections with certain nonsexually transmitted strains of *Chlamydia trachomatis*. Trachoma is common in dry, hot coun-

tries in North Africa, the Middle East, the Indian subcontinent, Australia, and Southeast Asia. In the United States, trachoma is rare, occurring occasionally among Native Americans and among immigrants from areas where trachoma is common.

The disease occurs mainly in children, particularly those between the ages of 3 and 6. Older children and adults are much less likely to have the disease because of increased immunity and better personal hygiene.

> **? Did You Know...**
> Trachoma is the leading preventable cause of blindness in the world.

Trachoma is contagious in its early stages and may be transmitted by eye-hand contact, by flies, or by sharing contaminated articles, such as towels, handkerchiefs, and eye makeup.

Symptoms

Trachoma usually affects both eyes. The conjunctivae become inflamed, red, and irritated, and the eyes water excessively. The eyelids swell. Sensitivity to bright light occurs.

In the later stages, blood vessels may gradually grow across the cornea (neovascularization), obstructing vision. In some people, the eyelid is scarred in such a way that the eyelashes turn inward (trichiasis). As the person blinks, the eyelashes rub against the cornea, causing infection and permanent damage. Impaired vision or blindness occurs in about 5% of people with trachoma.

Diagnosis

Doctors suspect trachoma based on the appearance of the eyes and on the duration of symptoms. The diagnosis can be confirmed by sending a sample from the eye to a laboratory, where the infecting organism is identified.

Prevention

Because the disease is contagious, reinfection commonly occurs. Regular hand and face washing helps prevent the spread of infection. Sharing towels, washcloths, bedding, and eye makeup should be avoided. Because flies can transfer the disease among people, places where flies can breed should be eliminated.

Treatment

Treatment consists of an antibiotic (such as azithromycin, doxycycline, or tetracycline) taken by mouth.

Alternatively, tetracycline or erythromycin can be applied as an ointment. Doctors often give antibiotics to entire neighborhoods where there are many people with trachoma. If the condition damages the eyelid, conjunctiva, or cornea, surgery may be needed.

Allergic Conjunctivitis

Allergic conjunctivitis is inflammation of the conjunctiva caused by an allergic reaction.

- Allergic reactions may inflame the conjunctiva.
- Redness, irritation, swelling, and discharge are common.
- Various eye drops may help decrease inflammation.

The conjunctiva contains a large number of cells from the immune system (mast cells) that release chemical substances (mediators) in response to a variety of stimuli (such as pollens or dust mites). These mediators cause inflammation in the eyes, which may be brief or long-lasting. About 20% of people have some degree of allergic conjunctivitis.

Seasonal allergic conjunctivitis and **perennial allergic conjunctivitis** are the most common types of allergic reaction in the eyes. Seasonal allergic conjunctivitis is often caused by tree or grass pollens, leading to its typical appearance in the spring and early summer. Weed pollens are responsible for symptoms of allergic conjunctivitis in the summer and early fall. Perennial allergic conjunctivitis occurs year-round and is most often caused by dust mites, animal dander, and feathers.

Vernal conjunctivitis is a more serious form of allergic conjunctivitis in which the stimulant (allergen) is not known. The condition is most common among boys, particularly those aged 5 to 20 years who also have eczema, asthma, or seasonal allergies. Vernal conjunctivitis typically reappears each spring and subsides in the fall and winter. Many children outgrow the condition by early adulthood.

Symptoms

People with all forms of allergic conjunctivitis develop intense itching and burning in both eyes. Although usually equal, occasionally one eye may be more affected than the other. The conjunctiva becomes red and sometimes swells, giving the surface of the eyeball a puffy appearance that many people find disturbing. With seasonal and perennial conjunctivitis, there is a large amount of thin, watery discharge. At times the discharge is stringy. Vision is seldom affected. Many people have a runny nose.

With vernal conjunctivitis, the eye discharge is thick and mucuslike. Unlike other types of allergic conjunctivitis, vernal conjunctivitis often affects the cornea, and painful ulcers develop. These ulcers cause deep eye pain with exposure to bright light and sometimes lead to a permanent decrease in vision.

Diagnosis and Treatment

Doctors recognize allergic conjunctivitis by its typical appearance and symptoms. The condition is treated with anti-allergy eye drops. Tear supplements can help reduce symptoms. Drops that combine an antihistamine, such as antazoline or pheniramine, and a drug that constricts the eye blood vessels, such as naphazoline, may be enough for mild cases. These drugs can be bought without a prescription. If they are ineffective, prescription anti-allergy eye drops may be effective. Nonsteroidal anti-inflammatory eye drops have anti-inflammatory properties and help relieve symptoms. Corticosteroid eye drops have more potent anti-inflammatory effects; however, they should not be used for more than a few weeks without close monitoring because they may cause increased pressure in the eyes (glaucoma), cataracts, and an increased risk of eye infections.

Episcleritis

Episcleritis is inflammation of the tissue lying between the sclera and the conjunctiva.

Episcleritis occurs in young adults and affects women more often than men. Usually, the inflammation affects only a small patch of the eyeball and causes a red, and sometimes slightly yellow, raised area. Symptoms include eye tenderness and irritation, with slightly increased watering of the eye and mildly increased sensitivity to bright light. The condition is not usually a sign of any other disease and tends to disappear and may recur. The diagnosis is based on the symptoms and on the appearance of the eye.

Treatment is often unnecessary. Eye drops that constrict blood vessels in the eye, such as tetrahydrozoline, can improve the appearance of the eyes but are not necessary. To shorten an attack, corticosteroid eye drops or an oral nonsteroidal anti-inflammatory drug can be used.

Scleritis

Scleritis is a deep, extremely painful inflammation and purple discoloration of the sclera (the white of the eye) that may severely damage vision.

Scleritis is most common among people aged 30 through 60 and affects women more often than men. In one third of cases, it affects both eyes. Scleritis may accompany rheumatoid arthritis, systemic lupus erythematosus, or another autoimmune disorder. About half of the cases of scleritis have no known cause.

Pinguecula and Pterygium

A pinguecula (left) is a growth next to the cornea. A pterygium (right) is a growth of the conjunctiva next to the cornea that spreads across the cornea. A pterygium may affect vision.

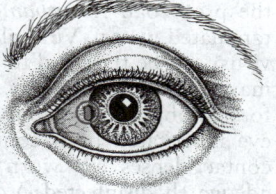 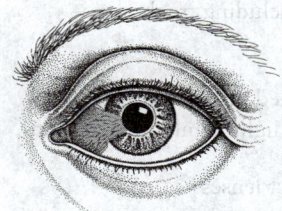

Symptoms include pain in the eye (typically a deep ache) that often interferes with sleep and reduces appetite. Other symptoms include eye tenderness, increased watering of the eye, and sensitivity to bright light. Redness occurs over part or all of the eye. Rarely, inflammation is severe enough to cause perforation of the eyeball and loss of the eye.

Doctors diagnose scleritis by its symptoms and appearance during a slit-lamp examination. Sometimes the area of inflammation is in the back part of the eye (posterior scleritis), and an ultrasound or computed tomography (CT) scan is needed to confirm the diagnosis.

Doctors treat scleritis with topical conrticosteroid eye drops. Sometimes, oral corticosteroids or nonsteroidal anti-inflammatory drugs taken by mouth are necessary. If the person has rheumatoid arthritis or does not respond to corticosteroids, drugs that suppress the immune system, such as cyclophosphamide or azathioprine, may be needed.

Noncancerous Growths

Two kinds of noncancerous (benign) growths commonly develop on the conjunctiva—pinguecula and pterygium. They both are more common among older people and probably occur as a result of long-term ultraviolet radiation exposure. Doctors easily recognize these growths by their typical appearance.

Pinguecula: This is a raised yellowish white growth next to, but not overlapping, the cornea (the translucent part of the eye). This growth can be unsightly, but it generally does not cause any significant problems and does not need to be removed.

Pterygium: This is a fleshy growth of the conjunctiva next to the cornea that spreads across the cornea. Most pterygia do not cause symptoms, but sometimes they cause irritation or distort the shape of the cornea, possibly causing a change in vision. Sometimes removal is appropriate to reduce irritation and to prevent changes in vision.

224 Corneal Disorders

The cornea is the domed, transparent covering in the front of the eye that protects the iris and lens and helps focus light on the retina. It is composed of cells, protein, and fluid. The cornea looks fragile but is almost as stiff as a fingernail. However, it is very sensitive to touch.

Corneal disease or damage can cause pain, tearing, and loss of vision. A slit lamp, which shows the cornea with magnification, is usually used to examine the cornea (see page 1423). A doctor may apply eye drops that contain a dye called fluorescein, which temporarily stains areas of the cornea where cells are damaged, making these areas easier to identify.

Superficial Punctate Keratitis

Superficial punctate keratitis is death of small groups of cells on the surface of the cornea.

- The eyes become red, watery, and sensitive to light.

- Most people recover fully.
- Symptoms can be relieved.

The cause of this disorder may be any of the following:

- A viral infection
- A bacterial infection (including trachoma— see page 1439)
- Dry eyes
- Strong chemicals splashed in the eye
- Exposure to ultraviolet light (sunlight, sunlamps, or welding arcs)
- Prolonged use of contact lenses
- An allergy to eye drops
- Blepharitis (eyelid inflammation)
- A side effect of certain drugs taken by mouth or vein (intravenously)

In superficial punctate keratitis, the eyes are usually painful, watery, sensitive to bright light, and bloodshot, and vision may be slightly blurred. Often there is a burning, gritty feeling or a feeling as if a foreign object is trapped in the eye. When ultraviolet light causes the disorder, symptoms usually do not occur until several hours after exposure and last for 1 to 2 days. When a virus causes the disorder, a lymph node in front of the ear on the affected side may be swollen and tender.

The diagnosis is based on the symptoms, on whether the person has been exposed to any of the known causes, and on an examination of the cornea with a slit lamp (a device used by a doctor to examine the eye with magnification—see page 1423).

Almost everyone who has this disorder recovers completely. When the cause is a virus (other than herpes simplex or herpes zoster [shingles]), no treatment is needed, and recovery usually occurs within 3 weeks. When the cause is a bacterial infection or prolonged use of contact lenses, antibiotics are used, and the wearing of contact lenses is temporarily discontinued. When the cause is dry eyes, ointments and artificial tears are effective. Artificial tears are eye drops prepared with substances that simulate real tears or with substances that when added to the person's tears coat the eye with more moisture. When the cause is exposure to ultraviolet light, an antibiotic ointment and an eye drop that dilates the pupil may provide relief. When the cause is a drug reaction or an allergy to eye drops, the drug or eye drops must be discontinued.

Corneal Ulcer

A corneal ulcer is an infected open sore on the cornea.

- Contact lenses, injuries, disorders, drugs, and nutritional deficiencies can cause open sores.

- Pain, foreign body sensation, redness, tearing, and light sensitivity are common.
- Antibiotic, antiviral, or antifungal drugs are usually given as soon as possible.

Corneal ulcers may begin with a corneal injury, which then becomes infected with bacteria, fungi, or the protozoan *Acanthamoeba* (which lives in contaminated water). Viral ulcers (often due to a herpes virus) can be triggered to recur by physical stress or may recur spontaneously. Ulcers can also occur if a foreign object lodges in the eye or, more often, if the eye is irritated by a contact lens, especially when contact lenses are worn during sleep or are not adequately disinfected. A deficiency of vitamin A and protein may lead to the formation of a corneal ulcer. However, such ulcers are rare in the United States.

When the eyelids do not close properly, the cornea may become dry and irritated. This kind of irritation can lead to injury and the development of a corneal ulcer. Corneal ulcers may also result from in-growing eyelashes (trichiasis), an inturned eyelid (entropion), or eyelid inflammation (blepharitis).

Symptoms

Corneal ulcers cause pain, usually a feeling like a foreign object is in the eye, with aching and sensitivity to bright light and increased tear production. The ulcer often appears as a white spot on the cornea. Sometimes, ulcers develop over the entire cornea and may penetrate deeply. Pus may accumulate behind the cornea, sometimes forming a white layer at the bottom of the cornea. The deeper the ulcer, the more severe the symptoms and complications. The conjunctiva usually is bloodshot, and a mucus-like white discharge is present.

Corneal ulcers may heal with treatment, but they may leave a cloudy scar that impairs vision. Other complications may include deep-seated infection, perforation of the cornea, displacement of the iris, and destruction of most or all of the tissue in the eye socket.

Diagnosis

To see an ulcer clearly, a doctor may apply eye drops that contain a dye called fluorescein, which temporarily stains the ulcer and allows it to be examined more clearly.

Treatment

A corneal ulcer is an emergency that should be treated immediately.

Treatment depends on the underlying cause. For instance, antibiotic, antiviral, or antifungal drugs are usually needed immediately. Corneal transplantation (keratoplasty) is sometimes needed (see box on page 1135).

Keratoconjunctivitis Sicca

Keratoconjunctivitis sicca (dry eye) is dryness of the conjunctiva and cornea.

- Too few tears may be produced, or tears may evaporate too quickly.
- The eyes become irritated and sensitive to light and usually burn and itch.
- Tear production may be measured by placing a strip of paper at the edge of the eyelid.
- Artificial tears help relieve symptoms.

Dry eyes may be due to inadequate tear production (aqueous tear-deficient dry eyes). With this type of dry eyes, the tear gland (lacrimal gland) does not produce enough tears to keep the entire conjunctiva and cornea covered by a complete layer of tears. This is the most common type among postmenopausal women. Dry eyes are common in Sjögren's syndrome (see page 577). Rarely, aqueous tear-deficient dry eyes may be a symptom of diseases such as rheumatoid arthritis or systemic lupus erythematosus (lupus).

Dry eyes may also be due to an abnormality of tear composition that results in rapid evaporation of the tears (evaporative dry eyes). Although the tear gland produces a sufficient amount of tears, the rate of evaporation is so rapid that the entire surface of the eye cannot be kept covered with a complete layer of tears during certain activities or in certain environments.

Symptoms

Symptoms of dry eyes include irritation, burning, itching, a pulling sensation, pressure behind the eye, and a feeling as if something is in the eye. Damage to the surface of the eye increases discomfort and sensitivity to bright light. Symptoms are worsened by

- Activities in which the rate of blinking is reduced, specifically those that involve prolonged use of the eyes, such as reading, working on a computer, driving, or watching television
- Drafty, dusty or smoky areas and dry environments, such as in airplanes or in shopping malls; areas with low humidity; and areas where air conditioners (especially in the car), fans, or heaters are being used
- The use of certain drugs, including isotretinoin and some tranquilizers, diuretics, antihypertensives, oral contraceptives, and antihistamines and other drugs with anticholinergic effects

Symptoms lessen during cool, rainy, or foggy weather and in humid places, such as in the shower. Even with the most severe dry eyes, it is rare that vision is lost. However, people sometimes feel that their blurred vision or eye irritation is so severe, frequent, and prolonged that it is difficult to function normally. In some people with severe dryness, the surface of the cornea can thicken, or ulcers and scars can develop. Occasionally, blood vessels can grow across the cornea. Scarring and blood vessel growth can impair vision.

Diagnosis

Although a doctor can usually diagnose dry eyes by the symptoms alone, a Schirmer test—in which a strip of filter paper is placed at the edge of the eyelid—can measure the amount of moisture bathing the eye. Doctors examine the eyes with a slit lamp (see page 1423) to determine whether the eye has been damaged.

Treatment

Artificial tears applied every few hours can generally control the problem. Artificial tears are eye drops prepared with substances that simulate real tears and help keep the eyes coated with moisture. Lubricating ointments applied before bed last longer than artificial tears and help prevent dryness in the morning. Such ointments are not usually used during the day because they may blur vision.

Eye drops that contain cyclosporine can decrease the inflammation associated with dryness. These drops sting and take months before an effect is noticed. Inflammation can lessen significantly, although the drops work only in a small number of people. Avoiding dry, drafty environments and smoke and using humidifiers can also help.

Minor surgery can be done to block the flow of tears through the tear duct into the nose. This way more tears are available to bathe the eyes. In people with extremely dry eyes, the eyelids may be partially sewn together to decrease tear evaporation.

Keratomalacia

Keratomalacia (also called xerophthalmia or xerotic keratitis) is drying and clouding of the cornea due to vitamin A deficiency and insufficient protein and calories in the diet.

The surface of the conjunctiva and cornea dries, sometimes leading to corneal ulcers and bacterial infections. The tear glands are also affected, resulting in an inadequate tear film and dry eyes. Night blindness (poor vision in the dark) may develop because of the effects of vitamin A deficiency on the retina. The diagnosis of keratomalacia is based on the presence of a dry or ulcerated cornea in an undernourished person.

Antibiotic eye drops or ointments can help cure an infection, but correcting the vitamin A deficiency and undernutrition with an improved diet or supplements is also important.

Herpes Simplex Keratitis

Herpes simplex keratitis is infection of the cornea caused by herpes simplex virus.

The herpes simplex virus (which causes cold sores—see page 1245) never leaves the body after an initial infection (primary infection). Instead, the virus remains in a dormant stage in the nerves. Sometimes, the virus reactivates and causes further symptoms.

Primary herpes simplex eye infections usually occur in children and cause a mild keratoconjunctivitis. Symptoms usually resemble those of common conjunctivitis, so the diagnosis of herpes simplex infection is not made. The infection resolves without treatment. However, if the infection reactivates, it can affect the cornea more seriously and cause more severe symptoms.

Symptoms of a reactivation include eye pain, tearing, redness, and sensitivity to bright light. Rarely, the infection worsens and the cornea swells, making vision hazy. The more often the infection recurs, the more likely is further damage to the surface of the cornea. Several recurrences may result in the formation of deep ulcers, permanent scarring, and a loss of feeling when the eye is touched. The herpes simplex virus can also cause blood vessels to grow onto the cornea and, occasionally, can lead to significant visual impairment. To diagnose a herpes simplex infection, a doctor examines the eye with a slit lamp (see page 1423). Sometimes, the doctor may take a sample from the infected area to identify the virus (viral culture).

The doctor may prescribe an antiviral eye drop, such as trifluridine. Acyclovir, another antiviral drug, can be taken by mouth. Treatment should be started as soon as possible. Deep infections that cause a lot of inflammation may require use of corticosteroid drops and drops that dilate the eye, such as atropine or scopolamine. Occasionally, to help speed healing, after numbing the eye, an ophthalmologist (a medical doctor who specializes in diagnosing and treating eye diseases and performing eye surgery) may have to gently swab the cornea with a soft cotton-tipped applicator to remove infected and damaged cells.

Herpes Zoster Ophthalmicus

Herpes zoster ophthalmicus is infection of the eye caused by varicella-zoster virus.

Varicella-zoster is the virus that causes chicken pox. Once people are infected, the virus remains in a dormant stage in the nerve roots. In some people, the virus reactivates and may spread to the skin, causing herpes zoster, also called shingles (see page 1247). If the forehead or nose becomes infected, the eye also becomes infected in about half of people, on the same side as the skin involvement.

The skin of the forehead and sometimes the tip of the nose are covered with small, extremely painful, red blisters. Infection of the eye causes pain, redness, light sensitivity, and eyelid swelling. Months and years later, the cornea can become swollen, severely damaged, and scarred. The structures behind the cornea can become inflamed (uveitis), the pressure in the eye can increase (glaucoma), and the cornea can become numb, which can lead to injuries. The appearance of active shingles, a history of the typical rash, or old scars from a shingles rash help a doctor make the diagnosis.

As with shingles anywhere in the body, early treatment with an antiviral drug such as acyclovir, valacyclovir, or famciclovir (which are taken by mouth) can reduce the duration of the painful rash. When herpes zoster infects the face and threatens the eye, treatment with an antiviral drug reduces the risk of eye complications. Corticosteroids, usually in eye drops, may also be needed if the eye is inflamed. Eye drops, such as atropine, are used to keep the pupil dilated, to help prevent a severe form of glaucoma, and to relieve pain.

Peripheral Ulcerative Keratitis

Peripheral ulcerative keratitis is inflammation and ulceration of the cornea that often occurs in people who have connective tissue disorders such as rheumatoid arthritis.

Peripheral ulcerative keratitis is probably caused by an autoimmune reaction (see page 1124). People develop blurred vision, increased sensitivity to bright light, and a sensation of a foreign object trapped in the eye. The ulcer is located in the periphery of the cornea and is usually oval in shape.

Of the people who have rheumatoid arthritis and peripheral ulcerative keratitis, about 40% die (mostly due to a heart attack) within 10 years of developing peripheral ulcerative keratitis unless they are treated. Treatment with drugs that suppress the immune system, such as oral or intravenous cyclophosphamide, reduces the death rate to about 8% in 10 years.

Keratoconus

Keratoconus is a gradual change in the shape of the cornea that causes it to become irregular and cone-shaped.

The condition usually begins between the ages of 10 and 25. Both eyes are usually affected, causing major changes in vision and requiring frequent changes in the prescription for eyeglasses or contact lenses. Contact lenses often correct the vision problems better than eyeglasses, but sometimes the change in corneal shape is so severe that contact lenses either cannot be worn or cannot correct vision. In severe cases, corneal transplantation (see box on page 1135) may be needed to restore vision. Some newer alternatives to transplantation, such as insertion of corneal ring segments (objects that change the shape of the cornea to help correct refraction) or ultraviolet light treatments that strengthen the cornea, may become more available in coming years.

Bullous Keratopathy

Bullous keratopathy is a blister-like swelling of the cornea.

Bullous keratopathy is most common among older people. Occasionally, bullous keratopathy occurs after eye surgery, such as cataract removal. The swelling leads to the formation of fluid-filled blisters on the surface of the cornea. The blisters can rupture, causing pain, often with the sensation of a foreign object trapped in the eye, and can impair vision.

The diagnosis is based on the typical appearance of a swollen, cloudy cornea with blisters on the surface.

Bullous keratopathy is treated by reducing the amount of fluid in the cornea. Salty eye drops (hypertonic saline) can be used to draw the excess fluid from the cornea. Soft contact lenses can be used to decrease discomfort by acting as a bandage to the cornea. If vision is reduced or discomfort is significant and prolonged, corneal transplantation (see box on page 1135) is often done.

CHAPTER

225 Cataract

A cataract is a clouding (opacity) of the lens of the eye that causes a progressive, painless loss of vision.

- Vision may be blurred, contrast may be lost, and halos may be visible around lights.
- Doctors can recognize cataracts by looking at the eye with an ophthalmoscope or slit lamp.
- Most cataracts can be removed and replaced with an artificial lens.

Cataracts are the leading cause of blindness worldwide. Cataracts are common in the United States, where they affect mostly older adults. Almost one in five people between the ages of 65 and 74 develops cataracts severe enough to reduce vision, and almost one in two people older than 75 has them. Fortunately, people in the United States can often have their cataracts treated before they cause blindness.

Cataracts usually develop without any apparent cause; however, contributing factors include the following:

- Injury to the eye
- Prolonged use of certain drugs (such as corticosteroids)
- Prolonged exposure to x-rays (such as with radiation therapy to the eye)
- Inflammatory and infectious eye diseases
- Diseases such as diabetes
- Dark eyes
- Prolonged exposure to direct sunlight
- Poor nutrition
- Smoking
- Alcohol use
- Heat from infrared exposure

People who have had a cataract in one eye are more likely to develop one later in the other eye. Sometimes cataracts can develop in both eyes at the same time. Babies can be born with them (congenital cataracts—see table on page 1709), and children can also develop cataracts, usually as a result of injury or illness.

Symptoms

Because all light entering the eye passes through the lens, clouding of the lens can block, distort, or diffuse light and cause poor vision. The first symptom of a cataract may be seeing halos and starbursts around lights (glare). Sometimes, the first symptom is blurred vision. Less commonly, double vision is an early symptom. A person may also notice that colors seem more yellow and less vibrant. Reading may become more difficult because of a worsening ability to distinguish the contrast between the light and dark of printed letters on a page.

How much vision is changed by a cataract depends on the intensity of light entering the eye and on the location of the cataract.

With a cataract near the back of the lens (posterior subcapsular cataract), visual acuity is worse when the pupil constricts (for example, in bright light or during reading). Posterior subcapsular cataracts are also more likely to cause loss of contrast, as well as glare from bright lights or car headlights

How Cataracts Affect Vision

On the left, a normal lens receives light and focuses it on the retina. On the right, a cataract blocks some light from reaching the lens and distorts the light being focused on the retina.

Lens   Retina

Normal Lens   **Lens With Cataract**

while driving at night. People with cataracts who take drugs that constrict their pupils (certain glaucoma eye drops, for example) may also have greater vision loss.

With a cataract in the center (inside) of the lens (nuclear cataract), distance vision worsens. However, near vision may at first improve because the cataract acts as a stronger lens, thus refocusing light. Older people, who generally have trouble seeing things that are close without eyeglasses, may discover that they can read again without eyeglasses, a phenomenon often described as gaining second sight. Unfortunately, a nuclear cataract eventually blocks and blurs light entering the eye and impairs vision.

Although cataracts almost never cause pain, rarely they can swell and increase the pressure in the eye (glaucoma), which can be painful.

> **? Did You Know...**
> Sometimes a cataract in a certain part of the lens can cause near vision to improve for a while, and a person can read again without needing reading glasses.

Diagnosis

A doctor can usually detect a cataract while examining the eye with an ophthalmoscope. A doctor can identify the exact location of the cataract and the extent to which it blocks light by using an instrument called a slit lamp, which allows examination of the lens and other parts of the eye in more detail.

Prevention

There are several things people can do to try to prevent cataracts. Consistent use of sunglasses with a

coating to filter ultraviolet (UV) light protects the eyes from bright sunlight and may help. Not smoking is useful and has other health advantages. People with diabetes should work with their doctor to be sure the level of sugar in their blood is well controlled. A diet high in vitamin C, vitamin A, and substances known as carotenoids (contained in vegetables such as spinach and kale) may protect against cataracts. Estrogen use by women after menopause may also be protective, but estrogen should not be used solely for this purpose. Finally, people who are taking corticosteroids for extended periods might discuss with their doctor the possibility of using a different drug.

Treatment

Until vision is significantly impaired, eyeglasses and contact lenses may improve a person's vision. Wearing sunglasses in bright light and using lamps that provide over-the-shoulder lighting may decrease glare and aid vision. Occasionally, drugs that keep the pupil dilated may be used to help vision if the cataract is small and located in the center of the lens.

The only treatment that provides a cure for cataracts is surgery. There are no eye drops or drugs that will make cataracts go away. Occasionally, cataracts cause changes (such as swelling of the cataract or glaucoma) that lead doctors to recommend the cataract be removed quickly. However, most times people should have surgery only when their vision is so impaired by cataracts that they feel unsafe, uncomfortable, or unable to perform daily tasks. There is no advantage to having cataracts removed before then.

Cataract surgery can be done on a person of any age and is generally safe even for people with illnesses such as heart disease and diabetes. Usually, the doctor makes a small incision in the eye and removes the cataract by breaking it up with ultrasound and taking the pieces out of the lens capsule (phacoemulsification). When all the cataract pieces have been removed, the surgeon usually places an artificial lens (intraocular lens) in the lens capsule. The intraocular lens cannot always be safely placed, however. When lens placement is not possible, people must wear thick eyeglasses or contact lenses after the cataract has been removed.

> **? Did You Know...**
> Cataracts are the leading cause of blindness worldwide.

Surgery to remove cataracts is almost always performed under local anesthesia, in which the eye surface is numbed with an injection or eye drops. Rarely, children or adults who cannot hold still during surgery require general anesthesia. The procedure normally takes about 30 minutes, and the person can go home the same day. No sutures are usually needed, because the incision into the eye is small and seals itself.

People should make arrangements in advance to get extra help at home for a few days after surgery because activity may be restricted (for example, bending over and heavy lifting may be prohibited), and vision changes, such as blurred vision and discomfort with bright light, may occur for a short time after surgery. For a few weeks after surgery, eye drops or ointments are used to prevent infection, reduce inflammation, and promote healing. A person is given eyeglasses or a plastic shield to wear while sleeping to protect the eye from injury until healing is complete, usually a few weeks. Rubbing the eye is avoided. The person visits the doctor the day after surgery and then typically one week and one month later. If a person has cataracts in both eyes, many doctors wait several months after the first eye has healed to remove a cataract from the other eye.

Many people notice improved distance vision within a few weeks after cataract surgery. Almost everyone will need eyeglasses for reading, and some people will need eyeglasses to obtain the best possible distance vision as well. Newer intraocular lenses with multiple focusing powers (multi-focal lenses) may allow a person to have good near and distance vision without needing glasses, although some people may experience glare and halos at night with these lenses. The doctor makes calculations before the surgery to decide how powerful the artificial lens should be. Thus, it is possible to go from wearing very thick eyeglasses before the surgery to wearing much thinner eyeglasses after it.

Complications after cataract surgery are rare. A person may develop an infection or serious bleeding in the eye, which can lead to a loss of vision. Eye pressure may become too high, which if left untreated, leads to glaucoma, or the implant can become displaced. The back of the eye (retina) can become swollen or detached (see page 1454). Rarely, people with retinal disorders, such as diabetic retinopathy, may notice their vision worsen after the operation. Proper follow-up with the doctor can lead to early detection and treatment of these unusual complications.

Sometimes people develop a haziness of the tissue (capsule) left behind in the eye after the original lens was removed (secondary cataract). This occurs in about one in four people who have had cataract surgery, months or even years after an artificial lens is implanted. Typically, it is treated by using a laser to make a small opening in the hazy capsule to let light through.

CHAPTER 226 Uveitis

Uveitis is inflammation anywhere in the pigmented inside lining of the eye, known as the uvea or uveal tract.

- The uvea may become inflamed because of infection, a bodywide autoimmune disorder (which causes the body to attack its own tissues), or for unknown reasons.
- Symptoms may include eye ache, eye redness, floaters, loss of vision, or a combination.
- Corticosteroids and drops that dilate and relax the pupil in the affected eye usually are prescribed.

The uveal tract consists of three structures: the iris, the ciliary body, and the choroid.

The iris, the colored ring around the black pupil, opens and closes to let more or less light into the eye, just like the shutter in a camera.

The ciliary body is the set of muscles that, by contracting, allows the lens to become thicker so the eye can focus on nearby objects. By relaxing, the ciliary body allows the lens to become thinner so the eye can focus on distant objects.

The choroid, the inner lining of the eyeball, extends from the edge of the ciliary muscles to the optic nerve at the back of the eye. The choroid lies between the retina on the inside and the sclera on the outside. The choroid contains layers of blood vessels that nourish the inside parts of the eye, particularly the retina.

Part or all of the uveal tract may become inflamed. Inflammation limited to part of the uvea is named, according to its location, as anterior uveitis, intermediate uveitis, posterior uveitis, or panuveitis (inflammation that affects the entire uveal tract). Sometimes, uveitis is referred to by the name of the specific part that is inflamed—for example, iritis (inflammation of the iris), choroiditis (inflammation of the choroid), or chorioretinitis (inflammation that involves both the choroid and the overlying retina). Inflammation of the uvea is limited to one eye in many people with uveitis but may involve both eyes.

The inflammation has many possible causes. Some causes are limited to the eye itself, and others are

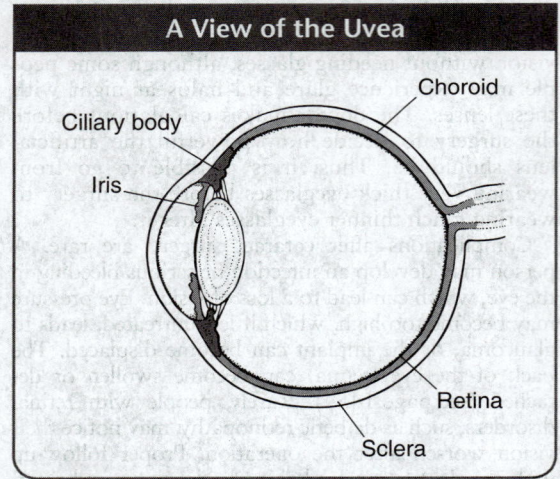

A View of the Uvea

Ciliary body

Choroid

Iris

Retina

Sclera

sensitivity to bright light, and a decrease in vision are typical. A doctor may be able to see prominent blood vessels on the surface of the eye near the edge of the cornea, white blood cells floating in the fluid that fills the front part of the eye (aqueous humor), and deposits of white blood cells on the inside surface of the cornea.

- Intermediate uveitis is typically painless. Vision may be decreased, and the person may see irregular floating black spots (floaters).

- Posterior uveitis typically causes decreased vision and floaters. There may also be retinal detachment (see page 1454—early symptoms may include flashing lights, loss of peripheral vision, and blurred vision) and inflammation of the optic nerve (see page 1459—symptoms include loss of vision, which may vary from a small blind spot to total blindness).

- Panuveitis may cause any combination of these symptoms.

Uveitis can rapidly damage the eye. It can cause long-term, vision-threatening complications, such as swelling of the macula, glaucoma, and cataracts. Many people have only one episode of uveitis. Others have periodic recurrences over months to years.

disorders that affect the entire body. In most people, no cause is identified, and they are said to have idiopathic uveitis. About 40% of people with uveitis have a disorder that also affects organs elsewhere in the body. These include inflammatory diseases, such as ankylosing spondylitis and juvenile idiopathic arthritis; sarcoidosis; and widespread infections, such as tuberculosis, syphilis, or Lyme disease. Other possible causes include infections that may affect only the eye, such as herpes (herpes simplex virus) infection, shingles (varicellazoster virus), toxoplasmosis, and cytomegalovirus—which occurs mainly in people infected by the human immunodeficiency virus (HIV).

Symptoms

The early symptoms of uveitis may be mild or severe, depending on which part of the uvea is affected and the amount of inflammation.

- Anterior uveitis has the most dramatic symptoms. Severe ache in the eye, redness of the conjunctiva,

Diagnosis and Treatment

A doctor makes the diagnosis based on the symptoms and a physical examination. If the doctor suspects a disorder that also affects other organs, appropriate tests are done.

Treatment must start early to prevent permanent damage. Treatment almost always includes using corticosteroids, usually given as eye drops. Drugs to dilate the pupils, such as scopolamine or homatropine drops, are also used. Other drugs may be used to treat specific causes of uveitis. For example, if infection is the cause, drugs may be given to eliminate the infecting organism.

CHAPTER

227 Glaucoma

Glaucoma is optic nerve damage (often, but not always, associated with increased eye pressure) that leads to progressive, irreversible loss of vision.

- Damage to the optic nerve can occur when pressure within the eye increases.

- The vision loss occurs so slowly that it may not be noticed for a long time.

- People at risk should have a complete eye examination, including measurement of eye pressures and testing of side (peripheral) vision.

- Eye pressure needs to be controlled throughout life, usually with eye drops but sometimes with eye surgery.

Almost 3 million people in the United States and 14 million people worldwide have glaucoma. Glaucoma is the third leading cause of blindness worldwide and the second leading cause of blindness in the United States, where it is the leading cause of blindness among blacks and Hispanics. In the United States, about one third of glaucoma occurs with eye pressures within the average range, a condition called low-tension glaucoma.

People at highest risk are those with any of the following:

- Age older than 40
- African-American race
- Family members who have (or had) the disease
- Farsightedness or nearsightedness
- Diabetes
- Long-term use of corticosteroid drugs
- Previous eye injury

Glaucoma occurs when an imbalance in production and drainage of fluid in the eye (aqueous humor) increases eye pressure to unhealthy levels. Normally the aqueous fluid, which nourishes the eye, is produced by the ciliary body behind the iris (in the posterior chamber) and flows through the pupil to the front of the eye (anterior chamber), where it exits into drainage canals between the iris and cornea (the "angle"). When functioning properly, the system works like a faucet (ciliary body) and sink (drainage canals). Balance between fluid production and drainage—between an open faucet and a properly draining sink—keeps the fluid flowing freely and prevents pressure in the eye from building up.

In glaucoma, the drainage canals become clogged, blocked, or covered. Fluid cannot leave the eye even though new fluid is being produced in the posterior chamber. In other words, the sink "backs up" while the faucet is still running. Because there is nowhere in the eye for the fluid to go, pressure in the eye increases. When the pressure becomes higher than the optic nerve can tolerate, damage to the optic nerve occurs. This damage is called glaucoma. Sometimes eye pressure increases within the range of normal but is nonetheless too high for the optic nerve to tolerate (called low-tension glaucoma).

There are many forms of adult and childhood glaucomas. Most glaucomas fall into two categories: open-angle or closed-angle glaucomas.

Open-angle glaucoma is more common. In open-angle glaucoma, the drainage canals in the eyes become clogged gradually over months or years. Pressure in the eye rises slowly because fluid is produced at a normal rate but drains sluggishly.

Closed-angle glaucoma is less common than open-angle glaucoma. In closed-angle glaucoma, the drainage canals in the eyes become blocked or covered because the angle between the iris and cornea is too narrow. The blockage can occur suddenly or slowly. If

Normal Fluid Drainage

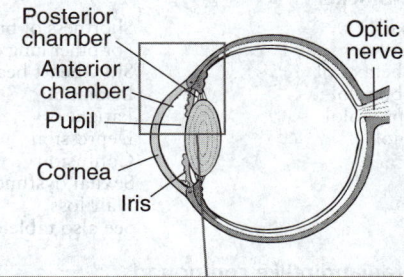

Fluid is produced in the ciliary body behind the iris (in the posterior chamber), passes into the front of the eye (anterior chamber), and then exits through the drainage canals.

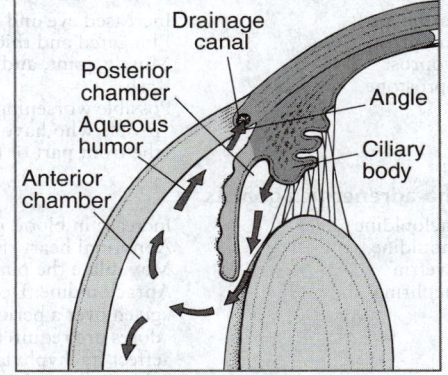

the blockage occurs suddenly, pressure in the eye rises rapidly. If the blockage occurs slowly, the pressure in the eye rises slowly like in open-angle glaucoma.

In most people, the cause of glaucoma is not known, although both open-angle and closed-angle glaucomas tend to run in families. In others, damage to the eye caused by infection, inflammation, tumor, large cataracts or surgery for cataracts, or other conditions keeps the fluid from draining freely and leads to increased eye pressure and optic nerve damage (secondary glaucoma).

Symptoms

Open-Angle Glaucoma: Open-angle glaucoma is painless and causes no early symptoms. The most important symptom of open-angle glaucoma is the development of blind spots, or patches of vision loss, over months to years. The blind spots slowly grow larger and coalesce. Peripheral vision is usually lost first. Vision loss occurs so gradually that it is often not noticed until much of it is lost. Because central vision is generally lost last, many people develop tunnel vision: they see straight ahead perfectly

℞ DRUGS USED TO TREAT GLAUCOMA

DRUG	SOME SIDE EFFECTS	COMMENTS
Beta-blockers		
Betaxolol Carteolol Levobetaxalol Levobunolol Metipranolol Timolol	Shortness of breath in people with asthma or other lung disorders that cause wheezing Slow heart beat Insomnia Fatigue Depression Confusion Sexual dysfunction Hair loss See also table on page 340	**How they work:** Decrease aqueous humor production **Given as:** Eye drops **Other comments:** These drops do not affect pupil size. Some side effects are worse in people with heart or blood vessel disease. Some side effects may develop slowly and may be mistakenly attributed to aging or other bodily processes.
Prostaglandin-like compounds		
Bimatoprost Latanoprost Travoprost Unoprostone	Increased eye and skin pigmentation Elongated and thickened eyelashes Muscle, joint, and back pain Rash Possible worsening of the disorder among people who have inflammation within the front part of the eye (uveitis)	**How they work:** Increase aqueous humor outflow **Given as:** Eye drops **Other comments:** These drops have few serious bodywide side effects.
Alpha-adrenergic agonists		
Apraclonidine Brimonidine Dipivefrin Epinephrine	Increase in blood pressure or heart rate Abnormal heart rhythm May dilate the pupil Apraclonidine: Decreased response if given over a period of time so that larger doses are required to have the same effect (tachyphylaxis) Brimonidine: May cause dry mouth and has a lower rate of allergic reactions than the other drugs Can be fatal in children less than 2 years of age Dipivefrin and epinephrine: May be less reliable and have more side effects than apraclonidine and brimonidine	**How they work:** Decrease aqueous humor production and increase aqueous humor outflow **Given as:** Eye drops
Carbonic anhydrase inhibitors		

Acetazolamide
Brinzolamide
Dorzolamide
Methazolamide
	Acetazolamide and methazolamide:
	  Fatigue
	  Altered taste
	  Loss of appetite
	  Depression
	  Kidney stones
	  Body salt (electrolyte) abnormalities
	  Numbness or tingling
	  Low or high blood cell counts (blood dyscrasias)
	  Weight loss
	  Nausea
	  Diarrhea
	Brinzolamide and dorzolamide:
	  Bad taste in the mouth
		How they work: Decrease aqueous humor production
		Given: For acetazolamide and methazolamide: By mouth or by vein
		For brinzolamide and dorzolamide: Eye drops

(Continued on the following page)

℞ DRUGS USED TO TREAT GLAUCOMA (*Continued*)

DRUG	SOME SIDE EFFECTS	COMMENTS
Cholinergic drugs		
Carbachol Demecarium Echothiophate Isoflurophate Neostigmine Physostigmine Pilocarpine	Hinder the eyes' ability to adapt to darkness Pupil constriction Blurred vision Demecarium, echothiophate, isoflurophate, neostigmine, and physostigmine: More likely to cause cataracts, retinal detachment, and bodywide side effects	**How they work:** Increase aqueous humor outflow **Given as:** Eye drops **Other comments:** People with darker pigmented pupils using carbachol and pilocarpine may need higher strengths.
Osmotic diuretics		
Glycerin Mannitol	Increase urine production Can have serious effects in some people (for example, dysfunction of the brain or nerves) by changing body salt (electrolyte) levels or may cause dehydration	**How they work:** Increase concentration of salts in the blood, which draws fluid from the eye by osmosis **Given:** By mouth or by vein **Other comments:** These drugs are used to treat acute closed-angle glaucoma.

but become blind in all other directions. If glaucoma is left untreated, eventually even tunnel vision is lost, and a person becomes totally blind.

Closed-Angle Glaucoma: If eye pressure rises rapidly in closed-angle glaucoma (acute closed-angle glaucoma), people typically notice an abrupt onset of severe eye pain and headache, redness, blurred vision, rainbow-colored halos around lights, and sudden loss of vision. They may also have nausea and vomiting as a response to the increase in eye pressure.

Acute closed-angle glaucoma is considered a medical emergency, because people can lose their vision as quickly as 2 to 3 hours after the appearance of symptoms if the condition is not treated.

People who have had open-angle or closed-angle glaucoma in one eye are likely to develop it in the other.

Screening and Diagnosis

Because the most common types of glaucoma can cause slow and silent loss of vision over years, early detection of the disease is extremely important. All people at high risk of glaucoma (see the bulleted list at the beginning of the chapter) should have a comprehensive eye examination every 1 to 2 years.

There are four parts to a comprehensive eye examination for glaucoma. First, pressure in the eye is measured. This measurement is taken painlessly with an instrument called a tonometer (see page 1423). In general, eye pressure readings of greater than 20 to 22 millimeters of mercury (mm Hg) are considered higher than normal.

But measuring eye pressure is not enough, because a third or more of people with glaucoma have eye pressure in the average range. So doctors also use an ophthalmoscope (see art on page 1422) and a slit lamp (see art on page 1423) to look for changes in the optic nerve that indicate damage caused by glaucoma.

In addition, visual field (peripheral vision) testing allows a doctor to detect blind spots. Most often, visual field testing is done with a machine that determines the person's ability to see small dots of light in all areas of the visual field (see page 1422).

Finally, doctors may also use a special lens to examine the drainage channels in the eye, a procedure known as gonioscopy. The gonioscope allows the doctor to determine whether the glaucoma is of the open-angle or closed-angle type.

? Did You Know...

Before older people take a drug with anticholinergic effects, their eyes should be checked to see whether development of closed-angle glaucoma is likely.

Treatment

Once a person loses vision because of glaucoma, the loss is permanent. But if glaucoma is detected, proper treatment can prevent further vision loss. So the goal of glaucoma treatment is to prevent the onset of vision loss or stop its progression.

Treatment of glaucoma is lifelong. It involves decreasing eye pressure by increasing fluid drainage out of the eyeball or by reducing the amount of fluid produced inside the eyeball. Some people with high eye pressure who do not have signs of optic nerve damage (known as glaucoma "suspects") can be monitored closely without treatment.

Eye drops and surgery are the main treatments for open-angle and closed-angle glaucomas.

Eye drops containing beta-blockers, prostaglandin-like compounds, alpha-adrenergic agonists, carbonic anhydrase inhibitors, or cholinergic drugs are commonly used to treat glaucoma. Most people with open-angle glaucoma respond well to these drugs. These drugs are also used for people with closed-angle glaucoma, although surgery, not eye drops, is the main treatment. Glaucoma eye drops are generally safe, but they may cause a variety of side effects. People need to use them for the rest of their lives, and regular check-ups are necessary to monitor eye pressure, optic nerves, and visual fields. Sometimes a kind of diuretic (osmotic diuretic) given by mouth or by vein is also used briefly to help decrease eye pressure rapidly in acute closed-angle glaucoma.

Surgery may be needed if eye drops cannot effectively control eye pressure, if a person cannot take eye drops, or if a person develops intolerable side effects from the eye drops. Laser surgery can be used to increase drainage in people with open-angle glaucoma (laser trabeculoplasty) or to make an opening in the iris (laser peripheral iridectomy or iridotomy) in people with acute closed-angle glaucoma. Laser surgery is done in the doctor's office or in a hospital or clinic. Anesthetic eye drops are used to prevent pain. People are usually able to go home the same day of any of these surgical procedures.

Glaucoma filtration surgery is the other form of surgery doctors use to treat glaucoma. With traditional glaucoma filtration surgery, doctors manually create a new drainage system (trabeculectomy or tube shunt) to allow fluid to bypass the clogged or blocked canals and filter out of the eye. Glaucoma filtration surgery is generally performed in a hospital. Newer filtration procedures (viscocanalostomy and Trabectome) remove only part of the drain to enhance the outflow of fluid. People are usually able to return home the day of the procedure.

The most common complication of glaucoma laser surgery is a temporary increase in eye pressure, which is treated with glaucoma eye drops. Rarely, the laser used in laser surgery may burn the cornea, but these burns usually heal quickly. With laser and glaucoma filtration surgery, inflammation and bleeding within the eye may occur but are usually short-lived. Glaucoma filtration surgery may occasionally lead to double vision, cataracts, or infection.

Because severe closed-angle glaucoma is a medical emergency, doctors may use very strong and fast-acting drugs that affect the eye pressure more rapidly than the standard eye drops or surgery. Doctors may use glycerin or acetazolamide pills or drugs given by vein (such as mannitol) if they think the eye is vulnerable to high pressure. Eye drops are also given as soon as possible. Emergency surgery is done if necessary.

The treatment of glaucoma caused by other disorders depends on the cause. For infection or inflammation, antibiotic, antiviral, or corticosteroid eye drops may provide a cure. A tumor obstructing fluid drainage should be treated, as should a cataract that is so large it causes eye pressure to rise. High eye pressure that results from cataract surgery is treated with glaucoma eye drops that reduce eye pressure. If eye drops do not work, glaucoma filtration surgery can be done.

CHAPTER 228 Retinal Disorders

The cornea and lens focus light onto the retina, the transparent, light-sensitive membrane on the inner surface of the back of the eye. The central area of the retina, called the macula, contains a high density of color-sensitive photoreceptor (light-sensing) cells. These cells, called cones, produce the sharpest visual images and are responsible for central and color vision. The peripheral area of the retina, which surrounds the macula, contains photoreceptor cells called rods, which respond to lower light levels but are not color sensitive. The rods are responsible for peripheral vision and night vision.

The optic nerve carries signals generated by the photoreceptors (cones and rods). Each photoreceptor is joined to the optic nerve by a tiny nerve branch. The optic nerve is connected to nerve cells that carry signals to the vision center of the brain, where they are interpreted as visual images.

Viewing the Retina

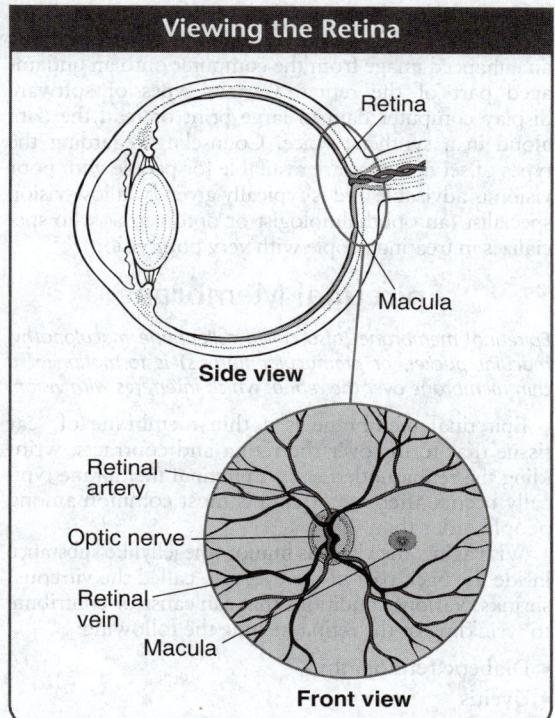

Side view

Retina

Macula

Front view

Retinal artery

Optic nerve

Retinal vein

Macula

The optic nerve and the retina have a rich supply of blood vessels that carry blood and oxygen. Part of this supply of blood vessels comes from the choroid, which is the layer of blood vessels that lies between the retina and the outer white coat of the eye (the sclera). The central retinal artery (the other major source of blood to the retina) reaches the retina near the optic nerve and then branches out within the retina. Blood drains from the retina into branches of the central retinal vein. The central retinal vein exits the eye near the optic nerve.

When examining a person's retina, a doctor puts drops in the eye to dilate the pupil. This allows the retina to be seen in much more detail with an ophthalmoscope.

Retinal disorders are often diagnosed and treated by an ophthalmologist (a medical doctor who specializes in diagnosing and treating eye diseases and performing eye surgery). Frequently, treatment is by an ophthalmologist who specializes in disorders of the retina.

Age-Related Macular Degeneration

Age-related macular degeneration (also called age-related maculopathy) causes progressive damage to the macula, the central and most vital area of the retina, resulting in gradual loss of central vision.

- Central vision becomes washed out and loses detail, and straight lines may appear wavy.
- Changes in the eye that characterize the disorder can usually be seen by a doctor using a hand-held ophthalmoscope.
- Dietary supplements may help slow progression of the disorder.
- Eye injections and laser treatments may be necessary for some people.

Age-related macular degeneration is the most common cause of irreversible loss of central vision in the elderly. It is equally common among men and women.

Causes

The following are risk factors for the disorder:

- Older age
- Smoking
- Fair skin
- Certain genetic abnormalities
- High blood pressure
- A diet low in omega-3 fatty acids (for example, in certain fish) and dark green leafy vegetables

Types: There are two forms of age-related macular degeneration:

- Dry (atrophic)
- Wet (neovascular or exudative)

Ninety percent of people with macular degeneration have the dry type. However, 90% of the blindness caused by macular degeneration occurs in the 10% of people who have the wet form.

In dry macular degeneration, the tissues of the macula thin as cells disappear. Both eyes may be affected simultaneously in the dry form. There is no evidence of scarring or of bleeding or other fluid leakage in the macula.

Wet macular degeneration starts off as the dry type. In wet macular degeneration, abnormal blood vessels develop under the macula. These vessels may leak fluid and blood under the retina (hence the description as "wet"). Eventually, a mound of scar tissue develops under the retina. The wet form develops in one eye first but eventually may affect both eyes.

Symptoms

In dry macular degeneration, central vision slowly and painlessly worsens. Objects may appear washed out, or fine detail may be lost.

In wet macular degeneration, loss of vision tends to progress quickly and may be sudden if one of the abnormal blood vessels bleeds. The first symptom may be distortion of vision in one eye, so that fine, straight lines appear wavy. Often, difficulty with reading or watching television results.

Age-related macular degeneration can severely damage vision, but it usually does not lead to complete blindness. Vision at the outer edges of the visual field (peripheral vision) is generally not affected. The dry type tends to cause slower vision loss.

Diagnosis

Doctors can usually diagnose macular degeneration by examining the eyes with an ophthalmoscope or a slit lamp. The retinal damage is almost always visible even before symptoms develop. Sometimes fluorescein angiography—a procedure in which a doctor injects dye into a vein and photographs the retina—is used to confirm the diagnosis. Optical coherence tomography, an imaging study, can sometimes help in making the diagnosis.

Treatment

No treatment is currently available to undo damage caused by the dry type. No treatment is currently recommended for mild disease.

Dietary Supplements: People with moderate to severe dry macular degeneration and those who have wet macular degeneration in one eye benefit from high doses of antioxidants (vitamin C, vitamin E, and beta-carotene [a form of vitamin A]) and zinc, with a small amount of copper. People who have used tobacco products within the past seven years should not take beta-carotene or vitamin A because these supplements can increase the risk of developing lung cancer. Controlling high blood pressure and eating more omega-3 fatty acids and dark green leafy vegetables may help slow progression of the disorder.

Drug Treatments and Laser Procedures: In the wet type of macular degeneration, drugs such as ranibizumab, bevacizumab, or pegaptanib can be injected into the eye to cause the new blood vessels to stop leaking. These injections need to be repeated every 1 to 2 months, but the injections can improve vision in some people, and one in three people regains reading vision. Another treatment is photodynamic therapy. In this treatment, a substance that sensitizes the retinal blood vessels to laser light is injected into a vein in the arm, and then a beam of laser light is used to destroy the abnormal new blood vessels. If the new blood vessels are not directly under the macula, a thermal laser can be used to destroy them before they do further harm. Corticosteroid drugs can sometimes be injected into the eye. Surgery is done only if these other treatments are not working.

Adjusting to Vision Loss: Magnifiers, reading glasses, telescopes, and closed-circuit television magnifying devices may help people with poor vision. Computer users can select from a variety of low-vision aids (see box on page 1426). For example, one device projects an enhanced image from the computer onto an undamaged part of the retina. Certain types of software display computer data in large print or read the data aloud in a synthetic voice. Counseling regarding the types of services that are available for people with poor vision is advisable and is typically given by a low-vision specialist (an ophthalmologist or optometrist who specializes in treating people with very poor vision).

Epiretinal Membrane

Epiretinal membrane (also called cellophane maculopathy, macular pucker, or premacular fibrosis) is formation of a thin membrane over the retina, which interferes with vision.

Epiretinal membrane is a thin membrane of scar tissue that forms over the retina and contracts, wrinkling the retina underneath. Epiretinal membrane typically occurs after age 50 and is most common among people older than 75.

With aging, the vitreous humor (the jellylike substance inside the back part of the eye; also called the vitreous) shrinks. Various conditions that can cause or contribute to wrinkling of the retina include the following:

- Diabetic retinopathy
- Uveitis
- Retinal detachment
- Injury to the eye

Most of the time, however, no clear cause can be identified.

Symptoms may include blurred vision or distorted vision (for example, straight lines may appear wavy). Many people say that it seems like they are looking through plastic wrap or cellophane. Doctors confirm the diagnosis by looking at the back of the eye with an ophthalmoscope. Fluorescein angiography and optical coherence tomography may also be helpful.

Most people need no treatment. If vision is poor, the membrane can be removed surgically, using a procedure called a membrane peel. This procedure can be done under local anesthesia in an operating room and usually takes about 30 minutes.

Detachment of the Retina

Retinal detachment is separation of the retina from the underlying layer to which it is attached.

- People notice a sudden increase in floaters, a sudden onset of flashing lights, a curtain or veil across vision, or sudden loss of vision.
- Doctors make the diagnosis by looking in the eye with an ophthalmoscope.
- Most retinal detachments can be repaired, resulting in improved vision if done soon after the detachment occurs.

A retinal detachment may begin in a small area, usually as the result of a retinal tear. If the small area is not soon reattached, the entire retina can detach. Retinal tears that can lead to retinal detachment are more likely to occur in people who have or have had the following:

- Severe nearsightedness (myopia)
- Cataract surgery
- An eye injury

When the retina detaches, it separates from part of its blood supply. Unless the retina is reattached, it may be permanently damaged by lack of blood. Fluid or blood from a damaged blood vessel may also collect between the retina and the underlying tissue, further worsening vision.

Symptoms and Diagnosis

A retinal detachment is painless. People usually see an increase in small, floating objects (floaters) or many flashes of bright light that last less than a second. Peripheral vision is typically lost first, and vision loss spreads as the detachment progresses. The loss of vision resembles a curtain or veil falling across the line of sight. If the macula becomes detached, vision rapidly deteriorates, and everything becomes blurred.

After applying eye drops to dilate the pupil, doctors examine the retina using an ophthalmoscope and can usually see a detachment. If the detachment is not visible, an ultrasound of the eye can reveal it.

Prognosis

Vision usually improves, except in the following conditions:

- The retina has been detached for several days or weeks.
- Bleeding or scarring has occurred.
- The macula has been detached or is damaged.

Treatment

Most retinal detachments can be repaired. The surgeon seals the tears with laser surgery or freezing therapy (cryopexy). Then the surgeon draws the retina and the eye wall together either by placing a band around the eye (a scleral buckle) or by removing the vitreous jelly behind the lens and in front of the retina with surgery called a vitrectomy. A gas bubble is often used to hold the retina is place.

Retinitis Pigmentosa

Retinitis pigmentosa is a rare, progressive degeneration of the retina that eventually causes moderate to severe vision loss.

Retinitis pigmentosa is often inherited. One form has a dominant pattern of inheritance, requiring only one abnormal gene from either parent. Other forms are recessive and require an abnormal gene from both parents. An X-linked recessive form occurs mainly in males who inherit one abnormal gene from their mother. In some people, mostly males, hearing loss may also be inherited (a disorder called Usher's syndrome).

The photoreceptors (light-sensing cells) of the retina that are responsible for vision when light is low (rods) gradually degenerate, so that vision becomes poor in the dark. The first symptoms often begin in early childhood. Over time, peripheral vision progressively deteriorates. In the late stages of the disease, the person typically has only a small area of central vision and possibly some peripheral vision remaining (tunnel vision).

When examining the retina with an ophthalmoscope, doctors see specific changes that suggest the diagnosis. Tests such as the electroretinogram, which evaluates the electrical response of the retina to light, may help to confirm the diagnosis.

Family members should be examined so that the inheritance pattern can be determined if possible. If the disorder is present in other family members, genetic counseling should be considered before having children.

No conventional treatment can reverse retinal damage. Vitamin A is recommended by some doctors in an attempt to slow the progression of the disorder. Gene therapy and implantable cells that make a compound to nourish the retina are under investigation.

Blockage of Central Retinal Arteries and Veins

A blood vessel in the retina may become blocked, causing sudden, painless loss of vision.

- Doctors typically make the diagnosis by looking in the eye with an ophthalmoscope and sometimes by performing tests.
- Treatment often is unsuccessful.

Blockage may occur in the main artery or vein in the retina (arteries supply blood, and veins drain blood away) or in their branches.

The central retinal artery, the main vessel that supplies blood to the retina, can become completely blocked by a particle, such as a piece of atherosclerotic plaque (see art on page 397) or a blood clot, that floats in the bloodstream (embolus) until it gets stuck in and blocks a vessel. Giant cell arteritis, an inflammation of the blood vessels, is also a possible cause of retinal artery blockage.

Retinal veins may become blocked in people with glaucoma, diabetes, or high blood pressure. Such blockage occurs mainly in older people.

Symptoms

If the central retinal artery is blocked, the affected eye has a sudden but painless loss of vision over the entire field of vision or sometimes only a part of it. Vision loss ranges from mild to severe.

Blockage of the central retinal vein causes similar symptoms except that vision loss sometimes is gradual, occurring over days or weeks. Recurrences are common.

Blockage of the central retinal artery or vein may also cause growth of abnormal blood vessels on the retina or iris. Sometimes these abnormal blood vessels bleed or cause glaucoma.

Diagnosis

Using an ophthalmoscope, doctors can see changes in blood vessels and the retina. If the central retinal artery is blocked, the retina may be pale. If the central retinal vein is blocked, the veins may be engorged or enlarged, and the front of the optic nerve may be swollen.

Fluorescein angiography—a procedure in which a doctor injects dye into a vein and then photographs the retina—helps determine the extent of damage to the retina and helps the doctor plan treatment. Doppler ultrasound scanning may sometimes be used to observe blood flow in the vessels.

If the artery has been blocked by an embolus, doctors need to search for a source. They often do tests such as echocardiography or carotid artery ultrasonography.

Treatment

Treatments for blockage of the main artery or vein or their branches tend not to be very effective. Preventing such blockages by controlling risk factors (for example, high blood pressure, diabetes, and other risk factors for atherosclerosis) is more effective.

Blockage of an Artery: Immediate treatment is often given in an attempt to unblock the retinal artery. However, treatments are rarely effective. Pressure inside the eye sometimes can be lowered by intermittently massaging the closed eyelids with the fingers. Alternatively, a procedure called anterior chamber paracentesis may help lower pressure inside the eye. In this procedure, drops are placed in the eye to numb the eye, and then a needle is inserted into the anterior chamber to withdraw a small amount of fluid, thereby rapidly lowering the pressure in the eye. Lowering the pressure inside the eye by massage or by anterior chamber paracentesis may

dislodge a blood clot or other embolus and allow it to enter a smaller branch of the vessel, thereby reducing the area of damage to the retina.

Vein Blockage of a Vein: Laser treatment of the leaking blood vessels can help improve vision for people with a blockage in a branch of the retinal vein. Injections of drugs into the eye are being investigated as treatments for vein blockage.

Abnormal Blood Vessel Growth: Laser treatment may be used to destroy abnormal blood vessels if they develop on the iris or angle.

Hypertensive Retinopathy

Hypertensive retinopathy is damage to the retina caused by high blood pressure.

When blood pressure becomes high (hypertension—see page 333), the retina may become damaged. Hypertension damages the small blood vessels in the retina, causing their walls to thicken, which decreases the amount of blood that can flow through them. As a result, the blood supply to the retina is reduced. Patches of the retina may become damaged because the blood supply is inadequate. As hypertensive retinopathy progresses, blood may leak into the retina. These changes lead to a gradual loss of vision, particularly if they affect the macula, the central part of the retina. Even mild hypertension may damage the retinal blood vessels if it goes untreated for years.

Using an ophthalmoscope, doctors can observe the typical appearance of the retina in people with high blood pressure. The amount of damage to the retinal blood vessels tends to correlate with the amount of damage to blood vessels in other organs affected by hypertension, such as the brain, heart, and kidneys. When blood pressure is extremely high, doctors may be able to see other changes in the eye, such as swelling of the front of the optic nerve.

> ### ? Did You Know...
> By looking into the eye with an ophthalmoscope, doctors can see the eye's arteries and veins. The appearance of these blood vessels can tell doctors how hypertension and atherosclerosis have affected other blood vessels in the body.

The goal of treatment is to lower blood pressure. When high blood pressure is severe and life threatening, treatment may be needed immediately to save vision and avoid other complications, including stroke, heart failure, kidney failure, and heart attack.

Diabetic Retinopathy

Diabetic retinopathy is damage to the retina as a result of diabetes.

- Blood vessels in the retina can leak.
- New blood vessels may develop, sometimes leading to bleeding (hemorrhage), scar formation, or retinal detachment.
- The diagnosis is based on an eye examination after the pupil is dilated with eye drops.
- Controlling blood sugar and blood pressure are important for people who have diabetic retinopathy or who are at risk of developing it.
- Laser treatments can sometimes prevent or delay further damage.

Diabetes mellitus is among the leading causes of blindness in the United States and other developed countries. Some retinal change occurs in virtually all people with diabetes, whether or not they use insulin therapy. People with diabetes who also have high blood pressure are at much higher risk of developing diabetic retinopathy because both conditions tend to damage the retina. Pregnancy can cause diabetic retinopathy to worsen.

High levels of sugar (glucose) in the blood make the walls of small blood vessels, including those in the retina, weaker and, therefore, more prone to damage. Damaged retinal blood vessels leak blood and fluid into the retina.

The extent of retinopathy and vision loss is related mostly to the following:

- How well blood sugar levels are controlled
- How well blood pressure is controlled
- How long the person has had diabetes

In general, retinopathy appears 5 years after people develop type 1 diabetes. Because diagnosis of type 2 diabetes may not occur for years, retinopathy may be present by the time people receive the diagnosis of type 2 diabetes.

Symptoms

Diabetes mellitus can cause two types of changes in the eye.

In **nonproliferative retinopathy**, small blood vessels in the retina leak fluid or blood and may develop small bulges. Areas of the retina affected by leakage may swell, causing damage to parts of the field of vision. At first, the effects on vision may be minimal, but gradually vision may become impaired. Blind spots may occur, although these may not be noticed by the person and are usually discovered only if testing is done. If leakage occurs near the macula, central vision may blur. Swelling of the macula (macular edema) due to leakage of fluid from blood vessels can eventually cause significant loss of vision.

In **proliferative retinopathy**, damage to the retina stimulates the growth of new blood vessels. The new blood vessels grow abnormally, sometimes leading to hemorrhage or scarring. Extensive scarring may cause retinal detachment. Proliferative retinopathy tends to result in greater loss of vision than does nonproliferative retinopathy. It can result in total or near-total blindness due to a large hemorrhage into the vitreous humor (the jellylike substance inside the back part of the eye) or to a type of retinal detachment called traction retinal detachment. Growth of new blood vessels can also lead to glaucoma. Macular edema with significant loss of vision can occur with proliferative diabetic retinopathy as well.

Diagnosis

Doctors diagnose nonproliferative and proliferative retinopathy by examining the retina with an ophthalmoscope or a slit lamp. Fluorescein angiography (see page 1424) helps to determine the location of the leakage, as well as areas of poor blood flow and the areas of new abnormal blood vessel formation.

Prevention

The best way to prevent diabetic retinopathy is to control diabetes and keep blood pressure at normal levels. People with diabetes should have an annual eye examination, in which the pupil is dilated with eye drops, so that retinopathy can be detected and any necessary treatment can be started early. Pregnant women with diabetes should have these eye examinations about once every 3 months.

Treatment

Treatment consists of laser photocoagulation, in which a laser beam is aimed into the eye at the retina to slow the growth of abnormal new retinal blood vessels and decrease leakage. Laser photocoagulation may need to be repeated. If bleeding from damaged vessels has been extensive, a procedure called vitrectomy may be needed. In this procedure, blood is removed from the cavity in which the vitreous humor lies. Vision often improves after vitrectomy for vitreous hemorrhage, and vision may improve after vitrectomy for traction retinal detachment. Laser treatment only rarely improves vision, but it commonly prevents further deterioration. Newer treatments that are being investigated involve injecting drugs into the eye. These treatments may help improve vision for some people with severe vision loss.

Endophthalmitis

Endophthalmitis is infection inside the eye.

- Eye surgery, eye injury, or infection in the bloodstream can cause the infection.

- Severe eye pain, eye redness, and loss of vision may occur.
- Cultures are taken of eye fluids, and antibiotics are given as soon as possible.

Endophthalmitis is uncommon. It is caused by organisms that have entered the eye through a surgical incision or an injury to the eyeball or, less often, have traveled through the bloodstream into the eye. Infection in the bloodstream has many possible causes, such as intravenous drug use, an abscess (a collection of pus), skin ulcers, infections such as pneumonia or sepsis, or surgery anywhere in the body. Infection is usually due to bacteria, but fungi or protozoa may also be responsible. Viruses can also cause extensive eye infections, but these are not usually classified as endophthalmitis.

Symptoms may be severe and include pain, redness in the white of the eye, extreme sensitivity to bright light, and partial or complete loss of vision. The diagnosis is based on the symptoms, an examination of the eye, cultures, and sometimes antibody or DNA testing. Cultures may be taken from the aqueous humor (fluid inside the front of the eye, also called the aqueous) and the vitreous humor (the jellylike substance inside the back part of the eye) to determine which organisms are responsible and which drugs are most active against them.

Endophthalmitis is a medical emergency. Immediate treatment with antibiotics is usually needed to preserve vision. A delay of even a few hours can result in irreversible vision loss in extreme cases. The choice of antibiotic may be adjusted depending on which organism is found to be causing the endophthalmitis. Antibiotics may be injected into the eye and given intravenously or orally. Oral corticosteroids may also be given for a few days after injection of antibiotics into the eye. Surgery may be needed to remove infected tissue from inside the eye, which may improve the chances of stopping the infection.

Cancers Affecting the Retina

Cancers affecting the retina usually occur in the choroid, a dense layer of blood vessels that supplies the retina. The choroid is sandwiched between the retina and the sclera (the outer white part of the eye). Because the retina depends on the choroid for its support and half of its blood supply, damage to the choroid by a cancer is likely to affect vision.

Choroidal Melanoma: Choroidal melanoma is a cancer that originates in the pigment-producing cells (melanocytes) of the choroid. Choroidal melanoma is the most common cancer originating in the eye. It is most common among people with fair complexions and blue eyes. In its early stages, the cancer usually does not interfere with vision. Later, it may cause blurred vision or retinal detachment, with symptoms such as flashes of light, a veil or curtain across the visual field, or a sudden increase or change in floaters. Melanomas, particularly if large, may extend into the orbit or spread through the bloodstream (metastasize) to other parts of the body and may be fatal.

Early diagnosis is important because smaller tumors are easier to cure. The diagnosis is made using an ophthalmoscope and performing tests, which may include ultrasound scanning, computed tomography (CT), and serial photographs.

If the melanoma is small, treatment with a laser, radiation, or an implant of radioactive materials may preserve vision and save the eye. If the cancer is large, the eye may have to be removed.

Choroidal Metastases: Choroidal metastases are cancers that have spread to the choroid from other parts of the body. Because of its rich blood supply, the choroid is often a place to which cancers from other parts of the body may spread. In women, breast cancer is the most common cause. In men, cancers of the lung or prostate are the most common causes.

Often, these cancers cause no symptoms until they are advanced. Symptoms, when they develop, are often loss of vision or symptoms of retinal detachment. Vision loss may be severe.

The diagnosis is sometimes made during a routine eye examination with an ophthalmoscope. The diagnosis is aided by ultrasound scanning. Confirmation of the diagnosis may involve using a fine needle to remove a sample of tissue for examination under a microscope (biopsy). Treatment is usually with chemotherapy and radiation therapy.

229 Optic Nerve Disorders

The small photoreceptors of the retina (the inner surface at the back of the eye) sense light and transmit impulses to the optic nerve. The optic nerve from each eye carries impulses to the brain, where visual information is interpreted. Damage to an optic nerve or damage to its pathways to the brain results in loss of vision. At a structure in the brain called the optic chiasm, each optic nerve splits, and half of its fibers cross over to the other side. Because of this anatomic arrangement, damage along the optic nerve pathway causes specific patterns of vision loss. By understanding the pattern of vision loss, a doctor can often determine where the problem is in the pathway.

Papilledema

Papilledema is a condition in which increased pressure in or around the brain causes the optic nerve to swell where it enters the eye.

- Symptoms may be fleeting disturbances in vision, headache, vomiting, or a combination.
- Doctors make the diagnosis by looking in the person's eye with a viewing instrument (ophthalmoscope).
- The disorder causing increased brain pressure is treated as soon as possible.

Causes

The condition is usually caused by the following:

- Brain tumor or abscess
- Head injury
- Bleeding in the brain
- Infection of the brain or its tissue coverings (meninges)
- Idiopathic intracranial hypertension (pseudotumor cerebri, which is not a tumor—see page 655)

These conditions typically result in papilledema in both eyes.

Symptoms

At first, papilledema may be present without affecting vision. Fleeting vision changes—blurred vision, double vision, flickering, or complete loss of vision—typically lasting seconds are characteristic of papilledema. Other symptoms may be caused by the elevated pressure in the brain. Headache, nausea, vomiting, or a combination may occur.

Diagnosis

An ophthalmologist (a medical doctor who specializes in diagnosing and treating eye diseases) uses an ophthalmoscope to diagnose papilledema. Magnetic resonance imaging (MRI) or computed tomography (CT) may be used to help determine the cause and monitor the effect of treatment. A spinal tap is often done to measure the pressure of the cerebrospinal fluid. A sample of the cerebrospinal fluid may be examined for evidence of a brain tumor or infection. Sometimes an ultrasound of the eye is done to distinguish between papilledema and other disorders that cause apparent swelling of the optic nerve.

Treatment

The disorder causing increased brain pressure is treated as soon as possible. For example, if the high pressure of the cerebrospinal fluid is caused by a brain tumor, corticosteroids may be given, but surgery to remove the tumor may be needed. Papilledema that occurs as a result of idiopathic intracranial hypertension can be treated with weight loss and a diuretic. An infection, if bacterial, can be treated with antibiotics. A brain abscess is drained, and antibiotics are given.

Optic Neuritis

Optic neuritis is inflammation of the optic nerve anywhere along its course.

- Multiple sclerosis is the most common cause.
- Loss of vision may develop, and moving the eye may hurt.
- Magnetic resonance imaging is done.
- If multiple sclerosis seems possible, corticosteroids may be given.

Optic neuritis is most often caused by multiple sclerosis. Some people who have optic neuritis later develop multiple sclerosis. Optic neuritis may also be caused by the following:

- Infections such as viruses (especially in children), meningitis, syphilis, sinusitis, tuberculosis, and human immunodeficiency virus (HIV)
- Tumors
- Chemicals or drugs such as lead, methyl alcohol, quinine, arsenic, and certain antibiotics
- Certain autoimmune diseases
- Intraocular inflammation (uveitis—see page 1447)

Rare causes include diabetes, pernicious anemia, Graves' disease, bee stings, vaccinations, and injuries. However, the cause of optic neuritis is often unknown.

Visual Pathways and the Consequences of Damage

Nerve signals travel along the optic nerve from each eye. The two optic nerves meet at the optic chiasm. There, the optic nerve from each eye divides, and half of the nerve fibers from each side cross to the other side. Because of this arrangement, the right side of the brain receives information from the left visual field of both eyes, and the left side of the brain receives information from the right visual field of both eyes. Damage to an eye or the visual pathway causes different types of vision loss depending on where the damage occurs.

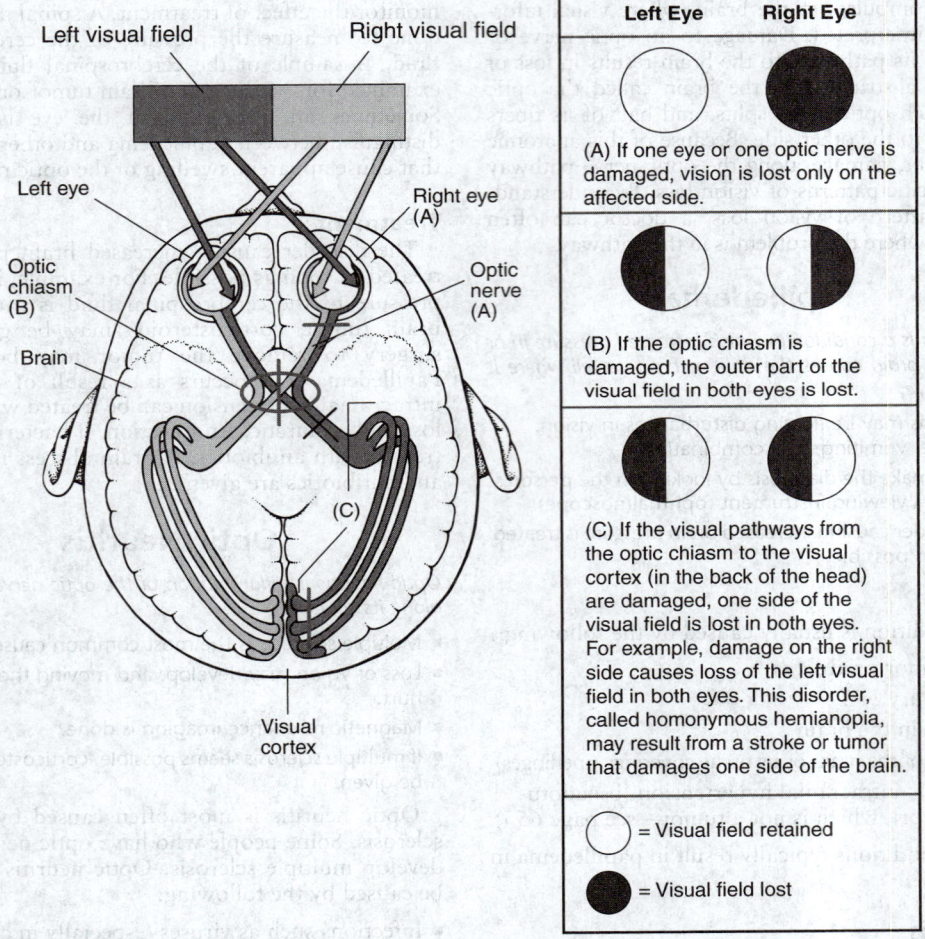

(A) If one eye or one optic nerve is damaged, vision is lost only on the affected side.

(B) If the optic chiasm is damaged, the outer part of the visual field in both eyes is lost.

(C) If the visual pathways from the optic chiasm to the visual cortex (in the back of the head) are damaged, one side of the visual field is lost in both eyes. For example, damage on the right side causes loss of the left visual field in both eyes. This disorder, called homonymous hemianopia, may result from a stroke or tumor that damages one side of the brain.

○ = Visual field retained

● = Visual field lost

Symptoms

Optic neuritis causes vision loss, which may be mild or severe and may occur in one or both eyes. Loss of vision may occur over days. Vision in the involved eye or eyes can range from almost normal to complete blindness. Color vision may be particularly affected, but the person may not realize this. There may be pain with eye movement. Depending on the cause, vision usually recovers within a few months. However, some people have repeat episodes of optic neuritis.

Diagnosis

Diagnosis involves examination of the reactions of the pupils and observing the back of the eyes with a viewing instrument (ophthalmoscope). The head of the optic nerve at the back of the eye (optic disk) may appear swollen. Testing the field of vision may reveal loss of a portion of the visual field. Magnetic resonance imaging (MRI) may show evidence of multiple sclerosis or, rarely, a tumor pressing on the optic nerve.

Treatment

In some instances, such as when multiple sclerosis seems possible, corticosteroids may be given by vein. These drugs may hasten recovery and reduce the chance of a recurrence. If a tumor is pressing on the optic nerve, vision usually improves once the pressure caused by the tumor is relieved.

Ischemic Optic Neuropathy

Ischemic optic neuropathy is damage of the optic nerve caused by a blockage of its blood supply.

- Blockage can occur with or without inflammation of the arteries (typically in association with a disorder called temporal arteritis).
- Vision may suddenly deteriorate.
- People with temporal arteritis may have pain when combing their hair and when chewing, generalized muscle aches and pains, fatigue, or a combination.
- Blood tests and sometimes removal of a piece of the artery (biopsy) are done to diagnose temporal arteritis.
- Temporal arteritis is treated with corticosteroids.

Causes

Blockage of the blood supply to the part of the optic nerve within the eye can lead to impaired function of optic nerve cells. Two types can occur: nonarteritic and arteritic.

Nonarteritic ischemic optic neuropathy usually occurs in people older than 50. Risk factors include high blood pressure, diabetes, and atherosclerosis. Rarely, it occurs in younger people with severe migraines. Arteritic ischemic optic neuropathy usually occurs in people older than 70. The blood supply to the optic nerve is blocked due to inflammation of the arteries (arteritis), most notably temporal arteritis (giant cell arteritis—see page 586).

Symptoms

Loss of vision may be rapid (over minutes, hours, or sometimes days). Depending on the cause, vision may be impaired in one or both eyes. Vision in the involved eye or eyes can range from almost normal to complete blindness. A small area of vision loss at the center of the visual field slowly enlarges and can progress to complete blindness. People with temporal arteritis tend to be older, and their loss of vision tends to be more severe. They may have pain when they chew, muscle aches and pains, and pain when they comb their hair.

About 40% of people with nonarteritic ischemic optic neuropathy spontaneously improve over time. In this condition, repeat episodes in the *same* eye are extremely rare. Involvement of the *other* eye is estimated to occur in about 20% of affected people over the next 5 years.

In people with arteritic ischemic optic neuropathy caused by temporal arteritis, loss of vision in the other eye occurs in 25 to 50% of people within days to weeks if treatment is not started.

Diagnosis

Diagnosis involves examination of the back of the eyes with a viewing instrument (ophthalmoscope). Determining the cause involves determining whether the person has any of the disorders known to be risk factors.

If temporal arteritis is suspected as a cause, blood tests and removal and examination of a temporal artery tissue sample under a microscope (biopsy) may be done to confirm the diagnosis. If a person has no symptoms of temporal arteritis, magnetic resonance imaging (MRI) or computed tomography (CT) of the brain may be done to make sure the optic nerve is not being compressed by a tumor.

Treatment

In people with nonarteritic ischemic optic neuropathy, treatment involves controlling blood pressure, diabetes, and other factors that affect the blood supply to the optic nerve. In people with arteritic ischemic optic neuropathy caused by temporal arteritis, high doses of corticosteroids are given to prevent loss of vision in the other eye. The role of aspirin in preventing involvement of the other eye is being investigated, although at this time there is no evidence to support its use.

Toxic Amblyopia

Toxic amblyopia (nutritional amblyopia) is damage to the optic nerve caused by undernutrition or by exposure to a substance that is harmful to the optic nerve, such as lead, wood alcohol, antifreeze, or certain drugs.

- A nutritional deficiency or toxic substance is often the cause of this disorder.
- Vision usually deteriorates gradually.
- People should avoid further exposure to toxic substances or take nutritional supplements.

Causes

Toxic amblyopia may be caused by a nutritional deficiency (sometimes called nutritional amblyopia), especially of vitamin B_{12}. Alcoholics are particularly susceptible to nutritional amblyopia. The actual cause is probably undernutrition rather than a toxic effect of alcohol. Rarely, toxic amblyopia is caused by drugs (such as chloramphenicol, isoniazid, ethambutol, and digoxin) or toxins such as lead, ethylene glycol (antifreeze), or methanol (wood alcohol or methyl alcohol).

Symptoms

Vision deteriorates over days to weeks. A blind spot may develop and gradually enlarge. It may not be noticed at first. If the disorder is caused by exposure to a toxin or to a nutritional deficiency, both eyes are usually affected. Ethylene glycol and particularly methanol poisoning can cause sudden, complete loss of vision. Both can cause other serious symptoms such as coma, difficulty breathing, vomiting, and abdominal pain.

> **? Did You Know...**
>
> Drinking antifreeze or wood alcohol can cause sudden and complete vision loss.

Diagnosis

Determining the cause involves obtaining a careful history of possible exposures to toxic substances. Sometimes testing for toxins or for a vitamin deficiency is done.

Treatment

People should avoid alcohol and other chemicals or drugs that may be toxic. If alcohol use or undernutrition is a cause, the person should eat a well-balanced diet and take vitamin supplements that include folate (folic acid) and B vitamins. However, if the cause is mainly vitamin B_{12} deficiency, treatment with dietary supplements alone is not enough. Vitamin B_{12} deficiency is typically treated with injections of vitamin B_{12}. If lead is the cause, chelating drugs (such as succimer or dimercaprol) help remove it from the body. If ethylene glycol or methanol poisoning is the cause, rapid treatment with hemodialysis (see page 266) and the drug fomepizole may help.

With treatment, most people recover some of the lost vision.

CHAPTER 230 Eye Socket Disorders

The eye sockets (orbits) are bony cavities that contain and protect the eyes and their supporting structures. Disorders affecting the orbits include fractures (see page 1430), infections, inflammation, vascular disorders, and tumors. Thyroid disease can also affect the orbit. Many eye socket disorders require treatment by a medical doctor who specializes in eye disorders (ophthalmologist).

Infections of the Orbit

Infections may involve the tissues around or within the eye. These infections are most common among children.

PRESEPTAL CELLULITIS

Preseptal cellulitis (periorbital cellulitis) is infection of the eyelid and skin and tissues around the front of the eye.

Preseptal cellulitis usually is caused by spread of an infection of the face or eyelid, an infected insect or animal bite, conjunctivitis, chalazion, or sinusitis.

Tissues around the eye become swollen, warm, tender, and usually red. Sometimes the eye is so swollen that it cannot be easily opened, but once opened, vision is not impaired. A fever may develop.

Doctors can often diagnose preseptal cellulitis by the person's symptoms, but sometimes orbital cellulitis may also be a possible diagnosis. If so, computed tomography (CT) or magnetic resonance imaging (MRI) is done.

Treatment consists of antibiotics (for example, amoxicillin with clavulanate). If people are very ill or cannot take pills, hospitalization is recommended. People should be monitored closely by an ophthalmologist.

ORBITAL CELLULITIS

Orbital cellulitis (postseptal cellulitis) is infection affecting the tissue within the orbit and around and behind the eye.

- Infection can spread to the orbit from sources such as the sinuses around the nose.
- Pain, swelling, red eye, impaired vision, and impaired eye movements can develop.
- Usually CT or MRI is done.
- Antibiotics are given by vein, and the person is admitted to the hospital.

What Is Cavernous Sinus Thrombosis?

The cavernous sinus is a large vein at the base of the brain, behind the eyes. The cavernous sinus is not one of the sinuses around the nose (the nasal sinuses). Cavernous sinus thrombosis is a very rare disorder in which this large vein becomes blocked by an infected blood clot.

Cavernous sinus thrombosis is usually caused by the spread of bacteria from a nasal sinus infection or from an infection in the eye or around the nose. Thus, infections in the area around the nose to the rim of the eyes are always considered serious.

Cavernous sinus thrombosis causes symptoms such as bulging eyes, severe headache or facial pain, impaired eye movements, double vision, loss of vision, drowsiness or coma, seizures, a high fever, and excessively dilated or uneven pupils. If bacteria spread to the brain, sleepiness, seizures, and abnormal sensations or muscle weakness in certain areas may develop. Computed tomography (CT) or magnetic resonance imaging (MRI) of the nasal sinuses, eyes, and brain is usually performed. To identify the bacteria, a blood sample and samples of fluid, mucus, or pus from the throat and nose are sent to a laboratory to be cultured.

High doses of antibiotics given by vein are started immediately. If the condition does not improve after 24 hours of antibiotic treatment, the infected nasal sinus may be drained surgically.

amination of the teeth and mouth and CT or MRI of the nasal sinuses. Often, doctors obtain samples from the nasal sinuses as well as blood samples and send them to a laboratory for testing. The samples are cultured (to grow organisms) to determine what organism is causing the infection, which areas are infected, and which antibiotic should be used. A person with orbital cellulitis is examined by an ophthalmologist.

Treatment

People are admitted to the hospital. Antibiotics are started as soon as possible, before the results of the laboratory testing are known. Antibiotics are usually given by vein initially. A few days later, once people recover, antibiotics are given by mouth. The antibiotic used at first may be changed if the culture results suggest that another antibiotic would be more effective. Sometimes surgery is needed to drain a collection of pus (abscess) or an infected nasal sinus, to correct impaired vision, to remove a foreign body or pus, or to treat the infection if antibiotics are not effective.

Inflammation of the Orbit

Any or all of the structures within the orbit may become inflamed.

Causes

Inflammation of the orbit can be the result of a bodywide (systemic) inflammatory disorder. Sometimes the inflammation affects only the eye.

Systemic inflammatory disorders that affect the eye include Wegener's granulomatosis, in which there is generalized inflammation of blood vessels (called vasculitis). Inflammatory disorders that affect only the eye include scleritis, in which the white coat of the eye (sclera) becomes inflamed. Eyelid disorders with inflammation are discussed elsewhere (see page 1434). Inflammation affecting the lacrimal gland, located at the upper outer edge of the orbit (see art on page 1434), is called inflammatory dacryoadenitis. Inflammation affects one of the muscles that move the eye is called myositis. Inflammation affecting the entire orbit and its contents is called inflammatory orbital pseudotumor (which is not really a tumor and is not a cancer) or nonspecific orbital inflammation.

Orbital cellulitis usually is caused by spread of an infection to the orbit from the sinuses around the nose (nasal sinuses), teeth, or bloodstream. An animal or insect bite or another wound can also spread infection and lead to orbital cellulitis.

Without adequate treatment, orbital cellulitis can lead to blindness. Infection can spread to the brain and spinal cord, or blood clots can form and spread from the veins around the eye to involve a large vein at the base of the brain (the cavernous sinus) and result in a serious disorder called cavernous sinus thrombosis.

Symptoms

Symptoms include pain, a bulging eye, red eye, reduced eye movement, double vision, swollen eyelids, and fever. The eyeball is swollen. Vision may be impaired.

Diagnosis

Doctors can usually recognize orbital cellulitis without diagnostic tests. However, CT or MRI usually is done to confirm the diagnosis. Also, determining the cause may require further assessment, including ex-

Symptoms

Symptoms vary depending on which structures are actually inflamed. In general, symptoms start rather suddenly, typically over a few days. Pain and redness of the eyeball or eyelid occur. Pain can be severe and incapacitating at times. Abnormal bulging of the eyes (proptosis), double vision, and vision loss are also possible.

Diagnosis

Computed tomography (CT) or magnetic resonance imaging (MRI) is done. A doctor may take a sample from the inflamed area for examination under a microscope (biopsy) to determine the cause.

Treatment

Many disorders causing inflammation are treated with a corticosteroid drug, which can be given by mouth. Corticosteroids can be given by vein (intravenously) if the inflammation is severe. Radiation therapy or drugs and treatments that change the body's immune responses (for example, methotrexate or cyclophosphamide) may sometimes be used.

Tumors of the Orbit

Rarely, tumors, either cancerous (malignant) or noncancerous (benign), occur in the tissues behind the eye. Tumors can form within these tissues, or cancerous tumors from elsewhere in the body can spread (metastasize) to these tissues.

These tumors can push the eye forward (a condition called proptosis or exophthalmos). Pain, double vision, and vision loss may also occur. Computed tomography (CT), magnetic resonance imaging (MRI), or both are done to obtain an image of the tumor and exclude other abnormalities. Usually a sample taken for examination under a microscope (biopsy) is needed to determine what type of tumor is present, and treatment depends on these results. Treatment may include surgical removal, radiation therapy, chemotherapy, or a combination of these treatments.

Proptosis

Proptosis (exophthalmos) is an abnormal bulging of one or both eyes.

- Disorders such as Graves' disease and orbital inflammation or tumors can push the eye outward.
- Testing may include measurement of the amount of bulging, computed tomography, magnetic resonance imaging, thyroid function tests, or a combination.
- The disorder causing the problem is treated.

Proptosis and exophthalmos have similar meaning. Exophthalmos is usually used when referring to the eye bulging that sometimes results from thyroid disease.

Causes

Many conditions can cause proptosis. Common causes include the following:

- Graves' disease
- Bleeding behind the eye
- Infection or inflammation of the orbit
- Tumors of the orbit
- Vascular disorders

In some types of thyroid disease, especially Graves' disease (see page 992), the tissues in the orbit may swell, pushing the eyeball forward. This is probably the most common cause of exophthalmos.

Proptosis can develop rapidly from bleeding behind the eye (for example, after a severe injury) or from inflammation in the orbit (see page 1463). Tumors, either cancerous (malignant) or noncancerous (benign), can form in the orbit behind the eyeball and push it forward. An unusual noncancerous accumulation of inflammatory and fibrous tissue (pseudotumor) may cause proptosis with pain and swelling. Cavernous sinus thrombosis causes swelling because blood in the veins cannot exit the eye. Abnormal connections between the arteries and veins (arteriovenous malformations) behind the eye may cause a pulsating proptosis, in which the eye bulges forward and pulses along with the heartbeat.

Symptoms

The protruding eye is less protected by the eyelids, and the cornea may become too dry. As a result, infected corneal ulcers may form. Prolonged proptosis can impair vision because the optic nerve is stretched. The increased pressure within the orbit also may compress the optic nerve, which also can impair vision.

Diagnosis

Not all people with protruding eyes have proptosis. Some people simply have prominent eyes with more white showing than normal. The extent of the protrusion can be measured with an ordinary ruler or with an instrument called an exophthalmometer. Further diagnostic tests may include computed tomography (CT), magnetic resonance imaging (MRI), or thyroid function tests.

Treatment

The treatment depends on the cause. If the problem is an abnormal connection between arteries and veins, a vascular procedure may be needed to close off certain blood vessels. Thyroid disease that is severe enough to cause exophthalmos may need to be treated. However, treating the thyroid condition usually does not relieve bulging of the eyes. Treatment of bleeding or inflammation involves treating the underlying disorder (see page 1463). Tumors (depending on type) are treated with chemotherapy, radiation therapy, or surgery. Corticosteroids may help the inflammation caused by a pseudotumor.

Treatment that relieves the symptoms of proptosis itself includes eyeshades and eye drops if symptoms are mild or corticosteroids, radiation therapy, or surgery if the condition is more severe.

Men's Health Issues

CHAPTER 231

Biology of the Male Reproductive System

The external structures of the male reproductive system include the penis and scrotum. The internal structures include the vas deferens, testes (testicles), urethra, prostate gland, and seminal vesicles.

Sperm, which carries the man's genes, is made in the testes and stored in the seminal vesicles. During ejaculation, sperm is transported along with a fluid called semen through the urethra.

Structure

▪ The penis and the urethra are part of the urinary and reproductive systems.

▪ The scrotum, testes, vas deferens, and prostate gland comprise the rest of the reproductive system.

The penis consists of the root (which is attached to the abdominal wall), the body (the middle portion), and the glans penis (the cone-shaped end). The opening of the urethra (the channel that transports semen and urine) is located at the tip of the glans penis. The base of the glans penis is called the corona. In uncircumcised males, the foreskin (prepuce) extends from the corona to cover the glans penis.

The body of the penis consists primarily of three cylindrical spaces (sinuses) of erectile tissue. The two larger ones, the corpora cavernosa, occur side

Male Reproductive Organs

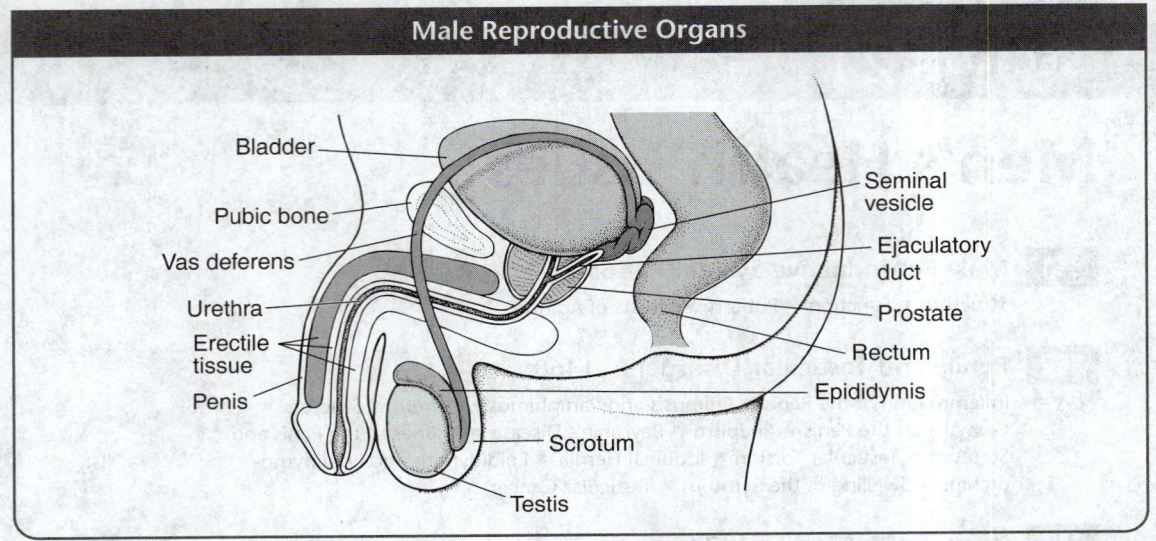

by side. The third sinus, the corpus spongiosum, surrounds the urethra and ends as the glans penis. When these spaces fill with blood, the penis becomes large and rigid (erect).

The scrotum is the thick-skinned sac that surrounds and protects the testes. The scrotum also acts as a climate-control system for the testes, because they need to be slightly cooler than body temperature for normal sperm development. The cremaster muscles in the wall of the scrotum relax or contract to allow the testes to hang farther from the body to cool or to be pulled closer to the body for warmth or protection.

The testes are oval bodies that average about 1.5 to 3 inches (4 to 7 centimeters) in length and 2 to 3 teaspoons (20 to 25 milliliters) in volume. Usually the left testis hangs slightly lower than the right one. The testes have two primary functions: producing sperm and producing testosterone (the primary male sex hormone). The epididymis is a coiled tube almost 20 feet (6 meters) long. It collects sperm from the testis and provides the space and environment for sperm to mature. One epididymis lies against each testis.

The vas deferens is a firm duct that transports sperm from the epididymis. One such duct travels from each epididymis to the back of the prostate and joins with the seminal vesicle. In the scrotum, other structures, such as blood vessels and nerves, also travel along with each vas deferens and together form an intertwined structure, the spermatic cord.

The urethra serves a dual function in males. This channel is the part of the urinary tract that transports urine from the bladder and the part of the reproductive system through which semen is ejaculated.

The prostate lies just under the bladder and surrounds the urethra. Walnut-sized in young men, the prostate enlarges with age. When the prostate enlarges too much, it can block urine flow through the urethra. The seminal vesicles, located above the prostate, join with the vas deferens to form the ejaculatory ducts. The prostate and the seminal vesicles produce fluid that nourishes the sperm. This fluid provides most of the volume of semen, the secretion in which the sperm is expelled during ejaculation. Other fluid that makes up a very small amount of the semen comes from the vas deferens and from mucous glands.

Function

- The penis becomes erect through a complex interaction of physiologic and psychologic factors.
- Contractions during ejaculation impel semen into the urethra and out of the penis.

During sexual activity, the penis becomes erect, enabling penetration during sexual intercourse. An erection results from a complex interaction of neurologic, vascular, hormonal, and psychologic actions. Pleasurable stimuli cause the brain to send nerve signals through the spinal cord to the penis. The arteries supplying blood to the corpora cavernosa and corpus spongiosum respond by dilating. The widened arteries dramatically increase blood flow to these erectile areas. At the same time, muscles around the veins that normally drain blood from the penis tighten, slowing the outflow of blood and elevating blood pressure in the penis. This combination of increased inflow and decreased outflow is what causes the penis to become engorged with blood and increase in length, diameter, and stiffness.

At the climax of sexual excitement (orgasm), ejaculation usually occurs, caused when friction on the glans penis and other stimuli send signals to the brain and spinal cord. Nerves stimulate muscle contractions along the seminal vesicles, prostate, and the ducts of the epididymis and vas deferens. These contractions force semen into the urethra. Contraction of the muscles around the urethra further propels the semen through and out of the penis. The neck (base) of the bladder also constricts to keep semen from flowing backward into the bladder.

Once ejaculation takes place—or the stimulation stops—the arteries constrict and the veins relax, reducing blood inflow, increasing blood outflow, and causing the penis to become limp (detumescence). After detumescence, erection cannot be obtained for a period of time (refractory period), commonly about 20 minutes in young men.

Puberty

- Puberty may begin as early as age 9 and continue until age 16.
- At puberty, the testes start to produce testosterone.
- Testosterone causes reproductive organs to mature, facial and pubic hair to appear, and the voice to deepen.

Puberty is the stage during which people reach full reproductive ability and develop the adult features of their gender. In boys, puberty usually occurs between the ages of 10 and 14 years. However, it is not unusual for puberty to begin as early as age 9 or to continue until age 16.

The pituitary gland, which is located in the brain, initiates puberty. The pituitary gland secretes luteinizing hormone and follicle-stimulating hormone, which stimulate the testes to produce testosterone. Testosterone is responsible for the development of secondary sex characteristics, features that distinguish the sexes but are not part of the reproductive system (such as facial hair growth and voice change).

Testosterone also produces many changes in the male reproductive organs, including

- Elongation and thickening of the penis
- Enlargement of the scrotum, testes, epididymis, and prostate
- Darkening of the skin of the scrotum
- Growth of pubic hair

Breast Disorders in Men

Breast disorders, which include breast enlargement and breast cancer, occur infrequently in men.

Breast Enlargement

Breast enlargement in males (gynecomastia) sometimes occurs during puberty. The enlargement is usually normal and transient, lasting a few months to a few years. Breast enlargement also commonly takes place after age 50.

Male breast enlargement may be caused by certain disorders (particularly liver disorders), certain drug therapies (including the use of female sex hormones and anabolic steroids), or heavy use of marijuana, beer, or heroin. Less commonly, male breast enlargement results from a hormonal imbalance, which can be caused by rare estrogen-producing tumors in the testes or adrenal glands.

One or both breasts may become enlarged. An enlarged breast may be tender. If tenderness is present, cancer is probably not the cause. Breast pain in men, as in women, is not usually a sign of cancer.

Generally, no specific treatment is needed. Breast enlargement often disappears on its own or after its cause is identified and treated. Surgical removal of excess breast tissue is effective but rarely necessary. Liposuction, a surgical technique that removes tissue through a suction tube inserted through a small incision, is the preferred surgical option and sometimes is followed by additional cosmetic surgery.

Breast Cancer

Men can develop breast cancer, although 99% of all breast cancers develop in women. Because male breast cancer is uncommon, it may not be suspected as a cause of symptoms. As a result, male breast cancer often progresses to an advanced stage before it is diagnosed. The prognosis is the same as that for a woman whose cancer is at the same stage.

Treatment options are generally the same as those used for women (surgery, radiation therapy, and chemotherapy), except that breast-conserving surgery is rarely used. Estrogen makes some breast cancers grow. Estrogen is the main female sex hormone, but it is present in males in low amounts. If an examination of tissue samples shows that estrogen is making the cancer grow, estrogen is suppressed with drugs such as tamoxifen.

Testosterone Replacement Therapy

Beginning at about age 30, the production of testosterone (the main male sex hormone) in men usually decreases an average of 1 to 2% per year. This decline is sometimes referred to as male menopause or andropause. However, the hormone decline in men differs greatly from what women experience in menopause, during which female hormones almost always decline rapidly over just a few years. The rate of testosterone decline varies greatly among men. Some men in their 70s have testosterone levels that match those of the average man in his 30s.

Whether young or old, men with low testosterone levels may develop certain characteristics associated with aging, including decreased libido, decreased muscle mass, increased abdominal fat, thin bones that easily fracture (osteoporosis), decreased energy level, slowed mathematical and spatial thinking, and a low blood count (anemia). It is not clear whether low testosterone levels increase the risk of coronary artery disease. Many men with normal testosterone levels are interested in taking testosterone to slow or reverse development of these characteristics, but currently testosterone replacement therapy is recommended only for men with low levels of testosterone.

The most worrisome side effect of testosterone replacement therapy is worsening of prostate disorders. Without knowing it, many men have small prostate cancers that would likely never produce symptoms or be lethal. The body's own testosterone can make prostate cancers grow, so testosterone replacement therapy, at least theoretically, could cause an unnoticed prostate cancer to produce symptoms or become lethal. Testosterone replacement also can worsen benign prostatic hyperplasia, a noncancerous enlargement of the prostate.

Thus, testosterone replacement therapy is recommended only for men whose blood tests show low testosterone levels and who have no prostate disorders. Men taking testosterone need to be checked frequently for prostate cancer. Such testing may detect cancers early, when they are more likely to be curable.

Sperm usually develops by age 14. Ejaculation first occurs during late puberty.

Effects of Aging

It is not clear whether aging itself or the disorders associated with aging cause the gradual changes that occur in men's sexual functioning. The frequency, duration, and rigidity of erections gradually decline throughout adulthood. Levels of the male sex hormone (testosterone) tend to decrease, reducing sex drive (libido). Blood flow to the penis decreases. Other changes include decreases in penile sensitivity and ejaculatory volume, reduced forewarning of ejaculation, orgasm without ejaculation, more rapid detumescence, and a longer refractory period.

CHAPTER

232 Penile and Testicular Disorders

The penis and testes (testicles) can be affected by inflammation, scar tissue, infection (including sexually transmitted diseases), or injury. Skin cancer can also develop on the penis. Birth defects can cause difficulty in urinating and in engaging in sexual intercourse. Disorders of the penis and testes can be psychologically disturbing as well as physically damaging. Disorders that affect only the skin of the penis do not affect sexual function or fertility. Disorders that affect the testes or that damage deeper parts of the penis may affect both.

Inflammation of the Penis

The foreskin of the penis and the glans penis (the cone-shaped end of the penis) can be inflamed.

- **Balanitis** is inflammation of the glans penis.
- **Posthitis** is inflammation of the foreskin.
- **Balanoposthitis** is inflammation of both the glans penis and the foreskin.

Inflammation of the penis can be caused by infections, such as yeast infections, sexually transmitted diseases (STDs), and scabies. Noninfectious causes include skin disorders, including balanitis xerotica obliterans. The inflammation causes pain, itching, redness, and swelling and can ultimately lead to a narrowing (stricture) of the urethra.

Balanoposthitis often begins with balanitis. It develops more often if the foreskin is tight or if a man has diabetes mellitus. Men who develop balanoposthitis have an increased chance of later developing balanitis xerotica obliterans, phimosis, paraphimosis, and penile cancer.

Diagnosis is usually by physical examination. Blood sugar may be measured to test for diabetes, and tests for yeast infections and STDs may be done. The cause of inflammation is treated.

Balanitis xerotica obliterans (also called lichen sclerosus et atrophicus) occurs when chronic inflammation causes the skin near the tip of the penis to harden and turn white. The opening of the urethra is often surrounded by this hard white tissue, which eventually blocks the flow of urine and semen. Antibacterial or anti-inflammatory creams may relieve the inflammation, but if the urethra must be reopened, it is done surgically.

Phimosis and Paraphimosis

Phimosis: In phimosis, the foreskin is tight and cannot be retracted over the glans penis (the cone-shaped end of the penis). This condition is normal in newborns and young boys and usually resolves without treatment by about age 5. In older men, phimosis may result from prolonged irritation or recurring balanoposthitis. The tightened foreskin can interfere with urination and sexual activity and may increase the risk of urinary tract infections. The usual treatment is circumcision. However, in children, sometimes the application of a corticosteroid cream 2 or 3 times daily and periodic gentle stretching of the foreskin are effective and spare the child a circumcision. The cream may be used for up to 3 months.

Paraphimosis: In paraphimosis, the retracted foreskin cannot be pulled forward to cover the glans penis. The condition most commonly develops when the foreskin is left retracted after a medical procedure (such as catheterization) or after cleaning the penis of a child. The glans penis swells, increasing pressure on the retracted foreskin, which then becomes trapped. The increasing pressure eventually prevents blood from reaching the penis, which could result in the destruction of penile tissue if the foreskin is not pulled forward. Immediate treatment involves squeezing the glans penis to shrink it so that the foreskin can be pulled forward. If this technique does not work, the penis is anesthetized and the foreskin is slit to relieve the constriction. Later, circumcision is done.

Urethral Stricture

A urethral stricture is scarring that narrows the urethra.

A urethral stricture most commonly results from a previous injury. Often no cause can be found. Prior infection is an infrequent cause. A less forceful urinary stream or a double stream usually occurs with mild strictures. Severe strictures may completely block the stream of urine. Pressure builds up behind the stricture and may cause passages from the urethra into the surrounding tissues (diverticula). By decreasing the frequency or completeness of urination, strictures often lead to urinary tract infections.

Urologists (doctors who specialize in the diagnosis and treatment of disorders of the urinary tract and male reproductive system) diagnose strictures by obtaining an x-ray after putting radiopaque dye into the urethra (retrograde urethrogram) or by looking directly into the urethra through a flexible viewing tube (cystoscope) after administering a lubricant containing a local anesthetic. To treat a stricture, urologists widen (dilate) the urethra by anesthetizing it and then inserting an instrument that forces the narrowing farther open. Or urologists can cut the stricture open (urethrotomy). Sometimes, scar tissue forms after strictures are treated, causing urethral strictures to recur. If strictures recur, the scar tissue may have to be removed surgically and the urethra may need to be rebuilt.

Growths on the Penis

Growths on the penis are sometimes caused by infections. One example is syphilis (see page 1271), which may cause flat pink or gray growths (condylomata lata). Also, certain viral infections can produce one or more small, firm, raised skin growths (genital warts, or condylomata acuminata) or small, firm, dimpled growths (molluscum contagiosum).

Skin cancer can occur anywhere on the penis, but it most commonly occurs at the glans penis (the cone-shaped end of the penis), especially its base. Cancers affecting the skin of the penis, uncommon in the United States, are even rarer in men who have been circumcised. The cause of cancer of the penis may be long-standing irritation, usually under the foreskin. Squamous cell carcinoma (see page 1334) occurs most commonly. Early forms of cancer that are less common include Bowen's disease (see page 1334), Paget's disease (see page 1337), and erythroplasia of Queyrat.

Cancer usually first appears as a painless, reddened area with sores that do not heal for weeks. Erythroplasia of Queyrat usually occurs in uncircumcised men. It produces a discrete, reddish, velvety area on the penis, usually on or at the base of the glans penis.

To diagnose cancer of the penis, doctors remove a tissue sample for examination under a microscope (biopsy).

To treat early or small cancers, doctors prescribe a cream containing fluorouracil or remove the cancer and some normal surrounding tissue with a laser or during surgery. For other cancers, doctors surgically remove the cancer, sparing as much of the penis as possible. When a lot of tissue is removed, the penis needs to be rebuilt surgically.

In most men, cancers are small and have not spread. These men survive for many years after treatment. Most men with cancer that has spread die within 5 years.

Priapism

Priapism is a painful, persistent erection unaccompanied by sexual desire or excitement.

Priapism probably results from abnormalities of the blood vessels and nerves that cause blood to become trapped in the erectile tissue (corpora cavernosa) of the penis. In most cases, priapism is caused by drugs taken to cause erection. Drugs may be those taken by mouth (for example, sildenafil, tadalafil, or vardenafil) or injected into the penis (for example, alprostadil). Other causes of priapism include blood clots, leukemia, sickle cell disease (particularly in children), a tumor in the pelvis, an injury to the penis or surrounding areas, dysfunction of the spinal cord, and use of other drugs, such as certain antidepressants, drugs used to treat other psychologic disorders, cocaine, and marijuana. Sometimes, however, no cause can be found.

Several symptoms help differentiate priapism from normal erections. Priapism lasts longer, usually several hours. Sexual excitement does not accompany priapism, and the erection is usually painful. Also, in priapism, the glans penis (the cone-shaped end of the penis) may be soft.

>
> **Did You Know...**
> A man with a prolonged, painful erection should see a doctor immediately.

Applying ice, climbing stairs, or both may help. These measures can be taken immediately and done easily. Any drug that appears to cause the priapism is stopped immediately. Injection into the penis of a drug that decreases erection (for example, phenylephrine) can relieve priapism, particularly priapism caused by injection of a drug into the penis. Spinal anesthesia may relieve priapism caused by a spinal cord injury.

When a blood clot is the probable cause, surgery to remove the clot or restore normal circulation in the penis is necessary. Usually, when other treatments are ineffective or the erection has lasted more than 4 hours, priapism can be treated by draining excess blood from the penis with a needle and syringe and using fluid to wash out any blood clots or other blockages from the blood vessels. One or more of many possible drugs may also be used, depending on the cause. Prolonged priapism usually impairs erectile function permanently.

Peyronie's Disease

Peyronie's disease is a fibrous thickening that contracts and deforms the penis, distorting the shape of an erection.

Many men have a small degree of curvature of their erect penis. Peyronie's disease produces a more severe curvature. Inflammation in the penis results in the formation of fibrous scar tissue that causes curvature in the erect penis, making penetration difficult or impossible. However, what causes the inflammation is not known with certainty.

The condition can make an erection painful. The scar tissue can extend into the erectile tissue (corpora cavernosa), preventing erection from occurring.

Minor curvature that does not impair sexual function does not require treatment. Peyronie's disease may resolve over several months without treatment. No treatment has proven clearly successful.

Vitamin E, which can aid wound healing and decrease scarring, may be taken by mouth. Para-aminobenzoate can also be taken by mouth but sometimes causes stomach pain or digestive problems and requires taking many pills each day. Corticosteroids or verapamil can be injected into the scar tissue to decrease inflammation and reduce scarring. Ultrasound treatments can stimulate blood flow, which may prevent further scarring. Radiation therapy may decrease pain but often worsens tissue damage. Surgery is not recommended unless the disease has progressed and the curvature has become too severe for successful intercourse. Surgery to remove the scar tissue shortens the penis and may worsen the disease or result in erectile dysfunction.

Injuries to the Penis and Scrotum

Several types of injuries can affect the penis.

Cuts to the Penis: Catching the penis in a pants zipper is common, but the resulting minor cut usually heals quickly. Cuts usually heal quickly if they are simply kept clean, but people may need to take antibiotics by mouth if the cuts become infected.

The penis can be partially or fully severed. Reattachment of a severed penis is sometimes possible, but full sensation and function are rarely recovered.

Urethral Injury: Injuries to the tube that carries urine through the penis (the urethra) are serious because they may result in scarring that obstructs the flow of urine. These injuries may result from blunt injury, such as a fall straddling a fence rail or bicycle handlebar, from deep cuts, or as a complication of surgical procedures. They typically require treatment by a urologist.

Fracture of the Penis: Excessive bending can fracture an erect penis. Such bending may occur during vigorous sexual intercourse if the penis is stubbed against the partner's pelvic bone. The "fracture" is actually a tear in one of the two tube-like structures in the penis (corpus cavernosum) that hold the extra blood flow that maintains erection.

The man has immediate pain and swelling, and the penis appears deformed. The injury often damages the structures that control erection and after the injury heals, the man may have difficulty with intercourse, urination, or both. Emergency surgery is usually necessary to repair such fractures to prevent abnormal curvature of the penis or permanent erectile dysfunction.

> **Did You Know...**
> The penis can fracture during vigorous sexual intercourse.

Injury of the Scrotum and Testes: The location of the scrotum makes it susceptible to injury. Blunt forces (for example, a kick or crushing blow) cause most injuries. However, occasionally gunshot or stab wounds penetrate the scrotum or testes. Rarely, the scrotum is torn off the testes. Testicular injury causes sudden, severe pain, usually with nausea and vomiting. Ultrasound examination may show whether the testes have ruptured. Ice packs, a jockstrap, and drugs for pain and nausea usually effectively treat bleeding in or around the testes. Ruptured testes require surgical repair. When the scrotum is torn off, the testes can die or lose their capacity for hormone or sperm production. Surgery to cover the testes by reconstructing the scrotum or simply by burying them under the skin of the thighs protects the testes.

Testicular Torsion

Testicular torsion is the twisting of a testis on its spermatic cord so that the testis's blood supply is blocked.

Testicular torsion usually occurs in men between puberty and about age 25, but it can occur at any age. Abnormal development of the spermatic cord or the membrane covering the testis makes testicular

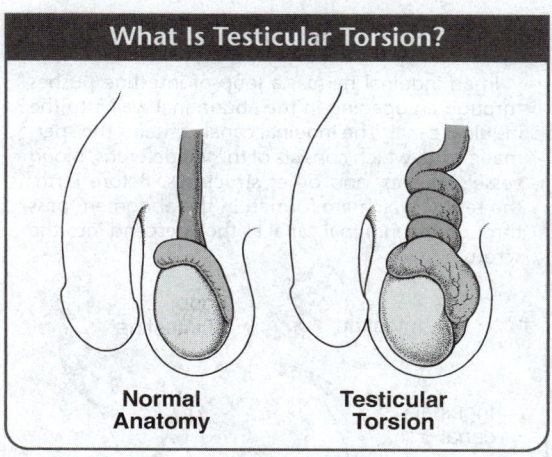

What Is Testicular Torsion?

Normal Anatomy

Testicular Torsion

torsion possible. With torsion, the testis usually dies within 6 to 12 hours after the blood supply is cut off unless the torsion is treated.

Severe pain and swelling develop suddenly in the testis. The pain may seem to come from the abdomen, and nausea and vomiting may develop. Doctors may diagnose the condition based on a description of the symptoms and the physical examination findings. Alternatively, doctors may use a scan, usually an ultrasound scan, for diagnosis.

Testicular torsion is an emergency because the testis will die unless it is untwisted rapidly. Doctors may try to untwist the testis without surgery by rotating it within the scrotum. Occasionally, this procedure is successful and surgery is done later. However, usually the procedure is unsuccessful, and surgery to untwist the spermatic cord is required immediately. During surgery, whether done immediately or later, urologists usually secure both testes to prevent future episodes of torsion.

Inguinal Hernia

An inguinal hernia is a protrusion of a piece of intestine through an opening in the abdominal wall in the groin.

An inguinal hernia extends into the groin and can extend into the scrotum. Other types of hernias (such as umbilical hernias and femoral hernias) occur at other locations (see page 202). With an inguinal hernia, the opening in the abdominal wall can be present from birth or develop later in life.

Inguinal hernias usually produce a painless bulge in the groin or scrotum. The bulge may enlarge when men stand and shrink when they lie down because the intestine slides back and forth with gravity. Sometimes a portion of the intestine is trapped in the

What Is an Inguinal Hernia?

In an inguinal hernia, a loop of intestine pushes through an opening in the abdominal wall into the inguinal canal. The inguinal canal contains the spermatic cord, which consists of the vas deferens, blood vessels, nerves, and other structures. Before birth, the testes, which are formed in the abdomen, pass through the inguinal canal as they descend into the scrotum.

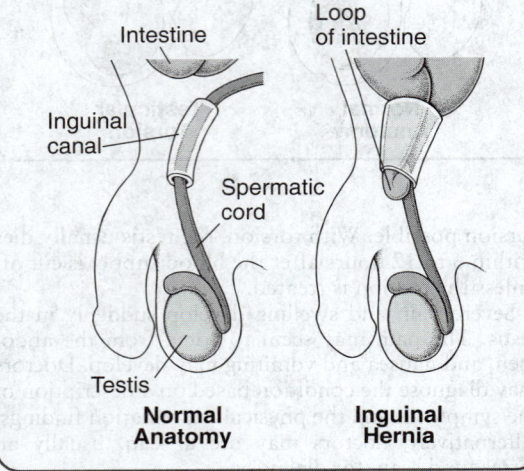

Normal Anatomy   **Inguinal Hernia**

scrotum (incarceration). If the intestine becomes trapped, the intestine's blood supply can be cut off (strangulation). Strangulated intestine may die (become gangrenous) within hours.

Surgical repair usually aims to tighten the opening so the hernia cannot slide back into the groin. Surgery usually relieves the symptoms of a hernia, depending on its size and the amount of discomfort it causes. For strangulated hernias, emergency surgery is needed to pull the intestine out of the inguinal canal and tighten the opening.

Epididymitis and Epididymo-orchitis

Epididymitis is inflammation of the epididymis (the coiled tube on top of the testis that provides the space and environment for sperm to mature), and epididymo-orchitis is inflammation of the epididymis and testes.

Epididymitis and epididymo-orchitis are usually caused by a bacterial infection. Infection can result from surgery, the insertion of a catheter into the bladder, or the spread of infections from elsewhere in the urinary tract. Sometimes, particularly in young men, the cause is a sexually transmitted disease. Rare causes include infection by certain viruses or fungi. Sometimes there is no infection of any kind. In such cases, doctors believe the epididymis becomes inflamed by reverse flow of urine into the epididymis, perhaps because of straining (as when men lift something very heavy).

Symptoms of epididymitis and epididymo-orchitis include swelling and tenderness of the affected area, pain that may become constant and severe, fluid around the testes (hydrocele), and sometimes a fever. Rarely, an abscess (collection of pus) that feels like a soft lump develops in the scrotum.

Epididymitis and epididymo-orchitis are diagnosed by physical examination, urinalysis, and sometimes Doppler ultrasonography, which assesses blood flow to the testes. These disorders are usually treated with antibiotics taken by mouth, bed rest, pain relievers, and ice packs applied to the scrotum. Immobilizing the scrotum with a jockstrap decreases pain from repetitive, minor bumps. Abscesses usually require surgical drainage.

Swelling in the Scrotum

The scrotum can swell for many reasons. Possible causes include cancer, testicular torsion, inguinal hernia, epididymitis, hydrocele, edema, orchitis, spermatocele, and varicocele.

Hydrocele: A hydrocele is a collection of fluid in the membrane that covers each testis. A hydrocele may be present at birth or develop later in life. It is most common after age 40. Usually the cause is unknown. However, the condition occasionally results from a testicular disorder (for example, injury, epididymitis, or cancer).

Usually, a hydrocele does not cause symptoms. It is found as a painless swelling surrounding the testis. Doctors may shine a bright light on the swelling (transillumination) to confirm the diagnosis. Ultrasound examination of the testis is done in unusual instances—for example, in a young man with no apparent cause for the hydrocele. The ultrasound scan may reveal an infection or tumor.

Most hydroceles need no treatment. However, unusually large hydroceles are sometimes removed surgically.

Edema: Edema is fluid retention involving the entire scrotum. Edema may result from salt and water retention or blockage of the flow of lymphatic fluid (see page 440). In both cases, men have no pain. Salt and water retention most commonly occurs because of heart failure, kidney failure, or chronic liver disease. Lymphedema results from blockage of lymph fluid most often because of compression of the abdominal or pelvic lymph vessels (for example, by a tumor or infection by certain kinds of parasites).

Doctors usually diagnose the cause of edema based on the man's symptoms and findings from a physical examination. Sometimes blood tests are done to evaluate liver and kidney function. Doctors treat edema by treating the cause.

Orchitis: Infection of the testes (orchitis) is usually caused by a virus, most often mumps. Mumps usually affects children. If a man contracts mumps, the testes can become painful and swollen and may sometimes later shrink and stop working (atrophy). Usually the diagnosis can be determined based on symptoms. Analgesics and cold or warm packs can help relieve pain. Infection usually resolves on its own without causing permanent problems. Sometimes mumps can permanently damage the ability of the testes to produce sperm, but mumps does not usually cause complete infertility unless it affects both testes.

Spermatocele: A spermatocele is a collection of sperm in a sac that develops next to the epididymis. Most spermatoceles are painless. While most need no treatment, a spermatocele that becomes large or bothersome can be removed surgically.

Varicocele: Varicocele is the development of varicose veins in the blood vessels that drain the testis. Veins contain valves that prevent blood from flowing backward. Faulty valves can result in a varicocele. Varicoceles usually develop on the left side of the scrotum and may produce no symptoms. Alternatively, varicoceles may cause a sense of fullness and aching and throbbing pain that become bothersome when a man stands. The varicocele feels like a bag of worms if the scrotum is touched when the man is standing. However, the swelling usually disappears and symptoms resolve when he reclines because blood flow to the enlarged veins decreases. Rarely, a varicocele impairs fertility.

If symptoms are severe, doctors may surgically tie off the affected veins.

Testicular Cancer

- Testicular cancer is common among young men.
- Usually a painless lump is present.
- Ultrasound scans and blood tests are done.
- The testis is removed, and sometimes radiation therapy or chemotherapy is given.

Most testicular cancers develop in men younger than age 40. It is one of the most common cancers in young men. Among the types of cancer that develop in the testes are seminoma, teratoma, embryonal carcinoma, and choriocarcinoma.

The cause of testicular cancer is not known, but men whose testes did not descend into the scrotum (cryptorchidism—see page 1735) by age 3 have a greater chance of developing testicular cancer than do men whose testes descended by that age. Cryptorchidism is best corrected surgically in childhood. Correcting cryptorchidism decreases the risk of testicular cancer. However, even if cryptorchidism is corrected, the risk of cancer is still higher than for men who never had cryptorchidism. Sometimes in adults, doctors recommend removal of a single undescended testis to reduce the risk of cancer.

Symptoms

Testicular cancer may cause an enlarged testis or a lump. A testis normally feels like a smooth oval, with the epididymis attached behind and on top. Testicular cancer produces a firm, growing lump in or attached to the testis. With cancer, the testis loses its normal shape, becoming large, irregular, or bumpy. Although testicular cancer is usually painless, the testis or lump may hurt when lightly touched and may even hurt without being touched. A firm lump on the testis requires prompt medical attention. Occasionally, blood vessels rupture within the tumor, yielding a suddenly enlarged, severely painful swelling.

Diagnosis

Physical examination and ultrasound scanning may indicate whether a lump is part of the testis and whether it is solid (and thus more likely to be cancer) or filled with fluid (cystic). Determining the blood levels of two proteins, alpha-fetoprotein and human chorionic gonadotropin, may help in making the diagnosis. The levels of these proteins often increase in men with testicular cancer. If cancer is suspected, surgery to remove the testis is done promptly. Most doctors recommend testicular self-examination.

> **? Did You Know...**
> Loss of one testis does not impair sex drive or the ability to have children or erections.

Treatment

The initial treatment for testicular cancer is surgical removal of the entire affected testis (radical orchiectomy). An artificial testis (prosthesis) can be placed if the man desires. The other testis is not removed, so men retain adequate levels of male hormones and remain fertile. Infertility sometimes occurs in men with testicular cancer, but fertility may return after treatment.

With certain types of cancers, lymph nodes in the abdomen are also removed (retroperitoneal lymph node dissection) because the cancer often spreads there first. Radiation therapy may also help, especially for a seminoma.

A combination of surgery and chemotherapy often cures testicular cancer that has spread. Blood levels of alpha-fetoprotein and human chorionic gonadotropin that were elevated at diagnosis decline after

successful treatment. If levels rise after treatment, the cancer may have recurred.

The prognosis for men with testicular cancer depends on the type and extent of the cancer but is usually excellent if the cancer has not spread. Even if the cancer has spread, cure is sometimes possible.

CHAPTER

233 Prostate Disorders

The prostate gland lies just under the bladder and surrounds the tube that carries urine from the bladder (the urethra). It produces the fluid in the semen that nourishes sperm. Walnut-sized in young men, the prostate gland enlarges with aging. Three common disorders affect the prostate: benign prostatic hyperplasia, prostate cancer, and prostatitis.

Benign Prostatic Hyperplasia

Benign prostatic hyperplasia (benign prostatic hypertrophy) is a noncancerous (benign) enlargement of the prostate gland that can make urination difficult.

- The prostate gland enlarges as men age.
- Men may have difficulty urinating and feel the need to urinate more often and more urgently.
- Usually, the diagnosis is based on results of a rectal examination, but a blood sample may be taken to check for prostate cancer.
- If needed, drugs to relax the muscles of the prostate and bladder (such as terazosin) or to shrink the prostate (such as finasteride) are used, but sometimes surgery is necessary.

Benign prostatic hyperplasia (BPH) becomes increasingly common as men age, especially after age 50. The precise cause is not known but probably involves changes induced by hormones, especially testosterone.

As the prostate enlarges, it gradually compresses the urethra and blocks the flow of urine (urinary obstruction). When men with BPH urinate, the bladder may not empty completely. Consequently, urine stagnates in the bladder, making men susceptible to urinary tract infections and bladder stones. Prolonged obstruction can damage the kidneys.

Drugs such as over-the-counter antihistamines and nasal decongestants can increase resistance to the flow of urine or reduce the bladder's ability to contract, causing temporary blockage of urine flow out of the bladder in men with BPH.

Symptoms

BPH first causes symptoms when the enlarged prostate begins to block the flow of urine. At first, men may have difficulty starting urination. Urination may also feel incomplete. Because the bladder does not empty completely, men have to urinate more frequently, often at night (nocturia). Also, the need to urinate may become more urgent. The volume and force of the urinary flow may diminish noticeably, and urine may dribble at the end of urination.

Complications: Other problems can develop, but these problems affect only a small number of men with BPH. Obstruction of urine flow with retention of some urine in the bladder may increase the pressure in the bladder and limit the flow of urine from the kidneys, putting increased stress on the kidneys. This increased pressure may impede kidney function, although the effect is usually temporary if the obstruction is relieved early. If obstruction is prolonged, the bladder may overstretch, causing overflow incontinence (see page 292). As the bladder stretches, small veins in the bladder and urethra also stretch. These veins sometimes burst when men strain to urinate, causing blood to enter the urine.

Complete blockage of urine flow out of the bladder (urinary retention) can develop, making urination impossible and usually leading to a full feeling and severe pain in the lower abdomen. However, occasionally urinary retention can occur with few or even no symptoms until retention is very severe. Urinary retention can be triggered by the following conditions:

- Being immobile (for example, when put on bed rest)
- Being exposed to cold
- Delaying urination for a long time
- Using certain anesthetics, alcohol, amphetamines, cocaine, opioids, or drugs with anticholinergic effects

What Happens When the Prostate Gland Enlarges?

In benign prostatic hyperplasia, the prostate gland enlarges. Normally the size of a walnut, the prostate gland may become as large as a tennis ball. The enlar-ging prostate gland squeezes the urethra, which carries urine out of the body. As a result, urine may flow through more slowly, or less urine may flow through.

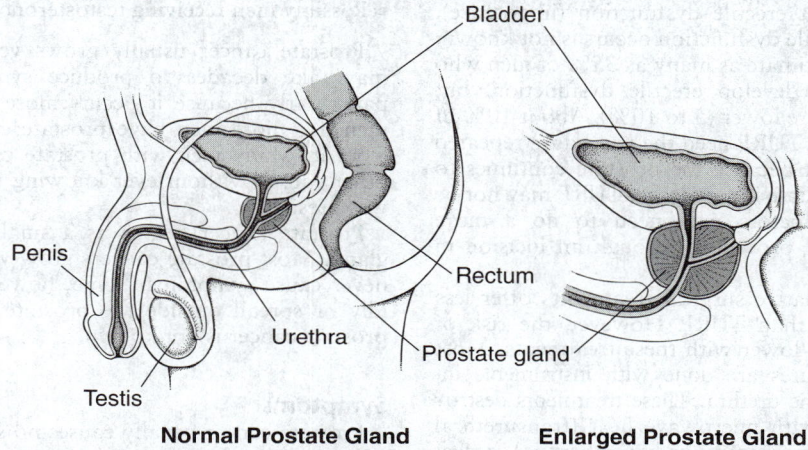

Normal Prostate Gland   **Enlarged Prostate Gland**

Diagnosis

By feeling the prostate during a rectal examination, doctors can usually determine if it is enlarged. Doctors insert a gloved and lubricated finger into the rectum. The prostate can be felt just in front of the rectum. A prostate affected by BPH feels enlarged, symmetrical, and smooth but is not painful to the touch.

A urine sample should be examined to make sure there is no infection or bleeding. Doctors usually also do a test to measure the level of prostate-specific antigen (PSA) in the blood in men who have an enlarged prostate on examination or who have symptoms of urine blockage. The PSA level can be elevated in men with BPH and also in men with prostate cancer. If the PSA level is elevated or the prostate is hard or lumpy to the touch, other tests may then be required to diagnose cancer (see page 1477).

Men who have symptoms of urine blockage may be asked to void into a device that measures the volume and rate of urine flow (a test called uroflowmetry). Immediately after the uroflowmetry, doctors do a bladder ultrasound examination to determine how completely the bladder has emptied. Both these tests help diagnose the presence and severity of urine blockage.

Treatment

Treatment is not necessary unless BPH causes especially bothersome symptoms or complications (such as urinary tract infections, impaired kidney function, blood in the urine, stones, or urinary retention). Drugs that can worsen symptoms, such as opioids and drugs with anticholinergic effects (for example, many antihistamines and some anti-depressants), should be stopped when possible.

Drugs: Drugs are usually tried first. Alpha-adrenergic blockers (such as terazosin, doxazosin, tamsulosin, or alfuzosin) relax certain muscles of the prostate and bladder and may improve the flow of urine. Some drugs (such as finasteride and dutasteride) may block the effects of the male hormones responsible for the prostate's growth, shrinking the prostate and preventing or delaying the need for surgery or other treatments. However, finasteride and dutasteride may need to be taken for 3 months or more before symptoms are relieved. Also, some men who take finasteride or dutasteride never experience relief of their symptoms. Men who have more severe symptoms may be treated with an alpha-adrenergic blocker plus either finasteride or dutasteride.

Surgery: If drugs are ineffective, surgery can be done. Surgery offers the greatest relief of symptoms but may cause complications. The most common surgical procedure is transurethral resection of the prostate (TURP), in which a doctor passes an endoscope (a viewing tube) up the urethra. Attached to the endoscope is a surgical instrument that is used to remove part of the prostate. The procedure spares men from an incision of the skin. Men who undergo TURP are usually given spinal anesthesia.

TURP can lead to such complications as infection and bleeding. Also, permanent incontinence develops in about 1 to 3% of men. The procedure also can cause permanent erectile dysfunction (impotence). How often erectile dysfunction occurs is not known. Some experts estimate as many as 35% of men who undergo TURP develop erectile dysfunction, but most estimates are lower (5 to 10%). About 10% of men undergoing TURP need the procedure repeated within 10 years, because the prostate continues to grow. If the prostate is very large, TURP may not be possible, and doctors may need to do a more invasive surgical procedure through an incision in the abdomen.

Various alternative surgical treatments offer less symptom relief than TURP. However, the risk of complications is lower with these treatments. Most of these procedures are done with instruments inserted through the urethra. These treatments destroy prostate tissue with microwave heat (transurethral microwave thermotherapy or hyperthermia), a needle (transurethral needle ablation), radiofrequency waves (radiofrequency vaporization), ultrasound (high intensity focused ultrasound), electric vaporization (transurethral electrovaporization), or lasers (laser therapy). Sometimes a channel can be inserted through the penis to widen the opening of the urethra (intraurethral stent).

Complications: Problems resulting from urine blockage may need treatment before BPH is definitively treated. Urinary retention can be treated by draining the bladder by means of a catheter inserted through the urethra. Infections can be treated with antibiotics.

Prostate Cancer

- The risk of prostate cancer increases as men age.
- Symptoms, such as difficulty urinating, a need to urinate frequently and urgently, and blood in the urine, usually occur only after the cancer is advanced.
- The cancer can spread, usually to the bone, kidneys, brain, or spinal cord.
- A digital rectal examination and a blood test may be done to check for prostate cancer in men without symptoms.
- If cancer is suspected, ultrasonography and a biopsy of prostate tissue are done.
- Treatment may involve watchful waiting, removal of the prostate gland, radiation therapy, or hormonal drugs to slow cancer growth.

Among men in the United States, prostate cancer is the most common cancer and one of the most common causes of cancer death. The chance of developing prostate cancer increases with age and is greater for

- Men who are black or Hispanic
- Men whose close relatives had the disease
- Possibly men receiving testosterone treatment

Prostate cancer usually grows very slowly and may take decades to produce symptoms. Thus, particularly because it occurs more often in older men, far more men have prostate cancer than die from it. Many men with prostate cancer die from other causes without ever knowing that the cancer was present.

Prostate cancer begins as a small bump in the gland. Most prostate cancers grow very slowly and never cause symptoms. Some, however, grow rapidly or spread outside the prostate. The cause of prostate cancer is not known.

Symptoms

Prostate cancer usually causes no symptoms until it reaches an advanced stage. Sometimes, symptoms similar to those of benign prostatic hyperplasia (BPH) develop, including difficulty urinating and a need to urinate frequently or urgently. However, these symptoms do not develop until after the cancer grows large enough to compress the urethra and partially block the flow of urine. Later, prostate cancer may cause bloody urine or a sudden inability to urinate.

> **? Did You Know...**
>
> Many men with prostate cancer die without ever knowing that they had the cancer.
>
> Whether men without symptoms should have a periodic blood test to check for prostate cancer is unclear.

In some men, symptoms of prostate cancer develop only after it spreads (metastasizes). The areas most often affected by cancer spread are bone (typically the pelvis, ribs, or vertebrae) and the kidneys. Bone cancer tends to be painful and may weaken the bone enough for it to easily fracture. Prostate cancer can also spread to the brain, which eventually causes seizures, confusion, headaches, weakness, or other neurologic symptoms. Spread to the spinal cord, which is also common, can cause pain, numbness, weakness, or urinary incontinence. After the cancer spreads, anemia is common.

Diagnosis

Doctors may suspect prostate cancer based on the symptoms, the results of a digital rectal examination, or the results of screening blood tests. The screening blood test is a measurement of prostate-specific antigen (PSA) levels. PSA is a substance produced only by prostate gland tissue.

If results of these tests suggest cancer, ultrasound scanning is usually done. In men with prostate cancer, ultrasound scans may or may not reveal the cancer but are used to guide biopsy of the prostate.

If the results of a digital rectal examination or PSA test suggest prostate cancer, tissue samples from the prostate are taken and analyzed (biopsy). When doing a biopsy, doctors usually first obtain images of the prostate by inserting an ultrasound probe (transducer) into the rectum (transrectal ultrasound). Doctors then insert a needle through the probe and use the needle to obtain tissue samples several times. Usually, 5 or 6 samples are taken from each side of the prostate to increase the likelihood of finding a small cancer. This procedure takes only a few minutes, and men are given local anesthesia.

Grading and staging help doctors determine the likely course and the best treatment of the cancer.

Grading: The Gleason scoring system is the most common way to grade prostate cancer. Based on the microscopic examination of tissues obtained from the biopsy, a number between 1 and 5 is assigned based on how distorted the cells appear. Because cancer cells often vary in their appearance, the number score for the most common abnormal cells is added to the number for the next most common abnormal cells to give a total score from 2 to 10. Scores between 6 and 7 are most common. The higher the number (high grade), the more aggressive the cancer is and the more likely it is that the cancer will spread.

Staging: Prostate cancers are staged according to three criteria:

- How far the cancer has spread within the prostate
- Whether the cancer has spread to lymph nodes in areas near the prostate
- Whether the cancer has spread to organs far from the prostate (metastatic cancer)

Testing to stage the cancer is often done when cancer is diagnosed. However, such testing may not be necessary when the likelihood of spread beyond the prostate is extremely low. Likelihood of spread is low when cancers have a Gleason score of 7 or less, the PSA level is less than 10 ng/mL, and the cancer has not penetrated the surface of the gland. Results of the digital rectal examination, ultrasound scan, and biopsy reveal how far the cancer has spread within the prostate.

If likelihood of spread is not low, doctors usually do a computed tomography (CT) scan or magnetic resonance imaging (MRI) of the abdomen and pelvis. Sometimes the MRI is done using a special coil inserted in the rectum. A bone scan may be done in people who have pain in their bones or who have a very high PSA level.

If spread to the brain or spinal cord is suspected, CT or MRI of those organs is done.

Screening: Because prostate cancer is common, many doctors check for it in men with no symptoms (screening). However, because screening tests are positive in many men who do not have cancer and because some men who do have cancer may not require treatment, experts disagree about whether and when screening is helpful. Screening is considered in men older than 50 and in those older than 40 who have risk factors, such as being black or having a family history of prostate cancer. Benefits of screening may decrease with age. For example, one professional organization recommends against screening men who are older than 75 or who are not expected to live at least 10 more years. Screening, once begun, is usually repeated yearly.

To screen for prostate cancer, doctors do a digital rectal examination and a blood test to measure PSA levels. If the prostate gland is hard, irregularly enlarged, or has a lump or if the PSA level is elevated, prostate cancer is more likely. However, PSA levels can be misleading. The PSA level can be normal when prostate cancer is present and can be elevated for reasons other than prostate cancer. PSA levels normally increase with age and with disorders such as BPH and prostatitis. Men with an elevated PSA level then require a transrectal prostate biopsy to identify those who have cancer. Because most men who have elevated PSA levels on screening tests do not have prostate cancer, many biopsies have negative results.

Some prostate cancers are aggressive and potentially fatal but may not cause symptoms until they are too advanced to be cured. Screening offers the advantage of finding such cancers early—when they might be cured. However, because many prostate cancers grow slowly and often never cause symptoms or death, screening may find cancers that would probably not hurt or kill a man even if they were never detected. The side effects of treating such a cancer can be more damaging than leaving the cancer untreated. Thus, it is not clear whether the benefits of screening outweigh the discomfort, stress, and possible harm from unnecessary testing and treatment.

Prognosis

Prognosis for most men with prostate cancer is very good. Most elderly men with prostate cancer tend to live as long as other men their age who have similar general health and do not have prostate cancer. For many men, long-term remission or even cure is possible. The prognosis depends upon the cancer's grade and stage. High-grade cancers have a poor prognosis unless treated very early. Cancers that have spread to surrounding tissues also have a poorer prognosis. Metastatic prostate cancer has no cure. Most men with metastatic cancer live about 1 to 3 years after diagnosis, but some live for many years.

Treatment

Choosing among treatment options can be complicated. Because studies have not directly compared one treatment to another, doctors are uncertain which treatment is most effective. Furthermore, for some men, doctors are not sure whether treatment will prolong life. Such men include those who are not expected to live very long (either because of old age or serious health problems) and those with low PSA levels who have low-grade cancers confined to the prostate. Thus, men often make their decision by balancing their degree of discomfort in living with a cancer that might or might not harm them against the possible side effects of treatment. Surgery, radiation therapy, and hormonal therapy may cause incontinence, erectile dysfunction (impotence), or other problems. For these reasons, men's preferences are a bigger consideration in choosing treatment for prostate cancer than they are for many other disorders.

Treatment for prostate cancer usually involves one of three strategies:

- Active surveillance
- Curative treatment
- Palliative treatment

Active surveillance (formerly called watchful waiting) means doctors give no treatment unless the cancer progresses. The advantage of this strategy is avoiding or postponing the potential side effects of treatment. Active surveillance should be considered mainly by elderly men (perhaps those over 70) whose cancers are unlikely to spread or cause symptoms. For example, most cancers that are confined to a small area within the prostate and have low Gleason scores grow very slowly and usually do not spread for many years. Thus, older men, particularly those who have other serious health problems, are far more likely to die of other causes before such cancers kill them or cause symptoms. In younger men, particularly those who are healthy, even a slow-growing cancer may eventually cause symptoms. In such men, active surveillance may be less preferred. During active surveillance, doctors periodically ask about symptoms, measure the PSA level, and do digital

rectal examinations to determine whether the cancer is causing symptoms, growing rapidly, or spreading. Younger men may also have periodic repeat biopsies. If testing shows growth or spread, doctors offer curative or palliative treatment.

Curative treatment aims to remove all of the cancer and includes

- Surgery
- Radiation therapy

Curative (also called definitive) treatment is a common strategy for men with cancers confined to the prostate that are likely to cause troublesome symptoms or death. Such cancers include those that are growing rapidly as well as some small, slowly growing cancers in men who are likely to live for some time (perhaps at least 10 or 15 years). Such men are typically those who are healthy, younger (particularly those under 60), or both. Curative treatment is not pursued if cancer has spread widely, but it can benefit some men with cancers that have spread to the area just outside the prostate. Such cancers are likely to cause symptoms within a relatively short period. However, curative treatment is most likely to be successful with cancers that are still confined to the area near the prostate. Curative treatment can prolong life and reduce or eliminate severe symptoms resulting from some cancers. However, some men experience side effects of curative treatment, most significantly erectile dysfunction and incontinence, which can impair quality of life.

Palliative treatment aims to treat the symptoms rather than cure the cancer. Palliative therapies include

- Hormonal therapy
- Chemotherapy
- Radiation beam therapy (mainly for cancer that has spread to the bones)

Palliative treatment is best suited to men with widespread prostate cancer, which is not curable. The growth or spread of such cancers can usually be slowed or temporarily reversed, relieving symptoms. Besides trying to slow the cancer's growth and spread, doctors may try to relieve symptoms resulting from the effects of cancer in other organs and tissues (such as the bones). However, because these treatments cannot cure the cancer, symptoms eventually worsen. Death from the disease eventually follows.

Surgery: Surgically removing the prostate (prostatectomy) is useful for cancer that is confined to the prostate. Prostatectomy is not done if staging tests show the cancer has spread. Prostatectomy is very effective in curing low-grade, slowly-growing cancers but is less effective in high-grade, fast-growing cancers. Such cancers are more likely to have spread even

COMMON METHODS AND STRATEGIES FOR TREATING PROSTATE CANCER

CHARACTERISTICS OF THE CANCER	TREATMENT STRATEGY	METHOD OF TREATMENT
Small, slow-growing cancer, confined to prostate in men expected to live many years	Curative treatment (to remove all traces of the cancer)	Surgery or radiation therapy
Small, slow-growing cancer, confined to prostate in men not expected to live many years	Active surveillance (to monitor and watch for symptoms)	No treatment
Large or fast-growing cancer, confined to prostate	Curative treatment	Surgery or radiation therapy
Cancer spread to areas around the prostate, but not to distant areas	Curative treatment	Radiation therapy
Widespread cancer	Palliative treatment (to relieve symptoms primarily rather than cure the cancer)	Hormonal therapy

if spread is not detectable with staging tests at the time of diagnosis.

Prostatectomy requires general or spinal anesthesia, an overnight hospital stay, and a surgical incision. Following surgery, men must have a catheter in their penis for a week or two until the connection between the bladder and urethra heals. Doctors do not routinely give radiation therapy, chemotherapy, or hormone therapy before or after surgery, but studies are being done to determine whether such treatments may benefit certain men.

Prostatectomy may lead to permanent erectile dysfunction and urinary incontinence. Erectile dysfunction may occur because the nerves to the penis that control erection run across the prostate and may be damaged during surgery. Incontinence may occur because part of the sphincter that closes the opening at the bottom of the bladder must be removed during surgery.

Techniques for doing prostatectomy include open radical prostatectomy and laparoscopic or robotic radical prostatectomy.

In open radical prostatectomy, the entire prostate, the seminal vesicles, and part of the vas deferens are removed through an incision in the lower abdomen or, rarely, in the area between the scrotum and anus. In the laparoscopic and robotic-assisted laparoscopic procedures, the same structures are removed, but these procedures are done through smaller incisions and result in less postoperative pain and blood loss.

Radical prostatectomy, irrespective of technique, is the surgery done when trying to cure prostate cancer. However, the procedure causes incontinence in about 3% of men and partial incontinence in more. Tempo-

rary incontinence develops in most men and may last for several months. Incontinence is less likely in younger men. A degree of erectile dysfunction commonly develops after radical prostatectomy and is more common in older men. Blockage of urine flow caused by narrowing of part of the bladder or scarring of the urethra (urethral stricture) develops in 7 to 20% of men. More than 90% of men with cancer confined to the prostate live at least 10 years after radical prostatectomy. Younger men who can otherwise expect to live at least 10 to 15 more years are most likely to benefit from radical prostatectomy. Usually prostatectomy can be done in such a way that some of the nerves needed to achieve erection are spared—this procedure is called nerve-sparing radical prostatectomy. This procedure cannot be used to treat cancer that has invaded the nerves and blood vessels of the prostate. Nerve-sparing radical prostatectomy is less likely than non–nerve-sparing radical prostatectomy to cause erectile dysfunction. Most men are diagnosed early and, thus, can be treated with nerve-sparing radical prostatectomy.

Radiation Therapy: Radiation therapy (see page 1087) may cure cancers that are confined to the prostate, as well as cancers that have invaded tissues around the prostate. Although radiation therapy cannot cure cancer that has spread to distant organs, it can help relieve the pain resulting from the spread of prostate cancer to bone. Combining radiation therapy and surgery does not seem to work better than either alone.

For many stages of prostate cancer, 10-year survival rates with radiation therapy are nearly as high as those achieved with surgery. More than 90% of men with cancer confined to the prostate live at least 10 years after undergoing radiation therapy. Radiation therapy can be delivered as

- External beam radiation therapy
- Radioactive implants

External beam radiation therapy uses a machine to send beams of radiation to the prostate and surrounding tissues. CT is often used to help focus the radiation beams more precisely on the cancer by precisely identifying the structures affected. This approach is called three-dimensional conformal radiation therapy. Treatments are usually given 5 days per week for 7 to 8 weeks. Although some degree of erectile dysfunction can occur in up to 40% of men, it is less likely to develop after radiation therapy than after prostatectomy. Incontinence is rare when three-dimensional conformal radiation therapy is used. Scars that narrow the urethra and impede the flow of urine (urethral strictures) develop in about 7% of men. Other troublesome but usually temporary side effects of external beam radiation therapy include burning during urination, having to urinate frequently, blood in the urine, diarrhea that is sometimes bloody, irritation of the rectum and diarrhea (radiation proctitis), and sudden urges to defecate. Other forms of external beam radiation therapy that are newer and may have fewer side effects include proton beam therapy and intensity modulated radiation therapy (IMRT).

Radioactive implants can be inserted into the prostate (brachytherapy). The implants are small, seedlike pieces of radioactive material. Doctors inject the implants into the prostate gland through the area between the scrotum and anus using guidance from ultrasound or CT scans. Brachytherapy can be done in less than 2 hours, does not require repeated treatment sessions, and uses only spinal anesthesia. Brachytherapy also can deliver high doses of radiation to the prostate while often sparing healthy surrounding tissues and producing fewer side effects. However, brachytherapy may cause urethral strictures in up to 10% of men. (Seeds may later be passed in the urine. They are radioactive, so they should be kept away from pregnant women, because the fetus may be susceptible to radiation-induced birth defects. The seeds can set off Homeland Security radiation detectors.) Cure rates 10 to 15 years after brachytherapy are similar to rates obtained with other treatments for some men. Combined treatment with brachytherapy and external beam radiation therapy is sometimes recommended for more aggressive cancers.

Hormonal Therapy: Because most prostate cancers require testosterone to grow or spread, treatments that block the effects of this hormone (hormonal therapy) can slow progression of the tumors. Hormonal therapy is commonly used to delay the spread of the cancer that has come back after surgery or radiation therapy or to treat widespread (metastatic) prostate cancer. Hormonal therapy is sometimes combined with other treatments. It is not curative. Hormonal therapy can prolong life as well as decrease symptoms. Eventually, however, hormonal therapy becomes ineffective, and the disease progresses.

Hormonal drugs used to treat prostate cancer in the United States include leuprolide, goserelin, and buserelin, which prevent the pituitary gland from stimulating the testes to make testosterone. These drugs are administered by injection in a doctor's office every 1, 3, 4, or 12 months, usually for the rest of the man's life. For some men, this treatment may only be given for a year or two and possibly resumed at a later time.

Drugs that block testosterone's effects (such as flutamide, bicalutamide, and nilutamide) may also be used. These drugs are taken daily by mouth.

Side effects of hormonal therapy may include hot flashes, osteoporosis, loss of energy, reduction in muscle mass, fluid weight gain, reduction of libido, decrease in body hair, erectile dysfunction, and breast enlargement (gynecomastia).

The oldest form of hormonal therapy involves the removal of both testes (bilateral orchiectomy). The effects of bilateral orchiectomy on testosterone level are equivalent to those produced by leuprolide, goserelin, and buserelin. The physical and psychologic effects of bilateral orchiectomy and other hormonal therapies make these therapies difficult for some men to accept.

Hormonal therapy usually becomes ineffective within 3 to 5 years in men with widespread prostate cancer. When cancer eventually progresses despite hormonal therapy, most men die within 1 or 2 years. When hormonal therapy fails (hormone resistance), alternative hormone drugs or chemotherapy may be tried.

Other Treatments: Chemotherapy is used in advanced cases when hormonal therapy has failed. Mitoxantrone, estramustine, and taxane drugs (such as docetaxel) can be used. Corticosteroids and the antifungal drug ketoconazole may also help relieve symptoms. Other treatments are being studied.

Follow-up: After all forms of treatment, PSA levels are measured at regular intervals (usually every 3 to 4 months for the first year, and then every 6 months for the rest of the man's life). By 1 month after surgery, PSA should not be detected. Following radiation therapy, PSA decreases more slowly and usually does not become undetectable but should remain stable at a low level. Increases in the PSA level may indicate that the cancer has recurred.

Digital rectal examination is done at the same time in men who have a prostate gland.

Prostatitis

Prostatitis is pain and swelling, inflammation, or both of the prostate gland.

- The cause is sometimes a bacterial infection.
- Pain can occur in the area between the scrotum and anus or in the lower back, penis, or testes.
- Men feel a frequent, urgent need to urinate, and urination, erection, ejaculation, and defecation may be painful.
- Urine and sometimes fluids expressed from the prostate gland are cultured.
- Bacterial infection is treated with antibiotics.
- Symptoms of prostatitis, regardless of the cause, may be treated with warm sitz baths, relaxation techniques, and drugs.

Prostatitis usually develops for unknown reasons. Prostatitis can result from a bacterial infection that spreads to the prostate from the urinary tract or from bacteria in the bloodstream. Bacterial infections may develop slowly and tend to recur (chronic bacterial prostatitis) or develop rapidly (acute bacterial prostatitis). Some people develop chronic prostatitis in the absence of bacterial infection. This type may or may not involve inflammation. Occasionally, prostatitis without bacterial infection causes inflammation but no symptoms.

Symptoms

In all types of prostatitis that cause symptoms, many of the symptoms are caused by spasm of the muscles in the bladder and pelvis, especially in the area between the scrotum and the anus (the perineum). Pain develops in the perineum, the lower back, and often the penis and testes. Men also may need to urinate frequently and urgently, and urinating may cause pain or burning. Pain may make obtaining an erection or ejaculating difficult or even painful. Constipation can develop, making defecation painful.

With acute bacterial prostatitis, symptoms tend to be more severe. Some symptoms tend to occur more often, such as fever, difficulty urinating, and blood in the urine. Bacterial prostatitis can result in a collection of pus (abscess) in the prostate or in epididymitis (inflammation of the epididymis).

Diagnosis

The diagnosis of prostatitis is usually based on the symptoms and a physical examination. The prostate, examined through the rectum by a doctor, may be swollen and tender to the touch, particularly with acute bacterial prostatitis. Samples of urine and, sometimes, of fluids expressed from the penis after massaging the prostate during the examination are taken for culture. Urine cultures reveal bacterial infections located anywhere in the urinary tract. In contrast, when infection is found by culturing fluid from the prostate, the prostate is clearly the cause of the infection. When prostatitis occurs without bacterial infection, urine cultures reveal no infection.

Treatment

No Infection: When cultures reveal no bacterial infection, prostatitis is usually difficult to cure. Most treatments for this kind of prostatitis relieve symptoms but may not cure the prostatitis. These treatments for symptoms can also be tried in chronic bacterial prostatitis. However, it is not clear how effective these treatments are.

Nondrug treatments may include periodic prostate massage (done by a doctor by placing a finger in the rectum) and sitting in a warm sitz bath. Relaxation techniques (biofeedback) to relieve spasm and pain of the pelvic muscles have also been used.

Among drug therapies, stool softeners can relieve painful defecation resulting from constipation. Analgesics and anti-inflammatory drugs may relieve pain and swelling regardless of its source. Alpha-adrenergic blockers (such as doxazosin, terazosin, tamsulosin, and alfuzosin) may help relieve symptoms by relaxing the muscles within the prostate. For reasons that are not understood, antibiotics sometimes relieve symptoms in nonbacterial prostatitis. If symptoms are severe despite other treatments, surgery, such as partial removal of the prostate, may be considered as a last resort. Destruction of the prostate by microwave or laser treatments is an alternative.

Infection: To treat acute bacterial prostatitis, an oral antibiotic that can penetrate prostate tissue (such as ofloxacin, levofloxacin, ciprofloxacin, or trimethoprim-sulfamethoxazole) is taken for 30 days. Taking antibiotics for less time may lead to a chronic infection. Chronic bacterial prostatitis can be difficult to cure. It is treated for at least 6 weeks with an antibiotic that can penetrate prostate tissue. If a prostate abscess occurs, surgical drainage is usually necessary.

CHAPTER 234

Sexual Dysfunction in Men

In men, sexual dysfunction refers to difficulties engaging in sexual intercourse. Sexual dysfunction encompasses a variety of disorders that affect sex drive (libido), the ability to achieve or maintain an erection (erectile dysfunction, or impotence), ejaculation, and the ability to achieve orgasm.

Sexual dysfunction may result from either physical or psychologic factors. Many sexual problems result from a combination of physical and psychologic factors. A physical problem may lead to psychologic problems (such as anxiety, fear, or stress), which can in turn aggravate the physical problem. Men sometimes pressure themselves or feel pressured by a partner to perform well sexually and become distressed when they cannot (performance anxiety). Performance anxiety can be troublesome and further worsen a man's ability to enjoy sexual relations.

> ### Did You Know...
>
> Sexual dysfunction may affect the sex drive or the ability to have an erection, to ejaculate, or to have an orgasm.
>
> How much of sexual dysfunction is due to physical factors and how much is due to psychologic factors can be difficult or impossible to discern.

Erectile dysfunction is the most common sexual dysfunction in men. Decreased libido also affects some men. Problems with ejaculation include uncontrolled ejaculation before or shortly after penetrating the vagina (premature ejaculation), ejaculation into the bladder (retrograde ejaculation), and inability to ejaculate (anejaculation).

Normal Sexual Function

Normal sexual function is a complex interaction involving both the mind (thoughts, memories, and emotions) and the body. The nervous, circulatory, and endocrine (hormonal) systems all interact with the mind to produce a sexual response. A delicate and balanced interplay among all parts of the nervous system controls the sexual response in men.

Desire (also called sex drive or libido) is the wish to engage in sexual activity. It may be triggered by thoughts, words, sights, smell, or touch. Desire leads to the first stage of the sexual response cycle, excitement. Excitement is sexual arousal. During excitement, the brain sends nerve signals through the spinal cord to the penis. The arteries supplying blood to the erectile tissues (corpora cavernosa and corpus spongiosum) respond by widening (dilating). The widened arteries dramatically increase blood flow to these areas, which become engorged with blood and expand. Muscles tighten around the veins that normally drain blood from the penis, slowing the outflow of blood and elevating blood pressure in the penis. This elevated blood pressure causes the penis to increase in length and diameter, producing an erection. Also, muscle tension increases throughout the body.

In the plateau stage, excitement and muscle tension are maintained or intensified. Orgasm is the peak or climax of sexual excitement. At orgasm, muscle tension throughout the body further increases. The man experiences contractions of the pelvic muscles followed by a release of muscle tension. Semen is usually, but not always, ejaculated from the penis. Ejaculation results when nerves stimulate muscle contractions in the male reproductive organs such as the seminal vesicles, prostate, and the ducts of the epididymis and vas deferens. These contractions force semen into the urethra. Contraction of the muscles around the urethra further propels the semen through and out of the penis. The neck of the bladder also constricts to keep semen from flowing backward into the bladder.

Although ejaculation and orgasm often occur nearly simultaneously, they are separate events. Ejaculation can occur without orgasm. Also, orgasm can occur in the absence of ejaculation, especially before puberty, or with the use of certain drugs (such as some antidepressants) or after surgery (such as removal of the prostate gland). Most men find orgasm highly pleasurable.

In resolution, a man returns to an unaroused state. Once ejaculation takes place or orgasm occurs, penile arteries constrict and the veins relax, reducing blood inflow, increasing blood outflow and causing the penis to become limp (detumescence). After orgasm, erection cannot be obtained for a period of time (refractory period), often as short as 20 minutes or less in young men but longer in older men. The time between erections generally increases as men age.

Decreased Libido

Decreased libido is a reduction in sex drive.

- Possible causes include psychologic factors (such as depression, anxiety, or relationship problems), drugs, and low levels of testosterone.
- Depending on the cause, doctors may suggest psychologic therapy, prescribe a different drug, or prescribe supplemental testosterone.

Sex drive (libido) varies greatly among men. And different men find different degrees of libido satisfactory. Libido may be decreased temporarily by conditions such as fatigue or anxiety. Libido also tends to gradually decrease as a man ages. Persistent low libido may cause a man and his sex partner distress.

Occasionally, libido can be low throughout a man's life. Lifelong low libido can result from traumatic childhood sexual experiences or from learned suppression of sexual thoughts. Most often, however, low libido develops after years of normal sexual desire. Psychologic factors, such as depression, anxiety, and relationship problems, are often the cause. Some drugs (such as those used to treat high blood pressure, depression, anxiety, or widespread prostate cancer) and decreased levels of testosterone can also lower libido.

A man with decreased libido thinks less about sex. He loses interest in sexual fantasy and masturbation and also in sexual activity. Even sexual stimulation, by sights, words, or touch, may fail to provoke interest. The man often retains the capacity for sexual function. Some men continue to engage in sexual activity to satisfy their partner.

A blood test can measure the level of testosterone in the blood. However, the diagnosis is usually based on the man's description of his symptoms.

If the cause is psychologic, various psychologic therapies, including behavioral therapies, such as the sensate focus technique (see page 1512), can help. Counseling can help address relationship issues. Men should also understand the role of stress and its impact on physical function. If the testosterone level is low, testosterone can be given, usually as a patch or gel applied to the skin or as an injection (see box on page 1468). If a drug appears to be the cause, a doctor can often try treating the man with a different drug.

Erectile Dysfunction

Erectile dysfunction (impotence) is the inability to achieve or maintain an erection adequate for penetration.

- The cause may be a disorder that reduces blood flow or damages nerves to the penis, a hormonal disorder, use of certain drugs, or psychologic issues.
- In many men, sex drive (libido) also decreases.
- A physical examination (including blood pressure measurement), blood tests, erection testing during sleep, and sometimes ultrasonography may detect a disorder contributing to erectile dysfunction.
- Drugs, taken by mouth or inserted or injected into the penis, may help, as may constriction and vacuum devices and psychologic therapy.

Psychologic Causes of Sexual Dysfunction

- Anger toward a partner
- Anxiety
- Depression
- Discord or boredom with a partner
- Fear of pregnancy, dependence on another person, or losing control
- Feelings of detachment from sexual activities or one's partner
- Guilt
- Inhibitions or ignorance about sexual behavior
- Performance anxiety (worrying about performance during intercourse)
- Previous traumatic sexual experiences (for example, rape, incest, sexual abuse, or previous sexual dysfunction)

Every man is occasionally unable to achieve an erection, which is normal. Erectile dysfunction occurs when the problem is frequent or continual.

Erectile dysfunction can range from mild to severe. A man with mild erectile dysfunction may occasionally achieve a full erection, but more often he achieves an erection that is inadequate for penetration or no erection at all. A man with severe erectile dysfunction is rarely able to achieve an erection.

Erectile dysfunction becomes more common with aging but is not part of the normal aging process. About half of men 65 years of age and three fourths of men 80 years of age have erectile dysfunction.

Causes

To achieve an erection, the penis needs an adequate inflow of blood, a slowing of blood outflow, and proper function of nerves leading to and from the penis. Disorders that narrow arteries and decrease blood inflow (such as atherosclerosis, diabetes, high blood pressure, and high blood cholesterol levels) or surgery affecting the blood vessels can cause erectile dysfunction. Also, abnormalities in the veins of the penis can sometimes drain blood back to the body so rapidly that erections cannot be sustained despite adequate blood inflow.

Damage to the nerves that lead to or from the penis can produce erectile dysfunction. Such damage could result from pelvic or abdominal surgery (particularly prostate surgery), radiation therapy, spinal disease, diabetes, multiple sclerosis, or peripheral nerve disorders.

Other risk factors include stroke, smoking, alcohol, and drugs. Drugs that commonly cause erectile dysfunction (particularly in older men) include

Sexual Activity and Heart Disease

Sexual activity is generally less taxing than moderate to heavy physical activity and is therefore usually safe for men with heart disease. Although the risk of a heart attack is higher during sexual activity than it is during rest, the risk is still very low during sexual activity.

Still, sexually active men with diseases of the heart and cardiovascular system (which include angina, high blood pressure, heart failure, abnormal rhythms of the heart, and blockage of the aortic valve [aortic stenosis]) need to consult their doctor. Usually, sexual activity is safe if the disease is mild, if it causes few symptoms, and if blood pressure is normal. If the disease is moderate in severity or if the man has other conditions that make a heart attack likely, testing may be necessary to determine how safe sexual activity is. If the disease is severe or if the man has an enlarged heart that blocks the flow of blood leaving the left ventricle (obstructive cardiomyopathy), sexual activity should be deferred until after treatment reduces the severity of the symptoms. Sexual activity should also be deferred until at least 2 to 6 weeks after a heart attack.

Use of sildenafil, vardenafil, and tadalafil may be dangerous in men taking nitroglycerin, who should not use these drugs.

Most often, testing to determine the safety of sexual activity involves monitoring the heart for signs of poor blood supply while the man is exercising on a treadmill. If the blood supply is adequate during exercise, a heart attack during sexual activity is very unlikely.

antihypertensives, antidepressants, some sedatives, cimetidine, digoxin, some diuretics, antipsychotics, and illicit drugs.

Occasionally, hormonal disturbances (such as abnormally low levels of testosterone) cause erectile dysfunction. Also, factors that decrease a man's energy level (such as illness, fatigue, and stress) can make it difficult to achieve an erection.

Psychologic issues that can cause sexual dysfunction (see box on page 1483) can impair the ability to achieve erections. Psychologic causes are more common in younger men. Any new stressful situation, such as a change of sex partners or problems with relationships or at work, can also contribute.

Symptoms

Sex drive (libido) often decreases in men with erectile dysfunction, although some men do maintain a normal libido. Regardless of whether libido changes, men with erectile dysfunction have difficulty engaging in intercourse either because the erect penis is not sufficiently hard, long, or elevated for penetration

or because the erection cannot be sustained. Some men stop having erections during sleep or upon awakening. Others may attain strong erections sometimes but be unable to attain or maintain erections other times.

When testosterone levels are low, the result is more likely to be a drop in libido than erectile dysfunction. In addition, low testosterone levels may lead to thinning of the bones, loss of energy, and loss of muscle mass.

Diagnosis

To diagnose the cause of erectile dysfunction, a doctor asks about disorders and conditions that may contribute to erectile dysfunction and drugs the man is taking. A general physical examination, including examination of the genital organs and prostate, is done. The doctor may assess the function of nerves that supply the genitals. Measuring the blood pressure in the legs and assessing the pulses in the legs and feet may reveal a problem with the arteries that supply blood to the penis.

A blood sample can be taken to measure the level of testosterone. Certain blood tests can help identify disorders that may lead to temporary or permanent erectile dysfunction, such as diabetes or infection.

If a problem with the arteries or veins is suspected, specialized tests may be done. For example, a device can be used at home to measure erections during sleep (when they normally occur). If erections are present during sleep, the cause may be mostly psychologic, whereas if erections are absent during sleep, the cause may be mostly physical. Ultrasonography also can be used to measure blood flow to the penis.

? Did You Know...

Occasional inability to achieve an erection is normal and does not mean that a man has erectile dysfunction.

About half of men older than 65 and one fourth of men older than 80 can usually have erections adequate for penetration.

Low levels of testosterone tend to decrease sex drive rather than cause erectile dysfunction.

Treatment

Measures that help prevent or control conditions that contribute to erectile dysfunction, such as high blood pressure, atherosclerosis, and diabetes, may also help improve erectile dysfunction, although the effect may be small. For example, losing excess weight, exercising, and stopping smoking may help.

Some men and their partners may choose not to pursue any treatment for erectile dysfunction. Physical contact without an erection may satisfy their needs for intimacy and fulfillment.

Sometimes, stopping use of a particular drug can improve erections.

Several folk remedies for erectile dysfunction exist, but none have proven to be effective.

For men who choose to pursue treatment, there are many choices.

Drug Treatment: Many drugs are used to treat erectile dysfunction. Most drugs that are given to treat erectile dysfunction increase blood flow to the penis. Most of these drugs are given by mouth, but some drugs can be applied locally—by injection or insertion into the penis.

Sildenafil, vardenafil, and tadalafil are known as phosphodiesterase inhibitors. These are the drugs most frequently used to treat erectile dysfunction. They are effective in about 60 to 75% of men with erectile dysfunction. These drugs are taken by mouth about 1 hour before sexual activity. Tadalafil is effective for about a day, longer than sildenafil and vardenafil, which are effective for about 4 to 6 hours. The drugs are effective only when the man is sexually aroused. Side effects of phosphodiesterase inhibitors include headache, flushing, stuffy nose, upset stomach, and vision problems. More serious side effects, including dangerously low blood pressure, can occur when phosphodiesterase inhibitors are taken with certain other drugs (such as nitroglycerin or amyl nitrite). Because of this risk, men should not take phosphodiesterase inhibitors if they take nitroglycerin. Rarely, men taking these drugs have experienced blindness, although it is possible that blindness had nothing to do with taking the drug. Phosphodiesterase inhibitors can cause a painful, prolonged erection, but this occurs very rarely.

Other oral drugs that have been used to treat erectile dysfunction are phentolamine, yohimbine, and testosterone. They have only limited effectiveness and can have significant side effects.

Drugs injected or inserted into the penis widen the arteries and increase blood flow to the penis. Men who cannot tolerate drugs taken by mouth can often be treated with these drugs. An example is alprostadil, in the form of a pellet (suppository), which can be inserted into the penis through the urethra. It may cause light-headedness, a burning sensation of the penis, or, occasionally, a prolonged, painful erection (priapism—see page 1470). Because these serious side effects occasionally occur, a man usually takes his first dose under observation in a doctor's office.

A man can also induce an erection by injecting drugs (such as alprostadil alone or a combination of alprostadil, papaverine, and phentolamine) into the shaft of his penis. Injection is one of the most effective ways to obtain an erection, producing erections in 80 to 90% of men with erectile dysfunction. However, many men are unwilling to inject their penis. Also, the injection is sometimes painful and occasionally causes priapism, and repeated injections may eventually produce scar tissue.

> **? Did You Know...**
>
> Combinations of drugs injected into the penis and devices that constrict or apply suction to the penis are highly effective and lack many of the side effects of oral drugs.
>
> Psychologic therapies can help even when erectile dysfunction has a physical cause.

Testosterone replacement therapy may help men whose erectile dysfunction is caused by abnormally low testosterone levels. Unlike other drugs, which work by increasing blood flow to the penis, testosterone works by correcting a hormonal deficiency. Testosterone can be taken in many forms, including patches, topical creams, and injections. Side effects can include liver dysfunction, increased red blood cell counts, and increased risk of stroke. Testosterone replacement alone is rarely adequate to restore erectile function. Whether testosterone increases risk of prostate cancer is unclear, but men taking testosterone should be closely monitored.

Constriction (Binding) and Vacuum Devices: Erectile dysfunction can often be managed with the use of a constriction device with or without a vacuum device. These devices enable a man to avoid the side effects that can occur with drug treatment. Constriction devices are among the least expensive treatments for erectile dysfunction. These devices (such as bands and rings made of metal, rubber, or leather) are placed at the base of the penis to slow the outflow of blood. These medically engineered devices can be purchased with a doctor's prescription in a pharmacy, but inexpensive versions (often called cock rings) can be purchased in stores that sell sexual paraphernalia. However, the devices are somewhat cumbersome and can cause penile pain, difficulty ejaculating, and bruising. Constriction devices should not be left on for longer than 30 minutes, or they may cause skin breakdown (ulceration).

Vacuum devices (which consist of a hollow chamber attached to a source of suction) fit over the penis, creating a seal. Mechanical suction applied to the chamber draws blood into the penis, producing an erection. Many vacuum devices have a constriction device that attaches to the base of the penis. If not, a constriction device can be applied separately.

Surgery: When erectile dysfunction does not respond to other treatments, a device that simulates an erection (prosthesis) can be surgically implanted in the penis.

A variety of prostheses are available. One type consists of a pair of firm rods, one inserted into each of the corpora cavernosa to create a permanently hard penis. Another prosthesis type is an inflatable balloon that is inserted into the penis. Before having intercourse, the man inflates the balloon with a small internal pump. Surgical implantation of a penile prosthesis requires at least a brief hospital stay and a 6-week recovery before intercourse is attempted.

Psychologic Therapy: Some types of psychologic therapy (which include behavior modification techniques, such as the sensate focus technique—see page 1512) can improve the mental and emotional factors that contribute to erectile dysfunction. Psychologic therapy can even help when the erectile dysfunction has a physical cause, because psychologic factors often compound the problem.

Specific therapies are selected based on the particular psychologic cause of the man's erectile dysfunction. For example, if the man is suffering from depression, psychotherapy may help with erectile dysfunction. Antidepressants may help erectile dysfunction by relieving depression, but antidepressants may themselves decrease libido and contribute to erectile dysfunction, so their effect may be difficult to predict. Sometimes psychotherapy can reduce anxiety about sexual performance in men with erectile dysfunction

from any cause. Improvement may take a long time, and many sessions are usually required. A man, and often his partner, must be highly motivated for psychotherapy to work.

Inability to Ejaculate

Inability to ejaculate (anejaculation) is usually caused by inability to reach orgasm. It usually occurs as part of erectile dysfunction. Causes, diagnosis, and treatment are the same as for erectile dysfunction (see page 1483). Retrograde ejaculation can sometimes result in absence of visible semen.

Premature Ejaculation

Premature ejaculation is ejaculation that occurs too early, usually before, upon, or shortly after penetration.

- The cause is most likely to be anxiety, other psychologic factors, or very sensitive penile skin.
- Behavior modification therapy, including strategies to delay ejaculation, helps most men.

Many males, especially adolescents, ejaculate sooner than they or their partners would like. Premature ejaculation is not just ejaculation that occurs before a man wants it to but rather ejaculation that occurs very soon—often within a minute or two—after penetration.

Many experts believe that premature ejaculation almost always results from anxiety or other psychologic causes. Others think that unusually sensitive penile skin may be a cause. Having intercourse less frequently than desired may worsen the problem by making the man even more sensitive. Premature ejaculation is rarely caused by a disease, although inflammation of the prostate gland or a nervous system disorder can cause the condition.

Premature ejaculation can distress a man and his partner. If the man ejaculates too early, the partner may be left unsatisfied sexually and may become resentful.

Behavior modification therapy can help most men overcome premature ejaculation. A therapist provides reassurance, explains why premature ejaculation occurs, and teaches the man strategies for delaying ejaculation.

Other methods that can help a man delay ejaculation include drug treatment (with a selective serotonin reuptake inhibitor, such as fluoxetine, paroxetine, or sertraline), application of an anesthetic to the penis, and use of condoms, which tend to decrease sensation. Sometimes a combination of drug treatment and behavior modification therapy enables a man to delay ejaculation even longer than he might be able to with only one of these treatments. When premature ejaculation is caused by more serious psychologic problems, psychologic therapy may help.

Learning to Delay Ejaculation

Two techniques are commonly used to treat premature ejaculation. They also help reduce the anxiety that often aggravates the problem. Each technique trains the man to experience high levels of excitement without ejaculating. Both involve self-stimulation of the penis (while masturbating) or stimulation by a partner until the man feels that he will soon ejaculate. When done with a partner, stimulation is at first by hand and later before or during intercourse.

In the **stop-and-start technique**, stimulation is stopped. With the **squeeze technique**, the man or his partner squeezes for 10 to 20 seconds the part of the penis where the head (glans) meets the shaft, preventing ejaculation and decreasing the strength of the erection. In both techniques, stimulation can resume after about 30 seconds. With practice, more than 95% of men learn to delay ejaculation for 5 to 10 minutes or even longer.

Retrograde Ejaculation

Retrograde ejaculation is a condition in which semen is ejaculated backward into the bladder rather than out through the penis.

In retrograde ejaculation, the part of the bladder that normally closes during ejaculation (the bladder neck) remains open, causing the semen to travel backward into the bladder. Common causes of retrograde ejaculation include diabetes, spinal cord injuries, certain drugs, and some surgical operations (including major abdominal or pelvic surgery—one of the most common causes is prostate surgery).

Men with retrograde ejaculation can still have orgasms. However, retrograde ejaculation decreases the amount of semen ejaculated out of the penis. Sometimes, no semen comes out. The condition can cause infertility but is otherwise not harmful.

A doctor makes the diagnosis of retrograde ejaculation by finding a large amount of sperm in a urine sample taken shortly after ejaculation. Men usually need no treatment unless infertility is an issue. About one third of men with retrograde ejaculation improve after treatment with drugs that close the bladder neck (such as pseudoephedrine, phenylephrine, chlorpheniramine, brompheniramine, or imipramine). However, most of these drugs can increase heart rate and blood pressure, which can be dangerous in men with high blood pressure or heart disease.

> **?** **Did You Know...**
> Insemination may be possible if infertility is caused by retrograde ejaculation.

If infertility requires treatment and drugs do not help, doctors can sometimes collect a man's sperm for insemination (see page 1588).

Women's Health Issues

235 Biology of the Female Reproductive System

The female reproductive system consists of the external and internal genital organs. The breasts are sometimes considered part of the reproductive system (see page 1546). However, other parts of the body also affect the development and functioning of the reproductive system. They include the hypothalamus (an area of the brain), the pituitary gland (located at the base of the brain, directly below the hypothalamus), and the adrenal glands (located on top of the kidneys). The hypothalamus orchestrates the interactions among the genital organs, pituitary gland, and adrenal glands (see art on page 980). These parts of the body interact with each other by releasing hormones. Hormones are chemical messengers that control and coordinate activities in the body. The hypothalamus produces gonadotropin-releasing hormone, which stimulates the pituitary gland to produce luteinizing hormone and follicle-stimulating hormone. These hormones stimulate the ovaries to produce the female sex hormones, estrogen and progesterone, and some male sex hormones (androgens). (Male sex hormones stimulate the growth of pubic and underarm hair at puberty and maintain muscle mass in girls as well as boys.) After childbirth, the hypothalamus signals the pituitary gland to produce prolactin, a hormone that stimulates milk production. The adrenal glands produce small amounts of female and male sex hormones.

> **? Did You Know...**
>
> Girls are born with over a million egg cells, but only about 400 are released during a lifetime of menstrual cycles.

External Genital Organs

The external genital organs include the mons pubis, labia majora, labia minora, Bartholin's glands, and clitoris. The area containing these organs is called the vulva. The external genital organs have three main functions:

- Enabling sperm to enter the body
- Protecting the internal genital organs from infectious organisms
- Providing sexual pleasure

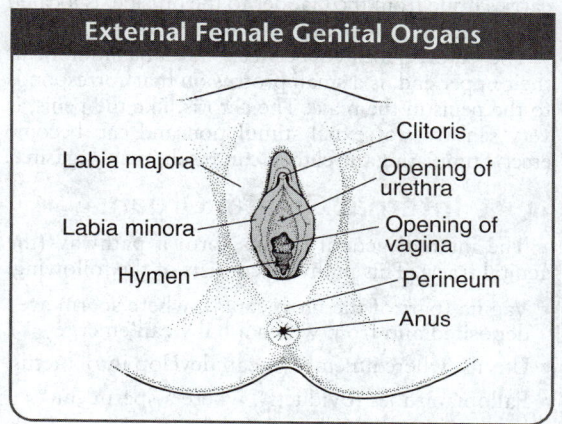

External Female Genital Organs

Labels: Labia majora, Labia minora, Hymen, Clitoris, Opening of urethra, Opening of vagina, Perineum, Anus

The mons pubis is a rounded mound of fatty tissue that covers the pubic bone. During puberty, it becomes covered with hair. The mons pubis contains oil-secreting (sebaceous) glands that release substances that are involved in sexual attraction (pheromones). The labia majora (literally, large lips) are relatively large, fleshy folds of tissue that enclose and protect the other external genital organs. They are comparable to the scrotum in males. The labia majora contain sweat and sebaceous glands, which produce lubricating secretions. After puberty, hair appears on the labia majora.

The labia minora (literally, small lips) can be very small or up to 2 inches wide. The labia minora lie just inside the labia majora and surround the openings to the vagina and urethra. A rich supply of blood vessels gives the labia minora a pink color. During sexual stimulation, these blood vessels become engorged with blood, causing the labia minora to swell and become more sensitive to stimulation.

The area between the vaginal opening and the anus, below the labia majora, is called the perineum. It varies in length from almost 1 to more than 2 inches (2 to 5 centimeters).

The labia majora and the perineum are covered with skin similar to that on the rest of the body. The skin is thick, dry, and sometimes scaly. In contrast, the labia minora are lined with a mucous membrane, whose surface is kept moist by fluid secreted by specialized cells.

The opening to the vagina is called the introitus. The vaginal opening is the entryway for the penis during sexual intercourse and the exit for menstrual blood and vaginal discharge as well as a baby. When stimulated, Bartholin's glands (located beside the vaginal opening) secrete a thick fluid that supplies lubrication for intercourse. The opening to the urethra, which carries urine from the bladder to the outside, is located above and in front of the vaginal opening.

The clitoris, located between the labia minora at their upper end, is a small protrusion that corresponds to the penis in the male. The clitoris, like the penis, is very sensitive to sexual stimulation and can become erect. Stimulating the clitoris can result in an orgasm.

Internal Genital Organs

The internal genital organs form a pathway (the genital tract). This pathway consists of the following:

- Vagina (part of the birth canal), where sperm are deposited and from which a baby can emerge
- Uterus, where an embryo can develop into a fetus
- Fallopian tubes (oviducts), where a sperm can fertilize an egg
- Ovaries, which produce and release eggs

Sperm can travel up the tract, and eggs down the tract.

At the beginning of the tract, just inside the opening of the vagina, is the hymen, a mucous membrane. In virgins, the hymen usually encircles the opening like a tight ring, but it may completely cover the opening. The hymen helps protect the genital tract but is not necessary for health. It may tear at the first attempt at sexual intercourse, or it may be so soft and pliable that no tearing occurs.

The hymen may also be torn during exercise or insertion of a tampon or diaphragm. Tearing usually causes slight bleeding. In women who have had intercourse, the hymen may be unnoticeable or may form small tags of tissue around the vaginal opening.

Vagina: The vagina is a narrow, muscular but elastic organ about 4 to 5 inches long in an adult woman. It connects the external genital organs to the uterus. The vagina is the main female organ of sexual intercourse. The penis is inserted into it. It is the passageway for sperm to the egg and for menstrual bleeding or a baby to the outside.

Usually, there is no space inside the vagina unless it is stretched open—for example, during an examination, sexual intercourse, or childbirth. The lower third of the vagina is surrounded by elastic muscles that control the diameter of its opening. These muscles contract rhythmically and involuntarily during orgasm.

The vagina is lined with a mucous membrane, kept moist by fluids oozing from cells on its surface and by secretions from glands in the cervix (the lower part of the uterus). A small amount of these fluids may pass to the outside as a clear or milky white vaginal discharge, which is normal. During a woman's reproductive years, the lining of the vagina has folds and wrinkles. Before puberty and after menopause (if the woman is not taking estrogen), the lining is smooth.

Uterus and Cervix: The uterus is a thick-walled, muscular, pear-shaped organ located in the middle of the pelvis, behind the bladder, and in front of the rectum. The uterus is anchored in position by several ligaments. The main function of the uterus is to sustain a developing fetus. The uterus consists of the cervix and the main body (corpus).

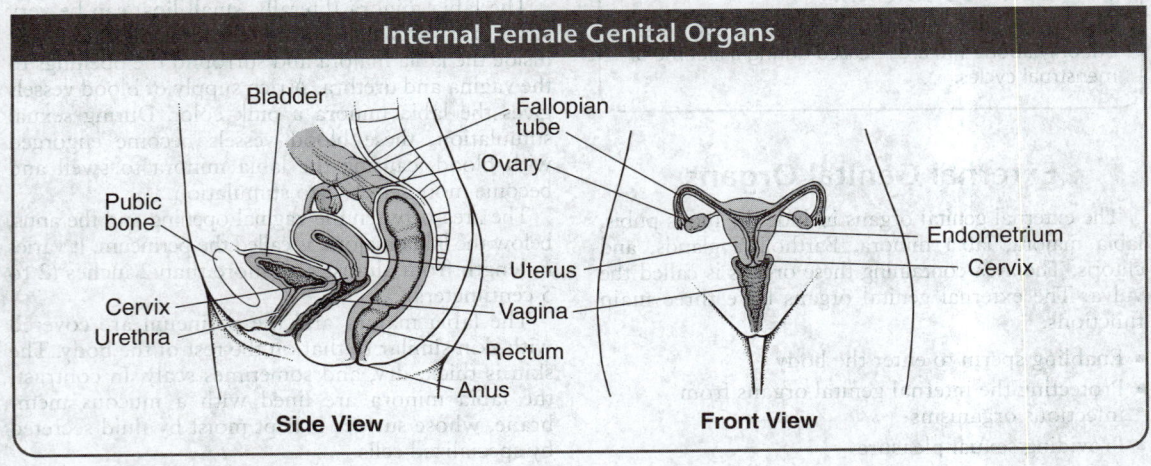

Internal Female Genital Organs

Bladder

Pubic bone

Cervix

Urethra

Fallopian tube

Ovary

Uterus

Vagina

Rectum

Anus

Side View

Endometrium

Cervix

Front View

The cervix is the lower part of the uterus, which protrudes into the upper end of the vagina. It can be seen during a pelvic examination. Like the vagina, the cervix is lined with a mucous membrane, but the mucous membrane of the cervix is smooth.

Sperm can enter and menstrual blood can exit the uterus through a channel in the cervix. The channel is usually narrow, but during labor, the channel widens to let the baby through. The cervix is usually a good barrier against bacteria, except around the time an egg is released by the ovaries (ovulation), during the menstrual period, or during labor. Bacteria that cause sexually transmitted diseases (see page 1264) can enter the uterus through the cervix during sexual intercourse.

The channel through the cervix is lined with glands that secrete mucus. This mucus is thick and impenetrable to sperm until just before ovulation. At ovulation, the consistency of the mucus changes so that sperm can swim through it and fertilization can occur. At this time, the mucus-secreting glands of the cervix can store live sperm for up to about 5 days, but occasionally slightly longer. These sperm can later move up through the corpus and into the fallopian tubes to fertilize an egg. Almost all pregnancies result from intercourse that occurs during the 3 days before ovulation. However, pregnancies sometimes result from intercourse that occurs up to 6 days before ovulation or during the 3 days after ovulation. For some women, the time between a menstrual period and ovulation varies from month to month. Consequently, pregnancy can occur at different times during a menstrual cycle.

The corpus of the uterus, which is highly muscular, can stretch to accommodate a growing fetus. Its muscular walls contract during labor to push the baby out through the cervix and the vagina. During the reproductive years, the corpus is twice as long as the cervix. After menopause, the reverse is true.

As part of a woman's reproductive cycle (which usually lasts about a month), the lining of the corpus (endometrium) thickens. If the woman does not become pregnant during that cycle, most of the endometrium is shed and bleeding occurs, resulting in the menstrual period.

Fallopian Tubes: The two fallopian tubes, which are about 2 to 3 inches (about 5 to 7 centimeters) long, extend from the upper edges of the uterus toward the ovaries. The tubes do not directly connect with the ovaries. Instead, the end of each tube flares into a funnel shape with fingerlike extensions (fimbriae). When an egg is released from an ovary, the fimbriae guide the egg into the relatively large opening of a fallopian tube.

The fallopian tubes are lined with tiny hairlike projections (cilia). The cilia and the muscles in the

---

How Many Eggs?

A baby girl is born with egg cells (oocytes) in her ovaries. Between 16 and 20 weeks of pregnancy, the ovaries of a female fetus contain 6 to 7 million oocytes. Most of the oocytes gradually waste away, leaving about 1 to 2 million present at birth. None develop after birth. At puberty, only about 300,000—more than enough for a lifetime of fertility—remain. Only a small percentage of oocytes mature into eggs. The many thousands of oocytes that do not mature degenerate. Degeneration progresses more rapidly in the 10 to 15 years before menopause. All are gone by menopause.

Only about 400 eggs are released during a woman's reproductive life, usually one during each menstrual cycle. Until released, an egg remains dormant in its follicle—suspended in the middle of a cell division. Thus, the egg is one of the longest-lived cells in the body. Because a dormant egg cannot perform the usual cellular repair processes, the opportunity for damage increases as a woman ages. A chromosomal or genetic abnormality is thus more likely when a woman conceives a baby later in life.

---

tube's wall propel an egg downward through the tube to the uterus. The egg may be fertilized by a sperm in the fallopian tube (see page 1617).

Ovaries: The ovaries are usually pearl-colored, oblong, and about the size of a walnut. They are attached to the uterus by ligaments. In addition to producing female sex hormones (estrogen and progesterone) and male sex hormones, the ovaries produce and release eggs. The developing egg cells (oocytes) are contained in fluid-filled cavities (follicles) in the wall of the ovaries. Each follicle contains one oocyte.

Puberty

Puberty is a sequence of events in which physical changes occur, resulting in adult physical characteristics and capacity to reproduce. These physical changes are regulated by changes in the levels of hormones that are produced by the pituitary gland—luteinizing hormone and follicle-stimulating hormone. At birth, levels of these hormones are high, but they decrease within a few months and remain low until puberty. Early in puberty, levels of luteinizing hormone and follicle-stimulating hormone increase, stimulating the production of sex hormones. The increased levels of sex hormones (primarily estrogen) result in physical changes, including maturation of the breasts, ovaries, uterus, and vagina. Normally, these changes occur sequentially during puberty, resulting in sexual maturity (see box on page 1752).

The first change of puberty is usually the start of breast development (breast budding). In girls who live in the United States, this change usually occurs around age 8 to 13. Shortly afterward, pubic and underarm hair begin to grow. The interval from breast budding to the first menstrual period is usually about 2½ years. In the United States, girls, on average, have their first period when they are almost 13. The girl's body shape changes, and the percentage of body fat increases.

The growth spurt accompanying puberty typically begins about when pubic and underarm hair begin to grow. Growth is fastest relatively early in puberty (before menstrual periods begin) and peaks at about age 12. Then growth slows considerably, usually stopping between the ages of 14 and 16.

Menstrual Cycle

Menstruation is the shedding of the lining of the uterus (endometrium) accompanied by bleeding. It occurs in approximately monthly cycles throughout a woman's reproductive life, except during pregnancy. Menstruation starts during puberty (at menarche) and stops permanently at menopause (see page 1514).

By definition, the menstrual cycle begins with the first day of bleeding, which is counted as day 1. The cycle ends just before the next menstrual period. Menstrual cycles normally range from about 25 to 36 days. Only 10 to 15% of women have cycles that are exactly 28 days. Usually, the cycles vary the most and the intervals between periods are longest in the years immediately after menarche and before menopause.

Menstrual bleeding lasts 3 to 7 days, averaging 5 days. Blood loss during a cycle usually ranges from ½ to 2½ ounces. A sanitary pad or tampon, depending on the type, can hold up to an ounce of blood. Menstrual blood, unlike blood resulting from an injury, usually does not clot unless the bleeding is very heavy.

The menstrual cycle is regulated by hormones. Luteinizing hormone and follicle-stimulating hormone, which are produced by the pituitary gland, promote ovulation and stimulate the ovaries to produce estrogen and progesterone. Estrogen and progesterone stimulate the uterus and breasts to prepare for possible fertilization. The cycle has three phases: follicular (before release of the egg), ovulatory (egg release), and luteal (after egg release).

Follicular Phase: This phase begins on the first day of menstrual bleeding (day 1). But the main event in this phase is the development of follicles in the ovaries.

At the beginning of the follicular phase, the lining of the uterus (endometrium) is thick with fluids and nutrients designed to nourish an embryo. If no egg has been fertilized, estrogen and progesterone levels are low. As a result, the top layers of the endometrium are shed, and menstrual bleeding occurs.

About this time, the pituitary gland slightly increases its production of follicle-stimulating hormone. This hormone then stimulates the growth of 3 to 30 follicles. Each follicle contains an egg. Later in the phase, as the level of this hormone decreases, only one of these follicles (called the dominant follicle) continues to grow. It soon begins to produce estrogen, and the other stimulated follicles begin to break down.

On average, the follicular phase lasts about 13 or 14 days. Of the three phases, this phase varies the most in length. It tends to become shorter near menopause. This phase ends when the level of luteinizing hormone increases dramatically (surges). The surge results in release of the egg (ovulation).

Ovulatory Phase: This phase begins when the level of luteinizing hormone surges. Luteinizing hormone stimulates the dominant follicle to bulge from the surface of the ovary and finally rupture, releasing the egg. The level of follicle-stimulating hormone increases to a lesser degree. The function of the increase in follicle-stimulating hormone is not understood.

The ovulatory phase usually lasts 16 to 32 hours. It ends when the egg is released.

About 12 to 24 hours after the egg is released, the surge in luteinizing hormone can be detected by measuring the level of this hormone in urine. This measurement can be used to determine when women are fertile. The egg can be fertilized for only up to about 12 hours after its release. Fertilization is more likely when sperm are present in the reproductive tract before the egg is released.

Around the time of ovulation, some women feel a dull pain on one side of the lower abdomen. This pain is known as mittelschmerz (literally, middle pain). The pain may last for a few minutes to a few hours. The pain is felt on the same side as the ovary that released the egg, but the precise cause of the pain is unknown. The pain may precede or follow the rupture of the follicle and may not occur in all cycles. Egg release does not alternate between the two ovaries and appears to be random. If one ovary is removed, the remaining ovary releases an egg every month.

Luteal Phase: This phase begins after ovulation. It lasts about 14 days (unless fertilization occurs) and ends just before a menstrual period. In this phase, the ruptured follicle closes after releasing the egg and forms a structure called a corpus luteum, which produces increasing quantities of progesterone. The corpus luteum prepares the uterus in case fertilization occurs. The progesterone produced by the corpus luteum causes the endometrium to thicken, filling with fluids and nutrients to nourish a potential

Changes During the Menstrual Cycle

The menstrual cycle is regulated by the complex interaction of hormones: luteinizing hormone, follicle-stimulating hormone, and the female sex hormones estrogen and progesterone.

The menstrual cycle begins with menstrual bleeding (menstruation), which marks the first day of the follicular phase. Bleeding occurs after estrogen and progesterone levels decrease at the end of the previous cycle. This decrease causes the top layers of thickened lining of the uterus (endometrium) to break down and be shed. About this time, the follicle-stimulating hormone level increases slightly, stimulating the development of several ovarian follicles. Each follicle contains an egg. Later, as the follicle-stimulating hormone level decreases, only one follicle continues to develop. This follicle produces estrogen.

The ovulatory phase begins with a surge in luteinizing hormone and follicle-stimulating hormone levels. Luteinizing hormone stimulates egg release (ovulation), which usually occurs 16 to 32 hours after the surge begins. The estrogen level peaks during the surge, and the progesterone level starts to increase.

During the luteal phase, luteinizing hormone and follicle-stimulating hormone levels decrease. The ruptured follicle closes after releasing the egg and forms a corpus luteum, which produces progesterone. During most of this phase, the estrogen level is high. Progesterone and estrogen cause the lining of the uterus to thicken more, to prepare for possible fertilization. If the egg is not fertilized, the corpus luteum degenerates and no longer produces progesterone, the estrogen level decreases, the top layers of the lining break down and are shed, and a new menstrual cycle begins.

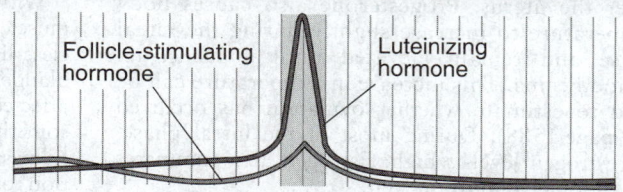

Pituitary Hormone Cycle

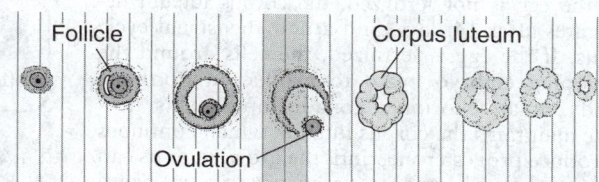

Ovarian Cycle

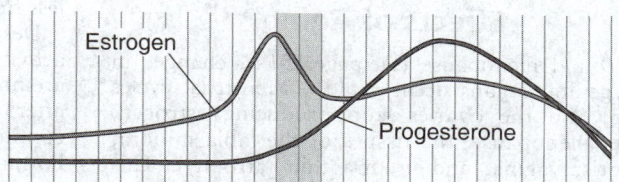

Sex Hormone Cycle

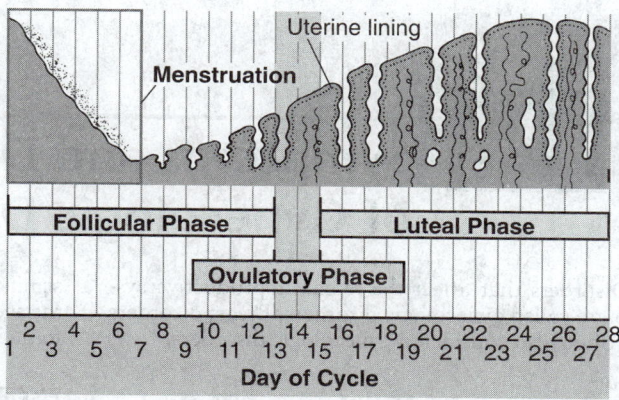

Endometrial Cycle

fetus. Progesterone causes the mucus in the cervix to thicken, so that sperm or bacteria are less likely to enter the uterus. Progesterone also causes body temperature to increase slightly during the luteal phase and remain elevated until a menstrual period begins. This increase in temperature can be used to estimate whether ovulation has occurred (see page 1588). During most of the luteal phase, the estrogen level is high. Estrogen also stimulates the endometrium to thicken.

The increase in estrogen and progesterone levels causes milk ducts in the breasts to widen (dilate). As a result, the breasts may swell and become tender.

If the egg is not fertilized, the corpus luteum degenerates after 14 days, and a new menstrual cycle begins. If the egg is fertilized, the cells around the developing embryo begin to produce a hormone called human chorionic gonadotropin. This hormone maintains the corpus luteum, which continues to produce progesterone, until the growing fetus can produce its own hormones. Pregnancy tests are based on detecting an increase in the human chorionic gonadotropin level.

Effects of Aging

Around menopause (see page 1514), changes in the genital organs occur rapidly. Menstrual cycles stop, and the ovaries stop producing estrogen. After menopause, the tissues of the labia minora, clitoris, vagina, and urethra thin (atrophy). This thinning can result in chronic irritation, dryness, and a discharge from the vagina. Vaginal infections are more likely to develop. Also after menopause, the uterus, fallopian tubes, and ovaries become smaller.

With aging, there is a decrease in the amount of muscle and connective tissue, including that in muscles, ligaments, and other tissues that support the bladder, uterus, vagina, and rectum. As a result, the affected organs may sag or drop down (prolapse), sometimes causing a feeling of pelvic pressure or fullness, difficulty urinating, loss of control of urination or bowel movements (incontinence), or pain during sexual intercourse. Women who have had many children are more likely to have such problems.

> ### ? Did You Know...
> Some women enjoy sexual intercourse more after menopause.

Because there is less estrogen to stimulate milk ducts, the breasts decrease in size and may sag. The connective tissue that supports the breasts also decreases, contributing to sagging. Fibrous tissue in the breasts is replaced with fat, making the breasts less firm.

Despite these changes, many women enjoy sexual activity more after menopause, possibly because they are no longer able to become pregnant. In addition, after menopause, the ovaries and adrenal glands continue to produce male sex hormones. Male sex hormones help maintain the sex drive, slow the loss of muscle tissue, and contribute to an overall sense of well-being.

CHAPTER
236 Symptoms and Diagnosis of Gynecologic Disorders

Disorders that affect the female reproductive system are called gynecologic disorders. Breast disorders are often also considered gynecologic disorders.

Symptoms

The most common symptoms of gynecologic disorders include vaginal itching, a vaginal discharge, abnormal bleeding from the vagina, pain in the pelvic area, and breast pain and lumps (see page 1547). The significance of gynecologic symptoms often depends on the age of the woman because symptoms may be related to the hormonal changes that occur with aging.

EXCESSIVE HAIRINESS

Excess body hair, particularly on the face (on the upper lip, chin, or sideburns area), trunk (around the nipples or on the chest or lower abdomen), and limbs, is called hirsutism. Excessive hairiness may not seem like a gynecologic disorder, but it is considered one because it usually results from high levels of male hormones. Sometimes other masculine traits, such as a deepened voice and increased muscle size, develop—a condition called virilization.

Causes

The most common cause of hirsutism is polycystic ovary syndrome (see page 1528). Hirsutism is common among postmenopausal women because levels of female hormones decrease. Rarely, hirsutism is due to a disorder of the pituitary gland or adrenal glands that results in overproduction of male hormones (such as testosterone). Rarely, hirsutism results from tumors in the ovaries, porphyria cutanea tarda (an enzyme deficiency that affects the skin), or use of certain drugs, such as anabolic steroids, corticosteroids, or minoxidil.

Evaluation and Treatment

Blood tests may be done to measure hormone levels.

The disorder causing hirsutism is treated when possible, often with hormone therapy such as oral contraceptives. Drugs that may be the cause are stopped.

Excess hair can be temporarily removed by shaving, plucking, waxing, and using depilatories. Eflornithine, a topical cream available by prescription, is sometimes helpful. It can slow the growth of hair, causing a gradual reduction of unwanted facial hair. Laser phototherapy is temporarily effective. The only safe permanent treatment is electrolysis, which destroys hair follicles.

PELVIC PAIN

Many women experience pelvic pain—pain that occurs in the lowest part of the abdomen, between the hipbones. The pain may be sharp, intermittent, or crampy (like menstrual cramps). It may be sudden and excruciating, or it may be dull, constant, or both. The pain may gradually increase in intensity, sometimes occurring in waves. Often, the pain is cyclical, occurring with menstrual periods or during ovulation. The pelvic area may feel tender to the touch. The pain may be accompanied by fever, nausea, or vomiting.

Causes

Pelvic pain may be caused by disorders related to any of the organs in the pelvis: the reproductive organs (uterus, fallopian tubes, ovaries, and vagina), bladder, rectum, or appendix. However, pelvic pain sometimes originates in organs outside the pelvis, such as the abdominal wall, intestine, kidneys, ureters, or lower part of the aorta. Psychologic factors, especially stress and depression, may contribute to any kind of pain (including pelvic pain) but, by themselves, rarely cause pelvic pain.

What Causes Pelvic Pain?

DISORDERS RELATED TO THE REPRODUCTIVE ORGANS

- Menstrual cramps (dysmenorrhea)
- Pregnancy that develops outside the uterus (ectopic pregnancy)
- Miscarriage
- Endometriosis
- Fibroids in the uterus
- Mittelschmerz (pain that occurs in the middle of the menstrual cycle and is caused by ovulation)
- A ruptured or twisted cyst in an ovary
- Pelvic inflammatory disease
- Tumors (cancerous or noncancerous) in gynecologic organs

DISORDERS NOT RELATED TO THE REPRODUCTIVE ORGANS

- Appendicitis
- Urinary tract infections, such as cystitis
- Diverticulitis
- Gastroenteritis
- Peptic ulcer disease
- Inflammatory bowel disease
- Irritable bowel syndrome
- Inflammation of the lymph nodes in the abdomen (mesenteric lymphadenitis)
- Stones in the urinary tract, such as kidney stones
- Pain in the abdominal wall (the muscles and connective tissue that surround the abdominal cavity)
- Tumors (cancerous or noncancerous) of the digestive tract

Evaluation and Treatment

When a woman has sudden, very severe pain in the lower abdomen or pelvis, doctors must quickly decide whether the cause requires emergency surgery. Examples of emergencies are appendicitis, a perforated ulcer, a bulge in the aorta (aortic aneurysm), a twisted ovarian cyst, a ruptured abscess (collection of pus) in the pelvis, or a pregnancy that develops outside of the uterus (ectopic pregnancy), usually in a fallopian tube.

Information about the pain, including its timing—when it occurs in relation to the menstrual cycle, eating, sleeping, sexual intercourse, activity, urination, and defecation—may help doctors determine the cause, as may information about any other factors that worsen or ease the pain.

COMMON CAUSES OF ABNORMAL VAGINAL BLEEDING

AGE GROUP	COMMON CAUSES
Infants	Exposure to estrogen from the mother before birth (causing minimal bleeding during the first 1 to 2 weeks of life)
Children	Injury (including sexual abuse) Infection (including that due to sexual abuse) Insertion of a foreign object (such as toilet paper or a toy) in the vagina Bulging (prolapse) of the urethra outside the body Puberty that occurs too early (precocious puberty) with premature menstrual periods

Women of reproductive age	Complications of pregnancy or labor:
	   Miscarriage (actual or threatened)
	   Pregnancy located outside the uterus (ectopic pregnancy)
	   Placental abnormalities, such as premature separation (abruptio placentae) or a location too near the cervix (placenta previa)
	   Incomplete delivery of the placenta
	 Hormonal dysfunction:
	   Dysfunctional uterine bleeding (the most common cause)
	   Brain dysfunction that affects regulation of the reproductive system
	   Thyroid disorders
	   Tumors of the adrenal gland or ovaries
	 Disorders of the reproductive organs:
	   Cancer
	   Noncancerous growths (such as polyps, fibroids, cysts, and benign uterine or ovarian tumors)
	   Endometriosis
	   Injuries
	   Infections (such as chlamydial infections and genital warts)
	   Pelvic inflammatory disease
	 Factors related to birth control methods:
	   Missed or skipped doses of oral contraceptives
	   Irregular bleeding during the first few months of taking oral contraceptives
	   Use of an intrauterine device (IUD)

Postmenopausal women	Cancer in a reproductive organ Noncancerous growths (such as polyps and tumors) in a reproductive organ Age-related thinning of the vagina Trauma during intercourse Thickening of the lining of the uterus (endometrial hyperplasia)

Doctors gently feel the entire abdomen and do a pelvic examination. This evaluation helps doctors determine which organs are affected and whether an infection is present. A pregnancy test is done. Depending on which disorders are suspected, other tests may include cultures (growing organisms in a laboratory) or other tests to check for infections such as gonorrhea and chlamydial infection, urinalysis and urine culture, ultrasonography, computed tomography (CT), and a complete blood cell count.

Sometimes surgery using a laparoscope (a viewing telescope to examine the interior of the abdomen and pelvis) is needed to identify the cause of the pain. A larger incision may also be required.

Treating the disorder causing the pain, if identified, may relieve the pain. If needed, analgesics can help relieve pain. Doctors may ask about stress, depression, and other psychologic factors to determine whether these factors may contribute to pain, especially when pain is persistent.

VAGINAL BLEEDING

Any vaginal bleeding that occurs before puberty, during pregnancy, or after menopause is considered abnormal. During the reproductive years, vaginal bleeding is usually from menstrual periods, although various disorders may cause bleeding or abnormal menstrual periods. Typically, menstrual periods last from 3 to 7 days and occur every 21 to 35 days. The interval in adolescents is somewhat more variable and may be as long as 45 days. Menstrual periods may be abnormal if they

- Become excessively heavy (saturating more than 1 or 2 tampons an hour)
- Last too long (more than 7 days)
- Occur too frequently (usually fewer than 21 days apart)
- Occur too infrequently (usually more than 90 days apart)

At any age, prolonged or excessive bleeding can result in iron deficiency and anemia.

Causes

Bleeding from the vagina may result from a disorder in the vagina or another reproductive organ, particularly the uterus. Common causes include disorders of the reproductive organs, injuries, complications of pregnancy or labor, changes in the normal hormonal control of ovulation (called dysfunctional uterine bleeding), and other hormonal disorders. For example, thyroid disorders can cause menstrual periods to be irregular, to be heavy and occur more frequently, or to occur less frequently (as well as to stop).

Some causes are more common among certain age groups. Bleeding in children, which is unusual, is most often due to a foreign object in the vagina or an injury. Dysfunctional uterine bleeding is more likely to occur in adolescents (when menstrual periods are just starting) or in women in their late 40s (when periods are nearing an end—see page 1526). Occasionally, pregnancy-related vaginal bleeding occurs in a woman who does not yet know she is pregnant. Cancer may cause bleeding in women of reproductive age, but not commonly. In postmenopausal women, cancer—of the cervix, vagina, or lining of the uterus (endometrial cancer)—is a more common cause of vaginal bleeding. However, bleeding may also result from age-related thinning of the vagina or thinning or thickening (hyperplasia) of the lining of the uterus.

Evaluation

In children, vaginal bleeding should be evaluated by a doctor. Women with very heavy bleeding (for example, more than 1 pad or tampon per hour), pain during bleeding, light-headedness, or difficulty breathing and those who are pregnant should see a doctor immediately.

Doctors ask about symptoms and do a pelvic examination. In women of reproductive age, a pregnancy test is done. If bleeding is prolonged, excessive, or frequent, a complete blood count may be done, and the iron level in blood may be measured. Other tests may be necessary, depending on the suspected cause.

A physical (including gynecologic) examination is done. Bleeding in children caused by precocious puberty (see box on page 1755) can be easily recognized because pubic hair and breasts also develop. Often, doctors can recognize disorders of the cervix or vagina during a physical examination.

Blood tests to evaluate thyroid function or to check for bleeding disorders may be done. Doctors often do ultrasonography, which may be done transabdominally or transvaginally (using an ultrasound device inserted into the vagina), to look for cancerous and noncancerous growths of the reproductive organs. Other procedures to identify cancer may include a Papanicolaou (Pap) test, a biopsy of the cervix, and dilation and curettage (D and C).

Treatment

Treatment varies depending on the cause. Oral contraceptives or other hormones may be used to treat dysfunctional uterine bleeding (see page 1526). Uterine polyps, fibroids, cancers, and some benign tumors may be surgically removed. Iron deficiency is treated with iron supplements.

VAGINAL DISCHARGE

A small amount of vaginal discharge is usually normal. The discharge consists of secretions (mucus) produced by the cervix and of fluid that seeps through the walls of the vagina. Estrogen stimulates this production. The discharge is usually milky white or thin and clear. Its amount and appearance may change as women age. Typically, the discharge has no odor. It is not accompanied by itching, burning, irritation, or rash.

Newborn girls normally have a vaginal discharge of mucus, often mixed with a small amount of blood. This discharge occurs because estrogen is absorbed from the mother through the placenta before birth. After birth, the level of estrogen decreases rapidly, causing a small amount of bleeding in the first 1 to 2 weeks of life. Normally, older infants and girls do not have any significant vaginal discharge until puberty, when estrogen levels increase.

During a woman's reproductive years, the amount and appearance of the normal vaginal discharge vary with the menstrual cycle. For example, at the middle of the cycle (at ovulation), the cervix produces more mucus and the mucus is thinner. Pregnancy, use of oral contraceptives, and sexual arousal also affect the amount and appearance of the discharge. After menopause, the estrogen level decreases, often reducing the amount of normal discharge.

A vaginal discharge is considered abnormal if it is

- Heavier than usual
- Thicker than usual
- Puslike
- White and clumpy (like cottage cheese)
- Grayish, greenish, yellowish, or blood-tinged
- Foul- or fishy-smelling
- Accompanied by itching, burning, a rash, or soreness

Causes

A discharge may indicate inflammation of the vagina (vaginitis), which may be due to an infection (see page 1536) or to irritation by a chemical (as for vaginal itching). In young girls, a foreign object in the vagina can cause inflammation of the vagina, with a discharge that may contain blood. Most commonly, the foreign object is a piece of toilet paper that has worked its way into the vagina. Sometimes it is a toy. Irritation may also result from spermicides, vaginal lubricants or creams, diaphragms, or, for women who are allergic to latex, latex condoms. After menopause, the vagina becomes thinner and dryer, increasing the chance of inflammation.

A white, gray, or yellowish cloudy discharge with a fishy odor is caused by bacterial vaginosis. A thick, white, and clumpy discharge (which looks like cottage cheese), often accompanied by itching, is typically caused by candidiasis, a yeast infection. A heavy, greenish yellow, frothy discharge that may have a bad odor is typically caused by trichomoniasis, a protozoan infection. A greenish or yellowish discharge may be due to cervical infection with gonorrhea or chlamydia. Gonorrhea, chlamydial infections, and trichomoniasis are sexually transmitted.

A watery, blood-tinged discharge may be caused by cancer of the vagina, cervix, or lining of the uterus (endometrium). Radiation therapy to the pelvis may also cause an abnormal discharge.

Evaluation

Clues to the cause of the abnormal discharge include its appearance, the woman's age, and other symptoms. A sample of the discharge is examined under a microscope to check for an infection and to identify it. Yeast infections and trichomoniasis can usually be diagnosed with this information alone. To diagnose gonorrhea and chlamydial infections, doctors have the sample cultured (grown in a laboratory) or tested for DNA, particularly for women who are sexually active and thus at risk of sexually transmitted diseases.

Treatment

Treatment depends on the cause. Changing underwear and bathing or showering daily may help relieve symptoms but do not eliminate the infection. If a product (such as a cream, powder, soap, or brand of condom) consistently causes irritation, it should not be used. Douching and using feminine hygiene sprays should be discouraged. These products do not eliminate the discharge and may make it worse, and douching may increase the risk of pelvic inflammatory disease (see page 1541).

VAGINAL ITCHING

Vaginal itching may involve the area containing the external genital organs (vulva) as well as the vagina. Many women have occasional vaginal itching that resolves without treatment. Itching is considered a problem only when it is persistent, is severe, recurs, or is accompanied by a discharge that looks or smells abnormal.

Causes

Vaginal itching may result from the following:

- **Infections:** Bacterial vaginosis, candidiasis (a yeast infection), and trichomoniasis (a protozoan infection) can cause itching (see page 1536). These infections tend to also cause a discharge.
- **Irritation:** Chemicals that come in contact with the vagina or vulva may irritate them. Examples are the chemicals in laundry detergents, bleaches, fabric softeners, synthetic fibers, bubble baths, soaps, feminine hygiene sprays, perfumes, menstrual pads, fabric dyes, toilet tissue, vaginal creams, douches, condoms, and contraceptive foams.
- **Changes in the skin or lining of the vagina:** Hormonal changes at menopause can cause vaginal dryness, which leads to itching. Skin disorders such as psoriasis or lichen sclerosus can cause itching. Lichen sclerosus is characterized by thin white areas on the vulva around the opening of the vagina. If untreated, lichen sclerosus can cause scarring and may increase the risk of cancer of the vulva.

Evaluation

Doctors can usually determine the cause by asking about symptoms and by examining the vulva and vagina. If the woman has a discharge, tests are needed.

Treatment

The cause is treated when possible. Changing underwear and bathing or showering once daily help keep the vagina and vulva clean. A nonallergenic soap should be used. These measures may minimize exposure to irritants that cause itching. More frequent washing may cause excessive dryness, which can increase itching. Using a mild (low-strength) corticosteroid cream such as hydrocortisone may provide temporary relief. For severe itching, an oral antihistamine may help temporarily. If a product (such as a cream, powder, soap, or brand of condom) consistently causes irritation and itching, it should not be used. Feminine hygiene sprays and douches should not be used.

Treatment of lichen sclerosus consists of a cream or an ointment containing a high-strength corticosteroid (such as clobetasol), available by prescription.

Gynecologic Evaluation

Preventive health care includes having regular gynecologic examinations, even when no symptoms are present, and screening tests. Screening tests are done before people have any symptoms to check for disorders that can be prevented or treated effectively if recognized early (see table on page 34). Women should have a gynecologic evaluation every year starting at about age 13 to 15. For all women who are sexually active, the evaluation should include a pelvic examination. For younger women who are not sexually active, this evaluation may not include a pelvic examination. Beginning about 3 years after first vaginal intercourse or at age 21, the pelvic examination should include cervical cytology testing (such as a Papanicolaou or Pap test) to detect precancerous changes of the cervix.

For gynecologic care, a woman should choose a health care practitioner with whom she can comfortably discuss sensitive topics, such as sex, birth control, pregnancy, and problems related to menopause. The practitioner may be a gynecologist, an internist, a nurse-midwife, or a general, family, or nurse practitioner.

Gynecologic evaluation of young and teenage girls can sometimes be done by their pediatrician. However, if the pediatrician cannot set aside time for the girl to speak privately about personal concerns or is reluctant to provide gynecologic care, another health care practitioner should be found for this care.

The gynecologic visit is the time to ask the practitioner questions about reproductive and sexual function and anatomy, including safe sex practices, such as the use of condoms to minimize the risks of sexually transmitted infections.

GYNECOLOGIC HISTORY

A gynecologic evaluation starts with a series of questions related to menstruation and reproductive function. These questions usually focus on the reason for the visit to the doctor's office. The answers form the gynecologic history. A complete gynecologic history includes the following information:

- The age at which menstrual bleeding began (menarche)
- Frequency, regularity, and duration of menstrual periods
- Amount of menstrual bleeding
- Dates of the last two menstrual periods
- Number of pregnancies, dates that they occurred, outcomes, and complications

Questions about abnormal bleeding—too much, too little, or between menstrual periods—are included.

A doctor usually asks about sexual activities to assess the risk of gynecologic infections, injuries, and pregnancy and to determine whether a woman has any sexual problems. A woman is asked whether she uses or wants to use birth control and whether she is interested in counseling or other information.

The doctor may ask the woman whether she has pain, cramps, or headaches during menstrual periods. She is asked whether she has pain during intercourse, in the middle of the menstrual cycle (which may indicate that the pain coincides with ovulation), or under other circumstances. If she has pain, she is asked how severe the pain is and what provides relief. The doctor also asks about breast problems, such as pain, lumps, areas of tenderness or redness, and discharge from the nipples. The woman is asked whether she examines her breasts, how often, and whether she needs any instruction on technique.

The doctor reviews the woman's history of past gynecologic disorders and usually obtains a general medical and surgical history that includes previous health problems. The doctor reviews all the drugs a woman is taking, including prescription and non-prescription drugs, illicit drugs, tobacco, and alcohol, because many of them affect gynecologic function. The woman is asked about mental, physical, or sexual abuse in the present and the past. Some questions about urination are asked to find out whether the woman has a urinary tract infection or has problems with leakage of urine (incontinence).

GYNECOLOGIC EXAMINATION

If a woman has any questions or fears about the gynecologic examination, she should talk with the doctor beforehand about her concerns. If any part of the examination causes pain, the woman should let the doctor know. The woman should empty her bladder before the physical examination and may be asked to collect a urine sample for analysis.

The doctor usually feels the neck and the thyroid gland to check for lumps and abnormalities. An enlarged, overactive thyroid gland can cause menstrual abnormalities. The doctor examines the skin for signs of acne, excessive hairiness (hirsutism), spots, and growths.

A breast examination is typically done before the pelvic examination. With the woman sitting, the doctor inspects the breasts for irregularities, dimpling, tightened skin, lumps, and a discharge. The woman then sits or lies down, with her arms above her head, while the doctor feels (palpates) each breast with a flat hand and examines each armpit for enlarged lymph nodes and for lumps and abnormalities. While performing the examination, the doctor may review the technique for breast self-examination with the woman (see art on page 1552).

The doctor may use a stethoscope to listen for activity of the intestine and to check for abnormal noises made by blood flowing through narrowed blood vessels. The doctor may tap areas of the abdomen with the fingers. The doctor gently feels the entire abdomen to check for abnormal growths or enlarged organs, especially the liver and spleen. Although the woman may experience some discomfort when the doctor presses deeply, the examination should not be painful.

During the pelvic examination, the woman lies on her back with her hips and knees bent and her buttocks moved to the edge of the examining table. Special pelvic examination tables have heel stirrups that help a woman maintain this position. If a woman wants to observe the pelvic examination, she should tell the doctor, who can provide a mirror. The doctor may explain the examination or review the findings before, during, or after the examination. For the examination, the doctor first inspects the external genital area and notes the distribution of hair and any abnormalities, discoloration, discharge, or inflammation. This examination may detect no abnormalities or may give clues to hormonal problems, cancer, infections, injury, or sexual abuse.

The doctor spreads the tissues around the opening of the vagina (labia) and examines the opening. Using a speculum (a metal or plastic instrument that spreads the walls of the vagina apart), the doctor examines the deeper areas of the vagina and the cervix. The cervix is examined closely for signs of irritation or cancer. The doctor may use a swab, brush, or small plastic spatula to obtain a sample for testing, usually a Papanicolaou (Pap) test or a variation of it. The doctor checks for protrusion of the bladder, rectum, or intestine into the vagina (see page 1543).

After removing the speculum, the doctor feels the vaginal wall to determine its strength and support. The doctor also feels for growths or tender areas within the vagina. After inserting the index and middle fingers of one gloved hand into the vagina,

the doctor places the fingers of the other hand on the lower abdomen above the pubic bone. Between the two hands, the uterus can usually be felt as a pear-shaped, smooth, firm structure, and its position, size, consistency, and degree of tenderness (if any) can be determined. Then the doctor attempts to feel the ovaries by moving the hand on the abdomen more to the side and exerting slightly more pressure. More pressure is required because the ovaries are small and much more difficult to feel than the uterus. The woman may find this part of the examination to be slightly uncomfortable, but it should not be painful. The doctor determines how large the ovaries are and whether they are tender.

A rectovaginal examination may be done. The doctor inserts the index finger into the vagina and the middle finger into the rectum to examine the back wall of the vagina for abnormal growths or thickness. In addition, the doctor can examine the rectum for hemorrhoids, fissures, polyps, and lumps. A small sample of stool can be obtained with a gloved finger and tested for unseen (occult) blood. A woman may be given a take-home kit to test for occult blood in the stool.

SCREENING TESTS

Two important screening tests for women are cervical cytology testing (such as the Papanicolaou [Pap] test) to check for cancer of the cervix and mammography to check for breast cancer (see page 1554). Women at risk of sexually transmitted diseases should be screened for these diseases. Other screening tests are done in pregnant women (see page 1624).

Screening for Cervical Cancer

Cervical cytology testing (such as the Pap test) involves collecting a sample of cells from the cervix and examining them under a microscope. There are two types of cervical cytology: the conventional test and the liquid-based test. Doctors collect the sample by inserting a speculum into the vagina to spread the walls of the vagina apart and using a plastic spatula (similar to a tongue depressor) to remove some cells from the surface and opening of the cervix. Then, a small bristle brush is inserted into the passageway through the cervix (cervical canal) to obtain cells from the wall of the canal. The sample is then sent to a laboratory, where it is examined under a microscope for abnormal cells, which may indicate precancerous changes or, rarely, cervical cancer. Usually, the Pap test feels scratchy or crampy, but it is not painful and takes only a few seconds.

Pap tests identify 80 to 85% of cervical cancers, even very early-stage cancer. They can also detect changes in cervical cells that can lead to cancer (precancerous changes). These changes, called cervical intraepithelial neoplasia (CIN), can be treated, thus helping prevent cancer.

Pap tests are most accurate if the woman is not having her period and does not douche or use vaginal creams for at least 24 hours before the test. Experts recommend that women have the first test about 3 years after they begin having vaginal intercourse but no later than age 21. How often the test is needed depends mainly on the woman's age and the results of previous Pap tests:

- Until age 30: Every year or every other year.
- After age 30: Every 2 to 3 years if test results have been normal for 3 years in a row. However, women with a high risk of cervical cancer need to be tested more frequently. Such women include those who have an HIV (human immunodeficiency virus) infection, who have a weakened immune system (which may result from taking a drug or having a disorder that suppresses the immune system), or who have had abnormal Pap test results.
- After age 65 or 70: No longer needed if test results have been normal for at least 3 years in a row and no result has been abnormal in the last 10 years. Pap tests should be resumed if the woman has a new sex partner or be continued if she has several sex partners.

Women who have had their uterus completely removed (total hysterectomy) and have not had any abnormal Pap test results do not need Pap tests.

Screening for Sexually Transmitted Diseases

Women at risk of sexually transmitted diseases should be screened yearly for these diseases, even if they have no symptoms. High-risk women include the following:

- Sexually active women aged 25 and younger
- Women who are just beginning sexual activity
- Women who have several sex partners
- Women whose partner has had several sex partners
- Women who have had a sexually transmitted disease
- Women who do not consistently use a barrier contraceptive (such as a condom) and are not in a mutually monogamous relationship or are unsure if the relationship is mutually monogamous
- Pregnant women
- Women who have a vaginal discharge

For most sexually transmitted diseases, the doctor uses a swab to obtain a small amount of cervical discharge from the cervix. The sample is sent to a

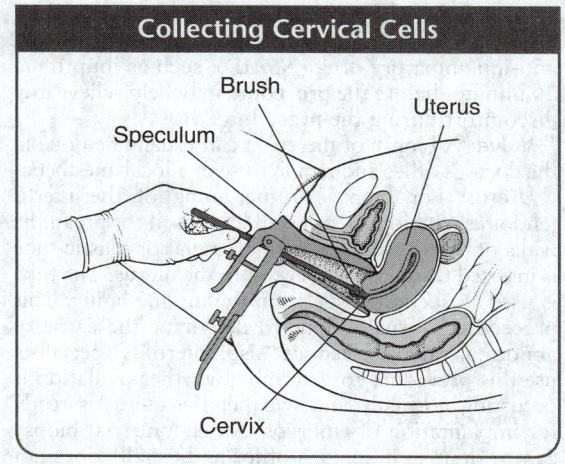

Collecting Cervical Cells

Brush

Uterus

Speculum

Cervix

laboratory for analysis. Women who think they may have one of these diseases can request screening. Testing for gonorrhea and chlamydial infection can also be done using a urine specimen.

A doctor may consider screening women for the human papillomavirus (HPV) if they are 30 years old or older or if a Pap test detected questionable abnormalities that may result from HPV infection. HPV can cause genital warts or cervical cancer. A sample of vaginal discharge, obtained with a swab, is also used for this test. Normal results of an HPV test indicate that cervical cancer and precancerous conditions are highly unlikely. For women at high risk of HPV, the HPV test can be done at the same time as a Pap test. If results of a Pap test and an HPV test are normal in women older than 30, neither test needs to be repeated for at least 3 years.

DIAGNOSTIC PROCEDURES

Occasionally, more extensive diagnostic procedures are needed.

Biopsy

A biopsy consists of removing a small sample of tissue for examination under a microscope. Biopsy of the vulva, vagina, cervix, or lining of the uterus can be done.

Cervix or Vagina: A cervical biopsy is done when a condition likely to eventually lead to cancer (precancerous condition) or cancer is suspected, usually because a Pap test result was abnormal. A biopsy of the cervix or vagina is usually done during colposcopy. During colposcopy, doctors can identify the area that looks most abnormal and take tissue samples from it. Usually, biopsy of the cervix or vagina does not require an anesthetic, although this procedure typically feels like a sharp pinch or a cramp. Taking a nonsteroidal anti-inflammatory drug (NSAID), such as ibuprofen, 20 minutes before the procedure may help relieve any discomfort during the procedure.

Vulva: A biopsy of the vulva can usually be done in the doctor's office and requires use of a local anesthetic.

Uterus: For biopsy of the lining of the uterus (endometrial biopsy), a speculum is used to spread the walls of the vagina, and a small metal or plastic tube is inserted through the cervix into the uterus. The tube is used to suction tissue from the uterine lining. This procedure is usually done to determine the cause of abnormal vaginal bleeding. Also, infertility specialists use this procedure to determine whether ovulation is occurring normally and whether the uterus is ready for implantation of embryos. An endometrial biopsy can be done in a doctor's office and usually does not require an anesthetic. Typically, it feels like strong menstrual cramps. Taking an NSAID, such as ibuprofen, 20 minutes before the procedure may help relieve discomfort during the procedure.

Colposcopy

Colposcopy is often done if results of a Papanicolaou (Pap) test are abnormal. For colposcopy, a speculum is used to spread the walls of the vagina and a binocular magnifying lens (similar to that of a microscope) is used to inspect the cervix for signs of cancer. Often, a sample of tissue is removed for examination under a microscope (biopsy). Colposcopy alone (without biopsy) is painless and thus requires no anesthetic. The biopsy procedure is typically described as causing a crampy sensation and also does not require an anesthetic. The procedure usually takes 10 to 15 minutes.

Endocervical Curettage

Endocervical curettage consists of inserting a small, sharp, scoop-shaped instrument (curet) into the passageway through the cervix (cervical canal) to obtain tissue. The curet is used to scrape a small amount of tissue from high inside the cervical canal. A cervical biopsy (to remove a smaller piece of tissue from the surface of the cervix) is typically done at the same time. The tissue samples are examined under a microscope by a pathologist.

Endocervical curettage is done when endometrial or cervical cancer is suspected or needs to be ruled out. Usually, it is done during colposcopy and does not require an anesthetic.

Dilation and Curettage

For dilation and curettage (D and C), a speculum is used to spread the walls of the vagina. Then, metal

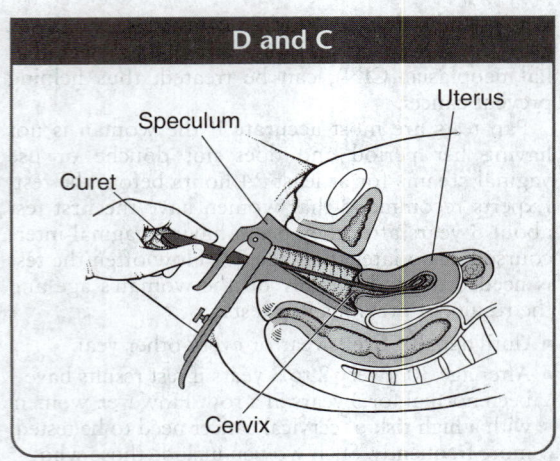

D and C

Uterus

Speculum

Curet

Cervix

rods are used to stretch open (dilate) the cervix so that a small, sharp, scoop-shaped instrument (curet) can be inserted to remove tissue from the lining of the uterus.

This procedure may be used to treat women who have had an incomplete (partial) miscarriage. D and C is sometimes used to identify abnormalities of the uterine lining when biopsy results are inconclusive, but it is no longer commonly used for this purpose because biopsies usually provide as much information and can be done in the doctor's office. D and C is often done in a hospital. Conscious sedation or a general anesthetic may be used. However, most women do not have to stay overnight in the hospital.

Hysterosalpingography

For hysterosalpingography, x-rays are taken after a radiopaque dye (which can be seen on x-rays) is injected through the cervix to outline the interior of the uterus and fallopian tubes.

The procedure is often used to help determine the cause of infertility or to confirm that a sterilization procedure to block the tubes is successful. The procedure is done in a place where x-rays can be taken, such as a hospital or the radiology suite of a doctor's office. Hysterosalpingography usually causes discomfort, such as cramps. Taking an NSAID, such as ibuprofen, 20 minutes before the procedure may help relieve discomfort.

Hysteroscopy

To view the interior of the uterus, doctors can insert a thin viewing tube (hysteroscope) through the vagina and cervix into the uterus. The tube is about 1/4 inch in diameter and contains cables that transmit light. Instruments used for a biopsy, electrocautery (heat), or surgery may be threaded through the tube. The site of abnormal bleeding or other abnormalities can usually be seen and can be sampled for a biopsy, sealed off using heat, or removed. This procedure may be done in a doctor's office or in a hospital with a general anesthetic at the same time as a dilation and curettage.

Laparoscopy

To directly examine the uterus, fallopian tubes, or ovaries, doctors use a viewing tube called a laparoscope. The laparoscope is attached to a thin cable containing flexible plastic or glass rods that transmit light. The laparoscope is inserted into the abdominal cavity through a small incision just below the navel. A probe is inserted through the vagina and into the uterus. The probe enables doctors to manipulate the organs for better viewing. Carbon dioxide is pumped through the laparoscope to inflate the abdomen, so that organs in the abdomen and pelvis can be seen clearly.

Often, laparoscopy is used to determine the cause of pelvic pain, infertility, and other gynecologic disorders. Instruments can be threaded through the laparoscope to perform some surgical procedures, such as biopsies, sterilization procedures, and removal of an ectopic pregnancy in a fallopian tube. Additional incisions may be required if surgical procedures, such as removal of an ovarian cyst or the uterus (hysterectomy), are needed.

Laparoscopy is done in a hospital and requires an anesthetic, usually a general anesthetic. An overnight stay in the hospital is usually not required. Laparoscopy may cause abdominal pain, but normal activities can usually be resumed in 3 to 5 days, depending on the extent of the procedure that is performed through the laparoscope.

Loop Electrical Excision Procedure

In a loop electrical excision procedure (LEEP), a thin wire loop that conducts an electrical current is used to remove a piece of tissue. Typically, this piece of tissue is larger than that obtained in a cervical biopsy.

This procedure may be done after an abnormal Pap test result to evaluate the abnormality more accurately or to remove the abnormal tissue. LEEP requires an anesthetic (often a local one), takes about 5 to 10 minutes, and can be done in a doctor's office. Afterward, women may feel mild to moderate discomfort and have a small amount of bleeding. Taking an NSAID, such as ibuprofen, 20 minutes before the procedure may help relieve discomfort during the procedure.

Sonohysterography

For sonohysterography, fluid is placed in the uterus through a thin tube (catheter) that is inserted through the vagina and then the cervix. Then ultrasonography is done. The fluid fills and stretches (distends) the uterus so that abnormalities inside the uterus, such as polyps or fibroids, can be more easily detected. The procedure is done in a doctor's office and may require a local anesthetic. Taking an NSAID, such as ibuprofen, 20 minutes before the procedure may help relieve discomfort.

Ultrasonography

Ultrasonography (see also page 2044) uses ultrasound waves, produced at a frequency too high to be heard. The ultrasound waves are emitted by a handheld device that is placed on the abdomen or inside the vagina. The waves reflect off internal structures, and the pattern of this reflection can be displayed on a monitor.

Ultrasonography can detect an ectopic pregnancy, tumors, cysts, and other abnormalities in the pelvic organs. It is commonly done during pregnancy to determine the condition and size of the fetus, to monitor the fetus, or to guide the placement of instruments during amniocentesis or chorionic villus sampling (see page 1613). Ultrasonography is painless and has no known risks.

Sexual Dysfunction in Women

Sexual dysfunction includes painful intercourse, painful contraction (spasm) of the vaginal muscles, or a problem with sexual desire, arousal, or orgasm that causes distress.

- Depression or anxiety, other psychologic factors, disorders, and drugs can contribute to sexual dysfunction, as can the situation.
- To identify a problem, doctors often talk to both partners separately and together, and a pelvic examination is often done to check the woman.

- Improving the relationship, communicating more clearly and openly, and arranging the best circumstances for sexual activities can often help, regardless of the cause of sexual dysfunction.

About 30 to 50% of women have sexual problems at some time during their life. If the problems are severe enough to cause distress, they may be considered sexual dysfunction. Sexual dysfunction can be described and diagnosed in terms of specific problems, such as lack of interest or desire, difficulty becoming aroused or reaching orgasm, pain during sexual activity, or involuntary tightening of the muscles around the vagina. However, these distinctions are not always useful. Almost all women with sexual dysfunction have features of more than one such specific problem. For example, women who have difficulty becoming aroused may enjoy sex less, have difficulty reaching orgasm, or even find sex painful. Women who have pain during sexual activity often understandably lose their interest and desire for sex.

Normal Sexual Function

Sexual function and responses involve mind (thoughts and emotions) and body (including the nervous, circulatory, and endocrine systems). Sexual response consists of the following:

- **Desire** is the wish to engage in or continue sexual activity. Desire may be triggered by thoughts, words, sights, smells, or touch. Desire may be obvious at the outset or may build once the woman is aroused.
- **Arousal** has a subjective element—sexual excitement that is felt and thought about. It also has a physical element—an increase in blood flow to the genital area. In women, the increased blood flow causes the clitoris (which corresponds to the penis in men) and vaginal walls to swell (a process called engorgement). The increased blood flow also causes vaginal secretions (which provide lubrication) to increase. As women age, blood flow may increase less. Blood flow also may increase without the woman being aware of it and without her feeling aroused.
- **Orgasm** is the peak or climax of sexual excitement. Just before orgasm, muscle tension throughout the body increases. As orgasm begins, the muscles around the vagina contract rhythmically.
- **Resolution** is a sense of well-being and widespread muscular relaxation. Resolution typically follows orgasm. However, resolution can occur slowly after highly arousing sexual activity without orgasm. Many women can respond to additional stimulation almost immediately after resolution.

Most people—men and women—engage in sexual activity for several reasons. For example, they may be attracted to a person or desire physical pleasure, affection, love, romance, or intimacy. However, women are more likely to have emotional motivations. Many women initiate or agree to sexual activity because they want one or more of the following:

- To experience emotional intimacy
- To increase their sense of well-being

- To confirm their desirability
- To please or placate a partner

Especially after a relationship has lasted a long time, women often have little or no desire for sex before sexual activity (initial desire), but desire can develop once sexual activity and stimulation begin. Desire before sexual activity typically lessens as women age but increases when women, regardless of their age, have a new partner. Some women may feel sexually satisfied whether they have an orgasm or not. Other women have much more sexual satisfaction with an orgasm.

> **? Did You Know...**
> Women in a long-term relationship often have little or no desire for sex until sexual activity and stimulation begin.

Causes

Many factors cause or contribute to various types of sexual dysfunction. Traditionally, causes are considered physical or psychologic. However, this distinction is not strictly accurate. Psychologic factors can cause physical changes in the brain, nerves, hormones, and, eventually, the genital organs. Physical changes can have psychologic effects, which, in turn, have more physical effects. Some factors are related more to the situation than to the woman.

Psychologic Factors: Depression and anxiety commonly contribute. Previous experiences can affect a woman's psychologic and sexual development, causing problems, as in the following:

- Harsh sexual or other experiences may lead to low self-esteem, shame, or guilt.
- Emotional, physical, or sexual abuse during childhood or adolescence can teach children to control and hide emotions—a useful defense mechanism. However, women who control and hide emotions may have difficulty expressing sexual feelings.
- If women lose a parent or another loved one during childhood, they may have difficulty becoming intimate with a sex partner because they are afraid of a similar loss—sometimes without being aware of it.

Various sexual worries can impair sexual function. For example, women may be worried about unwanted consequences of sex or about their or their partner's sexual performance.

Situational Factors: Factors related to the situation may involve the following:

	WHAT AFFECTS SEXUAL FUNCTION IN WOMEN?	
TYPE	**FACTOR**	
Psychologic factors	Abuse (emotional, physical, or sexual) during childhood or adolescence	
	Anxiety	
	Depression	
	Fear of intimacy	
	Fear of losing control	
	Fear of losing the partner	
	Low self-esteem	
	Worry about inability to have an orgasm or about sexual performance in a partner	
	Worry about unwanted consequences of sex (such as unwanted pregnancy or sexually transmitted diseases)	
Situational factors	Cultural background that restricts sexual expression or activity	
	Distractions	
	Relationship problems	
	Surroundings that are not conducive to sexual activity	
Physical factors	Atrophic vaginitis (thinning of tissues of the vagina)	
	Fatigue	
	Hyperprolactinemia (high levels of prolactin, a hormone produced by the pituitary gland)	
	Poor health	
	Surgical removal of both ovaries in premenopausal women	
	Underactive thyroid gland (hypothyroidism)	
	Some nerve disorders, such as multiple sclerosis	
Drugs	β-Blockers (used to treat hypertension or heart disorders)	
	Drugs that block the production and activity of testosterone (including the diuretic spironolactone)	
	Hormones (such as hormonal contraceptives or oral estrogen therapy)	
	Certain antidepressants, particularly selective serotonin reuptake inhibitors	

- The relationship: Women may not trust or have negative feelings about their sex partner. They may feel less attracted to their partner than earlier in their relationship.
- The surroundings: The setting may not be erotic, private, or safe enough for uninhibited sexual expression.
- The culture: Women may come from a culture that restricts sexual expression or activity. Cultures sometimes make women feel ashamed or guilty about sexuality. Women and their partners may come from cultures that view certain sexual practices differently.
- Distractions: Family, work, finances, or other things can preoccupy women and thus interfere with sexual arousal.

Physical Factors: Various physical conditions and drugs may lead or contribute to sexual dysfunction. Hormonal changes, which may occur with aging or result from a disorder, can interfere. For example, the tissues of the vagina can become thin, dry, and inelastic after menopause because estrogen levels decrease. This condition, called atrophic vaginitis, can make intercourse painful. Other conditions, such as the removal of both ovaries, can also cause estrogen levels to decrease and thus contribute to sexual dysfunction.

Selective serotonin reuptake inhibitors, a type of antidepressant, commonly cause problems. Estrogen therapy, if taken by mouth, sometimes used to control symptoms associated with menopause, can cause sexual dysfunction, but not always. In fact, estrogen therapy may enhance sexual function in postmenopausal women.

? **Did You Know...**

Taking a selective serotonin reuptake inhibitor (a type of antidepressant) can interfere with sexual function, but so can depression.

Diagnosis

Diagnosis often involves detailed questioning of both sex partners, alone and together. Doctors ask about symptoms, other disorders, drug use, the relationship between the partners, mood, self-esteem, childhood relationships, past sexual experiences, and personality traits.

Doctors also often need to do a pelvic examination. Doctors try to do this examination as gently as possible. They move slowly and often explain the examination procedures in detail. If the woman wishes, they may give her a mirror to observe her genitals. If she is fearful of anything entering her vagina, she can place her hand on the doctor's to control the internal examination. Usually, doctors do not need to use an instrument, such as a speculum, to diagnose sexual problems. Such instruments are needed to do a Papanicolaou (Pap) test.

If doctors suspect a sexually transmitted disease, tests are done.

Treatment

Certain treatments depend on the cause of dysfunction. However, some general measures can help regardless of the cause:

- Making time for and learning to focus on sexual activity: Women, who are used to multitasking, may be preoccupied with or distracted by other activities (involving work, household chores, children, and community). Making sexual activity a priority and recognizing how counterproductive distractions are may help. That is, women can concentrate their awareness (be mindful) during sexual activity and thus stay in the moment.

- Improving communication, including about sex, between the woman and her partner

- Choosing a good time and place for sexual activity: For example, late at night—when a woman is ready for sleep—is not a good time. Making sure the place is private can help if the woman is afraid of discovery or interruption. Enough time should be allowed, and a setting that encourages sexual feelings may help.

- Engaging in many types of sexual activities: For example, stroking and kissing responsive parts of the body and touching each other's genitals enough before initiating intercourse may enhance intimacy and lessen anxiety.

- Setting aside time together that does not involve sexual activity: Couples who talk to each other regularly are more likely to feel sexual desire.

- Encouraging trust, respect, and emotional intimacy between partners: These qualities should be cultivated with or without professional help. Women need them to respond sexually. Couples may need help learning to resolve conflicts, which can interfere with their relationship.

- Taking steps to prevent unwanted consequences: Such measures are particularly useful when fear of pregnancy or sexually transmitted diseases inhibits desire.

Often, more than one treatment is required because many women have more than one type of sexual dysfunction. Psychotherapy benefits some women, particularly when psychologic factors are prominent. However, just becoming aware of what is required for a healthy sexual response may be enough to help women change their thinking and behavior.

Because selective serotonin reuptake inhibitors (SSRIs) may contribute to several types of sexual dysfunction, substituting another antidepressant that impairs sexual response less may help. Such drugs may include bupropion, moclobemide, mirtazapine, and venlafaxine. Also, taking bupropion with an SSRI may be better for sexual response than taking the SSRI alone. Some evidence suggests that if women stopped having orgasms when they started taking SSRIs, sildenafil may help them have orgasms again.

Dyspareunia

Dyspareunia is pain when women try to begin sexual intercourse or pain during intercourse.

- The pain may be superficial or deep.
- It may result from vaginal dryness or disorders of the genital organs.
- The diagnosis is based on symptoms and a pelvic examination.
- Anesthetic ointments, lubricants, exercises to relax pelvic muscles, or a change in the position for intercourse may help.
- The cause, if identified, is treated.

The pain may be superficial, felt in the area around the opening of the vagina (genital area or vulva). Or the pain may be deep, felt within the pelvis when the penis or a dildo is thrust further inside. The pain may be burning, sharp, or cramping. Pelvic muscles tend to become tight, which increases the pain, whether it is superficial or deep.

Causes

Causes vary depending on whether the pain is superficial or deep.

Superficial Pain: Intercourse can be painful because the vagina does not secrete enough fluids. Then the vagina feels dry, and lubrication for intercourse is inadequate. Inadequate lubrication often results from insufficient foreplay. Also, as women age, the lining of the vagina thins and can become dry because estrogen levels decrease. This condition is called atrophic vaginitis. During breastfeeding, the vagina may become dry because estrogen levels are low. Taking antihistamines can cause slight, temporary dryness of the vagina.

Superficial pain may also result from the following:

- Increased sensitivity of the genital area to pain (provoked vestibulodynia—see page 1509), which is the most common cause

- Inflammation or infection in the genital area (including genital herpes), the vagina, or Bartholin's glands (the small glands on either side of the vaginal opening)

- Inflammation or infection of the urinary tract

- Injuries in the genital area
- An allergic reaction to contraceptive foams or jellies or to latex condoms
- Involuntary contraction of the vaginal muscles (vaginismus)
- Rarely, a congenital abnormality (such as an abnormal partition within the vagina)
- Surgery that narrows the vagina (for example, to repair tissues torn during childbirth or to correct a pelvic floor disorder—see page 1543)
- A hymen that interferes with entry of the penis

The hymen is a membrane that encircles or, in a very few women, covers the opening of the vagina. When women have sexual intercourse the first time, the hymen, if not previously stretched (for example, from tampon use or sexual stimulation with a finger inside the vagina), may tear, causing some pain and bleeding. A few women are born with an abnormally tight hymen.

Deep Pain: Deep pain during or after sexual intercourse may result from the following:

- Infection of the cervix, uterus, or fallopian tubes (pelvic inflammatory disease), which may cause collections of pus (abscesses) to form in the pelvis
- Endometriosis
- Growths in the pelvis (such as tumors and ovarian cysts)
- Bands of scar tissue (adhesions) between organs in the pelvis, which may form after an infection, surgery, or radiation therapy for cancer

Radiation therapy can cause both superficial and deep pain. The vagina can be less stretchable, and scarring around it can make it smaller and shorter.

Sometimes one of these disorders causes the uterus to get stuck in a bent-backward direction (retroversion). The ligaments, muscles, and other tissues that hold the uterus in place may weaken, resulting in the uterus dropping down toward the vagina (prolapse—see art on page 1544). Such changes can also cause deep pain.

Pain is greatly affected by emotions. For example, minor discomfort may feel like severe pain after a traumatic sexual experience, such as rape. Anger toward a sex partner, fear of intimacy or pregnancy, a negative self-image, or a belief that the pain will never go away may amplify pain.

Diagnosis

The diagnosis is based on the woman's description of the problem, including when and where the pain is felt, and on the results of a physical examination. The genital area is gently but thoroughly examined for possible causes, such as signs of inflammation or abnor-

malities. A doctor may touch the area gently with a cotton swab to determine where the pain occurs. The doctor checks the tightness of the pelvic muscles around the vagina by inserting one or two gloved fingers into the vagina. To check the uterus and ovaries, the doctor then places the other hand on the lower abdomen. A rectal examination may also be done.

Treatment

Couples are encouraged to find ways to attain mutual pleasure (including having orgasms and ejaculation) that do not involve penetration. Such means can include stimulation involving the mouth, hands, or a vibrator.

Pelvic muscle relaxation exercises may help relieve symptoms, regardless of the cause.

For superficial pain, applying an anesthetic ointment and taking sitz baths may help, as may liberally applying a lubricant before intercourse. Water-based lubricants rather than petroleum jelly or other oil-based lubricants are preferable. Oil-based lubricants tend to dry the vagina and can damage latex contraceptive devices such as condoms and diaphragms. Spending more time in foreplay may increase vaginal lubrication.

For deep pain, using a different position for intercourse may help. For example, being on top can give women more control of penetration, or another position may limit how deeply the penis can be thrust.

More specific treatment depends on the cause, as in the following:

- Thinning and drying of the vagina after menopause: Estrogen applied as cream, inserted into the vagina as a pill or in a ring, or taken by mouth (as part of hormone therapy)
- Infections: Antibiotics, antifungal drugs, or other drugs as appropriate (see table on page 1537)
- Cysts or abscesses: Surgical removal
- A rigid hymen or another congenital abnormality: Surgery to correct it
- Prolapse of the uterus: Insertion of a pessary, which resembles a diaphragm, into the vagina to support and reposition the uterus or sometimes surgery

PROVOKED VESTIBULODYNIA

Provoked vestibulodynia (vulvar vestibulitis) is increased sensitivity to pain in the area around the opening of the vagina (vestibule), making even gentle touch or stimulation painful.

Provoked vestibulodynia is the most common cause of dyspareunia that occurs when the penis enters the vagina or moves. The pain starts immediately, lessens when the penis stops moving, and resumes when the penis moves again.

Doctors are not sure why it happens, but the nerve pathways that conduct pain signals from the vulva and the parts of the brain that process those signals are physically changed (remodeled) and become more sensitive. As a result, touch that normally would seem mild is perceived as very painful. Muscles in the pelvis may also be tight, increasing pain. After intercourse, women may have a burning sensation in the genital area or burning after urination.

This disorder involves chronic pain and often occurs with other types of chronic pain, such as jaw pain or pain due to irritable bowel syndrome.

Treatment

Treatment may include anti-inflammatory creams or anesthetics applied to the area and drugs taken by mouth, such as certain antidepressants and anticonvulsants, given in low doses. These drugs may help reverse changes in the nerve pathways that increase sensitivity to pain. Which treatments are most effective is not clear.

Avoiding possible irritants, such as soap, bubble bath, panty liners, and tight jeans, may help. Pelvic muscle relaxation exercises, yoga, and general relaxation exercises can help relax pelvic (and other) muscles. Women may benefit from cognitive-behavioral therapy (which is used to treat chronic pain), particularly when they are also taught the skill of mindfulness (concentration of awareness in the moment). Psychotherapy and sex therapy can help some women.

Surgery to remove part of the area around the vaginal opening is sometimes advised. This procedure removes the hypersensitive nerve endings, but the nerves can regrow, and pain can recur.

Botulinum toxin (a bacterial toxin used to paralyze muscles or to treat wrinkles) may be given to deaden the pain nerves but is currently considered experimental.

Because this disorder involves chronic pain, treatments are becoming more comprehensive, including management of stress and emotional reactions to the pain.

Vaginismus

Vaginismus is involuntary contraction of muscles around the opening of the vagina in women with no abnormalities identified during examination. The tight muscle contraction makes sexual intercourse painful or impossible.

- Most women with vaginismus cannot tolerate sexual intercourse, and some cannot tolerate using tampons.
- Doctors base the diagnosis on symptoms and a subsequent pelvic examination, done as gently as possible.
- Women are taught how to touch their genital area, gradually moving closer to their vagina and becoming used to touching it without causing pain, and then to insert a finger, then progressively larger cones into the vagina.

- These exercises may enable women to have sexual intercourse without pain.

In vaginismus, vaginal muscles tighten involuntarily despite women's desire for sexual intercourse. Vaginismus usually begins when women first attempt to have sexual intercourse. However, it sometimes develops later, for example, when another factor makes intercourse painful for the first time or when women attempt intercourse while they are emotionally distressed. Because intercourse has become painful, women fear it. This fear makes muscles even tighter and attempts at sexual intercourse more painful. A reflex reaction develops so that when the vagina is pressed or sometimes even just touched, the vaginal muscles automatically (reflexively) tighten. Most women thus cannot tolerate sexual intercourse. Some women cannot tolerate the insertion of a tampon or have never wanted to try. However, most women with vaginismus enjoy sexual activity that does not involve penetration.

Diagnosis

The diagnosis is based on the woman's description of the problem and her medical and sexual history, including childhood and adolescence, and a subsequent pelvic examination.

To make the examination as tolerable as possible, doctors often move slowly and gently while they explain what they are doing in detail. They may offer women a mirror to see their genitals and, in some cases, to guide the doctor's hand or instruments into the vagina. Sometimes women must be treated before a pelvic examination can be done. Doctors look for scars, infections, or other abnormalities to determine whether they could be causing the symptoms. When vaginismus is the problem, no such abnormalities are found.

Treatment

Treatment aims to weaken the reflexive tightening of vaginal muscles and the fear of pain that occurs when the vagina and surrounding area are touched. To weaken this reflex, women are instructed to do certain touching exercises.

At first, women touch an area as close to the vaginal opening as they can without causing pain. Each day, they should move a little closer to the opening, slowly increasing how close they can come to the vagina without causing pain. When they can touch the tissues around the opening (called labia), they can practice opening the labia. Women are encouraged to use a mirror to see their genitals. They are taught to bear down (as when having a bowel movement), which makes the vaginal opening larger, so that it can be seen more easily. Once women can touch the vaginal opening without pain, they are instructed to insert their finger past the hymen, pushing or bearing down while inserting the finger to enlarge the opening and make insertion easier.

When they can do these exercises and experience no pain, they can start to use cone-shaped inserts, which are placed in the vagina. An insert is left in for 10 to 15 minutes. Then the vaginal muscles become used to pressure. As women become comfortable with an insert, they use progressively larger inserts, which gradually increase the pressure in the vagina. Eventually, women invite their partner to place an insert in the vagina. Thus, women learn to relax the vaginal muscles and override the reflexive tightening.

Only after completing these steps should the couple try intercourse again. Doctors usually recommend that women hold their partner's penis and place it partly or completely in their vagina in the same way that they placed the insert. Some women are more comfortable being on top during intercourse at this point. Some men may be overly cautious and too reluctant to push or may lose their erection. They may benefit from a phosphodiesterase inhibitor (such as sildenafil, tadalafil, or vardenafil).

Low Sexual Desire Disorder

Low sexual desire disorder (sexual desire/interest disorder) is lack of interest in sexual activity and sexual thoughts.

- Depression, anxiety, stress, relationship problems, past experiences, drugs, and, less often, hormonal changes can reduce sexual desire.
- Improving the relationship and the setting for sexual activity and identifying what stimulates the woman sexually can help.

A temporary reduction in sexual desire is common, often caused by temporary conditions, such as fatigue. In contrast, low sexual desire disorder causes sexual thoughts, fantasies, and desire for sexual activity to be decreased over a long period and more than would be expected for a woman's age and the length of the sexual relationship. Low sexual desire is considered a disorder only if it distresses women or their partner or if desire is absent throughout the sexual experience.

Causes

Depression, anxiety, stress, or problems in a relationship commonly reduce sexual desire. Having a poor sexual self-image also contributes.

Use of certain drugs, including antidepressants (particularly selective serotonin reuptake inhibitors), anticonvulsants (see table on page 716), chemotherapy drugs, beta-blockers (see table on page 340), and oral contraceptives, can reduce sexual desire, as can drinking excessive amounts of alcohol.

Because levels of sex hormones such as estrogen and testosterone decrease with aging, sexual desire might be expected to similarly decrease with aging. However, overall, low sexual desire disorder is as common among young healthy women as it is among older women. Still, changes in sex hormones sometimes cause low desire. For example, in young healthy women, sudden drops in levels of sex hormones may cause sexual desire to decrease. Similar reductions may occur during certain phases of the menstrual cycle and during the first few weeks after childbirth. In middle-aged and older women, sexual desire may decrease as testosterone production decreases, but the connection has not been proved. In younger women, removal of both ovaries (which make testosterone as well as estrogen) can reduce testosterone production. Even when such women take estrogen, sexual desire may be low. Oral contraceptives may reduce the effects of testosterone, as may oral estrogen taken as part of hormonal therapy by postmenopausal women.

Did You Know...

Young healthy women are as likely to have low sexual desire disorder as older women.

Desire most closely links to mood and relationship (rather than to hormones).

Diagnosis

Diagnosis is based on the woman's history and description of the problem. A pelvic examination may also be done.

Treatment

One of the most helpful measures is for women to identify and tell their partner which things stimulate them. Women may need to remind their partner that they need preparatory activities—which may involve touching or not—to get ready for sexual intercourse. For example, they may want to talk intimately, watch a romantic or erotic video, or dance. Women may want to kiss, hug, or cuddle. They may want their partner to touch various parts of their body, then the breasts or genitals (foreplay) before moving to sexual intercourse. Couples may experiment with different techniques or activities (including fantasy and sex toys) to find effective stimuli.

Measures recommended to treat sexual dysfunction in general (see page 1508) can also help increase sexual desire. Treatment often focuses on factors that contribute to a low sexual desire, such as depression, a poor sexual self-image, and problems in a relationship. Psychotherapy may benefit some women.

Other treatments depend on the cause. For example, if drugs may be contributing, they are stopped if possible. If loss of interest in sex is due to atrophic vaginitis, women may benefit from estrogen applied to the genital area as a cream, inserted into the vagina in a ring or as a tablet, or taken by mouth. For women who are taking oral contraceptives, doctors may recommend substituting contraceptive skin patches or using a barrier method (condom or diaphragm). For women taking estrogen therapy by mouth, doctors may recommend instead taking estrogen another way, such as a skin patch or gel.

Whether testosterone (taken by mouth or through a patch) is useful is being studied. Although it is not standard practice, some doctors occasionally prescribe it for postmenopausal women who are taking estrogen therapy and who have tried all other measures. Women who take testosterone must be evaluated regularly by their doctor because testosterone may have side effects and long-term safety is not known.

Sexual Arousal Disorders

Sexual arousal disorders involve a lack of response to sexual stimulation—mental or emotional (subjective), physical (such as swelling, tingling, or throbbing in the genital area or vaginal wetness), or both.

- Depression, low self-esteem, anxiety, stress, and relationship problems can interfere with sexual arousal.
- Improving the relationship and the settings for sexual activity and identifying what stimulates the woman sexually can help.

Usually, when women are sexually stimulated, they feel sexually excited mentally and emotionally. They may also be aware of certain physical changes. For example, the vagina releases secretions that provide lubrication (causing wetness). The tissues around the vaginal opening (labia) and the clitoris (which corresponds to the penis in men) swell, the breasts swell slightly, and these areas may tingle.

In sexual arousal disorders, the usual types of sexual stimulation (such as kissing, dancing, watching an erotic video, and touching the genitals) do not cause arousal—mentally or emotionally (subjectively), physically, or both.

In genital arousal disorder (a type of sexual arousal disorder), stimulation that does not involve the genitals (such as watching an erotic video) makes women feel aroused, but when the genitals are stimulated (including during intercourse), women are unaware of any physical responses or physical pleasure. As a result, sexual intercourse is unrewarding and possibly difficult and painful.

Sometimes physical responses occur, but women do not notice them because sensitivity in the area is reduced.

Causes

Sexual arousal disorders tend to have the same causes as low sexual desire disorder (see page 1511). For example, depression, low self-esteem, anxiety, stress, other psychologic factors (see page 1506), drugs, and relationship problems commonly interfere with sexual arousal. Inadequate sexual stimulation or the wrong setting for sexual activity can also contribute.

Genital arousal disorder may result from a low level of estrogen or testosterone as occurs during or after menopause, from infection of the vagina (vaginitis) or the bladder (cystitis), or from skin changes in the vulva. This disorder may develop when certain chronic disorders, such as diabetes and multiple sclerosis, damage nerves. The nerve damage leads to decreased sensation in the genital area.

Diagnosis

Diagnosis is based on the woman's history and description of the problem. A pelvic examination is also done.

Treatment

Measures that help couples with sexual dysfunction (see page 1508) can be particularly helpful. For example, treatment includes the following:

- Enhancing trust and intimacy in the couple's relationship
- Making the setting as conducive to sexual activity as possible
- Helping a woman learn to focus during sexual activity
- Identifying and communicating what stimulates the woman, as for low sexual desire disorder (see page 1511)

Couples may experiment with different stimuli, such as a vibrator, fantasy, or erotic videos. Couples may also try activities other than vaginal intercourse. For example, couples may do sensate focus exercises. For these exercises, partners take turns touching each other in pleasurable ways. At first, certain areas, including the genitals, are off limits, and the focus is sensual rather than sexual stimulation. The recipient guides the giver in the type of stimulation wanted. Partners focus on the sensations of the moment. They progress to touching other parts of the body sensually, then sexually and finally to genital stimulation. Such exercises can enhance intimacy and lessen anxiety before sexual activity.

SPOTLIGHT ON AGING

The main reason older women give up on sex is lack of a sexually functional partner. However, age-related changes, particularly those due to menopause, can make women more likely to experience sexual dysfunction. Also, disorders that can interfere with sexual function, such as diabetes, atherosclerosis, urinary tract infections, and arthritis, become more common as women age. However, these changes need not end sexual activity and pleasure, and not all sexual dysfunction in older women is caused by age-related changes.

In older women as in younger women, the most common problem is low sexual desire.

As women age, the ovaries produce smaller amounts of estrogen, progesterone, and testosterone. Some evidence suggests that these hormonal changes may reduce sexual desire, and the resulting changes in the reproductive organs can make sexual intercourse uncomfortable.

- The tissues around the vaginal opening (labia) and the walls of the vagina become less elastic and thinner (a disorder called atrophic vaginitis).
- Vaginal secretions are reduced, providing less lubrication during sexual intercourse.
- Less and less testosterone is produced starting when women are in their 30s and continuing through their 70s. Some evidence suggests that this decrease may lead to decreased sexual interest and response.
- The acidity of the vagina decreases, making the genitals more likely to become irritated and infected.

- Lack of estrogen may contribute to age-related weakening of muscles and other supportive tissues in the pelvis, sometimes allowing a pelvic organ (bladder, intestine, uterus, or rectum) to protrude into the vagina.
- Decreases in hormone levels and blood vessel disorders (such as atherosclerosis) reduce blood flow to the vagina, causing it to become shorter, narrower, and drier.

Other problems may interfere with sexual function. For example, older women may be distressed by changes in their body caused by disorders, surgery, or aging itself. They may think that sexual desire and fantasy are improper or shameful at an older age. They may be worried about the general health or sexual function of their partner or their own sexual performance. Many older women have sexual desire, but if their partner no longer responds to them, their desire may be slowly extinguished.

Older women should not assume that sexual dysfunction is normal for older age. If sexual dysfunction is bothering them, they should talk to their doctor. In many cases, treating a disorder (including depression), stopping or substituting a drug, learning more about sexual function, or talking to a health care practitioner or counselor can help.

If atrophic vaginitis is a problem, estrogen can be applied as a cream or inserted into the vagina as a pill or in a ring. Estrogen may be given by mouth or a patch or applied to an arm as a gel only if menopause occurred recently. Occasionally, testosterone is prescribed in addition to estrogen therapy if all other measures are ineffective, although testosterone is still considered experimental and long-term safety is unknown.

Drugs that are likely causes are stopped if possible. If a selective serotonin reuptake inhibitor (an antidepressant) is the cause, adding bupropion (a different type of antidepressant) may help. Or another antidepressant may be substituted.

For women who have atrophic vaginitis, doctors may prescribe estrogen, applied to the genital area as a cream, inserted into the vagina in a ring or as a tablet, or taken by mouth. For women who are taking oral contraceptives, doctors may recommend substituting contraceptive skin patches or using a barrier method (condom or diaphragm). For women taking estrogen therapy by mouth, doctors may recommend instead taking estrogen another way, such as a skin patch or gel.

Whether testosterone (taken by mouth or through a patch) is useful is being studied. Occasionally, some doctors prescribe testosterone, although it is considered experimental. Women who take tes-

tosterone must be evaluated regularly by their doctor because testosterone may have side effects and long-term safety is unknown.

Orgasmic Disorder

Orgasmic disorder is lack of or delay in sexual climax (orgasm) even though sexual stimulation is sufficient and the woman is sexually aroused.

- Women may not have an orgasm if lovemaking ends too soon, there is not enough foreplay, or they are afraid of losing control or letting go.
- Women are encouraged to use techniques, such as masturbation, to enhance pleasure and to learn about sexual function, and for some, psychotherapy is useful.

The amount and type of stimulation required for orgasm varies greatly from woman to woman. Most women can reach orgasm when the clitoris is stimulated, but less than half of women regularly reach orgasm during sexual intercourse. About 1 of 10 women never reaches orgasm, but many of them nonetheless consider sexual activity to be satisfactory.

Women with orgasmic disorder cannot have an orgasm under any circumstances, even when they masturbate and when they are highly aroused. However, not having an orgasm usually occurs because the woman is not sufficiently aroused and thus is not considered orgasmic disorder. Inability to have an orgasm is considered a disorder only when the lack of orgasm distresses the woman. Lovemaking without orgasm can cause frustration and may result in resentment and occasionally in distaste for anything sexual.

Causes

Situational and psychologic factors can contribute to orgasmic disorder. They include the following:

- Lovemaking that consistently ends (as when the man ejaculates) before the woman is aroused enough
- Insufficient foreplay
- Lack of understanding about how their genital organs function in one or both partners
- Poor communication about sex (for example, about what sort of stimulation a person enjoys)
- Problems in the relationship, such as unresolved conflicts and lack of trust
- Anxiety about sexual performance
- Fear of letting go, being vulnerable, and not being in control (possibly as part of a fear of not being in control of all aspects of their life or as part of a general tendency to keep emotions in check)

- A physically or emotionally traumatic experience, such as sexual abuse
- Psychologic disorders (such as depression)

Physical disorders can also contribute to orgasmic disorder. They include nerve damage (as results from diabetes, spinal cord injuries, or multiple sclerosis) and abnormalities in genital organs.

Certain drugs, particularly selective serotonin reuptake inhibitors (SSRIs—see table on page 868), may specifically inhibit orgasm.

Treatment

Techniques that may enhance pleasure, such as masturbation and relaxation techniques, may help, as may sensate focus exercises. In sensate focus exercises, partners take turns touching each other in pleasurable ways (see page 1512). Couples may try using more or different stimuli, such as a vibrator, fantasy, or erotic videos. A vibrator may be especially useful when there is nerve damage.

Education about sexual function may help. For some women, incorporating stimulation of the clitoris (which corresponds to the penis in men) may be all that is needed.

Psychotherapy may help women identify and manage fear of relinquishing control, fear of vulnerability, or issues of trusting a partner. Psychotherapy may be particularly useful for women who have been sexually abused or have psychologic disorders.

If an SSRI is the cause, adding bupropion (a different type of antidepressant) may help. Or another antidepressant may be substituted. Some evidence suggests that if women stopped having orgasms when they started taking SSRIs, sildenafil may help them have orgasms again.

CHAPTER

238 Menopause

Menopause is the permanent end of menstrual periods and thus of fertility.

- For up to several years before and just after menopause, estrogen levels fluctuate widely, periods become irregular, and symptoms (such as hot flashes) may occur.
- After menopause, bone density decreases.
- Menopause is usually obvious, but blood tests may be done to confirm it.
- Certain measures, including drugs, can lessen symptoms.

During the reproductive years, menstrual periods usually occur in approximately monthly cycles, with an egg released from the ovary (ovulation) about 2 weeks after the first day of a period. For this cycle to occur regularly, the ovaries must produce enough estrogen and progesterone (see page 1494). Menopause occurs because as women age, the ovaries stop producing estrogen and progesterone. During the years before menopause, production of estrogen and progesterone begins to decrease, and menstrual periods and ovulation occur less often. Eventually, menstrual periods and ovulation end permanently, and pregnancy is no longer possible. A woman's last period can be identified only later, after she has had no periods for at least 1 year. (Women who do not wish to become pregnant should use birth control until 1 year has passed since their last menstrual period.)

A distinctive transitional period called perimenopause occurs during the years before and the 1 year after the last menstrual period. How many years of perimenopause precede the last menstrual period varies greatly. During perimenopause, estrogen and progesterone levels fluctuate widely. These fluctuations are thought to cause the menopausal symptoms experienced by many women in their 40s.

In the United States, the average age for menopause is about 51. However, menopause may occur normally in women as young as 40. Menopause is considered premature when it occurs before age 40 (see page 1520). Premature menopause is also called premature ovarian failure.

 Did You Know...

Symptoms of menopause can start years before menstrual periods end.

The average age for menopause is about 51.

Symptoms

Perimenopause: During perimenopause, symptoms may be nonexistent, mild, moderate, or severe. Symptoms may last from 6 months to about 10 years.

Irregular menstrual periods may be the first symptom of perimenopause. Typically, periods occur more often, then less often, but any pattern is possible. Periods may be shorter or longer, lighter or heavier. They may not occur for months, then become regular again. In some women, periods occur regularly until menopause.

Hot flashes affect about three fourths of women and usually begin before periods stop. Most women have hot flashes for more than 1 year, and up to one half of women have them for more than 5 years. What causes hot flashes in unknown. They may be related to fluctuations in hormone levels and may be triggered by cigarette smoking, hot beverages, certain foods, alcohol, and possibly caffeine. During a hot flash, blood vessels near the skin surface widen (dilate). As a result, blood flow increases, causing the skin, especially on the head and neck, to become red and warm (flushed). Women feel warm or hot, and perspiration may be profuse. Hot flashes are sometimes called hot flushes because of this warming effect. A hot flash lasts from 30 seconds to 5 minutes and may be followed by chills. Night sweats are hot flashes that occur at night.

Other symptoms that may occur around the time of menopause include mood changes, depression, irritability, anxiety, nervousness, sleep disturbances (including insomnia), loss of concentration, headache, and fatigue. Many women experience these symptoms during perimenopause and assume that menopause is the cause. However, evidence supporting a connection between menopause and these symptoms is lacking. These symptoms are not directly related to the decreases in estrogen levels that occur with menopause. And many other factors (such as aging itself or a disorder) could explain the symptoms.

Night sweats may disturb sleep, contributing to fatigue, irritability, loss of concentration, and mood changes. In such cases, these symptoms may be indirectly (through night sweats) related to menopause. However, during menopause, sleep disturbances are common even among women who do not have hot flashes. Midlife stresses (such as struggles with adolescents, concerns about aging, caring for aging parents, and changes in marital relationship) may contribute to sleep disturbances. Thus, the relationship between fatigue, irritability, loss of concentration, and mood changes seems less clear.

After Menopause: Many of the symptoms that occur during perimenopause, although disturbing, become less frequent and less intense after menopause. However, the decrease in estrogen levels causes changes that can continue to negatively affect health (for example, increasing the risk of osteoporosis). These changes may worsen, unless measures to prevent them are taken.

- Reproductive tract: The lining of the vagina becomes thinner, drier, and less elastic (a condition called atrophic vaginitis). These changes may make sexual intercourse painful and may increase the risk of inflammation (vaginitis). Other genital organs—the labia minora, clitoris, uterus, and ovaries—decrease in size. Sex drive (libido) commonly decreases with aging. The effect of menopause on the ability to have an orgasm varies from woman to woman. In many women, the ability is unaffected. It improves in some women but is lost in others.

- Urinary tract: The lining of the urethra becomes thinner, and the urethra becomes shorter. Because of these changes, microorganisms can enter the body more easily, and some women develop urinary tract infections more easily. A woman with a urinary tract infection may feel a burning sensation when she urinates. The muscles that control the flow of urine out of the bladder become weaker. Many postmenopausal women have stress incontinence, in which small amounts of urine escape from the bladder during laughing, coughing, or other activities that put pressure on the bladder (see page 292). Some women develop urge incontinence, which is an abrupt, intense urge to urinate that cannot be suppressed. However, how much menopause contributes to incontinence is unclear. Many other factors, such as the effects of childbirth and the use of hormone therapy, contribute to incontinence.

- Skin: As estrogen decreases, the amount of collagen (a protein that makes skin strong) and elastin (a protein that makes skin elastic) also decrease. Thus, the skin may become thinner, drier, less elastic, and more vulnerable to injury.

- Bone: The decrease in estrogen often leads to a decrease in bone density and sometimes to osteoporosis (see page 544) because estrogen helps maintain bone. Bone becomes less dense and weaker, making fractures more likely. During the first 2 years after menopause, bone density decreases by about 3 to 5% each year. After that, it decreases by about 1 to 2% each year.

- Fat (lipid) levels: After menopause, levels of lipids, particularly low-density lipoprotein (LDL—the bad) cholesterol, increase in women. Levels of high-density lipoprotein (HDL—the good) cholesterol decrease. These changes in lipid levels may partly explain why atherosclerosis and thus coronary artery disease become more common among women after menopause. However, whether these changes result from aging or from the decrease in estrogen levels after menopause is unclear. Until menopause, the high estrogen levels may protect against coronary artery disease.

> **? Did You Know...**
> Many symptoms thought to be related to menopause—mood changes, depression, irritability, anxiety, nervousness, insomnia, loss of concentration, headache, and fatigue—probably are not.

Diagnosis

In about three fourths of women, menopause is obvious. Thus, laboratory tests are usually not needed. If menopause begins several years before age 50 or if symptoms are not clear-cut, tests may be done to check for disorders that can disrupt menstrual periods. Rarely, if menopause or perimenopause needs to be confirmed, blood tests are done to measure levels of estrogen and follicle-stimulating hormone (which stimulates the ovaries to produce estrogen and progesterone).

Before any treatment is started, doctors ask women about their medical and family history and perform a physical examination, including breast and pelvic examinations and measurement of blood pressure. Mammography is also done. Blood tests may be done, and bone density may be measured, particularly in women with risk factors for osteoporosis (see page 544). The information obtained helps doctors determine the woman's risk of developing certain disorders after menopause.

Treatment

Understanding what happens during perimenopause can help women cope with the symptoms. Talking with other women who have gone through menopause or with their doctor may also help.

General Measures: Noting which foods and beverages (such as coffee, tea, and spicy foods) seem to trigger hot flashes and not consuming them may help prevent this symptom. Not smoking and avoiding stress may help relieve hot flashes and improve sleep.

Wearing layers of clothing, which can be taken off when a woman feels hot and put on when she feels cold, can help her cope with hot flashes. Wearing clothing that breathes, such as cotton underwear and sleepwear, may enhance comfort.

Exercising regularly (particularly aerobic exercise) may help prevent or relieve hot flashes and improve sleep. Relaxation techniques, meditation, massage, and yoga may help prevent or relieve hot flashes and relieve depression, irritability, and fatigue. A technique called paced respiration, a type of slow, deep breathing exercise, may also help hot flashes. Weight-bearing exercise (such as walking, jogging, and weight lifting) and taking calcium and vitamin D supplements slow the loss of bone density. Regular exercise, particularly when combined with a diet lower in calories, fat, and cholesterol, also helps women lose weight, lower cholesterol levels, and reduce the risk of atherosclerosis, including coronary artery disease.

If vaginal dryness makes sexual intercourse painful, an over-the-counter vaginal lubricant may help. Staying sexually active also helps by stimulating blood flow to the vagina and the surrounding tissues and by keeping tissues flexible. Kegel exercises may help with bladder control (see page 1545). For these exercises, a woman tightens the pelvic muscles as if stopping urine flow.

Hormone Therapy: Hormone therapy can relieve moderate to severe symptoms such as hot flashes, night sweats, and vaginal dryness. However, hormone therapy may increase the risk of developing certain serious disorders. Whether to take hormone therapy is a difficult decision that must be made by a woman and her doctor based on the woman's individual situation. For many women, risks outweigh benefits, so this therapy is not recommended. However, for some women, depending on their medical conditions and risk factors, benefits may outweigh risks.

Hormone therapy can include estrogen and progestins, such as medroxyprogesterone acetate. The hormones used in hormone therapy are synthetic hormones, made in laboratories. They may or may not be identical to those made in the body, but the way they act in the body is very similar. Estradiol is the form of estrogen usually used. Progestins resemble progesterone, which is made by the body.

Women who have a uterus are usually given estrogen plus a progestin (combination hormone therapy) because taking estrogen alone increases the risk of cancer of the uterine lining (endometrial cancer). The progestin helps protect against this cancer. Women who no longer have a uterus may take estrogen alone.

The benefits and risks depend on whether the hormones are taken alone or together.

Estrogen has several benefits:

- Hot flashes and other symptoms: Estrogen is the most effective treatment for hot flashes. It also can prevent vaginal and urinary tract tissues from drying and thinning. Thus, it can reduce pain with sexual intercourse. However, topical therapy (for example, estrogen cream) would be recommended in this circumstance.
- Osteoporosis: Estrogen, with or without a progestin, helps prevent or slow the progression of osteoporosis. However, taking hormone therapy for the sole purpose of preventing osteoporosis is no longer recommended. Most women can take a bisphosphonate or raloxifene instead. These drugs increase bone mass by reducing the amount of bone the body breaks down as it re-forms bones (the amount broken down increases with aging).

Estrogen taken alone increases the risk of the following:

- Endometrial cancer: The risk increases from about 1 to about 4 in 1,000 women each year. The risk increases with higher doses and longer use of estrogen. Taking a progestin with estrogen almost eliminates the risk of endometrial cancer, reducing the risk below that for women who do not take hormone therapy. A woman whose uterus has been removed has no risk of developing this cancer and thus does not need to take a progestin. Usually, estrogen, with or without a progestin, is not prescribed for women who have had advanced endometrial cancer or who have vaginal bleeding (which can be a symptom of endometrial cancer) unless endometrial cancer has been ruled out. A progestin without estrogen may be prescribed for certain women who have endometrial cancer or breast cancer.
- Stroke
- Blood clots in the legs and lungs
- Blood clots in the eye

- Gallstones
- Urinary incontinence: Estrogen increases this risk and worsens preexisting incontinence.

Combination hormone therapy reduces the risk of the following:

- Osteoporosis
- Colorectal cancer

Combination hormone therapy increases the risk of the following:

- Breast cancer: The breast cancers that develop in women taking combination hormone therapy are larger and more likely to spread. Also, mammograms can be more difficult to interpret because hormone therapy increases breast density, making tumors harder to differentiate from breast tissue.
- Coronary artery disease: The risk of coronary artery disease almost doubles during the first year of therapy, even among women being treated with aspirin and statins.
- Stroke
- Blood clots in the legs or lungs
- Dementia
- Urinary incontinence: Combination therapy increases this risk and worsens preexisting incontinence.
- Ovarian cancer (possible increased risk)

Progestins have some benefits:

- Endometrial cancer: Taking a progestin with estrogen almost eliminates the risk of endometrial cancer in women who have a uterus.

Progestins may increase the risk of the following:

- Atherosclerosis and thus coronary artery disease: Progestins may increase this risk because they increase the LDL (the bad) cholesterol level and decrease the HDL (the good) cholesterol level. However, micronized progesterone appears to have fewer side effects and may not adversely affect cholesterol levels.

Estrogen taken alone does not increase or decrease the risk of coronary artery disease. Dementia risk may be increased with estrogen-alone therapy. The effect of estrogen alone or a progestin alone on the risk of breast cancer and blood clots in the lungs is also not clear. Estrogen and progestins, especially at high doses, may have side effects, including nausea, breast tenderness, headache, fluid retention, and mood changes.

Estrogen and a progestin can be taken in several ways:

- Tablets taken by mouth
- Estrogen skin patches (transdermal estrogen)
- Combination estrogen-progestin patches
- Estrogen creams, lotions, or gels
- Estrogen tablets inserted in the vagina
- Injections

℞ SOME DRUGS USED TO TREAT SYMPTOMS AND EFFECTS OF MENOPAUSE

DRUG	ADVANTAGES	DISADVANTAGES
Female hormones		
Estrogen	Relieves hot flashes, night sweats, and vaginal dryness Helps prevent osteoporosis	In women with a uterus, increases the risk of endometrial cancer if not taken with a progestin Increases the risk of stroke, urinary incontinence, and gallstones Has less clear effects on the risk of breast cancer, ovarian cancer, blood clots in the lungs, and colorectal cancer May increase the risk of blood clots in the eye, which can impair vision Possibly increases the risk of dementia
A progestin, such as medroxy-progesterone acetate	Reduces the risk of endometrial cancer associated with taking estrogen alone	Does not relieve vaginal dryness May have negative effects on cholesterol levels and thus may increase the risk of coronary artery disease Has less clear effects on the risk of breast cancer, blood clots in the lungs, dementia, and stroke Increases the risk of blood clots in the legs
Combination therapy (estrogen plus a progestin)	Helps relieve hot flashes Reduces the risk of osteoporosis and colorectal cancer	Increases the risk of coronary artery disease, stroke, breast cancer, blood clots in the legs or lungs, urinary incontinence, and dementia May increase the risk of ovarian cancer
Selective estrogen receptor modulators (SERMs)		
Raloxifene	Prevents and treats osteoporosis Does not appear to increase the risk of endometrial cancer In postmenopausal women with a high risk of breast cancer, reduces that risk	Increases the risk of blood clots in the legs or lungs May mildly worsen hot flashes May cause leg cramps
Bisphosphonates		
Alendronate (taken by mouth) Ibandronate (taken by mouth or given intravenously) Risedronate (taken by mouth) Zoledronic acid (given intravenously)	Prevent and treat osteoporosis	If taken by mouth, must be taken with 6 to 8 ounces of water after awakening, followed by 30 to 60 minutes without consuming any food, liquid, or drug and without lying down If taken incorrectly, can irritate the lining of the esophagus
Antidepressants		
Selective serotonin reuptake inhibitors (such as fluoxetine, sertraline, and sustained-release paroxetine) Serotonin-norepinephrine reuptake inhibitors (such as venlafaxine)	Relieve depression, anxiety, irritability, and insomnia May relieve hot flashes	Depending on the drug, can have side effects, such as sexual dysfunction, nausea, diarrhea, weight loss (in the short term), weight gain (in the long term), sedation, dry mouth, confusion, and increased or decreased blood pressure

(continued on the following page)

R℞ SOME DRUGS USED TO TREAT SYMPTOMS AND EFFECTS OF MENOPAUSE (Continued)

DRUG	ADVANTAGES	DISADVANTAGES
Lipid-lowering drugs		
Statins (such as atorvastatin, lovastatin, pravastatin, and simvastatin)	Prevent atherosclerosis (including coronary artery disease)	Depending on the drug, can have side effects, such as constipation, loose stools, abdominal pain, nausea, bloating, rash, muscle inflammation, increased levels of liver enzymes, and fatigue
Bile acid binders (such as cholestyramine and colestipol)		
Fibric acid derivatives (such as fenofibrate and gemfibrozil)		
Niacin		
Antihypertensive drug (only one type)		
Clonidine	May lessen hot flashes	Can have side effects, such as drowsiness, dry mouth, fatigue, an abnormally slow heart rate, rebound high blood pressure when the drug is stopped, and sexual dysfunction
Antiseizure drug (only one type)		
Gabapentin	May lessen frequency of hot flashes	Can have side effects, such as drowsiness, dizziness, rash, and leg swelling
Male hormone		
Testosterone, taken with estrogen	Lessens hot flashes	Decreases the HDL (the good) cholesterol level
		In high doses, may have some masculinizing effects, such as facial hair growth, acne, and weight gain
		May cause liver disorders
		Has not been studied extensively, so risks are unknown

HDL = high-density cholesterol.

As tablets taken by mouth, estrogen and a progestin may be taken as two tablets or as a combination tablet. Commonly, estrogen and a progestin are taken every day. This schedule typically causes irregular vaginal bleeding for the first year or more of therapy. Alternatively, estrogen may be taken daily, with a progestin taken for 12 to 14 days each month. With this schedule, most women have monthly vaginal bleeding.

Using an estrogen cream is as effective as taking estrogen by mouth for preventing or relieving drying or thinning of the vagina. The cream may be applied to the vagina, or an estrogen tablet or a ring containing estrogen (similar to a diaphragm) may be inserted into the vagina. Such treatment helps prevent intercourse from being painful. Some of the estrogen cream is absorbed into the bloodstream, particularly as the vaginal lining becomes healthier. The amount of estrogen absorbed into the bloodstream from the vagina depends on the type and dose of estrogen used. The amount of estrogen absorbed with creams is much higher than that with vaginal tablets or rings. Theoretically, estrogen absorbed through the vagina can increase the risk of endometrial cancer. Therefore, if women who have a uterus use estrogen creams, they should also take a progestin. Occasionally, women who have breast cancer or who have risk factors for it are offered a vaginal tablet or ring, but only after they have been evaluated by an oncologist.

Doctors prescribe the lowest hormone dose that controls symptoms. If women have symptoms while taking a high dose, the hormone level in the blood is measured to determine whether the hormone is being absorbed.

Selective Estrogen Receptor Modulators (SERMs): These drugs function like estrogen in some parts of the body. The only SERM currently used to prevent bone loss related to menopause is raloxifene. Like estrogen, raloxifene helps prevent bone density from decreasing in postmenopausal women and increases the risk of developing blood clots (from 1 to 10 in 10,000 women). Raloxifene also prevents fractures of the bones in the spine (vertebrae). However, raloxifene may have effects opposite to those of estrogen in other parts of the body. It does not relieve menopausal symptoms. Hot flashes worsen mildly and temporarily in about 1 in 10 women. Also, raloxifene does not appear to increase the risk of endometrial cancer. It inhibits the growth of breast tissue and reduces the risk of breast cancer.

Other Drugs: Several other types of drugs can help relieve some of the symptoms associated with menopause. Clonidine, which is used to treat high blood pressure, can reduce the intensity of hot flashes. It can be applied in a skin patch. Gabapentin, an antiseizure drug, may lessen the frequency of hot flashes. An antidepressant, such as fluoxetine, paroxetine, sertraline, or venlafaxine, may relieve hot flashes. Antidepressants may also help relieve depression, anxiety, and irritability (see page 866). A sleep aid can often relieve insomnia (see page 669).

Lipid-lowering drugs (see page 967) may be taken to lower cholesterol levels, reducing the risk of atherosclerosis and coronary artery disease. Women with risk factors for osteoporosis can take bisphosphonates to reduce that risk (see page 546). These drugs increase bone density and reduce the risk of some fractures.

Testosterone, the main male sex hormone, taken with estrogen is sometimes used to relieve some symptoms of menopause. This treatment is controversial because whether taking estrogen with testosterone is more effective than taking estrogen alone is unclear. Also, taking testosterone has risks and side effects, such as an increased risk of liver disorders and masculinizing effects.

Alternative Medicine: Some women take medicinal herbs (see page 2067) and other supplements to relieve hot flashes, irritability, mood changes, and memory loss. Examples are black cohosh, DHEA (dehydroepiandrosterone), dong quai, evening primrose, ginseng, and St. John's wort. However, such remedies are not regulated as drugs are. That is, their manufacturers are not required to show that they are safe or effective, and what their ingredients are and how much of each ingredient a product contains are not standardized (see page 2071). Also, none of these treatments has been shown to be effective, and some, such as black cohosh, vitamin E, and increased dietary soy protein, have been shown to be ineffective. Some (for example, kava) are harmful. Furthermore, some supplements can interact with other drugs and can worsen some disorders. Women who are considering taking such supplements are advised to discuss them with a doctor.

Premature Menopause

Premature menopause (premature ovarian failure) is the permanent end of menstrual periods before age 40 because ovulation stops and the ovaries become unable to produce hormones.

- Symptoms are the same as those of natural menopause.
- Tests are done to identify the cause.
- Various measures, including estrogen (used only for a few years) and other drugs, can relieve or reduce symptoms.
- The only way to become pregnant, if desired, is to have eggs from another woman implanted in the uterus.

Hormonally, premature menopause resembles natural menopause. The ovaries produce very little estrogen. Premature menopause has many causes:

- Genetic abnormalities: Chromosomes, including the sex chromosomes, may be abnormal. Sex chromosome abnormalities include Turner's syndrome and disorders that confer a Y chromosome (which normally occurs only in males).
- Autoimmune disorders: The body produces abnormal antibodies that attack the body's tissues, including the ovaries. Examples are thyroiditis, vitiligo, and myasthenia gravis.
- Metabolic disorders: Addison's disease and diabetes are examples.
- Viral infections: Mumps is an example.
- Chemotherapy for cancer
- Radiation therapy
- Surgical removal of the ovaries: Surgery to remove the uterus (hysterectomy) ends menstrual periods but does not cause menopause as long as the ovaries are functioning.
- Toxins: Tobacco is an example.

Premature menopause causes the same symptoms that occur with natural menopause, such as hot flashes and mood swings. Having a Y chromosome increases the risk of cancer of the ovaries.

Diagnosis

Doctors suspect premature menopause when women younger than 40 have menopausal symptoms. A pregnancy test is done, and levels of estrogen and follicle-stimulating hormone (which stimulates the ovaries to produce estrogen and progesterone) are measured on several occasions to confirm the diagnosis.

Additional tests may be done to help doctors identify the cause of premature menopause and thus evaluate a woman's health risks and recommend treatment.

For women younger than 35, a chromosome analysis may be done. If a chromosomal abnormality is detected, additional procedures and treatment may be required.

Treatment

Estrogen and other therapies used during natural menopause are used to treat symptoms.

If women with premature menopause wish to become pregnant, doctors recommend in vitro (test tube) fertilization (see page 1591). Another woman's eggs (donor eggs) are implanted in the uterus after they have been fertilized in the laboratory.

Estrogen and a progestin are also given to enable the uterus to support the pregnancy. This technique gives women up to a 50% chance of becoming pregnant. Otherwise the chance of becoming pregnant is less than a 10%.

Women who have a Y chromosome need to have their ovaries removed to decrease the risk of developing ovarian cancer.

---

239 Menstrual Disorders and Abnormal Vaginal Bleeding

Complex interactions among hormones control the start of menstruation during puberty, the rhythms and duration of menstrual cycles during the reproductive years, and the end of menstruation at menopause.

- Hormonal control of menstruation begins in the hypothalamus (the part of the brain that coordinates and controls hormonal activity).
- The hypothalamus releases gonadotropin-releasing hormone in pulses.
- Gonadotropin-releasing hormone stimulates the pituitary gland to produce two hormones called gonadotropins: luteinizing hormone and follicle-stimulating hormone.
- Luteinizing hormone and follicle-stimulating hormone stimulate the ovaries.
- The ovaries produce the female hormones estrogen and progesterone, which ultimately control menstruation (see page 1494).

Hormones produced by other glands, such as the adrenal glands and the thyroid gland, can also affect the functioning of the ovaries and menstruation.

During the reproductive years, vaginal bleeding may be abnormal when menstrual periods are too heavy or too light, last too long, occur too often, or are irregular. Any vaginal bleeding that occurs before puberty or after menopause is abnormal until proven otherwise.

Menstrual disorders include premenstrual syndrome, dysmenorrhea, dysfunctional uterine bleeding, and amenorrhea.

Premenstrual Syndrome

Premenstrual syndrome (PMS) is a group of physical and psychologic symptoms that start several days before and usually end a few hours after a menstrual period begins.

- PMS includes any combination of the following: becoming irritable, anxious, moody, or depressed or having headaches or sore, swollen breasts.

- Doctors base the diagnosis on symptoms, which are usually tracked in a monthly calendar.
- Consuming less sugar, salt, and caffeine and exercising may help relieve symptoms, as does taking certain supplements, pain relievers, birth control pills (sometimes), or antidepressants.

Because so many symptoms, such as a bad mood, irritability, bloating, and breast tenderness, have been ascribed to PMS, defining and identifying PMS can be difficult. PMS affects 20 to 50% of women. About 5% of women of reproductive age have a severe form of PMS called premenstrual dysphoric disorder.

PMS may occur partly because estrogen and progesterone levels fluctuate during the menstrual cycle. Some women are more sensitive to these fluctuations. Also, in some women with PMS, progesterone may be broken down differently. Progesterone is usually broken down into two components that have opposite effects on mood. Women with PMS may produce less of the component that tends to reduce anxiety and more of the component that tends to increase anxiety.

The fluctuations in estrogen and progesterone may affect other hormones, such as aldosterone, which helps regulate salt and water balance. Excess aldosterone can cause fluid retention and bloating.

Symptoms

The type and intensity of symptoms vary from woman to woman and from month to month in the same woman. The various physical and psychologic symptoms of PMS can temporarily upset a woman's life.

Symptoms may begin a few hours up to about 10 days before a menstrual period, and they often disappear completely a few hours after the period begins. Women

Symptoms That Can Occur in Premenstrual Syndrome

PHYSICAL

- Awareness of heartbeats (palpitations)
- Backache
- Bloating
- Breast fullness and pain
- Changes in appetite and cravings for certain foods
- Constipation
- Cramps, heaviness, or pressure in the lower abdomen
- Dizziness, including vertigo
- Easy bruising
- Fainting
- Fatigue
- Headaches
- Hot flashes
- Insomnia, including difficulty falling or staying asleep at night
- Joint and muscle pain
- Lack of energy
- Nausea and vomiting
- Pins-and-needles sensations in the hands and feet
- Skin problems, such as acne and localized scratch dermatitis
- Swelling of hands and feet
- Weight gain

PSYCHOLOGIC

- Agitation
- Anxiety
- Confusion
- Crying spells
- Depression
- Difficulty concentrating
- Emotional hypersensitivity
- Forgetfulness or memory loss
- Irritability
- Mood swings
- Nervousness
- Short temper
- Social withdrawal

Other disorders may worsen while PMS symptoms are occurring. They include the following:

- Seizure disorders, with more seizures than usual
- Connective tissue disorders (such as lupus or rheumatoid arthritis), with flare-ups
- Respiratory disorders (such as allergies and congestion of the nose and airways)

In **premenstrual dysphoric disorder**, premenstrual symptoms are so severe that they interfere with work, social activities, or relationships.

Diagnosis

The diagnosis is based on symptoms. To identify PMS, doctors ask a woman to keep a daily record of her symptoms. This record helps the woman be aware of changes in her body and moods and helps doctors identify any regular symptoms and determine what treatment is best. Premenstrual dysphoric disorder cannot be diagnosed until a woman has recorded her symptoms for at least two menstrual cycles. Doctors can distinguish premenstrual syndrome and premenstrual dysphoric disorder from mood disorders, such as depression, because the symptoms disappear soon after the menstrual period begins.

Treatment

Women can do the following to help relieve symptoms:

- Get enough rest and sleep
- Exercise regularly, which may help lessen bloating as well as irritability, anxiety, and insomnia
- Use stress reduction techniques (meditation or relaxation exercises)
- Avoid stressful activities
- Consume more protein and calcium and less sugar and caffeine (including that in chocolate)
- Consume less salt, which often reduces fluid retention and relieves bloating
- Take certain supplements: vitamin B complex (especially vitamin B_6), calcium (1,000 milligrams a day), vitamin D, and magnesium

Women should talk to their doctor before they take supplements, especially vitamin B_6, which may be harmful if taken in high doses. Nerve damage is possible with as little as 200 milligrams a day.

Doctors may prescribe diuretics (which help the kidneys eliminate salt and water from the body) to help reduce fluid retention.

Taking nonsteroidal anti-inflammatory drugs (NSAIDs—see page 644) may help relieve headaches, pain due to abdominal cramps, and joint pain. Taking combination oral contraceptives (birth control pills that contain estrogen and a progestin) reduces pain,

who are approaching menopause may have symptoms that persist through and after the menstrual period. The symptoms of PMS may be followed each month by a painful period (dysmenorrhea), particularly in teenagers.

breast tenderness, and changes in appetite in some women but worsens these symptoms in a few. Taking oral contraceptives that contain only a progestin does not help.

Women who have more severe symptoms may benefit from taking fluoxetine, paroxetine, or sertraline, which are antidepressants (see table on page 868). These drugs are used to prevent symptoms, and to be effective, they should be taken before symptoms begin. Taking these drugs after symptoms begin usually does not relieve symptoms as well as taking them before symptoms begin. They are most effective in reducing irritability, depression, and some other symptoms of PMS. Doctors may ask a woman to continue keeping a record of her symptoms so that they can judge the effectiveness of treatment.

Women who have premenstrual dysphoric disorder may benefit from taking antidepressants such as fluoxetine, paroxetine, or sertraline. Taking a gonadotropin-releasing hormone (GnRH) analogue (such as leuprolide or goserelin—see table on page 1532), given by injection, may control symptoms. This drug is a synthetic form of a hormone produced by the body. GnRH analogues cause the body to produce less estrogen and progesterone. Thus, these drugs are used with estrogen plus a progestin, taken in a low dose by mouth or patch.

Dysmenorrhea

Dysmenorrhea is pain in the lowest part of the abdomen (pelvis) during a menstrual period.

- The cause is unidentified in most women.
- Pain, usually crampy or sharp, starts a few days before a menstrual period and subsides after 2 or 3 days.
- Doctors base the diagnosis on symptoms and results of a physical examination.
- Nonsteroidal anti-inflammatory drugs or, if needed, low-dose birth control pills are used.

About three fourths of women have dysmenorrhea with no identifiable cause (primary dysmenorrhea). The rest have dysmenorrhea due to another condition (secondary dysmenorrhea).

Primary Dysmenorrhea: More than 50% of women may be affected, usually starting during adolescence. In about 5 to 15% of these women, primary dysmenorrhea is sometimes severe, interfering with daily activities and resulting in absence from school or work.

> **? Did You Know...**
> Taking birth control pills sometimes relieves symptoms but may make them worse.

DECIPHERING MEDICAL TERMS FOR MENSTRUAL DISORDERS*

TERM	DESCRIPTION
Amenorrhea	No periods
Dysmenorrhea	Painful periods
Hypomenorrhea	Unusually light periods
Menometrorrhagia	Prolonged bleeding that occurs at irregular intervals
Menorrhagia, or hypermenorrhea	Unusually long and heavy periods
Metrorrhagia	Bleeding that occurs at frequent, irregular intervals
Oligomenorrhea	Unusually infrequent periods
Polymenorrhea	Unusually frequent periods
Postmenopausal bleeding	Bleeding that occurs after menopause
Premenstrual syndrome (PMS)	Physical and psychologic symptoms that occur before the start of a period
Primary amenorrhea	No periods ever starting (at puberty)
Secondary amenorrhea	Periods that have stopped

*Breaking the words into their components helps decipher them: a = no; dys = painful (or abnormal); hypo = deficient (or below normal); men = month; metro = uterus; oligo = few or scanty; poly = many or much; post = after; pre = before; rhagia = to burst forth; rhea = flow.

Primary dysmenorrhea may become less severe with aging and after pregnancy.

In primary dysmenorrhea, the pain occurs only during menstrual cycles in which an egg is released. The pain is thought to result from prostaglandins released during menstruation. Prostaglandins are hormonelike substances that cause the uterus to contract, reduce the blood supply to the uterus, and increase the sensitivity of nerve endings in the uterus to pain. Women who have primary dysmenorrhea have higher levels of prostaglandins.

Secondary Dysmenorrhea: This type usually starts during adulthood. Common causes include the following:

- Endometriosis: Patches of endometrial tissue— normally occurring only in the lining of the uterus (endometrium)—appear outside the uterus.

Adenomyosis: Noncancerous Growth of the Uterus

In adenomyosis, glandular tissue from the lining of the uterus (endometrium) grows into the muscular wall of the uterus. The uterus becomes enlarged, sometimes doubling or tripling in size.

This common disorder causes symptoms in only a small percentage of women, usually those between the ages of 35 and 50. It is more common among women who have had children. The cause is unknown.

Symptoms include heavy and painful periods, bleeding between periods, vague pain in the pelvic area, and a feeling of pressure on the bladder and rectum. Sometimes sexual intercourse is painful.

Doctors suspect adenomyosis when they do a pelvic examination and discover that the uterus is enlarged, round, and softer than normal. Pelvic ultrasonography or magnetic resonance imaging (MRI) helps confirm the diagnosis. Sometimes when adenomyosis causes abnormal bleeding, a biopsy is done.

Usually, no treatment is effective, although oral contraceptives and gonadotropin-releasing hormone analogues (such as leuprolide or goserelin) may be tried. Analgesics may be taken for pain. In some women, a hysterectomy may be done.

- **Fibroids:** Noncancerous tumors composed of muscle and fibrous tissue grow in the uterus.
- **Adenomyosis:** The uterus enlarges when endometrial tissue grows into the muscular wall of the uterus.
- **Pelvic congestion syndrome:** Blood accumulates in the veins of the pelvis because these veins have widened and become convoluted.
- **Pelvic infection:** Symptoms can worsen before or during menstrual periods.
- **Cervical stenosis:** The passageway through the cervix (cervical canal) may be narrow at birth or may become narrow when polyps are removed or a precancerous condition (dysplasia) or cancer of the cervix is treated. In a few women, cervical stenosis causes pain during menstrual periods, as menstrual blood attempts to pass through the cervix but is partly blocked.

Symptoms

Pain occurs in the lowest part of the abdomen (pelvis) and may extend to the lower back or legs. The pain is usually crampy or sharp and comes and goes, but it may be a dull, constant ache. Usually, the pain starts 1 to 3 days before or during the menstrual period, peaks after 24 hours, and subsides after 2 or 3 days.

Other common symptoms include headache, nausea, constipation, diarrhea, and an urge to urinate frequently. Occasionally, vomiting occurs. Premenstrual irritability, nervousness, depression, and abdominal bloating may persist during part or all of the menstrual period. Sometimes the menstrual blood contains clumps of tissue.

Diagnosis

Diagnosis is based on symptoms and the results of a physical examination. To identify possible causes (such as fibroids), ultrasonography may be done. Also, doctors may examine the abdominal cavity using a viewing tube (laparoscope) inserted through a small incision just below the navel. They may examine the interior of the uterus using a similar tube (hysteroscope) inserted through the vagina and cervix. Other procedures may include magnetic resonance imaging (MRI) and removal of a tissue sample from the inside of the uterus for analysis (endometrial biopsy).

Treatment

Nonsteroidal anti-inflammatory drugs (NSAIDs) usually relieve pain effectively. NSAIDs may be more effective if started 1 or 2 days before a menstrual period begins and continued for 1 or 2 days after it begins. Nausea and vomiting usually disappear without treatment as the pain subsides. Applying heat to the lower abdomen, getting enough rest and sleep, and exercising regularly may also help relieve symptoms.

If the pain continues to interfere with daily activities, oral contraceptives that contain estrogen in a low dose plus a progestin may be prescribed to suppress the release of eggs from the ovaries (ovulation).

When dysmenorrhea results from another disorder, that disorder is treated if possible. A narrow cervical canal can be widened surgically. However, this operation usually relieves the pain only temporarily. If needed, fibroids or misplaced endometrial tissue (due to endometriosis) is surgically removed.

When other treatments are ineffective and the pain is severe, the nerves to the uterus may be cut surgically. However, this operation occasionally injures other pelvic organs, such as the ureters. Alternatively, hypnosis or acupuncture may be tried.

Amenorrhea

Amenorrhea is the absence of menstrual periods.

- Menstrual periods may never start, or they may start, then stop.
- Amenorrhea may result from various disorders or drugs that disrupt any part of the complex hormonal regulation of the menstrual cycle.

- Symptoms, such as excess body hair, headaches, hot flashes, and vaginal dryness, may accompany amenorrhea depending on the cause.
- The diagnosis is based on the woman's menstrual history, but information about symptoms, a physical examination, and sometimes other tests are needed to identify the cause.
- The disorder causing amenorrhea is treated if possible.
- Adolescent girls who have never had a period may be given hormones to start periods.

Some women never go through puberty, so periods never start. This disorder is called primary amenorrhea. In other women, periods start at puberty, then stop. This disorder is called secondary amenorrhea. Amenorrhea is normal only before puberty, during pregnancy, while breastfeeding, and after menopause.

Amenorrhea can also be classified based on other features:

- Whether an egg is released (ovulatory) or not (anovulatory)
- Where the abnormality occurs, such as the hypothalamus (which controls the hormones that regulate menstrual cycles), pituitary gland (which produces hormones that stimulate the ovaries), or ovaries (which produce the hormones that ultimately control menstrual cycles)
- What type of disorder is causing it—genetic, structural, hormonal, autoimmune, or something else

Most women have anovulatory amenorrhea (that is, no egg is released).

Amenorrhea also may indicate pregnancy (the most common cause of secondary amenorrhea) or be the first symptom of a serious disorder and should be evaluated.

Causes

Malfunction of any part of the complex hormonal system that regulates the menstrual cycle can cause amenorrhea. This system includes the hypothalamus, pituitary, ovaries, adrenal glands, and thyroid gland. Malfunction of these organs can cause primary or secondary amenorrhea, depending on when malfunction occurs. Various disorders (including genetic, hormonal, and autoimmune disorders), infections, tumors, injuries, radiation therapy, and drugs can cause malfunction.

Some conditions, such as the following, cause only primary amenorrhea:

- A birth defect of the uterus or fallopian tubes
- A chromosomal disorder, such as Turner's syndrome (in which the cells contain one X chromosome instead of the usual two)

In some genetic disorders, ovulation never begins, and puberty and secondary sexual characteristics do not develop normally.

What Is Pelvic Congestion Syndrome?

Sometimes pain that occurs before or during menstrual periods results from a problem with veins in the pelvis. The veins may widen (dilate) and become convoluted, and blood accumulates in them. The result is varicose veins in the pelvis—a disorder called pelvic congestion syndrome. Pain, sometimes debilitating, can result. Estrogen may contribute because it causes some of the veins supplying the ovaries and uterus to also dilate, so that blood can accumulate in these veins as well. Up to 15% of women of reproductive age have varicose veins in their pelvis, but not all of them have symptoms.

Typically, the pain is dull and aching, but it may be sharp or throbbing. It is worse at the end of the day (after a woman has been sitting or standing a long time) and is relieved when she lies down. The pain is also worse during or after sexual intercourse. It is often accompanied by low back pain, aches in the legs, abnormal menstrual bleeding, and an occasional clear or watery vaginal discharge. Some women have fatigue, mood swings, headaches, and abdominal bloating.

Doctors may suspect pelvic congestion syndrome when a woman has pelvic pain but a pelvic examination does not detect inflammation or another abnormality. Ultrasonography can help doctors confirm the diagnosis. Alternatively, the veins can be viewed with a viewing tube inserted through a small incision just below the navel in a procedure called laparoscopy.

Nonsteroidal anti-inflammatory drugs (NSAIDs) usually relieve the pain.

Some conditions, such as the following, usually cause only secondary amenorrhea:

- Polycystic ovary syndrome (characterized by irregular or no periods, obesity, high levels of male hormones, and often cysts in the ovaries)
- Hydatidiform mole (a tumor that develops from an abnormal fertilized egg or the placenta)
- Asherman's syndrome (scarring of the lining of the uterus due to an infection or surgery)
- Use of certain drugs (including hallucinogenic drugs, cocaine, opioids, chemotherapy drugs, antipsychotic drugs, antidepressants, and oral contraceptives) by women who have already started having menstrual periods

Some other disorders and stress due to internal or situational concerns can cause either type of amenorrhea. Stress interferes with the brain's control (through hormones) of the ovaries. For example, exercising too much or having eating disorders or undernutrition (as in anorexia nervosa, starvation, or excessive dieting) can cause the brain to signal the pituitary gland to decrease its production of the hormones that stimulate the ovaries. As a result, the ovaries produce less estrogen, and periods never begin or they stop. Psychiatric disorders, such as depression or obsessive-compulsive disorder, can also cause this stress.

Symptoms

Amenorrhea may or may not be accompanied by other symptoms, depending on the cause. Such symptoms may include acne, excess body hair (hirsutism), deepening of the voice, headaches, visual disturbances, hot flashes, vaginal dryness, and decreased sex drive.

If amenorrhea lasts a long time, it can cause problems usually associated with menopause, such as decreased bone density (osteoporosis) and an increased risk of heart and blood vessel disorders.

Diagnosis

Primary amenorrhea is diagnosed when periods have not started by age 16. Girls who have no signs of puberty (such as breast development, pubic hair, and a growth spurt) by age 13 or who have not started having periods within 5 years of starting puberty are evaluated for possible problems. For example, doctors try to determine whether any other family members have had delayed puberty or a genetic disorder.

Secondary amenorrhea is diagnosed when a woman of reproductive age (who is not pregnant, breastfeeding, or menopausal) has had no menstrual periods for at least 6 months whether periods had been regular or irregular previously. Sometimes secondary amenorrhea is diagnosed if such a woman has had no menstrual periods for only 3 months if periods had been regular previously. Doctors ask about use of drugs, exercise and eating habits, and other conditions that can cause amenorrhea.

In girls who have signs of puberty and in women of reproductive age, pregnancy tests are done to rule out pregnancy.

A physical examination can help doctors determine whether puberty has occurred or has occurred normally. Doctors examine the breasts and check for signs of puberty, such as pubic and underarm hair. They do a pelvic examination to determine whether the genital organs are developing normally and to check for abnormalities.

Other tests may be needed to confirm or identify the cause:

- Hormone levels in the blood may be measured.
- Magnetic resonance imaging (MRI) of the brain may be done to look for a pituitary tumor.

- Computed tomography (CT), MRI, or ultrasonography may be used to look for a tumor in the ovaries or adrenal glands.
- Hormones (estrogen and a progestin) may be given to try to trigger bleeding. The response may help doctors determine whether the abnormality is in the uterus or in the pituitary or hypothalamus.

Treatment

The underlying disorder is treated if possible. For example, a tumor is removed. Some disorders, such as Turner's syndrome and other genetic disorders, cannot be cured.

If a girl's periods have never started and all test results are normal, she is examined every 3 to 6 months to monitor the progression of puberty. A progestin and sometimes estrogen may be given to start her periods and to stimulate the development of secondary sexual characteristics, such as breasts.

Women who wish to become pregnant may be given hormones to induce release of an egg (see page 1589).

Problems associated with amenorrhea, such as osteoporosis or excess body hair, may require treatment.

Dysfunctional Uterine Bleeding

Dysfunctional uterine bleeding is abnormal bleeding resulting from changes in the hormonal control of menstruation.

- Bleeding occurs frequently or irregularly, lasts longer, or is heavier.
- This disorder is diagnosed when the physical examination, ultrasonography, and other tests have ruled out the usual causes of vaginal bleeding.
- An endometrial biopsy is usually done.
- The bleeding can usually be controlled with estrogen plus a progestin or sometimes with either alone.
- If the biopsy detects abnormal cells, treatment involves high doses of a progestin and sometimes removal of the uterus.

Dysfunctional uterine bleeding occurs most commonly at the beginning and end of the reproductive years: 20% of cases occur in adolescent girls, and more than 50% occur in women older than 45. In about 90% of cases, the ovaries do not release an egg (ovulate). Thus, pregnancy is impossible.

Dysfunctional uterine bleeding commonly results when the level of estrogen remains high instead of decreasing as it normally does after the egg is released and not fertilized. The high estrogen level is not balanced by an appropriate level of progesterone. In such cases, no egg is released. As a result, the lining of the uterus (endometrium) continues to thicken (instead of breaking down and being shed normally as a menstrual period). This condition is called endometrial hyperplasia. The lining is then shed incompletely and irregularly, causing bleeding. Bleeding is irregular, prolonged, and sometimes heavy. This type of bleeding is common among women who have polycystic ovary syndrome and occurs in some women with endometriosis. A high estrogen level not balanced by progesterone increases the risk of endometrial cancer, even in young women.

Dysfunctional uterine bleeding may be an early sign of menopause.

Symptoms

Bleeding may differ from typical menstrual periods in the following ways:

- Occur more frequently (less than 21 days apart—polymenorrhea)
- Last longer or involve more blood loss than menses (more than 7 days or more than about 3 ounces—menorrhagia)
- Occur frequently and irregularly between periods (metrorrhagia)

Bleeding during regular menstrual cycles may be abnormal, or bleeding may occur at unpredictable times. Some women have symptoms associated with menstrual periods, such as breast tenderness and bloating.

If bleeding continues, women may develop iron deficiency and sometimes anemia.

Diagnosis

Dysfunctional uterine bleeding is suspected when bleeding occurs at irregular times or in excessive amounts. It is diagnosed when all other possible causes of vaginal bleeding have been excluded. These causes include abnormalities of the genital organs (such as polycystic ovary syndrome), inflammation, blood clotting disorders, pregnancy, complications of pregnancy, and use of contraceptives or certain drugs.

To establish that bleeding is abnormal, doctors ask questions about the pattern of bleeding. To exclude other possible causes, they ask about other symptoms and possible causes (such as use of drugs, the presence of other disorders, fibroids, and complications during pregnancies). A physical examination is also done. A complete blood cell count can help doctors estimate how much blood has been lost and whether anemia is present.

Tests to check for possible causes may be done based on the findings during the interview and physical examination. For example, blood tests to determine how fast blood clots or to measure hormone levels may be done.

Transvaginal ultrasonography (using a thin probe inserted through the vagina and into the uterus) is often used to check for growths in the uterus and to determine whether the uterine lining is thickened.

If the risk of cancer of the uterine lining (endometrial cancer) is high, an endometrial biopsy is done before drug treatment is started. Risk is increased in women with the following:

- Age 35 or older
- Obesity
- Polycystic ovary syndrome
- High blood pressure
- Diabetes
- Bleeding that is persistent, irregular, or heavy despite treatment
- Thickening of the uterine lining (detected by ultrasonography)
- Inconclusive findings during ultrasonography

Most women with dysfunctional uterine bleeding have one or more of these conditions and thus require a biopsy.

Treatment

Treatment depends on how old the woman is, how heavy the bleeding is, whether the uterine lining is thickened, and whether the woman wishes to become pregnant. It focuses on controlling the bleeding and, if needed, preventing endometrial cancer.

When the uterine lining is thickened but its cells are normal, hormones may be used to control bleeding.

- For heavy bleeding, a combination oral contraceptive (a birth control pill with estrogen and a progestin) may be used.
- For very heavy bleeding, estrogen may be given intravenously until the bleeding stops. Sometimes a progestin is given by mouth at the same time or started 2 or 3 days later. Occasionally, bleeding is so heavy that fluids are given intravenously and a blood transfusion is needed. Very rarely, a catheter needs to be inserted into the uterus and inflated to put pressure on the bleeding vessels and thus stop the bleeding.

Bleeding usually stops in 12 to 24 hours. After bleeding stops, low doses of the oral contraceptive may then be prescribed for at least 3 months to prevent the bleeding from recurring.

Some women should not be treated with a combination oral contraceptive or estrogen. They include postmenopausal women and women with significant risk factors for a heart or blood vessel disorder. For these women, an intrauterine device (IUD) that contains a progestin may be used, or a progestin may be given alone by injection or by mouth. These treatments may also be used when those that include estrogen are ineffective.

If women wish to become pregnant and bleeding is not too heavy, they may be given clomiphene (a fertility drug) by mouth instead of hormones. It stimulates ovulation.

If the uterine lining remains thickened or the bleeding persists despite treatment with hormones, dilation and curettage (D and C) is usually needed. In this procedure, tissue from the uterine lining is removed by scraping. This procedure may reduce bleeding, but in some women, it causes scarring of the endometrium (Asherman's syndrome), which can cause menstrual bleeding to stop (amenorrhea).

If the uterine lining contains abnormal cells (particularly in women who are older than 35 and who do not want to become pregnant), treatment begins with a high dose of a progestin. A biopsy is done after 3 to 6 months of treatment. If it detects abnormal cells, a hysterectomy is done because the abnormal cells may become cancerous. If women are postmenopausal, a progestin is not used. Hysterectomy is done.

Polycystic Ovary Syndrome

Polycystic ovary syndrome involves disruption of the menstrual cycle and a tendency to have high levels of male hormones (androgens).

- Women are typically obese and have irregular or no menstrual periods, and in some, the voice deepens, breast size decreases, and acne and excess body hair develop.
- Doctors often base the diagnosis on symptoms, but blood tests to measure hormone levels and ultrasonography may also be done.
- Exercise, weight loss, and estrogen plus a progestin or a progestin alone may help reduce symptoms (including excess body hair) and normalize hormone levels.
- If women wish to become pregnant, losing weight and taking clomiphene, sometimes with metformin, may stimulate release of an egg.

Polycystic ovary syndrome affects about 5 to 10% of women. In the United States, it is the most common cause of infertility. It gets its name from the many fluid-filled sacs (cysts) that often develop in the ovaries, causing them to enlarge.

A common cause is excess production of luteinizing hormone by the pituitary gland. The excess luteinizing hormone increases the production of male hormones (androgens). High levels of male hormones increases the risk of metabolic syndrome (with high blood pressure, high cholesterol levels, and resistance to the effects of insulin). If male hormone levels remain high, the risk of diabetes, heart and blood vessel disorders, and high blood pressure is increased. Also, some of the male hormones may be converted to estrogen, increasing estrogen levels.

Not enough progesterone is produced to balance the increased level of estrogen. If this situation continues a long time, the lining of the uterus (endometrium) may become extremely thickened (a condition called endometrial hyperplasia). Also, the risk of cancer of the lining of the uterus (endometrial cancer) may be increased.

In many women, the body's cells resist the effects of insulin (called insulin resistance or sometimes prediabetes). Insulin helps sugar (glucose) pass into cells so that they can use it for energy. When cells resist its effects, sugar accumulates in the blood, and the pancreas produces more insulin to try to lower sugar levels in the blood. If insulin resistance becomes moderate or severe, diabetes is diagnosed.

> **? Did You Know...**
> Polycystic ovary syndrome is the most common cause of infertility in the United States.

Symptoms

Symptoms typically develop during puberty and worsen with time. Symptoms vary from woman to woman.

In some women, menstrual periods do not start at puberty. Irregular vaginal bleeding or amenorrhea is typical. Thus, these women are not releasing an egg from the ovaries (ovulating). These women also develop symptoms related to the high levels of male hormones—a process called masculinization or virilization. Symptoms include acne, a deepened voice, a decrease in breast size, and an increase in muscle size and in body hair (hirsutism). Hair grows as it does in men (for example, on the chest and face) and may thin at the temples.

Most women are obese. Producing too much insulin contributes to weight gain or makes losing weight difficult. Excess insulin may also cause skin in the armpits, on the nape of the neck, and in skinfolds to become dark and thick (a disorder called acanthosis nigricans).

Diagnosis

Often, the diagnosis is based on symptoms. Blood tests to measure levels of hormones such as follicle-stimulating hormone and male hormones are done. Ultrasonography is done to see whether the ovaries contain many cysts and to check for a tumor in an ovary or adrenal gland. These tumors can produce excess male hormones and thus cause the same symptoms as polycystic ovary syndrome.

In women with this syndrome, blood pressure and usually blood sugar levels are measured to check for metabolic syndrome. Tests to check Cushing's syndrome are also done. Often, a biopsy of the uterine lining (endometrial biopsy) is done to make sure no cancer is present.

Treatment

The choice of treatment depends on the type and severity of symptoms, the woman's age, and her plans regarding pregnancy.

If insulin levels are high, lowering them may help. Exercising (at least 30 minutes a day) and reducing consumption of carbohydrates (in breads, pasta, potatoes, and sweets) can help lower insulin levels. In some women, weight loss lowers insulin levels enough that ovulation can begin. Weight loss may help reduce hair growth and the risk of thickening of the uterine lining.

Metformin, which is used to treat type 2 diabetes, may be used to increase sensitivity to insulin so the body does not have to make as much insulin. This drug may help women lose weight, and ovulation and menstrual periods may resume. If women take metformin and do not wish to become pregnant, they should use birth control.

If women wish to become pregnant, losing weight may help. If not, clomiphene is tried. This drug stimulates ovulation. If clomiphene is ineffective and the woman has insulin resistance, metformin may help because lowering insulin levels may trigger ovulation. If these drugs are not effective, other fertility drugs may be tried. They include follicle-stimulating hormone (to stimulate the ovaries), a gonadotropin-releasing hormone agonist (to stimulate the release of follicle-stimulating hormone), and human chorionic gonadotropin (to trigger ovulation).

Women who do not wish to become pregnant may take a progestin by mouth or a combination oral contraceptive (a birth control pill that contains estrogen and a progestin). Either treatment may reduce the risk of endometrial cancer due to the high estrogen level and help lower the levels of male hormones. However, oral contraceptives are not given to women who have reached menopause or who have other significant risk factors for heart or blood vessel disorders.

Increased body hair can be bleached or removed by electrolysis, plucking, waxing, hair-removing liquids or creams (depilatories), or laser. No drug treatment for removing excess hair is ideal or completely effective. The following may help:

- Eflornithine cream may help remove unwanted facial hair.
- Oral contraceptives may help, but they must be taken for several months before any effect, which is often slight, can be seen.
- Spironolactone, a drug that blocks the production and action of male hormones, can reduce the amount of unwanted body hair. Side effects include increased urine production and low blood pressure (sometimes causing fainting). Spironolactone may not be safe for a developing fetus, so sexually active women taking the drug are advised to use effective birth control methods.
- Cyproterone, a strong progestin that blocks the action of male hormones, reduces the amount of unwanted body hair in 50 to 75% of affected women. It is used in many countries but is not approved in the United States.

Gonadotropin-releasing hormone agonists and antagonists are being studied as treatment for unwanted body hair. Both types of drugs inhibit the production of sex hormones by the ovaries. But both can cause bone loss and lead to osteoporosis.

CHAPTER 240 Endometriosis

Endometriosis is a noncancerous disorder in which patches of endometrial tissue—normally occurring only in the lining of the uterus (endometrium)—appear outside the uterus.

- Why endometrial tissue appears outside the uterus is unknown.
- Endometriosis can cause pain and bleeding, particularly before and during menstrual periods, but may cause no symptoms.

- Doctors check for endometrial tissue by inserting a thin viewing tube through a small incision near the navel (laparoscopy).
- Drugs are used to relieve pain and to slow the growth of the misplaced tissue.
- Surgery to remove the tissue may be done but may provide only temporary relief because the tissue may grow back, unless the ovaries are removed as well.

Endometriosis is a chronic disorder that may be painful. Exactly how many women have endometriosis is unknown because it can usually be diagnosed only by directly viewing the endometrial tissue (which requires a surgical procedure). Endometriosis probably affects about 10 to 15% of menstruating women aged 25 to 44. It can also affect teenagers.

Endometriosis sometimes runs in families and is more common among first-degree relatives (mothers, sisters, and children) of women with endometriosis. It is more likely to occur in women who have their first baby after age 30, who have never had a baby, who have short menstrual cycles (less than 27 days), or who have certain structural abnormalities of the uterus. Endometriosis seems to occur less often in women who have had several pregnancies, who use low-dose oral contraceptives, or who exercise regularly (especially if they started before age 15, exercise more than 7 hours a week, or both).

The cause of endometriosis is unclear, but there are several theories:

- Small pieces of the lining of the uterus (endometrium) that are shed during menstruation may flow backward through the fallopian tubes toward the ovaries into the abdominal cavity, rather than flow through the vagina and out of the body with the menstrual period.
- Cells from the endometrium (endometrial cells) may be transported through the blood or lymphatic vessels to another location.
- Cells located outside the uterus may change into endometrial cells.

Common locations of misplaced endometrial tissue (called implants) include the ovaries, the ligaments that support the uterus, the space between the rectum and vagina or cervix, and the fallopian tubes. Less common locations include the outer surface of the small and large intestines, the ureters (tubes leading from the kidneys to the bladder), the bladder, and the vagina. Rarely, endometrial tissue grows on the membranes covering the lungs (pleura), the sac that envelops the heart (pericardium), the vulva, the cervix, or surgical scars in the abdomen.

The misplaced endometrial tissue responds to hormones as normal endometrial tissue does. Thus, it can bleed and cause pain, particularly before and during menstrual periods. The severity of symptoms and the disorder's effects on fertility and on organ function vary greatly from woman to woman.

As the disorder progresses, the misplaced endometrial tissue tends to gradually increase in size. It may also spread to new locations. However, how much tissue is present and how quickly endometriosis progresses vary greatly. The tissue may remain on the surface of structures or may penetrate deeply (invade) and form nodules.

Endometriosis: Misplaced Tissue

In endometriosis, small or large patches of endometrial tissue, which is usually located only in the lining of the uterus (endometrium), appear in other parts of the body. How and why the tissue appears in other locations is unclear. The most common locations include the ovaries, fallopian tubes, and ligaments supporting the uterus. But the misplaced tissue may also appear in other locations in the pelvis and abdomen or, rarely, on the membranes that cover the lungs or heart. The misplaced endometrial tissue can irritate nearby tissues, causing bands of scar tissue (adhesions) to form between structures in the abdomen. The tissue can also block the fallopian tubes, causing infertility.

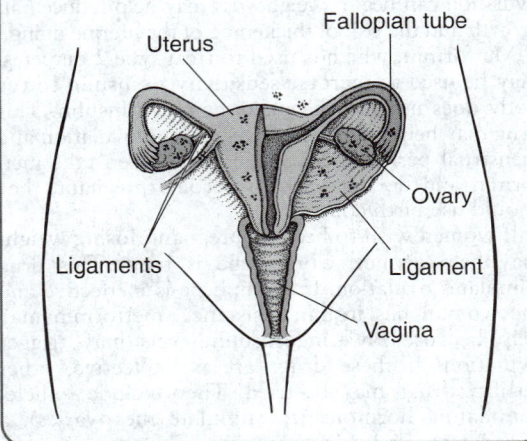

Symptoms

The main symptom is pain in the lower abdomen and pelvic area. The pain usually varies during the menstrual cycle, worsening before and during menstrual periods. Menstrual irregularities, such as heavy menstrual bleeding and spotting before menstrual periods, may occur. Misplaced endometrial tissue responds to the same hormones—estrogen and progesterone (produced by the ovaries)—as normal endometrial tissue in the uterus. Consequently, the misplaced tissue may bleed during menstruation and often causes cramps and pain.

The severity of symptoms does not depend on the amount of misplaced endometrial tissue. Some women with a large amount of tissue have no symptoms. Others, even some with a small amount, have incapacitating pain. In many women, endometriosis does not cause pain until it has been present for several years. For some women, sexual intercourse tends to be painful before or during menstruation.

Endometrial tissue attached to the large intestine may cause abdominal bloating, pain during bowel movements, or diarrhea, constipation, or rectal bleeding during menstruation. If the bladder is affected, women may feel pain above the pubic bone during urination, and urine may contain blood. Endometrial tissue may invade an ovary and form a blood-filled mass (endometrioma). Occasionally, an endometrioma ruptures or leaks, causing sudden, sharp abdominal pain.

The misplaced endometrial tissue and its bleeding may irritate nearby tissues. As a result, scar tissue may form, sometimes as bands of fibrous tissue (adhesions) between structures in the abdomen. The misplaced endometrial tissue and adhesions can interfere with the functioning of organs. Rarely, adhesions block the intestine.

Severe endometriosis may cause infertility when the misplaced tissue blocks the egg's passage from the ovary into the uterus. Mild endometriosis may also cause infertility, but how it does so is less clear. As many as 25 to 50% of infertile women have endometriosis.

During pregnancy, endometriosis may become inactive (go into remission) temporarily or sometimes permanently. Endometriosis tends to become inactive after menopause because estrogen levels decrease.

Diagnosis

A doctor may suspect endometriosis in a woman who has typical symptoms or unexplained infertility. Occasionally, during a pelvic examination, a woman may feel pain or tenderness, or a doctor may feel a mass of tissue behind the uterus or near the ovaries.

If endometriosis is suspected, a doctor examines the abdominal cavity with a thin, flexible viewing tube (called a laparoscope) to check for endometrial tissue. The laparoscope is inserted into the abdominal cavity through a small incision just above or below the navel. Carbon dioxide gas is injected into the abdominal cavity to distend it so that organs can be viewed more easily. The entire abdominal cavity is examined. If abnormal tissue is seen (particularly if the doctor is uncertain that the tissue is endometriosis), a biopsy may be done. A sample of the tissue is removed, using instruments inserted through the laparoscope. The sample is then examined using a microscope. Laparoscopy usually requires a general anesthetic, but an overnight stay in the hospital is usually required only if a very large amount of tissue is removed. Laparoscopy causes mild to moderate abdominal discomfort, but normal activities can usually be resumed in a few days.

Sometimes a biopsy is done during other procedures. A larger incision into the abdomen (laparotomy) may be required. Depending on the location of the misplaced tissue, the biopsy may be done when the vagina is inspected during a pelvic examination or when a flexible viewing tube is used to examine the lower part of the large intestine, rectum, and anus (sigmoidoscopy) or bladder (cystoscopy).

Other procedures may be used to determine the extent of endometriosis and follow its course, but their usefulness for diagnosis is limited. These tests include ultrasonography, x-rays taken after a barium enema, computed tomography (CT), and magnetic resonance imaging (MRI). Sometimes blood tests are done to measure levels of substances that increase when endometriosis is present. These substances (called markers) include cancer antigen 125 and antibodies to endometrial tissue. These markers cannot be used to confirm the diagnosis because they may be increased in several other disorders. Tests may be done to determine whether the endometriosis is affecting the woman's fertility (see page 1590).

Doctors classify endometriosis as minimal (stage I), mild (stage II), moderate (stage III), or severe (stage IV) based on the amount, location, density, and size of misplaced tissue and on the presence of adhesions.

Treatment

Treatment depends on a woman's symptoms, pregnancy plans, and age, as well as the stage of endometriosis.

Drugs: Usually, nonsteroidal anti-inflammatory drugs (NSAIDs—see page 644) are used to relieve pain. They may be all that is needed if symptoms are mild and women do not plan to become pregnant.

Other drugs can be used to suppress the activity of the ovaries and thus slow the growth of the misplaced endometrial tissue and reduce bleeding and pain. However, these drugs may not eliminate endometriosis, and even if they do, endometriosis often recurs after the drugs are stopped unless more radical treatment is used. These drugs include combination oral contraceptives (estrogen plus a progestin), progestins (such as medroxyprogesterone), danazol (a synthetic male hormone, or androgen), and gonadotropin-releasing hormone agonists (GnRH agonists—such as goserelin, leuprolide, and nafarelin).

Oral contraceptives are used primarily in women who do not plan to become pregnant soon. Oral contraceptives may also be used after treatment with danazol or a GnRH agonist. The oral contraceptives can be taken continuously, especially if pain is worse during menstrual periods.

GnRH agonists turn off the brain's signal to the ovaries to produce estrogen and progesterone. As a result, production of these hormones decreases. Continued use of GnRH agonists causes a decrease

℞ DRUGS COMMONLY USED TO TREAT ENDOMETRIOSIS

DRUG	SOME SIDE EFFECTS	COMMENTS
Combination estrogen-progestin oral contraceptives		
Ethinyl estradiol plus a progestin	Abdominal bloating, breast tenderness, increased appetite, ankle swelling, nausea, bleeding between periods (breakthrough bleeding), and deep vein thrombosis Possibly an increased risk of heart attack, stroke, and peripheral vascular disease	Oral contraceptives may be useful for women who wish to delay childbearing. They may be taken 3 weeks a month (cyclically) or every day (continuously).
Progestins		
Medroxyprogesterone acetate	Bleeding between periods, mood swings, depression, and atrophic vaginitis (drying and thinning of the vagina's lining) Possibly an increased risk of heart attack, stroke, and peripheral vascular disease	Progestins are drugs that resemble the hormone progesterone. They can be given by mouth or by injection into a muscle.
Androgen		
Danazol	Weight gain, acne, lowering of the voice, increased body hair, hot flashes, atrophic vaginitis, ankle swelling, muscle cramps, bleeding between periods, decreased breast size, mood swings, liver malfunction, carpal tunnel syndrome, and adverse effects on cholesterol levels in the blood	Danazol, a synthetic hormone related to testosterone, inhibits the activity of estrogen and progesterone. It is taken by mouth. The usefulness of danazol may be limited by its side effects.
GnRH agonists		
Goserelin Leuprolide Nafarelin	Hot flashes, atrophic vaginitis, a decrease in bone density, and mood swings	GnRH agonists may be injected under the skin or into a muscle once a month, used as a nasal spray, or implanted as a pellet under the skin. These drugs are often given with estrogen, a progestin, or both to reduce the effects of decreased estrogen levels, including decreased bone density. (This use of estrogen plus a progestin or of a progestin alone is called add-back therapy.)

GnRH = gonadotropin-releasing hormone.

in bone density and may lead to osteoporosis unless women also take small doses of oral contraceptives (estrogen plus a progestin or a progestin alone) or take a bisphosphonate (such as alendronate, ibandronate, or risedronate). Even when taken this way, GnRH agonists are not usually given for longer than 6 months.

New types of drugs, such as GnRH antagonists, antiprogestins, selective estrogen and progestin receptor modulators, aromatase inhibitors, and immune modulators (which stimulate the immune system) are being studied for the treatment of endometriosis.

Surgery: Surgery beyond diagnostic laparoscopy may be needed in the following situations:

- When patches of endometrial tissue are larger than 1½ to 2 inches (3½ to 5 centimeters) in diameter as observed at laparoscopy
- When adhesions in the lower abdomen or pelvis cause significant symptoms
- When endometrial tissue blocks one or both fallopian tubes
- When drugs cannot relieve severe lower abdominal or pelvic pain
- When endometriomas are present
- When endometriosis causes infertility

Often, misplaced endometrial tissue can be surgically removed during laparoscopy when the diagnosis is made. However, more extensive surgery requiring an incision into the abdomen (laparotomy) may be necessary.

If pain is persistent, the misplaced endometrial tissue may be removed, the nerve pathways that conduct pain sensation from the pelvis to the brain may be interrupted, or both may be done. Sometimes electrocautery (a device that uses an electrical current to produce heat), an argon beam coagulator (a device that uses argon gas to stop bleeding), an ultrasound device, or a laser is used to destroy or remove endometrial tissue during laparoscopic or abdominal surgery.

During surgery, doctors remove as much misplaced endometrial tissue as possible without damaging the ovaries. Thus, the woman's ability to have children may be preserved. Depending on the extent of the endometriosis, 40 to 70% of women who have surgery may become pregnant. If doctors cannot remove all of the tissue, women may be given an oral contraceptive or a GnRH agonist. This drug may increase their chances of becoming pregnant by further reducing the severity of endometriosis. Some women who have endometriosis can become pregnant by using assisted reproductive techniques, such as in vitro fertilization (see page 1592).

Surgical removal of misplaced endometrial tissue is only a temporary measure. After treatment, endometriosis recurs in most women, although the use of oral contraceptives or other drugs may slow its progression. These drugs may be started immediately after surgery.

Removal of both ovaries and the uterus (oophorectomy plus hysterectomy) is appropriate only when drugs do not relieve abdominal or pelvic pain in women who do not plan to become pregnant. Removal of the ovaries and uterus has the same effects as menopause because both result in decreased estrogen levels (see page 1514). Thus, women may be given estrogen to reduce the severity of menopausal symptoms. Most women are also given a progestin. A combination oral contraceptive (estrogen plus a progestin) may be used in young women of premenopausal age. The progestin is included to help suppress the progression of endometriosis. Estrogen may be started after surgery. If a large amount of endometrial tissue remains, estrogen may be delayed 4 to 6 months because it may stimulate growth of the remaining endometrial tissue. The delay gives the endometrial tissue time to decrease in size or disappear. A progestin alone can be given to reduce symptoms and to help remaining endometrial tissue regress.

CHAPTER

241 Fibroids

A fibroid is a noncancerous tumor composed of muscle and fibrous tissue.

- Fibroids can cause pain, vaginal bleeding, constipation, repeated miscarriages, and an urge to urinate frequently or urgently.
- Doctors do a pelvic examination and usually ultrasonography to confirm the diagnosis.
- Treatment is necessary only if fibroids cause problems.
- Usually, surgery or procedures to destroy the fibroids are needed to relieve symptoms or to make childbirth possible.

Fibroids are also called fibromyomas, fibromas, myofibromas, leiomyomas, and myomas.

Fibroids in the uterus are the most common noncancerous tumor of the female reproductive tract. By age 45, about 70% of women develop a fibroid. Many fibroids are small and cause no symptoms. But about one fourth of white women and one half of black women have fibroids that cause symptoms. Fibroids are more common among women who are overweight.

What causes fibroids to grow in the uterus is unknown. High estrogen and progesterone levels seem to stimulate their growth. Thus, fibroids often grow larger during pregnancy and, to a lesser extent, before menopause, and they shrink after menopause. If fibroids grow too large, they may not be able to get enough blood. As a result, they begin to degenerate.

Where Fibroids Grow

Fibroids can grow in the wall of the uterus, into the interior of the uterus (sometimes from a stalk), under the lining of the uterus, or on the outside of the uterus.

Pedunculated
submucosal fibroid

Intramural
fibroid

Pedunculated
subserous fibroid

Submucosal
fibroid

Uterus

Subserous
fibroid

Vagina

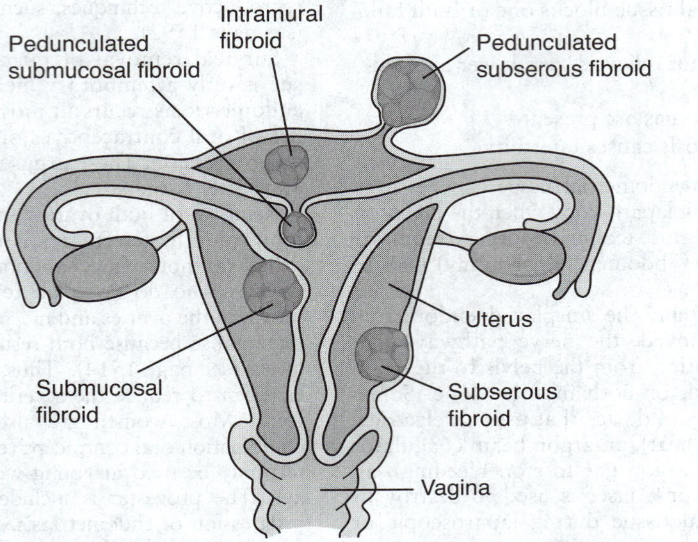

Fibroids may be microscopic or as large as a basketball. They may grow in different parts of the uterus, usually in the wall (which has three layers):

- Within the wall of the uterus (intramural fibroids)
- Just under the inside layer (lining or endometrium) of the uterus (submucosal fibroids)
- On the outside of the uterus (subserous fibroids)

Some fibroids grow from a stalk (called pedunculated fibroids). Fibroids that grow in the wall or just under the endometrium can distort the shape of the interior of the uterus. Usually, more than one fibroid is present.

Symptoms

Symptoms depend on the number of fibroids present, their size, and their location in the uterus. Many fibroids, even large ones, do not cause symptoms. Fibroids, particularly those just under the lining, commonly make menstrual bleeding heavier or last longer than usual. Anemia may result from the loss of blood. Less often, fibroids cause bleeding between menstrual periods, after sexual intercourse, or after menopause.

Large fibroids, particularly those that grow in the wall of the uterus, may cause pain, pressure, or a feeling of heaviness in the pelvic area during or between menstrual periods. Fibroids may press on the bladder, making a woman need to urinate more frequently or more urgently. They may press on the rectum, causing discomfort and constipation. Large fibroids may cause the abdomen to enlarge. A fibroid growing from a stalk inside the uterus may twist and cause severe pain. Fibroids that are growing or degenerating usually cause pressure or pain. Pain due to degenerating fibroids can last as long as they continue to degenerate.

Fibroids that cause no symptoms before pregnancy may cause problems during pregnancy. Problems include miscarriage, early (preterm) labor, abnormal positioning (presentation) of the baby before delivery, and excessive blood loss after delivery (postpartum hemorrhage).

Rarely, fibroids cause infertility by blocking the fallopian tubes or by distorting the shape of the uterus, making attachment to the lining of the uterus (implantation) of a fertilized egg difficult or impossible.

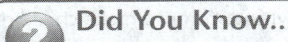
Did You Know...
By age 45, about 7 out of 10 women develop fibroids of the uterus.

Diagnosis

Doctors can often detect fibroids during a pelvic examination. Doctors also use other procedures to examine the uterus and confirm the diagnosis:

- Transvaginal ultrasonography: An ultrasound device is inserted into the vagina.
- Saline infusion sonohysterography: Ultrasonography is done after a small amount of fluid is infused into the uterus to outline its interior.

Sometimes magnetic resonance imaging (MRI) is also done. Occasionally, additional tests are necessary.

If bleeding (other than menstrual) has occurred, doctors may want to exclude cancer of the uterus. So they may do a Papanicolaou (Pap) test, biopsy of the uterine lining (endometrial biopsy), ultrasonography, sonohysterography, or hysteroscopy. For hysteroscopy, a flexible viewing tube is inserted through the vagina and cervix into the uterus. A local, regional, or general anesthetic is used.

Treatment

For most women who have fibroids but no bothersome symptoms or other problems, treatment is not required. They are reexamined every 6 to 12 months to determine whether fibroids are growing.

Several treatment options, including drugs and surgery, are available if bleeding or other symptoms worsen or if fibroids enlarge substantially.

Drugs: A few drugs may be used to relieve symptoms or to shrink fibroids, but their effects are only temporary. No drug can permanently shrink a fibroid.

Synthetic forms of a hormone produced by the body called gonadotropin-releasing hormone (GnRH) are most commonly used. These drugs are called GnRH agonists (see page 1531). Leuprolide and goserelin are most commonly used. They can shrink fibroids and reduce bleeding by causing the body to produce less estrogen (and progesterone). Because they shrink the fibroids and reduce bleeding, doctors may give GnRH agonists before surgery to make removal of fibroids easier, reduce blood loss, and thus reduce the risks of surgery. The drugs are injected once a month, used as a nasal spray, or implanted as a pellet under the skin. If taken for a long time, they may reduce bone density and increase the risk of osteoporosis. Estrogen may be given in low doses with GnRH agonists to help prevent these side effects.

Hormonal contraceptives, usually progestins (see page 1596), can control bleeding in some women. However, when women stop taking contraceptives, abnormal bleeding and pain tend to recur. Also, when some women are treated with contraceptives, the fibroids grow.

Raloxifene and related drugs (such as some selective estrogen receptor modulators, or SERMs) reverse some of estrogen's effects and can reduce fibroid growth.

Surgery: Surgery is usually considered for women who have any of the following:

- Symptoms, such as pain and bleeding, that remain severe enough to interfere with daily activities after other treatments have been tried
- Large fibroids that women can feel and that are bothersome
- For women who want to conceive, fibroids that have caused infertility or repeated miscarriages

Surgery traditionally involves one of the following:

- **Hysterectomy:** The entire uterus is removed, but the ovaries are not. Hysterectomy is the only permanent solution to fibroids. However, after hysterectomy, women cannot have children. Thus, hysterectomy is done only when women do not wish to become pregnant.
- **Myomectomy:** Only the fibroid or fibroids are removed. Unlike hysterectomy, most women who have a myomectomy can have children. Also, some women feel psychologically better if they keep their uterus. However, after myomectomy, new fibroids may grow, and about 25% of women need a hysterectomy about 4 to 8 years later.

For hysterectomy, surgeons may use one of the following methods:

- **Laparotomy:** They may make an incision that is several inches long in the abdomen.
- **Laparoscopy:** They may make one or a few small incisions just below the navel, then insert a viewing tube with surgical attachments through the incision. This procedure can be used to remove the entire uterus. Or only the main body of the uterus is removed, leaving the cervix in place (a procedure called laparoscopic supracervical hysterectomy).
- **Vaginal hysterectomy:** The entire uterus is removed through the vagina. An abdominal incision is not needed.

For myomectomy, surgeons may use laparotomy, laparoscopy (used to remove fibroids on the outer part of the uterus), or hysteroscopy. For hysteroscopy, they insert a telescope-like lighted device through the vagina into the uterus. This device can cut tissue and remove fibroids on the inside of the uterus. Which method is used depends on the size, number, and location of fibroids. Laparoscopy and hysteroscopy are outpatient procedures, and recovery is faster than recovery after an abdominal incision. However, laparoscopy often cannot be used to remove large fibroids, and the risk of complications after laparoscopy can be higher.

Other Treatments: Other treatments can be used to destroy rather than remove fibroids.

For **uterine artery embolization**, doctors use an anesthetic to numb a small area of the thigh and make a small puncture hole or incision there. Then, they insert a thin, flexible tube (catheter) through the incision into the main artery of the thigh (femoral artery). The catheter is threaded to the arteries that supply blood to the fibroid, and small synthetic particles are injected. The particles travel to the small arteries supplying the fibroid and block them. As a result, the fibroid dies, then shrinks. Most of the rest of the uterus appears to be unaffected. However, whether the fibroid will regrow (because blocked arteries reopen or new arteries form) and whether the woman can become pregnant are unknown. The most common problems after this procedure are pain and infection.

Other procedures to destroy fibroids involve heat (high-intensity focused ultrasonography or radiofrequency ablation) or cold (cryoablation) via needle insertion, ultrasonography, or both. In myolysis, a needle that transmits an electrical current or heat is inserted into the fibroid and used to destroy the core of the fibroid. In cryomyolysis (a type of cryoablation), a similar procedure, a cold probe is used to destroy the fibroid. Whether women who have one of these procedures can become pregnant is unknown.

After these treatments, fibroids may grow back. In such cases, another treatment or a hysterectomy may be done.

CHAPTER

242 Vaginal Infections

- Vaginal infections are caused by microorganisms, but women can take precautions, such as wearing loose, absorbent underwear, to reduce their risk of getting infections.

- Infections usually cause a discharge with itching, redness, and sometimes burning and soreness.

- Doctors examine a sample of fluids from the vagina or cervix to check for microorganisms that can cause infections.

- Treatment depends on the cause, but a sitz bath and antihistamines taken by mouth can help relieve itching.

In the United States, vaginal infections are one of the most common reasons women see their doctor, accounting for more than 10 million visits each year. Vaginal infections can cause discomfort, discharge, and vaginal odor. However, these symptoms do not necessarily indicate an infection. Instead, they may result from irritation of the vagina by chemicals or other materials such as hygiene products, bubble bath, laundry detergents, contraceptive foams and jellies, and synthetic underwear. The inflammation that results is called noninfectious vaginitis.

> **? Did You Know...**
>
> Children may get a vaginal infection when they move bacteria from the anus to the vagina by wiping from back to front.

Vaginal discharge may not be caused by a vaginal infection. A discharge can result from certain sexually transmitted diseases such as chlamydial infection (see page 1266) or gonorrhea (see page 1269). These diseases affect other reproductive organs, such as the cervix or uterus. Genital herpes (see page 1245), which can cause blisters on the vulva, in the vagina, and on the cervix, can also cause a vaginal discharge.

Causes

Vaginal infections may be caused by bacteria, yeast, and other microorganisms.

Certain conditions make infection more likely:

- **Reduced acidity (increased pH) in the vagina:** When acidity in the vagina is reduced, the number of protective bacteria that normally live in the vagina decreases, and the number of bacteria that can cause infection increases (see page 1539).

- **Poor hygiene:** When the genital area is not kept clean, the number of bacteria increases, making bacterial infections more likely.

- **Tight, nonabsorbent underwear:** This type of underwear may trap moisture, which encourages the growth of bacteria and yeast.

- **Tissue damage:** If tissues in the pelvis are damaged, the body's natural defenses are weakened. Damage can result from tumors, surgery, radiation therapy, or structural abnormalities such as birth defects or fistulas. Fistulas are abnormal connections between

SOME VAGINAL INFECTIONS

INFECTION	SYMPTOMS	COMPLICATIONS	TREATMENT
Bacterial vaginosis	A thin, white or gray cloudy discharge with a fishy odor, which may become stronger after sexual intercourse or during menstrual periods Itching and irritation	Pelvic inflammatory disease Infection of the membranes around the fetus Infections of the uterus after delivery of a baby or after an abortion Preterm labor and delivery	Clindamycin Metronidazole Tinidazole
Trichomonas vaginitis	A usually profuse, greenish yellow, frothy, fishy-smelling discharge Itching and soreness Pain during sexual intercourse and urination	Pelvic inflammatory disease Preterm labor and delivery	Metronidazole Tinidazole
Yeast infection (candidiasis)	Thick, white, clumpy discharge (like cottage cheese) Moderate to severe itching and burning (but not always) Redness and swelling of the genital area	No serious complications	Butoconazole Clotrimazole Fluconazole Miconazole Terconazole Tioconazole

organs, which may, for example, allow the intestine's contents to enter the vagina.

- **Irritation:** Irritation of vaginal tissues can lead to cracks or sores, which provide access to the bloodstream for bacteria and yeast.

Some specific causes of infection are more common among certain age groups.

Children: In children, vaginal infections are usually caused by bacteria from the anus. These bacteria may be moved to the vagina when girls, particularly those aged 2 to 6 years, wipe from back to front or do not adequately clean the genital area after bowel movements. Fingering the genital area, particularly if girls do not wash their hands after bowel movements, may also move these bacteria to the vagina. Fingering is often a response to itching.

Putting an object (such as a toy or toilet tissue) in the vagina is another common cause of vaginal infections. Pinworms may also cause vaginal infections.

Women of Reproductive Age: Hormonal changes shortly before and during menstrual periods or during pregnancy can reduce acidity in the vagina, as can frequent douching, use of spermicides, and semen. Reduced acidity encourages the growth of bacteria that cause disease.

Leaving tampons in too long can lead to infection, possibly because tampons provide a warm, moist environment where bacteria can thrive and because they can irritate the vagina.

Postmenopausal Women: After menopause, estrogen levels decrease. As a result, tissues in the vagina become thinner, drier, and more fragile. Cracks or sores may form, providing access for bacteria or yeast. Also, acidity in the vagina decreases.

Women who have urinary incontinence or are confined to bed may have difficulty keeping the genital area clean. Irritation from urine and stool can lead to infection.

> **? Did You Know...**
> Douching often can remove normal, protective bacteria from the vagina, increasing the risk of infection.

Symptoms

Typically, vaginal infections produce a vaginal discharge. This discharge differs from a normal one because it is accompanied by itching, redness, and sometimes burning or soreness in the genital area. A discharge may have a fishy odor. The appearance and amount of the discharge tend to vary depending on the cause. However, different disorders sometimes cause similar discharges.

Nearby Infections: Vulvitis and Bartholinitis

The vulva is the area surrounding the opening of the vagina and containing the external female genital organs. Bartholin's glands, which are external genital organs, are located on either side of the opening of the vagina.

Vulvitis: Vulvitis is inflammation of the vulva. When both the vulva and vagina are inflamed, the disorder is called vulvovaginitis. Vulvitis may result from allergic reactions to substances that come in contact with the vulva (such as soaps, bubble bath, fabrics, and perfumes), from skin disorders (such as dermatitis), or from infections, including yeast infections and sexually transmitted diseases (such as herpes). The vulva may be infested by pubic lice—a disorder called pediculosis pubis.

In children, infections of the vagina may also affect the vulva. These infections may be due to bacteria from the anus or other bacteria.

Urine or stool, if it remains in contact with the vulva, can irritate it and cause ongoing (chronic) vulvitis. Women who have incontinence or are confined to bed may have this problem.

Vulvitis causes itching, soreness, and redness. Rarely, the folds of skin around the vaginal and urethral openings (labia) become stuck together. Chronic vulvitis may result in sore, scaly, thickened, or whitish patches on the vulva. If chronic vulvitis does not respond to treatment, doctors usually do a biopsy to look for the cause, including skin disorders of the vulva (vulvar dystrophies, such as lichen sclerosus or squamous cell hyperplasia) or cancer.

Bartholinitis: Bartholinitis—infection of one or both glands or their ducts—may develop when bacteria from the vagina enter the glands. Rarely, bartholinitis is due to a sexually transmitted disease. Pus can accumulate in the gland, causing a painful, swollen abscess.

If the ducts to the gland become blocked, the gland may swell without causing pain—a disorder called Bartholin's cyst. A cyst may become infected.

Doctors can diagnose Bartholin's cyst and bartholinitis during a physical examination. In women 40 and older, a cyst is usually biopsied.

Cysts that cause no symptoms do not require treatment. Infections are treated with an antibiotic, which usually clears the infection in a few days if there is no abscess. However, the infection may recur. Analgesics may be taken to relieve pain.

Abscesses are usually drained.

Itching may interfere with sleep. Some infections can make sexual intercourse painful and make urination painful and more frequent. Rarely, the folds of skin around the vaginal and urethral openings become stuck together. However, sometimes symptoms are mild or do not occur.

Diagnosis

Girls or women who have a vaginal discharge with itching or who have other vaginal symptoms should see a doctor. To determine the cause, the doctor asks questions about the discharge (if present), about possible causes of the symptoms, and about hygiene. Questions may include the following:

- Have lotions or creams (including home remedies) been used to try to relieve the symptoms?
- When did the discharge begin?
- Was the discharge accompanied by itching, burning, pain, or a sore in the genital area?
- When do symptoms occur in relation to the menstrual period?
- Does the discharge come and go, or is it always present?
- Has an abnormal discharge occurred before, and if so, how did it respond to treatment?
- What kind of birth control has been and is being used?
- Is pain felt during sexual intercourse?
- Has the woman had previous vaginal infections?
- Does the sex partner have symptoms?

The doctor also asks about the possibility of sexually transmitted diseases. This information helps the doctor determine whether other people require treatment.

A pelvic examination is done. While examining the vagina, the doctor takes a sample of the discharge (if present) with a cotton-tipped swab. The sample is examined under a microscope. With this information, the doctor can usually determine whether the cause is bacterial vaginosis, trichomonas vaginitis, or a yeast infection. Usually, the doctor also uses a swab to take a sample of fluid from the cervix. The sample is tested for sexually transmitted diseases.

To determine whether there are other infections in the pelvis, the doctor checks the uterus and ovaries by inserting the index and middle fingers of one gloved hand into the vagina and pressing on the outside of the lower abdomen with the other hand. If this maneuver causes substantial pain or if a fever is present, other infections may be present.

Prevention

Keeping the genital area clean and dry can help prevent infections. Washing every day with a mild, nonscented soap (such as glycerin soap) and rinsing and drying thoroughly are recommended. Wiping from front to back after urinating or defecating prevents bacteria from the anus from being moved to the vagina. Young girls should be taught good hygiene.

Wearing loose, absorbent clothing, such as cotton or cotton-lined underpants, allows air to circulate and helps keep the genital area dry. Douching frequently and using medicated douches are discouraged. Douching can remove normal, protective bacteria from the vagina and reduce the acidity of the vagina, making infections, including pelvic inflammatory disease, more likely. Practicing sex safe and limiting the number of sex partners are important preventive measures.

Treatment

Measures used for prevention, such as keeping the genital area clean and dry, also help treat infections. Strong or scented soaps and unnecessary topical products (such as feminine hygiene sprays) should be avoided. Occasionally placing ice packs on the genital area, applying cool compresses, or sitting in a cool sitz bath (with or without baking soda or Epsom salts) may reduce soreness and itching. A sitz bath is taken in the sitting position with the water covering only the genital and rectal area. Flushing the genital area with lukewarm water squeezed from a water bottle may also provide relief.

If these measures do not relieve symptoms, drugs may be needed. For itching, a corticosteroid cream (such as hydrocortisone) can sometimes be applied to the vulva but not in the vagina. Antihistamines taken by mouth help relieve itching. They also cause drowsiness and may be useful if symptoms interfere with sleep.

Specific treatment depends on the cause.

Bacterial Vaginosis

Bacterial vaginosis is a vaginal infection that occurs when the balance of bacteria in the vagina is altered.

- Women who have a sexually transmitted disease, who have several sex partners, or who use an intrauterine device are more likely to get bacterial vaginosis.
- The thin, gray or white discharge may be profuse, smell fishy, and be accompanied by itching.
- Antibiotics applied as gels or creams or taken by mouth are effective.
- Bacterial vaginosis commonly recurs.

Causes

Many bacteria normally reside in the vagina. One type, called lactobacilli, maintains the normal acidity of the vagina. By doing so, lactobacilli help keep the lining of the vagina healthy and prevent the growth of certain bacteria that cause infections. Bacterial vaginosis, the most common vaginal infection, re-

sults when the number of protective lactobacilli decreases and the number of other bacteria that are normally present (such as *Gardnerella vaginalis* and *Peptostreptococcus* species) increases. Why these changes occur and whether the disorder is sexually transmitted are unknown. What is known is that bacterial vaginosis is more common among women who have a sexually transmitted disease, who have several sex partners, or who use an intrauterine device (IUD).

Symptoms

The vaginal discharge may be gray or white, thin, itchy, and profuse. Usually, the discharge has a fishy odor. The odor may become stronger after sexual intercourse and during menstrual periods.

The infection can lead to serious complications, such as pelvic inflammatory disease and, for pregnant women, infection of the membranes around the fetus, preterm labor and delivery, and infections of the uterus after delivery or after an abortion.

 Did You Know...

Some antibiotic creams used to treat vaginosis weaken latex condoms and diaphragms.

Treatment

Bacterial vaginosis is treated with an antibiotic (such as metronidazole or clindamycin) applied as a vaginal gel or cream. Metronidazole or tinidazole taken by mouth is also effective but may have bodywide side effects. Women who use clindamycin cream cannot rely on latex products (condoms or diaphragms) for birth control because the drug weakens latex.

Bacterial vaginosis usually resolves in a few days but commonly recurs. If it recurs often, antibiotics may have to be taken for a long time.

Trichomonas Vaginitis

Trichomonas vaginitis is a vaginal infection due to the protozoa Trichomonas vaginalis.

- The infection is usually sexually transmitted.
- The green or yellow discharge may be profuse, smell fishy, and be accompanied by itching.
- Always using a condom can prevent this infection.
- One dose of metronidazole or tinidazole taken by mouth cures most women.

The protozoa *Trichomonas vaginalis* can cause symptoms soon after they enter the vagina, or they can remain in the vagina or on the cervix for weeks or months without causing any symptoms. The bladder may also be infected. In men, the protozoa usually remain for only for a few days or weeks and may cause no symptoms.

Causes

Trichomonas genital infections (trichomoniasis—see page 1273) are almost always sexually transmitted. Women can be infected through sexual contact with men or women. But men can be infected through sexual contact only with women, not with men. Many people who have this infection have other sexually transmitted diseases. Because the protozoa can remain in women for a long time without causing symptoms, determining when the infection was acquired and thus from whom can be difficult or impossible.

This infection may occur in children. If it does, the cause may be sexual abuse.

Symptoms

Women may have a green or yellow vaginal discharge that is sometimes frothy, profuse, or both. It may smell fishy. The genital area may itch, and the vagina may be red and tender. As a result, sexual intercourse may be painful. Urination may also be painful if the bladder becomes infected.

The infection can lead to pelvic inflammatory disease and, in pregnant women, preterm labor and delivery.

Prevention and Treatment

Always using a condom during sexual intercourse can help prevent this infection from being transmitted.

A single dose of metronidazole or tinidazole taken by mouth cures up to 95% of women. Sex partners should be treated at the same time. People should not drink alcohol for at least 72 hours after they take metronidazole or tinidazole. Drinking alcohol while taking either drug can cause nausea, vomiting, cramps, flushing, and headaches.

During sexual intercourse, condoms should be used until the infection resolves to prevent transmission of the infection.

Yeast Infection

- The vagina may be infected by a yeast called *Candida*, usually *Candida albicans*, resulting in a yeast infection called candidiasis. Being pregnant or overweight or having diabetes or a weakened immune system increases the risk of yeast infections.
- The vagina and vulva itch, and women often have a thick, white, discharge resembling cottage cheese.

- Antifungal drugs—creams, vaginal suppositories, tablets, or capsules—are effective.

Causes

In women of reproductive age, yeast infections due to *Candida albicans* are particularly common. This yeast normally resides on the skin or in the intestine. From these areas, it can spread to the vagina. Yeast infections are not transmitted sexually. They are common among pregnant women, overweight women, and women who have diabetes. Yeast infections are more likely to occur just before menstrual periods. Yeast infections are also more likely to develop if the immune system is weakened—suppressed by drugs (such as corticosteroids or chemotherapy drugs) or impaired by a disorder (such as AIDS).

Antibiotics taken by mouth tend to kill the bacteria that normally reside in the vagina and that prevent yeast from growing. Thus, using antibiotics increases the risk of developing a yeast infection.

After menopause, yeast infections are uncommon except in women who take hormone therapy.

Symptoms

The vagina and vulva may itch or burn, particularly during intercourse. The genital area may become red and swollen. Women may have a white discharge, often thick and resembling cottage cheese. Symptoms may worsen the week before a menstrual period begins.

 Did You Know...

Yeast infections are not sexually transmitted.

Taking antibiotics increases the risk of yeast infections.

Prevention

Women who are at high risk of a yeast infection may need to take an antifungal drug by mouth to help prevent yeast infections. Such women include those with the following:

- A weakened immune system
- Diabetes
- A need to take antibiotics for a long time
- Repeated yeast infections

Treatment

Yeast infections are treated with antifungal drugs. They may be applied as a cream to the affected area, inserted into the vagina as a suppository, or taken

℞ DRUGS USED TO TREAT VAGINAL YEAST INFECTIONS

DRUG	DOSAGE
Creams or gels, available without a prescription	
Butoconazole	Applied as a cream once a day for 3 days
	Also available as a sustained-release cream that is applied once
Clotrimazole	Applied as a cream once a day for 7 to 14 days
	Also available as a vaginal tablet inserted once a day for 7 days or for 3 days or inserted only once, depending on the dose (number of milligrams per tablet)
Miconazole	Applied as a cream once a day for 7 days
	Also available as a vaginal suppository inserted once a day for 7 days or for 3 days, depending on the dose
Tioconazole	Applied as an ointment only once
Drugs taken by mouth, available by prescription	
Fluconazole	One tablet taken only once
Itraconazole	Available as a capsule, once or twice a day for up to 6 months

by mouth. Butoconazole, clotrimazole, miconazole, and tioconazole are available without a prescription. Oils in these creams and ointments weaken latex-based condoms (but not diaphragms), so women cannot rely on condoms for birth control.

Antifungal drugs (such as fluconazole and itraconazole) taken by mouth require a prescription. A single dose of fluconazole is as effective as the creams and ointments. However, if infections recur often, women may need to take several doses.

CHAPTER 243 Pelvic Inflammatory Disease

Pelvic inflammatory disease is an infection of the upper female reproductive organs.

- The infection is usually transmitted during sexual intercourse with an infected partner.
- Typically, women have pain in the lower abdomen, a vaginal discharge, and irregular vaginal bleeding.
- The diagnosis is based on symptoms, analysis of secretions from the cervix and vagina, and sometimes ultrasonography.
- Having sexual intercourse with only one partner and using barrier contraceptives (such as condoms) with spermicides reduces the risk of infection.
- Antibiotics can eliminate the infection.

Pelvic inflammatory disease may be an infection of the lining of the uterus (endometritis), the fallopian tubes (salpingitis), or both. If the infection is severe, it can spread to the ovaries (oophoritis) or produce a collection of pus in the fallopian tubes (tubo-ovarian abscess).

Pelvic inflammatory disease is the most common preventable cause of infertility in the United States. Infertility occurs in about one of five women with pelvic inflammatory disease. About one third of women who have had pelvic inflammatory disease develop the infection again.

Pelvic inflammatory disease usually occurs in sexually active women. It rarely affects girls before their first menstrual period (menarche) or women during pregnancy or after menopause. Risk is increased for the following women:

- Those who are younger than 24
- Those who do not use a barrier contraceptive (such as a condom or diaphragm)

- Those who have many sex partners
- Those who have a sexually transmitted disease or bacterial vaginosis
- Those who have had pelvic inflammatory disease before
- Those of lower socioeconomic status (who usually have less access to health care)

Causes

Pelvic inflammatory disease is usually caused by bacteria from the vagina. Most commonly, the bacteria are transmitted during sexual intercourse with a partner who has a sexually transmitted disease. These sexually transmitted bacteria are those that cause gonorrhea (*Neisseria gonorrhoeae*—see page 1269) or chlamydial infection (*Chlamydia trachomatis*—see page 1266). Gonorrhea and chlamydial infection typically spread from the vagina to the cervix, where they cause infection (cervicitis). These infections may remain in the cervix or spread upward, causing pelvic inflammatory disease.

Pelvic inflammatory disease is also commonly caused by the bacteria that cause bacterial vaginosis (see page 1539). These bacteria normally reside in the vagina. They cause symptoms and spread to other organs only if they increase in number (overgrow). They are not sexually transmitted.

Less commonly, women are infected during a vaginal delivery (see page 1670), an abortion, or a medical procedure, such as dilation and curettage (D and C) or gynecologic surgery—when bacteria are introduced into the vagina or when bacteria that normally reside in the vagina are moved into the uterus. Whether douching increases the risk of infection is unclear.

> **? Did You Know...**
>
> The most common preventable cause of infertility is pelvic inflammatory disease.

Symptoms

Symptoms commonly occur toward the end of the menstrual period or during the few days after it. For many women, the first symptom is mild to moderate pain (often aching) in the lower abdomen, which may be worse on one side. Other symptoms include irregular vaginal bleeding and a vaginal discharge, sometimes with a bad odor. As the infection spreads, pain in the lower abdomen becomes increasingly severe and may be accompanied by a low-grade fever (usually below 102° F [38.9° C]) and nausea or vomiting. Later, the fever may become higher, and the discharge often becomes puslike and yellow-green. Women may have pain during sexual intercourse or urination. The infection may be severe but cause mild or no symptoms. Symptoms due to gonorrhea tend to be more severe than those of a chlamydial infection, which may not cause a discharge or any other noticeable symptoms.

Sometimes infected fallopian tubes become blocked. Blocked tubes may swell because fluid is trapped. Women may feel pressure or have chronic pain in the lower abdomen.

The infection can spread to surrounding structures, including the membrane that lines the abdominal cavity and covers the abdominal organs (causing peritonitis). Peritonitis can cause sudden or gradual severe pain in the entire abdomen.

If infection of the fallopian tubes is due to gonorrhea or a chlamydial infection, it may spread to the tissues around the liver. Such an infection may cause pain in the upper right side of the abdomen. The pain resembles that of a gallbladder disorder or stones. This complication is called the Fitz-Hugh-Curtis syndrome.

An abscess forms in the fallopian tubes or ovaries of about 15% of women who have infected fallopian tubes, particularly if they have had the infection a long time. An abscess sometimes ruptures, and pus spills into the pelvic cavity (causing peritonitis). A rupture causes severe pain in the lower abdomen, quickly followed by nausea, vomiting, and very low blood pressure (shock). The infection may spread to the bloodstream (a condition called sepsis) and can be fatal.

Pelvic inflammatory disease often produces a pus-like fluid, which can result in formation of abnormal bands of scar tissue (adhesions) in the reproductive organs or between organs in the abdomen. Infertility and chronic pelvic pain may result. The longer and more severe the inflammation and the more often it recurs, the higher the risk of infertility and other complications. The risk increases each time a woman develops the infection.

Women who have had pelvic inflammatory disease are 6 to 10 times more likely to have a tubal pregnancy, in which the fetus grows in a fallopian tube rather than in the uterus. This type of pregnancy threatens the life of the woman, and the fetus cannot survive.

Diagnosis

Doctors suspect the disease if women have pain in the lower abdomen or if they have an unexplained discharge from the vagina, particularly if they are of reproductive age. A physical examination, including a pelvic examination, is done. Pain felt in the pelvic area during the pelvic examination supports the diagnosis.

Vaginal secretions may be checked for white blood cells. If the secretions do not contain white blood cells, pelvic inflammatory disease is unlikely. A sample of fluid (swab) is usually taken from the cervix and tested to determine whether the woman has gonorrhea or a chlamydial infection. A pregnancy test is done to see whether the woman may have a tubal pregnancy, which could be the cause of the symptoms. Other symptoms and laboratory test results help confirm the diagnosis. The white blood cell count in a sample of blood may be determined. It may be high.

Ultrasonography of the pelvis is done if pain prevents an adequate physical examination or if more information is needed. It can detect abscesses in the fallopian tubes or ovaries and a tubal pregnancy. If the diagnosis is still uncertain or if the woman does not respond to treatment, the doctor may insert a viewing tube (laparoscope) through a small incision near the navel to view the inside of the abdominal cavity and to obtain a sample of fluids for testing.

Prevention

Prevention of pelvic inflammatory disease is essential to the health and fertility of a woman. The only foolproof way to prevent the infection is abstaining from sex. However, if a woman has sexual intercourse with only one partner, the risk of pelvic inflammatory disease is very low, as long as neither person is infected with the bacteria that cause sexually transmitted diseases.

Barrier methods of birth control (such as condoms) and spermicides (such as vaginal foams) used with a barrier method can help prevent pelvic inflammatory disease.

Treatment

As soon as possible, antibiotics for gonorrhea and chlamydial infection are usually given by mouth or by injection into a muscle. If needed, the antibiotics are changed after test results are available. Most women are treated at home. However, hospitalization is usually necessary in the following situations:

- The infection does not lessen within 48 hours.
- Symptoms are severe.
- The woman may be pregnant.
- An abscess is detected.

In the hospital, antibiotics are given intravenously.

Abscesses that persist despite treatment with antibiotics may be drained. Often, a needle can be used. It is inserted through a small incision in the skin, and an imaging test, such as ultrasonography or computed tomography (CT), is used to guide the needle into the abscess. A ruptured abscess requires emergency surgery.

Women should refrain from sexual intercourse until antibiotic therapy is completed and a doctor confirms that the infection is completely eliminated, even if symptoms disappear. All recent sex partners should be tested for gonorrhea and chlamydial infection and treated. If pelvic inflammatory disease is diagnosed and treated promptly, a full recovery is more likely.

244 Pelvic Floor Disorders

Pelvic floor (pelvic support) disorders involve a dropping down (prolapse) of the bladder, urethra, small intestine, rectum, uterus, or vagina caused by weakness of or injury to the ligaments, connective tissue, and muscles of the pelvis.

- Women may feel pressure or a sense of fullness in the pelvis or have problems with urination or bowel movements.
- A pelvic examination is done while a woman bears down to make abnormalities more obvious.
- Pelvic muscle exercises and pessaries may help, but surgery may be needed.

Pelvic floor disorders occur only in women and become more common as women age. About 1 of 11 women needs surgery for a pelvic floor disorder during her lifetime.

The pelvic floor is a network of muscles, ligaments, and tissues that act like a hammock to support the organs of the pelvis: the uterus, vagina, bladder, urethra, and rectum. If the muscles become weak or the

> ### ? Did You Know...
> During their lifetime, about 1 of 11 women needs surgery to repair a pelvic floor disorder.

ligaments or tissues are stretched or damaged, the pelvic organs or small intestine may drop down and protrude into the vagina. If the disorder is severe, the organs may protrude all the way through the opening of the vagina and outside the body.

Pelvic floor disorders usually result from a combination of factors. Being pregnant and having a vaginal delivery may weaken or stretch some of the supporting structures in the pelvis. Pelvic floor disorders are more common among women who have had several vaginal deliveries, and the risk increases with each delivery. The delivery itself may damage nerves, leading to muscle weakness. The

When the Bottom Falls Out: Prolapse in the Pelvis

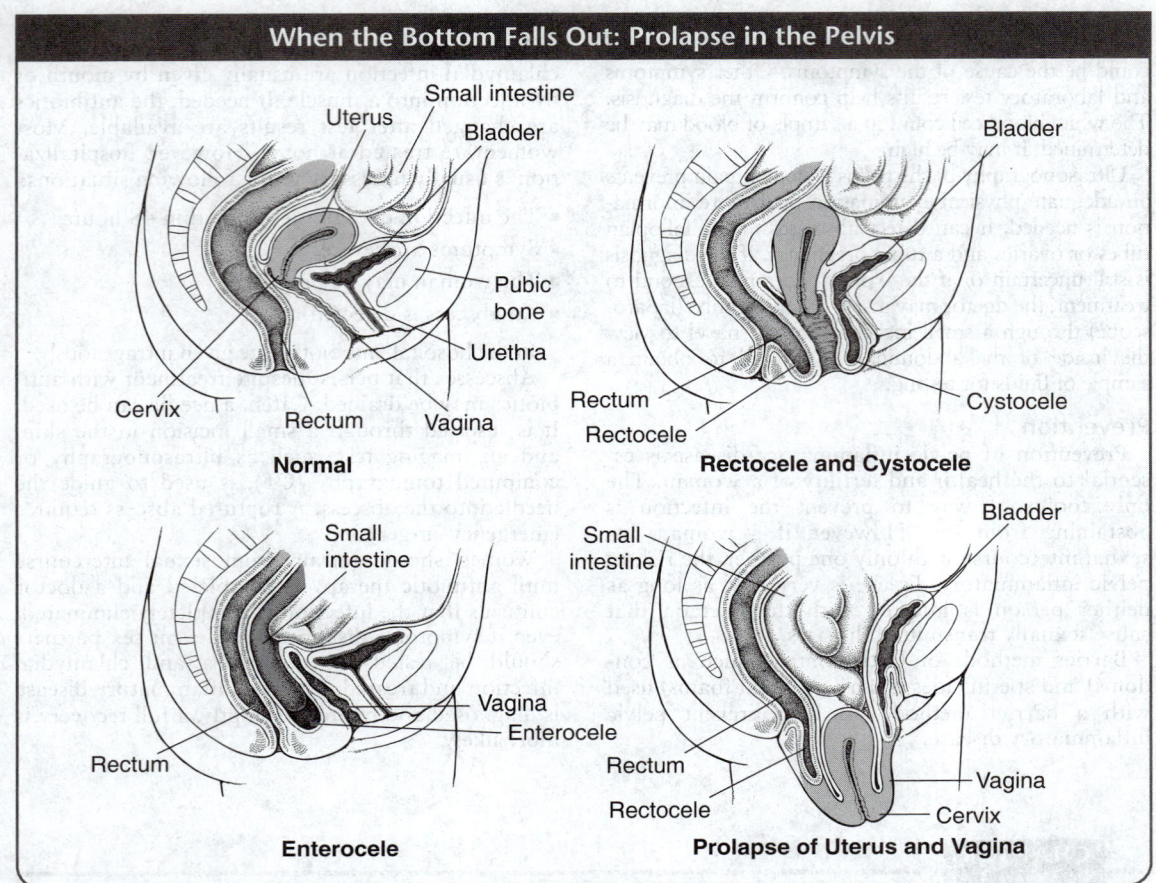

Normal

Uterus
Small intestine
Bladder
Pubic bone
Urethra
Cervix
Rectum
Vagina

Rectocele and Cystocele

Bladder
Rectum
Rectocele
Cystocele

Enterocele

Small intestine
Vagina
Enterocele
Rectum

Prolapse of Uterus and Vagina

Bladder
Small intestine
Rectum
Rectocele
Vagina
Cervix

risk of developing a pelvic floor may be less with a cesarean delivery than with a vaginal delivery.

Obesity, chronic coughing (for example, due to a lung disorder or smoking), frequent straining during bowel movements, and heavy lifting can also contribute to pelvic floor disorders. Other causes include disorders of nerves to the pelvic floor, injuries (including those due to surgery), and tumors. Some women have birth defects that affect this area or are born with weak pelvic tissues. As women age, the supporting structures in the pelvis may weaken, making pelvic floor disorders more likely to develop.

Types and Symptoms

All pelvic floor disorders are essentially hernias, in which organs protrude abnormally because supporting tissue is weakened. The different types of pelvic floor disorders are named according to the organ affected. Often, a woman has more than one type. In all types, the most common symptom is a feeling of heaviness or pressure in the area of the vagina—a feeling that the uterus, bladder, or rectum is dropping out.

Symptoms tend to occur when women are upright, straining, or coughing and to disappear when they are lying down and relaxing. For some women, sexual intercourse is painful. Mild cases may not cause symptoms until the woman becomes older.

Rectocele: A rectocele develops when the rectum drops down and protrudes into the back wall of the vagina. It results from weakening of the muscular wall of the rectum and the connective tissue around the rectum. A rectocele can make having a bowel movement difficult and may cause a sensation of constipation. Some women need to place a finger in the vagina and press against the rectum to have a bowel movement.

Enterocele: An enterocele develops when the small intestine and the lining of the abdominal cavity (peritoneum) bulge downward between the vagina and the rectum. It occurs most often after the uterus has been surgically removed. An enterocele results from weakening of the connective tissue and ligaments supporting the uterus. An enterocele often causes no symptoms. But some women feel a sense of fullness or pressure or pain in the pelvis. Pain may also be felt in the lower back.

Cystocele and Cystourethrocele: A cystocele develops when the bladder drops down and protrudes into the front wall of the vagina. It results from weakening of the connective tissue and supporting structures around the bladder. A cystourethrocele is similar but develops when the upper part of the urethra (bladder neck) also drops down. Women with either of these disorders may have stress incontinence (passage of urine during coughing, laughing, or any other maneuver that suddenly increases pressure within the abdomen) or overflow incontinence (passage of urine when the bladder becomes too full). After urination, the bladder may not feel completely empty. Sometimes a urinary tract infection develops. Because the nerves to the bladder or urethra can be damaged, women who have these disorders may develop urge incontinence (an intense, irrepressible urge to urinate, resulting in the passage of urine).

Prolapse of the Uterus: In prolapse of the uterus, the uterus drops down into the vagina. It usually results from weakening of the connective tissue and ligaments supporting the uterus. The uterus may bulge only into the upper part of the vagina, into the middle part, or all the way through the opening of the vagina, resulting in total uterine prolapse (procidentia). Prolapse of the uterus may cause pain in the lower back or over the tailbone, although many women have no symptoms. Total uterine prolapse can cause pain during walking. Sores may develop on the protruding cervix and cause bleeding, a discharge, and infection. Prolapse of the uterus may cause a kink in the urethra. A kink may hide urinary incontinence if present or make urinating difficult. Women with total uterine prolapse may also have difficulty having a bowel movement.

Prolapse of the Vagina: In prolapse of the vagina, the upper part of the vagina drops down into the lower part, so that the vagina turns inside out. The upper part may drop part way through the vagina or all the way through, protruding outside the body and causing total vaginal prolapse. Prolapse of the vagina occurs only in women who have had a hysterectomy. Total vaginal prolapse may cause pain while sitting or walking. Sores may develop on the protruding vagina and cause bleeding and a discharge. Prolapse of the vagina may cause a compelling or frequent need to urinate. Or it may cause a kink in the urethra. A kink may hide urinary incontinence if present or make urinating difficult. Having a bowel movement may also be difficult.

Diagnosis

Doctors can usually diagnose pelvic floor disorders by doing a pelvic examination with a speculum (an instrument that spreads the walls of the vagina apart). A doctor may insert one finger in the vagina and one finger in the rectum at the same time to determine how severe a rectocele or enterocele is.

A woman may be asked to bear down (as when having a bowel movement) or to cough. She may be examined while standing. The resulting pressure in the pelvis from coughing, standing, or both may make a pelvic floor disorder more obvious.

Procedures to determine how well the bladder and rectum are functioning may be done. For example, doctors often measure the amount of urine that the bladder can hold without leaking, the amount of urine left in the bladder after urination, and the rate of urine flow. If a woman has a problem with the passage of urine or urinary incontinence, doctors may use a flexible viewing tube to view the inside of the bladder (a procedure called cystoscopy) or the urethra (a procedure called urethroscopy). These procedures help doctors determine whether drugs or surgery is the best treatment. If the bladder is not functioning well, women are more likely to need surgery.

Treatment

Exercises: If prolapse is mild, Kegel exercises can help by strengthening the pelvic floor muscles. Kegel exercises target the muscles around the vagina, urethra, and rectum—the muscles used to stop a stream of urine. These muscles are tightly squeezed, held tight for about 1 or 2 seconds, then relaxed for about 10 seconds. Gradually, contractions are lengthened to about 10 seconds each. The exercise is repeated about 10 times in a row. Doing the exercises several times a day is recommended. Women can do Kegel exercises when sitting, standing, or lying down.

Some women have difficulty contracting the correct muscles. Learning the exercises can be made easier by using the following:

- Cone-shaped inserts placed in the vagina, which help women focus on contracting the correct muscle
- Biofeedback devices
- Electrical stimulation (a health care practitioner inserts a probe, which transmits an electrical current to make the correct muscle contract)

Pessaries: If prolapse is severe, a pessary may be used to support the pelvic organs. A pessary may be shaped like a diaphragm, cube, or doughnut. Pessaries are especially useful for women who are waiting for surgery or who cannot have surgery. A doctor fits the pessary to the woman by inserting and removing different sizes until the right one is found.

A pessary can be worn for many weeks before it needs to be removed and cleaned with soap and water. Women are taught how to insert and remove the pessary for monthly cleaning. If they prefer, they may go to the doctor's office periodically to have the pessary cleaned. Pessaries can irritate the vaginal tissues and cause a foul-smelling discharge. The discharge can be reduced by regular cleaning, nightly if possible. Some women choose to wear the pessary constantly, in which case the pessary should be changed every 2 to 3 weeks. They should also see their doctor every 6 to 12 months.

Surgery: Surgery is done if symptoms persist after women have tried Kegel exercises and a pessary. Surgery is usually done only after a woman has decided not to have any more children. The surgery usually involves inserting instruments into the vagina. The weakened area is located, and the tissues around it are built up to prevent the organ from dropping through the weakened area.

For severe prolapse of the uterus or vagina, the surgery may require an incision in the abdomen. The upper part of the vagina is attached with stitches to a nearby bone in the pelvis. Often, a catheter is inserted in the bladder to drain the urine for up to 24 hours. If urinary incontinence is present or would occur after prolapse of the uterus is repaired, surgery to correct incontinence can usually be done at the same time. Then the catheter to drain urine may need to remain in place longer. Heavy lifting, straining, and standing for a long time should be avoided for at least 3 months after surgery.

CHAPTER 245 Breast Disorders

Breast disorders may be noncancerous (benign) or cancerous (malignant). Most are noncancerous and not life threatening. Often, they do not require treatment. In contrast, breast cancer can mean loss of a breast or of life. Thus, for many women, breast cancer is their worst fear. However, potential problems can be detected early when women regularly examine their breasts themselves, are examined regularly by their doctor, and have mammograms as recommended. Early detection of breast cancer is essential to successful treatment.

Symptoms

Symptoms related to the breast are common. They include breast pain, lumps, and a discharge from the nipple. The breast's skin may become pitted, puckered, or dimpled. Breast symptoms do not necessarily mean that a woman has breast cancer or another serious disorder. For example, monthly breast tenderness that is related to hormonal changes before a menstrual period does not indicate a serious disorder. However, women should examine their breasts once a month (see art on page 1552) and should see their doctor if they observe any change in a breast, particularly any of the following:

- A lump that feels distinctly different from other breast tissue or that does not go away
- Swelling that does not go away
- Pitting, puckering, or dimpling in the skin of the breast
- Scaly skin around the nipple

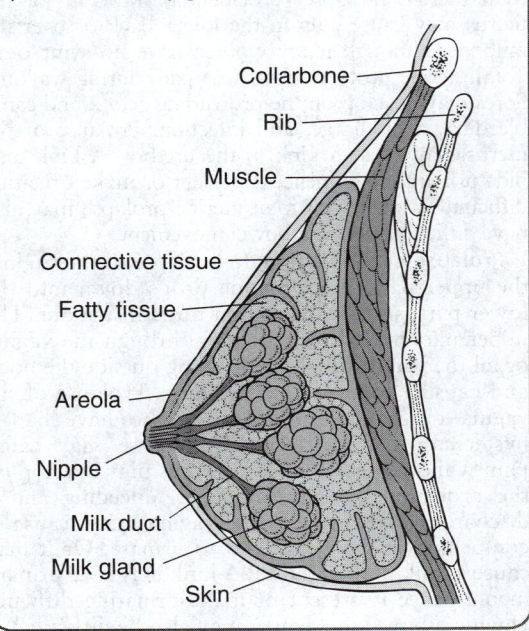

Inside the Breast

The female breast is composed of milk-producing glands (lobules) surrounded by fatty tissue and some connective tissue. Milk secreted by the glands flows through ducts to the nipple. Around the nipple is an area of pigmented skin called the areola.

Collarbone
Rib
Muscle
Connective tissue
Fatty tissue
Areola
Nipple
Milk duct
Milk gland
Skin

- Changes in the shape of the breast
- Changes in the nipple, such as turning inward
- Discharge from the nipple, especially if it is bloody

Breast Pain: Many women experience breast pain (mastalgia). Causes include the following:

- Hormonal changes
- Cysts
- Infection
- Fibrocystic changes
- Very rarely, cancer

Breast pain may be related to hormonal changes. For example, it may occur during or just before a menstrual period (as part of the premenstrual syndrome) or early in pregnancy. Women who take oral contraceptives or who take hormone therapy after menopause commonly have this kind of pain. When levels of the female hormones estrogen and progesterone increase (during the menstrual cycle or pregnancy or because of therapy), they cause the milk glands and ducts of the breasts to enlarge and the breasts to retain fluid. The breasts then become swollen and sometimes painful. Such pain is usually diffuse, making the breasts tender to touch. Pain related to the menstrual period may come and go for months or years.

Other causes of breast pain include breast cysts, infections, and abscesses. In these cases, breast pain is usually felt in a particular place. Fibrocystic changes (formerly called fibrocystic breast disease) may include breast pain. Pain is the first symptom in only about 5% of women with breast cancer. Breast pain that persists for more than 1 month should be evaluated.

Mild breast pain usually disappears eventually, even without treatment. Pain that occurs during menstrual periods can usually be relieved by taking acetaminophen or a nonsteroidal anti-inflammatory drug (NSAID).

For certain types of severe pain, danazol (a synthetic hormone related to testosterone) or tamoxifen (a drug used to treat breast cancer) may be used. These drugs inhibit the activity of estrogen and progesterone, which can make the breasts swell and be painful. Because long-term use of these drugs has side effects, the drugs are usually given for only a short time. Tamoxifen has fewer side effects than danazol. Tamoxifen is used mainly in postmenopausal women but may benefit younger women.

If a specific disorder is identified as the cause, the disorder is treated. For example, if a cyst is the cause, draining the fluid from the cyst usually relieves the pain.

Breast Lumps: Lumps in the breasts are relatively common and are usually not cancerous. Causes include the following:

- Cysts
- Fibroadenomas
- Scar tissue
- Rarely, cancer

But because lumps may be cancerous, they should be evaluated by a doctor without delay. Lumps may be fluid-filled sacs (cysts) or solid masses, which are usually fibroadenomas (see page 1548).

Other solid breast lumps include hardened glandular tissue (sclerosing adenosis) and scar tissue that has replaced injured fatty tissue (fat necrosis). Neither is cancerous. However, these lumps can be diagnosed only by biopsy. They require no treatment.

Nipple Discharge: One or both nipples sometimes discharge a fluid. A nipple discharge occurs normally during milk production (lactation) after childbirth. Or it can occur when the nipple is mechanically stimulated by fondling, suckling, or irritation from clothing or when women are sexually aroused. During the last weeks of pregnancy, the breasts may produce a milky discharge (colostrum). Stress can also result in a nipple discharge.

A normal nipple discharge is a thin, cloudy, whitish or almost clear fluid that is not sticky. However, during pregnancy or breastfeeding, a slightly bloody discharge sometimes occurs normally.

Several disorders can cause an abnormal discharge. Abnormal discharges vary in appearance depending on the cause:

- A bloody discharge may be caused by a noncancerous breast tumor (such as a tumor in a milk duct, called an intraductal papilloma) or, less commonly, by breast cancer. Among women who have an abnormal discharge, breast cancer is the cause in fewer than 10%.
- A greenish discharge is usually due to a fibroadenoma, which is a noncancerous solid lump.
- A discharge that contains pus and smells foul may result from a breast infection.
- A large amount of milky discharge in women who are not breastfeeding may represent galactorrhea (see page 989).

Disorders of the pituitary gland or brain, encephalitis (a brain infection), an underactive thyroid gland (hypothyroidism), kidney or liver disorders, and head or chest injuries can also cause a nipple discharge.

Taking certain drugs can cause a nipple discharge. These drugs include opioids, certain drugs used to treat stomach disorders (such as cimetidine, ranitidine, and metoclopramide), certain antidepressants, and certain antihypertensives (such as methyldopa, reserpine, and verapamil).

A discharge from one breast is likely to be caused by a problem with that breast, such as a noncancerous or cancerous breast tumor. A discharge from both breasts is more likely to be caused by a problem outside the breast, such as a hormonal disorder or use of certain drugs.

WHAT CAUSES NIPPLE DISCHARGE?	
TYPE	**EXAMPLES**
Breast disorders	Breast cancer
	Breast infections or abscesses
	Fibrocystic changes
	Most commonly, noncancerous milk duct tumors (intraductal papilloma)
Other disorders	Brain disorders
	Encephalitis (a brain infection)
	Head or chest injuries
	Kidney disorders
	Liver disorders
	Pituitary gland disorders
	An underactive thyroid gland (hypothyroidism)
Drugs	Certain antidepressants
	Certain antihypertensives, such as methyldopa, reserpine, and verapamil
	Older antipsychotic drugs such as chlorpromazine
	Certain drugs used to treat stomach disorders, such as cimetidine, ranitidine, and metoclopramide
	Opioids
	Oral contraceptives

If a nipple discharge persists for more than one menstrual cycle or seems unusual, women should see a doctor. Postmenopausal women who have a nipple discharge should see a doctor promptly. Doctors examine the breast, looking for abnormalities. Tests that may be done include ultrasonography of the breast, mammography, blood tests to measure hormone levels, and computed tomography (CT) or magnetic resonance imaging (MRI) of the head. Women are asked for a complete list of drugs they are taking. Sometimes a specific cause cannot be identified.

If a disorder is the cause, the disorder is treated. If a noncancerous tumor is causing a discharge from one breast, the duct that the discharge is coming from may be removed.

Breast Cysts

Breast cysts are fluid-filled sacs that develop in the breast.

Breast cysts are common. In some women, many cysts develop frequently, sometimes with other fibrocystic changes. The cause of breast cysts is unknown, although injury may be involved. Breast cysts can be tiny or several inches in diameter.

Cysts sometimes cause breast pain. To relieve the pain, a doctor may drain fluid from the cyst with a thin needle. Sometimes the fluid is examined under a microscope to check for cancer. The color and amount are noted. If the fluid is bloody, brown, or cloudy or if the cyst does not disappear or reappears within 12 weeks after it is drained, the entire cyst is removed surgically because cancer in the cyst wall, although rare, is possible.

Fibroadenomas

Fibroadenomas are small, solid, rubbery noncancerous lumps composed of fibrous and glandular tissue.

Fibroadenomas usually appear in young women, including teenagers. The cause is unknown.

The lumps are easy to move and have clearly defined edges that can be felt during self-examination. They may feel like small, slippery marbles. These characteristics indicate to a doctor that the lumps are less likely to be cancerous. Nonetheless, to be sure that they are not cancerous, the doctor usually removes the lumps. A local anesthetic is used.

Fibroadenomas often recur. If several lumps have been removed and found to be noncancerous, a woman and her doctor may decide against removing new lumps that develop.

Fibrocystic Changes

Fibrocystic changes (formerly called fibrocystic breast disease) include breast pain, cysts, and lumpiness that are not due to cancer.

Most women have some general lumpiness in the breasts, usually in the upper outer part, near the armpit. In the United States, many women have this kind of lumpiness, breast pain, breast cysts, or some combination of these symptoms—a condition called fibrocystic changes.

Normally, the levels of the female hormones estrogen and progesterone fluctuate during the menstrual cycle. Milk glands and ducts enlarge and breasts retain fluid when levels increase, and the breasts return to normal when levels decrease. (These fluctuations partly explain why breasts are swollen and more sensitive during a particular time of each menstrual cycle.) Fibrocystic changes may result from repeated stimulation by these hormones. The following increase the risk of these changes:

- Starting to menstruate at an early age
- Having a first baby at age 30 or later
- Never having a baby

Other breast disorders, such as infections, can cause these changes.

The lumpy areas may enlarge, causing a feeling of heaviness, discomfort, tenderness to the touch, or a burning pain. The symptoms tend to subside after menopause.

Most fibrocystic changes do not increase the risk of breast cancer, but a few of them do, although only slightly. These changes typically require a biopsy to rule out cancer and may make the breasts appear dense on mammograms. They include the following:

- **Complex fibroadenoma:** The cells that line the breast ducts and connective tissue in the breasts form a benign tumor with many types of changes in tissue.
- **Moderate or severe hyperplasia:** The cells that line the milk glands or ducts multiply too much, and their arrangement may become distorted (called atypical hyperplasia).
- **Sclerosing adenosis:** The number of milk glands increases, and scar tissue forms, distorting the arrangement of milk glands.
- **Papilloma:** Noncancerous, finger-like tumors develop in the cells that line the breast ducts.

Fibrocystic changes may make breast cancer more difficult to detect.

Treatment

Lumps, usually only one lump at a time, may be removed, and a biopsy may be done to rule out cancer. Sometimes the biopsy sample can be withdrawn with a needle, but sometimes it must be removed surgically.

Sometimes cysts are drained, but they tend to recur. No specific treatment is available or required, but certain measures may help relieve symptoms:

- Wearing a soft, supportive brassiere
- Taking pain relievers

If symptoms are severe, doctors may prescribe drugs, such as danazol (a synthetic male hormone) or tamoxifen (which blocks the effects of estrogen). Because side effects can occur with long-term use, the drugs are usually given for only a short time. Tamoxifen has fewer side effects than danazol.

Breast Infection and Abscess

A breast infection (mastitis) is rare, except around the time of childbirth (see page 1671) or after an injury or surgery. The most common symptom is a swollen, red area that feels warm and tender. An uncommon type of breast cancer called inflammatory breast cancer (see page 1551) can cause similar symptoms. A breast infection is treated with antibiotics.

A breast abscess, which is even rarer, is a collection of pus in the breast. An abscess may develop if a breast infection is not treated. An abscess is usually drained surgically and may be treated with antibiotics.

Breast Cancer

- Among women, breast cancer is the second most common cancer and the second most common cause of cancer deaths.
- Typically, the first symptom is a painless lump, usually noticed by the woman.
- Monthly self-examination, yearly breast examination by a doctor, and a yearly mammogram for women who are over 50 or at increased risk are recommended.
- If a solid lump is detected, a few cells are removed through a needle or the entire lump is surgically removed and examined (biopsied).
- Breast cancer almost always requires surgery, sometimes with radiation therapy, chemotherapy, other drugs, or a combination.
- Outcome is hard to predict and depends partly on the characteristics and spread of the cancer.

Breast cancer is the second most common cancer among women after skin cancer and, of cancers, is the second most common cause of death among women after lung cancer. In 2006, breast cancer was diagnosed in about 213,000 women in the United States. About one fifth of them will die of it.

Many women fear breast cancer, partly because it is common. However, some of the fear about breast cancer is based on misunderstanding. For example, the statement, "One of every eight women will get breast cancer," is misleading. That figure is an estimate based on women from birth to age 95. It means that theoretically, one of eight women who live to age 95 or older will develop breast cancer. However, a 40-year-old woman has only a 1 in 1,200 chance of developing breast cancer during the next year and about a 1 in 120 chance of developing it during the next decade. But as she ages, her risk increases.

Did You Know...

Fewer than 1% of women have the genes for breast cancer.

Several factors affect the risk of developing breast cancer. Thus, for some women, the risk is much higher or lower than average. Most factors that increase risk, such as age, cannot be modified. However, regular

WHAT ARE THE RISKS OF DEVELOPING OR DYING OF BREAST CANCER?

AGE (YEARS)	RISK (%)					
	IN 10 YEARS		IN 20 YEARS		IN 30 YEARS	
	DEVELOP	DIE	DEVELOP	DIE	DEVELOP	DIE
30	0.4	0.1	2.0	0.6	4.3	1.2
40	1.6	0.5	3.9	1.1	7.1	2.0
50	2.4	0.7	5.7	1.6	9.0	2.6
60	3.6	1.0	7.1	2.0	9.1	2.6
70	4.1	1.2	6.5	1.9	7.1	2.0

Based on information from Feuer EJ et al.: The lifetime risk of developing breast cancer. *Journal of the National Cancer Institute* 85(11):892–897, 1993.

exercise, particularly during adolescence and young adulthood, and possibly weight control may reduce the risk of developing breast cancer. Regularly drinking alcoholic beverages may increase the risk.

Far more important than trying to modify risk factors is being vigilant about detecting breast cancer so that it can be diagnosed and treated early, when it is more likely to be cured. Early detection is more likely when women have mammograms (see page 1554) and do breast self-examinations regularly (see art on page 1552).

Types

Breast cancer is usually classified by the extent of its spread and by the kind of tissue in which the cancer starts.

Carcinoma in situ means cancer in place. It is the earliest stage of breast cancer. Carcinoma in situ may be large and may even affect a substantial area of the breast, but it has not invaded the surrounding tissues or spread to other parts of the body. More than 15% of all breast cancers diagnosed in the United States are carcinoma in situ. It is usually detected during mammography.

Invasive cancer is further classified as follows.

- Localized: The cancer has invaded surrounding tissues but is confined to the breast.
- Regional: The cancer has invaded tissues near the breasts, such as the chest wall or lymph nodes.
- Distant (metastatic): The cancer has spread from the breast to other parts of the body. Cancer tends to move into the lymphatic vessels in the breast. Most lymphatic vessels in the breast drain into lymph nodes in the armpit (axillary lymph nodes). One function of lymph nodes is to filter out and

destroy abnormal or foreign cells, such as cancer cells. If cancer cells get past these lymph nodes, the cancer can spread anywhere in the body. Breast cancer can also spread through the bloodstream to other parts of the body. Breast cancer tends to spread to bones and the brain but can spread to any area, including the lungs, liver, skin, and scalp. Breast cancer can appear in these areas years or even decades after it is first diagnosed and treated. If the cancer has spread to one area, it probably has spread to other areas, even if it cannot be detected right away.

Breast cancer that starts in the milk ducts is called ductal carcinoma. About 90% of all breast cancers are this type. Breast cancer that starts in the milk-producing glands (lobules) is called lobular carcinoma. Breast cancer that starts in fatty or connective tissue, a rare type, is called sarcoma.

Ductal carcinoma in situ is confined to the milk ducts of the breast. It does not invade surrounding breast tissue, but it can spread along the ducts and gradually affect a substantial area of the breast. This type accounts for 20 to 30% of breast cancers. It is detected only during mammography. This type may become invasive.

Lobular carcinoma in situ develops within the milk-producing glands of the breast. It often occurs in several areas of both breasts. Women with this type have a 1 to 2% chance each year of developing invasive breast cancer in the affected or the other breast. This type accounts for 1 to 2% of breast cancers. Usually, lobular carcinoma in situ cannot be seen on a mammogram and is detected only by biopsy.

Invasive ductal carcinoma begins in the milk ducts but breaks through the wall of the ducts,

Risk Factors for Breast Cancer

AGE

Increasing age is an important risk factor. About 60% of breast cancers occur in women older than 60. Risk is greatest after age 75.

PREVIOUS BREAST CANCER

At highest risk are women who have had breast cancer. After the diseased breast is removed, the risk of developing cancer in the remaining breast is about 0.5 to 1.0% each year.

FAMILY HISTORY OF BREAST CANCER

Breast cancer in a first-degree relative (mother, sister, or daughter) increases a woman's risk by 2 to 3 times, but breast cancer in more distant relatives (grandmother, aunt, or cousin) increases the risk only slightly. Breast cancer in two or more first-degree relatives increases a woman's risk by 5 to 6 times.

BREAST CANCER GENE

Two separate genes for breast cancer (*BRCA1* and *BRCA2*) have been identified in two separate small groups of women. Fewer than 1% of women have these genes. They are most common among Ashkenazi Jews. If a woman has one of these genes, her chances of developing breast cancer are very high, possibly as high as 50 to 85% by age 80. However, if such a woman develops breast cancer, her chances of dying of breast cancer are not necessarily greater than those of any other woman with breast cancer. Women likely to have one of these genes are those who have several close, usually first-degree relatives who have had breast cancer. For this reason, routine screening for these genes does not appear necessary, except in women who have such a family history.

The risk of ovarian cancer is increased in families with both breast cancer genes. The risk of breast cancer in men is increased in families with the *BRCA2* gene.

Women with one of these genes may need to undergo more frequent testing for breast cancer. Or they may need to try to prevent cancer from developing by taking tamoxifen or raloxifene (which is similar to tamoxifen) or sometimes by even having a double mastectomy.

FIBROCYSTIC CHANGES

Having only certain types of fibrocystic changes seems to increase risk. These changes include those that require a biopsy to rule out breast cancer or those that make the breasts appear dense on a mammogram. For women with such changes, the risk is increased only slightly unless abnormal tissue structure (atypical hyperplasia) is detected during a biopsy or the women have a family history of breast cancer.

AGE AT FIRST MENSTRUAL PERIOD, AT FIRST PREGNANCY, AND AT MENOPAUSE

The earlier menstruation begins, the greater the risk of developing breast cancer. The risk is 1.2 to 1.4 times higher for women who first menstruated before age 12 than for those who first menstruated after age 14.

The later the first pregnancy occurs and the later menopause occurs, the higher the risk. Never having had a baby doubles the risk of developing breast cancer during a woman's lifetime.

These factors probably increase risk because they involve longer exposure to estrogen, which stimulates the growth of certain cancers. (Pregnancy, although it results in high estrogen levels, may reduce the risk of breast cancer.)

PROLONGED USE OF ORAL CONTRACEPTIVES OR ESTROGEN THERAPY

Taking oral contraceptives increases the risk of later developing breast cancer, but only very slightly. Also, the risk is increased mainly for women who started taking them at a young age (such as during their teens) and who have taken them for many years. After women stop taking contraceptives, the risk gradually decreases over the next 10 years to that for other women of the same age.

After menopause, taking combination hormone therapy (estrogen with a progestin) for a few years or more increases the risk of breast cancer.

OBESITY AFTER MENOPAUSE

Risk is somewhat higher for women who are obese after menopause. However, there is no proof that a high-fat diet contributes to the development of breast cancer or that changing the diet can decrease risk. Some studies suggest that obese women who are still menstruating are less likely to develop breast cancer.

RADIATION EXPOSURE

Radiation exposure (such as radiation therapy for cancer or significant exposure to x-rays) before age 30 increases risk.

---

invading the surrounding breast tissue. It can also spread to other parts of the body. It accounts for 65 to 80% of breast cancers.

Invasive lobular carcinoma begins in the milk-producing glands of the breast but invades surrounding breast tissue and spreads to other parts of the body. It is more likely than other types of breast cancer to occur in both breasts. It accounts for 10 to 15% of breast cancers.

Inflammatory breast cancer refers to the symptoms of the cancer rather than the affected tissue. This type is fast growing and often fatal. Cancer cells block the lymphatic vessels in the skin of the breast, causing the breast to appear inflamed: swollen,

How to Do a Breast Self-Examination

1. While standing in front of a mirror, look at the breasts. The breasts normally differ slightly in size. Look for changes in the size difference between the breasts and changes in the nipple, such as turning inward (an inverted nipple) or a discharge. Look for puckering or dimpling.

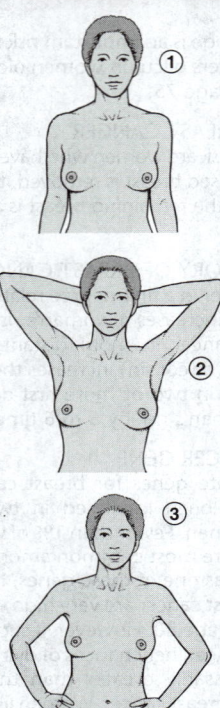

2. Watching closely in the mirror, clasp the hands behind the head and press them against the head. This position helps make subtle changes caused by cancer more noticeable. Look for changes in the shape and contour of the breasts, especially in the lower part of the breasts.

3. Place the hands firmly on the hips and bend slightly toward the mirror, pressing the shoulders and elbows forward. Again, look for changes in shape and contour.

Many women do the next part of the examination in the shower because the hand moves easily over wet, slippery skin.

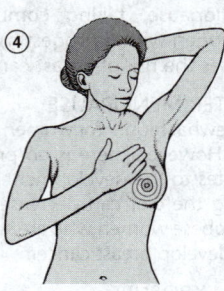

4. Raise the left arm. Using three or four fingers of the right hand, probe the left breast thoroughly with the flat part of the fingers. Moving the fingers in small circles around the breast, begin at the nipple and gradually move outward. Press gently but firmly, feeling for any unusual lump or mass under the skin. Be sure to check the whole breast. Also, carefully probe the armpit and the area between the breast and armpit for lumps.

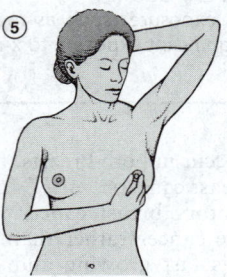

5. Squeeze the left nipple gently and look for a discharge. (See a doctor if a discharge appears at any time of the month, regardless of whether it happens during breast self-examination.)

(continued on the following page)

How to Do a Breast Self-Examination (*Continued*)

Repeat steps 4 and 5 for the right breast, raising the right arm and using the left hand.

6. Lie flat on the back with a pillow or folded towel under the left shoulder and with the left arm overhead. This position flattens the breast and makes it easier to examine. Examine the breast as in steps 4 and 5. Repeat for the right breast.

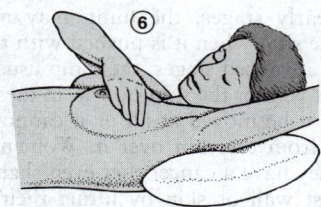

A woman should repeat this procedure at the same time each month. For menstruating women, 2 or 3 days after their period ends is a good time because the breasts are less likely to be tender and swollen. Postmenopausal women may choose any day of the month that is easy to remember, such as the first.

Adapted from a publication of the National Cancer Institute.

red, and warm. Usually, inflammatory breast cancer spreads to the lymph nodes in the armpit. The lymph nodes can be felt as hard lumps. However, often no lump may be felt in the breast itself because this cancer is dispersed throughout the breast. Inflammatory breast cancer accounts for about 1% of breast cancers.

Paget's disease of the nipple (see page 1337) is a ductal breast cancer. The first symptom is a crusty or scaly nipple sore or a discharge from the nipple. Slightly more than half of the women who have this cancer also have a lump in the breast that can be felt. Paget's disease may be in situ or invasive. Because this disease usually causes little discomfort, women may ignore it for a year or more before seeing a doctor. The prognosis depends on how invasive and how large the cancer is as well as whether it has spread to the lymph nodes.

Rare types of invasive ductal breast cancers include **medullary carcinoma, tubular carcinoma**, and **mucinous (colloid) carcinoma**. Mucinous carcinoma tends to develop in older women and to be slow growing. Women with these types of breast cancer have a much better prognosis than women with other types of invasive breast cancer.

Phyllodes breast tumors are relatively rare. About half are cancerous. They originate in breast tissue around milk ducts and milk-producing glands. The tumor spreads to other parts of the body in about 10 to 20% of women who have it.

Characteristics

All cells, including breast cancer cells, have molecules on their surfaces called receptors. A receptor has a specific structure that allows only particular substances to fit into it and thus affect the cell's activity. Whether breast cancer cells have certain receptors affects how quickly the cancer spreads and how it should be treated.

- **Estrogen and progesterone receptors:** Some breast cancer cells have receptors for estrogen. The resulting cancer, described as estrogen receptor–positive, grows or spreads when stimulated by estrogen. This type of cancer is more common among postmenopausal women than among younger women. Some breast cancer cells have receptors for progesterone. The resulting cancer, described as progesterone receptor–positive, is stimulated by progesterone. Breast cancers with estrogen receptors and possibly those with progesterone receptors grow more slowly than those that do not have these receptors, and the prognosis is better.

- **HER2 (HER2/neu) receptors:** Normal breast cells have HER2 receptors, which help them grow. (HER stands for human epithelial growth factor receptor, which is involved in multiplication, survival, and differentiation of cells.) In about 20 to 30% of breast cancers, cancer cells have too many HER2 receptors. Such cancers tend to be very fast growing.

Symptoms

At first, breast cancer causes no symptoms. Most commonly, the first symptom is a lump, which usually feels distinctly different from the surrounding breast tissue. In more than 80% of breast cancer cases, women discover the lump themselves. Usually, scattered lumpy changes in the breast, especially the upper outer region, are not cancerous and indicate fibrocystic changes. A firm, distinctive thickening that appears in one breast but not the other may indicate cancer.

In the early stages, the lump may move freely beneath the skin when it is pushed with the fingers.

In more advanced stages, the lump usually adheres to the chest wall or the skin over it. In these cases, the lump cannot be moved at all or it cannot be moved separately from the skin over it. Women can detect whether they have a cancer that even slightly adheres to the chest wall or skin by lifting their arms over their head while standing in front of a mirror. If a breast contains cancer that adheres to the chest wall or skin, this maneuver may make the skin pucker or one breast appear different from the other.

In very advanced cancer, swollen bumps or festering sores may develop on the skin. Sometimes the skin over the lump is dimpled and leathery and looks like the skin of an orange (peau d'orange) except in color.

The lump may be painful, but pain is an unreliable sign. Pain without a lump is rarely due to breast cancer.

Lymph nodes, particularly those in the armpit on the affected side, may feel like hard small lumps. The lymph nodes may be stuck together or adhere to the skin or chest wall. They are usually painless but may be slightly tender.

In inflammatory breast cancer, the breast is warm, red, and swollen, as if infected (but it is not). The skin of the breast may become dimpled and leathery, like the skin of an orange, or may have ridges. The nipple may turn inward (invert). A discharge from the nipple is common. Often, no lump can be felt in the breast.

Screening

Because breast cancer rarely causes symptoms in its early stages and because early treatment is more likely to be successful, screening is important. Screening is the hunt for a disorder before any symptoms occur.

Routine self-examination enables women to detect lumps at an early stage. However, self-examination alone does not reduce the death rate from breast cancer, and it does not detect as many early cancers as routine screening with mammography. Women who do not detect any lumps should continue to see their doctor for breast examinations and to have mammograms as recommended. When tumors are detected by self-examination, the prognosis is usually better, and breast-conserving surgery can usually be done rather than mastectomy.

A breast examination is a routine part of a physical examination. A doctor inspects the breasts for irregularities, dimpling, tightened skin, lumps, and a discharge. The doctor feels (palpates) each breast with a flat hand and checks for enlarged lymph nodes in the armpit—the area most breast cancers invade first—

and above the collarbone. Normal lymph nodes cannot be felt through the skin, so those that can be felt are considered enlarged. However, noncancerous conditions can also cause lymph nodes to enlarge. Lymph nodes that can be felt are checked to see if they adhere to the skin or chest wall and if they are matted together.

Mammography: For this test, x-rays are used to check for abnormal areas in the breast. A technician positions the woman's breast on top of an x-ray plate. An adjustable plastic cover is lowered on top of the breast, firmly compressing the breast. Thus, the breast is flattened so that the maximum amount of tissue can be imaged and examined. X-rays are aimed downward through the breast, producing an image on the x-ray plate. Two x-rays are taken of each breast in this position. Then plates may be placed vertically on either side of the breast, and x-rays are aimed from the side. This position produces a side view of the breast.

Mammography is one of the best ways to detect breast cancer early. Mammography is designed to be sensitive enough to detect the possibility of cancer at an early stage, sometimes years before it can be felt. Because mammography is so sensitive, it may indicate cancer when none is present—a false-positive result. About 90% of abnormalities detected during screening (that is, in women with no symptoms or lumps) are not cancer. Typically, when the result is positive,

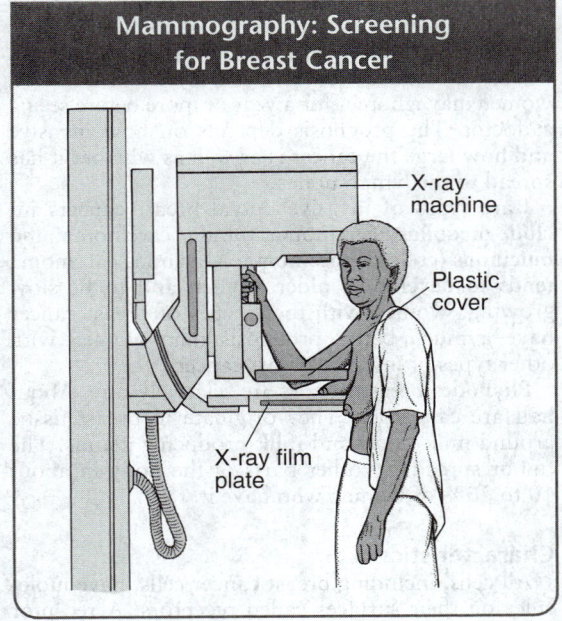

Mammography: Screening for Breast Cancer

X-ray machine

Plastic cover

X-ray film plate

more specific follow-up procedures, usually a breast biopsy, are scheduled to confirm the result. Mammography may miss up to 15% of breast cancers.

Having a mammogram every 1 to 2 years can reduce the rate of death due to breast cancer by 25 to 35% among women aged 50 and older. As yet, no study has shown that regularly having mammograms can reduce the death rate among women younger than 50. However, evidence may be harder to obtain because breast cancer is not common among younger women. Many experts recommend that women aged 40 to 49 have mammograms every 1 to 2 years. All experts recommend yearly mammograms for women aged 50 and older.

The dose of radiation used is very low and is considered safe. Mammography may cause some discomfort, but the discomfort lasts only a few seconds. Mammography should be scheduled at a time during the menstrual period when the breasts are less likely to be tender. Deodorants should not be used on the day of the procedure because they can interfere with the image obtained. The entire procedure takes about 15 minutes.

> ### ? Did You Know...
> Only about 10% of the abnormalities detected during routine screening with mammography turn out to be cancer.

Diagnosis

When a lump or another abnormality is detected in the breast during a physical examination or by a screening procedure, other procedures are necessary. Mammography is done first if it was not the way the abnormality was detected.

Ultrasonography is sometimes used to help distinguish between a fluid-filled sac (cyst) and a solid lump. This distinction is important because cysts are usually not cancerous. Cysts may be monitored (with no treatment) or drained with a small needle and syringe. Sometimes the fluid from the cyst is examined to check for cancer cells. Rarely, when cancer is suspected, cysts are removed.

If the abnormality is a solid lump, which is more likely to be cancerous, a mammogram followed by a biopsy is done. Often, an aspiration biopsy is used: Some cells are removed from the lump through a needle attached to a syringe. If this procedure detects cancer, the diagnosis is confirmed. If no cancer is detected, removal of an additional piece of tissue (incisional biopsy) or of the entire lump (excisional biopsy) is necessary to be sure that the aspiration biopsy did not miss the cancer. Most women do not need to be hospitalized for these procedures. Usually, only a local anesthetic is needed.

If Paget's disease of the nipple is suspected, a biopsy of nipple tissue is usually done. Sometimes this cancer can be diagnosed by examining a sample of the nipple discharge under a microscope.

A pathologist examines the biopsy samples under the microscope to determine whether cancer cells are present. Generally, a biopsy confirms cancer in only a few women with an abnormality detected during mammography. If cancer cells are detected, the sample is analyzed to determine the characteristics of the cancer cells, such as

- Whether the cancer cells have estrogen or progesterone receptors
- How many HER2 receptors are present
- How quickly the cancer cells are dividing

This information helps doctors estimate how rapidly the cancer may spread and which treatments are more likely to be effective.

A chest x-ray is taken and blood tests, including a complete blood cell count and liver function tests, are done to determine whether the cancer has spread. If the tumor is large, if the lymph nodes are enlarged, or if women have bone pain, imaging of bones throughout the body (a bone scan) may be done. Computed tomography (CT) of the abdomen is done if liver function is abnormal, if the liver is enlarged, or if the cancer has spread within the breast.

Magnetic resonance imaging (MRI) is often done to evaluate breast cancer after it is diagnosed because MRI can accurately determine how large the tumor is, whether the chest wall is involved, and how many tumors are present.

Staging

When cancer is diagnosed, a stage is assigned to it, based on how advanced it is. The stage helps doctors determine the most appropriate treatment and the prognosis. Stages of breast cancer may be described generally as in situ (not invasive) or invasive. Stages may be described in detail and designated by a number (0 through IV).

Prevention

Taking drugs that decrease the risk of breast cancer (chemoprevention) is recommended for the following women:

- Those over age 60
- Those who are over age 35 and have had a previous lobular carcinoma in situ
- Those who have *BRCA1* or *BRCA2* gene mutations
- Those who have a high risk of developing breast cancer based on the woman's current age, age at menarche, age at first live childbirth, number of first-degree relatives with breast cancer, and results of prior breast biopsies

STAGES OF BREAST CANCER

STAGE	DESCRIPTION
In situ carcinoma	
0	The tumor is confined, usually to a milk duct or milk-producing gland, and has not invaded surrounding breast tissue.
Localized and regional invasive cancer	
I	The tumor is less than ¾ inch (2 centimeters) in diameter and has not spread beyond the breast.
IIA	The tumor is ¾ inch or less in diameter, and it has spread to one to three lymph nodes in the armpit, microscopic amounts have spread to lymph nodes near the breastbone on the same side as the tumor, or both. *or* The tumor is larger than ¾ inch but smaller than 2 inches (5 centimeters) in diameter but has not spread beyond the breast.
IIB	The tumor is larger than ¾ inch but smaller than 2 inches in diameter, and it has spread to one to three lymph nodes in the armpit, microscopic amounts have spread to lymph nodes near the breastbone on the same side as the tumor, or both. *or* The tumor is larger than 2 inches in diameter but has not spread beyond the breast.
IIIA	The tumor is 2 inches or less in diameter and has spread to four to nine lymph nodes in the armpit or has enlarged at least one lymph node near the breastbone on the same side as the tumor. *or* The tumor is larger than 2 inches in diameter and has spread to up to nine lymph nodes in the armpit or to lymph nodes near the breastbone.
IIIB	The tumor has spread to the chest wall or skin or has caused breast inflammation (inflammatory breast cancer).
IIIC	The tumor can be any size plus at least one of the following: <ul><li>It has spread to 10 or more lymph nodes in the armpit.</li><li>It has spread to lymph nodes under or above the collar bone.</li><li>It has spread to lymph nodes in the armpit and has enlarged at least one lymph node near the breastbone on the same side as the tumor.</li><li>It has spread to four or more lymph nodes in the armpit, and microscopic amounts have spread to lymph nodes near the breastbone on the same side as the tumor.</li></ul>
Metastatic cancer	
IV	The tumor, regardless of size, has spread to distant organs or tissues, such as the lungs or bones, or to lymph nodes distant from the breast.

These drugs include tamoxifen and raloxifene. Women should ask their doctor about possible side effects before beginning chemoprevention. Risks of tamoxifen include cancer of the uterus (endometrial cancer), blood clots in the legs or lungs, and cataracts. These risks are higher for older women. Raloxifene appears to be about as effective as tamoxifen in postmenopausal women and to have a lower risk of blood clots and cataracts. Both drugs may also increase bone density and thus benefit women who have osteoporosis. For postmenopausal women, raloxifene is an alternative to tamoxifen.

TREATING CANCER BASED ON TYPE

TYPE	POSSIBLE TREATMENTS
Ductal carcinoma in situ	Mastectomy Wide excision with or without radiation therapy
Lobular carcinoma in situ	Observation plus regular examinations and mammograms Tamoxifen or, for some postmenopausal women, raloxifene to reduce the risk of invasive cancer Bilateral mastectomy (rarely) to prevent invasive cancers
Stages I and II (early-stage) cancer	Chemotherapy before surgery if the tumor is larger than 2 inches (5 centimeters) Breast-conserving surgery to remove the tumor and some surrounding tissue, usually followed by radiation therapy Sometimes mastectomy with breast reconstruction After surgery, chemotherapy, hormonal therapy, trastuzumab, or a combination, except in some postmenopausal women with tumors smaller than 0.4 inches (1 centimeter)
Stage III (locally advanced) cancer (including inflammatory breast cancer)	Chemotherapy or sometimes hormonal therapy before surgery to reduce the tumor's size Breast-conserving surgery or mastectomy if the tumor is small enough to be completely removed Mastectomy for inflammatory breast cancer Usually, radiation therapy after surgery Sometimes chemotherapy, hormonal therapy, or both after surgery
Stage IV (metastatic) cancer	If cancer causes symptoms and occurs in several sites, hormone therapy, ovarian ablation therapy,* or chemotherapy If the cancer cells have too many HER2 receptors, trastuzumab Radiation therapy for the following: ■ Metastases to the brain ■ Metastases that recur in the skin ■ Metastases that occur in one area of bone and that cause symptoms For metastases to bone, IV bisphosphonates (such as zoledronate or pamidronate) to reduce bone pain and bone loss
Paget's disease of the nipple	Usually, the same as for other types of breast cancer Occasionally, local excision only
Breast cancer that recurs in the breast or nearby structures	Radical or modified radical mastectomy sometimes preceded by chemotherapy or hormone therapy
Phyllodes tumors if they are cancerous	Wide excision Mastectomy if the tumor is large

*Ovarian ablation therapy involves removing the ovaries or using drugs to suppress estrogen production by the ovaries.

Treatment

Usually, treatment begins after the woman's condition has been thoroughly evaluated, about a week or more after the biopsy. Treatment options depend on the stage and type of breast cancer. However, treatment is complex because the different types of breast cancer differ greatly in growth rate, tendency to spread (metastasize), and response to treatment. Also, much is

Surgery for Breast Cancer

Surgery for breast cancer consists of two main options. In **breast-conserving surgery**, only the tumor and an area of normal tissue surrounding it are removed. Breast-conserving surgery includes the following:

- Lumpectomy: A small amount of surrounding normal tissue is removed.

- Wide excision (partial mastectomy): A somewhat larger amount of the surrounding normal tissue is removed.
- Quadrantectomy: One fourth of the breast is removed.

In **mastectomy**, all breast tissue is removed.

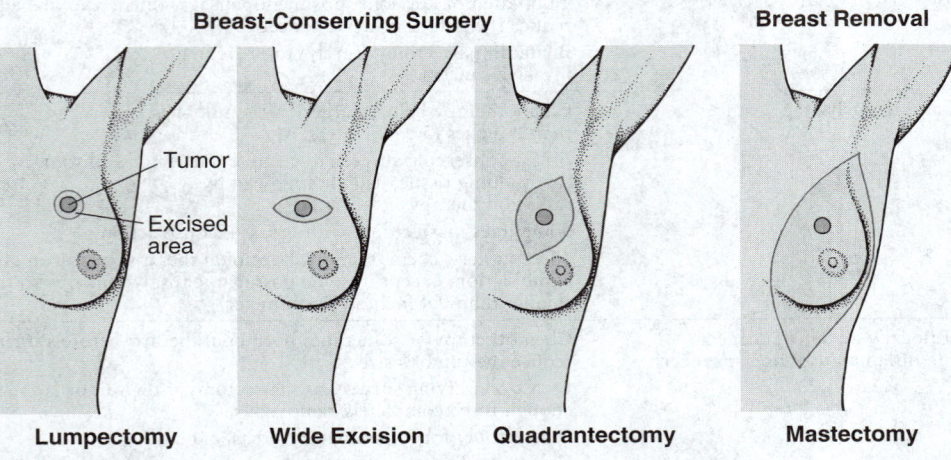

Breast-Conserving Surgery   **Breast Removal**

Tumor

Excised area

Lumpectomy   **Wide Excision**   **Quadrantectomy**   **Mastectomy**

still unknown about breast cancer. Consequently, doctors may have different opinions about the most appropriate treatment for a particular woman.

The preferences of a woman and her doctor affect treatment decisions. Women with breast cancer should ask for a clear explanation of what is known about the cancer and what is still unknown, as well as a complete description of treatment options. Then, they can consider the advantages and disadvantages of the different treatments and accept or reject the options offered. Losing some or all of a breast can be emotionally traumatic. Women must consider how they feel about this treatment, which can deeply affect their sense of wholeness and sexuality.

Doctors may ask women with breast cancer to participate in research studies investigating a new treatment. New treatments aim to improve the chances of survival or quality of life. All women who participate in a research study are treated because a new treatment is compared with other effective treatments. Women should ask their doctor to explain the risks and possible benefits of participation, so that they can make a well-informed decision.

Treatment usually involves surgery and may include radiation therapy, chemotherapy, or hormone-blocking drugs. Often, a combination of these treatments is used.

Surgery: The cancerous tumor and varying amounts of the surrounding tissue are removed. There are two main options for removing the tumor: breast-conserving surgery and removal of the breast (mastectomy). For women with invasive cancer (stage I or higher), mastectomy is no more effective than breast-conserving surgery plus radiation therapy as long as the entire tumor can be removed during breast-conserving surgery. Before surgery, chemotherapy may be used to shrink the tumor before removing it. This approach sometimes enables some women to have breast-conserving surgery rather than mastectomy.

Breast-conserving surgery leaves as much of the breast intact as possible. There are several types:

- Lumpectomy is removal of the tumor with a small amount of surrounding normal tissue.
- Wide excision or partial mastectomy is removal of the tumor and a somewhat larger amount of surrounding normal tissue.
- Quadrantectomy is removal of one fourth of the breast.

Removing the tumor with some normal tissue provides the best chance of preventing cancer from recurring within the breast. Breast-conserving surgery is usually combined with radiation therapy.

The major advantage of breast-conserving surgery is cosmetic: This surgery may help preserve body image. Thus, when the tumor is large in relation to the breast, this type of surgery is less likely to be useful. In such cases, removing the tumor plus some surrounding normal tissue means removing most of the breast. Breast-conserving surgery is usually more appropriate when tumors are small. In about 15% of women who have breast-conserving surgery, the amount of tissue removed is so small that little difference can be seen between the treated and untreated breasts. However, in most women, the treated breast shrinks somewhat and may change in contour.

Mastectomy is the other main surgical option. There are several types:

- Simple mastectomy consists of removing all breast tissue but leaving the muscle under the breast and enough skin to cover the wound. Reconstruction of the breast is much easier if these tissues are left. A simple mastectomy, rather than breast-conserving surgery, is usually done when there is a substantial amount of cancer in the milk ducts.
- Modified radical mastectomy consists of removing all breast tissue and some lymph nodes in the armpit but leaving the muscle under the breast. This procedure is usually done instead of a radical mastectomy.
- Radical mastectomy consists of removing all breast tissue plus the lymph nodes in the armpit and the muscle under the breast. This procedure is rarely done now.

Lymph node surgery (lymph node dissection) is also done if the cancer is or is suspected to be invasive. Nearby lymph nodes (usually about 10 to 20) are removed and examined to determine whether the cancer has spread to them. If cancer cells are detected in the lymph nodes, the cancer is more likely to have spread to other parts of the body. In such cases, additional treatment is needed. Removal of lymph nodes often causes problems because it affects the drainage of fluids in tissues. As a result, fluids may accumulate, causing persistent swelling (lymphedema) of the arm or hand. Arm and shoulder movement may be limited. Lymphedema may be treated by specially trained therapists. Women are taught how to massage the area, which may help the accumulated fluid drain, and how to apply a bandage, which helps keep fluid from reaccumulating. The affected arm should be used as normally as possible, except that the unaffected arm should be

What Is a Sentinel Lymph Node?

A network of lymphatic vessels and lymph nodes drain fluid from the tissue in the breast. The lymph nodes are designed to trap foreign or abnormal cells (such as bacteria or cancer cells) that may be contained in this fluid. Sometimes cancer cells pass through the nodes into the lymphatic vessels and spread to other parts of the body. Usually, the fluid from breast tissue drains through a single nearby lymph node first, but it may drain through more than one. Such lymph nodes are called sentinel lymph nodes.

Doctors can identify the sentinel lymph node by injecting blue dye or a radioactive substance into the fluid surrounding the breast cells. Doctors use a scanner to observe the dye or detect the radioactive substance when it reaches the first lymph nodes. The sentinel lymph node is then removed and examined to determine whether it contains cancer cells. If it does, other nearby lymph nodes are removed. If the sentinel lymph node does not contain cancer cells, the other lymph nodes are not removed. However, this biopsy is not completely reliable. In about 2 to 3% of women, cancer has spread to other lymph nodes when the sentinel lymph node is clear.

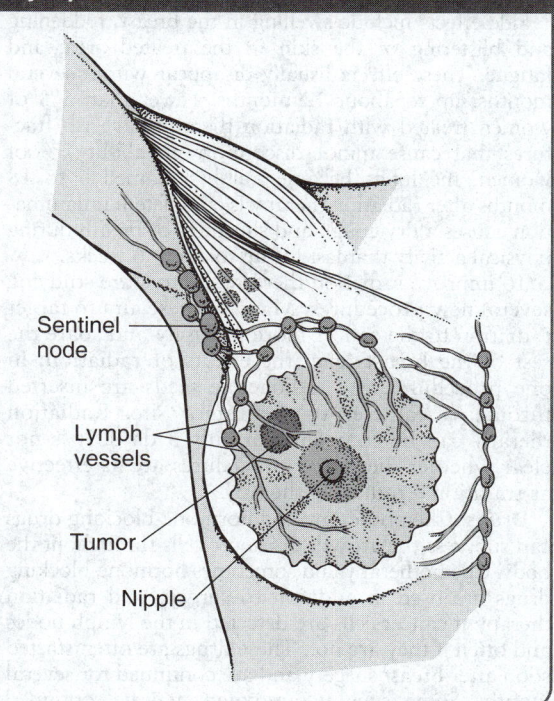

Sentinel node

Lymph vessels

Tumor

Nipple

used for heavy lifting. Women should exercise the affected arm daily as instructed and bandage it overnight indefinitely. Other problems include temporary or persistent numbness, a persistent burning sensation, and infection.

A **sentinel lymph node biopsy** is an alternative that may minimize or avoid the problems of lymph node surgery. This procedure involves locating and removing the first lymph node (or nodes) that the tumor drains into. If this node contains cancer cells, the other lymph nodes are removed. If it does not, the other lymph nodes are not removed. Whether this procedure is as effective as standard lymph node surgery is being studied.

Breast reconstruction surgery may be done at the same time as a mastectomy or later. A silicone or saline implant or tissue taken from other parts of the woman's body may be used. The safety of silicone implants, which sometimes leak, has been questioned. However, there is almost no evidence suggesting that silicone leakage has serious effects.

Radiation Therapy: This treatment is used to kill cancer cells at and near the site from which the tumor was removed, including nearby lymph nodes. Radiation therapy after mastectomy reduces the risk of cancer recurring near the site and in nearby lymph nodes. It may improve the chances of survival of women who have large tumors or cancer that has spread to several nearby lymph nodes.

Side effects include swelling in the breast, reddening and blistering of the skin in the treated area, and fatigue. These effects usually disappear within several months, up to about 12 months. Fewer than 5% of women treated with radiation therapy have rib fractures that cause minor discomfort. In about 1% of women, the lungs become mildly inflamed 6 to 18 months after radiation therapy is completed. Inflammation causes a dry cough and shortness of breath during physical activity that last for up to about 6 weeks.

To improve radiation therapy, doctors are studying several new procedures. Many of these aim to target radiation to the cancer more precisely and spare the rest of the breast from the effects of radiation. In one procedure, tiny radioactive seeds are inserted through a catheter to the tumor site. Radiation therapy can be completed in only 5 days. It is not clear whether these new procedures are as effective as traditional radiation therapy.

Drugs: Chemotherapy and hormone-blocking drugs can suppress the growth of cancer cells throughout the body. Chemotherapy and sometimes hormone-blocking drugs are used in addition to surgery and radiation therapy if cancer cells are detected in the lymph nodes and often if they are not. These drugs are often started soon after breast surgery and are continued for several months. Some, such as tamoxifen, may be continued for up to 5 years. These drugs delay the recurrence of cancer and prolong survival in most women. Analyzing the genetic material of the cancer (predictive genomic testing) may help predict which cancers are susceptible to chemotherapy or hormone-blocking drugs.

Chemotherapy is used to kill rapidly multiplying cells or slow their multiplication. Chemotherapy alone cannot cure breast cancer. It must be used with surgery or radiation therapy. Chemotherapy drugs are usually given intravenously in cycles. Sometimes they are given by mouth. Typically, a day of treatment is followed by several weeks of recovery. Using several chemotherapy drugs together is more effective than using a single drug. The choice of drugs depends partly on whether cancer cells are detected in nearby lymph nodes. Commonly used drugs include cyclophosphamide, doxorubicin, epirubicin, 5-fluorouracil, methotrexate, and paclitaxel (see table on page 1090). Side effects (such as vomiting, nausea, hair loss, and fatigue) vary depending on which drugs are used. Chemotherapy can cause infertility and early menopause by destroying the eggs in the ovaries. Chemotherapy may also suppress the production of blood cells by the bone marrow. So drugs, such as filgrastim or pegfilgrastim, may by used to stimulate the bone marrow.

Hormone-blocking drugs interfere with the actions of estrogen or progesterone, which stimulate the growth of cancer cells that have estrogen or progesterone receptors. These drugs may be used when cancer cells have these receptors.

- **Tamoxifen:** Tamoxifen, given by mouth, is a selective estrogen-receptor modulator. It binds with estrogen receptors and inhibits growth of breast tissue. In women who have estrogen receptor–positive cancer, tamoxifen increases the likelihood of survival during the first 10 years after diagnosis by about 20 to 25%. Tamoxifen, which is related to estrogen, has some of the benefits and risks of estrogen therapy taken after menopause (see page 1517). For example, it may decrease the risk of osteoporosis and fractures. It increases the risk of blood clots in the legs and lungs. It also substantially increases the risk of developing endometrial cancer. Thus, if women taking tamoxifen have spotting or bleeding from the vagina, they should see their doctor. However, the improvement in survival after breast cancer far outweighs the risk of endometrial cancer. Tamoxifen, unlike estrogen therapy, may worsen the vaginal dryness or hot flashes that occur after menopause. Tamoxifen is usually taken for 5 years.

- **Aromatase inhibitors:** These drugs (anastrozole, exemestane, and letrozole) inhibit aromatase (an enzyme that converts some hormones to estrogen) and thus may reduce the production of estrogen.

Rebuilding a Breast

After a general surgeon removes a breast tumor and the surrounding breast tissue (mastectomy), a plastic surgeon may reconstruct the breast. A silicone or saline implant may be used. Or in a more complex operation, tissue may be taken from other parts of the woman's body, usually the abdomen. Reconstruction may be done at the same time as the mastectomy—a choice that involves being under anesthesia for a longer time—or later—a choice that involves being under anesthesia a second time.

In many women, a reconstructed breast looks more natural than one that has been treated with radiation therapy, especially if the tumor was large.

If a silicone or saline implant is used and enough skin was left to cover it, the sensation in the skin over the implant is relatively normal. However, neither type of implant feels like breast tissue to the touch. If skin from other parts of the body is used to cover the breast, much of the sensation is lost. However, tissue from other parts of the body feels more like breast tissue than does a silicone or saline implant.

Silicone occasionally leaks out of its sack. As a result, an implant can become hard, cause discomfort, and appear less attractive. Also, silicone sometimes enters the bloodstream. Some women are concerned about whether the leaking silicone causes cancer in other parts of the body or rare diseases such as systemic lupus erythematosus (lupus). There is almost no evidence suggesting that silicone leakage has these serious effects, but because it might, the use of silicone implants has decreased, especially among women who have not had breast cancer.

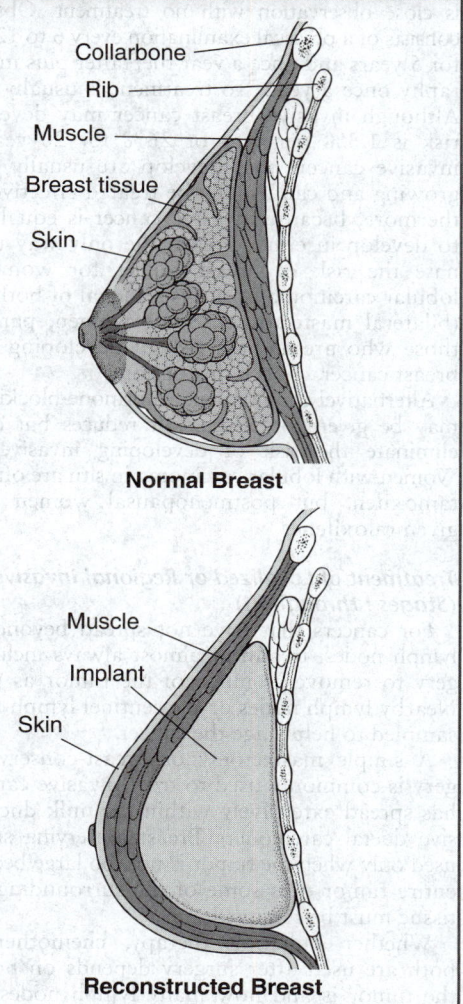

Normal Breast

Reconstructed Breast

In postmenopausal women, these drugs may be more effective than tamoxifen. These drugs may be given with tamoxifen or after tamoxifen has been used for 5 years. Aromatase inhibitors may increase the risk of osteoporosis.

Monoclonal antibodies are synthetic copies (or slightly modified versions) of natural substances that are part of the body's immune system. These drugs enhance the immune system's ability to fight cancer. Trastuzumab, a monoclonal antibody, is used with chemotherapy to treat metastatic breast cancer only when the cancer cells have too many HER2 receptors. This drug binds with HER2 receptors and thus helps prevent cancer cells from multiplying. Trastuzumab is usually taken for a year. It can weaken the heart muscle.

Treatment of Noninvasive Cancer (Stage 0)

For **ductal carcinoma in situ**, treatment usually consists of a simple mastectomy or wide excision with or without radiation therapy.

For **lobular carcinoma in situ,** treatment is less clear-cut. For many women, the preferred treatment is close observation with no treatment. Observation consists of a physical examination every 6 to 12 months for 5 years and once a year thereafter plus mammography once a year. No treatment is usually needed. Although invasive breast cancer may develop (the risk is 1.3% per year or 26% for 20 years), the invasive cancers that develop are usually not fast growing and can usually be treated effectively. Furthermore, because invasive cancer is equally likely to develop in either breast, the only way to eliminate the risk of breast cancer for women with lobular carcinoma in situ is removal of both breasts (bilateral mastectomy). Some women, particularly those who are at high risk of developing invasive breast cancer, choose this option.

Alternatively, tamoxifen, a hormone-blocking drug, may be given for 5 years. It reduces but does not eliminate the risk of developing invasive cancer. Women with lobular carcinoma in situ are often given tamoxifen, but postmenopausal women may be given raloxifene.

Treatment of Localized or Regional Invasive Cancer (Stages I through III)

For cancers that have not spread beyond nearby lymph nodes, treatment almost always includes surgery to remove as much of the tumor as possible. Nearby lymph nodes or the sentinel lymph node are sampled to help stage the cancer.

A simple mastectomy or breast-conserving surgery is commonly used to treat invasive cancer that has spread extensively within the milk ducts (invasive ductal carcinoma). Breast-conserving surgery is used only when the tumor is not too large because the entire tumor plus some of the surrounding normal tissue must be removed.

Whether radiation therapy, chemotherapy, or both are used after surgery depends on how large the tumor is and how many lymph nodes contain cancer cells. Breast-conserving surgery is usually followed by radiation therapy. Sometimes, when the tumor is too large for breast-conserving surgery, chemotherapy is given before surgery to reduce the size of the tumor. If chemotherapy reduces the size of the tumor enough, breast-conserving surgery may be possible. After surgery and radiation therapy, additional chemotherapy is usually given. If the cancer has estrogen receptors, women who are still menstruating are usually given tamoxifen, and postmenopausal women are given an aromatase inhibitor.

Treatment of Cancer That Has Spread (Stage IV)

Breast cancer that has spread beyond the lymph nodes is rarely cured, but most women who have it live at least 2 years, and a few live 10 to 20 years. Treatment extends life only slightly but may relieve symptoms and improve quality of life. However, some treatments have troublesome side effects. Thus, the decision of whether to be treated and, if so, which treatment to choose can be highly personal.

Most women are treated with chemotherapy or hormone-blocking drugs. However, chemotherapy, especially regimens that have uncomfortable side effects, are often postponed until symptoms (pain or other discomfort) develop or the cancer starts to worsen quickly. Pain is usually treated with analgesics. Other drugs may be given to relieve other symptoms. Chemotherapy or hormone-blocking drugs are given to relieve symptoms and improve quality of life rather than to prolong life. The most effective chemotherapy regimens for breast cancer that has spread include capecitabine, cyclophosphamide, docetaxel, doxorubicin, epirubicin, gemcitabine, paclitaxel, and vinorelbine.

Hormone-blocking drugs are preferred to chemotherapy in certain situations. For example, these drugs may be preferred when the cancer is estrogen receptor–positive, when cancer has not recurred for more than 2 years after diagnosis and initial treatment, or when cancer is not immediately life threatening. Different drugs are used in different situations:

- **Tamoxifen:** For women who are still menstruating, tamoxifen is usually the first hormone-blocking drug used because it has few side effects.
- **Aromatase inhibitors:** For postmenopausal women who have estrogen receptor–positive breast cancer, aromatase inhibitors (such as anastrozole, letrozole, and exemestane) may be more effective as a first treatment than tamoxifen.
- **Progestins:** These drugs, such as medroxyprogesterone or megestrol, may be used instead of aromatase inhibitors and tamoxifen and have almost as few side effects.
- **Fulvestrant:** This drug may be used when tamoxifen is no longer effective. It destroys the estrogen receptors in cancer cells. The most common side effect is stomach upset.

Alternatively, for women who are still menstruating, surgery to remove the ovaries, radiation to destroy them, or drugs to inhibit their activity (such as buserelin, goserelin, or leuprolide) may be used to stop estrogen production.

For cancers that have too many HER2 receptors and that have spread throughout the body, trastuzumab can be used alone or with chemotherapy such as paclitaxel. Trastuzumab can also be used with hormone-blocking drugs to treat women who have estrogen receptor–positive breast cancer.

In some situations, radiation therapy may be used instead of or before drugs. For example, if only one area of cancer is detected and that area is in a bone, radiation to that bone might be the only treatment used. Radiation therapy is usually the most effective treatment for cancer that has spread to bone, sometimes keeping it in check for years. It is also often the most effective treatment for cancer that has spread to the brain.

Surgery may be done to remove single tumors in other parts of the body (such as the brain) because such surgery can relieve symptoms.

Bisphosphonates (used to treat osteoporosis), such as pamidronate or zoledronate, reduce bone pain and bone loss and may prevent or delay bone problems that can result when cancer spreads to bone.

Treatment of Specific Types of Breast Cancer

For inflammatory breast cancer, treatment usually consists of both chemotherapy and radiation therapy. Mastectomy is usually done.

For Paget's disease of the nipple, treatment is usually similar to that of other types of breast cancer. It often involves simple mastectomy or breast-conserving surgery plus removal of the lymph nodes. Breast-conserving surgery is usually followed by radiation therapy. Less commonly, only the nipple with some surrounding normal tissue is removed.

For phyllodes tumors that are cancerous, treatment usually consists of wide excision. The tumor and a large amount of surrounding normal tissue are removed. If the tumor is large in relation to the breast, a simple mastectomy may be done. After surgical removal, about 20 to 35% of cancers recur near the same site.

Follow-up Care

After treatment is completed, follow-up physical examinations, including examination of the breasts, chest, neck, and armpits, are done every 3 months for 2 years, then every 6 months for 5 years from the date the cancer was diagnosed. Regular mammograms and breast self-examinations are also important. Women should promptly report certain symptoms to their doctor:

- Any changes in their breasts
- Pain
- Loss of appetite or weight
- Changes in menstruation
- Bleeding from the vagina (if not associated with menstrual periods)
- Blurred vision
- Any symptoms that seem unusual or that persist

Diagnostic procedures, such as chest x-rays, blood tests, bone scans, and computed tomography (CT), are not needed unless symptoms suggest the cancer has recurred.

The effects of treatment for breast cancer cause many changes in a woman's life. Support from family members and friends can help, as can support groups. Counseling may be helpful.

End-of-Life Issues

For women with metastatic breast cancer, quality of life may deteriorate, and the chances that further treatment will prolong life may be small. Staying comfortable may eventually become more important than trying to prolong life. Cancer pain can be adequately controlled with appropriate drugs (see page 61). So if women are having pain, they should ask their doctor for treatment to relieve it. Treatments can also relieve other troublesome symptoms, such as constipation, difficulty breathing, and nausea. Psychologic and spiritual counseling may also help.

Women with metastatic breast cancer should prepare advance directives indicating the type of care they desire in case they are no longer able to make such decisions (see page 69). Also, making or updating a will is important.

CHAPTER

246 Noncancerous Gynecologic Abnormalities

Noncancerous (benign) gynecologic growths include cysts, polyps, and myomas. Noncancerous growths can develop on the vulva or in the vagina, uterus, or ovaries. Occasionally, cysts or tumors in an ovary can cause the ovary to twist—a disorder called adnexal torsion. Rarely, certain growths become cancerous. Another abnormality is narrowing of the passageway through the lower part of the uterus (cervix) to the larger upper part (body)—a disorder called cervical stenosis.

Adnexal Torsion

Adnexal torsion is twisting of the ovary and sometimes the fallopian tube, cutting off the blood supply of these organs.

- Twisting causes sudden, severe pain and often vomiting.
- Doctors use an ultrasound device inserted into the vagina (transvaginal ultrasonography) to confirm the diagnosis.
- Surgery is done immediately to untwist the ovary and often to remove it.

An ovary and sometimes the fallopian tube twist on the ligament-like tissues that support them. Twisting of an ovary (adnexal torsion) is uncommon but is more likely to occur in women of reproductive age. It usually occurs when there is a problem with an ovary. The following conditions make it more likely to occur:

- Pregnancy
- Use of hormones to trigger ovulation (for infertility problems)
- Enlargement of the ovary, usually due to noncancerous (benign) tumors or cysts

Noncancerous tumors are more likely to cause twisting than cancerous ones.

Rarely, a normal ovary twists. Children are more likely to have this type of torsion.

Adnexal torsion usually occurs on only one side. Usually, only the ovary is involved, but occasionally, the fallopian tube also twists. Sometimes the blood supply to the ovary is cut off long enough to cause tissue in the ovary to die. Adnexal torsion can cause peritonitis—infection of the spaces in the abdomen (abdominal cavity) and the tissues lining it.

Symptoms

When an ovary twists, women have sudden, severe pain in the pelvic area. The pain is sometimes accompanied by nausea and vomiting. Before the sudden pain, women may have intermittent, crampy pain for days or occasionally even for weeks. This pain may occur because the ovary repeatedly twists, then untwists. The abdomen may feel tender.

Diagnosis

Doctors usually suspect the disorder based on symptoms and results of a physical examination. Ultrasonography using an ultrasound device inserted into the vagina (transvaginal ultrasonography) is done to confirm the diagnosis. This procedure can also usually determine whether blood flow to the ovary has been cut off.

> **? Did You Know...**
> The ovary sometimes twists, causing sudden, severe pain.

Treatment

If ultrasonography supports the diagnosis, women are treated immediately. One of the following procedures is used:

- **Laparoscopy:** Doctors may make a few small incisions in the abdomen. They then insert a flexible viewing tube (laparoscope) through the incision. Using instruments threaded through other incisions, they try to untwist the ovary and, if also twisted, the fallopian tube. Laparoscopy is done in a hospital and usually requires a general anesthetic, but it does not require an overnight stay.
- **Laparotomy:** Doctors make a larger incision in the abdomen. A laparoscope is not used because doctors can directly view the affected organs. Because the incision is larger, it requires an overnight stay in the hospital.

If the blood supply was cut off and tissue died, removal of the fallopian tubes and ovaries (salpingo-oophorectomy) is necessary. If an ovarian cyst is present, it is removed (called cystectomy). If an ovarian tumor is present, the entire ovary is removed (called oophorectomy).

Cervical Myomas

Cervical myomas are smooth, benign tumors in the cervix.

- A myoma may bleed, become infected, interfere with urinating, or cause pain during sexual intercourse.
- Doctors can see or feel most myomas during a pelvic examination.
- Myomas that cause symptoms can be removed surgically.

Myomas are benign tumors composed partly of muscle tissue. They seldom develop in the cervix, the lower part of the uterus. When they do, they are usually accompanied by myomas in the larger upper part of the uterus. Myomas in this part of the uterus are also called fibroids (see page 1533). Large cervical myomas may partially block the urinary tract or may protrude (prolapse) into the vagina. Sores sometimes develop on prolapsed myomas, which may become infected, bleed, or both. Prolapsed myomas can also block the flow of urine.

Symptoms

Most cervical myomas eventually cause symptoms. The most common symptom is bleeding from the vagina, which may be irregular or heavy. Heavy bleeding can cause anemia, with fatigue and weakness. Sexual intercourse may be painful.

If myomas become infected, they may cause pain, bleeding, or a discharge from the vagina. Rarely, prolapse causes symptoms such as a feeling of pressure or a lump in the abdomen.

If a myoma blocks the flow of urine, women may have a hesitant start when urinating, dribble at the end of urination, and retain urine. Urinary tract infections are more likely to develop.

Diagnosis

Doctors can often detect myomas during a physical examination. During a pelvic examination, doctors may see a myoma, particularly if prolapsed. Or doctors may feel a myoma when they check the size and shape of the uterus and cervix (with one gloved hand inside the vagina and the other on top of the abdomen).

If the diagnosis is uncertain, doctors may insert an ultrasound device through the vagina into the uterus to obtain an image of the area. This procedure, called transvaginal ultrasonography, is also done to check for blockage of urine flow and for additional myomas.

Blood tests are done to check for anemia. A Papanicolaou (Pap) test or variation of it (cervical cytology) is done to rule out cancer of the cervix.

Treatment

If myomas are small and do not cause any symptoms, no treatment is needed. If they cause symptoms, they are surgically removed if possible (a procedure called myomectomy). If only the myoma is removed, women can still bear children. However, if myomas are large, removal of the entire uterus (hysterectomy) may be necessary. Either procedure can be done by making a large incision in the abdomen (laparotomy). Sometimes these procedures can be done with instruments inserted through one or more small incisions near the navel (laparoscopy).

If a myoma prolapses, it is removed with instruments inserted through the vagina (transvaginally) if possible.

Cervical Stenosis

Cervical stenosis is narrowing of the passageway through the cervix (the lower part of the uterus).

- Infertility can occur, or the uterus can fill with blood or pus.
- The opening of the cervix can be widened to relieve symptoms.

In cervical stenosis, the passageway through the cervix (from the vagina to the main body of the uterus) is narrow or completely closed.

Some women are born with cervical stenosis. In others, cervical stenosis results from a disorder or another condition, such as the following:

- Cancer (cervical or endometrial)
- Surgery to treat precancerous changes of the cervix (dysplasia)
- Procedures that destroy or remove the lining of the uterus (endometrial ablation) in women who have persistent vaginal bleeding
- Radiation therapy to treat cancer of the cervix or of the lining of the uterus (endometrial cancer)
- Menopause, because the tissues in the cervix thin (atrophy)

Cervical stenosis may result in an accumulation of blood in the uterus (hematometra). In women who are still menstruating, menstrual blood mixed with cells from the uterus may flow backward into the pelvis, possibly causing endometriosis (see page 1529). If pus forms in the uterus (as it may in women with cervical or endometrial cancer), pus may accumulate in the uterus. Accumulation of pus in the uterus is called pyometra.

Symptoms

Before menopause, cervical stenosis may cause menstrual abnormalities, such as no periods (amenorrhea), painful periods (dysmenorrhea), and abnormal bleeding. Cervical stenosis can also cause infertility because sperm cannot pass through the cervix to fertilize the egg.

After menopause, cervical stenosis may be present but not cause symptoms.

A hematometra or pyometra can cause pain or cause the uterus to bulge. Sometimes women feel a lump in the pelvic area.

Diagnosis

Doctors suspect the diagnosis based on symptoms and circumstances, such as the following:

- When periods stop or become painful after surgery on the cervix
- When doctors cannot insert an instrument into the cervix to obtain a sample of tissue from the cervix for a Papanicolaou (Pap) test or a variation of it (cervical cytology) or from the lining of the uterus (an endometrial biopsy)

Doctors confirm the diagnosis by trying to pass a probe through the cervix into the uterus.

No further tests are needed for the following:

- Postmenopausal women who have never had abnormal Pap test results
- Women who have no symptoms, no hematometra, and no pyometra

If cervical stenosis causes symptoms, a hematometra, or a pyometra, tissue samples are taken and examined under a microscope to rule out cancer. After treatment (which widens the cervix), doctors take samples from the cervix and from the uterine lining.

Treatment

Cervical stenosis is treated only if women have symptoms, a hematometra, or a pyometra. Then, the cervix may be widened (dilated) by inserting small, lubricated metal rods (dilators) through its opening, then inserting progressively larger dilators. To try to keep the cervix open, doctors may place a tube (cervical stent) in the cervix for 4 to 6 weeks.

Cysts

Cysts are closed sacs that are separate from the tissue around them. They often contain fluid or semisolid material. Cysts that commonly occur in the genital organs include Bartholin's gland cysts, endometriomas, inclusion and epidermal cysts, and Skene's duct cysts.

BARTHOLIN'S GLAND CYSTS

Bartholin's gland cysts are mucus-filled sacs that can form when the glands located near the opening to the vagina are blocked.

- Cysts are usually painless, but if large, they can interfere with sitting, walking, and sexual intercourse.
- Cysts may become infected, forming a painful abscess.
- Doctors can usually see or feel the cysts during a pelvic examination.
- Doctors may create a permanent opening from the cyst to the outside or may surgically remove the cyst.

Bartholin's glands are very small, round glands that are located in the vulva on either side of the opening to the vagina. Because they are located deep under the skin, they cannot normally be felt. These glands may help provide fluids for lubrication during sexual intercourse.

If the duct to the gland is blocked, the gland becomes filled with mucus and enlarges. The result is a cyst. These cysts develop in about 2% of women, usually those in their 20s. As women age, they are less likely to have cysts and abscesses.

Typically, what causes the blockage is unknown. Rarely, cysts result from a sexually transmitted disease, such as gonorrhea.

Symptoms

Most cysts do not cause any symptoms. But if cysts become large, they can cause discomfort during sitting, walking, or sexual intercourse. Women may notice a painless lump near the opening of the vagina, making the vulva look lopsided.

Abscesses cause severe pain and sometimes fever. They are tender to the touch. The skin over them appears red. Women may have a discharge from the vagina, which is usually unrelated to the abscess.

Diagnosis

A woman should see a doctor in the following circumstances:

- The cyst continues to enlarge or persists after several days of immersing the area in hot water (in a tub or sitz bath).
- The cyst is painful (often indicating an abscess).
- A fever develops.
- The cyst interferes with walking or sitting.
- She is over 40.

If a cyst is large enough for a woman to notice it or for symptoms to develop, doctors can usually see or feel the cyst during a pelvic examination. Doctors can usually tell whether it is infected by its appearance. If a discharge is present, doctors may send a sample to be tested for other infections.

Because cancer of the vulva sometimes resembles a cyst, doctors may remove the cyst to examine under a microscope (biopsy). A biopsy is usually done if the cyst is irregular or bumpy or if the woman is over 40.

Treatment

If a cyst causes little or no pain, women may treat it themselves. They can use a sitz bath or soak in a few inches of warm water in a tub. Soaks should last 10 to 15 minutes and be done 3 or 4 times a day. Sometimes cysts disappear after a few days of such treatment. If the treatment is ineffective, women should see a doctor.

In women under 40, only cysts that cause symptoms require treatment. Draining the cysts is usually ineffective because they commonly recur. Thus, surgery may be done to make a permanent opening from the gland's duct to the surface of the vulva. Thus, if fluids refill the cyst, they can drain out. After a local anesthetic is injected to numb the site, one of the following procedures can be done:

- **Placement of a catheter:** A small incision is made in the cyst so that a small balloon-tipped tube (catheter) can be inserted into the cyst. Once in place, the balloon is inflated, and the catheter is left there for 4 to 6 weeks, so that a permanent opening can form. The catheter is inserted and removed in the doctor's office. Women can do their normal activities while the catheter is in place, although sexual intercourse may be uncomfortable.
- **Marsupialization:** Doctors make a small cut in the cyst and stitch the inside edges of the cyst to the

What Is Bartholin's Gland Cyst?

The small glands on either side of the vaginal opening, called Bartholin's glands, may become blocked. Fluids then accumulate, and the gland swells, forming a cyst. Cysts range from the size of a pea to that of a golf ball or larger. Most often, they occur only on one side. They may become infected, forming an abscess.

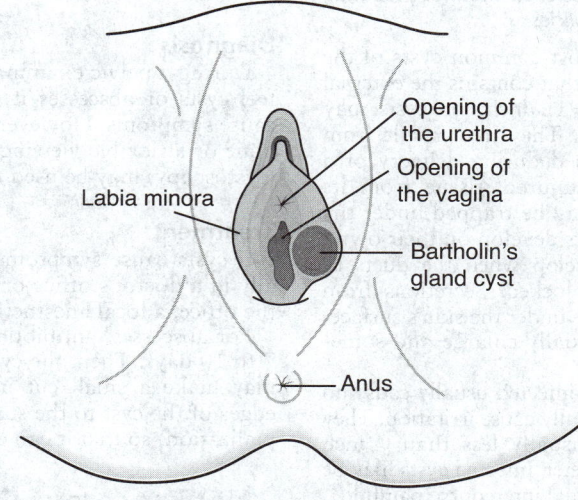

Labia minora

Opening of the urethra

Opening of the vagina

Bartholin's gland cyst

Anus

surface of the vulva. This procedure is done in an outpatient operating room. Sometimes general anesthesia is needed.

After these procedures, women may have a discharge for a few weeks. Usually, wearing panty liners is all that is needed. Taking sitz baths several times a day may help relieve any discomfort and help speed healing.

If cysts recur, they may be surgically removed. This procedure is done in an operating room.

In women over 40, all cysts must be treated. Treatment usually occurs during diagnosis, when doctors obtain a sample to check for cancer. Treatment involves surgically removing or marsupializing the cyst.

For an abscess, antibiotics are given by mouth for 7 to 10 days. A catheter can be inserted to drain the abscess or marsupialization may be done initially to treat the abscess or later to prevent the cyst from refilling.

Regardless of treatment, cysts sometimes recur.

ENDOMETRIOMAS OF THE VULVA

Vulvar endometriomas are rare, painful, blood-filled cysts that develop when tissue from the lining of the uterus (endometrial tissue) appears in the vulva.

For unknown reasons, patches of tissue from the lining of the uterus (endometrial tissue) sometimes appear outside the uterus. This disorder is called endometriosis (see page 1529). Endometriosis rarely occurs in the vulva. It is more common in other locations, such as the ovaries. Sometimes the endometrial tissue forms a cyst (endometrioma). Endometriomas often develop at the site of a previous operation, such as an episiotomy (an incision to widen the opening of the vagina to help with delivery of a baby).

Endometriomas may be painful, particularly during intercourse. Endometriomas respond to hormones just as normal endometrial tissue does. Thus, they can enlarge and cause pain, particularly before and during menstrual periods. Endometriomas are tender and may look blue. They can rupture, causing severe pain.

During a pelvic examination, doctors can usually see or feel endometriomas that cause symptoms.

Endometriomas in the vulva are surgically removed. This procedure is usually done in an operating room but may be done in a doctor's office. A local anesthetic is used. Doctors do a biopsy of the removed tissue to make sure it is not a melanoma, which can occur on the vulva and vagina.

INCLUSION AND EPIDERMAL CYSTS OF THE VULVA

Cysts that develop on the vulva include inclusion cysts and epidermal cysts. Vulvar inclusion cysts are small sacs that contain tissue from the surface of the vulva. Vulvar epidermal cysts are similar but contain secretions from oil-producing (sebaceous) glands near hair follicles.

Inclusion cysts are the most common cysts of the vulva. The vulva is the area that contains the external genital organs (see page 1491). Inclusion cysts may also develop in the vagina. They may result from injuries, such as tears caused during delivery of a baby. When the vulva is injured, tissue from its surface (epithelial tissue) may be trapped under the surface. Some inclusion cysts develop on their own.

Epidermal cysts may develop when the ducts to sebaceous glands become blocked. Secretions from these glands then accumulate under the skin's surface.

Both of these cysts eventually enlarge and sometimes become infected.

Cysts that do not become infected usually cause no symptoms, but they occasionally cause irritation. They are white or yellow and usually less than 1/2 inch (about 1 centimeter) in diameter. Infected cysts may be red and tender and make sexual intercourse painful.

Doctors can usually see or feel cysts during a pelvic examination.

If cysts cause symptoms, they are removed after a local anesthetic is injected to numb the site.

SKENE'S DUCT CYST

Skene's duct cysts develop near the opening of the urethra when the ducts to the glands are blocked.

- Large cysts may cause pain during sexual intercourse or problems urinating.
- Cysts that cause symptoms can be removed.

Skene's glands, also called periurethral or paraurethral glands, are located around the opening of the urethra. The tissue that surrounds them includes part of the clitoris. The glands may be involved in sexual stimulation and lubrication for sexual intercourse.

Cysts are uncommon. They form if the duct to the gland is blocked, usually because the gland is infected. These cysts occur mainly in adults. If cysts become infected, they may form an abscess.

Symptoms

Most cysts are less than 1/2 inch (about 1 centimeter) in diameter and do not cause any symptoms. Some cysts are larger and cause pain during sexual intercourse. Sometimes large cysts block the flow of urine through the urethra. In such cases, the first symptoms may be a hesitant start when urinating, dribbling at the end of urination, and retention of urine. Or a urinary tract infection may develop, causing a frequent, urgent need to urinate and painful urination.

Abscesses are tender, painful, and swollen. The skin over the ducts appears red. Most women do not have a fever.

Diagnosis

During a pelvic examination, doctors can usually feel cysts or abscesses if they are large enough to cause symptoms. However, ultrasonography may be done or a flexible viewing tube to view the bladder (cystoscopy) may be used to confirm the diagnosis.

Treatment

If cysts cause symptoms, they are removed, usually in a doctor's office or in an operating room. In the office, a local anesthetic is usually used.

For abscesses, antibiotics are given by mouth for 7 to 10 days. Then, the cyst is removed. Or doctors may make a small cut in the cyst and stitch the edges of the cyst to the surface of the vulva (marsupialization) so that it can drain.

Noncancerous Ovarian Growths

Noncancerous (benign) ovarian growths include functional cysts and tumors.

- Most noncancerous cysts and tumors do not cause any symptoms, but some cause pain or a feeling of heaviness in the pelvis.
- Doctors may detect growths during a pelvic examination, then use ultrasonography to confirm the diagnosis.
- Some cysts disappear on their own.
- Cysts or tumors may be removed through an incision in the abdomen, and sometimes the affected ovary must also be removed.

Functional Cysts: Functional cysts form from the fluid-filled cavities (follicles) in the ovaries. Each follicle contains one egg. Usually, during each menstrual cycle, one follicle releases one egg. About one third of women who are menstruating have cysts. Functional cysts seldom develop after menopause.

There are two types of functional cysts:

- **Follicular cysts:** These cysts form as the egg is developing in the follicle.
- **Corpus luteum cysts:** These cysts develop from the structure that forms after the follicle ruptures and releases its egg. This structure is called the corpus luteum. Corpus luteum cysts may bleed, causing the ovary to bulge or to rupture. If the cyst ruptures, fluids escape into spaces in the abdomen (the abdominal cavity) and may cause severe pain.

Most functional cysts are less than about 2/3 inch (1.5 centimeters) in diameter. A few reach or exceed about 2 inches (5 centimeters). Functional cysts usually disappear on their own after a few days or weeks.

Benign Tumors: Noncancerous (benign) ovarian tumors usually grow slowly and rarely become cancerous. The most common include the following:

- **Benign cystic teratomas (dermoid cysts):** These tumors usually develop from all three layers of tissue in the embryo (called germ cell layers). All organs form from these tissues. Thus, teratomas may contain tissues from other structures, such as nerve, glandular, and skin tissues.
- **Fibromas:** These tumors are solid masses composed of connective tissue (the tissues that hold structures together). Fibromas are slow-growing and are usually less than 3 inches (about 7 centimeters) in diameter. They usually occur on only one side.
- **Cystadenomas:** These fluid-filled cysts develop from the surface of the ovary and contain some tissue from glands in the ovaries.

Symptoms

Most functional cysts and noncancerous tumors do not cause any symptoms. Sometimes women have irregular periods and spotting. If corpus luteum cysts bleed, they may cause pain or tenderness in the pelvic area. If women have a fever, feel nauseated, and vomit, the spaces in the abdomen (abdominal cavity) and the tissues lining it may be infected (a disorder called peritonitis). Occasionally, sudden, severe abdominal pain occurs because a large cyst or mass causes the ovary to twist (a disorder called adnexal torsion).

Accumulation of fluid in the abdomen (ascites) can occur with fibromas and ovarian cancer. Ascites may cause a feeling of pressure or heaviness in the abdomen.

Diagnosis

Doctors usually detect cysts or tumors during a routine pelvic examination. But sometimes doctors suspect them based on symptoms.

A pregnancy test is done to rule out pregnancy, including pregnancy located outside the uterus (ectopic pregnancy). Ultrasonography using an ultrasound device inserted into the vagina (transvaginal ultrasonography) is done to confirm the diagnosis. If the diagnosis is still unclear, magnetic resonance imaging (MRI) or computed tomography (CT) may be done. If these tests suggest that the growth could be cancerous, doctors remove it and examine it under a microscope. They may also do blood tests to check for substances called markers, which may appear in the blood or may increase when some cancers are present.

Treatment

If ovarian cysts are less than 3 inches (about 7 centimeters) in diameter, they usually disappear without treatment. Ultrasonography is done periodically to check.

If a cyst or tumor needs to be removed, laparoscopy or laparotomy is done if possible. Laparoscopy requires two or three small incisions in the abdomen. It is done in a hospital and usually requires a general anesthetic. However, women do not have to stay overnight. Laparotomy is similar but requires a larger incision and an overnight stay in the hospital. Which procedure is used depends on how large the growth is and whether other organs are affected. Cystectomy (removal of the cyst) can usually be done for the following conditions:

- Most cysts that are larger than 3 inches and that persist for more than three menstrual cycles
- Cystic teratomas that are smaller than 4 inches (about 10 centimeters)
- Corpus luteum cysts if peritonitis develops

Removal of the affected ovary (oophorectomy) is necessary for the following:

- Fibromas and solid ovarian tumors
- Cystadenomas
- Cystic teratomas that are larger than 4 inches
- Cysts that cannot be surgically separated from the ovary
- Most cysts that are detected in postmenopausal women and are > 2 inches

Polyps of the Cervix

Cervical polyps are common fingerlike growths of tissue that protrude into the passageway through the cervix. Polyps are almost always benign (noncancerous).

About 2 to 5% of women have cervical polyps. They are probably caused by chronic inflammation or infection. They are rarely cancerous.

Most cervical polyps do not cause any symptoms. Some polyps bleed between menstrual periods or after intercourse. Some become infected, causing a puslike discharge from the vagina. Polyps are usually reddish pink and less than 1/2 inch (about 1 centimeter) in diameter.

Diagnosis and Treatment

Doctors can detect polyps when they do a pelvic examination.

Polyps that cause bleeding or a discharge are removed during the pelvic examination in the doctor's office. No anesthetic is needed. Rarely, bleeding occurs after polyps are removed. If it does, a caustic substance, such as silver nitrate, is applied to the affected area with a swab to stop the bleeding.

If symptoms (bleeding and a discharge) persist after polyps are removed, a Papanicolaou (Pap) test or a variation of it (cervical cytology) is done to rule out cancer of the cervix. Also, a sample of tissue from the lining of the uterus (endometrium) is taken and examined under a microscope (endometrial biopsy) to exclude endometrial cancer.

CHAPTER

247 Cancers of the Female Reproductive System

Cancers can occur in any part of the female reproductive system—the vulva, vagina, cervix, uterus, fallopian tubes, or ovaries. These cancers are called gynecologic cancers.

Gynecologic cancers can directly invade nearby tissues and organs or spread (metastasize) through the lymphatic vessels and lymph nodes (lymphatic system) or bloodstream to distant parts of the body.

Diagnosis

Regular pelvic examinations and Papanicolaou (Pap) tests or other similar tests (see page 1502) can lead to the early detection of certain gynecologic cancers, especially cancer of the cervix. Such examinations can sometimes prevent cancer by detecting precancerous changes (dysplasia) before they become cancer. Regular pelvic examinations can also detect early cancers of the vagina and vulva. However, cancers of the ovaries, uterus, and fallopian tubes are not easy for doctors to detect during a pelvic examination.

If cancer is suspected, a biopsy can confirm or rule out the diagnosis. If cancer is diagnosed, one or more procedures may be done to determine the stage of the cancer. The stage is based on how large the cancer is and how far it has spread. Some commonly used procedures include ultrasonography, computed tomography (CT), magnetic resonance imaging (MRI), chest x-rays, and bone scans using a radioactive substance.

Staging a cancer helps doctors choose the best treatment. Doctors often determine the stage of cancer after they remove the cancer and biopsy the surrounding tissues, including lymph nodes. For all gynecologic cancers, stages range from I (the earliest) to IV (advanced). For most cancers, further distinctions, designated by letters of the alphabet, are made within stages.

Treatment

The main treatment of endometrial or ovarian cancer is surgical removal of the tumor. Surgery may be followed by radiation therapy or chemotherapy. In women with cervical cancer, radiation therapy may be external (using a large machine) or internal (using radioactive implants placed directly on the cancer). External radiation therapy is usually given several days a week for several weeks. Internal radiation therapy involves staying in the hospital for several days while the implants are in place.

Chemotherapy may be given by injection or by mouth or by giving drugs through a catheter inserted into the abdomen (intraperitoneally). How often chemotherapy is given depends on the type of cancer. Sometimes women have to remain at the hospital while they receive chemotherapy.

When a gynecologic cancer is very advanced and a cure is not possible, radiation therapy or chemotherapy may still be recommended to reduce the size of the cancer or its metastases and to relieve pain and other symptoms. Women with incurable cancer should establish advance directives (see page 69). Because end-of-life care has improved, more and more women with incurable cancer are able to die comfortably at home (see page 60). Appropriate drugs can be used to relieve the anxiety and pain commonly experienced by people with incurable cancer.

Endometrial Cancer

Endometrial cancer of the uterus develops in the lining of the uterus (endometrium).

- Endometrial cancer usually affects women after menopause.
- It sometimes causes abnormal vaginal bleeding.
- To diagnosis this cancer, doctors remove a sample of tissue from the endometrium to be analyzed (biopsy).

STAGING CANCERS OF THE FEMALE REPRODUCTIVE SYSTEM*

TYPE	STAGE I	STAGE II	STAGE III	STAGE IV†
Endometrial (uterine) cancer	Only in the upper part of the uterus (not the cervix)	Spread to the cervix	Spread to nearby tissues, the vagina, or lymph nodes but still within the pelvis	Spread to the bladder or intestine (A) or distant organs (B)
Ovarian cancer	Only in one or both ovaries	Spread to the uterus, fallopian tubes, or nearby tissues within the pelvis	Spread outside the pelvis to the lymph nodes, the surface of the liver, the small intestine, or nearby tissues	Spread outside the abdomen or to the inside of the liver
Cervical cancer	Only in the cervix	Spread outside the cervix (including the upper part of the vagina) but still within the pelvis	Spread through-out the pelvis (including the lower part of the vagina), some-times blocking the ureters	Spread to the bladder or rectum (A) or distant organs (B)
Vulvar cancer	Only in the vulva and/or the area between the opening of the rectum and vagina (perineum) and ¾ inch (about 2 centimeters) or smaller	Only in the vulva and/or perineum, but larger than ¾ inch	In the vulva and/or perineum and spread to nearby tissues and/or lymph nodes	Spread beyond nearby tissues to the bladder, the intestine, or more distant lymph nodes
Vaginal cancer	Only in the vagina	Spread to nearby tissues but still within the pelvis	Spread throughout the pelvis	Spread to the bladder or rectum (A) or distant organs (B)
Fallopian tube cancer	Only in one or both fallopian tubes	Spread to nearby tissues but still within the pelvis	Spread to abdominal organs (such as the intestine and liver) or nearby lymph nodes	Spread to distant organs

*Simplified from the International Federation of Gynecology and Obstetrics Staging System.
†Stage IV is sometimes further classified as A or B depending on where the cancer has spread.

■ Usually, the uterus and fallopian tubes are removed, often followed by radiation therapy and sometimes by chemotherapy.

Cancer of the uterus begins in the lining of the uterus (endometrium) and is more precisely termed endometrial cancer (carcinoma). In the United States, it is the most common gynecologic cancer and the fourth most common cancer among women. One in 50 women gets endometrial cancer. This cancer usually develops after menopause, most often in women aged 50 to 65.

More than 80% of endometrial cancers are adenocarcinomas, which develop from gland cells. Fewer than 5% of cancers in the uterus are sarcomas. These cancers develop from connective tissue and tend to be more aggressive.

Causes

Endometrial cancer is more common in developed countries where the diet is high in fat.

The most important risk factors for endometrial cancer are

- Obesity
- Diabetes
- Hypertension

Other factors increase risk because they result in a high level of estrogen but not progesterone. They include the following:

- Having an early start of menstrual periods (menarche), menopause after age 52, or both
- Having menstrual problems (such as excessive bleeding, spotting between menstrual periods, or long intervals without periods)
- Not having any children
- Having tumors that produce estrogen
- Taking high doses of drugs that contain estrogen, such as estrogen therapy without a progestin (a synthetic drug similar to the hormone progesterone), after menopause
- Using tamoxifen for more than 5 years

Estrogen promotes the growth of tissue and rapid cell division in the lining of the uterus (endometrium). Progesterone helps balance the effects of estrogen. Levels of estrogen are high during part of the menstrual cycle. Thus, having more menstrual periods during a lifetime may increase the risk of endometrial cancer. Tamoxifen, a drug used to treat breast cancer, blocks the effects of estrogen in the breast, but it has the same effects as estrogen in the uterus. Thus, this drug may increase the risk of endometrial cancer. Taking oral contraceptives that contain estrogen and a progestin appears to reduce the risk of endometrial cancer.

Other risk factors include the following:

- Having had or having a family member who has had cancer of the breast, ovaries, or possibly the large intestine (colon) or lining of the uterus
- Having had radiation therapy directed at the pelvis

Symptoms

Abnormal bleeding from the vagina is the most common early symptom. Abnormal bleeding includes

- Bleeding after menopause
- Bleeding between menstrual periods
- Periods that are irregular, heavy, or longer than normal

One of three women with vaginal bleeding after menopause has endometrial cancer. Women who have vaginal bleeding after menopause should see a doctor promptly. A watery, blood-tinged discharge may also occur. Postmenopausal women may have a vaginal discharge for several weeks or months, followed by vaginal bleeding.

Diagnosis

Doctors may suspect endometrial cancer if women have typical symptoms or if results of a Papanicolaou (Pap) test, usually done as part of a routine examination, are abnormal. If cancer is suspected, doctors take a sample of tissue from the endometrium (endometrial biopsy) in their office and send it to a laboratory for analysis. This test accurately detects endometrial cancer more than 90% of the time. If the diagnosis is still uncertain, doctors scrape tissue from the uterine lining for analysis—a procedure called dilation and curettage (D and C—see page 1504). At the same time, doctors may view the interior of the uterus using a thin, flexible viewing tube inserted through the vagina and cervix into the uterus in a procedure called hysteroscopy. Alternatively, an ultrasound device may be inserted through the vagina into the uterus (transvaginal ultrasonography) to evaluate abnormalities.

If endometrial cancer is diagnosed, some or all of the following procedures may be done to determine whether the cancer has spread beyond the uterus: blood tests, kidney and liver function tests, and a chest x-ray. If results of the physical examination or other tests suggest that the cancer has spread beyond the uterus, computed tomography (CT) or magnetic resonance imaging (MRI) is done. Other procedures are sometimes required. Staging is based on information obtained from these procedures and during surgery to remove the cancer.

Prognosis

If endometrial cancer is detected early, nearly 70 to 95% of women who have it survive at least 5 years, and most are cured. The prognosis is better for women whose cancer has not spread beyond the uterus. If the cancer grows relatively slowly, the prognosis is also better. Less than one third of women who have this cancer die of it.

Treatment

Hysterectomy, surgical removal of the uterus, is the mainstay of treatment for women who have endometrial cancer. If the cancer has not spread beyond the uterus, removal of the uterus plus removal of the fallopian tubes and ovaries (salpingo-oophorectomy) almost always cures the cancer. Unless the cancer is very advanced, hysterectomy improves the prognosis. Nearby lymph nodes are usually removed at the same time. These tissues are examined by a pathologist to determine whether the cancer has spread and, if so, how far it has spread. With this information, doctors can determine whether additional treatment (chemotherapy, radiation therapy, or a progestin) is needed after surgery.

For very advanced cancer, treatment varies but usually involves a combination of surgery, radiation therapy, chemotherapy, and occasionally synthetic hormones.

Radiation therapy may be given after surgery in case some undetected cancer cells remain. More than half of women with cancer limited to the uterus do not need radiation therapy. However, if the cancer has spread to the cervix or beyond the uterus, radiation therapy is usually recommended after surgery.

If the cancer has spread beyond the uterus and cervix or recurs, chemotherapy drugs (such as carboplatin, cisplatin, cyclophosphamide, doxorubicin, and paclitaxel) may be used instead of or sometimes with radiation therapy. These drugs reduce the cancer's size and control its spread in more than half of women treated. However, these drugs are toxic and have many side effects.

If the cancer does not respond to chemotherapy, progestins (synthetic drugs similar to the hormone progesterone) may be used. These drugs are much less toxic than chemotherapy drugs. In 20 to 25% of women who have cancer that has spread or recurred, a progestin may reduce the cancer's size and control its spread for 2 to 3 years. Treatment is continued as long as the cancer responds to it.

If menopausal symptoms such as hot flashes and vaginal dryness become bothersome after the uterus is removed, hormones such as estrogen, a progestin, or both can taken to relieve them. This treatment is safe and does not increase the risk of developing cancer again.

Ovarian Cancer

- Ovarian cancer may not cause symptoms until it is large or has spread.
- If doctors suspect ovarian cancer, ultrasonography, magnetic resonance imaging, or computed tomography is done.
- Usually, both ovaries, both fallopian tubes, and the uterus are removed.
- Chemotherapy is often needed after surgery.

Cancer of the ovaries (ovarian carcinoma) develops most often in women aged 50 to 70. This cancer eventually develops in about 1 of 70 women. In the United States, it is the second most common gynecologic cancer. However, more women die of ovarian cancer than of any other gynecologic cancer. It is the fifth most common cause of cancer deaths in women.

Factors that increase the risk of ovarian cancer include the following:

Understanding Hysterectomy

A hysterectomy is the removal of the uterus. Usually, the uterus is removed through an incision in the lower abdomen. Sometimes the uterus can be removed through the vagina. Either method usually takes about 1 to 2 hours and requires a general anesthetic. Afterward, vaginal bleeding and pain may occur. The hospital stay is usually 2 to 3 days, and recovery may take up to 6 weeks. When the uterus is removed through the vagina, less bleeding occurs, recovery is faster, and there is no visible scar.

Because of advances in technology, hysterectomy may be done using laparoscopy or robotic surgery. Then, the hospital stay is only 1 day. Women usually have less pain after surgery and can return more quickly to normal activities.

In addition to treating certain gynecologic cancers, a hysterectomy may be used to treat prolapse of the uterus, endometriosis, or fibroids (if causing severe symptoms). Sometimes it is done as part of the treatment for cancer of the colon, rectum, or bladder.

There are several types of hysterectomy. The type used depends on the disorder being treated.

- **Subtotal (supracervical) hysterectomy:** Only the upper part of the uterus is removed, but the cervix is not. The fallopian tubes and ovaries may or may not be removed.
- **Total hysterectomy:** The entire uterus including the cervix is removed.
- **Radical hysterectomy:** The entire uterus plus the surrounding tissues, ligaments, and lymph nodes are removed. Both fallopian tubes and ovaries are usually also removed in women older than 45.

After a hysterectomy, menstruation stops. However, a hysterectomy does not cause menopause unless the ovaries are removed also. Removal of the ovaries has the same effects as menopause, so hormone therapy may be recommended (see page 1516). Many women anticipate feeling depressed or losing interest in sex after a hysterectomy. However, hysterectomy rarely has these effects unless the ovaries are also removed.

- Being older (the most important)
- Not having any children
- Having a first child late in life
- Starting menstruating early
- Having menopause late
- Having had or having a family member who had cancer of the uterus, breast, or large intestine (colon)

The risk of ovarian cancer is higher in developed countries because the diet tends to be high in fat. Use of oral contraceptives significantly decreases risk.

About 5 to 10% of cases are related to the *BRCA* gene, which is also involved in some breast cancers. In these cases, ovarian and breast cancer tends to run in families. This abnormal gene is most common among Ashkenazi Jewish women.

There are many types of ovarian cancer. They develop from the many different types of cells in the ovaries. Cancers that start on the surface of the ovaries (epithelial carcinomas) account for at least 80%. Most other ovarian cancers start from the cells that produce eggs (called germ cell tumors) or in connective tissue (called stromal cell tumors). Germ cell tumors are much more common among women younger than 30. Sometimes cancers from other parts of the body spread to the ovaries.

Ovarian cancer can spread directly to the surrounding area and through the lymphatic system to other parts of the pelvis and abdomen. It can also spread through the bloodstream, eventually appearing in distant parts of the body, mainly the liver and lungs.

Symptoms

Ovarian cancer causes the affected ovary to enlarge. In young women, enlargement of an ovary is likely to be caused by a noncancerous fluid-filled sac (cyst). However, after menopause, an enlarged ovary can be a sign of ovarian cancer.

Many women have no symptoms until the cancer is advanced. The first symptom may be vague discomfort in the lower abdomen, similar to indigestion. Other symptoms may include bloating, loss of appetite (because the stomach is compressed), gas pains, and backache. Ovarian cancer rarely causes vaginal bleeding.

Eventually, the abdomen may swell because the ovary enlarges or fluid accumulates in the abdomen. At this stage, pain in the pelvic area, anemia, and weight loss are common. Rarely, germ cell or stromal cell tumors produce estrogens, which can cause tissue in the uterine lining to grow excessively and breasts to enlarge. Or these tumors may produce male hormones (androgens), which can cause body hair to grow excessively, or hormones that resemble thyroid hormones, which can cause hyperthyroidism.

Diagnosis

Diagnosing ovarian cancer in its early stages is difficult because symptoms usually do not appear until the cancer is quite large or has spread beyond the ovaries and because many less serious disorders cause similar symptoms.

If doctors detect an enlarged ovary during a physical examination, ultrasonography is done first.

Sometimes computed tomography (CT) or magnetic resonance imaging (MRI) is used to help distinguish an ovarian cyst from a cancerous mass. If advanced cancer is suspected, CT or MRI is usually done before surgery to determine extent of the cancer.

If cancer seems unlikely, doctors reexamine the woman periodically.

If doctors suspect cancer or test results are unclear, the ovaries are examined using a thin, flexible viewing tube (laparoscope) inserted through a small incision just below the navel. Also, tissue samples are removed using instruments threaded through the laparoscope and examined (biopsied). In addition, blood tests are usually done to measure levels of substances that may indicate the presence of cancer (tumor markers), such as cancer antigen 125 (CA 125). Abnormal marker levels alone do not confirm the diagnosis of cancer, but when combined with other information, they can help confirm it.

If fluid has accumulated in the abdomen, it can be drawn out (aspirated) through a needle and tested to determine whether cancer cells are present.

If doctors suspect advanced cancer or cancer is confirmed, they make an incision in the abdomen to obtain a tissue sample. At the same time, they remove as much of the cancer as possible and determine how far the cancer has spread (its stage).

Prognosis

The prognosis is based on the stage (see table on page 1571). The percentages of women who are alive 5 years after diagnosis and treatment are

- Stage I: 70 to 100%
- Stage II: 50 to 70%
- Stage III: 20 to 50%
- Stage IV: 10 to 20%

The prognosis is worse when the cancer is more aggressive or when surgery cannot remove all visibly abnormal tissue. Cancer recurs in 70% of women who have had stage III or IV cancer.

Prevention

Some experts believe that if ovarian or breast cancer runs in the family, women should be tested for genetic abnormalities. If first- or second-degree relatives have such cancers, particularly among Ashkenazi Jewish families, women should discuss genetic testing for *BRCA* abnormalities with their doctors. Women with certain *BRCA* gene mutations may be offered the option of having both ovaries and tubes removed after they no longer wish to bear children, even when no cancer is present. This approach eliminates the risk of ovarian cancer and reduces the risk of breast cancer. These women should be evaluated by a gynecologist who special-

What Is an Ovarian Cyst?

An ovarian cyst is a fluid-filled sac in or on an ovary. Such cysts are relatively common. Most are noncancerous and disappear on their own. Cancerous cysts are more likely to occur in women older than 40.

Most noncancerous ovarian cysts do not cause symptoms. However, some cause pressure, aching, or a feeling of heaviness in the abdomen. Pain may be felt during sexual intercourse. If a cyst ruptures or becomes twisted, severe stabbing pain is felt in the abdomen. The pain may be accompanied by nausea and fever. Some cysts produce hormones that affect menstrual periods. As a result, periods may be irregular or heavier than normal. In postmenopausal women, such cysts may cause vaginal bleeding. Women who have any of these symptoms should see a doctor.

Doctors may find a cyst during a routine pelvic examination or occasionally suspect it based on symptoms. A pregnancy test is done to exclude that possibility. An ultrasound device may be inserted through the vagina into the uterus (transvaginal ultrasonography) to confirm the diagnosis.

If the cyst appears to be noncancerous, a woman may be asked to return periodically for pelvic examinations as long as the cyst remains. If the cyst could be cancerous, computed tomography (CT) or magnetic resonance imaging (MRI) may be done. If cancer still seems possible, the ovaries may be examined through a laparoscope, inserted through a small incision just below the navel. Blood tests can help confirm or rule out cancer.

For noncancerous cysts, no treatment is necessary. But if a cyst is larger than about 2 inches (5 centimeters) and persists, it may need to be removed. If cancer cannot be ruled out, the ovary is removed. Cancerous cysts plus the affected ovary and fallopian tube are removed.

Surgery may be done through a laparoscope (with only a small incision) or a larger incision in the abdomen.

izes in cancer (gynecologic oncologist). More information is available from the National Cancer Institute Cancer Information Service (1-800-4-CANCER) and the Women's Cancer Network (WCN) web site (www.wcn.org).

Treatment

The extent of surgery depends on the type of ovarian cancer and the stage. For most cancers, the ovaries, fallopian tubes, and uterus are removed. When cancer has spread beyond the ovary, nearby lymph nodes and surrounding structures that the cancer typically spreads to are also removed. If a woman has stage I cancer that affects only one ovary and she wishes to become pregnant, doctors may remove only the affected ovary and fallopian tube. For more advanced cancers that have spread to other parts of the body, removing as much of the cancer as possible prolongs survival.

After surgery, most women with stage I epithelial carcinomas usually require no further treatment. For other stage I cancers or for more advanced cancers, chemotherapy may be used to destroy any small areas of cancer that may remain. Typically, chemotherapy consists of paclitaxel combined with carboplatin, given 6 times. Most women with germ cell tumors can be cured with removal of the one affected ovary and fallopian tube plus combination chemotherapy, usually with bleomycin, cisplatin, and etoposide. Radiation therapy is rarely used.

Advanced ovarian cancer usually recurs. So after chemotherapy, doctors typically measure levels of cancer markers. If the cancer recurs, chemotherapy (using drugs such as carboplatin, doxorubicin, etoposide, gemcitabine, paclitaxel, or topotecan) is given.

Cervical Cancer

Cervical cancer develops in the cervix (the lower part of the uterus).

- Cervical cancer usually results from infection with the human papillomavirus, transmitted during sexual intercourse.
- Cervical cancer may cause irregular vaginal bleeding, but symptoms may not occur until the cancer has enlarged or spread.
- Papanicolaou (Pap) tests can usually detect abnormalities, which are then biopsied.
- Treatment usually involves removing the cancer and often surrounding tissue, often with radiation therapy and chemotherapy.
- Getting regular Pap tests and being vaccinated against HPV can prevent cervical cancer.

The cervix is the lower part of the uterus. It extends into the vagina. In the United States, cervical cancer (cervical carcinoma) is the third most common gynecologic cancer among all women and the most common among younger women. It usually affects women aged 35 to 55, but it can affect women as young as 20.

This cancer is usually caused by the human papillomavirus (HPV), which is transmitted during sexual intercourse. This virus also causes genital warts (see page 1267). The younger a woman was the first time she had sexual intercourse and the more sex partners she has had, the higher her risk of cervical cancer. Risk is also increased by having intercourse with men whose previous partners had cervical cancer, by smoking cigarettes, and by having a weakened immune system (due to a disorder such as cancer or AIDS or to drugs such as chemotherapy drugs or corticosteroids).

About 80 to 85% of cervical cancers are squamous cell carcinomas, which develop in the flat, skinlike cells covering the cervix. Most other cervical cancers are adenocarcinomas, which develop from gland cells.

Cervical cancer begins with slow, progressive changes in normal cells on the surface of the cervix. These changes, called dysplasia or cervical intraepithelial neoplasia (CIN), are considered precancerous. That means that if untreated, they may progress to cancer, sometimes after years.

Cervical cancer begins on the surface of the cervix and can penetrate deep beneath the surface. The cancer can spread directly to nearby tissues, including the vagina. Or it can enter the rich network of small blood and lymphatic vessels inside the cervix, then spread to other parts of the body.

Symptoms

Precancerous changes usually cause no symptoms. In the early stages, cervical cancer may cause no symptoms or cause abnormal bleeding from the vagina, most often after intercourse. Spotting or heavier bleeding may occur between periods, or periods may be unusually heavy. Large cancers are more likely to cause bleeding and may cause a foul-smelling discharge from the vagina and pain in the pelvic area.

If the cancer is widespread, it can cause lower back pain and swelling of the legs. The urinary tract may be blocked, and without treatment, kidney failure and death can result.

> ### ? Did You Know...
>
> Pap tests have reduced the number of deaths due to cervical cancer by more than 50%.
>
> If all women had Pap tests regularly, deaths due to this cancer could be virtually eliminated.

Diagnosis

Routine Pap tests or other similar tests can detect the beginnings of cervical cancer (see page 1502). Pap tests accurately detect up to 90% of cervical cancers, even before symptoms develop. They can also detect dysplasia. Women with dysplasia should be checked again in 3 to 4 months. Dysplasia can be treated, thus helping prevent cancer.

If a growth, a sore, or another abnormal area is seen on the cervix during a pelvic examination or if a Pap test detects dysplasia or cancer, a biopsy is done. Usually, doctors use an instrument with a binocular magnifying lens (colposcope), inserted through the vagina, to examine the cervix and to choose the best biopsy site. Two different types of biopsy are done:

- **Punch biopsy:** A tiny piece of the cervix, selected using the colposcope, is removed.
- **Endocervical curettage:** Tissue that cannot be viewed is scraped from inside the cervix.

These biopsies cause little pain and a small amount of bleeding. The two together usually provide enough tissue for pathologists to make a diagnosis.

If the diagnosis is not clear, a cone biopsy is done to remove a larger cone-shaped piece of tissue. Usually, a thin wire loop with an electrical current running through it is used. This procedure is called the loop electrosurgical excision procedure (LEEP). Alternatively, a laser (using a highly focused beam of light) can be used. Either procedure requires only a local anesthetic and can be done in the doctor's office. A cold (nonelectric) knife is sometimes used, but this procedure requires an operating room and an anesthetic.

If cervical cancer is diagnosed, its exact size and locations (its stage) are determined. Staging begins with a physical examination of the pelvis. Various procedures (such as cystoscopy, a chest x-ray, and sigmoidoscopy) can be used to determine whether the cancer has spread to nearby tissues or to distant parts of the body. Other procedures, such as computed tomography (CT), magnetic resonance imaging (MRI), a barium enema, bone and liver scans, and positron emission tomography (PET) may be done.

Prognosis

Prognosis depends on the stage of the cancer (see table on page 1571). The percentages of women who are alive 5 years after diagnosis and treatment are

- Stage I: 80 to 90% of women
- Stage II: 60 to 75%
- Stage III: 30 to 40%
- Stage IV: 15% or fewer

If the cancer is going to recur, it usually does so within 2 years.

Prevention

Pap Tests: The number of deaths due to cervical cancer has been reduced by more than 50% since Pap tests were introduced. Doctors often recommend that women have their first Pap test when they become sexually active or reach the age of 18 and that a Pap test be done once a year. If test results are normal for 3 consecutive years, women may schedule Pap tests every 2 or 3 years as long as they do not change their sexual lifestyle. Any woman who has had cervical cancer or dysplasia should continue to have Pap tests at least once a year. If all women had Pap tests on a regular basis, deaths due to this cancer could be virtually eliminated. However, in the United States, about 50% of women are not tested regularly.

HPV Vaccine: A newly developed vaccine targets the types of HPV that cause most cervical cancer (and genital warts). The vaccine can help prevent cervical cancer but does not treat it. Three doses of the vaccine are given (see page 1148). The first is followed by one 2 months and one 6 months after the first. Being vaccinated before becoming sexually active is best, but even if women are already sexually active, they should be vaccinated. (Using condoms during intercourse can help prevent spread of HPV.)

Treatment

Treatment depends on the stage of the cancer.

Early Stages: If only the surface of the cervix is involved, doctors can often completely remove the cancer by removing part of the cervix using the loop electrosurgical excision procedure, a laser, or a cold knife, done during a cone biopsy. These treatments preserve a woman's ability to have children. Because cancer can recur, doctors advise women to return for examinations and Pap tests every 3 months for the first year and every 6 months after that. Rarely, removal of the uterus (hysterectomy) is necessary.

If early-stage cancer involves more than the surface of the cervix, doctors usually do a hysterectomy and give radiation therapy and chemotherapy. If women with early-stage cervical cancer wish to preserve their ability to have children, a procedure called radical trachelectomy may be done. In this procedure, the cervix, the tissue next to the cervix, the upper part of the vagina, and the lymph nodes in the pelvis are removed. The uterus and vagina that remain are attached to each other. Thus, women still can become pregnant. However, babies must be delivered by cesarean section. This treatment appears to be as effective as other more invasive treatments for women with early-stage cervical cancer.

Initial Spread Within the Pelvis: Hysterectomy plus removal of surrounding tissues, ligaments, and lymph nodes (radical hysterectomy) is necessary. The ovaries may be removed. Normal, functioning ovaries in younger women are not removed. Radiation therapy may be used sometimes instead of hysterectomy. Radiation therapy may irritate the bladder or rectum. Later, as a result, the intestine may become blocked, and the bladder and rectum may be damaged. Also, the ovaries usually stop functioning. With either radical hysterectomy or radiation therapy, chemotherapy is usually also used, and about 85 to 90% of women are cured.

Further Spread Within the Pelvis or to Other Organs: Radiation therapy plus chemotherapy (with cisplatin) is preferred. A laparoscope may be used or surgery done to determine whether lymph nodes are involved and thus determine where radiation should be directed.

If the cancer remains in the pelvis after radiation therapy, doctors may recommend surgery to remove all pelvic organs (pelvic exenteration). This procedure cures up to 50% of women.

Extensive Spread or Recurrence: Chemotherapy, usually with cisplatin and topotecan, is sometimes recommended. However, chemotherapy reduces the cancer's size and controls its spread in only 15 to 25% of women treated, and this effect is usually only temporary.

Vulvar Cancer

Vulvar cancer, usually a skin cancer, develops in the area around the female genital organs.

- The cancer may appear to be a lump, an itchy area, or a sore that does not heal.
- A sample of the abnormal tissue is removed and examined (biopsied).
- All or part of the vulva and any other affected areas are removed surgically.
- Reconstructive surgery can help improve appearance and function.

The vulva refers to the area that contains the external female reproductive organs. In the United States, cancer of the vulva (vulvar carcinoma) is the fourth most common gynecologic cancer, accounting for 3 to 4% of these cancers. Vulvar cancer usually occurs after menopause. The average age at diagnosis is 70 years. As more women live longer, this cancer is likely to become more common.

The risk of developing vulvar cancer is increased by the following:

- Older age
- Precancerous changes (dysplasia) in vulvar tissues
- Lichen sclerosus, which causes persistent itching and scarring of the vulva
- Human papillomavirus (HPV) infection
- Cancer of the vagina or cervix
- Heavy cigarette smoking
- Chronic granulomatous disease (a hereditary disease that impairs the immune system)

Most vulvar cancers are skin cancers that develop near or at the opening of the vagina. About 90% of vulvar cancers are squamous cell carcinomas, and 5% are melanomas. The remaining 5% include adenocarcinomas, which develop from gland cells, basal cell carcinomas, and rare cancers such as Paget's disease and cancer of Bartholin's gland.

Vulvar cancer begins on the surface of the vulva. Most of these cancers grow slowly, remaining on the surface for years. However, some (for example, melanomas) grow quickly. Untreated, vulvar cancer can eventually invade the vagina, the urethra, or the anus and spread into lymph nodes in the area.

Symptoms

White, brown, or red patches on the vulva may be precancerous (indicating that cancer is likely to eventually develop). Vulvar cancer usually causes unusual lumps or flat, red sores that can be seen and felt and that do not heal. Sometimes the flat sores become scaly, discolored, or both. The surrounding tissue may contract and pucker. Melanomas may be bluish black or brown and raised. Some sores look like warts. Typically, vulvar cancer causes little discomfort, but itching is common. Eventually, the lump or sore may bleed or produce a watery discharge (weep). These symptoms should be evaluated promptly by a doctor.

About one fifth of women have no symptoms, at least at first.

Diagnosis

Doctors diagnose vulvar cancer by taking a sample of the abnormal skin and examining it (biopsy). The biopsy enables doctors to determine whether the abnormal skin is cancerous or just infected or irritated. The type of cancer, if present, can also be identified, helping doctors develop a treatment plan. If the skin abnormalities are not well-defined, doctors apply stains to the abnormal area to help determine where to take a sample of tissue for a biopsy. Alternatively, they may use instrument with a binocular magnifying lens (colposcope) to examine the surface of the vulva.

Prognosis

If vulvar cancer is detected and treated early, about 3 of 4 women have no sign of cancer 5 years after diagnosis. The percentage of women who are alive 5 years after diagnosis and treatment depends on whether the cancer has reached the lymph nodes. If it has not, 96% are still alive. If it has, only 66% are still alive.

Melanomas are more likely to spread than squamous cell carcinomas.

Treatment

Depending on the extent and type of the cancer, all or part of the vulva is surgically removed (a procedure called vulvectomy). Nearby lymph nodes are also removed. For early-stage cancers, such treatment is usually all that is needed.

For more advanced cancers, radiation therapy, often with chemotherapy (with cisplatin or fluorouracil), may be used before vulvectomy. Such treatment can shrink very large cancers, making them easier to remove. Sometimes the clitoris and other organs in the pelvis must be removed.

After the cancer is removed, surgery to reconstruct the vulva and other affected areas (such as the vagina) may be done. Such surgery can improve function and appearance.

Doctors work closely with the woman to develop a treatment plan that is best suited to her and takes into account her age, sexual lifestyle, and any other medical problems. Sexual intercourse is usually possible after vulvectomy.

Because basal cell carcinoma of the vulva does not tend to spread (metastasize) to distant sites, surgery usually involves removing only the cancer. The whole vulva is removed only if the cancer is extensive.

Vaginal Cancer

Cancer of the vagina, an uncommon cancer, is usually a squamous cell skin cancer (vaginal carcinoma), which typically develops in older women.

- Vaginal cancer may cause abnormal vaginal bleeding, particularly after sexual intercourse.
- If doctors suspect cancer, they remove and examine samples of tissue from the vagina (biopsy).
- The cancer is surgically removed, or radiation therapy is used.

In the United States, vaginal cancer accounts for only about 1% of gynecologic cancers. The average age at diagnosis is 60 to 65.

More than 95% of vaginal cancers are squamous cell carcinomas. Vaginal squamous cell carcinoma may be caused by human papillomavirus (HPV), the same virus that causes genital warts and cervical cancer. Having HPV infection or cervical or vulvar cancer increases the risk of developing vaginal cancer.

Most other vaginal cancers are adenocarcinomas. One rare type, clear cell carcinoma, occurs almost exclusively in women whose mothers took the drug diethylstilbestrol (DES), prescribed to prevent miscarriage during pregnancy. (In 1971, the drug was banned in the United States.)

Depending on the type, vaginal cancer may begin on the surface of the vaginal lining. If untreated, it continues to grow and invades surrounding tissue.

Eventually, it may enter blood and lymphatic vessels, then spread to other parts of the body.

Symptoms

The most common symptom is bleeding from the vagina, which may occur during or after sexual intercourse, between menstrual periods, or after menopause. Sores may form on the lining of the vagina. They may bleed and become infected. Other symptoms include a watery discharge and pain during sexual intercourse. A few women have no symptoms. Large cancers can also affect the bladder, causing a frequent urge to urinate and pain during urination. In advanced cancer, abnormal connections (fistulas) may form between the vagina and the bladder or rectum.

Diagnosis

Doctors may suspect vaginal cancer based on symptoms, abnormal areas seen during a routine pelvic examination, or an abnormal Papanicolaou (Pap) test result. Doctors may use an instrument with a binocular magnifying lens (colposcope) to examine the vagina. To confirm the diagnosis, doctors scrape cells from the vaginal wall to examine under a microscope. They also do a biopsy on any growth, sore, or other abnormal area seen during the examination.

Other tests, such as use of a viewing tube (endoscopy) to examine the bladder or rectum, a chest x-ray, and computed tomography (CT), may be done to determine whether the cancer has spread.

Prognosis

The prognosis depends on the stage of the cancer (see table on page 1571). If the cancer is limited to the vagina, about 65 to 70% of women survive at least 5 years after diagnosis. If the cancer has spread beyond the pelvis or to the bladder or rectum, only about 15 to 20% survive.

Treatment

Treatment also depends on the stage. For early-stage vaginal cancers, surgery to remove the vagina, uterus, and lymph nodes in the pelvis and the upper part of the vagina is the treatment of choice. Radiation therapy is used for most other cancers. It is usually a combination of internal (using radioactive implants placed inside the vagina) and external (directed at the pelvis from outside the body) radiation therapy.

Radiation therapy cannot be used if fistulas have developed. In such cases, the organs in the pelvis are removed.

Intercourse may be difficult or impossible after treatment for vaginal cancer, although sometimes a new vagina can be constructed with skin grafts or part of the intestine.

Fallopian Tube Cancer

Fallopian tube cancer develops in the tubes that lead from the ovaries to the uterus.

- Most cancers that affect the fallopian tubes have spread from other parts of the body.
- At first, women may have vague symptoms, such as abdominal discomfort or bloating, or no symptoms.
- Ultrasonography or computed tomography is done to check for abnormalities.
- Usually, the uterus, ovaries, and fallopian tubes are removed, followed by chemotherapy.

In the United States, fewer than 1% of gynecologic cancers are fallopian tube cancers. Most often, cancer that affects the fallopian tubes has spread from the ovaries rather than started in the fallopian tubes. Cancer that starts in the fallopian tubes usually affects women aged 50 to 60. It is more likely to develop in women who have had the following:

- Long-term inflammation of the fallopian tubes (chronic salpingitis)
- Disorders that cause inflammation in other parts of the body, such as tuberculosis
- Infertility

More than 95% of fallopian tube cancers are adenocarcinomas, which develop from gland cells. A few are sarcomas, which develop from connective tissue. Fallopian tube cancer spreads in much the same way as ovarian cancer: usually directly to the surrounding area or through the lymphatic system, eventually appearing in distant parts of the body.

Symptoms

Symptoms include vague abdominal discomfort, bloating, and pain in the pelvic area or abdomen. Some women have a watery or blood-tinged discharge from the vagina. When cancer is advanced, the abdominal cavity may fill with fluid (a condition called ascites), and women may feel a large mass in the pelvis.

Diagnosis

Fallopian tube cancer is seldom diagnosed early. Occasionally, it is diagnosed early when a mass or other abnormality is detected during a routine pelvic examination or an imaging test done for another reason. Usually, the cancer is not diagnosed until it is advanced, when it is obvious because a large mass or severe ascites is present.

If cancer is suspected, computed tomography (CT) is usually done. If the results suggest cancer, surgery is done to confirm the diagnosis, determine the extent of spread, and remove as much of the cancer as possible.

Prognosis and Treatment

The prognosis is similar to that for women who have ovarian cancer.

Treatment almost always consists of removal of the uterus (hysterectomy) and removal of the ovaries and fallopian tubes (salpingo-oophorectomy), adjacent lymph nodes, and surrounding tissues. Chemotherapy (as for ovarian cancer) is usually necessary after surgery. The most commonly used chemotherapy drugs are carboplatin and paclitaxel.

For some cancers, radiation therapy is useful. For cancer that has spread to other parts of the body, removing as much of the cancer as possible improves the prognosis.

Hydatidiform Mole

A hydatidiform mole is growth of an abnormal fertilized egg or an overgrowth of tissue from the placenta.

- Women appear to be pregnant, but the uterus enlarges much more rapidly than in a normal pregnancy.
- Most women have severe nausea and vomiting, vaginal bleeding, and very high blood pressure.
- Ultrasonography, blood tests to measure human chorionic gonadotropin (which is produced early during pregnancy) and a biopsy are done.
- Moles are removed using dilation and curettage with suction.
- If the disorder persists, chemotherapy is needed.

Most often, a hydatidiform mole is an abnormal fertilized egg that develops into a hydatidiform mole rather than a fetus (a condition called molar pregnancy). However, a hydatidiform mole can develop from cells that remain in the uterus after a miscarriage or a full-term pregnancy. Rarely, a hydatidiform mole develops when there is a living fetus. In such cases, the fetus typically dies, and a miscarriage often occurs.

Hydatidiform moles are most common among women under 17 or over 35. In the United States, they occur in about 1 in 2,000 pregnancies in the United States. For unknown reasons, moles are almost 10 times more common in Asian countries.

About 80% of hydatidiform moles are not cancerous. About 15 to 20% invade the surrounding tissue and tend to persist. About 2 to 3% become cancerous and spread throughout the body. They are then called choriocarcinomas. Choriocarcinomas can spread quickly through the lymphatic vessels or bloodstream. Hydatidiform moles and choriocarcinomas are types of gestational trophoblastic disease.

Symptoms

Women who have a hydatidiform mole feel as if they are pregnant. But because hydatidiform moles

Did You Know...

An abnormal fertilized egg or placental tissue can overgrow, causing symptoms similar to those of pregnancy, but the abdomen enlarges more rapidly.

grow much faster than a fetus, the abdomen becomes larger much faster than it does in a normal pregnancy. Severe nausea and vomiting are common, and vaginal bleeding may occur. As parts of the mole deteriorate, small amounts of tissue, which resemble a bunch of grapes, may pass through the vagina. These symptoms indicate the need for prompt evaluation by a doctor.

Hydatidiform moles can cause serious complications, including infections and very high blood pressure with increased protein in the urine (preeclampsia or eclampsia—see page 1649).

If choriocarcinoma develops, women may have other symptoms, caused by spread (metastasis) to other parts of the body.

Diagnosis

Often, doctors can diagnose a hydatidiform mole shortly after conception. The pregnancy test is positive, but no fetal movement and no fetal heartbeat are detected, and the uterus is much larger than expected.

Ultrasonography is done to be sure that the growth is a hydatidiform mole and not a fetus or amniotic sac (which contains the fetus and fluid around it). Blood tests to measure the level of human chorionic gonadotropin (hCG—a hormone normally produced early in pregnancy) are done. If a hydatidiform mole is present, the level is usually very high because the mole produces a large amount of this hormone. A sample of tissue is removed or obtained when it is passed, then examined under a microscope (biopsy) to confirm the diagnosis.

Prognosis

The cure rate for a hydatidiform mole is virtually 100% if the mole has not spread. The cure rate is 60 to 80% for choriocarcinoma that has spread widely. Most women can have children afterwards and do not have a higher risk of having complications, a miscarriage, or children with birth defects.

About 1% of women who have had a hydatidiform mole have another one. So if women have had a hydatidiform mole, ultrasonography is done early in subsequent pregnancies.

Treatment

A hydatidiform mole is completely removed, usually by dilation and curettage (D and C) with suction (see page 1504). Only rarely is removal of the uterus (hysterectomy) necessary.

A chest x-ray is done to see whether the mole has become cancerous (that is, a choriocarcinoma) and spread to the lungs. After surgery, the level of human chorionic gonadotropin in the blood is measured to determine whether the hydatidiform mole was completely removed. When removal is complete, the level returns to normal, usually within 10 weeks, and remains normal. If the level does not return to normal (called persistent disease), computed tomography (CT) of the brain, chest, abdomen, and pelvis is done to determine whether choriocarcinoma has developed and spread.

Hydatidiform moles do not require chemotherapy, but persistent disease does. Usually, only one drug (methotrexate or dactinomycin) is needed. Sometimes both drugs or another combination of chemotherapy drugs is needed.

Women who have had a hydatidiform mole removed are advised not to become pregnant for 1 year. Oral contraceptives are frequently recommended, but other effective contraceptive methods can be used.

CHAPTER

248 Violence Against Women

Violence against women is broadly defined as any act that is likely to cause physical, sexual, or psychologic harm or extreme suffering to a woman. Violence can occur in the home, workplace, or community. Two common forms of violence against women are domestic violence and rape.

Domestic Violence

- Domestic violence includes physical, sexual, and psychologic abuse between intimate partners.
- The victim is usually a woman.
- Physical injuries, psychologic problems, social isolation, loss of a job, financial difficulties, and even death can result.
- Keeping safe—for example, having a plan of escape—is the most important consideration.

Domestic violence includes physical, sexual, and psychologic abuse between people who live together, including intimate partners, parents and children, children and grandparents, and siblings. It occurs among people of all cultures, races, occupations, income levels, and ages. In the United States, as many as 30% of marriages are considered physically aggressive.

Women are more commonly victims of domestic violence than are men. About 95% of people who seek medical attention as a result of domestic violence are women, and perhaps 400,000 to 500,000 of women's visits to the emergency department each year are for injuries related to domestic violence. Women are more likely to be severely assaulted or killed by a male partner than by anyone else. Each year in the United States, about 2 million women are severely beaten by their partner.

Physical abuse is the most obvious form of domestic violence. It may include hitting, slapping, kicking, punching, breaking bones, pulling hair, pushing, and twisting arms. The victim may be deprived of food or sleep. Weapons, such as a gun or knife, may be used to threaten or cause injury.

Sexual assault is also common: 33 to 50% of women who are physically assaulted by their partner are also sexually assaulted by their partner. Sexual assault involves the use of threats or force to coerce sexual contact and includes unwanted touching, grabbing, or kissing.

Psychologic abuse may be even more common than physical abuse and may precede it. Psychologic abuse involves any nonphysical behavior that undermines or belittles the victim or that enables the perpetrator to control the victim. Psychologic abuse can include abusive language, social isolation, and financial control. Usually, the perpetrator uses language to demean, degrade, humiliate, intimidate, or threaten the victim in private or in public. The perpetrator may make the victim think she is crazy or make her feel guilty or responsible, blaming her for the abusive relationship. The perpetrator may also humiliate the victim in terms of her sexual performance, physical appearance, or both.

The perpetrator may try to partly or completely isolate the victim by controlling the victim's access to friends, relatives, and other people. Control may include forbidding direct, written, telephone, or e-mail contact with others. The perpetrator may use jealousy to justify his actions.

Often, the perpetrator withholds money to control the victim. The victim may depend on the perpetrator for most or all of her money. The perpetrator may maintain control by preventing the victim from getting a job, by keeping information about their finances from her, and by taking money from her.

After an incident of abuse, the perpetrator may beg for forgiveness and promise to change and stop the abusive behavior. However, typically, the abuse continues and often escalates.

> **Did You Know...**
>
> In the United States, about 2 million women are severely beaten by their partners each year.
>
> The abusing partner may try to control the victim by limiting her access to other people, even by telephone or e-mail, and to money.

Effects

A victim of domestic violence may be physically injured. Physical injuries can include bruises, black eyes, cuts, scratches, broken bones, lost teeth, and burns. Injuries may prevent the victim from going to work regularly, causing her to lose her job. Injuries, as well as the abusive situation, may embarrass the victim, causing her to isolate herself from family and friends. The victim may also have to move often—a financial burden—to escape the perpetrator. Sometimes the perpetrator kills the victim.

As a result of domestic violence, many victims have psychologic problems. Such problems include posttraumatic stress disorder, substance abuse, anxiety, and depression. About 60% of battered women are depressed. Women who are more severely battered are more likely to develop psychologic problems. Even when physical abuse decreases, psychologic abuse often continues, reminding the woman that she can be physically abused at any time. Abused women may feel that psychologic abuse is more damaging than physical abuse. Psychologic abuse increases the risk of depression and substance abuse.

Management

In cases of domestic violence, the most important consideration is safety. During a violent incident, the victim should try to move away from areas in which she can be trapped or in which the perpetrator can obtain weapons, such as the kitchen. If she can, the victim should promptly call 911 or the police

Children Who Witness Domestic Violence

Each year, at least 3.3 million children are estimated to witness physical or verbal abuse in their homes. These children may develop problems such as excessive anxiety or crying, fearfulness, difficulty sleeping, depression, social withdrawal, and difficulty in school. Also, children may blame themselves for the situation. Older children may run away from home. Boys who see their father abuse their mother may be more likely to become abusive adults. Girls who see their father abuse their mother may be more likely to tolerate abuse as adults. The perpetrator may also physically hurt the children. In homes where domestic violence is present, children are much more likely to be physically mistreated.

and leave the house. The victim should have any injuries treated and documented with photographs. She should teach her children not to get in the middle of a fight and when and how to call for help.

Developing a safety plan is important. It should include where to go for help, how to get away, and how to access money. The victim should also make and hide copies of official documents (such as children's birth certificates, social security cards, insurance cards, and bank account numbers). She should keep an overnight bag packed in case she needs to leave quickly.

Sometimes the only solution is to leave the abusive relationship permanently, because domestic violence tends to continue, especially among very aggressive men. Also, even when physical abuse decreases, psychologic abuse may persist. The decision to leave is not simple. After the perpetrator knows the victim has decided to leave, the victim's risk of serious harm and death may be greatest. At this time, the victim should take additional steps (such as obtaining a restraining or protection order) to protect herself and her children. Help is available through shelters for battered women, support groups, the courts, and a national hotline (1-800-799-SAFE or, for TTY, 1-800-787-3224).

Rape

Rape refers to unwanted penetration of the vagina, anus, or mouth.

- Victims may have tears in the vagina, cuts and bruises, upsetting emotions, and difficulty sleeping.
- Sexual transmitted diseases, including infection with the human immunodeficiency virus, and pregnancy are risks.

■ Women who are raped should be thoroughly evaluated in a center staffed by specially trained people (rape center).

■ Treatment of physical injuries, antibiotics to prevent infections, emergency contraception, and counseling or psychotherapy may be needed.

■ If possible, family members and close friends should meet with a member of the rape crisis team to discuss how to support a rape victim.

Rape is typically considered to be unwanted penetration of the victim's vagina, anus, or mouth. In victims younger than the age of consent, such penetration—whether wanted or not—is considered rape (statutory rape). Sexual assault is a broader term, including the use of force and threats to coerce any sexual contact and unwanted touching, grabbing, or kissing. The reported percentage of women who have been raped during their lifetime varies widely: from 2% to almost 30%. The reported percentage of children who are sexually abused is similarly high (see page 1880). Reported percentages are probably lower than the actual percentages because rape and sexual abuse are less likely to be reported to the police than are other crimes.

Typically, rape is an expression of aggression, anger, or the need for power rather than sexually motivated. About half of women who are raped are physically injured.

Men are also raped. Men are more likely than women to be physically injured and less likely to report the rape.

Symptoms

Physical injuries resulting from a rape may include tears in the upper part of the vagina and injuries to other parts of the body, such as bruises, black eyes, cuts, and scratches.

The psychologic effects of a rape are often more devastating than the physical. Shortly after a rape occurs, almost all women have symptoms of posttraumatic stress disorder, (which can occur after any stressful event (see page 861). Women feel fearful, anxious, and irritable. They may feel angry, depressed, embarassed, ashamed, or guilty (wondering whether they may have done something to provoke the rape or could have done something to avoid it). They may have intrusive, upsetting thoughts about or mental images of the assault, and they may relive the rape. Or they may stifle thoughts and feelings about the rape. They may avoid situations that remind them of the rape. Difficulty sleeping and nightmares are common. These symptoms may last for months, interfering with social activities and work. However, for most women, symptoms lessen substantially over a period of months.

After a rape, there is a risk of infection with sexually transmitted diseases (such as gonorrhea, chlamydial infection, and syphilis) and hepatitis B and C. Infection with the human immunodeficiency virus (HIV) is a particular concern, even though the chances of acquiring it in a single encounter are low. Rarely, a woman becomes pregnant.

> **? Did You Know...**
>
> Victims of domestic violence may develop depression, anxiety, or drug or alcohol abuse.
>
> Women are in greatest danger of serious harm after their partner knows they have decided to leave.

Evaluation

Having a thorough medical evaluation after a rape is important. Whenever possible, women who have been raped or sexually assaulted are taken to a sexual assault center that is staffed by trained, concerned support personnel. The center may be a hospital emergency department or a separate facility.

After a rape, doctors are required by law to notify the police and to examine the victim. The examination provides evidence for prosecution of the rapist and is necessary before medical care of the victim can begin. The best evidence is obtained when the rape victim goes to the hospital as soon as possible, without showering or washing, without brushing the teeth, without changing clothes, and, if possible, without even urinating. The medical record resulting from this examination is sometimes admissible in court as evidence. However, the medical record cannot be released unless the victim gives her consent in writing or a subpoena is issued. The record may also help the victim recall details of the rape if her testimony is required later.

Immediately after a rape, a woman may be afraid of undergoing a physical examination. If possible, a female doctor examines the woman. If not, a female nurse or volunteer is present to help allay any anxiety the woman may be feeling. Before beginning the examination, the doctor should ask the woman's permission to proceed. The woman should feel no pressure to consent, although consent is generally in her best interest. The woman can ask the doctor to explain what will happen during the examination so that she knows what to expect.

The doctor asks the woman to describe the events to help guide the examination and treatment. However, talking about the rape is often frightening for the woman. She may request to give a complete description later, after her immediate needs have been met. She may first need to be treated for injuries and to have some time for calming down.

To help determine the likelihood of pregnancy, the doctor asks the woman when her last menstrual period was and whether she uses a contraceptive. To help interpret the analysis of any sperm samples, the doctor asks the woman if she recently had sex before the rape and, if so, when.

The doctor notes physical injuries, such as cuts and scrapes, and may examine the vagina for injuries. Photographs of injuries are taken. Because some injuries such as bruises become apparent later, a second set of photographs may be taken later. A swab is used to take samples of semen and other body fluids for evidence. Other samples, such as samples of the perpetrator's hair, blood, or skin (sometimes found under the woman's nails), are collected. Sometimes DNA testing of the samples is done to identify the perpetrator. Some of the woman's clothing may be kept for evidence.

If the woman consents, blood tests are done to check for infections, including HIV infection. If the initial test results for gonorrhea, chlamydial infection, syphilis, and hepatitis are negative, the woman is tested again at 6 weeks. If results for syphilis and hepatitis are still negative, tests are repeated at 6 months. Blood tests for HIV infection may be repeated after 90 and 120 days. A Papanicalaou (Pap) test is done to check for human papillomavirus infection after 6 weeks.

Usually, a pregnancy test to measure the level of human chorionic gonadotropin in the urine (see page 1616) is done during the initial examination to detect any preexisting pregnancy. If the results are negative, the test is repeated within 6 weeks to check for pregnancy that may have resulted from the rape.

Treatment

After the examination, the woman is offered facilities to wash, change clothing, use mouthwash, and urinate if needed.

Any physical injuries are treated. For preventing infections, the woman is given antibiotics, typically one dose of ceftriaxone injected into a muscle, one dose of metronidazole given by mouth, and doxycycline given by mouth for 7 days. If test results for HIV were positive, treatment for HIV is started immediately (see page 1261).

If there is no preexisting pregnancy, emergency contraception may be used. A high dose of an oral contraceptive is given immediately, then repeated 12 hours later (see page 1599). This treatment is 99% effective if given within 72 hours of the rape. Inserting an intrauterine device (IUD) within 10 days of the rape is even more effective. If pregnancy results from the rape, abortion can be considered.

Common psychologic reactions to the rape (such as excessive anxiety or fear) are explained to the woman. As soon as feasible, a person trained in rape crisis intervention meets with her. The woman is referred to a rape crisis team if one is located in the area. This team can provide helpful medical, psychologic, and legal support. For the woman, talking about the rape and her feelings about it can help her recover. If symptoms of posttraumatic stress disorder persist, psychotherapy or antidepressants can be effective (see page 862). If necessary, the woman can be referred to a psychologist, social worker, or psychiatrist.

Family members and friends may have some of the same feelings as the victim: anxiety, anger, or guilt. They may irrationally blame the victim. Thus, in addition to her own feelings, the rape victim may have to handle negative, sometimes judgmental or derisive reactions of family members and friends, as well as those of officials. These reactions can interfere with the victim's recovery. Family members or close friends may benefit from meeting with a member of the rape crisis team or sexual assault evaluation unit to discuss their feelings and how they can help the victim. Usually, listening supportively to the victim and not expressing strong feelings about the rape are most helpful. Blaming or criticizing the victim may interfere with her recovery. A support network of health care practitioners, friends, and family members can be very helpful to the victim.

Infertility

Infertility is the inability of a couple to achieve a pregnancy after repeated intercourse without contraception for 1 year.

Frequent intercourse without birth control usually results in pregnancy:

- For 50% of couples within 3 months
- For 75% within 6 months
- For 90% within 1 year

To maximize the chance of pregnancy, couples should have frequent intercourse for the few days when egg release (ovulation) is most likely—usually in the middle of the menstrual cycle, which is about halfway between the first day of two periods. Women who have regular periods can estimate when ovulation occurs by measuring their temperature at rest (basal body temperature) each day before they get out of bed. A decrease suggests that ovulation is about to occur. An increase of 0.9° F (0.5° C) or more suggests ovulation has just occurred. Or women may use home ovulation predictor kits, which test urine or saliva. Use of caffeine and tobacco, which can impair fertility in women, is discouraged. Even with these measures, about one in five couples in the United States do not conceive for at least a year and are thus considered infertile.

The cause of infertility may be due to problems in the man, the woman, or both:

- Problems with sperm (in 35% of couples)
- Problems with ovulation (in 20%)
- Problems with the fallopian tubes in the pelvis (in 30%)
- Problems with mucus in the cervix (in 5% or fewer)
- Unidentified factors (in 10%)

Thus, the diagnosis of infertility problems requires a thorough assessment of both partners.

Age is a factor, especially for women. As women age, becoming pregnant becomes more difficult and the risk of complications during pregnancy increases. Also, women, particularly after age 35, have a limited time to resolve infertility problems before menopause.

Of the couples who have not conceived after a year of trying, more than 60% conceive eventually, with or without treatment. The goals of treatment are to treat the cause of infertility if possible, to make conception more likely, and to reduce the time needed to conceive.

Even when no cause of infertility can be identified, the couple may still be treated. In such cases, the woman may be given drugs that stimulate several eggs to mature and be released—so-called fertility drugs (see page 1589). Examples are clomiphene and human gonadotropins. A woman's chances of becoming pregnant are about 10 to 15% with each month of treatment. Alternatively, an artificial insemination technique that selects only the most active sperm may be tried.

While a couple is being treated for infertility, one or both partners may experience frustration, emotional stress, feelings of inadequacy, and guilt. They may alternate between hope and despair. Feeling isolated and unable to communicate, they may become angry at or resentful toward each other, family members, friends, or the doctor. The emotional stress can lead to fatigue, anxiety, sleep or eating disturbances, and an inability to concentrate. In addition, the financial burden and time commitment involved in diagnosis and treatment can cause marital strife.

These problems can be lessened if both partners are involved in and are given information about the treatment process (including how long it takes), regardless of which one has the diagnosed problem. Knowing what the chances of success are, as well as realizing that treatment may not be successful and cannot continue indefinitely, can help a couple cope with the stress. Information about when to end treatment, when to seek a second opinion, and when to consider adoption is also helpful. Ideally, couples should ask for this information before treatment is begun. Counseling and psychologic support, including support groups such as RESOLVE and the American Fertility Association, can help.

Problems With Sperm

Sperm may be too few in number, move too slowly, or be structurally abnormal, or their passage out of the body may be blocked or disrupted.

- An increase in the testes' temperature, certain disorders, injuries, and some drugs and toxins can cause problems with sperm.
- Semen is analyzed, and sometimes genetic tests are done.
- Clomiphene, a fertility drug, may increase the number of sperm, but assisted reproductive techniques may be needed.

To be fertile, a man must be able to deliver an adequate quantity of normal sperm to a woman's vagina, and sperm must be able to fertilize the egg. Conditions that interfere with this process can make a man less fertile.

WHAT CAUSES INFERTILITY IN MEN?

CAUSE	EXAMPLES
Reduced sperm production	
Increased temperature of the testes	Excessive heat Disorders that cause a prolonged fever
Hormonal disorders	Adrenal gland disorders (this gland produces testosterone and other hormones) Hyperprolactinemia Hypogonadism Hypothalamic disorders (this part of the brain controls the pituitary gland, which controls testosterone production) Hypothyroidism Pituitary gland disorders
Genetic disorders	Klinefelter's syndrome Other disorders that cause an abnormality in the sex chromosomes
Disorders of the testes	Infections Injury to the testes Mumps that affects the testes (mumps orchitis) Shrinking of the testes (as can occur when excess alcohol is regularly consumed) Undescended testes (testes that remain in the abdomen rather than move to the scrotum) Varicose veins in the testes (varicocele)
Drugs	Anabolic steroids Alcohol, when consumed in large amounts Androgens (such as testosterone) Aspirin when taken for a long time Chlorambucil (a chemotherapy drug) Cimetidine (used to treat stomach ulcers) Colchicine (used to treat gout) Corticosteroids taken by mouth (such as prednisone) Cotrimoxazole (an antibiotic) Cyclophosphamide (a chemotherapy drug) Drugs used to treat malaria Estrogens taken to treat prostate cancer Gonadotropin-releasing hormone (GnRH) analogs (used to treat prostate cancer) Marijuana Medroxyprogesterone (a synthetic female hormone) Methotrexate (a drug that suppresses the immune system) Monoamine oxidase inhibitors (MAOIs—a type of antidepressant) Nicotine Nitrofurantoin (an antibiotic) Opioids (narcotics) Spironolactone (a diuretic) Sulfasalazine (an antibiotic)

(continued on the following page)

WHAT CAUSES INFERTILITY IN MEN? (*Continued*)

CAUSE	EXAMPLES
Exposure to industrial or environmental toxins	Heavy metals, such as lead
	Pesticides (which can have effects similar to those of female hormones or decrease the effects of male hormones)
Absence of sperm in semen	
Disruption of the sperm's passage out of the body	Missing epididymides (which provide the space and environment for sperm to mature), usually in men with cystic fibrosis
	Blocked or missing vasa deferentia (tubes from the epididymides to the ejaculatory ducts), usually in men with cystic fibrosis
	Missing seminal vesicles (which provide nourishment for sperm)
	Blockage of both ejaculatory ducts
Retrograde ejaculation (semen travels back into the bladder rather than out of the penis)	Diabetes
	Nervous system dysfunction
	Pelvic surgery, such as prostate removal
	Removal of lymph nodes in the area behind the abdomen (as may be done to treat Hodgkin lymphoma)

Causes

Conditions that increase the temperature of the testes (where sperm are produced) can greatly reduce the number of sperm and the vigor of sperm movement and can increase the number of abnormal sperm. For example, taking a hot bath before sexual intercourse can negatively affect sperm. Some disorders of the testes, such as undescended testes and varicose veins, also increase the temperature of these organs. Effects of excessive or prolonged heat can last up to 3 months.

Certain hormonal or genetic disorders may interfere with sperm production, as can other disorders.

Exposure to industrial or environmental toxins and use of certain drugs can reduce sperm production. Taking anabolic steroids (such as testosterone) lowers production of the pituitary gland hormones that stimulate sperm production.

Some disorders result in the complete absence of sperm (azoospermia) in semen. They include serious disorders of the testes and blocked or missing vasa deferentia, missing seminal vesicles, and blockage of both ejaculatory ducts. The same genetic abnormality that causes cystic fibrosis can cause azoospermia, often by preventing both vasa deferentia from forming.

Azoospermia can also occur if semen, which contains the sperm, moves in the wrong direction (into the bladder instead of down the penis). This disorder is called retrograde ejaculation (see page 1487).

Diagnosis

Doctors ask the man about his medical history and do a physical examination to try to identify the cause. Doctors ask about past disorders and surgery, use of drugs, and possible exposure to toxins. They check for physical abnormalities, such as undescended testes, and for signs of hormonal or genetic disorders that can cause infertility. Levels of hormones (including testosterone) may be measured in the blood.

A semen analysis, the main screening procedure for male infertility, is needed. For this procedure, men are often asked not to ejaculate for 2 to 3 days before the analysis. The reason is to make sure the semen contains as many sperm as possible. Then they are asked to ejaculate by masturbation into a clean glass jar, preferably at the laboratory site. For men who have difficulty producing a semen sample this way, special condoms that have no lubricants or chemicals toxic to sperm can be used to collect semen during intercourse.

The volume of the semen sample is measured. Whether the color, consistency, thickness, and chemical composition of semen are normal is determined. The sperm are counted. A low sperm count may mean that fertility is reduced, but not always. Sperm are also examined under a microscope to determine whether they are abnormal in shape, size, or movement.

If the semen sample is abnormal, the analysis may be repeated because samples from the same man normally vary greatly. Two or three samples, obtained at least

> ### ❓ Did You Know...
>
> Taking a hot bath before sexual intercourse makes conception less likely.
>
> Using anabolic steroids can decrease sperm production.

1 week apart, provide more accurate results than a single sample. If the semen still seems to be abnormal, the doctor tries to identify the cause. If there are too few sperm, genetic testing is done. Also, urine may be checked for sperm after ejaculation to determine whether retrograde ejaculation is occurring.

Other tests can be done to evaluate sperm function and quality if routine tests of both partners do not explain infertility. These tests may

- Detect antibodies to sperm
- Determine whether sperm membranes are intact
- Determine the sperm's ability to bind to an egg and penetrate it

Sometimes a biopsy of the testes is done to obtain more detailed information about sperm production and the function of the testes.

Treatment

If possible, the disorder causing the problem is treated. For example, varicoceles can be treated with surgery. Sometimes fertility improves as a result.

Clomiphene, a drug used to trigger (induce) ovulation in women, may be used to try to increase sperm counts in men. However, whether clomiphene improves the sperm's ability to move or reduces the number of abnormal sperm is unclear. It has not been proved to increase fertility.

For men who have a low sperm count with normal-appearing motile sperm, artificial insemination may slightly increase their partner's chances of pregnancy. This technique uses the first portion of the ejaculated semen, which has the greatest concentration of sperm. A technique that selects only the most active sperm (washed sperm) is somewhat more successful. With washed semen, pregnancy usually occurs by the sixth attempt if it is going to occur. In vitro fertilization, often with intracytoplasmic sperm injection (the injection of one sperm into one egg), and gamete intrafallopian tube transfer (GIFT) are much more complex and costly procedures. They are successful in treating many types of male infertility.

For men who produce no sperm, inseminating the woman with sperm from another man (a donor) may be considered. Because of the danger of contracting sexually transmitted diseases, including infection with human immunodeficiency virus (HIV), fresh semen samples from donors are no longer used. Risk of disease transmission is minimized by freezing donor sperm for 6 months or more, then retesting donors for infection. If their test results remain negative, the sample is thawed and used.

Before artificial insemination or another technique is used, the partner of a man who has fertility problems may be treated with human gonadotropins to stimulate several eggs to mature and be released (see page 1589). This approach may make pregnancy more likely.

Problems With Ovulation

The ovaries do not release an egg each month (see page 1494).

- Ovulation problems can result from dysfunction of the part of the brain and the glands that control ovulation or dysfunction of the ovaries.
- Women can determine whether ovulation is occurring and estimate when it occurs by measuring body temperature or using home predictor kits.
- Doctors use ultrasonography or blood or urine tests to evaluate ovulation problems.
- Drugs, usually clomiphene, can often stimulate ovulation, but pregnancy does not always follow.

In women, a common cause of infertility is an ovulation problem.

Causes

Ovulation problems result when one part of the system that controls reproductive function malfunctions. This system includes the hypothalamus (an area of the brain), pituitary gland, ovaries, and other glands, such as the adrenal glands and thyroid gland. For example,

- The hypothalamus may not secrete gonadotropin-releasing hormone, which stimulates the pituitary gland to produce the hormones that stimulate the ovaries to trigger ovulation (luteinizing hormone and follicle-stimulating hormone).
- The pituitary gland may produce too little luteinizing hormone or follicle-stimulating hormone.
- The ovaries may produce too little estrogen.
- The pituitary gland may produce too much prolactin, a hormone that stimulates milk production. High levels of prolactin (hyperprolactinemia) may result in low levels of the hormones that trigger ovulation. Prolactin levels may be high because of a pituitary gland tumor (prolactinoma), which is almost always noncancerous.
- Other glands may malfunction. For example, the adrenal glands may overproduce male hormones (such as testosterone), or the thyroid glands can overproduce or underproduce thyroid hormones, which help keep the pituitary gland and ovaries in balance.

Ovulation problems may be due to many disorders. One of the most common causes is polycystic ovary syndrome, which is characterized by excess weight and excess production of male hormones by the ovaries. Other causes include diabetes and obesity. Problems may also result from excessive exercise, certain drugs (such as estrogens and progestins and antidepressants), weight loss, or psychologic stress. Sometimes the cause is early menopause—when the supply of eggs runs out early.

An ovulation problem is often the cause of infertility in women who have irregular periods or no periods (amenorrhea—see page 1524). An ovulation problem is sometimes the cause of infertility in women who have regular menstrual periods but do not have premenstrual symptoms, such as breast tenderness, lower abdominal swelling, and mood changes.

Diagnosis

To determine if or when ovulation is occurring, doctors may ask a woman to take her temperature at rest (basal body temperature) each day. If possible, she should use a basal body temperature thermometer (which is highly accurate) or, if it is unavailable, a mercury thermometer. Electronic thermometers are the least accurate. Usually, the best time is immediately after awakening. A decrease in basal body temperature suggests that ovulation is about to occur. An increase of more than 0.9° F (0.5° C) in temperature usually indicates that ovulation has just occurred. However, this method is inconvenient for many women and is not reliable or precise. At best, it predicts ovulation only within 2 days. A more accurate method is an ovulation predictor kit for use at home. This kit detects an increase in luteinizing hormone in the urine 24 to 36 hours before ovulation. Urine is tested on several consecutive days.

Doctors can accurately determine whether and when ovulation occurs. Methods include ultrasonography and measurement of the level of progesterone in the blood or saliva or the level of one of its by-products in the urine. A marked increase in these levels indicates that ovulation has occurred.

Doctors may do other tests to check for disorders that can cause ovulation problems. For example, they may measure testosterone levels in the blood to check for polycystic ovary syndrome.

Treatment

A drug to trigger ovulation, such as clomiphene or human gonadotropins, may be used. The particular drug is selected based on the specific problem. If the cause of infertility is early menopause, neither clomiphene nor human gonadotropins can stimulate ovulation.

Clomiphene Plus Medroxyprogesterone: If ovulation has not occurred for a long time, clomiphene with medroxyprogesterone is usually preferred. First, the woman takes medroxyprogesterone, usually by mouth, to trigger menstrual-like bleeding. This drug is taken for 5 to 10 days. A few days after bleeding begins, she takes clomiphene by mouth for 5 days. Usually, she ovulates 5 to 12 days after clomiphene is stopped and has a menstrual period 14 to 16 days after ovulation. Clomiphene is not effective for all causes of ovulation problems. It is most effective when the cause is polycystic ovary syndrome.

If a woman does not have a period after treatment with clomiphene, she takes a pregnancy test. If she is not pregnant, the treatment cycle is repeated. A higher dose of clomiphene is used in each cycle until ovulation occurs or the maximum dose is reached. When the dose that triggers ovulation is determined, the woman takes that dose for at least three or four more treatment cycles. Most women who become pregnant do so by the fourth cycle in which ovulation occurs. Although about 75 to 80% of women treated with clomiphene ovulate, only about 40 to 50% become pregnant. About 5% of pregnancies in women treated with clomiphene involve more than one fetus, primarily twins.

Side effects of clomiphene include hot flashes, abdominal bloating, breast tenderness, nausea, vision problems, and headaches. Fewer than 1% of women treated with clomiphene develop ovarian hyperstimulation syndrome. In this syndrome, the ovaries enlarge greatly and a large amount of fluid moves out the bloodstream into the abdomen. This syndrome may be life threatening. To try to prevent it, doctors prescribe the lowest effective dose of clomiphene, and if the ovaries enlarge, they stop the drug.

Human Gonadotropins: If a woman does not ovulate or become pregnant during treatment with clomiphene, hormonal therapy with human gonadotropins, injected into a muscle or under the skin, can be tried. Human gonadotropins stimulate the follicles of the ovaries to mature. Follicles are fluid-filled cavities, each of which contains an egg (see page 1493). Ultrasonography can detect when the follicles are mature. Then, the woman is given an injection of a different hormone, human chorionic gonadotropin, to trigger ovulation. When human gonadotropins are used appropriately, more than 95% of women treated with them ovulate, but only 50 to 75% become pregnant. About 10 to 30% of pregnancies in women treated with human gonadotropins involve more than one fetus, primarily twins.

Human gonadotropins can have severe side effects, so doctors closely monitor the woman during treatment. About 10 to 20% of women treated with human gonadotropins develop ovarian hyperstimulation syndrome. If hyperstimulation occurs, doctors may not give the woman human chorionic gonadotropin to trigger ovulation. Human gonadotropins are also expensive.

If the cause of infertility is early menopause, neither clomiphene nor human gonadotropins can stimulate ovulation.

Other Drugs: If the hypothalamus does not secrete gonadotropin-releasing hormone, a synthetic version of this hormone (called gonadorelin acetate), given intravenously, may be useful. This drug, like the natural hormone, stimulates the pituitary gland to produce the hormones that trigger ovulation. The risk of ovarian hyperstimulation is low with this treatment, so close monitoring is not needed. However, this drug is not available in the United States.

When the cause of infertility is high levels of the hormone prolactin, the best drug is one that acts like dopamine, called a dopamine agonist, such as bromocriptine or cabergoline. (Dopamine is a chemical messenger that generally inhibits the production of prolactin.)

Problems With the Fallopian Tubes

The fallopian tube may be blocked or damaged, preventing the egg from moving from the ovary to the uterus to be implanted.

- To identify the problem, doctors may use x-rays taken after a radiopaque dye is injected through the cervix or may directly view the organs through a viewing tube (laparoscope) inserted through an incision just below the navel.
- The fallopian tubes can sometimes be repaired, but in vitro fertilization is usually recommended.

Sometimes the fallopian tubes are blocked or damaged so that the egg cannot move from the ovary to the uterus. Causes include previous disorders and situations, such as the following:

- Pelvic infections (such as pelvic inflammatory disease)
- Use of an intrauterine device if it causes a pelvic infection (which is rare)
- A ruptured appendix
- Surgery in the pelvis or lower abdomen
- A mislocated (ectopic) pregnancy in the fallopian tubes

Current conditions may also block the tubes:

- Birth defects of the uterus and fallopian tubes
- Endometriosis
- Fibroids in the uterus
- Bands of scar tissue between normally unconnected structures (adhesions) in the uterus or pelvis

Diagnosis

Procedures used to determine whether the fallopian tubes are blocked include the following:

- **Hysterosalpingography:** X-rays are taken after a radiopaque dye is injected through the cervix. The dye outlines the interior of the uterus and fallopian tubes. This procedure is done a few days after a woman's menstrual period ends. This procedure can detect structural disorders that can block the fallopian tubes. However, in about 15% of cases, hysterosalpingography indicates that the fallopian tubes are blocked when they are not—called a false-positive result. After hysterosalpingography, fertility appears to be slightly improved even if the results are normal, possibly because the procedure temporarily widens (dilates) the tubes or clears the tubes of mucus. In such cases, doctors may wait to see if a woman becomes pregnant after this procedure before additional tests of fallopian tube function are done.

- **Sonohysterography:** A salt (saline) solution is injected into the interior of the uterus through the cervix during ultrasonography so that the interior is distended and abnormalities can be seen. If the solution flows into the fallopian tubes, the tubes are not blocked. This procedure is quick and does not require an anesthetic. It is considered safer than hysterosalpingography because it does not require radiation or injection of a dye. However, it is not as accurate.

If an abnormality within the uterus is detected, doctors examine the uterus with a viewing tube called a hysteroscope, which is inserted through the cervix into the uterus. If adhesions, a polyp, or a small fibroid is detected, instruments inserted through the hysteroscope may be used to dislodge or remove the abnormal tissue, increasing the chances that the woman will become pregnant.

If evidence suggests that the fallopian tubes are blocked or that a woman may have endometriosis, a small viewing tube called a laparoscope is inserted in the pelvic cavity through a small incision just below the navel. Usually, a general anesthetic is used. This procedure enables doctors to directly view the uterus, fallopian tubes, and ovaries. Instruments inserted through the laparoscope may also be used to dislodge or remove abnormal tissue in the pelvis.

Treatment

Treatment depends on the cause. Abnormal tissue is often dislodged or removed during diagnosis (using hysteroscopy or laparoscopy).

Surgery can be done to repair a fallopian tube damaged by an ectopic pregnancy or an infection. However, after such surgery, the chances of a normal pregnancy are small, and those of an ectopic pregnancy are higher than usual. Consequently, in vitro fertilization is often recommended instead.

Problems With Mucus in the Cervix

If mucus in the cervix is abnormal, it may prevent sperm from entering the uterus or may promote the destruction of sperm.

Normally, mucus in the cervix (the lower part of the uterus that opens into the vagina) is thick and impenetrable to sperm until just before release of an egg (ovulation). Then, just before ovulation, the mucus becomes clear and elastic (because the level of the hormone estrogen increases). As a result, sperm can move through the mucus into the uterus to the fallopian tubes, where fertilization can take place.

Abnormal mucus may do the following:

- Not change at ovulation (usually because of an infection), making pregnancy unlikely
- Allow bacteria in the vagina, usually those that cause infection in the cervix (cervicitis), to enter the uterus, sometimes resulting in the destruction of sperm
- Contain antibodies to sperm, which kill sperm before they can reach the egg

Usually, abnormal mucus causes infertility only if the abnormal mucus causes chronic cervicitis or if the cervix has been narrowed by treatment for a precancerous abnormality of the cervix (cervical dysplasia).

Did You Know...

Mucus in the cervix changes consistency to allow sperm to enter the uterus.

Diagnosis

Doctors examine women to see whether the cervix is narrow and to check for infection.

Tests to determine whether the mucus promotes sperm destruction are rarely used because these tests do not accurately predict the chances of pregnancy.

Treatment

Treatment may include placing semen directly in the uterus to bypass the mucus (intrauterine insemination). Drugs to thin the mucus, such as guaifenesin, may be used. However, there is no proof that either treatment increases the chances of pregnancy.

Problems With Eggs

The number of eggs may be low, or the quality may be poor.

The number and quality of eggs (ovarian reserve) may begin to decrease at age 30 or even earlier. They decrease rapidly after age 40. But age is not the only cause. Abnormalities in the ovaries can also cause such a decrease.

Diagnosis and Treatment

Doctors may evaluate the following women for problems with eggs:

- Those who are 35 or older
- Those who have had ovarian surgery

- Those who have responded poorly to fertility drugs (such as gonadotropins) that stimulate several eggs to mature and be released

Doctors can usually confirm the diagnosis by measuring levels of follicle-stimulating hormone (which triggers ovulation) and estrogen in the blood at a certain time during the menstrual cycle. Sometimes doctors give women clomiphene, a fertility drug, before measuring these levels.

If women are older than 42 or if the number or quality of eggs is decreased, using eggs from another woman (donor) may be the only way to achieve pregnancy.

Unidentified Factors

Unidentified factors are considered the explanation for infertility when semen in the man and ovulation and fallopian tubes in the woman are normal.

When no explanation for infertility is identified, the following approach is used:

- Women are given a fertility drug (clomiphene), which stimulates several eggs to mature and be released, and human chorionic gonadotropin (hCG), which triggers ovulation, for up to three menstrual cycles. This treatment may result in more than one fetus.
- Semen is placed directly in the uterus to bypass the mucus (intrauterine insemination) within 2 days after ovulation is triggered by treatment with fertility drugs.
- If pregnancy does not result, other assisted reproductive techniques, such as in vitro fertilization, are tried.

If clomiphene plus hCG is unsuccessful, women are sometimes given human gonadotropins (see page 1589) before assisted reproductive techniques are tried. Women have the same chance of pregnancy (about 65%) whether in vitro fertilization is done immediately after unsuccessful treatment with clomiphene plus hCG or whether human gonadotropins are given next, before in vitro fertilization is tried. However, women become pregnant more quickly if in vitro fertilization is done immediately after unsuccessful treatment with clomiphene plus hCG.

Assisted Reproductive Techniques

Assisted reproductive techniques involve manipulating sperm and eggs in a culture dish (in vitro) with the goal of producing an embryo.

If treatment has not resulted in pregnancy after four to six menstrual cycles, assisted reproductive techniques, such as in vitro fertilization or gamete intrafallopian tube transfer, may be considered. These techniques are more successful in women under age 35. In the United States, more than 43% of cycles of in vitro fertilization in women under 35 resulted in pregnancy, and almost 87% of the pregnancies ended in live births. In contrast, only about 18% of attempts in women aged 41to 42 resulted in pregnancy, and only about 60% of the pregnancies resulted in live births. For women over 42, using eggs from another woman (donor) is recommended.

Assisted reproductive techniques may result in more than one fetus but are less likely to do so than fertility drugs. If the risk of genetic abnormalities is high, the embryo can often be tested before it is implanted in the woman's uterus. This testing is called preimplantation genetic diagnosis.

> ### ❓ Did You Know...
>
> An embryo can be tested for genetic abnormalities before it is implanted in the woman.

In Vitro (Test Tube) Fertilization (IVF): This technique is used when infertility is due to certain problems with sperm, problems with the fallopian tubes, or abnormal mucus in the cervix and when women have endometriosis, as well as when the cause is unidentified. The technique involves the following:

- Stimulating the ovaries: Typically, a woman's ovaries are stimulated with clomiphene, human gonadotropins, or both. A gonadotropin-releasing hormone agonist or antagonist is often given to prevent ovulation from occurring until after several eggs have matured. As a result, many eggs usually mature. Then, human chorionic gonadotropin is given to trigger ovulation.
- Retrieving released eggs: Guided by ultrasonography, a doctor inserts a needle through the woman's vagina into the ovary and removes several eggs from the follicles. Sometimes the eggs are removed through a small tube (laparoscope) inserted through a small incision just below the navel.
- Fertilizing the eggs: The eggs are placed in a culture dish and fertilized with sperm selected as the most active.
- Growing the resulting embryos in a laboratory: After sperm are added, the eggs are allowed to grow for about 2 to 5 days.
- Implanting the embryos in the woman's uterus: One or a few of the resulting embryos are transferred from the culture dish into the woman's uterus through the vagina. The number of embryos implanted is determined by the woman's age and likelihood of response to treatment.

Additional embryos can be frozen in liquid nitrogen to be used later if pregnancy does not occur. Despite the implantation of several embryos, the chances of producing one full-term baby are only about 18 to 25% each time eggs are placed in the uterus. The chances of having a baby with in vitro fertilization depend on many factors, but the woman's age may be most important.

The greatest risk is having more than one fetus (multiple pregnancy). A multiple pregnancy can cause serious complications in the mother and the newborns: The mother may have excessive bleeding, the fetuses may die, or the babies may have a low birth weight. Because of these complications, doctors now transfer fewer embryos to the uterus at one time.

Intracytoplasmic Sperm Injection: This technique may be used when other techniques are likely to be unsuccessful or when the problem with sperm is severe. It resembles in vitro fertilization except that only one sperm is injected into only one egg.

Gamete Intrafallopian Tube Transfer (GIFT): This technique can be used if the fallopian tubes are functioning normally. Eggs and selected active sperm are obtained as for in vitro fertilization, but the eggs are not fertilized with sperm in the laboratory. Instead, the eggs and sperm are transferred to the far end of the woman's fallopian tube through a small incision in the abdomen (using a laparoscope) or through the vagina (guided by ultrasonography), so that the egg can be fertilized in the fallopian tube. Thus, this technique is more invasive than in vitro fertilization.

Other Techniques: These techniques include the following:

- Transfer of a more mature embryo (blastocyst transfer)
- Use of eggs from another woman (donor)
- Transfer of frozen embryos to a surrogate mother

These techniques raise moral and ethical issues, including questions about the disposal of stored embryos (especially in cases of death or divorce), legal parentage if a surrogate mother is involved, and selective reduction of the number of implanted embryos (similar to abortion) when more than three develop.

CHAPTER

250 Family Planning

Family planning involves using various methods to control the number and timing of pregnancies. A couple may use contraception to avoid pregnancy temporarily or sterilization to avoid pregnancy permanently. Abortion may be used to end an unwanted pregnancy when contraception has failed or not been used.

Contraception

Contraception is prevention of fertilization of an egg by a sperm (conception) or attachment of the fertilized egg to the lining of the uterus (implantation).

There are several methods of contraception. None is completely effective, but some methods are far more reliable than others. Effectiveness often depends on how closely people follow instructions. Following instructions for some methods is easier than for others. Thus, the difference in effectiveness between typical use (which is often inconsistent) and perfect use (following the instructions exactly) may vary greatly from one method to another. For example, oral contraceptives are very effective with perfect use. However, many women forget to take some doses. Thus, average use of oral contraceptives is much less effective than perfect use. In contrast, contraceptive implants, once inserted, require nothing more (and are thus used perfectly) until they need to be replaced. Thus, typical use is the same as perfect use (until implants need to be replaced). People tend to follow instructions more closely as they get used to

HOW EFFECTIVE IS CONTRACEPTION?		
METHOD	**PERCENTAGE OF WOMEN WHO BECOME PREGNANT DURING THE FIRST YEAR OF USE***	
	PERFECT USE	**TYPICAL USE**
Oral contraceptives	0.3	8
Implants	0.05	0.05
Skin patches and vaginal rings	0.3	8
Injections of medroxyprogesterone acetate	0.3	3
Condom	2	15
Diaphragm with spermicide	6	16
Cervical cap with spermicide	18 (women who have had children)	40 (women who have had children)
	9 (women who have not had children)	18 (women who have not had children)
Contraceptive sponge	26 (women who have had children)	32 (women who have had children)
	9 (women who have not had children)	16 (women who have not had children)
Intrauterine device (IUD)	0.1–0.8	0.1–0.8
Natural family planning (rhythm) methods	1–9	25
Withdrawal method	4	27

*About 85% of women become pregnant during 1 year of frequent intercourse if no contraception is used.

COMPARING CONTRACEPTIVE METHODS

METHOD	CONVENIENCE	SIDE EFFECTS	OTHER CONSIDERATIONS
Hormonal methods			
Oral contraceptives	Daily action is usually required. With combination oral contraceptives (estrogen plus a progestin), a woman typically takes the contraceptive every day for 3 weeks, followed by an inactive tablet every day for 1 week. Progestin-only oral contraceptives are taken every day. A visit to the doctor is required periodically to have the prescription renewed.	Irregular bleeding but only during the first few months Nausea, bloating, fluid retention, increased blood pressure, breast tenderness, migraine headaches, weight gain, acne, and nervousness Increased risk of blood clots and possibly cervical cancer	Women who are older than 35 and who smoke should not take oral contraceptives. Certain disorders also prohibit their use. Women who take oral contraceptives are less likely to have menstrual cramps, premenstrual syndrome, acne, and irregular bleeding and are less likely to develop osteoporosis and several types of cancer.
Implants	Implants require action only once every 3 years. They are inserted by a doctor.	Irregular or no menstrual periods during the first year Headaches and weight gain	Restrictions are similar to those of oral contraceptives. An incision is required to remove implants.
Skin patches	Women apply a patch once a week for 3 weeks. Then they do not wear one for a week. A visit to the doctor is required periodically to have the prescription renewed.	Similar to oral contraceptives, except irregular bleeding is uncommon	Restrictions are similar to those of oral contraceptives.
Vaginal rings	Women insert a ring once every 3 weeks. It is then removed and not used for 1 week. A new ring is used each month. A visit to the doctor is required periodically to have the prescription renewed.	Similar to oral contraceptives, except irregular bleeding is uncommon	Restrictions are similar to those of oral contraceptives. During the first week of use, a backup method of birth control should be used. Rings may be expelled. If they are expelled and then reinserted within 3 hours, no backup method of birth control is needed.
Injections of medroxyprogesterone acetate	An injection is given by a doctor every 3 months.	Irregular bleeding (which becomes less frequent with time) or no menstrual periods while injections are being used Slight weight gain, headache, and a temporary decrease in bone density	This method reduces the risk of uterine (endometrial) cancer, pelvic inflammatory disease, and iron deficiency anemia.

(continued on the following page)

COMPARING CONTRACEPTIVE METHODS (*Continued*)

METHOD	CONVENIENCE	SIDE EFFECTS	OTHER CONSIDERATIONS
Barrier methods			
Condom	Men apply a condom immediately before every act of sexual intercourse and discard it after one use. Condoms are available over the counter.	Allergic reactions and irritation	Latex condoms provide protection against common sexually transmitted diseases. Condoms must be used correctly to be effective. This method requires diligence by the sex partner.
Diaphragm with a contraceptive cream or jelly	Women insert a diaphragm before sexual intercourse. The diaphragm may be left in place for up to 24 hours. A doctor fits the diaphragm and checks the fit at least once a year. The contraceptive cream or jelly used with a diaphragm may make insertion messy.	Allergic reactions, irritation, and urinary tract infections	After initial insertion, additional cream or jelly should be inserted before each act of intercourse.
Contraceptive sponge	Women insert the sponge before sexual intercourse. The sponge can be inserted in advance and is effective for 24 hours. It is discarded after one use. Sponges are available over the counter.	Allergic reactions and vaginal dryness or irritation	Sponges may be difficult to remove. They must be removed after 30 hours.
Other methods			
Intrauterine device (IUD)	IUDs require action only once every 5 or 10 years, depending on the type used. They must be inserted and removed by a doctor.	Bleeding and pain Rarely, perforation of the uterus	Occasionally, the IUD is expelled.
Natural family planning (rhythm) methods	Women check their temperature, cervical mucus, other symptoms, or a combination almost every day.	None	This method requires diligence by women and abstinence from sexual intercourse several days a month. It is less effective for women with irregular menstrual cycles.
Withdrawal method	Men withdraw their penis from the vagina before ejaculation. Self-control and precise timing are required.	None	This method is unreliable because sperm may be released before ejaculation.

using a method. As a result, the difference between effectiveness with perfect use and that with typical use often decreases as time passes.

Did You Know...

The effectiveness of certain contraceptive measures, such as the pill or rhythm methods, depends a great deal on how well instructions are followed.

Besides its degree of effectiveness, each contraceptive method has other advantages and disadvantages. For example, hormonal methods have certain side effects and increase or decrease women's risk of developing certain disorders. Choice of method depends on lifestyle, preferences, and the degree of reliability needed.

HORMONAL METHODS

Contraceptive hormones can be taken by mouth, inserted into the vagina, applied to the skin, implanted under the skin, or injected into muscle. The hormones used to prevent conception include estrogen and progestins (drugs similar to the hormone progesterone). Hormonal methods prevent pregnancy mainly by stopping the ovaries from releasing eggs or by keeping mucus in the cervix thick so that sperm cannot pass through the cervix into the uterus. Thus, hormonal methods prevent the egg from being fertilized.

All hormonal methods can have similar side effects and restrictions on use.

Oral Contraceptives

Oral contraceptives, commonly known as birth control pills or just "the pill," contain hormones—either a combination of a progestin and estrogen or a progestin alone.

Combination tablets are typically taken once a day for 3 weeks, not taken for a week (allowing the menstrual period to occur), then started again. Inactive tablets may be included for the week when combination tablets are not taken to establish a routine of taking one tablet a day. One product is taken daily for 12 weeks, then not taken for 1 week. Thus, menstrual periods occur only 4 times a year. Another product involves taking an active tablet every day. With this product, there is no scheduled bleeding episode, but unscheduled bleeding episodes often occur. About 0.3% of women who take combination tablets as instructed become pregnant during the first year of use. However, the chances of becoming pregnant increase substantially if women skip or forget to take a tablet, especially the first ones in a monthly cycle.

The dose of estrogen in combination tablets varies. Usually, combination tablets with a low dose of estrogen (20 to 35 micrograms) are used because they have fewer serious side effects than those with a high dose (50 micrograms). Healthy women who do not smoke can take low-dose combination tablets without interruption until menopause.

Progestin-only tablets are taken every day of the month. They often cause irregular bleeding. Pregnancy rates are about the same as those with combination tablets. Progestin-only tablets are usually prescribed only when taking estrogen may be harmful. For example, these tablets may be prescribed for women who are breastfeeding because estrogen reduces the amount and quality of breast milk produced. Progestin-only tablets do not affect breast milk production.

Before starting oral contraceptives, a woman should have a physical examination, including measurement of blood pressure, to make sure she has no health problems that would make taking the contraceptives risky for her. Three months after starting oral contraceptives, the woman should have another examination to determine whether her blood pressure has changed. If it has not, she should then have an examination at least once a year.

If a woman has coronary artery disease or diabetes or has risk factors for them (such as a close relative with either disorder), a blood test is usually done to measure levels of cholesterol, other fats (lipids), and sugar (glucose). Even if these levels are abnormal, doctors may still prescribe a low-dose estrogen combination contraceptive. However, they periodically do blood tests to monitor the woman's lipid and sugar levels.

Also before starting oral contraceptives, a woman should talk with her doctor about the advantages and disadvantages of oral contraceptives for her situation.

Did You Know...

With one type of oral contraceptive, menstrual periods occur only 4 times a year.

Contraceptive hormones may have some health benefits.

Advantages: The main advantage is reliable, continuous contraception if oral contraceptives are taken as instructed. Also, taking oral contraceptives reduces the occurrence of menstrual cramps, premenstrual syndrome, acne, irregular bleeding, iron deficiency anemia, breast cysts, ovarian cysts, mislocated (ectopic) pregnancies (almost always in the fallopian tubes), and infections of the fallopian tubes. Also, women who have taken oral contraceptives are less likely to develop osteoporosis.

Taking oral contraceptives reduces the risk of developing several types of cancer, including uterine (endometrial) and ovarian. The risk is reduced for many years after the contraceptives are stopped.

When Taking Combination Oral Contraceptives Is Restricted*

A woman must not take oral contraceptives if any of the following situations apply:

- She smokes cigarettes and is older than 35.
- She has an active liver disorder or liver tumors.
- She has very high triglyceride levels (250 mg/dL or higher).
- She has untreated or poorly controlled high blood pressure.
- She has poorly controlled diabetes or diabetes that has resulted in poor circulation.
- She has kidney problems.
- She has had blood clots in her legs (deep vein thrombosis).
- She has an immobilized leg (as in a cast).
- She has coronary artery disease.
- She has had a stroke.
- She has had surgery within the preceding month or will have surgery within the next month.
- She has had cholestasis (reduced bile flow) of pregnancy or had jaundice while she was previously taking oral contraceptives.
- She has a type of breast or uterine (endometrial) cancer that grows in response to stimulation by estrogen.
- She has had a heart attack.
- She has abnormal vaginal bleeding with no known cause.
- She has active lupus (systemic lupus erythematosus).

A woman may take oral contraceptives but only with a doctor's supervision if any of the following situations apply:

- She is depressed.
- She has diabetes that is well controlled with treatment and that has not affected circulation.
- She has premenstrual syndrome.
- She has no menstrual periods (amenorrhea) for no identifiable reason.
- She frequently has migraine headaches (but no symptoms of nervous system dysfunction, such as numbness or weakness in the limbs or face).
- She smokes cigarettes but is younger than 35.
- She has had hepatitis or another liver disorder and has fully recovered.
- She has high blood pressure that is controlled with treatment.
- She has varicose veins.
- She has a seizure disorder that is being treated with drugs.
- She has fibroids in the uterus.
- She has been treated for precancerous abnormalities or cancer of the cervix.
- She is obese.
- She has close relatives who have had blood clots.

*These restrictions apply only to oral contraceptives that contain estrogen and a progestin.
mg/dL = milligrams per deciliter of blood.

Oral contraceptives taken early in a pregnancy do not harm the fetus. However, they should be stopped as soon as the woman realizes she is pregnant. Oral contraceptives do not have any long-term effects on fertility, although a woman may not release an egg (ovulate) for a few months after stopping the drugs. Doctors recommend that women wait 2 weeks after delivery before they start taking oral contraceptives.

Disadvantages: The disadvantages may include bothersome side effects. Irregular bleeding is common during the first few months of oral contraceptive use but usually stops as the body adjusts to the hormones. If irregular bleeding persists, doctors may suggest taking oral contraceptives every day, without any breaks, for several months to reduce the number of bleeding episodes.

Some side effects are related to the estrogen in the tablet. They may include nausea, bloating, fluid retention, an increase in blood pressure, breast tenderness, and migraine headaches. Others are related mostly to the type or dose of the progestin. They may include weight gain, acne, and nervousness. Some women who take oral contraceptives gain 3 to 5 pounds because of fluid retention. They may gain even more because appetite also increases. Many of these side effects are uncommon with the low-dose tablets.

In some women, oral contraceptives cause dark patches (melasma—see page 1309) on the face, similar to those that may occur during pregnancy. Exposure to the sun darkens the patches even more. If dark patches develop, women should discuss stopping the oral contraceptives with their doctor. The patches slowly fade after the contraceptives are stopped.

Taking oral contraceptives increases the risk of developing some disorders. The risk of developing blood clots in veins is higher for women who take combination oral contraceptives than for those who do not. The risk is 7 times higher with tablets containing a high dose of estrogen and 3 to 4 times higher with tablets containing a low dose of estrogen. However, this risk is still only half the risk of developing blood clots during pregnancy. Women with family members who have had blood clots should inform their doctor before taking oral contraceptives. Because surgery also increases the risk of developing blood clots, women must stop taking oral contraceptives a month before major elective surgery and not take them again until a month afterward. For healthy women who do not smoke, taking combination tablets with a low dose of estrogen does not increase the risk of having a stroke or heart attack.

Use of oral contraceptives, particularly for more than 5 years, may increase the risk of developing cervical cancer. Women who are taking oral contraceptives should have a Papanicolaou (Pap) test at least once a year. Such tests can detect precancerous changes in the cervix early—before they lead to cancer.

The current use of oral contraceptives does not increase overall risk of breast cancer, nor does former use in women aged 35 to 65. Also, use does not further increase breast cancer risk in high-risk groups (for example, women with certain benign breast disorders or a family history of breast cancer).

Taking oral contraceptives causes existing gallstones to grow faster but does not cause new stones to form. Thus, gallstones are diagnosed more often during the first few years of oral contraceptive use.

For women who are older than 35 and who smoke, using oral contraceptives increases their risk of having a heart attack. Typically, such women should not use oral contraceptives. However, if they are closely monitored by a health care practitioner, some of them may be able to take oral contraceptives.

Taking cyclophosphamide, certain antibiotics, or possibly certain antifungal drugs can make oral contraceptives less effective. If women taking oral contraceptives take one of these drugs, they should also use another contraceptive method until the beginning of their first period after stopping the drug.

Skin Patches and Vaginal Rings

Skin patches and vaginal rings that contain estrogen and a progestin are used for 3 of 4 weeks, then removed. In the 4th week, no contraception is used to allow the menstrual period to occur.

A contraceptive skin patch is placed on the skin once a week for 3 weeks. The patch is left in place for 1 week, then removed, and a new patch is placed on a different area of the skin. During the 4th week, no patch is used. Exercise and use of saunas or hot tubs do not displace the patches.

A vaginal ring is a small plastic device that is placed in the vagina and left there for 3 weeks. Then it is removed for 1 week. A woman can place and remove the vaginal ring herself. The ring comes in one size and can be placed anywhere in the vagina. Usually, the ring is not felt by the woman's partner during intercourse. A new ring is used each month.

Either method is effective, particularly with perfect use. Effectiveness is similar to that of oral contraceptives. Sometimes the patch is less effective in overweight women.

With either method, a woman has a regular menstrual period. Spotting or bleeding between periods (breakthrough bleeding) is uncommon. Side effects, effects on the risk of developing disorders, and restrictions on use are similar to those of combination oral contraceptives.

Contraceptive Implants

Contraceptive implants are a single rod containing a progestin. After numbing the skin with an anesthetic, a doctor uses a needle-like instrument (trocar) to place the implant under the skin of the inner arm above the elbow. No stitches are necessary. The implants release the progestin slowly into the bloodstream. The type of implant available in the United States is effective for 3 years.

The most common side effect is irregular or no menstrual periods during the first year of use. After that, periods frequently become regular. Headaches and weight gain may also occur. These side effects prompt some women to have the implant removed. Because the implant does not dissolve in the body, a doctor has to make an incision in the skin to remove it. Removal is more difficult than insertion because tissue under the skin thickens around the implant. As soon as the implant is removed, the ovaries return to their normal functioning, and women become fertile again.

Contraceptive Injections

A progestin called medroxyprogesterone acetate is injected by a health care practitioner once every 3 months. Two types of injections are available. One is injected into a muscle of the arm or buttock. The other is injected under the skin. Each type is very effective.

The progestin completely disrupts the menstrual cycle. About one third of women using this contraceptive have no menstrual bleeding during the 3 months after the first injection, and another third have irregular bleeding and spotting for more than 11 days each month. After this contraceptive is used for a while, irregular bleeding occurs less often. After 2 years, about 70% of the women have no bleeding at all. When the injections are stopped, a regular menstrual cycle resumes in about half of the women within 6 months and in about three fourths within 1 year. Fertility may not return for up to a year after injections are stopped.

Common side effects include a slight weight gain, headache, irregular or no menstrual periods, and a temporary decrease in bone density. Bones usually return to their previous density after the injections are stopped. People getting injections, particularly teenagers and young women, should take calcium and vitamin D supplements daily to help maintain bone density.

Medroxyprogesterone acetate does not increase the risk of developing any cancer, including breast cancer. It reduces the risk of developing uterine (endometrial) cancer, pelvic inflammatory disease (an infection of the upper female reproductive organs), and iron deficiency anemia. Interactions with other drugs are uncommon.

Emergency Contraception

Emergency contraception, the so-called morning-after pill, consists of synthetic hormones or drugs that affect hormones. It is used within 72 hours after one act of unprotected sexual intercourse or after one occasion when a contraceptive method fails (for example, when a condom breaks).

Emergency contraception decreases the chance of pregnancy after one act of unprotected intercourse, including when the act occurs near the time the egg is released (ovulation)—when conception is most likely. Near ovulation, the chance of pregnancy is about 8% without contraception. The sooner emergency contraception is taken, the more likely it is to be effective.

Two options are available:

- **Levonorgestrel:** This hormone, a progestin often taken in lower doses for contraception, is most commonly used. Usually, one dose is taken by mouth, followed by another dose 12 hours later. If the first dose is taken within 72 hours of intercourse, the chance of pregnancy decreases by almost 90%. If the first dose is taken within 24 hours of intercourse, the chance decreases by about 95%. Some doctors recommend taking both doses of levonorgestrel at the same time. This method seems to be just as effective. Each dose can be taken as one tablet or as 20 lower-dose tablets. These tablets are available without a prescription for women 18 years of age or older.

- **Combination oral contraceptives:** Two tablets of a combination oral contraceptive can be used. They are taken within 72 hours of unprotected intercourse. Then, two more tablets are taken 12 hours later. This option is slightly less effective in preventing pregnancy than levonorgestrel. As many as 50% of women have nausea, and 20% vomit. Antiemetic drugs can be taken to help prevent nausea and vomiting.

BARRIER CONTRACEPTIVES

Barrier contraceptives physically block the sperm's access to a woman's uterus. They include the condom, diaphragm, cervical cap, and contraceptive sponge.

Condoms: Condoms are thin protective sheaths that cover the penis. Condoms made of latex are the only contraceptives that provide protection against all common sexually transmitted diseases, including those due to bacteria (such as gonorrhea and syphilis) and those due to viruses (such as HPV—human papillomavirus—and HIV—human immunodeficiency virus). However, this protection, though considerable, is not complete. Condoms made of polyurethane also provide protection, but they are thinner and more likely to tear. Condoms made of lambskin do not protect against viral infections such as HIV infection.

Condoms must be used correctly to be effective (see box on page 1265). With some condoms, the tip needs to be positioned so that it extends about 1/2 inch (about 1¼ centimeters) beyond the penis to provide a space to collect semen. Other condoms have a reservoir at the tip for this purpose. Immediately after ejaculation, the penis should be withdrawn while the condom's rim is held firmly against the base of the penis to prevent the condom from slipping off and spilling semen. The condom should then be removed carefully. If semen is spilled, sperm could enter the vagina, resulting in pregnancy. A new condom should be used each time a person has sexual intercourse, and the condom should be discarded if its integrity is in doubt.

> **? Did You Know...**
> Latex condoms are the only contraceptive method that helps protect against all common sexually transmitted diseases, including HIV infection.

During the first year condoms are used, the chance of pregnancy is about 6% with perfect use and about 16% with typical use. A substance that kills sperm (spermicide), which may be included in the condom's lubricant or inserted separately into the vagina, increases the effectiveness of condoms.

Diaphragm: The diaphragm, a dome-shaped rubber cup with a flexible rim, is inserted into the vagina and positioned over the cervix. A diaphragm prevents sperm from entering the uterus.

Diaphragms come in various sizes and must be fitted by a health care practitioner, who also teaches the woman how to insert it. If a woman has gained or lost more than 10 pounds, has had

Blocking Access: Barrier Contraceptives

Barrier contraceptives prevent sperm from entering a woman's uterus. They include the condom, diaphragm, cervical cap, and contraceptive sponge. Some condoms contain spermicides. Spermicides should be used with condoms and other barrier contraceptives that do not already contain them.

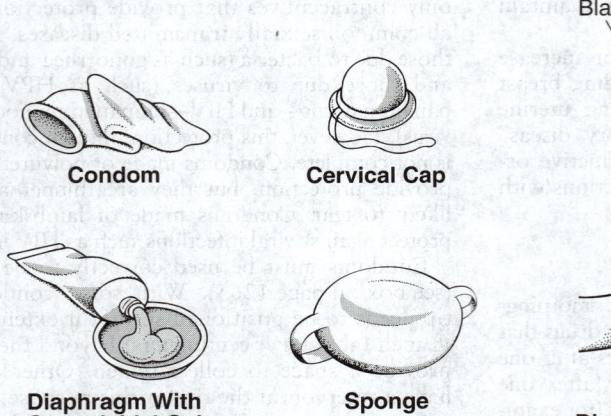

Condom

Cervical Cap

Diaphragm With Spermicidal Gel

Sponge

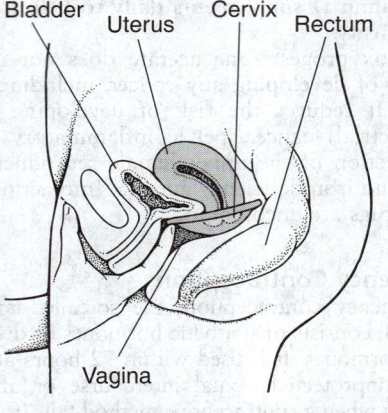

Bladder   Uterus   Cervix   Rectum

Vagina

Diaphragm in Place Over Cervix

a diaphragm for more than a year, or has had a baby or an abortion, she must be refitted for a diaphragm because the vagina's size and shape may have changed.

A diaphragm should cover the entire cervix without causing discomfort. Neither the woman nor her partner should notice its presence. A contraceptive cream or jelly (which kills sperm) should always be used with a diaphragm, in case the diaphragm is displaced during intercourse. The diaphragm is inserted before intercourse and should remain in place for at least 8 hours but no more than 24 hours afterward. If sexual intercourse is repeated while the diaphragm is in place, additional contraceptive cream or jelly should be inserted into the vagina to continue protection. A woman should inspect the diaphragm regularly for tears.

During the first year of diaphragm use, the percentage of women who become pregnant is about 6% with perfect use and about 16% with typical use.

Cervical Cap: The cervical cap resembles the diaphragm but is smaller and more rigid. It fits snugly over the cervix. It is not available in the United States.

Cervical caps must be fitted by a health care practitioner. A contraceptive cream or jelly should always be used with a cervical cap. The cap is inserted before intercourse and left in place for at least 8 hours after intercourse, up to 48 hours at a time.

During the first year of use by women who have not had children, pregnancy occurs in about 9% with perfect use and about 18% with typical use. About twice as many women who have had children become pregnant. Childbirth changes the cervix, making it more difficult to securely fit with a cap.

Contraceptive Sponge: In addition to blocking sperm from entering the uterus, the sponge contains a spermicide. It is available over the counter and does not need to be fitted by a health care practitioner.

The sponge can be inserted into the vagina by the woman up to 24 hours before sexual intercourse and provides protection through that period of time, regardless of how frequently intercourse is repeated. The sponge must be left in place for at least 6 hours after the last act of intercourse. It should not be left in place for more than 30 hours. Usually, neither partner is aware of its presence once it is inserted. It is less effective than the diaphragm.

Problems related to use are uncommon. They include allergic reactions, vaginal dryness or irritation, and difficulty removing the sponge.

SPERMICIDES

Spermicides are preparations that kill sperm on contact. They are available as vaginal foams, creams, gels, and suppositories and are placed in the vagina before sexual intercourse. These contraceptives also

Understanding Intrauterine Devices

Intrauterine devices (IUDs) are inserted by a doctor into a woman's uterus through the vagina. IUDs are made of molded plastic. One type releases copper from a copper wire wrapped around the base. The other type releases a progestin. A plastic string is attached, so that a woman can check to make sure the device is still in place.

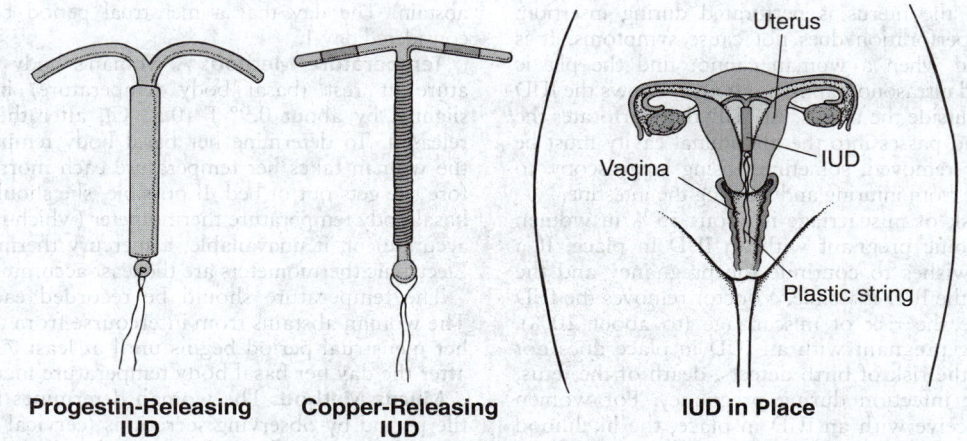

Progestin-Releasing IUD

Copper-Releasing IUD

IUD in Place

Uterus

Vagina

IUD

Plastic string

---

provide a physical barrier to sperm. No single type of preparation is more effective than another. Spermicides are best used with a barrier contraceptive, such as a condom or diaphragm.

INTRAUTERINE DEVICES

Intrauterine devices (IUDs) are small, flexible plastic devices that are inserted into the uterus. An IUD is left in place for 5 or 10 years, depending on the type, or until the woman wants the device removed. IUDs must be inserted and removed by a doctor or other health care practitioner. Insertion takes only a few minutes. Removal is also quick and usually causes minimal discomfort. IUDs prevent pregnancy in many ways:

- By killing or immobilizing sperm
- By preventing sperm from fertilizing the egg
- By preventing a fertilized egg from becoming implanted in the uterus

Two types of IUDs are currently available in the United States. One type, which releases a progestin (levonorgestrel), is effective for 5 years. During that time, only about 0.5% of women become pregnant. The other type, which releases copper, is effective for at least 10 years. During that time, less than 2% of women become pregnant. One year after removal of an IUD, 80 to 90% of women who try to conceive do so.

An IUD inserted up to 1 week after one act of unprotected sexual intercourse is nearly 100% effective as a method of emergency contraception. IUDs do not have any general, bodywide (systemic) effects.

The uterus is briefly contaminated with bacteria at the time of insertion, but an infection rarely results. IUD strings do not provide access for bacteria. An IUD increases the risk of a pelvic infection only during the first month of use.

Possible Problems: Bleeding and pain are the main reasons that women have an IUD removed, accounting for more than half of all removals before the usual replacement time. The copper-releasing IUD increases the amount of menstrual bleeding. In contrast, the progestin-releasing IUD reduces the amount, and after 1 year, menstrual bleeding stops completely in about 20% of women.

About 5% of IUDs are expelled during the first year after insertion, often during the first few weeks. Sometimes a woman does not notice the expulsion. A plastic string is attached to the IUD so that a woman can check every so often, especially after a menstrual period, to make sure that the IUD is still in place. If she cannot find the string, she should use another contraceptive method until she can see her health care practitioner to determine whether the IUD is still in place. If another IUD is inserted after one has been expelled, it usually stays in place.

? Did You Know...

Sperm can survive (and fertilize an egg) up to 5 days after intercourse.

Rarely, the uterus is perforated during insertion. Usually, perforation does not cause symptoms. It is discovered when a woman cannot find the plastic string and ultrasonography or an x-ray shows the IUD located outside the uterus. An IUD that perforates the uterus and passes into the abdominal cavity must be surgically removed, sometimes using laparoscopy, to prevent it from injuring and scarring the intestine.

The risk of miscarriage is about 55% in women who become pregnant with an IUD in place. If a woman wishes to continue the pregnancy and the string of the IUD is visible, a doctor removes the IUD to reduce the risk of miscarriage (to about 20%). Becoming pregnant with an IUD in place does not increase the risk of birth defects, death of the fetus, or pelvic infection during pregnancy. For women who conceive with an IUD in place, the likelihood of having a mislocated (ectopic) pregnancy is about 5%. Nonetheless, the overall risk of an ectopic pregnancy is much lower for women using IUDs than for those not using a contraceptive method because IUDs prevent pregnancy effectively.

Possible Benefits: In addition to providing effective birth control, IUDs may reduce the risk of uterine (endometrial) and cervical cancer.

TIMING METHODS

Some contraceptive methods depend on the timing of intercourse rather than on drugs or devices.

Natural Family Planning Methods

Natural family planning (rhythm) methods depend on abstinence from sexual intercourse during the woman's fertile time of the month. In most women, the ovary releases an egg about 14 days before the start of a menstrual period. Although the unfertilized egg survives only about 12 hours, sperm can survive for as long as 5 days after intercourse. Consequently, fertilization can result from intercourse that occurred up to 5 days before and 12 hours after the release of the egg.

There are several methods of natural family planning. Each method tries to estimate when the egg is released (ovulation). The calendar method is the least effective method. The temperature, mucus, and symptothermal methods more accurately estimate when ovulation occurs.

Calendar Method: This method is particularly ineffective for women who have irregular menstrual cycles. To calculate when to abstain from intercourse, a woman subtracts 18 days from the shortest and 11 days from the longest of her previous 12 menstrual cycles. For example, if cycles last from 26 to 29 days, she must abstain from intercourse from day 8 (26 minus 18) through day 18 (29 minus 11) of each cycle. The more the cycle length varies, the longer a woman must abstain. The day that a menstrual period begins is considered day 1.

Temperature Method: A woman's body temperature at rest (basal body temperature) increases slightly, by about 0.9° F (0.5° C), after the egg is released. To determine her basal body temperature, the woman takes her temperature each morning before she gets out of bed. If possible, she should use a basal body temperature thermometer (which is highly accurate) or, if unavailable, a mercury thermometer. Electronic thermometers are the least accurate.

The temperature should be recorded each day. The woman abstains from intercourse from the time her menstrual period begins until at least 72 hours after the day her basal body temperature increased.

Mucus Method: The woman determines her fertile period by observing secretions (cervical mucus) from the vagina, if possible, several times every day, starting the day after a menstrual period stops. There may be no mucus for a few days after the period stops, but then it appears and is cloudy and thick. Shortly before ovulation, more mucus is produced, and the mucus becomes thinner, elastic (stretching between the fingers), clearer, and more watery (like a raw egg white). Observations should be recorded.

Intercourse is avoided during the menstrual period because mucus cannot be checked during that time and mild vaginal bleeding may be confused with a period. Intercourse is permitted when mucus is absent but is restricted to every other day during this time because semen may be confused with mucus. Once mucus appears, intercourse is avoided until 3 or 4 days after the changes in mucus indicate ovulation. Intercourse is then permitted without restrictions on how often until the next period begins.

Women who use this method should not use douches or feminine hygiene sprays and creams because these products can change the mucus.

Symptothermal Method: This method combines the temperature, mucus, and calendar methods. The woman notes when cervical mucus increases in amount and becomes thinner, elastic, clearer, and more watery (as for the mucus method) and when temperature increases. She should abstain from intercourse from the first day requiring abstinence according to the calendar method until at least 72 hours after the day her basal body temperature increases (as for the temperature method) and cervical mucus changes.

All in the Timing: Natural Family Planning

Natural family planning involves abstaining from sexual intercourse when the woman may be fertile. Days to abstain may be based only on the timing of the menstrual period (calendar method), on the woman's temperature, on characteristics of cervical mucus (which change during the month), or on a combination of these methods (symptothermal method).

The exact days of abstinence vary from woman to woman because the length of a woman's cycle, the day her temperature increases, the pattern of changes in mucus, and the timing of other symptoms vary. The chart shown below gives only a general idea of how family planning methods are used. Having irregular menstrual periods makes using natural family planning methods more uncertain.

For the **calendar method** in the example below, 18 days were subtracted from the shortest cycle (26 – 18 = 8) and 11 days were subtracted from the longest (29 – 11 = 18). So the woman abstains from intercourse from day 8 through day 18.

For the **temperature method**, the woman abstains from intercourse from the beginning of her menstrual period until at least 72 hours after the day her basal body temperature increased.

For the **mucus method**, the woman abstains from intercourse during her menstrual period and from the time that cervical mucus appears until 4 days after she observes the largest amount of mucus and it becomes thinner, elastic, clearer, and more watery. She can have intercourse between the end of her menstrual period and the time mucus appears. But during this time, she should limit sexual intercourse to every other day so that she does not confuse semen with mucus from the cervix.

For the **symptothermal method**, the woman uses the temperature, mucus, and calendar methods. The woman notes when cervical mucus increases and changes in appearance and when basal body temperature increases. She abstains from intercourse starting the same day as determined by the calendar method until at least 72 hours after the day her temperature increases and the mucus changes, indicating ovulation.

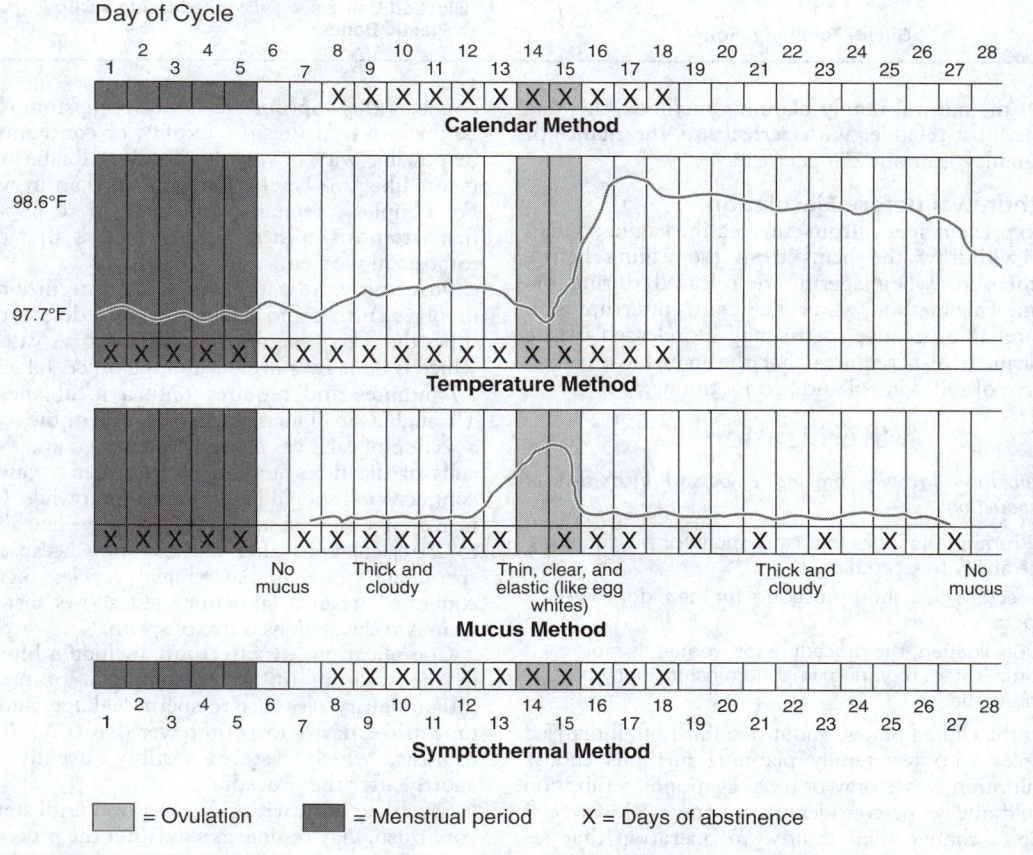

Disrupting the Tubes: Sterilization in Women

Both fallopian tubes (which carry the egg from the ovaries to the uterus) are cut, sealed, or blocked so that sperm cannot reach the egg to fertilize it.

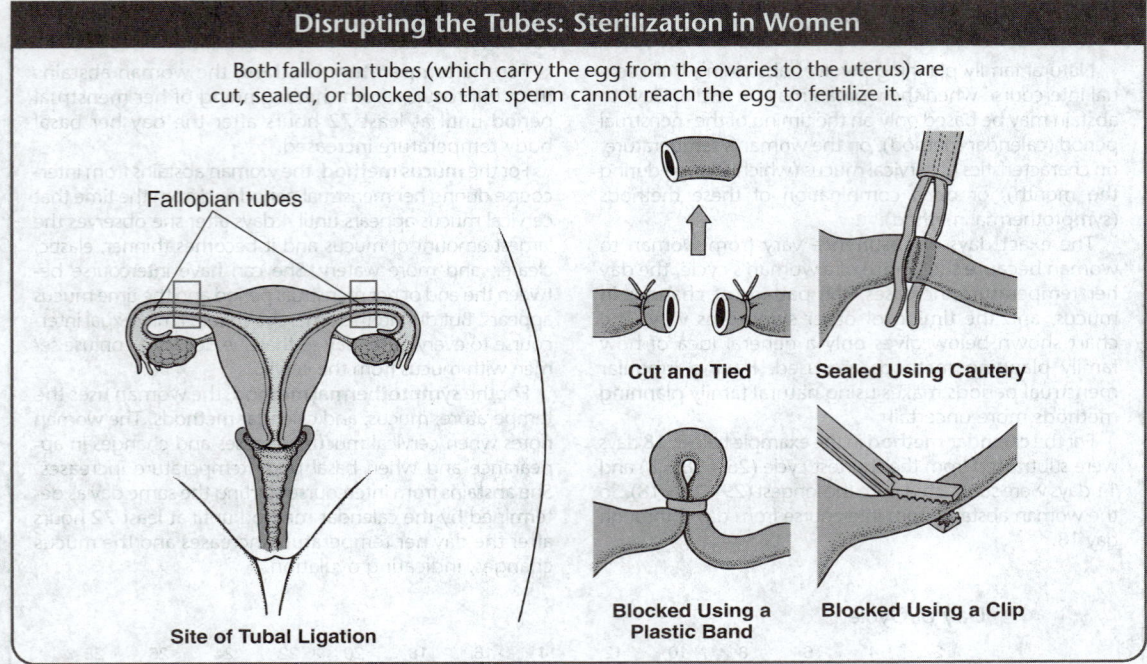

Fallopian tubes

Cut and Tied

Sealed Using Cautery

Blocked Using a Plastic Band

Blocked Using a Clip

Site of Tubal Ligation

Of the natural family planning methods, this one is the most reliable. With perfect use, the chance of pregnancy is about 2% per year.

Withdrawal Before Ejaculation

To prevent sperm from entering the vagina, a man can withdraw the penis from the vagina before ejaculation, when sperm are released during orgasm. This method, also called coitus interruptus, is not reliable because sperm may be released before orgasm. It also requires that the man have a high degree of self-control and precise timing.

Sterilization

Sterilization involves making a person incapable of reproduction.

- Disrupting the tubes that carry sperm or the egg ends the ability to reproduce.
- Vasectomy is a short procedure for men, done in the doctor's office.
- Tubal ligation, the procedure for women, is more complicated, requiring an abdominal incision and an anesthetic.

In the United States, about one third of all married couples who use family planning methods choose sterilization (vasectomy or tubal ligation). Sterilization should always be considered permanent. However, if couples change their minds, an operation that re-

connects the appropriate tubes (reanastomosis) can be done to try to restore fertility, or conception may be possible with in vitro fertilization. Reanastomosis is less likely to be effective in men than in women. For couples, pregnancy rates are 45 to 60% after reanastomosis in men and 50 to 80% after reanastomosis in women.

Vasectomy: Vasectomy is used to sterilize men. It involves cutting and sealing the vasa deferentia (the tubes that carry sperm from the testes). A vasectomy, which is done by a urologist in the office, takes about 20 minutes and requires only a local anesthetic. Through a small incision on each side of the scrotum, a section of each vas deferens is removed and the open ends of the tubes are sealed off. After a vasectomy, contraception should be continued for a while. Usually, men do not become sterile until they have had about 15 to 20 ejaculations after the operation because many sperm are stored in the seminal vesicles. Sterility is confirmed when a laboratory test shows that semen from two ejaculations is free of sperm.

Complications of vasectomy include a blood clot in the scrotum (in fewer than 5% of men), an inflammatory response to sperm leakage, and spontaneous reanastomosis (in fewer than 1%). Reanastomosis, which restores fertility, usually occurs shortly after the procedure.

Sexual activity, with contraception until sterility is confirmed, may resume as soon after the procedure as men wish. Fewer than 1% of women become pregnant after their partner is sterilized.

Tubal Ligation: Tubal ligation is used to sterilize women. It involves cutting and tying or blocking the fallopian tubes, which carry the egg from the ovaries to the uterus. More complicated than vasectomy, tubal ligation usually requires an abdominal incision and a general or regional anesthetic. Women who have just delivered a child can be sterilized immediately after childbirth or on the following day, without staying in the hospital any longer than usual. Sterilization may also be planned in advance and done as elective surgery.

Tubal ligation is often done using laparoscopy. Working through a thin tube inserted through a small incision in the woman's abdomen, a doctor may cut the fallopian tubes and tie off the cut ends. Or a doctor may use electrocautery (a device that produces an electrical current to cut through tissue) to seal off about 1 inch of each tube. The woman usually goes home the same day. After laparoscopy, up to 6% of women have minor complications, such as a skin infection at the incision site or constipation. Fewer than 1% have major complications, such as bleeding or punctures of the bladder or intestine.

Various mechanical devices, such as plastic bands and spring-loaded clips, can be used to block the fallopian tubes instead of cutting or sealing them. Sterilization is easier to reverse when these devices are used because they cause less tissue damage. However, reversal is successful in only about three fourths of the women.

Instead of laparoscopy, a doctor may use hysteroscopy, which involves inserting a flexible viewing tube through the vagina and uterus and into the fallopian tubes. Coils (microinserts) can be inserted into the fallopian tubes to seal them. No incisions are necessary. A local anesthetic is used, with or without drugs to make the woman drowsy (sedatives). About 3 months later, sterility is confirmed by x-rays taken after a radiopaque dye is injected through the vagina into the uterus and fallopian tubes (hysterosalpingography).

> **? Did You Know...**
>
> Sterilization, although considered permanent, can often be reversed.
>
> Contraception should be continued for a while after a vasectomy, until the sperm stored in the body are ejaculated.

About 2% of women become pregnant during the first 10 years after they are sterilized. About one third of these pregnancies are mislocated (ectopic) pregnancies that develop in the fallopian tubes.

Very rarely, tubal ligation causes complications, such as bleeding and injury of the intestine.

Surgical removal of the uterus (hysterectomy) also results in sterility. This procedure is usually done to treat a disorder rather than as a sterilization technique.

Abortion

Induced abortion is the intentional ending of a pregnancy by surgery or drugs.

- A pregnancy may be ended by surgically removing the contents of the uterus or by taking certain drugs.
- Complications are uncommon when an abortion is done by a trained health care practitioner in a hospital or clinic.

Worldwide, the status of abortion varies from being legally banned to being available on request. About two thirds of the women in the world have access to legal abortion. In the United States, elective abortion (abortion initiated by personal choice) is legal during the 1st trimester (up to 12 weeks). After 12 weeks, whether elective abortion is legal varies from state to state. In the United States, about 25% of all pregnancies are ended by elective abortion, making it one of the most common surgical procedures done.

Methods

Abortion methods include surgery (surgical evacuation) and drugs to stimulate contractions of the uterus. The method used depends in part on how long a woman has been pregnant. Ultrasonography is usually done to estimate the length of the pregnancy. Surgical evacuation can be used for most pregnancies. Drugs can be used for some pregnancies that are very early or late (more than 15 weeks). For abortions done early in the pregnancy, only a local anesthetic may be needed. For abortions done later, a general anesthetic may be needed.

Surgical Evacuation: The contents of the uterus are removed through the vagina. Surgical evacuation is used for more than 95% of abortions. Different techniques are used depending on the length of the pregnancy.

For pregnancies of less than 12 weeks, suction curettage is almost always used. Typically, doctors use a small, flexible tube attached to a vacuum source, usually a machine suction pump or hand pump but occasionally a vacuum syringe. The tube is inserted through the opening of the cervix into the interior of the uterus, which is then gently and thoroughly emptied. Sometimes this procedure does not terminate the pregnancy, especially when the procedure is done during the first week after a menstrual period is missed.

Sometimes doctors have to widen (dilate) the cervix to pass the suction tube through the cervix and into the uterus. For example, for pregnancies of

7 to 12 weeks, the cervix is usually dilated because a larger tube is used. For pregnancies of 4 to 6 weeks, a smaller tube is used, so little or no dilation is usually needed. To reduce the possibility of injuring the cervix during dilation, doctors may use natural substances that absorb fluids, such as dried seaweed stems (laminaria), rather than mechanical devices. Laminaria are inserted into the opening of the cervix and left in place for at least 4 to 5 hours, usually overnight. As the laminaria absorb large amounts of fluid from the body, they expand and stretch the opening of the cervix. Drugs such as prostaglandins can also be used to dilate the cervix.

For pregnancies of more than 12 weeks, dilation and evacuation is usually used. After the cervix is dilated, suction and forceps are used to remove the fetus and placenta. Then the uterus may be gently scraped to make sure everything has been removed. This technique results in fewer minor complications than do the drugs used to induce abortion. However, for pregnancies of more than 18 weeks, dilation and evacuation can cause serious complications, such as damage to the uterus or intestine.

> **? Did You Know...**
>
> Abortion is one of the most common surgical procedures done in the United States.

Drugs: Drugs to induce abortions may be used for pregnancies of less than 9 weeks or more than 15 weeks. Drugs are typically used for very early abortions, before the sac containing the embryo and placenta is clearly visible on an ultrasound scan. Options include mifepristone (RU-486) and prostaglandins, such as misoprostol.

Mifepristone, given by mouth, blocks the action of the hormone progesterone, which prepares the lining of the uterus to support the fetus. Mifepristone is used only for pregnancies of less than 9 weeks.

Prostaglandins are hormonelike substances that stimulate the uterus to contract. They may be used with mifepristone for pregnancies of less than 9 weeks or used alone for pregnancies of more than 15 weeks. Prostaglandins may be swallowed, held in the mouth (next to the cheek or under the tongue) until they dissolve, injected, or placed in the vagina. A prostaglandin is given after mifepristone when both are used. The most common regimen involves taking 1 to 3 tablets of mifepristone and, 2 days later, taking a prostaglandin (misoprostol) by mouth or vaginally. This regimen causes abortion in about 95% of women.

If abortion does not occur, surgical evacuation is done. For pregnancies of more than 15 weeks, two tablets placed in the vagina every 6 hours are almost 100% effective within 48 hours.

Complications

In general, abortion has a higher risk of complications than contraception or sterilization, especially for young women. However, complications from abortion are uncommon when it is done by a trained health care practitioner in a hospital or clinic. Serious complications occur in fewer than 1% of women.

The risk of complications is related to the length of the pregnancy: The longer a woman has been pregnant, the greater the risk. Risk is also related to the method used.

- **Surgical evacuation:** The uterus is perforated by a surgical instrument in 1 of 1,000 abortions. Less often, the intestine or another organ is injured. Severe bleeding occurs during or immediately after the procedure in 6 of 10,000 abortions. The instruments used can tear the cervix, especially in pregnancies of more than 12 weeks. Later, infections may develop. Very rarely, the procedure or a subsequent infection causes scar tissue to form in the lining of the uterus, resulting in sterility. This disorder is called Asherman's syndrome.

- **Drugs:** Mifepristone and the prostaglandin misoprostol have side effects. The most common are crampy pelvic pain, vaginal bleeding, and gastrointestinal problems such as nausea, vomiting, and diarrhea. Infection is less likely when drugs are used than when surgery is used.

- **Either method:** Bleeding and infection can occur if part of the placenta is left in the uterus. Later, particularly if the woman is inactive, blood clots may develop in the legs. If the fetus has Rh-positive blood, a woman who has Rh-negative blood may produce Rh antibodies—as in any pregnancy, miscarriage, or delivery. Such antibodies may endanger subsequent pregnancies. Giving the woman injections of $Rh_0(D)$ immune globulin prevents antibodies from developing (see page 1650).

Elective abortion probably does not increase risks for the fetus or woman during subsequent pregnancies.

Most women do not have psychologic problems after an abortion. However, problems are more likely to occur in women who had psychologic symptoms before pregnancy, who ended a desired pregnancy for health reasons, who were very ambivalent about the abortion, who are adolescents, who had a late abortion, or who obtained an abortion illegally.

CHAPTER

251 Detection of Genetic Disorders

■ Before women become pregnant, they and their partner should speak with their health care practitioner about their risk of having a baby with a genetic disorder.

■ Risk factors include older age in the woman, a family history of genetic abnormalities, a previous baby with a birth defect or miscarriage, and a chromosomal abnormality in one of the prospective parents.

■ Testing for genetic disorders is offered to all women but is particularly important if a couple's risk is higher than normal.

A big concern of prospective parents is whether their baby will be healthy. Some problems that occur in babies are due to genetic disorders. These disorders result from abnormalities in one or more genes or in chromosomes (see pages 8 and 1726). Some abnormalities are hereditary. That is, they are passed down from generation to generation. Others—said to occur spontaneously—result when genetic material in the parents' sperm or egg cells or in the cells of the developing embryo is damaged by chance or by drugs, chemicals, or other damaging substances (such as x-rays).

Couples who are thinking of having a baby should speak with their health care practitioner about the risks of genetic abnormalities (prenatal genetic counseling). They can discuss precautions that they can take to help prevent some genetic abnormalities. For example, women can take folate (folic acid) supplements and avoid exposure to toxic substances. Couples can also ask their doctor to determine whether their risk of having a baby with a hereditary genetic abnormality is higher than average. If so, tests that can help assess those risks more precisely (genetic screening) can be done. If these tests show a high risk of passing on a serious genetic abnormality, the couple can consider the following:

■ Contraception

■ Artificial insemination if the man has an abnormal gene

■ Use of an egg from another woman if the woman has an abnormal gene

■ In vitro (test tube) fertilization (see page 1592) with genetic diagnosis of the embryo before it is transferred to the woman's uterus

If the woman is already pregnant, the doctor explains what procedures can be used to test the fetus during the pregnancy (prenatal diagnostic testing). The doctor also explains what options are available if an abnormality is diagnosed. Abortion is one of these options. In some cases, the abnormality can be treated. Sometimes the couple is referred to a genetic specialist to discuss the issues.

Couples should take time to absorb the information and should ask any questions they have.

 Did You Know...

The chance of having a baby with Down syndrome at age 36 is about 1 in 300.

The chance of having a baby with Down syndrome at age 40 is about 1 in 100.

Risk Factors

All pregnancies involve some risk of genetic abnormalities. However, certain conditions increase risk.

Abnormalities Due to Several Factors: Some birth defects, such as cleft lip or palate, result from a combination of abnormalities in one or more genes and certain environmental exposures. The abnormal gene makes the fetus more likely to develop a birth defect, but the birth defect usually does not develop unless the fetus is exposed to specific substances, such as some drugs or alcohol. Many common birth defects, such as heart malformations, have this pattern of inheritance, which is called multifactorial.

Neural Tube Defects: Neural tube defects are birth defects of the brain or spinal cord (see page 1724). Examples are spina bifida (in which the spine does not completely close, sometimes exposing the spinal cord) and anencephaly (in which a large part of the brain and skull is missing). In the United States, neural tube defects occur in about 1 in 1,000 births. Most of these defects are caused by abnormalities in several genes (multifactorial). A few result from hereditary abnormalities in a single gene, from chromosomal abnormalities, or from exposure to drugs. The following also affect risk:

■ **Family history:** The risk of having a baby with a neural tube defect is increased by having a family member, including the couple's children, with such a defect (family history). For couples who have had a baby with spina bifida or anencephaly, the risk of having another baby with one of these defects is 2 to 3%. For couples who have had two children with one of these defects, the risk is 5 to 10%. However, about 95% of neural tube defects occur in families without a history of neural tube defects.

RISK OF HAVING A BABY WITH A CHROMOSOMAL ABNORMALITY

AGE OF WOMAN	RISK OF DOWN SYNDROME	RISK OF ANY CHROMO-SOMAL ABNORMALITY
20	1 in 1,667	1 in 526
22	1 in 1,429	1 in 500
24	1 in 1,250	1 in 476
26	1 in 1,176	1 in 476
28	1 in 1,053	1 in 435
30	1 in 952	1 in 384
32	1 in 769	1 in 323
34	1 in 500	1 in 238
36	1 in 294	1 in 156
38	1 in 175	1 in 102
40	1 in 106	1 in 66
42	1 in 64	1 in 42
44	1 in 38	1 in 26
46	1 in 23	1 in 16
48	1 in 14	1 in 10

Data based on information in Hook EB: Rates of chromosome abnormalities at different maternal ages. *Obstetrics and Gynecology* 58:282–285, 1981; and Hook EB, Cross PK, Schreinemachers DM: Chromosomal abnormality rates at amniocentesis and in live-born infants. *Journal of the American Medical Association* 249(15):2034–2038, 1983.

- **Folate deficiency:** Risk may also be increased by a diet that is low in folate. Folate supplements help prevent neural tube defects. Therefore, daily folate supplements are now routinely recommended for all women of childbearing age, particularly for pregnant women. Folate is usually included in prenatal vitamins.
- **Geographic location:** Risk also varies based on where a person lives. For example, risk is higher in the United Kingdom than in the United States.

Counseling about prenatal diagnosis by amniocentesis and ultrasonography is recommended for couples who have at least a 1% risk of having a baby with a neural tube defect.

Chromosomal Abnormalities: These abnormalities occur in about 1 of 200 live births and account for at least half of all miscarriages that occur during the 1st trimester. Most fetuses that have chromosomal abnormalities die before birth. Among live-born babies, Down syndrome is the most common chromosomal abnormality.

Several factors increase the risk of having a baby with a chromosomal abnormality:

- **Woman's age:** The risk of having a baby with Down syndrome increases with a woman's age—steeply after age 35.
- **Family history:** Having a family history (including the couple's children) of a chromosomal abnormality increases the risk. If a couple has had one baby with the most common form of Down syndrome (trisomy 21) and the woman is younger than 30, the risk of having another baby with a chromosomal abnormality is increased to about 1%.
- **Birth defect in a previous baby:** Having had a live-born baby with a birth defect or a stillborn baby—even when no one knows whether the baby had a chromosomal abnormality—increases the risk of having a baby with a chromosomal abnormality. About 30% of babies born with a birth defect and 5% of visibly normal stillborn babies have a chromosomal abnormality.
- **Previous miscarriages:** Having had several miscarriages may increase the risk of having a baby with a chromosomal abnormality. If the fetus in a first miscarriage has a chromosomal abnormality, a fetus in subsequent miscarriages is also likely to

have one, although not necessarily the same one. If a woman has had several miscarriages, the couple's chromosomes should be analyzed before they try to have another baby. If abnormalities are identified, the couple may choose to have prenatal diagnostic testing early in the next pregnancy.

- **Chromosomal abnormality in a prospective parent:** Rarely, a prospective parent has a structural chromosomal abnormality that increases the risk of having a baby with a structural chromosomal abnormality. A chromosomal abnormality in one or both parents increases the risk, even if the affected parent is healthy and has no physical sign of the abnormality. Doctors suspect such an abnormality when couples have had several miscarriages, problems with infertility, or a baby with a birth defect. For such couples, the risk of having a baby with a serious chromosomal abnormality is increased, as is the risk of miscarrying.

Single-Gene Disorders: In these disorders, only one pair of genes is involved. A gene may have a mutation, which interferes with its normal function, and can lead to disease or birth defects. The risk of such disorders depends on whether the disorder develops when only one gene in the pair has a mutation (such genes are dominant) or when both genes must have mutations (such genes are recessive—see page 12).

Risk also depends on whether the gene is located on the X chromosome. There are 23 pairs of chromosomes. One pair, the X and Y chromosomes (sex chromosomes), determines sex. All the rest of the chromosomes are called autosomal chromosomes. Women have two X chromosomes, and men have one X chromosome and one Y chromosome. If the abnormal gene is located on the X chromosome, the disorder it causes is called X-linked.

If the prospective mother and father are related, they are more likely to have the same mutation in one or more of the genes that cause autosomal recessive disorders. Thus, the risk of such disorders is increased.

Genetic Screening

- Screening involves assessing the couple's family history and, if needed, analysis of blood or tissue samples.

Genetic screening is used to determine whether a couple is at increased risk of having a baby with a hereditary genetic disorder. Any couple can request genetic screening, but screening is particularly recommended when one or both partners know they have a genetic abnormality, when family members have a genetic abnormality, or when partners belong to a high-risk ethnic group. Genetic screening involves assessing the couple's family history and sometimes undergoing blood tests or genetic tests.

Family History Assessment

To determine whether a couple has an increased risk of having a baby with a genetic disorder, doctors ask the couple about the following:

- Disorders that family members have had
- The cause of death in family members
- The health of all living first-degree relatives (parents, siblings, and children) and second-degree relatives (aunts, uncles, and grandparents)

WHEN ONE PARENT HAS AN ABNORMAL GENE

INHERITANCE PATTERN	CHANCE OF INHERITING THE DISORDER	CHANCE OF BEING A CARRIER[*]
Autosomal dominant	50% for sons and daughters	0%
Autosomal recessive	25% for sons and daughters	50%[†]
X-linked dominant	50% when the mother has the gene, usually only in daughters because the abnormal gene is often lethal in sons	0%
X-linked recessive	50% for sons when the mother has the gene	50% for daughters when the mother has the gene 100% for daughters when the father has the gene

[*]Carriers have only one abnormal gene and usually have no symptoms of the disorder that the gene causes.
[†]The 50% chance of being a carrier includes all children. Among unaffected children, the chance of being a carrier is, on average, 2 out of 3.

WHO SHOULD CONSIDER GENETIC SCREENING?

GROUP	DISORDER	SCREENING TESTS
All	Cystic fibrosis	DNA analysis of a sample of blood or of cells from the inside of the cheek
Ashkenazi Jews[*]	Canavan disease	DNA analysis of a sample of blood or of cells from the inside of the cheek
	Familial dysautonomia (hereditary dysfunction of the autonomic nervous system)	DNA analysis of a sample of blood or of cells from the inside of the cheek
	Tay-Sachs disease	Blood tests to measure the enzyme that is deficient in this disorder (hexosaminidase A)
		Possibly DNA analysis
Blacks	Sickle cell anemia	Blood tests to check for abnormal hemoglobin
Cajuns	Tay-Sachs disease	Blood tests to measure the enzyme that is deficient in this disorder (hexosaminidase A)
		Possibly DNA analysis
Mediterranean people	Beta-thalassemia	Blood tests to measure the average size of red blood cells (mean corpuscular volume)
Southeast Asians, Cambodians, Chinese, Filipinos, Laotians, and Vietnamese	Alpha-thalassemia	Blood tests to measure the average size of red blood cells
		If average size is small, blood tests to check for abnormal hemoglobin

[*]Most (90%) Jews are Ashkenazi. Thus, Jews who do not know whether they are Ashkenazi should be screened. Some experts also recommend screening for other disorders, such as Gaucher's disease, Niemann-Pick disease type A, and Fanconi anemia (syndrome) group C.

- Miscarriages, stillborn babies, or babies who have died soon after birth
- Babies with birth defects
- Intermarriages among relatives (which increases the risk of having the same abnormal gene)
- Ethnic background (certain groups are at higher risk of certain disorders)

Information about three generations is usually needed. If the family history is complicated, information about more distant relatives may be needed. Sometimes doctors review the medical records of relatives who may have had a genetic disorder.

Carrier Screening

Carriers are people who have an abnormal gene for a disorder but who do not have any symptoms or visible evidence of the disorder.

People can be carriers if the abnormal gene is recessive—that is, if two copies of the gene are needed to develop the disorder (see page 12).

Only women can carry an X-linked (sex-linked) recessive gene. Women have two X chromosomes. Thus, on the other X chromosome, the corresponding gene may be normal and protect women from developing the disorder. (Because men have only one X chromosome, all men who have an abnormal X-linked recessive gene have the resulting disorder, which is often fatal early in life.)

Carrier screening involves testing people who do not have symptoms but are at higher risk of carrying a recessive gene for a particular disorder. Risk is higher when one or both partners have a family history of certain disorders or have characteristics (such as ethnic background or racial or geographic group) that increase the risk of having certain disorders. However, screening is done only if the following criteria are also met:

- The disorder is very debilitating or lethal.
- A reliable screening test is available.
- The fetus can be treated, or reproductive options (such as abortion or elective sterilization) are available and acceptable to the parents.

In the United States, examples of disorders that meet these criteria include sickle cell anemia, the thalassemias, Tay-Sachs disease, and cystic fibrosis.

Carrier screening usually consists of analyzing the DNA from a blood sample. But sometimes a sample of cells from the inside of the cheek is analyzed. People provide the sample by swishing a special fluid in their mouth, then spitting it into a specimen container, or by rubbing a cotton swab inside their cheek.

If carrier screening indicates that both partners have a recessive gene for the same disorder, they may decide to have prenatal diagnostic testing. That is, the fetus may be tested for the disorder before birth. If the fetus has the disorder, treatment of the fetus may be possible, or termination of the pregnancy may be considered.

Prenatal Diagnostic Testing

- Measurement of certain substances in the pregnant woman's blood plus ultrasonography can help estimate the risk of genetic abnormalities in the fetus.

- These blood tests and ultrasonography may be done as part of routine care during pregnancy.
- If results of these tests suggest an increased risk, tests to analyze the genetic material of the fetus may be done.
- These genetic tests are invasive and have certain risks for the fetus.

Prenatal diagnostic testing involves testing the fetus before birth (prenatally) to determine whether the fetus has certain abnormalities, including certain hereditary or spontaneous genetic disorders. Some of these tests, such as ultrasonography and certain blood tests, are often part of routine prenatal care. Ultrasonography and blood tests are safe and sometimes help determine whether more invasive prenatal genetic tests (chorionic villus sampling, amniocentesis, and percutaneous umbilical blood sampling) are needed. Usually, these more invasive tests are done when couples have an increased risk of having a baby with a genetic abnormality (such as a neural tube defect) or a chromosomal abnormality (particularly when the woman is 35 or older). These tests have risks, although very small, particularly for the fetus.

Couples should discuss the risks with their health care practitioner and weigh the risks against their need to know. For example, they should think about whether not knowing the results of testing would cause anxiety and whether knowing that an abnormality was not found would be reassuring. They should think about whether they would pursue an abortion if an abnormality was found. If they would not, they

SOME GENETIC DISORDERS THAT CAN BE DETECTED BEFORE BIRTH		
DISORDER	**INCIDENCE**	**INHERITANCE PATTERN**
Cystic fibrosis	1 of 3,300 white people	Autosomal recessive
Congenital adrenal hyperplasia	1 of 10,000	Autosomal recessive
Duchenne's muscular dystrophy	1 of 3,500 male births	X-linked recessive
Hemophilia A	1 of 8,500 male births	X-linked recessive
Alpha- and beta-thalassemia	Varies widely by ethnic and racial group	Autosomal recessive
Fragile X syndrome	1 of 2,000 male births 1 of 4,000 female births	X-linked dominant
Polycystic kidney disease (adult type)	1 of 3,000	Autosomal dominant
Sickle cell anemia	1 of 400 blacks in the United States	Autosomal recessive
Tay-Sachs disease	1 of 3,600 Ashkenazi Jews and French Canadians 1 of 400,000 in other groups	Autosomal recessive

should consider whether they still want to know of an abnormality before birth (for example, to prepare psychologically) or whether knowing would only cause distress. For some couples, the risks outweigh the benefits of knowing whether their baby has a chromosomal abnormality, so they choose not to be tested.

If in vitro fertilization is done, genetic disorders can sometimes be diagnosed before the fertilized egg is transferred from the culture dish to the uterus. These tests are available only in specialized centers and are used primarily for couples with a high risk of certain genetic disorders (such as cystic fibrosis) or chromosomal abnormalities.

SCREENING OF THE PREGNANT WOMAN

Measuring levels of certain substances (called markers) in blood can help identify women with an increased risk of problems, such as having a baby with a brain or spinal cord defect (neural tube defect), Down syndrome, other chromosomal abnormalities, and some rarer genetic disorders. Knowing the woman's individual risk as precisely as possible can help the couple better assess the benefits of having invasive prenatal genetic testing. Doctors usually offer to measure these markers as part of routine prenatal care, although women can choose not to have these tests. For example, if couples can decide whether to have prenatal genetic testing without knowing the precise risk of a genetic or chromosomal abnormality, most parts of screening are unnecessary.

Markers are usually measured at 16 to 18 weeks of pregnancy (during the 2nd trimester), when these measurements are fairly accurate. Other markers can be measured during the 1st trimester.

First-Trimester Screening

Sometimes blood tests to estimate the risk of Down syndrome are done at about 11 to 14 weeks of pregnancy. These tests involve measuring levels of pregnancy-associated placental protein A (produced by the placenta) and beta-human chorionic gonadotropin in a pregnant woman's blood.

Also, ultrasonography is done to measure a fluid-filled space near the back of the fetus's neck (called fetal nuchal translucency). Abnormal ultrasound measurements indicate an increased risk of Down syndrome or another chromosomal abnormality in the fetus.

First-trimester blood tests plus ultrasonography provide results early. If results are abnormal and the couple wishes, chorionic villus sampling can then be done early to determine whether Down syndrome is present. Amniocentesis can also detect Down syndrome, but it is usually done later in pregnancy.

One advantage of 1st-trimester screening is that with earlier results, abortion, if desired, can be done earlier, when it is safer.

Second-Trimester Screening

During the 2nd trimester, markers in the pregnant woman's blood are measured and sometimes ultrasonography is done to identify women at increased risk of certain problems.

Important markers include the following:

- **Alpha-fetoprotein:** A protein produced by the fetus
- **Estriol:** A hormone formed from substances produced by the fetus
- **Human chorionic gonadotropin:** A hormone produced by the placenta
- **Inhibin A:** A hormone produced by the placenta

Alpha-fetoprotein levels: Alpha-fetoprotein is usually measured in all women, even those who have had 1st-trimester screening or chorionic villus sampling. A high level may indicate an increased risk of having any of the following:

- A baby with a neural tube defect of the brain (anencephaly) or spinal cord (spina bifida)
- A baby with a birth defect of the abdominal wall
- More than one fetus
- Pregnancy complications, such as miscarriage, slowed growth or death of the fetus, and premature detachment of the placenta (placental abruption)

If blood tests detect an abnormal alpha-fetoprotein level in a pregnant woman, ultrasonography is done. It can help by doing the following:

- Confirming the length of the pregnancy
- Determining whether more than one fetus is present
- Determining whether the fetus has died
- Detecting many birth defects

High-resolution or targeted ultrasonography, which can be done at some specialized centers, provides more detail and may be more accurate than standard ultrasonography, particularly for small birth defects.

If ultrasonography results are normal, a fetal problem is less likely, but certain conditions, such as neural tube defects, are still possible. Thus, whether ultrasonography results are normal or not, amniocentesis to measure the alpha-fetoprotein level in the fluid that surrounds the fetus (amniotic fluid) is recommended by many doctors. Also, the fetus's chromosomes may be analyzed and the amniotic fluid may be tested to determine whether it contains an enzyme called acetylcholinesterase. Levels of alpha-fetoprotein and acetylcholinesterase help doctors better assess risk:

- A high alpha-fetoprotein level plus acetylcholinesterase in the amniotic fluid indicates an increased risk of a neural tube defect, such as anencephaly or spina bifida.

■ A high alpha-fetoprotein level with or without acetylcholinesterase may indicate an increased risk of a neural tube defect and of abnormalities in other organs, such as the esophagus and the abdominal wall.

Sometimes the amniotic fluid sample is contaminated with blood from the fetus, resulting in an abnormal alpha-fetoprotein level. In such cases, the fetus may not have any abnormalities.

Triple and Quad Screening: Measuring other markers (estriol and beta-human chorionic gonadotropin) can help estimate the risk of Down syndrome and other chromosomal abnormalities. This testing may not be necessary for women who have had 1st-trimester screening. Measuring estriol and beta-human chorionic gonadotropin plus alpha-fetoprotein is called triple screening. Inhibin A may also be measured. Measuring these four markers is called quad screening.

Triple or quad screening is done around 15 to 20 weeks of pregnancy. It can help estimate the risk of Down syndrome in the fetus. If risk is high, amniocentesis is considered. Quad screening results are abnormal (positive) in almost 80% of Down syndrome cases. Triple screening detects almost as many cases.

At some medical centers, targeted ultrasonography (a genetic sonogram) is done during the 2nd trimester to help estimate the risk of a chromosomal abnormality. Targeted ultrasonography aims to identify certain structural birth defects that indicate an increased risk of a chromosomal abnormality. This test can also detect certain variations in organs that do not affect function but may indicate an increased risk of a chromosomal abnormality. However, normal results do not necessarily mean that the risk of a chromosomal abnormality is reduced.

Combined 1st- and 2nd-Trimester Screening: For the most accurate results, both groups of tests—1st-trimester tests and 2nd-trimester tests—are done, and results from both are analyzed together. However, if couples want information sooner, they can request a type of screening that provides results during the 1st trimester. Then screening is done in the 2nd trimester only if results of 1st-trimester screening did not require chorionic villus sampling or amniocentesis. Couples should remember that screening tests are not always accurate. They may miss abnormalities, or they may indicate abnormalities when none are present.

PROCEDURES

Several procedures can be used to detect genetic and chromosomal abnormalities. All, except ultrasonography, are invasive (that is, they require insertion of an instrument into the body) and have a slight risk for the fetus.

Ultrasonography

Ultrasonography is commonly done during pregnancy (see page 1625). It has no known risks for the woman or fetus. Ultrasonography can do the following:

■ Confirm the length of the pregnancy
■ Locate the placenta
■ Indicate whether the fetus is alive
■ After the third month, detect certain obvious structural birth defects, including those of the brain, spinal cord, heart, kidneys, stomach, abdominal wall, and bones
■ In the 2nd trimester, detect findings that tend to indicate a higher-than-normal chance of a chromosomal abnormality in the fetus (targeted ultrasonography)

Ultrasonography is often used to check for abnormalities in the fetus when a pregnant woman has abnormal results on a prenatal blood test or a family history of birth defects. However, normal results do not guarantee a normal baby because no test is completely accurate. Results of ultrasonography may suggest chromosomal abnormalities in the fetus, but ultrasonography cannot identify the specific problem. In such cases, amniocentesis may be recommended.

Ultrasonography is done before chorionic villus sampling and amniocentesis to confirm the length of the pregnancy so that these procedures can be done at the appropriate time during the pregnancy. During these procedures, ultrasonography is used to monitor the fetus and to guide placement of instruments.

At some specialized medical centers, targeted ultrasonography can be done. For this test, experts carefully assess the fetus to check for structural defects that may indicate an increased risk of a chromosomal abnormality. This test can provide greater detail than conventional ultrasonography. Thus, this test may detect smaller abnormalities, and abnormalities can be seen earlier, more accurately, or both.

Chorionic Villus Sampling

In chorionic villus sampling, a doctor removes a small sample of the chorionic villi, which are tiny projections that make up part of the placenta (see art on page 1618). This procedure is used to diagnose some disorders in the fetus, usually between 10 and 12 weeks of pregnancy. Chorionic villus sampling may be used instead of amniocentesis unless a sample of amniotic fluid is needed, as when the alpha-fetoprotein level in amniotic fluid must be measured.

The main advantage of chorionic villus sampling is that its results are available much earlier in the pregnancy than those of amniocentesis. Thus, if no abnormality is detected, the couple's anxiety can be relieved earlier. If an abnormality is detected earlier and if the couple decides to terminate the pregnancy, simpler, safer methods can be used. Also, early detection of an abnormality may enable doctors to treat the fetus appropriately before birth. For example, a pregnant woman may be given a corticosteroid to prevent male characteristics from developing in a female fetus that has congenital adrenal hyperplasia. In this hereditary disorder, the adrenal glands are enlarged and produce excessive amounts of male hormones (androgens).

Before the chorionic villus sampling, ultrasonography is done to determine whether the fetus is alive, to confirm the length of the pregnancy, to check for obvious abnormalities, and to locate the placenta.

A sample of the chorionic villi can be removed through the cervix (transcervically) or the abdominal wall (transabdominally). With both methods, ultrasonography is used for guidance and the tissue sample is suctioned through a needle or catheter with a syringe and then sent for laboratory analysis. Many women have light spotting for a day or two afterward.

- Through the cervix: The woman lies on her back with her hips and knees bent, usually supported by heel or knee stirrups, as for a pelvic examination. The doctor inserts a thin, flexible tube (catheter) through the vagina and cervix into the placenta. For most women, the procedure feels very similar to a Papanicolaou (Pap) test, but a few women find it more uncomfortable. This method cannot be used in women who have an active genital infection (such as genital herpes or gonorrhea), chronic inflammation of the cervix, or a placenta that covers the passage between the cervix and uterus.

- Through the abdominal wall: The doctor anesthetizes an area of skin over the abdomen and inserts a needle through the abdominal wall into the placenta. Most women do not find this procedure painful. But for some women, the area over the abdomen feels slightly sore for an hour or two afterward.

After chorionic villus sampling, most women who have Rh-negative blood and who do not have antibodies to Rh factor are given an injection of $Rh_0(D)$ immune globulin to prevent them from producing antibodies to Rh factor (see page 1650). A woman with Rh-negative blood may produce these antibodies if the fetus has Rh-positive blood and it comes into contact with her blood, as it may during chorionic villus sampling. These antibodies can cause problems in the fetus. The injection is not needed if the father also has Rh-negative blood because in such cases, the fetus always has Rh-negative blood.

The risks of chorionic villus sampling are comparable to those of amniocentesis. The most common

risk is that of miscarriage. In specialized centers, the risk of miscarriage is about 1 in 500 procedures. Rarely, the genetic diagnosis is unclear after chorionic villus sampling, and amniocentesis may be necessary. In general, the accuracy of the two procedures is comparable.

? Did You Know...

All pregnancies have a 2 to 3 % risk of miscarriage, and amniocentesis or chorionic villus sampling increases the risk by about 0.2%.

Amniocentesis

One of the most common procedures for detecting abnormalities before birth is amniocentesis. It is often offered to women over 35 to estimate their risk of having a baby with Down syndrome. However, it can be done for any woman who chooses, even if her risk is not higher than normal.

In this procedure, a sample of the fluid that surrounds the fetus (amniotic fluid) is removed and analyzed. Amniocentesis is usually done at 15 weeks of pregnancy or later. The fluid contains cells that have been shed by the fetus. These cells are grown in a laboratory so that the chromosomes in them can be analyzed. Amniocentesis enables doctors to measure the alpha-fetoprotein level in the amniotic fluid. This measurement more reliably indicates whether the fetus has a brain or spinal cord defect than does measurement of this level in the woman's blood.

Before the procedure, ultrasonography is done to evaluate the heart of the fetus, to confirm the length of the pregnancy, to locate the placenta and amniotic fluid, and to determine how many fetuses are present.

A doctor inserts a needle through the abdominal wall into the amniotic fluid. Sometimes a local anesthetic is first used to numb the site. During the procedure, ultrasonography is done so that the fetus can be monitored and the needle can be guided into place. Fluid is withdrawn, and the needle is removed. Results are usually available in about 1 to 2 weeks.

Occasionally, the amniotic fluid contains blood from the fetus. Such blood may increase the alpha-fetoprotein level, making the results hard to interpret.

Women who have Rh-negative blood are given $Rh_0(D)$ immune globulin after the procedure to prevent them from producing antibodies to Rh factor, which can cause problems in a fetus with Rh-positive blood (see page 1650).

Amniocentesis rarely causes any problems for the woman or the fetus. The following may occur:

- Soreness: Some women feel slightly sore for an hour or two afterward.

Detecting Abnormalities Before Birth

Chorionic villus sampling and amniocentesis are used to detect abnormalities in a fetus. During both procedures, ultrasonography is used for guidance.

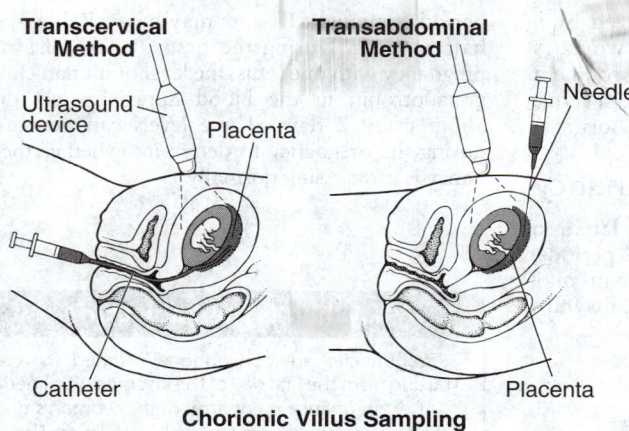

Transcervical Method

Ultrasound device

Placenta

Catheter

Transabdominal Method

Needle

Placenta

Chorionic Villus Sampling

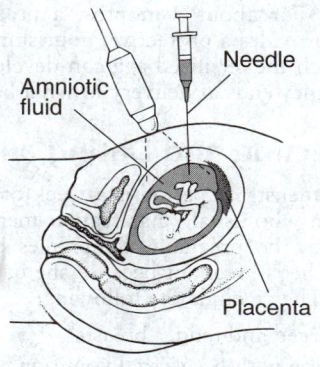

Needle

Amniotic fluid

Placenta

Amniocentesis

In chorionic villus sampling, a sample of chorionic villi (part of the placenta) is removed by one of two methods. In the transcervical method, a doctor inserts a thin, flexible tube (catheter) through the vagina and cervix into the placenta. In the transabdominal method, a doctor inserts a needle through the abdominal wall into the placenta. In both methods, a sample of the placenta is suctioned out with a syringe and analyzed.

In amniocentesis, a doctor inserts a needle through the abdominal wall into the amniotic fluid. A sample of fluid is withdrawn for analysis.

- Spotting of blood or leakage of amniotic fluid from the vagina: About 1 to 2% of the women have these problems, but the problems do not last long and usually stop without treatment.
- Miscarriage: The chance of miscarriage due to amniocentesis is about 1 in 500 to 1,000.
- Needle injuries to the fetus: These injuries are very rare.

Amniocentesis can usually be done when a woman is pregnant with twins or even more fetuses.

Percutaneous Umbilical Blood Sampling

Percutaneous umbilical blood sampling is used when rapid chromosome analysis is needed, particularly toward the end of pregnancy when ultrasonography has detected abnormalities in the fetus. Often, results can be available within 48 hours. It is occasionally done for other reasons—for example, when doctors suspect that a fetus has anemia. If the fetus has severe anemia, blood can be transfused to the fetus during percutaneous umbilical blood sampling.

The doctor first anesthetizes an area of skin over the abdomen. Guided by ultrasonography, the doctor then inserts a needle through the abdominal wall into the umbilical cord. A sample of the fetus's blood is withdrawn and analyzed, and the needle is removed.

Percutaneous umbilical blood sampling is an invasive procedure and has risks for the woman and fetus. Loss of the pregnancy as a result of this test occurs in about 1 in 100 procedures.

252   Normal Pregnancy

Pregnancy begins when an egg is fertilized by a sperm. For about 9 months, a pregnant woman's body provides a protective, nourishing environment in which the fertilized egg can develop into a fetus. Pregnancy ends at delivery, when a baby is born.

Detecting and Dating a Pregnancy

If a menstrual period is a week or more late in a woman who usually has regular menstrual periods, she may be pregnant. Sometimes a woman may guess she is pregnant because she has typical symptoms. They include the following:

- Enlarged and tender breasts
- Nausea with occasional vomiting
- A need to urinate frequently
- Unusual fatigue
- Changes in appetite

When a menstrual period is late, a woman may use a home pregnancy test to determine whether she is pregnant. Home pregnancy tests detect human chorionic gonadotropin (hCG) in urine. Human chorionic gonadotropin is a hormone produced by the placenta. Results of home pregnancy tests are accurate about 97% of the time. If results are negative but the woman still suspects she is pregnant, she should repeat the home pregnancy test a few days later. The first test may have been done too early (before the next menstrual period is expected to start). If results are positive, the woman should contact her doctor, who may do another pregnancy test to confirm the results.

Did You Know...

Results of home pregnancy tests are accurate about 97% of the time.

Doctors test a sample of blood or urine from the woman to determine whether she is pregnant. These tests are more than 99% accurate. One of these tests, called an enzyme-linked immunosorbent assay (ELISA), can quickly and easily detect even a low level of human chorionic gonadotropin in urine. Some tests can detect the very low level that is present several days after fertilization (before a menstrual period is missed). Results may be available in about half an hour. During the first 60 days of a normal pregnancy with one fetus, the level of human chorionic gonadotropin in the blood approximately doubles about every 2 days. These levels can be measured during the pregnancy to determine whether the pregnancy is progressing normally.

When Is the Baby Due?

Pregnancies are conventionally dated in weeks, starting from the first day of the last menstrual period.

After pregnancy is confirmed, the woman's doctor asks her when her last menstrual period was. The doctor calculates the approximate date of delivery by counting back 3 calendar months from the first day of the last menstrual period and adding 1 year and 7 days. For example, if the last menstrual period was January 1, the doctor counts back 3 months to October 1, then adds 1 year and 7 days. The calculated due date is October 8 the next year. Only 10% or fewer of pregnant women give birth on the calculated date, but 50% give birth within 1 week and almost 90% give birth within 2 weeks (before or after the date). Delivery between 3 weeks before and 2 weeks after the calculated date is considered normal.

Ovulation usually occurs about 2 weeks after a woman's menstrual period starts, and fertilization usually occurs shortly after ovulation. Consequently, the embryo is about 2 weeks younger than the number of weeks traditionally assigned to the pregnancy. In other words, a woman who is 4 weeks pregnant is carrying a 2-week-old embryo. If a woman's periods are irregular, the actual difference may be more or less than 2 weeks.

Pregnancy lasts an average of 266 days (38 weeks) from the date of fertilization (conception) or 280 days (40 weeks) from the first day of the last menstrual period if the woman has regular 28-day periods. Pregnancy is divided into three 3-month periods, based on the date of the last menstrual period:

- 1st trimester: 0 to 12 weeks of pregnancy
- 2nd trimester: 13 to 24 weeks
- 3rd trimester: 25 weeks to delivery

The most accurate way to determine when a baby is due is ultrasonography, particularly if it is done during the first 12 weeks.

From Egg to Embryo

Once a month, an egg is released from an ovary into a fallopian tube. After sexual intercourse, sperm move from the vagina through the cervix and uterus to the fallopian tubes, where one sperm fertilizes the egg. The fertilized egg (zygote) divides repeatedly as it moves down the fallopian tube to the uterus. First, the zygote becomes a solid ball of cells. Then it becomes a hollow ball of cells called a blastocyst.

Inside the uterus, the blastocyst implants in the wall of the uterus, where it develops into an embryo attached to a placenta and surrounded by fluid-filled membranes.

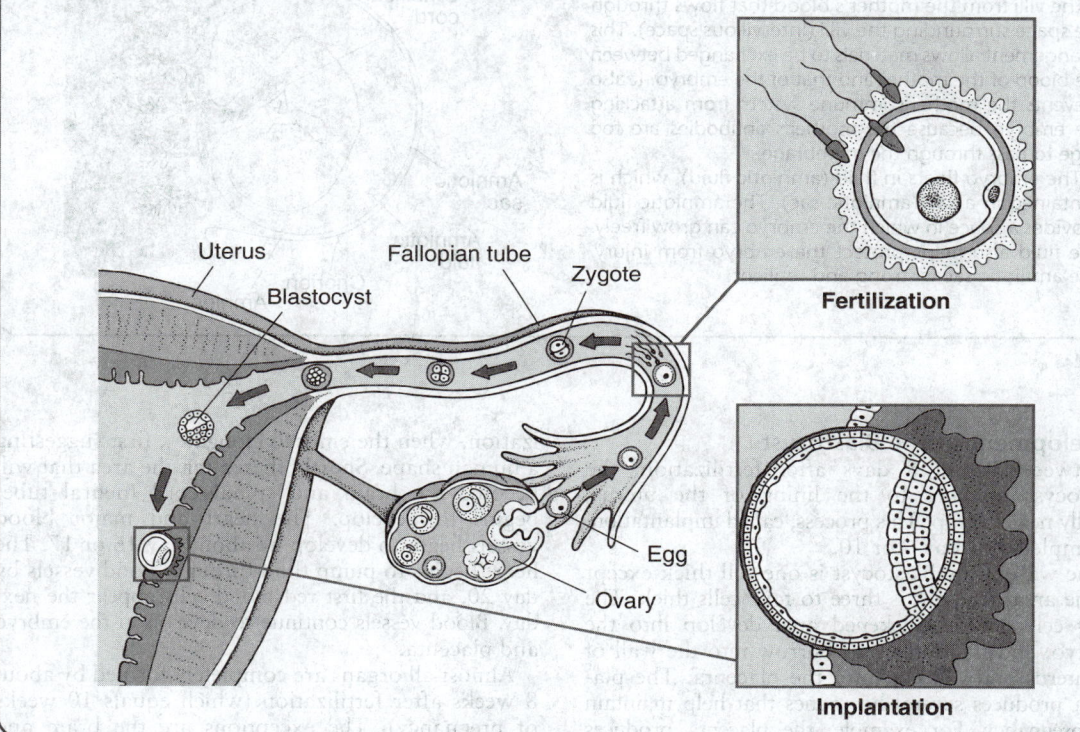

Stages of Development

A baby goes through several stages of development, beginning as a fertilized egg. The egg develops into a blastocyst, an embryo, then a fetus.

Fertilization

During each normal menstrual cycle, one egg (ovum) is usually released from one of the ovaries, about 14 days before the next menstrual period. Release of the egg is called ovulation. The egg is swept into the funnel-shaped end of one of the fallopian tubes.

At ovulation, the mucus in the cervix becomes more fluid and more elastic, allowing sperm to enter the uterus rapidly. Within 5 minutes, sperm may move from the vagina, through the cervix into the uterus, and to the funnel-shaped end of a fallopian tube—the usual site of fertilization. The cells lining the fallopian tube facilitate fertilization.

If a sperm penetrates the egg, fertilization results. Tiny hairlike cilia lining the fallopian tube propel the fertilized egg (zygote) through the tube toward the uterus. The cells of the zygote divide repeatedly as the zygote moves down the fallopian tube. The zygote enters the uterus in 3 to 5 days. In the uterus, the cells continue to divide, becoming a hollow ball of cells called a blastocyst. If fertilization does not occur, the egg degenerates and passes through the uterus with the next menstrual period.

If more than one egg is released and fertilized, the pregnancy involves more than one fetus, usually two (twins). Such twins are fraternal. Identical twins result when one fertilized egg separates into two embryos after it has begun to divide.

Placenta and Embryo at 8 Weeks

At 8 weeks of pregnancy, the placenta and fetus have been developing for 6 weeks. The placenta forms tiny hairlike projections (villi) that extend into the wall of the uterus. Blood vessels from the embryo, which pass through the umbilical cord to the placenta, develop in the villi. A thin membrane separates the embryo's blood in the villi from the mother's blood that flows through the space surrounding the villi (intervillous space). This arrangement allows materials to be exchanged between the blood of the mother and that of the embryo. It also prevents the mother's immune system from attacking the embryo because the mother's antibodies are too large to pass through the membrane.

The embryo floats in fluid (amniotic fluid), which is contained in a sac (amniotic sac). The amniotic fluid provides a space in which the embryo can grow freely. The fluid also helps protect the embryo from injury. The amniotic sac is strong and resilient.

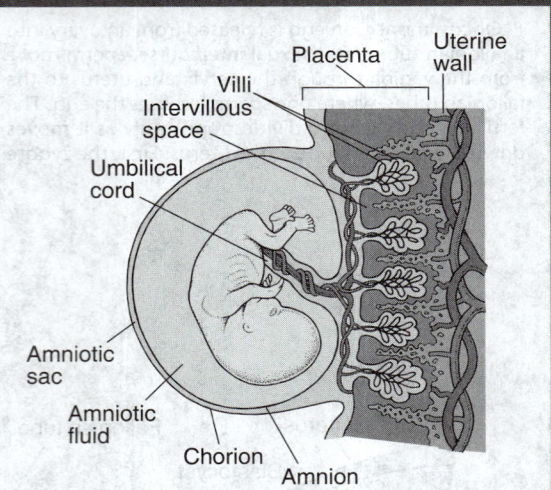

Development of the Blastocyst

Between 5 and 8 days after fertilization, the blastocyst attaches to the lining of the uterus, usually near the top. This process, called implantation, is completed by day 9 or 10.

The wall of the blastocyst is one cell thick except in one area, where it is three to four cells thick. The inner cells in the thickened area develop into the embryo, and the outer cells burrow into the wall of the uterus and develop into the placenta. The placenta produces several hormones that help maintain the pregnancy. For example, the placenta produces human chorionic gonadotropin, which prevents the ovaries from releasing eggs and stimulates the ovaries to produce estrogen and progesterone continuously. The placenta also carries oxygen and nutrients from mother to fetus and waste materials from fetus to mother.

Some of the cells from the placenta develop into an outer layer of membranes (chorion) surrounding the embryo. An inner layer of membranes (amnion) develops by about day 10 to 12, forming the amniotic sac. The amniotic sac fills with a clear liquid (amniotic fluid) and expands to envelop the developing embryo, which floats within it.

Development of the Embryo

The next stage in development is the embryo, which develops under the lining of the uterus on one side. This stage is characterized by the formation of most internal organs and external body structures. Organ formation begins about 3 weeks after fertil-

ization, when the embryo elongates, first suggesting a human shape. Shortly thereafter, the area that will become the brain and spinal cord (neural tube) begins to develop. The heart and major blood vessels begin to develop by about day 16 or 17. The heart begins to pump fluid through blood vessels by day 20, and the first red blood cells appear the next day. Blood vessels continue to develop in the embryo and placenta.

Almost all organs are completely formed by about 8 weeks after fertilization (which equals 10 weeks of pregnancy). The exceptions are the brain and spinal cord, which continue to mature throughout pregnancy. Most malformations (birth defects) occur during the period when organs are forming. During this period, the embryo is most vulnerable to the effects of drugs, radiation, and viruses. Therefore, a pregnant woman should not be given any live-virus vaccinations or take any drugs during this period unless they are considered essential to protect her health (see page 1636).

Development of the Fetus and Placenta

At the end of the 8th week after fertilization (10 weeks of pregnancy), the embryo is considered a fetus. During this stage, the structures that have already formed grow and develop. The following are markers during pregnancy:

- By 12 weeks of pregnancy: The fetus fills the entire uterus.
- By about 14 weeks: The sex can be identified.

- By about 16 to 20 weeks: Typically, the pregnant woman can feel the fetus moving. Women who have been pregnant before typically feel movements about 2 weeks earlier than women who are pregnant for the first time.
- By about 24 weeks: The fetus has a chance of survival outside the uterus.

The lungs continue to mature until near the time of delivery. The brain accumulates new cells throughout pregnancy and the first year of life after birth.

As the placenta develops, it extends tiny hairlike projections (villi) into the wall of the uterus. The projections branch and rebranch in a complicated treelike arrangement. This arrangement greatly increases the area of contact between the wall of the uterus and the placenta, so that more nutrients and waste materials can be exchanged. The placenta is fully formed by 18 to 20 weeks but continues to grow throughout pregnancy. At delivery, it weighs about 1 pound.

Physical Changes

Pregnancy causes many changes in a woman's body. Most of them disappear after delivery. These changes cause some symptoms, which are normal. However, certain disorders, such as gestational diabetes (see page 1630), develop during pregnancy, and some symptoms may indicate such a disorder.

Symptoms that should be immediately reported to a doctor if they occur during pregnancy include the following:

- Persistent or unusual headaches
- Persistent nausea and vomiting
- Dizziness
- Disturbances of eyesight
- Pain or cramps in the lower abdomen
- Contractions
- Vaginal bleeding
- Leakage of amniotic fluid (described as "the water breaks")
- Swelling of the hands or feet
- Decreased urine production
- Any illness or infection
- Tremor (shaking of the hands, feet, or both)
- Seizures
- Rapid heart rate
- Decreased movement of the fetus

General Health: Fatigue is common, especially in the first 12 weeks and again in late pregnancy. The woman may need to get more rest than usual.

Reproductive Tract: By 12 weeks of pregnancy, the enlarging uterus may cause the woman's abdomen to protrude slightly. The uterus continues to enlarge throughout pregnancy. The enlarging uterus extends to the level of the navel by 20 weeks and to the lower edge of the rib cage by 36 weeks.

The amount of normal vaginal discharge, which is clear or whitish, commonly increases. This increase is usually normal. However, if the discharge has an unusual color or smell or is accompanied by vaginal itching and burning, a woman should see her doctor. Such symptoms may indicate a vaginal infection. Some vaginal infections, such as trichomoniasis (a protozoan infection—see page 1539) and candidiasis (a yeast infection—see page 1540), are common during pregnancy and can be treated.

Breasts: The breasts tend to enlarge because hormones (mainly estrogen) are preparing the breasts for milk production. The glands that produce milk gradually increase in number and become able to produce milk. The breasts may feel firm and tender. Wearing a bra that fits properly and provides support may help.

During the last weeks of pregnancy, the breasts may produce a thin, yellowish or milky discharge (colostrum). Colostrum is also produced during the first few days after delivery, before breast milk is produced. This fluid, which is rich in minerals and antibodies, is the breastfed baby's first food.

Heart and Blood Flow: During pregnancy, the woman's heart must work harder because as the fetus grows, the heart must pump more blood to the uterus. By the end of pregnancy, the uterus is receiving one fifth of the woman's prepregnancy blood supply. During pregnancy, the amount of blood pumped by the heart (cardiac output) increases by 30 to 50%. As cardiac output increases, the heart rate at rest speeds up from a normal prepregnancy rate of about 70 beats per minute to 80 or 90 beats per minute. During exercise, cardiac output and heart rate increase more when a woman is pregnant than when she is not. During labor, cardiac output increases by an additional 10%. After delivery, cardiac output decreases rapidly at first, then more slowly. It returns to the prepregnancy level about 6 weeks after delivery.

Certain heart murmurs and irregularities in heart rhythm may appear because the heart is working harder. Sometimes a pregnant woman may feel these irregularities. Such changes are normal during pregnancy. However, other abnormal heart sounds and rhythms (for example, diastolic murmurs and tachyarrhythmias), which occur more often in pregnant women, may require treatment.

Blood pressure usually decreases during the 2nd trimester but may return to a normal prepregnancy level in the 3rd trimester.

The volume of blood increases by 50% during pregnancy. The amount of fluid in the blood increases more than the number of red blood cells (which carry oxygen). Thus, even though there are more red blood cells, blood tests indicate mild anemia, which is normal. For reasons not clearly understood, the number of white blood cells (which fight infection) increases slightly during pregnancy and markedly during labor and the first few days after delivery.

The enlarging uterus interferes with the return of blood from the legs and the pelvic area to the heart. As a result, swelling (edema) is common, especially in the legs. Varicose veins commonly develop in the legs and in the area around the vaginal opening (vulva). They sometimes cause discomfort. Clothing that is loose around the waist and legs is more comfortable and does not restrict blood flow. Some measures not only ease the discomfort but may also reduce leg swelling and make varicose veins more likely to disappear after delivery:

- Wearing elastic support hose
- Resting frequently with the legs elevated
- Lying on the left side

Urinary Tract: Like the heart, the kidneys work harder throughout pregnancy. They filter the increasing volume of blood. The volume of blood filtered by the kidneys reaches a maximum between 16 and 24 weeks and remains at the maximum until immediately before delivery. Then, pressure from the enlarging uterus may slightly decrease the blood supply to the kidneys.

Activity of the kidneys normally increases when a person lies down and decreases when a person stands. This difference is amplified during pregnancy—one reason a pregnant woman needs to urinate frequently while trying to sleep. Late in pregnancy, lying on the side, particularly the left side, increases kidney activity more than lying on the back. Lying on the left side relieves the pressure that the enlarged uterus puts on the main vein that carries blood from the legs. As a result, blood flow improves and kidney activity increases.

The uterus presses on the bladder, reducing its size so that it fills with urine more quickly than usual. This pressure also makes a pregnant woman need to urinate more often and more urgently.

Respiratory Tract: The high level of progesterone, a hormone produced continuously during pregnancy, signals the brain to lower the level of carbon dioxide in the blood. As a result, a pregnant woman breathes slightly faster and more deeply to exhale more carbon dioxide and keep the carbon dioxide level low. She may breathe deeper and faster also because the enlarging uterus limits how much the lungs can expand when she breathes in. The circumference of the woman's chest enlarges slightly.

Virtually every pregnant woman becomes somewhat more out of breath when she exerts herself, especially toward the end of pregnancy. During exercise, the breathing rate increases more when a woman is pregnant than when she is not.

Because more blood is being pumped, the lining of the airways receives more blood and swells somewhat, narrowing the airways. As a result, the nose occasionally feels stuffy, and the eustachian tubes (which connect the middle ear and back of the nose) may become blocked. These effects can slightly change the tone and quality of the woman's voice.

Digestive Tract: Nausea and vomiting, particularly in the mornings (morning sickness), are common. They may be caused by the high levels of estrogen and human chorionic gonadotropin, two hormones that help maintain the pregnancy. Nausea and vomiting may be relieved by changing the diet or patterns of eating. For example, drinking and eating small portions frequently, eating before getting hungry, and eating bland foods (such as bouillon, consommé, rice, and pasta) may help. Eating plain soda crackers and sipping a carbonated drink may relieve nausea. Keeping crackers by the bed and eating one or two before getting up may relieve morning sickness. No drugs specifically designed to treat morning sickness are currently available. If nausea and vomiting are so intense or persistent that dehydration, weight loss, or other problems develop, a woman may need to be treated with drugs that relieve nausea (antiemetic drugs) or to be hospitalized temporarily and given fluids intravenously (see page 1645).

Heartburn and belching are common, possibly because food remains in the stomach longer and because the ringlike muscle (sphincter) at the lower end of the esophagus tends to relax, allowing the stomach's contents to flow backward into the esophagus. Several measures can help relieve heartburn:

- Eating smaller meals
- Not bending or lying flat for several hours after eating
- Avoiding caffeine, tobacco, alcohol, and aspirin and related drugs (salicylates)
- Taking liquid antacids, but not antacids that contain sodium bicarbonate because they contain so much salt (sodium)

Heartburn during the night can be relieved by the following:

- Not eating for several hours before going to bed
- Raising the head of the bed or using pillows to raise the head and shoulders

The stomach produces less acid during pregnancy. Consequently, stomach ulcers rarely develop during pregnancy, and those that already exist often start to heal.

As pregnancy progresses, pressure from the enlarging uterus on the rectum and the lower part of the intestine may cause constipation. Constipation may be worsened because the high level of progesterone during pregnancy slows the automatic waves of muscular contractions in the intestine, which normally move food along. Eating a high-fiber diet, drinking plenty of fluids, and exercising regularly can help prevent constipation.

Hemorrhoids, a common problem, may result from pressure of the enlarging uterus or from constipation. Stool softeners, an anesthetic gel, or warm soaks can be used if hemorrhoids hurt.

Pica, a craving for strange foods or nonfoods (such as starch or clay), may develop.

Occasionally, pregnant women, usually those who also have morning sickness, have excess saliva. This symptom may be distressing but is harmless.

Skin: Mask of pregnancy (melasma) is a blotchy, brownish pigment that may appear on the skin of the forehead and cheeks. The skin surrounding the nipples (areolae) may also darken. A dark line commonly appears down the middle of the abdomen. These changes may occur because the placenta produces a hormone that stimulates melanocytes, the cells that make a dark brown skin pigment (melanin).

Pink stretch marks sometimes appear on the abdomen. This change probably results from rapid growth of the uterus and an increase in levels of adrenal hormones.

Small blood vessels may form a red spiderlike pattern on the skin, usually above the waist. These formations are called spider angiomas. Thin-walled, dilated capillaries may become visible, especially in the lower legs.

Hormones: Pregnancy affects virtually all hormones in the body, mostly because of the effects of hormones produced by the placenta. For example, the placenta produces a hormone that stimulates the woman's thyroid gland to become more active and produce larger amounts of thyroid hormones. When the thyroid gland becomes more active, the heart may beat faster, causing the woman to become aware of her heartbeat (have palpitations). Perspiration may increase, mood swings may occur, and the thyroid gland may enlarge. However, the disorder hyperthyroidism, in which the thyroid gland malfunctions and is overactive, develops in fewer than 0.1% of pregnancies.

Levels of estrogen and progesterone increase early during pregnancy because human chorionic gonadotropin, the main hormone the placenta produces, stimulates the ovaries to continuously produce them. After 9 to 10 weeks of pregnancy, the placenta itself produces large amounts of estrogen and progesterone. Estrogen and progesterone help maintain the pregnancy.

Skin Rashes During Pregnancy

Two intensely itchy rashes occur only during pregnancy.

Pruritic urticarial papules and plaques of pregnancy (urticaria of pregnancy): This rash is common. The cause is unknown.

Red, irregularly shaped, flat or slightly raised patches appear on the abdomen. The patches sometimes have tiny fluid-filled blisters in the center. Often, the skin around them is pale. The rash spreads to the thighs, buttocks, and occasionally the arms. Hundreds of itchy patches may develop. Itching is bothersome enough to keep the woman awake at night.

Typically, the rash appears during the last 2 to 3 weeks of pregnancy and occasionally during the last few days. However, it may occur at any time after the 24th week. Usually, the rash clears up promptly after delivery and does not recur during subsequent pregnancies.

Doctors may have difficulty making a definite diagnosis.

Herpes gestationis: The cause is thought to be abnormal antibodies that attack the body's own tissues—an autoimmune reaction.

The rash can begin as flat or raised red spots that often form on the abdomen first. Then blisters develop and the rash spreads. The blisters are small or large, irregularly shaped, and fluid-filled.

The rash can appear any time after the 12th week of pregnancy or immediately after delivery. Typically, the rash worsens soon after delivery and disappears within a few weeks or months. It often reappears during subsequent pregnancies and sometimes reappears if the woman later takes oral contraceptives. The baby may be born with a similar rash, which usually disappears without treatment within a few weeks.

This rash is diagnosed by removing a tiny piece of affected skin and testing it for abnormal antibodies.

Treatment: For either rash, applying a corticosteroid cream (such as triamcinolone acetonide) directly to the skin often helps. For more widespread rashes, a corticosteroid (such as prednisone) is given by mouth.

The placenta stimulates the adrenal glands to produce more aldosterone and cortisol (which help regulate how much fluid the kidneys excrete). As a result, more fluids are retained.

During pregnancy, changes in hormone levels affect how the body handles sugar. Early in pregnancy, the sugar (glucose) level in the blood may decrease slightly. But in the last half of pregnancy, the level may increase. More insulin (which controls the sugar level in the blood) is needed and is produced by the pancreas. Consequently, diabetes, if already present, may worsen during pregnancy. Diabetes can also begin during pregnancy. This disorder is called gestational diabetes (see page 1630).

Joints and Muscles: The joints and ligaments (fibrous cords and cartilage that connect bones) in the woman's pelvis loosen and become more flexible. This change helps make room for the enlarging uterus and prepare the woman for delivery of the baby. As a result, the woman's posture changes somewhat.

Backache in varying degrees is common because the spine curves more to balance the weight of the enlarging uterus. Avoiding heavy lifting, bending the knees (not the waist) to pick things up, and maintaining good posture can help. Wearing flat shoes with good

support or a lightweight maternity girdle may reduce strain on the back.

Medical Care

Ideally, a couple who is thinking of having a baby should see a doctor or other health care practitioner to discuss whether pregnancy is advisable. Usually, pregnancy is very safe. However, some disorders can become severe during pregnancy. Also, for some couples, the risk of having a baby with a hereditary disorder is increased.

If the couple decides to try to have a baby, they and the doctor discuss ways to make the pregnancy

---

Stages of Pregnancy

Although pregnancy involves a continuous process, it is divided into three 3-month periods called trimesters (weeks 0 to 12, 13 to 24, and 25 to delivery).

EVENTS	WEEKS OF PREGNANCY
1st Trimester	
The woman's last period before fertilization occurs.	0
Fertilization occurs. The fertilized egg (zygote) begins to develop into a hollow ball of cells called the blastocyst.	2
The blastocyst implants in the wall of uterus. The amniotic sac begins to form.	3
The area that will become the brain and spinal cord (neural tube) begins to develop.	5
The heart and major blood vessels are developing. The beating heart can be seen during ultrasonography.	6
The beginnings of arms and legs appear.	7
Bones and muscles form. The face and neck develop. Brain waves can be detected. The skeleton is formed. Fingers and toes are fully defined.	9
The kidneys begin to function. Almost all organs are completely formed. The fetus can move and respond to touch (when prodded through the woman's abdomen). The woman has gained some weight, and her abdomen may be slightly enlarged.	10

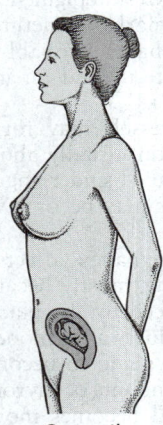

3 months

(continued on the following page)

Stages of Pregnancy (*Continued*)

EVENTS	WEEKS OF PREGNANCY
2nd Trimester	
The fetus's sex can be identified. The fetus can hear.	14
The fetus's fingers can grasp. The fetus moves more vigorously, so that the mother can feel it. The fetus's body begins to fill out as fat is deposited beneath the skin. Hair appears on the head and skin. Eyebrows and eyelashes are present.	16
The placenta is fully formed.	20
The fetus has a chance of survival outside the uterus. The woman begins to gain weight more rapidly.	24
3rd Trimester	
The fetus is active, changing positions often. The lungs continue to mature. The fetus's head moves into position for delivery. On average, the fetus is about 20 inches long and weighs about 7 pounds. The woman's enlarged abdomen causes the navel to bulge.	25
Delivery	37–42

6 months

9 months

as healthy as possible. The woman should ask the doctor about factors that could impair her health or the health of the developing fetus. Factors or situations to avoid include the following:

- Using tobacco or alcohol
- Being exposed to secondhand smoke, which may harm the fetus
- Having contact with cat litter or cat feces unless the cats are strictly confined to the home and are not exposed to other cats (such contact can transmit toxoplasmosis, an infection by a protozoan that can damage the fetus's brain)
- Having contact with people who have rubella (German measles) and some other infections, which can cause birth defects

- Having contact with people who have chickenpox or shingles unless the woman has had a test that shows she has had chickenpox and is immune to it

Chickenpox and shingles are caused by herpes viruses. During delivery, these viruses can be spread to the fetus and cause severe illness. The virus can also cause pneumonia, which is occasionally severe, in the woman.

Knowing about and dealing with such factors before pregnancy may help reduce the risk of problems during pregnancy (see page 1626). In addition, the woman can discuss her diet and her social, emotional, and medical concerns with the doctor.

When a woman sees a doctor or another health care practitioner before she is pregnant, she can be given any needed vaccines, such as the rubella vaccine. She can also start taking prenatal multivitamins containing folate (folic acid). If needed, genetic screening can be done to determine whether the woman and her partner are at increased risk of having a baby with a hereditary genetic disorder (see page 1609).

First Examination: After pregnancy is confirmed, the woman should have a physical examination, preferably between 6 and 8 weeks of pregnancy. At this time, the length of the pregnancy can be estimated and the date of delivery can be predicted as accurately as possible.

The first physical examination during pregnancy is very thorough. It includes the following:

- Measurement of weight, height, and blood pressure
- Pelvic examination: During this examination, the doctor notes the size and position of the uterus.
- Blood tests: A sample of blood is taken and analyzed. Analysis includes a complete blood cell count, tests for infectious diseases (such as syphilis, hepatitis, and human immunodeficiency virus [HIV]), and tests for evidence of immunity to rubella. Blood type, including Rh factor status (positive or negative), is determined.
- Urine tests: A sample of urine is taken, cultured, and analyzed.
- Papanicolaou (Pap) test or a variation of it: Samples of tissue from the cervix are taken to check for cancer of the cervix.
- Test for sexually transmitted diseases: Immediately after the Pap test, another sample of tissue from the cervix is taken to test for sexually transmitted diseases, such as gonorrhea and chlamydial infection.

Other tests may be done, depending on the woman's situation. If the woman has Rh-negative blood, it is tested for antibodies to the Rh factor (see page 1650). Having Rh antibodies can cause severe problems (even death) for a fetus that has Rh-positive blood. If antibodies in a pregnant woman's blood are detected early, the doctor can take measures to protect the fetus.

> **? Did You Know...**
> Things to avoid during pregnancy include tobacco, second-hand smoke, drugs, alcohol, cats, and contact with people who may have chickenpox or shingles.
>
> During the flu season, all pregnant women should get a flu shot.

Women of African descent are tested for sickle cell trait or disease if they have not been tested previously. Skin tests for tuberculosis are advisable for all women. X-rays are not routinely taken during pregnancy, but they can be taken safely when necessary. If an x-ray is required, the fetus is shielded by placing a lead-filled garment over the woman's lower abdomen to cover the uterus.

Follow-up Examinations: After the first examination, a pregnant woman should see her doctor every 4 weeks until 28 weeks of pregnancy, then every 2 weeks until 36 weeks, then once a week until delivery. At each examination, the woman's weight and blood pressure are usually recorded, and the size of the uterus is noted to determine whether the fetus is growing normally. The heartbeat of the fetus is also checked to determine whether it is normal. The woman's ankles are examined for swelling.

At each visit, urine is tested for sugar. Sugar in the urine may indicate diabetes. If the urine contains sugar, a blood test to check for diabetes is done as soon as possible. This test is also done as soon as possible and preferably before 20 weeks for women who

- Are severely overweight (> 250 pounds)
- Have had a history of gestational diabetes
- Have polycystic ovary syndrome with insulin resistance (see page 1528)

If the initial test is negative, these women should be retested at 26 to 30 weeks. All other women should have a screening blood test for diabetes at around 28 weeks of pregnancy.

At each visit, the urine is also tested for protein. Protein in urine may indicate preeclampsia (a type of high blood pressure that develops during pregnancy (see page 1649).

If women have a high risk of conceiving a baby with a genetic disorder, prenatal diagnostic testing can be done (see page 1611).

Most doctors believe that ultrasonography (see page 2044), the safest imaging procedure, should be done at least once during a pregnancy to make sure the fetus is normally formed and to verify the expected date of delivery. For the procedure, a device that produces sound waves (transducer) is placed on the woman's abdomen. The sound waves are processed to form an image that is displayed on a monitor. Sometimes, particularly during early pregnancy, the doctor uses an ultrasound device that can be inserted in the vagina. Ultrasonography produces high-quality images, including live-action images that show the fetus in motion. These images provide the doctor with useful information and can reassure a pregnant woman.

Ultrasonography can show the fetus's beating heart at 6 weeks of pregnancy and thus can confirm that the fetus is alive. Doctors may periodically use an ultrasound device to listen to the fetus's heartbeat. Or they may use a stethoscope designed to listen to a fetus's heartbeat (fetoscope). The fetoscope can detect the heartbeat as early as 18 to 20 weeks of pregnancy.

Ultrasonography can also be used to do the following:

- Identify the sex of the fetus at 14 weeks of pregnancy
- See whether a woman is carrying more than one fetus
- Identify abnormalities, such as a mislocated placenta (placenta previa) or an abnormal position of the fetus
- Date the pregnancy and thus help determine whether the pregnancy is progressing normally
- Identify birth defects (sometimes)
- Guide the placement of instruments during certain procedures, such as prenatal diagnostic testing

Toward the end of pregnancy, ultrasonography may be used to identify premature rupture of the fluid-filled membranes containing the fetus. Ultrasonography can provide information that helps doctors decide whether a cesarean delivery is needed.

Experts recommend that all pregnant women be vaccinated against the influenza virus during the influenza (flu) season.

Self-Care

There is much a pregnant woman can do to take care of herself during pregnancy. If she has any questions about diet, the use of drugs or nutritional supplements, physical activity, and sexual intercourse during pregnancy, she can talk with her doctor.

Diet and Weight: During pregnancy, the woman's diet should be adequate and nutritious. If she does not consume enough nutrients for herself and the fetus, nutrients first go to nourish the fetus. However, adding about 250 calories to the daily diet is usually enough to provide nourishment for both. Most of the extra calories should be protein. The diet should be well balanced and include fresh fruits, grains, and vegetables. Cereals that are high in fiber and low in sugar are a good choice.

In the United States, most women get enough salt in their diet, without adding salt to their food at the table. Commercially prepared foods often contain excessive amounts of salt and should be consumed sparingly.

Dieting to lose weight during pregnancy is not recommended, even for obese women, because some weight gain is essential for the fetus to develop normally. Dieting reduces the supply of nutrients to the fetus.

An average-size woman should gain about 25 to 30 pounds during pregnancy. Gaining more than 30 to 35 pounds puts fat on the woman and the fetus. Because controlling weight gain is more difficult later in pregnancy, a woman should try to avoid gaining too much weight during the first months. On the other hand, not gaining weight can hinder the growth and development of the fetus. A woman should try to gain between 2 and 3 pounds each month during early pregnancy.

Sometimes a pregnant woman gains weight because she is retaining fluid. Fluid may be retained because when she lies flat, the enlarging uterus interferes with blood flow from the legs back to the heart. Lying on one side, preferably the left side, for 30 to 45 minutes 2 or 3 times a day may relieve this problem. Wearing elastic support stockings may also help.

Drugs and Dietary Supplements: Generally, avoiding drugs during pregnancy is best. However, drugs must sometimes be used (see page 1636). A pregnant woman should check with her doctor before taking any drug—including nonprescription (over-the-counter) drugs, such as aspirin, or medicinal herbs—particularly during the first 3 months.

Pregnancy doubles the amount of iron needed. Most pregnant women need an iron supplement because the average woman does not absorb enough iron from food to meet the requirements of pregnancy. If a woman has anemia or develops anemia during pregnancy, she may need to take a larger dose of iron than other pregnant women. Iron supplements may cause mild stomach upset and constipation.

All pregnant women should take a folate (folic acid) supplement (usually included in prenatal vitamins) daily. Ideally, the folate supplement is begun before pregnancy. A deficiency of folate increases the risk of having a baby with a birth defect of the brain or spinal cord, such as spina bifida. Women who have had a baby with spina bifida should start taking a high dose of folate before they become pregnant. For some other women who may have a folate deficiency, the amount of folate in a standard prenatal vitamin is sufficient, even if the risk is somewhat increased. For example, women who are exposed to excessive ultraviolet (UV) light, particularly fair-skinned women, may have decreased folate levels. Also, women who have taken oral contraceptives within several months before conception are more likely to develop a folate deficiency, but there is no proof that they are more likely to have a baby with spina bifida.

> **? Did You Know...**
>
> Usually, exercise and sexual intercourse do not jeopardize a pregnancy.
>
> When traveling, pregnant women should always wear seat belts.

If the diet is adequate, other vitamin supplements may not be needed, although most doctors recommend that pregnant women take a prenatal multivitamin containing iron and folate daily.

Physical Activity: Many pregnant women are concerned about moderating their activities. However, most women can continue their usual activities and exercises throughout pregnancy. Mildly strenuous sports, such as swimming and brisk walking, are good choices. Vigorous activities, such as running and horseback riding, are also possible if done cautiously, to avoid injury, particularly to the abdomen. Contact sports should be avoided.

Sexual Intercourse: Sexual desire may increase or decrease during pregnancy. Sexual intercourse is safe throughout pregnancy unless a woman has vaginal bleeding, pain, leakage of amniotic fluid, or uterine contractions. In such cases, sexual intercourse should be avoided.

Preparing for Breastfeeding: Women who are planning to breastfeed do not need to do anything to prepare their nipples for breastfeeding during pregnancy (see page 1679). Expressing fluids from the breast manually before delivery may lead to an infection of the breast (mastitis) or even early labor. The body prepares the areola and nipple for breastfeeding by secreting a lubricant to protect the surface. This lubricant should not be rubbed off. Observing and talking with women who have breastfed successfully may be instructive and encouraging.

Travel During Pregnancy: The safest time to travel during pregnancy is between 14 and 28 weeks. Travel time should not exceed 6 hours a day. Women can obtain useful tips and information about travel from their doctor, so discussing their travel plans with the doctor is a good idea.

When traveling in a car, airplane, or other vehicle, pregnant women should always wear a seat belt. Placing the lap belt across the hips and under the expanding abdomen and placing the shoulder belt between the breasts can help make wearing seat belts more comfortable. The belts should be snug but not uncomfortably tight.

During any kind of travel, pregnant women should stretch and straighten their legs and ankles periodically.

Travel on airplanes is safe until about 36 weeks. The primary reason for this restriction at 36 weeks is the risk of labor and delivery in an unfamiliar environment.

CHAPTER 253 High-Risk Pregnancy

There is no formal or universally accepted definition of a "high-risk" pregnancy. Generally, however, a high-risk pregnancy involves at least one of the following:

- The woman or baby is more likely to become ill or die than usual.
- Complications before or after delivery are more likely to occur than usual.

Certain conditions or characteristics, called risk factors, make a pregnancy high risk. Doctors identify these factors to determine the degree of risk for a particular woman and baby and thus to provide better medical care.

Risk Factors Present Before Pregnancy

Some risk factors are present before women become pregnant. These risk factors include certain physical and social characteristics of women, problems that have occurred in previous pregnancies, and certain disorders women already have.

Physical Characteristics

The following characteristics of women affect risk during pregnancy.

Age: Girls aged 15 and younger are at increased risk of preeclampsia (a type of high blood pressure that develops during pregnancy). Young girls are also at increased risk of preterm labor and anemia. They are more likely to have babies who have anemia or who are underweight (small for gestational age).

Women aged 35 and older are at increased risk of problems such as high blood pressure, gestational diabetes (diabetes that develops during pregnancy), chromosomal abnormalities in the fetus, and stillbirth. Also, they are more likely to have complications during labor such as preeclampsia, a placenta that detaches too soon (placental abruption) or is mislocated (placenta previa), and difficult labor.

Weight: Women who weigh less than 100 pounds before becoming pregnant are more likely to have small, underweight babies.

Obese women are more likely to have very large babies, which may be difficult to deliver. Also, obese women are more likely to develop gestational diabetes, high blood pressure, or preeclampsia. They are more like to have a pregnancy that lasts 42 weeks or longer (postterm) and to need a cesarean delivery.

Height: Women shorter than 5 feet are more likely to have a small pelvis, which may make movement of the fetus through the pelvis and vagina (birth canal) difficult during labor. For example, the fetus's shoulder is more likely to lodge against the pubic bone. This complication is called shoulder dystocia (see page 1661). Also, short women are more likely to have preterm labor and a baby who has not grown as much as expected.

Reproductive Abnormalities: Structural abnormalities in the uterus or cervix increase the risk of having a difficult labor, a miscarriage, or a fetus in an abnormal position and of needing a cesarean delivery. These abnormalities include a double uterus or a weak (incompetent) cervix that tends to open (dilate) as the fetus grows.

Social Characteristics

Being unmarried or in a lower socioeconomic group increases the risk of problems during pregnancy. The reason these characteristics increase risk is unclear but is probably related to other characteristics that are more common among these women. For example, these women are more likely to smoke and less likely to consume a healthy diet and to obtain appropriate medical care.

Problems in a Previous Pregnancy

When women have had a problem in one pregnancy, they are more likely to have a problem, often the same one, in subsequent pregnancies. Such problems include having had any of the following:

- A premature baby
- An underweight baby
- A baby that weighed more than 10 pounds
- A baby with birth defects
- A previous miscarriage
- A late (postterm) delivery (after 42 weeks of pregnancy)
- Rh incompatibility that required a blood transfusion to the fetus
- Labor that required a cesarean delivery
- A baby who died shortly before or after birth (stillbirth)

Women may have a condition that tends to make the same problem recur. For example, women with diabetes are more likely to have babies that weigh more than 10 pounds at birth.

Women who had a baby with a genetic disorder or birth defect are more likely to have another baby with a similar problem. Genetic testing of the baby, even if stillborn, and of both parents may be appropriate before another pregnancy is attempted (see page 1609). If these women become pregnant again, tests such as high-resolution ultrasonography, chorionic villus sampling, and amniocentesis may help determine whether the fetus has a genetic disorder or birth defect. These women may be referred to a specialist.

Having had five or more pregnancies increases the risk of very rapid labor and excessive bleeding after delivery. Having had twins or more fetuses in one pregnancy (multiple births) increases the risk of a mislocated placenta (placenta previa—see page 1647).

Disorders Present Before Pregnancy

Before becoming pregnant, women may have a disorder that can increase the risk of problems during pregnancy (see page 1628). These women should talk with a doctor and try to get in the best physical condition possible before they become pregnant. After they become pregnant, they may need special care, often from an interdisciplinary team. The team may include an obstetrician (who may also be a specialist in the disorder), a specialist in the disorder, and other health care practitioners (such as nutritionists).

Risk Factors That Develop During Pregnancy

During pregnancy, a problem may occur or a condition may develop to make the pregnancy high risk. For example, pregnant women may be exposed to something that can cause birth defects (teratogens), such as radiation, certain chemicals, drugs, or infections. Or a disorder may develop. Some disorders are related to (are complications of) pregnancy. Other disorders are not directly related to pregnancy (see below). Certain disorders are more likely to occur during pregnancy because of the many changes pregnancy causes in a woman's body.

Drugs

Some drugs taken during pregnancy cause birth defects (see page 1636). Examples are isotretinoin (used to treat severe acne), some anticonvulsants, lithium, some antibiotics (such as streptomycin, kanamycin, and tetracycline), thalidomide, warfarin, and angiotensin-converting enzyme (ACE) inhibitors (if taken during the last two trimesters). Taking drugs that block the actions of folate (folic acid), such as the immunosuppressant methotrexate or the antibiotic trimethoprim, can also cause birth defects. A deficiency of folate increases the risk of having a baby with a birth defect. Early in pregnancy, women are asked if they are using any of these drugs.

Women are also asked if they use any recreational drugs. Of particular concern are alcohol, cocaine, and nicotine (in cigarette smoking). All of these drugs can cause miscarriage or cause the baby to be underweight or to have birth defects. These drugs have the following risks:

- **Alcohol:** The risk of mental retardation (intellectual disability) is increased. Fetal alcohol syndrome is also possible (see page 1642).
- **Cocaine:** The risk of premature detachment of the placenta (placental abruption), premature birth, and stillbirth is increased. The fetus may not grow as much as expected.
- **Smoking cigarettes:** The risk of stillbirth and pregnancy complications, such as premature labor, placenta previa, placental abruption, and premature rupture of membranes, is increased. The fetus may not grow as much as expected, and children are more likely to have behavioral problems and intellectual disability.

Pregnancy Complications

Pregnancy complications are problems that occur only during pregnancy (see page 1643). They may affect the woman, the fetus, or both and may occur at different times during the pregnancy. For example, complications such as a mislocated placenta (placenta previa) or premature detachment of the placenta from the uterus (placental abruption) can cause bleeding from the vagina during pregnancy. Women who have heavy bleeding are at risk of losing the baby or of going into shock and, if not promptly treated, of dying during labor and delivery.

CHAPTER 254 Pregnancy Complicated by Disease

Certain disorders, such as diabetes and high blood pressure, can increase the risk of problems during pregnancy. If women who have such a disorder wish to become pregnant, they should first talk with a doctor and try to get in the best physical condition possible before they become pregnant. After such women become pregnant, they may need special care, often from an interdisciplinary team. The team may include an obstetrician (who may also be a specialist in care of the disorder during pregnancy), a specialist in the disorder, and other health care practitioners (such as nutritionists).

Sometimes disorders that are not directly related to pregnancy develop during pregnancy. Some of them increase the risk of problems for pregnant women or the fetus. They include disorders that cause a high fever, infections, and disorders that require abdominal surgery.

Some disorders are more likely to occur during pregnancy because of the many changes pregnancy causes in a woman's body. Examples are thromboembolic disorders, anemia, and urinary tract infections.

Anemia

Anemia develops in most pregnant women to some degree. The most common cause is an iron deficiency.

For women who have a hereditary anemia (such as sickle cell disease, hemoglobin S-C disease, and some thalassemias), the risk of problems is increased during pregnancy. If women are at increased risk of having these disorders because of race, ethnic background, or family history, blood tests are routinely done before delivery to check for the disorders. Chorionic villus sampling or amniocentesis may be done to check for these disorders in the fetus.

Anemia Due to Nutritional Deficiencies: During pregnancy, iron deficiency commonly develops because women need twice as much iron as usual to make red blood cells in the fetus. Anemia often results. Anemia may also develop during pregnancy because of a folate (folic acid) deficiency. If folate is deficient, the risk of having a baby with a birth defect of the brain or spinal cord, such as spina bifida, is increased.

Anemia can usually be prevented or treated by taking iron and folate supplements during pregnancy. However, if anemia becomes severe and persists, the blood's capacity to carry oxygen is decreased, and the following may result:

- The fetus may not receive enough oxygen, which is needed for normal growth and development, especially of the brain.
- Pregnant women who have severe anemia may become excessively tired, short of breath, and light-headed.
- The risk of preterm labor is increased.

A normal amount of bleeding during labor and delivery can cause the anemia in these women to become dangerously severe. They are more likely to develop infections after delivery.

Sickle Cell Disease: In addition to causing symptoms of anemia, sickle cell disease increases the risk of the following during pregnancy:

- Infections: Pneumonia, urinary tract infections, and infections of the uterus are the most common.
- High blood pressure: About one third of pregnant women who have sickle cell disease develop high blood pressure during pregnancy.
- Heart failure
- Blockage of arteries of the lungs by blood clots (pulmonary embolism): This problem may be life threatening.
- Problems in the fetus: The fetus may grow slowly or not as much as expected. The fetus may even die.

A sudden, severe attack of pain, called sickle cell crisis, may occur during pregnancy as at any other time. The more severe sickle cell disease was before pregnancy, the higher the risk of health problems for pregnant women and the fetus, and the higher the risk of death for the fetus during pregnancy. Sickle cell anemia almost always worsens as pregnancy progresses.

With regular blood transfusions, women are less likely to have sickle cell crises, but they become more likely to reject the transfused blood. This condition, called alloimmunization, can be life threatening. Also, transfusions to pregnant women do not reduce risks for the fetus.

Asthma

The effect of pregnancy on asthma varies. Worsening of the disease is slightly more common than improvement, but most pregnant women do not have severe asthma attacks. The effect of asthma on pregnancy also varies, but risk of preterm delivery and poor fetal growth is increased.

Because asthma can change during pregnancy, doctors may ask women with asthma to use a peak flow meter to monitor their breathing more often. Pregnant women with asthma should see their doctor regularly so that treatment can be adjusted as needed. Maintaining good control of asthma is important. Inadequate treatment can result in serious problems.

Inhaled bronchodilators (such as albuterol) and inhaled corticosteroids (such as beclomethasone) can be taken during pregnancy. When inhaled, the drugs affect mainly the lungs and affect the whole body and the fetus less than when they are taken by mouth. Aminophylline (taken by mouth or given intravenously) and theophylline (taken by mouth) are not usually used during pregnancy. Corticosteroids taken by mouth are used only when other treatments are ineffective or after asthma suddenly worsens.

Being vaccinated against the influenza (flu) virus during the flu season is particularly important for pregnant women with asthma.

Autoimmune Disorders

Autoimmune disorders, including Graves' disease (see page 1635), are more common among women, particularly pregnant women. The abnormal antibodies produced in autoimmune disorders can cross the placenta and cause problems in the fetus. Pregnancy affects different autoimmune disorders in different ways.

Systemic Lupus Erythematosus (Lupus): Lupus may appear for the first time, worsen, or become less severe during pregnancy. How a pregnancy affects the course of lupus cannot be predicted, but the most common time for flare-ups is immediately after delivery.

Women who develop lupus often have a history of repeated miscarriages, fetuses that do not grow as much as expected, and preterm delivery. If women have complications due to lupus (such as kidney damage or high blood pressure), the risk of death for the fetus or newborn is increased.

In pregnant women, lupus antibodies may cross the placenta to the fetus. As a result, the fetus may have a very slow heart rate, anemia, a low platelet count, or a low white blood cell count. However, these antibodies gradually disappear over several weeks after the baby is born, and the problems they cause resolve except for the slow heart rate. Women with lupus may need to take prednisone (a corticosteroid) by mouth while they are pregnant.

Myasthenia Gravis: This disorder, which causes muscle weakness, does not usually cause serious or permanent complications during pregnancy. However, women may need to take higher doses of drugs (such as neostigmine) used to treat the disorder or may need to take corticosteroids or drugs that suppress the immune system (immunosuppressants). Very rarely during labor, women who have myasthenia gravis need help with breathing (assisted ventilation).

The antibodies that cause this disorder can cross the placenta. So about one of five babies born to women with myasthenia gravis is born with the disorder. However, the resulting muscle weakness in the baby is usually temporary because the antibodies from the mother gradually disappear and the baby does not produce antibodies of this type.

Immune (Idiopathic) Thrombocytopenic Purpura (ITP): In ITP, antibodies decrease the number of platelets (also called thrombocytes) in the bloodstream. Platelets are cell-like particles that help in the clotting process. Too few platelets (thrombocytopenia) can cause excessive bleeding in pregnant women and their babies. If not treated during pregnancy, the disorder tends to become more severe. Corticosteroids, usually prednisone given by mouth, can increase the number (count) of platelets and thus improve blood clotting in pregnant women with this disorder. However, prednisone increases the risk that the fetus will not grow as much as expected or will be born prematurely.

Women who have a dangerously low platelet count may be given high doses of immune globulin intravenously shortly before delivery. This treatment temporarily increases the platelet count and improves blood clotting. As a result, labor can proceed safely, and women can have a vaginal delivery without uncontrolled bleeding.

Pregnant women are given platelet transfusions only when a cesarean delivery is needed and when the platelet count is so low that severe bleeding may occur.

Rarely, when the platelet count remains dangerously low despite treatment, the spleen, which normally traps and destroys old blood cells and platelets, is removed. The best time for this surgery is during the 2nd trimester.

The antibodies that cause the disorder may cross the placenta to the fetus. However, they rarely affect the platelet count in the fetus.

Rheumatoid Arthritis: If arthritis has damaged the hip joints or lower (lumbar) spine, delivery may be difficult for the woman, but this disorder does not affect the fetus. The symptoms of rheumatoid arthritis may lessen during pregnancy, but they usually return to their original level after pregnancy.

Cancer

Because cancer tends to be life threatening and because delays in treatment may reduce the likelihood of successful treatment, cancer is usually treated the same way whether the woman is pregnant or not. Some of the usual treatments (surgery, chemotherapy drugs, and radiation therapy) may harm the fetus. Thus, some women may consider abortion. However, treatments can sometimes be timed so that risk to the fetus is reduced.

In some cancers, treatment may be modified during pregnancy.

- **Rectal cancer:** Removal of the uterus (hysterectomy) may be required. In such cases, cesarean delivery may be done as early as 28 weeks of pregnancy to save the baby.

- **Cervical cancer:** If the cancer is in a very early stage, treatment is usually postponed until after delivery. If more advanced cervical cancer is detected early in pregnancy, it is usually treated immediately as needed. If it is diagnosed late in pregnancy, doctors explain the risk of postponing treatment so that women can decide whether to postpone treatment until after the fetus is mature enough to be delivered. Cesarean delivery is usually done, but sometimes vaginal delivery is possible.

- **Other gynecologic cancers:** Cancer of the ovaries is hard to detect during pregnancy. It may require immediate treatment (removal of both ovaries). Cancer of the uterus (endometrial cancer) or fallopian tubes rarely occurs during pregnancy.

- **Breast cancer:** Breast cancer is hard to detect during pregnancy because the breasts enlarge. If any lump is detected, doctors evaluate it. Usually, breast cancer should be treated immediately.

Diabetes

For women who have diabetes before they become pregnant, the risks of complications during pregnancy depend on how long diabetes has been present and whether complications of diabetes, such as high blood pressure and kidney damage, are present.

Gestational Diabetes: About 1 to 3% of pregnant women develop diabetes during pregnancy. This disorder is called gestational diabetes. Unrecognized and untreated, gestational diabetes can increase the risk of health problems for pregnant women and their fetus and the risk of death for the fetus. Gestational diabetes is more common among obese women and among certain ethnic groups, particularly Native Americans, Pacific Islanders, and women of Mexican, Indian, or Asian descent. Most women with gestational diabetes develop it because they cannot produce enough insulin, as the need for insulin increases late in the pregnancy. More insulin is needed to control the increasing level of sugar (glucose) in the blood. Some women may have had diabetes before becoming pregnant, but the disease was not recognized until they became pregnant.

Most experts now recommend that doctors routinely screen all pregnant women for gestational diabetes. A blood test is used to measure the blood sugar level.

Risks of Diabetes During Pregnancy: If diabetes is poorly controlled early in the pregnancy, the risk of an early miscarriage and significant birth defects is increased. Babies born to diabetic women tend to be larger than those born to women without diabetes. If diabetes is poorly controlled, babies may be particularly large. A large fetus is less likely to pass easily through the vagina and is more likely to be injured during vaginal delivery. Consequently, cesarean delivery is often necessary. The fetus's lungs also tend to mature slowly. The risk of preeclampsia (a type of high blood pressure that occurs during pregnancy) is also increased for women with diabetes.

Newborns of women with diabetes are at increased risk of having low sugar, low calcium, and high bilirubin levels in the blood.

Treatment

The risk of complications during pregnancy can be reduced by controlling the level of sugar in the blood. The level should be kept as near normal as possible throughout pregnancy.

If women who have diabetes are planning to become pregnant, doctors advise them to immediately start taking steps to control the blood sugar level (such as following an appropriate diet, exercising, and, if needed, taking insulin) if they have not already done so (see page 1008). High-sugar foods are eliminated from the diet, and women should eat so that they do not gain excess weight during pregnancy.

Most pregnant women with diabetes are asked to measure their blood sugar level several times a day at home. Women who have gestational diabetes are usually taught to measure this level with a home blood sugar monitoring device. If blood sugar levels are high, women may need to take insulin.

Controlling diabetes is particularly important late in pregnancy. Then, the blood sugar level tends to increase as the body becomes less responsive to insulin. This effect occurs partly because the enlarging placenta makes hormones that counteract the effects of insulin. A higher dose of insulin is usually needed.

If an early delivery is being considered (for example, because the fetus is large), the doctor may remove and analyze a sample of the fluid that surrounds the fetus (amniotic fluid). This procedure, called amniocentesis,

helps the doctor determine whether the fetus's lungs are mature enough to breathe air.

In newborns of women with diabetes, hospital staff members measure blood levels of sugar, calcium, and bilirubin because these newborns often have abnormal levels. The newborns are also observed for symptoms of these abnormalities.

For women with diabetes, the requirement for insulin dramatically drops immediately after delivery. But the requirement usually returns to what it was before pregnancy within about 1 week.

After delivery, gestational diabetes usually disappears. However, many women who have gestational diabetes develop type 2 diabetes as they become older.

Fevers

A temperature higher than 103° F (39.5° C) during the 1st trimester increases the risk of a miscarriage and defects of the brain or spinal cord in the baby. Fever late in pregnancy increases the risk of preterm labor.

Fibroids

Fibroids in the uterus (see page 1533), which are relatively common noncancerous tumors, may increase the risk of preterm labor, abnormal presentation of the fetus, a mislocated placenta (placenta previa), and repeated miscarriages. Rarely, fibroids interfere with the movement of the fetus through the vagina during labor.

Heart Disorders

Most women who have heart disorders—including heart valve disorders (such as mitral valve prolapse) and some birth defects of the heart—can safely give birth to healthy children, without any permanent ill effects on heart function or life span. However, women who have moderate or severe heart failure before pregnancy are at considerable risk of problems.

Pregnancy requires the heart to work harder. Consequently, pregnancy may worsen a heart disorder or cause a heart disorder to produce symptoms for the first time. Usually, serious problems, including death of the woman or fetus, occur only when a heart disorder is severe before the woman becomes pregnant. About 1% of women who have a severe heart disorder before becoming pregnant die as a result of the pregnancy, usually because of heart failure.

The risk of problems increases throughout pregnancy as demands on the heart increase. Pregnant women with a heart disorder may become unusually tired and may need to limit their activities. Rarely, women with a severe heart disorder are advised to have an abortion early in pregnancy. Risk is also increased during labor and delivery. After delivery, women with a severe heart disorder may not be out of danger for at least 6 months, depending on the type of heart disorder.

A heart disorder in pregnant women may affect the fetus. The fetus may be born prematurely. Women with birth defects of the heart are more likely to have children with similar birth defects. Ultrasonography can detect some of these defects before the fetus is born. If a severe heart disorder in a pregnant woman suddenly worsens, the fetus may die.

During labor, women who have a severe heart disorder may be given an epidural anesthetic. This anesthetic blocks sensation in the lower spinal cord and prevents women from pushing. Pushing during labor strains the heart because it increases the amount of blood returning to the heart. Because pushing is not possible, the baby may have to be delivered with forceps. However, an epidural anesthetic should not be used if women have aortic valve stenosis.

For women with some types of heart disorders, pregnancy is inadvisable because it greatly increases the risk of death. Primary pulmonary hypertension and Eisenmenger's syndrome are examples. If women who have one of these disorders become pregnant, doctors advise them to terminate the pregnancy as early as possible.

Peripartum Cardiomyopathy: The heart's walls may be damaged late in pregnancy or after delivery, causing peripartum cardiomyopathy. The cause is unknown. This disorder tends to occur in women who have had several pregnancies, who are older, who are carrying twins, or who have preeclampsia. In some women, heart function does not return to normal after pregnancy. Peripartum cardiomyopathy tends to occur in subsequent pregnancies, particularly if heart function has not returned to normal. Thus, women who have had this disorder are often discouraged from becoming pregnant again.

Peripartum cardiomyopathy can result in heart failure (see page 352), which is treated as usual except that angiotensin-converting enzyme (ACE) inhibitors and aldosterone antagonists (spironolactone and eplerenone) are not used.

Heart Valve Disorders: Ideally, heart valve disorders are diagnosed and treated before the women become pregnant. Doctors often recommend surgical treatment for women with severe disorders.

The valves most often affected in pregnant women are the aortic and mitral valves. Disorders that cause the opening of a heart valve to narrow (stenosis) are particularly risky.

Women with mitral valve prolapse usually tolerate pregnancy well.

High Blood Pressure

High blood pressure (hypertension) during pregnancy is classified as one of the following:

- Chronic hypertension: Blood pressure was high before the pregnancy.
- Gestational hypertension: Blood pressure became high for the first time during pregnancy, usually after 20 weeks.

Preeclampsia causes high blood pressure to develop during pregnancy, but it is diagnosed and treated differently from other types of high blood pressure (see page 1649).

Women who have chronic hypertension are more likely to have potentially serious problems during pregnancy. These problems include the following:

- Preeclampsia
- Worsening of high blood pressure
- A fetus that does not grow as much as expected
- Premature detachment of the placenta from the uterus (placental abruption)
- Stillbirth

During pregnancy, women with high blood pressure are monitored closely to make sure blood pressure is well controlled, the kidneys are functioning normally, and the fetus is growing normally. However, premature detachment of the placenta cannot be prevented or anticipated. Often, a baby must be delivered early to prevent stillbirth or complications due to severe high blood pressure (such as stroke) in the woman.

Treatment

For most women with mild high blood pressure (140/90 to 150/100 millimeters of mercury [mm Hg]), treatment with antihypertensive drugs is often not recommended. Such treatment does not seem to reduce the risk of preeclampsia, premature detachment of the placenta, or a stillbirth or to improve the growth of the fetus. However, some women are treated to prevent pregnancy from causing episodes of even higher blood pressure, which require hospitalization.

For women whose blood pressure is higher than 150/100 mm Hg, treatment with antihypertensive drugs is recommended (see table on page 340). Treatment can reduce the risk of stroke and other complications due to very high blood pressure. Treatment is also recommended for women who have high blood pressure and a kidney disorder. If high blood pressure is not controlled well, the kidneys may be damaged further.

Most antihypertensive drugs used to treat high blood pressure can be used safely during pregnancy. However, angiotensin-converting enzyme (ACE) inhibitors are stopped during pregnancy, particularly during the last two trimesters. These drugs can cause severe kidney damage in the fetus. As a result, the baby may die shortly after birth. Aldosterone antagonists (spironolactone and eplerenone) are also stopped because they can cause a male fetus to develop feminine characteristics. Thiazide diuretics (such as hydrochlorothiazide) are usually stopped during pregnancy. These diuretics increase the risk that the fetus will not grow as much as expected.

> **? Did You Know...**
>
> Certain types of antihypertensive drugs—ACE inhibitors, aldosterone antagonists, and thiazide diuretics—are usually stopped during pregnancy.

Infections

Most common infections that occur during pregnancy, such as those of the skin and respiratory tract, cause no serious problems. However, some infections can be passed to the fetus before or during birth and damage the fetus or cause a miscarriage or premature birth.

Sexually transmitted diseases that can cause problems include the following:

- Chlamydial infection may cause preterm labor and premature rupture of the membranes. It can also cause eye inflammation (conjunctivitis) in newborns.
- Gonorrhea can also cause conjunctivitis in newborns.
- Syphilis can be transmitted from a mother to the fetus through the placenta. Syphilis can cause several birth defects.
- Human immunodeficiency virus (HIV) infection is transmitted to the fetus in one fourth of pregnant women who have the infection and are not treated (see page 1774). Experts recommend that women with HIV infection take one or more antiretroviral drugs during pregnancy. When pregnant women take zidovudine, the risk of transmitting HIV to the fetus is reduced to less than 7%. If women take several drugs, the risk can be reduced to as low as 2 to 3%. For some women with HIV infection, cesarean delivery, planned in advance, may further reduce the risk of transmitting HIV to the baby. Pregnancy does not seem to accelerate the progression of HIV infection in women.
- Genital herpes can be transmitted to the baby during a vaginal delivery. Babies who are infected with herpes can develop a life-threatening brain infection called herpes encephalitis. A herpes infection in babies can also damage other internal organs and cause skin and mouth sores, permanent brain damage, or even death. If women develop herpes sores in the genital area late in pregnancy or if herpes first developed during late pregnancy, women are usually advised to give birth by cesarean delivery, so that the virus is not transmitted to the baby. If no sores are present and herpes developed earlier, the risk of transmission is very low.

Infections that are not transmitted sexually and can cause problems include the following:

- German measles (rubella) can cause birth defects, particularly of the heart and inner ear.
- Cytomegalovirus infection can cross the placenta and damage the fetus's liver and brain.
- Chickenpox (varicella) increases the risk of a miscarriage. It may damage the eyes of the fetus or cause defects of the limbs, blindness, or mental retardation. The fetus's head may be smaller than normal.
- Toxoplasmosis, a protozoal infection, may cause a miscarriage, death of the fetus, and serious birth defects.
- Listeriosis, a bacterial infection, increases the risk of a premature birth, miscarriage, and stillbirth. Newborns may have the infection.
- Bacterial infections of the vagina (such as bacterial vaginosis) may lead to preterm labor or premature rupture of the membranes containing the fetus.
- Chronic viral hepatitis increases the risk of miscarriage and premature birth.

To determine whether to treat pregnant women with antimicrobial drugs, doctors weigh the risks of using the drug against the risks of the infection. Some antibacterial drugs, such as the penicillins, cephalosporins, and erythromycins, are generally considered safe for use during pregnancy. Other antibacterial drugs, including the tetracyclines and fluoroquinolones, may cause problems in the fetus (see table on page 1638).

Kidney Disorders

Women with a severe kidney disorder before pregnancy are more likely to have problems during pregnancy. If high blood pressure develops, kidney function may rapidly worsen during pregnancy. High blood pressure commonly occurs in people with a kidney disorder. Preeclampsia (a type of high blood pressure that develops during pregnancy) may also develop. The fetus may not grow as much as expected or may be stillborn.

In pregnant women who have a kidney disorder, kidney function and blood pressure are monitored closely, as is growth of the fetus. Often, the baby must be delivered early.

Women who have had a kidney transplant are usually able to safely give birth to healthy babies if they have the following:

- A transplant that has been in place for 2 or more years
- A kidney that is functioning normally

- No episodes of rejection
- Normal blood pressure

Women who have a kidney disorder that requires hemodialysis regularly often are at high risk of pregnancy complications, including miscarriage, stillbirth, preterm birth, and preeclampsia.

Liver and Gallbladder Disorders

Women who have chronic viral hepatitis or scarring of the liver (cirrhosis) are more likely to miscarry or to give birth prematurely. Cirrhosis can cause varicose veins to develop around the esophagus (esophageal varices). Pregnancy slightly increases the risk of massive bleeding from these veins, especially during the last 3 months of pregnancy.

Liver or gallbladder problems may result from hormonal changes during pregnancy. Some changes cause only minor, transient symptoms.

Cholestasis of Pregnancy: The normal hormonal effects of pregnancy can slow the movement of bile through the bile ducts. This slowing is called cholestasis. The most obvious symptom is itching all over the body (usually in the last few months of pregnancy). No rash develops. If itching is intense, cholestyramine may be given.

The disorder usually resolves after delivery but tends to recur in subsequent pregnancies.

Fatty Liver of Pregnancy: This rare disorder can develop toward the end of pregnancy. The cause is unknown. Symptoms include nausea, vomiting, abdominal discomfort, and jaundice. The disorder may rapidly worsen, and liver failure may develop.

Diagnosis is based on results of liver function tests and may be confirmed by a liver biopsy. The doctor may advise women to immediately end the pregnancy. The risk of death for pregnant women and the fetus is high in severe cases, but those who survive recover completely. Usually, the disorder does not recur in subsequent pregnancies.

Gallstones: Pregnant women who develop gallstones are closely monitored. If a gallstone blocks the gallbladder or causes an infection, surgery may be necessary. This surgery is usually safe for pregnant women and the fetus.

Seizure Disorders

Women who have seizures are slightly more likely to develop preeclampsia (a type of high blood pressure that develops during pregnancy) and to have a stillbirth or a fetus who does not grow as much as expected. On the other hand, taking anticonvulsants increases the risk of birth defects (see table on page 1638) and may slightly reduce intelligence in the baby. Thus, women who have a seizure disorder should discuss how to balance the risks with an expert in the field, preferably

before they become pregnant. Some women may be able to safely stop taking anticonvulsants during pregnancy, but most women should continue to take the drugs. The risk resulting from not taking the drugs—more frequent seizures, which can harm the fetus and the woman—usually outweighs the risks resulting from taking the drugs during pregnancy.

Disorders That Require Surgery

During pregnancy, a disorder that requires surgery involving the abdomen may develop. This type of surgery often slightly increases the risk of preterm labor and can cause a miscarriage, especially early in pregnancy. Thus, surgery is usually delayed if possible. However, if necessary, surgery should proceed without delay and is still usually reasonably safe.

Appendicitis: If appendicitis develops during pregnancy, surgery to remove the appendix (appendectomy) is done immediately because a ruptured appendix may be fatal. An appendectomy is not likely to harm the fetus or cause a miscarriage. However, appendicitis may be difficult to recognize during pregnancy. The cramping pain of appendicitis resembles uterine contractions, which are common during pregnancy. The appendix is pushed higher in the abdomen as the pregnancy progresses, so the location of pain due to appendicitis may not be what is expected.

Ovarian Cyst: If an ovarian cyst persists during pregnancy, surgery is usually postponed until after the 14th week of pregnancy. The cyst may be producing hormones that are supporting the pregnancy and often disappears without treatment. However, if a cyst or another mass is enlarging, is very tender, or has certain characteristics (seen on an ultrasound) surgery may be necessary before the 14th week. Such a mass may be cancerous.

Obstruction of the Intestine: During pregnancy, a blockage (obstruction) in the intestine can be very serious. If obstruction leads to gangrene of the intestine and peritonitis (inflammation of the membrane that lines the abdominal cavity), the woman may miscarry and her life is endangered. Exploratory surgery is usually done promptly when pregnant women have symptoms of intestinal obstruction, particularly if they have had abdominal surgery or an abdominal infection.

Thromboembolic Disorders

In the United States, thromboembolic disorders are the leading cause of death in pregnant women. In thromboembolic disorders, blood clots form in blood vessels. They may travel through the bloodstream and block an artery. The risk of developing a thromboembolic disorder is increased for about 6 to 8 weeks after delivery. Most complications due to blood clots result from injuries that occur during delivery. The risk is much higher after cesarean delivery than after vaginal delivery. Blood clots usually form in the superficial veins of the legs as thrombophlebitis or in the deep veins as deep vein thrombosis. Symptoms include swelling, pain in the calves, and tenderness. The severity of the symptoms does not correlate with the severity of the disease. Deep vein thrombosis may also develop in the pelvis. There, it may not cause symptoms. A clot can move from the deep veins of the legs or pelvis to the lungs. There, the clot may block one or more arteries. This blockage, called pulmonary embolism, can be life threatening.

Diagnosis and Treatment

During pregnancy, if women have symptoms suggesting a blood clot, Doppler ultrasonography (used to evaluate blood flow) may be done to check the legs for clots.

If pulmonary embolism (see page 488) is suspected, computed tomography (CT) may be done to confirm the diagnosis. CT is relatively safe during pregnancy. If the diagnosis of pulmonary embolism is still uncertain, a procedure called pulmonary angiography is required.

If a blood clot is detected, heparin (an anticoagulant) is started without delay. Heparin may be injected into a vein (intravenously) or under the skin (subcutaneously). Heparin does not cross the placenta and cannot harm the fetus. Treatment is continued for 6 to 8 weeks after delivery, when the risk of blood clots is high. After delivery, warfarin may be used instead of heparin. Warfarin can be taken by mouth, has a lower risk of complications than heparin, and can be taken by women who are breastfeeding.

Women who have had a blood clot during a previous pregnancy may be given heparin during subsequent pregnancies to prevent blood clots from forming.

Thyroid Disorders

Thyroid disorders may be present before women become pregnant, or they may develop during pregnancy. Being pregnant does not change the symptoms of thyroid disorders. How the fetus is affected depends on which thyroid disorder is present and which drugs are used for treatment. But generally, the following are risks:

- With an overactive thyroid gland (hyperthyroidism): Slow or less-than-expected growth in the fetus and stillbirth
- With an underactive thyroid gland (hypothyroidism): Impaired intellectual development in children and a miscarriage

The most common causes of hypothyroidism in pregnant women are Hashimoto's thyroiditis and treatment of Graves' disease.

If women have or have had a thyroid disorder, they and the baby are closely monitored during and after pregnancy. Doctors regularly check them for changes in symptoms and do blood tests to measure thyroid hormone levels.

Hashimoto's Thyroiditis: This chronic inflammation of the thyroid gland is caused by an autoimmune reaction—when the immune system malfunctions and attacks its own tissues. Because the immune system is suppressed during pregnancy, this disorder may become less evident. However, pregnant women sometimes develop hypothyroidism or hyperthyroidism that requires treatment.

Subacute Thyroiditis: This sudden inflammation of the thyroid gland is common during pregnancy. The thyroid gland may enlarge, forming a goiter, and become tender. The goiter usually develops during or after a respiratory infection. Hyperthyroidism may develop and cause symptoms, but it is temporary. Subacute thyroiditis usually requires no treatment.

Postdelivery Thyroiditis: In the first few weeks after delivery, the thyroid gland may become suddenly inflamed, making the thyroid temporarily overactive. This disorder may be caused by an autoimmune reaction. The disorder may persist, recur periodically, or steadily worsen.

Graves' Disease: Abnormal antibodies stimulate the thyroid gland to produce excess thyroid hormone. These antibodies can cross the placenta and stimulate the thyroid gland in the fetus. As a result, the fetus may have a rapid heart rate and may not grow as much as expected. The fetus's thyroid gland may enlarge, forming a goiter. Very rarely, a goiter is so large that it interferes with delivery through the vagina.

Usually during pregnancy, Graves' disease is treated with the lowest possible dose of propylthiouracil, taken by mouth. Physical examinations and measurements of thyroid hormone levels are done regularly because propylthiouracil crosses the placenta. The drug may slow the activity of the thyroid gland and prevent the fetus from producing enough thyroid hormone. It may also cause a goiter to form in the fetus. Synthetic thyroid hormones, usually also used to treat this disorder, are not used with propylthiouracil during pregnancy. These hormones may cover up problems that occur when doses of propylthiouracil are too high and may cause hypothyroidism in the fetus. Methimazole may be used instead of propylthiouracil.

Often, Graves' disease becomes less severe during the 3rd trimester, so the drug dose can be reduced or the drug can be stopped.

Radioactive iodine, used to diagnose or treat Graves' disease, is not used during pregnancy because it can damage the fetus's thyroid gland.

If a thyroid storm (sudden, extreme overactivity of the thyroid gland) occurs or symptoms become severe, women may be given beta-blockers (used to treat high blood pressure). If necessary, the thyroid gland of pregnant women may be removed during the 2nd trimester. Women thus treated must begin taking synthetic thyroid hormones 24 hours after surgery. For these women, taking these hormones causes no problems for the fetus.

Urinary Tract Infections

Urinary tract infections are common during pregnancy, probably because the enlarging uterus and hormones slow the flow of urine in the tubes that connect the kidneys to the bladder (ureters). When urine flow is slow, bacteria may not be flushed out of the urinary tract, increasing the risk of an infection. Urinary tract infections increase the risk of preterm labor and premature rupture of the membranes containing the fetus. Sometimes an infection in the bladder or ureters spreads up the urinary tract and reaches a kidney, causing an infection there (see page 1670). Bacteria may infect the urine without causing symptoms of urinary tract infections, so doctors usually check the urine for bacteria even in pregnant women without symptoms.

Treatment consists of antibiotics. Women who have had more than one infection or have had a kidney infection need to take antibiotics throughout pregnancy to prevent subsequent urinary tract infections.

CHAPTER

255 Pregnancy and Drug Use

More than 90% of pregnant women take prescription or nonprescription (over-the-counter) drugs or use social drugs (such as tobacco and alcohol) or illicit drugs at some time during pregnancy. In general, drugs should not be used during pregnancy unless absolutely necessary because many can harm the fetus. About 2 to 3% of all birth defects result from the use of drugs other than alcohol.

Sometimes drugs are essential for the health of the pregnant woman and the fetus. In such cases, a woman should talk with her doctor or other health care practitioner about the risks and benefits of taking the drugs. Before taking any drug (including over-the-counter drugs) or dietary supplement (including medicinal herbs), a pregnant woman should consult her health care practitioner. A health care practitioner may recommend that a woman take certain vitamins and minerals during pregnancy.

Drugs taken by a pregnant woman reach the fetus primarily by crossing the placenta, the same route

CATEGORIES OF RISK FOR DRUGS DURING PREGNANCY

CATEGORY	DESCRIPTION
A	These drugs are the safest. Well-designed studies in people show no risks to the fetus.
B	Studies in animals show no risk to the fetus, and no well-designed studies in people have been done. *or* Studies in animals show a risk to the fetus, but well-designed studies in people do not.
C	No adequate studies in animals or people have been done. *or* In animal studies, use of the drug resulted in harm to the fetus, but no information about how the drug affects the human fetus is available.
D	Evidence shows a risk to the human fetus, but benefits of the drug may outweigh risks in certain situations. For example, the mother may have a life-threatening disorder or a serious disorder that cannot be treated with safer drugs.
X	Risk to the fetus has been proved to outweigh any possible benefit.

How Drugs Cross the Placenta

Some of the fetus's blood vessels are contained in tiny hairlike projections (villi) of the placenta that extend into the wall of the uterus. The mother's blood passes through the space surrounding the villi (intervillous space). Only a thin membrane (placental membrane) separates the mother's blood in the intervillous space from the fetus's blood in the villi. Drugs in the mother's blood can cross this membrane into blood vessels in the villi and pass through the umbilical cord to the fetus.

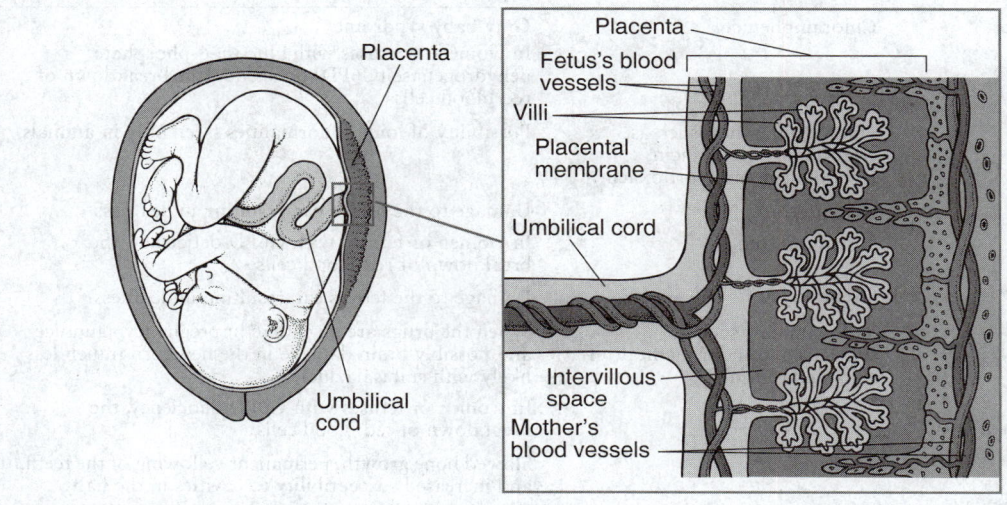

taken by oxygen and nutrients, which are needed for the fetus's growth and development. Drugs that a pregnant woman takes during pregnancy can affect the fetus in several ways:

- They can act directly on the fetus, causing damage, abnormal development (leading to birth defects), or death.
- They can alter the function of the placenta, usually by causing blood vessels to narrow (constrict) and thus reducing the supply of oxygen and nutrients to the fetus from the mother. Sometimes the result is a baby that is underweight and underdeveloped.
- They can cause the muscles of the uterus to contract forcefully, indirectly injuring the fetus by reducing its blood supply or triggering preterm labor and delivery.

How a drug affects a fetus depends on the fetus's stage of development and the strength and dose of the drug. Certain drugs taken early in pregnancy (within 20 days after fertilization) may act in an all-or-nothing fashion, killing the fetus or not affecting it at all. During this early stage, the fetus is highly resistant to birth defects. However, the fetus is particularly vulnerable to birth defects between the 3rd and the 8th week after fertilization, when its organs are developing. Drugs reaching the fetus during this stage may have no effect, or they may cause a miscarriage, an obvious birth defect, or a permanent but subtle defect that is noticed later in life. Drugs taken after organ development is complete are unlikely to cause obvious birth defects, but they may alter the growth and function of normally formed organs and tissues.

The Food and Drug Administration (FDA) classifies drugs according to the degree of risk they pose for the fetus if they are used during pregnancy. Some drugs are highly toxic and should never be used by pregnant women because they cause severe birth defects. One example is thalidomide. Several decades ago, this drug caused extreme underdevelopment of arms and legs and defects of the intestine, heart, and blood vessels in the babies of women who took the drug during pregnancy. Some drugs cause birth defects in animals, but the same effects have not been seen in people. One example is meclizine, frequently taken for motion sickness, nausea, and vomiting.

Often, a safer drug can be substituted for one that is likely to cause harm during pregnancy. For an overactive thyroid gland, propylthiouracil is usually preferred. For prevention of blood clots, the anticoagulant heparin is preferred. Several safe antibiotics, such as penicillin, are available.

SOME DRUGS THAT CAN CAUSE PROBLEMS DURING PREGNANCY*

TYPE	EXAMPLES	PROBLEM
Antianxiety drug	Diazepam	When the drug is taken late in pregnancy, depression, irritability, shaking, and exaggerated reflexes in the newborn
Antibiotics	Chloramphenicol	Gray baby syndrome
		In women or fetuses with glucose-6-phosphate dehydrogenase (G6PD) deficiency, the breakdown of red blood cells
	Fluoroquinolones (such as ciprofloxacin, ofloxacin, levofloxacin, and norfloxacin)	Possibility of joint abnormalities (seen only in animals)
	Kanamycin	Damage to the fetus's ear, resulting in deafness
	Nitrofurantoin	In women or fetuses with G6PD deficiency, the breakdown of red blood cells
	Streptomycin	Damage to the fetus's ear, resulting in deafness
	Sulfonamides (such as sulfasalazine and trimethoprim-sulfamethoxazole)	When the drugs are given late in pregnancy, jaundice and possibly brain damage in the newborn (much less likely with sulfasalazine)
		In women or fetuses with G6PD deficiency, the breakdown of red blood cells
	Tetracycline	Slowed bone growth, permanent yellowing of the teeth, and increased susceptibility to cavities in the baby
		Occasionally, liver failure in the pregnant woman
Anticoagulants	Heparin	When the drug is taken a long time, osteoporosis and a decrease in the number of platelets (which help blood clot) in the pregnant woman
	Warfarin	Birth defects
		Bleeding problems in the fetus and the pregnant woman
Anticonvulsants	Carbamazepine	Some risk of birth defects
		Bleeding problems in the newborn, which can be prevented if pregnant women take vitamin K by mouth every day for a month before delivery or if the newborn is given an injection of vitamin K soon after birth
	Phenobarbital	Same as those for carbamazepine
	Phenytoin	Same as those for carbamazepine
	Trimethadione	Increased risk of miscarriage
		High (70%) risk of birth defects, including a cleft palate and defects of the heart, face, skull, hands, and abdominal organs
	Valproate	Some (1%) risk of birth defects, including a cleft palate and defects of the heart, face, skull, spine, and limbs
Antihypertensives	Angiotensin-converting enzyme (ACE) inhibitors (see table on page 340)	When the drugs are taken late in pregnancy, kidney damage in the fetus, a reduction in the amount of fluid around the developing fetus (amniotic fluid), and defects of the face, limbs, and lungs
	Beta-blockers	When some beta-blockers are taken during pregnancy, a slowed heart rate and low blood sugar level in the fetus and possibly slowed growth

(continued on the following page)

SOME DRUGS THAT CAN CAUSE PROBLEMS DURING PREGNANCY* (Continued)

TYPE	EXAMPLES	PROBLEM
Antihypertensives (continued)	Thiazide diuretics	A decrease in the levels of oxygen, sodium, and potassium and in the number of platelets in the fetus's blood Slowed growth
Chemotherapy drugs	Actinomycin	Possibility of birth defects (seen only in animals)
	Busulfan	Birth defects such as underdevelopment of the lower jaw, cleft palate, abnormal development of the skull bones, spinal defects, ear defects, and clubfoot Slowed growth
	Chlorambucil	Same as those for busulfan
	Cyclophosphamide	Same as those for busulfan
	Mercaptopurine	Same as those for busulfan
	Methotrexate	Same as those for busulfan
	Vinblastine	Possibility of birth defects (seen only in animals)
	Vincristine	Possibility of birth defects (seen only in animals)
Mood-stabilizing drug	Lithium	Birth defects (mainly of the heart), lethargy, reduced muscle tone, poor feeding, underactivity of the thyroid gland, and nephrogenic diabetes insipidus in the newborn
Nonsteroidal anti-inflammatory drugs (NSAIDs)	Aspirin and other salicylates Ibuprofen Naproxen	When the drugs are taken in large doses, a delay in the start of labor, premature closing of the connection between the aorta and artery to the lungs (ductus arteriosus), jaundice, and (occasionally) brain damage in the fetus and bleeding problems in the woman during and after delivery and in the newborn When the drugs are taken late in pregnancy, a reduction in the amount of fluid around the developing fetus
Oral antihyperglycemic drugs	Chlorpropamide	A very low blood sugar level in the newborn Inadequate control of diabetes in the pregnant woman When the drug is taken early in pregnancy by a woman with type 2 diabetes, possibility of increased risk of birth defects
	Tolbutamide	Same as those for chlorpropamide
Sex hormones	Danazol	When this drug is taken very early in pregnancy, masculinization of a female fetus's genitals, sometimes requiring surgery to correct
	Diethylstilbestrol (DES)	Abnormalities of the uterus, menstrual problems, and an increased risk of vaginal cancer and complications during pregnancy in daughters Abnormalities of the penis in sons
	Synthetic progestins (but not the low doses used in oral contraceptives)	Same as those for danazol
Skin treatments	Etretinate	Birth defects, such as heart defects, small ears, and hydrocephalus (sometimes called water on the brain)
	Isotretinoin	Same as those for etretinate Mental retardation (intellectual disability) Risk of miscarriage

(continued on the following page)

SOME DRUGS THAT CAN CAUSE PROBLEMS DURING PREGNANCY* (*Continued*)

TYPE	EXAMPLES	PROBLEM
Thyroid drugs	Methimazole	An enlarged or underactive thyroid gland in the fetus
		Scalp defects in the newborn
	Propylthiouracil	An enlarged or underactive thyroid gland in the fetus
	Radioactive iodine	Destruction of the thyroid gland in the fetus
		When the drug is given near the end of the 1st trimester, very overactive and enlarged thyroid gland in the fetus
	Triiodothyronine	An overactive and enlarged thyroid gland in the fetus
Vaccines (live virus)	Vaccine for German measles (rubella) and chickenpox (varicella)	Potential infection of the placenta and developing fetus
	Vaccines for measles, mumps, polio, or yellow fever	Potential but unknown risks

* Unless absolutely necessary, drugs should not be used during pregnancy. However, drugs are sometimes essential for the health of the pregnant woman and the fetus. In such cases, a woman should talk with her health care practitioner about the risks and benefits of taking the drugs.

Some drugs can have effects after they are stopped. For example, isotretinoin, a drug used to treat skin disorders, is stored in fat beneath the skin and is released slowly. Isotretinoin can cause birth defects if women become pregnant within 2 weeks after the drug is stopped. Therefore, women are advised to wait at least 3 to 4 weeks after the drug is stopped before they become pregnant.

Vaccines made with a live virus (such as the rubella and varicella vaccines) are not given to women who are or might be pregnant. Other vaccines (such as those for cholera, hepatitis A and B, plague, rabies, tetanus, diphtheria, and typhoid) are given to pregnant women only if they are at substantial risk of developing that particular infection. However, all pregnant women who are in the 2nd or 3rd trimester during the influenza (flu) season should be vaccinated against the influenza virus.

Drugs to lower high blood pressure (antihypertensives) may be needed by pregnant women who have had high blood pressure before pregnancy or who develop it during pregnancy. Either type of high blood pressure increases the risk of problems for the woman and the fetus (see pages 1632 and 1649). However, antihypertensives can markedly reduce blood flow to the placenta if they lower blood pressure too rapidly in pregnant women. So pregnant women who have to take these drugs are closely monitored. Two types of antihypertensives—angiotensin-converting enzyme (ACE) inhibitors and thiazide diuretics—are usually not given to pregnant women because these drugs can cause serious problems in the fetus.

Digoxin, used to treat heart failure and some abnormal heart rhythms, readily crosses the placenta. But it typically has little effect on the baby before or after birth.

Most antidepressants appear to be relatively safe when used during pregnancy.

Social Drugs

Cigarette (Tobacco) Smoking: Although cigarette smoking harms both pregnant women and their fetus, only about 20% of women who smoke quit during pregnancy. The most consistent effect of smoking on the fetus during pregnancy is a reduction in birth weight: The more a woman smokes during pregnancy, the less the baby is likely to weigh. The average birth weight of babies born to women who smoke during pregnancy is 6 ounces less than that of babies born to women who do not smoke. The reduction in birth weight seems to be greater among the babies of older smokers.

Birth defects of the heart, brain, and face are more common among babies of smokers than among those of nonsmokers. Also, the risk of sudden infant death syndrome (SIDS) may be increased. A mislocated placenta (placenta previa), premature detachment of the placenta (abruptio placentae), premature rupture of the membranes (containing the fetus), preterm labor, uterine infections, miscarriages, stillbirths, and premature births are also more likely. In addition, children of women who smoke have slight but measurable deficiencies in physical growth and in intellectual and behavioral development. These effects

Taking Drugs While Breastfeeding

When mothers who are breastfeeding have to take a drug, they wonder whether they should stop breastfeeding. The answer depends on the following:

- How much of the drug passes into the milk
- Whether the drug is absorbed by the baby
- How the drug affects the baby
- How much milk the baby consumes, which depends on the baby's age and the amount of other foods and liquids in the baby's diet

Some drugs, such as epinephrine, heparin, and insulin, do not pass into breast milk and are thus safe to take. Most drugs pass into breast milk but usually in tiny amounts. However, even in tiny amounts, some drugs can harm the baby. Some drugs pass into breast milk, but the baby usually absorbs so little of them that they do not affect the baby. Examples are the antibiotics gentamicin, kanamycin, streptomycin, and tetracycline.

Drugs that are considered safe include most non-prescription (over-the-counter) drugs. Exceptions are antihistamines (commonly contained in cough and cold remedies, allergy drugs, motion sickness drugs, and sleep aids) and, if taken in large amounts for a long time, aspirin and other salicylates. Acetaminophen and ibuprofen, taken in usual doses, appear to be safe.

Drugs that are applied to the skin, eyes, or nose or that are inhaled are usually safe. Most antihypertensive drugs do not cause significant problems in breastfed babies. Women may take beta-blockers during breastfeeding, but the baby should be checked regularly for possible side effects, such as a slow heart rate and low blood pressure. Warfarin can be taken if the baby is full-term and healthy, but its use should be monitored.

Caffeine and theophylline do not harm breastfed babies but may make them irritable. The baby's heart and breathing rates may increase.

Even though some drugs are reportedly safe for breastfed babies, women who are breastfeeding should consult a health care practitioner before taking any drug, even an over-the-counter drug, or a medicinal herb. All drug labels should be checked to see whether they contain warnings against use during breastfeeding.

Some drugs require a doctor's supervision during their use. Taking them safely while breastfeeding may require adjusting the dose, limiting the length of time the drug is used, or timing when the drug is taken in relation to breastfeeding.

Most antianxiety drugs, antidepressants, and antipsychotic drugs require a doctor's supervision, even though they are unlikely to cause significant problems in the baby. However, these drugs stay in the body a long time. During the first few months of life, babies may have difficulty eliminating the drugs, and the drugs may affect the baby's nervous system. For example, the antianxiety drug diazepam (a benzodiazepine) causes lethargy, drowsiness, and weight loss in breastfed babies. Babies eliminate phenobarbital (an anticonvulsant and a barbiturate) slowly, so this drug may cause excessive drowsiness. Because of these effects, doctors reduce the dose of benzodiazepines and barbiturates as well as monitor their use by women who are breastfeeding.

Some drugs should not be taken by mothers who are breastfeeding. They include amphetamines, chemotherapy drugs (such as doxorubicin and methotrexate), chloramphenicol, ergotamine, lithium, radioactive drugs for diagnostic procedures, and illicit drugs such as cocaine, heroin, and phencyclidine (PCP). Drugs that may suppress milk production should not be taken. They include bromocriptine, estrogen, oral contraceptives that contain high-dose estrogen and a progestin, and levodopa.

If women who are breastfeeding must take a drug that may harm the baby, they must stop breastfeeding. But they can resume breastfeeding after they stop taking the drug. While taking the drug, women can maintain their milk supply by pumping breast milk, which is then discarded.

Women who smoke should not breastfeed within 2 hours of smoking and should never smoke in the presence of their baby whether they are breastfeeding or not. Smoking reduces milk production and interferes with normal weight gain in the baby.

Alcohol consumed in large amounts can make the baby drowsy and cause profuse sweating. The baby's length may not increase normally, and the baby may gain excess weight.

---

are thought to be caused by carbon monoxide and nicotine. Carbon monoxide may reduce the oxygen supply to the body's tissues. Nicotine stimulates the release of hormones that constrict the vessels supplying blood to the uterus and placenta, so that less oxygen and fewer nutrients reach the fetus.

Pregnant women should avoid exposure to secondhand smoke because it may similarly harm the fetus.

Alcohol: Drinking alcohol during pregnancy is the leading known cause of birth defects. Because the amount of alcohol required to cause fetal alcohol syndrome is unknown, pregnant women are advised to abstain from drinking any alcohol regularly or on binges. Avoiding alcohol altogether may be even safer. The range of effects of drinking during pregnancy is great.

The risk of miscarriage almost doubles for women who drink alcohol in any form during pregnancy, especially if they drink heavily. Often, the birth weight of babies born to women who drink regularly during pregnancy is substantially below normal. The average birth weight is about 4 pounds for babies exposed to large amounts of alcohol, compared with 7 pounds for all babies. Newborns of women who drank during pregnancy may not thrive and are more likely to die soon after birth.

Fetal alcohol syndrome is one of the most serious consequences of drinking during pregnancy. Binge drinking as few as three drinks a day can cause this syndrome. It occurs in about 2 of 1,000 live births. This syndrome includes inadequate growth before or after birth, facial defects, a small head (probably caused by inadequate growth of the brain), mental retardation (intellectual disability), and abnormal behavioral development. Less commonly, the position and function of the joints are abnormal and heart defects are present.

Babies or developing children of women who drank alcohol during pregnancy may have severe behavioral problems, such as antisocial behavior and attention deficit disorder. These problems can occur even when the baby has no obvious physical birth defects.

Caffeine: Whether consuming caffeine during pregnancy harms the fetus is unclear. Evidence seems to suggest that consuming caffeine in small amounts (for example, one cup of coffee a day) during pregnancy poses little or no risk to the fetus. Caffeine, which is contained in coffee, tea, some sodas, chocolate, and some drugs, is a stimulant that readily crosses the placenta to the fetus. Thus, it may stimulate the fetus, increasing the heart rate. Caffeine also may decrease blood flow across the placenta and decreases the absorption of iron (possibly increasing the risk of anemia (see page 1628). Some evidence suggests that drinking more than seven cups of coffee a day may increase the risk of having a stillbirth, premature birth, low-birth-weight baby, or miscarriage. Some experts recommend limiting coffee consumption and drinking decaffeinated beverages when possible.

Aspartame: Aspartame, an artificial sweetener, appears to be safe during pregnancy when it is consumed in small amounts, such as in amounts used in normal portions of artificially sweetened foods and beverages. Pregnant women with phenylketonuria, an unusual disorder, should not consume any aspartame.

Illicit Drugs

Use of illicit drugs (particularly opioids) during pregnancy can cause complications during pregnancy and serious problems in the developing fetus and the newborn. For pregnant women, injecting illicit drugs increases the risk of infections that can affect or be transmitted to the fetus. These infections include hepatitis and sexually transmitted diseases (including AIDS). Also, when pregnant women take illicit drugs, growth of the fetus is more likely to be inadequate, and premature births are more common.

Babies born to mothers who use cocaine often have problems, but whether cocaine is the cause of those problems is unclear. For example, the cause may be cigarette smoking, use of other illicit drugs, deficient prenatal care, or poverty.

Hallucinogens, such as methylenedioxymethamphetamine (MDMA, or Ecstasy), rohypnol, ketamine, methamphetamine, and LSD (lysergic acid diethylamide) may, depending on the drug, increase the risk of spontaneous miscarriage, premature delivery, or withdrawal syndrome in the fetus or newborn.

Opioids: Opioids, such as heroin, methadone, and morphine, readily cross the placenta. Consequently, the fetus may become addicted to them and may have withdrawal symptoms 6 hours to 8 days after birth (see page 2097). However, use of opioids rarely results in birth defects. Use of opioids during pregnancy increases the risk of complications during pregnancy, such as miscarriage, abnormal presentation of the baby, and preterm delivery. Babies of heroin users are more likely to be small.

Amphetamines: Use of amphetamines during pregnancy may result in birth defects, especially of the heart.

Marijuana: Whether use of marijuana during pregnancy can harm the fetus is unclear. The main component of marijuana, tetrahydrocannabinol, can cross the placenta and thus may affect the fetus. However, marijuana does not appear to increase the risk of birth defects or to slow the growth of the fetus. Marijuana does not cause behavioral problems in the newborn unless it is used heavily during pregnancy.

Drugs Used During Labor and Delivery

Local anesthetics, opioids, and other analgesics usually cross the placenta and can affect the newborn. For example, they can weaken the newborn's urge to breathe. Therefore, if these drugs are needed during labor, they are given in the smallest effective doses (see page 1654).

256 Complications of Pregnancy

Pregnancy complications are problems that occur only during pregnancy. They may affect the woman, the fetus, or both and may occur at different times during the pregnancy. For example, complications such as a mislocated placenta (placenta previa) or premature detachment of the placenta from the uterus (placental abruption) can cause bleeding from the vagina during the last 3 months of pregnancy. Women who bleed at this time are at risk of losing the baby or of bleeding excessively (hemorrhaging). There is also a very slight risk of dying during labor and delivery. However, most pregnancy complications can be effectively treated.

Problems With Amniotic Fluid

Amniotic fluid is the fluid that surrounds the fetus in the uterus. The fluid and fetus are contained in membranes called the amniotic sac. There may be too much or too little amniotic fluid.

Too much amniotic fluid (polyhydramnios or hydramnios) stretches the uterus and puts pressure on the diaphragm of pregnant women. This complication can lead to severe breathing problems for women or to labor that begins before 37 weeks of pregnancy (preterm labor).

Too much fluid may accumulate because of the following:

- Diabetes in the pregnant woman
- More than one fetus (multiple births)
- Rh antibodies to the fetus's blood produced by the pregnant woman (Rh incompatibility)
- Birth defects in the fetus, especially a blocked esophagus or defects of the brain and spinal cord (such as spina bifida)

However, about half the time, the cause is unknown.

Too little amniotic fluid (oligohydramnios) also can cause problems. If the amount of fluid is greatly reduced, the fetus's lungs may be immature and the fetus may be compressed, resulting in deformities. This combination of conditions is called Potter's syndrome.

There tends to be too little amniotic fluid in the following situations:

- The fetus has birth defects in the urinary tract.
- The fetus has not grown as much as expected.
- The fetus has died.
- The fetus has a chromosomal abnormality.

- The placenta is not functioning normally (as a result, the fetus may not grow as much as expected).
- The pregnancy has lasted too long (42 weeks or more).

Taking certain drugs such as angiotensin-converting enzyme (ACE) inhibitors (including enalapril or captopril) during the 2nd and 3rd trimesters can result in too little amniotic fluid. These drugs are usually avoided during pregnancy but sometimes may be needed to treat severe heart failure or high blood pressure. Taking nonsteroidal anti-inflammatory drugs (NSAIDs, such as aspirin or ibuprofen) late in pregnancy also can reduce the amount of amniotic fluid.

Doctors may suspect too much or too little amniotic fluid when the uterus is too large or too small for the length of the pregnancy. Sometimes the problem is incidentally detected during ultrasonography.

Cervical Incompetence

Cervical incompetence is painless opening of the cervix that results in delivery of the baby between 16 and 22 weeks of pregnancy.

- Connective tissue disorders present at birth and injuries can make tissues of the cervix weak.
- Cervical incompetence is identified only after a woman become pregnant.
- When the risk of cervical incompetence is high, the cervix is stitched closed to prevent early delivery of the baby.

Normally, the cervix dilates only when labor starts, in response to contractions of the uterus. However, in some women, tissues of the cervix (the lower part of the uterus) are weak. When the growing fetus and placenta put pressure on the weak tissues, the cervix may open (dilate) long before the baby is due. As a result, the baby may be delivered too early. If cervical incompetence has occurred, the risk that it will recur in a subsequent pregnancy is probably less than 30%. The risk is higher for women who have had three or more miscarriages during the 2nd trimester.

Causes

The cervix may be weak because of a connective tissue disorder present at birth (congenital), such as Ehlers-Danlos syndrome, or because of an injury. For example, injuries may occur when a large piece of tissue is removed from the cervix for a biopsy or when instruments are used to dilate the cervix (as can occur during dilation and curettage, or D & C).

The following also increase the risk of having a weak cervix:

- Use of fertility drugs such as clomiphene, which often results in more than one fetus (multiple births)
- Birth defects of the genital organs
- A short cervix, detected during ultrasonography
- Previous miscarriages during the 2nd trimester

Diagnosis and Treatment

Cervical incompetence is not identified until the woman becomes pregnant. It is suspected when a woman has had previous miscarriages during the 2nd trimester. Findings during ultrasonography may also suggest cervical incompetence. For example, if ultrasonography shows that a woman has a short cervix, particularly a woman who is at risk of cervical incompetence, doctors may closely watch for signs of premature labor. Doctors can detect early dilation of the cervix when they do routine examinations during pregnancy.

Doctors can place stitches around or through the cervix to keep it closed. Sometimes they close the cervix with tape or wires. Such procedures are called cervical cerclage. Cervical cerclage is done if the risk of cervical incompetence is high, such as when a woman has had previous episodes. Before cervical cerclage, the woman is given a general or regional anesthetic. Then doctors usually insert instruments through the vagina to place the stitches. Stitches are usually removed before delivery. Occasionally, they are left in place, and cesarean delivery is done.

Ectopic Pregnancy

Ectopic pregnancy is attachment (implantation) of a fertilized egg in an abnormal location.

- Women may have abdominal pain and vaginal bleeding.
- Ultrasonography is done, mainly to determine the location of the fetus.
- Usually, surgery is done to remove the fetus and placenta, but sometimes a single dose of methotrexate is used to end the ectopic pregnancy.

Normally, an egg is fertilized in the fallopian tube and becomes implanted in the uterus. However, if the tube is narrowed or blocked, the fertilized egg may never reach the uterus. Sometimes the fertilized egg implants in tissues outside of the uterus, resulting in an ectopic pregnancy. Ectopic pregnancies usually develop in one of the fallopian tubes (as a tubal pregnancy) but may develop in other locations.

A fetus in an ectopic pregnancy sometimes survives for several weeks. However because tissues outside the uterus are unable to provide the necessary blood supply and support, ultimately the fetus does not survive. The structure containing the fetus typically ruptures after about 6 to 16 weeks, long before the fetus is viable. When an ectopic pregnancy ruptures, bleeding may be severe and even life threatening. The later the tube ruptures, the worse the blood loss, and the higher the risk of death.

One of 100 to 200 pregnancies is an ectopic pregnancy. Risk factors for an ectopic pregnancy include having had a disorder of the fallopian tubes, pelvic inflammatory disease, a previous ectopic pregnancy, exposure to diethylstilbestrol as a fetus, or a tubal ligation (a sterilization procedure) that was unsuccessful or has been surgically reversed.

Symptoms

Symptoms include vaginal bleeding or spotting, cramping or pain in the lower abdomen, or both. If the fallopian tube ruptures, the woman usually feels severe, constant pain in the lower abdomen. If the woman has significant blood loss, she may faint, sweat, or feel light-headed.

Diagnosis

Doctors suspect an ectopic pregnancy in women who are of reproductive age and have lower abdominal pain or vaginal bleeding. In such women, a pregnancy test is done. If the pregnancy test is positive, ultrasonography is done using a probe inserted into the vagina. If ultrasonography detects a fetus in a location other than the uterus, the diagnosis is confirmed. If ultrasonography does not detect a fetus anywhere, ectopic pregnancy is still possible or the pregnancy may be in the uterus but at too early a stage to be seen. Doctors do blood tests to measure a hormone produced by the placenta. This test can help doctors determine whether the pregnancy is too early for the fetus to be visible in the uterus.

If needed to confirm the diagnosis, doctors may use a viewing tube called a laparoscope, inserted through a small incision just below the navel. This procedure enables them to view an ectopic pregnancy directly.

Treatment

An ectopic pregnancy must be ended as soon as possible to save the life of the woman. In most women, the fetus and placenta must be removed surgically, usually with a laparoscope but sometimes through an incision in the abdomen (in a procedure called laparotomy). Rarely, the uterus is so damaged that a hysterectomy is required.

Sometimes the drug methotrexate, usually given in a single injection, can be used instead of surgery. The drug causes the ectopic pregnancy to shrink and disappear. Occasionally, surgery is needed in addition to methotrexate.

Ectopic Pregnancy: A Mislocated Pregnancy

Normally, an egg is fertilized in the fallopian tube and becomes implanted in the uterus. However, if the tube is narrowed or blocked, the egg may move slowly or become stuck. The fertilized egg may never reach the uterus, resulting in an ectopic pregnancy. An ectopic pregnancy may be located in many different places, including a fallopian tube, an ovary, the cervix, and the abdomen.

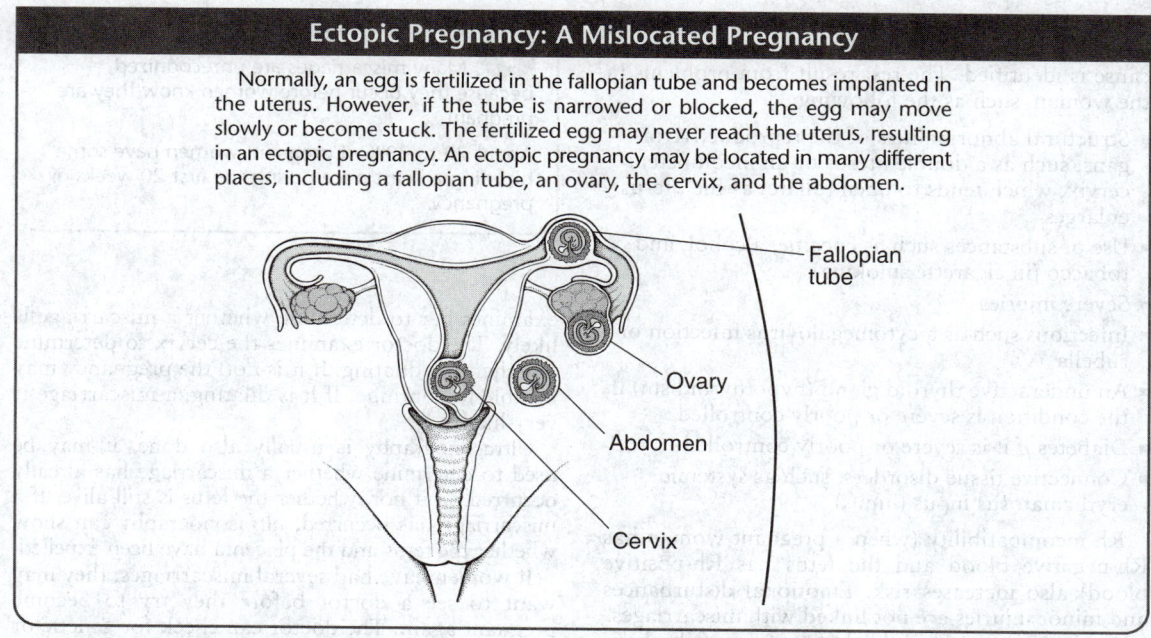

Fallopian tube

Ovary

Abdomen

Cervix

Hyperemesis Gravidarum

Hyperemesis gravidarum is extremely severe nausea and excessive vomiting during pregnancy.

Hyperemesis gravidarum differs from ordinary morning sickness. If women vomit often and have nausea to such an extent that they lose weight and become dehydrated, they have hyperemesis gravidarum. If women vomit occasionally but gain weight and are not dehydrated, they do not have hyperemesis gravidarum. The cause of hyperemesis gravidarum is unknown.

Diagnosis and Treatment

Doctors do blood and urine tests to determine whether dehydration is present and to check for electrolyte abnormalities, which may result from dehydration.

If hyperemesis gravidarum is confirmed, the woman is sometimes hospitalized for treatment because vomiting may persist for days. She is given fluids, sugar (glucose), electrolytes, and occasionally vitamins through an intravenous line inserted into a vein. She is not allowed to eat or drink anything for at least 24 hours. Sedatives, drugs used to relieve nausea (antiemetics), and other drugs are given as needed. After the woman is rehydrated and vomiting has subsided, she is given fluids to drink. If she can tolerate fluids, she can begin eating frequent, small portions of bland foods. The size of the portions is increased as they can tolerate more food.

If symptoms recur, the treatment is repeated. Rarely, if weight loss continues and symptoms persist despite

treatment, the woman is fed via a tube passed through the nose and down the throat to the small intestine for as long as necessary.

Miscarriage

A miscarriage (spontaneous abortion) is the loss of a fetus due to natural causes before 20 weeks of pregnancy.

- Miscarriages may occur because of a problem in the fetus or the woman (such as structural abnormalities, infections, certain disorders, use of cocaine or alcohol, cigarette smoking, or an injury), but the cause is often unknown.

- Bleeding and cramping may occur, particularly late in the pregnancy.

- Doctors examine the cervix and usually do ultrasonography.

- If any remnants of the pregnancy remain in the uterus after a miscarriage, they are removed.

Miscarriage is a common end to a high-risk pregnancy. A miscarriage occurs in about 15% of recognized pregnancies. Many more miscarriages are unrecognized because they occur before women know they are pregnant. About 85% of miscarriages occur during the first 12 weeks of pregnancy.

Causes

Most miscarriages that occur during the first 12 weeks of pregnancy are thought to occur because something was wrong with the fetus, such as a birth defect or a genetic disorder.

The remaining 15% of miscarriages occur during weeks 13 to 20. For many of these miscarriages, no cause is identified. The rest result from problems in the woman, such as the following:

- Structural abnormalities of the reproductive organs, such as a double uterus or an incompetent cervix, which tends to open (dilate) as the uterus enlarges
- Use of substances such as cocaine, alcohol, and tobacco (in cigarette smoking)
- Severe injuries
- Infections such as a cytomegalovirus infection or rubella
- An underactive thyroid gland (hypothyroidism) if the condition is severe or poorly controlled
- Diabetes if it is severe or poorly controlled
- Connective tissue disorders, such as systemic erythematosus lupus (lupus)

Rh incompatibility (when a pregnant woman has Rh-negative blood and the fetus has Rh-positive blood) also increases risk. Emotional disturbances and minor injuries are not linked with miscarriages.

A miscarriage is more likely for women who have had a miscarriage or preterm labor in a previous pregnancy. For women who have had three consecutive miscarriages during the 1st trimester, the chance of having another miscarriage is about 1 in 4.

Symptoms

A miscarriage is usually preceded by spotting or more obvious bleeding and a discharge from the vagina. The uterus contracts, causing cramps. However, about 20 to 30% of pregnant women have some bleeding at least once during the first 20 weeks of pregnancy. Fewer than half of these episodes result in a miscarriage.

Early in a pregnancy, the only sign of a miscarriage may be a small amount of vaginal bleeding. Later in a pregnancy, a miscarriage may cause profuse bleeding, and the blood may contain mucus or clots. Cramps become more severe until eventually, the uterus contracts enough to expel the fetus and placenta.

Sometimes the fetus dies but no symptoms of miscarriage occur. In such cases, the uterus does not enlarge. Rarely, the dead tissues in the uterus become infected before, during, or after a miscarriage. Such an infection may be serious, causing fever, chills, and a rapid heart rate. Affected women may become delirious, and blood pressure may fall.

Diagnosis

If a pregnant woman has bleeding and cramping during the first 20 weeks of pregnancy, a doctor

Did You Know...

Many miscarriages are unrecognized because they occur before women know they are pregnant.

About 20 to 30% of pregnant women have some bleeding at least once during the first 20 weeks of pregnancy.

examines her to determine whether a miscarriage is likely. The doctor examines the cervix to determine whether it is dilating. If it is not, the pregnancy may be able to continue. If it is dilating, a miscarriage is very likely.

Ultrasonography is usually also done. It may be used to determine whether a miscarriage has already occurred or, if not, whether the fetus is still alive. If a miscarriage has occurred, ultrasonography can show whether the fetus and the placenta have been expelled.

If women have had several miscarriages, they may want to see a doctor before they try to become pregnant again. The doctor can check for genetic or structural abnormalities and for other disorders that increase the risk of a miscarriage. For example, an imaging test (such as hysteroscopy or hysterosalpingography) may be done to look for structural abnormalities. If identified, some causes of a previous miscarriage can be treated, making a successful pregnancy possible.

Treatment

If the fetus is alive, bed rest may be advised to help reduce bleeding and cramping. If possible, the woman should not work but should stay off her feet at home. However, there is no clear evidence that bed rest is helpful. Refraining from sexual intercourse is advised, although intercourse has not been definitely connected with miscarriages.

If a miscarriage has occurred and the fetus and the placenta have been expelled, no treatment is needed.

If a miscarriage has occurred but some tissue from the fetus or placenta remains in the uterus, suction curettage (see page 1605) is done to remove them.

If the fetus dies during the first 13 weeks but remains in the uterus, suction curettage is usually used to remove the fetus and the placenta.

If the fetus dies later in the pregnancy, a drug that can induce labor (such as oxytocin) may be given intravenously. Oxytocin stimulates the uterus to contract and expel the fetus. Afterward, suction curettage may be needed to remove pieces of the placenta. Alternatively, a procedure similar to suction curettage called dilation and evacuation (D & E) may

Understanding the Language of Loss

Doctors may use the term *abortion* to refer to a miscarriage (spontaneous abortion) that occurs before 20 weeks of pregnancy as well as to intentional termination of pregnancy (induced abortion) for medical or other reasons. After 20 weeks of pregnancy, delivery of a fetus that has died is called a stillbirth. Terms for abortion include the following:

- **Therapeutic (induced) abortion:** An abortion that is brought about by medical means (drugs or surgery) because the woman's life or health is endangered or the fetus has major abnormalities
- **Threatened abortion:** Bleeding or cramping during the first 20 weeks of pregnancy, indicating that the fetus may be lost
- **Inevitable abortion:** Pain or bleeding with opening (dilation) of the cervix, indicating that the fetus will be lost
- **Complete abortion:** Expulsion of all of the fetus and placenta in the uterus
- **Incomplete abortion:** Expulsion of only part of the contents of the uterus
- **Missed abortion:** Retention of a dead fetus in the uterus
- **Septic abortion:** Infection of the contents of the uterus before, during, or after an abortion

be done. For D & E, labor does not need to be induced. However, this procedure may not be available because it requires special training.

Emotions After Miscarriage: After a miscarriage, women may feel grief, sadness, anger, guilt, or anxiety about subsequent pregnancies.

- **Grief:** Grief for a loss is a natural response and should not be suppressed or denied. Talking about their feelings with another person may help women deal with their feelings and gain perspective.
- **Guilt:** Women may think that they did something to cause the miscarriage. Usually, they have not. Women may recall taking a common over-the-counter drug early in pregnancy, drinking a glass of wine before they knew they were pregnant, or doing another everyday thing. These things are almost never the cause of a miscarriage, so women should not feel guilty about them.
- **Anxiety:** Women who have had a miscarriage may wish to talk with their doctor about the likelihood of a miscarriage in subsequent pregnancies and be tested if needed. Although having a miscarriage increases the risk of having another one, most women who have a miscarriage do not have problems in subsequent pregnancies.

Stillbirth

Stillbirth is death and delivery of a fetus after 20 weeks of pregnancy.

Stillbirth most commonly results when the placenta detaches from the placenta too early (placental abruption—see page 1648). It may occur when women have certain conditions, such as

- Diabetes that is poorly controlled
- Preeclampsia (a type of high blood pressure that develops during pregnancy)
- Use of substances such as cocaine, alcohol, or tobacco
- Injuries
- A clotting disorder

Sometimes stillbirth occurs when the fetus has a problem, such as a chromosomal or genetic abnormality, a birth defect, or an infection.

Doctors may suspect that the fetus is dead if the fetus stops moving, although movements often decrease as the growing fetus has less room to move. Tests, such as a nonstress test, ultrasonography, or electronic fetal monitoring, may be done to evaluate the fetus (see box on page 1654).

To try to identify the cause, doctors do genetic and blood tests (such as tests for infections and clotting disorders). Doctors also recommend evaluating the fetus to look for possible causes, such as infections and chromosomal abnormalities. The placenta and uterus are examined. Often, the cause cannot be determined.

If the dead fetus is not expelled, the woman may be given a drug such as a prostaglandin to cause the cervix to open (dilate). She is then usually given oxytocin, a drug that stimulates labor. If any tissue from the fetus or placenta remains in the uterus, suction curettage is done to remove it (see page 1605). Alternatively, dilation and evacuation (D & E) may be done to remove the dead fetus if a doctor with the special training required to do this procedure is available.

Changes that occur in women after a stillbirth are similar to those that occur after a miscarriage. Women typically feel grief at the loss and require emotional support and sometimes counseling. Whether a later pregnancy is likely to result in a stillbirth depends on the cause.

Placenta Previa

Placenta previa is attachment (implantation) of the placenta over or near the cervix, in the lower rather than the upper part of the uterus.

- Women may have painless, sometimes profuse bleeding late in the pregnancy.

- Ultrasonography can usually confirm the diagnosis.
- Bed rest may be all that is needed, but if bleeding continues or if the fetus's lungs are mature enough, cesarean delivery is usually done.

The placenta may completely or partially cover the opening of the cervix. Placenta previa occurs in 1 of 200 deliveries. As many as 15% of pregnant women have placenta previa during the 2nd trimester. The placenta previa may be visible on ultrasonography. However, it resolves on its own in more than 90% of women before they deliver. Risk is increased by the following:

- Having had more than one pregnancy
- Having had a cesarean delivery
- Having had twins, triplets, or other multiple births in a single pregnancy
- Having a structural abnormality of the uterus, such as fibroids
- Smoking

Placenta previa can cause painless bleeding from the vagina that suddenly begins late in pregnancy. The blood may be bright red. Bleeding may become profuse, endangering the life of the woman and the fetus.

When labor starts, the placenta tends to become detached very early, depriving the baby of oxygen. The lack of oxygen may result in brain damage or other problems in the baby.

Ultrasonography helps doctors identify placenta previa and distinguish it from a placenta that has detached too early (placental abruption).

Treatment

When bleeding is minor and occurs before about 34 weeks of pregnancy, doctors typically advise bed rest in the hospital until bleeding resolves. If the bleeding stops, the woman is usually encouraged to walk. If bleeding does not recur, she is usually sent home, provided that she can return to the hospital easily.

Delivery, typically cesarean, is usually done if bleeding is profuse or does not stop or if the fetus's lungs are mature enough for delivery (usually after 36 weeks). Doctors can determine whether the fetus's lungs are mature enough by taking a sample of amniotic fluid, usually from the vagina, and analyzing it. A cesarean delivery is done before labor starts. Women who bleed profusely may need repeated blood transfusions.

Placental Abruption

Placental abruption (abruptio placentae) is the premature detachment of a normally positioned placenta from the wall of the uterus.

- Women may have vaginal bleeding and severe abdominal pain and go into shock.

- Bed rest may be all that is needed, but if bleeding continues or if the pregnancy is near term, the baby is delivered as soon as possible.

The placenta may detach incompletely (sometimes just 10 to 20%) or completely. The cause is unknown. Detachment of the placenta occurs in 0.4 to 1.5% of all deliveries. The following increase risk:

- High blood pressure (including preeclampsia, a type of high blood pressure that develops during pregnancy)
- Use of cocaine
- Older age
- Vasculitis or other blood vessel disorders
- Previous placental abruption
- Abdominal injury
- Blood clotting disorders
- Use of tobacco

The uterus bleeds from the site where the placenta was attached. The blood may pass through the cervix and out the vagina as an external hemorrhage, or it may be trapped behind the placenta as a concealed hemorrhage. Thus, women may or may not have vaginal bleeding.

Symptoms and Diagnosis

Symptoms depend on the degree of detachment and the amount of blood lost (which may be massive). Symptoms may include sudden continuous or crampy abdominal pain, tenderness when the abdomen is pressed, and shock. Premature detachment of the placenta can lead to widespread clotting inside the blood vessels (disseminated intravascular coagulation), kidney failure, and bleeding into the walls of the uterus, especially in pregnant women who also have preeclampsia.

When the placenta detaches, the supply of oxygen and nutrients to the fetus may be reduced. If detachment occurs suddenly and greatly reduces the oxygen supply, the fetus may die. If it occurs gradually and less extensively, the fetus may not grow as much as expected or there may be too little amniotic fluid (oligohydramnios). Gradual detachment may cause less abdominal pain and a lower risk of shock than sudden detachment, but risk of preeclampsia and premature rupture of the membranes is increased.

Doctors suspect and usually diagnose premature detachment of the placenta on the basis of symptoms. Ultrasonography may help confirm the diagnosis.

Treatment

A woman with premature detachment of the placenta is hospitalized. The usual treatment is bed rest. If symptoms lessen, the woman is encouraged to walk and may be discharged from the hospital.

Problems With the Placenta

Normally, the placenta is located in the upper part of the uterus, firmly attached to the uterine wall until after delivery of the baby.

In placental abruption (abruptio placentae), the placenta detaches from the uterine wall prematurely, causing the uterus to bleed and reducing the fetus's supply of oxygen and nutrients. Women who have this complication are hospitalized, and the baby may be delivered early.

In placenta previa, the placenta is located over or near the cervix, in the lower part of the uterus. Placenta previa may cause painless bleeding that suddenly begins late in pregnancy. The bleeding may become profuse. The baby is usually delivered by cesarean.

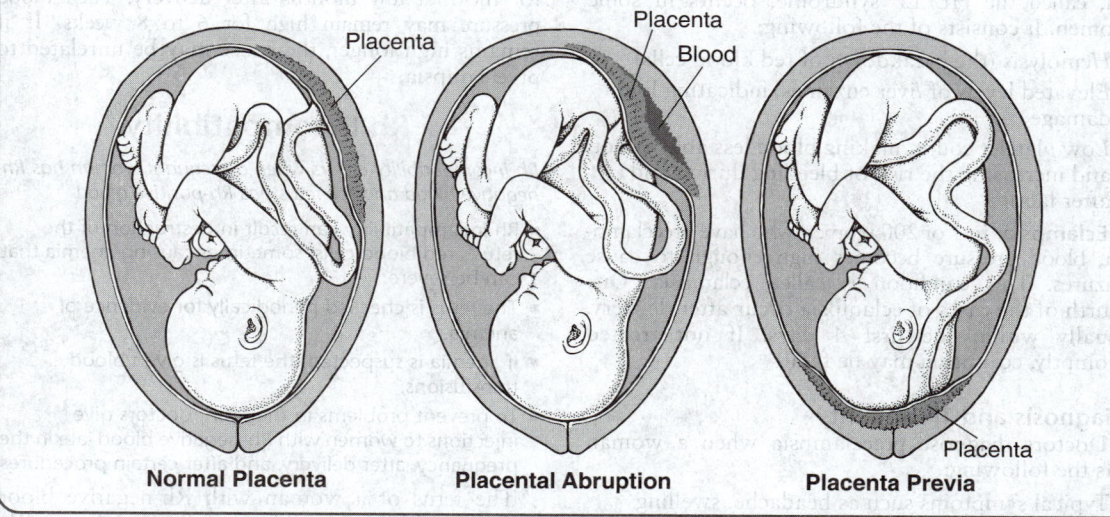

Normal Placenta **Placental Abruption** **Placenta Previa**

If bleeding continues or worsens (suggesting that the fetus is not getting enough oxygen) or if the pregnancy is near term, delivery as soon as possible is often best for the woman and the baby. If vaginal delivery is not possible, a cesarean delivery is done.

Preeclampsia

Preeclampsia is high blood pressure that is accompanied by protein in the urine and that develops after the 20th week of pregnancy.

- Preeclampsia can cause the placenta to detach and the baby to be born too early, increasing the risk that the baby will have problems soon after birth.
- The woman's hands and feet may swell, and if preeclampsia is severe, she may have seizures or organ damage.
- Depending on how severe preeclampsia is, treatment may involve bed rest, hospitalization, drugs to lower blood pressure, or delivery of the baby as soon as possible.

About 3 to 7% of pregnant women develop preeclampsia (toxemia of pregnancy). In this complication, an increase in blood pressure is accompanied by protein in the urine (proteinuria). Preeclampsia develops after the 20th week of pregnancy and usually before the end of the first week after delivery.

The cause of preeclampsia is unknown. But it is more common among women who

- Are pregnant for the first time
- Are carrying two or more fetuses
- Have had preeclampsia in a previous pregnancy
- Are obese
- Already have high blood pressure or a blood vessel disorder
- Have a blood clotting disorder
- Are younger than 20 or older than 35

Preeclampsia may lead to premature detachment of the placenta from the uterus (placental abruption). Babies may be small because the placenta malfunctions or because they are born prematurely. Babies of women with preeclampsia are 4 or 5 times more likely to have problems soon after birth than babies of women who do not have this complication.

Preeclampsia may cause fluids to accumulate (edema), resulting in swollen feet or hands. Women may gain excess weight. Tiny red dots (petechiae) may appear on the skin. Women may feel jittery. If severe, preeclampsia can damage organs, such as the brain, kidneys, lungs, or liver. Then women may have headaches, distorted vision, confusion, difficulty breathing, pain in the upper abdomen, vomiting, or other symptoms. A woman who has a new headache that does not resolve with acetaminophen or within 24 hours should call her doctor.

HELLP Syndrome: A variation of severe preeclampsia, called the HELLP syndrome, occurs in some women. It consists of the following:

- *H*emolysis (the breakdown of red blood cells)
- *E*levated *L*evels of *L*iver enzymes, indicating liver damage
- *L*ow *P*latelet count, making blood less able to clot and increasing the risk of bleeding during and after labor

Eclampsia: In 1 of 200 women who have preeclampsia, blood pressure becomes high enough to cause seizures. This condition is called eclampsia. One fourth of the cases of eclampsia occur after delivery, usually within the first 4 days. If not treated promptly, eclampsia may be fatal.

Diagnosis and Treatment

Doctors diagnose preeclampsia when a woman has the following:

- Typical symptoms such as headache, swelling around the eyes, and particularly swelling of the hands
- Increased blood pressure during the pregnancy
- Protein in the urine

Doctors may do blood and urine tests to confirm the diagnosis and to check for organ damage.

If mild preeclampsia develops early in the pregnancy, bed rest at home may be sufficient, but such women should see their doctor frequently. If preeclampsia worsens, women are usually hospitalized. There, they are kept in bed and monitored closely until the fetus is mature enough to be delivered safely. Drugs to lower blood pressure (antihypertensives) may be needed (see page 1640). A few hours before delivery, magnesium sulfate may be given intravenously to reduce the risk of seizures. If preeclampsia develops near the due date, labor is usually induced and the baby is delivered.

If preeclampsia is severe, the baby may be delivered by cesarean, which is the quickest way, unless the cervix is already opened (dilated) enough for a prompt vaginal delivery. A prompt delivery reduces the risk of complications for the woman and fetus. If blood pressure is high, drugs to lower blood pressure, such as hydralazine or labetalol, may be given intravenously before delivery is attempted. The HELLP syndrome is usually treated the same way.

After delivery, women who have had preeclampsia or eclampsia are closely monitored for 2 to 4 days because they are at increased risk of seizures. As their condition gradually improves, they are encouraged to walk. They may remain in the hospital for a few days, depending on the severity of the preeclampsia and its complications. After returning home, these women may need to take drugs to lower blood pressure. Typically, they have a checkup at least every 2 weeks for the first few months after delivery. Their blood pressure may remain high for 6 to 8 weeks. If it remains high longer, the cause may be unrelated to preeclampsia.

Rh Incompatibility

Rh incompatibility occurs when a pregnant woman has Rh-negative blood and the fetus has Rh-positive blood.

- Rh incompatibility can result in destruction of the fetus's red blood cells, sometimes causing anemia that can be severe.
- The fetus is checked periodically for evidence of anemia.
- If anemia is suspected, the fetus is given blood transfusions.
- To prevent problems in the fetus, doctors give injections to women with Rh-negative blood late in the pregnancy, after delivery, and after certain procedures.

The fetus of a woman with Rh-negative blood may have Rh-positive blood if the father has Rh-positive blood. In about 13% of marriages in the United States, the man has Rh-positive blood and the woman has Rh-negative blood.

 Did You Know...

Rh incompatibility does not cause problems in a first pregnancy.

The Rh factor is a molecule on the surface of red blood cells in some people. Blood is Rh-positive if red blood cells have the Rh factor and Rh-negative if they do not. Problems can occur if the fetus's Rh-positive blood enters the bloodstream of a woman with Rh-negative blood. The woman's immune system may recognize the fetus's red blood cells as foreign and produce antibodies, called Rh antibodies, to destroy Rh-positive blood cells. The production of these antibodies is called Rh sensitization.

During a first pregnancy, Rh sensitization is unlikely because no significant amount of the fetus's blood is likely to enter the woman's bloodstream until delivery. So the fetus or newborn rarely has problems. However, a woman becomes sensitized during delivery. Once she is sensitized, problems are more likely with each subsequent pregnancy when the fetus's blood is Rh-positive. In each pregnancy, the woman produces Rh antibodies earlier and in larger amounts.

If Rh antibodies cross the placenta to the fetus, they may destroy some of the fetus's red blood cells. If red blood cells are destroyed faster than the fetus can produce new ones, the fetus can develop anemia. Such destruction is called hemolytic disease of the fetus (erythroblastosis fetalis) or of the newborn (erythroblastosis neonatorum—see box on page 1703). In severe cases, the fetus may die. Miscarriage can occur.

Diagnosis

At the first visit to a doctor during a pregnancy, women are screened to determine whether they have Rh-positive or Rh-negative blood. If they have Rh-negative blood, their blood is checked for Rh antibodies and the father's blood type is determined. If he has Rh-positive blood, Rh sensitization is a risk. In such cases, the woman's blood is checked for Rh antibodies periodically during the pregnancy. The pregnancy can proceed as usual as long as no antibodies are detected.

If antibodies are detected, steps may be taken to protect the fetus, depending on how high the antibody level is. Doppler ultrasonography may be done periodically to evaluate blood flow in the fetus's brain. If it is abnormal, the fetus may have anemia. Then doctors anesthetize an area of skin over the woman's abdomen and use either of the following tests to check for anemia:

- **Amniocentesis:** A needle is inserted through the skin of the abdomen to withdraw fluid from the membranes that contain the fetus (amniotic sac). The level of bilirubin (a yellow pigment resulting from the normal breakdown of red blood cells) is measured in the fluid sample. If this level is high, anemia is likely.

- **Percutaneous umbilical blood sampling:** A needle is inserted through the abdomen into the umbilical cord. Blood from the fetus is then withdrawn and analyzed.

Prevention

As a precaution, women who have Rh-negative blood are given an injection of Rh antibodies at 28 weeks of pregnancy and within 72 hours after delivery of a baby who has Rh-positive blood, even after a miscarriage or an abortion. They are also given an injection after any episode of vaginal bleeding and after amniocentesis or chorionic villus sampling. The antibodies given are called $Rh_0(D)$ immune globulin. This treatment destroys any red blood cells from the baby that may have entered the woman's bloodstream. Thus, there are no red blood cells from the baby to trigger the production of antibodies by these women, and subsequent pregnancies are usually not endangered.

Treatment

If anemia is suspected, the fetus is given a blood transfusion. Usually, additional transfusions are given until the fetus is mature enough to be safely delivered. Then labor is induced. The baby may need additional transfusions after birth. Sometimes no transfusions are needed until after birth.

257 Normal Labor and Delivery

Although each labor and delivery is different, most follow a general pattern. Therefore, an expectant mother can have a general idea of what changes will occur in her body to enable her to deliver the baby and what procedures will be followed to help her. She also has several choices to make, such as whether to have a support person (such as the baby's father or another partner) present and where to have the baby.

An expectant mother may want her partner to remain with her during labor. The partner's encouragement and emotional support may help her relax, sometimes reducing her need for drugs to relieve pain. In addition, sharing the meaningful experience of childbirth has emotional and psychologic benefits, such as creating strong family bonds. On the other hand, an expectant mother may prefer privacy during labor, or the partner may not want to be present. Childbirth education classes prepare both mother and partner for the entire process.

In the United States, almost all babies are born in hospitals, but some women want to have their babies at home. However, unexpected complications can occur during or shortly after labor, even in women who had good prenatal care and no signs of any problems. Thus, most experts do not advise delivery at home. Women who prefer a homelike setting and fewer rules (for example, no limit on the number of visitors or on visiting hours) may choose birthing centers. Such centers provide an informal, personal experience of childbirth but are much safer than delivery at home. Birthing centers are part of a hospital or have an arrangement with a nearby hospital. Thus, birthing centers can provide a medical staff, emergency equipment, and full hospital facilities, if needed. If complications develop during labor, birthing centers immediately transfer the woman to the hospital.

Some hospitals have private rooms in which a woman stays from labor until discharge. These rooms are called LDRPs for labor, delivery, recovery, and postpartum (after delivery).

Regardless of the choices a woman makes, knowing what to expect helps prepare her for labor and delivery.

Labor

Labor is a series of rhythmic, progressive contractions of the uterus that gradually move the fetus through the lower part of the uterus (cervix) and birth canal (vagina) to the outside world.

Labor occurs in three main stages:

- First stage: This stage (which has two phases: initial and active) is labor proper. Contractions cause the cervix to open gradually (dilate) and to thin and pull back (efface) until it merges with the rest of the uterus. These changes enable the fetus to pass through the vagina.
- Second stage: The baby is delivered.
- Third stage: The placenta is delivered.

Labor usually starts within 2 weeks of (before or after) the estimated date of delivery. Exactly what causes labor to start is unknown. Toward the end of pregnancy (after 36 weeks), a doctor examines the cervix to try to predict when labor will start. On average, labor lasts 12 to 18 hours in a woman's first pregnancy and tends to be shorter, averaging 6 to 8 hours, in subsequent pregnancies.

Start of Labor

All pregnant women should know what the main signs of the start of labor are:

- Contractions in the lower abdomen at regular intervals
- Back pain

A woman who has had rapid deliveries in previous pregnancies should notify her doctor as soon as she thinks she is going into labor. When contractions in the lower abdomen first start, they may be weak, irregular, and far apart. They may feel like menstrual cramps. As time passes, abdominal contractions become longer, stronger, and closer together. Contractions and back pain may be preceded or accompanied by other clues, such as the following:

- **Bloody show:** A small discharge of blood mixed with mucus from the vagina is usually a clue that

labor is about to start. The bloody show may appear as early as 72 hours before contractions start.
- **Rupture of membranes:** Occasionally, the fluid-filled membranes that contain the fetus (amniotic sac) rupture before labor starts, and the amniotic fluid flows out through the vagina. This event is commonly described as "the water breaks."

When a woman's membranes rupture, she should contact her doctor or midwife immediately. About 80 to 90% of women whose membranes rupture before but near their due date go into labor spontaneously within 24 hours. If labor has not started after several hours and the baby is due, women are usually admitted to the hospital, where labor is artificially started (induced) to reduce the risk of infection. After the membranes rupture, bacteria from the vagina can enter the uterus more easily and cause an infection in the woman, the fetus, or both. Oxytocin (which causes the uterus to contract) or a similar drug, such as a prostaglandin, is used to induce labor. If the membranes rupture more than 3 weeks before the due date (prematurely), doctors do not induce labor until the fetus is more mature (see page 1657).

Admission to a Hospital or Birthing Center

When the membranes rupture or when strong contractions occur less than 6 minutes apart or last 30 seconds or more, a woman should go to a hospital or birthing center. If rupture of membranes is suspected or the cervix is dilated more than 1½ inches (4 centimeters), the woman is admitted. The strength, duration, and frequency of contractions are noted. Her weight, blood pressure, heart and breathing rates, and temperature are measured, and samples of urine and blood are taken for analysis. Her abdomen is examined to estimate how big the fetus is, whether the fetus is facing rearward or forward (position), and whether the head, face, buttocks, or shoulder is leading the way out (presentation).

Position and presentation of the fetus affect how the fetus passes through the vagina. The most common and safest combination consists of the following:

- Head first
- Facing rearward (facing down when the woman lies on her back)
- Face and body angled toward the right or left
- Neck bent forward
- Chin tucked in
- Arms folded across the chest (see art on page 1660)

Head first is called a vertex or cephalic presentation. During the last week or two before delivery, most fetuses turn so that the back of the head presents first. If the presentation is buttocks first (breech) or

Stages of Labor

FIRST STAGE

From the beginning of labor to the full opening (dilation) of the cervix—to about 4 inches (10 centimeters).

Initial (Latent) Phase

Contractions become progressively stronger and more rhythmic.

Discomfort is minimal.

The cervix begins to thin and opens to about 1½ inches (4 centimeters).

This phase lasts an average of 8½ hours (up to 20 hours) in a first pregnancy and 5 hours (up to 12 hours) in subsequent pregnancies.

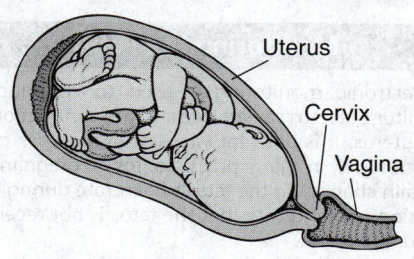

Active Phase

The cervix opens from about 1½ inches (4 centimeters) to the full 4 inches (10 centimeters). It thins and pulls back (effaces) until it merges with the rest of the uterus.

The presenting part of the baby, usually the head, begins to descend into the woman's pelvis.

The woman begins to feel the urge to push as the baby descends, but she should resist it.

This phase averages about 5 to 7 hours in a first pregnancy and 2 to 4 hours in subsequent pregnancies.

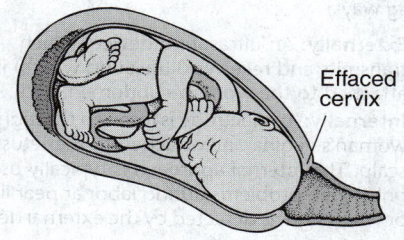

SECOND STAGE

From the complete opening of the cervix to delivery of the baby: This stage averages about 45 to 60 minutes in a first pregnancy and 15 to 30 minutes in subsequent pregnancies. During this stage, the woman pushes.

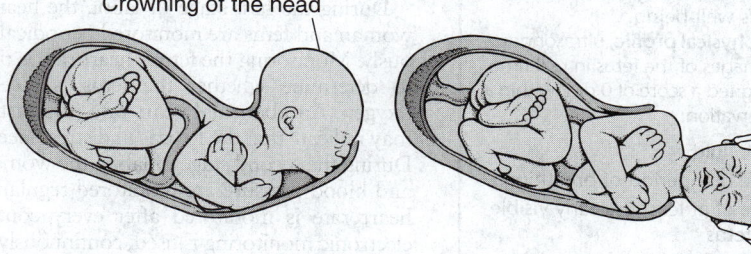

Crowning of the head

THIRD STAGE

From delivery of the baby to delivery of the placenta: This stage usually lasts only a few minutes but may last up to 30 minutes.

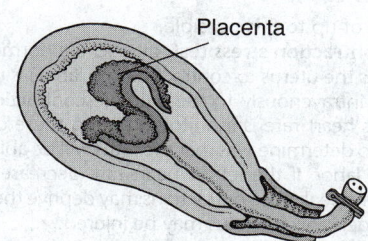

Placenta

shoulder first or the fetus is facing forward, delivery is considerably more difficult for the woman, fetus, and doctor. Cesarean delivery is recommended.

Monitoring the Fetus

Electronic monitoring is used to continuously monitor the fetus's heart rate and the contractions of the uterus. It is used for virtually all high-risk pregnancies and, in many practices, for all pregnancies. Certain changes in the fetus's heart rate during contractions can indicate that the fetus is not receiving enough oxygen.

The fetus's heart rate can be monitored in the following ways:

- **Externally:** An ultrasound device (which transmits and receives ultrasound waves) is attached to the woman's abdomen.
- **Internally:** An electrode is inserted through the woman's vagina and attached to the fetus's scalp. The internal approach is typically used only when problems during labor appear likely or when signals detected by the external device cannot be recorded.

In a high-risk pregnancy, electronic monitoring is sometimes used as part of a nonstress test, in which the fetus's heart rate is monitored as the fetus lies still and as it moves. If the heart rate does not increase with movement (is nonreactive), an ultrasound biophysical profile or a contraction stress test may be done. These tests check on the fetus's well-being.

For an **ultrasound biophysical profile**, ultrasonography is used to produce images of the fetus in real time, and the following are assigned a score of 0 or 2 within a 30-minute period of observation:

- Amount of amniotic fluid
- Presence or absence of a period of breathing
- Presence or absence of at least 3 clearly visible movements of the fetus
- Muscle tone of the fetus, indicated by certain back and forth changes in position of fingers, a limb, or the trunk

A score of up to 8 is possible.

For **a contraction stress test**, oxytocin (a hormone that causes the uterus to contract during labor) is usually given intravenously to start uterine contractions. The fetus's heart rate is monitored during these contractions to determine whether the fetus will be able to withstand labor. If the fetus's heart rate decreases as contractions peak, the contractions may deprive the fetus of oxygen and the fetus may be injured.

On the basis of such tests, a doctor may allow labor to continue or may do a cesarean delivery immediately.

A **vaginal examination** is done to determine whether the membranes have ruptured and how dilated and effaced the cervix is, but this examination may be omitted if the woman is bleeding or if the membranes have ruptured spontaneously. The color of the amniotic fluid is noted. The fluid should be clear and have no significant odor. If the membranes rupture and the amniotic fluid is green, the discoloration results from the fetus's first stool (fetal meconium).

An **intravenous line** is usually inserted into the woman's arm during labor in a hospital. This line is used to give the woman fluids to prevent dehydration and, if needed, to give drugs.

When fluids are given intravenously, the woman does not have to eat or drink during labor, although she may choose to drink some fluids and eat some light food early in labor. An empty stomach during delivery makes the woman less likely to vomit. Very rarely, vomit is inhaled. Inhaling vomit can cause inflammation of the lungs, which can be life threatening. Usually, the woman is given an antacid by mouth to neutralize stomach acid when she is admitted to the hospital and every 3 hours after that. Antacids reduce the risk of damage to the lungs if vomit is inhaled.

Fetal Monitoring

Soon after the woman is admitted to the hospital, the doctor or another health care practitioner listens to the fetus's heartbeat periodically using a handheld Doppler ultrasound device, or electronic fetal heart monitoring is used to continuously monitor heartbeats.

During the first stage of labor, the heart rates of the woman and fetus are monitored periodically or continuously. Monitoring the fetus's heart rate is the easiest way to determine whether the fetus is receiving enough oxygen. An abnormal heart rate (too fast or too slow) may indicate that the fetus is in distress (see page 1659). During the second stage of labor, the woman's heart rate and blood pressure are monitored regularly. The fetus's heart rate is monitored after every contraction or, if electronic monitoring is used, continuously.

Pain Relief

With the advice of her doctor or midwife, a woman usually plans an approach to pain relief long before labor starts. She may choose natural childbirth, which relies on relaxation and breathing techniques to deal with pain, or she may plan to use analgesics (given intravenously) or a particular type of anesthetic (local or regional) if needed. After labor starts, these plans may be modified, depending on how labor progresses, how the woman feels, and what the doctor or midwife recommends.

A woman's need for pain relief during labor varies considerably, depending to some extent on her level of anxiety. Attending childbirth preparation classes helps prepare the woman for labor and delivery. Such preparation and emotional support from the people attending the labor tend to lessen anxiety and often markedly reduce her need for drugs to relieve pain.

Analgesics may be used. If a woman requests analgesics during labor, they are usually given to her. However, because some of these drugs can slow (depress) breathing and other functions of the newborn, the amount given is as small as possible. Most commonly, fentanyl or morphine is given intravenously to relieve pain. These drugs may slow the initial phase of the first stage of labor, so they are usually given during the active phase of the first stage. In addition, because these drugs have the greatest effect during the first 30 minutes after they are given, the drugs are often not given when delivery is imminent. If they are given too close to delivery, the newborn may be overly sedated, making adjustment to life outside the uterus more difficult. To counteract the sedating effects of these drugs on the newborn, a doctor can give the newborn the drug naloxone immediately after delivery.

Local anesthesia numbs the vagina and the tissues around its opening. Commonly, this area is numbed by injecting a local anesthetic through the wall of the vagina into the area around the nerve that supplies sensation to the lower genital area (pudendal nerve). This procedure, called a pudendal block, is used only late in the second stage of labor, when the baby's head is about to emerge from the vagina. Another common but less effective procedure involves injecting a local anesthetic at the opening of the vagina. With both procedures, the woman can remain awake and push, and the fetus's functions are unaffected. These procedures are useful for deliveries that have no complications.

Regional anesthesia numbs a larger area. It may be used for women who want more complete pain relief. The following procedures can be used:

- **Lumbar epidural injection** is almost always used. It is used much more often than pudendal blocks. An anesthetic is injected in the lower back—into the space between the spine and the outer layer of tissue covering the spinal cord (epidural space). Alternatively, a catheter is placed in the epidural space, and an opioid, such as fentanyl or sufentanil, is continuously and slowly given through the catheter. A lumbar epidural injection for labor and delivery does not prevent the woman from pushing adequately.

- **Spinal injection** involves injecting an anesthetic into the space between the middle and inner layers of tissue covering the spinal cord (subarachnoid space). A spinal injection is typically used for cesarean delivery when there are no complications.

Natural Childbirth

Natural childbirth uses relaxation and breathing techniques to control pain during childbirth. Natural childbirth often helps reduce or eliminate the need for analgesics or anesthetics during labor and delivery.

To prepare for natural childbirth, a pregnant woman and her partner take childbirth classes, usually six to eight sessions over several weeks, to learn how to use the relaxation and breathing techniques. They also learn what happens in the various stages of labor and delivery.

The relaxation technique involves consciously tensing a part of the body and then relaxing it. This technique helps a woman relax the rest of her body while the uterus is contracting during labor and relax her whole body between contractions.

The breathing technique involves several types of breathing, which are used at different times during labor. During the first stage of labor, before the woman begins to push, the following types of breathing may help:

- Deep breathing with slow exhalation to help the woman relax at the beginning and end of a contraction
- Fast, shallow breathing (panting) in the upper chest at the peak of a contraction
- A pattern of panting and blowing to help the woman refrain from pushing when she has an urge to push before the cervix is completely dilated

In the second stage of labor, the woman alternates between pushing and panting.

The woman and her partner should practice relaxation and breathing techniques regularly during pregnancy. During labor, the woman's partner can help her by reminding her of what she should be doing at a particular stage and by noticing when she is tense, in addition to providing emotional support. The partner may massage the woman to help her relax more.

The most well-known method of natural childbirth is probably the Lamaze method. Another method, the Leboyer method, includes birth in a darkened room and immersion of the baby into lukewarm water immediately after delivery.

Occasionally, use of either an epidural or a spinal injection causes a fall in blood pressure. Consequently, if one of these procedures is used, the woman's blood pressure is measured frequently.

General anesthesia makes a woman temporarily unconscious. It is rarely necessary and infrequently used because it may slow the function of the fetus's heart, lungs, and brain. Although this effect is usually temporary, it can interfere with the newborn's adjustment to life outside the uterus. General anesthesia is typically used for emergency cesarean delivery because it is the quickest way to anesthetize the woman.

Delivery

Delivery is the passage of the fetus and placenta (afterbirth) from the uterus to the outside world.

For delivery in a hospital, a woman may be moved from a labor room to a birthing or delivery room, a room used only for deliveries. Usually, the father, partner, or other support people are encouraged to accompany her. If she is already in an LDRP (for labor, delivery, recovery, and postpartum), she remains there. The intravenous line remains in place.

When a woman is about to give birth, she may be placed in a semi-upright position, between lying down and sitting up. Her back can be supported by pillows or a backrest. The semi-upright position uses gravity: The downward pressure of the fetus helps the vagina and surrounding area stretch gradually, decreasing the risk of tearing. This position also puts less strain on the woman's back and pelvis. Some women prefer to deliver lying down. However, with this position, delivery may take longer.

Delivery of the Baby

As delivery progresses, the doctor or midwife examines the vagina to determine the position of the fetus's head. When the cervix is fully open (dilated) and thinned and pulled back (effaced), the woman is asked to bear down and push with each contraction to help move the fetus's head down through her pelvis and to widen the vaginal opening so that more and more of the head appears. When more than 1 inch (3 to 4 centimeters) of the head appears, the doctor or midwife places a hand over the fetus's head during a contraction to control the fetus's progress. As the head crowns (when the widest part of the head passes through the vaginal opening), the head and chin are eased out of the vaginal opening to prevent the woman's tissues from tearing.

Vacuum extraction can be used to assist in delivery of the head when the fetus is in distress or the woman is having difficulty pushing (see page 1664).

Forceps are sometimes used for the same reasons but are used less often than vacuum extractors.

Episiotomy is an incision that widens the opening of the vagina to make delivery of a baby easier. It is no longer done routinely. It is used only when necessary for immediate delivery. For this procedure, the doctor injects a local anesthetic to numb the area and makes an incision in the area between the openings of the vagina and anus (called the perineum). If the muscle around the opening of the anus (rectal sphincter) is damaged during an episiotomy or is torn during delivery, it usually heals well if the doctor repairs it immediately.

After the baby's head has emerged, the body is rotated sideways so that the shoulders can emerge easily, one at a time. The rest of the baby usually slips out quickly after the first shoulder comes out. Mucus and fluid are suctioned out of the baby's nose, mouth, and throat. The umbilical cord is clamped and cut. The baby is then dried, wrapped in a lightweight blanket, and placed on the woman's abdomen or in a warmed bassinet.

Delivery of the Placenta

After delivery of the baby, the doctor or midwife places a hand gently on the woman's abdomen to make sure the uterus is contracting. After delivery, the placenta usually detaches from the uterus within 3 to 10 minutes, and a gush of blood soon follows. Usually, the woman can push the placenta out on her own. If she cannot and particularly if she is bleeding excessively, the doctor or midwife applies firm downward pressure on the woman's abdomen, causing the placenta to detach from the uterus and come out. If the placenta has not been delivered within 45 to 60 minutes of delivery, the doctor or midwife may insert a hand into the uterus, separating the placenta from the uterus and removing it.

After the placenta is removed, it is examined for completeness. Fragments left in the uterus prevent the uterus from contracting. Contractions are essential to prevent further bleeding from the area where the placenta was attached to the uterus. So if fragments remain, bleeding can occur after delivery and may be substantial. Infections can also occur. If the placenta is incomplete, the doctor or midwife may remove the remaining fragments by hand. Sometimes fragments have to be surgically removed.

In many hospitals, as soon as the placenta is delivered or removed, the woman is given oxytocin (intravenously or intramuscularly), and her abdomen is periodically massaged to help the uterus contract.

After Delivery

The doctor stitches up any tears in the cervix, vagina, or nearby muscles and tissues and, if an episiotomy was done, the episiotomy incision. The woman is then moved to the recovery room or remains in the LDRP. Often, a baby who does not need further medical attention stays with the mother. Typically, the woman and her baby remain together in a warm, private area for 3 to 4 hours so that bonding can begin. Many women wish to begin breastfeeding soon after delivery. Later, the baby may be taken to the hospital nursery. In many hospitals, the woman may choose to have the baby remain with her—a practice called rooming-in. All hospitals with LDRPs require it. With rooming-in, the baby is usually fed on demand, and the woman is taught how to care for the baby before she leaves

the hospital. If a woman needs a rest, she may have the baby taken to the nursery.

Because most complications, particularly bleeding, occur within the first 24 hours after delivery, nurses and doctors carefully observe the woman and baby during this time.

258 Complications of Labor and Delivery

Usually, labor and delivery occur without any problems. Serious problems are relatively rare, and most can be anticipated and treated effectively. However, problems sometimes develop suddenly and unexpectedly. Regular visits to a doctor or certified midwife during pregnancy make anticipation of problems possible and improve the chances of having a healthy baby and safe delivery.

Labor and Timing Problems

- Labor may start too early (before the 37th week of pregnancy) or may start late (after the 42nd week of pregnancy).
- As a result, the health or life of the fetus may be endangered.
- Labor may start too early or late when the woman or fetus has a medical problem or the fetus is in an abnormal position.
- An ultrasound examination can help determine the length of a pregnancy.

No more than 10% of women deliver on their specified due date (usually estimated to be about 40 weeks of pregnancy). About 50% of women deliver within 1 week (before or after), and almost 90% deliver within 2 weeks of the due date.

Determining the length of pregnancy can be difficult because the precise date of conception often cannot be determined. Early in pregnancy, an ultrasound examination, which is safe and painless, can help determine the length of pregnancy. In mid to late pregnancy, ultrasound examinations are less reliable in determining the length of pregnancy.

> **Did You Know...**
> Only about 10% of women have their baby on their due date.

PREMATURE RUPTURE OF THE MEMBRANES

Premature rupture of the membranes is the leaking of amniotic fluid from around the fetus before labor starts.

- After the membranes rupture, labor often soon follows.
- If labor does not begin within 1 or 2 days, infections in the woman and fetus are a risk.
- The woman is usually hospitalized, given antibiotics, and monitored closely.
- If the fetus's lungs are mature, labor may be artificially started.

Usually, the fluid-filled membranes containing the fetus rupture during labor. But in about 10% of normal pregnancies, the membranes rupture before labor starts. The membranes may rupture near the due date (at 37 weeks or later, which is considered full term) or earlier (called preterm rupture at less than 37 weeks). If rupture is preterm, delivery is also likely to be too early (preterm). Regardless of when premature rupture occurs, it increases the risk of infection of the uterus and the fetus. The fetus is also more likely to be in an abnormal position, and the placenta is more likely to detach too soon (placental abruption).

After the membranes rupture, contractions usually begin within 12 to 48 hours when the woman is near term but can take 4 days or longer if rupture occurs before 34 weeks of pregnancy. Rupture of the membranes is commonly described as "the water breaks." The fluid within the membranes (amniotic fluid) then flows out from the vagina. The flow varies from a trickle to a gush. As soon as the membranes have ruptured, a woman should contact her doctor or midwife.

Using a speculum, the doctor or midwife examines the pelvis to confirm that the membranes have ruptured and to estimate how far the cervix (the lower part of the uterus) has opened (dilated).

If labor does not begin within 24 to 48 hours, the risk of infection of the uterus and fetus increases.

Therefore, a doctor or certified midwife usually artificially starts (induces) labor, depending on whether the fetus is mature enough for delivery. To determine whether the fetus's lungs are mature enough, the doctor may take a sample of amniotic fluid, usually from the vagina, and analyze it. If the lungs are mature enough, labor is induced and the baby is delivered. If they are not, the doctor usually does not induce labor.

If labor is delayed, the woman may be hospitalized so that she can be monitored closely. Her temperature and pulse rate are usually recorded at least 3 times daily. An increase in temperature or pulse rate may be an early sign of infection. If an infection develops, labor is promptly induced and the baby is delivered.

Very rarely, if the amniotic fluid stops leaking and contractions stop, the woman may be able to go home. Then, she may be required to stay in bed except for short showers and bathroom trips, or she may be allowed to lie or sit in bed or on the couch, but sexual activity is prohibited. In such cases, the woman should be seen by her doctor at least once a week.

Antibiotics are begun when rupture has been confirmed. Usually, antibiotics (such as erythromycin plus ampicillin or amoxicillin) are given intravenously, then by mouth for several days. They prolong the pregnancy and reduce the risk of infection in the newborn. If the membranes rupture before the 32nd week of pregnancy, corticosteroids are given to help the fetus's lungs mature.

PRETERM LABOR

Labor that occurs before 37 weeks of pregnancy is considered preterm.

- Measures such as rest and sometimes drugs may be used to delay labor.
- Antibiotics, corticosteroids, or drugs that slow labor may be needed.

What causes preterm labor is not well understood. However, certain conditions may make it more likely:

- Premature rupture of membranes
- Previous preterm deliveries
- Genital infections, including some sexually transmitted diseases
- Infections of the kidneys or the membranes containing the fetus
- Structural weakness of the cervix
- Pregnancy with more than one fetus
- Abnormalities in the placenta, uterus, or fetus

A healthy lifestyle during pregnancy can help, as can regular visits to the doctor or midwife, who can then identify potential problems early.

Because babies born prematurely can have serious health problems (see page 1689), doctors try to prevent or stop labor that begins before the 34th week of pregnancy. Preterm labor is difficult to stop. If vaginal bleeding occurs or the membranes rupture, allowing labor to continue is often best. If vaginal bleeding does not occur and the membranes are not leaking amniotic fluid (the fluid that surrounds the fetus in the uterus), the woman is advised to rest and to limit her activities as much as possible, preferably to sedentary ones. She is given fluids and may be given drugs that can slow labor. These measures can often delay labor for a brief time.

Samples may be taken from the cervix, vagina, and anus to culture. Analysis of these samples may suggest the cause of preterm labor.

Drugs that can slow labor include the following:

- **Magnesium sulfate:** This drug is often given intravenously to stop preterm labor. However, if the dose is too high, it may have an effect on the woman's heart and breathing rates.
- **Terbutaline:** This drug, given by injection under the skin, can also be used to stop preterm labor. However, it can increase the heart rate in the woman, fetus, or both. Doctors use caution when they give this drug to women who have diabetes.
- **Calcium channel blockers:** These drugs are usually used to treat high blood pressure. They sometimes cause headaches and low blood pressure in the woman.
- **Prostaglandin inhibitors:** These drugs may transiently reduce the amount of amniotic fluid. They are not used after the 32nd week of pregnancy because they may cause heart problems in the fetus.

Women may be given antibiotics until culture results are obtained. If results are negative, the antibiotics are then stopped.

If the cervix opens (dilates) more than 2 inches (5 centimeters), labor usually continues until the baby is born. If doctors think that premature delivery is inevitable, a woman may be given a corticosteroid such as betamethasone. The corticosteroid helps the fetus's lungs and other organs mature more quickly and reduces the risk that after birth, the baby will have difficulty breathing (neonatal respiratory distress syndrome) or other problems related to prematurity.

POSTTERM PREGNANCY AND POSTMATURITY

*A **postterm pregnancy** is one that lasts 42 weeks or more. In **postmaturity**, the placenta can no longer maintain a healthy environment for the fetus because the pregnancy has lasted too long.*

In most pregnancies that go a little beyond 41 to 42 weeks, no problems develop. However, beyond that time, problems may develop because the placenta often cannot continue to deliver adequate nutrients to the fetus. This condition is called postmaturity. Postterm pregnancies increase the risk of problems such as difficult labor, need for cesarean delivery, and passage of meconium (the fetus's first stool). Meconium can sometimes be inhaled before or during delivery, causing the baby to have difficulty breathing shortly after birth. In the postmature fetus, soft tissues, such as muscle, may waste away. The fetus or newborn may be deprived of oxygen, have low blood sugar, or die.

Typically, tests are started at 41 weeks to evaluate the fetus's movement and heart rate and the amount of amniotic fluid, which decreases markedly in postterm pregnancies. Doctors use ultrasonography and may use electronic fetal heart monitoring to monitor fetal status (see box on page 1654).

Typically, at 41 weeks or sometimes at 42 weeks, labor is induced. Sometimes cesarean delivery is required.

> **? Did You Know...**
> If a pregnancy lasts more than 42 weeks, the placenta may malfunction, causing problems for the fetus.

LABOR THAT PROGRESSES TOO SLOWLY

Labor that progresses too slowly may involve slow movement of the fetus through the birth canal because the fetus is too large or is abnormally positioned, the birth canal is too small, or the uterus contracts too weakly.

If labor is progressing too slowly, the fetus may be too big to move through the birth canal (pelvis and vagina). Or the fetus may be in an abnormal position. Sometimes the uterus cannot contract forcefully or often enough to keep the fetus moving.

Doctors estimate the size of the fetus and birth canal and check the fetus's position. They also check the strength and timing of contractions. These factors determine treatment.

If the birth canal is big enough for the fetus but labor is not progressing, the woman is given oxytocin intravenously to stimulate the uterus to contract more forcefully. If oxytocin is unsuccessful, a cesarean delivery is necessary. If the baby is already in position to be delivered, a vacuum extractor or forceps may be used instead. If the fetus is too big, cesarean delivery is done.

Fetus or Newborn Problems

If labor does not proceed normally, the fetus or newborn may have problems.

FETAL DISTRESS

Fetal distress refers to signs before and during childbirth indicating that the fetus is not well.

Fetal distress is an uncommon complication of labor. It typically occurs when the fetus has not been receiving enough oxygen. Fetal distress may occur when the pregnancy lasts too long (postmaturity) or when complications of pregnancy or labor occur.

Usually, doctors identify fetal distress based on an abnormal heart rate pattern in the fetus. Throughout labor, the fetus's heart rate is monitored. It is usually monitored continuously with electronic fetal heart monitoring. Or, a handheld Doppler ultrasound device may be used to check the heart rate every 15 minutes during early labor and after each contraction during late labor.

If a significant abnormality in the heart rate is detected, it can usually be corrected by the following:

- Giving the woman oxygen
- Increasing the amount of fluids given intravenously to the woman
- Turning the woman on her left side

If these measures are not effective, the baby is delivered as quickly as possible by a vacuum extractor, forceps, or cesarean delivery.

If the amniotic fluid appears green after the membranes have ruptured, the fetus may be in distress (but usually is not). This discoloration is caused by the fetus's first stool (called meconium). Meconium can sometimes be inhaled before labor or during delivery, causing the baby to have difficulty breathing shortly after birth.

> **? Did You Know...**
> An abnormal heart rate in a fetus may be the earliest sign of fetal distress.

BREATHING PROBLEMS

Rarely, a baby does not start to breathe at birth, even though no problems were detected before delivery. Then the baby requires resuscitation. Personnel skilled in resuscitating babies may attend the delivery for this reason.

ABNORMAL POSITION AND PRESENTATION OF THE FETUS

Position refers to whether the fetus is facing rearward (toward the woman's back, or face down when the woman lies on her back) or forward (face up). Presentation refers to the part of the fetus's body that leads the way out through the birth canal. The most common and safest combination consists of the following:

- Head first (called a vertex or cephalic presentation)
- Facing down
- Face and body angled toward the right or left
- Neck bent forward
- Chin tucked in
- Arms folded across the chest

If the fetus is in a different position or presentation, labor may be more difficult and delivery through the vagina may not be possible.

When a fetus faces forward (an abnormal position), the neck is often straightened rather than bent, and the head requires more space to pass through the birth canal. Delivery by a vacuum extractor or forceps or cesarean delivery may be necessary.

There are several abnormal presentations.

Breech Presentation: The buttocks present first. Breech presentation occurs in 2 to 3% of full-term deliveries. When delivered vaginally, babies that present buttocks first are more likely to be injured than those that present head first. Such injuries may occur before, during, or after birth and include death. Complications are less likely when breech presentation is detected before labor or delivery.

Sometimes the doctor can turn the fetus to present head first by pressing on the woman's abdomen before labor begins, usually at the 37th or 38th week of pregnancy. However, if labor begins and the fetus is in breech presentation, problems may occur. The passageway made by the buttocks in the birth canal

---

Position and Presentation of the Fetus

Toward the end of pregnancy, the fetus moves into position for delivery. Normally, the position of a fetus is facing rearward (toward the woman's back) with the face and body angled to one side and the neck flexed, and presentation is head first. An abnormal position is facing forward, and abnormal presentations include face, brow, breech, and shoulder.

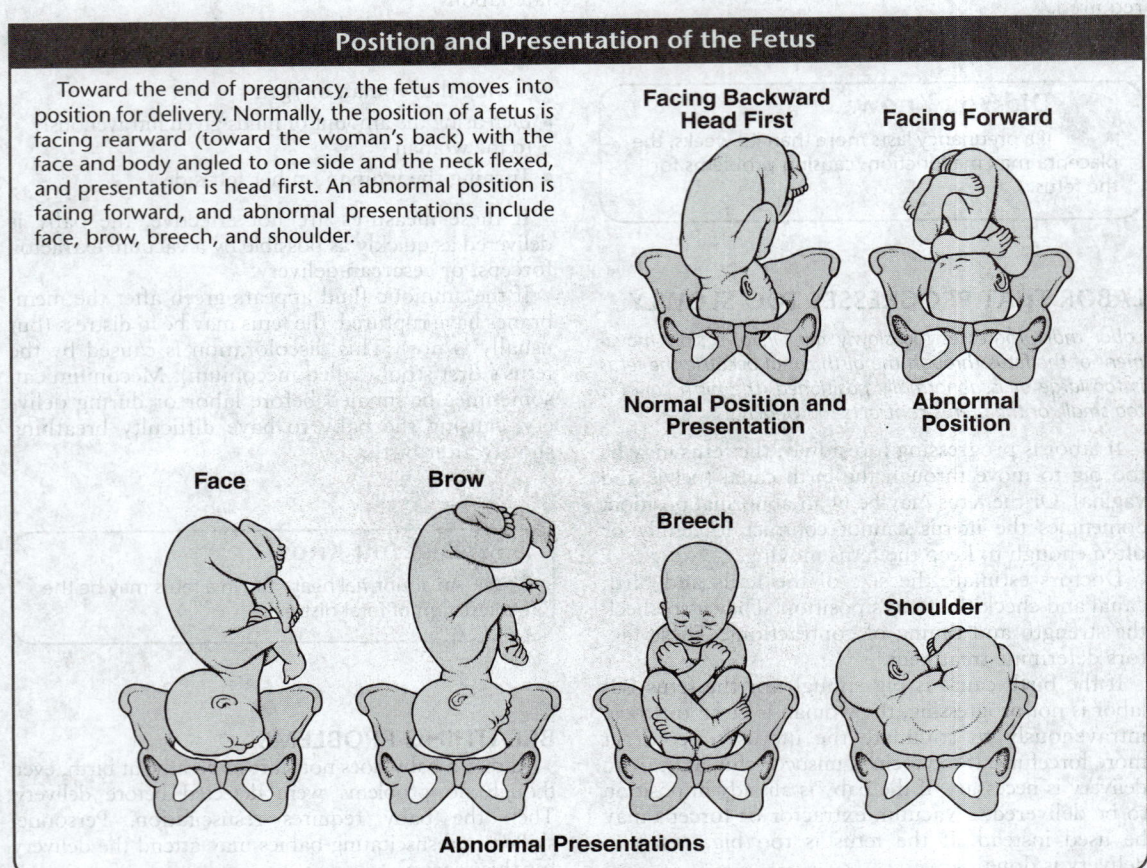

Facing Backward Head First

Facing Forward

Normal Position and Presentation

Abnormal Position

Face

Brow

Breech

Shoulder

Abnormal Presentations

may not be large enough for the head (which is wider) to pass through. In addition, when the head follows the buttocks, it cannot be molded to fit through the birth canal, as it normally is. Thus, the baby's body may be delivered and the head may be caught inside the woman. As a result, the spinal cord or other nerves may be stretched, leading to nerve damage. When the baby's navel is first seen outside the woman, the umbilical cord is compressed between the baby's head and the birth canal, so that very little oxygen can reach the baby. Brain damage due to lack of oxygen is more common among babies presenting buttocks first than among those presenting head first. In a first delivery, these problems are worse because the woman's tissues have not been stretched by previous deliveries. Because the baby could be injured or die, cesarean delivery is preferred when the fetus is in breech presentation.

Other Presentations: In face presentation, the neck arches back so that the face presents first. In brow presentation, the neck is moderately arched so that the brow presents first. Usually, fetuses do not stay in a face or brow presentation. They often correct themselves. If they do not, forceps, vacuum extractor, or cesarean delivery may be used.

Occasionally, a fetus lying horizontally (transversely) across the birth canal presents shoulder first. A cesarean delivery is done, unless the fetus is the second in a set of twins. In such a case, the fetus may be turned to be delivered through the vagina.

MULTIPLE BIRTHS

The term multiple births refers to the presence of more than one fetus in the uterus.

The number of twin, triplet, and other multiple births has been increasing during the last two decades. About 1 of 70 to 80 deliveries involves more than one fetus. The following make women more likely to become pregnant with more than one fetus:

- Taking fertility drugs
- Using assisted reproductive techniques
- Having had a pregnancy with more than one fetus
- Being older

Carrying more than one fetus overstretches the uterus, and an overstretched uterus tends to start contracting before the pregnancy reaches full term. As a result, the babies are usually born prematurely and are small. In some cases, the overstretched uterus does not contract well after delivery, causing bleeding in the woman after delivery. Because the fetuses can be in various positions and presentations, vaginal delivery can be complicated. Also, the contraction of the uterus after delivery of the first baby may shear away the placenta of the remaining baby or babies. As a result, the baby or babies that follow the first may have more problems during delivery.

Carrying more than one fetus also increases the risk of problems for the woman. They include high blood pressure plus protein in the urine (preeclampsia), gestational diabetes, excessive bleeding at delivery (postpartum hemorrhage), the need for cesarean delivery, small neonates (growth restriction), and preterm delivery.

During pregnancy, ultrasonography is done to confirm the number of fetuses.

Because problems can result from multiple births, doctors may decide in advance whether to deliver twins vaginally or by cesarean. If the first twin is in an abnormal position (anything other than head first), cesarean delivery is used. Occasionally, the first twin is delivered vaginally, but a cesarean delivery is considered safer for the second twin. For triplets and other multiple births, a cesarean delivery is usually done.

SHOULDER DYSTOCIA

Shoulder dystocia occurs when one shoulder of the fetus lodges against the woman's pubic bone, and the baby is therefore caught in the birth canal.

Because the fetus's shoulder is lodged against the woman's pubic bone, the fetus's head comes out, but it is pulled back tightly against the vaginal opening. The baby cannot breathe because the chest and umbilical cord are compressed by the birth canal. As a result, oxygen levels in the baby's blood decrease. Shoulder dystocia is more common with large fetuses, particularly when labor is difficult or when a vacuum extractor or forceps is used because the fetus's head has not fully moved down (descended) in the pelvis. It is also more common when women are obese, have diabetes, or have had a previous baby with shoulder dystocia.

When this complication occurs, the doctor quickly tries various techniques to free the shoulder so that the baby can be delivered vaginally. Sometimes when these techniques are tried, the baby's nerves are damaged or the baby's arm bone or collarbone may be broken. An episiotomy (an incision that widens the opening of the vagina) may be done to help with delivery. If these techniques are unsuccessful, the baby may be pushed back into the vagina and delivered by cesarean.

PROLAPSED UMBILICAL CORD

Prolapse of the umbilical cord means that the cord precedes the baby through the vagina.

A prolapsed umbilical cord occurs in about 1 of 1,000 deliveries. When the umbilical cord prolapses, the fetus's body may put pressure on the cord and thus cut off the fetus's blood supply. This uncommon complication may be obvious (overt) or not (occult).

Overt Prolapse: The membranes have ruptured, and the umbilical cord protrudes into or out of the vagina before the baby emerges. Overt prolapse usually occurs when a baby emerges feet or buttocks first (breech presentation). But it can occur when the baby emerges head first, particularly if the membranes rupture prematurely or the fetus has not moved down into the woman's pelvis. If the fetus has not moved down, the rush of fluid as the membranes rupture can carry the cord out ahead of the fetus.

If the cord prolapses, cesarean delivery must be done immediately to prevent the blood supply to the fetus from being cut off. Until surgery begins, a nurse or doctor holds the fetus's body off the cord so that the blood supply through the prolapsed cord is not cut off.

Occult Prolapse: The membranes are intact, and the cord is in front of the fetus or trapped in front of the fetus's shoulder. Usually, occult prolapse can be identified by an abnormal pattern in the fetus's heart rate. Changing the woman's position usually corrects the problem. Occasionally, a cesarean delivery is necessary.

NUCHAL CORD

A nuchal cord is an umbilical cord that is wrapped around the fetus's neck.

A nuchal cord occurs in about one fourth of deliveries. Normally, the baby is not harmed.

Before birth, a nuchal cord can sometimes be detected by ultrasonography, but no action is required. Doctors routinely check for it as they deliver the baby. If they feel it, they can slip the cord over the baby's head. Sometimes if the cord is tightly wrapped, it is clamped and cut before the shoulders are delivered.

Problems Affecting the Woman

Some complications of pregnancy also cause problems during labor or delivery. For example, preeclampsia (see page 1649), which involves high blood pressure accompanied by protein in the urine, can develop any time from the 20th week of pregnancy through the 6 weeks after delivery. Preeclampsia may lead to premature detachment of the placenta from the uterus (placental abruption—see page 1648) and problems in the newborn.

Other complications develop only after labor and delivery occur.

AMNIOTIC FLUID EMBOLISM

Very rarely, a volume of amniotic fluid—the fluid that surrounds the fetus in the uterus—enters the woman's bloodstream, usually during a particularly difficult labor. The fluid can cause a serious reaction that involves a rapid heart rate, irregular heart rhythm, collapse, shock, or even cardiac arrest and death (in about one fifth of women). Widespread blood clotting (disseminated intravascular coagulation), sometimes also with bleeding, is a common complication, requiring emergency care (see page 1046).

Prompt diagnosis and treatment are essential. Women may be given a blood transfusion. They may require assistance with breathing or drugs to help the heart contract.

EXCESSIVE UTERINE BLEEDING

Excessive bleeding from the uterus (postpartum hemorrhage) refers to loss of more than about 1 pint of blood immediately after vaginal delivery of a baby or loss of more than about 2 pints after cesarean delivery.

After the baby is delivered, excessive bleeding from the uterus is a major concern. Ordinarily, the woman loses about 1 pint of blood after delivery. Blood is lost because some blood vessels are opened when the placenta detaches from the uterus. The contractions of the uterus help close these vessels until the vessels can heal.

Loss of more than about 1 pint of blood during or after the third stage of labor (when the placenta is delivered) is considered excessive. Severe blood loss usually occurs soon after delivery but may occur as late as 1 month afterward.

Excessive bleeding may result when the contractions of the uterus after delivery are impaired. Then, the blood vessels that were opened when the placenta detached continue to bleed. Contractions may be impaired in the following situations:

- When the uterus has been stretched too much—for example, by too much amniotic fluid in the uterus, by several fetuses, or by a very large fetus
- When a piece of placenta remains inside the uterus after delivery
- When labor was prolonged or abnormal
- When a woman has delivered more than five babies
- When a muscle-relaxing anesthetic was used during labor and delivery

Excessive bleeding can also result in the following situations:

- When the vagina or cervix is torn or cut during delivery
- When the blood level of fibrinogen (which helps blood to clot) is low
- When a woman has a bleeding disorder that interferes with clotting
- Rarely, when the uterus ruptures or is turned inside out (inverted)

Excessive bleeding after one delivery may increase the risk of excessive bleeding after subsequent deliveries. Fibroids in the uterus may also increase the risk.

Prevention

Before a woman goes into labor, doctors take steps to prevent or to prepare for excessive bleeding after delivery. For example, they determine whether the woman has any conditions that increase the risk of bleeding (such as too much amniotic fluid). If the woman has an unusual blood type, doctors make sure that her blood type is available. Delivery should be slow and as gentle as possible. After delivery of the placenta, the woman is monitored for at least 1 hour to make sure that the uterus has contracted and to assess bleeding.

Treatment

If severe bleeding occurs, the woman's lower abdomen is massaged, and she is given oxytocin continuously through an intravenous line. These measures help the uterus contract. If bleeding continues, drugs that help the uterus contract can be injected into a muscle, placed as a tablet in the rectum, or, during cesarean delivery, injected into the uterus. The woman may need a blood transfusion.

Doctors look for the cause of excessive bleeding. The uterus may be examined to see whether any fragments of the placenta remain. Dilation and curettage may be done to remove these fragments. In this procedure, a small, sharp instrument (curet) is passed through the cervix (which is usually still open from the delivery— see page 1504). The curet is used to remove the retained fragments. This procedure requires an anesthetic. The cervix and vagina are examined for tears.

If the uterus cannot be stimulated to contract and bleeding continues, the arteries supplying blood to the uterus may have to be compressed to stop blood flow. For example, a balloon may be inserted into the uterus and inflated, packing may be inserted into the uterus, or a doctor may place stitches (sutures) around the bottom of the uterus. The procedures used usually do not cause infertility, abnormalities in menstruation, or other lasting problems. Removal of the uterus (hysterectomy) is rarely necessary to stop the bleeding.

INVERTED UTERUS

Very rarely, the uterus is turned inside out (inverted), so that it protrudes through the cervix and into or through the vagina. The uterus may be inverted if the placenta is firmly attached and doctors pull hard to remove it.

An inverted uterus is a medical emergency that must be treated promptly. Doctors return the uterus to its normal position (reinvert it) by hand. Pain relievers, sedatives, and sometimes a general anesthetic may be needed. Most women recover fully after this procedure. Occasionally, surgery is required to return the uterus to its normal position.

PLACENTA ACCRETA

Placenta accreta is a placenta with an abnormally firm attachment to the uterus.

When the placenta is too firmly attached, parts of the placenta may remain in the uterus after delivery. In these cases, delivery is delayed, and the risks of bleeding and infection in the uterus are increased. Bleeding may be life threatening.

This complication is more likely to occur in women

- Who have had a cesarean delivery
- Whose placenta covers the cervix
- Who are over 35
- Who have been pregnant several times
- Who have had fibroids surgically removed
- Who have disorders of the lining of the uterus (endometrium) such as Asherman's syndrome

Having a cesarean delivery greatly increases the risk of this complication. The more cesarean deliveries a woman has had, the higher the risk.

Diagnosis and Treatment

Before delivery, doctors can sometimes diagnose placenta accreta when ultrasonography or magnetic resonance imaging (MRI) is done. During delivery, the disorder is suspected if the placenta has not been delivered within 30 minutes after the baby's delivery, if doctors cannot separate the placenta from the uterus by hand, or if attempting to remove the placenta results in profuse bleeding.

Hysterectomy is the safest procedure. However, if future childbearing is important to the woman and if bleeding is not profuse, the abnormal area can sometimes be repaired.

UTERINE RUPTURE

Uterine rupture is a spontaneous tearing open of the uterus that may result in the fetus floating in the abdomen.

Rupture of the uterus is very rare. It is an emergency requiring immediate treatment.

The uterus can rupture before or during labor. Rupture is more likely in women who have had a cesarean delivery or who have had surgery on the uterus. The risk of uterine rupture for women who have had a cesarean delivery increases if they require induction of labor instead of have spontaneous labor. Rupture causes severe, constant pain in the abdomen and an abnormally slow heart rate in the fetus.

Using Forceps or a Vacuum Extractor

Forceps or a vacuum extractor may be used to help with delivery. Forceps are placed around the baby's head. A vacuum extractor uses suction to adhere to the baby's head. With either device, the baby is gently pulled out as the woman pushes.

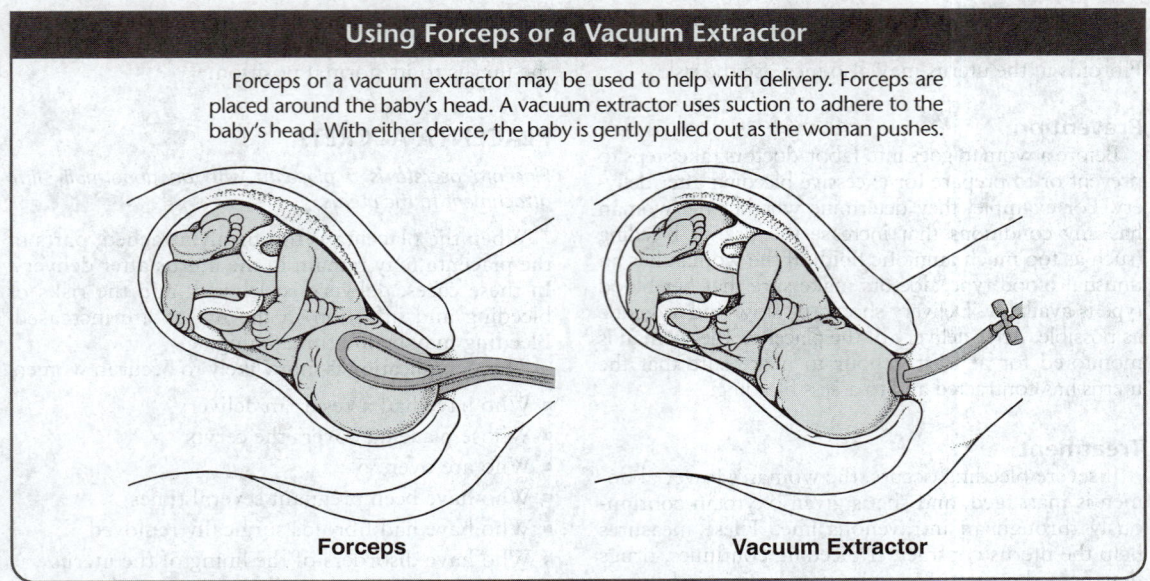

Forceps   **Vacuum Extractor**

The fetus must be delivered immediately. The uterus is repaired surgically.

Labor and Delivery Procedures

Induction of labor is the artificial starting of labor. Usually, labor is induced by giving the woman oxytocin, a hormone that makes the uterus contract more frequently and more forcefully. The oxytocin given is identical to the natural oxytocin produced by the pituitary gland. It is given intravenously with an infusion pump, so that the amount of drug given can be controlled precisely. Sometimes prostaglandins, which help the cervix open (dilate), are also given to help start labor. Alternatively, a tube (catheter) with a balloon attached can be inserted in the cervix. The balloon is then inflated to dilate the cervix.

Throughout induction and labor, the fetus's heart rate is monitored electronically. At first, a monitor is placed on the woman's abdomen. After the membranes are ruptured, an internal monitor may occasionally be inserted through the vagina and attached to the fetus's scalp. If induction is unsuccessful, the baby is delivered by cesarean.

Augmentation of labor is the artificial hastening of labor that is proceeding ineffectively or too slowly. Oxytocin is used to augment labor. Labor is augmented when women have contractions that are not effectively moving the fetus through the birth canal.

Slowing of labor is the artificial delaying of labor that is proceeding too forcefully. Very rarely, a woman has contractions that are too strong, too close together, or both. If contractions are caused by the use of

oxytocin, the drug is stopped immediately. The woman may be repositioned and given analgesics. If the contractions occur spontaneously, a drug that can slow labor (such as terbutaline or ritodrine) may be given to stop or slow the contractions.

A **vacuum extractor** consists of a small cup made of a rubberlike material that is connected to a vacuum. It is inserted into the vagina and uses suction to attach to the fetus's head. A vacuum extractor is occasionally used in a normal labor to ease delivery. If vacuum extraction delivery is tried and is unsuccessful, cesarean delivery is done. Rarely, a vacuum extractor bruises the baby's scalp or causes bleeding in the baby's eyes (retinal hemorrhage). The risk of shoulder dystocia and jaundice is also increased.

Forceps are metal surgical instruments with rounded edges that fit around the fetus's head. Forceps are occasionally used instead of a vacuum extractor in a normal labor to ease delivery. Rarely, using forceps bruises the baby's face or tears the woman's vagina.

Vacuum extraction or forceps delivery may be required in the following situations:

- When the fetus is in distress
- When the woman is having difficulty pushing
- When labor is prolonged
- When the woman has a disorder (such as some brain or heart disorders) that make vigorous pushing inadvisable

CESAREAN DELIVERY

Cesarean delivery is surgical delivery of a baby by incision through a woman's abdomen and uterus.

In the United States, about 2 to 3 in 10 deliveries are cesarean.

Doctors use a cesarean delivery when they think it is safer than vaginal delivery for the woman, the baby, or both, as in the following situations:

- When the woman has had a previous cesarean delivery
- When labor is prolonged
- When the fetus is in an abnormal position, such as breech presentation (buttocks first)
- When fetal distress requires quick delivery

An obstetrician, an anesthesiologist, nurses, and sometimes a pediatrician are involved in this surgical procedure. Use of anesthetics, intravenous drugs, antibiotics, and blood transfusions helps make a cesarean delivery safe. Having the woman walk around soon after surgery reduces the risk of blood clots forming in the legs or pelvis, traveling to the lungs, and blocking arteries there (pulmonary embolism). Cesarean delivery results in more overall pain afterward, a longer hospital stay, and a longer recovery time than vaginal delivery.

For a cesarean delivery, an incision can be made in the upper or lower part of the uterus.

- **Lower incision:** This type of incision is more common. The lower part of the uterus has fewer blood vessels and so less blood is usually lost. Also, the healed scar is stronger, so that it is less likely to open in subsequent deliveries. A lower incision may be horizontal or vertical.
- **Upper incision:** Usually, this incision is used when the placenta covers the cervix (a complication called placenta previa), when the fetus lies horizontally across the birth canal, when the fetus is in breech presentation, or when the fetus is very premature.

The choice of having a vaginal delivery or a repeat cesarean delivery is usually offered to women who have had a lower incision. Vaginal delivery is successful in about three fourths of these women. However, such women should plan to have their baby in facilities equipped to rapidly do a cesarean delivery because there is a very small chance that the incision from the previous cesarean section will open during labor.

CHAPTER 259 Postdelivery Period

The postdelivery (postpartum) period is the 6 weeks after delivery of a baby, when the mother's body returns to its prepregnancy state.

After delivery, the mother can expect to have some symptoms, but they are usually mild and temporary. Complications are rare. Nonetheless, the doctor, hospital staff members, or health care plan usually sets up a program of follow-up office or home visits.

The most common complications are the following:

- Excessive bleeding (postpartum hemorrhage— see page 1662)
- Infections of the uterus, bladder, kidneys, or breasts
- Problems with breastfeeding (see page 1679)
- Depression

Postpartum hemorrhage may occur soon after delivery but may occur up to 6 weeks later.

What to Expect at the Hospital

Immediately after delivery of a baby, the mother is monitored. If a general anesthetic was used during delivery, she is monitored for 2 to 3 hours after delivery, usually in a well-equipped recovery room with access to oxygen, intravenous fluids, and resuscitation equipment.

Staff members check the mother's pulse rate and temperature. Normally, within the first 24 hours, the mother's pulse rate (which increased during pregnancy) begins to decline toward normal and her temperature may increase slightly, usually returning to normal by the second day. After the first 24 hours, recovery is rapid.

Hospital staff members make every effort to minimize the new mother's pain and the risk of bleeding and infection.

Bleeding: Minimizing bleeding is the first priority. After delivery of the placenta (afterbirth), a nurse may periodically massage the mother's abdomen to help the uterus contract and remain contracted, thus preventing excessive bleeding. If needed, oxytocin is given to stimulate contraction of the uterus. The drug is injected into a muscle or given intravenously as a continuous infusion until the uterus is contracted.

Urination and Defecation: Urine production often increases greatly, but temporarily, after delivery. Because bladder sensation may be decreased after

AFTER DELIVERY: THE BODY'S RETURN TO NORMAL

AREA AFFECTED	WHAT HAPPENS
Discharge from the vagina	New mothers have a bloody discharge, occasionally with blood clots, for 3 or 4 days. The discharge becomes pale brown for about 10 to 12 days, then yellowish white. The discharge may continue for up to about 6 weeks after delivery. About a week or two after delivery, part of the remaining placenta may separate, causing vaginal bleeding of up to about a cup.
Breasts	During the early stages of milk production (lactation), the breasts become engorged with milk, sometimes making them feel tight and sore.
Heart rate	The heart rate, which increased during pregnancy, starts to decrease within the first 24 hours and returns to normal soon thereafter.
Temperature	Body temperature may increase slightly during the first 24 hours, usually returning to normal by the second day.
Uterus	After delivery, the uterus contracts, beginning to return to its prepregnancy size and position.
Genital area	The area around the vaginal opening is usually sore. Tears during delivery and repair may also make the area sore. The area may sting when women urinate.
Urination	Urine production often increases greatly, but temporarily, after delivery.
Bowel movements	The first bowel movement after delivery may be difficult, partly because the abdominal and pelvic muscles have been stretched and stressed. Also, the mother may be concerned about stitches or may have pain due to tearing or hemorrhoids.
Hemorrhoids	The pushing required for delivery can lead to or worsen hemorrhoids.
Abdomen	Muscle tone is low after delivery but gradually increases.
Skin	Stretch marks do not go away, but they may fade, turning from red to silver, but sometimes not for years. Other darkened areas of the skin may also fade.
Weight	Most new mothers lose only about 13 pounds after delivery. They at first look as if they are still pregnant. They may lose more during the first week as extra fluids are eliminated.
Mood	Many new mothers feel blue or mildly depressed. The sad mood or baby blues usually passes after about 2 weeks.

delivery, hospital staff members encourage a new mother to try to urinate regularly, at least every 4 hours. Doing so avoids overfilling the bladder and helps prevent bladder infections. Staff members may gently press on the mother's abdomen to check the bladder and determine whether it is being emptied. Occasionally, if the new mother cannot urinate on her own, a catheter must be inserted into the bladder to empty the urine. Hospital staff members try to avoid using a catheter, which increases the risk of bladder and kidney infections.

The new mother is also encouraged to defecate before leaving the hospital. But because hospital stays are so short, this expectation may not be practical. Doctors may recommend that if she has not defecated within 3 days, she take laxatives to avoid constipation, which can cause or worsen hemorrhoids. If the rectum or muscles around the anus were torn during delivery, doctors may prescribe stool softeners.

Diet and Exercise: A new mother can have a regular diet as soon as she wants it, sometimes shortly after delivery. She should get up and walk as soon as possible.

A new mother can start exercises to strengthen abdominal muscles, often after 1 day if delivery was vaginal and later if it was cesarean. Sit-ups with bent knees, done in bed, are effective. However, most women are too tired to start exercising so soon after delivery. Cesarean delivery is a major surgery and women should not begin exercising until they have had time to fully recover and allow healing, which typically takes about 6 weeks. Women can resume their prepregnancy exercise routine after approval from their doctor at their postpartum visit.

Vaccines and Immune Globulin: Before the mother leaves the hospital, she is given the German measles (rubella) vaccine if she has never had rubella or never been given this vaccine. If the mother has never received the tetanus, diphtheria, and pertussis (Tdap) vaccine and her last tetanus booster was at least 2 years ago, she should be given a Tdap vaccine before she is discharged.

If a new mother has Rh-negative blood and the baby has Rh-positive blood, she is usually given $Rh_0(D)$ immune globulin within 3 days of delivery. This drug masks any of the baby's red blood cells that may have passed to the mother so that they do not trigger the production of antibodies by the mother. Such antibodies may endanger subsequent pregnancies (see page 1650).

Before Discharge: Before a new mother leaves the hospital, she is examined. If mother and baby are healthy, they commonly leave the hospital within 24 to 48 hours after vaginal delivery and within 96 hours after a cesarean delivery. Sometimes discharge is even earlier than 24 hours if no general anesthetic was used and no problems occurred.

The mother is given information about changes to expect in her body and measures to take as her body recovers from having a baby. Regular follow-up visits are scheduled.

Continuing From Hospital to Home

Coping with some changes begins in the hospital, depending on how soon hospital discharge occurs, and continues at home.

Discharge From the Vagina: New mothers have a discharge from the vagina. Staff members give them pads to absorb it. Staff members also check the amount and color of the discharge. Usually, it appears bloody for 3 or 4 days. Then it becomes pale brown for about 10 to 12 days, then yellowish white. The discharge may continue for up to about 6 weeks after delivery.

About a week or two after delivery, part of the remaining placenta may separate, causing vaginal bleeding of up to about a cup. Sanitary pads, changed frequently, may be used to absorb this discharge. Comfortably fitting tampons, changed frequently, can also be used unless they interfere with healing of an episiotomy incision or of tears in the area between the vaginal opening and the anus (perineum).

Drugs: Mothers who are not breastfeeding may safely take drugs to help them sleep or to relieve pain. For women who are breastfeeding, acetaminophen and ibuprofen are relatively safe pain relievers. Many other drugs appear in breast milk (see box on page 1641).

Genital Area: The area around the vaginal opening is usually sore, and the area may sting during urination. Tears in the perineum or episiotomy repairs can contribute to the soreness and cause swelling.

Immediately after delivery and for the first 24 hours, ice or cold packs may be used to relieve the pain and swelling. Anesthetics can be applied to the skin. Washing the area around the vagina with warm water 2 or 3 times a day helps reduce tenderness. Warm sitz baths can help relieve pain. Sitz baths are taken in a sitting position with water covering only the perineum and buttocks. Women should be careful when sitting down and, if sitting is painful, use a doughnut-shaped pillow.

Hemorrhoids: Pushing during delivery can cause or worsen hemorrhoids. Pain caused by hemorrhoids can by relieved by warm sitz baths and applying a gel containing a local anesthetic.

> **? Did You Know...**
> When breasts are engorged, expressing milk between feedings temporarily relieves the pressure but overall tends to make engorgement worse.

Breast Engorgement: The breasts may be enlarged, tight, and sore because they are engorged with milk. Engorgement occurs during the early stages of milk production (lactation).

For mothers who are not going to breastfeed, the following can help:

- Wearing a snug-fitting bra to elevate the breasts and thus help suppress milk production
- Applying ice packs and taking analgesics (such as acetaminophen or ibuprofen) to help relieve discomfort until milk production stops on its own

For mothers who are breastfeeding, the following can help until milk production adjusts to the baby's needs:

- Feeding the baby regularly
- Wearing a comfortable nursing bra 24 hours a day
- If the breasts are swollen and very uncomfortable, expressing milk by hand in a warm shower or using a breast pump between feedings (however, this measure tends to stimulate milk production and prolong engorgement)

If the breasts are very swollen, the mother may have to express her milk just before breastfeeding to enable the baby's mouth to fit around the areola (the pigmented area of skin around the nipple).

Mood: Sadness is common during the days after delivery. New mothers should not be too concerned unless sadness is extreme or lasts more than 2 weeks.

What to Expect at Home

A new mother may resume normal daily activities when she feels ready. Eating a healthy diet and exercising regularly can help a new mother return to her prepregnancy weight.

She may resume sexual intercourse as soon as she desires it and it is comfortable. If delivery caused tearing or an episiotomy was done, sexual intercourse should be delayed until the area heals. A new mother may take showers or baths shortly after delivery, unless delivery was by cesarean.

If delivery was cesarean, nothing, including tampons and douches, should be put in the vagina for at least 2 weeks. Strenuous activity and heavy lifting should be avoided for about 6 weeks. Intercourse should also be avoided for 6 weeks. The incision site should be cared for in the same way as other surgical incisions. Showering can typically be resumed 24 hours after surgery. Care should be taken not to scrub the incision site. Baths should be avoided until the wound is completely closed and any staples or sutures have been removed. The incision site should be kept clean and dry. Any evidence of increasing redness or drainage from the incision should be brought to the doctor's attention. Pain around the incision site can last for a few months, and numbness can last even longer.

Abdomen: The uterus, still enlarged, continues to contract for some time, becoming progressively smaller during the next 2 weeks. These contractions are irregular and often painful. Contractions are intensified by breastfeeding. Breastfeeding triggers the production of the hormone oxytocin. Oxytocin stimulates the flow of milk (called the let-down reflex) and uterine contractions.

> **? Did You Know...**
> Women can become pregnant as early as 2 weeks after having a baby.

Normally, after 5 to 7 days, the uterus is firm and no longer tender but is still somewhat enlarged, extending to halfway between the pubic bone and the navel. By 2 weeks after delivery, the uterus returns close to its normal size. However, the new mother's abdomen does not become as flat as it was before the pregnancy for several months, even if she exercises.

Stretch marks do not go away, but they may fade, but sometimes not for a year.

Breastfeeding: Doctors recommend breastfeeding for at least 6 months, but some mothers cannot breastfeed or may not want to for various reasons. Bottle-feeding can be done instead (see page 1680).

Mothers who are breastfeeding need to learn how to position the baby during feeding (see art on page 1679). If the baby is not positioned well, the mother's nipples may become sore and cracked. Sometimes the baby draws in its lower lip and sucks it, irritating the nipple. In such cases, the mother can ease the baby's lip out of its mouth with her thumb. After a feeding, she should let the milk dry naturally on the nipples rather than wipe or wash them. If she wishes, she can dry her nipples with a hair dryer set on low. In very dry climates, hypoallergenic lanolin or ointment can be applied to the nipples.

When a mother breastfeeds, the breasts may leak milk. Pads can be worn to absorb the milk, but plastic bra liners can irritate the nipples and should be not be used.

While breastfeeding, mothers need to increase their caloric intake by about 500 calories per day. They should also increase their intake of most vitamins and minerals. Usually, eating a well-balanced diet, including enough dairy products and green, leafy vegetables, and continuing to take prenatal vitamins with additional folate (1 milligram) are all mothers need to do. They should drink enough fluids to ensure an adequate milk supply. Mothers on special diets should consult their doctor about the need for other vitamin and mineral supplements, such as vitamin B_{12} for vegetarians.

Family Planning: Use of contraceptives is recommended when intercourse resumes because pregnancy is possible as soon as the mother begins to release an egg from the ovary (ovulate) again. Mothers who are not breastfeeding usually begin to ovulate again about 4 to 6 weeks after delivery, before their first period. However, ovulation can occur earlier. Mothers who are solely breastfeeding tend to start ovulating and menstruating somewhat later, closer to 6 months after delivery. The interval depends on how much food other than breast milk the baby consumes. If more than four fifths of the baby's food is breast milk, ovulation is unlikely to occur. Occasionally, a mother who is breastfeeding ovulates, menstruates, and becomes pregnant as quickly as a mother who is not breastfeeding.

Full recovery after pregnancy takes about 1 to 2 years. So doctors usually advise a new mother to wait at least one year and optimally 18 months before becoming pregnant again (although she may choose not to follow that advice). At her first doctor's appointment after delivery, a new mother can discuss contraceptive options (see page 1593) with her doctor and choose one that suits her situation. Whether a mother is breastfeeding affects the method of contraception used. Oral contraceptives

AFTER DELIVERY: WHEN TO CALL THE DOCTOR

AREA	SYMPTOMS	POSSIBLE CAUSE
Discharge	If blood soaks a sanitary pad every hour for more than 2 hours If the discharge smells foul If the discharge contains very large clots (larger than a golf ball)	Infection of the uterus
Temperature	If the temperature is 100.4° F (38° C) or higher at any time during the first week	Infection
Urination	If urination hurts (not just stings) If the bladder cannot be emptied completely If urination occurs much more frequently than usual	Urinary tract infection
Lower abdomen	If pain or discomfort is felt in the lower abdomen (above the pubic area) after the first 5 days	Infection of the uterus or bladder
Back	If pain is felt in the back or side just under the rib cage, particularly if fever is also present or urination is painful	Kidney infection
Breast	If a firm lump is felt in the breast after engorgement has subsided	A blocked milk duct
	If the breast is painful, swollen, or red or feels hot or tender	Breast infection
Mood	If a very sad mood with fatigue and lack of energy lasts more than 2 weeks	Postpartum depression
Incision from a cesarean delivery	If soreness increases If this area turns red or becomes swollen or hard to the touch If there is any discharge from the incision	Wound infection
Leg or chest	If the leg is swollen or painful If a new mother has sudden, sharp chest pain or chest pain that worsens when she inhales If breathing becomes difficult	A blood clot in a leg or lung
General	If a new mother feels light-headed, faints, or feels short of breath	A blood clot in the lungs

that contain estrogen and progesterone can interfere with milk production and should not be used until milk production is well established. Progesterone-only contraceptives can be used, but methods that do not use drugs (such as barrier contraceptives) are even better. A diaphragm can be fitted only after the uterus has returned to normal, usually after about 6 to 8 weeks. Before that, foams, jellies, and condoms can be used. Intrauterine devices can be inserted about 6 weeks after pregnancy.

A new mother (or any woman) who has just been vaccinated against German measles (rubella) must wait at least 1 month before becoming pregnant again to avoid endangering the fetus.

Infections

Immediately after delivery, the woman's temperature often increases. A temperature of 101° F (38.3° C) or higher during the first 12 hours after delivery could indicate an infection but may not. Nonetheless, in such cases, the woman should be evaluated by her doctor or midwife. A postpartum infection is usually diagnosed after 24 hours have passed since delivery and the woman has had a temperature of 100.4° F (38° C) or higher on two occasions at least 6 hours apart. Postpartum infections seldom occur because doctors try to prevent or treat conditions that can lead to infections. However, infections, if they develop, may be serious. Thus, if a woman has a temperature of more than 100.4° F at any time during the first week after delivery, she should call the doctor.

Postpartum infections may be directly related to delivery (occurring in the uterus or the area around the uterus) or indirectly related (occurring in the kidneys, bladder, breasts, or lungs).

INFECTIONS OF THE UTERUS

- Bacteria can infect the uterus and surrounding areas soon after delivery.
- Such infections commonly cause pain in the lower abdomen, fever, and a foul-smelling discharge.
- Diagnosis is usually based on symptoms and results of a physical examination.
- Antibiotics usually cure the infection.

Postpartum infections usually begin in the uterus. Such infections may develop if membranes containing the fetus (amniotic sac) are infected and cause a fever during labor. They include infection of the uterine lining (endometritis), uterine muscle (myometritis), or areas around the uterus (parametritis).

Causes

Bacteria that normally live in the healthy vagina can cause an infection after delivery. Conditions that make a woman more likely to develop an infection include the following:

- Anemia
- Bacterial vaginosis
- Repeated vaginal examinations
- Internal monitoring of the fetus (which requires rupture of the membranes)
- A long delay (often more than 18 hours) between rupture of the membranes and delivery
- Prolonged labor
- Cesarean delivery
- Placental fragments remaining in the uterus after delivery
- Excessive bleeding after delivery (postpartum hemorrhage)
- Young age
- Low socioeconomic group

The chances of developing uterine infection depend mainly on the type of delivery:

- Normal vaginal deliveries: 1 to 3%
- Caesarean deliveries that have been scheduled and are done before labor starts: 5 to 15%
- Caesarean deliveries that are not scheduled and are done after labor starts: 15 to 20%

Symptoms

Symptoms commonly include pain in the lower abdomen or pelvis, fever (usually within 1 to 3 days after delivery), paleness, chills, a general feeling of illness or discomfort, and often headache and loss of appetite. The heart rate is often rapid. The uterus is swollen, tender, and soft. Typically, there is a malodorous discharge from the vagina, which varies in amount. But sometimes the only symptom is a low-grade fever.

When the tissues around the uterus are infected, they swell, causing significant discomfort. Women typically have severe pain and a high fever.

Some severe complications can occur but not often. They include the following:

- Inflammation of the membranes that line the abdomen (peritonitis)
- Blood clots in the pelvic veins (pelvic thrombophlebitis)
- A blood clot that travels to the lung and blocks an artery there (pulmonary embolism)
- High blood levels of poisonous substances (toxins) produced by the infecting bacteria, which lead to sepsis or toxic shock

In sepsis and toxic shock, blood pressure falls dramatically and the heart rate is very rapid. Severe kidney damage and even death may result. These complications are rare, especially when postpartum fever is diagnosed and treated promptly.

Diagnosis and Treatment

An infection may be diagnosed based mainly on results of a physical examination. Sometimes an infection is diagnosed when women have a fever and no other cause is identified.

Usually, doctors take a sample of urine and send it to be cultured and checked for bacteria. Occasionally, a blood sample is cultured.

If the uterus is infected, women are usually given antibiotics (usually clindamycin plus gentamicin) intravenously until they have had no fever for 48 hours. Afterward, most women do not need to take antibiotics by mouth.

BLADDER AND KIDNEY INFECTIONS

A bladder infection (cystitis) sometimes develops postpartum. The risk is increased when a catheter is placed in the bladder to relieve a buildup of urine during and after labor. A kidney infection (pyelonephritis) is caused by bacteria spreading from the bladder to the kidney after delivery. Sometimes a bladder or kidney infection develops because bacteria that were in the bladder during pregnancy cause no symptoms until after delivery.

Bladder and often kidney infections cause painful or frequent urination. Kidney and some bladder infections cause fever. Kidney infections may cause pain in the lower back or side, a general feeling of illness or discomfort, and constipation.

Diagnosis and Treatment

The diagnosis is based on examination and analysis of a urine sample. With kidney infections and some bladder infections, the sample may be cultured to identify the bacteria.

Typically, women are given an antibiotic intravenously for a kidney infection or by mouth for a bladder infection. If there is no evidence that the bladder infection has spread to the kidneys, antibiotics may be given for only a few days. If a kidney infection is suspected, antibiotics (such as ceftriaxone alone or ampicillin plus gentamicin) are given until the woman has had no fever for 48 hours. Often, antibiotics are given by mouth for an even longer period of time. After culture results are available, the antibiotic may be changed to one that is more effective against the bacteria present.

Drinking plenty of fluids helps keep the kidneys functioning well and flushes bacteria out of the urinary tract.

Another urine sample is cultured 6 to 8 weeks after delivery to verify that the infection is cured.

BREAST INFECTION

A breast infection (mastitis—see page 1549) can occur after delivery, usually during the first 6 weeks and almost always in women who are breastfeeding. If the baby is not positioned correctly during breastfeeding, cracking (and soreness) can develop. If the skin of or around the nipples becomes cracked, bacteria from the skin can enter the milk ducts and cause an infection.

An infected breast usually appears red and swollen and feels warm and tender. Only part of the breast may be red and sore. Women may have a fever. A fever that develops later than 10 days after delivery is often caused by a breast infection.

> **? Did You Know...**
> If a breast infection develops after delivery, women should usually continue to breastfeed.

Rarely, breast infections result in a collection of pus (abscess). The area around the abscess swells, and pus may drain from the nipple.

Doctors base the diagnosis on results of a physical examination.

Treatment

Breast infections are treated with antibiotics, such as dicloxacillin or erythromycin. Women are encouraged to drink plenty of fluids. Women who have a breast infection and are breastfeeding should continue to breastfeed because emptying of the breast helps with treatment and decreases the risk of a breast abscess.

Breast abscesses are treated with antibiotics and are usually drained surgically. This procedure can be done using a local anesthetic but may require sedatives given intravenously or a general anesthetic.

Blood Clots

The risk of developing blood clots (thrombophlebitis) is increased after delivery. Typically, blood clots occur in the legs or pelvis (a disorder called deep vein thrombosis—see page 433). Sometimes one of these clots breaks loose and travels through the bloodstream into the lungs, where it lodges in a blood vessel in the lung, blocking blood flow. This blockage is called pulmonary embolism (see page 488).

Symptoms

A fever that develops between 4 and 10 days after delivery may be caused by a blood clot. The affected part of the leg, often the calf, may be painful, tender to the touch, warm, and swollen. The first sign of pulmonary embolism may be shortness of breath.

Diagnosis

Diagnosis of deep vein thrombosis is usually based on results of ultrasonography. Occasionally, a blood test to measure D-dimer (a substance released from blood clots) is helpful. Diagnosis of pulmonary embolism is usually based on computed tomography (CT) of the chest.

Treatment

Treatment of a superficial blood clot in the leg consists of warm compresses (to reduce discomfort), compression bandages applied by a doctor or nurse, and bed rest with the leg elevated (by raising the foot of the bed 6 inches). Women with deep vein thrombosis or pulmonary embolism need to take drugs that make blood less likely to clot (anticoagulants).

Thyroid Disorders

In 4 to 7% of women, the thyroid gland malfunctions during the first 6 months after delivery. Thyroid hormone levels may be high or low, usually temporarily. Women who have a family history of thyroid disorders or diabetes are particularly susceptible. If women already have a thyroid disorder, such as a goiter or Hashimoto's thyroiditis, the disorder may become worse.

Treatment may be required.

Postpartum Depression

Postpartum depression is a feeling of extreme sadness and related psychologic disturbances during the first few weeks or months after delivery.

- Women who have had depression are more likely to develop postpartum depression.
- Women feel extremely sad, cry, become irritable and moody, and may lose interest in daily activities and the baby.
- A combination of counseling and antidepressants can help.

The baby blues—feeling sad or miserable within 3 days of delivery—is common after delivery. Women should not be overly concerned about these feelings because they usually disappear within 2 weeks. Postpartum depression is a more serious mood change. It lasts weeks or months and interferes with daily activities. About 10 to 15% of women are affected. Very rarely, an even more severe disorder called postpartum psychosis develops.

The causes of sadness or depression after delivery are unclear, but the following may contribute:

- Depression or another psychologic disorder that was present before or developed during pregnancy
- Close relatives who have depression (family history)
- The sudden decrease in levels of hormones (such as estrogen, progesterone, and thyroid hormones)
- Stresses of having and caring for a baby (such as difficulties during labor and delivery, lack of sleep, fatigue, loss of freedom, and feelings of isolation and incompetence)
- Lack of social support
- Marital discord
- Other significant life stressors such as financial difficulties or a recent move

If women have had depression before they became pregnant, they should tell their doctor or midwife. Such depression often evolves into postpartum depression. Depression during pregnancy is common and is an important risk factor for postpartum depression.

Symptoms

Symptoms may include frequent crying, mood swings, and irritability as well as feelings of extreme sadness. Less common symptoms include extreme fatigue, difficulty concentrating, sleep problems, loss of interest in sex and other activities, anxiety, appetite changes, and feelings of inadequacy or hopelessness. Women have difficulty functioning. They may have no interest in their baby.

In postpartum psychosis, depression may be combined with suicidal or violent thoughts, hallucinations, or bizarre behavior. Sometimes postpartum psychosis includes a desire to harm the baby.

Fathers may also become depressed, and marital stress may increase.

Without treatment, postpartum depression can last months or years, and women may not bond with their infant. As a result, the child may have emotional, social, and cognitive problems later. About one in three or four women who have had postpartum depression have it again.

Preventing Depression After Delivery

Women can take steps to combat feelings of sadness after having a baby:

- Getting as much rest as possible—for example, by napping when the baby naps
- Not trying to do everything—for example, by not trying to keep a spotless house and make home-cooked meals all the time
- Asking for help from family members and friends
- Talking to someone (husband or partner, family members, or friends) about their feelings.
- Showering and dressing each day
- Getting out of the house frequently—for example, to run an errand, meet with friends, or take a walk
- Spending time alone with their husband or partner
- Talking with other mothers about common experiences and feelings
- Joining a support group for women with depression

Diagnosis

Early diagnosis and treatment are important for women and their baby. Women should see their doctor if they continue to feel sad and have difficulty doing their usual activities for more than 2 weeks after delivery or if they have thoughts about harming themselves or the baby. If family members and friends notice symptoms, they should talk with the woman and encourage her to talk to a doctor.

Doctors may ask women to fill out a questionnaire designed to identify depression. They may also do blood tests to determine whether a disorder, such as a thyroid disorder, is causing the symptoms.

Treatment

If women feel sad, support from family members and friends is usually all that is needed. But if depression is diagnosed, professional help is also needed. Typically, a combination of counseling and antidepressants (see table on page 868) is recommended. Women who have postpartum psychosis may need to be hospitalized, preferably in a supervised unit that allows the baby to remain with them. They may need antipsychotic drugs (see table on page 894) as well as antidepressants.

Women who are breastfeeding should consult with their doctor before taking any of these drugs to determine whether they can continue to breastfeed (see box on page 1641). Many options that allow continuation of breastfeeding are available.

Children's Health Issues

CHAPTER

260 Newborns and Infants

The successful transition of a fetus, immersed in amniotic fluid and totally dependent on the placenta for nutrition and oxygen, to a squalling, air-breathing baby is a source of wonder. Healthy newborns (age birth to 1 month) and infants (age 1 month to 1 year) need good care to ensure their normal development and continued health.

Initial Care

Immediately after a baby is born, the doctor or nurse gently clears mucus and other material from the mouth, nose, and throat with a suction bulb. The newborn is then able to take a breath. Two clamps are placed on the newborn's umbilical cord, side by side, and the umbilical cord is then cut between the clamps. The newborn is dried and laid carefully on the mother's abdomen with skin-to-skin contact or on a sterile, warm blanket.

The doctor examines the newborn for any obvious abnormalities or signs of distress. A full physical examination comes later. The newborn's overall condition is recorded at 1 minute and at 5 minutes after birth using the Apgar score. A low Apgar score is a sign that the newborn is having difficulty and may need extra assistance with breathing or blood circulation. Once the newborn is stable and has breastfed, the nurses obtain the weight and length.

Keeping the newborn warm is critical. As soon as possible, the newborn is wrapped in lightweight clothing (swaddled), and the head is covered to reduce the loss of body heat. A few drops of an antibiotic are placed into the eyes to prevent infec-

tion from any harmful organisms that the newborn may have had contact with during delivery.

The mother and newborn usually recover together in the delivery room. If the delivery is in a birth center, the mother, father or mother's partner, and newborn remain together in the same room. Mothers who are breastfeeding put their newborn to their breast within the first 30 minutes. Once transported to the nursery, newborns are placed on their back in a small crib and kept warm. Because all babies are born with low levels of vitamin K, a doctor or nurse gives an injection of vitamin K to prevent bleeding (hemorrhagic disease of the newborn).

About 6 hours or more after birth, newborns are bathed. The nurse tries not to wash off the whitish greasy material (vernix caseosa) that covers most of the newborn's skin, because this material helps protect against infection.

Physical Examination

The doctor usually gives the newborn a thorough physical examination within the first 12 hours of life. The examination begins with a series of measurements, including weight, length, and head circumference. The

Cutting the Umbilical Cord

Soon after a baby is born, two clamps are placed on the umbilical cord, and the cord is cut between the clamps. The clamp on the cord's stump is removed within 24 hours after birth. The stump should be kept clean and dry. Some doctors recommend applying an alcohol solution to the stump daily. The stump falls off on its own in a week or two.

Cord Is Cut

Cord Is Clamped

APGAR SCORE

CHARACTERISTIC	MNEMONIC	SCORE*		
		0	1	2
Color of skin	Appearance	All blue, pale	Pink body, blue extremities	All pink
Heart rate	Pulse	Absent	< 100 beats/minute	> 100 beats/minute
Reflex response to nasal stimulation (by touch or a catheter)	Grimace	None	Grimace	Sneeze, cough
Muscle tone	Activity	Limp	Some flexion of extremities	Active
Breathing	Respiration	Absent	Irregular, slow	Good, crying

*The baby is given a score from 0 to 2 for each of 5 characteristics. A total score of 7 to 10 at 5 minutes is considered normal; 4 to 6, intermediate; and 0 to 3, low.

average weight at birth is 7 pounds, and the average length is 20 inches, although there is a wide range that is considered normal. Then the doctor examines the newborn's skin, head and face, heart and lungs, nervous system, abdomen, and genitals.

The skin is usually reddish, although the fingers and toes may have a bluish tinge because of poor blood circulation during the first few hours. Occasionally, the skin has several hard lumps (subcutaneous fat necrosis) where pressure from bones destroyed some fatty tissue. Such lumps are most common on the head, cheek, and neck, particularly if forceps were used during delivery. The lumps may break through to the skin surface, releasing a clear yellow fluid, but they usually heal fairly quickly.

A normal head-first delivery leaves the head slightly misshapen for several days. The bones that form the skull overlap, which allows the head to become compressed for delivery. Some swelling and bruising of the scalp is typical. Sometimes bleeding from one of the bones of the skull and its outer covering causes a small bump on the head that disappears in a few weeks. When the baby is delivered buttocks first (breech delivery), the head is usually not misshapen; however, the buttocks, genitals, or feet may be swollen and bruised. Delivery of a baby in the breech position is now usually avoided. When the baby is in the breech position, doctors usually recommend a cesarean or C section (surgical delivery of a baby by incision through a woman's abdomen and uterus), which minimizes danger to the baby.

Pressure during a vaginal delivery may bruise the newborn's face. In addition, compression through the birth canal may make the face initially appear asymmetrical. This asymmetry sometimes results when one of the nerves supplying the face muscles is damaged during delivery. Recovery is gradual over the next few weeks.

The doctor listens to the heart and lungs through a stethoscope to detect any abnormality. The doctor inspects the newborn's skin color and general condition for any sign of a problem. The strength of the pulse is checked.

The doctor looks for any abnormalities of the nerves and tests the newborn's reflexes. A newborn's most important reflexes are the Moro, rooting, and sucking reflexes.

Many serious disorders that are not apparent at birth can nonetheless be detected by blood tests in newborns. Because of this, all states require a number of blood tests in newborns. Early diagnosis and prompt treatment can reduce or prevent disorders that may interfere with an infant's healthy development.

The doctor examines the general shape of the abdomen and also checks the size, shape, and position of

Three Common Reflexes of Newborns

In the **Moro reflex**, when newborns are startled, their arms and legs swing out and forward in a slow movement with fingers outstretched.

In the **rooting reflex**, when either side of their mouth is touched, newborns turn their head toward that side. This reflex enables newborns to find the nipple.

In the **sucking reflex**, when an object is placed in their mouth, newborns begin sucking immediately.

internal organs, such as the kidneys, liver, and spleen. Enlarged kidneys may indicate an obstruction to the outflow of urine.

The doctor examines the flexibility and mobility of the arms, legs, and hips and checks to see whether the newborn has dislocated hips.

The doctor examines the genitals to ensure the urethra is open and in the proper location. In a boy, the testes should be present in the scrotum. In a girl, the labia are prominent because of exposure to the mother's hormones, and they remain swollen for the first few weeks. The doctor examines the anus to make sure the opening is not sealed shut.

First Few Days

Immediately after a normal birth, the mother and father are encouraged to hold their newborn. Breastfeeding should be initiated as soon after birth as possible if the mother plans to breastfeed. Breastfeeding stimulates oxytocin, a hormone that helps the mother's womb to heal and promotes development of the milk supply. Some experts believe that early physical contact with the newborn helps establish bonding. However, parents can bond well with their newborn even when the first hours are not spent together. Mother and baby spend a day or two in the hospital during which time new parents are taught to feed, bathe, and dress the baby and become familiar with the baby's activities, cues, and sounds. In the United States, discharge from the hospital within 24 to 48 hours is common.

Having a new baby in a household requires a great deal of adjustment for all involved. For a household that has had no children, changes in lifestyle may be dramatic. When other children are present, jealousy can be a problem. Preparing other children for the new baby and being careful to pay attention to them and include them in caring for the baby can ease the transition. Pets may also need some extra attention to help them adjust to the baby. In some cases, keeping pets away from the baby may be necessary.

Umbilical Cord: The plastic cord clamp on the umbilical cord is removed within 24 hours after birth. The stump should be kept clean and dry. The stump falls off on its own in a week or two. Rarely, the umbilical cord can become infected, so any signs of swelling or discharge should be checked by the doctor.

Circumcision: Circumcision, if desired, usually is performed within the first few days of life, often before the newborn is discharged. The decision about having a newborn circumcised usually depends on the parents' religious beliefs or personal preferences. The main medical reason for circumcision is to remove an unusually tight foreskin that is obstructing the flow of urine. Although circumcised males also have a lower risk of cancer of the penis and urinary tract infections, these risks can be minimized with proper hygiene and are not by themselves sufficient reasons to perform circumcision. About 2 to 20 boys per 1,000 have some complication, usually minor bleeding or local infection. However, serious infection, scarring, and, very rarely, accidental amputation of the penis tip can occur. An equal number of uncircumcised males require a circumcision later in life.

Circumcision should not be performed if the boy has not voided, or if the penis is abnormal in any way, because the foreskin may be used for any plastic surgical repair that may be needed later. Circumcision must be delayed if, during the pregnancy, the mother had been taking drugs that increase the risk of bleeding, such as anticoagulants or aspirin. The doctor waits until all such drugs have been eliminated from the newborn's circulation.

Skin: Most newborns have a mild skin rash sometime during the first week after birth. The rash usually appears in areas of the body rubbed by clothing—the arms, legs, and back—and rarely on the face. It tends to disappear without treatment. Applying lotions or powders, using perfumed soaps, and putting plastic pants over the diapers are likely to make the rash worse, especially in hot weather. Dryness and some skin peeling often occur after a few days, especially in the creases at the wrists and ankles.

Newborns who are otherwise normal may develop a yellow color to their skin (jaundice) after the first day. Jaundice occurs because the newborn's immature liver has not fully developed the ability to process waste products. However, jaundice that appears before 24 hours of age is of particular concern and may indicate more serious problems (see page 1701). If the newborn develops jaundice, the doctors usually do a blood test to measure the level of bilirubin, which is the main pigment in bile. If the level of bilirubin is above a certain point, treatment with phototherapy, in which the newborn is placed without clothes under fluorescent bilirubin lights, is begun. Rarely, a newborn with jaundice may need to be hospitalized for a day or two to receive phototherapy.

Urine and Bowel Movements: The first urine produced by a newborn is concentrated and often contains chemicals called urates, which can turn the diaper pink. If a newborn does not urinate within the first 24 hours of life, the doctor tries to find out why. Delay in starting to urinate is more common among boys.

The first bowel movement is a sticky greenish black substance (meconium). Every baby should pass meconium within the first 24 hours after birth. If a baby does not do so, the doctor may perform tests to determine whether there is a problem. Occasionally, for instance, a birth defect may cause a blockage of the intestines.

Feeding

A normal newborn has active rooting and sucking reflexes and can start feeding right away, so doctors recommend placing the newborn at the mother's breast immediately after birth. If this is not done, feedings are begun at least within 4 hours after birth.

Most babies swallow air along with the milk. Babies usually cannot burp on their own, so a parent needs to help. Babies should be held upright, leaning against the parent's chest, with their head against the parent's shoulder, while the parent pats them gently on their back. The combination of patting and pressure against the shoulder usually leads to an audible burp, often accompanied by spitting up of a small amount of milk.

Although babies may be fed breast milk or formula, doctors recommend exclusive breastfeeding for at least the first 6 months. However, breastfeeding is not always possible (for example, if the mother is taking certain drugs), and many healthy babies have been raised on formula feedings.

BREASTFEEDING

Benefits of Breastfeeding: Breast milk is the ideal food for newborns. Besides providing the necessary nutrients in the most easily digestible and absorbable form, breast milk contains antibodies and white blood cells that protect the baby against infection. Breast milk favorably changes the pH of the stool and intestinal flora, thus protecting the baby against bacterial diarrhea. Because of the protective qualities of breast milk, many types of infections occur less often in babies who are breastfed rather than bottle-fed. Breastfeeding also seems to protect against the development of certain chronic problems, such as allergies, diabetes, celiac sprue, and Crohn's disease.

Breastfeeding offers many advantages to the mother as well. For example, it helps her to bond and feel close to her baby in a way that bottle-feeding cannot. Mothers who breastfeed have a quicker recovery time after delivery and have some long-term health benefits, such as decreased risk of obesity, osteoporosis, breast cancer, and ovarian cancer. About 60% of mothers in the United States breastfeed their babies, and this proportion is steadily increasing. Mothers who work may breastfeed while at home and have the baby bottle-feed pumped breast milk or formula during the hours they are away. Most doctors recommend giving daily vitamin D supplements to breastfed infants after 2 months of age.

A thin yellow fluid, called colostrum, flows from the nipple before breast milk is produced. Colostrum is rich in calories, protein, and antibodies. The antibodies are absorbed directly into the body from the stomach, protecting the baby against many infections.

Positioning a Baby to Breastfeed

The mother settles into a comfortable, relaxed position. She may sit or lie almost flat, and she may hold the baby in several different positions. A mother should find the position that works best for her and her baby. She may wish to alternate among different positions.

A common position is holding the baby on the lap so that the baby is facing the mother, stomach to stomach. The mother supports the baby's neck and head with her left arm when the baby is feeding on the left breast. The baby is brought to the level of the breast, not the breast to the baby. Support for the mother and the baby is important. Pillows can be placed behind the mother's back or under her arm. Placing her feet on a footstool or coffee table may help keep her from leaning over the baby. Leaning over may strain her back and result in a poor latch. A pillow or folded blanket may be placed under the baby for added support.

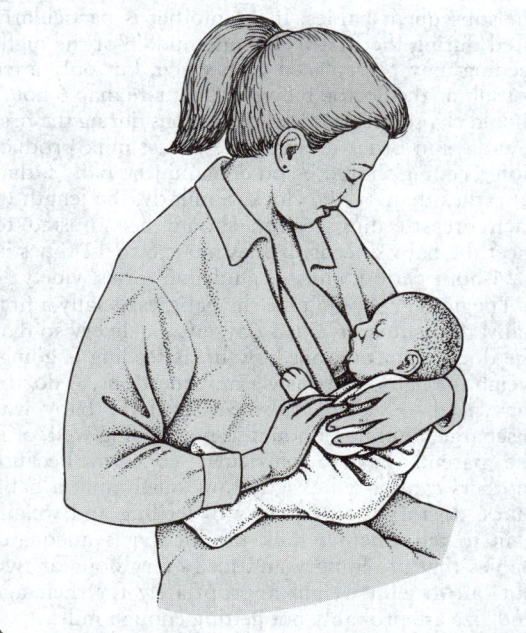

Breastfeeding Procedure: To begin breastfeeding, the mother settles into a comfortable, relaxed position, either seated or lying almost flat, and turns from one side to the other to offer each breast. The baby faces the mother. The mother supports her breast with her thumb and index finger on top and other fingers below and brushes her nipple against the middle of the baby's lower lip, which stimulates the baby's mouth to open (the rooting reflex) and grasp the breast. As the mother eases the nipple and areola into the baby's mouth, she makes sure the nipple is centered, which helps keep the nipple from becoming sore. Before removing the baby from the breast, the mother breaks the suction by inserting her finger into the baby's mouth and gently pressing the baby's chin down. Sore nipples result from poor positioning and are easier to prevent than to cure.

Initially, the baby tends to feed for several minutes at each breast. The resulting reflex (let-down reflex) in the mother triggers milk production. The production of milk depends on sufficient suckling time, so feeding times should be long enough for milk production to be fully established. During the first few weeks, the baby should be encouraged to nurse on both breasts with each feeding; however, some babies fall asleep while feeding at the first breast. The breast used last should be used first for the next feeding. For a first baby, full milk production is usually established in 72 to 96 hours. Less time is needed for subsequent babies. If the mother is particularly tired during the first night, one middle-of-the-night feeding may be replaced with water, but only after consulting the doctor. However, no more than 6 hours should elapse between feeding sessions during the first few days in order to stimulate breast milk production. Feeding should be on demand (the baby's, that is) rather than by the clock. Similarly, the length of each breastfeeding session should be adjusted to meet the baby's needs. Babies nurse 8 to 12 times in a 24-hour period, but this guideline varies widely.

The mother should take the baby, especially a first baby, to the doctor 3 to 5 days after delivery so that the doctor can find out how breastfeeding is going, weigh the baby, and answer any questions. A doctor may need to see the baby earlier if the baby was discharged within 24 hours, is not feeding well, or if the parents have a particular concern. Because mothers cannot tell exactly how much milk a baby takes, doctors use frequency of feeding and weight gain to tell whether milk production is adequate. Babies that are hungry and feed every hour or two but fail to gain weight appropriately for their age and size are probably not getting enough milk.

Weaning: When to stop breastfeeding (wean the infant) depends on the needs and desires of both mother and baby. The most desirable feeding combination is to breastfeed exclusively for at least 6 months, breastfeed along with solid foods until age 12 months, and then continue to breastfeed for as long as mother and child wish. Gradual weaning over weeks or months is easier for both the baby and mother than stopping suddenly. Mothers initially replace one to three breastfeeding sessions a day with a bottle or cup of fruit juice (fruit juice should not be used when weaning infants younger than 6 months old), expressed breast milk, or formula. Some feedings, particularly those at mealtimes, should be replaced with solid food. Learning to drink from a cup is an important developmental milestone, and weaning to a cup can be completed by age 10 months. Mothers gradually replace more and more breastfeedings, although many infants continue one or two breastfeedings daily until the age of 18 to 24 months or longer. When breastfeeding continues longer, the child should also be eating solid foods and drinking from a cup.

BOTTLE-FEEDING

In the hospital, newborns are usually fed shortly after delivery, then ideally on demand thereafter. During the first week after birth, babies take 1 or 2 ounces at a time, gradually increasing to 3 or 4 ounces about 6 to 8 times a day by the second week. Parents should not urge newborns to finish every bottle but, rather, allow them to take as much as they want whenever they are hungry. As infants grow, they drink larger amounts, consuming up to 6 to 8 ounces at a time by the third or fourth month. The proper position for babies who are bottle-feeding is semi-reclining or sitting up. Babies should not bottle-feed lying flat on their back because milk may flow into the nose or the eustachian tube. Older infants who are able to hold their own bottle should not be put to sleep holding the bottle because the continuous exposure to milk or juice can damage their teeth and lead to cavities.

Commercial baby formulas containing a proper balance of nutrients, calories, and vitamins are available in ready-to-feed, sterile bottles, cans of concentrated formula that must be diluted with water, and powder. Formulas are available both with and without an iron supplement. Most doctors recommend a formula that contains iron. Parents who use concentrated formula or powders must carefully follow the directions for preparation that are on the container. Formulas are usually made from cow's milk, although other special formulas are available for infants who cannot tolerate cow's milk. If an infant does not tolerate standard formula, the pediatrician will recommend an amino acid formula or a hydrolyzed formula. There are no long-term health differences in infants fed either standard or special formula. Plain cow's milk, however, is not an appropriate food during the first year of life.

To minimize the infant's exposure to microorganisms, formula must be fed from a sterile container. Disposable plastic liners eliminate the need to sterilize bottles. Nipples for the bottles should be sterilized in the dishwasher or in a pot of boiling water for 5 minutes. Parents should warm formula feedings to body temperature. Filled bottles (or formula containers, if disposable liners are used) are placed in a warm water bath and allowed to come to body temperature. Babies may be seriously burned if formula is too hot, so parents need to shake the bottle gently to even out the temperature and then check the temperature by placing a few drops on the sensitive skin inside their wrist. Formula at body temperature should feel neither warm nor cold to the touch. Microwave ovens may dangerously overheat formula and are not recommended for warming formula or baby food.

The size of the nipple opening is important. In general, formula should drip slowly out of a bottle held upside down. Larger, older infants want larger volumes of liquid and can tolerate a larger nipple opening.

STARTING SOLID FOODS

The time to start solid food depends on the infant's needs and readiness. Generally, infants need solids when they are large enough to need a more concentrated source of calories than formula. This need is recognized when an infant takes a full bottle and is satisfied, but then is hungry again in 2 or 3 hours. This typically occurs by the age of 6 months. Infants younger than this cannot easily swallow solid food, although some can swallow solids at younger ages if the food is placed on the back of the tongue. Some parents coax very young infants to eat large amounts of solid food in the hope that they will sleep through the night. This is unlikely to work, and forcing an infant to eat early can cause aspiration pneumonia and feeding problems later. Many infants take solids after a breastfeeding or bottle-feeding, which both satisfies their need to suck and quickly relieves their hunger.

Infants develop food allergies or intolerance easier than older children or adults. If many different foods are given in a brief period, it is difficult to tell which one may have been responsible for a reaction. Because of this difficulty, parents should introduce new foods one at a time, no more than one new food a week. Once it is clear a food is tolerated, another one may be introduced.

Single-grain cereals are begun first, followed by fruits and vegetables. Meats, which are a good source of protein, should be introduced later, after about 7 months. Many infants initially reject meat.

The food should be offered on a spoon so that the infant learns the new feeding technique. By age 6 to 9 months, infants are able to grasp food and bring it to their mouth, and they should be encouraged to help feed themselves. However, babies easily choke on food in small, hard bits (such as peanuts, raw carrots, candies, and small crackers), so these foods should be avoided. Pureed home foods are less expensive than commercial baby foods and offer adequate nutrition.

Although infants enjoy sweet foods, sugar is not an essential nutrient and should be given only in small quantities, if at all. Sweetened dessert baby foods have no benefit for babies. Honey must be avoided during the first year because it may contain the spores of *Clostridium botulinum*, which are harmless to older children and adults but can cause botulism in infants.

Stools and Urine

Infants typically urinate 15 to 20 times per day. The urine varies in color from nearly clear to dark yellow. Stools vary a great deal among infants in frequency, color, and consistency depending on the nature of the individual infants and the contents of their diet. The number of times infants defecate varies from once every other day to 6 or 8 times a day. Stool consistency ranges from firm and formed to soft and runny. Stool color ranges from mustard yellow to dark brown. The stool of breastfed infants tends to be softer and of lighter color than that of formula-fed infants.

Diapers must be changed often to keep the underlying skin dry. Wet skin chafes more easily than dry skin and is more likely to develop diaper rash. Modern, super-absorbent disposable diapers contain a layer of gel that absorbs liquid and keeps it away from the skin. These diapers keep skin drier than cloth diapers after small to moderate amounts of urine, but diapers of any type should be changed when the skin is exposed to wetness. Bacteria normally present in stool can break down urea, a substance in urine, resulting in an alkaline pH that irritates the skin, so diapers should be checked frequently for stool and changed immediately. There are several environmental considerations related to diapers. Disposable diapers consume larger amounts of material than cloth and contribute a significant volume of landfill waste. Cloth diapers consume large amounts of energy and chemicals in the laundering process.

Baby powders help keep skin dry when the infant is sweating slightly, but they do not help keep the skin dry from urine or stool and are not essential. Powder made of talcum may cause lung problems if inhaled by infants, so parents should purchase baby powders that contain cornstarch instead.

Sleeping

Because the nervous system of newborns is immature, newborns sleep a great deal, but only for an

An Infant's First Year: Physical Development

During the first year of life, an infant's weight and length are charted at each doctor's visit to make sure that growth is proceeding at a steady rate. Percentiles are a way of comparing infants of the same age. For an infant at the 10th percentile for weight, 10% of infants weigh less and 90% weigh more. For an infant at the 90th percentile, 90% of infants weigh less and 10% weigh more. For an infant at the 50th percentile, 50% of infants weigh less and 50% weigh more. Of more significance than the actual percentile is any significant change in percentile between doctor's visits.

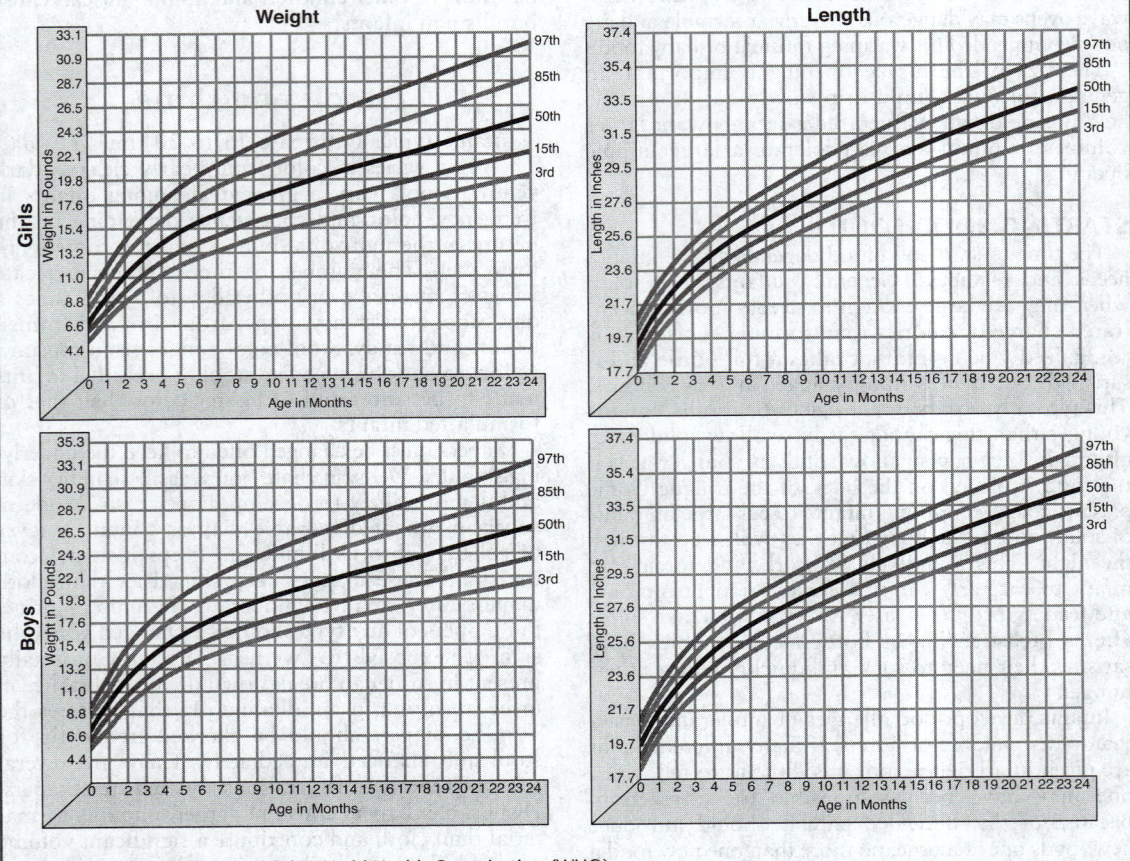

Adapted from a publication of the World Health Organization (WHO).

hour or two at a time, independent of day or night. By 4 to 6 weeks of age, many infants are on a cycle of waking for 4 hours and sleeping for 4 hours. Only by 2 to 3 months of age are infants capable of adopting a pattern of nighttime sleeping. By 1 year of age, most infants sleep 8 to 9 hours continuously through the night.

Parents can assist infants to sleep at night by handling and stimulating the child less in the late evening and keeping the child's room dark at night,

which is important in the development of normal vision. Infants should be encouraged at an early age to fall asleep on their own and not in a parent's arms. In this way, they will be able to quiet themselves when they wake in the middle of the night.

To minimize the risk of sudden infant death syndrome (SIDS—see page 1739), infants should sleep on their back, rather than on their stomach. This recommendation has helped reduce the incidence of SIDS in recent years. Also, infants should not sleep

AN INFANT'S FIRST YEAR: DEVELOPMENTAL MILESTONES

AGE	MILESTONE
1 month	Brings hands toward eyes and mouth Moves head from side to side when lying on stomach Follows an object moved in an arch about 6 inches (about 15 centimeters) above face to the midline (straight ahead) Responds to a noise in some way, such as startling, crying, or quieting May turn toward familiar sounds and voices Focuses on a face
3 months	Raises head 45 degrees (possibly 90 degrees) when lying on stomach Opens and shuts hands Pushes down when feet are placed on a flat surface Swings at and reaches for dangling toys Follows an object moved in an arch above face from one side to the other Watches faces intently Smiles at sound of mother's voice Begins to make speechlike sounds
5 months	Holds head steady when upright Rolls over one way, usually from stomach to back Reaches for objects Recognizes people at a distance Listens intently to human voices Smiles spontaneously Squeals in delight
7 months	Sits without support Bears some weight on legs when held upright Transfers objects from hand to hand Looks for dropped object Responds to own name Babbles, combining vowels and consonants Wiggles with excitement in anticipation of playing Plays peekaboo
9 months	Works to get a toy that is out of reach Objects if toy it taken away Crawls or creeps on hands and knees Pulls self up to standing position Stands holding on to someone or something Says "mama" or "dada" indiscriminately
12 months	Gets into a sitting position from stomach Walks by holding furniture; may walk one or two steps without support Stands for a few moments at a time Says "dada" and "mama" to the appropriate person Drinks from a cup Claps hands and waves bye-bye

with soft pillows, toys, or heavy blankets, which may obstruct their breathing. Putting an infant to bed with a pacifier also helps prevent SIDS (breastfed infants should be at least 1 month old or accustomed to breastfeeding before given a pacifier).

Physical Development

An infant's physical development depends on heredity, nutrition, and environment. Physical and psychologic abnormalities can also influence growth. Optimal growth requires optimal nutrition and health.

Newborns normally lose 5 to 7% of their birth weight during the first few days of life. Newborns who are breastfeeding can lose up to 7% of their birth weight. This weight is regained by the end of the first 2 weeks as newborns start to eat more. After this, newborns typically gain about 1 ounce per day during the first 2 months, and 1 pound per month after that. This weight gain generally results in a doubling of birth weight by age 5 months and a tripling by 1 year. A newborn's length increases about 30% by age 5 months and more than 50% by 1 year.

Different organs grow at different rates. For example, the reproductive system has a brief growth spurt just after birth, then changes very little until just before puberty. In contrast, the brain grows almost exclusively during the early years of life. At birth, the brain is one fourth of its future adult size. By 1 year, the brain is three fourths of its adult size. The kidneys function at the adult level by the end of the first year.

Lower front teeth usually begin to appear by the age of 5 to 9 months. Upper front teeth usually begin to appear by 8 to 12 months.

Behavioral, Social, and Intellectual Development

The rate of behavioral, social, and intellectual development varies considerably from infant to infant. Some infants develop faster, although certain patterns may run in families, such as late walking or talking. Environmental factors, such as lack of sufficient stimulation, can slow development. Conversely, stimulation can hasten development. Physical factors, such as deafness, can also slow development. Although a child's development is usually continuous, temporary pauses may occur in the development of a particular function, such as speech.

Crying is one means of communication. Infants cry because they are hungry, uncomfortable, distressed, and for many other reasons that may not be obvious. Infants cry most—typically 3 hours a day—at 6 weeks of age, usually decreasing to an hour a day by 3 months of age. Parents generally offer crying infants food, change their diaper, and look for a source of pain or discomfort. If this does not work, holding or walking with the infant sometimes helps. Occasionally nothing works. Parents should not force food on crying infants, who will readily eat if hunger is the cause of their distress.

Promoting Optimal Development

Babies obviously require appropriate food and shelter for their physical growth. If their physical needs are met regularly and consistently, babies quickly learn that their caretaker is a source of satisfaction, creating a firm bond of trust and attachment.

In addition to their physical needs, babies need affection and stimulation to develop emotionally and intellectually. Some parents provide a highly organized, structured environment for their baby using a variety of toys and gadgets. However, the particular content of the environment is less important than the existence of a pleasant, positive interaction enjoyed by both parent and baby. Parents who provide smiling faces, frequent amiable speech, physical contact, and love but who do not buy a variety of toys and gadgets are not shortchanging their baby's development.

Preventive Health Care Visits

Healthy infants should be seen by their doctor often during the first year of life. Visits typically take place by 1 to 2 weeks, and at 2, 4, 6, 9, and 12 months of age. During these visits, the doctor monitors the infant's growth and development by measuring the infant's length, weight, and head circumference, and asking the parents questions about various developmental milestones. The doctor also examines the infant for various abnormalities, including signs of hereditary disorders. Hearing and vision are tested. Premature infants (infants who spent less than 37 weeks in the uterus) are regularly examined for retinopathy of prematurity, an eye disease (see page 1699). Finally, on many visits, the doctor vaccinates the infant against various illnesses.

Health care visits also allow the doctor to educate the parents about eating, sleeping, behavior, child safety, and good health habits. In addition, the doctor advises the parents what changes to expect in their infant by the next visit.

Vaccinations

Children should be vaccinated to protect them against infectious diseases. Vaccines are preparations that

Vaccinating Infants and Children

Following the recommended vaccination schedule is important because it helps protect infants and children against infections that can be prevented. The schedule below is based on the one recommended by the Department of Health and Human Services and the Centers for Disease Control and Prevention. The schedule indicates which vaccines are needed, at what age, and how many doses (indicated by the numbers in the symbols).

There is a range of acceptable ages for many vaccines. A child's doctor can provide specific recommendations, which may vary depending on the child's known health conditions and other circumstances. Often, combination vaccines are used, so that children receive fewer injections. If children have not been vaccinated according to the schedule, catch-up vaccinations are recommended, and parents should contact a doctor or health department clinic to find out how to catch up. Parents should report any side effects after vaccinations to their child's doctor.

For more information about this schedule, parents should talk to a doctor or visit the Centers for Disease Control and Prevention's National Immunization Program site.

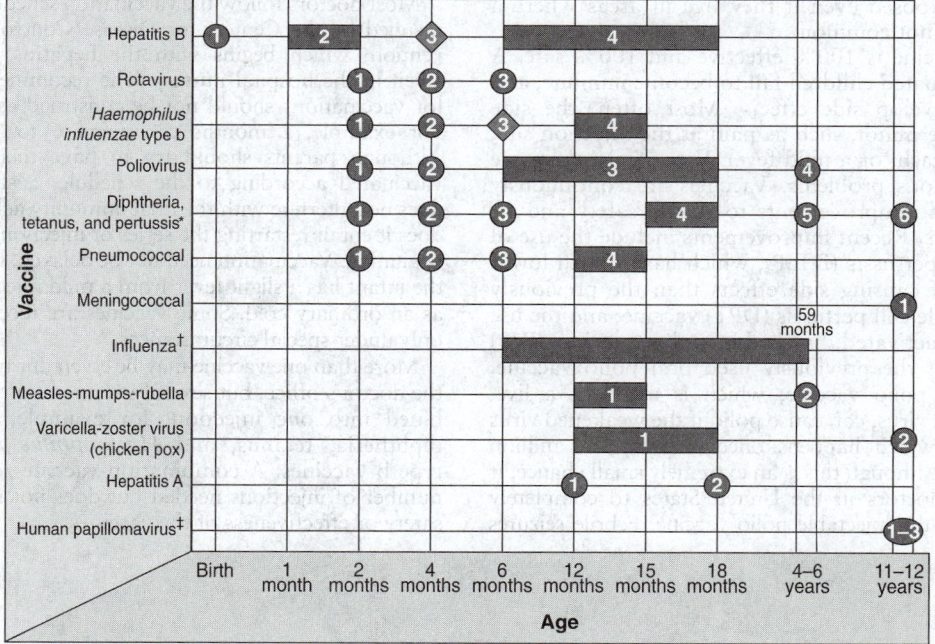

*Before age 11, children are given the diphtheria, tetanus, and pertussis (DTaP) preparation. An adolescent preparation of tetanus, diphtheria, and pertussis (Tdap) is recommended at age 11 to 12 years.

†Healthy children 6 to 59 months old should be given the influenza vaccine yearly, as should close contacts of infants up to 5 months old. Also, older children at high risk of developing influenza should be given the vaccine yearly. These children include those who have a heart or lung disorder (such as asthma), diabetes, kidney failure, or sickle cell disease or who have a weakened immune system (such as those who have HIV infection and those who are receiving chemotherapy).

‡The human papillomavirus vaccine is given to girls in 3 doses. The second dose is given 2 months after the first, and the third dose is given 4 months later.

contain either noninfectious fragments of bacteria or viruses or whole forms of these organisms that have been weakened so that they do not cause disease. Giving a vaccine (usually by injection) stimulates the body's immune system to defend against that disease. Vaccination is performed to produce a state of immunity to disease and is thus sometimes termed immunization.

Vaccines have eliminated smallpox and have nearly eliminated other infections, such as polio and measles, that were once common childhood scourges in the United States. Despite this success, it is important for health care practitioners to continue to vaccinate children. Many of the diseases prevented by vaccination are still present in the United States and remain common in other parts of the world. These diseases can spread rapidly among unvaccinated children, who, because of the ease of modern travel, can be exposed even if they live in areas where a disease is not common.

No vaccine is 100% effective and 100% safe. A few vaccinated children fail to become immune, and a few develop side effects. Most often, the side effects are minor, such as pain at the injection site, an itchy rash, or a mild fever. Very rarely, there are more serious problems. Vaccines are continuously undergoing improvements to ensure safety and effectiveness. Recent improvements include the use of acellular pertussis (DTaP), which has a much lower chance of causing side effects than the previously used whole-cell pertussis (DPT) vaccine, and the use of an inactivated, injectable polio vaccine (IVP) instead of the previously used oral polio vaccine. The oral polio vaccine, which is made of a live, weakened virus, can cause polio if the weakened virus mutates, which happens once in every 2.4 million children. Although this is an extremely small chance, it has led doctors in the United States to completely switch to the injectable polio vaccine. Febrile seizures

(seizures that are triggered by a fever) have occurred in about 3 in 10,000 children after receiving the measles-mumps-rubella vaccine. Although the public press has reported concerns that the measles-mumps-rubella vaccine may cause autism, scientific evidence shows that this does not happen.

To help people evaluate the risks of vaccination, the federal government requires doctors to give parents a Vaccine Information Statement each time a child is vaccinated. Also, a federal Vaccine Injury Compensation Program has been established to compensate anyone suffering permanent consequences of vaccination. This program was established because doctors and health authorities want as many children as possible to be protected from life-threatening diseases. When considering the risks of vaccination, parents must remember that the benefits of vaccination far outweigh the risks.

Most doctors follow the vaccination schedule recommended by the Centers for Disease Control and Prevention, which begins with the hepatitis B vaccine given in the hospital nursery. The recommended ages for vaccinations should not be construed as absolute. For example, 2 months can mean 6 to 10 weeks. Although parents should try to have their children vaccinated according to the schedule, a slight delay does not interfere with the final immunity achieved nor does it entail restarting the series of injections from the beginning. Vaccination need not be delayed, however, if the infant has a slight fever from a mild infection, such as an ordinary cold. Some vaccines are recommended only under special circumstances.

More than one vaccine may be given during a visit to the doctor's office, but several vaccines are often combined into one injection, for example, pertussis, diphtheria, tetanus, and *Haemophilus influenzae* type b vaccines. A combination vaccine reduces the number of injections needed but does not reduce the safety or effectiveness of the vaccines.

CHAPTER
261   Problems in Newborns

Although most infants are delivered at full term and have no problems, some infants may have medical problems related to factors that occur before birth, such as any health problems or habits of the mother. Examples of health problems are diabetes, high blood pressure, or preeclampsia (a condition that causes high blood pressure, swelling, and the presence of protein in the urine—see page 1649) that directly affect the growth of the fetus and the health of the newborn. Habits, such as smoking, use of alcohol, and use of illicit drugs also can affect the growth of the fetus and lead to problems

What Is a Neonatal Intensive Care Unit?

Often referred to as the NICU, this specialized facility brings together the medical team and technology needed to care for newborns with various disorders. Very premature newborns need the most care. Other newborns need care because of infection in the blood (sepsis) or pneumonia, respiratory disorders, heart problems, or birth defects that require surgery. These newborns are cared for in incubators to keep them warm while allowing the staff to observe them, or for short periods, they may be placed under overhead radiant warmers, which provide warmth while allowing the staff increased access to the newborn. Sick newborns may be attached to monitors that continuously measure their heart rate, breathing, blood pressure, and oxygen levels in the blood. They may have catheters placed inside an artery and the vein running inside the umbilical cord to permit continuous blood pressure monitoring, to allow repeated blood sampling, and to give fluids and drugs.

The NICU tends to be a very busy place. This busyness is sometimes at odds with the parents' need for time and privacy to become acquainted with their newborn; to learn the newborn's personality, likes, and dislikes; and ultimately to learn any special care that they will need to provide at home. Some NICUs have private (single-family) rooms and follow standards regarding noise control. Visiting hours have been greatly extended so that families can spend much more time with their newborn, and often hospitals arrange for on-site or nearby sleeping facilities for the parents.

Sometimes, parents feel that they have little to offer their newborn in a NICU. However, their presence, including stroking, speaking, and singing to their newborn, is very important. Newborns hear their mother's voice even before birth and are accustomed to it, and they often respond better to their own parents' attempts to calm them. Skin-to-skin contact (also called kangaroo care), in which the newborn is allowed to lie directly on the mother's or father's chest, is comforting to the newborn and enhances bonding. Increasing evidence indicates that premature newborns fed breast milk are significantly protected from developing necrotizing enterocolitis (a serious intestinal disorder) and infections, and that breastfeeding is otherwise beneficial.

Parents need to be kept informed of their newborn's condition and the doctor's plans, as well as the expected course and time of discharge. Regular meetings with the medical team are essential. Many NICUs also have social workers who help keep parents informed.

in the newborn. In addition to avoiding these substances, expectant mothers can improve the chances of having a healthy infant by getting care for medical problems, taking prenatal vitamins, receiving early prenatal care, and maintaining a healthy diet.

About 12% of infants are born before term (premature birth). The presence of more than one fetus (twins, triplets, quadruplets) and certain birth defects are likely to lead to early delivery. The earliest premature infants are likely to have problems with transition to newborn life, especially breathing problems caused by respiratory distress syndrome (see page 1694). Accelerated or diminished rates of fetal growth also directly impact the health of the newborn. Rarely, infants may have other problems such as birth defects, infections, or abnormal levels of sugar (glucose) in the blood. Doctors may be able to anticipate many problems by monitoring fetal growth and development, particularly by using ultrasonography (see page 1625). Newborns that are likely to have serious problems are often delivered in a hospital with a neonatal intensive care unit (NICU) where they can receive early, and if needed, intensive care from the time of birth.

Birth Injury

Birth injury is damage sustained during the birthing process, usually occurring during transit through the birth canal.

- Many newborns have minor injuries during birth.
- Infrequently, nerves are damaged or bones are broken.
- Most injuries resolve without treatment.

A difficult delivery, with the risk of injury to the fetus, may occur when the birth canal is too small or the fetus is too large (as sometimes occurs when the mother has diabetes). Injury is also more likely when the fetus is lying in an abnormal position in the uterus before birth. Overall, the rate of birth injuries is much lower now than in previous decades because of improved prenatal assessment with ultrasonography and because cesarean delivery may be done in certain circumstances.

? Did You Know...

Serious birth injuries are now quite rare as compared with a few decades ago.

Head and Brain Injury: In most births, the head is the first part to enter the birth canal and experiences much of the pressure during the delivery. Swelling of the scalp and bruising are common but not serious and resolve within a few days.

Blood may accumulate below the thick fibrous covering (periosteum) of one of the skull bones. This blood accumulation is called a cephalohematoma. Cephalohematomas feel soft and can increase in size initially after birth. Cephalohematomas do not need treatment and disappear over weeks to months.

Fracture of one of the bones of the skull may occur. Skull fractures are very rare. Unless the fracture forms an indentation (depressed fracture), it heals rapidly without treatment.

Bleeding in the brain (intracranial hemorrhage) is caused by the rupture of a blood vessel within the skull. Bleeding in the spaces around the brain results from deformity of the skull bones during delivery or from a lack of oxygen. Bleeding in the brain is much more common among very premature infants. It results from inadequate blood flow to the brain (ischemia) or a diminished amount of oxygen in the blood (hypoxia).

Most infants with bleeding do not have symptoms. But bleeding may cause sluggishness (lethargy), poor feeding, or seizures.

Bleeding can occur in several places within the skull.

- Subarachnoid hemorrhages occur below the innermost of the two membranes that cover the brain. They are the most common type of intracranial hemorrhage, usually occurring in full-term newborns. Newborns with subarachnoid hemorrhages may occasionally have seizures during the first few days of life but ultimately do well.

- Subdural hemorrhages, which occur between the outer and the inner layers of brain covering, are now much less common because of improved childbirth techniques. A subdural hemorrhage can put increased pressure on the surface of the brain. Newborns with subdural hemorrhages may develop problems, such as seizures or high levels of bilirubin in the blood.

- Intraventricular hemorrhages occur into the normal fluid-filled spaces (ventricles) in the brain. Intraparenchymal hemorrhages occur into the brain tissue itself. Intraventricular and intraparenchymal hemorrhages usually occur in very premature newborns and occur more typically as a result of an underdeveloped brain (see page 1690) rather than a birth injury.

All newborns who have a hemorrhage receive supportive measures, such as warmth, fluids given by vein (intravenously), and other treatments to maintain body functions, until they recover. Subdural hemorrhages should be treated by a surgeon.

Nerve Injury: Rarely, nerve injuries may occur. Pressure on the facial nerve caused by forceps used to assist delivery or by the fetus's head lying against the mother's pelvis can result in weakness of the muscles on one side of the face. This injury is evident when the newborn cries and the face appears asymmetric. No treatment is needed, and the weakness usually resolves by 2 to 3 months of age.

During a difficult delivery of a large infant, some of the larger nerves to one of the newborn's arms can be stretched and injured. Weakness or paralysis of the newborn's arm or hand results. Extreme movements at the shoulder should be avoided to allow the nerves to heal. Very rarely, the arm remains weak after several weeks. In this case, surgery may be needed to reattach torn nerves.

Occasionally, the nerve going to the diaphragm (the muscular sheath that separates the organs of the chest from those of the abdomen) is damaged, resulting in paralysis of the diaphragm on the same side. In this case, the newborn may have difficulty breathing. Injury of the nerves to the newborn's arm and diaphragm usually resolves completely within a few weeks.

Injuries to the spinal cord due to overstretching during delivery are extremely rare. These injuries can result in paralysis below where the injury occurred. Damage to the spinal cord is often permanent.

Perinatal Asphyxia: Perinatal asphyxia means that there has been some injury to the fetus or the newborn around the time of birth. It results when too little blood flows to the fetus's or newborn's tissues or when there is too little oxygen in the blood. There are many causes, and sometimes the exact cause cannot be identified. Some common causes include the following:

- Abnormal development of the fetus (for example, when there is a genetic abnormality)
- Infection in the fetus
- Exposure to certain drugs before birth
- Pressure on the umbilical cord or a clot in one of the blood vessels in the umbilical cord
- Sudden loss of blood

Asphyxia can also occur if the function of the placenta is inadequate and the placenta cannot provide enough oxygen to the fetus during labor.

Regardless of the cause, affected newborns appear pale and lifeless, breathe weakly or not at all, and have a very slow heart rate. If asphyxia results from rapid blood loss, newborns will be in shock. They are immediately given fluids into a vein and

Common Birthmarks and Minor Skin Markings in Newborns

There are several skin markings that are considered normal in newborns.

Bruises or marks caused by forceps may occur on the newborn's face and scalp. Bruising of the feet may occur after a breech delivery. Bruises typically resolve within just a few days.

Pink marks that are caused by dilated capillaries under the skin may occur on the forehead just above the nose, in the upper eyelids, or at the back of the neck (where they are called stork bites). This type of birthmark fades as the infant grows but sometimes remains as a faint mark that becomes brighter when the infant becomes excited or upset.

Milia are tiny, pearly white cysts that are normally found over the nose and cheeks. They are caused by plugged sweat gland ducts. Milia become smaller or disappear over a period of weeks.

White cysts are sometimes found on the gums or in the center of the roof of the mouth (Epstein's pearls). They are of no consequence.

Mongolian spots are bluish gray, flat areas that usually occur over the lower back or buttocks. At first glance, they appear to be bruises but are not and should not be mistaken for signs of abuse. They usually occur in black or Asian newborns, tend to appear less noticeable with age, and are of no consequence.

A **strawberry hemangioma** is a common birthmark. It starts as a flat, red or purplish area anywhere on the skin. Over a period of weeks, it becomes darker red and also becomes raised over the surface of the skin, appearing much like a strawberry. After several years, strawberry hemangiomas shrink and become fainter, so that by the time the child reaches school age, most are no longer visible. For this reason, surgery and other treatments are typically not needed.

then a blood transfusion. Newborns receive breathing and circulation support as needed. Newborns are kept warm, and blood sugar levels are monitored.

Asphyxiated newborns may show signs of injury to one or more organ systems. Brain function may be affected, and newborns may experience lethargy, seizures, or even coma. Kidney function and the output of urine can be affected by the lack of oxygen but do recover. There may also be problems with the lungs and breathing.

Many survivors will be completely normal, but others will have permanent signs of neurologic damage, ranging from mild learning disorders to delayed development to cerebral palsy. Some severely asphyxiated infants will not survive. Specific causes of perinatal asphyxia should be identified if possible and treated as appropriate. For example, antibiotics are given to treat blood infections, and blood transfusions are given when too much blood has been lost. Recently, it has been shown that cooling the full-term newborn's head for several hours beginning soon after birth offers some protection to the brain from injury and thus diminishes the neurologic damage.

Bone Injury: Rarely, bones may be broken (fractured) during a difficult delivery. A fracture of the collarbone (clavicle) is most common. The upper arm bone (humerus) or upper leg bone (femur) may break during a difficult delivery. However, arm or leg fractures are very unusual. A fractured bone in a newborn is kept from moving as much as possible by use of a sling or cast. Fractures in newborns almost always heal completely and rapidly.

Injury to the Skin and Soft Tissues: The newborn's skin may show some evidence of minor injury after delivery, especially those areas that receive pressure during contractions or emerge from the birth canal first during delivery. Swelling and bruising may occur around the orbits of the eyes and on the face during face-first deliveries and of the scrotum or labia after breech deliveries. Usually, no treatment is needed.

Prematurity

A premature newborn is delivered before 37 weeks of development in the uterus. A premature newborn has underdeveloped organs, which may not be ready to function outside of the uterus.

- A previous premature birth, multiple births, poor nutrition during pregnancy, late prenatal care, and severe high blood pressure increase the risk of a premature birth.

- Because many organs are underdeveloped, premature newborns may have difficulty breathing and feeding and are prone to bleeding in the brain, infections, and other problems.

- The earliest (smallest) premature newborns are at far greater risk of having problems, including developmental problems, but even so the majority of survivors have no permanent problems.

- Some premature newborns grow up with permanent problems.

- Early prenatal care reduces the risk of a premature birth.

- Premature birth can sometimes be delayed for a brief period by giving the mother drugs to slow or stop contractions.

- When an infant is expected to be delivered significantly early, doctors can give the mother injections of a corticosteroid to speed the development of the fetus's lungs and help prevent intraventricular hemorrhage.

Physical Features of a Premature Newborn

- Small size
- Large head relative to rest of the body
- Little fat under the skin
- Thin, shiny, pink skin
- Veins visible beneath the skin
- Few creases on soles of feet
- Scant hair
- Soft ears, with little cartilage
- Underdeveloped breast tissue
- Boys: Small scrotum with few folds; testes may be undescended in very premature newborns
- Girls: Labia majora not yet covering labia minora
- Rapid breathing with brief pauses (periodic breathing), apnea spells (pauses lasting longer than 20 seconds), or both
- Weak, poorly coordinated sucking and swallowing reflexes
- Reduced physical activity and muscle tone (a premature newborn tends not to draw up the arms and legs when at rest as does a full-term newborn)
- Sleeping for most of the time

Full-term pregnancy lasts 37 to 40 weeks. About 12% of newborns are born prematurely (preterm). Many of these newborns are born just a few weeks early and do not experience any problems related to their prematurity. However, the more prematurely newborns are born, the more they are prone to serious and even life-threatening complications. Extreme prematurity is the single most common cause of death in newborns. Also, newborns born very prematurely are at high risk of long-term problems, especially delayed development and learning disorders. Nonetheless, most infants who are born prematurely grow up with no long-term difficulties. The risk of premature birth is decreased with early prenatal care.

Causes

The reasons for premature birth are frequently unknown. However, the risk of premature birth is higher among adolescents and older women, women of lower socioeconomic status, women with inadequate prenatal care, and those with multiple fetuses (twins, triplets, quadruplets). Poor nutrition and untreated infections, such as urinary tract infections or sexually transmitted diseases, during pregnancy also increase the risk of premature birth. Other women at in-

creased risk of premature birth are those who have had a previous premature birth or who themselves have serious or life-threatening disorders, including heart disease, severe high blood pressure, kidney disease, preeclampsia or eclampsia (see page 1649), or infection of the uterus (chorioamnionitis).

Symptoms

Premature newborns usually weigh less than 5½ pounds (2.5 kilograms), and some weigh as little as 1 pound (½ kilogram). An ultrasound examination of the fetus done early in the pregnancy and physical features and examination of the newborn after delivery help doctors determine the gestational age (length of time spent in the uterus after the egg is fertilized).

Symptoms often depend on immaturity of various organs. For example, some organs, such as the lungs or brain, may not be fully developed. Premature newborns may also have difficulty regulating their body temperature and the level of sugar in the blood. The immune system is also underdeveloped.

Complications

Risk of complications increases with increasing prematurity and depends in part on the presence of certain causes of prematurity, such as infection, diabetes, high blood pressure, or preeclampsia in the mother.

Underdeveloped Brain: Several problems arise when an infant is born before the brain is fully developed. These problems include

- Inconsistent breathing: The part of the brain that controls regular breathing may be so immature that premature newborns breathe inconsistently, with short pauses in breathing or periods during which breathing stops completely for 20 seconds or longer (apnea—see page 1698).
- Difficulty coordinating feeding and breathing: The parts of the brain that control reflexes involving the mouth and throat are immature, so premature newborns may not be able to suck and swallow normally, resulting in difficulty coordinating feeding with breathing.
- Bleeding (hemorrhage) in the brain: Newborns born very prematurely are at increased risk of bleeding in the brain (see page 1688). Bleeding typically begins in an area of the brain called the germinal matrix and may extend into fluid-filled spaces within the brain called the ventricles. This form of hemorrhage is most likely to occur in newborns born very prematurely (before 28 weeks of pregnancy), when problems occur during labor or delivery, or when breathing problems (such as

respiratory distress syndrome) arise after birth. Most newborns with small brain hemorrhages have no symptoms, but some newborns with large hemorrhages may experience lethargy, seizures, or even coma. Newborns with small or moderate-sized hemorrhages usually develop normally. Newborns with very large hemorrhages are at higher risk of having developmental delay, cerebral palsy, or learning disorders, and a few may not survive. The final neurologic outcome is in large part determined by the amount and quality of the infant's interactions with the parents or caregivers (for example, holding, singing, playing with age-appropriate toys, and reading).

Underdeveloped Digestive Tract and Liver: An underdeveloped digestive tract and liver can cause several problems, including

- Frequent episodes of spitting-up: Initially, premature newborns may have difficulty with feedings. Not only do they have immature sucking and swallowing reflexes, but also their small stomach empties slowly, which can lead to frequent episodes of spitting up (reflux).

- Intestinal damage: Very premature newborns may develop a serious complication in which part of the intestine becomes severely damaged (called necrotizing enterocolitis—see page 1700).

- Jaundice: In premature newborns, the liver is slow in clearing bilirubin (the yellow bile pigment that results from the normal breakdown of red blood cells) from the blood. Thus, the yellow pigment accumulates, giving the skin and the whites of the eyes a yellow color (jaundice). Premature newborns tend to become jaundiced (see page 1700) in the first few days after birth. Usually, jaundice is mild and resolves as newborns take in larger amounts during feedings and have more frequent bowel movements (bilirubin is removed in the bowel movements and causes stools to be bright yellow at first). Rarely, very high levels of bilirubin accumulate and put newborns at risk of developing kernicterus. Kernicterus is a form of brain damage caused by deposits of bilirubin in the brain (see page 1701).

Underdeveloped Immune System: Infants born very prematurely have low levels of antibodies, substances in the bloodstream that help protect against infection. Antibodies cross the placenta (the organ that connects the fetus to the uterus and provides nourishment to the fetus) from mother to the fetus during the latter part of pregnancy. Therefore, the risk of developing infections, especially infection in the blood (sepsis), is higher in premature newborns. The use of special invasive devices for treatment, such as catheters in blood vessels and breathing (endotracheal) tubes, further increases the risk of developing serious infections.

Underdeveloped Kidneys: Before delivery, waste products produced in the fetus are removed by the placenta and then excreted by the mother's kidneys. After delivery, the newborn's kidneys must take over these functions. Kidney function is diminished in very premature newborns but improves as the kidneys mature. Newborns with underdeveloped kidneys may have difficulty regulating the amount of salt and water in the body.

Underdeveloped Lungs: The lungs of premature newborns may not have had enough time to fully develop before birth. Such newborns are likely to have respiratory distress syndrome, causing visibly labored breathing, flaring of the nostrils while breathing in, a grunting sound while breathing out, and a bluish discoloration to the skin (cyanosis) if oxygen levels in the blood are low (see page 1694). Respiratory distress syndrome occurs if the lungs are not mature enough to produce surfactant, a substance that coats the inside of the air sacs and allows the air sacs of the lungs to remain open.

Difficulty Regulating Blood Sugar Levels: Because premature newborns have difficulty feeding and maintaining normal blood sugar (glucose) levels, they are often treated with glucose (sugar) solutions given by vein (intravenously) or given small frequent feedings. Without regular feedings, newborns may develop low blood sugar levels (hypoglycemia—see page 1014). Most newborns with hypoglycemia do not develop symptoms. Others become listless with poor muscle tone, feed poorly, or become jittery. Rarely, seizures develop. Premature newborns are also prone to developing high blood sugar levels (hyperglycemia) if they receive too much sugar intravenously, but hyperglycemia rarely causes symptoms.

Difficulty Regulating Body Temperature: Because premature newborns have a large skin surface area relative to their weight compared to full-term newborns, they tend to lose heat rapidly and have difficulty maintaining normal body temperature, especially if they are in a cool room or if there is a draft. Therefore, their body temperature falls unless they are warmed in an incubator or by an overhead radiant warmer. If they are exposed to a cool environment, premature newborns generate extra body heat, markedly increasing their rate of metabolism and making it difficult for them to gain weight.

Prognosis

Over recent decades, the survival of premature newborns has improved dramatically. For most premature newborns, the long-term prognosis is very good, and they develop normally. However, risk of death and long-term problems begins to increase in infants born before 26 weeks of pregnancy and particularly in those born before 24 weeks. Risks include delayed development, cerebral palsy, and vision impairment. Many newborns who are extremely premature have normal intelligence, but some have learning disorders that eventually require special help in school.

Prevention

The best way for premature birth to be prevented is for the expectant mother to take good care of her own health. She should eat a nutritious diet and avoid alcohol, tobacco, and drugs unless they are needed to treat a medical condition. Ideally, expectant mothers should receive early and regular prenatal care so that any complications of pregnancy can be recognized early and treated.

If labor starts well before term, obstetricians may give drugs to the pregnant woman to slow or stop contractions for a short time. During that interval, corticosteroids, such as betamethasone, may be given to the mother to speed the development of the fetus's lungs to reduce the risk of the newborn developing respiratory distress syndrome and also to reduce the risk of brain hemorrhage.

Treatment

Treatment involves managing the complications of prematurity, such as respiratory distress syndrome and high bilirubin levels (hyperbilirubinemia). Very premature newborns are given nutrition into their veins until they can tolerate feedings into their stomach through a feeding tube and eventually feedings by mouth. The mother's breast milk is the best food for premature infants. Use of breast milk decreases the risk of developing necrotizing enterocolitis. Premature newborns may need to be hospitalized for days, weeks, or months.

Postmaturity

A postmature newborn is delivered after more than 42 weeks in the uterus.

- Near the end of a term pregnancy, placental function decreases, providing fewer nutrients and less oxygen to the fetus.
- Postmature newborns have dry, peeling, loose skin and may appear emaciated because they have not received sufficient nutrition.
- Some postmature newborns require resuscitation, but generally treatment focuses on providing good nutrition and general care.

Postmature (postterm) delivery is much less common than premature (preterm) delivery. Why a pregnancy continues beyond term is usually unknown.

Reduced function of the placenta (the organ that connects the fetus to the uterus and provides nourishment to the fetus) is the greatest risk to fetuses who go beyond term. Near the end of a term pregnancy, the placenta becomes smaller and less effective in providing oxygen and nutrients to the fetus. To compensate, the fetus begins to use its own fat and carbohydrates (sugars) to provide energy. As a result, its growth rate slows, and occasionally weight may even decrease. Postmature newborns are prone to developing low blood sugar levels (hypoglycemia) after delivery because they have exhausted their supply of stored fat and carbohydrates. If the placenta shrinks sufficiently, it may not provide adequate oxygen to the fetus, particularly during labor. A lack of adequate oxygen may result in fetal distress (see page 1659) and, in extreme cases, may result in injury to the brain and other organs. Fetal distress may cause the fetus to pass stools (meconium) into the amniotic fluid. The fetus may also reflexively take deep, gasping breaths triggered by the distress and thereby inhale the meconium-containing amniotic fluid into the lungs before birth. As a result, the newborn may have difficulty breathing after delivery (meconium aspiration syndrome—see page 1695).

Symptoms

Postmature newborns have dry, peeling, loose skin and may appear emaciated, especially if the function of the placenta was severely reduced. The fingernails and toenails are long. The umbilical cord and nails may be stained green if meconium was present in the amniotic fluid.

Treatment

Postmature newborns who experience low oxygen levels and fetal distress may need resuscitation at birth. If meconium is present in the amniotic fluid and the newborn is lethargic, a tube is passed into the windpipe (trachea) to suction as much meconium as possible from the respiratory tract. If meconium has been breathed into the lungs, a ventilator may be needed to support breathing. Sugar (glucose) solutions given by vein (intravenously) or frequent breast milk or formula feedings are given to prevent hypoglycemia.

If these problems do not occur, the major goal is to provide good nutrition so that postmature newborns can catch up to the weight that is appropriate for them.

Small for Gestational Age

A newborn, whether delivered preterm, term, or postterm, whose weight is less than that of 90% of newborns of the same gestational age at birth (below the 10th percentile) is considered small for gestational age.

- Newborns may be small because their parents are small, the placenta did not function normally, or the mother has a medical disorder or has used drugs or consumed alcohol during the pregnancy.

- Unless they are born with an infection or have a genetic disorder, most small-for-gestational-age newborns have no symptoms and do well.
- Some small newborns remain small as adults.

There are several causes for this condition. In many cases, newborns are small simply because of genetic factors, such as having small parents (less commonly, a specific genetic syndrome associated with small stature may be involved). In other cases, the placenta (the organ that connects the fetus to the uterus and provides nourishment to the fetus) may have functioned poorly so that the fetus did not receive adequate nutrients, impairing growth. A poorly functioning placenta may occur if the mother has high blood pressure, preeclampsia, kidney disease, or long-standing diabetes. A viral infection, such as cytomegalovirus infection acquired before birth, may be responsible. Fetal growth may also have been impaired if the mother smoked or used alcohol or illicit drugs during the pregnancy (see page 1641).

Small-for-gestational-age newborns who are not premature do not have the complications related to organ system immaturity that premature newborns of similar size have. They are, however, at increased risk of the following problems:

- Meconium aspiration (see page 1695)
- Excess red blood cells (polycythemia— see page 1703)
- Low blood sugar levels (hypoglycemia— see page 1014)
- Difficulty regulating body temperature (see page 1691)
- An impaired immune system

Unless they have a genetic syndrome or viral infection, most small-for-gestational-age newborns have no symptoms. If the fetal growth was impaired because of poor placental function and inadequate nutrition, growth may accelerate when newborns are provided with good nutrition after delivery. Depending on the cause and severity of growth impairment, some small-for-gestational-age newborns remain small as children and adults.

Large for Gestational Age

A newborn, whether delivered preterm, term, or postterm, whose weight is above that of 90% of newborns of the same gestational age at birth (above the 90th percentile) is considered large for gestational age.

- Newborns may be large because the parents are large or because the mother has diabetes.

- Large newborns born to mothers with diabetes are likely to be overweight as adults.
- Cesarean delivery is sometimes necessary.

Diabetes in mothers is the most common cause of large-for-gestational-age newborns. Women who are obese or who have previously had a large infant are also at risk of having large-for-gestational-age newborns. Some newborns are large for gestational age because of genetic factors, such as having rare syndromes (for example, Beckwith-Wiedemann syndrome or Sotos' syndrome).

The reason for excessive growth of the fetus varies but primarily results from an abundance of nutrients. In pregnant women with diabetes, a large amount of sugar (glucose) crosses the placenta (the organ that connects the fetus to the uterus and provides nourishment to the fetus) and results in high levels of glucose in the fetus's blood. The high levels of glucose trigger the release of increased amounts of insulin from the fetus's pancreas, resulting in accelerated growth of the fetus, including almost all organs except the brain, which grows normally.

Symptoms and Complications

Symptoms depend on which complications occur. Common complications include the following:

- **Excess amount of red blood cells (polycythemia— see page 1703):** Large-for-gestational-age newborns may have a ruddy complexion because too many red blood cells are produced. As the excess red blood cells are broken down, bilirubin is formed, which, along with poor feeding, results in jaundice.
- **Low blood sugar levels (hypoglycemia):** In newborns of mothers with diabetes, the oversupply of glucose from the placenta stops abruptly at delivery when the umbilical cord is cut and the continuing rapid production of insulin by the newborn's pancreas leads to low levels of sugar in the blood (hypoglycemia). Often hypoglycemia causes no symptoms. Sometimes, newborns are listless, limp, or jittery. Despite their large size, newborns of mothers with diabetes often do not feed well for the first few days.
- **Lung problems:** Lung development is delayed in newborns whose mothers have diabetes. When these newborns are delivered by cesarean, they are at risk of developing lung problems. Newborns born prematurely are more likely to have immature lungs and to develop respiratory distress syndrome (see page 1694), even when born only a few weeks before full term.
- **Increased risk of birth injuries:** Newborns who are large for gestational age are at increased risk of birth injuries such as stretching of the nerves in the shoulder (brachial plexus injuries) and collarbone (clavicle)

fractures. Vaginal delivery, especially breech deliveries, may be difficult when the fetus's head is large in comparison with the mother's pelvic measurements, which increases the risk of birth injury. Therefore, such a fetus may have to be delivered by caesarean.

Infants whose mother has diabetes also have a higher rate of birth defects than other newborns. Large-for-gestational-age newborns born to mothers with diabetes are likely to be significantly overweight later in childhood and as adults, which, along with their genetic predisposition, puts them at risk of developing type 2 diabetes (see page 1005).

Treatment

To treat hypoglycemia in newborns, glucose given by vein or frequent feedings by mouth or by tube into the stomach are often needed. Treatment of respiratory distress syndrome may require supplemental oxygen through a tube placed in the nose or intense intervention, such as respiratory support with a ventilator. Other complications may also requirement, such as phototherapy for jaundice.

Respiratory Distress Syndrome

Respiratory distress syndrome (hyaline membrane disease) is a breathing disorder of premature newborns in which the air sacs (alveoli) in a newborn's lungs do not remain open because the production of a substance that coats the alveoli (surfactant) is absent or insufficient.

- Little or no surfactant, as occurs in prematurity and in infants whose mother has diabetes, is a risk factor for respiratory distress syndrome.
- Affected infants have severe difficulty breathing and may appear blue due to a lack of oxygen in the blood.
- The diagnosis is based on symptoms, oxygen levels in the blood, and chest x-ray results.
- Without treatment, the syndrome may cause brain damage or death.
- If the fetus will be born preterm and presumably does not have enough surfactant before delivery, the mother may be given a corticosteroid by injection to speed up the fetus's production of surfactant.
- Oxygen is given, and a ventilator may be necessary.
- Treatment with surfactant given into the newborn's windpipe can provide the surfactant that is missing.

For newborns to be able to breathe easily, the air sacs (alveoli) in the lungs must be able to remain open and filled with air. Normally, the lungs produce a substance called surfactant. Surfactant coats the surface of the air sacs, where it lowers the surface tension and allows the air sacs to remain open throughout the respiratory cycle. Usually, production of surfactant begins after about 32 weeks of pregnancy. The more premature the newborn, the less

surfactant is available, and the greater the likelihood that respiratory distress syndrome will develop after birth. Respiratory distress syndrome occurs almost exclusively in premature newborns and is more common among newborns whose mother has diabetes. Rarely, the syndrome is inherited.

Symptoms and Diagnosis

In affected newborns, the lungs are stiff and the air sacs tend to collapse completely, emptying the lungs of air. In some very premature newborns, the lungs may be so stiff that the newborns are unable to begin breathing at birth. More commonly, newborns try to breathe, but because the lungs are so stiff, severe respiratory distress occurs. Respiratory distress is manifested by visibly labored breathing, including retractions of the chest below the rib cage, flaring of the nostrils during breathing in, and grunting while breathing out. Because much of the lung is airless, newborns have low levels of oxygen in the blood, which cause a bluish discoloration to the skin (cyanosis). Over a period of hours, the respiratory distress tends to become more severe as the muscles used for breathing tire, the small amount of surfactant in the lungs is used up, and increasing numbers of air sacs collapse. Eventually, without treatment, newborns may have damage to the brain and other organs from a lack of oxygen or may die.

Diagnosis of respiratory distress syndrome is based on the symptoms, levels of oxygen in the blood, and abnormal chest x-ray results.

Prevention and Treatment

The risk of respiratory distress syndrome is greatly reduced if delivery can be delayed until the fetus's lungs have produced sufficient surfactant. When premature birth cannot be avoided, obstetricians may give the mother injections of a corticosteroid (betamethasone). The corticosteroid goes into the fetus and accelerates the production of surfactant. Within 48 hours after the injections are started, the fetal lungs mature to the point that respiratory distress syndrome is less likely to develop after delivery or, if it does develop, is likely to be milder.

After delivery, newborns with mild respiratory distress syndrome may require only supplemental oxygen. The oxygen is given through prongs placed in the newborn's nostrils or through a small plastic hood (oxygen hood) filled with oxygen, which is placed over the head. Newborns with severe respiratory distress syndrome may require oxygen delivered by continuous positive airway pressure (CPAP)—a technique that allows newborns to breathe on their own while being given slightly pressurized oxygen or air given through prongs placed in both nostrils. In newborns with severe respiratory distress syndrome, a tube (endotracheal tube) may need to be passed into the windpipe (intubation), and the newborn's breathing may need to be supported with mechanical ventilation.

Use of a surfactant preparation can be lifesaving and reduces complications, such as rupture of the lungs (pneumothorax). The surfactant preparation acts in the same way that natural surfactant does. Surfactant can be given through an endotracheal tube and may be given immediately after birth in the delivery room to attempt to prevent respiratory distress syndrome before symptoms develop or in the early hours after birth to premature newborns who already have symptoms of this disorder.

Surfactant treatments may be repeated several times during the first days until respiratory distress syndrome resolves.

Transient Tachypnea

Transient tachypnea of the newborn (rapid breathing of the newborn, neonatal wet lung syndrome) is temporary difficulty with breathing and low blood oxygen levels due to excessive fluid in the lungs after birth.

- This disorder can occur after a scheduled caesarean delivery done before the onset of labor in newborns born a few weeks before term or at term.
- Affected newborns breathe rapidly and grunt when breathing out and may appear bluish if they are not getting enough oxygen into their blood.
- The diagnosis is based on symptoms and is confirmed by a chest x-ray.
- Almost all affected newborns recover completely in 2 to 3 days.
- Most affected newborns need treatment with oxygen, and some need assistance with breathing.

This disorder usually occurs in newborns born a few weeks before term or at term. It is more common after a cesarean delivery and is especially likely to occur if the mother has not been in labor before a cesarean delivery (for example, a mother who has a scheduled cesarean delivery).

Before birth, the air sacs (alveoli) of the lungs are filled with fluid. Immediately after birth, the fluid must be cleared from the lungs so that the air sacs can fill with air and the newborn can breathe normally. Some of the fluid is squeezed out of the lungs by pressure on the chest during a vaginal delivery. More of the fluid is rapidly reabsorbed directly by the cells lining the air sacs. Hormones released during labor cause the cells in the air sacs to begin absorbing fluid. If this fluid reabsorption does not occur rapidly, then the air sacs continue to be partially filled with fluid and newborns have difficulty breathing.

Newborns with transient tachypnea have respiratory distress with rapid breathing, drawing in of the chest wall during breathing in, and grunting during breathing out. They may develop a bluish discoloration of the skin (cyanosis) if the level of oxygen in the blood becomes low. A chest x-ray shows increased fluid in the lungs.

Most newborns with transient tachypnea recover completely within 2 to 3 days. Treatment with oxygen is usually needed. Rarely, some newborns may need continuous positive airway pressure (CPAP)—a technique that allows newborns to breathe on their own while being given slightly pressurized oxygen or air given through prongs placed in the nostrils—or even assistance with a ventilator.

Meconium Aspiration Syndrome

Meconium aspiration syndrome is respiratory distress in a newborn who has breathed (aspirated) meconium into the lungs before or around the time of birth.

- Fetuses may pass stools (meconium) in response to stress, such as a lack of oxygen.
- Stress may also cause fetuses to gasp reflexively, thus inhaling meconium into the lungs.
- Affected newborns have bluish skin, breathe rapidly, and grunt when breathing out.
- The diagnosis is based on meconium in the amniotic fluid at birth, respiratory distress in the newborn, and abnormal chest x-ray results.
- Affected infants require supplemental oxygen and may require assistance with a ventilator.
- Most affected newborns survive, but the syndrome can be fatal if severe.

Meconium is the dark green, sterile fecal material that is produced in the intestine before birth. Normally, meconium is expelled only after birth when newborns start to feed. However, in response to stress, such as an inadequate level of oxygen in the blood, the fetus may pass meconium into the amniotic fluid. Stress may also cause the fetus to take forceful gasps, so that the meconium-containing amniotic fluid is breathed (aspirated) into the lungs. After delivery, the aspirated meconium may block the airways and cause regions of the lungs to collapse. Sometimes airways are only partially blocked, allowing air to reach the parts of the lung beyond the block but preventing it from being breathed out. Thus, the involved lung may become over-expanded. Progressive over-expansion of a portion of the lung can result in rupture and then collapse of the lung. Air may then accumulate within the chest cavity around the lung (pneumothorax).

Meconium aspirated into the lungs also causes inflammation of the lungs (pneumonitis) and increases the risk of lung infection.

Meconium aspiration syndrome is often most severe in postmature newborns because they have a smaller volume of amniotic fluid so the meconium is concentrated in a smaller amount of amniotic fluid (see page 1692). Newborns with meconium aspiration syndrome are also at increased risk of persistent pulmonary hypertension (see below).

Symptoms and Diagnosis

Affected newborns have respiratory distress, in which they breathe rapidly, draw in their lower chest wall while breathing in, and grunt during breathing out. Their skin may be bluish (cyanotic) if the blood levels of oxygen are reduced, and they may also develop low blood pressure.

Doctors base the diagnosis on the presence of meconium in the amniotic fluid at the time of birth, respiratory distress in the newborn, and abnormal chest x-ray results.

Treatment

At delivery, if the newborn is covered with meconium and is limp and not breathing, doctors immediately suction the mouth, nose, and throat to remove any meconium. They then place a breathing tube into the windpipe (trachea) to suction out any meconium there.

Newborns are treated with antibiotics because of the risk of an infection and are given supplemental oxygen and are placed on a ventilator if necessary. Sometimes repeated suctioning is done to try to remove more of the meconium. Newborns on a ventilator are observed closely for serious complications, such as pneumothorax or persistent pulmonary hypertension.

Most newborns with meconium aspiration syndrome survive. However, if the disorder is severe, especially if it leads to persistent pulmonary hypertension, it can be fatal.

Persistent Pulmonary Hypertension

Persistent pulmonary hypertension is a serious disorder in which the arteries to the lungs remain narrowed (constricted) after delivery, thus limiting the amount of blood flow to the lungs and therefore the amount of oxygen in the bloodstream.

- This disorder is caused by severe respiratory distress in term or postterm newborns or by certain drugs taken by the mother before delivery.
- Breathing is rapid, and the skin is bluish.
- The diagnosis is confirmed by an echocardiogram.
- Treatment involves opening (dilating) the arteries to the lungs by giving oxygen, often while supporting the newborn's breathing with a ventilator.

- To help dilate the arteries in the lungs, sometimes nitric oxide is added to the gas that the newborn is breathing.
- Extracorporeal membrane oxygenation is sometimes used.

Normally, the blood vessels to the lungs are tightly constricted during fetal life. The lungs do not need much blood flow before birth because the placenta rather than the lungs eliminates carbon dioxide and transports oxygen to the fetus. Immediately after birth, the umbilical cord is cut and the newborn's lungs must take over the role of oxygenating the blood and removing carbon dioxide. To achieve this process, it is necessary for the fluid filling the air sacs (alveoli) to be replaced by air and for the pulmonary arteries, which bring blood to the lungs, to widen (dilate) so that an adequate amount of blood flows through the lungs.

In response to severe distress during delivery, to respiratory distress, or as a consequence of certain drugs taken by the mother before delivery (such as large doses of aspirin), the blood vessels to the lungs may not dilate as they normally should. As a result, blood pressure in the pulmonary arteries is too high (pulmonary hypertension), and blood flow to the lungs is insufficient. Because of this insufficient blood flow, not enough oxygen reaches the blood.

Causes

Persistent pulmonary hypertension is more common among newborns who are term or postterm and among newborns whose mother had taken very large doses of aspirin or indomethacin during pregnancy. In many newborns, the respiratory distress that initiates persistent pulmonary hypertension results from other lung disorders, such as meconium aspiration syndrome (see page 1695), pneumothorax, or pneumonia, but persistent pulmonary hypertension can also develop in newborns with no other lung disorder.

Symptoms and Diagnosis

Sometimes persistent pulmonary hypertension is present from birth. Other times, it develops over the first day or two. Breathing is usually rapid, and there may be severe respiratory distress if the newborn has an underlying lung disorder (see page 1694). The skin may have a bluish discoloration (cyanosis) due to low blood oxygen levels. Sometimes low blood pressure (hypotension) leads to symptoms, such as weak pulses and a pale, grayish hue to the skin.

Doctors may suspect persistent pulmonary hypertension if the mother used high doses of aspirin or indomethacin for a prolonged period during pregnancy or had a stressful delivery, or if the newborn has severe respiratory distress and oxygen levels are unexpectedly low. A chest x-ray may be entirely normal if there is no underlying lung disorder. A definitive diagnosis requires an echocardiogram to evaluate the pressure in the pulmonary arteries.

Treatment

Treatment involves placing newborns in an environment with 100% oxygen. In severe cases, a ventilator providing 100% oxygen may be needed. A high percentage of oxygen in the blood helps open the arteries going to the lungs.

In very severe cases, a very small concentration of the gas nitric oxide may be added to the oxygen that the newborn is breathing. Inhaled nitric oxide opens the arteries in the newborn's lungs and reduces pulmonary hypertension. This treatment may be needed for several days. Rarely, if all other treatments do not work, extracorporeal membrane oxygenation (ECMO) can be used. In this procedure, blood from the newborn is circulated through a machine that adds oxygen and removes carbon dioxide and then returns the blood to the newborn. ECMO has been lifesaving, allowing some newborns with pulmonary hypertension that does not respond to other treatments to survive until the pulmonary hypertension resolves.

Pneumothorax

Pneumothorax is a collection of air between the lung and the chest wall that develops when air leaks out of the lung.

- This disorder may develop in newborns who have lung disorders such as respiratory distress syndrome or meconium aspiration syndrome, who are treated with continuous positive airway pressure, or who are using a ventilator.
- The lung may collapse, breathing may be difficult, and blood pressure may decrease.
- The diagnosis is based on symptoms and the results of a chest x-ray.
- Newborns with symptoms are given oxygen, and air is removed from the chest cavity by using a needle and syringe.

Pneumothorax most often occurs in newborns with stiff lungs, such as newborns with respiratory distress syndrome (see page 1694) or meconium aspiration syndrome (see page 1695). Infrequently, it occurs as a complication from the use of continuous positive airway pressure (CPAP—a technique that allows newborns to breathe on their own while receiving slightly pressurized oxygen or air given through prongs placed in the nostrils) or a ventilator. If the pneumothorax is under pressure from CPAP or a ventilator, it can result in collapse of the lung and difficulty breathing. Also, if under pressure, the pneumothorax can compress the veins that bring blood to the heart. As a result, less blood fills the chambers of the heart, the output of the heart decreases, and the newborn's blood pressure decreases.

Air that leaks from the lungs into the tissues in the center of the chest is called **pneumomediastinum**. Unlike pneumothorax, this condition usually does not affect breathing.

Diagnosis and Treatment

Pneumothorax is suspected when newborns with underlying lung disorders or newborns receiving CPAP or on a ventilator develop worsening respiratory distress, a drop in blood pressure, or both. When examining these newborns, doctors may notice diminished sounds of air entering and leaving the lung on the side of the pneumothorax. In premature newborns, a fiber-optic light may be used to light up the affected side of the newborn's chest while in a darkened room (positive transillumination). This procedure is used to identify free air in the area surrounding the lungs (pleural cavity). A chest x-ray provides a definitive diagnosis.

No treatment is needed in newborns who do not have symptoms. Term newborns with mild symptoms may be placed in a small tent into which oxygen is pumped (an oxygen hood), so that they breathe air that contains more oxygen than does room air. However, if the newborn's breathing is labored or if the level of oxygen in the blood declines, and particularly if the circulation of blood is impaired, the air must be rapidly removed from the chest cavity. Air is removed from the chest cavity by using a needle and syringe. For newborns in significant distress, receiving CPAP, or on a ventilator, doctors may need to place a plastic tube into the chest cavity to continuously suction and remove air from the chest cavity. The tube can usually be removed after several days.

A pneumomediastinum can be seen on an x-ray and requires no treatment.

Bronchopulmonary Dysplasia

Bronchopulmonary dysplasia is a chronic lung disorder caused by repetitive lung injury.

- This disorder most often occurs in infants who were very premature, have severe lung disease, needed a ventilator, or have inadequately developed air sacs in the lungs.
- Breathing is rapid and may be labored, and the skin may be bluish.
- The diagnosis is based on symptoms, levels of oxygen in the blood, and a chest x-ray.
- Most infants with this disorder survive.

- Once discharged from the hospital, affected infants should not be exposed to cigarette smoke or fumes from a space heater or wood-burning stove and should be given palivizumab during the fall and winter months to protect against respiratory syncytial virus (RSV), a common respiratory infection.
- Giving supplemental oxygen, with a ventilator if necessary, and providing good nutrition are the mainstays of treatment.

Bronchopulmonary dysplasia is a chronic lung disorder that occurs most often in infants who were very premature and were born with a severe lung disorder (such as respiratory distress syndrome), particularly infants who needed treatment with a ventilator for more than a few weeks after birth. The delicate tissues of the lungs can be injured when the air sacs are over-stretched by the ventilator or when they are exposed to high oxygen levels for a time. As a result, the lungs become inflamed, and additional fluid accumulates within the lungs. Affected infants may not develop the normal number of air sacs. Full-term newborns who have lung disorders (such as pneumonia) occasionally develop bronchopulmonary dysplasia. Doctors now realize that bronchopulmonary dysplasia also may occur in some infants who were very premature but who did not have respiratory distress requiring a ventilator.

Symptoms and Diagnosis

Affected newborns usually breathe rapidly and may have respiratory distress, with drawing in of the lower chest while breathing in, and low levels of oxygen in the blood, causing a bluish discoloration of the skin (cyanosis). In some severely affected newborns, more than the usual amount of time is needed for air to leave the lungs during expiration, and this delay can lead to air trapping, in which the lungs become over-expanded.

The diagnosis of bronchopulmonary dysplasia is made in infants who were born prematurely, who have received ventilation for a prolonged time (generally for several weeks or months), and who have signs of respiratory distress and a prolonged need for supplemental oxygen. The diagnosis is supported by measurement of low levels of oxygen in the blood and results of a chest x-ray.

Prognosis

Although a few infants with very severe bronchopulmonary dysplasia die even after months of care, most infants survive. Over several months the seriousness of the lung injury diminishes as healthy lung tissue grows. However, later on, these children are at increased risk of developing asthma and viral pneumonia, such as that caused during winter months by RSV infection.

Prevention and Treatment

After discharge from the hospital, infants with bronchopulmonary dysplasia should not be exposed to cigarette smoke or fumes from a space heater or wood-burning stove. They should be protected as much as possible from exposure to people who have upper respiratory tract infections. These children should be protected from RSV infection by receiving doses of palivizumab, a specific antibody to that virus. This antibody must be injected monthly during the fall and winter when RSV infections occur in the community.

Ventilators are used only when absolutely necessary and then are used at the lowest possible settings to avoid injury to the lungs. Newborns are taken off ventilators as early as is safe.

In infants with bronchopulmonary dysplasia, supplemental oxygen provided through a small tube placed in the infant's nostrils may be needed initially to prevent cyanosis. Some infants with bronchopulmonary dysplasia need supplemental oxygen for months or longer.

Good nutrition is crucial to help the infant's lungs grow and to keep the new lung tissue healthy. Thus, the damaged areas of lung become less and less important relative to the overall size of the infant's lungs.

Because fluid tends to accumulate in the inflamed lungs, sometimes the daily intake of fluids is restricted, and diuretics may be used to increase the rate of excretion of fluid in the urine.

Apnea of Prematurity

Apnea of prematurity is a pause in breathing that lasts for more than 20 seconds.

- Apnea episodes occur in premature newborns whose respiratory center in the brain has not matured fully.
- Apnea may lower the amount of oxygen in the blood, resulting in a slow heart rate and bluish skin.
- This disorder is diagnosed by observation or by the alarm of a monitor attached to the newborn.
- As the respiratory center of the brain matures, apnea episodes become less frequent and then stop altogether.
- If gentle prodding does not cause the newborn to resume breathing, artificial respiration may be needed.
- Newborns with significant apnea are given caffeine to stimulate breathing.

Apnea of prematurity commonly occurs in infants who are born preterm, increasing in frequency and severity among the most prematurely born. In these newborns, the part of the brain that controls breathing (respiratory center) has not matured fully. As a result, newborns may have repeated episodes of normal breathing alternating with brief pauses in breathing. In tiny premature newborns, apnea can also be caused by temporary obstruction of the throat (pharynx) due to low muscle tone or a bending forward of the neck (obstructive apnea). Over time, as the respiratory center matures, episodes of apnea become less frequent, and by the time the newborn approaches term, they no longer occur.

Symptoms and Diagnosis

Premature newborns are routinely placed on a monitor that sounds an alarm if the newborn stops breathing for 20 seconds or if the heart rate slows. Depending on the length of the episodes, stoppage of breathing may decrease the oxygen levels in the blood, which results in a bluish discoloration of the skin (cyanosis). Low levels of oxygen in the blood may then slow the heart rate (bradycardia).

Apnea can sometimes be a sign of a disorder, such as infection in the blood (sepsis), low blood sugar (hypoglycemia), or a low body temperature (hypothermia). Therefore, doctors evaluate the newborn to rule out these disorders when there is a sudden or unexpected increase in frequency of apnea episodes. Doctors may obtain specimens of blood, urine, and cerebrospinal fluid to test for serious infections and test blood samples to determine whether the level of sugar is too low (hypoglycemia).

Treatment

When apnea is noticed, either by observation or monitor alarm, newborns are touched or prodded gently to stimulate breathing, which may be all that is required. Further treatment of apnea depends on the cause. Apnea caused by obstruction of the pharynx may be decreased by keeping newborns lying on their back or side with their head in a centered position. If episodes of apnea become frequent, and especially if newborns have cyanosis, they may be treated with a drug that stimulates the respiratory center, such as caffeine. If this treatment does not prevent frequent and severe episodes of apnea, newborns may need treatment with continuous positive airway pressure (CPAP)—a technique that allows newborns to breathe on their own while receiving slightly pressurized oxygen or air given through prongs placed in the nostrils—or with a ventilator.

Almost all premature newborns stop having episodes of apnea several weeks before they reach term.

Preterm birth is a risk factor for sudden infant death syndrome (SIDS—see page 1739), but an association between apnea and a later risk of SIDS has not been proved. Likewise, there is no proof that discharging a premature newborn from the hospital on an apnea monitor decreases the risk of SIDS.

Retinopathy of Prematurity

Retinopathy of prematurity is a disorder in which the small blood vessels in the back of the eye (retina) grow abnormally.

- Retinopathy of prematurity is strongly associated with premature birth, with most cases occurring in infants who are born after 26 or fewer weeks of pregnancy.
- In the most severe cases, the rapid abnormal growth of the small blood vessels makes them bleed, leading to scarring of the retina and vision loss.
- Because affected newborns have no symptoms, diagnosis depends on a careful examination by an eye specialist (ophthalmologist).
- This disorder is usually mild and resolves without treatment, but the eyes need to be monitored by an ophthalmologist until blood vessel growth is mature.
- If the disorder is severe, newborns require laser treatment to prevent vision loss.

In infants who were born very prematurely, growth of the blood vessels supplying the retina may stop growing for a time. When growth resumes, it occurs in a disorganized fashion. During disorganized rapid growth, the small blood vessels may bleed, which eventually leads to scarring. In the most severe cases, this process may ultimately result in detachment of the retina from the back of the eye and loss of vision.

Newborns who are developing retinopathy of prematurity do not have symptoms, and diagnosis depends on careful examination of the back of the eyes by an ophthalmologist. Routinely, therefore, an ophthalmologist examines the eyes of premature newborns who weigh less than 3 pounds (about 1,500 grams) at birth starting about 4 weeks after delivery. Eye examinations are repeated every 1 to 2 weeks as needed, until growth of the blood vessels in the retina is complete. Newborns with severe retinopathy must have eye examinations, at least yearly, for the rest of their life. If detected early, retinal detachment can be treated to attempt to avoid loss of vision in the affected eye.

Prevention and Treatment

In premature newborns who need oxygen, oxygen levels are monitored carefully so that the lowest amount of oxygen necessary can be used. Oxygen levels can be indirectly monitored using a pulse oximeter (an external sensor that measures the level of oxygen in the blood going through a finger or toe).

Retinopathy is usually mild and resolves spontaneously. For very severe retinopathy of prematurity, laser treatment is done on the outermost portions of the retina. This treatment stops the abnormal growth of blood vessels and decreases the risk of retinal detachment and loss of vision.

Necrotizing Enterocolitis

Necrotizing enterocolitis is injury to the inner surface of the intestine. This disorder occurs most often in very premature newborns.

- The abdomen may be swollen, stools may be bloody, and the newborn may vomit a greenish, yellow, or rust-colored fluid and appear very sick and sluggish.
- The diagnosis is confirmed by abdominal x-rays.
- About 60 to 80% of newborns with this disorder survive.
- Treatment involves stopping feedings, passing a suction tube into the stomach to relieve pressure, and giving antibiotics and fluids intravenously.
- In severe cases, drains are placed in the abdominal cavity, or part of the intestine that has lost its blood supply and is not viable is removed.

Eighty-five percent of cases of necrotizing enterocolitis (NEC) occur in premature newborns. The cause is not understood. Diminished blood flow to the intestine in a sick premature newborn may result in injury to the inner layers of the intestine, allowing bacteria that normally exist within the intestine to invade the damaged intestinal wall and then enter the infant's bloodstream, causing infection (sepsis). If the injury progresses through the entire thickness of the intestinal wall and the intestinal wall tears (perforates), intestinal contents leak into the abdominal cavity and cause inflammation and usually infection of the abdominal cavity and its lining (peritonitis).

Symptoms and Diagnosis

Newborns with NEC may develop swelling of the abdomen. They may vomit bile-stained intestinal fluid, and blood may be visible in the stools. These newborns soon appear very sick and sluggish (lethargic) and have a low body temperature and repeated pauses of breathing (apnea). The diagnosis of NEC is confirmed by abdominal x-rays, which show gas has formed in the intestinal wall (pneumatosis intestinalis) or that free air is in the abdominal cavity if the intestinal wall has perforated. Blood samples are taken to look for bacteria and other indicators of sepsis.

Prognosis

Intensive medical treatment and surgery when needed have improved the outcome for newborns with NEC. About 60 to 80% of such newborns survive.

Prevention and Treatment

Feeding premature newborns their mother's breast milk rather than formula seems to provide some protection.

If NEC is present, feedings are stopped. A suction tube is passed into the stomach to remove pressure from swallowed air and milk, thereby decompressing the intestine. Fluids are given by vein to maintain hydration, and antibiotics are given immediately.

About 70% of newborns with NEC do not need surgery. However, surgery is needed if there is intestinal perforation with peritonitis. Surgery may also be needed if the condition progressively worsens despite treatment. The surgery involves removing the part of the intestine that has not been receiving its blood supply. The ends of the healthy intestine are brought out to the skin surface to create a temporary opening for the excretion of stools (ostomy). Later, when the infant is healthy, the ends of the intestine are reattached and the entire intestine is put back into the abdominal cavity.

In the tiniest and sickest newborns with peritonitis who may not survive more extensive surgery, peritoneal drains are placed into the abdominal cavity on each side of the lower abdomen. Peritoneal drains allow stools and peritoneal fluid to drain from the abdominal cavity and, along with antibiotics, may lessen symptoms. The procedure helps stabilize many newborns so that an operation can be done at a later time when the newborns are in less critical condition. In some cases, newborns recover completely without needing additional surgery.

Hyperbilirubinemia

Hyperbilirubinemia is an abnormally high level of bilirubin (a pigment produced from the breakdown of red blood cells) in the blood.

- Severe hyperbilirubinemia is usually caused by illnesses that interfere with feeding, serious disorders such as sepsis, or the rapid breakdown of red blood cells.
- Bilirubin in the blood causes the skin and the whites of the eyes to appear yellow (jaundice).
- The diagnosis is based on the presence of jaundice and high levels of bilirubin measured in the blood.
- Newborns discharged from the hospital on the first day after birth should have their bilirubin level checked at home by a visiting nurse or in the doctor's office within a few days after discharge.
- When treatment is needed, newborns are treated with phototherapy and, for very severe cases, exchange blood transfusion.

Aging red blood cells are normally removed by the spleen, and the hemoglobin (the oxygen-carrying substance) from these red blood cells is broken down and recycled. The heme portion of the hemoglobin molecule is converted into a yellow pigment called bilirubin, which is carried in the blood to the liver where it is chemically modified and then excreted in the bile into the digestive tract. It is removed from the body when the newborn passes stools.

? Did You Know...
Mild hyperbilirubinemia is very common among healthy newborns and is not of concern.

In most newborns, the level of bilirubin in the blood increases in the first days after birth, and mild bilirubin elevations are considered normal. Bilirubin in the blood can cause the newborn's skin and the whites of the eyes to appear yellow (jaundice). If feedings are delayed for any reason, such as an illness or an intestinal problem, blood levels of bilirubin can become high. Also, breastfed newborns tend to have somewhat higher blood levels of bilirubin during the first week, but this increase also is usually of no concern. After several days, as the newborn takes more in feedings, the bilirubin level decreases.

Significant hyperbilirubinemia may occur when newborns have serious medical disorders, such as infection in the blood (sepsis). It may also be caused by the rapid breakdown of red blood cells (hemolysis), which occurs with Rh incompatibility (see page 1650) or ABO incompatibility (see box on page 1703).

In the large majority of cases, elevated levels of bilirubin in the blood are not serious. However, very high bilirubin levels can cause brain damage. Brain damage caused by hyperbilirubinemia is termed kernicterus. Very premature and critically ill newborns are at higher risk of developing kernicterus, but kernicterus usually can be avoided with appropriate treatment. However, newborns who are just a few weeks premature, who are breastfeeding, and who are discharged early from the hospital must be monitored closely for hyperbilirubinemia in the first few days after hospital discharge because they can develop kernicterus if the bilirubin level becomes very high. Premature newborns are at higher risk because they do not feed as vigorously as term infants and their mother's milk has not yet come in well.

Symptoms and Diagnosis

Newborns with hyperbilirubinemia have jaundice. It may be more difficult to recognize jaundice in dark-skinned newborns. Jaundice usually first appears on the newborn's face and then, as the bilirubin level increases, progresses downward to involve the chest, abdomen, and finally the legs and feet. But the appearance of jaundice does not provide an accurate measure of the bilirubin level.

The first symptoms of kernicterus are usually sluggishness (lethargy) and poor feeding. Newborns who have hyperbilirubinemia and these symptoms should be examined immediately by a doctor because they may need immediate treatment. The later stages of kernicterus involve irritability, muscle stiffening, arching of the back, seizures, and fever.

It is important that doctors assess the degree of jaundice in all newborns during the first days of life. Most doctors measure a newborn's bilirubin level before discharge from the hospital. Because bilirubin levels may take several days to rise to a dangerous level, newborns discharged from the hospital on the first day after birth should have their blood bilirubin levels checked at home by a visiting nurse or in the doctor's office within a few days after discharge. This testing is especially necessary for newborns born a few weeks prematurely who are breastfeeding.

Doctors first examine newborns under good lighting and then measure the level of bilirubin with a specialized piece of equipment held against the skin (transcutaneous bilirubinometer) or test a sample of blood.

Treatment

Mild hyperbilirubinemia does not require special treatment. Frequent breastfeedings accelerate the passage of stools, thus reducing the reabsorption of bilirubin from the intestinal contents and lowering the bilirubin level.

Moderate hyperbilirubinemia can be treated with phototherapy, in which newborns are undressed and placed under bilirubin lights. The light exposure alters the composition of the bilirubin in the newborn's skin, changing it to a form that is more readily excreted by the liver and kidneys. The newborn's eyes are shielded with a blindfold because the lights may damage the eyes. Newborns can also be treated at home by having them lie on a fiber-optic bilirubin blanket, which exposes their skin to bright light. Newborns being treated with bilirubin lights need to have their blood levels of bilirubin tested repeatedly until the levels decrease because jaundice may disappear even though the levels of bilirubin in the blood remain elevated.

? Did You Know...
It is normal for breastfed newborns to have slightly elevated levels of bilirubin during the first weeks after birth.

Very rarely, it may be necessary for a mother to change from breastfeeding to formula feeding for 1 or 2 days to ensure that the newborn is receiving enough with each feeding. The mother should resume breastfeeding as soon as the bilirubin levels start to decrease. Moderate hyperbilirubinemia sometimes continues for weeks in newborns who are breastfed, a normal phenomenon that poses no problems for the newborn.

If the newborn's bilirubin approaches a dangerous level even while phototherapy is used, the level can be lowered rapidly by doing an exchange blood transfusion. In this procedure, a sterile catheter is placed into the umbilical vein located in the cut surface of the umbilical cord. The newborn's bilirubin-containing blood is removed one syringe-full at a time and replaced with an equal volume of nonjaundiced blood provided by the blood bank.

Anemia in the Newborn

Anemia is a disorder in which there are too few red blood cells in the blood.

- Anemia can occur when red blood cells are broken down too rapidly, too much blood is lost, or the bone marrow does not produce enough red blood cells.
- If red blood cells are broken down too rapidly, levels of bilirubin increase, and the newborn's skin and the whites of the eyes appear yellow (jaundice).
- If a large amount of blood is lost very rapidly, the newborn may be in shock, appear pale, have a rapid heart rate, and have low blood pressure along with rapid, shallow breathing.
- If there is less severe blood loss or the blood is lost gradually, the newborn appears normal but pale.
- Treatment may involve fluids given by vein (intravenously) followed by a blood transfusion or an exchange blood transfusion.

Normally, the bone marrow does not produce new red blood cells between birth and 3 or 4 weeks of age, causing a slow drop in the red blood cell count (called physiologic anemia) over the first 2 to 3 months of life. Very premature newborns have a slightly greater drop in red blood cell count. More severe anemia can occur when

- Red blood cells are broken down too rapidly
- A lot of blood is taken from preterm infants for blood tests
- Too much blood is lost during labor or delivery
- The bone marrow does not produce blood cells

More than one of these processes can occur at the same time.

Severe red blood cell breakdown results in anemia and high levels of bilirubin in the blood (hyperbilirubinemia). Hemolytic disease of the newborn may cause the newborn's red blood cells to be destroyed rapidly. The red blood cells may also be rapidly destroyed if the newborn has a hereditary abnormality of the red blood cells. An example is hereditary spherocytosis, in which the red blood cells look like small spheres when viewed under a microscope. Another rare example occurs in some infants who lack a specific red blood cell enzyme (glucose-6-phosphate dehydrogenase [G6PD]). In these infants, exposure of the mother and fetus to certain drugs

used during pregnancy (such as aniline dyes, sulfa drugs, and many others) may result in rapid breakdown of red blood cells.

Infections acquired before birth, such as toxoplasmosis, rubella, cytomegalovirus infection, herpes simplex virus infection, or syphilis, may also rapidly destroy red blood cells, as can bacterial infections of the newborn acquired during or after birth.

Blood loss is another cause of anemia. Blood loss can occur in many ways. For example, blood is lost if there is a large transfusion of fetal blood across the placenta (the organ that connects the fetus to the uterus and provides nourishment to the fetus) and into the mother's circulation (fetal–maternal transfusion) or if too much blood gets trapped in the placenta at delivery, when the newborn is held above the mother's abdomen when the umbilical cord is clamped. Twin-to-twin transfusions, in which blood flows from one fetus to the other, can cause anemia in one twin and too much blood (polycythemia) in the other twin. The placenta may separate from the uterine wall before delivery (placental abruption), leading to hemorrhage of fetal blood.

Rarely, failure of the fetal bone marrow to produce red blood cells may result in anemia. Examples of this lack of production include rare genetic disorders such as Fanconi's anemia and Diamond-Blackfan anemia. Some infections (such as cytomegalovirus infection, syphilis, and HIV) also prevent the bone marrow from producing red blood cells.

Symptoms and Diagnosis

Most infants with mild or moderate anemia have no symptoms. Moderate anemia may result in sluggishness (lethargy), poor feeding, or no symptoms. Newborns who have suddenly lost a large amount of blood during labor or delivery may be in shock and appear pale and have a rapid heart rate and low blood pressure, along with rapid, shallow breathing. When the anemia is a result of rapid breakdown of red blood cells, there is also an increased production of bilirubin, and the newborn's skin and whites of the eyes appear yellow (jaundice). Diagnosis is based on symptoms and is confirmed with blood tests.

Treatment

Most infants have mild anemia and do not require any treatment.

Newborns who have rapidly lost large amounts of blood, often during labor and delivery, are treated with intravenous fluids followed by a blood transfusion. Very severe anemia caused by hemolytic disease may also require a blood transfusion, but the anemia is more often treated with an exchange blood transfusion, which lowers the bilirubin level as well as increases the red blood cell count. In an exchange

What Is Hemolytic Disease of the Newborn?

Hemolytic disease of the newborn (also called erythroblastosis fetalis or erythroblastosis neonatorum) is a condition in which red blood cells are broken down or destroyed more rapidly than normal, causing hyperbilirubinema, anemia, and, in the most severe forms, death. Hemolytic disease of the newborn may occur in Rh-positive babies born to Rh-negative mothers. It develops when the newborn's red blood cells are destroyed by anti-Rh antibodies that were produced by the mother and passed through the placenta from the mother's circulation into the fetal circulation before delivery. A mother who is Rh-negative can produce antibodies against Rh-positive blood cells if she was previously exposed to red blood cells from a fetus that was Rh-positive. Such exposure may occur during pregnancy or labor, but it may also occur if the mother had been accidentally transfused with Rh-positive blood at any time earlier in life.

The mother's body then responds to the "incompatible" blood by producing antibodies to destroy the "foreign" Rh-positive cells. These antibodies cross the placenta during a subsequent pregnancy. If the fetus she is carrying is Rh-negative, there is no consequence. However, if the fetus has Rh-positive red blood cells, the mother's antibodies attach to and start to destroy the fetal red blood cells, leading to anemia of varying degrees. The rapid breakdown of red blood cells begins in the fetus and continues after delivery.

Severe anemia caused by hemolytic disease of the newborn is treated in the same way as any other anemia. Doctors also observe the newborn for jaundice, which is likely to occur because hemoglobin from the red blood cells that are being rapidly broken down is converted to the yellow pigment bilirubin, giving the newborn's skin and whites of the eyes a yellow appearance. Jaundice can be treated by exposing the newborn to bright lights (phototherapy) or by having the newborn undergo an exchange blood transfusion. Very high levels of bilirubin in the blood can lead to brain damage (kernicterus), unless it is prevented by these measures.

To prevent sensitization of Rh-negative women, the Rh antigen, an $Rh_0(D)$ immune globulin preparation, is given by injection at about 28 weeks of pregnancy and again immediately after delivery. Injection of this immune globulin prevents the mother's immune system from producing anti-Rh antibodies, and it also rapidly coats any Rh-positive fetal red blood cells that have entered the mother's circulation so they are not recognized as Rh-positive cells by the mother's immune system. This treatment usually prevents hemolytic disease of the newborn from developing.

Sometimes other blood group incompatibilities may lead to similar (but milder) hemolytic diseases. For example, if the mother has blood type O and the fetus has blood type A or B, then the mother's body produces anti-A or anti-B antibodies that can cross the placenta, attach to fetal red blood cells, and cause their breakdown (hemolysis), leading to mild anemia and hyperbilirubinemia. Rh incompatibility usually leads to more severe anemia than ABO incompatibility.

---

transfusion, a small amount of the newborn's blood is gradually removed (one syringe at a time) and replaced with equal volumes of fresh donor blood.

Polycythemia in the Newborn

Polycythemia is an abnormally high concentration of red blood cells.

- This disorder may result from postmaturity (see page 1692), diabetes in the mother, or a low oxygen level in the fetal blood.
- A high concentration of red blood cells makes the blood thick (hyperviscosity) and may slow blood flow through small blood vessels.
- Most affected newborns do not have symptoms but occasionally have a ruddy or dusky color, are sluggish (lethargic), feed poorly, and very rarely may have seizures.
- The diagnosis is inferred from a test that measures the content of red blood cells in the blood.
- Usually no treatment is needed except to maintain normal hydration.

- When the newborn has symptoms, treatment with a partial exchange transfusion may be given to reduce the red blood cell concentration.

A markedly increased concentration of red blood cells may result in the blood being too thick, which slows the flow of blood through small blood vessels and interferes with the delivery of oxygen to tissues. A newborn who is born postmaturely or whose mother has diabetes, has severe high blood pressure, smokes, or lives at a high altitude is more likely to have polycythemia. Polycythemia may also result if the newborn receives too much blood from the placenta at birth, as may occur if the newborn is held below the level of the placenta for a time before the umbilical cord is clamped. Other causes include a low oxygen level in the blood (hypoxia), maternal diabetes, growth restriction in the womb, or a large transfusion of blood from one twin to another (twin-to-twin transfusion).

A newborn with severe polycythemia has a very ruddy or dusky color, is lethargic, feeds poorly, and may have seizures. If the newborn has such symptoms, and a blood test indicates too many red blood cells (high hematocrit), some of the newborn's blood is removed and replaced with an equal volume of saline solution, thus diluting the remaining red blood cells and correcting the polycythemia.

Thyroid Disorders in the Newborn

Thyroid disorders occur if the thyroid gland produces too little thyroid hormone (hypothyroidism) or too much thyroid hormone (hyperthyroidism).

HYPOTHYROIDISM IN THE NEWBORN

The most common cause of hypothyroidism in the newborn is complete absence or underdevelopment of the thyroid gland. Less commonly, the thyroid gland is present but does not produce normal amounts of thyroid hormones.

Initially, the newborn may have no symptoms. Later, the newborn may become sluggish (lethargic) and have a poor appetite, low muscle tone, constipation, a hoarse cry, and a bulging of the abdominal contents at the bellybutton (an umbilical hernia). Untreated infants will have delayed development, intellectual disability, and short stature. Eventually, the infant may develop coarse facial features and an enlarged tongue.

Because early treatment can prevent intellectual disability, all newborns receive a screening blood test in the hospital after birth to evaluate thyroid function. In affected newborns, the blood test shows an elevated level of thyroid-stimulating hormone and usually a lower level of thyroid hormone. Many newborns with hypothyroidism require thyroid hormone given by mouth for their entire life. Treatment is directed by a doctor who specializes in treating children with problems of the endocrine system (a pediatric endocrinologist).

HYPERTHYROIDISM IN THE NEWBORN

Rarely, a newborn may have hyperthyroidism, or neonatal Graves' disease. This condition usually occurs if the mother has Graves' disease during pregnancy or has been treated for it before pregnancy. In Graves' disease (see page 1635), the mother's body produces antibodies that stimulate the thyroid gland to produce increased amounts of thyroid hormone. These antibodies cross the placenta and similarly affect the fetus.

An affected newborn has a high metabolic rate, with rapid heart rate and breathing, irritability, and excessive appetite with poor weight gain. The newborn, like the mother, may have bulging eyes (exophthalmos). If the newborn has an enlarged thyroid gland (goiter), the gland may press against the windpipe and interfere with breathing at birth. A very rapid heart rate can lead to heart failure. Graves' disease is potentially fatal if not recognized and treated by a pediatric endocrinologist.

Doctors suspect hyperthyroidism based on the typical symptoms and confirm the diagnosis by detecting elevated levels of thyroid hormone and thyroid-stimulating antibodies from the mother in the newborn's blood. The results of a screening test of thyroid function done in all newborns may reveal hyperthyroidism.

Newborns with hyperthyroidism are treated with drugs, such as propylthiouracil, that slow the production of thyroid hormone by the thyroid gland. This treatment is needed only for a few months because the antibodies that cross the placenta from the mother eventually disappear from the infant's bloodstream.

Sepsis in the Newborn

Sepsis is bacterial infection in the blood.

- Newborns with sepsis are listless, do not feed well, and often have a low body temperature.
- The diagnosis is based on symptoms and the presence of bacteria in the blood.
- Most newborns who recover from sepsis do not have long-term problems.
- Treatment involves antibiotics, fluids given by vein (intravenously), and sometimes a ventilator to support breathing and drugs to support blood pressure.

Premature infants are at much higher risk of both early-onset and late-onset sepsis than are infants born at full term because of their immature immune system. Premature newborns lack certain antibodies against specific bacteria because these antibodies do not cross the placenta from the mother into the fetus's blood until late in pregnancy.

Other risk factors for and causes of sepsis differ depending on whether sepsis develops in the first few days of life (early-onset sepsis) or 7 days or more after birth (late-onset sepsis).

Early-Onset Sepsis: Risk factors include the following:

- Premature prolonged rupture of the fluid-filled membranes that surround the fetus
- Infection in the mother
- Presence of group B streptococcus (GBS) in the mother

The risk of sepsis is greater if the fluid-filled membranes that surround the fetus rupture more than 18 hours before birth or if the mother has an infection (particularly of the urinary tract or lining of the uterus).

SOME INFECTIONS OF NEWBORNS

INFECTION	TRANSMISSION	SYMPTOMS	TREATMENT AND PREVENTION
Conjunctivitis	The bacteria *Chlamydia* or *Neisseria gonorrhoeae* infect the fetus during delivery.	*Chlamydia*: Conjunctivitis usually begins 5 to 14 days after delivery but sometimes 6 weeks after. Newborns have swollen eyelids and a watery discharge from the eyes that contains increasing amounts of pus. *Neisseria gonorrhoeae*: Conjunctivitis usually begins 2 to 5 days after delivery. Newborns have severe inflammation of the eyelids and discharge of pus from the eyes. Without treatment, blindness may occur.	*Chlamydia*: Erythromycin is given as an eye ointment for prevention and by mouth for treatment. *Neisseria gonorrhoeae*: An eye ointment containing polymyxin and bacitracin, erythromycin, or tetracycline is used for prevention, and the antibiotic ceftriaxone is given by vein for treatment.
Cytomegalovirus infection	The virus is thought to cross the placenta from the mother during pregnancy or during delivery. After birth, newborns may become infected if breast milk contains the virus or if they are given a contaminated blood transfusion.	Most newborns do not have symptoms. About 10% of newborns infected at birth are premature and have a low birth weight, a small head, growth delay, jaundice, small bruises, inflammation of the lungs or eyes, and an enlarged liver and spleen. Newborns infected after birth can have an enlarged liver and spleen, hepatitis, a low platelet count, a high number of white blood cells, or all of these symptoms. Hearing loss, vision loss, and intellectual disability may occur.	The infection cannot be cured. Ganciclovir may help relieve some symptoms. Newborns should have repeated hearing evaluations during the first year.
Hepatitis B	The infection can occur during delivery if the mother is infected.	Chronic liver disease (such as chronic hepatitis or cirrhosis) develops but usually does not cause symptoms until young adulthood.	All newborns are given hepatitis B virus vaccine before hospital discharge. A newborn born to an infected mother is given hepatitis B virus vaccine and hepatitis B immune globulin within 12 hours of birth.
Herpes	Usually, the virus (herpes simplex) is transmitted during delivery through the mother's infected genital tract.	Usually, a rash of small fluid-filled blisters appears. Infection may be widespread, affecting many organs, such as the eyes, lungs, liver, brain, and skin. Other symptoms include sluggishness, diminished muscle tone, respiratory distress, pauses in breathing (apnea), and seizures.	The antiviral drug acyclovir is given by vein (intravenously). Eye infections are treated with trifluridine drops and acyclovir given intravenously.

(continued on the following page)

SOME INFECTIONS OF NEWBORNS (*Continued*)

INFECTION	TRANSMISSION	SYMPTOMS	TREATMENT AND PREVENTION
Human immunodeficiency virus (HIV) infection	The virus is transmitted from mother to fetus during pregnancy or to the newborn during labor and delivery or after birth through breastfeeding.	Symptoms range from none to very severe (AIDS). The lymph nodes may swell. Infection can affect many organs such as the liver, spleen, heart, kidneys, brain, and spinal cord. Symptoms can also include recurrent diarrhea, poor weight gain, invasive bacterial infections, and viral infections.	Antiretroviral drugs are used, and consultation with a specialist and enrollment in a clinical trial are advised. Early diagnosis and treatment of infections can help.
Human papillomavirus infection	Usually, newborns become infected during delivery.	Warts grow in the windpipe and can alter the newborn's cry and sometimes cause difficulty breathing or even block the airways. The lungs may become infected.	Warts are removed surgically. The drug interferon can reduce the risk of recurrent infections. Females aged 9 to 26 should be vaccinated.
Rubella	The virus may cross the placenta during pregnancy. Infection is now rare because vaccination is routine. Infection is more severe if the fetus is infected early in pregnancy.	Effects on the fetus range from death before birth to birth defects or to hearing loss without other symptoms. Newborns may have a low birth weight, brain inflammation, cataracts, damage to the retina, heart defects, an enlarged liver and spleen, bruising, bluish red spots, enlarged lymph nodes, and pneumonia.	No specific treatment is available. Vaccinating all women of childbearing age before pregnancy can prevent the infection. If an expectant mother who has not been immunized comes into close contact with an infected person early in pregnancy, she may be given an injection of immune globulin.
Syphilis	The bacteria (*Treponema pallidum*) cross the placenta during pregnancy if the mother acquires syphilis during pregnancy or if she has been inadequately treated for syphilis in the past.	Stillbirth or premature birth may occur. Newborns may have no symptoms. During the first month of life, large blisters or a flat copper-colored rash may develop on palms and soles. Raised bumps may develop around the nose and in the diaper area. Newborns may not grow well. They may have cracks around the mouth, or mucus, pus, or blood may run from the nose. Usually, the lymph nodes, liver, and spleen are enlarged. Rarely, inflammation of the eye or brain, seizures, meningitis, or intellectual disability occurs, but these symptoms may not appear until the child is age 2 years or older.	Before birth, the mother is treated with penicillin. After birth, the mother, if still infected, and newborn are treated with penicillin.

(continued on the following page)

SOME INFECTIONS OF NEWBORNS (*Continued*)

INFECTION	TRANSMISSION	SYMPTOMS	TREATMENT AND PREVENTION
Toxoplasmosis	The parasite (*Toxoplasma gondii*) may cross the placenta from the mother to the fetus during pregnancy. Infection is more severe if the fetus is infected early in pregnancy.	The fetus may grow slowly and be born prematurely. Newborns may have a small head, brain inflammation, jaundice, an enlarged liver and spleen, and inflammation of the heart, lungs, or eyes. Rashes may occur.	Avoiding handling cat litter during pregnancy is recommended. Transmission from the mother to the fetus may be prevented if the mother takes spiramycin. Pyrimethamine and sulfonamides may be taken later in pregnancy if the fetus is infected. Infected newborns with symptoms are treated with pyrimethamine, sulfadiazine, and leucovorin. Inflammation of the heart, lungs, or eyes is treated with corticosteroids.

The most common types of bacteria causing sepsis in the newborn around the time of birth are *Escherichia coli* and GBS, which are usually acquired during passage through the birth canal. Sepsis caused by GBS was the leading cause of early-onset sepsis until about a decade ago when screening of all expectant mothers for GBS became a routine part of prenatal care. If screening reveals GBS, the mother is given antibiotics when she goes into labor. The newborn, if delivered vaginally, is immediately given antibiotics.

Late-Onset Sepsis: Important risk factors include the following:

- Prolonged use of catheters in arteries, veins, or both
- Use of a breathing tube inserted through the nose or mouth (endotracheal tube) and attached to a ventilator to help support breathing
- Prolonged hospitalization

Sepsis that occurs later is more likely to be acquired from unwashed hands or the environment and may be caused by various organisms.

Symptoms and Diagnosis

Newborns with sepsis are usually listless, do not feed well, and often have a low body temperature. Other symptoms may include pauses in breathing (apnea), fever, pale color, and poor skin circulation, with cool extremities, abdominal swelling, vomiting, diarrhea, seizures, jitteriness, and jaundice. The diagnosis is suggested by the newborn's symptoms and the results of a complete blood count. A definite diagnosis is made only if bacteria are identified in a culture of the newborn's blood.

One of the most serious complications of sepsis is infection of the membranes surrounding the brain (meningitis). Newborns with meningitis may have extreme sluggishness (lethargy), coma, seizures, or bulging of the soft spot between the skull bones (fontanelle). Doctors can diagnose meningitis by doing a spinal tap (lumbar puncture), examining the cerebrospinal fluid, and culturing a sample of this fluid.

Prognosis and Treatment

Sepsis is the major cause of death in premature newborns after the first week. Newborns who recover from sepsis should not have long-term problems, except those with meningitis, who may have developmental delay, cerebral palsy, seizures, or hearing loss.

While awaiting blood culture results, doctors give intravenous antibiotics to newborns with suspected sepsis. Once the specific organism has been identified, the type of antibiotic can be adjusted. In addition to antibiotic therapy, other treatments may be needed, such as use of a ventilator, intravenous fluids, and support of blood pressure and circulation.

262 Birth Defects

Birth defects, also called congenital anomalies, are physical abnormalities that occur before a baby is born. They are usually obvious at birth or by 1 year of age.

- The cause of many birth defects is unknown, but infections, genetics, and certain environmental factors increase the risk.
- The diagnosis is based on the mother's risk factors, the results of an ultrasound, and sometimes blood tests, amniocentesis, or chorionic villus sampling.
- Some birth defects can be prevented by maintaining good nutrition while pregnant and avoiding alcohol, radiation, and certain drugs.
- Some birth defects can be corrected with surgery or drugs.

Birth defects can involve any part of any organ in the body. Some birth defects are more common than others. Birth defects are the leading cause of death in infants in the United States, and some cause the death of the fetus. A birth defect is evident in about 7.5% of all children by age 5 years, although many of these are minor. Major birth defects are evident in about 3 to 4% of newborns. Several birth defects can occur together in the same infant.

Causes and Risks

It is not surprising that birth defects are fairly common, considering the complexities involved in the development of a single fertilized egg into the millions of specialized cells that constitute a human being. Although the cause of most birth defects is unknown, certain genetic and environmental factors increase the chance of birth defects developing. These factors include exposure to radiation, certain drugs (see table on page 1638), alcohol, isotretinoin, nutritional deficiencies, certain infections in the mother, injuries, and hereditary disorders. Some risks are avoidable. Others occur no matter how strictly a pregnant woman adheres to healthful living practices.

Exposure to Harmful Substances (Teratogens): A teratogen is any substance that can cause or increase the chance of a birth defect. Radiation (including x-rays), certain drugs, and toxins (including alcohol) are teratogens. Most pregnant women who are exposed to teratogens have newborns without abnormalities. Whether a birth defect occurs depends on when, how much, and how long the pregnant woman was exposed to the teratogen. Exposure to a teratogen most commonly affects the

fetal organ that is developing most rapidly at the time of exposure. For example, exposure to a teratogen during the time that certain parts of the brain are developing is more likely to cause a defect in those areas than exposure before or after this critical period. Many birth defects develop before a woman knows she is pregnant.

Nutrition: Keeping a fetus healthy requires maintaining a nutritious diet. For example, insufficient folic acid (folate) in the diet increases the chance that a fetus will develop spina bifida or other abnormalities of the brain or spinal cord known as neural tube defects (see page 1724). Cleft lip or cleft palate is also more likely to develop. Maternal obesity also increases the risk of a neural tube defect.

Genetic and Chromosomal Factors: Chromosomes and genes may be abnormal. These abnormalities may be inherited from the parents, who can be affected by the condition or who can be carriers without symptoms (see box on page 12). However, many birth defects are caused by seemingly random and unexplained changes (mutations) in the genes of the child. Most birth defects caused by genetic factors include more than just the obvious malformation of a single body part.

Infections: Certain infections in pregnant women can cause birth defects. Whether an infection causes a birth defect depends on the age of the fetus. The infections that most often cause birth defects are cytomegalovirus, herpesvirus, parvovirus (fifth disease), rubella (German measles), varicella (chickenpox), toxoplasmosis (which can be transmitted in cat litter), and syphilis. A woman can have such an infection and not know it, because these infections can cause few or no symptoms in adults.

Diagnosis

During pregnancy, doctors assess whether a woman is at increased risk of having a baby with a birth defect (see page 1611). The chance is higher for women who are older than 35 years; have had frequent miscarriages; or have had other children with chromosomal abnormalities, birth defects, or who died for unknown reasons. These women may need special tests to find out whether their baby is developing normally.

Prenatal ultrasonography can often detect specific birth defects. Sometimes blood tests can also help. For example, a high level of alpha-fetoprotein in the mother's blood may indicate a defect of the brain or

OTHER BIRTH DEFECTS

MAJOR SYSTEM	BIRTH DEFECT	WHAT HAPPENS	TREATMENT
Heart	Hypoplastic left heart syndrome	Underdevelopment of the left ventricle, leading to inability to pump blood to the body	Separate operations to rebuild the left ventricle or a heart transplant
Digestive tract	Omphalocele and gastroschisis	Hole in or weakening of abdominal muscles, allowing internal abdominal organs to protrude externally	Surgery to close the abdomen
Musculoskeletal	Missing limb	Limb may not form or may be "amputated" in the womb	Artificial limb and therapy to help child adapt and be functional
	Prune-belly syndrome	Missing layers of abdominal muscles, causing the abdomen to bulge; urinary system defects often develop	Surgery if a urinary system defect blocks urine flow
Neurologic	Porencephaly	Brain tissue is missing and is replaced with fluid-filled sacs	No treatment is available; ventricular shunt may decrease pressure
	Hydranencephaly	Severe porencephaly with little remaining brain tissue	No treatment is available
Genital	Vanishing testes (bilateral anorchia; testicular regression)	Both testes are absent at birth	Supplemental male hormone (testosterone) beginning before puberty
Eye	Congenital glaucoma	Glaucoma is present at birth; pressure is raised in the eyeball (usually both); the eye may enlarge, and its usual appearance may be distorted	Surgery usually performed soon after birth; eye drops used until surgery; if the glaucoma is not treated, blindness can result
	Congenital cataracts	Cataracts (cloudy areas) in the lens of the eye are present at birth; usually vision is impaired	Surgery to remove the cataract as soon as possible is the best chance for normal vision

spinal cord (see page 1612). Amniocentesis (removing fluid from around the fetus) or chorionic villus sampling (removing tissue from the sac around the developing baby) may be necessary to confirm a suspected diagnosis. Increasingly, birth defects are being diagnosed before the baby is born.

Heart Defects

- Some heart defects are caused by an abnormal formation of the walls or valves of the heart.
- Detectable symptoms include trouble breathing, bluish skin, inability to grow or exercise normally, and heart failure.

- An ultrasound helps identify almost all heart defects.
- Treatment includes open-heart surgery for severe defects, use of a catheter with a balloon at its tip to open or widen valves or blood vessels, or drugs called prostaglandins.

One of 120 babies is born with a heart defect. Some are severe, but many are not. Defects may involve abnormal formation of the heart's walls or valves or of the blood vessels that enter or leave the heart.

Blood flow is different in the fetus than in children and adults. In children and adults, all blood returning to the heart (venous blood) goes through the right atrium and then through the right ventricle to the pulmonary artery, and from there it enters the

Normal Circulation in a Fetus

Blood flow through the heart in a fetus differs from that in children and adults. In children and adults, blood picks up oxygen in the lungs. But in a fetus, the blood that enters the heart already contains oxygen, supplied from the mother by the placenta. Only a small amount of blood goes through the lungs (which do not contain air). The rest of the blood bypasses the lungs through two structures: the foramen ovale, a hole between the right and left atria, and the ductus arteriosus, a blood vessel that connects the pulmonary artery and the aorta. Normally, these two structures close soon after birth.

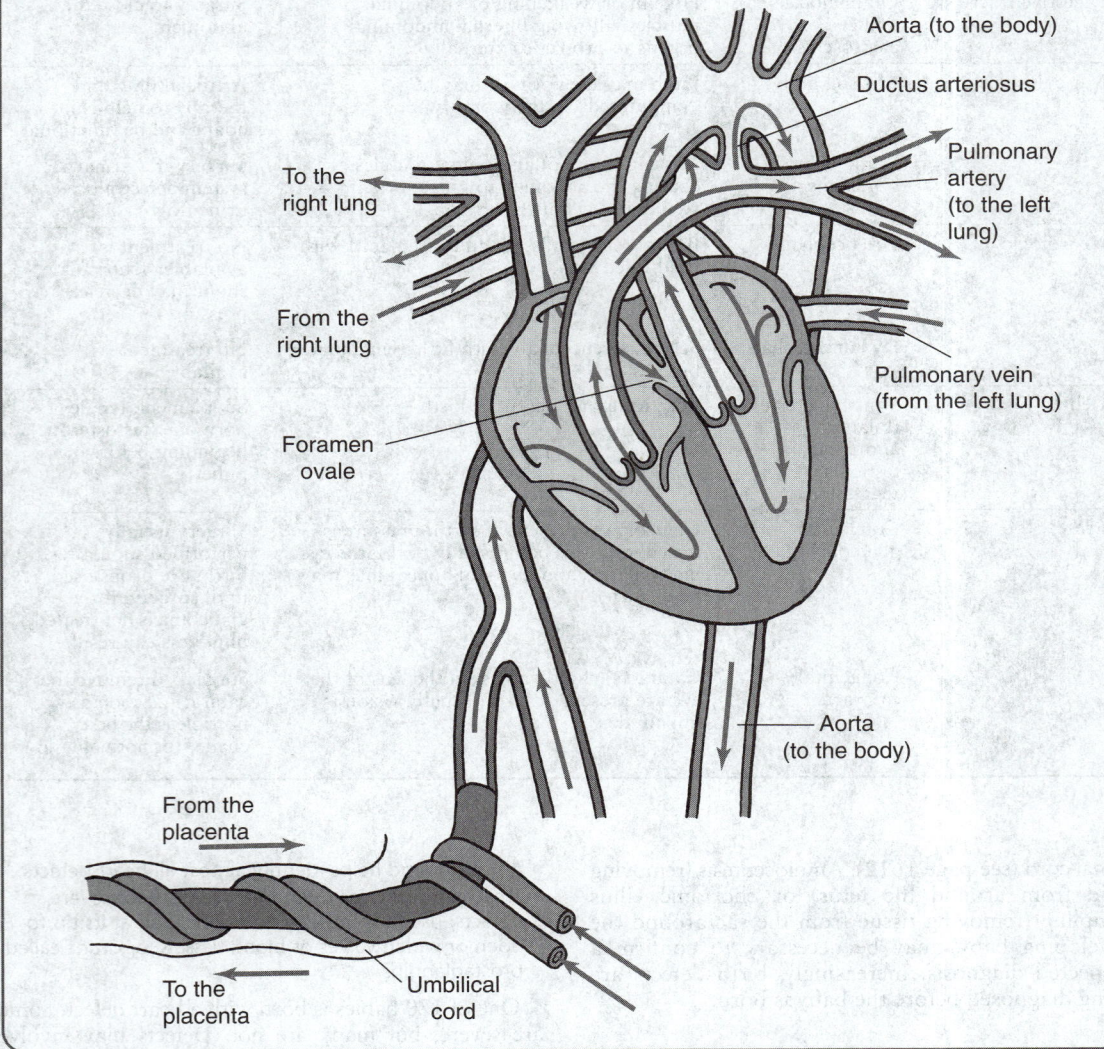

lungs. In the lungs, the blood picks up oxygen from the air sacs (alveoli) and also releases carbon dioxide (see art on page 446). The blood then returns from the lungs to the left atrium and left ventricle and

from there it is pumped out of the heart to the body (arterial blood) through a large artery called the aorta. However, because there is no air to breathe before birth, a fetus uses oxygen obtained from the mother's blood through the placenta. Because the fetus does not breathe, only a small amount of blood needs to go through the lungs, so the path by which blood circulates through the heart and lungs is different in the fetus.

Before birth, much of the venous blood coming to the right side of the heart bypasses the lungs and mixes in two different places with blood that has already traveled to the lungs. Such mixing occurs through the foramen ovale, a hole between the right and left atria. Mixing also occurs through the ductus arteriosus, a blood vessel connecting the pulmonary artery and the aorta. In the fetus, because blood arriving at the heart has already received oxygen from the placenta, both venous blood and arterial blood contain oxygen, so mixing arterial blood and venous blood does not affect how much oxygen gets pumped to the body. After birth, however, such mixing would severely limit the amount of oxygen in the blood, so the foramen ovale and ductus arteriosus normally close within days to a couple of weeks after birth.

Abnormally formed hearts alter the normal blood flow to the lungs and body. Either the flow of blood gets re-routed (shunted) or a defective heart valve or a blood vessel blocks the flow of blood.

Shunting can cause oxygen-poor blood to mix with oxygen-rich blood that is pumped to the body tissues (right-to-left shunt). The more oxygen-poor blood (which is blue) that flows to the body, the bluer the body appears, particularly the skin and lips. Many heart defects are characterized by a bluish discoloration of the skin (called cyanosis). Cyanosis indicates that not enough oxygen-rich blood is reaching the tissues where it is needed.

Shunting can also mix oxygen-rich blood, which is pumped under high pressures, with oxygen-poor blood being pumped through the pulmonary artery to the lungs (left-to-right shunt). Shunting makes the circulation inefficient and increases the pressure in the pulmonary artery. The high pressure damages the pulmonary artery and lungs. The shunt also eventually leads to an insufficient amount of blood being pumped to the body (heart failure).

In heart failure, blood also backs up, often in the lungs. Heart failure can also develop when the heart pumps too weakly (for example, when a baby is born with a weak heart muscle) or when blood is blocked from flowing to the baby's body.

Blockages may develop in the valves of the heart or in the blood vessels leading away from the heart. Blood may be impeded from flowing to the lungs because of narrowing of the pulmonary valve (pulmonary valve stenosis) or narrowing within the pulmonary artery itself (pulmonary artery stenosis). Blood may be impeded from flowing through the aorta to the body because of narrowing of the aortic valve (aortic valve stenosis) or blockage within the aorta itself (coarctation of the aorta).

Symptoms and Diagnosis

Often, heart defects cause few or no symptoms and are not detectable even during a physical examination of the child. Some mild defects cause symptoms only later in life. However, many heart defects do result in symptoms during childhood. Because oxygen-rich blood is necessary for normal growth, development, and activity, infants and children with heart defects may fail to grow or gain weight normally. They may not be able to exercise fully. In more severe cases, cyanosis may develop, and breathing or eating may be difficult. Abnormal blood flow through the heart usually causes an abnormal sound (murmur) that can be heard using a stethoscope; however, the vast majority of heart murmurs that occur during childhood are not caused by heart defects and are not indicative of any problems. Heart failure makes the heart beat rapidly and often causes fluid to collect in the lungs or liver. Some congenital heart defects (such as a hole in the atrium [patent foramen ovale]) increase the risk that a blood clot will form and block an artery in the brain, leading to a stroke.

Many heart defects can be diagnosed before birth by using ultrasonography. After birth, heart defects are suspected when symptoms develop or when particular heart murmurs are heard.

Diagnosing heart defects in children involves the same techniques used for diagnosing heart problems in adults (see page 320). A doctor may be able to diagnose the defect after asking the family specific questions and performing a physical examination, electrocardiography (ECG), and a chest x-ray. Ultrasonography (echocardiography) is used to diagnose almost all of the specific defects. Cardiac catheterization often can show small abnormalities that are not detected with echocardiography or can further illuminate the details of the abnormality.

 Did You Know...
One of 120 babies is born with a heart defect.

Treatment

Many significant heart defects are effectively repaired with open-heart surgery. When to perform the operation depends on the specific defect, its symptoms, and severity. For example, it may be better to postpone surgery until the child is a little older.

Patent Ductus Arteriosus: Failure to Close

The ductus arteriosus is a blood vessel that connects the pulmonary artery and the aorta. In the fetus, it enables blood to bypass the lungs. The fetus does not breathe air, and thus blood does not need to pass through the lungs to be oxygenated. After birth, blood does need to be oxygenated in the lungs, and normally the ductus arteriosus closes quickly, usually within days up to 2 weeks. In patent ductus arteriosus, this connection does not close, allowing some oxygenated blood, intended for the body, to return to the lungs. As a result, the blood vessels in the lungs may be overloaded and the body may not receive enough oxygenated blood.

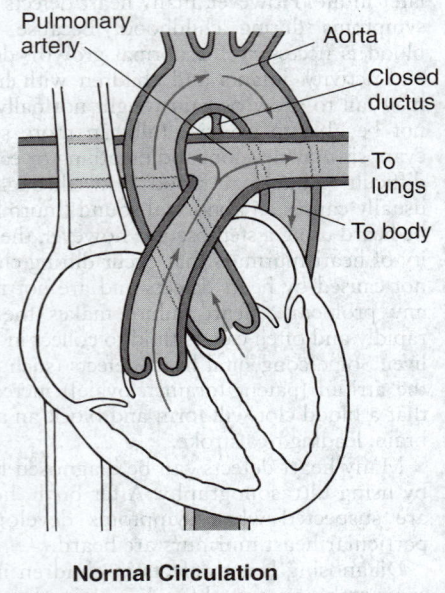

Normal Circulation

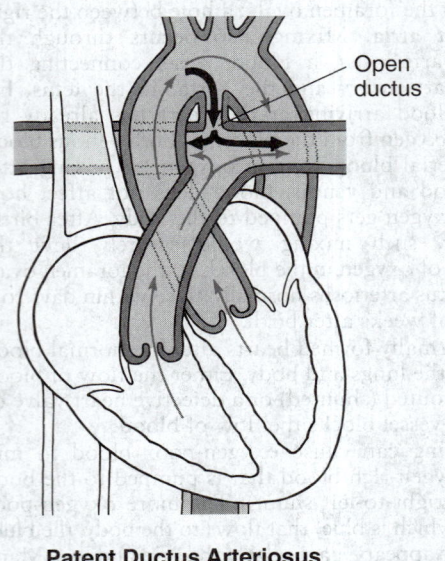

Patent Ductus Arteriosus

However, severe symptoms resulting from a heart defect are most effectively relieved with immediate surgery.

A narrowing can sometimes be relieved by passing a thin tube (catheter) through a blood vessel in the arm or leg into the narrowed area. A balloon attached to the catheter is inflated and widens the narrowing, usually in a valve (a procedure called balloon valvuloplasty) or blood vessel (a procedure called balloon angioplasty—see page 404). These balloon procedures spare the child from general anesthesia and open-heart surgery. However, balloon procedures are not usually as effective as surgery.

If the aorta or pulmonary artery is severely blocked, a temporary shunt can sometimes be created to keep an adequate amount of blood flowing. A shunt can be created with a catheter balloon (for example, between the right and left atria—balloon septostomy). Or drugs such as prostaglandin can be given to keep the ductus arteriosus open, shunting blood between the aorta and pulmonary artery. In rare cases, when no other treatment helps, a heart transplant is performed, but the lack of donor hearts limits the availability of this procedure.

Most children who have significant heart defects are at increased risk of developing life-threatening bacterial infections of the heart and its valves (endocarditis). They need to take antibiotics before certain treatments and procedures (see table on page 388).

PATENT DUCTUS ARTERIOSUS

In patent ductus arteriosus, the blood vessel connecting the pulmonary artery and the aorta (ductus arteriosus) fails to close as it usually does shortly after birth.

- Patent ductus arteriosus occurs when the normal channel between the pulmonary artery and the aorta does not close at birth.
- Often there are no symptoms.
- The diagnosis is based on a heart murmur.
- If the drug indomethacin does not close the defect, it must be closed surgically.

Septal Defect: A Hole in the Heart's Wall

A septal defect is a hole in the wall (septum) that separates the heart into the left and right sides. Atrial septal defects are located between the heart's upper chambers (atria). Ventricular septal defects are located between the lower chambers (ventricles). In both types, some oxygenated blood, intended for the body, is shortcircuited. It is returned to the lungs rather than pumped to the rest of the body.

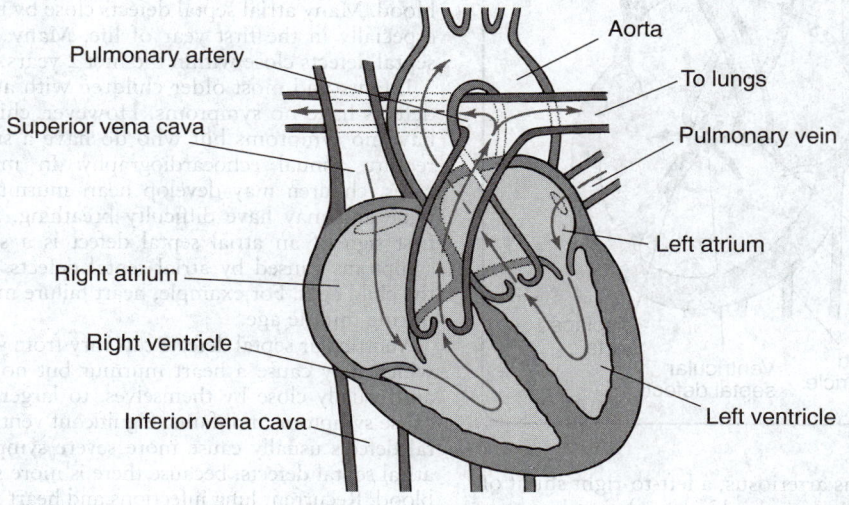

Pulmonary artery

Superior vena cava

Right atrium

Right ventricle

Inferior vena cava

Aorta

To lungs

Pulmonary vein

Left atrium

Left ventricle

Normal Circulation

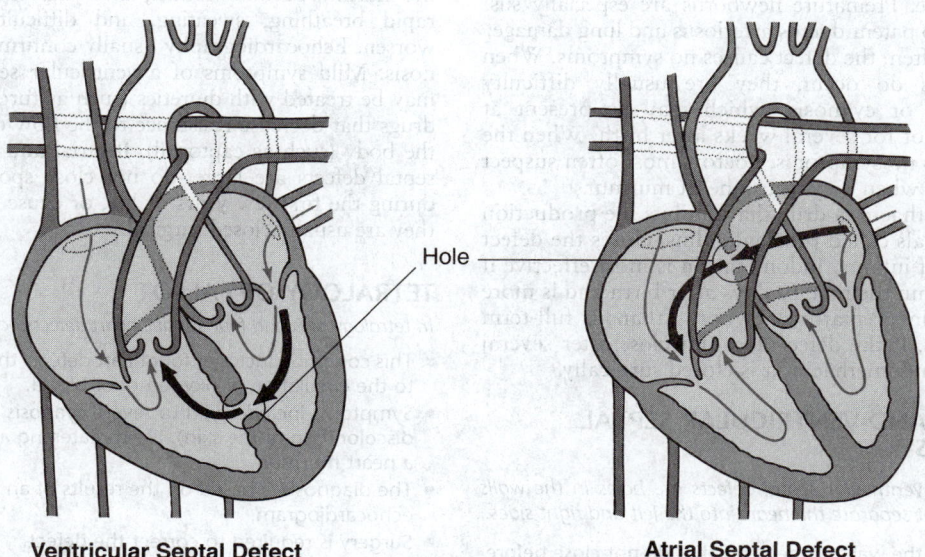

Hole

Ventricular Septal Defect

Atrial Septal Defect

Tetralogy of Fallot: Four Defects

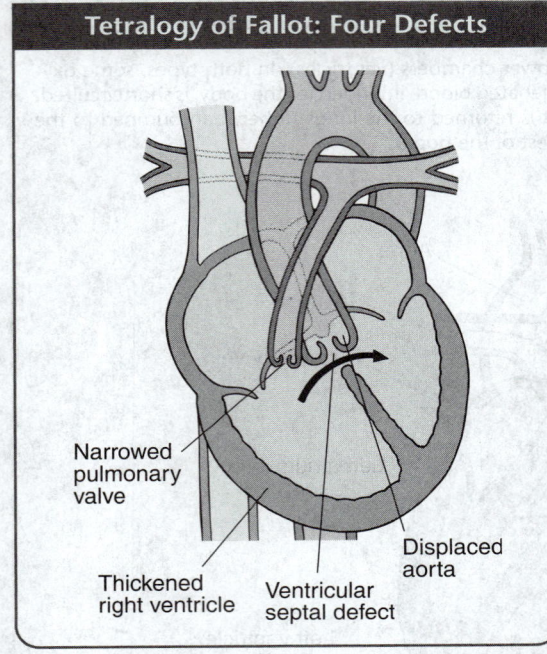

Narrowed pulmonary valve

Displaced aorta

Thickened right ventricle

Ventricular septal defect

- The diagnosis is based on detectable symptoms and echocardiography.
- Some large septal defects must be closed surgically.

Atrial septal defects are located between the heart's upper chambers (atria), which receive blood. Ventricular septal defects are located between the lower chambers (ventricles), which pump blood. These holes typically cause left-to-right shunting of blood. Many atrial septal defects close by themselves, especially in the first year of life. Many ventricular septal defects close within the first 2 years.

Infants and most older children with atrial septal defects have no symptoms. However, children who have no symptoms but who do have a small shunt require annual echocardiography. In more severe cases, children may develop heart murmurs and fatigue and may have difficulty breathing. Rarely, the first sign of an atrial septal defect is a stroke. The symptoms caused by atrial septal defects increase as the child ages. For example, heart failure may develop during middle age.

Ventricular septal defects can vary from small holes, which may cause a heart murmur but no symptoms and usually close by themselves, to larger holes that cause symptoms in infants. Significant ventricular septal defects usually cause more severe symptoms than atrial septal defects, because there is more shunting of blood. Recurrent lung infections and heart failure may develop. Because of the way lungs develop, shunting increases during the first 6 weeks after birth. Usually the murmur becomes louder, and symptoms, typically rapid breathing, sweating, and difficulty feeding, worsen. Echocardiography usually confirms the diagnosis. Mild symptoms of a ventricular septal defect may be treated with diuretics (such as furosemide) or drugs that decrease resistance to the flow of blood to the body (such as captopril). If atrial and ventricular septal defects are large, do not close spontaneously during the first few years of life, or cause symptoms, they are usually closed surgically.

In patent ductus arteriosus, a left-to-right shunt of blood from the aorta back into the pulmonary artery causes extra blood flow into the lungs, and high blood pressure in the lungs may damage the lung tissue. Premature newborns are especially susceptible to patent ductus arteriosus and lung damage.

Most often, the defect causes no symptoms. When symptoms do occur, they are usually difficulty breathing or cyanosis, which may be present at birth or not for several weeks after birth. When the infant has no symptoms, doctors most often suspect the defect when they hear a heart murmur.

Indomethacin, a drug that inhibits the production of chemicals called prostaglandins, closes the defect in 80% of infants. Indomethacin is most effective if given within the first 10 days after birth and is more effective in premature newborns than in full-term newborns. If the defect does not close after several doses of indomethacin, it is closed surgically.

ATRIAL AND VENTRICULAR SEPTAL DEFECTS

Atrial and ventricular septal defects are holes in the walls (septa) that separate the heart into the left and right sides.

- Holes in the walls of the heart that do not close before an infant is born are considered septal defects.
- Many defects are small, cause no symptoms, and close without treatment.

TETRALOGY OF FALLOT

In tetralogy of Fallot, four specific heart defects occur together.

- This condition includes four heart defects that can lead to the circulation of oxygen-poor blood.
- Symptoms include mild to severe cyanosis (a bluish discoloration of the skin), life-threatening attacks, and a heart murmur.
- The diagnosis is based on the results of an echocardiogram.
- Surgery is required to correct the defect.

The defects are a large ventricular septal defect, displacement of the aorta that allows oxygen-poor blood to flow directly from the right ventricle to the aorta (causing a right-to-left shunt), a narrowing of the outflow passage from the right side of the heart, and a thickening of the wall of the right ventricle.

In infants with tetralogy of Fallot, the narrowed passage from the right ventricle restricts blood flow to the lungs. The restricted blood flow causes the oxygen-poor blood in the right ventricle to pass through the septal defect to the left ventricle and into the aorta (right-to-left shunt). The main symptom is cyanosis, which can be mild or severe. Some infants have life-threatening attacks (hypercyanosis or "tet" spells), in which cyanosis suddenly worsens in response to activity, such as crying or having a bowel movement. The infant becomes very short of breath and may lose consciousness. Infants with tetralogy of Fallot usually have a heart murmur. Echocardiography confirms the diagnosis.

When an infant has a hypercyanotic spell, oxygen, morphine, and beta-blockers (such as propranolol) may provide quick relief. The infant may breathe more easily when the knees are close to the chest (knee-chest position). Giving fluids by vein or a drug such as phenylephrine, both of which increase resistance to the flow of blood to the body, may be helpful. A doctor may give the infant propranolol to prevent future spells until corrective surgery can be performed. In infants who have tetralogy with complete blockage of outflow from the right side of the heart (pulmonary atresia) and who depend on an open ductus arteriosus for survival, giving a prostaglandin such as alprostadil to maintain an open ductus arteriosus can be lifesaving.

Infants with tetralogy of Fallot eventually need surgery. If symptoms are frequent or severe, surgery is performed in early infancy but can be delayed until later in infancy if the child has few symptoms. To keep blood flowing to the lungs until corrective surgery can be performed, some doctors use less invasive procedures such as balloon valvulotomy, in which a long catheter with a balloon on its tip is passed through a vein into the heart. The balloon is inflated in the valve, widening the opening. During corrective surgery, the ventricular septal defect is closed, the narrowed passageway from the right ventricle and the narrowed pulmonary valve are widened, and any abnormal connections between the aorta and pulmonary artery are closed.

TRANSPOSITION OF THE GREAT ARTERIES

Transposition of the great arteries is a reversal of the normal connections of the aorta and the pulmonary artery with the heart.

- The aorta and pulmonary artery are reversed, which causes oxygen-poor blood to be circulated to the body and oxygen-rich blood to be circulated between the lungs and the heart and not to the body.

- Symptoms are apparent at birth and include great difficulty breathing and severe cyanosis (a bluish discoloration of the skin).
- The diagnosis is based on an examination, x-ray, electrocardiography, and echocardiography.
- Surgery is done during the first few days of life.

Oxygen-poor blood returning from the body flows from the right atrium to the right ventricle as usual, but then flows to the aorta and the body, bypassing the lungs. Oxygenated blood travels back and forth between the heart and lungs (from the lungs to the pulmonary vein, then left atrium and ventricle, then the pulmonary artery) but is not transported to the body. The body cannot survive without oxygen. However, infants with this defect may survive briefly after birth because the foramen ovale (a hole between the right and left atria) and the ductus arteriosus (a blood vessel connecting the pulmonary artery with the aorta—see art on page 1712) are still open at birth. These openings allow oxygen-rich blood to mix with oxygen-poor blood, sometimes supplying enough oxygen to the body to keep the infant alive. Transposition of the great arteries is often accompanied by a ventricular septal defect.

Transposition of the great arteries usually results in severe cyanosis and difficulty breathing, beginning at birth. A doctor performs a physical examination, x-ray, electrocardiography, and echocardiography to confirm the diagnosis. Usually, surgery is performed within the first few days of life. Surgery consists of attaching the aorta and pulmonary artery to the appropriate ventricles and reimplanting the heart's coronary arteries in the aorta after the aorta is repositioned. Giving alprostadil or performing a balloon septostomy can shunt the blood, which can keep the infant alive until surgery can be performed.

AORTIC VALVE STENOSIS

Aortic valve stenosis is a narrowing of the valve that opens to allow blood to flow from the left ventricle into the aorta and then to the body.

- This defect makes the heart work harder to pump blood to the rest of the body.
- For most children, the only symptom is a heart murmur, but some have fatigue, chest pain, and shortness of breath.
- The diagnosis is based on a murmur and symptoms.
- Surgery is needed to replace or widen the valve.

To propel blood through the narrowed aortic valve, the left ventricle must pump under very high pressures. Sometimes, not enough blood is pumped to supply the body with oxygenated blood.

Most children with aortic valve stenosis do not develop symptoms other than a heart murmur. In some older children, the defect causes fatigue, chest pain, shortness of breath, or fainting. In adolescents, severe aortic valve stenosis may lead to sudden death, presumably because of an erratic heart rhythm caused by poor blood flow through the coronary arteries to the heart. A few infants who have aortic valve stenosis develop irritability, an unnatural lack of color to the skin (pallor), low blood pressure, sweating, rapid heartbeat, and severe shortness of breath.

A doctor suspects aortic valve stenosis after detecting a particular murmur or if the child develops symptoms. Cardiac catheterization is often used to determine the severity of the narrowing.

For older children with severe narrowing or symptoms, the aortic valve must be replaced or widened. Usually the valve is opened surgically (using a procedure called balloon valvulotomy) or replaced with an artificial one. Children with an artificial valve must take an anticoagulant drug, such as warfarin, to prevent blood clots from forming. Infants with heart failure must have emergency treatment, usually including drugs and emergency surgery or balloon valvoplasty.

PULMONARY VALVE STENOSIS

Pulmonary valve stenosis is a narrowing of the pulmonary valve, which opens to allow blood to flow from the right ventricle to the lungs.

- The heart valve between the right ventricle and the artery to the lungs is narrowed.
- In most children, the only symptom is a heart murmur, but heart failure and cyanosis are possible.
- The diagnosis is based on symptoms and echocardiography.
- Balloon valvuloplasty to open the valve or surgery to reconstruct it is sometimes needed.

In most children with pulmonary valve stenosis, the valve is mildly to moderately narrowed, making the right ventricle pump harder and at a higher pressure to propel blood through the valve. Severe narrowing increases pressure in the right ventricle and prevents almost any blood from reaching the lungs. When pressure in the right ventricle becomes extremely high, oxygen-poor blood is forced through abnormal paths (usually a hole in the atrial wall [atrial septal defect]) instead of the pulmonary artery, causing right-to-left shunting.

Most children with pulmonary valve stenosis have no symptoms other than a heart murmur. However, severe cyanosis or heart failure is possible. Moderate symptoms, such as difficulty breathing with exertion and fatigue, may develop as the child gets older. Echocardiography is done to confirm the diagnosis. Occasionally, cardiac catheterization is needed to assess the severity of the narrowing.

If the valve is moderately narrowed, it may be opened with balloon valvuloplasty. If the valve is not well formed, it can be surgically reconstructed.

Severe disease that causes cyanosis in newborns is treated by giving a prostaglandin such as alprostadil, which opens the ductus arteriosus, until a surgeon can create another way to open or bypass the pulmonary valve. For some of these newborns, more surgery is needed when they are older.

COARCTATION OF THE AORTA

Coarctation of the aorta is a narrowing of the aorta, usually just before the point where the ductus arteriosus joins the aorta.

- The aorta narrows, causing decreased blood flow to the lower half of the body.
- Most infants have no symptoms or have a heart murmur and differences in blood pressures between the arms and legs.
- The diagnosis is based on symptoms, a chest x-ray, and echocardiography.
- Corrective surgery and sometimes drugs are needed.

Coarctation reduces blood flow to the lower half of the body; therefore, the blood pressure is lower than normal in the legs and tends to be higher than normal in the arms. Coarctation is a serious but treatable cause of high blood pressure. A heart murmur is sometimes present. Without treatment, coarctation eventually strains and enlarges the heart, causing heart failure; it also causes high blood pressure. Coarctation makes the child susceptible to rupture of the aorta, bacterial endocarditis, and bleeding in the brain. Children with coarctation often have other heart defects, such as aortic valve stenosis or an atrial or ventricular septal defect.

For most infants, mild or moderate coarctation does not cause symptoms. Rarely, children with coarctation have headaches or nosebleeds because of high blood pressure in the arms, or leg pains during exercise because of insufficient blood and oxygen to the legs.

With a severe coarctation in infancy, blood can flow only to the lower portion of the aorta (at a point past its narrowing) through the open connection between the aorta and the pulmonary artery, the ductus arteriosus. Symptoms usually do not occur until the ductus closes, usually when the newborn is a few days to about 2 weeks old. After the closure, the blood supplied through the ductus disappears, sometimes causing sudden loss of almost the entire blood supply to the lower body. Sudden, catastrophic heart failure and low blood pressure can result.

Coarctation is usually suspected only when a doctor notices a heart murmur or differences in pulses or blood pressures between the arms and legs when performing a physical examination. X-rays, electrocardiography, and echocardiography are usually used to confirm the diagnosis.

Coarctation that does not cause severe symptoms should be surgically repaired in early childhood, usually when the child is about 3 to 5 years old. Infants with severe symptoms from coarctation require emergency treatment, including giving a prostaglandin such as alprostadil to reopen the ductus arteriosus, other drugs to strengthen the heart's pumping, and emergency surgery to widen the narrowing. Some infants who undergo emergency surgery need more surgery when they are older. Sometimes, instead of surgery, doctors use balloon angioplasty and stents to relieve coarctation.

Urinary Tract Defects

- Defects can develop in the kidneys, ureters, bladder, or urethra.
- Many defects cause no symptoms, but others cause blood in the urine, urinary tract infections, or kidney stones.
- The diagnosis is based on ultrasonography, computed tomography, nuclear scanning, intravenous urography, and cystoscopy.
- If symptoms occur or pressure on the kidneys increases, surgery is needed.

Birth defects are more common in the kidney and urinary system than in any other system of the body. Defects can develop in the kidneys, the tubes that transport urine from the kidneys to the bladder (ureters), the bladder, or the tube that expels urine from the bladder (urethra). Any birth defect that blocks or slows the flow of urine can cause urine to stagnate, which can result in infections or formation of kidney stones. Blockage also results in an increase in urine pressure, which causes urine to flow backward from the bladder into the kidneys (reflux) and damages the kidneys and ureters over time. The combination of reflux and frequent infections is especially damaging to the kidneys.

Symptoms

Many urinary tract defects cause no symptoms. Some, such as kidney defects, may cause blood in the urine after minor injuries. Infections due to defects can develop anywhere in the urinary system and cause symptoms. Kidney damage results from blockage, but it usually causes symptoms only when very little kidney function remains. Then, kidney failure develops. Kidney stones may develop and cause severe, cramping pain in the side between the ribs and the hip (flank) or groin, or blood in the urine.

Did You Know...

Birth defects are more common in the kidney and urinary system than in any other system of the body.

Diagnosis and Treatment

The techniques used to diagnose abnormalities of the urinary tract include physical examination, ultrasonography, computed tomography (CT), nuclear scans, intravenous urography, and, rarely, cystoscopy (see page 257). Defects that cause symptoms or those that lead to increased pressure on the kidneys usually need to be surgically corrected.

KIDNEY AND URETER DEFECTS

A number of defects may result in abnormal kidneys. The kidneys may be in the wrong place (ectopia), in the wrong position (malrotation), joined together (horseshoe kidney), or missing (kidney agenesis). In Potter's syndrome, which causes death, both kidneys are missing. Kidney tissue may also develop abnormally. For example, a kidney may contain many cysts (fluid-filled sacs), as in polycystic kidney disease (see page 288). If an abnormality blocks an infant's urine flow, the affected kidney may swell so that it becomes visible and can be felt by a doctor.

Many birth defects involving the kidneys do not cause symptoms and are never detected. Some defects may interfere with the function of the kidneys, leading to kidney failure, which can require dialysis or kidney transplantation.

Abnormalities of the tubes that connect the kidneys to the bladder (ureters) include formation of extra ureters, misplaced ureters, and narrowed or widened ureters. A narrowed ureter prevents urine from passing normally from the kidney to the bladder.

BLADDER AND URETHRA DEFECTS

The bladder may not close completely, so that it opens out onto the surface of the abdomen (exstrophy). The wall of the bladder may develop outpouchings (diverticula) where urine can stagnate, sometimes causing urinary tract infections. The bladder outlet (the passageway from the bladder to the urethra) may be narrowed, causing the bladder to empty incompletely. In this case, the urine stream is weak.

The urethra may be abnormal or missing altogether. In posterior urethral valves, abnormal tissue blocks (usually partially) the flow of urine from the bladder. Affected infants have a weak urinary stream and are prone to urinary tract infections and possibly a widespread infection in the bloodstream (sepsis). They may fail to gain weight normally or may have anemia. Less severe defects may not cause symptoms until childhood. In this case, the symptoms that develop are also milder. Surgery to open the blockage must be performed in infants.

In boys, the opening of the urethra may be in the wrong place, such as on the underside of the penis (hypospadias). In boys with hypospadias, the penis may bend downward (chordee). Both hypospadias and chordee can be repaired surgically. The urethra in the penis may lie open as a channel rather than closed as a tube (epispadias). In both boys and girls, a narrowed urethra may obstruct the flow of urine.

Genital Defects

- Genital defects usually are caused by abnormal levels of sex hormones during fetal development.
- Sometimes the genitals are not clearly male or female (ambiguous).
- To determine the sex of an infant with ambiguous genitals, a physical examination and blood tests to analyze chromosomes and check hormone levels are done.
- Gender is then assigned, and hormones, surgery, or both may be needed.

Defects of the external genital organs (penis, testes, or clitoris) usually result from abnormal levels of sex hormones in the fetus before birth. Congenital adrenal hyperplasia (a metabolic disorder) and chromosomal abnormalities commonly cause genital defects.

A child may be born with genitals that are not clearly male or female (ambiguous genitals, or intersex state). Most children with ambiguous genitals are pseudohermaphrodites—that is, they have ambiguous external genital organs but either ovaries or testes (not both). Pseudohermaphrodites are genetically male or female.

Diagnostic evaluation of a child with ambiguous genitals includes physical examination and blood tests to analyze the chromosomes (the XY chromosome pattern is male and the XX chromosome pattern is female) and hormone levels (pituitary hormones and male sex hormones, or androgens, such as testosterone). X-rays and ultrasonography of the pelvis may help identify internal sex organs. Treatment with testosterone may help enlarge the penis so that assignment to a male sex is more realistic.

Most experts believe that the child's sex must be assigned quickly. Otherwise, bonding by the parents to the child may become more difficult, and the child may develop a gender identity disorder (see page 896). The decision to assign gender to a baby with ambiguous genitals depends on several factors. They include how much testosterone the fetus was exposed to, what the potential for sexual function is (as determined, for example, by how much erectile tissue the baby has), and the potential for reproduction. Environmental and psychologic factors, such as parents' perception of gender, also affect the decision. Surgery to correct the ambiguous genitals can be performed later, especially if the defect is complex. The underlying problem causing pseudohermaphroditism may also need treatment.

MALE GENITAL DEFECTS

Male and female sex organs develop from similar tissue in the embryo. When acted on by high levels of testosterone before birth (as in a normal male fetus), the genitals become the penis, scrotum, and penile urethra. Low or absent testosterone levels lead to the development of a clitoris, labia majora, and separate vaginal and urethral canals. Intermediate levels of testosterone cause ambiguous genitals: Genetic males have a small penis and testes that remain in the abdomen instead of descending into the scrotum (undescended testes, also known as cryptorchidism), and genetic females have an enlarged clitoris with fused labia. The appearance of the genitals in both sexes is very similar.

Pseudohermaphroditism in the male (better termed undervirilized 46,XY intersex), results in a genetic male who has female-appearing external genitals but has undescended testes. Pseudohermaphroditism may be caused by a prenatal deficiency of male sex hormones (androgens), an inability of the body's tissues to respond to androgens, exposure to female sex hormones (estrogens), or a chromosomal abnormality (see page 1726).

After they develop, the testes produce most of the male body's androgens. Absent or underdeveloped testes cause androgen deficiency.

Androgen deficiency during childhood causes incomplete sexual development. An affected boy retains a high-pitched voice and has poor muscle development for his age. The penis, testes, and scrotum are underdeveloped. Pubic and underarm hair is sparse, and the arms and legs are abnormally long.

Androgen deficiency can be treated with testosterone. The testosterone is usually given by injection or through a skin patch. Injection and skin application cause fewer side effects than taking testosterone by mouth. Testosterone stimulates growth, sexual development, and fertility.

> **? Did You Know...**
> Children may be born with genitals that are not clearly male or female.

FEMALE GENITAL DEFECTS

Female pseudohermaphroditism (also called virilization or overvirilized 46,XX intersex) is caused by exposure to high levels of male hormones. The most common cause is enlarged adrenal glands (congenital adrenal hyperplasia) that overproduce male hormones because an enzyme is missing. The male hormones cannot be converted to female hormones as occurs in normal females. Sometimes, male hormones enter the placenta from the mother's blood. For example, the mother may have been given drugs such as progesterone to prevent a miscarriage (some progesterone is changed into the male hormone testosterone by the fetus) or the mother may have had a hormone-producing tumor, although this is much less common.

A female pseudohermaphrodite has female internal organs but has an enlarged clitoris that resembles a small penis.

If the child is assigned to the female gender, surgery is performed to create female-appearing genitals. This surgery can include reduction of the clitoris, formation or repair of a vagina (vaginoplasty), and repair of the urethra.

Congenital adrenal hyperplasia can be life-threatening because it can cause serious abnormalities of electrolytes (sodium and potassium) in the blood. These are diagnosed with blood tests and treated with corticosteroids.

Digestive Tract Defects

- The digestive organs may be incompletely developed or abnormally positioned, causing blockages, or the muscles or nerves of the digestive tract may be defective.
- Symptoms include crampy abdominal pain, abdominal swelling, and vomiting.
- The diagnosis usually is based on x-rays.
- Surgery usually is required.

A birth defect can occur anywhere along the length of the digestive tract—in the esophagus, stomach, small intestine, large intestine, rectum, or anus. In many cases, an organ is not fully developed or is abnormally positioned, which often causes narrowing or blockage (obstruction). The internal or external muscles surrounding the abdominal cavity may weaken or develop holes. The nerves to the intestines may also fail to develop (Hirschsprung's disease, or congenital megacolon).

Blockages (obstructions) that develop in the intestines, rectum, or anus can cause rhythmic, crampy abdominal pain, abdominal swelling, and vomiting.

Most digestive tract defects require surgery. Generally, obstructions are surgically opened. Weakenings or holes in the muscles surrounding the abdominal cavity are sewn shut.

ESOPHAGEAL ATRESIA AND TRACHEOESOPHAGEAL FISTULA

In esophageal atresia, the esophagus narrows or comes to a blind end. Most newborns with esophageal atresia also have an abnormal connection between the esophagus and the trachea (tracheoesophageal fistula).

Normally, the esophagus, a long tubelike organ, connects the mouth to the stomach. In esophageal atresia, food is delayed or prevented from going from the esophagus to the stomach. A tracheoesophageal fistula is dangerous because it allows swallowed food and saliva to travel through the fistula to the lungs, leading to coughing, choking, difficulty breathing, and possibly pneumonia. Food or fluid in the lungs may impair oxygenation of blood, leading to a bluish discoloration of the skin (cyanosis). Characteristically, a newborn with esophageal atresia coughs and drools after attempting to swallow. Many children with esophageal atresia and tracheoesophageal fistula have other abnormalities, such as heart defects.

To detect a blockage, x-rays are taken as a tube is passed down the esophagus.

The first steps in treatment are withholding oral feedings and placing a tube in the upper esophagus to continuously suction out saliva before it can reach the lungs. The infant is fed by vein (intravenously). Surgery needs to be performed soon to establish a normal connection between the esophagus and stomach and to close the connection between the esophagus and the trachea.

ANAL ATRESIA

Anal atresia is narrowing or obstruction of the anus.

Most infants with anal atresia develop some type of abnormal connection (fistula) between the anus and either the urethra, the area between the urethra and anus (the perineum), the vagina, or the bladder.

Infants with anal atresia fail to defecate normally after birth. Eventually, intestinal obstruction develops. However, doctors often detect the abnormality by looking at the anus when they first examine the baby after birth, before symptoms develop.

Using x-rays, a radiologist can see the path of a fistula. Anal atresia usually requires immediate surgery to open a passage for feces and to close the fistula. Sometimes, a temporary colostomy (making a hole in the abdomen and connecting it to the colon to allow stool to flow into a plastic bag on the abdominal wall) may be necessary.

INTESTINAL MALROTATION

Intestinal malrotation (abnormal rotation of the intestines) is a potentially life-threatening defect in which the intestines develop incompletely or abnormally.

Atresia and Fistula: Defects in the Esophagus

In esophageal atresia, the esophagus narrows or comes to a blind end. It does not connect with the stomach as it normally does. A tracheoesophageal fistula is an abnormal connection between the esophagus and the trachea (which leads to the lungs).

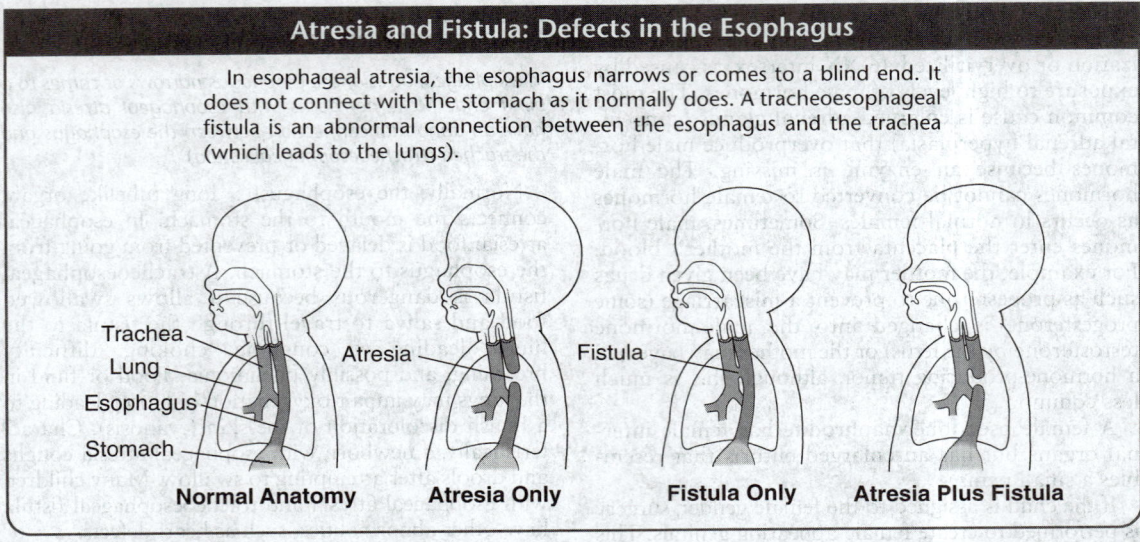

Trachea
Lung
Esophagus
Stomach

Atresia

Fistula

Normal Anatomy   **Atresia Only**   **Fistula Only**   **Atresia Plus Fistula**

Malrotation can cause the intestines to later twist (volvulus), cutting off their blood supply. Infants with intestinal malrotation can suddenly develop symptoms of vomiting, diarrhea, and abdominal swelling, and these symptoms can also come and go. If the blood supply to the middle of the intestine is completely cut off (midgut volvulus), sudden, severe pain and vomiting develop. Bile, a substance formed in the liver, may be vomited and appear yellow, green, or rust-colored. Eventually, the abdomen swells. X-rays may help the doctor determine the diagnosis. However, the volvulus can be seen only on x-rays taken after placing barium, a substance visible on the x-ray, in the rectum (barium enema).

Treatment, including intravenous fluids and usually emergency surgery, must begin within hours. If not treated rapidly, the defect can result in loss of intestinal tissue or death.

BILIARY ATRESIA

In biliary atresia, the bile ducts are destroyed—either partially or completely—so bile cannot reach the intestine.

- This defect causes bile to collect in the liver and can lead to irreversible liver damage.
- Typical symptoms include a yellowish discoloration of the skin (jaundice), dark urine, pale stools, and an enlarged liver.
- The diagnosis is based on blood tests, ultrasonography, and surgical examination of the liver and bile ducts.
- Surgery is needed to create new bile ducts.

Bile, a fluid secreted by the liver, carries away the liver's waste products and helps digest fats in the small intestine. Bile ducts within the liver collect the bile and carry it to the intestine. In biliary atresia, bile eventually accumulates in the liver and then escapes into the blood, causing a yellowish discoloration of the skin (jaundice). Progressive, irreversible scarring of the liver, called biliary cirrhosis, starts by the age of 2 months if the defect is not treated.

In infants with biliary atresia, the urine becomes dark, the stools become pale, and the skin becomes increasingly jaundiced. These symptoms and an enlarged, firm liver are usually first noticed about 2 weeks after birth. By the time infants are 2 to 3 months old, they may have stunted growth, be itchy and irritable, and have large veins visible on their abdomen, as well as a large spleen.

To prevent biliary cirrhosis, the diagnosis of biliary atresia must be made before the age of 2 months. To make the diagnosis, a doctor performs a series of blood tests. Ultrasonography may be helpful. If the defect is still suspected after these tests, surgery (which consists of examination of the liver and bile ducts and a liver biopsy) is performed to diagnose the defect.

Surgery is needed to create a path for bile to drain from the liver. Constructing replacement bile ducts that flow into the intestine is best, and this kind of operation is possible in 40 to 50% of infants. Most of the infants with replacement bile ducts can lead normal lives. Infants who cannot have replacement bile ducts constructed usually require liver transplantation by age 2 years.

DIAPHRAGMATIC HERNIA

A diaphragmatic hernia is a hole or weakening in the diaphragm that allows some of the abdominal organs to protrude into the chest.

Diaphragmatic hernias occur on the left side of the body 90% of the time. The stomach, loops of intestine, and even the liver and spleen can protrude through the hernia. If the hernia is large, the lung on the affected side is usually incompletely developed. Many children with diaphragmatic hernias also have heart defects.

After delivery, as the newborn cries and breathes, the loops of intestine quickly fill with air. This rapidly enlarging structure pushes against the heart, compressing the other lung and causing severe difficulty breathing, often right after birth. A chest x-ray usually shows the defect. The defect can also be detected before birth using ultrasound. Diagnosis before birth allows the doctor to prepare for treatment of the defect. Surgery is required to repair the diaphragm. Measures to deliver oxygen, such as a breathing tube and ventilator, may be needed.

HIRSCHSPRUNG'S DISEASE

In Hirschsprung's disease (congenital megacolon), a section of the large intestine is missing the nerve network that controls the intestine's rhythmic contractions. Symptoms of intestinal obstruction occur.

- This defect affects the large intestine so that normal bowel contractions do not occur.
- Typical symptoms include delayed passage of meconium in the newborn, vomiting, refusing to eat, and a swollen abdomen in later infancy.
- The diagnosis is based on a rectal biopsy and measurement of the pressure inside the rectum.
- Surgery is done to restore the normal passage of food through the intestines.

The large intestine depends on a network of nerves within its walls to synchronize rhythmic contractions and move digested material toward the anus, where the material is expelled as feces. In Hirschsprung's disease, the affected section of intestine cannot contract normally.

At the time of birth, newborns should pass a dark green fecal material (meconium). Delayed passage of meconium raises the suspicion of Hirschsprung's disease. Later in infancy, children with Hirschsprung's disease can have symptoms that suggest intestinal obstruction—bile-stained vomit, a swollen abdomen, and refusal to eat. If only a small section of the intestine is affected, a child may have milder symptoms and may not be diagnosed until later in childhood. These children may have ribbonlike stools and a swollen abdomen, and they often fail to gain weight. In rare cases, constipation is the only symptom.

Hirschsprung's disease can also lead to life-threatening toxic enterocolitis, which causes sudden fever, a swollen abdomen, and explosive and, at times, bloody diarrhea.

Rectal biopsy and measurement of the pressure inside the rectum (manometry) are the only tests that can reliably be used to diagnose Hirschsprung's disease. A barium enema may also be performed. During a barium enema, the doctor instills barium and air into the child's rectum and then takes x-rays.

Severe Hirschsprung's disease must be treated quickly to prevent toxic enterocolitis. Hirschsprung's disease is usually treated with surgery to remove the abnormal section of intestine and to connect the normal intestine to the rectum and anus. In some cases, for example, if the child is quite ill, the surgeon connects the lower end of the normal part of the intestine to an opening made in the abdominal wall (colostomy). Stool can thus pass through the opening into a collection bag, restoring normal movement of food through the intestines. The abnormal section of intestine is left disconnected from the rest of the intestine. When the child is older and healthier, the colostomy is closed, the abnormal section of intestine is removed, and the normal part of the intestine is reconnected to the rectum and anus in a so-called pull-through procedure.

Abdominal Wall Defects

Omphalocele: An omphalocele is caused by an opening (defect) in the middle of the abdominal wall at the bellybutton (umbilicus). The skin, muscle, and fibrous tissue are absent. The intestines protrude through the opening and are covered by fine membranes. The umbilical cord is in the center of the defect. An omphalocele is commonly associated with other birth defects (such as heart defects) and with specific genetic syndromes. Omphalocele is diagnosed with prenatal ultrasonography.

Surgical closure is the treatment of choice. However, the skin of the abdominal wall must often be stretched before surgery so there is enough tissue to cover the opening. Large defects sometimes also require skin flaps.

Gastroschisis: Gastroschisis is an abnormal opening of the abdominal wall, usually to the right of the umbilicus, which allows the uncovered intestines to spill out (herniate). The defect is diagnosed with prenatal ultrasonography.

In gastroschisis, the bowel may be damaged by compression and by exposure to amniotic fluid. Surgical closure is the treatment of choice. Large herniations may require the creation of a "silo," in which the exposed bowel is wrapped in a protective covering and suspended above the baby for several days or weeks. The silo is gradually compressed, forcing the intestines back into the abdomen.

Bone and Muscle Defects

Birth defects can occur in any bone or muscle, although the bones and muscles of the skull, face, spine, hips, legs, and feet are affected most often. Bones and muscles may develop incompletely. Also, structures that normally align together may be separated or misaligned. Usually, bone and muscle defects result in abnormal appearance and function of the affected part of the body. Most of these defects are repaired surgically if symptoms are troublesome. Often, the surgery is complex and involves reconstructing deformed or absent body parts.

FACIAL DEFECTS

The most common defects of the skull and face are cleft lip and cleft palate. **Cleft lip** is a separation of the upper lip, usually just below the nose. **Cleft palate** is a split in the roof of the mouth resulting in a passageway into the nose. Cleft lip and cleft palate often occur together.

Cleft lip is disfiguring and prevents infants from closing their lips around a nipple. A cleft palate interferes with eating and speech. A dental device can temporarily seal the roof of the mouth so infants can suckle better. Cleft lip and cleft palate

can be permanently corrected with surgery. The likelihood of cleft lip and cleft palate can be reduced if a woman takes folate (folic acid) before pregnancy and through the 1st trimester of pregnancy.

Another type of facial defect is a small lower jaw (mandible). Pierre Robin syndrome and Treacher Collins syndrome, which are characterized by several defects in the head and face, are among the causes of a small lower jaw. If the lower jaw is too small, the infant may have difficulty eating or breathing. Surgery may correct or diminish the problem.

LIMB AND JOINT DEFECTS

- Limb and joint defects may be caused by genetic abnormalities, growth restriction in the womb, or mechanical forces.
- The diagnosis is based on a physical examination, x-rays, and sometimes ultrasonography.
- Usually, surgery is needed to correct the defect.

Limbs or joints can be missing, deformed, or incompletely developed at birth. A child with one limb or joint abnormality is more likely to have another related abnormality. Limbs and joints may form abnormally. For example, bones in the hand and forearm may be missing because of a genetic defect. Normal development of a limb can also become disrupted in the womb. For example, a finger may stop growing because the finger gets constricted by fibers. Another cause of limb and joint abnormalities is mechanical force. For example, pressure may cause the hip to dislocate. Chromosomal abnormalities can cause limb and joint abnormalities. Sometimes the cause is unknown. The drug thalidomide, which was taken by some pregnant women in the late 1950s and early 1960s for morning sickness, caused a variety of limb defects—usually short, poorly functioning appendages developed in place of arms and legs.

Abnormalities of the arms and legs may occur in a horizontal fashion (for example, if the arm is shorter than normal) or in a lengthwise fashion (for example, the arm is abnormal on the thumb side [from the elbow to the thumb] but normal on the little finger side). Children often become very adept at using a malformed limb, and an artificial limb (prosthesis) can often be fitted (usually when the child is able to sit independently) to make the limb easier to use.

Hand defects are common. Sometimes a hand does not form completely, and part or all of the hand may be missing. For example, the person may have too few fingers. Sometimes a hand does not develop. For example, the fingers may not separate, producing a weblike hand. Some hand defects involve extra

Cleft Lip and Cleft Palate: Defects of the Face

Cleft Lip

Cleft Palate

fingers. The little fingers or thumbs are most commonly duplicated. Overgrowth may occur, in which the hands or individual fingers are too large. Surgery is usually done to correct the hand defect and provide as much function as possible.

In **developmental dysplasia of the hip,** formerly called congenital dislocation of the hip, the newborn's hip socket and the thighbone (femoral head), which normally form a joint, become separated, often because the hip has a socket that is not deep enough to hold the head of the femur. Dysplasia of the hip is more common among girls, among newborns born in a breech (buttocks-first) position, and among newborns who have close relatives with the defect. Newborn girls born in breech position should have ultrasonography of their hips. The right and left legs or hips often look different from each other in affected newborns.

The doctor may be able to detect the defect when examining the newborn. In infants younger than 4 months, ultrasonography of the hips can confirm the diagnosis. In infants older than 4 months, an x-ray can be used. The use of triple diapers (an older treatment) is not recommended. The best treatment is early use of the Pavlik harness. The Pavlik harness is a soft brace that holds the infant's knees spread outward and up toward the chest. However, if the defect persists past the age of 6 months, surgery to fix the hip in the normal position is usually needed.

Clubfoot (talipes equinovarus) is a defect in which the foot and ankle are twisted out of shape or position. The usual clubfoot is a down and inward turning of the hind foot and ankle, with twisting inward of the forefoot. Sometimes the foot only appears abnormal because it was held in an unusual position in the uterus (positional clubfoot). In contrast, true clubfoot is a structurally abnormal foot. With true clubfoot, the bones of the leg or foot or the muscles of the calf are often underdeveloped.

Positional clubfoot can be corrected by immobilizing the joints in a cast and by using physical therapy to stretch the foot and ankle. Early treatment with immobilization is beneficial for true clubfoot, but surgery, often complex, is also generally needed.

In **metatarsus adductus,** the foot appears turned inward. Mobility of the joints of the foot and ankle may be limited. Treatment depends on the severity of the deformity and immobility of the foot. Most mild cases resolve spontaneously. Corrective shoes or splints may be needed in more severe cases. Surgery is required only in exceptional instances.

In **arthrogryposis multiplex congenita,** many joints become "frozen" and consequently cannot bend. Many children with this defect have weakened muscles. It is likely that decreased movement of the muscles and joints before birth causes the decreased movement of the joints after birth. The cause is unknown. Sometimes

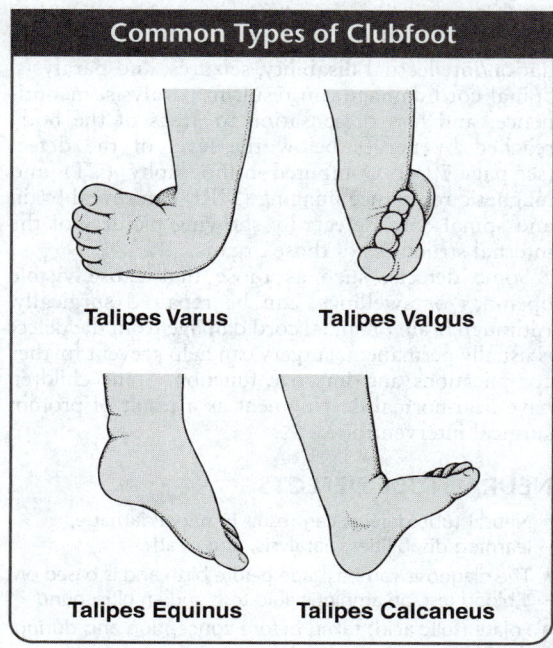

Common Types of Clubfoot

Talipes Varus

Talipes Valgus

Talipes Equinus

Talipes Calcaneus

the nerves that would normally move the bones in the affected joints are also impaired. Infants with the defect may also have dislocated hips, knees, or elbows. Placing the limbs in a cast and performing physical therapy, in which the stiff joints are carefully manipulated, may improve joint movements. Surgically freeing the bones from attached tissue sometimes results in more normal joint movement.

Brain and Spinal Cord Defects

- These defects can occur in early or late fetal development.
- Typical symptoms include intellectual disability, paralysis, incontinence, or loss of sensation in some parts of the body.
- The diagnosis is based on computed tomography and magnetic resonance imaging.
- Some defects can be repaired surgically, but brain or spinal cord damage is usually permanent.

Of the many possible defects in the brain and spinal cord, those known as neural tube defects develop within the first weeks of pregnancy. Others, such as porencephaly and hydranencephaly, develop later in pregnancy. Many brain and spinal cord defects result in visible abnormalities in the head or back.

Symptoms of brain or spinal cord damage may develop if the defect affects brain or spinal cord tissue. Brain damage can be fatal or result in mild or severe disabilities which may include mental retardation/intellectual disability, seizures, and paralysis. Spinal cord damage can result in paralysis, incontinence, and loss of sensation to areas of the body reached by nerves below the level of the defect (see page 795). Computed tomography (CT) and magnetic resonance imaging (MRI) can reveal brain and spinal cord defects by showing pictures of the internal structures of those organs.

Some defects, such as those that cause visible openings or swellings, can be repaired surgically. Although brain or spinal cord damage from the defect is usually permanent, surgery can help prevent further complications and improve function. Some children have near-normal development as a result of prompt surgical intervention.

NEURAL TUBE DEFECTS

- Neural tube defects can result in nerve damage, learning disabilities, paralysis, and death.
- The diagnosis can be made before birth and is based on a blood test, an amniotic fluid test, and an ultrasound.
- Folate (folic acid) taken before conception and during the first trimester can help prevent these defects.
- Surgery is needed to close neural tube defects.

The brain and spinal cord develop as a groove that folds over to become a tube (the neural tube). Layers of tissue that come from this tube normally become the brain and spinal cord and their covering tissues, including part of the spine and the meninges. Sometimes the neural tube does not develop normally, which may affect the brain, spinal cord, and meninges. In the most severe form of neural tube defect, the brain tissue may fail to develop (anencephaly); this defect is fatal. Another type of defect results when the neural tube fails to close completely and remains an open channel. In its mildest form, an open channel defect may affect only bone. For example, in spina bifida occulta (which means hidden spine split in two), the bony spine fails to close, but the spinal cord and meninges are unaffected. This common abnormality causes no symptoms. Sometimes, a meningocele develops in which the meninges and other tissue, such as brain tissue (meningoencephalocele) or spinal cord tissue (meningomyelocele), can protrude out of the opening. Sometimes the meninges are not involved when tissue protrudes from the brain (encephalocele) or spinal cord (myelocele). Damage to brain or spinal cord tissue is much more likely when tissue protrudes than when it does not.

In occult spinal dysraphism, newborns are born with visible abnormalities on their lower back. These include birthmarks, overly pigmented areas (hemangioma and flame nevus), tufts of hair, openings in the skin (dermal sinus), or small lumps (masses). The underlying spinal cord may be connected to the surface, which exposes it to bacteria, greatly increasing the chance for development of meningitis. The nerves of the spinal cord may become damaged as the child grows. Or, the spinal cord may have a fatty tumor (lipoma) on it, which also can lead to nerve damage. Therefore, newborns who have these abnormalities should have the underlying soft tissue and spinal cord evaluated using ultrasound or MRI.

> **? Did You Know...**
> Taking folate before and during pregnancy can decrease the risk of neural tube defects up to 50%.

Genetic factors can make neural tube defects more likely. The defect often develops before the mother knows she is pregnant. Most symptoms caused by neural tube defects result from brain or spinal cord damage. Meningoencephaloceles and meningomyeloceles cause severe disability. These include water on the brain (hydrocephalus), learning disabilities, paralysis with bone and joint abnormalities, decreased sensation of the skin, and bowel and urinary problems.

Many neural tube defects can be detected before birth. A high level of alpha-fetoprotein in the woman's blood or amniotic fluid may indicate a neural tube defect in the fetus (see page 1612). Ultrasonography performed late in pregnancy may show the defect or characteristic abnormalities. Folate (folic acid) taken before a woman gets pregnant and through the first three months of pregnancy can decrease the risk of neural tube defects by as much as 50%. For this reason, women of child-bearing age are encouraged to take folate if they think that they may become pregnant. Neural tube defects are usually closed surgically.

HYDROCEPHALUS

Hydrocephalus is an accumulation of extra fluid in the normal open spaces within the brain (ventricles), usually causing an enlarged head and developmental problems.

- Hydrocephalus occurs when the fluid in the normal spaces in the brain (ventricles) cannot drain.
- Typical symptoms include an abnormally large head and abnormal development.
- The diagnosis is based on CT, ultrasonography, or MRI.
- Surgery is needed to insert a drain (shunt) into the brain.

The fluid surrounding the brain (cerebrospinal fluid) is produced in spaces within the brain called

Spina Bifida: A Defect of the Spine

In spina bifida, the bones of the spine (vertebrae) do not form normally. Spina bifida can vary in severity. In one form, called occult **spinal dysraphism**, one or more vertebrae do not form normally, and the spinal cord and the layers of tissues (meninges) surrounding it may also be affected. The only symptom may be a tuft of hair, a dimpling, or a pigmented area on the skin over the defect. In a **meningocele**, the meninges protrude through the incompletely formed vertebrae, resulting in a fluid-filled bulge under the skin. The most severe type is a **meningomyelocele**, in which the spinal cord protrudes. The affected area appears raw and red, and the infant is likely to be severely impaired.

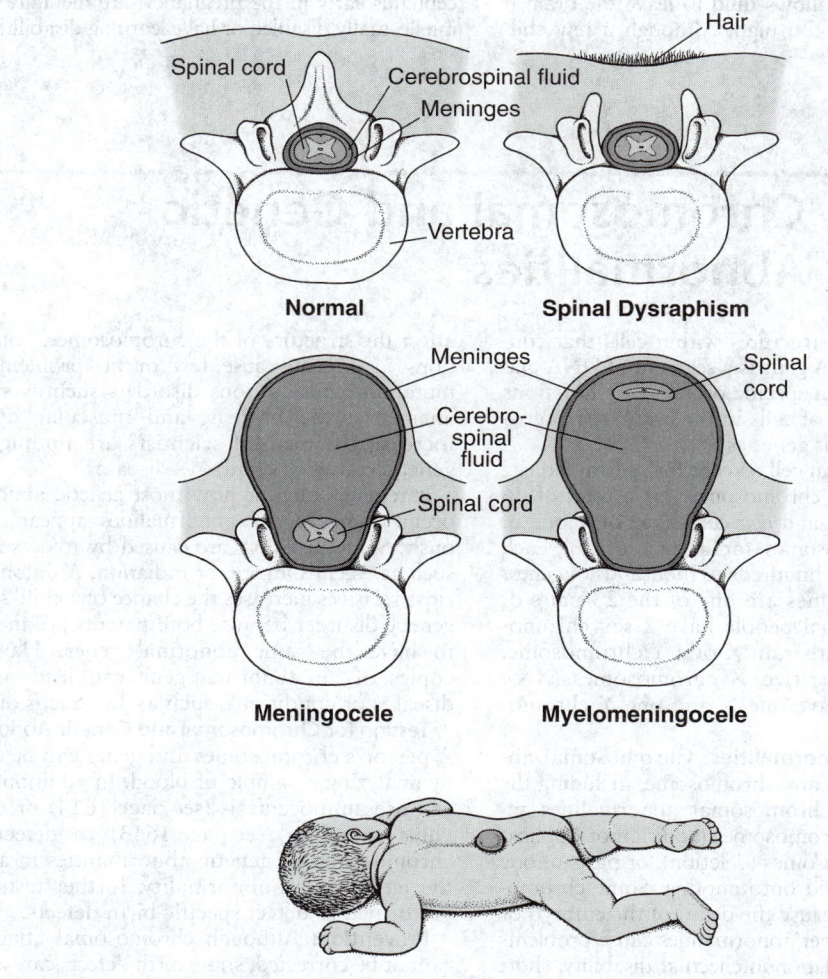

ventricles. The fluid must drain to a different area, where it is absorbed into the blood. When the fluid cannot drain, hydrocephalus (water on the brain) develops. Hydrocephalus often increases the pressure in the ventricles, which compresses the brain. Many conditions, such as a birth defect, bleeding within the brain (often associated with prematurity), or brain tumors, can block drainage and cause hydrocephalus.

An abnormally large head may be a symptom of untreated hydrocephalus. The infant usually does not develop normally. CT, ultrasonography, or MRI of the head reveals the diagnosis as well as the degree of brain compression.

The goal of treatment is to keep pressure normal within the brain. A permanent alternate drainage path (shunt) for cerebrospinal fluid decreases the pressure and volume of the fluid inside the brain. A doctor places the shunt in the ventricles in the brain and runs it under the skin from the head to another site, usually the abdomen (ventriculoperitoneal shunt). The shunt contains a valve that allows fluid to leave the brain if the pressure becomes too high. Although a few chil-dren can eventually do without the shunt as they get older, shunts are rarely removed. On occasion, a surgi-cal hole placed between the third and fourth ventricles (ventriculostomy) may treat the hydrocephalus.

If needed, pressure within the brain can often be temporarily reduced with repeated spinal taps (lumbar punctures) until a shunt is placed.

Some children with hydrocephalus develop normal intelligence. Others, especially those who develop hydro-cephalus early in the pregnancy, are mentally retarded/intellectually disabled or have learning disabilities.

263 Chromosomal and Genetic Abnormalities

Chromosomes are structures within cells that con-tain a person's genes. A gene is a segment of DNA and contains the code for a specific protein that functions in one or more types of cells in the body (see page 8 for a discussion about genetics).

Every normal human cell, except for sperm and egg cells, has 23 pairs of chromosomes for a total of 46 chromosomes. Sperm and egg cells have only one of each pair of chromosomes for a total of 23. Each chromosome contains hundreds to thousands of genes.

The sex chromosomes are one of the 23 pairs of chromosomes. Normal people have 2 sex chromo-somes, and each is either an X or a Y chromosome. Normal females have two X chromosomes (XX), and normal males have one X and one Y chromo-some (XY).

Chromosomal Abnormalities: Chromosomal ab-normalities can affect any chromosome, including the sex chromosomes. Chromosomal abnormalities in-clude having extra chromosomes (addition or duplica-tion), missing chromosomes (deletion), or parts of one chromosome misplaced onto another. Some chromo-somal abnormalities cause the death of the embryo or fetus before birth. Other abnormalities cause problems such as mental retardation/intellectual disability, short stature, seizures, heart problems, or a cleft palate.

The older a pregnant woman is, the greater the chance that her fetus will have a chromosomal abnor-mality (see table on page 1608). The same is not true of a man. As a man gets older, the chance of conceiving a baby with a chromosomal abnormality is only slightly increased.

Genetic Abnormalities: Small changes (mutations) may occur in a specific gene. These changes do not affect the structure of the chromosomes. Some muta-tions in a gene cause few or no problems. Other mutations cause serious disorders such as sickle cell anemia, cystic fibrosis, and muscular dystrophy. Increasingly, medical scientists are finding specific genetic causes of children's diseases.

It remains unclear how most genetic abnormalities occur. Some genetic abnormalities appear spontane-ously. Some probably are caused by toxic substances, such as Agent Orange, or radiation. A union between close relatives increases the chance of a child's having a genetic disorder because both parents are more likely to have the same abnormal genes. Having two copies of an abnormal gene can lead to serious diseases or conditions, such as Tay-Sachs disease.

Testing for Chromosomal and Genetic Abnormalities: A person's chromosomes and genes can be evaluated by analyzing a sample of blood. In addition, doctors can use amniocentesis (see page 1614) or chorionic villus sampling (see page 1613) to detect certain chromosomal or genetic abnormalities in a fetus. If the fetus has an abnormality, further tests may be performed to detect specific birth defects.

Prevention: Although chromosomal abnormalities cannot be corrected, some birth defects can sometimes be prevented (for example, taking folate [folic acid] to prevent neural tube defects or screening parents for carrier status of certain genetic abnormalities).

Down Syndrome

Down syndrome (trisomy 21, trisomy G) is a chromoso-mal disorder resulting in mental retardation/intellectual disability and physical abnormalities.

- Most cases of Down syndrome are caused by an extra copy of chromosome 21.
- Children with Down syndrome have delayed physical and mental development, specific head and facial features, and short stature.
- The diagnosis is suggested by the child's physical appearance and is confirmed by finding an extra copy of chromosome 21 in a blood sample.
- Most children with Down syndrome survive to adulthood.

An extra chromosome, making three of a kind, is called trisomy. The most common trisomy in a newborn is trisomy 21 (three copies of chromosome 21). Trisomy 21 causes about 95% of the cases of Down syndrome. The extra chromosome may come from the father; however, older mothers, especially those older than 35, more commonly contribute the extra chromosome. Yet, because most births occur to younger women, just 20% of infants with Down syndrome are born to mothers older than 35. Women who have Down syndrome have a 50% chance of having a child with Down syndrome. However, many affected fetuses abort spontaneously. Men with Down syndrome are usually infertile.

Symptoms

In Down syndrome, physical and mental development is delayed. Infants tend to be placid and passive. They rarely cry, and they have somewhat limp muscles. They tend to have a small head and a face that is broad and flat with slanting eyes and a short nose. However, some newborns appear normal at birth and then develop characteristic facial features during infancy. The tongue is large. There is extra skin around the back of the neck. The ears are small, rounded, and set low in the head. The hands are short and broad, with a single crease across the palm. The fingers are short, and the fifth finger, which often has two instead of three sections, curves inward. A space is visible between the first and second toes. Children with Down syndrome have a short stature.

The intelligence quotient (IQ) among children with Down syndrome varies but averages about 50, compared with normal children, whose average IQ is 100. Children with Down syndrome have better visual motor skills (such as drawing) than skills that require listening. Thus, their language skills typically develop slowly. Behavior suggestive of attention-deficit disorder (sometimes with hyperactivity) is often seen in childhood. Children with Down syndrome are at greater risk of autistic behavior, especially those with severe intellectual disability. Depression is also common among children and adults. Early intervention with educational and other services improves the functioning of young children with Down syndrome.

Children with Down syndrome often have heart defects. They are prone to hearing problems because of recurring ear infections and the associated accumulation of inner ear fluid (serous otitis). They are also prone to vision problems because of problems in their corneas and lenses. The joints in the neck may be unstable, which can lead to weakness or paralysis. Many people with Down syndrome develop thyroid disease. They are also at a higher risk of developing leukemia.

Did You Know...

Only 20% of infants with Down syndrome are born to mothers older than 35.

Diagnosis

Down syndrome may be suspected before birth based on physical defects detected during an ultrasound of the fetus or based on abnormal levels of certain proteins found in the mother's blood in the first 15 to 16 weeks of pregnancy. Screening for Down syndrome before 20 weeks of pregnancy is recommended for all women regardless of age.

An infant with Down syndrome has a physical appearance that suggests the diagnosis. A doctor confirms the diagnosis by testing the infant's blood for trisomy 21 or other disorders of the 21st chromosome. After the diagnosis is made, doctors use tests, such as ultrasound and blood tests, along with examinations by specialists, to detect abnormalities associated with Down syndrome. Treating such abnormalities can often prevent them from impairing health. Thus, these children should have regular screening for thyroid disease, vision problems, and hearing. The bony joints of their neck should be checked for instability by x-rays before they participate in Special Olympics or other sporting events.

Prognosis

The aging process seems to be accelerated, but most children with Down syndrome survive to adulthood. The average age at death is 49; however, many people reach their 50s or 60s. Symptoms of Alzheimer-like dementia, such as memory loss, further lowering of intellect, and personality changes, may develop at an early age. Heart abnormalities are often treatable with drugs or surgery. Heart disease and leukemia account for most deaths among children with Down syndrome.

When Part of a Chromosome Is Missing

A number of syndromes can occur in infants who are missing part of a chromosome. These syndromes are called **chromosome deletion syndromes**. They tend to cause severe birth defects and markedly retarded mental and physical development.

In the rare **cri du chat syndrome** (cat's cry syndrome), part of chromosome 5 is missing. An infant with this syndrome has a low birth weight; has a small head with many abnormal features, including a round face, small jaw, wide nose, widely separated eyes, crossed eyes (strabismus), and abnormally shaped ears set low in the head; and has a high-pitched cry that sounds like a kitten crying. Often the infant seems limp. The high-pitched cry occurs immediately after birth, lasts several weeks, and then disappears. Webbed fingers and toes (syndactyly) and heart defects are common. Mental and physical development is greatly retarded. Many children with cri du chat syndrome survive to adulthood but have substantial disabilities.

In **Prader-Willi syndrome**, another chromosomal deletion syndrome, mental retardation/intellectual disability is common. Many symptoms vary according to the child's age. Newborns with the defect feel limp, feed poorly, and gain weight slowly. Eventually these symptoms resolve. Then, between the ages of 1 and 6, appetite increases, often becoming insatiable. The hands and feet remain small. Obsessive-compulsive behaviors are common. The function of the reproductive organs is abnormally decreased, which retards growth and sexual development. Weight gain is excessive, which can lead to other health problems. Obesity can be severe enough to justify gastric bypass surgery.

Recent findings indicate that blacks with Down syndrome have a substantially shorter life span than whites. This finding may be the result of poor access to medical, educational, and other support services.

Fragile X Syndrome

Fragile X syndrome is a genetic abnormality in the X chromosome that leads to delayed development and other symptoms.

The symptoms of fragile X syndrome are caused by abnormalities in DNA on the X chromosome. Usually, affected boys inherit the genetic abnormality from their mother.

Many children with the syndrome have normal intelligence. However, the syndrome is the most commonly diagnosed inherited cause of mental retardation/intellectual disability among boys. The severity of symptoms, including mental retardation/intellectual disability, is worse in boys than in girls with the disorder. This is because boys have only one X chromosome. The second X chromosome in girls helps compensate for the fragile X chromosome. Symptoms, which are often subtle, include delayed development; large, protuberant ears; a prominent chin and forehead; and, in boys, large testes (most apparent after puberty). The joints may be abnormally flexible, and heart disease (mitral valve prolapse) may occur. Features of autism may develop. Women may experience menopause in their mid 30s.

The presence of abnormal DNA on the fragile X chromosome can be detected by tests before or after birth.

Early intervention, including speech and language therapy and occupational therapy, can help children with fragile X syndrome to maximize their abilities. Stimulants, antidepressants, and antianxiety drugs may be beneficial for some children.

Turner's Syndrome

In Turner's syndrome (gonadal dysgenesis), girls are born with one of their two X chromosomes partially or completely missing.

- Turner's syndrome is caused by the deletion of or partial formation of one of the two X chromosomes.
- Girls with the syndrome have a short stature, loose skin on the back of the neck, learning disabilities, and an inability to undergo puberty.
- The diagnosis is confirmed by analyzing the chromosomes.
- Treatment with hormones can stimulate growth and initiate puberty.

Turner's syndrome occurs in about 1 out of 4,000 live female births and is the most common sex chromosome abnormality in females. However, 99% of affected fetuses abort spontaneously.

Many newborns with Turner's syndrome have swelling (lymphedema) on the backs of their hands and tops of their feet. Swelling or loose folds of skin are often evident over the back of the neck. Other abnormalities often develop, including a webbed neck (wide skin attachment between the neck and shoulders) and a broad chest with wide-spaced nipples. Affected girls have a short stature compared with family members. Less common symptoms include drooping upper eyelids (ptosis), a low hairline at the back of the neck, moles (nevi), and poorly developed nails.

Girls with Turner's syndrome generally do not have menstrual periods (amenorrhea), and the breasts, vagina, and labia remain childlike rather than undergoing the changes of puberty. The ovaries usually do not contain developing eggs. A girl or woman with Turner's syndrome is virtually always short, and obesity is common.

Other disorders often develop. Heart defects include narrowing of part of the aorta (coarctation of the aorta—see page 1716). Kidney defects, diabetes mellitus, and thyroid diseases are common. Occasionally, abnormal blood vessels in the intestine cause bleeding. Hearing loss occurs, and crossed eyes (strabismus) and farsightedness (hyperopia) are common. Celiac disease occurs more frequently among girls with Turner's syndrome than among the general population.

Many girls with Turner's syndrome have attention-deficit/hyperactivity disorder and learning disabilities with difficulty assessing visual and spatial relationships, planning tasks, and paying attention. They tend to score poorly on certain performance tests and in mathematics, even if they achieve average or above-average scores on verbal intelligence tests. Mental retardation/intellectual disability is rare.

A doctor may suspect the diagnosis because of the newborn's abnormal appearance. However, they may not suspect the syndrome until the teenage years, when the girl has a short stature and does not mature sexually. Analysis of the chromosomes confirms the diagnosis.

Treatment with growth hormone can stimulate growth. Estrogen replacement therapy is usually needed to initiate puberty and is typically given at age 12 to 13. Treatment with the female hormone estrogen is usually not started until after satisfactory growth has been achieved. Estrogen treatment may improve the girl's ability to plan tasks, pay attention, and assess visual and spatial relationships as well as stimulate sexual maturation. Children with this syndrome should have regular hearing examinations, an eye examination by a pediatric ophthalmologist, regular thyroid function tests, and a screening test for celiac disease.

Noonan's Syndrome

Noonan's syndrome is a genetic defect that causes a number of physical abnormalities, including short stature, heart defects, and an abnormal appearance.

Noonan's syndrome can be inherited or can develop unpredictably from a spontaneous gene mutation in children whose parents have normal genes. It is relatively common, occurring in about 1 in 1,000 to 2,500 people. In the past, Noonan's syndrome was called male Turner's syndrome because of similarities in the two syndromes. However, the genetic defects causing the disorders are different. Boys or girls can be affected. The gene responsible for Noonan's syndrome has been localized to chromosome 12.

Children may have webbing of the neck, low-set ears, droopy eyelids, widely spaced eyes, shortened fourth (ring) fingers, a high-arched palate, and heart and blood vessel abnormalities. Hearing problems can occur, and intelligence may be impaired. Most affected people are short. Boys may have underdeveloped or undescended testes. In girls, the ovaries may be underactive or stop working. Puberty may be delayed, and young men with Noonan's syndrome may be infertile.

Growth may be improved by treatment with growth hormone. After satisfactory growth, testosterone treatment may help boys whose testes are underdeveloped. Testosterone stimulates the development of a more masculine appearance. As in Turner's syndrome, estrogen therapy may be necessary for young women to develop typical adult characteristics. Children suspected of having Noonan's syndrome should be screened for heart problems and hearing problems.

Triple X Syndrome

Triple X (trisomy X, XXX) syndrome is a rare disorder in which female infants are born with three X chromosomes.

Girls with triple X syndrome tend to have slightly lower intelligence and particular problems with verbal skills. Sometimes the syndrome causes menstrual irregularities and infertility, although some women with triple X syndrome have given birth to physically normal children who have normal chromosomes.

Extremely rare cases of infants with four or even five X chromosomes have been identified. The more X chromosomes the girl has, the greater the chance of mental retardation/intellectual disability and physical abnormalities.

Klinefelter's Syndrome

Klinefelter's syndrome is a disorder in which male infants are born with an extra X chromosome (XXY).

- Klinefelter's syndrome is caused by an extra X chromosome.
- Children may have learning disabilities, long arms and legs, small testes, and infertility.
- The diagnosis is suspected at puberty when most of the symptoms develop.
- Treatment with testosterone may be of benefit to some.

Klinefelter's syndrome is relatively common. Most boys with Klinefelter's syndrome have normal or slightly decreased intelligence. Many have speech and reading disabilities and difficulties with planning. Most have problems with language skills. Lack of insight, poor judgment, and impaired ability to learn from previous mistakes often cause these children to get into trouble. Although their physical characteristics can vary greatly, most are tall with long arms and legs but are otherwise normal in appearance.

Puberty usually occurs at the normal time, but the testes remain small. At puberty, growth of facial hair is often sparse, and the breasts may enlarge somewhat (gynecomastia). Men and boys with the syndrome are usually infertile. Men with Klinefelter's syndrome develop diabetes mellitus, chronic lung disease, varicose veins, hypothyroidism, and breast cancer more often than other men.

Some affected boys have 3, 4, and even 5 X chromosomes along with the Y. As the number of X chromosomes increases, the severity of mental retardation/intellectual disability and physical abnormalities also increases. Each extra X is associated with a 15- to 16-point reduction in intelligence quotient (IQ), with language most affected, particularly expressive language skills.

The syndrome is usually first suspected at puberty, when most of the symptoms develop. Analysis of the chromosomes confirms the diagnosis. Many men are diagnosed during an infertility assessment (probably all men with Klinefelter's syndrome are sterile).

Boys with Klinefelter's syndrome usually benefit from speech and language therapy and eventually can do well in school. Some men benefit by taking supplemental testosterone for life. The hormone improves bone density, making fractures less likely, and stimulates development of a more masculine appearance.

XYY Syndrome

The XYY syndrome is a disorder in which a male infant is born with an extra Y chromosome.

Boys with XYY syndrome tend to be tall and have difficulties with language. The intelligence quotient (IQ) tends to be slightly lower than that of other family members. Learning disabilities, hyperactivity, attention deficit disorder, and minor behavioral disorders can develop. The XYY syndrome was once thought to cause aggressive or violent criminal behavior, but this theory has been disproved.

Long QT Syndrome

Long QT syndrome is an abnormality of the heart's electrical system (see page 366), which may cause loss of consciousness or sudden death.

- Long QT syndrome can be caused by a genetic abnormality, drug use, or a disorder.

- This syndrome causes the heart to beat unusually fast, which can lead to sudden unconsciousness.
- Stress tests and electrocardiography can help confirm the diagnosis.
- Beta-blockers and pacemakers are the best forms of treatment, but some people may benefit from surgery.

The QT is an interval between two points on an electrocardiogram (see art on page 325). People with long QT syndrome have a prolongation of the QT interval. Long QT syndrome may affect as many as 1 of 7,000 people. In the United States, it may cause sudden death in 3,000 to 4,000 children and young adults each year. In children, this disorder is usually due to a genetic abnormality. Specific tests that evaluate for the most common genetic causes are now available. A person with the disorder may have family members who died suddenly and inexplicably. In most adults, long QT syndrome is caused by use of a drug or by a disorder.

People who have long QT syndrome are predisposed to developing an unusually fast heart rate, which often occurs during physical activity or emotional excitement. When the heart rate is too fast, the brain may not receive enough blood. The result is loss of consciousness and sometimes sudden death. Some people with long QT syndrome are also born deaf.

Doctors may recommend electrocardiography (ECG) for children or young adults who have suddenly and inexplicably lost consciousness. The procedure may be performed while the person is resting or after receiving drugs given by vein. The person also may be asked to walk on a treadmill or pedal an exercise bicycle in a procedure called exercise stress testing.

Beta-blockers are effective for most children and adults. For children and adults who do not respond to drugs, a pacemaker or a combination pacemaker-internal defibrillator may be tried. An internal defibrillator can shock the heart, reviving the person, whenever the heart develops a lethal rhythm abnormality. Occasionally, as an alternative, a nerve in the neck is cut in a procedure called cervicothoracic sympathectomy. Cutting this nerve can help prevent the fast heart rate that causes sudden death. For some children, restriction from competitive sports may be recommended.

CHAPTER
264

Problems in Infants and Very Young Children

Few children make it through their first years without minor problems. Crying, problems with feeding, rashes, and an occasional fever are common. These problems become health concerns only when they are extreme—for example, when children cry too much, when they are not growing well, or when they have high fevers that do not go away. Most childhood problems are not severe. Very rarely, families face the tragedy of sudden infant death syndrome (SIDS).

Fussiness, Excessive Crying, and Colic

Fussiness is the inability of an infant to settle down or be soothed. Excessive crying is hours-long periods of crying by a healthy infant whose basic needs are met. Colic is a pattern of weeks-long, excessive periods of crying that is loud, piercing, constant, and occurs in intervals, between which the infant acts normally.

- The cause of fussiness, excessive crying, and colic is usually unknown but can be due to conditions such as gastric reflux, infection, or injury.
- If no cause can be found, children are often diagnosed with excessive crying or colic.
- Unless a specific cause is found, there is no specific treatment.

Fussiness, excessive crying, and colic occur most commonly between the second week and third month of life. Their cause is usually unknown, but excessive crying is sometimes due to excess air in the digestive tract (for example, from not burping after eating or from swallowing air while crying) or to an infection, such as an ear or urinary tract infection. Rarely, excessive crying is a sign of a serious illness like intestinal obstruction or meningitis. Other causes of crying are gastroesophageal reflux (see page 1794), milk allergy, eruption of a tooth, a hair caught around a finger or toe (hair tourniquet), or a corneal abrasion.

Parents of children with excessive crying or colic should consult a doctor if there is nothing they can do to stop the child's crying or if the child has other symptoms, such as fever or poor feeding. Doctors try to diagnose and treat known causes of fussiness and crying. Infections may or may not require antibiotics. Gastroesophageal reflux can be treated by a number of strategies (see page 1795). Air in the digestive tract can be diminished by adequately burping the child. A change of formula may treat symptoms of milk allergy; however, parents should consult with their doctor before changing the formula. Crying from teething usually lessens with time. Mild analgesics and teething rings can be helpful. A hair tourniquet needs to be removed. Corneal abrasions are treated with an antibiotic ointment or drops to prevent infection.

If there is no readily identified reason for an infant's persistent crying, the doctor may diagnose excessive crying or colic. There is no specific treatment. If mothers who are breastfeeding notice that certain foods lead to increased crying in their infant, they should avoid eating those foods. Many infants get some relief from being held, rocked, or patted or from the white noise and vibration of a fan, washing machine, or car ride. A pacifier or swaddling clothes may also be comforting. Feeding sometimes soothes the child, but parents should avoid overfeeding in an attempt to stop the crying. Some children cry themselves to sleep.

Excessive crying and colic can be exhausting and stressful for parents. Parents should take advantage of nighttime crying interludes to lay infants on their back in their crib to encourage self-soothing and sleep. Emotional support from friends, family, neighbors, and doctors is key to coping. Parents should ask for whatever help they need (with siblings, errands, or child care) and share their feelings and fears. Overwhelmed parents can take comfort in the fact that despite the extreme distress the crying or colicky infant appears to be in, excessive crying and colic usually disappear by 3 to 4 months of age and cause no long-term harm.

Teething

A child's first tooth usually appears by 6 months of age, and a complete set of 20 primary or first teeth usually develops by age 3. Before a tooth appears, the child may cry, be irritable, and sleep and eat poorly. The child may drool, have red and tender gums, and chew constantly on food and objects during tooth eruption. During teething, the child may have a mildly elevated temperature (below 100° F or below 38° C). Children who have higher temperatures and those who are especially fussy should be evaluated by a doctor because these symptoms are not due to teething.

? Did You Know...

Despite popular belief, teething does not cause fever.

Teething infants get some relief from chewing on hard, cold objects, such as firm rubber teething rings. Massaging the child's gums with or without ice may help. Teething gels may provide relief for a few minutes. Parents should avoid the use of lidocaine gels. If a child is extremely uncomfortable, acetaminophen or ibuprofen is usually effective for pain.

Feeding Problems

- Feeding problems include gastroesophageal reflux, gastroenteritis, too much food, too little food, or fluid loss.
- Proper nutrition and feeding techniques can alleviate some feeding problems.
- Some feeding problems resolve without treatment but others require medical attention or hospitalization.

Feeding problems in infants and young children are usually minor but sometimes have serious consequences.

Spitting Up: Spitting up (burping up) is the effortless return of swallowed formula or breast milk through the mouth or nose after feeding. Almost all infants spit up, because infants cannot sit upright during and after feedings. Also, the valve (sphincter) that separates the esophagus and stomach is immature and does not keep all of the stomach's contents in place. Spitting up gets worse when an infant eats too fast or swallows air. Spitting up usually stops between the ages of 7 months and 12 months.

Spitting up can be reduced by feeding infants before they get very hungry, burping them every 4 to 5 minutes, placing them in an upright position during and after feeding, and making certain the bottle nipple lets out only a few drops with pressure or when the bottle is upside down. Spitting up that seems to cause an infant discomfort, interferes with feeding and growth, or persists into early childhood is called gastroesophageal reflux and may require medical attention (see page 1794). If the material that is spit up is green (indicating bile) or bloody or causes any coughing or choking, medical attention is needed.

Vomiting: Vomiting is the uncomfortable, forced throwing up of feedings. It is never normal. Vomiting in infants is most often the result of acute viral gastroenteritis. It can also be caused by infections elsewhere in the body, such as ear or urinary tract infections. Less commonly, vomiting occurs because of a serious medical disorder. Infants between the ages of 2 weeks and 4 months may rarely have forceful (projectile) vomiting after feedings because of a blockage at the stomach outlet (hypertrophic pyloric stenosis). Vomiting can also be caused by life-threatening disorders, such as meningitis, intestinal blockage, and appendicitis. These disorders usually cause severe pain, lethargy, and continuous vomiting that does not lessen with time.

Most vomiting caused by gastroenteritis stops without treatment. Giving the child fluids and electrolytes (such as sodium and chloride) from solutions available in stores or pharmacies prevents or treats dehydration. A child who is vomiting frequently may tolerate small amounts of solution given more often better than large amounts given less often. Older children can be given popsicles or gelatin, although red versions of these foods can be confused with blood if the child vomits again. A doctor should see any child who has severe abdominal pain, is unable to drink and retain fluids, has a high fever, is lethargic or acting extremely ill, vomits for more than 12 hours, vomits blood or green material (bile), or is unable to urinate. These symptoms may signal dehydration or a more severe condition.

Overfeeding: Overfeeding is the provision of more nutrition than a child needs for healthy growth. Overfeeding occurs when children are automatically fed as a response to crying, when they are given a bottle as a distraction or activity, or when they are allowed to keep a bottle with them at all times. Overfeeding also occurs when parents reward good behavior with food or expect children to finish their food even if they are not hungry. In the short term, overfeeding causes spitting up and diarrhea. In the long term, overfed children can become obese (see page 1756).

Underfeeding: Underfeeding is the provision of less nutrition than a child needs for healthy growth. It is one of many causes of failure to thrive (see page 1737) and may be related to the child or the caregiver. Underfeeding may result when a fussy or distracted infant does not sit well for feedings or has difficulty sucking or swallowing. Underfeeding can also result from improper feeding techniques and errors in formula preparation (see page 1680). Poverty and poor access to nutritious food are major reasons for underfeeding. Occasionally, abusive parents and parents with mental health disorders purposely withhold food from their children.

Community social agencies (such as the Women, Infants and Children [WIC] program) can help parents purchase formula and can teach them proper techniques for formula preparation and feeding. If an infant is so far below expected weight that supervised feedings are necessary, the doctor may admit the child to a hospital for evaluation. If the parents are abusive or neglectful, Child Protective Services may be called.

Treating Dehydration

Illnesses that cause vomiting and diarrhea can lead to dehydration in children. In infants, dehydration is treated by encouraging an infant to drink fluids that contain electrolytes. Breast milk contains all the fluids and electrolytes an infant needs and is the best treatment. If an infant is not breastfeeding, oral electrolyte rehydration solutions should be given. These can be bought as powders or liquids at drug or grocery stores without a prescription. The amount of solution to give a child depends on the child's age, but generally should be about 1½ to 2½ ounces of solution in a 24-hour period for each pound the child weighs—thus, a 20-pound infant should drink 30 to 50 ounces total.

Children older than 1 year may try small sips of clear soups, clear sodas or juice diluted to half-strength with water, or popsicles. Plain water, juice, and colas are not good for treating dehydration at any age because the salt content of water is too low and because juice and colas have a high sugar content and ingredients that irritate the digestive tract.

Treatment of dehydration at any age is more effective if children are first given small, frequent sips of fluids about every 10 minutes. The amount of fluid can slowly be increased and given at less frequent intervals if the child can keep the fluid down without vomiting or getting severe diarrhea. Infants who are able to digest fluids over 12 to 24 hours can then resume drinking formula from a bottle. Older children can try broths or soups and bland foods (for example, bananas, toast, and rice). Infants and young children who are unable to digest any fluids, or who develop listlessness and other serious signs of dehydration, may require more intensive treatment with fluids given by vein (intravenously) or electrolyte solutions given through a thin plastic tube (nasogastric tube) that is passed through the nose and down the throat until it reaches the stomach or small intestine.

Dehydration: Dehydration is usually caused by excess fluid loss, such as from vomiting and diarrhea, and occasionally by inadequate fluid intake, such as when an infant does not take in enough milk through breastfeeding. Children who are moderately dehydrated are less interactive or playful, cry without tears, have a dry mouth, and urinate fewer than 2 or 3 times a day. Children who are severely dehydrated become sleepy or lethargic. Sometimes dehydration causes the concentration of salt in the blood to fall or rise abnormally. Changes in salt concentration make the symptoms of dehydration worse and can worsen lethargy. In severe cases, the child can have seizures or suffer brain damage and die.

Dehydration is treated with fluids and electrolytes, such as sodium and chloride, given by mouth. In severe cases, fluids given by vein (intravenously) are needed.

Bowel Problems

- Bowel problems have many causes, including gastroenteritis, infection, lack of dietary fiber, antibiotics, and some specific disorders.
- Common symptoms of bowel problems include loose and watery stools (diarrhea) or hard and dry stools (constipation).
- Treatment depends on the cause and may include stopping antibiotics that cause diarrhea or constipation, giving fluids and electrolytes, adding more fiber to the diet, or taking drugs to ease chronic constipation.

The number and consistency of stools for a healthy child vary with age and diet. For example, infants who are breastfed normally have mustard-colored stools that are soft and seedy. However, repeated watery bowel movements for a time lasting longer than 12 hours are never normal.

Diarrhea: Diarrhea is frequent, watery bowel movements. Acute diarrhea starts suddenly and lessens in one to several days. Acute diarrhea is most often caused by viral gastroenteritis, which is especially likely when vomiting accompanies the diarrhea. Typically, vomiting occurs at the beginning of the illness and then tapers off, while diarrhea continues. Acute diarrhea can also be caused by a bacterial or parasitic infection; an infection elsewhere in the body, such as an ear or respiratory tract infection; and as a side effect from the use of antibiotics. Acute diarrhea is a concern mainly because it can cause dehydration. Therefore, the main treatment is giving fluids and electrolytes. Bacterial infections may be treated with antibiotics. Antibiotics that cause diarrhea may be discontinued, but only after consultation with a doctor.

Chronic diarrhea lasts for weeks or months. The most common causes of chronic diarrhea in infants and young children are relatively harmless conditions such as food allergy or sugar malabsorption (lactose intolerance). Serious disorders such as celiac disease and cystic fibrosis can also cause chronic diarrhea. In less developed countries, undernutrition and parasites are the most common causes of chronic diarrhea.

Constipation: Constipation is the infrequent passing of hard, dry stools (see page 1799). Constipation may be difficult to recognize because some infants and young children normally have bowel movements only once every 3 to 4 days. In general, children are constipated when they have not had a bowel movement in 5 or more days, when the stools are hard or cause pain, or when drops of blood are seen in the diaper or stool.

Did You Know...

It is normal for some infants and young children to have bowel movements only every 3 to 4 days.

Constipation in infants is usually caused by dehydration, insufficient fiber in the diet, or a change in feeding patterns. Rarely, medical disorders, such as an inadequate nerve supply to the large intestine (Hirschsprung's disease), low thyroid hormone levels, or calcium or potassium abnormalities, cause constipation. The use of certain drugs (such as antihistamines, anticholinergic drugs, and opioids) is another rare cause.

Treatment of constipation varies with the age of the child. Infants younger than 2 months of age who consume adequate amounts of formula or breast milk can be given a teaspoon of light corn syrup in their morning and evening bottles. Apple or prune juice is effective for infants between 2 months and 4 months of age. Infants between 4 months and 1 year can get relief from high-fiber cereals or from strained apricots, prunes, or plums. Children older than 1 year should be given high-fiber foods, such as fruits, peas, cereals, graham crackers, beans, and spinach. Parents should not give their child a laxative, suppository, or enema without first consulting a doctor. Doctors may prescribe various drugs to treat older children with severe constipation. Treatment of rare disorders includes surgery for Hirschsprung's disease, thyroid hormone replacement for low thyroid hormone levels, and calcium supplements for abnormal calcium levels.

Separation Anxiety

Separation anxiety is the fear young children have that their parents will leave them.

- Separation anxiety typically starts around age 8 months and is most intense between 10 months and 18 months.
- Separation anxiety begins to resolve as children age and begin to remember that parents return after leaving.
- Separation anxiety usually stops by age 2 years.

Children with separation anxiety panic and cry when a parent leaves them, even if only to go into an adjacent room. Separation anxiety is normal for infants at about 8 months of age, is most intense between 10 months and 18 months of age, and usually resolves by 2 years of age. The intensity and duration of a child's separation anxiety vary and depend partly on the child-parent relationship. Usually, separation anxiety in a child with a strong and healthy attachment to a parent resolves sooner than in a child whose connection is less strong.

Separation anxiety occurs at a time when infants start to become aware that their parents are unique individuals. Because they have incomplete memory and no sense of time, these young children fear any departure of their parents may be permanent. Separation anxiety resolves as a young child develops a sense of memory and keeps an image of the parents in mind when they are gone. The child recollects that in the past the parents returned.

Parents should not limit or forego separations in response to separation anxiety because doing so could compromise the child's maturation and development. When parents are ready to leave the home (or leave the child at a child care center), they should encourage the person with whom they are leaving the child to distract the child with toys, a game, or another activity. Then, the parents should leave without responding at length to the child's crying. If the parents are staying at home but in a different room, they should not return immediately in response to crying, but instead should call to the child from the other room. This teaches the child that parents are still present even though the child cannot see them. Separation anxiety may be worse when children are hungry or tired, so feeding children and letting them nap before leaving may also help.

Separation anxiety at the normal age causes no long-term harm to the child. Separation anxiety that lasts beyond age 2 may or may not be a problem depending on the extent to which it interferes with the child's development. It is normal for children to feel some fear when leaving for preschool or kindergarten. This feeling should diminish with time. Rarely, excessive fear of separations inhibits a child from attending child care or preschool or keeps a child from playing normally with peers. This anxiety is probably abnormal (separation anxiety disorder—see page 1871). In this case, the parents should seek medical attention for the child.

Rashes

- Known causes of rashes include irritation and bacterial, fungal, or viral infection.
- Symptoms include bright red rash; red or yellow scales; itching; and pearly pimples, bumps, or cysts.
- Rashes that require treatment can be helped by gentle cleansers, moisturizing ointments, antibiotic creams, and anti-itch drugs.

Skin rashes in infants and young children are not usually serious and can have various causes.

Diaper rash (diaper dermatitis) is a bright red rash caused by irritation from prolonged skin contact with urine or stool anywhere beneath a child's diaper. Typically, the areas of the skin that touch the diaper are most affected. Diaper rash can also be caused by infection with the fungus *Candida*, typically causing a bright red rash in the creases of the skin and small red spots. Less often, diaper rash is caused by bacteria. Diaper rash does not always bother the child. It can be prevented or minimized by using diapers that are made with an absorbent gel, by avoiding restrictive plastic diapers or pants that trap moisture, and by frequently changing diapers when they are soiled. Breastfed babies tend to have fewer diaper rashes because their stools contain fewer enzymes and other substances that can irritate the skin.

The main treatment for diaper rash is to frequently remove or change the child's diapers. The child's skin should be washed gently with mild soap and water. Often the rash clears up with these measures alone. Use of a skin moisturizer and barrier ointment, such as zinc, petroleum jelly, or vitamin A & D ointment, may help. Antifungal cream may be necessary if the doctor diagnoses a *Candida* infection. Antibiotic cream can be used if the rash is caused by bacteria.

Eczema (atopic dermatitis—see page 1286) is a red, scaly, dry rash that is most common where the arm and leg joints bend and tends to appear in patches that come and go, often worsening with cold, dry weather. Although the cause is unknown, eczema tends to run in families and in many cases is thought to be due to an allergy. Its origin may be similar to that of asthma. Most children outgrow eczema, but for others eczema is a life-long condition. Children with severe cases may intermittently develop infections of some particularly affected areas. Treatment includes use of skin moisturizers, gentle soaps, humidified air, corticosteroid creams, and anti-itch drugs. Efforts to control dust mites and other triggers of a child's allergies may occasionally help alleviate the condition.

Cradle cap (seborrheic dermatitis) is a red and yellow scaling, crusty rash that occurs on an infant's head and occasionally in the skin folds. The cause is not known. Cradle cap is harmless and disappears in most children by 6 months of age. Cradle cap can be treated by regularly shampooing and massaging mineral oil into the scalp. The scales may be worked off with a fine comb. Cradle cap that does not abate with these measures may need further treatment, such as selenium shampoo or corticosteroid creams.

Tinea is a fungal infection of the skin. In children, infections of the scalp (tinea capitis) and body (tinea corporis, or ringworm) are most common. The diagnosis and treatment of tinea are the same in children and adults (see page 1321). Some children have an inflammatory reaction to the fungal infection that leads to a scalp mass (kerion), which may require additional treatment.

Molluscum contagiosum is a cluster of flesh-colored pearly pimples or bumps caused by a viral skin infection (see page 1325) that usually disappears without treatment.

Milia are small pearly cysts on the face of newborns caused by the first secretions of the child's oil glands. Like newborn acne, milia require no treatment and disappear soon after birth.

Other skin rashes in young children are often caused by viral infections. Rashes caused by roseola and erythema infectiosum (fifth disease) are harmless and usually abate without treatment (see page 1774). Rashes caused by measles, rubella, and chickenpox are becoming less common because children are receiving vaccines.

Undescended and Retractile Testes

Undescended testes (cryptorchidism) are testes that remain in the abdomen instead of descending into the scrotum just before birth.

About 3 of every 100 boys have undescended testes at birth. Most testes descend on their own within about 6 months. Boys born prematurely are much more likely to have the condition as are boys whose family members had undescended testes. Half of the boys with the condition have an undescended testis only on the right side, and one fourth are affected on both sides.

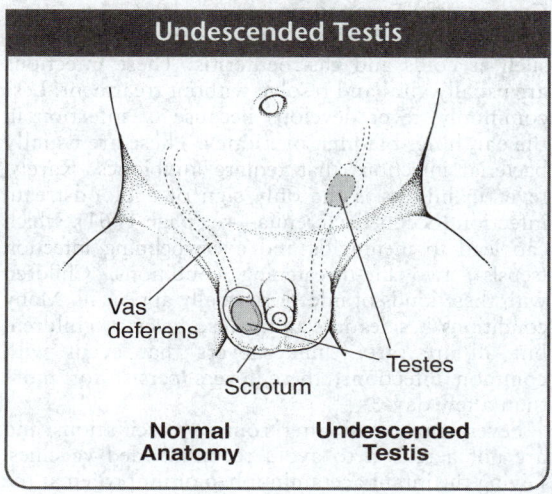

Undescended Testis

Vas deferens

Testes

Scrotum

Normal Anatomy

Undescended Testis

Undescended testes cause no symptoms. However, undescended testes can become twisted in the abdomen (testicular torsion—see page 1471), impair sperm production later in life, and increase the risk of hernia and testicular cancer. Surgery is usually performed to bring the testes down into the scrotum if the testes remain undescended at 1 year of age.

Retractile (hypermobile) testes are descended testes that easily move back and forth between the scrotum and the abdomen. Retractile testes do not lead to cancer or other complications. The testes usually stop retracting by puberty and do not require surgery or other treatment.

Fever

Fever is a rise in body temperature in response to infection, injury, or inflammation (see page 1142).

- Fever usually is caused by a viral infection such as a cold or gastroenteritis.
- Typically, children are irritable, disinterested, and do not feed or sleep well.
- The diagnosis is based on symptoms, a physical examination, and sometimes testing to determine the cause of the fever.
- Acetaminophen or ibuprofen can lower the fever and make the child feel better.

Body temperatures vary, and temperature elevations up to 100.3° F (about 38° C) can be normal in healthy children. Therefore, minor temperature elevations that do not distress a child do not require medical attention. Temperatures of 100.4° F (about 38° C) and higher are considered abnormal and usually deserve attention, particularly in infants younger than 3 months.

Causes and Symptoms

Fever is usually the result of common infections, such as colds and gastroenteritis. These infections are usually viral and resolve without treatment. Less commonly, fever develops because of infection in the ear, lung, bladder, or kidney. These are usually bacterial infections that require antibiotics. Rarely, fever in infants is the only sign of a bloodstream infection (occult bacteremia—see page 1761), which can lead to meningitis and overwhelming infection (sepsis), two life-threatening conditions. Children with these kinds of infection usually appear ill. Many conditions besides infection cause fever in children, but all are rare. Unlike fevers that occur with common infections, these fevers persist for more than a few days.

Fevers can occur after routine vaccinations and are not a reason to avoid recommended vaccines. Giving the infant acetaminophen or ibuprofen at the time of vaccination and afterward minimizes the risk of getting a fever or lowers the fever itself.

Infants with fever are usually irritable and may not sleep or feed well. Older children lose their interest in play, although sometimes children with high fevers appear surprisingly well. The irritability and disinterest that fever usually causes worsen the higher the fever gets. Occasionally, a rapidly rising fever can cause seizures (febrile seizures), and quite rarely, a fever gets so high that children become lethargic and unresponsive.

Diagnosis and Treatment

Detecting fever is not a challenge, but determining its cause can be. If the fever is low grade (100.3° F [about 38° C] or below) and of short duration, no testing or treatment may be needed. In other cases, knowledge of the child's symptoms and a thorough examination help doctors find the cause. In general, any infant with a temperature of 100.4° F (about 38° C) or higher should be seen by a doctor, as should older children with higher or recurring fevers or complaints of pain.

In infants younger than 2 months of age who have a fever, doctors may order blood and urine tests and perform a spinal tap (lumbar puncture—see art on page 635) to look for occult bacteremia, urinary tract infection, and meningitis. The reason for these tests is that in infants, the source of fever is difficult to determine. They are also at risk of serious infection compared with older children because of their immature immune system. Doctors may also order an x-ray if the infant's breathing is abnormal. For infants older than 2 months of age, testing may not be needed, but many doctors order blood and urine tests and perform a spinal tap if the source of the fever is not obvious and the child appears ill. For children 3 months of age and older, doctors rely more on the child's behavior and physical examination to determine which tests to order. Doctors may order blood and urine tests for children younger than 3 years old with high fevers if they cannot determine the source of fever after examining the child.

Most fevers do not require treatment except to make the child feel better and thus more willing to drink, avoiding dehydration. Acetaminophen and ibuprofen are used. Aspirin is not safe for lowering fever because it can interact with certain viral infections and cause a serious condition called Reye's syndrome (see box on page 1769). A warm (not cold) bath can sometimes make an older child feel better by reducing the fever. Rubbing the child down with alcohol or witch hazel is not recommended. Alcohol or witch hazel may have harmful fumes, come into contact with the eyes, or be accidentally ingested.

How to Take a Child's Temperature

A child's temperature can be taken from the rectum, the ear, the mouth, or the armpit. Rectal temperatures can be taken with a glass or digital thermometer. Thermometers containing mercury are no longer recommended because of the risk of breakage and exposure to mercury.

Rectal temperatures are most accurate; that is, they come closest to the child's true internal body temperature. To take a rectal temperature, a thermometer with a coat of petroleum jelly or another lubricant around the bulb should be gently inserted about 1/2 to 1 inch (about 1 1/4 to 2 1/2 centimeters) into the child's rectum while the child is lying face down. The child should be kept from moving. The thermometer should be kept in place for 2 to 3 minutes before removing it and taking a reading.

Ear temperatures are taken with a digital device that measures infrared radiation from the eardrum. Ear thermometers are unreliable in infants younger than 3 months of age. To take an ear temperature, the person should form a seal around the opening of the ear with the thermometer probe and press the start button. A digital readout provides the temperature.

Oral temperatures are taken by placing a glass or digital thermometer under the child's tongue for 2 to 3 minutes. Oral temperatures provide reliable readings but are difficult to take in young children, who usually cannot keep their mouth gently closed around the thermometer to get an accurate reading.

Armpit temperatures are taken by placing a glass or digital thermometer in the child's armpit for 4 to 5 minutes. Armpit temperatures are least accurate because the armpit is cooler than the rectum, ear, or mouth.

Additional treatment depends on the child's age and cause of the fever. Rarely, fevers persist and doctors are unable to determine the source even after extensive testing. This type of fever is called fever of unknown origin (see page 1143).

Failure to Thrive

Failure to thrive is a delay in physical growth and weight gain that can lead to delays in development and maturation.

- Medical disorders and a lack of access to proper nutrition are causes of failure to thrive.
- The diagnosis is based on a growth chart comparison, thorough examination, and parents' answers to specific questions about the child's health and environment.

- Children who are undernourished during the first year of life have developmental delays.
- Treatment depends on the cause.

Failure to thrive is a diagnosis given to children who are consistently underweight or who do not gain weight for unclear reasons. There are many causes. Most causes involve environmental and social factors that interact to keep the child from getting the nutrition the child needs. Occasionally, medical disorders prevent a child from growing normally.

Many environmental and social factors can be responsible. Parental neglect or abuse, parental mental health disorders, and chaotic family situations, in which routine, nutritious meals are insufficiently provided, may all blunt a child's appetite and intake of food. The amount of money a family has to spend on food and the nutritional value of the food they buy also affect growth. Inadequate intake of food may reflect inadequate parenting and environmental stimulation.

Sometimes failure to thrive is caused by a medical disorder in the child. The disorder can be as minor as difficulty chewing or swallowing (as with a cleft lip or cleft palate). Medical disorders, such as gastroesophageal reflux, narrowing of the esophagus, or intestinal malabsorption, may also affect a child's ability to retain, absorb, or process food. Infection, tumor, hormonal or metabolic disorders (such as diabetes or cystic fibrosis), heart disease, kidney disease, genetic disorders, and human immunodeficiency virus (HIV) infection are other physical reasons for failure to thrive.

Diagnosis

Doctors diagnose failure to thrive when a child's weight or rate of growth is well below what it should be when compared with past measurements or standard height-weight charts (see box on page 1741). If the rate of growth is adequate, the child may be small for his or her age but still growing normally.

To determine why a child may be failing to thrive, doctors ask parents specific questions about feeding; bowel habits; social, emotional, and financial stability of the family, which might affect the child's access to food; and illnesses that the child has had or that run in the family. The doctor examines the child, looking for signs of conditions that could explain the child's growth delay. The doctor makes decisions about blood and urine tests and x-rays based on this evaluation. More extensive testing is performed only if the doctor suspects an underlying disease.

Prognosis and Treatment

Because the first year of life is important for brain development, children who become undernourished during this time may fall permanently behind their peers, even if their physical growth improves. In about half of these children, mental development, especially verbal skills, remains below normal, and these children often have social and emotional problems in adulthood.

Treatment depends on the cause. If a medical disorder is found, specific treatment is given. Otherwise, treatment depends on how far below normal the child's weight is. Mild to moderate failure to thrive is treated with nutritious, high-calorie feedings given on a regular schedule. Parents may be counseled about family interactions that are damaging to the child and about financial and social resources available to them. Severe failure to thrive is treated in the hospital where social workers, nutritionists, feeding specialists, psychiatrists, and other specialists work together to determine the most likely causes of the child's failure to thrive and the best approach to feeding.

Apparent Life-Threatening Event

An apparent life-threatening event (ALTE) is the sudden occurrence of certain alarming symptoms such as prolonged periods of no breathing (apnea), change in color or muscle tone, coughing, and gagging in children under 1 year of age.

- Known causes include nervous system disorders and infections.
- The diagnosis is based on a discussion with caregivers, a physical examination, and the results of certain laboratory tests.
- The prognosis depends on the cause of the apparent life-threatening event.
- Treatment is aimed at specific causes when they can be identified.

ALTE is not a specific disorder. It is a group of symptoms that occur suddenly in young children.

Causes

The most common causes of ALTE include gastroesophageal reflux disease, nervous system disorders (such as seizures, meningitis, or brain tumors), and infections. Less common causes include heart disorders, metabolic disorders, child abuse, and narrowing or complete blockage of the airways. A cause cannot be determined in about 50% of cases.

Symptoms

An ALTE usually is characterized by an unexpected, sudden change in an infant's breathing that alarms the parent or caretaker. Features of an event include some or all of the following:

- Not breathing for 20 seconds or more
- Color change, usually blue or pale, but sometimes red

- Change in muscle tone, usually floppy
- Choking or gagging

Diagnosis

When an ALTE occurs, the doctor asks several key questions:

- What was observed by the caregiver who witnessed the event (including a description of changes in breathing, color, muscle tone, and eyes, noises made, and length of the episode)?
- What interventions were taken (such as gentle stimulation, mouth-to-mouth breathing, or cardiopulmonary resuscitation [CPR])?
- Has the mother used drugs while pregnant? Do members of the family currently use drugs, tobacco, and alcohol?
- What is the child's gestational age (length of time spent in the uterus after the egg is fertilized)? Were there any complications at birth?
- While feeding, does the child gag, cough, or vomit? Has poor weight gain been an issue?
- Has the child reached all age-appropriate developmental milestones?
- Has the child had an ALTE before or experienced a recent trauma?
- Have there been any other ALTEs in the family or early death?

The doctor does a physical examination to check for obvious defects, particularly nervous system abnormalities, such as being too stiff (posturing) or being too floppy (poor muscle tone), and signs of trauma.

The doctor may do laboratory tests (such as liver function, blood, stool, and urine tests), imaging tests (such as a chest x-ray or computed tomography [CT] of the head), electrocardiography, or a combination based on the examination findings. Tests (such as electroencephalography—see page 636) to check for other possible causes also may be done.

Prognosis

The prognosis depends on the cause. Some causes, such as neurologic disorders, are more dangerous than others. If the ALTE was not caused by a serious disorder, children do not seem to have any long-term consequences. The relationship of ALTE to sudden infant death syndrome (SIDS) is unclear. However, most doctors no longer think infants who had an ALTE are at increased risk of SIDS.

Treatment

The cause, if identified, is treated. Infants who have required CPR or have had any abnormalities identified during the examination or initial laboratory testing are hospitalized for monitoring and further evaluation.

Parents and caregivers should be trained in CPR for infants and in general safe infant care (such as putting infants to sleep on their back and eliminating exposure to tobacco smoke). Doctors sometimes recommend home apnea monitoring devices for a limited period of time. Monitors that can record the infants' breathing pattern and heart rate are preferred to those that simply sound an alarm. Recording monitors may help doctors distinguish false alarms from real events.

Sudden Infant Death Syndrome

Sudden infant death syndrome (SIDS) is the sudden, unexpected death of a seemingly healthy infant during sleep, in whom a thorough postmortem examination does not show a cause.

- The cause of SIDS is not known.
- Putting infants to sleep on their back; removing pillows, bumper guards, and toys from the crib; protecting infants from overheating; and preventing infants from breathing second-hand cigarette smoke may help prevent SIDS.
- Parents who have lost a child to SIDS should seek counseling and support groups.

Although SIDS (also called crib death) is rare overall (about 1 in 2,000), it is one of the most common causes of death in infants between the ages of 2 weeks and 1 year. It most often affects children between the second and fourth month of life. The syndrome occurs worldwide. SIDS is more common among premature infants, those who were small at birth, those that previously needed resuscitation, and those with upper respiratory tract infections. For unknown reasons, black and Native American infants are at higher risk. It is more common among infants in families with low incomes; whose mothers are single, less than 20 years old, or who have used cigarettes or illicit drugs during pregnancy; and who have had brothers or sisters who have also died of SIDS.

> **? Did You Know...**
> Although rare, sudden infant death syndrome is one of the most common causes of death in infants between the ages of 2 weeks and 1 year.

The cause of SIDS is unknown. It may be due to an abnormality in the control of breathing. Some infants with SIDS show signs of having had low levels of oxygen in their blood and having had periods when they stopped breathing. Laying infants down to sleep on their stomach and the use of soft bedding (such as pillows and lamb's wool blankets) have been linked to

Back to Sleep: Reducing the Risk of Sudden Infant Death Syndrome

- **Position:** Always place the infant on the infant's back to sleep, for naps and at night.
- **Surface:** Place the infant on a firm sleep surface, such as a safety-approved crib mattress, covered by a fitted sheet.
- **Bedding:** Keep soft objects, toys, blankets, and other loose bedding out of the infant's sleep area.
- **No smoking:** Do not allow smoking around the infant. Not smoking during pregnancy is also important.
- **Location:** Set up the infant's sleep area close to but separate from the sleep area of the parents and other children.
- **Pacifiers:** Consider offering the infant a clean, dry pacifier when placing the infant down to sleep.
- **Temperature:** Do not let the infant overheat during sleep.

Home monitors and products that claim to prevent sudden infant death syndrome do not seem helpful.

To help prevent flat spots from developing on the infant's head, infants should spend some time on their tummy when they are awake and someone is watching. Changing the direction that the infant lies in while in the crib each week and not leaving the infant in car seats, carriers, and bouncers too long also help.

Adapted from The National Institute of Child Health and Human Development, www.nichd.nih.gov.

SIDS. Sleeping together with an infant on a sofa, cushion, or soft bed also increases the risk of SIDS.

Despite the known risk factors for SIDS, there is no certain way to prevent it. However, certain measures seem to help, particularly putting infants to sleep on their back on a firm mattress. The number of SIDS deaths has decreased dramatically as more parents have put their infants to sleep on their back. Parents should also remove pillows, bumper guards, and toys that could block an infant's breathing. Protecting infants from overheating may also help, but this measure is not proved. Preventing infants from breathing second-hand cigarette smoke may help and clearly has other health benefits.

Most parents who have lost an infant to SIDS are grief-stricken and unprepared for the tragedy. They usually feel guilty. They may be further traumatized by investigations conducted by police, social workers, or others. Counseling and support from specially trained doctors and nurses and other parents who have lost an infant to SIDS are critical to helping parents cope with the tragedy. Specialists can recommend reading materials, web sites, and support groups to assist parents.

CHAPTER 265

Preschool and School-Aged Children

Between the ages of 1 and 13, children's physical, intellectual, and emotional capabilities expand tremendously. Children progress from barely tottering to running, jumping, and playing organized sports. At age 1, most children can utter only a few recognizable words. By age 10, most children can write book reports and use computers. Physical, intellectual, and social development, however, proceed at an individual pace.

Physical Development

Physical growth begins to slow at around age 1. As growth slows, children need fewer calories and parents may notice a decrease in appetite. Two-year-old children can have very erratic eating habits that sometimes make parents anxious. It seems as though some children eat virtually nothing yet continue to grow and thrive. Actually, they eat little one day and then make up for it by eating everything in sight the next day.

Children who are beginning to walk have an endearing physique, with the belly sticking forward and the back curved. They may also appear to be quite bow-legged. By 3 years of age, muscle tone increases and the proportion of body fat decreases, so the body begins to look leaner and more muscular. Most children are physically able to control their bowels and bladder at this time.

During the preschool and school years, growth in height and weight is steady. The next major growth spurt occurs in early adolescence. During the years of steady growth, most children follow a predictable pattern. Doctors report how the children are growing in relation to other children their age and monitor the children's weight gain compared to their height. Some children can become obese at an early age. Doubling the child's height at age 24 months fairly accurately predicts adult height.

Intellectual Development

At the age of 2, most children understand the concept of time in broad terms. Many 2- and 3-year-old children believe that anything that happened in the past happened "yesterday," and anything that will happen in

MILESTONES FROM AGES 18 MONTHS TO 6 YEARS		
AGE	**GROSS MOTOR SKILLS**	**FINE MOTOR SKILLS**
18 months	Walks well Walks upstairs holding on	Draws vertical stroke Makes a tower of 4 cubes
2 years	Runs with coordination Climbs on furniture	Handles a spoon well Turns single book pages Makes a tower of 7 cubes
2½ years	Jumps Walks upstairs and downstairs unaided	Scribbles in a circular pattern Opens doors
3 years	Mature gait in walking Rides tricycle	Favors using one hand over the other Copies a circle
4 years	Walks downstairs, alternating feet Hops on 1 foot Throws ball overhand	Copies a cross Dresses self
5 years	Skips Catches a bounced ball	Copies a square Draws a person in 6 parts
6 years	Walks along a straight line from heel to toe	Writes name

Height and Weight Charts for Boys and Girls

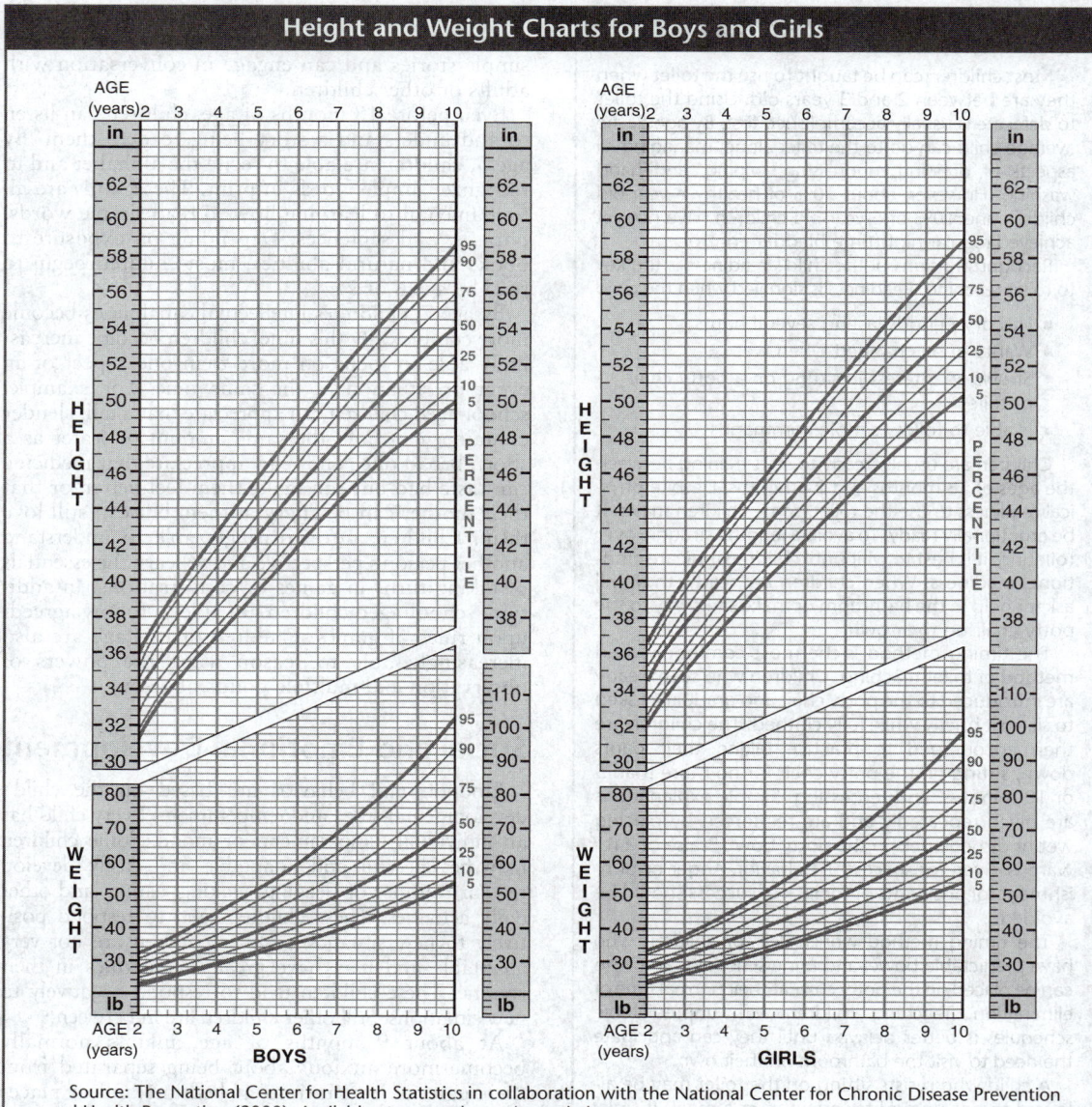

Source: The National Center for Health Statistics in collaboration with the National Center for Chronic Disease Prevention and Health Promotion (2000). Available at www.cdc.gov/growthcharts.

the future will happen "tomorrow." A child at this age has a vivid imagination but has difficulty distinguishing fantasy from reality. By age 4, most children have a more complicated understanding of time. They realize that the day is divided into morning, afternoon, and night. They can even appreciate the change in seasons.

From 18 months to 5 years of age, a child's vocabulary quickly expands from about 50 words to several thousand words. Children can begin to name and to actively ask about objects and events. By age 2, they begin to put two words together in short phrases, progressing to simple sentences by age 3. Pronunciation improves, with speech being

Toilet Teaching

Most children can be taught to use the toilet when they are between 2 and 3 years old. Using the toilet to defecate is usually accomplished first. By age 5, the average child can go to the toilet alone, managing all aspects of dressing, undressing, wiping, and hand washing. However, about 30% of healthy 4-year-old children and 10% of 6-year-old children have not yet achieved regular nighttime bladder control.

Recognizing signs of the child's readiness is the key to toilet teaching. Readiness is signaled when the child

- Has dry periods lasting several hours
- Wants to be changed when wet
- Shows an interest in sitting on a potty chair or toilet
- Is able to follow simple commands

Children are usually ready to start training between the ages of 18 months and 24 months. Despite physical readiness to use the toilet, some children may not be emotionally ready. To avoid a lengthy struggle over toileting, it is best to wait until children indicate emotional readiness. When children are ready, they will ask for help in the bathroom or make their way to the potty chair on their own.

The timing method is the most commonly used method of toilet teaching. Children who seem ready are introduced to the potty chair and gradually asked to sit on it briefly while fully clothed. The children are then encouraged to practice taking their pants down, sitting on the potty chair for no more than 5 or 10 minutes, and redressing. Simple explanations are given repeatedly and are reinforced by placing wet or dirty diapers in the potty bowl. Praise or a reward is given for successful behavior. Anger or punishment for accidents or for lack of success should be avoided.

The timing method works well for children who have predictable bowel and urine schedules and who can be placed on the potty chair at their normal time of elimination. Teaching children with unpredictable schedules is better delayed until they can anticipate the need to visit the bathroom on their own.

A child who resists sitting on the toilet may be allowed to get up and try again after a meal. If resistance continues for days, postponing the teaching for several weeks is the best strategy. Giving praise or a reward for sitting on the toilet and producing results is effective. Once the pattern is established, rewards can be given for every other success and then gradually withdrawn. Power struggles are unproductive and may strain the parent-child relationship.

half-understandable to a stranger by age 2 and fully understandable by age 4. A 4-year-old child can tell simple stories and can engage in conversation with adults or other children.

Even before 18 months of age, children can listen to and understand a story being read to them. By age 5, children are able to recite the alphabet and to recognize simple words in print. These skills are all fundamental to learning how to read simple words, phrases, and sentences. Depending on exposure to books and natural abilities, most children begin to read by age 6 or 7.

By age 7, children's intellectual capabilities become more complex. By this time, children become increasingly able to focus on more than one aspect of an event or situation at the same time. For example, school-aged children can appreciate that a tall, slender container can hold the same amount of water as a short, broad one. They can appreciate that medicine can taste bad but can make them feel better, or that their mother can be angry at them but can still love them. Children are increasingly able to understand another person's perspective and so learn the essentials of taking turns in games or conversations. In addition, school-aged children are able to follow agreed-upon rules of games. Children of this age are also increasingly able to reason using the powers of observation and multiple points of view.

Social and Emotional Development

Emotion and behavior are based on the child's developmental stage and temperament. Every child has an individual temperament, or mood. Some children may be cheerful and adaptable and easily develop regular routines of sleeping, waking, eating, and other daily activities. These children tend to respond positively to new situations. Other children are not very adaptable and may have great irregularities in their routine. These children tend to respond negatively to new situations. Still other children are in between.

At about 9 months of age, infants normally become more anxious about being separated from their parents. Separations at bedtime and at places like child care centers may be difficult and can be marked by temper tantrums. This behavior can last for many months. For many older children, a special blanket or stuffed animal serves at this time as a transitional object that acts as a symbol for the absent parent.

At 2 to 3 years of age, children begin to test their limits and do what they have been forbidden to do, simply to see what will happen. The frequent "nos" that children hear from parents reflect the struggle for independence at this age. Although distressing to parents and children, tantrums are normal because they help children express their frustration during a time when they cannot verbalize their feelings well. Parents can help decrease the number of tantrums by not letting their children become overtired or unduly frustrated and by knowing their children's behavior patterns and avoiding situations that are likely to induce tantrums. Rarely, temper tantrums need to be evaluated by a doctor (see page 1748). Some young children have particular difficulty controlling their impulses and need their parents to set stricter limits around which there can be some safety and regularity in their world.

At age 18 months to 2 years, children typically begin to establish gender identity (see page 896). During the preschool years, children also acquire a notion of gender role, of what boys and girls typically do. Exploration of the genitals is expected at this age and signals that children are beginning to make a connection between gender and body image.

Between 2 and 3 years of age, children begin to play more interactively with other children. Although they may still be possessive about toys, they may begin to share and even take turns in play. Asserting ownership of toys by saying, "That is mine!" helps establish the sense of self. Although children at this age strive for independence, they still need their parents nearby for security and support. For example, they may walk away from their parents when they feel curious only to later hide behind their parents when they are fearful.

At 3 to 5 years of age, many children become interested in fantasy play and imaginary friends. Fantasy play allows children to safely act out different roles and strong feelings in acceptable ways. Fantasy play also helps children grow socially. They learn to resolve conflicts with parents or other children in ways that help them vent frustrations and maintain self-esteem. Also at this time, typical childhood fears like that of "the monster in the closet" emerge. These fears are normal.

At 7 to 12 years of age, children work through numerous issues: self-concept, the foundation for which is laid by competency in the classroom; relationships with peers, which are determined by the ability to socialize and fit in well; and family relationships, which are determined in part by the approval children gain from parents and siblings. Although many children seem to place a high value on the peer group, they still look primarily to parents for support and guidance. Siblings can serve as role models and as valuable supports and critics in what can and cannot be done. This period of time is very active for children, who engage in many activities and are eager to explore new activities. At this age, children are eager learners and often respond well to advice about safety, healthy lifestyles, and avoidance of high-risk behaviors.

Promoting Optimal Health and Development

Parents can help their children achieve the best possible health. For example, they can help prevent obesity by establishing healthy eating patterns and promoting regular exercise. Children should consume a variety of healthy foods, including fruits and vegetables along with protein. Regular meals and small nutritious snacks encourage healthy eating in even a picky preschooler. Although children may avoid some healthy foods, such as broccoli or beans, for a period of time, it is important to continue to offer healthy foods. In addition, parents should limit intake of fruit juices, which, despite their apparent healthy origin, are mainly sugar water. Some children lose their appetite for food at mealtime if they drink too much fruit juice. Children who drink from a bottle should be weaned by about 1 year of age to prevent excess juice and milk intake and to avoid tooth decay.

Promoting optimal development in a child works best if approached with flexibility, keeping the individual child's age, temperament, developmental stage, and learning style in mind. A coordinated approach involving parents, teachers, and the child usually works best. Throughout these years, children need an environment that promotes lifelong curiosity and learning. The child should be provided with books and music. A routine of daily interactive reading, with parents asking as well as answering questions, helps children pay attention and read with comprehension and encourages their interest in learning activities. Limiting television and electronic games to less than 2 hours per day encourages more interactive play.

Playgroups and preschool have benefits for many young children. Children can learn important social skills, such as sharing. In addition, they may begin to recognize letters, numbers, and colors. Learning these skills makes the transition to school smoother. Importantly, in a structured preschool setting, potential developmental problems can be identified and addressed early.

Parents who are in need of child care may wonder what the best environment is and whether care by others may actually harm their child. Available information suggests that young children can do well both in their own home and in care out of the home, as long as the environment is loving and nurturing. By closely watching the child's response to a given child care setting, parents are better able to choose the best environment. Some children thrive in a child care environment where there are many children, whereas others may fare better in their own home or in a smaller group.

When the child begins to receive homework assignments, parents can help by showing interest in the child's work, by being available to sort through questions but not finishing the work themselves, by providing a quiet work environment at home for the child, and by communicating with the teacher about any concerns. As the school years progress, parents need to consider their child's needs when selecting extracurricular activities. Many children thrive when offered the opportunity to participate in team sports or learn a musical instrument. These activities may also provide a venue for improving social skills. On the other hand, some children become stressed if they are over-scheduled and expected to participate in too many activities. Children need to be encouraged and supported in their extracurricular activities without having unrealistic expectations placed on them.

Preventive Health Care Visits

Scheduled visits to the doctor provide parents with information about their child's growth and development. Such visits also give parents an opportunity to ask questions and seek advice. The American Academy of Pediatrics recommends that after the first year of life children should see their doctor for preventive health care visits at 15, 18, and 24 months of age and then yearly until age 6. It is then recommended that the child visit the doctor at age 8 and again at age 10. Visits can be made more often based on the advice of the doctor or the needs of the family.

A variety of measurements, screening procedures, and vaccinations are performed (see box on page 1685) at each visit. Height and weight are checked, and head circumference is measured until the child is about 18 months old. Good growth is one indicator that the child is generally healthy. The child's actual size is not nearly as important as whether the child stays at or near the same percentile on the height and weight charts at each visit. A child who is always in the 10th percentile is fine (although smaller than most children of the same age), whereas a child who drops from the 35th percentile to the 10th may have a medical problem. Beginning at age 3, blood pressure is measured at each visit.

Preventive visits should include a check of vision and hearing. Some children may need to have their blood checked for anemia or an increased level of lead (see page 2013). The age of the child and various other factors determine which tests are performed. Some doctors also recommend that the child's urine be checked, although the value of such testing has not been established.

The doctor also monitors how the child has progressed developmentally since the last visit. For example, the doctor may want to know whether an 18-month-old child has begun speaking or whether a 6-year-old child has begun reading a few words. In the same way, doctors often ask age-appropriate questions about the child's behavior. Does the 18-month-old child have tantrums? Does the 2-year-old child sleep through the night? Does the 6-year-old child wet the bed at night? Parents and doctors can discuss these types of behavioral and developmental issues during the preventive health care visits and together design approaches to any behavioral or developmental problems.

Child safety is discussed during preventive visits. Specific safety concerns are based on the age of the child. For a 6-month-old child, the doctor may wish to talk about childproofing the house to prevent unintentional poisonings or injury. For a 6-year-old child, the discussion might be focused on bicycle safety. The doctor may also emphasize other safety topics, such as the importance of installing and maintaining smoke alarms and the hazards of keeping guns in the home. Parents should take the opportunity to bring up topics that are most relevant to their unique family situation. As children get older, they can be active participants in these discussions.

Finally, the doctor performs a complete physical examination. In addition to examining the child from head to toe, including the heart, lungs, abdomen, genitals, and head and neck, the doctor may ask the child to perform some age-appropriate tasks. To check gross motor skills (such as walking and running), the doctor may ask a 4-year-old child to hop on one foot. To check fine motor skills (manipulating small objects with the hands), the child may be asked to draw a picture or copy some shapes.

266 Behavioral and Developmental Problems in Young Children

Children acquire many skills as they grow. Some skills, such as controlling urine and stool, depend mainly on the level of maturity of the child's nerves and brain. Others, such as behaving appropriately at home and in school, are the result of a complicated interaction between the child's physical and intellectual (cognitive) development, health, temperament, and relationship with parents, teachers, and caregivers.

Behavioral and developmental problems can become so troublesome that they threaten normal relationships between the child and others. Some behavioral problems, such as bed-wetting, can be mild and resolve quickly. Other behavioral problems, such as those that arise in children with attention-deficit/hyperactivity disorder (ADHD—see page 1849), can require ongoing treatment. Most of the problems described in this chapter arise out of developmentally normal habits that children easily acquire. The goal of treatment is to change undesirable habits by getting children to want to change their behavior. This goal often takes persistent changes in actions by the parents, which in turn result in improved behaviors by the children.

Eating Problems

Some eating problems are behavioral in nature. Parents of young children often are concerned that their children are not eating enough or eating too much, eating the wrong foods, refusing to eat certain foods, or engaging in inappropriate mealtime behavior (such as sneaking food to a pet or throwing or intentionally dropping food). Growth charts can help parents determine whether their children's growth rate is of concern.

Eating disorders (see page 876), such as anorexia nervosa and bulimia nervosa, typically do not occur until adolescence.

Undereating: A decrease in appetite, caused by a slowing growth rate, is common among children around 1 year of age. However, an eating problem may develop if a parent or caregiver tries to coerce the child to eat or shows too much concern about the child's appetite or eating habits. When parents coax and threaten, children with eating problems may refuse to eat the food in their mouth. Some children may even respond to parental attempts at force-feeding by vomiting.

Decreasing the tension and negative emotions surrounding mealtimes may be helpful. Emotional scenes can be avoided by putting food in front of the child and removing it 20 to 30 minutes later without comment. The child should be allowed to choose from whatever food is offered at mealtimes and scheduled snacks in the morning and afternoon. Food and fluids other than water should be restricted at all other times. Young children should be offered 3 meals and 2 to 3 snacks each day. Mealtimes should be scheduled at a time when other family members are eating. Distractions, such as television or pets, should be avoided. Sitting at a table is encouraged. Children should participate in cleaning up any food that is thrown or intentionally dropped on the floor. Using these techniques balances the child's appetite, amount of food eaten, and nutritional needs.

Overeating: Overeating is another problem. Overeating can lead to childhood obesity (see page 1756). Once fat cells form, they do not go away. Thus, obese children are more likely than children of normal weight to be obese as adults. Because childhood obesity can lead to adult obesity (see page 951), it should be prevented or treated.

Bed-Wetting

- The most common cause of bed-wetting is a slowly maturing bladder.
- Limiting fluids 2 to 3 hours before bed and restricting caffeine consumption may help prevent bed-wetting.
- Positive reinforcement, bed-wetting alarms, desmopressin, and imipramine help treat the disorder.

About 30% of children still wet the bed at age 4, 10% at age 6, 3% at age 12, and 1% at age 18. Bed-wetting is more common among boys and seems to run in families.

Bed-wetting is usually caused by slow maturation of the nerves that supply the bladder, so the child does not awaken appropriately when the bladder fills and needs emptying. Bed-wetting can accompany such sleep disorders as sleepwalking and night terrors (see page 1747). A physical disorder—usually a urinary tract infection—is found in only 1 to 2% of children who wet the bed. Other less common disorders, such as diabetes, also can cause bed-wetting. Bed-wetting occasionally is caused by psychologic problems, either in the child or in another family member, and is occasionally part of a constellation of symptoms that suggests the possibility of sexual abuse.

Behavioral Problems Due to Parenting Problems

Praise and reward can reinforce good behavior. Many busy parents give their children attention only for negative behavior, which can backfire when that is the only attention the children receive. Because most children prefer attention for inappropriate behavior to no attention at all, parents should create special times each day for pleasant interactions with their children.

A number of relatively minor problems of behavior may be due to parenting problems.

Child-parent interaction problems are difficulties in the relationship between children and their parents, which may begin during the first few months of life. The relationship may be strained because of a difficult pregnancy or delivery; because the mother has depression since the delivery or receives inadequate support from the father, relatives, or friends; or because the parents are disinterested. Contributing to the strain are a baby's unpredictable feeding and sleeping schedules. Most babies do not sleep through the night until 3 to 4 months of age. Poor relationships may slow development of mental and social skills and cause failure to thrive.

A doctor or nurse can discuss the temperament of an individual baby and offer the parents information on the development of babies and helpful tips for coping. The parents may then be able to develop more realistic expectations, accept their feelings of guilt and conflict as normal, and try to rebuild a healthy relationship. If the relationship is not repaired, the baby may continue to have problems later.

Unrealistic expectations contribute to the perception of behavioral problems. For example, parents who expect a 2-year-old child to pick up toys without help may mistakenly feel there is a behavioral problem. Parents may misinterpret other normal, age-related behaviors of a 2-year-old child, such as the refusal to follow an adult's request or rule.

A vicious circle pattern is a cycle of negative (inappropriate) behavior by the child that causes a negative (angry) response from the parent or caregiver, followed by further negative behavior by the child, leading to a further negative response from the parent. Vicious circles usually begin when a child is aggressive and resistant. The parents or caregivers respond by scolding, yelling, and spanking. Vicious circles also may result when parents react to a fearful, clinging, or manipulative child with overprotection and overpermissiveness.

The vicious circle pattern may be broken if parents learn to ignore inappropriate behavior that does not negatively affect others, such as temper tantrums or refusals to eat. Redirecting the child's attention to interesting activities allows for the rewarding of good behavior, which makes the child and parents feel successful. For behavior that cannot be ignored, distraction or a time-out procedure can be tried.

Discipline is more than just punishment. It is providing children with clear, structured, age-appropriate expectations that allow them to know what is expected. Discipline problems are inappropriate behaviors that develop when structure is ineffective. It is much easier and more satisfying to both parents and children to reward desirable behavior than to punish inappropriate behavior.

Efforts to control a child's behavior through scolding or physical punishments such as spanking may work briefly if used sparingly. However, these approaches generally tend not to alter the inappropriate behavior sufficiently and may reduce the child's sense of security and self-esteem. Moreover, spanking can get out of hand when the parent is angry. A time-out procedure can be helpful (see box on page 1749). However, punishments become ineffective when overused. Furthermore, threats that the parents will leave or send the child away can be psychologically damaging.

Sometimes bed-wetting stops and then begins again. The relapse usually follows a psychologically stressful event or condition, but a physical cause, especially a urinary tract infection, may be responsible.

Treatment

Parents and the child need to know that bed-wetting is quite common, that it can be corrected, and that nobody should feel guilty about it. An older child who wets the bed can take responsibility by

- Talking to a doctor
- Limiting fluids after dinner (especially caffeinated beverages)
- Urinating before going to bed
- Recording wet and dry nights
- Changing clothing and bedding when wet

Parents may choose to give the child age-appropriate rewards (positive reinforcement) for dry nights.

For children younger than 6, parents can avoid giving the child fluids 2 to 3 hours before bedtime and encourage the child to urinate just before going to bed. Caffeinated beverages should be strictly limited. In most children of this age, time and physical maturation solve the problem.

For children older than 6 to 7 years, some form of treatment is often indicated. Bed-wetting alarms, which awaken a child when a few drops of urine are detected, are the most effective treatment available. They can cure bed-wetting in about 70% of children, and only about 10 to 15% of children start wetting the bed again after the alarms are stopped. Alarms are relatively inexpensive and are easy to set up. In the first few weeks of use, the child awakens only after fully urinating. In the next few weeks, the child awakens after urinating a small amount and may wet the bed less often. Eventually, the need to urinate wakes the child before the bed is wet. Most parents find that the alarm can be removed after a 3-week dry period.

If bed-wetting persists in an older child after alarms and age-appropriate rewards have been tried, the doctor may prescribe drugs. An increasingly popular drug for bed-wetting is desmopressin in tablet form or, rarely, nasal spray form. This drug reduces the output of urine, which reduces bed-wetting. The drug is used for a 1- to 2-month period and then is stopped as soon as possible. It can be used intermittently, such as when the child goes to camp. Imipramine is an antidepressant drug used infrequently to treat bed-wetting because it relaxes the bladder and tightens the sphincter that blocks urine flow. It has become less popular in recent years because of side effects. To monitor side effects, doctors do an electrocardiogram before imipramine therapy is started and do blood tests periodically.

Encopresis

Encopresis is the accidental passing of bowel movements that is not caused by illness or physical abnormality.

Encopresis occurs in about 3% of 4-year-old children and becomes less common as age increases. It occurs most often in conjunction with toilet teaching or starting school. As children struggle to establish control of stooling, they sometimes block the urge to defecate too much, resulting in retention of stool. This retention leads to chronic constipation, which stretches the bowel wall and reduces the child's awareness of a full bowel, impairing muscle control. Stool leakage occurs when hard, dry stool is pushed out or when wet stool oozes around the impacted stool.

> 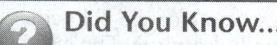 **Did You Know...**
>
> Accidental passage of bowel movements can be caused by constipation.

A doctor first tries to determine the cause. If the cause is constipation, a laxative is prescribed and other measures (such as changes to the child's toileting regimen, diet, environment, and behavior) are instituted to ensure regular bowel movements. Once regular bowel movements are achieved, the leakage often stops. Maintaining soft stools for several months can be necessary for the stretched bowel wall to return to normal and for awareness of rectal fullness to return. If these measures fail, diagnostic tests may be done, such as abdominal x-rays and

rarely a biopsy of the rectal wall, in which a tissue sample is taken and examined under a microscope. If a physical cause is found, it often can be treated. In the most severe cases, psychologic counseling may be needed for children whose encopresis is the result of emotional or behavioral problems.

Sleep Problems

Most children sleep for a stretch of at least 5 hours by age 3 months but then experience periods of night waking later in the first years of life, often associated with illness. As they get older, the amount of rapid eye movement (REM) sleep increases. Families vary in their attitudes about children sleeping with parents and other sleep habits. It is important that parents be open with each other about their preferences to avoid stress and mixed messages to their children.

For most children, sleep problems are intermittent or temporary and often do not need treatment.

Nightmares

Nightmares are frightening dreams that occur during REM sleep. Children having a nightmare can awaken fully and can vividly recall the details of the dream. Nightmares are not a cause for alarm, unless they occur very often. They can occur more often during times of stress, or even when children have seen a movie or television program containing frightening or aggressive content. If nightmares occur often, parents can keep a diary to see whether they can identify the cause.

Night Terrors and Sleepwalking

Night terrors are episodes of incomplete awakening with extreme anxiety shortly after falling asleep. They occur in non-REM sleep and are most common between the ages of 3 and 8. The child screams and appears frightened, with a rapid heart rate and rapid breathing. The child seems to be unaware of the parents' presence, may thrash around violently and does not respond to comforting, and may talk but be unable to answer questions. Usually, the child returns to sleep after a few minutes. Unlike with nightmares, the child cannot recall these episodes. Night terrors are dramatic because the child screams and is inconsolable during the episode. About one third of children with night terrors also experience sleepwalking (rising from bed and walking around while apparently asleep, also called somnambulism). About 15% of children between the ages of 5 and 12 have at least one episode of sleepwalking.

Night terrors and sleepwalking (see also page 676) almost always stop without treatment, although occasional episodes may occur for years. Usually, no treatment is needed, but if a disorder persists into adolescence or adulthood and is severe, treatment may be necessary. In children who need treatment, night terrors may sometimes respond to a sedative or certain antidepressants; however, these drugs are potent and can have side effects.

Resistance to Going to Bed

Children, particularly between the ages of 1 and 2, often resist going to bed due to separation anxiety (see page 1734), whereas older children may be attempting to control more aspects of their environment. Young children often cry when left alone in their crib, or they climb out and seek their parents. Another common cause of bedtime resistance is delayed sleep start time. These situations arise when children are allowed to stay up later and sleep later than usual for enough nights to reset their internal clock to a later sleep start time. It can be difficult to move bedtime earlier, but brief treatment with an over-the-counter antihistamine or melatonin can help children reset their clock.

Resistance to going to bed is not helped if parents stay in the room at length to provide comfort or let children get out of bed. In fact, these responses reinforce night waking, in which children attempt to reproduce the conditions under which they fell asleep. To avoid these problems, a parent may have to sit quietly in the hallway in sight of the child and make sure the child stays in bed. The child then establishes a sleep-onset routine of falling asleep alone and learns that getting out of bed is discouraged. The child also learns that the parents are available but will not provide more stories or play. Eventually, the child settles down and goes to sleep. Providing the child with an attachment object (like a teddy bear) is often helpful. A small night light, white noise, or both also can be comforting.

Awakening During the Night

Everyone awakens multiple times each night. Most, however, usually fall back to sleep on their own. Children often experience repeated night awakening after a move, an illness, or another stressful event. Sleeping problems may be worsened when children take long naps late in the afternoon or are overstimulated by playing before bedtime. Sleep sometimes is disrupted by restless leg syndrome (see page 674), and a few children, particularly those who thrash and snore, may have obstructive sleep apnea (see page 485).

Allowing the child to sleep with the parents because of the night awakening reinforces the behavior. Playing with or feeding the child during the night, spanking, and scolding also are counterproductive measures. Returning the child to bed with simple reassurance is usually more effective. A

bedtime routine that includes reading a brief story, offering a favorite doll or blanket, and using a small night-light (for children who are older than 3) is often helpful. To decrease the likelihood of the child awakening, it is important that the conditions under which the child awakens during the night are the same as those under which the child falls asleep. Parents and other caregivers should try to keep to a routine each night, so that the child learns what is expected. If children are physically healthy, allowing them to cry for a few minutes often allows them to settle down by themselves, which will diminish the night awakening.

Temper Tantrums

- Frustration, tiredness, and hunger are the most common causes.
- Children may scream, cry, thrash, and stomp their feet during a tantrum.
- If distraction does not stop the tantrum, the child may have to be removed from the situation.

Temper tantrums are common in childhood. They usually appear toward the end of the first year, are most common between ages 2 and 4, and are typically infrequent after age 5. If tantrums are frequent after age 5, they may persist throughout childhood.

Causes include frustration, tiredness, and hunger. Children also may have temper tantrums to seek attention, obtain something, or avoid doing something. Parents often place the blame on themselves (because of imagined poor parenting) when the real cause is often a combination of the child's personality, immediate circumstances, and developmentally normal behavior. An underlying mental, physical, or social problem may rarely be the cause and is more likely if a tantrum lasts for more than 15 minutes or if tantrums occur multiple times each day.

A child who is having a temper tantrum may shout, scream, cry, thrash about, roll on the floor, stomp, and throw things. Some of the behavior may be rage-like and potentially harmful. The child may become red in the face and hit or kick. Some children may voluntarily hold their breath for a few seconds and then resume normal breathing (unlike breath-holding spells, which also can occur after crying bouts caused by frustration—see page 1749).

Although providing a safe setting for children to compose themselves in (a time-out) is often effective, many children have difficulty stopping tantrums on their own. In most cases, addressing the source of the tantrum only prolongs it. It is therefore preferable to redirect and distract children by providing an alternative activity on which to focus. The child may benefit from being removed physically from the situation.

The Time-Out Technique

This disciplinary technique is best used when children are aware that their actions are incorrect or unacceptable and when they see withholding of attention as a punishment. Typically, children do not understand that withholding attention is a punishment linked to undesirable behavior until they are 2 years old. Care should be taken when this technique is used in group settings such as day care centers, because it can result in harmful humiliation.

The technique can be applied when a child misbehaves in a way that is known to result in a time-out. Usually, the child should receive verbal statements and reminders before the time-out technique is used.

- The inappropriate behavior is explained to the child, who is told to sit in the time-out chair or is led there if necessary.
- The child should sit in the chair for 1 minute for each year of age (a maximum of 5 minutes).
- A child who gets up from the chair before the allotted time is returned to the chair, and the time-out is restarted. Talking and eye contact are avoided.
- When it is time for the child to get up, the caregiver asks the reason for the time-out without anger and nagging. A child who does not recall the correct reason is briefly reminded. The child does not need to express remorse for the inappropriate behavior as long as it is clear that the child understands the reason for the time-out.

As soon as possible after the time-out, the caregiver should make an effort to identify good behavior and praise the child for it. Good behavior may be easier to achieve if the child is redirected to a new activity far from the scene of the inappropriate behavior.

Breath-Holding Spells

A breath-holding spell is an episode in which the child stops breathing and loses consciousness for a short period immediately after a frightening or emotionally upsetting event or a painful experience.

- Breath-holding spells usually are triggered by physically painful or emotionally upsetting events.
- Typical symptoms include paleness, stoppage of breathing, loss of consciousness, and seizures.
- Tantrums may be prevented by distracting the child and avoiding situations that trigger the spells.

Breath-holding spells occur in 5% of otherwise healthy children. They usually begin in the first year of life and peak at age 2. They disappear by age 4 in 50%

of children and by age 8 in about 83% of children. Breath-holding spells can take one of two forms.

The **cyanotic form** of breath-holding, which is most common, is initiated subconsciously by young children often as a component of a temper tantrum or in response to a scolding or other upsetting event. Episodes peak at about 2 years and are rare after 5 years. Typically, the child cries out (without necessarily being aware they are doing so), breathes out, and then stops breathing. Shortly afterward, the skin begins to turn blue, and the child becomes unconscious. A brief seizure may occur. After a few seconds, breathing resumes and normal skin color and consciousness return. It may be possible to interrupt the episode by placing a cold rag on the child's face when the spell begins. Despite the frightening nature of the episode, the parents must try to avoid reinforcing the initiating behavior. Parents should not avoid providing appropriate structure for children out of fear of causing spells. Distracting children and avoiding situations that lead to tantrums are the best ways of preventing and treating these spells. Cyanotic breath-holding spells respond to treatment with iron supplements, even when the child does not have iron-deficiency anemia, and to treatment for obstructive sleep apnea.

The **pallid form** typically follows a painful experience, such as falling and banging the head or being suddenly startled. The brain sends out a signal (via the vagus nerve) that severely slows the heart rate, causing loss of consciousness. Thus, in this form, the loss of consciousness and stoppage of breathing (which are both temporary) result from a nerve response to being startled that leads to slowing of the heart.

The child stops breathing, rapidly loses consciousness, and becomes pale and limp. A seizure and incontinence may occur. The heart typically beats very slowly during a spell. After the spell, the heart speeds up again, breathing restarts, and consciousness returns without any treatment. Because this form is rare, further diagnostic evaluation and treatment may be needed if the spells occur often.

School Avoidance

- Some psychologic and social factors may cause school avoidance.
- Children may fake illnesses and make up excuses to avoid going to school.
- Regular attendance at school; open communication among the child, parents, and school personnel; and sometimes psychologic therapy are ways to treat school avoidance.

School avoidance occurs in about 5% of all school-aged children and affects girls and boys equally. It usually occurs between ages 5 and 6 and between ages 10 and 11.

What Are Stress-Related Behaviors?

Each child handles stress differently. Certain behaviors that help children deal with stress include thumb sucking, nail biting, and, sometimes, head banging.

Thumb sucking (or sucking a pacifier) is a normal part of early childhood, and most children stop by the time they are 1 or 2 years old, but some continue into their school-age years. Occasional thumb sucking is normal at times of stress, but habitual sucking past the age of about 5 can alter the shape of the roof of the mouth, cause misalignment of teeth, and lead to teasing from other children. Occasionally, persistent thumb sucking can be the sign of an underlying emotional disorder.

All children eventually stop thumb sucking. Parents should intervene only if their child's dentist advises them to or if they feel their child's thumb sucking is socially unhealthy. Parents need to gently encourage the child to understand why it would be good to stop. Once the child signals a willingness to stop, gentle verbal reminders are a good start. These can be followed by symbolic rewards put directly on the thumb, such as a colored bandage, fingernail polish, or a star drawn with a nontoxic colored marker. Additional measures, such as a plastic guard over the thumb, overnight elbow splinting to prevent a child from bending it, or painting the thumbnail with a bitter substance can be used. However, none of these measures should be used against the child's will.

Nail biting is a common problem among young children. The habit usually disappears as the child gets older but is typically related to stress and anxiety. Children who are motivated to stop can be taught to substitute other habits (for example, twirling a pencil). A reward system in which the child keeps more rewards for avoiding the behavior reinforces desirable behavior. For instance, the child is given 10 pennies in the morning, and in the evening must return 1 penny for each nail that is bitten over the course of the day.

Head banging and **rhythmic rocking** are common among healthy toddlers. Although alarming to parents, the children do not seem to be in distress and actually seem to derive comfort from the activity.

Children usually outgrow rocking, rolling, and head banging between 18 months and 2 years of age, but repetitive actions sometimes still occur in older children and adolescents.

Children with autism and certain other developmental problems also may bang their head. However, these children have additional symptoms that make their diagnosis apparent.

Although children almost never damage themselves by these behaviors, this possibility (and the noise) can be reduced by pulling the crib away from the wall, taking off the wheels or placing carpet protectors under them, and applying a padded crib bumper to the inside of the crib.

The cause is often unclear, but psychologic factors (such as anxiety and depression) and social factors (such as having no friends, feeling rejected by peers, or being bullied) may contribute. Sensitive children may be overreacting with fear to a teacher's strictness or rebukes. Younger children tend to fake illness or make other excuses to avoid school. Children may complain of a stomachache, nausea, or other symptoms that justify staying home. Some children directly refuse to go to school. Alternatively, children may go to school without difficulty but become anxious or develop various symptoms during the school day, often going regularly to the nurse's office. This behavior is unlike that of adolescents, who may decide not to attend school (called truancy or "playing hooky"—see page 1757).

School avoidance tends to result in

- Poor academic performance
- Family difficulties
- Difficulties with peers

Most children recover from school avoidance, although some develop it again after a real illness or a vacation.

Home tutoring generally is not a solution. Children with school avoidance should return to school immediately, so that they do not fall behind in their schoolwork. If school avoidance is so intense that it interferes with the child's activity and if the child does not respond to simple reassurance by parents or teachers, referral to a mental health practitioner may be warranted.

Treatment should include communication between parents and school personnel, regular attendance at school, and sometimes therapy involving the family and child with a psychologist. Therapy includes treatment of underlying disorders as well as behavioral techniques to cope with the stresses at school.

CHAPTER
267 Adolescents

During adolescence (usually encompassing ages 10 to the late teens or early 20s), children become young adults. They mature socially and physically. Notably, they become sexually mature and socially independent. During this time, the adolescent develops a sense of who he or she is and learns to form intimate relationships with people who are not members of the family. Guiding adolescents through this intricate period of development can be a challenge for parents. Risk-taking (such as engaging in violence and binge drinking) is common among adolescents and causes acute health risks. Unhealthy behaviors such as smoking or drug use, which cause serious problems later in life, also typically begin in adolescence.

Physical and Sexual Development

Normal growth during adolescence includes both an increase in body size and sexual maturation (puberty). The timing and speed with which these changes occur vary and are affected by both heredity and environment. During adolescence, boys and girls reach adult height and weight. The growth spurt in boys occurs during mid-adolescence between the ages of 12 and 17 years. Boys grow about 4 inches (about 10 centimeters) during their year of maximum growth. The growth spurt in girls occurs in early adolescence between the ages of 9½ and 14½ years. Girls grow about 3½ inches (about 9 centimeters) during their year of maximum growth. In general, boys become heavier and taller than girls. By age 18, boys have about ¾ inch (about 2 centimeters) of growth remaining and girls have slightly less.

Puberty also occurs during adolescence. In boys, the first signs of puberty are enlargement of the scrotum and testes, followed by lengthening of the penis. Internally, the seminal vesicles and prostate gland enlarge. Next, pubic hair appears. Hair grows on the face and in the underarms about 2 years after it appears in the pubic area. Ejaculation may begin in mid-adolescence (around age 12½ to 14 years), about 1 year after the penis begins to lengthen. Fertility, however, is not attained until later in adolescence. Breast enlargement (gynecomastia) on one side or both is common among young adolescent boys and usually disappears within a year.

In the majority of girls, the first visible sign of puberty is breast budding, although in many girls the growth spurt can occur up to a year before. Soon after breast budding, pubic and underarm hair appears. The first menstrual period (menarche) occurs within a wide range (typically between ages 10 and 16 years), with most girls in the United States starting their periods at 12 or 13 years. Timing is influenced by genetics, ethnicity, nutrition, and other factors. Puberty begins earlier today than it did a century ago. For example, the average age of the first menstrual period (menarche) has decreased by about 3 years over the past 100 years. The reasons probably include improvements in nutrition, general health, and living conditions.

Even during normal adolescence, substantial emotional adjustments are required. If the timing is not typical, particularly in a boy whose physical development is delayed or a girl whose development occurs early, additional emotional stress is likely. Most boys who grow slowly eventually attain normal height. However, adolescents whose growth or sexual development is delayed should be evaluated to rule out diseases and other physical causes and given reassurance if the evaluation is negative.

Intellectual and Behavioral Development

In early adolescence, a child begins to develop the capacity for abstract, logical thought. This increased sophistication leads to an enhanced awareness of self and the ability to reflect on one's own being. Because of the many noticeable physical changes of adolescence, this self-awareness often turns into self-consciousness, with an accompanying feeling of awkwardness. The adolescent also has a preoccupation with physical appearance and attractiveness and a heightened sensitivity to differences from peers.

In mid adolescence, the weight of making decisions about a future career gets increasingly heavy, and most adolescents do not have a clearly defined goal, although they gradually realize their areas of interest and talent. Parents must be aware of the adolescent's capabilities and help the adolescent set realistic goals. Parents also must be prepared to identify roadblocks to learning, such as learning disabilities, attention problems, or inappropriate learning environments, which need to be corrected.

Adolescents also apply their new reflective capabilities to moral issues. Pre-adolescents understand right and wrong as fixed and absolute. Older adolescents often question standards of behavior and may reject traditions—to the consternation of parents. Ideally, this reflection culminates in the development and internalization of the adolescent's own moral code.

Milestones in Sexual Development

During puberty, sexual development occurs in a set sequence. However, when the changes begin and how quickly they occur vary from person to person. For girls, puberty begins at age 8½ to 10 years and lasts about 4 years. For boys, puberty begins at age 9½ to 10½ years and lasts about 3 years. The chart shows a typical sequence and normal range of development for the milestones of sexual development.

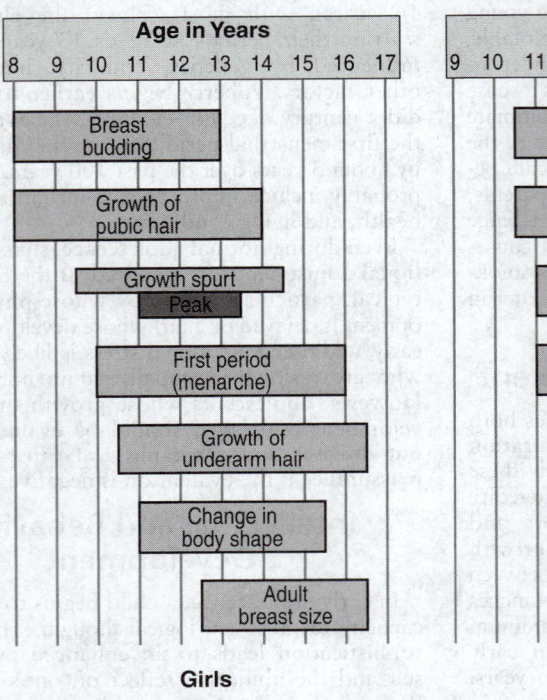

Girls

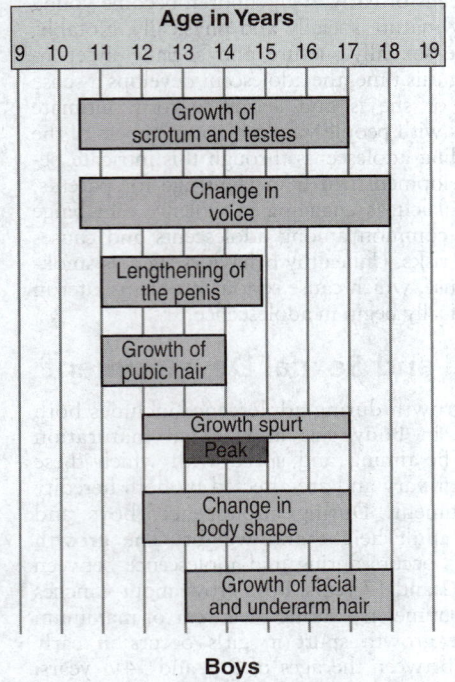

Boys

Many adolescents begin to engage in risky behaviors, such as fast driving. Many adolescents begin to experiment sexually, and some may engage in risky sexual practices. Some adolescents may engage in illegal activities, such as theft and alcohol and drug use. Experts speculate that these behaviors occur in part because adolescents tend to overestimate their own abilities in preparation for leaving their home. Recent studies of the nervous system also have shown that the parts of the brain that suppress impulses are not fully mature until early adulthood.

Emotional Development

During adolescence, the regions of the brain that control emotions develop and mature. This phase is characterized by seemingly spontaneous outbursts that can be challenging for parents and teachers who often receive the brunt. Adolescents gradually learn to sup-press inappropriate thoughts and actions and replace them with goal-oriented behaviors.

A typical area of conflict is the adolescent's normal desire to seek more freedom, which clashes with the parents' instincts to protect their children from harm. Frustration caused by trying to grow in many directions is common. Communication can be challenging as parents and adolescents renegotiate their relationship. All of these challenges are accentuated when families face other stresses or parents have emotional difficulties of their own because adolescents continue to need parenting. Doctors can help open lines of communication by offering adolescents and parents sensible, practical, supportive advice.

Social and Psychologic Development

The family is the center of social life for children. During adolescence, the peer group begins to replace the family as the child's primary social focus. Peer groups are often established because of distinctions in dress, appearance, attitudes, hobbies, interests, and other characteristics that may seem profound or trivial to outsiders. Initially, peer groups are usually same-sex but typically become mixed later in adolescence. These groups assume an importance to adolescents because they provide validation for the adolescent's tentative choices and support in stressful situations.

Adolescents who find themselves without a peer group may develop intense feelings of being different and alienated. Although these feelings usually do not have permanent effects, they may worsen the potential for dysfunctional or antisocial behavior. At the other extreme, the peer group can assume too much importance, also resulting in antisocial behavior. Gang membership is more common when the home and social environments are unable to counterbalance the dysfunctional demands of a peer group (see box on page 1758).

Doctors should screen all adolescents for mental health disorders, such as depression, bipolar disorder, and anxiety. Mental health disorders increase in incidence during this stage of life and may result in suicidal thinking or behavior. Psychotic disorders, such as schizophrenia, although rare, most often come to attention during late adolescence. Eating disorders, such as anorexia nervosa and bulimia nervosa (see page 876), are relatively common among girls and may be difficult to detect because adolescents go to great lengths to hide the behaviors and weight changes.

Substance use typically begins during adolescence. More than 70% of adolescents in the United States try alcohol before they graduate high school. Binge drinking is common and leads to both acute and chronic health risks. Research has shown that adolescents who start drinking alcohol at a young age are more likely to develop an alcohol use disorder as an adult. For example, adolescents who start drinking at age 13 are 5 times more likely to develop an alcohol use disorder than those who start drinking at age 21. Almost 50% of U.S. adolescents try cigarettes and more than 40% try marijuana while they are in high school. Use of other drugs is much less common, although misuse of prescription drugs, including drugs for pain and stimulants, is on the rise.

Parents can have a strong positive influence on their children by setting a good example (such as using alcohol in moderation and avoiding use of illicit drugs), sharing their values, and setting high expectations regarding staying away from drugs. Parents also should teach children that prescription drugs should be used only as directed by a doctor.

All adolescents should be confidentially screened for substance use. Appropriate advice should be given as part of routine health care because even very brief interventions by doctors and health care practitioners have been shown to decrease substance use by adolescents.

Development of Sexuality

The onset of sexual maturation (puberty) typically is accompanied by an interest in sexual anatomy, which may be a source of anxiety. As adolescents mature emotionally and sexually, they may begin to engage in sexual behaviors. Masturbation is common among girls and nearly universal among boys. Sexual experimentation with a partner often begins as touching or petting and may progress to oral, vaginal, or anal sex. By late adolescence, sexuality shifts from experimentation to being an expression of intimacy and sharing. Doctors should provide appropriate advice on safe-sex practices as part of routine health care and should screen all sexually active adolescents for sexually transmitted diseases.

Few elements of the human experience combine physical, intellectual, and emotional aspects as thoroughly as sexuality. Helping adolescents put sexuality into a healthy context, including issues of morality and the formation of a family, is extremely important. Parents should share their values and expectations openly with their adolescent children.

Some adolescents struggle with the issue of sexual identity. Many of those who explore homosexual relationships ultimately do not continue to be interested in same-sex relationships, whereas others never develop interest in opposite-sex relationships. Homosexuality is a normal variation of human sexuality and not a disorder (see page 896). Although it is not understood exactly why homosexual feelings develop, experts do not think homosexuality is something adolescents learn from their peers or the media or something they choose the same way they select an after-school activity or a career path.

Homosexual adolescents may face unique challenges as their sexuality develops. Adolescents may feel unwanted or unaccepted by family or peers if they express homosexual desires. Such pressure (especially during a time when social acceptance is critically important) can cause severe stress. Fear of abandonment by parents, sometimes real, may lead to dishonest or at least incomplete communication between adolescents and their parents. These adolescents also can be taunted and bullied by their peers. Threats of physical violence should be taken seriously and reported to school officials. The emotional development of homosexual and heterosexual adolescents is best helped by supportive friends and family members.

Preventive Health Care Visits

Annual health care visits allow doctors and other health care practitioners to monitor physical growth and sexual maturation and provide advice and counseling. Height, weight, and blood pressure should be monitored at every yearly health care visit. Overweight and obesity are common in the United States and are associated with heart disease and type 2 diabetes (formerly called non–insulin-dependent diabetes). Examination of the skin for acne, evaluation of the degree of sexual maturation, and examination of the back for scoliosis are particularly important in adolescence.

Routine health care also includes a review of the immunization record and administration of recommended vaccines (see box on page 1685). Screening tests, such as a blood cholesterol level test for obese adolescents or those with a family history of high cholesterol, also may be done. Tuberculosis testing may be done for adolescents with a history of exposure or for those who have traveled to areas of the world where tuberculosis is prevalent.

Most of a routine health care visit involves a psychosocial screening interview and counseling. The screening interview includes questions regarding the home environment, academic achievement and goals, activities and hobbies, engagement in risk-taking behaviors, and emotional health. Counseling revolves usually around physical and psychosocial development, healthy lifestyles, and injury prevention. Counseling typically includes wide-ranging topics such as

- The importance of wearing seatbelts
- The dangers of drinking and driving
- The danger of becoming drug or alcohol dependent
- Responsible sexual behavior
- Violence prevention

Doctors also may encourage activities such as participation in sports, the arts, and community service. Most doctors interview and examine adolescents privately, although parents may be invited to participate and share concerns and receive their own counseling and guidance at the beginning or end of the visit.

CHAPTER

268 Problems in Adolescents

The most common problems in adolescents relate to growth and development; childhood illnesses that continue into adolescence; mental health disorders; and the consequences of risky or illegal behaviors, including injury, legal consequences, pregnancy, and infectious diseases. Unintentional injuries resulting from motor vehicle crashes and injuries resulting from interpersonal violence are leading causes of death and disability among adolescents.

Mental health problems, such as mood disorders and schizophrenia (see page 1862), may develop or first become apparent during adolescence, leading to a risk of suicide. Eating disorders, such as anorexia nervosa and bulimia nervosa (see page 876), are particularly common among adolescent girls.

Delayed Puberty

Delayed puberty is defined as absence of the onset of sexual maturation at the expected time.

- Some causes of delayed puberty include disorders, radiation therapy or chemotherapy, excessive dieting or exercise, genetic disorders, tumors, and certain infections.

- Typical symptoms include a lack of testicular enlargement and pubic hair in boys and a lack of breasts and menstrual periods in girls.
- The diagnosis is based on the results of a physical, various laboratory tests, a bone scan, and, if needed, a chromosomal analysis and imaging studies.
- Treatment depends on the cause and may include hormone replacement therapy and, if needed, surgery.

The onset of sexual maturation (puberty) takes place when the hypothalamus gland begins to secrete a chemical signal called gonadotropin-releasing hormone. The pituitary gland responds to this signal by releasing hormones called gonadotropins, which stimulate the growth of the sex organs (the testes in boys and the ovaries in girls). The growing sex organs secrete the sex hormones testosterone in boys and estrogen in girls. These hormones cause the development of secondary sex characteristics, including facial hair and muscle mass in boys, breasts in girls, and pubic and underarm hair and sexual desire (libido) in both sexes.

Some adolescents do not start their sexual development at the usual age. In the majority of cases, the delay represents a normal variation, which may run

When Puberty Starts Too Early

Precocious puberty and pseudoprecocious puberty are sexual maturation that begins before age 9 in a boy or before age 7 or 8 in a girl.

True precocious puberty is caused by the early release of certain sex hormones (gonadotropins) from the pituitary gland. These hormones cause the ovaries or testes to develop and begin secreting other sex hormones, such as estrogen or testosterone, which trigger puberty. This early hormone release may be caused by a tumor or other abnormality in the pituitary gland or the hypothalamus (the region of the brain that controls the pituitary gland). Neurofibromatosis (a disorder where many fleshy growths of nerve tissue grow under the skin and in other parts of the body) and a few other rare disorders also have been linked to precocious puberty.

In **pseudoprecocious puberty**, high levels of testosterone or estrogen are produced by a tumor or other abnormality in the adrenal gland or in a testis or ovary. These hormones do not cause the testes or ovaries themselves to mature but do trigger secondary sex characteristics to develop, including pubic and underarm hair, adult body odor, acne, and changes in body shape. Boys develop facial hair, their penis lengthens, and they take on a masculine appearance. Girls develop breasts and may begin to menstruate, particularly in true precocious puberty. In both sexes, the growth spurt may be triggered, leading to a rapid height increase. This rapid height increase ends early, ultimately leaving these adolescents shorter as adults than would be expected.

In true precocious puberty, the sex glands (ovaries or testes) also mature and enlarge, whereas in pseudoprecocious puberty, the sex glands remain immature. Precocious puberty is 10 times more common among and much more likely to be of unknown cause (idiopathic) among girls.

Evaluation: Whenever a child has signs of premature, rapidly progressing, or disordered puberty, doctors take an x-ray of the hand and wrist to estimate bone maturity. If a child's bone age is very advanced, a more complete evaluation usually is indicated. Tests may include blood hormone levels to determine a cause, an ultrasound of the pelvis and adrenal glands to check for ovarian or adrenal tumors, and computed tomography or magnetic resonance imaging of the head to check for tumors of the hypothalamus or pituitary gland.

Treatment: Treatment is not needed for children who have only premature pubic and underarm hair growth or breast development, but regular reexamination is needed to check for later development of precocious puberty.

Treating an identifiable cause of precocious puberty, such as removing a tumor or cyst, may stop the progression of puberty. When no treatable cause is identified, drugs may slow the progression of puberty. Injections of a synthetic gonadotropin-releasing hormone (such as leuprolide acetate, deslorelin, or histrelin) may stop true precocious puberty by stopping the production of sex hormones. Pseudoprecocious puberty can be stopped by drugs that inhibit the action of the sex hormones.

in the family. These adolescents have a normal growth rate and are otherwise healthy. Although the growth spurt and puberty are delayed, they eventually proceed normally.

Various disorders, such as diabetes mellitus, inflammatory bowel disease, kidney disease, cystic fibrosis, and anemia, can delay or prevent sexual development. Development may be delayed in adolescents receiving radiation therapy or cancer chemotherapy. Adolescents, particularly girls, who become very thin because of excessive exercise or dieting often have delayed puberty, including an absence of menstruation.

There are many uncommon causes of delayed puberty. Chromosomal abnormalities, such as Turner's syndrome in girls (see page 1728) and Klinefelter's syndrome in boys (see page 1729), and other genetic disorders can affect production of hormones. A tumor that damages the pituitary gland or the hypothalamus can lower the levels of gonadotropins or stop production of the hormones altogether. A mumps infection can damage the testes and prevent puberty.

Symptoms

Delayed puberty is more common among boys and is defined as lack of testicular enlargement by age 14, lack of pubic hair by age 15, or a time lapse of more than 5 years from the start to the completion of genital enlargement. In girls, delayed puberty is defined as absence of breast development by age 13, a time lapse of more than 5 years from the beginning of breast growth to the first menstrual period, or failure to menstruate by age 16.

Although adolescents are typically uncomfortable about being different from their peers, boys in particular are likely to feel psychologic stress and embarrassment from delayed puberty. Girls who remain smaller and less sexually mature than their peers are not stigmatized as quickly as are boys.

Diagnosis

The initial evaluation of delayed puberty should consist of a complete history and physical, basic laboratory tests to look for signs of chronic disease, and hormone level tests. A bone age test also may be helpful. Boys under the age of 16 and girls under the age of 14 with delayed puberty who are otherwise healthy most likely have a normal or constitutional delay. For these adolescents, the doctor may elect to reassess at 6-month intervals to ensure that puberty begins and progresses normally. Sometimes a chromosomal analysis may be performed. Girls with severely delayed puberty should be evaluated for primary amenorrhea (see page 1524). Computed tomography (CT) or magnetic resonance imaging (MRI) may be performed to ensure that there is no brain tumor.

Treatment

The treatment for delayed puberty depends on its cause. An adolescent who is naturally late in developing needs no treatment, although if the adolescent is severely stressed by the lack of development or development is extremely delayed, some doctors may give supplemental sex hormones to begin the process sooner. If boys show no sign of puberty or bone maturation by age 15, they may be given a 4- to 8-month course of testosterone. At low doses, testosterone induces puberty, causes the development of some masculine characteristics (virilization), and does not jeopardize adult height potential. When an underlying disorder is the cause of delayed puberty, puberty usually proceeds once the disorder has been treated. Genetic disorders cannot be cured, although replacing hormones may help sex characteristics develop. Surgery may be needed for adolescents with tumors.

Short Stature

Short stature is defined as height below the 3rd percentile for the child's age (according to standard charts for age and height).

Most adolescents have short stature because their families are short, or because their growth spurt comes at the late end of the normal range of time for such development. However, some adolescents are short because of certain chronic illnesses or genetic and endocrine disorders. Such disorders include bone abnormalities and chronic illnesses that affect the heart, lungs, kidneys, or intestines.

The pituitary gland regulates the amount of growth hormone produced. If the pituitary gland does not produce enough growth hormone, abnormally slow growth and short stature with normal proportions (called hypopituitarism or pituitary dwarfism) can result. Hypopituitarism caused by a tumor can be treated surgically. Other causes of hypopituitarism are treated with growth hormone. Growth hormone also may be used to increase height in children who have short stature but normally functioning pituitary

glands, but this use is controversial. Some parents feel that short stature is a disorder, but most doctors do not approve of the use of growth hormone in these children. Regardless of the cause of short stature, pituitary hormone is effective only if given before the growth plates in the long bones become inactive. X-rays can help determine whether the growth plates are inactive.

Obesity

Obesity is defined as a body mass index (BMI) greater than the 95th percentile for age and gender.

- Although genetics and some disorders cause obesity, most adolescent obesity results from a lack of physical activity and overeating.
- The diagnosis is based on a BMI over the 95th percentile.
- Eating a nutritious diet, moving more, and going to counseling help treat obesity.

Obesity is twice as common among adolescents as it was 30 years ago. Although most of the complications of obesity occur in adulthood (see page 951), obese adolescents are more likely than their peers to have high blood pressure and type 2 diabetes. Although fewer than one third of obese adults were obese as adolescents, most obese adolescents remain obese in adulthood.

The factors that influence obesity among adolescents are the same as those among adults. Parents often are concerned that obesity is the result of some type of endocrine disease, such as hypothyroidism or hyperadrenocorticism, but such disorders are rarely the cause. Adolescents with weight gain caused by endocrine disorders are usually of small stature and have other signs of the underlying disorder. An adolescent who is short and has high blood pressure should be tested for Cushing's syndrome (see page 1001). Although genetic influences are common and responsible genes are now being identified, most obese adolescents simply consume more calories than they burn. Because of society's stigma against obesity, many obese adolescents have a poor self-image and become increasingly sedentary and socially isolated.

Intervention for obese adolescents should be focused on developing healthy eating and exercise habits rather than on losing a specific amount of weight. Caloric intake is reduced by

- Establishing a well-balanced diet of ordinary foods
- Making permanent changes in eating habits

Calorie burning is increased by

- Increasing physical activity

Summer camps for obese adolescents usually help them lose a significant amount of weight, but without continuing effort, the weight usually is regained. Counseling to help adolescents cope with their problems, including poor self-esteem, may be helpful.

Drugs that help reduce weight are generally not used during adolescence because of concerns about safety and possible abuse. One exception is for obese adolescents with a strong family history of type 2 diabetes. They are at high risk of developing diabetes. The drug metformin, which is used to treat diabetes, may help them lose weight and also lower their risk of becoming diabetic.

School Problems

School constitutes a large part of an adolescent's existence. Difficulties in almost any area of life often manifest as school problems.

Particular school problems include

- Fear of going to school
- Absenteeism without permission (truancy)
- Dropping out
- Academic underachievement

School problems during the adolescent years may be the result of

- Rebellion and a need for independence (most common)
- Mental health disorders, such as anxiety or depression
- Substance use
- Family conflict

Sometimes, inappropriate academic placement—particularly in adolescents with a learning disability or mild intellectual disability that was not recognized early in life—causes school problems.

Problems that developed earlier in childhood, such as attention-deficit/hyperactivity disorder (ADHD—see page 1849) and learning disorders (see page 1854), may continue to cause school problems for adolescents.

In general, adolescents with significant school problems should undergo educational testing and a mental health evaluation. Specific problems are treated as needed, and general support and encouragement are provided.

Between 1% and 5% of adolescents develop fear of going to school. This fear may be generalized or related to a particular person (a teacher or another student) or event at school (such as physical education class). The adolescent may develop physical symptoms, such as abdominal pain, or may simply refuse to go to school. School personnel and family members should identify the reason, if any, for the fear and encourage the adolescent to attend school.

Adolescents who are repeatedly truant or drop out of school have made a conscious decision to miss school. These adolescents generally have poor academic achievement and have had little success or satisfaction from school-related activities. They often have engaged in high-risk behaviors, such as having unprotected sex, taking drugs, and engaging in violence. Adolescents at risk of dropping out should be made aware of other educational options, such as vocational training and alternative programs. Changes in the learning environment and sometimes drug therapy can also be of great help to struggling adolescents.

Behavioral Problems

Adolescence is a time for developing independence. Typically, adolescents exercise their independence by questioning their parents' rules, which at times leads to rule breaking. Parents and doctors must distinguish occasional errors of judgment from a degree of misbehavior that requires professional intervention. The severity and frequency of infractions are guides. For example, drinking habitually, fighting often, frequent truancy, and theft are much more significant than isolated episodes of the same activities. Other warning signs include deterioration of performance at school and running away from home. Of particular concern are adolescents who cause serious injury or use a weapon in a fight.

Children occasionally engage in physical confrontation. During adolescence, the frequency and severity of violent interactions may increase. Although episodes of violence at school are highly publicized, adolescents are much more likely to be involved in violent episodes (or more often the threat of violence) at home and outside of school. Many factors contribute to an increased risk of violence for adolescents, including

- Developmental issues
- Gang membership
- Access to firearms
- Substance use
- Poverty

There is little evidence to suggest a relationship between violence and genetic defects or chromosomal abnormalities.

Because adolescents are much more independent and mobile than they were as children, they are often out of the direct physical control of adults. In these circumstances, adolescents' behavior is determined by their own moral and behavioral code. Parents guide rather than directly control the adolescents' actions. Adolescents who feel warmth and support from their parents are less likely to engage

Gang Membership and Violence

Gang membership has been linked with violent behavior. Youth gangs are self-formed associations made up of 3 or more members, typically ranging in age from 13 to 24. Gangs usually adopt a name and identifying symbols, such as a particular style of clothing, the use of certain hand signs, or graffiti. Some gangs require prospective members to perform random acts of violence before membership is granted.

Increasing youth gang violence has been blamed at least in part on gang involvement in drug distribution and drug use, particularly methamphetamines and heroin. Firearms and other weapons are frequent features of gang violence. In 2005, almost 16% of high school students in the United States reported carrying a weapon at least once during the month before they took part in a study about youth risks.

Violence prevention begins in early childhood with violence-free discipline. Limiting exposure to media violence may also help because exposure to these violent images has been shown to increase violence in school-age children. School-age children should have access to a safe school environment. Older children and adolescents should not have access to weapons and should be taught to avoid high-risk situations (such as places or settings where others have weapons or are using alcohol or drugs) and to use strategies to defuse tense situations.

All victims of gang violence should be encouraged to talk to parents, teachers, and even their doctor about problems they are experiencing.

in risky behaviors. Also, adolescents whose parents convey clear expectations regarding their children's behavior and show consistent limit setting and monitoring are less likely to engage in risky behaviors. Authoritative parenting is a parenting style in which children participate in establishing family expectations and rules. This parenting style, as opposed to harsh or permissive parenting, is most likely to promote mature behaviors.

Authoritative parents typically use a system of graduated privileges, in which adolescents initially are given small bits of responsibility and freedom (such as caring for a pet, doing household chores, picking out clothing, or decorating their room). If adolescents handle this responsibility well over a period of time, more privileges are granted. By contrast, poor judgment or lack of responsibility leads to loss of privileges. Each new privilege requires close monitoring by parents to make sure adolescents comply with the agreed-upon rules.

Some parents and their adolescents clash over almost everything. In these situations, the core issue is really control. Adolescents want to feel in control of their lives, and parents want adolescents to know the parents still make the rules. In these situations, everyone may benefit from the parents picking their battles and focusing their efforts on the adolescents' actions (such as attending school and complying with household responsibilities) rather than on expressions (such as dress, hairstyle, and preferred entertainment).

Adolescents whose behavior is dangerous or otherwise unacceptable despite their parents' best efforts may need professional intervention. Substance abuse is a common trigger of behavioral problems, and substance use disorders require specific treatment. Behavioral problems also may be a symptom of depression or other mental health disorders. Such disorders typically require treatment with drugs as well as counseling. If parents are not able to limit an adolescent's dangerous behavior, they may request help from the court system and be assigned to a probation officer who can help enforce reasonable household rules.

Drug and Substance Use and Abuse

Substance use among adolescents ranges from experimentation to dependence (see page 2078). The consequences range from none to minor to life threatening, depending on the substance, the circumstances, and the frequency of use. However, even occasional use can put adolescents at risk of significant harm, including overdose, motor vehicle collisions, violent behaviors, and consequences of sexual contact (such as pregnancy and sexually transmitted diseases). Although experimentation with alcohol and, to a lesser extent, marijuana is common, experimentation with other illicit drugs and misuse of prescription or over-the-counter drugs is uncommon. Adolescents who engage in these behaviors are at higher risk of harm. Parental attitudes and the examples that parents set regarding their own use of alcohol, tobacco, prescription drugs, and other substances are a powerful influence.

Alcohol

Alcohol is the substance most often used by adolescents. About 72% of high school seniors report having tried alcohol, although only 55% say they have ever been drunk. Society and the media portray drinking as acceptable or even fashionable. Despite these influences, parents can make a difference by conveying clear expectations to their adolescent regarding drinking, setting limits consistently, and monitoring. On the other hand, adolescents whose family members drink excessively may think this behavior is acceptable. Some adolescents who try alcohol go on to develop an alcohol use disorder, such as abuse or dependence. Risk factors for developing a disorder include starting drinking at a young age and genetics. Adolescents who have a family member with an alcohol use disorder should be made aware of their increased risk.

Tobacco

The majority of adults who smoke cigarettes begin smoking during adolescence. Children as young as age 10 experiment with cigarettes. Nearly one fifth of 9th graders report smoking regularly. In the United States, more than 2,000 people begin smoking every day. Of these new smokers, 31% are under age 16 and more than 50% are under age 18. If adolescents do not try cigarettes before age 19, they are very unlikely to become smokers as adults. Factors that increase the likelihood of an adolescent smoking are having parents who smoke (the single most predictive factor) or peers and role models (such as celebrities) who smoke. Risk factors often associated with smoking include

- Poor school performance
- High-risk behavior (such as excessive dieting, physical fighting, or use of alcohol or other drugs)
- Poor problem-solving abilities
- Poor self-esteem

Parents can help prevent their adolescent from smoking by being positive role models (that is, by not smoking), openly discussing the hazards of tobacco, and encouraging adolescents who already smoke to quit, including supporting them in seeking medical assistance if necessary.

Other Substances

Use of illicit substances other than tobacco and alcohol in adolescents, although decreasing overall in the last few years, remains high. In 2007, about 47% of 12th graders had used illicit drugs at some time in their life. Only about 25% had ever used an illicit drug other than marijuana.

About 2% of high school seniors have used anabolic steroids (see page 2090) in their lifetime. Although steroid use is more common among athletes, non-athletes are not immune. Use of anabolic steroids is associated with a number of side effects, including premature closure of the growth plates at the ends of bones, resulting in permanent short stature. Other side effects are common to both adolescents and adults.

Although use of most drugs is declining, there has been a notable increase in the misuse of prescription drugs, most notably narcotic pain drugs, antianxiety drugs, and stimulants. Over-the-counter (OTC) cough and cold drugs are also used by adolescents to get

high. These drugs are widely available and are considered safe by many adolescents and now serve as gateway drugs. Even young adolescents may try drugs, with some reporting drug use as early as age 12. Many adolescents who experiment with OTC, prescription, and illicit substances go on to develop substance use disorders.

Behaviors that should prompt parents to discuss their concerns with their child and doctor include

- Erratic behavior
- Depression or mood swings
- A change in friends
- Declining school performance
- Loss of interest in hobbies

Parents who find drugs or drug paraphernalia should discuss their concerns with their child.

During routine health care visits, parents should expect their child's doctor to give their child a questionnaire to screen for drug and alcohol use. Doctors can help assess whether an adolescent has a substance use disorder and implement an appropriate intervention. A drug test may be a useful part of an assessment, but this procedure has significant limitations. Results of a urine test may be negative in adolescents who use drugs if the drug is cleared from the body before the test is done, a drug not included on a standard testing panel has been used, or the specimen is adulterated. Given these limitations, a doctor with expertise in this area should determine whether a drug test is warranted in a given situation, and parents should respect their doctor's advice. When parents demand a drug test or demand information that would break their child's confidentiality, they may create an atmosphere of confrontation and inadvertently make it difficult for a doctor to obtain an accurate substance use history and form a therapeutic alliance with their child.

If the doctor thinks the adolescent has a substance use disorder, a referral for further assessment and treatment may be warranted. In general, the same behavioral therapies used for adults with substance use disorders (see page 2078) can also be used with adolescents. However, these therapies should be adapted. Adolescents should receive services from adolescent programs and therapists with expertise in treating adolescents with substance use disorders. In general, adolescents should not be treated in the same programs as adults.

Contraception and Adolescent Pregnancy

Many adolescents engage in sexual activity but may not be fully informed about contraception, pregnancy, and sexually transmitted diseases, including human immunodeficiency virus (HIV) infection. Impulsivity, lack of planning, and concurrent drug and alcohol use decrease the likelihood that adolescents will use birth control and barrier protection.

Any of the adult contraceptive methods may be used by adolescents (see page 1593), but the most common problem is adherence. For example, many adolescent girls forget to take daily oral contraceptives or stop using them entirely—often without substituting another form of birth control. Although male condoms are the most frequently used form of contraception, there are still perceptions that may inhibit consistent use (for example, that condom use decreases pleasure and interferes with "romantic love"). Some girls also are shy about asking male partners to use condoms during sex.

Pregnancy can be a source of significant emotional stress for adolescents. Pregnant adolescents and their partners tend to drop out of school or job training, thus worsening their economic status, lowering their self-esteem, and straining personal relationships. Pregnant adolescents (who account for 13% of all pregnancies in the United States) are less likely than adults to get prenatal care, resulting in poorer pregnancy outcomes, such as higher rates of premature birth. Pregnant adolescents, particularly the very young and those who are not receiving prenatal care, are more likely than women in their 20s to have medical problems such as anemia and toxemia. Infants of young mothers (especially mothers younger than 15 years) are more likely to be born prematurely and to have a low birth weight. However, with proper prenatal care, older adolescents have no higher risk of pregnancy problems than adults from similar backgrounds.

Having an abortion (see page 1605) does not remove the psychologic problems of an unwanted pregnancy—either for the adolescent girl or her partner. Emotional crises may occur when pregnancy is diagnosed, when the decision to have an abortion is made, immediately after the abortion is performed, when the baby would have been born, and on the anniversaries of that date. Family counseling and education about contraceptive methods, for both the girl and her partner, can be very helpful.

Parents may have different reactions when their daughter says she is pregnant or their son says he has impregnated someone. Emotions may range from apathy to disappointment and anger. It is important for parents to express their support and willingness to help the adolescent sort through his or her choices. Parents and adolescents need to communicate openly about abortion, adoption, and parenthood—all tough options for the adolescent to struggle with alone.

CHAPTER

269 Bacterial Infections

Bacteria are microscopic, single-celled organisms (see page 1151). Only some bacteria cause disease in people. The most common bacterial infections among children are skin infections (including impetigo), ear infections, and throat infections (strep throat). These and many other less common bacterial disorders are treated similarly in adults and children and are discussed elsewhere in the book. Other infections occur at all ages but have specific considerations in children. Several severe bacterial infections are preventable by routine immunization early in childhood.

Certain children are at particular risk of bacterial infections. These children include infants younger than 2 months, children who have no spleen or who have an immune system disorder, and children who have sickle cell disease.

Sometimes doctors diagnose bacterial infections by the typical symptoms they cause. Usually, however, bacteria must be identified in samples of tissue or body fluids, such as blood, urine, pus, or cerebrospinal fluid. Sometimes bacteria from these samples can be recognized under a microscope or identified with a rapid detection test. Usually, however, they are too few or too small to see, so doctors must try to grow (culture) them in the laboratory. It typically takes 24 to 48 hours to culture the bacteria. Cultures can also be used to test the susceptibility of particular bacteria to various antibiotics. The results can help a doctor determine which drug to use in treating an infected child. Doctors may treat certain

 Did You Know...
Not all bacteria cause disease or infections.

Bacterial Infections Preventable With Routine Immunization*

- Diphtheria
- Infection with *Haemophilus influenzae* type b (meningitis, epiglottitis, some severe eye infections, and occult bacteremia)
- Infection with *Streptococcus pneumoniae* (pneumonia, meningitis, occult bacteremia, and ear infections)
- Infection with *Neisseria meningitidis* (meningitis, sepsis, and occult bacteremia)
- Pertussis
- Tetanus

*Note: Many viral infections can also be prevented with routine immunization (see box on page 1685).

potentially serious childhood infections with antibiotics before they have the culture results. When results are obtained, the antibiotics are continued or changed as needed. If no bacteria are found, antibiotics may be stopped.

Occult Bacteremia

Occult (hidden) bacteremia is the presence of bacteria in the bloodstream of a child who has a fever but who may not appear particularly sick and who has no apparent other source of infection.

- Most commonly, occult bacteremia is caused by the bacteria *Streptococcus pneumoniae*.
- Typically, children have no symptoms other than fever.
- The diagnosis is based on blood tests.
- Antibiotics can eliminate the infection.

Children younger than 3 years commonly develop fevers. Most of the time, they have other symptoms, such as a cough and runny nose, which allow doctors to diagnose the cause. About one third of the time, children have no symptoms besides fever. Most of these children have viral infections that go away without treatment. However, about 3% of such children have bacteria circulating in the bloodstream (bacteremia). *Streptococcus pneumoniae* is the most common type of bacteria causing occult bacteremia. Circulating bacteria are almost never present in older children or adults with fever and no other symptoms. These circulating bacteria may attack various organs and result in serious illnesses, such as pneumonia or meningitis. Although only about 5 to 10% of children with occult bacteremia develop these serious problems, doctors perform blood cultures to identify the bacteria before such

problems develop. An elevated white blood cell count indicates a higher risk of bacterial infection. In this case, a doctor may choose to start antibiotics before blood culture results are available.

Because doctors cannot tell with certainty which children who have a fever have bacteremia, doctors may perform a complete blood cell count and blood cultures if children are younger than 3 years, have a temperature higher than 102° F (38.9° C), and do not have an apparent reason for their fever. Because occult bacteremia is much less common among children older than 3 years, these children do not usually require blood cultures.

If children may have occult bacteremia, doctors reevaluate them in 24 to 48 hours, when culture results are available. Children with positive culture results are given oral antibiotics at home if they do not appear very ill. Children who show signs of serious illness are typically given intravenous antibiotics in the hospital. Sometimes before obtaining culture results, doctors treat children who have a fever and who appear seriously ill or have risk factors for bacteremia (such as an elevated white blood cell count) with a single injection of an antibiotic, such as ceftriaxone.

The *Haemophilus influenzae* type b conjugate vaccine, now given to nearly all children in the United States, has nearly eliminated occult bacteremia due to *Haemophilus influenzae* type b. The relatively new conjugate vaccine against *Streptococcus pneumoniae*, given to infants, has greatly reduced the incidence of occult pneumococcal bacteremia. Newer conjugate vaccines against *Neisseria meningitidis* are being tested for use in young children. The use of these vaccines is expected to essentially eliminate occult bacteremia in children.

Meningitis

Bacterial meningitis is infection of the layers of tissue covering the brain and spinal cord (meninges).

- Bacterial meningitis usually results from a bacterial infection in the bloodstream (sepsis).
- Older children have a stiff neck with a fever, headache, and confusion, and infants are usually irritable, stop eating, vomit, or have other symptoms.
- The diagnosis is based on the results of a spinal tap and blood tests.
- Some children die of meningitis even after receiving appropriate treatment.
- Vaccination can help prevent certain bacterial infections that lead to meningitis.
- Antibiotics are given to treat the infection.

Meningitis can occur at any age. Meningitis is similar in older children, adolescents, and adults (see page 750) but different in newborns and infants.

Children at particular risk of meningitis include those with sickle cell disease and those lacking a spleen. Children with congenital deformities of the face and skull may have defects in the bones that allow bacteria access to the meninges. Children who have a weakened immune system, such as those with AIDS or those who have received chemotherapy, are more susceptible to meningitis.

Causes

Meningitis in newborns usually results from an infection of the bloodstream (sepsis). The infection is typically caused by bacteria acquired from the birth canal, most commonly group B streptococci, *Escherichia coli*, and *Listeria monocytogenes*. Older infants and children usually develop infection through contact with respiratory secretions from infected people. Bacteria that infect older infants and children include *Streptococcus pneumoniae* and *Neisseria meningitidis. Haemophilus influenzae* type b was the most common cause of meningitis, but widespread vaccination against that organism has now made it a rare cause. Current vaccines against *Streptococcus pneumoniae* and *Neisseria meningitidis* (pneumococcal and meningococcal conjugate vaccines) should also make these organisms rare causes of childhood meningitis.

Symptoms and Diagnosis

Older children and adolescents with meningitis typically have a few days of increasing fever, headache, confusion, and a stiff neck. They may have an upper respiratory tract infection that is unrelated to the meningitis. Newborns and infants rarely develop a stiff neck and are unable to communicate specific discomfort. These younger children become fussy and irritable (particularly when they are held) and stop feeding—important signs that should alert parents to a possibly serious problem. Sometimes newborns and infants have fever, vomiting, or a skin rash. One third have seizures. The nerves controlling some eye and facial movements may be damaged, causing an eye to turn inward or outward or the facial expression to become lopsided. In about 25% of newborns with meningitis, increased pressure of the fluid around the brain may make the fontanelles (the soft spots between the skull bones) bulge or feel firm. These symptoms usually develop over at least 1 to 2 days, but some infants, particularly those between birth and 3 or 4 months of age, become ill very rapidly, progressing from health to near death in less than 24 hours.

Rarely, pockets of pus (abscesses) form within the brain of infants with meningitis due to certain bacteria. As the abscesses grow, pressure on the brain increases, resulting in vomiting, head enlargement, and bulging fontanelles.

A doctor diagnoses bacterial meningitis by examining and culturing a sample of cerebrospinal fluid obtained through a spinal tap (lumbar puncture—see page 635). Doctors also order blood cultures to look for bacteria in the bloodstream. Ultrasonography or computed tomography (CT) may be used to determine if an abscess is present.

Prognosis

Even with timely, appropriate treatment, as many as 25% of newborns with bacterial meningitis die. In older infants and children, mortality rates vary from 3 to 5% when the cause is *Haemophilus influenzae* type b, 5 to 10% when the cause is *Neisseria meningitidis,* and 10 to 20% when the cause is *Streptococcus pneumoniae.*

Of the newborns who survive, 15 to 25% develop serious brain and nerve problems, such as enlargement of the ventricles (hydrocephalus), deafness, cerebral palsy, and mental retardation/intellectual disability. Up to 30% have mild residual problems, such as learning disorders, mild hearing loss, or occasional seizures. Older infants and children tend to have fewer of these complications.

Prevention

Health care practitioners and parents can help prevent bacterial meningitis by ensuring that all young children receive the *Haemophilus influenzae* type b and *Streptococcus pneumoniae* conjugate vaccines and that older children and adolescents receive either the *Neisseria meningitidis* polysaccharide or conjugate vaccine.

Treatment

Doctors give high doses of antibiotics by vein (intravenously) as soon as they suspect meningitis. Very sick children receive antibiotics even before a spinal tap is done. When culture results from the spinal tap become available, doctors change the antibiotics, if needed, based on the type of bacteria causing the meningitis. Children older than 6 weeks are often given corticosteroids to help prevent permanent neurologic problems. Sometimes a second culture and spinal tap are done to determine whether the antibiotics are working fast enough.

Diphtheria

Diphtheria is a contagious, sometimes fatal infection of the upper respiratory tract caused by the bacterium Corynebacterium diphtheriae.

- Diphtheria is caused by a bacterial infection that is now rare in developed countries.
- Typical symptoms include a sore throat, general feeling of illness, and fever, sometimes with swollen lymph nodes, and a tough, gray pseudomembrane forms in the throat.

- The diagnosis is based on symptoms, particularly a sore throat and the pseudomembrane.
- Vaccination can help prevent this infection.
- The child is hospitalized and given antibiotics to eliminate the infection.

Years ago, diphtheria was one of the leading causes of death among children. Today, diphtheria is rare in developed countries, primarily because of widespread vaccination. Fewer than five cases occur in the United States each year, but diphtheria bacteria still exist in the world and can cause outbreaks if vaccination is inadequate.

The bacteria that cause diphtheria are usually spread in droplets of moisture coughed into the air. Usually the bacteria multiply on or near the surface of the mucous membranes of the mouth or throat, where they cause inflammation. Some types of *Corynebacterium diphtheriae* release a potent toxin, which can damage the heart, kidneys, and nervous system. A milder form of diphtheria affects only the skin and occurs mainly in adults. This form is more common among people with poor hygiene (for example, homeless people).

Symptoms and Diagnosis

The illness begins 1 to 4 days after exposure to the bacteria. Symptoms begin over a few days, with sore throat, a general feeling of illness (malaise), and a fever up to 103° F (39.4° C). The child also may have a fast heart rate, nausea, vomiting, chills, and a headache. The lymph nodes in the neck may swell. The inflammation may make the throat swell, narrowing the airway and making breathing extremely difficult.

Typically, the bacteria form a tough, gray pseudomembrane—a sheet of material composed of dead white blood cells, bacteria, and other substances—near the tonsils or other parts of the throat. The pseudomembrane narrows the airway and may suddenly become detached and block the airway completely, preventing the child from being able to breathe. The toxin produced by diphtheria bacteria usually affects certain nerves, particularly those to the muscles of the face, throat, arms, and legs, causing symptoms such as difficulty swallowing or moving the eyes, arms, or legs. The bacterial toxin may also cause inflammation of the heart muscle (myocarditis), sometimes leading to abnormal heart rhythms, heart failure, and death.

A doctor suspects diphtheria in a sick child who has a sore throat with a pseudomembrane, particularly if muscles of the face or throat are paralyzed and if the child was not vaccinated. The diagnosis is confirmed by culture of material from the child's throat.

Prevention and Treatment

Children are routinely immunized against diphtheria (see box on page 1685). The diphtheria vaccine is usually combined with vaccines for tetanus and pertussis (whooping cough).

A child with symptoms of diphtheria is typically hospitalized in an intensive care unit and given antibodies (antitoxins) to neutralize the diphtheria toxin. Doctors also give antibiotics, such as penicillin or erythromycin, to kill the diphtheria bacteria. Antibiotics are given for 14 days. The child must be kept in isolation (to prevent other people from being exposed to infected secretions) until two cultures, taken after the antibiotics are stopped, confirm that the bacteria have been killed.

> **? Did You Know...**
> Routine vaccination can prevent many bacterial infections.

Retropharyngeal Abscess

A retropharyngeal abscess is a collection of pus in the lymph nodes at the back of the throat.

- A retropharyngeal abscess is caused by a bacterial infection.
- Symptoms include difficulty and pain when swallowing, a fever, stiff neck, and noisy breathing.
- The diagnosis is based on symptoms and x-rays and computed tomography of the neck.
- Children who receive prompt treatment do well.
- The abscess is drained surgically, and antibiotics are given to eliminate the infection.

Because the lymph nodes at the back of the throat disappear after childhood, retropharyngeal abscesses are more common among children than among adults. An abscess is usually caused by a bacterial infection that has spread from the tonsils, throat, sinuses, adenoids, nose, or middle ear. Many infections are caused by a combination of bacteria. An injury to the back of the throat from a sharp object, such as a fish bone, occasionally causes a retropharyngeal abscess.

Symptoms and Diagnosis

The main symptoms are difficulty and pain when swallowing, a fever, and enlargement of the lymph nodes in the neck. The voice is muffled, and children may drool. The neck may be stiff, and children may hold their head at an angle. The abscess can block the airway, making breathing difficult and noisy, particularly when children inhale (called stridor). Children may lie on their back, tilt their head and neck back, and raise their chin to make breathing easier.

Complications include bleeding around the abscess, rupture of the abscess into the airway (which can block the airway), and pneumonia. The voice box (larynx) may go into spasm and further interfere with breathing. Blood clots may form in the jugular veins of the neck. Infection may spread down into the chest. Sometimes widespread inflammation and infection of the bloodstream occurs, causing organs to malfunction (a condition called septic shock).

A doctor suspects the disorder in children who have a severe, unexplained sore throat, a stiff neck, and noisy breathing. X-rays and computed tomography (CT) scans of the neck can confirm the diagnosis.

Treatment

Most children do well with prompt treatment. Retropharyngeal abscesses often need to be drained surgically. A doctor cuts the abscess open allowing the pus to drain out. Penicillin plus metronidazole, clindamycin, ampicillin-sulbactam, cefoxitin, or other antibiotics are given, at first by vein and then by mouth.

Epiglottitis

Epiglottitis is a severe bacterial infection of the epiglottis, which can block the windpipe, obstructing air flow.

- Epiglottitis is caused by a bacterial infection.
- Typical symptoms include a sudden sore throat, a high fever, irritability, anxiety, and difficulties in swallowing and breathing.
- The diagnosis is based on symptoms and an x-ray of the neck.
- Vaccination can help prevent this infection.
- The child is hospitalized, measures are taken to keep the airway open, and antibiotics are given to eliminate the infection.

The epiglottis is a small flap of tissue that closes the entrance to the voice box (larynx) and windpipe (trachea) during swallowing. In the past, epiglottitis was most common among children 2 to 5 years old and was usually caused by the bacterium *Haemophilus influenzae* type b. Now that most children are vaccinated against *Haemophilus influenzae* type b, the disease is quite rare and is more common among adults (see page 1403). In adults, it is typically caused by *Streptococcus pneumoniae*, other streptococci, and staphylococci. Children with epiglottitis often have bacteria in the bloodstream (bacteremia), which sometimes spreads the infection to the lungs, the joints, the tissues covering the brain (meninges), the sac around the heart, or the tissue beneath the skin.

Symptoms

The infection usually begins suddenly and progresses rapidly. A previously healthy child develops a sore throat and often a high fever. The child may be irritable and anxious. Difficulties in swallowing and breathing are common. The child usually drools, breathes rapidly, and makes a loud noise while inhaling (called stridor). The difficulty in breathing often causes the child to lean forward while stretching the neck backward to try to increase the amount of air reaching the lungs. Labored breathing may lead to a buildup of carbon dioxide and low oxygen levels in the bloodstream, causing agitation and confusion followed by sluggishness (lethargy). The swollen epiglottis makes coughing up mucus difficult. Epiglottitis can quickly become fatal because swelling of the infected tissue may block the airway and cut off breathing.

Diagnosis

Epiglottitis is an emergency, and a child is hospitalized immediately when a doctor suspects it. If the child does not have all of the typical symptoms of epiglottitis and does not appear seriously ill, the doctor sometimes takes an x-ray of the neck, which can show an enlarged epiglottis. The doctor does not hold the child down or use a tongue depressor to look in the throat. These manipulations may cause throat spasm and complete airway blockage in a child with epiglottitis.

If an enlarged epiglottis is seen on x-ray or the child appears seriously ill, doctors examine the child under anesthesia in the operating room. The doctor inserts a thin flexible tube (laryngoscope) into the throat to directly view the larynx.

Prevention

Prevention of epiglottitis is better than treatment. Prevention is achieved by ensuring that all children receive the *Haemophilus influenzae* type b and *Streptococcus pneumoniae* conjugate vaccines.

Treatment

If the examination shows epiglottitis or triggers throat spasm, the doctor inserts a plastic tube (endotracheal tube) into the airway to keep it open. If the airway is too swollen to allow placement of an endotracheal tube, the doctor cuts an opening through the front of the neck (tracheostomy) and inserts the tube. This tube is left in place for several days until the swelling of the epiglottis goes down. The child also receives antibiotics, such as ceftriaxone or ampicillin-sulbactam. Once the child's airway is opened, the prognosis is good.

Pertussis

Pertussis (whooping cough) is a highly contagious infection caused by the bacterium Bordetella pertussis, *which results in fits of coughing that usually end in a prolonged, high-pitched, deeply indrawn breath (the whoop).*

- Pertussis is caused by a bacterial infection.
- Mild coldlike symptoms are followed by severe coughing fits, then gradual recovery.

- The diagnosis is based on the characteristic whoop-sounding cough and examination of the mucus in the nose and throat.
- Most children with pertussis recover slowly but completely.
- Vaccination can help prevent this infection.
- Very ill children usually are hospitalized and given antibiotics to eliminate the infection.

Pertussis, once rampant in the United States, is now better controlled although not eradicated. Local epidemics among unimmunized people occur every 2 to 4 years. Pertussis remains a major problem throughout the developing world.

People may develop pertussis at any age, but one third of cases occur in children younger than 10 years, and one third occur in adolescents 11 to 18 years of age. Pertussis is most serious in children younger than 2 years, and nearly all deaths occur in children younger than 6 months. One attack of pertussis does not always give full immunity for life, but a second attack, if it occurs, is usually mild and not always recognized as pertussis. In fact, some adults with "walking pneumonia" actually have pertussis.

An infected person spreads pertussis bacteria into the air in droplets of moisture produced by coughing. Anyone nearby may inhale these droplets and become infected. Pertussis usually is not contagious after the third week of the infection.

Symptoms

The illness lasts about 6 to 10 weeks, progressing through three stages: mild cold-like symptoms, severe coughing fits, and gradual recovery. Coldlike symptoms include sneezing, runny nose, a hacking cough at night, and a general feeling of illness (malaise). After 1 or 2 weeks, the person develops typical coughing fits. These fits typically consist of 5 or more rapidly consecutive forceful coughs followed by the whoop (a prolonged, high-pitched, deeply indrawn breath). After a fit, breathing is normal, but another coughing fit follows shortly thereafter. The cough often produces large amounts of thick mucus (usually swallowed by infants and children or seen as large bubbles from the nose). In younger children, vomiting often follows a prolonged fit of coughing. In infants, choking spells and pauses in breathing (apnea), possibly causing the skin to turn blue, may be more common than the whoops.

About one fourth of children develop pneumonia, resulting in difficulty breathing. Ear infections (otitis media) also frequently develop. Rarely, pertussis affects the brain in infants. Bleeding, swelling, or inflammation of the brain may cause seizures, confusion, brain damage, and mental retardation/intellectual disability.

After several weeks, the coughing fits gradually subside, but for many weeks or even months, children have a lingering, persistent cough.

Diagnosis and Prognosis

Doctors suspect pertussis because of the typical whooping cough or other symptoms. They confirm the diagnosis by culturing a sample of mucus from the back of the nose or throat. Culture results often are negative after several weeks of illness. Other diagnostic tests (such as a polymerase chain reaction or rapid detection test) performed on samples from the nose or throat may be helpful.

Most children with pertussis recover completely, although slowly. About 1 to 2% of the children younger than 1 year die.

Prevention and Treatment

Children are routinely vaccinated against pertussis. The pertussis vaccine is usually combined with vaccines for diphtheria and tetanus (see box on page 1685). The antibiotic erythromycin (or sometimes clarithromycin or azithromycin) is given as a preventive measure to children exposed to pertussis.

Severely ill infants are usually hospitalized because their breathing difficulty may become so severe that they require mechanical ventilation through a tube placed in their windpipe. Others may need extra oxygen and fluids given by vein. Seriously ill infants are usually kept in isolation (to prevent other people from being exposed to infected droplets in the air) until antibiotics have been given for 5 days. Older children who have mild disease are treated with antibiotics at home. Cough medicines are of questionable value and are not usually used.

The antibiotic erythromycin, clarithromycin, or azithromycin is usually used to eradicate the bacteria causing pertussis. Antibiotics are also used to treat infections that accompany the pertussis, such as pneumonia and ear infection.

Rheumatic Fever

Rheumatic fever is inflammation of the body's organ systems, especially the joints and the heart, resulting from a complication of streptococcal infection of the throat.

- This condition is a reaction to a streptococcal throat infection.
- Children may have a combination of joint pain, fever, chest pain or palpitations, jerky uncontrollable movements, a rash, and small bumps under the skin.
- The diagnosis is based on symptoms.
- Prompt and complete antibiotic treatment of any streptococcal throat infection is the best way to prevent rheumatic fever.
- Aspirin is given to alleviate pain, and antibiotics are given to eliminate the infection.

Although rheumatic fever follows a streptococcal throat infection (strep throat), it is not an infection.

Rather, it is an inflammatory reaction to the infection. The parts of the body most commonly affected by the inflammation include the joints, heart, skin, and nervous system. Most people with rheumatic fever recover, but the heart is permanently damaged in a small percentage of people.

In the United States, rheumatic fever rarely develops before age 3 or after age 40 and is much less common in developing countries, probably because antibiotics are widely used to treat streptococcal infections at an early stage. However, the incidence of rheumatic fever sometimes rises and falls in a particular area for unknown reasons. Overcrowded living conditions seem to increase the risk of rheumatic fever, and heredity seems to play a part. In the United States, a child who has a streptococcal throat infection but is not treated has only a 0.4 to 3% chance of developing rheumatic fever. About half of the children who have had rheumatic fever develop it again after another streptococcal throat infection if it is not treated. Rheumatic fever follows streptococcal infections of the throat but not those of the skin (impetigo) or other areas of the body. The reasons are not known.

Symptoms

Symptoms of rheumatic fever vary greatly, depending on which parts of the body become inflamed. Typically, symptoms begin several weeks after the disappearance of throat symptoms. The most common symptoms of rheumatic fever are joint pain, fever, chest pain or palpitations caused by heart inflammation (carditis), jerky uncontrollable movements (Sydenham's chorea), a rash, and small bumps (nodules) under the skin. A child may have one symptom or several.

Joints: Joint pain and fever are the most common first symptoms. One or several joints suddenly become painful and feel tender when touched. They may also be red, hot, and swollen and may contain fluid. Ankles, knees, elbows, and wrists are commonly affected. The shoulders, hips, and small joints of the hands and feet also may be affected. As pain in one joint abates, pain in another starts (migratory pain). Joint pains may be mild or severe and typically last 2 to 4 weeks. Rheumatic fever does not cause long-term joint damage.

Heart: Some children with heart inflammation have no symptoms, and the past inflammation is recognized years later when heart damage is discovered. Some children feel their heart beating rapidly. Others have chest pain caused by inflammation of the sac around the heart. Heart failure may develop, causing the child to feel tired and short of breath, with nausea, vomiting, stomachache, or a hacking, nonproductive cough.

Heart inflammation disappears gradually, usually within 5 months. However, it may permanently damage the heart valves, resulting in rheumatic heart disease. The likelihood of rheumatic heart disease varies with the severity of the initial heart inflammation. About 1% of people who had no heart inflammation develop rheumatic heart disease, compared with 30% who had mild inflammation and 70% who had severe inflammation. In rheumatic heart disease, the valve between the left atrium and ventricle (mitral valve) is most commonly damaged. The valve may become leaky (mitral valve regurgitation—see page 378), abnormally narrow (mitral valve stenosis—see page 381), or both. Valve damage causes the characteristic heart murmurs that enable a doctor to diagnose rheumatic fever. Later in life, usually in middle age, the valve damage may cause heart failure (see page 352) and atrial fibrillation, an abnormal heart rhythm (see page 366).

Skin: A flat, painless rash with a wavy edge (erythema marginatum) may appear as the other symptoms subside. It lasts for only a short time, sometimes less than a day. In children with heart or joint inflammation, small, hard nodules may form under the skin, typically near the affected joints. The nodules are usually painless.

Nervous System: Jerky uncontrollable movements (Sydenham's chorea) may begin gradually in children with rheumatic fever, but usually only after all other symptoms have subsided. A month may go by before the jerky movements become so intense that the child is taken to a doctor. By then, the child typically has rapid, purposeless, sporadic movements that disappear during sleep. The movements may involve any muscle except those of the eyes. They often begin in the hands and spread to the feet and face. Facial grimacing is common. In mild cases, children may seem clumsy and may have slight difficulties in dressing and eating. In severe cases, children may have to be protected from injuring themselves with their flailing arms or legs. The chorea lasts between 4 and 8 months.

Diagnosis

A doctor bases the diagnosis of rheumatic fever mainly on the characteristic combination of symptoms. Blood tests showing high levels of antibodies to streptococci may be helpful, but low levels of these antibodies are present in many children who do not have rheumatic fever. Abnormal heart rhythms caused by heart inflammation can be seen on an electrocardiogram (ECG—a recording of the heart's electrical activity). An echocardiogram (an image of structures in the heart produced by ultrasound waves) may be used to diagnose abnormalities of the heart valves.

? Did You Know...
Antibiotics can cure some bacterial infections.

Prevention and Treatment

The best way to prevent rheumatic fever is with prompt and complete antibiotic treatment of any streptococcal throat infection. In addition, children who have had rheumatic fever should be given penicillin by mouth every day or by monthly injections into the muscle to help prevent another streptococcal infection. How long this preventive treatment should be continued is unclear. It depends on the severity of the disease and is usually continued at least until adulthood. Some doctors recommend that it should be continued for life in certain people, such as those who have lasting heart damage, who had chorea, or who have close contact with young children (because the children may carry streptococcal bacteria, which could reinfect such people).

Treatment of rheumatic fever has three goals: eliminating any residual streptococcal infection; reducing inflammation, particularly in the joints and heart, and thus relieving symptoms; and limiting physical activity that might aggravate the inflamed structures.

Doctors give children with rheumatic fever an injection of a long-acting penicillin to eliminate any remaining infection. Aspirin is given in high doses to reduce inflammation and pain, particularly if inflammation has reached the joints and heart. Other nonsteroidal anti-inflammatory drugs (NSAIDs), such as naproxen, are as effective as aspirin. If heart inflammation is severe, corticosteroids such as prednisone may be given to further reduce inflammation.

Bed rest may help by avoiding stress on the painful, inflamed joints. When the heart is inflamed, strict bed rest (getting up only to go to the bathroom) is generally suggested.

If the heart valves become damaged, the risk of developing a valve infection (endocarditis) remains throughout life (see page 386). People who have heart valve damage must always take an antibiotic before any surgery, including dental surgery, throughout life.

Urinary Tract Infection

A urinary tract infection is a bacterial infection of the urinary bladder (cystitis) or the kidneys (pyelonephritis).

- Urinary tract infections are caused by a bacterial infection.
- Newborns and infants may have no symptoms other than a fever, whereas older children have pain or burning during urination, pain in the bladder region, and a need to urinate frequently.

- The diagnosis is based on an examination of the urine.
- Proper hygiene may help prevent UTIs.
- Antibiotics are given to eliminate the infection.

Urinary tract infections (UTIs) are common in childhood. Nearly all UTIs are caused by bacteria that enter the urethral opening and move upward to the urinary bladder and sometimes the kidneys. Rarely, in severe infections, bacteria may enter the bloodstream from the kidneys and cause infection of the bloodstream (sepsis) or of other organs.

During infancy, boys are more likely to develop UTIs. After infancy, girls are much more likely to develop them. UTIs are more common among girls because their short urethras make it easier for bacteria to move up the urinary tract. Uncircumcised infant boys (because bacteria tend to accumulate under the foreskin) and young children with severe constipation also are more prone to UTIs.

UTIs in older school-aged children and adolescents differ little from UTIs in adults (see page 302). Younger infants and children who have UTIs, however, more commonly have various structural abnormalities of their urinary system that make them more susceptible to urinary infection. These abnormalities include vesicoureteral reflux (an abnormality of the ureters—the tubes connecting the kidneys to the bladder—that allows urine to pass backward from the bladder up to the kidney) and a number of conditions that block the flow of urine. As many as 50% of newborns and infants with a UTI and 20 to 30% of school-aged children with a UTI have such abnormalities.

Up to 50% of infants and preschool children with a UTI—particularly those with fever—have both bladder and kidney infections. If the kidney is infected and reflux is severe, 5 to 20% of children go on to have some scarring of the kidneys. If there is little or no reflux, very few children have scarring of the kidneys. Scarring is a concern because it may lead to high blood pressure and impaired kidney function in adulthood.

Symptoms and Diagnosis

Newborns and infants with a UTI may have no symptoms other than a fever. Sometimes they do not eat well, are sluggish (lethargic), vomit, or have diarrhea. Older children with bladder infections usually have pain or burning during urination, a need to urinate frequently and urgently, and pain in the bladder region. They may have difficulty urinating or holding urine (incontinence). Urine may smell foul. Children with kidney infections typically have pain in the side or back over the affected kidney, fever, chills, and a general feeling of illness (malaise).

A doctor diagnoses a UTI by examining the urine. Toilet-trained children may provide a urine sample by urinating into a cup after thoroughly cleaning the urethral opening. Doctors obtain urine from younger children and infants by inserting a thin, flexible, sterile tube (catheter) through the urethral opening into the bladder. In infants, the doctor sometimes withdraws urine from the bladder with a needle inserted through the skin just above the pubic bone. Urine collected in plastic bags taped to the child's genital region is not helpful because it is often contaminated with bacteria and other material from the skin.

To detect white blood cells and bacteria in the urine, which occur in UTI, the laboratory examines the urine under a microscope and performs several chemical tests. The laboratory also performs a culture of the urine to grow and identify any bacteria present. The culture is the most significant of these tests.

In general, boys of all ages and girls younger than 2 years who develop even a single UTI need further tests to look for structural abnormalities of the urinary system. Older girls who have had recurring infections also need these tests. The tests include ultrasonography, which identifies kidney abnormalities and obstruction, and voiding cystourethrography, which further identifies abnormalities of the kidneys, ureters, and bladder and can identify when the flow of urine is partially reversed (reflux). For voiding cystourethrography, a catheter is passed through the urethra into the bladder, a dye is instilled through the catheter, and x-rays are taken before and after the child urinates. Another test, radionuclide cystourethrography, is similar to voiding cystourethrography, except that a radioactive agent is placed in the bladder and images are taken using a nuclear scanner. This procedure exposes the child's ovaries or testes to less radiation than voiding cystourethrography. However, radionuclide cystourethrography is much more useful for monitoring the healing of reflux than for diagnosing it, because the structures are not outlined as well as in voiding cystourethrography. Another type of nuclear scanning may be used to confirm the diagnosis of pyelonephritis and identify scarring of the kidneys.

Prevention and Treatment

Prevention of UTIs is difficult, but proper hygiene may help. Girls should be taught to wipe themselves from front to back (as opposed to back to front) after a bowel movement to minimize the chance of bacteria entering the urethral opening. Avoiding frequent bubble baths, which may irritate the skin around the urethral opening of both boys and girls, may help lessen the risk of UTIs. Circumcision of boys lowers their risk of UTIs during infancy by about 10 times, although it is not clear whether this advantage by itself is a sufficient reason for circumcision. Regular urination and regular bowel movements may lessen the risk of UTIs.

UTIs are treated with antibiotics. Children who appear very ill or whose initial test results suggest a UTI are given antibiotics before culture results are available. Otherwise, doctors wait for culture results to confirm the diagnosis. Children who are very ill and all newborns receive antibiotics by injection into either a muscle (intramuscularly) or a vein (intravenously). Other children are given antibiotics by mouth. Treatment typically lasts 7 to 14 days. Children who require tests to diagnose structural abnormalities often continue antibiotic treatment at a lower dose until tests are complete.

Some children with structural abnormalities of the urinary tract require surgery to correct the problem. Others need to take antibiotics daily to prevent infection. Certain mild abnormalities resolve without treatment.

270 Viral Infections

Viral infections are common among people of all ages but often seem to be concentrated in infants and children. Most childhood viral infections are not serious and include such diverse illnesses as colds with a sore throat, vomiting and diarrhea, and fever with a rash. Some viral illnesses that cause more serious disease, such as measles, are less common now due to widespread immunization. Several types of viral infections that children can acquire are discussed in the chapter on adult viral infections (see page 1236).

Most children with viral infections get better without treatment, and many viral infections are so distinctive that a doctor can diagnose them based on their symptoms. A doctor usually does not need to have a laboratory identify the specific virus involved.

Many viral infections result in fever and body aches or discomfort. Doctors treat these symptoms

What Is Reye's Syndrome?

Reye's syndrome is a very rare but life-threatening disorder that causes inflammation and swelling of the brain and degeneration of the liver.

The cause of Reye's syndrome is unknown, although it typically occurs after infection by certain viruses, such as influenza or varicella (chickenpox), particularly in children who take aspirin. Because of this increased risk of Reye's syndrome, aspirin is not recommended for children, except for the treatment of a few specific diseases. Now that aspirin use has declined—in large part because of the possibility of triggering Reye's syndrome—fewer than 20 children a year develop this disorder. The condition occurs mainly in children younger than 18. In the United States, most cases occur in late fall and winter.

Reye's syndrome begins with the symptoms of a viral infection, such as an upper respiratory tract infection, influenza, or chickenpox. After 5 to 7 days, the child suddenly develops very severe nausea and vomiting. Within a day, the child becomes confused, disoriented, and agitated. These changes in the child's mental condition are sometimes followed by seizures, coma, and death. Degeneration of the liver may lead to blood clotting problems and bleeding. The severity of illness varies greatly. Doctors do blood tests and often do a liver biopsy (the removal of tissue samples for examination) to confirm the diagnosis and to rule out other diseases.

The child's prognosis depends on the amount of swelling in the brain. The overall chances that the child will die are about 20%, but range from less than 2% among children with mild disease to more than 80% among those in a deep coma.

Children who survive the acute phase of the illness usually recover fully. Those with more severe symptoms may later show some evidence of brain damage, such as mental retardation/intellectual disability or a seizure disorder. Abnormal muscle movement or damage to specific nerves may also occur. Reye's syndrome rarely affects a child twice.

There is no specific treatment for Reye's syndrome. Children are placed in intensive care. Vitamin K or fresh frozen plasma is given to help prevent bleeding. Children in a deep coma may require placement of a tube into the windpipe to assist their breathing (endotracheal intubation). To alleviate the swelling and pressure on the brain, doctors restrict fluids, elevate the head of the bed, and give drugs that force the body to get rid of excess water (such as mannitol).

---

with acetaminophen or ibuprofen. Aspirin is not given to children or adolescents with these symptoms, because it increases the risk of Reye's syndrome in those who have certain viral infections. Generally, parents can discern whether their child is ill with a potentially serious infection and needs immediate medical care. This is particularly true for children beyond infancy.

Central Nervous System Infections

*Central nervous system infections are extremely serious. **Meningitis** affects the membranes surrounding the brain and spinal cord. **Encephalitis** affects the brain itself.*

- Central nervous system infections caused by viruses can cause meningitis and encephalitis.
- Symptoms usually start with fever and can progress to irritability, refusal to eat, and sometimes seizures.
- The diagnosis is based on a spinal tap.
- Many infections are mild, but others are severe and can cause death.
- Antiviral drugs are usually not effective so children need to receive supportive measures (such as warmth and plenty of fluids).

Viruses that infect the central nervous system (brain and spinal cord) include herpesviruses, arboviruses, coxsackieviruses, echoviruses, and enteroviruses. Some of these infections affect primarily the meninges (the tissues covering the brain and spinal cord) and result in meningitis. Others affect primarily the brain and result in encephalitis. Infections that affect both the meninges and brain result in meningoencephalitis. Meningitis is far more common among children than is encephalitis.

Viruses affect the central nervous system in two ways. They can directly infect and destroy cells in the central nervous system during the acute illness. After recovery from an infection—in the central nervous system or elsewhere in the body—the immune response to the infection sometimes causes secondary damage to the cells around the nerves. This secondary damage (postinfectious encephalomyelitis or acute disseminated encephalomyelitis) results in the child having symptoms several weeks after recovery from the acute illness.

Children acquire infections of the central nervous system through various routes. Newborns can develop herpesvirus infections through contact with infected secretions in the birth canal. Other viral infections are acquired by breathing air contaminated with virus-containing droplets exhaled by an infected person. Arbovirus infections are acquired from bites by infected insects.

SOME VIRAL INFECTIONS AT A GLANCE

INFECTION	PERIOD OF INCUBATION	PERIOD OF CON-TAGIOUSNESS	SITE OF RASH	NATURE OF RASH
Measles (rubeola)	7 to 14 days	From 2 to 4 days before the rash appears until 2 to 5 days after	Starts around the ears and on the face and neck In more severe cases, spreads over the trunk, arms, and legs	Irregular, flat, red areas that soon become raised Begins 3 to 5 days after the onset of symptoms and lasts 3 to 5 days
Rubella (German measles)	14 to 21 days	From shortly before the onset of symptoms until the rash disappears Infected newborns are usually contagious for many months	Starts on the face and neck Spreads to the trunk, arms, and legs	Fine, pinkish, flat rash Begins 1 or 2 days after the onset of symptoms and lasts 3 to 5 days
Roseola infantum (exanthem subitum or pseudorubella)	About 5 to 15 days	Unknown	Affects the chest and abdomen, with moderate involvement of the face, arms, and legs	Red and flat, possibly with raised areas Begins on about the 4th day, appearing as body temperature drops suddenly to normal, and lasts for a few hours to 2 days
Erythema infectiosum (fifth disease or parvovirus B19 infection)	4 to 14 days	From before the onset of the rash until a few days after	Starts on the cheeks Spreads to the arms, legs, and trunk	Red and flat with raised areas, often blotchy and with lacy patterns Begins shortly after the onset of symptoms and lasts 5 to 10 days May recur for several weeks
Chickenpox (varicella)	11 to 15 days	From a few days before the onset of symptoms until all spots have crusted	Usually appears first on the face and trunk Appears later on the neck, arms, legs, and scalp and infrequently on the palms and soles	Small, flat, red sores that become raised and form round, fluid-filled blisters against a red background before finally crusting Appears in crops, so various stages are present simultaneously Begins shortly after the onset of symptoms and lasts a few days to 2 weeks

The symptoms and treatment of viral meningitis (see page 756) and encephalitis (see page 760) in older children and adolescents are similar to those in adults. Because the immune system is still developing in newborns and infants, different infections can occur, and infants' inability to communicate directly makes it difficult to understand their symptoms. Usually, however, infants with central nervous system infections have some of the symptoms described below.

Symptoms

Viral central nervous system infections in newborns and infants usually begin with fever. Newborns may have no other symptoms and may initially not otherwise appear ill. Infants older than a month or so

Enteroviral Infections: Common in Childhood

The enteroviruses include numerous strains of coxsackievirus, echovirus, enterovirus, and poliovirus. These viruses are responsible for illness in 10 to 30 million people each year in the United States, primarily in the summer and fall. Infections are highly contagious and typically affect many people in a community, sometimes reaching epidemic proportions. Enteroviral infections are most common among children, particularly those living in conditions of poor hygiene.

The infection begins when material contaminated with the virus is swallowed. The virus then reproduces in the digestive tract. The body's immune defenses stop many infections at this stage, and the result is few or no symptoms. Colds and upper respiratory infections are common outcomes of infection with enteroviruses. Sometimes, the virus survives and spreads into the bloodstream, resulting in fever, headache, sore throat, and, at times, vomiting. People often refer to such illnesses as the "summer flu," although they are not influenza. Some strains of enterovirus also cause a generalized, nonitchy rash on the skin or sores inside the mouth. This type of illness is by far the most common enteroviral infection. Rarely, an enterovirus progresses from this stage to attack a particular organ. The virus can attack many different organs, and the symptoms and severity of disease depend on the specific organ infected. Several diseases are caused by enteroviruses:

- **Hand-foot-and-mouth disease** affects the skin and mucous membranes, causing painful sores to appear inside the mouth, on the hands and feet, and occasionally on the buttocks or genitals.
- **Herpangina** also affects the skin and mucous membranes, causing painful sores on the tongue and the back of the throat.
- **Aseptic meningitis** affects the membranes covering the brain and spinal cord (meninges), causing severe headache, stiff neck, and sensitivity to light.
- **Encephalitis** affects the brain, causing confusion, weakness, seizures, and coma.
- **Paralytic poliomyelitis** affects the nervous system, causing weakness of various muscles.
- **Myocarditis** affects the heart, causing weakness and shortness of breath with exertion.
- **Epidemic pleurodynia** (Bornholm disease) affects the muscles, causing severe intermittent pain in the wall of the lower chest (adults) or upper abdomen (children).
- **Hemorrhagic conjunctivitis** affects the eyes, causing painful, red, runny eyes; bleeding under the conjunctiva; and swollen eyelids.

Enteroviral infections usually resolve completely, but infections of the heart or central nervous system are occasionally fatal. There is no cure. Treatment is directed at relieving symptoms.

---

typically become irritable and fussy and refuse to eat. Vomiting is common. Sometimes the soft spot on top of a newborn's head (fontanelle) bulges, indicating an increase in pressure on the brain. Because irritation of the meninges is worsened by movement, an infant with meningitis may cry more, rather than calm down, when picked up and rocked. Some infants develop a strange, high-pitched cry. Infants with encephalitis often have seizures or make bizarre movements. Infants with severe encephalitis may become lethargic and comatose and then die. An infection with herpes simplex virus, which is often concentrated in only one part of the brain, may lead to seizures or weakness appearing in only one part of the body.

Postinfectious encephalomyelitis may cause many neurologic problems, depending on the part of the brain that is damaged. Children may have weakness of an arm or leg, vision or hearing loss, mental retardation/intellectual disability, or recurring seizures. These symptoms may not be apparent until the child is old enough for the problem to appear during testing. Often the symptoms resolve with time, but occasionally they are permanent.

Diagnosis

Doctors are concerned about the possibility of meningitis or encephalitis in every newborn who has a fever, as well as in an older infant who has a fever and is irritable or otherwise not acting normally. The infants undergo a spinal tap (lumbar puncture—see art on page 635) to obtain cerebrospinal fluid (CSF) for laboratory analysis. In viral infections, the number of lymphocytes (a type of white blood cell) is increased in the CSF, and no bacteria are seen. Immunologic tests that detect antibodies against viruses in samples of CSF may be performed, but these tests take days to complete. Polymerase chain reaction (PCR) techniques are used to identify organisms such as herpesviruses and enteroviruses.

A test of brain waves (electroencephalography—see page 636) can be used to help diagnose encephalitis caused by herpesvirus. Magnetic resonance imaging (MRI) and computed tomography (CT) may help confirm the diagnosis. Very rarely, a biopsy (the removal of tissue samples for examination) of brain tissue is needed to determine whether herpesvirus is the cause.

What Is Kawasaki Disease?

Kawasaki disease causes inflammation in the walls of blood vessels throughout the body. The cause is unknown, but evidence suggests a virus or other infectious organism triggers an abnormal immune system response in genetically predisposed children. Inflammation of blood vessels in the heart causes the most serious problems.

Most children with Kawasaki disease range in age from 1 to 8 years, although infants and adolescents can be affected. Roughly twice as many boys as girls are affected. The illness is more common among children of Japanese descent. Several thousand cases of Kawasaki disease are estimated to occur in the United States every year.

The illness begins with fever—usually above 102° F (38.9° C)—which rises and falls over 1 to 3 weeks. Within a day or two, the eyes become red but without any discharge. Within 5 days, a red, patchy rash usually appears over the trunk, around the diaper area, and on mucous membranes, such as the lining of the mouth or vagina. The child has a red throat; reddened, dry, cracked lips; and a strawberry-red tongue. Also, the palms and soles turn red or purplish red, and the hands and feet often swell. The skin on the fingers and toes begins to peel about 10 days after the illness starts. The lymph nodes in the neck are often swollen and slightly tender. The illness may last from 2 to 12 weeks or longer.

About 50% of children develop problems involving the heart, such as a rapid or irregular heart beat, usually beginning 1 to 4 weeks after the onset of illness. Half of the children with heart problems develop the most serious heart problem, coronary artery aneurysm (a bulge in the wall of a coronary artery). These aneurysms can rupture or provoke a blood clot, leading to a heart attack and sudden death. Other problems include inflammation of the tissues lining the brain (meningitis), joints, and gallbladder. These symptoms eventually resolve without causing permanent damage. Doctors perform an ultrasound of the heart to detect coronary artery aneurysms.

Children recover completely if their coronary arteries are not affected within the first 8 weeks of illness. For those with coronary artery problems, survival varies with the severity of disease. With treatment, fewer than 0.01% of children with Kawasaki disease in the United States die. Without treatment, the death rate may reach 1%. Of those who die, death typically occurs in the first few months but can occur decades afterward. About 50% of the aneurysms resolve within 1 year. Large aneurysms are less likely to resolve. However, even the ones that resolve may lead to an increased risk of heart problems in adulthood.

Treatment given within 10 days of symptoms significantly reduces the risk of coronary artery damage and speeds the resolution of fever, rash, and discomfort. For 1 to 4 days, high doses of immune globulin are given by vein, and high doses of aspirin are given by mouth. Once the fever is gone, a lower dose of aspirin is usually continued for at least 8 weeks. If there are no coronary artery aneurysms and signs of inflammation are gone, aspirin may be stopped. However, children with coronary artery abnormalities require continuous and long-term treatment with aspirin. An annual influenza vaccination is indicated for children (6 months of age or older) receiving long-term treatment with aspirin. If the child contracts influenza or chickenpox, dipyridamole is sometimes used temporarily instead of aspirin to lessen the risk of Reye's syndrome—see box on page 1769.

Children with large coronary aneurysms may be treated with anticoagulant drugs such as warfarin or dipyridamole. Some children may even require coronary artery bypass grafting or, rarely, a heart transplant.

Prognosis and Treatment

Prognosis varies greatly with the type of infection. Many types of viral meningitis and encephalitis are mild, and the child recovers quickly and completely. Other types are severe. Infection with herpes simplex virus is particularly grave. Even with treatment, 15% of newborns with herpes simplex infection of the brain die. If the herpes infection involves other parts of the body as well as the brain, mortality is as high as 50%. Nearly 30% of the survivors have permanent neurologic disability of some kind.

Most infants require only supportive care—they need to be kept warm and given plenty of fluids. Antiviral drugs are not effective for most central nervous system infections. However, infections caused by herpes simplex virus can be treated with acyclovir given by vein.

Chickenpox

Chickenpox (varicella) is a highly contagious infection with the varicella-zoster virus that causes a characteristic itchy rash, consisting of small, raised, blistered, or crusted spots.

- Chickenpox is caused by the varicella-zoster virus.
- Before the rash appears, children have a mild headache, moderate fever, loss of appetite, and a general feeling of illness.
- The diagnosis is based on symptoms, particularly the rash.
- Most children recover completely, although some children get very sick and can even die.
- Routine vaccination can prevent chickenpox.
- Usually, only the symptoms need to be treated.

Chickenpox is an infection that mostly affects children. Before the introduction of a vaccine in 1995, about 90% of children developed chickenpox by age 15. Now, the use of the vaccine has decreased the number of cases of chickenpox per year by about 70%. The disease is spread by airborne droplets of moisture containing the varicella-zoster virus. A person with chickenpox is most contagious just after symptoms start but remains contagious until the last blisters have crusted.

Although most people with chickenpox simply have sores on the skin and in the mouth, the virus sometimes infects the lungs, brain, heart, or joints. Such serious infections are more common among newborns, adults, and people with an impaired immune system.

A person who has had chickenpox develops immunity and cannot contract it again. However, the varicella-zoster virus remains dormant in the body after an initial infection with chickenpox, sometimes reactivating in later life, causing shingles. A vaccine against varicella-zoster is available for older adults, which may decrease the risk of developing shingles in later life.

Symptoms and Diagnosis

Symptoms begin 11 to 15 days after infection. They include mild headache, moderate fever, loss of appetite, and a general feeling of illness (malaise). Younger children often do not have these symptoms, but symptoms are often severe in adults.

About 24 to 36 hours after the first symptoms begin, a rash of small, flat, red spots appears. The spots usually begin on the trunk and face, later appearing on the arms and legs. Some children have only a few spots. Others have them almost everywhere, including on the scalp and inside the mouth. Within 6 to 8 hours, each spot becomes raised; forms an itchy, round, fluid-filled blister against a red background; and finally crusts. Spots continue to develop and crust for several days. The spots may become infected by bacteria, causing erysipelas, pyoderma, cellulitis, or bullous impetigo. New spots usually stop appearing by the fifth day, the majority are crusted by the sixth day, and most disappear in fewer than 20 days.

Spots in the mouth quickly rupture and form raw sores (ulcers), which often make swallowing painful. Raw sores may also occur on the eyelids and in the upper airways, rectum, and vagina. Spots in the voice box (larynx) and upper airways may occasionally cause severe difficulty in breathing. Lymph nodes at the side of the neck may become enlarged and tender. The worst part of the illness usually lasts 4 to 7 days.

Lung infection occurs in about 1 out of 400 people, especially adolescents and adults, resulting in cough and difficulty breathing. Brain infection (encephalitis) is less common and causes unsteadiness in walking, headache, dizziness, confusion, and seizures. Heart infection sometimes causes a heart murmur. Joint inflammation causes joint pain. Inflammation of the liver and problems with bleeding may also occur.

Reye's syndrome, a rare but very severe complication that occurs almost only in those younger than 18, may begin 3 to 8 days after the rash begins.

A doctor is usually certain of the diagnosis of chickenpox because the rash and the other symptoms are so typical. Measurement of the levels of antibodies in the blood and laboratory identification of the virus are rarely needed.

Prognosis

Healthy children nearly always recover from chickenpox without problems—only about 2 out of 100,000 children die. However, even this low rate means that before routine immunization, 100 children died annually in the United States because of complications of chickenpox. The infection is more severe in adults, of whom about 30 out of 100,000 die. Chickenpox is fatal in up to 15% of people with an impaired immune system.

Prevention

In the United States, children are routinely vaccinated against varicella-zoster beginning at 12 months of age, with a second dose given at 4 to 6 years of age (see box on page 1685). Older children without immunity also may be vaccinated. Susceptible people who are at high risk of complications (such as those with an impaired immune system and pregnant women) and who have been exposed to someone with chickenpox may be given antibodies against the varicella virus (varicella-zoster immune globulin). Isolation of an infected person helps prevent the spread of infection to people who have not had chickenpox. Children should not return to school and adults should not return to work until the final blisters have crusted.

Treatment

Mild cases of chickenpox require only the treatment of symptoms. Wet compresses on the skin help soothe itching, which may be intense, and prevent scratching, which may spread the infection and cause scars. Because of the risk of bacterial infection, the skin is bathed often with soap and water, the hands are kept clean, the nails are clipped to minimize scratching, and clothing is kept clean and dry. Drugs that relieve itching, such as antihistamines, are sometimes given by mouth. If a bacterial infection develops, antibiotics may be needed.

Doctors may prescribe antiviral drugs, such as acyclovir, valacyclovir, and famciclovir, for adolescents and adults as well as for groups at high risk of complications, such as people with skin disorders like eczema, people who are being treated with aspirin or corticosteroids, premature infants, and children with immune system disorders. The drugs must be given within 24 hours of the start of disease to be effective. These antiviral drugs are usually not given to pregnant women.

> **Did You Know...**
> Antibiotics cannot cure viral infections.

Erythema Infectiosum

Erythema infectiosum (fifth disease, parvovirus B19 infection) is a contagious viral infection that causes a blotchy or raised red rash with mild illness.

- Erythema infectiosum is caused by a virus.
- Symptoms include a mild fever; slapped-cheek red rash on the face; and a lacy rash on the arms, legs, and trunk.
- The diagnosis is based on the characteristic rash.
- Treatment aims to relieve symptoms.

Erythema infectiosum is caused by human parvovirus B19 and occurs most often during the spring months, often in geographically limited outbreaks among children and adolescents. Infection is spread mainly by breathing in small droplets that have been breathed out by an infected person. The infection can also be transmitted from mother to fetus during pregnancy, rarely resulting in stillbirth or severe anemia and excess fluid and swelling (edema) in the fetus (hydrops fetalis).

Symptoms begin about 4 to 14 days after infection but many children have none. However, some have a low fever and feel mildly ill for a few days. Seven to 10 days later, children develop red cheeks that often look like they have been slapped as well as a rash, especially on the arms, legs, and trunk but not usually on the palms or soles. The rash can be itchy and consists of raised, blotchy red areas and lacy patterns, particularly on areas of the arms not covered by clothing, because the rash may be worsened by exposure to sunlight.

The rash usually lasts 5 to 10 days. Over the next several weeks, the rash may temporarily reappear in response to sunlight, exercise, heat, fever, or emotional stress. In adolescents, mild joint pain and swelling may remain or come and go for weeks to months.

Erythema infectiosum can also manifest in a different way, particularly in children with sickle cell disease or in children with immunodeficiency diseases, such as acquired immunodeficiency syndrome (AIDS). The virus can affect the bone marrow and cause severe anemia.

A doctor bases the diagnosis on the characteristic appearance of the rash. Blood tests can help identify the virus, although these are rarely performed. Treatment is aimed at relieving the symptoms.

Human Immunodeficiency Virus Infection

Human immunodeficiency virus (HIV) infection is a viral infection that progressively destroys certain white blood cells and causes acquired immunodeficiency syndrome (AIDS).

- HIV infection is caused by the viruses HIV-1 and HIV-2 and, in young children, is typically acquired from the mother.
- Signs of infection include slowed growth, developmental delay, recurring bacterial infections, and lung inflammation.
- The diagnosis is based on special blood tests.
- Children who receive anti-HIV drug therapy can live to early adulthood.
- Infected mothers can prevent transmitting the infection to their newborns by taking anti-HIV drugs, formula feeding, and undergoing a cesarean delivery.
- Children are treated with the same drugs as adults.

Only about 2% of the people infected with HIV in the United States are children or adolescents. Worldwide, HIV is a much more common problem among children.

There are two human immunodeficiency viruses—HIV-1 and HIV-2. Both progressively destroy certain types of white blood cells called lymphocytes, which are an important part of the body's immune defenses. When these lymphocytes are destroyed, the body becomes susceptible to attack by many other infectious organisms. Many of the symptoms and complications of HIV infection, including death, are the result of these other infections and not of the HIV infection itself. HIV infection may lead to various troublesome infections with organisms that do not ordinarily infect healthy people. These are termed opportunistic infections, and they may result from viruses, parasites, and—in children, unlike in adults—bacteria.

Acquired immunodeficiency syndrome (AIDS) is the most severe form of HIV infection. A child with HIV infection is considered to have AIDS when at least one complicating illness develops or when there is a significant decline in the body's ability to defend itself from infection.

Transmission of Infection

In young children, HIV infection is nearly always acquired from the mother. Less than 7% of children now living with AIDS acquired the infection from other sources, including blood transfusion (from blood products used to treat hemophilia) or sexual abuse. Because of improved safety measures in blood and blood products, very few current infections result from these mechanisms.

As many as 7,000 HIV-infected women give birth each year in the United States. Without preventive measures, 25 to 33% of them would transmit the infection to their baby. The risk is highest in mothers who acquire the infection during pregnancy, who have more virus in their bodies, or who are severely ill. Transmission often takes place during labor and delivery.

The virus also can be transmitted in breast milk— 12 to 14% of babies not infected at birth acquire HIV infection if they breastfeed from an HIV-infected mother. Most often, transmission occurs in the first few weeks or months of life, although transmission may occur later. Transmission is more likely in mothers who acquire the infection while breastfeeding or who have infection of the breast (mastitis).

In adolescents, transmission is the same as in adults: through sexual intercourse—both heterosexual and homosexual—and through sharing of infected needles while injecting drugs.

The virus is *not* transmitted through food, water, household articles, or social contact in a home, workplace, or school. In very rare cases, HIV has been transmitted by contact with infected blood on the skin. In almost all such cases, the skin surface was broken by scrapes or open sores. Although saliva may contain the virus, transmission of infection by kissing or biting has never been confirmed.

Symptoms

Children born with HIV infection rarely have symptoms for the first few months. If the children remain untreated, only about 20% develop problems during the first or second year of life. For the remaining 80% of children, problems may not appear until age 3 or later even without treatment. With the use of effective anti-HIV drugs, children with HIV infection do not necessarily develop any symptoms of HIV infection. The symptoms of HIV infection acquired during adolescence are similar to those in adults (see page 1258).

The first signs of HIV infection in children are usually slowed growth and a delay of maturation, recurring diarrhea, lung infections, or a fungal infection of the mouth (thrush). Sometimes children have repeated episodes of bacterial infections, such as a middle ear infection (otitis media), sinusitis, or pneumonia.

A variety of symptoms and complications can appear as the child's immune system deteriorates. About one third of HIV-infected children develop lung inflammation (lymphocytic interstitial pneumonitis), with cough and difficulty breathing.

Children born with HIV infection commonly have at least one episode of *Pneumocystis* pneumonia in the first 15 months of life if they are not receiving anti-HIV drugs. More than half of untreated children infected with HIV develop the pneumonia at some time. *Pneumocystis* pneumonia is a major cause of death among children and adults with AIDS.

In a significant number of HIV-infected children, progressive brain damage prevents or delays developmental milestones, such as walking and talking. These children also may have impaired intelligence and a head that is small in relation to their body size. Up to 20% of untreated infected children progressively lose social and language skills and muscle control. They may become partially paralyzed or unsteady on their feet, or their muscles may become somewhat rigid.

Anemia (a low red blood cell count) is common among HIV-infected children and causes them to become weak and tire easily. About 20% of untreated children develop heart problems, such as rapid or irregular heartbeat, or heart failure.

Less commonly, untreated children develop inflammation of the liver (hepatitis) or inflammation of the kidneys (nephritis). Cancers are uncommon in children with AIDS, but non-Hodgkin lymphoma and lymphoma of the brain may occur somewhat more often than in uninfected children. Kaposi's sarcoma, an AIDS-related cancer that affects the skin and internal organs, is extremely rare in children.

Diagnosis

The diagnosis of HIV infection among children begins with the identification of HIV infection in pregnant women through routine prenatal screening. Newborns of mothers with HIV infection or of mothers who are at risk of HIV infection because of lifestyle should be tested. The infants should be tested at frequent intervals—typically in the first 2 days of life, at about 1 month of age, and between 4 months and 6 months of age. Such frequent testing identifies most HIV-infected infants by 6 months of age.

In infants, the standard adult blood tests for HIV antibodies are not helpful, because an infant's blood almost always contains HIV antibodies if the mother is HIV-infected (even if the infant is not). To definitively diagnose HIV infection in children younger than 18 months of age, special blood tests (DNA polymerase chain reaction test) that identify the virus in the blood are used. The standard blood tests are used to diagnose HIV infection in children older than 18 months and in adolescents.

Once HIV infection has been diagnosed, doctors monitor the course of the infection by frequently determining the number of CD4+ lymphocytes (CD4 count, which decreases with worsening infection) and by determining the number of virus particles in the blood (viral load, which increases with worsening infection).

Prognosis

With current drug therapy, most children born today with HIV infection live well beyond age 5 and about 50% live beyond age 10. More and more children are surviving well into adolescence and early adulthood. The prognosis is worse for those in whom the virus is detected early (within the first week of life) or who develop symptoms in the first year of life.

Prevention

The most effective means of preventing infection in newborns is for HIV-infected women to avoid pregnancy. If an infected woman does become pregnant, anti-HIV drugs are fairly effective at minimizing transmission. Women who do not meet criteria for combination therapy with three anti-HIV drugs are given zidovudine (ZDV, also called AZT) by mouth during the 2nd and 3rd trimesters (last 6 months) of pregnancy. ZDV is also given by vein (intravenously) during labor and delivery. ZDV is then given daily to the newborn for 6 weeks. This treatment reduces the rate of transmission from about 33% to about 8%. The rate is less than 2% in women receiving combination therapy. Also, cesarean delivery reduces the baby's risk of acquiring HIV infection.

In countries where good infant formulas and clean water are readily available, HIV-infected mothers should bottle-feed their babies and should be strongly discouraged from donating to milk banks. In countries where the risks of undernutrition or infectious diarrhea from unclean water are high, the benefits of breastfeeding outweigh the risk of HIV transmission.

Because a child's HIV status may not be known, all schools and day care centers should adopt special procedures for handling accidents, such as nosebleeds, and for cleaning and disinfecting surfaces contaminated with blood. During cleanup, personnel are advised to avoid having their skin come in contact with blood. Latex gloves should be routinely available, and hands should be washed after the gloves are removed. Contaminated surfaces should be cleaned and disinfected with a freshly prepared bleach solution containing 1 part of household bleach to 10 to 100 parts of water.

Prevention for adolescents is the same as for adults (see page 1260). All adolescents should have access to HIV testing and should be taught how HIV is transmitted and how it can be avoided, including abstaining from sex or using safe-sex practices.

Treatment

Drug Treatment: Children are treated with most of the same anti-HIV drugs as adults (see page 1261 and table on page 1262), typically a highly active antiretroviral therapy (HAART) combination of two or more reverse-transcriptase inhibitors and a protease inhibitor. However, not all of the drugs used for adults are available to small children, in part because some are not available in liquid form. It may be difficult for parents and children to follow complicated drug regimens, which can limit the effectiveness of therapy. In general, children develop the same types of side effects as adults but usually at a much lower rate. However, the side effects of drugs may also limit the treatment. A doctor monitors the effectiveness of treatment by regularly measuring the amount of virus present in the blood and the child's CD4$^+$ cell count (see page 1258). Increased numbers of virus in the blood may be a sign that the virus is developing resistance to the drugs or that the child is not taking the drugs. In either case, the doctor may need to change the drugs.

Prevention of Opportunistic Infections: To prevent *Pneumocystis* pneumonia, doctors give trimethoprim-sulfamethoxazole to all children with proven HIV infection and a significantly impaired immune system and to all infants born to HIV-infected women beginning at 4 to 6 weeks of age (continued until testing shows the infants are not infected). Children 5 years old and older who cannot tolerate trimethoprim-sulfamethoxazole can be given pentamidine. Dapsone is an alternative drug for children younger than 5 years who cannot tolerate trimethoprim-sulfamethoxazole.

Children with a significantly impaired immune system also are given azithromycin or clarithromycin to prevent *Mycobacterium avium* complex infection. Rifabutin is an alternative drug. Children with recurring bacterial infections may be given immune globulin by vein once a month.

Vaccination: Nearly all HIV-infected children should receive the routine childhood vaccinations, including diphtheria, tetanus, and pertussis (DTaP); inactivated polio vaccine; *Haemophilus influenzae*; *Streptococcus pneumoniae*; and hepatitis B. Vaccines containing live viruses such as the oral polio virus, varicella, and measles-mumps-rubella can cause a severe or fatal illness in children with HIV whose immune system is very impaired. However, the measles-mumps-rubella vaccine and varicella vaccine are recommended for children with HIV infection whose immune system is not severely impaired. Yearly influenza immunization is also recommended for all HIV-infected children over 6 months of age. However, the effectiveness of any vaccination will be less in children with HIV infection.

Social Issues: For children who need foster care, child care, or schooling, a doctor can help assess the child's risk of exposure to infectious diseases. In general, transmission of infections, such as chickenpox, to the HIV-infected child (or to any child with an impaired immune system) is more of a danger than is transmission of HIV from that child to others. A young child with HIV infection who has open skin sores or who engages in potentially dangerous behavior, such as biting, should not attend child care.

HIV-infected children should participate in as many routine childhood activities as their physical condition allows. Interaction with other children enhances social development and self-esteem. Because of the stigma associated with the illness and the fact that transmission of the infection to other children is extremely unlikely, there is no need for anyone other than the parents, the doctor, and perhaps the school nurse to be aware of the child's HIV status.

As a child's condition worsens, treatment is best given in the least restrictive environment possible. If home health care and social services are available, the child can spend more time at home rather than in a hospital.

Measles

Measles (rubeola, 9-day measles) is a highly contagious viral infection that causes various symptoms and a characteristic rash.

- Measles is caused by a virus.
- Symptoms include fever, runny nose, hacking cough, red eyes, and a red itchy rash.
- The diagnosis is based on typical symptoms and characteristic rash.
- Measles is rarely serious in healthy children, although occasionally it can be fatal or lead to brain damage.
- Routine vaccination can prevent the infection.
- Treatment aims to relieve symptoms.

Children become infected with measles by breathing in small airborne droplets of moisture coughed out by an infected person or by touching items contaminated by such droplets. Measles is contagious from several days before until several days after the rash appears.

Before vaccination became widely available, measles epidemics occurred every 2 or 3 years, particularly in preschool-aged and school-aged children. Small, localized outbreaks occurred during intervening years. Although measles is still common in other countries, only about 100 to 300 people a year in the United States develop measles. A woman who has had measles or has been vaccinated passes immunity (in the form of antibodies) to her child. This immunity lasts for most of the first year of life. Thereafter, however, susceptibility to measles is high unless vaccination is given. A person who has had measles develops immunity and cannot contract it again.

Symptoms and Diagnosis

The symptoms of measles begin about 7 to 14 days after infection. The infected child first develops a fever, runny nose, hacking cough, and red eyes. Sometimes the eyes are sensitive to bright light. Tiny white spots (Koplik's spots) appear inside the mouth 2 to 4 days later, and then the child develops a sore throat.

A mildly itchy rash appears 3 to 5 days after the start of symptoms. The rash begins in front of and below the ears and on the side of the neck as irregular, flat, red areas that soon become raised. The rash spreads within 1 to 2 days to the trunk, arms, palms, legs, and soles and begins to fade on the face.

At the peak of the illness, the child feels very sick and develops eye inflammation (conjunctivitis), the rash is extensive, and the temperature may exceed 104° F (40° C). In 3 to 5 days, the temperature falls, the child begins to feel better, and any remaining rash quickly fades. The diagnosis is based on the typical symptoms and characteristic rash.

Brain infection (encephalitis) occurs in about 1 out of 1,000 to 2,000 children with measles. If encephalitis occurs, it often starts with a high fever, headache, seizures, and coma, usually 2 days to 1 week after the rash appears. The illness may be brief, with recovery in about 1 week, or it may be prolonged, resulting in brain damage or death.

Secondary bacterial infections, such as pneumonia (especially in infants) or a middle ear infection (otitis media), occur fairly often. Rarely, blood platelet levels become so low that the child bruises and bleeds.

Prognosis

In healthy, well-nourished children, measles is rarely serious. However, secondary bacterial infections, particularly pneumonia, can occasionally be fatal. In rare cases, subacute sclerosing panencephalitis—a serious complication of measles—occurs months to years later, resulting in brain damage (see page 1783).

Prevention

Measles vaccine, one of the routine immunizations of childhood, is given between 12 and 15 months of age (see box on page 1685) but can be given to children as young as 6 months during a measles outbreak. Children (and adults) who are exposed to measles and do not have immunity may be protected by vaccination within 3 days of exposure. Pregnant women and infants younger than 1 year should not receive the vaccine in a non-outbreak situation and instead are given measles immune globulin for protection.

Treatment

There is no specific treatment for measles. Some doctors in the United States give vitamin A to children aged 6 months to 2 years who are hospitalized with measles, because vitamin A has reduced the number of deaths from measles in countries where vitamin A deficiency is common. Children with measles are kept warm and comfortable. Acetaminophen or ibuprofen may be given to reduce fever. If a secondary bacterial infection develops, an antibiotic is given.

Did You Know...

Routine vaccination can prevent many viral infections.

Mumps

Mumps (epidemic parotitis) is a contagious viral infection that causes painful enlargement of the salivary glands. The infection may also affect the testes, brain, and pancreas, especially in adults.

- Mumps is caused by a virus.
- Symptoms include chills, headache, poor appetite, fever, and a feeling of illness, followed by swelling of the salivary glands.
- The diagnosis is based on typical symptoms.
- Most children recover with no problems; however, infection can lead to meningitis or encephalitis.
- Routine vaccination can prevent the infection.
- Treatment aims to relieve symptoms.

Children become infected with mumps by breathing in small airborne droplets of moisture coughed out by an infected person or by having direct contact with objects contaminated by infected saliva. Mumps is less contagious than measles or chickenpox. In heavily populated areas, it occurs year-round but is most frequent in late winter and early spring. Epidemics may occur when people without immunity are crowded together. Although the infection may occur at any age, most cases occur in children 5 to 10 years old. The infection is unusual in children younger than 2 years. One infection with the mumps virus usually provides lifelong immunity.

Symptoms and Diagnosis

Symptoms begin 14 to 24 days after infection. Most children develop chills, headache, poor appetite, a general feeling of illness (malaise), and a low to moderate fever. These symptoms are followed in 12 to 24 hours by swelling of the salivary glands, which is most prominent on the second day and lasts 5 to 7 days. Some children simply have swelling of the salivary glands without the other symptoms. The swelling results in pain when chewing or swallowing, particularly when swallowing acidic liquids, such as citrus fruit juices. The glands are tender when touched. At this stage, the temperature usually rises to 103 or 104° F (about 39.4 or 40° C) and lasts 1 to 3 days.

About 20% of men who become infected after puberty develop inflammation of one or both testes (orchitis). Inflammation of the testes causes severe pain. Once healed, the affected testis may be smaller, but testosterone production and fertility are usually unaffected.

Mumps leads to inflammation of the layers of tissue covering the brain (meningitis) in 1 to 10% of people. Meningitis causes headache, vomiting, and a stiff neck. Mumps also causes inflammation of the brain (encephalitis) in 1 out of 1,000 to 5,000 people. Encephalitis causes drowsiness, coma, or seizures. Most people recover completely, but some have permanent nerve or brain damage, such as nerve deafness or paralysis of the facial muscles, usually affecting only one side of the body.

Inflammation of the pancreas (pancreatitis) may occur toward the end of the first week of infection. This disorder causes abdominal pain, nausea, and vomiting, which varies from mild to severe. These symptoms disappear in about a week, and the person recovers completely.

Doctors diagnose mumps based on the typical symptoms, particularly when they occur during an outbreak of mumps. Laboratory tests can identify the mumps virus and its antibodies, but such tests are rarely needed to make the diagnosis.

Prognosis

Almost all children with mumps recover fully without problems, but in rare cases symptoms may worsen again after about 2 weeks.

Prevention

Because vaccination against mumps is routine in childhood, beginning at 12 to 15 months of age (see box on page 1685), fewer than 300 cases usually occur each year. However, a 2006 mumps outbreak in the midwestern United States caused more than 2,500 cases in 4 months. Young adults had the highest infection rates, which highlighted the need for continued use of vaccination.

Treatment

Once the infection has started, it just has to run its course. To minimize discomfort, children should avoid foods that require much chewing or are acidic. Analgesics, such as acetaminophen and ibuprofen, may be used for headache and discomfort.

Boys or men with inflammation of the testes need bed rest. The scrotum may be supported with an athletic supporter or by an adhesive-tape bridge connected between the thighs. Ice packs may be applied to relieve pain.

If pancreatitis causes severe nausea and vomiting, fluids may be given by vein (intravenously), and intake by mouth should be avoided for a few days. Children with meningitis or encephalitis may need intravenous fluids and acetaminophen or ibuprofen for a fever or headache. If seizures develop, anticonvulsant drugs may be needed.

Polio

Polio (poliomyelitis, infantile paralysis) is a highly contagious, sometimes fatal, viral infection that affects nerves and can cause permanent muscle weakness, paralysis, and other symptoms.

- Polio is caused by a virus and is spread by digesting contaminated material.
- Serious symptoms include fever, headache, a stiff neck and back, deep muscle pain, and sometimes weakness or paralysis.
- The diagnosis is based on symptoms and the results of a stool culture.
- Some children recover completely, whereas others have permanent weakness.
- Routine vaccination can prevent the infection.
- There is no cure for polio.

Polio is caused by poliovirus, an enterovirus, which is spread by swallowing material contaminated by the virus. The infection spreads from the intestine to the parts of the brain and spinal cord that control the muscles.

In the early 20th century, polio was widespread throughout the United States. Today, because of extensive vaccination, polio outbreaks have largely disappeared, and most doctors have never seen a new polio infection. The last case of wild poliovirus infection in the United States occurred in 1979. The Western Hemisphere was certified polio-free in 1994. A global polio eradication program is under way, but cases still occur in sub-Saharan Africa and southern Asia. Unimmunized people of all ages are susceptible to polio. In the past, polio outbreaks occurred mainly in children and adolescents, because many older people had already been exposed to the virus and developed immunity.

Symptoms and Diagnosis

Fewer than 1 out of 60 to 100 infected people develop any symptoms. Of those with symptoms, 80 to 90% simply have fever, mild headache, sore throat, vomiting, and a general feeling of illness (malaise). These symptoms develop 5 to 9 days after exposure to the virus. The remaining 10 to 20% of people have more serious symptoms (major poliomyelitis). Major poliomyelitis is more likely to occur in older children and adults. The symptoms, which usually appear 7 to 14 days after infection, include fever, severe headache, a stiff neck and back, and deep muscle pain. Sometimes areas of skin develop odd sensations, such as pins and needles or unusual sensitivity to pain. Depending on which parts of the brain and spinal cord are affected, the disease may progress no further, or weakness or paralysis may develop in certain muscles. The person may have difficulty swallowing and may choke on saliva, food, or fluids. Sometimes fluids go up into the nose, and the voice may develop a nasal quality. Sometimes the part of the brain responsible for breathing is affected, causing weakness or paralysis of the chest muscles. Some people are completely unable to breathe.

A doctor can diagnose polio by its symptoms. Diagnosis is confirmed by identifying poliovirus in a stool sample or from a throat swab and by detecting high levels of antibodies to the virus in the blood.

Prognosis

People with minor polio completely recover. About two thirds of people with major polio have some permanent weakness. Some people, even those who apparently have recovered completely, develop a return or worsening of muscle weakness years or decades after an attack of polio. This condition (postpolio syndrome) often results in severe disability (see page 817).

Prevention

Polio vaccine is included among the routine childhood immunizations (see box on page 1685). Two types of vaccine are available worldwide: an inactivated poliovirus vaccine (Salk vaccine) given by injection and a live poliovirus vaccine (Sabin vaccine) taken by mouth. The live oral vaccine provides better immunity in a population but can mutate and cause polio in about 1 out of every 2.4 million children. Because polio has been eradicated in the United States, doctors recommend only the injected vaccine for children in this country. The oral vaccine is no longer available in the United States but is used in other parts of the world.

A first vaccination of people older than 18 is not routinely recommended because the risk of acquiring polio as an adult is extremely low in the United States. Adults who have never been vaccinated and who are traveling to an area where polio is still a health risk should receive the injected vaccine. Local and state health departments have information about which areas have polio.

Treatment

Polio cannot be cured, and available antiviral drugs do not affect the course of the disease. A ventilator may be needed if the muscles used in breathing are weakened. Often, the need for a ventilator is temporary.

Respiratory Tract Infections

Respiratory tract infections affect the nose, throat, and airways and may be caused by any of several different viruses.

- Common respiratory tract infections include the common cold and influenza.
- Typical symptoms include nasal congestion, a runny nose, scratchy throat, cough, and irritability.
- The diagnosis is based on symptoms.
- Good hygiene is the best way to prevent these infections, and routine vaccination can prevent influenza.
- Treatment aims to relieve symptoms.

Children develop on average six viral respiratory tract infections each year. Viral respiratory tract infections include the common cold (see page 1239) and influenza (see page 1240). Doctors often refer to these as upper respiratory infections (URIs), because they cause symptoms mainly in the nose and throat. In small children, viruses also commonly cause infections of the lower respiratory tract—the windpipe, airways, and lungs. These infections include croup, bronchiolitis, and pneumonia. Children sometimes have infections involving both the upper and lower respiratory tracts.

In children, rhinoviruses, influenza viruses (during annual winter epidemics), parainfluenza viruses, respiratory syncytial virus (RSV), enteroviruses, and certain strains of adenovirus are the main causes of viral respiratory infections.

Most often, viral respiratory tract infections spread when children's hands come into contact with nasal secretions from an infected person. These secretions contain viruses. When the children touch their mouth, nose, or eyes, the viruses gain entry and produce a new infection. Less often, infections spread when children breathe air containing droplets that were coughed or sneezed out by an infected person. For various reasons, nasal or respiratory secretions from children with viral respiratory tract infections contain more viruses than those from infected adults. This increased output of viruses, along with typically lesser attention to hygiene, makes children more likely to spread their infection to others. The possibility of transmission is further enhanced when many children are gathered together, such as in child care centers and schools. Contrary to what people may think, other factors, such as becoming chilled, wet, or tired, do not cause colds or increase a child's susceptibility to infection.

Symptoms and Complications

When viruses invade cells of the respiratory tract, they trigger inflammation and production of mucus. This situation leads to nasal congestion, a runny nose, scratchy throat, and cough, which may last up to 14 days. Fever, with a temperature as high as 101 to 102° F (about 38.3 to 38.9° C), is common. The child's temperature may even rise to 104° F (40° C). Other typical symptoms in children include decreased appetite, lethargy, and a general feeling of illness (malaise). Headaches and body aches develop, particularly with influenza. Infants and young children are usually not able to communicate their specific symptoms and just appear cranky and uncomfortable.

Because newborns and young infants prefer to breathe through their nose, even moderate nasal congestion can create difficulty breathing. Nasal congestion leads to feeding problems as well, because infants cannot breathe while suckling from the breast or bottle. Because infants are unable to spit out mucus that they cough up, they often gag and choke.

The small airways of young children can be significantly narrowed by inflammation and mucus, making breathing difficult. Children breathe rapidly and may develop a high-pitched noise heard on breathing out (wheezing) or a similar noise heard on breathing in (stridor). Severe airway narrowing may cause children to gasp for breath and turn blue (cyanosis). Such airway problems are most common with infection caused by parainfluenza viruses and RSV. Affected children need to be seen urgently by a doctor.

Some children with a viral respiratory tract infection also develop an infection of the middle ear (otitis media) or the lung tissue (pneumonia). Otitis media and pneumonia may be caused by the virus itself or by a bacterial infection that develops because the inflammation caused by the virus makes tissue more susceptible to invasion by other germs. In children with asthma, respiratory tract infections often lead to an asthma attack.

Diagnosis

Doctors and parents recognize respiratory tract infections by their typical symptoms. Generally, otherwise healthy children with mild upper respiratory tract symptoms do not need to see a doctor unless they have trouble breathing, are not drinking, or have a fever for more than a day or two. X-rays of the neck and chest may be taken in children who have difficulty breathing, stridor, wheezing, or audible lung congestion. Blood tests and tests of respiratory secretions are rarely helpful.

Prevention and Treatment

The best preventive measure is practicing good hygiene. An ill child and the people in the household should wash their hands frequently. In general, the more intimate physical contact (such as hugging, snuggling, or bed sharing) that takes place with an ill child, the greater the risk of spreading the infection to other family members. Parents must balance this risk with the need to comfort an ill child. Children should stay home from school or child care until the fever is gone and they feel well enough to attend.

Influenza is the only viral respiratory infection preventable by vaccination. All children aged 6 to 59 months should receive a yearly vaccination, as should older children with certain disorders. Such disorders include heart or lung disease (including cystic fibrosis and asthma), diabetes, kidney failure, and sickle cell disease. Additionally, children whose immune system is compromised (including children with human immunodeficiency virus [HIV] infection and those undergoing chemotherapy) should receive the vaccine.

Antibiotics are not necessary to treat viral respiratory tract infections. Children with respiratory tract infections need additional rest and should maintain normal fluid intake. Acetaminophen or nonsteroidal anti-inflammatory drugs (NSAIDs), such as ibuprofen, can be given for fever and aches. School-aged children may take a nonprescription (over-the-counter) decongestant for bothersome nasal congestion, although the drug often does not help. Infants and younger children are particularly sensitive to the side effects of decongestants and may experience agitation, confusion, hallucinations, lethargy, and rapid heart rate. In infants and young children, congestion may be relieved somewhat by using a cool-mist vaporizer to humidify the air and by suctioning the mucus from the nose with a rubber suction bulb.

RESPIRATORY SYNCYTIAL VIRUS

Respiratory syncytial virus causes upper and lower respiratory tract infections.

- Respiratory syncytial virus is a very common cause of respiratory infections in children.
- Typical symptoms include a runny nose, fever, cough, and wheezing, and a severe infection can lead to respiratory distress.
- The diagnosis is based on symptoms and their occurrence at expected times of year.
- Palivizumab is given to children at high risk of developing a severe infection.
- Oxygen and drugs are given only to children that develop breathing problems.

Respiratory syncytial virus (RSV) is a very common cause of respiratory tract infection, particularly in children. Nearly all children have been infected by age 4 years, many in the first year of life. Infection does not provide complete immunity, so reinfection is common, although usually less serious. Outbreaks typically occur in winter and early spring.

The first infection often involves the lower respiratory tract, most commonly causing bronchiolitis (see page 1786). Later infections usually involve only the upper respiratory tract. Children who have had bronchiolitis have an increased risk of developing asthma when they are older. Children with serious underlying disorders (such as congenital heart disease, asthma, cystic fibrosis, or immune system suppression) or who were born prematurely are at particular risk of developing serious illness. Adults are also infected with RSV, and the elderly may develop pneumonia.

Symptoms and Diagnosis

A runny nose and fever begin 3 to 5 days after infection. About half of children with a first infection also develop a cough and wheezing, indicating lower respiratory tract involvement. In infants younger than 6 months old, the first symptom may be a period of not breathing (apnea). Some children, usually young infants, develop severe respiratory distress, and a few die.

Doctors usually recognize RSV infection when the typical symptoms occur at the expected time of year or during an outbreak. Tests are usually not performed unless doctors are trying to identify an outbreak. When necessary, samples of nasal secretions are sent for a rapid antigen test.

Prevention and Treatment

Doctors may give monthly injections of palivizumab, which contains antibodies against RSV, to children who are at high risk of developing a severe RSV infection. Children who receive palivizumab are less likely to need hospitalization, but doctors are not sure whether this treatment prevents death or serious complications.

Children who have difficulty breathing are taken to a hospital. Depending on their condition, doctors may treat them with oxygen and drugs, such as albuterol or epinephrine, to open the airways (bronchodilators). Ribavirin, an antiviral drug, is no longer recommended except for children whose immune system is severely compromised.

Roseola Infantum

Roseola infantum (exanthem subitum, pseudorubella) is a viral infection of infants or very young children that causes a high fever followed by a rash.

Roseola infantum occurs throughout the year, sometimes in local outbreaks. The usual cause is herpesvirus 6, one of the many human herpesviruses. Most children who develop roseola infantum are between 6 months and 3 years of age.

Symptoms begin about 5 to 15 days after infection. A fever of 103 to 105° F (about 39.4 to 40.5° C) begins abruptly and lasts for 3 to 5 days. In 5 to 15% of children, seizures occur as a result of high fever, particularly as the fever begins and rises quickly. Despite the high fever, the child is usually alert and active. A few children have a mild runny nose, sore throat, or an upset stomach. The lymph nodes at the back of the head, the sides of the neck, and behind the ears may be enlarged. The fever usually disappears on the fourth day.

About 30% of children develop a rash within a few hours to, at most, a day after the temperature falls. The rash is red and flat, but it may have raised areas, mostly on the chest and abdomen and less extensively on the face, arms, and legs. The rash is not itchy and may last from a few hours to 2 days.

A doctor bases the diagnosis on the symptoms. Antibody tests and a culture of the virus are rarely needed.

Fever is treated with acetaminophen or ibuprofen. The seizures and rash do not require any specific treatment but because they are frightening, most parents bring their child to the doctor for evaluation. If the disease is severe in children with a compromised immune system, doctors may try treating them with the antiviral drugs foscarnet or ganciclovir.

Rotavirus Infection

Rotavirus is a common and contagious virus that causes vomiting and diarrhea.

Rotavirus is one of the most common causes of diarrhea in children. In the United States, about 50,000 children each year are hospitalized for diarrhea caused by rotavirus. Although hardly any children die in the United States from rotavirus, worldwide the virus causes over 600,000 deaths a year, mostly in developing countries. Infection is spread mainly by swallowing material contaminated by the virus. Adults can become infected, but serious illness is rare.

Symptoms begin with fever and vomiting, followed by watery diarrhea, which typically lasts 5 to 7 days. If fluid losses are not replaced, dehydration develops. Dehydration makes the child weak and listless, with a dry mouth and rapid pulse.

Doctors do not usually perform tests to detect rotavirus unless they are trying to identify an outbreak. When necessary, samples of stool are sent for a rapid antigen test.

Practicing good hygiene is the best preventive measure. A sick child and the people in the household should wash their hands frequently. In addition, an oral vaccine to prevent rotavirus infection is now recommended to be given at ages 2, 4, and 6 months.

There is no specific treatment for rotavirus. Most children get better with fluid replacement by mouth (see page 1794). Seriously ill children require fluids given by vein (intravenously).

Rubella

Rubella (German measles, 3-day measles) is a contagious viral infection that causes mild symptoms, such as joint pain and a rash.

- Rubella is caused by a virus and can cause severe birth defects if the mother is infected during pregnancy.
- Typical symptoms include swollen lymph nodes, rose-colored spots on the roof of the mouth, and a characteristic rash.
- The diagnosis is based on symptoms.
- Routine vaccination can prevent rubella.
- Treatment is aimed as relieving the symptoms.

Rubella is a typically mild childhood infection that may, however, have devastating consequences for infants infected before birth. A woman infected during the first 16 weeks (particularly the first 8 to 10 weeks) of pregnancy often passes the infection to the fetus. This fetal infection causes miscarriage, stillbirth, or severe birth defects (see page 1708).

Rubella was once common during spring, with major epidemics infecting millions of people every 6 to 9 years. The disease is now rare in the United States because of widespread vaccination. Nonetheless, some young adult women have never had rubella or rubella vaccination and are thus at risk of having children with serious birth defects if they become infected during early pregnancy.

Rubella is spread mainly by breathing in small virus-containing droplets of moisture that have been coughed into the air by an infected person. Close contact with an infected person can also spread the infection. The infection may be contagious from 7 days before until 14 days after the rash appears, although usually the period of maximal contagiousness is from a few days before symptoms begin until the rash disappears. An infant infected before birth can spread the infection for many months after birth.

Symptoms and Diagnosis

Symptoms begin about 14 to 21 days after infection. Some children feel mildly ill for a few days, with a runny nose, cough, and painless, rose-colored spots on the roof of the mouth. These spots later merge with each other into a red blush extending over the back of the throat. In most children, particularly older ones, the first sign of illness is the development of swollen lymph nodes in the neck and back of the head. A characteristic rash develops about a day later and lasts about 3 to 5 days. The rash begins on the face and neck and quickly spreads to the trunk, arms, and legs. As the rash appears, a mild reddening of the skin (flush) occurs, particularly on the face.

Adults, usually women, may develop arthritis or joint pain with rubella. In rare instances, a middle ear infection (otitis media) develops. Brain infection (encephalitis) is a very rare but occasionally fatal complication.

The diagnosis is based on the typical symptoms. A definite diagnosis, necessary during pregnancy, can be made by measuring levels of antibodies to rubella virus in the blood.

Prevention and Treatment

Rubella vaccine, one of the routine immunizations of childhood, is given beginning at 12 months of age (see box on page 1685). A person who has had rubella develops immunity and cannot contract it again.

Most children with rubella recover fully without treatment. A middle ear infection can be treated with antibiotics. No treatment is available for encephalitis, which must just run its course with supportive care.

Subacute Sclerosing Panencephalitis

Subacute sclerosing panencephalitis, a progressive and usually fatal disorder, is a rare complication of measles that appears months or years later and causes mental deterioration, muscle jerks, and seizures.

- Subacute sclerosing panencephalitis is caused by the measles virus.
- The first symptoms are usually poor school performance, forgetfulness, temper outbursts, distractibility, sleeplessness, and hallucinations.
- The diagnosis is based on symptoms.
- This disorder is usually fatal.
- There is no treatment.

Subacute sclerosing panencephalitis results from a long-term brain infection with the measles virus.

The virus sometimes enters the brain during a measles infection. It may cause immediate symptoms of brain infection (encephalitis), or it may remain in the brain for a long time without causing problems.

Subacute sclerosing panencephalitis occurs because the measles virus reactivates. In the United States, for reasons that are not known, the disorder occurs in about 65 to 110 people out of 1 million who had wild measles infection.

The number of people with subacute sclerosing panencephalitis is declining in the United States and Western Europe just as the number of people with wild measles infection has declined. Males are affected more often than females.

Symptoms and Diagnosis

The disorder usually begins in children or young adults, generally before age 20. The first symptoms may be poor performance in schoolwork, forgetfulness, temper outbursts, distractibility, sleeplessness, and hallucinations. Sudden muscular jerks of the arms, head, or body may occur. Eventually, seizures may occur, together with abnormal uncontrollable muscle movements. Intellect and speech continue to deteriorate. Later, the muscles become increasingly rigid, and swallowing may become difficult. The swallowing difficulty sometimes causes people to choke on their saliva, resulting in pneumonia. People may become blind. In the final phases, the body temperature may rise, and the blood pressure and pulse become abnormal.

A doctor bases the diagnosis on the symptoms. The diagnosis may be confirmed by a blood test that reveals high levels of antibody to the measles virus, by an abnormal electroencephalogram (EEG), or by magnetic resonance imaging (MRI) or computed tomography (CT) that shows brain abnormalities.

Prognosis and Treatment

The disease is nearly always fatal within 1 to 3 years. Although the cause of death is usually pneumonia, the pneumonia results from the extreme weakness and abnormal muscle control caused by the disease.

Nothing can be done to halt progression of the disease. Anticonvulsant drugs may be taken to control or reduce seizures.

271 Respiratory Disorders

Respiratory disorders commonly affect children. The most serious and common are asthma, bronchiolitis, and croup. An uncommon but very serious respiratory disorder is bacterial tracheitis.

Asthma

Asthma is a recurring inflammatory lung disorder in which certain stimuli (triggers) inflame the airways and cause them to temporarily narrow, resulting in difficulty breathing.

- Asthma triggers include smoke, perfume, pollen, mold, dust mites, and viral infections.
- Wheezing, cough, shortness of breath, chest tightness, and difficulty breathing are symptoms of asthma.
- The diagnosis is based on a child's repeated wheezing episodes and a family history of asthma.
- Most children with asthma outgrow the disorder.
- Asthma can be prevented by avoiding triggers.
- Treatment includes bronchodilators and inhaled corticosteroids.

Although asthma can develop at any age, it most commonly begins in children, particularly in the first 5 years of life. Some children continue to have asthma into the adult years. In other children, asthma resolves. Asthma has become much more common in recent decades. Doctors are not sure why this is so, but there are theories. More than 8.5% of children in the United States have been diagnosed with asthma, which is over a 100% increase in recent decades. The rate soars to 25% to 40% among some populations of urban children. Asthma is the leading cause of hospitalization for children and is the number one chronic condition causing elementary school absenteeism.

Most children with asthma are able to participate in normal childhood activities, except during flare-ups. A smaller number of children have moderate or severe asthma and need to take daily preventive drugs to enable them to engage in sports and normal play.

For unknown reasons, children with asthma respond to certain stimuli (triggers) in ways that children without asthma do not. There are many potential triggers, and most children respond to only a few. In some children, specific triggers for flare-ups cannot be identified.

These triggers all result in a similar response. Certain cells in the airways release chemical substances. These substances cause the airways to become inflamed and swollen and stimulate the muscle cells in the walls of the airways to contract. Repeated stimulation by these chemical substances increases mucus production in the airways, causes shedding of the cells lining the airways, and enlarges the muscle cells in the walls of the airways. Each of these responses contributes to a sudden narrowing of the airways (asthma attack). In most children, the airways return to normal between asthma attacks.

Risk Factors

Doctors do not completely understand why some children develop asthma, but a number of risk factors are recognized. A child with one parent who has asthma has a 25% risk of developing asthma. If both parents have asthma, the risk increases to 50%. Children whose mothers smoked during pregnancy are more likely to develop asthma. Asthma also has been linked to other factors related to the mother, such as young maternal age, poor maternal nutrition, and lack of breastfeeding. Prematurity and low birth weight are also risk factors.

In the United States, children in urban environments are more likely to develop asthma, particularly if they are from lower socioeconomic groups. Although it is not entirely understood, it is believed that poorer living conditions, greater potential exposure to triggers, and less access to health care contribute to the higher incidence of asthma in these groups. Although

COMMON ASTHMA TRIGGERS	
TRIGGERS	**EXAMPLES**
Allergens	Dust or house mites, molds, outdoor pollen, animal dander, cockroach feces, and feathers
Exercise	Cold air exposure
Infections	Respiratory viruses and common colds
Irritants	Firsthand and secondhand tobacco smoke, perfumes, wood smoke, cleaning products, scented candles, outdoor air pollution, strong odors, and irritating fumes
Other	Emotions (such as anxiety, anger, and excitement), aspirin, and gastroesophageal reflux

asthma affects a higher percentage of black children than white, the role that genetic aspects of race play in the increasing rate of asthma is controversial because black children are also more likely to live in urban areas.

Children who are exposed to high concentrations of allergens, such as dust mites or cockroach feces, at an early age are more likely to develop asthma. Children who have bronchiolitis (see page 1786) at an early age often wheeze with subsequent viral infections. The wheezing may at first be interpreted as asthma, but these children are no more likely than others to have asthma during adolescence.

Symptoms

As the airways narrow in an asthma attack, the child develops difficulty breathing, chest tightness, and coughing, typically accompanied by wheezing. Wheezing is a high-pitched noise heard when the child breathes out. Not all asthma attacks cause wheezing, however. Mild asthma, particularly in very young children, may result only in a cough. Some older children with mild asthma tend to cough only when exercising or when exposed to cold air. Also, children with extremely severe asthma may not wheeze because there is too little air flowing to make a noise. In a severe attack, breathing becomes visibly difficult, wheezing usually becomes louder, the child breathes faster and with greater effort, and the ribs stand out when the child breathes in (inspiration). With very severe attacks, the child gasps for breath and sits upright, leaning forward. The skin is sweaty and pale or blue-tinged. Children with frequent severe attacks sometimes have a slowing of their growth, but their growth usually catches up to that of other children by adulthood.

Diagnosis

A doctor suspects asthma in children who have repeated episodes of wheezing, particularly when family members are known to have asthma or allergies. Doctors usually take x-rays, and they sometimes do allergy testing to help determine the cause.

Children with frequent wheezing episodes may be tested for other disorders, such as cystic fibrosis or gastroesophageal reflux. Older children sometimes undergo pulmonary function tests (see page 454), although in most children, pulmonary function is normal between flare-ups.

Older children or adolescents known to have asthma often use a peak flow meter (a small device that records how fast a person can blow out air) to measure the degree of airway obstruction. Doctors and parents can use this measurement to assess the child's condition during an attack and between attacks. X-rays are not done during an attack in children known to have asthma unless doctors suspect another disorder such as pneumonia or a collapsed lung.

Did You Know...

One speck of dust can contain 40,000 dust mites, which are major triggers of asthma.

Prognosis and Prevention

One half or more of children with asthma outgrow the disorder. Those with more severe disease are more likely to have asthma as adults. Other risk factors for persistence and relapse include female sex, smoking, developing asthma at a younger age, and sensitivity to household dust mites.

Asthma flare-ups often can be prevented by avoiding whatever triggers a particular child's attacks. Parents of children with allergies usually are advised to remove feather pillows, carpets, drapes, upholstered furniture, stuffed toys, and other potential sources of dust mites and allergens from the child's room. Secondhand tobacco smoke often worsens symptoms in children with asthma, so it is important to eliminate smoking in areas where the child spends time. If a particular allergen cannot be avoided, a doctor may try to desensitize the child by using allergy shots, although the benefits of allergy shots for asthma are not well known. Because exercise is so important for a child's development, doctors usually encourage children to maintain physical activities, exercise, and sports participation and use an asthma drug immediately before exercising if needed.

Treatment

Treatment of an acute attack consists of

- Opening the airways (bronchodilation)
- Stopping inflammation

A variety of inhaled drugs open the airways (bronchodilators—see table on page 479). Typical examples are albuterol and ipratropium. Doctors do not recommend using long-acting bronchodilators, such as salmeterol and formoterol, as the only treatment for children. Older children and adolescents usually can take these drugs using a metered-dose inhaler. Children younger than 8 years or so often find it easier to use an inhaler with a spacer or holding chamber attached (see art on page 476). Infants and very young children sometimes can use an inhaler and spacer if an infant-sized mask is attached. Those who cannot use inhalers may receive inhaled drugs at home through a mask connected to a nebulizer (a small device that creates a mist of the drug by using compressed air). Inhalers and nebulizers are equally effective at delivering the drug. Albuterol also can be taken by mouth, although this route is less effective than inhalation and usually is used only in infants who do not have a nebulizer. Children with moderately severe attacks also may be given corticosteroids by mouth.

Children with very severe attacks are treated in the hospital with bronchodilators given in a nebulizer or an inhaler at least every 20 minutes initially. Sometimes doctors use injections of epinephrine (a bronchodilator) in children with very severe attacks if inhaled drugs are not effective. Doctors usually give corticosteroids by vein to children having a severe attack.

Children who have mild, infrequent attacks usually take drugs only during an attack. Children with more frequent or severe attacks also need to take drugs even when they are not having attacks. Different drugs are used depending on the frequency and severity of the attacks. Children with infrequent attacks that are not very severe usually use a low dose of an inhaled corticosteroid every day to help prevent attacks. These drugs reduce inflammation by blocking the release of the chemical substances that inflame the airways.

Children with more persistent asthma or those at risk of frequent or more severe attacks inhale a moderate or high dose of a corticosteroid daily, with or without an additional drug such as a leukotriene modifier (montelukast or zafirlukast), a long-acting bronchodilator, or cromolyn. Drugs are increased or decreased over time to achieve optimal control of the child's asthma symptoms and to prevent severe attacks. If these drugs do not prevent severe attacks, children may need to take corticosteroids by mouth. Children who experience attacks during exercise usually inhale a dose of bronchodilator just before exercising.

Because asthma is a long-term disorder with a variety of treatments, doctors work with parents and children to make sure they understand the disorder as well as possible. Adolescents and mature younger children should participate in developing their own asthma management plans and establishing their own goals for therapy to improve adherence to treatment. Parents and children should learn how to determine the severity of an attack, when to use drugs and a peak flow meter, when to call the doctor, and when to go to the hospital.

Parents and doctors should inform school nurses, child care providers, and others of the child's disorder and the drugs being used. Some children may be permitted to use inhalers in school as needed, and others must be supervised by the school nurse.

Bronchiolitis

Bronchiolitis is an infection that affects the lower respiratory tract of infants and young children under 24 months of age.

- Bronchiolitis usually is caused by viruses.
- Symptoms include runny nose, fever, cough, wheezing, and difficulty breathing.
- The diagnosis is based on symptoms and a physical examination.
- Most children do well at home and recover in a few days, but some need to be hospitalized.
- Treatment is primarily supporting the child through the illness with fluids and occasionally with oxygen.

Bronchiolitis is most often caused by respiratory syncytial virus and parainfluenza 3 virus, although other viruses, such as influenza, other forms of parainfluenza, metapneumovirus, and adenoviruses, are sometimes involved. Rare causes include rhinoviruses, enteroviruses, measles virus, and the bacteria *Mycoplasma*. Infection with these viruses causes inflammation of the airways. The inflammation causes the airways to narrow, obstructing the flow of air into and out of the lungs.

Bronchiolitis typically affects children younger than 24 months of age and is most common among infants younger than 6 months. During the first year of life, bronchiolitis affects about 11 of every 100 children, although during some epidemics a much higher proportion of infants are affected. Most cases occur between November and April, with a peak incidence during January and February. The infection may be more common among infants whose mothers smoke cigarettes, particularly those who smoked during pregnancy. The infection seems to be less common among breastfed infants. Parents and older siblings can be infected with the same virus, but for them the virus usually causes only a mild cold.

Symptoms and Diagnosis

Bronchiolitis starts with symptoms of a cold—runny nose, sneezing, mild fever, and some coughing. After several days, children develop difficulty breathing, with an increase in respiratory rate and a worsening cough. Usually children have a high-pitched sound on breathing out (wheezing). In most infants, the symptoms are mild. Even though infants may breathe somewhat rapidly and be very congested, they are alert, happy, and eating well. More severely affected infants breathe rapidly and shallowly, use a lot of their respiratory muscles to breathe, and have flaring of their nostrils. They seem fussy and anxious and can become dehydrated because of vomiting and difficulty with drinking. A fever usually is present but not always. Some children also develop an ear infection. Premature infants or infants younger than 2 months sometimes stop breathing temporarily. In very severe and unusual cases, the child may become blue around the mouth caused by a lack of oxygen.

A doctor bases the diagnosis on the symptoms and the physical examination. Sometimes the doctor swabs mucus from deep inside the nose to try to identify the virus in the laboratory. Other laboratory tests may be done, and sometimes a chest x-ray is needed.

Prognosis and Treatment

Most children recover at home in 3 to 5 days. During the illness, frequent small feedings of clear fluids may be given. Wheezing and cough may continue for 2 to 4 weeks. Increasing difficulty in breathing, bluish skin discoloration, fatigue, and dehydration indicate that the child should be hospitalized. Children with congenital heart or lung disease or an impaired immune system may be hospitalized sooner and are far more likely to become quite ill from bronchiolitis. With proper care, the chance of developing serious consequences due to bronchiolitis is low, even for children who need to be hospitalized.

Some children have repeated episodes of wheezing after having had bronchiolitis.

Most children can be treated at home with fluids and comfort measures. In the hospital, oxygen levels are monitored with a sensor attached to a finger or toe, and oxygen is given by an oxygen tent or face mask. A ventilator may be needed to assist breathing. Fluids are given by vein if the child cannot drink adequately. Inhaled drugs that open the airways (bronchodilators) may be tried, although their effectiveness in treating bronchiolitis is questionable. The antiviral drug ribavirin given by nebulizer is no longer given routinely but may be given to infants who are premature or who have other conditions that put them at high risk of severe breathing problems, such as congenital heart or lung disease, cystic fibrosis, or AIDS. Antibiotics are not helpful.

> **? Did You Know...**
> It takes 20 seconds, or the amount of time it takes to sing "Happy Birthday," to receive the full benefit of hand washing with regular soap, which is as good as or better than antibacterial soap.

Croup

Croup (laryngotracheobronchitis) is an inflammation of the windpipe (trachea) and voice box (larynx) typically caused by a contagious viral infection that causes cough, a loud

squeaking noise (stridor), and sometimes difficulty with breathing in (inspiration).

- Croup is caused by viruses.
- Symptoms include fever, runny nose, and a typical bark-like cough.
- The diagnosis is based on symptoms.
- Most children recover at home, but those who require hospitalization receive fluids, oxygen, and drugs.

Croup is caused by a viral infection that leads to swelling of the lining of the airways, particularly the area just below the voice box (larynx). Parainfluenza virus is the most common cause, but croup can be caused by other viruses, such as the respiratory syncytial virus or an influenza virus. Although croup is most common in the fall and winter, it occurs throughout the year. Croup primarily affects children 6 months to 3 years of age, although it occasionally affects those younger or older. Croup caused by an influenza virus may be particularly severe and may occur in a broader age range of children. The infection usually is spread by breathing in airborne droplets containing viruses or by having contact with objects contaminated by these droplets. Most children experience only a single episode of croup, but a few have repeated episodes (spasmodic croup) caused by viral infections that gradually decrease in frequency and severity.

Symptoms and Diagnosis

Croup usually starts with symptoms of a cold—runny nose, sneezing, mild fever, and some coughing. Then the child develops hoarseness and a frequent, unusual-sounding cough, which is described as brassy or barking. Croup ranges widely in its severity. Sometimes swelling of the airway causes difficulty breathing, which is most noticeable on breathing in (inspiration). In severe croup, there may be a loud squeaking noise (stridor) heard with each inspiration. About 50% of children have a fever. All symptoms are typically much worse at night and may awaken the child from sleep. The child's condition often improves in the morning and worsens again the next night.

A doctor distinguishes croup by its characteristic symptoms, especially the sound of the cough. The worst of the symptoms usually lasts 3 to 5 days, and the cough continues but changes to a looser-sounding cough. This change can cause concern for parents who think the infection has moved to the chest. However, it is the normal progression of the illness.

X-rays of the neck and chest help the doctor make a definitive diagnosis.

Treatment

If a child develops a croupy breathing pattern, the parents should contact the doctor because children with croup can become very ill very quickly. In general, a child who is mildly ill with croup may be cared for at home and usually recovers in 3 to 4 days. The child should be made comfortable, given plenty of fluids, and allowed to rest because fatigue and crying can worsen the condition. Home humidifying devices (for example, cool-mist vaporizers or humidifiers) may reduce drying of the upper airways and ease breathing. The humidity can be raised quickly by running a hot shower to steam up the bathroom. Carrying the child outside to breathe cold night air also may open the airways significantly.

For sicker children, the doctor may recommend a single dose of a corticosteroid to prevent worsening of symptoms. Children with continuous croup should be seen immediately by a doctor who will likely recommend corticosteroids and may hospitalize the child for observation and care. Children with increasing or continuing difficulty in breathing, rapid heart rate, fatigue, or bluish skin discoloration need to be given oxygen, as well as fluids by vein. Doctors usually treat the child with epinephrine given in a nebulizer and corticosteroids given by mouth or injection. These drugs help shrink swollen tissue in the airways. Children who improve with these treatments may be sent home, although children with more severe cases should remain in the hospital. Antibiotics are used only in the rare situation when a child with croup also develops a bacterial infection. Rarely, a ventilator is needed. Fortunately, the vast majority of children with croup recover completely.

 Did You Know...

Breathing cool air from the freezer can help lessen croup symptoms.

Bacterial Tracheitis

Bacterial tracheitis (pseudomembranous croup) is an infection of the windpipe (trachea) caused by bacteria.

Bacterial tracheitis is rare and can affect children of any age. The bacteria *Staphylococcus aureus* and streptococci are most frequently the cause. The infection develops suddenly and is characterized by a loud squeaking noise (stridor) when the child breathes in, high fever, and often large amounts of pus-filled secretions. Rarely, bacterial tracheitis may develop as a complication of croup.

A doctor bases the diagnosis on symptoms and an examination of the throat using an instrument (laryngoscope). X-rays often are taken of the throat to show the irregularities that distinguish bacterial tracheitis from croup.

With treatment, most children recover completely. Very ill children have a plastic breathing tube inserted through their mouth or nose into their trachea (endotracheal intubation). The tube keeps the airway from swelling shut. Antibiotics (such as cefuroxime or vancomycin) are given to treat the infection.

CHAPTER

272 Cystic Fibrosis

Cystic fibrosis is a hereditary disease that causes certain glands to produce abnormal secretions, resulting in tissue and organ damage, especially in the lungs and the digestive tract.

- Cystic fibrosis is caused by certain inherited genetic mutations that cause thick, sticky secretions to clog the lungs and other organs.
- Typical symptoms include vomiting and abdominal bloating in newborns, poor weight gain, coughing, wheezing, and frequent respiratory tract infections.
- The diagnosis is based on a sweat test.
- Half of the people with this disease live to their late 30s.
- Treatments include antibiotics, bronchodilators, drugs to thin lung secretions, chest therapy for respiratory problems, and supplements of pancreatic enzymes for digestive problems.
- Some people benefit from lung transplantation.

Cystic fibrosis is the most common inherited disease leading to a shortened life span among white people in the United States. It occurs in about 1 of 3,300 white infants and in 1 of 15,300 black infants. It is rare in Asians. Cystic fibrosis is equally common among boys and girls.

Causes

Abnormal Genes: Cystic fibrosis results when a person inherits two defective copies (mutations) of a particular gene. This gene controls the production of a protein that regulates the transport of chloride and sodium (salt) across cell membranes. Worldwide, about 3 of 100 white people carry one defective copy of the gene; thus, they are carriers but they themselves do not get sick. About 3 of 10,000 white people inherit two defective copies of the gene; thus, they develop cystic fibrosis. In these people, chloride and sodium transport is disrupted and dehydration and increased stickiness of secretions occur.

Abnormal Secretions: Cystic fibrosis affects many organs throughout the body and nearly all the glands that secrete fluids into a duct (exocrine glands). The organs most commonly affected are the lungs, the pancreas, the intestines, the liver and gallbladder, and the reproductive organs.

The lungs are normal at birth, but problems can develop at any time afterward as thick secretions begin to block the small airways (mucus plugging). The plugging leads to chronic bacterial infections and inflammation that cause permanent damage to the airways (termed bronchiectasis). These problems make breathing increasingly difficult and reduce the lungs' ability to transfer oxygen to the blood. People also have frequent bacterial respiratory tract infections.

Blockage of ducts in the pancreas prevents digestive enzymes from reaching the intestine. A lack of these enzymes leads to poor absorption of fats, proteins, and vitamins. This poor absorption, in turn, can lead to nutritional deficiencies and poor growth. Eventually, the pancreas can become scarred and no longer produce enough insulin, so some people develop diabetes.

The intestines can become blocked by thick secretions. This blockage is common immediately after birth (termed meconium ileus) but may occur later in life (distal intestinal obstruction syndrome).

The sweat glands secrete fluid containing more salt than normal, increasing the risk of dehydration.

Symptoms

About 15 to 20% of newborns who have cystic fibrosis have meconium ileus, which causes vomiting, abdominal enlargement (distention), and absence of bowel movements. Meconium ileus is sometimes complicated by perforation of the intestine, a dangerous condition causing peritonitis and, if untreated, shock and death. Some newborns have a twisting of the intestine on itself (volvulus) or incomplete development of the intestine. Newborns who have meconium ileus almost always develop other symptoms of cystic fibrosis later. Meconium can also temporarily obstruct the large intestine in some newborns with cystic fibrosis, so that a bowel movement may not occur until 1 to 2 days after birth.

The first symptom of cystic fibrosis in an infant who does not have meconium ileus is often a delay in regaining birth weight or poor weight gain at 4 to 6 weeks of age. This poor weight gain is due to inadequate amounts of pancreatic enzymes. The infant has frequent, bulky, foul-smelling, oily stools and may have a bloated (distended) abdomen and

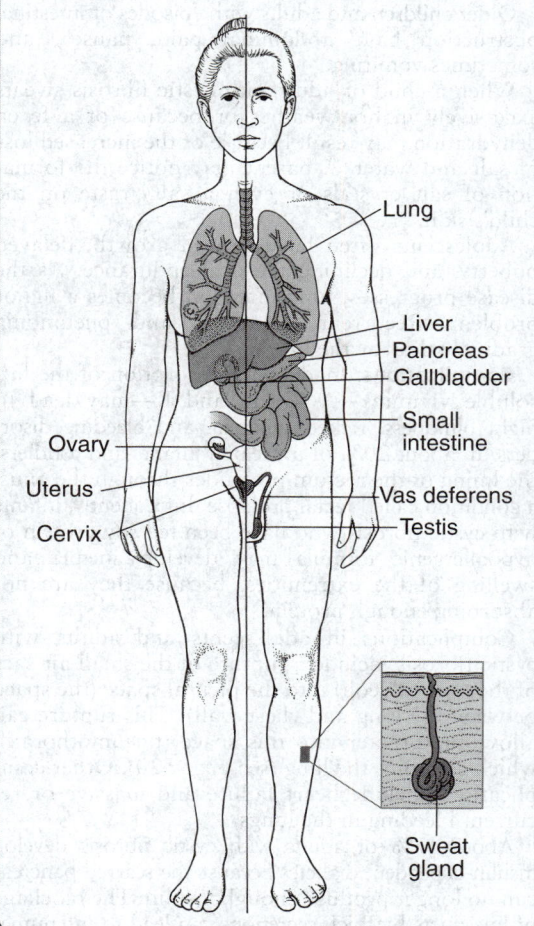

Cystic Fibrosis: Not Just a Lung Disease

In the lungs, thick bronchial secretions block the small airways, which become inflamed. As the disease progresses, the bronchial walls thicken, the airways fill with infected secretions, areas of the lung contract, and lymph nodes enlarge. In the liver, thick secretions block the bile ducts. Obstruction may also occur in the gallbladder. In the pancreas, thick secretions may block the gland completely so that digestive enzymes cannot reach the intestine. In the small intestine, intestinal blockage (meconium ileus) can result from thick secretions and requires surgery in some newborns. The reproductive organs are affected by cystic fibrosis in various ways, often resulting in infertility in males. The sweat glands in the skin secrete fluid containing more salt than normal.

Lung

Liver
Pancreas
Gallbladder

Small
intestine

Ovary

Uterus

Cervix

Vas deferens

Testis

Sweat
gland

small muscles. Without treatment, weight gain in infants and older children is slow despite a normal or large appetite.

Unless a diagnosis is made through newborn screening, about half the children with cystic fibrosis are first taken to the doctor because of frequent coughing, wheezing, and respiratory tract infections. Coughing, the most noticeable symptom, is often accompanied by gagging, vomiting, and disturbed sleep. Children may have difficulty breathing, wheezing, or both. As the disease progresses, symptoms tend to occur more frequently, the chest becomes barrel-shaped, and insufficient oxygen may make the fingers clubbed (see page 453) and the nail beds bluish. Polyps may form in the nose. The sinuses may fill with thick secretions, leading to chronic or recurrent sinus infections.

Older children and adults with episodes of intestinal obstruction have abdominal pain, nausea, and sometimes vomiting.

When a child or adult with cystic fibrosis sweats excessively in hot weather or because of a fever, dehydration may result because of the increased loss of salt and water. A parent may notice the formation of salt crystals or even a salty taste on the child's skin.

Adolescents often have slowed growth, delayed puberty, and declining physical endurance. As the disease progresses, lung infection becomes a major problem. Recurrent bronchitis and pneumonia gradually destroy the lungs.

Complications: Inadequate absorption of the fat-soluble vitamins—A, D, E, and K—may lead to night blindness, rickets, anemia, and bleeding disorders. In about 20% of untreated infants and toddlers, the lining of the rectum protrudes through the anus, a condition called rectal prolapse. Infrequently, infants with cystic fibrosis who have been fed soy protein or hypoallergenic formula may develop anemia and swelling of the extremities, because they are not absorbing enough protein.

Complications in adolescents and adults with cystic fibrosis include a rupture of the small air sacs of the lung (alveoli) into the pleural space (the space between the lung and chest wall). This rupture can allow air to enter into this space (pneumothorax), which collapses the lung (see page 520). Other complications include heart failure and massive or recurrent bleeding in the lungs.

About 17% of adults with cystic fibrosis develop insulin-dependent diabetes because the scarred pancreas can no longer produce enough insulin. The blockage of bile ducts by thick secretions can lead to inflammation of the liver and eventually to scarring of the liver (cirrhosis) in about 5% of people with cystic fibrosis (see page 222). Cirrhosis may increase the pressure in the veins entering the liver (portal hypertension—see page 217), leading to enlarged, fragile veins at the lower end of the esophagus (esophageal varices), which can rupture and bleed profusely. In almost all people with cystic fibrosis, the gallbladder is small and filled with thick bile and does not function well. About 10% of people develop gallstones, but only a small percentage develops symptoms. Surgical removal of the gallbladder is rarely needed.

People with cystic fibrosis often have impaired reproductive function. Almost all men have a low sperm count (which makes them sterile) because one of the ducts of the testis (the vas deferens) has developed abnormally and blocks the passage of sperm. In women, cervical secretions are too thick, causing decreased fertility. Otherwise, sexual function is not affected. Women with cystic fibrosis have a higher likelihood of complications during pregnancy (such as developing a lung infection or diabetes), but many women with cystic fibrosis have given birth.

Other complications may include osteoporosis, arthritis, kidney stones, anemia, and an increased risk of cancer of the bile ducts and intestines.

Diagnosis

If newborn screening is not done, the diagnosis of cystic fibrosis is usually confirmed in infancy or early childhood, but cystic fibrosis goes undetected until adolescence or early adulthood in about 10% of people with the disease.

The diagnosis is suggested by one or more of the typical symptoms and is confirmed by a sweat test. This test measures the amount of salt in sweat. The drug pilocarpine is placed on the skin to stimulate sweating, and filter paper or thin tubing is placed against the skin to collect the sweat. The concentration of salt in the sweat is then measured. A salt concentration higher than normal confirms the diagnosis in people who have symptoms of cystic fibrosis or who have a sibling with cystic fibrosis. Although the results of this test are valid any time after a newborn is 48 hours old, collecting a large enough sweat sample from a newborn younger than about 2 weeks old may be difficult. The sweat test, which can be performed on an outpatient basis, can also confirm the diagnosis in older children and young adults.

In newborns with cystic fibrosis, the level of trypsin (a digestive enzyme) in the blood is high. This enzyme level can be measured in a small drop of blood collected on a piece of filter paper. Measurement of this enzyme in combination with genetic testing is the basis of cystic fibrosis newborn screening programs performed in many parts of the world and in the United States. If the screening test is positive, newborns undergo sweat testing.

The diagnosis of cystic fibrosis can also be confirmed by genetic testing in a person who exhibits one or more typical symptoms or has a history of cystic fibrosis in a sibling. Finding two abnormal cystic fibrosis genes (mutations) confirms the diagnosis. However, because typical genetic testing does not look for all of the more than 1,500 different kinds of cystic fibrosis mutations, failure to detect two mutations does not guarantee the person does not have cystic fibrosis. The disease can be diagnosed prenatally by performing genetic testing on the fetus using chorionic villus sampling or amniocentesis (see page 1611).

Because cystic fibrosis can affect several organs, other tests may be helpful. If pancreatic enzyme levels are reduced, an analysis of the person's stool may reveal low or undetectable levels of the digestive enzymes elastase, trypsin, and chymotrypsin (secreted by the pancreas) or high levels of fat. If insulin secretion is reduced, blood sugar levels are high. Pulmonary function tests (see page 454) may show that breathing is compromised and are good indicators of how well the lungs are functioning. Also, chest x-rays and computed tomography (CT) may be helpful to document lung infection and the extent of lung damage.

Carrier testing can be performed for prospective parents. In particular, relatives of a child with cystic fibrosis may want to know whether they are likely to have children with the disease, and they should be offered genetic testing and counseling. A small blood sample is taken to help determine whether a person has a defective cystic fibrosis gene. Unless both prospective parents have at least one such gene, their children will not have cystic fibrosis. If both parents carry a defective cystic fibrosis gene, each pregnancy has a 25% chance of producing a child with cystic fibrosis, a 50% chance of producing a child who is a carrier, and a 25% chance of producing a child with no defective cystic fibrosis genes.

Prognosis

The severity of cystic fibrosis varies greatly from person to person regardless of age. The severity is determined largely by how much the lungs are affected. In the United States, half of the people with cystic fibrosis live about 37 years or longer. The outlook for longer survival has improved steadily over the past 50 years, mainly because treatments can now postpone some of the changes that occur in the lungs. Long-term survival is significantly better in people who do not develop pancreatic problems.

However, deterioration is inevitable, leading to loss of lung function and eventually death. People with cystic fibrosis usually die of respiratory failure after many years of deteriorating lung function. A small number, however, die of heart failure, liver disease, bleeding into the airways, or complications of surgery. Despite their many problems, people with cystic fibrosis usually attend school or work until shortly before death.

Treatment

A person with cystic fibrosis should have a comprehensive program of therapy directed by an experienced doctor—usually a pediatrician or an internist—along with a team of other doctors, nurses, a dietitian, social worker, genetics counselor, psychologist, and physical and respiratory therapists. The goals of therapy include long-term prevention and treatment of lung and digestive problems and other complications, maintenance of good nutrition, and encouragement of physical activity.

Children with cystic fibrosis need psychologic and social support because they may be unable to participate in normal childhood activities and may feel isolated. Much of the burden of treating a child with cystic fibrosis falls on the parents, who should receive adequate information and training so they can understand the disorder and the reasons for the treatments.

The treatment of lung problems focuses on preventing airway blockage and controlling infection. The person should receive all routine immunizations (see page 1145), particularly for those infections that cause respiratory infection, such as influenza and pneumococcus.

Respiratory therapy—consisting of postural drainage, percussion, hand vibration over the chest wall, and encouragement of coughing—is started at the first sign of lung problems (see page 461). Parents of a young child can learn these techniques and carry them out at home every day. Older children and adults can carry out respiratory therapy independently, using special breathing devices or a compression vest.

Often, people are given drugs that help prevent their airways from narrowing (bronchodilators). People with severe lung problems and a low level of oxygen in the blood may need supplemental oxygen therapy. In general, people with respiratory failure do not benefit from using a ventilator (breathing machine). However, occasional, short periods of mechanical ventilation in the hospital may help during an acute infection, after a surgical procedure, or while waiting for a lung transplant.

Aerosol (nebulized) drugs, such as dornase alfa (recombinant human deoxyribonuclease I) or a highly concentrated (hypertonic) salt solution, are widely used to help thin the pus-filled mucus. Such drugs make it easier to cough up sputum, improve lung function, and may also decrease the frequency of serious respiratory tract infections. Corticosteroids can relieve symptoms in infants with severe bronchial inflammation and in people who have narrowed airways that cannot be opened with bronchodilators. Sometimes, a nonsteroidal anti-inflammatory drug (NSAID—see page 644) is used to slow the deterioration of lung function.

Respiratory tract infections must be treated as early as possible with antibiotics. At the first sign of a respiratory tract infection, a sample of coughed-up sputum or a throat culture is collected and tested, so that the infecting organism can be identified and the doctor can choose the drugs most likely to control it. *Staphylococcus aureus* and *Pseudomonas* species are commonly found. An antibiotic often can be given by mouth (orally), or an antibiotic such as tobramycin can be given in an aerosol mist. However, if the infection is severe, antibiotics given by vein (intravenously) may be needed. This treatment often requires hospitalization but may be given at home. Taking an oral (azithromycin) or aerosol (tobramycin) antibiotic intermittently or continuously may help prevent recurrences of infection and slow the decline in lung function.

People who have pancreatic problems must take pancreatic enzyme replacements with each meal. A powder (for infants) and capsules are available. Special milk formulas containing protein and fats that are easy to digest may help infants who have pancreatic problems and poor growth.

The diet should provide enough calories and protein for normal growth. The proportion of fat should be normal to high. Because people with cystic fibrosis need more calories, they need to consume higher than normal amounts of fat to ensure adequate growth. People with cystic fibrosis should take double the usual recommended daily amount of fat-soluble vitamins (A, D, E, and K) in a special formulation that is more easily absorbed. When they exercise, have a fever, or are exposed to hot weather, they should increase their salt intake. Children who cannot absorb enough nutrients from food may need supplementary feedings through a tube inserted into the stomach or small intestine.

At some time, surgery may be needed to treat a pneumothorax, chronic sinus infection, severe chronic infection restricted to one area of the lung, bleeding from blood vessels in the esophagus, gallbladder disease, or obstruction of the intestine. Massive or recurrent bleeding in the lung can be treated by a procedure called embolization, which blocks off the bleeding artery.

Liver transplantation has been successful for severe liver damage. Double lung transplantation for severe lung disease is becoming more routine and more successful with experience and improved techniques. About 60% of people are alive 5 years after transplantation of both lungs, and their condition is much improved.

Gene therapy, in which normal cystic fibrosis genes are delivered directly to the airways, holds promise for treating cystic fibrosis. However, this therapy is only available in research trials. A number of new drugs, delivered by mouth or aerosol, are under investigation.

CHAPTER

273 Digestive Disorders

Children can develop a variety of digestive disorders. All digestive disorders involve varying degrees of pain, vomiting, or changes in appetite and bowel function. The challenge for parents is to provide information that will help doctors distinguish serious from nonserious disorders and, in some cases, to help their children adjust to chronic disorders that require fairly constant medical attention.

Gastroenteritis

Gastroenteritis is inflammation of the digestive tract that results in vomiting, diarrhea, or both and is sometimes accompanied by fever or abdominal cramps.

- Gastroenteritis is usually caused by a viral, bacterial, or parasitic infection.
- The infection causes a combination of vomiting, diarrhea, abdominal cramps, fever, and poor appetite, which can lead to dehydration.
- The child's symptoms and history of exposure help the doctor confirm the diagnosis.
- Gastroenteritis is best prevented by encouraging children to wash their hands and teaching them to avoid improperly stored foods.
- Fluids and rehydrating solutions are given, but sometimes children need to see a doctor.

Gastroenteritis, sometimes incorrectly called "stomach flu," is the most common digestive disorder among children (see page 145). About 1 billion episodes occur worldwide each year, most commonly in developing countries among children under 5 years of age. Severe gastroenteritis results in dehydration and in an imbalance of blood chemicals (electrolytes) because of a loss of body fluids in the vomit and stool. In developed countries where children are well nourished and have access to excellent medical care, gastroenteritis can cause discomfort and incapacitation but does not last long and only very rarely has serious consequences. In developing countries where children are more vulnerable and care is often not easy to access, millions of children die each year from diarrhea caused by gastroenteritis.

Causes

Viruses (such as rotavirus) are the most common cause of gastroenteritis in the United States. Children usually contract viral gastroenteritis from other children who have had it or who have been exposed to it, such as those in child care centers, schools, and other crowded settings. Viral gastroenteritis is generally spread from hand to mouth but can also be spread by sneezing and spitting. It spreads particularly easily because of the way children play—putting hands and fingers in and near their mouth and then touching toys and each other.

Bacteria (such as *Escherichia coli*, *Vibrio cholerae*, *Salmonella*, or *Shigella*) and parasites (such as *Giardia*) can also cause gastroenteritis (see table on page 146). Children can contract bacterial gastroenteritis from touching or eating contaminated foods, particularly raw or inadequately cooked meats or eggs, and drinking unpasteurized milk or juice. Bacteria may grow in many types of foods that have been left out and not refrigerated (potential problem situations include buffets and picnics). If *Staphylococcus* bacteria contaminate food, they may secrete a toxin that causes sudden vomiting and diarrhea. Gastroenteritis contracted from food containing microorganisms or bacterial toxins is sometimes called food poisoning (see page 151). Occasionally, some bacteria are transmitted by dogs or cats with diarrhea. Children can contract bacterial or parasitic gastroenteritis from eating shellfish; swallowing contaminated water, such as from wells, streams, and swimming pools; and while traveling in developing countries.

Occasionally, gastroenteritis results when children eat things they are not supposed to, such as plants and drugs. Rarely, gastroenteritis results because of an allergic condition (eosinophilic gastroenteritis) or from contact with animals at petting zoos.

Symptoms and Diagnosis

Symptoms are usually a combination of vomiting, diarrhea, abdominal cramps, fever, and poor appetite. Usually, vomiting predominates early in the illness, and diarrhea becomes more prominent later, but some children have both at the same time. With viral causes, watery diarrhea may be the main symptom. The stools may be bloody if certain bacteria are the cause. These symptoms eventually lessen in children who drink enough fluids. The most common complication of severe gastroenteritis is dehydration (see page 1733), which occurs when fluid is lost in vomit and stool. Children who are slightly dehydrated are thirsty, but seriously dehydrated children become listless, irritable, or sluggish (lethargic). Infants are much more likely than older children to become dehydrated and develop serious side effects. Dehydrated infants produce no tears when they cry. Older children have decreased urine output, dry mouth, and excessive thirst.

A doctor bases the diagnosis of gastroenteritis on the child's symptoms and on the parents' responses to questions about what the child has been exposed to. Diagnostic tests are not usually needed because most forms of gastroenteritis last a short time. However, general laboratory tests can help doctors pinpoint a cause of the gastroenteritis.

 Did You Know...

Millions of children die each year from diarrhea caused by gastroenteritis.

Prevention

The best way to prevent gastroenteritis is to encourage children to wash their hands and to teach them to avoid improperly stored foods. A good general guideline is to keep cold foods cold and hot foods hot. Food placed out for consumption should be consumed within an hour. Diaper-changing areas should be disinfected with a freshly prepared solution of household bleach (¼ cup bleach diluted in 1 gallon of water).

A vaccine to prevent rotavirus infection is available. The current rotavirus vaccine is not associated with intussusception (the serious problem of the intestine telescoping in on itself), as was the case with the original vaccine. Infants should receive three doses of the rotavirus vaccine, which is given by mouth at 2, 4, and 6 months of age.

Breastfeeding is another simple and effective way to prevent gastroenteritis. Children with diarrhea should not return to child care centers until their symptoms are gone.

Parents can help prevent dehydration by encouraging their child to drink fluids even if just in small, frequent amounts.

Treatment

Once a child has gastroenteritis, parents should monitor their child's hydration status. Infants are dehydrated and need medical care right away if

- The soft spot on their head is sunken
- Their eyes are sunken
- They have no tears when they cry
- Their mouth is dry
- They are not producing much urine

Children should be encouraged to drink fluids even if just in frequent, small amounts. Infants should continue to breastfeed or drink formula in addition to an oral electrolyte solution (rehydration solution—available as powders and liquids in pharmacies and some grocery stores). Juice, soda, carbonated beverages, teas, sports drinks, and beverages containing caffeine should not be given to infants and young children. These drinks may contain too much sugar, which can worsen diarrhea, and have too few salts (electrolytes), which are needed to replace those the body has lost. For older children, however, sports drinks are preferable to juice and soda because of their lower sugar content, but they still have lower amounts of electrolytes than oral electrolyte solutions.

For a vomiting child, frequent small amounts of fluid help prevent dehydration. Parents should offer the child a few sips of a liquid. If the liquid is not vomited, the sips are repeated every 10 or 15 minutes, increasing the amount given to an ounce or two after an hour or so and increased as tolerated. These larger amounts can be given less often, about every hour. Liquids are absorbed very quickly, so if the child vomits more than 10 minutes after drinking, most of the liquid has been absorbed and the liquids should be continued. The amount of liquid to give a child within a 24-hour period depends on the child's age but generally should be about $1\frac{1}{2}$ ounces of liquid for each pound the child weighs. If the child's vomiting or diarrhea lessens, parents may try resuming a more normal diet the next day. Electrolyte solutions should not be continued for longer than 24 hours because of potential problems associated with inadequate nutritional intake.

Children with diarrhea but little vomiting are fed their normal diet, with extra liquid given to make up for the fluid lost in the diarrhea. If there is significant diarrhea, the child's consumption of dairy products (which contain lactose) should probably be reduced. Severe gastroenteritis may decrease the child's ability to absorb lactose, resulting in even more diarrhea.

Children who cannot keep down even sips of liquid or who have signs of severe dehydration (such as lethargy, dry mouth, lack of tears, and no urine for 6 hours or more) are in danger and should see a doctor immediately. Children who do not have these signs should see a doctor if symptoms last more than 1 or 2 days. If the dehydration is severe, the doctor may give the child intravenous fluids.

Antidiarrheal drugs such as loperamide are not usually recommended for children. However, under the guidance of a doctor, certain drugs that prevent or relieve nausea or vomiting (such as ondansetron) can be given once the cause of vomiting has been determined. Antibiotics are of no value when a viral infection is the cause of gastroenteritis. Doctors give antibiotics only for certain bacteria that are known to respond to these drugs. Antiparasitic drugs may be given for a parasitic infection.

Gastroesophageal Reflux

Gastroesophageal reflux is the backward movement of food and acid from the stomach into the esophagus and sometimes into the mouth (see page 144).

- Reflux may be caused by the infant's position during feeding; overfeeding; exposure to caffeine, nicotine, and cigarette smoke; a food intolerance or allergy; or an abnormality of the digestive tract.
- Symptoms include vomiting, excessive spitting up, and feeding or breathing problems.
- Tests that help doctors diagnose the disorder include a barium study, an esophageal pH probe, a gastric emptying scan, and endoscopy.
- Treatment options include thickened formula for feedings, special positioning, frequent burping, histamine-2 (H_2) blockers, proton pump inhibitors, and, in certain cases, metoclopramide and surgery.

Nearly all infants have episodes of gastroesophageal reflux, which are characterized by wet burps, burping up, or spitting up. Wet burps typically occur shortly after eating and are considered normal. Gastroesophageal reflux becomes a concern when it

- Interferes with feeding and growth
- Damages the esophagus (esophagitis)
- Leads to breathing difficulties (such as coughing, wheezing, or stopping breathing)
- Continues beyond infancy into childhood

Causes

Healthy infants have reflux for many reasons. The circular band of muscle at the junction of the esophagus and stomach (the lower esophageal sphincter) normally keeps stomach contents from entering the esophagus. In infants, this muscle may be underdeveloped, or it may relax at inappropriate times, allowing stomach contents to move backward (reflux) into the esophagus. Being held flat during feeding or lying down after feeding promotes reflux because gravity is no longer able to help keep material in the stomach from flowing back up the esophagus. Overfeeding and drinking carbonated beverages predispose to reflux by increasing pressure in the stomach. Cigarette smoke (as secondhand smoke) and caffeine (in beverages or breast milk) relax the lower esophageal sphincter, allowing reflux to occur more readily. Caffeine and nicotine (in breast milk) also stimulate acid production so any reflux that does occur is more acidic. A food allergy or intolerance also can contribute to reflux, but this is a less common cause.

Anatomic abnormalities, such as narrowing of the esophagus, partial blocking of the stomach (pyloric stenosis), or abnormal positioning of the intestines (malrotation), can initially mimic reflux. However, these abnormalities are more serious and can progress to vomiting and other symptoms of obstruction, such as abdominal pain, listlessness, and dehydration.

Symptoms

The most obvious symptoms of gastroesophageal reflux in infants are vomiting and excessive spitting up. Reflux typically worsens in the first several months of life, peaks around 6 to 7 months of age, and then gradually lessens. Nearly all infants with reflux outgrow it by about 18 months of age.

In some infants, reflux causes complications and becomes known as gastroesophageal reflux disease (GERD). Such complications include irritability due to stomach discomfort, feeding problems that can result in poor growth, and "spells" of twisting and posturing that may be confused with seizures. Less commonly, small amounts of acid from the stomach may enter the windpipe (aspiration). Acid in the windpipe and breathing passages may result in coughing, wheezing, stopping breathing (apnea), or pneumonia. Many children with asthma also have reflux. Ear pain, hoarseness, hiccups, and sinusitis also can occur as a result of GERD. If the esophagus is significantly irritated (esophagitis), there may be some bleeding, resulting in iron deficiency anemia. In others, esophagitis can cause scar tissue, which can narrow the esophagus (stricture). Heartburn, a common symptom among adolescents and adults with GERD, is more commonly expressed as chest pain or abdominal pain among young children.

Diagnosis

Tests are often not needed to diagnose gastroesophageal reflux in infants who simply have mild symptoms such as frequent spit-ups. However, if symptoms are more complicated, various tests can be performed.

A **barium study** (see page 130) is the most common test. The child swallows barium, a liquid that outlines the digestive tract when x-rays are taken. This test can confirm the diagnosis of gastroesophageal reflux and also help the doctor identify some of the possible causes.

An **esophageal pH probe** is a thin flexible tube with a sensor at the tip that measures the degree of acidity (pH). Doctors pass the tube through the child's nose, down the throat, and into the end of the esophagus. The tube is usually left in place for 24 hours. Normally, children do not have acid in their esophagus, so if the sensor detects acid, it is a sign of reflux. Doctors sometimes use this test to see whether children with symptoms such as coughing or breathing difficulties have reflux.

In a **gastric emptying scan** (milk scan), the child drinks a beverage that contains a small amount of mildly radioactive material. This material is harmless to the child. A special camera or scanner that is highly sensitive to radiation can detect where the material is in the child's body. The camera can see how rapidly the material leaves the stomach and whether there is reflux, aspiration, or both.

In **upper endoscopy** (see page 129), the child is sedated, and a small flexible tube with a camera on the end (endoscope) is passed through the mouth into the esophagus and stomach. Doctors may perform upper endoscopy if they need to see whether there is an ulcer or irritation or if they need to obtain a sample for a biopsy. Bronchoscopy (see page 456) is a similar test in which doctors use an endoscope to examine the voice box (larynx) and airways. Bronchoscopy can help doctors decide whether reflux is a likely cause of lung or breathing problems.

Treatment

Treatment of reflux depends on the child's age and symptoms.

For infants who just have wet burps, doctors may recommend no treatment or may suggest measures such as thickening formula for feedings, special positioning, and frequent burping. Formula can be thickened by adding 1 to 3 teaspoons of rice cereal per ounce of formula. The nipple may have to be cross-cut to allow the formula to flow. Infants with reflux should be fed in an upright or semi-upright position and then maintained in an upright position for 30 minutes after eating.

For older children, the head of the bed can be elevated 6 inches (about 15¼ centimeters) to help reduce nighttime reflux. Older children also should avoid eating 2 to 3 hours before bedtime, drinking carbonated beverages or those that contain caffeine, taking certain drugs (such as those with anticholinergic effects), eating certain foods (such as chocolate), and overeating. All children should be kept away from tobacco smoke.

Drugs: If changes in feeding and positioning do not control symptoms, doctors may prescribe drugs. Several types of drugs are available for reflux:

- Those that neutralize acid
- Those that suppress acid production
- Those that improve the movement of the digestive tract

Antacids are drugs that neutralize gastric acid. These drugs work quickly to relieve symptoms such as heartburn.

For those with more severe disease, acid-suppressing drugs are required. By reducing stomach acid, these drugs lessen symptoms and allow the esophagus to heal. There are two types of acid-suppressing drugs, histamine-2 (H_2) blockers and proton pump inhibitors (PPIs). H_2 blockers do not suppress acid production quite as much as PPIs.

Promotility drugs stimulate the movement of contents through the esophagus, stomach, and intestines. These drugs (such as metoclopramide) may help increase the strength of the lower esophageal sphincter and increase the speed at which the stomach empties. Improved gastric emptying should decrease gastric pressure, making reflux less likely to occur. Doctors used to prescribe these drugs frequently for reflux but now think they are helpful only for certain children.

Surgery: Rarely, reflux does not respond to nonsurgical treatment and is so severe that doctors recommend surgery. The most common surgical procedure is a fundoplication. In fundoplication, the surgeon wraps the top of the stomach around the lower end of the esophagus to make that junction tighter and decrease reflux.

Peptic Ulcer

A peptic ulcer is erosion of the lining of the stomach or small intestine (duodenum) due to excess stomach acid, breakdown of the stomach's protective lining, or both.

Peptic ulcers are much less common among children than adults. As with adults, use of nonsteroidal anti-inflammatory drugs (NSAIDs) and infection with *Helicobacter pylori* bacteria can lead to the formation of peptic ulcers (see page 139). Children whose parents have peptic ulcers are more likely to have ulcers, as are those whose parents smoke. Adolescents who drink alcohol or smoke are also more likely to develop ulcers. Children of any age

can develop ulcers when they are extremely sick, such as after severe burns, injuries, and illnesses. These ulcers are referred to as stress ulcers.

Infants with ulcers may be fussy and irritable during and after feedings. Ulcers in older children usually cause abdominal pain. At any age, peptic ulcers can tear (perforate), bleed, or lead to blockage (obstruction). The diagnosis and treatment of peptic ulcers and their complications are the same for children and adults.

Hernia

A hernia is a protrusion of a piece of the intestine through an abnormal opening.

Diaphragmatic Hernia: Some infants are born with a diaphragmatic hernia (see page 1721). A diaphragmatic hernia is a hole or weakening in the diaphragm (the muscle that separates the chest from the abdomen and that helps in breathing). This opening allows some of the small intestine to push through the opening, creating a bulge. Sometimes the intestine becomes trapped (incarcerated) in the opening. Sometimes incarceration cuts off the blood supply to the trapped intestine (strangulation), which can lead to a tear (perforation) and peritonitis (inflammation and usually infection of the abdominal cavity and its lining), creating a surgical emergency. A diaphragmatic hernia that bulges through the opening that the esophagus normally passes through (the hiatus) is called a hiatus hernia (see page 156).

Umbilical Hernia: An umbilical hernia is a small opening in the abdominal wall near or at the belly button (umbilicus). The small intestine can protrude through the opening when the child coughs or strains during a bowel movement. The intestine rarely becomes trapped (incarcerated), and the hernia usually closes without treatment by the time the child is 5 years of age. If a large umbilical hernia does not close by that time, the doctor may advise surgery. Folk remedies such as taping a coin or other object over the hernia do not work and may irritate the skin.

Inguinal Hernia: A hernia in the groin is called an inguinal hernia (see page 1471). Inguinal hernias are more common among boys, particularly those who are premature. About 10% have hernias on both sides of the groin. Because inguinal hernias can become incarcerated, doctors usually advise surgery.

Hypertrophic Pyloric Stenosis

Hypertrophic pyloric stenosis is blockage of the passage out of the stomach due to overdevelopment (hypertrophy) of the muscle at the junction between the stomach and the intestines.

- For uncertain reasons, the passage that leads out of the stomach is blocked, preventing material from leaving the stomach.
- Infants feed well but vomit forcefully (projectile vomiting) shortly after eating.
- The diagnosis is based on results of abdominal ultrasonography.
- Typically, the problem is corrected by minor surgery.

The pylorus is the muscular sphincter located where the stomach joins the first part of the small intestine (duodenum). Normally, the pylorus contracts to keep food in the stomach for digestion and relaxes to let the food out into the intestine. For reasons that doctors do not fully understand, the pylorus sometimes closes off, blocking material from leaving the stomach. This blockage usually occurs in the first month or two of life and is much more common among boys, especially first-born boys. Rarely, some older children have pyloric stenosis caused by peptic ulcers or an uncommon disorder similar to a food allergy (such as eosinophilic gastroenteritis).

Symptoms and Diagnosis

An infant with pyloric stenosis is hungry and feeds well but vomits forcefully (projectile vomiting) shortly after eating. Until dehydration is severe, or infants become significantly undernourished, they otherwise appear well, unlike those with vomiting caused by other disorders. After several days, the infant begins to become dehydrated and loses weight. A few infants have a yellowish discoloration of the skin and the whites of the eyes (jaundice).

The doctor may be able to feel a small lump (about the size of an olive) in the infant's abdomen (the enlarged pylorus). Most commonly, the doctor does abdominal ultrasonography to confirm the diagnosis.

Treatment

Doctors give the infant intravenous fluids to treat the dehydration. Then, a surgeon cuts the thickened muscle to allow formula or breast milk to enter the small intestine more readily. This surgery is relatively minor, and most infants can eat within a day of the procedure.

Intussusception

Intussusception is a disorder in which one segment of the intestine slides into another, much like the parts of a telescope. The affected segments obstruct the bowel and block blood flow.

- The cause of intussusception is unknown.
- Symptoms include sudden stomach pain and vomiting.

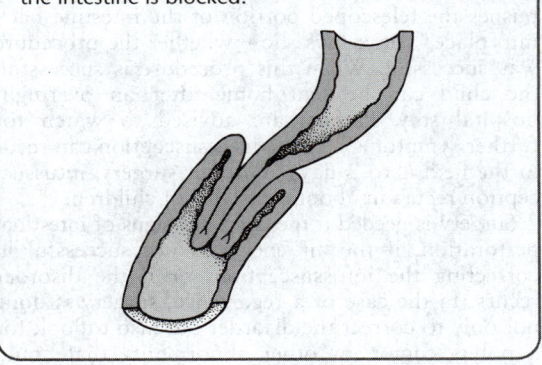

What Is Intussusception?

One part of the intestine slides into another, much like the parts of a collapsible telescope. As a result, the intestine is blocked.

- An air enema can confirm the diagnosis and also treat the condition.
- Sometimes surgery is needed.

Intussusception is the most common cause of intestinal blockage among children between the ages of 3 months and 3 years. Boys are affected slightly more than girls. In most cases, the cause is unknown. Intussusception occasionally affects older children, in whom it is often caused by something in the intestine such as a polyp or tumor. Sometimes, the sliding (telescoping) segments return to normal without treatment. If not, the telescoping segments obstruct the intestine and then shut off the blood flow to the affected area. If blood flow is shut off for more than a few hours, the affected intestine may die (develop gangrene). If a segment of the intestine dies, small holes (perforations) can develop, allowing bacteria to enter the abdominal cavity, resulting in a serious infection (peritonitis).

Symptoms

Intussusception usually causes sudden stomach pain and vomiting in a child who is otherwise healthy. The episodes of pain typically last 15 to 20 minutes. Some children become irritable or listless and apathetic between episodes. Without treatment, the pain becomes continuous, and some children pass currant jelly–like stools with blood and mucus or develop a fever. Children who have a perforation appear ill and have pain when their abdomen is touched.

Diagnosis and Treatment

A doctor may suspect intussusception based on the child's symptoms and a physical examination.

Ultrasonography can confirm the diagnosis. If ultrasonography confirms intussusception, an air enema is performed. With an air enema, the doctor puts air into the child's rectum through a small tube and then takes x-rays. The pressure of the air usually pushes the telescoped portion of the intestine back into place. The x-rays show whether the procedure was successful. When this procedure is successful, the child can be sent home after an overnight hospital stay. Parents are advised to watch for further symptoms because intussusception can recur in the next 1 to 2 days. Without surgery, intussusception recurs in about 5 to 10% of children.

Surgery is needed if the child has signs of intestinal perforation, if the air enema is not successful in correcting the intussusception, or if the disorder recurs. In the case of a recurrence, surgery is done not only to correct the disorder but also to look for a polyp, tumor, or other abnormality that could explain why the intussusception recurred.

Appendicitis

Appendicitis is inflammation and infection of the appendix.

- Appendicitis seems to develop when the appendix becomes blocked either by hard fecal material (called a fecalith) or swollen lymph nodes in the intestine that can occur with various infections.
- Pain—near the appendix or throughout the abdomen—may make children irritable or listless.
- Diagnosis is challenging and may require blood tests, x-rays, ultrasonography, computed tomography, or laparoscopy.
- An infected appendix is removed surgically.

The appendix is a small finger-length portion of intestine that does not clearly have any essential bodily function (see art on page 111). Appendicitis is a medical emergency that requires surgery. This disorder is rare in children younger than 1 year but becomes more common as children grow older and is most common among adolescents and those in their 20s.

Appendicitis seems to develop when the appendix becomes blocked either by hard fecal material (fecalith) or swollen lymph nodes in the intestine, which can occur with various infections. In either case, the appendix swells, and bacteria in it grow. Rarely, foreign bodies and worms can also cause appendicitis. If appendicitis is unrecognized or untreated, the appendix can rupture, creating a pocket of infection outside the intestine (abscess) or spilling contents of the intestines into the abdominal cavity, causing a serious infection (peritonitis). In about 25% of children with appendicitis, the appendix has already ruptured by the time they arrive at the hospital.

Symptoms and Diagnosis

Appendicitis almost always causes pain. The pain may start in the middle of the abdomen, near the navel, and gradually move to the lower right area of the abdomen. Pain, particularly in infants and children, may be widespread rather than confined to the right lower portion of the abdomen. Younger children may be less able to identify a specific location for the pain. After the pain has begun, many children develop vomiting and do not want to eat. A low-grade fever (100 to 101° F [37.7 to 38.3° C]) is a common symptom. This pattern is different from that in children who have viral gastroenteritis, in whom vomiting typically occurs first, and pain and diarrhea develop later.

The diagnosis of appendicitis in children can be challenging for many reasons. Many disorders can cause similar symptoms, including viral gastroenteritis, Meckel's diverticulum, intussusception, and Crohn's disease. Often, children do not have typical symptoms and physical examination findings, particularly when the appendix is not in its usual position in the right lower part of the abdomen.

Doctors who suspect appendicitis usually give intravenous fluids and antibiotics while waiting for results of blood tests and x-rays. They may do ultrasonography, computed tomography (CT), or laparoscopy (see page 130) to see inside the abdomen. Repeated physical examinations, especially in children whose pain is not typical of appendicitis, may help the doctor decide whether appendicitis is present.

Treatment

The best treatment for appendicitis is surgical removal of the inflamed appendix (appendectomy). Appendectomy is fairly simple and safe, requiring a hospital stay of 2 to 3 days in uncomplicated cases. If the appendix has ruptured, the doctor removes it and may wash out the abdomen with fluid, give antibiotics for several days, and watch for complications, such as infection and bowel blockage. About 10 to 20% of the time, surgeons discover a normal appendix while performing an appendectomy. This finding is not considered a medical error because the consequences of delaying surgery when appendicitis is suspected are serious. When the appendix is found to be normal, the surgeon looks within the abdomen for another cause of the pain. The doctor usually removes the normal appendix so that the child never develops appendicitis. Without surgery or antibiotics, more than 50% of people with appendicitis die.

Meckel's Diverticulum

Meckel's diverticulum is a saclike outpouching of the wall of the small intestine present in some children at birth.

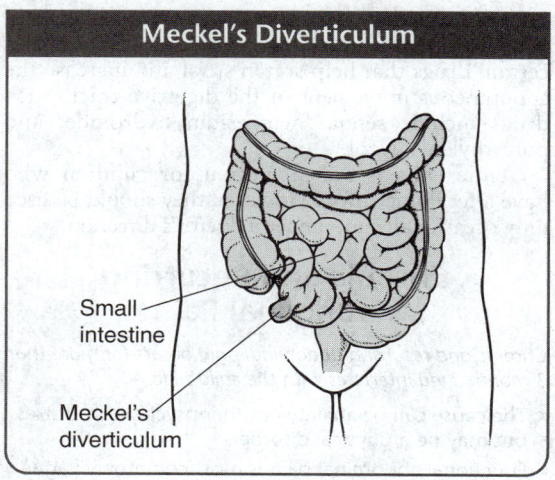

Meckel's Diverticulum

Small intestine

Meckel's diverticulum

- Most children do not have symptoms, but sometimes painless rectal bleeding occurs or the diverticulum becomes infected.
- Doctors base the diagnosis on symptoms, the results of a radionuclide scan, and sometimes ultrasonography.
- A bleeding diverticulum or one that causes symptoms must be surgically removed.

About 3% of infants are born with Meckel's diverticulum. People can live their whole lives without ever knowing they have Meckel's diverticulum, but occasionally the abnormality can cause problems.

Over half the time, the diverticulum contains tissue like that of the stomach, pancreas, or both. If stomach tissue is present, it can secrete acid just like the stomach does. This acid may cause ulcers and bleeding of the nearby intestine. A Meckel's diverticulum may also become inflamed (diverticulitis) or cause intussusception. Severe Meckel's diverticulitis can occur at any age, but older children are most affected.

Symptoms and Diagnosis

Most children with Meckel's diverticulum have no symptoms, and many adults learn they have the condition only after surgeons discover it while performing surgery for another reason. The most common symptom among children younger than 5 years is painless rectal bleeding, which comes from ulcers in the small intestine caused by acid secreted by the diverticulum. Because of the bleeding, stools may appear bright red or brick-colored or currant jelly–colored because of a mixture of blood and mucus. Sometimes, stool appears black because of the breakdown of blood. Only rarely is the bleeding so severe that the child needs emergency surgery.

Diverticulitis caused by a Meckel's diverticulum causes severe pain, abdominal tenderness, and sometimes vomiting and can easily be confused with appendicitis.

It is often difficult for doctors to diagnose Meckel's diverticulum. Blood tests, x-rays, computed tomography (CT), and barium enemas are not usually helpful. The best test is an imaging study called a Meckel's radionuclide scan, in which a small amount of a harmless radioactive substance is given by vein (intravenously). The substance is recognized by cells in the diverticulum, which can then be visualized using a radiation-sensing camera.

Treatment

No treatment is needed for a diverticulum that does not cause symptoms. A bleeding diverticulum or one that causes symptoms must be surgically removed. If a Meckel's diverticulum is found in a child during an operation being performed for another reason, it is generally removed to prevent future complications.

Constipation

Constipation refers to delay or difficulty in passing stool or an increase in the hardness and size of stool.

- Constipation is the result of behavior or a lack of fluids and fiber in the diet.
- Hard or large stools can cause abdominal discomfort and can tear the anus.
- Increased fluid and fiber in the diet, behavior modification, and sometimes enemas and laxatives can help ease the discomfort.

Parents often worry about their child's bowel movements. However, most constipation has no serious consequences and should be a concern only when passing stools becomes painful and leads to further withholding of stools or when constipation causes other symptoms.

Stool frequency and consistency is variable throughout childhood, and there is no single frequency and type of stool that is "normal." Newborn infants typically have four or more loose, yellow, and seedy stools per day. Breastfed infants typically have more stools than formula-fed infants and may defecate after each breastfeeding. After a month or two, some breastfed infants defecate less frequently, but the stools remain mushy or loose. After 1 year of age, most children have one to two stools a day that are soft and formed.

In older children, constipation is defined as the passing of hard stools that cause discomfort. It is most often caused by an insufficient amount of fiber in the diet. The condition also may be self-reinforcing, because discomfort while moving the bowels causes children to further withhold stool.

Constipation is extremely common among children. Although constipation rarely causes any serious severe problems, children who are defecating less than every other day, whose stools are hard or large, or who appear to have discomfort when defecating should be evaluated by a doctor. Chronic constipation can contribute to urinary problems such as urinary tract infections and bed wetting (enuresis).

Causes

The most common causes of constipation are dietary and behavior issues. Frequently, the child's diet contains insufficient amounts of fluid and fiber (such as from fruits, vegetables, and whole grains). Lack of fluid and fiber causes stool to become hard and difficult to pass. Such stools may cause abdominal discomfort, anal pain with defecation, or both. Also, passage of large hard stools may tear the anus (anal fissure), which is painful and may result in streaks of bright red blood on the outside of the stool or on the toilet paper. Because of these symptoms, or because the child does not want to take time to defecate, some children resist defecation (stool withholding behavior). As stool withholding behavior continues, constipation worsens, sometimes becoming a vicious circle. As a large amount of hard stool (fecal impaction) fills the rectum, it may enlarge, which can decrease the sensation of needing to defecate. Looser stool from above the hardened stool may then leak around this fecal mass into the child's underwear, which may cause parents to think the child has diarrhea when the actual problem is constipation.

Constipation that has existed since birth and constipation that does not go away after treatment suggest a physical defect, such as Hirschsprung's disease (see page 1721).

Treatment

Mild constipation can be treated by increasing the amount of fiber in the child's diet and ensuring good hydration. If the child will not consume a high-fiber diet, a fiber supplement (psyllium) can be given.

Behavior modification is also important. After eating a meal, the body has a reflex to pass stool. This is called the gastro-colic reflex. Frequently, a child ignores the signals from this reflex and puts off having a bowel movement. Putting off bowel movements contributes to the hardening of stool and subsequent constipation. Behavior modification techniques take advantage of this reflex. Having the child sit on the toilet for 5 to 10 minutes after meals helps retrain the digestive tract, develops a toilet routine, and encourages more regular defecation.

If constipation does not respond to diet and behavior modification, the doctor may recommend certain drugs that help soften stool and increase the spontaneous movement of the digestive tract. Such drugs include senna, magnesium hydroxide, and polyethylene glycol.

Gentle enemas are an option for children who have a fecal impaction. However, they should be used only occasionally and under a doctor's direction.

Chronic and Recurring Abdominal Pain

Chronic and recurring abdominal pain occurs for more than 3 months and interferes with the child's life.

- The cause can be anxiety or other psychologic distress but may be a physical disorder.
- Functional abdominal pain is most commonly vague and located around or above the navel.
- The diagnosis is based on symptoms and a physical examination.
- Pain in children who are under the age of 5 years or who are losing weight, bleeding, or producing severe vomiting or diarrhea is probably caused by a physical disorder.
- Physical causes are treated, or measures to relieve psychologic distress are taken.

Chronic and recurring abdominal pain affects about 10 to 15% of children between 5 and 16 years of age, particularly those between 8 and 12 years of age. It is uncommon among children under 5 years of age. It is somewhat more common among girls.

Causes

There are over 100 different causes of chronic abdominal pain in children, but the most common are functional pain, dairy (lactose) intolerance, constipation, and gastroesophageal reflux.

Functional Pain: Functional pain is real pain that results from stress or anxiety (from problems at school, home, or with friends) rather than from an underlying physical disorder. It is similar to a tension headache. In a tension headache, the pain is real, but there is no underlying problem such as a brain tumor or stroke. The headache is just how the body reacts to stress. Instead of a tension headache, children tend to have a tension stomachache. The pain can be severe and typically alters the child's life. For example, children who are very stressed by school are frequently absent. The exact mechanism of functional abdominal pain is unknown, but many doctors think the pain occurs when the nerves of the digestive tract become hypersensitive to stimuli (such as expansion or contraction of the intestines) that most people do not find uncomfortable. Why these nerves become hypersensitive is unclear but may involve a preceding infection or allergy. Genetic factors, life stresses, and the child's personality, social situation, and any underlying mental disorders (such as depression or anxiety) all may help cause functional pain.

Lactose Intolerance: Lactose is the predominant sugar found in milk and other dairy products. Lactase is an enzyme needed to break down lactose. Children who lack lactase cannot digest and absorb lactose, which leads to diarrhea and abdominal cramping (see page 164).

Constipation: Children who consume insufficient fluids or fiber are often constipated (see page 1799). A lack of fluid and fiber causes stool to become hard and difficult to pass. These stools may cause abdominal discomfort, pain with defecation, or both.

Gastroesophageal Reflux: The disorder that causes the backward movement of food and acid from the stomach into the esophagus and sometimes into the mouth is called gastroesophageal reflux (see page 1794). The reflux can cause abdominal pain, heartburn, and nausea.

Symptoms

The symptoms vary depending on the cause of the pain.

Functional Pain: For children with functional abdominal pain, the pain is most commonly vague and located around or above the navel. The further the pain is away from the navel the less likely it is to be functional. The intensity ranges from mild to severe. Pain most commonly lasts from minutes to several hours, but about 10% of children have pain that lasts all day. There are no obvious factors associated with the pain other than stress or anxiety, and the pain rarely wakes children from sleep. If school is the major problem, pain is commonly worse on weekdays and better on weekends and during vacations.

Children with functional pain may also show immaturity, unusual dependence on parents, anxiety or depression, apprehension, tension, and perfectionism. Often, parents see the child as special because of the position in the family (for instance, an only child, the youngest child, or the only boy or girl among a large group of siblings) or because of a medical problem.

Lactose Intolerance: Children with lactose intolerance commonly have pain similar to those with functional pain, except parents occasionally notice a relationship between the pain and the consumption of dairy products. The child may pass an excessive amount of gas (flatus). Passing gas or defecating relieves the pain. However, the pain may intensify before the child is able to defecate.

Some Causes of Chronic and Recurring Abdominal Pain

GASTROINTESTINAL DISORDERS

- Hiatal hernia
- Esophagitis
- Peptic ulcer disease*
- Liver disease (such as hepatitis)*
- Gallbladder disease (such as cholecystitis)*
- Pancreatic disease (such as pancreatitis)*
- Inflammatory bowel disease (such as Crohn's disease)*
- Meckel's diverticulum
- Appendicitis
- Intussusception
- Parasitic infection (such as giardiasis)*
- Tuberculosis of the intestine
- Celiac disease (such as celiac sprue)*
- Constipation*
- Lactose intolerance due to lactase deficiency*
- Functional pain*
- Gastroesophageal reflux*

GENITAL/URINARY DISORDERS

- Structural anomalies
- Urinary tract infection
- Kidney disease (such as kidney stone)*
- Normal monthly ovulation (in girls)
- Menstrual cramps (in girls)
- Pelvic inflammatory disease (in girls)
- Ovarian cysts (in girls)
- Endometriosis (in girls)

GENERAL ILLNESSES

- Heavy metal poisoning (lead)
- Henoch-Schönlein purpura
- Sickle cell disease
- Food allergy
- Musculoskeletal disease (such as bruised abdominal muscles or ribs)
- Porphyria
- Familial Mediterranean fever
- Hereditary angioedema
- Abdominal migraine

*Indicates the most common causes.

Constipation: Children whose pain is caused by chronic constipation have pain that is frequently crampy in nature and located in the lower abdomen. The pain is reduced by defecation.

Gastroesophageal Reflux: In children with gastroesophageal reflux, pain commonly is worse after eating (the most common time to reflux). The pain is burning in older children but may be vague in younger children. Most nonadolescent children feel the pain of gastroesophageal reflux just below the ribs, above the navel, or around the navel. Adolescents are more likely to describe the classic heartburn pain.

Diagnosis

The symptoms and physical examination suggest the cause and help doctors decide what tests, if any, are needed. Children with symptoms typical of functional pain may not require testing. Certain signs make the diagnosis of functional pain unlikely. These signs include weight loss, bleeding, significant vomiting or diarrhea, and age under 5 years. If these factors are present, or the cause is unclear, doctors usually perform basic blood and urine tests. Many doctors also perform tests for lactose intolerance (usually with a breath test) and for celiac disease with special blood tests. If needed, specific tests include x-rays, upper endoscopy, computed tomography (CT), and colonoscopy (see page 129).

Treatment

Physical causes of recurring abdominal pain are treated. When a physical cause for the child's symptoms cannot be found, a doctor may suspect a psychologic cause.

When the cause is functional pain, the parents are frequently concerned that something very serious is causing the pain. A doctor should provide reassurance that the pain, while real, is not serious. The child's pain should be acknowledged, both by parents and doctors, which helps build the child's confidence and trust. Having the doctor monitor the child's progress is important, and frequent visits may be necessary.

Pain symptoms are treated with acetaminophen or other mild analgesics. A high-fiber diet and fiber supplements can also help. Many drugs have been tried with varying success, including antispasmodics, peppermint oil, cyproheptadine, and acid-suppressing drugs.

Children are encouraged to fulfill their normal responsibilities, particularly attending school, despite pain. If pain is related to anxiety about school, then missing school may increase the child's anxiety and make the problem worse. Any other sources of stress or anxiety are dealt with when possible. If causes of anxiety cannot be eliminated, the doctor may prescribe antidepressants or antianxiety drugs. If the child is severely depressed or has significant psychologic or mental problems, consultation with a mental health practitioner is wise.

Giving children extra attention because of their pain may only reinforce any undesired behavior. Instead, children can be given rewards and attention for not having the pain. For example, for every day children do not have any abdominal pain, they can have special time with one or both of the parents.

CHAPTER 274 Neurologic Disorders

Neurologic disorders affect the brain, spinal cord, nerves, or a combination. These disorders include cerebral palsy (see page 1856), seizures, and disorders that also affect other parts of the body (such as the skin or eyes), such as neurofibromatosis, tuberous sclerosis, von Hippel-Lindau disease, and Sturge-Weber syndrome.

The approach to neurologic disorders in children often differs from that in adults because the brain and nervous system are still developing.

Seizures

Seizures are a periodic disturbance of the brain's electrical activity, resulting in some degree of temporary brain dysfunction.

Seizures are an abnormal, unregulated electrical discharge of nerve cells in the brain or part of the brain. This abnormal discharge can alter awareness or cause abnormal sensations, involuntary movements, or convulsions. Convulsions are rhythmic contractions of the muscles. In newborns, seizures may be difficult to recognize. Newborns may smack their lips or chew involuntarily. Their eyes may appear to gaze in different directions. They may periodically go limp. In older infants or young children, one part or all of the body may shake and jerk. The limbs may move without purpose. Children may stare or become confused.

SOME CAUSES OF SEIZURES IN NEWBORNS AND INFANTS

TYPE	DISORDER
General disorders	High fevers Lack of oxygen, as may occur during labor or delivery
Brain disorders	Birth defects of the brain Bleeding within the brain Brain malformations or tumors Head injury Infections, such as encephalitis or meningitis Stroke
Metabolic disorders	Hereditary disorders of amino acid processing (metabolism) Temporary abnormalities in blood levels of sugar (glucose), calcium, magnesium, vitamin B_6, or sodium
Drugs	Use of drugs (such as cocaine, heroin, or the sedative diazepam) by the mother during pregnancy

Epilepsy is not a specific disorder but refers to a tendency to have recurrent seizures that may or may not have an identifiable cause.

Seizures in children often have similar manifestations as in adults (see page 709). However, some types of seizures, such as febrile seizures and infantile spasms, occur only in children. Seizures caused by inherited disorders of metabolism typically start during infancy or childhood. Certain conditions in children, such as breath-holding (see page 1749) and night terrors (see page 1747), may resemble seizures but do not involve abnormal electrical activity in the brain and thus are not seizures.

In children, the condition causing the seizures may also affect their development. Brief, infrequent seizures do not seem to cause brain damage. Whether some types of recurrent seizures can affect the developing brain is debated. Seizures that last for hours may be associated with brain damage, especially if a high fever is also present, but seizures seldom last for hours.

> **Did You Know...**
> People should not put anything in the mouth of someone who is having a seizure.

Emergency Treatment: When children have a seizure, parents or other caregivers should try to make sure children do not hurt themselves by doing the following:

- Laying the child down on one side
- Keeping the child away from potential hazards (such as stairs or sharp objects)
- Not putting anything in the child's mouth or trying to hold the child's tongue

After the seizure ends, the following can help:

- Staying with the child until the child is fully awake
- Checking whether the child is breathing and if breathing is not apparent, starting mouth-to-mouth rescue breathing (attempting rescue breathing during a convulsive seizure is unnecessary and can injure the child or the rescuer)
- Not giving any food, liquid, or drug by mouth until the child is fully awake
- If the child has a fever, giving acetaminophen rectally

An ambulance should be called if the seizure lasts more than 5 minutes, if children are injured during the seizure, if they have difficulty breathing after the seizure, or if another seizure occurs immediately. All children should be taken to the hospital the first time they have a seizure. For children who are already known to have a seizure disorder, parents should discuss in advance with the doctor when, where, and how urgently evaluation is required if another seizure occurs.

FEBRILE SEIZURES

Febrile seizures (convulsive seizures) are seizures triggered by a fever.

Febrile seizures occur in about 2 to 5% of children younger than 6 years but most often occur in children aged 6 months to 3 years. Febrile seizures tend to run in families. Most children who have a febrile seizure have only one, and most seizures last less than 15 minutes.

Febrile seizures may be simple or complex.

- **Simple:** The entire body shakes (called a generalized seizure) for less than 15 minutes.
- **Complex:** The entire body shakes for more than 15 minutes, only one side of the body shakes (called a partial seizure), or seizures occur at least twice within 24 hours. Children who have complex febrile seizures are slightly more likely to develop a seizure disorder later in life.

Febrile seizures usually result from the fever itself. Most often, the fever is caused by an otherwise minor infection such as a viral respiratory infection. In such

Using Drugs to Treat Seizures in Children

When their child has had a seizure, parents are often concerned that the child may need to take a drug to control seizures (an anticonvulsant). Parents are concerned about side effects, and they know that getting children to take a drug on a regular basis is difficult.

Learning more about anticonvulsants can help parents better participate in decisions about treatment of their child.

Positives:

- Most children who have had only one seizure do not need to take anticonvulsants.
- Doctors can choose from more than 20 anticonvulsants in their search for one that is appropriate for a particular child.
- Anticonvulsants stop or control the seizures in 80% of children.
- Many children need to take only one anticonvulsant.
- Most children can eventually stop taking anticonvulsants.

Negatives:

- Most anticonvulsants have side effects, such as dizziness, nausea, unsteadiness, drowsiness, double vision, or rash.

- Some anticonvulsants may affect attention span and school performance while children are taking the drug.
- Some children who have taken anticonvulsants for a long time have mild problems with memory and attention.
- Children who take certain anticonvulsants must have regular blood tests to determine whether the dose is correct.
- Some newer anticonvulsants have not been tested in children (although these drugs often are used in children and results of that experience are published).

In weighing concerns, parents should remember that preventing further seizures is most important. To be sure drugs are taken on a regular schedule, parents can do the following:

- Use a pill box (which contains compartments for each day of the week, for different times of each day, or both).
- Refill prescriptions before they run out.
- Encourage the child to take responsibility for taking the drug.
- Discuss in advance with the doctor what to do if the child misses a dose.

---

cases, the infection and the seizure are harmless. However, life-threatening brain infections such as meningitis (see page 750) or encephalitis (see page 760) also sometimes cause seizures (as well as fever). Because parents cannot tell whether children have such a brain infection, children who have a fever and who have a seizure for the first time or are very sick should be taken to the emergency department for evaluation. Doctors examine the children and sometimes do tests to check for these disorders.

Did You Know...

Most children who have a febrile seizure have only one.

Treatment

Usually, seizures last less than 15 minutes, and no treatment is given other than drugs to reduce the fever. If seizures last 15 minutes or more, drugs such as the sedative lorazepam or the anticonvulsant fosphenytoin are given, usually by vein, to end them, and children are carefully monitored for problems with breathing and blood pressure.

Children who have had only a few simple febrile seizures are usually not given drugs to prevent additional seizures. Children who have had several febrile seizures or seizures lasting a long time may be given drugs.

INFANTILE SPASMS

In infantile spasms (salaam seizures), children who are lying on their back suddenly raise and bend their arms, bend their neck and upper body forward, and straighten their legs.

- Many children who have infantile spasms also develop abnormally or have intellectual disability.
- Electroencephalography and analysis of samples of blood, urine, and the fluid around the spinal cord as well as brain imaging help doctors diagnose the disorder and identify the cause.
- Injecting adrenocorticotropic hormone or a corticosteroid into the muscle often helps control the seizures.

Infantile spasms last for only a few seconds but may recur many times a day. They usually occur in children younger than 3 years. In many children, the spasms evolve into another type of seizure later in life.

Symptoms

Spasms usually consist of a sudden jerk, followed by stiffening. They typically occur after children wake up and rarely occur during sleep. In most affected children, intellectual development, including development of language skills, is slow, and intellectual disability is present. Children may lose developmental skills that they have learned, such as being able to sit up or roll over.

Diagnosis

Doctors base the diagnosis on symptoms. Electroencephalography (EEG) is done to check for abnormal electrical activity in the brain.

Samples of blood, urine, and the fluid around the spinal cord (cerebrospinal fluid) are usually analyzed to check for disorders that may be causing the seizures. Cerebrospinal fluid is obtained by doing a spinal tap (lumbar puncture). Magnetic resonance imaging (MRI) of the brain is usually done.

Treatment

Because early control of infantile spasms is associated with a better developmental outcome, early identification and treatment of seizures are essential. Sometimes adrenocorticotropic hormone, injected into a muscle once a day, or a corticosteroid (such as prednisone) is used.

Many anticonvulsants are not effective in stopping the spasms. However, clonazepam, nitrazepam, topiramate, valproate, vigabatrin, or zonisamide may help.

Neurofibromatosis

Neurofibromatosis is a genetic disorder in which many soft, fleshy growths of nerve tissue (neurofibromas) grow under the skin and in other parts of the body.

- People may have freckle-like spots on various parts of the body, lumps on or under the skin, weakness, abnormal sensation, or hearing or vision problems.
- Doctors do a physical examination and sometimes an imaging test to check for lumps and growths.
- No treatment can cure the disorder, but growths can be removed surgically.

Neurofibromas are flesh-colored growths of Schwann cells (which form a wrapping around peripheral nerve fibers) and other cells that support peripheral nerves. Neurofibromas, which can be felt under the skin as small lumps, usually start appearing after puberty.

Types: There are two types of neurofibromatosis:

- **Type 1** (also known as von Recklinghausen's disease) affects about 1 of 3,000 people. Neurofibromas develop along peripheral nerves (those outside the brain and spinal cord—for example, under or on the skin and just outside the spinal cord).

- **Type 2** affects about 1 of 40,000 people. It causes tumors of the auditory nerve (near the ear), called acoustic neuromas, and sometimes tumors in and around the brain.

Causes

About half the people with neurofibromatosis inherit it. Only one gene for neurofibromatosis—from one parent—is required for the disorder to develop, and each child of an affected parent has a 50% chance of inheriting the disorder. The genes for both types have been identified. In the rest of the people, neurofibromatosis results from a spontaneous gene mutation. Thus, these people have no family history of the disorder.

Symptoms

Type 1: About one third of people notice no symptoms, and the disorder is first suspected during a routine examination when doctors find lumps under the skin near nerves. Another third of people notice skin spots or bumps, and the remaining people notice neurologic symptoms such as weakness. In more than 90%, medium-brown (café au lait) spots develop on the skin of the chest, back, pelvis, and creases of the elbows and knees. These spots typically exist at birth or appear during infancy. Between ages 10 and 15, flesh-colored growths (neurofibromas) of varying sizes and shapes begin appearing on the skin. There may be fewer than 10 of these growths or thousands of them. Rarely, neurofibromas under the skin or an overgrowth of the bone under the neurofibroma causes structural abnormalities, such as an abnormally curved spine (kyphoscoliosis), rib deformities, enlarged long bones in the arms and legs, and bone defects of the skull. If the bone surrounding the eyeball is affected, the eyes bulge.

Neurofibromas may affect any nerve in the body but frequently grow on spinal nerve roots (the parts of the spinal nerve that emerge from the spinal cord through the spine). There, they often cause few or no problems. However, if they put pressure on (compress) the spinal cord, they can cause paralysis or disturbances in sensation in different parts of the body, depending on which part of the spinal cord is compressed. If neurofibromas compress peripheral nerves, the nerves may not function normally, and pain or weakness may result. Neurofibromas that affect nerves in the head can cause blindness, dizziness, deafness, noise in the ears (tinnitus), and incoordination.

Neurofibromatosis usually progresses slowly. As the number of neurofibromas increases, more neurologic problems may develop.

Type 2: Auditory nerve tumors develop on both sides of the body. The tumors may cause hearing loss and sometimes dizziness, as early as age 20. People may also have other types of tumors, including gliomas and meningiomas (see table on page 742), and some develop cataracts prematurely.

Diagnosis

Doctors base the diagnosis on findings during examination. They usually do computed tomography (CT) or magnetic resonance imaging (MRI) to check for growths in the head and near the spinal cord in people who have neurologic symptoms.

Genetic testing is not yet readily available.

Treatment

No known treatment can stop the progression of neurofibromatosis or cure it. Individual neurofibromas can usually be removed surgically or shrunk with radiation therapy. When they have grown close to a nerve, surgical removal often requires removing the nerve as well.

Because neurofibromatosis can be hereditary, genetic counseling is recommended when people with this disorder are considering having children. For people who have a child with the disorder but do not have the disorder themselves, the risk of having another child with the disorder is very small.

Sturge-Weber Syndrome

Sturge-Weber syndrome is a rare disorder affecting small blood vessels. It is characterized by a port-wine birthmark on the face, a blood vessel tumor (angioma) in the tissues that cover the brain, or both.

- This disorder can cause seizures, weakness, and increased pressure in an eye and can increase the risk of stroke.
- If children have a typical birthmark, doctors suspect the disorder and may do an imaging test to check for blood vessel tumors.
- Treatment focuses on relieving or preventing symptoms.

Sturge-Weber syndrome is present at birth but is not inherited. It affects blood vessels, particularly vessels in the skin, in the tissues that cover the brain, and in the eye. The port-wine birthmark is caused by an overgrowth of small blood vessels (capillaries) just under the skin. Tumors consisting of overgrown blood vessels (angiomas) may develop in the tissues that cover the brain, causing seizures or weakness on one side of the body. Abnormal blood vessels in the eye may cause glaucoma and affect vision. Abnormalities in the walls of arteries may increase the risk of strokes.

There are 3 types of Sturge-Weber syndrome:

- Type I: Port-wine birthmark and a brain angioma
- Type II: Port-wine birthmark but no brain angioma
- Type III: A brain angioma but no port-wine birthmark

Symptoms

The port-wine birthmark varies in size and color, ranging from light pink to deep purple. It usually appears on the forehead and upper eyelid of one eye but may also include the lower eyelid. If both eyelids are involved, people are much more likely to have a brain angioma.

Seizures occur in about 75 to 90% of people and typically start by the time children are 1 year old. Usually, seizures occur on only one side of the body, opposite the birthmark, but they may affect the whole body. About 25 to 50% of people have weakness or paralysis on the side opposite the birthmark. About 50% of people have some intellectual impairment. Impairment is more likely when seizures start before age 2 years and cannot be controlled with drugs. Development of motor and language skills may be delayed.

Pressure within the eye may damage the optic nerve, causing glaucoma, usually in the eye on the same side as the birthmark. Glaucoma may be present at birth or develop later. The eyeball may enlarge and bulge out.

Diagnosis

Doctors suspect the diagnosis in children with the characteristic birthmark. Computed tomography (CT) or magnetic resonance imaging (MRI) is used to check for brain angiomas. A neurologic examination is done to check for evidence of seizures or weakness.

Treatment

Treatment focuses on relieving symptoms. Anticonvulsants and drugs to treat glaucoma are used. Surgery for glaucoma may be required (see page 1452).

Aspirin may be given in low doses to reduce the risk of strokes.

Laser treatment may be used to lighten or remove the birthmark.

Tuberous Sclerosis

Tuberous sclerosis is a hereditary disorder that causes abnormalities in the brain, changes in the skin and sometimes tumors to develop in vital organs, such as the heart and lungs.

- Children may have abnormal skin growths, seizures, delayed development, learning disorders, or behavioral problems and may be intellectually impaired or autistic.
- Life expectancy is usually unaffected.
- Because the disorder is lifelong, people must be monitored for their entire life.
- Doctors suspect the disorder based on symptoms and do imaging tests to check for tumors and sometimes do genetic tests.
- Treatment focuses on relieving symptoms.

Tumors or other abnormal growths develop in several organs, such as the heart, lungs, kidneys, eyes, and skin. The tumors are usually noncancerous (benign). The disorder is named for the typical long and narrow tumors in the brain, which resemble roots or tubers.

Tuberous sclerosis is usually present at birth, but symptoms may be subtle or take time to develop, making the disorder difficult to recognize early.

Several genes involved in the disorder have been identified. If either parent has the disorder, children have a 50% chance of having it. However, tuberous sclerosis usually results from new mutations in the gene, rather than an inherited abnormal gene.

Symptoms

Tuberous sclerosis may cause seizures, mental retardation/intellectual disability, autism, delayed development of motor or language skills, learning disorders, or behavioral problems (such as hyperactivity and aggression).

The first symptom may be infantile spasms, a type of seizure (see page 1804). Some children have kidney tumors, which can cause high blood pressure, abdominal pain, and blood in the urine. Kidney cancer can also occur.

The skin is often affected, sometimes causing disfigurement:

- Light-colored, ash-leaf–shaped patches may appear on the skin during infancy or early childhood.
- Rough, raised patches resembling orange peel, usually on the back, may be present at birth.
- Medium-brown, freckle-like (café au lait) spots may also develop.
- Red lumps consisting of blood vessels and fibrous tissue (angiofibromas) may appear on the face later during childhood.
- Small fleshy bumps may grow around and under the toenails and fingernails at any time during childhood or early adulthood.

How well affected people do depends on how severe the symptoms are. If symptoms are mild, infants generally do well and grow up to live long, productive lives. If symptoms are severe, infants may have serious disabilities. Nonetheless, most children continue to develop, and life expectancy is not affected. Because tuberous sclerosis is a lifelong disorder, affected people must be closely monitored for the rest of their life.

Diagnosis

Doctors may suspect the diagnosis based on symptoms, such as seizures, delayed development, or typical skin growths. An eye examination (with ophthalmoscopy) is done to check for eye abnormalities. Magnetic resonance imaging (MRI) or ultrasonography is done to check for tumors in various organs.

Genetic testing may be done for the following reasons:

- To confirm the diagnosis when symptoms suggest it
- To determine whether people who have a family history of the disorder but who do not have symptoms have the abnormal gene
- To check for the disorder before birth (prenatal diagnosis) if the family history includes the disorder

Ultrasonography may be done before birth to check for heart or brain tumors in a fetus.

Treatment

Treatment focuses on relieving symptoms:

- For seizures: Anticonvulsants may be used. Sometimes if drugs are ineffective, surgery is done to remove a tumor or to remove a small part of the brain that is involved in causing the seizures.
- For high blood pressure: Antihypertensive drugs may be used, or surgery may be done to remove kidney tumors.
- For behavioral problems: Behavior management techniques (including time-outs and consistent use of appropriate consequences and praise) may help. Sometimes drugs are needed.
- For developmental delays: Special schooling or physical, occupational, or speech therapy may be recommended.
- For skin growths: They may be removed with dermabrasion (rubbing the skin with an abrasive metal instrument to remove the top layer) or lasers.

Genetic counseling is recommended for affected people and family members when they are considering having children.

Von Hippel–Lindau Disease

Von Hippel-Lindau disease is a rare hereditary disorder that causes tumors to develop in several organs.

- Children may have headaches, impaired vision, or high blood pressure and feel dizzy or weak.
- Doctors suspect the disorder based on the person's family history and results of a physical examination, then do imaging and other tests to check for tumors and other problems.
- Tumors are removed surgically, treated with radiation, or destroyed using a laser or application of extreme cold.

Tumors most commonly develop in the brain and retina of the eyes. These tumors, called angiomas, consist of blood vessels. Other types of tumors develop in other organs and include tumors in the adrenal glands (pheochromocytomas) and cysts in the kidneys, liver, or pancreas. As people with the disorder age, the risk of developing kidney cancer increases.

The gene that causes von Hippel-Lindau disease has been identified. Only one gene for the disorder—from one parent—is required for the disorder to develop. Each child of an affected parent has a 50% chance of inheriting the disorder. In 20% of people with this disorder, it results from a new mutation.

Symptoms

Typically, symptoms appear between ages 10 and 30, but they can appear earlier.

Symptoms depend on the size and location of the tumors. Children may have headaches and feel dizzy or weak. Vision may be impaired, and blood pressure may be high.

Tumors in the retina usually cause no symptoms, but if they enlarge, they can cause substantial loss of vision. When these tumors are present, the retina may become detached, fluid may accumulate on or under the macula (the central part of the retina), and the optic nerve may be damaged by increased pressure within the eye, resulting in glaucoma.

Without treatment, people may become blind, have brain damage, or die. Death usually results from complications of brain tumors or kidney cancer.

Diagnosis

Doctors determine whether any family members have the disorder and do a physical examination. If findings suggest the disorder, various tests are done to check for tumors and other abnormalities: computed tomography (CT) or magnetic resonance imaging (MRI) of the brain, an eye examination including ophthalmoscopy, and ultrasonography or CT of the abdomen. Hearing tests and blood tests are also done.

Von Hippel-Lindau disease is diagnosed when one of the following is present:

- More than one tumor in the brain or eye
- One tumor in the brain or eye plus one elsewhere in the body
- A family history of von Hippel-Lindau disease plus one tumor

If doctors detect one tumor typical of this disorder, they look for others.

Genetic testing is done to check for the abnormal gene in family members. If an abnormal gene is detected, family members are monitored for tumors for the rest of their life.

Treatment

Tumors are surgically removed, if possible, before they cause permanent damage. High-dose radiation therapy, focused on the tumor, can sometimes be used instead.

Typically, tumors of the retina are destroyed using laser therapy or application of extreme cold (cryotherapy). These procedures help preserve vision.

Tests used to detect tumors are repeated every 1 or 2 years because new tumors may develop.

CHAPTER

275 Ear, Nose, and Throat Disorders

Ear, nose, and throat disorders, particularly infections, are extremely common among children.

- Ear infections occur almost as often as the common cold. They can develop behind the eardrum (in the middle ear), called otitis media, or in front of the eardrum (in the outer ear), called otitis externa or external otitis (see page 1385).
- Throat infections are usually not serious, but they make children uncomfortable and can lead to missed school days and multiple visits to a doctor.

Other disorders, such as hearing impairment and neck masses, affect fewer children but are potentially serious. In general, any abnormality of a child's ear, nose, or throat that does not resolve within several days should be evaluated by a doctor.

Middle Ear Infections

Middle ear infection is infection of the space immediately behind the eardrum.

Middle ear infections (otitis media) may occur in older children and adults (see page 1388) but are extremely common between the ages of 3 months and 3 years and often accompany the common cold. Young children are particularly susceptible to middle ear infections for several reasons:

- Differences in the eustachian tube
- Increased susceptibility to infection in general
- Increased exposure to infection
- Use of a pacifier

Other important risk factors include

- Exposure to cigarette smoke
- Family history of frequent ear infections

The eustachian tube connects the middle ear with the nasal passages (see art on page 1389) and helps balance air pressure in the middle ear with that in the environment. In older children and adults, the tube is relatively vertical, wide, and rigid, and secretions that pass into it from the nasal passages drain easily. In infants and younger children, the eustachian tube is more horizontal, narrower, less rigid, and shorter. Thus, the tube is more likely to become blocked by secretions and to collapse, trapping the secretions in or close to the middle ear and preventing ventilation of the middle ear (that is, blocking air from reaching it). Also, the secretions may contain viruses or bacteria, which multiply and cause infection. Or viruses and bacteria can move back up the short eustachian tube of infants, causing middle ear infections.

At about the age of 6 months, infants become more susceptible to infection because they lose protection from their mother's antibodies, which they received through the placenta before birth. Breastfeeding seems to partially protect children from ear infections because breast milk contains the mother's antibodies.

Also at about this age, children become more sociable and may acquire viral infections after touching other children and objects, then putting their fingers in their mouth and nose. These infections may in turn lead to middle ear infections. Attendance at child care centers increases the risk of exposure to the common cold and hence to otitis media.

Using a pacifier may impair the function of the eustachian tube and thus interfere with air reaching the middle ear.

Middle ear infections can resolve relatively quickly (acute), or they can recur or persist over a long time (chronic).

ACUTE MIDDLE EAR INFECTION

Acute middle ear infection is a bacterial or viral infection of the middle ear, usually accompanying a cold.

- Children with ear infections may have a fever and trouble sleeping and may cry, become irritable, and pull on their ears.
- Doctors use a handheld light called an otoscope to check the eardrum for redness or bulging.
- Acetaminophen or ibuprofen can relieve fever and pain, and antibiotics are usually used when children do not get better quickly or get worse.

Acute middle ear infection (also called acute otitis media—see page 1388) is most often caused by the same viruses that cause the common cold. Acute infection may also be caused by bacteria that sometimes normally reside in the mouth and nose. These bacteria include *Streptococcus pneumoniae, Haemophilus influenzae,* and *Moraxella catarrhalis.* An infection initially caused by a virus sometimes leads to a bacterial infection.

Symptoms

Infants with acute middle ear infections have a fever and trouble sleeping. They cry or become irritable for no reason. They may also have a runny nose, cough, vomiting, and diarrhea. The ear is painful and hearing may be decreased. Infants and children who cannot communicate verbally may pull at their ears. Older children are usually able to tell parents that their ear hurts or that they cannot hear well.

Commonly, fluid accumulates behind the eardrum and remains after the acute infection has resolved. This disorder is called secretory otitis media (see page 1389).

 Did You Know...

Many ear infections resolve without use of antibiotics.

Complications: Rarely, acute middle ear infection leads to more serious complications. The eardrum may rupture, causing blood or fluid to drain from the ear. Also, nearby structures may become infected and cause symptoms:

- Infection of the bone surrounding the ear (mastoiditis): Pain
- Infection of the inner ear (labyrinthitis): Dizziness and deafness
- Infection of the tissues surrounding the brain (meningitis) or collections of pus (abscesses) in the brain: Headache, confusion, seizures, and other neurologic problems

If infections recur, abnormal skinlike tissue (a cholesteatoma) may grow through the eardrum. A cholesteatoma can damage the bones of the middle ear and cause hearing loss.

Diagnosis

Doctors diagnose acute middle ear infections by looking for bulging and redness of the eardrum with an otoscope. They may need to clean wax from the ear first so they can see more clearly. Doctors may use a rubber bulb and tube attached to the otoscope to squeeze air into the ear to see if the eardrum moves. If the eardrum does not move or moves only slightly, infection may be present.

Ventilating Tubes: Treating Recurring Ear Infections

Ventilating (tympanostomy) tubes are tiny, hollow plastic or metal tubes that are placed in the eardrum through a small slit. These tubes balance the pressure in the environment with that in the middle ear. Doctors recommend ventilating tubes for children who have had recurring ear infections (acute otitis media) or recurring or persistent collections of fluid in their middle ears (chronic secretory otitis media).

Placement of ventilating tubes is a common surgical procedure, done in a hospital or doctor's office. After the procedure, children usually go home within a few hours. The tubes usually fall out on their own after a few months, although some types stay in for a year or more.

Children with ventilating tubes may wash their hair and go swimming, but some doctors recommend that the children not submerge their head completely in water without using earplugs.

Drainage of fluid from the ears indicates an infection, and the doctor should be notified.

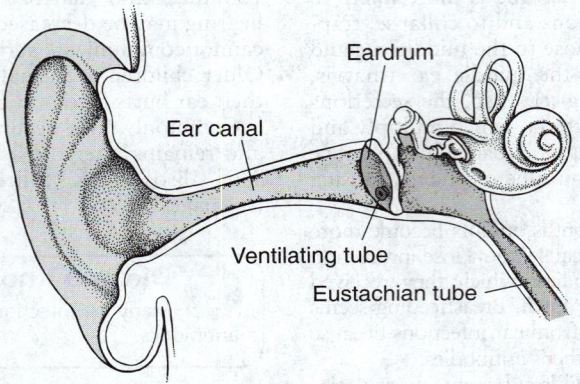

Treatment

Acetaminophen or ibuprofen is effective for fever and pain.

Many acute middle ear infections resolve without antibiotics. Thus, many doctors use antibiotics only when children do not improve after a brief period of time or when there are signs that the infection is getting worse. Antibiotics, such as amoxicillin (with or without clavulanate) or trimethoprim plus sulfamethoxazole, may be used.

Preparations that contain decongestants (such as pseudoephedrine) or antihistamines (such as brompheniramine or chlorpheniramine) are not helpful.

CHRONIC MIDDLE EAR INFECTION

Chronic middle ear infection results from recurring infections that damage the eardrum or lead to formation of a cholesteatoma, which in turn promotes more infection.

For children with chronic ear infection, doctors may recommend daily antibiotics for several months. If infection persists or recurs despite the use of antibiotics, doctors may recommend ventilating (tympanostomy) tubes. If the eardrum is damaged or a cholesteatoma has formed, surgery to repair the eardrum or to remove the cholesteatoma may be done.

Secretory Otitis Media

Secretory otitis media (serous otitis media) is fluid accumulation behind the eardrum (see page 1389).

- A previous ear infection is the usual cause, although some children may develop it as a result of gastroesophageal reflux disease or a blocked eustachian tube.
- Children have no pain, but fluid can impair hearing.
- Diagnosis involves physical examination of the eardrum and sometimes tympanometry.
- Secretory otitis media usually resolves without treatment, although some children need surgery to install a ventilating tube.

Secretory otitis media often occurs after acute otitis media. The fluid that has accumulated behind the eardrum during the acute infection remains after the infection resolves. Secretory otitis media may also occur without a preceding ear infection. It may be due to gastroesophageal reflux disease or a blockage of the eustachian tube by infection or enlarged adenoids. Allergies may also make secretory otitis media more likely to develop. Secretory otitis media is extremely common among children aged 3 months to 3 years.

Although this disorder is painless, the fluid often impairs hearing. Hearing may be impaired sufficiently to affect the understanding of speech, language development, learning, and behavior.

> ### Did You Know...
> After an ear infection, fluid may accumulate behind the eardrum, interfering with hearing but causing no pain.

Diagnosis

Doctors diagnose secretory otitis media by looking for changes in the color and appearance of the eardrum and by squeezing air into the ear to see whether the eardrum moves. If the eardrum does not move but there is no redness or bulging and the child has few symptoms, secretory otitis media is likely. If examination findings are unclear, doctors often do tympanometry. In tympanometry, a device containing a microphone and a sound source is placed snugly in the ear canal, and sound waves are bounced off the eardrum as the device varies the pressure in the ear canal.

Treatment

Secretory otitis media often does not resolve when treated with antibiotics or other drugs, such as decongestants, antihistamines, or nasal sprays. But it often resolves by itself after weeks or months.

If the disorder persists and children do not improve after 3 months, surgery may help. In the United States, myringotomy may be done. For this procedure, doctors make a tiny slit in the eardrum, remove the fluid, and insert a small ventilating (tympanostomy) tube in the slit to provide drainage from the middle to the outer ear. The adenoids (collections of lymphoid tissue located where the throat and nasal passage meet) are often removed at the same time. Sometimes a myringotomy is done to remove fluid but not to insert ventilating tubes. This procedure is called tympanocentesis.

Pharyngitis

Pharyngitis is infection of the throat (pharynx) and sometimes the tonsils.

- Pharyngitis is usually caused by a virus and resolves without treatment.
- Occasionally, it is caused by certain bacteria (particularly those called streptococci) and results in strep throat.
- The throat is sore and red, swallowing is painful, and the tonsils may be enlarged or coated white.

- The diagnosis is usually based on symptoms, but if strep throat is suspected, doctors may take a swab from the back of the throat and test it.
- Ibuprofen or acetaminophen and plenty of fluids are recommended for all sore throats, plus penicillin for strep throat.

Most pharyngitis is caused by the same viruses that cause the common cold. Like the common cold, viral pharyngitis resolves without treatment and is a problem only because it makes children miserable and causes them to miss school. *Streptococcus* bacteria (streptococci) are a less common but more serious cause of pharyngitis (strep throat). Strep throat is unusual in children younger than 2 years. Rarely, pharyngitis is caused by unusual infections, such as infectious mononucleosis (which is due to a virus) or, in countries with low vaccination rates, diphtheria.

The tonsils (patches of lymphoid tissue at the back of the throat) can also become infected in children with pharyngitis. A doctor may use the term tonsillitis when the tonsils are particularly enlarged. Occasionally, the tonsils remain infected, inflamed, or enlarged after an episode of pharyngitis.

Pharyngitis due to bacteria can cause the following:

- Persistent inflammation, infection, and enlargement of the tonsils (chronic tonsillitis)
- Pus within folds of the tonsils (cryptic tonsillitis)
- Abscesses in the tissues to the side of the pharynx (lateral pharyngeal abscesses), behind the pharynx (retropharyngeal abscesses), or around the tonsils (peritonsillar abscesses—see page 1402)

Rarely pharyngitis due to streptococci causes rheumatic fever (see page 1765), glomerulonephritis, or a life-threatening infection of the tissues (necrotizing fasciitis) or bloodstream (toxic shock syndrome).

Symptoms

All children with pharyngitis have a sore throat and some degree of pain when they swallow. The ears may be painful because the throat and ears share the same nerves. The back of the throat and tonsils are typically red, and the tonsils may be enlarged or coated with a white discharge.

Children with pharyngitis as part of a head cold have a runny nose, cough, and slight fever.

Children with strep throat may have tender, enlarged lymph nodes in the neck and a high fever. A few children with strep throat have symptoms of scarlet fever (see page 1180), which include bright white or red changes of the tongue (strawberry tongue) and a distinctive red skin rash (scarlatiniform rash).

Children with chronic tonsillitis may have a sore throat or discomfort or pain when they swallow.

Locating the Tonsils and Adenoids

The tonsils are two areas of lymphoid tissue located on either side of the throat. The adenoids, also lymphoid tissue, are located higher and further back, behind the palate, where the nasal passages connect with the throat. The adenoids are not visible through the mouth.

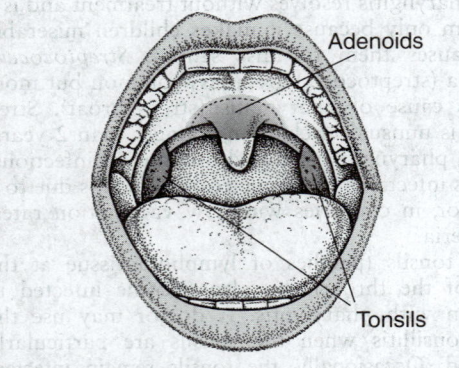

Adenoids

Tonsils

Diagnosis and Treatment

Doctors suspect pharyngitis when they see redness and a white discharge or pus in the back of the throat and when the lymph nodes in the neck are enlarged.

If doctors suspect strep throat, they may take a swab from the back of the throat and send it for two tests: rapid antigen testing and a bacterial culture. Rapid antigen testing can detect strep throat within minutes. If the result of a rapid test is positive, the bacterial culture is not needed. However, if the result of the rapid test is negative, a culture is usually done. Culture takes about 1 to 2 days for results.

Strep throat is usually treated with penicillin in a single injection or over 10 days by mouth. If children are allergic to penicillin, doctors may use erythromycin or another antibiotic. Treatment of strep throat and pharyngitis due to a virus includes giving ibuprofen or acetaminophen for pain and fever and encouraging children to drink fluids. Providing soup is a good way to keep children well hydrated and nourished when swallowing is painful and before their appetite has returned. Gargling with salt water or using an anesthetic throat spray may also help temporarily relieve pain.

Enlarged Tonsils and Adenoids

- Enlarged tonsils and adenoids in children may result from infections but may be normal.
- Enlargement usually causes no symptoms but can cause difficulty breathing or swallowing, a sore throat,

and sometimes recurring ear or sinus infections or obstructive sleep apnea.

- Antibiotics may be used if a bacterial infection is suspected, and sometimes the tonsils and adenoids are removed.

Tonsils and adenoids are collections of lymphoid tissue that help the body fight infection. They trap bacteria and viruses entering through the throat and produce antibodies. The tonsils are located on both sides of the back of the throat. The adenoids are located higher and further back, where the nasal passages connect with the throat. The tonsils are visible through the mouth, but the adenoids are not.

Some preschool and adolescent children have relatively large tonsils and adenoids that are not due to any problem. However, tonsils and adenoids can become enlarged because, for example, they become infected with bacteria that cause pharyngitis. When enlarged, tonsils sometimes interfere with breathing or swallowing, and adenoids may block the nose. Usually, tonsils and adenoids return to normal size once the infection is over. Sometimes they remain enlarged, particularly in children who have had frequent or chronic infections. Although extremely rare, cancer sometimes causes enlarged tonsils or adenoids in children.

Symptoms

Most enlarged tonsils and adenoids cause no symptoms. However, children with enlarged tonsils or adenoids may have a sore throat and discomfort or pain during swallowing. Enlarged adenoids can give the voice a pinched nose quality and change the shape of the palate and the position of the teeth.

Enlarged tonsils and adenoids are considered a problem when they cause more serious problems such as the following:

- Chronic ear infections and hearing loss: These problems result from blockage of the eustachian tube and fluid accumulation in the middle ear.
- Recurring sinus infections and nosebleeds
- Obstructive sleep apnea (see page 485): Some children with enlarged tonsils and adenoids snore and stop breathing for brief periods during sleep. As a result, oxygen levels in the blood may be low, and children may wake up frequently and be sleepy during the day. Rarely, obstructive sleep apnea caused by enlarged tonsils and adenoids has serious complications, such as high blood pressure in the lungs (pulmonary hypertension) and changes in the heart due to pulmonary hypertension (cor pulmonale—see box on page 523).
- Weight loss or lack of weight gain: Children may not eat sufficiently because of pain or because breathing takes constant physical effort.

Diagnosis

To determine whether the cause is an infection, doctors determine how many episodes of sore throat children have had during the past 1 to 3 years. This information is more helpful than the size of the tonsils alone. Enlarged tonsils are more likely to be the result of a disorder in children who have had frequent episodes of sore throat. Very large tonsils may be normal, and chronically infected tonsils may be normal-sized. Doctors also look for redness of the tonsils, enlargement of lymph nodes at the jaw and in the neck, and the effect of the tonsils on breathing.

Obstructive sleep apnea is suspected when parents report that the child stops breathing frequently during sleep. Doctors may also recommend polysomnography. For this test, oxygen levels in the blood are measured and the child is observed while sleeping.

> **? Did You Know...**
>
> Removing enlarged tonsils and adenoids is useful only when enlargement causes extreme discomfort, breathing problems, or recurrent infections.

Treatment

Doctors may give antibiotics if they think the cause may be a bacterial infection. If antibiotics are not effective or if doctors think antibiotics will not be useful, doctors may recommend surgical removal of the tonsils and adenoids (tonsillectomy and adenoidectomy).

Tonsillectomy and adenoidectomy used to be very common operations for children in the United States. But they are much less common now that doctors are more aware of which children will benefit from the operation. Children who benefit from surgery include those with the following:

- Obstructive sleep apnea
- Extreme discomfort when talking and breathing
- Multiple throat or ear infections (defined by some as seven or more infections in 1 year, five or more infections a year over 2 years, or three or more a year over 3 years)
- Cancer (rarely a cause)

Doctors may recommend adenoidectomy alone for the following:

- Ear infections
- Recurring nasal congestion
- Sinus infections

Tonsillectomy and adenoidectomy do not seem to decrease the frequency or severity of colds or cough.

Tonsillectomy and adenoidectomy are usually done on an outpatient basis. These operations should be done at least 3 weeks after any infection has cleared. The surgical complication rate is low, but postoperative pain and difficulty swallowing may last up to a week. Bleeding is a less common complication but may occur anytime from the first day of surgery to the tenth day after surgery.

Hearing Impairment

- Hearing loss usually results from genetic defects in newborns and from ear infections or earwax in older children.
- If children do not respond to sounds, have difficulty talking, or are slow starting to talk, their hearing may be impaired.
- A handheld device or a test that measures the brain's responses to sounds is used to test hearing in newborns, and various techniques are used for older children.
- If possible, the cause is treated, but hearing aids are usually needed.

Hearing impairment is relatively common among children:

- Severe impairment at birth in about 1 in 1,000
- Less severe impairment at birth in about 3 in 1,000
- Development of hearing impairment before adulthood in about 4 in 1,000 children with normal hearing at birth
- Some difficulty hearing in about 19 in 100 children aged 0 to 19 years
- Hearing loss (mild, moderate, or severe) in *one* ear in about 55 in 1,000 children

Not recognizing and treating impairment can seriously impair a child's ability to speak and understand language. The impairment can lead to failure in school, teasing by peers, social isolation, and emotional difficulties.

Causes

Genetic defects are the most common cause of hearing impairment in newborns. Ear infections, including secretory otitis media, and accumulation of earwax are the most common causes of hearing impairment in infants and older children. In older children, other causes include head injury, loud noise (including loud music), use of aminoglycoside antibiotics (such as gentamicin) or thiazide diuretics, certain viral infections (such as mumps), tumors or injuries that damage the auditory nerve, injury by pencils or other foreign objects that become stuck deep in the ear, and, rarely, autoimmune disorders.

Risk Factors for Hearing Impairment in Children

NEWBORNS

- Low birth weight (especially less than 3.3 pounds, or 1.5 kilograms)
- Low Apgar score (lower than 5 at 1 minute or lower than 7 at 5 minutes after birth)—this score reflects the newborn's overall condition
- Low blood oxygen levels or seizures resulting from a difficult delivery
- Infection with rubella, syphilis, herpes, cytomegalovirus, or toxoplasmosis before birth
- Abnormalities in the skull or face, especially those involving the outer ear and ear canal
- A high level of bilirubin (a waste product) in the blood
- Bacterial meningitis
- Bloodstream infection (sepsis)
- Use of a ventilator for a long time
- Use of certain drugs, such as aminoglycoside antibiotics and some diuretics
- History of early hearing loss in a parent or close relative

OLDER CHILDREN

All the above, plus the following:

- A head injury with a skull fracture or loss of consciousness
- Chronic otitis media with a cholesteatoma
- Some neurologic disorders, such as neurofibromatosis and neurodegenerative disorders
- Exposure to noise
- Perforation of the eardrum due to infection or injury

Symptoms

Parents may suspect severe hearing impairment if the child does not respond to sounds or if the child has difficulty talking or delayed speech.

Less severe hearing impairment can be more subtle and lead to behavior that is misinterpreted by parents and doctors, such as the following:

- Ignoring people who are talking to them some but not all of the time
- Being able to talk and hear well at home but not in school (mild or moderate hearing impairment may cause problems only in the midst of the background noise of a classroom)

In general, if children are developing well in one setting but have noticeable social, behavioral, language, or learning difficulties in a different setting, they should be screened for hearing impairment.

Screening and Diagnosis

Because hearing plays such an important role in a child's development, many doctors recommend that all newborns be tested for hearing impairment by the age of 3 months. This testing is required by law in many states.

Newborns are usually screened in two stages. First, children are tested for echoes produced by healthy ears in response to soft clicks made by a handheld device (evoked otoacoustic emissions testing). If this test raises questions about a child's hearing, a second test is done to measure electrical signals from the brain in response to sounds (the auditory brain stem response test, or ABR). The ABR is painless and usually done while children are sleeping. It can be used in children of any age. If results of the ABR are abnormal, the test is repeated in 1 month. If hearing loss is still detected, children may be fitted with hearing aids and may benefit from placement in an educational setting responsive to children with impaired hearing.

In older children, several techniques are used to diagnose hearing impairment:

- Asking a series of questions to detect delays in a child's normal development or to assess a parent's concern about language and speech development
- Examining the ears for abnormalities
- For children aged 6 months to 2 years, testing their response to various sounds
- Testing the response of the eardrum to a range of sound frequencies (tympanometry), which may indicate whether there is fluid in the middle ear
- After age 2 years, asking children to follow simple commands, which usually indicates whether they hear and understand speech or testing their responses to sounds using earphones

Did You Know...

If children ignore people who are talking to them some but not all of the time, their hearing may be impaired.

Treatment

Treating some causes of hearing loss can restore hearing. For example, ear infections can be treated with antibiotics or surgery, earwax can be manually removed or dissolved with ear drops, and cholesteatomas can be surgically removed.

Most often the cause of a child's hearing loss cannot be reversed, and treatment involves use of a hearing aid to compensate for the impairment as much as possible.

Hearing aids are available for infants as well as older children. Children with a mild or moderate hearing impairment in one ear usually need an FM radio system that transmits a teacher's voice directly to a set of speakers, hearing aids, or earphones. Cochlear implants (devices placed in the inner ear to stimulate the auditory nerve with an electrical current in response to sounds) are used for most children with severely impaired hearing (see art on page 1384).

People in deaf communities are proud of their rich culture and alternative forms of communication. Many people oppose the aggressive treatment of hearing impairment on the grounds that it denies children the opportunities available in those communities. Families who wish to consider this approach should discuss it with their doctor.

Objects in the Ears and Nose

Cotton, pieces of pencils, paper, pebbles, and beans are just a few of the many objects children put in their ears and nose. Insects sometimes crawl into ears and cause substantial pain.

In the Ear: Objects in the ear can be removed by flushing the ear canal with sterile water or saline or using suction, forceps, or other tools. Doctors may remove an insect by putting a topical anesthetic or mineral oil in the ear, which kills the insect, stops pain, and makes removal easier. Younger, more frightened children may need to be sedated or to be given a general anesthetic for these procedures.

Sharp objects, such as pencils, can pierce (perforate) the eardrum. Perforations require evaluation by an ear specialist, but most heal by themselves over time without loss of hearing.

In the Nose: Objects stuck up the nose are of particular concern because they can block the airway, cause infection, and be difficult to remove. Children are often scared to admit they put an object in their nose. Many parents become aware of the problem only when a child's nose bleeds persistently, is runny, or has a foul-smelling discharge or when the child has difficulty breathing on only one side of the nose.

Doctors use a topical anesthetic and attempt to remove the object using suction or forceps. If these measures do not work, doctors may need to sedate children or give them a general anesthetic to remove the object.

Neck Masses

Neck masses are swellings that change the shape of the neck.

Neck masses are extremely common among children. The most common cause is one or more enlarged lymph nodes (see box on page 1408). A lymph node may enlarge for the following reasons:

- It is infected (called lymphadenitis).
- There is an infection nearby, for example, in the throat.
- There is a general infection of the body (such as mononucleosis, tuberculosis, or HIV).

Sometimes neck masses are caused by a cyst (a fluid-filled sac) that has been present from birth but is noticed only after it has become inflamed or infected. Neck masses may also result from swelling due to a neck injury, inflammation of the salivary glands, or noncancerous (benign) tumors. Rarely, lymphoma, a thyroid tumor, or another cancerous (malignant) tumor is the cause.

Most neck masses cause no symptoms and are of greater concern to parents than to the children who have them. However, infected lymph nodes or cysts are tender and painful.

Diagnosis and Treatment

Because many neck masses are caused by viral infections and disappear without treatment, tests are usually not needed unless a mass persists for several weeks. However, doctors may take a swab from the back of the throat to test for a bacterial infection, or they may do blood tests to look for such disorders as infectious mononucleosis, leukemia, hyperthyroidism, or bleeding problems. Doctors may also take x-rays and use computed tomography (CT) to determine whether the mass is a tumor or a cyst and to determine more precisely how big it is and where it extends. A skin test may be done to check for tuberculosis, and a biopsy may be done to determine whether a cancerous tumor is present.

Treatment depends on the cause. Antibiotics are useful for infected lymph nodes and other bacterial infections. Masses caused by viral infections and swelling due to injury gradually disappear with time. Tumors and cysts usually require surgery.

Laryngeal Papillomas

Laryngeal papillomas are rare noncancerous (benign) tumors of the voice box (larynx).

Laryngeal papillomas are caused by human papillomavirus. Although papillomas can occur at any age, they most commonly affect children aged 1 to 4 years.

Papillomas are suspected when parents notice hoarseness, a weak cry, or other changes in the child's voice. Papillomas recur often and occasionally spread into the windpipe and lungs, blocking the airway. Rarely, they become cancerous (malignant).

Laryngeal papillomas are detected using a laryngoscope to view the voice box. Doctors do a biopsy of the papilloma to confirm the diagnosis.

Surgery is the usual treatment. Many children require numerous procedures through childhood to remove the tumors as they reappear. At puberty, some papillomas may disappear without treatment.

Juvenile Angiofibroma

Juvenile angiofibroma is a rare noncancerous (benign) tumor that grows in the back of the nose, in the same area where the adenoids are (see page 1812).

Juvenile angiofibroma occurs most commonly among adolescent boys. The tumor contains many blood vessels. It can grow slowly, spreading into the area around the brain and into the orbits of the eye.

Typically, the tumor causes a stuffy nose or headache, often with nosebleeds, which are sometimes very severe. The face may swell, or an eye may bulge. A mass may protrude from the nose, or the nose may become disfigured. If the tumor grows slowly, people may have few symptoms.

Doctors base the diagnosis on symptoms. It is confirmed by an imaging test such as computed tomography (CT) and usually angiography (x-rays of blood vessels taken after a dye is injected in the veins to outline them). A biopsy sample may be taken, but this can result in severe bleeding.

Usually, the tumor is surgically removed. Occasionally, radiation therapy is also used, especially if the tumor recurs.

Communication Disorders

A communication disorder can involve hearing, voice, speech, language, or a combination.

More than 10% of children have a communication disorder. There are several types:

Hearing Impairment: See page 1813.

Voice Disorders: More than 6% of school-age children have voice problems, such as hoarseness. Such problems may interfere with academic performance and socialization in school. These problems usually result from overusing or misusing the voice. As a result, small nodules can form on the vocal cords.

These nodules usually resolve with voice therapy and only rarely require surgery.

Speech Disorders: In these disorders, the production of a speech sound is difficult. As a result, children are less able to communicate meaningfully. About 5% of children entering the first grade have a speech disorder. Speech disorders include the following:

- Speaking through the nose, which may result from a cleft palate or other facial defect
- Stuttering
- Difficulty forming sounds because controlling and coordinating the muscles used to produce speech is difficult (articulation disorders)

Speech therapy is helpful in many of the disorders. A cleft palate is almost always repaired surgically. Speech therapy is often also needed.

Specific Language Impairment: The ability to use language—understanding or expressing it—is reduced in otherwise healthy children. Thus, the ability to communicate is greatly impaired, limiting educational, social, and vocational opportunities. This disorder occurs in about 5% of children and is more common among boys than girls. Abnormal genes appear to play a role in many cases.

Some children appear to recover on their own. Others need language therapy. Some respond poorly to therapy.

Diagnosis

To diagnose voice and speech disorders, doctors examine the mouth and look at the voice box with a mirror or a thin, flexible viewing tube (laryngoscope), which is inserted through the nose.

Language disorders are diagnosed by comparing the child's language with that expected for children of the same age.

Most important, parents or caretakers should be alert for communication problems in children and should contact a doctor if they suspect such a problem. Checklists of communication developmental landmarks are available and can help parents and caregivers detect a problem. For example, if children cannot say at least two words by their first birthday, they may have a communication disorder.

276 Eye Disorders

Congenital glaucoma and congenital cataracts (see table on page 1709) are uncommon disorders that can affect newborns and young children. Disorders that most often blur vision, such as nearsightedness, farsightedness, and astigmatism (all considered refractive errors), do occur in children and require prompt treatment to prevent amblyopia (a decrease in vision). Amblyopia affects about 2 to 3% of children and almost always develops before age 2. Misalignment of the eyes (strabismus) occurs in about 3% of children and can also cause loss of vision due to amblyopia.

In addition to doing a routine eye examination, doctors examine children at the earliest possible age for strabismus and refractive errors, which can cause amblyopia. Screening for this kind of visual problem should start by age 3 and continue during schooling.

Amblyopia

Amblyopia, a common cause of vision loss in children, is a decrease in vision that occurs because the brain ignores the image received from one eye. Vision loss may be irreversible if not diagnosed and treated before age 8.

- Amblyopia can be caused by farsightedness, astigmatism, misalignment of the eyes, or cataracts.
- Children can have no symptoms or symptoms that include squinting, covering one eye, or having one eye that does not look in the same direction as the other.
- The diagnosis is based on the results of vision testing.
- If diagnosed and treated early, amblyopia can be corrected.
- Treatment includes eyeglasses, an eye patch, or corrective surgery for cataracts.

Causes

A child's visual pathways are not fully developed at birth. The vision system and the brain need to be stimulated by clear, focused, properly aligned, overlapping images from both eyes to develop normally. This development takes place mainly in the first 3 years of life but is not complete until about 8 years of age. If the brain does not receive proper visual stimulation from an eye during the development period, it learns to ignore (suppress) the image from that eye, resulting in vision loss. If the suppression persists long enough, vision loss can be permanent. There are several reasons for lack of proper visual stimulation, each of which can cause a type of amblyopia.

Refractive Errors in Children

Refractive errors, such as nearsightedness (inability to see distant objects clearly), farsightedness (inability to see close objects clearly), and astigmatism (an irregular curvature of the focusing surfaces of the eye— see box on page 1418) result in blurring of vision. Blurring occurs because the eye cannot focus images precisely on the retina. If uncorrected, a decrease in vision (amblyopia) may develop.

Children are often not able to make their vision problems known. Sometimes a teacher or school nurse is the first to detect a vision problem.

All children should be screened for refractive errors and other eye problems. Children as young as 3 or 4 years old can view charts with pictures, figures, or letters used to test vision. Vision is tested in each eye separately to detect loss of vision that affects only one eye. The eye not being tested is covered.

Diagnosis is established by an eye examination and measurement of the refractive error. In young children, refractive errors are generally treated with eyeglasses. In older, more responsible children, refractive errors can be corrected with contact lenses. However, inadequate care and cleaning of contact lenses can lead to eye infections.

Refractive Amblyopia: Amblyopia may be caused by an uncorrected or unequal refractive error, usually farsightedness or astigmatism, particularly when there is a large difference between the two eyes.

Strabismic Amblyopia: Misalignment of the eyes (strabismus) can also cause amblyopia. The eyes produce two images—one from each eye—that normally are fused or united into a single image in the brain and then integrated to produce three-dimensional images and high levels of depth perception. The ability to fuse images develops during early childhood. If the two images are so misaligned that they cannot be fused together, the brain suppresses an image, ignoring the input from that eye. The brain is unaware of the image from the affected eye even though the eye may be structurally normal. In adults, because the visual pathways are already developed, seeing two different images results in double vision (diplopia) rather than in loss of vision.

Deprivation Amblyopia: A third type of amblyopia develops when a clouding or opacity of the lens of the eye (cataract) or the cornea reduces or distorts the light entering an eye.

Symptoms and Diagnosis

Children with amblyopia may be too young to describe symptoms. These children may squint, cover one eye, or have one eye that does not look in the same direction as the other, all of which may indicate a problem that requires examination. Children, however, often do not appear to have a problem. If one eye sees well and the other does not, children compensate well and do not seem to function differently from their peers. Thus, to detect problems in visual development, vision screening for all children should be started during early well-child examinations and continued throughout childhood. In some areas, preschool children are screened by volunteers and local and regional agencies. Once children reach school age, screening is done in school by health practitioners. If a problem is found during screening, the child should see an eye doctor, either an ophthalmologist or an optometrist.

> **? Did You Know...**
> Sometimes a teacher or school nurse is the first to notice a child has an eye disorder.

Treatment and Prognosis

Treating amblyopia involves forcing the brain to use the visual images from the problem eye. Sometimes this is accomplished simply by correcting refractive errors with eyeglasses. More often, doctors "handicap" the normal, stronger eye by putting a patch over it or using eye drops to blur its vision. If strabismus is the cause, it should be corrected (see below) after vision has been equalized between the eyes. A cataract or other opacity in the eye may require surgical treatment.

Treatment should be initiated promptly, preferably during the first 2 to 4 years of life. The earlier the treatment is initiated, the quicker the response will be. Regardless of the cause, amblyopia that has not been treated by age 8 usually cannot be fully reversed. Failure to effectively treat amblyopia may result in permanent blindness in the affected eye.

The sooner amblyopia or risk factors for amblyopia are detected, the more likely amblyopia can be prevented or corrected. For these reasons, vision screening programs for children should be supported by the community.

Strabismus

Strabismus (also called squint, cross-eye, lazy eye, or wandering eye) is an intermittent or constant misalignment of an eye so that its line of vision is not pointed at the same object as the other eye. If untreated, strabismus can cause amblyopia (a decrease in vision) and permanent loss of vision. Strabismus is treated with correction of any refractive error, a patch to equalize vision, and, in some cases, surgery.

- Strabismus is caused by an imbalance in the muscles that control the positioning of the eye.
- Symptoms include misalignment of the eyes, double vision, and paralysis of eye muscles.
- The diagnosis is based on an eye examination.
- Strabismus sometimes resolves on its own, but in most cases, eyeglasses, eye drops, or surgery is needed.

The causes of strabismus are varied and include an imbalance in the pull of muscles that control the position of the eyes and poor vision in one eye. Although not usually caused by a general medical or neurologic disorder, strabismus is a serious problem that should be evaluated and treated and not ignored or watched. Prompt examination by an eye doctor, either an ophthalmologist or an optometrist, is essential.

There are several types of strabismus. Some types are characterized by inward turning of the eye (esotropia or cross-eye) and some by outward turning of the eye (exotropia or walleye). Others are characterized by upward turning of the eye (hypertropia) or downward turning of the eye (hypotropia). The defect in alignment may be constant or intermittent and may be mild or severe.

Phoria is a tendency for misalignment of the eyes. The tendency is a minor defect that is easily corrected by the brain to maintain apparent alignment of the eyes and allow fusion of the images from both eyes. Thus, phorias usually do not cause symptoms and do not need treatment unless they are large and decompensate, producing double vision.

Tropia is a constant, visible deviation or misalignment of the eyes. An intermittent eye deviation that is frequent and poorly controlled by the brain is termed intermittent tropia.

Strabismus may cause double vision (diplopia) in older children or amblyopia in younger children.

Parents sometimes notice strabismus because the child squints or covers one eye. The defect may be detected by observing that the child's eyes appear to be positioned abnormally or do not move in unison.

Children should be examined periodically to measure vision and to detect strabismus starting at a few months of age. To examine an infant, a doctor shines a light into the eyes to see whether the light reflects back from the same location on each pupil.

Older children can be examined more thoroughly. Children may be asked to recognize objects or letters with one eye covered and to participate in tests to assess alignment of the eyes. All children with strabismus require examination by an eye doctor (ophthalmologist or optometrist).

Strabismus: A Misaligned Eye

There are several types of strabismus. In the most common types, an eye turns inward (esotropia or cross-eye) or outward (exotropia or walleye). In this illustration, the child's right eye is affected.

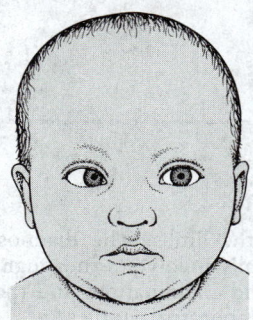

Esotropia

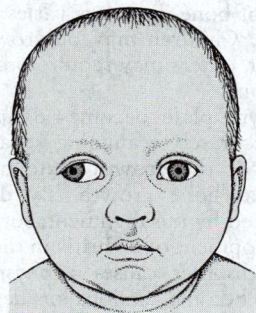

Exotropia

If the defect is minor or intermittent, treatment may not be needed. However, if strabismus is severe or is progressing, treatment is required. Treatment depends on the characteristics of the strabismus.

Infantile Esotropia: Infantile esotropia is a constant inward turning of the eyes that develops before 6 months of age. It often runs in families and tends to be severe. The eyes often begin to turn inward by 3 months of age. The degree of turning is large and easily noticeable.

Surgery, which is done by altering the pull of the eye muscles, is usually needed to realign the eyes. Repeated operations may be necessary. Even with the best possible treatment, strabismus may not be fully corrected. Occasionally, amblyopia develops, but it usually responds to treatment.

Accommodative Esotropia: Accommodative esotropia is inward turning of the eyes that develops between the ages of 6 months and 7 years, most often in children aged 2 to 3 years. It is related to optical focusing (accommodation) of the eyes.

The misalignment is the result of how the eyes move when focusing on nearby or distant objects. Children with accommodative esotropia are farsighted. Although everyone's eyes turn inward when focusing on very close objects, eyes that are farsighted also turn inward when looking at distant objects. In mild cases, the eyes may turn too far inward only when looking at nearby objects. In more severe cases, the eyes turn too far inward all the time. With treatment, accommodative esotropia can usually be corrected. Eyeglasses can help children focus on objects, reducing the tendency for the eyes to turn inward when viewing those objects. Many children outgrow farsightedness and eventually do not need eyeglasses.

Occasionally, drugs (such as echothiophate eye drops) are used to help the eyes to focus on nearby objects. If eyeglasses and eye drops fail to properly align the eyes, surgery may help. Amblyopia often develops in children with accommodative esotropia and sometimes in children with infantile esotropia.

 Did You Know...
Children as young as 3 can have their vision screened.

Intermittent Exotropia: Intermittent exotropia is outward turning of the eyes that occurs intermittently, usually when the child is looking at distant objects or when the child is tired or ill. Intermittent exotropia is detectable after the age of 6 months.

Intermittent exotropia that is of small magnitude, occurs infrequently, and does not cause symptoms may not require treatment because amblyopia does not usually develop. If symptoms of eye strain due to an uncorrected refractive error become troublesome or if attempting to bring the eyes into alignment becomes troublesome, eyeglasses may be used. In more severe cases, surgery may be needed.

Paralytic Strabismus: In paralytic strabismus, one or more of the eye muscles that move the eye in different directions become paralyzed. As a result, the muscles no longer work in balance. The eye muscle paralysis is usually caused by a disorder that affects the nerves to the eye muscles, such as certain viral infections, brain injuries, or brain tumors that increase pressure within the skull and compress these nerves.

In children with paralytic strabismus, movement of the affected eye is impaired only when the eye tries to move in a specific direction, not in all directions. Amblyopia or double vision may develop. The double vision is made worse by looking in directions normally controlled by the paralyzed eye muscles.

Paralytic strabismus may resolve by itself over time. However, it may need to be corrected with eyeglasses and covering of the unaffected eye. Sometimes eyeglasses with prisms are used. Alternatively, surgery may be needed. If paralytic strabismus results from another condition affecting the nerves, such as a brain tumor, the other condition also needs to be treated.

CHAPTER
277 Bone Disorders

- Bone disorders can be caused by injury or cancer, be inherited, occur as part of a child's growth, or occur for no known reason.
- Some bone disorders can cause pain and difficulties walking, whereas others cause no symptoms.
- Doctors base the diagnosis on a thorough history, close observation and examination, and the selective use of x-rays.
- Treatment depends on the disorder.

Children's bones grow continually and reshape (remodel) themselves extensively. Growth proceeds from a vulnerable part of the bone called the growth plate. In remodeling, old bone tissue is gradually replaced by new bone tissue (see page 535). Many bone disorders come from the changes that occur in a growing child's musculoskeletal system. These disorders may get better or worsen as the child grows. Other bone disorders may be inherited or occur in childhood for no known reason.

Causes

Bone disorders in children can result from such causes as injuries, cancer, and infections. Causes that affect mainly children typically involve the gradual misalignment of bones, which is caused by forces exerted on the growth plates as children are developing. A poor blood supply can also damage the growth plate, as can separation from the rest of the bone or even minor misalignment. Damage to the growth plate suppresses the growth of bones, distorts the joint, and can cause long-lasting joint damage (arthritis).

Certain rare hereditary disorders of connective tissue (see page 1825) can also affect the bones. They include Marfan syndrome, osteogenesis imperfecta, chondrodysplasias, and osteopetroses.

Symptoms and Diagnosis

Bone disorders sometimes cause painless deformities. Some deformities may affect a child's ability to walk or use the limbs. The diagnosis of a bone disorder typically involves a thorough history, close observation and examination, and the selective use of x-rays and laboratory studies.

Treatment

Treatment of bone disorders varies depending on the condition. Children may outgrow some disorders. However, others may require bracing or surgical intervention.

If the growth plate becomes damaged, surgery may help. Accurately realigning separated or misaligned ends of the growth plate may surgically restore normal bone growth. By decreasing the irritation caused by misalignment, surgery may prevent the development of arthritis in the joint.

If a bone disorder causes a physical deformity, children may become anxious or depressed. Some treatments for bone disorders may also be psychologically difficult to accept. For example, adolescents may be reluctant to wear a back brace for treatment of scoliosis because doing so makes them appear different from their peers. Professional counseling may relieve anxiety or depression. Counseling may also help children go through with difficult treatments.

Scoliosis

Scoliosis is abnormal curvature of the spine.

- Scoliosis can be present at birth or can develop during adolescence.
- Mild forms may cause only mild discomfort, but more severe forms can cause chronic pain or affect internal organs.
- The diagnosis is based on an examination and x-rays.
- Not all forms of scoliosis worsen, but those that do must be treated as soon as possible to prevent a severe deformity.
- Braces or surgery may be needed to straighten the spine.

Scoliosis is relatively common, especially among girls. It occurs in 2 to 4% of children aged 10 to 16 years. In girls, scoliosis is 60 to 80% more likely to progress and require bracing or surgery. Scoliosis may result from a birth defect or develop later in life, most often in early adolescence. Usually, the cause cannot be identified. The spine usually bulges toward the right when the curvature is in the upper back and to the left when it is in the lower back. The result is that the right shoulder is usually higher than the left. One hip may be higher than the other. Scoliosis often develops in children with kyphosis. The combination is called kyphoscoliosis.

Symptoms and Diagnosis

Mild scoliosis usually causes no symptoms. Sometimes the back becomes sore or stiff after the child sits or stands for a long period of time. Mild or more severe pain may eventually follow.

Mild scoliosis may be discovered during a routine physical examination. A parent, teacher, or doctor may suspect scoliosis when one of the child's shoulders seems higher than the other or when the child's clothes do not hang straight.

A number of factors contribute to the likelihood of scoliosis worsening. The more severe the curve, the greater the likelihood of it worsening, and curves tend to worsen in the early stages of puberty when growth is accelerated. Likewise, the more symptoms that develop, the greater the likelihood that scoliosis will worsen. Worsening scoliosis may eventually cause permanent problems, such as noticeable deformities or chronic pain. Severe scoliosis may even affect internal organs—for example, deforming and damaging the lungs. Sometimes scoliosis can worsen even if symptoms have not developed.

To diagnose the condition, a doctor asks the child to bend forward and views the spine from behind because the abnormal spinal curve can be seen more easily in this position. X-rays show the precise angles of curvature. If doctors think scoliosis may worsen, they may examine the child several times a year. Special devices may be used to measure the curve of the spine more precisely.

Prognosis and Treatment

In most children who have scoliosis, the curvature does not progress further but rather remains small. However, it needs to be monitored by a doctor regularly. Scoliosis that causes symptoms, is worsening, or is severe may need to be treated. The earlier treatment is begun, the better the chance of preventing a severe deformity.

A brace or object fashioned to hold the spine (orthosis) may be worn to keep the spine straight. In the most severe cases, the vertebrae need to be bonded together surgically (spinal fusion). A metal

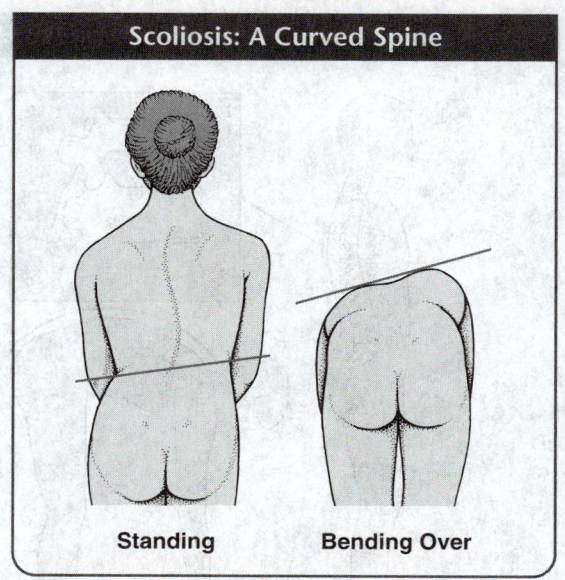

Scoliosis: A Curved Spine

Standing   Bending Over

rod may be inserted during surgery to keep the spine straight until the vertebrae have bonded permanently.

Scoliosis and its treatment often interfere with an adolescent's self-image and self-esteem. Counseling or psychotherapy may be needed.

Kyphosis

Kyphosis (Scheuermann's disease) is an abnormal curving of the spine that causes a humpback.

Some amount of kyphosis is common and begins in adolescence, affecting boys more often than girls. The cause is unknown, but kyphosis sometimes runs in families. The vertebrae curve forward on each other, usually in the upper back. As a result, the back develops a hump. Scoliosis also often develops in children with kyphosis (called kyphoscoliosis).

Kyphosis often causes no symptoms. Sometimes mild, persistent back pain develops. Kyphosis may be noticed only because it alters the body's appearance. The shoulders may appear rounded. The upper spine may appear more curved than normal, or a hump may be visible. Some people have an appearance similar to those with Marfan syndrome, in whom the limbs are much longer than the trunk.

Mild kyphosis that does not cause symptoms is sometimes detected only during a routine physical examination. A doctor confirms the diagnosis by taking x-rays of the spine, which show the curve and the deformity of the vertebrae.

Mild kyphosis can be treated by reducing weight-bearing stress and by avoiding strenuous activities.

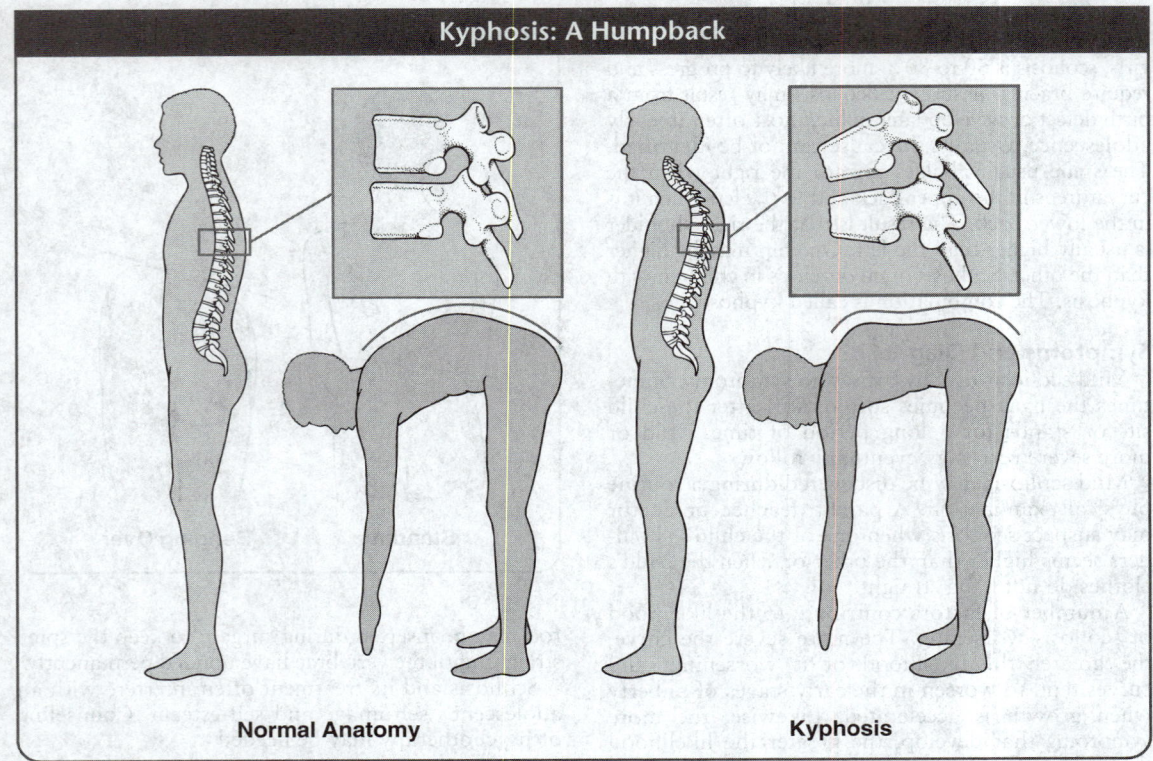

Kyphosis: A Humpback

Normal Anatomy

Kyphosis

The spine may straighten slightly with treatment, although symptoms may not lessen. It is unclear whether treating mild kyphosis prevents the curve from worsening. When kyphosis is more severe, treatment most often consists of wearing a spinal brace or sleeping on a rigid bed. Treatment may lessen symptoms and prevent the curve from worsening. Rarely, despite treatment, kyphosis worsens to such an extent that surgery is needed to straighten the spine.

Slipped Capital Femoral Epiphysis

Slipped capital femoral epiphysis is a separation within the thighbone (femur) at its growth plate in the hip joint.

Slipped capital femoral epiphysis usually develops in overweight adolescents, most commonly boys. The cause is not known. However, the disorder may result from a weakening in the growth plate, which can result from trauma or inflammation or from changes in levels of hormones in the blood, which normally occur around puberty. The separation causes the top part of the thighbone to eventually lose its blood supply, decay, and collapse.

The first symptom may be stiffness or mild pain in the hip. However, the pain may seem to come from the knee. The pain lessens with rest and worsens with walking or moving the hip. Later, a limp develops, followed by hip pain that extends down the inner thigh to the knee. The affected leg is usually twisted outward.

X-rays of the affected hip show slippage or separation of the head of the thighbone from the rest of the bone. Ultrasonography and magnetic resonance imaging (MRI) are also useful, especially if x-rays are normal. Early diagnosis is important because treatment becomes more difficult and gives less satisfactory results later.

Surgery is usually needed to align the separated ends of the thighbone and to fasten them together with metal pins. The hip is immobilized in a cast for several weeks to 2 months.

Legg-Calvé-Perthes Disease

Legg-Calvé-Perthes disease is destruction of the growth plate of the thighbone.

- This disease is caused by a poor blood supply to the upper growth plate of the thighbone.

- Typical symptoms include hip pain and trouble walking.
- The diagnosis is based on a bone scan or magnetic resonance imaging and x-rays.
- Treatment includes immobilization of the hip and bed rest.

Legg-Calvé-Perthes disease develops most commonly in boys between the ages of 5 and 10. It is caused by a poor blood supply to the upper growth plate of the thighbone. The reason for the poor blood supply is not known.

Legg-Calvé-Perthes disease can cause severe hip damage without causing significant symptoms at first. The severe damage may, however, lead to permanent arthritis of the hip. The first symptom is often pain in the hip joint and trouble walking (gait). Pain begins gradually and progresses slowly. The pain tends to worsen when moving the hip or walking. A limp can develop, sometimes before the child experiences much pain. Eventually, joint movement becomes restricted, and the thigh muscles may become wasted (atrophied) from lack of use.

The diagnosis is confirmed by a bone scan or an magnetic resonance imaging (MRI) scan. Later, x-rays may show changes around the growth plate, such as a fracture or destruction of the bone.

Treatment includes prolonged immobilization of the hip. Sometimes the partial immobilization provided by bed rest is sufficient. However, sometimes nearly total immobilization for 12 to 18 months is necessary, requiring traction, slings, plaster casts, or splints. Such treatments keep the legs rotated outward. Physical therapy is used to keep the muscles from contracting and wasting away. If a child is older than 6 and has moderate or severe bone destruction, surgery may be helpful. Regardless of how it is treated, Legg-Calvé-Perthes disease usually takes at least 2 to 3 years to heal. Doctors have recently found that treatment with bisphosphonates (drugs that help increase bone density) may reduce the need for surgery.

Osgood-Schlatter Disease

Osgood-Schlatter disease is inflammation of the bone and cartilage at the top of the shinbone (tibia).

Osgood-Schlatter disease develops between the ages of 10 and 15. The disease is usually more common among boys, but this situation is changing as girls become more active in sports programs. The cause is thought to be repetitive, excessive pulling by the tendon of the kneecap (patellar tendon) on its point of attachment at the top of the shinbone. This attachment point is called the tibial tubercle.

The major symptoms are pain, swelling, and tenderness at the tibial tubercle. The pain worsens

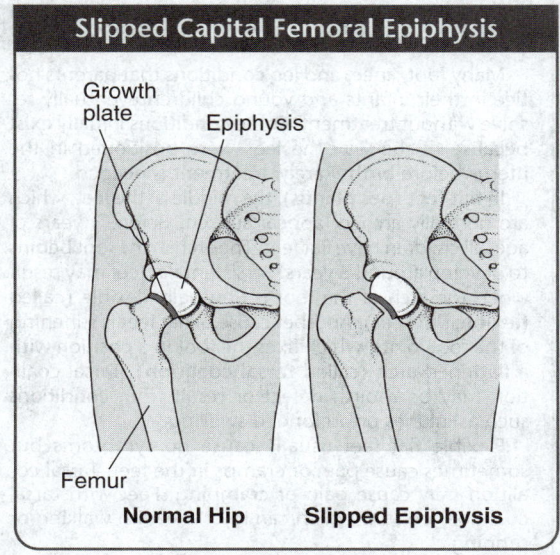

Slipped Capital Femoral Epiphysis

Growth plate

Epiphysis

Femur

Normal Hip   **Slipped Epiphysis**

with activity and is relieved with rest. Swelling and tenderness eventually develop at the site.

X-rays of the knee may show the tibial tubercle has enlarged or has broken into fragments. However, x-rays are not needed unless pain and swelling extend beyond the area over the tibial tubercle or unless pain is accompanied by redness and warmth. In such cases, x-rays are useful to rule out injuries or severe inflammatory conditions.

Avoiding sports and excessive exercise helps reduce pain. Avoiding deep knee bending is particularly helpful. However, doctors do allow children with Osgood-Schlatter disease to continue to participate in sports or exercise even when they are in pain. Use of nonsteroidal anti-inflammatory drugs (NSAIDs), stretching exercises, and application of ice on the affected knee may help relieve the pain. Symptoms usually resolve after several weeks or months.

Köhler's Bone Disease

Köhler's bone disease is inflammation of the tarsal navicular bone (a bone at the arch of the foot).

Köhler's bone disease usually affects children aged 3 to 5 years (more commonly boys) and affects only one foot. The foot becomes swollen and painful, and the arch of the foot is tender. Weight bearing and walking increase discomfort, and the child's manner of walking (gait) is impaired. X-rays show that the navicular bone is initially flattened and hardened and later breaks into fragments before healing and hardening back into

Common Foot, Knee, and Leg Conditions in Infants and Young Children

Many foot, knee, and leg conditions that parents notice in their infants and young children eventually resolve without treatment. Some conditions initially exist because of the way the legs were positioned in the uterus before birth. Rarely, treatment is needed.

In **flat feet (pes planus)**, the middle of the feet, which are normally arched, appear sunken. Before 3 years of age, all children have flat feet. The arch in the foot begins to develop around 3 years. Persistent flat feet may result when the arch of the foot is unusually flexible (called **flexible flat feet**). Another cause of flat feet is stiffening of the foot joints, which fixes the foot in a position with a flattened arch (called **tarsal coalition**). Tarsal coalition may be a birth defect or result from conditions such as injuries or prolonged swelling.

Flexible flat feet usually cause no symptoms but sometimes cause pain or cramps in the feet. Tarsal coalition may cause pain or cramping. Feet with tarsal coalition are stiff, which can interfere with walking or running.

Flexible flat feet usually do not require treatment. However, if an older child has pains or cramps in the feet, corrective shoes may be needed. Treatment for tarsal coalition often includes a cast. Sometimes surgically separating the stiffened foot joint restores mobility to the foot.

In **bowlegs** (physiologic genu varum), the knees appear rotated away from each other. This appearance is due to the position of the hips and inward curve of the lower leg (tibial torsion) created by the position of the legs in the uterus before birth. Typically, this condition corrects itself within the first 2 years as the child begins to walk.

Abnormal growth of the tibia can lead to a condition called **Blount disease** (tibia vara), in which the legs are bowed significantly. Blount disease can affect one or both legs. Most commonly, it appears after the first year. However, it can develop in adolescence. Children younger than 3 years may be treated with leg braces. Older children may be treated with surgery.

In **knock knees** (genu valgum), the knees point inward. Knock knees most often affect children aged 3 to 5 years. Usually, the condition corrects itself by the age of 10 without treatment. If the condition persists into adolescence, surgery may be required.

Femoral torsion is curving of the thighbone (femur). In internal femoral torsion, the thighs curve inward. The knees and usually the toes point toward each other. In external femoral torsion, the thighs curve outward. The knees and toes point away from each other. Internal femoral torsion develops much more often than external femoral torsion. Children with internal femoral torsion sometimes have abnormally flexible joints and ligaments.

Internal and external femoral torsion usually resolve without treatment when the child is older and begins to walk. Sometimes internal femoral torsion is corrected by making sure that the child sits straight. Maintaining a straight sitting position may not be possible until the child reaches school age. Rarely, when internal femoral torsion persists past the age of 10, surgically straightening the bone may be necessary. It can take years for internal or external femoral torsion to resolve.

---

bone. X-rays comparing the affected side with the unaffected side help assess how far the disease has progressed.

Köhler's bone disease rarely lasts beyond 2 years. Rest and pain relief are required, and excessive weight bearing must be avoided. This disease usually resolves without treatment and without any long-term consequences. In severe cases, having the child wear a below-knee walking plaster cast (well molded under the length of the arch of the foot) for a few weeks may help.

Sever's Disease

Sever's disease is inflammation of the heel bone (calcaneus).

The heel bone develops until about age 15. A child (usually aged 9 to 14) who is athletically active may develop Sever's disease if the calf muscle and tendon (Achilles) pull on their point of attachment to the immature heel bone.

Pain affects the sides or margins of the heel and is aggravated by standing on tip toes or running. Some children have warmth and swelling. Doctors base the diagnosis on the symptoms. X-rays are not helpful.

Heel pads relieve pain by reducing the pull of the Achilles tendon on the heel. Splints may be worn at night to passively stretch the calf muscles, helping maintain flexibility. In more severe cases, a cast may be recommended to immobilize the area. This treatment relieves pain and stretches the calf muscles. Symptoms may last several months.

Chondromalacia Patellae

Chondromalacia patellae (patellofemoral syndrome) is softening of the cartilage under the kneecap (patella).

Chondromalacia patellae typically develops in adolescents. Joggers are especially susceptible. The cause is probably a minor, repetitive injury resulting from misalignment of the kneecap. The misalignment causes the cartilage on the underside of the kneecap to grate against other bones when the knee bends.

Dull, aching pain is felt all around and behind the knee. Climbing (especially going up or down stairs), playing certain sports, sitting for a long time, and running usually worsen the pain.

A doctor makes the diagnosis based on the symptoms and physical examination and may recommend exercises to strengthen the quadriceps muscles, which straighten or extend the knee joint.

Increasing knee flexibility with stretching exercises helps. Activities that worsen the pain should be avoided. Ice and analgesics or nonsteroidal anti-inflammatory drugs (NSAIDs), such as ibuprofen or naproxen, can help relieve symptoms. Occasionally, the undersurface of the kneecap must be smoothed with a small (about the diameter of a pencil) fiberoptic scope (arthroscope), which allows the doctor to look inside the joint.

Osteopetroses

Osteopetroses are a group of rare disorders that increase the density of bones.

- These disorders occur when the body does not recycle old bone cells.
- Typical symptoms include impaired bone growth and thick bones that easily break.
- The diagnosis is based on symptoms and x-rays.
- Osteopetrosis that occurs in infancy is fatal if not treated.
- There is no cure, but some treatments can help relieve problems caused by the disorder.

In osteopetrosis (sometimes called marble bones), the body does not recycle old bone cells. The result is increased density or thickness of the bones and an alteration in how the bones are shaped. These changes make bones weaker than normal. The dense bone tissue also crowds out the bone marrow, which is where blood cells are formed.

Osteopetroses range from mild to severe and can even be life threatening. Symptoms may begin in infancy (early onset) or later in life (delayed onset).

Symptoms and Diagnosis

Although osteopetroses are different disorders, many of the same symptoms develop in most of them. Bone growth is usually impaired. Bones thicken and break easily. Formation of blood cells may be impaired because there is less bone marrow, leading to anemia, infection, or bleeding. Overgrowth of bone in the skull can compress nerves, causing facial paralysis or loss of vision or hearing, and can distort the face and teeth.

Doctors usually base the diagnosis on symptoms and on x-rays that show very dense bone. When the person has no symptoms, osteopetrosis is sometimes detected only by chance, after a doctor sees very dense bones on x-rays taken for an unrelated purpose.

Prognosis and Treatment

Early-onset osteopetrosis that is not treated with bone marrow transplantation usually causes death during infancy or early childhood. Death usually results from anemia, infection, or bleeding. Late-onset osteopetrosis is often very mild.

There is no cure. Corticosteroids, such as prednisone, decrease the formation of new bone cells and may increase the rate of removal of old bone cells, strengthening bones. Bone marrow transplantation seems to have cured some infants with early-onset disease. However, the long-term prognosis after transplantation is unknown.

Fractures, anemia, bleeding, and infection require treatment. If nerves going through the skull are compressed, surgery may be required to take pressure off the nerves. Orthodontic treatment may be needed to correct distorted teeth.

CHAPTER

278 Hereditary Connective Tissue Disorders

Muscles, bones, cartilage, ligaments, and tendons are built mostly of connective tissue. Connective tissue is also found in other parts of the body, such as the skin and internal organs. Connective tissue is strong and thus able to support weight and tension.

There are over 200 disorders that involve connective tissue. Some of these disorders have no clear cause, and some are inherited. Certain hereditary disorders cause connective tissue throughout the body to form abnormally. In general, hereditary connective tissue disorders develop in childhood but last throughout life.

Most hereditary connective tissue disorders are diagnosed based on their symptoms and findings during a physical examination. Analysis of genes, usually from a sample of a blood, may help doctors diagnose some hereditary disorders. A biopsy (removal of a tissue sample for examination under a microscope) can also help. The tissue is usually removed using a local anesthetic, which numbs the area. X-rays can reveal bone abnormalities that may be associated with a connective tissue disorder.

Cutis Laxa

Cutis laxa is a rare disorder of connective tissue that causes the skin to stretch easily and hang in loose folds.

In cutis laxa, the elastic fibers contained in the connective tissue become loose. Sometimes only the skin is affected, but connective tissues throughout the body can be affected. Cutis laxa is usually hereditary. In some kinds of cutis laxa, the abnormal genes cause problems unrelated to connective tissues—for example, mental retardation/intellectual disability.

Cutis laxa can be mild, affecting only a person's appearance, or severe, affecting the internal organs. The skin may be very loose at birth, or it may become loose later. The loose skin is often most noticeable on the face, resulting in a prematurely aged appearance. The lungs, heart, intestines, or arteries may be affected with a variety of severe impairments.

Although symptoms often become noticeable shortly after birth, they may begin suddenly in children and adolescents. Symptoms usually develop after a severe illness involving fever, inflammation of organs such as the lining of the lungs or heart, or erythema multiforme (patches of red, raised skin). In some people, symptoms develop gradually during adulthood.

A doctor can usually diagnose cutis laxa by examining the skin. Sometimes removal of a skin tissue sample for examination under a microscope (biopsy) is necessary. Severe impairments of the heart, lungs, arteries, or intestines can be fatal. Plastic surgery can often improve the appearance of the skin, although the improvement may be only temporary.

Ehlers-Danlos Syndrome

Ehlers-Danlos syndrome is a rare disorder of connective tissue that results in unusually flexible joints, very elastic skin, and fragile tissues.

- This syndrome is caused by a defect in one of the genes that controls the production of connective tissue.
- Typical symptoms include flexible joints, a humpback, flat feet, and elastic skin.
- The diagnosis is based on symptoms and results of a physical examination.
- Most people with this syndrome have a normal life span.
- There is no cure for Ehlers-Danlos syndrome.

Ehlers-Danlos syndrome is caused by an abnormality in one of the genes that controls the production of connective tissue. There are several variants (with widely varying severity) involving different genes and causing slightly different changes. The result is abnormally fragile connective tissue, which causes problems in joints and bones and may weaken internal organs.

Children with Ehlers-Danlos syndrome usually have very flexible joints. Some develop small, hard, round lumps under the skin, a humpback with an abnormal curve of the spine (kyphoscoliosis), or flat feet. The skin can be stretched up to several inches but returns to its normal position when released.

Ehlers-Danlos syndrome may alter the body's response to injuries. Minor injuries may result in wide gaping wounds. Although these wounds usually do not bleed excessively, they leave wide scars. Sprains and dislocations develop easily.

In a small number of children with Ehlers-Danlos syndrome, the blood clots poorly. Bleeding from minor wounds may be difficult to stop.

The intestines can bulge through the abdominal wall (called a hernia), and abnormal outpouchings (diverticula) can develop in the intestine. Rarely, a fragile intestine bleeds or ruptures (perforates).

If a pregnant woman has Ehlers-Danlos syndrome, delivery may be premature. If the fetus has Ehlers-Danlos syndrome, the amniotic sac may rupture early (premature rupture of membranes). A mother or baby who has Ehlers-Danlos syndrome can bleed excessively before, during, and after delivery.

A doctor bases the diagnosis on the symptoms and results of a physical examination. The doctor can try to confirm the diagnosis of some types of Ehlers-Danlos syndrome by taking a sample of skin to examine under a microscope (biopsy). Genetic and biochemical tests for some types are available at some research centers. Other tests are done to check for conditions that are associated with complications, such as problems with the heart or blood vessels.

Prognosis and Treatment

Despite the many and varied complications people with Ehlers-Danlos syndrome may have, their life span is usually normal. However, in a few people with one type of Ehlers-Danlos syndrome, complications (usually bleeding) are fatal. Genetic counseling for family members is suggested.

Special precautions should be taken to prevent injuries. For example, children with severe forms of Ehlers-Danlos syndrome can wear protective clothing and padding.

There is no way to cure Ehlers-Danlos syndrome or correct the abnormalities in the connective tissue. Injuries can be treated, but it may be difficult for a doctor to stitch cuts because stitches tend to tear out of the fragile tissue. Usually, using an adhesive tape or medical skin glue closes cuts more easily and leaves less scarring.

Surgery requires special techniques that minimize injury and ensure that a large supply of blood is available for transfusion. An obstetrician must supervise pregnancy and delivery.

Marfan Syndrome

Marfan syndrome is a rare disorder of connective tissue, resulting in abnormalities of the eyes, bones, heart, blood vessels, and central nervous system.

- This syndrome is caused by mutations in the gene that codes for a protein called fibrillin.
- Typical symptoms can range from mild to severe and include long arms and fingers, flexible joints, and heart and lung problems.
- The diagnosis is based on symptoms and family history.
- Most people with this syndrome live into their 60s.
- There is no cure for Marfan syndrome or any way to correct the abnormalities in the connective tissue.

Marfan syndrome is caused by mutations in the gene that encodes a protein called fibrillin. Fibrillin helps connective tissue maintain its strength, and therefore, some fibers and other parts of connective tissue undergo changes that ultimately weaken the tissue. The weakening affects bones and joints as well as internal structures, such as the heart, blood vessels, and eyes. Weakened tissues stretch, distort, and can even tear. For example, the aorta may weaken, bulge, or tear. Connective tissues that join structures may weaken or break, separa-ting formerly attached structures. For example, the eye's lens or retina may separate from its normal attachments.

Symptoms can range from mild to severe. Many people with Marfan syndrome never notice symptoms. In some people, symptoms may not become apparent until adulthood. People with Marfan syndrome are taller than expected for their age and family. Their arm span (the distance between fingertips when the arms are outstretched) is greater than their height. Their fingers are long and thin. Often, the breastbone (sternum) is deformed and pushed outward or inward. The joints may be very flexible. Flat feet and a humpback with an abnormal curve of the spine (kyphoscoliosis) are common, as are hernias. Usually, the person has little fat under the skin. The roof of the mouth is often high.

The most dangerous complications develop in the heart and lungs. Weakness may develop in the connective tissue of the wall of the body's main artery, the aorta. The weakened wall may result in blood seeping between the layers of the aorta's wall (aortic dissection—see page 431) or in a bulge (aneurysm—see page 427) that can rupture.

Pregnancy increases the risk of dissection. Delivery by caesarean is often recommended to minimize the risk.

If the aorta gradually widens, the aortic valve, which leads from the heart into the aorta, may begin to leak (called aortic regurgitation). The mitral valve, which is located between the left atrium and ventricle, may leak or bulge backward into the left atrium (prolapse—see page 380).

These heart valve abnormalities can impair the heart's ability to pump blood. Abnormal heart valves can also develop serious infections (infective endocarditis). Air-filled sacs (cysts) may develop in the lungs. The cysts may rupture, bringing air into the space that surrounds the lungs (pneumothorax—see page 520).

The lens of one or both eyes may be displaced (dislocated). The light-sensitive area at the back of the eye (retina) may detach from the rest of the eye. Displacement of the lens and detachment of the retina may cause permanent loss of vision.

Doctors may suspect the diagnosis if an unusually tall, thin person has any of the characteristic symptoms or if Marfan syndrome has been recognized in other family members.

Doctors monitor for complications that can cause serious symptoms. Echocardiography is used to evaluate the heart and aorta and is usually repeated yearly. Magnetic resonance imaging (MRI) can also be done to evaluate heart and brain problems. X-rays of the hand, spine, pelvis, chest, foot, and skull are done to check for abnormalities. The eyes are usually examined yearly. Echocardiography and eye examinations are also done whenever symptoms develop.

Prognosis and Treatment

Years ago, most people with Marfan syndrome died in their 30s. As of the late 1990s, most people with Marfan syndrome live until their 60s. Prevention of aortic dissection and rupture probably explains why the life span has been lengthened.

There is no cure for Marfan syndrome or any way to correct the abnormalities in the connective tissue. Treatment is aimed at preventing and fixing abnormalities before dangerous complications develop. Beta-blockers (such as atenolol and propranolol) are given to make blood flow more gently through the aorta. If the aorta has widened or developed an aneurysm, the affected section can be repaired or replaced surgically. Pregnant women are at especially high risk of complications with their aorta, so repair of the aorta before conception should be discussed. A displaced lens or retina can usually be reattached surgically.

Osteochondrodysplasias

Osteochondrodysplasias are a group of rare disorders of bone or cartilage that cause the skeleton to develop abnormally.

In osteochondrodysplasias, the growth plate, which contains cartilage, does not make new bone cells. Thus, growth of bone is impaired.

Each type of osteochondrodysplasia causes different symptoms. Osteochondrodysplasias usually cause short stature (dwarfism). Some cause more shortening of the limbs than the trunk (short-limbed dwarfism), whereas others cause more shortening of the trunk than the limbs. Some children and adults have short limbs, bowlegs, a bulky forehead, an unusually shaped nose (saddle nose), and an arched back. Sometimes joints do not develop their full range of motion.

A doctor usually makes the diagnosis based on the symptoms, physical examination, and x-rays of the bones. Sometimes the abnormal genes responsible for osteochondrodysplasias can be detected, usually by a blood test. Analyzing the genes is most helpful for predicting the disease before birth. Diagnosis of severe types before birth is also possible using other methods. In some cases, the fetus can be directly viewed with a flexible scope (fetoscopy), or ultrasonography is done. If joint movement is severely restricted, surgery may be needed to replace joints with artificial ones.

Because the inheritance pattern in most types is known, genetic counseling can be effective. Organizations such as Little People of America provide resources for affected people and act as advocates on their behalf. Similar societies are active in other countries.

Osteogenesis Imperfecta

Osteogenesis imperfecta is a group of disorders of bone formation that make the bones abnormally fragile.

- Typical symptoms include weak bones that break easily.
- The diagnosis is based on x-rays.
- The type that occurs in infancy is lethal.
- Certain drugs and injections can help strengthen bones.

Osteogenesis imperfecta (OI) is the best known of a group of disorders that disturb bone growth. These disorders are called osteodysplasias. In OI, synthesis of collagen, one of the normal components of bone, is impaired. The bones become weak and fracture easily. There are several types of OI.

OI can range from mild to severe. Most people with OI have fragile bones, and about 50% have hearing loss. Infants with severe OI are usually born with many broken bones. The skull may be so soft that the brain is not protected from pressure applied to the head during childbirth. This most severe type is lethal, and the infant can die either before childbirth or within the first few days or weeks of life. Another severe form of OI, which is not lethal, causes bones to often break after very minor injuries, usually when children begin to walk. Children with moderate OI may have few broken bones during childhood and even fewer after puberty, when bones strengthen. Sometimes heart or lung diseases develop in children with OI.

X-rays may show abnormal bone structure that suggests OI. The removal of a sample of skin for examination under a microscope (biopsy) or to grow a type of connective tissue cells (fibroblasts) in a culture dish is done to confirm the diagnosis. The most severe and lethal form of OI can be detected in pregnant women by an ultrasound. A test called audiometry is done often throughout childhood to monitor hearing.

Treatment

Bisphosphonates (such as pamidronate or alendronate) may strengthen bones. Growth hormone injections can also help children with certain types of OI. Treatment of broken bones is similar to that for children who do not have the disorder. However, broken bones can become deformed or fail to grow. As a result, body growth can become permanently stunted in children with many broken bones, and deformities are common. Bones may require stabilization with internal metal rods. Physical therapy and occupational therapy help prevent fractures and improve function. Taking measures to avoid even minor injuries can help prevent fractures.

Pseudoxanthoma Elasticum

Pseudoxanthoma elasticum is a disorder of connective tissue that causes abnormalities in the skin, eyes, and blood vessels.

Pseudoxanthoma elasticum stiffens the fibers that enable tissue to stretch and then spring back into place (elastic fibers). Elastic fibers are in the skin and various other tissues throughout the body, including blood vessels. The blood vessels may stiffen, losing their normal ability to expand and allow more blood to flow as needed. Stiffness also prevents the blood vessels from contracting.

The skin of the neck, underarms, and groin and around the navel eventually becomes thick, grooved, inflexible, and loose. Yellowish, pebbly bumps make the skin appear similar to an orange or a plucked chicken. The change in appearance may be mild and overlooked during early childhood but becomes more noticeable as the child ages.

Stiff blood vessels lead to high blood pressure. Nosebleeds and bleeding in the brain, uterus, and intestine may occur. Too little blood flow may result in chest pain (angina) and leg pain while walking (intermittent claudication). Bleeding may continue for prolonged periods. Damage to the back of the eye (retina) can cause severe loss of vision or blindness.

Prognosis and Treatment

There is no cure for pseudoxanthoma elasticum nor any way to correct the abnormalities in the connective tissue. Treatment is aimed at preventing complications. People should avoid drugs that may cause stomach or intestinal bleeding, such as aspirin, other nonsteroidal anti-inflammatory drugs (NSAIDs), and anticoagulants. People with pseudoxanthoma elasticum should avoid contact sports because injury to the eye is a risk. Complications often limit life span.

279 Juvenile Idiopathic Arthritis

Juvenile idiopathic arthritis is persistent or recurring inflammation of the joints similar to rheumatoid arthritis (see page 563) but beginning at or before age 16.

- Juvenile idiopathic arthritis may cause fever, rash, and lymph node swelling and may affect the heart.
- Diagnosis is based on the child's symptoms and a physical examination because there is no single definitive laboratory test to diagnose the disease.
- Children receive drugs to treat pain and inflammation.
- Flexibility exercises help enhance joint movement.

Juvenile idiopathic arthritis is an uncommon disease characterized by inflammation of joints or connective tissue. The cause is unknown. Although juvenile idiopathic arthritis is not considered a hereditary disorder, hereditary factors may increase a child's chance of developing it.

Symptoms

There are several types of juvenile idiopathic arthritis, each with different characteristics. The type is determined by which symptoms develop during the first 6 months of the disease and how many joints are affected.

In **pauciarticular juvenile idiopathic arthritis,** four or fewer joints, usually those of the leg (and often the jaw), are affected by pain and swelling. The knee is the most common joint affected. The hip and shoulder are usually spared. Occasionally, a single toe, a finger, or a wrist becomes stiff and swollen.

In **polyarthritis,** five or more (sometimes as many as 20 to 40) joints are affected. The inflammation usually affects the same joint on both sides of the body—for example, both knees or both hips. The jaw, neck joints, and wrists may be affected. Symptoms

may develop slowly. Inflammation may develop in the tendons and connective tissues around joints (tenosynovitis), causing pain, swelling, and warmth. Rarely, generally in adolescents, small lumps (rheumatoid nodules) may form over the elbows, fingers, or toes.

In **systemic disease** (Still's disease), inflammation occurs at sites other than the joints (which also may be affected). Children with systemic disease typically develop a high fever and rash that frequently appear before joint pain and swelling. The fever comes and goes, usually for at least 2 weeks. The temperature is usually highest in the afternoon or evening (often 103° F [39° C] or higher) and then returns rapidly to normal. A child with fever may feel tired and irritable. The rash is made up of flat, pink-colored or salmon-colored patches—mainly on the trunk and the upper part of the legs or arms. It appears for hours at a time (often in the evening with the fever) and does not always appear in the same spot. The liver, spleen, and lymph nodes may enlarge. Sometimes inflammation develops in the membranes surrounding the heart (pericarditis) or the lungs (pleuritis), causing chest pain. This inflammation may cause fluid to accumulate around the heart or lungs.

With any type of juvenile idiopathic arthritis, the joints may be stiff when the child awakens. Joints often become swollen and warm. Later, joints may become painful, but the pain may be milder than expected from the amount of swelling. Pain may become worse when the joint is moved. A child may be reluctant to walk or may limp. Joint pain persists for years if untreated.

Complications: Any type of juvenile idiopathic arthritis can interfere with physical growth. Joint deformities may develop if untreated. When juvenile idiopathic arthritis interferes with growth of the jaw, a small chin (micrognathia) can result. Long-standing (chronic) joint inflammation can eventually cause deformities or permanent damage of the affected joint.

Inflammation of the iris in the eye (iridocyclitis) can develop with any type of juvenile idiopathic arthritis, but most often iridocyclitis develops with pauciarticular juvenile idiopathic arthritis or polyarthritis. Iridocyclitis in juvenile idiopathic arthritis is asymptomatic (there is no pain or redness), but it can lead to permanent loss of vision if untreated.

Diagnosis

A doctor diagnoses juvenile idiopathic arthritis based on the child's symptoms and the results of a physical examination. There is no single, definitive laboratory test for juvenile idiopathic arthritis, but some blood tests are helpful. The erythrocyte sedimentation rate is usually very abnormal in the systemic form, less so in the polyarticular form, and usually normal in the pauciarticular form. Blood is tested for rheumatoid factor and antinuclear antibodies, which are present in some people with rheumatoid arthritis and related diseases (for example, autoimmune diseases, such as lupus, polymyositis, or scleroderma). However, many children with juvenile idiopathic arthritis do not have rheumatoid factor or antinuclear antibodies in their blood. An adolescent with polyarticular juvenile arthritis and a positive test result for rheumatoid factor has a form of arthritis that is very similar to rheumatoid arthritis in adults.

Children with juvenile idiopathic arthritis who have antinuclear antibodies in their blood are at a higher risk of developing iridocyclitis. X-rays eventually may show characteristic changes in the bones or joints. Children must be examined several times a year by an ophthalmologist for iridocyclitis regardless of whether symptoms are present. If children have systemic juvenile idiopathic arthritis, then an annual eye examination suffices.

Prognosis and Treatment

Symptoms of juvenile idiopathic arthritis may disappear over several years. At least half of children with pauciarticular juvenile idiopathic arthritis and slightly less than half of children with polyarthritis or systemic disease have a complete remission. With early treatment, most children function normally.

The types of juvenile idiopathic arthritis are treated similarly, and the drugs used to reduce pain and inflammation are the same as for rheumatoid arthritis (see page 564). Typically, nonsteroidal anti-inflammatory drugs (NSAIDs—see page 644) are used, but children with severe systemic disease may require corticosteroids (such as prednisone) given by mouth or by vein. When corticosteroids are necessary, the lowest possible dose is used to decrease the chance of long-term complications such as slowed growth, osteoporosis, and osteonecrosis (death of bone tissue). If just a few joints are inflamed, doctors may inject corticosteroids directly into the joint.

Sometimes, stronger drugs, such as methotrexate, are used for pauciarticular juvenile idiopathic arthritis and are usually needed to treat polyarticular and systemic juvenile idiopathic arthritis. Side effects include bone marrow depression and liver toxicity, so children taking these drugs require regular blood tests. Etanercept and infliximab, drugs that block tumor necrosis factor (a protein involved in inflammation), are effective and have improved the outcome for children with juvenile idiopathic arthritis significantly. Systemic juvenile arthritis is often treated with anakinra, a drug that blocks the inflammatory protein interleukin 1.

Iridocyclitis is treated with corticosteroid eye drops or ointments, which suppress inflammation. If this treatment is not enough, methotrexate is frequently used. Eye drops that widen (dilate) the pupil also help prevent permanent eye damage. Eye surgery may be needed if the eye has been damaged.

As in rheumatoid arthritis in adults, nondrug therapies are used for children. For example, physical therapy, splinting, and flexibility exercises help maintain strength and joint function.

CHAPTER 280

Diabetes Mellitus

Diabetes mellitus is a disorder in which blood sugar (glucose) levels are abnormally high because the body does not produce enough insulin.

- Diabetes is condition in which an insufficient amount of insulin is made.
- Typical symptoms include excessive thirst, urination, and fatigue.
- The diagnosis is based on symptoms and urine and blood tests.
- Treatment includes changes in diet, exercise, weight loss (if overweight), and insulin injections or drugs taken by mouth.

The symptoms, diagnosis, and treatment of diabetes are similar in children and adults (see page 1005).

Which Children Are at Risk of Type 2 Diabetes?

Children and adolescents meeting these criteria should be tested with a fasting blood sugar test every 2 years beginning at about age 10:

- Being overweight (weighing more than 85% of children of similar age, sex, and height **or** weighing more than 120% of the ideal weight for height)

Plus any two of the following factors:

- Having a close relative with type 2 diabetes
- Being Native American, black, Hispanic, or Asian/Pacific Islander
- Having high blood pressure, high blood levels of lipids (fats), or polycystic ovary syndrome

However, management of diabetes in children may be more complex. It must be tailored to the child's physical and emotional maturity level and to constant variations in food intake, physical activity, and stress.

Insulin is a hormone that is released by the pancreas. Insulin controls the amount of sugar (glucose) in the blood. A child with diabetes has high blood sugar levels either because the pancreas produces little or no insulin (type 1 diabetes, formerly called juvenile-onset diabetes) or because the body is insensitive to the amount of insulin that is produced (type 2 diabetes). In either case, the amount of insulin available is insufficient for the body's needs.

Type 1 diabetes can develop at any time during childhood, even during infancy, but it usually begins between ages 6 and 13 years. Type 2 diabetes occurs mainly in adolescents but is becoming increasingly common among overweight or obese children.

Up until the 1990s, more than 95% of children who developed diabetes had type 1 diabetes, usually because the immune system attacked the cells in the pancreas that make insulin (islet cells). Such an attack may be triggered by environmental factors in people whose genetic make-up leaves them susceptible. Recently, the number of children, especially adolescents, with type 2 diabetes has been steadily increasing. Today, 10 to 50% of children newly diagnosed with diabetes have type 2 diabetes. The increase in childhood type 2 diabetes has been particularly prominent among Native Americans, blacks, and Hispanics. Obesity and a family history of type 2 diabetes are major factors in the development of type 2 diabetes (but not type 1).

In newborns who are very underweight, blood sugar levels may be elevated transiently, usually because they are given intravenous infusions of glucose too rapidly. The infusions are given to increase the newborn's weight. This problem usually resolves without treatment.

Symptoms

High blood sugar levels are responsible for a variety of immediate symptoms and long-term complications.

Symptoms develop quickly in type 1 diabetes, usually over 2 to 3 weeks or less, and tend to be quite obvious. High blood sugar levels cause the child to urinate excessively. This fluid loss causes an increase in thirst and the consumption of fluids. Some children become dehydrated, resulting in weakness, lethargy, and a rapid pulse. Vision may become blurred.

Diabetic ketoacidosis occurs at the beginning of the disease in about one third of children with type 1 diabetes. Without insulin, cells cannot use the sugar that is in the blood. Cells switch to a back-up mechanism to obtain energy and break down fat, producing compounds called ketones as by-products. Ketones make the blood too acidic (ketoacidosis), causing nausea, vomiting, fatigue, and abdominal pain. The ketones make the child's breath smell like nail polish remover. Breathing becomes deep and rapid as the body attempts to correct the blood's acidity (see page 972). Some children develop a headache and may become confused or less alert. These symptoms may be caused by accumulation of fluid in the brain (cerebral edema). Diabetic ketoacidosis can progress to coma and death. Children with diabetic ketoacidosis are also dehydrated and often have other chemical imbalances in the blood, such as an abnormal level of potassium and high levels of lipids (fats).

Symptoms in children with type 2 diabetes are milder than those in type 1 diabetes and develop more slowly—over weeks or even a few months. Parents may notice an increase in the child's thirst and urination or only vague symptoms, such as fatigue. Typically, children with type 2 diabetes do not develop ketoacidosis or severe dehydration.

 Did You Know...
Type 2 diabetes is almost always associated with obesity.

Diagnosis

Doctors suspect diabetes when children have typical symptoms or when a urine test done during a routine physical examination reveals sugar. The diagnosis is confirmed by measurement of the blood sugar level. Preferably, the blood test is done after the child fasts overnight. A child is considered to

Breaking Down Sugar

There are many kinds of sugar. The white granules of table sugar are known as sucrose. Sucrose occurs naturally in sugar cane and sugar beets. Another kind of sugar, lactose, occurs in milk. Sucrose consists of two different simple sugars, glucose and fructose. Lactose consists of the simple sugars glucose and galactose. Sucrose and lactose must be broken down by the intestine into their simple sugars before they can be absorbed. Glucose is the main sugar the body uses for energy, so during and after absorption, most sugars are turned into glucose. Thus, when doctors talk about blood sugar, they are really talking about blood glucose.

have diabetes if the fasting blood sugar level is 126 milligrams per deciliter (mg/dL) or higher. Sometimes, doctors also do tests to see whether the blood is too acidic or contains ketones. Rarely, doctors do a blood test that detects antibodies to islet cells to help distinguish type 1 diabetes from type 2.

Because prompt measures (such as dietary changes, an increase in physical activity, and weight loss) may help prevent or delay the onset of type 2 diabetes, children at risk should be screened with a blood test. Nothing can be done to prevent type 1 diabetes.

Treatment

The main goal of treatment is to keep blood sugar levels as close to the normal range as can be done safely. To control blood sugar, children with type 1 diabetes take insulin, and children with type 2 diabetes take drugs given by mouth. Children with either type of diabetes need to change their diet, exercise regularly, and, if overweight, lose weight.

When type 1 diabetes is first diagnosed, children are usually hospitalized, and those with diabetic ketoacidosis are treated in an intensive care unit. Children with type 1 diabetes are given fluids (to treat dehydration) and insulin. They always require insulin because nothing else is effective. Those with ketoacidosis require insulin intravenously for a brief time. Those without ketoacidosis typically receive two or more daily injections of insulin, although some children may need to receive insulin continuously by a small infusion pump through a needle under the skin. Insulin treatment is usually begun in the hospital so that blood sugar levels can be tested often and doctors can change insulin dosage in response. Rarely, treatment is started at home.

Children with type 2 diabetes do not usually need to receive treatment in the hospital. They do require treatment with drugs to lower blood sugar levels

(antihyperglycemic drugs), which are taken by mouth. The drugs used for adults with type 2 diabetes (see table on page 1012) are safe for children, although some of the side effects—particularly diarrhea—cause more problems in children. Some children with type 2 diabetes need insulin. A few children who lose weight, improve their diet, and exercise regularly may be able to stop taking the drugs.

Nutritional management and education are particularly important for all children with diabetes. Because carbohydrates in food are turned into glucose by the body, variations in carbohydrate intake cause variations in blood sugar levels. Large amounts of sugar, as are present in soda, candy, and pastries, are discouraged because blood sugar may rise too high. Parents and older children are taught how to gauge the carbohydrate content of food and adjust what children eat as needed to maintain a consistent daily intake of carbohydrates. Children of all ages may find it difficult to consistently follow a properly balanced meal plan (consumed at regular intervals) and avoid the temptations of sugary snacks. Infants and preschool-aged children present a particular challenge to parents because of the concern arising from the dangers of frequent and very low blood levels sugar (hypoglycemia).

Adolescence: Adolescents may have particular problems controlling their blood sugar levels because of

- Hormonal changes during puberty: These changes affect how the body responds to insulin. As a result, higher doses are usually needed during this time.

- Adolescent lifestyle: Peer pressure, increased activities, erratic schedules, concern about body image, or eating disorders may interfere with the prescribed treatment regimen, particularly their meal plan.

- Experimentation with alcohol, cigarettes, and illicit drugs: Adolescents who experiment with these substances may neglect their treatment regimen.

- Conflicts with parents and other authority figures: Such conflicts may make adolescents less willing to follow their treatment regimen.

Thus, some adolescents need a parent or another adult to recognize these issues and give them the opportunity to discuss problems with a health care practitioner. The practitioner can make sure adolescents remain appropriately focused on keeping their blood sugar levels under control. Parents and health care practitioners should encourage adolescents to check their blood sugar levels frequently.

Support: Emotional issues affect children with diabetes and their families. The realization that they have a lifelong condition may cause some children to become sad or angry, and sometimes even deny that they have an illness. A doctor, psychologist, or counselor needs to address these emotions to secure the child's cooperation in adhering to the required regimen of meal plan, physical activity, blood sugar testing, and drugs. Failure to resolve these issues can lead to difficulties controlling blood sugar.

Summer camps for children with diabetes allow these children to share their experiences with one another while learning how to become personally more responsible for their condition.

For the treatment of diabetes, the child's primary care doctor usually enlists the aid of a team of other professionals, possibly including a pediatric endocrinologist, dietitian, diabetes educator, social worker, or psychologist. Family support groups may also help. The doctor may provide parents with information to bring to school so that school personnel understand their roles.

> **? Did You Know...**
> Children with type 1 diabetes always need insulin injections, regardless of whether they lose weight or change their diet.

Monitoring Treatment: Children and parents are taught to monitor the blood sugar level at least 4 times a day using a blood sample obtained by pricking a fingertip or the forearm with a small implement called a lancet. Once experience is gained, parents and many children can adjust the insulin dose as needed to achieve the best control. In general, by 10 years of age, children start to become interested in testing their own blood sugar levels and injecting insulin themselves. Parents should encourage this independence but make sure the child is being responsible. Doctors teach most children how to adjust their insulin dosage in accordance with the patterns of their home blood sugar records.

Children with diabetes typically see their doctor 4 times a year. The doctor evaluates their growth and development, reviews blood sugar records that the family member keeps, provides guidance and counseling about nutrition, and measures glycosylated hemoglobin (hemoglobin A_{1c})—a substance in the blood that reflects blood sugar levels over the long term. The doctor screens for long-term complications (see table on page 1008) once a year by measuring protein in the urine, assessing function of the thyroid gland, and performing neurologic and eye examinations.

Some children with diabetes do very well and control their diabetes without undue effort or conflict. In others, diabetes becomes a constant source of stress within the family, and control of the condition deteriorates. Adolescents in particular often find it difficult to follow the prescribed treatment regimen given the demands on their schedule and the limitations on their freedom that arise from diabetes. An adolescent benefits if the doctor considers the adolescent's desired schedule and activities and takes a flexible approach to problem solving—working with the adolescent rather than imposing solutions.

Complications of Treatment and Illness: No treatment completely maintains blood sugar at normal levels. The goal of treatment is to avoid blood sugar levels that are too high and too low. The complications of diabetes include coronary artery disease, kidney failure, blindness, peripheral vascular disease, and other serious disorders. Although these events take years to develop, the better the control of diabetes, the less likely that complications will ever occur.

Low blood sugar (hypoglycemia—see page 1014) occurs when too much insulin or too much of an antihyperglycemic drug is taken or when the child does not eat regularly or engages in unusually vigorous and sustained exercise. Hypoglycemia causes weakness, confusion, and even coma. In adults, adolescents, and older children, episodes of hypoglycemia rarely cause long-term problems. However, frequent episodes of hypoglycemia in children younger than 5 may permanently impair intellectual development. Also, young children may not be aware of the warning symptoms of hypoglycemia. To minimize the possibility of hypoglycemia, doctors and parents monitor young children with diabetes particularly closely and use a slightly higher target range for their blood sugar level.

Children and adolescents with type 1 diabetes who miss insulin injections may develop diabetic ketoacidosis within days. The long-term insufficient or inadequate use of insulin can lead to a syndrome of stunted growth, delayed puberty, and an enlarged liver (Mauriac syndrome).

CHAPTER 281   Hereditary Metabolic Disorders

Most of the foods and drinks people ingest are complex materials that the body must break down into simpler substances. This process may involve several steps. The simpler substances are then used as building blocks, which are assembled into the materials the body needs to sustain life. The process of creating these materials may also require several steps. The major building blocks are

- Carbohydrates
- Amino acids
- Fats (lipids)

This complicated process of breaking down and converting the substances ingested is called metabolism.

Metabolism is carried out by chemical substances called enzymes, which are made by the body. If a genetic abnormality affects the function of an enzyme or causes it to be deficient or missing altogether, various disorders can occur. The disorders usually result from an inability to break down some substance that should be broken down, allowing some intermediate substance that is often toxic to build up, or from an inability to produce some essential substance. Metabolic disorders are classified by the particular building block that is affected.

Some hereditary disorders of metabolism (such as phenylketonuria and lipidoses) can be diagnosed in the fetus by using amniocentesis or chorionic villus sampling (see page 1613). Usually, a hereditary metabolic disorder is diagnosed by using a blood test or examination of a tissue sample to determine whether a specific enzyme is deficient or missing.

Many of these disorders are now detected by routine screening tests done at birth. For a complete list of routine newborn screening tests by state, see the National Newborn Screening and Genetics Resource Center web site (http://genes-r-us.uthscsa.edu/).

Disorders of Carbohydrate Metabolism

Carbohydrates are sugars. Some sugars are simple, and others are more complex. Sucrose (table sugar) is made of two simpler sugars called glucose and fructose. Lactose (milk sugar) is made of glucose and galactose. Both sucrose and lactose must be broken down into their component sugars by enzymes before the body can absorb and use them. The carbohydrates in bread, pasta, rice, and other carbohydrate-containing foods are long chains of simple sugar molecules. These longer molecules must also be broken down by the body. If an enzyme needed to process a certain sugar is missing, the sugar can accumulate in the body, causing problems.

GLYCOGEN STORAGE DISEASES

Glycogen storage diseases occur when there is a defect in the enzymes that are involved in the metabolism of glycogen, resulting in growth abnormalities, weakness, and confusion.

- Glycogen storage diseases are caused by lack of an enzyme needed to change glucose into glycogen and break down glycogen into glucose.
- Typical symptoms include weakness, sweating, confusion, kidney stones, and stunted growth.
- The diagnosis is made by examining a piece of tissue under a microscope (biopsy).
- Treatment depends on the type of glycogen storage disease and usually involves regulating the intake of carbohydrates.

Glycogen is made of many glucose molecules linked together. The sugar glucose is the body's main source of energy for the muscles (including the heart) and brain. Any glucose that is not used immediately for energy is held in reserve in the liver, muscles, and kidneys in the form of glycogen and is released when needed by the body.

There are many different glycogen storage diseases (also called glycogenoses), each identified by a roman numeral. These diseases are caused by a hereditary lack of one of the enzymes that is essential to the process of forming glucose into glycogen and breaking down glycogen into glucose. About 1 in 20,000 infants has some form of glycogen storage disease.

Symptoms

Some of these diseases cause few symptoms. Others are fatal. The specific symptoms, age at which symptoms start, and their severity vary considerably among these diseases. For types II, V, and VII, the main symptom is usually weakness. For types I, III, and VI, symptoms are low levels of sugar in the blood and protrusion of the abdomen (because excess or abnormal glycogen may enlarge the liver). Low levels of sugar in the blood cause weakness, sweating, confusion, and sometimes seizures and coma. Other consequences for children may include stunted growth, frequent infections, and sores in the mouth and intestines.

TYPES AND CHARACTERISTICS OF GLYCOGEN STORAGE DISEASES

NAME	AFFECTED ORGANS, TISSUES, OR CELLS	SYMPTOMS
Type O	Liver or muscle	Episodes of low blood sugar levels (hypoglycemia) during fasting if the liver is affected
Von Gierke's disease (type IA)	Liver and kidney	Enlarged liver and kidney, slowed growth, very low blood sugar levels, and abnormally high levels of acid, fats, and uric acid in blood
Type IB	Liver and white blood cells	Same as in von Gierke's disease but may be less severe Low white blood cell count, recurring infections, and inflammatory bowel disease
Pompe's disease (type II)	All organs	Enlarged liver and heart and muscle weakness
Forbes' disease (type III)	Liver, muscle, and heart	Enlarged liver or cirrhosis, low blood sugar levels, muscle damage, heart damage, and weak bones in some people
Andersen's disease (type IV)	Liver, muscle, and most tissues	Cirrhosis, muscle damage, and delayed growth and development
McArdle disease (type V)	Muscle	Muscle cramps or weakness during physical activity
Hers' disease (type VI)	Liver	Enlarged liver Episodes of low blood sugar during fasting Often no symptoms
Tarui's disease (type VII)	Skeletal muscle and red blood cells	Muscle cramps during physical activity and red blood cell destruction (hemolysis)

Glycogen storage diseases tend to cause uric acid (a waste product) to accumulate in the joints, which can cause gout (see page 594), and in the kidneys, which can cause kidney stones (see page 299). In type I glycogen storage disease, kidney failure is common in the second decade of life or later.

Diagnosis and Treatment

The specific type of glycogen storage disease is diagnosed by examining a piece of muscle or liver tissue under a microscope (biopsy).

Treatment depends on the type of glycogen storage disease. For most types, eating many small carbohydrate-rich meals every day helps prevent blood sugar levels from dropping. For people who have glycogen storage diseases that cause low blood sugar levels, levels are maintained by giving uncooked cornstarch every 4 to 6 hours around the clock. For others, it is sometimes necessary to give carbohydrate solutions through a stomach tube all night to prevent low blood sugar levels from occurring at night.

GALACTOSEMIA

Galactosemia (a high blood level of galactose) is caused by lack of one of the enzymes necessary for metabolizing galactose, a sugar present in lactose (milk sugar). A metabolite that is toxic to the liver and kidneys builds up. The metabolite also damages the lens of the eye, causing cataracts.

- Galactosemia is caused by lack of one of the enzymes needed to metabolize the sugar in milk.
- Symptoms include vomiting, jaundice, diarrhea, and abnormal growth.
- The diagnosis is based on a blood test.
- Even with adequate treatment, affected children still develop mental and physical problems.
- Treatment involves completely eliminating milk and milk products from the diet.

Galactose is a sugar that is present in milk and in some fruits and vegetables. A deficient enzyme or liver dysfunction can alter the metabolism, which can lead to high levels of galactose in the blood (galactosemia). There are different forms of galactosemia, but the most common and the most severe form is referred to as classic galactosemia.

Symptoms

Newborns with galactosemia seem normal at first but, within a few days or weeks, lose their appetite, vomit, become jaundiced, have diarrhea, and stop growing normally. White blood cell function is affected, and serious infections can develop. If treatment is delayed, affected children remain short and become intellectually disabled or may die.

Diagnosis

Galactosemia is detectable with a blood test. This test is done as a routine screening test for newborns in all states in the United States. Before conception, adults with a sibling or child known to have the disorder can be tested to find out whether they carry the gene that causes the disease. If two carriers conceive a child, that child has a 1 in 4 chance of being born with the disease.

Prognosis

If galactosemia is recognized at birth and adequately treated, liver and kidney problems do not develop, and initial mental development is normal. However, even with adequate treatment, children with galactosemia may have a lower intelligence quotient (IQ) than their siblings, and they often have speech problems. Girls often have ovaries that do not function, and only a few are able to conceive naturally. Boys, however, have normal testicular function.

Treatment

Galactosemia is treated by completely eliminating milk and milk products—the source of galactose— from an affected child's diet. Galactose is also present in some fruits, vegetables, and sea products, such as seaweed. Doctors are not sure whether the small amounts in these foods cause problems in the long term. People who have the disorder must restrict galactose intake throughout life.

HEREDITARY FRUCTOSE INTOLERANCE

Hereditary fructose intolerance is caused by lack of the enzyme needed to metabolize fructose. Very small amounts of fructose cause low blood sugar levels and can lead to kidney and liver damage.

In this disorder, the body is missing an enzyme that allows it to use fructose, a sugar present in table sugar (sucrose) and many fruits. As a result, a by-product of fructose accumulates in the body, blocking the formation of glycogen and its conversion to glucose for use as energy. Ingesting more than tiny amounts of fructose or sucrose causes low blood sugar levels (hypoglycemia), with sweating, confusion, and sometimes seizures and coma. Children who continue to eat foods containing fructose develop kidney and liver damage, resulting in jaundice, vomiting, mental deterioration, seizures, and death. Chronic symptoms include poor eating, failure to thrive, digestive symptoms, liver failure, and kidney damage. For most types of this disorder, early diagnosis and dietary restrictions started early in infancy can help prevent these more serious problems.

The diagnosis is made when a chemical examination of a sample of liver tissue determines that the enzyme is missing. Treatment involves excluding fructose (generally present in sweet fruits), sucrose, and sorbitol (a sugar substitute) from the diet. Severe attacks of hypoglycemia respond to glucose given by vein. Milder attacks are treated with glucose tablets, which should be carried by anyone who has hereditary fructose intolerance.

MUCOPOLYSACCHARIDOSES

Mucopolysaccharidoses are a group of hereditary disorders in which complex sugar molecules are not broken down normally and accumulate in harmful amounts in the body tissues. The result is a characteristic facial appearance and abnormalities of the bones, eyes, liver, and spleen, sometimes accompanied by intellectual disability.

- Mucopolysaccharidoses occur when the body lacks enzymes needed to break down and store complex sugar molecules (mucopolysaccharides).
- Typically, symptoms include short stature, hairiness, stiff finger joints, and coarseness of the face.
- The diagnosis is based on symptoms and a physical examination.
- Although a normal life span is possible, some types cause premature death.
- A bone marrow transplant may help.

Complex sugar molecules called mucopolysaccharides are essential parts of many body tissues. In mucopolysaccharidoses, the body lacks enzymes needed to break down and store mucopolysaccharides. As a result, excess mucopolysaccharides enter the blood and are deposited in abnormal locations throughout the body.

During infancy and childhood, short stature, hairiness, and abnormal development become noticeable. The face may appear coarse. Some types of mucopolysaccharidoses cause intellectual disability to develop over several years. In some types, vision or hearing may become impaired. The arteries or heart valves can be affected. Finger joints are often stiff.

A doctor usually bases the diagnosis on the symptoms and a physical examination. The presence of a mucopolysaccharidosis in other family members also suggests the diagnosis. Urine tests may help but are sometimes inaccurate. X-rays may show characteristic bone abnormalities. Mucopolysaccharidoses can be diagnosed before birth by using amniocentesis or chorionic villus sampling (see page 1613).

Prognosis and Treatment

The prognosis depends on the type of mucopolysaccharidosis. A normal life span is possible. Some types, usually those that affect the heart, cause premature death.

In one type of mucopolysaccharidosis, attempts at replacing the abnormal enzyme have had limited, temporary success. Bone marrow transplantation may help some people. However, death or disability often results, and this treatment remains controversial.

DISORDERS OF PYRUVATE METABOLISM

Pyruvate metabolism disorders are caused by a lack of the ability to metabolize a substance called pyruvate. These disorders cause a buildup of lactic acid and a variety of neurologic abnormalities.

- A deficiency in any one of the enzymes involved in pyruvate metabolism leads to one of many disorders.
- Symptoms include seizures, intellectual disability, muscle weakness, and coordination problems.
- Some of these disorders are fatal.
- Some children are helped by diets that are either high in fat and low in carbohydrates or high in carbohydrates and low in protein.

Pyruvate is a substance that is formed in the processing of carbohydrates and proteins and that serves as an energy source for cells. Problems with pyruvate metabolism can limit a cell's ability to produce energy and allow a buildup of lactic acid, a waste product. Many enzymes are involved in pyruvate metabolism. A hereditary deficiency in any one of these enzymes results in one of a variety of disorders, depending on which enzyme is missing. Symptoms may develop any time between early infancy and late adulthood. Exercise and infections can worsen symptoms, leading to severe lactic acidosis. These disorders are diagnosed by measuring enzyme activity in cells from the liver or skin.

Pyruvate Dehydrogenase Complex Deficiency: This disorder is caused by a lack of a group of enzymes needed to process pyruvate. This deficiency results in a variety of symptoms, ranging from mild to severe. Some newborns with this deficiency have brain malformations. Other children appear normal at birth but develop symptoms, including weak muscles, seizures, poor coordination, and a severe balance problem, later in infancy or childhood. Intellectual disability is common.

This disorder cannot be cured, but some children are helped by a diet that is high in fat and low in carbohydrates.

Absence of Pyruvate Carboxylase: Pyruvate carboxylase is an enzyme. A lack of this enzyme causes a very rare condition that interferes with or blocks the production of glucose from pyruvate in the body. Lactic acid and ketones build up in the blood. Often, this disease is fatal. Children who survive have seizures and severe intellectual disability, although there are recent reports of children with milder symptoms. There is no cure, but some children are helped by eating frequent carbohydrate-rich meals and restricting dietary protein.

Disorders of Amino Acid Metabolism

Amino acids are the building blocks of proteins and have many functions in the body. Hereditary disorders of amino acid processing can result from defects either in the breakdown of amino acids or in the body's ability to get amino acids into cells. Because these disorders cause symptoms early in life, newborns are routinely screened for several common ones. In the United States, newborns are commonly screened for phenylketonuria, maple syrup urine disease, homocystinuria, tyrosinemia, and a number of other inherited disorders, although screening varies from state to state.

PHENYLKETONURIA

Phenylketonuria occurs in infants born without the ability to normally break down an amino acid called phenylalanine. Phenylalanine, which is toxic to the brain, builds up in the blood.

- Phenylketonuria is caused by lack of the enzyme needed to convert phenylalanine to tyrosine.
- Symptoms include intellectual disability, seizures, nausea, vomiting, an eczema-like rash, and a mousy body odor.
- The diagnosis is based on a blood test.
- A strict phenylalanine-restricted diet allows for normal growth and development.

Phenylketonuria (PKU) is a disorder that causes a buildup of the amino acid phenylalanine, which is an essential amino acid that cannot be synthesized in the body but is present in food. Excess phenylalanine is normally converted to tyrosine, another amino acid, and eliminated from the body. Without the enzyme that converts it to tyrosine, phenylalanine builds up in the blood and is toxic to the brain, causing intellectual disability.

Symptoms

Newborns with PKU rarely have symptoms right away, although sometimes they are sleepy or eat poorly. If not treated, affected infants progressively develop intellectual disability over the first few years of life, eventually becoming severe. Other symptoms include seizures, nausea and vomiting, an eczema-like rash, lighter skin and hair than their family members, aggressive or self-injurious behavior, hyperactivity, and sometimes psychiatric symptoms. Untreated children often give off a mousy body and urine odor as a result of a by-product of phenylalanine (phenylacetic acid) in their urine and sweat.

Diagnosis

PKU is usually diagnosed with a routine screening test.

PKU occurs in most ethnic groups. If PKU runs in the family and DNA is available from an affected family member, amniocentesis or chorionic villus sampling with DNA analysis can be done to determine whether a fetus has the disorder.

Parents and siblings of children with PKU can be tested to find out whether they carry the gene that causes the disease. If two carriers conceive a child, that child has a 1 in 4 chance of being born with the disease.

Prognosis

A phenylalanine-restricted diet, if started early and maintained well, allows for normal development. However, if very strict control of the diet is not maintained, affected children may begin to have difficulties in school. Dietary restrictions started after 2 to 3 years of age may control extreme hyperactivity and seizures and raise the child's eventual intelligence quotient (IQ) but do not reverse intellectual disability. Recent evidence suggests that some intellectually disabled adults with PKU (born before newborn screening tests were available) may function better when they follow the PKU diet.

A phenylalanine-restricted diet should continue for life, or intelligence may decrease and neurologic and mental problems may ensue.

Prevention and Treatment

To prevent intellectual disability, people must restrict phenylalanine intake (but not eliminate it altogether because people need some phenylalanine to live) beginning in the first few weeks of life. Because all natural sources of protein contain too much phenylalanine for children with PKU, affected children cannot have meat, milk, or other common foods that contain protein. Instead, they must eat a variety of processed foods, which are specially manufactured to be phenylalanine-free. Low-protein natural foods, such as fruits, vegetables, and restricted amounts of certain grain cereals, can be eaten.

Special nutritional products, including infant formula without phenylalanine, are also available. Future treatments may include cell transplantation and gene therapy.

MAPLE SYRUP URINE DISEASE

Maple syrup urine disease is caused by lack of the enzyme needed to metabolize amino acids. By-products of these amino acids cause the urine to smell like maple syrup.

Children with maple syrup urine disease are unable to metabolize certain amino acids. By-products of these amino acids build up, causing neurologic changes, including seizures and intellectual disability. These by-products also cause body fluids, such as urine and sweat, to smell like maple syrup. This disease is most common among Mennonite families.

There are many forms of maple syrup urine disease. In the most severe form, infants develop neurologic abnormalities, including seizures and coma, during the first week of life and can die within days to weeks. In the milder forms, children initially appear normal but during infection, surgery, or other physical stress, they can develop vomiting, staggering, confusion, and coma.

Since 2007, nearly every state in the United States has required that all newborns be screened for maple syrup urine disease with a blood test.

Infants with severe disease are treated with dialysis (see page 265). Some children with mild disease benefit from injections of vitamin B_1 (thiamin). After the disease has been brought under control, children must always consume a special artificial diet that is low in three amino acids (leucine, isoleucine, and valine). During times of physical stress or flare-ups, it may be necessary to monitor blood tests and give fluids by vein.

HOMOCYSTINURIA

Homocystinuria is caused by lack of the enzyme needed to metabolize homocysteine. This disorder can cause a number of symptoms, including decreased vision and skeletal abnormalities.

Children with homocystinuria are unable to metabolize the amino acid homocysteine, which, along with certain toxic by-products, builds up to cause a variety of symptoms. Symptoms may be mild or severe, depending on the particular enzyme defect.

Infants with this disorder are normal at birth. The first symptoms, including dislocation of the lens of the eye, causing severely decreased vision, usually begin after 3 years of age. Most children have skeletal abnormalities, including osteoporosis. Children are usually tall and thin with a curved spine, chest deformities, elongated limbs, and long, spiderlike fingers. Without early diagnosis and treatment, mental (psychiatric) and behavioral disorders and intellectual disability are common. Homocystinuria makes the blood more likely to clot spontaneously, resulting in strokes, high blood pressure, and many other serious problems.

Since 2008, nearly every state in the United States has required that all newborns be screened for homocystinuria with a blood test. A test measuring enzyme function in liver or skin cells confirms the diagnosis.

Some children with homocystinuria improve when given vitamin B_6 (pyridoxine) or vitamin B_{12} (cobalamin).

TYROSINEMIA

Tyrosinemia is caused by lack of the enzyme needed to metabolize tyrosine. The most common form of this disorder mostly affects the liver and the kidneys.

Children with tyrosinemia are unable to completely metabolize the amino acid tyrosine. By-products of this amino acid build up, causing a variety of symptoms. In some states, the disorder is detected with newborn screening tests.

There are two main types of tyrosinemia: type I and type II.

Type I tyrosinemia is most common among children of French-Canadian or Scandinavian descent. Children with this disorder typically become ill sometime within the first year of life with dysfunction of the liver, kidneys, and nerves, resulting in irritability, rickets, or even liver failure and death. Restriction of tyrosine in the diet is of little help. An experimental drug, which blocks production of toxic metabolites, may help children with type I tyrosinemia. Often, children with type I tyrosinemia require a liver transplant. Since 2007, nearly every state in the United States has required that all newborns be screened for type I tyrosinemia with a blood test.

Type II tyrosinemia is less common. Affected children sometimes have intellectual disability and frequently develop sores on the skin and eyes. Unlike type I tyrosinemia, restriction of tyrosine in the diet can prevent problems from developing.

Disorders of Lipid Metabolism

Fats (lipids) are an important source of energy for the body. The body's store of fat is constantly broken down and reassembled to balance the body's energy needs with the food available. Groups of specific enzymes help the body break down and process fats. Certain abnormalities in these enzymes can lead to the buildup of specific fatty substances that normally would have been broken down by the enzymes. Over time, accumulations of these sub-

---

Other Rare Hereditary Disorders of Lipid Metabolism

Wolman's disease results when specific types of cholesterol and glycerides accumulate in tissues. This disease causes enlargement of the spleen and liver. Calcium deposits in the adrenal glands cause them to harden, and fatty diarrhea (steatorrhea) also occurs. Infants with Wolman's disease usually die by 6 months of age.

Cerebrotendinous xanthomatosis occurs when cholestanol, a product of cholesterol metabolism, accumulates in tissues. This disease eventually leads to uncoordinated movements, dementia, cataracts, and fatty growths (xanthomas) on tendons. The disabling symptoms often appear after age 30. If started early, the drug chenodiol helps prevent progression of the disease, but it cannot undo any damage already done.

In **sitosterolemia**, fats from fruits and vegetables accumulate in blood and tissues. The buildup of fats leads to atherosclerosis, abnormal red blood cells, and xanthomas on tendons. Treatment consists of reducing the intake of foods that are rich in plant fats, such as vegetable oils, and taking cholestyramine resin.

In **Refsum's disease**, phytanic acid, which is a product of fat metabolism, accumulates in tissues. A buildup of phytanic acid leads to nerve and retinal damage, spastic movements, and changes in the bone and skin. Treatment involves avoiding eating green fruits and vegetables that contain chlorophyll. Plasmapheresis, in which phytanic acid is removed from the blood, may be helpful.

Disorders caused by the accumulation of lipids are called lipidoses. Other enzyme abnormalities prevent the body from converting fats into energy normally. These abnormalities are called fatty acid oxidation disorders.

GAUCHER'S DISEASE

Gaucher's disease is caused by a buildup of glucocerebrosides in tissues. Children who have the infantile form usually die within a year, but children and adults who develop the disease later in life may survive for many years.

In Gaucher's disease, glucocerebrosides, which are a product of fat metabolism, accumulate in tissues. Gaucher's disease is the most common lipidosis. The disease is most common among Ashkenazi (Eastern European) Jews. Gaucher's disease leads to an enlarged liver and spleen and a brownish pigmentation of the skin. Accumulations of glucocerebrosides in the eyes cause yellow spots called pingueculae to appear. Accumulations in the bone marrow can cause pain and destroy bone.

Type 1, the chronic form of Gaucher's disease, is the most common. It results in an enlarged liver and spleen and bone abnormalities. Most commonly diagnosed during adulthood, type 1 Gaucher's disease may lead to severe liver disease, including increased risk of bleeding from the stomach and esophagus and liver cancer. Neurologic problems can also occur.

Type 2, the infantile form, usually causes death in the first year of life. Affected infants have an enlarged spleen and severe neurologic problems.

Type 3, the juvenile form, can begin at any time during childhood. Children with type 3 disease have an enlarged liver and spleen, bone abnormalities, and slowly progressive neurologic problems. Children who survive to adolescence may live for many years.

Many people with Gaucher's disease can be treated with enzyme replacement therapy, in which enzymes are given by vein, usually every 2 weeks. Enzyme replacement therapy is most effective for people who do not have nervous system complications.

TAY-SACHS DISEASE

Tay-Sachs disease is caused by a buildup of gangliosides in the tissues. This disease results in early death.

In Tay-Sachs disease, gangliosides, which are products of fat metabolism, accumulate in tissues. The disease is most common among families of Eastern European Jewish origin. At a very early age, children with this disease become progressively intellectually disabled and appear to have floppy muscle tone. Spasticity develops and is followed by paralysis, dementia, and blindness. These children usually die by age 3 or 4. The disease cannot be treated or cured.

Before conception, parents can find out whether they carry the gene that causes the disease. During pregnancy, Tay-Sachs disease can be identified in the fetus by chorionic villus sampling or amniocentesis.

NIEMANN-PICK DISEASE

Niemann-Pick disease is caused by a buildup of sphingomyelin or cholesterol in the tissues. This disease causes many neurologic problems.

In Niemann-Pick disease, the deficiency of a specific enzyme results in the accumulation of sphingomyelin (a product of fat metabolism) or cholesterol. Niemann-Pick disease has several forms, depending on the severity of the enzyme deficiency, which determines how much sphingomyelin or cholesterol accumu-

lates. The most severe forms tend to occur in Jewish people. The milder forms occur in all ethnic groups.

In the most severe form (type A), children fail to grow normally and have several neurologic problems. These children usually die by age 3. Children with type B disease develop fatty growths in the skin, areas of dark pigmentation, and an enlarged liver, spleen, and lymph nodes. They may be intellectually disabled. Children with type C disease develop symptoms during childhood, with seizures and neurologic deterioration.

Some forms of Niemann-Pick disease can be diagnosed in the fetus by chorionic villus sampling or amniocentesis. After birth, the diagnosis can be made by a liver biopsy (removal of a tissue specimen for examination under a microscope). None of the types of Niemann-Pick disease can be cured, and children tend to die of infection or progressive dysfunction of the central nervous system. Currently, some therapies that may slow or halt the progression of symptoms in types B and C are being studied.

 Did You Know...
Fabry's disease affects only boys.

FABRY'S DISEASE

Fabry's disease is caused by a buildup of glycolipid in tissues. This disease causes skin growths, pain in the extremities, poor vision, recurrent episodes of fever, and kidney or heart failure.

In Fabry's disease, glycolipid, which is a product of fat metabolism, accumulates in tissues. Because the defective gene for this rare disorder is carried on the X chromosome, the full-blown disease occurs only in males (see page 13). The accumulation of glycolipid causes noncancerous (benign) skin growths (angiokeratomas) to form on the lower part of the trunk. The corneas become cloudy, resulting in poor vision. A burning pain may develop in the arms and legs, and children may have episodes of fever. Children with Fabry's disease eventually develop kidney failure and heart disease, although most often they live into adulthood. Kidney failure may lead to high blood pressure, which may result in stroke.

Fabry's disease can be diagnosed in the fetus by chorionic villus sampling or amniocentesis. The disease cannot be cured or even treated directly, but researchers are investigating a treatment in which the deficient enzyme is replaced by transfusion. Treatment consists of taking analgesics to help relieve pain and fever or anticonvulsants. People with kidney failure may need a kidney transplant.

FATTY ACID OXIDATION DISORDERS

Fatty acid oxidation disorders are caused by a lack or deficiency of the enzymes needed to break down fats, resulting in delayed mental and physical development.

Several enzymes help break down fats so that they may be turned into energy. An inherited defect or deficiency of one of these enzymes leaves the body short of energy and allows breakdown products, such as acyl-CoA, to accumulate. The enzyme most commonly deficient is medium chain acyl-CoA dehydrogenase (MCAD). Other enzyme deficiencies include short chain acyl-CoA-dehydrogenase deficiency (SCAD), long chain-3-hydroxyacyl-CoA-deficiency (LCHAD), and trifunctional protein deficiency (TFP).

MCAD Deficiency: This disorder is one of the most common inherited disorders of metabolism, particularly among people of Northern European descent.

Symptoms usually develop between birth and age 3. Children are most likely to develop symptoms if they go without food for a period of time (which depletes other sources of energy) or have an increased need for calories because of exercise or illness. The level of sugar in the blood drops significantly, causing confusion or coma. Children become weak and may have vomiting or seizures. Over the long term, children have delayed mental and physical development, an enlarged liver, heart muscle weakness, and an irregular heartbeat. Sudden death may occur.

Since 2007, nearly every state in the United States has required that all newborns be screened for MCAD with a blood test. Immediate treatment is with glucose given by vein. For long-term treatment, children must eat often, never skip meals, and consume a diet high in carbohydrates and low in fats. Supplements of the amino acid carnitine may be helpful. The long-term outcome is generally good.

282 Hereditary Periodic Fever Syndromes

Hereditary periodic fever syndromes are hereditary disorders that periodically cause episodes of fever and other symptoms that are not due to usual childhood infections or any other obvious disorder. The more common of these syndromes include

- Familial Mediterranean fever
- PFAPA (periodic fever, aphthous stomatitis, pharyngitis, and cervical adenitis) syndrome

Other less common syndromes include the following:

- Hereditary cryopyrinopathies: These include familial cold autoinflammatory syndrome, Muckle-Wells syndrome, and neonatal-onset multisystem inflammatory disease (NOMID). Episodes of fever, a rash, and joint pain are periodically triggered by cold temperatures.
- Hyper-IgD syndrome: This syndrome causes abdominal pain, vomiting or diarrhea, headache, joint pain, a rash, swollen lymph glands, and mouth and genital sores in addition to chills and fever.
- Tumor necrosis factor (TNF) receptor–associated periodic syndrome: This syndrome causes periodic attacks of muscle pain and swelling in the arms and legs, abdominal pain, joint pain, and rash in addition to fever.

- PAPA syndrome (pyogenic arthritis, pyoderma gangrenosum, and acne): This syndrome causes inflamed joints, skin ulcers, and acne.

Symptoms usually begin during childhood. Fewer than 10% of people develop symptoms after age 18. People periodically have attacks of fever and inflammation but feel well between attacks.

Familial Mediterranean Fever

Familial Mediterranean fever is a hereditary disorder characterized by episodes of high fever with abdominal pain or, less commonly, chest pain, joint pain, or a rash.

- Familial Mediterranean fever is caused by a gene inherited from both parents.
- Typically, most people have attacks of severe abdominal pain and a high fever.
- The diagnosis usually is based on symptoms.
- This disorder may cause amyloidosis if not adequately treated.
- Colchicine is taken to reduce or eliminate the number of painful attacks and eliminate the risk of kidney failure due to amyloidosis.

Familial Mediterranean fever occurs most commonly among people of Mediterranean origin (such as Sephardic Jews, Arabs, Armenians, and Turks). Most of these people have family members who have had the disorder (family history). However, in the United States, about 50% of people with familial Mediterranean fever have no known family history of the disorder.

Familial Mediterranean fever is caused by an abnormal recessive gene (see page 12). That is, to develop the disorder, people must have two copies of the abnormal gene, one from each parent. The abnormal gene results in the production of a defective form of pyrin, a protein that regulates inflammation.

If not treated adequately, some people with familial Mediterranean fever develop amyloidosis. In amyloidosis, an unusually shaped protein called amyloid is deposited in the kidneys and in many organs and tissues, impairing their function (see page 2107).

Symptoms

Symptoms usually begin between the ages of 5 and 15. Attacks of abdominal pain occur in about 95% of people. Attacks happen irregularly and are accompanied by fever as high as 104° F (40° C). The painful attacks usually last 24 to 72 hours but occasionally last as long as a week. Attacks may occur as often as twice a week or as seldom as once a year. The severity and frequency of the attacks tend to decrease with age and during pregnancy. Sometimes the attacks stop completely for a number of years, only to resume later. Some people have warning symptoms before the attacks begin.

The abdominal pain is caused by inflammation of the lining of the abdominal cavity (peritonitis). The pain usually starts in one part of the abdomen, then spreads throughout the entire abdomen. The severity of the pain may vary with each attack.

In the United States, certain symptoms are less common among affected people:

- **Chest pain:** About 30% of affected people have chest pain. Chest pain, which is typically triggered by breathing, is caused by inflammation of the membranes surrounding the lungs (pleuritis) or, rarely, by inflammation of the sac surrounding the heart (pericarditis).

- **Arthritis:** Only about 10% of people in the United States have inflammation of large joints (arthritis), such as the knees. The percentage is higher in other parts of the world, such as North Africa.

- **Rash:** A painful red rash that usually appears near the ankles may occur but is comparatively rare among affected people in the United States.

If amyloidosis affects the kidneys, people may retain fluids, feel weak, and lose their appetite.

About one third of women with the disorder are infertile or miscarry. The disorder can cause scar tissue to form in the abdomen. The scar tissue can interfere with conception.

Despite the severity of symptoms during attacks, people rapidly recover and remain free of illness until their next attack. However, without treatment, the amyloid deposits may damage the kidneys, eventually resulting in kidney failure.

Diagnosis

A doctor usually bases the diagnosis on typical symptoms. However, the abdominal pain of familial Mediterranean fever is virtually indistinguishable from that of other abdominal emergencies, particularly a ruptured appendix. Thus, some people with this disorder have urgent surgery before the correct diagnosis is made.

No routine laboratory test or imaging test is by itself diagnostic, but such tests can be useful in excluding other disorders. Blood tests can identify some of the abnormal genes that cause this disorder and can thus sometimes help with the diagnosis.

Prevention and Treatment

Taking colchicine daily by mouth eliminates or greatly reduces the number of painful attacks in about 85% of people. Also, it virtually eliminates the risk of kidney failure due to amyloidosis. If people have infrequent attacks preceded by warning symptoms, they can wait until symptoms start before they take colchicine, but they must then take it promptly.

Although mild analgesics, such as nonsteroidal anti-inflammatory drugs (NSAIDs) may relieve pain sufficiently, opioids, such as meperidine, are usually needed.

PFAPA Syndrome

PFAPA (periodic fevers with aphthous stomatitis, pharyngitis, and adenitis) syndrome causes recurrent episodes of fever that last 3 to 6 days, mouth sores (stomatitis), a sore throat (pharyngitis), and swollen lymph glands (adenitis). It typically starts between ages 2 and 5 years.

PFAPA syndrome is a relatively common periodic fever in children. Although a genetic cause has not been established, doctors tend to group PFAPA with hereditary fever syndromes. The syndrome typically starts between the ages of 2 and 5 years and tends to be more common among boys.

About once a month, children have a fever that lasts 3 to 6 days. The syndrome causes fatigue, chills, and occasionally abdominal pain and headache, as well as fever, sore throat, mouth ulcers, and swollen lymph glands. Children are healthy between episodes, and growth is normal. Children tend to outgrow the syndrome.

A doctor usually bases the diagnosis on symptoms and the pattern in which they occur. Blood tests may be done to measure substances that indicate inflammation (called markers).

No treatment is required, but children may be given corticosteroids to relieve symptoms. Cimetidine seems to cure the syndrome in some children, as may removing the tonsils (tonsillectomy).

Cancer is rare among children, occurring in only 1 of 5,000 children every year. The most common childhood cancers are leukemia (see page 1055), brain tumors, and lymphoma (see page 1061). Leukemia is responsible for about 33% of cases of childhood cancer, brain tumors for about 21%, and lymphomas for about 8%. Some of the more common cancers that occur mainly in children are Wilms' tumor, neuroblastoma, rhabdomyosarcoma, and retinoblastoma. Certain uncommon bone cancers—osteosarcoma and Ewing sarcoma (see page 553)—occur most often in children and young adults.

In contrast to many adult cancers, cancers in children tend to be much more curable. Over 75% of children with cancer survive at least 5 years. Nonetheless, in the United States, cancer kills over 2,000 children each year. Only injuries kill more children annually.

As in adults, doctors use a combination of treatments, including surgery, chemotherapy, and radiation therapy. However, because children are still growing, these treatments may have side effects that do not occur in adults. For example, in children, an arm or a leg treated with radiation may not grow to full size. If the brain is treated with radiation, intellectual development may not be normal.

Children who survive cancer also have more years than adults to develop long-term consequences of chemotherapy and radiation therapy, which include

- Infertility
- Poor growth
- Damage to the heart
- Development of second cancers, which occur in 3 to 12% of children who survive cancer

Because such severe consequences are possible and treatment is complex, children with cancer are best treated in centers with expertise in childhood cancers.

The impact of being diagnosed with cancer and the intensity of the treatment are overwhelming to the child and family. Maintaining a sense of normalcy for the child is difficult, especially because the child has to be hospitalized frequently and go to a doctor's office or outpatient center for treatment of the cancer and its complications. Overwhelming stress is typical, as parents struggle to continue to work, be attentive to siblings, and still attend to the many needs of the child with cancer (see page 1875). The situation is even more difficult when the child is being treated at a specialty center far from home.

A treatment team can help children and parents manage the difficult situation. The team should include the following:

- Pediatric cancer specialists (pediatric oncologist and radiation oncologist)
- Other needed specialists, such as a pediatric surgeon with expertise removing or biopsying childhood cancers, a pediatric radiologist with expertise reviewing imaging studies in children with cancer, and a pathologist with expertise diagnosing childhood cancers
- The primary care doctor
- A social worker, who can provide emotional support and help with financial aspects of care
- A teacher, who can work with the child, the school, and the health care team to make sure that the child's education continues
- A psychologist, who can help the child, siblings, and parents throughout treatment

Many centers also include a parent advocate—a parent who had a child with cancer and who can offer guidance to family members.

> **? Did You Know...**
> In the United States, cancer kills 2,000 children a year.

Brain Tumors

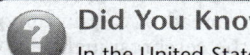

- The most common brain tumors in children are astrocytomas, medulloblastomas, and ependymomas.

- Brain tumors can cause various symptoms, including headaches, nausea, vomiting, vision problems, listlessness, and loss of coordination or balance.
- The diagnosis is usually based on results of magnetic resonance imaging and a biopsy.
- Treatment may involve surgery, radiation therapy, chemotherapy, or a combination.

Brain tumors (see also page 741) are the second most common cancer in children younger than 15 years (after leukemia) and the second leading cause of death from cancer. What causes brain tumors is usually unknown.

Symptoms

The first symptoms may result from increased pressure within the skull (intracranial pressure). Pressure may be increased because the tumor blocks the flow of cerebrospinal fluid within the brain or because the tumor takes up space. Increased pressure can cause the following:

- An enlarged head (hydrocephalus) in infants and very young children
- Headaches
- Nausea and vomiting (often when the child first awakens)
- Vision problems, such as double vision
- Difficulty turning the eyes upward
- Changes in mood or consciousness level, making the child irritable, listless, confused, or drowsy

Other symptoms vary depending on the specific part of the brain in which the tumor is located.

Diagnosis

Doctors suspect a brain tumor based on symptoms. To check for a brain tumor, doctors typically do an imaging test such as magnetic resonance imaging (MRI), which can usually detect the tumor. Before MRI is done, a contrast agent is usually injected into a vein. Contrast agents make the images clearer. If a brain tumor is suspected, a biopsy is done to confirm the diagnosis. Sometimes the tumor is removed at the time of the biopsy.

Sometimes a spinal tap (lumbar puncture—see art on page 635) is done to obtain cerebrospinal fluid for examination under a microscope. This procedure is done routinely to assess for spread of certain tumors that are known to invade the cerebrospinal fluid or when the diagnosis is unclear.

Treatment

Usually, treatment involves removing the tumor. Then, chemotherapy, radiation therapy, or both (see page 1092) are used. Treatment should be planned by a team of experts in treating brain tumors in children.

If the tumor is blocking the flow of cerebrospinal fluid, a small tube (catheter) may be used to drain the cerebrospinal fluid before the tumor is surgically removed. After a local or general anesthetic is used, the tube is inserted through a tiny opening drilled in the skull, and fluid is withdrawn to reduce the pressure within the skull. The tube is connected to a gauge that measures the pressure within the skull. After a few days, the tube is removed or converted to a permanent drain (shunt—see page 1726).

When possible, the tumor is removed surgically by opening the skull (called a craniotomy). Some brain tumors can be removed with little or no damage to the brain. After surgery, MRI may be done to determine whether any of the tumor is left and, if so, how much.

If the tumor cannot be removed surgically, additional treatment is usually required. In children younger than 5 to 10 years, depending on the tumor type, chemotherapy may be used first because radiation therapy can interfere with growth and brain development. If needed, radiation therapy may be used when children are older. Chemotherapy may also have serious side effects.

Because cancer is relatively rare in children, entry into a clinical trial (see page 2024) should be considered for all children with a brain tumor. In such trials, some children receive the standard treatment, and others receive the treatment being tested. The experimental treatment may involve new drugs, drugs used in new ways, or new surgical techniques. However, experimental treatments are not always effective, and side effects or complications may not be known.

ASTROCYTOMAS

Astrocytomas develop from star-shaped cells (astrocytes) that help nerve cells in the brain (or spinal cord) function. These tumors may be cancerous or not.

Astrocytomas are the most common brain tumors in children, accounting for up to 50%. These tumors are usually diagnosed between ages 5 and 9 years.

Symptoms and Diagnosis

Pressure within the skull increases, causing headaches (often when children first awaken), vomiting, and listlessness. Children may lose their coordination and have difficulty walking. Vision may be blurred or lost, and the eyes may bulge or involuntarily jerk in one direction, then drift back (nystagmus).

Astrocytomas in the spinal cord may cause back pain, difficulty walking, and muscle weakness.

MRI with a contrast agent is usually done. If it is unavailable, computed tomography (CT) is used, but it is less accurate. Then doctors must take a sample of tissue from the tumor and examine it under a microscope (biopsy) because treatment is based on how abnormal the tumor cells look (the tumor's grade). These tumors are typically classified as low-grade (for example, juvenile pilocytic astrocytoma), intermediate-grade, or high-grade (for example, glioblastoma).

Treatment

Most low-grade astrocytomas are surgically removed. Sometimes, separating the tumor from normal brain tissue is too difficult, or the tumor is inaccessible. In such cases, radiation therapy is used instead. Radiation therapy is also used if the tumor is likely to impair intellectual functioning or is progressing quickly. If children are younger than 10 years, chemotherapy may be used instead of radiation therapy because it can interfere with growth and brain development in young children. Most low-grade astrocytomas can be cured.

Intermediate-grade astrocytomas are somewhere between low-grade and high-grade astrocytomas. If they look more like high-grade tumors, they are treated more aggressively (radiation and chemotherapy). If they look more like low-grade astrocytomas, they are treated with surgery alone, surgery followed by radiation (older children), or chemotherapy (younger children).

High-grade astrocytomas are treated with a combination of surgery (if possible), radiation therapy, and chemotherapy. The outlook is worse for children with a high-grade tumor, in whom the overall survival is only 20 to 30%.

EPENDYMOMAS

Ependymomas are slow-growing tumors that develop from cells lining the spaces within the brain (ventricles).

Ependymomas are the third most common brain tumor in children, accounting for 10%. The majority of children diagnosed with ependymoma are younger than 8 years. About one third of cases occur in children younger than 3 years.

Most ependymomas develop in or near the back of the brain at the bottom of the skull (called the posterior fossa). This area is near the cerebellum (which helps control coordination and balance) and the brain stem (which controls critical body functions such as breathing). Ependymomas tend to spread to the brain stem. Sometimes ependymomas develop in the spinal cord.

Symptoms and Diagnosis

The first symptoms often result from increased pressure within the skull. They include headaches, vomiting, and listlessness. Infants may not meet developmental milestones. They may be irritable and

have no appetite. Mood or personality may change, and children may have difficulty concentrating. Children have problems with balance, coordination, and walking. Some children have seizures.

Ependymomas in the spinal cord may cause back pain, and children may have difficulty controlling urination and bowel movements.

The diagnosis is based on results of an MRI and a biopsy.

Prognosis and Treatment

How well children do after treatment depends partly on their age:

- About 25 to 46% of children aged 4 years and younger survive for 5 years.
- More than 70% of older children survive for 5 years.

How well children do also depends on how much of the tumor can be removed. Intellectual capacity may be affected in children who survive.

Initial therapy is removal of as much of the tumor as is safely possible. Radiation therapy, chemotherapy, or both are then required.

MEDULLOBLASTOMA

Medulloblastomas are rapidly growing tumors that develop in the cerebellum (the part of the brain that helps control coordination and balance).

Medulloblastomas account for about 20% of brain and spinal cord cancers in children. The peak incidence is in children 5 to 7 years old, but they can occur in infants and younger children and throughout adolescence. These tumors are more common among boys.

Medulloblastomas develop in the part of the brain that controls coordination and balance (cerebellum), which is located in the back of the brain below the cerebrum. Medulloblastomas tend to spread to other parts of the brain and to the spinal cord. Occasionally, they spread to other parts of the body.

What causes medulloblastomas is unclear. They sometimes occur in people with certain hereditary disorders (such as Gorlin's syndrome or Turcot's syndrome).

Symptoms and Diagnosis

In many children, the first symptom is frequent vomiting. Children may become clumsy, walk unsteadily, or have trouble maintaining their balance. They may have headaches, lethargy, and double vision.

The diagnosis is based on results of MRI with a contrast agent and a biopsy.

Prognosis

How well children do after treatment generally depends on whether they are categorized as having average-risk or high-risk disease. Risk is average if

- The tumor is at the very back of the brain.
- All or almost all of the tumor can be removed during surgery.
- The tumor has not spread to other parts of the body.

  Risk is high if

- The tumor is not at the very back of the brain.
- Some of the tumor cannot be removed during surgery.
- The tumor has spread to other parts of the brain, the spinal cord, or elsewhere in the body.

For children older than 3 years, the chances of surviving cancer-free for 5 years is about 80% if the tumor is average-risk and about 50 to 60% if it is high-risk. For children 3 years old and younger, outcome is harder to predict, but overall survival is poor. In about 40% of these children, the tumor has spread. When children are younger, intellectual development is more likely to be affected. For example, they may have difficulty learning, remembering, and making decisions.

Treatment

Medulloblastomas are best treated by removing the tumor and using chemotherapy, radiation therapy, or both. A few children (those younger than 3 years) may be effectively treated with chemotherapy alone.

Neuroblastoma

Neuroblastoma is a common childhood cancer that grows in parts of the nervous system.

- What causes neuroblastoma is not known.
- Symptoms depend on where neuroblastomas develop, such as the abdomen, chest, bone, skin, or spinal cord.
- Diagnosis usually involves an imaging test.
- Treatment involves surgery for tumors that have not spread, chemotherapy, and sometimes radiation therapy.

A neuroblastoma develops in a certain kind of nerve tissue located in many places of the body. It usually originates in nerves in the abdomen or chest, most commonly in the adrenal glands (located above each kidney). Very rarely, a neuroblastoma originates in the brain. In over half of the children, the cancer has spread to other parts of the body by the time a doctor is consulted.

Neuroblastoma is the most common cancer among infants and one of the most common tumors among children of any age. About 90% of all neuroblastomas occur in children younger than 5 years. The cause is not known. Rarely, neuroblastomas run in families.

Symptoms

The symptoms depend on where the neuroblastoma originated and whether and where it has spread, as in the following:

- Originating in the abdomen: The first symptoms include a large abdomen, a sensation of fullness, and abdominal pain.
- Originating in the chest: The child may cough or have difficulty breathing.
- Spread to the bones: The child has bone pain. If the cancer reaches the bone marrow, the number of various types of blood cells may be reduced. A reduced number of red blood cells (anemia) causes a weak and tired feeling. A reduced number of platelets causes easy bruising and tiny purple spots on the skin. A reduced number of white blood cells lowers the resistance to infection.
- Spread to the skin: Lumps appear.
- Spread to the spinal cord: The arms and legs may feel weak.

About 90 to 95% of neuroblastomas produce hormones, such as epinephrine, which sometimes increase the heart rate and cause anxiety.

Diagnosis

Early diagnosis of a neuroblastoma is not easy. If the cancer has grown large enough, a doctor may be able to feel a lump in the abdomen. A doctor who suspects a neuroblastoma may suggest ultrasonography, computed tomography (CT), or magnetic resonance imaging (MRI) of the chest and abdomen. A urine sample can be tested for excessive production of epinephrine-like hormones.

To see whether the cancer has spread, the doctor may do a bone scan, take x-rays of bones, or examine tissue samples from the liver, lungs, skin, bone marrow, or bone.

Prognosis and Treatment

Children younger than 1 year and children with small cancers have a very good prognosis. In children older than 1 year, the cure rate is low if the cancer has spread.

If the cancer has not spread, it can usually be removed by surgery. Most children are given chemotherapy drugs such as vincristine, cyclophosphamide, doxorubicin, etoposide, and cisplatin. Also, radiation therapy may be used in addition to surgery when chemotherapy is ineffective or when tumors are inoperable.

Retinoblastoma

Retinoblastoma is a cancer of the retina, the light-sensing area at the back of the eye.

- Retinoblastomas result from a genetic mutation.
- The child may have a white pupil or cross-eyes or occasionally vision problems.
- Doctors can diagnose retinoblastoma using indirect ophthalmoscopy.
- Treatment may involve surgery, chemotherapy, or sometimes radiation therapy.

Retinoblastomas represent about 3% of childhood cancers and almost always occur before age 4. They occur in both eyes at the same time in about 25% of children.

This cancer results from a mutation in certain genes that control eye development. Sometimes the mutation is inherited from a parent or occurs very early during development of the embryo. Children thus affected may pass the mutation on to their offspring, who may also develop retinoblastoma. Other times, the mutation occurs later in embryonic development and only in the embryo's eye cells. This mutation cannot be passed on to offspring. Retinoblastoma is hereditary in all children with cancer in both eyes and in 15 to 20% of children with cancer in one eye.

Retinoblastoma does not usually spread beyond the eye, but it occasionally spreads to the brain along the optic nerve (the nerve that leads from the eye to the brain). It may also spread to other organs, such as the bone marrow.

Symptoms and Diagnosis

Symptoms can include a white pupil or cross-eyes (strabismus). Large retinoblastomas may affect vision but tend to cause few other symptoms.

If a doctor suspects a retinoblastoma, the child is given a general anesthetic, and both eyes are examined. A light and a special lens (indirect ophthalmoscopy) are used to look through the lens and iris at the retina. A general anesthetic is necessary because small children are not able to cooperate during the careful, time-consuming examination required to diagnose retinoblastoma.

The cancer can also be identified by computed tomography (CT) or magnetic resonance imaging (MRI). Both tests help determine whether the cancer has spread to the brain. Doctors may also do a spinal tap (lumbar puncture) to look for cancer cells in a sample of cerebrospinal fluid. Finding cancer cells in this fluid is further evidence that the cancer has spread to the brain.

Because the cancer can spread to the bone marrow, a sample of bone marrow may be removed for examination.

Prognosis and Treatment

Without treatment, most children with retinoblastoma die within 2 years. However, with treatment, children with retinoblastoma are cured more than 90% of the time.

When only one eye is affected and that eye has little or no vision, doctors usually remove the entire eyeball along with part of the optic nerve. When children can see fairly well with the affected eye or when the cancer affects both eyes, doctors sometimes give chemotherapy and try to avoid surgery in an attempt to spare the eyeballs. Chemotherapy drugs include etoposide, carboplatin, vincristine, and cyclophosphamide. The chemotherapy may completely eliminate the cancer. If not, chemotherapy often shrinks the cancer enough that the remainder may be removed with lasers, freezing (cryogenic) probes, or patches containing radioactive material. If these treatments do not eliminate the cancer, doctors may remove the eyeball or give radiation therapy. Sometimes both eyeballs must be removed.

Chemotherapy is also used when the cancer has spread beyond the eye or when the cancer returns after initial treatment.

Radiation therapy to the eye has serious consequences, such as cataracts, decreased vision, chronic dry eye, and wasting of the tissue around the eye. The bones of the face may not grow normally, resulting in a deformed appearance.

After treatment, doctors reexamine the eyes every 2 to 4 months to determine whether the cancer has returned. Children with the hereditary type of retinoblastoma have a particularly high risk of having the cancer recur. Furthermore, within 30 years from the time of diagnosis, as many as 70% of people with a hereditary retinoblastoma develop a second cancer, such as soft-tissue sarcomas, melanomas, and osteosarcomas. Doctors recommend that immediate family members of any child with a retinoblastoma have regular eye examinations. Other young children in the family need to be checked for a retinoblastoma, and adults need to be checked for a retinocytoma, a noncancerous (benign) tumor caused by the same gene. Because family members may have the retinoblastoma gene but not develop the cancer, doctors may suggest that they have DNA analysis to check for the gene.

Rhabdomyosarcoma

Rhabdomyosarcoma is a fast-growing cancer that can develop in soft tissues (such as muscle) almost anywhere in the body.

- Rhabdomyosarcomas can develop anywhere, but the head and neck, genital or urinary tract, and limbs are the most common.
- Symptoms depend on where rhabdomyosarcomas develop.
- Diagnosis involves an imaging test and a biopsy.
- Treatment consists of surgery, chemotherapy, and sometimes radiation.

Rhabdomyosarcomas account for 3 to 4% of cancers in children. Two thirds of these cancers are diagnosed in children younger than 7 years. The cancer is slightly more common among boys than girls and is more common among whites than blacks, mainly because it is less common among black girls.

This cancer develops from cells that would normally develop into muscle cells. The cause is unknown.

Although rhabdomyosarcoma can occur almost anywhere, it tends to occur in the following:

- Head and neck (in 35 to 40% of cases), most common among school-aged children
- Genital or urinary tract, usually in the bladder, prostate, or vagina (in 25%), typically occurring in infants and toddlers
- Limbs (in 20%), most common among adolescents

Rhabdomyosarcoma can spread (metastasize) to other parts of the body. But it is usually diagnosed before the cancer has spread.

Symptoms

In most children, the first evidence of the cancer is a firm lump or problems related to an organ affected by the cancer, such as the following:

- Eyes: Tearing, eye pain, or a bulging eye
- Nose and throat: Nasal congestion, a change in the voice, or a nasal discharge that contains mucus and pus
- Genital or urinary tract: Abdominal pain, a lump in the abdomen that can be felt, difficulty urinating, and blood in the urine
- Limbs: Firm lumps on the arms or legs

Limb cancers frequently spread, especially to the lungs, bone marrow, and lymph nodes. Usually, this spread does not cause symptoms.

Diagnosis

If a lump is detected, computed tomography (CT) or sometimes magnetic resonance imaging (MRI) is done. The diagnosis is confirmed by taking a sample from the lump and examining it under a microscope (biopsy). Sometimes the entire lump is removed.

To determine whether the cancer has spread, CT of the chest and a bone scan (radionuclide scanning of bones—see page 2043) are done, and a sample of bone marrow is removed and examined.

Treatment

Treatment consists of surgery, chemotherapy, and sometimes radiation. The entire cancer is removed if possible. All children are treated with chemotherapy (most commonly, vincristine, actinomycin D, cyclophosphamide, doxorubicin, ifosfamide, and etoposide).

Radiation therapy is typically used if some cancer remains after surgery or if the cancer is considered high risk. Risk (and likelihood of a good outcome) depends on the following:

- Where the cancer is
- How much of the cancer can be removed
- Whether it has spread
- How old the child is
- What the cancer cells and tissue look like when examined under a microscope

Wilms' Tumor

Wilms' tumor (nephroblastoma) is a specific kind of kidney cancer.

- The cause of Wilms' tumor is not known, but some children may have a genetic abnormality.
- Children usually have a lump in the abdomen, and they may also have abdominal pain, fever, poor appetite, nausea, and vomiting.
- An imaging test is done to determine the nature and size of the lump.
- Treatment involves surgery and chemotherapy and sometimes radiation therapy.

Wilms' tumor usually develops in children younger than 5 years old, although it occasionally occurs in older children and rarely in adults. Very rarely, it develops before birth and appears in newborns. In about 4% of cases, Wilms' tumor occurs simultaneously in both kidneys.

The cause is not known, although a genetic abnormality may be involved in some cases. Wilms' tumor is more likely to develop in children with certain birth defect, for example, when both irises are missing or when one side of the body grows too much. Both of these defects may be caused by a genetic abnormality. However, most children with Wilms' tumor have no such recognizable abnormalities.

Symptoms

The first symptom is often a painless lump in the abdomen. The abdomen may enlarge, which parents may notice when children suddenly need a larger diaper size. Children may also have abdominal pain, fever, poor appetite, nausea, and vomiting. Blood appears in the urine in 15 to 20% of children. Because the kidneys are involved in controlling blood pressure, Wilms' tumor may cause high blood pressure.

This cancer can spread to other parts of the body, especially the lungs. If the lungs are involved, children may cough and be short of breath.

Diagnosis

Wilms' tumor is most often detected when parents notice a lump in the child's abdomen and take their child to a doctor. Or a doctor may feel such a lump during a routine examination. If the doctor suspects Wilms' tumor, ultrasonography, computed tomography (CT), or magnetic resonance imaging (MRI) is done to determine the nature and size of the lump.

Prognosis

In general, Wilms' tumor is very curable. About 60 to 95% of children survive, depending on how widespread the cancer is. The outcome is usually better in children who are

- Younger
- Have smaller tumors
- Have a tumor that has not spread

Even older children and children with widespread tumors have a very good prognosis. However, one type of Wilms' tumor (which accounts for less than 5% of cases) is more resistant to treatment. Children with this type of tumor, which is recognized by examining a sample of the tumor under a microscope, have a poorer prognosis.

Treatment

Doctors treat Wilms' tumor by removing the kidney that contains the tumor. During the operation, the other kidney is examined to determine whether it also has a tumor. After surgery, doctors give the child chemotherapy drugs—most commonly actinomycin D and vincristine. Other drugs such as doxorubicin, cyclophosphamide, and etoposide are sometimes used. Children with larger or widespread tumors are also treated with radiation therapy.

Sometimes the tumor cannot be removed initially. In such cases, children are first treated with chemotherapy and radiation therapy to shrink the tumor. Then the tumor is removed.

CHAPTER

284 Learning and Developmental Disorders

Developmental disorders, including attention-deficit/hyperactivity disorder, autism spectrum disorders, learning disabilities, and mental retardation/intellectual disability (see page 1858), are neurologically based conditions that can interfere with the acquisition, retention, or application of specific skills or sets of information. They may involve dysfunction in attention, memory, perception, language, problem-solving, or social interaction. These disorders may be mild and easily manageable with educational interventions, or they may be more severe and affected children may require more support.

Attention-Deficit/Hyperactivity Disorder

Attention-deficit/hyperactivity disorder (ADHD) is poor or short attention span and impulsiveness inappropriate for the child's age. Some children are also hyperactive.

- ADHD is a brain disorder that is present from birth or develops shortly after birth.
- Affected children have difficulty with sustained attention, concentration, and ability to complete tasks, and some children are also overactive and impulsive.
- Doctors use questionnaires completed by parents and teachers as well as observations of the child to make the diagnosis.

- Psychostimulant drugs plus structured environments, routines, a school intervention plan, and modified parenting techniques are often needed.

Although there is considerable controversy about the number of children affected, it is estimated that ADHD affects 5 to 15% of school-aged children and is diagnosed 10 times more often in boys than in girls. Many features of ADHD are often noticed before age 4 and invariably before age 7, but they may not interfere significantly with academic performance and social functioning until the middle school years. ADHD was previously called just attention deficit disorder (ADD). However, the common occurrence of hyperactivity in affected children—which is really a physical extension of attention deficit—led to a change in the current terminology.

ADHD can be inherited. Research indicates that the disorder is caused by abnormalities in neurotransmitters (substances that transmit nerve impulses within the brain). The symptoms of ADHD range from mild to severe and can become exaggerated or become a problem in certain environments, such as at home or at school. The constraints of school and organized lifestyles make ADHD a problem, whereas in prior generations, the symptoms may not have interfered significantly with children's

Signs of ADHD

All signs do not have to be present for a diagnosis of attention-deficit/hyperactivity disorder (ADHD). However, signs of inattention must always be present for a diagnosis. Signs must be present in two or more situations (for example, home and school) and must interfere with social or academic functioning.

SIGNS OF INATTENTION:

- Often fails to pay close attention to details
- Has difficulty sustaining attention in work and play
- Does not seem to listen when spoken to directly
- Often does not follow through on instructions and fails to finish tasks
- Often has difficulty organizing tasks and activities
- Often avoids, dislikes, or is reluctant to engage in tasks that require sustained mental effort
- Often loses things
- Is easily distracted by extraneous stimuli
- Is often forgetful

SIGNS OF HYPERACTIVITY:

- Often fidgets with hands or feet or squirms
- Often leaves seat in classroom and elsewhere
- Often runs about or climbs excessively
- Has difficulty playing or engaging in leisure activities quietly
- Is often on the go or acts as if "driven by a motor"
- Often talks excessively

SIGNS OF IMPULSIVITY:

- Often blurts out answers before questions have been completed
- Often has difficulty waiting to take turns
- Often interrupts or intrudes on others

Symptoms

ADHD is primarily a problem with sustained attention, concentration, and task persistence (ability to finish a task). Affected children may also be overactive and impulsive. Many preschool children are anxious, have problems communicating and interacting, and behave poorly. They seem inattentive. They may fidget and squirm. They may be impulsive and talk out of turn. During later childhood, such children may move their legs restlessly, move and fidget their hands, talk impulsively, and forget easily, and they may be disorganized. They are generally not aggressive.

From 20 to 60% of children with ADHD have learning disabilities, and about 80% have academic problems. Work may be messy, with careless mistakes and an absence of considered thought. Affected children often behave as if their mind is elsewhere and they are not listening. They often do not follow through on requests or complete schoolwork, chores, or other duties. There may be frequent shifts from one incomplete task to another.

About 40% of affected children may have issues with self-esteem, depression, anxiety, or opposition to authority by the time they reach adolescence. About 60% of young children have such problems as temper tantrums, and most older children have a low tolerance for frustration.

Diagnosis

The diagnosis is based on the number, frequency, and severity of symptoms. Symptoms must be present in at least two separate environments (typically, home and school)—occurrence of symptoms just at home or just at school and nowhere else does not qualify as ADHD. Symptoms must also be more pronounced than would be expected for the child's developmental level. Often, diagnosis is difficult because it depends on the judgment of the observer. Also, children who are primarily inattentive may escape notice until their academic performance becomes adversely affected.

There is no laboratory test for ADHD. Questionnaires about various aspects of behavior can help doctors and psychologists make the diagnosis. Because learning disabilities are common, many children receive psychologic testing both to help determine whether ADHD exists and to detect the presence of specific learning disabilities.

Prognosis and Treatment

Children with ADHD generally do not outgrow their inattentiveness, although children with hyperactivity tend to become somewhat less impulsive and hyperactive with age. However, most adolescents

functioning because such restraints were often much fewer. Although some of the symptoms of ADHD also occur in children without ADHD, they are more frequent and severe in children with ADHD.

Some people have raised concerns about whether food additives and sugar may cause ADHD. Although some children seem to become overactive or impulsive after eating foods containing sugar, studies have confirmed that ADHD is present at birth and that food and environmental factors do not cause the disorder.

and adults learn to adapt to their inattentiveness. Other problems that emerge or persist in adolescence and adulthood include poor academic achievement, disorganization (known as poor executive skills), low self-esteem, anxiety, depression, and difficulty in learning appropriate social behaviors. Importantly, the vast majority of children with ADHD become productive adults, and people who have ADHD seem to adjust better to work than to school situations. However, if the disorder is untreated in childhood, the risk of alcohol or substance abuse or suicide may increase.

To minimize the effects of ADHD, structures, routines, a school intervention plan, and modified parenting techniques are often needed. Some children who are not aggressive and who come from a stable and supportive home environment may benefit from drug treatment alone. Behavioral therapy conducted by a child psychologist is sometimes combined with drug treatment. Psychostimulant drugs are the most effective drug treatment.

Methylphenidate and other amphetamine-like drugs are the psychostimulants most often prescribed. They are equally effective and have similar side effects. A number of slow-release (longer-acting) preparations are available in addition to the regular forms and allow for once-daily dosing. Side effects include

- Sleep disturbances (such as insomnia)
- Appetite suppression
- Depression or sadness
- Headaches
- Stomachaches
- High blood pressure

Most children have no side effects except perhaps a decreased appetite. All side effects disappear when the drug is stopped. However, when taken in large doses for a long time, stimulants can occasionally slow children's growth, so doctors monitor weight and height.

A number of other drugs can be used to treat inattentiveness and behavioral symptoms. These drugs include clonidine, antidepressants, and antianxiety drugs. Sometimes, a combination of drugs is used.

Autism Spectrum Disorders

Autism spectrum disorders are disorders in which young children cannot develop normal social relationships, use language abnormally or not at all, behave in compulsive and ritualistic ways, and may fail to develop normal intelligence.

- Affected children have difficulty communicating with and relating to others and following rigid routines.
- Diagnosis is based on observation and the reports of parents and other caregivers.

ADHD: Epidemic or Over-Diagnosis?

An increasing number of children are diagnosed with attention-deficit/hyperactivity disorder (ADHD). However, there is concern among doctors and parents that many children are misdiagnosed. A high activity level may be completely normal and simply an exaggeration of normal childhood temperament. Alternatively, it may have a variety of causes, including emotional disorders or abnormalities of brain function, such as ADHD.

Generally, 2-year-olds are active and seldom stay still. A high activity and noise level is common until age 4. In these age groups, such behavior is normal. Active behavior can cause conflicts between parents and child and may worry parents. It also can create problems for others who supervise such children, including teachers.

Determining whether a child's activity level is abnormally high should not simply depend on how tolerant the annoyed person is. However, some children are clearly more active than average. If the high activity level is combined with short attention span and impulsivity, it may be defined as hyperactivity and considered part of ADHD.

Scolding and punishing children whose high activity level is within normal developmental limits usually backfires, increasing the child's activity level. Avoiding situations in which the child has to sit still for a long time or finding a teacher skilled in coping with such children may help. If simple measures do not help, a medical or psychologic evaluation may be useful to rule out an underlying disorder such as ADHD.

- Most children respond best to highly structured behavioral interventions.

Autism is one of several related disorders of brain development. These disorders, known as autism spectrum disorders (ASD) or pervasive developmental disorders, occur in 1 of 150 children. Classic autism is the most common of these disorders. Asperger's syndrome, Rett syndrome, childhood disintegrative disorder, and pervasive developmental disorder not otherwise specified (PDD-NOS) are the other ASD. Symptoms of ASD may appear in the first 2 years of life, but in milder forms symptoms may not be detected until school age. These disorders are 2 to 4 times more common among boys than girls. Autism is different from intellectual disability (previously called mental retardation), although many children with autism have both.

The specific causes of ASD are not fully understood, although they are clearly biologically determined. Several chromosomal abnormalities, such as fragile X syndrome, contribute to the development

COMPARING AUTISM SPECTRUM DISORDERS

DISORDER	EFFECTS	DESCRIPTION
Asperger's syndrome	Generally, language and cognitive skills are better than those in children with autism.	Children are socially isolated and often viewed as odd or eccentric. Children typically have repetitive patterns of behavior. They usually have specific, narrow, and obsessive interests and activities. Sensation may be unusual. For example, children may be very sensitive to noises, food odors or tastes, or clothing textures. Children tend to use and understand language concretely and literally. Thus, they have difficulty recognizing irony or jokes. Movements become clumsy.
Autism (autistic disorder)	It begins before age 3 years. Intellectual disability is impaired to some degree in many children, and severe regression of language and sociability occurs between age 18 and 24 months in about 25%.	Social interaction and communication are markedly impaired. Children may not make eye contact or be able to understand tone of voice or facial expressions. Children typically have repetitive stereotyped patterns of behavior.

Childhood disintegrative disorder	After 2 years of normal growth, a marked regression occurs in at least two of the following:
	  Social skills
	  Language
	  Bladder and bowel control
	  Motor skills
	Eventually, symptoms may become more severe than is typical in autism.
		Some characteristics may resemble those of autism (such as repetitive stereotyped behavior) or those of childhood schizophrenia (such as lack of response to emotional situations).

Other pervasive developmental disorders	Symptoms are less severe than those of autism.	These disorders include a wide range of intellectual, behavioral, and social problems that do not match the criteria needed to diagnose a specific disorder. Thus, these disorders are called pervasive developmental disorders not otherwise specified (PDD-NOS).
Rett syndrome	It begins after 6 months of normal development and causes severe intellectual disability. It is caused by a gene mutation and affects girls almost exclusively.	The brain and head do not grow as quickly as expected. Social interaction is impaired. Children lose the ability to speak. They become unable to use their hands purposefully and typically wring them compulsively. Seizures may occur, and coordination is lost. Some characteristics (for example, toe walking and body rocking) may resemble those of autism.

of autism. Prenatal infections, for example, viral infections such as rubella or cytomegalovirus, may also play a role. It is clear, however, that ASDs are *not* caused by poor parenting, adverse childhood conditions, or vaccination.

Symptoms

Children with ASD develop symptoms in at least 3 of the following areas:

- Social relationships
- Language

- Behavior
- Intelligence

Symptoms range from mild to severe and often keep children from functioning independently in school or society. In addition, about 20 to 40% of children with autism, particularly those with an intelligence quotient (IQ) less than 50, develop seizures before reaching adolescence. In about 25% of affected children, a regression in development occurs around the time of diagnosis and may be the initial indicator of a disorder.

Social Relationships: Often, infants with ASD do not cuddle and avoid eye contact. Although some affected infants become upset when separated from their parents, they may not turn to parents for security as do other children. Older children often prefer to play by themselves and do not form close personal relationships, particularly outside of the family. When interacting with other children, they may not use eye contact and facial expressions to establish social contact, and they are not able to interpret the moods and expressions of others.

Language: About 50% of children with classic autism never learn to speak. Those who learn do so much later than normal and use words in an unusual way. They often repeat words spoken to them (echolalia) or reverse the normal use of pronouns, particularly using *you* instead of *I* or *me* when referring to themselves. These children rarely have an interactive dialogue with others. They also often speak with an unusual rhythm and pitch.

Behavior: Children with ASD are very resistant to changes, such as new food, toys, furniture arrangement, and clothing. They often become excessively attached to particular inanimate objects. They often repeat certain acts, such as rocking, hand flapping, or spinning objects in a repetitive manner. Some may injure themselves through repetitive behaviors such as head banging or biting themselves.

Intelligence: About 70% of children with ASD have some degree of intellectual disability (an IQ less than 70). Their performance is uneven. They usually do better on tests of motor and spatial skills than on verbal tests. Some children with autism have idiosyncratic or splinter skills, such as the ability to carry out complex mental arithmetic or advanced musical skills. Unfortunately, such children often cannot use these skills in a productive or socially interactive way.

Diagnosis

The diagnosis is made by close observation of the child in a playroom setting and careful questioning of parents and teachers. Standardized tests, such as the Gilliam Autism Rating Scale or the more extensive Autism Diagnostic Observational Schedule, may help the evaluation. In addition to giving standardized tests, doctors do certain tests to look for underlying treatable or inherited medical disorders, such as hereditary metabolic disorders (see page 1834) and fragile X syndrome (see page 1728).

Prognosis and Treatment

The symptoms of autism generally persist throughout life. The prognosis is strongly influenced by how much usable language the child has acquired by age 7. Children with autism who have lower measured intelligence—for example, those who score below 50 on standard IQ tests—are likely to need more intensive support as adults.

Children with ASD often benefit from intensive behavioral modification techniques. Children with higher IQs are helped by therapy aimed at developing social skills. Individualized special education is crucial and often includes speech, occupational, physical, and behavioral therapy within a program equipped to manage children with autism.

Drug therapy cannot change the underlying disorder. However, the selective serotonin reuptake inhibitors (SSRIs), such as fluoxetine, paroxetine, and fluvoxamine, are often effective in reducing ritualistic behaviors of children with autism. Antipsychotic drugs, such as risperidone, may be used to reduce self-injurious behavior, although the risk of side effects (such as weight gain and movement disorders) must be considered.

Although some parents try special diets, gastrointestinal therapies, or immunologic therapies, currently there is no good evidence that any of these therapies helps children with autism.

ASPERGER'S SYNDROME AND PERVASIVE DEVELOPMENTAL DISORDER NOT OTHERWISE SPECIFIED

These autism spectrum disorders are closely related to classic autism but are less severe.

Children with Asperger's syndrome have impaired social interactions similar to those of children with autism, as well as stereotyped or repetitive behaviors and mannerisms and nonfunctional rituals. Their speech and language skills are normal, but they often have weakness in pragmatic (social) language. They have normal intelligence but also often have intense interests in narrow topics to the exclusion of other developmentally appropriate pursuits.

Children who have significantly impaired social interactions or stereotyped behaviors without all of the features of autism or Asperger's syndrome are considered to have pervasive developmental disorder not otherwise specified (abbreviated as PDD-NOS). Children with Asperger's syndrome or PDD-NOS tend to function at a higher level than children with classic autism and may be able to function independently. Children with Asperger's syndrome often respond well to psychotherapy.

RETT SYNDROME

Rett syndrome is a rare genetic disorder occurring almost only in girls that causes impaired social interactions, loss of language skills, and repetitive hand movements.

Girls with Rett syndrome appear to develop normally until some time between the age of 5 months and 4 years. When the disorder begins, head growth slows and language and social skills deteriorate. Typically, girls display repetitive hand motions resembling washing or wringing. Purposeful hand movements are lost, walking is impaired, and trunk movements are clumsy. Intellectual disability develops and is usually severe.

Slight spontaneous improvements in social interaction may occur in late childhood and early adolescence, but the language and behavior problems progress. Most girls with Rett syndrome need fulltime support and specialized educational programs. There is no cure.

CHILDHOOD DISINTEGRATIVE DISORDER

In childhood disintegrative disorder, apparently normal children begin to act younger (regress) after age 3.

In most children, physical and mental development occurs in spurts. It is common for children to take a step backward. For example, toilet-trained children occasionally wet themselves. Childhood disintegrative disorder, however, is a rare serious disorder in which children older than age 3 stop developing normally and regress to a much lower level of functioning, typically following a serious illness, such as an infection of the brain and nervous system.

Typical children with childhood disintegrative disorder develop normally until age 3 or 4, learning speech, becoming toilet trained, and displaying appropriate social behavior. Then, after a period of a few weeks or months during which time affected children are irritable and moody, they undergo obvious regression. Children may lose previously acquired language, motor, or social skills and may no longer have control over bladder or bowel function. In addition, children develop difficulties in social interaction and begin performing repetitive behaviors similar to those that occur in children with autism. Quite often children gradually deteriorate to a level of severe intellectual disability. Doctors make the diagnosis based on the symptoms and search for an underlying disorder. In cases of marked regression, a neurologic evaluation to look for treatable causes is essential.

Childhood disintegrative disorder cannot be specifically treated or cured, and most children, particularly those with more severe disability, need lifelong support.

Learning Disorders

Learning disorders involve an inability to acquire, retain, or broadly use specific skills or information, resulting from deficiencies in attention, memory, or reasoning and affecting academic performance.

- Affected children may be slow to learn names of colors or letters, to count, or to learn to read or write.
- Children take a series of academic and intelligence tests given by learning specialists.
- Treatment involves a learning plan tailored to the child's skills.

Learning disorders are quite different from intellectual disability (previously called mental retardation) and occur in children with normal or even high intellectual function. Learning disorders affect only certain functions, whereas in children with intellectual disability, difficulties affect cognitive functions broadly. Three common types of learning disorders are

- Reading disorders
- Disorders of written expression
- Mathematics disorders

Thus, children with learning disorders may have significant difficulty understanding and learning math, but have no difficulty reading, writing, and doing well in other subjects. Dyslexia is the best known of the learning disorders. Learning disorders do not include learning problems that are due primarily to problems of vision, hearing, coordination, or emotional disturbance.

Although the causes of learning disorders are not fully understood, they include abnormalities in the basic processes involved in understanding or in using spoken or written language or numerical and spatial reasoning.

An estimated 3 to 15% of school children in the United States may need special educational services to compensate for learning disorders. Boys with learning disorders may outnumber girls five to one, although girls are often not recognized or diagnosed as having learning disorders.

Many children with behavioral problems do poorly in school and are tested by educational psychologists for learning disorders. However, some children with certain types of learning disorders hide their deficits well, avoiding diagnosis, and therefore treatment, for a long time.

? **Did You Know...**
Learning disorders can occur in children with normal and high intellectual function.

Symptoms

Young children may be slow to learn the names of colors or letters, to assign words to familiar objects, to count, and to progress in other early learning skills. Learning to read and write may be delayed. Other symptoms may be a short attention span and distractibility (mimicking attention-deficit/hyperactivity disorder), halting speech, and a short memory span. Affected children may have difficulty with activities that require fine motor coordination, such as printing and copying.

Children with learning disorders may have difficulty communicating. Some children initially become frustrated and later develop behavioral problems, such as being easily distracted, hyperactive, withdrawn, shy, or aggressive.

Diagnosis and Treatment

Children who are not reading or learning at the grade level expected for their verbal or intellectual abilities should be evaluated. Testing of hearing and eyesight should be done, because problems with these senses can also interfere with reading and writing skills.

Doctors examine children for any physical disorders. Children take a series of intelligence tests, both verbal and nonverbal, and academic tests of reading, writing, and arithmetic skills. Often these tests can be done by specialists at the child's school, at the parents' request.

The most useful treatment for a learning disorder is education that is carefully tailored to the individual child. Measures such as eliminating food additives, taking large doses of vitamins, and analyzing the child's system for trace minerals are often tried but unproven. No drug treatment has much effect on academic achievement, intelligence, and general learning ability. Because some children with a learning disorder also have attention-deficit/hyperactive disorder, certain drugs, such as methylphenidate, may improve attention and concentration, enhancing their ability to learn.

DYSLEXIA

Dyslexia is a specific reading disorder involving difficulty separating single words from groups of words and parts of words (phonemes) within each word.

- Affected children may be late in speaking, have articulation problems, or have difficulty blending sounds or identifying sounds in words.

- Academic and intelligence tests are given.
- Treatment involves direct instruction in word recognition.

Dyslexia is a particular type of learning disorder that affects an estimated 3 to 5% of children. It is identified in more boys than girls; however, it may simply go unrecognized more often in girls. Dyslexia tends to run in families.

Dyslexia occurs when the brain has difficulty making the connection between sounds and symbols (letters). This difficulty is caused by poorly understood problems with certain connections in the brain. The problems are present from birth and may cause spelling and writing errors and reduced speed and accuracy when reading aloud. Although the letter reversals that often occur in children with dyslexia suggest visual problems, in most cases the problems are related to how sounds are perceived. People with dyslexia do not have problems understanding spoken language.

Symptoms and Diagnosis

Preschool children with dyslexia may be late in speaking, have speech articulation problems, and have difficulty remembering the names of letters, numbers, and colors. Dyslexic children often have difficulty blending sounds, rhyming words, identifying the positions of sounds in words, segmenting words into sounds, and identifying the number of sounds in words. Delays or hesitations in choosing words, making word substitutions, and naming letters and pictures are early indicators of dyslexia. Problems with short-term memory for sounds and for putting sounds in the correct order are common.

Many children with dyslexia confuse letters and words with similar ones. Reversing the letters while writing—for instance, *on* instead of *no,* and *saw* instead of *was*—or confusing letters—for instance, *b* instead of *d, w* instead of *m, n* instead of *h*—is common. However, many children without dyslexia reverse letters in kindergarten or first grade.

Children who are not progressing in word learning skills by the middle or end of first grade should be tested for dyslexia. Testing is usually conducted by school personnel and includes intelligence tests and tests of academic skills.

Treatment

The best treatment for word recognition is direct instruction that incorporates multisensory approaches. This type of treatment consists of teaching phonics with a variety of cues, usually separately and, when possible, as part of a reading program.

Indirect instruction for word recognition is also helpful. This instruction usually consists of training to improve word pronunciation or reading comprehension. Children are taught how to process sounds by blending sounds to form words, by separating words into segments, and by identifying the positions of sounds in words.

Component-skills instruction for word recognition is also helpful. It consists of training to blend sounds to form words, to segment words into word parts, and to identify the positions of sounds in words.

As children with dyslexia get older, compensatory strategies may be helpful. These strategies can include use of audio books, computer screen readers (available on most computers), and other technologic adaptations.

Indirect treatments, other than those for word recognition, may be used but are not recommended. Indirect treatments can include using tinted lenses that allow words and letters to be read more easily, eye movement exercises, or visual perceptual training. Drugs such as piracetam have also been tried. The benefits of most indirect treatments have not been proved and may provide unrealistic expectations and delay the teaching that is needed.

CHAPTER
285   Cerebral Palsy

Cerebral palsy refers to a group of symptoms including poor muscle control, spasticity, paralysis, and other neurologic problems resulting from brain injury before, during, or shortly after birth.

- Causes of cerebral palsy include birth injuries, oxygen deprivation, infections, and severe illnesses.
- Symptoms range from barely noticeable clumsiness to severe spasticity and may include intellectual disability, behavioral problems, difficulty seeing or hearing properly, and seizure disorders.
- The diagnosis is based on poor development, spasticity, and muscle weakness.
- Most children with cerebral palsy survive into adulthood.
- There is no cure for cerebral palsy, but physical therapy and special education can help children achieve their highest potential.

Cerebral palsy affects 2 to 4 of every 1,000 infants, but it is 10 times more common among premature infants. It is particularly common among infants of very low birth weight.

Cerebral palsy is not a disease. Rather, it is a constellation of symptoms that results from damage to the parts of the brain that control muscle movements (motor areas). Sometimes children who have cerebral palsy have damage to other parts of the brain as well. The brain damage that results in cerebral palsy may occur during pregnancy, during birth, after birth, or in early childhood. Once the brain damage has occurred, it does not get worse even though the symptoms may change as the child grows and matures. Brain damage occurring after age 5 is not considered cerebral palsy.

Causes

Many different types of injury to the brain can cause cerebral palsy, and often more than one cause is involved. Birth injuries and poor oxygen supply to the brain before, during, and immediately after birth cause 15 to 20% of cases. Prenatal infections, such as rubella, toxoplasmosis, or cytomegalovirus infection, sometimes result in cerebral palsy. Premature infants are particularly vulnerable, possibly in part because the blood vessels of the brain are poorly developed and bleed easily. High levels of bilirubin in the blood can lead to a form of brain damage called kernicterus. During the first years of life, severe illness, such as inflammation of the tissues covering the brain (meningitis), sepsis, trauma, and severe dehydration, can cause brain injury and result in cerebral palsy.

> **Did You Know...**
> Cerebral palsy is not a disease.

Symptoms

The symptoms of cerebral palsy can range from barely noticeable clumsiness to severe spasticity that contorts the child's arms and legs, requiring mobility aids, such as braces, crutches, and wheelchairs.

There are four main types of cerebral palsy: spastic, athetoid, ataxic, and mixed. In all forms of cerebral palsy, speech may be hard to understand because the child has difficulty controlling the muscles involved in speech. Because non-motor parts of the brain also may be affected, many children with cerebral palsy have other disabilities, such as mental retardation/intellectual disability, behavioral problems, difficulty seeing or hearing properly, and seizure disorders.

In the spastic type, which occurs in over 70% of children with cerebral palsy, the muscles are stiff and weak. The stiffness may affect both arms and both legs (quadriplegia), mainly the legs and lower part of the body (paraplegia or diplegia), or only the arm and leg on one side (hemiplegia). The affected arms and legs are poorly developed, stiff, and weak. Some children may walk in a criss-cross motion, where one leg swings over the other (scissors gait), and some may walk on their toes. Crossed, lazy, or wandering eyes (strabismus) and other vision problems may occur. Children with spastic quadriplegia are the most severely affected. They commonly have mental retardation/intellectual disability (sometimes severe) along with seizures and trouble swallowing. Trouble with swallowing makes these children prone to choking on secretions from the mouth and stomach (aspiration). Aspiration injures the lungs, causing difficulty breathing. Repeated aspiration can permanently damage the lungs. Children with spastic diplegia usually have normal mental development and rarely have seizures. About one fourth of children with spastic hemiplegia have below-normal intelligence, and one third of them have seizures.

In the athetoid type, which occurs in about 20% of children with cerebral palsy, the muscles spontaneously move slowly and without normal control. Movements of the arms, legs, and body may be writhing, abrupt, and jerky. Strong emotion makes the movements worse, and sleep makes them disappear. Children with the athetoid type usually have normal intelligence and rarely have seizures. Difficulty with articulating words clearly and normally is common and is often severe. Children with the athetoid type that is caused by kernicterus commonly have nerve deafness and difficulty looking upwards.

In the ataxic type, which occurs in about 5% of children with cerebral palsy, coordination is poor and movements are shaky. Children with the ataxic type also have muscle weakness and trembling. Children with this disorder have difficulty making rapid or fine movements and walk unsteadily, with their legs widely spaced.

In the mixed type, two of the above types, most often spastic and athetoid, are combined. This type occurs in many children with cerebral palsy. Children with mixed types may have severe mental retardation/intellectual disability.

Diagnosis

Cerebral palsy is difficult to diagnose during early infancy. As the baby matures, poor development, weakness, spasticity, or lack of coordination be-

comes noticeable. Although laboratory tests cannot identify cerebral palsy, a doctor may perform blood tests and computed tomography (CT) or magnetic resonance imaging (MRI) of the brain to clarify the nature of the brain damage and to look for other disorders. The doctor might recommend additional testing, such as electrical studies of nerves (nerve conduction) and muscles (electromyography) or a muscle biopsy (a small piece of muscle tissue is taken and examined under a microscope), if the child's symptoms appear to be evolving in a way not typical of cerebral palsy. The specific type of cerebral palsy often cannot be distinguished before the child is 2 years old.

 Did You Know...

After age 5, brain damage is not considered cerebral palsy.

Prognosis and Treatment

The prognosis usually depends on the type of cerebral palsy and on its severity. Most children with cerebral palsy survive into adulthood. Only the most severely affected—those incapable of any self-care—have a substantially shortened life expectancy.

Cerebral palsy cannot be cured, and its problems are lifelong. However, much can be done to improve a child's mobility and independence. Physical therapy, occupational therapy, and braces may improve muscle control and walking, particularly when rehabilitation is started as early as possible. Surgery may be performed to cut or lengthen tendons of the stiff muscles that limit motion. Sometimes cutting certain nerve roots coming from the spinal cord (dorsal rhizotomy) reduces the spasticity and may help a few children who were premature, as long as spasticity mostly affects the legs and mental development is good. Speech therapy may make speech much clearer and help with swallowing problems. Seizures can be treated with anticonvulsant drugs. Drugs taken by mouth, including baclofen, benzodiazepines (such as diazepam), tizanidine, and sometimes dantrolene, are sometimes used to help spasticity, but their benefits are limited by side effects. Some children with severe spasticity benefit from an implantable pump that provides a continuous infusion of baclofen around the spinal cord, although this technique is still experimental and not widely used. Botulinum toxin can be injected into spastic muscles.

Children with cerebral palsy grow normally and attend regular schools if they do not have severe intellectual and physical disabilities. Other children require extensive physical therapy, need special education, and are severely limited in activities of daily living, requiring some type of lifelong care and assistance. However, even severely affected children can benefit from education and training, which increases their independence and self-esteem and greatly reduces the burden for family members or other caretakers.

Information and counseling are available to parents to help them understand their child's condition and potential and to assist with problems as they arise. Loving parental care combined with assistance from public and private agencies, such as community health agencies, health organizations like the United Cerebral Palsy Association, and vocational rehabilitation organizations, can help children reach their highest potential.

286 Mental Retardation/ Intellectual Disability

Mental retardation/intellectual disability is significantly subaverage intellectual functioning present from birth or early infancy, causing limitations in the ability to conduct normal activities of daily living.

- Mental retardation/intellectual disability (MR/ID) can be genetic or the result of a disorder that interferes with brain development.
- Most children with MR/ID do not develop noticeable symptoms until they are in preschool.
- The diagnosis is based on the results of formal testing.
- A child's life expectancy is based on the extent of mental and physical problems.
- Proper prenatal care lowers the risk of having a child with MR/ID.
- Support from many specialists, therapy, and special education help children achieve the highest level of functioning possible.

The long-used term "mental retardation" has acquired an undesirable social stigma. Because of this stigma, doctors and health care practitioners have begun replacing it with the term "intellectual disability." Because this change is recent, the term "mental retardation/intellectual disability" (MR/ID) is used to mark the transition in terminology.

MR/ID is not a specific medical disorder like pneumonia or strep throat, and it is not a mental health disorder. People with MR/ID have significantly below average intellectual functioning that limits their ability to cope with two or more activities of normal daily living (adaptive skills). These activities include the ability to communicate; live at home; take care of oneself, including making decisions; participate in leisure, social, school, and work activities; and be aware of personal health and safety.

People with MR/ID have varying degrees of impairment. While recognizing each person's individuality, doctors find it helpful to classify a person's level of functioning. Intellectual functioning levels can be based on the results of developmental quotient (DQ) tests and intelligence quotient (IQ) tests or on the level of support needed. Support is categorized as intermittent, limited, extensive, or pervasive. Intermittent means occasional support; limited means support such as a day program in a sheltered workshop; extensive means daily, ongoing support; and pervasive means a high level of support for all activities of daily living, possibly including full-time nursing care.

Based only on IQ test scores, about 3% of the total population are considered to have MR/ID. However, if classification is based on the need for support, only about 1% of people are classified as having significant mental (cognitive) limitation.

Causes

A wide variety of medical and environmental conditions can cause MR/ID. Some are genetic; some are present before or at the time of conception; and others occur during pregnancy, during birth, or after birth. The common factor is that something interferes with the growth and development of the brain. However, doctors can identify a specific cause in only about one third of people with mild MR/ID and in two thirds of people with moderate to profound MR/ID.

Symptoms

Some children with MR/ID have abnormalities apparent at birth or shortly thereafter. These abnormalities may be physical as well as neurologic and may include unusual facial features, a head that is too large or too small, deformities of the hands or feet, and various other abnormalities. Sometimes children have an outwardly normal appearance but have other signs of serious illness, such as seizures,

LEVELS OF MENTAL RETARDATION/INTELLECTUAL DISABILITY

LEVEL	INTELLIGENCE QUOTIENT (IQ) RANGE	ABILITY AT PRESCHOOL AGE (BIRTH TO 6 YEARS)	ABILITY AT SCHOOL AGE (6 TO 20 YEARS)	ABILITY AT ADULT AGE (21 YEARS AND OLDER)
Mild	52–69	Can develop social and communication skills Slightly impaired motor coordination Often not diagnosed until later age	Can learn up to about the 6th-grade level by late teens Can be expected to learn appropriate social skills	Can usually achieve enough social and vocational skills for self-support May need guidance and assistance during times of unusual social or economic stress
Moderate	36–51	Can talk or learn to communicate Poor social awareness Fair motor coordination Can profit from training in self-help	Can learn some social and occupational skills Can progress to elementary school level in schoolwork May learn to travel alone in familiar places	May achieve self-support by doing unskilled or semiskilled work under sheltered conditions Needs supervision and guidance when under mild social or economic stress
Severe	20–35	Can say a few words Able to learn some self-help skills Has limited speech skills Poor motor coordination	Can talk or learn to communicate Can learn simple health habits Benefits from habit training	May contribute partially to self-care under complete supervision Can develop some useful self-protection skills in controlled environment
Profound	19 or below	Extreme cognitive limitation Little motor coordination May need nursing care	Some motor coordination Limited communication skills	May achieve very limited self-care Usually needs nursing care

lethargy, vomiting, abnormal urine odor, and failure to feed and grow normally. During their first year, many children with more severe MR/ID have delayed development of motor skills, and are slow to roll, sit, and stand.

However, most children with MR/ID do not develop symptoms that are noticeable until the preschool period. Symptoms become apparent at a younger age in those more severely affected. Usually, the first problem parents notice is a delay in language development. Children with MR/ID are slower to use words, put words together, and speak in complete sentences. Their social development is sometimes slow, because of cognitive impairment and language deficiencies. Children with MR/ID may be slow to learn to dress and feed themselves. Some parents may not consider the possibility of cognitive impairment until the child is in school or preschool and is unable to keep up with age-appropriate expectations.

Children with MR/ID are somewhat more likely than other children to have behavioral problems, such as explosive outbursts, temper tantrums, and physically aggressive behavior. These behaviors are often related to specific frustrating situations compounded by an impaired ability to communicate and control impulses. Older children may be gullible and easily taken advantage of or led into minor misbehavior.

About 10 to 40% of people with MR/ID also have a mental health disorder (dual diagnosis). In particular, anxiety and depression are common, especially in children who are aware that they are different from their peers or who are maligned and mistreated because of their disability.

Diagnosis

Many children are evaluated by teams of professionals, including a pediatric neurologist or developmental

Some Causes of Mental Retardation/Intellectual Disability

BEFORE OR AT CONCEPTION

- Inherited disorders (such as phenylketonuria, Tay-Sachs disease, neurofibromatosis, hypothyroidism, and fragile X syndrome)
- Chromosome abnormalities (such as Down syndrome)

DURING PREGNANCY

- Severe maternal undernutrition
- Infections with HIV, cytomegalovirus, herpes simplex, toxoplasmosis, rubella virus
- Toxins (such as alcohol, lead, and methylmercury)
- Drugs (such as phenytoin, valproate, isotretinoin, and cancer chemotherapy)
- Abnormal brain development (such as porencephalic cyst, grey matter heterotopia, and encephalocele)
- Preeclampsia and multiple births

DURING BIRTH

- Insufficient oxygen (hypoxia)
- Extreme prematurity

AFTER BIRTH

- Brain infections (such as meningitis and encephalitis)
- Severe head injury
- Undernutrition of the child
- Severe emotional neglect or abuse
- Toxins (such as lead and mercury)
- Brain tumors and their treatments

pediatrician, a psychologist, speech pathologist, occupational or physical therapist, special educator, social worker, or nurse.

Doctors evaluate a child suspected of having MR/ID by testing intellectual functioning and looking for a cause. Even though the cause of the child's MR/ID may be irreversible, identifying a disorder that caused the disability may allow doctors to predict the child's future course, prevent further loss of skills, plan any interventions that can increase the child's level of functioning, and counsel parents on the risk of having another child with that disorder.

Newborns with physical abnormalities or other symptoms suggestive of a condition associated with MR/ID often need laboratory tests to help detect metabolic and genetic disorders. Imaging tests, such as computed tomography (CT) or magnetic resonance imaging (MRI), may be performed to look for structural problems within the brain. An electroencephalogram (EEG) records the brain's electrical activity and is used to evaluate a child for possible seizures. A chromosome analysis, urine and blood tests, and x-rays of bones can also help rule out suspected causes of MR/ID.

Some children who are delayed in learning language and mastering social skills have conditions other than MR/ID. Because hearing problems interfere with language and social development, a hearing evaluation is typically performed. Emotional problems and learning disorders also can be mistaken for MR/ID. Children who have been severely deprived of normal love and attention (see page 1879) for long periods of time may seem to have MR/ID. A child with delays in sitting or walking (gross motor skills) or in manipulating objects (fine motor skills) may have a neurologic disorder not associated with MR/ID.

Because mild developmental problems are not always noticed by parents, doctors routinely perform developmental screening tests during well-child visits. Doctors use simple questionnaires, such as the Ages and Stages Questionnaires or Child Development Inventories, to quickly evaluate the child's cognitive, verbal, and motor skills. Parents can help the doctor determine the child's level of functioning by completing a Parents' Evaluation of Developmental Status (PEDS) test. Children who perform significantly below their age level on these screening tests are referred for formal testing.

Formal testing has three components: interviews with parents, observations of the child, and norm-referenced tests. Some tests, such as the Stanford-Binet Intelligence Test and the Wechsler Intelligence Scale for Children-IV, measure intellectual ability. Other tests, such as the Vineland Adaptive Behavior Scales, assess areas such as communication, daily living skills, social abilities, and motor skills. Generally, these formal tests accurately compare a child's intellectual and social abilities with those of others in the same age group. However, children of different cultural backgrounds, non–English-speaking families, and very low socioeconomic status are more likely to perform poorly on these tests. For these reasons, a diagnosis of MR/ID requires that the doctor integrate the test data with information obtained from parents and direct observations of the child. A diagnosis of MR/ID is appropriate only when both intellectual and adaptive skills are significantly below average.

Prognosis and Prevention

Because MR/ID sometimes coexists with serious physical problems, the life expectancy of children with MR/ID may be shortened, depending on the specific condition. In general, the more severe the cognitive disability and the more physical problems the child has, the shorter the life expectancy. However, a child with mild MR/ID has a relatively normal life expectancy, and health care is improving long-term health outcomes for people with all types of developmental disabilities. Many people with mild to moderate MR/ID can support themselves, can live independently, and can be successful at jobs that require basic intellectual skills.

Prevention applies to environmental, genetic, and infectious disorders as well as to accidental injuries. Fetal alcohol syndrome is a highly common and totally preventable cause of MR/ID. The March of Dimes and other groups concerned about the prevention of MR/ID focus much of their efforts on alerting women to the seriously damaging effects of drinking alcohol during pregnancy. Doctors may recommend genetic testing for people who have a family member or other child with a known inherited disorder, particularly ones related to MR/ID, such as phenylketonuria, Tay-Sachs disease, or fragile X syndrome. Identification of a gene for an inherited disorder allows genetic counselors to help parents evaluate the risk of having an affected child. Women who plan to get pregnant should receive necessary vaccinations, particularly against rubella. Women who are at risk of infectious disorders that may be harmful to a fetus, such as rubella and human immunodeficiency virus (HIV), should be tested before getting pregnant.

Proper prenatal care lowers the risk of having a child with MR/ID. Folate, a vitamin supplement, taken before conception and early in pregnancy can help prevent certain kinds of brain abnormalities. Advances in the practices of labor and delivery and in the care of premature infants have helped to reduce the rate of MR/ID related to prematurity.

Certain tests, such as ultrasound, amniocentesis, chorionic villus sampling, and various blood tests, can be performed during pregnancy to identify conditions that often result in MR/ID. Amniocentesis or chorionic villus sampling is often used for women at high risk of having a baby with Down syndrome, especially those aged 35 and older, and for women with family histories of metabolic disorders. Measuring maternal serum alpha-fetoprotein is a helpful screening test for neural tube defects, Down syndrome, and other abnormalities. A few conditions, such as hydrocephalus and severe Rh incompatibility (see page 1650), may be treated during pregnancy. Most conditions, however, cannot be treated, and early recognition can serve only to prepare the parents and allow them to consider the option of abortion.

Treatment

A child with MR/ID is best cared for by a multidisciplinary team consisting of the primary care doctor; social workers; speech, occupational, and physical therapists; neurologists or developmental pediatricians; psychologists; nutritionists; educators; and others. Together with the family, these people develop a comprehensive, individualized program for the child, which is begun as soon as the diagnosis of MR/ID is suspected. The parents and siblings of the child also need emotional support and sometimes counseling. The whole family should be an integral part of the program.

> **Did You Know...**
> A specific cause can be identified in only about a third of children with intellectual disability.

The full array of a child's strengths and weaknesses must be considered in determining what kind of support is needed. Factors such as physical disabilities, personality problems, mental illness, and interpersonal skills are all taken into consideration. Affected children with coexisting mental health disorders such as depression may be given appropriate drugs in dosages similar to those given to children without MR/ID. However, giving a child drugs without also instituting behavioral therapy and environmental changes is usually not helpful.

All children with MR/ID benefit from special education. The federal Individuals with Disabilities Education Act (IDEA) requires public schools to provide free and appropriate education to children and adolescents with MR/ID or other developmental disorders. Education must be provided in the least restrictive, most inclusive setting possible—where the children have every opportunity to interact with non-disabled peers and have equal access to community resources.

A child with MR/ID usually does best living at home. However, some families cannot provide care at home, especially for children with severe, complex disabilities. This decision is difficult and requires extensive discussion between the family and their entire support team. Having a child with severe disabilities at home requires dedicated care that some parents may not be able to provide. The family may need psychologic support. A social worker can organize services to assist the family. Help can be provided by day care centers, housekeepers, child caregivers, and respite care facilities. Most adults with MR/ID live in community-based residences that provide services appropriate to the person's needs, as well as work and recreational opportunities.

287 Mental Health Disorders

Several important mental health disorders, such as depression and eating disorders (see page 876), often develop during childhood and adolescence. Some disorders, such as autism, develop only during childhood.

With a few exceptions, symptoms of mental health disorders tend to be similar to feelings that every child experiences, such as sadness, anger, suspicion, excitement, withdrawal, and loneliness. The difference between a disorder and a normal feeling is the extent to which the feeling becomes so powerful as to overwhelm and interfere with the activities of normal life or cause the child to suffer. Thus, doctors must use a significant degree of judgment to determine when particular thoughts and emotions stop being a normal component of childhood experience and represent a disorder.

Some disorders affect mainly behavior, causing children to disturb others, including teachers, peers, and family members. These disorders, called disruptive behavioral disorders, include attention-deficit/hyperactivity disorder (the most common one—see page 1849), conduct disorder, and oppositional defiant disorder.

In children, some disorders affect both mental health and overall development. These disorders, called autism spectrum disorders (see page 1851), include autism, Asperger's syndrome, pervasive developmental disorder not otherwise specified, Rett syndrome, and childhood disintegrative disorder. The pervasive developmental disorders are a group of related conditions that all involve some combination of impaired social relationships, a restricted range of interests, abnormal language development and use, and, in some cases, intellectual impairment.

Childhood Schizophrenia

Childhood schizophrenia is a chronic disorder involving abnormal thought, perception, and social behavior.

- Schizophrenia is probably caused by chemical abnormalities in the brain and by problems during the brain's development.
- Adolescents withdraw, start having unusual emotions, and usually have hallucinations, delusions, and paranoia.
- Doctors do tests to rule out other possible causes.
- Antipsychotic drugs can help control symptoms, and counseling can help adolescents and family members learn how to manage the disorder.

Schizophrenia is quite rare in childhood. It typically develops during late adolescence and early adulthood (see page 889). When schizophrenia does develop during childhood, it usually begins between the age of 7 and the start of adolescence.

Schizophrenia probably occurs because of chemical abnormalities in the brain and problems during the brain's development. Doctors do not know what causes these abnormalities. However, experts agree that people can inherit a tendency to develop schizophrenia and that it is not caused by poor parenting or difficulties during childhood.

Symptoms

Children with schizophrenia typically become withdrawn and lose interest in activities. Thinking and perception are distorted. These symptoms may continue for some time before worsening. As with adults, children with schizophrenia are likely to have hallucinations, delusions, and paranoia, often fearing that others are planning to harm them or are controlling their thoughts. Their emotions are sometimes blunted. That is, their voice and facial expressions do not change in response to emotional situations. Events that normally make people laugh or cry may produce no response.

In adolescents, use of illicit drugs may cause symptoms similar to those of schizophrenia.

Diagnosis

There is no specific diagnostic test for schizophrenia. Doctors base the diagnosis on a thorough evaluation of symptoms over time and psychologic tests. They also do tests to check for other disorders (such as drug abuse or a brain tumor) that can cause similar symptoms.

> **? Did You Know...**
> Schizophrenia should not be blamed on poor parenting or difficulties during childhood.

Treatment

Schizophrenia cannot be cured, although hallucinations and delusions may be controlled with antipsychotic drugs, such as haloperidol, olanzapine, quetiapine, and risperidone (see table on page 894). Children are particularly susceptible to the side effects of antipsychotic drugs. Side effects may include tremors, slowed movements, movement disorders, and metabolic syndrome (which includes obesity, type 2 diabetes, and abnormal levels of fat in the blood—see page 960).

Social skills training, vocational rehabilitation, and psychologic and educational support for the child and counseling for family members are essential to help everyone cope with the disorder and its consequences. Doctors almost always refer children to psychiatrists who specialize in treating children.

Children may need to be hospitalized when symptoms worsen so that drug doses can be adjusted and they can be kept safe.

Depression

Depression is a feeling of sadness or irritability intense enough to interfere with functioning. It may follow a recent loss or other sad event but is out of proportion to that event and persists beyond an appropriate length of time (see page 863).

- Physical disorders, life experiences, and heredity can contribute to depression.
- Affected children and adolescents may be sad, disinterested, and sluggish or overactive, aggressive, and irritable.
- Doctors base the diagnosis on symptoms as reported by the child, parents, and teachers and do tests to check for other disorders that can be causing the symptoms.
- For adolescents, a combination of psychotherapy and antidepressants is usually most effective, but for younger children, psychotherapy alone is usually tried first.

Sadness and unhappiness are common human emotions, particularly in response to troubling situations. For children and adolescents, such situations may include the death of a parent, divorce, a friend moving away, difficulty adjusting to school, and difficulty making friends. However, feelings of sadness are sometimes out of proportion to the event or persist far longer than expected. In such cases, particularly if the feelings cause difficulties in day-to-day functioning, children may have depression. Like adults, some children become depressed even when no unhappy life events occur. Such children are more likely to have family members with mood disorders (a family history). Depression occurs in as many as 2% of children and 5% of adolescents.

Doctors do not know exactly what causes depression, but chemical abnormalities in the brain are probably involved. Some tendency to develop depression is inherited. A combination of factors, including life experiences and a genetic tendency (vulnerability), seems to contribute. Sometimes another disorder, such as an underactive thyroid gland or drug abuse, is part of the cause.

Did You Know...
Some children with depression are overactive and irritable rather than sad.

Symptoms

As in adults, the severity of depression in children varies greatly.

Children typically have feelings of overwhelming sadness or irritability, worthlessness, and guilt. They lose interest in activities that normally give them pleasure, such as playing sports, watching television, playing video games, or playing with friends. They may profess intense boredom. Many of these children also complain of physical problems, such as stomachache or headache.

Appetite may increase or decrease, often leading to substantial changes in weight. Sleep is usually disturbed. Children may have insomnia, sleep too much, or be troubled by frequent nightmares.

Depressed children are often not energetic or physically active. However, some, particularly younger children, have seemingly contradictory symptoms, such as overactivity and aggressive, very irritable behavior. Some children seem more irritable than sad.

Symptoms typically interfere with the ability to think and concentrate, and schoolwork usually suffers. Children may have suicidal thoughts, fantasies, and attempts.

Diagnosis

To diagnose depression, doctors rely on several sources of information, including an interview with the child or adolescent and information from parents and

Symptoms of Depression in Children

- Feeling sad or irritable
- Having no interest in favorite activities
- Withdrawing from friends and social situations
- Being unable to enjoy things
- Feeling rejected and unloved
- Not sleeping well and having nightmares or sleeping too much
- Blaming themselves
- Losing their appetite and weight
- Thinking about suicide
- Giving away valued possessions
- Complaining of new physical symptoms
- Making lower grades in school

teachers. Sometimes doctors use structured questionnaires (see page 866) to help distinguish depression from a normal reaction to an unhappy situation. Doctors try to find out whether family or social stresses may have precipitated the depression. Doctors also ask specifically about suicidal behavior, including thoughts and talk about suicide.

Doctors do tests to determine whether a physical disorder, such as an abnormal thyroid gland or drug abuse, is the cause.

Treatment

Treatment depends on the severity of symptoms. Any child who has suicidal thoughts should be closely supervised by experienced mental health care practitioners. If risk of suicide is high enough, children require brief hospitalization to keep them safe.

For most adolescents, a combination of psychotherapy and drugs is more effective than either alone. But for younger children, psychotherapy alone may be tried first, and drugs are used only if needed. Individual psychotherapy, group therapy, and family therapy may be beneficial.

Daily use of specialized artificial light (phototherapy) may be useful if depression is related to the seasons. In late fall and winter, the reduced amount of daylight causes hormonal changes that can contribute to depression. Phototherapy is most often used with drugs or psychotherapy in children and adolescents who have episodes of depression in winter.

Antidepressant drugs help correct chemical imbalances in the brain. Selective serotonin reuptake inhibitors (SSRIs), such as fluoxetine, sertraline, and paroxetine (see table on page 868), are the drugs most commonly prescribed for depressed children and adolescents. Tricyclic antidepressants, such as imipramine, are much less effective in children than adults and have more side effects, so they are rarely used in children.

Antidepressant Drugs and Suicide: Recently, there has been concern that antidepressants may increase the risk of suicidal thinking and behavior in children and adolescents, particularly during the first few weeks after the drugs are started. This concern has led to an overall decrease in the use of antidepressants in children. However, this decrease in the use of antidepressants has been associated with an increase in the rate of death by suicide, perhaps because depression is then not adequately treated in some children. Some experts hypothesize that antidepressants first cause agitation and anxiety before they relieve depression. During this initial period, children and adolescents may be more likely to talk about their suicidal feelings and sometimes even act on them. However, when depression is eventually relieved, the children are then less likely to commit suicide. Studies are being done to try to settle this issue, but doctors tend to agree that children with depression often benefit from drug treatment as long as they and family members are alert for worsening symptoms or suicidal thoughts.

Bipolar Disorder

In bipolar disorder (sometimes called manic-depressive illness), periods of intense elation and excitation (mania) alternate with periods of depression and despair. Mood may be normal in between these periods.

- Children may rapidly go from being excited, happy, and active to being depressed, withdrawn, and sluggish or full of rage and violent.
- Doctors base the diagnosis on symptoms and results of psychiatric tests.
- The diagnosis of bipolar disorder in young children is very controversial.
- Mood-stabilizing drugs to treat mania, antidepressants to treat depression, and psychotherapy can help.

Children normally have fairly rapid mood swings, going from happy and active to glum and withdrawn. These swings rarely indicate a mental health disorder. Bipolar disorder is far more severe than these normal mood changes, and the moods last much longer, often for weeks or months. Bipolar disorder is rare in children, although it is more common than previously thought. Some experts believe that young children (aged 4 to 11 years) who have intense mood swings many times a day may have a variation of bipolar disorder. This idea is a very controversial and is currently under study. Bipolar disorder typically begins during adolescence or early adulthood (see page 870). Bipolar disorder in adolescents is similar to bipolar disorder in adults.

The cause is unknown, but a tendency to develop bipolar disorder can be inherited. Chemical abnormalities in the brain may be involved. Bipolar disorder may begin after a stressful life event, such as incest, although the event itself does not cause the disorder. In children with the disorder, such an event may trigger an episode. Rarely, drugs with stimulant effects, such as amphetamines, which are sometimes used to treat attention-deficit/hyperactivity disorder (ADHD—see page 1849), cause symptoms similar to those of bipolar disorder. Also, certain other disorders, including ADHD and an overactive thyroid gland, can cause similar symptoms.

Symptoms

The main symptoms are episodes of feeling intense elation and excitement (mania). Sometimes there are episodes of depression. Mania is a state of elation, excitation, racing thoughts, irritability, and grandiosity (in which children feel they have some great talent or have made an important discovery). During manic episodes, sleep is disturbed, and children may become aggressive. School performance often deteriorates.

During an episode of depression, children with bipolar disorder, like those with depression alone, feel excessively sad and lose interest in their usual activities. They may think and move slowly and sleep more than usual. Feelings of hopelessness and guilt may overwhelm them.

Children with bipolar disorder appear normal between episodes, in contrast to children with ADHD, who are in a constant state of increased activity.

Diagnosis

Doctors base the diagnosis on a description of typical episodes by children and their parents. Because ADHD can cause similar symptoms, differentiating between the two is important. Doctors determine whether children are taking any drugs that could contribute to the symptoms. Doctors may also check for signs of other disorders that may contribute to or cause the symptoms. For example, they may do blood tests to check for an overactive thyroid gland.

Treatment

Bipolar disorder is treated with mood-stabilizing drugs, such as lithium and certain anticonvulsants such as carbamazepine and valproate. In most cases, an antipsychotic drug is also used.

Individual and family psychotherapy helps children and their families cope with the consequences of the disorder. Psychotherapy can help adolescents, who are prone to not follow their drug regimen, continue to do so.

Suicidal Behavior

Suicidal behavior is an action intended to harm oneself and includes suicide gestures, suicide attempts, and completed suicide.

- A stressful event may trigger suicide in children who have a mental health disorder such as depression.
- Children at risk of suicide may be depressed or anxious, withdraw from activities, talk about subjects related to death, or suddenly change their behavior.
- Family members and friends should take all suicide threats or attempts seriously.
- Health care practitioners try to determine how serious the risk of suicide is.
- Treatment may involve hospitalization if the risk is high, drugs to treat other mental health disorders, and individual and family counseling.

Suicide is rare in children before puberty and is mainly a problem of adolescence, particularly between the ages of 15 and 19, and of adulthood (see page 873). However, preadolescent children do commit suicide, and this potential problem must not be overlooked.

In the United States, suicide is the second or third leading cause of death in adolescents. It results in 2,000 deaths per year. It is also likely that a number of the deaths attributed to accidents, such as those due to motor vehicles and firearms, are actually suicides.

Many more young people attempt suicide than actually succeed. A survey done by the Centers for Disease Control and Prevention found that 28% of high school students had suicidal thoughts and 8.3% had attempted suicide. Frequently, suicide attempts involve at least some ambivalence about wishing to die and may be a cry for help.

Among adolescents in the United States, boys outnumber girls in completed suicide by more than 4 to 1. However, girls are 2 to 3 times more likely to attempt suicide.

Suicide gestures are acts of self-harm that are unlikely to result in death, such as taking an overdose of vitamins.

> **? Did You Know...**
> Suicide is the second or third leading cause of death among adolescents in the United States.

Risk Factors

Several factors typically interact before suicidal thoughts become suicidal behavior. Very often, there is an underlying mental health disorder and a stressful event that triggers the behavior. Stressful events include

- Death of a loved one
- A suicide in school or another group of peers
- Loss of a boyfriend or girlfriend
- A move from familiar surroundings (such as the school or neighborhood) or friends
- Humiliation by family members or friends
- Being bullied at school
- Failure at school
- Trouble with the law

However, such stressful events are fairly common among children and rarely lead to suicidal behavior if there are no other underlying problems. The most common underlying problems are the following:

- **Depression:** Adolescents with depression have feelings of hopelessness and helplessness that limit their ability to consider alternative solutions to immediate problems.

- **Alcohol or drug abuse:** The use of alcohol or drugs lowers inhibitions against dangerous actions and interferes with anticipation of consequences.
- **Poor impulse control:** Adolescents, particularly those who have a disruptive behavioral disorder such as conduct disorder, may act without thinking.

Children and adolescents attempting suicide are sometimes angry with family members or friends, are unable to tolerate the anger, and turn the anger against themselves. They may wish to manipulate or punish other people ("They will be sorry after I am dead").

Sometimes suicidal behavior results when a child imitates the actions of others. For example, a well-publicized suicide, such as that of a celebrity, is often followed by other suicides or suicide attempts. Similarly, copycat suicides sometimes occur in schools. Suicide is more likely in families in which mood disorders are common, especially if there is a family history of suicide or other violent behavior.

Diagnosis

Parents, doctors, teachers, and friends may be in a position to identify children who might attempt suicide, particularly those who have had any recent change in behavior. Children and adolescents often confide only in their peers, who must be strongly encouraged not to keep a secret that could result in the tragic death of the suicidal child. Children who express overt thoughts of suicide, such as "I wish I'd never been born" or "I'd like to go to sleep and never wake up," are at risk, but so are children with more subtle signs, such as social withdrawal, falling grades, or parting with favorite possessions. Health care practitioners have two key roles: evaluating a suicidal child's safety and need for hospitalization and treating underlying disorders, such as depression or substance abuse.

Prevention

Directly asking at-risk children about suicidal thoughts can bring out important issues that are contributing to the child's distress. Identifying these issues can, in turn, lead to meaningful interventions. Crisis hot lines, offering 24-hour assistance (see box on page 875), are available in many communities and provide ready access to a sympathetic person who can give immediate counseling and assistance in obtaining further care. Although it is difficult to prove that these services actually reduce the number of deaths from suicide, they are helpful in directing children and families to appropriate resources.

Treatment

Children who attempt suicide need urgent evaluation in a hospital emergency department. Any type of suicide attempt must be taken seriously, because

---

Risk Factors and Warning Signs of Suicide in Children and Adolescents

MENTAL AND PHYSICAL SYMPTOMS:

- Preoccupation with morbid themes
- Depression
- Dramatic changes in mood
- Changes in appetite
- Sleep disturbances
- Tension, anxiety, or nervousness
- Poor control of impulses

CHANGES IN BEHAVIOR:

- Poor hygiene and neglect of personal appearance (especially if it is an abrupt change)
- Withdrawal from social interactions
- A decline in grades
- An increase in violent behavior
- Giving away favorite possessions

CONVERSATION:

- Statements about feeling guilty
- Statements suggesting a wish to be dead, such as "I wish I'd never been born" or "I'd like to go to sleep and never wake up"
- Direct or indirect threats to commit suicide

CIRCUMSTANCES:

- Access to firearms or prescription drugs
- Family history of suicide
- A previous attempt at suicide
- Death of a loved one, especially by suicide
- Alcohol or drug abuse

---

one third of those who complete suicide have previously attempted it—sometimes an apparently trivial attempt, such as making a few shallow scratches to the wrist or swallowing a few pills. When parents or caregivers belittle or minimize an unsuccessful suicide attempt, children may see this response as a challenge, and the risk of subsequent suicide increases.

Once the immediate threat to life has been removed, the doctor decides whether the child should be hospitalized. The decision depends on the degree of risk in remaining at home and the family's capacity to provide support and physical safety for the child. The seriousness of a suicide attempt can be gauged by a number of factors, including the following:

- Whether the attempt was carefully planned rather than spontaneous—for example, leaving a suicide note indicates a planned attempt
- Whether steps were taken to prevent discovery

- What type of method used—for example, using a gun is more likely to cause death than taking pills
- Whether any injury was actually inflicted

It is critical to distinguish serious intent from actual consequences. For example, adolescents who ingest harmless pills that they believe to be lethal should be considered at extreme risk.

If hospitalization is not needed, families of children going home must ensure that firearms are removed from the home altogether and that drugs and sharp objects are removed or securely locked away. Even with these precautions, preventing suicide can be very difficult, and there are no proven measures for successfully preventing it.

If Suicide Occurs: Family members of children and adolescents who commit suicide have complicated reactions to the suicide, including grief, guilt, and depression. They may feel purposeless, detached from everyday activities, and bitter. They may have difficulty continuing with their life. Counseling can help them understand the psychiatric context of the suicide and reflect on and acknowledge the child's difficulties before the suicide. They may then be able to understand that the suicide was not their fault.

Conduct Disorder

A conduct disorder involves a repetitive pattern of behavior that violates the basic rights of others.

- Children with a conduct disorder are selfish and insensitive to the feelings of others and may bully, damage property, lie, or steal without guilt.
- Doctors base the diagnosis on the history of the child's behavior.
- Separating children from a troubled environment and providing a strictly structured setting, as in a mental health facility, may be the most effective treatment.

Although some children are better behaved than others, children who repeatedly and persistently violate rules and the rights of others in ways inappropriate for their age have a conduct disorder. Conduct disorder usually begins during late childhood or early adolescence and is more common among boys than girls.

Heredity and the environment probably influence the development of a conduct disorder. Children often have parents who have a mental health disorder, such as substance abuse, attention-deficit/hyperactivity disorder, a mood disorder, schizophrenia, or antisocial personality disorder. However, affected children may come from healthy families that function well.

Symptoms

In general, children with a conduct disorder are selfish, do not relate well to others, and lack an appropriate sense of guilt. They are insensitive to the feelings and well-being of others. They tend to misperceive the behavior of others as threatening and react aggressively. They may engage in bullying, threatening, and frequent fights and may be cruel to animals. Some children damage property, especially by setting fires. They may lie or steal.

The disorder affects boys and girls differently. Girls are less likely to be physically aggressive. Instead, girls typically run away, lie, abuse substances, and sometimes engage in prostitution. Boys tend to fight, steal, and vandalize.

Seriously violating rules is common and includes running away from home and frequently being truant from school. Children are likely to use and abuse illicit drugs and have difficulties in school. Suicidal thoughts may occur and must be taken seriously.

About half the children stop the inappropriate behaviors by adulthood. The younger a child is when conduct disorder begins, the more likely the behavior is to continue. If the behavior continues into adulthood, people often encounter legal trouble, chronically violate the rights of others, and are often diagnosed with antisocial personality disorder (see page 881). Some of these adults develop mood, anxiety, or other mental health disorders.

Diagnosis

Doctors base the diagnosis on the child's behavior. The symptoms or behavior must be troubling enough to impair functioning in relationships, at school, or at work.

The social environment is also considered. If misconduct develops as an adaptation to a very stressful environment (such as a war-torn area or area of civil unrest), it is not considered a conduct disorder.

Treatment

Treatment is very difficult because children with conduct disorder rarely perceive anything wrong with their behavior. Often, the most successful treatment is to separate children from the troubled environment and to provide a strictly structured setting, as in a mental health or a juvenile justice facility.

Certain drugs may be somewhat effective, especially if certain disorders, such as attention-deficit/hyperactivity disorder or depression, coexist. Treatment of such disorders can help lessen the symptoms of conduct disorder.

Oppositional Defiant Disorder

Oppositional defiant disorder is a recurring pattern of negative, defiant, and disobedient behavior, often directed at authority figures.

Children with oppositional defiant disorder are stubborn, difficult, and disobedient without being physically aggressive or actually violating the rights of others. Many preschool and early adolescent children occasionally display oppositional behaviors, but oppositional defiant disorder is diagnosed only if behaviors persist for 6 months or more and are serious enough to interfere with social or academic functioning. Most often, children develop this disorder by age 8.

Typical behaviors of these children include the following:

- Arguing with adults
- Losing their temper easily and often
- Actively defying rules and instructions
- Deliberately annoying people
- Blaming others for their own mistakes
- Being angry, resentful, and easily annoyed

These children do know the difference between right and wrong and feel guilty if they do anything that is seriously wrong.

Oppositional defiant disorder is best treated through behavior management techniques, which include a consistent approach to discipline and appropriate reinforcement of desired behavior. Parents and teachers can be instructed in these techniques by the child's counselor or therapist.

From time to time, children who have depression are mistakenly diagnosed with oppositional defiant disorder. This misdiagnosis most commonly happens when irritability is the main symptom of depression. Thus, when oppositional defiant disorder is diagnosed, all children should be carefully assessed for signs of depression, such as sleep or appetite disturbances.

Anxiety Disorders

Anxiety disorders are characterized by fear, worry, or dread that greatly impairs the ability to function and is out of proportion to the circumstances.

- There are many types of anxiety disorders, distinguished by the main focus of the fear or worry.
- Most commonly, children refuse to go to school, often using physical symptoms as the reason.
- Doctors usually base the diagnosis on symptoms but sometimes do tests to rule out disorders that could cause the physical symptoms often caused by anxiety.
- Behavioral therapy is often sufficient, but if anxiety is severe, drugs may be needed.

All children feel some anxiety sometimes. For example, 3- and 4-year-olds are often afraid of the dark or monsters. Older children and adolescents often become anxious when giving a book report in front of their classmates. Such fears and anxieties are not signs of a disorder. However, if children become so anxious that they cannot function or become greatly distressed, they may have an anxiety disorder. At some point during childhood, about 10 to 15% of children experience an anxiety disorder.

People can inherit a tendency to be anxious. Anxious parents tend to have anxious children.

Anxiety disorders include acute stress, generalized anxiety, obsessive-compulsive, panic, posttraumatic stress, and separation anxiety disorders, social phobia, and agoraphobia. Acute stress disorder is similar to posttraumatic stress disorder except that symptoms occur less than 1 month after the traumatic event. Agoraphobia—the fear of being trapped in places with no way to escape easily—often accompanies or results from panic disorder (see page 857).

Symptoms

Many children with an anxiety disorder refuse to go to school. They may have separation anxiety, social phobia, panic disorder, or a combination.

Some children talk specifically about their anxiety. For example, they may say "I am worried that I will never see you again" (separation anxiety) or "I am worried the kids will laugh at me" (social phobia). However, most children complain of physical symptoms, such as a stomachache. These children are often telling the truth because anxiety often causes an upset stomach, nausea, and headaches in children.

Many children who have an anxiety disorder struggle with anxiety into adulthood. However, with early treatment, many children learn how to control their anxiety.

Diagnosis

Doctors usually diagnose the disorder when the child or parents describe typical symptoms. However, doctors may be misled by the physical symptoms that anxiety can cause and do tests for physical disorders before an anxiety disorder is considered.

Treatment

If anxiety is mild, behavioral therapy alone is usually all that is needed. Therapists expose children to the situation that triggers anxiety and help the children remain in the situation. Thus, children gradually become desensitized and feel less anxiety. When appropriate, treating anxiety in parents at the same time often helps.

If anxiety is severe, drugs may be used. A type of antidepressant called a selective serotonin reuptake inhibitor (SSRI), such as fluoxetine, is usually the first choice (see table on page 868).

GENERALIZED ANXIETY DISORDER

Generalized anxiety disorder involves excessive, persistent nervousness, worry, and dread about many activities or events.

Children's worries are general and encompass many things and activities. Stress worsens the anxiety. These children often have difficulty paying attention and may be hyperactive and restless. They may also sleep poorly, sweat excessively, feel exhausted, and complain of physical symptoms, such as stomachache, muscle aches, and headache.

The diagnosis is based on symptoms: excessive worries that do not focus on a particular activity or situation or that include many activities and situations. The disorder is diagnosed when symptoms last more than 6 months.

If anxiety is mild, relaxation training or other types of counseling may be all that is needed.

If anxiety is severe or counseling is not effective, drugs that can reduce anxiety, usually selective serotonin reuptake inhibitors or sometimes buspirone, may be needed.

OBSESSIVE-COMPULSIVE DISORDER

Obsessive-compulsive disorder is characterized by recurring, unwanted, intrusive ideas, images, or impulses (obsessions) and unrelenting urges to act on the impulses (compulsions). The obsessions and compulsions cause great distress and interfere with school and relationships.

- Children with obsessive-compulsive disorder often worry or fear that they or loved ones will be harmed and feel compelled to do something to neutralize their fear.
- Behavioral therapy and drugs are often used in treatment.

What causes obsessive-compulsive disorder (OCD) is unclear. However, streptococcal infections may be involved in a few cases. In these cases, the disorder is called pediatric autoimmune neuropsychiatric disorder associated with streptococcus (PANDAS).

Symptoms

Typically, symptoms develop gradually, and most children can hide their symptoms at first.

Children are often obsessed with worries or fears of being harmed—for example, of contracting a deadly disease or of injuring themselves or others. They feel compelled to do something to balance or neutralize their worries and fears. For example, they may repeatedly do the following:

- Check to make sure they turned off their alarm or locked a door
- Wash their hands excessively
- Count various things (such as steps)

- Sit down and get up from a chair
- Constantly clean and arrange certain objects
- Make corrections in schoolwork
- Chew food a certain number of times
- Avoid touching certain things
- Make frequent requests for reassurance, sometimes dozens or even hundreds of times per day

Some obsessions and compulsions have a logical connection. For example, children may wash their hands to avoid disease. However, some are totally unrelated. For example, children may count to 50 over and over to prevent a grandparent from having a heart attack. If they resist the compulsions or are prevented from carrying them out, they become extremely anxious and concerned.

Most children have some idea that their obsessions and compulsions are abnormal and are often embarrassed by them and try to hide them. In most children, the disorder tends to be chronic.

Diagnosis and Treatment

Diagnosis is based on symptoms.

Behavioral therapy, if available, may be all that is needed if children are highly motivated. If needed, a combination of behavioral therapy and an SSRI is usually effective, enabling most children to function normally. Treatment usually needs to be continued indefinitely. A few children do not respond to treatment and remain greatly impaired.

If streptococcal infection is involved, antibiotics are used.

PANIC DISORDER

Panic disorder is characterized by panic attacks that occur at least once a week. A panic attack is a brief (5- to 20-minute) episode of intense anxiety that is usually accompanied by physical symptoms, such as a rapid heart beat, sweating, chest pain, and nausea.

- Panic disorder is diagnosed when children have panic attacks frequently enough to cause significant impairment or suffering.
- Panic disorder is usually treated with a combination of drugs and behavioral therapy.

Panic disorder is much more common among adolescents than among younger children. Sometimes children have separation anxiety or generalized anxiety when they are younger and then develop panic disorder as they go through puberty.

Panic attacks (see page 857) can occur in any anxiety disorder, usually in response to the focus of that disorder. For example, children with separation anxiety may have a panic attack when a parent leaves. Children who fear being trapped in places with no way to escape easily (agoraphobia) may have a panic attack when they are seated in the middle of a row in a crowded auditorium. Many children who have panic disorder also have agoraphobia. Physical disorders, such as asthma, can also trigger panic attacks.

Symptoms

During an attack, children feel great anxiety, which causes physical symptoms. The heart beats rapidly. Children may sweat profusely and feel short of breath. They may have chest pain or feel dizzy, nauseated, or numb. Children may feel like they are dying or going crazy. Things may seem unreal to them. Children worry about having other attacks. Panic attacks and the associated worries interfere with relationships and schoolwork.

In panic disorder, panic attacks usually occur on their own, with no specific trigger. But over time, children begin to avoid situations that they associate with the attacks. This avoidance can lead to agoraphobia, which makes children reluctant to go to school, visit the mall, or do other typical activities.

Panic disorder often worsens and lessens for no apparent reason. Symptoms may disappear on their own, then recur years later. Occasionally, adolescents with panic disorder may drop out of school, withdraw from society, and become reclusive and suicidal.

Diagnosis and Treatment

Usually, doctors do a physical examination to check for physical disorders that may be causing the symptoms. Doctors also consider other anxiety disorders, which may also cause panic attacks.

Usually, a combination of drugs and behavioral therapy is effective. In children, drugs are usually needed to control the panic attacks before behavioral therapy can begin. Benzodiazepines are the most effective drugs, but SSRIs are often preferred because benzodiazepines cause drowsiness (sedation) and may interfere with learning and memory. Behavioral therapy is especially useful for agoraphobia symptoms. However, drugs rarely help children with agoraphobia because children often continue to fear that they may have a panic attack, even long after attacks have been well controlled by drugs.

POSTTRAUMATIC STRESS DISORDER

Posttraumatic stress disorder causes recurring, intrusive memories of an overwhelming traumatic event as well as emotional numbness and increased tension or alertness (arousal).

- The disorder may develop after children witness or experience an act of violence, such as a dog attack, a school shooting, an accident, or a natural disaster.
- Children not only reexperience the event, but they also feel emotionally numb, extremely tense, and jittery.

- The diagnosis is based on symptoms that occur after a traumatic event.
- Treatment involves psychotherapy, behavioral therapy, and drugs.

Posttraumatic stress disorder (PTSD) may develop after children witness or experience an event that threatens their own or another's life or health. During the event, they typically feel intense fear, helplessness, or horror. These events include acts of violence, such as child abuse, school shootings, car accidents, attacks by a dog, fires, wars, natural disasters (such as hurricanes, tornados, or earthquakes), and deaths. In young children, domestic violence is the most common cause. Not all children who experience a severe traumatic event develop a stress disorder.

In posttraumatic stress disorder, symptoms may not appear until months or years later, and they last more than a month. If symptoms occur within a month of the stressful event and last less than a month, the disorder is called acute stress disorder. Children with acute stress disorder usually fare better than those with posttraumatic stress disorder, but they still benefit from early treatment.

> **? Did You Know...**
> Among young children, domestic violence is the most common cause of posttraumatic stress disorder.

Symptoms

Children constantly feel anxious. They usually fail in their attempts to avoid remembering the event. They may reexperience the traumatic event while they are awake (flashbacks) or asleep (as nightmares). Flashbacks are usually triggered by something associated with the original event. For example, seeing a dog may trigger a flashback in children who were attacked by a dog. During a flashback, children may be terrified and unaware of their surroundings. They may desperately try to hide or escape, acting as though they are in great danger. Less dramatically, children can reexperience the event in thoughts, mental images, or recollections, which are nonetheless greatly distressing.

Feeling emotionally numb is common. Children may lose interest in their usual activities, withdraw from other people, and worry about dying at a young age. They may feel extremely tense (called hyperarousal), making them jittery and unable to relax. They have difficulty sleeping.

Children may also feel guilty—for example, because they survived when others did not or because they could do nothing to stop the event.

Diagnosis and Treatment

Diagnosis is based on a history of a frightening, horrifying traumatic event followed by characteristic symptoms.

Supportive psychotherapy may help. Therapists reassure children that their response is valid but encourage them to face their memories (as a form of exposure therapy). Behavioral therapy can be used to systematically desensitize children to situations that cause them to reexperience the event.

SSRIs (a type of antidepressant) may help relieve some symptoms.

SEPARATION ANXIETY DISORDER

Separation anxiety disorder involves persistent, intense anxiety about being away from home or being separated from people to whom a child is attached, usually the mother.

- Most children feel some separation anxiety but usually grow out of it.
- Children often cry and plead with the person who is leaving and, after the person leaves, think only about being reunited.
- Doctors base the diagnosis on symptoms and their duration.
- Behavioral therapy is usually effective, and individual and family psychotherapy may help.
- Treatment aims to enable children to return to school as soon as possible.

Some degree of separation anxiety is normal and occurs in almost all children, especially in very young children (see page 1734). Children feel it when a person to whom they are attached leaves. That person is usually the mother, but it can be either parent or a caregiver. The anxiety typically stops as children learn that the person will return. In separation anxiety disorder, the anxiety is much more intense and goes beyond that expected for the child's age and developmental level. Separation anxiety disorder commonly occurs in younger children and is rare after puberty.

Some life stress, such as the death of a relative, friend, or pet or a geographic move or a change in schools, may trigger the disorder. Also, people can inherit a tendency to feel anxiety.

Symptoms

Children experience great distress when separated from home or from people to whom they are attached. Dramatic scenes commonly occur during goodbyes. Goodbye scenes are typically painful for both parent and child. Children often wail and plead with such desperation that the parent cannot leave, prolonging the scene and making separation even more difficult. If the parent is also anxious, children become more anxious, creating a vicious circle.

After the parent has left, children fixate on being reunited. They often need to know where the parent is and are preoccupied with fears that something terrible will happen to them or to their parent.

Traveling by themselves makes these children uncomfortable, and they may refuse to attend school or camp or to visit or sleep at friends' homes. Some children cannot stay alone in a room, clinging to a parent or shadowing the parent around the house.

Difficulty at bedtime is common. Children with separation anxiety disorder may insist that a parent or caregiver stay in the room until they fall asleep. Nightmares may disclose the children's fears, such as destruction of the family through fire or another catastrophe. Children often develop physical symptoms.

Children usually appear normal when a parent is present. As a result, the problem may seem less severe than it is. The longer the disorder lasts, the more severe it is.

Diagnosis

Doctors base the diagnosis on a description of the child's past behavior and sometimes on observation of goodbye scenes. The disorder is diagnosed only if symptoms last at least a month and cause substantial distress or greatly impair functioning.

Treatment

Behavioral therapy is used. It involves teaching parents and caregivers to keep the goodbye scenes as short as possible and coaching them to react to protestations matter-of-factly. Individual and family psychotherapy is also useful.

Enabling children to return to school is an immediate goal. It requires doctors, parents, and school personnel to work as a team. Helping children form an attachment to one of the adults in the preschool or school may help.

When the disorder is severe, drugs that can reduce anxiety, such as an SSRI, may help.

Children are prone to relapses after holidays and breaks from school. Thus, parents are often advised to plan regular separations during these periods to help children remain accustomed to being away from them.

SOCIAL PHOBIA

Social phobia (social anxiety disorder) involves a persistent fear of being embarrassed, ridiculed, or humiliated in social situations.

Sometimes social phobia develops after an embarrassing incident.

Usually, this disorder is first noticed when children or adolescents refuse to go to school. The reason they give is often a physical symptom, such as stomachache or headache.

Children are terrified that they will humiliate themselves in front of their peers by giving the wrong answer, saying something inappropriate, becoming embarrassed, or even vomiting. When the fear is excessive, children may refuse to talk on the telephone or to leave the house.

The diagnosis is based on symptoms.

Behavioral therapy is used most often. It involves not allowing children to miss school. Absence makes them even more reluctant to attend school.

If behavioral therapy is ineffective or children will not participate in it, a drug that can reduce anxiety, such as a selective serotonin reuptake inhibitor may help. The drug may reduce anxiety enough to enable children to participate in behavioral therapy.

Tic Disorders

Tics are rapid, repeated involuntary movements that are fundamentally purposeless.

One in four children may have a tic of some sort during a few months of their childhood. Such tics are much more likely to occur in boys than in girls. Common tics include repeated coughs or throat clearing, blinking or grimacing, shoulder shrugging, lip smacking, and various hand gestures. Stress and fatigue can make tics worse. Usually, tics occur only when children are awake. They can be voluntarily controlled for short periods of time but only with conscious effort.

Tics sometimes occur with other disorders such as obsessive-compulsive disorder or result from certain infections or certain drugs, especially drugs used to treat attention-deficit/hyperactivity disorder (ADHD), such as methylphenidate or amphetamine.

Eventually, most tics disappear without treatment. However, in fewer than 1% of children, tics persist. If they persist and cause problems (such as embarrassment), a tic disorder may be diagnosed. If the tics are all vocal (such as throat clearing), vocal tic disorder may be diagnosed. If the tics are all movements (such as eye blinking), motor tic disorder may be diagnosed. If children have a combination of vocal tics and tics involving movement, Tourette's syndrome may be diagnosed (see page 780).

In many cases, no treatment is needed other than reassurance. If tics persist and are bothersome, drugs may be used. Usually, antipsychotic drugs (such as haloperidol or risperidone) are very effective in controlling tics.

Somatoform Disorders

In somatoform disorders, an underlying psychologic problem causes distressing or disabling physical symptoms.

- There are several types of somatoform disorders.

- Symptoms may resemble those of a neurologic disorder (such as paralysis or loss of vision) or be vague (such as headache and nausea), or children may be obsessed with an imagined defect or be convinced that they have a serious disease.
- After doing tests to exclude physical disorders that could cause the symptoms, doctors base the diagnosis on symptoms.
- Individual and family psychotherapy, often using cognitive-behavioral techniques, can help.

Symptoms and treatment of somatoform disorders are very similar to those of anxiety disorders.

Children with a somatoform disorder may have a number of symptoms, including pain, difficulty breathing, and weakness, without evidence of a physical cause (see page 849). Often, children develop psychologically based physical symptoms when another family member is seriously ill. These physical symptoms are thought to develop unconsciously in response to a psychologic stress or problem (see box on page 851). The symptoms are not consciously fabricated, and children are actually experiencing the symptoms they describe.

Somatoform disorders include the following:

- **Conversion disorder (see also page 851):** Symptoms resemble those of a neurologic disorder. Children may seem to have a paralyzed arm or leg, become deaf or blind, or have shaking that may resemble seizures. These symptoms begin suddenly, usually after a distressing event, and may or may not resolve abruptly.

- **Somatization disorder (see also page 852):** Children develop numerous vague symptoms, such as headaches, abdominal pain (see page 1800), and nausea. Any part of the body may be affected. These symptoms may come and go for long periods of time.

- **Body dysmorphic disorder (see also page 850):** Children become preoccupied with an imagined defect in appearance, such as the size of their nose or ears, or become excessively concerned with a slight abnormality, such as a wart.

- **Hypochondriasis (see also page 852):** Children have no specific, ongoing symptoms but are obsessed with bodily functions, such as heartbeat, digestion, and sweating, and are convinced that they have a serious disease when nothing is wrong. They may also feel anxious and depressed.

Somatoform disorders are equally common among young boys and young girls but are more common among adolescent girls than adolescent boys.

Diagnosis

Doctors ask children about their symptoms and do a physical examination and sometimes tests to make sure that children do not have a physical disorder that could account for the symptoms.

However, extensive laboratory tests are generally avoided because they may further convince children that a physical problem exists and unnecessary diagnostic tests may themselves traumatize children.

If no physical problem can be identified, doctors may use standardized mental health tests to help determine whether symptoms are due to a somatoform disorder. Doctors also talk to the children and family members to try to identify underlying psychologic problems or troubled family relationships.

Treatment

Children may balk at the idea of visiting a psychotherapist because they think their symptoms are purely physical. However, individual and family psychotherapy, often using cognitive-behavioral techniques, can help children and family members recognize patterns of thought and behavior that perpetuate the symptoms. Therapists may use hypnosis, biofeedback, and relaxation therapy.

Psychotherapy is usually combined with a rehabilitation program that aims to help children get back into a normal routine. It can include physical therapy, which has the following benefits:

- It may treat actual physical effects, such as reduced mobility or loss of muscle, caused by a somatoform disorder.
- It makes children feel as if something concrete is being done to treat them.
- It enables children to participate actively in their treatment.

Drugs may be used to relieve pain or the anxiety or depression that can accompany these disorders.

CHAPTER 288 Social Issues Affecting Children and Their Families

To thrive, a child must experience the consistent and ongoing care by a loving, nurturing caregiver, whether that person is a parent or substitute caregiver. The security and support that such an adult can provide gives a child the self-confidence and resiliency to cope effectively with stress.

To mature emotionally and socially, children must interact with people outside the home. These interactions typically occur with close relatives; friends; neighbors; and people at child care sites, schools, churches, and sports teams or other activities. By coping with the minor stresses and conflicts inherent in these interactions, children gradually acquire the skills to handle more significant stressors. Children also learn by watching how the adults in their lives handle distress.

Certain major events, such as illness and divorce, may challenge a child's abilities to cope. These events may also interfere with the child's emotional and social development. For example, a chronic illness may prevent a child from participating in activities and also impair performance in school.

Events affecting the child may also have negative consequences for people close to the child. Everyone who cares for a sick child is under stress. The consequences of such stress vary with the nature and severity of the illness and with the family's emotional resources and other resources and supports.

Illness and Death in Infants

The medical needs of premature newborns or ill infants often require that they be separated from their parents temporarily. Although doctors may allow parents to hold their infant some of the time, medical care often sharply limits the opportunity for parents to interact with their infant. In addition, parents are usually emotionally distressed by their infant's condition. Separation and parental distress can reinforce feelings of inadequacy or guilt, particularly in severely ill infants who are hospitalized for a long time. Parents need to see, hold, and interact with their infant as soon as it is practical. Even with

---

? Did You Know...

Illness or death in an infant or a child often makes parents feel guilty, even when they are not at fault.

Sometimes children need to hear the same message about a difficult issue over and over.

Children who are bullied are often too frightened or embarrassed to tell an adult.

Talking With Children About Difficult Topics

Many life events, including illness or death of someone close, divorce, and bullying, are scary or unpleasant for children. Even events that do not directly affect the child, such as natural disasters, war, or terrorism, may cause anxiety. Fears about all of these, rational or irrational, can preoccupy a child.

Children often have difficulty talking about unpleasant topics. However, open discussion can help the child deal with difficult or embarrassing topics and dispel irrational fears. A child needs to know that anxiety is normal and anxious feelings will lessen over time.

Parents should discuss difficult topics during a quiet time, in a private place, and when the child is interested. Parents should remain calm, present factual information, and give the child undivided attention. Acknowledging what the child says with phrases such as "I understand" or with a quiet nod encourages the child to confide. Reflecting back what the child says is also encouraging. For example, if a child mentions anger about a divorce, a parent could say, "So, the divorce makes you angry" or "Tell me more about that." Asking how the child feels can also encourage discussion of sensitive emotions or fears—for example, fear of abandonment by the noncustodial parent during a divorce or guilt for causing the divorce.

By disclosing their own feelings, parents encourage children to acknowledge their fears and concerns. For example, about a divorce, a parent might say, "I am sad about the divorce, too. But, I also know it is the right thing for mommy and daddy to do. Even though we cannot live together anymore, we will both always love

you and take care of you." By doing this, parents are able to discuss their own feelings, offer reassurance, and explain that divorce is the right choice for them. Sometimes children, particularly younger ones, need to hear the same message repeatedly.

Sometimes a parent must raise a difficult topic with a child, such as telling the child about a serious illness in or death of a relative or friend. Although it might make sense to do so at the time, death should never be equated with "going to sleep and never waking up" because the child may become fearful of sleeping. If tragedy affects someone else, children may feel more confident, and less helpless, if they can contribute—for example, by picking flowers; writing or drawing a card; wrapping a present; or collecting food, clothing, money, or toys. When a child appears withdrawn or sad, refuses to engage in usual activities, or becomes aggressive, the parent should seek professional help.

A parent may also have to address a difficult aspect of the child's own behavior. For example, a parent who suspects the child or adolescent of using drugs or alcohol should address the issue directly with the child. A parent might say, "I am worried that you are using drugs. I feel this way because . . . ." The parent should then calmly list the worrisome behaviors, limiting the list to three or four behaviors. If the child denies there is a problem, the parent should restate the concerns calmly and explain to the child that there is a plan of action in place (such as an appointment with a pediatrician or counselor).

Throughout any discussion, parents should reassure their children that they are loved and will be supported.

---

severely ill infants, parents often can help to feed, bathe, and change their infant. Breastfeeding may be possible, even if the infant must be fed through a tube at first. Many neonatal nurseries help families store and use breast milk for their child.

> **? Did You Know...**
> Seeing and touching an infant who has died helps parents begin to grieve.

If an infant has a birth defect, parents may experience guilt, sadness, anger, or even horror. Many feel even more guilt because they have such feelings. Seeing and touching the child can help the parents look beyond the birth defect and see the infant as a whole person. This interaction helps reinforce the attachment to the child. Information

about the condition, possible treatments, and the infant's prognosis can help the parents adjust psychologically and plan for the best medical care.

Death of an infant is always emotionally traumatic for parents. However, if a newborn dies before being seen or touched by the parents, the parents may feel as though they never had a baby. Although painful, holding or seeing the dead baby can help parents begin to grieve and begin the process of closure. Parents of a stillborn baby sometimes find comfort from dressing the stillborn in baby clothes and taking pictures. This practice humanizes the infant and reinforces that the infant was a real part of their family. Emptiness, lost hopes and dreams, and fear may overwhelm parents, who may become depressed. Parents tend to feel guilty, blaming themselves even when they are not responsible for the death. The grief and guilt that follow may strain the relationship between parents. The grieving process may also mean that parents are unable to attend to the needs of other family members, including other children.

What Is Bullying?

Bullying is repeated physical or psychologic attacks that are performed to dominate or humiliate. Frequent teasing, threats, exclusion, intimidation, harassment, and violent assault are forms of bullying. Cyber-bullying is a newly described form in which bullies use e-mail and instant messaging to threaten their victims. Although bullying typically involves only two people, it can involve groups. Bullies often report that bullying inflates their sense of self-worth and creates feelings of power and control. Although bullying hurts and demeans the victim, bullies often unknowingly repel their friends and peers, thereby hurting themselves.

Even though they sometimes tell family members or friends, victims are often too embarrassed and frightened to disclose bullying to an adult. Teachers are often unaware that bullying is going on. Victims may refuse to go to school, appear sad or withdrawn, or become moody.

Victims need reassurance that bullying is always unacceptable. Parents can demonstrate ways a victim can respond to the bully—for example, telling an adult, walking away, changing their routines to avoid the bully, or engaging in counseling. Although it is usually not advisable (for safety reasons) to directly confront the bully, teaching the child to ignore and actually not be bothered by the bully will reduce the bully's satisfaction and eventually lessen the bullying. Praising the victim's courage for reporting bullying can begin to rebuild the victim's self-esteem.

If bullying occurs at school, parents should inform school officials. The victim's parents should also inform the bully's parents but should avoid confrontation, which could be counterproductive by making the bully's parents defensive. Victims may fear that telling the bully's parents will worsen bullying, but it often stops bullying, particularly if the discussion is positive and not accusatory, but instead focuses on the harmful behavior.

The bully's parents should make it clear to their child that bullying is not acceptable. Parents should insist that the bully apologize and make amends to the victim. Doing so can help the bully learn right from wrong, can make the bully more sensitive to the victim, and can make others see the bully more sympathetically. Adults should watch the child closely to ensure that bullying stops. Counseling is recommended for child who is doing the bullying. Often, bullies are expressing their unmet needs or modeling the aggressive behavior of a parent or older sibling.

Many families whose infants are severely ill or who have died can benefit from counseling from psychologic or religious personnel. Parent and family support groups also may help.

Illness in Children

Severe illness, even if temporary, can provoke a great deal of anxiety for children and their families. Chronic problems, such as asthma, diabetes, hearing or vision impairments, and cerebral palsy, or disability usually cause even more emotional distress.

Coping with illness may require coping with pain, undergoing tests, taking drugs, and changing diet and lifestyle. Chronic illness often interferes with a child's education because of frequent absences from school. The illness as well as side effects from treatments may impair the child's ability to learn. Even though parents and teachers may have lower academic expectations of ill children, it is important for them to maintain the challenges and encouragement children need to achieve their best.

Illness and hospitalization deprive children of opportunities to play with other children. Other children may even reject or taunt an ill child because of physical differences and limitations. Children can become self-conscious if illness changes their body, particularly when the changes occur during childhood or adolescence rather than being present from birth. Parents and family members may overprotect the child, discouraging independence.

Did You Know...

Sometimes one parent assumes the burden of the care and later resents it, while the other parent may feel isolated.

Chronic illness of a child places enormous psychologic, financial, emotional, and physical burdens on parents. Sometimes the parents become closer by working together to overcome these burdens. However, often the burdens can strain the relationship. Parents may feel guilty about the illness, particularly if it is genetic, resulted from complications during pregnancy, or was caused by an accident (such as a motor vehicle collision), or a behavior of a parent (such as smoking). In addition, medical care can be expensive and can cause the parents to miss work. Sometimes, one parent assumes the burden of the care, which can lead to feelings of resentment in the caregiving parent or feelings of isolation in the other. Parents may feel angry with health care providers, themselves, each other, or the child. Parents may also be in denial about the severity of their child's condition. The emotional distress involved in providing care can also make it difficult to form a deep attachment to a disabled or seriously ill child.

Parents who spend a lot of time with an ill child often have less time to devote to other children in the family. Siblings may resent the extra attention the ill child receives and then feel guilty for feeling that way. The ill child may feel guilty about hurting or burdening the family. Parents may be too lenient with the ill child, or they may enforce discipline inconsistently, particularly if the symptoms come and go.

Hospitalization is a frightening event for children even under the best circumstances, and it should be avoided whenever possible. If hospitalization is needed, it should be as brief as possible, preferably in a part of the hospital used exclusively for children. In most hospitals, parents are encouraged to stay with their children, even during painful or fear-provoking procedures. Despite their parents' presence, children may become clingy or dependent (regress) while in the hospital.

> **? Did You Know...**
> Parents may spend more time or be more lenient with the ill child than with siblings, who may then become resentful and feel guilty about their resentment.

Although a child's illness is always stressful for the entire family, there are several steps a parent can take to help lessen the impact. Parents should learn as much as possible about their child's illness from reliable sources, such as the child's doctors and reliable medical resources. Information obtained from some Internet sources is not always accurate, and parents should check with their doctors about the information they read. Doctors can often refer parents to a support group or another family that has already faced similar issues and can provide information and emotional support.

Services needed by the child may involve care by medical specialists, nurses, home health personnel, mental health personnel, and personnel from a variety of other services. A case manager may be needed to help coordinate medical care for children with complex chronic illness. The child's doctor, nurse, social worker, or other professional can serve as the case manager. The case manager can also ensure that the child receives training in social skills and that the family and child receive appropriate counseling, education, and psychologic and social support, such as respite care. Regardless of who coordinates services, the family and child must be partners in the process.

Divorce

Separation and divorce, and the events leading up to them, interrupt the stability and predictability that children need. Other than the death of an immediate family member, divorce is the most stressful event that can affect a family. Because the world as they know it has ended, children may feel a great loss as well as anxiety, anger, and sadness. Children may fear being abandoned or losing their parents' love. Also, for many reasons, parenting skills often worsen around the time of the divorce. Parents are usually preoccupied and may be angry and hostile toward each other. Children may feel guilty about causing the divorce. If parents ignore children or visit sporadically and unpredictably, children feel rejected.

Once parents decide to separate and divorce, family members move through several stages of adjustment. In the acute stage (the period when parents decide to separate, including the time preceding the divorce), turmoil is often maximal. This stage may last up to 2 years. During the transitional stage (the weeks around the actual divorce), the child is in an adjustment period to the new relationship between the parents, visitation, and the new relationship with the noncustodial parent. After the divorce (the post-divorce stage), a different type of stability should develop.

During the divorce, schoolwork may seem unimportant to children and adolescents, and school performance often worsens. Children may have fantasies that parents will reconcile. Children aged 2 to 5 years may have difficulty sleeping, temper tantrums, and separation anxiety. Toileting skills may deteriorate. Children aged 5 to 12 years can experience sadness, grief, intense anger, and irrational fears (phobias). Adolescents often feel insecure, lonely, and sad. Some engage in risk-taking behaviors, such as drug and alcohol use, sex, theft, and violence. Others may develop eating disorders, become defiant, skip school, or join peers who are engaging in risk-taking behaviors.

Children need to be able to express their feelings to an adult who listens attentively. Counseling can provide children with a caring adult who, unlike their parents, will not be upset by their feelings.

Children adjust best when parents cooperate with each other and focus on the child's needs. Parents must remember that a divorce only severs their relationship as husband and wife, not their relationship as parents of their children. Whenever possible, parents should live close to each other, treat each other respectfully in the child's presence, maintain the other's involvement in the child's life, and consider the child's wishes regarding visitation. Older children and adolescents should be given increasing say in living arrangements. Parents should never suggest

The Changing Structures of Families

Most people picture a traditional family as a married man and woman and their biologic children. However, a family may consist of a single parent, a gay couple, or unrelated adults who live and rear children together.

During the last several decades, increasing numbers of families have deviated from the traditional model. Divorce forces many children into single-parent families or blended families created by adults living together or remarriage. About 33% of children are born to single mothers, and about 10% of children are born to single teenage mothers. Many children are reared by grandparents or other relatives. Over 1 million children live with adoptive parents.

Even traditional families have changed. Often both parents work outside the home, requiring many children to receive regular care outside of the family setting. Because of school and career commitments, many couples postpone having children until their 30s and even 40s. Changing cultural expectations have resulted in fathers spending increasing amounts of time rearing children.

Conflicts develop in every family, but healthy families are strong enough to resolve conflicts or thrive despite them. Whatever their makeup, healthy families provide children with a sense of belonging and meet children's physical, emotional, developmental, and spiritual needs. Members of healthy families express emotion and support for each other in ways consistent within their own culture and family traditions.

before or after school. Sources of care include relatives, neighbors, licensed and unlicensed private homes, and child care centers. Care can also be provided in the home by a relative or nanny. Child care centers can be licensed, accredited, or both. Accreditation usually requires that the center meet higher standards than those required for licensing.

Care outside of the home varies in quality. Some care is excellent, some is poor. Care outside of the home can also have benefits. Children can benefit from the social and academic stimulation of quality child care.

 Did You Know...

Most preschool children receive care outside the home.

Child care outside the home can provide benefits: social interaction, physical and other activities, and opportunities to develop independence.

Early exposure to music, books, art, and language stimulates a child's intellectual and creative development. Group play stimulates social development. Outdoor play and occasional vigorous play help dissipate pent-up physical energy and stimulate muscle development. Opportunities to initiate their own activities help children develop independence. Nutritious meals or snacks should be available every few hours. Television and videos contribute little to the child's development and are best avoided. If they are used, the content should be age-appropriate and supervised by an adult. There are many resources available through local and national organizations that can help parents assess child care settings. The American Academy of Pediatrics supports materials provided at the Healthy Child Care America web site, which include checklists about good child care environments.

that their children take sides and should try not to express negative feelings about the other parent to their children. Parents should discuss issues openly, honestly, and calmly with their children; remain affectionate with them; continue to discipline consistently; and maintain normal expectations regarding chores and schoolwork. Most children regain a sense of security and support within about a year after divorce if the parents adjust and work to meet the child's needs.

For a child, remarriage of either parent can create new conflict but should restore a sense of stability and permanency if handled appropriately by all of the adults involved. Some children feel disloyal to one parent by accepting the other parent's new spouse.

Child Care

About 80% of children receive child care outside the home before they start school. Many children aged 5 to 12 also receive care outside the home

Foster Care

Foster care is care provided for children whose families are temporarily unable to care for them. The local government determines the process of arranging foster care. Foster care is surprisingly common in the United States—about 750,000 children are in the foster care system each year.

The foster parent assumes day-to-day care for the child. However, the birth parents usually remain the child's legal guardians. This means that the birth parents still make legal decisions for the child. For example, if the child needs an operation, only the birth parents can provide consent.

Most children in foster care are from poor families. About 70% of the children in foster care are put there by Child Protective Services because the child has been abused or neglected. Most of the remaining 30% are adolescents placed in care by the juvenile justice system. Very few children are placed voluntarily by their parents. Most children in foster care live with foster families, although many live with extended family and adolescents are likely to live in group homes or residential treatment facilities.

Did You Know...

Over half of children in foster care return to their birth families.

Removal from their family is enormously painful to children. In foster care, children may have frequent visits with their families or only limited, supervised visits. Children in foster care leave behind their neighborhoods, communities, schools, and most of their belongings. Many children and adolescents in foster care feel anxious, uncertain, and helpless to control their lives. Many feel angry, rejected, and pained by the separation or they develop a profound sense of loss. Some feel guilty, believing that they caused the disruption of their birth family. Peers often tease children about being in foster care, reinforcing perceptions that they are somehow different or unworthy. Children in foster care have more chronic illnesses and behavioral, emotional, and developmental problems than do other children. Yet, most children in foster care adjust well as long as the placement is stable and the foster family is skilled in nurturing the child's emotional needs. Most children in foster care benefit from counseling.

Over half of the children eventually return to their birth families. About 20% of children in foster care are eventually adopted, most often by their foster family. Other children return to a relative or become too old for foster care. A small number of children are later transferred to another foster care agency. Tragically, 18% of youth in foster care eventually age out of the system without a sense of belonging in any family.

Adoption

Adoption is the legal process of adding a person to an existing family. Adoption, unlike foster care, is meant to be permanent. The goal of adoption is to provide lifelong security to the child and the adoptive family.

Children who are orphaned are obvious candidates for adoption. In the United States, children can be adopted if the parents give up the child voluntarily or if the child is freed involuntarily through the court process known as termination of parental rights. International adoption (adoption of children from other countries, for example, from foreign orphanages) is also often possible.

Depending on the type, adoption can sometimes cost tens of thousands of dollars. Having experienced legal representation, often from a lawyer, helps the adoptive parents regardless of the type of adoption.

Sometimes, adoptive parents connect with birth parents. The parties may already be related in some way. For example, a stepparent can adopt a spouse's birth child or grandparents can adopt their grandchildren. In other cases, parents may connect through word of mouth or newspaper advertisements.

In some cases, birth parents may appreciate the chance to visit the child. A positive relationship with the birth parents may make adoptive parents less likely to worry that the birth parents will try to reclaim the child. Maintaining a relationship with the birth family usually benefits the child. All such issues are often best discussed with an expert (such as a mental health professional and a legal professional) before deciding whether or not to have an open adoption.

Did You Know...

Children should be told, ideally at or before age 7, that they were adopted.

Some states have a web site that enables birth parents and adopted children to connect with each other if both parties want to.

Most adopted children, including those previously in foster care or foreign orphanages, adjust well and develop few problems. However, as children age, they may develop feelings of rejection because they were given up by their birth family. During adolescence and young adulthood, in particular, adopted people may be very curious about their birth parents, even if they do not ask about them. Some adopted people seek information about, or seek out, their birth parents, and some birth parents seek out their birth children.

Not telling children they were adopted can hurt them later. Children adjust best if told at or before age 7. If asked, adoptive parents should tell the child about the birth parents in a comforting manner. For example, if the child was abused or neglected, parents can say the child was removed because the birth parent had problems or was ill and could not provide proper care. Alternatively, adoptive parents may say that the birth parent was not able to care for the child and gave the child to the adoptive parents so they could love and take care of him or her. Children need reassurance that they are loved and always will be loved. If children have contact with their birth families, it helps for parents to tell the children that two sets of parents love them.

If birth parents request anonymity, there is controversy about whether children should be able to find information about them. Some states provide a web site for birth parents and children to post their identity. If both do so, then they will be placed in touch with each other. Contact cannot be initiated unless both parties agree.

289 Child Neglect and Abuse

- Some factors that contribute to child neglect and abuse are poverty, drug and alcohol abuse, mental health disorders, and single parenthood.
- Children who are neglected or abused may appear tired or dirty or have physical injuries or emotional or mental health problems.
- Abuse is suspected when bruises suggest that the injury was not accidental, when injuries do not match the caregiver's explanation, or sometimes when both healed and new injuries are evident.
- Treatment of neglect and abuse includes protecting the child from further harm, counseling for parents and children, sometimes hospitalization, and often assisting the family in providing safe and appropriate care.

Children can be mistreated by having essential things withheld from them (neglect) or by having harmful things done to them (abuse). Neglect involves not meeting children's basic needs: physical, medical, educational, and emotional. Emotional neglect is a part of emotional abuse. Abuse can be physical, sexual, or emotional. The different forms of abuse sometimes occur together. Child neglect and abuse often occur together and with other forms of family violence, such as spousal abuse. In addition to immediate harm, neglect and abuse cause long-lasting problems, including mental health problems and substance abuse. Also, adults who were physically or sexually abused as children are more likely to abuse their own children.

In the United States, more than 896,000 children are neglected or abused every year, and about 1,400 of them die. Neglect is about 3 times more common than physical abuse.

Neglect and abuse result from a complex combination of individual, family, and social factors. Being a single parent, being poor, having problems with drug or alcohol abuse, or having a mental health problem (such as a personality disorder or low self-esteem) can make a parent more likely to neglect or abuse a child. Neglect is 12 times more common among children living in poverty.

Doctors and nurses are required by law to promptly report cases of suspected child neglect or abuse to a local Child Protective Services agency. Health professionals should, but are not required to, tell parents that a report is being made according to the law and that they will be contacted, interviewed, and possibly visited at their home. Depending on the circumstances, the local law enforcement agency may also be notified. Prompt reporting is also required from all people whose job places children younger than 18 in their care. Such people include teachers, child care workers, foster care providers, and police and legal services personnel. Anyone else who knows of or suspects neglect or abuse is encouraged to report it but is not required to do so.

All reported cases of child abuse are investigated by representatives of the local Child Protective Services agency, who determine the facts and make recommendations. Agency representatives may recommend social services (for the child and family members), temporary hospitalization, temporary foster care, or permanent termination of parental rights. Doctors and social workers help the representatives from the Child Protective Services agency decide what to do based on the immediate medical needs of the child, the seriousness of the harm, and the likelihood of further neglect or abuse.

Types

There are a number of different types of child neglect and abuse.

Physical Neglect: Not meeting a child's essential needs for food, clothing, and shelter is the most basic form of neglect. But there are many other forms. Parents may not obtain preventive dental or medical care for the child, such as vaccinations and routine physical examinations. Parents may delay obtaining medical care when the child is ill, putting the child at risk of more severe illness and even death. Parents may not make sure the child attends school or is privately schooled. Parents may leave a child in the care of a person who is known to be abusive, or they may leave a young child unattended.

Physical Abuse: Physically mistreating or harming a child, including inflicting excessive physical punishment, is physical abuse. Children of any age may be physically abused, but infants and toddlers are particularly vulnerable. Physical abuse is the most common cause of serious head injury in infants. In toddlers, physical abuse is more likely to result in abdominal injuries, which may be fatal. Physical abuse (including homicide) is among the 10 leading causes of death in children. Generally, a child's risk of physical abuse decreases during the early school years and increases during adolescence.

More than three fourths of perpetrators of abuse are the child's parents. Children who are born in poverty to a young, single parent are at highest risk. Family stress contributes to physical abuse. Stress may result from unemployment, frequent moves to another home, social isolation from friends or family members, or ongoing family violence. Children who are difficult (irritable, demanding, or hyperactive) or who have special needs (developmental or physical disabilities) may be more likely to be physically abused. Physical abuse is often triggered by a crisis in the midst of other stresses. A crisis may be a loss of a job, a death in the family, or a discipline problem.

Sexual Abuse: Any action with a child that is for the sexual gratification of an adult or a significantly older child is considered sexual abuse. It includes penetrating the child's vagina, anus, or mouth; touching the child with sexual intention but without penetration (molestation); exposing the genitals or showing pornography to a child; and using a child in the production of pornography. Sexual abuse does not include sexual play. In sexual play, children who are less than 4 years apart in age view or touch each other's genital area without force or coercion.

By the age of 18, about 12 to 25% of girls and 8 to 10% of boys have been sexually abused. Most perpetrators of sexual abuse are people known by the children, commonly a stepfather, an uncle, or the mother's boyfriend. Female perpetrators are less common.

Certain situations increase the risk of sexual abuse. For example, children who have several caregivers or a caregiver with several sex partners are at increased risk. Being socially isolated, having low self-esteem, having family members who are also sexually abused, or being associated with a gang also increases risk.

> **? Did You Know...**
> Neglect is 3 times more common than physical abuse.

Emotional Abuse: Using words or acts to psychologically mistreat a child is emotional abuse. Emotional abuse makes children feel that they are worthless, flawed, unloved, unwanted, in danger, or valuable only when they meet another person's needs.

Emotional abuse includes spurning, exploiting, terrorizing, isolating, and neglecting. Spurning means belittling the child's abilities and accomplishments. Exploiting means encouraging deviant or criminal behavior, such as committing crimes or abusing alcohol or drugs. Terrorizing means bullying, threatening, or frightening the child. Isolating means not allowing the child to interact with other adults or children. Emotionally neglecting a child means ignoring and not interacting with the child and not giving the child love and attention. Emotional abuse tends to occur over a long period of time.

Münchausen by Proxy: In this unusual type of child abuse, a caregiver, usually the mother, exaggerates, fakes, or causes an illness in the child (see box on page 850).

Symptoms

The symptoms of neglect and abuse vary depending partly on the nature and duration of the neglect or abuse, on the child, and on the particular circumstances. In addition to obvious physical injuries, symptoms include emotional and mental health problems. Such problems may develop immediately or later and may persist.

Physical Neglect: Physically neglected children may appear undernourished, tired, or dirty or may lack appropriate clothing. They may frequently be absent from school. In extreme cases, children may be found living alone or with siblings, without adult supervision. Physical and emotional development may be slow. Some neglected children die of starvation or exposure.

Physical Abuse: Bruises, burns, welts, or scrapes are common signs of physical abuse. These marks often have the shape of the object used to inflict them, such as a belt or lamp cord. Cigarette or scald burns may be visible on the arms or legs. Severe injuries to the mouth, eyes, brain, or other internal organs may be present but not visible. Children may have signs of old injuries, such as broken bones, which have healed. Sometimes injuries result in disfigurement.

Toddlers who have been intentionally dunked into a hot bathtub have scald burns. These burns may be located on the buttocks and may be shaped like a doughnut. The splash of hot water may cause small burns on other parts of the body.

Infants who are shaken may have shaken baby (shaken impact) syndrome. This syndrome is caused by violent shaking, often followed by throwing the infant. Infants who are shaken may have no visible signs of injury and may appear to be sleeping deeply. This sleepiness is due to brain damage and swelling, which may result from bleeding between the brain and skull (subdural hemorrhage). Infants may also have bleeding in the retina (retinal hemorrhage) at the back of the eye. Ribs and other bones may be broken.

Children who have been abused for a long time are often fearful and irritable. They often sleep poorly. They may be depressed and anxious. They are more likely to act in violent, criminal, or suicidal ways.

Sexual Abuse: Changes in behavior are common. Such changes may occur abruptly and may be extreme. Children may become aggressive or withdrawn or develop phobias or sleep disorders. Children who are sexually abused may behave in sexual ways inappropriate for their age. Children who are sexually abused by a parent or other family member may have conflicted feelings. They may feel emotionally close to the offender, yet betrayed.

Sexual abuse may also result in physical injuries. Children may have bruises, tears, or bleeding in areas around the genitals, rectum, or mouth. Injuries in the genital and rectal areas may make walking and sitting difficult. Girls may have a vaginal discharge. A sexually transmitted disease, such as gonorrhea, chlamydial infection, or sometimes human immunodeficiency virus (HIV) infection, may be present.

Emotional Abuse: In general, children who are emotionally abused tend to be insecure and anxious about their attachments to other people because they have not had their needs met consistently or predictably. Infants who are emotionally neglected may seem unemotional or uninterested in their surroundings. Their behavior may be mistaken for mental retardation/intellectual disability or a physical disorder. Children who are emotionally neglected may lack social skills or be slow to develop speech and language skills. Children who are spurned may have low self-esteem. Children who are exploited may commit crimes or abuse alcohol or drugs. Children who are terrorized may appear fearful and withdrawn. They may be distrustful, unassertive, and extremely anxious to please adults. They may inappropriately reach out to strangers. Children who are isolated may be awkward in social situations and have difficulty forming normal relationships. Older children may not attend school regularly or may not perform well when they do attend.

Diagnosis

Neglect and abuse are often difficult to recognize unless children appear severely undernourished or are obviously injured or unless neglect or abuse is witnessed by other people. Neglect and abuse may not be recognized for years. There are many reasons for this difficulty. Abused children may feel that abuse is a normal part of life and may not mention it. Physically and sexually abused children are often reluctant to volunteer information about their abuse because of shame, threats of retaliation, or even a feeling that they deserve the abuse. Physically abused children often describe what happened to them if asked directly, but sexually abused children may be sworn to secrecy or so traumatized that they are not able to talk about the abuse.

When doctors suspect neglect or any type of abuse, they look for signs of other types of abuse. They also fully evaluate the physical, environmental, emotional, and social needs of the child.

Physical Neglect: A neglected child is usually identified by health care practitioners or social workers during evaluation of an unrelated issue, such as an injury, an illness, or a behavioral problem. Doctors may notice that a child is not developing physically or emotionally at a normal rate or has missed many vaccinations or appointments. Teachers may identify a neglected child because of frequent unexplained absences from school. If neglect is suspected, doctors often check for anemia, infections, and lead poisoning, which are common among neglected children.

> **? Did You Know...**
> Most victims of sexual abuse know the perpetrator.

Physical Abuse: Physical abuse may be suspected when an infant who is not yet walking has bruises or serious injuries. Abuse may be suspected when a toddler or older child has certain types of bruises, such as bruises on the back of the legs, buttocks, and torso. When children are learning to walk, bruises often result, but such bruises typically occur on prominent bony areas on the front of the body, such as the knees, shins, forehead, chin, and elbows.

Abuse may also be suspected when parents seem to know little about their child's health or seem unconcerned about an obvious injury. Parents who abuse their child may be reluctant to describe to the doctor or friends how an injury occurred. The description may not fit the age and nature of the injury or may change each time the story is told.

If doctors suspect physical abuse, they obtain accurate drawings and photographs of the injuries. Sometimes x-rays are taken to look for signs of previous injuries. Often, if a child is younger than 2 years, x-rays of all bones are taken to check for fractures.

Sexual Abuse: Often, sexual abuse is diagnosed on the basis of the child's or a witness's account of the incident. However, because many children are reluctant to talk about sexual abuse, it may be suspected only because the child's behavior becomes abnormal. If a child has been sexually abused within 72 hours, doctors examine the child to collect legal evidence of sexual contact, such as swabs of body fluids and hair samples from the genital area. Photographs of any visible injuries are taken. In some communities, health care practitioners who are specially trained to evaluate sexual abuse of children perform this examination.

Emotional Abuse: Emotional abuse is usually identified during evaluation of another problem, such as poor performance in school or a behavioral problem. Children who are emotionally abused are checked for signs of physical and sexual abuse.

Treatment

A team of doctors, other health care practitioners, and social workers tries to deal with the causes and effects of neglect and abuse. The team helps family members understand the child's needs and helps them access local resources. For example, a child whose parents cannot afford health care may qualify for medical assistance from the state. Other community and government programs can provide assistance with food and shelter. Parents with substance abuse problems or mental health problems may be directed to appropriate treatment programs. Parenting programs are available in some areas.

All physical injuries and disorders are treated. Some children are hospitalized for treatment of injuries, severe undernutrition, or other disorders. Some severe injuries require surgery. Infants with shaken baby syndrome usually need to be admitted to a pediatric intensive care unit. Sometimes healthy children are hospitalized to protect them from further abuse until appropriate home care can be ensured.

Some children who have been sexually abused are given drugs to prevent sexually transmitted diseases, sometimes including HIV infection. Children who appear to be very upset need immediate counseling and support. Sexually abused children, even those who appear unaffected initially, are referred to a mental health care practitioner because long-lasting problems are common. Long-term psychologic counseling is

often needed. Doctors refer children with other types of abuse for counseling if behavioral or emotional problems develop.

The goal of treatment is to return children to a safe, healthy family environment. Depending on the nature of the abuse and the abuser, children may go home with their family members or may be removed from their home and placed with relatives or in foster care. This placement is often temporary, for example, until the parents obtain housing or employment or until regular home visits by a social worker are established. In severe cases of neglect or abuse, the parents' rights may be permanently terminated. In such cases, the child remains in foster care (see page 1877) until the child is adopted or becomes an adult.

Female Genital Mutilation

Female genital mutilation is ritual removal of part or all of the clitoris and labia.

Female genital mutilation is practiced routinely in parts of Africa (usually northern or central Africa), where it is deeply ingrained as part of some cultures. Women who experience sexual pleasure are considered impossible to control, are shunned, and cannot be married.

The average age of girls who undergo mutilation is 7 years, and mutilation is done without anesthesia. Mutilation may be limited to cutting out part of the clitoris, but in the most extreme form involves removal of the clitoris and labia (termed infibulation), usually followed by sewing the remaining tissue closed except for a small opening for menses and urine. The legs are often bound together for weeks afterward. Traditionally, infibulated females are cut open on their wedding night.

Consequences of genital mutilation include bleeding, infection (including tetanus), scarring, and psychologic problems. Infibulated women have increased susceptibility to AIDS, and childbirth may result in fatal hemorrhage.

Female genital mutilation may be decreasing due to the influence of religious leaders who have spoken out against the practice and growing opposition in some communities.

Older People's Health Issues

290   The Aging Body

Aging is a gradual, continuous process of spontaneous change that begins at birth and continues throughout all stages of life. It involves maturation and development for children, adolescents, and young adults. Then, during middle and late age, many bodily functions decline. Thus, aging has positive and negative aspects.

People do not become old or elderly at any specific age. Traditionally, age 65 has been designated as the beginning of old age. But the reason was based in history, not biology. Age 65 was chosen as the age for retirement in Germany, the first nation to establish a retirement program, and it continues to be the retirement age for most people in developed societies, although this tradition is changing.

When a person becomes old can be answered in different ways:

- **Chronologic age:** Chronologic age is based solely on the passage of time. It is a person's age in years. Chronologic age has limited significance in terms of health. Nonetheless, the likelihood of developing a health problem increases as people age. Because chronologic age helps predict many health problems, it has some legal and financial uses.
- **Biological age:** Biological age refers to changes in the body that commonly occur as people age. Because these changes affect some people sooner than others, some people are biologically old at 40, and others are biologically young at 60 and even older.
- **Psychologic age:** Psychologic age is based on how people act and feel. For example, an 80-year-old who works, plans, looks forward to future events, and participates in many activities is considered psychologically young.

Normal Aging: People often wonder whether what they are experiencing as they age is normal or abnormal. Although people age somewhat differently, many changes occur in almost everyone. Some of these changes seem to result from internal processes, that is, from aging itself. Thus, such changes, although undesired, are considered normal. They are to be expected and are generally unavoidable. For example, as people age, the lens of the eye thickens, stiffens, and becomes less able to focus on close objects, such as reading materials (a disorder called presbyopia). This change occurs in virtually all older people, and no cause or explanation has been identified other than aging itself. Thus, presbyopia is considered normal aging. Other terms used to describe these changes are usual aging and senescence.

Exactly what constitutes normal aging is not always clear. Changes that occur with normal aging make people more likely to develop certain disorders. However, people can sometimes take actions to compensate for these changes. For example, older people are more likely to lose teeth. But seeing a dentist regularly, eating fewer sweets, and brushing and flossing regularly may reduce the chances of tooth loss. Thus, tooth loss, although common with aging, may be an avoidable part of aging.

Also, functional decline that is part of aging sometimes seems similar to functional decline that is part of a disorder. For example, with advanced age, a decline in mental function is nearly universal and is considered normal aging. This decline includes increased difficulty learning new languages and increased forgetfulness. In contrast, the decline that occurs in dementia is much more severe. For example, people who are aging normally may misplace things or forget details, but people who have dementia may forget entire events. People with dementia also have difficulty doing normal daily tasks (such as driving, cooking, and handling finances) and understanding the environment, including knowing what year it is and where they are. Thus, dementia is considered a disorder, even though it is common in late life (see page 688). Certain kinds of dementia, such as Alzheimer's disease, differ from normal aging in other ways as well. For example, brain tissue (obtained during autopsy) in people with Alzheimer's disease looks different from that in older people without the disease. So the distinction between normal aging and dementia is clear.

> **? Did You Know...**
> Average life expectancy has increased a lot, but maximum life span has increased little if at all.

Sometimes the distinction between functional decline that is part of aging and functional decline that is part of a disorder seems arbitrary. For example, as people age, blood sugar levels increase more after eating carbohydrates than they do in younger people. This increase is considered normal aging. However, if the increase exceeds a certain level, diabetes, a disorder, is diagnosed (see page 1005). In this case, the difference is one of degree only.

Healthy (Successful) Aging: Healthy aging refers to postponement of or reduction in the undesired

Studying Aging

Gerontology is the study of the aging process including physical, mental, and social changes. The information is used to develop strategies and programs for improving the lives of older people. Some gerontologists have a medical degree and are also geriatricians.

Geriatrics is the branch of medicine that specializes in the care of older people, which often involves managing many disorders and problems at the same time. Geriatricians have studied the aging process so that they can better distinguish which changes result from aging itself and which indicate a disorder.

effects of aging. The goals of healthy aging are maintaining physical and mental health, avoiding disorders, and remaining active and independent. For most people, maintaining general good health requires more effort as they age. Developing certain healthy habits—following a nutritious diet, exercising regularly, and staying mentally active—can help. The sooner a person develops them, the better. However, it is never too late to begin. In this way, people can have some control over what happens to them as they age.

Some evidence suggests that in the United States, healthy aging is on the rise:

- A decrease in the percentage of older people residing in nursing homes (even though the percentage of people over age 65 and of those over age 85 has increased in the general population)
- A decrease in the percentage of people aged 75 to 84 who report impairments
- A decrease in the percentage of people over age 65 with debilitating disorders

Life Expectancy

The average life expectancy of Americans has been increasing dramatically over the past century. A male child born in 1900 could expect to live only 46 years, and a female child, 48 years. Today, however, a male child can expect to live more than 73 years, and a female child, nearly 80 years. Although much of this gain can be attributed to the significant decrease in childhood mortality, life expectancy at every age beyond 40 has also increased dramatically. For example, a 70-year-old man can now expect to live beyond age 83, and a 70-year-old woman, beyond age 85.

Despite the increase in average life expectancy, the maximum life span—the oldest age to which people can live—has changed little since records have been kept. Despite the best genetic makeup and health care, no one seems to live much beyond 125 years, although some experts suggest that this number may be slowly

increasing. Currently, a person has a 1 in 2 billion chance of living to the age of 120.

Several factors influence life expectancy:

- **Heredity:** Heredity influences whether a person will develop a disorder. For example, a person who inherits genes that increase the risk of developing high cholesterol levels is likely to have a shorter life. A person who inherits genes that protect against coronary artery disease and cancer is likely to have a longer life.

- **Lifestyle:** Avoiding smoking, not abusing drugs and alcohol, maintaining a healthy weight and diet, and exercising help people function well and avoid disorders.

- **Exposure to toxins in the environment:** Such exposure can shorten life expectancy even among people with the best genetic makeup.

- **Health care:** Preventing disorders or treating disorders after they are contracted, especially when the disorder can be cured (as with infections and sometimes cancer), helps increase life expectancy.

Changes in the Body

The body changes with aging because changes occur in individual cells and in whole organs. These changes result in changes in function and in appearance.

Aging Cells: As cells age, they function less well. Eventually, old cells must die, as a normal part of the body's functioning.

Old cells sometimes die because they are programmed to do so. The genes of cells program a process that, when triggered, results in death of the cell. This programmed death, called apoptosis, is a kind of cell suicide. The aging of a cell is one trigger. Old cells must die to make room for new cells. Other triggers include an excess number of cells and possibly damage to a cell.

Old cells also die because they can divide only a limited number of times. This limit is programmed by genes. When a cell can no longer divide, it grows larger, exists for a while, then dies. The mechanism that limits cell division involves a structure called a telomere. Telomeres are used to move the cell's genetic material in preparation for cell division. Every time a cell divides, the telomeres shorten a bit. Eventually, the telomeres become so short that the cell can no longer divide.

Sometimes damage to a cell directly causes its death. Cells may be damaged by harmful substances, such as radiation, sunlight, and chemotherapy drugs. Cells may also be damaged by certain by-products of their own normal activities. These by-products, called free radicals, are given off when cells produce energy.

Aging Organs: How well organs function depends on how well the cells within them function. Older cells function less well. Also, in some organs, cells die and are not replaced, so the number of cells decreases. The number of cells in the testes, ovaries, liver, and kidneys decreases markedly as the body ages. When the number of cells becomes too low, an organ cannot function normally. Thus, most organs function less well as people age. However, not all organs lose a large number of cells. The brain is one example. Healthy older people do not lose many brain cells. Substantial losses occur mainly in people who have had strokes or who have Alzheimer's disease or Parkinson's disease.

A decline in one organ's function, whether due to a disorder or to aging itself, can affect the function of another. For example, if atherosclerosis narrows blood vessels to the kidneys, the kidneys function less well because blood flow to them is decreased.

Often, the first signs of aging involve the musculoskeletal system. The eyes, followed by the ears, begin to change early in mid-life. Most internal functions also decline with aging. Most bodily functions peak shortly before age 30 and then begin a gradual but continuous decline. However, even with this decline, most functions remain adequate because most organs start with considerably more functional capacity than the body needs (functional reserve). For example, if half the liver is destroyed, the remaining tissue is more than enough to maintain normal function. Thus, disorders, rather than normal aging, usually account for most of the loss of function in old age.

Even though most functions remain adequate, the decline in function means that older people are less able to handle various stresses, including strenuous physical activity, extreme temperature changes in the environment, and disorders. This decline also means that older people are more likely to experience side effects from drugs.

Did You Know...
Disorders, not aging, usually account for most loss of function.

BONES AND JOINTS
Bones tend to become less dense. Thus, bones become weaker and more likely to break. In women, loss of bone density speeds up after menopause because less estrogen is produced. Estrogen helps prevent too much bone from being broken down during the body's normal process of forming, breaking down, and re-forming bone.

Bones become less dense partly because they contain less calcium (which gives bones strength). The amount of calcium decreases because the body absorbs less calcium from foods. Also, levels of vitamin D, which helps the body use calcium, decrease slightly. Certain bones are weakened more than others. Those most affected include the end of the thighbone (femur) at the hip, the ends of the arm bones (radius and ulna) at the wrist, and the bones of the spine (vertebrae).

Changes in vertebrae at the top of the spine cause the head to tip forward, compressing the throat. As a result, swallowing is more difficult, and choking is more likely. The vertebrae become less dense and the cushions of tissue (disks) between them lose fluid and become thinner, making the spine shorter. Thus, many older people become shorter.

The cartilage that lines the joints tends to thin, partly because of the wear and tear of years of movement. The surfaces of a joint may not slide over each other as well as they used to, and the joint may be slightly more susceptible to injury. Damage to the cartilage due to lifelong use of joints or repeated injury often leads to osteoarthritis, which is one of the most common disorders of later life.

Ligaments, which bind joints together, and tendons, which bind muscle to bone, tend to become less elastic, making joints feel tight or stiff. These tissues also weaken. Thus, most people become less flexible. Ligaments tend to tear more easily, and when they tear, they heal more slowly. These changes occur because the cells that maintain ligaments and tendons become less active.

MUSCLES AND BODY FAT
The amount of muscle tissue (muscle mass) and muscle strength tend to decrease. This process is called sarcopenia, which literally means loss of flesh. Loss of muscle mass begins around age 30 and continues throughout life. By age 75, the percentage of muscle mass is typically half of what it was during young adulthood. Muscle mass decreases possibly because the muscles are used less and begin to shrink. Also, the levels of growth hormone and testosterone, which stimulate muscle development, decrease. Muscles cannot contract as quickly because more fast-contracting (fast-twitch) muscle fibers are lost than slow-contracting (slow-twitch) muscle fibers.

Most older people retain enough muscle mass and strength for all necessary tasks. Many older people remain strong athletes. They compete in sports and enjoy vigorous physical activity. However, even the fittest notice some decline as they age.

? Did You Know...
To make up for the muscle mass lost during each day of strict bed rest, older people may need to exercise for up to 2 weeks.

Regular exercise to strengthen muscles can partially overcome or significantly delay loss of muscle mass and strength. In muscle-strengthening exercise, muscles contract against resistance provided by gravity (as in sit-ups or push-ups), weights, or rubber bands. If this type of exercise is done regularly, even people who have never exercised can increase muscle mass and strength. Conversely, physical inactivity, especially bed rest during an illness, can greatly accelerate the loss. During periods of inactivity, older people lose muscle mass and strength much more quickly than younger people do. For example, to make up for the muscle mass lost during each day of strict bed rest, people may need to exercise for up to 2 weeks.

By age 75, the percentage of body fat typically doubles compared with what it was during young adulthood. Too much body fat can increase the risk of health problems, such as diabetes. The distribution of fat also changes, changing the shape of the torso. A healthy diet and regular exercise can help older people keep body fat from increasing too much.

EYES

As people age, the following occurs:

- The lens stiffens, making focusing on close objects harder.
- The lens becomes denser, making seeing in dim light harder.
- The pupil reacts more slowly to changes in light.
- The lens yellows, changing the way colors are perceived.
- The number of nerve cells decrease, impairing depth perception.
- The eyes produce less fluid, making them feel dry.

A change in vision is often the first undeniable sign of aging.

Changes in the lens of the eyes can cause or contribute to the following:

- **Loss of near vision:** During their 40s, most people notice that seeing objects closer than 2 feet becomes difficult. This change in vision, called presbyopia, occurs because the lens in the eye stiffens. Normally, the lens changes its shape to help the eye focus. A stiffer lens makes focusing on close objects harder. Ultimately, almost everyone with presbyopia needs reading glasses. People who need glasses to

see distant objects may need to wear bifocals or glasses with variable-focus lenses.

- **Need for brighter light:** As people continue to age, seeing in dim light becomes more difficult because the lens tends to become less transparent. A denser lens means that less light passes through to the retina at the back of the eye. Also, the retina, which contains the cells that sense light, becomes less sensitive. So for reading, brighter light is needed. On average, 60-year-olds need 3 times more light to read than 20-year-olds.

- **Changes in color perception:** Colors are perceived differently, partly because the lens tends to yellow slightly with aging. Colors may look less bright and contrasts between different colors may be more difficult to see. Blues may look more gray, and blue print or background may look washed out. These changes are insignificant for most people. However, older people may have trouble reading black letters printed on a blue background or reading blue letters.

The pupil of the eye reacts more slowly to changes in light. The pupil widens and narrows to let more or less light in depending on the brightness of the surroundings. A slow-reacting pupil means that older people may be unable to see when they first enter a dark room. Or they may be temporarily blinded when they enter a brightly lit area. Older people may also become more sensitive to glare. However, increased sensitivity to glare is often due to darkened areas in the lens or to cataracts.

? Did You Know...
Most 60-year-olds need 3 times more light to read than 20-year-olds.

Fine details, including differences in shades and tones, become more difficult to discern. The reason is probably a decrease in the number of nerve cells that transmit visual signals from the eyes to the brain. This change affects the way depth is perceived, and judging distances becomes more difficult.

Older people may see more tiny black specks moving across their field of vision. These specks, called floaters, are bits of normal fluid in the eye that have solidified. Floaters do not significantly interfere with vision. Unless they suddenly increase in number, they are not a cause for concern.

The eyes tend to become dry. This change occurs because the number of cells that produce fluids to lubricate the eyes decreases. Tear production may decrease.

The appearance of the eyes changes in several ways:

- The whites (sclera) of the eyes may turn slightly yellow or brown. This change results from many years of exposure to ultraviolet light, wind, and dust.
- Random splotches of color may appear in the whites of the eyes, particularly in people with a dark complexion.
- A gray-white ring (arcus senilis) may appear on the surface of the eye. The ring is made of calcium and cholesterol salts. It does not affect vision.
- The lower eyelid may hang away from the eyeball because the muscles around the eye weaken and the tendons stretch. This condition (called ectropion) may interfere with lubricating the eyeball and contribute to dry eyes.
- The eye may appear to sink into the head because the amount of fat around the eye decreases.

EARS

Most changes in hearing are probably due as much to noise exposure as to aging. Exposure to loud noise over time damages the ear's ability to hear. Nonetheless, some changes in hearing occur as people age, regardless of their exposure to loud noise.

As people age, hearing high-pitched sounds becomes more difficult. This change is considered age-associated hearing loss (presbycusis). For example, violin music may sound less bright.

> ### ❓ Did You Know...
>
> Articulating consonants clearly may be more helpful than speaking more loudly to older people who have trouble understanding speech.
>
> High-pitched sounds are particularly hard for older people to hear.

The most frustrating consequence of presbycusis is that words become harder to understand. As a result, older people may think that other people are mumbling. Even when other people speak more loudly, older people still have difficulty understanding the words. The reason is that most consonants (such as k, t, s, p, and ch) are high-pitched, and consonants are the sounds that help people identify words. Because vowels are lower-pitched sounds, they are easier to hear. So older people may hear "Ell me exaly wha you wan oo ee," rather than "Tell me exactly what you want to keep." To help, other people need to articulate consonants more clearly, rather than simply speak louder. Understanding what women and children say may be more difficult than understanding

what men say because most women and children have higher-pitched voices. Gradually, hearing lower pitches also becomes more difficult.

Many older people have more trouble hearing in loud places or in groups because of the background noise. Also, earwax, which interferes with hearing, tends to accumulate more.

MOUTH AND NOSE

Generally, when people are in their 50s, the ability to taste and smell starts to gradually diminish. Both senses are needed to enjoy the full range of flavors in food. The tongue can identify only five basic tastes: sweet, sour, bitter, salt, and a relatively newly identified taste called umami (commonly described as meaty or savory). The sense of smell is needed to distinguish more subtle and complex flavors (such as raspberry).

As people age, taste buds on the tongue decrease in number and sensitivity. This change affects tasting sweet and salt more than bitter and sour. The ability to smell diminishes because the lining of the nose becomes thinner and drier and the nerve endings in the nose deteriorate. However, the change is slight, usually affecting only subtle smells. Because of these changes, many foods tend to taste bitter, and foods with subtle smells may taste bland.

The mouth tends to feel dry more often, partly because less saliva is produced. Dry mouth further reduces the ability to taste food.

As people age, the gums recede slightly. Consequently, the lower parts of the teeth are exposed to food particles and bacteria. Also, tooth enamel tends to wear away. These changes, as well as a dry mouth, make the teeth more susceptible to decay and cavities (caries) and thus make tooth loss more likely.

With aging, the nose tends to lengthen and thin, and the tip tends to droop.

SKIN

The skin tends to become thinner, less elastic, drier, and finely wrinkled. However, exposure to sunlight over the years greatly contributes to wrinkling and to making the skin rough and blotchy. People who have avoided exposure to sunlight often look much younger than their age.

The skin changes partly because the aging body produces less collagen (a tough, fibrous tissue that makes skin strong) and elastin (which makes skin flexible). As a result, the skin tears more easily.

The fat layer under the skin thins. This layer acts as a cushion for the skin, helping protect and support it. The fat layer also helps conserve body heat. When the layer thins, wrinkles are more likely to develop, and tolerance for cold decreases.

The number of nerve endings in the skin decreases. As a result, people become less sensitive to pain, temperature, and pressure, and injuries may be more likely.

The number of sweat glands and blood vessels decreases, and blood flow in the deep layers of the skin decreases. As a result, the body is less able to move heat from inside the body through blood vessels to the surface of the body. Less heat leaves the body, and the body cannot cool itself as well. Thus, the risk of heat-related disorders, such as heatstroke, is increased. Also, when blood flow is decreased, the skin tends to heal more slowly.

The number of pigment-producing cells (melanocytes) decreases. As a result, the skin has less protection against ultraviolet (UV) radiation, such as that from sunlight. Large, brown spots (age spots) develop on skin that has been exposed to sunlight, perhaps because the skin is less able to remove waste products.

The skin is less able to form vitamin D when it is exposed to sunlight. Thus, the risk of vitamin D deficiency increases.

BRAIN AND NERVOUS SYSTEM

The number of nerve cells in the brain typically decreases. However, the brain can partly compensate for this loss in several ways:

- As cells are lost, new connections are made between the remaining nerve cells.
- New nerve cells may form in some areas of the brain, even during old age.
- The brain has more cells than it needs to do most activities—a characteristic called redundancy.

Levels of the chemical substances involved in sending messages in the brain change. Most decrease, but some increase. Nerve cells may lose some of their receptors for messages. Blood flow to the brain decreases. Because of these age-related changes, the brain may function slightly less well. Older people may react and do tasks somewhat more slowly, but given time, they do these things accurately. Some mental functions—such as vocabulary, short-term memory, the ability to learn new material, and the ability to recall words—may be subtly reduced after age 70.

After about age 60, the number of cells in the spinal cord begins to decrease. Usually, this change does not affect strength or sensation.

> **? Did You Know...**
> The brain has ways to compensate for the loss of nerve cells that occurs with aging.

As people age, nerves may conduct signals more slowly. Usually, this change is so minimal that people do not notice it. Also, nerves may repair themselves more slowly and incompletely. Therefore, in older people with damaged nerves, sensation and strength may be decreased.

HEART AND BLOOD VESSELS

The heart and blood vessels become stiffer. The heart fills with blood more slowly. The stiffer arteries are less able to expand when more blood is pumped through them. Thus, blood pressure tends to increase.

Despite these changes, a normal older heart functions well. Differences between young and old hearts become apparent only when the heart has to work hard and pump more blood—for example, during exercise or an illness. An older heart cannot speed up as quickly or pump as fast or as much blood as a younger heart. Thus, older athletes are not able to perform as well as younger athletes. However, regular aerobic exercise can improve athletic performance in older people.

MUSCLES OF BREATHING AND THE LUNGS

The muscles used in breathing, such as the diaphragm, tend to weaken. The number of air sacs (alveoli) and capillaries in the lungs decreases. Thus, slightly less oxygen is absorbed from air that is breathed in. The lungs become less elastic. In people who do not smoke or have a lung disorder, these changes do not affect ordinary daily activities, but these changes may make exercising more difficult. Breathing at high altitudes (where there is less oxygen) may also be harder.

The lungs become less able to fight infection, partly because the cells that sweep debris containing microorganisms out of the airways are less able to do so. Cough, which also helps clear the lungs, tends to be weaker.

DIGESTIVE SYSTEM

Overall, the digestive system is less affected by aging than most parts of the body. The muscles of the esophagus contract less forcefully, but movement of food through the esophagus is not affected. Food is emptied from the stomach slightly more slowly, and the stomach cannot hold as much food because it is less elastic. But in most people, these changes are too slight to be noticed.

Certain changes cause problems in some people. The digestive tract may produce less lactase, an enzyme the body needs to digest milk. As a result, older people are more likely to develop intolerance of dairy products (lactose intolerance). People with

HOW THE BODY AGES: SOME NORMAL CHANGES

WHAT HAPPENS?	WHY?
Mental function	
Difficulty remembering or coming up with the right word Difficulty concentrating Difficulty learning new material	The nerve cells in the brain release different amounts of some chemical messengers (which send impulses from cell to cell), and the number of receptors on nerve cells may decrease. Thus, the brain does not send or process impulse as well or as quickly.
Physical activity	
Unsteadiness or loss of balance	Structures in the inner ear that help with balance stiffen and deteriorate slightly. The part of the brain that controls balance (cerebellum) may degenerate.
Dizziness or light-headedness when standing	The heart does not pump enough blood to the head because the heart is less able to respond to changes in position. The nervous system signals the heart to increase blood flow less effectively. The blood vessels do not constrict enough to maintain normal blood pressure when a person stands.
Loss of muscle strength	The number and size of muscle fibers decrease. The body produces less growth hormone and (in men) less testosterone, which help maintain muscles.
Difficulty moving Less flexibility	Less joint fluid is produced. The cartilage between bones in joints becomes stiffer and may erode. Tendons and ligaments become stiffer and weaker. Muscle tissue is lost, replaced by fatty or fibrous tissue, decreasing strength and making muscles stiffer.
Difficulty exercising strenuously	The heart cannot keep up with the demand for more blood during exercise. It cannot speed up as quickly or pump as fast as it used to, partly because the heart and blood vessels become stiffer and less elastic. Also, the heart does not respond as quickly or as well to chemical messengers that normally stimulate it to speed up. The lungs cannot keep up with the demand for oxygen during exercise. Less air is taken in with each breath, and the lungs do not absorb as much oxygen.
Eating problems	
Difficulty swallowing	The mouth is dry. The muscles involved in swallowing weaken, and coordination is impaired. People may not chew food enough because teeth are missing or dentures do not fit well. Then, chunks of food are too large to swallow. The bones at the top of the spine change, tipping the head forward and thus compressing the throat.
Disinterest in eating	Taste decreases, making food less appetizing. Smell decreases, making food less appetizing. The mouth is dry, leading to loss of taste. Chewing may be difficult because teeth are missing, jaw muscles are weak, or dentures do not fit well. Swallowing is difficult.
Sexual function	
Dryness of the vagina	Less estrogen is produced.
Erections do not last as long, are less rigid, or take more time	Less testosterone is produced. Blood flow to the penis decreases.

(continued on the following page)

HOW THE BODY AGES: SOME NORMAL CHANGES (*Continued*)

WHAT HAPPENS?	WHY?
The senses	
Need for reading glasses	The lens of the eye stiffens, making focusing on close objects more difficult.
Difficulty seeing in dim light	The retina of the eye becomes less sensitive to light. The lens of the eye becomes less transparent.
Difficulty adjusting to changes in light levels	The pupils react more slowly to changes in light. Darkened areas in the lens of the eye increase glare.
Dry eyes	The number of cells that produce fluids to lubricate the eyes decreases. The tear glands produce fewer tears.
Difficulty understanding words	Age-related hearing loss (presbycusis) develops, which often affects mainly high frequencies (which include consonants—the sounds that help people identify words).
Loss of hearing	Age-related hearing loss (presbycusis) develops. Earwax accumulates.
Loss of taste	Taste buds decrease in number and become less sensitive. People detect odors less well because the lining of the nose becomes thinner and drier and the nerve endings in the nose deteriorate.
Dry mouth	Less saliva is produced.
Skin and hair	
Wrinkles	The fat layer under the skin, which acts as a cushion, thins.
More tears in the skin	The body produces less collagen and elastin, which make the skin tough and elastic.
Dry skin	Glands in the skin produce less oil.
Bruises and broken blood vessels	Blood vessels in the skin become more fragile.
Slow healing of wounds	The number of blood vessels in the skin decreases. Cells responsible for healing wounds act more slowly and decrease in number.
Difficulty adjusting to changes in temperature	The fat layer under the skin, which helps conserve body heat, thins. The number of sweat glands decrease, and the sweat glands produce less sweat. Sweat helps cool the body. The number of blood vessels decreases, and blood flow in the deep layers of the skin decreases. As a result, the body cannot remove heat from body as well.
Decreased sensation and sensitivity to pain	The number of nerve endings in the skin decreases.
Gray or white hair	The hair follicles produce less pigment (melanin).
Thinning or loss of hair	Hairs, which must be replaced periodically, grow more slowly, and some hair follicles stop producing new hair.

lactose intolerance may feel bloated or have gas or diarrhea after they consume milk products.

In the large intestine, materials move through a little more slowly. In some people, this slowing contributes to constipation.

The liver tends to become smaller because the number of cells decreases. Less blood flows through it, and liver enzymes that help the body process drugs and other substances work less efficiently. As a result, the liver may be slightly less able to help remove drugs and other substances from the body. And the effects of drugs—intended and unintended—last longer.

KIDNEYS AND URINARY TRACT

The kidneys tend to become smaller because the number of cells decreases. Less blood flows through the kidneys and at about age 30, they begin to filter blood less well. As years pass, they may remove waste products from the blood less well. They may excrete too much water and too little salt, making dehydration more likely. Nonetheless, they almost always function well enough to meet the body's needs.

Certain changes in the urinary tract may make controlling urination more difficult:

- The maximum volume of urine that the bladder can hold decreases. Thus, older people may need to urinate more often.
- The bladder muscles may contract unpredictably (become overactive), regardless of whether people need to urinate.
- The bladder muscles weaken. As a result, they cannot empty the bladder as well, and more urine is left in the bladder after urination.
- The muscle that controls the passage of urine out of the body (urinary sphincter) is less able to close tightly and prevent leakage. Thus, older people have more difficulty postponing urination.

These changes are one reason that urinary incontinence (uncontrollable loss of urine) becomes more common as people age.

In women, the urethra (the tube through which urine leaves the body) shortens, and its lining becomes thinner. The decrease in the estrogen level that occurs with menopause may contribute to this and other changes in the urinary tract.

In men, the prostate gland tends to enlarge. In many men, it enlarges enough to interfere with the passage of urine and to prevent the bladder from emptying completely. As a result, older men tend to urinate with less force, to take longer to start the stream of urine, to dribble urine at the end of the stream, and to urinate more often. Older men are also more likely to be unable to urinate despite having a full bladder (called urinary retention).

REPRODUCTIVE ORGANS

Women: The effects of aging on sex hormone levels are more obvious in women than in men. In women, most of these effects are related to menopause, when the levels of female hormones (particularly estrogen) decrease, menstrual periods end permanently, and pregnancy is no longer possible. The decrease in female hormone levels causes the ovaries and uterus to shrink. The tissues of the vagina become thinner,

drier, and less elastic (a condition called atrophic vaginitis).

The breasts become less firm and more fibrous, and they tend to sag. This change makes finding lumps in the breasts more difficult.

> **Did You Know...**
> Because the breasts change with aging, finding lumps that could be cancer may be harder.

Some of the changes that begin at menopause (such as lower hormone levels and vaginal dryness) may interfere with sexual activity. However, for most women, aging does not greatly detract from enjoyment of sexual activity.

Men: In men, changes in sex hormone levels are less sudden. Levels of the male hormone testosterone decrease, resulting in fewer sperm and a decreased sex drive (libido), but the decrease is gradual. Although blood flow to the penis tends to decrease, many men can have erections and orgasms throughout life. However, erections may not last as long, may be slightly less rigid, or may require more stimulation to maintain. A second erection may require more time. Erectile dysfunction (impotence) becomes more common as men age.

ENDOCRINE SYSTEM

The levels and activity of some hormones, produced by endocrine glands, decrease.

- Growth hormone levels decrease, leading to decreased muscle mass.
- Aldosterone levels decrease, making dehydration more likely. This hormone signals the body to retain salt and therefore water.
- Insulin, which helps control the sugar level in blood, is less effective, and less insulin may be produced. Insulin enables sugar to move from the blood into cells, where it can be converted to energy. The changes in insulin mean that the sugar level increases more after a large meal and takes longer to return to normal.

For most people, the changes in the endocrine system have no noticeable effect on overall health. But in some, the changes may increase the risk of health problems. For example, the changes in insulin increase the risk of type 2 diabetes.

BLOOD PRODUCTION

The amount of active bone marrow, where blood cells are produced, decreases. Therefore, fewer blood cells are produced. Nonetheless, the bone marrow can usually produce enough blood cells throughout life. Problems may occur when the need for blood cells is greatly increased—for example, when anemia or an infection develops or bleeding occurs. In such cases, bone marrow is less able to increase its production of blood cells in response to the body's needs.

IMMUNE SYSTEM

The cells of the immune system act more slowly. These cells identify and destroy foreign substances such as bacteria, other infecting microbes, and probably cancer cells. This immune slowdown may partly explain several findings associated with aging:

- Cancer is more common among older people.
- Vaccines tend to be less protective in older people.
- Some infections, such as pneumonia and influenza, are more common among older people and result in death more often.
- Allergy symptoms may become less severe.

Despite the immune system slowdown, autoimmune disorders become more common. With aging, the immune system may become less able to distinguish the body's own cells from foreign substances that invade the body. Consequently, the immune system may be more likely to attack its own cells—an autoimmune reaction.

Disorders in Older People

Some disorders occur almost exclusively in older people. They are sometimes called geriatric syndromes (geriatric refers to the medical care of older people).

Other disorders affect people of all ages but may cause different symptoms or complications in older people. The following are some examples:

- **Underactive thyroid gland (hypothyroidism):** Usually, younger people gain weight and feel sluggish. In older people, the first or main symptom may be confusion.
- **Overactive thyroid gland (hyperthyroidism):** Usually, younger people become agitated and lose weight. In contrast, older people may become sleepy, withdrawn, depressed, and confused.
- **Depression:** Usually, younger people become tearful, withdrawn, and noticeably unhappy. Sometimes older people do not seem unhappy. Instead, they become confused, forgetful, and listless, lose interest in their usual activities, or seem lonely.
- **Heart attack:** Usually, younger people have chest pain. Older people may not have chest pain but may have difficulty breathing or abdominal pain.

They may sweat profusely, suddenly feel tired, pass out, or become confused.

- **Abdominal perforation:** An organ in the digestive tract, such as the stomach or intestine, occasionally tears (perforates), causing widespread serious infection in the abdominal cavity. Usually, younger people have severe abdominal pain and fever, and the abdomen feels tight. In contrast, older people may have none of these symptoms. Instead, they may become confused or feel very weak.

The confusion that these disorders cause in older people is often mistaken for dementia.

Older people often have more than one disorder at a time. Each disorder may affect the other. For example, depression may make dementia worse, and an infection may make diabetes worse.

However, disorders no longer have the same devastating or incapacitating effects that they once had in older people. Disorders that were once likely to result in death for older people, such as heart attacks, hip fractures, and pneumonia, can often be treated and controlled. With treatment, many people with chronic disorders, such as diabetes, kidney disorders, and coronary artery disease, can remain functional, active, and independent.

Indirect Influences on Health

- People who live alone have more health problems than those who live with someone.
- Having a limited income can make obtaining adequate, prompt health care difficult.
- The many changes that occur during old age can lead to or aggravate health problems.

Circumstances that may seem unrelated to health can affect the health of older people.

Social Relationships: Older people who maintain social contact, whether it be with a spouse, with friends, or through outside interests, have fewer health problems. For example, older people who are married or who live with a roommate tend to be in better health than those who live alone. Older people who live with someone also have lower rates of hospitalization and nursing home admissions than those who live alone.

When older people live alone, new problems and symptoms may not be reported because no one notices. These older people may have no one to help them take their drugs as instructed. They may not prepare and eat balanced meals because physical impairments interfere, because they are lonely, or because they cannot drive or walk to a grocery store. Also, older people living alone are more likely to be lonely and depressed.

Occasionally, living with a relative or another person causes problems. Older people may conceal

SOME DISORDERS THAT AFFECT MAINLY OLDER PEOPLE

DISORDER	DESCRIPTION
Alzheimer's disease and other dementias	Memory and other mental functions are progressively lost.
Aortic aneurysm	The wall of the aorta bulges. If untreated, an aneurysm can rupture and lead to death.
Atrophic urethritis and vaginitis	Tissues in the urethra thin, sometimes causing burning during urination. Tissues in the vagina thin, sometimes causing pain during intercourse.
Benign prostatic hyperplasia	The prostate gland enlarges, blocking the flow of urine out of the bladder.
Cataracts	The lens of the eye clouds, impairing vision.
Diabetes, type 2	The body does not respond to the insulin it produces. This disorder usually begins during middle age. Treatment with insulin may not be required.
Glaucoma	The optic nerve is damaged because pressure in part of the eye is elevated. Vision is progressively reduced, and blindness can result. Glaucoma usually begins during middle age.
Osteoarthritis	The cartilage that lines the joints degenerates, causing pain. Osteoarthritis usually begins during middle age.
Osteoporosis	Bones become less dense and more fragile. As a result, fractures are more likely.
Parkinson's disease	Nerve cells in the brain degenerate slowly and progressively, causing tremor, stiff (rigid) muscles, and difficulty moving and maintaining balance.
Pressure sores	The skin breaks down because prolonged pressure reduces blood flow to the affected area.
Prostate cancer	Cancer develops in the prostate gland and eventually interferes with the flow of urine.
Shingles (herpes zoster)	The chickenpox virus from an earlier infection is reactivated, causing blisters and sometimes long-lasting, excruciating pain.
Stroke	A blood vessel in the brain is blocked or ruptures. A stroke causes symptoms such as weakness or loss of sensation on one side of the body, problems with vision in one eye, difficulty speaking or understanding, loss of balance or coordination, or sudden severe headache.
Urinary incontinence	The flow of urine cannot be controlled, resulting in leakage.

or minimize health problems because they do not want to impose on or inconvenience the relative. If any member of the household is not pleased with the living arrangement, older people may be neglected or mistreated (psychologically or even physically).

Education: In people with higher levels of education, disorders tend to be detected earlier, and health outcomes tend to be better, even when a disorder is not detected early.

Finances: Poverty is more common among older people than among the general population, despite the financial help provided by Medicare, Social Security, and Medicaid. Medicare Part D (the prescription drug program), although imperfect, has

made drug costs more manageable for many older people with a low income. Yet, despite these programs, some older people do not have adequate health insurance and have difficulty paying for health care that is not covered, including drugs. When paying for drugs is difficult, otherwise treatable disorders often are untreated or are treated at a late stage.

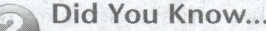 **Did You Know...**
People with higher education tend to have better health.

Response to Age-Related Changes: Older people may have difficulty coping with the many changes that occur with aging, such as retirement, loss of loved ones, and development of disorders (see page 1924). In response, older people may feel lonely, useless, powerless, or sad. They may lose their self-esteem. They may worry about becoming a burden to their family. They may become depressed, especially if they have a disorder that leads to temporary or permanent loss of independence or when they see their friends and loved ones die. These feelings may make older people less likely to see a health care practitioner, possibly delaying the diagnosis of a serious disorder.

Age-related changes and older people's responses to them can make treating disorders in older people complicated. Thus, older people often benefit from interdisciplinary care—care provided by a team of health care practitioners working together (see page 1903). This team may consist of doctors, nurses, social workers, therapists, pharmacists, and psychologists. Usually led by the person's primary care doctor, the team evaluates the person's needs and plans, coordinates, and implements care—including social services. Team members actively look for possible problems and take measures to correct or prevent them.

Disorders of Accelerated Aging

Certain disorders have some of the same effects as aging. Scientists study what happens in these disorders to try to learn what causes aging. For example, they identify the genes that are defective in these disorders and compare them with the same genes in older people.

Looking for the Fountain of Youth

Everyone wants to know how to stay young and live longer. Researchers are looking at genes, cells, hormones, eating patterns, and other factors for clues about what causes aging and how to prevent or slow it. Research has identified three strategies that may help people live longer:

- Exercising
- Following certain types of diets
- Eating fewer calories

People who exercise are healthier than those who do not. Exercise has many established health benefits: improving and maintaining the ability to do daily activities, maintaining a healthy weight, and helping prevent or postpone disorders such as coronary artery disease and diabetes.

People who eat a low-fat diet that includes lots of fruits and vegetables are healthier than people who eat more fat and starch. Also, people who live in Mediterranean countries and consume the so-called Mediterranean diet seem to live longer. This diet is generally thought to be healthier than northern European and American diets because it consists of more grains, fruits, vegetables, legumes, nuts, and fish and less red meat. In addition, the main fat consumed is olive oil. Olive oil contains many vitamins and is monounsaturated rather than saturated. Monounsaturated fats do not increase cholesterol the way saturated fats do.

Following a low-calorie diet for a lifetime may lead to longer life, possibly because it slows the body's metabolism, reduces the number of certain damaging substances in the body, or both. These damaging substances, called free radicals, are by-products of the normal activity of cells. The damage done to cells by free radicals is thought to contribute to aging and to disorders such as coronary artery disease and cancer. But no studies to test whether a low-calorie diet could prolong life have been done in people.

These three strategies would require a major change in lifestyle for most people. Consequently, many people look for other, less demanding ways to prevent or slow aging. For example, they may look for other ways to manage free radicals. Substances called antioxidants can neutralize free radicals and thus help prevent damage to cells. Vitamins C and E are antioxidants. So some people take large amounts of these vitamins as supplements in the hope of slowing the aging process. Other antioxidants, such as beta-carotene (a form of vitamin A), are sometimes taken as supplements. In theory, using antioxidants to prevent aging makes sense. However, no studies have shown that antioxidants taken as supplements prevent or slow aging. Evidence that they protect against disorders such cancer, heart attack, stroke, or cancer is inconclusive. Also, such supplements have not been proved to be harmless.

Levels of some hormones decrease as people age. Thus, people may try to delay or slow aging by taking supplements of these hormones. Examples are testosterone, estrogen, DHEA (dehydroepiandrosterone), human growth hormone, and melatonin. But whether hormonal supplements have any effect on aging is unknown, and some of them have known risks. Also, some experts believe that decreases in certain hormone levels may actually prolong life by slowing the body's metabolism.

Some people believe that Eastern practices, such as yoga, tai chi, and qigong, can prolong life. These practices are based on the principle that health involves the whole person (physical, emotional, mental, and spiritual) and balance within the body. The practices may include relaxation, breathing techniques, diet, and meditation as well as exercise. They are safe for older people and probably make them feel better. But whether these practices prolong life is difficult to prove.

PROGEROID SYNDROMES

Progeroid syndromes are rare disorders that cause premature aging and shorten life expectancy.

In progeroid syndromes, the aging process is greatly accelerated. Affected children develop all of the external signs of old age, including baldness, hunched posture, and dry, inelastic, and wrinkled skin. However, in contrast to normal aging, the ovaries or testes are inactive, resulting in sterility. Females have no menstrual periods. Affected children are unusually short. Thus, progeroid syndromes are not an exact model of accelerated aging.

There are several progeroid syndromes. In Hutchinson-Gilford syndrome and Werner's syndrome, the central nervous system and therefore the ability to do many daily activities are largely unaffected unless a stroke occurs.

Hutchinson-Gilford Syndrome (Progeria): This syndrome begins in early childhood. It is caused by a genetic abnormality but is usually not inherited. That is, the genetic abnormality (mutation) occurs on its own. It causes inelastic and wrinkled skin, baldness, and other problems usually associated with aging (such as disorders of the heart, kidneys, and lungs and osteoporosis). The body does not grow normally and thus appears too small for the head. Most children die in their teens. The cause is usually a heart attack or stroke. No treatment is available to reverse the condition, but complications can be treated as they are in older people.

Werner's Syndrome: This hereditary syndrome begins in adolescence or early adult life. It causes inelastic and wrinkled skin, baldness, and problems associated with aging, including atherosclerosis, cataracts, diabetes, osteoporosis, cataracts, muscle wasting, and cancer (including some types that are rare in other people).

DOWN SYNDROME

Down syndrome is much more common than progeroid syndromes (see page 1726). It also causes problems typical of old age in younger adults:

- Glucose intolerance
- Blood vessel disorders
- Cancer
- Hair loss
- Degenerative bone disease
- Premature death

In contrast to progeroid syndromes, Down syndrome greatly impairs the central nervous system. It usually causes mental retardation and, later in life, symptoms of Alzheimer's disease (see page 694). Also, brain tissue, obtained during an autopsy and examined under a microscope, has the same type of degeneration that is seen in people with Alzheimer's disease.

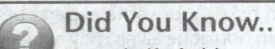

CHAPTER **291**   # Aging and Drugs

Drugs, the most common medical intervention, are an important part of medical care for older people. Without drugs, many older people would function less well or die at an earlier age.

> ### ? Did You Know...
> Up to half of older people do not take drugs as directed by their doctor.
>
> Older people are more susceptible to the effects (and side effects) of many drugs.

Older people tend to take more drugs than younger people because they are more likely to have chronic disorders such as high blood pressure, diabetes, and arthritis. Most drugs used by older people for chronic disorders are taken for years. Other drugs may be taken for only a short time to treat such problems as infections, some kinds of pain, and constipation. On average, older people take four or five prescription drugs and two nonprescription (over-the-counter, or OTC) drugs each day. Many OTC drugs are potentially hazardous for older people (see page 106).

Benefits and Risks

Many of the improvements in the health and function of older people during the past several decades can be attributed to drugs.

- Vaccines help prevent many infectious diseases (such as influenza and pneumonia) that once killed many older people.
- Antibiotics are often effective in treating pneumonia—once known as the killer of older people—and many other serious infections.

- Drugs to control high blood pressure (antihypertensives) help prevent strokes and heart attacks.
- Drugs to control blood sugar levels (antihyperglycemic drugs) enable millions of people with diabetes to lead normal lives. These drugs also reduce the risk of eye and kidney problems that diabetes can cause.
- Drugs to control pain and other symptoms enable millions of people with arthritis to continue to function.

However, drugs can have effects that are not intended or desired (side effects). Starting in late middle age, the risk of side effects from drugs increases. Older people are more than twice as susceptible to the side effects of drugs as younger people (see page 93). Side effects are also likely to be more severe, affecting quality of life and resulting in visits to the doctor and in hospitalization.

Older people are more susceptible to side effects for several reasons:

- As people age, the amount of water in the body decreases, and the percentage of fat tissue increases. Thus, in older people, drugs that dissolve in water reach higher concentrations because there is less water to dilute them, and drugs that dissolve in fat accumulate more because there is relatively more fat tissue to store them.
- As people age, the kidneys are less able to excrete drugs into urine, and the liver is less able to break down (metabolize) many drugs (see page 84). Thus, drugs are less readily removed from the body.
- Older people take more drugs and have more disorders.
- Fewer studies have been done in older people to help identify appropriate doses of drugs.

Because of these age-related changes, many drugs tend to stay in an older person's body much longer, prolonging the drug's effect and increasing the risk of side effects. Therefore, older people often need to take smaller doses of certain drugs or perhaps fewer daily doses. For example, digoxin, a drug commonly used to treat certain heart disorders, dissolves in water and is eliminated by the kidneys. Because the amount of water in the body decreases and the kidneys function less well as people age, digoxin concentrations in the body may be increased, resulting in side effects (such as nausea or abnormal heart rhythms). To prevent this problem, doctors may use a smaller dose. Or sometimes other drugs can be substituted.

Older people are more sensitive to the effects of many drugs. For example, older people tend to become sleepier and are more likely to become confused when taking antianxiety drugs or sleep aids to treat insomnia. Drugs that lower blood pressure by widening (dilating) arteries and reducing the amount of

Anticholinergic: What Does It Mean?

Anticholinergic effects are caused by drugs that block the action of acetylcholine. Acetylcholine is a neurotransmitter—a chemical messenger released by a nerve cell to transmit a nerve signal to a neighboring nerve cell or a target cell in a muscle or gland. Thus, acetylcholine helps cells talk to each other. Acetylcholine helps with memory, learning, and concentration. It also helps control the functioning of the heart, blood vessels, airways, and urinary and digestive organs. Acetylcholine acts on smooth (involuntary) muscle cells, such as those in the heart or airways, causing them to contract. Thus, drugs with anticholinergic effects can disrupt the normal functioning of these organs.

Many commonly used drugs have anticholinergic effects. Most of these drugs were not designed to have these effects, which are therefore usually considered undesirable side effects. Anticholinergic effects include the following:

- Confusion
- Blurred vision
- Constipation
- Dry mouth
- Light-headedness
- Difficulty starting and continuing to urinate
- Loss of bladder control

However, anticholinergic drugs can also have useful effects, such as helping control tremors and nausea.

Older people are more likely to experience anticholinergic effects because the amount of acetylcholine in the body decreases with age. Consequently, anticholinergic drugs block a higher percentage of acetylcholine, so that the aging body is less able to use what little acetylcholine is present. Also, cells in many parts of the body (such as the digestive tract) have fewer sites where acetylcholine can attach. As a result, doctors usually try to avoid using drugs with anticholinergic effects in older people, although doing so is not always possible.

work the heart has to do tend to lower blood pressure much more dramatically in older people than in the young. Knowing which drugs are particularly likely to cause problems in older people helps avoid side effects, such as dizziness, light-headedness, and falls. Older people who are taking these drugs can ask their doctor about changing to a different drug.

Many commonly used drugs have anticholinergic effects. These drugs include some antidepressants, many antihistamines (contained in OTC sleep aids, cold remedies, and allergy drugs), and diphenhydramine (used in the treatment of insomnia). Older people are particularly

Maximizing Benefits, Reducing Risks

Older people and the people who care for them can do many things to maximize the benefits and reduce the risks of taking drugs. Any questions about or problems with a drug should be discussed with the doctor or pharmacist. Taking drugs as instructed is essential for avoiding problems and promoting good health.

Know about the drugs and disorders being treated:

- Keep a list of all drugs being taken, including over-the-counter drugs and supplements, such as vitamins, minerals, and medicinal herbs.
- Learn why each drug is taken and what its effects are supposed to be.
- Learn what side effects each drug may have and what to do if a side effect occurs.
- Learn how to take each drug, including what time of day it should be taken, whether it can be taken at the same time as other drugs, and when to stop taking the drug.
- Learn what to do if a dose is missed.
- Write down information about how to take the drug or ask the doctor, nurse, or pharmacist to write it down (because such information can easily be forgotten).
- Keep a list of all disorders present.

Use drugs correctly:

- Take drugs as instructed.
- Use memory aids, such as weekly pill boxes, if needed to take drugs as instructed.
- Before stopping a drug, consult the doctor about any problems—for example, if side effects occur, if the drug does not seem to work, or if purchasing the drug is burdensome.
- Discard any unused drug from a previous prescription, unless instructed not to do so by a doctor, nurse, or pharmacist.
- When discarding a drug, follow the disposal instructions on the label, or mix the drug with kitty litter or coffee grounds, tightly wrap in plastic or a similar material, place in a sealable or watertight container or bag, and discard in the trash (most pharmacies do not dispose of left-over drugs).
- Do not take another person's drug, even if that person's problem seems similar.
- Check the expiration date on drugs, and do not use the drug if it has expired.

Work closely with the doctor and pharmacist:

- Get all prescriptions from the same pharmacy, preferably one that provides comprehensive services (including checking for possible drug interactions) and that maintains a complete drug profile for each person.
- Bring all drugs being taken to doctor appointments if requested to do so.
- Periodically discuss the list of drugs being taken and the list of disorders with the doctor, nurse, or pharmacist.
- Review the list of drugs with the doctor, nurse, or pharmacist every time any drug is changed (doctors and pharmacists can check for interactions between drugs).
- Make sure the doctor and pharmacist know about all over-the-counter drugs and supplements being taken, including vitamins, minerals, and medicinal herbs.
- Consult the doctor before taking any new drugs, including over-the-counter drugs and supplements.
- Report to the doctor or pharmacist any symptoms that might be related to the use of a drug.
- If the schedule of taking drugs is too complex to follow, ask the doctor about simplifying it.
- If seeing more than one doctor, make sure each doctor knows all the drugs being taken.
- Ask the pharmacist to print the label in large print, and check to make sure it can be read.
- Ask the pharmacist to package the drug in containers that are easy to hold and to open.

susceptible to anticholinergic effects, which include confusion, blurred vision, constipation, dry mouth, lightheadedness, difficulty starting and continuing to urinate, and loss of bladder control (urinary incontinence). Some anticholinergic effects, such as reduction of tremor (as in the treatment of Parkinson's disease) and reduction of nausea, are desirable, but most are not.

A drug may have a side effect because it interacts with

- A disease other than the one for which the drug is being taken (drug-disease interaction)

- Another drug (drug-drug interaction)
- Food (drug-food interaction)
- A medicinal herb (drug–medicinal herb interaction—see table on page 2068)

Because older people tend to have more diseases and take more drugs than younger people, they are more likely to have drug-disease and drug-drug interactions. Patients, doctors, and pharmacists can take steps to reduce the risk of these interactions (see box on page 91). Because OTC drugs and medicinal herbs

SOME DRUGS PARTICULARLY LIKELY TO CAUSE PROBLEMS IN OLDER PEOPLE

DRUG	USE	PROBLEM
Amitriptyline	To treat depression	Amitriptyline has strong anticholinergic effects.* It also causes excessive drowsiness.
Antihistamines that have anti-cholinergic effects (such as chlorpheniramine, cyproheptadine, dexchlorpheniramine, diphen-hydramine, hydroxyzine, orphen-adrine, promethazine, and tripelennamine)	To relieve allergy symptoms, to aid sleep, or to relieve cold symptoms	All nonprescription (over-the-counter) and many prescription antihistamines have strong anticholinergic effects.* Antihistamines are commonly included with other drugs in cough and cold preparations.
Antipsychotic drugs (such as chlorpromazine, haloperidol, mesoridazine, thioridazine, and thiothixene)	To treat loss of contact with reality (psychosis) or, somewhat controversially, to treat behavioral disturbances in people with dementia	Antipsychotic drugs can cause drowsiness, movement disorders (that resemble Parkinson's disease), and uncontrollable facial twitches. These drugs also have anticholinergic effects.* Some side effects are potentially fatal. Antipsychotic drugs should be used only when a psychotic disorder is present.
Barbiturates (such as phenobarbital and secobarbital)	To calm, to relieve anxiety, or to aid sleep	Barbiturates have more side effects than other drugs used to treat anxiety and insomnia. They also interact with many other drugs. Generally, older people should take barbiturates only as treatment for a seizure disorder.
Benzodiazepines that have long-lasting effects (such as chlordiaz-epoxide, clorazepate, diazepam, flurazepam, halazepam, nitrazepam, and quazepam)	To calm, to relieve anxiety, or to aid sleep	The effects of these drugs last a very long time (often more than several days) in older people. These drugs can cause prolonged drowsiness and loss of balance when a person is walking. Thus, the risk of falls and fractures is increased.
Chlorpropamide	To treat diabetes	This drug's effects last a long time. In older people, chlorpropamide can lower blood sugar levels (causing hypoglycemia) for several hours. This drug can also lower the sodium level in the blood (causing hyponatremia). A low sodium level can lead to changes in personality, confusion, and sluggishness (lethargy).
Cimetidine	To treat heartburn, indigestion, or ulcers	Typical doses of cimetidine, a histamine-2 (H_2) blocker, may have side effects, especially confusion.
Digoxin	To treat heart failure or abnormal heart rhythms (arrhythmias)	As people age, the kidneys are less able to excrete digoxin. Large doses of the drug can more easily reach harmful (toxic) levels. Side effects may include loss of appetite, nausea, and confusion.
Dipyridamole (immediate-release)[†]	To reduce the risk of blood clots or to improve blood flow	Dipyridamole frequently causes low blood pressure when older people stand up. It can also increase the risk of bleeding when it is taken with other drugs that make blood less likely to clot, such as aspirin or the antico-agulant warfarin.
Disopyramide	To treat abnormal heart rhythms	Disopyramide has strong anticholinergic effects.* It may cause heart failure in older people.

(continued on the following page)

SOME DRUGS PARTICULARLY LIKELY TO CAUSE PROBLEMS IN OLDER PEOPLE (*Continued*)

DRUG	USE	PROBLEM
Doxepin	To treat depression	Doxepin has strong anticholinergic effects.* It also causes excessive drowsiness.
Drugs that reduce or stop muscle spasms in the digestive tract (anti-spasmodic drugs, such as belladonna alkaloids, clidinium/chlordiazepoxide, dicyclomine, hyoscyamine, and propantheline)	To relieve abdominal cramps and pain	These drugs have strong anticholinergic effects* and are toxic in older people. Their usefulness—especially at the low doses tolerated by older people—is questionable.
Estrogens only (oral)	To help relieve menopausal symptoms, such as hot flashes, night sweats, and vaginal dryness	Estrogens increase the risk of breast and uterine (endometrial) cancer and may increase the risk of stroke and heart attack in older women.
Famotidine	To treat heartburn, indigestion, or ulcers	To some extent, high doses of famotidine, an H_2 blocker, may have side effects, especially confusion.
Fluoxetine	To treat depression	Fluoxetine's effects last a long time. It may cause sleep disturbances, restlessness, and increased agitation. It may also decrease appetite in some older people who do not need to lose weight.
Indomethacin	To relieve pain	Of all nonsteroidal anti-inflammatory drugs (NSAIDs), indomethacin affects the brain the most. It can cause confusion or dizziness.
Iron supplements (such as ferrous sulfate)	To provide supplemental iron	Doses higher than 325 milligrams daily do not greatly increase the amount of iron that is absorbed, and such doses are more likely to cause constipation.
Meperidine	To relieve pain	Meperidine, an opioid, often causes confusion. Like all opioids, it may cause constipation, retention of urine, drowsiness, and confusion. When taken by mouth, meperidine is not very effective.
Methyldopa	To lower high blood pressure	Methyldopa may slow the heart rate and worsen depression.
Muscle relaxants (such as carisoprodol, chlorzoxazone, cyclobenzaprine, metaxalone, methocarbamol, and oxybutynin)	To relieve muscle spasms	Most muscle relaxants have anticholinergic effects.* They also cause drowsiness and weakness. The usefulness of all muscle relaxants at the low doses tolerated by older people is questionable.
Nizatidine	To treat heartburn, indigestion, or ulcers	To some extent, high doses of nizatidine, an H_2 blocker, may have side effects, especially confusion.
Non–COX-selective nonsteroidal anti-inflammatory drugs (NSAIDs, such as naproxen, oxaprozin, and piroxicam)	To relieve pain and inflammation	Long-term use of the maximum dosage may cause kidney problems or bleeding from the stomach or intestine.
Pentazocine	To relieve pain	Pentazocine, an opioid, is more likely to cause confusion and hallucinations than other opioids. Like all opioids, it may cause constipation, retention of urine, drowsiness, and confusion.

(*continued on the following page*)

SOME DRUGS PARTICULARLY LIKELY TO CAUSE PROBLEMS IN OLDER PEOPLE (*Continued*)

DRUG	USE	PROBLEM
Propoxyphene and combination products that include it	To relieve pain	Propoxyphene, an opioid, provides no more pain relief than acetaminophen. Like all opioids, it may cause constipation, retention of urine, drowsiness, and confusion.
Ranitidine	To treat heartburn, indigestion, or ulcers	To some extent, high doses of ranitidine, an H$_2$ blocker, may have side effects, especially confusion.
Reserpine	To lower high blood pressure	Reserpine can cause dizziness when a person stands up, depression, drowsiness, and erectile dysfunction (impotence).
Trimethobenzamide	To relieve nausea	This drug can cause abnormal movements of the arms, legs, and other parts of the body. It is one of the least effective drugs for relieving nausea.

*Anticholinergic effects include confusion, blurred vision, constipation, dry mouth, light-headedness, difficulty starting and continuing to urinate, and loss of bladder control.

†Dipyridamole is also available in an extended-release formulation with aspirin. This product, which is used to prevent strokes in people who have had a stroke, is not included in this list.

can interact with other drugs, people should ask their doctor or pharmacist about these drugs as well as about prescription drugs.

Not following a doctor's directions for taking a drug (noncompliance or nonadherence) can be risky (see page 97). Old age alone does not make people less likely to take drugs as directed. However, up to half of older people do not do so. Not taking a drug, taking too little, or taking too much can cause problems. Taking less of a drug because it has side effects may seem reasonable, but people should talk to a doctor before they make any changes in the way they take a drug.

Remembering to Take Drugs

To benefit from taking drugs, people must remember not only to take the drugs but also to take them at the right time and in the right way. When several drugs are taken, the schedule for taking them can be complex. For example, drugs may have to be taken at different times throughout the day to avoid interactions. Some drugs may have to be taken with food. Other drugs have to be taken when no food is in the stomach. The more complex the schedule, the more likely people are to make mistakes following it. For example, bisphosphonates (such as alendronate and risedronate), which are used to increase bone density, need to be taken on an empty stomach and with only water (at least a full glass). If these drugs are taken with other liquids or food, they are not absorbed well and do not work effectively.

If older people have memory problems, following a complex schedule is even harder. Such people usually need help, often from family members. The doctor can be asked about simplifying the schedule. Often, doses can be rescheduled to make taking the drugs more convenient or reduce the total number of daily doses.

Memory aids can help older people remember to take their drugs. For example, using a drug can be associated with a specific daily task, such as eating a meal.

A pharmacist can provide containers that help people take drugs as instructed. Daily doses for 1 week or 2 weeks may be packaged in a plastic pack marked with the days or with the times of the day, so that people can keep track of doses taken by noting the empty spaces. Some pharmacies can package drugs in blister packs, so that the daily dose can be easily removed and kept track of. However, such packaging may cost a little more.

More elaborate containers with a computerized reminder system are available. These containers beep or flash at dosing time. Another alternative is a paging service with a beeper. This service is available from subscriber-based telecommunications companies.

292 Provision of Care

Providing medical care to older people can be complicated. People often have many different doctors at different locations. Travel and transportation issues become more difficult as people age. The drugs that are covered by the new Medicare prescription drug plan vary between insurance companies and change frequently. Assistance by a team of health care practitioners under the leadership of a primary care doctor or geriatrician is the best way to deal with these complexities. However, this ideal solution is often difficult to achieve.

Continuity of Care

Continuity of care is an ideal in which health care is provided for a person in a coordinated manner and without disruption despite involvement of different practitioners in different care settings. Also, all people involved in a person's health care, including the person receiving care, communicate and work with each other to coordinate health care and to set goals for health care.

Continuity of care is not always easy to accomplish, especially in the United States, where the health care system is complicated and fragmented. When continuity of care is missing, people may not adequately understand their health care problems and may not know which practitioner to talk to when they have problems or questions.

CHALLENGES TO CONTINUITY

Continuity of care is a particular concern for older people. Older people are particularly likely to have several doctors (each specializing in one organ system or problem) and thus to move from one care setting to another (called transition of care). They may receive care in several doctors' offices, in a hospital, in a rehabilitation facility, or in a long-term facility.

Many Practitioners: Having many practitioners at many places may disrupt the continuity of an older person's health care. For example, one health care practitioner may not have up-to-date, accurate information about the care provided or recommended by other practitioners. That practitioner may not know the names of the other practitioners involved or may not think to contact them. Information about care may be misremembered, miscommunicated, or misunderstood, particularly when older people have disorders affecting speech, vision, or cognition that make it more difficult for them to communicate effectively. An older person may mention an important detail to one practitioner and forget to mention it to the others.

To ensure that care is continuous (and optimal), all practitioners involved must have complete, up-to-date, and accurate information about what other practitioners have done—particularly about tests done and drugs prescribed. When this information is missing or miscommunicated, the following can result:

- Diagnostic tests may be needlessly repeated.
- Inappropriate drugs or other treatments may be prescribed.
- Preventive measures may not be taken because each practitioner assumes someone else has provided them.

Different practitioners may have different opinions about a person's health care. For example, practitioners in a hospital may disagree with a person's primary care doctor about whether surgery is required or about whether the person should go to a nursing home after being discharged. The person and family members may be overwhelmed and confused by differences of opinion among the various practitioners.

People taking many prescription drugs, as is common with older people, may fill their prescriptions at different pharmacies (for example, the one nearest each specialist's office). When different pharmacies are involved, each pharmacist may not know all the drugs people are taking and thus will not know when a newly prescribed drug might interact negatively with a current one.

Many Settings: Moving from one care setting to another, such as going from a hospital to a skilled nursing facility, increases the chance that errors in care may occur. New drugs may be prescribed in the hospital, and they may duplicate or negatively interact with the person's other drugs. Sometimes old, needed drugs may be unintentionally omitted. Even when changes in people's drugs are appropriate, the changes may not be communicated to all involved health care practitioners, such as the primary care doctor.

To prevent such problems, current regulations in the United States require health care organizations to do drug reconciliation whenever the care setting is changed and new drugs are ordered or existing orders are rewritten. Drug reconciliation involves comparing people's drug orders to all the drugs they were previously taking and thus make sure no drugs are duplicated or omitted. When changing care settings, older people or their caregiver need to ask one of the hospital staff members, such as a nurse, doctor, or social worker, whether drug reconciliation was done.

People should also be sure to obtain their own copy of the current drug regimen. They should then compare it with the list of drugs that they have been taking and check to make sure that no drugs are duplicated. If they have any questions, they should contact their primary care doctor. Making an appointment with the primary care doctor soon after discharge from the hospital is always a good idea. The doctor can then review all of the drugs and instructions recommended by the hospital.

Many Rules: The health care system has many rules that affect continuity of care. The rules may be made by the government, insurance companies, or professional organizations for health care practitioners. For example, some insurance companies limit which hospital people can go to. The person's doctor, if not on staff at that hospital, may be unable to provide care there. As a result, important information about the person may not be communicated.

Lack of Access to Care: Continuity of care may be disrupted when people do not have access to health care. For example, older people may miss a follow-up appointment because they do not have transportation to a doctor's office. They may not see a doctor or specialist because they do not have insurance and cannot afford to pay for health care themselves.

STRATEGIES TO IMPROVE CONTINUITY

Improving continuity of care requires efforts by the health care system, by the people receiving care, and by family members.

Health Care System

Managed care organizations and some government health care plans coordinate all health care and thus contribute to continuity of care. Also, the health care system has developed several strategies to improve continuity of care. Examples are

- Interdisciplinary care
- Geriatric care managers

Interdisciplinary Care: Interdisciplinary care is coordinated care provided by many types of practitioners, including doctors, nurses, pharmacists, dietitians, physical and occupational therapists, and social workers. These practitioners make a conscious, organized effort to communicate, cooperate, and agree with each other about a person's care. Interdisciplinary care aims to ensure that people move safely and easily from one care setting to another and from one health care practitioner to another. It also aims to ensure that the most qualified health care practitioner provides care for each problem and that care is not duplicated. Interdisciplinary care is not available everywhere.

Interdisciplinary care is particularly important when treatment is complex or when it involves movement from one care setting to another. People who are most likely to benefit include those who are very frail, those who have many disorders, those who need to see several different types of health care practitioners, and those who have side effects from drugs.

The practitioners who care for a particular person are called the interdisciplinary team. One practitioner, often the person's primary care doctor, coordinates care.

Sometimes the health care practitioners on an interdisciplinary team do not work together on a regular basis (an ad hoc team). They come together to meet a particular person's needs. In other situations, there is an established team with the same members who usually work together and who care for many people. Some nursing homes, hospitals, and hospice organizations have established teams.

Team members discuss plans for treatment and inform each other about changes in the person's health, changes in treatment, and results of examinations and tests. They make sure that the person's records are up-to-date and that the records accompany the person through the health care system. Such efforts help make changes in care setting or in health care practitioners smoother and less traumatic. Also, tests are less likely to be repeated unnecessarily, and mistakes or omissions in treatment are less likely.

The interdisciplinary team also includes the older person being cared for and family members or other caregivers. For effective interdisciplinary care, these people must actively participate in care and must communicate with the health care practitioners on the team.

Geriatric Care Managers: These people are specialists who make sure that an older person receives all the help and care needed. Most geriatric care managers are social workers or nurses. They may be members of an interdisciplinary team. Geriatric care managers can make arrangements for the services needed and supervise these arrangements. For example, care managers may arrange for a home nurse to visit or for an aide to help with housecleaning and preparation of meals. They may locate a pharmacy that delivers drugs or arrange for transportation to and from the doctor's office. Geriatric care managers are relatively uncommon.

People Receiving Care

To help improve the continuity of their care, older people or their caregivers can take a more active part in their care. For example, they can learn more about what can interfere with continuity, how the health care system works, and what tools are available (such as care managers or social workers) to improve continuity of care. Being familiar with their disorders and the details of their health insurance plan can also help.

Active participation begins with communication—giving and getting information. When older people have special health care needs or questions, they or their family members should tell their health care practitioners. For example, older people often need help determining which drugs are covered by their Medicare prescription drug plan.

When an interdisciplinary team or geriatric care manager is unavailable, people who are receiving care or their family members need to become proactive in care. For example, older people or their caregivers need to establish an ongoing relationship with at least one health care practitioner, usually the primary care doctor, to minimize the problems created by having several health care practitioners. Older people should make sure the primary doctor is aware of changes in their condition and their drugs, especially when a specialist has made a new diagnosis or changed a treatment regimen. They may need to ask one health care practitioner to call and talk with another to make sure that information is communicated clearly and that treatment is appropriate.

Active participation also includes seeing a health care practitioner (usually the primary care doctor) regularly and following the instructions of health care practitioners. It means asking questions about a disorder, treatment, or other aspect of care. It includes learning how to prevent disorders and taking the appropriate steps to do so.

For people who have a disorder, active participation may involve self-monitoring. For example, people with high blood pressure can regularly monitor their blood pressure. People with diabetes can regularly check the level of sugar in their blood.

Keeping a copy of their medical record can help people participate in their health care. They can often obtain a copy from their doctor. A copy of the medical record is useful as a reference for information about disorders present, drugs being taken, treatments and tests done, and payments made. This information can also help people explain a problem to a health care practitioner. File boxes, binders, computer software, and Internet programs have been designed for this purpose. When more than one doctor is involved, people can keep their own records of their care, including the type and date of examinations and procedures and a list of their diagnoses. At a minimum, people should keep a record of all drugs (prescription and nonprescription) they are currently taking, plus the doses and the reason they are taking the drug. They should bring this record with them each time they visit a doctor.

When people go to a hospital or to a new health care practitioner, they should check with someone at the new location to make sure that their medical record has been received.

Buying all drugs (prescription and nonprescription) at one pharmacy or through one mail order service and getting to know a pharmacist there are also important. Older people can ask their pharmacist questions about the drugs they are taking. They can also ask for containers that are easy to open and labels that are easy to read.

Care Providers: Practitioners

People, particularly older people, often need to see several types of health care practitioners. Sometimes a group of health care practitioners work together to provide care. This type of care is called interdisciplinary care (see page 1903).

Doctors: Older people may see many different kinds of doctors: family practice doctors, general internists, specialists in such areas as heart disorders (cardiologists) or cancer (oncologists), and surgeons. Sometimes general internists and different specialists work together in a group practice. A group practice makes referrals and communication among doctors easier, and people do not need to travel to many different locations.

Geriatricians are doctors, usually internists or family practice doctors, who are trained specifically to care for older people. A geriatrician may be the person's primary care doctor or may be called in for a short time for consultation. Geriatricians are trained to manage many disorders and problems at once. They have studied how the body changes as it ages, so that they can better distinguish when a symptom is due to a disorder rather than to aging itself. They evaluate older people in terms of social and emotional as well as physical needs. Then they can help older people live as independently as possible. The people most likely to benefit from seeing a geriatrician include those who

- Are very frail
- Have many disorders
- Need to see several different types of health care practitioners
- Take many drugs and are thus likely to have drug side effects

Nurses: Nurses may work in a doctor's office, a hospital, a rehabilitation or long-term care facility, or a senior center, or they may provide care in a person's home. Nurses may help coordinate care by communicating information to the different practitioners involved, the person, and family members. Also, they are often more readily available for questions that older people may have about their disorders or treatment. Nurses may teach older people about measures to help maintain good health, such as diet, safety, stress management, sleep, and exercise. Other duties include checking vital signs (blood pressure, pulse, and temperature), taking samples of blood, giving treatments, and teaching people how to care for themselves. Nurses may ask questions about the person's health (for the medical history) and home situation.

Registered nurses (RNs) often provide most of an older person's health care. RNs supervise care provided by licensed practical nurses (LPNs) and nurses' aides. RNs are taught to do a physical examination and check for changes that need to be evaluated by a doctor. They also can administer drugs to the person, as prescribed by a doctor. LPNs may do many functions but always under the supervision of an RN.

Nurse Practitioners: Nurse practitioners are registered nurses who receive additional training in diagnosis and treatment. Thus, these nurses have more responsibilities than RNs. They can write prescriptions and order tests for people. Some nurse practitioners, called geriatric nurse practitioners, are specially trained to care for older people.

Physician Assistants: Physician assistants (PAs) have some of the same functions as doctors and nurse practitioners but always under a doctor's supervision. Their functions include the following:

- Asking about the person's health (for the medical history)
- Doing physical examinations
- Ordering diagnostic tests
- Helping doctors develop treatment plans
- Assisting in surgery
- Doing routine procedures, such as giving shots and stitching up wounds
- Providing people with information about following their treatment plan and taking care of themselves (such as information about a healthy diet and exercise)

PAs work in most care settings, including long-term care facilities. They may provide health care in a person's home. Some PAs specialize in treating older people.

Pharmacists: In addition to dispensing drugs, pharmacists evaluate prescriptions to make sure that appropriate drugs are being used. Pharmacists can check to make sure that older people are not taking drugs that pose special risks for them. Pharmacists

also make sure that instructions are clear and include information about how much and how often a drug is to be used. They keep track of a person's prescriptions and refills. In this way, they can check for interactions between drugs.

Some pharmacists specialize in the care of older people. They are sometimes called consultant (senior care) pharmacists. They often work in nursing homes. They provide other practitioners with information about how to use drugs appropriately in older people.

Dietitians: Dietitians assess how well nutritional needs are being met. When needs are not being met, they provide specific recommendations about which foods to choose and how to prepare foods. About 1 in 6 older people are undernourished. Many older people can benefit from the assistance of a dietician.

Therapists: Different types of therapists may be needed, depending on the disorders and problems a person has.

Physical therapists (see page 48) evaluate and treat people who have difficulty moving—for example, difficulty walking, changing positions (standing up, sitting down, or lying down), transferring from bed to chair, lifting, or bending. They work with people who have had problems such as a stroke, amputation of a limb, or hip surgery. Treatments may include exercise, heat, and ultrasound.

Occupational therapists (see page 50) evaluate and treat people who have difficulty caring for themselves (for example, dressing or bathing), working, and doing other daily activities.

Speech therapists help people who have difficulty using and understanding language (see page 56).

Social Workers: Social workers help coordinate discharges from hospitals and transfers between institutions. They may help people fill out insurance and other forms. They help people identify services that can be provided in the home and community and often help arrange for these services. They also evaluate how people are responding to the care and services obtained.

Social workers may bring family members together for discussions about important health care issues. Many social workers counsel people with anxiety, depression, or difficulty coping with a disorder or disability.

Most social workers are familiar with the special needs of older people. But some are specially trained to counsel older people and to determine whether they need supervision or additional help.

Nurses' Aides: Nurses' aides care for people in hospitals, rehabilitation facilities, nursing homes, assisted living communities, or other medical facilities under the direction of nurses, doctors, and other medical staff members. They are sometimes trained to do some simple assessments of health. For example, an aide may measure temperature, pulse, and blood pressure.

Nurses' aides may respond to signal lights or bells indicating that someone needs help. They bathe, dress, and undress people. They serve and collect food trays and feed people who need help eating.

Home Health Aides: Employed by home health care agencies, home health aides do many of the same tasks that nurses' aides do, but in the home. They help with daily activities, especially with dressing and grooming. These aides may prepare meals, help the person out of a wheelchair, or take the person for a walk. They sometimes help with light housework. They may also do some simple health assessments under the supervision of a registered nurse.

Medical Ethicists: Medical ethicists help resolve conflicts about moral issues that come up during health care. For example, health care practitioners and family members may disagree about whether a treatment that appears to be ineffective should be stopped. Medical ethicists may be doctors, other health care practitioners, lawyers, or other people who have been specially trained in medical ethics. Some hospitals have a medical ethicist or a team of medical ethicists on staff.

Care Providers: Family and Friends

Some older people have family members, friends, or neighbors who are willing and able to provide help and care. Such people may be called caregivers. Occasionally, members of religious or other groups help or take over the role of caregiver altogether at no or low cost. Caregivers may provide help with basic activities (such as eating, dressing, and bathing) or with household chores (such as cooking, cleaning, shopping, paying bills, mowing the lawn, and taking drugs as prescribed).

Of the nearly 36 million people aged 65 or older in the United States, about 7 million need a caregiver's help on a daily basis. More than 22 million caregivers in the United States provide ongoing care for older people. They may provide care for a few hours a week or around the clock.

Most caregivers are the spouses or children of the people they care for, and most are women. About two thirds of caregivers work full- or part-time in addition to providing care.

Determining whether an older person needs care can be difficult. Most older people resist the idea that they need any help. Observing how well an older person is able to do the following can help concerned family members make this decision:

- **Eating:** Is clothing frequently stained by food? Is the person losing weight without an obvious explanation?

- **Getting in and out of a chair or bed:** Does the person rock back and forth several times before actually getting up? Are nearby furniture items or objects used for support? Does sitting down seem to involve falling backward into a chair?

- **Using the toilet:** Is clothing soiled or wet?

- **Bathing:** Are the person's skin and hair dirty?

- **Grooming:** Does the person look rumpled or disheveled?

- **Walking:** Does the person seem unsteady or have falls?

- **Taking prescribed drugs:** Do prescriptions last longer than they should? Are prescriptions used up faster than they should be? Are pills mixed together in one container?

- **Using the telephone:** Does the person seem to understand phone conversations? Is the phone consistently answered when the person is known to be home?

- **Managing money:** Are bills unpaid, leading to overdue notices? Has the person repeatedly been notified of overdrafts on accounts?

- **Preparing food:** Are food items kept past expiration dates? Do pots and pans seem to become scalded repeatedly? Has the stove been found left on?

- **Doing laundry:** Are clothes clean?

Rewards and Challenges

Caregiving can be very rewarding, even when it is hard work and causes stress. Many people choose to care for a spouse, partner, or parent out of love and respect. They find new meaning in their own life by making a difference in another person's life, even if their efforts are not always appreciated. However, no one can ever be fully prepared for the challenges of caregiving.

Physically, mentally, financially, and emotionally, caregiving can be demanding, as in the following situations:

- Caregivers may have to do all household tasks, dress and bathe the person, make sure the person follows the prescribed drug regimen, manage the person's finances, or a combination.

- They may spend their life's savings while they care for a dependent parent or spouse, or they may have to quit their job to care for the person.

- They may have to continually attend to the person's emotional needs.

- They may have to give up activities they enjoy.

- Family members may disagree or argue about who should provide or pay for the care and about other aspects of care.

The demands may be more trying when caregivers themselves are frail, have been thrust into their role

Avoiding Caregiver Burnout

Caregivers can help avoid burnout by doing the following:

- Learning about the cause, symptoms, and long-term effects of the older person's condition
- Anticipating changes in the older person and in the level of care the older person needs
- Letting the older person make decisions and solve problems as much as possible
- Knowing their own limits
- Not taking the older person's anger, frustration, or difficult behaviors personally (these behaviors may be symptoms of a disorder such as dementia)
- Avoiding arguments
- Discussing responsibilities with other family members and friends, then asking them to help when appropriate and possible
- Discussing feelings and experiences with a friend, someone who has had similar experiences, or people in a support group
- Eating and exercising regularly and getting enough sleep
- Scheduling regular time for relaxing, enjoyable activities
- Obtaining information about the older person's financial resources
- Avoiding depleting personal finances
- Contacting organizations that can provide information and referrals for caregivers
- Using day care or respite care to get a temporary break when needed
- Hiring a home health aide or health care practitioner, such as a licensed practical nurse (LPN) or nurse's aide, to help if needed
- Talking to a counselor, therapist, or clergyman if needed
- Remembering that an assisted living facility or a nursing home may be the best option

unexpectedly or reluctantly, or must care for someone who is uncooperative or combative.

The many responsibilities and conflicts that come with caring for an older person can isolate a caregiver, compromise relationships, and threaten job opportunities. They can lead to mounting anger, frustration, guilt, anxiety, stress, depression, and a sense of helplessness and exhaustion. These feelings are sometimes called caregiver burnout. Burnout can affect anyone at any time but is more likely when the person being cared for cannot be left alone or is

disruptive overnight. In the worst cases, when caregivers are unaware of or are unable to obtain help, burnout can lead to abandonment and even abuse of the older person (see page 1934).

To determine how to provide the help an older person needs and to avoid caregiver burnout, caregivers often need to talk with different practitioners, including doctors, nurses, physical and occupational therapists, social workers, and a care manager (a specialist trained in making sure that older people receive all the help and care they need—see page 1903). Caregivers can also use strategies to prepare themselves for caregiving and to avoid caregiver burnout.

Long-Distance Caregiving

In a modern, mobile society, family members sometimes live hundreds or even thousands of miles apart. Such distances complicate efforts to ensure that older family members receive the care that they need. Long-distance caregivers—usually adult children—have many challenges.

Good communication is often difficult to maintain. Family members may feel that they never get a complete or accurate impression of how the older person is managing or what is needed. Even when needs are understood, family members may feel there is little they can do for the older person unless they are there to do it.

Family members can take several steps to make helping from a distance less worrisome:

- Scheduling a regular time for phone calls, which can be reassuring for everyone
- Communicating by e-mail or Internet videoconferencing with a computer-mounted camera
- Finding a person who can visit their loved one regularly and who agrees to call them immediately if questions or concerns arise
- Arranging for participation in some type of meal program (such as Meals on Wheels) if shopping, meal preparation, and eating are concerns
- Installing a home security system if security is a concern
- Setting up a personal emergency response system (medical alert device) if falling is a concern

Also, family members should have copies of any advance directives, such as a living will or durable power of attorney for health care, so that they can help if their loved one needs emergency treatment.

Family members can get help from people who are familiar with resources in the community where the older person resides. The older person's primary care doctor may be helpful in arranging for local assistance. Or family members can arrange for a geriatric care manager to oversee the caregiving and health care. However, family members sometimes believe they have no other choice than to go and help directly. The Family Medical Leave Act permits people to keep their job while taking up to 12 weeks of unpaid leave to attend to a dependent family member. Only large employers are required to provide this protection, and there are other restrictions, such as those about employee eligibility.

Settings for Care

Health care practitioners may provide care for older people in a variety of settings.

Doctor's Office: Most older people receive medical care as outpatients. That is, they see their doctor in an office, then they go home. The office may be in a medical office building, a clinic, a hospital, or elsewhere. Diagnostic tests, such as blood tests or x-rays, are often done in a doctor's office. If not, they may be done at a nearby clinic. Some doctors' offices offer certain treatments, such as physical therapy.

Hospitals: Hospitals provide the most comprehensive medical care, usually to people who are very sick. Older people may enter the hospital through the emergency department, or they may be scheduled for admission by a doctor.

A doctor (who may be the person's primary care doctor, a specialist, or a staff doctor at the hospital) is in charge of the person's care in the hospital. Sometimes several other doctors are involved. Nurses, who are available 24 hours a day, provide much of the care. A nurse is always available, but doctors may come and go at more irregular times.

Many other people may help provide care in a hospital. They include pharmacists, dietitians, physical and occupational therapists, social workers, medical technicians, nurses' aides, and volunteers.

How long people stay in the hospital depends partly on how sick they are, what the diagnosis is, and, if needed, what arrangements for continuing care can be made after discharge. The health care practitioners involved determine whether and what type of continuing care is needed. This care may be provided in a rehabilitation facility, in a long-term care facility, or in the home by a visiting nurse.

> **? Did You Know...**
> Some senior centers have a nurse on duty for several days a week and provide physical and occupational therapy.

Surgical Centers: Surgical centers are places where same-day surgery may be done. Such surgery involves medical procedures that typically require anesthesia, that are too complicated to be done in a doctor's office, but that do not require an overnight stay in a hospital. Common examples are endoscopy, colonoscopy, and removal of cataracts. Surgical centers may be located in a hospital or be a separate, free-standing facility.

Many communities have surgical centers. Then, people can have procedures in their own community without needing to travel to a more distant hospital.

Rehabilitation Facilities: After discharge from the hospital, people with a severe disability may need to continue their recovery in a rehabilitation facility. A facility may be located in a hospital or a nursing home. These facilities provide skilled nursing care and physical, occupational, and speech therapy.

When people are discharged to a rehabilitation facility, doctors predetermine how long their stay will be. For older people, the stay ranges from several weeks to a few months. Goals for progress are set, and progress is evaluated every day. Thus, the types and amount of therapy can be adjusted as needed.

Some older people need to go to a rehabilitation facility for therapy but do not need to stay there.

Long-Term Care Facilities: When older people need more help than can be provided at home and need it for an indefinite time, a long-term care facility may be appropriate (see page 1917). Older people or family members can choose among several living arrangements that provide different services and levels of health care:

- **Board-and-care facilities** provide a room, meals, and some help with daily activities. Some facilities provide certain basic health care.

- **Assisted living communities** are similar to board-and-care facilities. However, they provide more health care, and most provide 24-hour supervision of the resident if needed. Some of these facilities have a registered nurse on site.

- **Nursing homes** provide nursing care, including giving residents their drugs, in addition to help with daily activities. Nursing homes have at least one registered nurse on site at all times. They also employ licensed practical nurses and nurses' aides. Some homes provide physical and occupational therapy.

- **Life-care communities** provide different levels of services and care, depending on need. For example, if people have early dementia, the community may provide only help with taking drugs and an environment where stimulation is minimized. As the dementia worsens, the community can provide help with all daily activities as needed. Life-care communities guarantee that people, regardless of their health, are cared for within the community for the rest of their life.

Home Health Care: After discharge from the hospital, many older people who are well enough to go home need some help with daily activities or with managing their health care. Home health care agencies provide this help. These agencies employ registered nurses, therapists, home health aides, and social workers.

Some people need home health care for a short time after they leave the hospital. For example, a nurse may be needed to change wound dressings. Other people, especially those with a chronic disorder, need home health care for a longer time. People with a heart or lung disorder may need a nurse to visit regularly and check whether they are worsening or improving. The nurse can also adjust a drug dose if needed. Or a nurse may regularly visit people with diabetes to make sure they are following their treatment plan, to monitor drug use, and to adjust doses as needed. A physical therapist may be needed to help people regain strength and balance or recover from a stroke. A home health aide may be needed to help with shopping, preparing meals, going out in a wheelchair, taking a walk, or bathing. A social worker can determine whether people are receiving the services they need and recommend additional services if needed. A social worker may help arrange for rides to and from medical appointments.

Community Services: In the United States, one source of support services and health care in the community is senior centers. In addition to social, recreational, and educational activities, some senior centers serve meals—an important service for people who cannot prepare their own. Often, senior centers are a place where family members who care for a person full-time can take the person and get a break from care (a service called respite care).

Many senior centers also provide some health care. For example, some senior centers have a nurse on duty at least a few days a week. The nurse can check blood pressure, make sure people are taking their drugs as instructed, and teach people about their disorders. The nurse also helps people with health problems determine whether they need to see a doctor. Sometimes the nurse contacts a person's doctor or family members. Some senior centers provide day care for people with mild to moderate dementia, and some provide physical and occupational therapy.

Other services available in the community include meal programs (such as Meals on Wheels), transportation services, help with daily activities, support groups, and respite care. Some religious communities provide many of these services. These services are usually inexpensive, and some are free.

Information about community services, including senior centers, can be obtained from the hospital discharge planning or case management department, home health care agencies, local health departments, and religious communities. Senior centers can also be found by looking in a local telephone book or on the Internet.

Day Hospitals: Day hospitals provide hospital care only during the day. They are usually located in a hospital. They enable people to have complex tests and treatments without having to check into an overnight (inpatient) hospital. Day hospitals are particularly useful for people who need rehabilitation over a period of time—for example, for people who have had a stroke or amputation of a leg. These hospitals also provide meals and transportation to and from medical appointments and therapy sessions.

The primary care doctor or a hospital may send a person to a day hospital. Day hospitals are usually used for a limited period of time (6 weeks to 6 months).

Hospice Care: For people who have a progressive, incurable disorder, hospice care provides the treatments and services needed to control symptoms, ease pain, and help people and their family members prepare for the death (see page 60). Hospice care may be provided in a person's home, in a nursing home, or in a hospice facility.

Hospice care usually involves a doctor, nurse, and social worker trained to care for dying people. Pharmacists, counselors, physical therapists, ethicists, and volunteers may also be involved. These practitioners are needed to make sure that all of the person's physical and psychologic needs are met as well as possible. Most people who receive hospice care do not have to go to a hospital before they die. Thus, they can die in a more comfortable, intimate environment, often with loved ones around them. Hospice care also involves helping family members prepare for the death and understand what to do when the person dies.

CHAPTER

293 Health Care Coverage for Older People

Dealing with the costs of a serious or chronic disorder can be as distressing as dealing with the disorder itself. The costs are often beyond the personal resources of most people. For older people, most health care expenses are paid for by the following:

- Medicare: It helps people who are age 65 or older, who are disabled, or who need kidney dialysis.
- Medicaid: It helps certain people who are poor or disabled.
- Other government programs such as the Department of Veterans Affairs (VA): The VA provides health care for honorably discharged veterans who meet certain eligibility requirements.

These programs are supplemented by private insurance or personal funds, including those of family members.

Understanding how Medicare, Medicaid, or other government programs work is complicated. What is completely paid for, what is partly paid for, who pays for how much of what, and how the payments are arranged can be difficult to understand. The programs change frequently, and for Medicaid, the regulations vary from state to state. The government and health care foundations provide current information about these programs on the Internet and in booklets available by mail. But part of the problem is the complexity and fragmented nature of the health care system and of the payment system for health care.

Health care can be paid for in two ways (see also page 23):

- **Fee-for-service:** Health care practitioners and institutions are paid for each hospital stay, each visit to a practitioner, each test, and each treatment.
- **Capitation:** Practitioners and institutions are paid a fixed amount to provide health care for a specific group of people regardless of how many visits, tests, or procedures those people have or how much they cost.

Some health care plans are managed. Managed care (see page 26) simply means that a health care plan gives directions to health care practitioners and institutions about what care should be provided and when. These directions are intended to help ensure better, more consistent care and to control costs. Managed care can include HMOs, preferred provider organizations (PPOs), point-of-service (POS) plans, or a combination.

Medicare

Medicare is a health insurance program that helps older people pay for health care services. It is funded by the federal government. About 45 million people are covered by Medicare. Of these, 38 million are age 65 and older and 7 million are younger but have certain permanent disabilities. Although it is funded by the government, Medicare is administered by private insurance companies, called intermediaries.

Medicare offers two types of health care plans: the original Medicare plan (Part A and Part B) and Medicare Part C, also known as Medicare Advantage. Medicare Part C offers alternative plans for health care, including managed care and fee-for-service care. Medicare Part D offers prescription drug coverage.

Medicare Eligibility: People generally are eligible for Medicare if they are

- Age 65 or older
- On kidney dialysis or have had a kidney transplant
- Under age 65 with certain disabilities

Deductibles and Copayments: Medicare pays only for services it considers appropriate (called covered services). For each covered service, Medicare has what is called an allowable charge. The allowable charge is the maximum amount Medicare will permit health care providers to charge people on Medicare for a service. However, Medicare does not pay for all of the allowable charges for covered services. The first time a certain service is needed, people must usually pay a small fixed amount (called a deductible) before Medicare pays anything. If people need the same service again after a specified time has passed, they have to pay another deductible. After the deductible has been paid, people usually also have to pay a certain percentage of the costs (called a copayment) each time they use a service. For example, in 2009, the deductible for outpatient services (such as a doctor's visit) was $135 for the calendar year, and the copayment for each use of most outpatient services was 20% of the allowable charges. This arrangement means that people pay the first $135 of their outpatient bills. Then, for the rest of the year, they pay 20% of the allowable charges each time they use a service, and Medicare pays 80%. When the calendar year is over, the process starts over, and people must pay another deductible for services used that year.

Who Needs Long-Term Care Insurance?

Because people are living longer, more people are likely to need long-term care. Long-term care involves helping people function as well as possible. It includes help with daily activities, such as preparing meals, bathing, and dressing, as well as help with health care. Long-term care may be provided in the home or a long-term care facility, such as a nursing home.

Long-term care is expensive and, as suggested by its name, is usually needed for a long time. Thus, many people need help paying for it. Many people mistakenly think that Medicare covers long-term care.

Whether to buy long-term care insurance depends on several things:

Need: Is long-term care insurance needed?

People who do not need this insurance include those

- Whose only income comes from Social Security and who have limited assets
- Who qualify for Medicaid or will qualify soon after they enter a nursing home that accepts Medicaid insurance
- Who have large financial reserves and can afford to pay for long-term care without insurance

People who should consider this insurance include those who are neither rich nor poor and

- Who want to protect their assets or those of a family member
- Who do not want to depend on a family member for care
- Who want to make sure they receive high-quality care
- Who want to have more control over when, how, and where they receive care—for example, in their home rather than in a nursing home

Costs: Will buying long-term care insurance cause financial hardship?

People should consider whether they can pay the premiums over the long-term, even if their income decreases.

They should find out how often and how much premiums increase and how many days a person has to pay for before the insurance pays (the elimination period).

Timing: Is it better to buy long-term care insurance now or later?

The younger people are, the more cheaply they can buy long-term care insurance. On the other hand, the younger people are when they start paying for it, the longer they are likely to pay before they need to use it. However, if people wait too long, they may develop disorders that make long-term care insurance difficult or impossible to obtain.

Coverage: People who have decided to buy long-term care insurance have to decide how many years of coverage they want (the benefit period). The average stay in a nursing home is 2 to 3 years, so most people choose a slightly longer time: 4 to 6 years.

People must also decide what maximum amount is needed to pay for each day of care (the daily benefit). The amount should be close to the average cost of care at local nursing homes.

Policies vary in many important details, so they must be carefully evaluated. For example, people must decide the following:

- Whether they want built-in inflation protection
- Whether they want a well-defined trigger for the start of benefits—for example, when they can no longer do a basic daily activity, such as bathing or dressing
- Whether benefits for home care are comparable with those for nursing home care
- Whether the policy has certain tax advantages, such as deduction of premiums from taxable income as medical expenses and exclusion of benefits from taxable income (called tax-qualified plans)

Supplemental Insurance: Some people have supplemental insurance to help pay for Medicare co-payments and other medical expenses that are not covered by Medicare. This insurance is sometimes provided by people's previous employer as part of a retirement benefit. Other people buy supplemental health insurance from private insurance companies. People who have low income and few assets may be eligible for supplemental coverage through the government-funded Medicaid program.

Some people buy supplemental insurance to pay for long-term care. The decision to buy long-term care insurance depends partly on whether people expect to need help paying for long-term care and on whether they can afford the long-term care insurance.

Original Medicare Plan

Available nationwide, the original Medicare plan operates on a fee-for-service basis. It has two parts:

- Part A (often referred to as hospital insurance) covers hospital services and some outpatient services commonly needed for a short time after a hospital stay.
- Part B (often referred to as medical insurance) covers outpatient services, including doctors' fees.

With the original Medicare plan, choice of doctor and hospital is not limited. However, some doctors require that people pay the bill and fill out the paperwork (file the claim) for reimbursement by Medicare. Other doctors file the claim themselves and receive payment directly from Medicare.

WHO PAYS FOR WHAT?

TYPE OF CARE	SERVICES	COVERED BY
Hospital care	Inpatient care, including mental health care General nursing and other hospital services and supplies Drugs used during hospitalization A semiprivate room (a private room only if medically necessary) Meals	Medicare Part A Medicare Part C (Medicare Advantage) Medicaid Department of Veterans Affairs (VA)*
Short-term care in a certified skilled nursing facility (nursing home)	Skilled nursing care Social services Drugs used in the facility Medical supplies and equipment used in the facility Dietary counseling Physical, occupational, and speech therapy (if needed) to meet the person's health goals Transportation by ambulance (when other transportation endangers health) to the nearest facility providing needed services unavailable at the skilled nursing facility A semiprivate room Meals	Medicare Part A if people need short-term care temporarily after a hospital stay Medicare Part C if people need short-term care temporarily after a hospital stay Medicaid VA*
Outpatient care	Doctor's, nurse practitioner's, and physician assistant's fees Emergency department visits Transportation by ambulance (when other transportation endangers health) Outpatient surgery (with no overnight stay in the hospital) Rehabilitation (physical, occupational, and speech therapy) Diagnostic tests, such as x-rays and laboratory tests Outpatient mental health care Outpatient dialysis A second opinion if surgery is recommended and a third opinion if opinions differ For people with diabetes, diabetes supplies, self-management training, eye examinations, and nutrition counseling Smoking cessation Durable medical equipment, such as wheelchairs, hospital beds, oxygen, and walkers	Medicare Part B Medicare Part C Medicaid VA*
Home health care	Personal care, including help with eating, bathing, going to the bathroom, dressing Part-time skilled nursing care Physical, occupational, and speech therapy Home health aide services Social services Medical supplies, such as wound dressings, but not prescription drugs	Medicare Part A if people are homebound and need part-time skilled nursing care or rehabilitation on a daily basis Medicare Part B Medicare Part C Medicaid VA

(continued on the following page)

WHO PAYS FOR WHAT? (*Continued*)

TYPE OF CARE	SERVICES	COVERED BY
Preventive care	Screening tests for prostate and colorectal cancer Mammography Papanicolaou (Pap) test Bone density measurements Glaucoma tests Influenza, pneumococcal, and hepatitis B vaccinations Diabetes screening Cholesterol screening	Medicare Part B Medicare Part C Medicaid VA*
Extra benefits	Prescription drugs Eyeglasses Hearing aids	Medicare Part C Medicare Part D (prescription drug plans) Medicaid in some states VA*
Long-term care in an assisted living community	Varies greatly from community to community Meals Help with daily activities Some social and recreational activities Some health care	Medicaid in a few states (partial coverage) VA* in some situations
Long-term care in a skilled nursing facility (nursing home)	Varies from state to state	Medicaid VA*
Hospice care	Physical care and counseling Room and meals only during inpatient respite care and short-term hospital stays	Medicare Part A Medicare Part C

*For the Veterans Administration, the rules of eligibility vary for different services and change frequently.

Some doctors do not accept Medicare payments as full payment (that is, they do not accept "assignment" from Medicare). They may charge more for a service than Medicare pays. (Medicare pays a set amount—what it considers a usual, customary, and reasonable amount—for each service it covers.) Generally, these doctors charge up to an extra 15% of the Medicare-approved amount. Paying any extra charges is the person's responsibility. So people should ask doctors in advance if they accept Medicare as full payment.

Part A: Enrollment in Part A is automatic for most people when they reach age 65. Anyone who is eligible for Social Security, Railroad Retirement, or Civil Service Retirement benefits has Part A. Such people are sent their Medicare card about 3 months before their 65th birthday. Part A is paid for by a federal tax that is automatically deducted each month from payroll checks (as for Social Security). Thus, people who are enrolled in Part A do not have to pay monthly fees for it. People who continue to work after age 65 should enroll in Part A during open enrollment (the 6-month period starting 3 months before their 65th birthday and ending 3 months after). Enrolling after this period often costs more. People who are not eligible may be able to purchase Part A.

Part A helps pay for the following:

- Hospital care
- Care in a skilled nursing facility but only if services are needed daily after a related minimum 3-day stay in a hospital
- Hospice care but only for people nearing the end of life

When hospice care is selected, the hospice organization manages all benefits from Medicare (and Medicaid).

For people who are homebound and need part-time skilled nursing care or rehabilitation, Part A helps pay for home health care, including help with personal care (such as bathing, going to the bathroom, and dressing). Part A does not pay for home health care or long-term care that does not involve skilled nursing care.

Part A pays for care on the basis of benefit periods. A benefit period begins when people are admitted to a hospital or skilled nursing facility and ends when they have been out of the facility for 60 days in a row. If they are readmitted after the 60 days, a new deductible must be paid. There is no limit to the number of benefit periods.

Part B: This part is optional. If people are eligible for Part A, they are eligible for Part B. People who choose to enroll can purchase Part B insurance for a fee paid each month. The fee is usually deducted from their Social Security, Railroad Retirement, or Civil Service Retirement check. The best time to sign up for Part B is during open enrollment. Otherwise, the rates may be higher. At age 65, some people are still working, or their spouse is still working. Many of these people have health insurance through their or their spouse's employer. These people have a delayed enrollment option, which enables them to enroll in Part B later but at the open-enrollment rate. The open-enrollment rate for Part B changes every year. In 2009, the rate was $96.40 a month per person, but it was higher if annual income was more than $85,000 for single people or more than $170,000 for married people who file a joint tax return. These rates range from $134.90 to $308.30, depending on people's income.

Part B helps pay for many services and supplies that are used on an outpatient basis and that are medically necessary, such as the following:

- Doctor's fees
- Emergency department visits
- Outpatient surgery (with no overnight stay in the hospital)
- Transportation by ambulance when other types of transportation are likely to be unsafe
- Rehabilitation
- Diagnostic tests
- Outpatient mental health care
- Reusable (durable) medical equipment, such as wheelchairs, for home use

Part B may pay for home health care for home-bound people when Part A does not. If surgery is recommended, Part B helps pay for a second opinion and, if opinions differ, a third opinion. For people with diabetes, Part B pays for some of the costs of monitoring sugar (glucose) levels in the blood. Part B helps pay for some preventive care. Examples are an annual influenza (flu) vaccine and screening tests such as mammography, Papanicolaou (Pap) tests, bone density measurements, and tests for prostate cancer and colorectal cancer. It helps pay for glaucoma tests for people who are at increased risk because they are black and over 50, have diabetes, or have a family history of glaucoma.

Limitations of Parts A and B: Neither Part A nor Part B covers the following:

- Private-duty nursing
- A telephone and television in the hospital
- A private hospital room (unless medically necessary)
- Most prescription drugs and all nonprescription drugs
- Personal care at home or in a nursing home unless people also need skilled nursing care or rehabilitation
- Hearing aids
- Vision care
- Dental care
- Care outside the United States, except in certain circumstances
- Experimental procedures
- Some preventive care
- Cosmetic surgery
- Most chiropractic services
- Acupuncture

Medicare Part C

Medicare Part C (Medicare Advantage) allows people to enroll in a private health insurance plan instead of the traditional fee-for-service Medicare (additional information is available at the Medicare web site). For this plan, Medicare makes arrangements with other organizations, such as insurance companies, hospital systems, or managed care organizations, to provide care. The Part C option is available in many areas of the United States. Part C plans vary from state to state.

Most Medicare Part C plans are managed care plans. However, some are unrestricted, private fee-for-service plans. In these fee-for-service plans, people can choose any doctor or hospital, and the plan pays for a share of the cost. However, a private company, not Medicare, decides how much a service costs, so costs may be higher than when the original Medicare plan is used.

Medicare managed care is handled by a health maintenance organization (HMO) or preferred provider organization (PPO).

- In HMOs, people choose a primary care doctor within the HMO's network. (The network includes doctors, medical clinics, and hospitals that the

HMO has selected and contracted with to care for its members.) The primary care doctor may refer people to other health care practitioners as needed. Practitioners must be part of the HMO network for the HMO to cover care. Emergency care when people are out of the area is an exception.

- In PPOs, people can, within some limits, choose doctors outside the PPO's network. But the monthly fee for PPOs is higher than that for HMOs.

Some HMOs offer a point-of-service (POS) option for an additional monthly fee. As in PPOs, people with this option can choose some doctors outside the HMO's network, and the HMO pays for part of the costs.

Medicare Part C provides all services covered by Parts A and B, including preventive care. Some plans offer coordination of care, lower or no deductibles and copayments, and benefits not covered by the original Medicare plan. For example, the plans may help pay for prescription drugs, eyeglasses, hearing aids, and assessment by an interdisciplinary team that specializes in caring for older people. People with Medicare Part C continue to pay a monthly fee for Part B and may have to pay an additional monthly fee for the extra benefits. The amount depends on the plan they choose. However, the additional fee is still usually less than that for a supplemental Medigap plan.

When deciding about Medicare options, people should consider what they want in terms of out-of-pocket costs, extra benefits, choice of doctors, convenience, and quality.

Medicare Part D

Medicare Part D helps cover costs of prescription drugs. To obtain Part D, people have to sign up for it (enroll) and pay the required monthly premium. Enrollment involves choosing a plan provided by an insurance or other company working with Medicare. There are over 1,600 plans available nationwide. The best time for people to enroll in Part D is when they first become eligible for Medicare. If they enroll later and they have not had another comparable plan for drug coverage during that time, their monthly premium is increased by an additional 1% for each month that they delay.

Covered Drugs: Each plan has a list of drugs it covers—called a formulary. The drugs covered by each plan vary, but the list must include at least two effective drugs in the categories and classes of drugs most commonly prescribed for people who use Medicare. Each plan may make changes to the list of drugs they cover. A plan that covered a person's drugs one year may not cover some of them the next year. Also, doctors may prescribe new drugs that are not

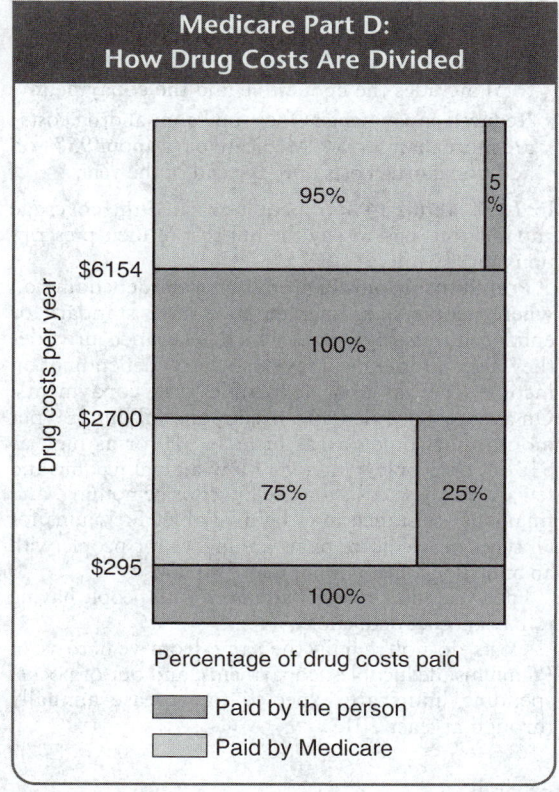

**Medicare Part D:
How Drug Costs Are Divided**

Drug costs per year

95%   5%

$6154

100%

$2700

75%   25%

$295

100%

Percentage of drug costs paid

▢ Paid by the person
▢ Paid by Medicare

covered by the plan. Thus, people must review their plan each year to ensure that the plan continues to meet their needs.

Standard Benefits: Medicare has defined a standard benefit plan. Companies must offer a plan that is at least equal in value. Many companies also offer enhanced plans that provide more coverage (such as a lower deductible or no deductible), but these plans have higher monthly premiums.

Medicare does not cover all drug costs. In 2009, the standard Part D benefit involves the following costs:

- **Annual deductible:** Before receiving any reimbursement, people must pay the first $295 of drug costs.

- **Copayments:** For the next $2405 of drug costs (after the $295 deductible), people must pay 25% of costs (the copayment) for each prescription themselves (out of pocket). Medicare pays the other 75%. Thus, the copayment for the first $2700 of drug costs is $601.25 in addition to the $295 deductible.

- **Coverage gap:** After the first $2700 of drug costs, people must pay all drug costs on the next $3154 of costs—that is, until total drug costs equal $6154. At this point, people will have spent a total of $4350 out of pocket. This out-of-pocket total includes the deductible and the copayment.

- **Reduced copayments:** Once total annual drug costs are more than $6154, Medicare pays about 95% of additional drug costs until the end of the year.

In 2007, about 14% of people reached the coverage gap and thus had to pay the full cost of their prescriptions for a while.

Premiums: Monthly premiums vary depending on where people live, whether they have standard or enhanced coverage, and which insurance provider they use. Premiums may also vary depending on income level, as may deductibles and copayments. On average, people pay a premium of about $30 per month, but some pay as little as $10 or as high as $136. For people with a very low annual income and few assets, these costs may be lower or be nothing, and financial assistance may be available. Premiums for all types of Medicare plans are higher for people with an annual income of more than $80,000.

Each year, the process starts over, with people having to pay another deductible.

Costs do not remain the same from year to year. Premiums, deductibles, copayments, and out-of-pocket spending limits are expected to increase annually through at least 2013.

PACE Program

The Program of All-Inclusive Care for the Elderly (PACE) is another Medicare option that is designed to provide more comprehensive, better-integrated health care for older people. This program uses funds from Medicare and Medicaid. As a type of managed care, it may require a monthly fee. PACE is available in 13 states.

PACE is designed for older people frail enough to need care in a nursing home. However, the goal of PACE is to enable older people to live at home as long as possible. In PACE, an interdisciplinary team assesses the participant's needs, develops a care plan, and provides all necessary health care. It includes medical and dental care, adult day care (including transportation to and from the facility), health and personal care at home, prescription drugs, social services, rehabilitation, meals, nutrition counseling, and hospital and long-term care when needed.

Medigap

Medigap is supplemental insurance designed to pay for medical care not covered by Medicare, including the deductibles and copayments required by Medicare

and extra charges by doctors who do not accept Medicare as full payment for a service. To obtain a Medigap policy, people must be enrolled in Medicare parts A and B and must not be enrolled in Medicare Part C. Medigap policies do not duplicate payment for services covered by Medicare Parts A and B. The best time to purchase Medigap insurance is during its enrollment period, which begins when Medicare Part B is purchased and ends 6 months later. At other times, Medigap may be unavailable or more expensive. Many insurance companies offer Medigap insurance.

There are 10 types of Medigap policies, labeled A through J. Each type offers a different set of benefits. But the benefits of a specific type are the same no matter which insurance company offers it. No Medigap policy covers payment for long-term personal care (at home or in a nursing home), vision or dental care, hearing aids, private-duty nursing, or all prescription drugs. However, additional insurance policies that cover such services can be purchased.

Medicaid

Medicaid is a program funded jointly by the federal and state governments to help pay for health care. It is intended for people of all ages who have a very low income and few assets. Eligibility requirements for Medicaid vary from state to state. People who are on Medicare may also qualify for Medicaid, which helps pay for some expenses not covered by Medicare.

If people have a very low income but have assets such as a home or stock investments, they may not qualify for Medicaid. To qualify, they may have to spend down. That is, they may have to sell their stocks and other assets and use the money to pay for health care until their income plus assets is low enough to qualify. To avoid having to spend down, some people give their assets away, often to family members. However, to qualify for Medicaid, they cannot have given these assets away within the 3 years before care was needed. In some states, people may be able to keep their home so that certain family members can remain there. However, when the family members leave, the government can sell the home to recover the money it has spent on care.

If people qualify for Medicaid and Medicare, most health care costs are covered.

Medicaid is the main public payer for long-term care, such as skilled nursing care (including that in a nursing home). For older people, Medicaid often pays for nursing home care. Medicaid is required to offer long-term care to eligible people who are 21 years or older and who participate in the Medicaid program. Medicaid also helps pay for the following:

- Hospital care
- Laboratory tests (such as blood and urine tests)
- Diagnostic tests (such as x-rays)
- Visits to the doctor
- Vaccinations
- Home health care

Because each state manages its own Medicaid program, the services covered vary from state to state. In some states, Medicaid helps pay for other items, such as prescription drugs, dental care, eyeglasses, and inter-mediate-level nursing care. Intermediate-level nursing care involves less care than skilled nursing care but more care than personal care. Its purpose is to maintain a person's condition and, if possible, to improve it.

Health care practitioners who provide care to people covered by Medicaid must accept what Medicaid pays as their full reimbursement. However, because this rate is often low, some practitioners choose not to provide care to people covered by Medicaid. Also, some nursing homes do not accept Medicaid insurance.

CHAPTER

294 Long-Term Care

The prospect of needing long-term care services concerns many older people. The likelihood of needing long-term care increases greatly as people age. Older people are more likely to develop chronic disorders and to have problems functioning. Learning about the many types of long-term care can help people choose the right time and place for this care. How long care is needed varies from weeks to years to indefinitely.

The focus of long-term care is on helping people function. It helps them do the activities necessary to care for themselves and to live as independently as possible. These activities include basic daily activities (such as eating, dressing, bathing, grooming, and walking) and other activities (such as shopping, balancing a checkbook, doing laundry, and cleaning). Long-term care usually includes help with health care. Most long-term care facilities also provide social and recreational activities.

Many people have their first experience with long-term care after a hospital stay. During an illness or after an injury, many older people lose some or all of the ability to care for themselves. Thus, although they may be well enough to leave the hospital, they may need to go to a long-term care facility for rehabilitation and recovery. This move can be physically and psychologically demanding. People have to adjust to many new faces and to new routines for sleeping, bathing, dressing, eating, and other daily activities. The move happens quickly, with little time to adjust.

Most people associate long-term care with a change in residence:

- To the home of a family member
- To a retirement community
- To an assisted living community
- To a board-and-care facility
- To a life-care community
- To a nursing home

However, only one third of older people who receive long-term care live in an institutional setting. The others receive care in their own home or in the home of a family member. People who receive care in institutions are usually those who have more physical and thinking (cognitive) problems, less social support from family members and friends, or both.

What type of arrangement is possible depends partly on a person's needs (medical, functional, social, and emotional). However, it also depends on a person's preference, finances, and social support (for example, family members' willingness and ability to help). One person may be able to live at home with the help of a spouse. Another person with similar problems but without family support may need to go to a nursing home.

After the type of arrangement needed is determined, a particular facility must be carefully chosen. Within each type, facilities differ considerably in environment, services (including health care), activities, living arrangements, and rules. Sometimes the difference is simply a matter of what people can afford, but even within a price range, quality varies.

Care in the Home

Care in the home is usually provided by family members, friends, or both. If needed, health care practitioners, such as visiting nurses, therapists, and home health aides, may come to the home to provide additional care. Home care is often coordinated by a community health agency after a period of acute hospitalization. Medicare provides time-limited

TYPES OF LONG-TERM CARE

TYPE	SERVICES	TYPICAL LIVING ARRANGEMENT	FUNDING
Assisted living communities	Meals (in a common dining room or in the person's room) Social and recreational activities Help with daily activities In some facilities, monitors for emergencies (such as intercoms and personal emergency response systems), services of nurses and physical therapists, and 24-hour supervision if needed	Apartments or occasionally just a bedroom with a private bath	Mostly private funds or long-term care insurance Help from Medicaid in some states
Board-and-care facilities	Meals (in a common dining room or in the person's room) Transportation to medical appointments or shops Social activities Help with personal care and sometimes some help with taking drugs (for example, reminding people to take their drugs)	Rooms on a common hallway	Mostly private funds
Life-care communities	Meals (usually in a common dining room, except for residents who need more care and who have meals in their room) Transportation Social and recreational activities As much help with daily activities and health care as needed	Varied arrangement according to need	Mostly private funds Help from Medicare and Medicaid for skilled nursing care when it is needed
Nursing homes	Meals Help with daily activities 24-hour skilled nursing care, rehabilitation (physical, occupational, respiratory, and speech therapy) Hospice care Oversight by a doctor	Rooms on a common hallway	Private funds Medicaid Medicare for skilled care for a short time in certified nursing homes if care is needed daily after a hospital stay lasting 3 days or more

coverage for services that are classified as skilled, such as wound care or the monitoring of active illnesses such as heart failure or diabetes. When people no longer need skilled care, they are usually responsible for the costs of any further nursing care. Long-term care insurance or Medicaid (for people who qualify) may cover home care services. Veterans may also qualify for home care services depending on their needs and disability rating.

Sometimes the primary doctor coordinates a team of health care practitioners who work together to provide better care for people living at home with a chronic disorder or disability. This arrangement is called a patient-centered home.

PACE: The program for all-inclusive care for the elderly (PACE) is a benefit provided under Medicare and Medicaid (see page 1916). This program is available (only in certain areas of the United States) to people who are at least 55 years old and who meet their state's standards for requiring care in a nursing home. Services provided by the PACE program allow nearly all participants to live at home, although nursing home care is provided if needed.

Delaying the Need for a Long-Term Care Facility

The idea of going to a long-term care facility, particularly a nursing home, does not appeal to most people. The following problems are common reasons for entering a long-term care facility. However, sometimes problems can be solved, and the need for a long-term care facility can be delayed or avoided.

Urinary incontinence: People with urinary incontinence may be hard to care for at home. However, urinary incontinence may be caused by a disorder that can be treated. Treating the disorder may cure the incontinence. People with urinary incontinence, their family members, or their caregivers should talk with a doctor to find out whether treatment is possible.

Problems with doing daily activities: Certain devices can help people function better. A physical or occupational therapist or a home health nurse can observe people in their home and can sometimes help them

choose appropriate devices that will enable them to continue to function safely at home.

Dementia: Taking care of people with dementia is difficult and frustrating. However, family members can learn ways of dealing with the behavior. For example, to deal with wandering, family members can place an identification bracelet on the person or purchase or rent a monitoring device. Learning more about how to care for people with dementia may delay the need for a long-term care facility.

Caregiver burnout: Strongly motivated family members can usually provide elaborate and detailed care. However, providing such care can wear them out physically and emotionally. Talking with health care practitioners can help. They can provide information about caregiving support groups and about groups that provide temporary (respite) care.

PACE involves an interdisciplinary team including doctors, nurses, physical and occupational therapists, social workers, dieticians, and drivers. The services are typically provided in an adult day health center and are available every day. The program provides transportation to the center. Some services may be provided in the home.

The Department of Health and Human Services web site explains PACE and provides an up-to-date list of participating health care practitioners.

Retirement Communities

Retirement communities are designed for people who can live independently but who need or want some help, mainly with caring for a home. Some older people choose to move to a retirement community before they need additional help. They may move because they do not want the responsibility of maintaining a large house and yard or because they have become lonely or isolated.

Retirement communities consist of a group of apartments, townhouses, or detached homes. These communities provide some services, such as transportation, entertainment facilities, some on-site nursing services, community meals, laundry services, and house cleaning and maintenance. Such services enable older people who are reasonably well to live independently. Retirement communities may arrange group activities, such as trips, game nights, or lectures by guest speakers. Some have recreational facilities, such as swimming pools and

golf courses. The homes are usually designed for older people. For example, they may have only one floor. Retirement communities enable some people to postpone a move to a facility that provides more intensive long-term care.

Some retirement communities are part of a life-care community (see page 1920). Life-care communities provide as much care as people need for the rest of their life.

Because retirement communities vary so much, people should ask questions to make sure the community they are considering is suitable for them.

- Is there an entrance fee in addition to the monthly fee? Which services, activities, and amenities are included in the monthly fee?
- What services, activities, and amenities are available? Is there a bank, beauty salon, post office, or general store? Is transportation readily available for trips to local shopping areas, doctors' offices, and other health care facilities? What social and physical activities are available?
- What is the minimum age to live in the community?
- Are the facilities well maintained? Are the living units and their setting pleasant? Is there enough parking?
- Are there service people to help?
- Are meals provided?

Financial Issues: People may rent or purchase their residence in retirement communities often in a condominium-type arrangement. Obtaining financing and conducting the sale or transfer of property are done as with any other private residence. When personal care services are needed, they are usually paid for privately or with long-term care insurance.

Assisted Living Communities

Assisted living communities are designed for people who can care for themselves if they have some help with daily activities. These communities can help older people who have problems with memory, who get confused, or who have physical problems. Some communities have special units for people with dementia where residents can be closely monitored. Assisted living communities may also provide help for couples who wish to continue to live together even though one or both partners require more assistance than the other can provide.

Assisted living communities vary from small and homey to large and elaborate. Residents usually have their own apartment or a bedroom with a bathroom. These communities provide meals, help with daily activities (including personal care), and offer some social and recreational activities. Residents can choose which activities and services they want. Most assisted living communities provide some health care, including 24-hour supervision if needed. Doctors and nurses may visit regularly, and physical therapists may be available. Services and activities offered vary greatly from community to community. Also, regulations for these communities differ from state to state.

When people need intensive treatment, they may have to move to another facility, such as a hospital or rehabilitation center. They may move back to the assisted living community if they are able. But to hold their living space while they are gone, they must continue to pay for it.

People who move to assisted living communities usually need help with daily activities because they have some health problems that limit their ability to function independently. Assisted living communities prefer people who do not need help moving (transferring), for example, from bed to chair. But even when people become relatively impaired, they may be able to stay in these communities because of the help provided. How much help is provided varies considerably from community to community. Generally, an assisted living community is not an alternative to a nursing home. More often, it is a transitional living arrangement that is followed by a move to a nursing home.

Financial Issues: Assisted living communities are usually less expensive than nursing homes because they provide less care. However, they can still be expensive. Although Medicare does not pay for assisted living communities, Medicaid sometimes provides financial support. Many long-term care insurance policies help pay for a significant part of assisted living costs.

Board-and-Care Facilities

Typically, board-and-care facilities are similar to assisted living communities. They are for people who need some help, particularly with personal care. Board-and-care facilities, sometimes also called rest homes, adult care homes, or personal care homes, provide a room, meals, help with daily activities, and occasionally some health care. In board-and-care facilities, people usually live in rooms, as in a college dormitory, rather than in apartments. Some facilities have a very homelike atmosphere.

Board-and-care facilities are not as closely regulated as nursing homes or even some assisted living communities. Many provide good care, but some do not. Some facilities attempt to care for people with very different needs. For example, younger people, many of whom have an untreated or a poorly treated mental disorder, live side by side with older people who do not have a mental disorder. In such an arrangement, the older people may feel uncomfortable or awkward.

Older people and their family members must carefully evaluate a board-and-care facility. They should ask what the facility does and does not provide and make sure that the staff members can meet the needs of the residents and treat them well.

Financial Issues: Typically, the cost of board-and-care facilities is modest when compared with other assisted living options or nursing homes. However, the cost varies widely, from several hundred dollars a month to several thousand, and is paid for with private funds or through Medicaid (for people who qualify).

 Did You Know...
Retirement and assisted living communities vary widely in the services and amenities they offer.

Life-Care Communities

Life-care communities (also called continuing care retirement communities) are for older people who want to move only once, to a place that will provide as much care as they need for the rest of their life. These communities guarantee that residents are cared for within the community regardless of their health. Life-care communities may also provide help for couples who wish to continue to live together or at least near one another even though one partner requires more assistance than the other can provide.

People may begin by living in a house or an apartment. But later, if health deteriorates, people can move to an assisted living community and finally to a nursing home, all on the same property. Life-care communities offer the security of continued care in one location, without having to move very far.

Financial Issues: Many life-care communities are expensive. Some require a large deposit as well as monthly payments and fees for additional services. Sometimes there is an upper limit (cap) for monthly payments and fees. But in many communities, costs increase when the level of services needed increases.

Medicare and Medicaid usually do not pay for residence in a life-care community but may help pay for skilled nursing care when it is needed. Long-term care insurance may provide reimbursement for monthly fees as well as for personal care services, whether provided in an independent living, an assisted living, or a nursing home setting within the life-care community.

Nursing Homes

Nursing homes are for people who need help with health care for chronic conditions but do not need to be hospitalized. The decision to move to a nursing home may be triggered by a change in circumstances. A disorder may suddenly worsen, or an injury may occur. Function may deteriorate suddenly or slowly but steadily. Family circumstances may change, making care at home difficult.

"Nursing home" is sometimes used as a general term for any long-term care facility. But it specifically refers to facilities licensed by the state that can provide both basic and skilled nursing care. "Skilled" indicates that some of the care included can be provided only by trained health care practitioners. "Nursing" indicates that nurses provide most of the care in the facility. Nurses give residents their drugs, monitor disorders, supervise treatments, consult with doctors about care, and organize most of the activities in the nursing home. The nursing staff includes registered nurses (the most highly trained), licensed practical nurses, nursing assistants, and a director of nursing, who oversees nursing care in the home.

Each nursing home also has a medical director, a doctor who oversees the medical care. In some nursing homes, the medical director is the only doctor who provides medical care. But in most nursing homes, several doctors, often working with nurse practitioners or physician assistants, provide care. Sometimes a doctor who has been taking care of the person before the move continues to provide care. Otherwise, the person chooses or is assigned a doctor. According to regulations, a doctor, nurse practitioner, or physician assistant must see every nursing home resident at least once every other month. Many residents see a health care practitioner more often because they need treatment for chronic disorders or they develop additional disorders, such as infections or confusion. Also, nurses may call a doctor to discuss problems and changes in treatments.

Many nursing homes provide other health care services, such as oxygen treatments and drugs or fluids given by vein (intravenous therapies). Almost all nursing homes provide rehabilitation, including physical, occupational, respiratory, and speech therapy. Many people are admitted to nursing homes specifically for rehabilitation, then are discharged to their home after several weeks.

Dentists and medical specialists, such as podiatrists, ophthalmologists, neurologists, or psychiatrists, may examine and treat residents on site. But most often, people with a specific problem have to be transported to a different site for treatment.

Some nursing homes have special units for people with dementia. These units are staffed by specially trained nurses. Many nursing homes provide hospice care for people who are dying.

Almost all nursing homes have a social worker on staff. Social workers help residents adjust to the home. They identify residents who are lonely and withdrawn and help residents, staff members, and family members communicate with each other. They may also help residents and family members make financial arrangements. For example, they may show family members how to apply for Medicare and Medicaid coverage.

Social workers often help coordinate the care provided by the different health care practitioners in a nursing home. These practitioners work together to enable each resident to function as well as possible and to have the best possible quality of life.

Although some nursing homes resemble hospitals rather than homes, many nursing homes are trying to change from a more institutional environment with rules and regulations to a more homelike environment that gives residents more control over their care. Some nursing homes permit pets, encourage residents to maintain existing hobbies or develop new ones, and provide many opportunities for contact between residents and people of all ages who live in the community around the nursing home. Providing this kind of environment is complicated because the residents of nursing homes are usually sick and frail. Many nursing homes have dining rooms, recreation rooms, beauty salons, patios, and gardens. All nursing homes provide recreational and social activities.

Nursing homes are highly regulated by the government. State health departments conduct surveys and inspections to monitor and evaluate quality in nursing homes. A copy of this evaluation is kept at the nursing home and can be reviewed by residents and their family members. Nursing homes also use other programs that monitor and help improve the quality of care.

Even though nursing homes are monitored and regulated by government, they vary considerably in quality, personality, and cost. So people or family

Choosing a Nursing Home

ENVIRONMENT

- Is the nursing home attractive, friendly, homelike, and relaxed?
- Are there any unpleasant odors? Is the nursing home clean and well maintained?
- Are the dining room and other common areas bright, cheery, and pleasant?
- How is the noise level in common areas monitored to prevent it from disturbing residents whose rooms are nearby?
- Are there safe, accessible walking paths on the grounds?
- Is there a garden or patio?
- Does the nursing home have appropriate safety devices, such as fire alarms and sprinklers? What are the plans for emergencies, such as fires?

RESIDENTS

- Is the nursing home accepting new residents?
- Do the residents seem reasonably happy and active, or are they wandering aimlessly or sitting and doing nothing?
- Are the residents clean and appropriately dressed?
- Are any of the residents restrained?

STAFF MEMBERS

- Do the staff members treat the residents with respect, patience, and friendliness?
- Are staff members experienced and qualified?
- Do the residents see the same staff members on a daily basis?
- Is there a high turnover in staff members?
- Do staff members respond to requests for help in a reasonable amount of time?
- What is the ratio of staff members to residents?

ROOMS

- Is there enough storage or closet space?
- Are the residents' rooms bright and cheery?
- Are private rooms available?
- How are roommates selected?
- How are private items stored or secured?
- Can residents have their own telephone and television?
- Is water available and within reach for residents?
- Can residents decorate their rooms with personal items?
- Are there safety features, such as grab bars and pull cords (to call for help)?
- Can residents keep food in their rooms?

MEALS

- What time are meals served?
- Are meals served hot?
- Are snacks available between meals?
- Can residents get from their room to the dining area easily?
- Can meals be provided in a resident's room if needed?
- Are the meals tasty and nutritious?
- How are special dining or menu requests handled? Are choices available at meals?
- Can the nursing home provide special diets when needed? Is there an additional cost?
- Are staff members available to help with feeding during meals?
- Is there a registered dietician on staff?

HEALTH CARE

- Can residents keep their own doctor rather than use the nursing home's doctor?
- How often is the nursing home's doctor available, and where?
- Does the nursing home have an arrangement with a nearby hospital?
- If residents have to be hospitalized, will a bed be available afterward?
- Are other health care practitioners (such as dentists, podiatrists, physical therapists, optometrists, counselors, and social workers) available?
- Are therapy programs (such as physical, occupational, or speech therapy) provided?
- Does the nursing home have special programs for people who have such disorders as Alzheimer's disease or HIV infection?
- What services does the nursing home provide for residents with a terminal disorder?
- How are prescription drugs ordered and given to residents? How is the use of drugs monitored?
- What is the policy on residents keeping nonprescription drugs?
- Are residents and family members encouraged to participate in developing a plan for care?

SERVICES

- Is help with daily dental care provided?
- How is personal laundry done?
- Is reading material available?

VISITING

- Is the nursing home conveniently located for frequent visits by family members and friends?
- Can family members visit any time?

(continued on the following page)

Choosing a Nursing Home (*Continued*)

ACTIVITIES

- What activities are offered?
- Are residents encouraged to participate? How are the residents informed of the activities?
- Is there an activity director?
- Does participation in activities cost extra?
- Are there rooms for other activities, such as a TV or game room?
- Are religious services held on the premises?

COSTS

- Are all the services that residents need covered in the basic charge?
- What services (such as beauty salons or laundry) cost extra, and what is the cost?

RESIDENTS' RIGHTS AND PRIVACY

- Does the nursing home have an active resident or family council or both?

- Are residents allowed to go in and out as they please?
- Are restraints used? When and why?
- Is there a lock on the door to private rooms? Do staff members knock before entering?
- Can married couples live together? Are they given privacy?
- Are the sexual needs of residents respected?
- How often are residents bathed? Can residents have a bath or shower whenever they want? Are bath and shower areas kept warm enough? How much privacy is provided in these areas?
- Are pets allowed? Can visitors bring pets?
- Can residents keep food or alcohol in their rooms?
- What is the nursing home's policy on lost or missing valuables?
- Who contacts family members in case of an emergency?
- If residents wish to leave, what are the policies on giving notice or refunds?

members who are interested in a nursing home should try to get as much information as possible. They can ask the administrator of the nursing home to see the state's evaluation of the home. Similar information is available on the Internet. One evaluation called the Quality Indicator Report looks at how well a nursing home handles specific problems. These problems commonly develop or worsen in residents of nursing homes but can be prevented with attentive care. They include a decline in the ability to do daily activities, undernutrition, weight loss, pressure sores, incontinence, constipation, infections, depression, and use of too many drugs. Whether these evaluations are valid is debated. Nonetheless, they provide information that can help people better compare nursing homes.

Other important questions to ask the administrator include whether the nursing home is certified to provide Medicare and Medicaid coverage, how often care of residents is reviewed, what type of medical care is available, and whether residents and

family members are included in the review of care. For some questions, the administrator may direct people to the nursing home's medical director or director of nursing.

Talking to other people who are familiar with the home is helpful. Such people include long-term care ombudsmen (who visit nursing homes and investigate complaints), doctors, clergy, family members of residents, residents, and employees of the nursing home. Some homes have resident organizations, consisting of family members and friends of residents who meet to discuss issues that come up in the nursing home. These organizations can provide family members of prospective residents with helpful information. However, making an unscheduled visit to a home for several hours is usually the best way to determine whether the quality of services is good and whether the home will be a good place for a loved one.

Financial Issues: In the United States, Medicaid and private funds pay for most nursing home care. Medicare pays for rehabilitative care for a short time in certified nursing homes if skilled care is needed daily after a hospital stay lasting 3 days or more. People are eligible for up to 100 days of Medicare coverage as long as they show continued improvement. Medicare pays all costs for 20 days, then requires a co-payment for the remaining 80 days. After 100 days, payment is either with private funds or, if the person is qualified, through Medicaid.

? Did You Know...
State departments of health regularly evaluate nursing homes, and nursing homes must make these evaluations available to residents and their family members.

295 Coping With Changes Related to Aging

As people grow older, they face many changes. With aging, the ability to do daily activities (functional ability) declines to some degree in every person. Also, older people, on average, tend to have more disorders and disability than do younger people. But the changes that accompany aging are more than just changes in health. As people age, they are often faced with events that can dramatically alter their lives. For example, they may retire from the workforce, lose a loved one, or change their living arrangements.

Whether the changes that accompany aging are viewed as a blessing or a curse may hinge on people's ability to cope with or adapt to change. Successful coping skills are often linked with how well older people stay connected with family and friends, with their community, and with their own values and sense of purpose. In general, older people are well able to cope with the many changes that occur in later life. These transitions can be substantially eased with planning and preparation as well as with outside help tailored to individual needs.

Life-Changing Events

Retirement

When people leave the workforce permanently, they lose one of the most obvious ways to measure their place in society. In addition, they are faced with the decision of what to do with the rest of their life. People who retire often go from a routine that fills much of their day to one with much more free time.

Whether retirement is viewed as a positive or negative event often depends on the reasons for retiring. Some people choose to retire, having looked forward to quitting unpleasant work or to pursuing more fulfilling interests. Others are forced to retire because of employment circumstances, family issues, or poor health.

About one third of retirees have difficulty coping with the consequences of retirement. People who retire unexpectedly because of illness or job loss or who tended to work long hours and bring work home with them may be most likely to experience difficulty. Spouses may have to adjust to seeing more of one another. Some retirees have difficulty coping with a reduced income. Others resent their diminished role in society. They may believe that they are unimportant

and powerless, with little left to contribute. Still others relish the time they now have to pursue their interests, to volunteer, and to enjoy friends and loved ones.

The transition from work to retirement can be eased through planning. Beginning to plan for retirement several years in advance is very helpful. Many employers offer retirement planning services, as do some community agencies. Retirement planning focuses on finding ways to meet financial needs and obligations and on identifying ways to fill available time through part-time employment, volunteer positions, leisure activities, or adoption of a pet. Counseling may help retirees and their families who experience difficulties.

> **? Did You Know...**
> Many employers and community agencies offer retirement planning services.

Losing a Loved One

The death of a loved one can weigh heavily on the heart and mind of an older person. When a spouse or partner or a close family member or friend dies, people feel a strong sense of loss and are reminded of their own mortality. In addition to a loss of companionship, older people may interact less with family and friends and experience a decline in social standing.

The death of a spouse or partner is perhaps the most striking loss older people confront. In some cases, the surviving spouse or partner dies soon afterward, usually when the survivor is the husband rather than the wife. Parents experiencing the death of a child, even in old age, also face a particularly difficult loss.

Older people may be confronted with the death of several loved ones or friends within a brief period of time. Many deaths occurring close together can be particularly difficult to cope with, causing older people to feel especially lonely and isolated. Each death may revive feelings of sadness and grief related to earlier losses.

When people are grieving over the loss of a loved one or friend, sadness is usually apparent. Sadness, a natural response to death, is not the same as depression and therefore does not necessarily indicate a need for treatment. People experience grief and sadness differently, and they may express grief in different ways. Some people are very vocal about their feelings. Others are more private. Some people need more time alone, while others seek out the company of others to help them. Some older people who are grieving are helped by joining a support group or discussing their feelings with a clergy member or counselor.

Feelings of intense sadness over an extended period of time or signs of declining health may indicate depression (see page 863). If grief is prolonged or overwhelming, if people become unable or unwilling to carry out even essential daily activities, or if they speak of suicide, evaluation and treatment by a doctor are necessary. If the doctor diagnoses depression, people may be referred to a mental health practitioner. At times, antidepressant drugs may be helpful. Some older people prefer to be counseled by a clergy member. They may view such counseling as less stigmatizing than that by a mental health practitioner. However, many clergy members do not have extensive training in mental health counseling.

Remarriage

Some older people choose to remarry or live with a new partner after a divorce or the death of a spouse because they desire companionship or intimacy. However, when older people marry, they may have to consider situations that do not usually arise when people marry at younger ages. For example, adult children may oppose a marriage, feeling their parent may be taken advantage of, for example, to care for an ill partner or provide economic support. Other adult children may be concerned about who will inherit their parent's money or personal property.

Some older people may choose not to remarry because marriage restricts their access to benefits (such as survivor's benefits, including medical benefits) from a spouse's pension or social security. Others may be concerned about taking on the role of caregiver.

Older people should ensure that they understand how remarriage will affect their benefits and finances. They may need to consult an attorney before the marriage. Open discussion of the changes in family and lifestyle may minimize conflicts after the marriage.

Changes in Living Arrangements

Living alone is a common situation for many older people and can present many challenges.

- People who live alone are more likely to be poor, and poverty is increasingly more likely the longer they live alone.

- Many older people who live alone describe feelings of loneliness and isolation.

- Because eating is a social activity for most people, some older people who live alone do not prepare full, balanced meals. Thus, undernutrition becomes a concern.

- Among people with health problems or difficulty seeing or hearing, it is all too easy for new or worsening symptoms of disease to go unnoticed.

- Many older people who live alone have problems following directions for prescribed treatments.

Despite these challenges and problems, most older people who live alone express a keen desire to maintain their independence. Many fear being overly dependent on others and wish to continue to live alone despite the challenges they face. Engaging in regular physical and mental activities and staying connected with others help older people who are living alone maintain their independence.

People returning home from a hospital stay, particularly after surgery, may benefit from having a discussion with a social worker or health care practitioner about any extra services that will be needed. Such services, which may include home health aides or visiting nurses, can help ensure that people resume living independently.

Alternative living arrangements may be an option when living alone is not. In some instances, someone may be willing to move into the dwelling of an increasingly dependent older person. That someone is most often an adult child, but it may be another family member or even a friend. The person moving in may provide companionship only or may undertake some caregiving responsibilities. This type of living arrangement may extend the time older people are able to remain in their own home and may be quite satisfying to all involved. However, expectations of each person regarding the arrangement should be clearly expressed and agreed on.

Relocation, or moving to another residence, sometimes becomes an attractive option or even a necessity for older people after retirement or the death of a spouse or relative. Older people may move when declining health uncovers a need for supervision or help with personal care. Alternatively, a decision to relocate may be made simply because older people are looking for better weather, more companionship, a greater sense of safety and security, or closer proximity to a family member. In other instances, older people relocate to reduce costs or to establish a simpler lifestyle. Usually the move is from a larger to a smaller dwelling. For example, older people may move from a family home to retirement housing and eventually to an assisted living community or nursing home.

People who respond poorly to relocation are more likely to have been living alone, socially isolated, impoverished, and depressed. Men respond more poorly than women do. Relocation can be very stressful. Much of the stress seems to arise when people feel they lack control over the move and do not know what to expect in the new environment. For older people who have memory loss, a move away from familiar surroundings may intensify confusion and dependence on others and lead to frustration.

Sometimes relocation involves moving into someone else's home. Older people may move into the home of an adult child. Less often, people move into the home of a sibling, another relative, or a friend. Even when older people have been independent or nearly so, choosing to live with another person can produce mixed results. Problems may develop if older people believe they are or might become a burden to others in the household. In some instances, not everyone in the household is pleased to have the older person move in. This situation may arise when adult children ask their parents to live with them out of a sense of guilt or obligation. An older person moving into the home of a relative may be vulnerable to mistreatment (see page 1934) or other problems if others in the household feel angry and frustrated with the arrangement.

On the other hand, relocation may lead to a very positive arrangement in which people provide services to one another as well as companionship and financial relief. Such relocations are most likely to go well when the older person is well prepared and when discussion regarding expectations and concerns is open and ongoing.

Many moves happen suddenly, but even a little preparation can help decrease the stress of relocating. Before a decision is made for an older person to move into someone else's home, every person already living in that home should have an opportunity to participate in a discussion about what to expect and how to handle problems. This type of discussion can help everyone involved to anticipate and possibly prevent conflicts. People who are moving should be acquainted with the new setting well in advance, if possible. The opportunity to tour future surroundings and meet potential neighbors can be very helpful.

Once a move has occurred, several actions help make the move successful. Older people should maintain or increase their level of physical activity to support good health. Getting involved in social activities in the new environment helps alleviate the stress of the move. Friends and family can help by being supportive and encouraging involvement in activities.

Intimacy

Intimacy takes many forms, including emotional intimacy, shared experiences, and physical intimacy, such as touching, cuddling, or sexual activity. The desire for intimacy does not diminish with aging. However, the health and emotional conditions that often accompany aging can complicate people's ability to develop and maintain an intimate relationship. In addition, aging can change the way in which intimacy is expressed in a relationship.

Sex is a physical expression of intimacy that is important to many older couples. There is no age at which sexual activity is inappropriate. However, many factors may contribute to the shift in emphasis from sex to other expressions of intimacy. Older people may lose their need for physical intimacy as passions mellow after years of living together. Many couples—most without being aware of it—grow comfortable with forms of intimacy other than sexual intercourse. These form allow them to express familiarity, caring, or engagement with their partner in ways that are equally meaningful and more natural to their daily lives and personalities. Also, levels of sex hormones decrease in men and women as they grow older. The resulting physical changes may reduce sex drive or may make sexual intercourse uncomfortable or difficult. Some medical conditions, as well as drugs, can hamper the ability to have and enjoy sexual intercourse. Sex and intimacy also require opportunities for privacy. Older poeple have fewer of these opportunities when they live with family members or in an assisted living community.

Intimacy–in all its forms—is sometimes lost. Some couples have difficulty maintaining closeness in the face of life's sometimes substantial challenges.

Many older people find a companionship that resembles intimacy in interactions with beloved pets. Caring for a pet engenders many of the same feelings present in human relationships. Providing a pet to an older person, if circumstances permit, can bring companionship and intimacy that greatly improves quality of life.

Staying Connected

Studies have shown that people who remain active and who interact with other people during old age live longer, happier, healthier lives. Volunteering, taking classes, joining social groups, engaging in hobbies, and pursuing some type of spiritual or religious practice are all ways of staying connected. Even people who are confined to their home because of illness can stay connected by having others visit them or by communicating over the telephone or by e-mail.

Volunteering: Volunteering allows older people to use skills and life experiences to contribute to the community and society. Hundreds of organizations across the United States welcome older volunteers. For example, the Retired and Senior Volunteer Program (RSVP) and the Foster Grandparent Program provide volunteer opportunities in many communities. Opportunities are almost limitless and include

- Working with children
- Working with older people
- Helping out in nonprofit organizations or municipal institutions such as libraries
- Assisting small businesses

Continuing Education: Being a life-long learner can be a very enjoyable and effective way of maintaining an active mind and of meeting and interacting with others who have similar interests. Many public school systems, colleges and universities, and municipalities offer continuing education classes for people of all ages as well as classes specifically developed with older adults in mind. Classes may range from practical topics (such as preparing tax returns, managing personal finances, or learning a new language) to more creative or entertaining topics (such as wine tasting and music appreciation).

Social Groups and Hobbies: For older people, hobbies can help maintain social connections as well as mental and physical fitness. People may develop new hobbies or rediscover hobbies from earlier years. Although many hobbies can be done in solitude, engaging in a hobby with another person or with a group can be more interesting and stimulating. Hobbies that involve physical activity, such as gardening or sports, can be particularly beneficial to people's health.

Spirituality and Religion: Spirituality and religion provide meaning, comfort, and a sense of belonging to many older people. Spirituality and religion are similar but not identical concepts. Religion is often associated with institutions, structure, and tradition, whereas spirituality is more associated with feelings, thoughts, and experiences. Most older people in the United States consider themselves both religious and spiritual.

Spirituality and religion may benefit older people in several ways:

- A positive and hopeful attitude about life and illness improves health.
- The social aspects of a religious community can help people feel connected to others.
- The meaning and purpose of life that religious beliefs convey and the effect of those beliefs can be steady and powerful influences, especially when people are facing difficult changes.

A religious community is often the largest source of social support for older people outside of the family, and involvement in religious organizations is the most common type of voluntary social activity—more common than all other forms of voluntary social activity combined. For many older people, their religion provides a foundation that enables them to cope with health problems and stresses, such as loss of a spouse.

296   Driving

Driving provides a sense of freedom, independence, and involvement with the world that many people take for granted in their earlier adulthood. But the privilege of driving is based on the ability to drive safely. Drivers aged 70 and over are among those at greatest risk of traffic violations and motor vehicle crashes per miles driven. Thus, impaired function due to age-related disorders should be viewed as a flashing yellow traffic signal—a warning that driving privileges should be reassessed.

Many factors can diminish the driving performance of older adults. Among these factors are age-related changes in reaction time and certain disorders that become more common with aging. Drugs that are commonly used to treat disorders in older people can also impair driving performance.

Some of these factors can be managed and modified.

 Did You Know...

Older people are more likely to get into motor vehicle crashes when making left turns.

Crash Rates and Traffic Violations

On average, older drivers actually have fewer crashes per year than do younger drivers. However, because they drive fewer miles than younger drivers do, older drivers average more crashes per mile driven. Crash rates begin to increase after about age 70, and they increase more rapidly after age 80. For every mile driven, older drivers have higher rates of traffic violations, crashes, and fatalities than do all other age groups over age 25. It should be noted that the current generation of older people are driving farther distances than previous generations, and this trend is expected to continue.

Failure to yield right-of-way is one of the more common traffic violations committed by older drivers. Also, older drivers have more difficulty merging into traffic and may have problems at intersections, particularly when making left turns. These difficulties have been attributed to

- Difficulty evaluating several pieces of information simultaneously (multitasking)
- Difficulty judging the speed of oncoming cars
- Reduction in field of view

Yet, older drivers are often more careful than younger drivers. They tend to avoid driving at night, during rush hour, or during inclement weather. Moreover, alcohol is much less likely to be a factor in crashes involving older drivers. Older drivers are also less likely to have crashes while driving on curved roads or at high speeds. For older drivers, crashes are less likely to involve a single vehicle. Multiple vehicles are more likely to be involved.

In a motor vehicle crash, older drivers are more likely to be injured than younger drivers. Crashes involving older drivers are also more likely to result in serious injuries and fatalities. The increased vulnerability of older drivers may be due to physical fragility. Also, older drivers are more likely to be involved in a crash while making a left-hand turn, and such turns leave drivers vulnerable. Older drivers who are killed as a result of motor vehicle crashes tend to have older cars that do not have air bags. Thus, for older drivers, fatality rates may decrease over the next decade as they switch to more modern vehicles.

Reasons for Problems

Driving involves the precise execution of simultaneous tasks (such as braking and steering). These tasks require several attributes, including the following:

- A clear mind
- Attention and mental focus
- Swift reaction time
- Coordination
- Adequate strength

- Good range of motion in the upper body (upper trunk, shoulders, and neck)
- Good vision and hearing
- Good judgment

Deficits in any of these attributes can greatly affect driving performance. Such deficits can result from several causes. Virtually all these attributes are impaired to some degree as people age.

Aging: Aging itself usually results in a gradual and subtle decline in strength, coordination, reaction time, ability to concentrate, and hearing. Older people may have less stamina and become fatigued more quickly, especially in situations that require concentration. Older people are less able to focus on more than one task at a time. However, most changes attributed to aging are modest and are often not the main reason for driving safety issues.

Disorders: Disorders that are more common among older people can be especially troublesome for older drivers. For example, the blood sugar level of drivers with diabetes may rise too high or drop too low. Such changes can interfere with clear thinking, attention and mental focus, vision, and sensation in the feet.

Older drivers with dementia (including Alzheimer's disease) can have poor judgment and concentration, a dangerous prospect when driving. Even when dementia is in its early stages, drivers may become more easily lost or more easily confused in congested traffic. Typically, reaction time and the ability to attend to items in all visual fields decrease in people with dementia.

Strokes or so-called ministrokes (transient ischemic attacks, or TIAs) can slow reaction time, cause muscle weakness, impair vision, and reduce coordination. Seizures can abruptly cause people to become unaware of their surroundings or even lose consciousness. A recent heart attack may increase the risk of fainting or experiencing light-headedness.

Arthritis causes joint pain and stiffness, limiting range of motion and possibly interfering with the ability to operate a car's controls. For example, pain and stiffness in the knees or hips may affect the ability to press the brake pedal or accelerator. Arthritis can make turning the head (as is necessary when turning or reversing a car) painful and difficult.

Glaucoma and macular degeneration are eye disorders that lead to problems when driving at twilight or at night. Glaucoma can also narrow the field of vision so that cars and other objects alongside the driver are difficult to see. Cataracts, which occur almost exclusively among older people, can cause glare from oncoming headlights or street lamps.

Drugs: Many older people take drugs that can have undesirable side effects. Side effects can include sleepiness, dizziness, confusion, and other symptoms that interfere with driving. Both prescription and nonprescription drugs can have these side effects. Drugs that may interfere with driving include the following:

- Alcohol
- Anticonvulsants
- Antiemetic drugs (used to manage nausea)
- Antipsychotics
- Benzodiazepines or antianxiety drugs
- Drugs used to treat glaucoma
- Muscle relaxants
- Nonprescription antihistamines
- Opioids
- Sleep aids
- Tricyclic antidepressants

Situations: Stress, particularly when driving in unfamiliar areas or in heavy traffic, may contribute to difficulty. Fatigue and distraction also decrease driving ability.

For some older adults, the only deficit in driving ability is simply a lack of driving experience. For example, an older person (usually a woman) may learn to drive only after a spouse dies.

Ways of Compensating

There are many strategies older drivers can adopt to compensate for factors that reduce performance and increase the risk of driving.

Avoiding Hazards: Older drivers can use their experience from years of driving to identify and avoid hazardous situations. For example, because stamina decreases with aging, older drivers may wish to drive shorter distances and take frequent breaks. They can avoid freeways and other areas where traffic is congested or known to be dangerous. They can avoid driving at night or twilight, when glare problems are most likely. They can avoid rush hour traffic and take fewer risks in traffic.

Avoiding Distractions: Avoiding distractions—an important consideration for all drivers—is essential for older drivers. Cell phones are an important safety feature for drivers who become stranded when a car unexpectedly needs repair. However, cell phone use (even hands-free models) while driving is strongly discouraged. In fact, it is illegal in some areas. Similarly, making adjustments to the stereo or another onboard system (such as climate control or seat position), eating or drinking, smoking (there are many other reasons not to smoke—at any age), applying make-up, reading maps, and even engaging in conversation with other passengers can be distracting. People should minimize distractions of all types.

Using Technology: Newer technology may assist older drivers. For example, advanced vision systems for night driving include curve lighting (lighting directed around a curve) and automatic dimming of headlights (high beams convert to low beams when there is oncoming traffic). Parking aids, which use cameras or infrared systems to help with backing up, parking, and other maneuvers, are especially helpful for people who have difficulty looking over their shoulders. Global positioning systems (GPS) may help older drivers locate destinations.

Other systems that are helpful to older drivers include cruise control, antilock brakes, and electronic stability devices that improve traction and steering. Some cars offer rearview mirrors that automatically dim when hit by blinding headlights, thus reducing glare. Car manufacturers are experimenting with infrared night vision technology to enhance night driving. Many are also redesigning handles and knobs to make them easier for people who have arthritis to operate. Other car design features, such as lower door thresholds, lumbar supports, extended visors, adjustable seats and steering wheels, are available to all drivers but may be particularly helpful for older drivers.

When crashes or other urgent situations occur, some emergency systems can automatically call and direct rescue teams to the car's location. Further innovations are anticipated in the future.

Driver Education: Another way that older drivers can help maintain or even improve their driving skills is through driver re-education programs. Several organizations—such as the American Association of Retired Persons (AARP) and American Automobile Association (AAA)—offer such programs to help older drivers adjust to the challenges of driving during old age. In addition, taking such programs can lower insurance rates.

Older drivers may also benefit from programs designed to ensure that their car fits them correctly. For example, they should have the right distance from their steering wheel and right seat height. Adjusting mirrors can help drivers compensate for blind spots.

Medical Care: Lifestyle and medical care can help older drivers avoid driving difficulties. There are many reasons to stay fit in older age. The ability to continue driving is one of them because strength and stamina affect driving performance. Doctors should regularly evaluate older people to identify any problems in vision, memory and thinking, or muscle strength that could impair their ability to drive.

Treatment of some disorders may improve driving performance. For example, cataract removal can be beneficial. Treatment of arthritis with drugs and physical therapy can improve flexibility and mobility. Good control of diabetes can prevent swings in the blood sugar level. Older drivers should review their

Warning Signs of Unsafe Driving

Older drivers and their family members may want to consider several factors as they determine whether it is still safe for them to drive. Things to consider include whether

- They get lost while driving
- Friends or family members worry about their driving or have stopped accepting rides
- They have had more near-misses lately
- They have difficulty seeing other cars and reading and reacting to road signs
- Traffic congestion, busy intersections, or left-hand turns make them anxious
- They feel other drivers drive too fast
- They find driving stressful or tiring
- The glare from oncoming headlights is bothersome
- They have trouble turning the steering wheel, pushing foot pedals, looking over their shoulder when backing up, or parking
- They have had accidents in which they were at fault in the past year, or they have been stopped by the police because of their driving
- They are too cautious when driving
- They sometimes forget to use mirrors or signals or check for oncoming traffic

Older drivers who are concerned about any of these issues may want to talk with their doctor or consult a driving rehabilitation specialist about ways to improve driving safety.

drugs with a doctor or pharmacist to make sure that driving performance will not be compromised by side effects.

Many states have laws that prohibit people from driving for a specified time after certain disorders are diagnosed. This waiting period (moratorium) provides time for the disorder to be stabilized with treatment. For example, some states require a 6-month moratorium on driving after a stroke or transient ischemic attack. A 3- to 6-month moratorium may be required after a heart attack or cardiac bypass surgery. For people who have had a seizure, some states require a seizure-free period of at least 6 months before driving can be resumed.

A Driving Decision

At some point, most older people face the decision to keep or give up a driver's license. A decline in the abilities required for safe driving may make driving dangerous. Also, some people drive less as they get older. They may find that maintaining a car for occasional use costs more than using public transportation. But giving up a driver's license may mean a loss of freedom and independence.

Sometimes the family doctor or a family member realizes that it is time for an older driver to give up the car keys. Dealing with these issues is always difficult, but ignoring them can bring even greater misery. There are some practical steps that may help older drivers feel more comfortable about giving up their car keys:

- Involve the driver in the decision to limit or stop driving
- Help find other ways to get around
- Investigate driving and delivery services
- Make sure the person has rides to usual activities
- Enlist the family doctor or a friend to discuss the issue

There are many publications and online resources that can help older drivers decide whether they should continue to drive. There are also resources available for family members and friends who may be concerned about an older driver.

Occupational therapists and people who teach driving skills (sometimes called driving education specialists) may develop expertise in evaluating older people who have impairments that may affect driving ability. These professionals are known as driving rehabilitation specialists. They are often located at hospitals or in universities, but some have private clinics. They may be able to evaluate drivers for safety, provide vehicle modification or adaptive equipment, and give mobility counseling or advice on alternative methods of transportation.

Most older drivers, sometimes with advice from family members or their doctors, can determine when to stop driving. However, some drivers, for example people with dementia, may lack insight into their driving ability and continue to drive even after a doctor has recommended they stop. One approach in this situation is to suggest that the older driver be tested by a driving rehabilitation specialist or the state agency that oversees or regulates licensure. Testing by the state can be requested by the driver, an immediate family member, or a doctor. It can include both written and on-road evaluations. In a few states, doctors are required to report any driver believed to be unsafe.

Laws regulating the possession and renewal of a driver's license by older drivers vary from country to country and from state to state.

CHAPTER

297 Falls

- Most falls occur when people with a physical condition that impairs mobility or balance encounter an environmental hazard.
- Although many people have no symptoms before a fall, some experience dizziness or other symptoms.
- After a fall, people may have broken bones or bruises.
- Doctors often do tests to evaluate whether an underlying condition contributed to the fall.
- Falls may be prevented by taking precautions around the home.
- After injuries are treated, people work with physical therapists to help reduce the risk of subsequent falls.

Many older people fear falling. And they have good reason to do so. Falls are common among older people. About one third of older people who live at home fall at least once a year, and people who live in a nursing home fall even more often.

Falls often cause injuries. Some of the injuries, such as a broken hip, can be serious. Older people are more likely to break bones in falls because many older people have porous, fragile bones (osteoporosis).

Fear of falling can lead to problems. People may worry about doing their usual activities and thus lose their self-confidence and even their independence. Older people can do many things to help overcome their fears and to reduce their risk of falling. Knowing what causes falls can help.

> **? Did You Know...**
> Although many older people fall, falls are not a normal part of growing older.

Causes

Falls can be caused by physical conditions that impair mobility or balance, hazards in the environment, or potentially hazardous situations. Most falls occur when several causes interact. For example, people with Parkinson's disease and impaired vision (a physical condition) may trip on an extension cord (an environmental hazard) while rushing to answer the telephone (a potentially hazardous situation).

People's physical condition is affected by changes due to aging itself, physical fitness, disorders present, and drugs used. The physical condition probably has a greater effect on the risk of falling than do environmental hazards and hazardous situations. Not only does a poor or impaired physical condition

increase the risk of falls, but it also affects how people respond to hazards and hazardous situations.

Physical impairments that increase the risk of falling include those involving

- Balance or walking
- Vision
- Sensation in the foot
- Muscle strength
- Cognition

Use of drugs that affect attention or lower blood pressure can also increase the risk of falling.

Hazards in the environment are involved in many falls. Falls may occur when people do not notice a hazard or do not respond quickly enough after a hazard is noticed.

Environmental hazards that increase the risk of falling include

- Inadequate lighting
- Throw rugs
- Slippery floors
- Electrical or extension cords or objects that are in the way of walking
- Uneven sidewalks and broken curbs

Most falls occur indoors. Some happen while people are standing still. But most occur while people are moving—getting in and out of bed or a chair, getting on or off a toilet seat, walking, or going up or down stairs. While moving, people may stumble or trip, or balance may be lost. Any movement can be hazardous. But if people are rushing or if their attention is divided, movement becomes even more hazardous. For example, rushing to the bathroom or to answer the telephone or talking on a cordless phone can make walking more hazardous.

Symptoms

Often before falling, people have no symptoms. When an environmental hazard or a hazardous situation results in a fall, there is little or no warning. However, if a fall is partly or completely due to a person's physical condition, symptoms may be noticed before falling. Symptoms may include dizziness, light-headedness, or irregular or rapid, pounding heartbeats (palpitations).

After a fall, injuries are common and tend to be more severe as people age. Over half of all falls result in at least a slight injury, such as a bruise, sprained ligament, or strained muscle. More serious injuries include broken bones, torn ligaments, deep cuts, and damage to organs such as a kidney or the liver. About 2% of falls result in a broken hip. Other bones (in the upper arm, wrist, back, and pelvis) are broken in about 5% of falls. Some falls result in loss of consciousness or a head injury.

Falls can cause even more problems if people cannot get up right away or summon help. Such a situation may be frightening and may make people feel helpless. Remaining on the floor, even for a few hours, can lead to problems such as dehydration, low body temperature (hypothermia), and skin sores due to pressure (pressure sores).

The effects of a fall may last a long time. About half of people who could walk before they fell and broke a hip cannot walk as well afterward, even after treatment and rehabilitation. People who have fallen may develop a fear of falling that robs them of their self-confidence. As a result, they may stay at home and give up activities, such as shopping, visiting friends, and cleaning. When people become less active, joints can become stiff and muscles can become weak. Stiff joints and weak muscles can further increase the risk of falling and make remaining active and independent more difficult. For all these reasons, falls can greatly reduce quality of life. Falls seem to be an important consideration in the decision of many people to move to a nursing home or an assisted living facility.

Rarely, falls result in death. Death may occur immediately—for example, when the head hits a hard surface and causes uncontrolled bleeding in the head. Much more commonly, death occurs later, resulting from complications of serious injuries caused by the fall.

Diagnosis

People who have fallen may be reluctant to discuss the problem with anyone, including a doctor, especially if they have not been injured. But even people who have been seriously injured during a fall and have been treated in an emergency department may be reluctant to admit they have fallen. People may be reluctant because they think falling is just part of getting older. And they do not want others to think they are helpless and now must move from their home into a more supervised environment such as a nursing home. Because of this reluctance, doctors should routinely ask all of their older patients whether they have fallen in the recent past.

If a person has fallen, doctors try to identify the cause of the fall. To do so, they ask about the circumstances of the fall, including any symptoms experienced just before the fall and any activities that may have contributed to the fall. Doctors also ask about the use of drugs—prescription and nonprescription—that may have contributed to the fall.

Doctors do a physical examination first to check for injuries and to obtain information about possible causes of the fall. Parts of the examination include the following:

- Blood pressure measurement: If blood pressure decreases when people stand up, the fall may be caused by orthostatic hypotension (see page 348).
- Heart sounds: With a stethoscope, doctors listen to the heart for evidence of a very slow heart rate, abnormal rhythms, and heart failure.
- Muscle strength and range of motion assessment: Doctors assess the back and legs and check for problems in the feet.
- Vision and nervous system assessment, including sense of position and balance

Doctors sometimes ask people to do some usual activities, such as sitting in a chair and then standing up or stepping up on a step. Observing these activities may help doctors identify conditions that contributed to the fall.

If the fall resulted from an environmental hazard and no major injury occurred, no tests may be done. However, when people's physical condition could have contributed to the fall, tests may be needed. For example, when the physical examination detects evidence of a heart problem, heart rate and rhythm may be recorded using electrocardiography (ECG). This test may take a few minutes and be done in the doctor's office. Or people may be asked to wear a portable ECG device (Holter monitor) for 1 or 2 days. Blood tests, such as a complete blood count and measurements of electrolyte levels, may be helpful in people who have been experiencing dizziness or light-headedness. If the nervous system appears to be malfunctioning, computed tomography (CT) or magnetic resonance imaging (MRI) of the head may be helpful.

Prevention

Older people can do many simple, practical things to help reduce the risk of falling.

- Exercising regularly: Weight training or resistance training may help strengthen weak legs and thus may improve steadiness during walking. Tai Chi and balancing exercises such as standing on one leg can help improve balance.
- Wearing appropriate shoes: Shoes that have firm, nonslip soles and low heels are best.
- Standing up slowly after sitting or lying down and taking a moment before starting to move: This strategy can help prevent dizziness because it gives the body time to adjust to the change in position.

- Learning a simple head maneuver: A simple head maneuver called the Epley maneuver may help some older people who feel dizzy when they move. It involves turning the head in specific ways. Doctors usually do the maneuver the first time, but people can learn how to do it themselves if it needs to be repeated.
- Reviewing drugs being taken: People can ask a doctor or another health care practitioner to review all prescription and nonprescription drugs being taken to see if any of the drugs could increase the risk of falling. If such drugs are being used, doctors may be able to lower the dose or people may be able to stop taking the drug.
- Having vision checked regularly: Getting the correct glasses and wearing them can help prevent falls. Treatment of glaucoma or cataracts, which limit vision, can also help.
- Consulting with a physical therapist about ways to reduce the risk of falling: Some older people need a physical therapist to train them to walk, particularly if they need to use a walker or cane.

Hazards in the environment can sometimes be removed or corrected.

- Lighting can be improved by increasing the number of lights or changing the types of lights.
- Light switches can be positioned so that they are easily reached. Or, lights that turn on when they are touched or when they detect nearby motion can be used.
- Adequate lighting for steps (inside and outside) and for outdoor areas used at night is particularly important. Steps should have sturdy, secure handrails.
- Electrical or extension cords that are in the way of walking can be eliminated by adding more electrical outlets, or the cords may be tacked over doorways.
- Items that clutter floors and stairways can be stored out of the way of walking.
- Grab bars can be installed next to toilets, tubs, and other places for people who need something to hold onto when they stand up. Grab bars must be installed correctly, so that they do not pull out of the wall.
- Raised toilet seats can help.
- Loose throw rugs can be removed or taped or tacked down.
- Nonslip mats should be used in the bathroom and kitchen.
- Frequently used household items can be stored in cabinets, cupboards, or other spaces between waist and eye level, so that they can be reached without stretching or bending.

Learning how to safely handle potentially hazardous situations may be more important than removing an

CHECKLIST FOR PREVENTING FALLS IN THE HOME	
All rooms	Reachable light switch
	No electrical or extension cords in the way of walking
	No throw rugs
	Cordless phone
Kitchen	Reachable cabinets (so that bending and stretching are unnecessary)
	Nonslip mats
Bedroom	Reachable bedside light
	Night-light
	Wall-to-wall carpet
Bathroom	Raised toilet seat
	Grab bars
	Nonslip mats
	Night-light
Living room	Tacked down or wall-to-wall carpet
Steps (inside and outside)	Good lighting
	Sturdy railing
	Nonslip treads

environmental hazard. Sometimes people need to pay more attention to potential hazards and think about ways to accomplish daily tasks more safely. For example, they can place cordless phones around the home so that they do not have to rush to answer phone calls.

Falls cannot always be prevented. So, people who are likely to fracture a hip—such as people who have osteoporosis—should maximize the strength of their bones by taking adequate calcium and vitamin D and taking additional prescription drugs to slow their bone loss. Some people may consider wearing a hip protector, an undergarment with a plastic and foam pad placed over the hip, which may prevent hip fractures if worn regularly.

Knowing what to do if a fall occurs can help older people be less afraid of falling. If they fall and cannot get up, they can turn onto their stomach, crawl to a piece of furniture (or other structure that can support their weight), and pull themselves up.

Older people should also have a good way to call for help. People who have fallen several times may keep a telephone in a place that can be reached from the floor. Another option is installing a personal emergency response system (a medical alert device) that signals someone to check in on them. Most of these systems include an alert button worn on a necklace. Pressing the button calls for help.

Treatment

The first priority is treatment of injuries, such as fractures, sprained ligaments, and strained muscles. The next priority is to prevent subsequent falls and injury due to falls.

Disorders that may have contributed to the fall are treated. For example, in people who have a very slow heart rate accompanied by light-headedness, a pacemaker for the heart may be implanted. If possible, potentially harmful drugs are stopped, the dose is reduced, or another drug is substituted.

Physical and occupational therapists can help improve people's walking and balance as well as their self-confidence after a fall. They can provide tips on how to avoid falling. Therapists can also encourage people to remain active. Physical therapy and supervised balance training and stretching can help reduce the risk of falling.

298 Elder Mistreatment

Elder mistreatment refers to harm or the threat of harm to an older person by another person. It includes abuse and neglect.

Older people can be mistreated by having harmful things done to them (abuse) or by having necessary things withheld from them (neglect). Elder mistreatment is a growing problem as the number of older people increases.

Each year in the United States, thousands of older people are mistreated. The perpetrator of mistreatment is usually a family member, most often an adult child or spouse who is the older person's caregiver. Sometimes professional caregivers, such as home health care workers or employees of nursing homes and other institutions, mistreat older people.

Any older person, regardless of health, can be mistreated. However, mistreatment is more likely when older people

- Are physically frail, often because of disabling chronic disorders
- Are socially isolated
- Have dementia or confusion

Mistreatment is also more likely when the perpetrators

- Are financially dependent on or living with the older person
- Abuse alcohol or drugs
- Have a psychologic disorder, such as schizophrenia
- Have been violent before
- Have stress, such as financial problems or a family death
- Lack skills and resources, making caregiving frustrating
- Have a disorder (such as dementia) that makes them (even if they were previously mild-mannered) agitated or violent

Caregivers are often overwhelmed by the demands of care, have inadequate preparation or resources, or do not know what is expected of them (see box on page 1907). They may also become increasingly socially isolated, sometimes increasing their resentment and making mistreatment more likely. Many caregivers do not intend to mistreat the person, and some may not even know that they are mistreating the person.

Many older people who are mistreated do not seek help for various reasons. They may be physically unable to do so. Or they may be afraid of being harmed further, of being abandoned, or of being forced into a nursing home. If the perpetrator is the caregiver, older people may feel too dependent on or want to protect the perpetrator, who may also be their adult child. They may feel ashamed.

The signs of mistreatment can be difficult to distinguish from other problems. For example, if an older person has a hip fracture, health care practitioners may be unable to distinguish whether the cause is physical abuse or osteoporosis, falls, or both (which are much more common causes). Also, if older people are confused, they may not have their complaints of abuse taken seriously, so the abuse goes unrecognized.

For all these reasons, doctors, nurses, social workers, friends, and family members often do not recognize mistreatment.

Types of Mistreatment

Older people may be abused, neglected, or both.

Abuse

Abuse can be physical, sexual, psychologic, or financial. Older people may be subjected to one or more of these types of abuse.

Physical abuse is the use of force to harm or to threaten harm. Examples are striking, shoving, shaking, beating, restraining, and force-feeding. Possible indications of physical abuse include unexplained injuries or injuries that are not treated adequately, rope burns and other rope marks, broken eyeglasses, and scratches, cuts, and bruises. A caregiver's refusal to allow an older person to have time alone with visitors or health care practitioners can raise concerns about physical abuse.

Sexual abuse is sexual contact without consent or by force or threat of force. Examples are intimate touching and rape. Bruises around the breasts and genital area or unexplained bleeding from the vagina or anus may indicate sexual abuse. However, sexual abuse does not always result in physical injuries.

Psychologic abuse is the use of words or actions to cause emotional stress or anguish. It may involve

- Issuing threats, insults, and harsh commands
- Ignoring the person (for example, by not speaking for a long time or after being spoken to)
- Treating the older person like a child (infantilization), sometimes with the goal of encouraging the person to become dependent on the perpetrator

People who are psychologically abused may become passive and withdrawn, anxious, or depressed.

Financial abuse is the exploitation of a person's possessions or funds. It includes

- Swindling
- Pressuring an older person to distribute assets
- Managing an older person's money irresponsibly

Caregivers may spend most of an older person's income on themselves and provide only a minimum amount for the older person.

Restricting an older person's freedom to make important life decisions, such as whom to socialize with and how to spend money, is sometimes considered another, more subtle form of abuse.

Neglect

Neglect is the failure to provide food, drugs, personal hygiene, or other necessities. Necessities may be withheld intentionally or simply be forgotten or overlooked by irresponsible or inattentive caregivers. Some caregivers are unaware that their treatment of an older person has crossed the line from being less than ideal to being mistreatment. These caregivers may lack a sense of what constitutes adequate and appropriate care, or they may have very different notions of what conduct is and is not acceptable.

Sometimes neglect results from desperate circumstances, such as financial difficulties, despite the caregiver's best intentions. Sometimes willing caregivers are unable to provide adequate care because of their

---

When to Suspect Mistreatment

When older people have certain problems or make certain changes, family members and friends, as well as health care practitioners, should be aware that mistreatment may be the cause. These problems include the following:

- Poor hygiene or an unpleasant odor
- Pressure sores
- Weight loss and a dry mouth
- Missing eyeglasses, hearing aids, or dentures
- Multiple bruises, bruises in places not usually injured by accident (such as the buttocks), or bruises in the shape of objects (such as an iron or belt)
- Rope marks
- Broken bones
- Scratches and cuts
- Anxiety, depression, or withdrawal and passivity
- Sudden financial changes (such as changes in a will, loss of money or other assets, or addition of names to an older person's bank card)

The caregiver's behavior may also suggest mistreatment, as in the following:

- Not letting the older person speak
- Treating the older person like a child
- Giving implausible explanations for injuries

---

own physical limitations or mental impairment. For example, caregivers may be unable to bathe the older person or to remember to give the person a drug.

Older people who are neglected may lose weight because of undernutrition, and their skin and mouth may become dry because of dehydration. They may have an unpleasant odor if they are inadequately cleaned. Pressure sores may develop on the buttocks or heels if people with limited mobility are left to sit or lie in one position too long. Necessary aids, such as eyeglasses, hearing aids, or dentures, may be missing. People may miss scheduled doctor appointments or not be taken for care when disorders are obviously worsening.

Prevention of Mistreatment

Older people who are worried about mistreatment can take steps to make it less likely to happen, such as the following:

- Not living with someone who has a history of violent behavior or substance abuse

When People Neglect Themselves

When people do not provide food, drugs, personal hygiene, or other necessities for themselves, the problem is called self-neglect.

Self-neglect occurs more often than mistreatment. Similar to mistreatment, self-neglect is most likely when older people

- Live alone and isolate themselves
- Have a disorder that impairs their judgment and memory (such as Alzheimer's disease)
- Have several chronic disorders
- Have severe depression

However, some people have no particular medical problems. Why such people neglect themselves is unclear.

Self-neglect can range from not keeping themselves or their clothing clean to not paying bills to not seeing a doctor when they have a life-threatening condition. People may eat too little and may become dehydrated and malnourished. If they see a doctor, they may refuse treatment, not fill their prescriptions, or skip follow-up visits. Their home may be filthy, in hazardous disrepair, or infested by animal or insect pests. Sometimes self-neglect endangers public health, for example, when people's behavior causes risk of fire.

Knowing where to draw the line between self-neglect and the right to autonomy and privacy can be very difficult for family members, friends, and health care practitioners. Older people may be making informed and capable choices. They may simply have decided to live in a way that others find undesirable. Often, a social worker is in the best position to make such a determination and can intervene if alerted by family members or friends.

If intervention is thought to be needed, help can be just a phone call away. Contacting the person's primary care doctor is a good way to start. Adult Protective Services or the state unit on aging (whose numbers are available through the Eldercare Locator at 800-677-1116) can also be contacted.

Responding to Mistreatment

Older people should never think that mistreatment is part of being old or dependent. Being mistreated threatens their personal dignity and sense of well-being and can even cost people their life.

Detecting mistreatment of older people can be difficult. Older people may be reluctant to tell others about it, or they may be unable to tell others because the perpetrator limits phone calls or access to visitors and health care practitioners.

If older people believe they are in danger, they can call an elder abuse hotline for immediate help. Such hotlines are listed in the local phone book, usually in the Blue Pages, or can be provided by a phone operator. A list of all state laws about elder mistreatment and telephone numbers to call to report mistreatment are available at the web site of the National Center for Elder Abuse. The local Area Agency on Aging is another good source of information and referral. If older people do not feel endangered but still want help, they can try talking about it with their doctor or other health care practitioner. However, many health care practitioners are unfamiliar with how to handle elder mistreatment because the topic has not traditionally been part of medical training and education.

Because mistreatment and its effects can vary greatly, interventions need to be tailored to each person's situation. Interventions may include the following:

- Medical assistance
- Education, such as information about mistreatment and available options, as well as help with devising safety plans
- Psychologic support, such as psychotherapy and support groups
- Law enforcement and legal intervention, such as arrest of the perpetrator, orders of protection, and legal advocacy
- Arrangement for alternative housing, such as housing that provides safe shelter with protection from the perpetrator

Relatives, friends, and acquaintances have a responsibility to help if they know of or strongly suspect mistreatment, as do health care practitioners. Directly confronting the perpetrator is not recommended because it can worsen mistreatment. Instead, the situation should be reported. Reporting suspected or confirmed abuse or neglect is mandatory in all states if the mistreatment occurs in an institution and in most states if it occurs in a home. Every state has laws that protect and provide services for vulnerable, incapacitated, or disabled people. Every

- Keeping in touch with friends and former neighbors, especially if an older person has to move to a caregiver's house
- Staying connected with social and community organizations (increasing the chances that mistreatment, if it occurs, is noticed)
- Insisting on legal advice before signing any documents related to where they will live or who controls their finances (the local Area Agency on Aging can refer people for legal help)

Family members and friends can help by maintaining close ties with an older person.

state also has laws protecting people who report suspected mistreatment from being sued for doing so. To report mistreatment, people can contact the following:

- In most states: The state social service department (Adult Protective Services)

- In a few states: The state unit on aging

- For abuse within an institution: The local long-term care ombudsman's office or the state department of health

Telephone numbers for these agencies and offices in any part of the United States can be found by calling the Eldercare Locator (800-677-1116) or the National Center on Elder Abuse (202-682-2470) and giving the person's county and city of residence or zip code.

Acetaminophen Poisoning ▪ Aspirin Poisoning ▪ Carbon Monoxide Poisoning ▪
Caustic Substances Poisoning ▪ Hydrocarbon Poisoning ▪ Insecticide Poisoning ▪
Iron Poisoning ▪ Lead Poisoning

CHAPTER

299   First Aid

The goal of first aid is to save life, to prevent an injury or illness from worsening, or to help speed recovery. First aid for cardiac arrest, choking, bleeding, minor wounds, and minor soft tissue injuries is discussed in this chapter. Other chapters discuss first aid for drowning, heatstroke, low body temperature (hypothermia), serious allergic reactions (anaphylaxis), spinal cord injuries, low blood sugar (hypoglycemia), poisoning, seizures, stings, bite wounds, burns, chemical burns of the eyes, fractures, frostbite, nosebleeds, sprains, and loose teeth.

Emergency First Aid Priorities

The first priority is to assess a person's airway, breathing, and circulation (the ABCs). A problem in any of these areas is always fatal if not corrected. The airway (A)—the passage through which air travels to the lungs—can become blocked. Various illnesses and injuries can cause breathing (B) to cease. Cardiac arrest—cessation of the heartbeat—stops blood from circulating (C) through the body.

The next priority is usually to get medical assistance by calling for emergency medical care (except in cases of choking and some instances of cardiac arrest, in which treatment should be started before calling for help). Most people in the United States access emergency medical care by calling 911. The caller should rapidly give the dispatcher a full description of the person's condition and how the injury or illness developed. The caller should not hang up until told to do so. If several lay people (rescuers) are present, one should call for help while another begins assessment and first aid.

After calling for medical assistance, the ABCs are corrected before any other treatment is started. Cardiopulmonary resuscitation (CPR—see page 1942) is provided, if necessary.

Basic First-Aid Supplies

The medicine chest or first-aid kit should be kept well stocked. The following basic supplies are useful to have on hand:

- Activated charcoal (a poison control center should be called before using)
- Adhesive tape
- Antihistamine
- Antiseptic ointment (such as bacitracin)
- Acetaminophen or ibuprofen
- Chewable baby aspirin (in case of symptoms of a heart attack; a doctor should be called before using)
- Cold pack or ice bag
- Cotton-tipped swabs
- Elastic wrap
- First-aid manual
- Gauze bandages in a roll, 2 or 3 inches (5 or 7 centimeters) wide
- Sharp scissors
- Soap or instant hand sanitizer
- Sterile adhesive bandages in several sizes
- Thermometer
- Thin, plastic gloves
- Tissues
- Tweezers

If many people are injured, the most seriously injured person should be treated first. Determining who is in most urgent need of treatment may be difficult, because someone screaming in pain may be less seriously injured than someone who cannot

Automated External Defibrillator: Jump-Starting the Heart

An automated external defibrillator (AED) is a device that can detect and correct a specific type of abnormal heart rhythm called ventricular fibrillation. Ventricular fibrillation causes cardiac arrest. If cardiac arrest occurs, an AED, if available, should be used immediately. An AED is used before calling for help and before attempting cardiopulmonary resuscitation (CPR) because an AED is more likely to save lives. If the AED detects ventricular fibrillation, it provides an electrical shock (defibrillation) that can restore normal heart rhythm and start the heart beating again. Emergency medical care should be obtained even if the heart has started beating again. If a person remains in cardiac arrest after an AED is used, CPR should be done.

AEDs are easy to use. The American Red Cross and other organizations provide training sessions on the use of AEDs. Most training sessions take only a few hours. Different AEDs have somewhat different instructions for use. The instructions that are written on the AED being used should be carefully followed. AEDs are available in many public gathering places, such as stadiums and concert halls. People who are told by their doctor that they are likely to develop ventricular fibrillation but who do not have an implanted defibrillator may want to purchase an AED for home use by family members.

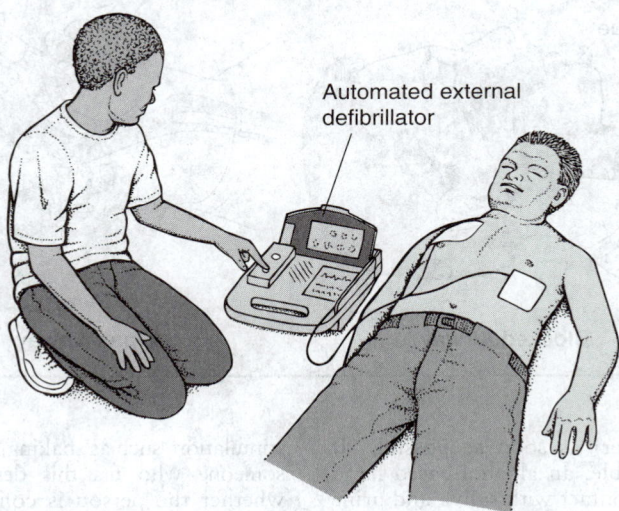

Automated external defibrillator

breathe or who is in a coma and, therefore, is quiet. Assessment should take less than 1 minute per injured person. In each case, the rescuer should consider whether the situation is life threatening, urgent but not life threatening, or not urgent. Difficulty breathing and massive bleeding are life threatening, but a broken arm can wait for treatment, no matter how painful. When there are many people with serious injuries and resources are limited, rescuers may need to provide treatment only to those people who rescuers believe have a chance of surviving.

If the injured person is unable to convey medical information, the information should be obtained in other ways. For example, if an unconscious person is found near an empty bottle of pills, the bottle should be given to the emergency medical personnel. A description of how a person became injured and other information from bystanders, family members, or rescuers can be essential to the person's treatment. After these steps have been taken, reassurance and simple measures, such as supplying a blanket and keeping the person calm and warm, can provide comfort.

Serious diseases, such as human immunodeficiency virus (HIV) infection and hepatitis B, can be transmitted through blood. Rescuers should avoid contact with blood from wounds, especially the blood of strangers whose medical history is unknown. Latex examination gloves afford the best protection. If gloves are not available, plastic can be used. For example, rescuers can place their hands inside plastic food storage bags or anything waterproof. If contaminated with blood, the hands—including the area under the fingernails—should be washed vigorously with soap and water or a mild solution of bleach (about 1 tablespoon of bleach per quart of water, or about 15 milliliters of

Opening an Airway in an Adult

After determining that a person is not breathing, the rescuer looks in the mouth and throat for any visible objects that may be blocking the airway and, if any are present, removes them. If the person does not start breathing, the tongue may be blocking the airway. The rescuer then tilts the person's head back slightly and lifts the chin, moving the tongue and thus opening the airway. If the person still does not start breathing, the rescuer begins artificial respiration. Opening the airway may be done as part of cardiopulmonary resuscitation (CPR).

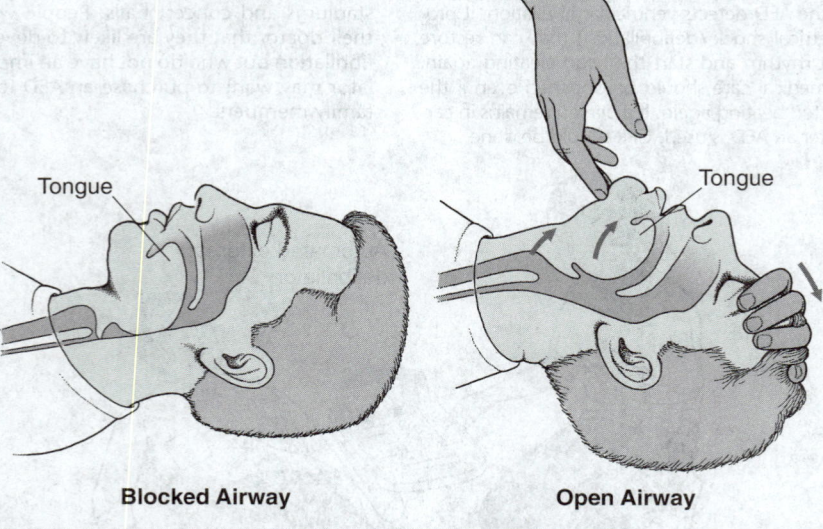

Tongue

Tongue

Blocked Airway   **Open Airway**

bleach per liter of water) as soon as possible. If neither is readily available, an alcohol-based hand sanitizer can be used. Contact with saliva and urine is much less likely to result in disease transmission than is contact with blood.

Cardiac Arrest

Cardiac arrest is what happens when a person dies. The heart does not beat and breathing ceases, which starves the body of oxygen. Sometimes a person can be revived during the first several minutes after cardiac arrest. However, the more time that passes, the less likely it is that the person can be revived and, if revived, the more likely it is that brain damage will have occurred. Brain damage is likely if cardiac arrest lasts for more than 5 minutes, and death is likely if cardiac arrest lasts for more than 10 minutes. Fewer than 5% of people who are not already hospitalized when they have a cardiac arrest survive to be discharged from the hospital, and many survivors have brain damage.

A person in cardiac arrest lies motionless without breathing and does not respond to questions or to stimulation, such as shaking. A rescuer who encounters someone who fits this description first determines whether the person is conscious by loudly asking, "Are you OK?" If there is no response, the rescuer turns the person face up and uses the "look, listen, and feel" approach to determine whether breathing has stopped:

- Looking to see whether the chest moves up and down
- Listening for sounds of breathing
- Feeling for air movement over the person's mouth

If the person is not breathing, the rescuer checks for airway blockage by looking into the mouth and throat for any visible objects.

First-Aid Treatment

First aid for cardiac arrest should proceed as quickly as possible. An automated external defibrillator (AED—a device that can start the heart beating again) should be used immediately if available. The next step is to call for emergency medical assistance. Next, if the person has not resumed breathing, cardiopulmonary resuscitation (CPR) should be started. CPR combines artificial respiration (mouth-to-mouth resuscitation, rescue breathing), which supplies oxygen to the lungs, with chest compressions, which circulate oxygen to the brain and other vital organs by forcing blood out of the heart.

Skill in CPR is best obtained through a training course. The American Heart Association, American Red Cross, and many local fire departments and hospitals offer CPR training courses. Because procedures may change over time, it is important to stay up to date on training and to repeat courses as recommended.

To begin CPR, the rescuer lays the person face up, rolling the head, body, and limbs at the same time. The rescuer then removes any object visibly blocking the airway. Next, the rescuer tilts the person's head back slightly and lifts the chin, which sometimes opens a blocked airway. If the person does not resume breathing, the rescuer's mouth is placed over the person's mouth and the rescuer begins artificial respiration by slowly exhaling air into the person's lungs (rescue breaths). To prevent air from escaping from the person's nose, the person's nose is pinched shut as the rescuer exhales into the mouth.

Artificial respiration is very similar in children and adults. However, with an infant, the rescuer's mouth is placed over the infant's mouth and nose. To prevent damaging the infant's smaller lungs, the rescuer exhales with less force than with adults.

Failure of the chest to rise after properly delivering rescue breaths indicates that the person's airway is blocked. If the chest rises, the rescuer gives two deep, slow breaths.

Next, chest compressions are done. The rescuer kneels to one side and, with arms held straight, leans over the person and places both hands, one on top of the other, on the lower part of the breastbone. The rescuer compresses the chest to a depth of 1 1/2 to 2 inches (4 to 5 centimeters) in an adult, less deeply in a child. For an infant, the rescuer uses two fingers to compress the infant's breastbone just below the nipples to a depth of 1/2 to 1 inch (1 to 2 1/2 centimeters). CPR can be done by one person (who alternately does rescue breaths and chest compressions) or by two people (one to do rescue breaths and one to do chest compressions). Chest compressions are done about 100 times per minute. Two breaths are given after each 30 compressions. Doing chest compressions can quickly tire a person, resulting in compressions that are too weak to be effective, so, if two rescuers are present, they should switch duties (the person doing chest compressions should now do rescue breathing and vice versa) about every 2 minutes. CPR is continued until medical assistance arrives, rescuers are too tired to continue, or the person recovers.

Performing Chest Compressions in an Adult

To perform chest compressions for cardiac pulmonary resuscitation (CPR), a rescuer kneels to one side and, with the arms held straight, leans over the person and places both hands, one on top of the other just above (about two finger widths) the lowest part of the breastbone (called the xiphoid process). The rescuer compresses the chest about 1 1/2 to 2 inches (4 to 5 centimeters) in adults. The chest is compressed about 100 times per minute.

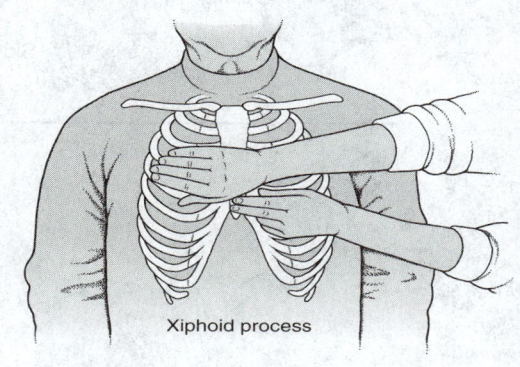

Xiphoid process

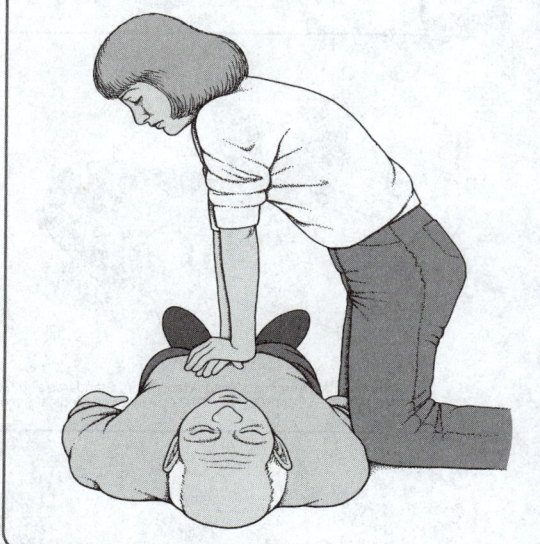

Performing Chest Compressions in a Child

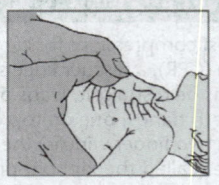

**Thumbs
Overlapping**

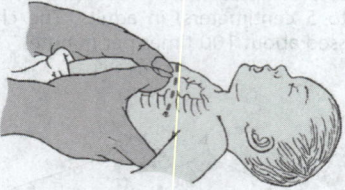

**Thumbs
Side by Side**

For newborns and small infants, the thumbs are placed side-by-side on the infant's breastbone just below an imaginary line between the nipples (indicated by the dotted line). Infants are small enough if their chest can be encircled with the hands. The thumbs should overlap if the newborn is very small.

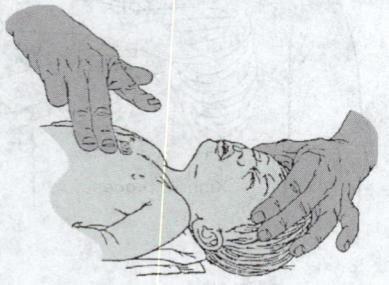

If an infant's chest cannot be encircled with the hands, two fingers are used. Fingers should be kept upright (nearly perpendicular to the chest) during compression. The rescuer compresses the chest about $1/2$ to 1 inch (1 to $2^1/2$ centimeters).

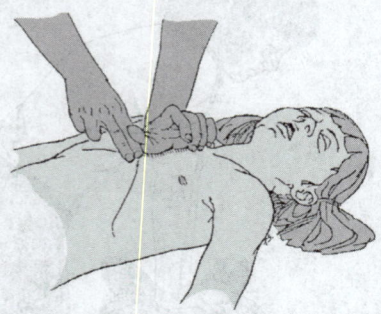

For children up to age 8 years, the heel of one hand is placed just above (by about two finger widths) the lowest part of the breastbone (called the xiphoid process). The rescuer presses straight down on the chest and compresses it about 1 inch ($2^1/2$ centimeters).

(Adapted from American Heart Association: Standards and Guidelines for CPR. Journal of the American Medical Association 1992;268:22512281. Copyright 1992, American Medical Association.)

Choking

Maneuvers to relieve choking are frequently life saving. Adults most often choke on a piece of food, such as a large piece of meat. Infants do not have well-developed swallowing reflexes and may choke if given small, rounded foods such as peanuts or hard candies. Children, especially toddlers, also may choke on balloons, toys, coins, other inedible objects that they place in their mouth, and foods (particularly rounded, smooth foods, such as hot dogs, round candies, nuts, and grapes).

Performing Abdominal Thrusts

The rescuer stands behind the person and encircles the person's abdomen with the arms. With one hand, the rescuer forms a fist and clasps the other hand around the fist. The rescuer places the hands halfway between the breastbone and navel and thrusts the hands inward and upward.

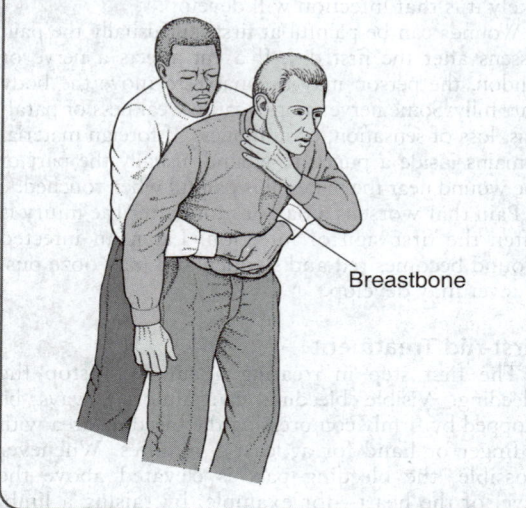

Breastbone

Coughing may be the first symptom and is often so severe that the person cannot ask for help. The person may grasp both hands near the throat. Breathing and speaking can become weak or stop. There can be high-pitched or snoring sounds. The person can turn blue, have a seizure, or faint.

First-Aid Treatment

Treatment for a person who is choking takes precedence over calling for emergency medical care.

A strong cough often expels the object from the airway. A person with a strong cough should be allowed to continue coughing. A person who can speak normally usually still has a strong cough. If a person who is choking cannot cough, the rescuer delivers abdominal thrusts (Heimlich maneuver). The abdominal thrusts increase pressure in the abdomen and chest, which expels the object.

If the person is conscious, the rescuer approaches from behind, using the arms to encircle the person's abdomen. The rescuer forms a fist, with the thumb pointing inward, and places it between the breastbone and navel, toward the person. The other hand is placed firmly over the fisted hand. The hands are then thrust inward and upward forcefully, 5 times in

succession. Less force should be used if the person is a child. Series of thrusts should be repeated until the object is expelled. If the person loses consciousness, the rescuer should stop the thrusts.

If the person loses consciousness, steps are taken to open the airway and provide artificial respiration (see art on page 1942). Failure of the chest to rise indicates that the airway is still blocked. The rescuer checks the airway for, and removes, visible objects. Artificial respiration is then resumed.

Clearing a Blocked Airway in an Infant

The infant is held face down with the chest resting on the rescuer's forearm. Then, the rescuer strikes the infant's back between the shoulder blades.

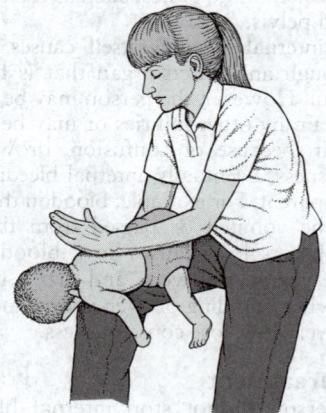

The infant is turned face up with the head lower than the body. Then, the rescuer places the second and third fingers on the infant's breastbone and thrusts inward and upward.

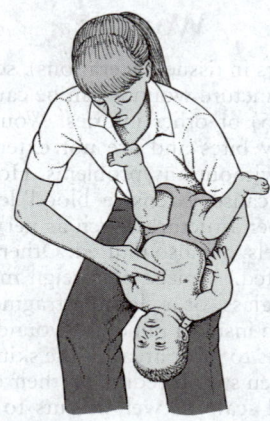

For an infant, abdominal thrusts are not done. Instead, the infant is turned face down, the chest resting on the rescuer's forearm, with the head lower than the body. The rescuer then strikes the infant between the shoulder blades 5 times using the heel of the hand (back blows). The strikes should be firm but not hard enough to cause injury. The rescuer then checks the mouth, removing any visible objects. If the airway remains blocked, the rescuer turns the infant face up with the head down, and using the second and third fingers, thrusts inward and upward on the infant's breastbone 5 times (chest thrusts). The rescuer then checks the mouth again.

Internal Bleeding

Heavy internal bleeding may occur in the abdominal cavity, chest cavity, digestive tract, or tissues surrounding broken large bones, such as the thigh bone (femur) and pelvis.

Initially, internal bleeding itself causes no symptoms, although an injured organ that is bleeding is often painful. However, the person may be distracted from this pain by other injuries or may be unable to express pain because of confusion, drowsiness, or unconsciousness. Eventually, internal bleeding usually becomes apparent. For example, blood in the digestive tract may be vomited or passed from the rectum. Extensive blood loss causes low blood pressure, making the person feel weak and dizzy. The person may faint when standing or even sitting and, if blood pressure is very low, lose consciousness.

First-Aid Treatment

A lay person cannot stop internal bleeding. If extensive bleeding causes light-headedness or symptoms of shock (see page 350), the person should be laid down and the legs elevated. Medical assistance should be summoned as quickly as possible.

Wounds

Cuts or tears in tissue (lacerations), scrapes (abrasions), and puncture wounds can be caused by bites (see page 2015) or other injuries. Wounds that are not caused by bites and are not extensive usually heal rapidly without any problems. However, some wounds can cause extensive blood loss. In some wounds, deeper structures, such as nerves, tendons, or blood vessels, are also injured. Other wounds can become infected. A piece of foreign material (such as a splinter, glass, or a clothing fragment) can also remain hidden inside a puncture wound.

Shallow cuts to most areas of the skin rarely bleed much and often stop bleeding on their own. Cuts to the hand and scalp as well as cuts to arteries and larger veins often bleed vigorously.

Infection can develop when a wound is contaminated with dirt and bacteria. Although any wound can become infected, infection is particularly likely in deep scrapes, which grind dirt into the skin, and in puncture wounds, which introduce contamination deep under the skin. Also, wounds that contain foreign material almost always become infected. The longer a wound remains contaminated, the more likely it is that infection will develop.

Wounds can be painful at first, but usually the pain lessens after the first day. If a cut affects a nerve or tendon, the person may be unable to move the body part fully. Some nerve injuries cause weakness or paralysis, loss of sensation, or numbness. If foreign material remains inside a puncture wound, usually the part of the wound near the material is painful when touched.

Pain that worsens a day or more after the injury is often the first sign of infection. Later, an infected wound becomes red and swollen and may ooze pus. A fever may develop.

First-Aid Treatment

The first step in treating a cut is to stop the bleeding. Visible bleeding can almost always be stopped by firmly compressing the bleeding area with a finger or hand for at least 5 minutes. Whenever possible, the bleeding part is elevated above the level of the heart—for example, by raising a limb. Because tourniquets shut off all blood flow to a body part and deprive it of oxygen, they are used only for very severe injuries (such as combat casualties).

To prevent infection, dirt and particles are removed and the wound is washed. Large, visible particles are picked off. Smaller dirt and particles that cannot be seen are removed by washing with mild soap and tap water. Dirt and particles that remain after washing often can be removed with a more highly pressured stream of warm tap water. Harsher agents, such as alcohol, iodine, and peroxide, are not recommended. These solutions can damage tissue, impairing the capacity to heal. Scrubbing is required to clean deep scrapes. If a wound is very small, it can be kept closed with certain commercially available tapes. Stitches may be needed for deep or large cuts. After cleaning and, if necessary, closing the wound, antibiotic ointment and a bandage are applied.

Medical assistance is needed under the following circumstances:

- If a cut is longer than about 1/3 inch (3/4 centimeter), is on the face, appears deep, or has edges that separate
- If bleeding does not stop on its own or within several minutes after pressure is applied
- If there are symptoms of a nerve or tendon injury, such as loss of sensation, loss of movement, or numbness

- If a scrape is deep or has dirt and particles that are difficult to remove
- If there is a puncture wound, particularly if foreign material in the wound is likely
- If the person has not had a tetanus vaccination within the past 5 years.

All wounds, whether treated at home or by health care practitioners, should be observed for symptoms of infection during the first several days after treatment. If any symptoms of infection develop, medical assistance should be sought within several hours. Most small wounds heal within a few days.

Soft Tissue Injuries

Soft tissue injuries include bumps and bruises (contusions) and small tears of muscles (minor strains) or of ligaments and tendons near joints (minor sprains).

Contusions, mild strains, and mild sprains produce mild to moderate pain and swelling. The swelling can become discolored, turning purple after a day and becoming yellow or brown days later. The person usually can continue using the body part. People with more severe symptoms, such as deformity, an inability to walk or use an injured part, or severe pain, may have a mild strain or sprain. However, they may also have a complete separation of bones that were attached within a joint (dislocation), partial separation of bones that were attached within a joint (subluxation), fracture (see page 1952), severe sprain or strain, or other severe injury. People with severe symptoms usually need medical care to determine the nature of the injury.

First-Aid Treatment

Contusions, mild strains, and mild sprains can be treated at home with *r*est, *i*ce, *c*ompression, and *e*levation (RICE—see page 1967), which speeds recovery and decreases pain and swelling. If a fracture, severe strain, severe sprain, subluxation (partial dislocation), or dislocation is a possibility, a splint should be applied until medical help is available.

Severed or Constricted Limbs or Digits

Body parts such as fingers and toes can become severed. Also, tissue may die because blood flow has been cut off by rings or other constricting devices. Rings cut off blood flow when parts of the body near the ring swell, often as the result of an injury or simply because of constriction by the ring.

Severed body parts, if properly preserved, can sometimes be reattached in the hospital. To prolong tissue life, the severed part should be put in a sealed,

Commonly Used Splints

A splint can be anything that prevents movement of a limb. A splint is used to prevent further damage and limit pain. To be effective, a splint must immobilize the joints above and below the injury.

Splints can be made from readily available objects, such as a magazine or stack of newspapers. But splints usually consist of a rigid, straight object, such as a board, strapped to the limb. A sling may be used with a splint to support the forearm when an arm, a wrist, or a collarbone is injured.

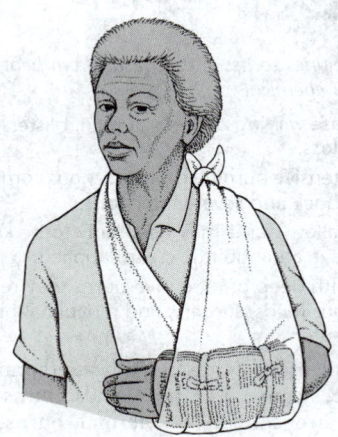

Splinted Arm in Sling

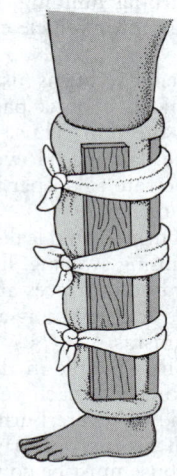

Splinted Leg

dry plastic bag, and the bag should be put in a container with ice. Dry ice should not be used. The severed part should not be placed in water.

An injured finger will probably swell. A ring on the finger should be removed as soon as possible, before swelling develops. Similarly, any other object that encircles a body part, such as a finger or toe or an arm or a leg, must be removed before the body part swells. Sustained, gentle traction can be used to remove rings. Soap and water may reduce friction, easing removal. Otherwise, prompt medical care is needed.

Burns are injuries to tissue that result from heat, electricity, radiation, or chemicals.

- Burns cause varying degrees of pain, blisters, swelling, and skin loss.
- Deep, extensive burns can cause serious complications, such as shock and severe infections.
- Small, shallow burns may need only to be kept clean and to have an antibiotic cream applied.
- People with deep or extensive burns may require intravenous fluids, surgery, and rehabilitation, often at a burn center.

Burns are usually caused by heat (thermal burns), such as fire, steam, tar, or hot liquids. Burns caused by chemicals are similar to thermal burns, whereas burns caused by radiation (see page 1984), sunlight (see page 1325), and electricity (see page 1990) differ significantly. Events associated with a burn, such as jumping from a burning building, being struck by debris, or being in a motor vehicle crash, may cause other injuries.

Thermal and chemical burns usually occur because heat or chemicals contact part of the body's surface, most often the skin. Thus, the skin usually sustains most of the damage. However, severe surface burns may penetrate to deeper body structures, such as fat, muscle, or bone.

When tissues are burned, fluid leaks into them from the blood vessels, causing swelling. In addition, damaged skin and other body surfaces are easily infected because they can no longer act as a barrier against invading microorganisms.

More than 2 million people in the United States require treatment for burns each year, and between 3,000 and 4,000 die of severe burns. Older people and young children are particularly vulnerable. In those age groups, abuse must be considered.

Classification

Doctors classify burns according to strict, widely accepted definitions. The definitions classify the burn's depth and the extent of tissue damage.

Burn Depth: The depth of injury from a burn is described as first, second, or third degree:

- **First-degree** burns are the most shallow (superficial). They affect only the top layer of skin (epidermis).
- **Second-degree** burns (also called partial-thickness burns) extend into the middle layer of skin (dermis). Second-degree burns are sometimes further described as superficial (involving the more superficial part of the dermis) or deep (involving both the superficial and the deep parts of the dermis).

When Chemicals Burn the Skin

Chemical burns are caused by caustic substances that contact the skin. Caustic substances are sometimes present in household products, including those containing lye (in drain cleaners and paint removers), phenols (in deodorizers, sanitizers, and disinfectants), sodium hypochlorite (in disinfectants and bleaches), and sulfuric acid (in toilet bowl cleaners). Many chemicals used in industry and during armed conflicts can cause burns. Wet cement left on the skin can cause severe burns as well.

The steps in stopping chemical burns are

- Remove contaminated clothing
- Brush away any dry powders or particles
- Rinse the area with large amounts of water.

Because chemicals can continue to inflict damage long after first contacting the skin, rinsing should continue for at least 30 minutes. In rare cases involving certain industrial chemicals (for example, metal sodium), water should not be used because it can actually worsen the burn. In addition, some chemicals have specific treatments that can further reduce skin damage. Further treatment of chemical burns is the same as that for thermal burns.

If more information is needed concerning treatment of a burn caused by a specific chemical, the local Poison Control Center can be contacted.

Estimating the Extent of a Burn

To determine the severity of a burn, doctors estimate what percentage of the body's surface has second- or third-degree burns. For adults, doctors use the rule of nines. This method divides almost all of the body into sections of 9% or of 2 times 9% (18%). For children, doctors use charts that adjust these percentages according to the child's age (Lund-Browder charts). Adjustment is needed because different areas of the body grow at different rates.

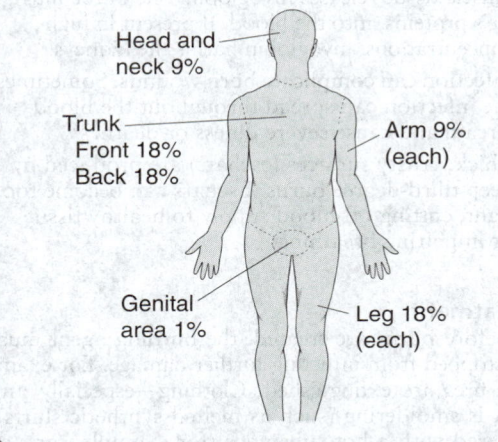

Head and neck 9%

Trunk
Front 18%
Back 18%

Arm 9% (each)

Genital area 1%

Leg 18% (each)

- **Third-degree** burns (also called full-thickness) involve all three layers of skin (epidermis, dermis, and fat layer). Usually, the sweat glands, hair follicles, and nerve endings are destroyed as well.

Burn Severity: Burns are classified as minor, moderate, or severe. These classifications may not correspond to a person's understanding of those terms. For example, doctors may classify a burn as minor even though it can cause the person significant pain and interfere with normal activities. The severity determines how they are predicted to heal and whether complications are likely. Doctors determine the severity of the burn by its depth and by the percentage of the body surface that has second- or third-degree burns. Special charts are used to show what percentage of the body surface various body parts comprise. For example, in an adult, the arm constitutes about 9% of the body. Separate charts are used for children because their body proportions are different.

- **Minor burns:** All first-degree burns as well as second-degree burns that involve less than 10% of the body surface usually are classified as minor.
- **Moderate and severe burns:** Burns involving the hands, feet, face, or genitals, second-degree burns

involving more than 10% of the body surface area, and all third-degree burns involving more than 1% of the body are classified as moderate or, more often, as severe.

Symptoms and Diagnosis

Symptoms of a burn wound vary with the burn's depth:

- **First-degree burns** are red, swollen, and painful. The burned area whitens (blanches) when lightly touched but does not develop blisters.
- **Second-degree burns** are pink or red, swollen, and painful, and they develop blisters that may ooze a clear fluid. The burned area may blanch when touched.
- **Third-degree burns** usually are not painful because the nerves have been destroyed. The skin becomes leathery and may be white, black, or bright red. The burned area does not blanch when touched, and hairs can easily be pulled from their roots without pain.

The appearance and symptoms of deep burns can worsen during the first hours or even days after the burn.

Doctors frequently examine hospitalized people for complications and assess burn wound depth and extent. In people with large burns, blood pressure, heart rate, and urine volume are measured often to help assess the extent of dehydration or shock and the need for intravenous fluids. Doctors do blood tests to monitor the body's electrolytes and blood count. Electrocardiography (ECG) and chest x-ray are also required. Tests of blood and urine are done to detect proteins caused by the destruction of muscle tissue (rhabdomyolysis) that sometimes occurs with deep third-degree burns.

? Did You Know...

The deepest burns may cause the least pain because the nerves that sense pain are destroyed.

Complications

Minor burns are usually superficial and do not cause complications. However, deep second-degree and third-degree burns swell and take more time to heal. In addition, deeper burns can cause scar tissue to form. This scar tissue shrinks (contracts) as it heals. If the scarring occurs in a limb or digit, the resulting contracture may restrict movement of nearby joints.

Severe burns and some moderate burns can cause serious complications due to extensive fluid loss and tissue damage. These complications may take hours

Smoke Inhalation

Many people who have been burned in fires have also inhaled smoke. Sometimes people inhale smoke without sustaining skin burns. Smoke inhalation often causes no serious, lasting effects. However, if the smoke contains certain poisonous chemicals or is unusually dense or if inhalation is prolonged, serious problems can develop.

Hot smoke sometimes burns the throat, resulting in swelling. As the swelling narrows this area, airflow into the lungs is obstructed. Breathing hot steam can burn the lungs as well as the throat, causing severe breathing problems.

Inhalation of chemicals released in the smoke, such as hydrogen chloride, phosgene, sulfur dioxide, and ammonia, can cause swelling and damage to the windpipe (trachea) and even the lungs. Eventually, the small airways leading to the lungs narrow, further obstructing airflow. Smoke can also contain chemicals that poison the body's cells, such as carbon monoxide (see page 2010) and cyanide.

Damage to the trachea or the lungs can cause shortness of breath, which can take up to 24 hours to develop. Obstruction of airflow due to swelling of the airways can produce difficulty breathing air in, wheezing, and shortness of breath. People may have soot in the mouth or nose, singed nasal hairs, or burns around the mouth. Lung damage may cause chest pain, coughing, and wheezing. If the oxygen supply is depleted due to smoke, people may pass out. High levels of carbon monoxide in the blood may cause confusion or disorientation or may even be fatal.

To assess the extent of injury due to smoke inhalation, doctors may pass a flexible viewing tube (bronchoscope) into the trachea. Doctors may assess lung damage with a chest x-ray or with a test that determines the level of oxygen in the blood.

People who have inhaled smoke are given oxygen through a face mask. If a tracheal burn is suspected, a breathing tube is inserted through the nose or mouth in case the trachea later swells and obstructs airflow. If people begin to wheeze, drugs that open small airways, such as albuterol, may be given, usually as a mist that is combined with oxygen and inhaled through a face mask. If lung damage causes shortness of breath that persists despite use of a face mask and albuterol, a ventilator may be necessary. Relieving the stress of breathing conserves people's energy and usually allows faster recovery.

- Dehydration eventually develops in people with widespread burns, because fluid seeps from the blood to the burned tissues and, if burns are deep and extensive enough, to the whole body.

- Shock develops if dehydration is severe (see page 350).

- Chemical imbalances can result from extensive burns.

- Destruction of muscle tissue (rhabdomyolysis) sometimes occurs with deep third-degree burns. The muscle tissue releases myoglobin, one of the muscle's proteins, into the blood. If present in high concentrations, myoglobin harms the kidneys.

- Infection can complicate burn wounds. Sometimes the infection can spread throughout the bloodstream and cause severe illness or death.

- Thick, crusty surfaces (eschars) are produced by deep third-degree burns. Eschars can become too tight, cutting off blood supply to healthy tissues or impairing breathing.

Treatment

Before burns are treated, the burning agent must be stopped from inflicting further damage. For example, fires are extinguished. Clothing—especially any that is smoldering (such as melted synthetic shirts), covered with a hot substance (for example, tar), or soaked with chemicals—is immediately removed.

Hospitalization is sometimes necessary for optimal care of burns. For example, elevating a severely burned arm or leg above the level of the heart to prevent swelling is more easily accommodated in a hospital. In addition, burns that prevent people from carrying out essential daily functions, such as walking or eating, make hospitalization necessary. Severe burns, deep second- and third-degree burns, burns occurring in the very young or the very old, and burns involving the hands, feet, face, or genitals are usually best treated at burn centers. Burn centers are hospitals that are specially equipped and staffed to care for burn victims.

Superficial Minor Burns: Superficial minor burns are immersed immediately in cool water if possible. The burn is carefully cleaned to prevent infection. If dirt is deeply embedded, doctors can give analgesics or numb the area by injecting a local anesthetic and then scrub the burn with a brush.

Often, the only treatment required is application of an antibiotic cream, such as silver sulfadiazine. The cream prevents infection and forms a seal to prevent further bacteria from entering the wound. A sterile bandage is then applied to protect the burned area from dirt and further injury. A tetanus vaccination is given if needed (see page 1150).

or days to develop. The deeper and more extensive the burn, the more severe are the problems it tends to cause. Young children and older adults tend to be more seriously affected by complications than other age groups. The following are some complications of some moderate and severe burns:

Care at home includes keeping the burn clean to prevent infection. In addition, many people are given analgesics, often opioids, for at least a few days. The burn can be covered with a nonstick bandage or with sterile gauze. The gauze can be removed without sticking by first being soaked in water.

Deep Minor Burns: As with more superficial burns, deep minor burns are treated with antibiotic cream. Any dead skin and broken blisters should be removed by a health care practitioner before the antibiotic cream is applied. In addition, keeping a deeply burned arm or leg elevated above the heart for the first few days reduces swelling and pain. The burn may require admission to a hospital or frequent re-examination at a hospital or doctor's office, possibly as often as daily for the first few days.

A **skin graft** may be needed. Some skin grafts replace burned skin that will not heal. Other skin grafts help by temporarily covering and protecting the skin as it heals on its own. In a skin grafting procedure, a piece of healthy skin is taken from an unburned area of the person's body (autograft), a dead person (allograft), or an animal (xenograft). After any dead tissue is removed and the wound is clean, a surgeon sews the skin graft over the burned area. Artificial skin can also be used. Autografts are permanent. Allografts and xenografts, however, are rejected after 10 to 14 days by the person's immune system and artificial skin is removed. These skin covers help by temporarily covering and protecting the skin as it begins to heal on its own. However, an autograft eventually must be placed. Burned skin can be replaced anytime within several days of the burn.

Physical and occupational therapy usually are needed to prevent immobility caused by scarring around the joints and to help people function if joint motion is limited. Stretching exercises are started within the first few days after the burn. Splints are applied to ensure that joints that are likely to be immobile rest in positions that are least likely to lead to contractures. The splints are left in place except when the joints are moved. If a skin graft has been used, however, therapy is not started for 3 to 5 days after the grafts are attached so that the healing graft is not disturbed. Bulky dressings that put pressure on the burn can prevent large scars from developing.

Severe Burns: Severe, life-threatening burns require immediate care. People who have gone into shock as a result of dehydration are given oxygen through a face mask.

Large amounts of intravenous fluids are given, beginning immediately, for people who have dehydration, shock, or burns that cover a large area of the body. Fluids are also given to people who devel-

---

Small, Shallow Burns

Most people who sustain small burns attempt to treat them at home rather than visit the doctor. Indeed, simple first-aid measures may be all that is necessary to treat small, shallow burns that are clean. In general, a clean burn is one that affects only clean skin and that does not contain any dirt particles or food. Running cold water over the burn can help relieve pain. Covering the burn with an over-the-counter antibiotic ointment and a nonstick, sterile bandage can help prevent infection.

Generally, a doctor's examination and treatment are recommended if a tetanus vaccination is needed. Likewise, a doctor should examine a burn if it has any of the following characteristics:

- Is larger than the size of the person's open hand
- Contains blisters
- Darkens or breaks the skin
- Involves the face, hand, foot, genitals, or skinfolds
- Is not completely clean
- Causes pain that is not relieved by acetaminophen
- Causes pain that does not improve within one day after the burn was sustained.

---

op destruction of muscle tissue. The fluids dilute the myoglobin in the blood, preventing extensive damage to the kidneys. Sometimes a chemical (sodium bicarbonate) is given intravenously to help dissolve myoglobin and thus also prevent further damage to the kidneys.

A **surgical procedure** to cut open eschars that cut off blood supply to a limb or that impair breathing may be needed. This procedure is called escharotomy. Escharotomy usually causes some bleeding, but because the burn causing the eschar has destroyed the nerve endings in the skin, there is little pain.

Skin care is extremely important. Keeping the burned area clean is essential, because the damaged skin is easily infected. Cleaning may be accomplished by gently running water over the burns periodically. Wounds are cleaned and bandages changed 1 to 3 times per day. Skin grafts are needed to cover burns that will not heal.

A **proper diet** that includes adequate amounts of calories, protein, and nutrients is important for healing. People who cannot consume enough calories may drink nutritional supplements or receive them by way of a tube inserted through the nose into the stomach (a nasogastric tube), or less often nutrition may be given intravenously. Additional vitamins and minerals are usually given.

Physical and occupational therapy are needed.

Depression is treated. Because severe burns take a long time to heal and can cause disfigurement, people can become depressed. Depression often can be relieved with drugs, psychotherapy, or both.

Prognosis

First- and some second-degree burns heal in days to weeks without scarring. Deep second-degree and small third-degree burns take weeks to heal and usually cause scarring. Most require skin grafting. Burns that involve more than 90% of the body surface, or more than 60% in an older person, are often fatal.

CHAPTER 301   Fractures

A fracture is a crack or break in a bone, usually accompanied by injury to the surrounding tissues.

- Fractures cause pain and swelling.
- Complications may involve damage to nerves, blood vessels, muscles, and internal organs and can be serious.
- Most fractures are diagnosed by x-rays, although some require repeat x-rays in 7 to 10 days or computed tomography or magnetic resonance imaging.
- Treatments range from mild restrictions on activity to casts or surgery.
- Rehabilitation is often helpful to build up strength and range of motion of the affected body part.

Fractures vary greatly in size, severity, and the treatment needed. They can range from a small, easily missed crack in a foot bone to a massive, life-threatening break of the pelvis. Serious injuries, including injuries to the skin, nerves, blood vessels, muscles, and organs, may occur at the same time as the fracture. These injuries can complicate treatment of the fracture, cause temporary or permanent problems, or both.

Trauma is the most common cause of fractures. Low-energy trauma, such as a fall on level ground, usually causes minor fractures. High-energy trauma, such as high-speed motor vehicle collisions and falls from buildings, can cause severe fractures that involve several bones.

Certain underlying disorders can weaken parts of the skeleton so that breaks are more likely to occur. Such disorders include certain infections, benign bone tumors, cancer, and osteoporosis.

Symptoms

Pain is the most obvious symptom. Fractures hurt, especially when force is applied, such as when a person tries to put weight on an injured limb. The area around the broken bone is also tender to touch. Swelling of soft tissue around the fracture begins within a few hours.

The limb may not function properly, so that an arm or a leg, hand, finger, or toe may move in only a limited range or in an abnormal direction. Moving is very painful. For a person who cannot speak (for example, a very young child, a person with a head injury, or an older person with dementia), refusal to move an extremity may be the only sign of a fracture. However, some fractures do not keep people from moving an injured extremity. Just because an extremity can move does not mean there is no fracture.

Complications

Internal bleeding may occur with a closed fracture (one in which the skin is not torn). The bleeding may occur from the bone itself or from surrounding soft tissues. The blood eventually works its way to the surface, forming a bruise (ecchymosis). At first, the bruise is purplish black, but it then slowly turns to green and yellow as the blood is broken down and reabsorbed back into the body. The blood can move quite a distance from the fracture, and it can take a few weeks for blood to be reabsorbed. The blood can cause temporary pain and stiffness in surrounding structures. Shoulder fractures, for instance, can bruise the entire arm and cause pain in the elbow and wrist. Some fractures, especially pelvic and femur fractures, can cause a person to lose quite a lot of blood into the surrounding tissues, resulting in low blood pressure.

Injury to an artery, vein, or nerve may occur. An open fracture (in which the skin is torn) can lead to a bone infection (osteomyelitis), which may be very difficult to cure. Fractures of long bones may release enough fat (and other substances in bone marrow) to travel through the veins, lodge in the lungs, and block a blood vessel there. Respiratory complications can result. Fractures that extend into joints usually damage cartilage (a smooth, tough, protective tissue

How Bones Heal

When most tissues, such as those of the skin, muscles, and internal organs, become injured, they tend to mend by having scar tissue replace the healthy tissue. The scar tissue often compromises the tissue's appearance or function in some way. In contrast, bone is unique in that it heals with its own tissue—bone—rather than with scar tissue. New bone made by the body to repair a fracture is called callus, and its formation and progress can be seen on x-rays. This unusual capacity for regeneration enables a mending bone to heal itself after a fracture, often so that the fracture eventually becomes virtually undetectable. Even shattered fragments of bone, with proper treatment, can often be restored to their normal function.

Fractures heal in three overlapping phases: inflammation, repair, and remodeling. Healing begins immediately with the **inflammatory phase**. In this phase, damaged soft tissue, bone fragments, and lost blood caused by the injury are removed by cells of the immune system. The region around the fracture becomes swollen and tender as cell activity and blood flow increase. The inflammatory phase reaches peak activity in a couple of days, but it takes weeks to subside. This process accounts for most of the early pain people experience with fractures.

The **repair phase** begins within days of the injury and lasts for weeks to months. New repaired bone, called the external callus, is formed during this phase. When first produced, the callus has no calcium. It is soft and rubbery and cannot be seen on an x-ray. This new bone is neither strong nor stable, so that during this period the fractured bone can easily collapse and become displaced (that is, slip out of its proper place). After 3 to 6 weeks, the callus calcifies and becomes much stiffer and stronger and becomes visible on x-rays.

The **remodeling phase** (in which the bone is built back to its normal state) lasts many months. The bulky external callus is slowly resorbed and replaced by stronger bone. During this phase, the normal contours and architecture of the bone are restored. It is not likely that the bone will fracture again during this phase. However, people may experience mild pain when pressure is applied to the bone that is rebuilding.

that reduces friction as joints move). Damaged cartilage tends to scar, causing osteoarthritis and impairing motion in the joints.

The person usually feels some discomfort with activities even after fractures have healed sufficiently to allow full weight bearing. For example, a fractured wrist may be strong enough to allow some use in about 2 months, but the bone is still being rebuilt (remodeled). Forceful gripping with the wrist will be painful for up to 1 year. The person may also notice increased pain and stiffness when the weather is damp, cold, or stormy.

Most fractures heal with few problems. However, some do not heal despite appropriate diagnosis and treatment. This failure to heal is called nonunion. Fractures may also heal very slowly (called delayed union) or incompletely (called malunion). Certain bones, such as the scaphoid bone of the hand and some parts of the hip, are prone to poor healing because the blood supply is often damaged when these areas are fractured.

Compartment Syndrome: Compartment syndrome is a very rare but serious limb-threatening condition caused by excessive swelling of injured muscles, such as may occur as a result of a fracture or crush injury to a limb. Certain muscle groups, such as those of the lower leg, are surrounded by a tight fibrous covering. This covering forms a closed space (compartment) that cannot expand to accommodate the normal swelling that occurs when muscles or bones inside that compartment are damaged. Instead, the swelling causes the pressure within the muscle tissue to increase. This increase in pressure decreases the blood flow that provides oxygen to the muscle. When the muscle is deprived of oxygen for too long, further injury to the muscle occurs, which leads to further swelling and higher tissue pressures. After only a few hours, irreversible injury and death of muscle and nearby soft tissues may result. A similar increase in muscle pressure and tissue damage can occur when a damaged limb is confined by a cast. Compartment syndrome is most common with fractures of the lower leg.

A doctor becomes concerned about compartment syndrome when people who have a fracture feel

- Increasing pain in an immobilized limb
- Pain when the fingers or toes of an immobilized limb are moved gently
- Numbness in the limb

The diagnosis of compartment syndrome can be confirmed by using a device that measures pressure in the muscles.

Pulmonary Embolism: Pulmonary embolism is the sudden blocking of blood flow in the lung when a blood clot that has formed in a vein breaks off (becoming an embolus) and travels to the lung (see page 488). Most of these clots come from the deep veins of the legs. In the lung, these clots cause many problems, including limiting blood flow to the heart, decreasing the lung's ability to put oxygen in the blood, and damaging lung tissue. Pulmonary embolism is the most common fatal complication of serious hip and pelvic fractures. People with hip

TYPES OF FRACTURES

TYPE	DESCRIPTION
Open	The skin and soft tissue covering the bone are torn, and the bone may be seen coming out of the skin. Dirt, debris, or bacteria can easily contaminate the wound.
Closed	The skin is not torn.
Avulsion	Small fragments of bone detach from where tendons or ligaments attach to bones. These fractures usually occur in the hand, foot, ankle, knee, or shoulder.
Osteoporotic	Osteoporosis weakens certain areas of the skeleton, making them more likely to break. These fractures occur in older people, usually in the hips, wrists, spine, shoulders, or pelvis.
Compression	The bone collapses into itself. These fractures occur in older people, very commonly in the spine.
Joint (intraarticular)	The fracture disrupts the part of a bone that makes up one of the joint surfaces, where two different bones contact each other. Joint fractures may lead to a loss of motion and gradually developing osteoarthritis.
Pathologic	An underlying disorder (such as infection, a noncancerous bone tumor, or cancer) weakens a bone, leading to a fracture.
Stress	A bone becomes stressed repeatedly over time because of certain activities, such as walking with a heavy pack or running. Stress fractures commonly occur in bones of the foot and lower leg.
Occult (hairline)	These fractures are difficult or impossible for a doctor to see on an initial x-ray. They may appear as dark or white lines days to weeks after injury, often only after new bone (callus) is formed during healing.
Greenstick	A partial crack and a bend occur in the bone, but the bone is not completely broken through. Greenstick fractures occur only in children.
Growth plate	The part of the bone that allows bones to lengthen (growth plate) is broken. The bone may then stop growing or grow crookedly. Growth plate fractures occur only in children.
Simple transverse	The break divides a bone cleanly across.
Displaced	The broken ends of the bones are separated.
Angulated	The broken ends of the bones are bent at an angle.
Nondisplaced	The normal shape and alignment of a bone are maintained despite cracks completely through the bone.
Spiral (torsion)	The bone is twisted apart, leaving sharp, triangular bone ends.
Comminuted	The bone is broken into many pieces, often because of high-energy trauma or weakening by osteoporosis.

fractures are at high risk of pulmonary embolism because of the combination of trauma to the leg, forced immobilization for hours or days, and swelling around the fracture site blocking blood flow in the veins. Of people with a hip fracture who die, about one third die of pulmonary embolism. Pulmonary embolism occurs much less commonly with fractures of the lower leg and very rarely with fractures of the arm.

Doctors may suspect pulmonary embolism based on a range of symptoms, including chest pain, cough, shortness of breath, extreme weakness, and fainting. An electrocardiogram (ECG), ultrasound scan, chest x-ray, or various other tests may suggest the presence of a blood clot in the lung. Confirmation usually involves computed tomography (CT) of the chest or lung scanning.

Pulmonary embolism may be prevented with drugs that reduce the tendency of the blood to clot. Such drugs include heparin, low-molecular-weight heparin, warfarin, and newer anticoagulants such as hirudin, danaparoid, and fondaparinux (a new drug similar to heparin). They are given to people with fractures that put them at risk of forming a pulmonary embolism. However, blood clots may form despite efforts to stop them.

Diagnosis

X-rays are the most important tool for diagnosing a fracture. X-rays are taken from several different angles to show how the fragments of bone are aligned. However, some small, nondisplaced fractures (called occult or hairline fractures) can be difficult or impossible to see on routine x-rays. Sometimes, additional x-rays taken at special angles reveal the fracture. Occasionally, such small fractures become visible on x-rays only days or weeks later, when the fracture begins to heal, revealing callus (new bone) formation. This course is particularly common with rib fractures. Stress fractures also may be undetectable on initial x-rays and visible only after callus formation begins. Fractures caused by disease (pathologic fractures) are diagnosed when x-rays show fractures in bones that have certain abnormalities, such as punched-out (lytic) areas caused by infection, noncancerous (benign) tumors, or cancer.

X-rays are usually the only test done to diagnose fractures. However, when findings strongly suggest a fracture but x-rays do not show one, doctors may do CT or magnetic resonance imaging (MRI). Alternatively, the doctor may apply a splint and re-examine the person days later and take another x-ray if symptoms are still significant. CT and MRI also are used to show details of fractures not seen on routine x-rays. CT can show the fine details of a fractured joint surface or can reveal areas of a fracture hidden by overlying bone. MRI shows the soft tissue around the bone, which helps to detect injury to nearby tendons and ligaments and joint structures, and can show evidence of cancer. MRI also shows injury (swelling or bruising) within the bone and can thus detect hidden or less visible (occult) fractures before they appear on x-rays.

Bone scanning (see page 543) is an imaging procedure that involves use of a radioactive substance (technetium-99m–labeled pyrophosphate) that is taken up by any healing bone. Occult fractures can be detected on bone scans 3 to 5 days after the injury. However, if doctors suspect an occult fracture, they usually order an MRI or CT scan rather than a bone scan.

Treatment

Fractures require immediate attention because they cause pain and loss of function. After initial emergency care, fractures usually require further treatment, such as immobilization with casts or fixation with surgery.

Fractures in children are often treated differently from those in adults because bones in children are smaller, more flexible and less brittle, and most importantly, still growing. Children's fractures heal much faster and more perfectly than adult fractures do. Several years after most fractures in children, the bone can look almost normal on x-ray. In addition, children develop less stiffness with cast treatment and are more likely to regain normal motion if a fracture involves a joint. Because of these factors and because surgery near a joint often risks damage to the part of the bone responsible for bone growth (the growth plate), treatment with casts is often preferred over surgery.

Initial Treatment: When a fracture is suspected, people typically should go to a hospital emergency department. Those who are unable to walk or who have multiple injuries must be transported by ambulance. Until they see the doctor, people can do the following:

- Immobilize and support the injured limb with a makeshift splint, sling, or a pillow
- Elevate the limb to the level of the heart to limit swelling
- Apply ice to control pain and swelling
- Take acetaminophen to relieve pain

Aspirin and other nonsteroidal anti-inflammatory drugs (NSAIDs) usually are no better than acetaminophen and in some people may worsen bleeding (see page 644).

Open fractures need to be treated immediately with surgery to carefully clean and close the wound. Massive open fractures with great losses of the skin, muscle, and blood supply to the bone are the most serious and difficult to treat.

For most closed fractures, treatment can be delayed up to 1 week without affecting the long-term result. However, there is usually no advantage to waiting, because until they are treated, people are troubled by pain and loss of function. People should keep an injured arm or leg elevated to control pain and swelling. For arm fractures, pillows are used for elevation. For leg fractures, people should lie flat with the leg on a pillow. The doctor compares the swelling of the injured limb with the normal appearance of the uninjured limb to help determine how long or often elevation is needed. During the later stages of healing, elastic stockings may be used during the daytime to help control swelling when the person is sitting or standing.

Immobilization: Fractures are immobilized with a splint, sling, or cast until they heal. Allowing the broken ends to move prevents healing and results in nonunion. Displaced fractures must be aligned (reduced) before being immobilized. Alignment

Commonly Used Techniques for Immobilizing a Joint

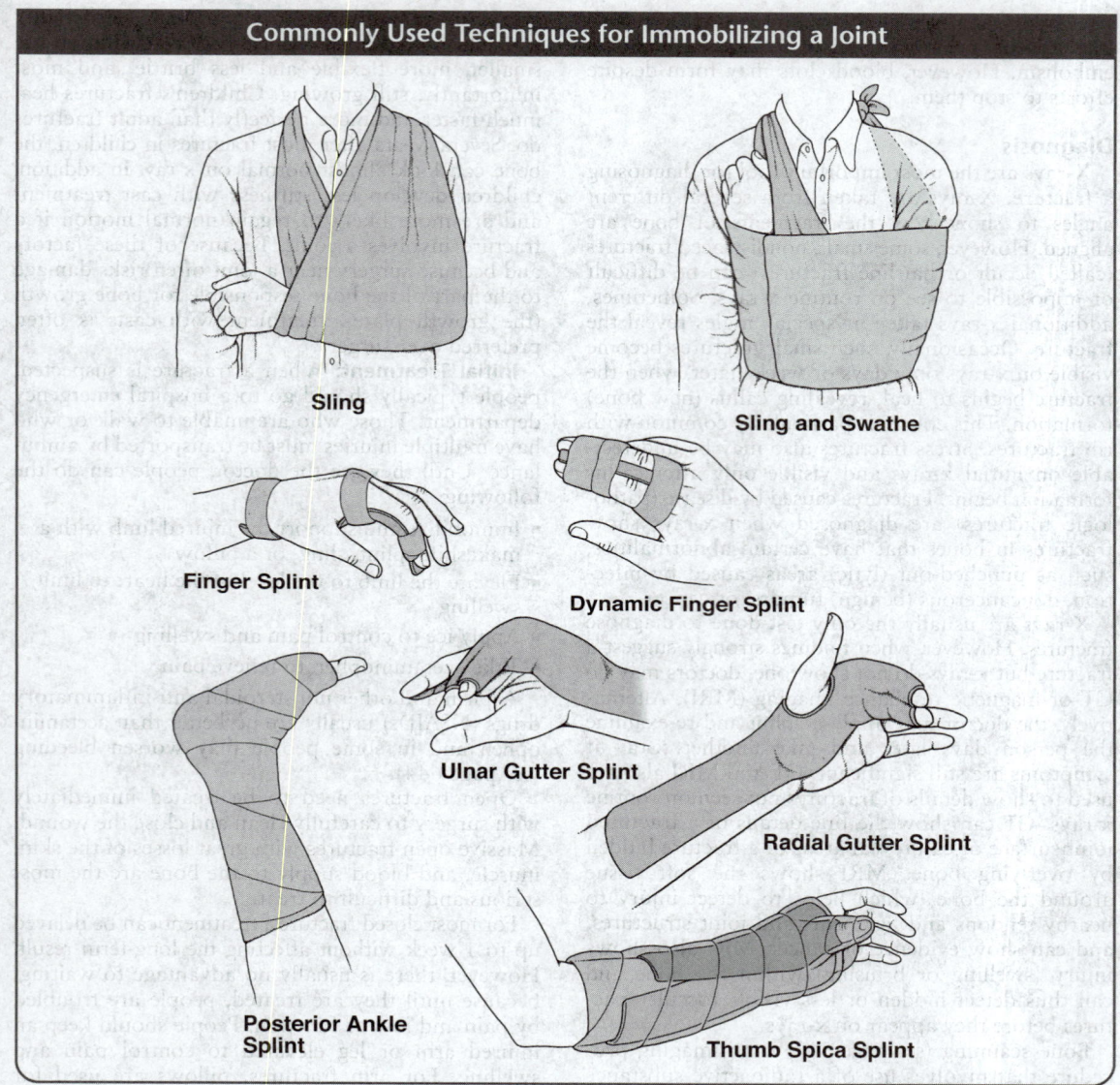

Sling

Sling and Swathe

Finger Splint

Dynamic Finger Splint

Ulnar Gutter Splint

Radial Gutter Splint

Posterior Ankle Splint

Thumb Spica Splint

without surgery is called closed reduction. Alignment with surgery is called open reduction. When minor fractures (such as those of the fingers or wrist) are reduced, people may need an injection of a local anesthetic, such as lidocaine, to prevent pain. When major fractures (such as those of the arm, shoulder, or lower leg) are reduced, people may need sedation and pain relievers given by vein, or general or spinal anesthesia.

A **splint** is a long, narrow slab of plaster, fiberglass, or aluminum applied with elastic wrap or tape. The slab does not completely encircle the limb, which allows for some expansion due to tissue swelling. For this reason, splints are often used for initial treatment of fractures. For finger fractures, aluminum splints lined with foam are commonly used.

A **sling** by itself provides sufficient support for many shoulder and elbow fractures. The weight of the arm pulling downward helps to keep many shoulder fractures well aligned. Cloth or a strap passing around behind the back can be added to keep the arm from swinging outward, especially at night. Slings permit some use of the hand.

A **cast** is made by wrapping rolls of plaster or fiberglass strips that harden once wetted. Plaster is often chosen for the initial cast when a displaced fracture is being treated. It molds well and has less of a tendency to cause painful contact points between the body and cast. Otherwise, fiberglass has the advantage of being stronger, lighter, and more durable. In either case, the cast is applied over a layer of soft cottony material to protect the skin from pressure and rubbing. If the cast becomes wet, it is often impossible to completely dry the lining. As a result, the skin can soften and break down (macerate). For partially healed fractures, a special, more expensive and less protective waterproof lining is sometimes substituted.

After a cast is applied (especially for the first 24 to 48 hours), it should be kept elevated as much as possible at or above the level of the heart to combat swelling. Regularly flexing and extending the fingers or wiggling the toes helps the blood to drain from the limb and also helps to prevent swelling. Pain, pressure, or numbness that remains constant or worsens over time should be reported to a doctor immediately. These conditions may be due to a developing pressure sore or compartment syndrome.

The combination of *rest*, *ice*, *compression* (for example, with a splint, cast, or sometimes an elastic bandage), and *elevation* is often called RICE therapy.

Surgical Treatment: Fractures sometimes require surgical treatment, as for the following:

- Open fractures: A doctor must explore and carefully clean these fractures to remove all traces of foreign material that may have contaminated the bone ends.

- Displaced fractures that cannot be aligned or kept aligned by closed reduction: When a bone fragment or a tendon is trapped in the bone ends, a doctor may not be able to reduce a displaced fracture. Sometimes the fracture can be reduced, but the natural pull of muscles on the fracture fragments keeps them from staying reduced.

- Comminuted fractures: Multiple pieces are often too unstable for a cast to keep them aligned against the forces of muscle contraction.

- Joint fractures: A near-perfect alignment of the joint surfaces is required to prevent people from developing arthritis later.

- Pathologic fractures: If possible, these fractures are stabilized surgically before they break further and become displaced. This approach avoids the pain, disability, and the more complex surgery involved with a displaced fracture.

Taking Care of a Cast

- When bathing, enclose the cast in a plastic bag and carefully seal the top with rubber bands or tape. Commercially available waterproof covers are convenient to use and are more fail-safe. If a cast becomes wet, the underlying padding may retain moisture. A hair dryer can remove some dampness. Otherwise, the cast must be changed to prevent the breakdown of skin.

- Never push a sharp or pointed object down inside the cast (for example, to scratch an itch).

- Check the skin around the cast every day, and apply lotion to any red or sore area.

- When resting, position the cast carefully, possibly using a small pillow or pad, to prevent the edge from pinching or digging into the skin. Chafing or pressure sores may develop where the skin is in contact with the edge of the cast. If the edge of the cast feels rough, it can be padded with soft adhesive tape, moleskin, tissues, or cloth.

- Elevate the cast regularly, as directed by the doctor, to control swelling.

- Contact a doctor immediately if the cast causes persistent pain or excessive tightness. Pressure sores or unexpected swelling may require immediate removal of the cast.

- Contact a doctor if an odor emanates from the cast or if the person has a fever. These symptoms may indicate an infection.

- Fractures of the thighbone (femur) and hip: If these fractures are not treated surgically, they require months of immobilization in bed before people are strong enough to bear weight. In contrast, surgical stabilization usually enables people to walk with crutches or a walker within days.

Surgery may also be needed to repair injury to ligaments, nerves, tendons, or major arteries.

Surgical stabilization involves first accurately reducing the fracture to restore the bone's original shape and length. The surgeon uses anesthesia to relax the muscles and x-ray equipment to help align the bones. A surgeon exposes the fracture to see and manipulate the fragments with special instruments. Then, the bone fragments are securely fixed using some combination of metal wires, pins, screws, rods, and plates. This procedure is called open reduction and internal fixation (ORIF). Metal plates are contoured and fixed to the outside of the bone with screws. Metal rods are inserted from one end of the bone into the marrow cavity. These implants are made of stainless steel, high-strength alloy metal, or titanium. All such implants made in the

SPOTLIGHT ON AGING

Older people are more likely to have fractures because of the following:

- Osteoporosis
- Frequent falls
- Impaired protective reflexes during falls

Age-related fractures often affect sections of the long bones. Fractures of the forearm, upper arm, leg, thigh, pelvis, and spine are common among older people.

Healing in older people is often slower than in younger adults. Also, because they typically have lower overall strength than younger people, it is harder for older people to compensate for the limitations caused by a fracture. Even minor fractures can significantly impair older people's ability to do normal daily activities, such as eating, dressing, bathing, and even walking, especially if they use a walker. Their strength, flexibility, and balance may already be reduced, making the return to daily activities more difficult. If muscles are not used, they can become stiff and weak, further impairing them. Nurses and caregivers must help older people regain their ability to do normal daily activities.

Older people with poor circulation are at risk of pressure sores (see page 1299) when an injured limb rests on the cast. Nurses and caregivers should pad and diligently inspect the areas where the skin touches the cast (contact points)—especially the heels—for any sign of skin breakdown. Nurses and caregivers should make sure older people periodically change position to avoid stiffness. For example, sitting for a long time can lead to the hip and knee becoming fixed in a bent position. To help to prevent stiffness, people should periodically stand and walk or, if bedridden, alternate between lying down with the legs straight and sitting with the knees bent. For older people who are confined to bed, the risk of blood clots leading to pulmonary embolism, pneumonia, and urinary infections is high. Bed rest can also lead to pressure sores unrelated to a cast.

When treating fractures in older people, doctors try to avoid or minimize immobilization (joint immobilization or bed rest), which causes more problems in older people. Thus, the goal is to rapidly return older people to daily activities rather than perfectly restoring limb alignment and length.

A **joint replacement procedure** (arthroplasty) may need to be done when fractures severely damage the upper end of the femur, which is part of the hip joint, or humerus, which is part of the shoulder joint.

Bone grafting, using chips of bone harvested from another part of the body such as the pelvis, may be done initially, if the gap between fragments is too large, or later, if the healing process has slowed (delayed union) or stopped (nonunion).

Treatment of Compartment Syndrome: Anything confining the limb, such as a splint or a cast, is removed immediately. If this does not relieve pressure in the muscle compartment, an emergency surgical procedure called fasciotomy must be done. In fasciotomy, the doctor makes an incision along the entire length of the thick fibrous tissue (fascia) that makes up the compartment. This incision relieves pressure and allows blood flow to return to the muscles. Otherwise, the muscles and nerves could die because of a lack of oxygen, and then the limb may need to be amputated. If left untreated, complications of compartment syndrome can cause death.

Rehabilitation and Prognosis

Healing time varies from weeks to months. The outcome depends on the nature and location of the fracture. For many fractures, people eventually recover full function and have few or no symptoms. Some fractures, particularly those that involve a joint, can leave residual pain, stiffness, or both.

Stiffness and loss of strength are natural consequences of immobilization. A joint of a fractured limb immobilized in a cast becomes progressively stiffer each week, eventually losing its ability to fully extend and flex. Wasting away of muscle (atrophy) also can be severe. For instance, after wearing a long leg cast for a few weeks, most people can insert their hand into the formerly tight space between the cast and their thigh. When the cast is removed, the weakness resulting from muscle atrophy is very apparent.

Daily exercise using range-of-motion and muscle-strengthening exercises (see page 48) helps people combat stiffness and regain strength. While the fracture is healing, the joints outside the cast can be exercised. The joints within the cast cannot be exercised until the fracture has healed sufficiently and the cast can be removed. When exercising, the person should pay attention to how the injured limb feels and avoid exercising too forcefully. Passive exercises in which a therapist applies external force (see page 49) must be used when muscles are too weak for effective motion and when strong muscle contractions might displace a fracture. Ultimately, active exercise (in which the person uses his own muscle force) against gravity or weight resistance is necessary to regain full strength of an injured limb.

last 20 years are compatible with the strong magnets that are used for MRI. Most will not set off security devices at airports. Some of the hardware used to repair a fracture is permanently left in place, and some is removed after healing has taken place.

Foot and Ankle Fractures

Fractures of the foot bones are common and are caused by falls, twisting injuries, or direct impact of the foot against hard objects. Foot fractures cause considerable pain, which is almost always made worse by attempting to walk or put weight on the foot.

Diagnosis is usually made by x-ray. Rarely, computed tomography (CT) or magnetic resonance imaging (MRI) is required. Treatment varies with the bone involved and the type of fracture but usually involves placing the foot and ankle in a cast.

Toe Fractures: Toe (phalanges) fractures can occur when an unprotected foot collides with a hard object. If the big toe is abnormally bent, it may need to be realigned. Simple fractures of the four smaller toes heal without a cast. Certain measures, including splinting the toe with tape or nylon fastening (Velcro) to the adjacent toes (known as buddy taping) for several weeks and wearing loose footwear, can provide comfort and protect the toe. Stiff-soled shoes support the fracture, and wide, soft shoes place less pressure on the swollen toe. If walking in shoes is too painful, the doctor can prescribe specially fabricated boots.

A fracture of the big toe (hallux) tends to be more severe than that of the other toes, causing more intense pain, swelling, and bleeding under the skin. A big toe can break when a person drops a heavy object onto it or occasionally when a person stubs it. Fractures that affect the joint of the big toe may require surgery.

Sesamoid Fractures: The sesamoids are two small round bones located within the flexor tendon under the big toe. These bones may fracture from running, hiking, and sports involving coming down too hard on the ball of the foot (such as basketball and tennis). Using padding or specially constructed orthoses (insoles) for the shoe helps relieve the pain. If pain continues, a sesamoid bone may need to be removed surgically.

Metatarsal Fractures: A stress fracture of the metatarsals (the bones in the middle of the foot) can occur when a person walks or runs excessively (see page 1976). Putting full weight on the foot causes increased pain. The affected area on the metatarsal bone is tender to touch. Stress fractures may not be seen on x-rays if they are small or new (in an early stage). Sometimes CT, MRI, or bone scanning shows the fracture when x-rays do not. When a developing stress fracture is recognized early, stopping activities that aggravate the fracture may be all that is necessary. In more advanced and severe cases, crutches and a cast are necessary.

A fracture and dislocation of the base of the 2nd metatarsal bone usually occurs when people fall in a way that causes the toes to bend or twist toward the sole of the foot. This injury, called Lisfranc's fracture-dislocation, is common among football players. The middle of the foot becomes painful, swollen, and tender. Lisfranc's fracture-dislocation is serious and can lead to chronic problems with strenuous activities, permanent pain, and arthritis. Surgery may be required but does not always restore the foot to its previous condition.

A fracture of the 5th metatarsal base (located at the outside edge of the middle of the foot) occurs commonly after the foot is injured by turning inward or is crushed. This fracture is sometimes called a dancer's fracture. The outside edge of the foot becomes tender, and a swollen bruise develops. The cause and symptoms may be similar to those of a sprained ankle. A cast is not usually necessary but can make walking easier. Crutches and a protective walking shoe may be needed for a few days. These fractures heal relatively quickly. Fractures of the shaft of the 5th metatarsal bone (Jones fractures) are less common than dancer's fractures and do not heal as easily.

Heel Fractures: A heel fracture can occur if people land on their feet after falling from a height. Sometimes the knees, spine, or both also are injured in such a fall. Heel fractures are very painful, and people are unable to bear weight on the foot. Surgery is sometimes needed.

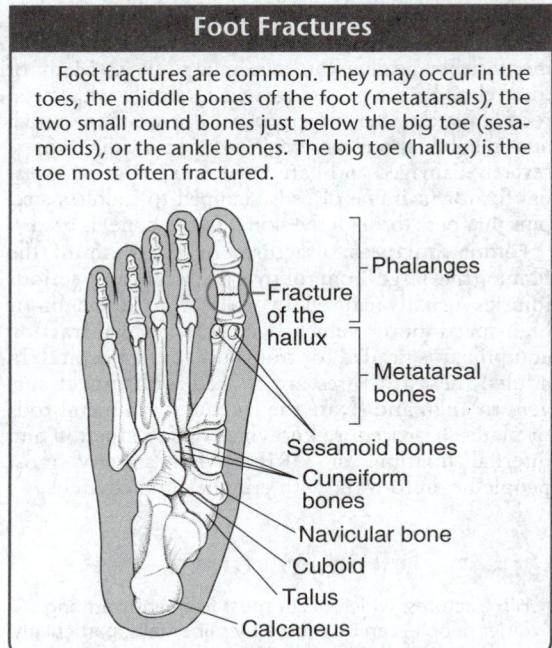

Foot Fractures

Foot fractures are common. They may occur in the toes, the middle bones of the foot (metatarsals), the two small round bones just below the big toe (sesamoids), or the ankle bones. The big toe (hallux) is the toe most often fractured.

Phalanges

Fracture of the hallux

Metatarsal bones

Sesamoid bones

Cuneiform bones

Navicular bone

Cuboid

Talus

Calcaneus

Ankle Fractures: The ankle may fracture when the foot rolls inward or outward during a fall or while running or jumping. Fractures usually involve the bony bump on the outside of the ankle (lateral malleolus), which is the end of the small bone of the lower leg (fibula). Less often, the bump on the inside of the ankle is involved. This bump is the end of the large bone of the lower leg (tibia). Sometimes both are affected, in which case there is usually significant ligament damage as well. Nondisplaced fractures of the ankle can be treated with a cast. Displaced fractures that cannot be realigned by the doctor or held in place with a cast require surgery.

Small chip (avulsion) fractures of the ligament attachments are similar to a severe sprain. This type of fracture is treated with a brace or cast for 6 weeks and usually heals well.

Leg Fractures

Tibia Fractures: Fractures of the **shaft of the tibia** (situated between the knee and the ankle) usually result from high-energy injuries, such as motor vehicle accidents, collisions, falls during skiing, and when pedestrians are struck by a car. This type of fracture can be very serious, particularly if the skin, muscle, nerves, or blood vessels are damaged. Such damage can lead to compartment syndrome (see page 1953).

For closed fractures of the tibia, an above-the-knee cast is needed until healing is under way and is then changed to a below-the-knee cast. The total time the person needs to wear these casts is usually about 3 months, but healing can take much longer. Many of these closed fractures are treated surgically with metal rods or plates. After surgery, usually no cast is required, and rehabilitation can begin sooner. If the skin is severely damaged and bare bone is exposed, an external fixator (a frame of rods clamped to stainless steel pins that pass through the skin into the bone) is used.

Femur Fractures: Fractures of the **shaft of the femur** (the large bone above the knee) are serious injuries usually caused by falls from a height or high-speed motor vehicle accidents. Special traction equipment is needed for transport to the hospital. In adults, these fractures are treated with urgent surgery to align and fixate the fracture with metal rods or plates (a procedure known as open reduction and internal fixation, or ORIF). After surgery, most people begin to walk with crutches immediately.

Hip Fractures

- Hip fractures, which occur most frequently among older people, can be caused by minor falls, particularly among people with osteoporosis.

- Most people with a hip fracture cannot move the leg, stand, or walk.
- Hip fractures are diagnosed with x-rays or sometimes other imaging tests.
- Surgery is usually done, and sometimes the joint is replaced.

More than 270,000 hip fractures occur in the United States each year, with about 90% of them occurring in people older than 60. Hip fractures are more common in older people because of osteoporosis and because older people are more likely to fall. Use of some drugs increases the risk of hip fractures in older people (see page 1896). One in 3 women and 1 in 6 men who reach age 90 will fracture a hip. Hip fractures in older people can lead to life-threatening complications, such as blood clots and pneumonia. Hip fractures sometimes change how people live. For example, people who have a hip fracture may need supervised care or have to move to a nursing home.

The upper end of the thighbone (femur) has large bony bumps (trochanters) where powerful muscles attach, then a short neck, and finally a spherical head that forms the outer half of the hip joint. Most hip fractures occur just below the spherical head (femoral neck or subcapital hip fractures) or through the trochanters (intertrochanteric hip fractures).

Femoral neck hip fractures are particularly problematic because the fracture often disrupts the blood supply to the femoral head, which forms the hip joint. Without a good blood supply, the bone cannot heal and eventually collapses and dies. These fractures can be caused by minimal force, such as walking, in people with osteoporosis and may be stress fractures.

Intertrochanteric hip fractures tend to create large broken bone surfaces that cause internal bleeding. These fractures usually result from a fall or direct blow.

Symptoms and Diagnosis

Most older people with fractured hips cannot move their leg, much less stand or walk. When a doctor examines the person, the leg may appear shortened and turned outward because of the unbalanced pull of muscles. Swelling and a purplish bruise may develop because of blood leaking from the fracture. Hip fractures can cause pain in the knee, called referred pain.

An x-ray usually shows an obvious fracture and can help a doctor confirm the diagnosis. However, faint fracture lines may not be seen initially on an x-ray. Thus, when a doctor still suspects a hip fracture or the person continues to have pain and is unable to stand a day or more after a fall, magnetic resonance imaging (MRI) or computed tomography (CT) may be done.

? **Did You Know...**

Surgery is the preferred treatment for hip fractures in older people because it allows people to walk sooner and avoid serious problems that can result from staying in bed too long.

Treatment

Most people with a hip fracture are treated with surgery. If people with hip fractures are forced by their injury to stay in bed, they are at increased risk of developing serious complications, such as pressure sores, blood clots leading to pulmonary embolism, mental confusion, and pneumonia. A great benefit of surgery is that it allows the person to get out of bed and begin walking as soon as possible. Usually, the person can take a few steps with a walker 1 to 2 days after the operation. Physical rehabilitation is started as soon as possible (see page 54).

The type of surgery depends on the type of fracture.

Femoral neck hip fractures may be repaired with metal pins or by removing the broken pieces and replacing the head of the femur with a metal implant (partial hip replacement). An implant may be needed when the blood supply to the femoral head has been damaged.

Intertrochanteric hip fractures are treated with a sliding compression screw and side plate, which holds the bone fragments in their proper position while the fracture heals. The fixation is usually strong enough to permit people to bear weight shortly after surgery. Although the bone fragments usually heal in a couple of months, most people need at least 6 months to fully regain their original level of comfort, strength, and walking ability.

Partial Hip Replacement: If partial hip replacement is needed, doctors use special metallic implants. These implants have a polished spherical surface to match the joint socket and a strong stem to fit within the central marrow canal of the thighbone. Some prosthetic implants are secured to the bone with a rapid-setting plastic cement. Others have special porous or ceramic coatings into which the surrounding living bone can grow and bond directly.

After joint replacement surgery, the person usually begins walking with crutches or a walker immediately and switches to a cane in 6 weeks. However, artificial joints do not last forever. The person, especially someone who is active or heavy, may need to undergo another operation 10 to 20 years later. Joint replacement is often advantageous for older people, because the likelihood that additional surgery will be needed is very low. In addition, older people benefit greatly from being able to walk almost immediately after surgery.

Sometimes the whole joint needs to be replaced. This procedure is commonly done to treat osteoarthritis. Whole-joint replacement is rarely used to treat fractures.

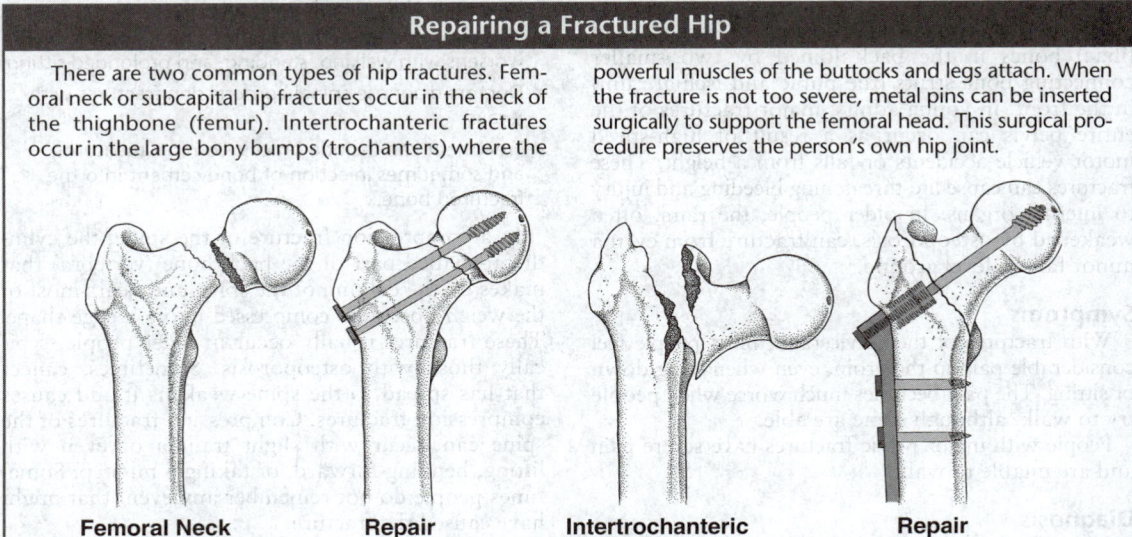

Repairing a Fractured Hip

There are two common types of hip fractures. Femoral neck or subcapital hip fractures occur in the neck of the thighbone (femur). Intertrochanteric fractures occur in the large bony bumps (trochanters) where the powerful muscles of the buttocks and legs attach. When the fracture is not too severe, metal pins can be inserted surgically to support the femoral head. This surgical procedure preserves the person's own hip joint.

Femoral Neck Fracture   **Repair**   **Intertrochanteric Fracture**   **Repair**

Replacing a Hip

When the topmost part (head) of the thighbone (femur) is badly damaged, it may be replaced with an artificial part (prosthesis), made of metal (usually a Moore prosthesis). This procedure is called partial hip replacement. Very rarely, the socket into which the femoral head fits (forming the hip joint) must also be replaced. The part used is a metal shell lined with durable plastic. This procedure is called total hip replacement.

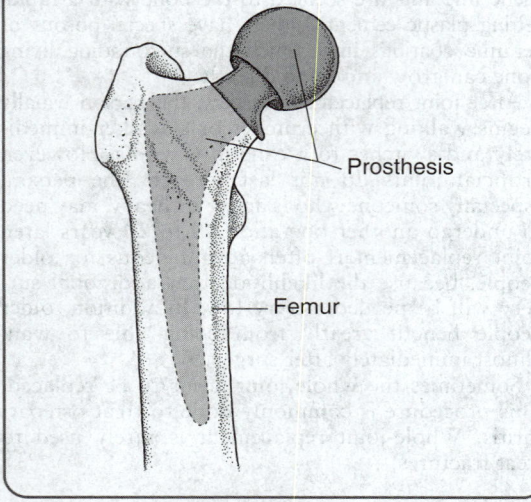

— Prosthesis

— Femur

Pelvis Fractures

The pelvis is made up of pairs of large broad (iliac) bones in the back joined by two smaller connecting bone struts (the pubic and ischial rami) in the front. In young adults, major fractures of the entire pelvis can occur as a result of high-speed motor vehicle accidents or falls from a height. These fractures can cause life-threatening bleeding and injury to internal organs. In older people, the rami, often weakened by osteoporosis, can fracture from even a minor fall on level ground.

Symptoms

With fractures of the pelvic rami, most people feel considerable pain in the groin, even when lying down or sitting. The pain becomes much worse when people try to walk, although some are able.

People with major pelvic fractures have severe pain and are unable to walk.

Diagnosis

Doctors suspect a pelvic fracture based on the symptoms and confirm the diagnosis using x-rays. Some-

times, computed tomography (CT) or magnetic resonance imaging (MRI) is required.

Prognosis and Treatment

People usually need to be admitted to a hospital or rehabilitation center.

Stable fractures of the pelvic rami typically heal without causing permanent disabilities and rarely require surgical treatment. Analgesics and nonsteroidal anti-inflammatory drugs (NSAIDs—see page 644) help relieve pain and inflammation. To avoid the weakness, stiffness, and other complications that occur with bed rest, walking and bearing weight fully should begin as soon as possible. People with fractures of the rami can try to walk without causing further injury to the area. Most people can walk short distances with a walker by 1 week and are moderately comfortable in 1 to 2 months.

Major pelvic fractures are often unstable and require immobilization. Doctors sometimes attach a rigid metal frame to the pelvis using screws driven into the bone. Permanent disability often results if the socket of the hip joint has been damaged. Because of the large amount of force required to cause a major pelvic fracture, internal organs are also often damaged. The mortality rate for this type of injury is high.

Compression Fractures of the Spine

- Compression fractures may occur with only slight trauma in older people with osteoporosis.
- The area around the fracture is painful, and the pain worsens with walking, standing, and prolonged sitting.
- Doctors diagnose spinal compression fractures with x-rays.
- Treatment can include braces, comfort measures, and sometimes injection of bone cement into the fractured bone.

In a compression fracture of the spine, the cylindrical-shaped part of the back bone (vertebra) that makes up the column of the spine and bears most of the weight, becomes compressed into a wedge shape. These fractures usually occur in older people, typically those with osteoporosis. Sometimes, cancer that has spread to the spine weakens it and causes compression fractures. Compression fractures of the spine can occur with slight trauma or even with lifting, bending forward, or taking a misstep. Sometimes people do not remember any event that might have caused the fracture.

Other fractures of the spine are discussed elsewhere (see page 798).

Symptoms

Compression fractures cause constant, dull back pain that may worsen with standing, walking, or prolonged sitting. When the doctor gently taps over the spine, the person feels discomfort. Because the spinal cord and nerve roots are contained within the spine, the cord or nerve roots very rarely may be injured, which may result in paralysis and a loss of sensation. Other symptoms of nerve injury include pain radiating into the leg, weakness of the leg muscles, and involuntary wetting or soiling of clothing with urine or stool (incontinence).

If compression fractures occur over time at several levels of the spine, a person can lose several inches of height, develop a humpback deformity, and be unable to stand up straight.

Diagnosis

Doctors use x-rays to confirm the diagnosis, check the spine for stability, and exclude the possibility of cancer.

Treatment

Braces are most effective for fractures located in the lower part of the spine. They can relieve pain and enable the person to more rapidly return to daily activities. Initially, bed rest may be required for a few days, but sitting up and walking for short periods as soon as possible can help prevent loss of function and further loss of bone density.

In older people, compression fractures of the spine that are not complicated by instability, nerve injury, or cancer heal on their own but slowly. Treatment often is limited to comfort measures.

Two minimally invasive procedures can sometimes be done to help relieve pain and possibly restore height and improve appearance:

- Vertebroplasty: A material called polymethyl-methacrylate—an acrylic bone cement—is injected into the collapsed vertebra. This procedure takes about an hour for each vertebra.
- Kyphoplasty: In this similar procedure, a balloon is inserted into the vertebra and is expanded to restore the vertebra to its normal shape. Then bone cement is injected.

Neither of these procedures reduces the risk of fractures in adjacent bones in the spine or ribs. This risk may even increase. Other risks may include leakage of the cement and possibly heart or lung problems.

Rib Fractures

Rib fractures usually result from a strong force, such as falls, motor vehicle accidents, or a hit with a baseball bat. However, sometimes in older people, only a slight force (such as a minor fall) is required. The fracture itself is rarely serious, although internal organs (such as the lung, liver, or spleen) are occasionally damaged by the force that causes the fracture. The more ribs that are injured, the more likely people are to have damage to the lung or other organs.

Rib fractures cause severe pain, particularly with deep breathing, and the pain lasts for weeks.

Some rib fractures are not visible on initial x-rays, especially if the bone is not displaced or if the person has osteoporosis.

Regardless of whether rib fractures are seen on imaging tests, treatment can be started. Opioid analgesics are usually used. Also, while awake, people with a rib fracture must cough or breathe deeply about once an hour. If they do not, small areas of the lung may collapse, possibly leading to pneumonia.

Clavicle Fractures

Clavicle fractures occur commonly after a fall on an outstretched arm or after a direct blow. Because the clavicle lies just under the skin and has little muscle covering, swelling and deformity are easily seen after a fracture. Most of these injuries involve the middle third of the bone and are immobilized with a sling. Surgery is occasionally needed.

Another clavicle injury involves partial or complete separation of the outer part of the clavicle from its attachment to the rest of the shoulder. This attachment is the acromioclavicular joint, so the injury is called an acromioclavicular separation or sprain or injury. It is sometimes called a shoulder separation. It usually results from a fall onto the outside of the shoulder. The injury is usually painful but not serious. No surgery is required unless it is severe. Sometimes the end of the clavicle sticks up from its attachment, resulting in a permanent bump that may be seen or felt.

Humerus Fractures

Fractures of the upper arm bone (humerus) usually occur near the shoulder. These fractures are common after a fall on an outstretched arm or after a direct blow. Symptoms include pain and an inability to raise the arm. Fractures of the middle of the humerus sometimes damage the radial nerve. Radial nerve damage leads to an inability to lift up the wrist. Most of these fractures can be treated with a sling and swathe. Surgery is needed if the fracture pieces are widely separated. If the fracture affects the shoulder joint, a prosthetic implant (partial shoulder replacement) may be needed.

Elbow Fractures

Elbow fractures can involve any of the three bones that make up the joint (radius, ulna, and humerus). Fractures of the radial head or neck (the upper end of the radius) occur commonly in active adults after a fall on an outstretched arm. The outer side of the elbow is painful, and people cannot fully straighten the arm. Fractures of the upper arm bone (humerus) are more serious, often affecting the nerves.

X-rays usually show a fracture, but sometimes the only sign is fluid around the elbow joint.

Most radial head fractures are mild and can be treated with a splint or a sling and early (within a few days) gentle range-of-motion exercises. Early motion helps prevent permanent stiffness. More severe radial head fractures may require surgical treatment.

Wrist Fractures

Wrist fractures involve the radius, and sometimes also the ulna. Certain types of wrist fractures are called Colles' fractures. These occur commonly after a fall on an outstretched arm, particularly in older people. People have pain, swelling, and tenderness, and often the wrist appears in an unnatural position.

For many fractures, closed reduction followed by casting is adequate. The cast may be worn for 3 to 6 weeks. Other wrist fractures require surgery, particularly if the joint surface is out of place, especially in active adults who need to be able to fully use their wrist. During surgery, an internal plate may be applied, or an external fixator (a frame of rods clamped to stainless steel pins that pass through the skin into the bone) is used.

Daily motion of the fingers, elbow (if free), and shoulder helps to avoid stiffness. Elevation of the hand is important to control swelling. Comfort, flexibility, and strength of the wrist continue to improve for 6 to 12 months after the fracture.

Hand Fractures

Hand fractures involve the bones that form part of the wrist (carpals), bones of the palm (metacarpals), or bones of the fingers and thumb (phalanges). Normal hand function results from a complex interaction of an intricate arrangement of muscles, tendons, ligaments, and joints, as well as bones. Thus, seemingly minor fractures can cause serious soft tissue injuries that, if not treated appropriately, can lead to disabling stiffness, weakness, or deformity.

Carpal Fractures: A carpal bone that is commonly fractured is the scaphoid bone (see box on page 604). A fracture of the scaphoid bone usually occurs with a fall on an outstretched hand. Symptoms include pain while rotating the palm and, particularly, tenderness at the hollow at the base of the thumb or pain when the thumb is pushed into the wrist. Because the initial x-ray is often normal, people who have a suspected fracture require splinting and re-examination in 7 to 10 days, or magnetic resonance imaging (MRI), which is more sensitive than an x-ray. The fracture may be treated with a thumb spica splint. Scaphoid bone fractures are prone to poor healing because the blood supply is often damaged when the bone is fractured. About 5% of the time, regardless of treatment, the bone eventually dies (called necrosis). If so, bone grafting may be necessary.

Metacarpal Fractures: Fractures of the ends of the 4th and 5th metacarpal bones (that attach to the ring finger and little finger) commonly occur from punching a hard object. This type of fracture, called a boxer's fracture, causes swelling and tenderness of the knuckle. These fractures are treated with a splint. Reduction is necessary only if the fracture is badly angled or rotated. Typically, good function of the finger returns.

Finger Fractures: Avulsion fractures occur commonly in the fingers at the site of tendon and joint capsule attachments. A mallet finger injury refers to the drooping of the fingertip that occurs when the tendon that extends the farthest part of the finger becomes detached (see page 598). A common cause is a baseball that strikes the fingertip (baseball finger). For simple mallet finger injuries, immobilization with a splint for 6 to 10 weeks is effective, but if avulsion fractures greatly disrupt the joint surface, surgery may be needed.

Fingertip fractures are usually the result of a crush injury, such as from a hammer blow. Blood may accumulate beneath the nail (subungual hematoma) from a tear in the nail bed and produce a very painful, blue-black discoloration. Most fingertip fractures are treated with a protective covering (such as commercially available aluminum and foam splint material) wrapped around the fingertip. Doctors can easily drain a subungual hematoma by making a small hole in the fingernail with a needle or a hot wire (electrocautery device).

Large, displaced finger fractures are repaired with surgery. An abnormal increase in sensitivity (hyperesthesia) frequently lasts long after a large fracture has healed. The person may require treatment to decrease hyperesthesia (desensitization therapy).

CHAPTER

302 Sports Injuries

Sports injuries are common among athletes and other people who participate in sports. Certain injuries that are traditionally considered sports injuries can also occur in people who do not participate in sports. For example, homemakers and factory workers often develop "tennis elbow," although they may never have played tennis.

Sports participation always carries the risk of injury. Sports injuries are more likely when people do not warm up properly (exercising muscles at a relaxed pace before an intense workout).

Muscles and ligaments are injured when subjected to forces greater than their inherent strength. For example, they may be injured if they are too weak or tight for the exercise being attempted. Joints are more prone to injury when the muscles and ligaments that support them are weak, as they are after a sprain.

Individual differences in body structure can make people susceptible to sports injuries by stressing parts of the body unevenly. For example, when legs are unequal in length, forces on the hips and knees are unequal and place more stress on one side of the body.

Excessive pronation—rolling onto the inside of the foot after it strikes the ground—can cause foot and knee pain. Some degree of pronation is normal and prevents injuries by helping distribute the foot's striking force throughout the foot. In people with excessive pronation, the feet are so flexible that the long arch flattens out, allowing the inner part of the foot to come close to touching the ground during walking or running and giving the appearance of flatfeet. Runners with excessive pronation may develop knee pain when running long distances because the knee caps tend to turn outward when the feet turn inward. This position in turn places excessive pressure across the front of the knee.

The opposite problem—too little pronation—can occur in people who have rigid ankles. In these people, the feet appear to have very high arches and do not absorb shock well, increasing the risk of developing small cracks in the bones (stress fractures—see page 1976) of the feet and legs.

The way in which the legs are aligned can produce pain, particularly in women with wide hips. Such women develop a tendency for the knee caps to be pushed outward from the midline. This force on the knee caps causes pain.

Generally, sports injuries can be divided into four categories:

- Overuse
- Blunt trauma (for example, falls and tackles)
- Fractures and dislocations
- Sprains (ligament injuries) and strains (muscle injuries)

Overuse: One of the most common causes of sports injuries is overuse (excessive wear and tear). Overuse injuries are generally due to faulty technique. An example of an improper technique is running along the same side of a banked road. Repeatedly hitting the slightly higher surface with the same foot results in different forces being applied to the right and left hips and knees. This difference in forces increases the risk of injury on the side striking the higher surface and changes the forces acting on the other leg, risking injury to it as well.

Some athletes increase the speed or intensity of their workouts too quickly, putting stress on the muscles. For example, some runners who increase speed or distance too quickly during training stress the legs, hips, or feet. This extra stress often leads to muscle sprains and stress fractures of the bones.

Some athletes overly train one set of muscles without equally strengthening the opposite group of muscles, resulting in imbalances that can contribute to injury.

Another factor contributing to overuse injuries is inadequate recovery after a workout. Also, some people do not stop exercising when pain develops (working through the pain). Continuing to exercise with pain injures more muscle or connective tissue, extending the damage and delaying recovery, whereas rest allows recovery.

> **Did You Know...**
> Not resting an injured body part (working through the pain) prolongs the time until recovery.

Blunt Trauma: Blunt athletic trauma can result in bruises, concussions, and fractures. This type of injury usually involves high-impact collisions with other athletes or objects (for example, being tackled in football or checked into the sideboards in hockey), falls, and direct blows (for example, in boxing and the martial arts).

Fractures and Dislocations: Fractured bones and dislocations of a joint are serious injuries that require

Children and Sports Injuries

About 3.5 million sports-related injuries involving children younger than 14 occur in the United States each year. As more children participate in organized athletic activities and begin participating at younger ages, they are at greater risk of sports injuries, particularly overuse injuries. This risk is particularly high for children who participate in a single sport year-round, move from one sports season to the next with no break between them, or play on elite-level teams. Some children may try to play when they are injured because they fear being dropped from a team.

In general, the same injury prevention guidelines apply to children as to adult athletes, including the need for proper warm-up and stretching techniques. Some experts believe children younger than 10 should participate in a wide range of activities rather than specialize in one sport. Specialization can lead children to train one group of muscles, increasing injury risk. Use of appropriate equipment that is properly fitted is important. Safety equipment, such as helmets, eye protection, mouth guards, and elbow and knee pads that are approved for the sport, can help prevent injury. Some sports have specific guidelines about the amount of time that child athletes can practice or play. For example, in baseball, pitch counts based on the pitcher's age have been established.

Pain during an activity or excessive pain after an activity may be clues to an overuse injury. The need for ice and pain-relieving drugs after exercise may also be a clue. If pain or soreness causes changes in gait, body mechanics, or sport technique, overuse may be a problem. Some children do not complain of pain but instead experience diminished success or enjoyment in sports participation and changes in mood or school performance.

In adolescent girls, a history of stress fractures may be a sign of the female athlete triad of osteoporosis, menstrual irregularities, and an inadequate diet. Although no athlete is immune from the consequences of inadequate nutrition, young women who participate in endurance activities or "appearance" sports, such as figure skating, gymnastics, or dance, are at particular risk.

monly during running, particularly with sudden changes of direction (for example, while dodging and avoiding competitors in football). Such injuries also are common in strength training, when people quickly drop or yank the load rather than moving slowly and smoothly with constant controlled tension.

Symptoms

Injury always causes pain, which can range from mild to severe. Injured tissue may have any combination of the following characteristics:

- Swelling
- Warmth
- Tenderness to touch
- Bruising
- Loss of normal range of motion

Diagnosis

To diagnose a sports injury, doctors ask when and how the injury happened, what recreational and occupational activities the person has recently or routinely been engaged in, and whether there has been a change in the intensity of the activity. Doctors also examine the injured area. People may be referred to a specialist for further testing. Diagnostic tests may include x-rays, computed tomography (CT), magnetic resonance imaging (MRI), ultrasonography, bone scanning, dual-energy x-ray absorptiometry (DEXA scanning—see page 543), and electromyography (EMG—see page 636).

Prevention

General measures that help increase safety during exercise are discussed elsewhere (see page 42). Exercise itself helps prevent injuries because tissues become more resilient to the stresses of vigorous activities.

Use of proper equipment can help prevent injuries. For example, wearing helmets and mouth guards can help prevent injuries while playing football. For running athletes, good running shoes are essential. Running shoes should have a rigid heel counter (the back part of the shoe that surrounds the heel) to control movement of the back of the foot, a support across the instep (saddle) to prevent excessive pronation, and a padded opening (collar) to support the ankle.

Shoe inserts (orthotics) can sometimes help correct problems such as excessive pronation. The inserts, which may be flexible, semirigid, or rigid and may vary in length, should be fitted into appropriate running shoes. The shoes must have adequate space for the inserts, which replace the inserts found in the shoes at the time of purchase.

Stopping exercise at the first sign of pain, which precedes most overuse injuries, limits the degree of injury to muscles and tendons.

immediate medical attention (see page 1952). People with these injuries often have deformity of a limb, intense pain, and dysfunction of the limb or joint and must be further evaluated with diagnostic tests, such as x-rays. When people suspect that they have a fracture or dislocated joint, they should splint the limb "as it lies" without moving it and go to the emergency department.

Sprains and Strains: Sprains and strains typically occur with sudden, forceful exertion, most com-

After sustaining a sports injury, athletes often want to know how quickly they can resume activity. Recovery time depends on the severity of the injury. Initially, exercise of previously injured areas should be of low intensity to strengthen weak muscles, tendons, and ligaments and prevent re-injury. Often, athletes need to adjust their technique to avoid re-injury. For example, a racquet sports player who has tennis elbow may need to alter technique for use of the racquet.

Treatment

Treatment of sports injuries is similar to treatment of non-sports injuries.

Initial Treatment: Immediate treatment for almost all injuries consists of *r*est, *i*ce, *c*ompression, and *e*levation (RICE). The injured part is rested immediately to minimize internal bleeding and swelling and to prevent further injury.

The injured part swells because fluid leaks from blood vessels. By causing the blood vessels to constrict, ice reduces their tendency to leak, thus limiting swelling. Ice also helps to reduce pain and muscle spasms and limit tissue damage.

Ice and cold packs should not be applied directly to the skin, because doing so could irritate or damage the skin. They should be enclosed (for example, in plastic) and placed over a towel or facecloth. An elastic bandage can be wrapped around the ice pack to keep it in place while the injured part is elevated. The ice is removed after 20 minutes, left off for 20 minutes or longer, and then reapplied for 20 minutes. This process can be repeated several times during the first 24 hours.

Whether or not ice is in place, wrapping the injured part with an elastic bandage compresses the injured tissue and limits internal bleeding and swelling. The wrap is thus kept on until the injury heals.

The injured area should be elevated above heart level so that gravity can help drain the accumulated fluid that causes swelling and pain. If possible, fluid should drain on an entirely downhill path from the injured area to the heart. For example, for a hand injury, the elbow, as well as the hand, should be elevated.

Did You Know...

An injured part should be rested in a position in which gravity can drain fluid from the injury in a direct downhill path to the heart.

Analgesics can be used to lessen pain. Acetaminophen is usually effective for pain but does not reduce inflammation. Nonsteroidal anti-inflammatory drugs

SPOTLIGHT ON AGING

Most older people can safely exercise. Exercise even improves some disorders, such as high blood pressure and diabetes. However, older people should check with their doctors before they start an exercise program. Exercise programs for older people should include activities to promote flexibility and agility as well as those for strengthening and aerobic conditioning. Older people are more likely to injure themselves than younger people who are participating in the same sport. Proper footwear and equipment are important.

People need to begin gradually and build up slowly. As with people of all ages, a careful warm-up period is key to reducing the chance of injury. Aging causes a decrease in flexibility because of changes in connective tissue. Older people are also more likely to have arthritis, which further decreases flexibility. Lack of flexibility means that joints bear greater stress during exercise, rather than spreading it to surrounding tissues, such as nearby muscles. This stress can gradually damage the joints. Extra warm-up and flexibility exercises can help prevent injury.

Older runners are subject to the same running-related sports injuries as younger runners. Older runners are also more likely to fall. Often, balance deteriorates in older people, so older athletes may want to consider adding balance exercises to their workouts. Dehydration can lead to episodes of confusion, which could possibly cause falls in older people.

(NSAIDs), such as ibuprofen or naproxen, can be used for pain and inflammation but have a slightly higher risk of side effects (most often stomach upset) than acetaminophen. If pain is severe or persists for more than 3 days, a medical evaluation is recommended.

Injections of corticosteroids into an injured joint or the surrounding tissues are sometimes used in addition to RICE to relieve pain and reduce swelling. However, corticosteroid injections can delay healing, increase the risk of tendon and cartilage damage, and enable a person to use an injured joint before it is fully healed, perhaps worsening the injury, and should only be done by a doctor.

Rehabilitation: After the initial injury has healed, the person should rehabilitate the injured area before resuming the activity that led to the injury. Rehabilitation may involve formal regimens carried out under the supervision of a physical therapist or athletic trainer or less formal strengthening and conditioning done without supervision. Sometimes, a physical therapist provides instructions for exercises that athletes can do on their own. Physical therapists may incorporate heat, cold, electricity, sound waves, traction, or water exercise into a treatment plan in addition to therapeutic exercises (see page 48). How long physical therapy is needed depends on the severity and complexity of the injury.

The activity or sport that caused the injury should be avoided or modified until the injury has healed. Complete inactivity causes muscles to lose mass, strength, and endurance. Therefore, substituting activities that do not stress the injured part is preferable to abstaining from all physical activity. Substitute activities include bicycling, swimming, and rowing when the leg or foot is injured. Swimming and bicycling are good substitutes when the lower back is injured.

Shoulder Injuries

Rotator cuff injuries and labral tears are the most common shoulder injuries.

ROTATOR CUFF INJURY

The muscles that help hold the upper arm in the shoulder joint (the rotator cuff muscles) can get pinched (shoulder impingement syndrome), become inflamed (tendinitis), or can tear partially or completely.

- The shoulder is painful when the arm is moved over the head and later, even when the arm is not moved.
- Exercises help.

Rotator cuff pinching (impingement) and tendinitis often occur in sports that require the arms to be moved over the head repeatedly, such as pitching in baseball, lifting heavy weights over the shoulder, serving the ball in racket sports, and swimming freestyle, butterfly, or backstroke. Repeatedly moving the arm over the head causes the top of the arm bone to pinch the rotator cuff muscles against the top part of the shoulder blade and results in inflammation and swelling of the muscles. If the movement is continued despite the inflammation, the tendon can weaken and tear.

Symptoms and Diagnosis

Shoulder pain is the main symptom. At first, the pain occurs only during activities that require lifting the arm over the head (impingement syndrome). Pain is worse when lifting the arm between 60 and 120 degrees away from the side. Unless effectively treated, the shoulder may later become painful at rest (tendinitis), often particularly at night, disrupting sleep. If the tendon tears, normal outward turning of the arm at the shoulder is weak or impossible.

Strengthening the Shoulders

EXERCISES FOR THE ROTATOR CUFF

- **External Rotation:** Lie on the left side and grasp a light dumbbell in the right hand with the elbow bent 90 degrees. Maintain this position throughout the set. Using the right elbow as a pivot point against the side of the waist, externally rotate the arm upward until it is as vertical as possible. Do 3 sets of 10 repetitions with a minute rest between each set. Repeat exercise using the opposite arm. As strength improves, increase the weight.

- **Internal Rotation:** Lie on the right side, and grasp a light dumbbell in the right hand with the right elbow bent at 90 degrees. Maintain this position throughout the set. Using the right elbow as a pivot point against the side of the waist, internally rotate the arm upward until it is vertical against the abdomen. Do 3 sets of repetitions with a minute rest between each set. Repeat exercise using the opposite arm. As strength improves, increase the weight.

EXERCISES FOR THE DELTOID MUSCLES

The deltoid muscles, which are part of the shoulder, must be included in overall shoulder-strengthening programs.

- **Anterior Deltoid:** Stand. Grasp a light dumbbell with the right hand and, with the palm facing down, raise the hand and arm away and in front of the body to shoulder level keeping the elbow straight. Do 3 sets of repetitions with a minute rest between each set. Repeat exercise using the opposite arm.

- **Middle Deltoid:** Stand. Grasp a light dumbbell with the right hand and, with the palm facing down, raise the hand and arm away and out to the side from the body to shoulder level keeping the elbow straight. Do 3 sets of repetitions with a minute rest between each set. Repeat exercise using the opposite arm.

Doctors make the diagnosis based on the person's symptoms and examination findings. Magnetic resonance imaging (MRI) sometimes is needed to rule out a tear of the rotator cuff muscles.

Treatment

The shoulder can be rested in a sling for a couple of days if pain is moderate or severe. Exercises that involve raising the arm above the level of the shoulder, especially against resistance, should be avoided. Once the shoulder can be moved through its range of motion without pain, the rotator cuff muscles are strengthened. Exercises to strengthen some of the muscles restore balance to the rotator cuff and decrease impingement during activities that involve reaching overhead. If the pain is severe, doctors sometimes inject a corticosteroid into the space above the rotator cuff (bursa).

Surgery is sometimes needed when the rotator cuff is torn or tendinitis does not resolve with other treatments. Surgery removes excess bone from the shoulder, creating a larger space for the rotator cuff and thus preventing pinching of the rotator cuff when the arm moves above the head. If the rotator cuff is torn, surgical repair is usually recommended.

LABRAL TEAR

The glenoid labrum, which cushions the shoulder joint, can tear as a result of injury.

The shoulders are ball and socket joints that allow the arms to have inward and outward rotation as well as forward, backward, and sideways movement. The shoulder tends to be unstable. It has been likened to a golf ball sitting on a tee because the socket (glenoid bone) is very shallow and small compared to the size of the ball (humeral head). To enhance stability, the socket is deepened by the labrum, a rubbery material attached around the lip of the glenoid bone. The labrum can tear during athletic activities, especially during throwing sports, or as a result of falling and landing on an outstretched arm.

When the labrum tears, the athlete feels pain deep in the shoulder during movement, for example, when pitching a baseball. This discomfort may be accompanied by a painful clicking or clunking sensation and a feeling of catching in the shoulder.

MRI may be necessary to make the diagnosis. Physical therapy is the usual initial treatment. If symptoms do not resolve, surgical repair is usually needed.

Elbow Injuries

Injuries can occur to the tendons that attach to the elbow.

LATERAL EPICONDYLITIS

Lateral epicondylitis (tennis elbow) is inflammation of the tendons that extend the hand backward and away from the palm.

- Pain develops in the outer aspect of the elbow and back side of the forearm.
- Ice, rest, analgesics, and exercises are usually effective.

The forearm muscles that are attached to the outer part of the elbow can become sore when stressed repetitively. Lateral epicondylitis can be caused by repetitive backhand returns in tennis. Other activities (for example, rowing and doing forearm curls while holding weights and repeatedly and forcefully turning a screwdriver) can also cause lateral epicondylitis.

Factors that increase the chance of developing lateral epicondylitis among tennis players include having weak shoulder and forearm muscles, playing with a racket that is too tightly strung or too short, hitting the ball off center on the racket (out of the sweet spot), and hitting heavy, wet balls. Hitting backhanded and allowing the wrist to bend increase the chance of developing lateral epicondylitis.

Symptoms and Diagnosis

Pain occurs in the outside of the forearm when the wrist is extended away from the palm. Pain can extend from around the elbow to the middle of the forearm. Continuing to stress the forearm muscles can worsen symptoms and result in pain, even at rest.

Doctors make the diagnosis based on the symptoms and results of a physical examination. The outer elbow hurts when the person places the arm and hand palm down on a table and tries to raise the hand against resistance by bending the wrist backward.

Treatment

Ice is applied to the outer elbow, and exercises that cause pain are avoided. Exercises that do not use the wrist extensor muscles primarily, such as jogging or cycling, can be substituted to maintain physical fitness. As pain decreases, elbow and wrist flexibility and strengthening exercises can be started. Use of a tennis elbow brace (usually for a few weeks) can be beneficial. When pain from lateral epicondylitis is severe, a health care practitioner may inject a corticosteroid into the outer elbow. Surgery is rarely needed.

MEDIAL EPICONDYLITIS

Medial epicondylitis (golfer's elbow) is inflammation of the tendons that flex or bend the wrist toward the palm, causing pain on the inner aspect of the elbow and forearm.

- An activity involving repeated stressful bending of the wrist toward the palm is the usual cause.
- Rest, ice, and analgesics help relieve pain.
- When pain subsides, stretching and strengthening exercises are done to help prevent recurrence.

This injury is caused by bending the wrist against resistance toward the palm repetitively. Actions that produce such force include serving with great force in tennis; using an overhand and a top spin serve; hitting heavy, wet balls; using a racket that is too heavy or that has a grip that is too small or has

When the Elbow Hurts

Tennis elbow and golfer's elbow cause pain in different areas of the elbow and forearm.

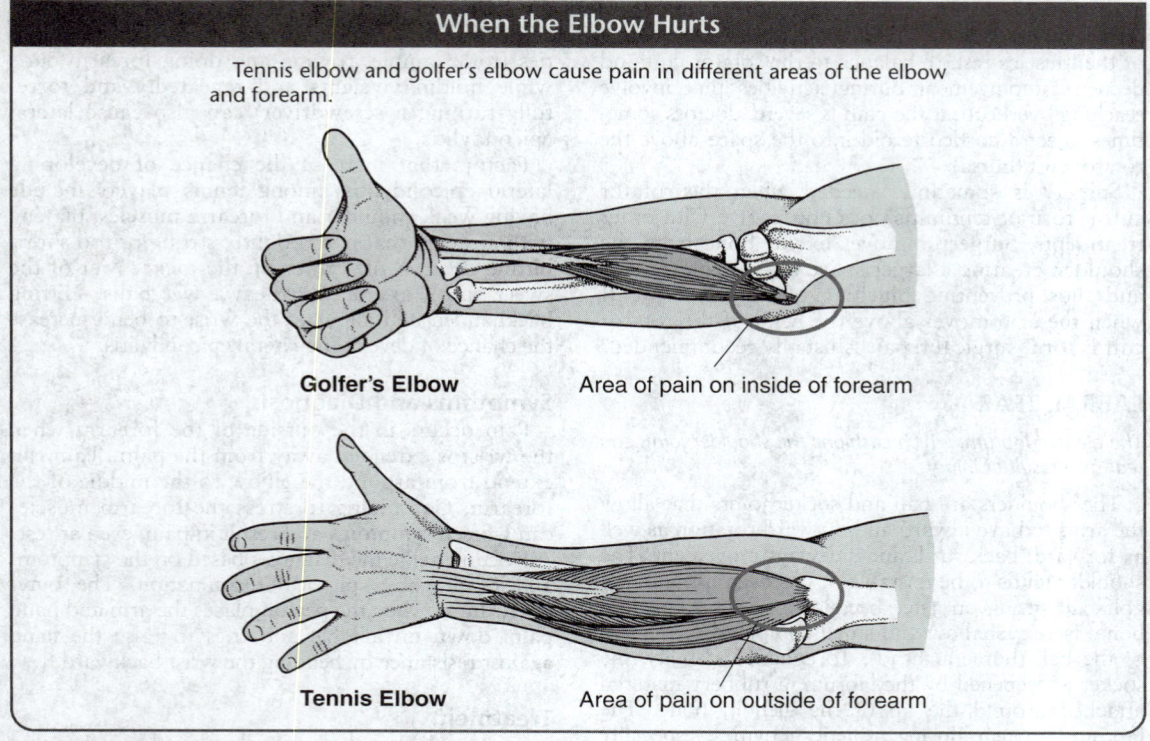

Golfer's Elbow   Area of pain on inside of forearm

Tennis Elbow   Area of pain on outside of forearm

strings that are too tight; pitching a baseball; and throwing a javelin. Poor technique when hitting the ball in golf can cause this inflammation as well—hence the term golfer's elbow. Injury occurs when "hitting from the top" and is basically forcefully bringing the club with the right arm (right-handed golfer) down from the top of the swing, placing extreme stress on the flexor muscles of the right elbow instead of pulling down the club with the left arm and the body. Nonathletic activities that may cause medial epicondylitis include bricklaying, hammering, and typing.

Pain is felt on the inner aspect of the elbow and forearm. It is worse when the wrist moves toward the palm.

Diagnosis

Doctors make the diagnosis based on the symptoms and results of an examination. The doctor asks the person to sit in a chair with the injured arm resting on a table, palm up. The doctor holds the wrist down and asks the person to raise the hand by bending the wrist. A person who has medial epicondylitis feels pain at the inner aspect of the elbow.

Treatment

Initial treatment includes avoiding any activity that causes pain when the wrist is bent toward the palm. Ice applied over the painful area and nonsteroidal anti-inflammatory drugs (NSAIDs) help relieve pain. After pain has decreased, an exercise program that strengthens the wrist and shoulder muscles is begun. Surgery is rarely needed.

Knee Injuries

Knee sprains, meniscal injuries, and runner's knee are common knee injuries.

KNEE SPRAINS AND MENISCAL INJURIES

Sprains of the external (medial and lateral collateral) or internal (anterior and posterior cruciate) knee ligaments usually result from twisting injuries while weight-bearing.

- Knee ligament injuries are often caused by bending or twisting of the knee when it is planted on the ground.
- Pain and swelling are common symptoms.
- Examination and sometimes magnetic resonance imaging or arthroscopy are needed to determine injury severity.

Strengthening the Wrist Muscles

These exercises are for lateral epicondylitis (tennis elbow).

- Sit on a chair next to a table. Place the injured forearm on the table, palm down, with the elbow straightened and the wrist and hand hanging over the edge. Hold a light weight in the hand. Slowly raise and lower the hand by bending and straightening the wrist. Repeat 10 times (1 set). Each set should last about 90 to 120 seconds for rehabilitation and about 50 to 70 seconds for general strength and conditioning. Rest 1 minute, then do 2 more sets of 10. If the exercise causes pain, stop immediately and try again the next day. Do this exercise every other day. Increase the weight as the exercise becomes easier.

- With the palms down and the arms outstretched in front of the body, hold a piece of wood the diameter of a broomstick with a 1-pound (about 1/2-kilogram) weight attached to it by a rope. Wind the weight up by rotating the stick. Repeat 10 times. Stop if any pain is felt. Do this exercise every other day. Gradually increase the weight but not the number of repetitions.

- Rest and immobilization are often enough, but sometimes surgery is needed for severe injuries.

Knee ligaments are often injured by a weight-bearing, twisting motion of the knee that occurs when the foot is planted on the ground and a force is applied to the outside of the knee, as when tackled in football (clipping injury). This motion often damages the anterior cruciate ligament inside the knee joint. Hyperextension of the knee (forceful straightening of the joint), if severe, typically damages the posterior cruciate ligament inside the joint. Weight-bearing and rotation at the time of injury can also injure the rubbery shock absorbers (menisci) inside the knee.

Symptoms

Symptoms depend on the severity of the injury. Swelling and pain can occur over the first few hours after a severe ligament injury or more than 24 hours later with a less severe injury. Sometimes, an athlete hears or feels a "pop" in the knee as the injury occurs. This pop usually indicates a ligament or meniscal tear.

A severe injury may cause muscle spasm, swelling, and stiffness within hours. After a severe ligament injury, the person may feel the knee is unstable and be reluctant to put weight on it, fearing that the knee will give way. Sometimes the knee becomes locked and cannot bend if a torn meniscus blocks knee movement.

Diagnosis

Doctors try and move the knee certain ways to determine whether ligaments are torn. However, muscle stiffness makes the knees stiff, preventing testing of normal joint motion. Sometimes, magnetic resonance imaging (MRI), arthroscopy (looking inside the joint with a flexible viewing tube), or both are needed. Sometimes just reexamining the person in 2 or 3 days, after muscle spasm has resolved, is all that is needed.

Treatment

If a large amount of fluid has built up in the knee, doctors can drain the fluid to help relieve pain. Most mild or moderate injuries can be treated initially with *rest*, *ice*, *compression*, and *elevation* (RICE) and immobilization of the knee. Severe injuries of ligaments or menisci usually require surgical repair.

PAIN IN THE FRONT OF THE KNEE

- Factors such as weak thigh muscles, excessive pronation, and tight leg muscles and tendons can cause pain in the front part of the knee.
- People may feel pain when running downhill but eventually may have pain during walking.

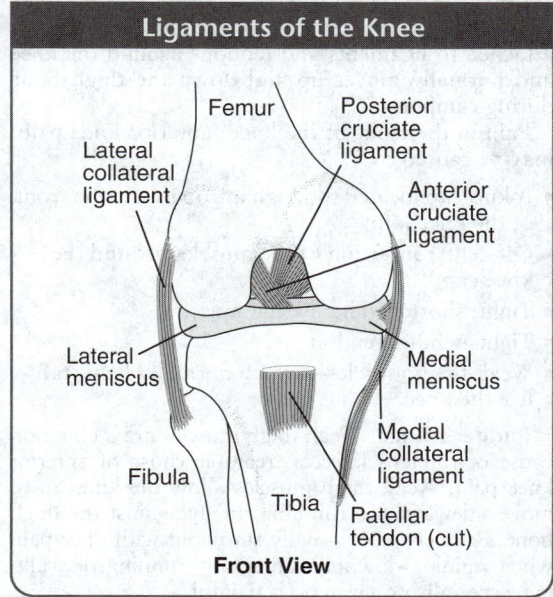

Ligaments of the Knee

Femur

Posterior cruciate ligament

Lateral collateral ligament

Anterior cruciate ligament

Lateral meniscus

Medial meniscus

Medial collateral ligament

Fibula

Tibia

Patellar tendon (cut)

Front View

When the Front of the Knee Hurts

Normally, the kneecap (patella) moves up and down the thigh bone during running. People may feel pain in the kneecap because thigh muscles are weak or the feet roll in too much (pronation). As a result, the kneecap rubs abnormally against the thigh bone, causing increased wear and tear.

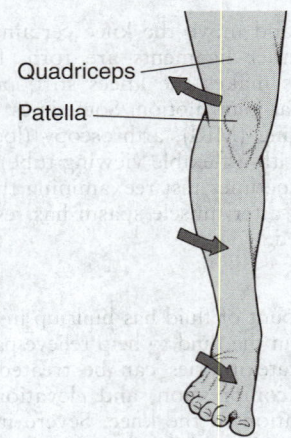

Quadriceps

Patella

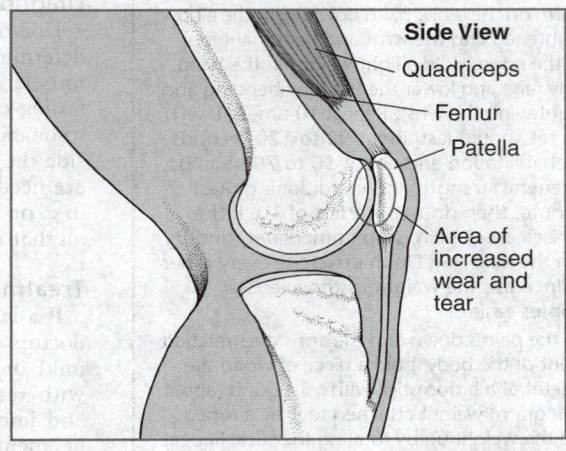

Side View

Quadriceps

Femur

Patella

Area of increased wear and tear

- Magnetic resonance imaging and arthroscopy may be needed for diagnosis.
- People should stop running until there is no pain and then use exercise to strengthen and balance muscles around the knee.
- If excessive pronation causes pain, shoe inserts can help.

The kneecap (patella) is a circular bone that is attached to ligaments and tendons around the knee and normally moves up and down the thigh bone during running.

Pain in the front of the knee (anterior knee pain) may be caused by

- A kneecap located too high or too low in the front of the knee joint
- Off-center insertion of the muscles around the knee cap
- Tight, shortened hamstring muscles
- Tight Achilles tendon
- Weak thigh muscles—which normally help stabilize the knee

Runner's Knee: Weak thigh muscles are a common cause of runner's knee, a treatable cause of anterior knee pain. Weak thigh muscles allow the kneecap to move sideways and rub abnormally against the thigh bone. Runner's knee usually starts out with knee pain when running downhill. Later, any running or walking, especially down steps, is painful.

Excessive Pronation: Excessive pronation of the foot when walking or running (rolling of the foot inward) can cause knee pain. Pronation forces the thigh muscles (quadriceps) to pull the kneecap outward and rub abnormally against the end of the thigh bone.

Diagnosis

Doctors ask about symptoms and examine the person. Sometimes MRI, arthroscopy (looking inside the joint with a flexible viewing tube), or both are needed.

Treatment

Running is avoided until it can be done without pain. Ice applied to the affected area, nonsteroidal anti-inflammatory drugs, and temporary use of a knee sleeve or elastic support also help. Other exercises, such as riding an exercise bike (with high seat position, low repetition, and low resistance) or swimming, can be done to protect the knee and maintain physical fitness during recovery. Exercises to strengthen and balance the muscles in the back (hamstrings) and front (quadriceps) of the thigh are helpful.

In runner's knee, stretching before exercise can help balance the abnormal forces caused by tight muscles and reduce injury.

A shoe insert can help correct excessive pronation.

Strengthening the Hamstrings

- Attach a 5-pound (2-kilogram) weight to the foot on the injured side and lie face down on a bed with the lower part of the body (from the waist down) off the bed and the toes touching the floor. Keeping the knee straight, slowly raise and lower the leg. Do 3 sets of 10 every other day. As strength returns, use increasingly heavier weights. This exercise strengthens primarily the upper part of the hamstrings.
- Attach a 5-pound (2-kilogram) weight to the foot on the injured side. Stand on the other leg. Slowly raise the weighted foot toward the buttocks by bending the knee, and lower it toward the floor by straightening the knee. Do 3 sets of 10 every other day. As strength returns, use increasingly heavier weights. This exercise strengthens primarily the lower part of the hamstrings.

Hamstring Injury

The muscles in the back of the thigh (hamstrings) can be strained (hamstring pull) in any running activity.

The hamstrings move the hip and knee backward. A hamstring injury often occurs when the hamstrings are contracted suddenly and violently, as can occur when a person sprints. It causes sudden pain in the back of the thigh. Hamstring injury can also develop more slowly, usually caused by inadequate flexibility training.

Doctors make the diagnosis based on the person's symptoms and results of a physical examination. Sometimes magnetic resonance imaging (MRI) is also needed.

Treatment

Ice and use of a thigh sleeve for compression and support are needed immediately after injury. Non-steroidal anti-inflammatory drugs (NSAIDs) or other analgesics are used to relieve pain. If walking is painful, the person may need crutches initially.

Once pain begins to resolve, the hamstrings should be gently stretched. When the pain has completely resolved, the quadriceps and hamstrings are gradually strengthened. The person should not run or jump until satisfactory muscle strength and range of motion have been regained. Recovery may occur in days or weeks, but a severe hamstring injury can often take up to several months to completely heal.

Lower Leg Injuries

Shin splints, ankle sprains, Achilles tendinitis, rupture of the Achilles tendon, and stress fractures of the foot are common injuries to the lower leg.

SHIN SPLINTS

Shin splints refers to pain in the lower legs that can be from various causes but that typically is caused by running or vigorous walking.

- Pain can occur in the front or back of the leg below the knee.
- Ice, analgesics, rest, and stretching exercises can help.

Repetitive impact forces in the legs during running or vigorous walking (such as hiking) can overload the muscles and tendons in the legs and cause shin pain. Excessive outward rotation of the foot on the leg (supination) may also cause or exacerbate shin splints.

Symptoms and Diagnosis

Pain can be in the front outer aspect of the leg or the back inner part of the leg. Shin splint pain typically begins at the start of activity but then lessens as activity continues. At first, the pain is felt only immediately after the heel strikes the ground during running or walking. If the person continues to run, the pain

---

Shin Splints

Shin splints may develop in the muscles in the front and outer parts of the shin (anterolateral shin splints) or in the muscles in the back and inner parts (posteromedial shin splints). Pain is felt in different areas, depending on which muscles are affected.

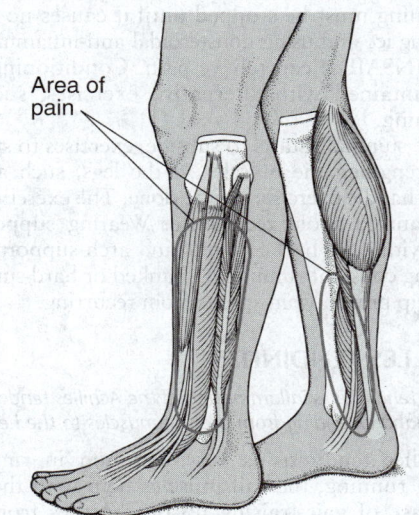

Area of pain

Anterolateral Shin Splint   **Posteromedial Shin Splint**

Strengthening the Shin Muscles

BUCKET-HANDLE EXERCISE

Wrap a towel around the handle of an empty water bucket. Sit on a table or other surface high enough to prevent the feet from touching the floor. Place the bucket handle over the front part of one shoe. Slowly raise and lower the bucket by bending the foot up and down. Do not move the lower leg, just lift with the foot. Repeat 10 times, then rest for a few seconds. Do 2 more sets of 10. To increase resistance, add water to the bucket—but not so much that the exercise is painful.

TOE RAISES

Stand up. Slowly rise up on the toes, then slowly lower the heels to the floor. Repeat 10 times, then rest for 1 minute. Do 2 more sets of 10. When this exercise becomes easy, do it while holding progressively heavier weights.

OUTWARD ROLLS

Stand up. Slowly roll the ankle out so that the inner part of the sole is raised off the floor. Slowly lower the sole back to the floor. Do 3 sets of 10.

---

occurs throughout each step, eventually becoming constant. Pain usually disappears with rest.

Doctors diagnose shin splints based on symptoms and the results of a physical examination.

Treatment

Running must be stopped until it causes no pain. Applying ice and using nonsteroidal anti-inflammatory drugs (NSAIDs) can relieve pain. Conditioning can be maintained with alternative exercises, such as swimming.

Once shin pain starts to subside, exercises to stretch and strengthen the muscles in the legs, such as the bucket-handle exercise, can be done. The exercises are important to avoid recurrence. Wearing supportive shoes with rigid heel counters and arch supports and avoiding constant running on banked or hard surfaces may help prevent shin splints from recurring.

ACHILLES TENDINITIS

Achilles tendinitis is inflammation of the Achilles tendon, the tough band extending from the calf muscles to the heel.

Achilles tendinitis is very common in runners. During running, the calf muscles help with the lift-off phase of gait (raising up on the toes from the foot being flat on the ground). Repetitive forces from running combined with insufficient recovery time from exercise can inflame the Achilles tendon.

Pain in the lower calf and back of the heel is usually the first symptom of tendinitis. Doctors diagnose Achilles tendinitis based on the symptoms and results of an examination.

Ice and NSAIDs relieve pain and inflammation. Refraining from running and from pedaling a bicycle as long as the pain persists is important. Exercises to stretch and strengthen the hamstring muscles can be started as soon as they can be done without pain. Other measures depend on what conditions are causing tendinitis. Measures may include wearing shoes with flexible soles or placing heel lifts in running shoes to reduce tension on the tendon and stabilize the heel. People should return to running gradually, stretch the tendon before running, and, at the beginning, apply ice after running.

ACHILLES TENDON RUPTURE

Athletic activity can cause a complete tear of the Achilles tendon, the tough band extending from the calf muscles to the heel.

Complete tears of the Achilles tendon are more common in middle-aged than in young athletes. It is particularly common among people who begin intense activity without sufficient conditioning, stretching, or both. Often rupture occurs during sudden cutting movements.

Symptoms are severe calf pain and inability to walk normally on the leg. Doctors can usually make the diagnosis based on an examination. Sometimes magnetic resonance imaging (MRI) is required. Surgical repair is usually recommended.

ANKLE SPRAIN

An ankle sprain is an injury to the ligaments (the tough elastic tissue that connects bone to bone) in the ankle.

- Usually, ankle sprains occur when people walk or run on uneven ground and the foot rolls inward, causing the ligaments of the ankle to stretch beyond their limits.
- Usually, the ankle is swollen, and walking is painful.
- Diagnosis is by examination and sometimes x-rays.
- Treatment includes *rest*, *ice*, compression with a bandage, and *elevation* of the leg (RICE) and often protection of the ankle with a brace or removable boot.

There are 25,000 ankle sprains reported a day in the United States. Sprains usually occur when the foot rolls inward, causing the sole of the foot to face the other foot. This type of movement is called inversion of the foot or sometimes rolling out of the ankle. This injury (sometimes called an inversion sprain) usually damages the ligaments on the outside of the ankle. It occurs when people walk on uneven ground, especially when they step on a rock or off the edge of a curb. The following tend to cause the ankle to roll outward and thus increase the risk of a sprain:

- Loose ligaments in the ankle from prior sprains
- Weakness or nerve damage in the leg muscles
- Certain types of shoes, such as spiked heels

Other ankle ligaments can be injured, and injuries are likely to be more severe than with a common inversion sprain. For example, the large, strong ligament on the inside of the ankle may be sprained, or the ligament that holds the two leg bones together above the ankle may be sprained (called a high ankle sprain).

Symptoms

The severity of the sprain depends on how much the ligaments are stretched or torn.

- **Mild:** The ligaments may stretch, but they do not actually tear, except microscopically. The ankle usually does not hurt or swell very much, but a mild sprain increases the risk of a repeat injury. Recovery can take hours to days.
- **Moderate:** A ligament tears partially. Obvious swelling and bruising are common, and walking is usually painful and difficult. Healing takes days to weeks. Moderate and severe sprains can impair proprioception (the ability of the brain to sense where the foot and ankle are without seeing them).
- **Severe:** A ligament tears completely, causing severe swelling and bruising. The ankle is unstable and unable to bear weight. Healing usually takes 6 to 8 weeks. When athletes return to unrestricted activity before healing is complete, they risk future injuries and difficulty walking on uneven surfaces. Also, in severe ankle sprains, damage to the smooth cartilaginous surfaces of the bones of the ankle joint (articular cartilage) can result in long-term pain, swelling, and occasionally catching (becoming stuck), giving way (involuntary buckling of the joint), and possibly arthritis of the ankle at an young age.

Diagnosis

Physical examination of the ankle can give clues to the extent of ligament damage. X-rays are often taken to determine whether a bone is broken, but they do not enable doctors to evaluate the ligaments. X-rays taken with the ankle in positions that stretch the ligaments (stress x-rays) may indicate the extent of ligament damage, as can MRI, but these tests are not necessary in most ankle sprains. Arthroscopy (use of a fiberoptic viewing tube to view inside the joint) sometimes is done if doctors suspect that the smooth surface of the ends of

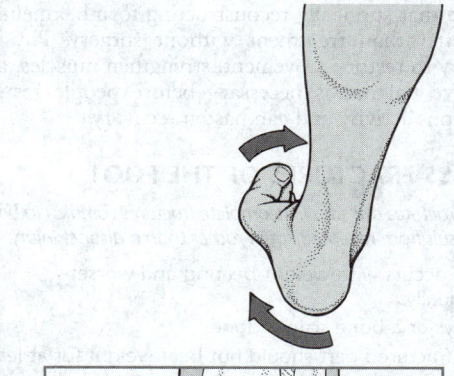

Spraining an Ankle

An ankle sprain may occur when the ankle rolls outward and the foot rolls inward (inversion), tearing the ligament along the outside of the ankle.

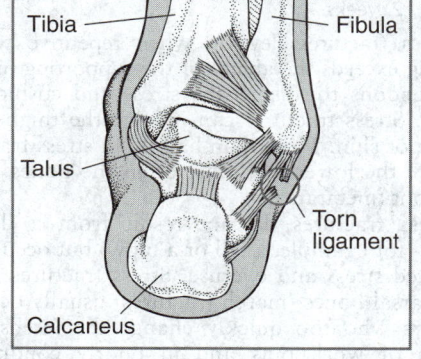

Tibia · Fibula · Talus · Torn ligament · Calcaneus

the bones in the ankle have been damaged, as when a sprain is very severe or fails to heal.

Treatment

Treatment consists of NSAIDs for pain control and RICE (*r*est, *i*ce, *c*ompression, and *e*levation). Other treatments depend on how severe the sprain is.

Usually, **mild sprains** are treated by applying ice packs to the area, wrapping the ankle and foot with an elastic bandage or tape, elevating the ankle, and, as the sprain heals, gradually increasing the amount of walking and exercise. For many people with mild sprains, walking and exercise can begin immediately as long as supportive footwear is worn.

For **moderate sprains**, a removable cast boot or ankle brace can be used initially. Physical therapy is important to help minimize swelling, maintain range of motion, maintain proprioception, and gradually increase the strength of the muscles around the ankle to prevent future ankle instability and recurrent sprains.

Severe sprains require immediate medical attention. Without treatment, they may result in long-term ankle instability and pain. The ankle should be immobilized in a brace or removable cast boot. Usually, people need crutches and are referred to a specialist. Whether surgery should be done is controversial. Most experts believe that surgically reconstructing torn ligaments is no better than treatment without surgery. Physical therapy to restore movement, strengthen muscles, and improve balance is necessary before people resume strenuous activity and can hasten recovery.

STRESS FRACTURES OF THE FOOT

Stress fractures are small, incomplete fractures (breaks) in bones that result from repeated stress rather than a distinct injury.

- Pain occurs with weight-bearing and worsens gradually.
- X-rays or a bone scan is done.
- The fractured part should not bear weight for at least 6 to 12 weeks.

Stress fractures develop when repetitive weight-bearing exceeds the ability of the supporting muscles and tendons to absorb the stress and cushion the bones. Stress fractures can involve the thigh bone, pelvis, or shin. More than half of all stress fractures involve the lower leg, most often the bones of the mid foot (metatarsals).

Stress fractures do not result from a distinct injury (for example, a fall or a blow) but occur after repeated stress and overuse. Stress fractures of the metatarsal bones (march fractures) usually occur in runners who too quickly change the intensity or length of work outs and in poorly conditioned people who walk long distances carrying a load (for example, newly recruited soldiers). Other risk factors include a high foot arch, shoes with inadequate shock-absorbing qualities, and thinning bones (osteoporosis).

Women and girls who exercise strenuously and do not eat an adequate diet (for example, some long distance runners and some athletes in sports that emphasize appearance) may be at risk of stress fractures. They may stop having menstrual periods (amenorrhea) and develop osteoporosis. This condition is known as the female athlete triad (amenorrhea, disordered eating habits, and osteoporosis).

> **? Did You Know...**
> Stress fractures of the bones of the foot are sometimes called march fractures because they commonly occur among newly recruited soldiers who have recently started marching long distances.

What Is a Stress Fracture?

Stress fractures are small cracks in a bone caused by repetitive impact. They commonly occur in the bones of the midfoot—the metatarsals.

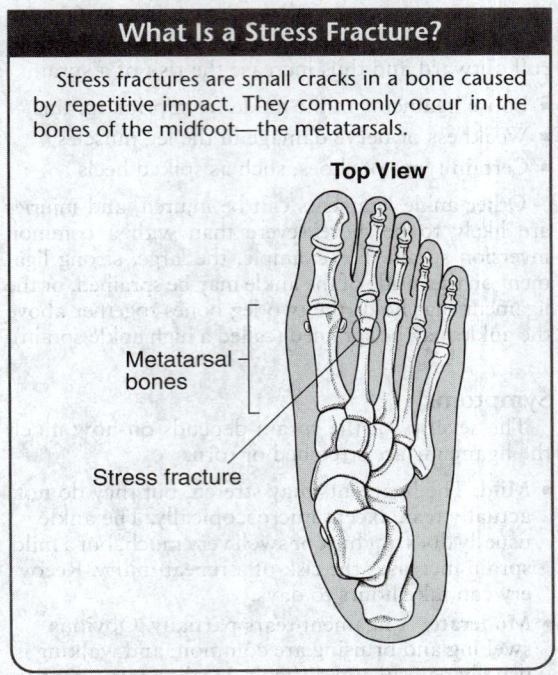

Top View

Metatarsal bones

Stress fracture

Symptoms

With metatarsal stress fractures, forefoot pain most often occurs after a long or intense workout, and then disappears shortly after stopping exercise. With subsequent exercise, onset of pain is earlier and may become so severe that it prevents exercise and persists even when not bearing weight.

Diagnosis

Standard x-rays are usually done but may be normal until about 2 to 3 weeks after the injury, when x-rays show that the bone is healing from the fracture. Earlier diagnosis is often possible by doing a bone scan. Women who have stress fractures should talk with their doctors about whether they should be tested for osteoporosis.

Treatment

Treatment includes reduction of weight-bearing on the involved foot. For a while, the person uses crutches and a wooden shoe or other commercially available supportive shoe or boot. Casts are sometimes needed. Healing can take up to 12 weeks. As with other injuries, people can maintain aerobic fitness by doing non-weight–bearing exercises (for example, swimming) until recovery is complete.

303 Heat Disorders

Humans, who are warm-blooded animals, maintain their body temperature within 1 or 2 degrees of 98.6° F (37° C) as measured by mouth and 100.4° F (38° C) as measured rectally, despite large fluctuations in external temperatures. This internal temperature range must be maintained for the body to function normally. Body temperature that gets too high or too low can result in serious injury to organs or death.

Temperature Regulation: The body regulates its temperature by balancing heat production and heat loss.

One way the body produces heat is through chemical reactions (metabolism) resulting mostly from the conversion of food into energy. Heat is also produced through the work of muscles during physical activity.

The body cools itself by losing heat, mainly through the processes of radiation and sweating. Radiation, in which heat flows from warmer to cooler areas, is the main source of heat loss when the body is warmer than its environment. Sweating, in which the sweat glands produce moisture that cools the skin as it evaporates, is the main source of heat loss when the environmental temperature approaches body temperature and during exercise. However, humidity (moisture in the air) slows water evaporation, decreasing the effectiveness of sweating. Therefore, heat loss may be difficult in hot, humid weather.

Heat Disorders: There are several types of heat disorder:

- Heat cramps
- Heat exhaustion
- Heatstroke (the most serious)

These types vary by their symptoms, whether (and by how much) body temperature is elevated, and by the severity of body fluid and salt depletion. Body fluid and salt depletion result from excessive sweating and can lead to low blood pressure and painful muscle contractions. Internal organs can be damaged if body temperature is very high for a long time.

Causes

Heat disorders are caused by excessive heat production, ineffective heat loss, or both.

Excessive heat production can be caused by the following:

- Infections that cause fever
- Increased thyroid activity, which speeds up the body's metabolism

- Strenuous muscle activity, which may occur during exercise or physical labor (particularly among obese people) or can result from disorders such as seizures, agitation, or alcohol or drug withdrawal
- Certain stimulant drugs, such as cocaine, amphetamines, methylenedioxymethamphetamine (MDMA, or Ecstasy), monoamine oxidase inhibitors (a type of antidepressant), and phencyclidine (angel dust)
- Overdoses of drugs that contain aspirin, because high doses of aspirin cause cells to produce excessive heat

Ineffective heat loss is most common in hot, humid conditions. The following also greatly interfere with heat loss:

- Heavy, tight, clothing that does not breathe (that is, does not allow air and moisture to pass through easily). Wearing such clothing prevents sweat from evaporating from the skin surface and cooling the body.
- Certain drugs, most often antipsychotic drugs and drugs with anticholinergic effects (see box on page 1897), may reduce sweating.
- Certain disorders that affect the skin interfere with sweating. These include cystic fibrosis, systemic sclerosis (formerly called scleroderma), psoriasis, eczema, and severe sunburns.
- Obesity interferes with heat loss because a thick layer of fat is a good insulator.
- Mental states that interfere with sensible responses to heat. For example, elderly people with dementia and intoxicated people who are in a hot environment may not move to a cool environment, remove heavy clothing, or turn on an air conditioner.

The chance of developing heat disorders increases when exposure to heat occurs suddenly, such as when a child is left in a closed car on a hot summer day. In hot weather, the interior of a closed car can heat from 80 to 120° F (27 to 49° C) in 15 minutes. When people are gradually exposed to longer periods of heat and humidity, the body adjusts and is better able to maintain normal body temperature. This process is called acclimatization. Acclimatization occurs more rapidly in young or physically active people than in older or physically inactive people.

Factors that increase vulnerability to the effects of most heat disorders include the following:

- Being very old or very young
- Having certain medical conditions, such as those that involve malfunction of the heart, lungs, kidneys, or liver
- Taking diuretics
- Having imbalances in blood chemistries (electrolytes)

Prevention

Using common sense is the best way to prevent heat disorders. For example, children (and pets too) should never be left in enclosed, poorly ventilated spaces, such as a hot car, even for a few minutes. During excessively hot weather, the very old and the young should not remain in unventilated residences without air-conditioning.

During hot, humid weather, it is best to wear light, loose-fitting clothing made of cloth that breathes, such as cotton. Fluids and salts lost through sweating can usually be replaced by consuming water or lightly salted foods and beverages, such as sports beverages, salted tomato juice, or cool bouillon. Alcoholic beverages are not a good fluid replacement.

Exertion in the Heat: Strenuous exertion in a very hot environment should be avoided. When exertion in a hot environment cannot be avoided, drinking

---

Ways to Help Prevent Heat Disorders

- Ensure adequate ventilation or air-conditioning during heat waves, particularly for people who are very old or very young.
- Avoid leaving children in automobiles in the hot sun, particularly with closed windows.
- Avoid strenuous exertion in hot environments and poorly ventilated spaces.
- Avoid inappropriately heavy, insulated clothing.
- If exertion in heat is unavoidable, wear open-mesh clothing, use a fan, and drink every few hours regardless of thirst.
- If 2% or more of body weight is lost during exercise or work, drink extra fluids.
- If 4% or more of body weight is lost during exercise or work, limit activity for 1 day.
- If large amounts of water are drunk, consume salts in fluids or food.
- If prolonged exertion in heat is unavoidable, starting 10 to 14 days before maximum exertion is required, begin with moderate activity done for about 15 minutes a day, slowly increasing the intensity of the activity and the time spent doing it.

---

plenty of fluids and frequently cooling the skin by misting or wetting it with cool water can help keep body temperature near normal. To replace adequate amounts of fluids, drinking must continue even after thirst is quenched. Weight loss after exercise or work can be used to monitor dehydration. People who lose 2 to 3% of their body weight should be reminded to drink extra fluids and should be within about 2 pounds (1 kilogram) of starting weight before the next day's exposure. People who lose at least 4% of their body weight should limit their activity for 1 day.

People engaged in outdoor activities who drink large quantities of water without salt may dilute the sodium in the blood (a condition called hyponatremia—see page 948), which may cause seizures and even death. Consuming salt, even in salty "junk" food, along with the water can alleviate this problem. Also, many commercially available drinks contain extra salt.

Slowly increasing the level and amount of work done in the heat eventually results in acclimatization, which enables people to work safely at temperatures that were previously dangerous. Progressing from 15 minutes per day of moderate activity (enough to stimulate sweating) during a hot time of day to 90 minutes of vigorous activity over 10 to 14 days is typically adequate.

Heat Cramps

Heat cramps are severe muscle spasms resulting from a combination of prolonged exercise, heavy sweating, and excessive water replacement in extreme heat.

During sweating, salts (electrolytes) and fluids are lost, but drinking large quantities of water dilutes the salts, causing cramps. Heavy sweating is most likely to occur on warm days, especially during strenuous exertion. Heat cramps are common among all of the following:

- Manual laborers, such as engine-room personnel, steelworkers, roofers, and miners
- Athletes, especially mountain climbers or skiers, whose many layers of clothing may keep them from noticing their heavy sweating, and tennis players and runners who do not take time to replace salts lost in sweat
- Military trainees

Heat cramps are strong contractions in muscles of the hands, calves, feet, thighs, or arms. The contractions cause muscles to become hard, tense, and painful. Pain can be intense. Fever does not occur.

Mild heat cramps can be treated by drinking beverages that contain salt or by eating salty food. Drinking 1 to 2 quarts (about 1 to 2 liters) of a sports drink or water containing 2 teaspoons of salt

SPOTLIGHT ON AGING

There are several reasons why older people have particular difficulty when the temperature is high. As people are exposed to long periods of high heat and humidity, their body gradually adjusts (acclimates) and is better able to maintain usual body temperatures. Older people, however, are not as able as younger people to acclimate to higher temperatures and humidity. Older people tend to have difficulty increasing the flow of blood to all skin surfaces, and thus their body does not cool itself as readily.

Certain drugs, such as antipsychotics and antidepressants, and some disorders that affect the skin, such as systemic sclerosis and psoriasis, can also interfere with sweating. Other disorders such as heart failure can interfere with the body's ability to cool itself. Aging also affects thirst; older people do not get thirsty as readily as younger people. Thus, older people tend to get dehydrated, which in turn means they are less able to sweat in warm surroundings.

is usually enough. Severe heat cramps are treated with fluids and salts given intravenously. Stretching the involved muscle often gives immediate relief of pain.

Heat Exhaustion

Heat exhaustion is excessive loss of salts (electrolytes) and fluids due to heat, leading to decreased blood volume that causes many symptoms, sometimes including fainting or collapse.

Heat exhaustion is more severe than heat cramps. Fluids and salts are more depleted, and symptoms are more severe.

Symptoms and Diagnosis

Dizziness, light-headedness, weakness, fatigue, headache, blurred vision, muscle aches, or nausea and vomiting may develop. Muscle cramps may occur but often do not. People may feel faint or even lose consciousness when standing. Drenching sweats are common. Mild confusion may develop. The heart rate and breathing rate may become rapid. Blood pressure may become low. Body temperature is usually normal and if it is high, it is not higher than 104° F (40° C).

Heat exhaustion usually is diagnosed on the basis of the symptoms and occurrence after exposure to heat.

Treatment

Treatment involves replacing fluids and salts, usually intravenously, and removing people from the hot environment. Removing or loosening clothing and applying wet cloths or ice packs to the skin also aid cooling.

After receiving fluids, people usually recover rapidly and fully. If left untreated, heat exhaustion can lead to heatstroke.

Heatstroke

Heatstroke is a life-threatening condition that results in very high body temperature and malfunction of many organ systems.

- Heatstroke can develop after hours of exertion in young athletes or after days of hot weather in rooms without air-conditioning in very old people.
- Body temperature is higher than 104° F (40° C), and the brain malfunctions.
- People should be cooled immediately.

Heatstroke is the most severe form of heat-induced illness. People with heatstroke are much sicker than people with other heat disorders. The following features in particular distinguish heatstroke from other heat disorders:

- Body temperature is usually higher than 104° F.
- Symptoms of brain malfunction develop.

Heatstroke may occur when people exert themselves in extreme heat or is in a closed, hot environment. For example, heatstroke can develop in young, healthy athletes, particularly those who are not acclimatized, after only hours of intense exertion in hot, humid weather. Heatstroke can also develop over days of hot weather when people, particularly older sedentary people, stay in rooms that are poorly ventilated and not air-conditioned. Older people, people who have certain medical conditions (such as those that involve malfunction of the heart, lungs, kidneys, or liver), and young children are most vulnerable to heatstroke.

Heatstroke occurs because the body cannot lose heat rapidly enough in conditions of extreme heat. Because the body cannot cool itself, body temperature continues to rise rapidly to dangerously high levels. Conditions that interfere with heat loss, including certain skin disorders, and drugs that decrease sweating increase the risk.

Heatstroke can temporarily or permanently damage vital organs, such as the heart, lungs, kidneys, liver, and brain. The higher the temperature, especially when higher than 106° F (41° C), the more rapidly problems develop. Death may occur.

Symptoms

Dizziness, light-headedness, weakness, fatigue, headache, blurred vision, muscle aches, nausea, and vomiting (which are also symptoms of heat exhaustion) are common warning symptoms. Affected people do not sense that body temperature is greatly elevated.

During heatstroke, the skin becomes hot, flushed, and dry. Sweating may not occur despite the heat. Because of brain malfunction, people may become confused and disoriented and may have seizures or go into a coma. The heart rate and breathing rate increase. The pulse rate is usually rapid. The blood pressure may be high or low. Body temperature usually exceeds 104° F and may be so high that it exceeds the markings on a typical thermometer.

Diagnosis

The diagnosis is usually evident. People have a high fever, symptoms of brain malfunction, and a history of being exposed to high heat and humidity. If the diagnosis is not evident, tests are done for other disorders that can cause similar symptoms, such as infections, stroke, and an overactive thyroid gland (hyperthyroidism).

Treatment

The body must be cooled immediately, and an ambulance should be called. While awaiting transportation to the hospital, people should be wrapped in cold, wet bedding or clothing; immersed in a lake, stream, or cool bathtub; or cooled by being immersed in ice-cold water. Misting the body with water and then blowing air across the body with a fan is also very effective. Using drugs (aspirin or acetaminophen) designed to treat a fever due to an infection is useless and should be avoided.

At the hospital, the body is usually cooled rapidly by removing the clothes and covering the exposed skin

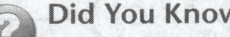

> **? Did You Know...**
> Drinking large amounts of plain water during exertion can dangerously dilute sodium in the bloodstream.

with water or occasionally ice. To speed evaporation and body cooling, a fan may be used to blow air on the body. Body temperature is measured frequently, often constantly. Cooled fluids may be given intravenously. To avoid overcooling, cooling is stopped when the body temperature is reduced to about 102° F (about 39° C).

Seizures, coma, and malfunction of other organs may also need treatment. Heatstroke is best treated in an intensive care unit of a hospital.

Prognosis

The risk of death from heatstroke climbs depending on the following factors:

- How old adults are
- How young children are
- How severe any conditions (such as heart, lungs, kidneys, or liver disorders) are
- What the highest body temperature is
- How long body temperature remains extremely high

In about 20% of people who survive, the brain may not fully recover, leaving a person with personality changes, clumsiness, or poor coordination. In some people, the kidneys do not fully recover. After recovery, body temperature may fluctuate abnormally for weeks.

CHAPTER

304   Cold Injuries

The skin and the tissues under it are kept at a constant temperature (about 98.6° F, or 37° C) by the circulating blood and other mechanisms. The blood gets its heat mainly from the energy given off by cells when they burn (metabolize) food—a process that requires a steady supply of food and oxygen. A normal body temperature is necessary for proper functioning of all the cells and tissues in the body. In a person with low body temperature, most organs, especially the heart and brain, become sluggish and eventually stop working.

Body temperature falls when the skin is exposed to colder surroundings. In response to this fall in temperature, the body uses several protective mechanisms to generate additional heat. For example, the muscles produce additional heat through shivering. Also, the small blood vessels in the skin narrow (constrict), so that more blood is diverted to vital organs, such as the heart and brain. However, as less warm blood reaches the skin, body parts such as the fingers, toes, ears, and nose cool more rapidly. If body temperature falls much below about

88° F (about 31° C), these protective mechanisms stop working, and the body cannot warm itself. If body temperature falls below 83° F (about 28° C), death is likely.

Cold injuries are less likely to occur, even in extremely cold weather, if the skin, fingers, toes, ears, and nose are well protected or are exposed only briefly. The risk of cold injuries increases when the flow of blood is too slow, when food intake is inadequate, or when insufficient oxygen is available, as occurs at high altitudes. Keeping warm in a cold environment requires several layers of clothing—preferably wool or synthetics such as polypropylene, because these materials insulate even when wet. Because the body loses a large amount of heat from the head, a warm hat is essential. Eating enough food and drinking enough fluids (particularly warm fluids) also help. Food provides fuel to be burned, and warm fluids directly provide heat and prevent dehydration. Alcoholic beverages should be avoided, because alcohol widens (dilates) blood vessels in the skin, which makes the body temporarily feel warm but actually causes greater heat loss.

Cold injuries include hypothermia, frostnip, chilblains, immersion foot, and frostbite. Other problems related to the cold include Raynaud's syndrome (see page 426) and allergic reactions to the cold (see page 1121).

?   Did You Know...

Drinking alcoholic beverages actually makes the body colder because the widening of blood vessels that makes a person feel warm allows more heat to escape from the body.

Hypothermia

Hypothermia is a dangerously low body temperature.

- Being surrounded by too cold of an environment, having certain disorders, being unable to move, or a combination can cause body temperature to become too low.
- The person shivers but then may become confused and lose awareness.
- Getting warm and dry can lead to recovery unless the body temperature is very low.
- If the body temperature is very low, doctors may warm the person with warmed oxygen and heated fluids given intravenously or passed into the abdominal or chest cavity through plastic tubes. Doctors also provide heat to the outside of the body.

Hypothermia results when the body loses more heat than can be replaced by increasing metabolism (through exercise) or by increasing warming from

SPOTLIGHT ON AGING

Aging takes a toll on the body's ability to adapt to the cold. With aging, the body becomes less efficient at shivering and at diverting blood away from the surface of the body. Also, the layer of fat just under the skin thins, so there is less insulation to prevent heat loss.

The body's ability to produce heat is decreased by disorders that commonly affect older people, such as hypothyroidism. The body's ability to retain heat is decreased by disorders such as diabetes. A person who is less able to move around because of an injury or a disorder such as a stroke or arthritis is also at a greater risk of dangerous cooling, because the decreased movement generates less heat-producing muscle activity. Alcohol and certain drugs, such as antidepressants, increase the risk as well.

Hypothermia is almost always preventable. Older people are advised to take the following precautions:

- Maintain a warm environment. Older people sometimes keep their home at a lower-than-desirable temperature as a means of saving money, but the thermostat should be set at 68° F or higher. It is especially important that the bedroom be kept warm. Fuel assistance programs and home winterization programs may help defray costs.

- Wear several layers of clothing. Clothing made of wool or synthetic materials such as polypropylene are especially useful because these materials insulate even when they become wet. Because the body loses a large amount of heat from the head, wearing a hat is important. Fingers and toes must also be protected.

- Eat warm foods and drink warm fluids. Food provides the body with fuel to be burned, and warm fluids provide heat and prevent dehydration.

- Avoid alcoholic beverages. Alcohol dilates blood vessels in the skin, which makes the body temporarily feel warm but actually causes greater heat loss.

- Exercise regularly. Exercise can increase the body's production of heat.

---

external sources, such as a fire or the sun. Wind increases heat loss, as does sitting or lying on a cold surface or being immersed in water. Sudden immersion in very cold water may cause fatal hypothermia in 5 to 15 minutes. However, a few people, mostly infants and young children, have survived for as long as 1 hour completely submerged in ice water. The shock can shut off all systems, essentially protecting the body. Hypothermia may also occur after prolonged exposure in only moderately cool water.

People at greatest risk are those who are lying immobile in a cold environment—such as people who have had a stroke or a seizure or who are unconscious from intoxication, a low blood sugar level, or an injury. Because they are not moving, these people generate less heat and also are unable to leave the cold environment. Such people are at risk of becoming hypothermic even when the surrounding temperature may be only as cold as 55 or 60° F (about 13 to 16° Celsius [C]). The very young and the very old are at particular risk. People in these age groups often do not compensate for cold as well as young adults and are dependent on others to anticipate their needs and keep them warm. Very old people quite often become hypothermic while indoors from sitting immobile in a cold room for hours. Infants lose body heat rapidly and are particularly susceptible to hypothermia. Sometimes a disorder, such as a widespread infection or an underfunctioning thyroid gland, causes or contributes to hypothermia.

Symptoms

Initial symptoms include intense shivering and teeth chattering. As body temperature falls further, shivering stops and movements become slow and clumsy, reaction time is longer, thinking is blurred, and judgment is impaired. These symptoms may develop so gradually that people, including companions of the affected person, do not realize what is happening. People may fall, wander off, or simply lie down to rest. When shivering stops, people become more sluggish and slip into a coma. The heart and breathing rates become slower and weaker. Eventually the heart stops.

The lower the body temperature is, the higher the risk of death. Death may occur at body temperatures below 88° F (about 31° C) but is most likely to occur below 83° F (about 28° C).

Diagnosis

Doctors diagnose hypothermia by measuring body temperature, typically with a rectal thermometer. Conventional thermometers do not record below 94° F (about 34° C). Thus, special thermometers are needed to measure temperatures in severe hypothermia. Blood and sometimes other tests are done to see whether a disorder caused hypothermia.

Treatment

In the early stages, drying the body, changing into warm dry clothing, being covered with warm blankets, and drinking hot beverages can bring about recovery. In people who are found unconscious, further heat loss is prevented by wrapping them in a warm dry blanket and, if possible, removing wet clothing and moving them to a warm place while arrangements are made for immediate transportation to a hospital. Cardiopulmonary resuscitation (CPR) is only recommended outside of a hospital after very careful consideration for the following reasons:

- It is difficult for untrained people to detect very faint respirations and heartbeats.
- Often, even if no pulse can be felt and no heartbeat can be heard, the heart may be beating. Applying chest compressions to a cold beating heart often disturbs heart rhythm, resulting in death.
- A severely hypothermic person must be handled gently, because a sudden jolt may cause an irregular heart rhythm, (arrhythmia) that could be fatal.

In the hospital, doctors warm the person with warmed oxygen and heated fluids given intravenously or passed into the abdominal or chest cavity through plastic tubes inserted into those areas. In addition, the blood may be warmed through the process of hemodialysis (in which the blood is pumped out of the body, through a filter with a heating attachment, and back into the body) or with a heart-lung machine (which pumps blood out of the body, heats the blood, adds oxygen, and then returns the blood to the body).

Because some people with hypothermia who have arrived at the hospital with no signs of life have recovered, doctors may continue resuscitation efforts until the person is warmed but still shows no signs of life. If certain blood test results are extremely abnormal, the person is already dead.

Nonfreezing Tissue Injuries

In nonfreezing tissue injuries, parts of the skin are chilled but not frozen.

Nonfreezing tissue injuries include frostnip, immersion foot, and chilblains.

Frostnip: Frostnip is a cold injury in which the chilled areas of skin become numb, swollen, and red. The only treatment needed is warming the area for a few minutes. During warming, the area may hurt or itch intensely. No permanent damage results, although sometimes the area is particularly sensitive to cold for months or years afterward.

Immersion Foot: Immersion foot (trench foot) is a cold injury that develops when a foot is kept in wet, cold socks and boots for several days. The foot is pale, clammy, swollen, and cold. After warming, the foot becomes red and painful to the touch. Sometimes blisters develop, which may open and become infected. The skin may become overly sensitive to changes in temperature. Treatment consists primarily of the following measures:

- Gently warming, drying, and cleaning the foot
- Elevating the foot
- Keeping the foot dry and warm

Some doctors give antibiotics to prevent infection. A tetanus booster is given if the person's tetanus vaccination is not current. Rarely, this type of injury occurs in the hands. Immersion foot can often be prevented by changing socks and drying the feet at least daily.

Chilblains: Chilblains (pernio) is an uncommon reaction that may occur with repeated exposure to cold. Symptoms include itching, pain, redness, swelling, and, in rare cases, discolored areas or blisters on the affected area (usually the leg or fingers). The condition is uncomfortable and recurrent but not serious. Preventing exposure to cold is the best treatment. The drug nifedipine, taken by mouth, sometimes relieves symptoms.

Frostbite

Frostbite is a cold injury in which an area of the body is frozen.

- Extreme cold may freeze tissues, destroying them and sometimes surrounding tissues.
- The area may be numb, white, swollen, blistered, or black and leathery.
- The area is rewarmed in warm water as soon as possible.
- Most areas heal over time, but sometimes surgery is required to remove dead tissue.

The damage caused by frostbite results from a combination of factors. Freezing kills some cells: others survive. Because cold causes blood vessels to narrow, tissue that is near the frozen area but not itself frozen may be damaged as a result of the decreased blood flow. Sometimes cold also causes clots to form in small blood vessels in this tissue. These clots may limit blood flow so much that the tissue dies. When blood flow returns to the affected area, the damaged tissues release a number of chemical substances that promote inflammation. Inflammation worsens the damage caused by the cold. In addition, toxic substances are released into the bloodstream as frozen tissue is warmed.

Exposure to below-freezing temperatures puts any part of the body at risk of frostbite. The risk of frostbite damage depends on how cold it is and how long the part was exposed. People at greatest risk of developing frostbite are those who have poor circulation because of diabetes or arteriosclerosis, blood vessel spasm (which may be caused by smoking,

some neurologic disorders, or certain drugs), or constriction of blood flow by gloves or boots that are too tight. Exposed hands and feet and an exposed face are most vulnerable. Contact with wetness or metal accelerates freezing and is particularly dangerous.

Symptoms

Symptoms vary with the depth and amount of tissue frozen. Shallow frostbite results in a numb white patch of skin that peels after warming. Slightly deeper frostbite causes blisters and swelling of the affected area. Deeper freezing causes the extremity to feel numb, cold, and hard. The area is pale and cold. Blisters often appear. Blisters filled with clear fluid indicate milder damage than do blisters filled with blood-stained fluid.

The extremity may become gray and soft (wet gangrene). If wet gangrene develops, in many cases the extremity must be amputated. More frequently, the area becomes black and leathery (dry gangrene).

Diagnosis

Frostbite is diagnosed by its typical appearance and occurrence after significant exposure to cold. Sometimes frostbite appears the same as nonfreezing injuries for the first few days. After a period of time, frostbitten tissue develops characteristics that differentiate it from nonfreezing injuries.

Treatment

Outside of the Hospital: People who have frostbite should be covered with a warm blanket because they may also have hypothermia. When possible, warming of the frostbitten area should begin immediately. The area is immersed in warm water that is no hotter than can be comfortably tolerated by the caregiver (100 to 104° F or about 40° Celsius [C]). Rubbing the area (particularly with snow) leads to further tissue damage. Because the area has no sensation, people cannot tell if a burn is developing. Thus, the area should not be warmed in front of a fire or with a heating pad or electric blanket.

It is more damaging to thaw and refreeze tissue than to allow it to remain frozen. Thus, if people with frostbite must be re-exposed to freezing conditions, particularly if they must walk on frostbitten feet, the tissue should not be thawed. Thawed feet are more vulnerable to damage from walking. If people must walk on frostbitten feet to reach help, the feet should not be thawed first. Also, every effort should be made to protect the damaged tissue from rubbing, constriction, or further damage. The feet are cleaned, dried, and covered. People are kept warm and given an analgesic if possible. They are taken to a hospital as soon as possible.

In the Hospital: In the hospital, warming is begun or continued. Full rewarming takes about 15 to 30 minutes. The frostbitten area becomes extremely painful as it is warmed, so an injection of an opioid analgesic may be necessary. Blisters should not be broken. If blisters break, they should be covered with antibiotic ointment.

Once the tissue is warmed, the frostbitten area should be gently washed, dried, wrapped in sterile bandages, and kept meticulously clean and dry to prevent infection. Anti-inflammatory drugs, such as ibuprofen by mouth, or aloe vera gel applied topically helps relieve the inflammation. Infection requires use of antibiotics, although some doctors try to prevent infection from occurring by giving antibiotics to all people with deep frostbite. Some doctors also use drugs given intravenously to improve circu-lation to the affected area, although these forms of treatment are beneficial only in the first few days after injury.

After Hospital Discharge: Whirlpool baths with warm water (about 98.6° F, or 37° C) three times per day followed by gentle drying, rest, and time are the best ongoing treatments. Most people slowly improve over several months, although amputation is sometimes necessary to remove the dead tissue. Because frostbite may appear to affect a larger area and to be more severe than it will weeks or months later, the decision to amputate is usually postponed for several months until the area has had time to heal. Sometimes an imaging test, such as magnetic resonance imaging (MRI), radionuclide scanning, microwave thermography, or a laser-Doppler flow study, helps determine which areas may recover and which will not. Areas that will not recover require amputation. Some people develop numbness or oversensitivity to cold after frostbite heals.

CHAPTER

305 Radiation Injury

Radiation injury is damage to tissues caused by exposure to ionizing radiation.

- Large doses of ionizing radiation can cause acute illness by reducing the production of blood cells and damaging the digestive tract.
- A very large dose of ionizing radiation can also damage the heart and blood vessels (cardiovascular system), brain, and skin.
- Ionizing radiation can increase the risk of cancer, and damage to sperm and egg cells can increase the risk of genetic defects in offspring.
- Doctors remove radioactive material from the person and treat symptoms and complications of radiation injury.

In general, ionizing radiation refers to high-energy electromagnetic waves (x-rays and gamma rays) and particles (alpha particles, beta particles, and neutrons) that are capable of stripping electrons from atoms (ionization). Ionization changes the chemistry of affected atoms and any molecules containing those atoms. By changing molecules in the highly ordered environment of the cell, ionizing radiation can disrupt and damage cells. Cellular damage can cause illness, increase the risk of developing cancer, or both.

Ionizing radiation is emitted by radioactive substances (radionuclides), such as uranium, radon, and plutonium. It is also produced by man-made devices, such as x-ray and radiation therapy machines.

Radio waves, such as from cell phones and AM and FM transmitters, and visible light also are forms of electromagnetic radiation. However, because of their lower energy, these forms of radiation are not ionizing, and thus public exposure levels from these common sources do not damage cells. In this discussion, "radiation" refers exclusively to ionizing radiation.

Measurement of Radiation: The amount of radiation is measured in several different units. The roentgen (R) is a measure of the ionizing ability of radiation in air and is commonly used to express the intensity of exposure to radiation. How much radiation people are exposed to and how much is deposited in their body may be very different. The gray (Gy) and sievert (Sv) are measures of the dose of radiation, which is the amount of radiation deposited in matter, and are the units used to measure dose in humans after exposure to radiation. The Gy and Sv are similar, except the Sv takes into account the effectiveness of different types of radiation to cause damage and the sensitivity of different tissues in the body to radiation. Low levels of exposure are measured in mGy (1 mGy = $1/1000$ Gy) and mSv (1 mSv = $1/1000$ Sv).

Contamination vs. Irradiation: The two main types of radiation exposure are contamination and irradiation. Many of the most significant radiation accidents have exposed people to both.

Contamination is contact with and retention of radioactive material, usually as a dust or liquid. External contamination is that on skin or clothing, from which some can fall or be rubbed off, contaminating other people and objects. Internal contamination is radioactive material deposited within the body, which it may enter by ingestion, inhalation, or through breaks in the skin. Once in the body, radioactive material may be transported to various sites, such as the bone marrow, where it continues to emit radiation, increasing the dose, until it is removed or emits all its energy (decays). Internal contamination is more difficult to remove than external contamination.

Irradiation is exposure to radiation but not to radioactive material, that is, no contamination is involved. A common example is diagnostic x-rays, such as for a broken bone. Radiation exposure can occur without direct contact between people and the source of radiation (such as radioactive material or an x-ray machine). When the source of the radiation is removed or turned off, irradiation ends. People who are irradiated but not contaminated are not radioactive, that is, they do not emit radiation, and their dose from that source of radiation does not continue to increase.

> ❓ **Did You Know...**
>
> The average person in the United States receives about the same dose of natural radiation as that from man-made sources of radiation (almost all of which is medical radiation used to diagnose or treat disease).

Sources of Radiation Exposure

People are exposed constantly to low levels of radiation, naturally occurring (background radiation), and intermittently to radiation from man-made sources. In the United States, people receive on average about 3 mSv per year from natural sources and 3 mSv per year from man-made sources, for a total of 6 mSv per year. However, in some parts of India, Iran, Brazil, and China, the average radiation dose from background is higher, between 5 and 10 mSv per year.

Background Radiation: Sources of background radiation include cosmic radiation from outer space and naturally occurring radioactive elements.

Cosmic radiation is significantly blocked by the earth's atmosphere but is concentrated at the north and south poles by the earth's magnetic field. Thus, exposure to cosmic radiation is greater for people living closer to the poles, living at high altitudes, and during airplane flights.

Radioactive elements, particularly uranium and the radioactive products into which it naturally decays (such as radon gas), are present in many rocks and minerals. These elements end up in various substances, including food, water, and construction materials. Radon exposure typically accounts for about two thirds of peoples' exposure to naturally occurring radiation. The doses from natural background radiation are far too low to cause radiation injury.

Man-Made Radiation: Most people's exposure to man-made sources of radiation involves medical imaging tests (particularly computed tomography [CT] and cardiac nuclear medicine scans). Medical diagnostic tests such as chest x-rays, mammograms, and dental x-rays do not deliver doses sufficient to cause radiation injury. People who are receiving radiation treatments for cancer may receive very high doses of radiation. However, every effort is made to deliver the radiation only to diseased tissues and to minimize the radiation to normal tissues.

Exposure also occurs from other sources, such as radiation accidents and fallout from nuclear weapons testing. However, these exposures represent a minor part of most people's annual exposure. Typically, radiation accidents involve people who work with radioactive materials and with x-ray sources, such as food irradiators and industrial x-ray machines. Such people may receive significant doses of radiation. These injuries commonly result from failure to follow safety procedures. Radiation exposure has also occurred from lost or stolen medical or industrial sources containing large amounts of radioactive material.

Rarely, radioactive material has been released from nuclear power plants, including the Three Mile Island plant in Pennsylvania in 1979 and the Chernobyl plant in the Ukraine in 1986. The Three Mile Island accident did not result in major radiation exposure. In fact, people living within 1 mile (1.6 kilometers) of the plant received only about 0.08 mSv additional radiation. However, people living near the Chernobyl plant received an average dose of about 300 mSv. More than 30 workers and emergency responders died, and many more were injured. There was low-level contamination from Chernobyl as far away as Europe, Asia, and even the United States. The average cumulative radiation dose for the general population in contaminated areas (various regions of Belarus, Russia, and Ukraine) over a 20-year period after the accident was estimated to be between 10 and 30 mSv. It should be noted that the average annual extra dose

ANNUAL RADIATION EXPOSURE IN THE UNITED STATES

SOURCE	AVERAGE EFFECTIVE DOSE (MILLISIEVERTS)
Naturally occurring sources	
Radon gas	2.00
Other terrestrial sources	0.28
Radiation from outer space	0.27
Natural radioactive material in the body	0.39
Subtotal	3.0
Man-made sources	
Diagnostic medical imaging*	3.0
Consumer products	0.10
Fallout from weapons testing	less than 0.01
Nuclear industry	less than 0.01
Subtotal	3.0
Total annual exposure	6.0
Other sources of exposure (per incident)	
Airline travel	0.005 mSv/hour of flight
Dental x-rays	0.005
Chest x-ray	0.02
Mammography	0.4
Computed tomography scan of the head	2
Computed tomography scan of the chest or abdomen	7
Barium enema	8

*Average value. Most people receive much lower doses each year, from examinations such as dental x-rays and mammograms, whereas a smaller number of ill or injured people require numerous imaging tests and thus receive much larger doses.

(0.5 to 1.5 mSv per year) received by residents of the territories contaminated by Chernobyl fallout is generally lower than typical background radiation in the United States.

Nuclear weapons release massive amounts of energy and radiation. These weapons have not been used against people since 1945. However, several nations now have nuclear weapons, and terrorist groups have also tried to obtain them or build their own, increasing the possibility that these weapons will again be used. The vast majority of the casualties from the detonation of a nuclear weapon result from the blast and thermal burns. A smaller fraction of the casualties (although still a high number) result from radiation-induced illness.

The possibility of intentional radiation exposure through terrorist activities includes the use of a device to contaminate an area by dispersing radioactive material (a radiation dispersal device that uses conventional explosives is referred to as a dirty bomb). Other terrorist scenarios include using a hidden radiation source to expose unsuspecting people to large doses of radiation, attacking a nuclear reactor or radioactive material storage facility, and detonating a nuclear weapon.

Effects of Radiation

The damaging effects of radiation depend on several factors:

- The amount (dose)

- How rapidly the dose is received
- How much of the body is exposed
- The sensitivity of particular tissues to radiation

A single, rapid dose of radiation to the entire body can be fatal, but the same total dose given over a period of weeks or months may have much less effect. The effects of radiation also depend on how much of the body is exposed. For example, more than 6 Gy is usually fatal when the radiation is distributed over the entire body. However, when concentrated in certain small areas and spread out over a period of weeks or months, as in radiation therapy for cancer, 10 or more times this amount can be given without serious harm.

Some parts of the body are more sensitive to radiation. Organs and tissues in which cells multiply quickly, such as the intestines and bone marrow, are harmed more easily by radiation than those in which cells multiply more slowly, such as muscles and brain cells. The thyroid gland is susceptible to cancer after being exposed to radioactive iodine because radioactive iodine concentrates in the thyroid gland.

Radiation and Children: Children are more susceptible to radiation injury because their cells typically divide more rapidly than those of adults.

The fetus is exceptionally sensitive to damage from radiation. In the fetus, exposure in excess of 300 mGy during 8 to 25 weeks after conception may cause reduced intelligence and poor school performance. Birth defects may occur due to exposure in the womb to high doses of radiation. However, at doses less than 100 mGy, particularly at the even lower doses used in imaging tests a pregnant woman might typically undergo, there is no apparent increase beyond the normal risk of having a birth defect.

> **? Did You Know...**
>
> Radiation is not as potent a cause of cancer or birth defects as people think.

Radiation and Cancer: A large radiation exposure increases the risk of cancer because of damage to the genetic material (DNA) in cells that survive the radiation. However, radiation is a weaker cause of cancer than people think. Even a whole-body dose of 1 Gy (over 300 times more than the average annual background radiation dose) increases a typical person's lifetime risk of dying from cancer from 25% to about 30%.

Children's risk of radiation-induced cancer is several times higher than that of adults. Children may be more susceptible because their cells divide more often and because they have a longer lifespan during which cancer may develop. The lifetime risk of cancer for a 1-year-old who has a CT scan of the abdomen is estimated to increase by 0.18%.

Radiation and Inherited Defects: In animals, irradiation of the ovaries or testes at high doses has been shown to lead to defective offspring (hereditary effects). However, no increase in the percentage of birth defects was observed in the children of survivors of the nuclear detonations in Japan. It may be that the radiation exposure was not high enough to cause a measurable increase.

Symptoms

Symptoms depend on whether radiation exposure involves the whole body or is limited to a small portion of the body. At high doses, whole-body exposure causes acute radiation illness, and partial-body exposure causes local radiation injury.

Acute Radiation Illness: Acute radiation illness typically occurs in people whose entire body has been exposed to very high doses of radiation all at once or over a short period of time. Doctors divide acute radiation syndromes into three groups based on the main organ system affected, although there is overlap among these groups:

- Hematopoietic syndrome
- Gastrointestinal syndrome
- Cerebrovascular syndrome

Acute radiation illness usually progresses through three stages:

- Early symptoms such as nausea, loss of appetite, vomiting, tiredness, and, when very high radiation doses are received, diarrhea (collectively called the prodrome)
- A symptom-free period (latent stage)
- Various patterns of symptoms (syndromes), depending on the amount of radiation received

Which syndrome develops, its severity, and its rate of progression depend on the radiation dose. As the dose increases, symptoms develop earlier, progress more rapidly (for example, from prodromal symptoms to the various organ system syndromes), and become more severe.

The severity and time course of the early symptoms are fairly consistent from person to person for a given amount of radiation exposure. Thus, doctors often can estimate a person's radiation exposure from the timing, nature, and severity of the early symptoms.

The **hematopoietic syndrome** is caused by the effects of radiation on the bone marrow, spleen, and lymph nodes—the primary sites of blood cell production (hematopoiesis). Loss of appetite (anorexia), lethargy, nausea, and vomiting may begin 1 to 6 hours after exposure to 1 to 6 Gy of radiation. These symptoms resolve within 24 to 48 hours after exposure, and people feel well for a week or more. During this symptom-free period, the blood-producing cells in the bone marrow, spleen, and lymph nodes begin to waste away and are not replaced, leading to a severe shortage of white blood cells, followed by a shortage of platelets and then red blood cells. The shortage of white blood cells can lead to severe infections. The shortage of platelets may cause uncontrolled bleeding. The shortage of red blood cells (anemia) causes fatigue, weakness, paleness, and difficulty breathing with physical exertion. After 4 to 5 weeks, if people survive, blood cells begin to be produced once more, but people feel weak and tired for months.

The **gastrointestinal syndrome** is due to the effects of radiation on the cells lining the digestive tract. Severe nausea, vomiting, and diarrhea may begin in less than 1 hour after exposure to 6 Gy or more of radiation. The symptoms may lead to severe dehydration, but they resolve within 2 days. During the next 4 or 5 days (latent stage), people feel well, but the cells lining the digestive tract, which normally act as a protective barrier, die and are shed. After this time, severe diarrhea—often bloody—returns, once more resulting in dehydration. Bacteria from the digestive tract may invade the body, producing severe infections. People who have received this much radiation also develop the hematopoietic syndrome, which results in bleeding and infection and increases their risk of death. After exposure to 6 Gy or more of radiation, death is common. However, with advanced medical support, about 50% of people may survive.

The **cerebrovascular syndrome** occurs when the total dose of radiation exceeds 20 to 30 Gy. People rapidly develop confusion, nausea, vomiting, bloody diarrhea, tremors, and shock. The latent phase is brief or absent. Within hours, blood pressure falls, accompanied by seizures and coma. The cerebrovascular syndrome is always fatal within a few hours to 1 or 2 days.

Local Radiation Injury: Radiation therapy for cancer is one of the most common causes of local radiation injuries. Other causes produce similar symptoms. Symptoms depend on the amount of radiation and the area of the body treated.

Nausea, vomiting, and loss of appetite may occur during or shortly after irradiation of the brain or abdomen. Large amounts of radiation to a limited area of the body often damage the skin over that area. Skin changes include hair loss, redness, peeling, sores, and, possibly eventual thinning of the skin and dilated blood vessels just beneath the skin's surface (spider veins). Radiation to the mouth and jaw can cause permanent dry mouth, resulting in an increased number of dental caries and damage to the jawbone. Radiation to the lungs can cause lung inflammation (radiation pneumonitis). Very high doses can result in severe scarring (fibrosis) of lung tissue, which can cause disabling shortness of breath and later death. The heart and its protective sac (pericardium) can become inflamed after extensive radiation to the chest, causing symptoms such as chest pain and shortness of breath. High accumulated doses of radiation to the spinal cord can cause catastrophic damage, leading to paralysis, incontinence, and loss of sensation. Extensive radiation to the abdomen (for lymph node, testicular, or ovarian cancer) can lead to chronic ulcers, scarring, and narrowing or perforation of the intestine, causing symptoms such as abdominal pain, vomiting, vomiting blood, and dark, tarry stools.

Occasionally, severe injuries develop long after the completion of radiation therapy. Kidney function may decline 6 months to a year after people have received extremely large amounts of radiation, resulting in anemia and high blood pressure. High accumulated doses of radiation to muscles may cause a painful condition that includes muscle wasting (atrophy) and calcium deposits in the irradiated muscle. Occasionally, radiation therapy may result in a new cancerous (malignant) tumor. These radiation-induced cancers typically occur 10 or more years after exposure.

Diagnosis

Exposure to radiation may be obvious from people's history. Radiation injury is suspected when people develop symptoms of illness or skin redness or sores after receiving radiation therapy or being exposed during a radiation accident. The time until symptoms develop can help doctors estimate the radiation dose. No specific tests are available to diagnose radiation exposure, although certain standard clinical tests may be used to detect infection, low blood counts, or organ malfunction. To help determine the severity of radiation exposure, doctors measure the number of lymphocytes (a type of white blood cell) in the blood. Typically, the lower the lymphocyte count 48 hours after exposure, the worse the radiation exposure.

Radioactive contamination, unlike irradiation, can be determined by surveying a person's body with a Geiger-Muller counter, a device that detects radiation. Swabs from the nose, throat, and any wounds also are checked for radioactivity.

The early symptoms of acute radiation illness—nausea, vomiting, and tremors—can also be caused by anxiety. Because anxiety is common after terrorist and nuclear incidents, people should not panic when such symptoms develop, particularly if the amount of radiation exposure is unknown and may have been small.

Prevention

Following widespread high-level environmental contamination from a nuclear power plant accident or the intentional release of radioactive material, people should follow the advice of public health officials. Such information is usually broadcast on TV and radio. The advice may be for people to evacuate the contaminated area or to take shelter where they are. Whether evacuation or sheltering is recommended depends on many factors, including time elapsed since the initial release, whether the release has stopped, weather conditions, availability of adequate shelters, and road and traffic conditions. If sheltering is recommended, sheltering in a concrete or metal structure, particularly one below grade (such as in a basement), is best. Half way between the top and bottom of a tall building, near the center away from windows, is best when no below-grade shelter is available.

Changing clothes and showering are recommended if people suspect they may have been contaminated with radioactive material. People can obtain potassium iodide (KI) tablets from local pharmacies and some public health agencies. However, potassium iodide is only useful if radioactive iodine is released. It does not provide protection from other radioactive materials. People with known iodine sensitivity and certain thyroid conditions should avoid potassium iodide. A doctor should be consulted if iodine sensitivity is suspected.

During imaging procedures that involve ionizing radiation and especially during radiation therapy for cancer, which involves high doses, the most susceptible parts of the body, such as the lenses of the eyes, female breasts, ovaries or testes, and thyroid gland, are shielded when possible (for example, by wearing a lead-filled covering).

> ### ? Did You Know...
>
> People living within 10 miles (16 kilometers) of a nuclear power plant should have ready access to potassium iodide tablets.
>
> Changing clothes and showing with warm water and regular shampoo are very effective in removing most external contamination.

Prognosis

The outcome depends on the radiation dose, dose rate (how quickly the exposure occurs), and the parts of the body that are affected. Other factors include people's state of health and whether they receive medical care. In general, without medical care, half of all people who receive more than 3 Gy of whole-body radiation at once die. Nearly all people who receive more than 6 Gy die. Nearly all those who receive less than 2 Gy fully recover within 1 month, although long-term complications such as cancer may occur. With medical care, about half of people survive 6 Gy of whole-body radiation. Some people have survived doses of up to 10 Gy.

Because doctors are unlikely to know the amount of radiation a person has received, they usually predict outcome based on the person's symptoms. The cerebrovascular syndrome is fatal within hours to a few days. The gastrointestinal syndrome generally is fatal within 3 to 10 days, although some people survive for a few weeks. Many people who receive proper medical care survive the hematopoietic syndrome, depending on radiation dose and their state of health. Those who do not survive typically die within 4 to 8 weeks after exposure.

Treatment

Physical injuries are treated before irradiation is treated because they are more immediately life-threatening. Irradiation has no emergency treatment, but doctors closely monitor people for the development of the various syndromes and treat the symptoms as they arise.

Contamination should be removed promptly to prevent the radioactive material from continuing to irradiate the person and to prevent the radioactive material from being taken up by the body. Contaminated wounds are treated before contaminated skin. Doctors decontaminate wounds by flushing them with a salt water solution and wiping them with a surgical sponge. After decontamination, wounds are covered to prevent recontamination as other sites are washed. Contaminated skin should be gently scrubbed with large amounts of soap and warm (not hot) water. Skin folds and nails need extra attention. Harsh chemicals, brushes, or scrubbing that may break the skin surface should be avoided. If hair cannot be decontaminated with soap and water, clipping it off with scissors is preferable to shaving. Shaving may cut the skin and allow contamination to enter the body. Skin and wound decontamination should continue until the Geiger-Muller counter shows that the radioactivity is gone or almost gone, until washing does not substantially reduce the amount of radioactivity measured, or until further cleaning risks damaging the skin. Burns should be gently rinsed but not scrubbed.

Certain measures can decrease internal contamination. If people have recently swallowed a significant amount of radioactive material, vomiting may be induced. Some radioactive materials have specific chemical treatments that can reduce their absorption after being swallowed or help speed their removal from the body. If administered shortly before or soon after internal contamination with radioactive iodine, potassium iodide very effectively prevents the thyroid gland from absorbing the radioactive iodine, thus reducing the risk of thyroid cancer and thyroid injury. Potassium iodide is effective only for radioactive iodine, not other radioactive elements. Other drugs, such as zinc or calcium diethylenetriamine penta-acetate (DTPA—for plutonium, yttrium, californium, and americium), calcium or aluminum phosphate solutions (for radioactive strontium), and Prussian blue (for radioactive cesium, rubidium and thallium), can be given intravenously to remove a fraction of certain radionuclides after they have entered the body. However, except for potassium iodide, which is very effective, drugs given to reduce internal contamination reduce exposure by only about 25 to 75%.

Nausea and vomiting can be reduced by taking drugs to prevent vomiting (antiemetics). Such drugs are routinely given to people undergoing radiation therapy or chemotherapy. Dehydration is treated with fluids given intravenously.

People with the gastrointestinal or hematopoietic syndrome are kept isolated to minimize their contact with infectious microorganisms. Blood transfusions and injections of growth factors that stimulate blood cell production (such as erythropoietin and colony-stimulating factor) are given to increase blood counts. This treatment helps decrease bleeding and anemia and helps fight infections. If the bone marrow is severely damaged, these growth factors are ineffective, and sometimes bone marrow transplantation is done, although the experience with this treatment for this condition is limited and the success rate is low.

People with the gastrointestinal syndrome require antiemetics, fluids given intravenously, and sedatives. Some people may be able to eat a bland diet. Antibiotics are given by mouth to kill bacteria in the intestine that may invade the body. Antibiotics as well as antifungal and antiviral drugs also are given intravenously when necessary.

Treatment for the cerebrovascular syndrome is geared toward providing comfort by relieving pain, anxiety, and breathing difficulties. Drugs are given to control seizures.

Pain caused by radiation-induced sores or ulcers is treated with analgesics. If these wounds fail to heal satisfactorily over time they may be repaired surgically with skin grafts or other procedures.

CHAPTER

306 Electrical and Lightning Injuries

Injuries can result from spontaneous atmospheric electricity (lightning injuries) or generated electricity, such as household or industrial electrical currents (electrical injuries). Electrical current passing through the body generates heat, which burns and destroys tissues. Burns can affect internal tissues as well as the skin. An electrical shock can short-circuit the body's own electrical systems, causing nerves to stop transmitting impulses or to transmit impulses erratically. Abnormal impulse transmission can affect the

- Muscles, causing them to contract violently
- Heart, causing it to stop beating (cardiac arrest)
- Brain, causing seizures, loss of consciousness, or other abnormalities

Electrical Injuries

An electrical injury occurs when a current passes through the body, interfering with the function of an internal organ or sometimes burning tissue.

- Often the main symptom is a skin burn, but not all people have visible injuries.
- Doctors check the person for abnormal heart rhythms, fractures, dislocations, and spinal cord or other injuries.
- Abnormal heart rhythms are monitored, burns are treated, and, if the burn caused extensive internal damage, intravenous fluids are given.

Electrical injury may result from contact with faulty electrical appliances or machinery or inadvertent contact with household wiring or electrical power lines. Getting shocked from touching an electrical outlet in the home or by a small appliance is rarely serious, but accidental exposure to high voltage causes about 400 deaths each year in the United States. The severity of the injury ranges from minor to fatal and is determined by the following factors:

- Intensity of the current
- Type of current
- Pathway of the current through the body

- Duration of exposure to the current
- Electrical resistance to the current

Intensity of the Current: The intensity of the current is measured in volts and amperes. Ordinary household current in the United States is 110 to 220 volts. Anything over 500 volts is considered high voltage. High voltage can jump (arc) through the air anywhere from an inch up to several feet, depending on the voltage. Thus, a person may be injured simply by coming too close to a high-voltage line. High voltage causes more severe injuries than low voltage and is more likely to cause internal damage.

Type of Current: Electrical current is categorized as direct current (DC) or alternating current (AC). Direct current, such as current generated by batteries, flows in the same direction constantly. Alternating current, such as current available through household wall sockets, changes direction 50 to 60 times per second. Alternating current, which is used in most households in the United States and Europe, is more dangerous than direct current. Direct current tends to cause a single muscle contraction often strong enough to force people away from the current's source. Alternating current causes a continuing muscle contraction, often preventing people from releasing their grip on the current's source. As a result, exposure may be prolonged. Even a small amount of alternating current—barely enough to be felt as a mild shock—may cause the grip to freeze. Slightly more alternating current can cause the chest muscles to contract, making breathing impossible. Even more current can cause deadly abnormal heart rhythms (arrhythmias).

Pathway of the Current: The path that the electricity takes through the body tends to determine which tissues are affected. Because alternating current continually reverses direction, the commonly used terms "entry" and "exit" are inappropriate. The terms "source" and "ground" are more precise. The most common source point for electricity is the hand, and the second most common is the head. The most common ground point is the foot. A current that travels from arm to arm or from arm to leg may go through the heart and is much more dangerous than a current that travels between a leg and the ground. A current that travels through the head may affect the brain.

Duration of Exposure: In general, the longer the person is exposed to the current, the worse the injury.

Resistance to the Current: Resistance is the ability to impede the flow of electricity. Most of the body's resistance is concentrated in the skin. The thicker the skin is, the greater its resistance. A thick, callused palm or sole, for example, is much more resistant to electrical current than an area of thin skin, such as an inner arm. The skin's resistance decreases when broken (for example, punctured or scraped) or when wet. If skin resistance is high, more of the damage is local, often causing only skin burns. If skin resistance is low, more of the damage affects the internal organs. Thus, the damage is mostly internal if people who are wet come in contact with electrical current, for example, when a hair dryer falls into a bathtub or people step in a puddle that is in contact with a downed electrical line.

Symptoms

Often, the main symptom of an electrical injury is a skin burn (see page 1948), although not all electrical injuries cause external damage. High-voltage injuries may cause massive internal burns. If muscle damage is extensive, a limb may swell so much that its arteries become compressed (compartment syndrome—see page 1953), cutting off blood supply to the limb. If a current travels close to the eyes, it may lead to cataracts. Cataracts can develop within days of the injury or years later. If large amounts of muscle are damaged (a disorder called rhabdomyolysis), a chemical substance, myoglobin, is released into the blood. The myoglobin can damage the kidneys.

Young children who bite or suck on extension cords can burn their mouth and lips. These burns may cause facial deformities and growth problems of the teeth, jaw, and face. An added danger is that severe bleeding from an artery in the lip may occur when the scab falls off, usually 7 to 10 days after the injury.

A minor shock may cause muscle pain and may trigger mild muscle contractions or startle people, causing a fall. Severe shocks can cause abnormal heart rhythms, ranging from inconsequential to immediately fatal. Severe shocks can also trigger powerful muscle contractions sufficient to throw people to the ground or to cause joint dislocations, bone fractures, and other blunt injuries.

The nerves and brain can be injured in various ways, causing seizures, bleeding (hemorrhage) in the brain, poor short-term memory, personality changes, irritability, or difficulty sleeping. Damage to the nerves in the body or spinal cord may cause weakness, paralysis, numbness, tingling, chronic pain, and erectile dysfunction (impotence).

Diagnosis

Doctors check people for burns, fractures, dislocations, and spinal cord or other injuries.

Most people who have no symptoms do not require testing or monitoring. An electrocardiogram (ECG) is done to monitor the heartbeat in some people. For some people, blood and urine tests may be needed. If people are unconscious, imaging tests such as computed tomography (CT) or magnetic resonance imaging (MRI) may be needed.

Prevention

Education about and respect for electricity are essential. Making sure that all electrical devices are properly designed, installed, and maintained helps prevent electrical injuries at home and work. Electrical wiring should be installed and serviced by properly trained people. Outlet guards reduce risk in homes with infants or young children.

Any electrical device that touches or may be touched by the body should be properly grounded. Three-pronged outlets are safest. Cutting off the lower (ground) prong of a power cord with three prongs (so that it will fit older two-pronged plugs) is dangerous and increases the chances of electrical injury. Circuit breakers that interrupt (trip) circuits when current as low as 5 milliamperes leaks are advisable in areas that get wet, such as kitchens and bathrooms and outdoors.

To avoid injury from current that jumps (arcing injury), poles and ladders should not be used near high-voltage power lines.

Treatment

First the person must be separated from the current's source. The safest way to do so is to shut off the current—for example, by throwing a circuit breaker or switch or by disconnecting the device from an electrical outlet. *No one should touch the person until the current has been shut off, particularly if high-voltage lines could be involved.*

High-voltage and low-voltage lines are difficult to distinguish, especially outdoors. Shutting off current to high-voltage lines is done by the local power company. Many well-meaning rescuers have been injured by electricity when trying to free a person.

Once the person can be safely touched, the rescuer should check to see if the person is breathing and has a pulse. If the person is not breathing and has no pulse, cardiopulmonary resuscitation (CPR) should be started immediately (see page 1942). Emergency medical assistance should be called for any person who has more than a minor injury. Because the extent of an electrical burn may be deceptive, medical assistance should be sought if any doubt exists regarding severity.

People with rhabdomyolysis may receive large amounts of fluids given intravenously. A tetanus shot is given if needed.

Skin burns are treated with burn cream (such as silver sulfadiazine, bacitracin, or sterile aloe vera) and sterile dressings. A person with only minor skin burns can usually be treated at home. If the injury is more severe, the person is admitted to the hospital, ideally a burn center. The person is kept in the hospital for 6 to 24 hours if any of the following exists:

- The results of an ECG are abnormal
- The person has lost consciousness
- The person has symptoms of a heart problem (for example, chest pain, shortness of breath, awareness of heartbeats [palpitations])
- The person has other severe injuries
- The person is pregnant (in many, but not necessarily all, cases)
- The person has a known heart problem (in many, but not necessarily all, cases)

Young children who bite or suck on extension cords should be referred to a children's orthodontist, an oral surgeon, or a surgeon who is experienced in the care of these injuries.

Lightning Injuries

A lightning injury occurs after brief exposure to the very intense current of the strike.

- About 10% of people who are struck by lightning die because the heart stops beating and breathing stops.
- In some people who survive severe lightning injury, an electrocardiogram is done to monitor the heartbeat, and blood or imaging tests are needed.
- Once the person is resuscitated, burns and other injuries are treated.

Lightning delivers a massive electrical pulse over a fraction of a millisecond. The brief duration of the exposure frequently limits the damage to the outer layer of skin. In addition, lightning is much less likely to cause internal burns than generated electricity. However, it can kill a person by instantaneously short-circuiting the heart or brain. Lightning is the second most frequent cause of storm-related deaths in the United States, resulting in about 30 to 50 deaths each year and nearly 10 times that many injuries, some of which result in permanent disability.

Lightning tends to strike tall or isolated objects, including trees, towers, shelters, flagpoles, bleachers, and fences. A person may be the tallest object in an open field. Metal objects and water do not attract lightning but easily transmit electricity once they are hit. Electricity from lightning can travel from outdoor power or telephone lines to electrical equipment or telephone lines inside a house.

Lightning can injure a person in several ways. Lightning can strike a person directly. In addition, electricity can reach a person who is touching or near an object that has been struck. Current can also reach a person through the ground. The shock can also throw a person, producing blunt injuries.

Symptoms

After a person has been struck by lightning, the heart may stop beating (cardiac arrest) or may beat erratically, and breathing often stops. The heart may beat again on its own, but if breathing has not restarted, the body is deprived of oxygen. The lack of oxygen and, possibly, neurologic damage can cause the heart to stop beating again.

Brain injury usually causes loss of consciousness. If brain damage is severe, coma may develop. Typically, the person awakens but does not remember what happened before the injury (amnesia). The person may be confused, think slowly, and have difficulty concentrating and remembering recent events. Personality changes may occur.

The eardrums are often perforated. Many eye injuries can develop, including cataracts. Often both legs become temporarily paralyzed, blue, and numb (keraunoparalysis). The skin may show no marks at all or may have minor burns that have a feathering, branching pattern, consist of clusters of tiny pinpoint spots like a cigarette burn, or consist of streaks where sweat has been turned into steam. Numbness, tingling, and weakness may develop because the nerves branching out from the spinal cord have been damaged (peripheral neuropathy).

Diagnosis

Lightning injuries are often witnessed, but they may also be suspected when a person is found unconscious or with amnesia outside during or shortly after a thunderstorm.

In the hospital, electrocardiography (ECG) may be done if injury is severe (for example, if a person collapsed and may have had a temporary cardiac arrest). The ECG, when done, determines whether the heart is beating normally. Sometimes blood tests or imaging tests, such as computed tomography (CT) or magnetic resonance imaging (MRI), are needed.

Prevention

During the thunderstorm season, listening to weather reports, which is particularly important for organizers of outdoor events, can help in deciding whether to cancel outdoor activities and in planning for any emergencies that may develop.

High winds, rain, and clouds may mean that a thunderstorm is imminent. By the time thunder is heard, the observers are already in danger and should be seeking safe shelter, such as a large habitable building or a fully enclosed metal vehicle (for example, a car, van, or truck) with the windows closed. Sheltering in a small open structure, such as a gazebo, is not safe. It is not safe to resume outdoor activities until 30 minutes after the last sound of thunder is heard or lightning is seen.

To prevent lightning injuries when indoors, people should avoid contact with plumbing or electrical wiring, talking on a hard-wired telephone, working on a computer, using a video game console, or using headsets attached by a cable to a sound system. Being away from windows and doors increases safety, as does turning off and unplugging electrical equipment before the thunderstorm arrives. Cellular telephones, personal digital assistants (PDAs), and MP3 players are safe because they do not attract lightning.

Prognosis

About 10% of people with lightning injuries die. The only cause of death is cardiac arrest and cessation of breathing at the time of the injury. People whose heartbeat and breathing resume survive. If memory of recent events is impaired or thinking is slow, the person may have permanent brain injury. Keraunoparalysis usually resolves within several hours, although the person may occasionally be left with weakness or clumsiness. People with nerve injury often have long-term problems, including chronic pain, sleep difficulties, and erectile dysfunction (impotence).

Treatment

A person struck by lightning does not retain electricity, so there is no danger in providing first aid. People without a heartbeat and who are not breathing need cardiopulmonary resuscitation (CPR) immediately (see page 1942). If an automated external defibrillator (AED) is available, it should be used. Emergency medical assistance should be called. Many people struck by lightning are in good general health and are more likely to recover if given timely CPR.

Burns and other injuries are treated as needed. If resuscitation efforts are not successful within the first 20 minutes, they are unlikely to be, so resuscitation efforts are then stopped.

CHAPTER

307   Drowning

Drowning occurs when submersion in liquid causes suffocation or interferes with breathing.

- During drowning, the body is deprived of oxygen, which can damage organs, particularly the lungs and brain.
- Doctors evaluate people for oxygen deprivation and problems that often accompany drowning (such as spinal injuries caused by diving).
- Treatment focuses on correcting oxygen deprivation and other problems.

Drowning may be nonfatal (previously described as near drowning) or fatal. Drowning is a leading cause of accidental death in the United States and the second leading cause in children ages 1 to 14 years. About four times as many people are hospitalized for nonfatal drowning as die from drowning. Drowning rates are higher for all of the following:

- Children 4 years or younger
- African American children and children from immigrant or impoverished families
- Males
- People who are intoxicated with alcohol or who use sedative drugs
- People who have conditions that cause temporary incapacitation, such as seizures, low blood sugar (hypoglycemia), stroke, heart attacks, and certain kinds of irregular heartbeat (arrhythmias)

Drowning is common in pools, hot tubs, and natural water settings. Children and toddlers are also at risk from even small amounts of water, such as in toilets, bathtubs, and buckets of water or other fluids, because they may be unable to escape after falling in.

Diving, particularly into shallow water, may cause spinal injuries and paralysis that increase the chances of drowning. People who intentionally hold their breath under water for extended periods may pass out and sometimes drown.

People swimming near an exhaust vent of a boat may develop carbon monoxide poisoning, which may cause unconsciousness and drowning.

Oxygen Deprivation: When people are submerged under water, water enters the lungs. The vocal cords may go into severe spasm, temporarily preventing water from reaching the lungs but also preventing breathing. In either case, the lungs cannot transfer oxygen to the blood. The decrease in the level of oxygen in the blood that results may lead to brain damage and death. Water in the lungs, particularly water that is contaminated by bacteria, algae, sand, dirt, chemicals, or vomit, can cause lung injury. Lung injury tends to cause continuing oxygen deprivation. Fresh water in the lungs is absorbed into the bloodstream. Absorbing large amounts of fresh water sometimes causes electrolyte abnormalities, such as a low sodium level in the blood.

Effects of Cold: Submersion in cold water has both good and bad effects. Cooling of the muscles makes swimming difficult, and dangerously low body temperature (hypothermia) can impair judgment. Cold, however, protects tissues from the ill effects of oxygen deprivation. In addition, cold water may stimulate the mammalian diving reflex, which may prolong survival in cold water. The diving reflex slows the heartbeat and redirects the flow of blood from the hands, feet, and intestines to the heart and brain, thus helping to preserve these vital organs. The diving reflex is more pronounced in children than in adults, so children have a greater chance of surviving prolonged submersion in cold water than do adults.

> **? Did You Know...**
> Children are more likely than adults to survive after prolonged submersion.

Symptoms

People who are drowning and struggling to breathe are usually unable to call for help. Children who are unable to swim may submerge in less than 1 minute. Adults may struggle longer.

People who are rescued may have a wide range of symptoms and findings. Some are only mildly anxious, whereas others are near death. They may be alert, drowsy, or comatose. Some people may not be breathing. People who are breathing may gasp for breath or vomit, cough, or wheeze. The skin may appear blue (cyanosis), indicating insufficient oxygen in the blood. In some cases, respiratory problems may not become evident for several hours after submersion.

Complications: Some people who are revived after prolonged submersion have permanent brain damage because of the lack of oxygen. People who inhale foreign particles may develop pneumonia or acute respiratory distress syndrome, causing prolonged difficulty breathing. People who drown in cold water often have hypothermia.

Diagnosis

Doctors diagnose drowning based on the events and the symptoms. Measurement of the level of oxygen in the blood and chest x-rays help reveal the extent of lung damage. Other tests, such as x-rays and computed tomography (CT) scans, may be done to diagnose head or spinal injuries. An electrocardiogram (ECG) and sometimes blood tests may be done to diganose disorders that may have contributed to drowning. For example, certain previously unrecognized heart arrhythmias can cause unconsciousness while swimming.

Prevention

Children: Swimming pools should be adequately fenced, because they are one of the most common sites of drowning accidents. In addition, all doors and gates leading to the pool area should be locked. Children in or near any body of water, including pools and bathtubs, need constant supervision, regardless of whether flotation devices are used. Because infants and young children can drown in only a few inches of water, even water-filled containers, such as buckets or ice chests are hazardous. Small children should wear life jackets when playing near bodies of water.

Swimming: People should not engage in swimming or boating when under the influence of alcohol or sedatives. Swimming should be curtailed if people feel or look very cold. People who have seizures that are well controlled need not avoid swimming, but they should be careful near water, whether boating, showering, or bathing.

To decrease the risk of drowning, people should not swim alone and should swim only in areas patrolled by lifeguards. Ocean swimmers should learn to escape rip currents (strong currents that pull away from the shore) by swimming parallel to the beach rather than by swimming toward the beach. Also, swimming near boat exhaust ports should be avoided.

> **? Did You Know...**
>
> People do not need to wait an hour after eating to return to swimming.

Other Measures: Wearing life jackets when in boats is encouraged for everyone and is required for nonswimmers and for small children. Spinal injuries can be prevented by not diving into shallow water.

Community swimming areas need to be supervised by trained lifeguards. Comprehensive community prevention programs should

- Target high-risk groups
- Teach as many adolescents and adults cardiopulmonary resuscitation (CPR) as possible
- Teach children to swim as soon as they are developmentally ready (around age 4 years)

However, even young children who have taken swimming lessons should be watched closely around water. Programs that teach infants and young children to swim have not been proven to decrease the risk of drowning.

Prognosis

The factors that most increase the chances of survival without permanent brain and lung damage are the following:

- Brief duration of submersion
- Cold water temperature
- Young age
- Rapid beginning of resuscitation (most important)

Survival is possible after submersion for as long as 40 minutes. Many people who need CPR can also recover fully, and almost all people who are alert and conscious upon their arrival at the hospital recover fully. People who have consumed alcoholic beverages before submersion are more likely to die or develop brain or lung damage.

Treatment

Out of the Hospital: Immediate on-site resuscitation is the key to increasing the chance of survival without brain damage. Attempts should be made to revive people even when the time under water is prolonged. Artificial respiration and CPR should be provided as necessary (see page 1942). The neck should be moved as little as possible if there is a chance of spinal injury. People who were submerged involuntarily or have any symptoms must be transported to a hospital, by ambulance if possible. People who were submerged but have only mild symptoms may be discharged to their home after several hours of observation in the emergency department. If symptoms persist for a few hours, or if the level of oxygen in the blood is low, people need to be admitted to the hospital.

In the Hospital: Most people need supplemental oxygen, sometimes in high concentrations or given via a ventilator at high pressures. If wheezing develops, bronchodilators can help. If an infection develops, antibiotics are given.

If the water was cold, people may have a dangerously low body temperature (hypothermia) and may need warming (see page 1982). Spinal injury requires special treatment (see page 798).

308 Diving and Compressed Air Injuries

People who engage in deep-sea or scuba diving are at risk of a number of injuries. Diving in cold water can rapidly lead to hypothermia (dangerously low body temperature), which causes clumsiness and poor judgment. Cold water can also rarely trigger fatal heartbeat irregularities in people with coronary artery disease. Other potential diving hazards include

- Drowning
- Bites and stings from various marine life
- Sunburn and heat disorders
- Cuts and bruises
- Motion sickness

Drugs (prescribed, recreational, and some over-the-counter) and alcohol may have unanticipated, dangerous effects at depth.

Most diving-related disorders, however, are caused by changes in pressure. These disorders also can affect people who work in underwater tunnels or caissons (watertight enclosures used for construction work). Such structures contain air under high pressure to keep out water.

High pressure under water is caused by the weight of the water above, just as barometric (atmospheric) pressure on land is caused by the weight of the air above. In diving, underwater pressure is often expressed in units of depth (feet or meters) or atmospheres absolute. Pressure in atmospheres absolute includes the weight of the water, which at about 33 feet (10 meters) is 1 atmosphere (14.7 pounds per square inch [72 kilograms per square meter]), plus the atmospheric pressure at the surface, which is 1 atmosphere. So a diver at a depth of 33 feet is exposed to a total pressure of 2 atmospheres absolute, or twice the atmospheric pressure at the surface. With each additional 33 feet of depth, the pressure increases by 1 atmosphere.

Diving disorders can be divided into various categories: Some result from expansion or compression of gas-filled spaces in the body (barotrauma), and others result from release of dissolved nitrogen in the blood and tissues (decompression sickness). Either process can cause bubbles in arteries to block blood flow to organs (arterial gas embolism). Gases such as oxygen and nitrogen can also cause disorders when breathed at high pressures, such as when people dive to very deep depths.

Diving disorders can result in drowning if they cause any of the following:

- Impaired thinking or drowsiness
- Unconsciousness
- Panic
- Loss of balance and disorientation

Barotrauma

Barotrauma is tissue injury caused by a change in pressure, which compresses or expands gas contained in various body structures.

- The lungs, mask (face mask), ears, or sinuses can be affected.
- Symptoms vary and may include breathing problems or chest pain (lung barotrauma), bloodshot eyes (mask barotrauma), vertigo or ear pain (ear barotrauma), and facial pain or a bloody nose (sinus barotrauma).
- Measures that can help prevent barotrauma include breathing during ascent (lung barotrauma), blowing out air from the nose into the mask and yawning or swallowing with the nostrils pinched (mask barotrauma), and taking a nasal decongestant (sinus and ear barotrauma).

Increased pressure outside the body is transmitted equally throughout the blood and body tissues, which do not compress because they are composed mainly of liquid. Thus, the leg, for example, does not feel squeezed as water pressure increases. However, gases (such as the air inside the lungs, sinuses, or middle ear or inside a face mask or goggles) compress or expand as outside pressure increases or decreases. This compression and expansion can cause pain and damage to tissue. Barotrauma most often affects the ears. However, barotrauma affecting the lungs (pulmonary barotrauma) is the most serious.

Pulmonary (Lung) Barotrauma: Because air under high pressure is compressed, each breath taken at depth contains many more molecules than a breath taken at the surface. At 33 feet (2 atmospheres absolute), for example, each breath contains twice as many molecules as a breath taken at the surface (and therefore depletes an air tank twice as rapidly). As pressure decreases, air expands—its volume increases. So, when divers fill their lungs with compressed air at 33 feet and ascend without freely exhaling, the volume of air doubles, causing the lungs to overinflate. Overinflation of the lungs can rupture small air sacs, allowing air to leak out. Air that leaks out of the lungs can be trapped in the space between the lungs and the chest wall and expand, causing the lungs to collapse (pneumothorax—

see page 520). Alternatively, air may be forced out of the lungs into the tissues surrounding the heart (pneumomediastinum), under the skin of the neck and upper chest (subcutaneous emphysema), or into the blood vessels. Air in the blood vessels typically travels to other parts of the body (air embolism—see page 1998), where it may block blood flow.

The most common cause of pulmonary barotrauma is breath-holding during an ascent from a scuba dive, typically resulting from running out of air at depth. In panic, divers may forget to exhale freely as air in the lungs expands during the ascent. Air embolism can occur in as little as 4 feet (about 1 meter) of water when people breathing pressurized air hold their breath while ascending rapidly. Pulmonary barotrauma can even happen in a pool when air is breathed in at the bottom of the pool (such as from an inverted bucket) and not exhaled during ascent.

Symptoms

Symptoms of barotrauma usually begin before or within minutes after divers reach the surface. Symptoms depend on which organ is affected. Divers often use the term "squeeze" for injuries other than those to the lungs caused by differences in pressure.

Pulmonary Barotrauma: Pneumothorax and pneumomediastinum cause chest pain and shortness of breath. Some people cough up blood or develop bloody froth at the mouth when lung tissue is injured. Air in the tissues of the neck can impair the vocal cords, causing the voice to sound different or hoarse. Subcutaneous emphysema causes crackling when the affected area of skin is touched.

Mask Barotrauma (Mask Squeeze): When divers do not properly equalize pressure in the face mask with the water pressure, the relatively lower pressure inside the mask causes it to act like a suction cup applied to the eyes and face. The difference in pressure inside and outside the mask causes blood vessels near the surface of the eyes (or on the face) to dilate, leak fluid, and finally burst and bleed. Although the eyes appear red and bloodshot, vision is not affected. Rarely, bleeding behind the eyes can occur, causing loss of vision. Bleeding of blood vessels in the face causes usually a bruised appearance.

Ear Barotrauma (Ear Squeeze): If pressure in the middle ear becomes lower than the water pressure, the resulting stress causes a painful inward bulge of the eardrum (see art on page 1389). When the pressure difference becomes high enough, the eardrum ruptures, resulting in a rush of cold water into the middle ear, causing vertigo (severe dizziness with a spinning sensation), disorientation, nausea, and sometimes vomiting. These symptoms may place divers at risk of drowning. The vertigo diminishes as the water in the ear reaches body temperature. A ruptured eardrum impairs hearing and may lead to a middle ear infection hours or days later, causing pain and producing discharge from the ear. The inner ear can be injured as well, causing a sudden loss of hearing, buzzing in the ear (tinnitus), and vertigo.

Sinus Barotrauma (Sinus Squeeze): Pressure differences have effects on the sinuses (air-filled pockets in the bones around the nose) that are similar to the effects of ear barotrauma. They cause facial pain, headaches, a feeling of congestion in the face or nose, or a bloody nose.

Dental Barotrauma (Tooth Squeeze): Pressure in the air spaces at the roots of teeth or next to fillings can cause toothache or damage teeth.

Eye Barotrauma (Eye Squeeze): Small air bubbles can form and become trapped behind hard contact lenses. The bubbles can damage the eyes and cause soreness, loss of vision, and the appearance of halos around lights.

Gastrointestinal Tract Barotrauma (Gut Squeeze): Breathing improperly from a regulator or using ear and sinus pressure-equalization techniques may cause divers to swallow small amounts of air during a dive. This air expands during ascent, causing abdominal fullness, cramps, pain, belching, and flatulence. These symptoms usually resolve on their own. Rarely, the stomach or intestine bursts, causing severe abdominal pain and severe illness.

Diagnosis

Doctors recognize barotrauma mainly by the nature of the symptoms and their onset in relation to diving. Depending on the symptoms, imaging tests may be done. For example, people with pulmonary barotrauma usually require chest x-rays.

Prevention

Pressure in the lungs and airways is automatically equalized with outside pressure when a supply of pressurized air is available at depth, as from a diving helmet or air tank. This pressurized air also equalizes pressure in the sinuses, as long as the openings to the sinuses are not narrowed, for example, by inflammation due to allergies or an upper respiratory tract infection.

Pressure in a face mask is equalized by blowing out air from the nose into the mask. Divers equalize pressure differences in the middle ear by yawning or swallowing with the nostrils pinched, which opens the tube connecting the middle ear and the back of the throat (eustachian tube).

Wearing earplugs or a tight-fitting wet suit hood creates a closed space between the earplug and the eardrum in which pressure cannot be equalized. The pressure inside goggles cannot be equalized either.

Therefore, neither earplugs nor goggles should be worn during diving. Tight-fitting wet suit hoods should be properly vented so that they do not block the external ear.

A decongestant (such as pseudoephedrine taken by mouth) is taken before diving by people with nasal congestion that could block nasal passages. Relief of congestion can facilitate equalization of pressures between the ears and sinuses, helping prevent sinus and ear barotrauma.

To prevent pulmonary barotrauma, people must freely exhale any air inhaled at depth—even the depth of a swimming pool—during ascent.

Treatment

Some people with pneumothorax require treatments such as inserting a plastic tube into the chest cavity to allow air to drain and the lung to re-expand. Treatment of pneumomediastinum and subcutaneous emphysema usually is bed rest and supplemental oxygen.

Ear and sinus barotrauma are treated with nasal decongestants (such as oxymetazoline nasal spray) or oral decongestants. Occasionally, when recovery is slow, corticosteroids may be given as a nasal spray or pills. A ruptured eardrum usually heals by itself, although a middle ear infection requires antibiotics given by mouth or as eardrops. A rupture between the middle and inner ear may require prompt surgical repair to prevent permanent damage. A rupture of the stomach or intestines requires surgical repair.

Air Embolism

Air embolism is blockage of blood supply to organs caused by bubbles in an artery.

- Within a few minutes of reaching the surface, divers can develop symptoms similar to those of a stroke.
- People are given oxygen, made recumbent, and sent as soon as possible to a recompression chamber.

Air bubbles can enter the blood after pulmonary barotrauma (see page 1997) or decompression sickness (see below) and travel to any organ in the body and block small blood vessels, most commonly those of the brain, but also of the heart, skin, and kidneys. A very large air embolism can block flow through the heart chambers or the large arteries.

Symptoms

Air embolism is a leading cause of death among divers. Symptoms of air embolism usually appear within a few minutes of reaching the surface. Air embolism to the brain often resembles a stroke, resulting in confusion and partial paralysis or loss of sensation. Some people have sudden loss of consciousness or seizures. Severe air embolism can lead to shock (see page 350) and death.

Diagnosis

Divers who lose consciousness during ascent or very shortly afterward are assumed to have air embolism. They must be treated promptly. Imaging tests are sometimes done but are not always reliable.

Treatment

People are immediately put in a recumbent position and given oxygen. They must be returned at once to a high-pressure environment, so that the air bubbles are compressed and forced to dissolve in the blood. Many medical centers have high-pressure (recompression or hyperbaric) chambers for this purpose.

Flying, even at a low altitude, reduces atmospheric pressure and allows bubbles to expand further, but it can be justified if it saves substantial time in getting people to a suitable chamber. If possible, people should fly in a plane pressurized to sea level, or the plane should not fly above 2,000 feet (610 meters).

Decompression Sickness

Decompression sickness (decompression illness, caisson disease, the bends) is a disorder in which nitrogen dissolved in the blood and tissues by high pressure forms bubbles as pressure decreases.

- Symptoms can include fatigue and pain in muscles and joints.
- In the more severe type, symptoms may be similar to those of stroke or can include difficulty breathing and chest pain.
- People are treated with oxygen and recompression (high-pressure or hyperbaric oxygen) therapy.
- Limiting the depth and duration of dives and the speed of ascent can help with prevention.

Air is composed mainly of nitrogen and oxygen. Because air under high pressure is compressed, each breath taken at depth contains many more molecules than a breath taken at the surface. Because oxygen is used continuously by the body, the extra oxygen molecules breathed under high pressure usually do not accumulate. However, the extra nitrogen molecules do accumulate in the blood and tissues. As outside pressure decreases during ascent from a dive or when leaving a caisson, the accumulated nitrogen that cannot be exhaled immediately forms bubbles in the blood and tissues. These bubbles may expand and injure tissue, or they may block blood vessels in many organs—either directly or by triggering small blood clots. This blood vessel blockage causes pain and various other symptoms (for example, sometimes similar to those of a stroke, such as sudden weakness on one side of the body, difficulty speaking, dizziness, or even flu-like symptoms). Nitrogen bubbles also cause inflammation, producing swelling and pain in muscles, joints, and tendons.

The risk of developing decompression sickness increases with many factors, such as the following:

- Certain heart defects
- Cold water
- Dehydration
- Flying after diving
- Exertion
- Fatigue
- Increasing pressure (that is, the depth of the dive)
- Length of time spent in a pressurized environment
- Obesity
- Older age
- Rapid ascent

Because excess nitrogen remains dissolved in the body tissues for at least 12 hours after each dive, repeated dives within 1 day are more likely to cause decompression sickness than a single dive. Flying immediately after diving (such as at the end of a vacation) exposes people to an even lower atmospheric pressure, making decompression sickness slightly more likely.

Nitrogen bubbles may form in small blood vessels or in the tissues themselves. Tissues with a high fat content, such as those in the brain and spinal cord, are particularly likely to be affected, because nitrogen dissolves very readily in fats.

Decompression sickness may affect a variety of organs and can range from mild to severe.

Symptoms

Symptoms of decompression sickness usually develop more slowly than do those of air embolism and pulmonary barotrauma. Only half of the people with decompression sickness have symptoms within 1 hour of surfacing, but 90% have symptoms by 6 hours. Symptoms commonly begin gradually and take some time to reach their maximum effect. The first symptoms may be fatigue, loss of appetite, headache, and a vague feeling of illness.

Type I (Less Severe): The less severe type (or musculoskeletal form) of decompression sickness, often called the bends, typically produces pain. The pain usually occurs in the joints of the arms or legs, back, or muscles. Sometimes the location is hard to pinpoint. The pain may be mild or intermittent at first but may steadily grow stronger and become severe. The pain may be sharp or may be described as "deep" or "like something boring into bone." It

is worse when moving. Less common symptoms include itching, skin mottling, swollen lymph nodes, rash, and extreme fatigue. These symptoms do not threaten life but may precede more dangerous problems.

Type II (More Severe): The more severe type of decompression sickness most commonly results in neurologic symptoms, which range from mild numbness to paralysis and death. The spinal cord is especially vulnerable. When the spinal cord is affected, symptoms can include numbness, tingling, weakness, or a combination in the arms, legs, or both. Mild weakness or tingling may progress over hours to irreversible paralysis. Inability to urinate or inability to control urination or defecation may also occur. Abdominal and back pain also is common. Symptoms of brain involvement, most of which are similar to those of air embolism, include headache, confusion, trouble speaking, and double vision. Loss of consciousness is rare.

The nerves of the inner ear may be affected, causing severe vertigo, ringing in the ears, and hearing loss. Gas bubbles that travel through the veins to the lungs produce cough, chest pain, and progressively worsening difficulty breathing (the chokes). Severe cases, which are rare, may result in shock and death.

Late Effects: Late effects of decompression sickness include the destruction of bone tissue (dysbaric osteonecrosis, avascular bone necrosis), especially in the shoulder and hip, which produces persistent pain and severe disability. These injuries do not occur among recreational divers but, rather, among people who work in a compressed-air environment and divers who work in underwater habitats. These workers are exposed to high pressure for prolonged periods and may have an undetected case of the bends. Technical divers, who dive to greater depths than recreational divers, may be at higher risk than recreational divers. Bone and joint injuries may gradually progress over months or years to severe, disabling arthritis. By the time severe joint damage has occurred, the only treatment may be joint replacement.

Permanent neurologic problems, such as partial paralysis, usually result from delayed or inadequate treatment of spinal cord symptoms. However, sometimes the damage is too severe to correct, even with appropriate treatment. Repeated treatments with oxygen in a high-pressure chamber seem to help some people recover from spinal cord damage.

Diagnosis

Doctors recognize decompression sickness by the nature of the symptoms and their onset in relation to diving. Tests such as computed tomography (CT) or magnetic resonance imaging (MRI) sometimes show brain or spinal cord abnormalities but are not reliable. However, recompression therapy is begun before the results of a CT or MRI scan are available, except in cases in which the diagnosis is uncertain or the diver's condition is stable. X-rays are needed to diagnose dysbaric osteonecrosis.

? Did You Know...

Flying within 15 hours after diving (common when vacationing) increases the risk of decompression sickness.

Prevention

Divers can usually prevent decompression sickness by restricting the total amount of gas the body absorbs. The amount can be restricted by limiting the depth and duration of dives to a range that does not need decompression stops during ascent (called no-stop limits by divers) or by ascending with decompression stops as specified in authoritative guidelines, such as the decompression table in the *United States Navy Diving Manual*. The table provides a schedule for ascent that usually allows excess nitrogen to escape without causing harm. Many divers wear a portable dive computer that continually tracks the diver's depth and time at depth. The computer calculates the decompression schedule for a safe return to the surface and indicates when decompression stops are needed.

In addition to following a table or computer guidelines for ascent, many divers make a safety stop of a few minutes at about 15 feet (4.5 meters) below the surface.

Following these procedures, however, does not eliminate the risk of decompression sickness. A small number of cases of decompression sickness develop after no-stop dives, and the incidence of decompression sickness has not declined despite the widespread use of dive computers. The inability to eliminate decompression sickness may be because the published tables and computer programs do not completely account for the variation in risk factors among different divers or because some people fail to obey the recommendations of the tables or computer.

Other precautions also are necessary:

- After several days of diving, a period of 12 to 24 hours at the surface is commonly recommended before flying or going to a higher altitude.
- People who have completely recovered from mild decompression sickness should refrain from diving for at least 2 weeks.

- People who have developed decompression sickness despite following dive table or computer recommendations should return to diving only after a thorough medical evaluation for underlying risk factors, such as a heart defect.

The Divers Alert Network (919-684-8111; www.diversalertnetwork.org) provides 24-hour consultation for diving-related problems.

Treatment

About 80% of people recover completely.

Divers having only itching, skin mottling, and fatigue usually do not need to undergo recompression, but they should be kept under observation, because more serious problems may follow. Breathing 100% oxygen from a close-fitting face mask may provide relief.

Recompression Therapy: Any other symptoms of decompression sickness indicate the need for treatment in a high-pressure (recompression or hyperbaric oxygen) chamber, because recompression restores normal blood flow and oxygen to affected tissues. After recompression, pressure is reduced gradually, with designated pauses, allowing time for excess gases to leave the body harmlessly. Because symptoms may reappear or worsen over the first 24 hours, even people with only mild or transient pain or neurologic symptoms are treated.

Recompression therapy is beneficial for up to 48 hours after diving and should be given even if reaching the nearest chamber requires significant travel. While awaiting transport and during transport, oxygen is administered with a close-fitting face mask, and fluids are given by mouth or intravenously. Long delays in treatment increase the risk of permanent injury.

Immersion Pulmonary Edema

Immersion pulmonary edema is sudden development of fluid in the lungs that typically occurs early during a dive and at depth.

Immersion pulmonary edema has become more common over the past two decades. A likely cause is malfunction of the regulator that controls gas flow, causing some suction forces to the airways. Immersion pulmonary edema is not related to lung barotrauma or decompression sickness. Cold water and a history of high blood pressure are risk factors.

Divers usually ascend rapidly and become very short of breath. A cough with frothy sputum is typical. Treatment includes diuretics that are effective immediately, such as intravenous furosemide, and oxygen, usually given under pressure by a mask. Mechanical ventilation may be necessary. Recompression therapy is not given.

Gas Toxicity

Problems during diving can result from toxic effects of gases such as nitrogen, oxygen, carbon dioxide, and carbon monoxide.

Air is a mixture of gases, mainly nitrogen and oxygen with very small amounts of other gases. Each gas has a partial pressure, based on its concentration in the air and on the atmospheric pressure. Both oxygen and nitrogen can have harmful effects at high partial pressures.

Oxygen Toxicity: Oxygen toxicity occurs in most people when the partial pressure of oxygen reaches 1.4 atmospheres, equivalent to slightly over 187 feet (57 meters) depth when breathing air. Although oxygen toxicity can rarely occur in a hyperbaric oxygen chamber, divers who use inappropriate concentrations of oxygen during deep dives are at higher risk.

Symptoms include tingling, focal seizures (such as facial, lip, or one-sided limb twitching), vertigo, nausea and vomiting, and constricted vision. About 10% of people have seizures or fainting, which typically results in drowning. To prevent oxygen toxicity during deep dives, special gas mixtures and special training are required.

Nitrogen Narcosis: Nitrogen narcosis (rapture of the deep) is caused by high partial pressures of nitrogen, and symptoms resemble those of alcohol intoxication. People show very poor judgment and become disoriented and often euphoric. They may fail to surface on time or even swim deeper, thinking they are going to the surface. This effect becomes noticeable at 100 feet (about 30 meters) in some divers breathing compressed air and is usually incapacitating at 300 feet (about 90 meters).

To minimize these effects, divers who must dive to great depths typically breathe a special mixture of gases rather than regular air. Low concentrations of oxygen are used, diluted with helium or hydrogen rather than nitrogen, because helium and hydrogen do not produce narcosis. However, substituting helium for nitrogen increases the risk of the high-pressure neurologic syndrome.

? Did You Know...

Hyperventilating before swimming underwater in an attempt to increase breath-holding time can increase the risk of drowning.

Carbon Dioxide Buildup: A buildup of carbon dioxide in the bloodstream is the body's signal to breathe. Divers, such as snorkelers, who hold their breath rather than use a breathing apparatus, often breathe vigorously (hyperventilate) before a dive,

breathing out a large amount of carbon dioxide but adding little oxygen to the blood. This maneuver allows them to hold their breath and swim under water longer because their carbon dioxide levels are low. However, this maneuver is also hazardous because divers can run out of oxygen and lose consciousness before the carbon dioxide reaches a level high enough to signal the need to return to the surface and breathe. This sequence of events is probably responsible for many unexplained drownings among spearfishing competitors and others who hold their breath while diving.

Some scuba divers have carbon dioxide buildup because they do not increase their breathing adequately during exertion. Others retain carbon dioxide because the compressed air at depth is denser and requires greater effort to move it through the airways and breathing apparatus. Regulator malfunction or contamination of the air supply with exhaled gases, an overly tight wetsuit, and overexertion are also possible causes. Symptoms may include headaches, difficulty breathing, nausea, vomiting, and flushing. High carbon dioxide levels can also lead to blackouts, increase the likelihood of seizures from oxygen toxicity, and worsen the severity of nitrogen narcosis. Divers who frequently have headaches after diving or who pride themselves on using air at a low rate may be retaining carbon dioxide.

Carbon Monoxide Poisoning: Carbon monoxide is a product on combustion. Carbon monoxide can enter a diver's air if the air compressor intake valve is placed too close to engine exhaust or if the lubricating oil in a malfunctioning compressor becomes hot enough to partially combust (flashing), producing carbon monoxide.

Symptoms include nausea, headache, weakness, clumsiness, and confusion. Severe cases can cause seizures, loss of consciousness, or coma. Diagnosis is with a blood test. As time passes, the results become less accurate, so the test should be done as soon as possible. The diver's air supply can also be tested for carbon monoxide.

People are given oxygen. High blood levels of oxygen help eliminate carbon monoxide from the blood but do not always cause organ damage to resolve. For people with severe poisoning, some experts recommend giving oxygen at high pressures in a high-pressure (hyperbaric) chamber, available at certain medical centers. Experts continue to debate the benefit of such treatment.

High-Pressure Neurologic Syndrome: A poorly understood set of neurologic symptoms can develop when people dive deeper than about 600 feet (180 meters), particularly when the dive is rapid and the diver breathes a mixture of helium and oxygen. Symptoms include nausea, vomiting, tremors,

Disorders Treated With Hyperbaric Oxygen Therapy

Treatment with hyperbaric oxygen therapy seems to benefit people with some disorders. These include

- Air embolism
- Clostridial infection (a severe bacterial infection of soft tissues)
- Decompression sickness
- Death of bone caused by radiation therapy (osteoradionecrosis)
- Poorly healing skin grafts
- Severe carbon monoxide poisoning

It is not clear whether treatment with hyperbaric oxygen therapy helps people with other disorders, and studies of recompression therapy in these disorders are still being done.

- Blockage of the large artery or vein that supplies the retina in the eye
- Brain abscess caused by actinomycosis
- Infection with "flesh-eating bacteria" (necrotizing fasciitis)
- Severe anemia in people with low blood pressure
- Severe bone infection (osteomyelitis)
- Severe crushing injury, usually of a limb
- Severe burns
- Soft tissue injury caused by radiation therapy
- Wounds in limbs that have poor blood supply

clumsiness, dizziness, fatigue, sleepiness, muscle jerks, stomach cramps, and confusion. The syndrome resolves on its own when people ascend or when the rate of descent is slowed.

Recompression Therapy

Recompression therapy (hyperbaric oxygen therapy) involves giving 100% oxygen for several hours in a sealed chamber at pressures higher than 1 atmosphere.

Recompression therapy has four effects on the blood that can be useful in treating diving injuries:

- Increasing the concentration of oxygen
- Decreasing the concentration of nitrogen
- Decreasing the concentration of carbon monoxide
- Decreasing the size of gas bubbles

Among divers, recompression therapy is used most often for decompression sickness and arterial gas embolism, but it also may occasionally be used to treat carbon monoxide poisoning. Recompression therapy is often referred to as hyperbaric oxygen therapy when it is given primarily to administer high concentrations of oxygen rather than to treat decompression sickness or arterial gas embolism. Hyperbaric oxygen therapy is used for several disorders unrelated to diving. Whether recompression therapy is effective for all these disorders is still being studied.

The sooner therapy is begun, the better the result is likely to be. Some chambers have room for more than one person and some have room for only one. Treatments are usually given once or twice daily for 45 to 300 minutes. Most often, 100% oxygen is given at 2.5 to 3 atmospheres of pressure.

Recompression therapy is relatively safe, but doctors try to avoid using it in people who have any of the following:

- Chronic lung disorders
- Sinus problems or colds
- Seizure disorders
- Claustrophobia
- Recent chest surgery
- Collapsed lung (pneumothorax)
- Recent ear surgery or injury
- Fever

Recompression therapy is usually avoided during pregnancy unless the mother's life is in danger because of possible harmful effects of high oxygen concentrations on the fetus. Recompression therapy can cause problems similar to those that occur with barotrauma (see page 1996). It can also cause temporary nearsightedness, low blood sugar levels, or, rarely, toxic effects on the lungs or seizures.

Information regarding the location of the nearest recompression chamber, the most rapid means of reaching it, and the most appropriate source to consult by telephone should be known by most divers. Such information is also available from the Divers Alert Network (919-684-8111; www.divers alertnetwork.org) 24 hours per day. The Undersea and Hyperbaric Medical Society (www.uhms.org) is another valuable information source.

Diving Precautions and Prevention of Diving Injuries

Diving is a relatively safe recreational activity for healthy people who have been appropriately trained and educated. Diving safety courses offered by national diving organizations are widely available.

Safety Precautions: Divers should take precautions that minimize the risk of barotrauma and decompression sickness.

The risk of barotrauma can be decreased by equalizing the pressure in various air spaces, including the face mask (by blowing out air from the nose into the mask) and the middle ear (for example, by yawning or swallowing). Divers should avoid holding their breath and breathe normally during ascent, which should be no faster than 0.5 to 1 feet/second, a rate that allows divers to gradually expel excess nitrogen and empty air-filled spaces (for example, the lungs and sinuses). Current recommendations also include a 3- to 5-minute safety stop at 15 feet (4.6 meters). Also, divers should not fly for 15 to 18 hours after diving.

Also, divers should be aware of and avoid certain diving conditions (for example, poor visibility or currents requiring excessive effort). Cold temperatures are a particular hazard because hypothermia can develop rapidly and compromise the diver's judgment and dexterity. Hypothermia can also cause potentially fatal abnormal heart rhythms in susceptible people. Diving alone is not recommended.

Recreational and sedative drugs and alcohol in any amount may have unpredictable or unanticipated effects at depth and should be strictly avoided. Nonsedating prescription drugs rarely interfere with recreational diving.

High Risk Factors for Diving: Because diving can involve heavy exertion, divers should have above-average aerobic capacity, that is, they should not be limited by heart or lung disorders. Disorders that can impair consciousness, alertness, or judgment, such as seizures and diabetes that is treated with insulin (because it can cause low blood sugar levels [hypoglycemia]) generally prohibit diving. Special programs for diabetic divers have been established. If there is any question, a doctor should be consulted. Although children younger than 10 years should not dive, programs that begin teaching children at age 8 have been successful. Most diving instructors are familiar with guidelines for teaching children to dive. Prospective divers should be evaluated for fitness and for factors that can increase

High Risk Factors for Diving
■ Alcohol or drug abuse
■ Chronic or short-term congestion of the nose and sinuses
■ Diabetes, type 1 or type 2, that is treated with insulin (usually)
■ Drugs that can cause drowsiness
■ Fainting spells
■ Gastroesophageal reflux if severe
■ Habitual air swallowing
■ Heart disorders, such as coronary artery disease, heart failure, irregular heart rhythms, valve disorders, and congenital heart defects that allow blood to leak from the venous to the arterial system
■ Inguinal hernia that has not been repaired
■ Impulsive behavior or being prone to accidents
■ Lung problems, such as asthma,* lung cysts, emphysema, previous pneumothorax
■ Obesity†
■ Older age†
■ Panic disorder
■ Physical disabilities
■ Poor cardiovascular fitness
■ Pregnancy
■ Ruptured eardrum
■ Seizures

* Possible higher risk of lung barotrauma.
† Higher risk of decompression sickness.

the risk of mishaps and injury during diving by doctors who are familiar with diving.

Professional divers may undergo additional medical tests, such as those for heart and lung function, exercise stress, hearing, and vision, as well as bone x-rays. In addition, adequate diver training is absolutely necessary.

CHAPTER
309 Altitude Illness

Altitude illness occurs because of a lack of oxygen at high altitudes.

■ Symptoms include headache, tiredness, irritability, and in more serious cases, shortness of breath, confusion, and even coma.
■ Doctors diagnose altitude illness primarily based on the symptoms.

■ Treatment includes rest, descending to a lower altitude, and sometimes drugs, extra oxygen, or both.
■ People may prevent this disorder by ascending slowly and sometimes by taking drugs.

As altitude increases, the atmospheric pressure decreases, thinning the air so that less oxygen is available. For example, compared with the air at sea level, the air at 19,000 feet (5,800 meters) contains only half the amount of oxygen. In Denver, which is located about 5,300 feet (1,615 meters) above sea level, the air contains 20% less oxygen.

Most people can ascend to 5,000 to 6,500 feet (1,500 to 2,000 meters) in one day without problems, but about 20% who ascend to 8,000 feet (2,500 meters) and 40% who ascend to 10,000 feet (3,000 meters) develop some form of altitude illness.

The organs most commonly affected by altitude illness are the

- Brain (causing acute mountain sickness and rarely high-altitude cerebral edema)
- Lungs (causing high-altitude pulmonary edema)

In the lungs, there is elevated pressure in the smallest blood vessels (capillaries). The capillaries also may leak fluid.

Risk Factors: Effects of high altitude vary greatly among individuals. But generally, risk is increased by

- Going too high too fast
- Undertaking too much exertion

Risk is greater in people who previously had altitude illness and in those who normally live at sea level or at very low altitude (below 3,000 feet [900 meters]). Young children and young adults also are probably more susceptible.

People who have disorders such as diabetes, coronary artery disease, and mild chronic obstructive pulmonary disease are not at increased risk for altitude illness. However, such people may have particular difficulties at high altitude because of the low oxygen levels (hypoxia). Physical fitness is not protective. Asthma does not generally seem to be worse at high altitudes. Also, spending less than a few weeks at higher altitudes (but below 10,000 feet) does not appear to be dangerous for a pregnant woman or the fetus.

Acclimatization: The body eventually adjusts (acclimatizes) to higher altitudes by increasing respiration and heart activity and by producing more red blood cells to carry oxygen to the tissues. Most people can adjust to altitudes of up to 10,000 feet in a few days. Adjusting to much higher altitudes takes many days or weeks, but some people can eventually carry out nearly normal activities at altitudes above 17,500 feet (about 5,300 meters). However, no one can fully acclimatize to long-term residence above that altitude.

> **? Did You Know...**
> Symptoms of acute mountain sickness may be mistaken for a hangover, physical exhaustion, a migraine, or a viral illness.

Symptoms

Acute Mountain Sickness: Acute mountain sickness is a mild form of altitude illness and is the most common form. It may develop at altitudes as low as 6,500 feet (2,000 meters). Symptoms usually develop within 6 to 10 hours of ascent and include headache and one or more other symptoms, such as lightheadedness, loss of appetite, nausea and vomiting, fatigue, weakness, irritability, or trouble sleeping. Some people describe the symptoms as similar to those of a hangover. Symptoms usually last 24 to 48 hours. Occasionally, acute mountain sickness progresses to more severe forms of altitude illness.

High-Altitude Pulmonary Edema (HAPE): HAPE usually develops 24 to 96 hours after a rapid ascent to over 8,000 feet (2,500 meters). HAPE is responsible for most deaths due to altitude illness. Respiratory infections, even minor ones, appear to increase the risk. Symptoms are worse at night and can quickly become more severe. Mild symptoms usually include a dry cough and shortness of breath after only mild exertion. Moderate symptoms include shortness of breath at rest; confusion; pink or bloody sputum; low-grade fever; and a bluish tinge to the skin, lips, and nails (cyanosis). Severe symptoms include gasping for breath and making gurgling sounds while breathing.

High-Altitude Cerebral Edema (HACE): HACE is a rare but potentially fatal condition. People with HACE have headache, confusion, walking that is unsteady and uncoordinated (ataxia), and coma. These symptoms may progress rapidly from mild to life-threatening within a few hours.

Other Symptoms: Swelling of the hands, the feet, and, on awakening, the face is common. The swelling causes little discomfort and usually goes away in a few days.

Retinal hemorrhages (small areas of bleeding in the retina at the back of the eye) may develop after ascent to altitudes of 9,000 feet (2,700 meters). These hemorrhages are common above 16,000 feet (5,000 meters). People usually have no symptoms unless the hemorrhage occurs in the part of the eye that is responsible for central vision (the macula). In such cases, people may notice a small blind spot. Retinal hemorrhages resolve rapidly without causing long-term problems.

Diagnosis

Doctors diagnose altitude illness based mainly on the symptoms. In people with HAPE, doctors can usually hear fluid in the lungs through a stethoscope. An x-ray of the chest and measurement of the amount of oxygen in the blood can help confirm the diagnosis.

Prevention

Rate of Ascent: The best way to prevent altitude illness is to ascend slowly. The altitude at which a person sleeps is more important than the maximum height reached during the day. On the first night, people should not sleep any higher than 8,000 to 10,000 feet (2,500 to 3,000 meters). Mountain climbers should sleep at that altitude for 2 to 3 nights before they sleep at any higher altitudes. Each day thereafter, sleeping altitude can be increased by about 1,000 feet (300 meters), although higher day hikes are acceptable as long as people return to the lower level for sleep.

People vary in their ability to ascend without developing symptoms. Thus, a climbing party should be paced for its slowest member. The pace of ascent should be slowed if symptoms of altitude illness develop.

Acclimatization reverses quickly. If acclimatized people have descended to low levels for more than a few days, they must once more follow a graded ascent.

Drugs: Acetazolamide taken at the start of the ascent can reduce the likelihood of altitude illness. If taken after the illness has begun, acetazolamide may help lessen symptoms. Acetazolamide should be continued for a few days after ascent. Some doctors believe that dexamethasone can also reduce the likelihood of altitude illness and lessen its symptoms.

People who have had previous episodes of HAPE should be alert for any symptoms of a recurrence and descend immediately if this occurs. Some doctors also recommend such people take the drug nifedipine by mouth or inhaled bronchodilators for prevention of HAPE.

General Measures: Avoiding strenuous exertion for a day or two after arrival may help prevent altitude illness, as may eating frequent, small meals that are high in easily digested carbohydrates (such as fruits, jams, and starches) instead of fewer large meals. People should drink plenty of noncaffeinated fluids. Alcohol and sedatives, which can cause symptoms similar to acute mountain sickness, should be avoided.

Although physical fitness enables greater exertion at altitude, it does not protect against any form of altitude illness.

Treatment

People with acute mountain sickness must stop their ascent and rest. They should not ascend to higher altitudes until symptoms disappear. Most people with acute mountain sickness improve within a day or two. Acetazolamide may help relieve symptoms. Acetaminophen or nonsteroidal anti-inflammatory drugs (NSAIDs—see page 644) help relieve headache.

What Is Chronic Mountain Sickness?

Most altitude sickness occurs in people who quickly ascend to high altitude. But some people develop altitude-related illness only after living a long time at high altitude.

Chronic mountain sickness (Monge's disease) is an uncommon illness that develops in some people who live at altitudes higher than 12,000 feet (about 3,600 meters) for many months or years. Symptoms include fatigue, shortness or breath, aches and pains, and a blue color to the lips and skin (cyanosis). In these people, the body overcompensates for the lack of oxygen by overproducing red blood cells. The extra red blood cells make the blood so thick that it is may form blood clots in the legs and lungs. It may become difficult for the heart to pump enough blood.

Periodic removal of a pint of blood (phlebotomy) provides temporary relief, but the only effective treatment is descent to a low altitude. Complete recovery can take months.

If symptoms are more severe, supplemental oxygen should be provided through a face mask. If supplemental oxygen is unavailable, or if symptoms persist or worsen despite treatment, the person should descend to a lower altitude, preferably at least 2,500 feet (760 meters) lower.

People with HAPE should descend to a low altitude as soon as possible. Oxygen should be given if it is available. The drug nifedipine may temporarily help by decreasing blood pressure in the arteries to the lungs.

If HACE develops, the person should descend as far down and as soon as possible. Oxygen and dexamethasone should be taken.

When prompt descent to a lower altitude is not possible and people are seriously ill, a hyperbaric bag can be used to buy time. This device consists of a lightweight, portable fabric bag large enough to completely contain a person and a manually operated pump. The person is sealed tightly in the bag, and the bag's internal pressure is then increased using the pump. The increased air pressure simulates a decrease in altitude. The person remains in the bag for 2 or 3 hours. The hyperbaric bag is as beneficial as supplemental oxygen, which often is not available when mountain climbing, but is not a substitute for descent.

CHAPTER

310 Poisoning

Poisoning is the harmful effect that occurs when a toxic substance is swallowed, is inhaled, or comes in contact with the skin, eyes, or mucous membranes, such as those of the mouth or nose.

- Possible poisonous substances include prescription and over-the-counter drugs, illicit drugs, gases, chemicals, vitamins, and food.
- Some poisons cause no damage, whereas others can cause severe damage or death.
- The diagnosis is based on symptoms, on information gleaned from the poisoned person and bystanders, and sometimes on blood and urine tests.
- Medications should always be kept in original child-proof containers and kept out of the reach of children.
- Treatment consists of supporting the person, preventing additional absorption of the poison, and sometimes increasing elimination of the poison.

Poisoning is the most common cause of nonfatal accidents in the home. More than 2 million people suffer some type of poisoning each year in the United States. Drugs—prescription, over the counter, and illicit—are the most common source of serious poisonings and poisoning-related deaths. Other common poisons include gases, household products, agricultural products, plants, industrial chemicals, vitamins, and foods (particularly certain species of mushrooms—see page 153—and fish—see page 155). However, almost any substance ingested in sufficiently large quantities can be toxic.

Young children are particularly vulnerable to accidental poisoning in the home, as are older people, often from confusion about their drugs. Also vulnerable to accidental poisoning are hospitalized people (from drug errors) and industrial workers (from exposure to toxic chemicals). Poisoning may also be a deliberate attempt to commit murder or suicide. Most adults who attempt suicide by poisoning take more than one drug and also consume alcohol.

The damage caused by poisoning depends on the poison, the amount taken, and the age and underlying health of the person who takes it. Some poisons are not very potent and cause problems only with prolonged exposure or repeated ingestion of large amounts. Other poisons are so potent that just a drop on the skin can cause severe damage.

Some poisons cause symptoms within seconds, whereas others cause symptoms only after hours or even days. Some poisons cause few obvious symptoms until they have damaged vital organs—such as the kidneys or liver—sometimes permanently.

Nontoxic Household Products*

Adhesives
Antacids
Bath oil†
Bathtub toys (floating)
Bleach (less than 5% sodium hypochlorite)
Body conditioners
Bubble bath soaps (detergents)†
Candles
Carboxymethylcellulose (dehydrating material packed with film, books, and other products)
Chalk (calcium carbonate)
Colognes
Cosmetics
Crayons
Deodorants
Deodorizers, spray and refrigerant
Fabric softeners
Hand lotions and creams
Hydrogen peroxide (3% medicinal)
Incense
Indelible markers
Ink (black, blue)
"Lead" pencils (which are really made of graphite)
Magic markers
Matches
Mineral oil†
Modeling clay
Newspaper
Perfumes
Petroleum jelly
Putty
Sachets (essential oils, powders)
Shaving creams and lotions
Soap and soap products
Suntan preparations
Sweetening agents (saccharin, aspartame)
Toothpaste with or without fluoride
Vitamins (children's multiple with or without iron)
Water colors
Wax or paraffin
Zinc oxide
Zirconium oxide

*Almost any substance can be toxic if ingested in sufficient amounts.
†Moderately viscous (thick) substances like oils and detergents are not toxic if ingested but can cause significant lung injury if they are inhaled or aspirated into the lungs.

First Aid

The first priority in helping a poisoned person is for bystanders not to become poisoned themselves. People exposed to a toxic gas should be removed from the source quickly, preferably out into fresh air, but rescue attempts should be done by professionals. Special training and precautions must be considered to avoid being overcome by the toxic gases or chemicals during rescue attempts.

In chemical spills, all contaminated clothing, including socks and shoes, and jewelry should be removed immediately. The skin should be thoroughly washed with soap and water. If the eyes have been exposed, they should be thoroughly flushed with water or saline. Rescuers must be careful to avoid contaminating themselves.

If the person appears very sick, emergency medical assistance (911 in most areas of the United States) should be called. Bystanders should do cardiopulmonary resuscitation (CPR) if needed (see page 1942). If the person does not appear very sick, bystanders can contact the nearest poison center for advice. In the United States, the local poison center can be reached at 800-222-1222. More information is available at the American Association of Poison Control Centers web site (www.aapcc.org). If the caller knows the identity of the poison and the amount ingested, treatment can often be initiated at home if this is recommended by the poison center.

Containers of the poisons and all drugs that might have been taken by the poisoned person (including over-the-counter products) should be saved and given to the doctor or rescue personnel. The poison center may recommend giving the poisoned person activated charcoal (see page 2008) before arrival at a hospital and, rarely, may recommend giving syrup of ipecac to induce vomiting, particularly if the person must travel far to reach the hospital. However, unless specifically instructed to, charcoal and syrup of ipecac should not be given in the home or by first responders (such as ambulance personnel). Syrup of ipecac has unpredictable effects, often causes prolonged vomiting, and may not remove substantial amounts of poison from the stomach.

Diagnosis

Identifying the poison is helpful to treatment. Labels on bottles and other information from the person, family members, or coworkers best enable the doctor or the poison center to identify poisons. Laboratory testing is much less likely to identify the poison, and many drugs and poisons cannot be readily identified or measured by the hospital. Sometimes, urine and blood tests may help in identification as well. Blood tests can sometimes reveal the severity of poisoning, but only with only a small number of poisons.

For certain poisonings, abdominal x-rays may show the presence and location of the ingested substances. Poisons that may be visible on x-rays include iron, lead, arsenic, other metals, and large packets of cocaine or other illicit drugs swallowed by so-called body packers or drug mules.

Prevention

In the United States, widespread use of child-resistant containers with safety caps has greatly reduced the number of poisoning deaths in children younger than age 5. To prevent accidental poisoning, drugs should be kept in their original containers. Toxic substances, such as insecticides and cleaning agents, should not be put in drink bottles or cups, even briefly. Other preventive measures include clearly labeling household products, storing drugs and toxic substances in cabinets that are locked and out of the reach of children, and using carbon monoxide detectors. Expired drugs should be disposed by mixing them with cat litter or some other nontempting substance and putting them in a trash container that is inaccessible to children. All labels should be read before taking or giving any drugs or using household products.

Limiting the amount of over-the-counter pain relievers in a single container reduces the severity of poisonings, particularly with acetaminophen, aspirin, or ibuprofen. The identifying marks printed on pills and capsules by the drug manufacturer can help prevent confusion and errors by people, pharmacists, and health care practitioners.

> **Did You Know...**
>
> In the United States, the local poison center can be reached by dialing 1-800-222-1222.

Treatment

Some people who have been poisoned must be hospitalized. With prompt medical care, most recover fully.

The principles for the treatment of all poisoning are the same:

- Support breathing and blood pressure
- Prevent additional absorption
- Increase elimination of the poison
- Give specific antidotes (substances that eliminate, inactivate, or counteract the effects of the poison), if available
- Prevent reexposure

The usual goal of hospital treatment is to keep people alive until the poison disappears or is inactivated by the body. Eventually, most poisons are inactivated by the liver or are passed into the urine. There are no specific antidotes for many serious poisonings.

Stomach emptying (stomach pumping), once commonly done, is now usually avoided because it removes only a small amount of the poison and can cause serious complications. Stomach emptying rarely improves a person's outcome. However, stomach emptying may be done if an unusually dangerous poison is involved or if the person appears very sick. In this procedure, a tube is inserted through the mouth or nose into the stomach. Water is poured into the stomach through the tube and is then drained out (gastric lavage). This procedure is repeated several times. If people are drowsy because of the poison, doctors usually first put a plastic breathing tube through the mouth into the windpipe (endotracheal intubation). Endotracheal intubation helps keep the gastric lavage liquid from running into the lungs. In the hospital, doctors do not give syrup of ipecac to empty the stomach because its effects are inconsistent.

For many swallowed poisons, hospital emergency departments may give activated charcoal. Activated charcoal binds to the poison that is still in the digestive tract, preventing its absorption into the blood. Charcoal is usually taken by mouth but may have to be given through a tube that is inserted through the nose into the stomach. Sometimes doctors give charcoal every 4 to 6 hours to help cleanse the body of the poison. Not all poisons are inactivated by charcoal. For example, charcoal does not bind alcohol, iron, or many household chemicals.

If a poisoning remains life threatening despite the use of charcoal and antidotes, more complicated treatments may be needed. The most common involve filtering poisons directly from the bloodstream—hemodialysis (which uses an artificial kidney [dialyzer] to filter the poisons—see page 266) or charcoal hemoperfusion (which uses charcoal to help eliminate the poisons). For either of these methods, small tubes (catheters) are inserted into blood vessels, one to drain blood from an artery and another to return blood to a vein. The blood is passed through special filters that remove the toxic substance before being returned to the body. Sometimes a solution containing sodium bicarbonate (the chemical in baking soda) is given by vein to make the urine more alkaline or basic (as opposed to acidic). This can increase the amount of certain drugs (such as aspirin and barbiturates) excreted in the urine.

Poisoning often requires additional treatment, termed supportive care, designed to stabilize the heart, blood pressure, and breathing until the poison disappears or is inactivated. For example, a person who becomes very drowsy or comatose may need a breathing tube inserted into the windpipe. The tube is then attached to a ventilator, which mechanically supports the person's breathing. The tube prevents vomit from entering the lungs, and the ventilator ensures adequate breathing. Treatment also may be needed to control seizures, fever, or vomiting.

If the kidneys stop working, hemodialysis is necessary. If liver damage is extensive, treatment for liver failure may be necessary. If the liver or kidneys sustain permanent, severe damage, organ transplantation may be needed.

People who attempt suicide by poisoning need mental health evaluation and appropriate treatment.

Acetaminophen Poisoning

- People sometimes ingest too many products that contain acetaminophen and accidentally poison themselves.
- Depending on the amount of acetaminophen in the blood, symptoms range from none at all to vomiting and abdominal pain to liver failure and death.
- The diagnosis is based on the amount of acetaminophen in the blood and results of liver function tests.
- Acetylcysteine is given to reduce the toxicity of the acetaminophen.

More than 100 products contain acetaminophen, a common over-the-counter pain reliever that is also present in many combination prescription drugs. If several similar products are consumed at a time, a person may inadvertently take too much acetaminophen. Many preparations intended for use in children are available in liquid, tablet, and capsule form, and a parent may try several preparations simultaneously or within several hours to treat a fever or pain, not realizing they all contain acetaminophen.

Acetaminophen usually is a very safe drug even in large doses, but it is not harmless. To cause poisoning, several times the recommended dose of acetaminophen must be taken. For example, a person who weighs 150 pounds generally needs to take about 30 325-milligram tablets before toxic effects due to a single overdose are possible. Death is extremely unlikely unless the person takes more than 40 325-milligram tablets. Toxicity also may develop if multiple smaller doses are taken over time. In toxic doses, acetaminophen can damage the liver. Liver failure can follow.

Symptoms and Diagnosis

Most overdoses cause no immediate symptoms. The level of acetaminophen in the blood, measured

2 to 4 hours after ingestion, may help predict the severity of the liver damage. If the overdose is very large, symptoms develop in four stages. In stage 1 (after several hours), the person may vomit but does not seem ill. Many people have no symptoms until stage 2 (after 24 to 72 hours), when nausea, vomiting, and abdominal pain may develop. At this stage, blood tests show that the liver is functioning abnormally. In stage 3 (after 3 to 4 days), vomiting becomes worse. Tests show that the liver is functioning poorly, and jaundice (yellowing of the eyes and skin) and bleeding develop. Sometimes the kidneys fail and the pancreas becomes inflamed (pancreatitis). In stage 4 (after 5 days), the person either recovers or experiences failure of the liver and often other organs, which may be fatal.

Treatment

If acetaminophen was taken within the previous several hours, activated charcoal may be given.

If the level of acetaminophen in the blood is high, acetylcysteine is generally given by mouth or by vein to reduce the toxicity of the acetaminophen. Acetylcysteine is given repeatedly, for one to several days. This antidote helps prevent liver injury but does not reverse injury that has already occurred. Therefore, acetylcysteine must be given before liver injury occurs. Treatment for liver failure or liver transplant may also be necessary.

Aspirin Poisoning

- Aspirin poisoning can occur acutely after taking a high dose or develop gradually after taking low doses repeatedly.
- Symptoms may include ringing in the ears, nausea, vomiting, drowsiness, confusion, and rapid breathing.
- The diagnosis is based on blood tests.
- Treatment involves giving activated charcoal by mouth or stomach tube, giving fluids and bicarbonate by vein, and, for severe poisoning, undergoing hemodialysis.

Ingestion of aspirin and similar drugs (salicylates) can lead to rapid poisoning due to an overdose. The dose necessary to cause acute poisoning, however, is quite large. A person weighing about 150 pounds would have to consume more than 30 325-miligram tablets to develop even mild poisoning. An acute aspirin overdose, therefore, is seldom accidental.

Gradual aspirin poisoning can develop unintentionally by taking aspirin repeatedly at much lower doses. Children with fever who are given only slightly higher than the prescribed dose of aspirin for several days may develop poisoning, although children are rarely given aspirin to treat fever because of the risk of development of Reye's syndrome (see box on page 1769). None of the over-the-counter cough and cold preparations sold in the United States for children contains aspirin; most contain either acetaminophen or ibuprofen. Adults, many of them elderly, can develop poisoning gradually after several weeks of use. The dosage of aspirin recommended to people with coronary artery disease to reduce the risk of heart attack (1 baby aspirin, 1/2 of an adult aspirin, or 1 full adult aspirin daily) is too small to cause gradual poisoning.

The most toxic form of salicylate is oil of wintergreen (methyl salicylate). Methyl salicylate is a component of products such as liniments and solutions used in hot vaporizers. A young child can die from swallowing less than 1 teaspoonful of pure methyl salicylate. Far less toxic are over-the-counter products containing bismuth subsalicylate (used to treat infections of the digestive tract), which can cause poisoning after several doses.

> **? Did You Know...**
>
> A young child can die from swallowing less than 1 teaspoonful of oil of wintergreen, which is found in solutions used in hot vaporizers.

Symptoms

The first symptoms of acute aspirin poisoning are usually nausea and vomiting followed by rapid breathing, ringing in the ears, and sweating. Later, if poisoning is severe, the person can develop lightheadedness, fever, drowsiness, hyperactivity, confusion, seizures, destroyed muscle tissue (rhabdomyolysis), kidney failure, and difficulty breathing.

The symptoms of gradual aspirin poisoning develop over days or weeks. Drowsiness, subtle confusion, and hallucinations are the most common symptoms. Lightheadedness, rapid breathing, shortness of breath, fever, dehydration, low blood pressure, a low oxygen level in the blood (hypoxia), a buildup of lactic acid in the blood (lactic acidosis), fluid in the lungs (pulmonary edema), seizures, and brain swelling can develop.

Diagnosis and Treatment

A blood sample is taken to measure the precise level of aspirin in the blood. Measurement of the blood pH (amount of acid in the blood) and the level of carbon dioxide or bicarbonate in the blood also can help doctors determine the severity of poisoning. Tests are usually repeated several times during treatment to reveal whether the person is recovering.

Activated charcoal is given as soon as possible and reduces aspirin absorption. For moderate or severe poisoning, fluids containing sodium bicarbonate are given by vein. Unless there is kidney damage, potassium is added to the fluid. This mixture moves aspirin from the bloodstream into the urine. If the person's condition is worsening despite other treatments, hemodialysis (which uses an artificial kidney [dialyzer] to filter the poisons—see page 266) can remove aspirin, other salicylates, and acids from the blood. Other symptoms such as fever or seizures are treated as necessary.

Carbon Monoxide Poisoning

- Carbon monoxide poisoning is common.
- Symptoms may include headache, nausea, drowsiness, and confusion.
- The diagnosis is based on blood tests.
- Carbon monoxide detectors and adequate venting of furnaces and other sources of indoor combustion help prevent carbon monoxide poisoning.
- Treatment includes fresh air and high concentrations of oxygen.

Carbon monoxide is a colorless, odorless gas that, when inhaled, prevents the blood from carrying oxygen and prevents the tissues from using oxygen effectively. Small amounts are not usually harmful, but poisoning occurs if levels of carbon monoxide in the blood become too high. Carbon monoxide disappears from the blood after several hours.

Smoke from fires commonly contains carbon monoxide, particularly when combustion of fuels is incomplete. If improperly vented, automobiles, furnaces, hot water heaters, gas heaters, kerosene heaters, and stoves (including wood stoves and stoves with charcoal briquettes) can cause carbon monoxide poisoning. Inhaling tobacco smoke produces carbon monoxide in the blood, but usually not enough to result in symptoms of poisoning.

> **? Did You Know...**
> Carbon monoxide is one of the most common causes of poisoning deaths.

Symptoms and Diagnosis

Mild carbon monoxide poisoning causes headache, nausea, dizziness, difficulty concentrating, vomiting, drowsiness, and poor coordination. Most people who develop mild carbon monoxide poisoning recover quickly when moved into fresh air. Moderate or severe carbon monoxide poisoning causes impaired judgment, confusion, unconsciousness, seizures, chest pain, shortness of breath, low blood pressure, and coma. Thus, most victims are not able to move themselves and must be rescued. Severe poisoning is often fatal. Rarely, weeks after apparent recovery from severe carbon monoxide poisoning, symptoms such as memory loss, poor coordination, and problems with vision (which are referred to as delayed neuropsychiatric symptoms) develop.

Carbon monoxide is dangerous because a person may not recognize drowsiness as a symptom of poisoning. Consequently, someone with mild poisoning can go to sleep and continue to breathe the carbon monoxide until severe poisoning or death occurs. Some people with long-standing, mild carbon monoxide poisoning caused by furnaces or heaters may mistake their symptoms for other conditions, such as the flu or other viral infections.

Carbon monoxide poisoning is diagnosed by measuring the level of carbon monoxide in the blood.

Prevention and Treatment

To prevent poisoning, indoor sources of combustion, such as gas space heaters and wood stoves, require proper installation and ventilation. If such ventilation is impractical, an open window can limit carbon monoxide accumulation by allowing it to escape from the building. Exhaust pipes attached to furnaces and other heating appliances need periodic inspections for cracks and leaks. Chemical detectors are available for the home that can sense carbon monoxide in the air and sound alarms when it is present. If carbon monoxide is suspected in a home, windows should be opened, and the home should be evacuated and evaluated for the source of the carbon monoxide. Constant monitoring with such detectors can identify carbon monoxide before poisoning develops. Like smoke detectors, carbon monoxide detectors are recommended for all homes.

For mild poisoning, fresh air may be all that is needed. To treat more severe poisoning, high concentrations of oxygen are given, usually through a face mask. Oxygen hastens the disappearance of carbon monoxide from the blood and relieves symptoms. The value of high-pressure oxygen treatment (in a hyperbaric chamber) remains uncertain.

Caustic Substances Poisoning

- When swallowed, caustic substances can burn all tissues they touch—from the lips to the stomach.
- Symptoms may include pain (particularly with swallowing), coughing, shortness of breath, and vomiting.
- A doctor inserts a flexible viewing tube (endoscope) down the esophagus to look for burns and determine the severity of the injury.
- Treatment is determined by the extent of the damage and may involve surgery.

Caustic substances (strong acids and alkalis), when swallowed, can burn the tongue, mouth, esophagus, and stomach. These burns may cause perforation (piercing) of the esophagus or stomach. Food and saliva leaking from a perforation cause severe, sometimes deadly infection within the chest (mediastinitis or empyema) or abdomen (peritonitis). Burns that do not perforate can result in scarring of the esophagus and stomach.

Industrial products are usually the most damaging because they are highly concentrated. However, some common household products, including drain and toilet bowl cleaners and some dishwasher detergents, contain damaging caustic substances, such as sodium hydroxide and sulfuric acid.

Caustic substances are available as solids and liquids. The burning sensation of a solid particle sticking to a moist surface (such as the lips) may prevent a person from consuming much of the product. Because liquids do not stick, it is easier to consume more of the product, and the entire esophagus can be damaged. Liquids also may be inhaled (aspirated) into the airways, leading to upper airway injury.

Symptoms

Pain in the mouth and throat develops rapidly, usually within minutes, and can be severe, particularly with swallowing. Coughing, drooling, an inability to swallow, vomiting, vomiting blood, and shortness of breath may occur. In severe cases involving strong caustic substances, a person may develop very low blood pressure (shock), difficulty breathing, or chest pain, possibly leading to death. Airway burns may cause coughing, rapid breathing, or shortness of breath.

Perforation of the esophagus or stomach may occur within hours, during the first week after ingestion, or any time in between, often after vomiting or severe coughing. The esophagus may perforate into the area between the lungs (the mediastinum) or into the area surrounding the lungs (the pleural cavity). Either circumstance causes severe chest pain, fever, rapid heart rate, rapid breathing, very low blood pressure, and the need for surgery. Peritonitis results in severe abdominal pain.

Scarring of the esophagus results in narrowing (stricture), which causes difficulty in swallowing. Strictures usually develop weeks after the burn, sometimes in burns that initially caused only mild symptoms. People with scars and damage to the esophagus often develop cancer of the esophagus years after the injury.

Diagnosis and Treatment

The mouth is examined for chemical burns. Because the esophagus and stomach may be burned without the mouth being burned, the doctor may insert an endoscope down the esophagus to look for burns, particularly if the person drools or has difficulty swallowing. Directly inspecting the area allows the doctor to determine the severity of the injury and possibly to predict the risk of subsequent narrowing and the possible need for surgical repair of the esophagus.

The extent of damage determines treatment. People with severe burns sometimes need immediate surgery to remove severely damaged tissue. Corticosteroids and antibiotics may be used to try to prevent strictures and infections, but whether these drugs are helpful is not clear.

Because caustic substances can cause as much damage returning up the esophagus as they did when swallowed, a person who has swallowed a caustic substance should not be made to vomit. Syrup of ipecac and charcoal are not given.

If burns are mild, the person may be encouraged to begin drinking milk or water fairly soon in order to dilute the corrosive liquid in the stomach. Drinking can begin at home or on the way to the hospital. If the person cannot drink, fluids are given by vein until drinking is possible. Perforations are treated with antibiotics and surgery. If strictures develop, a bypass tube (stent) may be placed in the narrowed portion of the esophagus to prevent esophageal closure and to allow for future widening (dilation). Repeated widening may be needed for months or years. For severe strictures, surgery to rebuild the esophagus may also be necessary.

Hydrocarbon Poisoning

- Sniffing glue or swallowing gasoline, paint thinners, some cleaning products, or kerosene can cause hydrocarbon poisoning.
- Swallowing or inhaling hydrocarbons can cause lung irritation, with coughing, choking, shortness of breath, and neurologic problems.
- Sniffing or breathing fumes can cause irregular heartbeats, rapid heart rate, or sudden death, particularly after exertion or stress.
- The diagnosis is based on a description of the events, the characteristic odor of petroleum on the person's breath or clothing, and sometimes a chest x-ray.
- Treatment involves removing contaminated clothing, washing the skin, and giving oxygen and antibiotics to people with breathing problems or pneumonia.

Petroleum products, cleaning products, and glues contain hydrocarbons (substances composed largely of hydrogen and carbon). Many children younger than age 5 are poisoned by swallowing petroleum products, such as gasoline, kerosene, and paint thinners, but most recover. At greater risk are adolescents who intentionally breathe the fumes of these products to become intoxicated, a type of drug abuse called huffing, bagging, sniffing, glue sniffing, or solvent inhalant abuse (see page 2099).

Swallowed hydrocarbons can enter and irritate the lungs, a serious condition in itself (chemical pneumonitis), and can lead to severe pneumonia. Lung involvement is a particular problem with thin, easy-flowing hydrocarbons such as mineral seal oil, which is used in furniture polish. Severe poisoning also can affect the brain, heart, bone marrow, and kidneys. Thick, less-runny hydrocarbons such as lamp oil and mineral oil are less likely to enter the lungs but can cause severe and persistent irritation if they do.

> ### ? Did You Know...
> A person who gets high by breathing hydrocarbon fumes may die suddenly.

Symptoms

A person usually coughs and chokes after swallowing hydrocarbons. A burning sensation can develop in the stomach, and the person may vomit. If the lungs are affected, the person continues to cough intensely. Breathing becomes rapid, and the skin may become bluish (cyanosis) because of low levels of oxygen in the blood. Young children may have cyanosis, hold their breath, and cough persistently.

Hydrocarbon ingestion also causes neurologic symptoms, including drowsiness, poor coordination, stupor or coma, and seizures. Inhalation of certain hydrocarbons may induce fatal irregular heartbeats or cardiac arrest, especially after exertion or stress.

Diagnosis and Treatment

Hydrocarbon poisoning is diagnosed based on a description of the events and the characteristic odor of petroleum on the person's breath or clothing or if a container is found near the person. Paint residue on the hands or around the mouth may suggest recent paint sniffing. Pneumonia and chemical pneumonitis are diagnosed with a chest x-ray and by measuring the level of oxygen in the blood (see page 455).

To treat poisoning, contaminated clothing should be removed, and the skin should be washed. If the person has stopped coughing and choking, particularly if the ingestion was small and accidental, treatment at home is possible. Home treatment should be discussed with someone at a poison center. People with breathing problems are hospitalized. If pneumonia or chemical pneumonitis develops, hospital treatment can include oxygen and, if severe, a ventilator.

Antibiotics help if pneumonia develops. Recovery from pneumonia typically takes about a week but may take much longer if thick, syrup-like hydrocarbons such as lamp oil or mineral oil have entered the lungs.

Insecticide Poisoning

- Many insecticides can cause poisoning after being swallowed, inhaled, or absorbed through the skin.
- Symptoms may include eye tearing, coughing, and breathing difficulties.
- The diagnosis is based on symptoms, blood tests, and a description of events surrounding the poisoning.
- Several drugs are effective in treating serious poisonings.

The properties that make insecticides deadly to insects can sometimes make them poisonous to humans. Most serious insecticide poisonings result from the organophosphate and carbamate types of insecticides, particularly when used in suicide attempts. Examples of organophosphates include malathion, parathion, diazinon, dichlorvos, chlorpyrifos, and sarin. Some of these compounds are derived from nerve gases. Pyrethrins and pyrethroids, which are other commonly used insecticides, are derived from flowers and usually are not poisonous to humans.

Many insecticides can cause poisoning after being swallowed, inhaled, or absorbed through the skin. Some insecticides are odorless, thus the person is unaware of being exposed to them. Organophosphate and carbamate insecticides make certain nerves "fire" erratically, causing many organs to become overactive and eventually to stop functioning. Pyrethrins can occasionally cause allergic reactions. Pyrethroids rarely cause any problems.

Symptoms

Organophosphates and carbamates cause eye tearing, blurred vision, salivation, sweating, coughing, vomiting, and frequent bowel movements and urination. Breathing may become difficult, and muscles twitch and become weak. Rarely, shortness of breath or muscle weakness is fatal. Symptoms last hours to days after exposure to carbamates but can last for weeks after exposure to organophosphates.

Pyrethrins can cause sneezing, eye tearing, coughing, and occasional difficulty breathing. Severe symptoms rarely develop.

Diagnosis and Treatment

The diagnosis of insecticide poisoning is based on the symptoms and on a description of the events surrounding the poisoning. Blood tests can confirm organophosphate or carbamate poisoning.

If an insecticide might have contacted the skin, clothing is removed and the skin is washed. Anyone with symptoms of organophosphate poisoning should see a doctor. Atropine, given by vein, can relieve most of the symptoms. Pralidoxime, given by vein, can speed up recovery of nerve function, eliminating the cause of the symptoms. Symptoms of carbamate poisoning also are relieved by atropine but usually not by pralidoxime. Symptoms of pyrethrin poisoning resolve without treatment.

Iron Poisoning

- Symptoms develop in stages and begin with vomiting, diarrhea, and abdominal pain.
- Liver failure can develop days later.
- The diagnosis is based on the person's history, symptoms, and the amount of iron in the blood.
- People with iron poisoning need to be hospitalized.

Pills containing iron are commonly used to treat certain kinds of anemia. Iron also is included in many multiple vitamin supplements. People—especially toddlers—who overdose on these pills may develop iron poisoning. Because many households contain adult multiple vitamin supplements that contain iron, iron overdose is common. However, overdose of iron-containing vitamins, particularly children's chewable vitamins, usually does not involve enough iron to cause serious poisoning. Overdose of pure iron supplements, however, may cause serious iron poisoning. Prenatal vitamins contain a lot of iron and may poison a small child.

Iron poisoning is the most common cause of fatal poisoning in children younger than age 5. It first irritates the stomach and digestive tract, sometimes causing bleeding. Within hours, iron poisons the cells, interfering with their internal chemical reactions. Within days, the liver can be damaged. Weeks after recovery, the stomach, digestive tract, and liver can develop scars due to the previous irritation.

Symptoms

Serious iron poisoning usually causes symptoms within 6 hours of the overdose. The symptoms of iron poisoning typically occur in 5 stages.

- In stage 1 (within 6 hours after the overdose), symptoms include vomiting, vomiting blood, diarrhea, abdominal pain, irritability, drowsiness, unconsciousness, and seizures. If poisoning is very serious, rapid breathing, a rapid heart rate, coma, and low blood pressure may develop.
- In stage 2 (6 to 48 hours after the overdose), the person's condition can appear to improve.
- In stage 3 (12 to 48 hours after the overdose), very low blood pressure (shock), fever, bleeding, jaundice, liver failure, and seizures can develop. Sugar levels in the blood can decrease.

- In stage 4 (2 to 5 days after the overdose), the liver fails, and people may die from shock, bleeding, and blood-clotting abnormalities. Confusion and sluggishness (lethargy) or coma may develop.
- In stage 5 (2 to 5 weeks after the overdose), the stomach or intestines can become blocked by constricting scars. Scarring in either organ can cause crampy abdominal pain and vomiting. Severe scarring of the liver (cirrhosis—see page 222) can develop later.

Diagnosis and Treatment

The diagnosis of iron poisoning is based on the person's history, symptoms, and the amount of iron in the blood. If many pills have been swallowed, they can sometimes be seen on x-rays of the stomach or intestines.

People with symptoms or high levels of iron in the blood need hospitalization. A large amount of iron can remain in the stomach even after vomiting. A special solution of polyethylene glycol may be given by mouth or through a stomach tube to wash the contents of the stomach and intestines (whole-bowel irrigation), although its effectiveness is unclear. Injections of deferoxamine, which binds iron in the blood, are given.

Lead Poisoning

- Some causes of lead poisoning are ingestion of lead paint and eating or drinking from certain imported, improperly lead-glazed ceramics.
- Very high levels of lead in the blood may cause personality changes, headaches, loss of sensation, weakness, a metallic taste in the mouth, uncoordinated walking, digestive problems, and anemia.
- The diagnosis is based on symptoms and a blood test.
- Testing household water, ceramics, and paint for lead can help identify potential sources of lead poisoning.
- Treatment consists of stopping exposure to lead and removing accumulated lead from the body.

Although it is far less common since paint containing lead pigment was banned in 1978 and lead was eliminated from most gasoline, lead poisoning (plumbism) is still a major public health problem in cities on the East Coast of the United States.

Workers in industries that handle lead are at risk of lead poisoning, as are children who live in older houses that contain peeling lead paint or lead pipes. During home remodeling, people may be exposed to significant amounts of lead in the form of particles scraped or sanded off during surface preparation for repainting. Young children may eat enough paint chips, particularly during remodeling, to develop symptoms of lead poisoning. Some ceramic glazes contain lead. Ceramic ware, such as pitchers, cups, and plates, made using these glazes (common outside the United

States) can leach lead, particularly when in contact with acidic substances (such as fruits, cola drinks, tomatoes, wine, and cider). Lead-contaminated moonshine whiskey and folk remedies are possible sources, as are occasional lead foreign objects in the stomach or tissues (such as bullets or curtain or fishing weights). Bullets lodged in soft tissues may increase levels of lead in the blood, but that process takes years to occur. Certain ethnic cosmetic products and imported herbal products and medicinal herbs contain lead and have caused cluster outbreaks of lead poisoning in immigrant communities.

Lead affects many parts of the body, including the brain, nerves, kidneys, liver, blood, digestive tract, and sex organs. Children are particularly susceptible because lead causes the most damage in nervous systems that are still developing.

If the level of lead in the blood is high for days, symptoms of sudden brain damage (encephalopathy) usually develop. Lower blood levels that are sustained for longer periods of time sometimes cause long-term intellectual deficits.

> ### ? Did You Know...
> Children living in communities where houses are old should be tested for lead poisoning, regardless of whether symptoms are present.

Symptoms and Diagnosis

Many people with mild lead poisoning have no symptoms. Symptoms that do occur usually develop over several weeks or longer. Sometimes symptoms flare up periodically.

Typical symptoms of lead poisoning include personality changes, headaches, loss of sensation, weakness, a metallic taste in the mouth, uncoordinated walking, poor appetite, vomiting, constipation, crampy abdominal pain, bone or joint pains, high blood pressure, and anemia. Kidney damage often develops without symptoms.

Young children may become cranky and their attention span and play activity may decrease over the course of several weeks. Encephalopathy can then begin suddenly and worsen over the next several days, resulting in persistent, forceful vomiting; confusion; sleepiness; and, finally, seizures and coma. Chronic lead poisoning in children may cause intellectual disability (mental retardation), seizure disorders, aggressive behavior disorders, developmental regression, chronic abdominal pain, and anemia.

Adults often develop loss of sex drive, infertility, and, in men, erectile dysfunction (impotence). Encephalopathy rarely develops in adults.

Some symptoms may diminish if exposure to lead is stopped, only to worsen again if exposure is resumed.

The diagnosis of lead poisoning is based on symptoms and a blood test. Adults whose jobs involve handling lead need frequent blood tests. Children living in communities with many older houses, where peeling lead-based paint is common, should also undergo blood tests for lead. In children, bone and abdominal x-rays often show evidence of lead poisoning.

Prevention

Commercially available kits can be used to test household paint, ceramics, and water supplies for lead content. Measures that reduce the risk of household poisoning include regular hand washing, regular washing of children's toys and pacifiers, and regular cleaning of household surfaces. Dusting affected windowsills weekly with a damp cloth removes some dust that could contain lead from paint. Chipped leaded paint should be repaired. Larger renovation projects to remove leaded paint can release large quantities of lead into the house and should be done professionally. Commercially available faucet filters can remove most lead from drinking water.

Adults exposed to lead dust at work should use appropriate personal protective equipment, change their clothing and shoes before going home, and shower before going to bed.

Treatment

Treatment consists of stopping exposure to lead and removing accumulated lead from the body. If an abdominal x-ray shows lead chips, a special solution of polyethylene glycol is given by mouth or through a stomach tube to wash the contents of the stomach and intestines (a process called whole-bowel irrigation).

Doctors remove lead from the body by giving drugs that bind with the lead (chelation therapy), allowing it to pass into the urine. All drugs that remove lead work slowly and can cause serious side effects.

People with mild lead poisoning are given succimer by mouth. People with more serious lead poisoning are treated in the hospital with injections of chelating drugs, such as dimercaprol, succimer, penicillamine, and edetate calcium disodium. Because chelating drugs also can remove beneficial minerals, such as zinc, copper, and iron, from the body, the person often is given supplements of these minerals.

Even after treatment, many children with encephalopathy develop some degree of permanent brain damage. Kidney damage is also sometimes permanent.

311 Bites and Stings

Many creatures, including humans, bite when frightened or provoked. Bites may cause injuries ranging from superficial scratches to extensive wounds and often become infected with bacteria from the mouth of the biting creature.

Certain animals can inject venom (poison) through mouthparts or a stinger. These venoms range in toxicity from mild to life threatening. Even mildly toxic venoms may cause serious allergic reactions.

Doctors diagnose most bites and stings by talking with and examining the person. If a wound is deep, x-rays or other imaging studies are sometimes done to look for teeth or other hidden foreign material. The most effective way to prevent infection and scarring is usually thorough cleaning and proper wound care, done as soon as possible.

Animal Bites

- Most animal bites in the United States are from dogs and cats.
- Wounds should be cleaned and cared for as soon as possible.

Although any animal may bite, dogs and, to a lesser extent, cats account for most bites in the United States. Owing to their popularity as household pets, dogs account for the majority of bites as a result of protecting their owners and territory. About 10 to 20 people, mostly children, die from dog bites each year. Cats do not defend territory and bite mainly when humans restrain them or attempt to intervene in a cat fight. Domestic animals, such as horses, cows, and pigs, bite infrequently, but their size and strength are such that serious wounds may result. Wild animal bites are rare.

Dog bites typically have a ragged, torn appearance. Cat bites involve deep puncture wounds that frequently become infected. Infected bites are painful, swollen, and red. Rabies (see page 757) may be transmitted from animals (most commonly bats, raccoons, foxes, and skunks) infected with that organism. Rabies is rare among pets in the United States because of vaccination. Squirrel, hamster, and rodent bites rarely transmit rabies.

Treatment

After receiving routine first-aid treatment (see page 1946), people who have been bitten by an animal should see a doctor immediately. If possible, the offending animal should be penned up by its owner. If the animal is loose, the person who has been bitten should not try to capture it. The police should be notified so that the proper authorities can observe the animal for signs of rabies.

Doctors clean an animal bite by flooding the wound with sterile salt water (saline) and cleansing it with soap and water. Sometimes tissue is trimmed from the edge of the bite wound, particularly if the tissue is crushed or ragged. Facial bite wounds are closed surgically (sutured). However, minor wounds, puncture wounds, and bite wounds to the hands are not closed. Antibiotics are sometimes given by mouth to prevent infection. Infected bites sometimes require surgical drainage, antibiotics given intravenously, or both.

Human Bites

- A human bite wound to the hand sustained by punching someone in the mouth often becomes infected.
- Wounds should be cleaned, and antibiotics should be given.

Because human teeth are not particularly sharp, most human bites cause a bruise and only a shallow tear (laceration), if any. Exceptions are on fleshy appendages, such as the ears, nose, and penis, which may be severed. The clenched-fist injury, or fight bite, which occurs on the knuckles of a person who punches another person in the mouth, is likely to become infected (see page 603). Hospitalization may be needed for administration of intravenous antibiotics. A clenched-fist cut frequently involves the finger tendon that passes over the knuckle. Sometimes the biting person transmits diseases, such as hepatitis. Transmission of the human immunodeficiency virus (HIV) is extremely unlikely because the concentration of the virus in saliva is lower than that in blood and because substances in saliva inhibit the virus's activity.

Symptoms

Bites are painful and usually produce a mark on the skin with the pattern of the teeth. Fight bites leave only a small, straight cut over a knuckle. A lacerated finger tendon often results in difficulty moving the finger in one direction. Infected bites become very painful, red, and swollen.

 Did You Know...

Transmission of HIV infection with a human bite wound is highly unlikely.

Treatment

Human bites are cleaned by flooding the wound with sterile salt water (saline) and cleansing it with soap and water. Severed parts can sometimes be reattached. Tears, except those involving the hand and those that have occurred many hours ago, are surgically closed. All people with human bites that have broken the skin are given antibiotics by mouth to prevent infection. Infected bites are treated with antibiotics and often must be opened surgically to examine and clean the wound. If the biting person is known or suspected to have a disease that may be spread by biting, preventive treatment may be necessary.

Snake Bites

- Venomous snakes in the United States include pit vipers (rattlesnakes, copperheads, and cottonmouths) and coral snakes.
- Severe envenomation can cause damage to the bitten extremity, bleeding, and vital organ damage.
- Venom antidote is given for serious bites.

Bites from nonpoisonous snakes rarely produce any serious problems. About 25 species of venomous (poisonous) snakes are native to the United States. The venomous snakes include pit vipers (rattlesnakes, copperheads, and cottonmouths) and coral snakes. Of the roughly 45,000 snakebites that occur in the United States each year, fewer than 8,000 are from venomous snakes, and about six people die. Fatal snakebites are much more common outside the United States.

In about 25% of all pit viper bites, venom is not injected. Most deaths occur in children, older people, and people who are untreated or treated too late or inappropriately. Rattlesnakes account for about 70% of poisonous snakebites in the United States and for almost all of the deaths. Copperheads and, to a lesser extent, cottonmouths account for most other poisonous snakebites. Coral snake bites and bites from imported snakes are much less common.

The venom of rattlesnakes and other pit vipers damages tissue around the bite. Venom may produce changes in blood cells, prevent blood from clotting, and damage blood vessels, causing them to leak. These changes can lead to internal bleeding and to heart, respiratory, and kidney failure. The venom of coral snakes affects nervous system activity but causes little damage to tissue around the bite. Most bites occur on the hand or foot.

> **Did You Know...**
> Snake bites can be terrifying but rarely cause deaths in the United States.

Symptoms

The symptoms of snake venom poisoning vary widely, depending on the following:

- The size and species of snake
- The amount and toxicity of the venom injected (related to the size and species of snake)
- The bite's location (the farther away from the head and trunk, the less dangerous)
- The person's age (very old and very young people are at higher risk)
- The person's underlying medical problems

Pit Vipers: Bites by most pit vipers rapidly cause pain. Redness and swelling usually follow within 20 to 30 minutes and can affect the entire leg or arm within several hours. People bitten by a rattlesnake may experience tingling and numbness in the fingers or toes or around the mouth and a metallic or rubbery taste in the mouth. Other symptoms include fever, chills, general weakness, faintness, sweating, anxiety, confusion, and nausea and vomiting. Some of these symptoms may be caused by terror rather than venom. Breathing difficulties can develop, particularly after Mojave rattlesnake bites. People may have a headache, blurred vision, drooping eyelids, and a dry mouth.

Moderate or severe pit viper poisoning commonly causes bruising of the skin 3 to 6 hours after the bite. The skin around the bite appears tight and discolored. Blisters, often filled with blood, may form in the bite area. Without treatment, tissue around the bite may be destroyed. The gums may bleed, and blood may appear in the person's vomit, stools, and urine.

Coral Snakes: Coral snake bites usually cause little or no immediate pain and swelling. More severe symptoms may take several hours to develop. The area around the bite may tingle, and nearby muscles may become weak. Muscle incoordination and severe general weakness may follow. Other symptoms may include double vision, blurred vision, confusion, drowsiness, increased saliva production, and speech and swallowing difficulties. Breathing problems, which may be extreme, may develop.

Diagnosis

Emergency medical personnel must try to determine whether the snake was poisonous, what species it was, and whether venom was injected. The bite marks sometimes suggest whether the snake was poisonous. The fangs of a poisonous snake usually produce one or two large punctures, whereas the teeth of nonpoisonous snakes usually leave multiple small rows of scratches. Without a detailed description of

Is That a Pit Viper?

Pit vipers have certain features that can help distinguish them from nonvenomous snakes:

- Triangular heads (like an arrowhead)
- Vertical slitlike pupils
- Pits between the eyes and nose
- Retractable fangs
- Rows of single scales across the underside of the tail

Nonvenomous snakes tend to have the following:

- Rounded heads
- Round pupils
- No pits
- No fangs
- Rows of double scales across the underside of the tail

If people see a snake with no fangs, they should not assume it is nonvenomous because the fangs may be retracted.

Pit Viper

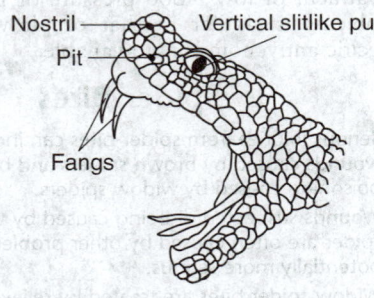

Nostril — Pit — Fangs — Vertical slitlike pupil

Nonvenomous Snake

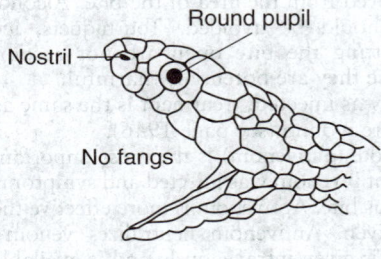

Nostril — Round pupil — No fangs

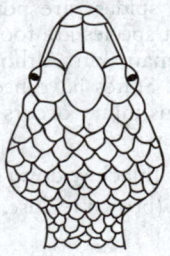

Triangular head

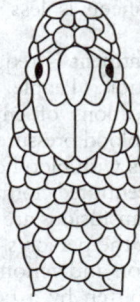

Rounded head

the snake, doctors may have difficulty determining the particular species that caused the bite. Envenomation is recognized by the development of characteristic symptoms. People who are bitten by a poisonous snake are generally kept in the hospital for observation for 6 to 8 hours to see if any symptoms develop. Doctors do various tests to assess the effects of the venom.

Treatment

First aid can be helpful before medical help arrives. People bitten by a poisonous snake should be moved beyond the snake's striking distance, kept as calm and still as possible, and taken to the nearest medical facility immediately. The bitten limb should be loosely immobilized and kept positioned just below heart level. Rings, watches, and tight clothing

---

What Is Serum Sickness?

Serum sickness is a reaction by the immune system against large amounts of foreign protein that have entered the bloodstream. A common source of such foreign protein is horse serum, an ingredient present in many venom antidotes (antivenoms) that are used to treat poisonous snake and spider bites and scorpion stings. Symptoms of serum sickness include fever, rash, and joint pains. Rarely, kidney damage and death can occur. Doctors treat serum sickness with antihistamines, such as diphenhydramine, and corticosteroids. Antivenoms that do not contain horse serum are unlikely to result in serum sickness.

---

should be removed from the area of the bite. Alcohol and caffeine should be avoided. Tourniquets, ice packs, and cutting the bite open are not recommended because they are potentially harmful.

If no venom was injected, treatment is the same as for any puncture wound (see page 1946).

Venom antidote (antivenom) is the most important part of treatment if venom was injected and symptoms indicate a serious bite. Antivenom is more effective the sooner it is given. Antivenom neutralizes venom's toxic effects. It is given intravenously and is available for all native poisonous snakes. Pit viper antivenom made from horse serum frequently causes serum sickness (an immune system reaction against foreign protein). Newer antivenom made of purified antibody fragments from sheep is less likely to cause serum sickness.

Intensive care unit treatment is required for people with severe envenomation. People are monitored closely, and the complications of envenomation are treated. People with low blood pressure are given fluids intravenously. If problems with blood clotting develop, fresh frozen plasma, concentrated clotting factors (cryoprecipitate), or platelet transfusions are given.

Prognosis depends on the person's age and overall health and on the location and venom content of the bite. Almost everyone bitten by a poisonous snake survives if treated early with appropriate amounts of antivenom.

Lizard Bites

The only two lizards known to be poisonous are the beaded lizard of Mexico and the Gila monster, present in Arizona; Sonora, Mexico; and adjacent areas. The venom of these lizards is somewhat similar in content and effect to that of some pit vipers, although symptoms tend to be much less severe, and bites are almost never fatal. Unlike most snakes, the Gila monster and beaded lizard clamp on firmly when they bite and chew the venom into the person rather than injecting it through fangs. The lizard may be difficult to dislodge.

Common symptoms include pain, swelling, and discoloration in the area around the bite as well as swollen lymph nodes. Weakness, sweating, thirst, headache, and ringing in the ears (tinnitus) may develop. In severe cases, blood pressure may fall.

Various suggestions for removing Gila monsters include the following:

- Forcing the jaws open with pliers
- Applying a flame under the lizard's chin
- Immersing the lizard and body extremity under water

Once the lizard has been detached, tooth fragments often remain in the skin and must be removed. Treatment of low blood pressure or blood clotting problems is similar to that of pit viper bites. A specific antivenom is not available.

Spider Bites

- Serious injuries from spider bites can include severe wounds caused by brown spiders and bodywide poisoning caused by widow spiders.
- Wounds suspected of being caused by the brown spider are often caused by other problems, some potentially more serious.
- Widow spider bites are treated by relieving symptoms and sometimes giving antivenom.
- Brown spider bites are treated by caring for the wound.

Almost all spiders are poisonous. However, the fangs of most species are too short or too fragile to penetrate human skin. Although at least 60 species in the United States have been implicated in biting people, serious injury occurs mainly from only two types of spiders:

- The widow (black widow) spider
- The brown (brown recluse, fiddleback, or violin) spider

Brown spiders are present in the Midwest and South Central United States, not in the coastal and Canadian border states, except when imported on clothing or luggage. Widow spiders are present throughout the United States. Although some people consider tarantulas dangerous, their bites do not seriously harm people. Spider bites cause fewer than three deaths a year in the United States, usually in children.

? Did You Know...

Although tarantulas are large and may appear frightening, their bites do not seriously harm people.

Symptoms

The bite of a **widow spider** usually causes a sharp pain, somewhat like a pinprick, followed by a dull, sometimes numbing, pain in the area around the bite. Cramping pain and muscle stiffness, which may be severe, develop in the abdomen or the shoulders, back, and chest. Other symptoms may include nausea, vomiting, sweating, restlessness, anxiety, headache, drooping and swelling of the eyelids, rash and itching, severe breathing problems, increased saliva production, and weakness.

The bite of a **brown spider** may cause little or no immediate pain, but some pain develops in the area around the bite within about an hour. Pain may be severe and may affect the entire injured area, which may become red and bruised and may itch. The rest of the body may itch as well. A blister forms, surrounded by a bruised area or by a more distinct red area that resembles a bull's-eye. Then the blister enlarges, fills with blood, and ruptures, forming an open sore (ulcer) that may leave a large crater-like scar. Uncommonly, nausea and vomiting, aches, fatigue, chills, sweats, blood disorders, and kidney failure develop.

Diagnosis

There is no way to identify a particular spider on the basis of its bite mark. Therefore, a specific diagnosis can be made only if the spider can be identified. Widow spiders are recognized by a red or orange hourglass-shaped marking on the abdomen. Brown spiders have a violin-shaped marking on their back. However, these identifying marks can be difficult to discern, and the spider is rarely retrieved intact, so the diagnosis is usually uncertain and based on symptoms. Many people mistake skin infections, some potentially serious (such as methicillin-resistant *Staphylococcus aureus* [MRSA] infections), or other disorders for spider bites.

Treatment

First-aid measures for a spider bite include cleaning the wound, placing an ice cube on the bite to reduce pain, and, if the bite is on an extremity, elevating the wound site.

For a **widow spider bite**, muscle pain and spasms can be relieved with muscle relaxants and analgesics. If the pain and spasms are severe, calcium given by vein (intravenously) may be required. Hot baths may relieve mild pain. Antivenom is given for severe poisoning. Hospitalization is usually required for people younger than 16 or older than 60 and for people with high blood pressure, heart disease, or severe symptoms.

> **? Did You Know...**
> Many people falsely assume that they were bitten by a spider when they really have another disorder, such as a skin infection.

Most **brown spider bites** heal without complications. Sores should be cleaned daily with a povidone-iodine solution and soaked 3 times a day in sterile salt water (saline). Moderately to severely damaged wounds may require surgical procedures.

Bee, Wasp, Hornet, and Ant Stings

- Stings by bees, wasps, hornets, and ants usually cause pain, redness, swelling, and itching.
- Allergic reactions are uncommon but may be serious.
- Stingers should be removed, and a cream or ointment can help relieve symptoms.

Stings by bees, wasps, and hornets are common throughout the United States. Some ants also sting. The average person can safely tolerate 10 stings for each pound of body weight. This means that the average adult could withstand more than 1,000 stings, whereas 500 stings could kill a child. However, one sting can cause death from an anaphylactic reaction (a life-threatening allergic reaction in which blood pressure falls and the airway closes—see page 1123) in a person who is allergic to such stings. In the United States, 3 or 4 times more people die from bee stings than from snakebites. A more aggressive type of honeybee, called the Africanized killer bee, has reached the southern and some southwestern states from South America. By attacking their victim in swarms, these bees cause a more severe reaction than do other bees.

In the South, particularly in the Gulf region, fire ants sting up to 40% of the people who live in infested areas each year, causing at least 30 deaths.

Symptoms

Bee, wasp, and hornet stings produce immediate pain and a red, swollen, sometimes itchy area about 1/2 inch (about 1 centimeter) across. In some people, the area swells to a diameter of 2 inches (5 centimeters) or more over the next 2 or 3 days. This swelling is sometimes mistaken for infection, which is unusual after bee stings. Allergic reactions may cause rash, itching all over, wheezing, trouble breathing, and shock.

The **fire ant sting** usually produces immediate pain and a red, swollen area, which disappears within 45 minutes. A blister then forms, rupturing in 2 to 3 days, and the area often becomes infected.

In some cases, a red, swollen, itchy patch develops instead of a blister. Isolated nerves may become inflamed, and seizures may occur.

Treatment

A bee may leave its stinger in the skin. The stinger should be removed as quickly as possible by scraping with a thin dull edge (for example, the edge of a credit card or a thin table knife). An ice cube placed over the sting reduces the pain. A cream or ointment containing an antihistamine, an anesthetic, a corticosteroid, or a combination of them is often useful. Severe allergic reactions are treated in the hospital with epinephrine, intravenous fluids, and other drugs.

People who are allergic to stings should always carry a preloaded syringe of epinephrine (available by prescription), which helps reverse anaphylactic or allergic reactions. Other stings are treated similarly to bee stings. People who have a history of anaphylactic reactions or a known allergy to insect bites should wear identification, such as a medical alert bracelet.

People who have had a severe allergic reaction to a bee sting sometimes undergo desensitization (allergen immunotherapy—see page 1114), which may help prevent future allergic reactions.

Puss Moth Caterpillar Stings

The venomous puss moth caterpillar (also called the asp) is present in the southern United States. It is teardrop shaped and has long silky hair, making it resemble a tuft of cotton or fur. When a puss moth caterpillar rubs or is pressed against a person's skin, its venomous hairs are embedded, usually causing severe burning and a rash. Pain usually subsides in about an hour. Occasionally, the reaction is more severe, causing swelling, nausea, and difficulty breathing.

People have gotten relief from puss moth caterpillar stings by putting tape on the site and pulling it off to remove embedded hairs. Use of a baking soda slurry or calamine lotion can be soothing, and an ice pack can ease pain. More severe reactions require immediate medical attention.

Insect Bites

Among the more common biting and sometimes bloodsucking insects in the United States are the following:

- Sand flies
- Horseflies
- Deerflies
- Blackflies
- Stable flies
- Mosquitoes
- Fleas
- Lice
- Bedbugs
- Kissing bugs
- Certain water bugs

None is venomous. The bites of these insects may be irritating because of the components of their saliva. Most bites result in nothing more than a small, red, itchy bump. Sometimes, people develop a large sore (ulcer), with swelling and pain. The most severe reactions occur in people who are allergic to the bites or who develop an infection after being bitten. Fleas can cause allergic reactions sometimes without biting.

The bite should be cleaned, and an ointment or cream containing an antihistamine, an anesthetic, a corticosteroid, or a combination may be applied to relieve itching, pain, and inflammation. People with multiple bites can take an antihistamine by mouth. People who are allergic to the bite should seek medical attention immediately or use an emergency allergy kit containing a preloaded syringe of epinephrine.

Tick and Mite Bites

Ticks carry many diseases. For example, deer ticks may carry the bacteria that cause Lyme disease (see page 1165). Other types of ticks may carry the bacteria that cause rickettsial or ehrlichial infections (see page 1202). The bites of pajaroello ticks, which are present in Mexico and the southwestern United States, produce pus-filled blisters that break, leaving open sores that develop scabs.

Mite infestations are common and are responsible for chiggers (an intensely itchy rash caused by mite larvae under the skin), scabies (see page 1312), other itchy rashes, and a number of other disorders. The effects on the tissues around the bite vary in severity.

Tick Paralysis

In North America, some tick species secrete a toxin that causes tick paralysis. A person with tick paralysis feels restless, weak, and irritable. After a few days, a progressive paralysis develops, usually moving up from the legs. The muscles that control breathing also may become paralyzed.

Tick paralysis is cured rapidly by finding and removing the tick or ticks. If breathing is impaired, oxygen therapy or a mechanical ventilator may be needed to assist with breathing.

Treatment

Ticks should be removed as soon as possible. Removal is best accomplished by grasping the tick with curved tweezers as close to the skin as possible and pulling it directly out. The tick's head, which may not come out with the body, should be removed, because it can cause prolonged inflammation. Most of the folk methods of removing a tick, such as applying alcohol, fingernail polish, or petroleum jelly or using a hot match, are ineffective and may cause the tick to expel infected saliva into the bite site.

Some mite infestations are treated by applying a cream containing permethrin or a solution of lindane. A cream containing a corticosteroid is sometimes used for a few days to reduce itching caused by mite infestations. If permethrin or lindane is used, it is given before the corticosteroid.

Centipede and Millipede Bites

Some of the larger centipedes can inflict a painful bite, causing swelling and redness. Symptoms rarely persist for more than 48 hours. Millipedes do not bite but may secrete a toxin that is irritating, particularly when accidentally rubbed into the eye.

An ice cube placed on a centipede bite usually relieves the pain. Toxic secretions of millipedes should be washed from the skin with large amounts of soap and water. If a skin reaction develops, a corticosteroid cream should be applied. Eye injuries should be flushed with water (irrigated) immediately.

Scorpion Stings

The stings of North American scorpions are rarely serious and usually result in pain, minimal swelling, tenderness, and warmth at the sting site. However, the bark scorpion (*Centruroides exilicauda* or *sculpturatus*), which is present in Arizona and New Mexico and on the California side of the Colorado River, has a much more toxic sting. The sting is painful, sometimes causing numbness or tingling in the area around the sting. Serious symptoms are more common in children and include

- Abnormal head, eye, and neck movements
- Increased saliva production
- Sweating
- Restlessness

Some people develop severe involuntary twitching and jerking of muscles. Breathing may become difficult.

The stings of most North American scorpions require no special treatment. Placing an ice cube on the wound reduces pain. A cream or ointment containing an antihistamine, an anesthetic, a corticosteroid, or a combination of them is often useful.

Centruroides stings that result in serious symptoms may require the use of sedatives, such as midazolam, given intravenously. *Centruroides* antivenom rapidly relieves symptoms, but it may cause a serious allergic reaction or serum sickness. The antivenom is available only in Arizona. It is given only if symptoms are severe.

In areas of the world where scorpions are more poisonous, such as Turkey, the Middle East, and India, stings are treated with drugs and methods that reduce symptoms and complications. Prazosin, an alpha-adrenergic blocking drug, is sometimes used. Antivenins to specific scorpion venoms are available, but their effectiveness has not been proven.

Marine Animal Stings and Bites

A variety of marine animals sting or bite.

STINGRAYS

Stingrays contain venom in spines located on the back of their tail. Injuries usually occur when a person steps on a stingray while wading in shallow ocean surf. The stingray thrusts its tail spine into the person's foot or leg, releasing venom. Fragments of the spine's covering may remain in the wound, increasing the risk of infection.

The wound from a stingray's spine is usually jagged and bleeds freely. Pain is immediate and severe, gradually diminishing over 6 to 48 hours. Many people with these wounds experience fainting spells, weakness, nausea, and anxiety. Vomiting, diarrhea, sweating, generalized cramps, breathing difficulties, and death are less common.

Treatment

Stingray injuries to an arm or leg should be gently flooded with salt water in an attempt to remove fragments of the tail spine. The spine should be removed only if it is at the skin surface and is not penetrating the neck, chest, or abdomen. Significant bleeding should be slowed by applying direct pressure. In the emergency department, doctors reexamine the wound for fragments of the spine. A tetanus shot may be needed, and the injured arm or leg should be elevated for several days. Some injured people are given antibiotics and may need surgery to close the wound.

JELLYFISH

Jellyfish belong to a group known as Cnidaria. Other Cnidaria include

- Sea anemones
- Corals
- Hydroids (such as the Portuguese man-of-war).

Cnidaria have stinging units (nematocysts) on their tentacles. A single tentacle may contain thousands of them. The severity of the sting depends on the type of animal. The sting of most species results in a painful, itchy rash, which may develop into blisters that fill with pus and then rupture. Other symptoms may include weakness, nausea, headache, muscle pain and spasms, runny eyes and nose, excessive sweating, and chest pain that worsens with breathing. Stings from the Portuguese man-of-war (in North America) and the box jellyfish (in Australia in the Indian and South Pacific oceans) have caused death.

Treatment

The first step in treating an injury caused by a jellyfish in the oceans of North America is rinsing with seawater to wash away venom from the skin. Any pieces of tentacles should be removed with tweezers or, after two pairs of gloves are put on, fingers. Vinegar should not be used as a rinse on injuries from the Portuguese man-of-war because it can cause additional venom to be released from nematocysts that have not yet stung ("unfired" nematocysts). In contrast, vinegar should be used for stopping additional "firings" of nematocysts from the more dangerous box jellyfish. Seawater should be used to rinse box jellyfish stings because fresh water will cause additional venom to be released.

For all types of stings, hot water or cold packs, whichever feels better to the person, can help relieve pain. At the slightest sign of breathing problems or altered awareness (including unconsciousness), medical help should be sought immediately.

MOLLUSKS

Mollusks include snails, octopuses, and bivalves (such as clams, oysters, and scallops). A few are venomous. The California cone (*Conus californicus*) is the only dangerous mollusk in North American waters. Its sting may cause pain, swelling, redness, and numbness in the area of the sting and may be followed by difficulty speaking, blurred vision, paralysis of muscles, respiratory failure, and cardiac arrest. The bites of North American octopuses are rarely serious. However, the bite of the blue-ringed octopus—present in Australian waters—although painless, produces weakness and paralysis that may be fatal.

Cone snails are a rare cause of envenomation among divers and shell collectors in the Indian and Pacific oceans. The snail injects its venom through a harpoon-like tooth when aggressively handled (for example, during shell cleaning or when placed in a pocket). The venom can cause temporary paralysis that is fatal on rare occasions.

Treatment

Cone snail stings can be immersed in warm water. First-aid measures seem to provide little help for injuries from California cone stings and blue-ringed octopus bites. If people with any type of mollusk envenomation develop trouble breathing, immediate medical help should be sought.

SEA URCHINS

Sea urchins are covered with long, sharp, venom-coated spines. Touching or stepping on these spines typically produces a painful puncture wound. The spines commonly break off in the skin and cause chronic pain and inflammation if not removed. Joint and muscle pain and rashes may develop.

Sea urchin spines should be removed immediately. Because vinegar dissolves most sea urchin spines, several vinegar soaks or compresses may be all that is needed to remove spines that have not penetrated deeply. Surgical removal may be required for imbedded spines. Because sea urchin venom is inactivated by heat, soaking the injured body part in hot water often relieves the pain.

Special Subjects

CHAPTER
312   The Science of Medicine and Clinical Trials

People expect doctors to use treatments that work well and to stop using those that do not. However, it is often difficult for doctors and other scientists to tell which treatments work. Making this distinction is part of the science of medicine and usually involves the conduction of clinical trials.

The Science of Medicine

Doctors have been treating people for many thousands of years. The earliest written description of medical treatment is from ancient Egypt and is over 3,500 years old. Even before that, healers and shamans were likely providing herbal and other remedies to the ill and injured. A few remedies, such as those used for some simple fractures and minor injuries, were effective. However, until very recently, many medical treatments did not work and some were actually harmful. Two hundred years ago, common remedies for a wide range of disorders included cutting open a vein to remove a pint or more of blood and giving various toxic substances to cause vomiting or diarrhea—all dangerous to a sick or injured person. A little over 100 years ago, along with mention of some useful drugs such as aspirin and digitalis, *The Merck Manual* mentioned cocaine as a treatment for alcoholism, arsenic and tobacco smoke as treatments for asthma, and sulfuric acid nasal spray as a treatment for colds. Doctors thought they were helping people. Of course, it is not fair to expect doctors in the past to have known what we know now, but why had doctors ever thought that tobacco smoke might benefit someone with asthma?

There were many reasons why doctors recommended ineffective (and sometimes harmful) treatments and why people accepted them. Typically, there were no alternatives. Doctors and sick people both often prefer doing something to doing nothing, people are comforted by turning problems over to an authority figure, and doctors often provide much-needed support and reassurance. Most importantly, however, doctors could not tell what treatments worked.

Cause and Effect: If one event comes immediately before another, people naturally assume the first is the cause of the second. For example, if a person pushes an unmarked button on a wall and a nearby elevator door opens, the person naturally assumes that the button controls the elevator. The ability to make such connections between events is a key part of human intelligence and is responsible for much of our understanding of the world. However, people often see connections where none exist. That is why athletes might continue to wear the "lucky" socks they had on when they won a big game or a student might insist on using the same "lucky" pencil to take exams. This way of thinking is also why some ineffective medical treatments were thought to work. For example, if an ill person's fever broke after the doctor drained a pint of blood or the shaman chanted a certain spell, people naturally assumed those actions must have been what caused the fever to break. To the person desperately seeking relief, getting better was all the proof necessary. Unfortunately, these apparent cause-and-effect relationships observed in early medicine were rarely correct, but they were enough to perpetuate centuries of ineffective remedies. How could this have happened?

People get better spontaneously. Unlike "sick" inanimate objects (such as a broken axe or a torn shirt), which remain damaged until repaired by someone, sick people often get well on their own (or despite their doctor's care) if the body heals itself or the disease runs its course. Colds are gone in a week, migraine headaches typically last a day or two, and food poisoning symptoms may stop in 12 hours. Many people even recover from life-threatening disorders, such as a heart attack or pneumonia, without treatment. Symptoms of chronic diseases (such as asthma or sickle cell disease) come and go. Thus, many treatments may seem to be effective if given enough time, and any treatment given near the time of spontaneous recovery may seem dramatically effective.

The placebo effect may be responsible. Belief in the power of treatment is often enough to make people feel better. Although belief cannot cause an underlying disorder, such as a broken bone or diabetes, to disappear, people who believe they are receiving a strong, effective treatment very often feel better. Pain, nausea, weakness, and many other symptoms can diminish. This effect happens even when the drug contains no active ingredients and can be of no possible benefit, as when a sugar pill (termed a placebo) is used (see page 77). What counts is the belief. An ineffective (or even harmful) treatment prescribed by a confident doctor to a trusting, hopeful person often results in remarkable improvement in the person. This improvement is termed the placebo effect. Thus, the person might see an *actual* (not simply misperceived) benefit from a treatment that has had no real effect on the disease itself.

Some people argue that the only important thing is whether a treatment makes people feel better. It does not matter whether the treatment actually "works," that is, affects the underlying disease. This argument may be reasonable when the symptom is the problem, as in many day-to-day aches and pains or in illnesses such as colds, which always go away on their own. In such cases, doctors do sometimes prescribe treatments for their placebo effect. However, when any dangerous or potentially serious disorder is present or when the treatment itself may have side effects, it is important for doctors not to miss an opportunity to prescribe a treatment that really does work.

How Doctors Try to Learn What Works

Because some doctors realized long ago that people can get better on their own, they tried to compare how different people with the same disease fared with or without treatment. However, until the middle of the 19th century, it was very difficult to make this comparison. Diseases were so poorly understood that it was difficult to tell when two or more people had the same disease. Doctors using a given term were often talking about different diseases entirely. For example, in the 18th and 19th centuries, the diagnosis of "dropsy" was given to people whose legs were swollen. We now know that swelling can result from heart failure, kidney failure, or severe liver disease—quite different diseases that do not respond to the same treatments. Similarly, numerous people who had fever and who were vomiting were diagnosed with "bilious fever." We now know that many different diseases cause fever and vomiting. Examples

are typhoid, malaria, and hepatitis. Only when accurate, scientifically based diagnoses became common—about 100 years ago—were doctors able to effectively evaluate treatments.

Comparing Apples to Apples: Even when doctors could reliably diagnose diseases, they still had to determine how to best evaluate a treatment.

Doctors realized they had to look at more than one sick person. One person getting better (or sicker) might be a coincidence. Achieving good results in a group of people is less likely to be due to chance. The larger the group, the more likely any observed effect is real. Thus, doctors typically compare results between a group of people who receives a study treatment (treatment group) and a group who receives an older treatment or no treatment at all (control group). Studies that involve a control group are called **controlled studies**.

At first, doctors simply gave all their patients with a certain illness a new treatment and then compared their results to those for people treated at an earlier time (either by the same or different doctors). For example, if doctors found that 80% of their patients survived malaria after receiving a new treatment, whereas previously only 70% survived, they would conclude that the new treatment was more effective. Studies that compare current treatment results to past results are called **retrospective or historical studies**.

A problem with historical studies is that the treatment group also has the benefit of other advances in medical care that had since been developed. It is not fair to compare the treatment results of people treated in 2006 with those treated in 1986. Medical advances in the intervening time may be responsible for any improvement in outcome. To avoid this problem with historical studies, doctors try to create treatment groups and control groups at the same time. Such studies are called **prospective studies**.

However, the biggest concern with all types of medical studies, including historical studies, is that similar groups of people should be compared. In the previous example, if the group of people who received the new treatment (treatment group) for malaria was made up of mostly young people who had mild disease and the previously treated (control) group was made up of older people who had severe disease, people in the treatment group may have fared better simply because they were younger and healthier. Thus, a new treatment could falsely appear to work better. Many other factors besides age and severity of illness also must be taken into account, such as

- The overall health of people being studied (people with chronic diseases such as diabetes or kidney failure tend to fare worse than healthier people)

- The specific doctor and hospital providing care (some may be more skilled and have better facilities than others)
- The percentages of men and women in the study groups (men and women may respond differently to treatment)
- The socioeconomic status of the people involved (people with more resources to help support them tend to fare better)

Doctors have tried many different methods to ensure that the groups being compared are as similar as possible. It might seem sensible to specifically choose people for treatment groups and control groups by matching them on various characteristics. For example, if a doctor was studying a new treatment for high blood pressure (hypertension), and one person in the treatment group was 42 years old and had diabetes, the doctor would try to ensure the placement of a 40-some-year-old person with hypertension and diabetes in the control group. These types of studies are called **case-control studies**. However, there are so many differences among people, including differences that the doctor does not even think of, that it is nearly impossible to intentionally create an exact match.

Perhaps surprisingly, the best way to ensure a match between groups is not to try at all. Instead, the doctor takes advantage of the laws of probability and randomly assigns (typically with the aid of a computer program) people who have the same disease to different groups. If a large enough group of people is divided randomly, the odds are that people in each group will have similar characteristics. Studies using such methods are called randomized. Prospective, **randomized studies** are the best way to make sure that a treatment or test is being compared between equivalent groups.

Eliminating Other Factors: Once doctors have created equivalent groups, they must make sure that the only difference they allow is the study treatment itself. That way, doctors can be sure that any difference in outcome is due to the treatment and not to some other factor, such as the quality or frequency of follow-up care.

Another factor relates to the placebo effect. People who know they are receiving an actual, new treatment rather than no treatment (or an older, presumably less effective treatment) often expect to feel better. Some people, on the other hand, may expect to experience more side effects from a new, experimental treatment. In either case, these expectations can exaggerate the effects of treatment, causing it to seem more effective or to have more complications than it really does.

To avoid the problems of the placebo effect, people in a study must not know whether they are receiving a new treatment. That is, they are "blinded." **Blinding** is usually accomplished by giving people in the control group an identical-appearing substance, usually a placebo—something with no medical effect. However, when an effective treatment for a disease already exists, giving the control group a placebo is not ethical. In those situations, the control group is given an established treatment. But whether a placebo or an established drug is used, the substance must appear identical to the study drug, except for the active ingredient. That is necessary so that people cannot tell whether they are taking the study drug. If the treatment group receives a red, bitter liquid, the control group should also receive a red, bitter liquid. If the treatment group receives a clear solution given by injection, the control group should receive a similar injection.

Because the doctor or nurse might accidentally let a person know what treatment they are receiving, it is better if all involved health care practitioners remain unaware of what is being given. This type of blinding is called **double-blinding**. Double-blinding usually requires a person separate from the study, such as a pharmacist, to prepare identical-appearing substances that are labeled only by a special number code. The number code is broken only after the study is completed.

An additional reason for double-blinding is that the placebo effect can even affect the doctor, who may unconsciously think a person receiving treatment is doing better than a person receiving no treatment, even if both are faring exactly the same. Not all medical studies can be double-blinded. For example, surgeons studying two different surgical procedures obviously know which procedure they are performing (although the people undergoing the procedures can be kept unaware). In such cases, doctors make sure that the people evaluating the outcome of treatment are blinded as to what has been done so they cannot unconsciously bias the results.

Choosing a Clinical Trial Design: The best type of clinical trial is prospective, randomized, placebo-controlled, and double-blinded. This design allows for the clearest determination of the effectiveness of a treatment. However, in some situations, this trial design may not be possible. For example, with very rare diseases, it is often hard to find enough people for a randomized trial. In those cases, retrospective case-control trials are often conducted.

What Participants Need to Know About Clinical Trials

Clinical trials are experiments designed to find out whether an intervention is safe and effective. The intervention is most often a drug but can also be a device, such as a pacemaker or stent, or a diagnostic tool, such as a blood test. Participation in a clinical trial is an option for many people who have serious illnesses, especially when no good treatments are available. Thousands of clinical trials are conducted each year and may take place at a variety of locations, including universities, hospitals, clinics, doctors' private offices, and professional clinical research sites.

The people who conduct clinical trials are called clinical researchers or investigators. Investigators are usually doctors who are paid to conduct the trials by the National Institutes of Health or by a pharmaceutical, biotechnologic, or medical device company. Investigators follow a detailed protocol that dictates who is eligible to participate in the trial, what interventions will be given or used, how often participants will be evaluated, and how data will be collected. Several thousand people typically participate in clinical trials for each new intervention before it becomes available to the general public.

Types of Clinical Trials: Clinical trial design can be complicated but typically follows the principles described above (see page 2025).

All interventions must be approved by the U.S. Food and Drug Administration (FDA) before they can be prescribed or used. The FDA's goal is to allow an intervention to be given to the general public only after that intervention has proved to be safe and effective in carefully designed clinical trials. The FDA requires three phases of clinical trials before approval is granted.

A phase I trial is the first time an intervention is used on people. Tests are conducted on a small group of healthy people to learn how the intervention acts in humans, including the side effects, and to learn what doses of drugs are safe. Because phase I trials involve healthy people, the participants receive no direct medical benefit, but their contribution to the health of others is significant.

If the intervention seems safe in a phase I trial, phase II trials are conducted. In phase II trials, the intervention is tested in a larger group of people who have the disease that the intervention is intended to treat. Phase II trials help researchers determine whether the intervention is safe for sick people and give an early determination of whether the intervention is effective. If the intervention is a drug, phase II trials help researchers determine what dose might be appropriate.

If safety is still satisfactory in phase II and the intervention seems effective, a phase III trial is conducted. In phase III trials, the intervention is given to or tested in a large group of people who have the disease being studied. In phase III, the new intervention is usually compared with the standard treatment, a placebo, or both.

Key Questions to Ask Before Participating in a Clinical Trial

- What is the main purpose of this trial?
- Does the trial involve a placebo or a treatment that is already on the market?
- How will the treatment be given to me?
- How long is the trial going to last?
- What will I be asked to do as a participant?
- What has already been learned about the trial treatment and have any trial results been published?
- Do I have to pay for any part of the trial? Will my insurance cover these costs?
- Is there any reimbursement for travel costs, parking, or child care?
- Will I be able to see my own doctor?
- If the treatment works for me, can I keep using it after the trial has ended?
- Can anyone find out whether I am participating in a clinical trial?
- Will I receive any follow-up care after the trial has ended?
- What will happen to my medical care if I stop participating in the trial?
- Do the trial doctor and investigator have any financial or special interest in the trial?
- What are the credentials and research experience of the trial doctor and trial staff?

Adapted from The Center for Information and Study on Clinical Research Participation, www.ciscrp.org.

It takes an average of 7 years for a promising drug to make its way through the clinical testing process. Many drugs, medical devices, and diagnostic tools never complete all 3 phases. Others do complete the 3 phases but are not approved for use because they fail to be effective or safe or both. Doctors also conduct clinical trials with interventions that have already been approved for use (sometimes termed phase IV trials). These trials may be done to compare two or more interventions or to test an intervention on a different disorder. In this case, 3 phases are not needed, but the clinical trial design is similar.

The Participation Experience

People have different reasons for wanting to participate in clinical trials. Some want the newest treatments, which they hope will be more effective than the current standard of care. Others participate

Elements of Informed Consent Documents

MAJOR ELEMENTS

- A statement explaining the trial's purpose, the procedures to be followed, the duration of participation, and any investigational treatments or procedures
- A description of foreseeable risks and discomforts to participants
- A description of benefits that the participant can reasonably expect
- A disclosure of any alternative treatments or procedures that might be advantageous to participants
- A statement about how participant confidentiality is maintained
- An explanation of compensation and whether medical treatments are available if injury occurs
- A list of contacts to answer trial-related questions and to help with research-related injuries
- A statement that participation is voluntary and that there is no penalty and no loss of benefits for refusing to participate

OTHER ELEMENTS WHEN APPROPRIATE

- A statement that there may be unforeseeable risks to the participant, embryo, or fetus—if the participant is or may become pregnant
- A list of circumstances under which the investigator may terminate a participant's enrollment
- A description of additional costs to the participant
- An explanation of the consequences and procedures if a participant decides to withdraw
- A statement that participants will be informed of significant new findings that might affect their willingness to participate
- The approximate number of participants enrolled in the trial

Adapted from The Food and Drug Administration, Code of Federal Regulations, Title 21, Section 50.25 (www.fda.gov).

certain minimum cholesterol or blood pressure level, a specific age range (between 40 and 65, for example), or the absence of pregnancy or certain diseases. Participants may be required to undergo an extensive screening process involving blood tests and other medical procedures.

Finding a Trial: Sometimes a person's doctor recommends participation in a clinical trial. This recommendation is particularly common for people who have cancer.

Trial recruitment ads run routinely in most major newspapers and on many local radio stations. Some local newspapers and newsletters now publish dedicated weekly sections listing clinical trials. Many communities have one or more research centers that consumers can call directly to get information or to get on a mailing list. Almost all clinical trials are listed at www.clinicaltrials.gov, a web site sponsored by the National Institutes of Health. Some web sites help match people to specific trials. For some top-rated organizations and web sites offering useful information about clinical trials, refer to Appendix IV (see page 2156).

In the Trial: Some people find it tedious to participate in a trial, especially if it lasts many months or requires frequent visits to the research site or frequent blood tests. Some trial protocols require participants to regularly telephone the trial nurse to report symptoms or to keep a medical diary at home as a condition of remaining in the trial.

Some trials are delayed, canceled by the sponsoring organization, or even stopped early once underway because certain participants do not fare well while taking or receiving the experimental treatment. Delays or cancellations can be hugely disappointing to people for whom the treatment brings relief. Also, after a clinical trial has ended, participants may no longer have access to an experimental treatment that was providing a real benefit.

Risks and Benefits

Deciding whether to participate in a clinical trial is an important and complicated decision. Both risks and benefits must be carefully considered.

Risks: First, participants should be aware that they are not guaranteed to receive the new treatment and may instead receive a placebo or older treatment.

A trial drug may have side effects and cause bad reactions ranging from headaches and sleeplessness to breathing difficulties or, on very rare occasions, even death. Although the researchers try to warn participants of all known side effects, unanticipated problems may develop.

The experimental treatment might not work as well as intended, possibly not even as well as standard treatment.

out of a desire to contribute to science. Still others may want access to free drugs and medical care.

Merely wanting to be in a clinical trial is not enough. Only people who are eligible for a particular trial can participate. Every trial has specific criteria that spell out the characteristics a participant must have to join, such as a type and stage of cancer, a

Benefits: There are also some very real benefits to clinical trial participation. If a treatment works as expected, participants could have a better outcome than with other treatments normally available to them. In some instances, participants have even been cured.

Volunteers typically receive excellent care in a manner that might otherwise cost thousands of dollars. Because participants are so well monitored, they tend to learn a great deal about their overall health and any underlying medical conditions. Sometimes there is an opportunity to build camaraderie with other participants, which may be particularly welcome by people who have rare or uncommon diseases. At a minimum, clinical trial participants can be sure that they are helping to advance medical science and public health.

Problems and Safeguards

In a very small fraction of situations, investigators in charge of clinical trials have acted unethically. One particularly shameful example is known as the Tuskegee experiments. Conducted around Tuskegee, Alabama, from 1932 to 1972, this study enrolled about 400 poor, mostly illiterate, African-American sharecroppers who had syphilis. These participants were not told that they had syphilis, and despite the widespread availability of the effective treatment penicillin, the Tuskegee investigators withheld penicillin and information about penicillin purely to continue to study how the disease progressed. Participants were also prevented from accessing syphilis treatment programs that were available to other people in the area. As a result of this horrendous breach of ethics and trust, several safeguards were put in place. Included in these safeguards are the establishment of Institutional Review Boards and the concept of informed consent.

Institutional Review Boards are specific committees in medical institutions that review proposed clinical trials involving humans. The purpose of these committees is to ensure that trials are conducted in an ethical manner and to avoid any unreasonable risks associated with the trial design. Only trials that have been approved by Institutional Review Boards are allowed to proceed.

Informed consent means that a person is given all the information needed to make an educated and informed decision as to whether to participate in a clinical trial. Information should describe all aspects of the trial, from its purpose to a statement about who pays for medical care to treat any research-related injuries. Informed consent documents tend to be lengthy (in some cases, dozens of pages long), technical, and hard to read. However, it is essential that participants read the documents carefully.

Participants should take the informed consent documents home, read them over several times, and discuss them with their personal doctor and family members. The doctor can help clarify some of the participation risks. Family members and friends particularly need to be involved if they will be providing transportation to the research center. After reviewing the informed consent documents carefully, participants should return to the investigator and trial coordinator and ask any further questions.

The protection of the safety and rights of clinical trial participants is a task shared by several government agencies as well as the Institutional Review Boards. However, to a large extent, participants—with the help of their doctor, family, and friends—must play an active part in their own protection. The Clinical Trial Participant's Bill of Rights can help people understand how to protect their rights during participation.

The Clinical Trial Participant's Bill of Rights

Any participant who gives consent to participate in a clinical trial or who is asked to give consent on behalf of another has the following rights:

- To be told the purpose of the clinical trial
- To be told about all the risks, side effects, or discomforts that might be reasonably expected
- To be told of any benefits that can be reasonably expected
- To be told what will happen during the trial and whether any procedures, drugs, or devices are different from those that are used as standard medical treatment
- To be told about available options and how such options may be better or worse than what is being studied in the clinical trial
- To be allowed to ask any questions about the trial before giving consent and at any time during the course of the trial
- To be allowed ample time, without pressure, to decide whether to consent to participate
- To refuse to participate, for any reason, before and after the trial has started
- To receive a signed and dated copy of the Informed Consent form
- To be told of any medical treatments available if complications occur during the trial

Adapted from The Center for Information and Study on Clinical Research Participation, www.ciscrp.org.

Clinical trial participants can always quit a trial if it proves to be uncomfortable or too inconvenient. In addition, a vigilant investigator and trial coordinator will insist that participants drop out if there are changes in their health—such as an allergic or strongly negative reaction to the trial intervention—that make the trial too risky for them to continue. Investigators may also stop a trial if participants in one of the groups seem to be having very positive or very negative outcomes compared with participants in the other group. For instance, if the trial intervention is very effective, the trial may be stopped so that all participants may receive the intervention and benefit. If the trial intervention is ineffective or harmful, the trial may be stopped so that no more of the participants are harmed.

313 Medical Decision Making

Making decisions about medical care is most effective when doctors and patients work together. The best and most appropriate decisions are reached when the doctor's experience and knowledge of medicine are combined with the patient's knowledge, wishes, and values. However, there are many challenges that can interfere.

Information Sources

Most doctors rely on their education and experience: what they have learned from their training, from their colleagues, and from diagnosing and treating people with similar problems. Doctors also read medical books and journals, consult with colleagues, and refer to other resources, such as authoritative health sites on the Internet, to get more information about specific problems and to keep up with new information generated by medical research. They also review recommendations (practice guidelines) published by groups of experts.

People who need health information rely on their doctors. But many people also turn to an ever-growing number of resources in print and on the Internet (see also page 23).

Research Studies: As new research findings are published, doctors evaluate the studies and consider how their findings might best be applied. Different types of studies provide different types of information.

- **A cross-sectional study** compares groups of people at the same point in time. Such a study may compare test results of people who do and do not have a given disease and is often used to evaluate how well tests help diagnose diseases.
- **A case-control study** compares the histories of people who do and do not have the condition that is being studied but otherwise seem to be similar. Such a study is often used to understand the cause or causes of an uncommon disease.

- In a **cohort study**, people are studied for a similar period of time, which varies from hours to decades, depending on what is being studied. A cohort study observes people with something in common (usually a disease) over time. This type of study may be used to determine the effect of a disease on people over time (prognosis).

A clinical trial is considered the most accurate type of study. In a controlled clinical trial, people entering the study are divided randomly (by chance) into two or more groups. One group of people receives a particular treatment or test, while the other groups (called control groups) receive different treatments or tests or no treatment or test at all. The random assignment ensures that the different groups are as similar as possible. That way, any difference in outcome is likely to be due to the treatment or test being studied rather than an underlying and potentially unknown difference between the groups (see page 2024).

 Did You Know...

Many of the resources doctors use are available to consumers.

A clinical trial in which people are randomly assigned to groups for evaluation is considered the most accurate type of research study.

Sometimes studies are done to compare the relative costs of different approaches to diagnosis and treatment. These studies are called cost-effectiveness or cost-benefit studies. They may help doctors consider the effects of decisions from society's perspective, but they may be less helpful when doctors are considering decisions for a particular person.

Because of differences in the way studies are planned and carried out, even studies that are intended to evaluate the same thing may produce conflicting results. One method to try to resolve these conflicts is to prepare a summary of the findings of all studies that pertain to the topic and rigorously compare and evaluate them. This type of study is called a systematic review. Another method that tries to resolve conflicting results of studies is called meta-analysis. A meta-analysis mathematically combines the results of many studies.

Medical Testing Decisions

Tests are done to screen for disease, diagnose disease, classify and measure the severity or stage of disease, and monitor the course of a disease, especially its response to treatment.

Screening Tests: Screening tests are used to try to detect a disease when there is no apparent evidence that a person has the disease. For example, most doctors recommend that women over 40 have a mammogram every year or every 2 years to look for breast cancer even if they have no breast lumps. Screening is based on the natural idea that outcome will be better if a disease is recognized and treated in its early stages. Although logical enough, this idea is not always correct. For some diseases, such as testicular cancer and ovarian cancer, there does not seem to be any difference in outcome between people whose disease is detected by screening and those whose disease is diagnosed after the first symptoms appear.

A further potential problem with screening tests is that the results usually require confirmation by a more definitive test. For example, women who have a mammogram with abnormal results need to have a breast biopsy. Such definitive tests are often invasive, uncomfortable, and sometimes a bit dangerous. For example, a lung biopsy can cause a collapsed lung. Because results of screening tests are sometimes abnormal in people without disease (which is common because no test is 100% accurate), some people undergo an unnecessary test that might harm them.

Clinical trials are necessary to tell which screening tests are effective and which people should undergo them. Despite these concerns, it is clear that for some diseases such as high blood pressure and cervical cancer, screening saves lives. To be useful, tests used for screening must be accurate, be relatively inexpensive, pose little risk, cause little or no discomfort, and improve outcomes.

> **? Did You Know...**
>
> A screening test may not be appropriate if early treatment does not make a difference in the outcome of the disease being screened for or if the disease is very rare.

Diagnostic, Classification, and Monitoring Tests: Diagnostic tests confirm or rule out a disease when a doctor suspects that a person has the disease. For example, a doctor who suspects serious heart disease might recommend cardiac catheterization. This test is a good diagnostic test but not a good screening test because it is expensive, can have serious side effects, and is uncomfortable. However, these drawbacks are outweighed by the need for this test when the presence or absence of disease must be confirmed.

Some tests are used to classify and measure the severity of a disease that has already been diagnosed. Results may lead to more specific and effective choices for treatment. For example, after a diagnosis of breast cancer is confirmed, additional tests are done to determine if and where the cancer has spread.

Tests are also used to monitor the course of a disease over time, often to determine the response to treatment. For example, blood tests are done periodically in people who take thyroid hormone to treat hypothyroidism to determine whether the hormone dose best meets their needs. A decision about how often such testing is needed is made based on the person's situation.

Doing Tests and Interpreting Results: When deciding whether to recommend testing for a disease, especially to make a diagnosis, doctors estimate how likely it is that a person has the disease (the pre-test probability of disease). In coming up with an estimate for a specific person, doctors may consider the following:

- Information about the disease in their practice area, including how common the disease is (prevalence) and how many new cases of the disease occur during a specific period of time (incidence)
- A person's particular characteristics (risk factors, such as family history of the disease) that increase or decrease the likelihood of being affected

With this information, doctors can then select the best test to screen for or confirm the presence of the disease.

Doctors must also be prepared to determine what test results may mean. Unfortunately, tests are not perfect. Results are sometimes normal in people who have the disease being tested for. That is, tests have false-negative results. Results are sometimes abnormal in people who do not have the disease being tested for. That is, tests have false-positive results. Therefore, important characteristics of a test are its sensitivity (the likelihood that results will be abnormal in people with the disease being tested for) and its specificity (the likelihood that results will be normal in people without the disease). Doctors can mathematically combine the pre-test

Does Everyone Need a Test?

In short, no. Although many people find medical tests reassuring, test results are not always right. Doctors must consider what they know about the disease they are testing for, what they know about the test itself, and what they know about the person.

For example, parents are concerned that their 4-year-old daughter might have a urinary tract infection (UTI) because she is walking holding her thighs together. In the office, the doctor discovers that the girl is not urinating more frequently or complaining of pain with urination. Her physical examination is normal. Based on these findings, the doctor thinks the likelihood of a UTI is very low, about 5%, and reassures the parents that nothing needs to be done unless other symptoms develop. The parents say they would feel better if the doctor did a test. Would a test help the doctor?

In this case, even a fairly accurate test may give confusing results. Suppose the doctor did a test that had a sensitivity of 90% and specificity of 90% for UTI (typical figures for many medical tests). Sensitivity of 90% means that done in 100 people *with* a UTI, the test will correctly be positive in 90. Specificity of 90% means that done in 100 people *without* a UTI, the test will correctly be negative in 90 but give a false-positive result in 10. This test seems very accurate (and is). But would it help this little girl? If the test result is positive, does that mean the child actually has a UTI? Suppose the doctor tests 1000 children who each have a 5% chance of having a UTI. The test's sensitivity and specificity (plus some simple arithmetic) tell the doctor that there will be 45 children who have true-positive test results, but 95 children who have false-positive results. That means that a positive result *in this particular child* is twice as likely to be false as it is to be true. Thus, even a positive test result should not change the doctor's decision not to treat. Because the doctor would not do anything different, it makes no sense to do the test in the first place.

It would be a different story if the doctor thought the likelihood of a UTI was 50-50. Because only 10% of test results (positive or negative) would be false, testing would be helpful.

Before doing a test, doctors weigh the potential harm of the test against the potential benefit of the information the test may provide. Doctors must also consider how the results will be used. It may not be useful to do a test if the results will not change the recommended treatment. For example, if a test is being considered to determine whether a particular treatment is an option for a person, but the person has already decided not to undergo that treatment, the test need not be done.

Treatment Decisions

Before recommending a course of action, doctors weigh the potential risk of harm from a treatment against its potential benefit.

Benefit: Sometimes the benefit of treatment is to decrease symptoms—for example, to reduce pain. Benefit may also be improved function—for example, being able to walk farther. At times, benefit is cure of a disease. At other times, a treatment reduces the likelihood of future undesirable events, such as complications of a disease.

For example, doctors may consider recommending a particular drug to reduce the risk of a stroke. They evaluate the results of a controlled clinical trial in which 2,000 people were studied. The results show that of 1,000 people given the drug, 20 have a stroke despite taking the drug. The study also shows that of the other 1,000 people in the study who are not given the drug (are given a placebo), 40 have a stroke. The results of the study could be expressed as showing that the drug cut the risk of stroke in half because 20 is half of 40 (50% decrease in *relative* risk). However, the results could also be expressed as showing that only 20 people of 1,000 benefited (2% decrease in *absolute* risk). It sounds much more impressive to say the risk of stroke is cut in half than to say there was a 2% decrease in risk.

Risk: Risk is the likelihood that a harmful outcome will occur. When describing risk of harm, absolute versus relative risk should be evaluated. In the example above, perhaps the drug that prevents stroke caused severe bleeding in 3% of people. Although 3% does not sound like much of a risk, it means that 30 people of every 1,000 who took the drug had severe bleeding.

People and their doctors must carefully choose which statistics they use to help make decisions. Obviously, contrasting "50% improvement" against "3% chance of serious harm" makes treatment sound like a good option. However, the same numbers also mean that the treatment benefited 20 of 1,000 people but harmed 30. Stated this way, the treatment does not sound like a good option. In this case, people

probability of disease with the results of the test and with information about the test's sensitivity and specificity to more accurately estimate the likelihood that the person has the disease (post-test probability).

Another characteristic of a test is its reliability. A highly reliable test gives the same result when a person undergoes the test more than once, unless the disease being tested for has actually lessened or worsened. Results from a less reliable test may change randomly.

must weigh the severity of the harm of treatment against the severity of the illness. For example, if a stroke is severe, leaving people unable to talk or care for themselves, and the drug-induced bleeding requires only some blood transfusions but no surgery and is not fatal, people may accept the higher risk of bleeding to avoid the lower but more serious risk of stroke.

> **? Did You Know...**
>
> Doctors weigh the potential risks against the potential benefits of treatment before they recommend a treatment.
>
> The results of research studies must be carefully evaluated to determine whether the results apply to a particular person.

Research studies provide information only about the average risk of harm and benefit. But average effects do not always tell doctors how a person will respond to a treatment. Because of this uncertainty, many scientific studies try to determine characteristics of people (such as age, other disorders they have, and blood test results) that can better identify those who are more likely to benefit from or be harmed by a treatment.

Participating in Decision Making

To participate fully in the medical decision making process, people need to work closely with their doctors. People may wish to obtain additional information about a recommended test or treatment before making a decision (see page 23). Information can be obtained from

- Pamphlets, brochures, and other materials doctors provide
- Publications, such as books, newsletters, and magazines, designed to explain medical information to consumers
- The Internet

People should read the information carefully, keeping in mind the potential sources of bias in the information. For example, anecdotal information may indicate a treatment is helpful, but the treatment may not be helpful for everyone. These resources may generate additional questions for people to discuss with their doctors (see page 19). People may

also want to consult with another doctor, particularly one who has additional expertise (that is, get a second opinion—see page 21).

People should also be clear in expressing their choices to their doctors, especially if they have conditions, such as a terminal illness, that may make it impossible for them to express their wishes at some point later on (see page 69).

Realities of Decision Making

Whenever a decision must be made about diagnosis or treatment, two tasks must be accomplished. The first is to choose information resources that are most appropriate to help determine the best course of action. The second is to apply what is learned to the person's situation.

There are several challenges. One challenge is time. Many decisions must be made quickly. Doctors and people with medical conditions may not have enough time to gather and evaluate all the information available. Another challenge is quality of information. Not all information or recommendations in books, web sites, and even published research studies are correct. Other information may be correct but apply only to some people and not to others. Doctors must help people weigh the quality of information. For example, doctors may feel that their personal experience merits more trust than information gleaned from some Internet sources.

Doctors must judge the potential effects of any diagnostic recommendations. They must help people weigh the consequences of overlooking a serious condition even if the diagnosis is unlikely.

The same type of reasoning is used in deciding about treatments. Doctors will probably not recommend treatments that may have serious side effects for people who have a mild condition. Conversely, if the condition is grave but cure is possible, potential side effects may be worth the risk.

Doctors and the people they are treating may not share the same perceptions of risk. A person who hears about a possible serious side effect of a drug may be very concerned, regardless of how rarely the side effect occurs. The doctor may not be as concerned if the possibility of that side effect is remote. Or the doctor may not understand that what might seem to be a relatively minor side effect for most people may cause great problems for a particular person. For example, a person who drives for a living may be more concerned about taking a drug that can cause drowsiness.

Often, the balance between the risk of the disease and its treatment is not clear-cut. A doctor may judge the risks and benefits of a treatment differently than the person being treated does. People should discuss these differences in judgment with their doctors. Understanding risks can also help a person weigh options. A doctor may outline several approaches and ask the person to help decide among them. By evaluating the relative and absolute risks of the various choices and then factoring in personal values, a person can make more informed choices about medical care.

CHAPTER

314 Common Imaging Tests

Imaging tests provide a picture of the body's interior—of the whole body or part of it. Most imaging tests are painless, relatively safe, and noninvasive (that is, they do not require an incision in the skin or the insertion of an instrument into the body).

Imaging tests may use the following:

- Radiation, as in x-rays, computed tomography (CT), and radionuclide scanning
- Sound waves, as in ultrasonography
- Magnetic fields, as in magnetic resonance imaging (MRI)
- Substances that are swallowed, injected, or inserted to highlight or outline the tissue or organ to be examined

Risks of Radiation

Radiation, usually as x-rays, is a valuable tool in diagnosis. Different diagnostic tests require different amounts of radiation, but most of them use low doses that are generally considered safe. For example, the radiation dose from one chest x-ray is more than 100 times lower than the average yearly dose of radiation from the environment (from cosmic radiation and natural isotopes—see page 1984). However, if people have many diagnostic tests that use low doses or several tests that use high doses, they may be exposed to a relatively large amount of radiation. Exposure to radiation is cumulative, regardless of the interval between tests. Such exposure increases the risk of cancer and sometimes damages tissues. When planning diagnostic tests, doctors consider a person's total (lifetime) exposure to radiation—the person's total radiation dose. However, the benefit of a diagnostic test often outweighs the potential risks.

About 70% of radiation exposure from imaging tests comes from CT. The radiation dose for CT is hundreds of times the dose for most plain x-rays. Still, even when CT is done, the risk is low for adults, and health is unlikely to be affected. However, the risk is higher in certain situations: during early childhood, during pregnancy (particularly early), and for certain tissues (such as breast tissue in young women, abdominal tissue, and the thyroid gland).

To minimize risks, doctors do the following:

- Use tests that do not require radiation, such as ultrasonography or MRI, when possible
- Recommend diagnostic tests that use radiation, particularly high doses (as in CT) and particularly in young children, only when such tests are necessary
- Take precautions to limit radiation exposure during tests (for example, shielding vulnerable parts of the body, such as the thyroid gland or a pregnant woman's abdomen) when possible

During Early Childhood: The risks from radiation are higher in young children because children live longer, giving cancers more time to develop. Also in children, cells are dividing more rapidly, and rapidly dividing cells are more susceptible to damage by radiation. About 18 of every 10,000 1-year-olds who have CT of the abdomen (which uses one of the highest doses of radiation) eventually develop cancer caused by the radiation.

When children require diagnostic tests, parents should talk to the doctor about the risks and about possible use of tests that do not require radiation. If tests that use radiation are necessary, parents can help minimize the risks by asking about the following:

- Using the lowest possible dose to make the diagnosis (for example, sometimes low-resolution scans, which use less radiation, can be used)
- Limiting exposure to the smallest possible area of the body
- Limiting the number of scans done

During Pregnancy: Pregnant women should be aware that radiation from imaging tests has risks for the fetus. If women need to have an imaging test, they should tell their doctor whether they are or may be pregnant. However, x-rays, if necessary, are done in pregnant women. During diagnostic tests, the examiner protects the fetus from exposure to radiation by covering the woman's abdomen with a lead apron.

COMPARING RADIATION DOSES FOR DIFFERENT TESTS[*]

IMAGING TEST	NUMBER OF CHEST X-RAYS NEEDED TO GET THE SAME DOSE	TIME NEEDED TO GET THE SAME DOSE FROM THE ENVIRONMENT
Chest x-ray (from front to back)	1	2.4 days
X-ray of the lumbar spine	35	84 days
CT of the head	100	243 days
CT of the abdomen	500	3.3 years
Mammography	15	30–60 days

[*]These doses account for how much radiation is delivered and how susceptible the body part exposed to radiation is to radiation damage.

The risk to the fetus depends on when during the pregnancy a test is done. The risk is greatest when organs are being formed, during the 5th to 10th weeks of pregnancy. At this time, radiation can cause birth defects. Earlier during pregnancy, the most likely problem to develop is a miscarriage. After the 10th week, miscarriages and birth defects are less likely.

The risk to the fetus also depends on what part of the mother's body is x-rayed. X-rays of body parts that are far away from the fetus, such as the wrists and ankles, expose the fetus to less radiation than x-rays of closer parts, such as the lower back. Also, x-rays of smaller body parts, such as fingers and toes, require less x-ray energy than x-rays of larger body parts, such as the back and pelvis. Because of these facts, plain x-rays that do not involve the abdomen have little risk, regardless of when they are done, particularly if a lead shield is worn over the uterus. Thus, if x-rays are necessary (for example, to evaluate a broken bone), the benefit usually outweighs the risk.

Contrast Agents

During imaging tests, contrast agents may be used to distinguish one tissue or structure from its surroundings or to provide greater detail. Contrast agents include substances that can be seen on x-rays (called radiopaque dyes) and substances that are used in magnetic resonance imaging (called paramagnetic contrast agents).

A radiopaque dye absorbs x-rays and thus appears white on x-rays. It is typically used to show blood vessels or the interior of the gastrointestinal, biliary, or urinary tract. Usually, the dye is injected into a vein (intravenous contrast), taken by mouth (oral contrast), or inserted through the anus (rectal contrast). With some tests, dye is injected into an artery through a catheter or into a joint through a needle. The dye used depends on what type of test is done and which body part is being evaluated.

Most radiopaque dyes that are injected into a vein contain iodine (iodinated contrast agents). Dyes that contain barium are used only in the gastrointestinal tract.

Before a test that uses a dye, people may be asked to refrain from eating for several hours and from drinking for 1 hour. After the test, drinking extra fluids for the rest of the day is recommended.

When some dyes are injected, people may feel a warm sensation throughout the body. Other dyes may cause a cold sensation at the injection site. Dyes taken by mouth may have an unpleasant taste.

Paramagnetic contrast agents change the magnetic properties of particles in a way that increases the contrast between different tissues, making the images clearer. These agents usually contain gadolinium.

Side Effects: Generally, radiopaque dyes are very safe. However, a few people have an allergic-type reaction or kidney damage after a dye is used, usually when it is given intravenously.

Allergic-type reactions vary in severity:

- Mild, such as nausea, flushing, or itching
- Moderate, such as a rash, vomiting, or chills
- Severe and life threatening (anaphylactoid), such as a swollen throat that interferes with breathing, wheezing, very low blood pressure, or an abnormal heart rate

At the first sign of a reaction, use of the contrast agent is stopped. Mild or moderate reactions are treated with the antihistamine diphenhydramine, given intravenously. Severe reactions may be treated with oxygen, fluids given intravenously, epinephrine, or other drugs, depending on the type of reaction.

Allergic-type reactions are most likely to occur in people who have many other allergies, who have asthma, or who have previously had allergic-type reactions after a radiopaque dye was used. If people have had several severe reactions to dyes, an imaging test that does not require a dye should be done instead. If a dye must be used, drugs (diphenhydramine and a corticosteroid) may be given before the test to prevent a reaction. People who previously have had a reaction to a contrast agent should tell their doctor before an imaging test is done.

Kidney damage (contrast nephropathy) may occur in people with certain conditions:

- Impaired kidney function
- Dehydration
- Age over 70
- Diabetes
- Heart failure
- High blood pressure (hypertension)
- Multiple myeloma
- Use of drugs that can damage the kidneys

In over 99% of people, the kidney damage causes no symptoms and goes away within 1 week or so. Fewer than 1% have lasting damage, and only some of those require kidney dialysis.

If tests that require radiopaque dyes must be used, people are given fluids intravenously before and after the dye is given. A low dose of the dye is used if possible. People who have had impaired kidney function for a long time may be given acetylcysteine the day before and the day the dye is given.

Paramagnetic contrast agents usually have no side effects. However, in a few people who have severe kidney disease or who are undergoing dialysis, these agents may cause a life-threatening disorder called nephrogenic systemic fibrosis.

Angiography

In angiography, x-rays are used to produce detailed images of blood vessels. It is sometimes called conventional angiography to distinguish it from computed tomography (CT) angiography and magnetic resonance angiography. During angiography, doctors can also treat disorders of blood vessels.

Angiography can provide still images or motion pictures (called cineangiography). Cineangiography can show how fast blood travels through blood vessels.

Angiography, although invasive, is relatively safe.

Procedure

Before the procedure, people are usually asked to refrain from eating and drinking for 12 hours. For the procedure, people lie on an x-ray table. Because the table may be tilted, straps may be applied across the chest and legs. X-ray cameras can be positioned as needed. Electrodes are placed on the chest to monitor the heart. Blood pressure and oxygen levels in blood are also monitored.

After injecting a local anesthetic, a doctor makes a small incision, typically in the arm or groin. Then a thin, flexible tube (catheter) is inserted, usually into an artery, and is threaded through blood vessels to the area being evaluated. When the catheter is in place, a radiopaque dye (which can be seen on x-rays) is injected. The dye flows through the blood vessels and outlines them. The images appear on a video screen and are recorded. Thus, doctors can assess the structure of blood vessels and identify any abnormalities present.

Before angiography, people are often given a sedative intravenously to help them relax and remain calm, but they remain conscious during the procedure. During the procedure, people may be asked to take deep breaths, hold their breath, or cough. People should report any discomfort they feel. Angiography may take less than an hour or several hours, depending on the area of the body being evaluated and the type of the examination or procedures being done. It is usually done as an outpatient procedure.

If the catheter is inserted into an artery, the insertion site must be steadily compressed for 10 to 20 minutes after all the instruments are removed. Compression reduces bleeding and bruises. People may need to lie flat for several hours after the procedure to help prevent bleeding. Sometimes they need to stay overnight in the hospital. For the remainder of the day, they are advised to rest and to drink extra fluids to help eliminate the dye from the body.

Uses

Angiography is used to check for abnormalities in blood vessels. Abnormalities may include blockages, narrowing, abnormal tangled clumps of arteries and veins (arteriovenous malformations), inflammation (vasculitis), bulges (aneurysms) in a weakened blood vessel wall, and tears (dissection) in a blood vessel wall.

During angiography, procedures to treat the abnormalities detected can sometimes be done:

- Narrowed arteries can be widened.
- Blockages can be removed.
- A tube made of wire mesh (stent) can be placed to keep an artery open.
- Tears or weakened areas in a blood vessel can be repaired.

Variations

Arteriography: This term refers to imaging of arteries. It is the most common type of angiography.

Venography: This term refers to imaging of veins.

Digital Subtraction Angiography: X-ray images of arteries are taken before and after a radiopaque dye is injected. Then a computer subtracts one image

COMMON TYPES OF ANGIOGRAPHY

TYPE	AREA TO BE EVALUATED	USES
Coronary angiography	Blood vessels of the heart With cardiac catheterization, the heart itself	To diagnose coronary artery disease and other heart disorders To determine whether angioplasty or coronary artery bypass surgery is feasible To determine the severity of a heart disorder To identify the cause of chest pain, shortness of breath, or certain other symptoms To clarify the specific structure of a person's heart before heart valve replacement surgery
Pulmonary angiography	Blood vessels of the lungs	To diagnose pulmonary embolism (blockage by blood clots in the pulmonary arteries, which lead from the heart to the lungs)
Aortography	Aorta	To check for the following: ▪ Bulges in a weakened wall (aneurysms) ▪ Tears in the lining (dissection) ▪ Leakage of the valve between the aorta and left ventricle (aortic regurgitation)
Cerebral angiography	Blood vessels of the brain	To check for the following: ▪ Narrowed or blocked blood vessels (which can cause a stroke) ▪ Aneurysms ▪ Abnormal tangled clumps of arteries and veins (arteriovenous malformations) ▪ Inflammation of blood vessels (vasculitis)
Fluorescein angiography	Blood vessels of the eye	To evaluate damage to the retina due to diabetes (diabetic retinopathy) or macular degeneration To evaluate the retina before laser therapy
Peripheral arteriography	Arteries of the arms, legs, and trunk, except the aorta and arteries of the heart	To check for the following: ▪ Narrowing or blockages ▪ Aneurysms ▪ Abnormal channels between an artery and a vein (arteriovenous fistulas) ▪ Abnormal tangled clumps of arteries and veins (arteriovenous malformations)

from the other. Images of structures other than arteries (such as bones) are thus eliminated. As a result, the arteries can be seen more clearly.

Disadvantages

For some people, the procedure is uncomfortable. In a few people, allergic-type reactions to the dye occur. The injection site may bleed, become infected, or be painful. Rarely, the catheter damages a blood vessel. Serious complications, such as shock, seizures, kidney damage, and sudden stopping of the heart's pumping (cardiac arrest), are very rare. Sometimes during cardiac catheterization, the heart skips beats or slows briefly. The risk of complications is higher in older people, although it is still low.

The dose of radiation used in angiography can vary, from about 77 to 263 times as much as that used in two plain x-rays of the chest.

Angiography is not always readily available. It must be done by highly skilled people.

Computed Tomography

In computed tomography (CT), an x-ray source and x-ray detector rotate around a person. In modern scanners, the x-ray detector usually has 4 to 64 or more rows of sensors that record the x-rays that pass through the body. Data from the sensors represent a series of x-ray images taken from multiple angles all around the person. However, the images are not viewed directly but are sent to a computer. The computer converts them into images that resemble 2-dimensional slices (cross-sections) of the body. (Tomo means slice in Greek.) The computer can also construct 3-dimensional images from the recorded images. CT used to be called CAT (computed axial tomography).

Procedure

For CT, a person lies on a motorized table that is moved through the opening of a doughnut-shaped scanner. The person is moved continuously through the scanner as these devices rotate around the person. For some CT scans, the table moves incrementally and stops when each scan (slice) is taken. For other CT scans, the table moves continuously during scanning. Because the person is moving in a straight line and the detectors are moving in a circle, the series of images appear to be taken in a spiral fashion around the person, hence the term spiral (helical) CT.

People should wear clothing that has no buttons, snaps, zippers, or other metal in it over the area to be scanned and should remove any jewelry. Such items are not dangerous but may block x-rays and distort the image. During the test, they must remain still and periodically hold their breath when the x-rays are taken so that the images are not blurred. People may hear whirring sounds during the procedure. The procedure, depending on the area examined and how modern the scanner is, usually takes from only a few seconds to a few minutes. CT of the chest takes less than a minute, and people have to hold their breath only once and only for a few seconds.

For CT, people may be given a contrast agent (see page 2035). Contrast agents are substances that can be seen on x-rays (called radiopaque dyes) and help distinguish one tissue from another. The dye may be injected into a vein, taken by mouth, or inserted through the anus. The dye used depends on what type of test is done and which body part is being evaluated.

CT can be done as an outpatient procedure. People can resume their usual activites immediately after the test.

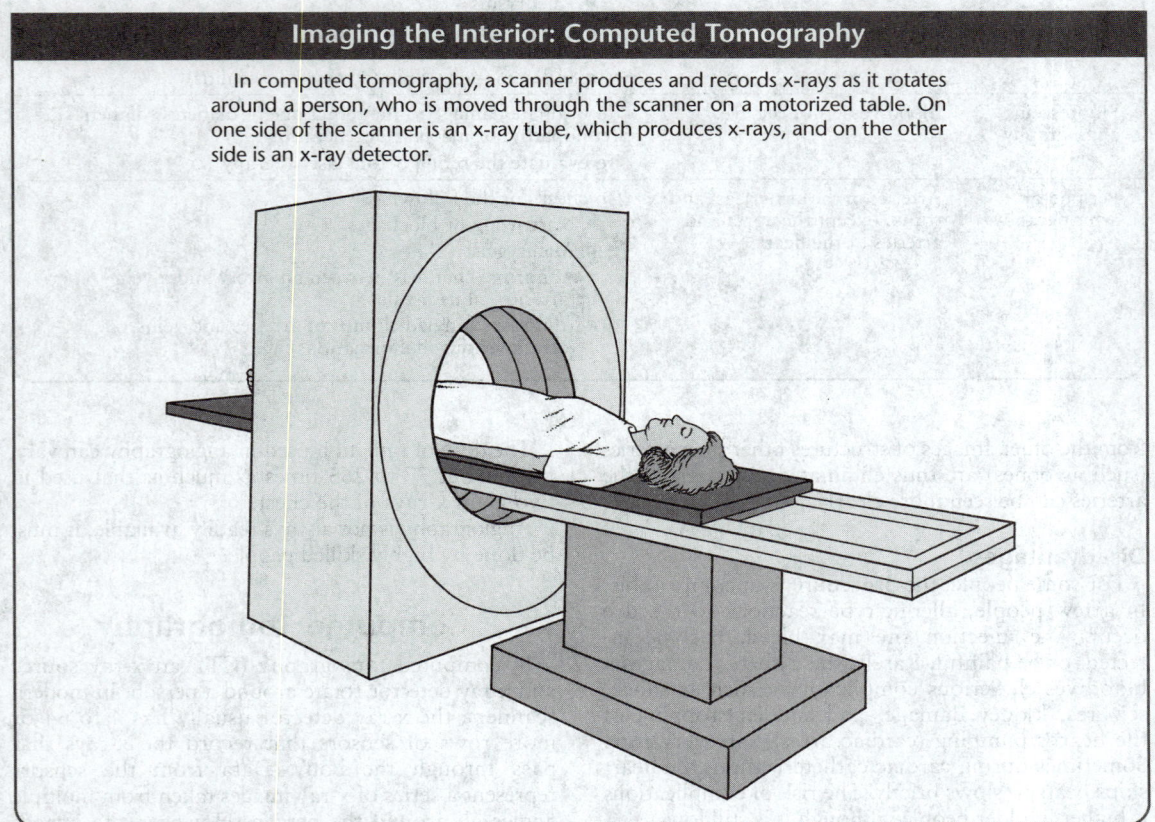

Imaging the Interior: Computed Tomography

In computed tomography, a scanner produces and records x-rays as it rotates around a person, who is moved through the scanner on a motorized table. On one side of the scanner is an x-ray tube, which produces x-rays, and on the other side is an x-ray detector.

SOME DISORDERS DETECTED BY COMPUTED TOMOGRAPHY

BODY SYSTEM	DISORDERS
Brain and spinal cord	Bleeding within the brain Birth defects Brain abscesses Brain tumors Hydrocephalus Strokes (ischemic) Ruptured or herniated disks Spinal fractures
Gastrointestinal tract	Appendicitis Blockages in the intestine Diverticulitis Pancreatitis Tumors
Eyes	A foreign body in the eye Infections in the eyeball and infections around the eye socket (orbit) Tumors of the eye socket or optic nerve
Heart and blood vessels	Aortic aneurysm Aortic dissection
Kidneys and urinary tract	Bleeding in or around the kidneys Stones in the kidneys or urinary tract Tumors in or around the kidneys
Liver	Fatty liver (excess fat in the liver) Liver tumors
Lungs	Bronchiectasis (widened airways) Emphysema Lung tumors Pneumonia Pulmonary embolism
Muscles and bones	Fractures (sometimes)

Uses

The highly detailed images provide more detail about tissue density and location of abnormalities than plain x-rays, so doctors can precisely locate structures and abnormalities. CT often enables the examiner to distinguish between different types of tissue, such as muscle, fat, and connective tissues. Thus, CT can provide detailed images of specific organs not visible on plain x-rays and is more useful for imaging most structures in the brain, head, neck, chest, and abdomen.

CT can detect and provide information about disorders in almost every part of the body. For example, doctors can use CT to detect a tumor, measure its size, precisely locate it, and determine how far it has spread into nearby tissues. CT can also help doctors monitor the effectiveness of treatment (such as antibiotics for a brain abscess or radiation therapy for a tumor).

Variations

CT Angiography: This procedure uses CT and a radiopaque dye to produce 2- and 3-dimensional images of blood vessels, including the arteries that supply the heart (coronary arteries). The dye is injected into a vein (not an artery as in conventional angiography), usually in the arm. Images are taken rapidly and are timed so that they show the dye flowing through the blood vessels being evaluated.

The computer digitally removes all tissues except blood vessels from the images.

CT angiography is used to detect the following:

- Narrowing or blockages (such as blood clots) in arteries
- Bulges (aneurysms) and tears (dissections) in large arteries
- Abnormal blood vessels that carry blood to tumors

CT angiography is commonly used instead of conventional angiography because it is safe and less invasive (it does not require insertion of a catheter in an artery). CT angiography shows abnormalities in blood vessels about as accurately as magnetic resonance angiography, but slightly less accurately than conventional angiography. CT angiography usually takes only 1 to 2 minutes.

? Did You Know...

Most radiation exposure in medicine comes from computed tomography (CT).

Before CT, people should discuss its risks and benefits with their doctors.

Disadvantages

Typically, CT of the abdomen uses about 500 times the amount of radiation used for a chest x-ray. CT now accounts for most exposure to man-made radiation in the general population and for about 70% of radiation exposure in medical practice. Therefore, the doctor and person should carefully weigh the benefit of each CT procedure against the risks (see page 2034). Generally, CT is avoided when possible in pregnant women unless there is no good alternative. Use of CT in children should be limited as much as possible.

The radiopaque dye used in CT angiography contains iodine. A few people have a mild to severe allergic reaction or kidney damage after such dyes are injected (see page 2035). People who have had reactions to radiopaque dyes should let their doctor know before CT angiography is done.

In some countries and in some areas of the United States, CT is not readily available.

Magnetic Resonance Imaging

In magnetic resonance imaging (MRI), a strong magnetic field and very high frequency radio waves are used to produce highly detailed images. MRI does not use x-rays and is usually very safe.

Procedure

For MRI, a person lies on a motorized table that is moved into the narrow interior of a large tubular scanner, which produces an extremely strong magnetic field. Normally, protons (positively charged parts of an atom) in tissues are in no particular arrangement. But when protons are surrounded by a strong magnetic field, as in an MRI scanner, they line up with the magnetic field. Then, the scanner emits a pulse of radio waves, which momentarily knocks all the protons out of line. As the protons line up with the magnetic field again, they release energy (called signals). The strength of the signal varies by tissue. The MRI scanner records these signals. A computer is used to analyze the signals and produce images.

Examiners can change how various tissues appear on a scan by varying the radio wave pulses, the strength and direction of the magnetic field, and other factors. For example, fat tissue appears dark on one type of scan and bright on another. These different scans provide complementary information, so more than one is often obtained.

A contrast agent containing gadolinium (a paramagnetic contrast agent) may be injected into a vein or a joint. Gadolinium agents change the magnetic field in a way that makes images clearer.

Before the test, people remove most or all of their clothing and are given a gown that has no buttons, snaps, zippers, or other metal on it to wear. All metal objects (such as keys and jewelry) and other objects that could be affected by the magnetic field (such as credit cards) should be left outside the MRI scanning room. People must lie still when images are taken and may have to hold their breath at times. Because the scanner makes loud banging noises, people may be given headphones or ear plugs to wear. A scan may take 20 to 60 minutes. After the test, people can resume their usual activities immediately.

Uses

MRI is preferred to computed tomography (CT) when doctors need more detail about soft tissues—for example, to image abnormalities in the brain, spinal cord, muscles, and liver. MRI is particularly useful for identifying tumors in these tissues. It can measure certain molecules in the brain that distinguish a brain tumor from a brain abscess. It can also identify abnormalities in female reproductive organs and fractures in the hip and pelvis. MRI helps doctors evaluate joint abnormalities (such as tears in ligaments or cartilage in the knee) and sprains. MRI helps doctors evaluate bleeding and infection.

MRI is also used when the risks of CT are high. For example, MRI may be preferred in people who have had a reaction to the radiopaque dye used in CT and in pregnant women (because of risks to the fetus).

MRI done after a gadolinium contrast agent is injected into a vein helps doctors evaluate inflammation, tumors, and blood vessels. Injecting this agent into a joint helps doctors get a clearer picture of joint abnormalities, particularly if they are complex (as in injuries or degeneration of ligaments and cartilages in the knee or a ruptured or herniated disk).

Variations

Functional MRI: This technique detects metabolic changes that occur when the brain is active. Thus, it can show which areas of the brain are active when a person does a specific task, such as reading, writing, remembering, calculating, or moving a limb.

Perfusion MRI: With this technique, doctors can estimate blood flow in a particular area. This information can be useful during a stroke, to determine whether parts of the brain are deprived of blood.

Diffusion-Weighted Imaging: This technique detects changes in water movement in brain cells that are not functioning normally. It is used primarily to identify early stroke.

Magnetic Resonance Spectroscopy: This technique uses radio waves that are emitted almost continuously rather than in pulses as in conventional MRI. Magnetic resonance spectroscopy is used to detect brain disorders, such as seizure disorders, Alzheimer's disease, and brain tumors and abscesses. It can distinguish between the dead debris inside an abscess and multiplying cells inside a tumor. This technique is also used to evaluate metabolic disorders in muscles and the nervous system.

Magnetic Resonance Angiography (MRA): MRA, like conventional angiography and CT angiography, can provide detailed images of blood vessels. However, it is safer and easier to do. Often, MRA can be done without injection of a contrast agent.

MRA can show blood flow through arteries and veins or blood flow only in one direction and thus show only arteries or only veins. As in CT angiography, a computer is used to remove all tissues except the blood vessels from the image.

Sometimes a gadolinium contrast agent is injected into a vein to outline blood vessels. The examiner carefully times the scanning so that the images are taken when gadolinium is concentrated in the blood vessels being evaluated.

MRA is used to evaluate blood vessels of the brain, heart, kidneys, arms, and legs. It is used to detect the following:

- Aortic aneurysms
- Aortic dissection

- Narrowed arteries in the limbs
- Blood clots in veins of the limbs and pelvis

Magnetic Resonance Venography: This term refers specifically to MRA of veins. It is often used to detect a blood clot in a vein that carries blood away from the brain (cerebral venous thrombosis) and to monitor the effect of treatment on this disorder.

Echo Planar Imaging: This ultrafast technique produces sequences of images in seconds. It can be used to image the brain, heart, and abdomen. Because it is fast, movement by the person being examined does not blur the images as much. Also, the technique can provide information about how tissues are functioning.

Disadvantages

MRI images usually take longer to produce than CT images. Thus, CT may be better in emergencies, such as serious injuries and stroke. MRI is also more expensive than CT.

Space in the MRI scanner is small and enclosed, making some people feel claustrophobic, even people who usually are not anxious about confined spaces. Some obese people have difficulty fitting within the scanner. Some MRI scanners (called open MRI scanners) have an open side and a larger interior. In them, people may feel less claustrophobic, and obese people may fit more easily. The images produced in open MRI scanners may be inferior to those produced by enclosed scanners depending on the magnet strength, but they can still be used to make a diagnosis. People who are anxious about MRI can be given an antianxiety drug, such as alprazolam or lorazepam, 15 to 30 minutes before scanning.

Usually, MRI is not used if people have certain materials (such as shrapnel) in specific parts of their body or implanted devices that can be affected by powerful magnetic fields. These devices include some cardiac pacemakers, defibrillators, cochlear implants, and magnetic metallic clips used to treat aneurysms. The magnetic field used in MRI can cause an implanted device to move, overheat, or malfunction. The device is more likely to be affected if it was implanted within the previous 6 weeks (because scar tissue, which can help hold the device in place, has not yet formed). These devices can also distort MRI images. Some devices, such as common dental implants, an artificial hip, or rods used to straighten the spine, are not affected by MRI. Before MRI is done, people who have any implanted devices should tell their doctor, who can determine whether imaging is safe.

The MRI magnetic field is very strong and always on. Thus, if a metal object (such as an oxygen tank or an IV pole) is near the entrance of the scanning room, the object may be pulled into the scanner at high speed. The person being evaluated may be injured, and separating the object from the magnet may be impossible.

Gadolinium contrast agents can cause headache, nausea, pain and a sensation of cold at the injection site, distortion of taste, and dizziness. These agents are much less likely to cause severe reactions than the radiopaque dyes used in conventional and CT angiography. However, gadolinium agents can cause a severe, life-threatening disorder called nephrogenic systemic fibrosis in people who already have severe kidney problems or who are undergoing dialysis. In nephrogenic systemic fibrosis, the skin, connective tissue, and organs thicken. As a result, red or dark patches may develop on the skin, the skin may feel tight, movement is difficult and limited, and organs may malfunction.

Plain X-Rays

X-rays are high-energy radiation waves that can penetrate most substances (to varying degrees). In low doses, x-rays are used to produce images that help doctors diagnose disease. In high doses, x-rays (radiation therapy) is used to treat cancer. X-rays may be used alone as plain x-rays or combined with other techniques, such as computed tomography (CT).

Procedure

For x-ray imaging, a person is positioned so that the body part to be evaluated is between the x-ray source and a device that records the image. The examiner goes behind a screen that blocks x-rays and runs the x-ray machine for only a few seconds. The person must remain still when the x-ray is taken. Several x-rays may be taken to obtain images from different angles.

An x-ray beam is passed through the part body to be evaluated. Different tissues block different amounts of the x-rays, depending on the tissue's density. The x-rays that pass through are recorded on a film or radiation detector plate, producing an image that shows the different levels of tissue density. The denser the tissue, the more x-rays it blocks and the whiter the image:

- Metal appears completely white (radiopaque).
- Bone appears almost white.
- Fat, muscle, and fluids appear as shades of gray.
- Air and gas appear black (radiolucent).

 Did You Know...
Radiation exposure from x-rays is very small.

Uses

Plain x-rays are typically the first imaging test done to evaluate the arms, spine, legs, or chest. These body parts contain important structures with very different densities that are easily distinguished on x-rays. Thus, x-rays are used to detect the following:

- Fractures: The almost white bone contrasts clearly with the gray muscles around it.
- Pneumonia: The black air in the lungs contrasts clearly with the white infected tissues, which block the x-rays.
- Blockages of the intestine: The black air in the blocked intestine contrasts clearly with the gray surrounding tissues.

Variations

X-Rays With a Radiopaque Dye: Plain x-rays can be done after a radiopaque dye (contrast agent) is given, usually by injection, by mouth, or into the rectum.

In conventional angiography, x-rays are taken after a dye is injected into blood vessels.

Before x-rays of the gastrointestinal tract, people may be asked to swallow barium or gastrografin (opaque substances) in a liquid or food. The x-rays then show the esophagus, stomach, and small intestine outlined by the barium or gastrografin. Or, an examiner may inject barium through a tube inserted into the anus (barium enema), then carefully pump air into the lower part of the intestine (colon) to expand it. Barium makes ulcers, tumors, blockages, polyps, and diverticulitis easier to see. A barium enema may cause mild to moderate crampy pain and an urge to defecate.

Fluoroscopy: This technique produces images that show motion, similar to those of a video camera. Fluoroscopy can show organs or structures as they function: the heart beating, the intestines moving food along, or the lungs inflating and deflating. Fluoroscopy is commonly used to determine whether a catheter is correctly placed in the heart during electrophysiologic testing (for abnormal heart rhythms) and during coronary catheterization. When the gastrointestinal tract is evaluated, a radiopaque dye, such as barium, is usually given by mouth.

Disadvantages

For plain x-rays, each image requires only a very small amount of radiation. For chest x-rays, the amount of radiation exposure with a single image is similar to the amount most people get from the environment in 2.4 days (background radiation exposure—see page 1984). However, some x-ray tests require several images, a high dose of radiation for each image, or both. As a result, the total radiation exposure is higher. For example, for x-rays of the lower back, done in a series, the amount of radiation equals about 3 months of background exposure. For mammography, the amount equals about 1 to 2 months of background exposure. Fluoroscopy usually requires high doses of radiation, so other imaging tests are done instead when possible.

Examiners take precautions to minimize a person's exposure to radiation. Women who are or could be pregnant should tell their doctor. Then, the examiner can take all possible precautions to shield the fetus from exposure. To evaluate the abdomen or pelvis of a pregnant woman, the doctor can sometimes substitute an imaging test that does not use radiation, such as ultrasonography. However, plain x-rays that do not involve the abdomen or pelvis usually expose the uterus to only very small amounts of radiation.

Some particular tests have other risks. For example, barium swallowed or inserted by enema may cause constipation.

Radionuclide Scanning

In radionuclide scanning, radionuclides are used to produce images. A radionuclide is an unstable atom that becomes more stable by releasing energy as radiation. Most radionuclides release high-energy photons as gamma rays (which are similar to x-rays). Radionuclides are also used to treat certain disorders, such as thyroid disorders.

Procedure

For scanning, a radionuclide is combined (or labeled) with a substance that accumulates in a specific part of the body. Different substances are used depending on which part of the body is to be evaluated. A substance may accumulate because the body uses (metabolizes) them, as for the following:

- Iodine is used to make thyroid hormones and thus accumulates in the thyroid gland.
- Diphosphonate accumulates where bone is repairing or rebuilding itself.

Or a substance may abnormally accumulate in a specific area, as for the following:

- Red blood cells accumulate in the intestine when the intestine is bleeding rapidly.
- White blood cells accumulate in areas that are inflamed or infected.

The combination of the radionuclide and the substance used to label it is called a radioactive tracer. With imaging, doctors can see where the tracer collects and gives off radiation, which is detected by special scanners or cameras, such as a gamma camera. The camera produces a flat image of where the tracer collects. Sometimes a computer analyzes the radiation to produce a series of 2-dimensional images that look like slices of the body.

Because the body metabolizes many of the substances used, radionuclide scanning can sometimes provide information about how a tissue is functioning, as well as what it looks like.

Usually, the tracer is injected in a vein, but for some tests, the tracer is swallowed, inhaled, or injected under the skin (subcutaneously) or into the joint. Imaging is done after the tracer has had time to move to the target tissues (which may be almost immediately or take up to several hours).

Before some tests (such as a gallbladder scan), the person is asked to refrain from eating and drinking for several hours. Clothing does not need to be removed. Sometimes the person lies on a motorized table, and the camera rotates around the person. The person must lie still during the scanning, which usually takes about 15 minutes. However, sometimes a scan needs to be repeated after a time, often hours later. After the test, drinking extra fluids to help the body eliminate the radionuclide is recommended. Normal activities can be resumed immediately.

Uses

Radionuclide scanning can be used to evaluate many parts of the body: thyroid gland, liver and gallbladder, lungs, urinary tract, bone, brain, and certain blood vessels. Various radionuclides are used to image different parts of the body or types of disorders, as for the following:

- **Blood flow to the heart:** Thallium is used to show blood flow through the arteries that carry blood to the heart. Thus, it can help doctors evaluate coronary artery disease. To determine how the heart functions when it is working hard, doctors sometimes use thallium during stress testing, usually by having the person walk or run on a treadmill. This test may also indicate how well the heart is pumping. The test can be done after a heart attack to help doctors estimate prognosis.
- **Bone:** Because technetium collects in bone, it is used to image the skeleton. It is used to check for cancer that has spread (metastasized) to bone and for bone infections.
- **Inflammation:** Technetium or other radionuclides are used to label white blood cells, which gather at sites of inflammation or infection. This test helps doctors identify inflammation and infection.
- **Bleeding:** Technetium is used to label red blood cells. This test helps doctors locate bleeding in the intestine.

Radionuclide scanning is also used to check for certain cancers, such as lung cancer that has spread to the liver, thyroid cancer, and colorectal cancer.

Variations

Single-Photon Emission Computed Tomography (SPECT): SPECT is similar to computed tomography but uses radionuclide emissions rather than x-rays. A rotating gamma camera takes images from many different angles (tomograms), each representing a slice of the body, and a computer is used to construct them into 2- and 3-dimensional images. These images help doctors more precisely locate structures and abnormalities.

Depending on the area being evaluated, people may be asked to restrict what they eat or drink before the test. The test usually takes 30 to 90 minutes.

Disadvantages

The amount of radiation exposure from radionuclide scanning depends on which radionuclide is used and how much is used. For example, with a lung scan, the dose is similar to that used in about 75 chest x-rays. Other scans may involve even more radiation.

Radionuclide scanning can take hours to do because of the need to wait between injection and scan. Sometimes the images are not very clear.

Because the radiation can affect a fetus, women who are pregnant or may be pregnant should tell their doctor.

POSITRON EMISSION TOMOGRAPHY

Positron emission tomography (PET) is a type of radionuclide scanning. In PET, a substance that the body uses (metabolizes), such as glucose or oxygen, is labeled with an atom (called a radionuclide) that releases positively charged particles of radiation called positrons. Positrons collect in a specific area of the body. The more active the tissue, the more positrons it collects and uses and the more radiation it gives off.

The PET scanner contains several rings of detectors that record the radiation released and produce color tomographic images of the area. The intensity of the color indicates how active the tissue is. The resulting scan shows different levels of activity in different intensities of color. Thus, PET can provide information about a tissue's function and can identify abnormal tissues, which may be more or less active than normal tissues. However, PET does not show anatomic and structural detail of tissues and organs as well as most other types of imaging tests.

Procedure

Before the procedure, people may be asked not to consume alcohol, caffeine, tobacco products, or any drugs that might affect mental function (such as sedatives).

For PET, a person lies on a table, and the labeled substance is injected in the person's vein. The substances take about 30 to 60 minutes to reach the area being evaluated. The table is then positioned so that area being evaluated is within the large circular opening of the PET scanner.

The person is asked to lie flat during most of the test, which may take 45 to 60 minutes. Depending on the area of the body being evaluated, the person may be asked to do certain activities, such as mental tasks to stimulate activity in the brain.

Uses

PET is used to evaluate blood flow and activity in the heart and brain. PET can show how well the heart functions, which can help determine whether a person is a candidate for coronary artery bypass graft surgery or a heart transplant. A PET scan of the brain can also show which areas of the brain are most active during certain activities—for example, during mathematical calculations.

PET can show where a cancer is and where it has spread. PET helps doctors evaluate lung cancer, colorectal cancer, esophageal cancer, head and neck cancer, lymphoma, and melanoma. It helps doctors determine whether enlarged lymph nodes in people with cancer are due to the spread (metastasis) of the cancer or to another abnormality.

PET is used in research to provide information about seizure disorders and to help doctors diagnose Alzheimer's disease, Parkinson's disease, transient ischemic attacks, and strokes.

Variations

PET Computed Tomography (PET-CT): This procedure provides detailed 2-dimensional images showing anatomy (via CT) and function (via PET). The two images (CT and PET images) can be viewed separately, or one may be overlaid on top of the other. This technique is particularly useful for cancers in body parts that have many different tissues close together, such as the neck and pelvis. It helps precisely locate the cancer and can detect early recurrences. This test usually takes less than 1 hour.

Disadvantages

The amount of radiation exposure from PET is similar to that from CT.

Because radionuclides used in PET give off radiation for only a short time, PET can be done only if the radionuclide is produced at a nearby location and can be obtained quickly. PET is relatively expensive and not widely available.

Ultrasonography

Ultrasonography uses high-frequency sound (ultrasound) waves to produce images of internal organs and other tissues. A device called a transducer converts electrical current into sound waves, which are sent into the body's tissues. Sound waves bounce off structures in the body and are reflected back to the transducer, which converts the waves into electrical signals. A computer converts the pattern of electrical signals into an image, which is displayed on a monitor and recorded on film, on videotape, or as a digital computer image. No x-rays are used.

Ultrasonography is painless, relatively inexpensive, and considered very safe, even during pregnancy.

Procedure

If the abdomen is being examined, people may be asked to refrain from eating and drinking for several hours before the test.

Usually, the examiner places thick gel on the area to ensure good sound transmission, and a handheld transducer is placed on the skin and moved over the area to be evaluated. To evaluate some body parts, the examiner inserts the transducer into the body—for example, into the anus to image the prostate gland or into the vagina to better image the uterus and ovaries. To evaluate the heart, the examiner sometimes attaches the transducer to a viewing tube called an endoscope and passes it down the throat into the esophagus. This procedure is called transesophageal echocardiography.

After the test, usual activites can usually be resumed immediately.

> **? Did You Know...**
> Ultrasonography and magnetic resonance imaging (MRI) do not use radiation.

Uses

Ultrasound images are acquired rapidly enough to show the motion of organs and structures in the body in real time (as in a movie). For example, the motion of the beating heart can be seen, even in a fetus. Ultrasonography is effectively used to check for growths and foreign objects that are close to the body's surface, such as those in the thyroid gland, breasts, testes, and limbs, as well as some lymph nodes. Because sound waves are blocked by gas (for example, in the lungs or intestine) and by bone, using ultrasonography to image structures deeper in the body is more difficult. It can be done only when there is no gas or bone between the transducer and the area being evaluated.

Ultrasonography is commonly used to evaluate the following:

- **Heart:** For example, to detect abnormalities in the way the heart beats, structural abnormalities such as defective heart valves, and abnormal enlarge-

ment of the heart's chambers or walls (ultrasonography of the heart is called echocardiography)
- **Gallbladder and biliary tract:** For example, to detect gallstones and blockages in the bile ducts
- **Urinary tract:** For example, to distinguish benign cysts from solid masses (which may be cancer) in the kidneys or to detect blockages such as stones or other structural abnormalities in the kidneys, ureters, or bladder
- **Female reproductive organs:** For example, to detect tumors and inflammation in the ovaries, fallopian tubes, or uterus
- **Pregnancy:** For example, to evaluate the growth and development of the fetus and to detect abnormalities of the placenta (such as a misplaced placenta, called placenta previa)

Ultrasonography can also be used to guide doctors when they remove a sample of tissue for a biopsy. Ultrasonography can show the position of the biopsy instrument, as well as the area to be biopsied (such as a mass). Thus, doctors can see where to insert the instrument and can guide it directly to its target.

Variations

Doppler Ultrasonography: This procedure uses changes that occur in the frequency of sound waves when they are reflected from a moving object (called the Doppler effect). In this case, the moving objects are red blood cells in the blood. Thus, Doppler ultrasonography can be used to evaluate blood flow—how fast it flows, which direction it flows in, and whether blood is flowing through blood vessels. It can detect blocked blood vessels, especially in leg veins, and narrowed arteries, especially the carotid arteries in the neck, which carry blood to the brain.

Color Doppler Ultrasonography: For this test, color is superimposed on the shades-of-gray image of blood flow produced by Doppler ultrasonography. The color indicates direction of blood flow. Red indicates flow toward and blue indicates flow away from the transducer.

Color Doppler ultrasonography can help assess the risk of stroke because it helps doctors identify and evaluate narrowing or blockage of arteries in the neck and head. The procedure is useful for evaluating people who have had a transient ischemic attack or stroke and people who have risk factors for atherosclerosis but no symptoms.

Disadvantages

Insertion of the transducer into the body may cause some discomfort. Rarely, when a transducer is inserted, tissue is damaged, causing bleeding or infection.

315 Hospital Care

People may be admitted to a hospital when they have a serious or life-threatening problem (such as a heart attack) or when a disorder (such as heart failure) suddenly worsens. They may go to the hospital's emergency department when a less serious problem (such as a sprained ankle) requires immediate attention. Or they may be scheduled for admission to a hospital by a doctor because they need certain tests, intensive treatment, or surgery.

A hospital can be a frightening and confusing place. Often, care occurs quickly and without explanation. Knowing what to expect can help people cope and actively participate in their care during their stay. Understanding more about what hospitals do and why they do it can help people feel less intimidated by their hospital experience, more in control, and more confident about their health when they are discharged home.

The Emergency Department: For many people, hospital care begins with a visit to the emergency department. When and how to go to an emergency department are important (see page 19). When people do go to the emergency department, they should bring their medical information. Of particular importance is a list of all drugs being taken, including over-the-counter drugs, prescription drugs, and dietary supplements (such as vitamins, minerals, and medicinal herbs). A copy of their most recent medical summary and records of recent hospital stays are also helpful, although many people do not have these records. In such cases, the emergency department staff typically obtains the information from the primary care doctor, the hospital records department, or both.

Being Admitted to the Hospital

People are admitted to a hospital only when appropriate treatment cannot be provided in another place (such as at home or in an outpatient surgery center). The main goal of hospitalization is to restore or improve health so that people can return home. Thus, hospital stays are intended to be relatively short and to enable people to be safely discharged to home or to another health care setting where treatment can be completed. A doctor—the primary care doctor, a specialist, or an emergency department doctor—determines whether people have a medical problem serious enough to warrant admission to the hospital.

The first step in admission is registration. Sometimes registration can be done before arriving at the hospital. Registration involves filling out forms that provide the following:

- Basic information (such as name and address)
- Health insurance information
- Telephone numbers of family members or friends to contact in case of an emergency
- Consent to be treated
- Consent to release information to insurance companies
- Agreement to pay the charges

People are given an identification bracelet to be worn on the wrist. They should check to make sure the information on it is correct and should wear it at all times. That way, when tests or procedures are done, staff members can make sure that they have the right person.

After admission, people may be taken for blood tests or x-rays or go immediately to a hospital room. Hospital rooms may be private (one bed) or shared (more than one bed). Even in a private room,

---

What to Bring to the Hospital

People should bring a list of the drugs and doses they are taking and any written instructions from the doctor. Hospitals recommend that people also bring advance directives (see page 69). All of this information should be given to the nurse responsible for getting them settled into a hospital room. People should also bring the following:

- Toiletries
- A robe
- Sleepwear
- Slippers
- Eyeglasses, hearing aids, and dentures (if they are used at home)
- A few personal items, such as photographs of loved ones, to make them feel more comfortable

If a child is being hospitalized, parents should bring a comforting object, such as a favorite blanket or stuffed toy. All personal items should be marked or labeled.

Prescription drugs and any valuables (such as a wedding ring or other jewelry, credit cards, or large sums of money) should be left at home.

Special Care Units: When People Need Special Care

People who need specific types of care may be put in special care units.

Intensive care units (ICUs) are for people who are seriously ill. These people include those who have had a sudden, general malfunction (failure) of an organ, such as the liver, lungs (requiring assistance with breathing), or kidneys (requiring dialysis). People who are in shock, who have a severe infection, or who have had major surgery are likely to be placed in an ICU. Large hospitals may have a special pediatric intensive care unit (PICU) for children.

Some hospitals also have a type of intensive care unit for people who are too sick to go to a regular hospital bed but are more stable than people in the ICU. These units may be called step-down units or intermediate care units.

Coronary care units are for people who are having or have had a heart attack. People who are likely to have a heart attack (such as people with angina or an abnormal heart rhythm) and people with heart failure may be admitted to a coronary care unit or, if it is unavailable, to an ICU.

Intensive care and coronary care units have equipment to support and constantly monitor vital functions:

- A machine to monitor heart rate (electrocardiography, or ECG), blood pressure, and breathing rate is connected to people by various lines or wires.

- A flexible catheter inserted into a vein (an intravenous line) is used to give people drugs, fluids, and sometimes nutrients.

- Ventilators to help people with breathing and defibrillators to restore heart rhythm to normal are available.

Visiting hours and rules are more restrictive in these units.

Isolation is used to prevent a person from infecting others. Isolation may be complete (when a disorder can be transmitted through the air). Or it may be incomplete (when a disorder is transmitted only by contact with the skin, blood, or stool). Incomplete isolation requires fewer precautions.

Reverse isolation is used to prevent a person from being infected by others. Reverse isolation is needed when a person's immune system is not functioning well—for example, after bone marrow transplantation. Either type of isolation may involve the following:

- The person is placed in a single room.
- Anyone who goes into the room must wear a mask, gown, cap, and gloves, which are sterilized or burned after use.
- All items that come in contact with the person are also sterilized.
- The air in the room may be filtered.
- Visitors are usually limited to the immediate family.

---

privacy is limited. Staff members frequently go in and out of the room, and although they usually knock, they may enter before people can respond.

Various tests, such as blood or urine tests, may be done to check for other problems. Staff members may ask questions to determine whether people are likely to develop problems in the hospital or to need extra help after discharge from the hospital. People may be asked about eating habits, mood, vaccinations, and drugs taken. They may be asked a standard series of questions to evaluate mental function (see table on page 632).

During the hospital stay, people are examined by a doctor at least once a day. Nurses and other staff members usually come in several times a day and provide most of the care. Physical therapists may come in regularly to help with exercise. If people need extra help, such as help with eating or getting to the toilet, family members may provide this care. Family members can also talk with a social worker at the hospital about making arrangements for extra help. Children may require a parent or other caregiver to stay at the hospital most of the time.

Problems Due to Hospitalization

Just being in the hospital can cause certain problems, such as infections, pressure sores, and depression. Many hospital-related problems are caused by having to stay in bed for long periods. Others may result from being in unfamiliar surroundings or being given drugs to relieve pain or to treat a disorder. Sometimes one problem leads to another. When hospitalized, certain people—those who are confused, depressed, or undernourished or who are older—often become less able to take care of themselves. People who cannot adequately care for themselves are more likely to have longer stays in hospital and end up being sent to a nursing home after discharge.

If the person or family members anticipate problems, they should discuss preventive measures with staff members. For example, if communicating is a problem because English is not the person's first language or if hearing is impaired, family members should tell hospital staff members. Staff members can take measures to help, such as arranging for someone to translate.

Hospital-Acquired Infections

People who are admitted to the hospital are at risk of acquiring an infection there. Such infections are called nosocomial infections. In the United States, about 5% to 10% of people who are hospitalized get a nosocomial infection, and about 90,000 of these people die each year. The risk of infection is higher for infants, older people, and people with a weakened immune system.

These infections may be caused by bacteria or fungi. Bacterial and fungal infections can be dangerous and deadly.

Organisms that are acquired in hospitals are often resistant to many common antibiotics. The frequent use of antibiotics in hospitals encourages resistant strains to develop.

Hospital-acquired infections include pneumonia, urinary tract infections, infection of surgical incisions, and blood infections.

Lung Infections: People who stay in bed do not use their lungs as much, and the muscles that control breathing may weaken. Then, taking a deep breath may become difficult, and if mucus accumulates in the airways, people may not be able to cough forcefully enough to clear the mucus out. When mucus accumulates, bacteria cannot be cleared from the airways very well, and pneumonia may develop (see page 463).

The risk of lung infections is increased by the following:

- Using a ventilator, which makes the risk very high
- Having had antibiotic treatment previously
- Having other disorders, such as heart, lung, liver, or kidney disorders
- Being older than 70
- Living in a nursing home
- Having had abdominal or chest surgery

Deep breathing and coughing exercises can help prevent lung infections. These exercises can help keep the lungs open and prevent breathing muscles from weakening.

Urinary Tract Infections: Sometimes people in the hospital have a drainage tube placed in their bladder (urinary catheter). A catheter may be inserted when doctors need to closely monitor how much urine people produce—for example, in those who are critically ill. In the past, doctors placed urinary catheters in people who were incontinent. However, catheters significantly increase the risk of a urinary tract infection because they make it easy for bacteria to enter the bladder. Thus, to prevent urinary tract infections, doctors try to use these catheters as seldom as possible. When catheters are used, they must be carefully cleaned and regularly examined. If people are incontinent, diapers that are changed as often as needed are a better choice than a urinary catheter.

Prevention: General measures that hospital staff members use to help prevent hospital-acquired infections include the following:

- Frequent hand washing
- Frequent use of alcohol-based hand sanitizers
- Use of protective gear such as gloves and gowns when procedures are done

To prevent development of resistant bacteria, many hospitals have programs to limit the use of antibiotics.

Problems Due to Bed Rest

Staying in bed for a long time without regular physical activity can cause many problems.

Blood Clots: A leg injury, leg surgery, or bed rest may prevent people from using their legs. When the legs are not being used, blood moves more slowly from the leg veins to the heart. Blood clots are more likely to form in this slow-moving blood (see page 433). Blood clots sometimes travel from the leg veins to the lungs and block a blood vessel. These clots, called pulmonary emboli, can be life threatening (see page 488).

Pneumatic compression stockings may be used to prevent blood clots. Powered by an electric pump, these stockings repeatedly squeeze the calves and move blood into and through the veins. People at high risk of developing blood clots may be given an anticoagulant (such as heparin), which helps keep blood from clotting.

Constipation: When people stay in bed or are less active, stool (feces) moves more slowly through the intestine and rectum and out of the body. Thus, constipation is more likely to occur. Also, people may be taking drugs that cause constipation.

To prevent constipation, staff members encourage people to drink plenty of fluids, and extra fiber is included as part of meals or as a supplement. Stool softeners or laxatives may be prescribed.

Depression: Many people who stay in bed for a long time become depressed. Having less contact with other people and feeling helpless may also contribute to depression.

Pressure Sores: When people stay in one position in bed for too long, pressure is put on the areas of skin that touch the bed. The pressure cuts off the blood supply to those areas. If the blood supply is cut off too long, tissue breaks down, resulting in a pressure sore (also called pressure ulcer or bedsore—see page 1299). Pressure sores can begin to form in as few as 2 hours. Pressure sores are more likely to develop in people who are undernourished or who leak urine involuntarily (are incontinent). Being undernourished makes the skin thin, dry, inelastic, and more likely to tear or break. Being incontinent exposes the skin to urine, which softens it, causing it to break open. Pressure sores usually occur on the lower back, tailbone, heels, elbows, and hips. Pressure sores can be serious, leading to infection that spreads to the bloodstream (sepsis).

If people have difficulty moving, staff members periodically change their position in bed to help prevent pressure sores from forming. The skin is inspected for any sign of pressure sores. Pads may be placed over parts of the body that are in contact with the bed, such as the heels, to protect them.

Weak Bones: When bones do not bear weight regularly (that is, when people do not spend enough time standing or walking), bones become weak and more prone to fractures.

Weak Muscles and Stiff Joints: When muscles are not used, they become weak. Staying in bed can make joints—muscles and the tissues around them (ligaments and tendons)—stiff. Over time, stiff joints can become permanently bent—called a contracture. A vicious circle may result: People stay in bed because of a disorder or surgery, resulting in weak muscles and stiff joints, which make moving (including standing and walking) even more difficult.

Prevention: Steps to prevent problems related to bed rest may seem bothersome or too demanding, but they are necessary for a good recovery. Moving as soon and as much as possible can help prevent most problems, including constipation. People are encouraged to get out of bed as soon as they can. If people cannot get out of bed, they should sit up, move, or do exercises in bed. Flexing and relaxing muscles in bed can help keep muscles from weakening. For people who cannot exercise on their own, a physical therapist or another staff member moves their limbs for them. Furnishings, such as handrails, grab bars in the bathroom, raised toilet seats, low beds, and carpeting, can make movement easier.

For children, hospitals frequently have playrooms to encourage activity and to prevent boredom or depression.

Undernutrition

People who are hospitalized may eat less for several reasons:

- Illness or drugs may cause loss of appetite.
- Food may be unfamiliar and unappetizing.
- Some people are on a restricted diet, such as a low-fat or low-salt diet, which they may not enjoy.
- Meals are served and removed at set times.
- People may be served foods they do not like or cannot eat for philosophical or religious reasons (for example, because the foods are not kosher).

- For some people, eating in a hospital bed with a tray is difficult.
- Some people need help or more time while eating. Often, by the time someone arrives to help with eating, the food has cooled and is even less appetizing.
- If dentures are left at home, are misplaced, or do not fit right, chewing can be difficult.
- Water may be difficult to reach from a hospital bed.

Undernutrition is a serious problem, particularly for older people and people who have chronic disorders. People who are undernourished cannot fight off infections. Sores and wounds heal more slowly, and recovery is less likely. Vitamin D deficiency is particularly common among people who are hospitalized. This deficiency increases the risk of fractures caused by falls.

Prevention: Hospital staff members can make sure that restrictive diets are changed as soon as possible and can check how much people eat each day. At hospital admission, people or their family members can let staff members know what foods are preferred or not eaten. Hospital diets can be modified to some degree. Family members may bring in favorite foods. Having family members present at meals helps because people tend to eat more when they eat with others. Family or staff members should make sure that people who wear dentures have and wear them.

A pitcher of fresh water should be placed within easy reach from the bed unless fluids must be limited because of a disorder. Family and staff members should encourage people to drink by regularly offering them something to drink.

If people cannot take food by mouth, a fluid containing nutrients can be given through a tube inserted into the stomach (through the nose or through a small hole in the wall of the abdomen—see page 916) or, less often, a vein (intravenously—see page 917). Such feedings may be necessary for a short time until people can safely eat enough food by mouth. If people cannot take food by mouth (even if only temporarily), family members should check with staff members to make sure adequate nutrition is provided.

Confusion and Decline in Mental Function

Being ill, particularly when it involves taking drugs for pain or anxiety, can make anyone confused. The hospital environment adds to the problem. There, people give up their personal effects and clothing—marks of their identity—for a hospital gown. They are in a strange place without familiar landmarks and usual routines. Often, hospitals provide little stimulation (such as sights, sounds, and interaction with other people). People may be alone or with an

SPOTLIGHT ON AGING

More than one third of people admitted to the hospital are older people. And at any time, almost half of people in the hospital are 65 or older. Almost half of older people seen in an emergency department are admitted to the hospital.

When many older people leave the hospital, they are in worse shape than before they became ill. Part of the reason for the decline is that older people tend to have serious and debilitating disorders when they enter the hospital. Many hospitals do not adequately deal with the physical needs of older people. However, part of the reason is just being in a hospital, which can cause problems, regardless of age. Older people are more likely to already have or to develop these problems, and the consequences are more likely to be serious for the following reasons:

- **Confusion:** Changes that occur as people age make them more likely to become suddenly and noticeably confused (delirious—see page 682).
- **Dehydration:** Older people tend to feel thirsty less quickly or less intensely than younger people. They thus are inclined to drink less, especially when circumstances make getting water more difficult, as occurs in a hospital.
- **Falls:** Older people are more likely to fall and, if they fall, more likely to have a serious injury such as a broken bone.
- **Incontinence:** Older people may have particular difficulty getting out of a high hospital bed after they have had surgery, when they have a serious disorder, or when they have various equipment attached to them. As a result, they may not get to a toilet in time.
- **Loss of independence:** During a hospital stay, older people may become unable to take care of themselves because staff members provide this care (such as bathing).
- **Loss of muscle tissue:** When they spend a lot of time in bed or are immobilized, older people tend to lose more muscle tissue and lose it more quickly.
- **Pressure sores:** Older people are prone to pressure sores because they tend to have less fat under the skin and blood flow to the skin is decreased. If they develop pressures sores, they may be sent to a nursing home rather than their own home after they are discharged from the hospital.
- **Side effects of drugs:** Before entering the hospital, many older people are taking several drugs. In the hospital, more drugs may be prescribed. The more drugs people take, the greater the chance for side effects and drug interactions. Also, older people are more sensitive to the effects of certain drugs.

- **Undernutrition:** Physical age-related changes may reduce appetite or absorption of nutrients (see box on page 916), as may certain disorders (including dental problems) and drugs.

Many older people have difficulty bouncing back psychologically and physically from the experience of being in a hospital as well as from the disorder they have had.

PREVENTIVE STRATEGIES

Some hospitals have developed strategies to prevent problems that can result when older people are hospitalized. These strategies are designed to help older people continue to function as well as they did before they became ill.

- **An interdisciplinary team:** This team consists of health care practitioners who work together to care for an older person. Team members evaluate the person's needs and coordinate the person's hospital care. Team members look for possible problems and correct or prevent them.
- **A one-focus team:** This team focuses on preventing and managing one specific problem, such as undernutrition or pressure sores. Such teams are often led by a nurse, who checks the person for the problem and develops a care plan.
- **Geriatricians:** These doctors are trained specifically to care for older people and can help prevent problems common among them. For example, geriatricians avoid prescribing drugs that are particularly likely to cause problems.
- **Guidelines:** Hospitals may also follow guidelines for care (protocols) developed specifically for older people.
- **An assigned nurse:** Sometimes one nurse is assigned to have primary responsibility for and to monitor a person's care. This nurse makes sure that other staff members understand the treatment plan for the person.

Geriatric nursing units: These units are designed for older people and staffed with people trained in caring for older people. In these units, older people are encouraged to get out of bed as soon and as much as possible. They are encouraged to dress each morning, to follow their usual daily routine as much as possible, and to eat in a group dining room. If older people are going to be in the hospital a long time, they are encouraged to personalize their room with photographs, pillows, and other familiar items. Staff members encourage family members and friends to participate in care.

(continued on the following page)

TREATMENT

How aggressively a disorder is treated in a hospital should not depend on age. Family members and older people should talk with a doctor to make sure options for treatment are based on the severity of the disorder, not on age. However, less aggressive treatments are sometimes appropriate for older people, depending on their wishes and sometimes appropriate for older people, depending on their wishes and outlook—that is, how the disorder is expected to progress and how long they are expected to live. Having advance directives, which state what sort of care people want, is particularly important for older people.

uncommunicative roommate in a room that has blank white walls and bland, institutionalized furnishings. For most of the time, there may be no one to talk with. The only sound available may be that from a television.

Hospital procedures and schedules can be disorienting. For example, people may be awakened frequently during the night, depriving them of needed sleep. They may be unable to get their bearings in an unfamiliar, dimly lit room. The many tests and the complicated equipment may be overwhelming.

Intensive care units (ICUs) can be even more confusing. People in ICUs are alone, sometimes with no windows or clocks to help them orient themselves. The beeping of electronic monitors, constant bright light, and frequent interruptions to take blood, to change intravenous (IV) tubes, or to give drugs may interfere with sleeping. People who are tired are more easily confused and disoriented. Sometimes confusion is so severe that people develop a type of delirium called ICU psychosis (see page 683).

If people become unusually confused while staying in a hospital, family members should tell staff members. Delirium can usually be cured if its cause (a disorder, drug, or stressful situation) is corrected.

Prevention: Staff and family members can help keep people oriented by doing the following:

- Making sure that the lighting in the room is adequate
- Encouraging people to get out of bed, walk regularly, and do as many usual daily activities as possible
- Talking with people about what is going on outside the hospital to keep their mind active
- Explaining tests and treatments to help people understand what is happening and why
- Making sure people who wear glasses or a hearing aid have and wear these items
- Making sure that people consume enough fluids and food (dehydration can cause delirium)

Incontinence

In the hospital, people may involuntarily leak urine (urinary incontinence) or pass stool (fecal inconti-

nence). In these cases, incontinence may result from the environment rather than from people's physical condition. The following may make incontinence more likely:

- Being restricted to bed rest
- Being given diuretics, which cause the bladder to fill quickly with urine
- Having trouble getting out of bed because the bed is too high or because people are weak or ill
- Having a disorder or having had surgery that makes walking difficult or painful
- Having equipment, such as IV or oxygen lines, heart monitors, and catheters, in the way

Thus, getting to a toilet becomes complicated and may take more time and planning than usual.

One alternative—bedpans—may be hard to use or uncomfortable. Help may be needed to use the bedpan or to get to a toilet. People who have dementia, who suddenly become confused, or who have had a stroke may be unable to use a call bell to request help. After the call bell is pushed, help may be delayed. Such delays may result in incontinence. Also, some drugs and disorders can make incontinence more likely to develop.

Prevention: Staff members can set up regular times to help people go to the toilet. Placing a toilet chair (commode) by the bed is sometimes useful. Lowering a bed or rearranging medical equipment may help. Having access to a urinal is helpful for men. Making sure people are familiar with the path from bed to toilet and making the toilet easy to identify may also help prevent incontinence.

Falls

Conditions in a hospital can increase the risk of falling, particularly for older people. After being in bed a long time (bed rest), leg muscles can become weak and less able to squeeze the leg veins and thus force blood toward the heart. Thus, blood pools in the legs when people stand up, causing blood pressure to drop and making people feel dizzy or light-headed (a disorder called orthostatic hypotension). Also, people may be given drugs that make them feel dizzy, drowsy, or confused. A bed may be too high or have rails, making getting out of bed more difficult. Lighting may be dim, so people may not see obstacles. People who are confused or disoriented are more likely to fall.

Because being in the hospital disrupts usual routines, parents who are staying in the hospital to care for a sick infant or small child may forget their usual precautions, such as keeping the crib rails up when the infant is in bed.

Prevention: If people who are hospitalized or their family members realize what can cause falls in a hospital, they can take steps to prevent them. For example, to counter weak muscles, people can get out of bed as soon as possible and exercise. Family or staff members can accompany people while they walk down hospital corridors until muscle strength is regained.

Most falls occur when people get out of bed. So family or staff members can help by doing the following:

- If a bed has rails or is too high, asking whether the rails are needed and whether the bed can be lowered
- Making sure people know how high the hospital bed is
- Encouraging people to be careful and move slowly when getting out of bed
- Making sure people are wearing slippers or shoes with nonskid soles
- Showing people where the toilet is and how to get there (to prevent missteps and bumping into furniture)
- Showing people how to call for help
- For infants and small children, making sure the crib rails are raised

Often, staff members try to identify and provide extra help to people who are likely to fall. Staff members may check on them at regular intervals or put them in rooms near the nursing station.

Family members can ask a doctor to check the drugs being taken and identify any that can increase the risk of falling. If such a drug is being used, family members can ask the doctor about possibly changing the drug or reducing the dose.

Being Discharged From the Hospital

When people have recovered sufficiently or can be appropriately treated elsewhere, they are discharged from the hospital. Staff members may ask questions to determine whether people are likely to need extra help after discharge. A discharge planner or a social worker at the hospital can anticipate which problems are likely, then make suggestions about and arrange for needed services. However, people and their family members should be involved in the plans to make sure they are appropriate.

If further care is needed temporarily or permanently after a hospital stay, people are often sent to another facility. They may go to a rehabilitation facility or a nursing home (skilled nursing facility). Sometimes care can be continued at home (see page 1909).

Before leaving the hospital, people or their family members should make sure that that they receive detailed instructions for follow-up care and that they understand the instructions. They should get a written schedule for using all their drugs and for follow-up appointments. If people are being discharged to another facility, a written summary of their hospital evaluation and treatment plan (called a transition care record) should be sent with them and another copy faxed to the facility. Information in this record should include the following:

- The reason for the hospitalization
- Major procedures or tests done
- The main diagnosis at discharge
- Instructions for follow-up care
- A list of current drugs, including how long they should be taken

<table>
<tr><td>**CHAPTER**
316</td><td># Surgery</td></tr>
</table>

Surgery is the term traditionally used for treatments that involve cutting or stitching tissue. However, advances in surgical techniques have made the definition more complicated. Sometimes lasers, rather than scalpels, are used to cut tissue, and wounds may be closed without stitches. In modern medical care,

distinguishing between a surgical and medical procedure is not always easy. However, making that distinction is not important as long as the doctor doing the procedure is well trained and experienced.

Surgery is a broad area of care and involves many different techniques. In some surgical procedures, tissue is removed. In others, blockages are opened. In still others, arteries and veins are attached in new places to provide additional blood flow to areas that do not receive enough. Grafts, sometimes made of artificial materials, may be implanted to replace blood vessels or connective tissue, and metal rods may be inserted into bone to replace broken parts.

A diagnosis is sometimes accomplished by doing surgery. A biopsy, in which a piece of tissue is removed for examination under a microscope, is the most common type of diagnostic surgery. In some emergencies, in which there is no time for diagnostic tests, surgery is used for both diagnosis and treatment. For example, surgery may be needed to quickly identify and repair organs that are bleeding from a gunshot wound.

The urgency of surgery is often described by three categories—emergency, urgent, and elective. Emergency surgery, such as stopping rapid internal bleeding, is done as soon as possible because minutes can make a difference. Urgent surgery, such as removal of an inflamed appendix, is best done within hours. Elective surgery, such as replacement of a knee joint, can be delayed for some period of time, until everything has been done to optimize a person's chances of doing well during and after the surgical procedure.

Anesthesia

Because surgery is generally painful, it is almost always preceded by the administration of some type of anesthetic. Anesthetics blocks the perception of pain. Anesthesia may be local, regional, or general. Anesthetics are typically given by health care practitioners specially trained and certified in providing anesthesia. These practitioners may be doctors (anesthesiologists) or nurse practitioners (nurse anesthetists). Nurse anesthetists practice under the direction of an anesthesiologist.

Local and Regional Anesthesia: These types of anesthesia consist of injections of drugs (such as lidocaine or bupivacaine) that numb only specific parts of the body. In local anesthesia, the drug is injected under the skin of the site to be cut, numbing only that site. In regional anesthesia, which numbs a larger area of the body, the drug is injected around one or more nerves and numbs an area of the body supplied by those nerves. For example, injecting a drug around certain nerves can numb fingers, toes, or large parts of limbs. One type of regional anesthesia involves injecting a drug into a vein (intravenous regional anesthesia). A device such as a woven elastic bandage or blood pressure cuff compresses the area where the limb joins the body, trapping the drug within the veins of that limb. Intravenous regional anesthesia can numb an entire limb.

Cosmetic Surgery

Cosmetic surgery involves a wide variety of operations, including removing facial and neck wrinkles (rhytidectomy); removing fat and wrinkles from the abdomen (abdominoplasty); enlarging or reducing breasts (mammoplasty); restoring scalp hair (hair replacement surgery); altering the appearance of facial features, such as the jaw (mandibuloplasty), eyelids (blepharoplasty), and nose (rhinoplasty); removing body fat (liposuction); and eliminating varicose veins (sclerotherapy).

Popular and tempting as cosmetic surgery may be, there are certain drawbacks and precautions:

- It is expensive.
- It poses risks, including serious health risks as well as the possibility that appearance may be less pleasing to the person than it was originally.
- Because obtaining the best results requires close adherence to instructions after the operation, cosmetic surgery is recommended only for highly motivated people.
- A person should choose a doctor who has met a medical specialty's standards for practice (board certification) and who has extensive experience doing the procedure.

During local and regional anesthesia, the person remains awake. However, doctors sometimes give antianxiety drugs intravenously to calm and relax the person. Rarely, numbness, tingling, or pain can persist in the numbed area for days or even weeks after the surgical procedure.

Spinal anesthesia and epidural anesthesia are specific types of regional anesthesia in which a drug is injected around the spinal cord in the lower back. Depending on the site of the injection and position of the body, a large area (such as from the waist to the toes) can be numbed. These types of anesthesia are useful for operations of the lower body, such as hernia repairs and prostate, rectal, bladder, leg, and some gynecologic operations. Spinal and epidural anesthesia also can be useful for childbirth. Headaches occasionally develop in the days after spinal anesthesia but usually can be treated effectively.

General Anesthesia: In general anesthesia, a drug that circulates throughout the bloodstream is given, rendering the person unconscious. The drug can be given intravenously or inhaled. Because a general anesthetic slows breathing, the anesthesiologist inserts a breathing tube in the windpipe (a ventilator breathes for the person if the operation is long). For short operations, however, such a tube may not be necessary. Instead, the anesthesiologist can support breathing by using a handheld breathing mask.

Surgery Through a Keyhole

Technical advances now make it possible to do surgery with smaller incisions and less tissue disruption than occurs with traditional surgery. To do this surgery, surgeons insert tiny lights, video cameras, and surgical instruments through keyhole-sized incisions. The surgeons can then do procedures using the images transmitted to video monitors as guides for manipulating the surgical instruments. This kind of surgery has various names depending on where it is done: laparoscopy in the abdomen, arthroscopy in joints, and thoracoscopy in the chest.

Because it causes less tissue damage than traditional surgery, keyhole surgery has several advantages, including the following:

- A briefer hospital stay (in most cases)
- Often, less pain after the operation
- Earlier return to work
- A tendency toward smaller scars

However, the difficulties of keyhole surgery are often underestimated by people undergoing the surgery and sometimes by surgeons. Because surgeons are using a video monitor, they are seeing only a two-dimensional view of the site on which they are operating. Also, the surgical instruments used have long handles and are controlled from outside of the person's body, so the surgeon may find that using them feels less natural than using traditional surgical instruments. For these reasons, keyhole surgery has potential disadvantages:

- Keyhole surgery often takes longer than traditional surgery.
- More importantly, especially when a procedure is new, errors are more likely to occur than with traditional approaches because of the complexity of keyhole surgery.

People also should know that although keyhole surgery may cause less pain than traditional surgery, pain still occurs, often more than anticipated.

Because keyhole surgery is technically difficult, people should do the following:

- Choose a highly experienced surgeon
- Establish that surgery is necessary
- Ask the surgeon how pain will be treated

General anesthetics affect vital organs, so the anesthesiologist closely monitors the heart rate, heart rhythm, breathing, body temperature, and blood pressure until the drugs wear off. Serious side effects are very rare.

Major and Minor Surgery

A distinction is sometimes made between major and minor surgery, although many surgical procedures have characteristics of both.

Major Surgery: Major surgery often involves opening one of the major body cavities—the abdomen (laparotomy), the chest (thoracotomy), or the skull (craniotomy)—and can stress vital organs. The surgery usually is done using general anesthesia in a hospital operating room by a team of doctors. A stay of at least one night in the hospital usually is needed after major surgery.

Minor Surgery: In minor surgery, major body cavities are not opened. Minor surgery can involve the use of local, regional, or general anesthesia and may be done in an emergency department, an ambulatory surgical center, or a doctor's office. Vital organs usually are not stressed, and surgery can be done by a single doctor, who may or may not be a surgeon. Usually, the person can return home on the same day that minor surgery is done.

> **?** **Did You Know...**
> Improved technologies and procedures have made serious side effects of general anesthesia very rare.

Surgical Risk

The risks of surgery (that is, how likely surgery is to cause death or a serious problem) depend on the type of surgery and characteristics of the person.

Types of surgery that have the highest risk include

- Heart or lung surgery
- Prostate gland removal
- Major operations on the bones and joints (for example, hip replacement)

Generally, the poorer the person's overall health, the higher the risks of surgery. Some particular health problems that increase surgical risk include

- Severe chest pain (angina)
- Recent heart attack
- Severe heart failure
- Undernutrition (common among older people who live in institutions)
- Severe disorders of the lungs or liver
- Chronic kidney disease
- Chronic lung disease (often smoking-related)
- Weakened immune system (for example, because of long-term corticosteroid treatment)
- Diabetes (especially if poorly controlled)

Risks are often higher among older people (see box on page 2058). However, risks are determined more by general health than by age. Chronic disorders that increase surgical risk and other treatable dis-orders, such as dehydration, infections, and imbalances in body fluids and electrolytes, should be controlled with treatment as well as possible before an operation.

Second Opinion

The choice to undergo surgery is not always clear. There may be nonsurgical options for treatment, and there may be several possible surgical procedures. Thus, a person may seek the opinion of more than one doctor. Some health insurance plans require a second opinion for elective surgery. However, experts may disagree on which doctor should give the second opinion.

- Some experts advise obtaining a second opinion from a doctor who is not a surgeon to eliminate any bias toward surgery when nonsurgical treatment is an option.

- Others advise that another surgeon give the second opinion, believing that a surgeon knows more about the advantages and disadvantages of surgery than would a doctor who is not a surgeon.

- Some experts recommend establishing up front that any surgeon giving a second opinion will not do the surgical procedure, so that there is no conflict of interest.

Preparing for the Day of Surgery

Various preparations are made in the days and weeks before surgery. It is often recommended that physical conditioning and nutrition be improved as much as possible because good general health helps a person recover from the stress of surgery. Valuables should be left at home.

Alcohol and Tobacco Use: Eliminating or minimizing alcohol and tobacco use before undergoing surgery that involves general anesthesia can increase safety. Recent tobacco use makes abnormal heart rhythms more likely to develop during general anesthesia and impairs lung function. Excessive alcohol consumption can damage the liver, causing heavy bleeding during surgery and unpredictably increasing or decreasing the effect of the drugs used for general anesthesia. Alcohol consumption should be decreased gradually, however, because a sudden decrease before undergoing general anesthesia can have harmful effects, such as fever and abnormalities of blood pressure or heart rhythm.

Doctors' Evaluations: The surgeon performs a physical examination and takes a medical history, which includes the person's recent symptoms, past medical conditions, past reactions to anesthetics (if any), use of tobacco and alcohol, infections, risk factors for blood clots, problems pertaining to the heart and lungs (such as cough or chest pain), and allergies. The person is also asked to list all drugs currently being taken. Nonprescription as well as prescription drugs must be disclosed because serious health problems could result. For example, the use of aspirin, which a person may consider too trivial to mention, can increase bleeding during surgery. Additionally, the use of supplements or medicinal herbs (for example, ginkgo biloba or St. John's wort) should be mentioned as well because they may have effects during or after surgery.

The anesthesiologist may meet the person before the operation to review test results and identify any medical conditions that might affect the choice of anesthetic. The safest and most effective types of anesthesia may be discussed as well.

Tests: Tests done before surgery (preoperative testing) may include blood and urine tests, an electrocardiogram, x-rays, and tests of lung capacity (pulmonary function tests). These tests can help determine how well the vital organs are functioning. If organs are functioning poorly, the stress of surgery or anesthesia can cause problems. Preoperative tests occasionally also reveal an inapparent temporary illness, such as an infection, which requires the postponement of surgery.

Blood Storage for Transfusion: People may wish to store their own blood in case a blood transfusion is needed during surgery. Using stored blood (autologous blood transfusion—see page 1029) eliminates the risk of infections and most transfusion reactions. A pint of blood can be withdrawn from the person and preserved until surgery. Blood should be withdrawn no more often than once weekly, and the last donation should probably be at least 2 weeks before surgery. The body replaces the missing blood during the weeks after the blood donation.

Decision Making: Sometime before the surgery, the surgeon obtains the person's permission to perform the operation, a process called informed consent. The surgeon discusses risks and benefits of the operation, as well as alternative treatments, and answers questions. The person reads and signs a form documenting consent. In cases of emergency surgery in which the person is unable to provide informed consent, doctors try to contact the family. Rarely, emergency surgery must proceed before the family is contacted.

A durable power of attorney for health care and a living will (see page 70) should be prepared before surgery in case the person becomes unable to communicate or becomes incapacitated after surgery.

Preparing the Digestive Tract: Because some of the drugs given during surgery may cause vomiting, people should generally not eat or drink anything for at least 8 hours beforehand. For outpatient surgery, people should not eat or drink anything after midnight. Specific guidelines should be given and vary depending on the kind of surgery. People should ask the doctor which of their regularly prescribed drugs should be taken before surgery. People undergoing surgery involving the intestines are given laxatives for a day or two before the operation.

Fingernails: Because the device that monitors the level of oxygen in the blood is attached to a finger, nail polish and artificial nails should be removed before going to the hospital. Then, this device can perform more accurately.

The Day of Surgery

Before most operations, a person removes all clothing, jewelry, hearing aids, false teeth, and contact lenses or eyeglasses and puts on a hospital gown. The person is taken to a specially designated room (the holding area) or to the operating room itself for final preparations before surgery. The skin that will be cut (operative site) is scrubbed with an antiseptic, which minimizes the number of bacteria and helps prevent infection. A health care practitioner may shave the operative site. A plastic tube (catheter) is inserted in one of the veins of the hand or arm. Fluids and drugs are given through the catheter. A drug may be given intravenously for sedation. If an operation involves the mouth, intestinal tract, lungs or respiratory tract, or urinary tract, people are given one or more antibiotics within the hour before the operation to prevent infection (prophylaxis). This therapy also applies to people undergoing some other operations in which infections are particularly problematic (for example, joint or heart valve replacement).

If the final preparations are done in the holding area, the person is then taken to the operating room. At this point, the person may still be awake, although groggy, or may already be asleep. The person is moved to the operating table, lit by specially designed surgical lights. Doctors, nurses, and other personnel who will be near or touching the operative site thoroughly scrub their hands with antiseptic soap, which minimizes the number of bacteria and viruses in the operating room. For surgery, they also wear scrub suits, caps, masks, shoe covers, sterile gowns, and sterile gloves. Before the surgery begins, a time out is held during which the surgical team confirms the following:

- The person's identity
- The correct procedure and side (if applicable)
- Availability of all needed equipment

- Prophylaxis to prevent infection or blood clots (if needed)

Local, regional, or general anesthesia is used.

After Surgery

After the operation is completed and anesthesia begins to wear off, the person is taken to a recovery room to be closely watched for about 1 or 2 hours. Most people feel groggy when awakening, particularly after major surgery. Some people are nauseated for a short while. Some feel cold.

Depending on the nature of the surgery and the type of anesthesia, a person may go home directly from the recovery room or be admitted to the hospital, sometimes in an intensive care unit (ICU).

Direct Discharge Home: A person being sent home must be

- Thinking clearly
- Breathing normally
- Able to drink fluids
- Able to urinate
- Able to walk
- Free of severe pain

People who have been given sedatives and then discharged need to be accompanied home by someone else and are not permitted to drive themselves. The operative site should be free of bleeding and unexpected swelling.

Hospitalization: People who are admitted to the hospital after surgery may awaken to find many tubes and devices in and on them. For example, there may be a breathing tube in the throat, adhesive pads on the chest to monitor the heartbeat, a tube in the bladder, a device attached to a finger to measure the level of oxygen in the blood, a dressing on the operative site, a tube in the nose or mouth, and one or more tubes in the veins.

Pain is expected after most operations and can almost always be relieved. Drugs that relieve pain (analgesics) can be given intravenously, by mouth, or by injection into the muscle or can be applied to the skin as a patch. If epidural anesthesia was used, the plastic tube used to give the anesthetic may be left in the person's back. Opioid analgesics, such as morphine, can be injected through the tube. People staying in the hospital may be given a device that continuously injects an opioid analgesic into a vein, which also can deliver a small additional amount of analgesic when people press a button (patient-controlled analgesia). If pain persists, additional treatment can be requested. Repeated use of opioid analgesics often causes constipation. To prevent constipation, doctors may give the person a stimulant laxative or stool softener.

In the Operating Room

The operating room provides a sterile environment in which the operating team can do surgery. The operating team consists of the following:

- Chief surgeon, who directs the surgery
- One or more assistant surgeons, who help the chief surgeon
- Anesthesiologist, who controls the supply of anesthetic and monitors the person closely
- Scrub nurse, who passes instruments to the surgeon
- Circulating nurse, who provides extra equipment to the operating team

The operating room typically contains a monitor that displays vital signs, an instrument table, and an operating lamp. Anesthetic gases are piped into the anesthetic machine. A catheter attached to a suction machine removes excess blood and other fluids, which can prevent surgeons from seeing the tissues clearly. Fluids given by vein, started before the person enters the operating room, are continued.

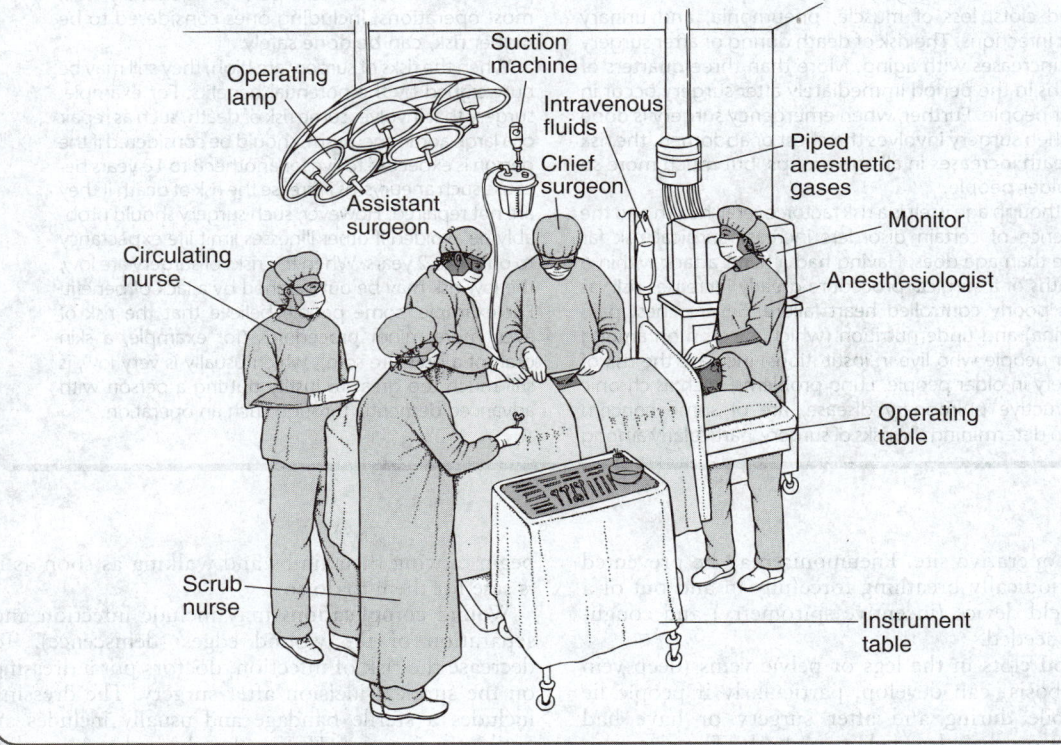

Good nutrition is critical for rapid healing and minimizing the chance of infection. Nutritional needs increase after major surgery. If surgery makes eating impossible for more than several days, an alternative source of nutrition can speed recovery and prevent problems. People whose digestive tracts are functioning but who are otherwise unable to eat may be given nutrients through a tube placed into the stomach. Such a tube may be passed through the nose, mouth, or an incision in the abdominal wall. Rarely, people who have had surgery of the digestive tract and cannot eat for extended periods may be given nutrients through a catheter inserted in one of the body's large veins (parenteral nutrition—see page 917).

Complications: Complications such as fever, blood clots, wound problems, confusion, difficulty urinating or defecating, and muscle loss can develop during the days after surgery.

Fever has several common causes, including an inflammatory response to the trauma of an operation; a high metabolic rate that occurs with the stress of an operation, which causes the body to burn more calories and generate more heat; and infections, such as pneumonia, urinary tract infections, and infections

In the mid-1900s, surgeons often hesitated to do even simple operations on people over age 50. Times have changed. Now, more than one third of all operations in the United States are done on people aged 65 or over.

However, aging does increase the risk of complications during and after surgery. For example, older people are much more likely than younger people to develop delirium after surgery. They are also more likely to experience serious complications from bed rest, which may occur after surgery. These complications include blood clots, loss of muscle, pneumonia, and urinary tract infections. The risk of death during or after surgery also increases with aging. More than three quarters of deaths in the period immediately after surgery occur in older people. Further, when emergency surgery is done or when surgery involves the chest or abdomen, the risk of death increases in all age groups, but much more so for older people.

Although age itself is a risk factor, overall health and the presence of certain disorders increase surgical risk far more than age does. Having had a heart attack within 6 months of a surgical procedure greatly increases risk, as does poorly controlled heart failure. Severe chest pain (angina) and undernutrition (which is common among older people who live in institutions) increase the risk of surgery in older people. Lung problems, such as chronic obstructive pulmonary disease, are of some concern when determining the risks of surgery, particularly among smokers. Impaired kidney function and problems with mental function, such as dementia, may also increase the risk.

Certain surgical procedures pose more risk than others. For example, surgery involving the abdomen or chest, removal of the prostate, and major surgery on a joint (such as hip replacement) rank high on the list of risky procedures. Many procedures that older people commonly undergo, such as cataract surgery and surgery on small joints, pose lower risk. If an older person is generally well, most operations, including ones considered to be higher risk, can be done safely.

When the risks of surgery are high, they still may be outweighed by the potential benefits. For example, surgery that involves some risk of death, such as repair of a large aortic aneurysm, should be considered if the person is expected to live for another 8 to 10 years because such aneurysms increase the risk of death if they are not repaired. However, such surgery should probably be avoided if other illnesses limit life expectancy to only 1 to 2 years. When the risks of surgery are low, the low risk may be outweighed by a lack of benefit. For example, some people believe that the risk of even more minor procedures (for example, a skin graft of a pressure sore), which usually is very low, is still much too great to justify putting a person with advanced dementia through such an operation.

---

at the operative site. Pneumonia may be prevented by periodically breathing forcefully in and out of a handheld device (incentive spirometry) and coughing as needed.

Blood clots in the legs or pelvic veins (deep vein thrombosis) can develop, particularly if people lie immobile during and after surgery or have had surgery on their leg, pelvis, or both. The clots can dislodge and travel through the bloodstream to the lungs, where they can block blood from circulating through the lungs (causing pulmonary embolism). As a result, the oxygen supply to the rest of the body may be decreased, and sometimes blood pressure may fall. For operations that make blood clots particularly likely and for people who are likely to have to lie still without much movement, doctors give drugs that keep blood from clotting (anticoagulants), such as low-molecular-weight heparin, or put compression stockings on the person's legs to improve blood circulation. However, anticoagulants may not be recommended for operations in which these drugs may substantially increase bleeding. People should begin moving their limbs and walking as soon as it is safe for them to do so.

Wound complications may include infection and separation of the wound edges (dehiscence). To decrease the risk of infection, doctors put a dressing on the surgical incision after surgery. The dressing includes a sterile bandage and usually includes an antibiotic ointment. The bandage keeps bacteria away from the incision and absorbs fluids that ooze from the incision. Because these fluids can encourage bacteria to grow and infect the incision, the dressing is changed often, usually daily. The wound is examined whenever the dressing is changed, sometimes more often. Occasionally, infection develops despite the best wound care. An infected site becomes increasingly painful 1 or more days after surgery and can become red and warm or drain pus or fluid. Fever can develop. If any of these symptoms develop, the doctor should be seen as soon as possible.

Delirium (confusion and agitation) can develop, particularly among older people. Drugs with anticholinergic effects (such as confusion, blurred vision, and loss of bladder control), opioids, sedatives, or histamine-2 (H_2) blockers may contribute, as may too little oxygen in the blood. Drugs that can cause confusion should be avoided in older people when possible.

Difficulty urinating and difficulty defecating (constipation) can develop after surgery. Factors that contribute can include use of drugs with anticholinergic effects or opioids, inactivity, and not eating or drinking. Urine flow may become completely blocked, stretching the bladder. Blockage can lead to urinary tract infections. Sometimes pressing on the lower abdomen while trying to urinate relieves the blockage, but often a catheter needs to be inserted into the bladder. The catheter may be left in place or may be removed as soon as the bladder is emptied. Frequently sitting up may help prevent blockage. People who develop constipation and whose surgery did not involve the intestinal tract can be given laxatives that stimulate the intestines, such as bisacodyl, senna, or cascara. Stool softeners such as docusate do not help.

Loss of muscle (sarcopenia) and strength occur in all people who need bed rest for a long time. With complete bed rest, young adults lose about 1% of their muscle per day, but older people lose up to 5% per day because they have lower levels of growth hormone, which is responsible for maintaining muscle tissue. Adequate amounts of muscle are important for recovery. Thus, people should sit up in bed, move, stand, and exercise as soon as and as much as is safe for them.

Discharge Home After Hospitalization: Before leaving the hospital, people are responsible for

- Scheduling a follow-up visit with the doctor
- Knowing what drugs to take
- Knowing what activities to avoid or limit

Examples of activities that may need to be avoided temporarily include climbing stairs, driving a car, lifting heavy objects, and having sexual intercourse. A person should know what symptoms necessitate contacting the doctor before the scheduled follow-up visit.

Resuming normal activity during recovery from surgery should occur gradually. Some people need rehabilitation (see page 45), which involves special exercises and activities, to improve strength and flexibility. For example, rehabilitation after hip replacement surgery can involve learning ways to walk, stretch, and exercise.

CHAPTER

317 Complementary and Alternative Medicine

Complementary and alternative medicine (CAM) includes a variety of healing approaches and therapies that are taken from around the world and that historically have not been included in conventional Western medicine. Many aspects of CAM are rooted in ancient, indigenous systems of healing, such as those of China, India, Tibet, Africa, and the Americas. Many of these treatments and health care practices are popular, and now some are used in hospitals and are reimbursed by insurance companies. Acupuncture and some chiropractic treatments are examples. Because interest in and use of CAM are increasing, more and more medical schools are including information about CAM treatments, such as acupuncture, herbal medicine, chiropractic treatments, and homeopathy.

- **Complementary medicine:** CAM practices are used with conventional medicine.
- **Alternative medicine:** CAM is used alone.

Integrative medicine refers to the use of all appropriate therapeutic approaches (conventional and alternative) in a framework that focuses on the whole person and that reaffirms the relationship between doctor and patient.

Although the distinction between conventional medicine and alternative medicine is not always easy to determine, a basic philosophical difference exists. Conventional medicine generally defines health as the absence of disease or dysfunction. The main causes of disease and dysfunction are usually considered to be isolated factors, such as bacteria or viruses, biochemical imbalances, and aging, and treatment often involves drugs or surgery. In contrast, alternative medicine practices often define health holistically, that is, as a balance of systems—physical, emotional, and spiritual—involving the whole person. Disharmony among these systems is thought to cause illness. Treatment involves strengthening the body's own defenses and restoring these balances.

Acceptance and Use

An increasing number of people in Western countries are exploring alternative medicine as part of their medical care. In 1997, Americans made more than 629 million visits to alternative medicine practitioners—a 47% increase since 1990. This number substantially exceeds the 386 million visits made to all primary care doctors in the same year. In 2007, 38% of Americans 18 years of age or older used some form of alternative medicine. The conditions for which people are most likely to seek alternative therapies include the following:

- Musculoskeletal problems (for example, chronic low back pain, neck pain, or joint pain)
- Anxiety
- High blood cholesterol levels
- Head or chest colds
- Headaches
- Sleep problems

Additionally, many people facing life-challenging illnesses, such as cancer, seek alternative therapies when conventional treatment offers little hope, especially at the end of life.

> **? Did You Know...**
>
> Americans now make more visits to alternative medicine practitioners than to primary care doctors.

Effectiveness and Safety

In 1992, the Office of Alternative Medicine within the National Institutes of Health (NIH) was formed to research the effectiveness and safety of alternative therapies. In 1999, this office became the National Center for Complementary and Alternative Medicine (NCCAM—visit their website at www.nccam.nih.gov).

Effectiveness: The effectiveness of alternative therapies is an important consideration. Some therapies have been shown to be effective for specific conditions, although these therapies are applied more broadly. Many forms of alternative medicine have not undergone rigorous scientific evaluation. However, a lack of scientific studies does not mean that a therapy is ineffective. A large number of alternative therapies have been practiced for thousands of years. They include acupuncture, meditation, yoga, therapeutic diets, massage, and herbal medicine. However, it can be difficult to do scientific research studies on them. Barriers to doing research on CAM therapies include the following:

- Lack of interest among medical researchers
- Limited availability of research funds
- Difficulties applying conventional research methods to studying alternative therapies

An example is acupuncture. Medical researchers often have little scientific interest in acupuncture because its theory depends on nonscientific notions such as vital energy. Commercial research funds are limited because acupuncture cannot be patented. Thus, there is no profit motive. Government research funds are limited because the scientific community remains skeptical of acupuncture theory and the validity of its method.

Applying conventional research methods to study CAM is difficult for many reasons, including

- Conventional research design requires that the same treatment be given to every person in the study (subject). However, many CAM therapies treat the unique and particular imbalances of individual people. For example, acupuncture needles are placed at points on the body according to a person's unique needs, or people with the same medical diagnosis may be prescribed completely different homeopathic or herbal medicines.
- Conventional research design compares active treatment with a placebo (an intervention that is made to resemble a drug or treatment but does not include an active drug or treatment—see page 77). Some CAM therapies, such as homeopathy and herbal medicine, lend themselves to placebo design. However, designing a placebo acupuncture or chiropractic treatment is difficult. Designing a placebo for meditation is impossible.
- Conventional research design uses the method of double blinding (preventing research subjects and researchers who work directly with them from knowing which people are receiving a new treatment—see page 2026). Double blinding reduces the bias of people who receive an active treatment expecting or being expected to do better than the control group. Placebos are used to blind subjects, but placebo design may be limited in CAM. Researcher blinding may also be limited. For example, a Reiki practitioner would know whether a real energy treatment is being administered.

If an alternative therapy has been proved ineffective, its use cannot be further advocated scientifically.

Safety: Safety is another important consideration. Although some CAM therapies can have risky side effects, the greatest risk occurs when a person is treated with an unproven CAM therapy instead of a proven conventional medicine approach. Regarding the risk of CAM therapies themselves, some are clearly safe. Examples are using meditation for pain management, acupuncture to treat nausea, yoga to improve balance, or ginger tea to aid digestion. Others may conceivably be harmful. Because herbal medicines and other dietary supplements (which are used in many alternative therapies) are not regulated as drugs by the Food and Drug Administration (FDA), their manufacturers do not have to prove their safety (see page 2070).

Some general risks include the following:

- Some substances may interact dangerously with prescription drugs.
- Although highly purified dietary supplements are readily available in the United States and many countries in Europe, products produced in other countries may contain dangerous contaminants, toxic ingredients, or other drugs.
- Harm can be done by alternative therapies that involve manipulation of the body or other nonchemical interventions (for example, manipulation that injures vulnerable parts of the body).

In many cases of alternative medicine, harm has neither been established nor excluded, but in some cases, potential harm has been shown. Sometimes the potential for harm is widely discounted by people who advocate use of the alternative product or therapy.

Types of Alternative Medicine

Alternative medicine can be classified into five major categories of practice: whole medical systems, mind-body techniques, biologically based therapies, manipulative and body-based therapies, and energy therapies. The category names only partially describe their components. Some approaches are understandable within the concepts of modern science, whereas other approaches are not. Many types overlap with others.

Whole Medical Systems

Whole medical systems are complete systems of diagnosis and practice. Examples are traditional Chinese medicine, Ayurveda, and unconventional Western practices of natural healing.

Traditional Chinese Medicine

Originating in China more than 2,000 years ago, this system is based on the theory that illness results from the improper flow of the life force (qi, pronounced chee) through the body. Qi is restored by balancing the opposing forces of yin and yang, which manifest in the body as heat and cold, external and internal, and deficiency and excess. Various practices are used to preserve and restore qi and thus health. They include diet, medicinal herbs, massage, meditative exercise called qi gong, and acupuncture.

Traditional Chinese medicine uses formulas containing mixtures of herbs to treat various ailments. For example, Chinese herbs seem to effectively treat common forms of arthritis and have few side effects. One herbal combination, sho-saiko-to, may reduce scarring in the liver and protect people with cirrhosis against liver cancer. One problem with traditional Chinese medicine is that standardization and quality control are almost nonexistent. For example, some traditional Chinese medicines have been laced with drugs or contaminated with toxic heavy metals.

Acupuncture: Acupuncture, a therapy within traditional Chinese medicine, is one of the most widely accepted alternative medicine techniques in the Western world. Licensed practitioners do not necessarily have a medical degree, although some medical doctors, often pain specialists, are trained and licensed to perform acupuncture. Acupuncture involves stimulating specific points on the body, usually by inserting very fine needles into the skin and underlying tissues. Stimulating these specific points is believed to unblock the flow of qi along energy pathways or meridians (there are more than 350 of these points along the meridians) and thus restore balance between yin and yang. Sometimes stimulation is increased by twisting or warming the needle. Acupuncture points may also be stimulated by pressure (called acupressure), lasers, ultrasound, or a very low-voltage electrical current (called electroacupuncture) applied to the needle. The procedure is not painful but may cause a tingling sensation.

Research has shown that acupuncture releases various chemical messengers in the brain (neurotransmitters) that serve as natural painkillers, including endorphins. Acupuncture has also been used to relieve pain after surgical or dental procedures. Besides its potential effectiveness as a pain reliever, acupuncture may help relieve the nausea and vomiting that commonly occur with pregnancy or after surgery or chemotherapy. As part of a comprehensive treatment plan (sometimes as accompanying treatment), acupuncture may be useful in treating addiction, carpal tunnel syndrome, fibromyalgia, headache, low back pain, osteoarthritis, and dry mouth (in people with advanced cancer). Acupuncture may also aid in stroke rehabilitation and may improve the success rates of in vitro fertilization. It is not clear whether acupuncture can help improve lung function in people with asthma or decrease pain and improve joint function in people with rheumatoid arthritis. Acupuncture is ineffective in helping people stop smoking or lose weight.

Millions of people are treated with acupuncture every day. Side effects are rare if the technique is done correctly, but the following should be noted:

- Temporary worsening of symptoms may occur.
- Infection is extremely rare because most health care practitioners use disposable needles. Reusable needles must be sterilized correctly.
- As with any medical treatment involving needles, some people may feel faint and need to lie down.
- Acupuncture may cause bruising or bleeding in people who have severe bleeding disorders or who take warfarin, an anticoagulant.
- People who have a pacemaker or an implanted defibrillator should not undergo electroacupuncture.
- Acupuncture has many proposed uses in pregnancy, such as the control of nausea, the reversal of breech presentation, and regulation of labor. However, because acupuncture may stimulate uterine contractions, it should only be administered by a specially trained practitioner.
- Rarely, deep needle placement can cause a collapsed lung and internal injury.

Ayurveda

Ayurveda is the traditional medical system of India, originating more than 4,000 years ago. It is based on the theory that illness results from the imbalance of the body's life force or prana. The balancing of this life force is determined by the equilibrium of the three bodily qualities called doshas: vata, pitta, and kapha. Most people have a dominant dosha, and the specific balance among the three doshas is unique to each person.

Health care practitioners evaluate people by questioning them about symptoms, behavior, and lifestyle; observing their overall appearance, including the eyes, tongue, and skin; and taking their pulse and checking their urine and stool. After determining the balance of doshas, health care practitioners design a treatment specifically tailored to each person. Ayurveda uses diet, herbs, massage, meditation, yoga, and internal cleansing (therapeutic elimination). Cleansing typically involves injecting fluid into the rectum to cause a bowel movement (an enema) or washing out the nose with water (nasal lavage) to restore balance within the body and with nature.

Few well-designed studies of Ayurvedic practices have been done.

In some of the herbal combinations used, heavy metals (mainly lead, mercury, and arsenic) are included because they are thought to have therapeutic effects. However, heavy metal poisoning has occurred in some people.

Homeopathy

Homeopathy, which was developed in Germany in the late 1700s, is based on the principle that like cures like (thus the name homeo [Greek for "like"] and patho [Greek for "disease"]). In other words, a substance that in large doses causes illness is believed to cure the same illness if given in minute doses. The minute dose is thought to stimulate the body's healing mechanisms. Treatments are based on a person's unique characteristics, including personality and lifestyle as well as symptoms and general health.

The remedies used in homeopathy are derived from naturally occurring substances, such as plant and animal extracts and minerals. These substances are used to stimulate the body's innate capacity to heal. Remedies are prepared by diluting these substances over and over and rapid shaking of the resulting solution. The more chemically dilute the homeopathic medicine, the more potent it is considered to be. Many homeopathic remedies are diluted so much that none of the original substance is present. However, many other homeopathic remedies do retain some pharmacologic activity.

 Did You Know...
Some homeopathic medicines may contain none of the active ingredient.

No scientific explanation for how ultradiluted remedies used in homeopathy might cure illness has been proved. There are few risks associated with homeopathy. However, side effects, such as allergic reactions and toxic reactions, can occur.

In the United States, homeopathic medicines are classified by the Food and Drug Administration as over-the-counter or prescription drugs. Quality testing for consistency of ingredients and potency is limited. Homeopathic medicines may contain alcohol, which is sometimes used to dilute the drug. The label is required to have the following:

- The word "homeopathic"
- The manufacturer's name
- Mention of at least one way the drug can be used
- Instructions for safe use
- The active ingredient and amount of dilution (unless specifically exempted)

Some homeopathic drugs are available by prescription only.

Homeopathy has not been established as effective treatment for any specific disorder.

Naturopathy

Naturopathy, which draws on practices from many cultures, began as a formal health care system in the United States in the early 1900s. Founded on the notion of the healing power of nature, naturopathy emphasizes prevention and treatment of disease through a healthy lifestyle, treatment of the whole person, and use of the body's natural healing abilities. This system also focuses on finding the cause of the disease rather than merely treating symptoms. Some of this system's principles are not that different from those of modern Western medicine.

Naturopathy uses a combination of therapies, including the following:

- Diet and nutritional supplementation
- Medicinal herbs
- Homeopathy
- Physical therapies (such as heat or cold therapy, ultrasonography, and massage)
- Mind-body therapies
- Exercise therapy
- Counseling on diet, lifestyle, and stress management
- Natural childbirth
- Hydrotherapy (agitated warm water or cold water applications)

Few clinical trials have been conducted specifically on naturopathy.

Mind-Body Techniques

Mind-body techniques are based on the theory that mental and emotional factors can influence physical health. Behavioral, psychologic, social, and spiritual methods are used to preserve health and prevent or cure disease.

Because of the abundance of scientific evidence backing the benefits of mind-body techniques, many of the approaches are now considered mainstream. Methods include the following:

- Meditation
- Relaxation techniques
- Guided imagery
- Hypnotherapy (hypnosis)
- Biofeedback

Mind-body techniques can be used to treat anxiety and panic disorders, chronic pain, coronary artery disease, depression, headaches, difficulty sleeping (insomnia), and loss of urinary control (incontinence). Mind-body methods are also used as an aid in childbirth, in coping with the disease-related and treatment-related symptoms of cancer, and in preparing people for surgery. The effectiveness of mind-body techniques in treating people with asthma, high blood pressure, and ringing in the ears (tinnitus) is not as clear.

There are few known risks associated with the use of mind-body techniques.

Meditation

In meditation, people regulate their attention or systematically focus on particular aspects of inner or outer experience. Meditation usually involves sitting or resting quietly, often with the eyes closed. Sometimes it involves the repetitive sounding of a phrase (a mantra) meant to help the person focus. The most highly studied forms of meditation are transcendental meditation and mindfulness meditation.

Meditation has been shown to have favorable effects on heart and blood vessel (cardiovascular) function, immunity, and brain activity, such as increasing activity in parts of the brain associated with mental clarity. Meditation often induces physical relaxation, mental calmness, and favorable emotional states such as loving-kindness and even-temperedness. Meditation fosters the capacity for metacognitive awareness (the ability to stand back from and witness the contents of consciousness). Metacognitive awareness interrupts habitual and reflexive responses to stress and improves tolerance of and coping with emotional distress.

Most meditation practices were developed within a religious or spiritual context and held as their ultimate goal some type of spiritual growth, personal transformation, or transcendental experience. As a health care intervention, however, meditation may be effective regardless of people's cultural or religious background. Meditation has been shown to offer numerous health benefits, including relieving stress, anxiety, depression, insomnia, pain, and symptoms of chronic disorders such as cancer or cardiovascular disorders. Meditation is also used to promote wellness.

Relaxation Techniques

Relaxation techniques are practices specifically designed to relieve tension and stress. The specific technique may be aimed at reducing activity of the nerves that control the stress response (sympathetic nervous system), lowering blood pressure, easing muscle tension, slowing metabolic processes, or altering brain wave activity. Relaxation techniques may be used with other techniques, such as meditation, guided imagery, or hypnotherapy.

Guided Imagery

Guided imagery involves the use of mental images to promote relaxation and wellness, reduce pain, or facilitate healing of a particular ailment, such as cancer or psychologic trauma. The images can involve any of the senses and may be self-directed or guided by a practitioner, sometimes in a group setting. For example, a person with cancer might be told to imagine an army of white blood cells fighting against the cancer cells.

Guided imagery has not been thoroughly scientifically studied, but many people claim to have had success with it.

Hypnotherapy

This alternative therapy is derived from Western practice. In hypnotherapy (hypnosis), people are guided into an advanced state of relaxation and heightened attention. Hypnotized people become absorbed in the images suggested by the hypnotherapist and are able to suspend disbelief. Because their attention is more focused and they are more open to suggestion, hypnotherapy can be used to help people change their behavior and thus improve their health. Hypnotherapy can be used to treat or help treat purely psychologic symptoms.

Hypnotherapy may also be helpful in treating many conditions and symptoms in which psychologic factors can influence physical symptoms:

- Phobias
- Certain pain syndromes
- Smoking cessation
- Conversion disorders (in which apparent physical illness is actually caused mainly by psychologic stress and conflict)
- Irritable bowel syndrome
- Headaches
- Asthma
- Some skin disorders (such as warts and psoriasis)
- High blood pressure
- Nausea and vomiting caused by chemotherapy, particularly the nausea some people get before chemotherapy (anticipatory nausea)
- Anxiety and diminished quality of life in people who have cancer

Hypnotherapy has been used with some success to help people stop smoking and lose weight. Some people are able to learn to hypnotize themselves.

The mechanism of hypnotherapy is poorly understood from a scientific standpoint.

Biofeedback

Biofeedback is a method of bringing unconscious biologic processes under conscious control. Biofeedback involves the use of electronic devices to measure and report back to the conscious mind information such as heart rate, blood pressure, muscle tension, and brain surface electrical activity. With the help of a therapist or with training, people then can understand why these functions change and can learn how to regulate them.

Typically, biofeedback is used to treat pain, including headache and chronic abdominal pain (see page 648), stress, insomnia, fecal or urinary incontinence, attention-deficit/hyperactivity disorder, mild cognitive impairment, tinnitus, and Raynaud's syndrome.

Biofeedback has been shown to be clinically effective in treating certain problems (for example, headaches, incontinence, and attention-deficit/hyperactivity disorder).

Biologically Based Therapies

Biologically based therapies use naturally occurring substances and include individual biologic therapies (such as using shark cartilage to treat cancer and glucosamine to treat osteoarthritis), diet therapy, herbal medicine, orthomolecular medicine, and chelation therapy. Many biologically based therapies have not been shown to be effective (for example, shark cartilage for cancer).

Diet Therapy

Diet therapy uses specialized dietary regimens (such as Gerson therapy, a macrobiotic diet, and the Pritikin diet) to treat or prevent a specific disease (such as cancer or cardiovascular disorders) or generally to promote wellness. Some diets (such as the Mediterranean diet) are widely accepted and encouraged in traditional Western medicine. The Ornish diet, a very low-fat vegetarian diet, can help reverse arterial blockages that cause coronary artery disease and may help prevent or slow the progression of prostate and other cancers. Some people following a macrobiotic diet have reported cancer remission, but a well-controlled clinical research study has not been conducted.

Because benefits usually take months or years to be realized, diet therapy is more likely to be effective if started early. When beginning a therapeutic diet that involves a dramatically different way of eating, people should receive some expert supervision so that they can avoid nutritional deficiencies.

Herbal Medicine

Herbal medicine or herbalism, the oldest known form of health care, uses plants and plant extracts to treat disease and promote wellness. Either a single herb or a mixture of different herbs can be used. Chinese herbal medicine mixtures can also contain minerals and animal parts. Unlike conventional drugs, in which a single, active chemical may be extracted and isolated, herbal medicine usually makes use of the medicinal plant in its whole form. Common herbal remedies include the following:

- Garlic
- Peppermint
- Chamomile
- St. John's wort
- Ginkgo biloba
- Valerian
- Ginseng

Herbal medicines (medicinal herbs—see page 2067) are available as extracts (solutions obtained by steeping or soaking a substance, usually in water), tinctures (usually alcohol-based preparations, with the alcohol acting as a natural preservative), infusions (the most common method of internal herbal preparation, usually referred to as a tea), decoctions (similar to an infusion), pills, powders, and injectables. Some herbal medicines are spread on a moistened cloth and applied to the skin. Potential problems include the following:

- **Impurities:** In the United States, the government has very little oversight of herbal products and places few regulations on the industry (see page 2070). (In contrast, in the European Union and Australia, government agencies regulate plant medicines as drugs.)
- **Interactions:** Some herbal medicines interact with drugs (for example, ginseng causes bleeding when used with warfarin—see table on page 2068) or foods (for example, St. John's wort causes dangerously high blood pressure when consumed with aged cheeses, Chianti wine, or other foods high in tyramine).
- **Side effects:** Some herbal medicines have side effects (for example, ginseng increases blood pressure, and garlic reduces blood clotting and increases blood sugar) that can be harmful for certain people.

People should tell their doctors all of the herbal medicines that they take. Recent clinical studies of several herbal medicines have shown them to be effective in treating various disorders.

? Did You Know...

There are many possible, potentially serious interactions between herbal medicines and drugs or foods.

Orthomolecular Medicine

Orthomolecular medicine uses combinations of vitamins, minerals, and amino acids normally found in the body to treat specific conditions and to maintain health. Nutrition comes first in diagnosis and treatment. Sometimes referred to as nutritional medicine, orthomolecular therapy emphasizes supplementing the diet with high-dose combinations of vitamins, minerals, enzymes, hormones (such as melatonin), and amino acids. Dosages often far exceed the amounts normally consumed in the diet.

A common form of orthomolecular medicine is megavitamin therapy, often with doses well above the recommended daily allowances (RDAs). Orthomolecular medicine practitioners contend these RDAs are inadequate to maintain health or to treat disease. While most treatments lack scientific evidence, conventional medicine does use some of highly concentrated micronutrients. For example, high doses of antioxidant substances are a conventionally used treatment for delaying the progression of macular degeneration, but recent studies have shown they are not effective in preventing cancer.

Sometimes orthomolecular medicine involves reducing the amount of a natural substance in the body. In certain specific disorders (such as vitamin deficiencies and metabolic disorders), treatments that could be considered orthomolecular are scientifically proven. However, for many uses, orthomolecular methods have no proven benefit and in some cases are potentially toxic.

Chelation Therapy

In this therapy, a drug is used to bind with and remove excess or toxic amounts of a metal or mineral (such as lead, copper, iron, or calcium) from the bloodstream. In conventional Western medicine, chelation therapy is a widely accepted way to treat lead poisoning and other heavy metal poisonings. Copper chelation has been under investigation as a cancer treatment. Chelation therapy with ethylenediaminetetraacetic acid (EDTA) is used as a complementary and alternative medicine therapy to remove calcium and thus treat atherosclerosis. The effectiveness and safety of this therapy are currently being evaluated scientifically. Side effects can be serious or rarely fatal.

Manipulative and Body-Based Therapies

Manipulative and body-based therapies treat various conditions through bodily manipulation. These therapies include chiropractic, massage, rolfing, reflexology, and postural reeducation.

Chiropractic

In chiropractic, the relationship between the structure of the spine and the function of the nervous system is seen as key to maintaining or restoring health. The main method for correcting this relationship is spinal manipulation. Chiropractors may also provide physical therapies (such as heat and cold, electrical stimulation, and rehabilitation strategies), massage, or acupressure or recommend exercises or lifestyle changes.

Chiropractic is being actively studied. Problems treated by chiropractic include low back pain, various headache disorders (although effectiveness is not always clear), neck pain, and pain caused by compressed nerves.

Past clinical trials have shown chiropractic to be as effective as conventional medical treatment in providing short-term relief of low back pain. Conventional medical practice guidelines include chiropractic as a treatment option for sudden low back pain that persists despite measures people take on their own. Treatments continued beyond 3 months may not provide added benefit. The usefulness of manipulation for conditions not directly related to the musculoskeletal system has not been established.

Serious complications resulting from spinal manipulation, such as low back pain, damage to cervical nerves, and damage to arteries in the neck, are rare. Other side effects may include discomfort, headache, and fatigue, which usually disappear within 24 hours. Spinal manipulation is not recommended for people who have any of the following:

- Osteoporosis
- Symptoms of neuropathy (for example, loss of sensation or strength in one or more limbs)
- Previous spinal surgery
- Stroke
- Blood vessel disorders

Massage Therapy

Massage therapy is the manipulation of body tissues to promote wellness and reduce pain and stress. It involves a variety of light-touch and deep-touch techniques, from stroking and kneading (as used in Swedish massage) to applying pressure to specific points (as used in Shiatsu, acupressure, and neuromuscular massage). Massage therapists claim to help the musculoskeletal, nervous, and circulatory systems of the body. Other healing effects of massage include the benefits of caring and human touch, basic needs that are unmet in the lives of many people.

Massage has been shown to be helpful in the following:

- Relieving pain, such as that caused by back injuries, muscle soreness, fibromyalgia, and anxiety
- Treating fatigue, pain, nausea, and vomiting in people with cancer

- Helping the brain, nerves, and behavior of low-birth-weight infants develop normally
- Preventing injury to the mother's genitals during childbirth
- Relieving chronic constipation
- Controlling asthma

Massage may lower stress and anxiety.

Precautions for massage therapy and other therapies that involve forceful manipulation include the following:

- Bare skin should not be massaged in people who have infectious or contagious skin diseases, open wounds, burns, high fever, or tumors.
- Massage can cause bruising and bleeding in people who have a low platelet count or a bleeding disorder.
- Massage should not stress bones affected by osteoporosis or cancer that has spread to the bones (metastatic cancer).

Rolfing

Rolfing, also called structural integration, is based on the theory that good health depends on correct body alignment. It is a form of deep tissue massage that is typically done over a series of sessions. Correct alignment of bone and muscle is achieved by manipulating and stretching the fibrous tissue that surrounds certain body organs (fascia), such as muscles. The effectiveness of rolfing has not been scientifically proven.

Reflexology

In reflexology, manual pressure is applied to specific areas of the foot that are believed to correspond to different organs or systems of the body. Stimulation of these areas is believed to eliminate the blockage of energy responsible for pain or disease in the corresponding body part. Reflexology may help relieve anxiety in people who have cancer.

Postural Reeducation

Postural reeducation uses movement and touch to help people relearn healthy posture, move more easily, and become more aware of their body. The therapies involved seek to release habitual, harmful ways of holding the body by focusing on awareness through movement. The effectiveness of postural reeducation is not clear.

Energy Therapies

Energy therapies focus on the energy fields thought to exist in and around the body (biofields). They also encompass the use of external energy sources (electromagnetic fields) to influence health and healing. All energy therapies are based on a core belief in the existence of a universal life force or subtle energy that resides in and around the body. Energy therapies include magnets, Reiki, therapeutic touch, yoga, Ayurveda (see page 2062), acupuncture (see page 2061), and qi gong.

Practitioners of energy therapies typically place their hands on or near the body and use their energy to affect the energy field of the person.

Magnets

Magnet-based therapies use static magnetic fields, pulsed electrical fields, or alternating-current or direct-current fields. Magnets, in particular, have become a popular treatment for various musculoskeletal conditions. Magnets have been marketed in clothing, jewelry, and mattresses to relieve pain.

Static magnet therapy remains scientifically unproven, especially for pain relief, which is one of the most common applications. Research studies of the effectiveness of static magnets have been inconclusive. Research studies of electromagnetic therapy for treating osteoarthritis and other pain conditions have been more promising. Using pulsating electromagnetic fields to speed healing of fractures that have stopped healing is well-established. A magnetic device is used in conventional psychiatry to deliver magnetic pulses through the skull as a treatment for depression.

It is not clear whether magnet therapy is safe for the following people:

- Pregnant women (the effects on the fetus are unknown)
- People who have implanted cardiac devices
- People who use an insulin pump
- People who take a drug by patch

Reiki

Reiki is of Japanese origin. In it, practitioners channel energy through their hands and transfer it into the person's body to promote healing. Practitioners complete a course of training with the intention of developing the ability to direct healing energy to others. Reiki is safe. Practitioners either do not touch the client or make very light contact with finger tips. Its effectiveness is not proven.

Therapeutic Touch

Therapeutic touch, sometimes referred to as a laying on of hands, uses the therapist's healing energy to identify and repair imbalances in a person's biofield. Unlike in Reiki, therapists usually do not touch the person. Instead, therapists move their hands back and forth over the person. Therapeutic touch has been used to lessen anxiety and improve the sense of well-being in people who have cancer, but these effects have not been studied rigorously. Therapeutic touch has gained acceptance by many holistic nurses who integrate this therapy into their hospital work routine. Therapeutic touch is safe.

CHAPTER

318 Medicinal Herbs and Nutraceuticals

Medicinal herbs are plant parts, sometimes ground, extracted, or otherwise prepared, used for health benefits. Nutraceuticals, a more recent and more general term, are a group of natural substances that includes certain herbs and such products as cholesterol-lowering margarines and psyllium-fortified products that are used as dietary supplements and regulated as foods.

Traditional systems of medicine have been used throughout the world for centuries. Certain ancient systems, such as traditional Chinese medicine, Ayurveda (the holistic system of medicine from India), and Tibetan medicine, are still used extensively, particularly in their country of origin. In the United States, interest in the therapies of such systems, particularly for the treatment of chronic illness, is growing. These therapies, usually referred to as complementary or

alternative medicine (see page 2059), range from medicinal herbs to acupuncture to massage. Most of them have not been studied scientifically, and nearly all are unregulated.

The most commonly used alternative therapy is **dietary supplements**, which include medicinal herbs and nutraceuticals. Because the use of dietary supplements is widespread, the United States government passed the Dietary Supplement Health and Education Act (DSHEA) in 1994. It defines a dietary supplement as any product (besides tobacco) that contains a vitamin, mineral, herb, or amino acid and that is intended as a supplement to the normal diet. The act requires that the label of a dietary supplement identify it as such. The label must state that the claims for

SOME POSSIBLE MEDICINAL HERB–DRUG INTERACTIONS

MEDICINAL HERB	AFFECTED DRUGS	INTERACTION
Chamomile	Anticoagulants (drugs that prevent blood clots, such as warfarin)	Chamomile taken with anticoagulants may increase the risk of bleeding.
	Sedatives (such as barbiturates and benzodiazepines)	Chamomile may intensify or prolong the effects of sedatives.
	Iron	Chamomile may reduce iron absorption.
Echinacea	Drugs that can damage the liver (such as anabolic steroids, amiodarone, methotrexate, and ketoconazole)	Echinacea taken for more than 8 weeks may damage the liver. When echinacea is taken with another drug that can damage the liver, the risk of liver damage may be increased.
	Immunosuppressants (drugs that intentionally suppress the immune system, such as corticosteroids and cyclosporine)	By stimulating the immune system, echinacea may negate the effects of immunosuppressants.
Ephedra*	Stimulant drugs (such as caffeine, epinephrine, phenylpropanolamine, and pseudoephedrine)	Ephedra contains ephedrine, which is a stimulant that increases the stimulant effects of other drugs, increasing the risk of irregular or rapid heart rate and high blood pressure.
	Monoamine oxidase inhibitors (MAOIs, a type of antidepressant)	Ephedrine may intensify the effects of these drugs and increase the risk of side effects, such as headache, tremors, irregular or rapid heart rate, and high blood pressure.
Feverfew	Anticoagulants (such as warfarin)	Feverfew taken with anticoagulants may increase the risk of bleeding.
	Iron	Feverfew may reduce iron absorption.
	Drugs used to manage migraine headaches (such as ergotamine)	Feverfew may increase heart rate and blood pressure when it is taken with drugs used to manage migraine headaches.
	Nonsteroidal anti-inflammatory drugs (NSAIDs)	NSAIDs reduce the effectiveness of feverfew in preventing and managing migraine headaches.
Garlic	Anticoagulants (such as warfarin)	Garlic taken with anticoagulants may increase the risk of bleeding.
	Drugs that decrease blood sugar levels (hypoglycemic drugs, such as insulin and glipizide)	Garlic may intensify the effects of these drugs, causing an excessive decrease in blood sugar levels (hypoglycemia).
	Protease inhibitors (such as indinavir or saquinavir), which are used to treat human immunodeficiency virus (HIV) infection	Garlic decreases blood levels of protease inhibitors, making them less effective.
Ginger	Anticoagulants (such as warfarin)	Ginger taken with anticoagulants may increase the risk of bleeding.
Ginkgo	Anticoagulants (such as warfarin), aspirin, and other NSAIDs	Ginkgo taken with anticoagulants or with aspirin or other NSAIDs may increase the risk of bleeding.
	Anticonvulsants (such as phenytoin)	Ginkgo may reduce the effectiveness of anticonvulsants in preventing seizures.
	Monoamine oxidase inhibitors (MAOIs, a type of antidepressant)	Ginkgo may intensify the effects of these drugs and increase the risk of side effects, such as headache, tremors, and manic episodes.

(continued on the following page)

SOME POSSIBLE MEDICINAL HERB–DRUG INTERACTIONS (*Continued*)

MEDICINAL HERB	AFFECTED DRUGS	INTERACTION
Ginseng	Anticoagulants (such as warfarin), aspirin, and other NSAIDs	Ginseng taken with anticoagulants or with aspirin or other NSAIDs may increase the risk of bleeding.
	Drugs that decrease blood sugar levels (hypoglycemic drugs)	Ginseng may intensify the effects of these drugs, causing an excessive decrease in blood sugar levels (hypoglycemia).
	Corticosteroids	Ginseng may intensify the side effects of corticosteroids.
	Digoxin	Ginseng may increase digoxin levels.
	Estrogen therapy	Ginseng may intensify the side effects of estrogen.
	MAOIs	Ginseng can cause headache, tremors, and manic episodes when it is taken with MAOIs.
	Opioids (narcotics)	Ginseng may reduce the effectiveness of opioids.
Goldenseal	Anticoagulants (such as warfarin)	Goldenseal may oppose the effects of anticoagulants and may increase the risk of blood clots.
Green tea	Warfarin	Green tea may cause warfarin to be less effective.
Kava	Sedatives (such as barbiturates and benzodiazepines)	Kava may intensify or prolong the effects of sedatives.
Licorice (glycyrriza glabra)†	Antihypertensives	Licorice may increase salt and water retention and increase blood pressure, making antihypertensives less effective.
	Antiarrhythmics	Licorice may increase the risk of an abnormal heart rhythm, making antiarrhythmic therapy less effective.
	Digoxin	Because licorice increases urine formation, it can result in low levels of potassium, which is excreted in urine. When licorice is taken with digoxin, the low potassium levels increase the risk of digoxin toxicity.
	Diuretics	Licorice may intensify the effects of most diuretics, causing increased, rapid loss of potassium. Licorice may interfere with the effectiveness of potassium-sparing diuretics, such as spironolactone, making these diuretics less effective.
	MAOIs	Licorice may intensify the effects of these drugs and increase the risk of side effects, such as headache, tremors, and manic episodes.
Milk thistle	Drugs that decrease blood sugar levels (hypoglycemic drugs)	Milk thistle may intensify the effects of these drugs, causing an excessive decrease in blood sugar levels.
	Protease inhibitors (such as indinavir or saquinavir), which are used to treat HIV infection	Milk thistle decreases blood levels of protease inhibitors, making them less effective.
Saw palmetto	Estrogen therapy and oral contraceptives	Saw palmetto may intensify the effects of these drugs.

(*continued on the following page*)

SOME POSSIBLE MEDICINAL HERB–DRUG INTERACTIONS (*Continued*)

MEDICINAL HERB	AFFECTED DRUGS	INTERACTION
St. John's wort	Benzodiazepines	St. John's wort may reduce the effectiveness of these drugs in reducing anxiety and may increase the risk of side effects such as drowsiness.
	Cyclosporine	St. John's wort may reduce blood levels of cyclosporine, making it less effective, with potentially dangerous results (such as rejection of an organ transplant).
	Digoxin	St. John's wort may reduce blood levels of digoxin, making it less effective, with potentially dangerous results.
	Iron	St. John's wort may reduce iron absorption.
	MAOIs	St. John's wort may intensify the effects of MAOIs, possibly causing very high blood pressure that requires emergency treatment.
	Nonnucleoside reverse transcriptase inhibitors	St. John's wort increases the metabolism of these drugs, reducing their effectiveness.
	Oral contraceptives	St. John's wort increases the metabolism of these drugs, reducing their effectiveness.
	Photosensitizing drugs (such as lansoprazole, omeprazole, piroxicam, and sulfonamide antibiotics)	When taken with these drugs, St. John's wort may increase the risk of sun sensitivity.
	Protease inhibitors (such as indinavir or saquinavir), which are used to treat HIV infection	St. John's wort may reduce blood levels of protease inhibitors, making them less effective.
	Selective serotonin reuptake inhibitors (such as fluoxetine, paroxetine, and sertraline)	St. John's wort may intensify the effects of these drugs.
	Warfarin	St. John's wort may reduce blood levels of warfarin, making it less effective and clot formation more likely.
Valerian	Anesthetics	Valerian may prolong sedation time.
	Sedatives (such as barbiturates and benzodiazepines)	Valerian may intensify or prolong the effects of sedatives, causing excessive sedation.

*Sale of supplements containing ephedra is banned in the United States.
†True, natural licorice, not the more common, artificially flavored licorice candy.

the dietary supplement have not been evaluated by the Food and Drug Administration (FDA). The label must also list each ingredient by name, quantity, and total weight and must identify the plant parts from which each ingredient is derived.

Most dietary supplements used in alternative medicine are derived from plants, and some are derived from animals. Because such dietary supplements are natural, some people assume that they are safe to use. However, a substance is not necessarily safe just because it is natural. For example, many potent poisons, such as hemlock, are derived from plants, and some, such as snake venoms, are derived from animals. Furthermore, almost all substances that affect the body, whether dietary supplements or drugs approved for medical use by the FDA (see page 76), can have unwanted side effects.

Safety and Effectiveness

Because dietary supplements are not regulated as drugs by the FDA, their manufacturers are not required to prove that supplements are safe and effective (although they must have a history of safety). Consequently, few supplements have been studied rigorously for safety and effectiveness (although some may eventually be shown to be safe and effective). Furthermore, because the need to evaluate supplements in humans has been recognized only recently, much of the available information has not been gathered systematically or scientifically and so is difficult to evaluate. In contrast, both prescription and nonprescription (over-the-counter) drugs have been extensively and systematically studied by researchers and reviewed for safety and effectiveness by the FDA (see page 77). These studies include those in animals to detect the development of cancer and organ damage and those in humans to detect any signs of toxicity.

The amount and quality of evidence supporting the effectiveness of supplements varies greatly. For some supplements, evidence supporting their effectiveness is convincing. However, for most, scientific studies have not been designed well enough to provide clear, reliable answers. For some supplements, the only evidence suggesting effectiveness is reports about individual people or studies conducted in animals.

Purity and Standardization

Other areas of concern are the purity and standardization of supplements. Supplements, unlike drugs, are not regulated to ensure that they are pure or that they contain the ingredients or the amount of active ingredient they claim to contain. As a result, the supplement may contain other substances, including, in some cases, prescription or nonprescription drugs and even dangerous substances such as mercury.

The amount of active ingredient in a dose of a supplement may vary, especially when whole herbs are ground or made into extracts to produce a tablet, capsule, or solution. The buyer is at risk of getting less, more, or, in some cases, none of the active ingredient in a supplement. Standardization requires that each individual dosage form of the product contains a precise amount of its active ingredient or ingredients. However, most herbal products are mixtures of several substances, and which ingredient is the most active is not always known. Therefore, determining which ingredient or ingredients should be considered active and thus subject to standardization can be difficult. Some supplements, particularly those produced in Europe, have been standardized and may include a designation of standardization on the label.

Advice on how to choose a pure, standardized product varies from expert to expert. Most experts recommend buying from a well-known manufacturer, and many recommend buying products made in Germany because oversight of supplements is stricter there than in the United States.

Although the content of a supplement is not standardized, the way in which it is manufactured has been standardized. In 2007, the FDA created current good manufacturing practices (GMPs) that standardize the manufacturing, packaging, labeling, and storing of dietary supplements. These GMPs help ensure the quality of dietary supplements and help protect the public health.

Interactions With Drugs

Supplements can interact with prescription and nonprescription drugs. Such interactions may intensify or reduce the effectiveness of a drug or cause a serious side effect. Before taking supplements, people should consult their doctor, so that such interactions can be avoided. Few well-designed studies have been conducted to investigate supplement-drug interactions, so most information about these interactions comes from sporadic individual reports of interactions.

Black Cohosh

Black cohosh is a plant. The underground stem of this plant is available in powder, tablet, or liquid form.

Medicinal Claims: People most often take black cohosh for menopausal symptoms (such as hot flashes, night sweats, mood swings, rapid heart rate, and vaginal dryness). People sometimes take black cohosh to treat arthritis, to induce labor, or to treat menstrual symptoms.

Scientific evidence regarding benefit in relieving menstrual symptoms is conflicting. There are few reliable data on the effectiveness of black cohosh for other disorders and symptoms.

Possible Side Effects: Side effects are uncommon. The most likely are headache and stomach discomfort. There is no evidence that black cohosh interferes with any drugs.

Black cohosh may cause headaches, dizziness, excessive sweating, nervous system problems, and vision disturbances (if high doses are taken). Other side effects include low blood pressure, constipation, loss of bone mass, muscle damage, digestive tract discomfort, liver toxicity, reduced pulse rate, nausea, and vomiting.

People who are sensitive to aspirin or have a seizure disorder, liver disease, hormone-sensitive cancers (for example, certain kinds of breast cancer), stroke, or high blood pressure probably should not take black cohosh. The U.S. Pharmacopeia (USP) has recommended that black cohosh products should be labeled with a warning declaring that they may be toxic to the liver.

Chamomile

The daisy-like flower of this herb is dried and used as tea or in an extract.

Medicinal Claims: People most often take chamomile as a mild sedative. People sometimes take chamomile by mouth to relieve stomach cramps and indigestion or apply a compress of chamomile extract to soothe irritated skin.

Possible Side Effects: Chamomile is generally considered safe. The most likely side effect is an allergic reaction. Allergic reactions may include skin irritation, itchy eyes, sneezing, and runny nose. People very rarely have a severe and life-threatening allergic reaction (anaphylaxis). In high doses, chamomile may lead to drowsiness, sedation, and vomiting.

Chamomile may reduce the absorption of drugs taken by mouth. Chamomile may also increase the effects of drugs that prevent blood clots (anticoagulants) and sedatives (including alcohol) and decrease the absorption of iron supplements.

Chondroitin Sulfate

Chondroitin sulfate is a natural component of cartilage. It is extracted from shark or cow cartilage or manufactured synthetically. It is frequently combined with glucosamine.

Medicinal Claims: People most often take chondroitin sulfate by mouth for osteoarthritis. For arthritis, it is frequently taken along with glucosamine (see page 2075). Scientific evidence shows no benefit when chondroitin sulfate is taken by itself. However, evidence suggests that combined with glucosamine, it may reduce joint pain and improve joint mobility.

Possible Side Effects: Chondroitin sulfate seems to have no serious side effects. Among the most common side effects are stomach pain, nausea, and other digestive tract symptoms. Other side effects include heart rate problems and swelling.

Chondroitin sulfate may also affect the action of drugs that prevent blood clots (anticoagulants) such as warfarin. Chondroitin sulfate is safe for most, but people who have asthma, blood-clotting disorders, or prostate cancer should use caution when taking it.

Chromium

Chromium is a mineral required in small quantities by the body. It enables insulin to function. Whole-grain products are good sources of chromium. Picolinate is often paired with chromium in supplements.

Medicinal Claims: Although chromium deficiency impairs insulin function, supplementation has not been shown to enhance the function of insulin. Nor has it been shown to promote weight loss, build muscle, or reduce body fat. Chromium supplements may lower levels of cholesterol and low-density lipoprotein (LDL)—the bad—cholesterol, as well as raise levels of high-density lipoprotein (HDL)—the good—cholesterol. Chromium supplements interfere with iron absorption.

Possible Side Effects: The maximum safe level of chromium intake is not known. Some evidence suggests that chromium damages chromosomes and consequently may be harmful or perhaps cause cancer.

Coenzyme Q10

Coenzyme Q10 (ubiquinone) is an enzyme that is naturally produced in the body. It participates in the energy-managing processes of cells and has an antioxidant effect. Antioxidants protect cells against damage by free radicals, which are highly chemically active by-products of normal cell activity. The levels of coenzyme Q10 seem to be lower in older people and in people with chronic diseases, such as heart problems, cancer, Parkinson's disease, diabetes, human immunodeficiency virus (HIV) infection or AIDS, and muscular dystrophies. However, it is not known whether these low levels contribute to these disorders.

Medicinal Claims: Coenzyme Q10 is being studied for use in people with heart failure and degenerative neurologic disorders, such as Parkinson's disease, Huntington's disease, and amyotrophic lateral sclerosis (ALS). It may provide some relief for people who develop muscle pains caused by certain drugs that lower lipid levels in the blood (statins). Coenzyme Q10 may also help protect the heart from the toxic effects of certain cancer chemotherapy drugs (such as doxorubicin and daunorubicin). Although some preliminary studies suggest coenzyme Q10 may be useful in treating these disorders, results are unclear and more testing is needed.

Possible Side Effects: Coenzyme Q10 may decrease response to the anticoagulant warfarin, which prevents blood clots. Side effects are uncommon, but some people have digestive symptoms, such as abdominal pain, nausea, heartburn, diarrhea, and vomiting, and central nervous system symptoms, such as dizziness, light sensitivity, irritability, and headache. Other side effects include skin itching, rash, loss of appetite, fatigue, and flu-like symptoms. Coenzyme Q10 is not recommended for people who exercise vigorously.

Cranberry

Cranberries are fruit that can be consumed whole or made into food products such as jellies and juices.

Medicinal Claims: People most often take cranberries to help prevent and relieve the symptoms of urinary tract infections. The effectiveness of cranberries in preventing urinary tract infections has been documented. Natural unprocessed cranberry juice contains anthocyanidins, which prevent *Escherichia coli* (the bacteria that usually cause urinary tract infections) from attaching to the urinary tract wall.

Some people take cranberry juice to reduce fever and treat certain cancers. However, there is no scientific proof that it is effective for these uses.

Possible Side Effects: No side effects are known. However, because most cranberry juice is highly sweetened to offset its tart taste, people with diabetes should not consume cranberry juice unless it is artificially sweetened. People who have kidney stones should consult their doctor before taking cranberry products. Cranberry products may increase the effects of drugs that prevent blood clots (such as the anticoagulant warfarin), causing severe bleeding. Therefore, people who take warfarin should not consume cranberry juice at the same time.

Creatine

Creatine is an amino acid made in the liver and stored in muscles. When combined with phosphate, it is a readily available source of energy in the body. In the diet, creatine is found in milk, red meat, and some fish.

Medicinal Claims: People take supplements of creatine to improve physical or athletic performance and to decrease fatigue. Its use is associated with weight gain. A few studies indicate that creatine can increase the amount of work performed with a short maximal effort (for example, in sprinting). However, a few others indicate no improvement in this type of activity.

Possible Side Effects: Creatine supplements may elevate levels of creatine in the urine and blood and cause kidney dysfunction. People who have diabetes or a history of kidney dysfunction or who take drugs that are toxic to the kidneys should avoid creatine supplements.

Dehydroepiandrosterone

Dehydroepiandrosterone (DHEA) is a steroid produced in the adrenal glands and converted into sex hormones (estrogens and androgens). DHEA's effects on the body are similar to those of testosterone. DHEA can be extracted from the Mexican yam.

Medicinal Claims: People take DHEA supplements to improve mood, energy, sense of well-being, and the ability to function well under stress. Other uses include deepening nightly sleep, lowering cholesterol levels, and decreasing body fat. It is also claimed to reverse aging and improve brain function in people with Alzheimer's disease. The medicinal claims of DHEA have not been proved. Many athletes claim that DHEA builds muscle and enhances athletic performance.

Possible Side Effects: Theoretically, DHEA may result in breast enlargement in men and hairiness in women and may stimulate the growth of prostate,

ovarian, breast, and other hormone-sensitive cancers. However, these effects have not been substantiated. DHEA should not be used by children. Other known side effects are agitation, insomnia, nervousness, irritability, and psychosis.

Echinacea

Echinacea is a perennial herb, which contains echinacoside and several other active substances. Various parts of the plant are used medicinally.

Medicinal Claims: People take echinacea mostly to help prevent or treat viral infections in the upper respiratory tract, such as the common cold. Some people apply echinacea as a cream or ointment to treat skin disorders and promote healing of wounds.

Many studies have evaluated the effects of echinacea on colds, but none is considered conclusive. One problem is that there are many different preparations of echinacea, and there is no standard dosage. However, several of the better-designed studies show no benefit from echinacea in cold prevention or treatment.

Possible Side Effects: No dangerous side effects have been identified. In children, risk of rash may be increased.

Echinacea may interact with drugs that can cause liver damage, thereby increasing the risk of liver damage. Echinacea may negate the effects of immunosuppressants, which are used, for example, to prevent rejection of organ transplants. People who have type 1 diabetes, autoimmune diseases (such as rheumatoid arthritis and multiple sclerosis), or an impaired immune system (for example, by AIDS or tuberculosis) should consult their doctor before they take echinacea.

Feverfew

Feverfew is a bushy perennial herb. The dried leaves are used in capsules, tablets, and liquid extracts. Parthenolide and glycosides are thought to be its active components.

Medicinal Claims: People take feverfew mostly to prevent migraine headaches. Evidence from three of four relatively small but well-designed studies supports these claims, but the largest and best designed of these studies did not. Differences in study findings may reflect the different formulations of feverfew used. In studies of people with arthritis, feverfew did not relieve symptoms. It has also been used to treat fevers, toothaches, insect bites, infertility, psoriasis, allergies, ringing in the ears (tinnitus), dizziness, nausea, vomiting, and problems during childbirth.

Possible Side Effects: Mouth ulcers and skin inflammation (dermatitis) may occur. Taste may be altered, and heart rate may be increased. Feverfew may interact with drugs that prevent blood clots (anticoagulants), drugs used to manage migraine headaches, and nonsteroidal anti-inflammatory drugs (NSAIDs). It may reduce the normal clotting tendency of particles in the blood that help stop bleeding (platelets) and may reduce the absorption of iron. Feverfew is not recommended for children or for women who are pregnant or breastfeeding. In addition, feverfew may cause allergic rashes.

Fish Oil

Fish oil may be extracted directly or concentrated and put in capsule form. Active ingredients are omega-3 fatty acids (eicosapentaenoic acid [EPA] and docosahexaenoic acid [DHA]). Western diets typically are low in omega-3 fatty acids.

Medicinal Claims: Fish oil is used for the prevention and treatment of atherosclerotic cardiovascular disease (see page 396). Strong scientific evidence suggest that the fatty acids in fish oil reduce the risk of heart attack and death caused by abnormal heart rhythms in people who have coronary artery disease and are taking traditional drugs. These fatty acids also reduce triglycerides and slightly lower blood pressure. Fish oil helps prevent toxicity to the kidneys caused by the drug cyclosporine. Fish oil supplements are also used to treat rheumatoid arthritis. However, scientific evidence supporting any benefit is inconclusive. For infants, intake of omega-3 fatty acids must be adequate to help the brain develop. Thus, breastfeeding mothers must consume sufficient amounts of omega-3 fatty acids.

Possible Side Effects: Fishy-tasting belching, acne exacerbation, nausea, and diarrhea may occur. A few studies suggest that too much fish oil can cause bleeding, but others do not show a relationship. Although some fish contain excess amounts of mercury, laboratory testing does not consistently show excess mercury in fish oil supplements. Even so, based on documented side effects, pregnant or breastfeeding women should not take omega-3 fatty acid supplements extracted from fish and should limit eating certain types and amounts of fish because of the potential risk of mercury contamination.

Garlic

Garlic has long been used in cooking and in medicine. When a garlic bulb is cut or crushed, an amino acid byproduct called allicin is released. Allicin is responsible for garlic's strong odor and medicinal properties.

Medicinal Claims: Garlic reduces the normal clotting tendency of particles in the blood that help stop bleeding (platelets). Because garlic stops microorganisms (such as bacteria) from reproducing, it can be used as an antiseptic and antibacterial. In large doses, garlic can slightly reduce blood pressure, overactivity of the intestine, and blood sugar levels. Advocates suggest that garlic lowers levels of low-density lipoprotein (LDL)—the bad—cholesterol. However, at least one well-designed study did not support this beneficial effect. Most studies have used aged garlic extracts. Preparations formulated to have little or no odor may be inactive and need to be studied.

Possible Side Effects: Garlic usually has no harmful effects other than making the breath, body, and breast milk smell like garlic. However, consuming large amounts can cause nausea and burning in the mouth, esophagus, and stomach.

Garlic may interact with drugs that prevent blood clots (such as warfarin), increasing risk of bleeding. Thus, garlic should not be eaten or taken as a supplement 1 week before surgery or before a dental procedure.

Ginger

Like garlic, ginger has long been used in cooking and in medicine. The stem of this herb contains substances called gingerols, which give ginger its flavor and odor.

Medicinal Claims: Many people take ginger to relieve pregnancy-related nausea and vomiting. Scientific studies suggest ginger is effective for this purpose, but results are mixed on whether ginger is effective for nausea caused by motion, chemotherapy, or surgery. It is unclear whether ginger is effective in treating rheumatoid arthritis, osteoarthritis, or joint and muscle pain.

Possible Side Effects: Ginger is usually not harmful, although some people experience a burning sensation when they eat it. It may also cause digestive discomfort and cause a disagreeable taste in the mouth. Ginger may increase the risk of bleeding. Therefore, people who take ginger and drugs that prevent blood clots may need to be monitored.

Ginkgo

Ginkgo is derived from the leaves of the ginkgo tree (commonly planted for ornamental purposes). The leaves contain numerous biologically active substances. Ginkgo is one of the most commonly used herbal supplements.

The fruit of the ginkgo tree is not used in ginkgo products. Contact with the fruit pulp, which may be encountered under ginkgo trees, can cause severe skin inflammation (dermatitis). The seeds of the fruit are toxic and can cause seizures and, in large amounts, death.

Medicinal Claims: Ginkgo reduces the clotting tendency of particles in the blood that help stop bleeding by forming clots (platelets), dilates blood vessels (thereby improving blood flow), and reduces inflammation. People take ginkgo for many reasons, such as improving blood flow to the lower legs in people with atherosclerotic vascular disease of the arteries in the legs (peripheral arterial disease) and treating dementia (as in Alzheimer's disease). Scientific studies clearly show ginkgo benefits people with peripheral arterial disease. Ginkgo increased the distance that affected people could walk without pain. Benefit for people with dementia seems unlikely based on findings from a large clinical trial. In this clinical trial, ginkgo was not effective in reducing the development of dementia and Alzheimer's disease in older people. However, a previous large U.S. clinical trial indicated that ginkgo temporarily stabilized mental and social function in people with mild to moderate dementia.

Studies show ginkgo does not seem to alleviate memory loss, ringing in the ears (tinnitus), or altitude sickness. Ginkgo may prevent damage to the kidneys caused by the drug cyclosporine, which suppresses the immune system.

Possible Side Effects: Although ginkgo leaf extracts usually have no side effects except mild digestive upset, the use of ginkgo should be supervised by a doctor because it is not suitable for self-medication. Ginkgo may interact with drugs that prevent blood clots, aspirin, and other nonsteroidal anti-inflammatory drugs (NSAIDs). It may increase the risk of bleeding, although a large clinical trial found no evidence for increased risk of bleeding among people taking ginkgo. Ginkgo may also reduce the effectiveness of anticonvulsants.

Ginseng

Ginseng is usually derived from two different species of plant: American ginseng and Asian ginseng. American ginseng is milder than Asian ginseng. Ginseng is available in many forms, such as fresh and dried roots, extracts, solutions, capsules, tablets, cosmetics, sodas, and teas. The active components are panaxosides in American ginseng and ginsenosides in Asian ginseng.

Siberian ginseng is not really ginseng and contains different active components, but it has antistress effects similar to those of American ginseng and Asian ginseng.

Ginseng products vary considerably in quality because many contain little or no detectable active ingredient. In very few cases, some ginseng products from Asia have been purposefully mixed with mandrake root, which has been used to induce vomiting,

or with phenylbutazone or aminopyrine—drugs that have been removed from the market in the United States because of unacceptable side effects.

Medicinal Claims: People take ginseng mostly to enhance physical and mental performance and to increase energy and resistance to the harmful effects of stress and aging. Many take it to enhance sexual performance, including treating erectile dysfunction. Ginseng seems to reduce blood sugar levels and increase levels of high-density lipoprotein (HDL)—the good—cholesterol. It may also increase hemoglobin and protein levels in the blood.

Evaluating some of ginseng's effects is difficult because measuring an increase in energy and other quality-of-life effects is difficult. In one small study of people with diabetes, ginseng reduced blood sugar levels and, according to a subjective report, improved mood and energy. In one large but short study, ginseng improved quality of life, according to a subjective report.

Possible Side Effects: Ginseng has a reasonably good safety record. However, some authorities recommend limiting the use of ginseng to 3 months because of the possible development of side effects. The most common side effects are nervousness and excitability, which usually decrease after the first few days. The ability to concentrate may be decreased, and blood sugar may decrease to abnormally low levels (causing hypoglycemia). Other side effects may include headaches, allergic reactions, and sleep and digestive problems, breast tenderness, and menstrual irregularities. Because ginseng has an estrogen-like effect, women who are pregnant or breastfeeding should not take it, nor should children. Occasionally, there have been reports of more serious side effects, such as asthma attacks, increased blood pressure, palpitations, and, in postmenopausal women, uterine bleeding. To many people, ginseng tastes unpleasant.

Ginseng can interact with drugs that prevent blood clots, aspirin, other nonsteroidal anti-inflammatory drugs (NSAIDs), corticosteroids, digoxin, estrogen therapy, monoamine oxidase inhibitors (MAOIs, used to treat depression), and drugs that decrease blood sugar levels (hypoglycemic drugs, used to treat diabetes).

Glucosamine

Glucosamine is extracted from a material (chitin) present in the shells of crabs, oysters, and shrimp. Glucosamine is taken in tablet or capsule form, usually as glucosamine sulfate, but sometimes as glucosamine hydrochloride. Glucosamine often is taken with chondroitin sulfate (see page 2072).

Medicinal Claims: People take glucosamine mostly to treat osteoarthritis of the knee. Its role in treating osteoarthritis in other locations is less well defined. Evidence is conflicting. Some evidence suggests it has both pain-relieving and disease-modifying effects, whereas other large and well-designed studies show it to be of no benefit. One very large study has shown that glucosamine hydrochloride is beneficial only when combined with chondroitin sulfate.

Possible Side Effects: Glucosamine is safe for most people. Common side effects are itching and mild digestive problems such as heartburn, diarrhea, vomiting, and nausea. People who have a shellfish allergy and take glucosamine extracted from shellfish may have an allergic reaction. Glucosamine may increase blood sugar in people with diabetes. Reports say that glucosamine increases the effects of warfarin (a drug that prevents blood clots) and thus increases the risk of bleeding. It may also reduce the effectiveness of such drugs as acetaminophen and some drugs that treat cancer and diabetes.

Goldenseal

Goldenseal, an endangered plant, is related to the buttercup. Its active components are hydrastine and berberine, which have antiseptic activity. Berberine is also active against diarrhea.

Medicinal Claims: Goldenseal is used as an antiseptic wash for mouth sores, inflamed and sore eyes, wounds, and irritated skin and as a douche for vaginal infections. It has been combined with echinacea as a cold remedy, but the effectiveness of goldenseal as a cold remedy has not been proved. Goldenseal is also used as a remedy for indigestion and diarrhea. In two relatively well-designed studies, berberine isolated from goldenseal reduced diarrhea.

Possible Side Effects: Goldenseal can cause many side effects, including digestive irritation and upset, contractions of the uterus, jaundice in newborns, and worsening of high blood pressure (hypertension). If taken in large amounts, goldenseal can cause seizures and respiratory failure and may affect contraction of the heart. Goldenseal may interact with drugs that prevent blood clots (such as warfarin). Women who are pregnant or breastfeeding, newborns, and people who have heart disease, a seizure disorder, or problems with blood clotting should not take goldenseal.

Green Tea

Green tea is made from the dried leaves of the same plant as traditional tea. However, traditional tea leaves are fermented, and green tea leaves are steamed but unfermented. Green tea may be brewed and drunk or ingested in tablet or capsule form. It is thought to have effects that protect cells from damage by oxygen, mutations, and cancer. Green tea contains caffeine, but many extracts have been decaffeinated. It is high in flavonoids and catechins.

Medicinal Claims: Green tea is said to have multiple health benefits, but none are supported by strong scientific evidence. People take green tea for many reasons, including prevention of cancer, coronary artery disease, and tooth decay. Other reasons are protection of skin from the sun, reduction of fat (lipid) levels in the blood, relief of osteoarthritis pain and menopausal symptoms, and enhancement of weight loss, memory, and longevity.

Possible Side Effects: Side effects are related to the effects of caffeine. They include insomnia, anxiety, frequent urination, nausea, diarrhea, irritability, upset stomach, rapid heart rate (tachycardia), and mild tremor. Pregnant women should avoid excessive caffeine. Caffeine in high doses may lead to high blood pressure, delirium, seizures, and irregular heart rhythms.

Kava

Kava comes from the root of a shrub that grows in the South Pacific. It is ingested as a tea or in capsule form.

Medicinal Claims: People use kava mostly to reduce anxiety, restlessness, or stress and to aid sleep. Some people use kava for asthma, menopausal symptoms, and urinary tract infections.

Possible Side Effects: Over 20 people in Europe developed liver toxicity (including liver failure) after taking kava. Thus, the Food and Drug Administration (FDA) has required a warning label on kava products, and safety is under continuing surveillance.

When kava is prepared traditionally (as tea) and used in high doses or over long periods of time, a scaly skin rash (kava dermopathy), vision problems, changes in blood (such as an increased number of red blood cells), and changes in movement disorders (such as worsening of Parkinson's disease) may occur. Also, kava may prolong the effect of other sedatives (such as barbiturates) and affect driving or other activities requiring alertness.

Licorice

Natural licorice, which has a very sweet taste, is extracted from the root of a shrub and used medicinally as a capsule, tablet, or liquid extract. Most licorice candy made in the United States is artificially flavored and does not contain natural licorice. Glycyrrhizin is the active ingredient in natural licorice. For people who are particularly sensitive to the effects of glycyrrhizin, licorice products that are specially treated to contain a much lower amount of glycyrrhizin (about one tenth of the usual amount) are available. These products are called deglycyrrhizinated licorice.

Medicinal Claims: People most often take licorice to suppress coughs, to soothe a sore throat, and to relieve stomach upset. Applied externally, it is thought to soothe skin irritation (for example, eczema).

Possible Side Effects: Glycyrrhizin causes the kidneys to retain salt and water, possibly leading to high blood pressure. It also causes the kidneys to excrete potassium, possibly causing low potassium levels in the blood. Increased potassium secretion can be a particular problem for people who have heart disease and for those who take digoxin or diuretics that increase potassium excretion in urine. Such people and those who have high blood pressure should avoid taking licorice.

Licorice may increase the risk of premature delivery. Thus, pregnant women should avoid licorice.

Melatonin

Melatonin, a hormone produced by the pineal gland (located in the middle of the brain), regulates the sleep-wake cycle. Melatonin used in supplements is derived from animals or produced artificially. In some countries, melatonin is considered a drug and is regulated as such.

Medicinal Claims: People use melatonin mostly to treat insomnia and to help minimize the effects of jet lag or of shift work. People who are traveling across time zones may take melatonin on the day or night of departure and for 2 or 3 nights after arrival. People who rotate work shifts may take melatonin before going to bed.

Evidence suggests that melatonin supplements can affect the sleep-wake cycle. However, in one large well-designed study, melatonin supplements did not relieve symptoms of jet lag, and only a few small studies suggest that these supplements can treat insomnia.

Possible Side Effects: Drowsiness may occur 30 minutes after taking melatonin and lasts for about 1 hour. Otherwise, melatonin seems to have few short-term side effects, although headache and temporary depression have been reported. Whether melatonin is safe when used long-term is unknown. Theoretically, a viral or prion infection (see page 765) could result from taking melatonin derived from animal brains but not from taking artificially produced melatonin. In people who are depressed, melatonin may worsen symptoms. Melatonin is best taken under medical supervision.

Milk Thistle

The main active ingredient, silymarin, is found in the seeds of this prickly leafed, purple-flowered plant.

Medicinal Claims: Milk thistle is claimed to protect the liver from damage by viruses, toxic substances (such as alcohol and the toxins from death cap mushrooms), and certain drugs (such as acetaminophen). Thus, people take milk thistle to prevent and treat mushroom poisoning and other liver disorders, such as cirrhosis and hepatitis C.

Well-designed scientific studies do not show that milk thistle significantly benefits people with a liver disorder. In reports that have collected information about many individuals with mushroom poisoning, milk thistle reduced the death rate.

Possible Side Effects: Brief stomach upset and mild allergies but no serious side effects have been reported. Milk thistle may intensify the effects of drugs that decrease blood sugar levels (hypoglycemic drugs).

Women who have hormone-sensitive conditions (such as breast, uterine, or ovarian cancer; endometriosis; and uterine fibroids) should avoid the above-ground parts of milk thistle.

S-Adenosyl-L-Methionine

S-adenosyl-L-methionine (SAMe) is a naturally occurring agent in the human body and is manufactured synthetically as a supplement.

Medicinal Claims: SAMe is said to be effective in treating depression, osteoarthritis, and liver disorders, but scientific studies so far do not confirm this claim. More research is needed to verify its effectiveness.

Possible Side Effects: No serious side effects have been reported. People with a bipolar disorder should not use SAMe because it can cause manic episodes.

Saw Palmetto

The plant's berries can be made into tea. Saw palmetto is also available as tablets, capsules, and a liquid extract.

Medicinal Claims: Saw palmetto opposes the actions of testosterone. People take saw palmetto mostly to treat benign enlargement of the prostate gland (benign prostatic hyperplasia). In a number of studies, saw palmetto relieved the symptoms of an enlarged prostate gland, such as the frequent urge to urinate. However, a large, well-designed study did not show any benefit.

Claims that it increases sperm production, breast size, or sexual vigor are unproved.

Possible Side Effects: Headache and diarrhea occasionally occur. Because saw palmetto may have hormonal effects, women who are pregnant or who may become pregnant should not take it. Women taking hormone therapy should consult their doctor before they take saw palmetto. Saw palmetto may interact with estrogen therapy and oral contraceptives and may affect the blood clot–preventing effects of warfarin.

St. John's Wort

The reddish substance in the plant's flowers contains numerous biologically active compounds, including hypericin and hyperforin.

Medicinal Claims: People take St. John's wort mostly to relieve symptoms of depression. Study results vary, but there may be a benefit in treating mild to moderate short-term depression. However, a large, well-designed study found that St. John's wort is ineffective in treating severe (major) depression.

St. John's wort has been used in the treatment of vitiligo, but its effectiveness in treating this disorder is unproved.

Possible Side Effects: St. John's wort may cause increased sensitivity to sunlight. Other side effects include digestive tract symptoms, fatigue, and headache. Pregnant women should not take this supplement because it increases muscle tone in the uterus and thus may increase the risk of a miscarriage.

One of the larger problems with St. John's wort is that it may interact negatively with drugs people take (see table on page 2070). These interactions may lead to toxic reactions or ineffectiveness of the drug.

Valerian

The plant's dried root contains valepotriates, which may have calming effects.

Medicinal Claims: People take valerian mostly as a sedative and sleep aid, especially in parts of Europe. In two relatively well-designed studies, valerian improved sleep quality and shortened the time needed to fall asleep.

Some people take valerian for headaches, depression, irregular heartbeat, and trembling. It is usually used for short periods of time (4 to 6 weeks). There is not enough scientific evidence to determine whether valerian is effective for these conditions.

Possible Side Effects: Headaches, excitability, uneasiness, and heart disturbances have been reported. People who are driving or doing other activities requiring alertness should not take it. Other side effects include upset stomach, dizziness, and tiredness.

Valerian may prolong the effect of other sedatives (such as barbiturates) when it is taken with them.

Valerian is not recommended for women who are pregnant or breastfeeding.

Zinc

Zinc, a mineral, is required in small quantities for many metabolic processes. Dietary sources include oysters, beef, and fortified cereals.

Medicinal Claims: People most often take zinc in the form of lozenges to reduce the duration of cold symptoms. Scientific studies are inconsistent, but if zinc has an effect, it probably is small and occurs only when it is taken very soon after cold symptoms develop.

Some people take zinc to help heal wounds because zinc deficiency delays wound healing. Mild zinc deficiency impairs growth in children and can be corrected with zinc supplementation. For more on zinc deficiency, see page 950.

Possible Side Effects: Zinc is generally safe, but toxicity can develop if high doses are taken. The common side effects of zinc lozenges include nausea, vomiting, diarrhea, mouth irritation, mouth sores, and bad taste. Because zinc is a trace metal and can remove other necessary metals from the body, zinc lozenges should not be taken for more than 14 days. Zinc sprays may cause nose and throat irritation. The effects of certain antibiotics may be lowered by the consumption of zinc supplements.

CHAPTER

319 Drug Use and Abuse

Drugs are an integral part of everyday life for many people—legitimately and illegitimately—and drug use among adolescents remains high (see page 1758).

The legality and social acceptance of a particular drug often depend on what it is used for, what its effects are, and who is using it. For example, many abused drugs have legitimate medical uses:

- Amphetamines: To treat attention-deficit/hyperactivity disorder

- Barbiturates and benzodiazepines: To treat anxiety and insomnia

- Cocaine: To numb surfaces of the body (as a topical anesthetic)

- Ketamine: To provide anesthesia
- Marijuana: To treat nausea due to advanced cancer
- Opioids: To relieve pain and provide anesthesia

However, use of these drugs for pleasure is illegal and dangerous. Legality and social acceptance of a drug often vary among different societies or countries. Legality and acceptance may also change within a society or country over time, as happened with alcohol in the United States.

Many drugs, some legal and some not, alter the mind. Some mind-altering (psychoactive) drugs affect brain function each time they are used, regardless of how much is used. Others affect brain function only if a large amount is used or if the drug is used continually. Some drugs affect the brain in such a way that people want or feel a need to use the drug again and again (craving). Some cause symptoms, such as euphoria (a high).

Narcotics are often thought of when drug abuse is discussed. This term refers to drugs that cause loss of feeling, a sense of numbness, and drowsiness. The term often refers specifically to opioids (drugs that bind to opiate receptors on cells). However, the term narcotics is also used in a broader (and inaccurate) sense to include any drug that is illegal or used illegitimately.

Did You Know...
Some people who abuse drugs are not dependent on them.

Definitions

Different terms are used to indicate the problems caused by using mind-altering drugs. However, doctors and other experts sometimes disagree about the exact meaning of these terms.

Tolerance: This term means that people need more and more of a drug to feel the effects originally produced by a smaller amount. People can develop tremendous tolerance to drugs such as opioids and alcohol.

Intoxication: This term refers to the immediate and temporary effects of a specific drug. When people are intoxicated, mental function and judgment are impaired, and mood may be altered. Depending on the drug, people may feel a sense of excitement, an exaggerated feeling of well-being, or euphoria, or they may feel more calm, relaxed, and sleepy. Many drugs impair physical functioning, with decreased coordination, leading to falls and vehicle crashes. Some drugs trigger aggressive behavior, leading to fighting. As larger amounts of the drug are used, adverse effects become more obvious (called an overdose), with serious complications and risk of death.

Drug Dependence: Drug dependence refers to factors that make it difficult for a person to stop taking a drug. These factors include craving and withdrawal. Drug dependence may be psychologic or physical.

Psychologic dependence refers to a compelling desire to repeat the experience of taking a mind-altering drug (craving) or to avoid the discontent of not using the drug (withdrawal). Desiring the drug experience may be the only obvious reason for compulsive use. Drugs that cause psychologic dependence often produce one or more of the following:

- Reduced anxiety and tension
- Elation, euphoria, or other pleasurable mood changes
- Feelings of increased mental and physical ability
- Feeling a temporary escape from reality
- Altered perceptions of the environment (for example, auditory or visual hallucinations)

The intense desire and compulsion to use a drug lead to using it in larger amounts, more frequently, or over a longer period than at first intended. People who are psychologically dependent on a drug give up social and other activities because of drug use. They also continue to use the drug even though they know that the drug is physically harmful or interferes with other aspects of their life, including family and work.

Physical dependence means that stopping the drug results in unpleasant, sometimes painful physical symptoms (withdrawal). Symptoms occur because the body adapts to the continuous presence of a drug.

People going through withdrawal feel sick and may have various unpleasant symptoms depending on the drug involved. Withdrawal from some drugs (such as alcohol or barbiturates) can be serious and even life threatening.

How drug dependence develops is complex and unclear. It depends on interaction of the following:

- **Drug:** Drugs vary in how likely they are to make people dependent on them.
- **User:** The user's personality, health, physical characteristics (including genetic makeup), and emotional circumstances affect whether the user is likely to become dependent. For example, the presence of constant pain may drive a person to use drugs inappropriately, as may emotional distress. However, research has not identified any clear-cut biochemical or physical differences in people to explain why some become dependent and others do not.
- **Cultural and social factors:** Peer or group pressure and stress (for example, due to work or family obligations) may contribute to dependency, as may the mass media's portrayal of prescription drugs as safely relieving all distress.

Drug Abuse: Drug abuse can be defined in terms of society's disapproval and the effect the drug has on the person's social and emotional well-being. Drug abuse may involve the following:

- Using drugs, usually illegal drugs, recreationally (not for medical reasons)
- Using mind-altering drugs to relieve medical problems or symptoms without a health care practitioner's recommendation
- Using drugs because of a strong psychologic or physical compulsion (dependence) to use them

Use of illegal drugs is often considered abuse largely because the drugs are illegal. But drugs that are abused are not necessarily illegal, and they may or may not alter the mind. They include prescription drugs, alcohol, and substances in products not considered drugs (such as glue or paint), as well as illegal drugs. People of all socioeconomic groups abuse drugs.

Some people who abuse drugs use an amount large enough or over a period long enough to threaten their quality of life, health, or safety or those of other people. But many people control their abuse of drugs so that it does not adversely affect their health or functioning, making the effects less obvious. Drug abuse does not necessarily include dependence.

Recreational Drug Use: The recreational use of drugs involves using drugs occasionally in relatively small doses and thus often without harm to users. That is, users do not develop tolerance or become physically dependent, and the drug does not physically harm them (at least in the short term). Drugs usually considered recreational include opium, alcohol, nicotine, marijuana, caffeine, hallucinogenic mushrooms, and cocaine.

Recreational drugs are usually taken by mouth or inhaled.

Drug Addiction: Drug addiction has no universally accepted definition. It is characterized by an intense craving for the drug and compulsive, uncontrolled use of the drug despite harm done to the user or other people. People who are addicted spend more and more time obtaining the drug, using the drug, or recovering from its effects. Thus, addiction usually interferes with the ability to work, study, or interact normally with family and friends. Because there is a risk of harm, addiction implies the need to stop drug use, regardless of whether the addict understands and agrees.

Addiction can involve illegal or legal drugs. However, obtaining and using an illegal drug is very different from obtaining and using a legal drug, which may involve simply going to the doctor, getting a prescription, and going to the pharmacy. Obtaining an illegal drug (or a legal drug used without medical need) may involve lying and stealing. For example, people may falsify symptoms to a doctor or visit several doctors with the same symptoms to obtain several prescriptions. When people with severe pain due to advanced cancer become dependent (psychologically and physically) on an opioid such as morphine, their ongoing need for that drug is not usually considered an addiction. However, when people become dependent on heroin, steal to get money to buy heroin, and lie to family members and friends, their behavior is considered an addiction.

At times, family members or friends may behave in ways that allow an addict to continue to use drugs or alcohol. These people are called enablers. They are considered codependents when their own needs are intertwined with perpetuating the addict's use of the addictive substance. Enablers may call in sick for an addict or make excuses for the addict's behavior. Enablers may plead with the addict to stop using drugs or alcohol but rarely do anything else to help the addict stop.

A pregnant addict exposes her fetus to the drugs she is using. Often, a pregnant addict does not admit to her doctor that she is using drugs or alcohol. The fetus may become dependent and may develop serious defects as a result of the mother's drug use (see page 1708). Soon after delivery, the newborn can experience severe or even fatal withdrawal, particularly when the doctor is unaware of the mother's addiction.

Methods of Use

Drugs may be swallowed, smoked, inhaled through the nose as a powder (snorted), or injected. When drugs are injected, their effects may occur more quickly, be stronger, or both.

Drugs may be injected into a vein (intravenously), a muscle (intramuscularly), or under the skin (subcutaneously). Veins in the arms are typically used for intravenous injections, but if these areas become too scarred, drugs may be injected into veins anywhere in the body, including those of the thigh, neck, or armpit.

Complications From Drug Injection: Injecting drugs has more risks than other methods. People are exposed not only to the side effects of the drug but also to problems related to injection itself, such as the following:

- **Adulterants:** Adulterants are substances that are added to a drug to alter its physical qualities. They are usually added, without the user's knowledge, to reduce costs or to make the drug easier to use. Thus, users do not know what they are injecting. In street drugs such as heroin and cocaine, adulterants may also be added to enhance mind-altering properties or

Other Drugs of Abuse

Drug abuse typically involves mind-altering drugs, but it may involve drugs taken for other purposes, usually losing weight or enhancing athletic performance. Taking these drugs without medical need and medical supervision can endanger the quality of life, health, or safety of the user. Using a drug this way is considered drug abuse. Anabolic steroids are probably the most commonly abused drugs in this group (see page 2090).

Growth Hormone

Growth hormone is produced by the pituitary gland to help the body control how proteins, carbohydrates, and fats are used to stimulate growth. Growth hormone is also manufactured as a drug and is sometimes given to children of small stature when their body is unable to make enough growth hormone. Some athletes abuse growth hormone because they believe it can increase muscle growth and strength while decreasing body fat.

Use of growth hormone without medical need over a long period can cause an increase in fat levels in the blood, diabetes, and an increase in heart size, which may result in heart failure.

Laboratory tests to identify growth hormone not made by the person's own body are not routinely available.

Erythropoietin and Darbepoetin

Erythropoietin is a hormone produced by the kidneys. It stimulates bone marrow to produce red blood cells. Erythropoietin is also manufactured as a drug. Darbepoetin is a drug similar to erythropoietin. Both drugs are used to increase production of red blood cells in people with certain kinds of anemia. These drugs may be taken by athletes because they believe that with more red blood cells, more oxygen can get to their muscles, enabling them to perform better.

Using erythropoietin or darbepoetin without medical need may change the body's regulation of red cell production, so that the number of red blood cells suddenly decreases when these drugs are stopped.

Diuretics

Diuretics are drugs that speed the elimination of salt and water by the kidneys. Diuretics are used to treat a variety of disorders, including high blood pressure and heart failure. However, some people, including athletes and people with eating disorders such as anorexia nervosa, take diuretics to help them lose weight quickly. Inappropriate use of diuretics may cause dehydration and severe deficiencies of electrolytes such as potassium. Such deficiencies can lead to severe illness or death.

Ipecac Syrup

Ipecac syrup is a drug that triggers vomiting. It is sometimes used to treat children who have swallowed chemicals or poisons. However, people with eating disorders such as anorexia nervosa often take ipecac syrup to help them lose weight. Inappropriate use of ipecac may cause diarrhea, severe deficiencies of electrolytes, weakness, irregular heart rhythms, and heart failure.

Laxatives

Laxatives are drugs that speed the passage of substances through the digestive tract and that are used to treat constipation. However, people who falsely believe they must have frequent bowel movements as part of being healthy often abuse laxatives. In addition, people with eating disorders such as anorexia nervosa sometimes take laxatives because they believe doing so can help them lose weight.

Laxatives used often and without medical need may cause dehydration and severe deficiencies of electrolytes. Regular use of laxatives can also interfere with absorption of other drugs, causing them to stop working. Inappropriate use of laxatives over a long period can damage the muscle layers of the large intestine. Severe constipation and other intestinal disorders (such as diverticulosis) may result.

---

to substitute for the drug. Quinine, a common heroin adulterant, can cause double vision, paralysis, and other symptoms of nerve injury, including Guillain-Barré syndrome (see page 828).

- **Fillers:** Some people crush tablets of prescription drugs, dissolve them, and inject the solution intravenously. These people are injecting the fillers that tablets commonly contain (such as cellulose, talc, and cornstarch). Fillers can become trapped in the lungs, causing inflammation. Fillers can also damage heart valves, increasing the risk of infection there (endocarditis).
- **Bacteria and viruses:** Injecting drugs with unsterilized needles, particularly needles used by someone else, can introduce bacteria and viruses into the

body. As a result, abscesses may develop near the injection site, or bacteria or viruses may travel through the bloodstream to other parts of the body, such as the lungs, heart, brain, or bones, and cause infection. Infection of the heart valves (endocarditis—see page 386) is a common serious consequence of injecting drugs contaminated with bacteria or using dirty needles. Sharing needles can spread serious infections, such as hepatitis B and C and human immunodeficiency virus (HIV) infection.

- **Injuries due to needle use:** Drug abuser's elbow (myositis ossificans) is caused by repeated, inept needle punctures. The muscle around the elbow is replaced with scar tissue. Subcutaneous injections (those given under the skin, also called skin popping) can cause skin sores. Intravenous injections lead to scarring of veins (tracks), which makes the veins more and more difficult to inject and impairs blood flow.

Screening

Screening involves checking for drug abuse in people who do not necessarily have any symptoms of drug abuse. It may be done systematically or randomly in people such as the following:

- Certain groups of people, such as students, athletes, and prisoners
- People who are applying for or who already hold certain types of jobs (such as pilots or commercial truck drivers)
- People who have been involved in motor vehicle or boating accidents or accidents at work
- People who have attempted suicide by unclear means
- People in a court-ordered treatment program for drug abuse or with terms of probation or parole requiring abstinence—to monitor compliance
- People in a substance abuse treatment program— to detect continuing substance abuse and thus better plan treatment

Tricks of the Trade: Body Packing

To smuggle drugs across borders or other security checkpoints, people may voluntarily swallow packets filled with drugs. This tactic is called body packing.

Body packing often involves drugs with a high street value (primarily heroin or cocaine). The drugs may be placed in condoms or in packets wrapped in several layers of polyethylene or latex and sometimes covered with an outer layer of wax. After body packers (mules) swallow several packets, they typically take drugs to slow the movement of substances through the digestive tract until the packets can be retrieved.

If a packet tears, a drug overdose may occur, sometimes causing serious symptoms. Symptoms may include repeated seizures, high blood pressure, a very high body temperature, difficulty breathing, and coma. Packets may block or tear the intestine. If the intestine tears, its contents may leak into the abdominal cavity and cause infection—a disorder called peritonitis.

Body stuffing is similar to body packing. It occurs when people swallow drug packets to avoid being caught by law enforcement. Sometimes packets are hidden in the rectum or vagina. The amounts of drugs are smaller than those in body packing. But the drugs are usually less securely wrapped, so overdose is still a concern.

Typically, people have to give consent for screening except in certain circumstances, such as car accidents. Screening cannot determine how often a substance is used and thus cannot distinguish casual users from those with more serious problems. Also, drug screening targets only some substances and thus misses many others. Substances most commonly targeted include alcohol, marijuana, cocaine, opioids, amphetamines, phencyclidine, benzodiazepines, and barbiturates.

A sample of urine, blood, breath, saliva, sweat, or hair may be tested. Urine testing is most common because it is noninvasive, quick, inexpensive, and able to detect many drugs. It can detect drugs that were used within 1 to 4 days, sometimes longer, depending on the drug used. Hair testing is not as widely available but can detect some drugs if they were used in the previous 100 days. Health care practitioners may directly observe the collection of the sample and seal it so that they can be sure the sample has not been tampered with.

Diagnosis

Sometimes drug abuse is diagnosed when people go to a health care practitioner because they want help stopping use of the drug. Other people try to hide their drug use.

Practitioners may suspect problems with drug use when they notice changes in mood or behavior in a person. They may then do a thorough physical examination. Signs of drug abuse may be apparent. For example, repeatedly injecting drugs intravenously produces track marks. Track marks are lines of tiny, dark dots (needle punctures) surrounded by an area of darkened or discolored skin. Injecting drugs under the skin produces circular scars or ulcers. Addicts may claim other reasons for the marks, such as frequent blood donations, bug bites, or other injuries.

Health care practitioners also use other methods (such as questionnaires) to identify abuse of some drugs and other substances and to determine the extent of abuse and its effects. Urine and sometimes blood tests may be done to check for the presence of drugs.

If a drug use problem is identified, especially if the drugs are injected, people are thoroughly evaluated for hepatitis, HIV infection, and other infections common in people who use these drugs.

Treatment

Specific treatment depends on the drug being used, but it typically involves counseling and sometimes involves use of other drugs. Family support and support groups help people remain committed to stopping use of the drug.

Treatment of complications is the same as that for similar complications with other causes. For example, abscesses may be drained, and antibiotics may be used to treat infections.

Because sharing needles is a common cause of HIV infection, a harm-reduction movement was started. Its purpose is to reduce the harm of drug use in users who cannot stop. Thus, users are provided clean needles and syringes so they do not reuse other abusers' needles. This strategy helps reduce the spread (and the cost to society) of HIV infection and hepatitis.

Alcohol

- Genetics and personal characteristics may play a part in the development of alcohol use disorders.
- Drinking too much alcohol may make people sleepy or aggressive, impair coordination and mental function, and interfere with work, family, and other activities.
- Drinking too much alcohol for a long time can make people dependent on alcohol and damage the liver, brain, and heart.
- Doctors may use questionnaires or determine the blood alcohol level to help identify people with an alcohol use disorder.
- Immediate treatment may include assistance with breathing, fluids, thiamin, other vitamins, and, for withdrawal, benzodiazepines.

- Detoxification and rehabilitation programs can help people with severe alcohol use disorders.

About 45 to 50% of adults currently drink alcohol, 20% are former drinkers, and 30 to 35% are lifetime abstainers. Drinking large amounts of alcohol (more than 2 to 6 drinks per day) for extended periods can damage a number of organs, especially the liver, heart, and brain. However, drinking a moderate amount of alcohol may reduce the risk of death from heart and blood vessel (cardiovascular) disorders. Nonetheless, drinking alcohol for this purpose is not recommended, especially when other safer, more effective preventive measures are available.

Alcohol Abuse: Most people do not consume enough alcohol or consume it often enough to impair their health or interfere with their activities. However, 7 to 10% of adults in the United States have a problem with alcohol use (alcohol use disorder). Disorders include at-risk drinking (defined solely by amount consumed), alcohol abuse, and alcohol dependence (the most severe alcohol use disorder). Alcoholism is an imprecise term. It typically refers to excessive drinking, unsuccessful attempts at stopping drinking, and continued drinking despite adverse social and occupational consequences. Men are 2 to 4 times more likely than women to become alcoholics.

CLASSIFYING ALCOHOL USE DISORDERS

DISORDER	DESCRIPTION
At-risk drinking	Defined by the amount and frequency of drinking: ■ More than 14 drinks* a week or 4 drinks per occasion for men ■ More than 7 drinks a week or 3 drinks per occasion for women
Alcohol abuse	Drinking that does any of the following but without evidence of dependence: ■ Prevents people from fulfilling their obligations ■ Is done in physically dangerous situations (such as driving) ■ Results in legal, social, or interpersonal problems
Alcohol dependence	Frequent consumption of large amounts of alcohol causing more than three of the following problems: ■ People need to drink more and more alcohol to produce the same effects (tolerance). ■ Stopping the drug results in unpleasant, sometimes painful physical symptoms (withdrawal). ■ People drink more than they intended. ■ People want to reduce use but cannot. ■ People have spent a lot of time getting or drinking alcohol or recovering from its effects. ■ People have missed important events or activities (such as work, a wedding, or a graduation) because of drinking. ■ People continue to drink even though drinking is causing physical or psychologic problems.

*One drink is equivalent to 12 ounces of beer, 5 ounces of wine, or 1½ ounces of liquor, such as whiskey.

Generally, people who become alcoholics have been regularly using alcohol in excessive amounts for a long time and are dependent on alcohol. The amount of alcohol people consume on an average day before they develop alcohol problems varies widely. But it may be as little as 2 drinks per day for women and 3 drinks for men (one drink is equivalent to 12 ounces of beer, 5 ounces of wine, or 1½ ounces of liquor, such as whiskey). Many people with alcohol problems are also binge drinkers—that is, men who drink 5 or more drinks and women who drink 4 or more drinks per occasion. Binge drinking may go on for many days, followed by drinking little or none for a few days. Binge drinking is a particular problem among younger people.

> ### ? Did You Know...
> Drinking very large amounts of alcohol can quickly cause death.

Alcoholism leads to many destructive behaviors. Drunkenness may disrupt family and social relationships. Married couples often divorce. Extreme absenteeism from work can lead to unemployment. Alcoholics often cannot control their behavior, tend to drive while drunk, and experience physical injury from falls, fights, or motor vehicle accidents. Some alcoholics become violent. Alcoholism in men is often associated with domestic violence against women (see page 1581).

Special Populations: Very young children who drink alcohol (typically accidentally) are at significant risk of very low blood sugar and coma. Women may be more sensitive to the effects of alcohol than men, even on a per-weight basis. Older people may be more sensitive than younger adults. Drinking during pregnancy increases the risk of fetal alcohol syndrome (see page 1641).

Although sensitivity to the effects of alcohol may vary, people of all ages are susceptible to alcohol use disorders. Increasingly, adolescents are having alcohol problems, with especially disastrous consequences (see page 1758). Those who start drinking at an early age (particularly the preteen years) are much more likely to become dependent on alcohol as adults.

Causes

Alcohol use disorders involve heredity to some extent. Blood relatives of alcoholics are more likely to have alcohol use disorders than people in the general population, and alcohol use disorders are more likely to develop in biologic children of alcoholics than in adopted children. Some research suggests that

people at risk of alcoholism are less easily intoxicated than people who are not alcoholics. That is, their brains are less sensitive to the effects of alcohol. Blood relatives of alcoholics may have this trait.

Certain background and personality traits may predispose people to alcohol use disorders. Alcoholics frequently come from broken homes, and relationships with their parents are often disturbed. Alcoholics tend to feel isolated, lonely, shy, depressed, or hostile. They may act self-destructively and may be sexually immature. Whether such traits are the cause of alcoholism or the result is not certain.

Symptoms

Alcohol causes three basic types of problems:

- Those that occur immediately when people drink too much at a particular time (intoxication and overdose)
- Those that occur over a long period of time when people regularly consume excessive amounts
- Those that occur when heavy, long-term use is stopped suddenly (withdrawal)

Immediate Effects: Alcohol has almost immediate effects because it is absorbed faster than it is processed (metabolized) and eliminated from the body. As a result, alcohol levels in the blood rise rapidly. Effects can occur within a few minutes of drinking.

Effects vary greatly from person to person. For example, people who drink regularly (2 or more drinks per day) are less affected by a given amount of alcohol than those who normally do not drink or who drink only socially, a phenomenon termed tolerance. People who have developed tolerance to alcohol may also be tolerant of other drugs that slow brain function, such as barbiturates and benzodiazepines.

Effects vary depending on the level of alcohol in the bloodstream, which is usually expressed in terms of milligrams per deciliter (1/10 liter) of blood, abbreviated mg/dL. Actual blood levels required to produce given symptoms vary greatly with tolerance, but in typical users who have not developed tolerance, the following symptoms are typical:

- 20 to 50 mg/dL: Tranquility, mild drowsiness, some decrease in fine motor coordination, and some impairment of driving ability
- 50 to 100 mg/dL: Impaired judgment and a further decrease in coordination
- 100 to 150 mg/dL: Unsteady gait, slurred speech, loss of behavioral inhibitions, and memory impairment
- 150 to 300 mg/dL: Delirium and lethargy (likely)
- 300 to 400 mg/dL: Often unconsciousness
- ≥ 400 mg/dL: Possibly fatal

EFFECTS OF PROLONGED ALCOHOL USE

TYPE OF PROBLEM	EFFECTS
Nutritional	
Low folate (folic acid) levels	Anemia (fatigue, weakness, and light-headedness) Birth defects
Low iron levels	Anemia
Low niacin levels	Pellagra (skin damage, diarrhea, and depression)
Gastrointestinal	
Esophagus	Cancer Inflammation (esophagitis)
Stomach	Cancer Inflammation (gastritis) Ulcers
Liver	A bleeding tendency (coagulopathy) Cancer Fatty liver Inflammation (hepatitis) Severe scarring (cirrhosis)
Pancreas	Inflammation (pancreatitis) Low blood sugar levels (hypoglycemia)
Cardiovascular	
Heart	Disturbance of the heart's rhythm (arrhythmia) Heart failure
Blood vessels	Atherosclerosis High blood pressure Stroke
Neurologic	
Brain	Confusion Poor short-term memory (poor recall of recent events) Psychosis (loss of contact with reality) Reduced coordination
Nerves	Deterioration of the nerves in arms and legs that control movements (reduced ability to walk)
Genitourinary	
Reproductive organs	Decreased sex drive In men, enlarged breasts, smooth skin, and shrinking of the testes

Vomiting is common with moderate to severe intoxication. Because people may be very drowsy, vomited material may enter the lungs (be aspirated), sometimes leading to pneumonia and death. Drinking large amounts can also cause low blood pressure and low blood sugar levels.

In most U.S. states, the legal definition of intoxication is a blood alcohol content (BAC) of 80 mg/dL or higher. The effects of a particular blood level differ in chronic drinkers. Many seem unaffected and appear to function normally with relatively high levels (such as 300 to 400 mg/dL).

Long-Term Effects: Prolonged use of excessive amounts of alcohol damages many organs of the body, particularly the liver (alcoholic liver disease). Because people may not eat an adequate diet, they may also develop severe vitamin and other nutritional deficiencies.

Alcoholic liver disease includes liver inflammation (hepatitis), fatty liver, and cirrhosis (see page 222). An alcohol-damaged liver is less able to rid the body of toxic waste products, which can cause brain dysfunction (hepatic encephalopathy). People developing hepatic encephalopathy become dull, sleepy, stuporous, and confused and may lapse into a coma. Usually, they also have liver flap (asterixis): When the arms and hands are outstretched, the hands suddenly drop, then resume their original position. Liver flap resembles but is not a tremor. Hepatic coma is life threatening and needs to be treated immediately. With cirrhosis of the liver, pressure builds up in the blood vessels around the liver (portal hypertension—see page 217). These blood vessels can bleed heavily, causing people to vomit blood. This bleeding is a particular problem because the damaged liver does not produce enough of the substances that make blood clot.

Excessive alcohol use can cause inflammation of the pancreas (pancreatitis). People develop severe abdominal pain with vomiting.

Excessive alcohol use can damage the nerves and parts of the brain. People may develop a chronic tremor. Damage to the part of the brain that coordinates movement (cerebellum) can lead to poorly controlled movement of the arms and legs. It can also damage the lining (myelin sheath) of nerves in the brain, resulting in a rare disorder called Marchiafava-Bignami disease. People with this disorder become agitated, confused, and demented. Some develop seizures and go into a coma before dying.

Severe alcoholism can cause a severe deficiency of thiamin, a B vitamin. This deficiency can lead to Wernicke's encephalopathy (see page 2088), which, if not promptly treated, may result in Korsakoff's syndrome (see page 2089), coma, or even death.

Drinking alcohol may worsen existing depression, and alcoholics are more likely to become depressed than people who are not alcoholics. Because alcoholism, especially binge drinking, often causes deep feelings of remorse during dry periods, alcoholics are prone to suicide even when they are not drinking.

In pregnant women, alcohol use can cause severe problems in the developing fetus, including low birth weight, short body length, small head size, heart damage, muscle damage, and low intelligence or intellectual disability (mental retardation). These effects are called the fetal alcohol syndrome (see page 1641). Avoidance of alcohol is therefore recommended during pregnancy.

Withdrawal Symptoms: If people who drink continually for a period of time suddenly stop drinking, withdrawal symptoms are likely. For example, withdrawal can occur during hospitalization (for example, for elective surgery) because drinkers are unable to obtain alcohol.

Withdrawal symptoms vary from mild to severe. Severe untreated alcohol withdrawal can be fatal.

Mild withdrawal usually begins 12 to 24 hours after drinking stops. Mild symptoms include tremor, headache, weakness, sweating, and nausea. Some people have seizures (called alcoholic epilepsy or rum fits).

Alcoholic hallucinosis may occur in heavy drinkers who stop drinking. They hear voices that seem accusatory and threatening, causing apprehension and terror. Alcoholic hallucinosis may last for days and can be controlled with antipsychotic drugs, such as chlorpromazine or thioridazine.

Delirium tremens (DTs) is the most serious group of withdrawal symptoms. Usually, delirium tremens does not begin immediately. Rather, it appears about 48 to 72 hours after the drinking stops. People are initially anxious. Later, they become increasingly confused, do not sleep well, have frightening nightmares, sweat excessively, and become very depressed. The pulse rate tends to speed up. Fever typically develops. The episode may escalate to include fleeting hallucinations, illusions that arouse fear and restlessness, and disorientation with visual hallucinations that may be terrifying. Objects seen in dim light may be particularly terrifying, and the people become extremely confused. Their balance is impaired, sometimes making them think the floor is moving, the walls are falling, or the room is rotating. As the delirium progresses, a persistent tremor develops in the hands and sometimes extends to the head and body. Most people become severely uncoordinated. Delirium tremens can be fatal, particularly when untreated.

Diagnosis

Acute alcohol intoxication is usually apparent based on what people or their friends tell the doctor and on results of the physical examination. If it is not clear why a person is acting abnormally, doctors may do tests to rule out other possible causes of symptoms, such as low blood sugar or head injury. Tests may include tests to determine the amount of alcohol in the blood and the blood sugar level, urine tests for certain toxic substances, and computed tomography (CT) of the head. Doctors do not assume that simply because people have alcohol on their breath that nothing else could be wrong.

For legal purposes (for example, when people are in vehicle crashes or are acting abnormally at work), alcohol levels can be measured in the blood or estimated by measuring the amount in a sample of exhaled breath.

In people with a long-term alcohol use disorder, blood tests may be done to check for abnormalities in liver function and evidence of other organ damage. If symptoms are very severe, an imaging test such as CT may be done to rule out a brain injury or infection.

Screening for Alcohol Abuse: Some people may not know that their amount of drinking could be a problem. Others know but do not want to admit that they have an alcohol problem. Therefore, health care practitioners do not wait for people to ask for help. They may suspect an alcohol use disorder in people whose behavior changes inexplicably or whose behavior becomes self-destructive. They may also suspect an alcohol use disorder when medical problems, such as high blood pressure or stomach inflammation (gastritis), do not respond to usual treatment.

Many practitioners periodically screen people for alcohol-related problems by asking about their use of alcohol. Questions may include the following:

- On average, how many days per week do you drink alcohol?
- On a typical day when you drink, how many drinks do you have?
- What is the maximum number of drinks you had on any given occasion in the past month?

If doctors suspect alcoholism, they may ask more specific questions about consequences of drinking, such as the following:

- Have you ever felt you should cut down on your drinking?
- Does criticism of your drinking annoy you?
- Have you ever felt guilty about drinking?
- Have you ever had an "eye opener" (a drink first thing in the morning) to steady your nerves or to get rid of a hangover?

Two or more "yes" answers to these questions indicate a probable alcohol problem.

Treatment

Treatment may occur in the following situations:

- People come because they do not want to continue drinking.
- People are brought in because they have symptoms related to high blood alcohol levels.
- People come because they have intolerable withdrawal symptoms. However, alcoholics who develop withdrawal symptoms usually treat themselves by drinking.

Emergency Treatment: Emergency treatment is needed when very large amounts of alcohol or alcohol withdrawal causes severe symptoms.

There is no specific antidote for acute intoxication. Coffee and other home remedies do not reverse the effects of alcohol. However, if people are in a coma, they may need to have a tube inserted in their airway to keep them from choking on vomit and secretions. If their breathing is suppressed, they may need to be placed on a ventilator.

If needed to prevent or treat dehydration or low blood pressure, fluids are given intravenously, and thiamin is given to prevent Wernicke's encephalopathy. Often, doctors also add magnesium (which helps the body process thiamin) and multivitamins (for possible vitamin deficiencies) to the fluids.

For withdrawal symptoms, doctors often prescribe a benzodiazepine (a mild sedative) for a few days. It reduces agitation and helps prevent some withdrawal symptoms, seizures, and delirium tremens. Because people can become dependent on benzodiazepines, these drugs are used for only a short time. Antipsychotic drugs are sometimes given to people with alcoholic hallucinosis.

Delirium tremens can be life threatening and is treated aggressively to control the high fever and severe agitation. People are treated in an intensive care unit if possible. Treatment usually includes the following:

- High doses of benzodiazepines, given intravenously
- High doses of vitamins (especially thiamin)
- Fluids given intravenously
- Drugs that lower fever (such as acetaminophen)
- Drugs that control heart rate and blood pressure
- Treatment of complications (such as pancreatitis, pneumonia, and seizures)

With such treatment, delirium tremens usually begins to clear within 12 to 24 hours of its beginning, but severe cases may last for 5 to 7 days. Most people do not remember events during severe withdrawal after it resolves.

After any urgent medical problems are resolved, further treatment depends on how severe the alcohol use disorder is. If people have not become dependent on alcohol, doctors may discuss the serious consequences of alcoholism with them, recommend ways to reduce or stop their drinking, and schedule follow-up visits to check on how well they are doing.

For people with more severe disorders, a detoxification and rehabilitation program should be started.

Detoxification and Rehabilitation: In the first phase, alcohol is completely withdrawn, and any withdrawal symptoms are treated. Then alcoholics have to learn ways to modify their behavior. Without help, most alcoholics relapse within a few days or weeks. Rehabilitation programs, which combine psychotherapy with medical supervision, can help.

Alcoholics Anonymous: A Path to Recovery

No approach has benefited so many alcoholics as effectively as Alcoholics Anonymous (AA). AA is an international fellowship of people who want to stop drinking. There are no dues or fees. The program operates on the basis of the "Twelve Steps," which offers the alcoholic a new way of living without alcohol. Members of the fellowship typically work with a sponsor—a fellow member who is abstaining from alcohol use—who offers guidance and support. AA operates within a spiritual context but is not affiliated with any specific ideology or religious doctrine. However, alternative organizations, such as LifeRing Recovery (Secular Organizations for Sobriety), exist for those seeking a more secular approach.

AA helps its members in other ways as well. It provides a place where recovering alcoholics can socialize away from the tavern and with friends who do not drink and who are always available for support when the urge to start drinking again becomes strong. In meetings, alcoholics hear other people relate—to the entire group—how they are struggling every day to avoid taking a drink. By providing a means to help others, AA builds self-esteem and confidence formerly found only in drinking alcohol. Most metropolitan areas have many AA meetings available day and night, 7 days a week. Alcoholics are encouraged to try several different meetings and to attend those at which they feel most comfortable.

People are warned about how difficult stopping is. They are also taught ways to enhance the motivation to stop and to avoid situations that are likely to trigger drinking. Treatment is tailored to the individual. These programs also enlist the support of family members and friends. Self-help groups, such as Alcoholics Anonymous, can also help.

Sometimes certain drugs (disulfiram, naltrexone, and acamprosate) can help alcoholics avoid drinking alcohol. However, drugs can typically help only if people are motivated and cooperative and if the drugs are used as part of an ongoing intensive counseling regimen. Results vary.

Disulfiram deters drinking because it interferes with alcohol metabolism, causing acetaldehyde (a substance that results from the breakdown of alcohol) to build up in the bloodstream. Acetaldehyde makes people feel ill. It causes facial flushing, a throbbing headache, a rapid heart rate, rapid breathing, and sweating within 5 to 15 minutes after people drink alcohol. Nausea and vomiting may follow 30 to 60 minutes later. These uncomfortable and potentially dangerous reactions last 1 to 3 hours. The discomfort from drinking alcohol after taking disulfiram is so intense that few people risk drinking alcohol—even the small amount in some over-the-counter cough and cold preparations or some foods. Disulfiram must be taken every day. If people stop taking disulfiram, its effectiveness in treating alcohol dependence is limited. Pregnant women, people who have a serious illness, and older people should not use disulfiram.

Naltrexone alters the effects of alcohol on certain chemicals made by the brain (endorphins), which may be associated with alcohol craving and consumption. This drug is effective in most people who take it consistently. A long-acting form can be given by injection once a month. Naltrexone, unlike disulfiram, does not make people sick. Thus, people taking naltrexone can continue to drink. Naltrexone should not be taken by people who have hepatitis or certain other liver disorders.

WERNICKE'S ENCEPHALOPATHY

Wernicke's encephalopathy causes confusion, eye problems, and loss of balance and results from thiamin deficiency.

Wernicke's encephalopathy is caused by a severe deficiency of thiamin, a B vitamin (see page 923). In people who have only a small amount of thiamin stored in the body, it may be triggered by consuming carbohydrates.

Wernicke's encephalopathy often develops in people with severe alcoholism because the long-term use of excess amounts of alcohol interferes with the absorption of thiamin. Also, alcoholics often do not consume an adequate diet and thus not enough thiamin. Wernicke's encephalopathy may result from other conditions that cause prolonged undernutrition or vitamin deficiencies. These conditions include dialysis, severe vomiting, starvation, cancer, and AIDS.

Symptoms

Wernicke's encephalopathy causes confusion, drowsiness, involuntary eye movements (nystagmus), partial paralysis of the eyes (ophthalmoplegia), and loss of balance. To maintain balance, people walk with their feet far apart and take slow, short steps.

Internal body processes may malfunction, causing tremor, agitation, a cold body temperature, a sudden and excessive decrease in blood pressure when people stand (orthostatic hypotension), and fainting. If untreated, Wernicke's encephalopathy can lead to Korsakoff's syndrome (see page 2089), coma, or death. The combination is called Wernicke-Korsakoff syndrome.

Diagnosis

Doctors suspect the diagnosis in people who have the characteristic symptoms and undernutrition or a thiamin deficiency, especially if they are alcoholics.

Tests, such as blood tests to measure blood sugar levels, a complete blood cell count, liver function tests, and imaging, are usually done to rule out other causes. Thiamin levels are not routinely measured.

Prognosis

The prognosis depends on how quickly the disorder is diagnosed and treated. Prompt treatment may correct all abnormalities. However, loss of balance and confusion may persist days to months. Without treatment, about 10 to 20% of people die.

Treatment

Thiamin is given immediately by injection into a vein or muscle. It is continued daily for at least 3 to 5 days. Magnesium, which helps the body process thiamin, is also given by injection or by mouth. Fluids and multivitamins are given, and if levels of electrolytes (such as potassium) are abnormal, they are corrected. Some people may require hospitalization.

People with Wernicke's syndrome must stop drinking alcohol. Thiamin supplements, taken by mouth, may need to be continued after the initial treatment.

KORSAKOFF'S SYNDROME

Korsakoff's syndrome (Korsakoff's amnestic syndrome) causes memory loss for recent events, confusion, and apathy.

Korsakoff's syndrome occurs in 80% of people with untreated Wernicke's encephalopathy. Korsakoff's syndrome is sometimes triggered by a severe bout of delirium tremens, whether Wernicke's encephalopathy is present or not. Other causes include head injuries, stroke, bleeding within the brain, and, rarely, certain brain tumors.

People with Korsakoff's syndrome lose memory for recent events. Memory is so poor that they often makes up stories, sometimes very convincingly, to try to cover up the inability to remember (called confabulation). They lose all sense of time. People become confused and apathetic and may not respond to events, even frightening ones. About 1 in 5 people with the syndrome do not completely recover. Some require care in an institution.

Doctors base the diagnosis on symptoms, particularly confabulation, in people with conditions that can cause Korsakoff's syndrome.

Treatment consists of thiamin and fluids given intravenously. Thiamin supplements, taken by mouth, may need to be continued after the initial treatment.

Recovery depends on the cause. If the cause is a head injury or bleeding in the brain, people who are treated often improve. If the cause is Wernicke's encephalopathy, the chances of recovery are worse: Only about 20% recover completely, and about 25% of

people require institutional care. Improvement may take months and continue for up to 2 years or longer.

Amphetamines

- Amphetamines increase alertness, enhance physical performance, and produce euphoria and a sense of well-being.
- An overdose can cause extreme agitation, delirium, and a life-threatening heart attack or stroke.
- Urine tests can detect most amphetamines.
- For most people, treatment involves reassurance and a calm environment, but sedatives such as benzodiazepines may be needed.

Amphetamines include amphetamine and its many variants such as methamphetamine (speed or crystal meth) and methylenedioxymethamphetamine (MDMA, Ecstasy, or Adam). Methamphetamine is the most commonly used amphetamine in the United States. Use of MDMA is growing in popularity. Amphetamines are usually taken by mouth but can be snorted, smoked, or injected.

Because some amphetamines are widely used as treatment for attention-deficit/hyperactivity disorder, obesity, and narcolepsy, there is a ready supply that can be diverted to illegal use. Some amphetamines are not approved for medical use and are manufactured and used illegally.

Some amphetamine users are depressed and seek the mood-elevating effects of these stimulants to temporarily relieve the depression. Others use them during high-energy activities. Amphetamines cause more dopamine to be released in the brain. (Dopamine is a neurotransmitter, a substance that helps nerve cells communicate.) This effect is the likely cause of mood elevation. MDMA differs from other amphetamines in that it also interferes with the reuptake of serotonin (another neurotransmitter) in the brain. Amphetamine users frequently develop dependence.

 Did You Know...
High doses of amphetamines may raise body temperature to dangerous levels.

Symptoms

Immediate Effects: Amphetamines increase alertness, reduce fatigue, heighten concentration, decrease appetite, and enhance physical performance. They may produce a feeling of well-being, euphoria, and loss of inhibitions. Also, people sweat profusely, and the pupils are dilated. High doses (overdose) increase blood pressure and heart rate. These increases may be life threatening. People may become extremely paranoid, violent, and out of control.

Binge usage (perhaps over several days) eventually causes extreme exhaustion and a need for sleep.

Complications: People may become delirious. Heart attacks have occurred, even in healthy young athletes. Blood pressure may become so high that a blood vessel in the brain ruptures, causing a stroke. Other effects include dizziness, nausea, vomiting, diarrhea, seizures, and a life-threatening high body temperature (hyperthermia).

Complications are more likely in the following situations:

- When drugs such as MDMA are used in warm rooms with little ventilation
- When the user is very active physically (for example, when dancing fast)
- When the user sweats heavily and does not drink enough water to restore lost fluids, resulting in dehydration

Long-Term Effects: People who habitually use amphetamines rapidly develop tolerance as part of dependence. They need to use more and more to get the same effect. The amount ultimately used may be more than several times the original dose. Most people using very high doses become confused and psychotic because amphetamines can cause severe anxiety, paranoia, and a distorted sense of reality. Psychotic reactions include hearing and seeing things that are not there (auditory and visual hallucinations) and false beliefs (delusions), such as a feeling of having unlimited power (omnipotence) or of being persecuted (paranoia). Memory may be affected. Confusion, memory loss, and delusions may last for months. Although these effects can occur in any user, people with a mental health disorder, such as schizophrenia, are more vulnerable to them.

Users have a high rate of severe tooth decay affecting numerous teeth. The causes include decreased salivation, corrosive substances in the smoke, and poor oral hygiene—called meth mouth.

Withdrawal Symptoms: When an amphetamine is suddenly stopped, symptoms vary. People dependent on amphetamines become tired or sleepy—an effect that may last for 2 or 3 days after stopping the drug. As a result, they are more likely to be injured. Some people are extremely anxious and restless, and some, especially those with a tendency toward depression, become depressed when they stop. They may become suicidal but may lack the energy to attempt suicide for several days.

Diagnosis

Doctors base the diagnosis on symptoms in people known to have taken amphetamines. If the diagnosis is unclear, urine tests may be done, but the test usually does not detect MDMA. Other tests, such as electrocardiography, computed tomography, and blood tests, may be done to check for complications.

Treatment

For most people, treatment involves reassurance and a calm environment.

For people with severe symptoms such as high blood pressure, extreme agitation, or seizures, doctors usually give benzodiazepines (sedative drugs), such as lorazepam, intravenously. If blood pressure remains high, nitrates or other antihypertensive drugs are given intravenously.

Treatment may be needed to correct dehydration, hyperthermia, and other complications.

During drug withdrawal, long-term users may need to be hospitalized so that they can be observed for suicidal behavior. Antidepressants may be given if depression persists. Otherwise, no treatment is generally needed for people experiencing withdrawal.

Cognitive-behavioral therapy (a form of psychotherapy) helps some people stay free of amphetamines.

Anabolic Steroids

- Users of anabolic steroids are often athletes who are looking to promote muscle growth and increase their strength and energy.
- Anabolic steroids increase muscle size, but their use can also have many side effects, including mood swings, aggressive behavior, irritability, and acne.
- These substances can be detected in urine for up to 6 months.
- Treatment involves stopping use.

Anabolic steroids include the hormone testosterone and related drugs. Anabolic steroids have many physical effects, including promoting muscle growth and increasing strength and energy. Thus, these drugs are often used illegitimately to gain a competitive edge in sports. Users are often athletes, typically football players, wrestlers, or weight lifters, and most users are male. Anabolic steroids are used medically to treat low testosterone levels (hypogonadism) and sometimes to prevent muscles from wasting away in people who are confined to bed or who have severe burns, cancer, or AIDS.

The drugs may be taken by mouth, injected into a muscle, or applied to a skin as a gel or in a patch.

Athletes may take steroids for a certain period, stop, then start again several times a year. This process is called cycling. Athletes also often use many steroids at the same time (a practice called stacking), and they take them by different routes (by mouth, injection, or patch). They may also increase the dose through a cycle (called pyramiding). Pyramiding may result in very high doses. Cycling, stacking, and pyramiding are intended to enhance desired effects and minimize harmful effects, but little evidence supports these benefits.

At doses used to treat disorders, anabolic steroids cause few problems. However, athletes may take doses 10 to 50 times these doses.

Symptoms

Steroids increase muscle size. How much muscles increase depends directly on how much of the drug is taken.

Steroids have several psychologic effects (usually only with very high doses):

- Wide and erratic mood swings
- Irrational behavior
- Increased aggressiveness (steroid or roid rage)
- Irritability
- Increased sex drive (libido) in men and sometimes in women
- Depression

Increased acne is common in both sexes. Libido may increase or, less commonly, decrease. Aggressiveness and appetite may increase. In males, breast tissue may enlarge (gynecomastia), and testes may shrink and sperm count decrease. In females, masculinizing effects such as loss of head hair, excess body hair (hirsutism), an enlarged clitoris, and a deepened voice are common. Also, breast size may decrease, and tissues lining the vagina may thin and become less elastic (atrophy). Menstruation may change or stop. Gynecomastia in men and masculinizing effects in women may be irreversible.

In younger adolescents, steroids can interfere with the development of arm and leg bones.

Long-term use can cause production of excess red blood cells and abnormal levels of fats (lipids) in the blood. Low density lipoprotein (LDL)—the bad—cholesterol levels increase, and high density lipoprotein (HDL)—the good—cholesterol levels decrease.

Diagnosis

Urine tests are done to check for breakdown products of anabolic steroids. These products can be detected up to 6 months after use is stopped.

Prevention

Adolescents and young adults should be taught about the risks of taking steroids starting in middle school. Also, programs that teach alternative, healthy ways to increase muscle size and improve performance may be useful. Such programs emphasize good nutrition and weight training techniques.

Classifying the Abuse Potential of Prescription Drugs

Prescription drugs that can cause dependency are subject to restrictions dictated by United States government regulations. All prescription drugs regulated under the Controlled Substances Act are assigned a schedule or class number that determines how they may be prescribed:

- Schedule I: Drugs are considered to have a high potential for abuse, no accepted medical use, and no acceptable safety data. Heroin is an example.
- Schedule II: Drugs have a high potential for abuse but have some appropriate medical uses. Morphine is an example.
- Schedules III, IV, and V: Drugs have progressively less potential for abuse and have accepted medical uses. Schedule V drugs have the least potential for abuse.

Treatment

The main treatment is stopping use. Although physical dependence does not occur, psychologic dependence, particularly in competitive bodybuilders, may exist. Gynecomastia may require surgical reduction.

Antianxiety and Sedative Drugs

- Using prescription drugs to relieve anxiety or help with sleeping can cause dependence.
- An overdose can cause drowsiness, confusion, and slowed respiration.
- Stopping a drug after using it for a long time causes anxiety, irritability, and sleep problems.
- If people become dependent on a drug, they are gradually weaned off the drug by reducing the dose.

Prescription drugs used to treat anxiety (antianxiety drugs) and induce sleep (sedatives or sleep aids) can cause dependence. These drugs include benzodiazepines (such as diazepam and lorazepam) and barbiturates. Each works in a different way, and each has a different potential for dependency and tolerance.

Severe or life-threatening symptoms are less likely with benzodiazepines than with barbiturates because for benzodiazepines, the difference between prescribed doses and dangerous doses (called the margin of safety) is large. People can take relatively large amounts of benzodiazepines without dying.

Most people dependent on antianxiety drugs and sedatives started out taking them for a medical reason. Dependency can develop within as little as 2 weeks of continual use.

Symptoms

Immediate Effects: Antianxiety drugs and sedatives decrease alertness and can result in slurred speech, poor coordination, confusion, and slowed breathing. These effects are magnified when people take alcohol. These drugs may make people alternately depressed and anxious. Some people experience memory loss, faulty judgment, a shortened attention span, and frightening shifts in their emotions. People may speak slowly and have difficulty thinking and understanding others. People may have involuntary eye movements (nystagmus).

In older people, symptoms may be more severe and may include dizziness, disorientation, delirium, and loss of balance. Falls may occur, resulting in broken bones, especially hip fractures.

Higher doses cause more severe symptoms, including stupor (people can be aroused only temporarily and with difficulty), very slow and shallow breathing, and, mainly with barbiturates, eventually death.

Withdrawal Symptoms: When withdrawal symptoms occur and how they progress vary from drug to drug and depend on the dose of the drug. Symptoms may begin within 12 to 24 hours.

People who have used sedatives for more than a few days often feel that they cannot sleep without them. When they stop the drugs, they may have mild withdrawal symptoms:

- Anxiety and nervousness at bedtime
- Poor sleep
- Disturbing dreams
- Irritability when they awaken

If high doses have been taken, abrupt withdrawal can produce a severe, frightening, and potentially life-threatening reaction, much like alcohol withdrawal. Seizures may occur after withdrawal.

Other effects include dehydration, delirium, insomnia, confusion, and frightening visual and auditory hallucinations (seeing and hearing things that are not there). Serious withdrawal reactions can occur with barbiturates and benzodiazepines. People are usually hospitalized during the withdrawal process because a severe reaction is possible.

Treatment

Emergency Treatment: People who have taken an overdose require immediate medical evaluation. An overdose of barbiturates is more dangerous than an overdose of benzodiazepines. If people who take a dangerous overdose of antianxiety drugs or sedatives have significant respiratory, heart, or blood pressure problems, they should be hospitalized, usually in an intensive care unit or another area where they can be monitored.

Benzodiazepines have an antidote, flumazenil, which can reverse a serious overdose.

Supportive care may include fluids given intravenously, drugs if blood pressure drops, and a ventilator.

Detoxification and Rehabilitation: People with mild withdrawal symptoms require social and psychologic support to help them overcome a strong urge to begin using the drug again to stop the feelings of anxiety.

People with severe withdrawal symptoms usually need to be treated in a hospital, sometimes in an intensive care unit, and be closely supervised. They are given low doses of the drug intravenously. The dose is decreased gradually over days or weeks and then stopped. Sometimes another similar drug that is easier to gradually withdraw is substituted. Even with the best treatment, people may not feel normal for a month or more.

Cocaine

- Cocaine is a strong stimulant that increases alertness, causes euphoria, and makes people feel powerful.
- High doses can cause serious, life-threatening disorders, such as a heart attack or stroke.
- The diagnosis can be confirmed by urine tests.
- Sedatives such as lorazepam given intravenously can relieve many symptoms.
- People who stop using the drug must be closely supervised because they may be suicidal and they require much help to remain free of the drug.

Cocaine has effects similar to those of amphetamines. It may be snorted, injected directly into a vein, or heated and inhaled. When boiled with sodium bicarbonate, cocaine is converted into a freebase form called crack cocaine. Heating crack cocaine releases cocaine vapor that can be inhaled. Inhaling the vapor is usually referred to as smoking, but the crack is not actually burned. Crack cocaine acts almost as fast as cocaine injected intravenously.

Heavy regular users and people who inject the drug intravenously or smoke it are most likely to become dependent. Light occasional users and people who snort the drug nasally are less likely to become dependent. Cocaine may contain many fillers, adulterants, and contaminants, which, when injected, can cause complications such as infections.

Symptoms

Immediate Effects: Cocaine produces a sense of extreme alertness, euphoria, and great power when it is injected intravenously or inhaled. These feelings are less intense when cocaine is snorted. Because cocaine's effects may last only a short time, users may inject, smoke, or snort it every 15 to 30 minutes. Binges, often over several days, lead to exhaustion and a need for sleep.

Complications: Acute cocaine toxicity can be fatal. Cocaine increases blood pressure and heart rate and narrows (constricts) blood vessels. Heart rhythm may be disturbed (called arrhythmias). Cocaine's effects on the heart can cause chest pain, a heart attack (even in healthy young athletes), or sudden death. Cocaine can also cause kidney failure, stroke, and lung problems.

High doses (overdose) can impair judgment and cause tremors, extreme nervousness, seizures, hallucinations, insomnia, paranoid delusions, delirium, and violent behavior. People sweat profusely and the pupils are dilated. Very high doses can cause a life-threatening high body temperature (hyperthermia).

Long-Term Effects: Long-term users may develop tolerance, requiring more and more of the drug to get the same effects. Long-term use may damage the tissue separating the two halves of the nose (septum), causing sores (ulcerations) that may require surgery. Heavy use may impair mental function, including attention and memory.

If women use cocaine during pregnancy, the fetus is more likely to have problems. However, such women usually have many other risk factors for problems in the fetus, including tobacco and alcohol use, poor nutrition, and lack of prenatal care. Doctors now think that these other risk factors are more responsible for problems than the cocaine.

Withdrawal Symptoms: Withdrawal reactions include extreme fatigue and depression—the opposite of the drug's effects. Appetite is increased, and people have trouble concentrating. Suicidal urges emerge when addicts stop taking the drug. After several days, when mental and physical strength has returned, addicts may attempt suicide.

 Did You Know...
Using cocaine can cause sudden death.

Diagnosis

Doctors usually base the diagnosis on symptoms in people known to use the drug. Urine testing can detect evidence of the drug for 2 to 3 days after its use.

Treatment

Emergency Treatment: Cocaine is a very short-acting drug, so treatment of uncomfortable reactions is usually not necessary. People who are very agitated or delirious or who have seizures or high blood pressure are given benzodiazepines (sedatives), such as lorazepam, intravenously. Nitrates or other antihypertensive drugs may be given intravenously to lower blood pressure or heart rate. Hyperthermia may also need to be treated.

Detoxification and Rehabilitation: Stopping long-term cocaine use may require close supervision because people can become depressed and suicidal. Entering a hospital or a drug treatment center may be necessary. The most effective method of treating cocaine addiction is psychotherapy. Many self-help groups and cocaine hotlines are available to help people remain free of the drug.

Sometimes the mental health disorders common to cocaine addicts, such as depression, are treated with the appropriate drugs for those disorders.

Gamma Hydroxybutyrate

Gamma hydroxybutyrate (GHB or G) is taken by mouth. It is similar to ketamine or alcohol in its effects, but its effects last longer and GHB is much more dangerous.

Symptoms

GHB produces feelings of relaxation and tranquility. It may also cause fatigue and feelings of being uninhibited.

At higher doses, GHB may cause dizziness, loss of coordination, nausea, and vomiting. GHB can slow breathing and cause seizures and coma, sometimes leading to respiratory failure and death. Combining GHB and any other sedative, especially alcohol, is extremely dangerous. Most deaths have occurred when GHB was taken with alcohol.

Withdrawal symptoms occur if GHB is not taken for several days after previous frequent use.

Diagnosis and Treatment

No readily available tests can confirm the use of GHB. Treatment is needed only for overdose. A ventilator may be needed if breathing is affected. Most people recover rapidly.

Hallucinogens

- Hallucinogens distort and intensify sensations, but the actual effects can depend on the user's mood and expectations.
- The chief dangers are the psychologic effects and impaired judgment they cause.
- A dark, quiet room and calm, nonthreatening talk can help users who are experiencing a bad trip.

Hallucinogens include LSD (lysergic acid diethylamide), psilocybin (mushroom), mescaline (peyote), dimethyltryptamine (DMT) and 2,5-dimethoxy-4-methylamphetamine (DOM or STP), an amphetamine derivative. Many new compounds are being synthesized, and the list of hallucinogens is growing.

These drugs may be taken various ways. LSD is taken by mouth using tablets or blotter paper. DMT can be smoked.

People may become psychologically dependent on hallucinogens, but physical dependence, which results in unpleasant symptoms (withdrawal) when the drug is stopped, is not typical.

Symptoms

Hallucinogens distort and intensify auditory and visual sensations. For example, people may feel as if they are seeing sounds and hearing colors. People feel as if they are not real (called depersonalization) or are detached from their environment (called dissociation). Many hallucinogens cause nausea and vomiting. LSD causes blurred vision, sweating, palpitations, and impaired coordination.

The actual effect can depend on the user's mood and expectations when the drug is taken and the setting in which the drug is taken. For example, users who were depressed before the drug was taken are likely to feel sadder when the drug takes effect. The chief dangers of using these drugs are the psychologic effects and impaired judgment they cause, which can lead to dangerous decisions or accidents. For example, users may think they can fly and may even jump out a window to prove it.

The user's ability to cope with the visual and auditory distortions also affects the experience—or "trip." Inexperienced, frightened users are less able to cope than someone who is more experienced and not afraid of the trip. Users under the influence of a hallucinogen, usually LSD, can become extremely anxious and begin to panic, resulting in a bad trip. They may want to stop the trip, which is not possible.

Some users remain out of touch with reality (psychotic) for many days or longer after the drug's effects have worn off. A prolonged psychosis is more likely in users with a preexisting mental health disorder.

Some people—especially long-term or repeated users of hallucinogens, particularly LSD—may experience flashbacks after they stop using the drugs. Flashbacks are similar to but generally less intense than the original experience. Typically, flashbacks disappear over 6 to 12 months but can recur as long as 5 years after the last use of LSD, especially in users who still have an anxiety or another mental health disorder.

Diagnosis and Treatment

Doctors usually base the diagnosis on symptoms. Tests are not available to confirm the use of many of these drugs.

Most users do not seek treatment. A quiet, dark room and calm, nonthreatening talk can help users who are having a bad trip. They need reassurance that the effects are caused by the drug and will end. If anxiety is severe, benzodiazepines (sedatives), such as lorazepam, may help. People who experience a prolonged psychosis may need mental health treatment.

Ketamine

Ketamine is a drug used for anesthesia. People who use it illicitly may snort it or inject it intravenously, into a muscle, or under the skin.

Symptoms

Ketamine reduces pain perception and causes giddiness and euphoria, which are often followed by bursts of anxiety. With high doses (overdose), users have a distorted perception of their body, the environment, and time. They feel scattered or as if they are not real (called depersonalization), and they feel detached from their environment (called dissociation).

At even higher doses, hallucinations and paranoid delusions may occur, and the sense of detachment from the world intensifies. Ketamine users often refer to these experiences as a k-hole. People may become combative. Coordination may be lost, and muscles tremble and jerk.

Very high doses may cause a life-threatening high body temperature (hyperthermia), a fast heart rate, very high blood pressure, seizures, and coma. Ketamine can also disrupt memory for several hours.

Diagnosis and Treatment

No test can rapidly confirm the presence of ketamine in the body.

Usually, reassurance and a quiet, nonthreatening environment help people recover. Benzodiazepines (sedatives) can be used to control seizures. Ketamine's effects usually abate in about 30 minutes.

Marijuana

- Marijuana produces a dreamy state, a sense of well-being, and distorted perceptions.
- Stopping the drug causes only mild symptoms.
- Marijuana can be detected in urine for days to weeks after it was used.
- Treatment involves counseling, which is effective only when people are motivated to stop.

Marijuana (cannabis) use is widespread. Surveys of high school students have shown periodic variation in its use.

In the United States, marijuana is commonly smoked in the form of cigarettes (joints) made from the stems, leaves, and flowering tops of the dried plant (*Cannabis sativa* or *Cannabis indica*). Marijuana is also used as hashish, the pressed resin (tarry substance) of the plant. The active ingredient of marijuana is tetrahydrocannabinol (THC), which occurs in many variations. The most active variation is delta-9-THC. Dronabinol, a synthetic form of delta-9-THC, is used to relieve nausea and vomiting caused by chemotherapy drugs and to enhance appetite in people with AIDS.

Most people use marijuana intermittently and without developing noticeable social or psychologic dysfunction or dependence. However, some people become dependent on marijuana.

Symptoms

Marijuana slows brain activity, producing a dreamy state in which ideas seem disconnected and free-flowing. It is mildly psychedelic, causing time, color, and spatial perceptions to distort and be enhanced. Colors may seem brighter, sounds may seem louder, and appetite may be increased. Marijuana generally relieves tension and provides a sense of well-being. The sense of exaltation, excitement, and inner joyousness (a high) seems to be related to the setting in which the drug is taken—such as whether the smoker is alone or in a group and what the prevailing mood is. Coordination, reaction time, depth perception, and concentration may be impaired during marijuana use, so driving or operating heavy equipment is dangerous. Other effects include an increased heart rate, bloodshot eyes, and dry mouth. Effects usually last 4 to 6 hours after inhalation.

Some people, especially those who have not used marijuana before, experience anxiety or feel panicky or paranoid. If people have a psychosis (loss of contact with reality) such as schizophrenia, using marijuana may make symptoms worse or trigger new symptoms.

Complications: People who use large quantities of marijuana for a long time may develop breathing problems, such as bronchitis, wheezing, coughing, and increased phlegm. However, even daily smokers do not develop obstructive airway disease. There is no evidence of increased risk of head and neck or airway cancers, as there is with tobacco.

Pregnant women who use marijuana may have smaller babies than nonusers, but the effect seems small. Delta-9-THC passes into breast milk, but no harmful effects have been detected. Nonetheless, women who are pregnant or breastfeeding are advised not to use it.

Withdrawal Symptoms: Marijuana is eliminated from the body slowly over several weeks, so withdrawal symptoms tend to be mild. After a few weeks of heavy, frequent use, abruptly stopping causes symptoms that begin about 12 hours later and last up to 7 days. Symptoms include insomnia, irritability, depression, nausea, and loss of appetite.

Diagnosis and Treatment

A urine test can detect marijuana for several days or weeks after it is used, even in casual users. In regular users, the test may detect the drug for even longer while the drug is slowly released from body fat. Urine testing is an effective means of identifying marijuana use, but a positive result means only that a person has used marijuana. It does not prove that the user is currently impaired (intoxicated).

For people who want to stop using marijuana, counseling, behavior modification, and drug treatment programs may be helpful. However, success relies heavily on their motivation to stop and, for some users, on their willingness to disassociate from their social circle of regular users.

Nicotine

- People who stop using nicotine may become irritable, anxious, and restless.
- Smoking harms almost every organ in the body.
- Counseling, behavior modification, nicotine replacement products, and certain drugs can help people quit.

Nicotine is the substance in tobacco (present in cigarettes, cigars, and pipe and chewing tobacco) that users become dependent on. It is also the active ingredient in some drug products used to help people quit smoking.

Most nicotine exposure is from smoking tobacco, although children may accidentally eat it (usually cigarettes or butts left in ashtrays or sometimes nicotine gum or patches). In the United States, about 45 million adults smoke, and smoking is the leading cause of death. About one half of current smokers will die prematurely of a disorder caused by smoking. Smoking is so deadly because smokers inhale hundreds of other substances, including ones that can cause cancer.

About 70% of smokers acknowledge that they desire to quit smoking but are unable to do so. Of people who quit, 90% do so on their own, but only about 3 to 4% successfully quit in any given year.

Symptoms

Immediate Effects: Nicotine, when obtained through smoking, usually has few noticeable effects. Some people experience flushing. People who handle large amounts of tobacco leaves may absorb nicotine through their skin and develop nausea, vomiting, diarrhea, sweating, and weakness. This illness has been termed green tobacco sickness. Children who eat tobacco products can develop similar symptoms, along with agitation and confusion, sometimes from as little as one cigarette. However, serious or fatal toxicity in children is uncommon, probably because the vomiting empties the stomach.

Long-Term Effects: Because smoking involves inhaling many harmful substances, it has many serious consequences. It harms nearly every organ in the body. Smoking increases the risk of coronary artery disease, lung cancer, chronic lung disorders, stroke, other cancers (such as bladder, esophageal, kidney, throat, and stomach cancers), and pneumonia. Smoking during pregnancy can cause problems such as preterm birth, a low birth weight, and sudden infant death syndrome.

Withdrawal Symptoms: Nicotine withdrawal may result in many unpleasant symptoms, including a craving for nicotine, irritability, anxiety, poor concentration, restlessness, trembling (tremor), depression, headaches, drowsiness, and stomach upset. Many people gain weight while trying to stop smoking. Withdrawal is most troublesome in severely dependent people.

Treatment

Emergency treatment is rarely required except for children who have eaten products that contain nicotine. Doctors usually give them activated charcoal by mouth to absorb any drug remaining in the gastrointestinal tract. Sometimes drugs such as diazepam are used.

Smoking Cessation: Most issues regarding nicotine use involve efforts to quit smoking. Most smokers who quit do so for health or economic reasons. People who want to quit smoking can get help from health care practitioners, who can provide advice and support and recommend ways to modify behavior. Other sources for help include the Internet and package inserts in nicotine replacement products.

Quitting smoking abruptly (cold turkey) is generally preferable to tapering off. Selection of a quit date is very helpful. The quit date may be random or on a special occasion (such as a holiday or anniversary). A stressful time, such as when a deadline (for example, a tax deadline) needs to be met, is not a good time to try to quit.

Behavior modification can help people change the habits that cue smoking during normal daily activities. These cues may be phone conversations, coffee breaks, meals, sexual activity, boredom, traffic problems, or other frustrations. People who recognize smoking cues may modify the cues (for example, taking a walk in place of a coffee break) or substitute another oral activity (such as sucking on candy, chewing on a toothpick, or chewing gum).

Substituting a nonsmoked version of nicotine for a time helps many people break the habit of smoking. Many nonprescription (over-the-counter) and prescription nicotine replacement products are available. They include nicotine chewing gum, a nicotine patch, nicotine nasal spray, and a nicotine inhaler.

Using the patch with the gum or spray is more effective than any one product alone. These products have a few cautions:

- People with jaw (temporomandibular) disorders should not use the gum.
- People with severe skin sensitivity should not use the patch.
- These products may have harmful effects in pregnant or breastfeeding women and in adolescents.
- People who have had certain types of heart attacks recently should talk to their doctor before using one of these products.

Bupropion can be used with a nicotine replacement product. Together, they have a higher success rate than either alone. The results of both drugs are best when used with a behavior modification program.

A newer drug, varenicline, helps lessen craving and withdrawal symptoms and helps some people quit smoking. Nicotine replacement products and varenicline should not be used together.

If people who are depressed attempt to quit smoking, they should receive counseling. Bupropion is an antidepressant, making it particularly useful for people who are depressed or at risk of depression. Nortriptyline, another antidepressant, may be used instead.

Nicotine suppresses appetite and slightly increases the rate at which calories are burned. Thus, people who quit smoking often gain weight, which is particularly a concern among women. Exercise helps prevent weight gain and may reduce the craving for nicotine.

Support from family members and friends can help. Many U.S. states have telephone quitlines that can provide additional support for smokers trying to quit.

In the United States, about 20 million people try to quit each year. More than 90% of them return to smoking within days, weeks, or months. Receiving counseling or taking drugs improves the chances of success. About 20 to 30% of people who receive such help quit successfully. The more often people make a serious attempt to quit smoking, the more likely they are to ultimately succeed. Many people fail several times before they succeed.

Opioids

- Opioids are used to relieve pain, but they also cause an exaggerated sense of well-being and, if used too much, dependence and addiction.
- Taking too much of an opioid can be fatal, usually because breathing stops.
- Urine tests can be done to check for opioids.
- Treatment may involve stopping the drug abruptly, substituting another drug and gradually reducing its

dose to nothing, or substituting another drug that is taken indefinitely.

- Ongoing counseling and support are essential to controlling opioid addition.

Opioids have a legitimate medical use as powerful pain relievers (see page 642). They include codeine (which has a low potential for dependence), oxycodone (alone and in various combinations, such as oxycodone plus acetaminophen), meperidine, morphine, pentazocine, and hydromorphone. Methadone taken by mouth and fentanyl taken by a skin patch are used for chronic severe pain. Heroin, which is illegal in the United States but is used in very limited treatment applications in other countries, is one of the strongest opioids.

Opioids are common drugs of abuse because they are widely available and cause an exaggerated sense of well-being. People can become dependent on any opioid.

Although many people who use opioids to relieve pain for more than several days feel some symptoms of withdrawal when they stop, serious dependence and addiction rarely occur when opioid use is medically supervised.

Tolerance can develop after 2 to 3 days of continued opioid use. That is, people need more and more of a drug to feel the effects originally produced by a smaller amount. People may become more tolerant of some effects than of others. People who have developed tolerance may show few signs of drug use and function normally in their usual activities as long as they have access to drugs.

Did You Know...

Taking opioids to relieve the pain of an immediate injury, if supervised by a doctor, rarely leads to addiction.

Taking opioids during pregnancy can cause addiction in the fetus and withdrawal symptoms in the newborn.

Symptoms

Immediate Effects: Opioids are strong sedating drugs, causing people to become drowsy and quiet. Opioids may also cause euphoria. They dull pain and may enhance sexual pleasure. Other effects, such as constipation, nausea, vomiting, and itching, are less desirable. Opioids may cause confusion, especially in older people. In larger doses, they cause lethargy or sleep and may slow the heart rate and breathing rate.

The products that result from the breakdown (metabolism) of the opioid meperidine can cause seizures.

When taken with certain other drugs, some opioids can cause a serious disorder called serotonin syndrome. This syndrome is characterized by confusion, tremors, involuntary muscle spasms or twitching, agitation, excessive sweating, and a high body temperature.

Taking too much of an opioid at once (overdose) is life threatening. Breathing becomes dangerously slow and shallow, and the lungs may fill with fluid. Blood pressure, heart rate, and body temperature may decrease, and pupils constrict (becoming like pinpoints). People may become unconscious or die, usually because breathing stops.

Long-Term Effects: Opioids themselves do not cause many long-term complications other than dependence. However, many complications can result from sharing needles with another person and from unknowingly injecting other substances with the opioid (see page 2080).

Withdrawal Symptoms: Withdrawal is uncomfortable but not life threatening. Symptoms can appear as early as 4 hours after opioid use stops and generally peak within 48 to 72 hours. They usually subside after about a week, although the time frame can vary considerably depending on which opioid is used. Each opioid is eliminated from the body at a different rate, which alters how quickly withdrawal progresses and stops. Withdrawal symptoms are worse in people who have used large doses for a long time.

At first, people feel anxious and crave the drug. Breathing becomes rapid, usually accompanied by yawning, perspiration, watery eyes, a runny nose, dilated pupils, and stomach cramps. Later, people may become hyperactive and agitated and have a heightened sense of alertness. Heart rate increases. Other symptoms include gooseflesh, tremors, muscle twitching, fever and chills, aching muscles, loss of appetite, and diarrhea.

Opioid use during pregnancy is especially serious because heroin and methadone easily cross the placenta into the fetus. Because babies born to addicted mothers have been exposed to the drugs their mothers have taken, they may quickly develop withdrawal symptoms, including tremors, high-pitched crying, jitters, seizures, and rapid breathing. If mothers take opioids immediately before labor and delivery, the baby's breathing may be weak.

Diagnosis

Doctors base the diagnosis on symptoms and urine tests to check for the drug. Other tests may be done to check for complications.

Treatment

An opioid overdose requires emergency treatment. The ultimate and difficult goal of treatment is to help addicts control their addiction. Detoxification can help people get through the initial period of drug withdrawal, but further assistance is usually required to prevent people from returning to using drugs. Those who continually return to using opioids may require maintenance treatment.

Emergency Treatment: An opioid overdose is a medical emergency that must be treated quickly to prevent death. Breathing may require support, sometimes with a ventilator, if the overdose has suppressed breathing. A drug called naloxone is given intravenously as an antidote to the opioid, rapidly reversing all adverse effects. Because some people briefly become agitated and delirious before they become fully conscious, physical restraints may be applied for a short time. Because naloxone precipitates withdrawal symptoms in people who are dependent on opioids, it is used only when clearly necessary (as when breathing is weak).

People recovering from an overdose should be observed for several hours until the effects of naloxone have worn off to be sure that no adverse effects of the opioid remain. If people took an opioid with long-lasting effects (such as methadone or slow-release forms of other opioids), they are usually observed for a longer time.

If symptoms redevelop, people may be given another dose of naloxone, be admitted to the hospital, or both.

Detoxification: There are two basic approaches:

- Stopping the opioid and allowing withdrawal to run its course (cold turkey detoxification)
- Substituting a similar but less potent drug, then gradually decreasing the dose and stopping the drug

With detoxification, treatment is usually needed to lessen the symptoms of withdrawal. Clonidine usually provides some relief. However, clonidine may cause low blood pressure and drowsiness. Stopping clonidine may cause restlessness, insomnia, irritability, a fast heartbeat, and headaches. Sometimes drugs that block the effects of opioids, such as naltrexone, are needed to help people remain free of the opioid after they are fully detoxified.

Drugs that can be substituted, then stopped include methadone and buprenorphine. Methadone is an opioid that is taken by mouth. It blocks withdrawal symptoms and the craving for other opioids, especially heroin. Because methadone's effects last much longer than those of other opioids, it can be taken less frequently, usually once a day. The dose can then be decreased slowly. Doctors can begin the substitution, but then the use of methadone must be supervised in a licensed methadone treatment program, usually at a clinic.

Buprenorphine is a partial opioid agonist. That means it has some of the effects of opioids but blocks some of the effects of opioids. It does not require supervision in a special program, and thus doctors who are trained in its use can prescribe it in their office. In many countries, buprenorphine has replaced methadone in detoxification programs.

Maintenance: For people who continually return to using opioids (called chronic, relapsing opioid addiction), another approach—called maintenance—is often preferred. It involves substituting a prescribed drug that the user takes for a long time. Methadone, buprenorphine, or naltrexone may be used.

Maintaining addicts with regular doses of one of these drugs for months or years enables them to be socially productive because they do not have to spend time getting the opioid and because the drugs used do not interfere with functioning the way that illicit drug use does. For some addicts, the treatment works. For many addicts, lifelong maintenance is necessary.

Methadone suppresses withdrawal symptoms and the craving for the opioid without making addicts overly drowsy or elated. However, addicts must appear regularly, up to once a day, at a clinic, where methadone is dispensed in the amount that prevents severe withdrawal symptoms from developing, minimizes craving, and supports daily functioning.

Buprenorphine is being used more and more because it can be prescribed by doctors in their office. Thus, addicts do not have to go to a special clinic.

Naltrexone is a drug that blocks the effects of opioids (opioid antagonist). Before starting naltrexone, people must be fully detoxified from opioids, or a severe withdrawal reaction can occur. Depending on the dose, naltrexone's effects last from 24 to 72 hours. Thus, the drug can be taken once a day or as few as 3 times a week. Because this drug has no opioid effects, some addicts do not want to use it. This drug is most useful for addicts who are strongly motivated to remain free of opioids and who are not severely dependent on opioids.

Rehabilitation: Regardless of which approach is used, ongoing counseling and support is essential. Support may include specially trained doctors, nurses, counselors, opioid maintenance programs, family members, friends, and other people with the same addiction (support groups).

The therapeutic community concept emerged nearly 25 years ago in response to the problems of heroin addiction. Daytop Village and Phoenix House pioneered this nondrug approach. Addicts live in a communal, residential center for an extended period of time. These programs help addicts build new lives through training, education, and redirection. The programs have helped many people, but initial dropout rates are high. Questions about precisely how well these programs have worked and how widely they should be applied remain unanswered. Because these programs require a lot of resources to run, many people may be unable to afford them.

Phencyclidine

Phencyclidine (PCP or angel dust) is most often smoked after being sprinkled on plant material, such as parsley, mint leaves, tobacco, or marijuana. Occasionally, PCP is taken by mouth or injected.

Symptoms

PCP depresses brain function, and users usually become confused and disoriented shortly after taking the drug. They may not know where they are, who they are, or what time or day it is. They may go into a trance as if hypnotized. PCP users can be combative, and because they do not feel pain, they may continue fighting even when they are hit hard. Salivation, sweating, blood pressure, and heart rate also increase. Muscle tremors (shaking) are common.

High doses (overdose) can cause hallucinations, seizures, a life-threatening high body temperature (hyperthermia), coma, and possibly death. Long-term PCP use may damage the brain, kidneys, and muscles.

Treatment

When PCP users become agitated (as most do when brought for treatment), they are put in a quiet room and allowed to relax. Their blood pressure, heart rate, and breathing are monitored frequently. Soothing talk does not help. In fact, they may

---

Abused Inhalants With Medical Uses

Amyl nitrite: This inhalant widens (dilates) the arteries of the heart, allowing more oxygen to reach the heart muscle. Thus, it is used to relieve chest pain caused by coronary artery disease. Amyl nitrite is sold only by prescription.

Two closely related drugs, butyl nitrite and isobutyl nitrite, are not used medically. They can be sold legally for commercial purposes related to their use as air-fresheners, but other use is banned.

All three of these nitrite drugs briefly lower blood pressure, produce dizziness, and cause flushing, followed by a rapid heartbeat. These effects combined may produce a sense of excitement and euphoria. People also use these drugs because they believe that they enhance sexual pleasure. When used with sildenafil (used to treat erectile dysfunction), these nitrite drugs may greatly lower blood pressure, which can cause fainting, heart attack, or stroke.

Nitrous oxide: This gas (laughing gas) is used as an anesthetic. It is also used as a propellant in cans and dispensers of whipped cream. Nitrous oxide is sometimes abused because it produces a sense of euphoria and a pleasant dreamlike state. Prolonged exposure to nitrous oxide can cause numbness and weakness in the legs and arms, which can be permanent.

---

become even more agitated. If quiet surroundings do not calm agitated people, the doctor may give them a sedative such as lorazepam.

Solvent Inhalants

Adolescents use inhalants more frequently than cocaine or LSD but less frequently than marijuana or alcohol. In the United States, about 10% of adolescents have inhaled solvents. Inhalant use is particularly a problem among children aged 12 and younger. Inhalants are found in many common household products. Thus, children and adolescents can easily obtain them.

The product may be sprayed into a plastic bag and inhaled (bagging, sniffing, or snorting), or a cloth soaked with the product may be placed next to the nose or in the mouth (huffing).

Symptoms

Users rapidly become intoxicated. They may become dizzy, drowsy, and confused. Speech may be slurred. They may have difficulty standing and walking, resulting in an unsteady gait. Users may also become excited—but not because the solvents are stimulants. Later, perceptions and sense of reality may be distorted, resulting in illusions, hallucinations, and delusions. Users experience a euphoric, dreamy high, culminating in a short period of sleep. They

---

Common Products That Contain Solvent Inhalants

ADHESIVES
Airplane glue
Rubber cement
Polyvinyl chloride cement

AEROSOLS
Spray paint
Hair spray

SOLVENTS AND GASES
Nail polish remover
Paint remover
Paint thinner
Typing correction fluid and thinner
Fuel gas
Cigarette lighter fluid
Gasoline

CLEANING AGENTS
Dry cleaning fluid
Spot remover
Degreaser

may become delirious and confused, with mood swings. Thinking and coordination may be impaired. Intoxication can last anywhere from a few minutes to more than an hour.

Death can occur suddenly, even the first time one of these products is directly inhaled, because breathing becomes very slow and shallow or because heart rhythm is disturbed (called arrhythmia).

With chronic use, people become somewhat tolerant of the solvent's effects. People may become psychologically dependent on solvents, with a strong urge to continue using the solvents. But physical dependence does not occur. That is, stopping the drug does not cause unpleasant symptoms (withdrawal).

Chronic use or exposure to solvents (including exposure in the workplace) can severely damage the brain, heart, kidneys, liver, and lungs. In addition, bone marrow may be damaged, impairing red blood cell production and causing anemia.

Treatment

Treating children and adolescents who use inhalants involves evaluating any organ damage. Education and counseling to improve mental health and social skills and to manage sociologic problems may help. Recovery rates from inhalant use are among the poorest for any mood-altering substance. However, most users stop by the end of adolescence.

CHAPTER

320 Travel and Health

Travel preparation is crucial, even for healthy people. Proper preparations are inexpensive relative to the costs of getting sick or injured while away from home.

Travel Kits

Travel kits containing first-aid supplies, pain relievers (such as acetaminophen or nonsteroidal anti-inflammatory drugs), decongestants, antacids, antibiotics, and loperamide for traveler's diarrhea are useful for minor injuries and illnesses. Also, topical drugs, such as hydrocortisone 1% cream, an over-the-counter antifungal cream, and an antibiotic ointment, should be considered. Travelers should carry their travel kit, prescription drugs, extra eyeglasses or other corrective lenses (as well as a current written prescription for either), and hearing-aid batteries in a carry-on bag in case their checked baggage is delayed, lost, or stolen. Major problems can often be prevented with common-sense precautions.

Health and Travel Insurance

Health insurance is important for travelers. Even with domestic travel, some plans limit coverage for health care away from home. Thus, travelers should know the limitations of their policies.

Coverage is more often a problem for international travel. Some domestic insurance plans limit coverage for vaccinations and preventive drugs for international travel, even though some vaccinations are required for entry into certain countries. Likewise, Medicare and most commercial health insurance plans do not cover the cost of any treatment given

outside the United States. In addition, a cash deposit or payment in full may be required in international hospitals before care is provided.

To avoid high costs or inability to obtain care, travelers should determine in advance what international coverage, if any, their health plan offers, how to seek prior authorization for international care, and how to make a claim after an emergency. Travel health insurance, including insurance for emergency evacuation, is available through many commercial agencies, travel services, and credit card companies. Travelers may want to purchase insurance for services such as emergency care, transportation for care within foreign countries, transportation back to the United States for care, medical equipment and personnel during transport, dental care, prenatal or postnatal care, lost or stolen prescription drugs, and medical translators.

The International Association for Medical Assistance to Travellers (IAMAT), a nonprofit organization, maintains a list of English-speaking doctors in cities around the world (www.iamat.org). Other directories listing English-speaking doctors in foreign countries are available from several organizations and web sites (see page 2164). United States consulates may help travelers identify and secure emergency medical services.

Vaccinations

Vaccinations are important for travel to most developing countries and are required by some countries for entry. Ideally, travelers should visit their usual

VACCINES FOR INTERNATIONAL TRAVEL*†‡

INFECTION	REGIONS WHERE THE VACCINE IS RECOMMENDED	COMMENTS
Hepatitis A	Throughout the developing world	Two doses are given at least 6 months apart. Protection is full after the first dose for 6–12 months and after the second dose for life.
Hepatitis B	Throughout the developing world (hepatitis B is particularly common in China)	This vaccine is recommended for extended-stay travelers and all health care workers.
Influenza	Year-round in the tropics, between October and April in the Northern hemisphere, and between April and September in the Southern hemisphere	This vaccine is recommended for adult travelers to these destinations and for people traveling to any destination in large groups.
Japanese B encephalitis	Rural areas throughout most of Asia, particularly in areas with rice and pig farming	Three doses are given over 28 days.
Meningococcus	Northern Sub-Saharan Africa from Mali to Ethiopia (the meningitis belt)	Risk is higher during the dry season (December through June). This vaccine is required for entry into Saudi Arabia during Hajj or Umrah.
Rabies	All countries, including the United States	This vaccine is recommended for travelers at risk of animal bites, including rural campers, veterinarians, and field workers. It does not eliminate the need for additional vaccinations after an animal bite (for added protection).
Typhoid fever	Throughout the developing world, especially in South Asia (including India)	Two forms of the vaccine are available. Single injection form: It protects for 2 years and is safe for pregnant women. Pill form: One pill is taken every other day for a total of 4 pills. This form protects for 5 years and is not safe for pregnant women.
Yellow fever	Tropical South America and tropical Africa	The disease is rare, but many countries require vaccination for entry. This vaccine is not safe for pregnant women.

*See also the Immunization chapter on page 1144.

†In addition to the listed vaccinations, travelers should be up to date on vaccinations for measles, mumps, rubella, tetanus, diphtheria, polio, pneumococcal disease, and varicella.

‡All recommendations are subject to change. For the latest recommendations, consult the Centers for Disease Control and Prevention (www.cdc.gov).

health care practitioners at least 6 to 8 weeks before their travels. An International Certificate of Vaccination is the best place to document the names and dates of all vaccinations. The certificate is easy to carry and can be obtained from many travel clinics or from the Superintendent of Documents at the U.S. Government Printing Office.

Traveling With Medical Conditions

Traveling with a medical condition requires special preparation. People with a medical condition should visit their doctor before departure to ensure that their condition is stable and to determine whether any changes in drugs are needed. Detailed written medical information, including information about vaccinations, drugs, results of major diagnostic tests, and types and dates of treatments, may be the most valuable thing a person can have in a medical emergency. People should consider asking their doctor to prepare such information in a letter. Medical identification bracelets or necklaces are essential for people with conditions that can cause rapid, life-threatening symptoms, confusion, or unconsciousness (such as diabetes, seizures, and severe allergic reactions). Travelers should also carry proof of medical insurance. Travelers with heart disorders should travel with a copy of a recent electrocardiogram (ECG).

Drugs should remain in their original bottles so that the precise names of the drugs and the instructions for taking them can be reviewed in an emergency. The generic name of a drug is more useful than its brand name because brand names differ among countries.

Travelers should also pack an extra supply of drugs in carry-on bags in case checked bags get lost, stolen, or delayed in transit or the return trip is delayed. Because opioids, syringes, and large amounts of any drug are likely to raise the suspicions of security or customs officers, travelers should have a doctor's note explaining the medical need for the supplies. In addition, syringes should be packed together with the drugs that are dispensed in them. Travelers should also check with airports, airlines, or embassies to determine what additional documentation is helpful in making travel with these supplies go smoothly.

Problems in Transit

Several conditions are common even among healthy people while in transit.

Motion Sickness

Motion sickness during air, sea, rail, bus, or car travel occurs when the brain receives conflicting signals about movement (see page 663). Motion sickness is often triggered by turbulence and vibration and made worse by warmth, anxiety, hunger, or overeating. The main symptoms are stomach upset, nausea, vomiting, sweating, and dizziness (vertigo).

Motion sickness can be minimized by the following:

- Moderating intake of food, fluids, and alcohol (before and during travel)
- Fixing the eyes on a stationary object or on the horizon
- Lying down and keeping the eyes closed
- Choosing a seat where motion is felt least (for example, in the center of an airplane, over the wing)
- Refraining from reading
- Sitting by an open window or an air vent if possible

A cabin in the middle of a ship close to water level may reduce motion sickness in some people. A scopolamine patch (which requires a prescription) or nonprescription (over-the-counter) or prescription antihistamines are often useful, especially if taken before travel. However, these drugs often cause drowsiness, light-headedness, and dry mouth and can result in confusion, falls, and other problems in older people.

Blood Clots

Blood clots can occur when people sit for long periods during air, rail, bus, or car travel. Blood clots (deep vein thrombosis—see page 433) are more common in people who

- Are older
- Are overweight
- Smoke cigarettes
- Have varicose veins
- Are taking estrogen
- Are pregnant
- Have recently had surgery
- Have had blood clots
- Have been inactive or immobile

Blood clots form in leg or pelvic veins and occasionally dislodge and travel to the lungs (called pulmonary emboli—see page 488). Some blood clots in the legs do not cause symptoms, whereas others cause cramping, swelling, and color changes of the calves and feet. Pulmonary emboli are much more serious than blood clots in the legs. People may first develop a sensation of not feeling well, followed by shortness of breath, chest pain, or fainting. Pulmonary emboli are sometimes fatal.

The risk of developing blood clots can be reduced by changing positions frequently, straightening and moving the legs frequently while seated, drinking enough fluids, and getting up to walk and stretch every 1 to 2 hours. Prolonged leg crossing may decrease leg circulation and should be avoided. Avoiding caffeine and alcohol and wearing elastic support stockings also reduce risk.

Ear and Sinus Pressure

Ear and sinus pressure while flying is the result of changes in air pressure in the airplane (cabin pressure). Normally, as an airplane takes off and climbs (ascends), cabin pressure decreases, and small pockets of air trapped in the sinuses and middle ear expand, leading to ear pressure, ear popping, or both and to mild sinus pressure or discomfort. As an airplane descends, ca-bin pressure increases, and similar symp-toms occur. These mild sensations usually disappear as air pressure in the sinuses and ears equalizes with cabin pressure. Untreated dental problems or teeth that were subjected to recent dental procedures may also become painful when air pressure changes.

Swallowing (particularly while holding the nose closed) frequently or yawning during ascent and descent helps equalize pressure. Some people suck on hard candies during descent. These actions are normally sufficient to relieve minor ear and sinus discomfort. With allergies, sinus problems, and head colds, however, the passages that connect the ears and sinuses to the nose and mouth become inflamed and sometimes blocked by mucus, which prevents air pressure from equalizing normally. People with these problems may experience significant discomfort. They may benefit from taking decongestants before flying or by blowing hard against a closed mouth and pinched nostrils to equalize air pressure.

Children are particularly susceptible to the pain of unequal air pressure. They should chew gum, suck hard candy, or be given something to drink during ascent and descent to encourage swallowing. Babies can be breastfed or given a bottle or pacifier.

Sleep Disturbance

Sleep disturbance after air travel (jet lag) is common when people travel across more than 3 time zones. Sleep disturbance does not occur with sea, rail, or car travel because travelers have time to adjust to time zone changes. The most obvious symptom is fatigue on arrival. Other symptoms include irritability, difficulty sleeping (insomnia), headache, and difficulty concentrating. Jet lag can be minimized by starting to adjust sleep and wake times 1 or 2 days before departure to coincide with those of the destination time zone. In flight, a person should drink plenty of fluids and avoid smoking, caffeine, and excessive alcohol. Managing exposure to light can also help travelers adjust to a new time zone.

Westward Travel: People traveling westward tend to awaken earlier and feel tired earlier than they should by local time. For example, if people who normally wake up at 7 AM and go to bed at 11 PM travel 3 time zones *west*, they tend to awaken at 4 AM local time and feel the need for sleep by 8 PM. To adjust, people should try to get bright sunlight in the late afternoon and try to stay up until the appropriate bedtime.

Eastward Travel: People traveling eastward tend to awaken later and stay awake longer than they should by local time. For example, if people who normally wake up at 7 AM and go to bed at 11 PM travel 3 time zones *east*, they tend to awaken at 10 AM local time and not feel the need for sleep until 2 AM. To adjust, people should get bright sunlight in the early morning. Those who had an overnight flight should try to remain physically active until evening and try not to nap.

Short-acting sedatives may help people fall asleep at the appropriate local time after eastward travel. However, sedatives may have side effects, such as daytime drowsiness, amnesia, and nighttime insomnia. Long-acting sedatives, such as diazepam, can cause confusion and falls in older people and should be avoided.

The hormone melatonin regulates the sleep-wake cycle. Some doctors have recommended using melatonin supplements after eastward travel to reset the body's internal clock for sleep. Although some travelers report melatonin is beneficial, its effectiveness and safety have not been thoroughly proved.

Dehydration

Dehydration while flying is common because of the low humidity in airplanes. Dehydration tends to affect older people and people who have certain medical conditions, such as diabetes or who take drugs used to increase sodium and water excretion in the urine (diuretics). The main symptoms are light-headedness, drowsiness, confusion, and, occasionally, fainting.

Dehydration can be prevented by drinking fluids and by avoiding alcohol and caffeine. Dry skin can be treated with moisturizers.

Spread of Infection

Spread of infection on airplanes and cruise ships often receives media attention but is relatively uncommon. Concern is greatest for influenza, viral diarrhea, and bacterial meningitis. Travelers can minimize their risk of influenza by making sure they have received the most current influenza vaccine. They can minimize their risk of diarrhea by washing their hands frequently. There is no reliable way to prevent bacterial meningitis. Some cruise ships offer antibiotics to passengers who have been in close contact with passengers who have these infections.

Minor Injuries

Minor injuries are common. Unaccustomed lifting of heavy luggage is a common cause of shoulder injuries. Luggage falling out of overhead storage bins can cause other significant injuries. During ship travel, injuries can be prevented by wearing shoes that provide good traction on wet surfaces, using handrails and removing sunglasses before entering ship stairwells, and remaining alert in unfamiliar surroundings. A flashlight is useful for preventing falls at night.

Anxiety

Anxiety affects many people who travel. Fear of flying, fear of confined spaces, and worries about medical conditions worsening during flight are common sources of anxiety. Anxiety can cause insomnia, making jet lag worse. People may hyperventilate, often with symptoms such as chest pain, trouble breathing, muscle spasms, and tingling in the arms and hands and around the mouth. The company of a seasoned traveler or caregiver may help relieve anxiety. Cognitive therapy and desensitization programs or hypnosis may also help. Sedatives or antianxiety drugs, such as zolpidem or alprazolam, may be of benefit (see table on page 855).

Specific Medical Conditions and Travel

People with certain medical conditions encounter special problems in transit.

Heart Disease

If people with angina pectoris, heart failure, or rhythm disturbances have symptoms during rest or with minimal exertion, they should not travel. If people have had a heart attack within the past 4 weeks or a heart attack causing shock or heart failure within the past 6 weeks, they are advised not to travel. People with severe or worsening angina should avoid flying. Their symptoms may worsen because less oxygen is available at high altitudes.

All travelers with heart disease should carry a copy of a recent electrocardiogram. People with pacemakers, implantable defibrillators, or coronary stents should carry a card or doctor's letter documenting the presence, type, location, and electronic characteristics of the implanted device. An implanted metal device may trigger an alarm as the person passes through electronic security. Electronic security devices do not generally affect implantable defibrillators, but travelers are advised to avoid standing in walk-through metal detectors for more than 15 seconds. Hand-held metal detectors are also safe for people with defibrillators, but prolonged contact, such as holding the detector over the defibrillator for more than 5 seconds, should be avoided.

If given 24 hours' notice, most major airlines can provide low-sodium, low-fat meals on flights with regular meal service. If notified in advance, many cruise lines can also provide these meals.

> ### ? Did You Know...
> At high altitudes, symptoms of certain heart and lung disorders and sickle cell anemia can worsen because less oxygen is available.

Lung Disease

Travelers with lung cysts, severe emphysema, a large collection of fluid around the lungs (pleural effusion), or recent lung collapse or who have had recent chest surgery can develop complications caused by airplane pressure changes. They should not fly without approval from their doctor.

Other travelers with lung disease may need supplemental oxygen while they are aboard an airplane. A doctor determines a person's need for in-flight oxygen by measuring the level of oxygen in the blood. Airlines will provide in-flight oxygen if they are given a doctor's prescription and 48 hours' notice. Travelers are not allowed to carry oxygen in any form aboard an airplane. Travelers who need oxygen during airport layovers must make their own arrangements, although most oxygen vendors will assist their regular customers without charge if they have services in the destination city. Other respiratory equipment, such as continuous positive airway pressure devices, can be accommodated on an airplane provided the equipment does not exceed the size allowed for carry-on luggage. However, travelers who need this equipment should allow extra time for security checks.

Ground travel at high altitudes may present special problems because less oxygen is available than at sea level. In general, people with mild or moderate lung problems do not experience any difficulty at altitudes below 5000 feet, but the higher the altitude, the greater the chance of problems. People with lung disease traveling in or through such areas should take the same precautions that they would if they were flying.

Bus, train, car, and ship travel is safe for people with lung disease but requires planning to ensure a supply of oxygen. Commercial services can coordinate oxygen deliveries for travelers anywhere in the world.

People with asthma, emphysema, or bronchitis may find that their symptoms worsen in cities where air pollution is significant. They may need additional treatment with their inhalers or additional drugs, such as corticosteroids, to control symptoms adequately.

Diabetes

Blood sugar levels are best managed in transit by frequent testing, with adjustments of food intake and drug doses as needed. Travelers with diabetes should pack sugar (glucose) supplements in their carry-on bags or carry juice, crackers, and fruit for when blood sugar levels are low. If travel plans incur time changes of more than a few hours, people with diabetes, especially those taking insulin, should consult with a doctor about how best to schedule their drugs. Insulin can be stored without refrigeration for many days but should be kept out of extreme heat.

If given 24 hours' notice, most major airlines provide special meals for people with diabetes. Measures to prevent dehydration while in flight are important.

> **Did You Know...**
> When people with diabetes are traveling, target blood sugar levels should be slightly higher than when not traveling.

Blood sugar levels should be monitored frequently on arrival because activities and diet often differ from those at home. Because controlling blood sugar levels precisely is more difficult while traveling, levels tend to vary more than usual. Trying to keep levels very close to normal thus increases the risk that levels may sometimes become too low. For this reason, target blood sugar levels should be somewhat higher than ideal while traveling. Diabetic travelers should adhere to established diets despite temptations to try new foods and to eat more frequently or off schedule. They should wear comfortable socks and shoes, check their feet daily, and avoid walking barefoot to prevent minor injuries that may become infected or be slow to heal.

Pregnancy

Pregnancy is generally not affected by travel. However, pregnant women who are close to their due date (over 36 weeks) and those at risk of miscarriage, premature delivery, or placental abruption should avoid flying and traveling long distances. Most airlines have policies regarding travel for pregnant women, and these policies should be checked before tickets are purchased. Pregnant women traveling long distances should take precautions to reduce the risk of blood clots (such as getting up often when traveling by airplane and stopping to take short walks when traveling by car) and dehydration. Seat belts should be fastened below the abdomen and across the hips to prevent injury to the fetus.

Vaccines containing a virus that has been weakened but not killed—for example, yellow fever and measles-mumps-rubella—are not safe for pregnant women.

Pregnant women should avoid prolonged use of water purification tablets that contain iodine because iodine can affect development of the thyroid gland in the fetus.

Pregnant women who cannot postpone travel to regions of the world where malaria is common must weigh the risks of taking protective drugs whose effects on pregnancy are not well known against those of traveling without adequate protection. Malarial infection is more likely to be serious and life threatening among pregnant women than among women who are not pregnant, even when preventive drugs are used.

Pregnant women are also at risk of contracting hepatitis E infection, a viral liver infection rare in the United States but common in Asia, the Middle East, North Africa, and Mexico (see table on page 229). Miscarriage, liver failure, or death may result. There is no treatment, so postponing travel to regions where hepatitis E is common should be considered. Women who cannot postpone travel should be vigilant about hand washing.

Other Conditions

Travel and transit also affect other medical conditions.

Some travelers with sickle cell disease are at risk of experiencing pain (sickle cell crisis) when exposed to the low humidity and low oxygen levels in airplane cabins. This risk can be minimized with adequate hydration and oxygen.

Drugs used to treat human immunodeficiency virus (HIV) infection or AIDS may interact with drugs frequently taken by international travelers to prevent malaria and traveler's diarrhea. So affected travelers should discuss the risk of such interactions with their doctors and pharmacist.

People with a colostomy should wear a large bag or bring extra supplies because fecal output may increase with expansion of intestinal gas during flight. Because gas expands in flight, water should be substituted for air in devices secured by air-filled cuffs or balloons, such as feeding tubes and urinary catheters.

People who wear contact lenses may want to wear eyeglasses en route or wet their lenses frequently with artificial tears to compensate for low humidity in the airplane. Artificial tears may be helpful for people with dry eyes. In general, bringing an extra set of eyeglasses or lenses or a prescription in case replacements are necessary is a good idea. Extra batteries for hearing aids may also be useful.

Travelers with serious mental health disorders, such as poorly controlled schizophrenia, may pose a risk to themselves or others and should be accompanied by a responsible attendant. Sedating drugs may be recommended also.

Most airlines provide disabled travelers with wheelchairs and stretchers on commercial flights. Some airlines accommodate travelers who need special equipment, such as intravenous lines or ventilators, as long as trained personnel accompany them and arrangements have been made in advance.

General advice about traveling with various medical conditions can be obtained from the medical departments of major airlines, from the Federal Aviation Administration (www.faa.gov), from online travel information sources (see page 2164), or from local travel clinics.

Problems at the Destination

Problems after arrival are especially important to prevent and avoid in international settings. Though many people are most concerned about infection when considering a trip overseas, heart disease is the most common cause of death among international travelers. Heart disease is the most common cause of death among nontravelers as well, suggesting that attention to health before leaving home is the best way to prevent illness while away.

Injuries

Injuries are the most common cause of death among younger and middle-aged travelers. The most common are due to motor vehicle or water accidents. Common-sense measures can be taken to prevent many such injuries. For example, people uncomfortable with unfamiliar traffic patterns (such as driving on the left side of the road in England versus the right side in the United States) can take public transportation or hire drivers familiar with local roads and traffic laws. Travelers should avoid overcrowded taxis, ferries, or other transports and avoid nighttime driving and swimming in poorly lit areas. People should wear seat belts even as passengers and should use a helmet when cycling. Travelers should avoid motorcycles and mopeds and avoid riding on bus roofs or in open truck beds. Also, alcohol should never be consumed before driving or swimming, even where laws do not formally prohibit such actions or where laws that do exist are not enforced.

Many cities are unsafe after dark, and some are unsafe even during the day. A traveler should avoid walking alone on ill-lit or deserted streets in such cities, especially in countries where the traveler is obviously a stranger.

 Did You Know...

The most common cause of death among younger and middle-aged travelers is injury.

Traveler's Diarrhea

Traveler's diarrhea (see page 152) is the most common infectious disease among international travelers.

The risk of traveler's diarrhea may be reduced by the following measures:

- Drinking and brushing teeth with bottled, filtered, boiled, or chlorinated water
- Avoiding ice

- Eating freshly prepared foods only if they have been heated to steaming temperatures
- Eating only fruits and vegetables that people peel or shell themselves
- Avoiding food from street vendors
- Washing hands frequently
- Avoiding all foods likely to have been exposed to flies

Taking certain antibiotics can also prevent traveler's diarrhea. However, such use has a risk of side effects and may increase the chances that bacteria will develop resistance to antibiotics. Thus, many doctors recommend preventive antibiotics only for people who have an immune deficiency disorder.

In most cases, traveler's diarrhea subsides by itself and requires only the steady intake of fluids to prevent dehydration. Ordinary clear liquids (without caffeine or alcohol) are adequate for most people. Young children and older people may benefit from powdered rehydration mixes or an oral rehydration solution. Other measures, though not always necessary, may be helpful.

People who have moderate to severe symptoms (3 or more unformed stools over 8 hours) should consider taking an antibiotic, especially if they have vomiting, fever, abdominal cramps, or blood in the stool. For most destinations, the appropriate antibiotic is ciprofloxacin or ofloxacin. Azithromycin is appropriate for Southeast Asia and the Indian subcontinent. People should contact their doctor for an antibiotic prescription before travel. If people are older than 6 years of age and have no bloody stools, fever, or abdominal pain, they can also be treated with the antidiarrheal drug loperamide (which is available without a prescription).

For older adults and young children, powdered rehydration mixes are available for travel. If these mixes are unavailable, rehydration solutions can be made with small amounts of salt, baking soda, and sugar or honey mixed in water. However, solutions should be prepared carefully because young children can become seriously ill or die if they drink much of a solution that has been incorrectly mixed (for example, if a rehydration mix has not been fully diluted).

Malaria

Malaria (see page 1218) is common throughout the tropics. Malaria is prevented by avoiding mosquito bites and taking an antimalarial drug. Mosquito bites are prevented by the following measures:

- Wearing long-sleeved shirts and long trousers (especially at dawn and dusk, when mosquitoes are most active)
- Sleeping under a mosquito net

- Wearing clothing impregnated with permethrin
- Using insect repellants that contain diethyltoluamide (DEET)

Insect repellants can also help prevent other mosquito-borne diseases such as dengue and yellow fever. Even with these measures, taking an antimalarial drug (such as mefloquine, chloroquine, or atovaquone/proguanil) is necessary.

Schistosomiasis

Schistosomiasis is a common and potentially serious infection caused by a parasite that lives in fresh water in Africa, Southeast Asia, China, and eastern South America. Schistosomiasis can be prevented by avoiding freshwater activities in areas in which schistosomiasis is common (see page 1222).

Lice and Scabies

Lice and scabies are common in crowded accomodations, underdeveloped areas, and places where hygiene measures are poor (see page 1312). Infestations can be treated with permethrin, malathion, or lindane lotions. However, these lotions should not be used to prevent infestations.

Sexually Transmitted Infections

Sexually transmitted infections, including human immunodeficiency virus (HIV) infection, gonorrhea, syphilis, trichomoniasis, and hepatitis B, are more common in developing countries. All can be prevented through abstinence or with correct, consistent use of a condom (see box on page 1265). Because HIV and hepatitis B also are transmitted through blood and needles, an international traveler should not accept a blood transfusion without assurance that the blood has been tested for infection. Also, injections should be accepted only through one-time-only disposable needles.

Problems After Travel

Symptoms or problems that develop during travel and that do not subside by the time a person returns home warrant medical attention.

Travel-related problems can also develop after travel. For example, nitrogen narcosis (the bends) can occur after a diver gets on the plane to go home (see page 1998). Some symptoms may develop weeks or months after a person has returned. Fever after international travel is especially common. For example, malaria often causes fever days after exposure. Although the connection between travel and new symptoms often is not apparent, information about recent travel can be the key element in making a diagnosis. Therefore, people should tell their doctor about any recent travel when they experience any medical problem.

Both the International Society of Travel Medicine (www.istm.org) and the American Society of Tropical Medicine and Hygiene (www.astmh.org) have lists of travel clinics on their web sites. Many of these clinics specialize in assisting travelers who are ill after they return home.

CHAPTER
321 Amyloidosis

Amyloidosis is a rare disease in which a protein called amyloid accumulates in various tissues and organs, impairing normal function.

- The symptoms and severity of amyloidosis depend on which organs are affected.
- Diagnosis is made by examining a small piece of tissue under a microscope.
- Drugs can rarely reduce symptoms.
- Organ transplantation can treat some types of amyloidosis.

Amyloidosis causes few or no symptoms in some people but causes severe symptoms and fatal complications in other people. The severity of the disease depends on which organs are affected by amyloid deposits. Amyloidosis is twice as common among men as women and is more common among older people.

Many forms of amyloidosis exist, and the disease can be classified into four groups: primary amyloidosis, secondary amyloidosis, hereditary amyloidosis, and amyloidosis associated with normal aging.

Primary amyloidosis (light chain amyloidosis) occurs with abnormalities of plasma cells, and some people with primary amyloidosis also have multiple myeloma (cancer of the plasma cells—see page 1051). Typical sites of amyloid buildup in primary amyloidosis are the heart, lungs, skin, tongue, thyroid gland, intestines, liver, kidneys, and blood vessels.

Secondary amyloidosis may develop in response to various diseases that cause persistent infection or

EFFECTS OF AMYLOID BUILDUP

ORGAN OR SYSTEM AFFECTED	POSSIBLE CONSEQUENCES
Blood and blood vessels	Easy bruising
Brain	Alzheimer's disease
Digestive system	Enlarged tongue Intestinal obstruction Poor nutrient absorption
Heart	Abnormal heart rhythms (arrhythmias) Enlarged heart Heart failure
Kidneys	Fluid accumulation in tissues, causing swelling (edema) Kidney failure
Liver	Enlarged liver
Lungs	Difficulty breathing
Lymph nodes	Enlarged lymph nodes
Musculoskeletal system	Carpal tunnel syndrome
Nervous system	Numbness Tingling Weakness
Skin	Bruises Papules
Thyroid gland	Enlarged thyroid gland

inflammation (such as tuberculosis, rheumatoid arthritis, and familial Mediterranean fever) and certain types of cancer. Typical sites of amyloid buildup in secondary amyloidosis are the spleen, liver, kidneys, adrenal glands, and lymph nodes.

Hereditary amyloidosis has been noted in some families, particularly those from Portugal, Sweden, and Japan. The amyloid-producing defect occurs because of mutations in specific proteins in the blood. Typical sites for amyloid buildup in hereditary amyloidosis are the nerves, heart, blood vessels, and kidneys.

Amyloidosis associated with normal aging usually affects the heart. What causes amyloid to build up in the heart, other than age, is usually not known. Amyloid also accumulates in the brain of people with Alzheimer's disease and is thought to play a role in causing Alzheimer's disease.

Symptoms and Diagnosis

The accumulation of large amounts of amyloid can disturb the normal functioning of many organs.

Many people have few symptoms, whereas others develop severe, life-threatening disease. Common symptoms are fatigue and weight loss. Other symptoms of amyloidosis depend on where the amyloid builds up.

Amyloidosis is sometimes difficult for doctors to recognize because it causes so many different problems. However, doctors may suspect amyloidosis when

- Several organs fail
- Fluid accumulates in the tissues, causing swelling (edema)
- Unexplained bleeding occurs, especially in the skin

The hereditary form is suspected when an inherited peripheral nerve disorder is discovered in a family.

The diagnosis is generally made by testing a small amount of abdominal fat obtained through a needle inserted near the navel. Alternatively, doctors can do a biopsy by taking a sample of tissue from the skin, rectum, gums, kidney, or liver and examining it under a microscope with the use of special stains.

Prognosis and Treatment

There is no cure for amyloidosis. However, in secondary amyloidosis, treating the underlying disease usually slows or reverses the amyloidosis. Primary amyloidosis with or without multiple myeloma has a bleak prognosis. Most people who have both diseases die within 1 to 2 years. People who have amyloidosis and who develop heart failure have a poor prognosis as well.

Treatment to decrease or control symptoms and complications of amyloidosis has been only modestly successful for most people. Chemotherapy (prednisone and melphalan, sometimes combined with colchicine) and stem cell transplantation offer relief to some people. Colchicine alone may help relieve amyloidosis that is triggered by familial Mediterranean fever. Accumulations of amyloid in a specific area of the body can sometimes be removed surgically.

Organ transplants (for example, a kidney or the heart) have extended the lives of a small number of people with organ failure due to amyloidosis. However, the disease usually continues to progress, and eventually the transplanted organ accumulates amyloid. The exception is liver transplantation (see page 1132), which usually stops progression of the hereditary form of amyloidosis.

---

322 Disorders of Unknown Cause

Many people have disorders for which no specific cause has been identified. Some doctors believe that some of these disorders of unknown cause are due to psychologic factors. Others believe that the disorders are caused by infections (such as viral infections), toxic chemicals, or abnormalities of the immune system. Although a cause has not been proved for any of these disorders, many people undergo considerable testing and try unproved treatments in time-consuming and costly attempts to diagnose and relieve their symptoms. Some people thought to have disorders of unknown cause actually have common disorders that are in the early stages (before the typical symptoms have developed) or that have unusual symptoms.

Chronic Fatigue Syndrome

Chronic fatigue syndrome refers to long-standing severe and disabling fatigue without a proven physical or psychologic cause.

- Unexplained fatigue lasts for 6 months or longer.
- Sometimes symptoms begin with a coldlike illness.
- No treatments have proved to be effective, but symptoms may lessen over time.

Chronic fatigue syndrome may occur in up to 38 of 100,000 people in the United States. However, a recent telephone survey found the prevalence to be many times higher. Chronic fatigue syndrome affects people primarily between the ages of 20 and 50 and is about 1½ times more common among women than men.

Causes

Despite considerable research, the cause of chronic fatigue syndrome remains unknown. Controversy exists as to whether there is a single cause or many causes and whether the cause is physical or psychologic.

Some studies have suggested infection with the Epstein-Barr virus, rubella virus, herpesvirus, or human immunodeficiency virus (HIV) as a possible cause of chronic fatigue syndrome. However, current research indicates that these viral infections probably do not cause this syndrome. It is unclear whether other infections are related to the syndrome.

Some evidence suggests abnormalities of the immune system as possible causes. Other suggested causes include allergies (about 65% of people with chronic fatigue syndrome report previous allergies), hormonal abnormalities, decreased blood flow to the brain, and lack of certain nutrients in the diet.

Chronic fatigue syndrome seems to run in families, possibly supporting an infectious agent as a cause. Alternatively, members of the same family may respond similarly to physical and psychosocial stress.

Some researchers have suggested that prolonged bed rest during convalescence from an illness may play a role in causing this disorder.

Some researchers believe the syndrome ultimately will prove to have several causes, including genetic predisposition and exposure to microbes, toxins, and other physical and emotional factors.

Symptoms and Diagnosis

The main symptom is fatigue that usually lasts at least 6 months and that is severe enough to interfere with daily activities. Severe fatigue is present even on awake-ning and persists throughout the day. The fatigue often worsens with physical exertion or psychologic stress. However, evidence of muscle weakness or

Diagnosis of Chronic Fatigue Syndrome

According to the Centers for Disease Control and Prevention, diagnosis of chronic fatigue syndrome requires the following:

1. Medically unexplained persistent or recurring fatigue of at least 6 months' duration that is all of the following:

   - Is new or has a definite beginning
   - Is not due to exercise
   - Is not substantially relieved by rest
   - Substantially interferes with work-related, educational, social, or personal activities

2. At least four of the following symptoms for at least 6 months:

   - Poor short-term memory or reduced concentration severe enough to interfere with work-related, educational, social, or personal activities
   - Sore throat
   - Low-grade fever
   - Tender lymph nodes in the neck or armpits
   - Muscle pain
   - Abdominal pain
   - Pain in more than one joint without joint swelling or tenderness
   - Headaches that differ from previous headaches in type, pattern, or severity
   - Unrefreshing sleep
   - Persistent feeling of illness for at least 24 hours after exercise

These symptoms must have been present persistently or recurrently during, but not before, the period of fatigue.

However, not all doctors agree that these criteria should be applied strictly with every person. The criteria are more useful as a common definition in research studies.

of joint or nerve abnormalities is rare. Symptoms may begin after a coldlike illness that involves tender or painful swollen lymph nodes. In these people, extreme fatigue may begin with a fever and runny nose. However, in many people, fatigue begins without any preceding coldlike illness. Other symptoms that may occur are difficulty concentrating and sleeping, sore throat, headache, joint pains, muscle pains, and abdominal pain.

No laboratory tests are available to confirm a diagnosis of chronic fatigue syndrome. Doctors therefore must rule out other diseases that may cause similar symptoms, such as thyroid disease, psychologic problems, alcoholism, or the early stage of a liver, inflammatory, or kidney disorder. The diagnosis of chronic fatigue syndrome is made only if no other cause, including side effects of drugs, is found to explain the fatigue.

Treatment

In most cases, symptoms of chronic fatigue syndrome lessen over time.

Excessive periods of prolonged rest cause deconditioning and may worsen symptoms of chronic fatigue syndrome. Gradual introduction of regular aerobic exercise, such as walking, swimming, cycling, or jogging, under close medical supervision may reduce fatigue and improve physical function. Formal, structured physical rehabilitation programs may be best. Psychotherapy, including individual and group behavior therapy, may be helpful as well.

Many different drugs and alternative therapies have been tried. Although many treatments, such as antidepressants and corticosteroids, seem to make a few people feel better, none are clearly effective for all. It is hard for people and doctors to tell what treatments work because symptoms are different in different people and because symptoms may come and go on their own.

Controlled clinical trials are the best way to test therapies, and no drug therapy has been shown to be effective in controlled trials. A number of treatments directed at possible causes, including use of interferons, intravenous injections of immune globulin, and antiviral drugs, have been mostly disappointing. Dietary supplements, such as evening primrose oil, fish oil supplements, and high-dose vitamins, are commonly used, but their benefits remain unproved. Other alternative treatments (for example, essential fatty acids, animal liver extracts, exclusion diets, and removal of dental fillings) have also been ineffective.

Gulf War Syndrome

Gulf War syndrome consists of a group of symptoms experienced by more than 100,000 American, British, and Canadian veterans of the 1992 Persian Gulf War.

- Some Gulf War veterans have developed various symptoms.
- Although the veterans have been exposed to many different possibly harmful agents, the cause is unknown.
- Most symptoms involve the nervous system.
- The syndrome does not seem to increase the need for hospitalization or lead to earlier death.

Gulf War syndrome is poorly understood. Within a few months of returning from the Persian Gulf, veterans from different military units in the United States, Britain, and Canada began reporting a variety of symptoms, including headache, fatigue, difficulty sleeping, joint pain, chest pain, skin rashes, and diarrhea. In most cases, however, the symptoms reported by the person, such as headache and nausea, could not be objectively confirmed by a doctor. Even when symptoms, such as a skin rash, could be confirmed, no specific cause could be identified.

The cause of Gulf War syndrome is unknown. Gulf War veterans have often been exposed to a number of potentially toxic substances, including chemical weapons, depleted uranium weapons, insecticides, and smoke from burning oil wells. Veterans may also have been exposed to irritating petroleum products, decontamination solutions, and a variety of airborne substances that may have caused allergies. Vaccination with the anthrax vaccine, which was given to U.S. military personnel involved in the Gulf War as protection against biological warfare, has also been proposed as a cause, although this vaccine has not caused symptoms in other recipients. The use of pyridostigmine tablets to help prevent the lethal effects of chemical weapons has been suggested as a possible cause as well. However, none of these agents has been convincingly linked to Gulf War syndrome. Many exposed people have not developed symptoms, and many people with symptoms have had no identifiable exposure.

Symptoms

Symptoms predominantly involve the nervous system. They include problems with memory, reasoning, concentration, and attention and difficulty falling asleep, depression, fatigue, and headache. Other symptoms may include disorientation, dizziness, erectile dysfunction (impotence), muscle pains, muscle fatigue, weakness, pins-and-needles sensations, diarrhea, skin rashes, cough, and chest pain.

Diagnosis, Prognosis, and Treatment

Diagnosis and treatment have not been established. Therefore, doctors focus on relieving the symptoms.

Veterans who have Gulf War syndrome do not have a higher hospitalization or death rate than anyone else of the same age.

Multiple Chemical Sensitivity Syndrome

Multiple chemical sensitivity syndrome seems to be triggered by exposure to low levels of several identifiable or unidentifiable substances commonly present in the environment.

- Symptoms may include rapid heart rate, chest pain, sweating, shortness of breath, fatigue, flushing, and dizziness.
- Tests may be done to rule out allergic disorders.
- Treatment may involve psychotherapy, avoidance of certain substances, or both.

Multiple chemical sensitivity syndrome is more common among women than men. In addition, 40% of people with chronic fatigue syndrome and 16% of people with fibromyalgia also have multiple chemical sensitivity syndrome.

Reported Triggers for Multiple Chemical Sensitivity Syndrome

- Alcohol and drugs
- Caffeine and food additives
- Carpet and furniture odors
- Fuel odors and engine exhaust
- Painting materials
- Perfume and other scented products
- Pesticides and herbicides

Some doctors consider this disorder to be psychologic in cause, probably a type of anxiety disorder similar to agoraphobia (fear of going out in public) or a panic attack (see page 857). Others believe the disorder may be a type of allergic reaction (see page 1112). Various changes in the immune system may occur, supporting the idea of an allergic reaction. However, there is no consistent pattern of such changes among people who have this syndrome, and the cause remains unknown.

Symptoms and Diagnosis

Some people start having symptoms after a single exposure to high levels of various toxic substances. People blame their symptoms on exposure to these substances, but evidence is usually lacking.

Symptoms may include a rapid heart rate, chest pain, sweating, shortness of breath, fatigue, flushing, dizziness, nausea, choking, trembling, numbness, coughing, hoarseness, and difficulty concentrating.

A doctor bases the diagnosis of multiple chemical sensitivity on the symptoms. The diagnosis is supported if the symptoms

- Recur after repeated exposure to the chemical substance
- Recur after exposure to levels much lower than those that have been tolerated previously or that are commonly tolerated by others
- Subside when the person leaves the offending environment
- Develop in response to a wide variety of unrelated chemical substances

Tests, including blood and skin prick tests, may be done to diagnose allergic disorders.

Treatment

Treatment usually involves trying to avoid the toxic substances thought to cause the symptoms. However, avoidance may be difficult because many of these substances are widespread. People should avoid too much social isolation. Psychotherapy is sometimes helpful, not necessarily because the disorder is psychologic, but because it helps people cope with their symptoms.

Appendixes

APPENDIX

I   Weights and Measures

In medicine, precise measurements are necessary—for example, when various substances are measured in laboratory tests to evaluate health or make a diagnosis. Different units of measure may be used depending on the substance. Usually, the metric system, based on multiples of 10, is used to measure the following:

- **Mass:** Grams measure mass, the amount of matter in an object. Mass is similar to weight, but weight is affected by gravity.

- **Volume:** Liters measure volume, the amount of space an object occupies.

- **Length:** Meters measure length.

Prefixes, indicating which multiple of 10 is meant, can be attached to the basic unit, such as meter (m), liter (L), or gram (g). Using prefixes helps make a number more readable. Commonly used prefixes include kilo (k), deci (d), centi (c), milli (m), and micro (μ).

Other units measure different properties of a substance. For example, a mole (mol) is the amount of a substance that contains the same number of particles (molecules or ions) that is in 12 grams of carbon. Thus, regardless of the substance, 1 mole always contains the same number of particles. However, the number of grams in 1 mole varies greatly from substance to substance. One mole equals the molecular (atomic) weight of a substance in grams. For example, the molecular weight of sodium is 23, so 1 mole of sodium equals 23 grams. A molecule of table salt (sodium chloride) consists of one atom of sodium and one atom of chlorine (which has a molecular weight of 35 grams). Thus, one mole of sodium chloride weighs 23 grams + 35 grams = 58 grams.

Osmolarity is a measure of the number of particles in a liter of liquid, and osmolality is a measure of the number of particles in a kilogram (kg) of liquid. Because 1 liter of water weighs 1 kg, osmolarity and osmolality are the same for substances dissolved in water. An osmole is the amount of a substance that dissolves in liquid to form 1 mole. For example, because table salt dissolves into sodium and chloride in water, one mole of table salt dissolved in 1 liter of water results in 1 mole of sodium and 1 mole of chloride. Thus, its osmolarity is 2 osmoles per liter, and its osmolality is 2 osmoles per kg.

Equivalents (Eq) and milliequivalents (mEq) measure a substance's ability to combine with another substance. A milliequivalent is roughly equivalent to a milliosmole.

Formulas are used to convert a measurement from one unit to another. The same amount can be expressed in terms of different units. For example, the concentration of calcium in the blood is normally about 10 milligrams in a deciliter (mg/dL), 2.5 millimoles in a liter (mmol/L), or 5 milliequivalents in a liter (mEq/L).

The units used for medical tests vary depending on the substance being measured. The units that are traditionally used in the United States are called conventional units. Conventional units usually express concentration as weight per volume, and the volume can vary. The International System of Units (SI units) always expresses concentration as moles per liter.

PREFIXES IN THE METRIC SYSTEM

PREFIX	MULTIPLE OF 10	COMPARISON	
kilo (k)	1000	1 kilometer (km) = 1000 meters (m)	1 meter = 0.001 kilometer
deci (d)	0.1	1 deciliter (dL) = 0.1 liter (L)	1 liter = 10 deciliters
centi (c)	0.01	1 centimeter (cm) = 0.01 meter	1 meter = 100 centimeters
milli (m)	0.001	1 milliliter (mL) = 0.001 liter	1 liter = 1000 milliliters
micro (μ)	0.000001	1 microliter (μL) = 0.000001 liter	1 liter = 1 million microliters
pico (p)	0.000000000001	1 picoliter (pL) = 0.000000000001 liter	1 liter = 1 trillion picoliters

EQUIVALENTS FOR WEIGHT, VOLUME, AND LENGTH

NONMETRIC TO METRIC	METRIC TO NONMETRIC
Weight	
1 pound (lb) = 16 ounces (oz) = 0.454 kilogram (kg)	1 kilogram = 2.2 pounds
1 ounce = 28.35 grams (g)	1 gram = 0.035 ounce
Volume	
1 gallon (gal) = 4 quarts (qt) = 3.785 liters (L)	1 liter = 1.057 quarts
1 quart = 2 pints (pt) = 0.946 liter	
1 pint = 16 fluid ounces (fl oz) = 0.473 liter	
1 cup = 8 fluid ounces = 16 tablespoons (tbsp)	
1 fluid ounce = 29.573 milliliters (mL)	
1 tablespoon = 1/2 fluid ounce = 3 teaspoons (tsp)	
Length	
1 mile (mi) = 1,760 yards (yd) = 1.609 kilometers (km)	1 kilometer = 0.62 mile
1 yard = 3 feet (ft) = 0.914 meter (m)	1 meter = 39.37 inches (in)
1 foot = 12 inches = 30.48 centimeters (cm)	1 centimeter = 0.39 inch
1 inch = 2.54 centimeters	1 millimeter (mm) = 0.039 inch

EQUIVALENTS FOR HEIGHT AND WEIGHT

HEIGHT		WEIGHT	
ft-in	cm	lb	kg
4'10"	147.3	100	45.4
4'11"	149.9	110	49.9
5'0"	152.4	120	54.5
5'1"	154.9	130	59.0
5'2"	157.5	140	63.6
5'3"	160.0	150	68.1
5'4"	162.6	160	72.6
5'5"	165.1	170	77.2
5'6"	167.6	180	81.7
5'7"	170.2	190	86.3
5'8"	172.7	200	90.8
5'9"	175.3	210	95.3
5'10"	177.8	220	99.9
5'11"	180.3	230	104.4
6'0"	182.9	240	109.0
6'1"	185.4	250	113.5
6'2"	188.0	260	118.0
6'3"	190.5	270	122.6
6'4"	193.0	280	127.1

EQUIVALENTS FOR TEMPERATURE

To convert Fahrenheit to centigrade: Subtract 32, then multiply by 5/9 or 0.555.

To convert centigrade to Fahrenheit: Multiply by 9/5 or 1.8, then add 32.

COMMON TEMPERATURES	DEGREES	
	Centigrade (C)	Fahrenheit (F)
Freezing	0	32.0
Body temperature range	36.0	96.8
	36.5	97.7
	37.0	98.6
	37.5	99.5
	38.0	100.4
	38.5	101.3
	39.0	102.2
	39.5	103.1
	40.0	104.0
	40.5	104.9
	41.0	105.8
	41.5	106.7
	42.0	107.6
Boiling	100.0	212.0

APPENDIX II

Common Medical Tests

A large number of tests are widely available. Many tests are specialized for a particular disorder or group of related disorders (which are usually described with the appropriate disorders in this book). Other tests are commonly used for a wide range of disorders.

Tests are done for a variety of reasons, including

- Screening
- Diagnosing a disorder
- Evaluating the severity of a disorder so that treatment can be planned
- Monitoring the response to treatment

Sometimes a test is used for more than one purpose. A blood test may show that a person has too few red blood cells (anemia). The same test may be repeated after treatment to determine whether the number of red blood cells has returned to normal. Sometimes a disorder can be treated at the same time a screening or diagnostic test is done. For example, when colonoscopy (examination of the inside of the large intestine with a flexible viewing tube) detects growths (polyps), they can be removed before colonoscopy is completed.

Types of Tests

There are different types of medical tests but the lines that separate them often become blurred. For example, endoscopy of the stomach enables the examiner to view the inside of the stomach as well as obtain tissue samples for examination in a laboratory. Tests are usually one of the six following types.

Analysis of Body Fluids: The most commonly analyzed fluids are

- Blood
- Urine
- Fluid that surrounds the spinal cord and brain (cerebrospinal fluid)
- Fluid within a joint (synovial fluid)

Less often, sweat, saliva, and fluid from the digestive tract (such as gastric juices) are analyzed. Sometimes the fluids analyzed are present only if a disorder is present, as when fluid collects in the abdomen, causing ascites, or in the space between the two-layered membrane covering the lungs and lining the chest wall (pleura), causing pleural effusion.

Imaging: These tests provide a picture of the inside of the body—in its entirety or only of certain parts (see page 2034). Ordinary x-rays are the most common imaging tests. Others include ultrasonog-raphy, radioisotope (nuclear) scanning, computed tomography (CT), magnetic resonance imaging (MRI), positron emission tomography (PET), and angiography.

Endoscopy: A viewing tube (endoscope) is used to directly observe the inside of body organs or spaces (cavities). Most often, a flexible endoscope is used, but in some cases, a rigid one is more useful. The tip of the endoscope is usually equipped with a light and a camera, so that the examiner can watch the images on a television monitor rather than look directly through the endoscope. Tools are often passed through a channel in the endoscope. One type of tool is used to cut and remove tissue samples.

In endoscopy, the viewing tube is usually passed through an existing body opening, such as the following:

- Nose: To examine the voice box (laryngoscopy) or the lungs (bronchoscopy)
- Mouth: To examine the esophagus (esophagoscopy), stomach (gastroscopy), or small intestine (upper gastrointestinal endoscopy)
- Anus: To examine the large intestine, rectum, and anus (coloscopy)
- Urethra: To examine the bladder (cystoscopy)
- Vagina: To examine the uterus (hysteroscopy)

However, sometimes an opening in the body must be created. A small cut (incision) is made through the skin and the layers of tissue beneath the skin, so that the endoscope can be passed into a body cavity. Such incisions are used to view the inside of the following:

- Joints (arthroscopy)
- Abdominal cavity (laparoscopy)
- Area of the chest between the lungs (mediastinoscopy)
- Lungs and pleura (thoracoscopy)

Measurement of Body Functions: Often, body functions are measured by recording and analyzing the activity of various organs. For example, electrical activity of the heart is measured with electrocardiography (ECG), and electrical activity of the brain is measured with electroencephalography (EEG). The lungs' ability to hold air, to move air in and out, and to exchange oxygen and carbon dioxide is measured with pulmonary function tests.

Biopsy: Tissue samples are removed and examined, usually with a microscope. The examination often focuses on finding abnormal cells that may provide evidence of inflammation or of a disorder, such as cancer. Tissues that are commonly examined include skin, breast, lung, liver, kidney, and bone.

Analysis of Genetic Material (Genetic Testing): Usually, cells from skin, blood, or bone marrow are analyzed. Cells are examined to check for abnormalities of chromosomes, genes (including DNA), or both. Genetic testing may be done in the following:

- Fetuses: To determine whether they have a genetic disorder

- Children and young adults: To determine whether they have a disorder or are at risk of developing a disorder

- Adults: Sometimes to help determine the likelihood that their relatives, such as children or grandchildren, will develop certain disorders

Risks and Results

Every test has some risk. The risk may be the possibility of injury during the test, or it may be the need for further testing if the result is abnormal. Further testing is often more expensive, dangerous, or both. Doctors weigh the risk of a test against the usefulness of the information it will provide.

Normal test values are expressed as a range, which is based on the average values in a healthy population. That is, 95% of healthy people have values within this range. However, average values are slightly different for women and men and may vary by age. For some tests, these values also vary among laboratories. Thus, when doctors get a laboratory test result, the laboratory also gives them its own normal range for that test. The table below lists some typical normal results. However, because values vary by laboratory, people should consult their doctor about the significance of their own test results rather than refer to this table.

BLOOD TESTS*

TEST	REFERENCE VALUES (CONVENTIONAL UNITS†)
Acidity (pH)	7.35–7.45
Alcohol (ethanol)	0 mg/dL (more than 0.1 mg/dL usually indicates intoxication)
Ammonia	15–50 units/L
Amylase	53–123 units/L
Antinuclear antibodies (ANA)‡	0 (a negative result)
Ascorbic acid	0.4–1.5 mg/dL
Bicarbonate (carbon dioxide content)	18–23 mEq/L
Bilirubin	*Direct:* Up to 0.4 mg/dL *Total:* Up to 1.0 mg/dL
Blood volume	8.5–9.1% of body weight
Calcium	8.5–10.5 mg/dL (slightly higher in children)
Carbon dioxide pressure§	35–45 mm Hg
Carboxyhemoglobin (carbon monoxide in hemoglobin)	Less than 5% of total hemoglobin
CD4 cell count	500–1500 cells/μL
Ceruloplasmin	15–60 mg/dL
Chloride	98–106 mEq/L
Complete blood cell count (CBC)	*See individual tests:* Hemoglobin, hematocrit, mean corpuscular hemoglobin, mean corpuscular hemoglobin concentration, mean corpuscular volume, platelet count, and white blood cell count

(continued on the following page)

BLOOD TESTS* (Continued)

TEST	REFERENCE VALUES (CONVENTIONAL UNITS†)
Copper	70–150 µg/dL
Creatine kinase (CK), also called creatine phosphokinase (CPK)	*Male:* 38–174 units/L *Female:* 96–140 units/L
Creatine kinase (CK) in its different forms (isoenzymes)	5% or less of CK-MB (the form of CK that occurs mainly in heart muscle)
Creatinine	0.6–1.2 mg/dL
Electrolytes	*See individual tests:* Calcium, chloride, magnesium, potassium, and sodium (which are routinely tested)
Erythrocyte sedimentation rate (ESR)	*Male:* 1–13 mm/hour *Female:* 1–20 mm/hour
Glucose	*Fasting:* 70–110 mg/dL
Hematocrit	*Male:* 45–52% *Female:* 37–48%
Hemoglobin	*Male:* 13–18 g/dL *Female:* 12–16 g/dL
Iron	60–160 µg/dL (higher in males)
Iron-binding capacity	250–460 µg/dL
Lactate (lactic acid)	*Venous:* 4.5–19.8 mg/dL *Arterial:* 4.5–14.4 mg/dL
Lactic dehydrogenase	50–150 units/L
Lead	20 µg/dL or less (much lower in children)
Lipase	10–150 units/L
Lipids: Cholesterol, total	Less than 225 mg/dL for people aged 40–49 yr (increases with age)
High-density lipoprotein (HDL)	30–70 mg/dL
Low-density lipoprotein (LDL)	60 mg/dL
Triglycerides	40–200 mg/dL (higher in males)
Liver function tests	Include bilirubin (total), phosphatase (alkaline), protein (total and albumin), transaminases (alanine and aspartate), and prothrombin
Magnesium	1.5–2.0 mg/dL
Mean corpuscular hemoglobin (MCH)	27–32 pg/cell
Mean corpuscular hemoglobin concentration (MCHC)	32–36% hemoglobin/cell
Mean corpuscular volume (MCV)	76–100 cubic µm
Osmolality	280–296 mOsm/kg plasma
Oxygen pressure§	83–100 mm Hg
Oxygen saturation (arterial)	96–100%

(continued on the following page)

BLOOD TESTS* (*Continued*)

TEST	REFERENCE VALUES (CONVENTIONAL UNITS[†])
Partial thromboplastin time (PTT)	30–45 seconds
Phosphatase (alkaline)	50–160 units/L (higher in infants and adolescents, lower in females)
Phosphorus	3.0–4.5 mg/dL
Platelet count	150,000–350,000/mL
Potassium	3.5–5.0 mEq/L
Prostate-specific antigen (PSA)	0–4 ng/mL (increases with age)

Protein:
  Total
  Albumin
  Globulin
	
	6.0–8.4 g/dL
	3.5–5.0 g/dL
	2.3–3.5 g/dL

Prothrombin time (PT)	10–13 seconds
Red blood cell (RBC) count	4.2–5.9 million/mL
Sodium	135–145 mEq/L
Thyroid-stimulating hormone (TSH)	0.5–5.0 milliunits/L

Transaminases (liver enzymes):
  Alanine (ALT)
  Aspartate (AST)
	
	1–21 units/L
	7–27 units/L

Troponin in its different forms:
  I
  T
	
	Less than 1.6 ng/mL
	Less than 0.1 ng/mL

Urea nitrogen (BUN)	7–18 mg/dL
Uric acid	3.0–7.0 mg/dL
Vitamin A[‖]	30–65 µg/dL
White blood cell (WBC) count	4,300–10,800 /mL

*Blood can be tested for many other substances as well.

[†]Units are explained in Appendix I. Conventional units can be converted to international units by using a conversion factor. International units (IU), a different system, are sometimes used by laboratories.

[‡]Other antibodies can also be identified.

[§]Expressed as a comparison with the level of mercury (Hg) in a tube, which results from air pressure at sea level.

[‖]Other vitamins can also be measured.

DIAGNOSTIC PROCEDURES

PROCEDURE	BODY AREA OR SAMPLE TESTED	DESCRIPTION
Amniocentesis	Fluid from the sac surrounding the fetus	Analysis of fluid, removed by a needle inserted through the abdominal wall, to detect an abnormality in the fetus
Arteriography (angiography)	Any artery in the body, commonly in the brain, heart, kidneys, aorta, or legs	X-ray study using radiopaque dye injected through a thin tube (catheter), which is threaded to the artery being studied, to detect and outline or highlight a blockage or defect in an artery
Audiometry	Ears	Assessment of the ability to hear and distinguish sounds at specific pitches and volumes using headphones
Auscultation	Heart	Listening with a stethoscope for abnormal heart sounds
Barium x-ray studies	Esophagus, stomach, intestine, or rectum	X-ray study to detect ulcers, tumors, or other abnormalities
Biopsy	Any tissue in the body	Removal and examination of a tissue sample under a microscope to check for cancer or another abnormality
Blood pressure measurement	Usually an arm	Test for high or low blood pressure, usually using an inflatable cuff wrapped around the arm
Blood tests	Usually a blood sample from an arm	Measurement of substances in the blood to evaluate organ function and to help diagnose and monitor various disorders
Bone marrow aspiration	Hipbone or breastbone	Removal of a bone marrow sample by a needle for examination under a microscope to check for abnormalities in blood cells
Bronchoscopy	Airways of the lungs	Direct examination with a viewing tube to check for a tumor or other abnormality
Cardiac catheterization	Heart	Study of heart function and structure using a catheter inserted into a blood vessel and threaded to the heart
Chorionic villus sampling	Placenta	Removal of a sample for examination under a microscope to check for abnormalities in the fetus
Chromosomal analysis	Blood	Examination under a microscope to detect a genetic disorder or to determine a fetus's sex
Colonoscopy	Large intestine	Direct examination with a viewing tube to check for a tumor or other abnormality
Colposcopy	Cervix	Direct examination of the cervix with a magnifying lens
Computed tomography (CT)	Any part of the body	Computer-enhanced x-ray study to detect structural abnormalities
Cone biopsy	Cervix	Removal and examination of a cone-shaped piece of tissue, usually using a heated wire loop or a laser
Culture	A sample from any area of the body (usually a fluid such as blood or urine)	Growth and examination of microorganisms from the sample to identify infection with bacteria or fungi

(continued on the following page)

DIAGNOSTIC PROCEDURES (*Continued*)

PROCEDURE	BODY AREA OR SAMPLE TESTED	DESCRIPTION
Dilation and curettage (D and C)	Cervix and uterus	Examination of a sample under a microscope to check for abnormalities in the uterine lining using a small, sharp instrument (curet)
Dual x-ray absorptiometry (DEXA)	Skeleton, focusing on specific regions, usually the hip, spine, and wrist	Low-dose x-ray study to determine the density of bones
Echocardiography	Heart	Study of heart structure and function using sound waves
Electrocardiography (ECG)	Heart	Study of the heart's electrical activity using electrodes attached to the arms, legs, and chest
Electroencephalography (EEG)	Brain	Study of the brain's electrical function using electrodes attached to the scalp
Electromyography	Muscles	Recording of a muscle's electrical activity using small needles inserted into the muscle
Electrophysiologic testing	Heart	Test to evaluate rhythm or electrical conduction abnormalities using a catheter inserted into a blood vessel and threaded to the heart
Endoscopic retrograde cholangiopancreatography (ERCP)	Biliary tract	X-ray study of the biliary tract done after injection of a radiopaque dye and using a flexible viewing tube
Endoscopy	Digestive tract	Direct examination of internal structures using a flexible viewing tube
Enzyme-linked immunosorbent assay (ELISA)	Usually blood	Test that involves mixing the sample of blood with substances that can trigger allergies (allergens) or with microorganisms to test for the presence of specific antibodies
Fluoroscopy	Digestive tract, heart, or lungs	A continuous x-ray study that enables a doctor to see the inside of an organ as it functions
Hysteroscopy	Uterus	Direct examination of the inside of the uterus with a flexible viewing tube
Intravenous urography	Kidneys and urinary tract	X-ray study of the kidneys and urinary tract after a radiopaque dye is injected into a vein (intravenously)
Joint aspiration	Joints, especially those of the shoulders, elbows, fingers, hips, knees, ankles, and toes	Removal and examination of fluid from the space within joints to check for blood cells, crystals formed from minerals, and microorganisms
Laparoscopy	Abdomen	Direct examination using a viewing tube inserted through an incision in the abdomen to diagnose and treat abnormalities in the abdomen
Magnetic resonance imaging (MRI)	Any part of the body	Imaging test using a strong magnetic field and radio waves to check for structural abnormalities
Mammography	Breasts	X-ray study to check for breast cancer

(continued on the following page)

DIAGNOSTIC PROCEDURES (*Continued*)

PROCEDURE	BODY AREA OR SAMPLE TESTED	DESCRIPTION
Mediastinoscopy	Chest	Direct examination of the area of the chest between the lungs using a viewing tube inserted through a small incision just above the breastbone
Myelography	Spinal column	Simple or computer-enhanced x-ray study of the spinal column after injection of a radiopaque dye
Nerve conduction study	Nerves	Test to determine how fast a nerve impulse travels using electrodes or needles inserted along the path of the nerve
Occult blood test	Large intestine	Test to detect blood in stool
Ophthalmoscopy	Eyes	Direct examination using a handheld device that shines light into the eye to detect abnormalities inside the eye
Papanicolaou (Pap) test	Cervix	Examination of cells scraped from the cervix under a microscope to detect cancer
Paracentesis	Abdomen	Insertion of a needle into the abdominal cavity to remove fluid for examination
Percutaneous transhepatic cholangiography	Liver and biliary tract	X-ray study of the liver and biliary tract after a radiopaque dye is injected into the liver
Positron emission tomography (PET)	Brain and heart	Imaging test using particles that release radiation (positrons) to detect abnormalities in function
Pulmonary function tests	Lungs	Tests to measure the lungs' capacity to hold air, to move air in and out of the body, and to exchange oxygen and carbon dioxide as people blow into a measuring device
Radionuclide imaging	Many organs	Imaging test using particles that release radiation (radionuclides) to detect abnormalities in blood flow, structure, or function
Reflex tests	Tendons	Tests using a physical stimulus (such as a light tap) to detect abnormalities in nerve function
Retrograde urography	Bladder and ureters	X-ray study of the bladder and ureters after a radiopaque dye is inserted into the ureter
Sigmoidoscopy	Rectum and last portion of the large intestine	Direct examination using a viewing tube to detect tumors or other abnormalities
Skin allergy tests	Usually an arm or the back	Tests for allergies done by placing a solution containing a possible allergen on the skin, then pricking the skin with a needle
Spinal tap (lumbar puncture)	Spinal canal	Removal of spinal fluid, using a needle inserted into the hipbone, to check for abnormalities in spinal fluid
Spirometry	Lungs	Test of lung function that involves blowing into a measuring device
Stress testing	Heart	Test of heart function during exertion using a treadmill or other exercise machine and electrocardiography (if people cannot exercise, a drug is used to simulate exercise's effects)

(*continued on the following page*)

DIAGNOSTIC PROCEDURES (*Continued*)

PROCEDURE	BODY AREA OR SAMPLE TESTED	DESCRIPTION
Thoracentesis	Pleural space (the space between the pleura, a two-layered membrane that covers the lungs and lines the chest wall)	Removal of fluid from this space with a needle to detect abnormalities
Thoracoscopy	Lungs	Examination of the lung surfaces, pleura, and pleural space through a viewing tube
Tympanometry	Ears	Measurement of the resistance to pressure (impedance) in the middle ear using a device inserted in the ear and sound waves to help determine the cause of hearing loss
Ultrasonography (ultrasound scanning)	Any part of the body	Imaging using sound waves to detect structural or functional abnormalities
Urinalysis	Kidneys and urinary tract	Chemical analysis of a urine sample to detect protein, sugar, ketones, and blood cells
Venography	Veins	X-ray study using a radiopaque dye (similar to arteriography) to detect blockage of a vein

APPENDIX III

Drug Names: Generic and Trade

Most prescription drugs placed on the market are given trade names (also called proprietary, brand, or specialty names) to distinguish them as being produced and marketed exclusively by a particular manufacturer. In the United States, these names are usually registered as trademarks with the Patent Office; this gives the registrant certain legal rights with respect to use of the name. A trade name may be registered for a product containing a single active ingredient, with or without additives, or for one containing two or more active ingredients.

A drug marketed by several companies may have several trade names. A drug manufactured in one country and marketed in many countries may have different trade names in each country.

Throughout this book, generic (nonproprietary) names have been used whenever possible. However, because trade names are commonly used and may be more readily recognized, the generic drugs mentioned in

this book are listed below in alphabetic order along with many of their trade names. A second table follows, listing the trade names in alphabetic order along with their generic name.

With few exceptions, the trade names in these tables are limited to those marketed in the United States. These tables are by no means all-inclusive, and no effort has been made to list every trade name in current use for each drug. The inclusion of a drug in these tables does not indicate approval of a drug's use, nor does it imply that a drug is effective or safe. Many drugs are marketed almost exclusively under their generic name. Including a trade name of such a drug in these tables does not indicate an endorsement or a preference for the trade name version over the generic version.

Whether it is best to use a trade or a generic version of a drug may be a complex decision. It is best to discuss such matters with a doctor or pharmacist.

SOME TRADE NAMES OF GENERIC DRUGS*

GENERIC NAME	TRADE NAME	GENERIC NAME	TRADE NAME
Abacavir	ZIAGEN	Adenosine	ADENOCARD
Abatacept	ORENCIA	Albendazole	ALBENZA
Abciximab	ReoPro	Albuterol	PROVENTIL HFA
Acarbose	PRECOSE		VENTOLIN HFA
Acebutolol	SECTRAL	Alclometasone	ACLOVATE
Acetaminophen	TYLENOL	Alemtuzumab	CAMPATH
Acetazolamide	DIAMOX	Alendronate	FOSAMAX
Acetylcysteine	ACETADOTE	Alfuzosin	UROXATRAL
Acetylsalicylic acid	See Aspirin	Allopurinol	LOPURIN
ACTH	See Corticotropin		ZYLOPRIM
Acitretin	SORIATANE	All-*trans*-retinoic acid	See Tretinoin
Actinomycin	SEE DACTINOMYCIN	Almotriptan	AXERT
Acyclovir	ZOVIRAX	Alosetron	LOTRONEX
Adalimumab	HUMIRA	Alprazolam	XANAX
Adapalene	DIFFERIN	Alprostadil	CAVERJECT
Adefovir	HEPSERA		PROSTIN VR

SOME TRADE NAMES OF GENERIC DRUGS*

GENERIC NAME	TRADE NAME	GENERIC NAME	TRADE NAME
Aluminum chloride	DRYSOL XERAC AC	Atorvastatin	LIPITOR
		Atovaquone	MEPRON
Aluminum hydroxide	ALU-CAP AMPHOGEL GAVISCON	Atovaquone-proguanil	MALARONE
		Atropine	ATROPEN
Amantadine	SYMMETREL	Auranofin	RIDAURA
Ambrisentan	LETAIRIS	Azacitidine	VIDAZA
Aminocaproic acid	AMICAR	Azathioprine	IMURAN
Amiodarone	CORDARONE	Azelaic acid	AZELEX FINACEA
Amlexanox	APHTHASOL		
		Azelastine	OPTIVAR
Amlodipine	NORVASC	Azithromycin	ZITHROMAX
Amorolfine†	LOCERYL	Aztreonam	AZACTAM
Amoxicillin	AMOXIL TRIMOX	Bacitracin	BACIIM
		Baclofen	LIORESAL
Amoxicillin/clavulanate	AUGMENTIN	Balsalazide	COLAZAL
Amphetamine	ADDERALL	Basiliximab	SIMULECT
Amphotericin B	FUNGIZONE	Beclomethasone	BECONASE AQ
Ampicillin	PRINCIPEN	Benazepril	LOTENSIN
Ampicillin-sulbactam	UNASYN	Benzathine penicillin G	BICILLIN L-A
Amprenavir	AGENERASE	Benznidazole†	RADANIL
Anagrelide	AGRYLIN	Benzocaine	ANBESOL CEPACOL LANACANE
Anakinra	KINERET		
Anastrozole	ARIMIDEX		
Anidulafungin	ERAXIS	Benzafibrate†	BEZALIP
Anistreplase	EMINASE	Benzonatate	TESSALON
Antazoline	VASOCON-A	Benzoyl peroxide	BENZAC
Anthralin	ANTHRA-DERM	Benzphetamine	DIDREX
Apomorphine	APOKYN	Bepridil†	VASCOR
Apraclonidine	IOPIDINE	Benztropine	COGENTIN
Argatroban	ARGATROBAN	Betamethasone	CELESTONE
Aripiprazole	ABILIFY	Betaxolol	KERLONE
Arsenic trioxide	TRISENOX	Bethanechol	URECHOLINE
Artemether-lumefantrine	COARTEM	Bevacizumab	AVASTIN
Asparaginase	ELSPAR	Bicalutamide	CASODEX
Aspirin	BAYER	Bimatoprost	LUMIGAN
Atenolol	TENORMIN	Bisacodyl	DULCOLAX

SOME TRADE NAMES OF GENERIC DRUGS*

GENERIC NAME	TRADE NAME	GENERIC NAME	TRADE NAME
Bismuth subsalicylate	PEPTO-BISMOL	Carbamazepine	TEGRETOL
Bisoprolol	ZEBETA	Carbenicillin	GEOCILLIN
Bithionol	BITIN LOROTHIDOL	Carbidopa	LODOSYN
		Carbimazole	NEO-MERCAZOLE
Bivalirudin	ANGIOMAX	Carboplatin	PARAPLATIN
Bleomycin	BLENOXANE	Carisoprodol	SOMA
Bortezomib	VELCADE	Carteolol	OCUPRESS
Bosentan	TRACLEER	Carvedilol	COREG
Botulinum toxin	BOTOX	Caspofungin	CANCIDAS
Brimonidine	ALPHAGAN P	Cefadroxil	DURICEF
Brinzolamide	AZOPT	Cefazolin	ANCEF KEFZOL
Bromocriptine	PARLODEL		
Budesonide	RHINOCORT	Cefdinir	OMNICEF
Bumetanide	BUMEX	Cefditoren	SPECTRACEF
Buprenorphine	BUPRENEX	Cefepime	MAXIPIME
Bupropion	WELLBUTRIN	Cefixime	SUPRAX
Buserelin	ETILAMIDE	Cefotaxime	CLAFORAN
Buspirone	BUSPAR	Cefoxitin	MEFOXIN
Busulfan	MYLERAN	Cefpodoxime	VANTIN
Butenafine	MENTAX	Cefprozil	CEFZIL
Butoconazole	GYNAZOLE-1	Ceftazidime	FORTAZ TAZICEF
Butorphanol	STADOL		
Calcitonin	MIACALCIN	Ceftibuten	CEDAX
Calcipotriene	DOVONEX	Ceftizoxime	CEFIZOX
Calcitriol	ROCALTROL	Ceftobiprole†	ZEFTERA ZEVTERA
Calcium carbonate	CALTRATE OS-CAL TUMS		
		Ceftriaxone	ROCEPHIN
Candesartan	ATACAND	Cefuroxime	CEFTIN ZINACEF
Cantharidin	CANTHARONE		
Capecitabine	XELODA	Celecoxib	CELEBREX
Capsaicin	CAPSIN CAPZASIN ZOSTRIX	Celiprolol†	CELECTOL
		Cephalexin	KEFLEX
		Cetirizine	ZYRTEC
		Cevimeline	EVOXAC
Captopril	CAPOTEN	Chlorambucil	LEUKERAN
Carbachol	MIOSTAT	Chloramphenicol	CHLORAMPHENICOL

SOME TRADE NAMES OF GENERIC DRUGS*

GENERIC NAME	TRADE NAME	GENERIC NAME	TRADE NAME
Chlordiazepoxide	LIBRIUM	Cloxacillin	CLOXAPEN
Chlorhexidine	HIBICLENS	Clozapine	CLOZARIL
2-Chlorodeoxyadenosine	LEUSTATIN	Coal tar	DENOREX
Chloroquine	ARALEN		NEUTROGENA T/GEL
Chlorothiazide	DIURIL	Colesevelam	WELCHOL
Chlorpheniramine	CHLOR-TRIMETON	Colestipol	COLESTID
Chlorpropamide	DIABINESE	Colistin	COLY-MYCIN M
Chlorthalidone	THALITONE	Corticotropin (ACTH)	H. P. ACTHAR GEL
Chlorzoxazone	PARAFON FORTE	Cortisol	CORTEF
Cholestyramine	QUESTRAN	Cotrimoxazole	See Trimethoprim-sulfamethoxazole
Ciclopirox	LOPROX		
Cidofovir	VISTIDE	Cromolyn	CROLOM
Cilostazol	PLETAL		INTAL
Cimetidine	TAGAMET	Cyclizine	MAREZINE
Ciprofibrate†	MODALIM	Cyclobenzaprine	FLEXERIL
Ciprofloxacin	CILOXAN	Cyclopentolate	CYCLOGYL
	CIPRO	Cyclophosphamide	LYOPHILIZED CYTOXAN
Cisplatin	PLATINOL		
Citalopram	CELEXA	Cycloserine	SEROMYCIN
Cladribine	See 2-Chlorodeoxyadenosine	Cyclosporine	NEORAL SANDIMMUNE
		Cyproterone†	ANDROCUR
Clarithromycin	BIAXIN	Cytarabine (cytosine arabinoside)	CYTOSAR-U DEPOCYT
Clemastine	TAVIST-1		
Clindamycin	CLEOCIN	Dacarbazine	DTIC-DOME
Clobetasol	CLOBEX TEMOVATE	Daclizumab	ZENAPAX
		Dactinomycin	COSMEGEN
Clocortolone	CLODERM	Dalfopristin	See Quinapristin
Clofazimine	LAMPRENE	Danaparoid†	ORGARAN
Clomiphene	CLOMID SEROPHENE	Dantrolene	DANTRIUM
		Dapsone	ACZONE
Clomipramine	ANAFRANIL	Daptomycin	CUBICIN
Clonazepam	KLONOPIN	Darbepoetin	ARANESP
Clonidine	CATAPRES	Darifenacin	ENABLEX
Clopidogrel	PLAVIX	Darunavir	PREZISTA
Clorazepate	TRANXENE	Daunorubicin	CERUBIDINE
Clotrimazole	LOTRIMIN AF MYCELEX	Deferoxamine	DESFERAL

SOME TRADE NAMES OF GENERIC DRUGS[*]

GENERIC NAME	TRADE NAME	GENERIC NAME	TRADE NAME
Delavirdine	RESCRIPTOR	Dirithromycin[†]	DYNABAC
Demeclocycline	DECLOMYCIN	Disopyramide	NORPACE
Deoxycoformycin	See Pentostatin	Disulfiram	ANTABUSE
Desipramine	NORPRAMIN	Divalproex	DEPAKOTE
Desloratadine	CLARINEX	Docetaxel	TAXOTERE
Desmopressin	DDAVP	Docosanol	ABREVA
	STIMATE	Docusate	COLACE
Desonide	DESOWEN	Donepezil	ARICEPT
Desoximetasone	TOPICORT	Doripenem	DORIBAX
Dexbrompheniramine	DRIXORAL	Dornase alfa	PULMOZYME
Dextroamphetamine	DEXEDRINE	Dorzolamide	TRUSOPT
Dextromethorphan	DELSYM	Doxazosin	CARDURA
Diazepam	DIASTAT	Doxepin	SINEQUAN
	VALIUM		ZONALON
Diazoxide	PROGLYCEM	Doxorubicin	DOXIL
Dibromopropamidine[†]	BROLENE	Doxycycline	VIBRAMYCIN
Diclofenac	CATAFLAM	Doxylamine	UNISOM
	VOLTAREN	Dronabinol	MARINOL
Dicyclomine	BENTYL	Drotrecogin alfa	XIGRIS
Didanosine (ddI)	VIDEX	(activated protein C)	
Diethylpropion	TENUATE	Duloxetine	CYMBALTA
Diflorasone	PSORCON	Dutasteride	AVODART
Digitoxin[†]	DIGITALINE	Dyclonine	SUCRETS
Digoxin	LANOXIN	Dyphylline	LUFYLLIN
Dihydroergotamine	D.H.E. 45	Echothiophate	PHOSPHOLINE
	MIGRANAL	Eculizumab	SOLIRIS
Diloxanide[†]	ENTAMIDE	Edetate calcium	CALCIUM DISODIUM
Diltiazem	CARDIZEM	disodium	VERSENATE
	DILACOR XR	Edrophonium	TENSILON
Dimercaprol	BAL	Efavirenz	SUSTIVA
Dimethyl sulfoxide	RIMSO-50	Eflornithine	VANIQA
Diphenhydramine	BENADRYL	Eletriptan	RELPAX
Diphenoxylate with	LOMOTIL	Emedastine	EMADINE
atropine		Emtricitabine	EMTRIVA
Dipivefrin	AKPro	Enalapril	VASOTEC
	PROPINE	Enfuvirtide	FUZEON
Dipyridamole	PERSANTINE		

SOME TRADE NAMES OF GENERIC DRUGS*

GENERIC NAME	TRADE NAME	GENERIC NAME	TRADE NAME
Enoxaparin	LOVENOX	Felbamate	FELBATOL
Entacapone	COMTAN	Felodipine	PLENDIL
Entecavir	BARACLUDE	Fenofibrate	FENOGLIDE
Epirubicin	ELLENCE		LIPOFEN
Eplerenone	INSPRA	Fenoldopam	CORLOPAM
Epoprostenol	FLOLAN	Fentanyl	SUBLIMAZE
Eprosartan	TEVETEN	Fexofenadine	ALLEGRA
Eptifibatide	INTEGRILIN	Filgrastim	NEUPOGEN
Ergocalciferol	DRISDOL	Finasteride	PROSCAR
Ergotamine	ERGOMAR	5-Fluorouracil	EFUDEX
Erlotinib	TARCEVA	Flecainide	TAMBOCOR
Ertapenem	INVANZ	Fluconazole	DIFULCAN
Erythromycin	E-MYCIN	Flucytosine	ANCOBON
	ERYTHROCIN	Fludarabine	FLUDARA
Erythropoietin	EPOGEN/PROCRIT	Flumazenil	ROMAZICON
Escitalopram	LEXAPRO	Flunisolide	AeroBid
Esomeprazole	NEXIUM	Fluocinolone	SYNALAR
Estradiol	CLIMARA	Fluocinonide	LIDEX
	MENOSTAR	Fluorouracil	CARAC
Estramustine	EMCYT	Fluoxetine	PROZAC
Estrogens	PREMARIN	Flurandrenolide	CORDRAN
Eszopiclone	LUNESTA	Flurazepam	DALMANE
Etanercept	ENBREL	Flurbiprofen	ANSAID
Ethacrynic acid	EDECRIN		OCUFEN
Ethambutol	MYAMBUTOL	Fluticasone	CUTIVATE
Ethosuximide	ZARONTIN		FLONASE
			FLOVENT
Etidronate	DIDRONEL	Fluvastatin	LESCOL
Etoposide	VePesid	Fluvoxamine	LUVOX
Etravirine	INTELENCE	Fomepizole	ANTIZOL
Everolimus†	CERTICAN	Fondaparinux	ARIXTRA
Exemestane	AROMASIN	Formoterol	FORADIL
Exenatide	BYETTA	Fosamprenavir	LEXIVA
Ezetimibe	ZETIA	Foscarnet	FOSCAVIR
Famciclovir	FAMVIR	Fosfomycin	MONUROL
Famotidine	PEPCID	Fosinopril	MONOPRIL

SOME TRADE NAMES OF GENERIC DRUGS*

GENERIC NAME	TRADE NAME	GENERIC NAME	TRADE NAME
Fosphenytoin	CEREBYX	Hydrocodone-acetaminophen	ANEXSIA VICODIN
Fulvestrant	FASLODEX		
Furosemide	LASIX	Hydrocodone-ibuprofen	VICOPROFEN
Gabapentin	NEURONTIN	Hydrocortisone	See Cortisol
Galantamine	RAZADYNE	Hydromorphone	DILAUDID
Gallium nitrate	GANITE	Hydroquinone	TRI-LUMA
Ganciclovir	CYTOVENE	Hydroxychloroquine	PLAQUENIL
Gatifloxacin	ZYMAR	Hydroxyurea	HYDREA
Gemcitabine	GEMZAR	Hydroxyzine	VISTARIL
Gemfibrozil	LOPID	Hyoscyamine	ANASPAZ
Gefitinib	IRESSA		LEVBID
Gemtuzumab ozogamicin	MYLOTARG		LEVSIN
Glatiramer	COPAXONE	Ibandronate	BONIVA
Glimepiride	AMARYL	Ibuprofen	ADVIL MOTRIN
Glipizide	GLUCOTROL	Ibutilide	CORVERT
Glyburide	DIABETA MICRONASE	Ifosfamide	IFEX
		Iloprost	VENTAVIS
Gold	See Auranofin	Imatinib	GLEEVEC
Gonadorelin	FACTREL	Imipenem-cilastatin	PRIMAXIN
Goserelin	ZOLADEX	Imipramine	TOFRANIL
Granisetron	KYTRIL	Imiquimod	ALDARA
Griseofulvin	GRIS-PEG	Indinavir	CRIXIVAN
Growth hormone (somatropin)	GENOTROPIN NUTROPIN	Indomethacin	INDOCIN
		Infliximab	REMICADE
Guaifenesin	MUCINEX	Insulin	HUMULIN NOVOLIN
Guanfacine	TENEX		
Halcinonide	HALOG	Interferon alfacon-1	INFERGEN
Halobetasol	ULTRAVATE	Interferon-alfa-2A	ROFERON A
Haloperidol	HALDOL	Interferon-alfa-2A, pegylated	PEGASYS
Hexachlorophene	PHisoHex		
Histrelin	SUPPRELIN LA	Interferon-alfa-2B	INTRON A
Homatropine	TUSSIGON	Interferon-alfa-2B, pegylated	See Peginterferon alfa-2B
Hyaluronate	HYALGAN SYNVISC	Interferon-alfa-N3	ALFERON N
Hydrochlorothiazide	ORETIC	Interferon-beta-1A	AVONEX REBIF

SOME TRADE NAMES OF GENERIC DRUGS*

GENERIC NAME	TRADE NAME	GENERIC NAME	TRADE NAME
Interferon-beta-1B	BETASERON	Levonorgestrel†	NORPLANT
Interferon-gamma-1B	ACTIMMUNE	Levorphanol	LEVO-DROMORAN
Iodoquinol	YODOXIN	Levothyroxine sodium	SYNTHROID
Ipratropium	ATROVENT	Lidocaine	XYLOCAINE
Irbesartan	AVAPRO	Linezolid	ZYVOX
Irinotecan	CAMPTOSAR	Lisinopril	PRINIVIL
Isocarboxazid	MARPLAN	Lithium	LITHOBID
Isoflurane	FORANE	Lomefloxacin†	MAXAQUIN
Isoproterenol	ISUPREL	Loperamide	IMODIUM
Isosorbide dinitrate	ISORDIL	Lopinavir-ritonavir	KALETRA
Isosorbide mononitrate	ISMO	Loracarbef†	LORABID
Isotretinoin	ACCUTANE	Loratadine	CLARITIN
Itraconazole	SPORANOX	Lorazepam	ATIVAN
Ivermectin	STROMECTOL	Losartan	COZAAR
Kaolin-pectin	KAPECTOLIN	Lovastatin	MEVACOR
Ketoconazole	NIZORAL	Lubiprostone	AMITIZA
Ketorolac	ACULAR	Mafenide	SULFAMYLON
Labetalol	TRANDATE	Magnesium carbonate	RENACIDIN
Lactulose	CONSTULOSE	Malathion	OVIDE
Lamivudine (3TC)	EPIVIR	Maraviroc	SELZENTRY
Lamotrigine	LAMICTAL	α-Mecaptopropionyl-glycine	TIOPRONIN
Lansoprazole	PREVACID	Mechlorethamine (nitrogen mustard)	MUSTARGEN
Latanoprost	XALATAN		
Leflunomide	ARAVA	Meclizine	ANTIVERT
Lenalidomide	REVLIMID	Medroxyprogesterone acetate	PROVERA
Lepirudin	REFLUDAN		
Letrozole	FEMARA	Mefenamic acid	PONSTEL
Leuprolide	LUPRON	Megestrol	MEGACE
Levalbuterol	XOPENEX	Meglumine antimoniate†	GLUCANTIME
Levetiracetam	KEPPRA	Melarsoprol†	ARSOBAL
Levobunolol	BETAGAN	Meloxicam	MOBIC
Levocetirizine	XYZAL	Melphalan	ALKERAN
Levodopa-carbidopa	SINEMET	Memantine	NAMENDA
Levofloxacin	LEVAQUIN QUIXIN	Mercaptopurine	PURINETHOL
		Meropenem	MERREM

SOME TRADE NAMES OF GENERIC DRUGS[*]

GENERIC NAME	TRADE NAME	GENERIC NAME	TRADE NAME
Merperidine	DEMEROL	Mitoxantrone	NOVANTRONE
Mesalamine	ASACOL	Moclobemide[†]	AURORIX
	CANASA	Modafinil	PROVIGIL
Metaxalone	SKELAXIN	Moexipril	UNIVASC
Metformin	GLUCOPHAGE	Molindone	MOBAN
Methadone	DOLOPHINE	Mometasone	ELOCON
Methamphetamine	DESOXYN		NASONEX
Methenamine	HIPREX	Montelukast	SINGULAIR
Methimazole	TAPAZOLE	Moricizine[†]	ETHMOZINE
Methocarbamol	ROBAXIN	Morphine	MS CONTIN
Methotrexate	TREXALL		ORAMORPH
Methoxsalen	OXSORALEN	Moxifloxacin	AVELOX
Methylphenidate	CONCERTA	Mupirocin	BACTROBAN
	METHYLIN	Muromonab (OKT3)	ORTHOCLONE OKT3
	RITALIN	Mycophenolate mofetil	CELLCEPT
Methylprednisolone	MEDROL	Nadolol	CORGARD
Methyltestosterone	VIRILON	Nafarelin	SYNAREL
Metipranolol	OPTIPRANOLOL	Naftifine	NAFTIN
Metoclopramide	REGLAN	Naltrexone	REVIA
Metolazone	ZAROXOLYN	Naphazoline	NAPHCON-A
Metoprolol	LOPRESSOR	Naproxen	ALEVE
	TOPROL-XL		ANAPROX
Metronidazole	FLAGYL		NAPROSYN
Metyrapone	METOPIRONE	Naratriptan	AMERGE
Micafungin	MYCAMINE	Natalizumab	TYSABRI
Miconazole	MONISTAT	Nateglinide	STARLIX
Midodrine	PROAMATINE	Nedocromil	ALOCRIL
Mifepristone (RU-486)	MIFEPREX	Nelfinavir	VIRACEPT
Miglitol	GLYSET	Neomycin	NEO-RX
Miltefosine[†]	IMPAVIDO	Neostigmine	PROSTIGMIN
	MILTEX	Nevirapine	VIRAMUNE
Minocycline	MINOCIN	Niacin	NIASPAN
Minoxidil	ROGAINE	Nicardipine	CARDENE
Mirtazapine	REMERON	Nicotine	NICORETTE
Misoprostol	CYTOTEC		NICOTROL
Mitomycin	MUTAMYCIN	Nicotinic acid	See Niacin

SOME TRADE NAMES OF GENERIC DRUGS*

GENERIC NAME	TRADE NAME	GENERIC NAME	TRADE NAME
Nifedipine	PROCARDIA	Oxycodone-acetaminophen	PERCOCET
Nifurtimox†	LAMPIT		ROXICET
Nilutamide	NILANDRON		TYLOX
Nitazoxanide	ALINIA	Oxymetazoline	AFRIN
Nitrazepam†	MOGADON		DRISTAN 12-Hr NASAL SPRAY
Nitrofurantoin	FURADANTIN		OCUCLEAR
	MACRODANTIN	Oxymetholone	ANADROL
Nitrogen mustard	See Mechlorethamine	Oxymorphone	OPANA
Nitroglycerin	NITROLINGUAL	Oxytocin	PITOCIN
Nitroprusside	NITROPRESS	Paclitaxel	ABRAXANE
Nizatidine	AXID		TAXOL
Norepinephrine	LEVOPHED	Paliperidone	INVEGA
Norfloxacin	NOROXIN	Palivizumab	SYNAGIS
Nortriptyline	AVENTYL	Pamidronate	AREDIA
Nystatin	MYCOSTATIN	Pantoprazole	PROTONIX
	NILSTAT	Papaverine	PAVABID
Octreotide	SANDOSTATIN	Para-aminobenzoate	POTABA
Ofloxacin	FLOXIN	Paroxetine	PAXIL
	OCUFLOX	Pegaptanib	MACUGEN
Olanzapine	ZYPREXA	Pegfilgrastim	NEULASTA
Olmesartan	BENICAR	Peginterferon alfa-2B	PEGINTRON
Olopatadine	PATANOL	Pegvisomant	SOMAVERT
Olsalazine	DIPENTUM	Pemirolast	ALAMAST
Omalizumab	XOLAIR	Penbutolol	LEVATOL
Omeprazole	PRILOSEC	Penciclovir	DENAVIR
Ondansetron	ZOFRAN	Penicillamine	CUPRIMINE
Orlistat	XENICAL	Penicillin G benzathine	BICILLIN L-A
Orphenadrine	INVAGESIC	Penicillin V	VEETIDS
Oseltamivir	TAMIFLU	Pentamidine	NEBUPENT
Oxacillin	BACTOCILL	Pentazocine	TALWIN
Oxaliplatin	ELOXATIN	Pentobarbital	NEMBUTAL
Oxaprozin	DAYPRO	Pentosan polysulfate	ELMIRON
Oxcarbazepine	TRILEPTAL	Pentostatin	NIPENT
Oxiconazole	OXISTAT	Pentoxifylline	TRENTAL
Oxybutynin	DITROPAN	Perindopril	ACEON
Oxycodone	OxyContin	Permethrin	NIX

SOME TRADE NAMES OF GENERIC DRUGS*

GENERIC NAME	TRADE NAME	GENERIC NAME	TRADE NAME
Phenazopyridine	PYRIDIUM PLUS	Procarbazine	MATULANE
Phendimetrazine	BONTRIL	Progesterone	CRINONE
Phenelzine	NARDIL		ENDOMETRIN
Pheniramine	TUSSIONEX	Propafenone	RYTHMOL
	PENNKINETIC	Proparacaine	OPHTHAINE
Phenobarbital	LUMINAL	Propoxyphene	DARVON
Phenoxybenzamine	DIBENZYLINE	Propranolol	INDERAL
Phenylbutazone†	BUTAZOLIDINE	Protriptyline	VIVACTIL
Phentermine	ADIPEX-P	Prussian blue	RADIOGARDASE
Phentolamine	REGITINE	Pseudoephedrine	AFRINOL
Phenylephrine	PROMETH VC PLAIN		SUDAFED
Phenytoin	DILANTIN	Psyllium	METAMUCIL
Physostigmine	ANTILIRIUM	Pyrantel pamoate	PIN-X
Pilocarpine	SALAGEN		REESE'S PINWORM
Pimecrolimus	ELIDEL		MEDICINE
Pimozide	ORAP	Pyrazinamide	RIFATER
Pioglitazone	ACTOS	Pyridostigmine	MESTINON
Piperacillin-tazobactam	ZOSYN	Pyrimethamine	DARAPRIM
Piracetam	NOOTROPIL	Quazepam	DORAL
Pirbuterol	MAXAIR	Quetiapine	SEROQUEL
Piroxicam	FELDENE	Quinacrine	ATABRINE
Podophyllin	PODOFIN	Quinapril	ACCUPRIL
Polycarbophil	FiberCon	Quinine	QUALAQUIN
Polyethylene glycol	TriLyte	Quinupristin-dalfopristin	SYNERCID
Polymyxin B-bacitracin-neomycin	NEOSPORIN	Rabeprazole	ACIPHEX
		Raloxifene	EVISTA
Posaconazole	NOXAFIL	Raltegravir	ISENTRESS
Potassium citrate	UROCIT-K	Ramelteon	ROZEREM
Potassium iodide	ThyroSafe	Ramipril	ALTACE
Pramlintide	SYMLIN	Ranibizumab	LUCENTIS
Pramipexole	MIRAPEX	Ranitidine	ZANTAC
Pravastatin	PRAVACHOL	Rasagiline	AZILECT
Praziquantel	BILTRICIDE	Repaglinide	PRANDIN
Prazosin	MINIPRESS	Reteplase	RETAVASE
Pregabalin	LYRICA	Retinoic acid	SEE TRETINOIN
Primidone	MYSOLINE	Ribavirin	VIRAZOLE

SOME TRADE NAMES OF GENERIC DRUGS*

GENERIC NAME	TRADE NAME	GENERIC NAME	TRADE NAME
Rifabutin	MYCOBUTIN	Sitagliptin	JANUVIA
Rifampin	RIFADIN RIMACTANE	Sodium oxybate	XYREM
		Solifenacin	VESICARE
Rifaximin	XIFAXAN	Sorafenib	NEXAVAR
Riluzole	RILUTEK	Sotalol	BETAPACE
Rimantadine	FLUMADINE	Spectinomycin	TROBICIN
Risedronate	ACTONEL	Spiramycin†	ROVAMYCINE
Risperidone	RISPERDAL	Spironolactone	ALDACTONE
Ritonavir	NORVIR	Stavudine (d4T)	ZERIT
Rituximab	RITUXAN	Streptokinase	STREPTASE
Rivastigmine	EXELON	Streptozocin	ZANOSAR
Rizatriptan	MAXALT	Succimer	CHEMET
Ropinirole	REQUIP	Succinylcholine	QUELICIN
Rosiglitazone	AVANDIA	Sucralfate	CARAFATE
Rosuvastatin	CRESTOR	Sufentanil	SUFENTA
Rotigotine†	NEUPRO	Sulconazole	EXELDERM
Salmeterol	SEREVENT	Sulfacetamide	BLEPH-10
Salmeterol-fluticasone	ADVAIR	Sulfadoxine-pyrimethamine	FANSIDAR
Salsalate	DISALCID SALFLEX	Sulfamethoxazole	See Trimethoprim-sulfamethoxazole
Saquinavir	INVIRASE	Sulfasalazine	AZULFIDINE
Scopolamine	TRANSDERM SCOP	Sulfinpyrazone†	APO-SULFINPYRAZONE
Secobarbital	SECONAL		
Selegiline	ELDEPRYL	Sulfisoxazole	LIPO GANTRISIN
Selenium sulfide	SELSUN	Sulindac	CLINORIL
Senna	SENOKOT	Sumatriptan	IMITREX
Sertraline	ZOLOFT	Sunitinib	SUTENT
Sevelamer	RENAGEL	Suramin†	ANTRYPOL
Sevoflurane	SOJOURN	Tacrine	COGNEX
Sibutramine	MERIDIA	Tacrolimus	PROGRAF
Sildenafil	VIAGRA	Tadalafil	CIALIS
Silver sulfadiazine	SILVADENE	Tamsulosin	FLOMAX
Simethicone	MYLICON PHAZYME	Tazarotene	TAZORAC
		Telbivudine	TYZEKA
Simvastatin	ZOCOR	Telithromycin	KETEK
Sirolimus	RAPAMUNE		

SOME TRADE NAMES OF GENERIC DRUGS*

GENERIC NAME	TRADE NAME	GENERIC NAME	TRADE NAME
Telmisartan	MICARDIS	Tizanidine	ZANAFLEX
Temazepam	RESTORIL	Tobramycin	TOBREX
Temsirolimus	TORISEL	Tolcapone	TASMAR
Tenecteplase	TNKase	Tolmetin	TOLECTIN
Tenofovir	VIREAD	Tolnaftate	TINACTIN
Terazosin	HYTRIN	Tolterodine	DETROL
Terbinafine	LAMISIL AT	Topiramate	TOPAMAX
Terconazole	TERAZOL	Topotecan	HYCAMTIN
Teriparatide	FORTEO	Torsemide	DEMADEX
Testosterone	ANDRODERM DELATESTRYL	Tramadol	RYZOLT ULTRAM
Tetrabenazine	XENAZINE	Trandolapril	MAVIK
Tetracycline	SUMYCIN	Tranylcypromine	PARNATE
Tetrahydrozoline	TYZINE	Trastuzumab	HERCEPTIN
Thalidomide	THALOMID	Travoprost	TRAVATAN
Theophylline	THEOLAIR	Tretinoin	AVITA RENOVA RETIN-A
Thiabendazole	MINTEZOL		
Thiothixene	NAVANE	Triamcinolone	KENALOG
Thyroid hormone, synthetic	See Levothyroxine sodium	Triamcinolone hexacetonide	ARISTOSPAN
Thyrotropin	THYROGEN	Triamterene	DYRENIUM
Tiagabine	GABITRIL	Triazolam	HALCION
Ticarcillin-clavulanate	TIMENTIN	Trichloroacetic acid	TRI-CHLOR
Ticlopidine	TICLID	Triclabendazole†	FASINEX
Tigecycline	TYGACIL	Trifluridine	VIROPTIC
Tiludronate	SKELID	Triiodothyronine	THYROLAR
Timolol	TIMOPTIC	Trimethadione	TRIDIONE
Tinidazole	TINDAMAX	Trimethobenzamide	TIGAN
Tioconazole	VAGISTAT-1	Trimethoprim-polymyxin	POLYTRIM
Tiopronin (α-mecapto-propionylglycine)	TIOPRONIN	Trimethoprim-sulfamethoxazole	BACTRIM SEPTRA
Tiotropium	SPIRIVA	Trimipramine	SURMONTIL
Tipranavir	APTIVUS	Tropicamide	MYDRIACYL
Tirofiban	AGGRASTAT	Trospium	SANCTURA
Tissue plasminogen activator (alteplase)	ACTIVASE	Undecylenate	DESENEX

SOME TRADE NAMES OF GENERIC DRUGS[*]

GENERIC NAME	TRADE NAME	GENERIC NAME	TRADE NAME
Unoprostone[†]	RESCULA	Vitamin D	See Ergocalciferol
Ursodeoxycholic acid	ACTIGALL	Voriconazole	VFEND
Ursodiol	See Ursodeoxycholic acid	Warfarin	COUMADIN
Valacyclovir	VALTREX	Xylometazoline	OTRIVIN
Valganciclovir	VALCYTE	Yohimbine	YOCON
Valproate	DEPACON	Zafirlukast	ACCOLATE
Valsartan	DIOVAN	Zaleplon	SONATA
Vancomycin	VANCOCIN	Zanamivir	RELENZA
Vardenafil	LEVITRA	Zidovudine (AZT)	RETROVIR
Varenicline	CHANTIX	Zileuton	ZYFLO
Venlafaxine	EFFEXOR	Ziprasidone	GEODON
Verapamil	CALAN	Zoledronic acid	ZOMETA
	ISOPTIN SR	Zoledronate	See Zoledronic acid
Vigabatrin[†]	SABRIL	Zolmitriptan	ZOMIG
Vinorelbine	NAVELBINE	Zolpidem	AMBIEN
Vitamin A	AQUASOL A	Zonisamide	ZONEGRAN
Vitamin B$_3$	See Niacin		

[*]Some drugs mentioned in this book are manufactured only as generics and therefore have no trade name and are not included in this table.
[†]Not available in the United States.

GENERIC NAMES OF SOME TRADE NAME DRUGS[*]

TRADE	GENERIC	TRADE	GENERIC
ABILIFY	Aripiprazole	ALFERON N	Interferon-alpha-N3
ABRAXANE	Paclitaxel	ALINIA	Nitazoxanide
ABREVA	Docosanol	ALKERAN	Melphalan
ACCOLATE	Zafirlukast	ALLEGRA	Fexofenadine
ACCUPRIL	Quinapril	ALOCRIL	Nedocromil
ACCUTANE	Isotretinoin	ALPHAGAN P	Brimonidine
ACEON	Perindopril	ALTACE	Ramipril
ACETADOTE	Acetylcysteine	ALU-CAP	Aluminum hydroxide
ACIPHEX	Rabeprazole	AMARYL	Glimepiride
ACLOVATE	Alclometasone	AMBIEN	Zolpidem
ACTIGALL	Ursodeoxycholic acid	AMERGE	Naratriptan
ACTIMMUNE	Interferon-gamma-1B	AMICAR	Aminocaproic acid
ACTIVASE	Tissue plasminogen activator (alteplase)	AMIKIN	Amikacin
		AMITIZA	Lubiprostone
ACTONEL	Risedronate	AMOXIL	Amoxicillin
ACTOS	Pioglitazone	AMPHOGEL	Aluminum hydroxide
ACULAR	Ketorolac	ANADROL	Oxymetholone
ACZONE	Dapsone	ANAFRANIL	Clomipramine
ADDERALL	Amphetamine	ANAPROX	Naproxen
ADENOCARD	Adenosine	ANASPAZ	Hyoscyamine
ADIPEX-P	Phentermine	ANBESOL	Benzocaine
ADVAIR	Salmeterol-fluticasone	ANCEF	Cefazolin
ADVIL	Ibuprofen	ANCOBON	Flucytosine
AEROBID	Flunisolide	ANDROCUR[†]	Cyproterone
AFRIN	Oxymetazoline	ANDRODERM	Testosterone
AFRINOL	Pseudoephedrine	ANEXSIA	Hydrocodone-acetaminophen
AGENERASE	Amprenavir	ANGIOMAX	Bivalirudin
AGGRASTAT	Tirofiban	ANSAID	Flurbiprofen
AGRYLIN	Anagrelide	ANTABUSE	Disulfiram
AKPro	Dipivefrin	ANTHRA-DERM	Anthralin
ALAMAST	Pemirolast	ANTILIRIUM	Physostigmine
ALBENZA	Albendazole	ANTIVERT	Meclizine
ALDACTONE	Spironolactone	ANTIZOL	Fomepizole
ALDARA	Imiquimod	ANTRYPOL[†]	Suramin
ALEVE	Naproxen		

GENERIC NAMES OF SOME TRADE NAME DRUGS*

TRADE	GENERIC	TRADE	GENERIC
APHTHASOL	Amlexanox	AXID	Nizatidine
APOKYN	Apomorphine	AZACTAM	Aztreonam
APO-SULFINPYRAZONE†	Sulfinpyrazone	AZELEX	Azelaic acid
APTIVUS	Tipranavir	AZILECT	Rasagiline
AQUASOL A	Vitamin A	AZOPT	Brinzolamide
ARALEN	Chloroquine	AZULFIDINE	Sulfasalazine
ARANESP	Darbepoetin	BACIIM	Bacitracin
ARAVA	Leflunomide	BACTOCILL	Oxacillin
AREDIA	Pamidronate	BACTRIM	Trimethoprim-sulfamethoxazole
ARGATROBAN	Argatroban	BACTROBAN	Mupirocin
ARICEPT	Donepezil	BAL	Dimercaprol
ARIMIDEX	Anastrozole	BARACLUDE	Entecavir
ARISTOSPAN	Triamcinolone hexacetonide	BAYER	Aspirin
ARIXTRA	Fondaparinux	BECONASE AQ	Beclomethasone
AROMASIN	Exemestane	BENADRYL	Diphenhydramine
ARSOBAL†	Melarsoprol	BENICAR	Olmesartan
ASACOL	Mesalamine	BENTYL	Dicyclomine
ASENDIN	Amoxapine	BENZAC	Benzoyl peroxide
ATABRINE	Quinacrine	BETAGAN	Levobunolol
ATACAND	Candesartan	BETAPACE	Sotalol
ATIVAN	Lorazepam	BETASERON	Interferon-beta-1B
ATROPEN	Atropine	BEZALIP†	Benzafibrate
ATROVENT	Ipratropium	BIAXIN	Clarithromycin
AUGMENTIN	Amoxicillin-clavulanate	BICILLIN L-A	Benzathine penicillin G
AURORIX†	Moclobemide	BILTRICIDE	Praziquantel
AVANDIA	Rosiglitazone	BITIN	Bithionol
AVAPRO	Irbesartan	BLENOXANE	Bleomycin
AVASTIN	Bevacizumab	BLEPH-10	Sulfacetamide
AVELOX	Moxifloxacin	BONIVA	Ibandronate
AVENTYL	Nortriptyline	BONTRIL	Phendimetrazine
AVITA	Tretinoin	BOTOX	Botulinum toxin
AVODART	Dutasteride	BROLENE†	Dibromopropamidine
AVONEX	Interferon-beta-1A	BUMEX	Bumetanide
AXERT	Almotriptan	BUPRENEX	Buprenorphine

GENERIC NAMES OF SOME TRADE NAME DRUGS*

TRADE	GENERIC	TRADE	GENERIC
BUSPAR	Buspirone	CERUBIDINE	Daunorubicin
BUTAZOLIDINE†	Phenylbutazone	CHANTIX	Varenicline
BYETTA	Exenatide	CHEMET	Succimer
CALCIUM DISODIUM VERSENATE	Edetate calcium disodium	CHLOR-TRIMETON	Chlorpheniramine
CALAN	Verapamil	CIALIS	Tadalafil
CALTRATE	Calcium carbonate	CILOXAN	Ciprofloxacin
CAMPATH	Alemtuzumab	CIPRO	Ciprofloxacin
CAMPTOSAR	Irinotecan	CLAFORAN	Cefotaxime
CANASA	Mesalamine	CLARINEX	Desloratadine
CANCIDAS	Caspofungin	CLARITIN	Loratadine
CANTHARONE	Cantharidin	CLEOCIN	Clindamycin
CAPOTEN	Captopril	CLIMARA	Estradiol
CAPSIN	Capsaicin	CLINORIL	Sulindac
CAPZASIN	Capsaicin	CLOBEX	Clobetasol
CARAC	Fluorouracil	CLODERM	Clocortolone
CARAFATE	Sucralfate	CLOMID	Clomiphene
CARDIZEM	Diltiazem	CLOXAPEN	Cloxacillin
CARDURA	Doxazosin	CLOZARIL	Clozapine
CASODEX	Bicalutamide	COARTEM	Artemether-lumefantrine
CATAFLAM	Diclofenac	COGENTIN	Benztropine
CATAPRES	Clonidine	COGNEX	Tacrine
CAVERJECT	Alprostadil	COLACE	Docusate
CEDAX	Ceftibuten	COLAZAL	Balsalazide
CEFIZOX	Ceftizoxime	COLESTID	Colestipol
CEFTIN	Cefuroxime	COLY-MYCIN M	Colistin
CEFZIL	Cefprozil	COMTAN	Entacapone
CELEBREX	Celecoxib	CONCERTA	Methylphenidate
CELECTOL†	Celiprolol	CONSTULOSE	Lactulose
CELESTONE	Betamethasone	COPAXONE	Glatiramer
CELEXA	Citalopram	CORDARONE	Amiodarone
CELLCEPT	Mycophenolate mofetil	CORDRAN	Flurandrenolide
CEPACOL	Benzocaine	COREG	Carvedilol
CEREBYX	Fosphenytoin	CORGARD	Nadolol
CERTICAN†	Everolimus	CORLOPAM	Fenoldopam
		CORTEF	Cortisol

GENERIC NAMES OF SOME TRADE NAME DRUGS*

TRADE	GENERIC	TRADE	GENERIC
CORVERT	Ibutilide	DESFERAL	Deferoxamine
COSMEGEN	Dactinomycin	DESOWEN	Desonide
COUMADIN	Warfarin	DESOXYN	Methamphetamine
COZAAR	Losartan	DESQUAM	Benzoyl peroxide
CRESTOR	Rosuvastatin	DETROL	Tolterodine
CRINONE	Progesterone	DEXEDRINE	Dextroamphetamine
CRIXIVAN	Indinavir	D.H.E. 45	Dihydroergotamine
CROLOM	Cromolyn	DIABETA	Glyburide
CUBICIN	Daptomycin	DIABINESE	Chlorpropamide
CUPRIMINE	Penicillamine	DIAMOX	Acetazolamide
CUTIVATE	Fluticasone	DIASTAT	Diazepam
CYCLOCORT	Amcinonide	DIBENZYLINE	Phenoxybenzamine
CYCLOGYL	Cyclopentolate	DIDREX	Benzphetamine
CYMBALTA	Duloxetine	DIDRONEL	Etidronate
CYTOSAR-U	Cytarabine (cytosine arabinoside)	DIFFERIN	Adapalene
CYTOTEC	Misoprostol	DIFULCAN	Fluconazole
CYTOVENE	Ganciclovir	DIGITALINE†	Digitoxin
DALMANE	Flurazepam	DILACOR XR	Diltiazem
DANTRIUM	Dantrolene	DILANTIN	Phenytoin
DARAPRIM	Pyrimethamine	DILAUDID	Hydromorphone
DARVON	Propoxyphene	DIOVAN	Valsartan
DAYPRO	Oxaprozin	DIPENTUM	Olsalazine
DDAVP	Desmopressin	DISALCID	Salsalate
DECLOMYCIN	Demeclocycline	DITROPAN	Oxybutynin
DELATESTRYL	Testosterone	DIURIL	Chlorothiazide
DELSYM	Dextromethorphan	DOLOPHINE	Methadone
DEMADEX	Torsemide	DORAL	Quazepam
DEMEROL	Meperidine	DORIBAX	Doripenem
DENAVIR	Penciclovir	DOVONEX	Calcipotriene
DENOREX	Coal tar	DOXIL	Doxorubicin
DEPACON	Valproate	DRISDOL	Ergocalciferol
DEPAKOTE	Divalproex	DRISTAN 12-Hr NASAL SPRAY	Oxymetazoline
DEPOCYT	Cytarabine (cytosine arabinoside)	DRIXORAL	Dexbrompheniramine
DESENEX	Undecylenate	DRYSOL	Aluminum chloride

GENERIC NAMES OF SOME TRADE NAME DRUGS*

TRADE	GENERIC	TRADE	GENERIC
DTIC-DOME	Dacarbazine	EXELON	Rivastigmine
DULCOLAX	Bisacodyl	FACTREL	Gonadorelin
DURICEF	Cefadroxil	FAMVIR	Famciclovir
DYMELOR	Acetohexamide	FANSIDAR	Sulfadoxine-pyrimethamine
DYNABAC†	Dirithromycin		
DYRENIUM	Triamterene	FASINEX†	Triclabendazole
EDECRIN	Ethacrynic acid	FASLODEX	Fulvestrant
EFFEXOR	Venlafaxine	FELBATOL	Felbamate
EFUDEX	5-Fluorouracil	FELDENE	Piroxicam
ELDEPRYL	Selegiline	FEMARA	Letrozole
ELIDEL	Pimecrolimus	FENOGLIDE	Fenofibrate
ELLENCE	Epirubicin	FiberCon	Polycarbophil
ELMIRON	Pentosan polysulfate	FINACEA	Azelaic acid
ELOCON	Mometasone	FLAGYL	Metronidazole
ELOXATIN	Oxaliplatin	FLEXERIL	Cyclobenzaprine
ELSPAR	Asparaginase	FLOLAN	Epoprostenol
EMADINE	Emedastine	FLOMAX	Tamsulosin
EMCYT	Estramustine	FLONASE	Fluticasone
EMINASE	Anistreplase	FLOVENT	Fluticasone
EMTRIVA	Emtricitabine	FLOXIN	Ofloxacin
E-MYCIN	Erythromycin	FLUDARA	Fludarabine
ENABLEX	Darifenacin	FLUMADINE	Rimantadine
ENBREL	Etanercept	FORADIL	Formoterol
ENDOMETRIN	Progesterone	FORANE	Isoflurane
ENTAMIDE†	Diloxanide	FORTAZ	Ceftazidime
EPIVIR	Lamivudine (3TC)	FORTEO	Teriparatide
EPOGEN-PROCRIT	Erythropoietin	FOSAMAX	Alendronate
ERAXIS	Anidulafungin	FOSCAVIR	Foscarnet
ERGOMAR	Ergotamine	FUNGIZONE	Amphotericin B
ERYTHROCIN	Erythromycin	FUZEON	Enfuvirtide
ETHMOZINE†	Moricizine	GABITRIL	Tiagabine
ETILAMIDE	Buserelin	GANITE	Gallium nitrate
EVISTA	Raloxifene	GAVISCON	Aluminum hydroxide
EVOXAC	Cevimeline	GEMZAR	Gemcitabine
EXELDERM	Sulconazole	GENOTROPIN	Growth hormone

GENERIC NAMES OF SOME TRADE NAME DRUGS*

TRADE	GENERIC	TRADE	GENERIC
GEOCILLIN	Carbenicillin	INTRON A	Interferon-alfa-2B
GEODON	Ziprasidone	INVAGESIC	Orphenadrine
GLEEVEC	Imatinib	INVANZ	Ertapenem
GLUCANTIME†	Meglumine antimoniate	INVEGA	Paliperidone
GLUCOPHAGE	Metformin	INVIRASE	Saquinavir
GLUCOTROL	Glipizide	IOPIDINE	Apraclonidine
GLYSET	Miglitol	IRESSA	Gefitinib
Gris-PEG	Griseofulvin	ISENTRESS	Raltegravir
GYNAZOLE-1	Butoconazole	ISMO	Isosorbide mononitrate
HALCION	Triazolam	ISOPTIN SR	Verapamil
HALDOL	Haloperidol	ISORDIL	Isosorbide dinitrate
HALOG	Halcinonide	ISUPREL	Isoproterenol
HEPSERA	Adefovir	JANUVIA	Sitagliptin
HERCEPTIN	Trastuzumab	KALETRA	Lopinavir-ritonavir
HIBICLENS	Chlorhexidine	KAPECTOLIN	Kaolin-pectin
HIPREX	Methenamine	KEFLEX	Cephalexin
H.P. ACTHAR GEL	Corticotropin (ACTH)	KEFZOL	Cefazolin
HUMIRA	Adalimumab	KENALOG	Triamcinolone
HUMULIN	Insulin	KEPPRA	Levetiracetam
HYALGAN	Hyaluronate	KERLONE	Betaxolol
HYCAMTIN	Terazosin	KETEK	Telithromycin
HYDREA	Hydroxyurea	KINERET	Anakinra
HYTRIN	Topotecan	KLONOPIN	Clonazepam
IFEX	Ifosfamide	KYTRIL	Granisetron
IMITREX	Sumatriptan	LAMICTAL	Lamotrigine
IMODIUM	Loperamide	LAMISIL AT	Terbinafine
IMPAVIDO†	Miltefosine	LAMPIT†	Nifurtimox
IMURAN	Azathioprine	LAMPRENE	Clofazimine
INDERAL	Propranolol	LANACANE	Benzocaine
INDOCIN	Indomethacin	LANOXIN	Digoxin
INFERGEN	Interferon alfacon-1	LASIX	Furosemide
INSPRA	Eplerenone	LESCOL	Fluvastatin
INTAL	Cromolyn	LETAIRIS	Ambrisentan
INTEGRILIN	Eptifibatide	LEUKERAN	Chlorambucil
INTELENCE	Etravirine	LEUSTATIN	2-Chlorodeoxyadenosine

GENERIC NAMES OF SOME TRADE NAME DRUGS*

TRADE	GENERIC	TRADE	GENERIC
LEVAQUIN	Levofloxacin	LUPRON	Leuprolide
LEVATOL	Penbutolol	LUVOX	Fluvoxamine
LEVBID	Hyoscyamine	LYOPHILIZED CYTOXAN	Cyclophosphamide
LEVITRA	Vardenafil		
LEVO-DROMORAN	Levorphanol	LYRICA	Pregabalin
LEVOPHED	Norepinephrine	MACUGEN	Pegaptanib
LEVSIN	Hyoscyamine	MALARONE	Atovaquone-proguanil
LEXAPRO	Escitalopram	MAREZINE	Cyclizine
LEXIVA	Fosamprenavir	MARINOL	Dronabinol
LIBRIUM	Chlordiazepoxide	MARPLAN	Isocarboxazid
LIDEX	Fluocinonide	MATULANE	Procarbazine
LIORESAL	Baclofen	MAVIK	Trandolapril
LIPITOR	Atorvastatin	MAXAIR	Pirbuterol
LIPOFEN	Fenofibrate	MAXALT	Rizatriptan
LIPO GANTRISIN	Sulfisoxazole	MAXAQUIN†	Lomefloxacin
LITHOBID	Lithium	MAXIPIME	Cefepime
LOCERYL†	Amorolfine	MEFOXIN	Cefoxitin
LODOSYN	Carbidopa	MEGACE	Megestrol
LOMOTIL	Diphenoxylate with atropine	MENOSTAR	Estradiol
		MENTAX	Butenafine
LOPID	Gemfibrozil	MEPRON	Atovaquone
LOPRESSOR	Metoprolol	MERIDIA	Sibutramine
LOPROX	Ciclopirox	MERREM	Meropenem
LOPURIN	Allopurinol	MESTINON	Pyridostigmine
LORABID†	Loracarbef	METAMUCIL	Psyllium
LOROTHIDOL	Bithionol	METHYLIN	Methylphenidate
LOTENSIN	Benazepril	METOPIRONE	Metyrapone
LOTRIMIN AF	Clotrimazole	MEVACOR	Lovastatin
LOTRONEX	Alosetron	MIACALCIN	Calcitonin
LOVENOX	Enoxaparin	MICARDIS	Telmisartan
LUCENTIS	Ranibizumab	MICRONASE	Glyburide
LUFYLLIN	Dyphylline	MIDAMOR	Amiloride
LUMIGAN	Bimatoprost	MIFEPREX	Mifepristone (RU-486)
LUMINAL	Phenobarbital	MIGRANAL	Dihydroergotamine
LUNESTA	Eszopiclone	MILTEX†	Miltefosine

GENERIC NAMES OF SOME TRADE NAME DRUGS*

TRADE	GENERIC	TRADE	GENERIC
MINIPRESS	Prazosin	NAVELBINE	Vinorelbine
MINOCIN	Minocycline	NEBUPENT	Pentamidine
MINTEZOL	Thiabendazole	NEMBUTAL	Pentobarbital
MIOSTAT	Carbachol	NEO-MERCAZOLE	Carbimazole
MIRAPEX	Pramipexole	NEORAL	Cyclosporine
MOBAN	Molindone	NEO-RX	Neomycin
MOBIC	Meloxicam	NEOSPORIN	Polymyxin B-bacitracin-neomycin
MODALIM†	Ciprofibrate		
MOGADON†	Nitrazepam	NEULASTA	Pegfilgrastim
MONISTAT	Miconazole	NEUPOGEN	Filgrastim
MONOPRIL	Fosinopril	NEUPRO†	Rotigotine
MONUROL	Fosfomycin	NEURONTIN	Gabapentin
MOTRIN	Ibuprofen	NEUTROGENA T/GEL	Coal tar
MS CONTIN	Morphine	NEXAVAR	Sorafenib
MUCINEX	Guaifenesin	NEXIUM	Esomeprazole
MUSTARGEN	Mechlorethamine (nitrogen mustard)	NIASPAN	Niacin
		NICORETTE	Nicotine
MUTAMYCIN	Mitomycin	NICOTROL	Nicotine
MYAMBUTOL	Ethambutol	NILANDRON	Nilutamide
MYCAMINE	Micafungin	NILSTAT	Nystatin
MYCELEX	Clotrimazole	NIPENT	Pentostatin
MYCOBUTIN	Rifabutin	NITROLINGUAL	Nitroglycerin
MYCOSTATIN	Nystatin	NITROPRESS	Nitroprusside
MYDRIACYL	Tropicamide	NIX	Permethrin
MYLERAN	Busulfan	NIZORAL	Ketoconazole
MYLICON	Simethicone	NOOTROPIL	Piracetam
MYLOTARG	Gemtuzumab ozogamicin	NOROXIN	Norfloxacin
MYSOLINE	Primidone	NORPACE	Disopyramide
NAFTIN	Naftifine	NORPLANT†	Levonorgestrel
NAMENDA	Memantine	NORPRAMIN	Desipramine
NAPHCON-A	Naphazoline	NORVASC	Amlodipine
NAPROSYN	Naproxen	NORVIR	Ritonavir
NARDIL	Phenelzine	NOVANTRONE	Mitoxantrone
NASONEX	Mometasone	NOVOLIN	Insulin
NAVANE	Thiothixene	NOXAFIL	Posaconazole

GENERIC NAMES OF SOME TRADE NAME DRUGS*

TRADE	GENERIC	TRADE	GENERIC
NUTROPIN	Growth hormone	PERSANTINE	Dipyridamole
OCUCLEAR	Oxymetazoline	PHAZYME	Simethicone
OCUFEN	Flurbiprofen	PHisoHex	Hexachlorophene
OCUFLOX	Ofloxacin	PHOSPHOLINE	Echothiophate
OCUPRESS	Carteolol	PIN-X	Pyrantel pamoate
OMNICEF	Cefdinir	PITOCIN	Oxytocin
OPANA	Oxymorphone	PLAQUENIL	Hydroxychloroquine
OPHTHAINE	Proparacaine	PLATINOL	Cisplatin
OPTIMINE	Azatadine	PLAVIX	Clopidogrel
OPTIPRANOLOL	Metipranolol	PLENDIL	Felodipine
OPTIVAR	Azelastine	PLETAL	Cilostazol
ORAMORPH	Morphine	PODOFIN	Podophyllin
ORAP	Pimozide	POLYTRIM	Trimethoprim-polymyxin
ORENCIA	Abatacept		
ORETIC	Hydrochlorothiazide	PONSTEL	Mefenamic acid
ORGARAN†	Danaparoid	POTABA	Para-aminobenzoate
ORTHOCLONE OKT3	Muromonab (OKT3)	PRANDIN	Repaglinide
OS-CAL	Calcium carbonate	PRAVACHOL	Pravastatin
OTRIVIN	Xylometazoline	PRECOSE	Acarbose
OVIDE	Malathion	PREMARIN	Estrogens
OXISTAT	Oxiconazole	PREVACID	Lansoprazole
OxyContin	Oxycodone	PREZISTA	Darunavir
PARAFON FORTE	Chlorzoxazone	PRILOSEC	Omeprazole
PARAPLATIN	Carboplatin	PRIMAXIN	Imipenem-cilastatin
PARLODEL	Bromocriptine	PRINCIPEN	Ampicillin
PARNATE	Tranylcypromine	PRINIVIL	Lisinopril
PATANOL	Olopatadine	PROAMATINE	Midodrine
PAVABID	Papaverine	PROCARDIA	Nifedipine
PAXIL	Paroxetine	PROGLYCEM	Diazoxide
PEGASYS	Interferon-alfa-2A, pegylated	PROGRAF	Tacrolimus
		PROMETH VC PLAIN	Phenylephrine
PEGINTRON	Interferon-alfa-2B, pegylated	PROPINE	Dipivefrin
		PROSCAR	Finasteride
PEPCID	Famotidine	PROSTIGMIN	Neostigmine
PEPTO-BISMOL	Bismuth subsalicylate	PROSTIN VR	Alprostadil
PERCOCET	Oxycodone-acetaminophen	PROTONIX	Pantoprazole

GENERIC NAMES OF SOME TRADE NAME DRUGS*

TRADE	GENERIC	TRADE	GENERIC
PROVENTIL	Albuterol	RETIN-A	Tretinoin
PROVERA	Medroxyprogesterone acetate	RETROVIR	Zidovudine (AZT)
PROVIGIL	Modafinil	REVIA	Naltrexone
PROZAC	Fluoxetine	REVLIMID	Lenalidomide
PSORCON	Diflorasone	RHINOCORT	Budesonide
PULMOZYME	Dornase alfa	RIDAURA	Auranofin
PURINETHOL	Mercaptopurine	RIFADIN	Rifampin
PYRIDIUM PLUS	Phenazopyridine	RIFATER	Pyrazinamide
QUALAQUIN	Quinine	RILUTEK	Riluzole
QUELICIN	Succinylcholine	RIMACTANE	Rifampin
QUESTRAN	Cholestyramine	RIMSO-50	Dimethyl sulfoxide
QUIXIN	Levofloxacin	RISPERDAL	Risperidone
RADANIL†	Benznidazole	RITALIN	Methylphenidate
RADIOGARDASE	Prussian blue	RITUXAN	Rituximab
RAPAMUNE	Sirolimus	ROCALTROL	Calcitriol
RAZADYNE	Galantamine	ROCEPHIN	Ceftriaxone
REBIF	Interferon-beta-1A	ROFERON A	Interferon-alfa-2A
REESE'S PINWORM MEDICINE	Pyrantel pamoate	ROGAINE	Minoxidil
REFLUDAN	Lepirudin	ROMAZICON	Flumazenil
REGITINE	Phentolamine	ROVAMYCINE†	Spiramycin
REGLAN	Metoclopramide	ROXICET	Oxycodone-acetaminophen
RELENZA	Zanamivir	ROZEREM	Ramelteon
RELPAX	Eletriptan	RYTHMOL	Propafenone
REMERON	Mirtazapine	RYZOLT	Tramadol
REMICADE	Infliximab	SABRIL†	Vigabatrin
RENACIDIN	Magnesium carbonate	SALAGEN	Pilocarpine
RENAGEL	Sevelamer	SALFLEX	Salsalate
RENOVA	Tretinoin	SANCTURA	Trospium
ReoPro	Abciximab	SANDIMMUNE	Cyclosporine
REQUIP	Ropinirole	SANDOSTATIN	Octreotide
RESCRIPTOR	Delavirdine	SECONAL	Secobarbital
RESCULA†	Unoprostone	SECTRAL	Acebutolol
RESTORIL	Temazepam	SELSUN	Selenium sulfide
RETAVASE	Reteplase	SELZENTRY	Maraviroc

GENERIC NAMES OF SOME TRADE NAME DRUGS*

TRADE	GENERIC	TRADE	GENERIC
SENOKOT	Senna	SUPRAX	Cefixime
SEPTRA	Trimethoprim-sulfamethoxazole	SURMONTIL	Trimipramine
		SUSTIVA	Efavirenz
SEREVENT	Salmeterol	SUTENT	Sunitinib
SEROMYCIN	Cycloserine	SYMLIN	Pramlintide
SEROPHENE	Clomiphene	SYMMETREL	Amantadine
SEROQUEL	Quetiapine	SYNAGIS	Palivizumab
SILVADENE	Silver sulfadiazine	SYNALAR	Fluocinolone
SIMULECT	Basiliximab	SYNAREL	Nafarelin
SINEMET	Levodopa-carbidopa	SYNERCID	Quinupristin-dalfopristin
SINEQUAN	Doxepin	SYNTHROID	Levothyroxine sodium
SINGULAIR	Montelukast	SYNVISC	Hyaluronate
SKELAXIN	Metaxalone	TAGAMET	Cimetidine
SKELID	Tiludronate	TALWIN	Pentazocine
SOJOURN	Sevoflurane	TAMBOCOR	Flecainide
SOLIRIS	Eculizumab	TAMIFLU	Oseltamivir
SOMA	Carisoprodol	TARCEVA	Erlotinib
SOMAVERT	Pegvisomant	TASMAR	Tolcapone
SONATA	Zaleplon	TAVIST-1	Clemastine
SORIATANE	Acitretin	TAXOL	Paclitaxel
SPECTRACEF	Cefditoren	TAXOTERE	Docetaxel
SPIRIVA	Tiotropium	TAZICEF	Ceftazidime
SPORANOX	Itraconazole	TAZORAC	Tazarotene
STADOL	Butorphanol	TEGRETOL	Carbamazepine
STARLIX	Nateglinide	TEMOVATE	Clobetasol
STIMATE	Desmopressin	TENEX	Guanfacine
STREPTASE	Streptokinase	TENORMIN	Atenolol
STROMECTOL	Ivermectin	TENSILON	Edrophonium
SUBLIMAZE	Fentanyl	TENUATE	Diethylpropion
SUCRETS	Dyclonine	TERAZOL	Terconazole
SUDAFED	Pseudoephedrine	TESSALON	Benzonatate
SUFENTA	Sufentanil	TEVETEN	Eprosartan
SULFAMYLON	Mafenide	THALITONE	Chlorthalidone
SUMYCIN	Tetracycline	THALOMID	Thalidomide
SUPPRELIN LA	Histrelin	THEOLAIR	Theophylline

GENERIC NAMES OF SOME TRADE NAME DRUGS*

TRADE	GENERIC	TRADE	GENERIC
THYROGEN	Thyrotropin	TUMS	Calcium carbonate
THYROLAR	Triiodothyronine	TUSSIGON	Homatropine
ThyroSafe	Potassium iodide	TUSSIONEX PENNKINETIC	Pheniramine
TICLID	Ticlopidine	TYGACIL	Tigecycline
TIGAN	Trimethobenzamide	TYLENOL	Acetaminophen
TIMENTIN	Ticarcillin-clavulanate	TYLOX	Oxycodone-acetaminophen
TIMOPTIC	Timolol
TINACTIN	Tolnaftate	TYSABRI	Natalizumab
TINDAMAX	Tinidazole	TYZEKA	Telbivudine
TIOPRONIN	α-Mecaptopropionyl-glycine	TYZINE	Tetrahydrozoline
		ULTRAM	Tramadol
TNKase	Tenecteplase	ULTRAVATE	Halobetasol
TOBREX	Tobramycin	UNASYN	Ampicillin-sulbactam
TOFRANIL	Imipramine	UNISOM	Doxylamine
TOLECTIN	Tolmetin	UNIVASC	Moexipril
TOPAMAX	Topiramate	URECHOLINE	Bethanechol
TOPICORT	Desoximetasone	UROCIT-K	Potassium citrate
TOPROL-XL	Metoprolol	UROXATRAL	Alfuzosin
TORISEL	Temsirolimus	VAGISTAT-1	Tioconazole
TRACLEER	Bosentan	VALCYTE	Valganciclovir
TRANDATE	Labetalol	VALIUM	Diazepam
TRANSDERM SCOP	Scopolamine	VALTREX	Valacyclovir
TRANXENE	Clorazepate	VANCOCIN	Vancomycin
TRAVATAN	Travoprost	VANIQA	Eflornithine
TRENTAL	Pentoxifylline	VANTIN	Cefpodoxime
TREXALL	Methotrexate	VASCOR†	Bepridil
TRI-CHLOR	Trichloroacetic acid	VASOCON-A	Antazoline
TRIDIONE	Trimethadione	VASOTEC	Enalapril
TRILEPTAL	Oxcarbazepine	VEETIDS	Penicillin V
TRI-LUMA	Hydroquinone	VELCADE	Bortezomib
TriLyte	Polyethylene glycol	VENTAVIS	Iloprost
TRIMOX	Amoxicillin	VENTOLIN	Albuterol
TRISENOX	Arsenic trioxide	VePesid	Etoposide
TROBICIN	Spectinomycin	VESICARE	Solifenacin
TRUSOPT	Dorzolamide	VFEND	Voriconazole

GENERIC NAMES OF SOME TRADE NAME DRUGS[*]

TRADE	GENERIC	TRADE	GENERIC
VIAGRA	Sildenafil	YODOXIN	Iodoquinol
VIBRAMYCIN	Doxycycline	ZANAFLEX	Tizanidine
VICODIN	Hydrocodone-acetaminophen	ZANOSAR	Streptozocin
		ZANTAC	Ranitidine
VICOPROFEN	Hydrocodone-ibuprofen	ZARONTIN	Ethosuximide
VIDAZA	Azacitidine	ZAROXOLYN	Metolazone
VIDEX	Didanosine (ddI)	ZEBETA	Bisoprolol
VIRACEPT	Nelfinavir	ZEFTERA[†]	Ceftobiprole
VIRAMUNE	Nevirapine	ZENAPAX	Daclizumab
VIRAZOLE	Ribavirin	ZERIT	Stavudine (d4T)
VIREAD	Tenofovir	ZETIA	Ezetimibe
VIRILON	Methyltestosterone	ZEVTERA[†]	Ceftobiprole
VIROPTIC	Trifluridine	ZIAGEN	Abacavir
VISTARIL	Hydroxyzine	ZINACEF	Cefuroxime
VISTIDE	Cidofovir	ZITHROMAX	Azithromycin
VIVACTIL	Protriptyline	ZOCOR	Simvastatin
VOLTAREN	Diclofenac	ZOFRAN	Ondansetron
WELCHOL	Colesevelam	ZOLADEX	Goserelin
WELLBUTRIN	Bupropion	ZOLOFT	Sertraline
XALATAN	Latanoprost	ZOMETA	Zoledronic acid
XANAX	Alprazolam	ZOMIG	Zolmitriptan
XELODA	Capecitabine	ZONALON	Doxepin
XENAZINE	Tetrabenazine	ZONEGRAN	Zonisamide
XENICAL	Orlistat	ZOSTRIX	Capsaicin
XERAC AC	Aluminum chloride	ZOSYN	Piperacillin-tazobactam
XIFAXAN	Rifaximin	ZOVIRAX	Acyclovir
XIGRIS	Drotrecogin alfa (activated protein C)	ZYFLO	Zileuton
XOLAIR	Omalizumab	ZYLOPRIM	Allopurinol
XOPENEX	Levalbuterol	ZYMAR	Gatifloxacin
XYLOCAINE	Lidocaine	ZYPREXA	Olanzapine
XYREM	Sodium oxybate	ZYRTEC	Cetirizine
XYZAL	Levocetirizine	ZYVOX	Linezolid
YOCON	Yohimbine		

[*]Some drugs mentioned in this book are manufactured only as generics and therefore have no trade name and are not included in this table.

[†]Not available in the United States.

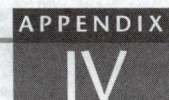

APPENDIX IV

Resources for Help and Information

ADOPTION

Adoption.Com
800-FOR-ADOPT (800-367-2367)
www.adoption.com

National Adoption Center
Philadelphia, PA
800-TO-ADOPT (800-862-3678)
www.adopt.org/assembled/home.html

AGING

Administration on Aging
Washington, DC
202-619-0724
800-438-4380 (information on Alzheimer's disease)
800-677-1116 (Eldercare locator)
800-877-8339 (TTY)
www.aoa.gov

American Association of Retired People (AARP)
Washington, DC
888-OUR-AARP (888-687-2277)
www.aarp.org

Benefits Check Up
The National Council on Aging
www.benefitscheckup.org

Health and Age
Boomerang Pharmaceutical Communications
www.healthandage.com

Infoaging.org
American Federation for Aging Research (AFAR)
New York, NY
212-703-9977
www.infoaging.org

National Association of Area Agencies on Aging
Washington, DC
202-872-0888
www.n4a.org

National Council on Aging
Washington, DC
202-479-1200
202-479-6674 (TDD)
www.ncoa.org

National Institute on Aging
Bethesda, MD
800-222-2225
800-222-4225 (TTY)
www.nia.nih.gov

Older Women's League
Washington, DC
800-825-3695
www.owl-national.org

AIDS

AIDS Action
Washington, DC
202-530-8030
www.aidsaction.org

AIDSinfo
U.S. Department of Health and Human Services
800-HIV-0440 (800-448-0440)
www.aidsinfo.nih.gov

The American Foundation for AIDS Research (amFAR)
New York, NY
212-806-1600
www.amfar.org

American Social Health Association (ASHA)
Research Triangle Park, NC
919-361-8400
www.ashastd.org

CDC-INFO
Atlanta, GA
800-CDC-INFO (800-232-4636)
888-232-6348 (TTY)

Gay Men's Health Crisis
New York, NY
800-AIDS-NYC (800-243-7692)
212-367-1000
www.gmhc.org

Metropolitan Community Churches Global HIV/ AIDS Ministry
www.mccgham.org

National Association for People with AIDS
Silver Spring, MD
866-846-9366
240-247-0880
www.napwa.org

National HIV/AIDS Treatment Hotline
800-822-7422
415-558-9051

Project Inform
San Francisco, CA
415-558-8669
www.projinf.org

Women Alive
Los Angeles, CA
800-554-4876
323-965-1564
www.women-alive.org

ALCOHOLISM

(See also Drug Abuse)

Al-Anon/Alateen Family Group Headquarters
Virginia Beach, VA
888-4AL-ANON (888-425-2666)
757-563-1600
www.al-anon.org

Alcoholics Anonymous
New York, NY
212-870-3400
www.aa.org

LifeRing Recovery
Oakland, CA
800-811-4142
510-763-0779
www.lifering.org

National Clearinghouse for Alcohol & Drug Information
Rockville, MD
800-729-6686
800-487-4889 (TDD)
www.ncadi.samhsa.gov

National Council on Alcoholism & Drug Dependence
New York, NY
800-NCA-CALL (800-622-2255)
212-269-7797
www.ncadd.org

ALLERGY & ASTHMA

Allergy and Asthma Network/Mothers of Asthmatics, Inc.
Fairfax, VA
800-878-4403
www.aanma.org

American Academy of Allergy, Asthma, and Immunology
Milwaukee, WI
414-272-6071
www.aaaai.org

Asthma & Allergy Foundation of America
Washington, DC
800-7-ASTHMA (800-727-8462)
www.aafa.org

ALZHEIMER'S DISEASE & OTHER DEMENTIAS

Alzheimer's Association
Chicago, IL
800-272-3900
312-335-8700
www.alz.org

Alzheimer's Disease Education & Referral Center
Silver Spring, MD
800-438-4380
www.nia.nih.gov/alzheimers.org

The Alzheimer's Society
London, UK
www.alzheimers.org.uk

AMPUTATION

(See also Disabilities and Rehabilitation)

American Amputee Foundation (AAF)
North Little Rock, AR
501-835-9290
www.americanamputee.org

National Amputation Foundation
Malverne, NY
516-887-3600
www.nationalamputation.org

AMYLOIDOSIS

Amyloidosis Network International, Inc.
Clarkston, MI
877-AMYLOID (877-269-5643)
www.amyloidosis.org

AMYOTROPHIC LATERAL SCLEROSIS (ALS; LOU GEHRIG'S DISEASE)

The ALS Association
Calabasas Hills, CA
818-880-9007
www.alsa.org

ANKYLOSING SPONDYLITIS

Spondylitis Association of America
Sherman Oaks, CA
800-777-8189
818-981-1616
www.spondylitis.org

ARTHRITIS

Arthritis Foundation
Atlanta, GA
800-283-7800
www.arthritis.org

Juvenile Arthritis Alliance
Atlanta, GA
800-283-7800
www.arthritis.org/ja-alliance-main.php

ASTHMA

(See Allergy & Asthma)

ATTENTION–DEFICIT/HYPERACTIVITY DISORDER

(See also Learning Disorders)

Attention Deficit Disorder Association (ADDA)
Wilmington, DE
800-939-1019
www.add.org

Children and Adults With Attention–Deficit/ Hyperactivity Disorder (CHADD)
Landover, MD
800-233-4050
301-306-7070
www.chadd.org

Learning Disabilities Association of America
Pittsburgh, PA
412-341-1515
www.ldanatl.org

AUTISM

(See also Learning Disorders)

Autism Research Institute (ARI)
San Diego, CA
866-366-3361
www.autism.com

Autism Society of America
Bethesda, MD
800-3AUTISM (800-328-8476)
301-657-0881
www.autism-society.org

Autism Speaks
New York, NY
212-252-8584
www.autismspeaks.org

National Autism Association (NAA)
Nixa, MO
877-NAA-AUTISM (877-622-3884)
www.nationalautismassociation.org

BALDING

National Alopecia Areata Foundation
San Rafael, CA
415-472-3780
www.naaf.org

BEREAVEMENT

(See Death and Bereavement)

BIRTH DEFECTS

(See also Cleft Palate; Spina Bifida)

Federation for Children With Special Needs
Boston, MA
617-236-7210
www.fcsn.org

March of Dimes Birth Defects Foundation
White Plains, NY
888-663-4637
914-997-4481
www.marchofdimes.com

Mount Sinai Center for Jewish Genetic Diseases, Inc.
New York, NY
212-659-6774
www.mssm.edu/jewish_genetics

BLINDNESS AND VISION PROBLEMS

American Association of the Deaf-Blind
Silver Spring, MD
800-735-2258 (Maryland relay)
301-495-4403
301-495-4402 (TTY)
www.aadb.org

American Council of the Blind
Arlington, VA
800-424-8666
202-467-5081
www.acb.org

American Foundation for the Blind
New York, NY
800-AFB-LINE (800-232-5463)
212-502-7600
www.afb.org

Association for Education & Rehabilitation of the Blind & Visually Impaired
Alexandria, VA
877-492-2708
703-671-4500
www.aerbvi.org

Association for Macular Diseases, Inc.
New York, NY
212-605-3719
www.macula.org

The Foundation Fighting Blindness
Owings Mills, MD
800-683-5555
410-568-0150
800-683-5551 (TDD)
www.blindness.org

Glaucoma Research Foundation
San Francisco, CA
800-826-6693
415-986-3162
www.glaucoma.org

Helen Keller Services for the Blind
Sands Point, NY
516-944-8900
www.helenkeller.org

National Association for Visually Handicapped
New York, NY
212-889-3141
www.navh.org

Prevent Blindness America
Chicago, IL
800-331-2020
www.preventblindness.org

BLOOD DISORDERS

Cooley's Anemia Foundation (Thalessemia)
New York, NY
800-522-7222
www.thalessemia.org

The Leukemia & Lymphoma Society
White Plains, NY
800-955-4572
914-949-5213
www.leukemia.org

National Hemophilia Foundation
New York, NY
212-328-3700
www.hemophilia.org

Sickle Cell Disease Association of America, Inc. (SCDAA)
Baltimore, MD
800-421-8453
410-528-1555
www.sicklecelldisease.org

BRAIN DISORDERS

(See also Cancer & Other Tumors; Alzheimer's Disease & Other Dementias; Epilepsy)

Brain Injury Association of America
Vienna, VA
800-444-6443
703-761-0750
www.biausa.org

National Institute of Neurological Disorders & Stroke
Bethesda, MD
800-352-9424
301-468-5981 (TTY)
www.ninds.nih.gov

BULLYING

Bullying.org
www.bullying.org

Stop Bullying Now
www.stopbullyingnow.hrsa.gov/index.asp?area=main

Stop Cyberbullying
201-463-8663
www.stopcyberbullying.org

CANCER & OTHER TUMORS

American Cancer Society
Atlanta, GA
800-ACS-2345 (800-227-2345)
866-228-4327 (TTY)
www.cancer.org

CancerCare
New York, NY
800-813-HOPE (800-813-4673)
212-712-8400
www.cancercare.org

National Cancer Institute
Bethesda, MD
800-4-CANCER (800-422-6237)
www.cancer.gov

National Coalition for Cancer Survivorship
Silver Spring, MD
888-650-9127
301-650-9127
www.canceradvocacy.org

BRAIN

Acoustic Neuroma Association (ANA)
Cumming, GA
877-200-8211
770-205-8211
www.anausa.org

American Brain Tumor Association
Des Plains, IL
800-886-2282
847-827-9910
www.abta.org

The Children's Brain Tumor Foundation
New York, NY
866-228-4673
www.cbtf.org

National Brain Tumor Society
Watertown, MA
800-770-8287
617-924-9997
www.braintumor.org

Pituitary Network Association
Thousand Oaks, CA
805-499-9973
www.pituitary.org

BREAST

Breast Cancer Network of Strength
Chicago, IL
800-221-2141
312-986-8338
www.networkofstrength.org

National Alliance of Breast Cancer Organizations (NABCO)
New York, NY
888-806-2226

Susan G. Komen for the Cure
Dallas, TX
877-GO-KOMEN (877-465-6636)
www.ww5.komen.org

PROSTATE

US-TOO International
Downers Grove, IL
800-80-USTOO (800-808-7866)
630-795-1002
www.ustoo.com

Zero–The Project to End Prostate Cancer
Washington, DC
888-245-9455
202-463-9455
www.zerocancer.org

SKIN

The Skin Cancer Foundation
New York, NY
212-725-5176
www.skincancer.org

CARDIOVASCULAR DISORDERS

American Heart Association
Dallas, TX
800-AHA-USA1 (800-242-8721)
www.americanheart.org

Heart and Stroke Foundation of Canada
Ottawa, ON
613-569-4361
www.heartandstroke.com

National Heart, Lung, and Blood Institute
Bethesda, MD
301-592-8573
240-629-3255 (TTY)
www.nhlbi.nih.gov

National Stroke Association
Centennial, CO
800-STROKES (800-787-6537)
www.stroke.org

Sister Kenny Rehabilitation Institute
Allina Hospitals and Clinics
Minneapolis, MN
866-880-3550
www.sisterkennyinstitute.com

Vascular Disease Foundation (VDF)
Lakewood, CO
888-VDF-4463 (888-833-4463)
303-949-0500
www.vdf.org

CEREBRAL PALSY

United Cerebral Palsy (UCP)
Washington, DC
800-872-5827
202-776-0406
www.ucp.org

CHILD ABUSE & NEGLECT

American Humane, Protecting Children
Denver, CO
800-227-4645
303-792-9900
www.americanhumane.org

The Kempe Center and Foundation
Aurora, CO
303-864-5300
www.kempe.org

CHILDBIRTH/PREGNANCY

(See also Adoption; Family Planning; Infertility)

American Pregnancy Helpline
866-942-6466
www.thehelpline.org

Childbirth Connection
New York, NY
212-777-5000
www.childbirthconnection.org

CLEFT PALATE

Cleft Palate Foundation
Chapel Hill, NC
800-24-CLEFT (800-242-5338)
www.cleftline.org

Wide Smiles
Stockton, CA
209-942-2812
www.widesmiles.org

CLINICAL TRIALS

The Center for Information and Study on Clinical Research Participation (CISCRP)
Dedham, MA
888-CISCRP3 (888-247-2773)
www.ciscrp.org

ClinicalTrials.gov
National Institutes of Health
800-411-1222
www.clinicaltrials.gov

CYSTIC FIBROSIS

Cystic Fibrosis Foundation
Bethesda, MD
800-344-4823
301-951-4422
www.cff.org

DEAFNESS & HEARING DISORDERS

Alexander Graham Bell Association for the Deaf and Hard of Hearing
Washington, DC
800-432-7543
202-337-5220
202-337-5221 (TTY)
www.agbell.org

American Association of the Deaf-Blind
Silver Spring, MD
800-735-2258 (Maryland relay)
301-495-4403
301-495-4402 (TTY)
www.aadb.org

American Society for Deaf Children (ASDC)
Camp Hill, PA
866-895-4206
717-703-0073
www.deafchildren.org

American Tinnitus Association (ATA)
Portland, OR
800-634-8978
503-248-9985
www.ata.org

Deafness Research Foundation (DRF)
New York, NY
866-454-3924
212-328-9840
888-435-3924 (TTY)
www.drf.org

The Ear Foundation
Nashville, TN
800-545-HEAR (800-545-4327)
615-329-7849
www.hearinglossweb.com

Helen Keller National Center for Deaf-Blind Youths and Adults (HKNC)
Sands Point, NY
516-944-8900
www.hknc.org

National Association of the Deaf (NAD)
Silver Spring, MD
301-587-1788
301-587-1789 (TTY)
www.nad.org

DEATH & BEREAVEMENT

Aiding Mothers and Fathers Experiencing Neonatal Death (AMEND)
St. Louis, MO
314-487-7582
www.amendgroup.com

Caring Connections
800-658-8898
www.caringinfo.org

Compassion and Choices
Denver, CO
800-247-7421
www.compassionandchoices.org

The Compassionate Friends
Oak Brook, IL
877-969-0010
630-990-0010
www.compassionatefriends.org

Hospice Education Institute
Machiasport, ME
800-331-1620
207-255-8800
www.hospiceworld.org

National Hospice Foundation
Alexandria, VA
703-516-4928
www.nationalhospicefoundation.org

DEMENTIA

(See Alzheimer's and Other Dementias)

DEPRESSION

(See also Psychiatric Disease)

Depression and Bipolar Support Alliance (DBSA)
Chicago, IL
800-826-3632
www.ndmda.org

International Foundation for Reasearch and Education on Depression (iFred)
Baltimore, MD
410-268-0044
www.ifred.org

National Alliance for Research on Schizophrenia and Depression (NARSAD)
Great Neck, NY
800-829-8289
www.narsad.org

DIABETES

American Diabetes Association
Alexandria, VA
800-DIABETES (800-342-2383)
www.diabetes.org

Juvenile Diabetes Research Foundation International (JDRF)
New York, NY
800-533-CURE (800-533-2873)
www.jdrf.org

National Institute of Diabetes and Digestive and Kidney Diseases (NIDDK)
Bethesda, MD
301-496-3583
www.niddk.nih.gov

DIGESTIVE DISORDERS

Crohn's & Colitis Foundation of America (CCFA)
New York, NY
800-932-2423
www.ccfa.org

Digestive Disease National Coalition (DDNC)
Washington, DC
202-544-7497
www.ddnc.org

International Foundation for Functional Gastrointestinal Disorders (IFFGD)
Milwaukee, WI
888-964-2001
414-964-1799
www.iffgd.org

Intestinal Disease Foundation
Pittsburgh, PA
877-587-9606
412-261-5888
www.intestinalfoundation.org

National Institute of Diabetes and Digestive and Kidney Diseases (NIDDK)
Bethesda, MD
301-496-3583
www.niddk.nih.gov

United Ostomy Associations of America, Inc. (UOAA)
Fairview, TN
800-826-0826
www.uoa.org

DISABILITIES & REHABILITATION

(See also Amputation; Mental Retardation/ Intellectual Disability)

Disabled American Veterans (DAV)
Cold Spring, KY
877-I-AM-A-VET (877-426-2838)
859-441-7300
www.dav.org

Easter Seals
Chicago, IL
800-221-6827
312-726-6200
312-726-4258 (TTY)
www.easterseals.com

National Organization on Disability (NOD)
Washington, DC
202-293-5960
202-293-5968 (TTY)
www.nod.org

The National Rehabilitation Association (NRA)
Alexandria, VA
888-258-4295
703-836-0850
703-836-0849 (TDD)
www.nationalrehab.org

National Rehabilitation Information Center (NARIC)
Landover, MD
800-346-2742
301-459-5900
301-459-5984 (TTY)
www.naric.com

Paralyzed Veterans of America (PVA)
Washington, DC
800-424-8200
202-872-1300
www.pva.org

DOMESTIC VIOLENCE

National Domestic Violence Hotline
Austin, TX
800-799-SAFE (800-799-7233)
800-787-3224 (TTY)
www.ndvh.org

DOWN SYNDROME

Association for Children with Down Syndrome (ACDS)
Plainview, NY
516-933-4700
www.acds.org

National Down Syndrome Congress (NDSC)
Atlanta, GA
800-232-NDSC (800-232-6372)
770-604-9500
www.ndsccenter.org

National Down Syndrome Society (NDSS)
New York, NY
800-221-4602
www.ndss.org

DRUG ABUSE

(See also Alcoholism)

Cocaine Anonymous World Service (CA)
Los Angeles, CA
800-347-8998
310-559-5833
www.ca.org

Hazelden
Center City, MN
800-257-7810
651-213-4200
www.hazelden.org

Narcotics Anonymous World Services (NA)
Van Nuys, CA
818-773-9999
www.na.org

EAR

(See Deafness and Hearing Disorders)

EATING DISORDERS

National Association of Anorexia Nervosa and Associated Disorders (ANAD)
Highland Park, IL
847-831-3438
847-831-3763
www.anad.org

Overeaters Anonymous (OA)
Rio Rancho, NM
505-891-2664
www.oa.org

ENDOCRINE DISORDERS

(See also Diabetes)

National Adrenal Diseases Foundation (NADF)
Great Neck, NY
516-487-4992
www.nadf.us

EPILEPSY

Epilepsy Foundation
Landover, MD
800-332-1000
www.epilepsyfoundation.org

ERECTILE DYSFUNCTION (IMPOTENCE)

Impotence Anonymous (IA)
800-669-1603

The Impotence Institute of America
Maryville, TN
800-669-1603

EYE

(See Blindness and Vision Problems)

FAMILY PLANNING

(See also Adoption; Childbirth/Pregnancy; Infertility)

Planned Parenthood
New York, NY
800-230-PLAN (800-230-7526)
212-541-7800
www.plannedparenthood.org

FIBROMYALGIA

Fibromyalgia Support
Houston, TX
www.fibromyalgia-support.org

National Fibromyalgia Association (NFA)
Anaheim, CA
714-921-0150
www.fmaware.org

GAUCHER'S DISEASE

National Gaucher Foundation (NGF)
Tucker, GA
800-504-3189
www.gaucherdisease.org

GENERAL

American Academy of Neurology (AAN)
Saint Paul, MN
800-879-1960
651-695-2717
www.aan.com

American Academy of Pediatrics (AAP)
Elm Grove Village, IL
847-434-4000
www.aap.org

American Medical Association (AMA)
Chicago, IL
800-621-8335
www.ama-assn.org

Centers for Disease Control and Prevention (CDC)
Atlanta, GA
800-CDC-INFO (800-232-4636)
888-232-6348 (TTY)
www.cdc.gov

FamilyDoctor.org
www.familydoctor.org

Kids Health
The Nemours Foundation
Wilmington, DE
302-651-4046
www.kidshealth.org/parent

The Merck Manuals
Whitehouse Station, NJ
908-423-1000
www.merckmanuals.com

National Institutes of Health (NIH)
Bethesda, MD
301-496-4000
310-402-9612 (TTY)
www.nih.gov

U.S. Department of Health and Human Services (HHS)
Washington, DC
877-696-6775
202-619-0257
www.os.dhhs.gov

U.S. Food and Drug Administration (FDA)
Silver Spring, MD
888-INFO-FDA (888-463-6332)
www.fda.gov

GENETIC DISEASES

(See also Birth Defects)

Genetic Alliance
Washington, DC
202-966-5557
www.geneticalliance.org

HAND DISORDERS

American Society for Surgery of the Hand (ASSH)
Rosemont, IL
847-384-8300
www.assh.org

HEADACHE

American Headache Society (AHS)
Mt. Royal, NJ
800-255-2243
856-423-0043
www.americanheadachesociety.org

National Headache Foundation (NHF)
Chicago, IL
888-NHF-5552 (888-643-5552)
www.headaches.org

HEAD INJURY

(See Brain Disorders)

HEARING

(See Deafness and Hearing Disorders)

HEART DISORDERS

(See Cardiovascular Disorders)

HEMOCHROMATOSIS

American Hemochromatosis Society (AHS)
Lake Mary, FL
407-829-4488
www.americanhs.org

The Hemochromatosis Information Center
Taylors, SC
1-888-565-4766
1-864-292-1175
www.hemochromatosis.org

Iron Disorders Institute
Greenville, SC
888-565-IRON (888-565-4766)
www.irondisorders.org

Iron Overload Diseases Association (IOD)
West Palm Beach, FL
866-768-8629
561-586-8246
www.ironoverload.org

HOME CARE

National Association for Home Care and Hospice
Washington, DC
202-547-7424
www.nahc.org

HOSPICE

(See Death and Bereavement; Home Care)

IMMUNIZATION

(See Vaccination)

IMPOTENCE

(See Erectile Dysfunction [Impotence])

INCONTINENCE

National Association for Continence (NAFC)
Charleston, SC
800-BLADDER (800-252-3337)
843-377-0905
www.nafc.org

The Simon Foundation for Continence
Wilmette, IL
800-23SIMON (800-237-4666)
www.simonfoundation.org

INFERTILITY

(See also Adoption; Childbirth/Pregnancy;
Family Planning)

**American Society for Reproductive Medicine
(ASRM)**
Birmingham, AL
205-978-5000
www.asrm.org

Ferre Institute
Binghamton, NY
607-724-4308
www.ferre.org

Resolve: The National Infertility Association
McLean, VA
703-556-7172
www.resolve.org

IRON OVERLOAD

(See Hemochromatosis)

KIDNEY DISORDERS

American Association of Kidney Patients (AAKP)
Tampa, FL
800-749-2257
www.aakp.org

American Kidney Fund
Rockville, MD
800-638-8299
www.akfinc.org

National Kidney Foundation
New York, NY
800-622-9010
212-889-2210
www.kidney.org

**National Kidney and Urologic Diseases Information
Clearinghouse (NKUDIC)**
Bethesda, MD
800-891-5390
866-569-1162 (TTY)
www.kidney.niddk.nih.gov

LABORATORY TESTS

Lab Tests Online
Washington, DC
www.labtestsonline.org

LEARNING DISORDERS

(See Attention–Deficit/Hyperactivity Disorder)

**American Association on Intellectual and
Developmental Disabilities (AAIDD)**
Washington, DC
800-424-3688
202-387-1968
www.aaidd.org

Learning Disabilities Association of America (LDA)
Pittsburgh, PA
412-341-1515
www.ldanatl.org

National Center for Learning Disabilities (NCLD)
New York, NY
888-575-7373
212-545-7510
www.ncld.org

LEPROSY

American Leprosy Foundation
Rockville, MD
301-984-1336
users.erols.com/lwm-alf/

LIVER DISORDERS

American Liver Foundation
New York, NY
800-GO-LIVER (800-465-4837)
212-668-1000
www.liverfoundation.org

LUNG DISORDERS

(See Respiratory [Lung] Disorders)

LUPUS

Lupus Foundation of America, Inc.
Washington, DC
800-558-0121
202-349-1155
www.lupus.org

MEDIC ALERT

MedicAlert
Turlock, CA
888-633-4298
209-668-3333
www.medicalert.org

MENTAL HEALTH

(See Depression; Psychiatric Disease)

MENTAL RETARDATION/INTELLECTUAL DISABILITY

(See also Learning Disorders)

The Arc of the United States
Silver Spring, MD
800-433-5255
301-565-3842
www.thearc.org

FRAXA Research Foundation
Newburyport, MA
978-462-1866
www.fraxa.org

The Joseph P. Kennedy, Jr. Foundation
Washington, DC
202-393-1250
www.jpkf.org

National Association of Councils on Developmental Disabilities (NACDD)
Washington, DC
202-506-5813
www.nacdd.org

Voice of the Retarded (VOR)
Elk Grove Village, IL
877-399-4VOR (877-399-4867)
www.vor.net

MOVEMENT DISORDERS

(See also Parkinson's Disease)

We Move
New York, NY
www.wemove.org

MULTIPLE SCLEROSIS

Multiple Sclerosis Association of America (MSAA)
Cherry Hill, NJ
800-532-7667
856-488-4500
www.msassociation.org

National Multiple Sclerosis Society
New York, NY
800-344-4867
www.nationalmssociety.org

MUSCULAR DYSTROPHY

Muscular Dystrophy Association (MDA)
Tucson, AZ
800-572-1717
www.mda.org

MYASTHENIA GRAVIS

Myasthenia Gravis Foundation of America, Inc. (MGFA)
New York, NY
800-541-5454
212-297-2156
www.myasthenia.org

NEURAL TUBE DEFECTS

(See Birth Defects; Spina Bifida)

NUTRITION

American Dietetic Association (ADA)
Chicago, IL
800-877-1600
www.eatright.org

ORGAN DONATION

(See Transplantation)

OSTEOPOROSIS

National Osteoporosis Foundation (NOF)
Washington, DC
800-231-4222
202-223-2226
www.nof.org

PAGET'S DISEASE

The Paget Foundation
New York, NY
800-23-PAGET (800-237-2438)
212-509-5335
www.paget.org

PAIN RELIEF

American Pain Foundation
Baltimore, MD
888-615-PAIN (888-615-7246)
www.painfoundation.org

PARKINSON'S DISEASE

American Parkinson Disease Association, Inc. (APDA)
Staten Island, NY
800-223-2732
718-981-8001
www.apdaparkinson.org

National Parkinson Foundation (NPF)
Miami, FL
800-327-4545
305-243-6666
www.parkinson.org

Parkinson's Action Network (PAN)
Washington, DC
800-850-4726
202-638-4101
www.parkinsonsaction.org

Parkinson's Disease Foundation (PDF)
New York, NY
800-457-6676
212-923-4700
www.pdf.org

POSTPARTUM DEPRESSION

(See also Depression; Psychiatric Disease)

Postpartum Support International (PSI)
Santa Barbara, CA
800-944-4PPD (800-944-4773)
805-967-7636
www.postpartum.net

POSTTRAUMATIC STRESS DISORDER

(See also Depression; Psychiatric Disease)

Hope For Healing.org
www.hopeforhealing.org/ptsd.html

National Center for Posttraumatic Stress Disorder
White River Junction, VT
802-296-6300
www.ncptsd.va.gov/ncmain/index.jsp

PRADER-WILLI SYNDROME

Prader-Willi Syndrome Association (USA)
Sarasota, FL
800-926-4797
941-312-0400
www.pwsausa.org

PREGNANCY

(See Childbirth/Pregnancy)

PROSTATE DISORDERS

(See also Cancer and Other Tumors)

Prostatitis Foundation
Smithshire, IL
888-891-4200
309-325-7184
www.prostatitis.org

PSORIASIS

National Psoriasis Foundation
Portland, OR
800-723-9166
503-244-7404
www.psoriasis.org

PSYCHIATRIC DISEASE

(See also Depression)

Mental Health America
Alexandria, VA
800-969-6642
703-684-7722
800-443-5959 (TTY)
www.nmha.org

National Alliance on Mental Illness (NAMI)
Arlington, VA
800-950-NAMI (800-950-6264)
703-524-7600
www.nami.org

National Institute of Mental Health (NIMH)
Bethesda, MD
866-615-6464
301-443-4513
866-415-8051 (TTY)
www.nimh.nih.gov

RARE DISORDERS

National Organization for Rare Disorders (NORD)
Danbury, CT
800-999-6673
203-744-0100
203-797-9590 (TDD)
www.rarediseases.org

RESPIRATORY (LUNG) DISORDERS

American Lung Association
Washington, DC
800-LUNGUSA (800-586-4872)
212-315-8700
www.lungusa.org

Asthma & Allergy Foundation of America (AAFA)
Washington, DC
800-7-ASTHMA (800-727-8462)
www.aafa.org

REYE'S SYNDROME

National Reye's Syndrome Foundation
Bryan, OH
800-233-7393
www.reyessyndrome.org

SJÖGREN'S SYNDROME

Sjögren's Syndrome Foundation
Bethesda, MD
800-475-6473
301-530-4420
www.sjogrens.org

SLEEP DISORDERS

American Sleep Apnea Association (ASAA)
Washington, DC
202-293-3650
www.sleepapnea.org

SPINA BIFIDA

Spina Bifida Association
Washington, DC
800-621-3141
202-944-3285
www.spinabifidaassociation.org

SPINAL CORD INJURY

The National Spinal Cord Injury Association (NSCIA)
Rockville, MD
800-962-9629
www.spinalcord.org

STROKE

(See Brain Disorders; Cardiovascular Disorders)

STUTTERING & OTHER SPEECH DISORDERS

National Council on Stuttering
Skokie, IL
708-677-8280

National Stuttering Association (NSA)
New York, NY
800-WESTUTTER (800-937-8888)
www.nsastutter.org

Stuttering Foundation
Memphis, TN
800-992-9392
901-452-7343
www.stutteringhelp.org

SUDDEN INFANT DEATH SYNDROME (SIDS)

American SIDS Institute
Marietta, GA
800-232-SIDS
770-426-8746
www.sids.org

First Candle (formerly Sudden Infant Death Syndrome Alliance)
Baltimore, MD
800-221-7437
410-653-8226
www.firstcandle.org

Sudden Infant Death Syndrome and Other Infant Death (SIDS/OID) Information Web Site
Ledyard, CT
www.sids-network.org

SUICIDE

Metanoia
800-SUICIDE (800-784-2433)
www.metanoia.org/suicide

Suicide Awareness Voices of Education (SAVE)
Bloomington, MN
952-946-7998
800-273-TALK (800-273-8255)
www.save.org

Survivors of Suicide
www.survivorsofsuicide.com

TAY-SACHS DISEASE

National Tay-Sachs & Allied Diseases Association, Inc. (NTSAD)
Boston, MA
800-906-8723
www.ntsad.org

TRANSPLANTATION

OrganDonor.gov
Washington, DC
877-696-6775
202-619-0257
www.organdonor.gov

Transplant Living
888-894-6361
www.transplantliving.org

United Network for Organ Sharing (UNOS)
Richmond, VA
888-894-6361
804-782-4800
www.unos.org

TRAVEL HEALTH

Centers for Disease Control and Prevention (CDC) Travelers' Health
Atlanta, GA
800-CDC-INFO (800-232-4636)
888-232-6348 (TTY)
www.cdc.gov/travel

Federal Aviation Administration (FAA)
Washington, DC
866-TELL-FAA (866-835-5322)
www.faa.gov

International Association for Medical Assistance to Travelers (IAMAT)
Niagara Falls, NY
716-754-4883
www.iamat.org

International Society of Travel Medicine (ISTM)
Snellville, GA
770-736-7060
www.istm.org

International SOS
Trevose, PA
800-523-8930
215-942-8000
www.internationalsos.org

Travel Health Online
www.tripprep.com

U.S. Department of State
Washington, DC
888-407-4747
202-501-4444
www.travel.state.gov

World Health Organization (WHO)
Geneva, Switzerland
+41 22 791 21 11
www.who.int/ith

VACCINATION

Centers for Disease Control and Prevention (CDC) Vaccines and Immunizations
Atlanta, GA
800-CDC-INFO (800-232-4636)
888-232-6348 (TTY)
www.cdc.gov/vaccines/

Institute for Vaccine Safety
Baltimore, MD
www.vaccinesafety.edu

Vaccine Information for the Public and Health Professionals
St. Paul, MN
651-647-9009
www.vaccineinformation.org

WOMEN'S HEALTH

(See also Aging)

American College of Obstetricians and Gynecologists (ACOG)
Washington, DC
202-638-5577
www.acog.org

National Women's Health Network (NWHN)
Washington, DC
202-682-2640
www.nwhn.org

INDEX

Note: Page numbers in *italics* refer to illustrations, tables, or sidebars.

A

Abacavir *1262*
Abatacept 1127
  in rheumatoid arthritis *567, 568*
Abdomen 110–114, *111*
  abscess of 201–202, 1153
  birth defects of 1721
  examination of
    in aortic aneurysm 429
    in ascites 218
    in digestive system disorders 128
    in gynecologic disorders 1502
    in heart disease 326
    in high blood pressure 337
    in newborn 1677
    in superior mesenteric artery disease 420
  fluid in (ascites) 218
    removal of (paracentesis) 131, 218
  pain in 114–117, *115, 116,* 128
    in appendicitis 203, 1798
    in Crohn's disease 169
    in familial Mediterranean fever 1842
    in infants 1732
    in intestinal obstruction 205
    in intussusception 1797
    in ischemic colitis 206
    in pancreatic cancer 199
    in pancreatitis 159, 161
    in peptic ulcers 140, *141*
    recurring, in children 1800–1802, *1801*
    in ruptured spleen 1074
    in splenic enlargement 1072
  radiation injury to 1988
  stretch marks on, during pregnancy 1621
Abdominal aorta, aneurysm of 428–429, *428*
Abdominal cavity 110
Abdominal wall, hernia of 202–203
Abducens nerve 837, *838*
Abetalipoproteinemia *969*
ABO incompatibility *1703*
Abortion 1605–1606, *1647*
  for adolescent 1760
  spontaneous (*see* Miscarriage)
Abrasions 1946–1947
Abraxane *1090*
Abruptio placentae 1648–1649, *1649*

Abscess
  abdominal 201–202, 1153
  anus and rectum 184
  Bartholin's gland *1538*
  brain 763–764
    coma with *704*
    with ear infection 1809
    headache with *650*
    in meningitis 1762
  breast 1177, 1549
  chest 1153
  face 1153
  fallopian tube 1542
  hand 604–605
  jaw 1153
  lacrimal sac 1436
  lung 465, 472–473, 1177
  pelvic 1153
  pharyngeal 1811
  pilonidal 187
  retroperitoneal 201
  skin 1177, 1316–1317
    in acne 1296
  sweat gland 1317
  throat (retropharyngeal) 1763–1764, 1811
  tonsillar 1402–1403, 1811
  tooth 1361
  urethral 303, 1568
Absence (petit mal) seizures 712, *714*
Abuse
  child 1270, 1879–1882
    foster care for 1877–1878
    information resources on 2155
  domestic 1581–1582, *1582*
    information resources on 2158
  drug (*see* Drugs, abuse of)
  elder 1934–1937, *1935*
  financial 1935
  psychologic 1581, 1935
  sexual 1581, 1582–1584, 1880, 1881
Acalculous cholecystitis 245, 246
Acarbose *1012*
Accessory nerve *839*
Accidents (*see* Injury)
Acclimatization 1977
Accommodative esotropia 1819
ACE (*see* Angiotensin-converting enzyme)

H

T

NOTES

THE ONE-PAGE MERCK MANUAL OF HEALTH

People think healthy living involves rare treasures and dark secrets—the exotic plant from a Tibetan meadow, the secret advice from a sage in a remote village—or years of intense study and practice. Actually, the truth is hidden in plain sight, and it's pretty simple (though seldom easy). That's why The Merck Manual of Health requires only *one* sheet of paper.

DIET AND NUTRITION

- Eat less (yes, this means you), particularly less sugars, simple carbohydrates, trans fats, and saturated fats
- Eat more fruits, vegetables, and whole grains
- Vary your diet
- If your medical condition requires a special diet, *follow it*

VITAMINS AND SUPPLEMENTS

- If you're a breastfed baby, take vitamin D; if you're a bottle-fed baby, use formula with iron
- If you're over 50 years old, take calcium and vitamin D
- If you're pregnant (or thinking of becoming pregnant), take prenatal vitamins

SUBSTANCE USE

- Don't smoke (and if you do, *don't* smoke in bed)
- Drink alcohol only in moderation (if that's hard for you, don't drink at all)
- Don't take any drugs that aren't intended to treat a medical problem

EXERCISE AND SLEEP

- Do 30 to 60 minutes of structured exercise (aerobic *and* resistance) that is appropriate for your age and medical condition (fun is good) *at least* 3 times per week
- Walk more—and take the stairs
- Keep as regular a sleep schedule as possible

INFECTIONS

- Wash your hands before eating and cooking
- Store, prepare, and cook foods (particularly meats) appropriately
- Drink only clean or treated water
- Practice safe sex
- Wash minor wounds with soap and water and keep covered
- Use appropriate clothing and insect repellent when mosquito or tick exposure is likely
- Don't do intravenous drugs, and if you do, don't share needles

INJURIES AND GENERAL SAFETY

- Wear a seatbelt; if you're a child, use a car seat
- Wear a helmet while riding a bicycle or motorcycle and use other protective gear as appropriate for the activity (recreation or occupation)
- Store and handle firearms safely
- Follow the accepted safety procedures for your job and recreational activities
- Don't operate vehicles or power equipment while intoxicated, overly sleepy, or distracted
- Look before crossing or entering a road, changing lanes, or merging
- Wear a life vest while boating, don't dive into shallow water, and learn to swim
- Have working smoke and carbon monoxide detectors in your home

MENTAL HEALTH

- Treat others as you would be treated
- Accept responsibility for your actions
  - Also take responsibility for someone or something besides yourself
- Make *and keep* friends
- Act nicer
  - Don't speak ill to or about others
- Practice mind-calming techniques (for example, meditation or prayer)
- Don't sweat the small stuff and be sensible about what's small
- With adversity, change what you can, live with what you can't, and try to know the difference
- When you do something, do your best (but don't expect more from yourself than your best)
- Do something useful for your family and community
- Understand that you will die (yes, you) and you will experience pain and loss

HEALTH CARE

- Brush your teeth at least twice a day
- See a dentist regularly for cleaning and examination
- See a health care practitioner regularly for age-appropriate and sex-appropriate screening and vaccinations
  - Blood pressure, glucose, and lipid levels
  - Pap smears, mammograms, and colon cancer screening
  - Prenatal screening
- Be cautious about sun exposure and wear sunscreen
- If something feels wrong physically or mentally, see appropriate practitioners
  - If you trust them, do what they advise
  - If you don't trust them, or if what they say seems too good to be true or doesn't make sense, don't ignore the issue, get another opinion

If you do all of these things but think you need something more, take the time, effort, and money you'd spend looking for a better supplement, diet, or exercise and instead read a book to a child or help those in your community who are in need.

Yours in Good Health,

Robert S. Porter, MD

Editor-in-Chief, The Merck Manuals